2014

Educational ICD-9-CM
Volumes 1, 2 & 3
and HCPCS Level II

D1450236

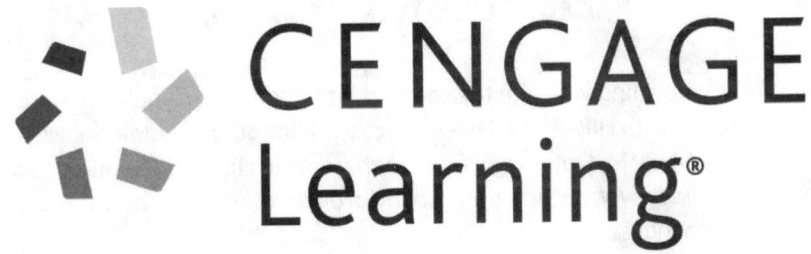

PUBLISHER'S NOTICE

All codes, indexes, and other material in the ICD-9-CM are compiled from official ICD-9-CM codes and instructions as well as the Medicare regulations and manuals issued or authorized by the Centers for Medicare and Medicaid Services. The code book is designed to provide accurate and authoritative information in regard to the subject covered, and every reasonable effort has been made to ensure the accuracy of the information within these pages. However, the ultimate responsibility for correct coding lies with the provider of services.

Optum, its employees, agents and staff make no representation, warranty or guarantee that this compilation of codes and narratives is error-free or that the use of this code book will prevent differences of opinion or disputes with Medicare or other third-party payers as to the codes that are accepted or the amounts that will be paid to providers for services, and will bear no responsibility or liability for the results or consequences of the use of this code book.

CODE UPDATE INFORMATION

We are committed to providing you with the code update information you need to code accurately and to be in compliance with HIPAA regulations. In case of adoption of additional ICD-9-CM code changes effective April 1, 2014, Optum will provide these code changes to you at no additional cost! Just check back at **http://www.optumcoding.com/productalerts** to review the latest information concerning any new changes.

In case of HCPCS Level II code changes. Just check back at
http:\\www.optumcoding.com/productalerts and look for the HCPCS Level II update file.

Contents

HCPCS Level II

Preface

Providers are required by law under the Health Insurance Portability and Accountability Act of 1996 (HIPAA) to document and report healthcare services provided to Medicare beneficiares using standard code sets. The standard code set for documenting and reporting diagnoses and reasons for health care encounters in all settings is ICD-9-CM. For acute care hospital admissions, ICD-9-CM is required for documenting and reporting procedures and services. The HCPCS (Healthcare Common Procedure Coding System) Level II code set is the standard code set for reporting medical services and supplies.

Educational ICD-9-CM Volumes 1, 2 & 3 and HCPCS Level II has been designed with the coder in mind. All volumes of the most recent official government versions have been combined into one book.

Our technical experts have drawn upon their extensive hands-on experience to enhance the government's book with valuable features essential to correct coding and reimbursement. Additional coding information and self-test(s) are designed to enhance the learning experience. This coding resource is designed to function not only as a training tool, but also as a professional guide to both ICD-9-CM and HCPCS Level II code sets.

As you review the content, you'll find the following:

- ICD-9-CM official guidelines for coding and reporting, published by the U.S. Department of Health and Human Services and approved by the cooperating parties (American Hospital Association (AHA), American Health Information Management Association (AHIMA), Centers for Medicare and Medicaid Services and National Center for Health Statisics (NCHS))
- All the official ICD-9-CM codes
- Symbols that alert coders to codes requiring a fourth- or fifth-digit assignment
- An explanation of the basic ICD-9-CM coding conventions
- The 10 steps to Correct Coding feature
- All official HCPCS Level II code and descriptions
- Enhanced index to HCPCS Level II
- Medicare manual references
- HCPCS modifiers
- Enhanced table of drugs and chemicals

Please review "How to Use ICD-9-CM (Volumes 1, 2 & 3)" in this section to learn about the features that will help you assign and report correct codes.

Use of Official Sources

The ICD-9-CM for Hospitals contains the official U.S. Department of Health and Human Services, Ninth Revision, Seventh Edition ICD-9-CM codes, effective for the current year.

Technical Editors

Regina Magnani, RHIT, *Clinical/Technical Editor, Optum*
Ms. Magnani has more than 30 years of experience in the health care industry in both health information management and patient financial services. Her areas of expertise include facility revenue cycle management, patient financial services, CPT/HCPCS and ICD-9-CM coding, the outpatient prospective payment system (OPPS), and chargemaster development and maintenance. She is an active member of the Healthcare Financial Management Association (HFMA), the American Health Information Management Association (AHIMA), and the American Association of Healthcare Administrative Management (AAHAM).

Trudy Whitehead, CPC-H, CMAS, *Clinical/Technical Editor, Optum*
Ms. Whitehead has more than 20 years of experience in hospital and physician coding and reimbursement. Recently she developed an APC review system for the postpayment review of Medicare FFS APC claims, including workflow, training, and development of an instruction manual as director of ambulatory review systems. She has conducted hospital and insurance bill auditing, managed facility claims processing and claims negotiations, developed outpatient repricer and rules engines, performed hospital chargemaster reviews, and worked on software development. Ms. Whitehead is a member of the AAPC and the American Association of Medical Audit Specialists.

Anita C. Hart, RHIA, CCS, CCS-P, *Product Manager, Optum*
Ms. Hart's experience includes 15 years conducting and publishing research in clinical medicine and human genetics for Yale University, Massachusetts General Hospital, and Massachusetts Institute of Technology. Her research conclusions have been published in several peer-reviewed journals. In addition, Ms. Hart has supervised medical records management, health information management, coding and reimbursement, and workers' compensation issues as the office manager for a physical therapy rehabilitation clinic. Ms. Hart is an expert in physician and facility coding, reimbursement systems, and compliance issues. She is also the author of the several Optum publications and has served as subject matter advisor on numerous other publications for hospital and physician practices. Ms. Hart is the ICD-9-CM and ICD-10-CM/PCS subject matter expert for Optum, has served as the product manager for that product line for 15 years, and has presented at numerous national conferences. Ms. Hart is a member of the American Academy of Professional Coders (AAPC) and a fully credentialed active member of the American Health Information Management Association (AHIMA). Ms Hart is a current AHIMA Approved ICD-10-CM/PCS Trainer and leads the training initiatives within Optum Coding Solutions business unit.

Anita Schmidt, BS, RHIT, *Clinical/Technical Editor, Optum*
Ms. Schmidt has expertise in level I adult and pediatric trauma hospital coding, specializing in ICD-9-CM, DRG, and CPT coding. Her experience includes analysis of medical record documentation and assignment of ICD-9-CM codes and DRGs, and CPT code assignments for same-day surgery cases. She has conducted coding training and auditing including DRG validation, conducted electronic health record training, and worked with clinical documentation specialists to identify documentation needs and potential areas for physician education. Ms. Schmidt is an active member of the American Health Information Management Association (AHIMA) and the Minnesota Health Information Management Association (MNHIMA).

In addition to the editors, the following people have contributed to this book:

Stacy Perry, *Manager, Desktop Publishing*
Tracy Betzler, *Senior Desktop Publishing Specialist*
Hope M. Dunn, *Senior Desktop Publishing Specialist*
Katie Russell, *Desktop Publishing Specialist*
Kate Holden, *Editor*

Introduction

History and Future of ICD-9-CM

The International Classification of Diseases, Ninth Revision, Clinical Modification (ICD-9-CM) is based on the official version of the World Health Organization's Ninth Revision, International Classification of Diseases (ICD-9). ICD-9 classifies morbidity and mortality information for statistical purposes, and for the indexing of hospital records by disease and operations, for data storage and retrieval.

This modification of ICD-9 supplants the Eighth Revision International Classification of Diseases, Adapted for Use in the United States (ICDA-8) and the Hospital Adaptation of ICDA (H-ICDA).

The concept of extending the International Classification of Diseases for use in hospital indexing was originally developed in response to a need for a more efficient basis for storage and retrieval of diagnostic data. In 1950, the U.S. Public Health Service and the Veterans Administration began independent tests of the International Classification of Diseases for hospital indexing purposes. The following year, the Columbia Presbyterian Medical Center in New York City adopted the International Classification of Diseases, Sixth Revision, with some modifications for use in its medical record department. A few years later, the Commission on Professional and Hospital Activities (CPHA) in Ann Arbor, Mich., adopted the International Classification of Diseases with similar modifications for use in hospitals participating in the Professional Activity Study.

The problem of adapting ICD for indexing hospital records was taken up by the U.S. National Committee on Vital and Health Statistics through its subcommittee on hospital statistics. The subcommittee reviewed the modifications made by the various users of ICD and proposed that uniform changes be made. This was done by a small working party.

In view of the growing interest in the use of the International Classification of Diseases for hospital indexing, a study was undertaken in 1956 by the American Hospital Association and the American Medical Record Association (then the American Association of Medical Record Librarians) of the relative efficiencies of coding systems for diagnostic indexing. This study indicated the International Classification of Diseases provided a suitable and efficient framework for indexing hospital records. The major users of the International Classification of Diseases for hospital indexing purposes then consolidated their experiences, and an adaptation was first published in December 1959. A revision was issued in 1962 and the first "Classification of Operations and Treatments" was included.

In 1966, the international conference for revising the International Classification of Diseases noted the eighth revision of ICD had been constructed with hospital indexing in mind and considered the revised classification suitable, in itself, for hospital use in some countries. However, it was recognized that the basic classification might provide inadequate detail for diagnostic indexing in other countries. A group of consultants was asked to study the eighth revision of ICD (ICD-8) for applicability to various users in the United States. This group recommended that further detail be provided for coding of hospital and morbidity data. The American Hospital Association was requested to develop the needed adaptation proposals. This was done by an advisory committee (the Advisory Committee to the Central Office on ICDA). In 1968 the United States Public Health Service published the product, Eighth Revision International Classification of Diseases, Adapted for Use in the United States. This became commonly known as ICDA-8, and beginning in 1968 it served as the basis for coding diagnostic data for both official morbidity and mortality statistics in the United States.

In 1968, the CPHA published the Hospital Adaptation of ICDA (H-ICDA) based on both the original ICD-8 and ICDA-8. In 1973, CPHA published a revision of H-ICDA, referred to as H-ICDA-2. Hospitals throughout the United States were divided in their use of these classifications until January 1979, when ICD-9-CM was made the single classification intended primarily for use in the United States, replacing these earlier related, but somewhat dissimilar, classifications.

Physicians have been required by law to submit diagnosis codes for Medicare reimbursement since the passage of the Medicare Catastrophic Coverage Act of 1988. This act requires physician offices to include the appropriate diagnosis codes when billing for services provided to Medicare beneficiaries on or after April 1, 1989. The Centers for Medicare and Medicaid Services (formerly known as Health Care Financing Administration) designated ICD-9-CM as the coding system physicians must use.

The ICD-10-CM classification system was developed by the National Center for Health Statistics (NCHS) as a clinical modification to the ICD-10 system developed by the World Health Organization (WHO), primarily as a unique system for use in the United States for morbidity and mortality reporting. Although ICD-10-CM has not yet been implemented for use in the United States, ICD-10 has been adopted for use in the coding and classification of mortality data from death certificates. ICD-10 replaced ICD-9 for this purpose as of January 1, 1999. The Department of Health and Human Services (HHS) published the final rule regarding the adoption of both ICD-10-CM and ICD-10-PCS in the January 16, 2009 *Federal Register* (45 CFR part 162[CMS—0013—F]). On April 17, 2012, the Department of Health and Human Services released a notice postponing the date by which certain health care entities must comply with diagnosis and procedure codes from the International Classification of Diseases, 10th edition (ICD-10). The compliance date for implementing ICD-10-CM and ICD-10-PCS as a replacement for ICD-9-CM is October 1, 2014.

ICD-9-CM Background

In February 1977, a steering committee was convened by the National Center for Health Statistics to provide advice and counsel in developing a clinical modification of ICD-9. The organizations represented on the steering committee included the following:

- American Association of Health Data Systems
- American Hospital Association
- American Medical Record Association
- Association for Health Records
- Council on Clinical Classifications
- Centers for Medicare and Medicaid Services, Department of Health and Human Services
- WHO Center for Classification of Diseases for North America, sponsored by the National Center for Health Statistics, Department of Health and Human Services

The Council on Clinical Classifications was sponsored by the following:

- American Academy of Pediatrics
- American College of Obstetricians and Gynecologists
- American College of Physicians
- American College of Surgeons
- American Psychiatric Association
- Commission on Professional and Hospital Activities

The steering committee met periodically in 1977. Clinical guidance and technical input were provided by task forces on classification from the Council on Clinical Classification's sponsoring organizations.

ICD-9-CM is a clinical modification of the World Health Organization's ICD-9. The term "clinical" is used to emphasize the modification's intent: to serve as a useful tool to classify morbidity data for indexing medical records, medical care review, and ambulatory and other medical care programs, as well as for basic health statistics. To describe the clinical picture of the patient, the codes must be more precise than those needed only for statistical groupings and trend analysis.

CHARACTERISTICS OF ICD-9-CM

ICD-9-CM far exceeds its predecessors in the number of codes provided. The disease classification has been expanded to include health-related conditions and to provide greater specificity at the fifth-digit level of detail. These fifth digits are not optional; they are intended for use in recording the information substantiated in the clinical record.

Volume I (Tabular List) of ICD-9-CM contains four appendices:

Appendix A: Morphology of Neoplasms

Appendix B: Deleted Effective October 1, 2004

Appendix C: Classification of Drugs by American Hospital Formulary Service List Number and Their ICD-9-CM Equivalents

Appendix D: Classification of Industrial Accidents According to Agency

Appendix E: List of Three-digit Categories

These appendices are included as a reference to provide further information about the patient's clinical picture, to further define a diagnostic statement, to aid in classifying new drugs or to reference three-digit categories.

Volume 2 (Alphabetic Index) of ICD-9-CM contains many diagnostic terms that do not appear in Volume I since the index includes most diagnostic terms currently in use.

Volume 3 (Procedure Index and Procedure Tabular) of ICD-9-CM contains codes for operations and procedures. The format for the tabular is the same as Volume 1 disease tabular, except the codes consist of two digits with one or two digits following the decimal point. Conventions in the index follow Volume 2 conventions except some subterms appear immediately below the main term rather than following alphabetizing rules.

THE DISEASE CLASSIFICATION

ICD-9-CM is totally compatible with its parent system, ICD-9, thus meeting the need for comparability of morbidity and mortality statistics at the international level. A few fourth-digit codes were created in existing three-digit rubrics only when the necessary detail could not be accommodated by the use of a fifth-digit subclassification. To ensure that each rubric of ICD-9-CM collapses back to its ICD-9 counterpart the following specifications governed the ICD-9-CM disease classification:

Specifications for the Tabular List:

1. Three-digit rubrics and their contents are unchanged from ICD-9.

2. The sequence of three-digit rubrics is unchanged from ICD-9.

3. Three-digit rubrics are not added to the main body of the classification.

4. Unsubdivided three-digit rubrics are subdivided where necessary to

   • add clinical detail

   • isolate terms for clinical accuracy.

5. The modification in ICD-9-CM is accomplished by adding a fifth digit to existing ICD-9 rubrics, except as noted under #7 below.

6. The optional dual classification in ICD-9 is modified.

   • Duplicate rubrics are deleted:
     – four-digit manifestation categories duplicating etiology entries
     – manifestation inclusion terms duplicating etiology entries

   • Manifestations of disease are identified, to the extent possible, by creating five-digit codes in the etiology rubrics.

   • When the manifestation of a disease cannot be included in the etiology rubrics, provision for its identification is made by retaining the ICD-9 rubrics used for classifying manifestations of disease.

7. The format of ICD-9-CM is revised from that used in ICD-9.

   • American spelling of medical terms is used.

   • Inclusion terms are indented beneath the titles of codes.

   • Codes not to be used for primary tabulation of disease are printed in italics with the notation, "code first underlying disease."

Specifications for the Alphabetic Index:

1. The format of the Alphabetic Index follows that of ICD-9.

2. When two codes are required to indicate etiology and manifestation, the manifestation code appears in brackets (e.g., diabetic cataract 250.5 *[366.41]*).

THE ICD-9-CM COORDINATION AND MAINTENANCE COMMITTEE

The ICD-9-CM Coordination and Maintenance Committee, a federal committee, was created as a forum for proposals to update the International Classification of Diseases, Ninth Revision, Clinical Modification, Sixth Edition (ICD-9-CM). A representative from the National Center for Health Statistics (NCHS) and one from the Centers for Medicare and Medicaid Services (CMS) co-chair the ICD-9-CM Coordination and Maintenance Committee Meetings. Responsibility for maintaining ICD-9-CM is divided between the two agencies, with NCHS classifying diagnoses (volumes 1 and 2) and CMS classifying procedures (volume 3).

Proposals for changes to the ICD-9-CM classification system are submitted and discussed in two open forum meetings held in March and September of each year at the Headquarters of the Centers for Medicare and Medicaid Services (CMS) in Baltimore, Maryland. Comments received during and after the meetings are then discussed by the Committee. A notice of the new codes and code revisions approved by the Committee are published in the Federal Register as part of the proposed and final rule for the changes to the inpatient prospective payment system. All final decisions are made by the director of NCHS and the administrator of CMS. The complete official document of changes to the classification system is released as the Addenda for the International Classification of Diseases, Ninth Revision, Clinical Modification, Sixth Edition, Volumes 1, 2 and 3.

This educational edition of *ICD-9-CM Volumes 1, 2 & 3* is based on the official version of the International Classification of Diseases, Ninth Revision, Clinical Modification, Sixth Edition, issued by the U.S. Department of Health and Human Services. Annual code changes are implemented by the government and are effective Oct. 1 and valid through Sept. 30 of the following year. If a convincing case is made that a new code is required to capture new technology or an emerging disease, this new code may be implemented on April 1 of the following year.

How to Use the ICD-9-CM (Volumes 1, 2 & 3)

The code book is totally compatible with its parent system, ICD-9, thus meeting the need for comparability of morbidity and mortality statistics at the international level.

This book is consistent with the content of the government's version of ICD-9-CM. However, to accommodate the coder's approach to coding, the Alphabetic Index has been placed before the Tabular List in both the disease and procedure classifications. This allows the user to locate the correct codes in a logical, natural manner by locating the term in the index, then confirming the accuracy of the code in the Tabular List.

STEPS TO CORRECT CODING

1. Look up the main term in the Alphabetic Index and scan the subterm entries as appropriate. Follow any cross-references such as "*see*" and "*see also.*" Do not code from the Alphabetic Index without verifying the accuracy of the code in the Tabular List.

2. Locate the code in the numerically arranged Tabular List.

3. Observe the punctuation, footnotes, cross-references, color-coded prompts and other conventions described in the 'Conventions' section.

4. To determine the appropriateness of the code selection, read all instructional material:

   - "includes" and "*excludes*" notes
   - "*see*," "*see also*" and "*see category*" cross-references
   - "use additional code" and "*code first underlying disease*" instructions
   - "code also" and "*omit code*" notes
   - fourth- and fifth-digit requirements

5. Consult definitions, relevant illustrations, color coding and the check fourth- and fifth-digit symbols.

6. Consult the official ICD-9-CM guidelines for coding and reporting, and refer to the AHA's *Coding Clinic for ICD-9-CM* for coding guidelines governing the use of specific codes.

7. Confirm and transcribe the correct code.

ORGANIZATION

Introduction
The introductory material in this book includes the history and future of ICD-9-CM as well as an overview of the classification system.

Official ICD-9-CM Conventions
This section provides a full explanation of all the official footnotes, symbols, instructional notes, and conventions found in the official government version.

Additional Conventions
Exclusive color-coding, symbols, and notations have been included in the *Educational ICD-9-CM Volumes 1, 2, & 3 and HCPCS Level II* to alert coders to important coding issues, such as identification of manifestation codes and notification when additional digits are required for valid code assignment. This section provides a full explanation of the additional conventions used throughout this book.

Coding Guidelines
Included in this book are the official ICD-9-CM coding guidelines as approved by the four cooperating parties of the ICD-9-CM Coordination and Maintenance Committee. Failure to comply with the official coding guidelines may result in denied or delayed claims.

10 Steps to Correct Coding
This resource takes the coder through the coding process step by step. Detailed explanations are accompanied by coding examples demonstrating the practical application of ICD-9-CM conventions and coding guidelines.

Disease Classification: Alphabetic Index to Diseases
The Alphabetic Index to Diseases is separated by tabs labeled with the letters of the alphabet, contains diagnostic terms for illnesses, injuries and reasons for encounters with health care professionals. The Table of Drugs and Chemicals is easily located with the tab in this section.

The warning statement at the bottom of every page of the index, ▽ Subterms under main terms may continue to next column or page, is a reminder to always check for additional subterms before making final selection.

Disease Classification: Tabular List of Diseases
The Tabular List of Diseases arranges the ICD-9-CM codes and descriptors numerically. The side tabs divide this section into chapters, identified by the code range on the tab.

The Tabular List includes two supplementary classifications:

- V Codes—Supplementary Classification of Factors Influencing Health Status and Contact with Health Services (V01–V91)
- E Codes—Supplementary Classification of External Causes of Injury and Poisoning (E000–E999)

ICD-9-CM includes four official appendixes:

- Appendix A: Morphology of Neoplasms
- Appendix B: Deleted Effective October 1, 2004
- Appendix C: Classification of Drugs by AHFS List
- Appendix D: Classification of Industrial Accidents According to Agency
- Appendix E: List of Three-digit Categories

These appendices are included as a reference to provide further information about the patient's circumstances, help further define a diagnostic statement, maintain a tumor registry and aid in classifying new drugs.

Procedure Classification: Alphabetic Index to Procedures
The Alphabetic Index to Procedures lists common surgical and procedural terminology.

The warning statement at the bottom of every page of the index, ▽ Subterms under main terms may continue to next column or page, is a reminder to always check for additional subterms before making final selection.

Procedure Classification: Tabular List of Procedures
The Tabular List of Procedures numerically arranges the procedure codes and their descriptors.

ICD-9-CM Official Conventions

ICD-9-CM Footnotes, Symbols, Instructional Notes and Conventions

This ICD-9-CM text preserves all symbols, instructional notes and conventions found in the government's official version. Accurate coding depends upon understanding the meaning of these elements.

The following appear in the disease Tabular List, unless otherwise noted.

ICD-9-CM Conventions Used in the Tabular List

In addition to the symbols above, the ICD-9-CM disease tabular has certain abbreviations, punctuation, symbols and other conventions. This ICD-9-CM text preserves these conventions. Proper use of the conventions will lead to efficient and accurate coding.

Abbreviations

NEC   Not elsewhere classifiable
This abbreviation is used when the ICD-9-CM system does not provide a code specific for the patient's condition.

NOS   Not otherwise specified
This abbreviation is the equivalent of 'unspecified' and is used only when the coder lacks the information necessary to code to a more specific four-digit subcategory.

[ ]   Brackets enclose synonyms, alternative terminology or explanatory phrases.
Brackets that appear beneath a code indicate the fifth digits that are considered valid fifth digits for the code. This convention is applied for those instances in ICD-9-CM where not all common fifth digits are considered valid for each subcategory within a category.

[]   Slanted brackets that appear in the Alphabetic Indexes indicate mandatory multiple coding. Both codes must be assigned to fully describe the condition and are sequenced in the order listed.

( )   Parentheses enclose supplementary words, called nonessential modifiers, that may be present in the narrative description of a disease without affecting the code assignment.

:   Colons are used in the Tabular List after an incomplete term that needs one or more of the modifiers that follow in order to make it assignable to a given category.

}   Braces enclose a series of terms, each of which is modified by the statement appearing to the right of the brace.

Other Conventions

Boldface   Boldface type is used for all codes and titles in the Tabular List.

Italicized   Italicized type is used for all exclusion notes and to identify codes that should not be used for describing the primary diagnosis.

Instructional Notes Used in the Tabular

These notes appear only in the Tabular List of Diseases:

Includes: An includes note further defines or clarifies the content of the chapter, subchapter, category, sub-category or subclassification.

EXCLUDES   Terms following the word "Excludes" are not classified to the chapter, subchapter, category, subcategory or specific subclassification code under which it is found. The note also may provide the location of the excluded diagnosis. Excludes notes are italicized.

Use additional code:
This instruction signals the coder that an additional code should be used if the information is available to provide a more complete picture of that diagnosis.

There are coding circumstances outside of the etiology/manifestation convention when multiple coding for a single condition is required. The "Use additional code" note will be found under the associated condition code in the tabular. In the index, the multiple coding requirement is indicated by the use of the slanted bracket. The two codes are to be sequenced as listed in the index.

Code first underlying disease:
The "Code first underlying disease" instructional note found under certain codes is a sequencing rule. Most often this sequencing rule applies to the etiology/manifestation convention and is found under the manifestation code. The manifestation code may never be used alone or as a principal or first-listed diagnosis (i.e., sequenced first). The instructional note, the code and its descriptor appear in italics in the Tabular List.

Not all codes with a "Code first underlying disease" instructional note are part of the etiology/manifestation convention. The "Code first" note will appear, but the title of the code and the instructional note will not be in italics. These codes may be reported alone or as the secondary diagnosis.

Code, if applicable, any causal condition first:
A code with this note indicates that this code may be assigned as a principal diagnosis when the causal condition is unknown or not applicable. If a causal condition is known, then the code for that condition should be sequenced as the principal or first-listed diagnosis.

Instructional Notes Used in the Index

Omit code:
"Omit code" is used to instruct the coder that no code is to be assigned. When this instruction is found in the Alphabetic Index to Diseases the medical term should not be coded as a diagnosis.

When used in Volume 3, 'omit code' is meant to indicate procedures that do not merit separate code assignments, such as minor procedures preformed in conjunction with more extensive procedures or procedures that represent an operative approach.

See Condition:
The "see condition" note found in the Alphabetic Index to Disease instructs the coder to refer to a main term for the condition. This note will follow index terms that are nouns for anatomical sites or adjectival forms of disease term.

Morphology Codes
For each neoplastic disease listed in the index, a morphology code (M code) is provided that identifies histological type and behavior.

The histology is identified by the first four digits and the behavior is identified by the digit following the slash. Appendix A of Volume 1 contains a listing of morphology codes. This appendix is helpful when the pathology report identifies the neoplasm by using an M code. The coder may refer to Appendix A to determine the nomenclature of the neoplasm that will be the main term to search in the Index.

Additional Conventions

ADDITIONAL DIGITS REQUIRED

√3ʳ   This symbol indicates that the code requires a third digit.

√4ᵗ   This symbol indicates that the code requires a fourth digit.

√5ᵗ   This symbol indicates that a code requires a fifth digit.

☑   This symbol found only in the Alphabetic Index sections and the Table of Drugs and Chemicals indicates that an additional digit is required. Referring to the tabular section is essential to locate the appropriate additional digit.

DEFINITIONS

DEF: This symbol indicates a definition of disease or procedure term. The definition will appear in red type in the Disease and Procedure Tabular Lists.

Color Coding

Manifestation Code

These codes will appear in italic type as well as with a red color bar over the code title. A manifestation code is not allowed to be reported as a principal or first-listed diagnosis because each describes a manifestation of some other underlying disease, not the disease identified. This is referred to as mandatory multiple coding of etiology and manifestation. Code the underlying disease first. A 'Code first underlying disease' instructional note will appear with underlying disease codes identified. In the Alphabetic Index these codes are listed as the secondary code in slanted brackets with the code for the underlying disease listed first.

Other Notations

Alphabetic Indexes

▽   **Subterms under main terms may continue to next column or page.**
This warning statement is a reminder to always check for additional subterms and information that may continue onto the next page or column before making a final selection.

Official ICD-9-CM Guidelines for Coding and Reporting

Effective October 1, 2011

Note: Since no official ICD-9-CM addenda to the guidelines were released since 2013, the guidelines included in this book stand as the official guidelines effective October 1, 2013, through September 30, 2014.

The Centers for Medicare and Medicaid Services (CMS) and the National Center for Health Statistics (NCHS), two departments within the U.S. Federal Government's Department of Health and Human Services (DHHS) provide the following guidelines for coding and reporting using the International Classification of Diseases, 9th Revision, Clinical Modification (ICD-9-CM). These guidelines should be used as a companion document to the official version of the ICD-9-CM as published on CD-ROM by the U.S. Government Printing Office (GPO).

These guidelines have been approved by the four organizations that make up the Cooperating Parties for the ICD-9-CM: the American Hospital Association (AHA), the American Health Information Management Association (AHIMA), CMS, and NCHS. These guidelines are included on the official government version of the ICD-9-CM, and also appear in "Coding Clinic for ICD-9-CM" published by the AHA.

These guidelines are a set of rules that have been developed to accompany and complement the official conventions and instructions provided within the ICD-9-CM itself. The instructions and conventions of the classification take precedence over guidelines. These guidelines are based on the coding and sequencing instructions in Volumes I, II and III of ICD-9-CM, but provide additional instruction. Adherence to these guidelines when assigning ICD-9-CM diagnosis and procedure codes is required under the Health Insurance Portability and Accountability Act (HIPAA). The diagnosis codes (Volumes 1-2) have been adopted under HIPAA for all healthcare settings. Volume 3 procedure codes have been adopted for inpatient procedures reported by hospitals. A joint effort between the healthcare provider and the coder is essential to achieve complete and accurate documentation, code assignment, and reporting of diagnoses and procedures. These guidelines have been developed to assist both the healthcare provider and the coder in identifying those diagnoses and procedures that are to be reported. The importance of consistent, complete documentation in the medical record cannot be overemphasized. Without such documentation accurate coding cannot be achieved. The entire record should be reviewed to determine the specific reason for the encounter and the conditions treated.

The term encounter is used for all settings, including hospital admissions. In the context of these guidelines, the term provider is used throughout the guidelines to mean physician or any qualified health care practitioner who is legally accountable for establishing the patient's diagnosis. Only this set of guidelines, approved by the Cooperating Parties, is official.

The guidelines are organized into sections. Section I includes the structure and conventions of the classification and general guidelines that apply to the entire classification, and chapter-specific guidelines that correspond to the chapters as they are arranged in the classification. Section II includes guidelines for selection of principal diagnosis for non-outpatient settings. Section III includes guidelines for reporting additional diagnoses in non-outpatient settings. Section IV is for outpatient coding and reporting.

Section I. Conventions, general coding guidelines and chapter specific guidelines

A. Conventions for the ICD-9-CM
1. Format:
2. Abbreviations
   a. Index abbreviations
   b. Tabular abbreviations
3. Punctuation

4. Includes and Excludes Notes and Inclusion terms
5. Other and Unspecified codes
   a. "Other" codes
   b. "Unspecified" codes
6. Etiology/manifestation convention ("code first", "use additional code" and "in diseases classified elsewhere" notes)
7. "And"
8. "With"
9. "See" and "See Also"

B. General Coding Guidelines
1. Use of Both Alphabetic Index and Tabular List
2. Locate each term in the Alphabetic Index
3. Level of Detail in Coding
4. Code or codes from 001.0 through V91.99
5. Selection of codes 001.0 through 999.9
6. Signs and symptoms
7. Conditions that are an integral part of a disease process
8. Conditions that are not an integral part of a disease process
9. Multiple coding for a single condition
10. Acute and Chronic Conditions
11. Combination Code
12. Late Effects
13. Impending or Threatened Condition
14. Reporting Same Diagnosis Code more than Once
15. Admissions/Encounters for Rehabilitation
16. Documentation for BMI and Pressure Ulcer Stages
17. Syndromes
18. Documentation of Complications of Care

C. Chapter-Specific Coding Guidelines
1. Chapter 1: Infectious and Parasitic Diseases (001-139)
   a. Human Immunodeficiency Virus (HIV) Infections
   b. Septicemia, Systemic Inflammatory Response Syndrome (SIRS), Sepsis, Severe Sepsis and Septic Shock
   c. Methicillin Resistant *Staphylococcus aureus* (MRSA) Conditions
2. Chapter 2: Neoplasms (140-239)
   a. Treatment directed at the malignancy
   b. Treatment of secondary site
   c. Coding and sequencing of complications
   d. Primary malignancy previously excised
   e. Admissions/Encounters involving chemotherapy, immunotherapy and radiation therapy
   f. Admission/encounter to determine extent of malignancy
   g. Symptoms, signs, and ill-defined conditions listed in Chapter 16 associated with neoplasms
   h. Admission/encounter for pain control/management
   i. Malignant neoplasm associated with transplanted organ
3. Chapter 3: Endocrine, Nutritional, and Metabolic Diseases and Immunity Disorders (240-279)
   a. Diabetes mellitus
4. Chapter 4: Diseases of Blood and Blood Forming Organs (280-289)
   a. Anemia of chronic disease

Section III. Reporting Additional Diagnoses

A. Previous conditions

B. Abnormal findings

C. Uncertain diagnosis

Section IV. Diagnostic Coding and Reporting Guidelines for Outpatient Services

A. Selection of first-listed condition

    1. Outpatient Surgery

    2. Observation Stay

B. Codes from 001.0 through V91.99

C. Accurate reporting of ICD-9-CM diagnosis codes

D. Selection of codes 001.0 through 999.9

E. Codes that describe symptoms and signs

F. Encounters for circumstances other than a disease or injury

G. Level of Detail in Coding

    1. ICD-9-CM codes with 3, 4, or 5 digits

    2. Use of full number of digits required for a code

H. ICD-9-CM code for the diagnosis, condition, problem, or other reason for encounter/visit

I. Uncertain diagnosis

J. Chronic diseases

K. Code all documented conditions that coexist

L. Patients receiving diagnostic services only

M. Patients receiving therapeutic services only

N. Patients receiving preoperative evaluations only

O. Ambulatory surgery

P. Routine outpatient prenatal visits

Appendix I: Present on Admission Reporting Guidelines

Section I. Conventions, general coding guidelines and chapter specific guidelines

The conventions, general guidelines and chapter-specific guidelines are applicable to all health care settings unless otherwise indicated. The conventions and instructions of the classification take precedence over guidelines.

A. Conventions for the ICD-9-CM

The conventions for the ICD-9-CM are the general rules for use of the classification independent of the guidelines. These conventions are incorporated within the index and tabular of the ICD-9-CM as instructional notes. The conventions are as follows:

1. Format:

The ICD-9-CM uses an indented format for ease in reference

2. Abbreviations

    a. Index abbreviations

    NEC "Not elsewhere classifiable"

    This abbreviation in the index represents "other specified" when a specific code is not available for a condition the index directs the coder to the "other specified" code in the tabular.

    b. Tabular abbreviations

    NEC "Not elsewhere classifiable"

This abbreviation in the tabular represents "other specified". When a specific code is not available for a condition the tabular includes an NEC entry under a code to identify the code as the "other specified" code.

(See Section I.A.5.a. "Other" codes").

NOS "Not otherwise specified"

This abbreviation is the equivalent of unspecified.

(See Section I.A.5.b., "Unspecified" codes)

3. Punctuation

[ ] Brackets are used in the tabular list to enclose synonyms, alternative wording or explanatory phrases. Brackets are used in the index to identify manifestation codes. *(See Section I.A.6. "Etiology/manifestations")*

( ) Parentheses are used in both the index and tabular to enclose supplementary words that may be present or absent in the statement of a disease or procedure without affecting the code number to which it is assigned. The terms within the parentheses are referred to as nonessential modifiers.

: Colons are used in the Tabular list after an incomplete term which needs one or more of the modifiers following the colon to make it assignable to a given category.

4. Includes and Excludes Notes and Inclusion terms

Includes: This note appears immediately under a three-digit code title to further define, or give examples of, the content of the category.

Excludes: An excludes note under a code indicates that the terms excluded from the code are to be coded elsewhere. In some cases the codes for the excluded terms should not be used in conjunction with the code from which it is excluded. An example of this is a congenital condition excluded from an acquired form of the same condition. The congenital and acquired codes should not be used together. In other cases, the excluded terms may be used together with an excluded code. An example of this is when fractures of different bones are coded to different codes. Both codes may be used together if both types of fractures are present.

Inclusion terms: List of terms is included under certain four and five digit codes. These terms are the conditions for which that code number is to be used. The terms may be synonyms of the code title, or, in the case of "other specified" codes, the terms are a list of the various conditions assigned to that code. The inclusion terms are not necessarily exhaustive. Additional terms found only in the index may also be assigned to a code.

5. Other and Unspecified codes

    a. "Other" codes

    Codes titled "other" or "other specified" (usually a code with a 4th digit 8 or fifth-digit 9 for diagnosis codes) are for use when the information in the medical record provides detail for which a specific code does not exist. Index entries with NEC in the line designate "other" codes in the tabular. These index entries represent specific disease entities for which no specific code exists so the term is included within an "other" code.

    b. "Unspecified" codes

    Codes (usually a code with a 4th digit 9 or 5th digit 0 for diagnosis codes) titled "unspecified" are for use when the information in the medical record is insufficient to assign a more specific code.

6. **Etiology/manifestation convention ("code first", "use additional code" and "in diseases classified elsewhere" notes)**

   Certain conditions have both an underlying etiology and multiple body system manifestations due to the underlying etiology. For such conditions, the ICD-9-CM has a coding convention that requires the underlying condition be sequenced first followed by the manifestation. Wherever such a combination exists, there is a "use additional code" note at the etiology code, and a "code first" note at the manifestation code. These instructional notes indicate the proper sequencing order of the codes, etiology followed by manifestation.

   In most cases the manifestation codes will have in the code title, "in diseases classified elsewhere." Codes with this title are a component of the etiology/ manifestation convention. The code title indicates that it is a manifestation code. "In diseases classified elsewhere" codes are never permitted to be used as first listed or principal diagnosis codes. They must be used in conjunction with an underlying condition code and they must be listed following the underlying condition.

   There are manifestation codes that do not have "in diseases classified elsewhere" in the title. For such codes a "use additional code" note will still be present and the rules for sequencing apply.

   In addition to the notes in the tabular, these conditions also have a specific index entry structure. In the index both conditions are listed together with the etiology code first followed by the manifestation codes in brackets. The code in brackets is always to be sequenced second.

   The most commonly used etiology/manifestation combinations are the codes for Diabetes mellitus, category 250. For each code under category 250 there is a use additional code note for the manifestation that is specific for that particular diabetic manifestation. Should a patient have more than one manifestation of diabetes, more than one code from category 250 may be used with as many manifestation codes as are needed to fully describe the patient's complete diabetic condition. The category 250 diabetes codes should be sequenced first, followed by the manifestation codes.

   "Code first" and "Use additional code" notes are also used as sequencing rules in the classification for certain codes that are not part of an etiology/ manifestation combination.
   See - Section I.B.9. "Multiple coding for a single condition".

7. **"And"**

   The word "and" should be interpreted to mean either "and" or "or" when it appears in a title.

8. **"With"**

   The word "with" should be interpreted to mean "associated with" or "due to" when it appears in a code title, the Alphabetic Index, or an instructional note in the Tabular List.

   The word "with" in the alphabetic index is sequenced immediately following the main term, not in alphabetical order.

9. **"See" and "See Also"**

   The "see" instruction following a main term in the index indicates that another term should be referenced. It is necessary to go to the main term referenced with the "see" note to locate the correct code.

   A "see also" instruction following a main term in the index instructs that there is another main term that may also be referenced that may provide additional index entries that may be useful. It is not necessary to follow the "see also" note when the original main term provides the necessary code.

B. **General Coding Guidelines**

1. **Use of Both Alphabetic Index and Tabular List**

   Use both the Alphabetic Index and the Tabular List when locating and assigning a code. Reliance on only the Alphabetic Index or the Tabular List leads to errors in code assignments and less specificity in code selection.

2. **Locate each term in the Alphabetic Index**

   Locate each term in the Alphabetic Index and verify the code selected in the Tabular List. Read and be guided by instructional notations that appear in both the Alphabetic Index and the Tabular List.

3. **Level of Detail in Coding**

   Diagnosis and procedure codes are to be used at their highest number of digits available.

   ICD-9-CM diagnosis codes are composed of codes with 3, 4, or 5 digits. Codes with three digits are included in ICD-9-CM as the heading of a category of codes that may be further subdivided by the use of fourth and/or fifth digits, which provide greater detail.

   A three-digit code is to be used only if it is not further subdivided. Where fourth-digit subcategories and/or fifth-digit subclassifications are provided, they must be assigned. A code is invalid if it has not been coded to the full number of digits required for that code. For example, Acute myocardial infarction, code 410, has fourth digits that describe the location of the infarction (e.g., 410.2, Of inferolateral wall), and fifth digits that identify the episode of care. It would be incorrect to report a code in category 410 without a fourth and fifth digit.

   ICD-9-CM Volume 3 procedure codes are composed of codes with either 3 or 4 digits. Codes with two digits are included in ICD-9-CM as the heading of a category of codes that may be further subdivided by the use of third and/or fourth digits, which provide greater detail.

4. **Code or codes from 001.0 through V91.99**

   The appropriate code or codes from 001.0 through V91.99 must be used to identify diagnoses, symptoms, conditions, problems, complaints or other reason(s) for the encounter/visit.

5. **Selection of codes 001.0 through 999.9**

   The selection of codes 001.0 through 999.9 will frequently be used to describe the reason for the admission/encounter. These codes are from the section of ICD-9-CM for the classification of diseases and injuries (e.g., infectious and parasitic diseases; neoplasms; symptoms, signs, and ill-defined conditions, etc.).

6. **Signs and symptoms**

   Codes that describe symptoms and signs, as opposed to diagnoses, are acceptable for reporting purposes when a related definitive diagnosis has not been established (confirmed) by the provider. Chapter 16 of ICD-9-CM, Symptoms, Signs, and Ill-defined conditions (codes 780.0 - 799.9) contain many, but not all codes for symptoms.

7. **Conditions that are an integral part of a disease process**

   Signs and symptoms that are associated routinely with a disease process should not be assigned as additional codes, unless otherwise instructed by the classification.

8. **Conditions that are not an integral part of a disease process**

   Additional signs and symptoms that may not be associated routinely with a disease process should be coded when present.

9. **Multiple coding for a single condition**

   In addition to the etiology/manifestation convention that requires two codes to fully describe a single condition that affects multiple body systems, there are other single conditions that also require more than one code. "Use additional code" notes are found in the tabular at codes that are not part of an etiology/manifestation pair where a secondary code is useful to fully describe a condition. The sequencing rule is the same as the etiology/manifestation pair - "use additional code" indicates that a secondary code should be added.

For example, for infections that are not included in chapter 1, a secondary code from category 041, Bacterial infection in conditions classified elsewhere and of unspecified site, may be required to identify the bacterial organism causing the infection. A "use additional code" note will normally be found at the infectious disease code, indicating a need for the organism code to be added as a secondary code.

"Code first" notes are also under certain codes that are not specifically manifestation codes but may be due to an underlying cause. When a "code first" note is present and an underlying condition is present the underlying condition should be sequenced first.

"Code, if applicable, any causal condition first", notes indicate that this code may be assigned as a principal diagnosis when the causal condition is unknown or not applicable. If a causal condition is known, then the code for that condition should be sequenced as the principal or first-listed diagnosis.

Multiple codes may be needed for late effects, complication codes and obstetric codes to more fully describe a condition. See the specific guidelines for these conditions for further instruction.

10. Acute and Chronic Conditions

If the same condition is described as both acute (subacute) and chronic, and separate subentries exist in the Alphabetic Index at the same indentation level, code both and sequence the acute (subacute) code first.

11. Combination Code

A combination code is a single code used to classify:

- Two diagnoses, or
- A diagnosis with an associated secondary process (manifestation)
- A diagnosis with an associated complication

Combination codes are identified by referring to subterm entries in the Alphabetic Index and by reading the inclusion and exclusion notes in the Tabular List.

Assign only the combination code when that code fully identifies the diagnostic conditions involved or when the Alphabetic Index so directs. Multiple coding should not be used when the classification provides a combination code that clearly identifies all of the elements documented in the diagnosis. When the combination code lacks necessary specificity in describing the manifestation or complication, an additional code should be used as a secondary code.

12. Late Effects

A late effect is the residual effect (condition produced) after the acute phase of an illness or injury has terminated. There is no time limit on when a late effect code can be used. The residual may be apparent early, such as in cerebrovascular accident cases, or it may occur months or years later, such as that due to a previous injury. Coding of late effects generally requires two codes sequenced in the following order: The condition or nature of the late effect is sequenced first. The late effect code is sequenced second.

Exceptions to the above guidelines are those instances the late effect code has been expanded (at the fourth and fifth-digit

levels) to include the manifestation(s) or the classification instructs otherwise. The code for the acute phase of an illness or injury that led to the late effect is never used with a code for the late effect.

13. Impending or Threatened Condition

Code any condition described at the time of discharge as "impending" or "threatened" as follows:

> If it did occur, code as confirmed diagnosis.
> If it did not occur, reference the Alphabetic Index to determine if the condition has a subentry term for "impending" or "threatened" and also reference main term entries for "Impending" and for "Threatened."
> If the subterms are listed, assign the given code.
> If the subterms are not listed, code the existing underlying condition(s) and not the condition described as impending or threatened.

14. Reporting Same Diagnosis Code More than Once

Each unique ICD-9-CM diagnosis code may be reported only once for an encounter. This applies to bilateral conditions or two different conditions classified to the same ICD-9-CM diagnosis code.

15. Admissions/Encounters for Rehabilitation

When the purpose for the admission/encounter is rehabilitation, sequence the appropriate V code from category V57, Care involving use of rehabilitation procedures, as the principal/first-listed diagnosis. The code for the condition for which the service is being performed should be reported as an additional diagnosis.

Only one code from category V57 is required. Code V57.89, Other specified rehabilitation procedures, should be assigned if more than one type of rehabilitation is performed during a single encounter. A procedure code should be reported to identify each type of rehabilitation therapy actually performed.

16. Documentation for BMI and Pressure Ulcer Stages

For the Body Mass Index (BMI) and pressure ulcer stage codes, code assignment may be based on medical record documentation from clinicians who are not the patient's provider (i.e., physician or other qualified healthcare practitioner legally accountable for establishing the patient's diagnosis), since this information is typically documented by other clinicians involved in the care of the patient (e.g., a dietitian often documents the BMI and nurses often documents the pressure ulcer stages). However, the associated diagnosis (such as overweight, obesity, or pressure ulcer) must be documented by the patient's provider. If there is conflicting medical record documentation, either from the same clinician or different clinicians, the patient's attending provider should be queried for clarification.

The BMI and pressure ulcer stage codes should only be reported as secondary diagnoses. As with all other secondary diagnosis codes, the BMI and pressure ulcer stage codes should only be assigned when they meet the definition of a reportable additional diagnosis (see Section III, Reporting Additional Diagnoses).

17. Syndromes

Follow the Alphabetic Index guidance when coding syndromes. In the absence of index guidance, assign codes for the documented manifestations of the syndrome.

18. Documentation of complications of care

Code assignment is based on the provider's documentation of the relationship between the condition and the care or procedure. The guideline extends to any complications of care, regardless of the chapter the code is located in. It is important to note that not all conditions that occur during or following medical care or surgery are classified as complications. There must be a cause-and-effect relationship between the care provided and the condition, and an indication in the documentation that it is a complication. Query the provider for clarification, if the complication is not clearly documented.

C. Chapter-Specific Coding Guidelines

In addition to general coding guidelines, there are guidelines for specific diagnoses and/or conditions in the classification. Unless otherwise indicated, these guidelines apply to all health care settings. Please refer to Section II for guidelines on the selection of principal diagnosis.

1. Chapter 1: Infectious and Parasitic Diseases (001-139)

a. Human Immunodeficiency Virus (HIV) Infections

1) Code only confirmed cases

Code only confirmed cases of HIV infection/illness. This is an exception to the hospital inpatient guideline Section II, H.

In this context, "confirmation" does not require documentation of positive serology or culture for HIV; the provider's diagnostic statement that the patient is HIV positive, or has an HIV-related illness is sufficient.

2) Selection and sequencing of HIV codes

(a) Patient admitted for HIV-related condition

If a patient is admitted for an HIV-related condition, the principal diagnosis should be 042, followed by additional diagnosis codes for all reported HIV-related conditions.

(b) Patient with HIV disease admitted for unrelated condition

If a patient with HIV disease is admitted for an unrelated condition (such as a traumatic injury), the code for the unrelated condition (e.g., the nature of injury code) should be the principal diagnosis. Other diagnoses would be 042 followed by additional diagnosis codes for all reported HIV-related conditions.

(c) Whether the patient is newly diagnosed

Whether the patient is newly diagnosed or has had previous admissions/encounters for HIV conditions is irrelevant to the sequencing decision.

(d) Asymptomatic human immunodeficiency virus

V08 Asymptomatic human immunodeficiency virus [HIV] infection, is to be applied when the patient without any documentation of symptoms is listed as being "HIV positive," "known HIV," "HIV test positive," or similar terminology. Do not use this code if the term "AIDS" is used or if the patient is treated for any HIV-related illness or is described as having any condition(s) resulting from his/her HIV positive status; use 042 in these cases.

(e) Patients with inconclusive HIV serology

Patients with inconclusive HIV serology, but no definitive diagnosis or manifestations of the illness, may be assigned code 795.71, Inconclusive serologic test for Human Immunodeficiency Virus [HIV].

(f) Previously diagnosed HIV-related illness

Patients with any known prior diagnosis of an HIV-related illness should be coded to 042. Once a patient has developed an HIV-related illness, the patient should always be assigned code 042 on every subsequent admission/encounter. Patients previously diagnosed with any HIV illness (042) should never be assigned to 795.71 or V08.

(g) HIV Infection in Pregnancy, Childbirth and the Puerperium

During pregnancy, childbirth or the puerperium, a patient admitted (or presenting for a health care encounter) because of an HIV-related illness should receive a principal diagnosis code of 647.6x, Other specified infectious and parasitic diseases in the mother classifiable elsewhere, but complicating the pregnancy, childbirth or the puerperium, followed by 042 and the code(s) for the HIV-related illness(es). Codes from Chapter 15 always take sequencing priority.

Patients with asymptomatic HIV infection status admitted (or presenting for a health care encounter) during pregnancy, childbirth, or the puerperium should receive codes of 647.6x and V08.

(h) Encounters for testing for HIV

If a patient is being seen to determine his/her HIV status, use code V73.89, Screening for other specified viral disease. Use code V69.8, Other problems related to lifestyle, as a secondary code if an asymptomatic patient is in a known high risk group for HIV. Should a patient with signs or symptoms or illness, or a confirmed HIV related diagnosis be tested for HIV, code the signs and symptoms or the diagnosis. An additional counseling code V65.44 may be used if counseling is provided during the encounter for the test.

When a patient returns to be informed of his/her HIV test results use code V65.44, HIV counseling, if the results of the test are negative.

If the results are positive but the patient is asymptomatic use code V08, Asymptomatic HIV infection. If the results are positive and the patient is symptomatic use code 042, HIV infection, with codes for the HIV related symptoms or diagnosis. The HIV counseling code may also be used if counseling is provided for patients with positive test results.

b. Septicemia, Systemic Inflammatory Response Syndrome (SIRS), Sepsis, Severe Sepsis, and Septic Shock

1) SIRS, Septicemia, and Sepsis

(a) The terms *septicemia* and *sepsis* are often used interchangeably by providers, however they are not considered synonymous terms. The following descriptions are provided for reference but do not preclude querying the provider for clarification about terms used in the documentation:

(i) Septicemia generally refers to a systemic disease associated with the presence of pathological microorganisms or toxins in the blood, which can include bacteria, viruses, fungi or other organisms.

(ii) Systemic inflammatory response syndrome (SIRS) generally refers to the systemic response to infection, trauma/burns, or other insult (such as cancer) with symptoms including fever, tachycardia, tachypnea, and leukocytosis.

(iii) Sepsis generally refers to SIRS due to infection.

(iv) Severe sepsis generally refers to sepsis with associated acute organ dysfunction.

(b) The Coding of SIRS, sepsis and severe sepsis

The coding of SIRS, sepsis and severe sepsis requires a minimum of 2 codes: a code for the underlying cause (such as infection or trauma) and a code from subcategory 995.9 Systemic inflammatory response syndrome (SIRS).

(i) The code for the underlying cause (such as infection or trauma) must be sequenced before the code from subcategory 995.9 Systemic inflammatory response syndrome (SIRS).

(ii) Sepsis and severe sepsis require a code for the systemic infection (038.xx, 112.5, etc.) and either code 995.91, Sepsis, or 995.92, Severe sepsis. If the causal organism is not documented, assign code 038.9, Unspecified septicemia.

(iii) Severe sepsis requires additional code(s) for the associated acute organ dysfunction(s).

(iv) If a patient has sepsis with multiple organ dysfunctions, follow the instructions for coding severe sepsis.

(v) Either the term sepsis or SIRS must be documented to assign a code from subcategory 995.9.

(vi) *See Section I.C.17.g), Injury and poisoning, for information regarding systemic inflammatory response syndrome (SIRS) due to trauma/burns and other non-infectious processes.*

(c) Due to the complex nature of sepsis and severe sepsis, some cases may require querying the provider prior to assignment of the codes.

2) Sequencing sepsis and severe sepsis

(a) Sepsis and severe sepsis as principal diagnosis

If sepsis or severe sepsis is present on admission, and meets the definition of principal diagnosis, the systemic infection code (e.g., 038.xx, 112.5, etc) should be assigned as the principal diagnosis, followed by code 995.91, Sepsis, or 995.92, Severe sepsis, as required by the sequencing rules in the Tabular List. Codes from subcategory 995.9 can never be assigned as a principal diagnosis. A code should also be assigned for any localized infection, if present.

If the sepsis or severe sepsis is due to a postprocedural infection, see Section I.C.1.b.10 for guidelines related to sepsis due to postprocedural infection.

(b) Sepsis and severe sepsis as secondary diagnoses

When sepsis or severe sepsis develops during the encounter (it was not present on admission), the systemic infection code and code 995.91 or 995.92 should be assigned as secondary diagnoses.

(c) Documentation unclear as to whether sepsis or severe sepsis is present on admission

Sepsis or severe sepsis may be present on admission but the diagnosis may not be confirmed until sometime after admission. If the documentation is not clear whether the sepsis or severe sepsis was present on admission, the provider should be queried.

3) Sepsis/SIRS with Localized Infection

If the reason for admission is both sepsis, severe sepsis, or SIRS and a localized infection, such as pneumonia or cellulitis, a code for the systemic infection (038.xx, 112.5, etc) should be assigned first, then code 995.91 or 995.92, followed by the code for the localized infection. If the patient is admitted with a localized infection, such as pneumonia, and sepsis/SIRS doesn't develop until after admission, see guideline I.C.1.b.2.b).

If the localized infection is postprocedural, *see Section I.C.1.b.10 for guidelines related to sepsis due to postprocedural infection.*

Note: The term urosepsis is a nonspecific term. If that is the only term documented then only code 599.0 should be assigned based on the default for the term in the ICD-9-CM index, in addition to the code for the causal organism if known.

4) Bacterial Sepsis and Septicemia

In most cases, it will be a code from category 038, Septicemia, that will be used in conjunction with a code from subcategory 995.9 such as the following:

(a) Streptococcal sepsis

If the documentation in the record states streptococcal sepsis, codes 038.0, Streptococcal septicemia, and code 995.91 should be used, in that sequence.

(b) Streptococcal septicemia

If the documentation states streptococcal septicemia, only code 038.0 should be assigned, however, the provider should be queried whether the patient has sepsis, an infection with SIRS.

5) Acute organ dysfunction that is not clearly associated with the sepsis

If a patient has sepsis and an acute organ dysfunction, but the medical record documentation indicates that the acute organ dysfunction is related to a medical condition other than the sepsis, do not assign code 995.92, Severe sepsis. An acute organ dysfunction must be associated with the sepsis in order to assign the severe sepsis code. If the documentation is not clear as to whether an acute organ dysfunction is related to the sepsis or another medical condition, query the provider.

6) Septic shock

(a) Sequencing of septic shock

Septic shock generally refers to circulatory failure associated with severe sepsis, and, therefore, it represents a type of acute organ dysfunction.

For cases of septic shock, the code for the systemic infection should be sequenced first, followed by codes 995.92, Severe sepsis and 785.52, Septic shock or 998.02, Postoperative septic shock. Any additional codes for other acute organ dysfunctions should also be assigned. As noted in the sequencing instructions in the Tabular List, the code for septic shock cannot be assigned as a principal diagnosis.

(b) Septic Shock without documentation of severe sepsis

Since septic shock indicates the presence of severe sepsis, code 995.92, Severe sepsis, can be assigned with code 785.52, Septic shock, or code 998.02 Postoperative shock, septic, even if the term severe sepsis is not documented in the record.

7) Sepsis and septic shock complicating abortion and pregnancy

Sepsis and septic shock complicating abortion, ectopic pregnancy, and molar pregnancy are classified to category codes in Chapter 11 (630-639).

See section I.C.11.i.7. for information on the coding of puerperal sepsis.

8) Negative or inconclusive blood cultures

Negative or inconclusive blood cultures do not preclude a diagnosis of septicemia or sepsis in patients with clinical evidence of the condition, however, the provider should be queried.

9) Newborn sepsis

See Section I.C.15.j for information on the coding of newborn sepsis.

10) Sepsis due to a Postprocedural Infection

(a) Documentation of causal relationship

As with all postprocedural complications, code assignment is based on the provider's documentation of the relationship between the infection and the procedure.

(b) Sepsis due to postprocedural infection

In cases of postprocedural sepsis, the complication code, such as code 998.59, Other postoperative infection, or 674.3x, Other complications of obstetrical surgical wounds should be coded first followed by the appropriate sepsis codes (systemic infection code and either code 995.91or 995.92). An additional code(s) for any acute organ dysfunction should also be assigned for cases of severe sepsis.

See Section I.C.1.b.6 if the sepsis or severe sepsis results in postprocedural septic shock.

(c) Postprocedural infection and postprocedural septic shock

In cases where a postprocedural infection has occurred and has resulted in severe sepsis and postprocedural septic shock, the code for the precipitating complication such as code 998.59, Other postoperative infection, or 674.3x, Other complications of obstetrical surgical wounds should be coded first followed by the appropriate sepsis codes (systemic infection code and code 995.92). Code 998.02, Postoperative septic shock, should be assigned as an additional code. In cases of severe sepsis, an additional code(s) for any acute organ dysfunction should also be assigned.

11) External cause of injury codes with SIRS

Refer to Section I.C.19.a.7 for instruction on the use of external cause of injury codes with codes for SIRS resulting from trauma.

12) Sepsis and Severe Sepsis Associated with Non-infectious Process

In some cases, a non-infectious process, such as trauma, may lead to an infection which can result in sepsis or severe sepsis. If sepsis or severe sepsis is documented as associated with a non-infectious condition, such as a burn or serious injury, and this condition meets the definition for principal diagnosis, the code for the non-infectious condition should be sequenced first, followed by the code for the systemic infection and either code 995.91, Sepsis, or 995.92, Severe sepsis. Additional codes for any associated acute organ dysfunction(s) should also be assigned for cases of severe sepsis. If the sepsis or severe sepsis meets the definition of principal diagnosis, the systemic infection and sepsis codes should be sequenced before the non-infectious condition. When both the associated non-infectious condition and the sepsis or severe sepsis meet the definition of principal diagnosis, either may be assigned as principal diagnosis.

See Section I.C.1.b.2.a. for guidelines pertaining to sepsis or severe sepsis as the principal diagnosis.

Only one code from subcategory 995.9 should be assigned. Therefore, when a non-infectious condition leads to an infection resulting in sepsis or severe sepsis, assign either code 995.91 or 995.92. Do not additionally assign code 995.93, Systemic inflammatory response syndrome due to non-infectious process without acute organ dysfunction, or 995.94, Systemic inflammatory response syndrome with acute organ dysfunction.

See Section I.C.17.g for information on the coding of SIRS due to trauma/burns or other non-infectious disease processes.

c. Methicillin Resistant Staphylococcus aureus (MRSA) Conditions

1) Selection and sequencing of MRSA codes

(a) Combination codes for MRSA infection

When a patient is diagnosed with an infection that is due to methicillin resistant *Staphylococcus aureus* (MRSA), and that infection has a combination code that includes the causal organism (e.g., septicemia, pneumonia) assign the appropriate code for the condition (e.g., code 038.12, Methicillin resistant Staphylococcus aureus septicemia or code 482.42, Methicillin resistant pneumonia due to Staphylococcus aureus). Do not assign code 041.12, Methicillin resistant Staphylococcus aureus, as an additional code because the code includes the type of infection and the MRSA organism. Do not assign a code from subcategory V09.0, Infection with microorganisms resistant to penicillins, as an additional diagnosis.

See Section C.1.b.1 for instructions on coding and sequencing of septicemia.

(b) Other codes for MRSA infection

When there is documentation of a current infection (e.g., wound infection, stitch abscess, urinary tract infection) due to MRSA, and that infection does not have a combination code that includes the causal organism, select the appropriate code to identify the condition along with code 041.12, Methicillin resistant

Staphylococcus aureus, for the MRSA infection. Do not assign a code from subcategory V09.0, Infection with microorganisms resistant to penicillins.

(c) Methicillin susceptible Staphylococcus aureus (MSSA) and MRSA colonization

The condition or state of being colonized or carrying MSSA or MRSA is called colonization or carriage, while an individual person is described as being colonized or being a carrier. Colonization means that MSSA or MSRA is present on or in the body without necessarily causing illness. A positive MRSA colonization test might be documented by the provider as "MRSA screen positive" or "MRSA nasal swab positive".

Assign code V02.54, Carrier or suspected carrier, Methicillin resistant Staphylococcus aureus, for patients documented as having MRSA colonization. Assign code V02.53, Carrier or suspected carrier, Methicillin susceptible Staphylococcus aureus, for patient documented as having MSSA colonization. Colonization is not necessarily indicative of a disease process or as the cause of a specific condition the patient may have unless documented as such by the provider.

Code V02.59, Other specified bacterial diseases, should be assigned for other types of staphylococcal colonization (e.g., S. *epidermidis, S. saprophyticus)*. Code V02.59 should not be assigned for colonization with any type of *Staphylococcus aureus* (MRSA, MSSA).

(d) MRSA colonization and infection

If a patient is documented as having both MRSA colonization and infection during a hospital admission, code V02.54, Carrier or suspected carrier, Methicillin resistant *Staphylococcus aureus*, and a code for the MRSA infection may both be assigned.

2. Chapter 2: Neoplasms (140-239)

General guidelines

Chapter 2 of the ICD-9-CM contains the codes for most benign and all malignant neoplasms. Certain benign neoplasms, such as prostatic adenomas, may be found in the specific body system chapters. To properly code a neoplasm it is necessary to determine from the record if the neoplasm is benign, in-situ, malignant, or of uncertain histologic behavior. If malignant, any secondary (metastatic) sites should also be determined.

The neoplasm table in the Alphabetic Index should be referenced first. However, if the histological term is documented, that term should be referenced first, rather than going immediately to the Neoplasm Table, in order to determine which column in the Neoplasm Table is appropriate. For example, if the documentation indicates "adenoma," refer to the term in the Alphabetic Index to review the entries under this term and the instructional note to "see also neoplasm, by site, benign." The table provides the proper code based on the type of neoplasm and the site. It is important to select the proper column in the table that corresponds to the type of neoplasm. The tabular should then be referenced to verify that the correct code has been selected from the table and that a more specific site code does not exist.

See Section I. C. 18.d.4. for information regarding V codes for genetic susceptibility to cancer.

a. Treatment directed at the malignancy

If the treatment is directed at the malignancy, designate the malignancy as the principal diagnosis.

The only exception to this guideline is if a patient admission/encounter is solely for the administration of chemotherapy, immunotherapy or radiation therapy, assign the appropriate V58.x code as the first-listed or principal diagnosis, and the diagnosis or problem for which the service is being performed as a secondary diagnosis.

b. Treatment of secondary site

When a patient is admitted because of a primary neoplasm with metastasis and treatment is directed toward the secondary site only, the secondary neoplasm is designated as the principal diagnosis even though the primary malignancy is still present.

c. Coding and sequencing of complications

Coding and sequencing of complications associated with the malignancies or with the therapy thereof are subject to the following guidelines:

1) Anemia associated with malignancy

When admission/encounter is for management of an anemia associated with the malignancy, and the treatment is only for anemia, the appropriate anemia code (such as code 285.22, Anemia in neoplastic disease) is designated as the principal diagnosis and is followed by the appropriate code(s) for the malignancy.

Code 285.22 may also be used as a secondary code if the patient suffers from anemia and is being treated for the malignancy.

If anemia in neoplastic disease and anemia due to antineoplastic chemotherapy are both documented, assign codes for both conditions.

2) Anemia associated with chemotherapy, immunotherapy and radiation therapy

When the admission/encounter is for management of an anemia associated with chemotherapy, immunotherapy or radiotherapy and the only treatment is for the anemia, the anemia is sequenced first. The appropriate neoplasm code should be assigned as an additional code.

3) Management of dehydration due to the malignancy

When the admission/encounter is for management of dehydration due to the malignancy or the therapy, or a combination of both, and only the dehydration is being treated (intravenous rehydration), the dehydration is sequenced first, followed by the code(s) for the malignancy.

4) Treatment of a complication resulting from a surgical procedure

When the admission/encounter is for treatment of a complication resulting from a surgical procedure, designate the complication as the principal or first-listed diagnosis if treatment is directed at resolving the complication.

d. Primary malignancy previously excised

When a primary malignancy has been previously excised or eradicated from its site and there is no further treatment directed to that site and there is no evidence of any existing primary malignancy, a code from category V10, Personal history of malignant neoplasm, should be used to indicate the former site of the malignancy. Any mention of extension, invasion, or metastasis to another site is coded as a secondary malignant neoplasm to that site. The secondary site may be the principal or first-listed with the V10 code used as a secondary code.

e. **Admissions/Encounters involving chemotherapy, immunotherapy and radiation therapy**

1) **Episode of care involves surgical removal of neoplasm**

When an episode of care involves the surgical removal of a neoplasm, primary or secondary site, followed by adjunct chemotherapy or radiation treatment during the same episode of care, the neoplasm code should be assigned as principal or first-listed diagnosis, using codes in the 140-198 series or where appropriate in the 200-203 series.

2) **Patient admission/encounter solely for administration of chemotherapy, immunotherapy and radiation therapy**

If a patient admission/encounter is solely for the administration of chemotherapy, immunotherapy or radiation therapy assign code V58.0, Encounter for radiation therapy, or V58.11, Encounter for antineoplastic chemotherapy, or V58.12, Encounter for antineoplastic immunotherapy as the first-listed or principal diagnosis. If a patient receives more than one of these therapies during the same admission more than one of these codes may be assigned, in any sequence.

The malignancy for which the therapy is being administered should be assigned as a secondary diagnosis.

3) **Patient admitted for radiotherapy/chemotherapy and immunotherapy and develops complications**

When a patient is admitted for the purpose of radiotherapy, immunotherapy or chemotherapy and develops complications such as uncontrolled nausea and vomiting or dehydration, the principal or first-listed diagnosis is V58.0, Encounter for radiotherapy, or V58.11, Encounter for antineoplastic chemotherapy, or V58.12, Encounter for antineoplastic immunotherapy followed by any codes for the complications.

f. **Admission/encounter to determine extent of malignancy**

When the reason for admission/encounter is to determine the extent of the malignancy, or for a procedure such as paracentesis or thoracentesis, the primary malignancy or appropriate metastatic site is designated as the principal or first-listed diagnosis, even though chemotherapy or radiotherapy is administered.

g. **Symptoms, signs, and ill-defined conditions listed in Chapter 16 associated with neoplasms**

Symptoms, signs, and ill-defined conditions listed in Chapter 16 characteristic of, or associated with, an existing primary or secondary site malignancy cannot be used to replace the malignancy as principal or first-listed diagnosis, regardless of the number of admissions or encounters for treatment and care of the neoplasm.

h. **Admission/encounter for pain control/management**

See Section I.C.6.a.5 for information on coding admission/encounter for pain control/management.

i. **Malignant neoplasm associated with transplanted organ**

A malignant neoplasm of a transplanted organ should be coded as a transplant complication. Assign first the appropriate code from subcategory 996.8, Complications of transplanted organ, followed by code 199.2, Malignant neoplasm associated with transplanted organ. Use an additional code for the specific malignancy.

3. **Chapter 3: Endocrine, Nutritional, and Metabolic Diseases and Immunity Disorders (240-279)**

a. **Diabetes mellitus**

Codes under category 250, Diabetes mellitus, identify complications/manifestations associated with diabetes mellitus. A fifth-digit is required for all category 250 codes to identify the type of diabetes mellitus and whether the diabetes is controlled or uncontrolled.

See I.C.3.a.7 for secondary diabetes

1) **Fifth-digits for category 250:**

The following are the fifth-digits for the codes under category 250:

0   type II or unspecified type, not stated as uncontrolled

1   type I, [juvenile type], not stated as uncontrolled

2   type II or unspecified type, uncontrolled

3   type I, [juvenile type], uncontrolled

The age of a patient is not the sole determining factor, though most type I diabetics develop the condition before reaching puberty. For this reason type I diabetes mellitus is also referred to as juvenile diabetes.

2) **Type of diabetes mellitus not documented**

If the type of diabetes mellitus is not documented in the medical record the default is type II.

3) **Diabetes mellitus and the use of insulin**

All type I diabetics must use insulin to replace what their bodies do not produce. However, the use of insulin does not mean that a patient is a type I diabetic. Some patients with type II diabetes mellitus are unable to control their blood sugar through diet and oral medication alone and do require insulin. If the documentation in a medical record does not indicate the type of diabetes but does indicate that the patient uses insulin, the appropriate fifth-digit for type II must be used. For type II patients who routinely use insulin, code V58.67, Long-term (current) use of insulin, should also be assigned to indicate that the patient uses insulin. Code V58.67 should not be assigned if insulin is given temporarily to bring a type II patient's blood sugar under control during an encounter.

4) **Assigning and sequencing diabetes codes and associated conditions**

When assigning codes for diabetes and its associated conditions, the code(s) from category 250 must be sequenced before the codes for the associated conditions. The diabetes codes and the secondary codes that correspond to them are paired codes that follow the etiology/manifestation convention of the classification *(See Section I.A.6., Etiology/manifestation convention).* Assign as many codes from category 250 as needed to identify all of the associated conditions that the patient has. The corresponding secondary codes are listed under each of the diabetes codes.

(a) Diabetic retinopathy/diabetic macular edema

Diabetic macular edema, code 362.07, is only present with diabetic retinopathy. Another code from subcategory 362.0, Diabetic retinopathy, must be used with code 362.07. Codes under subcategory 362.0 are diabetes manifestation codes, so they must be used following the appropriate diabetes code.

5) Diabetes mellitus in pregnancy and gestational diabetes

(a) For diabetes mellitus complicating pregnancy, *see Section I.C.11.f., Diabetes mellitus in pregnancy.*

(b) For gestational diabetes, *see Section I.C.11, g., Gestational diabetes.*

6) Insulin pump malfunction

(a) Underdose of insulin due insulin pump failure

An underdose of insulin due to an insulin pump failure should be assigned 996.57, Mechanical complication due to insulin pump, as the principal or first listed code, followed by the appropriate diabetes mellitus code based on documentation.

(b) Overdose of insulin due to insulin pump failure

The principal or first listed code for an encounter due to an insulin pump malfunction resulting in an overdose of insulin, should also be 996.57, Mechanical complication due to insulin pump, followed by code 962.3, Poisoning by insulins and antidiabetic agents, and the appropriate diabetes mellitus code based on documentation.

7) Secondary Diabetes Mellitus

Codes under category 249, Secondary diabetes mellitus, identify complications/manifestations associated with secondary diabetes mellitus. Secondary diabetes is always caused by another condition or event (e.g., cystic fibrosis, malignant neoplasm of pancreas, pancreatectomy, adverse effect of drug, or poisoning).

(a) Fifth-digits for category 249:

A fifth-digit is required for all category 249 codes to identify whether the diabetes is controlled or uncontrolled.

(b) Secondary diabetes mellitus and the use of insulin

For patients who routinely use insulin, code V58.67, Long-term (current) use of insulin, should also be assigned. Code V58.67 should not be assigned if insulin is given temporarily to bring a patient's blood sugar under control during an encounter.

(c) Assigning and sequencing secondary diabetes codes and associated conditions

When assigning codes for secondary diabetes and its associated conditions (e.g. renal manifestations), the code(s) from category 249 must be sequenced before the codes for the associated conditions. The secondary diabetes codes and the diabetic manifestation codes that correspond to them are paired codes that follow the etiology/manifestation convention of the classification. Assign as many codes from category 249 as needed to identify all of the associated conditions that the patient has. The corresponding codes for the associated conditions are listed under each of the secondary diabetes codes. For example, secondary diabetes with diabetic nephrosis is assigned to code 249.40, followed by 581.81.

(d) Assigning and sequencing secondary diabetes codes and its causes

The sequencing of the secondary diabetes codes in relationship to codes for the cause of the diabetes is based on the reason for the encounter, applicable ICD-9-CM sequencing conventions, and chapter- specific guidelines.

If a patient is seen for treatment of the secondary diabetes or one of its associated conditions, a code from category 249 is sequenced as the principal or first-listed diagnosis, with the cause of the secondary diabetes (e.g. cystic fibrosis) sequenced as an additional diagnosis.

If, however, the patient is seen for the treatment of the condition causing the secondary diabetes (e.g., malignant neoplasm of pancreas), the code for the cause of the secondary diabetes should be sequenced as the principal or first-listed diagnosis followed by a code from category 249.

(i) Secondary diabetes mellitus due to pancreatectomy

For postpancreatectomy diabetes mellitus (lack of insulin due to the surgical removal of all or part of the pancreas), assign code 251.3, Postsurgical hypoinsulinemia. Assign a code from subcategory 249, Secondary diabetes mellitus and a code from subcategory V88.1, Acquired absence of pancreas as additional codes. Code also any diabetic manifestations (e.g. diabetic nephrosis 581.81).

(ii) Secondary diabetes due to drugs

Secondary diabetes may be caused by an adverse effect of correctly administered medications, poisoning or late effect of poisoning.

See section I.C.17.e for coding of adverse effects and poisoning, and section I.C.19 for E code reporting.

4. Chapter 4: Diseases of Blood and Blood Forming Organs (280-289)

a. Anemia of chronic disease

Subcategory 285.2, Anemia in chronic illness, has codes for anemia in chronic kidney disease, code 285.21; anemia in neoplastic disease, code 285.22; and anemia in other chronic illness, code 285.29. These codes can be used as the principal/first listed code if the reason for the encounter is to treat the anemia. They may also be used as secondary codes if treatment of the anemia is a component of an encounter, but not the primary reason for the encounter. When using a code from subcategory 285 it is also necessary to use the code for the chronic condition causing the anemia.

1) **Anemia in chronic kidney disease**

When assigning code 285.21, Anemia in chronic kidney disease, it is also necessary to assign a code from category 585, Chronic kidney disease, to indicate the stage of chronic kidney disease.

See I.C.10.a. Chronic kidney disease (CKD).

2) **Anemia in neoplastic disease**

When assigning code 285.22, Anemia in neoplastic disease, it is also necessary to assign the neoplasm code that is responsible for the anemia. Code 285.22 is for use for anemia that is due to the malignancy, not for anemia due to antineoplastic chemotherapy drugs. Assign the appropriate code for anemia due to antineoplastic chemotherapy.

See I.C.2.c.1 Anemia associated with malignancy.

See I.C.2.c.2 Anemia associated with chemotherapy, immunotherapy and radiation therapy.

5. **Chapter 5: Mental, Behavioral and Neurodevelopmental Disorders (290-319)**

Reserved for future guideline expansion

6. **Chapter 6: Diseases of Nervous System and Sense Organs (320-389)**

a. **Pain - Category 338**

1) **General coding information**

Codes in category 338 may be used in conjunction with codes from other categories and chapters to provide more detail about acute or chronic pain and neoplasm-related pain, unless otherwise indicated below.

If the pain is not specified as acute or chronic, do not assign codes from category 338, except for post-thoracotomy pain, postoperative pain, neoplasm related pain, or central pain syndrome.

A code from subcategories 338.1 and 338.2 should not be assigned if the underlying (definitive) diagnosis is known, unless the reason for the encounter is pain control/ management and not management of the underlying condition.

(a) **Category 338 Codes as Principal or First-Listed Diagnosis**

Category 338 codes are acceptable as principal diagnosis or the first-listed code:

- When pain control or pain management is the reason for the admission/encounter (e.g., a patient with displaced intervertebral disc, nerve impingement and severe back pain presents for injection of steroid into the spinal canal). The underlying cause of the pain should be reported as an additional diagnosis, if known.

- When an admission or encounter is for a procedure aimed at treating the underlying condition (e.g., spinal fusion, kyphoplasty), a code for the underlying condition (e.g., vertebral fracture, spinal stenosis) should be assigned as the principal diagnosis. No code from category 338 should be assigned.

- When a patient is admitted for the insertion of a neurostimulator for pain control, assign the appropriate pain code as the principal or first listed diagnosis. When an admission or encounter is for a procedure aimed at treating the underlying condition and a neurostimulator is inserted for pain control during the same admission/encounter, a code for the underlying condition should be assigned as the principal diagnosis and the appropriate pain code should be assigned as a secondary diagnosis.

(b) **Use of Category 338 Codes in Conjunction with Site Specific Pain Codes**

(i) **Assigning Category 338 Codes and Site-Specific Pain Codes**

Codes from category 338 may be used in conjunction with codes that identify the site of pain (including codes from chapter 16) if the category 338 code provides additional information. For example, if the code describes the site of the pain, but does not fully describe whether the pain is acute or chronic, then both codes should be assigned.

(ii) **Sequencing of Category 338 Codes with Site-Specific Pain Codes**

The sequencing of category 338 codes with site-specific pain codes (including chapter 16 codes), is dependent on the circumstances of the encounter/admission as follows:

- If the encounter is for pain control or pain management, assign the code from category 338 followed by the code identifying the specific site of pain (e.g., encounter for pain management for acute neck pain from trauma is assigned code 338.11, Acute pain due to trauma, followed by code 723.1, Cervicalgia, to identify the site of pain).

- If the encounter is for any other reason except pain control or pain management, and a related definitive diagnosis has not been established (confirmed) by the provider, assign the code for the specific site of pain first, followed by the appropriate code from category 338.

2) **Pain due to devices, implants and grafts**

Pain associated with devices, implants or grafts left in a surgical site (for example painful hip prosthesis) is assigned to the appropriate code(s) found in Chapter 17, Injury and Poisoning. Use additional code(s) from category 338 to identify acute or chronic pain due to presence of the device, implant or graft (338.18-338.19 or 338.28-338.29).

3) **Postoperative Pain**

Post-thoracotomy pain and other postoperative pain are classified to subcategories 338.1 and 338.2, depending on whether the pain is acute or chronic. The default for post-thoracotomy and other postoperative pain not specified as acute or chronic is the code for the acute form.

Routine or expected postoperative pain immediately after surgery should not be coded.

(a) **Postoperative pain not associated with specific postoperative complication**

Postoperative pain not associated with a specific postoperative complication is assigned to the appropriate postoperative pain code in category 338.

(b) Postoperative pain associated with specific postoperative complication

Postoperative pain associated with a specific postoperative complication (such as painful wire sutures) is assigned to the appropriate code(s) found in Chapter 17, Injury and Poisoning. If appropriate, use additional code(s) from category 338 to identify acute or chronic pain (338.18 or 338.28). If pain control/management is the reason for the encounter, a code from category 338 should be assigned as the principal or first-listed diagnosis in accordance with *Section I.C.6.a.1.a above.*

(c) Postoperative pain as principal or first-listed diagnosis

Postoperative pain may be reported as the principal or first-listed diagnosis when the stated reason for the admission/encounter is documented as postoperative pain control/management.

(d) Postoperative pain as secondary diagnosis

Postoperative pain may be reported as a secondary diagnosis code when a patient presents for outpatient surgery and develops an unusual or inordinate amount of postoperative pain.

The provider's documentation should be used to guide the coding of postoperative pain, as well as *Section III. Reporting Additional Diagnoses and Section IV. Diagnostic Coding and Reporting in the Outpatient Setting.*

See Section II.I.2 for information on sequencing of diagnoses for patients admitted to hospital inpatient care following post-operative observation.

See Section II.J for information on sequencing of diagnoses for patients admitted to hospital inpatient care from outpatient surgery.

See Section IV.A.2 for information on sequencing of diagnoses for patients admitted for observation.

4) Chronic pain

Chronic pain is classified to subcategory 338.2. There is no time frame defining when pain becomes chronic pain. The provider's documentation should be used to guide use of these codes.

5) Neoplasm Related Pain

Code 338.3 is assigned to pain documented as being related, associated or due to cancer, primary or secondary malignancy, or tumor. This code is assigned regardless of whether the pain is acute or chronic.

This code may be assigned as the principal or first-listed code when the stated reason for the admission/encounter is documented as pain control/pain management. The underlying neoplasm should be reported as an additional diagnosis.

When the reason for the admission/encounter is management of the neoplasm and the pain associated with the neoplasm is also documented, code 338.3 may be assigned as an additional diagnosis.

See Section I.C.2 for instructions on the sequencing of neoplasms for all other stated reasons for the admission/encounter (except for pain control/pain management).

6) Chronic pain syndrome

This condition is different than the term "chronic pain," and therefore this code should only be used when the provider has specifically documented this condition.

b. Glaucoma

1) Glaucoma

For types of glaucoma classified to subcategories 365.1-365.6, an additional code should be assigned from subcategory 365.7, Glaucoma stage, to identify the glaucoma stage. Codes from 365.7, Glaucoma stage, may not be assigned as a principal or first-listed diagnosis.

2) Bilateral glaucoma with same stage

When a patient has bilateral glaucoma and both are documented as being the same type and stage, report only the code for the type of glaucoma and one code for the stage.

3) Bilateral glaucoma stage with different stages

When a patient has bilateral glaucoma and each eye is documented as having a different stage, assign one code for the type of glaucoma and one code for the highest glaucoma stage.

4) Bilateral glaucoma with different types and different stages

When a patient has bilateral glaucoma and each eye is documented as having a different type and a different stage, assign one code for each type of glaucoma and one code for the highest glaucoma stage.

5) Patient admitted with glaucoma and stage evolves during the admission

If a patient is admitted with glaucoma and the stage progresses during the admission, assign the code for highest stage documented.

6) Indeterminate stage glaucoma

Assignment of code 365.74, Indeterminate stage glaucoma, should be based on the clinical documentation. Code 365.74 is used for glaucoma whose stage cannot be clinically determined. This code should not be confused with code 365.70, Glaucoma stage, unspecified. Code 365.70 should be assigned when there is no documentation regarding the stage of the glaucoma.

7. Chapter 7: Diseases of Circulatory System (390-459)

a. Hypertension

Hypertension Table

The Hypertension Table, found under the main term, "Hypertension", in the Alphabetic Index, contains a complete listing of all conditions due to or associated with hypertension and classifies them according to malignant, benign, and unspecified.

1) Hypertension, Essential, or NOS

Assign hypertension (arterial) (essential) (primary) (systemic) (NOS) to category code 401 with the appropriate fourth digit to indicate malignant (.0), benign (.1), or unspecified (.9). Do not use either .0 malignant or .1 benign unless medical record documentation supports such a designation.

2) Hypertension with Heart Disease

Heart conditions (425.8, 429.0-429.3, 429.8, 429.9) are assigned to a code from category 402 when a causal relationship is stated (due to hypertension) or implied (hypertensive). Use an additional code from category 428 to identify the type of heart failure in those patients with heart failure. More than one code from category 428 may be assigned if the patient has systolic or diastolic failure and congestive heart failure.

The same heart conditions (425.8, 429.0-429.3, 429.8, 429.9) with hypertension, but without a stated causal relationship, are coded separately. Sequence according to the circumstances of the admission/encounter.

3) Hypertensive Chronic Kidney Disease

Assign codes from category 403, Hypertensive chronic kidney disease, when conditions classified to category 585 or code 587 are present with hypertension. Unlike hypertension with heart disease, ICD-9-CM presumes a cause-and-effect relationship and classifies chronic kidney disease (CKD) with hypertension as hypertensive chronic kidney disease.

Fifth digits for category 403 should be assigned as follows:

- 0 with CKD stage I through stage IV, or unspecified.
- 1 with CKD stage V or end stage renal disease.

The appropriate code from category 585, Chronic kidney disease, should be used as a secondary code with a code from category 403 to identify the stage of chronic kidney disease.

See Section I.C.10.a for information on the coding of chronic kidney disease.

4) Hypertensive Heart and Chronic Kidney Disease

Assign codes from combination category 404, Hypertensive heart and chronic kidney disease, when both hypertensive kidney disease and hypertensive heart disease are stated in the diagnosis. Assume a relationship between the hypertension and the chronic kidney disease, whether or not the condition is so designated. Assign an additional code from category 428, to identify the type of heart failure. More than one code from category 428 may be assigned if the patient has systolic or diastolic failure and congestive heart failure.

Fifth digits for category 404 should be assigned as follows:

- 0 without heart failure and with chronic kidney disease (CKD) stage I through stage IV, or unspecified
- 1 with heart failure and with CKD stage I through stage IV, or unspecified
- 2 without heart failure and with CKD stage V or end stage renal disease
- 3 with heart failure and with CKD stage V or end stage renal disease

The appropriate code from category 585, Chronic kidney disease, should be used as a secondary code with a code from category 404 to identify the stage of kidney disease.

See Section I.C.10.a for information on the coding of chronic kidney disease.

5) Hypertensive Cerebrovascular Disease

First assign codes from 430-438, Cerebrovascular disease, then the appropriate hypertension code from categories 401-405.

6) Hypertensive Retinopathy

Two codes are necessary to identify the condition. First assign the code from subcategory 362.11,

Hypertensive retinopathy, then the appropriate code from categories 401-405 to indicate the type of hypertension.

7) Hypertension, Secondary

Two codes are required: one to identify the underlying etiology and one from category 405 to identify the hypertension. Sequencing of codes is determined by the reason for admission/encounter.

8) Hypertension, Transient

Assign code 796.2, Elevated blood pressure reading without diagnosis of hypertension, unless patient has an established diagnosis of hypertension. Assign code 642.3x for transient hypertension of pregnancy.

9) Hypertension, Controlled

Assign appropriate code from categories 401-405. This diagnostic statement usually refers to an existing state of hypertension under control by therapy.

10) Hypertension, Uncontrolled

Uncontrolled hypertension may refer to untreated hypertension or hypertension not responding to current therapeutic regimen. In either case, assign the appropriate code from categories 401-405 to designate the stage and type of hypertension. Code to the type of hypertension.

11) Elevated Blood Pressure

For a statement of elevated blood pressure without further specificity, assign code 796.2, Elevated blood pressure reading without diagnosis of hypertension, rather than a code from category 401.

b. Cerebral infarction/stroke/cerebrovascular accident (CVA)

The terms stroke and CVA are often used interchangeably to refer to a cerebral infarction. The terms stroke, CVA, and cerebral infarction NOS are all indexed to the default code 434.91, Cerebral artery occlusion, unspecified, with infarction.

Additional code(s) should be assigned for any neurologic deficits associated with the acute CVA, regardless of whether or not the neurologic deficit resolves prior to discharge.

See Section I.C.18.d.3 for information on coding status post administration of tPA in a different facility within the last 24 hours.

c. Postoperative cerebrovascular accident

A cerebrovascular hemorrhage or infarction that occurs as a result of medical intervention is coded to 997.02, Iatrogenic cerebrovascular infarction or hemorrhage. Medical record documentation should clearly specify the cause- and-effect relationship between the medical intervention and the cerebrovascular accident in order to assign this code. A secondary code from the code range 430-432 or from a code from subcategories 433 or 434 with a fifth digit of "1" should also be used to identify the type of hemorrhage or infarct.

This guideline conforms to the use additional code note instruction at category 997. Code 436, Acute, but ill-defined, cerebrovascular disease, should not be used as a secondary code with code 997.02.

d. **Late Effects of Cerebrovascular Disease**

1) **Category 438, Late Effects of Cerebrovascular disease**

Category 438 is used to indicate conditions classifiable to categories 430-437 as the causes of late effects (neurologic deficits), themselves classified elsewhere. These "late effects" include neurologic deficits that persist after initial onset of conditions classifiable to 430-437. The neurologic deficits caused by cerebrovascular disease may be present from the onset or may arise at any time after the onset of the condition classifiable to 430-437.

Codes in category 438 are only for use for late effects of cerebrovascular disease, not for neurologic deficits associated with an acute CVA.

2) **Codes from category 438 with codes from 430-437**

Codes from category 438 may be assigned on a health care record with codes from 430-437, if the patient has a current cerebrovascular accident (CVA) and deficits from an old CVA.

3) **Code V12.54**

Assign code V12.54, Transient ischemic attack (TIA), and cerebral infarction without residual deficits (and not a code from category 438) as an additional code for history of cerebrovascular disease when no neurologic deficits are present.

e. **Acute myocardial infarction (AMI)**

1) **ST elevation myocardial infarction (STEMI) and non ST elevation myocardial infarction (NSTEMI)**

The ICD-9-CM codes for acute myocardial infarction (AMI) identify the site, such as anterolateral wall or true posterior wall. Subcategories 410.0-410.6 and 410.8 are used for ST elevation myocardial infarction (STEMI). Subcategory 410.7, Subendocardial infarction, is used for non ST elevation myocardial infarction (NSTEMI) and nontransmural MIs.

2) **Acute myocardial infarction, unspecified**

Subcategory 410.9 is the default for the unspecified term acute myocardial infarction. If only STEMI or transmural MI without the site is documented, query the provider as to the site, or assign a code from subcategory 410.9.

3) **AMI documented as nontransmural or subendocardial but site provided**

If an AMI is documented as nontransmural or subendocardial, but the site is provided, it is still coded as a subendocardial AMI. If NSTEMI evolves to STEMI, assign the STEMI code. If STEMI converts to NSTEMI due to thrombolytic therapy, it is still coded as STEMI.

See Section I.C.18.d.3 for information on coding status post administration of tPA in a different facility within the last 24 hours.

8. **Chapter 8: Diseases of Respiratory System (460-519)**

See I.C.17.f. for ventilator-associated pneumonia.

a. **Chronic Obstructive Pulmonary Disease [COPD] and Asthma**

1) **Conditions that comprise COPD and Asthma**

The conditions that comprise COPD are obstructive chronic bronchitis, subcategory 491.2, and emphysema, category 492. All asthma codes are under category 493, Asthma. Code 496, Chronic airway

obstruction, not elsewhere classified, is a nonspecific code that should only be used when the documentation in a medical record does not specify the type of COPD being treated.

2) **Acute exacerbation of chronic obstructive bronchitis and asthma**

The codes for chronic obstructive bronchitis and asthma distinguish between uncomplicated cases and those in acute exacerbation. An acute exacerbation is a worsening or a decompensation of a chronic condition. An acute exacerbation is not equivalent to an infection superimposed on a chronic condition, though an exacerbation may be triggered by an infection.

3) **Overlapping nature of the conditions that comprise COPD and asthma**

Due to the overlapping nature of the conditions that make up COPD and asthma, there are many variations in the way these conditions are documented. Code selection must be based on the terms as documented. When selecting the correct code for the documented type of COPD and asthma, it is essential to first review the index, and then verify the code in the tabular list. There are many instructional notes under the different COPD subcategories and codes. It is important that all such notes be reviewed to assure correct code assignment.

4) **Acute exacerbation of asthma and status asthmaticus**

An acute exacerbation of asthma is an increased severity of the asthma symptoms, such as wheezing and shortness of breath. Status asthmaticus refers to a patient's failure to respond to therapy administered during an asthmatic episode and is a life threatening complication that requires emergency care. If status asthmaticus is documented by the provider with any type of COPD or with acute bronchitis, the status asthmaticus should be sequenced first. It supersedes any type of COPD including that with acute exacerbation or acute bronchitis. It is inappropriate to assign an asthma code with 5th digit 2, with acute exacerbation, together with an asthma code with 5th digit 1, with status asthmatics. Only the 5th digit 1 should be assigned.

b. **Chronic Obstructive Pulmonary Disease [COPD] and Bronchitis**

1) **Acute bronchitis with COPD**

Acute bronchitis, code 466.0, is due to an infectious organism. When acute bronchitis is documented with COPD, code 491.22, Obstructive chronic bronchitis with acute bronchitis, should be assigned. It is not necessary to also assign code 466.0. If a medical record documents acute bronchitis with COPD with acute exacerbation, only code 491.22 should be assigned. The acute bronchitis included in code 491.22 supersedes the acute exacerbation. If a medical record documents COPD with acute exacerbation without mention of acute bronchitis, only code 491.21 should be assigned.

c. **Acute Respiratory Failure**

1) **Acute respiratory failure as principal diagnosis**

Code 518.81, Acute respiratory failure, may be assigned as a principal diagnosis when it is the condition established after study to be chiefly responsible for occasioning the admission to the hospital, and the selection is supported by the Alphabetic Index and Tabular List. However, chapter-specific coding guidelines (such as obstetrics, poisoning, HIV, newborn) that provide sequencing direction take precedence.

2) Acute respiratory failure as secondary diagnosis

Respiratory failure may be listed as a secondary diagnosis if it occurs after admission, or if it is present on admission, but does not meet the definition of principal diagnosis.

3) Sequencing of acute respiratory failure and another acute condition

When a patient is admitted with respiratory failure and another acute condition, (e.g., myocardial infarction, cerebrovascular accident, aspiration pneumonia), the principal diagnosis will not be the same in every situation. This applies whether the other acute condition is a respiratory or nonrespiratory condition. Selection of the principal diagnosis will be dependent on the circumstances of admission. If both the respiratory failure and the other acute condition are equally responsible for occasioning the admission to the hospital, and there are no chapter-specific sequencing rules, the guideline regarding two or more diagnoses that equally meet the definition for principal diagnosis *(Section II, C.)* may be applied in these situations.

If the documentation is not clear as to whether acute respiratory failure and another condition are equally responsible for occasioning the admission, query the provider for clarification.

d. Influenza due to certain identified viruses

Code only confirmed cases of avian influenza (codes 488.01-488.02, 488.09, Influenza due to identified avian influenza virus), 2009 H1N1 influenza virus (codes 488.11-488.12, 488.19), or novel influenza A (codes 488.81-488.82, 488.89, Influenza due to identified novel influenza A virus). This is an exception to the hospital inpatient guideline Section II, H. (Uncertain Diagnosis).

In this context, "confirmation" does not require documentation of positive laboratory testing specific for avian, 2009 H1N1 or novel influenza A virus. However, coding should be based on the provider's diagnostic statement that the patient has avian influenza, 2009 H1N1 influenza, or novel influenza A.

If the provider records "suspected" or "possible" or "probable" avian, 2009 H1N1, or novel influenza A, the appropriate influenza code from category 487, Influenza should be assigned. A code from category 488, Influenza due to certain identified influenza viruses, should not be assigned.

9. Chapter 9: Diseases of Digestive System (520-579)

Reserved for future guideline expansion

10. Chapter 10: Diseases of Genitourinary System (580-629)

a. Chronic kidney disease

1) Stages of chronic kidney disease (CKD)

The ICD-9-CM classifies CKD based on severity. The severity of CKD is designated by stages I-V. Stage II, code 585.2, equates to mild CKD; stage III, code 585.3, equates to moderate CKD; and stage IV, code 585.4, equates to severe CKD. Code 585.6, End stage renal disease (ESRD), is assigned when the provider has documented end-stage-renal disease (ESRD).

If both a stage of CKD and ESRD are documented, assign code 585.6 only.

2) Chronic kidney disease and kidney transplant status

Patients who have undergone kidney transplant may still have some form of CKD, because the kidney transplant may not fully restore kidney function. Therefore, the presence of CKD alone does not constitute a transplant complication. Assign the appropriate 585 code for the patient's stage of CKD and code V42.0. If a transplant complication such as failure or rejection is documented, see section I.C.17.f.2.b for information on coding complications of a kidney transplant. If the documentation is unclear as to whether the patient has a complication of the transplant, query the provider.

3) Chronic kidney disease with other conditions

Patients with CKD may also suffer from other serious conditions, most commonly diabetes mellitus and hypertension. The sequencing of the CKD code in relationship to codes for other contributing conditions is based on the conventions in the tabular list.

See I.C.3.a.4 for sequencing instructions for diabetes.
See I.C.4.a.1 for anemia in CKD.
See I.C.7.a.3 for hypertensive chronic kidney disease.
See I.C.17.f.2.b, Kidney transplant complications, for instructions on coding of documented rejection or failure.

11. Chapter 11: Complications of Pregnancy, Childbirth, and the Puerperium (630-679)

a. General Rules for Obstetric Cases

1) Codes from chapter 11 and sequencing priority

Obstetric cases require codes from chapter 11, codes in the range 630-679, Complications of Pregnancy, Childbirth, and the Puerperium. Chapter 11 codes have sequencing priority over codes from other chapters. Additional codes from other chapters may be used in conjunction with chapter 11 codes to further specify conditions. Should the provider document that the pregnancy is incidental to the encounter, then code V22.2 should be used in place of any chapter 11 codes. It is the provider's responsibility to state that the condition being treated is not affecting the pregnancy.

2) Chapter 11 codes used only on the maternal record

Chapter 11 codes are to be used only on the maternal record, never on the record of the newborn.

3) Chapter 11 fifth-digits

Categories 640-648, 651-676 have required fifth-digits, which indicate whether the encounter is antepartum, postpartum and whether a delivery has also occurred.

4) Fifth-digits, appropriate for each code

The fifth-digits, which are appropriate for each code number, are listed in brackets under each code. The fifth-digits on each code should all be consistent with each other. That is, should a delivery occur all of the fifth-digits should indicate the delivery.

b. Selection of OB Principal or First-listed Diagnosis

1) Routine outpatient prenatal visits

For routine outpatient prenatal visits when no complications are present codes V22.0, Supervision of normal first pregnancy, and V22.1, Supervision of other normal pregnancy, should be used as the first-listed diagnoses. These codes should not be used in conjunction with chapter 11 codes.

2) Prenatal outpatient visits for high-risk patients

For routine prenatal outpatient visits for patients with high-risk pregnancies, a code from category V23, Supervision of high-risk pregnancy, should be used as the first-listed diagnosis. Secondary chapter 11 codes may be used in conjunction with these codes if appropriate.

3) Episodes when no delivery occurs

In episodes when no delivery occurs, the principal diagnosis should correspond to the principal complication of the pregnancy, which necessitated the encounter. Should more than one complication exist, all of which are treated or monitored, any of the complications codes may be sequenced first.

4) When a delivery occurs

When a delivery occurs, the principal diagnosis should correspond to the main circumstances or complication of the delivery. In cases of cesarean delivery, the selection of the principal diagnosis should be the condition established after study that was responsible for the patient's admission. If the patient was admitted with a condition that resulted in the performance of a cesarean procedure, that condition should be selected as the principal diagnosis. If the reason for the admission/encounter was unrelated to the condition resulting in the cesarean delivery, the condition related to the reason for the admission/encounter should be selected as the principal diagnosis, even if a cesarean was performed.

5) Outcome of delivery

An outcome of delivery code, V27.0-V27.9, should be included on every maternal record when a delivery has occurred. These codes are not to be used on subsequent records or on the newborn record.

c. Fetal Conditions Affecting the Management of the Mother

1) Codes from categories 655 and 656

Codes from categories 655, Known or suspected fetal abnormality affecting management of the mother, and 656, Other known or suspected fetal and placental problems affecting the management of the mother, are assigned only when the fetal condition is actually responsible for modifying the management of the mother, i.e., by requiring diagnostic studies, additional observation, special care, or termination of pregnancy. The fact that the fetal condition exists does not justify assigning a code from this series to the mother's record.

See I.C.18.d. for suspected maternal and fetal conditions not found

2) In utero surgery

In cases when surgery is performed on the fetus, a diagnosis code from category 655, Known or suspected fetal abnormalities affecting management of the mother, should be assigned identifying the fetal condition. Procedure code 75.36, Correction of fetal defect, should be assigned on the hospital inpatient record.

No code from Chapter 15, the perinatal codes, should be used on the mother's record to identify fetal

conditions. Surgery performed in utero on a fetus is still to be coded as an obstetric encounter.

d. HIV Infection in Pregnancy, Childbirth and the Puerperium

During pregnancy, childbirth or the puerperium, a patient admitted because of an HIV-related illness should receive a principal diagnosis of 647.6x, Other specified infectious and parasitic diseases in the mother classifiable elsewhere, but complicating the pregnancy, childbirth or the puerperium, followed by 042 and the code(s) for the HIV-related illness(es).

Patients with asymptomatic HIV infection status admitted during pregnancy, childbirth, or the puerperium should receive codes of 647.6x and V08.

e. Current Conditions Complicating Pregnancy

Assign a code from subcategory 648.x for patients that have current conditions when the condition affects the management of the pregnancy, childbirth, or the puerperium. Use additional secondary codes from other chapters to identify the conditions, as appropriate.

f. Diabetes mellitus in pregnancy

Diabetes mellitus is a significant complicating factor in pregnancy. Pregnant women who are diabetic should be assigned code 648.0x, Diabetes mellitus complicating pregnancy, and a secondary code from category 250, Diabetes mellitus, or category 249, Secondary diabetes to identify the type of diabetes.

Code V58.67, Long-term (current) use of insulin, should also be assigned if the diabetes mellitus is being treated with insulin.

g. Gestational diabetes

Gestational diabetes can occur during the second and third trimester of pregnancy in women who were not diabetic prior to pregnancy. Gestational diabetes can cause complications in the pregnancy similar to those of pre-existing diabetes mellitus. It also puts the woman at greater risk of developing diabetes after the pregnancy. Gestational diabetes is coded to 648.8x, Abnormal glucose tolerance. Codes 648.0x and 648.8x should never be used together on the same record.

Code V58.67, Long-term (current) use of insulin, should also be assigned if the gestational diabetes is being treated with insulin.

h. Normal Delivery, Code 650

1) Normal delivery

Code 650 is for use in cases when a woman is admitted for a full-term normal delivery and delivers a single, healthy infant without any complications antepartum, during the delivery, or postpartum during the delivery episode. Code 650 is always a principal diagnosis. It is not to be used if any other code from chapter 11 is needed to describe a current complication of the antenatal, delivery, or perinatal period. Additional codes from other chapters may be used with code 650 if they are not related to or are in any way complicating the pregnancy.

2) Normal delivery with resolved antepartum complication

Code 650 may be used if the patient had a complication at some point during her pregnancy, but the complication is not present at the time of the admission for delivery.

3) V27.0, Single liveborn, outcome of delivery

V27.0, Single liveborn, is the only outcome of delivery code appropriate for use with 650.

i. The Postpartum and Peripartum Periods

1) Postpartum and peripartum periods

The postpartum period begins immediately after delivery and continues for six weeks following delivery. The peripartum period is defined as the last month of pregnancy to five months postpartum.

2) Postpartum complication

A postpartum complication is any complication occurring within the six-week period.

3) Pregnancy-related complications after 6 week period

Chapter 11 codes may also be used to describe pregnancy-related complications after the six-week period should the provider document that a condition is pregnancy related.

4) Postpartum complications occurring during the same admission as delivery

Postpartum complications that occur during the same admission as the delivery are identified with a fifth digit of "2." Subsequent admissions/encounters for postpartum complications should be identified with a fifth digit of "4."

5) Admission for routine postpartum care following delivery outside hospital

When the mother delivers outside the hospital prior to admission and is admitted for routine postpartum care and no complications are noted, code V24.0, Postpartum care and examination immediately after delivery, should be assigned as the principal diagnosis.

6) Admission following delivery outside hospital with postpartum conditions

A delivery diagnosis code should not be used for a woman who has delivered prior to admission to the hospital. Any postpartum conditions and/or postpartum procedures should be coded.

7) Puerperal sepsis

Code 670.2x, Puerperal sepsis, should be assigned with a secondary code to identify the causal organism (e.g., for a bacterial infection, assign a code from category 041, Bacterial infections in conditions classified elsewhere and of unspecified site). A code from category 038, Septicemia, should not be used for puerperal sepsis. Do not assign code 995.91, Sepsis, as code 670.2x describes the sepsis. If applicable, use additional codes to identify severe sepsis (995.92) and any associated acute organ dysfunction.

j. Code 677, Late effect of complication of pregnancy

1) Code 677

Code 677, Late effect of complication of pregnancy, childbirth, and the puerperium is for use in those cases when an initial complication of a pregnancy develops a sequelae requiring care or treatment at a future date.

2) After the initial postpartum period

This code may be used at any time after the initial postpartum period.

3) Sequencing of Code 677

This code, like all late effect codes, is to be sequenced following the code describing the sequelae of the complication.

k. Abortions

1) Fifth-digits required for abortion categories

Fifth-digits are required for abortion categories 634-637. Fifth digit assignment is based on the status of the patient at the beginning (or start) of the encounter. Fifth-digit 1, incomplete, indicates that all of the products of conception have not been expelled from the uterus. Fifth-digit 2, complete, indicates that all products of conception have been expelled from the uterus.

2) Code from categories 640-648 and 651-659

A code from categories 640-648 and 651-659 may be used as additional codes with an abortion code to indicate the complication leading to the abortion.

Fifth digit 3 is assigned with codes from these categories when used with an abortion code because the other fifth digits will not apply. Codes from the 660-669 series are not to be used for complications of abortion.

3) Code 639 for complications

Code 639 is to be used for all complications following abortion. Code 639 cannot be assigned with codes from categories 634-638.

4) Abortion with Liveborn Fetus

When an attempted termination of pregnancy results in a liveborn fetus assign code 644.21, Early onset of delivery, with an appropriate code from category V27, Outcome of Delivery. The procedure code for the attempted termination of pregnancy should also be assigned.

5) Retained Products of Conception following an abortion

Subsequent admissions for retained products of conception following a spontaneous or legally induced abortion are assigned the appropriate code from category 634, Spontaneous abortion, or 635 Legally induced abortion, with a fifth digit of "1" (incomplete). This advice is appropriate even when the patient was discharged previously with a discharge diagnosis of complete abortion.

12. Chapter 12: Diseases Skin and Subcutaneous Tissue (680-709)

a. Pressure ulcer stage codes

1) Pressure ulcer stages

Two codes are needed to completely describe a pressure ulcer: A code from subcategory 707.0, Pressure ulcer, to identify the site of the pressure ulcer and a code from subcategory 707.2, Pressure ulcer stages.

The codes in subcategory 707.2, Pressure ulcer stages, are to be used as an additional diagnosis with a code(s) from subcategory 707.0, Pressure Ulcer. Codes from 707.2, Pressure ulcer stages, may not be assigned as a principal or first-listed diagnosis. The pressure ulcer stage codes should only be used with pressure ulcers and not with other types of ulcers (e.g., stasis ulcer).

The ICD-9-CM classifies pressure ulcer stages based on severity, which is designated by stages I-IV and unstageable.

2) Unstageable pressure ulcers

Assignment of code 707.25, Pressure ulcer, unstageable, should be based on the clinical documentation. Code 707.25 is used for pressure ulcers whose stage cannot be clinically determined (e.g., the ulcer is covered by eschar or has been treated with a skin or muscle graft) and pressure ulcers that are documented as deep tissue injury but not documented as due to trauma. This code should not be confused with code 707.20, Pressure ulcer, stage unspecified. Code 707.20 should be assigned when there is no documentation regarding the stage of the pressure ulcer.

3) Documented pressure ulcer stage

Assignment of the pressure ulcer stage code should be guided by clinical documentation of the stage or documentation of the terms found in the index. For clinical terms describing the stage that are not found in the index, and there is no documentation of the stage, the provider should be queried.

4) Bilateral pressure ulcers with same stage

When a patient has bilateral pressure ulcers (e.g., both buttocks) and both pressure ulcers are documented as being the same stage, only the code for the site and one code for the stage should be reported.

5) Bilateral pressure ulcers with different stages

When a patient has bilateral pressure ulcers at the same site (e.g., both buttocks) and each pressure ulcer is documented as being at a different stage, assign one code for the site and the appropriate codes for the pressure ulcer stage.

6) Multiple pressure ulcers of different sites and stages

When a patient has multiple pressure ulcers at different sites (e.g., buttock, heel, shoulder) and each pressure ulcer is documented as being at different stages (e.g., stage 3 and stage 4), assign the appropriate codes for each different site and a code for each different pressure ulcer stage.

7) Patients admitted with pressure ulcers documented as healed

No code is assigned if the documentation states that the pressure ulcer is completely healed.

8) Patients admitted with pressure ulcers documented as healing

Pressure ulcers described as healing should be assigned the appropriate pressure ulcer stage code based on the documentation in the medical record. If the documentation does not provide information about the stage of the healing pressure ulcer, assign code 707.20, Pressure ulcer stage, unspecified.

If the documentation is unclear as to whether the patient has a current (new) pressure ulcer or if the patient is being treated for a healing pressure ulcer, query the provider.

9) Patient admitted with pressure ulcer evolving into another stage during the admission

If a patient is admitted with a pressure ulcer at one stage and it progresses to a higher stage, assign the code for highest stage reported for that site.

13. Chapter 13: Diseases of Musculoskeletal and Connective Tissue (710-739)

a. Coding of Pathologic Fractures

1) Acute Fractures vs. Aftercare

Pathologic fractures are reported using subcategory 733.1, when the fracture is newly diagnosed. Subcategory 733.1 may be used while the patient is receiving active treatment for the fracture. Examples of active treatment are: surgical treatment, emergency department encounter, evaluation and treatment by a new physician.

Fractures are coded using the aftercare codes (subcategories V54.0, V54.2, V54.8 or V54.9) for encounters after the patient has completed active treatment of the fracture and is receiving routine care for the fracture during the healing or recovery phase. Examples of fracture aftercare are: cast change or removal, removal of external or internal fixation device, medication adjustment, and follow up visits following fracture treatment.

Care for complications of surgical treatment for fracture repairs during the healing or recovery phase should be coded with the appropriate complication codes.

Care of complications of fractures, such as malunion and nonunion, should be reported with the appropriate codes.

See Section I. C. 17.b for information on the coding of traumatic fractures.

14. Chapter 14: Congenital Anomalies (740-759)

a. Codes in categories 740-759, Congenital Anomalies

Assign an appropriate code(s) from categories 740-759, Congenital Anomalies, when an anomaly is documented. A congenital anomaly may be the principal/first listed diagnosis on a record or a secondary diagnosis.

When a congenital anomaly does not have a unique code assignment, assign additional code(s) for any manifestations that may be present.

When the code assignment specifically identifies the congenital anomaly, manifestations that are an inherent component of the anomaly should not be coded separately. Additional codes should be assigned for manifestations that are not an inherent component.

Codes from Chapter 14 may be used throughout the life of the patient. If a congenital anomaly has been corrected, a personal history code should be used to identify the history of the anomaly. Although present at birth, a congenital anomaly may not be identified until later in life. Whenever the condition is diagnosed by the physician, it is appropriate to assign a code from codes 740-759.

For the birth admission, the appropriate code from category V30, Liveborn infants, according to type of birth should be sequenced as the principal diagnosis, followed by any congenital anomaly codes, 740-759.

15. Chapter 15: Newborn (Perinatal) Guidelines (760-779)

For coding and reporting purposes the perinatal period is defined as before birth through the 28th day following birth. The following guidelines are provided for reporting purposes. Hospitals may record other diagnoses as needed for internal data use.

a. General Perinatal Rules

1) Chapter 15 Codes

They are never for use on the maternal record. Codes from Chapter 11, the obstetric chapter, are never permitted on the newborn record. Chapter 15 code may be used throughout the life of the patient if the condition is still present.

2) Sequencing of perinatal codes

Generally, codes from Chapter 15 should be sequenced as the principal/first-listed diagnosis on the newborn record, with the exception of the appropriate V30 code for the birth episode, followed by codes from any other chapter that provide additional detail. The "use additional code" note at the beginning of the chapter supports this guideline. If the index does not provide a specific code for a perinatal condition, assign code 779.89, Other specified conditions originating in the perinatal period, followed by the code from another chapter that specifies the condition. Codes for signs and symptoms may be assigned when a definitive diagnosis has not been established.

3) Birth process or community acquired conditions

If a newborn has a condition that may be either due to the birth process or community acquired and the documentation does not indicate which it is, the default is due to the birth process and the code from Chapter 15 should be used. If the condition is community-acquired, a code from Chapter 15 should not be assigned.

4) Code all clinically significant conditions

All clinically significant conditions noted on routine newborn examination should be coded. A condition is clinically significant if it requires:

- clinical evaluation; or
- therapeutic treatment; or
- diagnostic procedures; or
- extended length of hospital stay; or
- increased nursing care and/or monitoring; or
- has implications for future health care needs

Note: The perinatal guidelines listed above are the same as the general coding guidelines for "additional diagnoses", except for the final point regarding implications for future health care needs. Codes should be assigned for conditions that have been specified by the provider as having implications for future health care needs. Codes from the perinatal chapter should not be assigned unless the provider has established a definitive diagnosis.

b. Use of codes V30-V39

When coding the birth of an infant, assign a code from categories V30-V39, according to the type of birth. A code from this series is assigned as a principal diagnosis, and assigned only once to a newborn at the time of birth.

c. Newborn transfers

If the newborn is transferred to another institution, the V30 series is not used at the receiving hospital.

d. Use of category V29

1) Assigning a code from category V29

Assign a code from category V29, Observation and evaluation of newborns and infants for suspected conditions not found, to identify those instances when a healthy newborn is evaluated for a suspected condition that is determined after study not to be present. Do not use a code from category V29 when the patient has identified signs or symptoms of a suspected problem; in such cases, code the sign or symptom.

A code from category V29 may also be assigned as a principal code for readmissions or encounters when the V30 code no longer applies. Codes from category V29 are for use only for healthy newborns and infants for which no condition after study is found to be present.

2) V29 code on a birth record

A V29 code is to be used as a secondary code after the V30, Outcome of delivery, code.

e. Use of other V codes on perinatal records

V codes other than V30 and V29 may be assigned on a perinatal or newborn record code. The codes may be used as a principal or first-listed diagnosis for specific types of encounters or for readmissions or encounters when the V30 code no longer applies.

See Section I.C.18 for information regarding the assignment of V codes.

f. Maternal Causes of Perinatal Morbidity

Codes from categories 760-763, Maternal causes of perinatal morbidity and mortality, are assigned only when the maternal condition has actually affected the fetus or newborn. The fact that the mother has an associated medical condition or experiences some complication of pregnancy, labor or delivery does not justify the routine assignment of codes from these categories to the newborn record.

g. Congenital Anomalies in Newborns

For the birth admission, the appropriate code from category V30, Liveborn infants according to type of birth, should be used, followed by any congenital anomaly codes, categories 740-759. Use additional secondary codes from other chapters to specify conditions associated with the anomaly, if applicable.

Also, see Section I.C.14 for information on the coding of congenital anomalies.

h. Coding Additional Perinatal Diagnoses

1) Assigning codes for conditions that require treatment

Assign codes for conditions that require treatment or further investigation, prolong the length of stay, or require resource utilization.

2) Codes for conditions specified as having implications for future health care needs

Assign codes for conditions that have been specified by the provider as having implications for future health care needs.

Note: This guideline should not be used for adult patients.

3) Codes for newborn conditions originating in the perinatal period

Assign a code for newborn conditions originating in the perinatal period (categories 760-779), as well as complications arising during the current episode of care classified in other chapters, only if the diagnoses have been documented by the responsible provider at the time of transfer or discharge as having affected the fetus or newborn.

i. Prematurity and Fetal Growth Retardation

Providers utilize different criteria in determining prematurity. A code for prematurity should not be assigned unless it is documented. The 5th digit assignment for codes from category 764 and subcategories 765.0 and 765.1 should be based on the recorded birth weight and estimated gestational age.

A code from subcategory 765.2, Weeks of gestation, should be assigned as an additional code with category 764 and codes from 765.0 and 765.1 to specify weeks of gestation as documented by the provider in the record.

j. Newborn sepsis

Code 771.81, Septicemia [sepsis] of newborn, should be assigned with a secondary code from category 041, Bacterial infections in conditions classified elsewhere and of unspecified site, to identify the organism. A code from category 038, Septicemia, should not be used on a newborn record. Do not assign code 995.91, Sepsis, as code 771.81 describes the sepsis. If applicable, use additional codes to identify severe sepsis (995.92) and any associated acute organ dysfunction.

16. Chapter 16: Symptoms, Signs, and Ill-Defined Conditions (780-799)

Reserved for future guideline expansion

17. Chapter 17: Injury and Poisoning (800-999)

a. Coding of Injuries

When coding injuries, assign separate codes for each injury unless a combination code is provided, in which case the combination code is assigned. Multiple injury codes are provided in ICD-9-CM, but should not be assigned unless information for a more specific code is not available. These traumatic injury codes are not to be used for normal, healing surgical wounds or to identify complications of surgical wounds.

The code for the most serious injury, as determined by the provider and the focus of treatment, is sequenced first.

1) Superficial injuries

Superficial injuries such as abrasions or contusions are not coded when associated with more severe injuries of the same site.

2) Primary injury with damage to nerves/blood vessels

When a primary injury results in minor damage to peripheral nerves or blood vessels, the primary injury is sequenced first with additional code(s) from categories 950-957, Injury to nerves and spinal cord, and/or 900-904, Injury to blood vessels. When the primary injury is to the blood vessels or nerves, that injury should be sequenced first.

b. Coding of Traumatic Fractures

The principles of multiple coding of injuries should be followed in coding fractures. Fractures of specified sites are coded individually by site in accordance with both the provisions within categories 800-829 and the level of detail furnished by medical record content. Combination categories for multiple fractures are provided for use when there is insufficient detail in the medical record (such as trauma cases transferred to another hospital), when the reporting form limits the number of codes that can be used in reporting pertinent clinical data, or when there is insufficient specificity at the fourth-digit or fifth-digit level. More specific guidelines are as follows:

1) Acute Fractures vs. Aftercare

Traumatic fractures are coded using the acute fracture codes (800-829) while the patient is receiving active treatment for the fracture. Examples of active treatment are: surgical treatment, emergency department encounter, and evaluation and treatment by a new physician.

Fractures are coded using the aftercare codes (subcategories V54.0, V54.1, V54.8, or V54.9) for encounters after the patient has completed active treatment of the fracture and is receiving routine care for the fracture during the healing or recovery phase. Examples of fracture aftercare are: cast change or removal, removal of external or internal fixation device, medication adjustment, and follow up visits following fracture treatment.

Care for complications of surgical treatment for fracture repairs during the healing or recovery phase should be coded with the appropriate complication codes.

Care of complications of fractures, such as malunion and nonunion, should be reported with the appropriate codes.

Pathologic fractures are not coded in the 800-829 range, but instead are assigned to subcategory 733.1. *See Section I.C.13.a for additional information.*

2) Multiple fractures of same limb

Multiple fractures of same limb classifiable to the same three-digit or four-digit category are coded to that category.

3) Multiple unilateral or bilateral fractures of same bone

Multiple unilateral or bilateral fractures of same bone(s) but classified to different fourth-digit subdivisions (bone part) within the same three-digit category are coded individually by site.

4) Multiple fracture categories 819 and 828

Multiple fracture categories 819 and 828 classify bilateral fractures of both upper limbs (819) and both lower limbs (828), but without any detail at the fourth-digit level other than open and closed type of fractures.

5) Multiple fractures sequencing

Multiple fractures are sequenced in accordance with the severity of the fracture. The provider should be asked to list the fracture diagnoses in the order of severity.

c. Coding of Burns

Current burns (940-948) are classified by depth, extent and by agent (E code). Burns are classified by depth as first degree (erythema), second degree (blistering), and third degree (full-thickness involvement).

1) Sequencing of burn and related condition codes

Sequence first the code that reflects the highest degree of burn when more than one burn is present.

a. When the reason for the admission or encounter is for treatment of external multiple burns, sequence first the code that reflects the burn of the highest degree.

b. When a patient has both internal and external burns, the circumstances of admission govern the selection of the principal diagnosis or first-listed diagnosis.

c. When a patient is admitted for burn injuries and other related conditions such as smoke inhalation and/or respiratory failure, the circumstances of admission govern the selection of the principal or first-listed diagnosis.

2) Burns of the same local site

Classify burns of the same local site (three-digit category level, 940-947) but of different degrees to the subcategory identifying the highest degree recorded in the diagnosis.

3) Non-healing burns

Non-healing burns are coded as acute burns.

Necrosis of burned skin should be coded as a non-healed burn.

4) Code 958.3, Posttraumatic wound infection

Assign code 958.3, Posttraumatic wound infection, not elsewhere classified, as an additional code for any documented infected burn site.

5) Assign separate codes for each burn site

When coding burns, assign separate codes for each burn site. Category 946 Burns of Multiple specified sites, should only be used if the location of the burns are not documented.

Category 949, Burn, unspecified, is extremely vague and should rarely be used.

6) Assign codes from category 948, Burns

Burns classified according to extent of body surface involved, when the site of the burn is not specified or when there is a need for additional data. It is advisable to use category 948 as additional coding when needed to provide data for evaluating burn mortality, such as that needed by burn units. It is also advisable to use category 948 as an additional code for reporting purposes when there is mention of a third-degree burn involving 20 percent or more of the body surface.

In assigning a code from category 948:

Fourth-digit codes are used to identify the percentage of total body surface involved in a burn (all degree).

Fifth-digits are assigned to identify the percentage of body surface involved in third-degree burn.

Fifth-digit zero (0) is assigned when less than 10 percent or when no body surface is involved in a third-degree burn.

Category 948 is based on the classic "rule of nines" in estimating body surface involved: head and neck are assigned nine percent, each arm nine percent, each leg 18 percent, the anterior trunk 18 percent, posterior trunk 18 percent, and genitalia one percent. Providers may change these percentage assignments where necessary to accommodate infants and children who have proportionately larger heads than adults and patients who have large buttocks, thighs, or abdomen that involve burns.

7) Encounters for treatment of late effects of burns

Encounters for the treatment of the late effects of burns (i.e., scars or joint contractures) should be coded to the residual condition (sequelae) followed by the appropriate late effect code (906.5-906.9). A late effect E code may also be used, if desired.

8) Sequelae with a late effect code and current burn

When appropriate, both a sequelae with a late effect code, and a current burn code may be assigned on the same record (when both a current burn and sequelae of an old burn exist).

d. Coding of Debridement of Wound, Infection, or Burn

Excisional debridement involves surgical removal or cutting away, as opposed to a mechanical (brushing, scrubbing, washing) debridement.

For coding purposes, excisional debridement is assigned to code 86.22.

Nonexcisional debridement is assigned to code 86.28.

e. Adverse Effects, Poisoning and Toxic Effects

The properties of certain drugs, medicinal and biological substances or combinations of such substances, may cause toxic reactions. The occurrence of drug toxicity is classified in ICD-9-CM as follows:

1) Adverse Effect

When the drug was correctly prescribed and properly administered, code the reaction plus the appropriate code from the E930-E949 series. Codes from the E930-E949 series must be used to identify the causative substance for an adverse effect of drug, medicinal and biological substances, correctly prescribed and properly administered. The effect, such as tachycardia, delirium, gastrointestinal hemorrhaging, vomiting, hypokalemia, hepatitis, renal failure, or respiratory failure, is coded and followed by the appropriate code from the E930-E949 series.

Adverse effects of therapeutic substances correctly prescribed and properly administered (toxicity, synergistic reaction, side effect, and idiosyncratic reaction) may be due to (1) differences among patients, such as age, sex, disease, and genetic factors, and (2) drug-related factors, such as type of drug, route of administration, duration of therapy, dosage, and bioavailability.

2) Poisoning

(a) Error was made in drug prescription

Errors made in drug prescription or in the administration of the drug by provider, nurse, patient, or other person, use the appropriate poisoning code from the 960-979 series.

(b) Overdose of a drug intentionally taken

If an overdose of a drug was intentionally taken or administered and resulted in drug toxicity, it would be coded as a poisoning (960-979 series).

(c) Nonprescribed drug taken with correctly prescribed and properly administered drug

If a nonprescribed drug or medicinal agent was taken in combination with a correctly prescribed and properly administered drug, any drug toxicity or other reaction resulting from the interaction of the two drugs would be classified as a poisoning.

(d) Interaction of drug(s) and alcohol

When a reaction results from the interaction of a drug(s) and alcohol, this would be classified as poisoning.

(e) Sequencing of poisoning

When coding a poisoning or reaction to the improper use of a medication (e.g., wrong dose, wrong substance, wrong route of administration) the poisoning code is sequenced first, followed by a code for the manifestation. If there is also a diagnosis of drug abuse or dependence to the substance, the abuse or dependence is coded as an additional code.

See Section I.C.3.a.6.b. if poisoning is the result of insulin pump malfunctions and Section I.C.19 for general use of E-codes.

3) Toxic Effects

(a) Toxic effect codes

When a harmful substance is ingested or comes in contact with a person, this is classified as a toxic effect. The toxic effect codes are in categories 980-989.

(b) Sequencing toxic effect codes

A toxic effect code should be sequenced first, followed by the code(s) that identify the result of the toxic effect.

(c) External cause codes for toxic effects

An external cause code from categories E860-E869 for accidental exposure, codes E950.6 or E950.7 for intentional self-harm, category E962 for assault, or categories E980-E982, for undetermined, should also be assigned to indicate intent.

f. Complications of care

1) Complications of care

(a) Documentation of complications of care

See Section I.B.18. for information on documentation of complications of care.

(b) Use additional code to identify nature of complication

An additional code identifying the complication should be assigned with codes in categories 996-999, Complications of Surgical and Medical Care NEC, when the additional code provides greater specificity as to the nature of the condition. If the complication code fully describes the condition, no additional code is necessary.

2) Transplant complications

(a) Transplant complications other than kidney

Codes under subcategory 996.8, Complications of transplanted organ, are for use for both complications and rejection of transplanted organs. A transplant complication code is only assigned if the complication affects the function of the transplanted organ. Two codes are required to fully describe a transplant complication, the appropriate code from subcategory 996.8 and a secondary code that identifies the complication.

Pre-existing conditions or conditions that develop after the transplant are not coded as complications unless they affect the function of the transplanted organs.

See I.C.18.d.3 for transplant organ removal status

See I.C.2.i for malignant neoplasm associated with transplanted organ.

(b) Chronic kidney disease and kidney transplant complications

Patients who have undergone kidney transplant may still have some form of chronic kidney disease (CKD) because the kidney transplant may not fully restore kidney function. Code 996.81 should be assigned for documented complications of a kidney transplant, such as transplant failure or rejection or other transplant complication. Code 996.81 should not be assigned for post kidney transplant patients who have chronic kidney (CKD) unless a transplant complication such as transplant failure or rejection is documented. If the documentation is unclear as to whether the patient has a complication of the transplant, query the provider.

Conditions that affect the function of the transplanted kidney, other than CKD, should be assigned code 996.81, Complications of transplanted organ, Kidney, and a secondary code that identifies the complication.

For patients with CKD following a kidney transplant, but who do not have a complication such as failure or rejection, *see section I.C.10.a.2, Chronic kidney disease and kidney transplant status.*

3) Ventilator associated pneumonia

(a) Documentation of Ventilator associated Pneumonia

As with all procedural or postprocedural complications, code assignment is based on the provider's documentation of the relationship between the condition and the procedure.

Code 997.31, Ventilator associated pneumonia, should be assigned only when the provider has documented ventilator associated pneumonia (VAP). An additional code to identify the organism (e.g., Pseudomonas aeruginosa, code 041.7) should also be assigned. Do not assign an additional code from categories 480-484 to identify the type of pneumonia.

Code 997.31 should not be assigned for cases where the patient has pneumonia and is on a mechanical ventilator but the provider has not specifically stated that the pneumonia is ventilator-associated pneumonia.

If the documentation is unclear as to whether the patient has a pneumonia that is a complication attributable to the mechanical ventilator, query the provider.

(b) Patient admitted with pneumonia and develops VAP

A patient may be admitted with one type of pneumonia (e.g., code 481, Pneumococcal pneumonia) and subsequently develop VAP. In this instance, the principal diagnosis would be the appropriate code from categories 480-484 for the pneumonia diagnosed at the time of admission. Code 997.31, Ventilator associated pneumonia, would be assigned as an additional diagnosis when the provider has also documented the presence of ventilator associated pneumonia.

g. SIRS due to Non-infectious Process

The systemic inflammatory response syndrome (SIRS) can develop as a result of certain non-infectious disease processes, such as trauma, malignant neoplasm, or pancreatitis. When SIRS is documented with a noninfectious condition, and no subsequent infection is documented, the code for the underlying condition, such as an injury, should be assigned, followed by code 995.93, Systemic inflammatory response syndrome due to noninfectious process without acute organ dysfunction, or 995.94, Systemic inflammatory response syndrome due to non-infectious process with acute organ dysfunction. If an acute organ dysfunction is documented, the appropriate code(s) for the associated acute organ dysfunction(s) should be assigned in addition to code 995.94. If acute organ dysfunction is documented, but it cannot be determined if the acute organ dysfunction is associated with SIRS or due to another condition (e.g., directly due to the trauma), the provider should be queried.

When the non-infectious condition has led to an infection that results in SIRS, *see Section I.C.1.b.12 for the guideline for sepsis and severe sepsis associated with a non-infectious process.*

18. Classification of Factors Influencing Health Status and Contact with Health Service (Supplemental V01-V91)

Note: The chapter specific guidelines provide additional information about the use of V codes for specified encounters.

a. Introduction

ICD-9-CM provides codes to deal with encounters for circumstances other than a disease or injury. The Supplementary Classification of Factors Influencing Health Status and Contact with Health Services (V01.0 - V91.99) is provided to deal with occasions when circumstances other than a disease or injury (codes 001-999) are recorded as a diagnosis or problem.

There are four primary circumstances for the use of V codes:

1) A person who is not currently sick encounters the health services for some specific reason, such as to act as an organ donor, to receive prophylactic care, such as inoculations or health screenings, or to receive counseling on health related issues.

2) A person with a resolving disease or injury, or a chronic, long-term condition requiring continuous care, encounters the health care system for specific aftercare of that disease or injury (e.g., dialysis for renal disease; chemotherapy for malignancy; cast change). A diagnosis/symptom code should be used whenever a current, acute, diagnosis is being treated or a sign or symptom is being studied.

3) Circumstances or problems influence a person's health status but are not in themselves a current illness or injury.

4) Newborns, to indicate birth status

b. V codes use in any healthcare setting

V codes are for use in any healthcare setting. V codes may be used as either a first listed (principal diagnosis code in the inpatient setting) or secondary code, depending on the circumstances of the encounter. Certain V codes may only be used as first listed, others only as secondary codes.

See Section I.C.18.e, V Codes That May Only be Principal/First-Listed Diagnosis.

c. V Codes indicate a reason for an encounter

They are not procedure codes. A corresponding procedure code must accompany a V code to describe the procedure performed.

d. Categories of V Codes

1) Contact/Exposure

Category V01 indicates contact with or exposure to communicable diseases. These codes are for patients who do not show any sign or symptom of a disease but have been exposed to it by close personal contact with an infected individual or are in an area where a disease is epidemic. These codes may be used as a first listed code to explain an encounter for testing, or, more commonly, as a secondary code to identify a potential risk.

Codes V15.84 – V15.86 describe contact with or (suspected) exposure to asbestos, potentially hazardous body fluids, and lead.

Subcategories V87.0 – V87.3 describe contact with or (suspected) exposure to hazardous metals, aromatic compounds, other potentially hazardous chemicals, and other potentially hazardous substances.

2) Inoculations and vaccinations

Categories V03-V06 are for encounters for inoculations and vaccinations. They indicate that a patient is being seen to receive a prophylactic inoculation against a disease. The injection itself must be represented by the appropriate procedure code. A code from V03-V06 may be used as a secondary code if the inoculation is given as a routine part of preventive health care, such as a well-baby visit.

3) Status

Status codes indicate that a patient is a carrier of a disease, has the sequelae or residual of a past disease or condition, or has another factor influencing a person's health status. This includes such things as the presence of prosthetic or mechanical devices resulting from past treatment. A status code is informative, because the status may affect the course of treatment and its outcome. A status code is distinct from a history code. The history code indicates that the patient no longer has the condition.

A status code should not be used with a diagnosis code from one of the body system chapters, if the diagnosis code includes the information provided by the status code. For example, code V42.1, Heart transplant status, should not be used with code 996.83, Complications of transplanted heart. The status code does not provide additional information. The complication code indicates that the patient is a heart transplant patient.

The status V codes/categories are:

V02   Carrier or suspected carrier of infectious diseases

Carrier status indicates that a person harbors the specific organisms of a disease without manifest symptoms and is capable of transmitting the infection.

V07.5x   Use of agents affecting estrogen receptors and estrogen level

This code indicates when a patient is receiving a drug that affects estrogen receptors and estrogen levels for prevention of cancer.

V08   Asymptomatic HIV infection status

This code indicates that a patient has tested positive for HIV but has manifested no signs or symptoms of the disease.

V09   Infection with drug-resistant microorganisms

This category indicates that a patient has an infection that is resistant to drug treatment. Sequence the infection code first.

V21   Constitutional states in development

V22.2   Pregnant state, incidental

This code is a secondary code only for use when the pregnancy is in no way complicating the reason for visit. Otherwise, a code from the obstetric chapter is required.

V26.5x   Sterilization status

V42   Organ or tissue replaced by transplant

V43   Organ or tissue replaced by other means

V44   Artificial opening status

V45   Other postsurgical states

Assign code V45.87, Transplant organ removal status, to indicate that a transplanted organ has been previously removed. This code should not be assigned for the encounter in which the transplanted organ is removed. The complication necessitating removal of the transplant organ should be assigned for that encounter.

See section I.C17.f.2. for information on the coding of organ transplant complications.

Assign code V45.88, Status post administration of tPA (rtPA) in a different facility within the last 24 hours prior to admission to the current facility, as a secondary diagnosis when a patient is received by transfer into a facility and documentation indicates they were administered tissue plasminogen activator (tPA) within the last 24 hours prior to admission to the current facility.

This guideline applies even if the patient is still receiving the tPA at the time they are received into the current facility.

The appropriate code for the condition for which the tPA was administered (such as cerebrovascular disease or myocardial infarction) should be assigned first.

Code V45.88 is only applicable to the receiving facility record and not to the transferring facility record.

V46   Other dependence on machines

V49.6   Upper limb amputation status

V49.7   Lower limb amputation status

Note: Categories V42-V46, and subcategories V49.6, V49.7 are for use only if there are no complications or malfunctions of the organ or tissue replaced, the amputation site or the equipment on which the patient is dependent.

V49.81   Asymptomatic postmenopausal status (age-related) (natural)

V49.82   Dental sealant status

V49.83   Awaiting organ transplant status

V49.86   Do not resuscitate status

This code may be used when it is documented by the provider that a patient is on do not resuscitate status at any time during the stay.

V49.87   Physical restraint status

This code may be used when it is documented by the provider that a patient has been put in restraints during the current encounter. Please note that this code should not be reported when it is documented by the provider that a patient is temporarily restrained during a procedure.

V58.6x   Long-term (current) drug use

Codes from this subcategory indicate a patient's continuous use of a prescribed drug (including such things as aspirin therapy) for the long-term treatment of a condition or for prophylactic use. It is not for use for patients who have addictions to drugs. This subcategory is not for use of medications for detoxification or maintenance programs to prevent withdrawal symptoms in patients with drug dependence (e.g., methadone maintenance for opiate dependence). Assign the appropriate code for the drug dependence instead.

Assign a code from subcategory V58.6, Long-term (current) drug use, if the patient is receiving a medication for an extended period as a prophylactic measure (such as for the prevention of deep vein thrombosis) or as treatment of a chronic condition (such as arthritis) or a disease requiring a lengthy course of treatment (such as cancer). Do not assign a code from subcategory V58.6 for medication being administered for a brief period of time to treat an acute illness or injury (such as a course of antibiotics to treat acute bronchitis).

V83   Genetic carrier status

Genetic carrier status indicates that a person carries a gene, associated with a particular disease, which may be passed to offspring who may develop that disease. The person does not have the disease and is not at risk of developing the disease.

V84   Genetic susceptibility status

Genetic susceptibility indicates that a person has a gene that increases the risk of that person developing the disease.

Codes from category V84, Genetic susceptibility to disease, should not be used as principal or first-listed codes. If the patient has the condition to which he/she is susceptible, and that condition is the reason for the encounter, the code for the current condition should be sequenced first. If the patient is being seen for follow-up after completed treatment for this condition, and the condition no longer exists, a follow-up code should be sequenced first, followed by the appropriate personal history and genetic susceptibility codes. If the purpose of the encounter is genetic counseling associated with procreative management, a code from subcategory V26.3, Genetic counseling and testing, should be assigned as the first-listed code, followed by a code from category V84. Additional codes should be assigned for any applicable family or personal history.

See Section I.C. 18.d.14 for information on prophylactic organ removal due to a genetic susceptibility.

V85   Body Mass Index (BMI)

V86   Estrogen receptor status

V88   Acquired absence of other organs and tissue

V90   Retained foreign body

4) History (of)

There are two types of history V codes, personal and family. Personal history codes explain a patient's past medical condition that no longer exists and is not receiving any treatment, but that has the potential for recurrence, and therefore may require continued monitoring. The exceptions to this general rule are category V14, Personal history of allergy to medicinal agents, and subcategory V15.0, Allergy, other than to medicinal agents. A person who has had an allergic episode to a substance or food in the past should always be considered allergic to the substance.

Family history codes are for use when a patient has a family member(s) who has had a particular disease that causes the patient to be at higher risk of also contracting the disease.

Personal history codes may be used in conjunction with follow-up codes and family history codes may be used in conjunction with screening codes to explain the need for a test or procedure. History codes are also acceptable on any medical record regardless of the reason for visit. A history of an illness, even if no longer present, is important information that may alter the type of treatment ordered.

The history V code categories are:

V10   Personal history of malignant neoplasm

V12   Personal history of certain other diseases

V13   Personal history of other diseases

Except: V13.4, Personal history of arthritis, and subcategory V13.6, Personal history of congenital (corrected) malformations. These conditions are life-long so are not true history codes.

V14   Personal history of allergy to medicinal agents

V15   Other personal history presenting hazards to health

Except: Codes V15.7, Personal history of contraception; V15.84, Contact with and (suspected) exposure to asbestos; V15.85, Contact with and (suspected) exposure to potentially hazardous body fluids; V15.86, Contact with and (suspected) exposure to lead.

V16   Family history of malignant neoplasm

V17   Family history of certain chronic disabling diseases

V18   Family history of certain other specific diseases

V19   Family history of other conditions

V87   Other specified personal exposures and history presenting hazards to health

Except: Subcategories V87.0, Contact with and (suspected) exposure to hazardous metals; V87.1, Contact with and (suspected) exposure to hazardous aromatic compounds; V87.2, Contact with and (suspected) exposure to other potentially hazardous chemicals; and V87.3, Contact with and (suspected) exposure to other potentially hazardous substances.

5) Screening

Screening is the testing for disease or disease precursors in seemingly well individuals so that early detection and treatment can be provided for those who test positive for the disease. Screenings that are recommended for many subgroups in a population include: routine mammograms for women over 40, a fecal occult blood test for everyone over 50, an amniocentesis to rule out a fetal anomaly for pregnant women over 35, because the incidence of breast cancer and colon cancer in these subgroups is higher than in the general population, as is the incidence of Down's syndrome in older mothers.

The testing of a person to rule out or confirm a suspected diagnosis because the patient has some sign or symptom is a diagnostic examination, not a screening. In these cases, the sign or symptom is used to explain the reason for the test.

A screening code may be a first listed code if the reason for the visit is specifically the screening exam. It may also be used as an additional code if the screening is done during an office visit for other health problems. A screening code is not necessary if the screening is inherent to a routine examination, such as a pap smear done during a routine pelvic examination.

Should a condition be discovered during the screening then the code for the condition may be assigned as an additional diagnosis.

The V code indicates that a screening exam is planned. A procedure code is required to confirm that the screening was performed.

The screening V code categories:

V28　　　　Antenatal screening

V73-V82　Special screening examinations

6) Observation

There are three observation V code categories. They are for use in very limited circumstances when a person is being observed for a suspected condition that is ruled out. The observation codes are not for use if an injury or illness or any signs or symptoms related to the suspected condition are present. In such cases the diagnosis/symptom code is used with the corresponding E code to identify any external cause. The observation codes are to be used as principal diagnosis only. The only exception to this is when the principal diagnosis is required to be a code from the V30, Live born infant, category. Then the V29 observation code is sequenced after the V30 code. Additional codes may be used in addition to the observation code but only if they are unrelated to the suspected condition being observed.

Codes from subcategory V89.0, Suspected maternal and fetal conditions not found, may either be used as a first listed or as an additional code assignment depending on the case. They are for use in very limited circumstances on a maternal record when an encounter is for a suspected maternal or fetal condition that is ruled out during that encounter (for example, a maternal or fetal condition may be suspected due to an abnormal test result). These codes should not be used when the condition is confirmed. In those cases, the confirmed condition should be coded. In addition, these codes are not for use if an illness or any signs or symptoms related to the suspected condition or problem are present. In such cases the diagnosis/symptom code is used.

Additional codes may be used in addition to the code from subcategory V89.0, but only if they are unrelated to the suspected condition being evaluated.

Codes from subcategory V89.0 may not be used for encounters for antenatal screening of mother. *See Section I.C.18.d., Screening.*

For encounters for suspected fetal condition that are inconclusive following testing and evaluation, assign the appropriate code from category 655, 656, 657 or 658.

The observation V code categories:

V29　　　Observation and evaluation of newborns for suspected condition not found

　　　　　For the birth encounter, a code from category V30 should be sequenced before the V29 code.

V71　　　Observation and evaluation for suspected condition not found

V89　　　Suspected maternal and fetal conditions not found

7) Aftercare

Aftercare visit codes cover situations when the initial treatment of a disease or injury has been performed and the patient requires continued care during the healing or recovery phase, or for the long-term consequences of the disease. The aftercare V code should not be used if treatment is directed at a current, acute disease or injury. The diagnosis code is to be used

in these cases. Exceptions to this rule are codes V58.0, Radiotherapy, and codes from subcategory V58.1, Encounter for chemotherapy and immunotherapy for neoplastic conditions. These codes are to be first listed, followed by the diagnosis code when a patient's encounter is solely to receive radiation therapy or chemotherapy for the treatment of a neoplasm. Should a patient receive both chemotherapy and radiation therapy during the same encounter code V58.0 and V58.1 may be used together on a record with either one being sequenced first.

The aftercare codes are generally first listed to explain the specific reason for the encounter. An aftercare code may be used as an additional code when some type of aftercare is provided in addition to the reason for admission and no diagnosis code is applicable. An example of this would be the closure of a colostomy during an encounter for treatment of another condition.

Aftercare codes should be used in conjunction with any other aftercare codes or other diagnosis codes to provide better detail on the specifics of an aftercare encounter visit, unless otherwise directed by the classification. The sequencing of multiple aftercare codes is discretionary.

Certain aftercare V code categories need a secondary diagnosis code to describe the resolving condition or sequelae, for others, the condition is inherent in the code title.

Additional V code aftercare category terms include fitting and adjustment, and attention to artificial openings.

Status V codes may be used with aftercare V codes to indicate the nature of the aftercare. For example code V45.81, Aortocoronary bypass status, may be used with code V58.73, Aftercare following surgery of the circulatory system, NEC, to indicate the surgery for which the aftercare is being performed. Also, a transplant status code may be used following code V58.44, Aftercare following organ transplant, to identify the organ transplanted. A status code should not be used when the aftercare code indicates the type of status, such as using V55.0, Attention to tracheostomy with V44.0, Tracheostomy status.

See Section I. B.16 Admissions/Encounter for Rehabilitation

The aftercare V category/codes:

V51.0　　Encounter for breast reconstruction following mastectomy

V52　　　Fitting and adjustment of prosthetic device and implant

V53　　　Fitting and adjustment of other device

V54　　　Other orthopedic aftercare

V55　　　Attention to artificial openings

V56　　　Encounter for dialysis and dialysis catheter care

V57　　　Care involving the use of rehabilitation procedures

V58.0　　Radiotherapy

V58.11　Encounter for antineoplastic chemotherapy

V58.12　Encounter for antineoplastic immunotherapy

V58.3x　Attention to dressings and sutures

V58.41	Encounter for planned post-operative wound closure
V58.42	Aftercare, surgery, neoplasm
V58.43	Aftercare, surgery, trauma
V58.44	Aftercare involving organ transplant
V58.49	Other specified aftercare following surgery
V58.7x	Aftercare following surgery
V58.81	Fitting and adjustment of vascular catheter
V58.82	Fitting and adjustment of non-vascular catheter
V58.83	Monitoring therapeutic drug
V58.89	Other specified aftercare

8) Follow-up

The follow-up codes are used to explain continuing surveillance following completed treatment of a disease, condition, or injury. They imply that the condition has been fully treated and no longer exists. They should not be confused with aftercare codes that explain current treatment for a healing condition or its sequelae. Follow-up codes may be used in conjunction with history codes to provide the full picture of the healed condition and its treatment. The follow-up code is sequenced first, followed by the history code.

A follow-up code may be used to explain repeated visits. Should a condition be found to have recurred on the follow-up visit, then the diagnosis code should be used in place of the follow-up code.

The follow-up V code categories:

| V24 | Postpartum care and evaluation |
| V67 | Follow-up examination |

9) Donor

Category V59 is the donor codes. They are used for living individuals who are donating blood or other body tissue. These codes are only for individuals donating for others, not for self donations. They are not for use to identify cadaveric donations.

10) Counseling

Counseling V codes are used when a patient or family member receives assistance in the aftermath of an illness or injury, or when support is required in coping with family or social problems. They are not necessary for use in conjunction with a diagnosis code when the counseling component of care is considered integral to standard treatment.

The counseling V categories/codes:

V25.0	General counseling and advice for contraceptive management
V26.3	Genetic counseling
V26.4	General counseling and advice for procreative management
V61.x	Other family circumstances
V65.1	Person consulted on behalf of another person
V65.3	Dietary surveillance and counseling
V65.4	Other counseling, not elsewhere classified

11) Obstetrics and related conditions

See Section I.C.11., the Obstetrics guidelines for further instruction on the use of these codes.

V codes for pregnancy are for use in those circumstances when none of the problems or complications included in the codes from the Obstetrics chapter exist (a routine prenatal visit or postpartum care). Codes V22.0, Supervision of normal first pregnancy, and V22.1, Supervision of other normal pregnancy, are always first listed and are not to be used with any other code from the OB chapter.

The outcome of delivery, category V27, should be included on all maternal delivery records. It is always a secondary code.

V codes for family planning (contraceptive) or procreative management and counseling should be included on an obstetric record either during the pregnancy or the postpartum stage, if applicable.

Obstetrics and related conditions V code categories:

V22	Normal pregnancy
V23	Supervision of high-risk pregnancy
	Except: V23.2, Pregnancy with history of abortion. Code 646.3, Recurrent pregnancy loss, from the OB chapter is required to indicate a history of abortion during a pregnancy.
V24	Postpartum care and evaluation
V25	Encounter for contraceptive management
	Except V25.0x
	(See Section I.C.18.d.11, Counseling)
V26	Procreative management
	Except: V26.5x, Sterilization status, V26.3 and V26.4
	(See Section I.C.18.d.11., Counseling)
V27	Outcome of delivery
V28	Antenatal screening
	(See Section I.C.18.d.6., Screening)
V91	Multiple gestation placenta status

12) Newborn, infant and child

See Section I.C.15, the Newborn guidelines for further instruction on the use of these codes.

Newborn V code categories:

V20	Health supervision of infant or child
V29	Observation and evaluation of newborns for suspected condition not found
	(See Section I.C.18.d.7, Observation)
V30-V39	Liveborn infant according to type of birth

13) Routine and administrative examinations

The V codes allow for the description of encounters for routine examinations, such as, a general check-up, or examinations for administrative purposes, such as a pre-employment physical. The codes are not to be used if the examination is for diagnosis of a suspected condition or for treatment purposes. In such cases the diagnosis code is used. During a routine exam, should a diagnosis or condition be discovered, it should be coded as an additional code. Pre-existing and chronic conditions and history codes may also be included as additional codes as long as the examination is for administrative purposes and not focused on any particular condition.

Pre-operative examination and pre-procedural laboratory examination V codes are for use only in those situations when a patient is being cleared for a procedure or surgery and no treatment is given.

The V codes categories/code for routine and administrative examinations:

V20.2 Routine infant or child health check

Any injections given should have a corresponding procedure code.

V70 General medical examination

V72 Special investigations and examinations

Codes V72.5 and V72.62 may be used if the reason for the patient encounter is for routine laboratory/radiology testing in the absence of any signs, symptoms, or associated diagnosis. If routine testing is performed during the same encounter as a test to evaluate a sign, symptom, or diagnosis, it is appropriate to assign both the V code and the code describing the reason for the non-routine test.

14) Miscellaneous V codes

The miscellaneous V codes capture a number of other health care encounters that do not fall into one of the other categories. Certain of these codes identify the reason for the encounter, others are for use as additional codes that provide useful information on circumstances that may affect a patient's care and treatment.

Prophylactic Organ Removal

For encounters specifically for prophylactic removal of breasts, ovaries, or another organ due to a genetic susceptibility to cancer or a family history of cancer, the principal or first listed code should be a code from subcategory V50.4, Prophylactic organ removal, followed by the appropriate genetic susceptibility code and the appropriate family history code.

If the patient has a malignancy of one site and is having prophylactic removal at another site to prevent either a new primary malignancy or metastatic disease, a code for the malignancy should also be assigned in addition to a code from subcategory V50.4. A V50.4 code should not be assigned if the patient is having organ removal for treatment of a malignancy, such as the removal of the testes for the treatment of prostate cancer.

Miscellaneous V code categories/codes:

V07 Need for isolation and other prophylactic or treatment measures

Except V07.5X, Use of agents affecting estrogen receptors and estrogen levels

V40.31 Wandering in diseases classified elsewhere

V50 Elective surgery for purposes other than remedying health states

V58.5 Orthodontics

V60 Housing, household, and economic circumstances

V62 Other psychosocial circumstances

V63 Unavailability of other medical facilities for care

V64 Persons encountering health services for specific procedures, not carried out

V66 Convalescence and Palliative Care

V68 Encounters for administrative purposes

V69 Problems related to lifestyle

15) Nonspecific V codes

Certain V codes are so non-specific, or potentially redundant with other codes in the classification, that there can be little justification for their use in the inpatient setting. Their use in the outpatient setting should be limited to those instances when there is no further documentation to permit more precise coding. Otherwise, any sign or symptom or any other reason for visit that is captured in another code should be used.

Nonspecific V code categories/codes:

V11 Personal history of mental disorder

A code from the mental disorders chapter, with an in remission fifth-digit, should be used.

V13.4 Personal history of arthritis

V13.6 Personal history of congenital malformations

V15.7 Personal history of contraception

V23.2 Pregnancy with history of abortion

V40 Mental and behavioral problems

Exception: V40.31 Wandering in diseases classified elsewhere

V41 Problems with special senses and other special functions

V47 Other problems with internal organs

V48 Problems with head, neck, and trunk

V49 Problems with limbs and other problems

Exceptions:

V49.6 Upper limb amputation status

V49.7 Lower limb amputation status

V49.81 Asymptomatic postmenopausal status (age-related) (natural)

V49.82 Dental sealant status

V49.83 Awaiting organ transplant status

V49.86 Do not resuscitate status

V49.87 Physical restraints status

V51.8 Other aftercare involving the use of plastic surgery

V58.2 Blood transfusion, without reported diagnosis

V58.9 Unspecified aftercare

See Section IV.K. and Section IV.L. of the Outpatient guidelines.

e. V Codes That May Only be Principal/First-Listed Diagnosis

The list of V codes/categories below may only be reported as the principal/first-listed diagnosis, except when there are multiple encounters on the same day and the medical records for the encounters are combined or when there is more than one V code that meets the definition of principal diagnosis (e.g., a patient is admitted to home healthcare for both aftercare and rehabilitation and they equally meet the definition of principal diagnosis). These codes should not be reported if they do not meet the definition of principal or first-listed diagnosis.

See Section II and Section IV.A for information on selection of principal and first-listed diagnosis.

See Section II.C for information on two or more diagnoses that equally meet the definition for principal diagnosis.

V20.x	Health supervision of infant or child
V22.0	Supervision of normal first pregnancy
V22.1	Supervision of other normal pregnancy
V24.x	Postpartum care and examination
V26.81	Encounter for assisted reproductive fertility procedure cycle
V26.82	Encounter for fertility preservation procedure
V30.x	Single liveborn
V31.x	Twin, mate liveborn
V32.x	Twin, mate stillborn
V33.x	Twin, unspecified
V34.x	Other multiple, mates all liveborn
V35.x	Other multiple, mates all stillborn
V36.x	Other multiple, mates live- and stillborn
V37.x	Other multiple, unspecified
V39.x	Unspecified
V46.12	Encounter for respirator dependence during power failure
V46.13	Encounter for weaning from respirator [ventilator]
V51.0	Encounter for breast reconstruction following mastectomy
V56.0	Extracorporeal dialysis
V57.x	Care involving use of rehabilitation procedures
V58.0	Radiotherapy
V58.11	Encounter for antineoplastic chemotherapy
V58.12	Encounter for antineoplastic immunotherapy
V59.x	Donors
V66.0	Convalescence and palliative care following surgery
V66.1	Convalescence and palliative care following radiotherapy
V66.2	Convalescence and palliative care following chemotherapy
V66.3	Convalescence and palliative care following psychotherapy and other treatment for mental disorder
V66.4	Convalescence and palliative care following treatment of fracture
V66.5	Convalescence and palliative care following other treatment
V66.6	Convalescence and palliative care following combined treatment
V66.9	Unspecified convalescence
V68.x	Encounters for administrative purposes
V70.0	Routine general medical examination at a health care facility
V70.1	General psychiatric examination, requested by the authority
V70.2	General psychiatric examination, other and unspecified
V70.3	Other medical examination for administrative purposes
V70.4	Examination for medicolegal reasons
V70.5	Health examination of defined subpopulations
V70.6	Health examination in population surveys
V70.8	Other specified general medical examinations
V70.9	Unspecified general medical examination
V71.x	Observation and evaluation for suspected conditions not found

19. **Supplemental Classification of External Causes of Injury and Poisoning (E-codes, E000-E999)**

Introduction: These guidelines are provided for those who are currently collecting E codes in order that there will be standardization in the process. If your institution plans to begin collecting E codes, these guidelines are to be applied. The use of E codes is supplemental to the application of ICD-9-CM diagnosis codes.

External causes of injury and poisoning codes (categories E000 and E800-E999) are intended to provide data for injury research and evaluation of injury prevention strategies. Activity codes (categories E001-E030) are intended to be used to describe the activity of a person seeking care for injuries as well as other health conditions, when the injury or other health condition resulted from an activity or the activity contributed to a condition. E codes capture how the injury, poisoning, or adverse effect happened (cause), the intent (unintentional or accidental; or intentional, such as suicide or assault), the person's status (e.g. civilian, military), the associated activity and the place where the event occurred.

Some major categories of E codes include:

transport accidents

poisoning and adverse effects of drugs, medicinal substances and biologicals

accidental falls

accidents caused by fire and flames

accidents due to natural and environmental factors

late effects of accidents, assaults or self injury

assaults or purposely inflicted injury

suicide or self inflicted injury

These guidelines apply for the coding and collection of E codes from records in hospitals, outpatient clinics, emergency departments, other ambulatory care settings and provider offices, and nonacute care settings, except when other specific guidelines apply.

a. **General E Code Coding Guidelines**

1) **Used with any code in the range of 001-V91**

An E code from categories E800-E999 may be used with any code in the range of 001-V91, which indicates an injury, poisoning, or adverse effect due to an external cause.

An activity E code (categories E001-E030) may be used with any code in the range of 001-V91 that indicates an injury, or other health condition that resulted from an activity, or the activity contributed to a condition.

2) **Assign the appropriate E code for all initial treatments**

Assign the appropriate E code for the initial encounter of an injury, poisoning, or adverse effect of drugs, not for subsequent treatment.

External cause of injury codes (E-codes) may be assigned while the acute fracture codes are still applicable.

See Section I.C.17.b.1 for coding of acute fractures.

3) **Use the full range of E codes**

Use the full range of E codes (E800 – E999) to completely describe the cause, the intent and the place of occurrence, if applicable, for all injuries, poisonings, and adverse effects of drugs.

See a.1.), j.), and k.) in this section for information on the use of status and activity E codes.

4) **Assign as many E codes as necessary**

Assign as many E codes as necessary to fully explain each cause.

5) **The selection of the appropriate E code**

The selection of the appropriate E code is guided by the Index to External Causes, which is located after the alphabetical index to diseases and by Inclusion and Exclusion notes in the Tabular List.

6) **E code can never be a principal diagnosis**

An E code can never be a principal (first listed) diagnosis.

7) **External cause code(s) with systemic inflammatory response syndrome (SIRS)**

An external cause code is not appropriate with a code from subcategory 995.9, unless the patient also has another condition for which an E code would be appropriate (such as an injury, poisoning, or adverse effect of drugs.

8) **Multiple Cause E Code Coding Guidelines**

More than one E-code is required to fully describe the external cause of an illness, injury or poisoning. The assignment of E-codes should be sequenced in the following priority:

If two or more events cause separate injuries, an E code should be assigned for each cause. The first listed E code will be selected in the following order:

E codes for child and adult abuse take priority over all other E codes.

See Section I.C.19.e., Child and Adult abuse guidelines.

E codes for terrorism events take priority over all other E codes except child and adult abuse.

E codes for cataclysmic events take priority over all other E codes except child and adult abuse and terrorism.

E codes for transport accidents take priority over all other E codes except cataclysmic events, child and adult abuse and terrorism.

Activity and external cause status codes are assigned following all causal (intent) E codes.

The first-listed E code should correspond to the cause of the most serious diagnosis due to an assault, accident, or self-harm, following the order of hierarchy listed above.

9) **If the reporting format limits the number of E codes**

If the reporting format limits the number of E codes that can be used in reporting clinical data, report the code for the cause/intent most related to the principal diagnosis. If the format permits capture of additional E codes, the cause/intent, including medical misadventures, of the additional events should be reported rather than the codes for place, activity or external status.

b. **Place of Occurrence Guideline**

Use an additional code from category E849 to indicate the Place of Occurrence. The Place of Occurrence describes the place where the event occurred and not the patient's activity at the time of the event.

Do not use E849.9 if the place of occurrence is not stated.

c. **Adverse Effects of Drugs, Medicinal and Biological Substances Guidelines**

1) **Do not code directly from the Table of Drugs**

Do not code directly from the Table of Drugs and Chemicals. Always refer back to the Tabular List.

2) **Use as many codes as necessary to describe**

Use as many codes as necessary to describe completely all drugs, medicinal or biological substances.

If the reporting format limits the number of E codes, and there are different fourth digit codes in the same three digit category, use the code for "Other specified" of that category of drugs, medicinal or biological substances. If there is no "Other specified" code in that category, use the appropriate "Unspecified" code in that category.

If the reporting format limits the number of E codes, and the codes are in different three digit categories, assign the appropriate E code for other multiple drugs and medicinal substances.

3) **If the same E code would describe the causative agent**

If the same E code would describe the causative agent for more than one adverse reaction, assign the code only once.

4) **If two or more drugs, medicinal or biological substances**

If two or more drugs, medicinal or biological substances are reported, code each individually unless the combination code is listed in the Table of Drugs and Chemicals. In that case, assign the E code for the combination.

5) **When a reaction results from the interaction of a drug(s)**

When a reaction results from the interaction of a drug(s) and alcohol, use poisoning codes and E codes for both.

6) **Codes from the E930-E949 series**

Codes from the E930-E949 series must be used to identify the causative substance for an adverse effect of drug, medicinal and biological substances, correctly prescribed and properly administered. The effect, such as tachycardia, delirium, gastrointestinal hemorrhaging, vomiting, hypokalemia, hepatitis, renal failure, or respiratory failure, is coded and followed by the appropriate code from the E930-E949 series.

d. Child and Adult Abuse Guideline

1) Intentional injury

When the cause of an injury or neglect is intentional child or adult abuse, the first listed E code should be assigned from categories E960-E968, Homicide and injury purposely inflicted by other persons, (except category E967). An E code from category E967, Child and adult battering and other maltreatment, should be added as an additional code to identify the perpetrator, if known.

2) Accidental intent

In cases of neglect when the intent is determined to be accidental E code E904.0, Abandonment or neglect of infant and helpless person, should be the first listed E code.

e. Unknown or Suspected Intent Guideline

1) If the intent (accident, self-harm, assault) of the cause of an injury or poisoning is unknown

If the intent (accident, self-harm, assault) of the cause of an injury or poisoning is unknown or unspecified, code the intent as undetermined E980-E989.

2) If the intent (accident, self-harm, assault) of the cause of an injury or poisoning is questionable

If the intent (accident, self-harm, assault) of the cause of an injury or poisoning is questionable, probable or suspected, code the intent as undetermined E980-E989.

f. Undetermined Cause

When the intent of an injury or poisoning is known, but the cause is unknown, use codes: E928.9, Unspecified accident, E958.9, Suicide and self-inflicted injury by unspecified means, and E968.9, Assault by unspecified means.

These E codes should rarely be used, as the documentation in the medical record, in both the inpatient outpatient and other settings, should normally provide sufficient detail to determine the cause of the injury.

g. Late Effects of External Cause Guidelines

1) Late effect E codes

Late effect E codes exist for injuries and poisonings but not for adverse effects of drugs, misadventures and surgical complications.

2) Late effect E codes (E929, E959, E969, E977, E989, or E999.1)

A late effect E code (E929, E959, E969, E977, E989, or E999.1) should be used with any report of a late effect or sequela resulting from a previous injury or poisoning (905-909).

3) Late effect E code with a related current injury

A late effect E code should never be used with a related current nature of injury code.

4) Use of late effect E codes for subsequent visits

Use a late effect E code for subsequent visits when a late effect of the initial injury or poisoning is being treated. There is no late effect E code for adverse effects of drugs.

Do not use a late effect E code for subsequent visits for follow-up care (e.g., to assess healing, to receive rehabilitative therapy) of the injury or poisoning when no late effect of the injury has been documented.

h. Misadventures and Complications of Care Guidelines

1) Code range E870-E876

Assign a code in the range of E870-E876 if misadventures are stated by the provider. When applying the E code guidelines pertaining to sequencing, these E codes are considered causal codes.

2) Code range E878-E879

Assign a code in the range of E878-E879 if the provider attributes an abnormal reaction or later complication to a surgical or medical procedure, but does not mention misadventure at the time of the procedure as the cause of the reaction.

i. Terrorism Guidelines

1) Cause of injury identified by the Federal Government (FBI) as terrorism

When the cause of an injury is identified by the Federal Government (FBI) as terrorism, the first-listed E-code should be a code from category E979, Terrorism. The definition of terrorism employed by the FBI is found at the inclusion note at E979. The terrorism E-code is the only E-code that should be assigned. Additional E codes from the assault categories should not be assigned.

2) Cause of an injury is suspected to be the result of terrorism

When the cause of an injury is suspected to be the result of terrorism a code from category E979 should not be assigned. Assign a code in the range of E codes based circumstances on the documentation of intent and mechanism.

3) Code E979.9, Terrorism, secondary effects

Assign code E979.9, Terrorism, secondary effects, for conditions occurring subsequent to the terrorist event. This code should not be assigned for conditions that are due to the initial terrorist act.

4) Statistical tabulation of terrorism codes

For statistical purposes these codes will be tabulated within the category for assault, expanding the current category from E960-E969 to include E979 and E999.1.

j. Activity Code Guidelines

Assign a code from category E001-E030 to describe the activity that caused or contributed to the injury or other health condition.

Unlike other E codes, activity E codes may be assigned to indicate a health condition (not just injuries) resulted from an activity, or the activity contributed to the condition.

The activity codes are not applicable to poisonings, adverse effects, misadventures or late effects.

Do not assign E030, Unspecified activity, if the activity is not stated.

k. External cause status

A code from category E000, External cause status, should be assigned whenever any other E code is assigned for an encounter, including an Activity E code, except for the events noted below. Assign a code from category E000, External cause status, to indicate the work status of the person at the time the event occurred. The status code indicates whether the event occurred during military activity, whether a non-military person was at work, whether an individual including a student or volunteer was involved in a non-work activity at the time of the causal event.

A code from E000, External cause status, should be assigned, when applicable, with other external cause codes, such as transport accidents and falls. The external cause status codes are not applicable to poisonings, adverse effects, misadventures or late effects.

Do not assign a code from category E000 if no other E codes (cause, activity) are applicable for the encounter.

Do not assign code E000.9, Unspecified external cause status, if the status is not stated.

Section II. Selection of Principal Diagnosis

The circumstances of inpatient admission always govern the selection of principal diagnosis. The principal diagnosis is defined in the Uniform Hospital Discharge Data Set (UHDDS) as "that condition established after study to be chiefly responsible for occasioning the admission of the patient to the hospital for care."

The UHDDS definitions are used by hospitals to report inpatient data elements in a standardized manner. These data elements and their definitions can be found in the July 31, 1985, Federal Register (Vol. 50, No, 147), pp. 31038-40.

Since that time the application of the UHDDS definitions has been expanded to include all non-outpatient settings (acute care, short term, long term care and psychiatric hospitals; home health agencies; rehab facilities; nursing homes, etc).

In determining principal diagnosis the coding conventions in the ICD-9-CM, Volumes I and II take precedence over these official coding guidelines.

(See Section I.A., Conventions for the ICD-9-CM)

The importance of consistent, complete documentation in the medical record cannot be overemphasized. Without such documentation the application of all coding guidelines is a difficult, if not impossible, task.

A. Codes for symptoms, signs, and ill-defined conditions

Codes for symptoms, signs, and ill-defined conditions from Chapter 16 are not to be used as principal diagnosis when a related definitive diagnosis has been established.

B. Two or more interrelated conditions, each potentially meeting the definition for principal diagnosis.

When there are two or more interrelated conditions (such as diseases in the same ICD-9-CM chapter or manifestations characteristically associated with a certain disease) potentially meeting the definition of principal diagnosis, either condition may be sequenced first, unless the circumstances of the admission, the therapy provided, the Tabular List, or the Alphabetic Index indicate otherwise.

C. Two or more diagnoses that equally meet the definition for principal diagnosis

In the unusual instance when two or more diagnoses equally meet the criteria for principal diagnosis as determined by the circumstances of admission, diagnostic workup and/or therapy provided, and the Alphabetic Index, Tabular List, or another coding guidelines does not provide sequencing direction, any one of the diagnoses may be sequenced first.

D. Two or more comparative or contrasting conditions.

In those rare instances when two or more contrasting or comparative diagnoses are documented as "either/or" (or similar terminology), they are coded as if the diagnoses were confirmed and the diagnoses are sequenced according to the circumstances of the admission. If no further determination can be made as to which

diagnosis should be principal, either diagnosis may be sequenced first.

E. A symptom(s) followed by contrasting/comparative diagnoses

When a symptom(s) is followed by contrasting/comparative diagnoses, the symptom code is sequenced first. All the contrasting/comparative diagnoses should be coded as additional diagnoses.

F. Original treatment plan not carried out

Sequence as the principal diagnosis the condition, which after study occasioned the admission to the hospital, even though treatment may not have been carried out due to unforeseen circumstances.

G. Complications of surgery and other medical care

When the admission is for treatment of a complication resulting from surgery or other medical care, the complication code is sequenced as the principal diagnosis. If the complication is classified to the 996-999 series and the code lacks the necessary specificity in describing the complication, an additional code for the specific complication should be assigned.

H. Uncertain Diagnosis

If the diagnosis documented at the time of discharge is qualified as "probable", "suspected", "likely", "questionable", "possible", or "still to be ruled out", or other similar terms indicating uncertainty, code the condition as if it existed or was established. The bases for these guidelines are the diagnostic workup, arrangements for further workup or observation, and initial therapeutic approach that correspond most closely with the established diagnosis.

Note: This guideline is applicable only to inpatient admissions to short-term, acute, long-term care and psychiatric hospitals.

I. Admission from Observation Unit

1. Admission Following Medical Observation

When a patient is admitted to an observation unit for a medical condition, which either worsens or does not improve, and is subsequently admitted as an inpatient of the same hospital for this same medical condition, the principal diagnosis would be the medical condition which led to the hospital admission.

2. Admission Following Post-Operative Observation

When a patient is admitted to an observation unit to monitor a condition (or complication) that develops following outpatient surgery, and then is subsequently admitted as an inpatient of the same hospital, hospitals should apply the Uniform Hospital Discharge Data Set (UHDDS) definition of principal diagnosis as "that condition established after study to be chiefly responsible for occasioning the admission of the patient to the hospital for care."

J. Admission from Outpatient Surgery

When a patient receives surgery in the hospital's outpatient surgery department and is subsequently admitted for continuing inpatient care at the same hospital, the following guidelines should be followed in selecting the principal diagnosis for the inpatient admission:

- If the reason for the inpatient admission is a complication, assign the complication as the principal diagnosis.

- If no complication, or other condition, is documented as the reason for the inpatient admission, assign the reason for the outpatient surgery as the principal diagnosis.

- If the reason for the inpatient admission is another condition unrelated to the surgery, assign the unrelated condition as the principal diagnosis.

Section III. Reporting Additional Diagnoses
GENERAL RULES FOR OTHER (ADDITIONAL) DIAGNOSES

For reporting purposes the definition for "other diagnoses" is interpreted as additional conditions that affect patient care in terms of requiring:

> clinical evaluation; or
>
> therapeutic treatment; or
>
> diagnostic procedures; or
>
> extended length of hospital stay; or
>
> increased nursing care and/or monitoring.

The UHDDS item #11-b defines Other Diagnoses as "all conditions that coexist at the time of admission, that develop subsequently, or that affect the treatment received and/or the length of stay. Diagnoses that relate to an earlier episode which have no bearing on the current hospital stay are to be excluded." UHDDS definitions apply to inpatients in acute care, short-term, long term care and psychiatric hospital setting. The UHDDS definitions are used by acute care short-term hospitals to report inpatient data elements in a standardized manner. These data elements and their definitions can be found in the July 31, 1985, Federal Register (Vol. 50, No, 147), pp. 31038-40.

Since that time the application of the UHDDS definitions has been expanded to include all non-outpatient settings (acute care, short term, long term care and psychiatric hospitals; home health agencies; rehab facilities; nursing homes, etc).

The following guidelines are to be applied in designating "other diagnoses" when neither the Alphabetic Index nor the Tabular List in ICD-9-CM provide direction. The listing of the diagnoses in the patient record is the responsibility of the attending provider.

A. Previous conditions

If the provider has included a diagnosis in the final diagnostic statement, such as the discharge summary or the face sheet, it should ordinarily be coded. Some providers include in the diagnostic statement resolved conditions or diagnoses and status-post procedures from previous admission that have no bearing on the current stay. Such conditions are not to be reported and are coded only if required by hospital policy.

However, history codes (V10-V19) may be used as secondary codes if the historical condition or family history has an impact on current care or influences treatment.

B. Abnormal findings

Abnormal findings (laboratory, x-ray, pathologic, and other diagnostic results) are not coded and reported unless the provider indicates their clinical significance. If the findings are outside the normal range and the attending provider has ordered other tests to evaluate the condition or prescribed treatment, it is appropriate to ask the provider whether the abnormal finding should be added.

Please note: This differs from the coding practices in the outpatient setting for coding encounters for diagnostic tests that have been interpreted by a provider.

C. Uncertain Diagnosis

If the diagnosis documented at the time of discharge is qualified as "probable", "suspected", "likely", "questionable", "possible", or "still to be ruled out" or other similar terms indicating uncertainty, code the condition as if it existed or was established. The bases for these guidelines are the diagnostic workup, arrangements for further workup or observation, and initial therapeutic approach that correspond most closely with the established diagnosis.

Note: This guideline is applicable only to inpatient admissions to short-term, acute, long-term care and psychiatric hospitals.

Section IV. Diagnostic Coding and Reporting Guidelines for Outpatient Services

These coding guidelines for outpatient diagnoses have been approved for use by hospitals/ providers in coding and reporting hospital-based outpatient services and provider-based office visits.

Information about the use of certain abbreviations, punctuation, symbols, and other conventions used in the ICD-9-CM Tabular List (code numbers and titles), can be found in Section IA of these guidelines, under "Conventions Used in the Tabular List." Information about the correct sequence to use in finding a code is also described in Section I.

The terms encounter and visit are often used interchangeably in describing outpatient service contacts and, therefore, appear together in these guidelines without distinguishing one from the other.

Though the conventions and general guidelines apply to all settings, coding guidelines for outpatient and provider reporting of diagnoses will vary in a number of instances from those for inpatient diagnoses, recognizing that:

> The Uniform Hospital Discharge Data Set (UHDDS) definition of principal diagnosis applies only to inpatients in acute, short-term, long-term care and psychiatric hospitals.
>
> Coding guidelines for inconclusive diagnoses (probable, suspected, rule out, etc.) were developed for inpatient reporting and do not apply to outpatients.

A. Selection of first-listed condition

In the outpatient setting, the term first-listed diagnosis is used in lieu of principal diagnosis.

In determining the first-listed diagnosis the coding conventions of ICD-9-CM, as well as the general and disease specific guidelines take precedence over the outpatient guidelines.

Diagnoses often are not established at the time of the initial encounter/visit. It may take two or more visits before the diagnosis is confirmed.

The most critical rule involves beginning the search for the correct code assignment through the Alphabetic Index. Never begin searching initially in the Tabular List as this will lead to coding errors.

1. Outpatient Surgery

When a patient presents for outpatient surgery, code the reason for the surgery as the first-listed diagnosis (reason for the encounter), even if the surgery is not performed due to a contraindication.

2. Observation Stay

When a patient is admitted for observation for a medical condition, assign a code for the medical condition as the first-listed diagnosis.

When a patient presents for outpatient surgery and develops complications requiring admission to observation, code the reason for the surgery as the first reported diagnosis (reason for the encounter), followed by codes for the complications as secondary diagnoses.

B. Codes from 001.0 through V91.99

The appropriate code or codes from 001.0 through V91.99 must be used to identify diagnoses, symptoms, conditions, problems, complaints, or other reason(s) for the encounter/visit.

C. Accurate reporting of ICD-9-CM diagnosis codes

For accurate reporting of ICD-9-CM diagnosis codes, the documentation should describe the patient's condition, using terminology which includes specific diagnoses as well as symptoms, problems, or reasons for the encounter. There are ICD-9-CM codes to describe all of these.

D. Selection of codes 001.0 through 999.9

The selection of codes 001.0 through 999.9 will frequently be used to describe the reason for the encounter. These codes are from the section of ICD-9-CM for the classification of diseases and injuries (e.g. infectious and parasitic diseases; neoplasms; symptoms, signs, and ill-defined conditions, etc.).

E. Codes that describe symptoms and signs

Codes that describe symptoms and signs, as opposed to diagnoses, are acceptable for reporting purposes when a diagnosis has not been established (confirmed) by the provider. Chapter 16 of ICD-9-CM, Symptoms, Signs, and Ill-defined conditions (codes 780.0 - 799.9) contain many, but not all codes for symptoms.

F. Encounters for circumstances other than a disease or injury

ICD-9-CM provides codes to deal with encounters for circumstances other than a disease or injury. The Supplementary Classification of factors Influencing Health Status and Contact with Health Services (V01.0- V91.99) is provided to deal with occasions when circumstances other than a disease or injury are recorded as diagnosis or problems. *See Section I.C. 18 for information on V-codes.*

G. Level of Detail in Coding

1. ICD-9-CM codes with 3, 4, or 5 digits

ICD-9-CM is composed of codes with either 3, 4, or 5 digits. Codes with three digits are included in ICD-9-CM as the heading of a category of codes that may be further subdivided by the use of fourth and/or fifth digits, which provide greater specificity.

2. Use of full number of digits required for a code

A three-digit code is to be used only if it is not further subdivided. Where fourth-digit subcategories and/or fifth-digit subclassifications are provided, they must be assigned. A code is invalid if it has not been coded to the full number of digits required for that code.

See also discussion under Section I.b.3., General Coding Guidelines, Level of Detail in Coding.

H. ICD-9-CM code for the diagnosis, condition, problem, or other reason for encounter/visit

List first the ICD-9-CM code for the diagnosis, condition, problem, or other reason for encounter/visit shown in the medical record to be chiefly responsible for the services provided. List additional codes that describe any coexisting conditions. In some cases the first-listed diagnosis may be a symptom when a diagnosis has not been established (confirmed) by the physician.

I. Uncertain diagnosis

Do not code diagnoses documented as "probable", "suspected," "questionable," "rule out," or "working diagnosis" or other similar terms indicating uncertainty. Rather, code the condition(s) to the highest degree of certainty for that encounter/visit, such as symptoms, signs, abnormal test results, or other reason for the visit.

Please note: This differs from the coding practices used by short-term, acute care, long-term care and psychiatric hospitals.

J. Chronic diseases

Chronic diseases treated on an ongoing basis may be coded and reported as many times as the patient receives treatment and care for the condition(s)

K. Code all documented conditions that coexist

Code all documented conditions that coexist at the time of the encounter/visit, and require or affect patient care treatment or management. Do not code conditions that were previously treated and no longer exist. However, history codes (V10-V19) may be used as secondary codes if the historical condition or family history has an impact on current care or influences treatment.

L. Patients receiving diagnostic services only

For patients receiving diagnostic services only during an encounter/visit, sequence first the diagnosis, condition, problem, or other reason for encounter/visit shown in the medical record to be chiefly responsible for the outpatient services provided during the encounter/visit. Codes for other diagnoses (e.g., chronic conditions) may be sequenced as additional diagnoses.

For encounters for routine laboratory/radiology testing in the absence of any signs, symptoms, or associated diagnosis, assign V72.5 and/or a code from subcategory V72.6. If routine testing is performed during the same encounter as a test to evaluate a sign, symptom, or diagnosis, it is appropriate to assign both the V code and the code describing the reason for the non-routine test.

For outpatient encounters for diagnostic tests that have been interpreted by a physician, and the final report is available at the time of coding, code any confirmed or definitive diagnosis(es) documented in the interpretation. Do not code related signs and symptoms as additional diagnoses.

Please note: This differs from the coding practice in the hospital inpatient setting regarding abnormal findings on test results.

M. Patients receiving therapeutic services only

For patients receiving therapeutic services only during an encounter/visit, sequence first the diagnosis, condition, problem, or other reason for encounter/visit shown in the medical record to be chiefly responsible for the outpatient services provided during the encounter/visit. Codes for other diagnoses (e.g., chronic conditions) may be sequenced as additional diagnoses.

The only exception to this rule is that when the primary reason for the admission/encounter is chemotherapy, radiation therapy, or rehabilitation, the appropriate V code for the service is listed first, and the diagnosis or problem for which the service is being performed listed second.

N. Patients receiving preoperative evaluations only

For patients receiving preoperative evaluations only, sequence first a code from category V72.8, Other specified examinations, to describe the pre-op consultations. Assign a code for the condition to describe the reason for the surgery as an additional diagnosis. Code also any findings related to the pre-op evaluation.

O. Ambulatory surgery

For ambulatory surgery, code the diagnosis for which the surgery was performed. If the postoperative diagnosis is known to be different from the preoperative diagnosis at the time the diagnosis is confirmed, select the postoperative diagnosis for coding, since it is the most definitive.

P. Routine outpatient prenatal visits

For routine outpatient prenatal visits when no complications are present, codes V22.0, Supervision of normal first pregnancy, or V22.1, Supervision of other normal pregnancy, should be used as the principal diagnosis. These codes should not be used in conjunction with chapter 11 codes.

APPENDIX I. PRESENT ON ADMISSION REPORTING GUIDELINES

Introduction

These guidelines are to be used as a supplement to the *ICD-9-CM Official Guidelines for Coding and Reporting* to facilitate the assignment of the Present on Admission (POA) indicator for each diagnosis and external cause of injury code reported on claim forms (UB-04 and 837 Institutional).

These guidelines are not intended to replace any guidelines in the main body of the *ICD-9-CM Official Guidelines for Coding and Reporting*. The

POA guidelines are not intended to provide guidance on when a condition should be coded, but rather, how to apply the POA indicator to the final set of diagnosis codes that have been assigned in accordance with Sections I, II, and III of the official coding guidelines. Subsequent to the assignment of the ICD-9-CM codes, the POA indicator should then be assigned to those conditions that have been coded.

As stated in the Introduction to the ICD-9-CM Official Guidelines for Coding and Reporting, a joint effort between the healthcare provider and the coder is essential to achieve complete and accurate documentation, code assignment, and reporting of diagnoses and procedures. The importance of consistent, complete documentation in the medical record cannot be overemphasized. Medical record documentation from any provider involved in the care and treatment of the patient may be used to support the determination of whether a condition was present on admission or not. In the context of the official coding guidelines, the term "provider" means a physician or any qualified healthcare practitioner who is legally accountable for establishing the patient's diagnosis.

These guidelines are not a substitute for the provider's clinical judgment as to the determination of whether a condition was/was not present on admission. The provider should be queried regarding issues related to the linking of signs/symptoms, timing of test results, and the timing of findings.

General Reporting Requirements

All claims involving inpatient admissions to general acute care hospitals or other facilities that are subject to a law or regulation mandating collection of present on admission information.

Present on admission is defined as present at the time the order for inpatient admission occurs -- conditions that develop during an outpatient encounter, including emergency department, observation, or outpatient surgery, are considered as present on admission.

POA indicator is assigned to principal and secondary diagnoses (as defined in Section II of the Official Guidelines for Coding and Reporting) and the external cause of injury codes.

Issues related to inconsistent, missing, conflicting or unclear documentation must still be resolved by the provider.

If a condition would not be coded and reported based on UHDDS definitions and current official coding guidelines, then the POA indicator would not be reported.

Reporting Options

Y - Yes

N - No

U - Unknown

W – Clinically undetermined

Unreported/Not used (or "1" for Medicare usage) – (Exempt from POA reporting)

Reporting Definitions

Y = present at the time of inpatient admission

N = not present at the time of inpatient admission

U = documentation is insufficient to determine if condition is present on admission

W = provider is unable to clinically determine whether condition was present on admission or not

Timeframe for POA Identification and Documentation

There is no required timeframe as to when a provider (per the definition of "provider" used in these guidelines) must identify or document a condition to be present on admission. In some clinical situations, it may not be possible for a provider to make a definitive diagnosis (or a condition may not be recognized or reported by the

patient) for a period of time after admission. In some cases it may be several days before the provider arrives at a definitive diagnosis. This does not mean that the condition was not present on admission. Determination of whether the condition was present on admission or not will be based on the applicable POA guideline as identified in this document, or on the provider's best clinical judgment.

If at the time of code assignment the documentation is unclear as to whether a condition was present on admission or not, it is appropriate to query the provider for clarification.

ASSIGNING THE POA INDICATOR

Condition is on the "Exempt from Reporting" list

Leave the "present on admission" field blank if the condition is on the list of ICD-9-CM codes for which this field is not applicable. This is the only circumstance in which the field maybe left blank.

POA explicitly documented

Assign Y for any condition the provider explicitly documents as being present on admission.

Assign N for any condition the provider explicitly documents as not present at the time of admission.

Conditions diagnosed prior to inpatient admission

Assign "Y" for conditions that were diagnosed prior to admission (example: hypertension, diabetes mellitus, asthma)

Conditions diagnosed during the admission but clearly present before admission

Assign "Y" for conditions diagnosed during the admission that were clearly present but not diagnosed until after admission occurred.

Diagnoses subsequently confirmed after admission are considered present on admission if at the time of admission they are documented as suspected, possible, rule out, differential diagnosis, or constitute an underlying cause of a symptom that is present at the time of admission.

Condition develops during outpatient encounter prior to inpatient admission

Assign Y for any condition that develops during an outpatient encounter prior to a written order for inpatient admission.

Documentation does not indicate whether condition was present on admission

Assign "U" when the medical record documentation is unclear as to whether the condition was present on admission. "U" should not be routinely assigned and used only in very limited circumstances. Coders are encouraged to query the providers when the documentation is unclear.

Documentation states that it cannot be determined whether the condition was or was not present on admission

Assign "W" when the medical record documentation indicates that it cannot be clinically determined whether or not the condition was present on admission.

Chronic condition with acute exacerbation during the admission

If the code is a combination code that identifies both the chronic condition and the acute exacerbation, see POA guidelines pertaining to combination codes.

If the combination code only identifies the chronic condition and not the acute exacerbation (e.g., acute exacerbation of chronic leukemia), assign "Y."

Conditions documented as possible, probable, suspected, or rule out at the time of discharge

If the final diagnosis contains a possible, probable, suspected, or rule out diagnosis, and this diagnosis was based on signs, symptoms or clinical findings suspected at the time of inpatient admission, assign "Y."

If the final diagnosis contains a possible, probable, suspected, or rule out diagnosis, and this diagnosis was based on signs, symptoms or clinical findings that were not present on admission, assign "N".

Conditions documented as impending or threatened at the time of discharge

If the final diagnosis contains an impending or threatened diagnosis, and this diagnosis is based on symptoms or clinical findings that were present on admission, assign "Y".

If the final diagnosis contains an impending or threatened diagnosis, and this diagnosis is based on symptoms or clinical findings that were not present on admission, assign "N".

Acute and chronic conditions

Assign "Y" for acute conditions that are present at time of admission and N for acute conditions that are not present at time of admission.

Assign "Y" for chronic conditions, even though the condition may not be diagnosed until after admission.

If a single code identifies both an acute and chronic condition, see the POA guidelines for combination codes.

Combination codes

Assign "N" if any part of the combination code was not present on admission (e.g., obstructive chronic bronchitis with acute exacerbation and the exacerbation was not present on admission; gastric ulcer that does not start bleeding until after admission; asthma patient develops status asthmaticus after admission)

Assign "Y" if all parts of the combination code were present on admission (e.g., patient with diabetic nephropathy is admitted with uncontrolled diabetes).

If the final diagnosis includes comparative or contrasting diagnoses, and both were present, or suspected, at the time of admission, assign "Y".

For infection codes that include the causal organism, assign "Y" if the infection (or signs of the infection) was present on admission, even though the culture results may not be known until after admission (e.g., patient is admitted with pneumonia and the provider documents pseudomonas as the causal organism a few days later).

Same diagnosis code for two or more conditions

When the same ICD-9-CM diagnosis code applies to two or more conditions during the same encounter (e.g. bilateral condition, or two separate conditions classified to the same ICD-9-CM diagnosis code):

Assign "Y" if all conditions represented by the single ICD-9-CM code were present on admission (e.g. bilateral fracture of the same bone, same site, and both fractures were present on admission)

Assign "N" if any of the conditions represented by the single ICD-9-CM code was not present on admission (e.g. dehydration with hyponatremia is assigned to code 276.1, but only one of these conditions was present on admission).

Obstetrical conditions

Whether or not the patient delivers during the current hospitalization does not affect assignment of the POA indicator. The determining factor for POA assignment is whether the pregnancy complication or obstetrical condition described by the code was present at the time of admission or not.

If the pregnancy complication or obstetrical condition was present on admission (e.g., patient admitted in preterm labor), assign "Y".

If the pregnancy complication or obstetrical condition was not present on admission (e.g., 2nd degree laceration during delivery, postpartum hemorrhage that occurred during current hospitalization, fetal distress develops after admission), assign "N".

If the obstetrical code includes more than one diagnosis and any of the diagnoses identified by the code were not present on admission assign "N". (e.g., Code 642.7, Pre-eclampsia or eclampsia superimposed on pre-existing hypertension).

If the obstetrical code includes information that is not a diagnosis, do not consider that information in the POA determination. (e.g. Code 652.1x, Breech or other malpresentation successfully converted to cephalic presentation should be reported as present on admission if the fetus was breech on admission but was converted to cephalic presentation after admission (since the conversion to cephalic presentation does not represent a diagnosis, the fact that the conversion occurred after admission has no bearing on the POA determination).

Perinatal conditions

Newborns are not considered to be admitted until after birth. Therefore, any condition present at birth or that developed in utero is considered present at admission and should be assigned "Y". This includes conditions that occur during delivery (e.g., injury during delivery, meconium aspiration, exposure to streptococcus B in the vaginal canal).

Congenital conditions and anomalies

Assign "Y" for congenital conditions and anomalies, **except for categories 740-759, Congenital anomalies, which are on the exempt list.** Congenital conditions are always considered present on admission.

External cause of injury codes

Assign "Y" for any E code representing an external cause of injury or poisoning that occurred prior to inpatient admission (e.g., patient fell out of bed at home, patient fell out of bed in emergency room prior to admission)

Assign "N" for any E code representing an external cause of injury or poisoning that occurred during inpatient hospitalization (e.g., patient fell out of hospital bed during hospital stay, patient experienced an adverse reaction to a medication administered after inpatient admission)

CATEGORIES AND CODES EXEMPT FROM DIAGNOSIS PRESENT ON ADMISSION REQUIREMENT

Note: *"Diagnosis present on admission" for these code categories are exempt because they represent circumstances regarding the healthcare encounter or factors influencing health status that do not represent a current disease or injury or are always present on admission.*

Categories or subcategories listed are inclusive of all codes within those categories or subcategories, unless otherwise indicated. In order to streamline the POA exempt list and make it easier to read, where all of the codes in a code range are POA exempt, only the code range is shown, rather than listing each of the individual codes in the range.

| 137-139 | Late effects of infectious and parasitic diseases |
| 268.1 | Rickets, late effect |

326	Late effects of intracranial abscess or pyogenic infection		V46	Other dependence on machines and devices
412	Old myocardial infarction		V49.60-V49.77	Upper and lower limb amputation status
438	Late effects of cerebrovascular disease		V49.81-V49.85	Other specified conditions influencing health status
650	Normal delivery		V50	Elective surgery for purposes other than remedying health states
660.7	Failed forceps or vacuum extractor, unspecified		V51	Aftercare involving the use of plastic surgery
677	Late effect of complication of pregnancy, childbirth, and the puerperium		V52	Fitting and adjustment of prosthetic device and implant
740-759	Congenital anomalies		V53	Fitting and adjustment of other device
905-909	Late effects of injuries, poisonings, toxic effects, and other external causes		V54	Other orthopedic aftercare
V02	Carrier or suspected carrier of infectious diseases		V55	Attention to artificial openings
V03	Need for prophylactic vaccination and inoculation against bacterial diseases		V56	Encounter for dialysis and dialysis catheter care
V04	Need for prophylactic vaccination and inoculation against certain viral diseases		V57	Care involving use of rehabilitation procedures
V05	Need for other prophylactic vaccination and inoculation against single diseases		V58	Encounter for other and unspecified procedures and aftercare
V06	Need for prophylactic vaccination and inoculation against combinations of diseases		V59	Donors
V07	Need for isolation and other prophylactic or treatment measures		V60	Housing, household, and economic circumstances
			V61	Other family circumstances
V10	Personal history of malignant neoplasm		V62	Other psychosocial circumstances
V11	Personal history of mental disorder		V64	Persons encountering health services for specific procedures, not carried out
V12	Personal history of certain other diseases		V65	Other persons seeking consultation
V13	Personal history of other diseases		V66	Convalescence and palliative care
V14	Personal history of allergy to medicinal agents		V67	Follow-up examination
V15	Other personal history presenting hazards to health		V68	Encounters for administrative purposes
V16	Family history of malignant neoplasm		V69	Problems related to lifestyle
V17	Family history of certain chronic disabling diseases		V70	General medical examination
V18	Family history of certain other specific conditions		V71	Observation and evaluation for suspected condition not found
V19	Family history of other conditions		V72	Special investigations and examinations
V20	Health supervision of infant or child		V73	Special screening examination for viral and chlamydial diseases
V21	Constitutional states in development		V74	Special screening examination for bacterial and spirochetal diseases
V22	Normal pregnancy		V75	Special screening examination for other infectious diseases
V23	Supervision of high-risk pregnancy			
V24	Postpartum care and examination		V76	Special screening for malignant neoplasms
V25	Encounter for contraceptive management		V77	Special screening for endocrine, nutritional, metabolic, and immunity disorders
V26	Procreative management		V78	Special screening for disorders of blood and blood-forming organs
V27	Outcome of delivery		V79	Special screening for mental disorders and developmental handicaps
V28	Antenatal screening			
V29	Observation and evaluation of newborns for suspected condition not found		V80	Special screening for neurological, eye, and ear diseases
V30-V39	Liveborn infants according to type of birth		V81	Special screening for cardiovascular, respiratory, and genitourinary diseases
V42	Organ or tissue replaced by transplant		V82	Special screening for other conditions
V43	Organ or tissue replaced by other means		V83	Genetic carrier status
V44	Artificial opening status			
V45	Other postprocedural states			

Code	Description
V84	Genetic susceptibility to disease
V85	Body Mass Index
V86	Estrogen receptor status
V87.32	Contact with and (suspected) exposure to algae bloom
V87.4	Personal history of drug therapy
V88	Acquired absence of other organs and tissue
V89	Suspected maternal and fetal conditions not found
V90	Retained foreign body
V91	Multiple gestation placenta status
E000	External cause status
E001-E030	Activity
E800-E807	Railway accidents
E810-E819	Motor vehicle traffic accidents
E820-E825	Motor vehicle nontraffic accidents
E826-E829	Other road vehicle accidents
E830-E838	Water transport accidents
E840-E845	Air and space transport accidents
E846-E848	Vehicle accidents not elsewhere classifiable
E849	Place of occurrence (Except E849.7)
E883.1	Accidental fall into well
E883.2	Accidental fall into storm drain or manhole
E884.0	Fall from playground equipment
E884.1	Fall from cliff
E885.0	Fall from (nonmotorized) scooter
E885.1	Fall from roller skates
E885.2	Fall from skateboard
E885.3	Fall from skis
E885.4	Fall from snowboard
E886.0	Fall on same level from collision, pushing, or shoving, by or with other person, In sports
E890.0-E890.9	Conflagration in private dwelling
E893.0	Accident caused by ignition of clothing, from controlled fire in private dwelling
E893.2	Accident caused by ignition of clothing, from controlled fire not in building or structure
E894	Ignition of highly inflammable material
E895	Accident caused by controlled fire in private dwelling
E897	Accident caused by controlled fire not in building or structure
E917.0	Striking against or struck accidentally by objects or persons, in sports without subsequent fall
E917.1	Striking against or struck accidentally by objects or persons, caused by a crowd, by collective fear or panic without subsequent fall
E917.2	Striking against or struck accidentally by objects or persons, in running water without subsequent fall
E917.5	Striking against or struck accidentally by objects or persons, object in sports with subsequent fall
E917.6	Striking against or struck accidentally by objects or persons, caused by a crowd, by collective fear or panic with subsequent fall
E919	Accident caused by machinery (Except E919.2)
E921	Accident caused by explosion of pressure vessel
E922	Accident caused by firearm and air gun missile
E926.2	Visible and ultraviolet light sources
E928.0-E928.8	Other and unspecified environmental and accidental causes
E929.0-E929.9	Late effects of accidental injury
E959	Late effects of self-inflicted injury
E970-E978	Legal intervention
E979	Terrorism
E981	Poisoning by gases in domestic use, undetermined whether accidentally or purposely inflicted
E982	Poisoning by other gases, undetermined whether accidentally or purposely inflicted
E985	Injury by firearms, air guns and explosives, undetermined whether accidentally or purposely inflicted
E987.0	Falling from high place, undetermined whether accidentally or purposely inflicted, residential premises
E987.2	Falling from high place, undetermined whether accidentally or purposely inflicted, natural sites
E989	Late effects of injury, undetermined whether accidentally or purposely inflicted
E990-E999	Injury resulting from operations of war

10 Steps to Correct Coding

Follow the 10 steps below to correctly code encounters for healthcare services.

Step 1: Identify the reason for the visit or encounter (i.e., a sign, symptom, diagnosis and/or condition).

The medical record documentation should accurately reflect the patient's condition, using terminology that includes specific diagnoses and symptoms, or clearly states the reasons for the encounter.

Choosing the main term that best describes the reason chiefly responsible for the service provided is the most important step in coding.

For outpatient services, if symptoms are present and documented but a definitive diagnosis has not yet been determined, code the symptoms. **For outpatient services, do not code conditions that are referred to as "rule out," "suspected," "probable" or "questionable."** Diagnoses often are not established at the time of the initial encounter/visit. Two or more visits may be necessary to establish the diagnosis. Code only what is documented in the available records and only to the highest degree of certainty known at the time of the patient's visit unless it is an inpatient medical record, in which case uncertain diagnoses may be reported.

The Uniform Hospital Discharge Data Set (UHDDS) provides definitions of required data elements for the reporting of nonoutpatient services (e.g., acute care, short term, long term care and psychiatric hospital; home health agencies; rehab facilities, nursing homes). These data elements include the definition of principal diagnosis as "that condition established after study to be chiefly responsible for occasioning admission of the patient to the hospital for care."

When determining the first-listed or principal diagnosis, the coding conventions in the ICD-9-CM text take precedence over other coding guidelines or advice.

Step 2: After selecting the reason for the encounter, always consult the Alphabetic Index, Volume 2, before verifying code selection in the Tabular section.

The most critical rule is to begin the code selection process in the Alphabetic Index. Never turn first to the Tabular List (Volume 1). The Index provides cross references, essential and non-essential modifiers, and inclusion terms not found in the Tabular List. To prevent coding errors, always use both the Alphabetic Index and the Tabular List when locating and assigning a code. Always verify the code found in the Alphabetic Index in the Tabular List. First, the Index does not include the important instructional notes found in the Tabular. Second, the advantage of a classification system is that like items are grouped together. A quick scan of the Tabular might provide coding options for the coder that would have been missed.

Step 3: Locate the main term entry.

The Alphabetic Index is a listing of conditions. Conditions may be expressed as nouns or eponyms, with critical use of adjectives. Some conditions have multiple entries under synonyms. Reasons for encounters may be located under general terms such as admission, encounter, and examination. Other general terms such as history of or status post are used to locate factors influencing health.

Step 4: Read and interpret any notes listed with the main term or the subterm.

Notes such as common fifth-digit references and cross references are identified by italicized type. Always check any cross-references to ensure that all alternative terms are researched.

Step 5: Review entries for modifiers.

Nonessential modifiers are the terms located within parentheses following the main term entry. These parenthetical terms are supplementary words or explanatory information that may either be present or absent in the diagnostic statement and do not affect code selection. The subterms listed under the main term are essential modifiers that do affect coding assignment. Each line of indent represents a more specific code entry.

Step 6: Interpret abbreviations, cross-references, fifth digits, and brackets.

The cross-references used are "see," "see category" and "see also" which indicate alternative term choices for code searches. The abbreviation NEC may follow main terms or subterms. NEC (not elsewhere classified) indicates that there is no specific code for the condition even though the medical

documentation may be very specific. Is a fifth digit required? You MUST refer to the Tabular List to discover the correct code. Italicized brackets [ ] enclose a second code that must be used along with the code immediately preceding it, with the bracketed code sequenced as the secondary code. This is a mandatory multiple code situation. Both the underlying condition and the manifestation (code in the slanted bracket) must be reported.

Step 7: Choose a potential code and locate it in the Tabular List.

The coder must follow any Includes, Excludes notes, and other instructional notes, such as "Code first" and "Use additional code," listed in the Tabular for the chapter, category, subcategory, and subclassification level of code selection which direct the coder to use a different or additional code.

Any codes in the Tabular range, 001.0 through 999.9, may be used to identify the diagnostic reason for the encounter. The Tabular encompasses many codes describing disease and injury classifications (e.g., infectious and parasitic diseases, neoplasms, symptoms, signs and ill-defined conditions, etc.).

Codes that describe symptoms and signs, as opposed to definitive diagnoses, should be used for reporting purposes when an established diagnosis has not been made (confirmed) by the physician. Chapter 16 of the ICD-9-CM code book, "Symptoms, Signs, and Ill-Defined Conditions" (codes 780.01-799.9) contains many, but not all, codes for symptoms.

ICD-9-CM classifies encounters with health care providers for circumstances other than a disease or injury using codes in the Supplementary Classification of Factors Influencing Health Status and Contact with Health Services (V01.0-V91.99). There are many occasions when circumstances other than a disease or injury are recorded as chiefly responsible for the encounter.

Step 8: Determine whether the code is at the highest level of specificity.

A code is invalid if it has not been coded to the full number of digits (greatest level of specificity) required. A three-digit code is to be used only if the category is not further subdivided. Assign four-digit codes (subcategory codes) only if there are no five-digit codes for that category. Assign five-digit codes (fifth-digit subclassification codes) for those categories mandating the use of five digits.

Step 9: Assign the code.

Having reviewed all relevant information concerning the possible code choices, assign the code that most completely describes the condition.

Repeat steps one through nine for all additional documented conditions that meet the following criteria:

- Conditions that currently exist at the time of the visit
- Conditions that require or affect patient care, treatment or management.

Step 10: Sequence codes correctly

Sequencing is defined as the order in which the codes are listed on the claim. List first the ICD-9-CM code for the diagnosis, condition, problem or other reason for the encounter/visit, which is shown in the medical record to be chiefly responsible for the services provided. List additional codes that describe any coexisting conditions. Follow the official coding guidelines (See Section IV Diagnostic Coding and reporting Guidelines for Outpatient Services) concerning proper sequencing of codes.

Coding Examples

Diagnosis: Anorexia
- Step 1: The reason for the encounter was the condition, anorexia.
- Step 2. Consult the Index to Diseases.
- Step 3: Locate the main term "Anorexia."
- Step 4: There are no italicized instructional notes to interpret.
- Step 5: Note that there are two possible subterms (essential modifiers), "hysterical" and "nervosa," neither of which is documented in this instance and therefore cannot be used in code selection. The code listed next to the main term is called the default code selection.
- Step 6: There are no abbreviations, cross-references, fifth-digit notations, or brackets.
- Step 7: Turn to code 783.0 in the Tabular List and read the instructional notes. In this case the "Excludes" note indicates that anorexia

determined to be of non-organic origin should be coded to Chapter 5. The diagnostic statement does not indicate non-organic origin.

- Step 8: There is no further division of the category past the fourth digit subcategory. Therefore, the subcategory code level is the highest level of specificity.

- Step 9: The default code, 783.0 is the correct code selection.

- Step 10: Since anorexia is listed as the chief reason for the healthcare encounter, the primary or principal diagnosis is 783.0.

Diagnosis: Acute bronchitis
- Step 1: The reason for the encounter was the condition, acute bronchitis.

- Step 2. Consult the Alphabetic Index to Diseases.

- Step 3: Locate the main term "Bronchitis."

- Step 4: There are no italicized instructional notes to interpret.

- Step 5: Review entries for modifiers. Since "acute" is not listed as a nonessential modifier, read past the "with" modifier until you find the subterm "acute or subacute" with code 466.0.

- Step 6: There are no abbreviations, cross-references, fifth-digit notations, or brackets.

- Step 7: Since there are no more appropriate subterms, turn to code 466.0 in the Tabular List. The Includes note under category 466.0 does refer to possible infective organism and other alternative terms for acute bronchitis. Note that the inclusion term list is not exhaustive but is only a representative selection of diagnoses included in the subcategory. At the beginning of chapter 8, "Diseases of the Respiratory System," you will notice the "use additional code" note that instructs the user to assign a code to identify the infectious organism. This instructional note applies to the entire chapter.

- Step 8: There is no further division of the category past the fourth-digit subcategory, which is the highest level of specificity.

- Step 9: Assign code 466.0.

- Step 10: Repeat steps 1 through 9 for any additional code assignments.

Diagnosis: Acute bronchitis due to staphylococcus
- Step 1: The reason for the encounter was the condition, acute bronchitis due to staphylococcus.

- Step 2: Follow the steps listed in the example above for the diagnosis of acute bronchitis. Then start the search for a code identifying the underlying infectious organism, which in this case is staphylococcus.

- Step 3. Consult the Index to Diseases.

- Step 4: Locate the main term "Staphylococcus, staphylococcal."

- Step 5: The italicized instructional notes instruct the user to "see condition." Locate the main term "Infection, infected, infective."

- Step 6: Review entries for modifiers. Locate the subterm "staphylococcal NEC," which references code 041.10. The abbreviation NEC could prompt the coder to review the medical record for documentation concerning the specific type of staphylococcus.

- Step 7: Verify code 041.10 in the Tabular List. The code title is "Staphylococcus, unspecified." If there is additional information identifying the organism as aureus or other, assign the appropriate code, 041.11 or 041.19. Otherwise, assign code 041.10 Staphylococcus, unspecified, as an additional code.

- Step 8: There is no further division of the category past the fifth-digit subclassification level, which is the highest level of specificity. The final code assignment would be 041.10.

- Step 9: Assign code 041.10.

- Step 10: Sequence codes as directed by the instructional note for category 466. Code first 466.0, and assign code 041.10 as an additional diagnosis.

Diagnosis: Traveler's diarrhea
- Step 1: The reason for the encounter was the condition, Traveler's diarrhea.

- Step 2: Consult the Index to Diseases.

- Step 3: Locate the main term "Diarrhea" in the Alphabetic Index.

- Step 4: There are no italicized instructional notes to interpret.

- Step 5: Review entries for modifiers. Note that the nonessential modifiers (in parentheses) after the main term do not include the term "Traveler's," which means that the coder should search the subterms for the term "Traveler's." The subterm "Traveler's" has a possible code selection, 009.2, and suggests the subterm "due to specified organism NEC 008.8." The diagnostic statement does not include the infectious agent; therefore, code 008.8 does not apply.

- Step 6: There are no abbreviations, cross-references, fifth-digit notations, or brackets.

- Step 7: Locate code 009.2 in the Tabular List and read all instructional notes under the main category and subcategories. The Includes notes does not list the term "Traveler's" under code 009.2. As instructed by the Alphabetic Index, you should code the condition to 009.2. The ICD-9-CM code book implies that "Traveler's diarrhea" is the same as infectious diarrhea when it is not attributed to any specified infectious agent.

- Step 8: There is no further division of the category past the fourth-digit subcategory level. Therefore, the subcategory code level is the highest level of specificity. The final code assignment would be 009.2.

- Step 9: Assign code 009.2.

- Step 10: Since infectious diarrhea is listed as the chief reason for the healthcare encounter, the primary or principal diagnosis is 009.2.

Diagnosis: Ingrown toenail, infected
- Step 1: The reason for the encounter was the condition, infected ingrown toenail.

- Step 2. Consult the Index to Diseases.

- Step 3: First you must decide what the searchable main term should be. Reminder: search for condition, not anatomical site. The Alphabetic Index helps you determine the main term. Refer to "toenail" in the Alphabetic Index; the closest match is "Toe," which includes the instruction "see condition." Locate the main term "Infection" in the Alphabetic Index. The subterm toe has a subterm "nail" which refers the coder to category 681, Cellulitis and abscess of finger and toe. This does not indicate the condition ingrown toenail. The main term, therefore, is "Ingrown." A review of the Alphabetic Index takes you to "Ingrowing."

- Step 4: There are no italicized instructional notes to interpret.

- Step 5: Review the subterms. The subterm "nail" appears and lists nonessential modifiers (in parentheses) as "finger," "toe" and "infected." These nonessential modifiers complete the diagnostic statement.

- Step 6: There are no abbreviations, cross-references, fifth-digit notations, or brackets.

- Step 7: Verify code 703.0 in the Tabular List before assigning the code, review all instructional notes under category 703 and under code 703.0. The note, "Excludes: infection, nail NOS (681.9)," can be ignored because the diagnostic statement specifies the infection is due to the ingrowing nail.

- Step 8: Therefore, the subcategory code level is the highest level of specificity. The final code assignment would be 703.0.

- Step 9: The correct code choice is 703.0, Ingrowing nail with infection.

- Step 10: Since infectious infected ingrown toenail is listed as the chief reason for the healthcare encounter, the primary or principal diagnosis is 703.0.

ICD-9-CM Self Test

PART I ICD-9-CM DIAGNOSIS

1. A 55-year-old woman is brought to the emergency department by family members after developing symptoms that include high fever, confusion, muscle weakness, and severe headaches. Family members inform the staff that she recently returned from a visit to relatives in Colorado where she spent time outdoors camping. Family members are now concerned since the patient had made a remark about the number of bug bites she suffered while camping there. A blood sample is drawn and the physician also performs a spinal tap. Laboratory tests confirm the presence of the West Nile virus in both samples and the physician admits the patient with a diagnosis of encephalomyelitis due to West Nile virus infection.

2. A health care worker presents with symptoms of jaundice, nausea, and dark urine. The doctor orders an HCV enzyme linked immunosorbent assay blood test, which returns positive and is later confirmed by a recombinant immunoblot assay. The health care worker is diagnosed with acute hepatitis C and the decision to begin therapy with interferon and/or ribavarin is deferred until a quantitative HCV polymerase chain reaction test can be done to determine the titer level and the genotype of the C virus.

3. A 28-year-old patient presents for evaluation exhibits prominent psychiatric/behavioral symptoms painful distortion of sense of touch, ataxia and a non-diagnostic diffusely abnormal electroencephalogram. The physician makes a clinical determination of variant Creutzfeldt-Jakob disease (vCJD) with behavioral disturbances.

4. A patient with eczema was treated for fever and diffuse rash over 80 percent of the body associated with exposure to a family member who was recently vaccinated for smallpox.

5. A 34-year-old female presents post-assessment and treatment of associated glandular conditions by her endocrinologist. Diagnosis is consistent with bilateral medullary carcinoma, secondary hypertension, and hyperparathyroidism diagnosed as multiple endocrine neoplasia (MEN) syndrome, Type IIA. The tumor is localized in the upper central lobe of the thyroid. The patient will be admitted for total substernal thyroidectomy.

6. A 2-year-old female is brought to the urgent care center by her mother, who says the child has been running intermittent fevers over the past three days. She also reports that she was appearing somewhat sluggish earlier in the day. Upon examination, the child is currently afebrile and is alert and playful. CBC, however, reveals bandemia. She will be referred to her primary care pediatrician for further workup to rule out bacterial infection.

7. The husband of a young mother of three observed her suddenly falling asleep for no apparent reason while feeding the youngest child. She appeared to be in a state of unconsciousness for several minutes. Alarmed, the husband was checking for heart beat and pulse, and instructing the older child to call 911, when the wife suddenly became alert. The wife behaved as if she had just simply awakened from sleep. After reporting this episode to her physician, who found no other underlying reason for these episodes to occur, the physician asked the patient to keep a sleep diary for two weeks. The diary indicated that episodes of sudden uncontrollable sleepiness occurred again and again during the daytime. The physician then ordered a multiple sleep latency test (MSLT). The result indicated a diagnosis of narcolepsy.

8. A 16-year-old girl came to the physician's office with her outer ear severely abscessed and the surrounding tissue beginning to show signs of vascular compromise. Recently, she had multiple ear piercings around her ear that did not heal properly. She tried a topical antiseptic, but the condition worsened. A culture was taken that revealed a *Pseudomonas aeruginosa* infection. The physician recommended that she be hospitalized for care including drain insertion, wound debridement, and intravenous antibiotic therapy of amikacin sulfate. A diagnosis of chondritis of the pinna with *Pseudomonas aeruginosa* infection was established.

9. A patient is admitted to an acute care hospital experiencing sudden numbness or weakness of the left arm, sudden confusion, loss of balance and coordination, and a severe headache. CT scan indicates an occlusion and the patient is given a course of tPA. The patient is discharged a few days later with all symptoms resolved prior to release from the hospital. Final physician diagnosis of cerebrovascular accident is documented.

10. A 45-year-old woman, noted to be about 30 pounds overweight, who recently returned from India via a long plane journey presents to her physician's office complaining of pain and tenderness in her right leg. The physician notes swelling and redness developing in the lower half of her upper thigh. Since deep vein thrombosis is suspected, with a greater risk of developing pulmonary embolism, the physician orders a Doppler ultrasound and venography. A thrombus in the femoral vein is confirmed. She is admitted, the leg is held in elevated position, and the administration of intravenous heparin is initiated.

11. A 68-year-old patient presents with biopsy-confirmed metastatic carcinoid lesions of the liver from her co-existing primary carcinoid transverse colon malignancy.

12. An adult male, age 67, with mild form of COPD was admitted to the hospital with a fever, productive cough, and signs of bronchial obstruction, such as wheezing and dyspnea on exertion. The patient was in obvious distress. Sputum cultures exhibited normal flora. The physician ruled out pneumonia. The physician determined that the patient was experiencing an acute bronchitis in addition to the chronic bronchitis. The patient was provided an Albuterol inhaler to relieve the bronchospasms and IV hydration.

13. A 19-year-old boy presents to his dentist for his semiannual oral exam after the recent removal of his orthodontic braces. The dentist discovers initial decay and white spots on the buccal smooth surface of his lower canines where the edge of the metal braces had been secured to the teeth for the last two years. He is advised to practice good brushing habits and informed that the initial decay will progress very slowly and not require filling for a while yet.

14. A 45-year-old man with irregular brushing habits comes to the dentist having noticed that some of his teeth are appearing much longer and he is experiencing some bleeding from gums when brushing. The dentist notes that the gums are receding above his maxillary canines and premolars but does not note redness or swelling. The dentist educates the patient about the possible dangerous progression of bacterial infection and gingivitis when the gums have begun to recede and informs the patient that at this stage, he has minimal gingival recession.

15. A patient post liver transplant currently on glucocorticoid immunosuppressant drug therapy develops mononucleosis-like illness with lymphadenopathy. Laryngeal examination revealed hypopharyngeal and supraglottic mucosal hyperplasia. Immunostaining of laryngeal biopsy was positive for latent membrane protein-1 (LMP1). A diagnosis of post transplant lymphoproliferative disorder (PTLD) was established.

16. A 29-year-old female presents in premature labor at 35 weeks for delivery of dichorionic/diamniotic twin pregnancy, with spontaneous rupture of membranes post-onset of labor. Fetal lung maturity has been assessed, and the twins are determined ready for delivery. The pregnancy has been complicated by moderate pre-eclampsia and threatened premature labor. The patient was mildly pre-eclamptic on admission. At 12 weeks' gestation, the patient underwent an elective fetal reduction procedure to sustain pregnancy. Two viable twin males were delivered without complication via spontaneous vaginal delivery, with episiotomy.

17. A patient is admitted with diabetic neuropathy due to secondary diabetes from chronic therapeutic adrenocorticosteroid use.

18. A 47-year-old male presents for a physical exam. The patient complains of intermittent recurrent low back pain bilaterally, but worse on the right. The patient states that he injured his back last year and has had to limit his physical activity due to the injury. Physical exam reveals no acute injury. BP is slightly elevated at 144/100, cholesterol is elevated at 272. Diagnoses on exam are borderline HTN, hypercholesterolemia, and chronic low back pain. Antihypertensive and cholesterol-lowering medications have been discussed with the patient; however, he was urged to first try managing his diet. Treatment options were discussed with the patient to manage his low back pain.

19. A 58-year-old male presents with a seven-year history of acute gout attacks and periods of relative remission. He is currently being monitored for hyperuricemia and intermittent joint swelling and stiffness due to tophi. Diagnosis is consistent with Stage IV chronic tophaceous gout.

20. A type II diabetic patient presents with blurring of vision. Upon eye exam, multiple vascular hemorrhages and areas of ischemic changes were noted bilaterally in multiple quadrants of the retina consistent with severe nonproliferative diabetic retinopathy with retinal edema. No revascularizations were noted on this exam.

21. A 62-year-old male with longstanding hypertensive renal disease is admitted with progressive exacerbation of renal symptoms with indicative BUN and creatinine compromise. Management is focused on assessment of renal function and control of underlying hypertensive disease. GFR is assessed at 22, and the nephrologist elects to initiate dialysis. The patient is diagnosed with Stage IV chronic kidney disease and imminent renal failure.

22. A 55-year-old man diagnosed with Lou Gehrig's disease experienced rapid progression of muscle weakness and paralysis and opted for placement of an esophagostomy for tube feeding. The patient now presents with an infected esophagostomy site. The physician documentation confirms cultures positive for methicillin susceptible *Staphylococcus aureus*.

23. An otherwise healthy 55-year-old woman was admitted with a recent history of flu-like syndrome with fever, chills, cough, and myalgia. On admission, she had dyspnea, nonproductive cough, and rales in both lungs. Diagnostic imaging showed diffuse alveolar infiltration of both lungs, without pleural effusion. Sputum cultures were obtained on admission and empirical antibiotic treatment was initiated with Vancomycin due to suspected bacterial pneumonia. Due to her progressive respiratory failure, mechanical ventilation was initiated on day two. Sputum cultures identified *S. aureus* with an antimicrobial drug resistance profile.

24. A 37-year-old woman who gave birth one year ago is experiencing sensations of bladder fullness, incomplete emptying after urination, and urine leakage or incontinence upon changing position. Upon physical examination, the physician notes bulging in the anterior vaginal wall, some loss of normal vaginal rugae, but the lateral vaginal sulcus is intact. The physician documents a diagnosis of central defect cystocele with overflow incontinence.

25. Patient with diffuse large mediastinal B-cell lymphoma presents with progressive dyspnea. Diagnostic imaging and pleurocentesis confirms malignant pleural effusion.

26. A patient is admitted in acute renal failure associated with tumor lysis syndrome after initiation of chemotherapy for hairy cell leukemia.

27. A patient is admitted with high fever, nausea, and vomiting. The site of a recently placed PICC-line is slightly reddened and sore. The catheter is cultured and removed. Etiology of symptoms is determined to be PICC-line associated *Staphylococcus aureus* septicemia. The patient is treated with IV antibiotics.

28. A patient presents for local infection characterized by swelling, tenderness, and erythema at the upper extremity injection site following hepatitis B vaccination.

29. An HIV-positive male presents for anal Papanicolaou smear, which is positive for histologically-confirmed anal intraepithelial neoplasia (AIN I).

30. An 87-year-old man with uncomplicated vascular dementia has been bedridden for months and is now discovered to have a stage III decubitus ulcer appearing over the ischial area of the right buttock, affecting the subcutaneous layer, which are beginning to necrose and appearing with craterization. Appropriate wound debridement and protective dressing is carried out.

31. A patient develops signs and symptoms of acute respiratory distress, pulmonary edema, and hypotension within 2 hours of receiving a transfusion for a chronic anemia. Upon admission, labs revealed an increased white blood cell (WBC) count. Clinical presentation was felt to be consistent with TRALI. Investigation has been initiated into the blood products in question. Of primary importance is stopping of the offending transfusion. The patient responded positively to treatment with continuous positive airway pressure and added oxygen and hemodynamic support with no sequelae.

32. A 6-year-old patient presents with erythema multiform minor due to amoxicillin prescribed for otitis media. The patient has approximately 13 percent body surface exfoliation, primarily on limbs.

33. This 4-year-old female presents for ophthalmologic evaluation. The mother reports squinting and avoidance of light, and has noticed at times that the child seems unaware of people or objects in the periphery. Direct examination reveals bilateral optic nerves to be underdeveloped. The ophthalmologist documents a diagnosis of optic nerve hypoplasia. Further testing will be undertaken to determine the degree of impairment.

34. A 45-year-old female presents with low-back pain, leg weakness, sensory symptoms, and sphincter involvement. She has had multiple exacerbations of shingles over the years, and a lower back rash appeared three weeks ago. MRI revealed no mass lesion outside or within the spinal cord, and presumptive diagnosis was made of herpes zoster myelitis. The patient was placed on corticosteroids.

35. A patient presents to the emergency room with dermatitis, conjunctivitis, and pharyngitis. The patient is an avid swimmer who persisted with his morning workout in the bay, despite red tide warnings. Due to onset of symptoms associated with exposure, diagnosis is consistent with effects of red tide.

36. A 50-year-old female with a long history of refractory temporal lobe epilepsy presents for follow-up MRI to assess neurological changes. MRI reveals scarring consistent with mesial temporal sclerosis.

37. A patient presents with subclavian vein PICC line in situ with acute, complicating subclavian vein thrombus.

38. A newborn infant presents for observation and evaluation after apparent life-threatening event (ATLE). The patient sustained an observed spontaneous episode of seizure followed by an apneic episode characterized by breathing cessation, cyanosis, and bradycardia.

39. A frail, elderly patient with atrial fibrillation controlled on Coumadin presents with fracture of the femur for ORIF repair. However, his INR was 2.9 on admission, so the patient received two units of FFP to reverse anticoagulation. He then received four additional units over a five-hour period for a total of six units FFP, approximately 1,200 mL. The patient then developed acute respiratory distress, hypertension, tachycardia, elevated central venous and pulmonary artery wedge pressure, and jugular venous distension or S3 gallop on physical exam, consistent with transfusion-associated circulatory overload. He responded rapidly with supportive care and diuresis.

40. A 42-year-old barrel-chested obese male presents with a BMI of 45.2 for evaluation of chronic hypoxia, fatigue, and daytime somnolence. Sleep studies and PFTs ($PaCO_2 > 45$ mmHg) are positive for obstructive sleep apnea. Based on diagnostic testing and clinical examination, a diagnosis of Pickwickian syndrome due to morbid obesity is established.

41. A patient presents with an acute onset of fever, cough, and respiratory distress. The patient has recently been treated for RSV pneumonia. Pulmonary infiltrates present on exam are consistent with pneumonia. The patient has recently returned to work. He is a zoological worker who regularly handles exotic avian species transported from Asia. Laboratory testing is positive for low pathogenic avian influenza A (H7N2) virus. The physician documents avian influenza pneumonia superimposed on persistent, unresolved RSV pneumonia.

42. A 28-year-old female with poor obstetric history presents for MRI. Findings are consistent with unicornuate uterus and cervical hypoplasia.

43. A middle-aged, overweight patient presents for evaluation of mandibular jaw pain. Physical exam and diagnostic imaging of TMJ structures reveal no abnormalities. Family history is positive for cardiovascular disease, resulting in the early demise of the patient's father at the age of 52. The physician documents the diagnosis of jaw pain, etiology undetermined, and schedules the patient for further studies to rule out cardiovascular origin.

44. A patient with sickle cell anemia develops tachycardia, tachypnea, and hypotension following blood transfusion. The transfusion was aborted. The patient was placed on IV saline, furosemide, and low-dose dopamine to improve renal support and prevent shock due to acute hemolytic transfusion reaction. Donor blood was re-typed and crossed, resulting in identification of ABO incompatibility as a clerical error at the blood bank, resulting in mislabeling.

45. A 60-year-old male presents for evaluation of dementia. Over the past six months, he has had increased episodes of wandering from home and subsequently becoming disoriented and lost. He is accompanied by his daughter, who has responded to calls to retrieve and relocate him after these wandering episodes. As a veteran with a remote history of closed head trauma, previous imaging studies were inconclusive. Follow-up imaging studies and laboratory and cognitive tests have been ordered to rule out or otherwise identify causal pathology. Diagnosis: Wandering due to dementia, etiology undetermined.

46. A 52-year-old male presents with a recent onset of visual disturbances. Over the past five years, he has postponed regular eye exams, since he had no perceived changes in his vision until a few months ago, when he began to experience "blind spots" in his peripheral field of vision. Examination revealed high IOP, despite free flow of aqueous and atrophic cupping of the optic disc. Findings are consistent with moderate primary open angle glaucoma. The patient was prescribed topical combination pharmacotherapy.

47. A lung cancer patient presents with pleuritic chest pain and shortness of breath. Chest x-ray reveals spontaneous pneumothorax due to recurrence of primary LLL neoplasm.

48. A 46-year-old female presents five weeks post gastric banding procedure with nausea, vomiting, and epigastric pain. She has lost 20 lbs in 5 weeks but is dehydrated with compromise of intake. She denies gastrointestinal bleeding, or fever. Physical exam is significant for a normal, healing scar of the abdomen. The abdomen is soft and nontender. Endoscopy revealed a stricture of the stomach proximal to the gastric band with gastric bezoar, which was removed. The stricture was dilated endoscopically with a balloon dilator.

49. A patient with atrial septal defect, hypertrophic cardiomyopathy, and pulmonary artery stenosis associated with Noonan's syndrome is admitted for surgical correction of his atrial septal defect.

50. During a laparoscopic cholecystectomy procedure for cholecystitis, the surgeon inadvertently perforates the intestine, requiring emergent open abdominal repair.

PART II ICD-9-CM PROCEDURE CODING

1. Prior to a cardiac stenting procedure, the interventional cardiologist uses a fiber-optic, catheter-based near-infrared intravascular spectroscopy system to assess coronary plaques in the coronary vessels in order to determine whether a drug eluting or metal stent is the most appropriate type of stent. The final diagnosis is arteriosclerotic heart disease due to lipid rich plaque.

2. A 63-year-old male is hospitalized for sepsis due to septicemia from a gram negative bacteria. Shortly after admission, he developed acute respiratory failure and is now noted to be in septic shock. He was placed on mechanical ventilators, with a heart rate of over 90 beats/min, a fever of 103 Fahrenheit, and severe hypotension. In an attempt to restore hemodynamic stability and control hypotension, the patient is also given fluid resuscitation with hypertonic saline and IV infusion of norepinephrine. The patient was extubated 48 hours after initiation of mechanical ventilation with improved respiratory function.

3. A 63-year-old man was admitted to the hospital with a history of eight hours of chest pain associated with nausea, diaphoresis, and dyspnea. His electrocardiogram revealed 4-5 mm ST-segment elevation in the inferior leads with reciprocal ST-depression and was diagnosed with inferior myocardial infarction. Oxygen, aspirin, and morphine were administered. 50 mg tPA was administered per the Global Utilization of Streptokinase and Tissue Plasminogen Activator for Occluded Coronary Arteries (GUSTO) trial protocol and eptifibatide was also initiated. The patient was intubated, stabilized, and brought to the O.R. for PTCA with drug-eluting stent insertion. Diagnostic left heart cardiac catheterization indicated the left anterior descending branch of the main coronary artery to have a major obstruction. Rotational atherectomy was performed to reduce the size of the blockage followed by PTCA with drug-eluting stent insertion. IVUS was used to visualize the lumen of the descending branch, determine the patency of the vessel prior to insertion of the stent. After stent placement, IVUS was used to determine if the stent was positioned fully against the wall of the artery.

4. An 81-year-old man fell from the front steps of his home. He has a fracture of the right femur neck at the head and requires total hip replacement. The surgeon uses CT-based preoperative planning and navigational tools to precisely measure pelvic position on the O.R. table and the acetabular alignment of the implant.

5. A 70-year-old white male with arteriosclerosis of the carotid artery is diagnosed with stenosis or occlusion of the carotid artery. The patient is admitted for carotid artery atherectomy and insertion of non-drug-eluting stent. This is done now in an attempt to reduce his risk of cerebrovascular accident. The patient undergoes percutaneous angioplasty with tPA infusion of the area in question within the carotid artery before a non-drug-eluting stent deployment is carried out with cerebral protection from a thrombus or emboli also being used.

6. A patient is admitted with severe emphysema and undergoes bronchoscopy to determine the most appropriate treatment (e.g., endobronchial valve therapy or lung volume reduction surgery). The physician views the airway using a bronchoscope that is inserted through the oral cavity and advanced past the larynx to inspect the bronchus. The physician also assesses the patient's intrapulmonary air flow using intrapulmonary balloon catheters inserted into diseased portions of the lung during the bronchoscopy.

7. A 45-year-old male with loud snoring suffers from fatigue, irritability, and high blood pressure. Previous overnight exam in the sleep lab helped determine that he has severe obstructive sleep apnea. He presents at the hospital for a scheduled uvulopalatopharyngolplasty with the implantation of a palatal implant to remain in the soft palate.

8. Seventy six year-old male patient with congestive heart failure due to malignant hypertension is admitted for the implantation of the DeBakey axial flow ventricular assist device (VAD).

9. The physician repairs an umbilical hernia in a 5-year-old patient. The physician makes an umbilical incision and the laparoscope is placed through the umbilical port. Additional trocars are placed through small incisions in the lower abdomen. The hernia sac is identified and reduced and mesh is placed to reinforce the defect.

10. A 40-year-old female with a 3 inch discrepancy in the length of her legs has walked for years with specially made platform shoes that equalize her shorter leg and keep her hips aligned. In childhood, she suffered a fracture of the right femur that developed a bone infection. This interference with the natural growth opportunity of the bone resulted in one leg being shorter than the other. She has previously refused to undergo limb lengthening with the external frame device method and has opted now to have the internal limb lengthening device implanted to gradually elongate her short leg with distraction.

11. A patient is admitted for surgical removal and treatment of malignant neoplasm of the breast. Immediately after lumpectomy for removal of the tumor, the radiation oncologist delivers a specialized high dose of focal radiation directly to the tumor bed while normal tissues are protected.

12. A patient with metastatic, overlapping brain tumors is admitted to the interventional radiology suite for chemotherapy. After an infusion of Mannitol into the carotid artery, chemotherapy is infused into the same artery.

13. A 9-year-old patient with cerebral palsy reports to the operating suite for surgical correction of congenital planovalgus flat foot deformity. Subtalar arthroereisis is performed with implant of a Vitallium staple across the lateral subtalar joint.

14. A closed fracture reduction with external fixation of the proximal tibial plateau is performed in the operating suite. A Sheffield ring external fixation device is affixed with the assistance of tensioned Kirchner wires. Adequate alignment confirmed radiologically.

15. The physician repairs a defect in a vertebral disc after a lumbar discectomy for degenerative disc disease. Sutures are fastened to the vertebral disc and a mesh device is positioned adjacent to the defect. Tension is applied to the sutures, which are then attached to hold the mesh adjacent the defect.

16. A patient with cancer throughout the colon is admitted for treatment. The physician makes an abdominal incision, removes the entire colon and rectum, strips the mucosa from the distal rectum, and performs an anastomosis between the terminal ileum and anus.

17. A patient with chronic liver disease undergoes a liver biopsy. Using imaging guidance, the radiologist inserts a catheter into the jugular vein in the neck and directs it into the primary vein in the liver. A small biopsy needle is then inserted through the tube and into the liver to obtain a sample of tissue.

18. This 75-year-old male was admitted through the emergency room with slurred speech and unilateral weakness, which has worsened in severity over the past five hours. MRI and CT revealed acute ischemic cerebral thrombosis.

    Once the location of the stroke-inducing thrombus was identified using angiography, the balloon guide catheter was inserted employing standard catheterization techniques via a femoral artery approach. Under x-ray guidance, the catheter was maneuvered to the carotid artery. A guidewire and the microcatheter were deployed through the balloon guide catheter and then placed just beyond the clot in the appropriate intracranial artery. The retriever device was deployed in order to engage and ensnare the thrombus. Upon capture of the thrombus, the balloon guide catheter was inflated to momentarily halt forward flow during this maneuver. The thrombus was pulled into the balloon guide catheter and completely out of the body. The balloon was then deflated, and blood flow was restored. The patient was taken to the floor in stable condition.

19. A 75-year-old active female who is fourteen years status post total hip replacement with ceramic-on-polyethylene bearing surface complains of increasing pain and inflammation. Radiographic studies reveal wear of the articular bearing surface of the prosthetic joint, necessitating revision of the acetabular component. The same type of bearing surface was used as in her previous surgery and was carried out without complications.

20. A 47-year-old male with coronary atherosclerosis was taken to the angioplasty suite where percutaneous transluminal coronary angioplasty (PTCA) was performed on lesions in the left anterior descending artery (LAD) main branch and the diagonal and the circumflex/obtuse marginal bifurcation. A drug-eluting stent in the main branch of the LAD and angioplasty with two additional stents were placed in the branch vessels of the circumflex and obtuse marginal bifurcation of this vessel utilizing a crush technique.

21. A patient with chronic systolic and diastolic congestive heart failure with a pre-existing AICD is admitted for implantation of a cardiac contractility modulation system implantation to improve heart function. The patient received a total Optimizer III® system. During the procedure, a catheter-based transducer was introduced for hemodynamic measurements during the positioning of three standard pacemaker leads—two placed in the right ventricular septum and one in the right atrium. The leads were connected to the implantable pulse generator (IPG) which was placed in a subcutaneous pectoral pocket. Intraoperative testing of the device was performed to ensure appropriate function.

22. A patient is admitted for treatment of medulloblastoma in the fourth ventricle, between the brain stem and the cerebellum. After a 1 cm burr hole is drilled through the skull at the location of the tumor, the physician uses the AutoLITT™ workstation in the MRI control room to monitor and control the thermal ablation in real time. A standard MRI scanner guides the placement of the MRI compatible laser probe through the transcranial burr hole. The laser is used to thermally ablate the tumor tissue while simultaneously cooling the surrounding tissue to prevent that tissue from being damaged. The physician repositions the probe to treat different areas of the tumor. After the treatment is completed, the physician withdraws the probe and the burr hole is closed.

23. A patient is admitted for surgical treatment of an acute bowel obstruction. The physician inserts a colonic stent using endoscopic visualization with fluoroscopy. After the patient is sedated, the physician inserts the endoscope, visualizes the obstruction, and measures the length of the obstruction. Contrast is injected, and a guidewire is placed through the scope and beyond the level of the obstruction. A Colonic Z-Stent® designed to fit through the scope is inserted over the guidewire and deployed under endoscopic visualization with fluoroscopic confirmation.

24. A 59-year-old patient with atherosclerotic PVD of the SFA presents for balloon angioplasty of the SFA with insertion of drug-eluting stent. Upon adequate dilation of the vessel, the DES was threaded over the guidewire and deployed into the SFA.

25. A patient with medically refractory localization-related epilepsy with complex partial seizures presents for implantation of an RNS. Via premeasured craniectomy, the ferrule was inserted into the cranium, upon which the neurostimulator and intracranial leads were fitted into place into the skull. Implanted intracranial leads were connected to the neurostimulator, and the neurostimulator was placed in the ferrule and anchored to the skull with bone screws. The scalp was replaced over the skull, covering the implanted neurostimulator, and the surgical site was sutured closed.

26. A patient presents for treatment of hypertensive cardiovascular disease with diastolic heart failure by implantation of the Rheos carotid sinus baroreflex activation system. The total system was placed by inserting the generator under the skin near the collarbone. The electrodes were placed on the carotid arteries, with the leads tunneled under the skin and connected to the device. The programmer system was retested and activated.

27. A patient with noncommunicating, obstructive hydrocephalus presents for the placement of an internal ventriculocisternostomy shunt. The scalp was incised and retracted posterior to the ear. A burr hole was created through the skull, and a shunt tube was placed through the lateral ventricle with endoscopic assistance. The flow of fluid was tested, and the distal end of the shunt was directed toward the cisterna magna with free flow of fluid. The ends were connected, and patency was retested. The dura and scalp were closed in layers.

28. A patient with severe aortic valve stenosis presents for TAVR (transcatheter aortic valve replacement). The procedure was performed via an endovascular approach, utilizing a transfemoral vein approach. Balloon valvuloplasty was performed adjunct to the deployment of a bioprosthetic aortic valve. Once optimal placement was achieved, the catheters were removed and the groin access site was closed.

29. A patient presents for uterine artery embolization of two large intramural uterine fibroids. Under local anesthesia, the femoral artery was accessed, and a catheter was advanced through the femoral artery into the uterine artery under imaging guidance. Contrast arteriogram was performed, and the uterine arteries were selected for embolization. Polyvinyl microspheres were injected into each selected site, with successful occlusion of the circulation to both uterine fibroids. The catheter was withdrawn, and the access sites were closed without incident.

30. A patient presents for modified radical mastectomy for left upper outer quadrant adenocarcinoma of the breast. A sentinel node biopsy is performed in addition to the mastectomy procedure.

31. A patient presents for an arthroscopic-assisted open reduction and internal fixation (ORIF) of tibial plateau fracture.

Answer Key can be found in the back of the book.

A

AAT (alpha-1 antitrypsin) deficiency 273.4
AAV (disease) (illness) (infection) — *see* Human immunodeficiency virus (disease) (illness) (infection)
Abactio — *see* Abortion, induced
Abactus venter — *see* Abortion, induced
Abarognosis 781.99
Abasia (-astasia) 307.9
  atactica 781.3
  choreic 781.3
  hysterical 300.11
  paroxysmal trepidant 781.3
  spastic 781.3
  trembling 781.3
  trepidans 781.3
Abderhalden-Kaufmann-Lignac syndrome (cystinosis) 270.0
Abdomen, abdominal — *see also* condition
  accordion 306.4
  acute 789.0 ☑
  angina 557.1
  burst 868.00
  convulsive equivalent (*see also* Epilepsy) 345.5 ☑
  heart 746.87
  muscle deficiency syndrome 756.79
  obstipum 756.79
Abdominalgia 789.0 ☑
  periodic 277.31
Abduction contracture, hip or other joint — *see* Contraction, joint
Abercrombie's syndrome (amyloid degeneration) 277.39
Aberrant (congenital) — *see also* Malposition, congenital
  adrenal gland 759.1
  blood vessel NEC 747.60
    arteriovenous NEC 747.60
    cerebrovascular 747.81
    gastrointestinal 747.61
    lower limb 747.64
    renal 747.62
    spinal 747.82
    upper limb 747.63
  breast 757.6
  endocrine gland NEC 759.2
  gastrointestinal vessel (peripheral) 747.61
  hepatic duct 751.69
  lower limb vessel (peripheral) 747.64
  pancreas 751.7
  parathyroid gland 759.2
  peripheral vascular vessel NEC 747.60
  pituitary gland (pharyngeal) 759.2
  renal blood vessel 747.62
  sebaceous glands, mucous membrane, mouth 750.26
  spinal vessel 747.82
  spleen 759.0
  testis (descent) 752.51
  thymus gland 759.2
  thyroid gland 759.2
  upper limb vessel (peripheral) 747.63
Aberratio
  lactis 757.6
  testis 752.51
Aberration — *see also* Anomaly
  chromosome — *see* Anomaly, chromosome(s)
  distantial 368.9
  mental (*see also* Disorder, mental, nonpsychotic) 300.9
Abetalipoproteinemia 272.5
Abionarce 780.79
Abiotrophy 799.89
Ablatio
  placentae — *see* Placenta, ablatio
  retinae (*see also* Detachment, retina) 361.9
Ablation
  pituitary (gland) (with hypofunction) 253.7
  placenta — *see* Placenta, ablatio
  uterus 621.8
Ablepharia, ablepharon, ablephary 743.62
Ablepsia — *see* Blindness
Ablepsy — *see* Blindness

Ablutomania 300.3
Abnormal, abnormality, abnormalities — *see also* Anomaly
  acid-base balance 276.4
    fetus or newborn — *see* Distress, fetal
  adaptation curve, dark 368.63
  alveolar ridge 525.9
  amnion 658.9 ☑
    affecting fetus or newborn 762.9
  anatomical relationship NEC 759.9
  apertures, congenital, diaphragm 756.6
  auditory perception NEC 388.40
  autosomes NEC 758.5
    13 758.1
    18 758.2
    21 or 22 758.0
    D_1 758.1
    E_3 758.2
    G 758.0
  ballistocardiogram 794.39
  basal metabolic rate (BMR) 794.7
  biosynthesis, testicular androgen 257.2
  blood level (of)
    cobalt 790.6
    copper 790.6
    iron 790.6
    lead 790.6
    lithium 790.6
    magnesium 790.6
    mineral 790.6
    zinc 790.6
  blood pressure
    elevated (without diagnosis of hypertension) 796.2
    low (*see also* Hypotension) 458.9
      reading (incidental) (isolated) (nonspecific) 796.3
  blood sugar 790.29
  bowel sounds 787.5
  breathing behavior — *see* Respiration
  caloric test 794.19
  cervix (acquired) NEC 622.9
    congenital 752.40
    in pregnancy or childbirth 654.6 ☑
      causing obstructed labor 660.2 ☑
        affecting fetus or newborn 763.1
  chemistry, blood NEC 790.6
  chest sounds 786.7
  chorion 658.9 ☑
    affecting fetus or newborn 762.9
  chromosomal NEC 758.89
    analysis, nonspecific result 795.2
    autosomes (*see also* Abnormal, autosomes NEC) 758.5
    fetal, (suspected) affecting management of pregnancy 655.1 ☑
    sex 758.81
  clinical findings NEC 796.4
  communication — *see* Fistula
  configuration of pupils 379.49
  coronary
    artery 746.85
    vein 746.9
  cortisol-binding globulin 255.8
  course, Eustachian tube 744.24
  creatinine clearance 794.4
  dentofacial NEC 524.9
    functional 524.50
    specified type NEC 524.89
  development, developmental NEC 759.9
    bone 756.9
    central nervous system 742.9
  direction, teeth 524.30
  Dynia (*see also* Defect, coagulation) 286.9
  Ebstein 746.2
  echocardiogram 793.2
  echoencephalogram 794.01
  echogram NEC — *see* Findings, abnormal, structure
  electrocardiogram (ECG) (EKG) 794.31
  electroencephalogram (EEG) 794.02
  electromyogram (EMG) 794.17
    ocular 794.14
  electro-oculogram (EOG) 794.12
  electroretinogram (ERG) 794.11
  erythrocytes 289.9

Abnormal, abnormality, abnormalities — *see also* Anomaly — *continued*
  erythrocytes — *continued*
    congenital, with perinatal jaundice 282.9 [774.0]
  Eustachian valve 746.9
  excitability under minor stress 301.9
  fat distribution 782.9
  feces 787.7
  fetal heart rate — *see* Distress, fetal
  fetus NEC
    affecting management of pregnancy — *see* Pregnancy, management affected by, fetal
    causing disproportion 653.7 ☑
      affecting fetus or newborn 763.1
      causing obstructed labor 660.1 ☑
        affecting fetus or newborn 763.1
    findings without manifest disease — *see* Findings, abnormal
  fluid
    amniotic 792.3
    cerebrospinal 792.0
    peritoneal 792.9
    pleural 792.9
    synovial 792.9
    vaginal 792.9
  forces of labor NEC 661.9 ☑
    affecting fetus or newborn 763.7
  form, teeth 520.2
  function studies
    auditory 794.15
    bladder 794.9
    brain 794.00
    cardiovascular 794.30
    endocrine NEC 794.6
    kidney 794.4
    liver 794.8
    nervous system
      central 794.00
      peripheral 794.19
    oculomotor 794.14
    pancreas 794.9
    placenta 794.9
    pulmonary 794.2
    retina 794.11
    special senses 794.19
    spleen 794.9
    thyroid 794.5
    vestibular 794.16
  gait 781.2
    hysterical 300.11
  gastrin secretion 251.5
  globulin
    cortisol-binding 255.8
    thyroid-binding 246.8
  glucagon secretion 251.4
  glucose 790.29
    in pregnancy, childbirth, or puerperium 648.8 ☑
    fetus or newborn 775.0
    non-fasting 790.29
  gravitational (G) forces or states 994.9
  hair NEC 704.2
  hard tissue formation in pulp 522.3
  head movement 781.0
  heart
    rate
      fetus, affecting liveborn infant
        before the onset of labor 763.81
        during labor 763.82
        unspecified as to time of onset 763.83
      intrauterine
        before the onset of labor 763.81
        during labor 763.82
        unspecified as to time of onset 763.83
      newborn
        before the onset of labor 763.81
        during labor 763.82
        unspecified as to time of onset 763.83
    shadow 793.2
    sounds NEC 785.3

Abnormal, abnormality, abnormalities — *see also* Anomaly — *continued*
  hemoglobin (*see also* Disease, hemoglobin) 282.7
    trait — *see* Trait, hemoglobin, abnormal
  hemorrhage, uterus — *see* Hemorrhage, uterus
  histology NEC 795.4
  increase
    in
      appetite 783.6
      development 783.9
  involuntary movement 781.0
  jaw closure 524.51
  karyotype 795.2
  knee jerk 796.1
  laboratory findings — *see* Findings, abnormal
  labor NEC 661.9 ☑
    affecting fetus or newborn 763.7
  length, organ or site, congenital — *see* Distortion
  liver function test 790.6
  loss of height 781.91
  loss of weight 783.21
  lung shadow 793.19
  mammogram 793.80
    calcification 793.89
    calculus 793.89
    microcalcification 793.81
  Mantoux test 795.51
  membranes (fetal)
    affecting fetus or newborn 762.9
    complicating pregnancy 658.8 ☑
  menstruation — *see* Menstruation
  metabolism (*see also* condition) 783.9
  movement 781.0
    disorder NEC 333.90
      sleep related, unspecified 780.58
      specified NEC 333.99
    head 781.0
    involuntary 781.0
    specified type NEC 333.99
  muscle contraction, localized 728.85
  myoglobin (Aberdeen) (Annapolis) 289.9
  narrowness, eyelid 743.62
  optokinetic response 379.57
  organs or tissues of pelvis NEC
    in pregnancy or childbirth 654.9 ☑
      affecting fetus or newborn 763.89
      causing obstructed labor 660.2 ☑
        affecting fetus or newborn 763.1
  origin — *see* Malposition, congenital
  palmar creases 757.2
  Papanicolaou (smear)
    anus 796.70
      with
        atypical squamous cells
          cannot exclude high grade squamous intraepithelial lesion (ASC-H) 796.72
          of undetermined significance (ASC-US) 796.71
        cytologic evidence of malignancy 796.76
        high grade squamous intraepithelial lesion (HGSIL) 796.74
        low grade squamous intraepithelial lesion (LGSIL) 796.73
        glandular 796.70
        specified finding NEC 796.79
    cervix 795.00
      with
        atypical squamous cells
          cannot exclude high grade squamous intraepithelial lesion (ASC-H) 795.02
          of undetermined significance (ASC-US) 795.01
        cytologic evidence of malignancy 795.06
        high grade squamous intraepithelial lesion (HGSIL) 795.04

Abnormal, abnormality, abnormalities — *see also* Anomaly — *continued*
  Papanicolaou — *continued*
    cervix — *continued*
      with — *continued*
        low grade squamous intraepithelial lesion (LGSIL) 795.03
        nonspecific finding NEC 795.09
    other site 796.9
    vagina 795.10
      with
        atypical squamous cells
          cannot exclude high grade squamous intraepithelial lesion (ASC-H) 795.12
          of undetermined significance (ASC-US) 795.11
        cytologic evidence of malignancy 795.16
        high grade squamous intraepithelial lesion (HGSIL) 795.14
        low grade squamous intraepithelial lesion (LGSIL) 795.13
    glandular 795.10
    specified finding NEC 795.19
  parturition
    affecting fetus or newborn 763.9
    mother — *see* Delivery, complicated
  pelvis (bony) — *see* Deformity, pelvis
  percussion, chest 786.7
  periods (grossly) (*see also* Menstruation) 626.9
  phonocardiogram 794.39
  placenta — *see* Placenta, abnormal
  plantar reflex 796.1
  plasma protein — *see* Deficiency, plasma, protein
  pleural folds 748.8
  position (*see also* Malposition)
    gravid uterus 654.4 ☑
      causing obstructed labor 660.2 ☑
        affecting fetus or newborn 763.1
  posture NEC 781.92
  presentation (fetus) — *see* Presentation, fetus, abnormal
  product of conception NEC 631.8
  puberty — *see* Puberty
  pulmonary
    artery 747.39
    function, newborn 770.89
    test results 794.2
    ventilation, newborn 770.89
      hyperventilation 786.01
  pulsations in neck 785.1
  pupil reflexes 379.40
  quality of milk 676.8 ☑
  radiological examination 793.99
    abdomen NEC 793.6
    biliary tract 793.3
    breast 793.89
      mammogram NOS 793.80
      mammographic
        calcification 793.89
        calculus 793.89
        microcalcification 793.81
    gastrointestinal tract 793.4
    genitourinary organs 793.5
    head 793.0
    image test inconclusive due to excess body fat 793.91
    intrathoracic organ NEC 793.2
    lung (field) 793.19
    musculoskeletal system 793.7
    retroperitoneum 793.6
    skin and subcutaneous tissue 793.99
    skull 793.0
  red blood cells 790.09
    morphology 790.09
    volume 790.09
  reflex NEC 796.1
  renal function test 794.4
  respiration signs — *see* Respiration
  response to nerve stimulation 794.10
  retinal correspondence 368.34
  rhythm, heart (*see also* Arrhythmia)

Abnormal, abnormality, abnormalities — *see also* Anomaly — *continued*
  rhythm, heart (*see also* Arrhythmia) — *continued*
    fetus — *see* Distress, fetal
  saliva 792.4
  scan
    brain 794.09
    kidney 794.4
    liver 794.8
    lung 794.2
    thyroid 794.5
  secretion
    gastrin 251.5
    glucagon 251.4
  semen 792.2
  serum level (of)
    acid phosphatase 790.5
    alkaline phosphatase 790.5
    amylase 790.5
    enzymes NEC 790.5
    lipase 790.5
  shape
    cornea 743.41
    gallbladder 751.69
    gravid uterus 654.4 ☑
      affecting fetus or newborn 763.89
      causing obstructed labor 660.2 ☑
        affecting fetus or newborn 763.1
    head (*see also* Anomaly, skull) 756.0
    organ or site, congenital NEC — *see* Distortion
  sinus venosus 747.40
  size
    fetus, complicating delivery 653.5 ☑
      causing obstructed labor 660.1 ☑
    gallbladder 751.69
    head (*see also* Anomaly, skull) 756.0
    organ or site, congenital NEC — *see* Distortion
    teeth 520.2
  skin and appendages, congenital NEC 757.9
  soft parts of pelvis — *see* Abnormal, organs or tissues of pelvis
  spermatozoa 792.2
  sputum (amount) (color) (excessive) (odor) (purulent) 786.4
  stool NEC 787.7
    bloody 578.1
      occult 792.1
    bulky 787.7
    color (dark) (light) 792.1
    content (fat) (mucus) (pus) 792.1
    occult blood 792.1
  synchondrosis 756.9
  test results without manifest disease — *see* Findings, abnormal
  thebesian valve 746.9
  thermography — *see* Findings, abnormal, structure
  threshold, cones or rods (eye) 368.63
  thyroid-binding globulin 246.8
  thyroid product 246.8
  toxicology (findings) NEC 796.0
  tracheal cartilage (congenital) 748.3
  transport protein 273.8
  ultrasound results — *see* Findings, abnormal, structure
  umbilical cord
    affecting fetus or newborn 762.6
    complicating delivery 663.9 ☑
    specified NEC 663.8 ☑
  union
    cricoid cartilage and thyroid cartilage 748.3
    larynx and trachea 748.3
    thyroid cartilage and hyoid bone 748.3
  urination NEC 788.69
    psychogenic 306.53
    stream
      intermittent 788.61
      slowing 788.62
      splitting 788.61
      weak 788.62
    urgency 788.63
  urine (constituents) NEC 791.9

Abnormal, abnormality, abnormalities — *see also* Anomaly — *continued*
  uterine hemorrhage (*see also* Hemorrhage, uterus) 626.9
    climacteric 627.0
    postmenopausal 627.1
  vagina (acquired) (congenital)
    in pregnancy or childbirth 654.7 ☑
      affecting fetus or newborn 763.89
      causing obstructed labor 660.2 ☑
        affecting fetus or newborn 763.1
  vascular sounds 785.9
  vectorcardiogram 794.39
  visually evoked potential (VEP) 794.13
  vulva (acquired) (congenital)
    in pregnancy or childbirth 654.8 ☑
      affecting fetus or newborn 763.89
      causing obstructed labor 660.2 ☑
        affecting fetus or newborn 763.1
  weight
    gain 783.1
      of pregnancy 646.1 ☑
        with hypertension — *see* Toxemia, of pregnancy
    loss 783.21
  x-ray examination — *see* Abnormal, radiological examination

Abnormally formed uterus — *see* Anomaly, uterus

Abnormity (any organ or part) — *see* Anomaly

ABO
  hemolytic disease 773.1
  incompatibility (due to transfusion of blood or blood products)
    with hemolytic transfusion reaction (HTR) (not specified as acute or delayed) 999.61
      24 hours or more after transfusion 999.63
      acute 999.62
      delayed 999.63
      less than 24 hours after transfusion 999.62
      unspecified time after transfusion 999.61
    reaction 999.60
      specified NEC 999.69

Abocclusion 524.20

Abolition, language 784.69

Aborter, habitual or recurrent NEC
  without current pregnancy 629.81
  current abortion (*see also* Abortion, spontaneous) 634.9 ☑
    affecting fetus or newborn 761.8
  observation in current pregnancy 646.3 ☑

Abortion (complete) (incomplete) (inevitable) (with retained products of conception) 637.9 ☑

> *Note* — Use the following fifth-digit subclassification with categories 634–637:
>
> 0   unspecified
>
> 1   incomplete
>
> 2   complete

  with
    complication(s) (any) following previous abortion — *see* category 639 ☑
    damage to pelvic organ (laceration) (rupture) (tear) 637.2 ☑
    embolism (air) (amniotic fluid) (blood clot) (pulmonary) (pyemic) (septic) (soap) 637.6 ☑
    genital tract and pelvic infection 637.0 ☑
    hemorrhage, delayed or excessive 637.1 ☑
    metabolic disorder 637.4 ☑
    renal failure (acute) 637.3 ☑
    sepsis (genital tract) (pelvic organ) 637.0 ☑
      urinary tract 637.7 ☑
    shock (postoperative) (septic) 637.5 ☑
    specified complication NEC 637.7 ☑

Abortion — *continued*
  with — *continued*
    toxemia 637.3 ☑
    unspecified complication(s) 637.8 ☑
    urinary tract infection 637.7 ☑
  accidental — *see* Abortion, spontaneous
  artificial — *see* Abortion, induced
  attempted (failed) — *see* Abortion, failed
  criminal — *see* Abortion, illegal
  early — *see* Abortion, spontaneous
  elective — *see* Abortion, legal
  failed (legal) 638.9
    with
      damage to pelvic organ (laceration) (rupture) (tear) 638.2
      embolism (air) (amniotic fluid) (blood clot) (pulmonary) (pyemic) (septic) (soap) 638.6
      genital tract and pelvic infection 638.0
      hemorrhage, delayed or excessive 638.1
      metabolic disorder 638.4
      renal failure (acute) 638.3
      sepsis (genital tract) (pelvic organ) 638.0
        urinary tract 638.7
      shock (postoperative) (septic) 638.5
      specified complication NEC 638.7
      toxemia 638.3
      unspecified complication(s) 638.8
      urinary tract infection 638.7
  fetal indication — *see* Abortion, legal
  fetus 779.6
  following threatened abortion — *see* Abortion, by type
  habitual or recurrent (care during pregnancy) 646.3 ☑
    with current abortion (*see also* Abortion, spontaneous) 634.9 ☑
      affecting fetus or newborn 761.8
    without current pregnancy 629.81
  homicidal — *see* Abortion, illegal
  illegal 636.9 ☑
    with
      damage to pelvic organ (laceration) (rupture) (tear) 636.2 ☑
      embolism (air) (amniotic fluid) (blood clot) (pulmonary) (pyemic) (septic) (soap) 636.6 ☑
      genital tract and pelvic infection 636.0 ☑
      hemorrhage, delayed or excessive 636.1 ☑
      metabolic disorder 636.4 ☑
      renal failure 636.3 ☑
      sepsis (genital tract) (pelvic organ) 636.0 ☑
        urinary tract 636.7 ☑
      shock (postoperative) (septic) 636.5 ☑
      specified complication NEC 636.7 ☑
      toxemia 636.3 ☑
      unspecified complication(s) 636.8 ☑
      urinary tract infection 636.7 ☑
    fetus 779.6
  induced 637.9 ☑
    illegal — *see* Abortion, illegal
    legal indications — *see* Abortion, legal
    medical indications — *see* Abortion, legal
    therapeutic — *see* Abortion, legal
  late — *see* Abortion, spontaneous
  legal (legal indication) (medical indication) (under medical supervision) 635.9 ☑
    with
      damage to pelvic organ (laceration) (rupture) (tear) 635.2 ☑
      embolism (air) (amniotic fluid) (blood clot) (pulmonary) (pyemic) (septic) (soap) 635.6 ☑
      genital tract and pelvic infection 635.0 ☑
      hemorrhage, delayed or excessive 635.1 ☑

Abortion — *continued*
legal — *continued*
with — *continued*
metabolic disorder 635.4 ☑
renal failure (acute) 635.3 ☑
sepsis (genital tract) (pelvic organ) 635.0 ☑
urinary tract 635.7 ☑
shock (postoperative) (septic) 635.5 ☑
specified complication NEC 635.7 ☑
toxemia 635.3 ☑
unspecified complication(s) 635.8 ☑
urinary tract infection 635.7 ☑
fetus 779.6
medical indication — *see* Abortion, legal
mental hygiene problem — *see* Abortion, legal
missed 632
operative — *see* Abortion, legal
psychiatric indication — *see* Abortion, legal
recurrent — *see* Abortion, spontaneous
self-induced — *see* Abortion, illegal
septic — *see* Abortion, by type, with sepsis
spontaneous 634.9 ☑
with
damage to pelvic organ (laceration) (rupture) (tear) 634.2 ☑
embolism (air) (amniotic fluid) (blood clot) (pulmonary) (pyemic) (septic) (soap) 634.6 ☑
genital tract and pelvic infection 634.0 ☑
hemorrhage, delayed or excessive 634.1 ☑
metabolic disorder 634.4 ☑
renal failure 634.3 ☑
sepsis (genital tract) (pelvic organ) 634.0 ☑
urinary tract 634.7 ☑
shock (postoperative) (septic) 634.5 ☑
specified complication NEC 634.7 ☑
toxemia 634.3 ☑
unspecified complication(s) 634.8 ☑
urinary tract infection 634.7 ☑
fetus 761.8
threatened 640.0 ☑
affecting fetus or newborn 762.1
surgical — *see* Abortion, legal
therapeutic — *see* Abortion, legal
threatened 640.0 ☑
affecting fetus or newborn 762.1
tubal — *see* Pregnancy, tubal
voluntary — *see* Abortion, legal
Abortus fever 023.9
Aboulomania 301.6
Abrachia 755.20
Abrachiatism 755.20
Abrachiocephalia 759.89
Abrachiocephalus 759.89
Abrami's disease (acquired hemolytic jaundice) 283.9
Abramov-Fiedler myocarditis (acute isolated myocarditis) 422.91
Abrasion — *see also* Injury, superficial, by site
cornea 918.1
dental 521.20
extending into
dentine 521.22
pulp 521.23
generalized 521.25
limited to enamel 521.21
localized 521.24
teeth, tooth (dentifrice) (habitual) (hard tissues) (occupational) (ritual) (traditional) (wedge defect) (*see also* Abrasion, dental) 521.20
Abrikossov's tumor (M9580/0) — *see also* Neoplasm, connective tissue, benign
malignant (M9580/3) — *see* Neoplasm, connective tissue, malignant
Abrism 988.8
Abruption, placenta — *see* Placenta, abruptio
Abruptio placentae — *see* Placenta, abruptio

Abscess (acute) (chronic) (infectional) (lymphangitic) (metastatic) (multiple) (pyogenic) (septic) (with lymphangitis) — *see also* Cellulitis 682.9
abdomen, abdominal
cavity 567.22
wall 682.2
abdominopelvic 567.22
accessory sinus (chronic) (*see also* Sinusitis) 473.9
adrenal (capsule) (gland) 255.8
alveolar 522.5
with sinus 522.7
ambic 006.3
bladder 006.8
brain (with liver or lung abscess) 006.5
liver (without mention of brain or lung abscess) 006.3
with
brain abscess (and lung abscess) 006.5
lung abscess 006.4
lung (with liver abscess) 006.4
with brain abscess 006.5
seminal vesicle 006.8
specified site NEC 006.8
spleen 006.8
anaerobic 040.0
ankle 682.6
anorectal 566
antecubital space 682.3
antrum (chronic) (Highmore) (*see also* Sinusitis, maxillary) 473.0
anus 566
apical (tooth) 522.5
with sinus (alveolar) 522.7
appendix 540.1
areola (acute) (chronic) (nonpuerperal) 611.0
puerperal, postpartum 675.1 ☑
arm (any part, above wrist) 682.3
artery (wall) 447.2
atheromatous 447.2
auditory canal (external) 380.10
auricle (ear) (staphylococcal) (streptococcal) 380.10
axilla, axillary (region) 682.3
lymph gland or node 683
back (any part) 682.2
Bartholin's gland 616.3
with
abortion — *see* Abortion, by type, with sepsis
ectopic pregnancy (*see also* categories 633.0–633.9) 639.0
molar pregnancy (*see also* categories 630–632) 639.0
complicating pregnancy or puerperium 646.6 ☑
following
abortion 639.0
ectopic or molar pregnancy 639.0
bartholinian 616.3
Bezold's 383.01
bile, biliary, duct or tract (*see also* Cholecystitis) 576.8
bilharziasis 120.1
bladder (wall) 595.89
amebic 006.8
bone (subperiosteal) (*see also* Osteomyelitis) 730.0 ☑
accessory sinus (chronic) (*see also* Sinusitis) 473.9
acute 730.0 ☑
chronic or old 730.1 ☑
jaw (lower) (upper) 526.4
mastoid — *see* Mastoiditis, acute
petrous (*see also* Petrositis) 383.20
spinal (tuberculous) (*see also* Tuberculosis) 015.0 ☑ *[730.88]*
nontuberculous 730.08
bowel 569.5
brain (any part) 324.0
amebic (with liver or lung abscess) 006.5
cystic 324.0
late effect — *see* category 326

Abscess — *see also* Cellulitis — *continued*
brain — *continued*
otogenic 324.0
tuberculous (*see also* Tuberculosis) 013.3 ☑
breast (acute) (chronic) (nonpuerperal) 611.0
newborn 771.5
puerperal, postpartum 675.1 ☑
tuberculous (*see also* Tuberculosis) 017.9 ☑
broad ligament (chronic) (*see also* Disease, pelvis, inflammatory) 614.4
acute 614.3
Brodie's (chronic) (localized) (*see also* Osteomyelitis) 730.1 ☑
bronchus 519.19
buccal cavity 528.3
bulbourethral gland 597.0
bursa 727.89
pharyngeal 478.29
buttock 682.5
canaliculus, breast 611.0
canthus 372.20
cartilage 733.99
cecum 569.5
with appendicitis 540.1
cerebellum, cerebellar 324.0
late effect — *see* category 326
cerebral (embolic) 324.0
late effect — *see* category 326
cervical (neck region) 682.1
lymph gland or node 683
stump (*see also* Cervicitis) 616.0
cervix (stump) (uteri) (*see also* Cervicitis) 616.0
cheek, external 682.0
inner 528.3
chest 510.9
with fistula 510.0
wall 682.2
chin 682.0
choroid 363.00
ciliary body 364.3
circumtonsillar 475
cold (tuberculous) (*see also* Tuberculosis, abscess)
articular — *see* Tuberculosis, joint
colon (wall) 569.5
colostomy or enterostomy 569.61
conjunctiva 372.00
connective tissue NEC 682.9
cornea 370.55
with ulcer 370.00
corpus
cavernosum 607.2
luteum (*see also* Salpingo-oophoritis) 614.2
Cowper's gland 597.0
cranium 324.0
cul-de-sac (Douglas') (posterior) (*see also* Disease, pelvis, inflammatory) 614.4
acute 614.3
dental 522.5
with sinus (alveolar) 522.7
dentoalveolar 522.5
with sinus (alveolar) 522.7
diaphragm, diaphragmatic 567.22
digit NEC 681.9
Douglas' cul-de-sac or pouch (*see also* Disease, pelvis, inflammatory) 614.4
acute 614.3
Dubois' 090.5
ductless gland 259.8
ear
acute 382.00
external 380.10
inner 386.30
middle — *see* Otitis media
elbow 682.3
endamebic — *see* Abscess, amebic
entamebic — *see* Abscess, amebic
enterostomy 569.61
epididymis 604.0
epidural 324.9
brain 324.0

Abscess — *see also* Cellulitis — *continued*
epidural — *continued*
late effect — *see* category 326
spinal cord 324.1
epiglottis 478.79
epiploon, epiploic 567.22
erysipelatous (*see also* Erysipelas) 035
esophagostomy 530.86
esophagus 530.19
ethmoid (bone) (chronic) (sinus) (*see also* Sinusitis, ethmoidal) 473.2
external auditory canal 380.10
extradural 324.9
brain 324.0
late effect — *see* category 326
spinal cord 324.1
extraperitoneal — *see* Abscess, peritoneum
eye 360.00
eyelid 373.13
face (any part, except eye) 682.0
fallopian tube (*see also* Salpingo-oophoritis) 614.2
fascia 728.89
fauces 478.29
fecal 569.5
femoral (region) 682.6
filaria, filarial (*see also* Infestation, filarial) 125.9
finger (any) (intrathecal) (periosteal) (subcutaneous) (subcuticular) 681.00
fistulous NEC 682.9
flank 682.2
foot (except toe) 682.7
forearm 682.3
forehead 682.0
frontal (sinus) (chronic) (*see also* Sinusitis, frontal) 473.1
gallbladder (*see also* Cholecystitis, acute) 575.0
gastric 535.0 ☑
genital organ or tract NEC
female 616.9
with
abortion — *see* Abortion, by type, with sepsis
ectopic pregnancy (*see also* categories 633.0–633.9) 639.0
molar pregnancy (*see also* categories 630–632) 639.0
following
abortion 639.0
ectopic or molar pregnancy 639.0
puerperal, postpartum, childbirth 670.8 ☑
male 608.4
genitourinary system, tuberculous (*see also* Tuberculosis) 016.9 ☑
gingival 523.30
gland, glandular (lymph) (acute) NEC 683
glottis 478.79
gluteal (region) 682.5
gonorrheal NEC (*see also* Gonococcus) 098.0
groin 682.2
gum 523.30
hand (except finger or thumb) 682.4
head (except face) 682.8
heart 429.89
heel 682.7
helminthic (*see also* Infestation, by specific parasite) 128.9
hepatic 572.0
amebic (*see also* Abscess, liver, amebic) 006.3
duct 576.8
hip 682.6
tuberculous (active) (*see also* Tuberculosis) 015.1 ☑
ileocecal 540.1
ileostomy (bud) 569.61
iliac (region) 682.2
fossa 540.1
iliopsoas 567.31
nontuberculous 728.89
tuberculous (*see also* Tuberculosis) 015.0 ☑ *[730.88]*
infraclavicular (fossa) 682.3

☑ **Additional Digit Required — Refer to the Tabular List for Digit Selection**
▽ **Subterms under main terms may continue to next column or page**
2014 ICD-9-CM   **49**

Index

Abscess — Abscess

Abscess — *see also* Cellulitis — *continued*
  inguinal (region) 682.2
    lymph gland or node 683
  intersphincteric (anus) 566
  intestine, intestinal 569.5
    rectal 566
  intra-abdominal (*see also* Abscess, peritoneum) 567.22
    postoperative 998.59
  intracranial 324.0
    late effect — *see* category 326
  intramammary — *see* Abscess, breast
  intramastoid (*see also* Mastoiditis, acute) 383.00
  intraorbital 376.01
  intraperitoneal 567.22
  intraspinal 324.1
    late effect — *see* category 326
  intratonsillar 475
  iris 364.3
  ischiorectal 566
  jaw (bone) (lower) (upper) 526.4
    skin 682.0
  joint (*see also* Arthritis, pyogenic) 711.0 ✓
    vertebral (tuberculous) (*see also* Tuberculosis) 015.0 ✓ [730.88]
      nontuberculous 724.8
  kidney 590.2
    with
      abortion — *see* Abortion, by type, with urinary tract infection
      calculus 592.0
      ectopic pregnancy (*see also* categories 633.0–633.9) 639.8
      molar pregnancy (*see also* categories 630–632) 639.8
      complicating pregnancy or puerperium 646.6 ✓
        affecting fetus or newborn 760.1
      following
        abortion 639.8
        ectopic or molar pregnancy 639.8
  knee 682.6
    joint 711.06
    tuberculous (active) (*see also* Tuberculosis) 015.2 ✓
  labium (majus) (minus) 616.4
    complicating pregnancy, childbirth, or puerperium 646.6 ✓
  lacrimal (passages) (sac) (*see also* Dacryocystitis) 375.32
    caruncle 375.30
    gland (*see also* Dacryoadenitis) 375.00
  lacunar 597.0
  larynx 478.79
  lateral (alveolar) 522.5
    with sinus 522.7
  leg, except foot 682.6
  lens 360.00
  lid 373.13
  lingual 529.0
    tonsil 475
  lip 528.5
  Littre's gland 597.0
  liver 572.0
    amebic 006.3
      with
        brain abscess (and lung abscess) 006.5
        lung abscess 006.4
      due to Entamoeba histolytica 006.3
    dysenteric (*see also* Abscess, liver, amebic) 006.3
    pyogenic 572.0
    tropical (*see also* Abscess, liver, amebic) 006.3
  loin (region) 682.2
  lumbar (tuberculous) (*see also* Tuberculosis) 015.0 ✓ [730.88]
    nontuberculous 682.2
  lung (miliary) (putrid) 513.0
    amebic (with liver abscess) 006.4
      with brain abscess 006.5
  lymphangitic, acute — *see* Cellulitis
  lymph, lymphatic, gland or node (acute) 683
    any site, except mesenteric 683

Abscess — *see also* Cellulitis — *continued*
  lymph, lymphatic, gland or node — *continued*
    mesentery 289.2
  malar 526.4
  mammary gland — *see* Abscess, breast
  marginal (anus) 566
  mastoid (process) (*see also* Mastoiditis, acute) 383.00
    subperiosteal 383.01
  maxilla, maxillary 526.4
    molar (tooth) 522.5
      with sinus 522.7
    premolar 522.5
    sinus (chronic) (*see also* Sinusitis, maxillary) 473.0
  mediastinum 513.1
  meibomian gland 373.12
  meninges (*see also* Meningitis) 320.9
  mesentery, mesenteric 567.22
  mesosalpinx (*see also* Salpingo-oophoritis) 614.2
  milk 675.1 ✓
  Monro's (psoriasis) 696.1
  mons pubis 682.2
  mouth (floor) 528.3
  multiple sites NEC 682.9
  mural 682.2
  muscle 728.89
    psoas 567.31
  myocardium 422.92
  nabothian (follicle) (*see also* Cervicitis) 616.0
  nail (chronic) (with lymphangitis) 681.9
    finger 681.02
    toe 681.11
  nasal (fossa) (septum) 478.19
    sinus (chronic) (*see also* Sinusitis) 473.9
  nasopharyngeal 478.29
  nates 682.5
  navel 682.2
    newborn NEC 771.4
  neck (region) 682.1
    lymph gland or node 683
  nephritic (*see also* Abscess, kidney) 590.2
  nipple 611.0
    puerperal, postpartum 675.0 ✓
  nose (septum) 478.19
    external 682.0
  omentum 567.22
  operative wound 998.59
  orbit, orbital 376.01
  ossifluent — *see* Abscess, bone
  ovary, ovarian (corpus luteum) (*see also* Salpingo-oophoritis) 614.2
  oviduct (*see also* Salpingo-oophoritis) 614.2
  palate (soft) 528.3
    hard 526.4
  palmar (space) 682.4
  pancreas (duct) 577.0
  paradontal 523.30
  parafrenal 607.2
  parametric, parametrium (chronic) (*see also* Disease, pelvis, inflammatory) 614.4
    acute 614.3
  paranephric 590.2
  parapancreatic 577.0
  parapharyngeal 478.22
  pararectal 566
  parasinus (*see also* Sinusitis) 473.9
  parauterine (*see also* Disease, pelvis, inflammatory) 614.4
    acute 614.3
  paravaginal (*see also* Vaginitis) 616.10
  parietal region 682.8
  parodontal 523.30
  parotid (duct) (gland) 527.3
    region 528.3
  parumbilical 682.2
    newborn 771.4
  pectoral (region) 682.2
  pelvirectal 567.22
  pelvis, pelvic
    female (chronic) (*see also* Disease, pelvis, inflammatory) 614.4
      acute 614.3

Abscess — *see also* Cellulitis — *continued*
  pelvis, pelvic — *continued*
    male, peritoneal (cellular tissue) — *see* Abscess, peritoneum
    tuberculous (*see also* Tuberculosis) 016.9 ✓
  penis 607.2
    gonococcal (acute) 098.0
      chronic or duration of 2 months or over 098.2
  perianal 566
  periapical 522.5
    with sinus (alveolar) 522.7
  periappendiceal 540.1
  pericardial 420.99
  pericecal 540.1
  pericemental 523.30
  pericholecystic (*see also* Cholecystitis, acute) 575.0
  pericoronal 523.30
  peridental 523.30
  perigastric 535.0 ✓
  perimetric (*see also* Disease, pelvis, inflammatory) 614.4
    acute 614.3
  perinephric, perinephritic (*see also* Abscess, kidney) 590.2
  perineum, perineal (superficial) 682.2
    deep (with urethral involvement) 597.0
    urethra 597.0
  periodontal (parietal) 523.31
    apical 522.5
  periosteum, periosteal (*see also* Periostitis) 730.3 ✓
    with osteomyelitis (*see also* Osteomyelitis) 730.2 ✓
      acute or subacute 730.0 ✓
      chronic or old 730.1 ✓
  peripleuritic 510.9
    with fistula 510.0
  periproctic 566
  periprostatic 601.2
  perirectal (staphylococcal) 566
  perirenal (tissue) (*see also* Abscess, kidney) 590.2
  perisinuous (nose) (*see also* Sinusitis) 473.9
  peritoneum, peritoneal (perforated) (ruptured) 567.22
    with
      abortion — *see* Abortion, by type, with sepsis
      appendicitis 540.1
      ectopic pregnancy (*see also* categories 633.0–633.9) 639.0
      molar pregnancy (*see also* categories 630–632) 639.0
    following
      abortion 639.0
      ectopic or molar pregnancy 639.0
    pelvic, female (*see also* Disease, pelvis, inflammatory) 614.4
      acute 614.3
    postoperative 998.59
    puerperal, postpartum, childbirth 670.8 ✓
    tuberculous (*see also* Tuberculosis) 014.0 ✓
  peritonsillar 475
  perityphlic 540.1
  periureteral 593.89
  periurethral 597.0
    gonococcal (acute) 098.0
      chronic or duration of 2 months or over 098.2
  periuterine (*see also* Disease, pelvis, inflammatory) 614.4
    acute 614.3
  perivesical 595.89
  pernicious NEC 682.9
  petrous bone — *see* Petrositis
  phagedenic NEC 682.9
    chancroid 099.0
  pharynx, pharyngeal (lateral) 478.29
  phlegmonous NEC 682.9
  pilonidal 685.0
  pituitary (gland) 253.8

Abscess — *see also* Cellulitis — *continued*
  pleura 510.9
    with fistula 510.0
  popliteal 682.6
  postanal 566
  postcecal 540.1
  postlaryngeal 478.79
  postnasal 478.19
  postpharyngeal 478.24
  posttonsillar 475
  posttyphoid 002.0
  Pott's (*see also* Tuberculosis) 015.0 ✓ [730.88]
  pouch of Douglas (chronic) (*see also* Disease, pelvis, inflammatory) 614.4
  premammary — *see* Abscess, breast
  prepatellar 682.6
  prostate (*see also* Prostatitis) 601.2
    gonococcal (acute) 098.12
      chronic or duration of 2 months or over 098.32
  psoas 567.31
    nontuberculous 728.89
    tuberculous (*see also* Tuberculosis) 015.0 ✓ [730.88]
  pterygopalatine fossa 682.8
  pubis 682.2
  puerperal — *see* Puerperal, abscess, by site
  pulmonary — *see* Abscess, lung
  pulp, pulpal (dental) 522.0
    finger 681.01
    toe 681.10
  pyemic — *see* Septicemia
  pyloric valve 535.0 ✓
  rectovaginal septum 569.5
  rectovesical 595.89
  rectum 566
  regional NEC 682.9
  renal (*see also* Abscess, kidney) 590.2
  retina 363.00
  retrobulbar 376.01
  retrocecal 567.22
  retrolaryngeal 478.79
  retromammary — *see* Abscess, breast
  retroperineal 682.2
  retroperitoneal 567.38
    postprocedural 998.59
  retropharyngeal 478.24
    tuberculous (*see also* Tuberculosis) 012.8 ✓
  retrorectal 566
  retrouterine (*see also* Disease, pelvis, inflammatory) 614.4
    acute 614.3
  retrovesical 595.89
  root, tooth 522.5
    with sinus (alveolar) 522.7
  round ligament (*see also* Disease, pelvis, inflammatory) 614.4
    acute 614.3
  rupture (spontaneous) NEC 682.9
  sacrum (tuberculous) (*see also* Tuberculosis) 015.0 ✓ [730.88]
    nontuberculous 730.08
  salivary duct or gland 527.3
  scalp (any part) 682.8
  scapular 730.01
  sclera 379.09
  scrofulous (*see also* Tuberculosis) 017.2 ✓
  scrotum 608.4
  seminal vesicle 608.0
    amebic 006.8
  septal, dental 522.5
    with sinus (alveolar) 522.7
  septum (nasal) 478.19
  serous (*see also* Periostitis) 730.3 ✓
  shoulder 682.3
  side 682.2
  sigmoid 569.5
  sinus (accessory) (chronic) (nasal) (*see also* Sinusitis) 473.9
    intracranial venous (any) 324.0
      late effect — *see* category 326
  Skene's duct or gland 597.0
  skin NEC 682.9

✓ Additional Digit Required — Refer to the Tabular List for Digit Selection

▽ᵂ Subterms under main terms may continue to next column or page

Abscess — *see also* Cellulitis — *continued*
skin — *continued*
   tuberculous (primary) (*see also* Tuberculosis) 017.0 ☑
sloughing NEC 682.9
specified site NEC 682.8
   amebic 006.8
spermatic cord 608.4
sphenoidal (sinus) (*see also* Sinusitis, sphenoidal) 473.3
spinal
   cord (any part) (staphylococcal) 324.1
      tuberculous (*see also* Tuberculosis) 013.5 ☑
   epidural 324.1
spine (column) (tuberculous) (*see also* Tuberculosis) 015.0 ☑ *[730.88]*
   nontuberculous 730.08
spleen 289.59
   amebic 006.8
staphylococcal NEC 682.9
stitch 998.59
stomach (wall) 535.0 ☑
strumous (tuberculous) (*see also* Tuberculosis) 017.2 ☑
subarachnoid 324.9
   brain 324.0
   cerebral 324.0
   late effect — *see* category 326
   spinal cord 324.1
subareolar (*see also* Abscess, breast)
   puerperal, postpartum 675.1 ☑
subcecal 540.1
subcutaneous NEC 682.9
subdiaphragmatic 567.22
subdorsal 682.2
subdural 324.9
   brain 324.0
   late effect — *see* category 326
   spinal cord 324.1
subgaleal 682.8
subhepatic 567.22
sublingual 528.3
   gland 527.3
submammary — *see* Abscess, breast
submandibular (region) (space) (triangle) 682.0
   gland 527.3
submaxillary (region) 682.0
   gland 527.3
submental (pyogenic) 682.0
   gland 527.3
subpectoral 682.2
subperiosteal — *see* Abscess, bone
subperitoneal 567.22
subphrenic (*see also* Abscess, peritoneum) 567.22
   postoperative 998.59
subscapular 682.2
subungual 681.9
suburethral 597.0
sudoriparous 705.89
suppurative NEC 682.9
supraclavicular (fossa) 682.3
suprahepatic 567.22
suprapelvic (*see also* Disease, pelvis, inflammatory) 614.4
   acute 614.3
suprapubic 682.2
suprarenal (capsule) (gland) 255.8
sweat gland 705.89
syphilitic 095.8
teeth, tooth (root) 522.5
   with sinus (alveolar) 522.7
   supporting structures NEC 523.30
temple 682.0
temporal region 682.0
temporosphenoidal 324.0
   late effect — *see* category 326
tendon (sheath) 727.89
testicle — *see* Orchitis
thecal 728.89
thigh (acquired) 682.6
thorax 510.9
   with fistula 510.0
throat 478.29

Abscess — *see also* Cellulitis — *continued*
thumb (intrathecal) (periosteal) (subcutaneous) (subcuticular) 681.00
thymus (gland) 254.1
thyroid (gland) 245.0
toe (any) (intrathecal) (periosteal) (subcutaneous) (subcuticular) 681.10
tongue (staphylococcal) 529.0
tonsil(s) (lingual) 475
tonsillopharyngeal 475
tooth, teeth (root) 522.5
   with sinus (alveolar) 522.7
   supporting structure NEC 523.30
trachea 478.9
trunk 682.2
tubal (*see also* Salpingo-oophoritis) 614.2
tuberculous — *see* Tuberculosis, abscess
tubo-ovarian (*see also* Salpingo-oophoritis) 614.2
tunica vaginalis 608.4
umbilicus NEC 682.2
   newborn 771.4
upper arm 682.3
upper respiratory 478.9
urachus 682.2
urethra (gland) 597.0
urinary 597.0
uterus, uterine (wall) (*see also* Endometritis) 615.9
   ligament (*see also* Disease, pelvis, inflammatory) 614.4
      acute 614.3
   neck (*see also* Cervicitis) 616.0
uvula 528.3
vagina (wall) (*see also* Vaginitis) 616.10
vaginorectal (*see also* Vaginitis) 616.10
vas deferens 608.4
vermiform appendix 540.1
vertebra (column) (tuberculous) (*see also* Tuberculosis) 015.0 ☑ *[730.88]*
   nontuberculous 730.0 ☑
vesical 595.89
vesicouterine pouch (*see also* Disease, pelvis, inflammatory) 614.4
vitreous (humor) (pneumococcal) 360.04
vocal cord 478.5
von Bezold's 383.01
vulva 616.4
   complicating pregnancy, childbirth, or puerperium 646.6 ☑
vulvovaginal gland (*see also* Vaginitis) 616.3
web-space 682.4
wrist 682.4
Absence (organ or part) (complete or partial)
acoustic nerve 742.8
adrenal (gland) (congenital) 759.1
   acquired V45.79
albumin (blood) 273.8
alimentary tract (complete) (congenital) (partial) 751.8
   lower 751.5
   upper 750.8
alpha-fucosidase 271.8
alveolar process (acquired) 525.8
   congenital 750.26
anus, anal (canal) (congenital) 751.2
aorta (congenital) 747.22
aortic valve (congenital) 746.89
appendix, congenital 751.2
arm (acquired) V49.60
   above elbow V49.66
   below elbow V49.65
   congenital (*see also* Deformity, reduction, upper limb) 755.20
      lower — *see* Absence, forearm, congenital
      upper (complete) (partial) (with absence of distal elements, incomplete) 755.24
      with
         complete absence of distal elements 755.21
         forearm (incomplete) 755.23
artery (congenital) (peripheral) NEC (*see also* Anomaly, peripheral vascular system) 747.60

Absence — *continued*
artery (*see also* Anomaly, peripheral vascular system) — *continued*
   brain 747.81
   cerebral 747.81
   coronary 746.85
   pulmonary 747.31
   umbilical 747.5
atrial septum 745.69
auditory canal (congenital) (external) 744.01
auricle (ear) (with stenosis or atresia of auditory canal), congenital 744.01
bile, biliary duct (common) or passage (congenital) 751.61
bladder (acquired) V45.74
   congenital 753.8
bone (congenital) NEC 756.9
   marrow 284.9
      acquired (secondary) 284.89
      congenital 284.09
      hereditary 284.09
      idiopathic 284.9
   skull 756.0
bowel sounds 787.5
brain 740.0
   specified part 742.2
breast(s) (acquired) V45.71
   congenital 757.6
broad ligament (congenital) 752.19
bronchus (congenital) 748.3
calvarium, calvaria (skull) 756.0
canaliculus lacrimalis, congenital 743.65
carpal(s) (congenital) (complete) (partial) (with absence of distal elements, incomplete) (*see also* Deformity, reduction, upper limb) 755.28
   with complete absence of distal elements 755.21
cartilage 756.9
caudal spine 756.13
cecum (acquired) (postoperative) (posttraumatic) V45.72
   congenital 751.2
cementum 520.4
cerebellum (congenital) (vermis) 742.2
cervix (acquired) (uteri) V88.01
   with remaining uterus V88.03
   and uterus V88.01
   congenital 752.43
chin, congenital 744.89
cilia (congenital) 743.63
   acquired 374.89
circulatory system, part NEC 747.89
clavicle 755.51
clitoris (congenital) 752.49
coccyx, congenital 756.13
cold sense (*see also* Disturbance, sensation) 782.0
colon (acquired) (postoperative) V45.72
   congenital 751.2
congenital
   lumen — *see* Atresia
   organ or site NEC — *see* Agenesis
   septum — *see* Imperfect, closure
corpus callosum (congenital) 742.2
cricoid cartilage 748.3
diaphragm (congenital) (with hernia) 756.6
   with obstruction 756.6
digestive organ(s) or tract, congenital (complete) (partial) 751.8
   acquired V45.79
   lower 751.5
   upper 750.8
ductus arteriosus 747.89
duodenum (acquired) (postoperative) V45.72
   congenital 751.1
ear, congenital 744.09
   acquired V45.79
   auricle 744.01
   external 744.01
   inner 744.05
   lobe, lobule 744.21
   middle, except ossicles 744.03
      ossicles 744.04
   ossicles 744.04

Absence — *continued*
ejaculatory duct (congenital) 752.89
endocrine gland NEC (congenital) 759.2
epididymis (congenital) 752.89
   acquired V45.77
epiglottis, congenital 748.3
epileptic (atonic) (typical) (*see also* Epilepsy) 345.0 ☑
erythrocyte 284.9
erythropoiesis 284.9
   congenital 284.01
esophagus (congenital) 750.3
Eustachian tube (congenital) 744.24
extremity (acquired)
   congenital (*see also* Deformity, reduction) 755.4
   lower V49.70
   upper V49.60
extrinsic muscle, eye 743.69
eye (acquired) V45.78
   adnexa (congenital) 743.69
   congenital 743.00
   muscle (congenital) 743.69
eyelid (fold), congenital 743.62
   acquired 374.89
face
   bones NEC 756.0
   specified part NEC 744.89
fallopian tube(s) (acquired) V45.77
   congenital 752.19
femur, congenital (complete) (partial) (with absence of distal elements, incomplete) (*see also* Deformity, reduction, lower limb) 755.34
   with
      complete absence of distal elements 755.31
      tibia and fibula (incomplete) 755.33
fibrin 790.92
fibrinogen (congenital) 286.3
   acquired 286.6
fibula, congenital (complete) (partial) (with absence of distal elements, incomplete) (*see also* Deformity, reduction, lower limb) 755.37
   with
      complete absence of distal elements 755.31
      tibia 755.35
         with
            complete absence of distal elements 755.31
            femur (incomplete) 755.33
               with complete absence of distal elements 755.31
finger (acquired) V49.62
   congenital (complete) (partial) (*see also* Deformity, reduction, upper limb) 755.29
      meaning all fingers (complete) (partial) 755.21
      transverse 755.21
fissures of lungs (congenital) 748.5
foot (acquired) V49.73
   congenital (complete) 755.31
forearm (acquired) V49.65
   congenital (complete) (partial) (with absence of distal elements, incomplete) (*see also* Deformity, reduction, upper limb) 755.25
      with
         complete absence of distal elements (hand and fingers) 755.21
         humerus (incomplete) 755.23
fovea centralis 743.55
fucosidase 271.8
gallbladder (acquired) V45.79
   congenital 751.69
gamma globulin (blood) 279.00
genital organs
   acquired V45.77
   congenital
      female 752.89
         external 752.49

☑ **Additional Digit Required** — Refer to the Tabular List for Digit Selection   ▽ **Subterms under main terms may continue to next column or page**

2014 ICD-9-CM   **51**

Absence — *continued*
  genital organs — *continued*
    congenital — *continued*
      female — *continued*
        internal NEC 752.89
      male 752.89
        penis 752.69
  genitourinary organs, congenital NEC 752.89
  glottis 748.3
  gonadal, congenital NEC 758.6
  hair (congenital) 757.4
    acquired — *see* Alopecia
  hand (acquired) V49.63
    congenital (complete) (*see also* Deformity, reduction, upper limb) 755.21
  heart (congenital) 759.89
    acquired — *see* Status, organ replacement
  heat sense (*see also* Disturbance, sensation) 782.0
  humerus, congenital (complete) (partial) (with absence of distal elements, incomplete) (*see also* Deformity, reduction, upper limb) 755.24
    with
      complete absence of distal elements 755.21
      radius and ulna (incomplete) 755.23
  hymen (congenital) 752.49
  ileum (acquired) (postoperative) (posttraumatic) V45.72
    congenital 751.1
  immunoglobulin, isolated NEC 279.03
    IgA 279.01
    IgG 279.03
    IgM 279.02
  incus (acquired) 385.24
    congenital 744.04
  internal ear (congenital) 744.05
  intestine (acquired) (small) V45.72
    congenital 751.1
    large 751.2
    large V45.72
      congenital 751.2
  iris (congenital) 743.45
  jaw — *see* Absence, mandible
  jejunum (acquired) V45.72
    congenital 751.1
  joint (acquired) (following prior explantation of joint prosthesis) (with or without presence of antibiotic-impregnated cement spacer) NEC V88.29
    congenital NEC 755.8
    hip V88.21
    knee V88.22
  kidney(s) (acquired) V45.73
    congenital 753.0
  labium (congenital) (majus) (minus) 752.49
  labyrinth, membranous 744.05
  lacrimal apparatus (congenital) 743.65
  larynx (congenital) 748.3
  leg (acquired) V49.70
    above knee V49.76
    below knee V49.75
    congenital (partial) (unilateral) (*see also* Deformity, reduction, lower limb) 755.31
      lower (complete) (partial) (with absence of distal elements, incomplete) 755.35
        with
          complete absence of distal elements (foot and toes) 755.31
          thigh (incomplete) 755.33
            with complete absence of distal elements 755.31
      upper — *see* Absence, femur
  lens (congenital) 743.35
    acquired 379.31
  ligament, broad (congenital) 752.19
  limb (acquired)
    congenital (complete) (partial) (*see also* Deformity, reduction) 755.4
      lower 755.30

Absence — *continued*
  limb — *continued*
    congenital (*see also* Deformity, reduction) — *continued*
      lower — *continued*
        complete 755.31
        incomplete 755.32
        longitudinal — *see* Deficiency, lower limb, longitudinal
        transverse 755.31
      upper 755.20
        complete 755.21
        incomplete 755.22
        longitudinal — *see* Deficiency, upper limb, longitudinal
        transverse 755.21
    lower NEC V49.70
    upper NEC V49.60
  lip 750.26
  liver (congenital) (lobe) 751.69
  lumbar (congenital) (vertebra) 756.13
    isthmus 756.11
    pars articularis 756.11
  lumen — *see* Atresia
  lung (bilateral) (congenital) (fissure) (lobe) (unilateral) 748.5
    acquired (any part) V45.76
  mandible (congenital) 524.09
  maxilla (congenital) 524.09
  menstruation 626.0
  metacarpal(s), congenital (complete) (partial) (with absence of distal elements, incomplete) (*see also* Deformity, reduction, upper limb) 755.28
    with all fingers, complete 755.21
  metatarsal(s), congenital (complete) (partial) (with absence of distal elements, incomplete) (*see also* Deformity, reduction, lower limb) 755.38
    with complete absence of distal elements 755.31
  muscle (congenital) (pectoral) 756.81
    ocular 743.69
  musculoskeletal system (congenital) NEC 756.9
  nail(s) (congenital) 757.5
  neck, part 744.89
  nerve 742.8
  nervous system, part NEC 742.8
  neutrophil 288.00
  nipple (congenital) 757.6
    acquired V45.71
  nose (congenital) 748.1
    acquired 738.0
  nuclear 742.8
  ocular muscle (congenital) 743.69
  organ
    of Corti (congenital) 744.05
    or site
      acquired V45.79
      congenital NEC 759.89
  osseous meatus (ear) 744.03
  ovary (acquired) V45.77
    congenital 752.0
  oviduct (acquired) V45.77
    congenital 752.19
  pancreas (congenital) 751.7
    acquired (postoperative) (posttraumatic) V88.11
    partial V88.12
    total V88.11
  parathyroid gland (congenital) 759.2
  parotid gland(s) (congenital) 750.21
  patella, congenital 755.64
  pelvic girdle (congenital) 755.69
  penis (congenital) 752.69
    acquired V45.77
  pericardium (congenital) 746.89
  perineal body (congenital) 756.81
  phalange(s), congenital 755.4
    lower limb (complete) (intercalary) (partial) (terminal) (*see also* Deformity, reduction, lower limb) 755.39
      meaning all toes (complete) (partial) 755.31

Absence — *continued*
  phalange(s), congenital — *continued*
    lower limb (*see also* Deformity, reduction, lower limb) — *continued*
      transverse 755.31
    upper limb (complete) (intercalary) (partial) (terminal) (*see also* Deformity, reduction, upper limb) 755.29
      meaning all digits (complete) (partial) 755.21
      transverse 755.21
  pituitary gland (congenital) 759.2
  postoperative — *see* Absence, by site, acquired
  prostate (congenital) 752.89
    acquired V45.77
  pulmonary
    artery 747.31
    trunk 747.31
    valve (congenital) 746.01
    vein 747.49
  punctum lacrimale (congenital) 743.65
  radius, congenital (complete) (partial) (with absence of distal elements, incomplete) 755.26
    with
      complete absence of distal elements 755.21
      ulna 755.25
        with
          complete absence of distal elements 755.21
          humerus (incomplete) 755.23
  ray, congenital 755.4
    lower limb (complete) (partial) (*see also* Deformity, reduction, lower limb) 755.38
      meaning all rays 755.31
      transverse 755.31
    upper limb (complete) (partial) (*see also* Deformity, reduction, upper limb) 755.28
      meaning all rays 755.21
      transverse 755.21
  rectum (congenital) 751.2
    acquired V45.79
  red cell 284.9
    acquired (secondary) 284.81
    congenital 284.01
    hereditary 284.01
    idiopathic 284.9
  respiratory organ (congenital) NEC 748.9
  rib (acquired) 738.3
    congenital 756.3
  roof of orbit (congenital) 742.0
  round ligament (congenital) 752.89
  sacrum, congenital 756.13
  salivary gland(s) (congenital) 750.21
  scapula 755.59
  scrotum, congenital 752.89
  seminal tract or duct (congenital) 752.89
    acquired V45.77
  septum (congenital) (*see also* Imperfect, closure, septum)
    atrial 745.69
      and ventricular 745.7
    between aorta and pulmonary artery 745.0
    ventricular 745.3
      and atrial 745.7
  sex chromosomes 758.81
  shoulder girdle, congenital (complete) (partial) 755.59
  skin (congenital) 757.39
  skull bone 756.0
    with
      anencephalus 740.0
      encephalocele 742.0
      hydrocephalus 742.3
        with spina bifida (*see also* Spina bifida) 741.0 ☑
      microcephalus 742.1
  spermatic cord (congenital) 752.89
  spinal cord 742.59
  spine, congenital 756.13

Absence — *continued*
  spleen (congenital) 759.0
    acquired V45.79
  sternum, congenital 756.3
  stomach (acquired) (partial) (postoperative) V45.75
    with postgastric surgery syndrome 564.2
    congenital 750.7
  submaxillary gland(s) (congenital) 750.21
  superior vena cava (congenital) 747.49
  tarsal(s), congenital (complete) (partial) (with absence of distal elements, incomplete) (*see also* Deformity, reduction, lower limb) 755.38
  teeth, tooth (congenital) 520.0
    with abnormal spacing 524.30
    acquired 525.10
      with malocclusion 524.30
      due to
        caries 525.13
        extraction 525.10
        periodontal disease 525.12
        trauma 525.11
  tendon (congenital) 756.81
  testis (congenital) 752.89
    acquired V45.77
  thigh (acquired) 736.89
  thumb (acquired) V49.61
    congenital 755.29
  thymus gland (congenital) 759.2
  thyroid (gland) (surgical) 246.8
    with hypothyroidism 244.0
    cartilage, congenital 748.3
    congenital 243
  tibia, congenital (complete) (partial) (with absence of distal elements, incomplete) (*see also* Deformity, reduction, lower limb) 755.36
    with
      complete absence of distal elements 755.31
      fibula 755.35
        with
          complete absence of distal elements 755.31
          femur (incomplete) 755.33
            with complete absence of distal elements 755.31
  toe (acquired) V49.72
    congenital (complete) (partial) 755.39
      meaning all toes 755.31
      transverse 755.31
    great V49.71
  tongue (congenital) 750.11
  tooth, teeth (congenital) 520.0
    with abnormal spacing 524.30
    acquired 525.10
      with malocclusion 524.30
      due to
        caries 525.13
        extraction 525.10
        periodontal disease 525.12
        trauma 525.11
  trachea (cartilage) (congenital) (rings) 748.3
  transverse aortic arch (congenital) 747.21
  tricuspid valve 746.1
  ulna, congenital (complete) (partial) (with absence of distal elements, incomplete) (*see also* Deformity, reduction, upper limb) 755.27
    with
      complete absence of distal elements 755.21
      radius 755.25
        with
          complete absence of distal elements 755.21
          humerus (incomplete) 755.23
  umbilical artery (congenital) 747.5
  ureter (congenital) 753.4
    acquired V45.74
  urethra, congenital 753.8
    acquired V45.74
  urinary system, part NEC, congenital 753.8
    acquired V45.74

☑ **Additional Digit Required** — Refer to the Tabular List for Digit Selection   ▽ **Subterms under main terms may continue to next column or page**

52   **2014 ICD-9-CM**

Absence — continued
uterus (acquired) V88.01
with remaining cervical stump V88.02
and cervix V88.01
congenital 752.31
uvula (congenital) 750.26
vagina, congenital 752.45
acquired V45.77
vas deferens (congenital) 752.89
acquired V45.77
vein (congenital) (peripheral) NEC (see also
Anomaly, peripheral vascular system)
747.60
brain 747.81
great 747.49
portal 747.49
pulmonary 747.49
vena cava (congenital) (inferior) (superior)
747.49
ventral horn cell 742.59
ventricular septum 745.3
vermis of cerebellum 742.2
vertebra, congenital 756.13
vulva, congenital 752.49
Absentia epileptica — see also Epilepsy
345.0 ✓
Absinthemia — see also Dependence 304.6 ✓
Absinthism — see also Dependence 304.6 ✓
Absorbent system disease 459.89
Absorption
alcohol, through placenta or breast milk
760.71
antibiotics, through placenta or breast milk
760.74
anticonvulsants, through placenta or breast
milk 760.77
antifungals, through placenta or breast milk
760.74
anti-infective, through placenta or breast
milk 760.74
antimetabolics, through placenta or breast
milk 760.78
chemical NEC 989.9
specified chemical or substance — see
Table of Drugs and Chemicals
through placenta or breast milk (fetus
or newborn) 760.70
alcohol 760.71
anticonvulsants 760.77
antifungals 760.74
anti-infective agents 760.74
antimetabolics 760.78
cocaine 760.75
"crack" 760.75
diethylstilbestrol [DES] 760.76
hallucinogenic agents 760.73
medicinal agents NEC 760.79
narcotics 760.72
obstetric anesthetic or analgesic drug
763.5
specified agent NEC 760.79
suspected, affecting management of
pregnancy 655.5 ✓
cocaine, through placenta or breast milk
760.75
drug NEC (see also Reaction, drug)
through placenta or breast milk (fetus
or newborn) 760.70
alcohol 760.71
anticonvulsants 760.77
antifungals 760.74
anti-infective agents 760.74
antimetabolics 760.78
cocaine 760.75
"crack" 760.75
diethylstilbestrol [DES] 760.76
hallucinogenic agents 760.73
medicinal agents NEC 760.79
narcotics 760.72
obstetric anesthetic or analgesic drug
763.5
specified agent NEC 760.79
suspected, affecting management of
pregnancy 655.5 ✓
fat, disturbance 579.8

Absorption — continued
hallucinogenic agents, through placenta or
breast milk 760.73
immune sera, through placenta or breast
milk 760.79
lactose defect 271.3
medicinal agents NEC, through placenta or
breast milk 760.79
narcotics, through placenta or breast milk
760.72
noxious substance — see Absorption,
chemical
protein, disturbance 579.8
pus or septic, general — see Septicemia
quinine, through placenta or breast milk
760.74
toxic substance — see Absorption, chemical
uremic — see Uremia
Abstinence symptoms or syndrome
alcohol 291.81
drug 292.0
neonatal 779.5
Abt-Letterer-Siwe syndrome (acute histiocytosis X) (M9722/3) 202.5 ✓
Abulia 799.89
Abulomania 301.6
Abuse
adult 995.80
emotional 995.82
multiple forms 995.85
neglect (nutritional) 995.84
physical 995.81
psychological 995.82
sexual 995.83
alcohol — see also Alcoholism 305.0 ✓
dependent 303.9 ✓
non-dependent 305.0 ✓
child 995.50
counseling
perpetrator
non-parent V62.83
parent V61.22
victim V61.21
emotional 995.51
multiple forms 995.59
neglect (nutritional) 995.52
physical 995.54
shaken infant syndrome 995.55
psychological 995.51
sexual 995.53
drugs, nondependent 305.9 ✓

Note — Use the following fifth-digit
subclassification with the following
codes: 305.0, 305.2–305.9:

0   unspecified

1   continuous

2   episodic

3   in remission

---

amphetamine type 305.7 ✓
antidepressants 305.8 ✓
anxiolytic 305.4 ✓
barbiturates 305.4 ✓
caffeine 305.9 ✓
cannabis 305.2 ✓
cocaine type 305.6 ✓
hallucinogens 305.3 ✓
hashish 305.2 ✓
hypnotic 305.4 ✓
inhalant 305.9 ✓
LSD 305.3 ✓
marijuana 305.2 ✓
mixed 305.9 ✓
morphine type 305.5 ✓
opioid type 305.5 ✓
phencyclidine (PCP) 305.9 ✓
sedative 305.4 ✓
specified NEC 305.9 ✓
tranquilizers 305.4 ✓
spouse 995.80
tobacco 305.1
Acalcerosis 275.40
Acalcicosis 275.40
Acalculia 784.69

Acalculia — continued
developmental 315.1
Acanthocheilonemiasis 125.4
Acanthocytosis 272.5
Acanthokeratodermia 701.1
Acantholysis 701.8
bullosa 757.39
Acanthoma (benign) (M8070/0) — see also
Neoplasm, by site, benign
malignant (M8070/3) — see Neoplasm, by
site, malignant
Acanthosis (acquired) (nigricans) 701.2
adult 701.2
benign (congenital) 757.39
congenital 757.39
glycogenic
esophagus 530.89
juvenile 701.2
tongue 529.8
Acanthrocytosis 272.5
Acapnia 276.3
Acarbia 276.2
Acardia 759.89
Acardiacus amorphus 759.89
Acardiotrophia 429.1
Acardius 759.89
Acariasis 133.9
sarcoptic 133.0
Acaridiasis 133.9
Acarinosis 133.9
Acariosis 133.9
Acarodermatitis 133.9
urticarioides 133.9
Acarophobia 300.29
Acatalasemia 277.89
Acatalasia 277.89
Acatamathesia 784.69
Acataphasia 784.59
Acathisia 781.0
due to drugs 333.99
Acceleration, accelerated
atrioventricular conduction 426.7
idioventricular rhythm 427.89
Accessory (congenital)
adrenal gland 759.1
anus 751.5
appendix 751.5
atrioventricular conduction 426.7
auditory ossicles 744.04
auricle (ear) 744.1
autosome(s) NEC 758.5
21 or 22 758.0
biliary duct or passage 751.69
bladder 753.8
blood vessels (peripheral) (congenital) NEC
(see also Anomaly, peripheral vascular system) 747.60
cerebral 747.81
coronary 746.85
bone NEC 756.9
foot 755.67
breast tissue, axilla 757.6
carpal bones 755.56
cecum 751.5
cervix 752.44
chromosome(s) NEC 758.5
13-15 758.1
16-18 758.2
21 or 22 758.0
autosome(s) NEC 758.5
D₁ 758.1
E₃ 758.2
G 758.0
sex 758.81
coronary artery 746.85
cusp(s), heart valve NEC 746.89
pulmonary 746.09
cystic duct 751.69
digits 755.00
ear (auricle) (lobe) 744.1
endocrine gland NEC 759.2
external os 752.44
eyelid 743.62
eye muscle 743.69
face bone(s) 756.0
fallopian tube (fimbria) (ostium) 752.19

Accessory — continued
fingers 755.01
foreskin 605
frontonasal process 756.0
gallbladder 751.69
genital organ(s)
female 752.89
external 752.49
internal NEC 752.89
male NEC 752.89
penis 752.69
genitourinary organs NEC 752.89
heart 746.89
valve NEC 746.89
pulmonary 746.09
hepatic ducts 751.69
hymen 752.49
intestine (large) (small) 751.5
kidney 753.3
lacrimal canal 743.65
leaflet, heart valve NEC 746.89
pulmonary 746.09
ligament, broad 752.19
liver (duct) 751.69
lobule (ear) 744.1
lung (lobe) 748.69
muscle 756.82
navicular of carpus 755.56
nervous system, part NEC 742.8
nipple 757.6
nose 748.1
organ or site NEC — see Anomaly, specified
type NEC
ovary 752.0
oviduct 752.19
pancreas 751.7
parathyroid gland 759.2
parotid gland (and duct) 750.22
pituitary gland 759.2
placental lobe — see Placenta, abnormal
preauricular appendage 744.1
prepuce 605
renal arteries (multiple) 747.62
rib 756.3
cervical 756.2
roots (teeth) 520.2
salivary gland 750.22
sesamoids 755.8
skin tags 757.39
spleen 759.0
sternum 756.3
submaxillary gland 750.22
tarsal bones 755.67
teeth, tooth 520.1
causing crowding 524.31
tendon 756.89
thumb 755.01
thymus gland 759.2
thyroid gland 759.2
toes 755.02
tongue 750.13
tragus 744.1
ureter 753.4
urethra 753.8
urinary organ or tract NEC 753.8
uterus 752.2
vagina 752.49
valve, heart NEC 746.89
pulmonary 746.09
vertebra 756.19
vocal cords 748.3
vulva 752.49
Accident, accidental — see also condition
birth NEC 767.9
cardiovascular (see also Disease, cardiovascular) 429.2
cerebral (see also Disease, cerebrovascular,
acute) 434.91
cerebrovascular (current) (CVA) (see also
Disease, cerebrovascular, acute)
434.91
aborted 434.91
embolic 434.11
healed or old V12.54
hemorrhagic — see Hemorrhage, brain

Accident, accidental — *see also* condition — *continued*
cerebrovascular (*see also* Disease, cerebrovascular, acute) — *continued*
impending 435.9
ischemic 434.91
late effect — *see* Late effect(s) (of) cerebrovascular disease
postoperative 997.02
thrombotic 434.01
coronary (*see also* Infarct, myocardium) 410.9 ☑
craniovascular (*see also* Disease, cerebrovascular, acute) 436
during pregnancy, to mother, affecting fetus or newborn 760.5
heart, cardiac (*see also* Infarct, myocardium) 410.9 ☑
intrauterine 779.89
vascular — *see* Disease, cerebrovascular, acute
Accommodation
disorder of 367.51
drug-induced 367.89
toxic 367.89
insufficiency of 367.4
paralysis of 367.51
hysterical 300.11
spasm of 367.53
Accouchement — *see* Delivery
Accreta placenta (without hemorrhage) 667.0 ☑
with hemorrhage 666.0 ☑
Accretio cordis (nonrheumatic) 423.1
Accretions on teeth 523.6
Accumulation secretion, prostate 602.8
Acephalia, acephalism, acephaly 740.0
Acephalic 740.0
Acephalobrachia 759.89
Acephalocardia 759.89
Acephalocardius 759.89
Acephalochiria 759.89
Acephalochirus 759.89
Acephalogaster 759.89
Acephalostomus 759.89
Acephalothorax 759.89
Acephalus 740.0
Acetonemia 790.6
diabetic 250.1 ☑
due to secondary diabetes 249.1 ☑
Acetonglycosuria 982.8
Acetonuria 791.6
Achalasia 530.0
cardia 530.0
digestive organs congenital NEC 751.8
esophagus 530.0
pelvirectal 751.3
psychogenic 306.4
pylorus 750.5
sphincteral NEC 564.89
Achard-Thiers syndrome (adrenogenital) 255.2
Ache(s) — *see* Pain
Acheilia 750.26
Acheiria 755.21
Achillobursitis 726.71
Achillodynia 726.71
Achlorhydria, achlorhydric 536.0
anemia 280.9
diarrhea 536.0
neurogenic 536.0
postvagotomy 564.2
psychogenic 306.4
secondary to vagotomy 564.2
Achloroblepsia 368.52
Achloropsia 368.52
Acholia 575.8
Acholuric jaundice (familial) (splenomegalic) — *see also* Spherocytosis 282.0
acquired 283.9
Achondroplasia 756.4
Achrestic anemia 281.8
Achroacytosis, lacrimal gland 375.00
tuberculous (*see also* Tuberculosis) 017.3 ☑
Achroma, cutis 709.00
Achromate (congenital) 368.54

Achromatopia 368.54
Achromatopsia (congenital) 368.54
Achromia
congenital 270.2
parasitica 111.0
unguium 703.8
Achylia
gastrica 536.8
neurogenic 536.3
psychogenic 306.4
pancreatica 577.1
Achylosis 536.8
Acid
burn (*see also* Burn, by site)
from swallowing acid — *see* Burn, internal organs
deficiency
amide nicotinic 265.2
amino 270.9
ascorbic 267
folic 266.2
nicotinic (amide) 265.2
pantothenic 266.2
intoxication 276.2
peptic disease 536.8
stomach 536.8
psychogenic 306.4
Acidemia 276.2
arginosuccinic 270.6
fetal
affecting management of pregnancy 656.3 ☑
before onset of labor, in liveborn infant 768.2
during labor and delivery in liveborn infant 768.3
intrauterine 656.3 ☑
unspecified as to time of onset, in liveborn infant 768.4
newborn 775.81
pipecolic 270.7
Acidity, gastric (high) (low) 536.8
psychogenic 306.4
Acidocytopenia 288.59
Acidocytosis 288.3
Acidopenia 288.59
Acidosis 276.2
diabetic 250.1 ☑
due to secondary diabetes 249.1 ☑
fetal, affecting management of pregnancy 656.8 ☑
fetal, affecting newborn 775.81
kidney tubular 588.89
newborn 775.81
lactic 276.2
metabolic NEC 276.2
with respiratory acidosis 276.4
of newborn 775.81
late, of newborn 775.7
newborn 775.81
renal
hyperchloremic 588.89
tubular (distal) (proximal) 588.89
respiratory 276.2
complicated by
metabolic acidosis 276.4
of newborn 775.81
metabolic alkalosis 276.4
Aciduria 791.9
arginosuccinic 270.6
beta-aminoisobutyric (BAIB) 277.2
glutaric
type I 270.7
type II (type IIA, IIB, IIC) 277.85
type III 277.86
glycolic 271.8
methylmalonic 270.3
with glycinemia 270.7
organic 270.9
orotic (congenital) (hereditary) (pyrimidine deficiency) 281.4
Acladiosis 111.8
skin 111.8
Aclasis
diaphyseal 756.4
tarsoepiphyseal 756.59

Acleistocardia 745.5
Aclusion 524.4
Acmesthesia 782.0
Acne (pustular) (vulgaris) 706.1
agminata (*see also* Tuberculosis) 017.0 ☑
artificialis 706.1
atrophica 706.0
cachecticorum (Hebra) 706.1
conglobata 706.1
conjunctiva 706.1
cystic 706.1
decalvans 704.09
erythematosa 695.3
eyelid 706.1
frontalis 706.0
indurata 706.1
keloid 706.1
lupoid 706.0
necrotic, necrotica 706.0
miliaris 704.8
neonatal 706.1
nodular 706.1
occupational 706.1
papulosa 706.1
rodens 706.0
rosacea 695.3
scorbutica 267
scrofulosorum (Bazin) (*see also* Tuberculosis) 017.0 ☑
summer 692.72
tropical 706.1
varioliformis 706.0
Acneiform drug eruptions 692.3
Acnitis (primary) — *see also* Tuberculosis 017.0 ☑
Acomia 704.00
Acontractile bladder 344.61
Aconuresis — *see also* Incontinence 788.30
Acosta's disease 993.2
Acousma 780.1
Acoustic — *see* condition
Acousticophobia 300.29
Acquired — *see* condition
Acquired immune deficiency syndrome — *see* Human immunodeficiency virus (disease) (illness) (infection)
Acquired immunodeficiency syndrome — *see* Human immunodeficiency virus (disease) (illness) (infection)
Acragnosis 781.99
Acrania 740.0
Acroagnosis 781.99
Acroangiodermatitis 448.9
Acroasphyxia, chronic 443.89
Acrobrachycephaly 756.0
Acrobystiolith 608.89
Acrobystitis 607.2
Acrocephalopolysyndactyly 755.55
Acrocephalosyndactyly 755.55
Acrocephaly 756.0
Acrochondrohyperplasia 759.82
Acrocyanosis 443.89
newborn 770.83
meaning transient blue hands and feet — *omit code*
Acrodermatitis 686.8
atrophicans (chronica) 701.8
continua (Hallopeau) 696.1
enteropathica 686.8
Hallopeau's 696.1
perstans 696.1
pustulosa continua 696.1
recalcitrant pustular 696.1
Acrodynia 985.0
Acrodysplasia 755.55
Acrohyperhidrosis — *see also* Hyperhidrosis 780.8
Acrokeratosis verruciformis 757.39
Acromastitis 611.0
Acromegaly, acromegalia (skin) 253.0
Acromelalgia 443.82
Acromicria, acromikria 756.59
Acronyx 703.0
Acropachyderma 757.39
Acropachy, thyroid — *see also* Thyrotoxicosis 242.9 ☑

Acroparesthesia 443.89
simple (Schultz's type) 443.89
vasomotor (Nothnagel's type) 443.89
Acropathy thyroid — *see also* Thyrotoxicosis 242.9 ☑
Acrophobia 300.29
Acroposthitis 607.2
Acroscleriasis — *see also* Scleroderma 710.1
Acroscleroderma — *see also* Scleroderma 710.1
Acrosclerosis — *see also* Scleroderma 710.1
Acrosphacelus 785.4
Acrosphenosyndactylia 755.55
Acrospiroma, eccrine (M8402/0) — *see* Neoplasm, skin, benign
Acrostealgia 732.9
Acrosyndactyly — *see also* Syndactylism 755.10
Acrotrophodynia 991.4
Actinic — *see also* condition
cheilitis (due to sun) 692.72
chronic NEC 692.74
due to radiation, except from sun 692.82
conjunctivitis 370.24
dermatitis (due to sun) (*see also* Dermatitis, actinic) 692.70
due to
roentgen rays or radioactive substance 692.82
ultraviolet radiation, except from sun 692.82
sun NEC 692.70
elastosis solare 692.74
granuloma 692.73
keratitis 370.24
ophthalmia 370.24
reticuloid 692.73
Actinobacillosis, general 027.8
Actinobacillus
lignieresii 027.8
mallei 024
muris 026.1
Actinocutitis NEC — *see also* Dermatitis, actinic 692.70
Actinodermatitis NEC — *see also* Dermatitis, actinic 692.70
Actinomyces
israelii (infection) — *see* Actinomycosis
muris-ratti (infection) 026.1
Actinomycosis, actinomycotic 039.9
with
pneumonia 039.1
abdominal 039.2
cervicofacial 039.3
cutaneous 039.0
pulmonary 039.1
specified site NEC 039.8
thoracic 039.1
Actinoneuritis 357.89
Action, heart
disorder 427.9
postoperative 997.1
irregular 427.9
postoperative 997.1
psychogenic 306.2
Active — *see* condition
Activity decrease, functional 780.99
Acute — *see also* condition
abdomen NEC 789.0 ☑
gallbladder (*see also* Cholecystitis, acute) 575.0
Acyanoblepsia 368.53
Acyanopsia 368.53
Acystia 753.8
Acystinervia — *see* Neurogenic, bladder
Acystineuria — *see* Neurogenic, bladder
Adactylia, adactyly (congenital) 755.4
lower limb (complete) (intercalary) (partial) (terminal) (*see also* Deformity, reduction, lower limb) 755.39
meaning all digits (complete) (partial) 755.31
transverse (complete) (partial) 755.31
upper limb (complete) (intercalary) (partial) (terminal) (*see also* Deformity, reduction, upper limb) 755.29

Adactylia, adactyly — continued
upper limb (see also Deformity, reduction, upper limb) — continued
meaning all digits (complete) (partial) 755.21
transverse (complete) (partial) 755.21
Adair-Dighton syndrome (brittle bones and blue sclera, deafness) 756.51
Adamantinoblastoma (M9310/0) — see Ameloblastoma
Adamantinoma (M9310/0) — see Ameloblastoma
Adamantoblastoma (M9310/0) — see Ameloblastoma
Adams-Stokes (-Morgagni) disease or syndrome (syncope with heart block) 426.9
Adaptation reaction — see also Reaction, adjustment 309.9
Addiction — see also Dependence
absinthe 304.6 ✓
alcoholic (ethyl) (methyl) (wood) 303.9 ✓
complicating pregnancy, childbirth, or puerperium 648.4 ✓
affecting fetus or newborn 760.71
suspected damage to fetus affecting management of pregnancy 655.4 ✓
drug (see also Dependence) 304.9 ✓
ethyl alcohol 303.9 ✓
heroin 304.0 ✓
hospital 301.51
methyl alcohol 303.9 ✓
methylated spirit 303.9 ✓
morphine (-like substances) 304.0 ✓
nicotine 305.1
opium 304.0 ✓
tobacco 305.1
wine 303.9 ✓
Addison's
anemia (pernicious) 281.0
disease (bronze) (primary adrenal insufficiency) 255.41
tuberculous (see also Tuberculosis) 017.6 ✓
keloid (morphea) 701.0
melanoderma (adrenal cortical hypofunction) 255.41
Addison-Biermer anemia (pernicious) 281.0
Addison-Gull disease — see Xanthoma
Addisonian crisis or melanosis (acute adrenocortical insufficiency) 255.41
Additional — see also Accessory
chromosome(s) 758.5
13-15 758.1
16-18 758.2
21 758.0
autosome(s) NEC 758.5
sex 758.81
Adduction contracture, hip or other joint — see Contraction, joint
ADEM (acute disseminated encephalomyelitis) (postinfectious) 136.9 [323.61]
infectious 136.9 [323.61]
noninfectious 323.81
Adenasthenia gastrica 536.0
Aden fever 061
Adenitis — see also Lymphadenitis 289.3
acute, unspecified site 683
epidemic infectious 075
axillary 289.3
acute 683
chronic or subacute 289.1
Bartholin's gland 616.89
bulbourethral gland (see also Urethritis) 597.89
cervical 289.3
acute 683
chronic or subacute 289.1
chancroid (Ducrey's bacillus) 099.0
chronic (any lymph node, except mesenteric) 289.1
mesenteric 289.2
Cowper's gland (see also Urethritis) 597.89
epidemic, acute 075
gangrenous 683
gonorrheal NEC 098.89

Adenitis — see also Lymphadenitis — continued
groin 289.3
acute 683
chronic or subacute 289.1
infectious 075
inguinal (region) 289.3
acute 683
chronic or subacute 289.1
lymph gland or node, except mesenteric 289.3
acute 683
chronic or subacute 289.1
mesenteric (acute) (chronic) (nonspecific) (subacute) 289.2
mesenteric (acute) (chronic) (nonspecific) (subacute) 289.2
due to Pasteurella multocida (P. septica) 027.2
parotid gland (suppurative) 527.2
phlegmonous 683
salivary duct or gland (any) (recurring) (suppurative) 527.2
scrofulous (see also Tuberculosis) 017.2 ✓
septic 289.3
Skene's duct or gland (see also Urethritis) 597.89
strumous, tuberculous (see also Tuberculosis) 017.2 ✓
subacute, unspecified site 289.1
sublingual gland (suppurative) 527.2
submandibular gland (suppurative) 527.2
submaxillary gland (suppurative) 527.2
suppurative 683
tuberculous — see Tuberculosis, lymph gland
urethral gland (see also Urethritis) 597.89
venereal NEC 099.8
Wharton's duct (suppurative) 527.2
Adenoacanthoma (M8570/3) — see Neoplasm, by site, malignant
Adenoameloblastoma (M9300/0) 213.1
upper jaw (bone) 213.0
Adenocarcinoma (M8140/3) — see also Neoplasm, by site, malignant

Note — The list of adjectival modifiers below is not exhaustive. A description of adenocarcinoma that does not appear in this list should be coded in the same manner as carcinoma with that description. Thus, "mixed acidophil-basophil adenocarcinoma," should be coded in the same manner as "mixed acidophil-basophil carcinoma," which appears in the list under "Carcinoma."

Except where otherwise indicated, the morphological varieties of adenocarcinoma in the list below should be coded by site as for "Neoplasm, malignant."

with
apocrine metaplasia (M8573/3)
cartilaginous (and osseous) metaplasia (M8571/3)
osseous (and cartilaginous) metaplasia (M8571/3)
spindle cell metaplasia (M8572/3)
squamous metaplasia (M8570/3)
acidophil (M8280/3)
specified site — see Neoplasm, by site, malignant
unspecified site 194.3
acinar (M8550/3)
acinic cell (M8550/3)
adrenal cortical (M8370/3) 194.0
alveolar (M8251/3)
and
epidermoid carcinoma, mixed (M8560/3)
squamous cell carcinoma, mixed (M8560/3)
apocrine (M8401/3)
breast — see Neoplasm, breast, malignant
specified site NEC — see Neoplasm, skin, malignant

Adenocarcinoma — see also Neoplasm, by site, malignant — continued
apocrine — continued
unspecified site 173.99
basophil (M8300/3)
specified site — see Neoplasm, by site, malignant
unspecified site 194.3
bile duct type (M8160/3)
liver 155.1
specified site NEC — see Neoplasm, by site, malignant
unspecified site 155.1
bronchiolar (M8250/3) — see Neoplasm, lung, malignant
ceruminous (M8420/3) 173.29
chromophobe (M8270/3)
specified site — see Neoplasm, by site, malignant
unspecified site 194.3
clear cell (mesonephroid type) (M8310/3)
colloid (M8480/3)
cylindroid type (M8200/3)
diffuse type (M8145/3)
specified site — see Neoplasm, by site, malignant
unspecified site 151.9
duct (infiltrating) (M8500/3)
with Paget's disease (M8541/3) — see Neoplasm, breast, malignant
specified site — see Neoplasm, by site, malignant
unspecified site 174.9
embryonal (M9070/3)
endometrioid (M8380/3) — see Neoplasm, by site, malignant
eosinophil (M8280/3)
specified site — see Neoplasm, by site, malignant
unspecified site 194.3
follicular (M8330/3)
and papillary (M8340/3) 193
moderately differentiated type (M8332/3) 193
pure follicle type (M8331/3) 193
specified site — see Neoplasm, by site, malignant
trabecular (M8332/3) 193
unspecified type 193
well differentiated type (M8331/3) 193
gelatinous (M8480/3)
granular cell (M8320/3)
Hürthle cell (M8290/3) 193
in
adenomatous
polyp (M8210/3)
polyposis coli (M8220/3) 153.9
polypoid adenoma (M8210/3)
tubular adenoma (M8210/3)
villous adenoma (M8261/3)
infiltrating duct (M8500/3)
with Paget's disease (M8541/3) — see Neoplasm, breast, malignant
specified site — see Neoplasm, by site, malignant
unspecified site 174.9
inflammatory (M8530/3)
specified site — see Neoplasm, by site, malignant
unspecified site 174.9
in situ (M8140/2) — see Neoplasm, by site, in situ
intestinal type (M8144/3)
specified site — see Neoplasm, by site, malignant
unspecified site 151.9
intraductal (noninfiltrating) (M8500/2)
papillary (M8503/2)
specified site — see Neoplasm, by site, in situ
unspecified site 233.0
specified site — see Neoplasm, by site, in situ
unspecified site 233.0

Adenocarcinoma — see also Neoplasm, by site, malignant — continued
islet cell (M8150/3)
and exocrine, mixed (M8154/3)
specified site — see Neoplasm, by site, malignant
unspecified site 157.9
pancreas 157.4
specified site NEC — see Neoplasm, by site, malignant
unspecified site 157.4
lobular (M8520/3)
specified site — see Neoplasm, by site, malignant
unspecified site 174.9
medullary (M8510/3)
mesonephric (M9110/3)
mixed cell (M8323/3)
mucinous (M8480/3)
mucin-producing (M8481/3)
mucoid (M8480/3) (see also Neoplasm, by site, malignant)
cell (M8300/3)
specified site — see Neoplasm, by site, malignant
unspecified site 194.3
nonencapsulated sclerosing (M8350/3) 193
oncocytic (M8290/3)
oxyphilic (M8290/3)
papillary (M8260/3)
and follicular (M8340/3) 193
intraductal (noninfiltrating) (M8503/2)
specified site — see Neoplasm, by site, in situ
unspecified site 233.0
serous (M8460/3)
specified site — see Neoplasm, by site, malignant
unspecified site 183.0
papillocystic (M8450/3)
specified site — see Neoplasm, by site, malignant
unspecified site 183.0
pseudomucinous (M8470/3)
specified site — see Neoplasm, by site, malignant
unspecified site 183.0
renal cell (M8312/3) 189.0
sebaceous (M8410/3)
serous (M8441/3) (see also Neoplasm, by site, malignant)
papillary
specified site — see Neoplasm, by site, malignant
unspecified site 183.0
signet ring cell (M8490/3)
superficial spreading (M8143/3)
sweat gland (M8400/3) — see Neoplasm, skin, malignant
trabecular (M8190/3)
tubular (M8211/3)
villous (M8262/3)
water-clear cell (M8322/3) 194.1
Adenofibroma (M9013/0)
clear cell (M8313/0) — see Neoplasm, by site, benign
endometrioid (M8381/0) 220
borderline malignancy (M8381/1) 236.2
malignant (M8381/3) 183.0
mucinous (M9015/0)
specified site — see Neoplasm, by site, benign
unspecified site 220
prostate
with
other lower urinary tract symptoms (LUTS) 600.21
urinary
obstruction 600.21
retention 600.21
serous (M9014/0)
specified site — see Neoplasm, by site, benign
unspecified site 220
specified site — see Neoplasm, by site, benign

Adenofibroma — *continued*
  unspecified site 220
Adenofibrosis
  breast 610.2
  endometrioid 617.0
Adenoiditis 474.01
  acute 463
  chronic 474.01
    with chronic tonsillitis 474.02
Adenoids (congenital) (of nasal fossa) 474.9
  hypertrophy 474.12
  vegetations 474.2
Adenolipomatosis (symmetrical) 272.8
Adenolymphoma (M8561/0)
  specified site — *see* Neoplasm, by site, benign
  unspecified 210.2
Adenomatosis (M8220/0)
  endocrine (multiple) (M8360/1)
    single specified site — *see* Neoplasm, by site, uncertain behavior
    two or more specified sites 237.4
    unspecified site 237.4
  erosive of nipple (M8506/0) 217
  pluriendocrine — *see* Adenomatosis, endocrine
  pulmonary (M8250/1) 235.7
    malignant (M8250/3) — *see* Neoplasm, lung, malignant
  specified site — *see* Neoplasm, by site, benign
  unspecified site 211.3
Adenomatous
  cyst, thyroid (gland) — *see* Goiter, nodular
  goiter (nontoxic) (*see also* Goiter, nodular) 241.9
    toxic or with hyperthyroidism 242.3 ☑
Adenoma (sessile) (M8140/0) — *see also* Neoplasm, by site, benign

Note — Except where otherwise indicated, the morphological varieties of adenoma in the list below should be coded by site as for "Neoplasm, benign."

  acidophil (M8280/0)
    specified site — *see* Neoplasm, by site, benign
    unspecified site 227.3
  acinar (cell) (M8550/0)
  acinic cell (M8550/0)
  adrenal (cortex) (cortical) (functioning) (M8370/0) 227.0
    clear cell type (M8373/0) 227.0
    compact cell type (M8371/0) 227.0
    glomerulosa cell type (M8374/0) 227.0
    heavily pigmented variant (M8372/0) 227.0
    mixed cell type (M8375/0) 227.0
  alpha cell (M8152/0)
    pancreas 211.7
    specified site NEC — *see* Neoplasm, by site, benign
    unspecified site 211.7
  alveolar (M8251/0)
  apocrine (M8401/0)
    breast 217
    specified site NEC — *see* Neoplasm, skin, benign
    unspecified site 216.9
  basal cell (M8147/0)
  basophil (M8300/0)
    specified site — *see* Neoplasm, by site, benign
    unspecified site 227.3
  beta cell (M8151/0)
    pancreas 211.7
    specified site NEC — *see* Neoplasm, by site, benign
    unspecified site 211.7
  bile duct (M8160/0) 211.5
  black (M8372/0) 227.0
  bronchial (M8140/1) 235.7
    carcinoid type (M8240/3) — *see* Neoplasm, lung, malignant
    cylindroid type (M8200/3) — *see* Neoplasm, lung, malignant
  ceruminous (M8420/0) 216.2

Adenoma — *see also* Neoplasm, by site, benign — *continued*
  chief cell (M8321/0) 227.1
  chromophobe (M8270/0)
    specified site — *see* Neoplasm, by site, benign
    unspecified site 227.3
  clear cell (M8310/0)
  colloid (M8334/0)
    specified site — *see* Neoplasm, by site, benign
    unspecified site 226
  cylindroid type, bronchus (M8200/3) — *see* Neoplasm, lung, malignant
  duct (M8503/0)
  embryonal (M8191/0)
  endocrine, multiple (M8360/1)
    single specified site — *see* Neoplasm, by site, uncertain behavior
    two or more specified sites 237.4
    unspecified site 237.4
  endometrioid (M8380/0) (*see also* Neoplasm, by site, benign)
    borderline malignancy (M8380/1) — *see* Neoplasm, by site, uncertain behavior
  eosinophil (M8280/0)
    specified site — *see* Neoplasm, by site, benign
    unspecified site 227.3
  fetal (M8333/0)
    specified site — *see* Neoplasm, by site, benign
    unspecified site 226
  follicular (M8330/0)
    specified site — *see* Neoplasm, by site, benign
    unspecified site 226
  hepatocellular (M8170/0) 211.5
  Hürthle cell (M8290/0) 226
  intracystic papillary (M8504/0)
  islet cell (functioning) (M8150/0)
    pancreas 211.7
    specified site NEC — *see* Neoplasm, by site, benign
    unspecified site 211.7
  liver cell (M8170/0) 211.5
  macrofollicular (M8334/0)
    specified site NEC — *see* Neoplasm, by site, benign
    unspecified site 226
  malignant, malignum (M8140/3) — *see* Neoplasm, by site, malignant
  mesonephric (M9110/0)
  microfollicular (M8333/0)
    specified site — *see* Neoplasm, by site, benign
    unspecified site 226
  mixed cell (M8323/0)
  monomorphic (M8146/0)
  mucinous (M8480/0)
  mucoid cell (M8300/0)
    specified site — *see* Neoplasm, by site, benign
    unspecified site 227.3
  multiple endocrine (M8360/1)
    single specified site — *see* Neoplasm, by site, uncertain behavior
    two or more specified sites 237.4
    unspecified site 237.4
  nipple (M8506/0) 217
  oncocytic (M8290/0)
  oxyphilic (M8290/0)
  papillary (M8260/0) (*see also* Neoplasm, by site, benign)
    intracystic (M8504/0)
  papillotubular (M8263/0)
  Pick's tubular (M8640/0)
    specified site — *see* Neoplasm, by site, benign
    unspecified site
      female 220
      male 222.0
  pleomorphic (M8940/0)
  polypoid (M8210/0)
  prostate (benign) 600.20

Adenoma — *see also* Neoplasm, by site, benign — *continued*
  prostate — *continued*
    with
      other lower urinary tract symptoms (LUTS) 600.21
      urinary
        obstruction 600.21
        retention 600.21
  rete cell 222.0
  sebaceous, sebaceum (gland) (senile) (M8410/0) (*see also* Neoplasm, skin, benign)
    disseminata 759.5
  Sertoli cell (M8640/0)
    specified site — *see* Neoplasm, by site, benign
    unspecified site
      female 220
      male 222.0
  skin appendage (M8390/0) — *see* Neoplasm, skin, benign
  sudoriferous gland (M8400/0) — *see* Neoplasm, skin, benign
  sweat gland or duct (M8400/0) — *see* Neoplasm, skin, benign
  testicular (M8640/0)
    specified site — *see* Neoplasm, by site, benign
    unspecified site
      female 220
      male 222.0
  thyroid 226
  trabecular (M8190/0)
  tubular (M8211/0) (*see also* Neoplasm, by site, benign)
    papillary (M8460/3)
    Pick's (M8640/0)
      specified site — *see* Neoplasm, by site, benign
      unspecified site
        female 220
        male 222.0
  tubulovillous (M8263/0)
  villoglandular (M8263/0)
  villous (M8261/1) — *see* Neoplasm, by site, uncertain behavior
  water-clear cell (M8322/0) 227.1
  wolffian duct (M9110/0)
Adenomyoma (M8932/0) — *see also* Neoplasm, by site, benign
  prostate 600.20
    with
      other lower urinary tract symptoms (LUTS) 600.21
      urinary
        obstruction 600.21
        retention 600.21
Adenomyometritis 617.0
Adenomyosis (uterus) (internal) 617.0
Adenopathy (lymph gland) 785.6
  inguinal 785.6
  mediastinal 785.6
  mesentery 785.6
  syphilitic (secondary) 091.4
  tracheobronchial 785.6
    tuberculous (*see also* Tuberculosis) 012.1 ☑
      primary, progressive 010.8 ☑
  tuberculous (*see also* Tuberculosis, lymph gland) 017.2 ☑
    tracheobronchial 012.1 ☑
      primary, progressive 010.8 ☑
Adenopharyngitis 462
Adenophlegmon 683
Adenosalpingitis 614.1
Adenosarcoma (M8960/3) 189.0
Adenosclerosis 289.3
Adenosis
  breast (sclerosing) 610.2
  vagina, congenital 752.49
Adentia (complete) (partial) — *see also* Absence, teeth 520.0
Adherent
  labium (minus) 624.4
  pericardium (nonrheumatic) 423.1

Adherent — *continued*
  pericardium — *continued*
    rheumatic 393
  placenta 667.0 ☑
    with hemorrhage 666.0 ☑
  prepuce 605
  scar (skin) NEC 709.2
  tendon in scar 709.2
Adhesion(s), adhesive (postinfectional) (postoperative)
  abdominal (wall) (*see also* Adhesions, peritoneum) 568.0
  amnion to fetus 658.8 ☑
    affecting fetus or newborn 762.8
  appendix 543.9
  arachnoiditis — *see* Meningitis
  auditory tube (Eustachian) 381.89
  bands (*see also* Adhesions, peritoneum)
    cervix 622.3
    uterus 621.5
  bile duct (any) 576.8
  bladder (sphincter) 596.89
  bowel (*see also* Adhesions, peritoneum) 568.0
  cardiac 423.1
    rheumatic 398.99
  cecum (*see also* Adhesions, peritoneum) 568.0
  cervicovaginal 622.3
    congenital 752.49
    postpartal 674.8 ☑
      old 622.3
  cervix 622.3
  clitoris 624.4
  colon (*see also* Adhesions, peritoneum) 568.0
  common duct 576.8
  congenital (*see also* Anomaly, specified type NEC)
    fingers (*see also* Syndactylism, fingers) 755.11
    labium (majus) (minus) 752.49
    omental, anomalous 751.4
    ovary 752.0
    peritoneal 751.4
    toes (*see also* Syndactylism, toes) 755.13
    tongue (to gum or roof of mouth) 750.12
  conjunctiva (acquired) (localized) 372.62
    congenital 743.63
    extensive 372.63
  cornea — *see* Opacity, cornea
  cystic duct 575.8
  diaphragm (*see also* Adhesions, peritoneum) 568.0
  due to foreign body — *see* Foreign body
  duodenum (*see also* Adhesions, peritoneum) 568.0
    with obstruction 537.3
  ear, middle — *see* Adhesions, middle ear
  epididymis 608.89
  epidural — *see* Adhesions, meninges
  epiglottis 478.79
  Eustachian tube 381.89
  eyelid 374.46
    postoperative 997.99
      surgically created V45.69
  gallbladder (*see also* Disease, gallbladder) 575.8
  globe 360.89
  heart 423.1
    rheumatic 398.99
  ileocecal (coil) (*see also* Adhesions, peritoneum) 568.0
  ileum (*see also* Adhesions, peritoneum) 568.0
  intestine (postoperative) (*see also* Adhesions, peritoneum) 568.0
    with obstruction 560.81
      with hernia (*see also* Hernia, by site, with obstruction)
        gangrenous — *see* Hernia, by site, with gangrene
  intra-abdominal (*see also* Adhesions, peritoneum) 568.0
  iris 364.70
    to corneal graft 996.79

☑ **Additional Digit Required** — Refer to the Tabular List for Digit Selection   ⏎ **Subterms under main terms may continue to next column or page**

56   **2014 ICD-9-CM**

Adhesion(s), adhesive — *continued*
joint (*see also* Ankylosis) 718.5 ☑
kidney 593.89
labium (majus) (minus), congenital 752.49
liver 572.8
lung 511.0
mediastinum 519.3
meninges 349.2
  cerebral (any) 349.2
    congenital 742.4
  congenital 742.8
  spinal (any) 349.2
    congenital 742.59
  tuberculous (cerebral) (spinal) (*see also*
    Tuberculosis, meninges) 013.0 ☑
mesenteric (*see also* Adhesions, peritoneum)
  568.0
middle ear (fibrous) 385.10
  drum head 385.19
    to
      incus 385.11
      promontorium 385.13
      stapes 385.12
  specified NEC 385.19
nasal (septum) (to turbinates) 478.19
nerve NEC 355.9
  spinal 355.9
    root 724.9
      cervical NEC 723.4
      lumbar NEC 724.4
      lumbosacral 724.4
      thoracic 724.4
ocular muscle 378.60
omentum (*see also* Adhesions, peritoneum)
  568.0
organ or site, congenital NEC — *see*
  Anomaly, specified type NEC
ovary 614.6
  congenital (to cecum, kidney, or omen-
    tum) 752.0
parauterine 614.6
parovarian 614.6
pelvic (peritoneal)
  female (postoperative) (postinfection)
    614.6
  male (postoperative) (postinfection) (*see
    also* Adhesions, peritoneum)
    568.0
  postpartal (old) 614.6
  tuberculous (*see also* Tuberculosis)
    016.9 ☑
penis to scrotum (congenital) 752.69
periappendiceal (*see also* Adhesions, peritoneum) 568.0
pericardium (nonrheumatic) 423.1
  rheumatic 393
  tuberculous (*see also* Tuberculosis)
    017.9 ☑ [420.0]
pericholecystic 575.8
perigastric (*see also* Adhesions, peritoneum)
  568.0
periovarian 614.6
periprostatic 602.8
perirectal (*see also* Adhesions, peritoneum)
  568.0
perirenal 593.89
peritoneum, peritoneal (fibrous) (postoperative) 568.0
  with obstruction (intestinal) 560.81
    with hernia (*see also* Hernia, by site,
      with obstruction)
      gangrenous — *see* Hernia, by site,
        with gangrene
    duodenum 537.3
  congenital 751.4
  female (postoperative) (postinfective)
    614.6
  pelvic, female 614.6
  pelvic, male 568.0
  postpartal, pelvic 614.6
  to uterus 614.6
peritubal 614.6
periureteral 593.89
periuterine 621.5
perivesical 596.89
perivesicular (seminal vesicle) 608.89

Adhesion(s), adhesive — *continued*
pleura, pleuritic 511.0
  tuberculous (*see also* Tuberculosis,
    pleura) 012.0 ☑
pleuropericardial 511.0
postoperative (gastrointestinal tract) (*see
  also* Adhesions, peritoneum) 568.0
  eyelid 997.99
    surgically created V45.69
  pelvic female 614.9
  pelvic male 568.0
  urethra 598.2
postpartal, old 624.4
preputial, prepuce 605
pulmonary 511.0
pylorus (*see also* Adhesions, peritoneum)
  568.0
Rosenmüller's fossa 478.29
sciatic nerve 355.0
seminal vesicle 608.89
shoulder (joint) 726.0
sigmoid flexure (*see also* Adhesions, peritoneum) 568.0
spermatic cord (acquired) 608.89
  congenital 752.89
spinal canal 349.2
  nerve 355.9
    root 724.9
      cervical NEC 723.4
      lumbar NEC 724.4
      lumbosacral 724.4
      thoracic 724.4
stomach (*see also* Adhesions, peritoneum)
  568.0
subscapular 726.2
tendonitis 726.90
  shoulder 726.0
testicle 608.89
tongue (congenital) (to gum or roof of
  mouth) 750.12
  acquired 529.8
trachea 519.19
tubo-ovarian 614.6
tunica vaginalis 608.89
ureter 593.89
uterus 621.5
  to abdominal wall 614.6
    in pregnancy or childbirth 654.4 ☑
      affecting fetus or newborn 763.89
vagina (chronic) (postoperative) (postradiation) 623.2
vaginitis (congenital) 752.49
vesical 596.89
vitreomacular adhesion 379.27
vitreous 379.29
Adie (-Holmes) syndrome (tonic pupillary reaction) 379.46
Adiponecrosis neonatorum 778.1
Adiposa dolorosa 272.8
Adiposalgia 272.8
Adiposis
  cerebralis 253.8
  dolorosa 272.8
  tuberosa simplex 272.8
Adiposity 278.02
  heart (*see also* Degeneration, myocardial)
    429.1
  localized 278.1
Adiposogenital dystrophy 253.8
Adjustment
  prosthesis or other device — *see* Fitting of
  reaction — *see* Reaction, adjustment
Administration, prophylactic
  antibiotics, long-term V58.62
    short-term use — *omit code*
  antitoxin, any V07.2
  antivenin V07.2
  chemotherapeutic agent NEC V07.39
  chemotherapy NEC V07.39
  diphtheria antitoxin V07.2
  fluoride V07.31
  gamma globulin V07.2
  immune sera (gamma globulin) V07.2
  passive immunization agent V07.2
  RhoGAM V07.2

Admission (encounter)
as organ donor — *see* Donor
by mistake V68.9
for
  adequacy testing (for)
    hemodialysis V56.31
    peritoneal dialysis V56.32
  adjustment (of)
    artificial
      arm (complete) (partial) V52.0
      eye V52.2
      leg (complete) (partial) V52.1
    brain neuropacemaker V53.02
    breast
      implant V52.4
        exchange (different material)
          (different size) V52.4
      prosthesis V52.4
    cardiac device V53.39
      defibrillator, automatic im-
        plantable (with syn-
        chronous cardiac pacemak-
        er) V53.32
      pacemaker V53.31
        carotid sinus V53.39
    catheter
      non-vascular V58.82
      vascular V58.81
    cerebral ventricle (communicating)
      shunt V53.01
    colostomy belt V55.3
    contact lenses V53.1
    cystostomy device V53.6
    dental prosthesis V52.3
    device, unspecified type V53.90
      abdominal V53.59
      cardiac V53.39
        defibrillator, automatic im-
          plantable (with syn-
          chronous cardiac pace-
          maker V53.32
        pacemaker V53.31
      carotid sinus V53.39
      cerebral ventricle (communicat-
        ing) shunt V53.01
      gastrointestinal NEC V53.59
      insulin pump V53.91
      intestinal V53.50
      nervous system V53.09
      orthodontic V53.4
      other device V53.99
      prosthetic V52.9
        breast V52.4
        dental V52.3
        eye V52.2
        specified type NEC V52.8
      special senses V53.09
      substitution
        auditory V53.09
        nervous system V53.09
        visual V53.09
      urinary V53.6
    dialysis catheter
      extracorporeal V56.1
      peritoneal V56.2
    diaphragm (contraceptive) V25.02
    gastric lap band V53.51
    gastrointestinal appliance and device
      NEC V53.59
    growth rod V54.02
    hearing aid V53.2
    ileostomy device V55.2
    intestinal appliance and device
      V53.50
    neuropacemaker (brain) (peripheral
      nerve) (spinal cord) V53.02
    orthodontic device V53.4
    orthopedic (device) V53.7
      brace V53.7
      cast V53.7
      shoes V53.7
    pacemaker
      brain V53.02
      cardiac V53.31
      carotid sinus V53.39
      peripheral nerve V53.02

Admission — *continued*
for — *continued*
  adjustment — *continued*
    pacemaker — *continued*
      spinal cord V53.02
    prosthesis V52.9
      arm (complete) (partial) V52.0
      breast V52.4
      dental V52.3
      eye V52.2
      leg (complete) (partial) V52.1
      specified type NEC V52.8
    spectacles V53.1
    wheelchair V53.8
  adoption referral or proceedings V68.89
  aftercare (*see also* Aftercare) V58.9
    cardiac pacemaker V53.31
    chemotherapy (oral) (intravenous)
      V58.11
    dialysis
      extracorporeal (renal) V56.0
      peritoneal V56.8
      renal V56.0
    fracture (*see also* Aftercare, fracture)
      V54.9
    medical NEC V58.89
    organ transplant V58.44
    orthopedic V54.9
      following explanation of joint
        prosthesis (for joint pros-
        thesis insertion) (staged
        procedure) V54.82
      specified care NEC V54.89
    pacemaker device
      brain V53.02
      cardiac V53.31
      carotid sinus V53.39
      nervous system V53.02
      spinal cord V53.02
    postoperative NEC V58.49
      wound closure, planned V58.41
    postpartum
      immediately after delivery V24.0
      routine follow-up V24.2
    postradiation V58.0
    radiation therapy V58.0
    removal of
      non-vascular catheter V58.82
      vascular catheter V58.81
    specified NEC V58.89
    surgical NEC V58.49
      wound closure, planned V58.41
  antineoplastic
    chemotherapy (oral) (intravenous)
      V58.11
    immunotherapy V58.12
  artificial insemination V26.1
  assisted reproductive fertility procedure
    cycle V26.81
  attention to artificial opening (of) V55.9
    artificial vagina V55.7
    colostomy V55.3
    cystostomy V55.5
    enterostomy V55.4
    gastrostomy V55.1
    ileostomy V55.2
    jejunostomy V55.4
    nephrostomy V55.6
    specified site NEC V55.8
      intestinal tract V55.4
      urinary tract V55.6
    tracheostomy V55.0
    ureterostomy V55.6
    urethrostomy V55.6
  battery replacement
    cardiac pacemaker V53.31
  blood typing V72.86
    Rh typing V72.86
  boarding V65.0
  breast
    augmentation or reduction V50.1
    implant exchange (different material)
      (different size) V52.4
    reconstruction following mastectomy
      V51.0

Admission — continued
  for — continued
    breast — continued
      removal
        prophylactic V50.41
        tissue expander without synchronous insertion of permanent implant V52.4
    change of
      cardiac pacemaker (battery) V53.31
      carotid sinus pacemaker V53.39
      catheter in artificial opening — see Attention to, artificial, opening
      drains V58.49
      dressing
        wound V58.30
          nonsurgical V58.30
          surgical V58.31
      fixation device
        external V54.89
        internal V54.01
      Kirschner wire V54.89
      neuropacemaker device (brain) (peripheral nerve) (spinal cord) V53.02
      nonsurgical wound dressing V58.30
      pacemaker device
        brain V53.02
        cardiac V53.31
        carotid sinus V53.39
        nervous system V53.02
      plaster cast V54.89
      splint, external V54.89
      Steinmann pin V54.89
      surgical wound dressing V58.31
      traction device V54.89
      wound packing V58.30
        nonsurgical V58.30
        surgical V58.31
  checkup only V70.0
  chemotherapy, (oral) (intravenous) antineoplastic V58.11
  circumcision, ritual or routine (in absence of medical indication) V50.2
  clinical research investigation (control) (normal comparison) (participant) V70.7
  closure of artificial opening — see Attention to, artificial, opening
  contraceptive
    counseling V25.09
      emergency V25.03
      postcoital V25.03
    management V25.9
      specified type NEC V25.8
  convalescence following V66.9
    chemotherapy V66.2
    psychotherapy V66.3
    radiotherapy V66.1
    surgery V66.0
    treatment (for) V66.5
      combined V66.6
      fracture V66.4
      mental disorder NEC V66.3
      specified condition NEC V66.5
  cosmetic surgery NEC V50.1
    breast reconstruction following mastectomy V51.0
    following healed injury or operation V51.8
  counseling (see also Counseling) V65.40
    without complaint or sickness V65.49
    contraceptive management V25.09
      emergency V25.03
      postcoital V25.03
    dietary V65.3
    exercise V65.41
    fertility preservation (prior to cancer therapy) (prior to surgical removal of gonads) V26.42
    for
      nonattending third party V65.19

Admission — continued
  for — continued
    counseling (see also Counseling) — continued
      for — continued
        pediatric
          pre-adoption visit for adoptive parent(s) V65.11
          pre-birth visit for expectant parent(s) V65.11
        victim of abuse
          child V61.21
          partner or spouse V61.11
      genetic V26.33
      gonorrhea V65.45
      HIV V65.44
      human immunodeficiency virus V65.44
      injury prevention V65.43
      insulin pump training V65.46
      natural family planning
        procreative V26.41
        to avoid pregnancy V25.04
      procreative management V26.49
        using natural family planning V26.41
      sexually transmitted disease NEC V65.45
        HIV V65.44
      specified reason NEC V65.49
      substance use and abuse V65.42
      syphilis V65.45
      victim of abuse
        child V61.21
        partner or spouse V61.11
    desensitization to allergens V07.1
    dialysis V56.0
      catheter
        fitting and adjustment
          extracorporeal V56.1
          peritoneal V56.2
        removal or replacement
          extracorporeal V56.1
          peritoneal V56.2
      extracorporeal (renal) V56.0
      peritoneal V56.8
      renal V56.0
    dietary surveillance and counseling V65.3
    drug monitoring, therapeutic V58.83
    ear piercing V50.3
    elective surgery V50.9
      breast
        augmentation or reduction V50.1
        reconstruction following mastectomy V51.0
        removal, prophylactic V50.41
      circumcision, ritual or routine (in absence of medical indication) V50.2
      cosmetic NEC V50.1
        breast reconstruction following mastectomy V51.0
        following healed injury or operation V51.8
      ear piercing V50.3
      face-lift V50.1
      hair transplant V50.0
      plastic
        breast reconstruction following mastectomy V51.0
        cosmetic NEC V50.1
        following healed injury or operation V51.8
      prophylactic organ removal V50.49
        breast V50.41
        ovary V50.42
      repair of scarred tissue (following healed injury or operation) V51.8
      specified type NEC V50.8
    end-of-life care V66.7
    examination (see also Examination) V70.9
      administrative purpose NEC V70.3
      adoption V70.3

Admission — continued
  for — continued
    examination (see also Examination) — continued
      allergy V72.7
      antibody response V72.61
      at health care facility V70.0
      athletic team V70.3
      camp V70.3
      cardiovascular, preoperative V72.81
      clinical research investigation (control) (participant) V70.7
      dental V72.2
      developmental testing (child) (infant) V20.2
      donor (potential) V70.8
      driver's license V70.3
      ear V72.19
      employment V70.5
      eye V72.0
      fertility preservation (prior to cancer therapy) (prior to surgical removal of gonads) V26.82
      follow-up (routine) — see Examination, follow-up
      for admission to
        old age home V70.3
        school V70.3
      general V70.9
        specified reason NEC V70.8
      gynecological V72.31
      health supervision
        child (over 28 days old) V20.2
        infant (over 28 days old) V20.2
        newborn
          8 to 28 days old V20.32
          under 8 days old V20.31
      hearing V72.19
        following failed hearing screening V72.11
      immigration V70.3
      infant
        8 to 28 days old V20.32
        over 28 days old, routine V20.2
        under 8 days old V20.31
      insurance certification V70.3
      laboratory V72.60
        ordered as part of a routine general medical examination V72.62
        pre-operative V72.63
        pre-procedural V72.63
        specified NEC V72.69
      marriage license V70.3
      medical (general) (see also Examination, medical) V70.9
      medicolegal reasons V70.4
      naturalization V70.3
      pelvic (annual) (periodic) V72.31
      postpartum checkup V24.2
      pregnancy (possible) (unconfirmed) V72.40
        negative result V72.41
        positive result V72.42
      preoperative V72.84
        cardiovascular V72.81
        respiratory V72.82
        specified NEC V72.83
      preprocedural V72.84
        cardiovascular V72.81
        general physical V72.83
        respiratory V72.82
        specified NEC V72.83
      prior to chemotherapy V72.83
      prison V70.3
      psychiatric (general) V70.2
        requested by authority V70.1
      radiological NEC V72.5
      respiratory, preoperative V72.82
      school V70.3
      screening — see Screening
      skin hypersensitivity V72.7
      specified type NEC V72.85
      sport competition V70.3
      vision V72.0
      well baby and child care V20.2

Admission — continued
  for — continued
    exercise therapy V57.1
    face-lift, cosmetic reason V50.1
    fertility preservation (prior to cancer therapy) (prior to surgical removal of gonads) V26.82
    fitting (of)
      artificial
        arm (complete) (partial) V52.0
        eye V52.2
        leg (complete) (partial) V52.1
      biliary drainage tube V58.82
      brain neuropacemaker V53.02
      breast V52.4
        implant V52.4
        prosthesis V52.4
      cardiac pacemaker V53.31
      catheter
        non-vascular V58.82
        vascular V58.81
      cerebral ventricle (communicating) shunt V53.01
      chest tube V58.82
      colostomy belt V55.2
      contact lenses V53.1
      cystostomy device V53.6
      dental prosthesis V52.3
      device, unspecified type V53.90
        abdominal V53.59
        cerebral ventricle (communicating) shunt V53.01
        gastrointestinal NEC V53.59
        insulin pump V53.91
        intestinal V53.50
        intrauterine contraceptive
          insertion V25.11
          removal V25.12
            and reinsertion V25.13
          replacement V25.13
        nervous system V53.09
        orthodontic V53.4
        other device V53.99
        prosthetic V52.9
          breast V52.4
          dental V52.3
          eye V52.2
        special senses V53.09
        substitution
          auditory V53.09
          nervous system V53.09
          visual V53.09
      diaphragm (contraceptive) V25.02
      fistula (sinus tract) drainage tube V58.82
      gastric lap band V53.51
      gastrointestinal appliance and device NEC V53.59
      growth rod V54.02
      hearing aid V53.2
      ileostomy device V55.2
      intestinal appliance and device V53.50
      intrauterine contraceptive device
        insertion V25.11
        removal V25.12
          and reinsertion V25.13
        replacement V25.13
      neuropacemaker (brain) (peripheral nerve) (spinal cord) V53.02
      orthodontic device V53.4
      orthopedic (device) V53.7
        brace V53.7
        cast V53.7
        shoes V53.7
      pacemaker
        brain V53.02
        cardiac V53.31
        carotid sinus V53.39
        spinal cord V53.02
      pleural drainage tube V58.82
      portacath V58.81
      prosthesis V52.9
        arm (complete) (partial) V52.0
        breast V52.4
        dental V52.3

☑ Additional Digit Required — Refer to the Tabular List for Digit Selection   ▽ Subterms under main terms may continue to next column or page

58   2014 ICD-9-CM

Admission — continued
for — continued
  fitting — continued
    prosthesis — continued
      eye V52.2
      leg (complete) (partial) V52.1
      specified type NEC V52.8
    spectacles V53.1
    wheelchair V53.8
  follow-up examination (routine) (following) V67.9
    cancer chemotherapy V67.2
    chemotherapy V67.2
    high-risk medication NEC V67.51
    injury NEC V67.59
    psychiatric V67.3
    psychotherapy V67.3
    radiotherapy V67.1
    specified surgery NEC V67.09
    surgery V67.00
      vaginal pap smear V67.01
    treatment (for) V67.9
      combined V67.6
      fracture V67.4
      involving high-risk medication NEC V67.51
      mental disorder V67.3
      specified NEC V67.59
  hair transplant, for cosmetic reason V50.0
  health advice, education, or instruction V65.4 ☑
  hearing conservation and treatment V72.12
  hormone replacement therapy (postmenopausal) V07.4
  hospice care V66.7
  immunizations (childhood) appropriate for age V20.2
  immunotherapy, antineoplastic V58.12
  insertion (of)
    intrauterine contraceptive device V25.11
    subdermal implantable contraceptive V25.5
  insulin pump titration V53.91
  insulin pump training V65.46
  intrauterine device
    insertion V25.11
    management V25.42
    removal V25.12
      and reinsertion V25.13
    replacement V25.13
  investigation to determine further disposition V63.8
  in vitro fertilization cycle V26.81
  isolation V07.0
  issue of
    disability examination certificate V68.01
    medical certificate NEC V68.09
    repeat prescription NEC V68.1
      contraceptive device NEC V25.49
  kidney dialysis V56.0
  lengthening of growth rod V54.02
  mental health evaluation V70.2
    requested by authority V70.1
  natural family planning counseling and advice
    procreative V26.41
    to avoid pregnancy V25.04
  nonmedical reason NEC V68.89
  nursing care evaluation V63.8
  observation (without need for further medical care) (see also Observation) V71.9
    accident V71.4
    alleged rape or seduction V71.5
    criminal assault V71.6
    following accident V71.4
      at work V71.3
    foreign body ingestion V71.89
    growth and development variations, childhood V21.0
    inflicted injury NEC V71.6

Admission — continued
for — continued
  observation (see also Observation) — continued
    ingestion of deleterious agent or foreign body V71.89
    injury V71.6
    malignant neoplasm V71.1
    mental disorder V71.09
    newborn — see Observation, suspected, condition, newborn
    rape V71.5
    specified NEC V71.89
    suspected
      abuse V71.81
      accident V71.4
        at work V71.3
      benign neoplasm V71.89
      cardiovascular V71.7
      disorder V71.9
      exposure
        anthrax V71.82
        biological agent NEC V71.83
        SARS V71.83
      heart V71.7
      inflicted injury NEC V71.6
      malignant neoplasm V71.1
      maternal and fetal problem not found
        amniotic cavity and membrane V89.01
        cervical shortening V89.05
        fetal anomaly V89.03
        fetal growth V89.04
        oligohydramnios V89.01
        other specified NEC V89.09
        placenta V89.02
        polyhydramnios V89.01
      mental NEC V71.09
      neglect V71.81
      specified condition NEC V71.89
      tuberculosis V71.2
    tuberculosis V71.2
  occupational therapy V57.21
  organ transplant, donor — see Donor
  ovary, ovarian removal, prophylactic V50.42
  palliative care V66.7
  Papanicolaou smear
    cervix V76.2
      for suspected malignant neoplasm V76.2
      no disease found V71.1
      routine, as part of gynecological examination V72.31
      to confirm findings of recent normal smear following initial abnormal smear V72.32
    vaginal V76.47
      following hysterectomy for malignant condition V67.01
  passage of sounds or bougie in artificial opening — see Attention to, artificial, opening
  paternity testing V70.4
  peritoneal dialysis V56.32
  physical therapy NEC V57.1
  plastic surgery
    breast reconstruction following mastectomy V51.0
    cosmetic NEC V50.1
    following healed injury or operation V51.8
  postmenopausal hormone replacement therapy V07.4
  postpartum observation
    immediately after delivery V24.0
    routine follow-up V24.2
  poststerilization (for restoration) V26.0
  procreative management V26.9
    assisted reproductive fertility procedure cycle V26.81
    in vitro fertilization cycle V26.81
    specified type NEC V26.89

Admission — continued
for — continued
  prophylactic
    administration of
      antibiotics, long-term V58.62
        short-term use — omit code
      antitoxin, any V07.2
      antivenin V07.2
      chemotherapeutic agent NEC V07.39
      chemotherapy NEC V07.39
      diphtheria antitoxin V07.2
      fluoride V07.31
      gamma globulin V07.2
      immune sera (gamma globulin) V07.2
      RhoGAM V07.2
      tetanus antitoxin V07.2
    breathing exercises V57.0
    chemotherapy NEC V07.39
      fluoride V07.31
    measure V07.9
      specified type NEC V07.8
    organ removal V50.49
      breast V50.41
      ovary V50.42
  psychiatric examination (general) V70.2
    requested by authority V70.1
  radiation management V58.0
  radiotherapy V58.0
  reconstruction following mastectomy V51.0
  reforming of artificial opening — see Attention to, artificial, opening
  rehabilitation V57.9
    multiple types V57.89
    occupational V57.21
    orthoptic V57.4
    orthotic V57.81
    physical NEC V57.1
    specified type NEC V57.89
    speech (-language) V57.3
    vocational V57.22
  removal of
    breast tissue expander without synchronous insertion of permanent implant V52.4
    cardiac pacemaker V53.31
    cast (plaster) V54.89
    catheter from artificial opening — see Attention to, artificial, opening
    cerebral ventricle (communicating) shunt V53.01
    cystostomy catheter V55.5
    device
      cerebral ventricle (communicating) shunt V53.01
      fixation
        external V54.89
        internal V54.01
        intrauterine contraceptive V25.12
        traction, external V54.89
    drains V58.49
    dressing
      wound V58.30
        nonsurgical V58.30
        surgical V58.31
    fixation device
      external V54.89
      internal V54.01
    intrauterine contraceptive device V25.12
    Kirschner wire V54.89
    neuropacemaker (brain) (peripheral nerve) (spinal cord) V53.02
    nonsurgical wound dressing V58.30
    orthopedic fixation device
      external V54.89
      internal V54.01
    pacemaker device
      brain V53.02
      cardiac V53.31
      carotid sinus V53.39
      nervous system V53.02
    plaster cast V54.89

Admission — continued
for — continued
  removal of — continued
    plate (fracture) V54.01
    rod V54.01
    screw (fracture) V54.01
    splint, traction V54.89
    staples V58.32
    Steinmann pin V54.89
    subdermal implantable contraceptive V25.43
    surgical wound dressing V58.31
    sutures V58.32
    traction device, external V54.89
    ureteral stent V53.6
    wound packing V58.30
      nonsurgical V58.30
      surgical V58.31
  repair of scarred tissue (following healed injury or operation) V51.8
  replacement of intrauterine contraceptive device V25.13
  reprogramming of cardiac pacemaker V53.31
  respirator [ventilator] dependence during
    mechanical failure V46.14
    power failure V46.12
    for weaning V46.13
  restoration of organ continuity (poststerilization) (tuboplasty) (vasoplasty) V26.0
  Rh typing V72.86
  routine infant and child vision and hearing testing V20.2
  sensitivity test (see also Test, skin)
    allergy NEC V72.7
    bacterial disease NEC V74.9
    Dick V74.8
    Kveim V82.89
    Mantoux V74.1
    mycotic infection NEC V75.4
    parasitic disease NEC V75.8
    Schick V74.3
    Schultz-Charlton V74.8
  social service (agency) referral or evaluation V63.8
  speech (-language) therapy V57.3
  sterilization V25.2
  suspected disorder (ruled out) (without need for further care) — see Observation
  terminal care V66.7
  tests only — see Test
  therapeutic drug monitoring V58.83
  therapy
    blood transfusion, without reported diagnosis V58.2
    breathing exercises V57.0
    chemotherapy, antineoplastic V58.11
      prophylactic NEC V07.39
      fluoride V07.31
    dialysis (intermittent) (treatment)
      extracorporeal V56.0
      peritoneal V56.8
      renal V56.0
      specified type NEC V56.8
    exercise (remedial) NEC V57.1
      breathing V57.0
    immunotherapy, antineoplastic V58.12
    long-term (current) (prophylactic) drug use NEC V58.69
      antibiotics V58.62
        short-term use — omit code
      anticoagulants V58.61
      anti-inflammatories, non-steroidal (NSAID) V58.64
      antiplatelets V58.63
      antithrombotics V58.63
      aspirin V58.66
      bisphosphonates V58.68
      high-risk medications NEC V58.69
      insulin V58.67
      methadone for pain control V58.69

☑ Additional Digit Required — Refer to the Tabular List for Digit Selection   ▽ Subterms under main terms may continue to next column or page

2014 ICD-9-CM   59

Admission — continued
for — continued
therapy — continued
long-term drug use — continued
opiate analgesic V58.69
steroids V58.65
occupational V57.21
orthoptic V57.4
physical NEC V57.1
radiation V58.0
speech (-language) V57.3
vocational V57.22
toilet or cleaning
of artificial opening — see Attention
to, artificial, opening
of non-vascular catheter V58.82
of vascular catheter V58.81
treatment
measure V07.9
specified type NEC V07.8
tubal ligation V25.2
tuboplasty for previous sterilization
V26.0
ultrasound, routine fetal V28.3
vaccination, prophylactic (against)
arthropod-borne virus, viral NEC
V05.1
disease NEC V05.1
encephalitis V05.0
Bacille Calmette Guérin (BCG) V03.2
BCG V03.2
chickenpox V05.4
cholera alone V03.0
with typhoid-paratyphoid
(cholera + TAB) V06.0
common cold V04.7
dengue V05.1
diphtheria alone V03.5
diphtheria-tetanus-pertussis (DTP)
(DTaP) V06.1
with
poliomyelitis (DTP + polio)
V06.3
typhoid-paratyphoid (DTP +
TAB) V06.2
diphtheria-tetanus [Td] [DT] without
pertussis V06.5
disease (single) NEC V05.9
bacterial NEC V03.9
specified type NEC V03.89
combinations NEC V06.9
specified type NEC V06.8
specified type NEC V05.8
viral NEC V04.89
encephalitis, viral, arthropod-borne
V05.0
Hemophilus influenzae, type B [Hib]
V03.81
hepatitis, viral V05.3
human papillomavirus (HPV) V04.89
immune sera (gamma globulin)
V07.2
influenza V04.81
with
Streptococcus pneumoniae
[pneumococcus] V06.6
Leishmaniasis V05.2
measles alone V04.2
measles-mumps-rubella (MMR) V06.4
mumps alone V04.6
with measles and rubella (MMR)
V06.4
not done because of contraindication
V64.09
pertussis alone V03.6
plague V03.3
pneumonia V03.82
poliomyelitis V04.0
with diphtheria-tetanus-pertussis
(DTP+ polio) V06.3
rabies V04.5
respiratory syncytial virus (RSV)
V04.82
rubella alone V04.3
with measles and mumps (MMR)
V06.4

Admission — continued
for — continued
vaccination, prophylactic — continued
smallpox V04.1
specified type NEC V05.8
Streptococcus pneumoniae [pneumo-
coccus] V03.82
with
influenza V06.6
tetanus toxoid alone V03.7
with diphtheria [Td] [DT] V06.5
and pertussis (DTP) (DTaP)
V06.1
tuberculosis (BCG) V03.2
tularemia V03.4
typhoid alone V03.1
with diphtheria-tetanus-pertussis
(TAB + DTP) V06.2
typhoid-paratyphoid alone (TAB)
V03.1
typhus V05.8
varicella (chicken pox) V05.4
viral encephalitis, arthropod-borne
V05.0
viral hepatitis V05.3
yellow fever V04.4
vasectomy V25.2
vasoplasty for previous sterilization
V26.0
vision examination V72.0
vocational therapy V57.22
waiting period for admission to other
facility V63.2
undergoing social agency investigation V63.8
well baby and child care V20.2
x-ray of chest
for suspected tuberculosis V71.2
routine V72.5
Adnexitis (suppurative) — see also Salpingo-
oophoritis 614.2
Adolescence NEC V21.2
Adoption
agency referral V68.89
examination V70.3
held for V68.89
Adrenal gland — see condition
Adrenalism 255.9
tuberculous (see also Tuberculosis) 017.6 ☑
Adrenalitis, adrenitis 255.8
meningococcal hemorrhagic 036.3
Adrenarche, precocious 259.1
Adrenocortical syndrome 255.2
Adrenogenital syndrome (acquired) (congen-
ital) 255.2
iatrogenic, fetus or newborn 760.79
Adrenoleukodystrophy 277.86
neonatal 277.86
x-linked 277.86
Adrenomyeloneuropathy 277.86
Adventitious bursa — see Bursitis
Adynamia (episodica) (hereditary) (periodic)
359.3
Adynamic
ileus or intestine (see also Ileus) 560.1
ureter 753.22
Aeration lung, imperfect, newborn 770.5
Aerobullosis 993.3
Aerocele — see Embolism, air
Aerodermectasia
subcutaneous (traumatic) 958.7
surgical 998.81
surgical 998.81
Aerodontalgia 993.2
Aeroembolism 993.3
Aerogenes capsulatus infection — see also
Gangrene, gas 040.0
Aero-otitis media 993.0
Aerophagy, aerophagia 306.4
psychogenic 306.4
Aerosinusitis 993.1
Aerotitis 993.0
Affection, affections — see also Disease
sacroiliac (joint), old 724.6
shoulder region NEC 726.2

Afibrinogenemia 286.3
acquired 286.6
congenital 286.3
postpartum 666.3 ☑
African
sleeping sickness 086.5
tick fever 087.1
trypanosomiasis 086.5
Gambian 086.3
Rhodesian 086.4
Aftercare V58.9
amputation stump V54.89
artificial openings — see Attention to, artificial, opening
blood transfusion without reported diagnosis V58.2
breathing exercise V57.0
cardiac device V53.39
defibrillator, automatic implantable
(with synchronous cardiac pacemaker) V53.32
pacemaker V53.31
carotid sinus V53.39
carotid sinus pacemaker V53.39
cerebral ventricle (communicating) shunt
V53.01
chemotherapy (oral) (intravenous) session
(adjunctive) (maintenance) V58.11
defibrillator, automatic implantable cardiac
(with synchronous cardiac pacemak-
er) V53.32
exercise (remedial) (therapeutic) V57.1
breathing V57.0
extracorporeal dialysis (intermittent)
(treatment) V56.0
following surgery NEC V58.49
for
injury V58.43
neoplasm V58.42
organ transplant V58.44
trauma V58.43
joint
explantation of prosthesis (staged
procedure) V54.82
replacement V54.81
of
circulatory system V58.73
digestive system V58.75
genital organs V58.76
genitourinary system V58.76
musculoskeletal system V58.78
nervous system V58.72
oral cavity V58.75
respiratory system V58.74
sense organs V58.71
skin V58.77
subcutaneous tissue V58.77
teeth V58.75
urinary system V58.76
spinal — see Aftercare, following
surgery, of, specified body system
wound closure, planned V58.41
fracture V54.9
healing V54.89
pathologic
ankle V54.29
arm V54.20
lower V54.22
upper V54.21
finger V54.29
foot V54.29
hand V54.29
hip V54.23
leg V54.24
lower V54.26
upper V54.25
pelvis V54.29
specified site NEC V54.29
toe(s) V54.29
vertebrae V54.27
wrist V54.29
traumatic
ankle V54.19
arm V54.10
lower V54.12
upper V54.11

Aftercare — continued
fracture — continued
healing — continued
traumatic — continued
finger V54.19
foot V54.19
hand V54.19
hip V54.13
leg V54.14
lower V54.16
upper V54.15
pelvis V54.19
specified site NEC V54.19
toe(s) V54.19
vertebrae V54.17
wrist V54.19
removal of
external fixation device V54.89
internal fixation device V54.01
specified care NEC V54.89
gait training V57.1
for use of artificial limb(s) V57.81
internal fixation device V54.09
involving
dialysis (intermittent) (treatment)
extracorporeal V56.0
peritoneal V56.8
renal V56.0
gait training V57.1
for use of artificial limb(s) V57.81
growth rod
adjustment V54.02
lengthening V54.02
internal fixation device V54.09
orthoptic training V57.4
orthotic training V57.81
radiotherapy session V58.0
removal of
drains V58.49
dressings
wound V58.30
nonsurgical V58.30
surgical V58.31
fixation device
external V54.89
internal V54.01
fracture plate V54.01
nonsurgical wound dressing V58.30
pins V54.01
plaster cast V54.89
rods V54.01
screws V58.32
staples V58.32
surgical wound dressings V58.31
sutures V58.32
traction device, external V54.89
wound packing V58.30
nonsurgical V58.30
surgical V58.31
neuropacemaker (brain) (peripheral nerve)
(spinal cord) V53.02
occupational therapy V57.21
orthodontic V58.5
orthopedic V54.9
change of external fixation or traction
device V54.89
following joint
explantation of prosthesis (staged
procedure) V54.82
replacement V54.81
internal fixation device V54.09
removal of fixation device
external V54.89
internal V54.01
specified care NEC V54.89
orthoptic training V57.4
orthotic training V57.81
pacemaker
brain V53.02
cardiac V53.31
carotid sinus V53.39
peripheral nerve V53.02
spinal cord V53.02
peritoneal dialysis (intermittent) (treatment)
V56.8
physical therapy NEC V57.1

Aftercare — *continued*
  physical therapy — *continued*
    breathing exercises V57.0
  radiotherapy session V58.0
  rehabilitation procedure V57.9
    breathing exercises V57.0
    multiple types V57.89
    occupational V57.21
    orthoptic V57.4
    orthotic V57.81
    physical therapy NEC V57.1
    remedial exercises V57.1
    specified type NEC V57.89
    speech (-language) V57.3
    therapeutic exercises V57.1
    vocational V57.22
  renal dialysis (intermittent) (treatment) V56.0
  specified type NEC V58.89
    removal of non-vascular catheter V58.82
    removal of vascular catheter V58.81
  speech (-language) therapy V57.3
  stump, amputation V54.89
  vocational rehabilitation V57.22
After-cataract 366.50
  obscuring vision 366.53
  specified type, not obscuring vision 366.52
Agalactia 676.4 ☑
Agammaglobulinemia 279.00
  with lymphopenia 279.2
  acquired (primary) (secondary) 279.06
  Bruton's X-linked 279.04
  infantile sex-linked (Bruton's) (congenital) 279.04
  Swiss-type 279.2
Aganglionosis (bowel) (colon) 751.3
Age (old) — *see also* Senile 797
Agenesis — *see also* Absence, by site, congenital
  acoustic nerve 742.8
  adrenal (gland) 759.1
  alimentary tract (complete) (partial) NEC 751.8
    lower 751.2
    upper 750.8
  anus, anal (canal) 751.2
  aorta 747.22
  appendix 751.2
  arm (complete) (partial) (*see also* Deformity, reduction, upper limb) 755.20
  artery (peripheral) NEC (*see also* Anomaly, peripheral vascular system) 747.60
    brain 747.81
    coronary 746.85
    pulmonary 747.31
    umbilical 747.5
  auditory (canal) (external) 744.01
  auricle (ear) 744.01
  bile, biliary duct or passage 751.61
  bone NEC 756.9
  brain 740.0
    specified part 742.2
  breast 757.6
  bronchus 748.3
  canaliculus lacrimalis 743.65
  carpus NEC (*see also* Deformity, reduction, upper limb) 755.28
  cartilage 756.9
  cecum 751.2
  cerebellum 742.2
  cervix 752.43
  chin 744.89
  cilia 743.63
  circulatory system, part NEC 747.89
  clavicle 755.51
  clitoris 752.49
  coccyx 756.13
  colon 751.2
  corpus callosum 742.2
  cricoid cartilage 748.3
  diaphragm (with hernia) 756.6
  digestive organ(s) or tract (complete) (partial) NEC 751.8
    lower 751.2
    upper 750.8
  ductus arteriosus 747.89

Agenesis — *see also* Absence, by site, congenital — *continued*
  duodenum 751.1
  ear NEC 744.09
    auricle 744.01
    lobe 744.21
  ejaculatory duct 752.89
  endocrine (gland) NEC 759.2
  epiglottis 748.3
  esophagus 750.3
  Eustachian tube 744.24
  extrinsic muscle, eye 743.69
  eye 743.00
    adnexa 743.69
  eyelid (fold) 743.62
  face
    bones NEC 756.0
    specified part NEC 744.89
  fallopian tube 752.19
  femur NEC (*see also* Absence, femur, congenital) 755.34
  fibula NEC (*see also* Absence, fibula, congenital) 755.37
  finger NEC (*see also* Absence, finger, congenital) 755.29
  foot (complete) (*see also* Deformity, reduction, lower limb) 755.31
  gallbladder 751.69
  gastric 750.8
  genitalia, genital (organ)
    female 752.89
      external 752.49
      internal NEC 752.89
    male 752.89
      penis 752.69
  glottis 748.3
  gonadal 758.6
  hair 757.4
  hand (complete) (*see also* Deformity, reduction, upper limb) 755.21
  heart 746.89
    valve NEC 746.89
      aortic 746.89
      mitral 746.89
      pulmonary 746.01
  hepatic 751.69
  humerus NEC (*see also* Absence, humerus, congenital) 755.24
  hymen 752.49
  ileum 751.1
  incus 744.04
  intestine (small) 751.1
    large 751.2
  iris (dilator fibers) 743.45
  jaw 524.09
  jejunum 751.1
  kidney(s) (partial) (unilateral) 753.0
  labium (majus) (minus) 752.49
  labyrinth, membranous 744.05
  lacrimal apparatus (congenital) 743.65
  larynx 748.3
  leg NEC (*see also* Deformity, reduction, lower limb) 755.30
  lens 743.35
  limb (complete) (partial) (*see also* Deformity, reduction) 755.4
    lower NEC 755.30
    upper 755.20
  lip 750.26
  liver 751.69
  lung (bilateral) (fissures) (lobe) (unilateral) 748.5
  mandible 524.09
  maxilla 524.09
  metacarpus NEC 755.28
  metatarsus NEC 755.38
  muscle (any) 756.81
  musculoskeletal system NEC 756.9
  nail(s) 757.5
  neck, part 744.89
  nerve 742.8
  nervous system, part NEC 742.8
  nipple 757.6
  nose 748.1
  nuclear 742.8

Agenesis — *see also* Absence, by site, congenital — *continued*
  organ
    of Corti 744.05
    or site not listed — *see* Anomaly, specified type NEC
  osseous meatus (ear) 744.03
  ovary 752.0
  oviduct 752.19
  pancreas 751.7
  parathyroid (gland) 759.2
  patella 755.64
  pelvic girdle (complete) (partial) 755.69
  penis 752.69
  pericardium 746.89
  perineal body 756.81
  pituitary (gland) 759.2
  prostate 752.89
  pulmonary
    artery 747.31
    trunk 747.31
    vein 747.49
  punctum lacrimale 743.65
  radioulnar NEC (*see also* Absence, forearm, congenital) 755.25
  radius NEC (*see also* Absence, radius, congenital) 755.26
  rectum 751.2
  renal 753.0
  respiratory organ NEC 748.9
  rib 756.3
  roof of orbit 742.0
  round ligament 752.89
  sacrum 756.13
  salivary gland 750.21
  scapula 755.59
  scrotum 752.89
  seminal duct or tract 752.89
  septum
    atrial 745.69
    between aorta and pulmonary artery 745.0
    ventricular 745.3
  shoulder girdle (complete) (partial) 755.59
  skull (bone) 756.0
    with
      anencephalus 740.0
      encephalocele 742.0
      hydrocephalus 742.3
        with spina bifida (*see also* Spina bifida) 741.0 ☑
      microcephalus 742.1
  spermatic cord 752.89
  spinal cord 742.59
  spine 756.13
    lumbar 756.13
      isthmus 756.11
      pars articularis 756.11
  spleen 759.0
  sternum 756.3
  stomach 750.7
  tarsus NEC 755.38
  tendon 756.81
  testicular 752.89
  testis 752.89
  thymus (gland) 759.2
  thyroid (gland) 243
    cartilage 748.3
  tibia NEC (*see also* Absence, tibia, congenital) 755.36
  tibiofibular NEC 755.35
  toe (complete) (partial) (*see also* Absence, toe, congenital) 755.39
  tongue 750.11
  trachea (cartilage) 748.3
  ulna NEC (*see also* Absence, ulna, congenital) 755.27
  ureter 753.4
  urethra 753.8
  urinary tract NEC 753.8
  uterus 752.31
  uvula 750.26
  vagina (total) (partial) 752.45
  vas deferens 752.89
  vein(s) (peripheral) NEC (*see also* Anomaly, peripheral vascular system) 747.60

Agenesis — *see also* Absence, by site, congenital — *continued*
  vein(s) (*see also* Anomaly, peripheral vascular system) — *continued*
    brain 747.81
    great 747.49
    portal 747.49
    pulmonary 747.49
    vena cava (inferior) (superior) 747.49
  vermis of cerebellum 742.2
  vertebra 756.13
    lumbar 756.13
      isthmus 756.11
      pars articularis 756.11
  vulva 752.49
Ageusia — *see also* Disturbance, sensation 781.1
Aggressiveness 301.3
Aggressive outburst — *see also* Disturbance, conduct 312.0 ☑
  in children or adolescents 313.9
Aging skin 701.8
Agitated — *see* condition
Agitation 307.9
  catatonic (*see also* Schizophrenia) 295.2 ☑
Aglossia (congenital) 750.11
Aglycogenosis 271.0
Agnail (finger) (with lymphangitis) 681.02
Agnosia (body image) (tactile) 784.69
  verbal 784.69
    auditory 784.69
      secondary to organic lesion 784.69
    developmental 315.8
    secondary to organic lesion 784.69
  visual 368.16
    object 368.16
Agoraphobia 300.22
  with panic disorder 300.21
Agrammatism 784.69
Agranulocytopenia — *see also* Agranulocytosis 288.09
Agranulocytosis — *see also* Neutropenia 288.09
  chronic 288.09
  cyclical 288.02
  due to infection 288.04
  genetic 288.01
  infantile 288.01
  periodic 288.02
  pernicious 288.09
Agraphia (absolute) 784.69
  with alexia 784.61
  developmental 315.39
Agrypnia — *see also* Insomnia 780.52
Ague — *see also* Malaria 084.6
  brass-founders' 985.8
  dumb 084.6
  tertian 084.1
Agyria 742.2
AHTR (acute hemolytic transfusion reaction) — *see* Complications, transfusion
Ahumada-del Castillo syndrome (nonpuerperal galactorrhea and amenorrhea) 253.1
AIDS 042
AIDS-associated retrovirus (disease) (illness) 042
  infection — *see* Human immunodeficiency virus, infection
AIDS-associated virus (disease) (illness) 042
  infection — *see* Human immunodeficiency virus, infection
AIDS-like disease (illness) (syndrome) 042
AIDS-related complex 042
AIDS-related conditions 042
AIDS-related virus (disease) (illness) 042
  infection — *see* Human immunodeficiency virus, infection
AIDS virus (disease) (illness) 042
  infection — *see* Human immunodeficiency virus, infection
Ailment, heart — *see* Disease, heart
Ailurophobia 300.29
Ainhum (disease) 136.0
AIN I (anal intraepithelial neoplasia I) (histologically confirmed) 569.44

☑ **Additional Digit Required — Refer to the Tabular List for Digit Selection**   ▽ **Subterms under main terms may continue to next column or page**

2014 ICD-9-CM   **61**

AIN II (anal intraepithelial neoplasia II) (histologically confirmed) 569.44
AIN III (anal intraepithelial neoplasia III) 230.6
   anal canal 230.5
AIPHI (acute idiopathic pulmonary hemorrhage in infants (over 28 days old)) 786.31
Air
   anterior mediastinum 518.1
   compressed, disease 993.3
   embolism (any site) (artery) (cerebral) 958.0
      with
         abortion — see Abortion, by type, with embolism
         ectopic pregnancy (see also categories 633.0–633.9) 639.6
         molar pregnancy (see also categories 630–632) 639.6
      due to implanted device — see Complications, due to (presence of) any device, implant, or graft classified to 996.0–996.5 NEC
      following
         abortion 639.6
         ectopic or molar pregnancy 639.6
      infusion, perfusion, or transfusion 999.1
      in pregnancy, childbirth, or puerperium 673.0 ☑
      traumatic 958.0
   hunger 786.09
      psychogenic 306.1
   leak (lung) (pulmonary) (thorax) 512.84
      iatrogenic 512.1
      persistent 512.84
      postoperative 512.2
   rarefied, effects of — see Effect, adverse, high altitude
   sickness 994.6
Airplane sickness 994.6
Akathisia, acathisia 781.0
   due to drugs 333.99
   neuroleptic-induced acute 333.99
Akinesia algeria 352.6
Akiyami 100.89
Akureyri disease (epidemic neuromyasthenia) 049.8
Alacrima (congenital) 743.65
Alactasia (hereditary) 271.3
Alagille syndrome 759.89
Alalia 784.3
   developmental 315.31
      receptive-expressive 315.32
   secondary to organic lesion 784.3
Alaninemia 270.8
Alastrim 050.1
Albarrán's disease (colibacilluria) 791.9
Albers-Schönberg's disease (marble bones) 756.52
Albert's disease 726.71
Albinism, albino (choroid) (cutaneous) (eye) (generalized) (isolated) (ocular) (oculocutaneous) (partial) 270.2
Albinismus 270.2
Albright (-Martin) (-Bantam) disease (pseudohypoparathyroidism) 275.49
Albright (-McCune) (-Sternberg) syndrome (osteitis fibrosa disseminata) 756.59
Albuminous — see condition
Albuminuria, albuminuric (acute) (chronic) (subacute) 791.0
   Bence-Jones 791.0
   cardiac 785.9
   complicating pregnancy, childbirth, or puerperium 646.2 ☑
      with hypertension — see Toxemia, of pregnancy
      affecting fetus or newborn 760.1
   cyclic 593.6
   gestational 646.2 ☑
   gravidarum 646.2 ☑
      with hypertension — see Toxemia, of pregnancy
      affecting fetus or newborn 760.1
   heart 785.9
   idiopathic 593.6
   orthostatic 593.6

Albuminuria, albuminuric — continued
   postural 593.6
   pre-eclamptic (mild) 642.4 ☑
      affecting fetus or newborn 760.0
      severe 642.5 ☑
         affecting fetus or newborn 760.0
   recurrent physiologic 593.6
   scarlatinal 034.1
Albumosuria 791.0
   Bence-Jones 791.0
   myelopathic (M9730/3) 203.0 ☑
Alcaptonuria 270.2
Alcohol, alcoholic
   abstinence 291.81
   acute intoxication 305.0 ☑
      with dependence 303.0 ☑
   addiction (see also Alcoholism) 303.9 ☑
      maternal
         with suspected fetal damage affecting management of pregnancy 655.4 ☑
         affecting fetus or newborn 760.71
   amnestic disorder, persisting 291.1
   anxiety 291.89
   brain syndrome, chronic 291.2
   cardiopathy 425.5
   chronic (see also Alcoholism) 303.9 ☑
   cirrhosis (liver) 571.2
   delirium 291.0
      acute 291.0
      chronic 291.1
      tremens 291.0
      withdrawal 291.0
   dementia NEC 291.2
   deterioration 291.2
   drunkenness (simple) 305.0 ☑
   hallucinosis (acute) 291.3
   induced
      circadian rhythm sleep disorder 291.82
      hypersomnia 291.82
      insomnia 291.82
      mental disorder 291.9
         anxiety 291.89
         mood 291.89
         sexual 291.89
         sleep 291.82
         specified type 291.89
      parasomnia 291.82
      persisting
         amnestic disorder 291.1
         dementia 291.2
      psychotic disorder
         with
            delusions 291.5
            hallucinations 291.3
      sleep disorder 291.82
   insanity 291.9
   intoxication (acute) 305.0 ☑
      with dependence 303.0 ☑
      pathological 291.4
   jealousy 291.5
   Korsakoff's, Korsakov's, Korsakow's 291.1
   liver NEC 571.3
      acute 571.1
      chronic 571.2
   mania (acute) (chronic) 291.9
   mood 291.89
   paranoia 291.5
   paranoid (type) psychosis 291.5
   pellagra 265.2
   poisoning, accidental (acute) NEC 980.9
      specified type of alcohol — see Table of Drugs and Chemicals
   psychosis (see also Psychosis, alcoholic) 291.9
      Korsakoff's, Korsakov's, Korsakow's 291.1
   polyneuritic 291.1
      with
         delusions 291.5
         hallucinations 291.3
   related disorder 291.9
   withdrawal symptoms, syndrome NEC 291.81
      delirium 291.0
      hallucinosis 291.3

Alcoholism 303.9 ☑

Note — Use the following fifth-digit subclassification with category 303:

0   unspecified
1   continuous
2   episodic
3   in remission

   with psychosis (see also Psychosis, alcoholic) 291.9
   acute 303.0 ☑
   chronic 303.9 ☑
      with psychosis 291.9
   complicating pregnancy, childbirth, or puerperium 648.4 ☑
      affecting fetus or newborn 760.71
   history V11.3
   Korsakoff's, Korsakov's, Korsakow's 291.1
   suspected damage to fetus affecting management of pregnancy 655.4 ☑
Alder's anomaly or syndrome (leukocyte granulation anomaly) 288.2
Alder-Reilly anomaly (leukocyte granulation) 288.2
Aldosteronism (primary) 255.10
   congenital 255.10
   familial type I 255.11
   glucocorticoid-remediable 255.11
   secondary 255.14
Aldosteronoma (M8370/1) 237.2
Aldrich (-Wiskott) syndrome (eczema-thrombocytopenia) 279.12
Aleppo boil 085.1
Aleukemic — see condition
Aleukia
   congenital 288.09
   hemorrhagica 284.9
      acquired (secondary) 284.89
      congenital 284.09
      idiopathic 284.9
   splenica 289.4
Alexia (congenital) (developmental) 315.01
   secondary to organic lesion 784.61
Algoneurodystrophy 733.7
Algophobia 300.29
Alibert-Bazin disease (M9700/3) 202.1 ☑
Alibert's disease (mycosis fungoides) (M9700/3) 202.1 ☑
Alice in Wonderland syndrome 293.89
Alienation, mental — see also Psychosis 298.9
Alkalemia 276.3
Alkalosis 276.3
   metabolic 276.3
      with respiratory acidosis 276.4
   respiratory 276.3
Alkaptonuria 270.2
Allen-Masters syndrome 620.6
Allergic bronchopulmonary aspergillosis 518.6
Allergy, allergic (reaction) 995.3
   air-borne substance — see also Fever, hay 477.9
      specified allergen NEC 477.8
   alveolitis (extrinsic) 495.9
      due to
         Aspergillus clavatus 495.4
         cryptostroma corticale 495.6
         organisms (fungal, thermophilic actinomycete, other) growing in ventilation (air conditioning systems) 495.7
      specified type NEC 495.8
   anaphylactic reaction or shock 995.0
      due to food — see Anaphylactic reaction or shock, due to, food
   angioderma 995.1
   angioneurotic edema 995.1
   animal (cat) (dog) (epidermal) 477.8
      dander 477.2
      hair 477.2
   arthritis (see also Arthritis, allergic) 716.2 ☑
   asthma — see Asthma
   bee sting (anaphylactic shock) 989.5
   biological — see Allergy, drug

Allergy, allergic — continued
   bronchial asthma — see Asthma
   conjunctivitis (eczematous) 372.14
   dander, animal (cat) (dog) 477.2
   dandruff 477.8
   dermatitis (venenata) — see Dermatitis
   diathesis V15.09
   drug, medicinal substance, and biological (any) (correct medicinal substance properly administered) (external) (internal) 995.27
      wrong substance given or taken NEC 977.9
         specified drug or substance — see Table of Drugs and Chemicals
   dust (house) (stock) 477.8
   eczema — see Eczema
   endophthalmitis 360.19
   epidermal (animal) 477.8
   existing dental restorative material
   feathers 477.8
   food (any) (ingested) 693.1
      atopic 691.8
      in contact with skin 692.5
   gastritis 535.4 ☑
   gastroenteritis 558.3
   gastrointestinal 558.3
   grain 477.0
   grass (pollen) 477.0
      asthma (see also Asthma) 493.0 ☑
      hay fever 477.0
   hair, animal (cat) (dog) 477.2
   hay fever (grass) (pollen) (ragweed) (tree) (see also Fever, hay) 477.9
   history (of) V15.09
      to
         arachnid bite V15.06
         eggs V15.03
         food additives V15.05
         insect bite V15.06
         latex V15.07
         milk products V15.02
         nuts V15.05
            peanuts V15.01
         radiographic dye V15.08
         seafood V15.04
         specified food NEC V15.05
         spider bite V15.06
   horse serum — see Allergy, serum
   inhalant 477.9
      dust 477.8
      pollen 477.0
      specified allergen other than pollen 477.8
   kapok 477.8
   medicine — see Allergy, drug
   migraine 339.00
   milk protein 558.3
   pannus 370.62
   pneumonia 518.3
   pollen (any) (hay fever) 477.0
      asthma (see also Asthma) 493.0 ☑
   primrose 477.0
   primula 477.0
   purpura 287.0
   ragweed (pollen) (Senecio jacobae) 477.0
      asthma (see also Asthma) 493.0 ☑
      hay fever 477.0
   respiratory (see also Allergy, inhalant) 477.9
      due to
         drug — see Allergy, drug
         food — see Allergy, food
   rhinitis (see also Fever, hay) 477.9
      due to food 477.1
   rose 477.0
   Senecio jacobae 477.0
   serum (prophylactic) (therapeutic) 999.59
      anaphylactic reaction or shock 999.49
   shock (anaphylactic) (due to adverse effect of correct medicinal substance properly administered) 995.0
      food — see Anaphylactic reaction or shock, due to, food
      from
         administration of blood and blood products 999.41

☑ **Additional Digit Required** — Refer to the Tabular List for Digit Selection   ▽ **Subterms under main terms may continue to next column or page**

62   **2014 ICD-9-CM**

Allergy, allergic — *continued*
  shock — *continued*
    from — *continued*
      immunization 999.42
      serum NEC 999.49
  sinusitis (*see also* Fever, hay) 477.9
  skin reaction 692.9
    specified substance — *see* Dermatitis, due to
  tree (any) (hay fever) (pollen) 477.0
    asthma (*see also* Asthma) 493.0 ☑
  upper respiratory (*see also* Fever, hay) 477.9
  urethritis 597.89
  urticaria 708.0
  vaccine — *see* Allergy, serum
Allescheriosis 117.6
Alligator skin disease (ichthyosis congenita) 757.1
  acquired 701.1
Allocheiria, allochiria — *see also* Disturbance, sensation 782.0
Almeida's disease (Brazilian blastomycosis) 116.1
Alopecia (atrophicans) (pregnancy) (premature) (senile) 704.00
  adnata 757.4
  areata 704.01
  celsi 704.01
  cicatrisata 704.09
  circumscripta 704.01
  congenital, congenitalis 757.4
  disseminata 704.01
  effluvium (telogen) 704.02
  febrile 704.09
  generalisata 704.09
  hereditaria 704.09
  marginalis 704.01
  mucinosa 704.09
  postinfectional 704.09
  seborrheica 704.09
  specific 091.82
  syphilitic (secondary) 091.82
  telogen effluvium 704.02
  totalis 704.09
  toxica 704.09
  universalis 704.09
  x-ray 704.09
Alpers' disease 330.8
Alpha-lipoproteinemia 272.4
Alpha thalassemia 282.43
Alphos 696.1
Alpine sickness 993.2
Alport's syndrome (hereditary hematuri-anephropathy-deafness) 759.89
ALPS (autoimmune lymphoproliferative syndrome) 279.41
ALTE (apparent life threatening event) **in newborn and infant** 799.82
Alteration (of), altered
  awareness 780.09
    transient 780.02
  consciousness 780.09
    persistent vegetative state 780.03
    transient 780.02
  mental status 780.97
    amnesia (retrograde) 780.93
    memory loss 780.93
Alternaria (infection) 118
Alternating — *see* condition
Altitude, high (effects) — *see* Effect, adverse, high altitude
Aluminosis (of lung) 503
Alvarez syndrome (transient cerebral ischemia) 435.9
Alveolar capillary block syndrome 516.64
Alveolus, alveolar — *see* condition
Alymphocytosis (pure) 279.2
Alymphoplasia, thymic 279.2
Alzheimer's
  dementia (senile)
    with behavioral disturbance 331.0 *[294.11]*
    without behavioral disturbance 331.0 *[294.10]*
  disease or sclerosis 331.0

Alzheimer's — *continued*
  disease or sclerosis — *continued*
    with dementia — *see* Alzheimer's, dementia
Amastia — *see also* Absence, breast 611.89
Amaurosis (acquired) (congenital) — *see also* Blindness 369.00
  fugax 362.34
  hysterical 300.11
  Leber's (congenital) 362.76
  tobacco 377.34
  uremic — *see* Uremia
Amaurotic familial idiocy (infantile) (juvenile) (late) 330.1
Ambisexual 752.7
Amblyopia (acquired) (congenital) (partial) 368.00
  color 368.59
    acquired 368.55
  deprivation 368.02
  ex anopsia 368.00
  hysterical 300.11
  nocturnal 368.60
    vitamin A deficiency 264.5
  refractive 368.03
  strabismic 368.01
  suppression 368.01
  tobacco 377.34
  toxic NEC 377.34
  uremic — *see* Uremia
Ameba, amebic (histolytica) — *see also* Amebiasis
  abscess 006.3
    bladder 006.8
    brain (with liver and lung abscess) 006.5
    liver 006.3
      with
        brain abscess (and lung abscess) 006.5
        lung abscess 006.4
    lung (with liver abscess) 006.4
      with brain abscess 006.5
    seminal vesicle 006.8
    spleen 006.8
  carrier (suspected of) V02.2
  meningoencephalitis
    due to Naegleria (gruberi) 136.29
    primary 136.29
Amebiasis NEC 006.9
  with
    brain abscess (with liver or lung abscess) 006.5
    liver abscess (without mention of brain or lung abscess) 006.3
    lung abscess (with liver abscess) 006.4
      with brain abscess 006.5
  acute 006.0
  bladder 006.8
  chronic 006.1
  cutaneous 006.6
  cutis 006.6
  due to organism other than Entamoeba histolytica 007.8
  hepatic (*see also* Abscess, liver, amebic) 006.3
  nondysenteric 006.2
  seminal vesicle 006.8
  specified
    organism NEC 007.8
    site NEC 006.8
Ameboma 006.8
Amelia 755.4
  lower limb 755.31
  upper limb 755.21
Ameloblastoma (M9310/0) 213.1
  jaw (bone) (lower) 213.1
    upper 213.0
  long bones (M9261/3) — *see* Neoplasm, bone, malignant
  malignant (M9310/3) 170.1
    jaw (bone) (lower) 170.1
      upper 170.0
  mandible 213.1
  tibial (M9261/3) 170.7
Amelogenesis imperfecta 520.5
  nonhereditaria (segmentalis) 520.4

Amenorrhea (primary) (secondary) 626.0
  due to ovarian dysfunction 256.8
  hyperhormonal 256.8
Amentia — *see also* Disability, intellectual 319
  Meynert's (nonalcoholic) 294.0
    alcoholic 291.1
  nevoid 759.6
American
  leishmaniasis 085.5
  mountain tick fever 066.1
  trypanosomiasis — *see* Trypanosomiasis, American
Ametropia — *see also* Disorder, accommodation 367.9
Amianthosis 501
Amimia 784.69
Amino acid
  deficiency 270.9
    anemia 281.4
  metabolic disorder (*see also* Disorder, amino acid) 270.9
Aminoaciduria 270.9
  imidazole 270.5
Amnesia (retrograde) 780.93
  auditory 784.69
    developmental 315.31
    secondary to organic lesion 784.69
  dissociative 300.12
  hysterical or dissociative type 300.12
  psychogenic 300.12
  transient global 437.7
Amnestic (confabulatory) **syndrome** 294.0
  alcohol-induced persisting 291.1
  drug-induced persisting 292.83
  posttraumatic 294.0
Amniocentesis screening (for) V28.2
  alphafetoprotein level, raised V28.1
  chromosomal anomalies V28.0
Amnion, amniotic — *see also* condition
  nodosum 658.8 ☑
Amnionitis (complicating pregnancy) 658.4 ☑
  affecting fetus or newborn 762.7
Amoral trends 301.7
Amotio retinae — *see also* Detachment, retina 361.9
Ampulla
  lower esophagus 530.89
  phrenic 530.89
Amputation
  any part of fetus, to facilitate delivery 763.89
  cervix (supravaginal) (uteri) 622.8
    in pregnancy or childbirth 654.6 ☑
      affecting fetus or newborn 763.89
  clitoris — *see* Wound, open, clitoris
  congenital
    lower limb 755.31
    upper limb 755.21
  neuroma (traumatic) (*see also* Injury, nerve, by site)
    surgical complication (late) 997.61
  penis — *see* Amputation, traumatic, penis
  status (without complication) — *see* Absence, by site, acquired
  stump (surgical) (posttraumatic)
    abnormal, painful, or with complication (late) 997.60
    healed or old NEC (*see also* Absence, by site, acquired)
      lower V49.70
      upper V49.60
  traumatic (complete) (partial)

> *Note* — "Complicated" includes traumatic amputation with delayed healing, delayed treatment, foreign body, or infection.

    arm 887.4
      at or above elbow 887.2
        complicated 887.3
      below elbow 887.0
        complicated 887.1
      both (bilateral) (any level(s)) 887.6
        complicated 887.7
      complicated 887.5
      finger(s) (one or both hands) 886.0
        with thumb(s) 885.0
        complicated 885.1

Amputation — *continued*
  traumatic — *continued*
    finger(s) — *continued*
      complicated 886.1
    foot (except toe(s) only) 896.0
      and other leg 897.6
        complicated 897.7
      both (bilateral) 896.2
        complicated 896.3
      complicated 896.1
      toe(s) only (one or both feet) 895.0
        complicated 895.1
    genital organ(s) (external) NEC 878.8
      complicated 878.9
    hand (except finger(s) only) 887.0
      and other arm 887.6
        complicated 887.7
      both (bilateral) 887.6
        complicated 887.7
      complicated 887.1
      finger(s) (one or both hands) 886.0
        with thumb(s) 885.0
          complicated 885.1
        complicated 886.1
      thumb(s) (with fingers of either hand) 885.0
        complicated 885.1
    head 874.9
    late effect — *see* Late, effects (of), amputation
    leg 897.4
      and other foot 897.6
        complicated 897.7
      at or above knee 897.2
        complicated 897.3
      below knee 897.0
        complicated 897.1
      both (bilateral) 897.6
        complicated 897.7
      complicated 897.5
    lower limb(s) except toe(s) — *see* Amputation, traumatic, leg
    nose — *see* Wound, open, nose
    penis 878.0
      complicated 878.1
    sites other than limbs — *see* Wound, open, by site
    thumb(s) (with finger(s) of either hand) 885.0
      complicated 885.1
    toe(s) (one or both feet) 895.0
      complicated 895.1
    upper limb(s) — *see* Amputation, traumatic, arm
Amputee (bilateral) (old) — *see also* Absence, by site, acquired V49.70
Amusia 784.69
  developmental 315.39
  secondary to organic lesion 784.69
Amyelencephalus 740.0
Amyelia 742.59
Amygdalitis — *see* Tonsillitis
Amygdalolith 474.8
Amyloid disease or degeneration 277.30
  heart 277.39 *[425.7]*
Amyloidosis (familial) (general) (generalized) (genetic) (primary) 277.30
  with lung involvement 277.39 *[517.8]*
  cardiac, hereditary 277.39
  heart 277.39 *[425.7]*
  nephropathic 277.39 *[583.81]*
  neuropathic (Portuguese) (Swiss) 277.39 *[357.4]*
  pulmonary 277.39 *[517.8]*
  secondary 277.39
  systemic, inherited 277.39
Amylopectinosis (brancher enzyme deficiency) 271.0
Amylophagia 307.52
Amyoplasia, congenita 756.89
Amyotonia 728.2
  congenita 358.8
Amyotrophia, amyotrophy, amyotrophic 728.2
  congenita 756.89
  diabetic 250.6 ☑ *[353.5]*

☑ Additional Digit Required — Refer to the Tabular List for Digit Selection   Subterms under main terms may continue to next column or page

2014 ICD-9-CM   63

Index

Amyotrophia, amyotrophy, amyotrophic — Anemia

Amyotrophia, amyotrophy, amyotrophic — *continued*
  diabetic — *continued*
    due to secondary diabetes 249.6 ☑ *[353.5]*
  lateral sclerosis (syndrome) 335.20
  neuralgic 353.5
  sclerosis (lateral) 335.20
  spinal progressive 335.21
Anacidity, gastric 536.0
  psychogenic 306.4
Anaerosis of newborn 770.88
Analbuminemia 273.8
Analgesia — *see also* Anesthesia 782.0
Analphalipoproteinemia 272.5
Anaphylactic reaction or shock (correct substance properly administered) 995.0
  due to
    administration of blood and blood products 999.41
    chemical — *see* Table of Drugs and Chemicals
    correct medicinal substance properly administered 995.0
    drug or medicinal substance
      correct substance properly administered 995.0
      overdose or wrong substance given or taken 977.9
      specified drug — *see* Table of Drugs and Chemicals
    following sting(s) 989.5
    food 995.60
      additives 995.66
      crustaceans 995.62
      eggs 995.68
      fish 995.65
      fruits 995.63
      milk products 995.67
      nuts (tree) 995.64
      peanuts 995.61
      seeds 995.64
      specified NEC 995.69
      tree nuts 995.64
      vegetables 995.63
    immunization 999.42
    overdose or wrong substance given or taken 977.9
      specified drug — *see* Table of Drugs and Chemicals
    serum NEC 999.49
  following sting(s) 989.5
  purpura 287.0
  serum NEC 999.49
Anaphylactoid reaction or shock — *see* Anaphylactic reaction or shock
Anaphylaxis — *see* Anaphylactic reaction or shock
Anaplasia, cervix 622.10
Anaplasmosis, human 082.49
Anarthria 784.51
Anarthritic rheumatoid disease 446.5
Anasarca 782.3
  cardiac (*see also* Failure, heart) 428.0
  fetus or newborn 778.0
  lung 514
  nutritional 262
  pulmonary 514
  renal (*see also* Nephrosis) 581.9
Anaspadias 752.62
Anastomosis
  aneurysmal — *see* Aneurysm
  arteriovenous, congenital NEC (*see also* Anomaly, arteriovenous) 747.60
    ruptured, of brain (*see also* Hemorrhage, subarachnoid) 430
  intestinal 569.89
    complicated NEC 997.49
      involving urinary tract 997.5
  retinal and choroidal vessels 743.58
    acquired 362.17
Anatomical narrow angle (glaucoma) 365.02
Ancylostoma (infection) (infestation) 126.9
  americanus 126.1
  braziliense 126.2
  caninum 126.8

Ancylostoma — *continued*
  ceylanicum 126.3
  duodenale 126.0
  Necator americanus 126.1
Ancylostomiasis (intestinal) 126.9
  ancylostoma
    americanus 126.1
    caninum 126.8
    ceylanicum 126.3
    duodenale 126.0
  braziliense 126.2
  Necator americanus 126.1
Anders' disease or syndrome (adiposis tuberosa simplex) 272.8
Andersen's glycogen storage disease 271.0
Anderson's disease 272.7
Andes disease 993.2
Andrews' disease (bacterid) 686.8
Androblastoma (M8630/1)
  benign (M8630/0)
    specified site — *see* Neoplasm, by site, benign
    unspecified site
      female 220
      male 222.0
  malignant (M8630/3)
    specified site — *see* Neoplasm, by site, malignant
    unspecified site
      female 183.0
      male 186.9
  specified site — *see* Neoplasm, by site, uncertain behavior
  tubular (M8640/0)
    with lipid storage (M8641/0)
      specified site — *see* Neoplasm, by site, benign
      unspecified site
        female 220
        male 222.0
    specified site — *see* Neoplasm, by site, benign
    unspecified site
      female 220
      male 222.0
  unspecified site
    female 236.2
    male 236.4
Android pelvis 755.69
  with disproportion (fetopelvic) 653.3 ☑
    affecting fetus or newborn 763.1
    causing obstructed labor 660.1 ☑
      affecting fetus or newborn 763.1
Anectasis, pulmonary (newborn or fetus) 770.5
Anemia 285.9
  with
    disorder of
      anaerobic glycolysis 282.3
      pentose phosphate pathway 282.2
    koilonychia 280.9
  6-phosphogluconic dehydrogenase deficiency 282.2
  achlorhydric 280.9
  achrestic 281.8
  Addison's (pernicious) 281.0
  Addison-Biermer (pernicious) 281.0
  agranulocytic 288.09
  amino acid deficiency 281.4
  antineoplastic chemotherapy induced 285.3
  aplastic 284.9
    acquired (secondary) 284.89
    congenital 284.01
    constitutional 284.01
    due to
      antineoplastic chemotherapy 284.89
      chronic systemic disease 284.89
      drugs 284.89
      infection 284.89
      radiation 284.89
    idiopathic 284.9
    myxedema 244.9
    of or complicating pregnancy 648.2 ☑
    red cell (acquired) (adult) (with thymoma) 284.81
      congenital 284.01

Anemia — *continued*
  aplastic — *continued*
    red cell — *continued*
      pure 284.01
      specified type NEC 284.89
      toxic (paralytic) 284.89
  aregenerative 284.9
    congenital 284.01
  asiderotic 280.9
  atypical (primary) 285.9
  autohemolysis of Selwyn and Dacie (type I) 282.2
  autoimmune hemolytic 283.0
  Baghdad Spring 282.2
  Balantidium coli 007.0
  Biermer's (pernicious) 281.0
  blood loss (chronic) 280.0
    acute 285.1
  bothriocephalus 123.4
  brickmakers' (*see also* Ancylostomiasis) 126.9
  cerebral 437.8
  childhood 282.9
  chlorotic 280.9
  chronic 285.9
    blood loss 280.0
    hemolytic 282.9
      idiopathic 283.9
    simple 281.9
  chronica congenita aregenerativa 284.01
  combined system disease NEC 281.0 *[336.2]*
    due to dietary deficiency 281.1 *[336.2]*
  complicating pregnancy or childbirth 648.2 ☑
  congenital (following fetal blood loss) 776.5
    aplastic 284.01
    due to isoimmunization NEC 773.2
    Heinz-body 282.7
    hereditary hemolytic NEC 282.9
    nonspherocytic
      Type I 282.2
      Type II 282.3
    pernicious 281.0
    spherocytic (*see also* Spherocytosis) 282.0
  Cooley's (erythroblastic) 282.44
  crescent — *see* Disease, sickle-cell
  cytogenic 281.0
  Dacie's (nonspherocytic)
    type I 282.2
    type II 282.3
  Davidson's (refractory) 284.9
  deficiency 281.9
    2, 3 diphosphoglycurate mutase 282.3
    2, 3 PG 282.3
    6-PGD 282.2
    6-phosphogluronic dehydrogenase 282.2
    amino acid 281.4
    combined B_{12} and folate 281.3
    enzyme, drug-induced (hemolytic) 282.2
    erythrocytic glutathione 282.2
    folate 281.2
      dietary 281.2
      drug-induced 281.2
    folic acid 281.2
      dietary 281.2
      drug-induced 281.2
    G-6-PD 282.2
    GGS-R 282.2
    glucose-6-phosphate dehydrogenase (G-6-PD) 282.2
    glucose-phosphate isomerase 282.3
    glutathione peroxidase 282.2
    glutathione reductase 282.2
    glyceraldehyde phosphate dehydrogenase 282.3
    GPI 282.3
    G SH 282.2
    hexokinase 282.3
    iron (Fe) 280.9
      specified NEC 280.8
    nutritional 281.9
      with
        poor iron absorption 280.9
        specified deficiency NEC 281.8

Anemia — *continued*
  deficiency — *continued*
    nutritional — *continued*
      due to inadequate dietary iron intake 280.1
      specified type NEC 281.8
    of or complicating pregnancy 648.2 ☑
    pentose phosphate pathway 282.2
    PFK 282.3
    phosphofructo-aldolase 282.3
    phosphofructokinase 282.3
    phosphoglycerate kinase 282.3
    PK 282.3
    protein 281.4
    pyruvate kinase (PK) 282.3
    TPI 282.3
    triosephosphate isomerase 282.3
    vitamin B_{12} NEC 281.1
      dietary 281.1
      pernicious 281.0
  Diamond-Blackfan (congenital hypoplastic) 284.01
  dibothriocephalus 123.4
  dimorphic 281.9
  diphasic 281.8
  diphtheritic 032.89
  Diphyllobothrium 123.4
  drepanocytic (*see also* Disease, sickle-cell) 282.60
  due to
    antineoplastic chemotherapy 285.3
    blood loss (chronic) 280.0
      acute 285.1
    chemotherapy, antineoplastic 285.3
    defect of Embden-Meyerhof pathway glycolysis 282.3
    disorder of glutathione metabolism 282.2
    drug — *see* Anemia, by type (*see also* Table of Drugs and Chemicals)
      chemotherapy, antineoplastic 285.3
    fetal blood loss 776.5
    fish tapeworm (D. latum) infestation 123.4
    glutathione metabolism disorder 282.2
    hemorrhage (chronic) 280.0
      acute 285.1
    hexose monophosphate (HMP) shunt deficiency 282.2
    impaired absorption 280.9
    loss of blood (chronic) 280.0
      acute 285.1
    myxedema 244.9
    Necator americanus 126.1
    prematurity 776.6
    selective vitamin B_{12} malabsorption with proteinuria 281.1
  Dyke-Young type (secondary) (symptomatic) 283.9
  dyserythropoietic (congenital) (types I, II, III) 285.8
  dyshemopoietic (congenital) 285.8
  Egypt (*see also* Ancylostomiasis) 126.9
  elliptocytosis (*see also* Elliptocytosis) 282.1
  enzyme deficiency, drug-induced 282.2
  epidemic (*see also* Ancylostomiasis) 126.9
  EPO resistant 285.21
  erythroblastic
    familial 282.44
    fetus or newborn (*see also* Disease, hemolytic) 773.2
    late 773.5
  erythrocytic glutathione deficiency 282.2
  erythropoietin-resistant (EPO resistant anemia) 285.21
  essential 285.9
  Faber's (achlorhydric anemia) 280.9
  factitious (self-induced blood letting) 280.0
  familial erythroblastic (microcytic) 282.44
  Fanconi's (congenital pancytopenia) 284.09
  favism 282.2
  fetal 678.0 ☑
    following blood loss, affecting newborn 776.5

☑ **Additional Digit Required** — Refer to the Tabular List for Digit Selection   ▽ **Subterms under main terms may continue to next column or page**

64   **2014 ICD-9-CM**

Anemia — *continued*
fetus or newborn
  due to
    ABO
      antibodies 773.1
      incompatibility, maternal/fetal 773.1
      isoimmunization 773.1
    Rh
      antibodies 773.0
      incompatibility, maternal/fetal 773.0
      isoimmunization 773.0
  following fetal blood loss 776.5
fish tapeworm (D. latum) infestation 123.4
folate (folic acid) deficiency 281.2
  dietary 281.2
  drug-induced 281.2
folate malabsorption, congenital 281.2
folic acid deficiency 281.2
  dietary 281.2
  drug-induced 281.2
G-6-PD 282.2
general 285.9
glucose-6-phosphate dehydrogenase deficiency 282.2
glutathione-reductase deficiency 282.2
goat's milk 281.2
granulocytic 288.09
Heinz-body, congenital 282.7
hemoglobin deficiency 285.9
hemolytic 283.9
  acquired 283.9
    with hemoglobinuria NEC 283.2
    autoimmune (cold type) (idiopathic) (primary) (secondary) (symptomatic) (warm type) 283.0
    due to
      cold reactive antibodies 283.0
      drug exposure 283.0
      warm reactive antibodies 283.0
    fragmentation 283.19
    idiopathic (chronic) 283.9
    infectious 283.19
      autoimmune 283.0
      non-autoimmune 283.10
    toxic 283.19
    traumatic cardiac 283.19
  acute 283.9
    due to enzyme deficiency NEC 282.3
    fetus or newborn (*see also* Disease, hemolytic) 773.2
      late 773.5
    Lederer's (acquired infectious hemolytic anemia) 283.19
  autoimmune (acquired) 283.0
  chronic 282.9
    idiopathic 283.9
  cold type (secondary) (symptomatic) 283.0
  congenital (spherocytic) (*see also* Spherocytosis) 282.0
    nonspherocytic — *see* Anemia, hemolytic, nonspherocytic, congenital
  drug-induced 283.0
    enzyme deficiency 282.2
  due to
    cardiac conditions 283.19
    drugs 283.0
    enzyme deficiency NEC 282.3
      drug-induced 282.2
    presence of shunt or other internal prosthetic device 283.19
    thrombotic thrombocytopenic purpura 446.6
  elliptocytotic (*see also* Elliptocytosis) 282.1
  familial 282.9
  hereditary 282.9
    due to enzyme deficiency NEC 282.3
    specified NEC 282.8
  idiopathic (chronic) 283.9
  infectious (acquired) 283.19
  mechanical 283.19
  microangiopathic 283.19

Anemia — *continued*
hemolytic — *continued*
  non-autoimmune NEC 283.10
  nonspherocytic
    congenital or hereditary NEC 282.3
      glucose-6-phosphate dehydrogenase deficiency 282.2
      pyruvate kinase (PK) deficiency 282.3
      type I 282.2
      type II 282.3
    type I 282.2
    type II 282.3
  of or complicating pregnancy 648.2 ☑
  resulting from presence of shunt or other internal prosthetic device 283.19
  secondary 283.19
    autoimmune 283.0
  sickle-cell — *see* Disease, sickle-cell
  Stransky-Regala type (Hb-E) (*see also* Disease, hemoglobin) 282.7
  symptomatic 283.19
    autoimmune 283.0
  toxic (acquired) 283.19
  uremic (adult) (child) 283.11
  warm type (secondary) (symptomatic) 283.0
hemorrhagic (chronic) 280.0
  acute 285.1
HEMPAS 285.8
hereditary erythroblast multinuclearity-positive acidified serum test 285.8
Herrick's (hemoglobin S disease) 282.61
hexokinase deficiency 282.3
high A$_2$ 282.46
hookworm (*see also* Ancylostomiasis) 126.9
hypochromic (idiopathic) (microcytic) (normoblastic) 280.9
  with iron loading 285.0
  due to blood loss (chronic) 280.0
    acute 285.1
  familial sex linked 285.0
  pyridoxine-responsive 285.0
hypoplasia, red blood cells 284.81
  congenital or familial 284.01
hypoplastic (idiopathic) 284.9
  congenital 284.01
  familial 284.01
  of childhood 284.09
idiopathic 285.9
  hemolytic, chronic 283.9
in (due to) (with)
  chronic illness NEC 285.29
  chronic kidney disease 285.21
  end-stage renal disease 285.21
  neoplastic disease 285.22
infantile 285.9
infective, infectional 285.9
intertropical (*see also* Ancylostomiasis) 126.9
iron (Fe) deficiency 280.9
  due to blood loss (chronic) 280.0
    acute 285.1
  of or complicating pregnancy 648.2 ☑
  specified NEC 280.8
Jaksch's (pseudoleukemia infantum) 285.8
Joseph-Diamond-Blackfan (congenital hypoplastic) 284.01
labyrinth 386.50
Lederer's (acquired infectious hemolytic anemia) 283.19
leptocytosis (hereditary) 282.40
leukoerythroblastic 284.2
macrocytic 281.9
  nutritional 281.2
  of or complicating pregnancy 648.2 ☑
  tropical 281.2
malabsorption (familial), selective B$_{12}$ with proteinuria 281.1
malarial (*see also* Malaria) 084.6
malignant (progressive) 281.0
malnutrition 281.9
marsh (*see also* Malaria) 084.6
Mediterranean 282.40
  with hemoglobinopathy 282.49
megaloblastic 281.9

Anemia — *continued*
megaloblastic — *continued*
  combined B$_{12}$ and folate deficiency 281.3
  nutritional (of infancy) 281.2
  of infancy 281.2
  of or complicating pregnancy 648.2 ☑
  refractory 281.3
  specified NEC 281.3
megalocytic 281.9
microangiopathic hemolytic 283.19
microcytic (hypochromic) 280.9
  due to blood loss (chronic) 280.0
    acute 285.1
  familial 282.49
  hypochromic 280.9
microdrepanocytosis 282.41
miners' (*see also* Ancylostomiasis) 126.9
myelopathic 285.8
myelophthisic (normocytic) 284.2
newborn (*see also* Disease, hemolytic) 773.2
  due to isoimmunization (*see also* Disease, hemolytic) 773.2
  late, due to isoimmunization 773.5
  posthemorrhagic 776.5
nonregenerative 284.9
nonspherocytic hemolytic — *see* Anemia, hemolytic, nonspherocytic
normocytic (infectional) (not due to blood loss) 285.9
  due to blood loss (chronic) 280.0
    acute 285.1
  myelophthisic 284.2
nutritional (deficiency) 281.9
  with
    poor iron absorption 280.9
    specified deficiency NEC 281.8
  due to inadequate dietary iron intake 280.1
  megaloblastic (of infancy) 281.2
of childhood 282.9
of chronic
  disease NEC 285.29
  illness NEC 285.29
of or complicating pregnancy 648.2 ☑
  affecting fetus or newborn 760.8
of prematurity 776.6
orotic aciduric (congenital) (hereditary) 281.4
osteosclerotic 289.89
ovalocytosis (hereditary) (*see also* Elliptocytosis) 282.1
paludal (*see also* Malaria) 084.6
pentose phosphate pathway deficiency 282.2
pernicious (combined system disease) (congenital) (dorsolateral spinal degeneration) (juvenile) (myelopathy) (neuropathy) (posterior sclerosis) (primary) (progressive) (spleen) 281.0
  of or complicating pregnancy 648.2 ☑
pleochromic 285.9
  of sprue 281.8
portal 285.8
posthemorrhagic (chronic) 280.0
  acute 285.1
  newborn 776.5
postoperative
  due to (acute) blood loss 285.1
    chronic blood loss 280.0
  other 285.9
postpartum 648.2 ☑
pressure 285.9
primary 285.9
profound 285.9
progressive 285.9
  malignant 281.0
  pernicious 281.0
protein-deficiency 281.4
pseudoleukemica infantum 285.8
puerperal 648.2 ☑
pure red cell 284.81
  congenital 284.01
pyridoxine-responsive (hypochromic) 285.0
pyruvate kinase (PK) deficiency 282.3
refractoria sideroblastica 238.72

Anemia — *continued*
refractory (primary) 238.72
  with
    excess
      blasts-1 (RAEB-1) 238.72
      blasts-2 (RAEB-2) 238.73
      hemochromatosis 238.72
      ringed sideroblasts (RARS) 238.72
  due to
    drug 285.0
    myelodysplastic syndrome 238.72
    toxin 285.0
  hereditary 285.0
  idiopathic 238.72
  megaloblastic 281.3
  sideroblastic 238.72
    hereditary 285.0
  sideropenic 280.9
Rietti-Greppi-Micheli (thalassemia minor) 282.46
scorbutic 281.8
secondary (to) 285.9
  blood loss (chronic) 280.0
    acute 285.1
  hemorrhage 280.0
    acute 285.1
  inadequate dietary iron intake 280.1
semiplastic 284.9
septic 285.9
sickle-cell (*see also* Disease, sickle-cell) 282.60
sideroachrestic 285.0
sideroblastic (acquired) (any type) (congenital) (drug-induced) (due to disease) (hereditary) (primary) (secondary) (sex-linked hypochromic) (vitamin B$_6$ responsive) 285.0
  refractory 238.72
  congenital 285.0
  drug-induced 285.0
  hereditary 285.0
  sex-linked hypochromic 285.0
  vitamin B$_6$-responsive 285.0
sideropenic (refractory) 280.9
  due to blood loss (chronic) 280.0
    acute 285.1
simple chronic 281.9
specified type NEC 285.8
spherocytic (hereditary) (*see also* Spherocytosis) 282.0
splenic 285.8
  familial (Gaucher's) 272.7
splenomegalic 285.8
stomatocytosis 282.8
syphilitic 095.8
target cell (oval) 285.8
  with thalassemia — *see* Thalassemia
thalassemia 282.40
thrombocytopenic (*see also* Thrombocytopenia) 287.5
toxic 284.89
triosephosphate isomerase deficiency 282.3
tropical, macrocytic 281.2
tuberculous (*see also* Tuberculosis) 017.9 ☑
vegan's 281.1
vitamin
  B$_6$-responsive 285.0
  B$_{12}$ deficiency (dietary) 281.1
    pernicious 281.0
von Jaksch's (pseudoleukemia infantum) 285.8
Witts' (achlorhydric anemia) 280.9
Zuelzer (-Ogden) (nutritional megaloblastic anemia) 281.2
Anencephalus, anencephaly 740.0
fetal, affecting management of pregnancy 655.0 ☑
Anergasia — *see also* Psychosis, organic 294.9
senile 290.0
Anesthesia, anesthetic 782.0
complication or reaction NEC 995.22
  due to
    correct substance properly administered 995.22

☑ **Additional Digit Required** — Refer to the Tabular List for Digit Selection   ▽ **Subterms under main terms may continue to next column or page**

2014 ICD-9-CM   **65**

Anesthesia, anesthetic — *continued*
  complication or reaction — *continued*
    due to — *continued*
      overdose or wrong substance given 968.4
      specified anesthetic — *see* Table of Drugs and Chemicals
  cornea 371.81
  death from
    correct substance properly administered 995.4
    during delivery 668.9 ☑
    overdose or wrong substance given 968.4
    specified anesthetic — *see* Table of Drugs and Chemicals
  eye 371.81
  functional 300.11
  hyperesthetic, thalamic 338.0
  hysterical 300.11
  local skin lesion 782.0
  olfactory 781.1
  sexual (psychogenic) 302.72
  shock
    due to
      correct substance properly administered 995.4
      overdose or wrong substance given 968.4
      specified anesthetic — *see* Table of Drugs and Chemicals
  skin 782.0
  tactile 782.0
  testicular 608.9
  thermal 782.0
Anetoderma (maculosum) 701.3
Aneuploidy NEC 758.5
Aneurin deficiency 265.1
Aneurysm (anastomotic) (artery) (cirsoid) (diffuse) (false) (fusiform) (multiple) (ruptured) (saccular) (varicose) 442.9
  abdominal (aorta) 441.4
    ruptured 441.3
    syphilitic 093.0
  aorta, aortic (nonsyphilitic) 441.9
    abdominal 441.4
      dissecting 441.02
      ruptured 441.3
      syphilitic 093.0
    arch 441.2
      ruptured 441.1
    arteriosclerotic NEC 441.9
      ruptured 441.5
    ascending 441.2
      ruptured 441.1
    congenital 747.29
    descending 441.9
      abdominal 441.4
        ruptured 441.3
      ruptured 441.5
      thoracic 441.2
        ruptured 441.1
    dissecting 441.00
      abdominal 441.02
      thoracic 441.01
      thoracoabdominal 441.03
    due to coarctation (aorta) 747.10
    ruptured 441.5
    sinus, right 747.29
    syphilitic 093.0
    thoracoabdominal 441.7
      ruptured 441.6
    thorax, thoracic (arch) (nonsyphilitic) 441.2
      dissecting 441.01
      ruptured 441.1
      syphilitic 093.0
    transverse 441.2
      ruptured 441.1
    valve (heart) (*see also* Endocarditis, aortic) 424.1
  arteriosclerotic NEC 442.9
    cerebral 437.3
      ruptured (*see also* Hemorrhage, subarachnoid) 430

Aneurysm — *continued*
  arteriovenous (congenital) (peripheral) NEC (*see also* Anomaly, arteriovenous) 747.60
    acquired NEC 447.0
      brain 437.3
        ruptured (*see also* Hemorrhage, subarachnoid) 430
      coronary 414.11
      pulmonary 417.0
    brain (cerebral) 747.81
      ruptured (*see also* Hemorrhage, subarachnoid) 430
    coronary 746.85
    pulmonary 747.32
    retina 743.58
    specified site NEC 747.89
      acquired 447.0
    traumatic (*see also* Injury, blood vessel, by site) 904.9
  basal — *see* Aneurysm, brain
  berry (congenital) (ruptured) (*see also* Hemorrhage, subarachnoid) 430
    nonruptured 437.3
  brain 437.3
    arteriosclerotic 437.3
      ruptured (*see also* Hemorrhage, subarachnoid) 430
    arteriovenous 747.81
      acquired 437.3
        ruptured (*see also* Hemorrhage, subarachnoid) 430
      ruptured (*see also* Hemorrhage, subarachnoid) 430
    berry (congenital) (ruptured) (*see also* Hemorrhage, subarachnoid) 430
      nonruptured 437.3
    congenital 747.81
      ruptured (*see also* Hemorrhage, subarachnoid) 430
    meninges 437.3
      ruptured (*see also* Hemorrhage, subarachnoid) 430
    miliary (congenital) (ruptured) (*see also* Hemorrhage, subarachnoid) 430
    mycotic 421.0
      ruptured (*see also* Hemorrhage, subarachnoid) 430
    nonruptured 437.3
    ruptured (*see also* Hemorrhage, subarachnoid) 430
      syphilitic 094.87
    syphilitic (hemorrhage) 094.87
    traumatic — *see* Injury, intracranial
  cardiac (false) (*see also* Aneurysm, heart) 414.10
  carotid artery (common) (external) 442.81
    internal (intracranial portion) 437.3
      extracranial portion 442.81
      ruptured into brain (*see also* Hemorrhage, subarachnoid) 430
    syphilitic 093.89
      intracranial 094.87
  cavernous sinus (*see also* Aneurysm, brain) 437.3
    arteriovenous 747.81
      ruptured (*see also* Hemorrhage, subarachnoid) 430
    congenital 747.81
      ruptured (*see also* Hemorrhage, subarachnoid) 430
  celiac 442.84
  central nervous system, syphilitic 094.89
  cerebral — *see* Aneurysm, brain
  chest — *see* Aneurysm, thorax
  circle of Willis (*see also* Aneurysm, brain) 437.3
    congenital 747.81
      ruptured (*see also* Hemorrhage, subarachnoid) 430
    ruptured (*see also* Hemorrhage, subarachnoid) 430
  common iliac artery 442.2
  congenital (peripheral) NEC 747.60
    brain 747.81

Aneurysm — *continued*
  congenital — *continued*
    brain — *continued*
      ruptured (*see also* Hemorrhage, subarachnoid) 430
      cerebral — *see* Aneurysm, brain, congenital
    coronary 746.85
    gastrointestinal 747.61
    lower limb 747.64
    pulmonary 747.32
    renal 747.62
    retina 743.58
    specified site NEC 747.89
    spinal 747.82
    upper limb 747.63
  conjunctiva 372.74
  conus arteriosus (*see also* Aneurysm, heart) 414.10
  coronary (arteriosclerotic) (artery) (vein) (*see also* Aneurysm, heart) 414.11
    arteriovenous 746.85
    congenital 746.85
    syphilitic 093.89
  cylindrical 441.9
    ruptured 441.5
    syphilitic 093.9
  dissecting 442.9
    aorta 441.00
      abdominal 441.02
      thoracic 441.01
      thoracoabdominal 441.03
    syphilitic 093.9
  ductus arteriosus 747.0
  embolic — *see* Embolism, artery
  endocardial, infective (any valve) 421.0
  femoral 442.3
  gastroduodenal 442.84
  gastroepiploic 442.84
  heart (chronic or with a stated duration of over 8 weeks) (infectional) (wall) 414.10
    acute or with a stated duration of 8 weeks or less (*see also* Infarct, myocardium) 410.9 ☑
    congenital 746.89
    valve — *see* Endocarditis
  hepatic 442.84
  iliac (common) 442.2
  infective (any valve) 421.0
  innominate (nonsyphilitic) 442.89
    syphilitic 093.89
  interauricular septum (*see also* Aneurysm, heart) 414.10
  interventricular septum (*see also* Aneurysm, heart) 414.10
  intracranial — *see* Aneurysm, brain
  intrathoracic (nonsyphilitic) 441.2
    ruptured 441.1
    syphilitic 093.0
  jugular vein (acute) 453.89
    chronic 453.76
  lower extremity 442.3
  lung (pulmonary artery) 417.1
  malignant 093.9
  mediastinal (nonsyphilitic) 442.89
    syphilitic 093.89
  miliary (congenital) (ruptured) (*see also* Hemorrhage, subarachnoid) 430
  mitral (heart) (valve) 424.0
  mural (arteriovenous) (heart) (*see also* Aneurysm, heart) 414.10
  mycotic, any site 421.0
    without endocarditis — *see* Aneurysm by site
    ruptured, brain (*see also* Hemorrhage, subarachnoid) 430
  myocardium (*see also* Aneurysm, heart) 414.10
  neck 442.81
  pancreaticoduodenal 442.84
  patent ductus arteriosus 747.0
  peripheral NEC 442.89
    congenital NEC (*see also* Aneurysm, congenital) 747.60
  popliteal 442.3

Aneurysm — *continued*
  pulmonary 417.1
    arteriovenous 747.32
      acquired 417.0
    syphilitic 093.89
    valve (heart) (*see also* Endocarditis, pulmonary) 424.3
  racemose 442.9
    congenital (peripheral) NEC 747.60
  radial 442.0
  Rasmussen's (*see also* Tuberculosis) 011.2 ☑
  renal 442.1
  retinal (acquired) 362.17
    congenital 743.58
    diabetic 250.5 ☑ *[362.01]*
      due to secondary diabetes 249.5 ☑ *[362.01]*
  sinus, aortic (of Valsalva) 747.29
  specified site NEC 442.89
  spinal (cord) 442.89
    congenital 747.82
    syphilitic (hemorrhage) 094.89
  spleen, splenic 442.83
  subclavian 442.82
    syphilitic 093.89
  superior mesenteric 442.84
  syphilitic 093.9
    aorta 093.0
    central nervous system 094.89
    congenital 090.5
    spine, spinal 094.89
  thoracoabdominal 441.7
    ruptured 441.6
  thorax, thoracic (arch) (nonsyphilitic) 441.2
    dissecting 441.01
    ruptured 441.1
    syphilitic 093.0
  traumatic (complication) (early) — *see* Injury, blood vessel, by site
  tricuspid (heart) (valve) — *see* Endocarditis, tricuspid
  ulnar 442.0
  upper extremity 442.0
  valve, valvular — *see* Endocarditis
  venous 456.8
    congenital NEC (*see also* Aneurysm, congenital) 747.60
  ventricle (arteriovenous) (*see also* Aneurysm, heart) 414.10
  visceral artery NEC 442.84
Angiectasis 459.89
Angiectopia 459.9
Angiitis 447.6
  allergic granulomatous 446.4
  hypersensitivity 446.20
    Goodpasture's syndrome 446.21
    specified NEC 446.29
  necrotizing 446.0
  Wegener's (necrotizing respiratory granulomatosis) 446.4
Angina (attack) (cardiac) (chest) (effort) (heart) (pectoris) (syndrome) (vasomotor) 413.9
  abdominal 557.1
  accelerated 411.1
  agranulocytic 288.03
  aphthous 074.0
  catarrhal 462
  crescendo 411.1
  croupous 464.4
  cruris 443.9
    due to atherosclerosis NEC (*see also* Arteriosclerosis, extremities) 440.20
  decubitus 413.0
  diphtheritic (membranous) 032.0
  equivalent 413.9
  erysipelatous 034.0
  erythematous 462
  exudative, chronic 476.0
  faucium 478.29
  gangrenous 462
    diphtheritic 032.0
  infectious 462
  initial 411.1
  intestinal 557.1
  ludovici 528.3
  Ludwig's 528.3

☑ **Additional Digit Required** — Refer to the Tabular List for Digit Selection   ▽ **Subterms under main terms may continue to next column or page**

66   **2014 ICD-9-CM**

Angina — *continued*
  malignant 462
    diphtheritic 032.0
  membranous 464.4
    diphtheritic 032.0
  mesenteric 557.1
  monocytic 075
  nocturnal 413.0
  phlegmonous 475
    diphtheritic 032.0
  preinfarctional 411.1
  Prinzmetal's 413.1
  progressive 411.1
  pseudomembranous 101
  psychogenic 306.2
  pultaceous, diphtheritic 032.0
  scarlatinal 034.1
  septic 034.0
  simple 462
  stable NEC 413.9
  staphylococcal 462
  streptococcal 034.0
  stridulous, diphtheritic 032.3
  syphilitic 093.9
    congenital 090.5
  tonsil 475
  trachealis 464.4
  unstable 411.1
  variant 413.1
  Vincent's 101
Angioblastoma (M9161/1) — *see* Neoplasm, connective tissue, uncertain behavior
Angiocholecystitis — *see also* Cholecystitis, acute 575.0
Angiocholitis — *see also* Cholecystitis, acute 576.1
Angiodysgensis spinalis 336.1
Angiodysplasia (intestinalis) (intestine) 569.84
  with hemorrhage 569.85
  duodenum 537.82
    with hemorrhage 537.83
  stomach 537.82
    with hemorrhage 537.83
Angioedema (allergic) (any site) (with urticaria) 995.1
  hereditary 277.6
Angioendothelioma (M9130/1) — *see also* Neoplasm, by site, uncertain behavior
  benign (M9130/0) (*see also* Hemangioma, by site) 228.00
  bone (M9260/3) — *see* Neoplasm, bone, malignant
  Ewing's (M9260/3) — *see* Neoplasm, bone, malignant
  nervous system (M9130/0) 228.09
Angiofibroma (M9160/0) — *see also* Neoplasm, by site, benign
  juvenile (M9160/0) 210.7
    specified site — *see* Neoplasm, by site, benign
    unspecified site 210.7
Angiohemophilia (A) (B) 286.4
Angioid streaks (choroid) (retina) 363.43
Angiokeratoma (M9141/0) — *see also* Neoplasm, skin, benign
  corporis diffusum 272.7
Angiokeratosis
  diffuse 272.7
Angioleiomyoma (M8894/0) — *see* Neoplasm, connective tissue, benign
Angioleucitis 683
Angiolipoma (M8861/0) — *see also* Lipoma, by site 214.9
  infiltrating (M8861/1) — *see* Neoplasm, connective tissue, uncertain behavior
Angioma (M9120/0) — *see also* Hemangioma, by site 228.00
  capillary 448.1
  hemorrhagicum hereditaria 448.0
  malignant (M9120/3) — *see* Neoplasm, connective tissue, malignant
  pigmentosum et atrophicum 757.33
  placenta — *see* Placenta, abnormal
  plexiform (M9131/0) — *see* Hemangioma, by site
  senile 448.1

Angioma — *see also* Hemangioma, by site — *continued*
  serpiginosum 709.1
  spider 448.1
  stellate 448.1
Angiomatosis 757.32
  bacillary 083.8
  corporis diffusum universale 272.7
  cutaneocerebral 759.6
  encephalocutaneous 759.6
  encephalofacial 759.6
  encephalotrigeminal 759.6
  hemorrhagic familial 448.0
  hereditary familial 448.0
  heredofamilial 448.0
  meningo-oculofacial 759.6
  multiple sites 228.09
  neuro-oculocutaneous 759.6
  retina (Hippel's disease) 759.6
  retinocerebellosa 759.6
  retinocerebral 759.6
  systemic 228.09
Angiomyolipoma (M8860/0)
  specified site — *see* Neoplasm, connective tissue, benign
  unspecified site 223.0
Angiomyoliposarcoma (M8860/3) — *see* Neoplasm, connective tissue, malignant
Angiomyoma (M8894/0) — *see* Neoplasm, connective tissue, benign
Angiomyosarcoma (M8894/3) — *see* Neoplasm, connective tissue, malignant
Angioneurosis 306.2
Angioneurotic edema (allergic) (any site) (with urticaria) 995.1
  hereditary 277.6
Angiopathia, angiopathy 459.9
  diabetic (peripheral) 250.7 ☑ [443.81]
    due to secondary diabetes 249.7 ☑ [443.81]
  peripheral 443.9
    diabetic 250.7 ☑ [443.81]
      due to secondary diabetes 249.7 ☑ [443.81]
    specified type NEC 443.89
  retinae syphilitica 093.89
  retinalis (juvenilis) 362.18
    background 362.10
    diabetic 250.5 ☑ [362.01]
      due to secondary diabetes 249.5 ☑ [362.01]
    proliferative 362.29
    tuberculous (*see also* Tuberculosis) 017.3 ☑ [362.18]
Angiosarcoma (M9120/3) — *see* Neoplasm, connective tissue, malignant
Angiosclerosis — *see* Arteriosclerosis
Angioscotoma, enlarged 368.42
Angiospasm 443.9
  brachial plexus 353.0
  cerebral 435.9
  cervical plexus 353.2
  nerve
    arm 354.9
      axillary 353.0
      median 354.1
      ulnar 354.2
    autonomic (*see also* Neuropathy, peripheral, autonomic) 337.9
    axillary 353.0
    leg 355.8
      plantar 355.6
    lower extremity — *see* Angiospasm, nerve, leg
    median 354.1
    peripheral NEC 355.9
    spinal NEC 355.9
    sympathetic (*see also* Neuropathy, peripheral, autonomic) 337.9
    ulnar 354.2
    upper extremity — *see* Angiospasm, nerve, arm
  peripheral NEC 443.9
  traumatic 443.9
    foot 443.9
    leg 443.9

Angiospasm — *continued*
  vessel 443.9
Angiospastic disease or edema 443.9
Angle's
  class I 524.21
  class II 524.22
  class III 524.23
Anguillulosis 127.2
Angulation
  cecum (*see also* Obstruction, intestine) 560.9
  coccyx (acquired) 738.6
    congenital 756.19
  femur (acquired) 736.39
    congenital 755.69
  intestine (large) (small) (*see also* Obstruction, intestine) 560.9
  sacrum (acquired) 738.5
    congenital 756.19
  sigmoid (flexure) (*see also* Obstruction, intestine) 560.9
  spine (*see also* Curvature, spine) 737.9
  tibia (acquired) 736.89
    congenital 755.69
  ureter 593.3
  wrist (acquired) 736.09
    congenital 755.59
Angulus infectiosus 686.8
Anhedonia 780.99
Anhidrosis (lid) (neurogenic) (thermogenic) 705.0
Anhydration 276.51
  with
    hypernatremia 276.0
    hyponatremia 276.1
Anhydremia 276.52
  with
    hypernatremia 276.0
    hyponatremia 276.1
Anidrosis 705.0
Aniridia (congenital) 743.45
Anisakiasis (infection) (infestation) 127.1
Anisakis larva infestation 127.1
Aniseikonia 367.32
Anisocoria (pupil) 379.41
  congenital 743.46
Anisocytosis 790.09
Anisometropia (congenital) 367.31
Ankle — *see* condition
Ankyloblepharon (acquired) (eyelid) 374.46
  filiforme (adnatum) (congenital) 743.62
  total 743.62
Ankylodactly — *see also* Syndactylism 755.10
Ankyloglossia 750.0
Ankylosis (fibrous) (osseous) 718.50
  ankle 718.57
  any joint, produced by surgical fusion V45.4
  cricoarytenoid (cartilage) (joint) (larynx) 478.79
  dental 521.6
  ear ossicle NEC 385.22
    malleus 385.21
  elbow 718.52
  finger 718.54
  hip 718.55
  incostapedial joint (infectional) 385.22
  joint, produced by surgical fusion NEC V45.4
  knee 718.56
  lumbosacral (joint) 724.6
  malleus 385.21
  multiple sites 718.59
  postoperative (status) V45.4
  sacroiliac (joint) 724.6
  shoulder 718.51
  specified site NEC 718.58
  spine NEC 724.9
  surgical V45.4
  teeth, tooth (hard tissues) 521.6
  temporomandibular joint 524.61
  wrist 718.53
Ankylostoma — *see* Ancylostoma
Ankylostomiasis (intestinal) — *see* Ancylostomiasis
Ankylurethria — *see also* Stricture, urethra 598.9
Annular — *see also* condition
  detachment, cervix 622.8

Annular — *see also* condition — *continued*
  organ or site, congenital NEC — *see* Distortion
  pancreas (congenital) 751.7
Anodontia (complete) (partial) (vera) 520.0
  with abnormal spacing 524.30
  acquired 525.10
    causing malocclusion 524.30
    due to
      caries 525.13
      extraction 525.10
      periodontal disease 525.12
      trauma 525.11
Anomaly, anomalous (congenital) (unspecified type) 759.9
  abdomen 759.9
  abdominal wall 756.70
  acoustic nerve 742.9
  adrenal (gland) 759.1
  Alder (-Reilly) (leukocyte granulation) 288.2
  alimentary tract 751.9
    lower 751.5
    specified type NEC 751.8
    upper (any part, except tongue) 750.9
      tongue 750.10
        specified type NEC 750.19
  alveolar 524.70
    ridge (process) 525.8
    specified type NEC 524.79
  ankle (joint) 755.69
  anus, anal (canal) 751.5
  aorta, aortic 747.20
    arch 747.21
    coarctation (postductal) (preductal) 747.10
    cusp or valve NEC 746.9
    septum 745.0
    specified type NEC 747.29
  aorticopulmonary septum 745.0
  apertures, diaphragm 756.6
  appendix 751.5
  aqueduct of Sylvius 742.3
    with spina bifida (*see also* Spina bifida) 741.0 ☑
  arm 755.50
    reduction (*see also* Deformity, reduction, upper limb) 755.20
  arteriovenous (congenital) (peripheral) NEC 747.60
    brain 747.81
    cerebral 747.81
    coronary 746.85
    gastrointestinal 747.61
      acquired — *see* Angiodysplasia
    lower limb 747.64
    renal 747.62
    specified site NEC 747.69
    spinal 747.82
    upper limb 747.63
  artery (*see also* Anomaly, peripheral vascular system) NEC 747.60
    brain 747.81
    cerebral 747.81
    coronary 746.85
    eye 743.9
    pulmonary 747.39
    renal 747.62
    retina 743.9
    umbilical 747.5
  arytenoepiglottic folds 748.3
  atrial
    bands 746.9
    folds 746.9
    septa 745.5
  atrioventricular
    canal 745.69
    common 745.69
    conduction 426.7
    excitation 426.7
    septum 745.4
  atrium — *see* Anomaly, atrial
  auditory canal 744.3
    specified type NEC 744.29
      with hearing impairment 744.02
  auricle
    ear 744.3

Angina — Anomaly, anomalous

Anomaly, anomalous — *continued*
  auricle — *continued*
    ear — *continued*
      causing impairment of hearing 744.02
    heart 746.9
      septum 745.5
  autosomes, autosomal NEC 758.5
  Axenfeld's 743.44
  back 759.9
  band
    atrial 746.9
    heart 746.9
    ventricular 746.9
  Bartholin's duct 750.9
  biliary duct or passage 751.60
    atresia 751.61
  bladder (neck) (sphincter) (trigone) 753.9
    specified type NEC 753.8
  blood vessel 747.9
    artery — *see* Anomaly, artery
    peripheral vascular — *see* Anomaly, peripheral vascular system
    vein — *see* Anomaly, vein
  bone NEC 756.9
    ankle 755.69
    arm 755.50
    chest 756.3
    cranium 756.0
    face 756.0
    finger 755.50
    foot 755.67
    forearm 755.50
    frontal 756.0
    head 756.0
    hip 755.63
    leg 755.60
    lumbosacral 756.10
    nose 748.1
    pelvic girdle 755.60
    rachitic 756.4
    rib 756.3
    shoulder girdle 755.50
    skull 756.0
      with
        anencephalus 740.0
        encephalocele 742.0
        hydrocephalus 742.3
          with spina bifida (*see also* Spina bifida) 741.0 ☑
        microcephalus 742.1
    toe 755.66
  brain 742.9
    multiple 742.4
    reduction 742.2
    specified type NEC 742.4
    vessel 747.81
  branchial cleft NEC 744.49
    cyst 744.42
    fistula 744.41
    persistent 744.41
    sinus (external) (internal) 744.41
  breast 757.6
  broad ligament 752.10
    specified type NEC 752.19
  bronchus 748.3
  bulbar septum 745.0
  bulbus cordis 745.9
    persistent (in left ventricle) 745.8
  bursa 756.9
  canal of Nuck 752.9
  canthus 743.9
  capillary NEC (*see also* Anomaly, peripheral vascular system) 747.60
  cardiac 746.9
    septal closure 745.9
      acquired 429.71
    valve NEC 746.9
      pulmonary 746.00
      specified type NEC 746.89
  cardiovascular system 746.9
    complicating pregnancy, childbirth, or puerperium 648.5 ☑
  carpus 755.50
  cartilage, trachea 748.3
  cartilaginous 756.9

Anomaly, anomalous — *continued*
  caruncle, lacrimal, lachrymal 743.9
  cascade stomach 750.7
  cauda equina 742.59
  cecum 751.5
  cerebral (*see also* Anomaly, brain vessels) 747.81
  cerebrovascular system 747.81
  cervix (uterus) 752.40
    with doubling of vagina and uterus 752.2
    in pregnancy or childbirth 654.6 ☑
      affecting fetus or newborn 763.89
      causing obstructed labor 660.2 ☑
        affecting fetus or newborn 763.1
  Chédiak-Higashi (-Steinbrinck) (congenital gigantism of peroxidase granules) 288.2
  cheek 744.9
  chest (wall) 756.3
  chin 744.9
    specified type NEC 744.89
  chordae tendineae 746.9
  choroid 743.9
    plexus 742.9
  chromosomes, chromosomal 758.9
    13 (13-15) 758.1
    18 (16-18) 758.2
    21 or 22 758.0
    autosomes NEC (*see also* Abnormal, autosomes) 758.5
      deletion 758.39
      Christchurch 758.39
      D₁ 758.1
      E₃ 758.2
      G 758.0
    mitochondrial 758.9
    mosaics 758.89
    sex 758.81
      complement, XO 758.6
      complement, XXX 758.81
      complement, XXY 758.7
      complement, XYY 758.81
      gonadal dysgenesis 758.6
      Klinefelter's 758.7
      Turner's 758.6
    trisomy 21 758.0
  cilia 743.9
  circulatory system 747.9
    specified type NEC 747.89
  clavicle 755.51
  clitoris 752.40
  coccyx 756.10
  colon 751.5
  common duct 751.60
  communication
    coronary artery 746.85
    left ventricle with right atrium 745.4
  concha (ear) 744.3
  connection
    renal vessels with kidney 747.62
    total pulmonary venous 747.41
  connective tissue 756.9
    specified type NEC 756.89
  cornea 743.9
    shape 743.41
    size 743.41
    specified type NEC 743.49
  coronary
    artery 746.85
    vein 746.89
  cranium — *see* Anomaly, skull
  cricoid cartilage 748.3
  cushion, endocardial 745.60
    specified type NEC 745.69
  cystic duct 751.60
  dental arch 524.20
    specified NEC 524.29
  dental arch relationship 524.20
    angle's class I 524.21
    angle's class II 524.22
    angle's class III 524.23
    articulation
      anterior 524.27
      posterior 524.27
      reverse 524.27

Anomaly, anomalous — *continued*
  dental arch relationship — *continued*
    disto-occlusion 524.22
      division I 524.22
      division II 524.22
    excessive horizontal overlap 524.26
    interarch distance (excessive) (inadequate) 524.28
    mesio-occlusion 524.23
    neutro-occlusion 524.21
    open
      anterior occlusal relationship 524.24
      posterior occlusal relationship 524.25
    specified NEC 524.29
  dentition 520.6
  dentofacial NEC 524.9
    functional 524.50
    specified type NEC 524.89
  dermatoglyphic 757.2
  Descemet's membrane 743.9
    specified type NEC 743.49
  development
    cervix 752.40
    vagina 752.40
    vulva 752.40
  diaphragm, diaphragmatic (apertures) NEC 756.6
  digestive organ(s) or system 751.9
    lower 751.5
    specified type NEC 751.8
    upper 750.9
  distribution, coronary artery 746.85
  ductus
    arteriosus 747.0
    Botalli 747.0
  duodenum 751.5
  dura 742.9
    brain 742.4
    spinal cord 742.59
  ear 744.3
    causing impairment of hearing 744.00
      specified type NEC 744.09
    external 744.3
      causing impairment of hearing 744.02
      specified type NEC 744.29
    inner (causing impairment of hearing) 744.05
    middle, except ossicles (causing impairment of hearing) 744.03
      ossicles 744.04
    ossicles 744.04
    prominent auricle 744.29
    specified type NEC 744.29
      with hearing impairment 744.09
  Ebstein's (heart) 746.2
    tricuspid valve 746.2
  ectodermal 757.9
  Eisenmenger's (ventricular septal defect) 745.4
  ejaculatory duct 752.9
    specified type NEC 752.89
  elbow (joint) 755.50
  endocardial cushion 745.60
    specified type NEC 745.69
  endocrine gland NEC 759.2
  epididymis 752.9
  epiglottis 748.3
  esophagus 750.9
    specified type NEC 750.4
  Eustachian tube 744.3
    specified type NEC 744.24
  eye (any part) 743.9
    adnexa 743.9
      specified type NEC 743.69
    anophthalmos 743.00
    anterior
      chamber and related structures 743.9
        angle 743.9
          specified type NEC 743.44
        specified type NEC 743.44
      segment 743.9
        combined 743.48
        multiple 743.48
        specified type NEC 743.49
    cataract (*see also* Cataract) 743.30

Anomaly, anomalous — *continued*
  eye — *continued*
    glaucoma (*see also* Buphthalmia) 743.20
    lid 743.9
      specified type NEC 743.63
    microphthalmos (*see also* Microphthalmos) 743.10
    posterior segment 743.9
      specified type NEC 743.59
      vascular 743.58
      vitreous 743.9
        specified type NEC 743.51
    ptosis (eyelid) 743.61
    retina 743.9
      specified type NEC 743.59
    sclera 743.9
      specified type NEC 743.47
    specified type NEC 743.8
  eyebrow 744.89
  eyelid 743.9
    specified type NEC 743.63
  face (any part) 744.9
    bone(s) 756.0
    specified type NEC 744.89
  fallopian tube 752.10
    specified type NEC 752.19
  fascia 756.9
    specified type NEC 756.89
  femur 755.60
  fibula 755.60
  finger 755.50
    supernumerary 755.01
    webbed (*see also* Syndactylism, fingers) 755.11
  fixation, intestine 751.4
  flexion (joint) 755.9
    hip or thigh (*see also* Dislocation, hip, congenital) 754.30
  folds, heart 746.9
  foot 755.67
  foramen
    Botalli 745.5
    ovale 745.5
  forearm 755.50
  forehead (*see also* Anomaly, skull) 756.0
  form, teeth 520.2
  fovea centralis 743.9
  frontal bone (*see also* Anomaly, skull) 756.0
  gallbladder 751.60
  Gartner's duct 752.41
  gastrointestinal tract 751.9
    specified type NEC 751.8
    vessel 747.61
  genitalia, genital organ(s) or system
    female 752.9
      external 752.40
        specified type NEC 752.49
      internal NEC 752.9
    male (external and internal) 752.9
      epispadias 752.62
      hidden penis 752.65
      hydrocele, congenital 778.6
      hypospadias 752.61
      micropenis 752.64
      testis, undescended 752.51
        retractile 752.52
      specified type NEC 752.89
  genitourinary NEC 752.9
  Gerbode 745.4
  globe (eye) 743.9
  glottis 748.3
  granulation or granulocyte, genetic 288.2
    constitutional 288.2
    leukocyte 288.2
  gum 750.9
  gyri 742.9
  hair 757.9
    specified type NEC 757.4
  hand 755.50
  hard tissue formation in pulp 522.3
  head (*see also* Anomaly, skull) 756.0
  heart 746.9
    auricle 746.9
    bands 746.9
    fibroelastosis cordis 425.3
    folds 746.9

Anomaly, anomalous — *continued*
  heart — *continued*
    malposition 746.87
    maternal, affecting fetus or newborn 760.3
    obstructive NEC 746.84
    patent ductus arteriosus (Botalli) 747.0
    septum 745.9
      acquired 429.71
      aortic 745.0
      aorticopulmonary 745.0
      atrial 745.5
      auricular 745.5
      between aorta and pulmonary artery 745.0
      endocardial cushion type 745.60
        specified type NEC 745.69
      interatrial 745.5
      interventricular 745.4
        with pulmonary stenosis or atresia, dextraposition of aorta, and hypertrophy of right ventricle 745.2
        acquired 429.71
      specified type NEC 745.8
      ventricular 745.4
        with pulmonary stenosis or atresia, dextraposition of aorta, and hypertrophy of right ventricle 745.2
        acquired 429.71
    specified type NEC 746.89
    tetralogy of Fallot 745.2
    valve NEC 746.9
      aortic 746.9
        atresia 746.89
        bicuspid valve 746.4
        insufficiency 746.4
        specified type NEC 746.89
        stenosis 746.3
          subaortic 746.81
          supravalvular 747.22
      mitral 746.9
        atresia 746.89
        insufficiency 746.6
        specified type NEC 746.89
        stenosis 746.5
      pulmonary 746.00
        atresia 746.01
        insufficiency 746.09
        stenosis 746.02
          infundibular 746.83
          subvalvular 746.83
      tricuspid 746.9
        atresia 746.1
        stenosis 746.1
    ventricle 746.9
  heel 755.67
  Hegglin's 288.2
  hemianencephaly 740.0
  hemicephaly 740.0
  hemicrania 740.0
  hepatic duct 751.60
  hip (joint) 755.63
  hourglass
    bladder 753.8
    gallbladder 751.69
    stomach 750.7
  humerus 755.50
  hymen 752.40
  hypersegmentation of neutrophils, hereditary 288.2
  hypophyseal 759.2
  ileocecal (coil) (valve) 751.5
  ileum (intestine) 751.5
  ilium 755.60
  integument 757.9
    specified type NEC 757.8
  interarch distance (excessive) (inadequate) 524.28
  intervertebral cartilage or disc 756.10
  intestine (large) (small) 751.5
    fixational type 751.4
  iris 743.9
    specified type NEC 743.46
  ischium 755.60

Anomaly, anomalous — *continued*
  jaw-cranial base relationship 524.10
    specified NEC 524.19
  jaw NEC 524.9
    closure 524.51
    size (major) NEC 524.00
    specified type NEC 524.89
  jejunum 751.5
  joint 755.9
    hip
      dislocation (*see also* Dislocation, hip, congenital) 754.30
      predislocation (*see also* Subluxation, congenital, hip) 754.32
      preluxation (*see also* Subluxation, congenital, hip) 754.32
      subluxation (*see also* Subluxation, congenital, hip) 754.32
    lumbosacral 756.10
      spondylolisthesis 756.12
      spondylosis 756.11
    multiple arthrogryposis 754.89
    sacroiliac 755.69
  Jordan's 288.2
  kidney(s) (calyx) (pelvis) 753.9
    vessel 747.62
  Klippel-Feil (brevicollis) 756.16
  knee (joint) 755.64
  labium (majus) (minus) 752.40
  labyrinth, membranous (causing impairment of hearing) 744.05
  lacrimal
    apparatus, duct or passage 743.9
      specified type NEC 743.65
    gland 743.9
      specified type NEC 743.64
  Langdon Down (mongolism) 758.0
  larynx, laryngeal (muscle) 748.3
    web, webbed 748.2
  leg (lower) (upper) 755.60
    reduction NEC (*see also* Deformity, reduction, lower limb) 755.30
  lens 743.9
    shape 743.36
    specified type NEC 743.39
  leukocytes, genetic 288.2
    granulation (constitutional) 288.2
  lid (fold) 743.9
  ligament 756.9
    broad 752.10
    round 752.9
  limb, except reduction deformity 755.9
    lower 755.60
      reduction deformity (*see also* Deformity, reduction, lower limb) 755.30
      specified type NEC 755.69
    upper 755.50
      reduction deformity (*see also* Deformity, reduction, upper limb) 755.20
      specified type NEC 755.59
  lip 750.9
    harelip (*see also* Cleft, lip) 749.10
    specified type NEC 750.26
  liver (duct) 751.60
    atresia 751.69
  lower extremity 755.60
    vessel 747.64
  lumbosacral (joint) (region) 756.10
  lung (fissure) (lobe) NEC 748.60
    agenesis 748.5
    specified type NEC 748.69
  lymphatic system 759.9
  Madelung's (radius) 755.54
  mandible 524.9
    size NEC 524.00
  maxilla 524.9
    size NEC 524.00
  May (-Hegglin) 288.2
  meatus urinarius 753.9
    specified type NEC 753.8
  meningeal bands or folds, constriction of 742.8
  meninges 742.9
    brain 742.4

Anomaly, anomalous — *continued*
  meninges — *continued*
    spinal 742.59
  meningocele (*see also* Spina bifida) 741.9 ☑
    acquired 349.2
  mesentery 751.9
  metacarpus 755.50
  metatarsus 755.67
  middle ear, except ossicles (causing impairment of hearing) 744.03
    ossicles 744.04
  mitral (leaflets) (valve) 746.9
    atresia 746.89
    insufficiency 746.6
    specified type NEC 746.89
    stenosis 746.5
  mouth 750.9
    specified type NEC 750.26
  multiple NEC 759.7
    specified type NEC 759.89
  muscle 756.9
    eye 743.9
      specified type NEC 743.69
    specified type NEC 756.89
  musculoskeletal system, except limbs 756.9
    specified type NEC 756.9
  nail 757.9
    specified type NEC 757.5
  narrowness, eyelid 743.62
  nasal sinus or septum 748.1
  neck (any part) 744.9
    specified type NEC 744.89
  nerve 742.9
    acoustic 742.9
      specified type NEC 742.8
    optic 742.9
      specified type NEC 742.8
    specified type NEC 742.8
  nervous system NEC 742.9
    brain 742.9
      specified type NEC 742.4
    specified type NEC 742.8
  neurological 742.9
  nipple 757.6
  nonteratogenic NEC 754.89
  nose, nasal (bone) (cartilage) (septum) (sinus) 748.1
  ocular muscle 743.9
  omphalomesenteric duct 751.0
  opening, pulmonary veins 747.49
  optic
    disc 743.9
      specified type NEC 743.57
    nerve 742.9
  opticociliary vessels 743.9
  orbit (eye) 743.9
    specified type NEC 743.66
  organ
    of Corti (causing impairment of hearing) 744.05
    or site 759.9
      specified type NEC 759.89
  origin
    both great arteries from same ventricle 745.11
    coronary artery 746.85
    innominate artery 747.69
    left coronary artery from pulmonary artery 746.85
    pulmonary artery 747.39
    renal vessels 747.62
    subclavian artery (left) (right) 747.21
  osseous meatus (ear) 744.03
  ovary 752.0
  oviduct 752.10
  palate (hard) (soft) 750.9
    cleft (*see also* Cleft, palate) 749.00
  pancreas (duct) 751.7
  papillary muscles 746.9
  parathyroid gland 759.2
  paraurethral ducts 753.9
  parotid (gland) 750.9
  patella 755.64
  Pelger-Huët (hereditary hyposegmentation) 288.2
  pelvic girdle 755.60

Anomaly, anomalous — *continued*
  pelvic girdle — *continued*
    specified type NEC 755.69
  pelvis (bony) 755.60
    complicating delivery 653.0 ☑
    rachitic 268.1
      fetal 756.4
  penis (glans) 752.69
  pericardium 746.89
  peripheral vascular system NEC 747.60
    gastrointestinal 747.61
    lower limb 747.64
    renal 747.62
    specified site NEC 747.69
    spinal 747.82
    upper limb 747.63
  Peter's 743.44
  pharynx 750.9
    branchial cleft 744.41
    specified type NEC 750.29
  Pierre Robin 756.0
  pigmentation 709.00
    congenital 757.33
    specified NEC 709.09
  pituitary (gland) 759.2
  pleural folds 748.8
  portal vein 747.40
  position tooth, teeth 524.30
    crowding 524.31
    displacement 524.30
      horizontal 524.33
      vertical 524.34
    distance
      interocclusal
        excessive 524.37
        insufficient 524.36
      excessive spacing 524.32
    rotation 524.35
    specified NEC 524.39
  preauricular sinus 744.46
  prepuce 752.9
  prostate 752.9
  pulmonary 748.60
    artery 747.39
    circulation 747.39
    specified type NEC 748.69
    valve 746.00
      atresia 746.01
      insufficiency 746.09
      specified type NEC 746.09
      stenosis 746.02
        infundibular 746.83
        subvalvular 746.83
    vein 747.40
    venous
      connection 747.49
        partial 747.42
        total 747.41
      return 747.49
        partial 747.42
        total (TAPVR) (complete) (subdiaphragmatic) (supradiaphragmatic) 747.41
  pupil 743.9
  pylorus 750.9
    hypertrophy 750.5
    stenosis 750.5
  rachitic, fetal 756.4
  radius 755.50
  rectovaginal (septum) 752.40
  rectum 751.5
  refraction 367.9
  renal 753.9
    vessel 747.62
  respiratory system 748.9
    specified type NEC 748.8
  rib 756.3
    cervical 756.2
  Rieger's 743.44
  rings, trachea 748.3
  rotation (*see also* Malrotation)
    hip or thigh (*see also* Subluxation, congenital, hip) 754.32
  round ligament 752.9
  sacroiliac (joint) 755.69
  sacrum 756.10

Anomaly, anomalous — *continued*
saddle
  back 754.2
  nose 754.0
    syphilitic 090.5
salivary gland or duct 750.9
  specified type NEC 750.26
scapula 755.50
sclera 743.9
  specified type NEC 743.47
scrotum 752.9
sebaceous gland 757.9
seminal duct or tract 752.9
sense organs 742.9
  specified type NEC 742.8
septum
  heart — *see* Anomaly, heart, septum
  nasal 748.1
sex chromosomes NEC (*see also* Anomaly,
    chromosomes) 758.81
shoulder (girdle) (joint) 755.50
  specified type NEC 755.59
sigmoid (flexure) 751.5
sinus of Valsalva 747.29
site NEC 759.9
skeleton generalized NEC 756.50
skin (appendage) 757.9
  specified type NEC 757.39
skull (bone) 756.0
  with
    anencephalus 740.0
    encephalocele 742.0
    hydrocephalus 742.3
      with spina bifida (*see also* Spina
        bifida) 741.0 ☑
    microcephalus 742.1
specified type NEC
  adrenal (gland) 759.1
  alimentary tract (complete) (partial)
    751.8
    lower 751.5
    upper 750.8
  ankle 755.69
  anus, anal (canal) 751.5
  aorta, aortic 747.29
    arch 747.21
  appendix 751.5
  arm 755.59
  artery (peripheral) NEC (*see also*
    Anomaly, peripheral vascular
    system) 747.60
    brain 747.81
    coronary 746.85
    eye 743.58
    pulmonary 747.39
    retinal 743.58
    umbilical 747.5
  auditory canal 744.29
    causing impairment of hearing
      744.02
  bile duct or passage 751.69
  bladder 753.8
    neck 753.8
  bone(s) 756.9
    arm 755.59
    face 756.0
    leg 755.69
    pelvic girdle 755.69
    shoulder girdle 755.59
    skull 756.0
      with
        anencephalus 740.0
        encephalocele 742.0
        hydrocephalus 742.3
          with spina bifida (*see also*
            Spina bifida)
            741.0 ☑
        microcephalus 742.1
  brain 742.4
  breast 757.6
  broad ligament 752.19
  bronchus 748.3
  canal of Nuck 752.89
  cardiac septal closure 745.8
  carpus 755.59
  cartilaginous 756.9

Anomaly, anomalous — *continued*
specified type — *continued*
  cecum 751.5
  cervix 752.49
  chest (wall) 756.3
  chin 744.89
  ciliary body 743.46
  circulatory system 747.89
  clavicle 755.51
  clitoris 752.49
  coccyx 756.19
  colon 751.5
  common duct 751.69
  connective tissue 756.89
  cricoid cartilage 748.3
  cystic duct 751.69
  diaphragm 756.6
  digestive organ(s) or tract 751.8
    lower 751.5
    upper 750.8
  duodenum 751.5
  ear 744.29
    auricle 744.29
      causing impairment of hearing
        744.02
    causing impairment of hearing
      744.09
    inner (causing impairment of hear-
      ing) 744.05
    middle, except ossicles 744.03
      ossicles 744.04
  ejaculatory duct 752.89
  endocrine 759.2
  epiglottis 748.3
  esophagus 750.4
  Eustachian tube 744.24
  eye 743.8
    lid 743.63
    muscle 743.69
  face 744.89
    bone(s) 756.0
  fallopian tube 752.19
  fascia 756.89
  femur 755.69
  fibula 755.69
  finger 755.59
  foot 755.67
  fovea centralis 743.55
  gallbladder 751.69
  Gartner's duct 752.89
  gastrointestinal tract 751.8
  genitalia, genital organ(s)
    female 752.89
      external 752.49
      internal NEC 752.89
    male 752.89
      penis 752.69
      scrotal transposition 752.81
  genitourinary tract NEC 752.89
  glottis 748.3
  hair 757.4
  hand 755.59
  heart 746.89
    valve NEC 746.89
      pulmonary 746.09
  hepatic duct 751.69
  hydatid of Morgagni 752.89
  hymen 752.49
  integument 757.8
  intestine (large) (small) 751.5
    fixational type 751.4
  iris 743.46
  jejunum 751.5
  joint 755.8
  kidney 753.3
  knee 755.64
  labium (majus) (minus) 752.49
  labyrinth, membranous 744.05
  larynx 748.3
  leg 755.69
  lens 743.39
  limb, except reduction deformity 755.8
    lower 755.69
      reduction deformity (*see also* De-
        formity, reduction, lower
        limb) 755.30

Anomaly, anomalous — *continued*
specified type — *continued*
  limb, except reduction deformity —
    continued
    upper 755.59
      reduction deformity (*see also* De-
        formity, reduction, upper
        limb) 755.20
  lip 750.26
  liver 751.69
  lung (fissure) (lobe) 748.69
  meatus urinarius 753.8
  metacarpus 755.59
  mouth 750.26
  Müllerian
    cervix 752.49
    uterus 752.39
    vagina 752.49
  muscle 756.89
    eye 743.69
  musculoskeletal system, except limbs
    756.9
  nail 757.5
  neck 744.89
  nerve 742.8
    acoustic 742.8
    optic 742.8
  nervous system 742.8
  nipple 757.6
  nose 748.1
  organ NEC 759.89
    of Corti 744.05
  osseous meatus (ear) 744.03
  ovary 752.0
  oviduct 752.19
  pancreas 751.7
  parathyroid 759.2
  patella 755.64
  pelvic girdle 755.69
  penis 752.69
  pericardium 746.89
  peripheral vascular system NEC (*see also*
    Anomaly, peripheral vascular
    system) 747.60
  pharynx 750.29
  pituitary 759.2
  prostate 752.89
  radius 755.59
  rectum 751.5
  respiratory system 748.8
  rib 756.3
  round ligament 752.89
  sacrum 756.19
  salivary duct or gland 750.26
  scapula 755.59
  sclera 743.47
  scrotum 752.89
    transposition 752.81
  seminal duct or tract 752.89
  shoulder girdle 755.59
  site NEC 759.89
  skin 757.39
  skull (bone(s)) 756.0
    with
      anencephalus 740.0
      encephalocele 742.0
      hydrocephalus 742.3
        with spina bifida (*see also*
          Spina bifida) 741.0 ☑
      microcephalus 742.1
  specified organ or site NEC 759.89
  spermatic cord 752.89
  spinal cord 742.59
  spine 756.19
  spleen 759.0
  sternum 756.3
  stomach 750.7
  tarsus 755.67
  tendon 756.89
  testis 752.89
  thorax (wall) 756.3
  thymus 759.2
  thyroid (gland) 759.2
    cartilage 748.3
  tibia 755.69
  toe 755.66

Anomaly, anomalous — *continued*
specified type — *continued*
  tongue 750.19
  trachea (cartilage) 748.3
  ulna 755.59
  urachus 753.7
  ureter 753.4
    obstructive 753.29
  urethra 753.8
    obstructive 753.6
  urinary tract 753.8
  uterus (Müllerian) 752.39
  uvula 750.26
  vagina 752.49
  vascular NEC (*see also* Anomaly, periph-
    eral vascular system) 747.60
    brain 747.81
  vas deferens 752.89
  vein(s) (peripheral) NEC (*see also*
    Anomaly, peripheral vascular
    system) 747.60
    brain 747.81
    great 747.49
    portal 747.49
    pulmonary 747.49
    vena cava (inferior) (superior) 747.49
  vertebra 756.19
  vulva 752.49
spermatic cord 752.9
spine, spinal 756.10
  column 756.10
  cord 742.9
    meningocele (*see also* Spina bifida)
      741.9 ☑
    specified type NEC 742.59
    spina bifida (*see also* Spina bifida)
      741.9 ☑
    vessel 747.82
  meninges 742.59
  nerve root 742.9
spleen 759.0
Sprengel's 755.52
sternum 756.3
stomach 750.9
  specified type NEC 750.7
submaxillary gland 750.9
superior vena cava 747.40
talipes — *see* Talipes
tarsus 755.67
  with complete absence of distal ele-
    ments 755.31
teeth, tooth NEC 520.9
  position 524.30
    crowding 524.31
    displacement 524.30
      horizontal 524.33
      vertical 524.34
    distance
      interocclusal
        excessive 524.37
        insufficient 524.36
    excessive spacing 524.32
    rotation 524.35
    specified NEC 524.39
    spacing 524.30
tendon 756.9
  specified type NEC 756.89
termination
  coronary artery 746.85
testis 752.9
thebesian valve 746.9
thigh 755.60
  flexion (*see also* Subluxation, congenital,
    hip) 754.32
thorax (wall) 756.3
throat 750.9
thumb 755.50
  supernumerary 755.01
thymus gland 759.2
thyroid (gland) 759.2
  cartilage 748.3
tibia 755.60
  saber 090.5
toe 755.66
  supernumerary 755.02

Anomaly, anomalous — *continued*
toe — *continued*
webbed (*see also* Syndactylism, toes)
755.13
tongue 750.10
specified type NEC 750.19
trachea, tracheal 748.3
cartilage 748.3
rings 748.3
tragus 744.3
transverse aortic arch 747.21
trichromata 368.59
trichromatopsia 368.59
tricuspid (leaflet) (valve) 746.9
atresia 746.1
Ebstein's 746.2
specified type NEC 746.89
stenosis 746.1
trunk 759.9
Uhl's (hypoplasia of myocardium, right
ventricle) 746.84
ulna 755.50
umbilicus 759.9
artery 747.5
union, trachea with larynx 748.3
unspecified site 759.9
upper extremity 755.50
vessel 747.63
urachus 753.7
specified type NEC 753.7
ureter 753.9
obstructive 753.20
specified type NEC 753.4
obstructive 753.29
urethra (valve) 753.9
obstructive 753.6
specified type NEC 753.8
urinary tract or system (any part, except
urachus) 753.9
specified type NEC 753.8
urachus 753.7
uterus 752.39
with only one functioning horn 752.33
in pregnancy or childbirth 654.0 ☑
affecting fetus or newborn 763.89
causing obstructed labor 660.2 ☑
affecting fetus or newborn 763.1
uvula 750.9
vagina 752.40
valleculae 748.3
valve (heart) NEC 746.9
formation, ureter 753.29
pulmonary 746.00
specified type NEC 746.89
vascular NEC (*see also* Anomaly, peripheral
vascular system) 747.60
ring 747.21
vas deferens 752.9
vein(s) (peripheral) NEC (*see also* Anomaly,
peripheral vascular system) 747.60
brain 747.81
cerebral 747.81
coronary 746.89
great 747.40
specified type NEC 747.49
portal 747.40
pulmonary 747.40
retina 743.9
vena cava (inferior) (superior) 747.40
venous — *see* Anomaly, vein
venous return (pulmonary) 747.49
partial 747.42
total 747.41
ventricle, ventricular (heart) 746.9
bands 746.9
folds 746.9
septa 745.4
vertebra 756.10
vesicourethral orifice 753.9
vessels NEC (*see also* Anomaly, peripheral
vascular system) 747.60
optic papilla 743.9
vitelline duct 751.0
vitreous humor 743.9
specified type NEC 743.51
vulva 752.40

Anomaly, anomalous — *continued*
wrist (joint) 755.50
Anomia 784.69
Anonychia 757.5
acquired 703.8
Anophthalmos, anophthalmus (clinical)
(congenital) (globe) 743.00
acquired V45.78
Anopsia (altitudinal) (quadrant) 368.46
Anorchia 752.89
Anorchism, anorchidism 752.89
Anorexia 783.0
hysterical 300.11
nervosa 307.1
Anosmia — *see also* Disturbance, sensation
781.1
hysterical 300.11
postinfectional 478.9
psychogenic 306.7
traumatic 951.8
Anosognosia 780.99
Anosphrasia 781.1
Anosteoplasia 756.50
Anotia 744.09
Anovulatory cycle 628.0
Anoxemia 799.02
newborn 770.88
Anoxia 799.02
altitude 993.2
cerebral 348.1
with
abortion — *see* Abortion, by type,
with specified complication
NEC
ectopic pregnancy (*see also* categories 633.0–633.9) 639.8
molar pregnancy (*see also* categories
630–632) 639.8
complicating
delivery (cesarean) (instrumental)
669.4 ☑
ectopic or molar pregnancy 639.8
obstetric anesthesia or sedation
668.2 ☑
during or resulting from a procedure
997.01
following
abortion 639.8
ectopic or molar pregnancy 639.8
newborn (*see also* Distress, fetal, liveborn
infant) 770.88
due to drowning 994.1
fetal, affecting newborn 770.88
heart — *see* Insufficiency, coronary
high altitude 993.2
intrauterine
fetal death (before onset of labor) 768.0
during labor 768.1
liveborn infant — *see* Distress, fetal,
liveborn infant
myocardial — *see* Insufficiency, coronary
newborn 768.9
mild or moderate 768.6
severe 768.5
pathological 799.02
Anteflexion — *see* Anteversion
Antenatal
care, normal pregnancy V22.1
first V22.0
sampling
chorionic villus V28.89
screening of mother (for) V28.9
based on amniocentesis NEC V28.2
chromosomal anomalies V28.0
raised alphafetoprotein levels V28.1
chromosomal anomalies V28.0
fetal growth retardation using ulatrasonics V28.4
genomic V28.89
isoimmunization V28.5
malformations using ulatrasonics V28.3
proteomic V28.89
raised alphafetoprotein levels in amniotic fluid V28.1
risk
pre-term labor V28.82

Antenatal — *continued*
screening of mother — *continued*
specified condition NEC V28.89
Streptococcus B V28.6
survey
fetal anatomic V28.81
testing
nuchal translucency V28.89
Antepartum — *see* condition
Anterior — *see also* condition
spinal artery compression syndrome 721.1
Antero-occlusion 524.24
Anteversion
cervix — *see* Anteversion, uterus
femur (neck), congenital 755.63
uterus, uterine (cervix) (postinfectional)
(postpartal, old) 621.6
congenital 752.39
in pregnancy or childbirth 654.4 ☑
affecting fetus or newborn 763.89
causing obstructed labor 660.2 ☑
affecting fetus or newborn 763.1
Anthracosilicosis (occupational) 500
Anthracosis (lung) (occupational) 500
lingua 529.3
Anthrax 022.9
with pneumonia 022.1 [484.5]
colitis 022.2
cutaneous 022.0
gastrointestinal 022.2
intestinal 022.2
pulmonary 022.1
respiratory 022.1
septicemia 022.3
specified manifestation NEC 022.8
Anthropoid pelvis 755.69
with disproportion (fetopelvic) 653.2 ☑
affecting fetus or newborn 763.1
causing obstructed labor 660.1 ☑
affecting fetus or newborn 763.1
Anthropophobia 300.29
Antibioma, breast 611.0
Antibodies
maternal (blood group) (*see also* Incompatibility) 656.2 ☑
anti-D, cord blood 656.1 ☑
fetus or newborn 773.0
Antibody
anticardiolipin 795.79
with
hemorrhagic disorder 286.53
hypercoagulable state 289.81
antiphosphatidylglycerol 795.79
with
hemorrhagic disorder 286.53
hypercoagulable state 289.81
antiphosphatidylinositol 795.79
with
hemorrhagic disorder 286.53
hypercoagulable state 289.81
antiphosphatidylserine 795.79
with
hemorrhagic disorder 286.53
hypercoagulable state 289.81
antiphospholipid 795.79
with
hemorrhagic disorder 286.53
hypercoagulable state 289.81
deficiency syndrome
agammaglobulinemic 279.00
congenital 279.04
hypogammaglobulinemic 279.00
Anticoagulant
intrinsic, circulating, causing hemorrhagic
disorder (*see also* Circulating, anticoagulants) 286.59
lupus (LAC) 795.79
with
hemorrhagic disorder 286.53
hypercoagulable state 289.81
Antimongolism syndrome 758.39
Antimonial cholera 985.4
Antisocial personality 301.7
Antithrombinemia — *see also* Circulating anticoagulants 286.59

Antithromboplastinemia — *see also* Circulating anticoagulants 286.59
Antithromboplastinogenemia — *see also*
Circulating anticoagulants 286.59
Antitoxin complication or reaction — *see*
Complications, vaccination
Anton (-Babinski) syndrome (hemiasomatognosia) 307.9
Antritis (chronic) 473.0
maxilla 473.0
acute 461.0
stomach 535.4 ☑
Antrum, antral — *see* condition
Anuria 788.5
with
abortion — *see* Abortion, by type, with
renal failure
ectopic pregnancy (*see also* categories
633.0–633.9) 639.3
molar pregnancy (*see also* categories
630–632) 639.3
calculus (impacted) (recurrent) 592.9
kidney 592.0
ureter 592.1
congenital 753.3
due to a procedure 997.5
following
abortion 639.3
ectopic or molar pregnancy 639.3
newborn 753.3
postrenal 593.4
puerperal, postpartum, childbirth 669.3 ☑
specified as due to a procedure 997.5
sulfonamide
correct substance properly administered
788.5
overdose or wrong substance given or
taken 961.0
traumatic (following crushing) 958.5
Anus, anal — *see also* condition
high risk human papillomavirus (HPV) DNA
test positive 796.75
low risk human papillomavirus (HPV) DNA
test positive 796.79
Anusitis 569.49
Anxiety (neurosis) (reaction) (state) 300.00
alcohol-induced 291.89
depression 300.4
drug-induced 292.89
due to or associated with physical condition
293.84
generalized 300.02
hysteria 300.20
in
acute stress reaction 308.0
transient adjustment reaction 309.24
panic type 300.01
separation, abnormal 309.21
syndrome (organic) (transient) 293.84
Aorta, aortic — *see* condition
Aortectasia — *see also* Ectasia, aortic 447.70
with aneurysm 441.9
Aortitis (nonsyphilitic) 447.6
arteriosclerotic 440.0
calcific 447.6
Döhle-Heller 093.1
luetic 093.1
rheumatic (*see also* Endocarditis, acute,
rheumatic) 391.1
rheumatoid — *see* Arthritis, rheumatoid
specific 093.1
syphilitic 093.1
congenital 090.5
Apathetic 799.25
thyroid storm (*see also* Thyrotoxicosis)
242.9 ☑
Apathy 799.25
Apepsia 536.8
achlorhydric 536.0
psychogenic 306.4
Aperistalsis, esophagus 530.0
Apert-Gallais syndrome (adrenogenital) 255.2
Apertognathia 524.20
Apert's syndrome (acrocephalosyndactyly)
755.55
Aphagia 787.20

Aphagia — *continued*
psychogenic 307.1
Aphakia (acquired) (bilateral) (postoperative) (unilateral) 379.31
congenital 743.35
Aphalangia (congenital) 755.4
lower limb (complete) (intercalary) (partial) (terminal) 755.39
meaning all digits (complete) (partial) 755.31
transverse 755.31
upper limb (complete) (intercalary) (partial) (terminal) 755.29
meaning all digits (complete) (partial) 755.21
transverse 755.21
Aphasia (amnestic) (ataxic) (auditory) (Broca's) (choreatic) (classic) (expressive) (global) (ideational) (ideokinetic) (ideomotor) (jargon) (motor) (nominal) (receptive) (semantic) (sensory) (syntactic) (verbal) (visual) (Wernicke's) 784.3
developmental 315.31
syphilis, tertiary 094.89
uremic — *see* Uremia
Aphemia 784.3
uremic — *see* Uremia
Aphonia 784.41
clericorum 784.49
hysterical 300.11
organic 784.41
psychogenic 306.1
Aphthae, aphthous — *see also* condition
Bednar's 528.2
cachectic 529.0
epizootic 078.4
fever 078.4
oral 528.2
stomatitis 528.2
thrush 112.0
ulcer (oral) (recurrent) 528.2
genital organ(s) NEC
female 616.50
male 608.89
larynx 478.79
Apical — *see* condition
Apical ballooning syndrome 429.83
Aplasia — *see also* Agenesis
alveolar process (acquired) 525.8
congenital 750.26
aorta (congenital) 747.22
aortic valve (congenital) 746.89
axialis extracorticalis (congenital) 330.0
bone marrow (myeloid) 284.9
acquired (secondary) 284.89
congenital 284.01
idiopathic 284.9
brain 740.0
specified part 742.2
breast 757.6
bronchus 748.3
cementum 520.4
cerebellar 742.2
congenital (pure) red cell 284.01
corpus callosum 742.2
erythrocyte 284.81
congenital 284.01
extracortical axial 330.0
eye (congenital) 743.00
fovea centralis (congenital) 743.55
germinal (cell) 606.0
iris 743.45
labyrinth, membranous 744.05
limb (congenital) 755.4
lower NEC 755.30
upper NEC 755.20
lung (bilateral) (congenital) (unilateral) 748.5
nervous system NEC 742.8
nuclear 742.8
ovary 752.0
Pelizaeus-Merzbacher 330.0
prostate (congenital) 752.89
red cell (with thymoma) 284.81
acquired (secondary) 284.81
due to drugs 284.81

Aplasia — *see also* Agenesis — *continued*
red cell — *continued*
adult 284.81
congenital 284.01
hereditary 284.01
of infants 284.01
primary 284.01
pure 284.01
due to drugs 284.81
round ligament (congenital) 752.89
salivary gland 750.21
skin (congenital) 757.39
spinal cord 742.59
spleen 759.0
testis (congenital) 752.89
thymic, with immunodeficiency 279.2
thyroid 243
uterus 752.39
ventral horn cell 742.59
Apleuria 756.3
Apnea, apneic (spells) 786.03
newborn, neonatorum 770.81
essential 770.81
obstructive 770.82
primary 770.81
sleep 770.81
specified NEC 770.82
psychogenic 306.1
sleep, unspecified 780.57
with
hypersomnia, unspecified 780.53
hyposomnia, unspecified 780.51
insomnia, unspecified 780.51
sleep disturbance 780.57
central, in conditions classified elsewhere 327.27
obstructive (adult) (pediatric) 327.23
organic 327.20
other 327.29
primary central 327.21
Apneumatosis newborn 770.4
Apodia 755.31
Aponeurosis 726.90
Apophysitis (bone) — *see also* Osteochondrosis 732.9
calcaneus 732.5
juvenile 732.6
Apoplectiform convulsions — *see also* Disease, cerebrovascular, acute 436
Apoplexia, apoplexy, apoplectic — *see also* Disease, cerebrovascular, acute 436
abdominal 569.89
adrenal 036.3
attack 436
basilar (*see also* Disease, cerebrovascular, acute) 436
brain (*see also* Disease, cerebrovascular, acute) 436
bulbar (*see also* Disease, cerebrovascular, acute) 436
capillary (*see also* Disease, cerebrovascular, acute) 436
cardiac (*see also* Infarct, myocardium) 410.9 ☑
cerebral (*see also* Disease, cerebrovascular, acute) 436
chorea (*see also* Disease, cerebrovascular, acute) 436
congestive (*see also* Disease, cerebrovascular, acute) 436
newborn 767.4
embolic (*see also* Embolism, brain) 434.1 ☑
fetus 767.0
fit (*see also* Disease, cerebrovascular, acute) 436
healed or old V12.54
heart (auricle) (ventricle) (*see also* Infarct, myocardium) 410.9 ☑
heat 992.0
hemiplegia (*see also* Disease, cerebrovascular, acute) 436
hemorrhagic (stroke) (*see also* Hemorrhage, brain) 432.9
ingravescent (*see also* Disease, cerebrovascular, acute) 436

Apoplexia, apoplexy, apoplectic — *see also* Disease, cerebrovascular, acute — *continued*
late effect — *see* Late effect(s) (of) cerebrovascular disease
lung — *see* Embolism, pulmonary
meninges, hemorrhagic (*see also* Hemorrhage, subarachnoid) 430
neonatorum 767.0
newborn 767.0
pancreatitis 577.0
placenta 641.2 ☑
progressive (*see also* Disease, cerebrovascular, acute) 436
pulmonary (artery) (vein) — *see* Embolism, pulmonary
sanguineous (*see also* Disease, cerebrovascular, acute) 436
seizure (*see also* Disease, cerebrovascular, acute) 436
serous (*see also* Disease, cerebrovascular, acute) 436
spleen 289.59
stroke (*see also* Disease, cerebrovascular, acute) 436
thrombotic (*see also* Thrombosis, brain) 434.0 ☑
uremic — *see* Uremia
uteroplacental 641.2 ☑
Appendage
fallopian tube (cyst of Morgagni) 752.11
intestine (epiploic) 751.5
preauricular 744.1
testicular (organ of Morgagni) 752.89
Appendicitis 541
with
perforation, peritonitis (generalized), or rupture 540.0
with peritoneal abscess 540.1
peritoneal abscess 540.1
acute (catarrhal) (fulminating) (gangrenous) (inflammatory) (obstructive) (retrocecal) (suppurative) 540.9
with
perforation, peritonitis, or rupture 540.0
with peritoneal abscess 540.1
peritoneal abscess 540.1
amebic 006.8
chronic (recurrent) 542
exacerbation — *see* Appendicitis, acute
fulminating — *see* Appendicitis, acute
gangrenous — *see* Appendicitis, acute
healed (obliterative) 542
interval 542
neurogenic 542
obstructive 542
pneumococcal 541
recurrent 542
relapsing 542
retrocecal 541
subacute (adhesive) 542
subsiding 542
suppurative — *see* Appendicitis, acute
tuberculous (*see also* Tuberculosis) 014.8 ☑
Appendiclausis 543.9
Appendicolithiasis 543.9
Appendicopathia oxyurica 127.4
Appendix, appendicular — *see also* condition
Morgagni (male) 752.89
fallopian tube 752.11
Appetite
depraved 307.52
excessive 783.6
psychogenic 307.51
lack or loss (*see also* Anorexia) 783.0
nonorganic origin 307.59
perverted 307.52
hysterical 300.11
Apprehension, apprehensiveness (abnormal) (state) 300.00
specified type NEC 300.09
Approximal wear 521.10
Apraxia (classic) (ideational) (ideokinetic) (ideomotor) (motor) 784.69
oculomotor, congenital 379.51

Apraxia — *continued*
verbal 784.69
Aptyalism 527.7
Aqueous misdirection 365.83
Arabicum elephantiasis — *see also* Infestation, filarial 125.9
Arachnidism 989.5
Arachnitis — *see* Meningitis
Arachnodactyly 759.82
Arachnoidism 989.5
Arachnoiditis (acute) (adhesive) (basic) (brain) (cerebrospinal) (chiasmal) (chronic) (spinal) — *see also* Meningitis 322.9
meningococcal (chronic) 036.0
syphilitic 094.2
tuberculous (*see also* Tuberculosis, meninges) 013.0 ☑
Araneism 989.5
Arboencephalitis, Australian 062.4
Arborization block (heart) 426.6
Arbor virus, arbovirus (infection) NEC 066.9
ARC 042
Arches — *see* condition
Arcuate uterus 752.36
Arcuatus uterus 752.36
Arcus (cornea)
juvenilis 743.43
interfering with vision 743.42
senilis 371.41
Arc-welders' lung 503
Arc-welders' syndrome (photokeratitis) 370.24
Areflexia 796.1
Areola — *see* condition
Argentaffinoma (M8241/1) — *see also* Neoplasm, by site, uncertain behavior
benign (M8241/0) — *see* Neoplasm, by site, benign
malignant (M8241/3) — *see* Neoplasm, by site, malignant
syndrome 259.2
Argentinian hemorrhagic fever 078.7
Arginosuccinicaciduria 270.6
Argonz-Del Castillo syndrome (nonpuerperal galactorrhea and amenorrhea) 253.1
Argyll-Robertson phenomenon, pupil, or syndrome (syphilitic) 094.89
atypical 379.45
nonluetic 379.45
nonsyphilitic 379.45
reversed 379.45
Argyria, argyriasis NEC 985.8
conjunctiva 372.55
cornea 371.16
from drug or medicinal agent
correct substance properly administered 709.09
overdose or wrong substance given or taken 961.2
Arhinencephaly 742.2
Arias-Stella phenomenon 621.30
Ariboflavinosis 266.0
Arizona enteritis 008.1
Arm — *see* condition
Armenian disease 277.31
Arnold-Chiari obstruction or syndrome — *see also* Spina bifida 741.0 ☑
type I 348.4
type II (*see also* Spina bifida) 741.0 ☑
type III 742.0
type IV 742.2
Arousals
confusional 327.41
Arrest, arrested
active phase of labor 661.1 ☑
affecting fetus or newborn 763.7
any plane in pelvis
complicating delivery 660.1 ☑
affecting fetus or newborn 763.1
bone marrow (*see also* Anemia, aplastic) 284.9
cardiac 427.5
with
abortion — *see* Abortion, by type, with specified complication NEC

Arrest, arrested — *continued*
cardiac — *continued*
with — *continued*
ectopic pregnancy (*see also* categories 633.0–633.9) 639.8
molar pregnancy (*see also* categories 630–632) 639.8
complicating
anesthesia
correct substance properly administered 427.5
obstetric 668.1 ☑
overdose or wrong substance given 968.4
specified anesthetic — *see* Table of Drugs and Chemicals
delivery (cesarean) (instrumental) 669.4 ☑
ectopic or molar pregnancy 639.8
surgery (nontherapeutic) (therapeutic) 997.1
fetus or newborn 779.85
following
abortion 639.8
ectopic or molar pregnancy 639.8
personal history, successfully resuscitated V12.53
postoperative (immediate) 997.1
long-term effect of cardiac surgery 429.4
cardiorespiratory (*see also* Arrest, cardiac) 427.5
deep transverse 660.3 ☑
affecting fetus or newborn 763.1
development or growth
bone 733.91
child 783.40
fetus 764.9 ☑
affecting management of pregnancy 656.5 ☑
tracheal rings 748.3
epiphyseal 733.91
granulopoiesis 288.09
heart — *see* Arrest, cardiac
respiratory 799.1
newborn 770.87
sinus 426.6
transverse (deep) 660.3 ☑
affecting fetus or newborn 763.1
Arrhenoblastoma (M8630/1)
benign (M8630/0)
specified site — *see* Neoplasm, by site, benign
unspecified site
female 220
male 222.0
malignant (M8630/3)
specified site — *see* Neoplasm, by site, malignant
unspecified site
female 183.0
male 186.9
specified site — *see* Neoplasm, by site, uncertain behavior
unspecified site
female 236.2
male 236.4
Arrhinencephaly 742.2
due to
trisomy 13 (13-15) 758.1
trisomy 18 (16-18) 758.2
Arrhythmia (auricle) (cardiac) (cordis) (gallop rhythm) (juvenile) (nodal) (reflex) (sinus) (supraventricular) (transitory) (ventricle) 427.9
bigeminal rhythm 427.89
block 426.9
bradycardia 427.89
contractions, premature 427.60
coronary sinus 427.89
ectopic 427.89
extrasystolic 427.60
postoperative 997.1
psychogenic 306.2
vagal 780.2

Arrillaga-Ayerza syndrome (pulmonary artery sclerosis with pulmonary hypertension) 416.0
Arsenical
dermatitis 692.4
keratosis 692.4
pigmentation 985.1
from drug or medicinal agent
correct substance properly administered 709.09
overdose or wrong substance given or taken 961.1
Arsenism 985.1
from drug or medicinal agent
correct substance properly administered 692.4
overdose or wrong substance given or taken 961.1
Arterial — *see* condition
Arteriectasis 447.8
Arteriofibrosis — *see* Arteriosclerosis
Arteriolar sclerosis — *see* Arteriosclerosis
Arteriolith — *see* Arteriosclerosis
Arteriolitis 447.6
necrotizing, kidney 447.5
renal — *see* Hypertension, kidney
Arteriolosclerosis — *see* Arteriosclerosis
Arterionephrosclerosis — *see also* Hypertension, kidney 403.90
Arteriopathy 447.9
Arteriosclerosis, arteriosclerotic (artery) (deformans) (diffuse) (disease) (endarteritis) (general) (obliterans) (obliterative) (occlusive) (senile) (with calcification) 440.9
with
gangrene 440.24
psychosis (*see also* Psychosis, arteriosclerotic) 290.40
ulceration 440.23
aorta 440.0
arteries of extremities — *see* Arteriosclerosis, extremities
basilar (artery) (*see also* Occlusion, artery, basilar) 433.0 ☑
brain 437.0
bypass graft
coronary artery 414.05
autologous artery (gastroepiploic) (internal mammary) 414.04
autologous vein 414.02
nonautologous biological 414.03
of transplanted heart 414.07
extremity 440.30
autologous vein 440.31
nonautologous biological 440.32
cardiac — *see* Arteriosclerosis, coronary
cardiopathy — *see* Arteriosclerosis, coronary
cardiorenal (*see also* Hypertension, cardiorenal) 404.90
cardiovascular (*see also* Disease, cardiovascular) 429.2
carotid (artery) (common) (internal) (*see also* Occlusion, artery, carotid) 433.1 ☑
central nervous system 437.0
cerebral 437.0
late effect — *see* Late effect(s) (of) cerebrovascular disease
cerebrospinal 437.0
cerebrovascular 437.0
coronary (artery) 414.00
due to
calcified coronary lesion (severely) 414.4
lipid rich plaque 414.3
graft — *see* Arteriosclerosis, bypass graft
native artery 414.01
of transplanted heart 414.06
extremities (native artery) NEC 440.20
bypass graft 440.30
autologous vein 440.31
nonautologous biological 440.32
claudication (intermittent) 440.21
and
gangrene 440.24
rest pain 440.22

Arteriosclerosis, arteriosclerotic — *continued*
extremities — *continued*
claudication — *continued*
and — *continued*
rest pain — *continued*
and
gangrene 440.24
ulceration 440.23
and gangrene 440.24
ulceration 440.23
and gangrene 440.24
gangrene 440.24
rest pain 440.22
and
gangrene 440.24
ulceration 440.23
and gangrene 440.24
specified site NEC 440.29
ulceration 440.23
and gangrene 440.24
heart (disease) (*see also* Arteriosclerosis, coronary)
valve 424.99
aortic 424.1
mitral 424.0
pulmonary 424.3
tricuspid 424.2
iliac 440.8
kidney (*see also* Hypertension, kidney) 403.90
labyrinth, labyrinthine 388.00
medial NEC (*see also* Arteriosclerosis, extremities) 440.20
mesentery (artery) 557.1
Mönckeberg's (*see also* Arteriosclerosis, extremities) 440.20
myocarditis 429.0
nephrosclerosis (*see also* Hypertension, kidney) 403.90
peripheral (of extremities) — *see* Arteriosclerosis, extremities
precerebral 433.9 ☑
specified artery NEC 433.8 ☑
pulmonary (idiopathic) 416.0
renal (*see also* Hypertension, kidney) 403.90
arterioles (*see also* Hypertension, kidney) 403.90
artery 440.1
retinal (vascular) 440.8 [362.13]
specified artery NEC 440.8
with gangrene 440.8 [785.4]
spinal (cord) 437.0
vertebral (artery) (*see also* Occlusion, artery, vertebral) 433.2 ☑
Arteriospasm 443.9
Arteriovenous — *see* condition
Arteritis 447.6
allergic (*see also* Angiitis, hypersensitivity) 446.20
aorta (nonsyphilitic) 447.6
syphilitic 093.1
aortic arch 446.7
brachiocephalica 446.7
brain 437.4
syphilitic 094.89
branchial 446.7
cerebral 437.4
late effect — *see* Late effect(s) (of) cerebrovascular disease
syphilitic 094.89
coronary (artery) (*see also* Arteriosclerosis, coronary)
rheumatic 391.9
chronic 398.99
syphilitic 093.89
cranial (left) (right) 446.5
deformans — *see* Arteriosclerosis
giant cell 446.5
necrosing or necrotizing 446.0
nodosa 446.0
obliterans (*see also* Arteriosclerosis)
subclaviocarotica 446.7
pulmonary 417.8
retina 362.18
rheumatic — *see* Fever, rheumatic

Arteritis — *continued*
senile — *see* Arteriosclerosis
suppurative 447.2
syphilitic (general) 093.89
brain 094.89
coronary 093.89
spinal 094.89
temporal 446.5
young female, syndrome 446.7
Artery, arterial — *see* condition
Arthralgia — *see also* Pain, joint 719.4 ☑
allergic (*see also* Pain, joint) 719.4 ☑
in caisson disease 993.3
psychogenic 307.89
rubella 056.71
Salmonella 003.23
temporomandibular joint 524.62
Arthritis, arthritic (acute) (chronic) (subacute) 716.9 ☑
meaning Osteoarthritis — *see* Osteoarthrosis

Note — Use the following fifth-digit subclassification with categories 711–712, 715–716:
0   site unspecified
1   shoulder region
2   upper arm
3   forearm
4   hand
5   pelvic region and thigh
6   lower leg
7   ankle and foot
8   other specified sites
9   multiple sites

allergic 716.2 ☑
ankylosing (crippling) (spine) 720.0
sites other than spine 716.9 ☑
atrophic 714.0
spine 720.9
back (*see also* Arthritis, spine) 721.90
Bechterew's (ankylosing spondylitis) 720.0
blennorrhagic 098.50
cervical, cervicodorsal (*see also* Spondylosis, cervical) 721.0
Charcôt's 094.0 [713.5]
diabetic 250.6 ☑ [713.5]
due to secondary diabetes 249.6 ☑ [713.5]
syringomyelic 336.0 [713.5]
tabetic 094.0 [713.5]
chylous (*see also* Filariasis) 125.9 [711.7] ☑
climacteric NEC 716.3 ☑
coccyx 721.8
cricoarytenoid 478.79
crystal (-induced) — *see* Arthritis, due to crystals
deformans (*see also* Osteoarthrosis) 715.9 ☑
spine 721.90
with myelopathy 721.91
degenerative (*see also* Osteoarthrosis) 715.9 ☑
idiopathic 715.09
polyarticular 715.09
spine 721.90
with myelopathy 721.91
dermatoarthritis, lipoid 272.8 [713.0]
due to or associated with
acromegaly 253.0 [713.0]
actinomycosis 039.8 [711.4] ☑
amyloidosis 277.39 [713.7]
bacterial disease NEC 040.89 [711.4] ☑
Behçet's syndrome 136.1 [711.2] ☑
blastomycosis 116.0 [711.6] ☑
brucellosis (*see also* Brucellosis) 023.9 [711.4] ☑
caisson disease 993.3
coccidioidomycosis 114.3 [711.6] ☑
coliform (Escherichia coli) 711.0 ☑
colitis, ulcerative (*see also* Colitis, ulcerative) 556.9 [713.1]

☑ **Additional Digit Required** — Refer to the Tabular List for Digit Selection   ▽ **Subterms under main terms may continue to next column or page**

2014 ICD-9-CM   73

Arrest, arrested — Arthritis, arthritic

Arthritis, arthritic — *continued*
   due to or associated with — *continued*
      cowpox 051.01 *[711.5]* ☑
      crystals (*see also* Gout)
         dicalcium phosphate
            275.49 *[712.1]* ☑
         pyrophosphate 275.49 *[712.2]* ☑
         specified NEC 275.49 *[712.8]* ☑
      dermatoarthritis, lipoid 272.8 *[713.0]*
      dermatological disorder NEC
         709.9 *[713.3]*
      diabetes 250.6 ☑ *[713.5]*
         due to secondary diabetes
            249.6 ☑ *[713.5]*
      diphtheria 032.89 *[711.4]* ☑
      dracontiasis 125.7 *[711.7]* ☑
      dysentery 009.0 *[711.3]* ☑
      endocrine disorder NEC 259.9 *[713.0]*
      enteritis NEC 009.1 *[711.3]* ☑
         infectious (*see also* Enteritis, infectious) 009.0 *[711.3]* ☑
         specified organism NEC
            008.8 *[711.3]* ☑
         regional (*see also* Enteritis, regional)
            555.9 *[713.1]*
         specified organism NEC
            008.8 *[711.3]* ☑
      epiphyseal slip, nontraumatic (old)
         716.8 ☑
      erysipelas 035 *[711.4]* ☑
      erythema
         epidemic 026.1
         multiforme 695.10 *[713.3]*
         nodosum 695.2 *[713.3]*
      Escherichia coli 711.0 ☑
      filariasis NEC 125.9 *[711.7]* ☑
      gastrointestinal condition NEC
         569.9 *[713.1]*
      glanders 024 *[711.4]* ☑
      Gonococcus 098.50
      gout 274.00
      helminthiasis NEC 128.9 *[711.7]* ☑
      hematological disorder NEC 289.9 *[713.2]*
      hemochromatosis 275.03 *[713.0]*
      hemoglobinopathy NEC (*see also* Disease, hemoglobin) 282.7 *[713.2]*
      hemophilia (*see also* Hemophilia)
         286.0 *[713.2]*
      Hemophilus influenzae (H. influenzae)
         711.0 ☑
      Henoch (-Schönlein) purpura
         287.0 *[713.6]*
      H. influenzae 711.0 ☑
      histoplasmosis NEC (*see also* Histoplasmosis) 115.99 *[711.6]* ☑
      human parvovirus 079.83 *[711.5]* ☑
      hyperparathyroidism 252.00 *[713.0]*
      hypersensitivity reaction NEC
         995.3 *[713.6]*
      hypogammaglobulinemia (*see also* Hypogamma-globulinemia)
         279.00 *[713.0]*
      hypothyroidism NEC 244.9 *[713.0]*
      infection (*see also* Arthritis, infectious)
         711.9 ☑
      infectious disease NEC 136.9 *[711.8]* ☑
      leprosy (*see also* Leprosy)
         030.9 *[711.4]* ☑
      leukemia NEC (M9800/3) 208.9 *[713.2]*
      lipoid dermatoarthritis 272.8 *[713.0]*
      Lyme disease 088.81 *[711.8]* ☑
      Mediterranean fever, familial
         277.31 *[713.7]*
      meningococcal infection 036.82
      metabolic disorder NEC 277.9 *[713.0]*
      multiple myelomatosis (M9730/3) 203.0
         [713.2]
      mumps 072.79 *[711.5]* ☑
      mycobacteria 031.8 *[711.4]* ☑
      mycosis NEC 117.9 *[711.6]* ☑
      neurological disorder NEC 349.9 *[713.5]*
      ochronosis 270.2 *[713.0]*
      O'Nyong Nyong 066.3 *[711.5]* ☑
      parasitic disease NEC 136.9 *[711.8]* ☑

Arthritis, arthritic — *continued*
   due to or associated with — *continued*
      paratyphoid fever (*see also* Fever, paratyphoid) 002.9 *[711.3]* ☑
      parvovirus B19 079.83 *[711.5]* ☑
      Pneumococcus 711.0 ☑
      poliomyelitis (*see also* Poliomyelitis)
         045.9 ☑ *[711.5]* ☑
      Pseudomonas 711.0 ☑
      psoriasis 696.0
      pyogenic organism (E. coli) (H. influenzae) (Pseudomonas) (Streptococcus) 711.0 ☑
      rat-bite fever 026.1 *[711.4]* ☑
      regional enteritis (*see also* Enteritis, regional) 555.9 *[713.1]*
      Reiter's disease 099.3 *[711.1]* ☑
      respiratory disorder NEC 519.9 *[713.4]*
      reticulosis, malignant (M9720/3) 202.3
         [713.2]
      rubella 056.71
      salmonellosis 003.23
      sarcoidosis 135 *[713.7]*
      serum sickness 999.59 *[713.6]*
      Staphylococcus 711.0 ☑
      Streptococcus 711.0 ☑
      syphilis (*see also* Syphilis)
         094.0 *[711.4]* ☑
      syringomyelia 336.0 *[713.5]*
      thalassemia (*see also* Thalassemia)
         282.40 *[713.2]*
      tuberculosis (*see also* Tuberculosis, arthritis) 015.9 ☑ *[711.4]* ☑
      typhoid fever 002.0 *[711.3]* ☑
      ulcerative colitis (*see also* Colitis, ulcerative) 556.9 *[713.1]*
      urethritis
         nongonococcal (*see also* Urethritis, nongonococcal)
            099.40 *[711.1]* ☑
         nonspecific (*see also* Urethritis, nongonococcal) 099.40 *[711.1]* ☑
         Reiter's 099.3
      viral disease NEC 079.99 *[711.5]* ☑
   erythema epidemic 026.1
   gonococcal 098.50
   gouty 274.00
      acute 274.01
   hypertrophic (*see also* Osteoarthrosis)
      715.9 ☑
      spine 721.90
         with myelopathy 721.91
   idiopathic, blennorrheal 099.3
   in caisson disease 993.3 *[713.8]*
   infectious or infective (acute) (chronic)
      (subacute) NEC 711.9 ☑
      nonpyogenic 711.9 ☑
      spine 720.9
   inflammatory NEC 714.9
   juvenile rheumatoid (chronic) (polyarticular)
      714.30
      acute 714.31
      monoarticular 714.33
      pauciarticular 714.32
   lumbar (*see also* Spondylosis, lumbar) 721.3
   meningococcal 036.82
   menopausal NEC 716.3 ☑
   migratory — *see* Fever, rheumatic
   neuropathic (Charcôt's) 094.0 *[713.5]*
      diabetic 250.6 ☑ *[713.5]*
         due to secondary diabetes
            249.6 ☑ *[713.5]*
      nonsyphilitic NEC 349.9 *[713.5]*
      syringomyelic 336.0 *[713.5]*
      tabetic 094.0 *[713.5]*
   nodosa (*see also* Osteoarthrosis) 715.9 ☑
      spine 721.90
         with myelopathy 721.91
   nonpyogenic NEC 716.9 ☑
      spine 721.90
         with myelopathy 721.91
   ochronotic 270.2 *[713.0]*
   palindromic (see also Rheumatism, palindromic) 719.3 ☑
   pneumococcal 711.0 ☑

Arthritis, arthritic — *continued*
   postdysenteric 009.0 *[711.3]* ☑
   postrheumatic, chronic (Jaccoud's) 714.4
   primary progressive 714.0
      spine 720.9
   proliferative 714.0
      spine 720.0
   psoriatic 696.0
   purulent 711.0 ☑
   pyogenic or pyemic 711.0 ☑
   reactive 099.3
   rheumatic 714.0
      acute or subacute — *see* Fever, rheumatic
      chronic 714.0
      spine 720.9
   rheumatoid (nodular) 714.0
      with
         splenoadenomegaly and leukopenia
            714.1
         visceral or systemic involvement
            714.2
      aortitis 714.89
      carditis 714.2
      heart disease 714.2
      juvenile (chronic) (polyarticular) 714.30
         acute 714.31
         monoarticular 714.33
         pauciarticular 714.32
      spine 720.0
   rubella 056.71
   sacral, sacroiliac, sacrococcygeal (*see also* Spondylosis, sacral) 721.3
   scorbutic 267
   senile or senescent (*see also* Osteoarthrosis)
      715.9 ☑
      spine 721.90
         with myelopathy 721.91
   septic 711.0 ☑
   serum (nontherapeutic) (therapeutic)
      999.59 *[713.6]*
   specified form NEC 716.8 ☑
   spine 721.90
      with myelopathy 721.91
      atrophic 720.9
      degenerative 721.90
         with myelopathy 721.91
      hypertrophic (with deformity) 721.90
         with myelopathy 721.91
      infectious or infective NEC 720.9
      Marie-Strümpell 720.0
      nonpyogenic 721.90
         with myelopathy 721.91
      pyogenic 720.9
      rheumatoid 720.0
      traumatic (old) 721.7
      tuberculous (*see also* Tuberculosis)
         015.0 ☑ *[720.81]*
   staphylococcal 711.0 ☑
   streptococcal 711.0 ☑
   suppurative 711.0 ☑
   syphilitic 094.0 *[713.5]*
      congenital 090.49 *[713.5]*
   syphilitica deformans (Charcôt) 094.0 *[713.5]*
   temporomandibular joint 524.69
   thoracic (*see also* Spondylosis, thoracic)
      721.2
   toxic of menopause 716.3 ☑
   transient 716.4 ☑
   traumatic (chronic) (old) (post) 716.1 ☑
      current injury — *see* nature of injury
   tuberculous (*see also* Tuberculosis, arthritis)
      015.9 ☑ *[711.4]* ☑
   urethritica 099.3 *[711.1]* ☑
   urica, uratic 274.00
   venereal 099.3 *[711.1]* ☑
   vertebral (*see also* Arthritis, spine) 721.90
   villous 716.8 ☑
   von Bechterew's 720.0
Arthrocele — *see also* Effusion, joint 719.0 ☑
Arthrochondritis — *see* Arthritis
Arthrodesis status V45.4
Arthrodynia — *see also* Pain, joint 719.4 ☑
   psychogenic 307.89
Arthrodysplasia 755.9

Arthrofibrosis joint — *see also* Ankylosis
   718.5 ☑
Arthrogryposis 728.3
   multiplex, congenita 754.89
Arthrokatadysis 715.35
Arthrolithiasis 274.00
Arthro-onychodysplasia 756.89
Arthro-osteo-onychodysplasia 756.89
Arthropathy — *see also* Arthritis 716.9 ☑

> Note — Use the following fifth-digit subclassification with categories 711–712, 716:
>
> | | |
> |---|---|
> | 0 | site unspecified |
> | 1 | shoulder region |
> | 2 | upper arm |
> | 3 | forearm |
> | 4 | hand |
> | 5 | pelvic region and thigh |
> | 6 | lower leg |
> | 7 | ankle and foot |
> | 8 | other specified sites |
> | 9 | multiple sites |

   Behçet's 136.1 *[711.2]* ☑
   Charcôt's 094.0 *[713.5]*
      diabetic 250.6 ☑ *[713.5]*
         due to secondary diabetes
            249.6 ☑ *[713.5]*
      syringomyelic 336.0 *[713.5]*
      tabetic 094.0 *[713.5]*
   crystal (-induced) — *see* Arthritis, due to crystals
   gouty 274.00
      acute 274.01
      chronic (without mention of tophus
         (tophi)) 274.02
         with tophus (tophi) 274.03
   neurogenic, neuropathic (Charcôt's) (tabetic) 094.0 *[713.5]*
      diabetic 250.6 ☑ *[713.5]*
         due to secondary diabetes
            249.6 ☑ *[713.5]*
      nonsyphilitic NEC 349.9 *[713.5]*
      syringomyelic 336.0 *[713.5]*
   postdysenteric NEC 009.0 *[711.3]* ☑
   postrheumatic, chronic (Jaccoud's) 714.4
   psoriatic 696.0
   pulmonary 731.2
   specified NEC 716.8 ☑
   syringomyelia 336.0 *[713.5]*
   tabes dorsalis 094.0 *[713.5]*
   tabetic 094.0 *[713.5]*
   transient 716.4 ☑
   traumatic 716.1 ☑
   uric acid 274.00
Arthrophyte — *see also* Loose, body, joint
   718.1 ☑
Arthrophytis 719.80
   ankle 719.87
   elbow 719.82
   foot 719.87
   hand 719.84
   hip 719.85
   knee 719.86
   multiple sites 719.89
   pelvic region 719.85
   shoulder (region) 719.81
   specified site NEC 719.88
   wrist 719.83
Arthropyosis — *see also* Arthritis, pyogenic
   711.0 ☑
Arthroscopic surgical procedure converted to open procedure V64.43
Arthrosis (deformans) (degenerative) — *see also* Osteoarthrosis 715.9 ☑
   Charcôt's 094.0 *[713.5]*
   polyarticular 715.09
   spine (*see also* Spondylosis) 721.90
Arthus phenomenon 995.21

Arthus phenomenon — *continued*
 due to
  correct substance properly administered 995.21
  overdose or wrong substance given or taken 977.9
   specified drug — *see* Table of Drugs and Chemicals
  serum 999.59
Articular — *see also* condition
 disc disorder (reducing or non-reducing) 524.63
 spondylolisthesis 756.12
Articulation
 anterior 524.27
 posterior 524.27
 reverse 524.27
Artificial
 device (prosthetic) — *see* Fitting, device
 insemination V26.1
 menopause (states) (symptoms) (syndrome) 627.4
 opening status (functioning) (without complication) V44.9
  anus (colostomy) V44.3
  colostomy V44.3
  cystostomy V44.50
   appendico-vesicostomy V44.52
   cutaneous-vesicostomy V44.51
   specified type NEC V44.59
  enterostomy V44.4
  gastrostomy V44.1
  ileostomy V44.2
  intestinal tract NEC V44.4
  jejunostomy V44.4
  nephrostomy V44.6
  specified site NEC V44.8
  tracheostomy V44.0
  ureterostomy V44.6
  urethrostomy V44.6
  urinary tract NEC V44.6
  vagina V44.7
  vagina status V44.7
ARV (disease) (illness) (infection) — *see* Human immunodeficiency virus (disease) (illness) (infection)
Arytenoid — *see* condition
Asbestosis (occupational) 501
Asboe-Hansen's disease (incontinentia pigmenti) 757.33
Ascariasis (intestinal) (lung) 127.0
Ascaridiasis 127.0
Ascaridosis 127.0
Ascaris 127.0
 lumbricoides (infestation) 127.0
 pneumonia 127.0
Ascending — *see* condition
ASC-H (atypical squamous cells cannot exclude high grade squamous intraepithelial lesion)
 anus 796.72
 cervix 795.02
 vagina 795.12
Aschoff's bodies — *see also* Myocarditis, rheumatic 398.0
Ascites 789.59
 abdominal NEC 789.59
 cancerous (M8000/6) 789.51
 cardiac 428.0
 chylous (nonfilarial) 457.8
  filarial (*see also* Infestation, filarial) 125.9
 congenital 778.0
 due to S. japonicum 120.2
 fetal, causing fetopelvic disproportion 653.7 ☑
 heart 428.0
 joint (*see also* Effusion, joint) 719.0 ☑
 malignant (M8000/6) 789.51
 pseudochylous 789.59
 syphilitic 095.2
 tuberculous (*see also* Tuberculosis) 014.0 ☑
Ascorbic acid (vitamin C) **deficiency** (scurvy) 267
ASC-US (atypical squamous cells of undetermined significance)
 anus 796.71

ASC-US — *continued*
 cervix 795.01
 vagina 795.11
ASCVD (arteriosclerotic cardiovascular disease) 429.2
Aseptic — *see* condition
Asherman's syndrome 621.5
Asialia 527.7
Asiatic cholera — *see also* Cholera 001.9
Asocial personality or trends 301.7
Asomatognosia 781.8
Aspergillosis 117.3
 with pneumonia 117.3 [484.6]
 allergic bronchopulmonary 518.6
 nonsyphilitic NEC 117.3
Aspergillus (flavus) (fumigatus) (infection) (terreus) 117.3
Aspermatogenesis 606.0
Aspermia (testis) 606.0
Asphyxia, asphyxiation (by) 799.01
 antenatal — *see* Distress, fetal
 bedclothes 994.7
 birth (*see also* Asphyxia, newborn) 768.9
 bunny bag 994.7
 carbon monoxide 986
 caul (*see also* Asphyxia, newborn) 768.9
 cave-in 994.7
  crushing — *see* Injury, internal, intrathoracic organs
 constriction 994.7
 crushing — *see* Injury, internal, intrathoracic organs
 drowning 994.1
 fetal, affecting newborn 768.9
 food or foreign body (in larynx) 933.1
  bronchioles 934.8
  bronchus (main) 934.1
  lung 934.8
  nasopharynx 933.0
  nose, nasal passages 932
  pharynx 933.0
  respiratory tract 934.9
   specified part NEC 934.8
  throat 933.0
  trachea 934.0
 gas, fumes, or vapor NEC 987.9
  specified — *see* Table of Drugs and Chemicals
 gravitational changes 994.7
 hanging 994.7
 inhalation — *see* Inhalation
 intrauterine
  fetal death (before onset of labor) 768.0
   during labor 768.1
  liveborn infant — *see* Distress, fetal, liveborn infant
 local 443.0
 mechanical 994.7
  during birth (*see also* Distress, fetal) 768.9
 mucus 933.1
  bronchus (main) 934.1
  larynx 933.1
  lung 934.8
  nasal passages 932
  newborn 770.18
  pharynx 933.0
  respiratory tract 934.9
   specified part NEC 934.8
  throat 933.0
  trachea 934.0
  vaginal (fetus or newborn) 770.18
 newborn 768.9
  with neurologic involvement 768.5
  blue 768.6
  livida 768.6
  mild or moderate 768.6
  pallida 768.5
  severe 768.5
  white 768.5
 pathological 799.01
 plastic bag 994.7
 postnatal (*see also* Asphyxia, newborn) 768.9
  mechanical 994.7
 pressure 994.7
 reticularis 782.61

Asphyxia, asphyxiation — *continued*
 strangulation 994.7
 submersion 994.1
 traumatic NEC — *see* Injury, internal, intrathoracic organs
 vomiting, vomitus — *see* Asphyxia, food or foreign body
Aspiration
 acid pulmonary (syndrome) 997.39
  obstetric 668.0 ☑
 amniotic fluid 770.13
  with respiratory symptoms 770.14
 bronchitis 507.0
 clear amniotic fluid 770.13
  with
   pneumonia 770.14
   pneumonitis 770.14
   respiratory symptoms 770.14
 contents of birth canal 770.17
  with respiratory symptoms 770.18
 fetal 770.10
  blood 770.15
   with
    pneumonia 770.16
    pneumonitis 770.16
   pneumonitis 770.18
 food, foreign body, or gasoline (with asphyxiation) — *see* Asphyxia, food or foreign body
 meconium 770.11
  with
   pneumonia 770.12
   pneumonitis 770.12
   respiratory symptoms 770.12
  below vocal cords 770.11
   with respiratory symptoms 770.12
 mucus 933.1
  into
   bronchus (main) 934.1
   lung 934.8
   respiratory tract 934.9
    specified part NEC 934.8
   trachea 934.0
  newborn 770.17
  vaginal (fetus or newborn) 770.17
 newborn 770.10
  with respiratory symptoms 770.18
  blood 770.15
   with
    pneumonia 770.16
    pneumonitis 770.16
    respiratory symptoms 770.16
  pneumonia 507.0
   fetus or newborn 770.18
    meconium 770.12
  pneumonitis 507.0
   fetus or newborn 770.18
    meconium 770.12
  obstetric 668.0 ☑
 postnatal stomach contents 770.85
  with
   pneumonia 770.86
   pneumonitis 770.86
   respiratory symptoms 770.86
 syndrome of newborn (massive) 770.18
  meconium 770.12
 vernix caseosa 770.12
Asplenia 759.0
 with mesocardia 746.87
Assam fever 085.0
Assimilation, pelvis
 with disproportion 653.2 ☑
  affecting fetus or newborn 763.1
  causing obstructed labor 660.1 ☑
   affecting fetus or newborn 763.1
Assmann's focus — *see also* Tuberculosis 011.0 ☑
Astasia (-abasia) 307.9
 hysterical 300.11
Asteatosis 706.8
 cutis 706.8
Astereognosis 780.99
Asterixis 781.3
 in liver disease 572.8
Asteroid hyalitis 379.22
Asthenia, asthenic 780.79

Asthenia, asthenic — *continued*
 cardiac (*see also* Failure, heart) 428.9
  psychogenic 306.2
 cardiovascular (*see also* Failure, heart) 428.9
  psychogenic 306.2
 heart (*see also* Failure, heart) 428.9
  psychogenic 306.2
 hysterical 300.11
 myocardial (*see also* Failure, heart) 428.9
  psychogenic 306.2
 nervous 300.5
 neurocirculatory 306.2
 neurotic 300.5
 psychogenic 300.5
 psychoneurotic 300.5
 psychophysiologic 300.5
 reaction, psychoneurotic 300.5
 senile 797
 Stiller's 780.79
 tropical anhidrotic 705.1
Asthenopia 368.13
 accommodative 367.4
 hysterical (muscular) 300.11
 psychogenic 306.7
Asthenospermia 792.2
Asthma, asthmatic (bronchial) (catarrh) (spasmodic) 493.9 ☑

> Note — Use the following fifth-digit subclassification with codes 493.0–493.2, 493.9:
>
> 0   without mention of status asthmaticus or acute exacerbation or unspecified
>
> 1   with status asthmaticus
>
> 2   with acute exacerbation

 with
  chronic obstructive pulmonary disease (COPD) 493.2 ☑
  hay fever 493.0 ☑
  rhinitis, allergic 493.0 ☑
 allergic 493.9 ☑
  stated cause (external allergen) 493.0 ☑
 atopic 493.0 ☑
 cardiac (*see also* Failure, ventricular, left) 428.1
 cardiobronchial (*see also* Failure, ventricular, left) 428.1
 cardiorenal (*see also* Hypertension, cardiorenal) 404.90
 childhood 493.0 ☑
 Colliers' 500
 cough variant 493.82
 croup 493.9 ☑
 detergent 507.8
 due to
  detergent 507.8
  inhalation of fumes 506.3
  internal immunological process 493.0 ☑
 endogenous (intrinsic) 493.1 ☑
 eosinophilic 518.3
 exercise induced bronchospasm 493.81
 exogenous (cosmetics) (dander or dust) (drugs) (dust) (feathers) (food) (hay) (platinum) (pollen) 493.0 ☑
 extrinsic 493.0 ☑
 grinders' 502
 hay 493.0 ☑
 heart (*see also* Failure, ventricular, left) 428.1
 IgE 493.0 ☑
 infective 493.1 ☑
 intrinsic 493.1 ☑
 Kopp's 254.8
 late-onset 493.1 ☑
 meat-wrappers' 506.9
 Millar's (laryngismus stridulus) 478.75
 millstone makers' 502
 miners' 500
 Monday morning 504
 New Orleans (epidemic) 493.0 ☑
 platinum 493.0 ☑
 pneumoconiotic (occupational) NEC 505
 potters' 502
 psychogenic 316 [493.9] ☑

☑ **Additional Digit Required** — Refer to the Tabular List for Digit Selection   ▽ **Subterms under main terms may continue to next column or page**

2014 ICD-9-CM   **75**

Asthma, asthmatic — *continued*
  pulmonary eosinophilic 518.3
  red cedar 495.8
  Rostan's (*see also* Failure, ventricular, left) 428.1
  sandblasters' 502
  sequoiosis 495.8
  stonemasons' 502
  thymic 254.8
  tuberculous (*see also* Tuberculosis, pulmonary) 011.9 ☑
  Wichmann's (laryngismus stridulus) 478.75
  wood 495.8
Astigmatism (compound) (congenital) 367.20
  irregular 367.22
  regular 367.21
Astroblastoma (M9430/3)
  nose 748.1
  specified site — *see* Neoplasm, by site, malignant
  unspecified site 191.9
Astrocytoma (cystic) (M9400/3)
  anaplastic type (M9401/3)
    specified site — *see* Neoplasm, by site, malignant
    unspecified site 191.9
  fibrillary (M9420/3)
    specified site — *see* Neoplasm, by site, malignant
    unspecified site 191.9
  fibrous (M9420/3)
    specified site — *see* Neoplasm, by site, malignant
    unspecified site 191.9
  gemistocytic (M9411/3)
    specified site — *see* Neoplasm, by site, malignant
    unspecified site 191.9
  juvenile (M9421/3)
    specified site — *see* Neoplasm, by site, malignant
    unspecified site 191.9
  nose 748.1
  pilocytic (M9421/3)
    specified site — *see* Neoplasm, by site, malignant
    unspecified site 191.9
  piloid (M9421/3)
    specified site — *see* Neoplasm, by site, malignant
    unspecified site 191.9
  protoplasmic (M9410/3)
    specified site — *see* Neoplasm, by site, malignant
    unspecified site 191.9
  specified site — *see* Neoplasm, by site, malignant
  subependymal (M9383/1) 237.5
    giant cell (M9384/1) 237.5
  unspecified site 191.9
Astroglioma (M9400/3)
  nose 748.1
  specified site — *see* Neoplasm, by site, malignant
  unspecified site 191.9
Asymbolia 784.60
Asymmetrical breathing 786.09
Asymmetry — *see also* Distortion
  breast, between native and reconstructed 612.1
  chest 786.9
  face 754.0
  jaw NEC 524.12
    maxillary 524.11
  pelvis with disproportion 653.0 ☑
    affecting fetus or newborn 763.1
    causing obstructed labor 660.1 ☑
      affecting fetus or newborn 763.1
Asynergia 781.3
Asynergy 781.3
  ventricular 429.89
Asystole (heart) — *see also* Arrest, cardiac 427.5
Ataxia, ataxy, ataxic 781.3
  acute 781.3
  brain 331.89

Ataxia, ataxy, ataxic — *continued*
  cerebellar 334.3
    hereditary (Marie's) 334.2
    in
      alcoholism 303.9 ☑ *[334.4]*
      myxedema (*see also* Myxedema) 244.9 *[334.4]*
      neoplastic disease NEC 239.9 *[334.4]*
  cerebral 331.89
  family, familial 334.2
    cerebral (Marie's) 334.2
    spinal (Friedreich's) 334.0
  Friedreich's (heredofamilial) (spinal) 334.0
  frontal lobe 781.3
  gait 781.2
    hysterical 300.11
  general 781.3
  hereditary NEC 334.2
    cerebellar 334.2
    spastic 334.1
    spinal 334.0
  heredofamilial (Marie's) 334.2
  hysterical 300.11
  locomotor (progressive) 094.0
    diabetic 250.6 ☑ *[337.1]*
      due to secondary diabetes 249.6 ☑ *[337.1]*
  Marie's (cerebellar) (heredofamilial) 334.2
  nonorganic origin 307.9
  partial 094.0
  postchickenpox 052.7
  progressive locomotor 094.0
  psychogenic 307.9
  Sanger-Brown's 334.2
  spastic 094.0
    hereditary 334.1
    syphilitic 094.0
  spinal
    hereditary 334.0
    progressive locomotor 094.0
  telangiectasia 334.8
Ataxia-telangiectasia 334.8
Atelectasis (absorption collapse) (complete) (compression) (massive) (partial) (postinfective) (pressure collapse) (pulmonary) (relaxation) 518.0
  newborn (congenital) (partial) 770.5
    primary 770.4
  primary 770.4
  tuberculous (*see also* Tuberculosis, pulmonary) 011.9 ☑
Ateleiosis, ateliosis 253.3
Atelia — *see* Distortion
Ateliosis 253.3
Atelocardia 746.9
Atelomyelia 742.59
Athelia 757.6
Atheroembolism
  extremity
    lower 445.02
    upper 445.01
  kidney 445.81
  specified site NEC 445.89
Atheroma, atheromatous — *see also* Arteriosclerosis 440.9
  aorta, aortic 440.0
    valve (*see also* Endocarditis, aortic) 424.1
  artery — *see* Arteriosclerosis
  basilar (artery) (*see also* Occlusion, artery, basilar) 433.0 ☑
  carotid (artery) (common) (internal) (*see also* Occlusion, artery, carotid) 433.1 ☑
  cerebral (arteries) 437.0
  coronary (artery) — *see* Arteriosclerosis, coronary
  degeneration — *see* Arteriosclerosis
  heart, cardiac — *see* Arteriosclerosis, coronary
  mitral (valve) 424.0
  myocardium, myocardial — *see* Arteriosclerosis, coronary
  pulmonary valve (heart) (*see also* Endocarditis, pulmonary) 424.3
  skin 706.2
  tricuspid (heart) (valve) 424.2
  valve, valvular — *see* Endocarditis

Atheroma, atheromatous — *see also* Arteriosclerosis — *continued*
  vertebral (artery) (*see also* Occlusion, artery, vertebral) 433.2 ☑
Atheromatosis — *see also* Arteriosclerosis
  arterial, congenital 272.8
Atherosclerosis — *see* Arteriosclerosis
Athetosis (acquired) 781.0
  bilateral 333.79
  congenital (bilateral) 333.6
  double 333.71
  unilateral 781.0
Athlete's
  foot 110.4
  heart 429.3
Athletic team examination V70.3
Athrepsia 261
Athyrea (acquired) — *see also* Hypothyroidism 244.9
  congenital 243
Athyreosis (congenital) 243
  acquired — *see* Hypothyroidism
Athyroidism (acquired) — *see also* Hypothyroidism 244.9
  congenital 243
Atmospheric pyrexia 992.0
Atonia, atony, atonic
  abdominal wall 728.2
  bladder (sphincter) 596.4
    neurogenic NEC 596.54
      with cauda equina syndrome 344.61
  capillary 448.9
  cecum 564.89
    psychogenic 306.4
  colon 564.89
    psychogenic 306.4
  congenital 779.89
  dyspepsia 536.3
    psychogenic 306.4
  intestine 564.89
    psychogenic 306.4
  stomach 536.3
    neurotic or psychogenic 306.4
    psychogenic 306.4
  uterus 661.2 ☑
    with hemorrhage (postpartum) 666.1 ☑
    without hemorrhage
      intrapartum 661.2 ☑
      postpartum 669.8 ☑
  vesical 596.4
Atopy NEC V15.09
Atransferrinemia, congenital 273.8
Atresia, atretic (congenital) 759.89
  alimentary organ or tract NEC 751.8
    lower 751.2
    upper 750.8
  ani, anus, anal (canal) 751.2
  aorta 747.22
    with hypoplasia of ascending aorta and defective development of left ventricle (with mitral valve atresia) 746.7
    arch 747.11
    ring 747.21
  aortic (orifice) (valve) 746.89
    arch 747.11
  aqueduct of Sylvius 742.3
    with spina bifida (*see also* Spina bifida) 741.0 ☑
  artery NEC (*see also* Atresia, blood vessel) 747.60
    cerebral 747.81
    coronary 746.85
    eye 743.58
    pulmonary 747.31
    umbilical 747.5
  auditory canal (external) 744.02
  bile, biliary duct (common) or passage 751.61
    acquired (*see also* Obstruction, biliary) 576.2
  bladder (neck) 753.6
  blood vessel (peripheral) NEC 747.60
    cerebral 747.81
    gastrointestinal 747.61
    lower limb 747.64

Atresia, atretic — *continued*
  blood vessel — *continued*
    pulmonary artery 747.31
    renal 747.62
    spinal 747.82
    upper limb 747.63
  bronchus 748.3
  canal, ear 744.02
  cardiac
    valve 746.89
      aortic 746.89
      mitral 746.89
      pulmonary 746.01
      tricuspid 746.1
  cecum 751.2
  cervix (acquired) 622.4
    congenital 752.43
    in pregnancy or childbirth 654.6 ☑
      affecting fetus or newborn 763.89
      causing obstructed labor 660.2 ☑
        affecting fetus or newborn 763.1
  choana 748.0
  colon 751.2
  cystic duct 751.61
    acquired 575.8
      with obstruction (*see also* Obstruction, gallbladder) 575.2
  digestive organs NEC 751.8
  duodenum 751.1
  ear canal 744.02
  ejaculatory duct 752.89
  epiglottis 748.3
  esophagus 750.3
  Eustachian tube 744.24
  fallopian tube (acquired) 628.2
    congenital 752.19
  follicular cyst 620.0
  foramen of
    Luschka 742.3
      with spina bifida (*see also* Spina bifida) 741.0 ☑
    Magendie 742.3
      with spina bifida (*see also* Spina bifida) 741.0 ☑
  gallbladder 751.69
  genital organ
    external
      female 752.49
      male NEC 752.89
        penis 752.69
    internal
      female 752.89
      male 752.89
  glottis 748.3
  gullet 750.3
  heart
    valve NEC 746.89
      aortic 746.89
      mitral 746.89
      pulmonary 746.01
      tricuspid 746.1
  hymen 752.42
    acquired 623.3
    postinfective 623.3
  ileum 751.1
  intestine (small) 751.1
    large 751.2
  iris, filtration angle (*see also* Buphthalmia) 743.20
  jejunum 751.1
  kidney 753.3
  lacrimal, apparatus 743.65
    acquired — *see* Stenosis, lacrimal
  larynx 748.3
  ligament, broad 752.19
  lung 748.5
  meatus urinarius 753.6
  mitral valve 746.89
    with atresia or hypoplasia of aortic orifice or valve, with hypoplasia of ascending aorta and defective development of left ventricle 746.7
  nares (anterior) (posterior) 748.0
  nasolacrimal duct 743.65
  nasopharynx 748.8

Atresia, atretic — *continued*
nose, nostril 748.0
acquired 738.0
organ or site NEC — *see* Anomaly, specified type NEC
osseous meatus (ear) 744.03
oviduct (acquired) 628.2
congenital 752.19
parotid duct 750.23
acquired 527.8
pulmonary (artery) 747.31
valve 746.01
vein 747.49
pulmonic 746.01
pupil 743.46
rectum 751.2
salivary duct or gland 750.23
acquired 527.8
sublingual duct 750.23
acquired 527.8
submaxillary duct or gland 750.23
acquired 527.8
trachea 748.3
tricuspid valve 746.1
ureter 753.29
ureteropelvic junction 753.21
ureterovesical orifice 753.22
urethra (valvular) 753.6
urinary tract NEC 753.29
uterus 752.31
acquired 621.8
vagina (acquired) 623.2
congenital (total) (partial) 752.45
postgonococcal (old) 098.2
postinfectional 623.2
senile 623.2
vascular NEC (*see also* Atresia, blood vessel) 747.60
cerebral 747.81
vas deferens 752.89
vein NEC (*see also* Atresia, blood vessel) 747.60
cardiac 746.89
great 747.49
portal 747.49
pulmonary 747.49
vena cava (inferior) (superior) 747.49
vesicourethral orifice 753.6
vulva 752.49
acquired 624.8
Atrichia, atrichosis 704.00
congenital (universal) 757.4
Atrioventricularis commune 745.69
At risk for falling V15.88
Atrophia — *see also* Atrophy
alba 709.09
cutis 701.8
idiopathica progressiva 701.8
senilis 701.8
dermatological, diffuse (idiopathic) 701.8
flava hepatis (acuta) (subacuta) (*see also* Necrosis, liver) 570
gyrata of choroid and retina (central) 363.54
generalized 363.57
senilis 797
dermatological 701.8
unguium 703.8
congenita 757.5
Atrophoderma, atrophodermia 701.9
diffusum (idiopathic) 701.8
maculatum 701.3
et striatum 701.3
due to syphilis 095.8
syphilitic 091.3
neuriticum 701.8
pigmentosum 757.33
reticulatum symmetricum faciei 701.8
senile 701.8
symmetrical 701.8
vermiculata 701.8
Atrophy, atrophic
adrenal (autoimmune) (capsule) (cortex) (gland) 255.41
with hypofunction 255.41
alveolar process or ridge (edentulous) 525.20

Atrophy, atrophic — *continued*
alveolar process or ridge — *continued*
mandible 525.20
minimal 525.21
moderate 525.22
severe 525.23
maxilla 525.20
minimal 525.24
moderate 525.25
severe 525.26
appendix 543.9
Aran-Duchenne muscular 335.21
arm 728.2
arteriosclerotic — *see* Arteriosclerosis
arthritis 714.0
spine 720.9
bile duct (any) 576.8
bladder 596.89
blanche (of Milian) 701.3
bone (senile) 733.99
due to
disuse 733.7
infection 733.99
tabes dorsalis (neurogenic) 094.0
posttraumatic 733.99
brain (cortex) (progressive) 331.9
with dementia 290.10
Alzheimer's 331.0
with dementia — *see* Alzheimer's, dementia
circumscribed (Pick's) 331.11
with dementia
with behavioral disturbance 331.11 [294.11]
without behavioral disturbance 331.11 [294.10]
congenital 742.4
hereditary 331.9
senile 331.2
breast 611.4
puerperal, postpartum 676.3 ☑
buccal cavity 528.9
cardiac (brown) (senile) (*see also* Degeneration, myocardial) 429.1
cartilage (infectional) (joint) 733.99
cast, plaster of Paris 728.2
cerebellar — *see* Atrophy, brain
cerebral — *see* Atrophy, brain
cervix (endometrium) (mucosa) (myometrium) (senile) (uteri) 622.8
menopausal 627.8
Charcôt-Marie-Tooth 356.1
choroid 363.40
diffuse secondary 363.42
hereditary (*see also* Dystrophy, choroid) 363.50
gyrate
central 363.54
diffuse 363.57
generalized 363.57
senile 363.41
ciliary body 364.57
colloid, degenerative 701.3
conjunctiva (senile) 372.89
corpus cavernosum 607.89
cortical (*see also* Atrophy, brain) 331.9
Cruveilhier's 335.21
cystic duct 576.8
dacryosialadenopathy 710.2
degenerative
colloid 701.3
senile 701.3
Déjérine-Thomas 333.0
diffuse idiopathic, dermatological 701.8
disuse
bone 733.7
muscle 728.2
pelvic muscles and anal sphincter 618.83
Duchenne-Aran 335.21
ear 388.9
edentulous alveolar ridge 525.20
mandible 525.20
minimal 525.21
moderate 525.22
severe 525.23
maxilla 525.20

Atrophy, atrophic — *continued*
edentulous alveolar ridge — *continued*
maxilla — *continued*
minimal 525.24
moderate 525.25
severe 525.26
emphysema, lung 492.8
endometrium (senile) 621.8
cervix 622.8
enteric 569.89
epididymis 608.3
eyeball, cause unknown 360.41
eyelid (senile) 374.50
facial (skin) 701.9
facioscapulohumeral (Landouzy-Déjérine) 359.1
fallopian tube (senile), acquired 620.3
fatty, thymus (gland) 254.8
gallbladder 575.8
gastric 537.89
gastritis (chronic) 535.1 ☑
gastrointestinal 569.89
genital organ, male 608.89
glandular 289.3
globe (phthisis bulbi) 360.41
gum (*see also* Recession, gingival) 523.20
hair 704.2
heart (brown) (senile) (*see also* Degeneration, myocardial) 429.1
hemifacial 754.0
Romberg 349.89
hydronephrosis 591
infantile 261
paralysis, acute (*see also* Poliomyelitis, with paralysis) 045.1 ☑
intestine 569.89
iris (generalized) (postinfectional) (sector shaped) 364.59
essential 364.51
progressive 364.51
sphincter 364.54
kidney (senile) (*see also* Sclerosis, renal) 587
with hypertension (*see also* Hypertension, kidney) 403.90
congenital 753.0
hydronephrotic 591
infantile 753.0
lacrimal apparatus (primary) 375.13
secondary 375.14
Landouzy-Déjérine 359.1
laryngitis, infection 476.0
larynx 478.79
Leber's optic 377.16
lip 528.5
liver (acute) (subacute) (*see also* Necrosis, liver) 570
chronic (yellow) 571.8
yellow (congenital) 570
with
abortion — *see* Abortion, by type, with specified complication NEC
ectopic pregnancy (*see also* categories 633.0–633.9) 639.8
molar pregnancy (*see also* categories 630–632) 639.8
chronic 571.8
complicating pregnancy 646.7 ☑
following
abortion 639.8
ectopic or molar pregnancy 639.8
from injection, inoculation or transfusion (onset within 8 months after administration) — *see* Hepatitis, viral
healed 571.5
obstetric 646.7 ☑
postabortal 639.8
postimmunization — *see* Hepatitis, viral
posttransfusion — *see* Hepatitis, viral
puerperal, postpartum 674.8 ☑
lung (senile) 518.89
congenital 748.69
macular (dermatological) 701.3
syphilitic, skin 091.3

Atrophy, atrophic — *continued*
macular — *continued*
syphilitic, skin — *continued*
striated 095.8
muscle, muscular 728.2
disuse 728.2
Duchenne-Aran 335.21
extremity (lower) (upper) 728.2
familial spinal 335.11
general 728.2
idiopathic 728.2
infantile spinal 335.0
myelopathic (progressive) 335.10
myotonic 359.21
neuritic 356.1
neuropathic (peroneal) (progressive) 356.1
peroneal 356.1
primary (idiopathic) 728.2
progressive (familial) (hereditary) (pure) 335.21
adult (spinal) 335.19
infantile (spinal) 335.0
juvenile (spinal) 335.11
spinal 335.10
adult 335.19
hereditary or familial 335.11
infantile 335.0
pseudohypertrophic 359.1
spinal (progressive) 335.10
adult 335.19
Aran-Duchenne 335.21
familial 335.11
hereditary 335.11
infantile 335.0
juvenile 335.11
syphilitic 095.6
myocardium (*see also* Degeneration, myocardial) 429.1
myometrium (senile) 621.8
cervix 622.8
myotatic 728.2
myotonia 359.21
nail 703.8
congenital 757.5
nasopharynx 472.2
nerve (*see also* Disorder, nerve)
abducens 378.54
accessory 352.4
acoustic or auditory 388.5
cranial 352.9
first (olfactory) 352.0
second (optic) (*see also* Atrophy, optic nerve) 377.10
third (oculomotor) (partial) 378.51
total 378.52
fourth (trochlear) 378.53
fifth (trigeminal) 350.8
sixth (abducens) 378.54
seventh (facial) 351.8
eighth (auditory) 388.5
ninth (glossopharyngeal) 352.2
tenth (pneumogastric) (vagus) 352.3
eleventh (accessory) 352.4
twelfth (hypoglossal) 352.5
facial 351.8
glossopharyngeal 352.2
hypoglossal 352.5
oculomotor (partial) 378.51
total 378.52
olfactory 352.0
peripheral 355.9
pneumogastric 352.3
trigeminal 350.8
trochlear 378.53
vagus (pneumogastric) 352.3
nervous system, congenital 742.8
neuritic (*see also* Disorder, nerve) 355.9
neurogenic NEC 355.9
bone
tabetic 094.0
nutritional 261
old age 797
olivopontocerebellar 333.0

Atrophy, atrophic — *continued*

optic nerve (ascending) (descending) (infectional) (nonfamilial) (papillomacular bundle) (postretinal) (secondary NEC) (simple) 377.10

associated with retinal dystrophy 377.13

dominant hereditary 377.16

glaucomatous 377.14

hereditary (dominant) (Leber's) 377.16

Leber's (hereditary) 377.16

partial 377.15

postinflammatory 377.12

primary 377.11

syphilitic 094.84

congenital 090.49

tabes dorsalis 094.0

orbit 376.45

ovary (senile), acquired 620.3

oviduct (senile), acquired 620.3

palsy, diffuse 335.20

pancreas (duct) (senile) 577.8

papillary muscle 429.81

paralysis 355.9

parotid gland 527.0

patches skin 701.3

senile 701.8

penis 607.89

pharyngitis 472.1

pharynx 478.29

pluriglandular 258.8

polyarthritis 714.0

prostate 602.2

pseudohypertrophic 359.1

renal (*see also* Sclerosis, renal) 587

reticulata 701.8

retina (*see also* Degeneration, retina) 362.60

hereditary (*see also* Dystrophy, retina) 362.70

rhinitis 472.0

salivary duct or gland 527.0

scar NEC 709.2

sclerosis, lobar (of brain) 331.0

with dementia

with behavioral disturbance 331.0 *[294.11]*

without behavioral disturbance 331.0 *[294.10]*

scrotum 608.89

seminal vesicle 608.89

senile 797

degenerative, of skin 701.3

skin (patches) (senile) 701.8

spermatic cord 608.89

spinal (cord) 336.8

acute 336.8

muscular (chronic) 335.10

adult 335.19

familial 335.11

juvenile 335.10

paralysis 335.10

acute (*see also* Poliomyelitis, with paralysis) 045.1 ☑

spine (column) 733.99

spleen (senile) 289.59

spots (skin) 701.3

senile 701.8

stomach 537.89

striate and macular 701.3

syphilitic 095.8

subcutaneous 701.9

due to injection 999.9

sublingual gland 527.0

submaxillary gland 527.0

Sudeck's 733.7

suprarenal (autoimmune) (capsule) (gland) 255.41

with hypofunction 255.41

tarso-orbital fascia, congenital 743.66

testis 608.3

thenar, partial 354.0

throat 478.29

thymus (fat) 254.8

thyroid (gland) 246.8

with

cretinism 243

myxedema 244.9

Atrophy, atrophic — *continued*

thyroid — *continued*

congenital 243

tongue (senile) 529.8

papillae 529.4

smooth 529.4

trachea 519.19

tunica vaginalis 608.89

turbinate 733.99

tympanic membrane (nonflaccid) 384.82

flaccid 384.81

ulcer (*see also* Ulcer, skin) 707.9

upper respiratory tract 478.9

uterus, uterine (acquired) (senile) 621.8

cervix 622.8

due to radiation (intended effect) 621.8

vagina (senile) 627.3

vascular 459.89

vas deferens 608.89

vertebra (senile) 733.99

vulva (primary) (senile) 624.1

Werdnig-Hoffmann 335.0

yellow (acute) (congenital) (liver) (subacute) (*see also* Necrosis, liver) 570

chronic 571.8

resulting from administration of blood, plasma, serum, or other biological substance (within 8 months of administration) — *see* Hepatitis, viral

Attack

akinetic (*see also* Epilepsy) 345.0 ☑

angina — *see* Angina

apoplectic (*see also* Disease, cerebrovascular, acute) 436

benign shuddering 333.93

bilious — *see* Vomiting

cataleptic 300.11

cerebral (*see also* Disease, cerebrovascular, acute) 436

coronary (*see also* Infarct, myocardium) 410.9 ☑

cyanotic, newborn 770.83

epileptic (*see also* Epilepsy) 345.9 ☑

epileptiform 780.39

heart (*see also* Infarct, myocardium) 410.9 ☑

hemiplegia (*see also* Disease, cerebrovascular, acute) 436

hysterical 300.11

jacksonian (*see also* Epilepsy) 345.5 ☑

myocardium, myocardial (*see also* Infarct, myocardium) 410.9 ☑

myoclonic (*see also* Epilepsy) 345.1 ☑

panic 300.01

paralysis (*see also* Disease, cerebrovascular, acute) 436

paroxysmal 780.39

psychomotor (*see also* Epilepsy) 345.4 ☑

salaam (*see also* Epilepsy) 345.6 ☑

schizophreniform (*see also* Schizophrenia) 295.4 ☑

sensory and motor 780.39

syncope 780.2

toxic, cerebral 780.39

transient ischemic (TIA) 435.9

unconsciousness 780.2

hysterical 300.11

vasomotor 780.2

vasovagal (idiopathic) (paroxysmal) 780.2

Attention to

artificial opening (of) V55.9

digestive tract NEC V55.4

specified site NEC V55.8

urinary tract NEC V55.6

vagina V55.7

colostomy V55.3

cystostomy V55.5

dressing

wound V58.30

nonsurgical V58.30

surgical V58.31

gastrostomy V55.1

ileostomy V55.2

jejunostomy V55.4

nephrostomy V55.6

Attention to — *continued*

surgical dressings V58.31

sutures V58.32

tracheostomy V55.0

ureterostomy V55.6

urethrostomy V55.6

Attrition

gum (*see also* Recession, gingival) 523.20

teeth (hard tissues) 521.10

excessive 521.10

extending into

dentine 521.12

pulp 521.13

generalized 521.15

limited to enamel 521.11

localized 521.14

Atypical — *see also* condition

cells

endocervical 795.00

endometrial 795.00

glandular

anus 796.70

cervical 795.00

vaginal 795.10

distribution, vessel (congenital) (peripheral) NEC 747.60

endometrium 621.9

kidney 593.89

Atypism, cervix 622.10

Audible tinnitus — *see also* Tinnitus 388.30

Auditory — *see* condition

Audry's syndrome (acropachyderma) 757.39

Aujeszky's disease 078.89

Aura

jacksonian (*see also* Epilepsy) 345.5 ☑

persistent migraine 346.5 ☑

with cerebral infarction 346.6 ☑

without cerebral infarction 346.5 ☑

Aurantiasis, cutis 278.3

Auricle, auricular — *see* condition

Auriculotemporal syndrome 350.8

Australian

Q fever 083.0

X disease 062.4

Autism, autistic (child) (infantile) 299.0 ☑

Autodigestion 799.89

Autoerythrocyte sensitization 287.2

Autographism 708.3

Autoimmune

cold sensitivity 283.0

disease NEC 279.49

hemolytic anemia 283.0

inhibitors to clotting factors 286.52

lymphoproliferative syndrome (ALPS) 279.41

thyroiditis 245.2

Autoinfection, septic — *see* Septicemia

Autointoxication 799.89

Automatism 348.89

with temporal sclerosis 348.81

epileptic (*see also* Epilepsy) 345.4 ☑

paroxysmal, idiopathic (*see also* Epilepsy) 345.4 ☑

Autonomic, autonomous

bladder 596.54

neurogenic 596.54

with cauda equina 344.61

dysreflexia 337.3

faciocephalalgia (*see also* Neuropathy, peripheral, autonomic) 337.9

hysterical seizure 300.11

imbalance (*see also* Neuropathy, peripheral, autonomic) 337.9

Autophony 388.40

Autosensitivity, erythrocyte 287.2

Autotopagnosia 780.99

Autotoxemia 799.89

Autumn — *see* condition

Avellis' syndrome 344.89

Aversion

oral 783.3

newborn 779.31

nonorganic origin 307.59

Aviators

disease or sickness (*see also* Effect, adverse, high altitude) 993.2

Aviators — *continued*

ear 993.0

effort syndrome 306.2

Avitaminosis (multiple NEC) — *see also* Deficiency, vitamin 269.2

A 264.9

B 266.9

with

beriberi 265.0

pellagra 265.2

B_1 265.1

B_2 266.0

B_6 266.1

B_{12} 266.2

C (with scurvy) 267

D 268.9

with

osteomalacia 268.2

rickets 268.0

E 269.1

G 266.0

H 269.1

K 269.0

multiple 269.2

nicotinic acid 265.2

P 269.1

Avulsion (traumatic) 879.8

blood vessel — *see* Injury, blood vessel, by site

cartilage (*see also* Dislocation, by site)

knee, current (*see also* Tear, meniscus) 836.2

symphyseal (inner), complicating delivery 665.6 ☑

complicated 879.9

diaphragm — *see* Injury, internal, diaphragm

ear — *see* Wound, open, ear

epiphysis of bone — *see* Fracture, by site

external site other than limb — *see* Wound, open, by site

eye 871.3

fingernail — *see* Wound, open, finger

fracture — *see* Fracture, by site

genital organs, external — *see* Wound, open, genital organs

head (intracranial) NEC (*see also* Injury, intracranial, with open intracranial wound)

complete 874.9

external site NEC 873.8

complicated 873.9

internal organ or site — *see* Injury, internal, by site

joint (*see also* Dislocation, by site)

capsule — *see* Sprain, by site

ligament — *see* Sprain, by site

limb (*see also* Amputation, traumatic, by site)

skin and subcutaneous tissue — *see* Wound, open, by site

muscle — *see* Sprain, by site

nerve (root) — *see* Injury, nerve, by site

scalp — *see* Wound, open, scalp

skin and subcutaneous tissue — *see* Wound, open, by site

symphyseal cartilage (inner), complicating delivery 665.6 ☑

tendon (*see also* Sprain, by site)

with open wound — *see* Wound, open, by site

toenail — *see* Wound, open, toe(s)

tooth 873.63

complicated 873.73

Awaiting organ transplant status V49.83

Awareness of heart beat 785.1

Axe grinders' disease 502

Axenfeld's anomaly or syndrome 743.44

Axilla, axillary — *see also* condition

breast 757.6

Axonotmesis — *see* Injury, nerve, by site

Ayala's disease 756.89

Ayerza's disease or syndrome (pulmonary artery sclerosis with pulmonary hypertension) 416.0

☑ **Additional Digit Required** — Refer to the Tabular List for Digit Selection   ▽ **Subterms under main terms may continue to next column or page**

2014 ICD-9-CM   **79**

Biting — *continued*
nail 307.9
Black
death 020.9
eye NEC 921.0
hairy tongue 529.3
heel 924.20
lung disease 500
palm 923.20
Blackfan-Diamond anemia or syndrome
(congenital hypoplastic anemia) 284.01
Blackhead 706.1
Blackout 780.2
Blackwater fever 084.8
Bladder — *see* condition
Blast
blindness 921.3
concussion — *see* Blast, injury
injury 869.0
with open wound into cavity 869.1
abdomen or thorax — *see* Injury, internal, by site
brain (*see also* Concussion, brain) 850.9
with skull fracture — *see* Fracture, skull
ear (acoustic nerve trauma) 951.5
with perforation, tympanic membrane — *see* Wound, open, ear, drum
lung (*see also* Injury, internal, lung) 861.20
otitic (explosive) 388.11
Blastomycosis, blastomycotic (chronic) (cutaneous) (disseminated) (lung) (pulmonary) (systemic) 116.0
Brazilian 116.1
European 117.5
keloidal 116.2
North American 116.0
primary pulmonary 116.0
South American 116.1
Bleb(s) 709.8
emphysematous (bullous) (diffuse) (lung) (ruptured) (solitary) 492.0
filtering, eye (postglaucoma) (status) V45.69
with complication 997.99
postcataract extraction (complication) 997.99
lung (ruptured) 492.0
congenital 770.5
subpleural (emphysematous) 492.0
Bleeder (familial) (hereditary) — *see* Defect, coagulation 286.9
nonfamilial 286.9
Bleeding — *see also* Hemorrhage 459.0
anal 569.3
anovulatory 628.0
atonic, following delivery 666.1 ☑
capillary 448.9
due to subinvolution 621.1
puerperal 666.2 ☑
ear 388.69
excessive, associated with menopausal onset 627.0
familial (*see also* Defect, coagulation) 286.9
following intercourse 626.7
gastrointestinal 578.9
gums 523.8
hemorrhoids — *see* Hemorrhoids, bleeding
intermenstrual
irregular 626.6
regular 626.5
intraoperative 998.11
irregular NEC 626.4
menopausal 627.0
mouth 528.9
nipple 611.79
nose 784.7
ovulation 626.5
postclimacteric 627.1
postcoital 626.7
postmenopausal 627.1
following induced menopause 627.4
postoperative 998.11
preclimacteric 627.0
puberty 626.3

Bleeding — *see also* Hemorrhage — *continued*
puberty — *continued*
excessive, with onset of menstrual periods 626.3
rectum, rectal 569.3
tendencies (*see also* Defect, coagulation) 286.9
throat 784.8
umbilical stump 772.3
umbilicus 789.9
unrelated to menstrual cycle 626.6
uterus, uterine 626.9
climacteric 627.0
dysfunctional 626.8
functional 626.8
unrelated to menstrual cycle 626.6
vagina, vaginal 623.8
functional 626.8
vicarious 625.8
Blennorrhagia, blennorrhagic — *see* Blennorrhea
Blennorrhea (acute) 098.0
adultorum 098.40
alveolaris 523.40
chronic or duration of 2 months or over 098.2
gonococcal (neonatorum) 098.40
inclusion (neonatal) (newborn) 771.6
neonatorum 098.40
Blepharelosis — *see also* Entropion 374.00
Blepharitis (eyelid) 373.00
angularis 373.01
ciliaris 373.00
with ulcer 373.01
marginal 373.00
with ulcer 373.01
scrofulous (*see also* Tuberculosis) 017.3 ☑ *[373.00]*
squamous 373.02
ulcerative 373.01
Blepharochalasis 374.34
congenital 743.62
Blepharoclonus 333.81
Blepharoconjunctivitis — *see also* Conjunctivitis 372.20
angular 372.21
contact 372.22
Blepharophimosis (eyelid) 374.46
congenital 743.62
Blepharoplegia 374.89
Blepharoptosis 374.30
congenital 743.61
Blepharopyorrhea 098.49
Blepharospasm 333.81
due to drugs 333.85
Blessig's cyst 362.62
Blighted ovum 631.8
Blind
bronchus (congenital) 748.3
eye (*see also* Blindness)
hypertensive 360.42
hypotensive 360.41
loop syndrome (postoperative) 579.2
sac, fallopian tube (congenital) 752.19
spot, enlarged 368.42
tract or tube (congenital) NEC — *see* Atresia
Blindness (acquired) (congenital) (both eyes) 369.00
with deafness V49.85
blast 921.3
with nerve injury — *see* Injury, nerve, optic
Bright's — *see* Uremia
color (congenital) 368.59
acquired 368.55
blue 368.53
green 368.52
red 368.51
total 368.54
concussion 950.9
cortical 377.75
day 368.10
acquired 368.10
congenital 368.10
hereditary 368.10

Blindness — *continued*
day — *continued*
specified type NEC 368.10
due to
injury NEC 950.9
refractive error — *see* Error, refractive
eclipse (total) 363.31
emotional 300.11
face 368.16
hysterical 300.11
legal (both eyes) (USA definition) 369.4
with impairment of better (less impaired) eye
near-total 369.02
with
lesser eye impairment 369.02
near-total 369.04
total 369.03
profound 369.05
with
lesser eye impairment 369.05
near-total 369.07
profound 369.08
total 369.06
severe 369.21
with
lesser eye impairment 369.21
blind 369.11
near-total 369.13
profound 369.14
severe 369.22
total 369.12
total
with lesser eye impairment
total 369.01
mind 784.69
moderate
both eyes 369.25
with impairment of lesser eye (specified as)
blind, not further specified 369.15
low vision, not further specified 369.23
near-total 369.17
profound 369.18
severe 369.24
total 369.16
one eye 369.74
with vision of other eye (specified as)
near-normal 369.75
normal 369.76
near-total
both eyes 369.04
with impairment of lesser eye (specified as)
blind, not further specified 369.02
total 369.03
one eye 369.64
with vision of other eye (specified as)
near-normal 369.65
normal 369.66
night 368.60
acquired 368.62
congenital (Japanese) 368.61
hereditary 368.61
specified type NEC 368.69
vitamin A deficiency 264.5
nocturnal — *see* Blindness, night
one eye 369.60
with low vision of other eye 369.10
profound
both eyes 369.08
with impairment of lesser eye (specified as)
blind, not further specified 369.05
near-total 369.07
total 369.06
one eye 369.67
with vision of other eye (specified as)
near-normal 369.68
normal 369.69
psychic 784.69
severe
both eyes 369.22

Blindness — *continued*
severe — *continued*
both eyes — *continued*
with impairment of lesser eye (specified as)
blind, not further specified 369.11
low vision, not further specified 369.21
near-total 369.13
profound 369.14
total 369.12
one eye 369.71
with vision of other eye (specified as)
near-normal 369.72
normal 369.73
snow 370.24
sun 363.31
temporary 368.12
total
both eyes 369.01
one eye 369.61
with vision of other eye (specified as)
near-normal 369.62
normal 369.63
transient 368.12
traumatic NEC 950.9
word (developmental) 315.01
acquired 784.61
secondary to organic lesion 784.61
Blister — *see also* Injury, superficial, by site
beetle dermatitis 692.89
due to burn — *see* Burn, by site, second degree
fever 054.9
fracture — *omit code*
multiple, skin, nontraumatic 709.8
Bloating 787.3
Bloch-Siemens syndrome (incontinentia pigmenti) 757.33
Bloch-Stauffer dyshormonal dermatosis 757.33
Bloch-Sulzberger disease or syndrome (incontinentia pigmenti) (melanoblastosis) 757.33
Block
alveolar capillary 516.8
arborization (heart) 426.6
arrhythmic 426.9
atrioventricular (AV) (incomplete) (partial) 426.10
with
2:1 atrioventricular response block 426.13
atrioventricular dissociation 426.0
first degree (incomplete) 426.11
second degree (Mobitz type I) 426.13
Mobitz (type) II 426.12
third degree 426.0
complete 426.0
congenital 746.86
congenital 746.86
Mobitz (incomplete)
type I (Wenckebach's) 426.13
type II 426.12
partial 426.13
auriculoventricular (*see also* Block, atrioventricular) 426.10
complete 426.0
congenital 746.86
congenital 746.86
bifascicular (cardiac) 426.53
bundle branch (complete) (false) (incomplete) 426.50
bilateral 426.53
left (complete) (main stem) 426.3
with right bundle branch block 426.53
anterior fascicular 426.2
with
posterior fascicular block 426.3
right bundle branch block 426.52
hemiblock 426.2
incomplete 426.2

☑ **Additional Digit Required** — Refer to the Tabular List for Digit Selection   ▽ **Subterms under main terms may continue to next column or page**

2014 ICD-9-CM   81

Block — *continued*
　bundle branch — *continued*
　　left — *continued*
　　　incomplete — *continued*
　　　　with right bundle branch block 426.53
　　　　posterior fascicular 426.2
　　　　with
　　　　　anterior fascicular block 426.3
　　　　　right bundle branch block 426.51
　　　right 426.4
　　　　with
　　　　　left bundle branch block (incomplete) (main stem) 426.53
　　　　　left fascicular block 426.53
　　　　　　anterior 426.52
　　　　　　posterior 426.51
　　　　Wilson's type 426.4
　cardiac 426.9
　conduction 426.9
　　complete 426.0
　Eustachian tube (*see also* Obstruction, Eustachian tube) 381.60
　fascicular (left anterior) (left posterior) 426.2
　foramen Magendie (acquired) 331.3
　　congenital 742.3
　　　with spina bifida (*see also* Spina bifida) 741.0 ☑
　heart 426.9
　　first degree (atrioventricular) 426.11
　　second degree (atrioventricular) 426.13
　　third degree (atrioventricular) 426.0
　　bundle branch (complete) (false) (incomplete) 426.50
　　　bilateral 426.53
　　　left (*see also* Block, bundle branch, left) 426.3
　　　right (*see also* Block, bundle branch, right) 426.4
　　complete (atrioventricular) 426.0
　　congenital 746.86
　　incomplete 426.13
　　intra-atrial 426.6
　　intraventricular NEC 426.6
　　sinoatrial 426.6
　　specified type NEC 426.6
　hepatic vein 453.0
　intraventricular (diffuse) (myofibrillar) 426.6
　　bundle branch (complete) (false) (incomplete) 426.50
　　　bilateral 426.53
　　　left (*see also* Block, bundle branch, left) 426.3
　　　right (*see also* Block, bundle branch, right) 426.4
　kidney (*see also* Disease, renal) 593.9
　　postcystoscopic 997.5
　myocardial (*see also* Block, heart) 426.9
　nodal 426.10
　optic nerve 377.49
　organ or site (congenital) NEC — *see* Atresia
　parietal 426.6
　peri-infarction 426.6
　portal (vein) 452
　sinoatrial 426.6
　sinoauricular 426.6
　spinal cord 336.9
　trifascicular 426.54
　tubal 628.2
　vein NEC 453.9
Blocq's disease or syndrome (astasia-abasia) 307.9
Blood
　constituents, abnormal NEC 790.6
　disease 289.9
　　specified NEC 289.89
　donor V59.01
　　other blood components V59.09
　　stem cells V59.02
　　whole blood V59.01
　dyscrasia 289.9
　　with
　　　abortion — *see* Abortion, by type, with hemorrhage, delayed or excessive

Blood — *continued*
　dyscrasia — *continued*
　　with — *continued*
　　　ectopic pregnancy (*see also* categories 633.0–633.9) 639.1
　　　molar pregnancy (*see also* categories 630–632) 639.1
　　following
　　　abortion 639.1
　　　ectopic or molar pregnancy 639.1
　　newborn NEC 776.9
　　puerperal, postpartum 666.3 ☑
　flukes NEC (*see also* Infestation, Schistosoma) 120.9
　in
　　feces (*see also* Melena) 578.1
　　　occult 792.1
　　urine (*see also* Hematuria) 599.70
　mole 631.8
　occult 792.1
　poisoning (*see also* Septicemia) 038.9
　pressure
　　decreased, due to shock following injury 958.4
　　fluctuating 796.4
　　high (*see also* Hypertension) 401.9
　　　borderline 796.2
　　　incidental reading (isolated) (nonspecific), without diagnosis of hypertension 796.2
　　low (*see also* Hypotension) 458.9
　　　incidental reading (isolated) (nonspecific), without diagnosis of hypotension 796.3
　spitting (*see also* Hemoptysis) 786.30
　staining cornea 371.12
　transfusion
　　without reported diagnosis V58.2
　　donor V59.01
　　　stem cells V59.02
　　reaction or complication — *see* Complications, transfusion
　tumor — *see* Hematoma
　vessel rupture — *see* Hemorrhage
　vomiting (*see also* Hematemesis) 578.0
Blood-forming organ disease 289.9
Bloodgood's disease 610.1
Bloodshot eye 379.93
Bloom (-Machacek) (-Torre) syndrome 757.39
Blotch, palpebral 372.55
Blount-Barber syndrome (tibia vara) 732.4
Blount's disease (tibia vara) 732.4
Blue
　baby 746.9
　bloater 491.20
　　with
　　　acute bronchitis 491.22
　　　exacerbation (acute) 491.21
　diaper syndrome 270.0
　disease 746.9
　dome cyst 610.0
　drum syndrome 381.02
　sclera 743.47
　　with fragility of bone and deafness 756.51
　toe syndrome 445.02
Blueness — *see also* Cyanosis 782.5
Blurring, visual 368.8
Blushing (abnormal) (excessive) 782.62
BMI (body mass index)
　adult
　　25.0-25.9 V85.21
　　26.0-26.9 V85.22
　　27.0-27.9 V85.23
　　28.0-28.9 V85.24
　　29.0-29.9 V85.25
　　30.0-30.9 V85.30
　　31.0-31.9 V85.31
　　32.0-32.9 V85.32
　　33.0-33.9 V85.33
　　34.0-34.9 V85.34
　　35.0-35.9 V85.35
　　36.0-36.9 V85.36
　　37.0-37.9 V85.37
　　38.0-38.9 V85.38
　　39.0-39.9 V85.39

BMI — *continued*
　adult — *continued*
　　40.0-44.9 V85.41
　　45.0-49.9 V85.42
　　50.0-59.9 V85.43
　　60.0-69.9 V85.44
　　70 and over V85.45
　　between 19-24 V85.1
　　less than 19 V85.0
　pediatric
　　5th percentile to less than 85th percentile for age V85.52
　　85th percentile to less than 95th percentile for age V85.53
　　greater than or equal to 95th percentile for age V85.54
　　less than 5th percentile for age V85.51
Boarder, hospital V65.0
　infant V65.0
Bockhart's impetigo (superficial folliculitis) 704.8
Bodechtel-Guttmann disease (subacute sclerosing panencephalitis) 046.2
Boder-Sedgwick syndrome (ataxia-telangiectasia) 334.8
Body, bodies
　Aschoff (*see also* Myocarditis, rheumatic) 398.0
　asteroid, vitreous 379.22
　choroid, colloid (degenerative) 362.57
　　hereditary 362.77
　cytoid (retina) 362.82
　drusen (retina) (*see also* Drusen) 362.57
　　optic disc 377.21
　fibrin, pleura 511.0
　foreign — *see* Foreign body
　Hassall-Henle 371.41
　loose
　　joint (*see also* Loose, body, joint) 718.1 ☑
　　　knee 717.6
　　knee 717.6
　　sheath, tendon 727.82
　Mallory's 034.1
　mass index (BMI)
　　adult
　　　25.0-25.9 V85.21
　　　26.0-26.9 V85.22
　　　27.0-27.9 V85.23
　　　28.0-28.9 V85.24
　　　29.0-29.9 V85.25
　　　30.0-30.9 V85.30
　　　31.0-31.9 V85.31
　　　32.0-32.9 V85.32
　　　33.0-33.9 V85.33
　　　34.0-34.9 V85.34
　　　35.0-35.9 V85.35
　　　36.0-36.9 V85.36
　　　37.0-37.9 V85.37
　　　38.0-38.9 V85.38
　　　39.0-39.9 V85.39
　　　40.0-44.9 V85.41
　　　45.0-49.9 V85.42
　　　50.0-59.9 V85.43
　　　60.0-69.9 V85.44
　　　70 and over V85.45
　　　between 19-24 V85.1
　　　less than 19 V85.0
　　pediatric
　　　5th percentile to less than 85th percentile for age V85.52
　　　85th percentile to less than 95th percentile for age V85.53
　　　greater than or equal to 95th percentile for age V85.54
　　　less than 5th percentile for age V85.51
　Mooser 081.0
　Negri 071
　rice (joint) (*see also* Loose, body, joint) 718.1 ☑
　　knee 717.6
　rocking 307.3
Boeck's
　disease (sarcoidosis) 135
　lupoid (miliary) 135

Boeck's — *continued*
　sarcoid 135
Boerhaave's syndrome (spontaneous esophageal rupture) 530.4
Boggy
　cervix 622.8
　uterus 621.8
Boil — *see also* Carbuncle 680.9
　abdominal wall 680.2
　Aleppo 085.1
　ankle 680.6
　anus 680.5
　arm (any part, above wrist) 680.3
　auditory canal, external 680.0
　axilla 680.3
　back (any part) 680.2
　Baghdad 085.1
　breast 680.2
　buttock 680.5
　chest wall 680.2
　corpus cavernosum 607.2
　Delhi 085.1
　ear (any part) 680.0
　eyelid 373.13
　face (any part, except eye) 680.0
　finger (any) 680.4
　flank 680.2
　foot (any part) 680.7
　forearm 680.3
　Gafsa 085.1
　genital organ, male 608.4
　gluteal (region) 680.5
　groin 680.2
　hand (any part) 680.4
　head (any part, except face) 680.8
　heel 680.7
　hip 680.6
　knee 680.6
　labia 616.4
　lacrimal (*see also* Dacryocystitis) 375.30
　　gland (*see also* Dacryoadenitis) 375.00
　　passages (duct) (sac) (*see also* Dacryocystitis) 375.30
　leg, any part, except foot 680.6
　multiple sites 680.9
　natal 085.1
　neck 680.1
　nose (external) (septum) 680.0
　orbit, orbital 376.01
　partes posteriores 680.5
　pectoral region 680.2
　penis 607.2
　perineum 680.2
　pinna 680.0
　scalp (any part) 680.8
　scrotum 608.4
　seminal vesicle 608.0
　shoulder 680.3
　skin NEC 680.9
　specified site NEC 680.8
　spermatic cord 608.4
　temple (region) 680.0
　testis 608.4
　thigh 680.6
　thumb 680.4
　toe (any) 680.7
　tropical 085.1
　trunk 680.2
　tunica vaginalis 608.4
　umbilicus 680.2
　upper arm 680.3
　vas deferens 608.4
　vulva 616.4
　wrist 680.4
Bold hives — *see also* Urticaria 708.9
Bolivian hemorrhagic fever 078.7
Bombé, iris 364.74
Bomford-Rhoads anemia (refractory) 238.72
Bone — *see* condition
Bonnevie-Ullrich syndrome 758.6
Bonnier's syndrome 386.19
Bonvale Dam fever 780.79
Bony block of joint 718.80
　ankle 718.87
　elbow 718.82
　foot 718.87

☑ **Additional Digit Required** — Refer to the Tabular List for Digit Selection

▽ **Subterms under main terms may continue to next column or page**

Bony block of joint — *continued*
  hand 718.84
  hip 718.85
  knee 718.86
  multiple sites 718.89
  pelvic region 718.85
  shoulder (region) 718.81
  specified site NEC 718.88
  wrist 718.83
BOOP (bronchiolitis obliterans organized
  pneumonia) 516.8
Borderline
  diabetes mellitus 790.29
  hypertension 796.2
  intellectual functioning V62.89
  osteopenia 733.90
  pelvis 653.1 ☑
    with obstruction during labor 660.1 ☑
     affecting fetus or newborn 763.1
  psychosis (*see also* Schizophrenia) 295.5 ☑
    of childhood (*see also* Psychosis, child-
     hood) 299.8 ☑
  schizophrenia (*see also* Schizophrenia)
    295.5 ☑
Borna disease 062.9
Bornholm disease (epidemic pleurodynia)
  074.1
Borrelia vincentii (mouth) (pharynx) (tonsils)
  101
Bostock's catarrh — *see also* Fever, hay 477.9
Boston exanthem 048
Botalli, ductus (patent) (persistent) 747.0
Bothriocephalus latus infestation 123.4
Botulism 005.1
  food poisoning 005.1
  infant 040.41
  non-foodborne 040.42
  wound 040.42
Bouba — *see also* Yaws 102.9
Bouffée délirante 298.3
Bouillaud's disease or syndrome (rheumatic
  heart disease) 391.9
Bourneville's disease (tuberous sclerosis)
  759.5
Boutonneuse fever 082.1
Boutonniere
  deformity (finger) 736.21
  hand (intrinsic) 736.21
Bouveret (-Hoffmann) disease or syndrome
  (paroxysmal tachycardia) 427.2
Bovine heart — *see* Hypertrophy, cardiac
Bowel — *see* condition
Bowen's
  dermatosis (precancerous) (M8081/2) —
    see Neoplasm, skin, in situ
  disease (M8081/2) — *see* Neoplasm, skin,
    in situ
  epithelioma (M8081/2) — *see* Neoplasm,
    skin, in situ
  type
    epidermoid carcinoma in situ (M8081/2)
     — *see* Neoplasm, skin, in situ
    intraepidermal squamous cell carcinoma
     (M8081/2) — *see* Neoplasm, skin,
     in situ
Bowing
  femur 736.89
    congenital 754.42
  fibula 736.89
    congenital 754.43
  forearm 736.09
    away from midline (cubitus valgus)
     736.01
    toward midline (cubitus varus) 736.02
  leg(s), long bones, congenital 754.44
  radius 736.09
    away from midline (cubitus valgus)
     736.01
    toward midline (cubitus varus) 736.02
  tibia 736.89
    congenital 754.43
Bowleg(s) 736.42
  congenital 754.44
  rachitic 268.1
Boyd's dysentery 004.2
Brachial — *see* condition

Brachman-de Lange syndrome (Amsterdam
  dwarf, intellectual disabilities, and
  brachycephaly) 759.89
Brachycardia 427.89
Brachycephaly 756.0
Brachymorphism and ectopia lentis 759.89
Bradley's disease (epidemic vomiting) 078.82
Bradycardia 427.89
  chronic (sinus) 427.81
  newborn 779.81
  nodal 427.89
  postoperative 997.1
  reflex 337.09
  sinoatrial 427.89
    with paroxysmal tachyarrhythmia or
     tachyarrhythmia 427.81
    chronic 427.81
  sinus 427.89
    with paroxysmal tachyarrhythmia or
     tachycardia 427.81
    chronic 427.81
    persistent 427.81
    severe 427.81
  tachycardia syndrome 427.81
  vagal 427.89
Bradykinesia 781.0
Bradypnea 786.09
Brailsford's disease 732.3
  radial head 732.3
  tarsal scaphoid 732.5
Brailsford-Morquio disease or syndrome
  (mucopolysaccharidosis IV) 277.5
Brain — *see also* condition
  death 348.82
  syndrome (acute) (chronic) (nonpsychotic)
    (organic) (with neurotic reaction)
    (with behavioral reaction) (*see also*
    Syndrome, brain) 310.9
    with
     presenile brain disease 290.10
     psychosis, psychotic reaction (*see al-
      so* Psychosis, organic) 294.9
    congenital (*see also* Disability, intellectu-
     al) 319
Branched-chain amino-acid disease 270.3
Branchial — *see* condition
Brandt's syndrome (acrodermatitis enteropath-
  ica) 686.8
Brash (water) 787.1
Brass-founders' ague 985.8
Bravais-Jacksonian epilepsy — *see also*
  Epilepsy 345.5 ☑
Braxton Hicks contractions 644.1 ☑
Braziers' disease 985.8
Brazilian
  blastomycosis 116.1
  leishmaniasis 085.5
BRBPR (bright red blood per rectum) 569.3
Break
  cardiorenal — *see* Hypertension, cardiorenal
  retina (*see also* Defect, retina) 361.30
Breakbone fever 061
Breakdown
  device, implant, or graft — *see* Complica-
    tions, mechanical
  nervous (*see also* Disorder, mental, nonpsy-
    chotic) 300.9
  perineum 674.2 ☑
Breast — *see also* condition
  buds 259.1
    in newborn 779.89
  dense 793.82
  nodule 793.89
Breast feeding difficulties 676.8 ☑
Breath
  foul 784.99
  holder, child 312.81
  holding spells 786.9
  shortness 786.05
Breathing
  asymmetrical 786.09
  bronchial 786.09
  exercises V57.0
  labored 786.09
  mouth 784.99
    causing malocclusion 524.59

Breathing — *continued*
  periodic 786.09
    high altitude 327.22
  tic 307.20
Breathlessness 786.09
Breda's disease — *see also* Yaws 102.9
Breech
  delivery, affecting fetus or newborn 763.0
  extraction, affecting fetus or newborn 763.0
  presentation (buttocks) (complete) (frank)
    652.2 ☑
    with successful version 652.1 ☑
    before labor, affecting fetus or newborn
     761.7
    during labor, affecting fetus or newborn
     763.0
Breisky's disease (kraurosis vulvae) 624.09
Brennemann's syndrome (acute mesenteric
  lymphadenitis) 289.2
Brenner's
  tumor (benign) (M9000/0) 220
    borderline malignancy (M9000/1) 236.2
    malignant (M9000/3) 183.0
    proliferating (M9000/1) 236.2
Bretonneau's disease (diphtheritic malignant
  angina) 032.0
Breus' mole 631.8
Brevicollis 756.16
Bricklayers' itch 692.89
Brickmakers' anemia 126.9
Bridge
  myocardial 746.85
Bright's
  blindness — *see* Uremia
  disease (*see also* Nephritis) 583.9
    arteriosclerotic (*see also* Hypertension,
     kidney) 403.90
Bright red blood per rectum (BRBPR) 569.3
Brill's disease (recrudescent typhus) 081.1
  flea-borne 081.0
  louse-borne 081.1
Brill-Symmers disease (follicular lymphoma)
  (M9690/3) 202.0 ☑
Brill-Zinsser disease (recrudescent typhus)
  081.1
Brinton's disease (linitis plastica) (M8142/3)
  151.9
Brion-Kayser disease — *see also* Fever,
  paratyphoid 002.9
Briquet's disorder or syndrome 300.81
Brissaud's
  infantilism (infantile myxedema) 244.9
  motor-verbal tic 307.23
Brissaud-Meige syndrome (infantile
  myxedema) 244.9
Brittle
  bones (congenital) 756.51
  nails 703.8
    congenital 757.5
Broad — *see also* condition
  beta disease 272.2
  ligament laceration syndrome 620.6
Brock's syndrome (atelectasis due to enlarged
  lymph nodes) 518.0
Brocq's disease 691.8
  atopic (diffuse) neurodermatitis 691.8
  lichen simplex chronicus 698.3
  parakeratosis psoriasiformis 696.2
  parapsoriasis 696.2
Brocq-Duhring disease (dermatitis herpetiformis) 694.0
Brodie's
  abscess (localized) (chronic) (*see also* Os-
    teomyelitis) 730.1 ☑
  disease (joint) (*see also* Osteomyelitis)
    730.1 ☑
Broken
  arches 734
    congenital 755.67
  back — *see* Fracture, vertebra, by site
  bone — *see* Fracture, by site
  compensation — *see* Disease, heart
  heart syndrome 429.83
  implant or internal device — *see* listing un-
    der Complications, mechanical
  neck — *see* Fracture, vertebra, cervical

Broken — *continued*
  nose 802.0
    open 802.1
  tooth, teeth 873.63
    complicated 873.73
Bromhidrosis 705.89
Bromidism, bromism
  acute 967.3
    correct substance properly administered
     349.82
    overdose or wrong substance given or
     taken 967.3
  chronic (*see also* Dependence) 304.1 ☑
Bromidrosiphobia 300.23
Bromidrosis 705.89
Bronchi, bronchial — *see* condition
Bronchiectasis (cylindrical) (diffuse) (fusiform)
  (localized) (moniliform) (postinfectious)
  (recurrent) (saccular) 494.0
  with acute exacerbation 494.1
  congenital 748.61
  tuberculosis (*see also* Tuberculosis) 011.5 ☑
Bronchiolectasis — *see* Bronchiectasis
Bronchiolitis (acute) (infectious) (subacute)
  466.19
  with
    bronchospasm or obstruction 466.19
    influenza, flu, or grippe (*see also* Influen-
     za) 487.1
  catarrhal (acute) (subacute) 466.19
  chemical 506.0
    chronic 506.4
  chronic (obliterative) 491.8
  due to external agent — *see* Bronchitis,
    acute, due to
  fibrosa obliterans 491.8
  influenzal (*see also* Influenza) 487.1
  obliterans 491.8
    with organizing pneumonia (BOOP)
     516.8
    status post lung transplant 996.84
  obliterative (chronic) (diffuse) (subacute)
    491.8
    due to fumes or vapors 506.4
  respiratory syncytial virus 466.11
  vesicular — *see* Pneumonia, broncho-
Bronchitis (diffuse) (hypostatic) (infectious)
  (inflammatory) (simple) 490
  with
    emphysema — *see* Emphysema
    influenza, flu, or grippe (*see also* Influen-
     za) 487.1
    obstruction airway, chronic 491.20
     with
      acute bronchitis 491.22
      exacerbation (acute) 491.21
    tracheitis 490
     acute or subacute 466.0
      with bronchospasm or obstruc-
       tion 466.0
     chronic 491.8
  acute or subacute 466.0
    with
     bronchiectasis 494.1
     bronchospasm 466.0
     obstruction 466.0
     tracheitis 466.0
    chemical (due to fumes or vapors) 506.0
    due to
     fumes or vapors 506.0
     radiation 508.8
  allergic (acute) (*see also* Asthma) 493.9 ☑
  arachidic 934.1
  aspiration 507.0
    due to fumes or vapors 506.0
  asthmatic (acute) 493.90
    with
     acute exacerbation 493.92
     status asthmaticus 493.91
    chronic 493.2 ☑
  capillary 466.19
    with bronchospasm or obstruction
     466.19
    chronic 491.8
  caseous (*see also* Tuberculosis) 011.3 ☑
  Castellani's 104.8

☑ Additional Digit Required — Refer to the Tabular List for Digit Selection ▼ Subterms under main terms may continue to next column or page

Bronchitis — *continued*
- catarrhal 490
  - acute — *see* Bronchitis, acute
  - chronic 491.0
- chemical (acute) (subacute) 506.0
  - chronic 506.4
  - due to fumes or vapors (acute) (subacute) 506.0
    - chronic 506.4
- chronic 491.9
  - with
    - tracheitis (chronic) 491.8
  - asthmatic 493.2 ☑
  - catarrhal 491.0
  - chemical (due to fumes and vapors) 506.4
  - due to
    - fumes or vapors (chemical) (inhalation) 506.4
    - radiation 508.8
    - tobacco smoking 491.0
  - mucopurulent 491.1
  - obstructive 491.20
    - with
      - acute bronchitis 491.22
      - exacerbation (acute) 491.21
  - purulent 491.1
  - simple 491.0
  - specified type NEC 491.8
- croupous 466.0
  - with bronchospasm or obstruction 466.0
  - due to fumes or vapors 506.0
- emphysematous 491.20
  - with
    - acute bronchitis 491.22
    - exacerbation (acute) 491.21
- exudative 466.0
- fetid (chronic) (recurrent) 491.1
- fibrinous, acute or subacute 466.0
  - with bronchospasm or obstruction 466.0
- grippal (*see also* Influenza) 487.1
- influenzal (*see also* Influenza) 487.1
- membranous, acute or subacute 466.0
  - with bronchospasm or obstruction 466.0
- moulders' 502
- mucopurulent (chronic) (recurrent) 491.1
  - acute or subacute 466.0
- obliterans 491.8
- obstructive (chronic) 491.20
  - with
    - acute bronchitis 491.22
    - exacerbation (acute) 491.21
- pituitous 491.1
- plastic (inflammatory) 466.0
- pneumococcal, acute or subacute 466.0
  - with bronchospasm or obstruction 466.0
- pseudomembranous 466.0
- purulent (chronic) (recurrent) 491.1
  - acute or subacute 466.0
    - with bronchospasm or obstruction 466.0
- putrid 491.1
- scrofulous (*see also* Tuberculosis) 011.3 ☑
- senile 491.9
- septic, acute or subacute 466.0
  - with bronchospasm or obstruction 466.0
- smokers' 491.0
- spirochetal 104.8
- suffocative, acute or subacute 466.0
- summer (*see also* Asthma) 493.9 ☑
- suppurative (chronic) 491.1
  - acute or subacute 466.0
- tuberculous (*see also* Tuberculosis) 011.3 ☑
- ulcerative 491.8
  - Vincent's 101
- Vincent's 101
- viral, acute or subacute 466.0

Bronchoalveolitis 485
Bronchoaspergillosis 117.3
Bronchocele
- meaning
  - dilatation of bronchus 519.19
  - goiter 240.9

Bronchogenic carcinoma 162.9
Bronchohemisporosis 117.9
Broncholithiasis 518.89

Broncholithiasis — *continued*
- tuberculous (*see also* Tuberculosis) 011.3 ☑
Bronchomalacia 748.3
Bronchomoniliasis 112.89
Bronchomycosis 112.89
Bronchonocardiosis 039.1
Bronchopleuropneumonia — *see* Pneumonia, broncho-
Bronchopneumonia — *see* Pneumonia, broncho-
Bronchopneumonitis — *see* Pneumonia, broncho-
Bronchopulmonary — *see* condition
Bronchopulmonitis — *see* Pneumonia, broncho-
Bronchorrhagia 786.30
- newborn 770.3
- tuberculous (*see also* Tuberculosis) 011.3 ☑
Bronchorrhea (chronic) (purulent) 491.0
- acute 466.0
Bronchospasm 519.11
- with
  - asthma — *see* Asthma
  - bronchiolitis, acute 466.19
    - due to respiratory syncytial virus 466.11
  - bronchitis — *see* Bronchitis
  - chronic obstructive pulmonary disease (COPD) 496
  - emphysema — *see* Emphysema
    - due to external agent — *see* Condition, respiratory, acute, due to
- acute 519.11
- exercise induced 493.81
Bronchospirochetosis 104.8
Bronchostenosis 519.19
Bronchus — *see* condition
Bronze, bronzed
- diabetes 275.01
- disease (Addison's) (skin) 255.41
  - tuberculous (*see also* Tuberculosis) 017.6 ☑
Brooke's disease or tumor (M8100/0) — *see* Neoplasm, skin, benign
Brown enamel of teeth (hereditary) 520.5
Brown-Séquard's paralysis (syndrome) 344.89
Brown's tendon sheath syndrome 378.61
Brow presentation complicating delivery 652.4 ☑
Brucella, brucellosis (infection) 023.9
- abortus 023.1
- canis 023.3
- dermatitis, skin 023.9
- melitensis 023.0
- mixed 023.8
- suis 023.2
Bruck-de Lange disease or syndrome (Amsterdam dwarf, intellectual disabilities, and brachycephaly) 759.89
Bruck's disease 733.99
Brugada syndrome 746.89
Brug's filariasis 125.1
Brugsch's syndrome (acropachyderma) 757.39
Bruhl's disease (splenic anemia with fever) 285.8
Bruise (skin surface intact) — *see also* Contusion
- with
  - fracture — *see* Fracture, by site
  - open wound — *see* Wound, open, by site
  - internal organ (abdomen, chest, or pelvis) — *see* Injury, internal, by site
  - umbilical cord 663.6 ☑
    - affecting fetus or newborn 762.6
Bruit 785.9
- arterial (abdominal) (carotid) 785.9
- supraclavicular 785.9
Brushburn — *see* Injury, superficial, by site
Bruton's X-linked agammaglobulinemia 279.04
Bruxism 306.8
- sleep related 327.53
Bubbly lung syndrome 770.7
Bubo 289.3
- blennorrhagic 098.89

Bubo — *continued*
- chancroidal 099.0
- climatic 099.1
- due to Hemophilus ducreyi 099.0
- gonococcal 098.89
- indolent NEC 099.8
- inguinal NEC 099.8
  - chancroidal 099.0
  - climatic 099.1
  - due to H. ducreyi 099.0
- scrofulous (*see also* Tuberculosis) 017.2 ☑
- soft chancre 099.0
- suppurating 683
- syphilitic 091.0
  - congenital 090.0
- tropical 099.1
- venereal NEC 099.8
- virulent 099.0
Bubonic plague 020.0
Bubonocele — *see* Hernia, inguinal
Buccal — *see* condition
Buchanan's disease (juvenile osteochondrosis of iliac crest) 732.1
Buchem's syndrome (hyperostosis corticalis) 733.3
Buchman's disease (osteochondrosis, juvenile) 732.1
Bucket handle fracture (semilunar cartilage) — *see also* Tear, meniscus 836.2
Budd-Chiari syndrome (hepatic vein thrombosis) 453.0
Budgerigar-fanciers' disease or lung 495.2
Büdinger-Ludloff-Läwen disease 717.89
Buds
- breast 259.1
- in newborn 779.89
Buerger's disease (thromboangiitis obliterans) 443.1
Bulbar — *see* condition
Bulbus cordis 745.9
- persistent (in left ventricle) 745.8
Bulging fontanels (congenital) 756.0
Bulimia 783.6
- nervosa 307.51
- nonorganic origin 307.51
Bulky uterus 621.2
Bulla(e) 709.8
- lung (emphysematous) (solitary) 492.0
Bullet wound — *see also* Wound, open, by site
- fracture — *see* Fracture, by site, open
- internal organ (abdomen, chest, or pelvis) — *see* Injury, internal, by site, with open wound
- intracranial — *see* Laceration, brain, with open wound
Bullis fever 082.8
Bullying — *see also* Disturbance, conduct 312.0 ☑
Bundle
- branch block (complete) (false) (incomplete) 426.50
  - bilateral 426.53
  - left (*see also* Block, bundle branch, left) 426.3
    - hemiblock 426.2
  - right (*see also* Block, bundle branch, right) 426.4
- of His — *see* condition
- of Kent syndrome (anomalous atrioventricular excitation) 426.7
Bungpagga 040.81
Bunion 727.1
Bunionette 727.1
Bunyamwera fever 066.3
Buphthalmia, buphthalmos (congenital) 743.20
- associated with
  - keratoglobus, congenital 743.22
  - megalocornea 743.22
  - ocular anomalies NEC 743.22
- isolated 743.21
- simple 743.21
Bürger-Grütz disease or syndrome (essential familial hyperlipemia) 272.3
Buried roots 525.3

Burke's syndrome 577.8
Burkitt's
- tumor (M9750/3) 200.2 ☑
- type malignant, lymphoma, lymphoblastic, or undifferentiated (M9750/3) 200.2 ☑
Burn (acid) (cathode ray) (caustic) (chemical) (electric heating appliance) (electricity) (fire) (flame) (hot liquid or object) (irradiation) (lime) (radiation) (steam) (thermal) (x-ray) 949.0

Note — Use the following fifth-digit subclassification with category 948 to indicate the percent of body surface with third degree burn:
0   Less than 10% or unspecified
1   10–19%
2   20–29%
3   30–39%
4   40–49%
5   50–59%
6   60–69%
7   70–79%
8   80–89%
9   90% or more of body surface

- with
  - blisters — *see* Burn, by site, second degree
  - erythema — *see* Burn, by site, first degree
  - skin loss (epidermal) (*see also* Burn, by site, second degree)
    - full thickness (*see also* Burn, by site, third degree)
      - with necrosis of underlying tissues — *see* Burn, by site, third degree, deep
- first degree — *see* Burn, by site, first degree
- second degree — *see* Burn, by site, second degree
- third degree — *see* Burn, by site, third degree
  - deep — *see* Burn, by site, third degree, deep
- abdomen, abdominal (muscle) (wall) 942.03
  - with
    - trunk — *see* Burn, trunk, multiple sites
  - first degree 942.13
  - second degree 942.23
  - third degree 942.33
    - deep 942.43
      - with loss of body part 942.53
- ankle 945.03
  - with
    - lower limb(s) — *see* Burn, leg, multiple sites
  - first degree 945.13
  - second degree 945.23
  - third degree 945.33
    - deep 945.43
      - with loss of body part 945.53
- anus — *see* Burn, trunk, specified site NEC
- arm(s) 943.00
  - first degree 943.10
  - second degree 943.20
  - third degree 943.30
    - deep 943.40
      - with loss of body part 943.50
  - lower — *see* Burn, forearm(s)
  - multiple sites, except hand(s) or wrist(s) 943.09
    - first degree 943.19
    - second degree 943.29
    - third degree 943.39
      - deep 943.49
        - with loss of body part 943.59
  - upper 943.03
    - first degree 943.13
    - second degree 943.23
    - third degree 943.33

☑ **Additional Digit Required** — Refer to the Tabular List for Digit Selection   ☖ **Subterms under main terms may continue to next column or page**

Burn — *continued*
  arm(s) — *continued*
    upper — *continued*
      third degree — *continued*
        deep 943.43
          with loss of body part 943.53
  auditory canal (external) — *see* Burn, ear
  auricle (ear) — *see* Burn, ear
  axilla 943.04
    with
      upper limb(s), except hand(s) or wrist(s) — *see* Burn, arm(s), multiple sites
    first degree 943.14
    second degree 943.24
    third degree 943.34
      deep 943.44
        with loss of body part 943.54
  back 942.04
    with
      trunk — *see* Burn, trunk, multiple sites
    first degree 942.14
    second degree 942.24
    third degree 942.34
      deep 942.44
        with loss of body part 942.54
  biceps
    brachii — *see* Burn, arm(s), upper
    femoris — *see* Burn, thigh
  breast(s) 942.01
    with
      trunk — *see* Burn, trunk, multiple sites
    first degree 942.11
    second degree 942.21
    third degree 942.31
      deep 942.41
        with loss of body part 942.51
  brow — *see* Burn, forehead
  buttock(s) — *see* Burn, back
  canthus (eye) 940.1
    chemical 940.0
  cervix (uteri) 947.4
  cheek (cutaneous) 941.07
    with
      face or head — *see* Burn, head, multiple sites
    first degree 941.17
    second degree 941.27
    third degree 941.37
      deep 941.47
        with loss of body part 941.57
  chest wall (anterior) 942.02
    with
      trunk — *see* Burn, trunk, multiple sites
    first degree 942.12
    second degree 942.22
    third degree 942.32
      deep 942.42
        with loss of body part 942.52
  chin 941.04
    with
      face or head — *see* Burn, head, multiple sites
    first degree 941.14
    second degree 941.24
    third degree 941.34
      deep 941.44
        with loss of body part 941.54
  clitoris — *see* Burn, genitourinary organs, external
  colon 947.3
  conjunctiva (and cornea) 940.4
    chemical
      acid 940.3
      alkaline 940.2
  cornea (and conjunctiva) 940.4
    chemical
      acid 940.3
      alkaline 940.2
  costal region — *see* Burn, chest wall
  due to ingested chemical agent — *see* Burn, internal organs
  ear (auricle) (canal) (drum) (external) 941.01

Burn — *continued*
  ear — *continued*
    with
      face or head — *see* Burn, head, multiple sites
    first degree 941.11
    second degree 941.21
    third degree 941.31
      deep 941.41
        with loss of a body part 941.51
  elbow 943.02
    with
      hand(s) and wrist(s) — *see* Burn, multiple specified sites
      upper limb(s), except hand(s) or wrist(s) (*see also* Burn, arm(s), multiple sites)
    first degree 943.12
    second degree 943.22
    third degree 943.32
      deep 943.42
        with loss of body part 943.52
  electricity, electric current — *see* Burn, by site
  entire body — *see* Burn, multiple, specified sites
  epididymis — *see* Burn, genitourinary organs, external
  epigastric region — *see* Burn, abdomen
  epiglottis 947.1
  esophagus 947.2
  extent (percent of body surface)
    less than 10 percent 948.0 ☑
    10-19 percent 948.1 ☑
    20-29 percent 948.2 ☑
    30-39 percent 948.3 ☑
    40-49 percent 948.4 ☑
    50-59 percent 948.5 ☑
    60-69 percent 948.6 ☑
    70-79 percent 948.7 ☑
    80-89 percent 948.8 ☑
    90 percent or more 948.9 ☑
  extremity
    lower — *see* Burn, leg
    upper — *see* Burn, arm(s)
  eye(s) (and adnexa) (only) 940.9
    with
      face, head, or neck 941.02
        first degree 941.12
        second degree 941.22
        third degree 941.32
          deep 941.42
            with loss of body part 941.52
      other sites (classifiable to more than one category in 940–945) — *see* Burn, multiple, specified sites
      resulting rupture and destruction of eyeball 940.5
    specified part — *see* Burn, by site
  eyeball (*see also* Burn, eye)
    with resulting rupture and destruction of eyeball 940.5
  eyelid(s) 940.1
    chemical 940.0
  face — *see* Burn, head
  finger (nail) (subungual) 944.01
    with
      hand(s) — *see* Burn, hand(s), multiple sites
      other sites — *see* Burn, multiple, specified sites
      thumb 944.04
        first degree 944.14
        second degree 944.24
        third degree 944.34
          deep 944.44
            with loss of body part 944.54
    first degree 944.11
    second degree 944.21
    third degree 944.31
      deep 944.41
        with loss of body part 944.51
  multiple (digits) 944.03

Burn — *continued*
  finger — *continued*
    multiple — *continued*
      with thumb — *see* Burn, finger, with thumb
      first degree 944.13
      second degree 944.23
      third degree 944.33
        deep 944.43
          with loss of body part 944.53
  flank — *see* Burn, abdomen
  foot 945.02
    with
      lower limb(s) — *see* Burn, leg, multiple sites
    first degree 945.12
    second degree 945.22
    third degree 945.32
      deep 945.42
        with loss of body part 945.52
  forearm(s) 943.01
    with
      upper limb(s), except hand(s) or wrist(s) — *see* Burn, arm(s), multiple sites
    first degree 943.11
    second degree 943.21
    third degree 943.31
      deep 943.41
        with loss of body part 943.51
  forehead 941.07
    with
      face or head — *see* Burn, head, multiple sites
    first degree 941.17
    second degree 941.27
    third degree 941.37
      deep 941.47
        with loss of body part 941.57
  fourth degree — *see* Burn, by site, third degree, deep
  friction — *see* Injury, superficial, by site
  from swallowing caustic or corrosive substance NEC — *see* Burn, internal organs
  full thickness — *see* Burn, by site, third degree
  gastrointestinal tract 947.3
  genitourinary organs
    external 942.05
      with
        trunk — *see* Burn, trunk, multiple sites
      first degree 942.15
      second degree 942.25
      third degree 942.35
        deep 942.45
          with loss of body part 942.55
    internal 947.8
  globe (eye) — *see* Burn, eyeball
  groin — *see* Burn, abdomen
  gum 947.0
  hand(s) (phalanges) (and wrist) 944.00
    first degree 944.10
    second degree 944.20
    third degree 944.30
      deep 944.40
        with loss of body part 944.50
    back (dorsal surface) 944.06
      first degree 944.16
      second degree 944.26
      third degree 944.36
        deep 944.46
          with loss of body part 944.56
    multiple sites 944.08
      first degree 944.18
      second degree 944.28
      third degree 944.38
        deep 944.48
          with loss of body part 944.58
  head (and face) 941.00
    first degree 941.10
    second degree 941.20
    third degree 941.30
      deep 941.40
        with loss of body part 941.50

Burn — *continued*
  head — *continued*
    eye(s) only 940.9
      specified part — *see* Burn, by site
    multiple sites 941.09
      with eyes — *see* Burn, eyes, with face, head, or neck
      first degree 941.19
      second degree 941.29
      third degree 941.39
        deep 941.49
          with loss of body part 941.59
  heel — *see* Burn, foot
  hip — *see* Burn, trunk, specified site NEC
  iliac region — *see* Burn, trunk, specified site NEC
  infected 958.3
  inhalation (*see also* Burn, internal organs) 947.9
  internal organs 947.9
    from caustic or corrosive substance (swallowing) NEC 947.9
    specified NEC (*see also* Burn, by site) 947.8
  interscapular region — *see* Burn, back
  intestine (large) (small) 947.3
  iris — *see* Burn, eyeball
  knee 945.05
    with
      lower limb(s) — *see* Burn, leg, multiple sites
    first degree 945.15
    second degree 945.25
    third degree 945.35
      deep 945.45
        with loss of body part 945.55
  labium (majus) (minus) — *see* Burn, genitourinary organs, external
  lacrimal apparatus, duct, gland, or sac 940.1
    chemical 940.0
  larynx 947.1
  late effect — *see* Late, effects (of), burn
  leg 945.00
    first degree 945.10
    second degree 945.20
    third degree 945.30
      deep 945.40
        with loss of body part 945.50
    lower 945.04
      with other part(s) of lower limb(s) — *see* Burn, leg, multiple sites
      first degree 945.14
      second degree 945.24
      third degree 945.34
        deep 945.44
          with loss of body part 945.54
    multiple sites 945.09
      first degree 945.19
      second degree 945.29
      third degree 945.39
        deep 945.49
          with loss of body part 945.59
    upper — *see* Burn, thigh
  lightning — *see* Burn, by site
  limb(s)
    lower (including foot or toe(s)) — *see* Burn, leg
    upper (except wrist and hand) — *see* Burn, arm(s)
  lip(s) 941.03
    with
      face or head — *see* Burn, head, multiple sites
    first degree 941.13
    second degree 941.23
    third degree 941.33
      deep 941.43
        with loss of body part 941.53
  lumbar region — *see* Burn, back
  lung 947.1
  malar region — *see* Burn, cheek
  mastoid region — *see* Burn, scalp
  membrane, tympanic — *see* Burn, ear
  midthoracic region — *see* Burn, chest wall
  mouth 947.0
  multiple (*see also* Burn, unspecified) 949.0

☑ Additional Digit Required — Refer to the Tabular List for Digit Selection   ▽ Subterms under main terms may continue to next column or page

2014 ICD-9-CM   85

Burn — continued

multiple (see also Burn, unspecified) — continued
  specified sites classifiable to more than one category in
    940-945 ☑, 946.0
    first degree 946.1
    second degree 946.2
    third degree 946.3
      deep 946.4
        with loss of body part 946.5
muscle, abdominal — see Burn, abdomen
nasal (septum) — see Burn, nose
neck 941.08
  with
    face or head — see Burn, head, multiple sites
  first degree 941.18
  second degree 941.28
  third degree 941.38
    deep 941.48
      with loss of body part 941.58
nose (septum) 941.05
  with
    face or head — see Burn, head, multiple sites
  first degree 941.15
  second degree 941.25
  third degree 941.35
    deep 941.45
      with loss of body part 941.55
occipital region — see Burn, scalp
orbit region 940.1
  chemical 940.0
oronasopharynx 947.0
palate 947.0
palm(s) 944.05
  with
    hand(s) and wrist(s) — see Burn, hand(s), multiple sites
  first degree 944.15
  second degree 944.25
  third degree 944.35
    deep 944.45
      with loss of a body part 944.55
parietal region — see Burn, scalp
penis — see Burn, genitourinary organs, external
perineum — see Burn, genitourinary organs, external
periocular area 940.1
  chemical 940.0
pharynx 947.0
pleura 947.1
popliteal space — see Burn, knee
prepuce — see Burn, genitourinary organs, external
pubic region — see Burn, genitourinary organs, external
pudenda — see Burn, genitourinary organs, external
rectum 947.3
sac, lacrimal 940.1
  chemical 940.0
sacral region — see Burn, back
salivary (ducts) (glands) 947.0
scalp 941.06
  with
    face or neck — see Burn, head, multiple sites
  first degree 941.16
  second degree 941.26
  third degree 941.36
    deep 941.46
      with loss of body part 941.56
scapular region 943.06
  with
    upper limb(s), except hand(s) or wrist(s) — see Burn, arm(s), multiple sites
  first degree 943.16
  second degree 943.26
  third degree 943.36
    deep 943.46
      with loss of body part 943.56
sclera — see Burn, eyeball

Burn — continued

scrotum — see Burn, genitourinary organs, external
septum, nasal — see Burn, nose
shoulder(s) 943.05
  with
    hand(s) and wrist(s) — see Burn, multiple, specified sites
    upper limb(s), except hand(s) or wrist(s) — see Burn, arm(s), multiple sites
  first degree 943.15
  second degree 943.25
  third degree 943.35
    deep 943.45
      with loss of body part 943.55
skin NEC (see also Burn, unspecified) 949.0
skull — see Burn, head
small intestine 947.3
sternal region — see Burn, chest wall
stomach 947.3
subconjunctival — see Burn, conjunctiva
subcutaneous — see Burn, by site, third degree
submaxillary region — see Burn, head
submental region — see Burn, chin
sun — see Sunburn
supraclavicular fossa — see Burn, neck
supraorbital — see Burn, forehead
temple — see Burn, scalp
temporal region — see Burn, scalp
testicle — see Burn, genitourinary organs, external
testis — see Burn, genitourinary organs, external
thigh 945.06
  with
    lower limb(s) — see Burn, leg, multiple sites
  first degree 945.16
  second degree 945.26
  third degree 945.36
    deep 945.46
      with loss of body part 945.56
thorax (external) — see Burn, chest wall
throat 947.0
thumb(s) (nail) (subungual) 944.02
  with
    finger(s) — see Burn, finger, with other sites, thumb
    hand(s) and wrist(s) — see Burn, hand(s), multiple sites
  first degree 944.12
  second degree 944.22
  third degree 944.32
    deep 944.42
      with loss of body part 944.52
toe (nail) (subungual) 945.01
  with
    lower limb(s) — see Burn, leg, multiple sites
  first degree 945.11
  second degree 945.21
  third degree 945.31
    deep 945.41
      with loss of body part 945.51
tongue 947.0
tonsil 947.0
trachea 947.1
trunk 942.00
  first degree 942.10
  second degree 942.20
  third degree 942.30
    deep 942.40
      with loss of body part 942.50
  multiple sites 942.09
    first degree 942.19
    second degree 942.29
    third degree 942.39
      deep 942.49
        with loss of body part 942.59
  specified site NEC 942.09
    first degree 942.19
    second degree 942.29
    third degree 942.39
      deep 942.49

Burn — continued

trunk — continued
  specified site — continued
    third degree — continued
      deep — continued
        with loss of body part 942.59
tunica vaginalis — see Burn, genitourinary organs, external
tympanic membrane — see Burn, ear
tympanum — see Burn, ear
ultraviolet 692.82
unspecified site (multiple) 949.0
  with extent of body surface involved specified
    less than 10 percent 948.0 ☑
    10-19 percent 948.1 ☑
    20-29 percent 948.2 ☑
    30-39 percent 948.3 ☑
    40-49 percent 948.4 ☑
    50-59 percent 948.5 ☑
    60-69 percent 948.6 ☑
    70-79 percent 948.7 ☑
    80-89 percent 948.8 ☑
    90 percent or more 948.9 ☑
    first degree 949.1
    second degree 949.2
    third degree 949.3
      deep 949.4
        with loss of body part 949.5
uterus 947.4
uvula 947.0
vagina 947.4
vulva — see Burn, genitourinary organs, external
wrist(s) 944.07
  with
    hand(s) — see Burn, hand(s), multiple sites
  first degree 944.17
  second degree 944.27
  third degree 944.37
    deep 944.47
      with loss of body part 944.57
Burnett's syndrome (milk-alkali) 275.42
Burnier's syndrome (hypophyseal dwarfism) 253.3
Burning
feet syndrome 266.2
sensation (see also Disturbance, sensation) 782.0
tongue 529.6
Burns' disease (osteochondrosis, lower ulna) 732.3
Bursa — see also condition
pharynx 478.29
Bursitis NEC 727.3
Achilles tendon 726.71
adhesive 726.90
  shoulder 726.0
ankle 726.79
buttock 726.5
calcaneal 726.79
collateral ligament
  fibular 726.63
  tibial 726.62
Duplay's 726.2
elbow 726.33
finger 726.8
foot 726.79
gonococcal 098.52
hand 726.4
hip 726.5
infrapatellar 726.69
ischiogluteal 726.5
knee 726.60
occupational NEC 727.2
olecranon 726.33
pes anserinus 726.61
pharyngeal 478.29
popliteal 727.51
prepatellar 726.65
radiohumeral 727.3
scapulohumeral 726.19
  adhesive 726.0
shoulder 726.10
  adhesive 726.0

Bursitis — continued

subacromial 726.19
  adhesive 726.0
subcoracoid 726.19
subdeltoid 726.19
  adhesive 726.0
subpatellar 726.69
syphilitic 095.7
Thornwaldt's, Tornwaldt's (pharyngeal) 478.29
toe 726.79
trochanteric area 726.5
wrist 726.4
Burst stitches or sutures (complication of surgery) (external) (see also Dehiscence) 998.32
internal 998.31
Buruli ulcer 031.1
Bury's disease (erythema elevatum diutinum) 695.89
Buschke's disease or scleredema (adultorum) 710.1
Busquet's disease (osteoperiostitis) — see also Osteomyelitis 730.1 ☑
Busse-Buschke disease (cryptococcosis) 117.5
Buttock — see condition
Button
Biskra 085.1
Delhi 085.1
oriental 085.1
Buttonhole hand (intrinsic) 736.21
Bwamba fever (encephalitis) 066.3
Byssinosis (occupational) 504
Bywaters' syndrome 958.5

C

Cacergasia 300.9
Cachexia 799.4
cancerous (see also Neoplasm, by site, malignant) 799.4
cardiac — see Disease, heart
dehydration 276.51
  with
    hypernatremia 276.0
    hyponatremia 276.1
due to malnutrition 799.4
exophthalmic 242.0 ☑
heart — see Disease, heart
hypophyseal 253.2
hypopituitary 253.2
lead 984.9
  specified type of lead — see Table of Drugs and Chemicals
malaria 084.9
malignant (see also Neoplasm, by site, malignant) 799.4
marsh 084.9
nervous 300.5
old age 797
pachydermic — see Hypothyroidism
paludal 084.9
pituitary (postpartum) 253.2
renal (see also Disease, renal) 593.9
saturnine 984.9
  specified type of lead — see Table of Drugs and Chemicals
senile 797
Simmonds' (pituitary cachexia) 253.2
splenica 289.59
strumipriva (see also Hypothyroidism) 244.9
tuberculous NEC (see also Tuberculosis) 011.9 ☑
Café au lait spots 709.09
Caffey's disease or syndrome (infantile cortical hyperostosis) 756.59
Caisson disease 993.3
Caked breast (puerperal, postpartum) 676.2 ☑
Cake kidney 753.3
Calabar swelling 125.2
Calcaneal spur 726.73
Calcaneoapophysitis 732.5
Calcaneonavicular bar 755.67
Calcareous — see condition
Calcicosis (occupational) 502
Calciferol (vitamin D) **deficiency** 268.9

☑ Additional Digit Required — Refer to the Tabular List for Digit Selection   ▽ Subterms under main terms may continue to next column or page

86   2014 ICD-9-CM

Calciferol (vitamin D) **deficiency** —
   continued
  with
    osteomalacia 268.2
    rickets (*see also* Rickets) 268.0
Calcification
  adrenal (capsule) (gland) 255.41
    tuberculous (*see also* Tuberculosis)
      017.6 ☑
  aorta 440.0
  artery (annular) — *see* Arteriosclerosis
  auricle (ear) 380.89
  bladder 596.89
    due to S. hematobium 120.0
  brain (cortex) — *see* Calcification, cerebral
  bronchus 519.19
  bursa 727.82
  cardiac (*see also* Degeneration, myocardial)
    429.1
  cartilage (postinfectional) 733.99
  cerebral (cortex) 348.89
    artery 437.0
  cervix (uteri) 622.8
  choroid plexus 349.2
  conjunctiva 372.54
  corpora cavernosa (penis) 607.89
  cortex (brain) — *see* Calcification, cerebral
  dental pulp (nodular) 522.2
  dentinal papilla 520.4
  disc, intervertebral 722.90
    cervical, cervicothoracic 722.91
    lumbar, lumbosacral 722.93
    thoracic, thoracolumbar 722.92
  fallopian tube 620.8
  falx cerebri — *see* Calcification, cerebral
  fascia 728.89
  gallbladder 575.8
  general 275.40
  heart (*see also* Degeneration, myocardial)
    429.1
    valve — *see* Endocarditis
  intervertebral cartilage or disc (postinfection-
    al) 722.90
    cervical, cervicothoracic 722.91
    lumbar, lumbosacral 722.93
    thoracic, thoracolumbar 722.92
  intracranial — *see* Calcification, cerebral
  intraspinal ligament 728.89
  joint 719.80
    ankle 719.87
    elbow 719.82
    foot 719.87
    hand 719.84
    hip 719.85
    knee 719.86
    multiple sites 719.89
    pelvic region 719.85
    shoulder (region) 719.81
    specified site NEC 719.88
    wrist 719.83
  kidney 593.89
    tuberculous (*see also* Tuberculosis)
      016.0 ☑
  larynx (senile) 478.79
  lens 366.8
  ligament 728.89
    intraspinal 728.89
    knee (medial collateral) 717.89
  lung 518.89
    active 518.89
    postinfectional 518.89
    tuberculous (*see also* Tuberculosis, pul-
      monary) 011.9 ☑
  lymph gland or node (postinfectional) 289.3
    tuberculous (*see also* Tuberculosis,
      lymph gland) 017.2 ☑
  mammographic 793.89
  massive (paraplegic) 728.10
  medial NEC (*see also* Arteriosclerosis, extrem-
    ities) 440.20
  meninges (cerebral) 349.2
  metastatic 275.40
  Mönckeberg's — *see* Arteriosclerosis
  muscle 728.10
    heterotopic, postoperative 728.13

Calcification — *continued*
  myocardium, myocardial (*see also* Degener-
    ation, myocardial) 429.1
  ovary 620.8
  pancreas 577.8
  penis 607.89
  periarticular 728.89
  pericardium (*see also* Pericarditis) 423.8
  pineal gland 259.8
  pleura 511.0
    postinfectional 518.89
    tuberculous (*see also* Tuberculosis,
      pleura) 012.0 ☑
  pulp (dental) (nodular) 522.2
  renal 593.89
  Rider's bone 733.99
  sclera 379.16
  semilunar cartilage 717.89
  spleen 289.59
  subcutaneous 709.3
  suprarenal (capsule) (gland) 255.41
  tendon (sheath) 727.82
    with bursitis, synovitis or tenosynovitis
      727.82
  trachea 519.19
  ureter 593.89
  uterus 621.8
  vitreous 379.29
Calcified — *see also* Calcification
  hematoma NEC 959.9
Calcinosis (generalized) (interstitial) (tumoral)
  (universalis) 275.49
  circumscripta 709.3
  cutis 709.3
  intervertebralis 275.49 [722.90]
  Raynaud's phenomenonsclerodactylytelang-
    iectasis (CRST) 710.1
Calciphylaxis — *see also* Calcification, by site
  275.49
Calcium
  blood
    high (*see also* Hypercalcemia) 275.42
    low (*see also* Hypocalcemia) 275.41
  deposits (*see also* Calcification, by site)
    in bursa 727.82
    in tendon (sheath) 727.82
      with bursitis, synovitis or tenosynovi-
        tis 727.82
  salts or soaps in vitreous 379.22
Calciuria 791.9
Calculi — *see* Calculus
Calculosis, intrahepatic — *see* Choledocholithiasis
Calculus, calculi, calculous 592.9
  ampulla of Vater — *see* Choledocholithiasis
  anuria (impacted) (recurrent) 592.0
  appendix 543.9
  bile duct (any) — *see* Choledocholithiasis
  biliary — *see* Cholelithiasis
  bilirubin, multiple — *see* Cholelithiasis
  bladder (encysted) (impacted) (urinary)
    594.1
    diverticulum 594.0
  bronchus 518.89
  calyx (kidney) (renal) 592.0
    congenital 753.3
  cholesterol (pure) (solitary) — *see*
    Cholelithiasis
  common duct (bile) — *see* Choledocholithi-
    asis
  conjunctiva 372.54
  cystic 594.1
    duct — *see* Cholelithiasis
  dental 523.6
    subgingival 523.6
    supragingival 523.6
  epididymis 608.89
  gallbladder (*see also* Cholelithiasis)
    congenital 751.69
  hepatic (duct) — *see* Choledocholithiasis
  intestine (impaction) (obstruction) 560.39
  kidney (impacted) (multiple) (pelvis) (recur-
    rent) (staghorn) 592.0
    congenital 753.3
  lacrimal (passages) 375.57
  liver (impacted) — *see* Choledocholithiasis

Calculus, calculi, calculous — *continued*
  lung 518.89
  mammographic 793.89
  nephritic (impacted) (recurrent) 592.0
  nose 478.19
  pancreas (duct) 577.8
  parotid gland 527.5
  pelvis, encysted 592.0
  prostate 602.0
  pulmonary 518.89
  renal (impacted) (recurrent) 592.0
    congenital 753.3
  salivary (duct) (gland) 527.5
  seminal vesicle 608.89
  staghorn 592.0
  Stensen's duct 527.5
  sublingual duct or gland 527.5
    congenital 750.26
  submaxillary duct, gland, or region 527.5
  suburethral 594.8
  tonsil 474.8
  tooth, teeth 523.6
  tunica vaginalis 608.89
  ureter (impacted) (recurrent) 592.1
  urethra (impacted) 594.2
  urinary (duct) (impacted) (passage) (tract)
    592.9
    lower tract NEC 594.9
      specified site 594.8
  vagina 623.8
  vesical (impacted) 594.1
  Wharton's duct 527.5
Caliectasis 593.89
California
  disease 114.0
  encephalitis 062.5
Caligo cornea 371.03
Callositas, callosity (infected) 700
Callus (infected) 700
  bone 726.91
  excessive, following fracture (*see also* Late,
    effect (of), fracture)
Calvé (-Perthes) disease (osteochondrosis,
  femoral capital) 732.1
Calvities — *see also* Alopecia 704.00
Cameroon fever — *see also* Malaria 084.6
Camptocormia 300.11
Camptodactyly (congenital) 755.59
Camurati-Engelmann disease (diaphyseal
  sclerosis) 756.59
Canal — *see* condition
Canaliculitis (lacrimal) (acute) 375.31
  Actinomyces 039.8
  chronic 375.41
Canavan's disease 330.0
Cancer (M8000/3) — *see also* Neoplasm, by
  site, malignant

> Note — The term "cancer" when modi-
> fied by an adjective or adjectival phrase
> indicating a morphological type should
> be coded in the same manner as "carci-
> noma" with that adjective or phrase.
> Thus, "squamous-cell cancer" should be
> coded in the same manner as "squa-
> mous-cell carcinoma," which appears in
> the list under "Carcinoma."

  bile duct type (M8160/3), liver 155.1
  hepatocellular (M8170/3) 155.0
Cancerous (M8000/3) — *see* Neoplasm, by site,
  malignant
Cancerphobia 300.29
Cancrum oris 528.1
Candidiasis, candidal 112.9
  with pneumonia 112.4
  balanitis 112.2
  congenital 771.7
  disseminated 112.5
  endocarditis 112.81
  esophagus 112.84
  intertrigo 112.3
  intestine 112.85
  lung 112.4
  meningitis 112.83
  mouth 112.0
  nails 112.3
  neonatal 771.7

Candidiasis, candidal — *continued*
  onychia 112.3
  otitis externa 112.82
  otomycosis 112.82
  paronychia 112.3
  perionyxis 112.3
  pneumonia 112.4
  pneumonitis 112.4
  skin 112.3
  specified site NEC 112.89
  systemic 112.5
  urogenital site NEC 112.2
  vagina 112.1
  vulva 112.1
  vulvovaginitis 112.1
Candidiosis — *see* Candidiasis
Candiru infection or infestation 136.8
Canities (premature) 704.3
  congenital 757.4
Canker (mouth) (sore) 528.2
  rash 034.1
Cannabinosis 504
Canton fever 081.9
Cap
  cradle 690.11
Capillariasis 127.5
Capillary — *see* condition
Caplan-Colinet syndrome 714.81
Caplan's syndrome 714.81
Capsule — *see* condition
Capsulitis (joint) 726.90
  adhesive (shoulder) 726.0
  hip 726.5
  knee 726.60
  labyrinthine 387.8
  thyroid 245.9
  wrist 726.4
Caput
  crepitus 756.0
  medusae 456.8
  succedaneum 767.19
Carapata disease 087.1
Carate — *see* Pinta
**Carbohydrate-deficient glycoprotein syn-
  drome** (CGDS) 271.8
Carboxyhemoglobinemia 986
Carbuncle 680.9
  abdominal wall 680.2
  ankle 680.6
  anus 680.5
  arm (any part, above wrist) 680.3
  auditory canal, external 680.0
  axilla 680.3
  back (any part) 680.2
  breast 680.2
  buttock 680.5
  chest wall 680.2
  corpus cavernosum 607.2
  ear (any part) (external) 680.0
  eyelid 373.13
  face (any part, except eye) 680.0
  finger (any) 680.4
  flank 680.2
  foot (any part) 680.7
  forearm 680.3
  genital organ (male) 608.4
  gluteal (region) 680.5
  groin 680.2
  hand (any part) 680.4
  head (any part, except face) 680.8
  heel 680.7
  hip 680.6
  kidney (*see also* Abscess, kidney) 590.2
  knee 680.6
  labia 616.4
  lacrimal
    gland (*see also* Dacryoadenitis) 375.00
    passages (duct) (sac) (*see also* Dacryocys-
      titis) 375.30
  leg, any part except foot 680.6
  lower extremity, any part except foot 680.6
  malignant 022.0
  multiple sites 680.9
  neck 680.1
  nose (external) (septum) 680.0
  orbit, orbital 376.01

☑ **Additional Digit Required** — Refer to the Tabular List for Digit Selection   ▽ **Subterms under main terms may continue to next column or page**

2014 ICD-9-CM   **87**

Index

Carbuncle — Carcinoma

Carbuncle — *continued*
  partes posteriores 680.5
  pectoral region 680.2
  penis 607.2
  perineum 680.2
  pinna 680.0
  scalp (any part) 680.8
  scrotum 608.4
  seminal vesicle 608.0
  shoulder 680.3
  skin NEC 680.9
  specified site NEC 680.8
  spermatic cord 608.4
  temple (region) 680.0
  testis 608.4
  thigh 680.6
  thumb 680.4
  toe (any) 680.7
  trunk 680.2
  tunica vaginalis 608.4
  umbilicus 680.2
  upper arm 680.3
  urethra 597.0
  vas deferens 608.4
  vulva 616.4
  wrist 680.4
Carbunculus — *see also* Carbuncle 680.9
Carcinoid (tumor) (M8240/1) — *see* Tumor, carcinoid
Carcinoidosis 259.2
Carcinomaphobia 300.29
Carcinomatosis
  peritonei (M8010/6) 197.6
  specified site NEC (M8010/3) — *see* Neoplasm, by site, malignant
  unspecified site (M8010/6) 199.0
Carcinoma (M8010/3) — *see also* Neoplasm, by site, malignant

Note — *Except where otherwise indicated, the morphological varieties of carcinoma in the list below should be coded by site as for "Neoplasm, malignant."*

  with
    apocrine metaplasia (M8573/3)
    cartilaginous (and osseous) metaplasia (M8571/3)
    osseous (and cartilaginous) metaplasia (M8571/3)
    productive fibrosis (M8141/3)
    spindle cell metaplasia (M8572/3)
    squamous metaplasia (M8570/3)
  acidophil (M8280/3)
    specified site — *see* Neoplasm, by site, malignant
    unspecified site 194.3
  acidophil-basophil, mixed (M8281/3)
    specified site — *see* Neoplasm, by site, malignant
    unspecified site 194.3
  acinar (cell) (M8550/3)
  acinic cell (M8550/3)
  adenocystic (M8200/3)
  adenoid
    cystic (M8200/3)
    squamous cell (M8075/3)
  adenosquamous (M8560/3)
  adnexal (skin) (M8390/3) — *see* Neoplasm, skin, malignant
  adrenal cortical (M8370/3) 194.0
  alveolar (M8251/3)
    cell (M8250/3) — *see* Neoplasm, lung, malignant
  anaplastic type (M8021/3)
  apocrine (M8401/3)
    breast — *see* Neoplasm, breast, malignant
    specified site NEC — *see* Neoplasm, skin, malignant
    unspecified site 173.99
  basal cell (pigmented) (M8090/3) (*see also* Neoplasm, skin, malignant) 173.91
    fibro-epithelial type (M8093/3) — *see* Neoplasm, skin, malignant
    morphea type (M8092/3) — *see* Neoplasm, skin, malignant

Carcinoma — *see also* Neoplasm, by site, malignant — *continued*
  basal cell (*see also* Neoplasm, skin, malignant) — *continued*
    multicentric (M8091/3) — *see* Neoplasm, skin, malignant
  basaloid (M8123/3)
  basal-squamous cell, mixed (M8094/3) — *see* Neoplasm, skin, malignant
  basophil (M8300/3)
    specified site — *see* Neoplasm, by site, malignant
    unspecified site 194.3
  basophil-acidophil, mixed (M8281/3)
    specified site — *see* Neoplasm, by site, malignant
    unspecified site 194.3
  basosquamous (M8094/3) — *see* Neoplasm, skin, malignant
  bile duct type (M8160/3)
    and hepatocellular, mixed (M8180/3) 155.0
    liver 155.1
    specified site NEC — *see* Neoplasm, by site, malignant
    unspecified site 155.1
  branchial or branchiogenic 146.8
  bronchial or bronchogenic — *see* Neoplasm, lung, malignant
  bronchiolar (terminal) (M8250/3) — *see* Neoplasm, lung, malignant
  bronchiolo-alveolar (M8250/3) — *see* Neoplasm, lung, malignant
  bronchogenic (epidermoid) 162.9
  C cell (M8510/3)
    specified site — *see* Neoplasm, by site, malignant
    unspecified site 193
  ceruminous (M8420/3) 173.29
  chorionic (M9100/3)
    specified site — *see* Neoplasm, by site, malignant
    unspecified site
      female 181
      male 186.9
  chromophobe (M8270/3)
    specified site — *see* Neoplasm, by site, malignant
    unspecified site 194.3
  clear cell (mesonephroid type) (M8310/3)
  cloacogenic (M8124/3)
    specified site — *see* Neoplasm, by site, malignant
    unspecified site 154.8
  colloid (M8480/3)
  cribriform (M8201/3)
  cylindroid type (M8200/3)
  diffuse type (M8145/3)
    specified site — *see* Neoplasm, by site, malignant
    unspecified site 151.9
  duct (cell) (M8500/3)
    with Paget's disease (M8541/3) — *see* Neoplasm, breast, malignant
    infiltrating (M8500/3)
      specified site — *see* Neoplasm, by site, malignant
      unspecified site 174.9
  ductal (M8500/3)
  ductular, infiltrating (M8521/3)
  embryonal (M9070/3)
    and teratoma, mixed (M9081/3)
    combined with choriocarcinoma (M9101/3) — *see* Neoplasm, by site, malignant
    infantile type (M9071/3)
    liver 155.0
    polyembryonal type (M9072/3)
  endometrioid (M8380/3)
  eosinophil (M8280/3)
    specified site — *see* Neoplasm, by site, malignant
    unspecified site 194.3
  epidermoid (M8070/3) (*see also* Carcinoma, squamous cell)

Carcinoma — *see also* Neoplasm, by site, malignant — *continued*
  epidermoid (*see also* Carcinoma, squamous cell) — *continued*
    and adenocarcinoma, mixed (M8560/3)
    in situ, Bowen's type (M8081/2) — *see* Neoplasm, skin, in situ
    intradermal — *see* Neoplasm, skin, in situ
  fibroepithelial type basal cell (M8093/3) — *see* Neoplasm, skin, malignant
  follicular (M8330/3)
    and papillary (mixed) (M8340/3) 193
    moderately differentiated type (M8332/3) 193
    pure follicle type (M8331/3) 193
    specified site — *see* Neoplasm, by site, malignant
    trabecular type (M8332/3) 193
    unspecified site 193
    well differentiated type (M8331/3) 193
  gelatinous (M8480/3)
  giant cell (M8031/3)
    and spindle cell (M8030/3)
  granular cell (M8320/3)
  granulosa cell (M8620/3) 183.0
  hepatic cell (M8170/3) 155.0
  hepatocellular (M8170/3) 155.0
    and bile duct, mixed (M8180/3) 155.0
  hepatocholangiolitic (M8180/3) 155.0
  Hürthle cell (thyroid) 193
  hypernephroid (M8311/3)
  in
    adenomatous
      polyp (M8210/3)
      polyposis coli (M8220/3) 153.9
    pleomorphic adenoma (M8940/3)
    polypoid adenoma (M8210/3)
    situ (M8010/3) — *see* Carcinoma, in situ
    tubular adenoma (M8210/3)
    villous adenoma (M8261/3)
  infiltrating duct (M8500/3)
    with Paget's disease (M8541/3) — *see* Neoplasm, breast, malignant
    specified site — *see* Neoplasm, by site, malignant
    unspecified site 174.9
  inflammatory (M8530/3)
    specified site — *see* Neoplasm, by site, malignant
    unspecified site 174.9
  in situ (M8010/2) (*see also* Neoplasm, by site, in situ)
    epidermoid (M8070/2) (*see also* Neoplasm, by site, in situ)
      with questionable stromal invasion (M8076/2)
        specified site — *see* Neoplasm, by site, in situ
        unspecified site 233.1
      Bowen's type (M8081/2) — *see* Neoplasm, skin, in situ
    intraductal (M8500/2)
      specified site — *see* Neoplasm, by site, in situ
      unspecified site 233.0
    lobular (M8520/2)
      specified site — *see* Neoplasm, by site, in situ
      unspecified site 233.0
    papillary (M8050/2) — *see* Neoplasm, by site, in situ
    squamous cell (M8070/2) (*see also* Neoplasm, by site, in situ)
      with questionable stromal invasion (M8076/2)
        specified site — *see* Neoplasm, by site, in situ
        unspecified site 233.1
    transitional cell (M8120/2) — *see* Neoplasm, by site, in situ
  intestinal type (M8144/3)
    specified site — *see* Neoplasm, by site, malignant
    unspecified site 151.9

Carcinoma — *see also* Neoplasm, by site, malignant — *continued*
  intraductal (noninfiltrating) (M8500/2)
    papillary (M8503/2)
      specified site — *see* Neoplasm, by site, in situ
      unspecified site 233.0
    specified site — *see* Neoplasm, by site, in situ
    unspecified site 233.0
  intraepidermal (M8070/2) (*see also* Neoplasm, skin, in situ)
    squamous cell, Bowen's type (M8081/2) — *see* Neoplasm, skin, in situ
  intraepithelial (M8010/2) (*see also* Neoplasm, by site, in situ)
    squamous cell (M8072/2) — *see* Neoplasm, by site, in situ
  intraosseous (M9270/3) 170.1
    upper jaw (bone) 170.0
  islet cell (M8150/3)
    and exocrine, mixed (M8154/3)
      specified site — *see* Neoplasm, by site, malignant
      unspecified site 157.9
    pancreas 157.4
    specified site NEC — *see* Neoplasm, by site, malignant
    unspecified site 157.4
  juvenile, breast (M8502/3) — *see* Neoplasm, breast, malignant
  Kulchitsky's cell (carcinoid tumor of intestine) 259.2
  large cell (M8012/3)
    squamous cell, non-keratinizing type (M8072/3)
  Leydig cell (testis) (M8650/3)
    specified site — *see* Neoplasm, by site, malignant
    unspecified site 186.9
      female 183.0
      male 186.9
  liver cell (M8170/3) 155.0
  lobular (infiltrating) (M8520/3)
    non-infiltrating (M8520/3)
      specified site — *see* Neoplasm, by site, in situ
      unspecified site 233.0
    specified site — *see* Neoplasm, by site, malignant
    unspecified site 174.9
  lymphoepithelial (M8082/3)
  medullary (M8510/3)
    with
      amyloid stroma (M8511/3)
        specified site — *see* Neoplasm, by site, malignant
        unspecified site 193
      lymphoid stroma (M8512/3)
        specified site — *see* Neoplasm, by site, malignant
        unspecified site 174.9
  Merkel cell 209.36
    buttock 209.36
    ear 209.31
    eyelid, including canthus 209.31
    face 209.31
    genitals 209.36
    lip 209.31
    lower limb 209.34
    neck 209.32
    nodal presentation 209.75
    scalp 209.32
    secondary (any site) 209.75
    specified site NEC 209.36
    trunk 209.35
    unknown primary site 209.75
    upper limb 209.33
    visceral metastatic presentation 209.75
  mesometanephric (M9110/3)
  mesonephric (M9110/3)
  metastatic (M8010/6) — *see* Metastasis, cancer
  metatypical (M8095/3) — *see* Neoplasm, skin, malignant

Carcinoma — *see also* Neoplasm, by site, malignant — *continued*
  morphea type basal cell (M8092/3) — *see* Neoplasm, skin, malignant
  mucinous (M8480/3)
  mucin-producing (M8481/3)
  mucin-secreting (M8481/3)
  mucoepidermoid (M8430/3)
  mucoid (M8480/3)
    cell (M8300/3)
      specified site — *see* Neoplasm, by site, malignant
      unspecified site 194.3
  mucous (M8480/3)
  neuroendocrine
    high grade (M8240/3) 209.30
    malignant poorly differentiated (M8240/3) 209.30
  nonencapsulated sclerosing (M8350/3) 193
  noninfiltrating
    intracystic (M8504/2) — *see* Neoplasm, by site, in situ
    intraductal (M8500/2)
      papillary (M8503/2)
        specified site — *see* Neoplasm, by site, in situ
        unspecified site 233.0
      specified site — *see* Neoplasm, by site, in situ
      unspecified site 233.0
    lobular (M8520/2)
      specified site — *see* Neoplasm, by site, in situ
      unspecified site 233.0
  oat cell (M8042/3)
    specified site — *see* Neoplasm, by site, malignant
    unspecified site 162.9
  odontogenic (M9270/3) 170.1
    upper jaw (bone) 170.0
  onocytic (M8290/3)
  oxyphilic (M8290/3)
  papillary (M8050/3)
    and follicular (mixed) (M8340/3) 193
    epidermoid (M8052/3)
    intraductal (noninfiltrating) (M8503/2)
      specified site — *see* Neoplasm, by site, in situ
      unspecified site 233.0
  serous (M8460/3)
    specified site — *see* Neoplasm, by site, malignant
    surface (M8461/3)
      specified site — *see* Neoplasm, by site, malignant
      unspecified site 183.0
    unspecified site 183.0
  squamous cell (M8052/3)
  transitional cell (M8130/3)
  papillocystic (M8450/3)
    specified site — *see* Neoplasm, by site, malignant
    unspecified site 183.0
  parafollicular cell (M8510/3)
    specified site — *see* Neoplasm, by site, malignant
    unspecified site 193
  pleomorphic (M8022/3)
  polygonal cell (M8034/3)
  prickle cell (M8070/3)
  pseudoglandular, squamous cell (M8075/3)
  pseudomucinous (M8470/3)
    specified site — *see* Neoplasm, by site, malignant
    unspecified site 183.0
  pseudosarcomatous (M8033/3)
  regaud type (M8082/3) — *see* Neoplasm, nasopharynx, malignant
  renal cell (M8312/3) 189.0
  reserve cell (M8041/3)
  round cell (M8041/3)
  Schmincke (M8082/3) — *see* Neoplasm, nasopharynx, malignant
  Schneiderian (M8121/3)
    specified site — *see* Neoplasm, by site, malignant

Carcinoma — *see also* Neoplasm, by site, malignant — *continued*
  Schneiderian — *continued*
    unspecified site 160.0
  scirrhous (M8141/3)
  sebaceous (M8410/3) — *see* Neoplasm, skin, malignant
  secondary (M8010/6) — *see* Neoplasm, by site, malignant, secondary
  secretory, breast (M8502/3) — *see* Neoplasm, breast, malignant
  serous (M8441/3)
    papillary (M8460/3)
      specified site — *see* Neoplasm, by site, malignant
      unspecified site 183.0
    surface, papillary (M8461/3)
      specified site — *see* Neoplasm, by site, malignant
      unspecified site 183.0
  Sertoli cell (M8640/3)
    specified site — *see* Neoplasm, by site, malignant
    unspecified site 186.9
  signet ring cell (M8490/3)
    metastatic (M8490/6) — *see* Neoplasm, by site, secondary
  simplex (M8231/3)
  skin appendage (M8390/3) — *see* Neoplasm, skin, malignant
  small cell (M8041/3)
    fusiform cell type (M8043/3)
    squamous cell, non-keratinizing type (M8073/3)
  solid (M8230/3)
    with amyloid stroma (M8511/3)
      specified site — *see* Neoplasm, by site, malignant
      unspecified site 193
  spheroidal cell (M8035/3)
  spindle cell (M8032/3)
    and giant cell (M8030/3)
  spinous cell (M8070/3)
  squamous (cell) (M8070/3)
    adenoid type (M8075/3)
    and adenocarcinoma, mixed (M8560/3)
    intraepidermal, Bowen's type — *see* Neoplasm, skin, in situ
    keratinizing type (large cell) (M8071/3)
    large cell, non-keratinizing type (M8072/3)
    microinvasive (M8076/3)
      specified site — *see* Neoplasm, by site, malignant
      unspecified site 180.9
    non-keratinizing type (M8072/3)
    papillary (M8052/3)
    pseudoglandular (M8075/3)
    skin (*see also* Neoplasm, skin, malignant) 173.92
    small cell, non-keratinizing type (M8073/3)
    spindle cell type (M8074/3)
    verrucous (M8051/3)
  superficial spreading (M8143/3)
  sweat gland (M8400/3) — *see* Neoplasm, skin, malignant
  theca cell (M8600/3) 183.0
  thymic (M8580/3) 164.0
  trabecular (M8190/3)
  transitional (cell) (M8120/3)
    papillary (M8130/3)
    spindle cell type (M8122/3)
  tubular (M8211/3)
  undifferentiated type (M8020/3)
  urothelial (M8120/3)
  ventriculi 151.9
  verrucous (epidermoid) (squamous cell) (M8051/3)
  villous (M8262/3)
  water-clear cell (M8322/3) 194.1
  wolffian duct (M9110/3)
Carcinosarcoma (M8980/3) — *see also* Neoplasm, by site, malignant
  embryonal type (M8981/3) — *see* Neoplasm, by site, malignant

Cardiac — *see also* condition
  death — *see* Disease, heart
  device
    defibrillator, automatic implantable (with synchronous cardiac pacemaker) V45.02
    in situ NEC V45.00
    pacemaker
      cardiac
        fitting or adjustment V53.31
        in situ V45.01
      carotid sinus
        fitting or adjustment V53.39
        in situ V45.09
  pacemaker — *see* Cardiac, device, pacemaker
  tamponade 423.3
Cardia, cardial — *see* condition
Cardialgia — *see also* Pain, precordial 786.51
Cardiectasis — *see* Hypertrophy, cardiac
Cardiochalasia 530.81
Cardiomalacia — *see also* Degeneration, myocardial 429.1
Cardiomegalia glycogenica diffusa 271.0
Cardiomegaly — *see also* Hypertrophy, cardiac 429.3
  congenital 746.89
  glycogen 271.0
  hypertensive (*see also* Hypertension, heart) 402.90
  idiopathic 429.3
Cardiomyoliposis — *see also* Degeneration, myocardial 429.1
Cardiomyopathy (congestive) (constrictive) (familial) (infiltrative) (obstructive) (restrictive) (sporadic) 425.4
  alcoholic 425.5
  amyloid 277.39 *[425.7]*
  beriberi 265.0 *[425.7]*
  cobalt-beer 425.5
  congenital 425.3
  due to
    amyloidosis 277.39 *[425.7]*
    beriberi 265.0 *[425.7]*
    cardiac glycogenosis 271.0 *[425.7]*
    Chagas' disease 086.0
    Friedreich's ataxia 334.0 *[425.8]*
    hypertension — *see* Hypertension, with, heart involvement
    mucopolysaccharidosis 277.5 *[425.7]*
    myotonia atrophica 359.21 *[425.8]*
    progressive muscular dystrophy 359.1 *[425.8]*
    sarcoidosis 135 *[425.8]*
  glycogen storage 271.0 *[425.7]*
  hypertensive — *see* Hypertension, with, heart involvement
  hypertrophic 425.18
    nonobstructive 425.18
    obstructive 425.11
      congenital 746.84
  idiopathic (concentric) 425.4
  in
    Chagas' disease 086.0
    sarcoidosis 135 *[425.8]*
  ischemic 414.8
  metabolic NEC 277.9 *[425.7]*
    amyloid 277.39 *[425.7]*
    thyrotoxic (*see also* Thyrotoxicosis) 242.9 ☑ *[425.7]*
  thyrotoxicosis (*see also* Thyrotoxicosis) 242.9 ☑ *[425.7]*
  newborn 425.4
    congenital 425.3
  nutritional 269.9 *[425.7]*
    beriberi 265.0 *[425.7]*
  obscure of Africa 425.2
  peripartum 674.5 ☑
  postpartum 674.5 ☑
  primary 425.4
  secondary 425.9
  stress induced 429.83
  takotsubo 429.83
  thyrotoxic (*see also* Thyrotoxicosis) 242.9 ☑ *[425.7]*
  toxic NEC 425.9

Cardiomyopathy — *continued*
  tuberculous (*see also* Tuberculosis) 017.9 ☑ *[425.8]*
Cardionephritis — *see* Hypertension, cardiorenal
Cardionephropathy — *see* Hypertension, cardiorenal
Cardionephrosis — *see* Hypertension, cardiorenal
Cardioneurosis 306.2
Cardiopathia nigra 416.0
Cardiopathy — *see also* Disease, heart 429.9
  hypertensive (*see also* Hypertension, heart) 402.90
  idiopathic 425.4
  mucopolysaccharidosis 277.5 *[425.7]*
Cardiopericarditis — *see also* Pericarditis 423.9
Cardiophobia 300.29
Cardioptosis 746.87
Cardiorenal — *see* condition
Cardiorrhexis — *see also* Infarct, myocardium 410.9 ☑
Cardiosclerosis — *see* Arteriosclerosis, coronary
Cardiosis — *see* Disease, heart
Cardiospasm (esophagus) (reflex) (stomach) 530.0
  congenital 750.7
Cardiostenosis — *see* Disease, heart
Cardiosymphysis 423.1
Cardiothyrotoxicosis — *see* Hyperthyroidism
Cardiovascular — *see* condition
Carditis (acute) (bacterial) (chronic) (subacute) 429.89
  Coxsackie 074.20
  hypertensive (*see also* Hypertension, heart) 402.90
  meningococcal 036.40
  rheumatic — *see* Disease, heart, rheumatic
  rheumatoid 714.2
Care (of)
  child (routine) V20.1
  convalescent following V66.9
    chemotherapy V66.2
    medical NEC V66.5
    psychotherapy V66.3
    radiotherapy V66.1
    surgery V66.0
    surgical NEC V66.0
    treatment (for) V66.5
      combined V66.6
      fracture V66.4
      mental disorder NEC V66.3
      specified type NEC V66.5
  end-of-life V66.7
  family member (handicapped) (sick)
    creating problem for family V61.49
    provided away from home for holiday relief V60.5
    unavailable, due to
      absence (person rendering care) (sufferer) V60.4
      inability (any reason) of person rendering care V60.4
  holiday relief V60.5
  hospice V66.7
  lack of (at or after birth) (infant) (child) 995.52
    adult 995.84
  lactation of mother V24.1
  palliative V66.7
  postpartum
    immediately after delivery V24.0
    routine follow-up V24.2
  prenatal V22.1
    first pregnancy V22.0
    high-risk pregnancy V23.9
      inconclusive fetal viability V23.87
      specified problem NEC V23.89
  terminal V66.7
  unavailable, due to
    absence of person rendering care V60.4
    inability (any reason) of person rendering care V60.4
  well baby V20.1

☑ **Additional Digit Required** — Refer to the Tabular List for Digit Selection   ⧖ **Subterms under main terms may continue to next column or page**

2014 ICD-9-CM 89

Caries (bone) — *see also* Tuberculosis, bone
  015.9 ☑ *[730.8]* ☑
  arrested 521.04
  cementum 521.03
  cerebrospinal (tuberculous)
    015.0 ☑ *[730.88]*
  dental (acute) (chronic) (incipient) (infected)
    521.00
    with pulp exposure 521.03
    extending to
      dentine 521.02
      pulp 521.03
    other specified NEC 521.09
    pit and fissure 521.06
    primary
      pit and fissure origin 521.06
      root surface 521.08
      smooth surface origin 521.07
    root surface 521.08
    smooth surface 521.07
  dentin (acute) (chronic) 521.02
  enamel (acute) (chronic) (incipient) 521.01
  external meatus 380.89
  hip (*see also* Tuberculosis) 015.1 ☑ *[730.85]*
  initial 521.01
  knee 015.2 ☑ *[730.86]*
  labyrinth 386.8
  limb NEC 015.7 ☑ *[730.88]*
  mastoid (chronic) (process) 383.1
  middle ear 385.89
  nose 015.7 ☑ *[730.88]*
  orbit 015.7 ☑ *[730.88]*
  ossicle 385.24
  petrous bone 383.20
  sacrum (tuberculous) 015.0 ☑ *[730.88]*
  spine, spinal (column) (tuberculous)
    015.0 ☑ *[730.88]*
  syphilitic 095.5
    congenital 090.0 *[730.8]* ☑
  teeth (internal) 521.00
    initial 521.01
  vertebra (column) (tuberculous)
    015.0 ☑ *[730.88]*

Carini's syndrome (ichthyosis congenita) 757.1
Carious teeth 521.00
Carneous mole 631.8
Carnosinemia 270.5
Carotid body or sinus syndrome 337.01
Carotidynia 337.01
Carotinemia (dietary) 278.3
Carotinosis (cutis) (skin) 278.3
Carpal tunnel syndrome 354.0
Carpenter's syndrome 759.89
Carpopedal spasm — *see also* Tetany 781.7
Carpoptosis 736.05
Carrier (suspected) **of**
  amebiasis V02.2
  bacterial disease (meningococcal, staphylo-
    coccal) NEC V02.59
  cholera V02.0
  cystic fibrosis gene V83.81
  defective gene V83.89
  diphtheria V02.4
  dysentery (bacillary) V02.3
    amebic V02.2
  Endamoeba histolytica V02.2
  gastrointestinal pathogens NEC V02.3
  genetic defect V83.89
  gonorrhea V02.7
  group B streptococcus V02.51
  HAA (hepatitis Australian-antigen) V02.61
  hemophilia A (asymptomatic) V83.01
    symptomatic V83.02
  hepatitis V02.60
    Australian-antigen (HAA) V02.61
    B V02.61
    C V02.62
    serum V02.61
    specified type NEC V02.69
    viral V02.60
  infective organism NEC V02.9
  malaria V02.9
  paratyphoid V02.3
  Salmonella V02.3
    typhosa V02.1
  serum hepatitis V02.61

Carrier (suspected) **of** — *continued*
  Shigella V02.3
  Staphylococcus NEC V02.59
    methicillin
      resistant Staphylococcus aureus
        V02.54
      susceptible Staphylococcus aureus
        V02.53
  Streptococcus NEC V02.52
    group B V02.51
  typhoid V02.1
  venereal disease NEC V02.8
Carrión's disease (Bartonellosis) 088.0
Car sickness 994.6
Carter's
  relapsing fever (Asiatic) 087.0
Cartilage — *see* condition
Caruncle (inflamed)
  abscess, lacrimal (*see also* Dacryocystitis)
    375.30
  conjunctiva 372.00
    acute 372.00
  eyelid 373.00
  labium (majus) (minus) 616.89
  lacrimal 375.30
  urethra (benign) 599.3
  vagina (wall) 616.89
Cascade stomach 537.6
Caseation lymphatic gland — *see also* Tuberculosis 017.2 ☑
Caseous
  bronchitis — *see* Tuberculosis, pulmonary
  meningitis 013.0 ☑
  pneumonia — *see* Tuberculosis, pulmonary
Cassidy (-Scholte) syndrome (malignant carcinoid) 259.2
Castellani's bronchitis 104.8
Castleman's tumor or lymphoma (mediastinal lymph node hyperplasia) 785.6
Castration, traumatic 878.2
  complicated 878.3
Casts in urine 791.7
Catalepsy 300.11
  catatonic (acute) (*see also* Schizophrenia)
    295.2 ☑
  hysterical 300.11
  schizophrenic (*see also* Schizophrenia)
    295.2 ☑
Cataphasia — *see also* Disorder, fluency 315.35
Cataplexy (idiopathic) — *see* Narcolepsy
Cataract (anterior cortical) (anterior polar)
  (black) (capsular) (central) (cortical) (hypermature) (immature) (incipient) (mature) 366.9
  anterior
    and posterior axial embryonal 743.33
    pyramidal 743.31
    subcapsular polar
      infantile, juvenile, or presenile 366.01
      senile 366.13
  associated with
    calcinosis 275.40 *[366.42]*
    craniofacial dysostosis 756.0 *[366.44]*
    galactosemia 271.1 *[366.44]*
    hypoparathyroidism 252.1 *[366.42]*
    myotonic disorders 359.21 *[366.43]*
    neovascularization 366.33
  blue dot 743.39
  cerulean 743.39
  complicated NEC 366.30
  congenital 743.30
    capsular or subcapsular 743.31
    cortical 743.32
    nuclear 743.33
    specified type NEC 743.39
    total or subtotal 743.34
    zonular 743.32
  coronary (congenital) 743.39
    acquired 366.12
  cupuliform 366.14
  diabetic 250.5 ☑ *[366.41]*
    due to secondary diabetes
      249.5 ☑ *[366.41]*
  drug-induced 366.45
  due to
    chalcosis 360.24 *[366.34]*

Cataract — *continued*
  due to — *continued*
    chronic choroiditis (*see also* Choroiditis)
      363.20 *[366.32]*
    degenerative myopia 360.21 *[366.34]*
    glaucoma (*see also* Glaucoma)
      365.9 *[366.31]*
    infection, intraocular NEC 366.32
    inflammatory ocular disorder NEC 366.32
    iridocyclitis, chronic 364.10 *[366.33]*
    pigmentary retinal dystrophy
      362.74 *[366.34]*
    radiation 366.46
  electric 366.46
  glassblowers' 366.46
  heat ray 366.46
  heterochromic 366.33
  in eye disease NEC 366.30
  infantile (*see also* Cataract, juvenile) 366.00
  intumescent 366.12
  irradiational 366.46
  juvenile 366.00
    anterior subcapsular polar 366.01
    combined forms 366.09
    cortical 366.03
    lamellar 366.03
    nuclear 366.04
    posterior subcapsular polar 366.02
    specified NEC 366.09
    zonular 366.03
  lamellar 743.32
    infantile, juvenile, or presenile 366.03
  morgagnian 366.18
  myotonic 359.21 *[366.43]*
  myxedema 244.9 *[366.44]*
  nuclear 366.16
  posterior, polar (capsular) 743.31
    infantile, juvenile, or presenile 366.02
    senile 366.14
  presenile (*see also* Cataract, juvenile) 366.00
  punctate
    acquired 366.12
    congenital 743.39
  secondary (membrane) 366.50
    obscuring vision 366.53
    specified type, not obscuring vision
      366.52
  senile 366.10
    anterior subcapsular polar 366.13
    combined forms 366.19
    cortical 366.15
    hypermature 366.18
    immature 366.12
    incipient 366.12
    mature 366.17
    nuclear 366.16
    posterior subcapsular polar 366.14
    specified NEC 366.19
    total or subtotal 366.17
  snowflake 250.5 ☑ *[366.41]*
    due to secondary diabetes
      249.5 ☑ *[366.41]*
  specified NEC 366.8
  subtotal (senile) 366.17
    congenital 743.34
  sunflower 360.24 *[366.34]*
  tetanic NEC 252.1 *[366.42]*
  total (mature) (senile) 366.17
    congenital 743.34
    localized 366.21
    traumatic 366.22
  toxic 366.45
  traumatic 366.20
    partially resolved 366.23
    total 366.22
  zonular (perinuclear) 743.32
    infantile, juvenile, or presenile 366.03
Cataracta 366.10
  brunescens 366.16
  cerulea 743.39
  complicata 366.30
  congenita 743.30
  coralliformis 743.39
  coronaria (congenital) 743.39
    acquired 366.12
  diabetic 250.5 ☑ *[366.41]*

Cataracta — *continued*
  diabetic — *continued*
    due to secondary diabetes
      249.5 ☑ *[366.41]*
  floriformis 360.24 *[366.34]*
  membranacea
    accreta 366.50
    congenita 743.39
  nigra 366.16
Catarrh, catarrhal (inflammation) — *see also*
  condition 460
  acute 460
  asthma, asthmatic (*see also* Asthma)
    493.9 ☑
  Bostock's (*see also* Fever, hay) 477.9
  bowel — *see* Enteritis
  bronchial 490
    acute 466.0
    chronic 491.0
    subacute 466.0
  cervix, cervical (canal) (uteri) — *see* Cervicitis
  chest (*see also* Bronchitis) 490
  chronic 472.0
  congestion 472.0
  conjunctivitis 372.03
  due to syphilis 095.9
    congenital 090.0
  enteric — *see* Enteritis
  epidemic (*see also* Influenza) 487.1
  Eustachian 381.50
  eye (acute) (vernal) 372.03
  fauces (*see also* Pharyngitis) 462
  febrile 460
  fibrinous acute 466.0
  gastroenteric — *see* Enteritis
  gastrointestinal — *see* Enteritis
  gingivitis 523.00
  hay (*see also* Fever, hay) 477.9
  infectious 460
  intestinal — *see* Enteritis
  larynx (*see also* Laryngitis, chronic) 476.0
  liver 070.1
    with hepatic coma 070.0
  lung (*see also* Bronchitis) 490
    acute 466.0
    chronic 491.0
  middle ear (chronic) — *see* Otitis media,
    chronic
  mouth 528.00
  nasal (chronic) (*see also* Rhinitis) 472.0
    acute 460
  nasobronchial 472.2
  nasopharyngeal (chronic) 472.2
    acute 460
  nose — *see* Catarrh, nasal
  ophthalmia 372.03
  pneumococcal, acute 466.0
  pulmonary (*see also* Bronchitis) 490
    acute 466.0
    chronic 491.0
  spring (eye) 372.13
  suffocating (*see also* Asthma) 493.9 ☑
  summer (hay) (*see also* Fever, hay) 477.9
  throat 472.1
  tracheitis 464.10
    with obstruction 464.11
  tubotympanal 381.4
    acute (*see also* Otitis media, acute, non-
      suppurative) 381.00
    chronic 381.10
  vasomotor (*see also* Fever, hay) 477.9
  vesical (bladder) — *see* Cystitis
Catarrhus aestivus — *see also* Fever, hay 477.9
Catastrophe, cerebral — *see also* Disease,
  cerebrovascular, acute 436
Catatonia, catatonic (acute) 781.99
  with
    affective psychosis — *see* Psychosis, af-
      fective
  agitation 295.2 ☑
  dementia (praecox) 295.2 ☑
  due to or associated with physical condition
    293.89
  excitation 295.2 ☑
  excited type 295.2 ☑
  in conditions classified elsewhere 293.89

☑ **Additional Digit Required** — Refer to the Tabular List for Digit Selection

▽ **Subterms under main terms may continue to next column or page**

Catatonia, catatonic — *continued*
　schizophrenia 295.2 ☑
　stupor 295.2 ☑
Cat's ear 744.29
Cat-scratch — *see also* Injury, superficial
　disease or fever 078.3
Cauda equina — *see also* condition
　syndrome 344.60
Cauliflower ear 738.7
Caul over face 768.9
Causalgia 355.9
　lower limb 355.71
　upper limb 354.4
Cause
　external, general effects NEC 994.9
　not stated 799.9
　unknown 799.9
Caustic burn — *see also* Burn, by site
　from swallowing caustic or corrosive sub-
　　stance — *see* Burn, internal organs
Cavare's disease (familial periodic paralysis)
　359.3
Cave-in, injury
　crushing (severe) (*see also* Crush, by site)
　　869.1
　suffocation 994.7
Cavernitis (penis) 607.2
　lymph vessel — *see* Lymphangioma
Cavernositis 607.2
Cavernous — *see* condition
Cavitation of lung — *see also* Tuberculosis
　011.2 ☑
　nontuberculous 518.89
　primary, progressive 010.8 ☑
Cavity
　lung — *see* Cavitation of lung
　optic papilla 743.57
　pulmonary — *see* Cavitation of lung
　teeth 521.00
　vitreous (humor) 379.21
Cavovarus foot, congenital 754.59
Cavus foot (congenital) 754.71
　acquired 736.73
Cazenave's
　disease (pemphigus) NEC 694.4
　lupus (erythematosus) 695.4
CDGS (carbohydrate-deficient glycoprotein
　syndrome) 271.8
Cecitis — *see* Appendicitis
Cecocele — *see* Hernia
Cecum — *see* condition
Celiac
　artery compression syndrome 447.4
　disease 579.0
　infantilism 579.0
Cell, cellular — *see also* condition
　anterior chamber (eye) (positive aqueous
　　ray) 364.04
Cellulitis (diffuse) (with lymphangitis) — *see
　also* Abscess 682.9
　abdominal wall 682.2
　anaerobic (*see also* Gas gangrene) 040.0
　ankle 682.6
　anus 566
　areola 611.0
　arm (any part, above wrist) 682.3
　auditory canal (external) 380.10
　axilla 682.3
　back (any part) 682.2
　breast 611.0
　　postpartum 675.1 ☑
　broad ligament (*see also* Disease, pelvis, in-
　　flammatory) 614.4
　　acute 614.3
　buttock 682.5
　cervical (neck region) 682.1
　cervix (uteri) (*see also* Cervicitis) 616.0
　cheek, external 682.0
　　internal 528.3
　chest wall 682.2
　chronic NEC 682.9
　colostomy 569.61
　corpus cavernosum 607.2
　digit 681.9

Cellulitis — *see also* Abscess — *continued*
　Douglas' cul-de-sac or pouch (chronic) (*see
　　also* Disease, pelvis, inflammatory)
　　614.4
　　acute 614.3
　drainage site (following operation) 998.59
　ear, external 380.10
　enterostomy 569.61
　erysipelar (*see also* Erysipelas) 035
　esophagostomy 530.86
　eyelid 373.13
　face (any part, except eye) 682.0
　finger (intrathecal) (periosteal) (subcuta-
　　neous) (subcuticular) 681.00
　flank 682.2
　foot (except toe) 682.7
　forearm 682.3
　gangrenous (*see also* Gangrene) 785.4
　genital organ NEC
　　female — *see* Abscess, genital organ,
　　　female
　　male 608.4
　glottis 478.71
　gluteal (region) 682.5
　gonococcal NEC 098.0
　groin 682.2
　hand (except finger or thumb) 682.4
　head (except face) NEC 682.8
　heel 682.7
　hip 682.6
　jaw (region) 682.0
　knee 682.6
　labium (majus) (minus) (*see also* Vulvitis)
　　616.10
　larynx 478.71
　leg, except foot 682.6
　lip 528.5
　mammary gland 611.0
　mouth (floor) 528.3
　multiple sites NEC 682.9
　nasopharynx 478.21
　navel 682.2
　　newborn NEC 771.4
　neck (region) 682.1
　nipple 611.0
　nose 478.19
　　external 682.0
　orbit, orbital 376.01
　palate (soft) 528.3
　pectoral (region) 682.2
　pelvis, pelvic
　　with
　　　abortion — *see* Abortion, by type,
　　　　with sepsis
　　　ectopic pregnancy (*see also* cate-
　　　　gories 633.0–633.9) 639.0
　　　molar pregnancy (*see also* categories
　　　　630–632) 639.0
　　female (*see also* Disease, pelvis, inflam-
　　　matory) 614.4
　　　acute 614.3
　　　following
　　　　abortion 639.0
　　　　ectopic or molar pregnancy 639.0
　　　male 567.21
　　　puerperal, postpartum, childbirth
　　　　670.8 ☑
　penis 607.2
　perineal, perineum 682.2
　perirectal 566
　peritonsillar 475
　periurethral 597.0
　periuterine (*see also* Disease, pelvis, inflam-
　　matory) 614.4
　　acute 614.3
　pharynx 478.21
　phlegmonous NEC 682.9
　rectum 566
　retromammary 611.0
　retroperitoneal (*see also* Peritonitis)
　　567.2 ☑, 567.38
　round ligament (*see also* Disease, pelvis, in-
　　flammatory) 614.4
　　acute 614.3
　scalp (any part) 682.8
　　dissecting 704.8

Cellulitis — *see also* Abscess — *continued*
　scrotum 608.4
　seminal vesicle 608.0
　septic NEC 682.9
　shoulder 682.3
　specified sites NEC 682.8
　spermatic cord 608.4
　submandibular (region) (space) (triangle)
　　682.0
　　gland 527.3
　submaxillary 528.3
　　gland 527.3
　submental (pyogenic) 682.0
　　gland 527.3
　suppurative NEC 682.9
　testis 608.4
　thigh 682.6
　thumb (intrathecal) (periosteal) (subcuta-
　　neous) (subcuticular) 681.00
　toe (intrathecal) (periosteal) (subcutaneous)
　　(subcuticular) 681.10
　tonsil 475
　trunk 682.2
　tuberculous (primary) (*see also* Tuberculosis)
　　017.0 ☑
　tunica vaginalis 608.4
　umbilical 682.2
　　newborn NEC 771.4
　vaccinal 999.39
　vagina — *see* Vaginitis
　vas deferens 608.4
　vocal cords 478.5
　vulva (*see also* Vulvitis) 616.10
　wrist 682.4
Cementoblastoma, benign (M9273/0) 213.1
　upper jaw (bone) 213.0
Cementoma (M9273/0) 213.1
　gigantiform (M9275/0) 213.1
　　upper jaw (bone) 213.0
　upper jaw (bone) 213.0
Cementoperiostitis 523.40
　acute 523.33
　apical 523.40
Cephalgia, cephalagia — *see also* Headache
　784.0
　histamine 339.00
　nonorganic origin 307.81
　other trigeminal autonomic (TACS) 339.09
　psychogenic 307.81
　tension 307.81
Cephalhematocele, cephalematocele
　due to birth injury 767.19
　fetus or newborn 767.19
　traumatic (*see also* Contusion, head) 920
Cephalhematoma, cephalematoma (calci-
　fied)
　due to birth injury 767.19
　fetus or newborn 767.19
　traumatic (*see also* Contusion, head) 920
Cephalic — *see* condition
Cephalitis — *see* Encephalitis
Cephalocele 742.0
Cephaloma — *see* Neoplasm, by site, malig-
　nant
Cephalomenia 625.8
Cephalopelvic — *see* condition
Cercomoniasis 007.3
Cerebellitis — *see* Encephalitis
Cerebellum (cerebellar) — *see* condition
Cerebral — *see* condition
Cerebritis — *see* Encephalitis
Cerebrohepatorenal syndrome 759.89
Cerebromacular degeneration 330.1
Cerebromalacia — *see also* Softening, brain
　348.89
　due to cerebrovascular accident 438.89
Cerebrosidosis 272.7
Cerebrospasticity — *see* Palsy, cerebral
Cerebrospinal — *see* condition
Cerebrum — *see* condition
Ceroid storage disease 272.7
Cerumen (accumulation) (impacted) 380.4
Cervical — *see also* condition
　auricle 744.43
　high risk human papillomavirus (HPV) DNA
　　test positive 795.05

Cervical — *see also* condition — *continued*
　intraepithelial glandular neoplasia 233.1
　low risk human papillomavirus (HPV) DNA
　　test positive 795.09
　rib 756.2
　shortening — *see* Short, cervical
Cervicalgia 723.1
Cervicitis (acute) (chronic) (nonvenereal)
　(subacute) (with erosion or ectropion)
　616.0
　with
　　abortion — *see* Abortion, by type, with
　　　sepsis
　　ectopic pregnancy (*see also* categories
　　　633.0–633.9) 639.0
　　molar pregnancy (*see also* categories
　　　630–632) 639.0
　　ulceration 616.0
　chlamydial 099.53
　complicating pregnancy or puerperium
　　646.6 ☑
　　affecting fetus or newborn 760.8
　following
　　abortion 639.0
　　ectopic or molar pregnancy 639.0
　gonococcal (acute) 098.15
　　chronic or duration of 2 months or more
　　　098.35
　senile (atrophic) 616.0
　syphilitic 095.8
　trichomonal 131.09
　tuberculous (*see also* Tuberculosis) 016.7 ☑
Cervicoaural fistula 744.49
Cervicocolpitis (emphysematosa) — *see also*
　Cervicitis 616.0
Cervix — *see* condition
Cesarean delivery, operation or section NEC
　669.7 ☑
　affecting fetus or newborn 763.4
　(planned) occurring after 37 completed
　　weeks of gestation but before 39
　　completed weeks gestation due to
　　(spontaneous) onset of labor
　　649.8 ☑
　post mortem, affecting fetus or newborn
　　761.6
　previous, affecting management of pregnan-
　　cy 654.2 ☑
Céstan-Chenais paralysis 344.89
Céstan-Raymond syndrome 433.8 ☑
Céstan's syndrome 344.89
Cestode infestation NEC 123.9
　specified type NEC 123.8
Cestodiasis 123.9
CGF (congenital generalized fibromatosis)
　759.89
Chabert's disease 022.9
Chacaleh 266.2
Chafing 709.8
Chagas' disease — *see also* Trypanosomiasis,
　American 086.2
　with heart involvement 086.0
Chagres fever 084.0
Chalasia (cardiac sphincter) 530.81
Chalazion 373.2
Chalazoderma 757.39
Chalcosis 360.24
　cornea 371.15
　crystalline lens 360.24 [366.34]
　retina 360.24
Chalicosis (occupational) (pulmonum) 502
Chancre (any genital site) (hard) (indurated)
　(infecting) (primary) (recurrent) 091.0
　congenital 090.0
　conjunctiva 091.2
　Ducrey's 099.0
　extragenital 091.2
　eyelid 091.2
　Hunterian 091.0
　lip (syphilis) 091.2
　mixed 099.8
　nipple 091.2
　Nisbet's 099.0
　of
　　carate 103.0
　　pinta 103.0

☑ **Additional Digit Required** — Refer to the Tabular List for Digit Selection　　　　　　　　　　▽ **Subterms under main terms may continue to next column or page**

Chancre — continued
  of — continued
    yaws 102.0
    palate, soft 091.2
    phagedenic 099.0
    Ricord's 091.0
    Rollet's (syphilitic) 091.0
    seronegative 091.0
    seropositive 091.0
    simple 099.0
    soft 099.0
      bubo 099.0
    urethra 091.0
    yaws 102.0
Chancriform syndrome 114.1
Chancroid 099.0
  anus 099.0
  penis (Ducrey's bacillus) 099.0
  perineum 099.0
  rectum 099.0
  scrotum 099.0
  urethra 099.0
  vulva 099.0
Chandipura fever 066.8
Chandler's disease (osteochondritis dissecans, hip) 732.7
Change(s) (of) — see also Removal of —
  arteriosclerotic — see Arteriosclerosis
  battery
    cardiac pacemaker V53.31
  bone 733.90
    diabetic 250.8 ☑ [731.8]
      due to secondary diabetes
        249.8 ☑ [731.8]
    in disease, unknown cause 733.90
  bowel habits 787.99
  cardiorenal (vascular) (see also Hypertension, cardiorenal) 404.90
  cardiovascular — see Disease, cardiovascular
  circulatory 459.9
  cognitive or personality change of other type, nonpsychotic 310.1
  color, teeth, tooth
    during formation 520.8
    extrinsic 523.6
    intrinsic posteruptive 521.7
  contraceptive device V25.42
  cornea, corneal
    degenerative NEC 371.40
    membrane NEC 371.30
    senile 371.41
  coronary (see also Ischemia, heart) 414.9
  degenerative
    chamber angle (anterior) (iris) 364.56
    ciliary body 364.57
    spine or vertebra (see also Spondylosis) 721.90
  dental pulp, regressive 522.2
  drains V58.49
  dressing
    wound V58.30
      nonsurgical V58.30
      surgical V58.31
  fixation device V54.89
    external V54.89
    internal V54.01
  heart (see also Disease, heart)
  hip joint 718.95
  hyperplastic larynx 478.79
  hypertrophic
    nasal sinus (see also Sinusitis) 473.9
    turbinate, nasal 478.0
    upper respiratory tract 478.9
  inflammatory — see Inflammation
  joint (see also Derangement, joint) 718.90
    sacroiliac 724.6
  Kirschner wire V54.89
  knee 717.9
  macular, congenital 743.55

Change(s) — see also Removal of —
  continued
  malignant (M— —/3) (see also Neoplasm, by site, malignant)

Note — for malignant change occurring in a neoplasm, use the appropriate M code with behavior digit /3 e.g., malignant change in uterine fibroid — M8890/3. For malignant change occurring in a nonneoplastic condition (e.g., gastric ulcer) use the M code M8000/3.

  mental (status) NEC 780.97
    due to or associated with physical condition — see Syndrome, brain
  myocardium, myocardial — see Degeneration, myocardial
  of life (see also Menopause) 627.2
  pacemaker battery (cardiac) V53.31
  peripheral nerve 355.9
  personality (nonpsychotic) NEC 310.1
  plaster cast V54.89
  refractive, transient 367.81
  regressive, dental pulp 522.2
  retina 362.9
    myopic (degenerative) (malignant) 360.21
    vascular appearance 362.13
  sacroiliac joint 724.6
  scleral 379.19
    degenerative 379.16
  senile (see also Senility) 797
  sensory (see also Disturbance, sensation) 782.0
  skin texture 782.8
  spinal cord 336.9
  splint, external V54.89
  subdermal implantable contraceptive V25.5
  suture V58.32
  traction device V54.89
  trophic 355.9
    arm NEC 354.9
    leg NEC 355.8
    lower extremity NEC 355.8
    upper extremity NEC 354.9
  vascular 459.9
  vasomotor 443.9
  voice 784.49
    psychogenic 306.1
  wound packing V58.30
    nonsurgical V58.30
    surgical V58.31
Changing sleep-work schedule, affecting sleep 327.36
Changuinola fever 066.0
Chapping skin 709.8
Character
  depressive 301.12
Charcôt's
  arthropathy 094.0 [713.5]
  cirrhosis — see Cirrhosis, biliary
  disease 094.0
    spinal cord 094.0
  fever (biliary) (hepatic) (intermittent) — see Choledocholithiasis
  joint (disease) 094.0 [713.5]
    diabetic 250.6 ☑ [713.5]
      due to secondary diabetes
        249.6 ☑ [713.5]
    syringomyelic 336.0 [713.5]
  syndrome (intermittent claudication) 443.9
    due to atherosclerosis 440.21
Charcôt-Marie-Tooth disease, paralysis, or syndrome 356.1
CHARGE association (syndrome) 759.89
Charleyhorse (quadriceps) 843.8
  muscle, except quadriceps — see Sprain, by site
Charlouis' disease — see also Yaws 102.9
Chauffeur's fracture — see Fracture, ulna, lower end
Cheadle (-Möller) (-Barlow) disease or syndrome (infantile scurvy) 267
Checking (of)
  contraceptive device (intrauterine) V25.42
  device
    fixation V54.89

Checking — continued
  device — continued
    fixation - continued
      external V54.89
      internal V54.09
      traction V54.89
    Kirschner wire V54.89
    plaster cast V54.89
    splint, external V54.89
Checkup
  following treatment — see Examination
  health V70.0
  infant (over 28 days old) (not sick) V20.2
  newborn, routine
    8 to 28 days old V20.32
    over 28 days old, routine V20.2
    under 8 days old V20.31
    weight V20.32
  pregnancy (normal) V22.1
    first V22.0
    high-risk pregnancy V23.9
      inconclusive fetal viability V23.87
      specified problem NEC V23.89
Chédiak-Higashi (-Steinbrinck) anomaly, disease, or syndrome (congenital gigantism of peroxidase granules) 288.2
Cheek — see also condition
  biting 528.9
Cheese itch 133.8
Cheese washers' lung 495.8
Cheilitis 528.5
  actinic (due to sun) 692.72
    chronic NEC 692.74
      due to radiation, except from sun 692.82
    due to radiation, except from sun 692.82
  acute 528.5
  angular 528.5
  catarrhal 528.5
  chronic 528.5
  exfoliative 528.5
  gangrenous 528.5
  glandularis apostematosa 528.5
  granulomatosa 351.8
  infectional 528.5
  membranous 528.5
  Miescher's 351.8
  suppurative 528.5
  ulcerative 528.5
  vesicular 528.5
Cheilodynia 528.5
Cheilopalatoschisis — see also Cleft, palate, with cleft lip 749.20
Cheilophagia 528.9
Cheiloschisis — see also Cleft, lip 749.10
Cheilosis 528.5
  with pellagra 265.2
  angular 528.5
  due to
    dietary deficiency 266.0
    vitamin deficiency 266.0
Cheiromegaly 729.89
Cheiropompholyx 705.81
Cheloid — see also Keloid 701.4
Chemical burn — see also Burn, by site
  from swallowing chemical — see Burn, internal organs
Chemodectoma (M8693/1) — see Paraganglioma, nonchromaffin
Chemoprophylaxis NEC V07.39
Chemosis, conjunctiva 372.73
Chemotherapy
  convalescence V66.2
  encounter (for) (oral) (intravenous) V58.11
  maintenance (oral) (intravenous) V58.11
  prophylactic NEC V07.39
    fluoride V07.31
Cherubism 526.89
Chest — see condition
Cheyne-Stokes respiration (periodic) 786.04
Chiari's
  disease or syndrome (hepatic vein thrombosis) 453.0
  malformation
    type I 348.4
    type II (see also Spina bifida) 741.0 ☑

Chiari's — continued
  malformation — continued
    type III 742.0
    type IV 742.2
    network 746.89
Chiari-Frommel syndrome 676.6 ☑
Chicago disease (North American blastomycosis) 116.0
Chickenpox — see also Varicella 052.9
  exposure to V01.71
  vaccination and inoculation (prophylactic) V05.4
Chiclero ulcer 085.4
Chiggers 133.8
Chignon 111.2
  fetus or newborn (from vacuum extraction) 767.19
Chigoe disease 134.1
Chikungunya fever 066.3
Chilaiditi's syndrome (subphrenic displacement, colon) 751.4
Chilblains 991.5
  lupus 991.5
Child
  behavior causing concern V61.20
    adopted child V61.24
    biological child V61.23
    foster child V61.25
Childbed fever 670.8 ☑
Childbirth — see also Delivery
  puerperal complications — see Puerperal
Childhood, period of rapid growth V21.0
Chill(s) 780.64
  with fever 780.60
  without fever 780.64
  congestive 780.99
    in malarial regions 084.6
  septic — see Septicemia
  urethral 599.84
Chilomastigiasis 007.8
Chin — see condition
Chinese dysentery 004.9
Chiropractic dislocation — see also Lesion, nonallopathic, by site 739.9
Chitral fever 066.0
Chlamydia, chlamydial — see condition
Chloasma 709.09
  cachecticorum 709.09
  eyelid 374.52
    congenital 757.33
    hyperthyroid 242.0 ☑
  gravidarum 646.8 ☑
  idiopathic 709.09
  skin 709.09
  symptomatic 709.09
Chloroma (M9930/3) 205.3 ☑
Chlorosis 280.9
  Egyptian (see also Ancylostomiasis) 126.9
  miners' (see also Ancylostomiasis) 126.9
Chlorotic anemia 280.9
Chocolate cyst (ovary) 617.1
Choked
  disk or disc — see Papilledema
  on food, phlegm, or vomitus NEC (see also Asphyxia, food) 933.1
  phlegm 933.1
  while vomiting NEC (see also Asphyxia, food) 933.1
Chokes (resulting from bends) 993.3
Choking sensation 784.99
Cholangiectasis — see also Disease, gallbladder 575.8
Cholangiocarcinoma (M8160/3)
  and hepatocellular carcinoma, combined (M8180/3) 155.0
  liver 155.1
  specified site NEC — see Neoplasm, by site, malignant
  unspecified site 155.1
Cholangiohepatitis 575.8
  due to fluke infestation 121.1
Cholangiohepatoma (M8180/3) 155.0
Cholangiolitis (acute) (chronic) (extrahepatic) (gangrenous) 576.1
  intrahepatic 575.8

Cholangiolitis — continued
    paratyphoidal (see also Fever, paratyphoid) 002.9
    typhoidal 002.0
Cholangioma (M8160/0) 211.5
    malignant — see Cholangiocarcinoma
Cholangitis (acute) (ascending) (catarrhal) (chronic) (infective) (malignant) (primary) (recurrent) (sclerosing) (secondary) (stenosing) (suppurative) 576.1
    chronic nonsuppurative destructive 571.6
    nonsuppurative destructive (chronic) 571.6
Cholecystdocholithiasis — see Choledocholithiasis
Cholecystitis 575.10
    with
        calculus, stones in
            bile duct (common) (hepatic) — see Choledocholithiasis
            gallbladder — see Cholelithiasis
    acute 575.0
    acute and chronic 575.12
    chronic 575.11
    emphysematous (acute) (see also Cholecystitis, acute) 575.0
    gangrenous (see also Cholecystitis, acute) 575.0
    paratyphoidal, current (see also Fever, paratyphoid) 002.9
    suppurative (see also Cholecystitis, acute) 575.0
    typhoidal 002.0
Choledochitis (suppurative) 576.1
Choledocholith — see Choledocholithiasis
Choledocholithiasis 574.5 ☑

Note — Use the following fifth-digit subclassification with category 574:

0   without mention of obstruction
1   with obstruction

    with
        cholecystitis 574.4 ☑
            acute 574.3 ☑
            chronic 574.4 ☑
        cholelithiasis 574.9 ☑
            with
                cholecystitis 574.7 ☑
                    acute 574.6 ☑
                        and chronic 574.8 ☑
                    chronic 574.7 ☑
Cholelithiasis (impacted) (multiple) 574.2 ☑

Note — Use the following fifth-digit subclassification with category 574:

0   without mention of obstruction
1   with obstruction

    with
        cholecystitis 574.1 ☑
            acute 574.0 ☑
            chronic 574.1 ☑
        choledocholithiasis 574.9 ☑
            with
                cholecystitis 574.7 ☑
                    acute 574.6 ☑
                        and chronic 574.8 ☑
                    chronic cholecystitis 574.7 ☑
Cholemia — see also Jaundice 782.4
    familial 277.4
    Gilbert's (familial nonhemolytic) 277.4
Cholemic gallstone — see Cholelithiasis
Choleperitoneum, choleperitonitis — see also Disease, gallbladder 567.81
Cholera (algid) (Asiatic) (asphyctic) (epidemic) (gravis) (Indian) (malignant) (morbus) (pestilential) (spasmodic) 001.9
    antimonial 985.4
    carrier (suspected) of V02.0
    classical 001.0
    contact V01.0
    due to
        Vibrio
            cholerae (Inaba, Ogawa, Hikojima serotypes) 001.0
            El Tor 001.1

Cholera — continued
    El Tor 001.1
        exposure to V01.0
        vaccination, prophylactic (against) V03.0
Cholerine — see also Cholera 001.9
Cholestasis 576.8
    due to total parenteral nutrition (TPN) 573.8
Cholesteatoma (ear) 385.30
    attic (primary) 385.31
    diffuse 385.35
    external ear (canal) 380.21
    marginal (middle ear) 385.32
        with involvement of mastoid cavity 385.33
        secondary (with middle ear involvement) 385.33
    mastoid cavity 385.30
    middle ear (secondary) 385.32
        with involvement of mastoid cavity 385.33
    postmastoidectomy cavity (recurrent) 383.32
    primary 385.31
    recurrent, postmastoidectomy cavity 383.32
    secondary (middle ear) 385.32
        with involvement of mastoid cavity 385.33
Cholesteatosis (middle ear) — see also Cholesteatoma 385.30
    diffuse 385.35
Cholesteremia 272.0
Cholesterin
    granuloma, middle ear 385.82
    in vitreous 379.22
Cholesterol
    deposit
        retina 362.82
        vitreous 379.22
    elevated (high) 272.0
        with elevated (high) triglycerides 272.2
    imbibition of gallbladder (see also Disease, gallbladder) 575.6
Cholesterolemia 272.0
    essential 272.0
    familial 272.0
    hereditary 272.0
Cholesterosis, cholesterolosis (gallbladder) 575.6
    with
        cholecystitis — see Cholecystitis
        cholelithiasis — see Cholelithiasis
        middle ear (see also Cholesteatoma) 385.30
Cholocolic fistula — see also Fistula, gallbladder 575.5
Choluria 791.4
Chondritis (purulent) 733.99
    auricle 380.03
    costal 733.6
        Tietze's 733.6
    patella, posttraumatic 717.7
    pinna 380.03
    posttraumatica patellae 717.7
    tuberculous (active) (see also Tuberculosis) 015.9 ☑
        intervertebral 015.0 ☑ [730.88]
Chondroangiopathia calcarea seu punctate 756.59
Chondroblastoma (M9230/0) — see also Neoplasm, bone, benign
    malignant (M9230/3) — see Neoplasm, bone, malignant
Chondrocalcinosis (articular) (crystal deposition) (dihydrate) — see also Arthritis, due to, crystals 275.49 [712.3] ☑
    due to
        calcium pyrophosphate 275.49 [712.2] ☑
        dicalcium phosphate crystals 275.49 [712.1] ☑
        pyrophosphate crystals 275.49 [712.2] ☑
Chondrodermatitis nodularis helicis 380.00
Chondrodysplasia 756.4
    angiomatose 756.4
    calcificans congenita 756.59
    epiphysialis punctata 756.59
    hereditary deforming 756.4

Chondrodysplasia — continued
    rhizomelic punctata 277.86
Chondrodystrophia (fetalis) 756.4
    calcarea 756.4
    calcificans congenita 756.59
    fetalis hypoplastica 756.59
    hypoplastica calcinosa 756.59
    punctata 756.59
    tarda 277.5
Chondrodystrophy (familial) (hypoplastic) 756.4
    myotonic (congenital) 359.23
Chondroectodermal dysplasia 756.55
Chondrolysis 733.99
Chondroma (M9220/0) — see also Neoplasm, cartilage, benign
    juxtacortical (M9221/0) — see Neoplasm, bone, benign
    periosteal (M9221/0) — see Neoplasm, bone, benign
Chondromalacia 733.92
    epiglottis (congenital) 748.3
    generalized 733.92
    knee 717.7
    larynx (congenital) 748.3
    localized, except patella 733.92
    patella, patellae 717.7
    systemic 733.92
    tibial plateau 733.92
    trachea (congenital) 748.3
Chondromatosis (M9220/1) — see Neoplasm, cartilage, uncertain behavior
Chondromyxosarcoma (M9220/3) — see Neoplasm, cartilage, malignant
Chondro-osteodysplasia (Morquio-Brailsford type) 277.5
Chondro-osteodystrophy 277.5
Chondro-osteoma (M9210/0) — see Neoplasm, bone, benign
Chondropathia tuberosa 733.6
Chondrosarcoma (M9220/3) — see also Neoplasm, cartilage, malignant
    juxtacortical (M9221/3) — see Neoplasm, bone, malignant
    mesenchymal (M9240/3) — see Neoplasm, connective tissue, malignant
Chordae tendineae rupture (chronic) 429.5
Chordee (nonvenereal) 607.89
    congenital 752.63
    gonococcal 098.2
Chorditis (fibrinous) (nodosa) (tuberosa) 478.5
Chordoma (M9370/3) — see Neoplasm, by site, malignant
Chorea (gravis) (minor) (spasmodic) 333.5
    with
        heart involvement — see Chorea with rheumatic heart disease
        rheumatic heart disease (chronic, inactive, or quiescent) (conditions classifiable to 393–398) (see rheumatic heart condition involved)
            active or acute (conditions classifiable to 391) 392.0
    acute — see Chorea, Sydenham's
    apoplectic (see also Disease, cerebrovascular, acute) 436
    chronic 333.4
    electric 049.8
    gravidarum — see Eclampsia, pregnancy
    habit 307.22
    hereditary 333.4
    Huntington's 333.4
    posthemiplegic 344.89
    pregnancy — see Eclampsia, pregnancy
    progressive 333.4
        chronic 333.4
        hereditary 333.4
    rheumatic (chronic) 392.9
        with heart disease or involvement — see Chorea, with rheumatic heart disease
    senile 333.5
    Sydenham's 392.9
        with heart involvement — see Chorea, with rheumatic heart disease

Chorea — continued
    Sydenham's — continued
        nonrheumatic 333.5
        variabilis 307.23
Choreoathetosis (paroxysmal) 333.5
Chorioadenoma (destruens) (M9100/1) 236.1
Chorioamnionitis 658.4 ☑
    affecting fetus or newborn 762.7
Chorioangioma (M9120/0) 219.8
Choriocarcinoma (M9100/3)
    combined with
        embryonal carcinoma (M9101/3) — see Neoplasm, by site, malignant
        teratoma (M9101/3) — see Neoplasm, by site, malignant
    specified site — see Neoplasm, by site, malignant
    unspecified site
        female 181
        male 186.9
Chorioencephalitis, lymphocytic (acute) (serous) 049.0
Chorioepithelioma (M9100/3) — see Choriocarcinoma
Choriomeningitis (acute) (benign) (lymphocytic) (serous) 049.0
Chorionepithelioma (M9100/3) — see Choriocarcinoma
Chorionitis — see also Scleroderma 710.1
Chorioretinitis 363.20
    disseminated 363.10
        generalized 363.13
        in
            neurosyphilis 094.83
            secondary syphilis 091.51
        peripheral 363.12
        posterior pole 363.11
        tuberculous (see also Tuberculosis) 017.3 ☑ [363.13]
    due to
        histoplasmosis (see also Histoplasmosis) 115.92
        toxoplasmosis (acquired) 130.2
            congenital (active) 771.2
    focal 363.00
        juxtapapillary 363.01
        peripheral 363.04
        posterior pole NEC 363.03
    juxtapapillaris, juxtapapillary 363.01
    progressive myopia (degeneration) 360.21
    syphilitic (secondary) 091.51
        congenital (early) 090.0 [363.13]
        late 090.5 [363.13]
        late 095.8 [363.13]
    tuberculous (see also Tuberculosis) 017.3 ☑ [363.13]
Choristoma — see Neoplasm, by site, benign
Choroid — see condition
Choroideremia, choroidermia (initial stage) (late stage) (partial or total atrophy) 363.55
Choroiditis — see also Chorioretinitis 363.20
    leprous 030.9 [363.13]
    senile guttate 363.41
    sympathetic 360.11
    syphilitic (secondary) 091.51
        congenital (early) 090.0 [363.13]
        late 090.5 [363.13]
        late 095.8 [363.13]
    Tay's 363.41
    tuberculous (see also Tuberculosis) 017.3 ☑ [363.13]
Choroidopathy NEC 363.9
    degenerative (see also Degeneration, choroid) 363.40
    hereditary (see also Dystrophy, choroid) 363.50
    specified type NEC 363.8
Choroidoretinitis — see Chorioretinitis
Choroidosis, central serous 362.41
Choroidretinopathy, serous 362.41
Christian's syndrome (chronic histiocytosis X) 277.89
Christian-Weber disease (nodular nonsuppurative panniculitis) 729.30
Christmas disease 286.1

☑ **Additional Digit Required — Refer to the Tabular List for Digit Selection**   ▽ **Subterms under main terms may continue to next column or page**

Chromaffinoma (M8700/0) — *see also* Neoplasm, by site, benign
  malignant (M8700/3) — *see* Neoplasm, by site, malignant
Chromatopsia 368.59
Chromhidrosis, chromidrosis 705.89
Chromoblastomycosis 117.2
Chromomycosis 117.2
Chromophytosis 111.0
Chromotrichomycosis 111.8
Chronic — *see* condition
Churg-Strauss syndrome 446.4
Chyle cyst, mesentery 457.8
Chylocele (nonfilarial) 457.8
  filarial (*see also* Infestation, filarial) 125.9
  tunica vaginalis (nonfilarial) 608.84
    filarial (*see also* Infestation, filarial) 125.9
Chylomicronemia (fasting) (with hyperprebe-talipoproteinemia) 272.3
Chylopericardium (acute) 420.90
Chylothorax (nonfilarial) 457.8
  filarial (*see also* Infestation, filarial) 125.9
Chylous
  ascites 457.8
  cyst of peritoneum 457.8
  hydrocele 603.9
  hydrothorax (nonfilarial) 457.8
    filarial (*see also* Infestation, filarial) 125.9
Chyluria 791.1
  bilharziasis 120.0
  due to
    Brugia (malayi) 125.1
    Wuchereria (bancrofti) 125.0
      malayi 125.1
  filarial (*see also* Infestation, filarial) 125.9
  filariasis (*see also* Infestation, filarial) 125.9
  nonfilarial 791.1
Cicatricial (deformity) — *see* Cicatrix
Cicatrix (adherent) (contracted) (painful) (vicious) 709.2
  adenoid 474.8
  alveolar process 525.8
  anus 569.49
  auricle 380.89
  bile duct (*see also* Disease, biliary) 576.8
  bladder 596.89
  bone 733.99
  brain 348.89
  cervix (postoperative) (postpartal) 622.3
    in pregnancy or childbirth 654.6 ☑
      causing obstructed labor 660.2 ☑
  chorioretinal 363.30
    disseminated 363.35
    macular 363.32
    peripheral 363.34
    posterior pole NEC 363.33
  choroid — *see* Cicatrix, chorioretinal
  common duct (*see also* Disease, biliary) 576.8
  congenital 757.39
  conjunctiva 372.64
  cornea 371.00
    tuberculous (*see also* Tuberculosis) 017.3 ☑ [371.05]
  duodenum (bulb) 537.3
  esophagus 530.3
  eyelid 374.46
    with
      ectropion — *see* Ectropion
      entropion — *see* Entropion
  hypopharynx 478.29
  knee, semilunar cartilage 717.5
  lacrimal
    canaliculi 375.53
    duct
      acquired 375.56
      neonatal 375.55
    punctum 375.52
    sac 375.54
  larynx 478.79
  limbus (cystoid) 372.64
  lung 518.89
  macular 363.32
    disseminated 363.35
    peripheral 363.34
  middle ear 385.89

Cicatrix — *continued*
  mouth 528.9
  muscle 728.89
  nasolacrimal duct
    acquired 375.56
    neonatal 375.55
  nasopharynx 478.29
  palate (soft) 528.9
  penis 607.89
  prostate 602.8
  rectum 569.49
  retina 363.30
    disseminated 363.35
    macular 363.32
    peripheral 363.34
    posterior pole NEC 363.33
  semilunar cartilage — *see* Derangement, meniscus
  seminal vesicle 608.89
  skin 709.2
    infected 686.8
    postinfectional 709.2
    tuberculous (*see also* Tuberculosis) 017.0 ☑
  specified site NEC 709.2
  throat 478.29
  tongue 529.8
  tonsil (and adenoid) 474.8
  trachea 478.9
  tuberculous NEC (*see also* Tuberculosis) 011.9 ☑
  ureter 593.89
  urethra 599.84
  uterus 621.8
  vagina 623.4
    in pregnancy or childbirth 654.7 ☑
      causing obstructed labor 660.2 ☑
  vocal cord 478.5
  wrist, constricting (annular) 709.2
CIDP (chronic inflammatory demyelinating polyneuropathy) 357.81
CIN I (cervical intraepithelial neoplasia I) 622.11
CIN II (cervical intraepithelial neoplasia II) 622.12
CIN III (cervical intraepithelial neoplasia III) 233.1
Cinchonism
  correct substance properly administered 386.9
  overdose or wrong substance given or taken 961.4
Circine herpes 110.5
Circle of Willis — *see* condition
Circular — *see also* condition
  hymen 752.49
Circulating anticoagulants, antibodies, or inhibitors — *see also* Anticoagulants 286.59
  extrinsic 287.8
  following childbirth 666.3 ☑
  intrinsic, causing hemorrhagic disorder 286.59
    with
      acquired hemophilia 286.52
      antiphospholipid antibody 286.53
  postpartum 666.3 ☑
Circulation
  collateral (venous), any site 459.89
  defective 459.9
    congenital 747.9
    lower extremity 459.89
  embryonic 747.9
  failure 799.89
    fetus or newborn 779.89
    peripheral 785.59
  fetal, persistent 747.83
  heart, incomplete 747.9
Circulatory system — *see* condition
Circulus senilis 371.41
Circumcision
  in absence of medical indication V50.2
  ritual V50.2
  routine V50.2
  status (post), female 629.20
Circumscribed — *see* condition

Circumvallata placenta — *see* Placenta, abnormal
Cirrhosis, cirrhotic 571.5
  with alcoholism 571.2
  alcoholic (liver) 571.2
  atrophic (of liver) — *see* Cirrhosis, portal
  Baumgarten-Cruveilhier 571.5
  biliary (cholangiolitic) (cholangitic) (cholestatic) (extrahepatic) (hypertrophic) (intrahepatic) (nonobstructive) (obstructive) (pericholangiolitic) (posthepatic) (primary) (secondary) (xanthomatous) 571.6
    due to
      clonorchiasis 121.1
      flukes 121.3
  brain 331.9
  capsular — *see* Cirrhosis, portal
  cardiac 571.5
    alcoholic 571.2
  central (liver) — *see* Cirrhosis, liver
  Charcôt's 571.6
  cholangiolitic — *see* Cirrhosis, biliary
  cholangitic — *see* Cirrhosis, biliary
  cholestatic — *see* Cirrhosis, biliary
  clitoris (hypertrophic) 624.2
  coarsely nodular 571.5
  congestive (liver) — *see* Cirrhosis, cardiac
  Cruveilhier-Baumgarten 571.5
  cryptogenic (of liver) 571.5
    alcoholic 571.2
  dietary (*see also* Cirrhosis, portal) 571.5
  due to
    bronzed diabetes 275.01
    congestive hepatomegaly — *see* Cirrhosis, cardiac
    cystic fibrosis 277.00
    hemochromatosis (*see also* Hemochromatosis) 275.03
    hepatolenticular degeneration 275.1
    passive congestion (chronic) — *see* Cirrhosis, cardiac
    Wilson's disease 275.1
    xanthomatosis 272.2
  extrahepatic (obstructive) — *see* Cirrhosis, biliary
  fatty 571.8
    alcoholic 571.0
  florid 571.2
  Glisson's — *see* Cirrhosis, portal
  Hanot's (hypertrophic) — *see* Cirrhosis, biliary
  hepatic — *see* Cirrhosis, liver
  hepatolienal — *see* Cirrhosis, liver
  hobnail — *see* Cirrhosis, portal
  hypertrophic (*see also* Cirrhosis, liver)
    biliary — *see* Cirrhosis, biliary
    Hanot's — *see* Cirrhosis, biliary
  infectious NEC — *see* Cirrhosis, portal
  insular — *see* Cirrhosis, portal
  intrahepatic (obstructive) (primary) (secondary) — *see* Cirrhosis, biliary
  juvenile (*see also* Cirrhosis, portal) 571.5
  kidney (*see also* Sclerosis, renal) 587
  Laennec's (of liver) 571.2
    nonalcoholic 571.5
  liver (chronic) (hepatolienal) (hypertrophic) (nodular) (splenomegalic) (unilobar) 571.5
    with alcoholism 571.2
    alcoholic 571.2
    congenital (due to failure of obliteration of umbilical vein) 777.8
    cryptogenic 571.5
      alcoholic 571.2
    fatty 571.8
      alcoholic 571.0
    macronodular 571.5
      alcoholic 571.2
    micronodular 571.5
      alcoholic 571.2
    nodular, diffuse 571.5
      alcoholic 571.2
    pigmentary 275.01
    portal 571.5
      alcoholic 571.2

Cirrhosis, cirrhotic — *continued*
  liver — *continued*
    postnecrotic 571.5
      alcoholic 571.2
    syphilitic 095.3
  lung (chronic) (*see also* Fibrosis, lung) 515
  macronodular (of liver) 571.5
    alcoholic 571.2
  malarial 084.9
  metabolic NEC 571.5
  micronodular (of liver) 571.5
    alcoholic 571.2
  monolobular — *see* Cirrhosis, portal
  multilobular — *see* Cirrhosis, portal
  nephritis (*see also* Sclerosis, renal) 587
  nodular — *see* Cirrhosis, liver
  nutritional (fatty) 571.5
  obstructive (biliary) (extrahepatic) (intrahepatic) — *see* Cirrhosis, biliary
  ovarian 620.8
  paludal 084.9
  pancreas (duct) 577.8
  pericholangiolitic — *see* Cirrhosis, biliary
  periportal — *see* Cirrhosis, portal
  pigment, pigmentary (of liver) 275.01
  portal (of liver) 571.5
    alcoholic 571.2
  posthepatic (*see also* Cirrhosis, postnecrotic) 571.5
  postnecrotic (of liver) 571.5
    alcoholic 571.2
  primary (intrahepatic) — *see* Cirrhosis, biliary
  pulmonary (*see also* Fibrosis, lung) 515
  renal (*see also* Sclerosis, renal) 587
  septal (*see also* Cirrhosis, postnecrotic) 571.5
  spleen 289.51
  splenomegalic (of liver) — *see* Cirrhosis, liver
  stasis (liver) — *see* Cirrhosis, liver
  stomach 535.4 ☑
  Todd's (*see also* Cirrhosis, biliary) 571.6
  toxic (nodular) — *see* Cirrhosis, postnecrotic
  trabecular — *see* Cirrhosis, postnecrotic
  unilobar — *see* Cirrhosis, liver
  vascular (of liver) — *see* Cirrhosis, liver
  xanthomatous (biliary) (*see also* Cirrhosis, biliary) 571.6
    due to xanthomatosis (familial) (metabolic) (primary) 272.2
Cistern, subarachnoid 793.0
Citrullinemia 270.6
Citrullinuria 270.6
Ciuffini-Pancoast tumor (M8010/3) (carcinoma, pulmonary apex) 162.3
Civatte's disease or poikiloderma 709.09
CJD (Creutzfeldt-Jakob disease) 046.19
  variant (vCJD) 046.11
CLABSI (central line-associated bloodstream infection) 999.32
Clam diggers' itch 120.3
Clap — *see* Gonorrhea
Clarke-Hadfield syndrome (pancreatic infantilism) 577.8
Clark's paralysis 343.9
Clastothrix 704.2
Claude Bernard-Horner syndrome — *see also* Neuropathy, peripheral, autonomic 337.9
Claude's syndrome 352.6
Claudication, intermittent 443.9
  cerebral (artery) (*see also* Ischemia, cerebral, transient) 435.9
  due to atherosclerosis 440.21
  spinal cord (arteriosclerotic) 435.1
    syphilitic 094.89
  spinalis 435.1
  venous (axillary) 453.89
Claudicatio venosa intermittens 453.89
Claustrophobia 300.29
Clavus (infected) 700
Clawfoot (congenital) 754.71
  acquired 736.74
Clawhand (acquired) 736.06
  congenital 755.59
Clawtoe (congenital) 754.71

☑ **Additional Digit Required** — Refer to the Tabular List for Digit Selection   ▽ **Subterms under main terms may continue to next column or page**

94   2014 ICD-9-CM

Chromaffinoma — Clawtoe

Clawtoe — *continued*
  acquired 735.5
Clay eating 307.52
Clay shovelers' fracture — *see* Fracture, vertebra, cervical
Cleansing of artificial opening — *see also* Attention to artificial opening V55.9
Cleft (congenital) — *see also* Imperfect, closure
  alveolar process 525.8
  branchial (persistent) 744.41
    cyst 744.42
  clitoris 752.49
  cricoid cartilage, posterior 748.3
  facial (*see also* Cleft, lip) 749.10
  lip 749.10
    with cleft palate 749.20
      bilateral (lip and palate) 749.24
        with unilateral lip or palate 749.25
          complete 749.23
          incomplete 749.24
        unilateral (lip and palate) 749.22
          with bilateral lip or palate 749.25
            complete 749.21
            incomplete 749.22
      bilateral 749.14
        with cleft palate, unilateral 749.25
          complete 749.13
          incomplete 749.14
      unilateral 749.12
        with cleft palate, bilateral 749.25
          complete 749.11
          incomplete 749.12
  nose 748.1
  palate 749.00
    with cleft lip 749.20
      bilateral (lip and palate) 749.24
        with unilateral lip or palate 749.25
          complete 749.23
          incomplete 749.24
        unilateral (lip and palate) 749.22
          with bilateral lip or palate 749.25
            complete 749.21
            incomplete 749.22
      bilateral 749.04
        with cleft lip, unilateral 749.25
          complete 749.03
          incomplete 749.04
      unilateral 749.02
        with cleft lip, bilateral 749.25
          complete 749.01
          incomplete 749.02
  penis 752.69
  posterior, cricoid cartilage 748.3
  scrotum 752.89
  sternum (congenital) 756.3
  thyroid cartilage (congenital) 748.3
  tongue 750.13
  uvula 749.02
    with cleft lip (*see also* Cleft, lip, with cleft palate) 749.20
  water 366.12
Cleft hand (congenital) 755.58
Cleidocranial dysostosis 755.59
Cleidotomy, fetal 763.89
Cleptomania 312.32
Clérambault's syndrome 297.8
  erotomania 302.89
Clergyman's sore throat 784.49
Click, clicking
  systolic syndrome 785.2
Clifford's syndrome (postmaturity) 766.22
Climacteric — *see also* Menopause 627.2
  arthritis NEC (*see also* Arthritis, climacteric) 716.3 ☑
  depression (*see also* Psychosis, affective) 296.2 ☑
  disease 627.2
    recurrent episode 296.3 ☑
    single episode 296.2 ☑
  female (symptoms) 627.2
  male (symptoms) (syndrome) 608.89
  melancholia (*see also* Psychosis, affective) 296.2 ☑
    recurrent episode 296.3 ☑

Climacteric — *see also* Menopause — *continued*
  melancholia (*see also* Psychosis, affective) — *continued*
    single episode 296.2 ☑
  paranoid state 297.2
  paraphrenia 297.2
  polyarthritis NEC 716.39
    male 608.89
  symptoms (female) 627.2
Clinical research investigation (control) (participant) V70.7
Clinodactyly 755.59
Clitoris — *see* condition
Cloaca, persistent 751.5
Clonorchiasis 121.1
Clonorchiosis 121.1
Clonorchis infection, liver 121.1
Clonus 781.0
Closed bite 524.20
Closed surgical procedure converted to open procedure
  arthroscopic V64.43
  laparoscopic V64.41
  thoracoscopic V64.42
Closure
  artificial opening (*see also* Attention to artificial opening) V55.9
  congenital, nose 748.0
  cranial sutures, premature 756.0
  defective or imperfect NEC — *see* Imperfect, closure
  fistula, delayed — *see* Fistula
  fontanelle, delayed 756.0
  foramen ovale, imperfect 745.5
  hymen 623.3
  interauricular septum, defective 745.5
  interventricular septum, defective 745.4
  lacrimal duct 375.56
    congenital 743.65
    neonatal 375.55
  nose (congenital) 748.0
    acquired 738.0
  primary angle without glaucoma damage 365.06
  vagina 623.2
  valve — *see* Endocarditis
  vulva 624.8
Clot (blood)
  artery (obstruction) (occlusion) (*see also* Embolism) 444.9
  atrial appendage 429.89
  bladder 596.7
  brain (extradural or intradural) (*see also* Thrombosis, brain) 434.0 ☑
    late effect — *see* Late effect(s) (of) cerebrovascular disease
  circulation 444.9
  heart (*see also* Infarct, myocardium) 410.9 ☑
    without myocardial infarction 429.89
  vein (*see also* Thrombosis) 453.9
Clotting defect NEC — *see also* Defect, coagulation 286.9
Clouded state 780.09
  epileptic (*see also* Epilepsy) 345.9 ☑
  paroxysmal (idiopathic) (*see also* Epilepsy) 345.9 ☑
Clouding
  corneal graft 996.51
Cloudy
  antrum, antra 473.0
  dialysis effluent 792.5
Clouston's (hidrotic) ectodermal dysplasia 757.31
Clubbing of fingers 781.5
Clubfinger 736.29
  acquired 736.29
  congenital 754.89
Clubfoot (congenital) 754.70
  acquired 736.71
  equinovarus 754.51
  paralytic 736.71
Club hand (congenital) 754.89
  acquired 736.07
Clubnail (acquired) 703.8

Clubnail — *continued*
  congenital 757.5
Clump kidney 753.3
Clumsiness 781.3
  syndrome 315.4
Cluttering — *see also* Disorder, fluency 315.35
Clutton's joints 090.5
Coagulation, intravascular (diffuse) (disseminated) — *see also* Fibrinolysis 286.6
  newborn 776.2
Coagulopathy — *see also* Defect, coagulation 286.9
  consumption 286.6
  intravascular (disseminated) NEC 286.6
    newborn 776.2
Coalition
  calcaneoscaphoid 755.67
  calcaneus 755.67
  tarsal 755.67
Coal miners'
  elbow 727.2
  lung 500
Coal workers' lung or pneumoconiosis 500
Coarctation
  aorta (postductal) (preductal) 747.10
  pulmonary artery 747.31
Coated tongue 529.3
Coats' disease 362.12
Cocainism — *see also* Dependence 304.2 ☑
Coccidioidal granuloma 114.3
Coccidioidomycosis 114.9
  with pneumonia 114.0
  cutaneous (primary) 114.1
  disseminated 114.3
  extrapulmonary (primary) 114.1
  lung 114.5
    acute 114.0
    chronic 114.4
    primary 114.0
  meninges 114.2
  primary (pulmonary) 114.0
    acute 114.0
  prostate 114.3
  pulmonary 114.5
    acute 114.0
    chronic 114.4
    primary 114.0
  specified site NEC 114.3
Coccidioidosis 114.9
  lung 114.5
    acute 114.0
    chronic 114.4
    primary 114.0
  meninges 114.2
Coccidiosis (colitis) (diarrhea) (dysentery) 007.2
Cocciuria 791.9
Coccus in urine 791.9
Coccydynia 724.79
Coccygodynia 724.79
Coccyx — *see* condition
Cochin-China
  diarrhea 579.1
    anguilluliasis 127.2
  ulcer 085.1
Cockayne's disease or syndrome (microcephaly and dwarfism) 759.89
Cockayne-Weber syndrome (epidermolysis bullosa) 757.39
Cocked-up toe 735.2
Cock's peculiar tumor 706.2
Codman's tumor (benign chondroblastoma) (M9230/0) — *see* Neoplasm, bone, benign
Coenurosis 123.8
Coffee workers' lung 495.8
Cogan's syndrome 370.52
  congenital oculomotor apraxia 379.51
  nonsyphilitic interstitial keratitis 370.52
Coiling, umbilical cord — *see* Complications, umbilical cord
Coitus, painful (female) 625.0
  male 608.89
  psychogenic 302.76
Cold 460
  with influenza, flu, or grippe (*see also* Influenza) 487.1

Cold — *continued*
  abscess (*see also* Tuberculosis, abscess)
    articular — *see* Tuberculosis, joint
  agglutinin
    disease (chronic) or syndrome 283.0
      hemoglobinuria 283.0
        paroxysmal (cold) (nocturnal) 283.2
  allergic (*see also* Fever, hay) 477.9
  bronchus or chest — *see* Bronchitis
    with grippe or influenza (*see also* Influenza) 487.1
  common (head) 460
    vaccination, prophylactic (against) V04.7
  deep 464.10
  effects of 991.9
    specified effect NEC 991.8
  excessive 991.9
    specified effect NEC 991.8
  exhaustion from 991.8
  exposure to 991.9
    specified effect NEC 991.8
  grippy (*see also* Influenza) 487.1
  head 460
  injury syndrome (newborn) 778.2
  intolerance 780.99
  on lung — *see* Bronchitis
  rose 477.0
  sensitivity, autoimmune 283.0
  virus 460
Coldsore — *see also* Herpes, simplex 054.9
Colibacillosis 041.49
  generalized 038.42
Colibacilluria 791.9
Colic (recurrent) 789.7
  abdomen 789.7
    psychogenic 307.89
  appendicular 543.9
  appendix 543.9
  bile duct — *see* Choledocholithiasis
  biliary — *see* Cholelithiasis
  bilious — *see* Cholelithiasis
  common duct — *see* Choledocholithiasis
  Devonshire NEC 984.9
    specified type of lead — *see* Table of Drugs and Chemicals
  flatulent 787.3
  gallbladder or gallstone — *see* Cholelithiasis
  gastric 536.8
  hepatic (duct) — *see* Choledocholithiasis
  hysterical 300.11
  in
    adult 789.0 ☑
    child over 12 months old 789.0 ☑
    infant 789.7
  infantile 789.7
  intestinal 789.7
  kidney 788.0
  lead NEC 984.9
    specified type of lead — *see* Table of Drugs and Chemicals
  liver (duct) — *see* Choledocholithiasis
  mucous 564.9
    psychogenic 316 [564.9]
  nephritic 788.0
  painter's NEC 984.9
  pancreas 577.8
  psychogenic 306.4
  renal 788.0
  saturnine NEC 984.9
    specified type of lead — *see* Table of Drugs and Chemicals
  spasmodic 789.7
  ureter 788.0
  urethral 599.84
    due to calculus 594.2
  uterus 625.8
    menstrual 625.3
  vermicular 543.9
  virus 460
  worm NEC 128.9
Colicystitis — *see also* Cystitis 595.9
Colitis (acute) (catarrhal) (croupous) (cystica superficialis) (exudative) (hemorrhagic) (noninfectious) (phlegmonous) (presumed noninfectious) 558.9
  adaptive 564.9

☑ **Additional Digit Required** — Refer to the Tabular List for Digit Selection   ▽ **Subterms under main terms may continue to next column or page**

2014 ICD-9-CM   **95**

Colitis — continued
  allergic 558.3
  amebic (see also Amebiasis) 006.9
    nondysenteric 006.2
  anthrax 022.2
  bacillary (see also Infection, Shigella) 004.9
  balantidial 007.0
  chronic 558.9
    ulcerative (see also Colitis, ulcerative)
      556.9
  coccidial 007.2
  dietetic 558.9
  due to radiation 558.1
  eosinophilic 558.42
  functional 558.9
  gangrenous 009.0
  giardial 007.1
  granulomatous 555.1
  gravis (see also Colitis, ulcerative) 556.9
  infectious (see also Enteritis, due to, specific
      organism) 009.0
    presumed 009.1
  ischemic 557.9
    acute 557.0
    chronic 557.1
    due to mesenteric artery insufficiency
      557.1
  membranous 564.9
    psychogenic 316 [564.9]
  mucous 564.9
    psychogenic 316 [564.9]
  necrotic 009.0
  polyposa (see also Colitis, ulcerative) 556.9
  protozoal NEC 007.9
  pseudomembranous 008.45
  pseudomucinous 564.9
  regional 555.1
  segmental 555.1
  septic (see also Enteritis, due to, specific or-
      ganism) 009.0
  spastic 564.9
    psychogenic 316 [564.9]
  Staphylococcus 008.41
    food 005.0
  thromboulcerative 557.0
  toxic 558.2
  transmural 555.1
  trichomonal 007.3
  tuberculous (ulcerative) 014.8 ☑
  ulcerative (chronic) (idiopathic) (nonspecific)
      556.9
    entero- 556.0
    fulminant 557.0
    ileo- 556.1
    left-sided 556.5
    procto- 556.2
    proctosigmoid 556.3
    psychogenic 316 [556] ☑
    specified NEC 556.8
    universal 556.6
Collagen disease NEC 710.9
  nonvascular 710.9
  vascular (allergic) (see also Angiitis, hyper-
      sensitivity) 446.20
Collagenosis — see also Collagen disease 710.9
  cardiovascular 425.4
  mediastinal 519.3
Collapse 780.2
  adrenal 255.8
  cardiorenal (see also Hypertension, cardiore-
      nal) 404.90
  cardiorespiratory 785.51
    fetus or newborn 779.85
  cardiovascular (see also Disease, heart)
      785.51
    fetus or newborn 779.85
  circulatory (peripheral) 785.59
    with
      abortion — see Abortion, by type,
        with shock
      ectopic pregnancy (see also cate-
        gories 633.0–633.9) 639.5
      molar pregnancy (see also categories
        630–632) 639.5
    during or after labor and delivery
      669.1 ☑

Collapse — continued
  circulatory — continued
    fetus or newborn 779.85
    following
      abortion 639.5
      ectopic or molar pregnancy 639.5
    during or after labor and delivery 669.1 ☑
      fetus or newborn 779.89
    during or resulting from a surgical proce-
      dure 998.00
  external ear canal 380.50
    secondary to
      inflammation 380.53
      surgery 380.52
      trauma 380.51
  general 780.2
  heart — see Disease, heart
  heat 992.1
  hysterical 300.11
  labyrinth, membranous (congenital) 744.05
  lung (massive) (see also Atelectasis) 518.0
    pressure, during labor 668.0 ☑
  myocardial — see Disease, heart
  nervous (see also Disorder, mental, nonpsy-
      chotic) 300.9
  neurocirculatory 306.2
  nose 738.0
  postoperative (cardiovascular) 998.09
  pulmonary (see also Atelectasis) 518.0
    fetus or newborn 770.5
      partial 770.5
      primary 770.4
  thorax 512.89
    iatrogenic 512.1
    postoperative 512.1
  trachea 519.19
  valvular — see Endocarditis
  vascular (peripheral) 785.59
    with
      abortion — see Abortion, by type,
        with shock
      ectopic pregnancy (see also cate-
        gories 633.0–633.9) 639.5
      molar pregnancy (see also categories
        630–632) 639.5
    cerebral (see also Disease, cerebrovascu-
      lar, acute) 436
    during or after labor and delivery
      669.1 ☑
    fetus or newborn 779.89
    following
      abortion 639.5
      ectopic or molar pregnancy 639.5
  vasomotor 785.59
  vertebra 733.13
Collateral — see also condition
  circulation (venous) 459.89
  dilation, veins 459.89
Colles' fracture (closed) (reversed) (separation)
    813.41
  open 813.51
Collet-Sicard syndrome 352.6
Collet's syndrome 352.6
Colliculitis urethralis — see also Urethritis
    597.89
Colliers'
  asthma 500
  lung 500
  phthisis (see also Tuberculosis) 011.4 ☑
Collodion baby (ichthyosis congenita) 757.1
Colloid milium 709.3
Coloboma NEC 743.49
  choroid 743.59
  fundus 743.52
  iris 743.46
  lens 743.36
  lids 743.62
  optic disc (congenital) 743.57
    acquired 377.23
  retina 743.56
  sclera 743.47
Coloenteritis — see Enteritis
Colon — see condition
Colonization
  MRSA (methicillin resistant Staphylococcus
    aureus) V02.54

Colonization — continued
  MSSA (methicillin susceptible Staphylococ-
    cus aureus) V02.53
Coloptosis 569.89
Color
  amblyopia NEC 368.59
    acquired 368.55
  blindness NEC (congenital) 368.59
    acquired 368.55
Colostomy
  attention to V55.3
  fitting or adjustment V55.3
  malfunctioning 569.62
  status V44.3
Colpitis — see also Vaginitis 616.10
Colpocele 618.6
Colpocystitis — see also Vaginitis 616.10
Colporrhexis 665.4 ☑
Colpospasm 625.1
Column, spinal, vertebral — see condition
Coma 780.01
  apoplectic (see also Disease, cerebrovascu-
    lar, acute) 436
  diabetic (with ketoacidosis) 250.3 ☑
    due to secondary diabetes 249.3 ☑
    hyperosmolar 250.2 ☑
      due to secondary diabetes 249.2 ☑
  eclamptic (see also Eclampsia) 780.39
  epileptic 345.3
  hepatic 572.2
  hyperglycemic 250.3 ☑
    due to secondary diabetes 249.3 ☑
  hyperosmolar (diabetic) (nonketotic)
    250.2 ☑
    due to secondary diabetes 249.2 ☑
  hypoglycemic 251.0
    diabetic 250.3 ☑
      due to secondary diabetes 249.3 ☑
  insulin 250.3 ☑
    due to secondary diabetes 249.3 ☑
    hyperosmolar 250.2 ☑
      due to secondary diabetes 249.2 ☑
    non-diabetic 251.0
    organic hyperinsulinism 251.0
  Kussmaul's (diabetic) 250.3 ☑
    due to secondary diabetes 249.3 ☑
  liver 572.2
  newborn 779.2
  prediabetic 250.2 ☑
    due to secondary diabetes 249.2 ☑
  uremic — see Uremia
Combat fatigue — see also Reaction, stress,
    acute 308.9
Combined — see condition
Comedo 706.1
Comedocarcinoma (M8501/3) — see also
    Neoplasm, breast, malignant
  noninfiltrating (M8501/2)
    specified site — see Neoplasm, by site,
      in situ
    unspecified site 233.0
Comedomastitis 610.4
Comedones 706.1
  lanugo 757.4
Comma bacillus, carrier (suspected) of V02.3
Comminuted fracture — see Fracture, by site
Common
  aortopulmonary trunk 745.0
  atrioventricular canal (defect) 745.69
  atrium 745.69
  cold (head) 460
    vaccination, prophylactic (against) V04.7
  truncus (arteriosus) 745.0
  ventricle 745.3
Commotio (current)
  cerebri (see also Concussion, brain) 850.9
    with skull fracture — see Fracture, skull,
      by site
  retinae 921.3
  spinalis — see Injury, spinal, by site
Commotion (current)
  brain (without skull fracture) (see also Con-
    cussion, brain) 850.9
    with skull fracture — see Fracture, skull,
      by site
  spinal cord — see Injury, spinal, by site

Communication
  abnormal (see also Fistula)
    between
      base of aorta and pulmonary artery
        745.0
      left ventricle and right atrium 745.4
      pericardial sac and pleural sac 748.8
      pulmonary artery and pulmonary
        vein 747.39
      congenital, between uterus and anterior
        abdominal wall 752.39
        bladder 752.39
        intestine 752.39
        rectum 752.39
    left ventricular — right atrial 745.4
    pulmonary artery-pulmonary vein 747.39
Compartment syndrome — see Syndrome,
    compartment
Compensation
  broken — see Failure, heart
  failure — see Failure, heart
  neurosis, psychoneurosis 300.11
Complaint — see also Disease
  bowel, functional 564.9
    psychogenic 306.4
  intestine, functional 564.9
    psychogenic 306.4
  kidney (see also Disease, renal) 593.9
  liver 573.9
  miners' 500
Complete — see condition
Complex
  cardiorenal (see also Hypertension, cardiore-
    nal) 404.90
  castration 300.9
  Costen's 524.60
  ego-dystonic homosexuality 302.0
  Eisenmenger's (ventricular septal defect)
    745.4
  homosexual, ego-dystonic 302.0
  hypersexual 302.89
  inferiority 301.9
  jumped process
    spine — see Dislocation, vertebra
  primary, tuberculosis (see also Tuberculosis)
    010.0 ☑
  regional pain syndrome 355.9
    type I 337.20
      lower limb 337.22
      specified site NEC 337.29
      upper limb 337.21
    type II
      lower limb 355.71
      upper limb 354.4
  Taussig-Bing (transposition, aorta and
    overriding pulmonary artery) 745.11
Complications
  abortion NEC — see categories 634-639 ☑
  accidental puncture or laceration during a
    procedure 998.2
  amniocentesis, fetal 679.1 ☑
  amputation stump (late) (surgical) 997.60
    traumatic — see Amputation, traumatic
  anastomosis (and bypass) (see also Compli-
    cations, due to (presence of) any de-
    vice, implant, or graft classified to
    996.0–996.5 NEC)
    hemorrhage NEC 998.11
    intestinal (internal) NEC 997.49
      involving urinary tract 997.5
    mechanical — see Complications, me-
      chanical, graft
    urinary tract (involving intestinal tract)
      997.5
  anesthesia, anesthetic NEC (see also Anes-
    thesia, complication) 995.22
    in labor and delivery 668.9 ☑
      affecting fetus or newborn 763.5
      cardiac 668.1 ☑
      central nervous system 668.2 ☑
      pulmonary 668.0 ☑
      specified type NEC 668.8 ☑
  aortocoronary (bypass) graft 996.03
    atherosclerosis — see Arteriosclerosis,
      coronary
    embolism 996.72

Complications — continued
- aortocoronary graft — continued
  - occlusion NEC 996.72
  - thrombus 996.72
- arthroplasty (see also Complications, prosthetic joint) 996.49
- artificial opening
  - cecostomy 569.60
  - colostomy 569.60
  - cystostomy 596.83
    - infection 596.81
    - mechanical 596.82
    - specified complication NEC 596.83
  - enterostomy 569.60
  - esophagostomy 530.87
    - infection 530.86
    - mechanical 530.87
  - gastrostomy 536.40
  - ileostomy 569.60
  - jejunostomy 569.60
  - nephrostomy 997.5
  - tracheostomy 519.00
  - ureterostomy 997.5
  - urethrostomy 997.5
- bariatric surgery
  - gastric band procedure 539.09
    - infection 539.01
  - specified procedure NEC 539.89
    - infection 539.81
- bile duct implant (prosthetic) NEC 996.79
  - infection or inflammation 996.69
  - mechanical 996.59
- bleeding (intraoperative) (postoperative) 998.11
- blood vessel graft 996.1
  - aortocoronary 996.03
    - atherosclerosis — see Arteriosclerosis, coronary
    - embolism 996.72
    - occlusion NEC 996.72
    - thrombus 996.72
  - atherosclerosis — see Arteriosclerosis, extremities
    - embolism 996.74
    - occlusion NEC 996.74
    - thrombus 996.74
  - bone growth stimulator NEC 996.78
    - infection or inflammation 996.67
  - bone marrow transplant 996.85
  - breast implant (prosthetic) NEC 996.79
    - infection or inflammation 996.69
    - mechanical 996.54
  - bypass (see also Complications, anastomosis)
    - aortocoronary 996.03
      - atherosclerosis — see Arteriosclerosis, coronary
      - embolism 996.72
      - occlusion NEC 996.72
      - thrombus 996.72
    - carotid artery 996.1
      - atherosclerosis — see Arteriosclerosis, extremities
      - embolism 996.74
      - occlusion NEC 996.74
      - thrombus 996.74
  - cardiac (see also Disease, heart) 429.9
    - device, implant, or graft NEC 996.72
      - infection or inflammation 996.61
      - long-term effect 429.4
      - mechanical (see also Complications, mechanical, by type) 996.00
        - valve prosthesis 996.71
          - infection or inflammation 996.61
    - postoperative NEC 997.1
      - long-term effect 429.4
  - cardiorenal (see also Hypertension, cardiorenal) 404.90
  - carotid artery bypass graft 996.1
    - atherosclerosis — see Arteriosclerosis, extremities
    - embolism 996.74
    - occlusion NEC 996.74
    - thrombus 996.74
  - cataract fragments in eye 998.82

Complications — continued
- catheter device NEC (see also Complications, due to (presence of) any device, implant, or graft classified to 996.0–996.5 NEC)
  - mechanical — see Complications, mechanical, catheter
- cecostomy 569.60
- cesarean section wound 674.3 ☑
- chemotherapy (antineoplastic) 995.29
- chin implant (prosthetic) NEC 996.79
  - infection or inflammation 996.69
  - mechanical 996.59
- colostomy (enterostomy) 569.60
  - specified type NEC 569.69
- contraceptive device, intrauterine NEC 996.76
  - infection 996.65
  - inflammation 996.65
  - mechanical 996.32
- cord (umbilical) — see Complications, umbilical cord
- cornea
  - due to
    - contact lens 371.82
- coronary (artery) bypass (graft) NEC 996.03
  - atherosclerosis — see Arteriosclerosis, coronary
  - embolism 996.72
  - infection or inflammation 996.61
  - mechanical 996.03
  - occlusion NEC 996.72
  - specified type NEC 996.72
  - thrombus 996.72
- cystostomy 596.83
  - infection 596.81
  - mechanical 596.82
  - specified complication NEC 596.83
- delivery 669.9 ☑
  - procedure (instrumental) (manual) (surgical) 669.4 ☑
  - specified type NEC 669.8 ☑
- dialysis (hemodialysis) (peritoneal) (renal) NEC 999.9
  - catheter NEC (see also Complications, due to (presence of) any device, implant, or graft classified to 996.0–996.5 NEC)
    - infection or inflammation 996.62
      - peritoneal 996.68
    - mechanical 996.1
      - peritoneal 996.56
- drug NEC 995.29
- due to (presence of) any device, implant, or graft classified to 996.0–996.5 NEC 996.70
  - with infection or inflammation — see Complications, infection or inflammation, due to (presence of) any device, implant, or graft classified to 996.0–996.5 NEC
  - arterial NEC 996.74
    - coronary NEC 996.03
      - atherosclerosis — see Arteriosclerosis, coronary
      - embolism 996.72
      - occlusion NEC 996.72
      - specified type NEC 996.72
      - thrombus 996.72
    - renal dialysis 996.73
  - arteriovenous fistula or shunt NEC 996.74
  - bone growth stimulator 996.78
  - breast NEC 996.79
  - cardiac NEC 996.72
    - defibrillator 996.72
    - pacemaker 996.72
    - valve prosthesis 996.71
  - catheter NEC 996.79
    - spinal 996.75
    - urinary, indwelling 996.76
    - vascular NEC 996.74
      - renal dialysis 996.73
    - ventricular shunt 996.75
  - coronary (artery) bypass (graft) NEC 996.03

Complications — continued
- due to any device, implant, or graft classified to 996.0–996.5 — continued
  - coronary bypass — continued
    - atherosclerosis — see Arteriosclerosis, coronary
    - embolism 996.72
    - occlusion NEC 996.72
    - thrombus 996.72
  - electrodes
    - brain 996.75
    - heart 996.72
  - esophagostomy 530.87
  - gastrointestinal NEC 996.79
  - genitourinary NEC 996.76
  - heart valve prosthesis NEC 996.71
  - infusion pump 996.74
  - insulin pump 996.57
  - internal
    - joint prosthesis 996.77
    - orthopedic NEC 996.78
    - specified type NEC 996.79
  - intrauterine contraceptive device NEC 996.76
  - joint prosthesis, internal NEC 996.77
  - mechanical — see Complications, mechanical
  - nervous system NEC 996.75
  - ocular lens NEC 996.79
  - orbital NEC 996.79
  - orthopedic NEC 996.78
    - joint, internal 996.77
  - renal dialysis 996.73
  - specified type NEC 996.79
  - urinary catheter, indwelling 996.76
  - vascular NEC 996.74
  - ventricular shunt 996.75
- during dialysis NEC 999.9
- ectopic or molar pregnancy NEC 639.9
- electroshock therapy NEC 999.9
- enterostomy 569.60
  - specified type NEC 569.69
- esophagostomy 530.87
  - infection 530.86
  - mechanical 530.87
- external (fixation) device with internal component(s) NEC 996.78
  - infection or inflammation 996.67
  - mechanical 996.49
- extracorporeal circulation NEC 999.9
- eye implant (prosthetic) NEC 996.79
  - infection or inflammation 996.69
  - mechanical
    - ocular lens 996.53
    - orbital globe 996.59
- fetal, from amniocentesis 679.1 ☑
- gastrointestinal, postoperative NEC (see also Complications, surgical procedures) 997.49
- gastrostomy 536.40
  - specified type NEC 536.49
- genitourinary device, implant or graft NEC 996.76
  - erosion of implanted vaginal mesh 629.31
  - exposure of implanted vaginal mesh 629.32
  - infection or inflammation 996.65
    - urinary catheter, indwelling 996.64
  - mechanical (see also Complications, mechanical, by type) 996.30
    - specified NEC 996.39
- graft (bypass) (patch) (see also Complications, due to (presence of) any device, implant, or graft classified to 996.0–996.5 NEC)
  - bone marrow 996.85
  - corneal NEC 996.79
    - infection or inflammation 996.69
    - rejection or reaction 996.51
    - retroprosthetic membrane 996.51
  - mechanical — see Complications, mechanical, graft
  - organ (immune or nonimmune cause) (partial) (total) 996.80
    - bone marrow 996.85

Complications — continued
- graft (see also Complications, due to any device, implant, or graft classified to 996.0–996.5) — continued
  - organ — continued
    - heart 996.83
    - intestines 996.87
    - kidney 996.81
    - liver 996.82
    - lung 996.84
    - pancreas 996.86
    - specified NEC 996.89
  - skin NEC 996.79
    - infection or inflammation 996.69
    - rejection 996.52
      - artificial 996.55
      - decellularized allodermis 996.55
- heart (see also Disease, heart transplant (immune or nonimmune cause)) 996.83
- hematoma (intraoperative) (postoperative) 998.12
- hemorrhage (intraoperative) (postoperative) 998.11
- hyperalimentation therapy NEC 999.9
- immunization (procedure) — see Complications, vaccination
- implant (see also Complications, due to (presence of) any device, implant, or graft classified to 996.0–996.5 NEC)
  - dental placement, hemorrhagic 525.71
  - mechanical — see Complications, mechanical, implant
- infection and inflammation
  - due to (presence of) any device, implant or graft classified to 996.0–996.5 NEC 996.60
    - arterial NEC 996.62
      - coronary 996.61
      - renal dialysis 996.62
    - arteriovenous fistula or shunt 996.62
    - artificial heart 996.61
    - bone growth stimulator 996.67
    - breast 996.69
    - cardiac 996.61
    - catheter NEC 996.69
      - central venous 999.31
        - bloodstream 999.32
        - localized 999.33
      - Hickman 999.31
        - bloodstream 999.32
        - localized 999.33
      - peripherally inserted central (PICC) 999.31
        - bloodstream 999.32
        - localized 999.33
      - peritoneal 996.68
      - portacath (port-a-cath) 999.31
        - bloodstream 999.32
        - localized 999.33
      - spinal 996.63
      - triple lumen 999.31
        - bloodstream 999.32
        - localized 999.33
      - umbilical venous 999.31
        - bloodstream 999.32
        - localized 999.33
      - urinary, indwelling 996.64
      - vascular (arterial) (dialysis) (peripheral venous) NEC 996.62
      - ventricular shunt 996.63
    - central venous catheter 999.31
      - bloodstream 999.32
      - localized 999.33
    - coronary artery bypass 996.61
    - electrodes
      - brain 996.63
      - heart 996.61
    - gastrointestinal NEC 996.69
    - genitourinary NEC 996.65
      - indwelling urinary catheter 996.64
    - heart assist device 996.61
    - heart valve 996.61
    - Hickman catheter 999.31

☑ Additional Digit Required — Refer to the Tabular List for Digit Selection   ▽ Subterms under main terms may continue to next column or page

2014 ICD-9-CM   97

Complications — continued
  infection and inflammation — contin-
      ued
    due to any device, implant or graft classi-
        fied to 996.0–996.5 — contin-
        ued
      Hickman catheter — continued
        bloodstream 999.32
        localized 999.33
      infusion pump 996.62
      insulin pump 996.69
      intrauterine contraceptive device
          996.65
      joint prosthesis, internal 996.66
      ocular lens 996.69
      orbital (implant) 996.69
      orthopedic NEC 996.67
        joint, internal 996.66
      peripherally inserted central catheter
          (PICC) 999.31
        bloodstream 999.32
        localized 999.33
      portacath (port-a-cath) 999.31
        bloodstream 999.32
        localized 999.33
      specified type NEC 996.69
      triple lumen catheter 999.31
        bloodstream 999.32
        localized 999.33
      umbilical venous catheter 999.31
        bloodstream 999.32
        localized 999.33
      urinary catheter, indwelling 996.64
      ventricular shunt 996.63
  infusion (procedure) 999.88
    blood — see Complications, transfusion
    infection NEC 999.39
    sepsis NEC 999.39
  inhalation therapy NEC 999.9
  injection (procedure) 999.9
    drug reaction (see also Reaction, drug)
        995.27
    infection NEC 999.39
    sepsis NEC 999.39
    serum (prophylactic) (therapeutic) —
        see Complications, vaccination
    vaccine (any) — see Complications, vac-
        cination
  inoculation (any) — see Complications,
      vaccination
  insulin pump 996.57
  internal device (catheter) (electronic) (fixa-
      tion) (prosthetic) (see also Complica-
      tions, due to (presence of) any de-
      vice, implant, or graft classified to
      996.0–996.5 NEC)
    mechanical — see Complications, me-
        chanical
  intestinal pouch, specified NEC 569.79
  intestinal transplant (immune or nonim-
      mune cause) 996.87
  intraoperative bleeding or hemorrhage
      998.11
  intrauterine contraceptive device (see also
      Complications, contraceptive device)
      996.76
    with fetal damage affecting manage-
        ment of pregnancy 655.8 ☑
    infection or inflammation 996.65
  in utero procedure
    fetal 679.1 ☑
    maternal 679.0 ☑
  jejunostomy 569.60
  kidney transplant (immune or nonimmune
      cause) 996.81
  labor 669.9 ☑
    specified condition NEC 669.8 ☑
  liver transplant (immune or nonimmune
      cause) 996.82
  lumbar puncture 349.0
  mechanical
    anastomosis — see Complications, me-
        chanical, graft
    artificial heart 996.09
    bypass — see Complications, mechani-
        cal, graft

Complications — continued
  mechanical — continued
    catheter NEC 996.59
      cardiac 996.09
      cystostomy 596.82
      dialysis (hemodialysis) 996.1
        peritoneal 996.56
      during a procedure 998.2
      urethral, indwelling 996.31
    colostomy 569.62
    device NEC 996.59
      balloon (counterpulsation), intra-
          aortic 996.1
      cardiac 996.00
        automatic implantable defibrilla-
            tor 996.04
        long-term effect 429.4
        specified NEC 996.09
      contraceptive, intrauterine 996.32
      counterpulsation, intra-aortic 996.1
      fixation, external, with internal com-
          ponents 996.49
      fixation, internal (nail, rod, plate)
          996.40
      genitourinary 996.30
        specified NEC 996.39
      insulin pump 996.57
      nervous system 996.2
      orthopedic, internal 996.40
        prosthetic joint (see also Compli-
            cations, mechanical, de-
            vice, orthopedic, prosthet-
            ic, joint) 996.47
    prosthetic NEC 996.59
      joint 996.47
        articular bearing surface wear
            996.46
        aseptic loosening 996.41
        breakage 996.43
        dislocation 996.42
        failure 996.47
        fracture 996.43
          around prosthetic 996.44
          peri-prosthetic 996.44
        instability 996.42
        loosening 996.41
        peri-prosthetic osteolysis
            996.45
        subluxation 996.42
        wear 996.46
      umbrella, vena cava 996.1
      vascular 996.1
    dorsal column stimulator 996.2
    electrode NEC 996.59
      brain 996.2
      cardiac 996.01
      spinal column 996.2
    enterostomy 569.62
    esophagostomy 530.87
    fistula, arteriovenous, surgically created
        996.1
    gastrostomy 536.42
    graft NEC 996.52
      aortic (bifurcation) 996.1
      aortocoronary bypass 996.03
      blood vessel NEC 996.1
      bone 996.49
      cardiac 996.00
      carotid artery bypass 996.1
      cartilage 996.49
      corneal 996.51
      coronary bypass 996.03
      decellularized allodermis 996.55
      genitourinary 996.30
        specified NEC 996.39
      muscle 996.49
      nervous system 996.2
      organ (immune or nonimmune
          cause) 996.80
        heart 996.83
        intestines 996.87
        kidney 996.81
        liver 996.82
        lung 996.84
        pancreas 996.86
        specified NEC 996.89

Complications — continued
  mechanical — continued
    graft — continued
      orthopedic, internal 996.49
      peripheral nerve 996.2
      prosthetic NEC 996.59
      skin 996.52
        artificial 996.55
      specified NEC 996.59
      tendon 996.49
      tissue NEC 996.52
      tooth 996.59
      ureter, without mention of resection
          996.39
      vascular 996.1
    heart valve prosthesis 996.02
      long-term effect 429.4
    implant NEC 996.59
      cardiac 996.00
        automatic implantable defibrilla-
            tor 996.04
        long-term effect 429.4
        specified NEC 996.09
      electrode NEC 996.59
        brain 996.2
        cardiac 996.01
        spinal column 996.2
      genitourinary 996.30
      nervous system 996.2
      orthopedic, internal 996.49
      prosthetic NEC 996.59
        in
          bile duct 996.59
          breast 996.54
          chin 996.59
          eye
            ocular lens 996.53
            orbital globe 996.59
      vascular 996.1
    insulin pump 996.57
    nonabsorbable surgical material 996.59
    pacemaker NEC 996.59
      brain 996.2
      cardiac 996.01
      nerve (phrenic) 996.2
    patch — see Complications, mechanical,
        graft
    prosthesis NEC 996.59
      bile duct 996.59
      breast 996.54
      chin 996.59
      ocular lens 996.53
      reconstruction, vas deferens 996.39
    reimplant NEC 996.59
      extremity (see also Complications,
          reattached, extremity) 996.90
      organ (see also Complications, trans-
          plant, organ, by site) 996.80
    repair — see Complications, mechanical,
        graft
    respirator [ventilator] V46.14
    shunt NEC 996.59
      arteriovenous, surgically created
          996.1
      ventricular (communicating) 996.2
    stent NEC 996.59
    tracheostomy 519.02
    vas deferens reconstruction 996.39
    ventilator [respirator] V46.14
  medical care NEC 999.9
    cardiac NEC 997.1
    gastrointestinal NEC 997.49
    nervous system NEC 997.00
    peripheral vascular NEC 997.2
    respiratory NEC 997.39
    urinary NEC 997.5
    vascular
      mesenteric artery 997.71
      other vessels 997.79
      peripheral vessels 997.2
      renal artery 997.72
  nephrostomy 997.5
  nervous system
    device, implant, or graft NEC 349.1
      mechanical 996.2
    postoperative NEC 997.00

Complications — continued
  obstetric 669.9 ☑
    procedure (instrumental) (manual) (sur-
        gical) 669.4 ☑
      specified NEC 669.8 ☑
      surgical wound 674.3 ☑
  ocular lens implant NEC 996.79
    infection or inflammation 996.69
    mechanical 996.53
  organ transplant — see Complications,
      transplant, organ, by site
  orthopedic device, implant, or graft
    internal (fixation) (nail) (plate) (rod) NEC
        996.78
      infection or inflammation 996.67
      joint prosthesis 996.77
        infection or inflammation 996.66
      mechanical 996.40
  pacemaker (cardiac) 996.72
    infection or inflammation 996.61
    mechanical 996.01
  pancreas transplant (immune or nonim-
      mune cause) 996.86
  perfusion NEC 999.9
  perineal repair (obstetrical) 674.3 ☑
    disruption 674.2 ☑
  pessary (uterus) (vagina) — see Complica-
      tions, contraceptive device
  phototherapy 990
  postcystoscopic 997.5
  postmastoidectomy NEC 383.30
  postoperative — see Complications, surgical
      procedures
  pregnancy NEC 646.9 ☑
    affecting fetus or newborn 761.9
  prosthetic device, internal (see also Compli-
      cations, due to (presence of) any de-
      vice, implant or graft classified to
      996.0–996.5 NEC)
    mechanical NEC (see also Complications,
        mechanical) 996.59
  puerperium NEC (see also Puerperal)
      674.9 ☑
  puncture, spinal 349.0
  pyelogram 997.5
  radiation 990
  radiotherapy 990
  reattached
    body part, except extremity 996.99
    extremity (infection) (rejection) 996.90
      arm(s) 996.94
        digit(s) (hand) 996.93
          foot 996.95
        finger(s) 996.93
        foot 996.95
        forearm 996.91
        hand 996.92
        leg 996.96
        lower NEC 996.96
        toe(s) 996.95
        upper NEC 996.94
  reimplant NEC (see also Complications, due
      to (presence of) any device, implant,
      or graft classified to 996.0–996.5
      NEC)
    bone marrow 996.85
    extremity (see also Complications, reat-
        tached, extremity) 996.90
      due to infection 996.90
    mechanical — see Complications, me-
        chanical, reimplant
    organ (immune or nonimmune cause)
        (partial) (total) (see also Complica-
        tions, transplant, organ, by site)
        996.80
  renal allograft 996.81
  renal dialysis — see Complications, dialysis
  respirator [ventilator], mechanical V46.14
  respiratory 519.9
    device, implant or graft NEC 996.79
      infection or inflammation 996.69
      mechanical 996.59
    distress syndrome, adult, following
        trauma and surgery 518.52
    insufficiency, acute, postoperative
        518.52

Complications — *continued*
 respiratory — *continued*
  postoperative NEC 997.39
  therapy NEC 999.9
 sedation during labor and delivery 668.9 ☑
  affecting fetus or newborn 763.5
  cardiac 668.1 ☑
  central nervous system 668.2 ☑
  pulmonary 668.0 ☑
  specified type NEC 668.8 ☑
 seroma (intraoperative) (postoperative) (noninfected) 998.13
  infected 998.51
 shunt (*see also* Complications, due to (presence of) any device, implant, or graft classified to 996.0–996.5 NEC)
  mechanical — *see* Complications, mechanical, shunt
 specified body system NEC
  device, implant, or graft — *see* Complications, due to (presence of) any device, implant, or graft classified to 996.0–996.5 NEC
  postoperative NEC 997.99
 spinal puncture or tap 349.0
 stoma, external
  gastrointestinal tract
   colostomy 569.60
   enterostomy 569.60
   esophagostomy 530.87
    infection 530.86
    mechanical 530.87
   gastrostomy 536.40
  urinary tract 997.5
 stomach banding 539.09
 stomach stapling 539.89
 surgical procedures 998.9
  accidental puncture or laceration 998.2
  amputation stump (late) 997.60
  anastomosis — *see* Complications, anastomosis
  burst stitches or sutures (external) (*see also* Dehiscence) 998.32
   internal 998.31
  cardiac 997.1
   long-term effect following cardiac surgery 429.4
  cataract fragments in eye 998.82
  catheter device — *see* Complications, catheter device
  cecostomy malfunction 569.62
  colostomy malfunction 569.62
  cystostomy malfunction 596.82
   infection 596.81
   mechanical 596.82
   specified complication NEC 596.83
  dehiscence (of incision) (external) (*see also* Dehiscence) 998.32
   internal 998.31
  dialysis NEC (*see also* Complications, dialysis) 999.9
  disruption (*see also* Dehiscence)
   anastomosis (internal) — *see* Complications, mechanical, graft
   internal suture (line) 998.31
   wound (external) 998.32
    internal 998.31
  dumping syndrome (postgastrectomy) 564.2
  elephantiasis or lymphedema 997.99
   postmastectomy 457.0
  emphysema (surgical) 998.81
  enterostomy malfunction 569.62
  esophagostomy malfunction 530.87
  evisceration 998.32
  fistula (persistent postoperative) 998.6
  foreign body inadvertently left in wound (sponge) (suture) (swab) 998.4
  from nonabsorbable surgical material (Dacron) (mesh) (permanent suture) (reinforcing) (Teflon) — *see* Complications, due to (presence of) any device, implant, or graft classified to 996.0–996.5 NEC
  gastrointestinal NEC 997.49
  gastrostomy malfunction 536.42

Complications — *continued*
 surgical procedures — *continued*
  hematoma 998.12
  hemorrhage 998.11
  ileostomy malfunction 569.62
  internal prosthetic device NEC (*see also* Complications, internal device) 996.70
   hemolytic anemia 283.19
   infection or inflammation 996.60
   malfunction — *see* Complications, mechanical
   mechanical complication — *see* Complications, mechanical
   thrombus 996.70
  jejunostomy malfunction 569.62
  nervous system NEC 997.00
  obstruction, internal anastomosis — *see* Complications, mechanical, graft
  other body system NEC 997.99
  peripheral vascular NEC 997.2
  postcardiotomy syndrome 429.4
  postcholecystectomy syndrome 576.0
  postcommissurotomy syndrome 429.4
  postgastrectomy dumping syndrome 564.2
  postmastectomy lymphedema syndrome 457.0
  postmastoidectomy 383.30
   cholesteatoma, recurrent 383.32
   cyst, mucosal 383.31
   granulation 383.33
   inflammation, chronic 383.33
  postvagotomy syndrome 564.2
  postvalvulotomy syndrome 429.4
  reattached extremity (infection) (rejection) (*see also* Complications, reattached, extremity) 996.90
  respiratory NEC 997.39
  seroma 998.13
  shock (endotoxic) (septic) 998.02
   hypovolemic 998.09
  shunt, prosthetic (thrombus) (*see also* Complications, due to (presence of) any device, implant, or graft classified to 996.0–996.5 NEC)
   hemolytic anemia 283.19
   specified complication NEC 596.83
  specified complication NEC 998.89
  stitch abscess 998.59
  transplant — *see* Complications, graft
  ureterostomy malfunction 997.5
  urethrostomy malfunction 997.5
  urinary NEC 997.5
  vascular
   mesenteric artery 997.71
   other vessels 997.79
   peripheral vessels 997.2
   renal artery 997.72
  wound infection 998.59
 therapeutic misadventure NEC 999.9
  surgical treatment 998.9
 tracheostomy 519.00
 transfusion (blood) (lymphocytes) (plasma) 999.80
  acute lung injury (TRALI) 518.7
  atrophy, liver, yellow, subacute (within 8 months of administration) — *see* Hepatitis, viral
  bone marrow 996.85
  embolism
   air 999.1
   thrombus 999.2
  febrile nonhemolytic reaction (FNHTR) 780.66
  hemolysis NEC 999.89
   bone marrow 996.85
  hemolytic reaction, incompatibility unspecified 999.83
   acute 999.84
   delayed 999.85
  hepatitis (serum) (type B) (within 8 months after administration) — *see* Hepatitis, viral
  incompatibility reaction
   ABO 999.60

Complications — *continued*
 transfusion — *continued*
  incompatibility reaction — *continued*
   ABO — *continued*
    with hemolytic transfusion reaction (HTR) (not specified as acute or delayed) 999.61
     acute 999.62
     delayed 999.63
    specified type NEC 999.69
   minor blood group 999.89
   non-ABO (minor antigens) (Duffy) (Kell) (Kidd) (Lewis) (M) (N) (P) (S) 999.75
    with hemolytic transfusion reaction (HTR) (not specified as acute or delayed) 999.76
     acute 999.77
     delayed 999.78
    specified type NEC 999.79
   Rh antigen (C) (c) (D) (E) (e) (factor) 999.70
    with hemolytic transfusion reaction (HTR) (not specified as acute or delayed) 999.71
     acute 999.72
     delayed 999.73
    specified type NEC 999.74
  infection 999.39
   acute 999.34
  jaundice (serum) (within 8 months after administration) — *see* Hepatitis, viral
  sepsis 999.39
  shock or reaction NEC 999.89
   bone marrow 996.85
  specified reaction NEC 999.89
  subacute yellow atrophy of liver (within 8 months after administration) — *see* Hepatitis, viral
  thromboembolism 999.2
 transplant NEC (*see also* Complications, due to (presence of) any device, implant, or graft classified to 996.0–996.5 NEC)
  bone marrow 996.85
  organ (immune or nonimmune cause) (partial) (total) 996.80
   bone marrow 996.85
   heart 996.83
   intestines 996.87
   kidney 996.81
   liver 996.82
   lung 996.84
   pancreas 996.86
   specified NEC 996.89
  stem cell(s) 996.88
   from
    peripheral blood 996.88
    umbilical cord 996.88
 trauma NEC (early) 958.8
 ultrasound therapy NEC 999.9
 umbilical cord
  affecting fetus or newborn 762.6
  complicating delivery 663.9 ☑
   affecting fetus or newborn 762.6
   specified type NEC 663.8 ☑
 urethral catheter NEC 996.76
  infection or inflammation 996.64
  mechanical 996.31
 urinary, postoperative NEC 997.5
 vaccination 999.9
  anaphylaxis NEC 999.42
  cellulitis 999.39
  encephalitis or encephalomyelitis 323.51
  hepatitis (serum) (type B) (within 8 months after administration) — *see* Hepatitis, viral
  infection (general) (local) NEC 999.39
  jaundice (serum) (within 8 months after administration) — *see* Hepatitis, viral
  meningitis 997.09 *[321.8]*
  myelitis 323.52
  protein sickness 999.52

Complications — *continued*
 vaccination — *continued*
  reaction (allergic) 999.52
   serum 999.52
  sepsis 999.39
  serum intoxication, sickness, rash, or other serum reaction NEC 999.52
  shock (allergic) (anaphylactic) 999.49
  subacute yellow atrophy of liver (within 8 months after administration) — *see* Hepatitis, viral
  vaccinia (generalized) 999.0
   localized 999.39
 vascular
  device, implant, or graft NEC 996.74
   infection or inflammation 996.62
   mechanical NEC 996.1
    cardiac (*see also* Complications, mechanical, by type) 996.00
  following infusion, perfusion, or transfusion 999.2
  postoperative NEC 997.2
   mesenteric artery 997.71
   other vessels 997.79
   peripheral vessels 997.2
   renal artery 997.72
 ventilation therapy NEC 999.9
 ventilator [respirator], mechanical V46.14
Compound presentation, complicating delivery 652.8 ☑
 causing obstructed labor 660.0 ☑
Compressed air disease 993.3
Compression
 with injury — *see* specific injury
 arm NEC 354.9
 artery 447.1
  celiac, syndrome 447.4
 brachial plexus 353.0
 brain (stem) 348.4
  due to
   contusion, brain — *see* Contusion, brain
   injury NEC (*see also* Hemorrhage, brain, traumatic)
    birth — *see* Birth, injury, brain
   laceration, brain — *see* Laceration, brain
  osteopathic 739.0
 bronchus 519.19
 by cicatrix — *see* Cicatrix
 cardiac 423.9
 cauda equina 344.60
  with neurogenic bladder 344.61
 celiac (artery) (axis) 447.4
 cerebral — *see* Compression, brain
 cervical plexus 353.2
 cord (umbilical) — *see* Compression, umbilical cord
 cranial nerve 352.9
  second 377.49
  third (partial) 378.51
   total 378.52
  fourth 378.53
  fifth 350.8
  sixth 378.54
  seventh 351.8
 divers' squeeze 993.3
 duodenum (external) (*see also* Obstruction, duodenum) 537.3
 during birth 767.9
 esophagus 530.3
  congenital, external 750.3
 Eustachian tube 381.63
 facies (congenital) 754.0
 fracture — *see* Fracture, by site
 heart — *see* Disease, heart
 intestine (*see also* Obstruction, intestine) 560.9
  with hernia — *see* Hernia, by site, with obstruction
 laryngeal nerve, recurrent 478.79
 leg NEC 355.8
 lower extremity NEC 355.8
 lumbosacral plexus 353.1
 lung 518.89

☑ Additional Digit Required — Refer to the Tabular List for Digit Selection
🔻 Subterms under main terms may continue to next column or page
2014 ICD-9-CM
99

Index
Complications — Compression

Compression — *continued*
　lymphatic vessel 457.1
　medulla — *see* Compression, brain
　nerve NEC (*see also* Disorder, nerve)
　　arm NEC 354.9
　　autonomic nervous system (*see also*
　　　Neuropathy, peripheral, autonom-
　　　ic) 337.9
　　axillary 353.0
　　cranial NEC 352.9
　　due to displacement of intervertebral
　　　disc 722.2
　　　with myelopathy 722.70
　　　cervical 722.0
　　　　with myelopathy 722.71
　　　lumbar, lumbosacral 722.10
　　　　with myelopathy 722.73
　　　thoracic, thoracolumbar 722.11
　　　　with myelopathy 722.72
　　iliohypogastric 355.79
　　ilioinguinal 355.79
　　leg NEC 355.8
　　lower extremity NEC 355.8
　　median (in carpal tunnel) 354.0
　　obturator 355.79
　　optic 377.49
　　plantar 355.6
　　posterior tibial (in tarsal tunnel) 355.5
　　root (by scar tissue) NEC 724.9
　　　cervical NEC 723.4
　　　lumbar NEC 724.4
　　　lumbosacral 724.4
　　　thoracic 724.4
　　saphenous 355.79
　　sciatic (acute) 355.0
　　sympathetic 337.9
　　traumatic — *see* Injury, nerve
　　ulnar 354.2
　　upper extremity NEC 354.9
　peripheral — *see* Compression, nerve
　spinal (cord) (old or nontraumatic) 336.9
　　by displacement of intervertebral disc
　　　— *see* Displacement, interverte-
　　　bral disc
　　nerve
　　　root NEC 724.9
　　　　postoperative 722.80
　　　　　cervical region 722.81
　　　　　lumbar region 722.83
　　　　　thoracic region 722.82
　　　　traumatic — *see* Injury, nerve,
　　　　　spinal
　　　traumatic — *see* Injury, nerve, spinal
　　spondylogenic 721.91
　　　cervical 721.1
　　　lumbar, lumbosacral 721.42
　　　thoracic 721.41
　　traumatic (*see also* Injury, spinal, by site)
　　　with fracture, vertebra — *see* Frac-
　　　　ture, vertebra, by site, with
　　　　spinal cord injury
　spondylogenic — *see* Compression, spinal
　　cord, spondylogenic
　subcostal nerve (syndrome) 354.8
　sympathetic nerve NEC 337.9
　syndrome 958.5
　thorax 512.89
　　iatrogenic 512.1
　　postoperative 512.1
　trachea 519.19
　　congenital 748.3
　ulnar nerve (by scar tissue) 354.2
　umbilical cord
　　affecting fetus or newborn 762.5
　　　cord prolapsed 762.4
　　complicating delivery 663.2 ☑
　　　cord around neck 663.1 ☑
　　　cord prolapsed 663.0 ☑
　upper extremity NEC 354.9
　ureter 593.3
　urethra — *see* Stricture, urethra
　vein 459.2
　vena cava (inferior) (superior) 459.2
　vertebral NEC — *see* Compression, spinal
　　(cord)

Compulsion, compulsive
　eating 307.51
　neurosis (obsessive) 300.3
　personality 301.4
　states (mixed) 300.3
　swearing 300.3
　　in Gilles de la Tourette's syndrome
　　　307.23
　tics and spasms 307.22
　water drinking NEC (syndrome) 307.9
Concato's disease (pericardial polyserositis)
　423.2
　peritoneal 568.82
　pleural — *see* Pleurisy
Concavity, chest wall 738.3
Concealed
　hemorrhage NEC 459.0
　penis 752.65
Concentric fading 368.12
Concern (normal) **about sick person in family**
　V61.49
Concrescence (teeth) 520.2
Concretio cordis 423.1
　rheumatic 393
Concretion — *see also* Calculus
　appendicular 543.9
　canaliculus 375.57
　clitoris 624.8
　conjunctiva 372.54
　eyelid 374.56
　intestine (impaction) (obstruction) 560.39
　lacrimal (passages) 375.57
　prepuce (male) 605
　　female (clitoris) 624.8
　salivary gland (any) 527.5
　seminal vesicle 608.89
　stomach 537.89
　tonsil 474.8
Concussion (current) 850.9
　with
　　loss of consciousness 850.5
　　　brief (less than one hour)
　　　　30 minutes or less 850.11
　　　　31-59 minutes 850.12
　　　moderate (1-24 hours) 850.2
　　　prolonged (more than 24 hours)
　　　　(with complete recovery)
　　　　(with return to pre-existing
　　　　conscious level) 850.3
　　　　without return to pre-existing
　　　　conscious level 850.4
　　mental confusion or disorientation
　　　(without loss of consciousness)
　　　850.0
　　　with loss of consciousness — *see*
　　　　Concussion, with, loss of con-
　　　　sciousness
　without loss of consciousness 850.0
　blast (air) (hydraulic) (immersion) (underwa-
　　ter) 869.0
　　with open wound into cavity 869.1
　　abdomen or thorax — *see* Injury, inter-
　　　nal, by site
　　brain — *see* Concussion, brain
　　ear (acoustic nerve trauma) 951.5
　　　with perforation, tympanic mem-
　　　　brane — *see* Wound, open,
　　　　ear drum
　　thorax — *see* Injury, internal, intratho-
　　　racic organs NEC
　brain or cerebral (without skull fracture)
　　850.9
　　with
　　　loss of consciousness 850.5
　　　　brief (less than one hour)
　　　　　30 minutes or less 850.11
　　　　　31-59 minutes 850.12
　　　　moderate (1-24 hours) 850.2
　　　　prolonged (more than 24 hours)
　　　　　(with complete recovery)
　　　　　(with return to pre-exist-
　　　　　ing conscious level) 850.3
　　　　　without return to pre-existing
　　　　　conscious level 850.4

Concussion — *continued*
　brain or cerebral — *continued*
　　with — *continued*
　　　mental confusion or disorientation
　　　　(without loss of conscious-
　　　　ness) 850.0
　　　with loss of consciousness — *see*
　　　　Concussion, brain, with,
　　　　loss of consciousness
　　　skull fracture — *see* Fracture, skull,
　　　　by site
　　without loss of consciousness 850.0
　cauda equina 952.4
　cerebral — *see* Concussion, brain
　conus medullaris (spine) 952.4
　hydraulic — *see* Concussion, blast
　internal organs — *see* Injury, internal, by
　　site
　labyrinth — *see* Injury, intracranial
　ocular 921.3
　osseous labyrinth — *see* Injury, intracranial
　spinal (cord) (*see also* Injury, spinal, by site)
　　due to
　　　broken
　　　　back — *see* Fracture, vertebra, by
　　　　　site, with spinal cord injury
　　　　neck — *see* Fracture, vertebra,
　　　　　cervical, with spinal cord
　　　　　injury
　　　fracture, fracture dislocation, or
　　　　compression fracture of spine
　　　　or vertebra — *see* Fracture,
　　　　vertebra, by site, with spinal
　　　　cord injury
　syndrome 310.2
　underwater blast — *see* Concussion, blast
Condition — *see also* Disease
　fetal hematologic 678.0 ☑
　psychiatric 298.9
　respiratory NEC 519.9
　　acute or subacute NEC 519.9
　　　due to
　　　　external agent 508.9
　　　　　specified type NEC 508.8
　　　　fumes or vapors (chemical) (in-
　　　　　halation) 506.3
　　　　radiation 508.0
　　chronic NEC 519.9
　　　due to
　　　　external agent 508.9
　　　　　specified type NEC 508.8
　　　　fumes or vapors (chemical) (in-
　　　　　halation) 506.4
　　　　radiation 508.1
　　due to
　　　external agent 508.9
　　　　specified type NEC 508.8
　　　fumes or vapors (chemical) (inhala-
　　　　tion) 506.9
　　　smoke inhalation 508.2
Conduct disturbance — *see also* Disturbance,
　conduct 312.9
　adjustment reaction 309.3
　hyperkinetic 314.2
Condyloma NEC 078.11
　acuminatum 078.11
　gonorrheal 098.0
　latum 091.3
　syphilitic 091.3
　　congenital 090.0
　venereal, syphilitic 091.3
Confinement — *see* Delivery
Conflagration — *see also* Burn, by site
　asphyxia (by inhalation of gases, fumes, or
　　vapors) 987.9
　specified agent — *see* Table of Drugs
　　and Chemicals
Conflict
　family V61.9
　　specified circumstance NEC V61.8
　interpersonal NEC V62.81
　marital V61.10
　　involving
　　　divorce V61.03
　　　estrangement V61.09
　parent (guardian)-child V61.20

Conflict — *continued*
　parent-child — *continued*
　　adopted child V61.24
　　biological child V61.23
　　foster child V61.25
　partner V61.10
Confluent — *see* condition
Confusional arousals 327.41
Confusion, confused (mental) (state) — *see*
　also State, confusional 298.9
　acute 293.0
　epileptic 293.0
　postoperative 293.9
　psychogenic 298.2
　reactive (from emotional stress, psycholog-
　　ical trauma) 298.2
　subacute 293.1
Congelation 991.9
Congenital — *see also* condition
　aortic septum 747.29
　generalized fibromatosis (CGF) 759.89
　intrinsic factor deficiency 281.0
　malformation — *see* Anomaly
Congestion, congestive
　asphyxia, newborn 768.9
　bladder 596.89
　bowel 569.89
　brain (*see also* Disease, cerebrovascular NEC)
　　437.8
　　malarial 084.9
　breast 611.79
　bronchi 519.19
　bronchial tube 519.19
　catarrhal 472.0
　cerebral — *see* Congestion, brain
　cerebrospinal — *see* Congestion, brain
　chest 786.9
　chill 780.99
　　malarial (*see also* Malaria) 084.6
　circulatory NEC 459.9
　conjunctiva 372.71
　due to disturbance of circulation 459.9
　duodenum 537.3
　enteritis — *see* Enteritis
　eye 372.71
　fibrosis syndrome (pelvic) 625.5
　gastroenteritis — *see* Enteritis
　general 799.89
　glottis 476.0
　heart (*see also* Failure, heart) 428.0
　hepatic 573.0
　hypostatic (lung) 514
　intestine 569.89
　intracranial — *see* Congestion, brain
　kidney 593.89
　labyrinth 386.50
　larynx 476.0
　liver 573.0
　lung 786.9
　　active or acute (*see also* Pneumonia) 486
　　　congenital 770.0
　　chronic 514
　　hypostatic 514
　　idiopathic, acute 518.52
　　passive 514
　malaria, malarial (brain) (fever) (*see also*
　　Malaria) 084.6
　medulla — *see* Congestion, brain
　nasal 478.19
　nose 478.19
　orbit, orbital 376.33
　　inflammatory (chronic) 376.10
　　　acute 376.00
　ovary 620.8
　pancreas 577.8
　pelvic, female 625.5
　pleural 511.0
　prostate (active) 602.1
　pulmonary — *see* Congestion, lung
　renal 593.89
　retina 362.89
　seminal vesicle 608.89
　spinal cord 336.1
　spleen 289.51
　　chronic 289.51
　stomach 537.89

☑ Additional Digit Required — Refer to the Tabular List for Digit Selection   ▼ Subterms under main terms may continue to next column or page

100   2014 ICD-9-CM

Congestion, congestive — *continued*
  trachea 464.11
  urethra 599.84
  uterus 625.5
    with subinvolution 621.1
  viscera 799.89
Congestive — *see* Congestion
Conical
  cervix 622.6
  cornea 371.60
  teeth 520.2
Conjoined twins 759.4
  causing disproportion (fetopelvic) 678.1 ☑
  fetal 678.1 ☑
Conjugal maladjustment V61.10
  involving
    divorce V61.03
    estrangement V61.09
Conjunctiva — *see* condition
Conjunctivitis (exposure) (infectious)
  (nondiphtheritic) (pneumococcal) (pustular) (staphylococcal) (streptococcal)
  NEC 372.30
  actinic 370.24
  acute 372.00
    atopic 372.05
    chemical 372.06
    contagious 372.03
    follicular 372.02
    hemorrhagic (viral) 077.4
    toxic 372.06
  adenoviral (acute) 077.3
  allergic (chronic) 372.14
    with hay fever 372.05
  anaphylactic 372.05
  angular 372.03
  Apollo (viral) 077.4
  atopic 372.05
  blennorrhagic (neonatorum) 098.40
  catarrhal 372.03
  chemical 372.06
    allergic 372.05
    meaning corrosion — *see* Burn, conjunc-
    tiva
  chlamydial 077.98
    due to
      Chlamydia trachomatis — *see* Tra-
      choma
      paratrachoma 077.0
  chronic 372.10
    allergic 372.14
    follicular 372.12
    simple 372.11
    specified type NEC 372.14
    vernal 372.13
  diphtheritic 032.81
  due to
    dust 372.05
    enterovirus type 70 077.4
    erythema multiforme 695.10 *[372.33]*
    filariasis (*see also* Filariasis) 125.9 *[372.15]*
    mucocutaneous
      disease NEC 372.33
      leishmaniasis 085.5 *[372.15]*
    Reiter's disease 099.3 *[372.33]*
    syphilis 095.8 *[372.10]*
    toxoplasmosis (acquired) 130.1
      congenital (active) 771.2
    trachoma — *see* Trachoma
  dust 372.05
  eczematous 370.31
  epidemic 077.1
    hemorrhagic 077.4
  follicular (acute) 372.02
    adenoviral (acute) 077.3
    chronic 372.12
  glare 370.24
  gonococcal (neonatorum) 098.40
  granular (trachomatous) 076.1
    late effect 139.1
  hemorrhagic (acute) (epidemic) 077.4
  herpetic (simplex) 054.43
    zoster 053.21
  inclusion 077.0
  infantile 771.6
  influenzal 372.03

Conjunctivitis — *continued*
  Koch-Weeks 372.03
  light 372.05
  medicamentosa 372.05
  membranous 372.04
  meningococcic 036.89
  Morax-Axenfeld 372.02
  mucopurulent NEC 372.03
  neonatal 771.6
    gonococcal 098.40
  Newcastle's 077.8
  nodosa 360.14
  of Beal 077.3
  parasitic 372.15
    filariasis (*see also* Filariasis) 125.9 *[372.15]*
    mucocutaneous leishmaniasis
      085.5 *[372.15]*
  Parinaud's 372.02
  petrificans 372.39
  phlyctenular 370.31
  pseudomembranous 372.04
    diphtheritic 032.81
  purulent 372.03
  Reiter's 099.3 *[372.33]*
  rosacea 695.3 *[372.31]*
  serous 372.01
    viral 077.99
  simple chronic 372.11
  specified NEC 372.39
  sunlamp 372.04
  swimming pool 077.0
  toxic 372.06
  trachomatous (follicular) 076.1
    acute 076.0
    late effect 139.1
  traumatic NEC 372.39
  tuberculous (*see also* Tuberculosis)
    017.3 ☑ *[370.31]*
  tularemic 021.3
  tularensis 021.3
  vernal 372.13
    limbar 372.13 *[370.32]*
  viral 077.99
    acute hemorrhagic 077.4
    specified NEC 077.8
Conjunctivochalasis 372.81
Conjunctoblepharitis — *see* Conjunctivitis
Connective tissue — *see* condition
Conn (-Louis) syndrome (primary aldosteronism) 255.12
Conradi (-Hünermann) syndrome or disease
  (chondrodysplasia calcificans congenita)
  756.59
Consanguinity V19.7
Consecutive — *see* condition
Consolidated lung (base) — *see* Pneumonia,
  lobar
Constipation 564.00
  atonic 564.09
  drug induced
    correct substance properly administered
      564.09
    overdose or wrong substance given or
      taken 977.9
      specified drug — *see* Table of Drugs
      and Chemicals
  neurogenic 564.09
  other specified NEC 564.09
  outlet dysfunction 564.02
  psychogenic 306.4
  simple 564.00
  slow transit 564.01
  spastic 564.09
Constitutional — *see also* condition
  arterial hypotension (*see also* Hypotension)
    458.9
  obesity 278.00
    morbid 278.01
  psychopathic state 301.9
  short stature in childhood 783.43
  state, developmental V21.9
    specified development NEC V21.8
  substandard 301.6
Constitutionally substandard 301.6
Constriction
  anomalous, meningeal bands or folds 742.8

Constriction — *continued*
  aortic arch (congenital) 747.10
  asphyxiation or suffocation by 994.7
  bronchus 519.19
  canal, ear (*see also* Stricture, ear canal, ac-
    quired) 380.50
  duodenum 537.3
  gallbladder (*see also* Obstruction, gallblad-
    der) 575.2
    congenital 751.69
  intestine (*see also* Obstruction, intestine)
    560.9
  larynx 478.74
    congenital 748.3
  meningeal bands or folds, anomalous 742.8
  organ or site, congenital NEC — *see* Atresia
  prepuce (congenital) 605
  pylorus 537.0
    adult hypertrophic 537.0
    congenital or infantile 750.5
    newborn 750.5
  ring (uterus) 661.4 ☑
    affecting fetus or newborn 763.7
  spastic (*see also* Spasm)
    ureter 593.3
    urethra — *see* Stricture, urethra
  stomach 537.89
  ureter 593.3
  urethra — *see* Stricture, urethra
  visual field (functional) (peripheral) 368.45
Constrictive — *see* condition
Consultation
  without complaint or sickness V65.9
    feared complaint unfounded V65.5
    specified reason NEC V65.8
  medical (*see also* Counseling, medical)
    specified reason NEC V65.8
Consumption — *see* Tuberculosis
Contact — *see also* Exposure (suspected)
  with
    AIDS virus V01.79
    anthrax V01.81
    asbestos V15.84
    cholera V01.0
    communicable disease V01.9
      specified type NEC V01.89
      viral NEC V01.79
    Escherichia coli (E. coli) V01.83
    German measles V01.4
    gonorrhea V01.6
    HIV V01.79
    human immunodeficiency virus V01.79
    lead V15.86
    meningococcus V01.84
    parasitic disease NEC V01.89
    poliomyelitis V01.2
    potentially hazardous body fluids V15.85
    rabies V01.5
    rubella V01.4
    SARS-associated coronavirus V01.82
    smallpox V01.3
    syphilis V01.6
    tuberculosis V01.1
    varicella V01.71
    venereal disease V01.6
    viral disease NEC V01.79
  dermatitis — *see* Dermatitis
Contamination, food — *see also* Poisoning,
  food 005.9
Contraception, contraceptive
  advice NEC V25.09
    family planning V25.09
    fitting of diaphragm V25.02
    prescribing or use of
      oral contraceptive agent V25.01
      specified agent NEC V25.02
  counseling NEC V25.09
    emergency V25.03
    family planning V25.09
    fitting of diaphragm V25.02
    prescribing or use of
      oral contraceptive agent V25.01
        emergency V25.03
        postcoital V25.03
      specified agent NEC V25.02
  device (in situ) V45.59

Contraception, contraceptive —
  continued
  device — *continued*
    causing menorrhagia 996.76
    checking V25.42
    complications 996.32
    insertion V25.11
    intrauterine V45.51
    reinsertion V25.13
    removal V25.12
      and reinsertion V25.13
    replacement V25.13
    subdermal V45.52
  fitting of diaphragm V25.02
  insertion
    intrauterine contraceptive device V25.11
    subdermal implantable V25.5
  maintenance V25.40
    examination V25.40
      oral contraceptive V25.41
      specified method NEC V25.49
      subdermal implantable V25.43
        intrauterine device V25.42
    intrauterine device V25.42
    oral contraceptive V25.41
    specified method NEC V25.49
    subdermal implantable V25.43
  management NEC V25.49
  prescription
    oral contraceptive agent V25.01
      emergency V25.03
      postcoital V25.03
      repeat V25.41
    specified agent NEC V25.02
      repeat V25.49
  sterilization V25.2
  surveillance V25.40
    intrauterine device V25.42
    oral contraceptive agent V25.41
      subdermal implantable V25.43
    specified method NEC V25.49
Contraction, contracture, contracted
  Achilles tendon (*see also* Short, tendon,
    Achilles) 727.81
  anus 564.89
  axilla 729.90
  bile duct (*see also* Disease, biliary) 576.8
  bladder 596.89
    neck or sphincter 596.0
  bowel (*see also* Obstruction, intestine) 560.9
  Braxton Hicks 644.1 ☑
  breast implant, capsular 611.83
  bronchus 519.19
  burn (old) — *see* Cicatrix
  capsular, of breast implant 611.83
  cecum (*see also* Obstruction, intestine) 560.9
  cervix (*see also* Stricture, cervix) 622.4
    congenital 752.49
  cicatricial — *see* Cicatrix
  colon (*see also* Obstruction, intestine) 560.9
  conjunctiva trachomatous, active 076.1
    late effect 139.1
  Dupuytren's 728.6
  eyelid 374.41
  eye socket (after enucleation) 372.64
  face 729.90
  fascia (lata) (postural) 728.89
    Dupuytren's 728.6
    palmar 728.6
    plantar 728.71
  finger NEC 736.29
    congenital 755.59
    joint (*see also* Contraction, joint) 718.44
  flaccid, paralytic
    joint (*see also* Contraction, joint)
      718.4 ☑
    muscle 728.85
    ocular 378.50
  gallbladder (*see also* Obstruction, gallblad-
    der) 575.2
  hamstring 728.89
    tendon 727.81
  heart valve — *see* Endocarditis
  Hicks' 644.1 ☑
  hip (*see also* Contraction, joint) 718.4 ☑

☑ Additional Digit Required — Refer to the Tabular List for Digit Selection   ⬙ Subterms under main terms may continue to next column or page

2014 ICD-9-CM   **101**

Contraction, contracture, contracted — *continued*
hourglass
  bladder 596.89
    congenital 753.8
  gallbladder (*see also* Obstruction, gall-
    bladder) 575.2
    congenital 751.69
  stomach 536.8
    congenital 750.7
    psychogenic 306.4
  uterus 661.4 ☑
    affecting fetus or newborn 763.7
hysterical 300.11
infantile (*see also* Epilepsy) 345.6 ☑
internal os (*see also* Stricture, cervix) 622.4
intestine (*see also* Obstruction, intestine)
  560.9
joint (abduction) (acquired) (adduction)
  (flexion) (rotation) 718.40
  ankle 718.47
  congenital NEC 755.8
    generalized or multiple 754.89
      lower limb joints 754.89
    hip (*see also* Subluxation, congenital,
      hip) 754.32
    lower limb (including pelvic girdle)
      not involving hip 754.89
    upper limb (including shoulder gir-
      dle) 755.59
  elbow 718.42
  foot 718.47
  hand 718.44
  hip 718.45
  hysterical 300.11
  knee 718.46
  multiple sites 718.49
  pelvic region 718.45
  shoulder (region) 718.41
  specified site NEC 718.48
  wrist 718.43
kidney (granular) (secondary) (*see also*
  Sclerosis, renal) 587
  congenital 753.3
  hydronephritic 591
  pyelonephritic (*see also* Pyelitis, chronic)
    590.00
  tuberculous (*see also* Tuberculosis)
    016.0 ☑
ligament 728.89
  congenital 756.89
liver — *see* Cirrhosis, liver
muscle (postinfectional) (postural) NEC
  728.85
  congenital 756.89
    sternocleidomastoid 754.1
  extraocular 378.60
  eye (extrinsic) (*see also* Strabismus) 378.9
    paralytic (*see also* Strabismus, paralyt-
      ic) 378.50
  flaccid 728.85
  hysterical 300.11
  ischemic (Volkmann's) 958.6
  paralytic 728.85
  posttraumatic 958.6
  psychogenic 306.0
    specified as conversion reaction
      300.11
myotonic 728.85
neck (*see also* Torticollis) 723.5
  congenital 754.1
  psychogenic 306.0
ocular muscle (*see also* Strabismus) 378.9
  paralytic (*see also* Strabismus, paralytic)
    378.50
organ or site, congenital NEC — *see* Atresia
outlet (pelvis) — *see* Contraction, pelvis
palmar fascia 728.6
paralytic
  joint (*see also* Contraction, joint)
    718.4 ☑
  muscle 728.85
    ocular (*see also* Strabismus, paralytic)
      378.50
pelvis (acquired) (general) 738.6
  affecting fetus or newborn 763.1

Contraction, contracture, contracted — *continued*
pelvis — *continued*
  complicating delivery 653.1 ☑
    causing obstructed labor 660.1 ☑
    generally contracted 653.1 ☑
      causing obstructed labor
        660.1 ☑
    inlet 653.2 ☑
      causing obstructed labor
        660.1 ☑
    midpelvic 653.8 ☑
      causing obstructed labor
        660.1 ☑
    midplane 653.8 ☑
      causing obstructed labor
        660.1 ☑
    outlet 653.3 ☑
      causing obstructed labor
        660.1 ☑
plantar fascia 728.71
premature
  atrial 427.61
  auricular 427.61
  auriculoventricular 427.61
  heart (junctional) (nodal) 427.60
  supraventricular 427.61
  ventricular 427.69
prostate 602.8
pylorus (*see also* Pylorospasm) 537.81
rectosigmoid (*see also* Obstruction, intestine) 560.9
rectum, rectal (sphincter) 564.89
  psychogenic 306.4
ring (Bandl's) 661.4 ☑
  affecting fetus or newborn 763.7
scar — *see* Cicatrix
sigmoid (*see also* Obstruction, intestine)
  560.9
socket, eye 372.64
spine (*see also* Curvature, spine) 737.9
stomach 536.8
  hourglass 536.8
    congenital 750.7
  psychogenic 306.4
tendon (sheath) (*see also* Short, tendon)
  727.81
toe 735.8
ureterovesical orifice (postinfectional) 593.3
urethra 599.84
uterus 621.8
  abnormal 661.9 ☑
    affecting fetus or newborn 763.7
  clonic, hourglass or tetanic 661.4 ☑
    affecting fetus or newborn 763.7
  dyscoordinate 661.4 ☑
    affecting fetus or newborn 763.7
  hourglass 661.4 ☑
    affecting fetus or newborn 763.7
  hypotonic NEC 661.2 ☑
    affecting fetus or newborn 763.7
  incoordinate 661.4 ☑
    affecting fetus or newborn 763.7
  inefficient or poor 661.2 ☑
    affecting fetus or newborn 763.7
  irregular 661.2 ☑
    affecting fetus or newborn 763.7
  tetanic 661.4 ☑
    affecting fetus or newborn 763.7
vagina (outlet) 623.2
vesical 596.89
  neck or urethral orifice 596.0
visual field, generalized 368.45
Volkmann's (ischemic) 958.6
Contusion (skin surface intact) 924.9
with
  crush injury — *see* Crush
  dislocation — *see* Dislocation, by site
  fracture — *see* Fracture, by site
  internal injury (*see also* Injury, internal,
    by site)
    heart — *see* Contusion, cardiac
    kidney — *see* Contusion, kidney
    liver — *see* Contusion, liver
    lung — *see* Contusion, lung
    spleen — *see* Contusion, spleen

Contusion — *continued*
with — *continued*
  intracranial injury — *see* Injury, intracra-
    nial
  nerve injury — *see* Injury, nerve
  open wound — *see* Wound, open, by
    site
abdomen, abdominal (muscle) (wall) 922.2
  organ(s) NEC 868.00
adnexa, eye NEC 921.9
ankle 924.21
  with other parts of foot 924.20
arm 923.9
  lower (with elbow) 923.10
  upper 923.03
    with shoulder or axillary region
      923.09
auditory canal (external) (meatus) (and
  other part(s) of neck, scalp, or face,
  except eye) 920
auricle, ear (and other part(s) of neck, scalp,
  or face except eye) 920
axilla 923.02
  with shoulder or upper arm 923.09
back 922.31
bone NEC 924.9
brain (cerebral) (membrane) (with hemorrhage) 851.8 ☑

> Note — Use the following fifth–digit
> subclassification with categories
> 851–854:
>
> 0   unspecified state of consciousness
>
> 1   with no loss of consciousness
>
> 2   with brief [less than one hour]
>   loss of consciousness
>
> 3   with moderate [1–24 hours] loss
>   of consciousness
>
> 4   with prolonged [more than 24
>   hours] loss of consciousness and
>   return to pre–existing conscious
>   level
>
> 5   with prolonged [more than 24
>   hours] loss of consciousness,
>   without return to pre–existing
>   conscious level
>
> Use fifth–digit 5 to designate when a
> patient is unconscious and dies before
> regaining consciousness, regardless of
> the duration of the loss of consciousness
>
> 6   with loss of consciousness of un-
>   specified duration
>
> 9   with concussion, unspecified

  with
    open intracranial wound 851.9 ☑
    skull fracture — *see* Fracture, skull,
      by site
  cerebellum 851.4 ☑
    with open intracranial wound
      851.5 ☑
  cortex 851.0 ☑
    with open intracranial wound
      851.1 ☑
  occipital lobe 851.4 ☑
    with open intracranial wound
      851.5 ☑
  stem 851.4 ☑
    with open intracranial wound
      851.5 ☑
breast 922.0
brow (and other part(s) of neck, scalp, or
  face, except eye) 920
buttock 922.32
canthus 921.1
cardiac 861.01
  with open wound into thorax 861.11
cauda equina (spine) 952.4
cerebellum — *see* Contusion, brain, cerebellum
cerebral — *see* Contusion, brain
cheek(s) (and other part(s) of neck, scalp, or
  face, except eye) 920

Contusion — *continued*
chest (wall) 922.1
chin (and other part(s) of neck, scalp, or face,
  except eye) 920
clitoris 922.4
conjunctiva 921.1
conus medullaris (spine) 952.4
cornea 921.3
corpus cavernosum 922.4
cortex (brain) (cerebral) — *see* Contusion,
  brain, cortex
costal region 922.1
ear (and other part(s) of neck, scalp, or face
  except eye) 920
elbow 923.11
  with forearm 923.10
epididymis 922.4
epigastric region 922.2
eyeball 921.3
eyelid(s) (and periocular area) 921.1
eye NEC 921.9
face (and neck, or scalp, any part, except
  eye) 920
femoral triangle 922.2
fetus or newborn 772.6
finger(s) (nail) (subungual) 923.3
flank 922.2
foot (with ankle) (excluding toe(s)) 924.20
forearm (and elbow) 923.10
forehead (and other part(s) of neck, scalp,
  or face, except eye) 920
genital organs, external 922.4
globe (eye) 921.3
groin 922.2
gum(s) (and other part(s) of neck, scalp, or
  face, except eye) 920
hand(s) (except fingers alone) 923.20
head (any part, except eye) (and face) (and
  neck) 920
heart — *see* Contusion, cardiac
heel 924.20
hip 924.01
  with thigh 924.00
iliac region 922.2
inguinal region 922.2
internal organs (abdomen, chest, or pelvis)
  NEC — *see* Injury, internal, by site
interscapular region 922.33
iris (eye) 921.3
kidney 866.01
  with open wound into cavity 866.11
knee 924.11
  with lower leg 924.10
labium (majus) (minus) 922.4
lacrimal apparatus, gland, or sac 921.1
larynx (and other part(s) of neck, scalp, or
  face, except eye) 920
late effect — *see* Late, effects (of), contusion
leg 924.5
  lower (with knee) 924.10
lens 921.3
lingual (and other part(s) of neck, scalp, or
  face, except eye) 920
lip(s) (and other part(s) of neck, scalp, or
  face, except eye) 920
liver 864.01
  with
    laceration — *see* Laceration, liver
    open wound into cavity 864.11
lower extremity 924.5
  multiple sites 924.4
lumbar region 922.31
lung 861.21
  with open wound into thorax 861.31
malar region (and other part(s) of neck,
  scalp, or face, except eye) 920
mandibular joint (and other part(s) of neck,
  scalp, or face, except eye) 920
mastoid region (and other part(s) of neck,
  scalp, or face, except eye) 920
membrane, brain — *see* Contusion, brain
midthoracic region 922.1
mouth (and other part(s) of neck, scalp, or
  face, except eye) 920
multiple sites (not classifiable to same three-
  digit category) 924.8

☑ **Additional Digit Required — Refer to the Tabular List for Digit Selection**
        Subterms under main terms may continue to next column or page

102   **2014 ICD-9-CM**

Contusion — continued
- multiple sites — continued
  - lower limb 924.4
  - trunk 922.8
  - upper limb 923.8
- muscle NEC 924.9
- myocardium — see Contusion, cardiac
- nasal (septum) (and other part(s) of neck, scalp, or face, except eye) 920
- neck (and scalp or face, any part, except eye) 920
- nerve — see Injury, nerve, by site
- nose (and other part(s) of neck, scalp, or face, except eye) 920
- occipital region (scalp) (and neck or face, except eye) 920
  - lobe — see Contusion, brain, occipital lobe
- orbit (region) (tissues) 921.2
- palate (soft) (and other part(s) of neck, scalp, or face, except eye) 920
- parietal region (scalp) (and neck, or face, except eye) 920
  - lobe — see Contusion, brain
- penis 922.4
- pericardium — see Contusion, cardiac
- perineum 922.4
- periocular area 921.1
- pharynx (and other part(s) of neck, scalp, or face, except eye) 920
- popliteal space (see also Contusion, knee) 924.11
- prepuce 922.4
- pubic region 922.4
- pudenda 922.4
- pulmonary — see Contusion, lung
- quadriceps femoralis 924.00
- rib cage 922.1
- sacral region 922.32
- salivary ducts or glands (and other part(s) of neck, scalp, or face, except eye) 920
- scalp (and neck, or face any part, except eye) 920
- scapular region 923.01
  - with shoulder or upper arm 923.09
- sclera (eye) 921.3
- scrotum 922.4
- shoulder 923.00
  - with upper arm or axillar regions 923.09
- skin NEC 924.9
- skull 920
- spermatic cord 922.4
- spinal cord (see also Injury, spinal, by site)
  - cauda equina 952.4
  - conus medullaris 952.4
- spleen 865.01
  - with open wound into cavity 865.11
- sternal region 922.1
- stomach — see Injury, internal, stomach
- subconjunctival 921.1
- subcutaneous NEC 924.9
- submaxillary region (and other part(s) of neck, scalp, or face, except eye) 920
- submental region (and other part(s) of neck, scalp, or face, except eye) 920
- subperiosteal NEC 924.9
- supraclavicular fossa (and other part(s) of neck, scalp, or face, except eye) 920
- supraorbital (and other part(s) of neck, scalp, or face, except eye) 920
- temple (region) (and other part(s) of neck, scalp, or face, except eye) 920
- testis 922.4
- thigh (and hip) 924.00
- thorax 922.1
  - organ — see Injury, internal, intrathoracic
- throat (and other part(s) of neck, scalp, or face, except eye) 920
- thumb(s) (nail) (subungual) 923.3
- toe(s) (nail) (subungual) 924.3
- tongue (and other part(s) of neck, scalp, or face, except eye) 920
- trunk 922.9
  - multiple sites 922.8

Contusion — continued
- trunk — continued
  - specified site — see Contusion, by site
  - tunica vaginalis 922.4
- tympanum (membrane) (and other part(s) of neck, scalp, or face, except eye) 920
- upper extremity 923.9
  - multiple sites 923.8
- uvula (and other part(s) of neck, scalp, or face, except eye) 920
- vagina 922.4
- vocal cord(s) (and other part(s) of neck, scalp, or face, except eye) 920
- vulva 922.4
- wrist 923.21
  - with hand(s), except finger(s) alone 923.20

Conus (any type) (congenital) 743.57
- acquired 371.60
- medullaris syndrome 336.8

Convalescence (following) V66.9
- chemotherapy V66.2
- medical NEC V66.5
- psychotherapy V66.3
- radiotherapy V66.1
- surgery NEC V66.0
- treatment (for) NEC V66.5
  - combined V66.6
  - fracture V66.4
  - mental disorder NEC V66.3
  - specified disorder NEC V66.5

Conversion
- closed surgical procedure to open procedure
  - arthroscopic V64.43
  - laparoscopic V64.41
  - thoracoscopic V64.42
- hysteria, hysterical, any type 300.11
- neurosis, any 300.11
- reaction, any 300.11

Converter, tuberculosis (test reaction) 795.51
Convulsions (idiopathic) 780.39
- apoplectiform (see also Disease, cerebrovascular, acute) 436
- brain 780.39
- cerebral 780.39
- cerebrospinal 780.39
- due to trauma NEC — see Injury, intracranial
- eclamptic (see also Eclampsia) 780.39
- epileptic (see also Epilepsy) 345.9 ☑
- epileptiform (see also Seizure, epileptiform) 780.39
- epileptoid (see also Seizure, epileptiform) 780.39
- ether
  - anesthetic
    - correct substance properly administered 780.39
    - overdose or wrong substance given 968.2
    - other specified type — see Table of Drugs and Chemicals
- febrile (simple) 780.31
  - complex 780.32
- generalized 780.39
- hysterical 300.11
- infantile 780.39
  - epilepsy — see Epilepsy
- internal 780.39
- jacksonian (see also Epilepsy) 345.5 ☑
- myoclonic 333.2
- newborn 779.0
- paretic 094.1
- pregnancy (nephritic) (uremic) — see Eclampsia, pregnancy
- psychomotor (see also Epilepsy) 345.4 ☑
- puerperal, postpartum — see Eclampsia, pregnancy
- recurrent 780.39
  - epileptic — see Epilepsy
- reflex 781.0
- repetitive 780.39
  - epileptic — see Epilepsy
- salaam (see also Epilepsy) 345.6 ☑
- scarlatinal 034.1

Convulsions — continued
- spasmodic 780.39
- tetanus, tetanic (see also Tetanus) 037
- thymic 254.8
- uncinate 780.39
- uremic 586

Convulsive — see also Convulsions
- disorder or state 780.39
  - epileptic — see Epilepsy
- equivalent, abdominal (see also Epilepsy) 345.5 ☑

Cooke-Apert-Gallais syndrome (adrenogenital) 255.2
Cooley's anemia (erythroblastic) 282.44
Coolie itch 126.9
Cooper's
- disease 610.1
- hernia — see Hernia, Cooper's

Coordination disturbance 781.3
Copper wire arteries, retina 362.13
Copra itch 133.8
Coprolith 560.39
Coprophilia 302.89
Coproporphyria, hereditary 277.1
Coprostasis 560.32
- with hernia (see also Hernia, by site, with obstruction)
  - gangrenous — see Hernia, by site, with gangrene

Cor
- biloculare 745.7
- bovinum — see Hypertrophy, cardiac
- bovis (see also Hypertrophy, cardiac)
- pulmonale (chronic) 416.9
  - acute 415.0
- triatriatum, triatrium 746.82
- triloculare 745.8
  - biatriatum 745.3
  - biventriculare 745.69

Corbus' disease 607.1
Cord — see also condition
- around neck (tightly) (with compression)
  - affecting fetus or newborn 762.5
  - complicating delivery 663.1 ☑
    - without compression 663.3 ☑
      - affecting fetus or newborn 762.6
- bladder NEC 344.61
  - tabetic 094.0
- prolapse
  - affecting fetus or newborn 762.4
  - complicating delivery 663.0 ☑

Cord's angiopathy — see also Tuberculosis 017.3 ☑ [362.18]
Cordis ectopia 746.87
Corditis (spermatic) 608.4
Corectopia 743.46
Cori type glycogen storage disease — see Disease, glycogen storage
Cork-handlers' disease or lung 495.3
Corkscrew esophagus 530.5
Corlett's pyosis (impetigo) 684
Corn (infected) 700
Cornea — see also condition
- donor V59.5
- guttata (dystrophy) 371.57
- plana 743.41

Cornelia de Lange's syndrome (Amsterdam dwarf, intellectual disabilities, and brachycephaly) 759.89
Cornual gestation or pregnancy — see Pregnancy, cornual
Cornu cutaneum 702.8
Coronary (artery) — see also condition
- arising from aorta or pulmonary trunk 746.85

Corpora — see also condition
- amylacea (prostate) 602.8
- cavernosa — see condition

Corpulence — see Obesity
Corpus — see condition
Corrigan's disease — see Insufficiency, aortic
Corrosive burn — see Burn, by site
Corsican fever — see also Malaria 084.6
Cortical — see also condition
- blindness 377.75
- necrosis, kidney (bilateral) 583.6

Corticoadrenal — see condition
Corticosexual syndrome 255.2
Coryza (acute) 460
- with grippe or influenza (see also Influenza) 487.1
- syphilitic 095.8
  - congenital (chronic) 090.0

Costen's syndrome or complex 524.60
Costiveness — see also Constipation 564.00
Costochondritis 733.6
Cotard's syndrome (paranoia) 297.1
Cot death 798.0
Cotia virus 059.8
Cotungo's disease 724.3
Cough 786.2
- with hemorrhage (see also Hemoptysis) 786.39
- affected 786.2
- bronchial 786.2
  - with grippe or influenza (see also Influenza) 487.1
- chronic 786.2
- epidemic 786.2
- functional 306.1
- hemorrhagic 786.39
- hysterical 300.11
- laryngeal, spasmodic 786.2
- nervous 786.2
- psychogenic 306.1
- smokers' 491.0
- tea tasters' 112.89

Counseling NEC V65.40
- without complaint or sickness V65.49
- abuse victim NEC V62.89
  - child V61.21
  - partner V61.11
  - spouse V61.11
- child abuse, maltreatment, or neglect V61.21
- contraceptive NEC V25.09
  - device (intrauterine) V25.02
    - maintenance V25.40
      - intrauterine contraceptive device V25.42
    - oral contraceptive (pill) V25.41
    - specified type NEC V25.49
    - subdermal implantable V25.43
  - management NEC V25.9
  - oral contraceptive (pill) V25.01
    - emergency V25.03
    - postcoital V25.03
  - prescription NEC V25.02
    - oral contraceptive (pill) V25.01
      - emergency V25.03
      - postcoital V25.03
      - repeat prescription V25.41
    - repeat prescription V25.40
  - subdermal implantable V25.43
  - surveillance NEC V25.40
- dietary V65.3
- exercise V65.41
- expectant parent(s)
  - pediatric pre-adoption visit V65.11
  - pediatric pre-birth visit V65.11
- explanation of
  - investigation finding NEC V65.49
  - medication NEC V65.49
- family planning V25.09
  - natural
    - procreative V26.41
    - to avoid pregnancy V26.04
- for nonattending third party V65.19
- genetic V26.33
- gonorrhea V65.45
- health (advice) (education) (instruction) NEC V65.49
- HIV V65.44
- human immunodeficiency virus V65.44
- injury prevention V65.43
- insulin pump training V65.46
- marital V61.10
- medical (for) V65.9
  - boarding school resident V60.6
  - condition not demonstrated V65.5
  - feared complaint and no disease found V65.5

☑ **Additional Digit Required** — Refer to the Tabular List for Digit Selection   ▽ Subterms under main terms may continue to next column or page

2014 ICD-9-CM   103

Counseling — *continued*
  medical — *continued*
    institutional resident V60.6
    on behalf of another V65.19
    person living alone V60.3
  natural family planning
    procreative V26.41
    to avoid pregnancy V25.04
  parent (guardian)-child conflict V61.20
    adopted child V61.24
    biological child V61.23
    foster child V61.25
    specified problem NEC V61.29
  partner abuse
    perpetrator V61.12
    victim V61.11
  pediatric
    pre-adoption visit for adoptive parent(s) V65.11
    pre-birth visit for expectant parents V65.11
  perpetrator of
    child abuse V62.83
      parental V61.22
    partner abuse V61.12
    spouse abuse V61.12
  procreative V65.49
  sex NEC V65.49
    transmitted disease NEC V65.45
      HIV V65.44
  specified reason NEC V65.49
  spousal abuse
    perpetrator V61.12
    victim V61.11
  substance use and abuse V65.42
  syphilis V65.45
  victim (of)
    abuse NEC V62.89
    child abuse V61.21
    partner abuse V61.11
    spousal abuse V61.11
Coupled rhythm 427.89
Couvelaire uterus (complicating delivery) — *see* Placenta, separation
Cowper's gland — *see* condition
Cowperitis — *see also* Urethritis 597.89
  gonorrheal (acute) 098.0
    chronic or duration of 2 months or over 098.2
Cowpox (abortive) 051.01
  due to vaccination 999.0
  eyelid 051.01 *[373.5]*
    postvaccination 999.0 *[373.5]*
Coxa
  plana 732.1
  valga (acquired) 736.31
    congenital 755.61
    late effect of rickets 268.1
  vara (acquired) 736.32
    congenital 755.62
    late effect of rickets 268.1
Coxae malum senilis 715.25
Coxalgia (nontuberculous) 719.45
  tuberculous (*see also* Tuberculosis) 015.1 ☑ *[730.85]*
Coxalgic pelvis 736.30
Coxitis 716.65
Coxsackie (infection) (virus) 079.2
  central nervous system NEC 048
  endocarditis 074.22
  enteritis 008.67
  meningitis (aseptic) 047.0
  myocarditis 074.23
  pericarditis 074.21
  pharyngitis 074.0
  pleurodynia 074.1
  specific disease NEC 074.8
Crabs, meaning pubic lice 132.2
Crack baby 760.75
Cracked
  nipple 611.2
    puerperal, postpartum 676.1 ☑
  tooth 521.81
Cradle cap 690.11
Craft neurosis 300.89
Craigiasis 007.8

Cramp(s) 729.82
  abdominal 789.0 ☑
  bathing 994.1
  colic 789.7
    infantile 789.7
    psychogenic 306.4
  due to immersion 994.1
  extremity (lower) (upper) NEC 729.82
  fireman 992.2
  heat 992.2
  hysterical 300.11
  immersion 994.1
  intestinal 789.0 ☑
    psychogenic 306.4
  linotypist's 300.89
    organic 333.84
  muscle (extremity) (general) 729.82
    due to immersion 994.1
    hysterical 300.11
  occupational (hand) 300.89
    organic 333.84
  psychogenic 307.89
  salt depletion 276.1
  sleep related leg 327.52
  stoker 992.2
  stomach 789.0 ☑
  telegraphers' 300.89
    organic 333.84
  typists' 300.89
    organic 333.84
  uterus 625.8
    menstrual 625.3
  writers' 333.84
    organic 333.84
    psychogenic 300.89
Cranial — *see* condition
Cranioclasis, fetal 763.89
Craniocleidodysostosis 755.59
Craniofenestria (skull) 756.0
Craniolacunia (skull) 756.0
Craniopagus 759.4
Craniopathy, metabolic 733.3
Craniopharyngeal — *see* condition
Craniopharyngioma (M9350/1) 237.0
Craniorachischisis (totalis) 740.1
Cranioschisis 756.0
Craniostenosis 756.0
Craniosynostosis 756.0
Craniotabes (cause unknown) 733.3
  rachitic 268.1
  syphilitic 090.5
Craniotomy, fetal 763.89
Cranium — *see* condition
Craw-craw 125.3
CRBSI (catheter-related bloodstream infection) 999.31
Creaking joint 719.60
  ankle 719.67
  elbow 719.62
  foot 719.67
  hand 719.64
  hip 719.65
  knee 719.66
  multiple sites 719.69
  pelvic region 719.65
  shoulder (region) 719.61
  specified site NEC 719.68
  wrist 719.63
Creeping
  eruption 126.9
  palsy 335.21
  paralysis 335.21
Crenated tongue 529.8
Creotoxism 005.9
Crepitus
  caput 756.0
  joint 719.60
    ankle 719.67
    elbow 719.62
    foot 719.67
    hand 719.64
    hip 719.65
    knee 719.66
    multiple sites 719.69
    pelvic region 719.65
    shoulder (region) 719.61

Crepitus — *continued*
  joint — *continued*
    specified site NEC 719.68
    wrist 719.63
Crescent or conus choroid, congenital 743.57
Cretin, cretinism (athyrotic) (congenital) (endemic) (metabolic) (nongoitrous) (sporadic) 243
  goitrous (sporadic) 246.1
  pelvis (dwarf type) (male type) 243
    with disproportion (fetopelvic) 653.1 ☑
      affecting fetus or newborn 763.1
      causing obstructed labor 660.1 ☑
        affecting fetus or newborn 763.1
  pituitary 253.3
Cretinoid degeneration 243
Creutzfeldt-Jakob disease (CJD) (syndrome) 046.19
  with dementia
    with behavioral disturbance 046.19 *[294.11]*
    without behavioral disturbance 046.19 *[294.10]*
  familial 046.19
  iatrogenic 046.19
  specified NEC 046.19
  sporadic 046.19
  variant (vCJD) 046.11
    with dementia
      with behavioral disturbance 046.11 *[294.11]*
      without behavioral disturbance 046.11 *[294.10]*
Crib death 798.0
Cribriform hymen 752.49
Cri-du-chat syndrome 758.31
Crigler-Najjar disease or syndrome (congenital hyperbilirubinemia) 277.4
Crimean hemorrhagic fever 065.0
Criminalism 301.7
Crisis
  abdomen 789.0 ☑
  addisonian (acute adrenocortical insufficiency) 255.41
  adrenal (cortical) 255.41
  asthmatic — *see* Asthma
  brain, cerebral (*see also* Disease, cerebrovascular, acute) 436
  celiac 579.0
  Dietl's 593.4
  emotional NEC 309.29
    acute reaction to stress 308.0
    adjustment reaction 309.9
    specific to childhood or adolescence 313.9
  gastric (tabetic) 094.0
  glaucomatocyclitic 364.22
  heart (*see also* Failure, heart) 428.9
  hypertensive — *see* Hypertension
  nitritoid
    correct substance properly administered 458.29
    overdose or wrong substance given or taken 961.1
  oculogyric 378.87
    psychogenic 306.7
  Pel's 094.0
  psychosexual identity 302.6
  rectum 094.0
  renal 593.81
  sickle cell 282.62
  stomach (tabetic) 094.0
  tabetic 094.0
  thyroid (*see also* Thyrotoxicosis) 242.9 ☑
  thyrotoxic (*see also* Thyrotoxicosis) 242.9 ☑
  vascular — *see* Disease, cerebrovascular, acute
Crocq's disease (acrocyanosis) 443.89
Crohn's disease — *see also* Enteritis, regional 555.9
Cronkhite-Canada syndrome 211.3
Crooked septum, nasal 470
Cross
  birth (of fetus) complicating delivery 652.3 ☑
    with successful version 652.1 ☑

Cross — *continued*
  birth complicating delivery — *continued*
    causing obstructed labor 660.0 ☑
  bite, anterior or posterior 524.27
  eye (*see also* Esotropia) 378.00
Crossed ectopia of kidney 753.3
Crossfoot 754.50
Croup, croupous (acute) (angina) (catarrhal) (infective) (inflammatory) (laryngeal) (membranous) (nondiphtheritic) (pseudomembranous) 464.4
  asthmatic (*see also* Asthma) 493.9 ☑
  bronchial 466.0
  diphtheritic (membranous) 032.3
  false 478.75
  spasmodic 478.75
    diphtheritic 032.3
  stridulous 478.75
    diphtheritic 032.3
Crouzon's disease (craniofacial dysostosis) 756.0
Crowding, teeth 524.31
CRST syndrome (cutaneous systemic sclerosis) 710.1
Cruchet's disease (encephalitis lethargica) 049.8
Cruelty in children — *see also* Disturbance, conduct 312.9
Crural ulcer — *see also* Ulcer, lower extremity 707.10
Crush, crushed, crushing (injury) 929.9
  abdomen 926.19
    internal — *see* Injury, internal, abdomen
  ankle 928.21
    with other parts of foot 928.20
  arm 927.9
    lower (and elbow) 927.10
    upper 927.03
      with shoulder or axillary region 927.09
  axilla 927.02
    with shoulder or upper arm 927.09
  back 926.11
  breast 926.19
  buttock 926.12
  cheek 925.1
  chest — *see* Injury, internal, chest
  ear 925.1
  elbow 927.11
    with forearm 927.10
  face 925.1
  finger(s) 927.3
    with hand(s) 927.20
      and wrist(s) 927.21
  flank 926.19
  foot, excluding toe(s) alone (with ankle) 928.20
  forearm (and elbow) 927.10
  genitalia, external (female) (male) 926.0
    internal — *see* Injury, internal, genital organ NEC
  hand, except finger(s) alone (and wrist) 927.20
  head — *see* Fracture, skull, by site
  heel 928.20
  hip 928.01
    with thigh 928.00
  internal organ (abdomen, chest, or pelvis) — *see* Injury, internal, by site
  knee 928.11
    with leg, lower 928.10
  labium (majus) (minus) 926.0
  larynx 925.2
  late effect — *see* Late, effects (of), crushing
  leg 928.9
    lower 928.10
      and knee 928.11
    upper 928.00
  limb
    lower 928.9
      multiple sites 928.8
    upper 927.9
      multiple sites 927.8
  multiple sites NEC 929.0
  neck 925.2
  nerve — *see* Injury, nerve, by site

Crush, crushed, crushing — *continued*
  nose 802.0
    open 802.1
  penis 926.0
  pharynx 925.2
  scalp 925.1
  scapular region 927.01
    with shoulder or upper arm 927.09
  scrotum 926.0
  shoulder 927.00
    with upper arm or axillary region 927.09
  skull or cranium — *see* Fracture, skull, by site
  spinal cord — *see* Injury, spinal, by site
  syndrome (complication of trauma) 958.5
  testis 926.0
  thigh (with hip) 928.00
  throat 925.2
  thumb(s) (and fingers) 927.3
  toe(s) 928.3
    with foot 928.20
      and ankle 928.21
  tonsil 925.2
  trunk 926.9
    chest — *see* Injury, internal, intrathoracic organs NEC
    internal organ — *see* Injury, internal, by site
    multiple sites 926.8
    specified site NEC 926.19
  vulva 926.0
  wrist 927.21
    with hand(s), except fingers alone 927.20
Crusta lactea 690.11
Crusts 782.8
Crutch paralysis 953.4
Cruveilhier-Baumgarten cirrhosis, disease, or syndrome 571.5
Cruveilhier's disease 335.21
Cruz-Chagas disease — *see also* Trypanosomiasis 086.2
Crying
  constant, continuous
    adolescent 780.95
    adult 780.95
    baby 780.92
    child 780.95
    infant 780.92
    newborn 780.92
  excessive
    adolescent 780.95
    adult 780.95
    baby 780.92
    child 780.95
    infant 780.92
    newborn 780.92
Cryofibrinogenemia 273.2
Cryoglobulinemia (mixed) 273.2
Crypt (anal) (rectal) 569.49
Cryptitis (anal) (rectal) 569.49
Cryptococcosis (European) (pulmonary) (systemic) 117.5
Cryptococcus 117.5
  epidermicus 117.5
  neoformans, infection by 117.5
Cryptopapillitis (anus) 569.49
Cryptophthalmos (eyelid) 743.06
Cryptorchid, cryptorchism, cryptorchidism 752.51
Cryptosporidiosis 007.4
  hepatobiliary 136.8
  respiratory 136.8
Cryptotia 744.29
Crystallopathy
  calcium pyrophosphate (*see also* Arthritis) 275.49 *[712.2]* ☑
  dicalcium phosphate (*see also* Arthritis) 275.49 *[712.1]* ☑
  gouty 274.00
  pyrophosphate NEC (*see also* Arthritis) 275.49 *[712.2]* ☑
  uric acid 274.00
Crystalluria 791.9
Csillag's disease (lichen sclerosis et atrophicus) 701.0
Cuban itch 050.1

Cubitus
  valgus (acquired) 736.01
    congenital 755.59
    late effect of rickets 268.1
  varus (acquired) 736.02
    congenital 755.59
    late effect of rickets 268.1
Cultural deprivation V62.4
Cupping of optic disc 377.14
Curling esophagus 530.5
Curling's ulcer — *see* Ulcer, duodenum
Curschmann (-Batten) (-Steinert) disease or syndrome 359.21
Curvature
  organ or site, congenital NEC — *see* Distortion
  penis (lateral) 752.69
  Pott's (spinal) (*see also* Tuberculosis) 015.0 ☑ *[737.43]*
  radius, idiopathic, progressive (congenital) 755.54
  spine (acquired) (angular) (idiopathic) (incorrect) (postural) 737.9
    congenital 754.2
    due to or associated with
      Charcôt-Marie-Tooth disease 356.1 *[737.40]*
      mucopolysaccharidosis 277.5 *[737.40]*
      neurofibromatosis 237.71 *[737.40]*
      osteitis
        deformans 731.0 *[737.40]*
        fibrosa cystica 252.01 *[737.40]*
      osteoporosis (*see also* Osteoporosis) 733.00 *[737.40]*
      poliomyelitis (*see also* Poliomyelitis) 138 *[737.40]*
      tuberculosis (Pott's curvature) (*see also* Tuberculosis) 015.0 ☑ *[737.43]*
    kyphoscoliotic (*see also* Kyphoscoliosis) 737.30
    kyphotic (*see also* Kyphosis) 737.10
    late effect of rickets 268.1 *[737.40]*
    Pott's 015.0 ☑ *[737.40]*
    scoliotic (*see also* Scoliosis) 737.30
    specified NEC 737.8
    tuberculous 015.0 ☑ *[737.40]*
Cushing's
  basophilism, disease, or syndrome (iatrogenic) (idiopathic) (pituitary basophilism) (pituitary dependent) 255.0
  ulcer — *see* Ulcer, peptic
Cushingoid due to steroid therapy
  correct substance properly administered 255.0
  overdose or wrong substance given or taken 962.0
Cut (external) — *see* Wound, open, by site
Cutaneous — *see also* condition
  hemorrhage 782.7
  horn (cheek) (eyelid) (mouth) 702.8
  larva migrans 126.9
Cutis — *see also* condition
  hyperelastic 756.83
    acquired 701.8
  laxa 756.83
    senilis 701.8
  marmorata 782.61
  osteosis 709.3
  pendula 756.83
    acquired 701.8
  rhomboidalis nuchae 701.8
  verticis gyrata 757.39
    acquired 701.8
Cyanopathy, newborn 770.83
Cyanosis 782.5
  autotoxic 289.7
  common atrioventricular canal 745.69
  congenital 770.83
  conjunctiva 372.71
  due to
    endocardial cushion defect 745.60
    nonclosure, foramen botalli 745.5
    patent foramen botalli 745.5

Cyanosis — *continued*
  due to — *continued*
    persistent foramen ovale 745.5
    enterogenous 289.7
  fetus or newborn 770.83
  ostium primum defect 745.61
  paroxysmal digital 443.0
  retina, retinal 362.10
Cycle
  anovulatory 628.0
  menstrual, irregular 626.4
Cyclencephaly 759.89
Cyclical vomiting 536.2
  associated with migraine 346.2 ☑
  psychogenic 306.4
Cyclitic membrane 364.74
Cyclitis — *see also* Iridocyclitis 364.3
  acute 364.00
    primary 364.01
    recurrent 364.02
  chronic 364.10
    in
      sarcoidosis 135 *[364.11]*
      tuberculosis (*see also* Tuberculosis) 017.3 ☑ *[364.11]*
  Fuchs' heterochromic 364.21
  granulomatous 364.10
  lens induced 364.23
  nongranulomatous 364.00
  posterior 363.21
  primary 364.01
  recurrent 364.02
  secondary (noninfectious) 364.04
    infectious 364.03
  subacute 364.00
    primary 364.01
    recurrent 364.02
Cyclokeratitis — *see* Keratitis
Cyclophoria 378.44
Cyclopia, cyclops 759.89
Cycloplegia 367.51
Cyclospasm 367.53
Cyclosporiasis 007.5
Cyclothymia 301.13
Cyclothymic personality 301.13
Cyclotropia 378.33
Cyesis — *see* Pregnancy
Cylindroma (M8200/3) — *see also* Neoplasm, by site, malignant
  eccrine dermal (M8200/0) — *see* Neoplasm, skin, benign
  skin (M8200/0) — *see* Neoplasm, skin, benign
Cylindruria 791.7
Cyllosoma 759.89
Cynanche
  diphtheritic 032.3
  tonsillaris 475
Cynorexia 783.6
Cyphosis — *see* Kyphosis
Cyprus fever — *see also* Brucellosis 023.9
Cyriax's syndrome (slipping rib) 733.99
Cyst (mucus) (retention) (serous) (simple)

> *Note — In general, cysts are not neoplastic and are classified to the appropriate category for disease of the specified anatomical site. This generalization does not apply to certain types of cysts which are neoplastic in nature, for example, dermoid, nor does it apply to cysts of certain structures, for example, branchial cleft, which are classified as developmental anomalies.*
>
> *The following listing includes some of the most frequently reported sites of cysts as well as qualifiers which indicate the type of cyst. The latter qualifiers usually are not repeated under the anatomical sites. Since the code assignment for a given site may vary depending upon the type of cyst, the coder should refer to the listings under the specified type of cyst before consideration is given to the site.*

  accessory, fallopian tube 752.11

Cyst — *continued*
  adenoid (infected) 474.8
  adrenal gland 255.8
    congenital 759.1
  air, lung 518.89
  allantoic 753.7
  alveolar process (jaw bone) 526.2
  amnion, amniotic 658.8 ☑
  anterior chamber (eye) 364.60
    exudative 364.62
    implantation (surgical) (traumatic) 364.61
    parasitic 360.13
  anterior nasopalatine 526.1
  antrum 478.19
  anus 569.49
  apical (periodontal) (tooth) 522.8
  appendix 543.9
  arachnoid, brain 348.0
  arytenoid 478.79
  auricle 706.2
  Baker's (knee) 727.51
    tuberculous (*see also* Tuberculosis) 015.2 ☑
  Bartholin's gland or duct 616.2
  bile duct (*see also* Disease, biliary) 576.8
  bladder (multiple) (trigone) 596.89
  Blessig's 362.62
  blood, endocardial (*see also* Endocarditis) 424.90
  blue dome 610.0
  bone (local) 733.20
    aneurysmal 733.22
    jaw 526.2
      developmental (odontogenic) 526.0
      fissural 526.1
      latent 526.89
    solitary 733.21
    unicameral 733.21
  brain 348.0
    congenital 742.4
    hydatid (*see also* Echinococcus) 122.9
    third ventricle (colloid) 742.4
  branchial (cleft) 744.42
  branchiogenic 744.42
  breast (benign) (blue dome) (pedunculated) (solitary) (traumatic) 610.0
    involution 610.4
    sebaceous 610.8
  broad ligament (benign) 620.8
    embryonic 752.11
  bronchogenic (mediastinal) (sequestration) 518.89
    congenital 748.4
  buccal 528.4
  bulbourethral gland (Cowper's) 599.89
  bursa, bursal 727.49
    pharyngeal 478.26
  calcifying odontogenic (M9301/0) 213.1
    upper jaw (bone) 213.0
  canal of Nuck (acquired) (serous) 629.1
    congenital 752.41
  canthus 372.75
  carcinomatous (M8010/3) — *see* Neoplasm, by site, malignant
  cartilage (joint) — *see* Derangement, joint
  cauda equina 336.8
  cavum septi pellucidi NEC 348.0
  celomic (pericardium) 746.89
  cerebellopontine (angle) — *see* Cyst, brain
  cerebellum — *see* Cyst, brain
  cerebral — *see* Cyst, brain
  cervical lateral 744.42
  cervix 622.8
    embryonal 752.41
    nabothian (gland) 616.0
  chamber, anterior (eye) 364.60
    exudative 364.62
    implantation (surgical) (traumatic) 364.61
    parasitic 360.13
  chiasmal, optic NEC (*see also* Lesion, chiasmal) 377.54
  chocolate (ovary) 617.1
  choledochal (congenital) 751.69
    acquired 576.8

☑ **Additional Digit Required — Refer to the Tabular List for Digit Selection**   ▽ **Subterms under main terms may continue to next column or page**

2014 ICD-9-CM   **105**

Cyst — *continued*
  choledochus 751.69
  chorion 658.8 ☑
  choroid plexus 348.0
  chyle, mesentery 457.8
  ciliary body 364.60
    exudative 364.64
    implantation 364.61
    primary 364.63
  clitoris 624.8
  coccyx (*see also* Cyst, bone) 733.20
  colloid
    third ventricle (brain) 742.4
    thyroid gland — *see* Goiter
  colon 569.89
  common (bile) duct (*see also* Disease, biliary) 576.8
  congenital NEC 759.89
    adrenal glands 759.1
    epiglottis 748.3
    esophagus 750.4
    fallopian tube 752.11
    kidney 753.10
      multiple 753.19
      single 753.11
    larynx 748.3
    liver 751.62
    lung 748.4
    mediastinum 748.8
    ovary 752.0
    oviduct 752.11
    pancreas 751.7
    periurethral (tissue) 753.8
    prepuce NEC 752.69
      penis 752.69
    sublingual 750.26
    submaxillary gland 750.26
    thymus (gland) 759.2
    tongue 750.19
    ureterovesical orifice 753.4
    vulva 752.41
  conjunctiva 372.75
  cornea 371.23
  corpora quadrigemina 348.0
  corpus
    albicans (ovary) 620.2
    luteum (ruptured) 620.1
  Cowper's gland (benign) (infected) 599.89
  cranial meninges 348.0
  craniobuccal pouch 253.8
  craniopharyngeal pouch 253.8
  cystic duct (*see also* Disease, gallbladder) 575.8
  Cysticercus (any site) 123.1
  Dandy-Walker 742.3
    with spina bifida (*see also* Spina bifida) 741.0 ☑
  dental 522.8
    developmental 526.0
    eruption 526.0
    lateral periodontal 526.0
    primordial (keratocyst) 526.0
    root 522.8
  dentigerous 526.0
    mandible 526.0
    maxilla 526.0
  dermoid (M8084/0) (*see also* Neoplasm, by site, benign)
    with malignant transformation (M9084/3) 183.0
    implantation
      external area or site (skin) NEC 709.8
      iris 364.61
      skin 709.8
      vagina 623.8
      vulva 624.8
    mouth 528.4
    oral soft tissue 528.4
    sacrococcygeal 685.1
      with abscess 685.0
  developmental of ovary, ovarian 752.0
  dura (cerebral) 348.0
    spinal 349.2
  ear (external) 706.2
  echinococcal (*see also* Echinococcus) 122.9

Cyst — *continued*
  embryonal
    cervix uteri 752.41
    genitalia, female external 752.41
    uterus 752.39
    vagina 752.41
  endometrial 621.8
    ectopic 617.9
  endometrium (uterus) 621.8
    ectopic — *see* Endometriosis
  enteric 751.5
  enterogenous 751.5
  epidermal (inclusion) (*see also* Cyst, skin) 706.2
  epidermoid (inclusion) (*see also* Cyst, skin) 706.2
    mouth 528.4
    not of skin — *see* Cyst, by site
    oral soft tissue 528.4
  epididymis 608.89
  epiglottis 478.79
  epiphysis cerebri 259.8
  epithelial (inclusion) (*see also* Cyst, skin) 706.2
  epoophoron 752.11
  eruption 526.0
  esophagus 530.89
  ethmoid sinus 478.19
  eye (retention) 379.8
    congenital 743.03
    posterior segment, congenital 743.54
  eyebrow 706.2
  eyelid (sebaceous) 374.84
    infected 373.13
    sweat glands or ducts 374.84
  falciform ligament (inflammatory) 573.8
  fallopian tube 620.8
    congenital 752.11
  female genital organs NEC 629.89
  fimbrial (congenital) 752.11
  fissural (oral region) 526.1
  follicle (atretic) (graafian) (ovarian) 620.0
    nabothian (gland) 616.0
  follicular (atretic) (ovarian) 620.0
    dentigerous 526.0
  frontal sinus 478.19
  gallbladder or duct 575.8
  ganglion 727.43
  Gartner's duct 752.41
  gas, of mesentery 568.89
  gingiva 523.8
  gland of moll 374.84
  globulomaxillary 526.1
  graafian follicle 620.0
  granulosal lutein 620.2
  hemangiomatous (M9121/0) (*see also* Hemangioma) 228.00
  hydatid (*see also* Echinococcus) 122.9
    fallopian tube (Morgagni) 752.11
    liver NEC 122.8
    lung NEC 122.9
    Morgagni 752.89
      fallopian tube 752.11
    specified site NEC 122.9
  hymen 623.8
    embryonal 752.41
  hypopharynx 478.26
  hypophysis, hypophyseal (duct) (recurrent) 253.8
    cerebri 253.8
  implantation (dermoid)
    anterior chamber (eye) 364.61
    external area or site (skin) NEC 709.8
    iris 364.61
    vagina 623.8
    vulva 624.8
  incisor, incisive canal 526.1
  inclusion (epidermal) (epithelial) (epidermoid) (mucous) (squamous) (*see also* Cyst, skin) 706.2
    not of skin — *see* Neoplasm, by site, benign
  intestine (large) (small) 569.89
  intracranial — *see* Cyst, brain
  intraligamentous 728.89
    knee 717.89

Cyst — *continued*
  intrasellar 253.8
  iris (idiopathic) 364.60
    exudative 364.62
    implantation (surgical) (traumatic) 364.61
    miotic pupillary 364.55
    parasitic 360.13
  Iwanoff's 362.62
  jaw (bone) (aneurysmal) (extravasation) (hemorrhagic) (traumatic) 526.2
    developmental (odontogenic) 526.0
    fissural 526.1
  keratin 706.2
  kidney (congenital) 753.10
    acquired 593.2
    calyceal (*see also* Hydronephrosis) 591
    multiple 753.19
    pyelogenic (*see also* Hydronephrosis) 591
    simple 593.2
    single 753.11
    solitary (not congenital) 593.2
  labium (majus) (minus) 624.8
    sebaceous 624.8
  lacrimal
    apparatus 375.43
    gland or sac 375.12
  larynx 478.79
  lens 379.39
    congenital 743.39
  lip (gland) 528.5
  liver 573.8
    congenital 751.62
    hydatid (*see also* Echinococcus) 122.8
      granulosis 122.0
      multilocularis 122.5
  lung 518.89
    congenital 748.4
    giant bullous 492.0
  lutein 620.1
  lymphangiomatous (M9173/0) 228.1
  lymphoepithelial
    mouth 528.4
    oral soft tissue 528.4
  macula 362.54
  malignant (M8000/3) — *see* Neoplasm, by site, malignant
  mammary gland (sweat gland) (*see also* Cyst, breast) 610.0
  mandible 526.2
    dentigerous 526.0
    radicular 522.8
  maxilla 526.2
    dentigerous 526.0
    radicular 522.8
  median
    anterior maxillary 526.1
    palatal 526.1
  mediastinum (congenital) 748.8
  meibomian (gland) (retention) 373.2
    infected 373.12
  membrane, brain 348.0
  meninges (cerebral) 348.0
    spinal 349.2
  meniscus knee 717.5
  mesentery, mesenteric (gas) 568.89
    chyle 457.8
    gas 568.89
  mesonephric duct 752.89
  mesothelial
    peritoneum 568.89
    pleura (peritoneal) 568.89
  milk 611.5
  miotic pupillary (iris) 364.55
  Morgagni (hydatid) 752.89
    fallopian tube 752.11
  mouth 528.4
  Müllerian duct 752.89
    appendix testis 608.89
    cervix (embryonal) 752.41
    fallopian tube 752.11
    prostatic utricle 599.89
    vagina (embryonal) 752.41
  multilocular (ovary) (M8000/1) 239.5
  myometrium 621.8

Cyst — *continued*
  nabothian (follicle) (ruptured) 616.0
  nasal sinus 478.19
  nasoalveolar 528.4
  nasolabial 528.4
  nasopalatine (duct) 526.1
    anterior 526.1
  nasopharynx 478.26
  neoplastic (M8000/1) (*see also* Neoplasm, by site, unspecified nature)
    benign (M8000/0) — *see* Neoplasm, by site, benign
    uterus 621.8
  nervous system — *see* Cyst, brain
  neuroenteric 742.59
  neuroepithelial ventricle 348.0
  nipple 610.0
  nose 478.19
    skin of 706.2
  odontogenic, developmental 526.0
  omentum (lesser) 568.89
    congenital 751.8
  oral soft tissue (dermoid) (epidermoid) (lymphoepithelial) 528.4
  ora serrata 361.19
  orbit 376.81
  ovary, ovarian (twisted) 620.2
    adherent 620.2
    chocolate 617.1
    corpus
      albicans 620.2
      luteum 620.1
    dermoid (M9084/0) 220
    developmental 752.0
    due to failure of involution NEC 620.2
    endometrial 617.1
    follicular (atretic) (graafian) (hemorrhagic) 620.0
    hemorrhagic 620.2
    in pregnancy or childbirth 654.4 ☑
      affecting fetus or newborn 763.89
      causing obstructed labor 660.2 ☑
        affecting fetus or newborn 763.1
    multilocular (M8000/1) 239.5
    pseudomucinous (M8470/0) 220
    retention 620.2
    serous 620.2
    theca lutein 620.2
    tuberculous (*see also* Tuberculosis) 016.6 ☑
    unspecified 620.2
  oviduct 620.8
  palatal papilla (jaw) 526.1
  palate 526.1
    fissural 526.1
    median (fissural) 526.1
  palatine, of papilla 526.1
  pancreas, pancreatic 577.2
    congenital 751.7
    false 577.2
    hemorrhagic 577.2
    true 577.2
  paralabral
    hip 718.85
    shoulder 840.7
  paramesonephric duct — *see* Cyst, Müllerian duct
  paranephric 593.2
  para ovarian 752.11
  paraphysis, cerebri 742.4
  parasitic NEC 136.9
  parathyroid (gland) 252.8
  paratubal (fallopian) 620.8
  paraurethral duct 599.89
  paroophoron 752.11
  parotid gland 527.6
    mucous extravasation or retention 527.6
  parovarian 752.11
  pars planus 364.60
    exudative 364.64
    primary 364.63
  pelvis, female
    in pregnancy or childbirth 654.4 ☑
      affecting fetus or newborn 763.89
      causing obstructed labor 660.2 ☑
        affecting fetus or newborn 763.1

☑ Additional Digit Required — Refer to the Tabular List for Digit Selection   ▽ Subterms under main terms may continue to next column or page

106   2014 ICD-9-CM

Cyst — Cyst   Index

Cyst — continued
  penis (sebaceous) 607.89
  periapical 522.8
  pericardial (congenital) 746.89
    acquired (secondary) 423.8
  pericoronal 526.0
  perineural (Tarlov's) 355.9
  periodontal 522.8
    lateral 526.0
  peripancreatic 577.2
  peripelvic (lymphatic) 593.2
  peritoneum 568.89
    chylous 457.8
  pharynx (wall) 478.26
  pilar 704.41
  pilonidal (infected) (rectum) 685.1
    with abscess 685.0
    malignant (M9084/3) 173.59
  pituitary (duct) (gland) 253.8
  placenta (amniotic) — see Placenta, abnormal
  pleura 519.8
  popliteal 727.51
  porencephalic 742.4
    acquired 348.0
  postanal (infected) 685.1
    with abscess 685.0
  posterior segment of eye, congenital 743.54
  postmastoidectomy cavity 383.31
  preauricular 744.47
  prepuce 607.89
    congenital 752.69
  primordial (jaw) 526.0
  prostate 600.3
  pseudomucinous (ovary) (M8470/0) 220
  pudenda (sweat glands) 624.8
  pupillary, miotic 364.55
    sebaceous 624.8
  radicular (residual) 522.8
  radiculodental 522.8
  ranular 527.6
  Rathke's pouch 253.8
  rectum (epithelium) (mucous) 569.49
  renal — see Cyst, kidney
  residual (radicular) 522.8
  retention (ovary) 620.2
  retina 361.19
    macular 362.54
    parasitic 360.13
    primary 361.13
    secondary 361.14
  retroperitoneal 568.89
  sacrococcygeal (dermoid) 685.1
    with abscess 685.0
  salivary gland or duct 527.6
    mucous extravasation or retention 527.6
  Sampson's 617.1
  sclera 379.19
  scrotum (sebaceous) 706.2
    sweat glands 706.2
  sebaceous (duct) (gland) 706.2
    breast 610.8
    eyelid 374.84
    genital organ NEC
      female 629.89
      male 608.89
      scrotum 706.2
  semilunar cartilage (knee) (multiple) 717.5
  seminal vesicle 608.89
  serous (ovary) 620.2
  sinus (antral) (ethmoidal) (frontal) (maxillary) (nasal) (sphenoidal) 478.19
  Skene's gland 599.89
  skin (epidermal) (epidermoid, inclusion) (epithelial) (inclusion) (retention) (sebaceous) 706.2
    breast 610.8
    eyelid 374.84
    genital organ NEC
      female 629.89
      male 608.89
    neoplastic 216.3
      scrotum 706.2
    sweat gland or duct 705.89
  solitary
    bone 733.21

Cyst — continued
  solitary — continued
    kidney 593.2
  spermatic cord 608.89
  sphenoid sinus 478.19
  spinal meninges 349.2
  spine (see also Cyst, bone) 733.20
  spleen NEC 289.59
    congenital 759.0
    hydatid (see also Echinococcus) 122.9
  spring water (pericardium) 746.89
  subarachnoid 348.0
    intrasellar 793.0
  subdural (cerebral) 348.0
    spinal cord 349.2
  sublingual gland 527.6
    mucous extravasation or retention 527.6
  submaxillary gland 527.6
    mucous extravasation or retention 527.6
  suburethral 599.89
  suprarenal gland 255.8
  suprasellar — see Cyst, brain
  sweat gland or duct 705.89
  sympathetic nervous system 337.9
  synovial 727.40
    popliteal space 727.51
  Tarlov's 355.9
  tarsal 373.2
  tendon (sheath) 727.42
  testis 608.89
  theca-lutein (ovary) 620.2
  Thornwaldt's, Tornwaldt's 478.26
  thymus 254.8
  thyroglossal (duct) (infected) (persistent) 759.2
  thyroid (gland) 246.2
    adenomatous — see Goiter, nodular
    colloid (see also Goiter) 240.9
  thyrolingual duct (infected) (persistent) 759.2
  tongue (mucous) 529.8
  tonsil 474.8
  tooth (dental root) 522.8
  trichilemmal (proliferating) 704.42
  tubo-ovarian 620.8
    inflammatory 614.1
  tunica vaginalis 608.89
  turbinate (nose) (see also Cyst, bone) 733.20
  Tyson's gland (benign) (infected) 607.89
  umbilicus 759.89
  urachus 753.7
  ureter 593.89
  ureterovesical orifice 593.89
    congenital 753.4
  urethra 599.84
  urethral gland (Cowper's) 599.89
  uterine
    ligament 620.8
      embryonic 752.11
    tube 620.8
  uterus (body) (corpus) (recurrent) 621.8
    embryonal 752.39
  utricle (ear) 386.8
    prostatic 599.89
  utriculus masculinus 599.89
  vagina, vaginal (squamous cell) (wall) 623.8
    embryonal 752.41
    implantation 623.8
    inclusion 623.8
  vallecula, vallecular 478.79
  ventricle, neuroepithelial 348.0
  verumontanum 599.89
  vesical (orifice) 596.89
  vitreous humor 379.29
  vulva (sweat glands) 624.8
    congenital 752.41
    implantation 624.8
    inclusion 624.8
    sebaceous gland 624.8
  vulvovaginal gland 624.8
  wolffian 752.89
Cystadenocarcinoma (M8440/3) — see also Neoplasm, by site, malignant
  bile duct type (M8161/3) 155.1
  endometrioid (M8380/3) — see Neoplasm, by site, malignant

Cystadenocarcinoma — see also Neoplasm, by site, malignant — continued
  mucinous (M8470/3)
    papillary (M8471/3)
      specified site — see Neoplasm, by site, malignant
      unspecified site 183.0
    specified site — see Neoplasm, by site, malignant
    unspecified site 183.0
  papillary (M8450/3)
    mucinous (M8471/3)
      specified site — see Neoplasm, by site, malignant
      unspecified site 183.0
    pseudomucinous (M8471/3)
      specified site — see Neoplasm, by site, malignant
      unspecified site 183.0
    serous (M8460/3)
      specified site — see Neoplasm, by site, malignant
      unspecified site 183.0
    specified site — see Neoplasm, by site, malignant
    unspecified 183.0
  pseudomucinous (M8470/3)
    papillary (M8471/3)
      specified site — see Neoplasm, by site, malignant
      unspecified site 183.0
    specified site — see Neoplasm, by site, malignant
    unspecified site 183.0
  serous (M8441/3)
    papillary (M8460/3)
      specified site — see Neoplasm, by site, malignant
      unspecified site 183.0
    specified site — see Neoplasm, by site, malignant
    unspecified site 183.0
Cystadenofibroma (M9013/0)
  clear cell (M8313/0) — see Neoplasm, by site, benign
  endometrioid (M8381/0) 220
    borderline malignancy (M8381/1) 236.2
    malignant (M8381/3) 183.0
  mucinous (M9015/0)
    specified site — see Neoplasm, by site, benign
    unspecified site 220
  serous (M9014/0)
    specified site — see Neoplasm, by site, benign
    unspecified site 220
  specified site — see Neoplasm, by site, benign
  unspecified site 220
Cystadenoma (M8440/0) — see also Neoplasm, by site, benign
  bile duct (M8161/0) 211.5
  endometrioid (M8380/0) (see also Neoplasm, by site, benign)
    borderline malignancy (M8380/1) — see Neoplasm, by site, uncertain behavior
    malignant (M8440/3) — see Neoplasm, by site, malignant
  mucinous (M8470/0)
    borderline malignancy (M8470/1)
      specified site — see Neoplasm, uncertain behavior
      unspecified site 236.2
    papillary (M8471/0)
      borderline malignancy (M8471/1)
        specified site — see Neoplasm, by site, uncertain behavior
        unspecified site 236.2
      specified site — see Neoplasm, by site, benign
      unspecified site 220
    specified site — see Neoplasm, by site, benign
    unspecified site 220

Cystadenoma — see also Neoplasm, by site, benign — continued
  papillary (M8450/0)
    borderline malignancy (M8450/1)
      specified site — see Neoplasm, by site, uncertain behavior
      unspecified site 236.2
    lymphomatosum (M8561/0) 210.2
    mucinous (M8471/0)
      borderline malignancy (M8471/1)
        specified site — see Neoplasm, by site, uncertain behavior
        unspecified site 236.2
      specified site — see Neoplasm, by site, benign
      unspecified site 220
    pseudomucinous (M8471/0)
      borderline malignancy (M8471/1)
        specified site — see Neoplasm, by site, uncertain behavior
        unspecified site 236.2
      specified site — see Neoplasm, by site, benign
      unspecified site 220
    serous (M8460/0)
      borderline malignancy (M8460/1)
        specified site — see Neoplasm, by site, uncertain behavior
        unspecified site 236.2
      specified site — see Neoplasm, by site, benign
      unspecified site 220
    specified site — see Neoplasm, by site, benign
    unspecified site 220
  pseudomucinous (M8470/0)
    borderline malignancy (M8470/1)
      specified site — see Neoplasm, by site, uncertain behavior
      unspecified site 236.2
    papillary (M8471/0)
      borderline malignancy (M8471/1)
        specified site — see Neoplasm, by site, uncertain behavior
        unspecified site 236.2
      specified site — see Neoplasm, by site, benign
      unspecified site 220
    specified site — see Neoplasm, by site, benign
    unspecified site 220
  serous (M8441/0)
    borderline malignancy (M8441/1)
      specified site — see Neoplasm, by site, uncertain behavior
      unspecified site 236.2
    papillary (M8460/0)
      borderline malignancy (M8460/1)
        specified site — see Neoplasm, by site, uncertain behavior
        unspecified site 236.2
      specified site — see Neoplasm, by site, benign
      unspecified site 220
    specified site — see Neoplasm, by site, benign
    unspecified site 220
  thyroid 226
Cystathioninemia 270.4
Cystathioninuria 270.4
Cystic — see also condition
  breast, chronic 610.1
  corpora lutea 620.1
  degeneration, congenital
    brain 742.4
    kidney (see also Cystic, disease, kidney) 753.10
  disease
    breast, chronic 610.1
    kidney, congenital 753.10
      medullary 753.16
      multiple 753.19
      polycystic — see Polycystic, kidney
      single 753.11
      specified NEC 753.19
    liver, congenital 751.62

☑ **Additional Digit Required** — Refer to the Tabular List for Digit Selection   ⬙ **Subterms under main terms may continue to next column or page**

2014 ICD-9-CM   107

Cyst — Cystic

Cystic — *see also* condition — *continued*
  disease — *continued*
    lung 518.89
      congenital 748.4
    pancreas, congenital 751.7
    semilunar cartilage 717.5
  duct — *see* condition
  eyeball, congenital 743.03
  fibrosis (pancreas) 277.00
    with
      manifestations
        gastrointestinal 277.03
        pulmonary 277.02
        specified NEC 277.09
      meconium ileus 277.01
      pulmonary exacerbation 277.02
  hygroma (M9173/0) 228.1
  kidney, congenital 753.10
    medullary 753.16
    multiple 753.19
    polycystic — *see* Polycystic, kidney
    single 753.11
    specified NEC 753.19
  liver, congenital 751.62
  lung 518.89
    congenital 748.4
  mass — *see* Cyst
  mastitis, chronic 610.1
  ovary 620.2
  pancreas, congenital 751.7
Cysticerciasis 123.1
Cysticercosis (mammary) (subretinal) 123.1
Cysticercus 123.1
  cellulosae infestation 123.1
Cystinosis (malignant) 270.0
Cystinuria 270.0
Cystitis (bacillary) (colli) (diffuse) (exudative)
  (hemorrhagic) (purulent) (recurrent)
  (septic) (suppurative) (ulcerative) 595.9
  with
    abortion — *see* Abortion, by type, with
      urinary tract infection
    ectopic pregnancy (*see also* categories
      633.0–633.9) 639.8

Cystitis — *continued*
  with — *continued*
    fibrosis 595.1
    leukoplakia 595.1
    malakoplakia 595.1
    metaplasia 595.1
    molar pregnancy (*see also* categories
      630–632) 639.8
  actinomycotic 039.8 *[595.4]*
  acute 595.0
    of trigone 595.3
  allergic 595.89
  amebic 006.8 *[595.4]*
  bilharzial 120.9 *[595.4]*
  blennorrhagic (acute) 098.11
    chronic or duration of 2 months or more
      098.31
  bullous 595.89
  calculous 594.1
  chlamydial 099.53
  chronic 595.2
    interstitial 595.1
    of trigone 595.3
  complicating pregnancy, childbirth, or
    puerperium 646.6 ☑
    affecting fetus or newborn 760.1
  cystic(a) 595.81
  diphtheritic 032.84
  echinococcal
    granulosus 122.3 *[595.4]*
    multilocularis 122.6 *[595.4]*
  emphysematous 595.89
  encysted 595.81
  follicular 595.3
  following
    abortion 639.8
    ectopic or molar pregnancy 639.8
  gangrenous 595.89
  glandularis 595.89
  gonococcal (acute) 098.11
    chronic or duration of 2 months or more
      098.31
  incrusted 595.89
  interstitial 595.1

Cystitis — *continued*
  irradiation 595.82
  irritation 595.89
  malignant 595.89
  monilial 112.2
  of trigone 595.3
  panmural 595.1
  polyposa 595.89
  prostatic 601.3
  radiation 595.82
  Reiter's (abacterial) 099.3
  specified NEC 595.89
  subacute 595.2
  submucous 595.1
  syphilitic 095.8
  trichomoniasis 131.09
  tuberculous (*see also* Tuberculosis) 016.1 ☑
  ulcerative 595.1
Cystocele
  female (without uterine prolapse) 618.01
    with uterine prolapse 618.4
      complete 618.3
      incomplete 618.2
    lateral 618.02
    midline 618.01
    paravaginal 618.02
  in pregnancy or childbirth 654.4 ☑
    affecting fetus or newborn 763.89
    causing obstructed labor 660.2 ☑
      affecting fetus or newborn 763.1
  male 596.89
Cystoid
  cicatrix limbus 372.64
  degeneration macula 362.53
Cystolithiasis 594.1
Cystoma (M8440/0) — *see also* Neoplasm, by
  site, benign
  endometrial, ovary 617.1
  mucinous (M8470/0)
    specified site — *see* Neoplasm, by site,
      benign
    unspecified site 220

Cystoma — *see also* Neoplasm, by site, benign
  — *continued*
  serous (M8441/0)
    specified site — *see* Neoplasm, by site,
      benign
    unspecified site 220
  simple (ovary) 620.2
Cystoplegia 596.53
Cystoptosis 596.89
Cystopyelitis — *see also* Pyelitis 590.80
Cystorrhagia 596.89
Cystosarcoma phyllodes (M9020/1) 238.3
  benign (M9020/0) 217
  malignant (M9020/3) — *see* Neoplasm,
    breast, malignant
Cystostomy status V44.50
  with complication 596.83
    infection 596.81
    mechanical 596.82
    specified complication NEC 596.83
  appendico-vesicostomy V44.52
  cutaneous-vesicostomy V44.51
  specified type NEC V44.59
Cystourethritis — *see also* Urethritis 597.89
Cystourethrocele — *see also* Cystocele
  female (without uterine prolapse) 618.09
    with uterine prolapse 618.4
      complete 618.3
      incomplete 618.2
  male 596.89
Cytomegalic inclusion disease 078.5
  congenital 771.1
Cytomycosis, reticuloendothelial — *see also*
  Histoplasmosis, American 115.00
Cytopenia 289.9
  refractory
    with
      multilineage dysplasia (RCMD)
        238.72
      and ringed sideroblasts (RCMD-
        RS) 238.72

☑ Additional Digit Required — Refer to the Tabular List for Digit Selection

▽ Subterms under main terms may continue to next column or page

108

2014 ICD-9-CM

Cystic — Cytopenia

Index

D

Daae (-Finsen) disease (epidemic pleurodynia) 074.1

Dabney's grip 074.1

Da Costa's syndrome (neurocirculatory asthenia) 306.2

Dacryoadenitis, dacryadenitis 375.00
acute 375.01
chronic 375.02

Dacryocystitis 375.30
acute 375.32
chronic 375.42
neonatal 771.6
phlegmonous 375.33
syphilitic 095.8
congenital 090.0
trachomatous, active 076.1
late effect 139.1
tuberculous (see also Tuberculosis) 017.3 ☑

Dacryocystoblennorrhea 375.42

Dacryocystocele 375.43

Dacryolith, dacryolithiasis 375.57

Dacryoma 375.43

Dacryopericystitis (acute) (subacute) 375.32
chronic 375.42

Dacryops 375.11

Dacryosialadenopathy, atrophic 710.2

Dacryostenosis 375.56
congenital 743.65

Dactylitis
bone (see also Osteomyelitis) 730.2 ☑
sickle-cell 282.62
Hb-C 282.64
Hb-SS 282.62
specified NEC 282.69
syphilitic 095.5
tuberculous (see also Tuberculosis) 015.5 ☑

Dactylolysis spontanea 136.0

Dactylosymphysis — see also Syndactylism 755.10

Damage
arteriosclerotic — see Arteriosclerosis
brain 348.9
anoxic, hypoxic 348.1
during or resulting from a procedure 997.01
ischemic, in newborn 768.70
mild 768.71
moderate 768.72
severe 768.73
child NEC 343.9
due to birth injury 767.0
minimal (child) (see also Hyperkinesia) 314.9
newborn 767.0
cardiac (see also Disease, heart)
cardiorenal (vascular) (see also Hypertension, cardiorenal) 404.90
central nervous system — see Damage, brain
cerebral NEC — see Damage, brain
coccyx, complicating delivery 665.6 ☑
coronary (see also Ischemia, heart) 414.9
eye, birth injury 767.8
heart (see also Disease, heart)
valve — see Endocarditis
hypothalamus NEC 348.9
liver 571.9
alcoholic 571.3
medication 995.20
myocardium (see also Degeneration, myocardial) 429.1
pelvic
joint or ligament, during delivery 665.6 ☑
organ NEC
with
abortion — see Abortion, by type, with damage to pelvic organs
ectopic pregnancy (see also categories 633.0–633.9) 639.2
molar pregnancy (see also categories 630–632) 639.2
during delivery 665.5 ☑

Damage — continued
pelvic — continued
organ — continued
following
abortion 639.2
ectopic or molar pregnancy 639.2
renal (see also Disease, renal) 593.9
skin, solar 692.79
acute 692.72
chronic 692.74
subendocardium, subendocardial (see also Degeneration, myocardial) 429.1
vascular 459.9

Dameshek's syndrome (erythroblastic anemia) 282.49

Dana-Putnam syndrome (subacute combined sclerosis with pernicious anemia) 281.0 [336.2]

Danbolt (-Closs) syndrome (acrodermatitis enteropathica) 686.8

Dandruff 690.18

Dandy fever 061

Dandy-Walker deformity or syndrome (atresia, foramen of Magendie) 742.3
with spina bifida (see also Spina bifida) 741.0 ☑

Dangle foot 736.79

Danielssen's disease (anesthetic leprosy) 030.1

Danlos' syndrome 756.83

Darier's disease (congenital) (keratosis follicularis) 757.39
due to vitamin A deficiency 264.8
meaning erythema annulare centrifugum 695.0

Darier-Roussy sarcoid 135

Dark area on retina 239.81

Darling's
disease (see also Histoplasmosis, American) 115.00
histoplasmosis (see also Histoplasmosis, American) 115.00

Dartre 054.9

Darwin's tubercle 744.29

Davidson's anemia (refractory) 284.9

Davies-Colley syndrome (slipping rib) 733.99

Davies' disease 425.0

Dawson's encephalitis 046.2

Day blindness — see also Blindness, day 368.60

Dead
fetus
retained (in utero) 656.4 ☑
early pregnancy (death before 22 completed weeks gestation) 632
late (death after 22 completed weeks gestation) 656.4 ☑
syndrome 641.3 ☑
labyrinth 386.50
ovum, retained 631.8

Deaf and dumb NEC 389.7

Deaf mutism (acquired) (congenital) NEC 389.7
endemic 243
hysterical 300.11
syphilitic, congenital 090.0

Deafness (acquired) (complete) (congenital) (hereditary) (middle ear) (partial) 389.9
with
blindness V49.85
blue sclera and fragility of bone 756.51
auditory fatigue 389.9
aviation 993.0
nerve injury 951.5
boilermakers' 951.5
central 389.14
with conductive hearing loss 389.20
bilateral 389.22
unilateral 389.21
conductive (air) 389.00
with sensorineural hearing loss 389.20
bilateral 389.22
unilateral 389.21
bilateral 389.06
combined types 389.08
external ear 389.01

Deafness — continued
conductive — continued
inner ear 389.04
middle ear 389.03
multiple types 389.08
tympanic membrane 389.02
unilateral 389.05
emotional (complete) 300.11
functional (complete) 300.11
high frequency 389.8
hysterical (complete) 300.11
injury 951.5
low frequency 389.8
mental 784.69
mixed conductive and sensorineural 389.20
bilateral 389.22
unilateral 389.21
nerve
with conductive hearing loss 389.20
bilateral 389.22
unilateral 389.21
bilateral 389.12
unilateral 389.13
neural
with conductive hearing loss 389.20
bilateral 389.22
unilateral 389.21
bilateral 389.12
unilateral 389.13
noise-induced 388.12
nerve injury 951.5
nonspeaking 389.7
perceptive 389.10
with conductive hearing loss 389.20
bilateral 389.22
unilateral 389.21
central 389.14
neural
bilateral 389.12
unilateral 389.13
sensorineural 389.10
asymmetrical 389.16
bilateral 389.18
unilateral 389.15
sensory
bilateral 389.11
unilateral 389.17
psychogenic (complete) 306.7
sensorineural (see also Deafness, perceptive) 389.10
asymmetrical 389.16
bilateral 389.18
unilateral 389.15
sensory
with conductive hearing loss 389.20
bilateral 389.22
unilateral 389.21
bilateral 389.11
unilateral 389.17
specified type NEC 389.8
sudden NEC 388.2
syphilitic 094.89
transient ischemic 388.02
transmission — see Deafness, conductive
traumatic 951.5
word (secondary to organic lesion) 784.69
developmental 315.31

Death
after delivery (cause not stated) (sudden) 674.9 ☑
anesthetic
due to
correct substance properly administered 995.4
overdose or wrong substance given 968.4
specified anesthetic — see Table of Drugs and Chemicals
during delivery 668.9 ☑
brain 348.82
cardiac (sudden) (SCD) — code to underlying condition
family history of V17.41
personal history of, successfully resuscitated V12.53
cause unknown 798.2

Death — continued
cot (infant) 798.0
crib (infant) 798.0
fetus, fetal (cause not stated) (intrauterine) 779.9
early, with retention (before 22 completed weeks gestation) 632
from asphyxia or anoxia (before labor) 768.0
during labor 768.1
late, affecting management of pregnancy (after 22 completed weeks gestation) 656.4 ☑
from pregnancy NEC 646.9 ☑
instantaneous 798.1
intrauterine (see also Death, fetus) 779.9
complicating pregnancy 656.4 ☑
maternal, affecting fetus or newborn 761.6
neonatal NEC 779.9
sudden (cause unknown) 798.1
cardiac (SCD)
family history of V17.41
personal history of, successfully resuscitated V12.53
during delivery 669.9 ☑
under anesthesia NEC 668.9 ☑
infant, syndrome (SIDS) 798.0
puerperal, during puerperium 674.9 ☑
unattended (cause unknown) 798.9
under anesthesia NEC
due to
correct substance properly administered 995.4
overdose or wrong substance given 968.4
specified anesthetic — see Table of Drugs and Chemicals
during delivery 668.9 ☑
violent 798.1

de Beurmann-Gougerot disease (sporotrichosis) 117.1

Debility (general) (infantile) (postinfectional) 799.3
with nutritional difficulty 269.9
congenital or neonatal NEC 779.9
nervous 300.5
old age 797
senile 797

Débove's disease (splenomegaly) 789.2

Decalcification
bone (see also Osteoporosis) 733.00
teeth 521.89

Decapitation 874.9
fetal (to facilitate delivery) 763.89

Decapsulation, kidney 593.89

Decay
dental 521.00
senile 797
tooth, teeth 521.00

Decensus, uterus — see Prolapse, uterus

Deciduitis (acute)
with
abortion — see Abortion, by type, with sepsis
ectopic pregnancy (see also categories 633.0–633.9) 639.0
molar pregnancy (see also categories 630–632) 639.0
affecting fetus or newborn 760.8
following
abortion 639.0
ectopic or molar pregnancy 639.0
in pregnancy 646.6 ☑
puerperal, postpartum 670.1 ☑

Deciduoma malignum (M9100/3) 181

Deciduous tooth (retained) 520.6

Decline (general) — see also Debility 799.3

Decompensation
cardiac (acute) (chronic) (see also Disease, heart) 429.9
failure — see Failure, heart
cardiorenal (see also Hypertension, cardiorenal) 404.90
cardiovascular (see also Disease, cardiovascular) 429.2
heart (see also Disease, heart) 429.9

Decompensation — *continued*
  heart (*see also* Disease, heart) — *continued*
    failure — *see* Failure, heart
    hepatic 572.2
    myocardial (acute) (chronic) (*see also* Disease, heart) 429.9
      failure — *see* Failure, heart
    respiratory 519.9
Decompression sickness 993.3
Decrease, decreased
  blood
    platelets (*see also* Thrombocytopenia) 287.5
    pressure 796.3
      due to shock following
        injury 958.4
        operation 998.00
    white cell count 288.50
      specified NEC 288.59
  cardiac reserve — *see* Disease, heart
  estrogen 256.39
    postablative 256.2
  fetal movements 655.7 ☑
  fragility of erythrocytes 289.89
  function
    adrenal (cortex) 255.41
      medulla 255.5
    ovary in hypopituitarism 253.4
    parenchyma of pancreas 577.8
    pituitary (gland) (lobe) (anterior) 253.2
      posterior (lobe) 253.8
  functional activity 780.99
  glucose 790.29
  haptoglobin (serum) NEC 273.8
  leukocytes 288.50
  libido 799.81
  lymphocytes 288.51
  platelets (*see also* Thrombocytopenia) 287.5
  pulse pressure 785.9
  respiration due to shock following injury 958.4
  sexual desire 799.81
  tear secretion NEC 375.15
  tolerance
    fat 579.8
    salt and water 276.9
  vision NEC 369.9
  white blood cell count 288.50
Decubital gangrene — *see also* Ulcer, pressure 707.00 [785.4]
Decubiti — *see also* Ulcer, pressure 707.00
Decubitus (ulcer) — *see also* Ulcer, pressure 707.00
  with gangrene 707.00 [785.4]
  ankle 707.06
  back
    lower 707.03
    upper 707.02
  buttock 707.05
  coccyx 707.03
  elbow 707.01
  head 707.09
  heel 707.07
  hip 707.04
  other site 707.09
  sacrum 707.03
  shoulder blades 707.02
Deepening acetabulum 718.85
Defect, defective 759.9
  3-beta-hydroxysteroid dehydrogenase 255.2
  11-hydroxylase 255.2
  21-hydroxylase 255.2
  abdominal wall, congenital 756.70
  aorticopulmonary septum 745.0
  aortic septal 745.0
  atrial septal (ostium secundum type) 745.5
    acquired 429.71
    ostium primum type 745.61
    sinus venosus 745.8
  atrioventricular
    canal 745.69
    septum 745.4
      acquired 429.71
  atrium secundum 745.5
    acquired 429.71

Defect, defective — *continued*
  auricular septal 745.5
    acquired 429.71
  bilirubin excretion 277.4
  biosynthesis, testicular androgen 257.2
  bridge 525.60
  bulbar septum 745.0
  butanol-insoluble iodide 246.1
  chromosome — *see* Anomaly, chromosome
  circulation (acquired) 459.9
    congenital 747.9
    newborn 747.9
  clotting NEC (*see also* Defect, coagulation) 286.9
  coagulation (factor) (*see also* Deficiency, coagulation factor) 286.9
    with
      abortion — *see* Abortion, by type, with hemorrhage
      ectopic pregnancy (*see also* categories 634–638) 639.1
      molar pregnancy (*see also* categories 630–632) 639.1
    acquired (any) 286.7
    antepartum or intrapartum 641.3 ☑
      affecting fetus or newborn 762.1
    causing hemorrhage of pregnancy or delivery 641.3 ☑
    complicating pregnancy, childbirth, or puerperium 649.3 ☑
    due to
      liver disease 286.7
      vitamin K deficiency 286.7
    newborn, transient 776.3
    postpartum 666.3 ☑
    specified type NEC 286.9
  conduction (heart) 426.9
    bone (*see also* Deafness, conductive) 389.00
  congenital, organ or site NEC (*see also* Anomaly)
    circulation 747.9
    Descemet's membrane 743.9
      specified type NEC 743.49
    diaphragm 756.6
    ectodermal 757.9
    esophagus 750.9
    pulmonic cusps — *see* Anomaly, heart valve
    respiratory system 748.9
      specified type NEC 748.8
  crown 525.60
  cushion endocardial 745.60
  dental restoration 525.60
  dentin (hereditary) 520.5
  Descemet's membrane (congenital) 743.9
    acquired 371.30
    specific type NEC 743.49
  deutan 368.52
  developmental (*see also* Anomaly, by site)
    cauda equina 742.59
    left ventricle 746.9
      with atresia or hypoplasia of aortic orifice or valve, with hypoplasia of ascending aorta 746.7
      in hypoplastic left heart syndrome 746.7
    testis 752.9
    vessel 747.9
  diaphragm
    with elevation, eventration, or hernia — *see* Hernia, diaphragm
    congenital 756.6
      with elevation, eventration, or hernia 756.6
      gross (with elevation, eventration, or hernia) 756.6
  ectodermal, congenital 757.9
  Eisenmenger's (ventricular septal defect) 745.4
  endocardial cushion 745.60
    specified type NEC 745.69
  esophagus, congenital 750.9
  extensor retinaculum 728.9
  fibrin polymerization (*see also* Defect, coagulation) 286.3

Defect, defective — *continued*
  filling
    biliary tract 793.3
    bladder 793.5
    dental 525.60
    gallbladder 793.3
    kidney 793.5
    stomach 793.4
    ureter 793.5
  fossa ovalis 745.5
  gene, carrier (suspected) of V83.89
  Gerbode 745.4
  glaucomatous, without elevated tension 365.89
  Hageman (factor) (*see also* Defect, coagulation) 286.3
  hearing (*see also* Deafness) 389.9
  high grade 317
  homogentisic acid 270.2
  interatrial septal 745.5
    acquired 429.71
  interauricular septal 745.5
    acquired 429.71
  interventricular septal 745.4
    with pulmonary stenosis or atresia, dextraposition of aorta, and hypertrophy of right ventricle 745.2
    acquired 429.71
    in tetralogy of Fallot 745.2
  iodide trapping 246.1
  iodotyrosine dehalogenase 246.1
  kynureninase 270.2
  learning, specific 315.2
  major osseous 731.3
  mental (*see also* Disability, intellectual) 319
  osseous, major 731.3
  osteochondral NEC 738.8
  ostium
    primum 745.61
    secundum 745.5
  pericardium 746.89
  peroxidase-binding 246.1
  placental blood supply — *see* Placenta, insufficiency
  platelet (qualitative) 287.1
    constitutional 286.4
  postural, spine 737.9
  protan 368.51
  pulmonic cusps, congenital 746.00
  renal pelvis 753.9
    obstructive 753.29
    specified type NEC 753.3
  respiratory system, congenital 748.9
    specified type NEC 748.8
  retina, retinal 361.30
    with detachment (*see also* Detachment, retina, with retinal defect) 361.00
    multiple 361.33
      with detachment 361.02
    nerve fiber bundle 362.85
    single 361.30
      with detachment 361.01
  septal (closure) (heart) NEC 745.9
    acquired 429.71
    atrial 745.5
    specified type NEC 745.8
  speech NEC 784.59
    developmental 315.39
    late effect of cerebrovascular disease — *see* Late effect(s) (of) cerebrovascular disease, speech and language deficit
    secondary to organic lesion 784.59
  Taussig-Bing (transposition, aorta and overriding pulmonary artery) 745.11
  teeth, wedge 521.20
  thyroid hormone synthesis 246.1
  tritan 368.53
  ureter 753.9
    obstructive 753.29
  vascular (acquired) (local) 459.9
    congenital (peripheral) NEC 747.60
      gastrointestinal 747.61
      lower limb 747.64
      renal 747.62
      specified NEC 747.69

Defect, defective — *continued*
  vascular — *continued*
    congenital — *continued*
      spinal 747.82
      upper limb 747.63
    ventricular septal 745.4
      with pulmonary stenosis or atresia, dextraposition of aorta, and hypertrophy of right ventricle 745.2
      acquired 429.71
      atrioventricular canal type 745.69
      between infundibulum and anterior portion 745.4
      in tetralogy of Fallot 745.2
      isolated anterior 745.4
  vision NEC 369.9
  visual field 368.40
    arcuate 368.43
    heteronymous, bilateral 368.47
    homonymous, bilateral 368.46
    localized NEC 368.44
    nasal step 368.44
    peripheral 368.44
    sector 368.43
  voice and resonance 784.40
  wedge, teeth (abrasion) 521.20
Defeminization syndrome 255.2
Deferentitis 608.4
  gonorrheal (acute) 098.14
    chronic or duration of 2 months or over 098.34
Defibrination syndrome — *see also* Fibrinolysis 286.6
Deficiency, deficient
  3-beta-hydroxysteroid dehydrogenase 255.2
  6-phosphogluconic dehydrogenase (anemia) 282.2
  11-beta-hydroxylase 255.2
  17-alpha-hydroxylase 255.2
  18-hydroxysteroid dehydrogenase 255.2
  20-alpha-hydroxylase 255.2
  21-hydroxylase 255.2
  AAT (alpha-1 antitrypsin) 273.4
  abdominal muscle syndrome 756.79
  accelerator globulin (Ac G) (blood) (*see also* Defect, coagulation) 286.3
  AC globulin (congenital) (*see also* Defect, coagulation) 286.3
    acquired 286.7
  activating factor (blood) (*see also* Defect, coagulation) 286.3
  adenohypophyseal 253.2
  adenosine deaminase 277.2
  aldolase (hereditary) 271.2
  alpha-1-antitrypsin 273.4
  alpha-1-trypsin inhibitor 273.4
  alpha-fucosidase 271.8
  alpha-lipoprotein 272.5
  alpha-mannosidase 271.8
  amino acid 270.9
  anemia — *see* Anemia, deficiency
  aneurin 265.1
    with beriberi 265.0
  antibody NEC 279.00
  antidiuretic hormone 253.5
  antihemophilic
    factor (A) 286.0
      B 286.1
      C 286.2
    globulin (AHG) NEC 286.0
  antithrombin III 289.81
  antitrypsin 273.4
  argininosuccinate synthetase or lyase 270.6
  ascorbic acid (with scurvy) 267
  autoprothrombin
    I (*see also* Defect, coagulation) 286.3
    II 286.1
    C (*see also* Defect, coagulation) 286.3
  bile salt 579.8
  biotin 266.2
  biotinidase 277.6
  bradykinase-1 277.6
  brancher enzyme (amylopectinosis) 271.0
  calciferol 268.9
    with
      osteomalacia 268.2

Deficiency, deficient — *continued*
calciferol — *continued*
  with — *continued*
    rickets (*see also* Rickets) 268.0
calcium 275.40
  dietary 269.3
calorie, severe 261
carbamyl phosphate synthetase 270.6
cardiac (*see also* Insufficiency, myocardial) 428.0
carnitine 277.81
  due to
    hemodialysis 277.83
    inborn errors of metabolism 277.82
    valproic acid therapy 277.83
  iatrogenic 277.83
  palmitoyltransferase (CPT1, CPT2) 277.85
  palmityl transferase (CPT1, CPT2) 277.85
  primary 277.81
  secondary 277.84
carotene 264.9
Carr factor (*see also* Defect, coagulation) 286.9
central nervous system 349.9
ceruloplasmin 275.1
cevitamic acid (with scurvy) 267
choline 266.2
Christmas factor 286.1
chromium 269.3
citrin 269.1
clotting (blood) (*see also* Defect, coagulation) 286.9
coagulation factor NEC 286.9
  with
    abortion — *see* Abortion, by type, with hemorrhage
    ectopic pregnancy (*see also* categories 634–638) 639.1
    molar pregnancy (*see also* categories 630–632) 639.1
  acquired (any) 286.7
  antepartum or intrapartum 641.3 ☑
    affecting fetus or newborn 762.1
  complicating pregnancy, childbirth, or puerperium 649.3 ☑
  due to
    liver disease 286.7
    vitamin K deficiency 286.7
  newborn, transient 776.3
  postpartum 666.3 ☑
  specified type NEC 286.3
color vision (congenital) 368.59
  acquired 368.55
combined glucocorticoid and mineralocorticoid 255.41
combined, two or more coagulation factors (*see also* Defect, coagulation) 286.9
complement factor NEC 279.8
contact factor (*see also* Defect, coagulation) 286.3
copper NEC 275.1
corticoadrenal 255.41
craniofacial axis 756.0
cyanocobalamin (vitamin B_{12}) 266.2
debrancher enzyme (limit dextrinosis) 271.0
desmolase 255.2
diet 269.9
dihydrofolate reductase 281.2
dihydropteridine reductase 270.1
dihydropyrimidine dehydrogenase (DPD) 277.6
disaccharidase (intestinal) 271.3
disease NEC 269.9
ear(s) V48.8
edema 262
endocrine 259.9
enzymes, circulating NEC (*see also* Deficiency, by specific enzyme) 277.6
ergosterol 268.9
  with
    osteomalacia 268.2
    rickets (*see also* Rickets) 268.0
erythrocytic glutathione (anemia) 282.2
eyelid(s) V48.8
factor (*see also* Defect, coagulation) 286.9
  I (congenital) (fibrinogen) 286.3

Deficiency, deficient — *continued*
factor (*see also* Defect, coagulation) — *continued*
  I — *continued*
    antepartum or intrapartum 641.3 ☑
      affecting fetus or newborn 762.1
    newborn, transient 776.3
    postpartum 666.3 ☑
  II (congenital) (prothrombin) 286.3
  V (congenital) (labile) 286.3
  VII (congenital) (stable) 286.3
  VIII (congenital) (functional) 286.0
    with
      functional defect 286.0
      vascular defect 286.4
  IX (Christmas) (congenital) (functional) 286.1
  X (congenital) (Stuart-Prower) 286.3
  XI (congenital) (plasma thromboplastin antecedent) 286.2
  XII (congenital) (Hageman) 286.3
  XIII (congenital) (fibrin stabilizing) 286.3
  Hageman 286.3
  multiple (congenital) 286.9
    acquired 286.7
fibrinase (*see also* Defect, coagulation) 286.3
fibrinogen (congenital) (*see also* Defect, coagulation) 286.3
  acquired 286.6
fibrin-stabilizing factor (congenital) (*see also* Defect, coagulation) 286.3
finger — *see* Absence, finger
fletcher factor (*see also* Defect, coagulation) 286.9
fluorine 269.3
folate, anemia 281.2
folic acid (vitamin B_c) 266.2
  anemia 281.2
follicle-stimulating hormone (FSH) 253.4
fructokinase 271.2
fructose-1, 6-diphosphate 271.2
fructose-1-phosphate aldolase 271.2
FSH (follicle-stimulating hormone) 253.4
fucosidase 271.8
galactokinase 271.1
galactose-1-phosphate uridyl transferase 271.1
gamma globulin in blood 279.00
glass factor (*see also* Defect, coagulation) 286.3
glucocorticoid 255.41
glucose-6-phosphatase 271.0
glucose-6-phosphate dehydrogenase anemia 282.2
glucuronyl transferase 277.4
glutathione-reductase (anemia) 282.2
glycogen synthetase 271.0
growth hormone 253.3
Hageman factor (congenital) (*see also* Defect, coagulation) 286.3
head V48.0
hemoglobin (*see also* Anemia) 285.9
hepatophosphorylase 271.0
hexose monophosphate (HMP) shunt 282.2
HGH (human growth hormone) 253.3
HG-PRT 277.2
homogentisic acid oxidase 270.2
hormone (*see also* Deficiency, by specific hormone)
  anterior pituitary (isolated) (partial) NEC 253.4
    growth (human) 253.3
  follicle-stimulating 253.4
  growth (human) (isolated) 253.3
  human growth 253.3
  interstitial cell-stimulating 253.4
  luteinizing 253.4
  melanocyte-stimulating 253.4
  testicular 257.2
human growth hormone 253.3
humoral 279.00
  with
    hyper-IgM 279.05
      autosomal recessive 279.05
      X-linked 279.05
    increased IgM 279.05

Deficiency, deficient — *continued*
humoral — *continued*
  congenital hypogammaglobulinemia 279.04
    non-sex-linked 279.06
  selective immunoglobulin NEC 279.03
    IgA 279.01
    IgG 279.03
    IgM 279.02
      increased 279.05
  specified NEC 279.09
hydroxylase 255.2
hypoxanthine-guanine phosphoribosyltransferase (HG-PRT) 277.2
ICSH (interstitial cell-stimulating hormone) 253.4
immunity NEC 279.3
  cell-mediated 279.10
    with
      hyperimmunoglobulinemia 279.2
      thrombocytopenia and eczema 279.12
    specified NEC 279.19
  combined (severe) 279.2
    syndrome 279.2
  common variable 279.06
  humoral NEC 279.00
    IgA (secretory) 279.01
    IgG 279.03
    IgM 279.02
immunoglobulin, selective NEC 279.03
  IgA 279.01
  IgG 279.03
  IgM 279.02
inositol (B complex) 266.2
interferon 279.49
internal organ V47.0
interstitial cell-stimulating hormone (ICSH) 253.4
intrinsic factor (Castle's) (congenital) 281.0
intrinsic (urethral) sphincter (ISD) 599.82
invertase 271.3
iodine 269.3
iron, anemia 280.9
labile factor (congenital) (*see also* Defect, coagulation) 286.3
  acquired 286.7
lacrimal fluid (acquired) 375.15
  congenital 743.64
lactase 271.3
Laki-Lorand factor (*see also* Defect, coagulation) 286.3
lecithin-cholesterol acyltranferase 272.5
LH (luteinizing hormone) 253.4
limb V49.0
  lower V49.0
    congenital (*see also* Deficiency, lower limb, congenital) 755.30
  upper V49.0
    congenital (*see also* Deficiency, upper limb, congenital) 755.20
lipocaic 577.8
lipoid (high-density) 272.5
lipoprotein (familial) (high density) 272.5
liver phosphorylase 271.0
long chain 3-hydroxyacyl CoA dehydrogenase (LCHAD) 277.85
long chain/very long chain acyl CoA dehydrogenase (LCAD, VLCAD) 277.85
lower limb V49.0
  congenital 755.30
    with complete absence of distal elements 755.31
    longitudinal (complete) (partial) (with distal deficiencies, incomplete) 755.32
      with complete absence of distal elements 755.31
      combined femoral, tibial, fibular (incomplete) 755.33
      femoral 755.34
      fibular 755.37
      metatarsal(s) 755.38
      phalange(s) 755.39
        meaning all digits 755.31
      tarsal(s) 755.38

Deficiency, deficient — *continued*
lower limb — *continued*
  congenital — *continued*
    longitudinal — *continued*
      tibia 755.36
      tibiofibular 755.35
    transverse 755.31
luteinizing hormone (LH) 253.4
lysosomal alpha-1, 4 glucosidase 271.0
magnesium 275.2
mannosidase 271.8
medium chain acyl CoA dehydrogenase (MCAD) 277.85
melanocyte-stimulating hormone (MSH) 253.4
menadione (vitamin K) 269.0
  newborn 776.0
mental (familial) (hereditary) (*see also* Disability, intellectual) 319
methylenetetrahydrofolate reductase (MTHFR) 270.4
mineralocorticoid 255.42
mineral NEC 269.3
molybdenum 269.3
moral 301.7
multiple, syndrome 260
myocardial (*see also* Insufficiency, myocardial) 428.0
myophosphorylase 271.0
NADH-diaphorase or reductase (congenital) 289.7
NADH (DPNH)-methemoglobin-reductase (congenital) 289.7
neck V48.1
niacin (amide) (-tryptophan) 265.2
nicotinamide 265.2
nicotinic acid (amide) 265.2
nose V48.8
number of teeth (*see also* Anodontia) 520.0
nutrition, nutritional 269.9
  specified NEC 269.8
ornithine transcarbamylase 270.6
ovarian 256.39
oxygen (*see also* Anoxia) 799.02
pantothenic acid 266.2
parathyroid (gland) 252.1
phenylalanine hydroxylase 270.1
phosphoenolpyruvate carboxykinase 271.8
phosphofructokinase 271.2
phosphoglucomutase 271.0
phosphohexosisomerase 271.0
phosphomannomutase 271.8
phosphomannose isomerase 271.8
phosphomannosyl mutase 271.8
phosphorylase kinase, liver 271.0
pituitary (anterior) 253.2
  posterior 253.5
placenta — *see* Placenta, insufficiency
plasma
  cell 279.00
  protein (paraproteinemia) (pyroglobulinemia) 273.8
    gamma globulin 279.00
  thromboplastin
    antecedent (PTA) 286.2
    component (PTC) 286.1
platelet NEC 287.1
  constitutional 286.4
polyglandular 258.9
potassium (K) 276.8
proaccelerin (congenital) (*see also* Defect, congenital) 286.3
  acquired 286.7
proconvertin factor (congenital) (*see also* Defect, coagulation) 286.3
  acquired 286.7
prolactin 253.4
protein 260
  anemia 281.4
  C 289.81
  plasma — *see* Deficiency, plasma, protein
  S 289.81
prothrombin (congenital) (*see also* Defect, coagulation) 286.3
  acquired 286.7

Deficiency, deficient — *continued*
  Prower factor (*see also* Defect, coagulation) 286.3
  PRT 277.2
  pseudocholinesterase 289.89
  psychobiological 301.6
  PTA 286.2
  PTC 286.1
  purine nucleoside phosphorylase 277.2
  pyracin (alpha) (beta) 266.1
  pyridoxal 266.1
  pyridoxamine 266.1
  pyridoxine (derivatives) 266.1
  pyruvate carboxylase 271.8
  pyruvate dehydrogenase 271.8
  pyruvate kinase (PK) 282.3
  riboflavin (vitamin B_2) 266.0
  saccadic eye movements 379.57
  salivation 527.7
  salt 276.1
  secretion
    ovary 256.39
    salivary gland (any) 527.7
    urine 788.5
  selenium 269.3
  serum
    antitrypsin, familial 273.4
    protein (congenital) 273.8
  short chain acyl CoA dehydrogenase (SCAD) 277.85
  short stature homeobox gene (SHOX)
    with
      dyschondrosteosis 756.89
      short stature (idiopathic) 783.43
      Turner's syndrome 758.6
  smooth pursuit movements (eye) 379.58
  sodium (Na) 276.1
  SPCA (*see also* Defect, coagulation) 286.3
  specified NEC 269.8
  stable factor (congenital) (*see also* Defect, coagulation) 286.3
    acquired 286.7
  Stuart (-Prower) factor (*see also* Defect, coagulation) 286.3
  sucrase 271.3
  sucrase-isomaltase 271.3
  sulfite oxidase 270.0
  syndrome, multiple 260
  thiamine, thiaminic (chloride) 265.1
  thrombokinase (*see also* Defect, coagulation) 286.3
    newborn 776.0
  thrombopoieten 287.39
  thymolymphatic 279.2
  thyroid (gland) 244.9
  tocopherol 269.1
  toe — *see* Absence, toe
  tooth bud (*see also* Anodontia) 520.0
  trunk V48.1
  UDPG-glycogen transferase 271.0
  upper limb V49.0
    congenital 755.20
      with complete absence of distal elements 755.21
      longitudinal (complete) (partial) (with distal deficiencies, incomplete) 755.22
        carpal(s) 755.28
        combined humeral, radial, ulnar (incomplete) 755.23
        humeral 755.24
        metacarpal(s) 755.28
        phalange(s) 755.29
          meaning all digits 755.21
        radial 755.26
        radioulnar 755.25
        ulnar 755.27
      transverse (complete) (partial) 755.21
  vascular 459.9
  vasopressin 253.5
  viosterol (*see also* Deficiency, calciferol) 268.9
  vitamin (multiple) NEC 269.2
    A 264.9
      with
        Bitôt's spot 264.1

Deficiency, deficient — *continued*
  vitamin — *continued*
    A — *continued*
      with — *continued*
        Bitôt's spot — *continued*
          corneal 264.2
            with corneal ulceration 264.3
        keratomalacia 264.4
        keratosis, follicular 264.8
        night blindness 264.5
        scar of cornea, xerophthalmic 264.6
        specified manifestation NEC 264.8
          ocular 264.7
        xeroderma 264.8
        xerophthalmia 264.7
        xerosis
          conjunctival 264.0
            with Bitôt's spot 264.1
          corneal 264.2
            with corneal ulceration 264.3
    B_1 NEC 265.1
      beriberi 265.0
    B_2 266.0
    B_6 266.1
    B_{12} 266.2
    B_c (folic acid) 266.2
    B (complex) NEC 266.9
      with
        beriberi 265.0
        pellagra 265.2
      specified type NEC 266.2
    C (ascorbic acid) (with scurvy) 267
    D (calciferol) (ergosterol) 268.9
      with
        osteomalacia 268.2
        rickets (*see also* Rickets) 268.0
    E 269.1
    folic acid 266.2
    G 266.0
    H 266.2
    K 269.0
      of newborn 776.0
    nicotinic acid 265.2
    P 269.1
    PP 265.2
    specified NEC 269.1
  zinc 269.3
Deficient — *see also* Deficiency
  blink reflex 374.45
  craniofacial axis 756.0
  number of teeth (*see also* Anodontia) 520.0
  secretion of urine 788.5
Deficit
  attention 799.51
  cognitive communication 799.52
  concentration 799.51
  executive function 799.55
  frontal lobe 799.55
  neurologic NEC 781.99
    due to
      cerebrovascular lesion (*see also* Disease, cerebrovascular, acute) 436
      late effect — *see* Late effect(s) (of) cerebrovascular disease
      transient ischemic attack 435.9
    ischemic
      reversible (RIND) 434.91
        history of (personal) V12.54
      prolonged (PRIND) 434.91
        history of (personal) V12.54
  oxygen 799.02
  psychomotor 799.54
  visuospatial 799.53
Deflection
  radius 736.09
  septum (acquired) (nasal) (nose) 470
  spine — *see* Curvature, spine
  turbinate (nose) 470
Defluvium
  capillorum (*see also* Alopecia) 704.00
  ciliorum 374.55

Defluvium — *continued*
  unguium 703.8
Deformity 738.9
  abdomen, congenital 759.9
  abdominal wall
    acquired 738.8
    congenital 756.70
    muscle deficiency syndrome 756.79
  acquired (unspecified site) 738.9
    specified site NEC 738.8
  adrenal gland (congenital) 759.1
  alimentary tract, congenital 751.9
    lower 751.5
      specified type NEC 751.8
    upper (any part, except tongue) 750.9
      specified type NEC 750.8
      tongue 750.10
        specified type NEC 750.19
  ankle (joint) (acquired) 736.70
    abduction 718.47
    congenital 755.69
    contraction 718.47
    specified NEC 736.79
  anus (congenital) 751.5
    acquired 569.49
  aorta (congenital) 747.20
    acquired 447.8
    arch 747.21
      acquired 447.8
    coarctation 747.10
  aortic
    arch 747.21
      acquired 447.8
    cusp or valve (congenital) 746.9
      acquired (*see also* Endocarditis, aortic) 424.1
    ring 747.21
  appendix 751.5
  arm (acquired) 736.89
    congenital 755.50
  arteriovenous (congenital) (peripheral) NEC 747.60
    gastrointestinal 747.61
    lower limb 747.64
    renal 747.62
    specified NEC 747.69
    spinal 747.82
    upper limb 747.63
  artery (congenital) (peripheral) NEC (*see also* Deformity, vascular) 747.60
    acquired 447.8
    cerebral 747.81
    coronary (congenital) 746.85
      acquired (*see also* Ischemia, heart) 414.9
    retinal 743.9
    umbilical 747.5
  atrial septal (congenital) (heart) 745.5
  auditory canal (congenital) (external) (*see also* Deformity, ear) 744.3
    acquired 380.50
  auricle
    ear (congenital) (*see also* Deformity, ear) 744.3
      acquired 380.32
    heart (congenital) 746.9
  back (acquired) — *see* Deformity, spine
  Bartholin's duct (congenital) 750.9
  bile duct (congenital) 751.60
    acquired 576.8
      with calculus, choledocholithiasis, or stones — *see* Choledocholithiasis
  biliary duct or passage (congenital) 751.60
    acquired 576.8
      with calculus, choledocholithiasis, or stones — *see* Choledocholithiasis
  bladder (neck) (sphincter) (trigone) (acquired) 596.89
    congenital 753.9
  bone (acquired) NEC 738.9
    congenital 756.9
    turbinate 738.0
  boutonniere (finger) 736.21
  brain (congenital) 742.9

Deformity — *continued*
  brain — *continued*
    acquired 348.89
    multiple 742.4
    reduction 742.2
    vessel (congenital) 747.81
  breast (acquired) 611.89
    congenital 757.6
    reconstructed 612.0
  bronchus (congenital) 748.3
    acquired 519.19
  bursa, congenital 756.9
  canal of Nuck 752.9
  canthus (congenital) 743.9
    acquired 374.89
  capillary (acquired) 448.9
    congenital NEC (*see also* Deformity, vascular) 747.60
  cardiac — *see* Deformity, heart
  cardiovascular system (congenital) 746.9
  caruncle, lacrimal (congenital) 743.9
    acquired 375.69
  cascade, stomach 537.6
  cecum (congenital) 751.5
    acquired 569.89
  cerebral (congenital) 742.9
    acquired 348.89
  cervix (acquired) (uterus) 622.8
    congenital 752.40
  cheek (acquired) 738.19
    congenital 744.9
  chest (wall) (acquired) 738.3
    congenital 754.89
    late effect of rickets 268.1
  chin (acquired) 738.19
    congenital 744.9
  choroid (congenital) 743.9
    acquired 363.8
    plexus (congenital) 742.9
      acquired 349.2
  cicatricial — *see* Cicatrix
  cilia (congenital) 743.9
    acquired 374.89
  circulatory system (congenital) 747.9
  clavicle (acquired) 738.8
    congenital 755.51
  clitoris (congenital) 752.40
    acquired 624.8
  clubfoot — *see* Clubfoot
  coccyx (acquired) 738.6
    congenital 756.10
  colon (congenital) 751.5
    acquired 569.89
  concha (ear) (congenital) (*see also* Deformity, ear) 744.3
    acquired 380.32
  congenital, organ or site not listed (*see also* Anomaly) 759.9
  cornea (congenital) 743.9
    acquired 371.70
  coronary artery (congenital) 746.85
    acquired (*see also* Ischemia, heart) 414.9
  cranium (acquired) 738.19
    congenital (*see also* Deformity, skull, congenital) 756.0
  cricoid cartilage (congenital) 748.3
    acquired 478.79
  cystic duct (congenital) 751.60
    acquired 575.8
  Dandy-Walker 742.3
    with spina bifida (*see also* Spina bifida) 741.0 ☑
  diaphragm (congenital) 756.6
    acquired 738.8
  digestive organ(s) or system (congenital) NEC 751.9
    specified type NEC 751.8
  ductus arteriosus 747.0
  duodenal bulb 537.89
  duodenum (congenital) 751.5
    acquired 537.89
  dura (congenital) 742.9
    brain 742.4
      acquired 349.2
    spinal 742.59
      acquired 349.2

Index

Deficiency, deficient — Deformity

Deformity — continued
ear (congenital) 744.3
  acquired 380.32
  auricle 744.3
    causing impairment of hearing 744.02
  causing impairment of hearing 744.00
  external 744.3
    causing impairment of hearing 744.02
  internal 744.05
  lobule 744.3
  middle 744.03
    ossicles 744.04
  ossicles 744.04
ectodermal (congenital) NEC 757.9
  specified type NEC 757.8
ejaculatory duct (congenital) 752.9
  acquired 608.89
elbow (joint) (acquired) 736.00
  congenital 755.50
  contraction 718.42
endocrine gland NEC 759.2
epididymis (congenital) 752.9
  acquired 608.89
  torsion 608.24
epiglottis (congenital) 748.3
  acquired 478.79
esophagus (congenital) 750.9
  acquired 530.89
Eustachian tube (congenital) NEC 744.3
  specified type NEC 744.24
extremity (acquired) 736.9
  congenital, except reduction deformity 755.9
    lower 755.60
    upper 755.50
  reduction — see Deformity, reduction
eye (congenital) 743.9
  acquired 379.8
  muscle 743.9
eyebrow (congenital) 744.89
eyelid (congenital) 743.9
  acquired 374.89
  specified type NEC 743.62
face (acquired) 738.19
  congenital (any part) 744.9
    due to intrauterine malposition and pressure 754.0
fallopian tube (congenital) 752.10
  acquired 620.8
femur (acquired) 736.89
  congenital 755.60
fetal
  with fetopelvic disproportion 653.7 ☑
    affecting fetus or newborn 763.1
    causing obstructed labor 660.1 ☑
      affecting fetus or newborn 763.1
  known or suspected, affecting management of pregnancy 655.9 ☑
finger (acquired) 736.20
  boutonniere type 736.21
  congenital 755.50
  flexion contracture 718.44
  swan neck 736.22
flexion (joint) (acquired) 736.9
  congenital NEC 755.9
  hip or thigh (acquired) 736.39
    congenital (see also Subluxation, congenital, hip) 754.32
foot (acquired) 736.70
  cavovarus 736.75
    congenital 754.59
  congenital NEC 754.70
    specified type NEC 754.79
  valgus (acquired) 736.79
    congenital 754.60
      specified type NEC 754.69
  varus (acquired) 736.79
    congenital 754.50
      specified type NEC 754.59
forearm (acquired) 736.00
  congenital 755.50
forehead (acquired) 738.19
  congenital (see also Deformity, skull, congenital) 756.0

Deformity — continued
frontal bone (acquired) 738.19
  congenital (see also Deformity, skull, congenital) 756.0
gallbladder (congenital) 751.60
  acquired 575.8
gastrointestinal tract (congenital) NEC 751.9
  acquired 569.89
  specified type NEC 751.8
genitalia, genital organ(s) or system NEC
  congenital 752.9
  female (congenital) 752.9
    acquired 629.89
    external 752.40
    internal 752.9
  male (congenital) 752.9
    acquired 608.89
globe (eye) (congenital) 743.9
  acquired 360.89
gum (congenital) 750.9
  acquired 523.9
gunstock 736.02
hand (acquired) 736.00
  claw 736.06
  congenital 755.50
  minus (and plus) (intrinsic) 736.09
  pill roller (intrinsic) 736.09
  plus (and minus) (intrinsic) 736.09
  swan neck (intrinsic) 736.09
head (acquired) 738.10
  congenital (see also Deformity, skull, congenital) 756.0
  specified NEC 738.19
heart (congenital) 746.9
  auricle (congenital) 746.9
  septum 745.9
    auricular 745.5
    specified type NEC 745.8
    ventricular 745.4
  valve (congenital) NEC 746.9
    acquired — see Endocarditis
    pulmonary (congenital) 746.00
    specified type NEC 746.89
  ventricle (congenital) 746.9
heel (acquired) 736.76
  congenital 755.67
hepatic duct (congenital) 751.60
  acquired 576.8
    with calculus, choledocholithiasis, or stones — see Choledocholithiasis
hip (joint) (acquired) 736.30
  congenital NEC 755.63
  flexion 718.45
    congenital (see also Subluxation, congenital, hip) 754.32
hourglass — see Contraction, hourglass
humerus (acquired) 736.89
  congenital 755.50
hymen (congenital) 752.40
hypophyseal (congenital) 759.2
ileocecal (coil) (valve) (congenital) 751.5
  acquired 569.89
ileum (intestine) (congenital) 751.5
  acquired 569.89
ilium (acquired) 738.6
  congenital 755.60
integument (congenital) 757.9
intervertebral cartilage or disc (acquired) (see also Displacement, intervertebral disc)
  congenital 756.10
intestine (large) (small) (congenital) 751.5
  acquired 569.89
iris (acquired) 364.75
  congenital 743.9
  prolapse 364.89
ischium (acquired) 738.6
  congenital 755.60
jaw (acquired) (congenital) NEC 524.9
  due to intrauterine malposition and pressure 754.0
joint (acquired) NEC 738.8
  congenital 755.9

Deformity — continued
joint — continued
  contraction (abduction) (adduction) (extension) (flexion) — see Contraction, joint
kidney(s) (calyx) (pelvis) (congenital) 753.9
  acquired 593.89
  vessel 747.62
    acquired 459.9
Klippel-Feil (brevicollis) 756.16
knee (acquired) NEC 736.6
  congenital 755.64
labium (majus) (minus) (congenital) 752.40
  acquired 624.8
lacrimal apparatus or duct (congenital) 743.9
  acquired 375.69
larynx (muscle) (congenital) 748.3
  acquired 478.79
  web (glottic) (subglottic) 748.2
leg (lower) (upper) (acquired) NEC 736.89
  congenital 755.60
  reduction — see Deformity, reduction, lower limb
lens (congenital) 743.9
  acquired 379.39
lid (fold) (congenital) 743.9
  acquired 374.89
ligament (acquired) 728.9
  congenital 756.9
limb (acquired) 736.9
  congenital, except reduction deformity 755.9
    lower 755.60
      reduction (see also Deformity, reduction, lower limb) 755.30
    upper 755.50
      reduction (see also Deformity, reduction, upper limb) 755.20
  specified NEC 736.89
lip (congenital) NEC 750.9
  acquired 528.5
  specified type NEC 750.26
liver (congenital) 751.60
  acquired 573.8
  duct (congenital) 751.60
    acquired 576.8
      with calculus, choledocholithiasis, or stones — see Choledocholithiasis
lower extremity — see Deformity, leg
lumbosacral (joint) (region) (congenital) 756.10
  acquired 738.5
lung (congenital) 748.60
  acquired 518.89
  specified type NEC 748.69
lymphatic system, congenital 759.9
Madelung's (radius) 755.54
maxilla (acquired) (congenital) 524.9
meninges or membrane (congenital) 742.9
  brain 742.4
    acquired 349.2
  spinal (cord) 742.59
    acquired 349.2
mesentery (congenital) 751.9
  acquired 568.89
metacarpus (acquired) 736.00
  congenital 755.50
metatarsus (acquired) 736.70
  congenital 754.70
middle ear, except ossicles (congenital) 744.03
  ossicles 744.04
mitral (leaflets) (valve) (congenital) 746.9
  acquired — see Endocarditis, mitral
  Ebstein's 746.89
  parachute 746.5
  specified type NEC 746.89
  stenosis, congenital 746.5
mouth (acquired) 528.9
  congenital NEC 750.9
    specified type NEC 750.26
multiple, congenital NEC 759.7

Deformity — continued
multiple, congenital — continued
  specified type NEC 759.89
muscle (acquired) 728.9
  congenital 756.9
    specified type NEC 756.89
    sternocleidomastoid (due to intrauterine malposition and pressure) 754.1
musculoskeletal system, congenital NEC 756.9
  specified type NEC 756.9
nail (acquired) 703.9
  congenital 757.9
nasal — see Deformity, nose
neck (acquired) NEC 738.2
  congenital (any part) 744.9
    sternocleidomastoid 754.1
nervous system (congenital) 742.9
nipple (congenital) 757.6
  acquired 611.89
nose, nasal (cartilage) (acquired) 738.0
  bone (turbinate) 738.0
  congenital 748.1
    bent 754.0
    squashed 754.0
  saddle 738.0
    syphilitic 090.5
  septum 470
    congenital 748.1
  sinus (wall) (congenital) 748.1
    acquired 738.0
  syphilitic (congenital) 090.5
    late 095.8
ocular muscle (congenital) 743.9
  acquired 378.60
opticociliary vessels (congenital) 743.9
orbit (congenital) (eye) 743.9
  acquired NEC 376.40
    associated with craniofacial deformities 376.44
    due to
      bone disease 376.43
      surgery 376.47
      trauma 376.47
organ of Corti (congenital) 744.05
ovary (congenital) 752.0
  acquired 620.8
oviduct (congenital) 752.10
  acquired 620.8
palate (congenital) 750.9
  acquired 526.89
  cleft (congenital) (see also Cleft, palate) 749.00
  hard, acquired 526.89
  soft, acquired 528.9
pancreas (congenital) 751.7
  acquired 577.8
parachute, mitral valve 746.5
parathyroid (gland) 759.2
parotid (gland) (congenital) 750.9
  acquired 527.8
patella (acquired) 736.6
  congenital 755.64
pelvis, pelvic (acquired) (bony) 738.6
  with disproportion (fetopelvic) 653.0 ☑
    affecting fetus or newborn 763.1
    causing obstructed labor 660.1 ☑
      affecting fetus or newborn 763.1
  congenital 755.60
  rachitic (late effect) 268.1
penis (glans) (congenital) 752.9
  acquired 607.89
pericardium (congenital) 746.9
  acquired — see Pericarditis
pharynx (congenital) 750.9
  acquired 478.29
Pierre Robin (congenital) 756.0
pinna (acquired) 380.32
  congenital 744.3
pituitary (congenital) 759.2
pleural folds (congenital) 748.8
portal vein (congenital) 747.40
posture — see Curvature, spine
prepuce (congenital) 752.9
  acquired 607.89

☑ Additional Digit Required — Refer to the Tabular List for Digit Selection
▽ Subterms under main terms may continue to next column or page

2014 ICD-9-CM
113

Deformity — *continued*
- prostate (congenital) 752.9
  - acquired 602.8
- pulmonary valve — *see* Endocarditis, pulmonary
- pupil (congenital) 743.9
  - acquired 364.75
- pylorus (congenital) 750.9
  - acquired 537.89
- rachitic (acquired), healed or old 268.1
- radius (acquired) 736.00
  - congenital 755.50
    - reduction — *see* Deformity, reduction, upper limb
- rectovaginal septum (congenital) 752.40
  - acquired 623.8
- rectum (congenital) 751.5
  - acquired 569.49
- reduction (extremity) (limb) 755.4
  - brain 742.2
  - lower limb 755.30
    - with complete absence of distal elements 755.31
    - longitudinal (complete) (partial) (with distal deficiencies, incomplete) 755.32
      - with complete absence of distal elements 755.31
      - combined femoral, tibial, fibular (incomplete) 755.33
      - femoral 755.34
      - fibular 755.37
      - metatarsal(s) 755.38
      - phalange(s) 755.39
        - meaning all digits 755.31
      - tarsal(s) 755.38
      - tibia 755.36
      - tibiofibular 755.35
    - transverse 755.31
  - upper limb 755.20
    - with complete absence of distal elements 755.21
    - longitudinal (complete) (partial) (with distal deficiencies, incomplete) 755.22
      - with complete absence of distal elements 755.21
      - carpal(s) 755.28
      - combined humeral, radial, ulnar (incomplete) 755.23
      - humeral 755.24
      - metacarpal(s) 755.28
      - phalange(s) 755.29
        - meaning all digits 755.21
      - radial 755.26
      - radioulnar 755.25
      - ulnar 755.27
    - transverse (complete) (partial) 755.21
- renal — *see* Deformity, kidney
- respiratory system (congenital) 748.9
  - specified type NEC 748.8
- rib (acquired) 738.3
  - congenital 756.3
    - cervical 756.2
- rotation (joint) (acquired) 736.9
  - congenital 755.9
  - hip or thigh 736.39
    - congenital (*see also* Subluxation, congenital, hip) 754.32
- sacroiliac joint (congenital) 755.69
  - acquired 738.5
- sacrum (acquired) 738.5
  - congenital 756.10
- saddle
  - back 737.8
  - nose 738.0
    - syphilitic 090.5
- salivary gland or duct (congenital) 750.9
  - acquired 527.8
- scapula (acquired) 736.89
  - congenital 755.50
- scrotum (congenital) 752.9
  - acquired 608.89
- sebaceous gland, acquired 706.8
- seminal tract or duct (congenital) 752.9
  - acquired 608.89

Deformity — *continued*
- septum (nasal) (acquired) 470
  - congenital 748.1
- shoulder (joint) (acquired) 736.89
  - congenital 755.50
    - specified type NEC 755.59
  - contraction 718.41
- sigmoid (flexure) (congenital) 751.5
  - acquired 569.89
- sinus of Valsalva 747.29
- skin (congenital) 757.9
  - acquired NEC 709.8
- skull (acquired) 738.19
  - congenital 756.0
    - with
      - anencephalus 740.0
      - encephalocele 742.0
      - hydrocephalus 742.3
        - with spina bifida (*see also* Spina bifida) 741.0 ☑
      - microcephalus 742.1
    - due to intrauterine malposition and pressure 754.0
- soft parts, organs or tissues (of pelvis)
  - in pregnancy or childbirth NEC 654.9 ☑
    - affecting fetus or newborn 763.89
    - causing obstructed labor 660.2 ☑
      - affecting fetus or newborn 763.1
- spermatic cord (congenital) 752.9
  - acquired 608.89
    - torsion 608.22
      - extravaginal 608.21
      - intravaginal 608.22
- spinal
  - column — *see* Deformity, spine
  - cord (congenital) 742.9
    - acquired 336.8
    - vessel (congenital) 747.82
  - nerve root (congenital) 742.9
    - acquired 724.9
- spine (acquired) NEC 738.5
  - congenital 756.10
    - due to intrauterine malposition and pressure 754.2
  - kyphoscoliotic (*see also* Kyphoscoliosis) 737.30
  - kyphotic (*see also* Kyphosis) 737.10
  - lordotic (*see also* Lordosis) 737.20
  - rachitic 268.1
  - scoliotic (*see also* Scoliosis) 737.30
- spleen
  - acquired 289.59
  - congenital 759.0
- Sprengel's (congenital) 755.52
- sternum (acquired) 738.3
  - congenital 756.3
- stomach (congenital) 750.9
  - acquired 537.89
- submaxillary gland (congenital) 750.9
  - acquired 527.8
- swan neck (acquired)
  - finger 736.22
  - hand 736.09
- talipes — *see* Talipes
- teeth, tooth NEC 520.9
- testis (congenital) 752.9
  - acquired 608.89
    - torsion 608.20
- thigh (acquired) 736.89
  - congenital 755.60
- thorax (acquired) (wall) 738.3
  - congenital 754.89
  - late effect of rickets 268.1
- thumb (acquired) 736.20
  - congenital 755.50
- thymus (tissue) (congenital) 759.2
- thyroid (gland) (congenital) 759.2
  - cartilage 748.3
    - acquired 478.79
- tibia (acquired) 736.89
  - congenital 755.60
  - saber 090.5
- toe (acquired) 735.9
  - congenital 755.66
  - specified NEC 735.8
- tongue (congenital) 750.10

Deformity — *continued*
- tongue — *continued*
  - acquired 529.8
- tooth, teeth NEC 520.9
- trachea (rings) (congenital) 748.3
  - acquired 519.19
- transverse aortic arch (congenital) 747.21
- tricuspid (leaflets) (valve) (congenital) 746.9
  - acquired — *see* Endocarditis, tricuspid
  - atresia or stenosis 746.1
  - specified type NEC 746.89
- trunk (acquired) 738.3
  - congenital 759.9
- ulna (acquired) 736.00
  - congenital 755.50
- upper extremity — *see* Deformity, arm
- urachus (congenital) 753.7
- ureter (opening) (congenital) 753.9
  - acquired 593.89
- urethra (valve) (congenital) 753.9
  - acquired 599.84
- urinary tract or system (congenital) 753.9
  - urachus 753.7
- uterus (congenital) 752.39
  - acquired 621.8
- uvula (congenital) 750.9
  - acquired 528.9
- vagina (congenital) 752.40
  - acquired 623.8
- valve, valvular (heart) (congenital) 746.9
  - acquired — *see* Endocarditis
  - pulmonary 746.00
  - specified type NEC 746.89
- vascular (congenital) (peripheral) NEC 747.60
  - acquired 459.9
  - gastrointestinal 747.61
  - lower limb 747.64
  - renal 747.62
  - specified site NEC 747.69
  - spinal 747.82
  - upper limb 747.63
- vas deferens (congenital) 752.9
  - acquired 608.89
- vein (congenital) NEC (*see also* Deformity, vascular) 747.60
  - brain 747.81
  - coronary 746.9
  - great 747.40
- vena cava (inferior) (superior) (congenital) 747.40
- vertebra — *see* Deformity, spine
- vesicourethral orifice (acquired) 596.89
  - congenital NEC 753.9
    - specified type NEC 753.8
- vessels of optic papilla (congenital) 743.9
- visual field (contraction) 368.45
- vitreous humor (congenital) 743.9
  - acquired 379.29
- vulva (congenital) 752.40
  - acquired 624.8
- wrist (joint) (acquired) 736.00
  - congenital 755.50
  - contraction 718.43
  - valgus 736.03
    - congenital 755.59
  - varus 736.04
    - congenital 755.59

Degeneration, degenerative
- adrenal (capsule) (gland) 255.8
  - with hypofunction 255.41
  - fatty 255.8
  - hyaline 255.8
  - infectional 255.8
  - lardaceous 277.39
- amyloid (any site) (general) 277.39
- anterior cornua, spinal cord 336.8
- anterior labral 840.8
- aorta, aortic 440.0
  - fatty 447.8
  - valve (heart) (*see also* Endocarditis, aortic) 424.1
- arteriovascular — *see* Arteriosclerosis
- artery, arterial (atheromatous) (calcareous) (*see also* Arteriosclerosis)
  - amyloid 277.39

Degeneration, degenerative — *continued*
- artery, arterial (*see also* Arteriosclerosis) — *continued*
  - lardaceous 277.39
  - medial NEC (*see also* Arteriosclerosis, extremities) 440.20
- articular cartilage NEC (*see also* Disorder, cartilage, articular) 718.0 ☑
  - elbow 718.02
  - knee 717.5
  - patella 717.7
  - shoulder 718.01
  - spine (*see also* Spondylosis) 721.90
- atheromatous — *see* Arteriosclerosis
- bacony (any site) 277.39
- basal nuclei or ganglia NEC 333.0
- bone 733.90
- brachial plexus 353.0
- brain (cortical) (progressive) 331.9
  - arteriosclerotic 437.0
  - childhood 330.9
    - specified type NEC 330.8
  - congenital 742.4
  - cystic 348.0
    - congenital 742.4
  - familial NEC 331.89
  - grey matter 330.8
  - heredofamilial NEC 331.89
  - in
    - alcoholism 303.9 ☑ *[331.7]*
    - beriberi 265.0 *[331.7]*
    - cerebrovascular disease 437.9 *[331.7]*
    - congenital hydrocephalus 742.3 *[331.7]*
      - with spina bifida (*see also* Spina bifida) 741.0 ☑ *[331.7]*
    - Fabry's disease 272.7 *[330.2]*
    - Gaucher's disease 272.7 *[330.2]*
    - Hunter's disease or syndrome 277.5 *[330.3]*
    - lipidosis
      - cerebral 330.1
      - generalized 272.7 *[330.2]*
    - mucopolysaccharidosis 277.5 *[330.3]*
    - myxedema (*see also* Myxedema) 244.9 *[331.7]*
    - neoplastic disease NEC (M8000/1) 239.9 *[331.7]*
    - Niemann-Pick disease 272.7 *[330.2]*
    - sphingolipidosis 272.7 *[330.2]*
    - vitamin B_{12} deficiency 266.2 *[331.7]*
  - motor centers 331.89
  - senile 331.2
  - specified type NEC 331.89
- breast — *see* Disease, breast
- Bruch's membrane 363.40
- bundle of His 426.50
  - left 426.3
  - right 426.4
- calcareous NEC 275.49
- capillaries 448.9
  - amyloid 277.39
  - fatty 448.9
  - lardaceous 277.39
- cardiac (brown) (calcareous) (fatty) (fibrous) (hyaline) (mural) (muscular) (pigmentary) (senile) (with arteriosclerosis) (*see also* Degeneration, myocardial) 429.1
  - valve, valvular — *see* Endocarditis
- cardiorenal (*see also* Hypertension, cardiorenal) 404.90
- cardiovascular (*see also* Disease, cardiovascular) 429.2
  - renal (*see also* Hypertension, cardiorenal) 404.90
- cartilage (joint) — *see* Derangement, joint
- cerebellar NEC 334.9
  - primary (hereditary) (sporadic) 334.2
- cerebral — *see* Degeneration, brain
- cerebromacular 330.1
- cerebrovascular 437.1
  - due to hypertension 437.2
  - late effect — *see* Late effect(s) (of) cerebrovascular disease
- cervical plexus 353.2

Degeneration, degenerative — *continued*
cervix 622.8
  due to radiation (intended effect) 622.8
    adverse effect or misadventure 622.8
changes, spine or vertebra (*see also* Spondylosis) 721.90
chitinous 277.39
chorioretinal 363.40
  congenital 743.53
  hereditary 363.50
choroid (colloid) (drusen) 363.40
  hereditary 363.50
  senile 363.41
  diffuse secondary 363.42
cochlear 386.8
collateral ligament (knee) (medial) 717.82
  lateral 717.81
combined (spinal cord) (subacute) 266.2 *[336.2]*
  with anemia (pernicious) 281.0 *[336.2]*
    due to dietary deficiency 281.1 *[336.2]*
    due to vitamin B$_{12}$ deficiency anemia (dietary) 281.1 *[336.2]*
conjunctiva 372.50
  amyloid 277.39 *[372.50]*
cornea 371.40
  calcarous 371.44
  familial (hereditary) (*see also* Dystrophy, cornea) 371.50
    macular 371.55
    reticular 371.54
  hyaline (of old scars) 371.41
  marginal (Terrien's) 371.48
  mosaic (shagreen) 371.41
  nodular 371.46
  peripheral 371.48
  senile 371.41
cortical (cerebellar) (parenchymatous) 334.2
  alcoholic 303.9 ☑ *[334.4]*
  diffuse, due to arteriopathy 437.0
corticobasal 331.6
corticostriatal-spinal 334.8
cretinoid 243
cruciate ligament (knee) (posterior) 717.84
  anterior 717.83
cutis 709.3
  amyloid 277.39
dental pulp 522.2
disc disease — *see* Degeneration, intervertebral disc
dorsolateral (spinal cord) — *see* Degeneration, combined
endocardial 424.90
extrapyramidal NEC 333.90
eye NEC 360.40
  macular (*see also* Degeneration, macula) 362.50
    congenital 362.75
    hereditary 362.76
fatty (diffuse) (general) 272.8
  liver 571.8
    alcoholic 571.0
  localized site — *see* Degeneration, by site, fatty
  placenta — *see* Placenta, abnormal
globe (eye) NEC 360.40
  macular — *see* Degeneration, macula
grey matter 330.8
heart (brown) (calcareous) (fatty) (fibrous) (hyaline) (mural) (muscular) (pigmentary) (senile) (with arteriosclerosis) (*see also* Degeneration, myocardial) 429.1
  amyloid 277.39 *[425.7]*
  atheromatous — *see* Arteriosclerosis, coronary
  gouty 274.82
  hypertensive (*see also* Hypertension, heart) 402.90
  ischemic 414.9
  valve, valvular — *see* Endocarditis
hepatolenticular (Wilson's) 275.1
hepatorenal 572.4
heredofamilial
  brain NEC 331.89

Degeneration, degenerative — *continued*
heredofamilial — *continued*
  spinal cord NEC 336.8
hyaline (diffuse) (generalized) 728.9
  localized (*see also* Degeneration, by site)
    cornea 371.41
    keratitis 371.41
hypertensive vascular — *see* Hypertension
infrapatellar fat pad 729.31
internal semilunar cartilage 717.3
intervertebral disc 722.6
  with myelopathy 722.70
  cervical, cervicothoracic 722.4
    with myelopathy 722.71
  lumbar, lumbosacral 722.52
    with myelopathy 722.73
  thoracic, thoracolumbar 722.51
    with myelopathy 722.72
intestine 569.89
  amyloid 277.39
  lardaceous 277.39
iris (generalized) (*see also* Atrophy, iris) 364.59
  pigmentary 364.53
  pupillary margin 364.54
ischemic — *see* Ischemia
joint disease (*see also* Osteoarthrosis) 715.9 ☑
  multiple sites 715.09
  spine (*see also* Spondylosis) 721.90
kidney (*see also* Sclerosis, renal) 587
  amyloid 277.39 *[583.81]*
  cyst, cystic (multiple) (solitary) 593.2
    congenital (*see also* Cystic, disease, kidney) 753.10
  fatty 593.89
  fibrocystic (congenital) 753.19
  lardaceous 277.39 *[583.81]*
  polycystic (congenital) 753.12
    adult type (APKD) 753.13
    autosomal dominant 753.13
    autosomal recessive 753.14
    childhood type (CPKD) 753.14
    infantile type 753.14
  waxy 277.39 *[583.81]*
Kuhnt-Junius (retina) 362.52
labyrinth, osseous 386.8
lacrimal passages, cystic 375.12
lardaceous (any site) 277.39
lateral column (posterior), spinal cord (*see also* Degeneration, combined) 266.2 *[336.2]*
lattice 362.63
lens 366.9
  infantile, juvenile, or presenile 366.00
  senile 366.10
lenticular (familial) (progressive) (Wilson's) (with cirrhosis of liver) 275.1
  striate artery 437.0
lethal ball, prosthetic heart valve 996.02
ligament
  collateral (knee) (medial) 717.82
    lateral 717.81
  cruciate (knee) (posterior) 717.84
    anterior 717.83
liver (diffuse) 572.8
  amyloid 277.39
  congenital (cystic) 751.62
  cystic 572.8
    congenital 751.62
  fatty 571.8
    alcoholic 571.0
  hypertrophic 572.8
  lardaceous 277.39
  parenchymatous, acute or subacute (*see also* Necrosis, liver) 570
  pigmentary 572.8
  toxic (acute) 573.8
  waxy 277.39
lung 518.89
lymph gland 289.3
  hyaline 289.3
  lardaceous 277.39
macula (acquired) (senile) 362.50
  atrophic 362.51
  Best's 362.76

Degeneration, degenerative — *continued*
macula — *continued*
  congenital 362.75
  cystic 362.54
  cystoid 362.53
  disciform 362.52
  dry 362.51
  exudative 362.52
  familial pseudoinflammatory 362.77
  hereditary 362.76
  hole 362.54
  juvenile (Stargardt's) 362.75
  nonexudative 362.51
  pseudohole 362.54
  wet 362.52
medullary — *see* Degeneration, brain
membranous labyrinth, congenital (causing impairment of hearing) 744.05
meniscus — *see* Derangement, joint
microcystoid 362.62
mitral — *see* Insufficiency, mitral
Mönckeberg's (*see also* Arteriosclerosis, extremities) 440.20
moral 301.7
motor centers, senile 331.2
mural (*see also* Degeneration, myocardial) 429.1
  heart, cardiac (*see also* Degeneration, myocardial) 429.1
  myocardium, myocardial (*see also* Degeneration, myocardial) 429.1
muscle 728.9
  fatty 728.9
  fibrous 728.9
  heart (*see also* Degeneration, myocardial) 429.1
  hyaline 728.9
muscular progressive 728.2
myelin, central nervous system NEC 341.9
myocardium, myocardial (brown) (calcareous) (fatty) (fibrous) (hyaline) (mural) (muscular) (pigmentary) (senile) (with arteriosclerosis) 429.1
  with rheumatic fever (conditions classifiable to 390) 398.0
    active, acute, or subacute 391.2
      with chorea 392.0
    inactive or quiescent (with chorea) 398.0
  amyloid 277.39 *[425.7]*
  congenital 746.89
  fetus or newborn 779.89
  gouty 274.82
  hypertensive (*see also* Hypertension, heart) 402.90
  ischemic 414.8
  rheumatic (*see also* Degeneration, myocardium, with rheumatic fever) 398.0
  syphilitic 093.82
nasal sinus (mucosa) (*see also* Sinusitis) 473.9
  frontal 473.1
  maxillary 473.0
nerve — *see* Disorder, nerve
nervous system 349.89
  amyloid 277.39 *[357.4]*
  autonomic (*see also* Neuropathy, peripheral, autonomic) 337.9
  fatty 349.89
  peripheral autonomic NEC (*see also* Neuropathy, peripheral, autonomic) 337.9
nipple 611.9
nose 478.19
oculoacousticocerebral, congenital (progressive) 743.8
olivopontocerebellar (familial) (hereditary) 333.0
osseous labyrinth 386.8
ovary 620.8
  cystic 620.2
  microcystic 620.2
pallidal, pigmentary (progressive) 333.0
pancreas 577.8

Degeneration, degenerative — *continued*
pancreas — *continued*
  tuberculous (*see also* Tuberculosis) 017.9 ☑
papillary muscle 429.81
paving stone 362.61
penis 607.89
peritoneum 568.89
pigmentary (diffuse) (general)
  localized — *see* Degeneration, by site
  pallidal (progressive) 333.0
  secondary 362.65
pineal gland 259.8
pituitary (gland) 253.8
placenta (fatty) (fibrinoid) (fibroid) — *see* Placenta, abnormal
popliteal fat pad 729.31
posterolateral (spinal cord) (*see also* Degeneration, combined) 266.2 *[336.2]*
pulmonary valve (heart) (*see also* Endocarditis, pulmonary) 424.3
pulp (tooth) 522.2
pupillary margin 364.54
renal (*see also* Sclerosis, renal) 587
  fibrocystic 753.19
  polycystic 753.12
    adult type (APKD) 753.13
    autosomal dominant 753.13
    autosomal recessive 753.14
    childhood type (CPKD) 753.14
    infantile type 753.14
reticuloendothelial system 289.89
retina (peripheral) 362.60
  with retinal defect (*see also* Detachment, retina, with retinal defect) 361.00
  cystic (senile) 362.50
  cystoid 362.53
  hereditary (*see also* Dystrophy, retina) 362.70
    cerebroretinal 362.71
    congenital 362.75
    juvenile (Stargardt's) 362.75
    macula 362.76
  Kuhnt-Junius 362.52
  lattice 362.63
  macular (*see also* Degeneration, macula) 362.50
  microcystoid 362.62
  palisade 362.63
  paving stone 362.61
  pigmentary (primary) 362.74
    secondary 362.65
  posterior pole (*see also* Degeneration, macula) 362.50
  secondary 362.66
  senile 362.60
    cystic 362.53
    reticular 362.64
saccule, congenital (causing impairment of hearing) 744.05
sacculocochlear 386.8
senile 797
  brain 331.2
  cardiac, heart, or myocardium (*see also* Degeneration, myocardial) 429.1
  motor centers 331.2
  reticule 362.64
  retina, cystic 362.50
  vascular — *see* Arteriosclerosis
silicone rubber poppet (prosthetic valve) 996.02
sinus (cystic) (*see also* Sinusitis) 473.9
  polypoid 471.1
skin 709.3
  amyloid 277.39
  colloid 709.3
spinal (cord) 336.8
  amyloid 277.39
  column 733.90
  combined (subacute) (*see also* Degeneration, combined) 266.2 *[336.2]*
    with anemia (pernicious) 281.0 *[336.2]*
  dorsolateral (*see also* Degeneration, combined) 266.2 *[336.2]*
  familial NEC 336.8

Degeneration, degenerative — *continued*
　spinal — *continued*
　　fatty 336.8
　　funicular (*see also* Degeneration, com-
　　　bined) 266.2 *[336.2]*
　　heredofamilial NEC 336.8
　　posterolateral (*see also* Degeneration,
　　　combined) 266.2 *[336.2]*
　　subacute combined — *see* Degenera-
　　　tion, combined
　　tuberculous (*see also* Tuberculosis)
　　　013.8 ☑
　spine 733.90
　spleen 289.59
　　amyloid 277.39
　　lardaceous 277.39
　stomach 537.89
　　lardaceous 277.39
　strionigral 333.0
　sudoriparous (cystic) 705.89
　suprarenal (capsule) (gland) 255.8
　　with hypofunction 255.41
　sweat gland 705.89
　synovial membrane (pulpy) 727.9
　tapetoretinal 362.74
　　adult or presenile form 362.50
　testis (postinfectional) 608.89
　thymus (gland) 254.8
　　fatty 254.8
　　lardaceous 277.39
　thyroid (gland) 246.8
　tricuspid (heart) (valve) — *see* Endocarditis,
　　tricuspid
　tuberculous NEC (*see also* Tuberculosis)
　　011.9 ☑
　turbinate 733.90
　uterus 621.8
　　cystic 621.8
　vascular (senile) (*see also* Arteriosclerosis)
　　hypertensive — *see* Hypertension
　vitreoretinal (primary) 362.73
　　secondary 362.66
　vitreous humor (with infiltration) 379.21
　wallerian NEC — *see* Disorder, nerve
　waxy (any site) 277.39
　Wilson's hepatolenticular 275.1
Deglutition
　paralysis 784.99
　　hysterical 300.11
　pneumonia 507.0
Degos' disease or syndrome 447.8
**Degradation disorder, branched-chain
　amino acid** 270.3
Dehiscence
　anastomosis — *see* Complications, anasto-
　　mosis
　cesarean wound 674.1 ☑
　closure of
　　cornea 998.32
　　fascia, superficial or muscular 998.31
　　internal organ 998.31
　　mucosa 998.31
　　muscle or muscle flap 998.31
　　ribs or rib cage 998.31
　　skin 998.32
　　skull or craniotomy 998.31
　　sternum or sternotomy 998.31
　　subcutaneous tissue 998.32
　　tendon or ligament 998.31
　　traumatic laceration (external) (internal)
　　　998.31
　episiotomy 674.2 ☑
　operation wound 998.32
　　deep 998.31
　　external 998.32
　　internal 998.31
　　superficial 998.32
　perineal wound (postpartum) 674.2 ☑
　postoperative 998.32
　　abdomen 998.32
　　　internal 998.31
　　internal 998.31
　traumatic injury wound repair 998.33
　uterine wound 674.1 ☑
Dehydration (cachexia) 276.51

Dehydration — *continued*
　with
　　hypernatremia 276.0
　　hyponatremia 276.1
　newborn 775.5
Deiters' nucleus syndrome 386.19
Déjérine's disease 356.0
Déjérine-Klumpke paralysis 767.6
Déjérine-Roussy syndrome 338.0
Déjérine-Sottas disease or neuropathy (hy-
　pertrophic) 356.0
Déjérine-Thomas atrophy or syndrome 333.0
de Lange's syndrome (Amsterdam dwarf, in-
　tellectual disabilities, and brachycephaly)
　759.89
Delay, delayed
　adaptation, cones or rods 368.63
　any plane in pelvis
　　affecting fetus or newborn 763.1
　　complicating delivery 660.1 ☑
　birth or delivery NEC 662.1 ☑
　　affecting fetus or newborn 763.89
　　second twin, triplet, or multiple mate
　　　662.3 ☑
　closure (*see also* Fistula)
　　cranial suture 756.0
　　fontanel 756.0
　coagulation NEC 790.92
　conduction (cardiac) (ventricular) 426.9
　delivery NEC 662.1 ☑
　　second twin, triplet, etc. 662.3 ☑
　　　affecting fetus or newborn 763.89
　development
　　in childhood 783.40
　　　physiological 783.40
　　intellectual NEC 315.9
　　learning NEC 315.2
　　reading 315.00
　　sexual 259.0
　　speech 315.39
　　　and language due to hearing loss
　　　　315.34
　　　associated with hyperkinesis 314.1
　　spelling 315.09
　gastric emptying 536.8
　menarche 256.39
　　due to pituitary hypofunction 253.4
　menstruation (cause unknown) 626.8
　milestone in childhood 783.42
　motility — *see* Hypomotility
　passage of meconium (newborn) 777.1
　primary respiration 768.9
　puberty 259.0
　separation of umbilical cord 779.83
　sexual maturation, female 259.0
　vaccination V64.00
Del Castillo's syndrome (germinal aplasia)
　606.0
Déleage's disease 359.89
Deletion syndrome
　5p 758.31
　22q11.2 758.32
　autosomal NEC 758.39
　constitutional 5q deletion 758.39
Delhi (boil) (button) (sore) 085.1
Delinquency (juvenile) 312.9
　group (*see also* Disturbance, conduct)
　　312.2 ☑
　neurotic 312.4
Delirium, delirious 780.09
　acute 780.09
　　due to conditions classified elsewhere
　　　293.0
　alcoholic 291.0
　　acute 291.0
　　chronic 291.1
　alcoholicum 291.0
　chronic (*see also* Psychosis) 293.89
　　due to or associated with physical condi-
　　　tion — *see* Psychosis, organic
　drug-induced 292.81
　due to conditions classified elsewhere 293.0
　eclamptic (*see also* Eclampsia) 780.39
　exhaustion (*see also* Reaction, stress, acute)
　　308.9
　hysterical 300.11

Delirium, delirious — *continued*
　in
　　presenile dementia 290.11
　　senile dementia 290.3
　induced by drug 292.81
　manic, maniacal (acute) (*see also* Psychosis,
　　affective) 296.0
　　recurrent episode 296.1 ☑
　　single episode 296.0 ☑
　puerperal 293.9
　senile 290.3
　subacute (psychotic) 293.1
　thyroid (*see also* Thyrotoxicosis) 242.9 ☑
　traumatic (*see also* Injury, intracranial)
　　with
　　　lesion, spinal cord — *see* Injury,
　　　　spinal, by site
　　　shock, spinal — *see* Injury, spinal, by
　　　　site
　tremens (impending) 291.0
　uremic — *see* Uremia
　withdrawal
　　alcoholic (acute) 291.0
　　　chronic 291.1
　　drug 292.0

Delivery

*Note — Use the following fifth-digit
subclassification with categories
640–649, 651–676:*

0　*unspecified as to episode of care*

1　*delivered, with or without men-
　tion of antepartum condition*

2　*delivered, with mention of postpar-
　tum complication*

3　*antepartum condition or complica-
　tion*

4　*postpartum condition or complica-
　tion*

　breech (assisted) (buttocks) (complete)
　　(frank) (spontaneous) 652.2 ☑
　　affecting fetus or newborn 763.0
　　extraction NEC 669.6 ☑
　cesarean (for) 669.7 ☑
　　abnormal
　　　cervix 654.6 ☑
　　　pelvic organs or tissues 654.9 ☑
　　　pelvis (bony) (major) NEC 653.0 ☑
　　　presentation or position 652.9 ☑
　　　　in multiple gestation 652.6 ☑
　　　size, fetus 653.5 ☑
　　　soft parts (of pelvis) 654.9 ☑
　　　uterus, congenital 654.0 ☑
　　　vagina 654.7 ☑
　　　vulva 654.8 ☑
　　abruptio placentae 641.2 ☑
　　acromion presentation 652.8 ☑
　　affecting fetus or newborn 763.4
　　anteversion, cervix or uterus 654.4 ☑
　　atony, uterus 661.2 ☑
　　　with hemorrhage 666.1 ☑
　　bicornis or bicornuate uterus 654.0 ☑
　　breech presentation (buttocks) (com-
　　　plete) (frank) 652.2 ☑
　　brow presentation 652.4 ☑
　　cephalopelvic disproportion (normally
　　　formed fetus) 653.4 ☑
　　chin presentation 652.4 ☑
　　cicatrix of cervix 654.6 ☑
　　contracted pelvis (general) 653.1 ☑
　　　inlet 653.2 ☑
　　　outlet 653.3 ☑
　　cord presentation or prolapse 663.0 ☑
　　cystocele 654.4 ☑
　　deformity (acquired) (congenital)
　　　pelvic organs or tissues NEC 654.9 ☑
　　　pelvis (bony) NEC 653.0 ☑
　　displacement, uterus NEC 654.4 ☑
　　disproportion NEC 653.9 ☑
　　distress
　　　fetal 656.8 ☑
　　　maternal 669.0 ☑
　　eclampsia 642.6 ☑

Delivery — *continued*
　cesarean — *continued*
　　face presentation 652.4 ☑
　　failed
　　　forceps 660.7 ☑
　　　trial of labor NEC 660.6 ☑
　　　vacuum extraction 660.7 ☑
　　　ventouse 660.7 ☑
　　fetal deformity 653.7 ☑
　　fetal-maternal hemorrhage 656.0 ☑
　　fetus, fetal
　　　distress 656.8 ☑
　　　prematurity 656.8 ☑
　　fibroid (tumor) (uterus) 654.1 ☑
　　footling 652.8 ☑
　　　with successful version 652.1 ☑
　　hemorrhage (antepartum) (intrapartum)
　　　NEC 641.9 ☑
　　hydrocephalic fetus 653.6 ☑
　　incarceration of uterus 654.3 ☑
　　incoordinate uterine action 661.4 ☑
　　inertia, uterus 661.2 ☑
　　　primary 661.0 ☑
　　　secondary 661.1 ☑
　　lateroversion, uterus or cervix 654.4 ☑
　　mal lie 652.9 ☑
　　malposition
　　　fetus 652.9 ☑
　　　　in multiple gestation 652.6 ☑
　　　pelvic organs or tissues NEC 654.9 ☑
　　　uterus NEC or cervix 654.4 ☑
　　malpresentation NEC 652.9 ☑
　　　in multiple gestation 652.6 ☑
　　maternal
　　　diabetes mellitus (conditions classifi-
　　　　able to 249 and 250) 648.0 ☑
　　　heart disease NEC 648.6 ☑
　　meconium in liquor 656.8 ☑
　　　staining only 792.3
　　oblique presentation 652.3 ☑
　　oversize fetus 653.5 ☑
　　pelvic tumor NEC 654.9 ☑
　　placental insufficiency 656.5 ☑
　　placenta previa 641.0 ☑
　　　with hemorrhage 641.1 ☑
　　(planned) occurring after 37 completed
　　　weeks of gestation but before 39
　　　completed weeks gestation due
　　　to (spontaneous) onset of labor
　　　649.8 ☑
　　poor dilation, cervix 661.0 ☑
　　pre-eclampsia 642.4 ☑
　　　severe 642.5 ☑
　　previous
　　　cesarean delivery, section 654.2 ☑
　　　surgery (to)
　　　　cervix 654.6 ☑
　　　　gynecological NEC 654.9 ☑
　　　　rectum 654.8 ☑
　　　　uterus NEC 654.9 ☑
　　　　　previous cesarean delivery,
　　　　　　section 654.2 ☑
　　　　vagina 654.7 ☑
　　prolapse
　　　arm or hand 652.7 ☑
　　　uterus 654.4 ☑
　　prolonged labor 662.1 ☑
　　rectocele 654.4 ☑
　　retroversion, uterus or cervix 654.3 ☑
　　rigid
　　　cervix 654.6 ☑
　　　pelvic floor 654.4 ☑
　　　perineum 654.8 ☑
　　　vagina 654.7 ☑
　　　vulva 654.8 ☑
　　sacculation, pregnant uterus 654.4 ☑
　　scar(s)
　　　cervix 654.6 ☑
　　　cesarean delivery, section 654.2 ☑
　　　uterus NEC 654.9 ☑
　　　　due to previous cesarean delivery,
　　　　　section 654.2 ☑
　　Shirodkar suture in situ 654.5 ☑
　　shoulder presentation 652.8 ☑

☑ **Additional Digit Required — Refer to the Tabular List for Digit Selection**

▽ **Subterms under main terms may continue to next column or page**

Delivery — *continued*
  cesarean — *continued*
    stenosis or stricture, cervix 654.6 ☑
    transverse presentation or lie 652.3 ☑
    tumor, pelvic organs or tissues NEC 654.4 ☑
    umbilical cord presentation or prolapse 663.0 ☑
  completely normal case — *see* category 650
  complicated (by) NEC 669.9 ☑
    abdominal tumor, fetal 653.7 ☑
      causing obstructed labor 660.1 ☑
    abnormal, abnormality of
      cervix 654.6 ☑
        causing obstructed labor 660.2 ☑
      forces of labor 661.9 ☑
      formation of uterus 654.0 ☑
      pelvic organs or tissues 654.9 ☑
        causing obstructed labor 660.2 ☑
      pelvis (bony) (major) NEC 653.0 ☑
        causing obstructed labor 660.1 ☑
      presentation or position NEC 652.9 ☑
        causing obstructed labor 660.0 ☑
      size, fetus 653.5 ☑
        causing obstructed labor 660.1 ☑
      soft parts (of pelvis) 654.9 ☑
        causing obstructed labor 660.2 ☑
      uterine contractions NEC 661.9 ☑
      uterus (formation) 654.0 ☑
        causing obstructed labor 660.2 ☑
      vagina 654.7 ☑
        causing obstructed labor 660.2 ☑
    abnormally formed uterus (any type) (congenital) 654.0 ☑
      causing obstructed labor 660.2 ☑
    acromion presentation 652.8 ☑
      causing obstructed labor 660.0 ☑
    adherent placenta 667.0 ☑
      with hemorrhage 666.0 ☑
    adhesions, uterus (to abdominal wall) 654.4 ☑
    advanced maternal age NEC 659.6 ☑
      multigravida 659.6 ☑
      primigravida 659.5 ☑
    air embolism 673.0 ☑
    amnionitis 658.4 ☑
    amniotic fluid embolism 673.1 ☑
    anesthetic death 668.9 ☑
    annular detachment, cervix 665.3 ☑
    antepartum hemorrhage — *see* Delivery, complicated, hemorrhage
    anteversion, cervix or uterus 654.4 ☑
      causing obstructed labor 660.2 ☑
    apoplexy 674.0 ☑
      placenta 641.2 ☑
    arrested active phase 661.1 ☑
    asymmetrical pelvis bone 653.0 ☑
      causing obstructed labor 660.1 ☑
    atony, uterus with hemorrhage (hypotonic) (inertia) 666.1 ☑
      hypertonic 661.4 ☑
    Bandl's ring 661.4 ☑
    battledore placenta — *see* Placenta, abnormal
    bicornis or bicornuate uterus 654.0 ☑
      causing obstructed labor 660.2 ☑
    birth injury to mother NEC 665.9 ☑
    bleeding (*see also* Delivery, complicated, hemorrhage) 641.9 ☑
    breech presentation (assisted) (buttocks) (complete) (frank) (spontaneous) 652.2 ☑
      with successful version 652.1 ☑
    brow presentation 652.4 ☑

Delivery — *continued*
  complicated — *continued*
    cephalopelvic disproportion (normally formed fetus) 653.4 ☑
      causing obstructed labor 660.1 ☑
    cerebral hemorrhage 674.0 ☑
    cervical dystocia 661.2 ☑
    chin presentation 652.4 ☑
      causing obstructed labor 660.0 ☑
    cicatrix
      cervix 654.6 ☑
        causing obstructed labor 660.2 ☑
      vagina 654.7 ☑
        causing obstructed labor 660.2 ☑
    coagulation defect 649.3 ☑
    colporrhexis 665.4 ☑
      with perineal laceration 664.0 ☑
    compound presentation 652.8 ☑
      causing obstructed labor 660.0 ☑
    compression of cord (umbilical) 663.2 ☑
      around neck 663.1 ☑
      cord prolapsed 663.0 ☑
    contraction, contracted pelvis 653.1 ☑
      causing obstructed labor 660.1 ☑
      general 653.1 ☑
        causing obstructed labor 660.1 ☑
      inlet 653.2 ☑
        causing obstructed labor 660.1 ☑
      midpelvic 653.8 ☑
        causing obstructed labor 660.1 ☑
      midplane 653.8 ☑
        causing obstructed labor 660.1 ☑
      outlet 653.3 ☑
        causing obstructed labor 660.1 ☑
    contraction ring 661.4 ☑
    cord (umbilical) 663.9 ☑
      around neck, tightly or with compression 663.1 ☑
        without compression 663.3 ☑
      bruising 663.6 ☑
      complication NEC 663.9 ☑
        specified type NEC 663.8 ☑
      compression NEC 663.2 ☑
      entanglement NEC 663.3 ☑
        with compression 663.2 ☑
      forelying 663.0 ☑
      hematoma 663.6 ☑
      marginal attachment 663.8 ☑
      presentation 663.0 ☑
      prolapse (complete) (occult) (partial) 663.0 ☑
      short 663.4 ☑
      specified complication NEC 663.8 ☑
      thrombosis (vessels) 663.6 ☑
      vascular lesion 663.6 ☑
      velamentous insertion 663.8 ☑
    Couvelaire uterus 641.2 ☑
    cretin pelvis (dwarf type) (male type) 653.1 ☑
      causing obstructed labor 660.1 ☑
    crossbirth 652.3 ☑
      with successful version 652.1 ☑
      causing obstructed labor 660.0 ☑
    cyst (Gartner's duct) 654.7 ☑
    cystocele 654.4 ☑
      causing obstructed labor 660.2 ☑
    death of fetus (near term) 656.4 ☑
      early (before 22 completed weeks gestation) 632
    deformity (acquired) (congenital)
      fetus 653.7 ☑
        causing obstructed labor 660.1 ☑
      pelvic organs or tissues NEC 654.9 ☑
        causing obstructed labor 660.2 ☑
      pelvis (bony) NEC 653.0 ☑

Delivery — *continued*
  complicated — *continued*
    deformity — *continued*
      pelvis — *continued*
        causing obstructed labor 660.1 ☑
    delay, delayed
      delivery in multiple pregnancy 662.3 ☑
      due to locked mates 660.5 ☑
      following rupture of membranes (spontaneous) 658.2 ☑
        artificial 658.3 ☑
    depressed fetal heart tones 659.7 ☑
    diastasis recti 665.8 ☑
    dilatation
      bladder 654.4 ☑
        causing obstructed labor 660.2 ☑
      cervix, incomplete, poor or slow 661.0 ☑
    diseased placenta 656.7 ☑
    displacement uterus NEC 654.4 ☑
      causing obstructed labor 660.2 ☑
    disproportion NEC 653.9 ☑
      causing obstructed labor 660.1 ☑
    disruptio uteri — *see* Delivery, complicated, rupture, uterus
    distress
      fetal 656.8 ☑
      maternal 669.0 ☑
    double uterus (congenital) 654.0 ☑
      causing obstructed labor 660.2 ☑
    dropsy amnion 657.0 ☑
    dysfunction, uterus 661.9 ☑
      hypertonic 661.4 ☑
      hypotonic 661.2 ☑
        primary 661.0 ☑
        secondary 661.1 ☑
      incoordinate 661.4 ☑
    dystocia
      cervical 661.2 ☑
      fetal — *see* Delivery, complicated, abnormal, presentation
      maternal — *see* Delivery, complicated, prolonged labor
      pelvic — *see* Delivery, complicated, contraction pelvis
      positional 652.8 ☑
      shoulder girdle 660.4 ☑
    eclampsia 642.6 ☑
    ectopic kidney 654.4 ☑
      causing obstructed labor 660.2 ☑
    edema, cervix 654.6 ☑
      causing obstructed labor 660.2 ☑
    effusion, amniotic fluid 658.1 ☑
    elderly multigravida 659.6 ☑
    elderly primigravida 659.5 ☑
    embolism (pulmonary) 673.2 ☑
      air 673.0 ☑
      amniotic fluid 673.1 ☑
      blood clot 673.2 ☑
      cerebral 674.0 ☑
      fat 673.8 ☑
      pyemic 673.3 ☑
      septic 673.3 ☑
    entanglement, umbilical cord 663.3 ☑
      with compression 663.2 ☑
      around neck (with compression) 663.1 ☑
    eversion, cervix or uterus 665.2 ☑
    excessive
      fetal growth 653.5 ☑
        causing obstructed labor 660.1 ☑
      size of fetus 653.5 ☑
        causing obstructed labor 660.1 ☑
    face presentation 652.4 ☑
      causing obstructed labor 660.0 ☑
      to pubes 660.3 ☑
    failure, fetal head to enter pelvic brim 652.5 ☑
      causing obstructed labor 660.0 ☑

Delivery — *continued*
  complicated — *continued*
    female genital mutilation 660.8 ☑
    fetal
      acid-base balance 656.8 ☑
      death (near term) NEC 656.4 ☑
        early (before 22 completed weeks gestation) 632
      deformity 653.7 ☑
        causing obstructed labor 660.1 ☑
      distress 656.8 ☑
      heart rate or rhythm 659.7 ☑
      reduction of multiple fetuses reduced to single fetus 651.7 ☑
    fetopelvic disproportion 653.4 ☑
      causing obstructed labor 660.1 ☑
    fever during labor 659.2 ☑
    fibroid (tumor) (uterus) 654.1 ☑
      causing obstructed labor 660.2 ☑
    fibromyomata 654.1 ☑
      causing obstructed labor 660.2 ☑
    forelying umbilical cord 663.0 ☑
    fracture of coccyx 665.6 ☑
    hematoma 664.5 ☑
      broad ligament 665.7 ☑
      ischial spine 665.7 ☑
      pelvic 665.7 ☑
      perineum 664.5 ☑
      soft tissues 665.7 ☑
      subdural 674.0 ☑
      umbilical cord 663.6 ☑
      vagina 665.7 ☑
      vulva or perineum 664.5 ☑
    hemorrhage (uterine) (antepartum) (intrapartum) (pregnancy) 641.9 ☑
      accidental 641.2 ☑
      associated with
        afibrinogenemia 641.3 ☑
        coagulation defect 641.3 ☑
          hyperfibrinolysis 641.3 ☑
          hypofibrinogenemia 641.3 ☑
      cerebral 674.0 ☑
      due to
        low-lying placenta 641.1 ☑
        placenta previa 641.1 ☑
        premature separation of placenta (normally implanted) 641.2 ☑
        retained placenta 666.0 ☑
        trauma 641.8 ☑
        uterine leiomyoma 641.8 ☑
      marginal sinus rupture 641.2 ☑
      placenta NEC 641.9 ☑
      postpartum (atonic) (immediate) (within 24 hours) 666.1 ☑
        with retained or trapped placenta 666.0 ☑
      delayed 666.2 ☑
      secondary 666.2 ☑
      third stage 666.0 ☑
    hourglass contraction, uterus 661.4 ☑
    hydramnios 657.0 ☑
    hydrocephalic fetus 653.6 ☑
      causing obstructed labor 660.1 ☑
    hydrops fetalis 653.7 ☑
      causing obstructed labor 660.1 ☑
    hypertension — *see* Hypertension, complicating pregnancy
    hypertonic uterine dysfunction 661.4 ☑
    hypotonic uterine dysfunction 661.2 ☑
    impacted shoulders 660.4 ☑
    incarceration, uterus 654.3 ☑
      causing obstructed labor 660.2 ☑
    incomplete dilation (cervix) 661.0 ☑
    incoordinate uterus 661.4 ☑
    indication NEC 659.9 ☑
      specified type NEC 659.8 ☑
    inertia, uterus 661.2 ☑
      hypertonic 661.4 ☑
      hypotonic 661.2 ☑
      primary 661.0 ☑
      secondary 661.1 ☑

☑ Additional Digit Required — Refer to the Tabular List for Digit Selection   ⟱ Subterms under main terms may continue to next column or page

2014 ICD-9-CM   117

Delivery — Delivery

Delivery — *continued*
  complicated — *continued*
    infantile
      genitalia 654.4 ☑
        causing obstructed labor
          660.2 ☑
      uterus (os) 654.4 ☑
        causing obstructed labor
          660.2 ☑
    injury (to mother) NEC 665.9 ☑
    intrauterine fetal death (near term) NEC
      656.4 ☑
      early (before 22 completed weeks
        gestation) 632
    inversion, uterus 665.2 ☑
    kidney, ectopic 654.4 ☑
      causing obstructed labor 660.2 ☑
    knot (true), umbilical cord 663.2 ☑
    labor
      onset (spontaneous) after 37 complet-
        ed weeks of gestation but be-
        fore 39 completed weeks
        gestation with delivery by
        (planned) cesarean section
        649.8 ☑
      premature (before 37 completed
        weeks gestation) 644.2 ☑
    laceration 664.9 ☑
      anus (sphincter) (healed) (old)
        654.8 ☑
        with mucosa 664.3 ☑
          not associated with third-degree
            perineal laceration
            664.6 ☑
      bladder (urinary) 665.5 ☑
      bowel 665.5 ☑
      central 664.4 ☑
      cervix (uteri) 665.3 ☑
      fourchette 664.0 ☑
      hymen 664.0 ☑
      labia (majora) (minora) 664.0 ☑
      pelvic
        floor 664.1 ☑
        organ NEC 665.5 ☑
      perineum, perineal 664.4 ☑
        first degree 664.0 ☑
        second degree 664.1 ☑
        third degree 664.2 ☑
        fourth degree 664.3 ☑
        central 664.4 ☑
        extensive NEC 664.4 ☑
        muscles 664.1 ☑
        skin 664.0 ☑
        slight 664.0 ☑
      peritoneum (pelvic) 665.5 ☑
      periurethral tissue 664.8 ☑
      rectovaginal (septum) (without per-
        ineal laceration) 665.4 ☑
        with perineum 664.2 ☑
          with anal or rectal mucosa
            664.3 ☑
      skin (perineum) 664.0 ☑
      specified site or type NEC 664.8 ☑
      sphincter ani (healed) (old) 654.8 ☑
        with mucosa 664.3 ☑
          not associated with third-degree
            perineal laceration
            664.6 ☑
      urethra 665.5 ☑
      uterus 665.1 ☑
        before labor 665.0 ☑
      vagina, vaginal (deep) (high) (sulcus)
        (wall) (without perineal lacer-
        ation) 665.4 ☑
        with perineum 664.0 ☑
        muscles, with perineum 664.1 ☑
      vulva 664.0 ☑
    lateroversion, uterus or cervix 654.4 ☑
      causing obstructed labor 660.2 ☑
    locked mates 660.5 ☑
    low implantation of placenta — *see* De-
      livery, complicated, placenta,
      previa
    mal lie 652.9 ☑

Delivery — *continued*
  complicated — *continued*
    malposition
      fetus NEC 652.9 ☑
        causing obstructed labor
          660.0 ☑
      pelvic organs or tissues NEC 654.9 ☑
        causing obstructed labor
          660.2 ☑
      placenta 641.1 ☑
        without hemorrhage 641.0 ☑
      uterus NEC or cervix 654.4 ☑
        causing obstructed labor
          660.2 ☑
    malpresentation 652.9 ☑
      causing obstructed labor 660.0 ☑
    marginal sinus (bleeding) (rupture)
      641.2 ☑
    maternal hypotension syndrome
      669.2 ☑
    meconium in liquor 656.8 ☑
    membranes, retained — *see* Delivery,
      complicated, placenta, retained
    mentum presentation 652.4 ☑
      causing obstructed labor 660.0 ☑
    metrorrhagia (myopathia) — *see* Deliv-
      ery, complicated, hemorrhage
    metrorrhexis — *see* Delivery, complicat-
      ed, rupture, uterus
    multiparity (grand) 659.4 ☑
    myelomeningocele, fetus 653.7 ☑
      causing obstructed labor 660.1 ☑
    Nägele's pelvis 653.0 ☑
      causing obstructed labor 660.1 ☑
    nonengagement, fetal head 652.5 ☑
      causing obstructed labor 660.0 ☑
    oblique presentation 652.3 ☑
      causing obstructed labor 660.0 ☑
    obstetric
      shock 669.1 ☑
      trauma NEC 665.9 ☑
    obstructed labor 660.9 ☑
      due to
        abnormality of pelvic organs or
          tissues (conditions classifi-
          able to 654.0–654.9)
          660.2 ☑
        deep transverse arrest 660.3 ☑
        impacted shoulders 660.4 ☑
        locked twins 660.5 ☑
        malposition and malpresentation
          of fetus (conditions classi-
          fiable to 652.0–652.9)
          660.0 ☑
        persistent occipitoposterior
          660.3 ☑
        shoulder dystocia 660.4 ☑
    occult prolapse of umbilical cord
      663.0 ☑
    oversize fetus 653.5 ☑
      causing obstructed labor 660.1 ☑
    pathological retraction ring, uterus
      661.4 ☑
    pelvic
      arrest (deep) (high) (of fetal head)
        (transverse) 660.3 ☑
      deformity (bone) (*see also* Deformity,
        pelvis, with disproportion)
        soft tissue 654.9 ☑
          causing obstructed labor
            660.2 ☑
      tumor NEC 654.9 ☑
        causing obstructed labor
          660.2 ☑
    penetration, pregnant uterus by instru-
      ment 665.1 ☑
    perforation — *see* Delivery, complicated,
      laceration
    persistent
      hymen 654.8 ☑
        causing obstructed labor
          660.2 ☑
      occipitoposterior 660.3 ☑

Delivery — *continued*
  complicated — *continued*
    placenta, placental
      ablatio 641.2 ☑
      abnormality 656.7 ☑
        with hemorrhage 641.2 ☑
      abruptio 641.2 ☑
      accreta 667.0 ☑
        with hemorrhage 666.0 ☑
      adherent (without hemorrhage)
        667.0 ☑
        with hemorrhage 666.0 ☑
      apoplexy 641.2 ☑
      battledore placenta — *see* Placenta,
        abnormal
      detachment (premature) 641.2 ☑
      disease 656.7 ☑
      hemorrhage NEC 641.9 ☑
      increta (without hemorrhage)
        667.0 ☑
        with hemorrhage 666.0 ☑
      low (implantation) 641.1 ☑
        without hemorrhage 641.0 ☑
      malformation 656.7 ☑
        with hemorrhage 641.2 ☑
      malposition 641.1 ☑
        without hemorrhage 641.0 ☑
      marginal sinus rupture 641.2 ☑
      percreta 667.0 ☑
        with hemorrhage 666.0 ☑
      premature separation 641.2 ☑
      previa (central) (lateral) (marginal)
        (partial) 641.1 ☑
        without hemorrhage 641.0 ☑
      retained (with hemorrhage) 666.0 ☑
        without hemorrhage 667.0 ☑
      rupture of marginal sinus 641.2 ☑
      separation (premature) 641.2 ☑
      trapped 666.0 ☑
        without hemorrhage 667.0 ☑
      vicious insertion 641.1 ☑
    polyhydramnios 657.0 ☑
    polyp, cervix 654.6 ☑
      causing obstructed labor 660.2 ☑
    precipitate labor 661.3 ☑
    premature
      labor (before 37 completed weeks
        gestation) 644.2 ☑
      rupture, membranes 658.1 ☑
        delayed delivery following
          658.2 ☑
    presenting umbilical cord 663.0 ☑
    previous
      cesarean delivery, section 654.2 ☑
      surgery
        cervix 654.6 ☑
          causing obstructed labor
            660.2 ☑
        gynecological NEC 654.9 ☑
          causing obstructed labor
            660.2 ☑
        perineum 654.8 ☑
        rectum 654.8 ☑
        uterus NEC 654.9 ☑
          due to previous cesarean de-
            livery, section 654.2 ☑
        vagina 654.7 ☑
          causing obstructed labor
            660.2 ☑
        vulva 654.8 ☑
    primary uterine inertia 661.0 ☑
    primipara, elderly or old 659.5 ☑
    prolapse
      arm or hand 652.7 ☑
        causing obstructed labor
          660.0 ☑
      cord (umbilical) 663.0 ☑
      fetal extremity 652.8 ☑
      foot or leg 652.8 ☑
        causing obstructed labor
          660.0 ☑
      umbilical cord (complete) (occult)
        (partial) 663.0 ☑
      uterus 654.4 ☑

Delivery — *continued*
  complicated — *continued*
    prolapse — *continued*
      uterus — *continued*
        causing obstructed labor
          660.2 ☑
    prolonged labor 662.1 ☑
      first stage 662.0 ☑
      second stage 662.2 ☑
      active phase 661.2 ☑
      due to
        cervical dystocia 661.2 ☑
        contraction ring 661.4 ☑
        tetanic uterus 661.4 ☑
        uterine inertia 661.2 ☑
          primary 661.0 ☑
          secondary 661.1 ☑
      latent phase 661.0 ☑
    pyrexia during labor 659.2 ☑
    rachitic pelvis 653.2 ☑
      causing obstructed labor 660.1 ☑
    rectocele 654.4 ☑
      causing obstructed labor 660.2 ☑
    retained membranes or portions of pla-
      centa 666.2 ☑
      without hemorrhage 667.1 ☑
    retarded (prolonged) birth 662.1 ☑
    retention secundines (with hemorrhage)
      666.2 ☑
      without hemorrhage 667.1 ☑
    retroversion, uterus or cervix 654.3 ☑
      causing obstructed labor 660.2 ☑
    rigid
      cervix 654.6 ☑
        causing obstructed labor
          660.2 ☑
      pelvic floor 654.4 ☑
        causing obstructed labor
          660.2 ☑
      perineum or vulva 654.8 ☑
        causing obstructed labor
          660.2 ☑
      vagina 654.7 ☑
        causing obstructed labor
          660.2 ☑
    Robert's pelvis 653.0 ☑
      causing obstructed labor 660.1 ☑
    rupture (*see also* Delivery, complicated,
      laceration)
      bladder (urinary) 665.5 ☑
      cervix 665.3 ☑
      marginal sinus 641.2 ☑
      membranes, premature 658.1 ☑
      pelvic organ NEC 665.5 ☑
      perineum (without mention of other
        laceration) — *see* Delivery,
        complicated, laceration, per-
        ineum
      peritoneum (pelvic) 665.5 ☑
      urethra 665.5 ☑
      uterus (during labor) 665.1 ☑
        before labor 665.0 ☑
    sacculation, pregnant uterus 654.4 ☑
    sacral teratomas, fetal 653.7 ☑
      causing obstructed labor 660.1 ☑
    scar(s)
      cervix 654.6 ☑
        causing obstructed labor
          660.2 ☑
      cesarean delivery, section 654.2 ☑
        causing obstructed labor
          660.2 ☑
      perineum 654.8 ☑
        causing obstructed labor
          660.2 ☑
      uterus NEC 654.9 ☑
        causing obstructed labor
          660.2 ☑
        due to previous cesarean delivery,
          section 654.2 ☑
      vagina 654.7 ☑
        causing obstructed labor
          660.2 ☑
      vulva 654.8 ☑

☑ **Additional Digit Required** — Refer to the Tabular List for Digit Selection

▽ **Subterms under main terms may continue to next column or page**

Delivery — *continued*
  complicated — *continued*
    scar(s) — *continued*
      vulva — *continued*
        causing obstructed labor
          660.2 ☑
    scoliotic pelvis 653.0 ☑
      causing obstructed labor 660.1 ☑
    secondary uterine inertia 661.1 ☑
    secundines, retained — *see* Delivery,
      complicated, placenta, retained
    separation
      placenta (premature) 641.2 ☑
      pubic bone 665.6 ☑
      symphysis pubis 665.6 ☑
    septate vagina 654.7 ☑
      causing obstructed labor 660.2 ☑
    shock (birth) (obstetric) (puerperal)
      669.1 ☑
    short cord syndrome 663.4 ☑
    shoulder
      girdle dystocia 660.4 ☑
      presentation 652.8 ☑
        causing obstructed labor
          660.0 ☑
    Siamese twins 678.1 ☑
    slow slope active phase 661.2 ☑
    spasm
      cervix 661.4 ☑
      uterus 661.4 ☑
    spondylolisthesis, pelvis 653.3 ☑
      causing obstructed labor 660.1 ☑
    spondylolysis (lumbosacral) 653.3 ☑
      causing obstructed labor 660.1 ☑
    spondylosis 653.0 ☑
      causing obstructed labor 660.1 ☑
    stenosis or stricture
      cervix 654.6 ☑
        causing obstructed labor
          660.2 ☑
      vagina 654.7 ☑
        causing obstructed labor
          660.2 ☑
    sudden death, unknown cause 669.9 ☑
    tear (pelvic organ) (*see also* Delivery,
      complicated, laceration) 664.9 ☑
      anal sphincter (healed) (old) 654.8 ☑
        not associated with third-degree
          perineal laceration
          664.6 ☑
    teratomas, sacral, fetal 653.7 ☑
      causing obstructed labor 660.1 ☑
    tetanic uterus 661.4 ☑
    tipping pelvis 653.0 ☑
      causing obstructed labor 660.1 ☑
    transverse
      arrest (deep) 660.3 ☑
      presentation or lie 652.3 ☑
        with successful version 652.1 ☑
        causing obstructed labor
          660.0 ☑
    trauma (obstetrical) NEC 665.9 ☑
      periurethral 664.8 ☑
    tumor
      abdominal, fetal 653.7 ☑
        causing obstructed labor
          660.1 ☑
      pelvic organs or tissues NEC 654.9 ☑
        causing obstructed labor
          660.2 ☑
    umbilical cord (*see also* Delivery, compli-
      cated, cord) 663.9 ☑
      around neck tightly, or with compres-
        sion 663.1 ☑
      entanglement NEC 663.3 ☑
        with compression 663.2 ☑
      prolapse (complete) (occult) (partial)
        663.0 ☑
    unstable lie 652.0 ☑
      causing obstructed labor 660.0 ☑
    uterine
      inertia (*see also* Delivery, complicat-
        ed, inertia, uterus) 661.2 ☑
      spasm 661.4 ☑

Delivery — *continued*
  complicated — *continued*
    vasa previa 663.5 ☑
    velamentous insertion of cord 663.8 ☑
    young maternal age 659.8 ☑
  delayed NEC 662.1 ☑
    following rupture of membranes (spon-
      taneous) 658.2 ☑
      artificial 658.3 ☑
    second twin, triplet, etc. 662.3 ☑
  difficult NEC 669.9 ☑
    previous, affecting management of
      pregnancy or childbirth V23.49
    specified type NEC 669.8 ☑
  early onset (spontaneous) 644.2 ☑
  footling 652.8 ☑
    with successful version 652.1 ☑
  forceps NEC 669.5 ☑
    affecting fetus or newborn 763.2
  missed (at or near term) 656.4 ☑
  multiple gestation NEC 651.9 ☑
    with fetal loss and retention of one or
      more fetus(es) 651.6 ☑
    following (elective) fetal reduction
      651.7 ☑
    specified type NEC 651.8 ☑
      with fetal loss and retention of one
        or more fetus(es) 651.6 ☑
      following (elective) fetal reduction
        651.7 ☑
  nonviable infant 656.4 ☑
  normal — *see* category 650
  precipitate 661.3 ☑
    affecting fetus or newborn 763.6
  premature NEC (before 37 completed weeks
    gestation) 644.2 ☑
    previous, affecting management of
      pregnancy V23.41
  quadruplet NEC 651.2 ☑
    with fetal loss and retention of one or
      more fetus(es) 651.5 ☑
    following (elective) fetal reduction
      651.7 ☑
  quintuplet NEC 651.8 ☑
    with fetal loss and retention of one or
      more fetus(es) 651.6 ☑
    following (elective) fetal reduction
      651.7 ☑
  sextuplet NEC 651.8 ☑
    with fetal loss and retention of one or
      more fetus(es) 651.6 ☑
    following (elective) fetal reduction
      651.7 ☑
  specified complication NEC 669.8 ☑
  stillbirth (near term) NEC 656.4 ☑
    early (before 22 completed weeks gesta-
      tion) 632
  term pregnancy (live birth) NEC — *see* cate-
    gory 650
    stillbirth NEC 656.4 ☑
  threatened premature 644.2 ☑
  triplets NEC 651.1 ☑
    with fetal loss and retention of one or
      more fetus(es) 651.4 ☑
    delayed delivery (one or more mates)
      662.3 ☑
    following (elective) fetal reduction
      651.7 ☑
    locked mates 660.5 ☑
  twins NEC 651.0 ☑
    with fetal loss and retention of one fetus
      651.3 ☑
    delayed delivery (one or more mates)
      662.3 ☑
    following (elective) fetal reduction
      651.7 ☑
    locked mates 660.5 ☑
  uncomplicated — *see* category 650
  vacuum extractor NEC 669.5 ☑
    affecting fetus or newborn 763.3
  ventouse NEC 669.5 ☑
    affecting fetus or newborn 763.3
Dellen, cornea 371.41
Delusions (paranoid) 297.9

Delusions — *continued*
  grandiose 297.1
  parasitosis 300.29
  systematized 297.1
Dementia 294.20
  with behavioral disturbance (aggressive)
    (combative) (violent) 294.21
  alcohol-induced persisting (*see also* Psy-
    chosis, alcoholic) 291.2
  Alzheimer's — *see* Alzheimer's, dementia
  arteriosclerotic (simple type) (uncomplicat-
    ed) 290.40
    with
      acute confusional state 290.41
      delirium 290.41
      delusions 290.42
      depressed mood 290.43
    depressed type 290.43
    paranoid type 290.42
  Binswanger's 290.12
  catatonic (acute) (*see also* Schizophrenia)
    295.2 ☑
  congenital (*see also* Disability, intellectual)
    319
  degenerative 290.9
    presenile-onset — *see* Dementia, prese-
      nile
    senile-onset — *see* Dementia, senile
  developmental (*see also* Schizophrenia)
    295.9 ☑
  dialysis 294.8
    transient 293.9
  drug-induced persisting (*see also* Psychosis,
    drug) 292.82
  due to or associated with condition(s) clas-
    sified elsewhere
    Alzheimer's
      with behavioral disturbance
        331.0 *[294.11]*
      without behavioral disturbance
        331.0 *[294.10]*
    cerebral lipidoses
      with behavioral disturbance
        330.1 *[294.11]*
      without behavioral disturbance
        330.1 *[294.10]*
    epilepsy
      with behavioral disturbance
        345.9 ☑ *[294.11]*
      without behavioral disturbance
        345.9 ☑ *[294.10]*
    hepatolenticular degeneration
      with behavioral disturbance
        275.1 *[294.11]*
      without behavioral disturbance
        275.1 *[294.10]*
    HIV
      with behavioral disturbance
        042 *[294.11]*
      without behavioral disturbance
        042 *[294.10]*
    Huntington's chorea
      with behavioral disturbance
        333.4 *[294.11]*
      without behavioral disturbance
        333.4 *[294.10]*
    Jakob-Creutzfeldt disease (CJD)
      with behavioral disturbance
        046.19 *[294.11]*
      without behavioral disturbance
        046.19 *[294.10]*
      variant (vCJD) 046.11
        with dementia
          with behavioral disturbance
            046.11 *[294.11]*
          without behavioral disbur-
            bance 046.11 *[294.10]*
    Lewy bodies
      with behavioral disturbance
        331.82 *[294.11]*
      without behavioral disturbance
        331.82 *[294.10]*
    multiple sclerosis
      with behavioral disturbance
        340 *[294.11]*

Dementia — *continued*
  due to or associated with condition(s) classi-
    fied elsewhere — *continued*
    multiple sclerosis — *continued*
      without behavioral disturbance
        340 *[294.10]*
    neurosyphilis
      with behavioral disturbance
        094.9 *[294.11]*
      without behavioral disturbance
        094.9 *[294.10]*
    Parkinsonism
      with behavioral disturbance
        331.82 *[294.11]*
      without behavioral disturbance
        331.82 *[294.10]*
    Parkinson's disease
      with behavioral disturbance
        332.0 *[294.11]*
      without behavioral disturbance
        332.0 *[294.10]*
    Pelizaeus-Merzbacher disease
      with behavioral disturbance
        333.0 *[294.11]*
      without behavioral disturbance
        333.0 *[294.10]*
    Pick's disease
      with behavioral disturbance
        331.11 *[294.11]*
      without behavioral disturbance
        331.11 *[294.10]*
    polyarteritis nodosa
      with behavioral disturbance
        446.0 *[294.11]*
      without behavioral disturbance
        446.0 *[294.10]*
    syphilis
      with behavioral disturbance
        094.1 *[294.11]*
      without behavioral disturbance
        094.1 *[294.10]*
    Wilson's disease
      with behavioral disturbance
        275.1 *[294.11]*
      without behavioral disturbance
        275.1 *[294.10]*
  frontal 331.19
    with behavioral disturbance
      331.19 *[294.11]*
    without behavioral disturbance
      331.19 *[294.10]*
  frontotemporal 331.19
    with behavioral disturbance
      331.19 *[294.11]*
    without behavioral disturbance
      331.19 *[294.10]*
  hebephrenic (acute) 295.1 ☑
  Heller's (infantile psychosis) (*see also* Psy-
    chosis, childhood) 299.1 ☑
  idiopathic 290.9
    presenile-onset — *see* Dementia, prese-
      nile
    senile-onset — *see* Dementia, senile
  in
    arteriosclerotic brain disease 290.40
    senility 290.0
  induced by drug 292.82
  infantile, infantilia (*see also* Psychosis,
    childhood) 299.0 ☑
  Lewy body 331.82
    with behavioral disturbance
      331.82 *[294.11]*
    without behavioral disturbance
      331.82 *[294.10]*
  multi-infarct (cerebrovascular) (*see also* De-
    mentia, arteriosclerotic) 290.40
  old age 290.0
  paralytica, paralytic 094.1
    juvenilis 090.40
    syphilitic 094.1
      congenital 090.40
    tabetic form 094.1
  paranoid (*see also* Schizophrenia) 295.3 ☑
  paraphrenic (*see also* Schizophrenia)
    295.3 ☑
  paretic 094.1

☑ **Additional Digit Required — Refer to the Tabular List for Digit Selection**   ◥ **Subterms under main terms may continue to next column or page**

2014 ICD-9-CM   119

Dementia — *continued*
  praecox (*see also* Schizophrenia) 295.9 ☑
  presenile 290.10
    with
      acute confusional state 290.11
      delirium 290.11
      delusional features 290.12
      depressive features 290.13
    depressed type 290.13
    paranoid type 290.12
    simple type 290.10
    uncomplicated 290.10
  primary (acute) (*see also* Schizophrenia) 295.0 ☑
  progressive, syphilitic 094.1
  puerperal — *see* Psychosis, puerperal
  schizophrenic (*see also* Schizophrenia) 295.9 ☑
  senile 290.0
    with
      acute confusional state 290.3
      delirium 290.3
      delusional features 290.20
      depressive features 290.21
    depressed type 290.21
    exhaustion 290.0
    paranoid type 290.20
  simple type (acute) (*see also* Schizophrenia) 295.0 ☑
  simplex (acute) (*see also* Schizophrenia) 295.0 ☑
  syphilitic 094.1
  uremic — *see* Uremia
  vascular 290.40
    with
      delirium 290.41
      delusions 290.42
      depressed mood 290.43
Demerol dependence — *see also* Dependence 304.0 ☑
Demineralization, ankle — *see also* Osteoporosis 733.00
Demodex folliculorum (infestation) 133.8
Demoralization 799.25
de Morgan's spots (senile angiomas) 448.1
Demyelinating
  polyneuritis, chronic inflammatory 357.81
Demyelination, demyelinization
  central nervous system 341.9
    specified NEC 341.8
  corpus callosum (central) 341.8
  global 340
Dengue (fever) 061
  sandfly 061
  vaccination, prophylactic (against) V05.1
  virus hemorrhagic fever 065.4
Dens
  evaginatus 520.2
  in dente 520.2
  invaginatus 520.2
Dense
  breast(s) 793.82
Density
  increased, bone (disseminated) (generalized) (spotted) 733.99
  lung (nodular) 518.89
Dental — *see also* condition
  examination only V72.2
Dentia praecox 520.6
Denticles (in pulp) 522.2
Dentigerous cyst 526.0
Dentin
  irregular (in pulp) 522.3
  opalescent 520.5
  secondary (in pulp) 522.3
  sensitive 521.89
Dentinogenesis imperfecta 520.5
Dentinoma (M9271/0) 213.1
  upper jaw (bone) 213.0
Dentition 520.7
  abnormal 520.6
  anomaly 520.6
  delayed 520.6
  difficult 520.7
  disorder of 520.6
  precocious 520.6

Dentition — *continued*
  retarded 520.6
Denture sore (mouth) 528.9
Dependence

> Note — Use the following fifth-digit subclassification with category 304:
>
> 0   unspecified
> 1   continuous
> 2   episodic
> 3   in remission

  with
    withdrawal symptoms
      alcohol 291.81
      drug 292.0
  14-hydroxy-dihydromorphinone 304.0 ☑
  absinthe 304.6 ☑
  acemorphan 304.0 ☑
  acetanilid(e) 304.6 ☑
  acetophenetidin 304.6 ☑
  acetorphine 304.0 ☑
  acetyldihydrocodeine 304.0 ☑
  acetyldihydrocodeinone 304.0 ☑
  Adalin 304.1 ☑
  Afghanistan black 304.3 ☑
  agrypnal 304.1 ☑
  alcohol, alcoholic (ethyl) (methyl) (wood) 303.9 ☑
    maternal, with suspected fetal damage affecting management of pregnancy 655.4 ☑
  allobarbitone 304.1 ☑
  allonal 304.1 ☑
  allylisopropylacetylurea 304.1 ☑
  alphaprodine (hydrochloride) 304.0 ☑
  Alurate 304.1 ☑
  Alvodine 304.0 ☑
  amethocaine 304.6 ☑
  amidone 304.0 ☑
  amidopyrine 304.6 ☑
  aminopyrine 304.6 ☑
  amobarbital 304.1 ☑
  amphetamine(s) (type) (drugs classifiable to 969.7) 304.4 ☑
  amylene hydrate 304.6 ☑
  amylobarbitone 304.1 ☑
  amylocaine 304.6 ☑
  Amytal (sodium) 304.1 ☑
  analgesic (drug) NEC 304.6 ☑
    synthetic with morphine-like effect 304.0 ☑
  anesthetic (agent) (drug) (gas) (general) (local) NEC 304.6 ☑
  Angel dust 304.6 ☑
  anileridine 304.0 ☑
  antipyrine 304.6 ☑
  anxiolytic 304.1 ☑
  aprobarbital 304.1 ☑
  aprobarbitone 304.1 ☑
  atropine 304.6 ☑
  Avertin (bromide) 304.6 ☑
  barbenyl 304.1 ☑
  barbital(s) 304.1 ☑
  barbitone 304.1 ☑
  barbiturate(s) (compounds) (drugs classifiable to 967.0) 304.1 ☑
  barbituric acid (and compounds) 304.1 ☑
  benzedrine 304.4 ☑
  benzylmorphine 304.0 ☑
  Beta-chlor 304.1 ☑
  bhang 304.3 ☑
  blue velvet 304.0 ☑
  Brevital 304.1 ☑
  bromal (hydrate) 304.1 ☑
  bromide(s) NEC 304.1 ☑
  bromine compounds NEC 304.1 ☑
  bromisovalum 304.1 ☑
  bromoform 304.1 ☑
  Bromo-seltzer 304.1 ☑
  bromural 304.1 ☑
  butabarbital (sodium) 304.1 ☑
  butabarpal 304.1 ☑

Dependence — *continued*
  butallylonal 304.1 ☑
  butethal 304.1 ☑
  buthalitone (sodium) 304.1 ☑
  Butisol 304.1 ☑
  butobarbitone 304.1 ☑
  butyl chloral (hydrate) 304.1 ☑
  caffeine 304.4 ☑
  cannabis (indica) (sativa) (resin) (derivatives) (type) 304.3 ☑
  carbamazepine 304.6 ☑
  Carbrital 304.1 ☑
  carbromal 304.1 ☑
  carisoprodol 304.6 ☑
  Catha (edulis) 304.4 ☑
  chloral (betaine) (hydrate) 304.1 ☑
  chloralamide 304.1 ☑
  chloralformamide 304.1 ☑
  chloralose 304.1 ☑
  chlordiazepoxide 304.1 ☑
  Chloretone 304.1 ☑
  chlorobutanol 304.1 ☑
  chlorodyne 304.1 ☑
  chloroform 304.6 ☑
  Cliradon 304.0 ☑
  coca (leaf) and derivatives 304.2 ☑
  cocaine 304.2 ☑
    hydrochloride 304.2 ☑
    salt (any) 304.2 ☑
  codeine 304.0 ☑
  combination of drugs (excluding morphine or opioid type drug) NEC 304.8 ☑
    morphine or opioid type drug with any other drug 304.7 ☑
  croton-chloral 304.1 ☑
  cyclobarbital 304.1 ☑
  cyclobarbitone 304.1 ☑
  dagga 304.3 ☑
  Delvinal 304.1 ☑
  Demerol 304.0 ☑
  desocodeine 304.0 ☑
  desomorphine 304.0 ☑
  desoxyephedrine 304.4 ☑
  DET 304.5 ☑
  dexamphetamine 304.4 ☑
  dexedrine 304.4 ☑
  dextromethorphan 304.0 ☑
  dextromoramide 304.0 ☑
  dextronorpseudoephedrine 304.4 ☑
  dextrorphan 304.0 ☑
  diacetylmorphine 304.0 ☑
  Dial 304.1 ☑
  diallylbarbituric acid 304.1 ☑
  diamorphine 304.0 ☑
  diazepam 304.1 ☑
  dibucaine 304.6 ☑
  dichloroethane 304.6 ☑
  diethyl barbituric acid 304.1 ☑
  diethylsulfone-diethylmethane 304.1 ☑
  difencloxazine 304.0 ☑
  dihydrocodeine 304.0 ☑
  dihydrocodeinone 304.0 ☑
  dihydrohydroxycodeinone 304.0 ☑
  dihydroisocodeine 304.0 ☑
  dihydromorphine 304.0 ☑
  dihydromorphinone 304.0 ☑
  dihydroxcodeinone 304.0 ☑
  Dilaudid 304.0 ☑
  dimenhydrinate 304.6 ☑
  dimethylmeperidine 304.0 ☑
  dimethyltriptamine 304.5 ☑
  Dionin 304.0 ☑
  diphenoxylate 304.6 ☑
  dipipanone 304.0 ☑
  d-lysergic acid diethylamide 304.5 ☑
  DMT 304.5 ☑
  Dolophine 304.0 ☑
  DOM 304.2 ☑
  Doriden 304.1 ☑
  dormiral 304.1 ☑
  Dormison 304.1 ☑
  Dromoran 304.0 ☑
  drug NEC 304.9 ☑

Dependence — *continued*
  drug — *continued*
    analgesic NEC 304.6 ☑
    combination (excluding morphine or opioid type drug) NEC 304.8 ☑
      morphine or opioid type drug with any other drug 304.7 ☑
    complicating pregnancy, childbirth, or puerperium 648.3 ☑
      affecting fetus or newborn 779.5
    hallucinogenic 304.5 ☑
    hypnotic NEC 304.1 ☑
    narcotic NEC 304.9 ☑
    psychostimulant NEC 304.4 ☑
    sedative 304.1 ☑
    soporific NEC 304.1 ☑
    specified type NEC 304.6 ☑
    suspected damage to fetus affecting management of pregnancy 655.5 ☑
    synthetic, with morphine-like effect 304.0 ☑
    tranquilizing 304.1 ☑
  duboisine 304.6 ☑
  ectylurea 304.1 ☑
  Endocaine 304.6 ☑
  Equanil 304.1 ☑
  Eskabarb 304.1 ☑
  ethchlorvynol 304.1 ☑
  ether (ethyl) (liquid) (vapor) (vinyl) 304.6 ☑
  ethidene 304.6 ☑
  ethinamate 304.1 ☑
  ethoheptazine 304.6 ☑
  ethyl
    alcohol 303.9 ☑
    bromide 304.6 ☑
    carbamate 304.6 ☑
    chloride 304.6 ☑
    morphine 304.0 ☑
  ethylene (gas) 304.6 ☑
    dichloride 304.6 ☑
  ethylidene chloride 304.6 ☑
  etilfen 304.1 ☑
  etorphine 304.0 ☑
  etoval 304.1 ☑
  eucodal 304.0 ☑
  euneryl 304.1 ☑
  Evipal 304.1 ☑
  Evipan 304.1 ☑
  fentanyl 304.0 ☑
  ganja 304.3 ☑
  gardenal 304.1 ☑
  gardenpanyl 304.1 ☑
  gelsemine 304.6 ☑
  Gelsemium 304.6 ☑
  Gemonil 304.1 ☑
  glucochloral 304.1 ☑
  glue (airplane) (sniffing) 304.6 ☑
  glutethimide 304.1 ☑
  hallucinogenics 304.5 ☑
  hashish 304.3 ☑
  headache powder NEC 304.6 ☑
  Heavenly Blue 304.5 ☑
  hedonal 304.1 ☑
  hemp 304.3 ☑
  heptabarbital 304.1 ☑
  Heptalgin 304.0 ☑
  heptobarbitone 304.1 ☑
  heroin 304.0 ☑
    salt (any) 304.0 ☑
  hexethal (sodium) 304.1 ☑
  hexobarbital 304.1 ☑
  Hycodan 304.0 ☑
  hydrocodone 304.0 ☑
  hydromorphinol 304.0 ☑
  hydromorphinone 304.0 ☑
  hydromorphone 304.0 ☑
  hydroxycodeine 304.0 ☑
  hypnotic NEC 304.1 ☑
  Indian hemp 304.3 ☑
  inhalant 304.6 ☑
  intranarcon 304.1 ☑
  Kemithal 304.1 ☑

☑ **Additional Digit Required — Refer to the Tabular List for Digit Selection**   ▽ **Subterms under main terms may continue to next column or page**

Dependence — *continued*
- ketobemidone 304.0 ☑
- khat 304.4 ☑
- kif 304.3 ☑
- Lactuca (virosa) extract 304.1 ☑
- lactucarium 304.1 ☑
- laudanum 304.0 ☑
- Lebanese red 304.3 ☑
- Leritine 304.0 ☑
- lettuce opium 304.1 ☑
- Levanil 304.1 ☑
- Levo-Dromoran 304.0 ☑
- levo-iso-methadone 304.0 ☑
- levorphanol 304.0 ☑
- Librium 304.1 ☑
- Lomotil 304.6 ☑
- Lotusate 304.1 ☑
- LSD (-25) (and derivatives) 304.5 ☑
- Luminal 304.1 ☑
- lysergic acid 304.5 ☑
  - amide 304.5 ☑
- maconha 304.3 ☑
- magic mushroom 304.5 ☑
- marihuana 304.3 ☑
- MDA (methylene dioxyamphetamine) 304.4 ☑
- Mebaral 304.1 ☑
- Medinal 304.1 ☑
- Medomin 304.1 ☑
- megahallucinogenics 304.5 ☑
- meperidine 304.0 ☑
- mephobarbital 304.1 ☑
- meprobamate 304.1 ☑
- mescaline 304.5 ☑
- methadone 304.0 ☑
- methamphetamine(s) 304.4 ☑
- methaqualone 304.1 ☑
- metharbital 304.1 ☑
- methitural 304.1 ☑
- methobarbitone 304.1 ☑
- methohexital 304.1 ☑
- methopholine 304.6 ☑
- methyl
  - alcohol 303.9 ☑
  - bromide 304.6 ☑
  - morphine 304.0 ☑
  - sulfonal 304.1 ☑
- methylaparafynol 304.1 ☑
- methylated spirit 303.9 ☑
- methylbutinol 304.6 ☑
- methyldihydromorphinone 304.0 ☑
- methylene
  - chloride 304.6 ☑
  - dichloride 304.6 ☑
  - dioxyamphetamine (MDA) 304.4 ☑
- methylphenidate 304.4 ☑
- methyprylone 304.1 ☑
- metopon 304.0 ☑
- Miltown 304.1 ☑
- morning glory seeds 304.5 ☑
- morphinan(s) 304.0 ☑
- morphine (sulfate) (sulfite) (type) (drugs classifiable to 965.00–965.09) 304.0 ☑
- morphine or opioid type drug (drugs classifiable to 965.00–965.09) with any other drug 304.7 ☑
- morphinol(s) 304.0 ☑
- morphinon 304.0 ☑
- morpholinylethylmorphine 304.0 ☑
- mylomide 304.1 ☑
- myristicin 304.5 ☑
- narcotic (drug) NEC 304.9 ☑
- nealbarbital 304.1 ☑
- nealbarbitone 304.1 ☑
- Nembutal 304.1 ☑
- Neonal 304.1 ☑
- Neraval 304.1 ☑
- Neravan 304.1 ☑
- neurobarb 304.1 ☑
- nicotine 305.1 ☑
- Nisentil 304.0 ☑
- nitrous oxide 304.6 ☑

Dependence — *continued*
- Noctec 304.1 ☑
- Noludar 304.1 ☑
- nonbarbiturate sedatives and tranquilizers with similar effect 304.1 ☑
- noptil 304.1 ☑
- normorphine 304.0 ☑
- noscapine 304.0 ☑
- Novocaine 304.6 ☑
- Numorphan 304.0 ☑
- nunol 304.1 ☑
- Nupercaine 304.6 ☑
- Oblivon 304.1 ☑
- on
  - aspirator V46.0
  - hemodialysis V45.11
  - hyperbaric chamber V46.8
  - iron lung V46.11
  - machine (enabling) V46.9
    - specified type NEC V46.8
  - peritoneal dialysis V45.11
  - Possum (Patient-Operated-Selector-Mechanism) V46.8
  - renal dialysis machine V45.11
  - respirator [ventilator] V46.11
    - encounter
      - during
        - mechanical failure V46.14
        - power failure V46.12
      - for weaning V46.13
  - supplemental oxygen V46.2
  - wheelchair V46.3
- opiate 304.0 ☑
- opioids 304.0 ☑
- opioid type drug 304.0 ☑
  - with any other drug 304.7 ☑
- opium (alkaloids) (derivatives) (tincture) 304.0 ☑
- ortal 304.1 ☑
- Oxazepam 304.1 ☑
- oxycodone 304.0 ☑
- oxymorphone 304.0 ☑
- Palfium 304.0 ☑
- Panadol 304.6 ☑
- pantopium 304.0 ☑
- pantopon 304.0 ☑
- papaverine 304.0 ☑
- paracetamol 304.6 ☑
- paracodin 304.0 ☑
- paraldehyde 304.1 ☑
- paregoric 304.0 ☑
- Parzone 304.0 ☑
- PCP (phencyclidine) 304.6 ☑
- Pearly Gates 304.5 ☑
- pentazocine 304.0 ☑
- pentobarbital 304.1 ☑
- pentobarbitone (sodium) 304.1 ☑
- Pentothal 304.1 ☑
- Percaine 304.6 ☑
- Percodan 304.0 ☑
- Perichlor 304.1 ☑
- Pernocton 304.1 ☑
- Pernoston 304.1 ☑
- peronine 304.0 ☑
- pethidine (hydrochloride) 304.0 ☑
- petrichloral 304.1 ☑
- peyote 304.5 ☑
- Phanodron 304.1 ☑
- phenacetin 304.6 ☑
- phenadoxone 304.0 ☑
- phenaglycodol 304.1 ☑
- phenazocine 304.0 ☑
- phencyclidine 304.6 ☑
- phenmetrazine 304.4 ☑
- phenobal 304.1 ☑
- phenobarbital 304.1 ☑
- phenobarbitone 304.1 ☑
- phenomorphan 304.0 ☑
- phenonyl 304.1 ☑
- phenoperidine 304.0 ☑
- pholcodine 304.0 ☑
- piminodine 304.0 ☑
- Pipadone 304.0 ☑
- Pitkin's solution 304.6 ☑

Dependence — *continued*
- Placidyl 304.1 ☑
- polysubstance 304.8 ☑
- Pontocaine 304.6 ☑
- pot 304.3 ☑
- potassium bromide 304.1 ☑
- Preludin 304.4 ☑
- Prinadol 304.0 ☑
- probarbital 304.1 ☑
- procaine 304.6 ☑
- propanal 304.1 ☑
- propoxyphene 304.6 ☑
- psilocibin 304.5 ☑
- psilocin 304.5 ☑
- psilocybin 304.5 ☑
- psilocyline 304.5 ☑
- psilocyn 304.5 ☑
- psychedelic agents 304.5 ☑
- psychostimulant NEC 304.4 ☑
- psychotomimetic agents 304.5 ☑
- pyrahexyl 304.3 ☑
- Pyramidon 304.6 ☑
- quinalbarbitone 304.1 ☑
- racemoramide 304.0 ☑
- racemorphan 304.0 ☑
- Rela 304.6 ☑
- scopolamine 304.6 ☑
- secobarbital 304.1 ☑
- Seconal 304.1 ☑
- sedative NEC 304.1 ☑
  - nonbarbiturate with barbiturate effect 304.1 ☑
- Sedormid 304.1 ☑
- sernyl 304.1 ☑
- sodium bromide 304.1 ☑
- Soma 304.6 ☑
- Somnal 304.1 ☑
- Somnos 304.1 ☑
- Soneryl 304.1 ☑
- soporific (drug) NEC 304.1 ☑
- specified drug NEC 304.6 ☑
- speed 304.4 ☑
- spinocaine 304.6 ☑
- Stovaine 304.6 ☑
- STP 304.5 ☑
- stramonium 304.6 ☑
- Sulfonal 304.1 ☑
- sulfonethylmethane 304.1 ☑
- sulfonmethane 304.1 ☑
- Surital 304.1 ☑
- synthetic drug with morphine-like effect 304.0 ☑
- talbutal 304.1 ☑
- tetracaine 304.6 ☑
- tetrahydrocannabinol 304.3 ☑
- tetronal 304.1 ☑
- THC 304.3 ☑
- thebacon 304.0 ☑
- thebaine 304.0 ☑
- thiamil 304.1 ☑
- thiamylal 304.1 ☑
- thiopental 304.1 ☑
- tobacco 305.1 ☑
- toluene, toluol 304.6 ☑
- tranquilizer NEC 304.1 ☑
  - nonbarbiturate with barbiturate effect 304.1 ☑
- tribromacetaldehyde 304.6 ☑
- tribromethanol 304.6 ☑
- tribromomethane 304.6 ☑
- trichloroethanol 304.6 ☑
- trichoroethyl phosphate 304.1 ☑
- triclofos 304.1 ☑
- Trional 304.1 ☑
- Tuinal 304.1 ☑
- Turkish Green 304.3 ☑
- urethan(e) 304.6 ☑
- Valium 304.1 ☑
- Valmid 304.1 ☑
- veganin 304.0 ☑
- veramon 304.1 ☑
- Veronal 304.1 ☑
- versidyne 304.6 ☑

Dependence — *continued*
- vinbarbital 304.1 ☑
- vinbarbitone 304.1 ☑
- vinyl bitone 304.1 ☑
- vitamin B₆ 266.1
- wine 303.9 ☑
- Zactane 304.6 ☑

Dependency
- passive 301.6
- reactions 301.6

Depersonalization (episode, in neurotic state) (neurotic) (syndrome) 300.6

Depletion
- carbohydrates 271.9
- complement factor 279.8
- extracellular fluid 276.52
- plasma 276.52
- potassium 276.8
  - nephropathy 588.89
- salt or sodium 276.1
  - causing heat exhaustion or prostration 992.4
  - nephropathy 593.9
- volume 276.50
  - extracellular fluid 276.52
  - plasma 276.52

Deployment (military)
- personal history of V62.22
- returned from V62.22
- status V62.21

Deposit
- argentous, cornea 371.16
- bone, in Boeck's sarcoid 135
- calcareous, calcium — *see* Calcification
- cholesterol
  - retina 362.82
  - skin 709.3
  - vitreous (humor) 379.22
- conjunctival 372.56
- cornea, corneal NEC 371.10
  - argentous 371.16
  - in
    - cystinosis 270.0 *[371.15]*
    - mucopolysaccharidosis 277.5 *[371.15]*
- crystalline, vitreous (humor) 379.22
- hemosiderin, in old scars of cornea 371.11
- metallic, in lens 366.45
- skin 709.3
- teeth, tooth (betel) (black) (green) (materia alba) (orange) (soft) (tobacco) 523.6
- urate, in kidney (*see also* Disease, renal) 593.9

Depraved appetite 307.52

Depression 311
- acute (*see also* Psychosis, affective) 296.2 ☑
  - recurrent episode 296.3 ☑
  - single episode 296.2 ☑
- agitated (*see also* Psychosis, affective) 296.2 ☑
  - recurrent episode 296.3 ☑
  - single episode 296.2 ☑
- anaclitic 309.21
- anxiety 300.4
- arches 734
  - congenital 754.61
- autogenous (*see also* Psychosis, affective) 296.2 ☑
  - recurrent episode 296.3 ☑
  - single episode 296.2 ☑
- basal metabolic rate (BMR) 794.7
- bone marrow 289.9
- central nervous system 799.1
  - newborn 779.2
- cerebral 331.9
  - newborn 779.2
- cerebrovascular 437.8
  - newborn 779.2
- chest wall 738.3
- endogenous (*see also* Psychosis, affective) 296.2 ☑
  - recurrent episode 296.3 ☑
  - single episode 296.2 ☑
- functional activity 780.99
- hysterical 300.11

☑ **Additional Digit Required** — Refer to the Tabular List for Digit Selection   ▽ **Subterms under main terms may continue to next column or page**

2014 ICD-9-CM   **121**

Dependence — Depression

Depression — *continued*
  involutional, climacteric, or menopausal (*see also* Psychosis, affective) 296.2 ☑
    recurrent episode 296.3 ☑
    single episode 296.2 ☑
  major 296.2 ☑
    recurrent episode 296.3 ☑
    single episode 296.2 ☑
  manic (*see also* Psychosis, affective) 296.80
  medullary 348.89
    newborn 779.2
  mental 300.4
  metatarsal heads — *see* Depression, arches
  metatarsus — *see* Depression, arches
  monopolar (*see also* Psychosis, affective) 296.2 ☑
    recurrent episode 296.3 ☑
    single episode 296.2 ☑
  nervous 300.4
  neurotic 300.4
  nose 738.0
  postpartum 648.4 ☑
  psychogenic 300.4
    reactive 298.0
  psychoneurotic 300.4
  psychotic (*see also* Psychosis, affective) 296.2 ☑
    reactive 298.0
    recurrent episode 296.3 ☑
    single episode 296.2 ☑
  reactive 300.4
    neurotic 300.4
    psychogenic 298.0
    psychoneurotic 300.4
    psychotic 298.0
  recurrent 296.3 ☑
  respiratory center 348.89
    newborn 770.89
  scapula 736.89
  senile 290.21
  situational (acute) (brief) 309.0
    prolonged 309.1
  skull 754.0
  sternum 738.3
  visual field 368.40
Depressive reaction — *see also* Reaction, depressive
  acute (transient) 309.0
    with anxiety 309.28
  prolonged 309.1
  situational (acute) 309.0
    prolonged 309.1
Deprivation
  cultural V62.4
  emotional V62.89
    affecting
      adult 995.82
      infant or child 995.51
  food 994.2
    specific substance NEC 269.8
  protein (familial) (kwashiorkor) 260
  sleep V69.4
  social V62.4
    affecting
      adult 995.82
      infant or child 995.51
  symptoms, syndrome
    alcohol 291.81
    drug 292.0
  vitamins (*see also* Deficiency, vitamin) 269.2
  water 994.3
de Quervain's
  disease (tendon sheath) 727.04
  syndrome 259.51
  thyroiditis (subacute granulomatous thyroiditis) 245.1
Derangement
  ankle (internal) 718.97
    current injury (*see also* Dislocation, ankle) 837.0
    recurrent 718.37
  cartilage (articular) NEC (*see also* Disorder, cartilage, articular) 718.0 ☑
    knee 717.9
      recurrent 718.36
    recurrent 718.3 ☑

Derangement — *continued*
  collateral ligament (knee) (medial) (tibial) 717.82
    current injury 844.1
      lateral (fibular) 844.0
    lateral (fibular) 717.81
      current injury 844.0
  cruciate ligament (knee) (posterior) 717.84
    anterior 717.83
      current injury 844.2
    current injury 844.2
  elbow (internal) 718.92
    current injury (*see also* Dislocation, elbow) 832.00
    recurrent 718.32
  gastrointestinal 536.9
  heart — *see* Disease, heart
  hip (joint) (internal) (old) 718.95
    current injury (*see also* Dislocation, hip) 835.00
    recurrent 718.35
  intervertebral disc — *see* Displacement, intervertebral disc
  joint (internal) 718.90
    ankle 718.97
    current injury (*see also* Dislocation, by site)
      knee, meniscus or cartilage (*see also* Tear, meniscus) 836.2
    elbow 718.92
    foot 718.97
    hand 718.94
    hip 718.95
    knee 717.9
    multiple sites 718.99
    pelvic region 718.95
    recurrent 718.30
      ankle 718.37
      elbow 718.32
      foot 718.37
      hand 718.34
      hip 718.35
      knee 718.36
      multiple sites 718.39
      pelvic region 718.35
      shoulder (region) 718.31
      specified site NEC 718.38
      temporomandibular (old) 524.69
      wrist 718.33
    shoulder (region) 718.91
    specified site NEC 718.98
    spine NEC 724.9
    temporomandibular 524.69
    wrist 718.93
  knee (cartilage) (internal) 717.9
    current injury (*see also* Tear, meniscus) 836.2
    ligament 717.89
      capsular 717.85
      collateral — *see* Derangement, collateral ligament
      cruciate — *see* Derangement, cruciate ligament
      specified NEC 717.85
    recurrent 718.36
  low back NEC 724.9
  meniscus NEC (knee) 717.5
    current injury (*see also* Tear, meniscus) 836.2
    lateral 717.40
      anterior horn 717.42
      posterior horn 717.43
      specified NEC 717.49
    medial 717.3
      anterior horn 717.1
      posterior horn 717.2
    recurrent 718.3 ☑
    site other than knee — *see* Disorder, cartilage, articular
  mental (*see also* Psychosis) 298.9
  rotator cuff (recurrent) (tear) 726.10
    current 840.4
  sacroiliac (old) 724.6
    current — *see* Dislocation, sacroiliac
  semilunar cartilage (knee) 717.5
    current injury 836.2

Derangement — *continued*
  semilunar cartilage — *continued*
    current injury — *continued*
      lateral 836.1
      medial 836.0
    recurrent 718.3 ☑
  shoulder (internal) 718.91
    current injury (*see also* Dislocation, shoulder) 831.00
    recurrent 718.31
  spine (recurrent) NEC 724.9
    current — *see* Dislocation, spine
  temporomandibular (internal) (joint) (old) 524.69
    current — *see* Dislocation, jaw
Dercum's disease or syndrome (adiposis dolorosa) 272.8
Derealization (neurotic) 300.6
Dermal — *see* condition
Dermaphytid — *see* Dermatophytosis
Dermatergosis — *see* Dermatitis
Dermatitis (allergic) (contact) (occupational) (venenata) 692.9
  ab igne 692.82
  acneiform 692.9
  actinic (due to sun) 692.70
    acute 692.72
    chronic NEC 692.74
    other than from sun NEC 692.82
  ambustionis
    due to
      burn or scald — *see* Burn, by site
      sunburn (*see also* Sunburn) 692.71
  amebic 006.6
  ammonia 691.0
  anaphylactoid NEC 692.9
  arsenical 692.4
  artefacta 698.4
    psychogenic 316 [698.4]
  asthmatic 691.8
  atopic (allergic) (intrinsic) 691.8
    psychogenic 316 [691.8]
  atrophicans 701.8
    diffusa 701.8
    maculosa 701.3
  autoimmune progesterone 279.49
  berlock, berloque 692.72
  blastomycetic 116.0
  blister beetle 692.89
  Brucella NEC 023.9
  bullosa 694.9
    striata pratensis 692.6
  bullous 694.9
    mucosynechial, atrophic 694.60
      with ocular involvement 694.61
    seasonal 694.8
  calorica
    due to
      burn or scald — *see* Burn, by site
      cold 692.89
      sunburn (*see also* Sunburn) 692.71
  caterpillar 692.89
  cercarial 120.3
  combustionis
    due to
      burn or scald — *see* Burn, by site
      sunburn (*see also* Sunburn) 692.71
  congelationis 991.5
  contusiformis 695.2
  diabetic 250.8 ☑
  diaper 691.0
  diphtheritica 032.85
  due to
    acetone 692.2
    acids 692.4
    adhesive plaster 692.4
    alcohol (skin contact) (substances classifiable to 980.0–980.9) 692.4
      taken internally 693.8
    alkalis 692.4
    allergy NEC 692.9
    ammonia (household) (liquid) 692.4
    animal
      dander (cat) (dog) 692.84
      hair (cat) (dog) 692.84
    arnica 692.3

Dermatitis — *continued*
  due to — *continued*
    arsenic 692.4
      taken internally 693.8
    blister beetle 692.89
    cantharides 692.3
    carbon disulphide 692.2
    caterpillar 692.89
    caustics 692.4
    cereal (ingested) 693.1
      contact with skin 692.5
    chemical(s) NEC 692.4
      internal 693.8
      irritant NEC 692.4
      taken internally 693.8
    chlorocompounds 692.2
    coffee (ingested) 693.1
      contact with skin 692.5
    cold weather 692.89
    cosmetics 692.81
    cyclohexanes 692.2
    dander, animal (cat) (dog) 692.84
    deodorant 692.81
    detergents 692.0
    dichromate 692.4
    drugs and medicinals (correct substance properly administered) (internal use) 693.0
      external (in contact with skin) 692.3
      wrong substance given or taken 976.9
        specified substance — *see* Table of Drugs and Chemicals
      wrong substance given or taken 977.9
        specified substance — *see* Table of Drugs and Chemicals
    dyes 692.89
      hair 692.89
    epidermophytosis — *see* Dermatophytosis
    esters 692.2
    external irritant NEC 692.9
      specified agent NEC 692.89
    eye shadow 692.81
    fish (ingested) 693.1
      contact with skin 692.5
    flour (ingested) 693.1
      contact with skin 692.5
    food (ingested) 693.1
      in contact with skin 692.5
    fruit (ingested) 693.1
      contact with skin 692.5
    fungicides 692.3
    furs 692.84
    glycols 692.2
    greases NEC 692.1
    hair, animal (cat) (dog) 692.84
    hair dyes 692.89
    hot
      objects and materials — *see* Burn, by site
      weather or places 692.89
    hydrocarbons 692.2
    infrared rays, except from sun 692.82
      solar NEC (*see also* Dermatitis, due to, sun) 692.70
    ingested substance 693.9
      drugs and medicinals (*see also* Dermatitis, due to, drugs and medicinals) 693.0
      food 693.1
      specified substance NEC 693.8
    ingestion or injection of chemical 693.8
      drug (correct substance properly administered) 693.0
        wrong substance given or taken 977.9
          specified substance — *see* Table of Drugs and Chemicals
    insecticides 692.4
    internal agent 693.9
      drugs and medicinals (*see also* Dermatitis, due to, drugs and medicinals) 693.0

☑ **Additional Digit Required** — Refer to the Tabular List for Digit Selection

▽ **Subterms under main terms may continue to next column or page**

Dermatitis — *continued*
  due to — *continued*
    internal agent — *continued*
      food (ingested) 693.1
        in contact with skin 692.5
        specified agent NEC 693.8
    iodine 692.3
    iodoform 692.3
    irradiation 692.82
    jewelry 692.83
    keratolytics 692.3
    ketones 692.2
    lacquer tree (Rhus verniciflua) 692.6
    light (sun) NEC (*see also* Dermatitis, due to, sun) 692.70
      other 692.82
    low temperature 692.89
    mascara 692.81
    meat (ingested) 693.1
      contact with skin 692.5
    mercury, mercurials 692.3
    metals 692.83
    milk (ingested) 693.1
      contact with skin 692.5
    Neomycin 692.3
    nylon 692.4
    oils NEC 692.1
    paint solvent 692.2
    pediculocides 692.3
    petroleum products (substances classifiable to 981) 692.4
    phenol 692.3
    photosensitiveness, photosensitivity (sun) 692.72
      other light 692.82
    plants NEC 692.6
    plasters, medicated (any) 692.3
    plastic 692.4
    poison
      ivy (Rhus toxicodendron) 692.6
      oak (Rhus diversiloba) 692.6
      plant or vine 692.6
      sumac (Rhus venenata) 692.6
      vine (Rhus radicans) 692.6
    preservatives 692.89
    primrose (primula) 692.6
    primula 692.6
    radiation 692.82
      sun NEC (*see also* Dermatitis, due to, sun) 692.70
      tanning bed 692.82
    radioactive substance 692.82
    radium 692.82
    ragweed (Senecio jacobae) 692.6
    Rhus (diversiloba) (radicans) (toxicodendron) (venenata) (verniciflua) 692.6
    rubber 692.4
    scabicides 692.3
    Senecio jacobae 692.6
    solar radiation — *see* Dermatitis, due to, sun
    solvents (any) (substances classifiable to 982.0–982.8) 692.2
      chlorocompound group 692.2
      cyclohexane group 692.2
      ester group 692.2
      glycol group 692.2
      hydrocarbon group 692.2
      ketone group 692.2
      paint 692.2
    specified agent NEC 692.89
    sun 692.70
      acute 692.72
      chronic NEC 692.74
      specified NEC 692.79
    sunburn (*see also* Sunburn) 692.71
    sunshine NEC (*see also* Dermatitis, due to, sun) 692.70
    tanning bed 692.82
    tetrachlorethylene 692.2
    toluene 692.2
    topical medications 692.3
    turpentine 692.2
    ultraviolet rays, except from sun 692.82

Dermatitis — *continued*
  due to — *continued*
    ultraviolet rays, except from sun — *continued*
      sun NEC (*see also* Dermatitis, due to, sun) 692.70
    vaccine or vaccination (correct substance properly administered) 693.0
      wrong substance given or taken
        bacterial vaccine 978.8
          specified — *see* Table of Drugs and Chemicals
        other vaccines NEC 979.9
          specified — *see* Table of Drugs and Chemicals
    varicose veins (*see also* Varicose, vein, inflamed or infected) 454.1
    x-rays 692.82
  dyshydrotic 705.81
  dysmenorrheica 625.8
  eczematoid NEC 692.9
    infectious 690.8
  eczematous NEC 692.9
  epidemica 695.89
  erysipelatosa 695.81
  escharotica — *see* Burn, by site
  exfoliativa, exfoliative 695.89
    generalized 695.89
    infantum 695.81
    neonatorum 695.81
  eyelid 373.31
    allergic 373.32
    contact 373.32
    eczematous 373.31
    herpes (zoster) 053.20
      simplex 054.41
    infective 373.5
      due to
        actinomycosis 039.3 *[373.5]*
        herpes
          simplex 054.41
          zoster 053.20
        impetigo 684 *[373.5]*
        leprosy (*see also* Leprosy) 030.0 *[373.4]*
        lupus vulgaris (tuberculous) (*see also* Tuberculosis) 017.0 ☑ *[373.4]*
        mycotic dermatitis (*see also* Dermatomycosis) 111.9 *[373.5]*
        vaccinia 051.02 *[373.5]*
          postvaccination 999.0 *[373.5]*
        yaws (*see also* Yaws) 102.9 *[373.4]*
  facta, factitia 698.4
    psychogenic 316 *[698.4]*
  ficta 698.4
    psychogenic 316 *[698.4]*
  flexural 691.8
  follicularis 704.8
  friction 709.8
  fungus 111.9
    specified type NEC 111.8
  gangrenosa, gangrenous (infantum) (*see also* Gangrene) 785.4
  gestationis 646.8 ☑
  gonococcal 098.89
  gouty 274.89
  harvest mite 133.8
  heat 692.89
  herpetiformis (bullous) (erythematous) (pustular) (vesicular) 694.0
    juvenile 694.2
    senile 694.5
  hiemalis 692.89
  hypostatic, hypostatica 454.1
    with ulcer 454.2
  impetiginosa 684
  infantile (acute) (chronic) (intertriginous) (intrinsic) (seborrheic) 690.12
  infectiosa eczematoides 690.8
  infectious (staphylococcal) (streptococcal) 686.9
    eczematoid 690.8
  infective eczematoid 690.8
  Jacquet's (diaper dermatitis) 691.0

Dermatitis — *continued*
  leptus 133.8
  lichenified NEC 692.9
  lichenoid, chronic 701.0
  lichenoides purpurica pigmentosa 709.1
  meadow 692.6
  medicamentosa (correct substance properly administered) (internal use) (*see also* Dermatitis, due to, drugs or medicinals) 693.0
    due to contact with skin 692.3
  mite 133.8
  multiformis 694.0
    juvenile 694.2
    senile 694.5
  napkin 691.0
  neuro 698.3
  neurotica 694.0
  nummular NEC 692.9
  osteatosis, osteatotic 706.8
  papillaris capillitii 706.1
  pellagrous 265.2
  perioral 695.3
  perstans 696.1
  photosensitivity (sun) 692.72
    other light 692.82
  pigmented purpuric lichenoid 709.1
  polymorpha dolorosa 694.0
  primary irritant 692.9
  pruriginosa 694.0
  pruritic NEC 692.9
  psoriasiform nodularis 696.2
  psychogenic 316
  purulent 686.00
  pustular contagious 051.2
  pyococcal 686.00
  pyocyaneus 686.09
  pyogenica 686.00
  radiation 692.82
  repens 696.1
  Ritter's (exfoliativa) 695.81
  Schamberg's (progressive pigmentary dermatosis) 709.09
  schistosome 120.3
  seasonal bullous 694.8
  seborrheic 690.10
    infantile 690.12
  sensitization NEC 692.9
  septic (*see also* Septicemia) 686.00
    gonococcal 098.89
  solar, solare NEC (*see also* Dermatitis, due to, sun) 692.70
  stasis 454.1
    due to
      postphlebitic syndrome 459.12
        with ulcer 459.13
      varicose veins — *see* Varicose
    ulcerated or with ulcer (varicose) 454.2
  sunburn (*see also* Sunburn) 692.71
  suppurative 686.00
  traumatic NEC 709.8
  trophoneurotica 694.0
  ultraviolet, except from sun 692.82
    due to sun NEC (*see also* Dermatitis, due to, sun) 692.82
  varicose 454.1
    with ulcer 454.2
  vegetans 686.8
  verrucosa 117.2
  xerotic 706.8

Dermatoarthritis, lipoid 272.8 *[713.0]*
Dermatochalasia, dermatochalasis 374.87
Dermatofibroma (lenticulare) (M8832/0) — *see* Neoplasm, skin, benign
  protuberans (M8832/1) — *see* Neoplasm, skin, uncertain behavior
Dermatofibrosarcoma (protuberans) (M8832/3) — *see* Neoplasm, skin, malignant
Dermatographia 708.3
Dermatolysis (congenital) (exfoliativa) 757.39
  acquired 701.8
  eyelids 374.34
  palpebrarum 374.34
  senile 701.8
Dermatomegaly NEC 701.8

Dermatomucomyositis 710.3
Dermatomycosis 111.9
  furfuracea 111.0
  specified type NEC 111.8
Dermatomyositis (acute) (chronic) 710.3
Dermatoneuritis of children 985.0
Dermatophiliasis 134.1
Dermatophytide — *see* Dermatophytosis
Dermatophytosis (Epidermophyton) (infection) (microsporum) (tinea) (Trichophyton) 110.9
  beard 110.0
  body 110.5
  deep seated 110.6
  fingernails 110.1
  foot 110.4
  groin 110.3
  hand 110.2
  nail 110.1
  perianal (area) 110.3
  scalp 110.0
  scrotal 110.8
  specified site NEC 110.8
  toenails 110.1
  vulva 110.8
Dermatopolyneuritis 985.0
Dermatorrhexis 756.83
  acquired 701.8
Dermatosclerosis — *see also* Scleroderma 710.1
  localized 701.0
Dermatosis 709.9
  Andrews' 686.8
  atopic 691.8
  Bowen's (M8081/2) — *see* Neoplasm, skin, in situ
  bullous 694.9
    specified type NEC 694.8
  erythematosquamous 690.8
  exfoliativa 695.89
  factitial 698.4
  gonococcal 098.89
  herpetiformis 694.0
    juvenile 694.2
    senile 694.5
  hysterical 300.11
  linear IgA 694.8
  menstrual NEC 709.8
  neutrophilic, acute febrile 695.89
  occupational (*see also* Dermatitis) 692.9
  papulosa nigra 709.8
  pigmentary NEC 709.00
    progressive 709.09
      Schamberg's 709.09
      Siemens-Bloch 757.33
  progressive pigmentary 709.09
  psychogenic 316
  pustular subcorneal 694.1
  Schamberg's (progressive pigmentary) 709.09
  senile NEC 709.3
  specified NEC 702.8
  Unna's (seborrheic dermatitis) 690.10
Dermographia 708.3
Dermographism 708.3
Dermoid (cyst) (M9084/0) — *see also* Neoplasm, by site, benign
  with malignant transformation (M9084/3) 183.0
Dermopathy
  infiltrative, with thyrotoxicosis 242.0 ☑
  nephrogenic fibrosing 701.8
  senile NEC 709.3
Dermophytosis — *see* Dermatophytosis
Descemet's membrane — *see* condition
Descemetocele 371.72
Descending — *see* condition
Descensus uteri (complete) (incomplete) (partial) (without vaginal wall prolapse) 618.1
  with mention of vaginal wall prolapse — *see* Prolapse, uterovaginal
Desensitization to allergens V07.1
Desert
  rheumatism 114.0
  sore (*see also* Ulcer, skin) 707.9

☑ **Additional Digit Required — Refer to the Tabular List for Digit Selection**   ▽ **Subterms under main terms may continue to next column or page**

2014 ICD-9-CM   **123**

Desertion (child) (newborn) 995.52
  adult 995.84
Desmoid (extra-abdominal) (tumor) (M8821/1)
  — see also Neoplasm, connective tissue,
  uncertain behavior
  abdominal (M8822/1) — see Neoplasm,
  connective tissue, uncertain behavior
Despondency 300.4
Desquamative dermatitis NEC 695.89
Destruction
  articular facet (see also Derangement, joint)
    718.9 ☑
    vertebra 724.9
  bone 733.90
    syphilitic 095.5
  joint (see also Derangement, joint) 718.9 ☑
    sacroiliac 724.6
  kidney 593.89
  live fetus to facilitate birth NEC 763.89
  ossicles (ear) 385.24
  rectal sphincter 569.49
  septum (nasal) 478.19
  tuberculous NEC (see also Tuberculosis)
    011.9 ☑
  tympanic membrane 384.82
  tympanum 385.89
  vertebral disc — see Degeneration, interver-
    tebral disc
Destructiveness — see also Disturbance, con-
    duct 312.9
  adjustment reaction 309.3
Detachment
  cartilage (see also Sprain, by site)
    knee — see Tear, meniscus
  cervix, annular 622.8
    complicating delivery 665.3 ☑
  choroid (old) (postinfectional) (simple)
    (spontaneous) 363.70
    hemorrhagic 363.72
    serous 363.71
  knee, medial meniscus (old) 717.3
    current injury 836.0
  ligament — see Sprain, by site
  placenta (premature) — see Placenta, sepa-
    ration
  retina (recent) 361.9
    with retinal defect (rhegmatogenous)
      361.00
      giant tear 361.03
      multiple 361.02
      partial
        with
          giant tear 361.03
          multiple defects 361.02
          retinal dialysis (juvenile)
            361.04
          single defect 361.01
        retinal dialysis (juvenile) 361.04
        single 361.01
        subtotal 361.05
        total 361.05
    delimited (old) (partial) 361.06
    old
      delimited 361.06
      partial 361.06
      total or subtotal 361.07
    pigment epithelium (RPE) (serous)
      362.42
      exudative 362.42
      hemorrhagic 362.43
    rhegmatogenous (see also Detachment,
      retina, with retinal defect) 361.00
    serous (without retinal defect) 361.2
    specified type NEC 361.89
    traction (with vitreoretinal organization)
      361.81
  vitreous humor 379.21
Detergent asthma 507.8
Deterioration
  epileptic
    with behavioral disturbance
      345.9 ☑ [294.11]
    without behavioral disturbance
      345.9 ☑ [294.10]
  heart, cardiac (see also Degeneration, my-
    ocardial) 429.1

Deterioration — continued
  mental (see also Psychosis) 298.9
  myocardium, myocardial (see also Degener-
    ation, myocardial) 429.1
  senile (simple) 797
  transplanted organ — see Complications,
    transplant, organ, by site
de Toni-Fanconi syndrome (cystinosis) 270.0
Deuteranomaly 368.52
Deuteranopia (anomalous trichromat) (com-
    plete) (incomplete) 368.52
Deutschländer's disease — see Fracture, foot
Development
  abnormal, bone 756.9
  arrested 783.40
    bone 733.91
    child 783.40
    due to malnutrition (protein-calorie)
      263.2
    fetus or newborn 764.9 ☑
    tracheal rings (congenital) 748.3
  defective, congenital (see also Anomaly)
    cauda equina 742.59
    left ventricle 746.9
      with atresia or hypoplasia of aortic
        orifice or valve with hypopla-
        sia of ascending aorta 746.7
      in hypoplastic left heart syndrome
        746.7
  delayed (see also Delay, development)
    783.40
    arithmetical skills 315.1
    language (skills) 315.31
      and speech due to hearing loss
        315.34
      expressive 315.31
      mixed receptive-expressive 315.32
    learning skill, specified NEC 315.2
    mixed skills 315.5
    motor coordination 315.4
    reading 315.00
    specified
      learning skill NEC 315.2
      type NEC, except learning 315.8
    speech 315.39
      and language due to hearing loss
        315.34
      associated with hyperkinesia 314.1
      phonological 315.39
    spelling 315.09
    written expression 315.2
  imperfect, congenital (see also Anomaly)
    heart 746.9
    lungs 748.60
  improper (fetus or newborn) 764.9 ☑
  incomplete (fetus or newborn) 764.9 ☑
    affecting management of pregnancy
      656.5 ☑
    bronchial tree 748.3
    organ or site not listed — see Hypoplasia
    respiratory system 748.9
  sexual, precocious NEC 259.1
  tardy, mental (see also Disability, intellectu-
    al) 319
Developmental — see condition
Devergie's disease (pityriasis rubra pilaris)
    696.4
Deviation
  conjugate (eye) 378.87
    palsy 378.81
    spasm, spastic 378.82
  esophagus 530.89
  eye, skew 378.87
  mandible, opening and closing 524.53
  midline (jaw) (teeth) 524.29
    specified site NEC — see Malposition
  occlusal plane 524.76
  organ or site, congenital NEC — see Malpo-
    sition, congenital
  septum (acquired) (nasal) 470
    congenital 754.0
  sexual 302.9
    bestiality 302.1
    coprophilia 302.89
    ego-dystonic
      homosexuality 302.0

Deviation — continued
  sexual — continued
    ego-dystonic — continued
      lesbianism 302.0
    erotomania 302.89
      Clérambault's 297.8
    exhibitionism (sexual) 302.4
    fetishism 302.81
      transvestic 302.3
    frotteurism 302.89
    homosexuality, ego-dystonic 302.0
      pedophilic 302.2
    lesbianism, ego-dystonic 302.0
    masochism 302.83
    narcissism 302.89
    necrophilia 302.89
    nymphomania 302.89
    pederosis 302.2
    pedophilia 302.2
    sadism 302.84
    sadomasochism 302.84
    satyriasis 302.89
    specified type NEC 302.89
    transvestic fetishism 302.3
    transvestism 302.3
    voyeurism 302.82
    zoophilia (erotica) 302.1
  teeth, midline 524.29
  trachea 519.19
  ureter (congenital) 753.4
Devic's disease 341.0
Device
  cerebral ventricle (communicating) in situ
    V45.2
  contraceptive — see Contraceptive, device
  drainage, cerebrospinal fluid V45.2
Devil's
  grip 074.1
  pinches (purpura simplex) 287.2
Devitalized tooth 522.9
Devonshire colic 984.9
  specified type of lead — see Table of Drugs
    and Chemicals
Dextraposition, aorta 747.21
  with ventricular septal defect, pulmonary
    stenosis or atresia, and hypertrophy
    of right ventricle 745.2
  in tetralogy of Fallot 745.2
Dextratransposition, aorta 745.11
Dextrinosis, limit (debrancher enzyme defi-
    ciency) 271.0
Dextrocardia (corrected) (false) (isolated)
    (secondary) (true) 746.87
  with
    complete transposition of viscera 759.3
    situs inversus 759.3
Dextroversion, kidney (left) 753.3
Dhobie itch 110.3
DHTR (delayed hemolytic transfusion reaction)
    — see Complications, transfusion
Diabetes, diabetic (brittle) (congenital) (famil-
    ial) (mellitus) (severe) (slight) (without
    complication) 250.0 ☑

*Note — Use the following fifth-digit
subclassification with category 250:*

0 *type II or unspecified type, not
   stated as uncontrolled*

*Fifth-digit 0 is for use for type II pa-
tients, even if the patient requires insulin*

1 *type I [juvenile type], not stated
   as uncontrolled*

2 *type II or unspecified type, uncontrolled*

*Fifth-digit 2 is for use for type II pa-
tients, even if the patient requires insulin*

3 *type I [juvenile type], uncontrolled*

  with
    coma (with ketoacidosis) 250.3 ☑
      due to secondary diabetes 249.3 ☑
    hyperosmolar (nonketotic) 250.2 ☑
      due to secondary diabetes
        249.2 ☑

Diabetes, diabetic — continued
  with — continued
    complication NEC 250.9 ☑
      due to secondary diabetes 249.9 ☑
      specified NEC 250.8 ☑
        due to secondary diabetes
          249.8 ☑
    gangrene 250.7 ☑ [785.4]
      due to secondary diabetes
        249.7 ☑ [785.4]
    hyperglycemia — code to Diabetes, by
      type, with 5th digit for not stated
      as uncontrolled
    hyperosmolarity 250.2 ☑
      due to secondary diabetes 249.2 ☑
    ketosis, ketoacidosis 250.1 ☑
      due to secondary diabetes 249.1 ☑
    loss of protective sensation (LOPS) —
      see Diabetes, neuropathy
    osteomyelitis 250.8 ☑ [731.8]
      due to secondary diabetes
        249.8 ☑ [731.8]
    specified manifestations NEC 250.8 ☑
      due to secondary diabetes 249.8 ☑
  acetonemia 250.1 ☑
    due to secondary diabetes 249.1 ☑
  acidosis 250.1 ☑
    due to secondary diabetes 249.1 ☑
  amyotrophy 250.6 ☑ [353.5]
    due to secondary diabetes
      249.6 ☑ [353.5]
  angiopathy, peripheral 250.7 ☑ [443.81]
    due to secondary diabetes
      249.7 ☑ [443.81]
  asymptomatic 790.29
  autonomic neuropathy (peripheral)
    250.6 ☑ [337.1]
    due to secondary diabetes
      249.6 ☑ [337.1]
  bone change 250.8 ☑ [731.8]
    due to secondary diabetes
      249.8 ☑ [731.8]
  borderline 790.29
  bronze, bronzed 275.01
  cataract 250.5 ☑ [366.41]
    due to secondary diabetes
      249.5 ☑ [366.41]
  chemical induced — see Diabetes, sec-
    ondary
  complicating pregnancy, childbirth, or
    puerperium 648.0 ☑
  coma (with ketoacidosis) 250.3 ☑
    due to secondary diabetes 249.3 ☑
    hyperglycemic 250.3 ☑
      due to secondary diabetes 249.3 ☑
    hyperosmolar (nonketotic) 250.2 ☑
      due to secondary diabetes 249.2 ☑
    hypoglycemic 250.3 ☑
      due to secondary diabetes 249.3 ☑
    insulin 250.3 ☑
      due to secondary diabetes 249.3 ☑
  complicating pregnancy, childbirth, or
    puerperium (maternal) (conditions
    classifiable to 249 and 250) 648.0 ☑
    affecting fetus or newborn 775.0
  complication NEC 250.9 ☑
    due to secondary diabetes 249.9 ☑
    specified NEC 250.8 ☑
      due to secondary diabetes 249.8 ☑
  dorsal sclerosis 250.6 ☑ [340]
    due to secondary diabetes
      249.6 ☑ [340]
  drug-induced — see also Diabetes, sec-
    ondary
    overdose or wrong substance given or
      taken — see Table of Drugs and
      Chemicals
  due to
    cystic fibrosis — see Diabetes, secondary
    infection — see Diabetes, secondary
  dwarfism-obesity syndrome 258.1
  gangrene 250.7 ☑ [785.4]
    due to secondary diabetes
      249.7 ☑ [785.4]

Diabetes, diabetic — *continued*
gastroparesis 250.6 ☑ *[536.3]*
  due to secondary diabetes
    249.6 ☑ *[536.3]*
gestational 648.8 ☑
  complicating pregnancy, childbirth, or
    puerperium 648.8 ☑
glaucoma 250.5 *[365.44]*
  due to secondary diabetes
    249.5 *[365.44]*
glomerulosclerosis (intercapillary)
  250.4 ☑ *[581.81]*
  due to secondary diabetes
    249.4 ☑ *[581.81]*
glycogenosis, secondary 250.8 ☑ *[259.8]*
  due to secondary diabetes
    249.8 ☑ *[259.8]*
hemochromatosis (*see also* Hemochromatosis) 275.03
hyperosmolar coma 250.2 ☑
  due to secondary diabetes 249.2 ☑
hyperosmolarity 250.2 ☑
  due to secondary diabetes 249.2 ☑
hypertension-nephrosis syndrome
  250.4 ☑ *[581.81]*
  due to secondary diabetes
    249.4 ☑ *[581.81]*
hypoglycemia 250.8 ☑
  due to secondary diabetes 249.8 ☑
hypoglycemic shock 250.8 ☑
  due to secondary diabetes 249.8 ☑
inadequately controlled — code to Diabetes, by type, with 5th digit for not stated as uncontrolled
insipidus 253.5
  nephrogenic 588.1
  pituitary 253.5
  vasopressin-resistant 588.1
intercapillary glomerulosclerosis
  250.4 ☑ *[581.81]*
  due to secondary diabetes
    249.4 ☑ *[581.81]*
iritis 250.5 ☑ *[364.42]*
  due to secondary diabetes
    249.5 ☑ *[364.42]*
ketosis, ketoacidosis 250.1 ☑
  due to secondary diabetes 249.1 ☑
Kimmelstiel (-Wilson) disease or syndrome
  (intercapillary glomerulosclerosis)
  250.4 ☑ *[581.81]*
  due to secondary diabetes
    249.4 ☑ *[581.81]*
Lancereaux's (diabetes mellitus with marked
  emaciation) 250.8 ☑ *[261]*
  due to secondary diabetes
    249.8 ☑ *[261]*
latent (chemical) — *see* Diabetes, secondary
  complicating pregnancy, childbirth, or
    puerperium 648.0 ☑
lipoidosis 250.8 ☑ *[272.7]*
  due to secondary diabetes
    249.8 ☑ *[272.7]*
macular edema 250.5 ☑ *[362.07]*
  due to secondary diabetes
    249.5 ☑ *[362.07]*
maternal
  with manifest disease in the infant 775.1
  affecting fetus or newborn 775.0
microaneurysms, retinal 250.5 ☑ *[362.01]*
  due to secondary diabetes
    249.5 ☑ *[362.01]*
mononeuropathy 250.6 ☑ *[355.9]*
  due to secondary diabetes
    249.6 ☑ *[355.9]*
neonatal, transient 775.1
nephropathy 250.4 ☑ *[583.81]*
  due to secondary diabetes
    249.4 ☑ *[583.81]*
nephrosis (syndrome) 250.4 ☑ *[581.81]*
  due to secondary diabetes
    249.4 ☑ *[581.81]*
neuralgia 250.6 ☑ *[357.2]*
  due to secondary diabetes
    249.6 ☑ *[357.2]*

Diabetes, diabetic — *continued*
neuritis 250.6 ☑ *[357.2]*
  due to secondary diabetes
    249.6 ☑ *[357.2]*
neurogenic arthropathy 250.6 ☑ *[713.5]*
  due to secondary diabetes
    249.6 ☑ *[713.5]*
neuropathy 250.6 ☑ *[357.2]*
  autonomic (peripheral) 250.6 ☑ *[337.1]*
    due to secondary diabetes
      249.6 ☑ *[337.1]*
  due to secondary diabetes
    249.6 ☑ *[357.2]*
nonclinical 790.29
osteomyelitis 250.8 ☑ *[731.8]*
  due to secondary diabetes
    249.8 ☑ *[731.8]*
out of control — code to Diabetes, by type,
  with 5th digit for uncontrolled
peripheral autonomic neuropathy
  250.6 ☑ *[337.1]*
  due to secondary diabetes
    249.6 ☑ *[337.1]*
phosphate 275.3
polyneuropathy 250.6 ☑ *[357.2]*
  due to secondary diabetes
    249.6 ☑ *[357.2]*
poorly controlled — code to Diabetes, by
  type, with 5th digit for not stated as
  uncontrolled
renal (true) 271.4
retinal
  edema 250.5 ☑ *[362.07]*
    due to secondary diabetes
      249.5 ☑ *[362.07]*
  hemorrhage 250.5 ☑ *[362.01]*
    due to secondary diabetes
      249.5 ☑ *[362.01]*
  microaneurysms 250.5 ☑ *[362.01]*
    due to secondary diabetes
      249.5 ☑ *[362.01]*
retinitis 250.5 ☑ *[362.01]*
  due to secondary diabetes
    249.5 ☑ *[362.01]*
retinopathy 250.5 ☑ *[362.01]*
  background 250.5 ☑ *[362.01]*
    due to secondary diabetes
      249.5 ☑ *[362.01]*
  due to secondary diabetes
    249.5 ☑ *[362.01]*
  nonproliferative 250.5 ☑ *[362.03]*
    due to secondary diabetes
      249.5 ☑ *[362.03]*
  mild 250.5 ☑ *[362.04]*
    due to secondary diabetes
      249.5 ☑ *[362.04]*
  moderate 250.5 ☑ *[362.05]*
    due to secondary diabetes
      249.5 ☑ *[362.05]*
  severe 250.5 ☑ *[362.06]*
    due to secondary diabetes
      249.5 ☑ *[362.06]*
  proliferative 250.5 ☑ *[362.02]*
    due to secondary diabetes
      249.5 ☑ *[362.02]*
secondary (chemical-induced) (due to
  chronic condition) (due to infection)
  (drug-induced) 249.0 ☑
  with
    coma (with ketoacidosis) 249.3 ☑
      hyperosmolar (nonketotic)
        249.2 ☑
    complication NEC 249.9 ☑
      specified NEC 249.8 ☑
    gangrene 249.7 ☑ *[785.4]*
    hyperosmolarity 249.2 ☑
    ketosis, ketoacidosis 249.1 ☑
    osteomyelitis 249.8 ☑ *[731.8]*
    specified manifestations NEC
      249.8 ☑
  acetonemia 249.1 ☑
  acidosis 249.1 ☑
  amyotrophy 249.6 ☑ *[353.5]*
  angiopathy, peripheral 249.7 ☑ *[443.81]*

Diabetes, diabetic — *continued*
secondary — *continued*
  autonomic neuropathy (peripheral)
    249.6 ☑ *[337.1]*
  bone change 249.8 ☑ *[731.8]*
  cataract 249.5 ☑ *[366.41]*
  coma (with ketoacidosis) 249.3 ☑
    hyperglycemic 249.3 ☑
    hyperosmolar (nonketotic) 249.2 ☑
    hypoglycemic 249.3 ☑
    insulin 249.3 ☑
  complicating pregnancy, childbirth, or
    puerperium (maternal) 648.0 ☑
  affecting fetus or newborn 775.0
  complication NEC 249.9 ☑
    specified NEC 249.8 ☑
  dorsal sclerosis 249.6 ☑ *[340]*
  due to overdose or wrong substance
    given or taken — *see* Table of
    Drugs and Chemicals
  gangrene 249.7 ☑ *[785.4]*
  gastroparesis 249.6 ☑ *[536.3]*
  glaucoma 249.5 ☑ *[365.44]*
  glomerulosclerosis (intercapillary)
    249.4 ☑ *[581.81]*
  glycogenosis, secondary 249.8 ☑ *[259.8]*
  hyperosmolar coma 249.2 ☑
  hyperosmolarity 249.2 ☑
  hypertension-nephrosis syndrome
    249.4 ☑ *[581.81]*
  hypoglycemia 249.8 ☑
  hypoglycemic shock 249.8 ☑
  intercapillary glomerulosclerosis
    249.4 ☑ *[581.81]*
  iritis 249.5 ☑ *[364.42]*
  ketosis, ketoacidosis 249.1 ☑
  Kimmelstiel (-Wilson) disease or syn-
    drome (intercapillary glomeru-
    losclerosis) 249.4 ☑ *[581.81]*
  Lancereaux's (diabetes mellitus with
    marked emaciation)
    249.8 ☑ *[261]*
  lipoidosis 249.8 ☑ *[272.7]*
  macular edema 249.5 ☑ *[362.07]*
  maternal
    with manifest disease in the infant
      775.1
    affecting fetus or newborn 775.0
  microaneurysms, retinal
    249.5 ☑ *[362.01]*
  mononeuropathy 249.6 ☑ *[355.9]*
  nephropathy 249.4 ☑ *[583.81]*
  nephrosis (syndrome) 249.4 ☑ *[581.81]*
  neuralgia 249.6 ☑ *[357.2]*
  neuritis 249.6 ☑ *[357.2]*
  neurogenic arthropathy 249.6 ☑ *[713.5]*
  neuropathy 249.6 ☑ *[357.2]*
    autonomic (peripheral)
      249.6 ☑ *[337.1]*
  osteomyelitis 249.8 ☑ *[731.8]*
  peripheral autonomic neuropathy
    249.6 ☑ *[337.1]*
  polyneuropathy 249.6 ☑ *[357.2]*
  retinal
    edema 249.5 ☑ *[362.07]*
    hemorrhage 249.5 ☑ *[362.01]*
    microaneurysms 249.5 ☑ *[362.01]*
    retinitis 249.5 ☑ *[362.01]*
  retinopathy 249.5 ☑ *[362.01]*
    background 249.5 ☑ *[362.01]*
    nonproliferative 249.5 ☑ *[362.03]*
      mild 249.5 ☑ *[362.04]*
      moderate 249.5 ☑ *[362.05]*
      severe 249.5 ☑ *[362.06]*
    proliferative 249.5 ☑ *[362.02]*
  ulcer (skin) 249.8 ☑ *[707.9]*
    lower extemity 249.8 ☑ *[707.10]*
      ankle 249.8 ☑ *[707.13]*
      calf 249.8 ☑ *[707.12]*
      foot 249.8 ☑ *[707.15]*
      heel 249.8 ☑ *[707.14]*
      knee 249.8 ☑ *[707.19]*
      specified site NEC
        249.8 ☑ *[707.19]*

Diabetes, diabetic — *continued*
secondary — *continued*
  ulcer — *continued*
    lower extemity — *continued*
      thigh 249.8 ☑ *[707.11]*
      toes 249.8 ☑ *[707.15]*
    specified site NEC 249.8 ☑ *[707.8]*
    xanthoma 249.8 ☑ *[272.2]*
  steroid induced — *see also* Diabetes, sec-
    ondary
  overdose or wrong substance given or
    taken 962.0
stress 790.29
subclinical 790.29
subliminal 790.29
sugar 250.0 ☑
ulcer (skin) 250.8 ☑ *[707.9]*
  due to secondary diabetes
    249.8 ☑ *[707.9]*
  lower extremity 250.8 ☑ *[707.10]*
    ankle 250.8 ☑ *[707.13]*
      due to secondary diabetes
        249.8 ☑ *[707.13]*
    calf 250.8 ☑ *[707.12]*
      due to secondary diabetes
        249.8 ☑ *[707.12]*
    due to secondary diabetes
      249.8 ☑ *[707.10]*
    foot 250.8 ☑ *[707.15]*
      due to secondary diabetes
        249.8 ☑ *[707.15]*
    heel 250.8 ☑ *[707.14]*
      due to secondary diabetes
        249.8 ☑ *[707.14]*
    knee 250.8 ☑ *[707.19]*
      due to secondary diabetes
        249.8 ☑ *[707.19]*
    specified site NEC 250.8 ☑ *[707.19]*
      due to secondary diabetes
        249.8 ☑ *[707.19]*
    thigh 250.8 ☑ *[707.11]*
      due to secondary diabetes
        249.8 ☑ *[707.11]*
    toes 250.8 ☑ *[707.15]*
      due to secondary diabetes
        249.8 ☑ *[707.15]*
  specified site NEC 250.8 ☑ *[707.8]*
    due to secondary diabetes
      249.8 ☑ *[707.8]*
  xanthoma 250.8 ☑ *[272.2]*
    due to secondary diabetes
      249.8 ☑ *[272.2]*
Diacyclothrombopathia 287.1
Diagnosis deferred 799.9
Dialysis (intermittent) (treatment)
  anterior retinal (juvenile) (with detachment)
    361.04
  extracorporeal V56.0
  hemodialysis V56.0
    status only V45.11
  peritoneal V56.8
    status only V45.11
  renal V56.0
    status only V45.11
  specified type NEC V56.8
Diamond-Blackfan anemia or syndrome
  (congenital hypoplastic anemia) 284.01
Diamond-Gardener syndrome (autoerythrocyte sensitization) 287.2
Diaper rash 691.0
Diaphoresis (excessive) NEC — *see also* Hyperhidrosis) 780.8
Diaphragm — *see* condition
Diaphragmalgia 786.52
Diaphragmitis 519.4
Diaphyseal aclasis 756.4
Diaphysitis 733.99
Diarrhea, diarrheal (acute) (autumn) (bilious)
  (bloody) (catarrhal) (choleraic) (chronic)
  (gravis) (green) (infantile) (lienteric)
  (noninfectious) (presumed noninfectious) (putrefactive) (secondary) (sporadic) (summer) (symptomatic) (thermic)
  787.91
  achlorhydric 536.0

☑ **Additional Digit Required** — Refer to the Tabular List for Digit Selection

🔺 **Subterms under main terms may continue to next column or page**

Diarrhea, diarrheal — *continued*
allergic 558.3
amebic (*see also* Amebiasis) 006.9
   with abscess — *see* Abscess, amebic
   acute 006.0
   chronic 006.1
   nondysenteric 006.2
bacillary — *see* Dysentery, bacillary
bacterial NEC 008.5
balantidial 007.0
bile salt-induced 579.8
cachectic NEC 787.91
chilomastix 007.8
choleriformis 001.1
coccidial 007.2
Cochin-China 579.1
   anguilluliasis 127.2
   psilosis 579.1
Dientamoeba 007.8
dietetic 787.91
due to
   achylia gastrica 536.8
   Aerobacter aerogenes 008.2
   Bacillus coli — *see* Enteritis, E. coli
   bacteria NEC 008.5
   bile salts 579.8
   Capillaria
      hepatica 128.8
      philippinensis 127.5
   Clostridium perfringens (C) (F) 008.46
   Enterobacter aerogenes 008.2
   enterococci 008.49
   Escherichia coli — *see* Enteritis, E. coli
   Giardia lamblia 007.1
   Heterophyes heterophyes 121.6
   irritating foods 787.91
   Metagonimus yokogawai 121.5
   Necator americanus 126.1
   Paracolobactrum arizonae 008.1
   Paracolon bacillus NEC 008.47
      Arizona 008.1
   Proteus (bacillus) (mirabilis) (Morganii)
      008.3
   Pseudomonas aeruginosa 008.42
   S. japonicum 120.2
   specified organism NEC 008.8
      bacterial 008.49
      viral NEC 008.69
   Staphylococcus 008.41
   Streptococcus 008.49
      anaerobic 008.46
   Strongyloides stercoralis 127.2
   Trichuris trichiuria 127.3
   virus NEC (*see also* Enteritis, viral) 008.69
dysenteric 009.2
   due to specified organism NEC 008.8
dyspeptic 787.91
endemic 009.3
   due to specified organism NEC 008.8
epidemic 009.2
   due to specified organism NEC 008.8
fermentative 787.91
flagellate 007.9
Flexner's (ulcerative) 004.1
functional 564.5
   following gastrointestinal surgery 564.4
   psychogenic 306.4
giardial 007.1
Giardia lamblia 007.1
hill 579.1
hyperperistalsis (nervous) 306.4
infectious 009.2
   due to specified organism NEC 008.8
   presumed 009.3
inflammatory 787.91
   due to specified organism NEC 008.8
malarial (*see also* Malaria) 084.6
mite 133.8
mycotic 117.9
nervous 306.4
neurogenic 564.5
parenteral NEC 009.2
postgastrectomy 564.4
postvagotomy 564.4
prostaglandin induced 579.8
protozoal NEC 007.9

Diarrhea, diarrheal — *continued*
psychogenic 306.4
septic 009.2
   due to specified organism NEC 008.8
specified organism NEC 008.8
   bacterial 008.49
   viral 008.69
Staphylococcus 008.41
Streptococcus 008.49
   anaerobic 008.46
toxic 558.2
travelers' 009.2
   due to specified organism NEC 008.8
trichomonal 007.3
tropical 579.1
tuberculous 014.8 ☑
ulcerative (chronic) (*see also* Colitis, ulcerative) 556.9
viral (*see also* Enteritis, viral) 008.8
zymotic NEC 009.2
Diastasis
cranial bones 733.99
   congenital 756.0
joint (traumatic) — *see* Dislocation, by site
muscle 728.84
   congenital 756.89
recti (abdomen) 728.84
   complicating delivery 665.8 ☑
   congenital 756.79
Diastema, teeth, tooth 524.30
Diastematomyelia 742.51
Diataxia, cerebral, infantile 343.0
Diathesis
allergic V15.09
bleeding (familial) 287.9
cystine (familial) 270.0
gouty 274.9
hemorrhagic (familial) 287.9
   newborn NEC 776.0
oxalic 271.8
scrofulous (*see also* Tuberculosis) 017.2 ☑
spasmophilic (*see also* Tetany) 781.7
ulcer 536.9
uric acid 274.9
Diaz's disease or osteochondrosis 732.5
Dibothriocephaliasis 123.4
   larval 123.5
Dibothriocephalus (infection) (infestation)
   (latus) 123.4
   larval 123.5
Dicephalus 759.4
Dichotomy, teeth 520.2
Dichromat, dichromata (congenital) 368.59
Dichromatopsia (congenital) 368.59
Dichuchwa 104.0
Dicroceliasis 121.8
Didelphys, didelphic — *see also* Double uterus 752.2
Didymitis — *see also* Epididymitis 604.90
Died — *see also* Death
   without
      medical attention (cause unknown) 798.9
   sign of disease 798.2
Dientamoeba diarrhea 007.8
Dietary
inadequacy or deficiency 269.9
surveillance and counseling V65.3
Dietl's crisis 593.4
Dieulafoy lesion (hemorrhagic)
   of
      duodenum 537.84
      esophagus 530.82
      intestine 569.86
      stomach 537.84
Difficult
birth, affecting fetus or newborn 763.9
delivery NEC 669.9 ☑
Difficulty
feeding 783.3
   adult 783.3
   breast 676.8 ☑
   child 783.3
   elderly 783.3
   infant 783.3
   newborn 779.31

Difficulty — *continued*
feeding — *continued*
   nonorganic (infant) NEC 307.59
mechanical, gastroduodenal stoma 537.89
reading 315.00
specific, spelling 315.09
swallowing (*see also* Dysphagia) 787.20
walking 719.7
Diffuse — *see* condition
Diffused ganglion 727.42
Di George's syndrome (thymic hypoplasia) 279.11
Digestive — *see* condition
Di Guglielmo's disease or syndrome (M9841/3) 207.0 ☑
Dihydropyrimidine dehydrogenase disease (DPD) 277.6
Diktyoma (M9051/3) — *see* Neoplasm, by site, malignant
Dilaceration, tooth 520.4
Dilatation
anus 564.89
   venule — *see* Hemorrhoids
aorta (focal) (general) (*see also* Ectasia, aortic) 447.70
   with aneurysm 441.9
   congenital 747.29
   infectional 093.0
   ruptured 441.5
   syphilitic 093.0
appendix (cystic) 543.9
artery 447.8
bile duct (common) (congenital) 751.69
   acquired 576.8
bladder (sphincter) 596.89
   congenital 753.8
   in pregnancy or childbirth 654.4 ☑
      causing obstructed labor 660.2 ☑
      affecting fetus or newborn 763.1
blood vessel 459.89
bronchus, bronchi 494.0
   with acute exacerbation 494.1
calyx (due to obstruction) 593.89
capillaries 448.9
cardiac (acute) (chronic) (*see also* Hypertrophy, cardiac) 429.3
   congenital 746.89
      valve NEC 746.89
         pulmonary 746.09
   hypertensive (*see also* Hypertension, heart) 402.90
cavum septi pellucidi 742.4
cecum 564.89
   psychogenic 306.4
cervix (uteri) (*see also* Incompetency, cervix)
   incomplete, poor, slow
      affecting fetus or newborn 763.7
      complicating delivery 661.0 ☑
         affecting fetus or newborn 763.7
colon 564.7
   congenital 751.3
   due to mechanical obstruction 560.89
   psychogenic 306.4
common bile duct (congenital) 751.69
   acquired 576.8
      with calculus, choledocholithiasis, or stones — *see* Choledocholithiasis
cystic duct 751.69
   acquired (any bile duct) 575.8
duct, mammary 610.4
duodenum 564.89
esophagus 530.89
   congenital 750.4
   due to
      achalasia 530.0
      cardiospasm 530.0
Eustachian tube, congenital 744.24
fontanel 756.0
gallbladder 575.8
   congenital 751.69
gastric 536.8
   acute 536.1
   psychogenic 306.4
heart (acute) (chronic) (*see also* Hypertrophy, cardiac) 429.3

Dilatation — *continued*
heart (*see also* Hypertrophy, cardiac) — *continued*
   congenital 746.89
   hypertensive (*see also* Hypertension, heart) 402.90
   valve (*see also* Endocarditis)
      congenital 746.89
ileum 564.89
   psychogenic 306.4
inguinal rings — *see* Hernia, inguinal
jejunum 564.89
   psychogenic 306.4
kidney (calyx) (collecting structures) (cystic) (parenchyma) (pelvis) 593.89
lacrimal passages 375.69
lymphatic vessel 457.1
mammary duct 610.4
Meckel's diverticulum (congenital) 751.0
meningeal vessels, congenital 742.8
myocardium (acute) (chronic) (*see also* Hypertrophy, cardiac) 429.3
organ or site, congenital NEC — *see* Distortion
pancreatic duct 577.8
pelvis, kidney 593.89
pericardium — *see* Pericarditis
pharynx 478.29
prostate 602.8
pulmonary
   artery (idiopathic) 417.8
      congenital 747.39
   valve, congenital 746.09
pupil 379.43
rectum 564.89
renal 593.89
saccule vestibularis, congenital 744.05
salivary gland (duct) 527.8
sphincter ani 564.89
stomach 536.8
   acute 536.1
   psychogenic 306.4
submaxillary duct 527.8
trachea, congenital 748.3
ureter (idiopathic) 593.89
   congenital 753.20
   due to obstruction 593.5
urethra (acquired) 599.84
vasomotor 443.9
vein 459.89
ventricular, ventricle (acute) (chronic) (*see also* Hypertrophy, cardiac) 429.3
   cerebral, congenital 742.4
   hypertensive (*see also* Hypertension, heart) 402.90
venule 459.89
   anus — *see* Hemorrhoids
vesical orifice 596.89
Dilated, dilation — *see* Dilatation
Diminished
hearing (acuity) (*see also* Deafness) 389.9
pulse pressure 785.9
vision NEC 369.9
vital capacity 794.2
Diminuta taenia 123.6
Diminution, sense or sensation (cold) (heat) (tactile) (vibratory) — *see also* Disturbance, sensation 782.0
Dimitri-Sturge-Weber disease (encephalocutaneous angiomatosis) 759.6
Dimple
parasacral 685.1
   with abscess 685.0
pilonidal 685.1
   with abscess 685.0
postanal 685.1
   with abscess 685.0
Dioctophyma renale (infection) (infestation) 128.8
Dipetalonemiasis 125.4
Diphallus 752.69
Diphtheria, diphtheritic (gangrenous) (hemorrhagic) 032.9
carrier (suspected) of V02.4
cutaneous 032.85
cystitis 032.84

☑ Additional Digit Required — Refer to the Tabular List for Digit Selection   ⵠ Subterms under main terms may continue to next column or page

126   2014 ICD-9-CM

Diphtheria, diphtheritic — *continued*
faucial 032.0
infection of wound 032.85
inoculation (anti) (not sick) V03.5
laryngeal 032.3
myocarditis 032.82
nasal anterior 032.2
nasopharyngeal 032.1
neurological complication 032.89
peritonitis 032.83
specified site NEC 032.89
Diphyllobothriasis (intestine) 123.4
larval 123.5
Diplacusis 388.41
Diplegia (upper limbs) 344.2
brain or cerebral 437.8
congenital 343.0
facial 351.0
congenital 352.6
infantile or congenital (cerebral) (spastic) (spinal) 343.0
lower limbs 344.1
syphilitic, congenital 090.49
Diplococcus, diplococcal — *see* condition
Diplomyelia 742.59
Diplopia 368.2
refractive 368.15
Dipsomania — *see also* Alcoholism 303.9 ☑
with psychosis (*see also* Psychosis, alcoholic) 291.9
Dipylidiasis 123.8
intestine 123.8
Direction, teeth, abnormal 524.30
Dirt-eating child 307.52
Disability, disabilities
heart — *see* Disease, heart
intellectual 319
borderline V62.89
mild, IQ 50-70 317
moderate, IQ 35-49 318.0
profound, IQ under 20 318.2
severe, IQ 20-34 318.1
learning NEC 315.2
special spelling 315.09
Disarticulation — *see also* Derangement, joint 718.9 ☑
meaning
amputation
status — *see* Absence, by site
traumatic — *see* Amputation, traumatic
dislocation, traumatic or congenital — *see* Dislocation
Disaster, cerebrovascular — *see also* Disease, cerebrovascular, acute 436
Discharge
anal NEC 787.99
breast (female) (male) 611.79
conjunctiva 372.89
continued locomotor idiopathic (*see also* Epilepsy) 345.5 ☑
diencephalic autonomic idiopathic (*see also* Epilepsy) 345.5 ☑
ear 388.60
blood 388.69
cerebrospinal fluid 388.61
excessive urine 788.42
eye 379.93
nasal 478.19
nipple 611.79
patterned motor idiopathic (*see also* Epilepsy) 345.5 ☑
penile 788.7
postnasal — *see* Sinusitis
sinus, from mediastinum 510.0
umbilicus 789.9
urethral 788.7
bloody 599.84
vaginal 623.5
Discitis 722.90
cervical, cervicothoracic 722.91
lumbar, lumbosacral 722.93
thoracic, thoracolumbar 722.92
Discogenic syndrome — *see* Displacement, intervertebral disc

Discoid
kidney 753.3
meniscus, congenital 717.5
semilunar cartilage 717.5
Discoloration
mouth 528.9
nails 703.8
teeth 521.7
due to
drugs 521.7
metals (copper) (silver) 521.7
pulpal bleeding 521.7
during formation 520.8
extrinsic 523.6
intrinsic posteruptive 521.7
Discomfort
chest 786.59
visual 368.13
Discomycosis — *see* Actinomycosis
Discontinuity, ossicles, ossicular chain 385.23
Discrepancy
centric occlusion
maximum intercuspation 524.55
of teeth 524.55
leg length (acquired) 736.81
congenital 755.30
uterine size-date 649.6 ☑
Discrimination
political V62.4
racial V62.4
religious V62.4
sex V62.4
Disease, diseased — *see also* Syndrome
Abrami's (acquired hemolytic jaundice) 283.9
absorbent system 459.89
accumulation — *see* Thesaurismosis
acid-peptic 536.8
Acosta's 993.2
Adams-Stokes (-Morgagni) (syncope with heart block) 426.9
Addison's (bronze) (primary adrenal insufficiency) 255.41
anemia (pernicious) 281.0
tuberculous (*see also* Tuberculosis) 017.6 ☑
Addison-Gull — *see* Xanthoma
adenoids (and tonsils) (chronic) 474.9
adrenal (gland) (capsule) (cortex) 255.9
hyperfunction 255.3
hypofunction 255.41
specified type NEC 255.8
ainhum (dactylolysis spontanea) 136.0
akamushi (scrub typhus) 081.2
Akureyri (epidemic neuromyasthenia) 049.8
Albarrán's (colibacilluria) 791.9
Albers-Schönberg's (marble bones) 756.52
Albert's 726.71
Albright (-Martin) (-Bantam) 275.49
Alibert's (mycosis fungoides) (M9700/3) 202.1 ☑
Alibert-Bazin (M9700/3) 202.1 ☑
alimentary canal 569.9
alligator skin (ichthyosis congenita) 757.1
acquired 701.1
Almeida's (Brazilian blastomycosis) 116.1
Alpers' 330.8
alpine 993.2
altitude 993.2
alveoli, teeth 525.9
Alzheimer's — *see* Alzheimer's
amyloid (any site) 277.30
anarthritic rheumatoid 446.5
Anders' (adiposis tuberosa simplex) 272.8
Andersen's (glycogenosis IV) 271.0
Anderson's (angiokeratoma corporis diffusum) 272.7
Andes 993.2
Andrews' (bacterid) 686.8
angiospastic, angiospasmodic 443.9
cerebral 435.9
with transient neurologic deficit 435.9
vein 459.89

Disease, diseased — *see also* Syndrome — *continued*
anterior
chamber 364.9
horn cell 335.9
specified type NEC 335.8
antral (chronic) 473.0
acute 461.0
anus NEC 569.49
aorta (nonsyphilitic) 447.9
syphilitic NEC 093.89
aortic (heart) (valve) (*see also* Endocarditis, aortic) 424.1
apollo 077.4
aponeurosis 726.90
appendix 543.9
aqueous (chamber) 364.9
arc-welders' lung 503
Armenian 277.31
Arnold-Chiari (*see also* Spina bifida) 741.0 ☑
arterial 447.9
occlusive (*see also* Occlusion, by site) 444.22
with embolus or thrombus — *see* Occlusion, by site
due to stricture or stenosis 447.1
specified type NEC 447.8
arteriocardiorenal (*see also* Hypertension, cardiorenal) 404.90
arteriolar (generalized) (obliterative) 447.9
specified type NEC 447.8
arteriorenal — *see* Hypertension, kidney
arteriosclerotic (*see also* Arteriosclerosis)
cardiovascular 429.2
coronary — *see* Arteriosclerosis, coronary
heart — *see* Arteriosclerosis, coronary
vascular — *see* Arteriosclerosis
artery 447.9
cerebral 437.9
coronary — *see* Arteriosclerosis, coronary
specified type NEC 447.8
arthropod-borne NEC 088.9
specified type NEC 088.89
Asboe-Hansen's (incontinentia pigmenti) 757.33
atticoantral, chronic (with posterior or superior marginal perforation of ear drum) 382.2
auditory canal, ear 380.9
Aujeszky's 078.89
auricle, ear NEC 380.30
Australian X 062.4
autoimmune NEC 279.49
hemolytic (cold type) (warm type) 283.0
parathyroid 252.1
thyroid 245.2
aviators' (*see also* Effect, adverse, high altitude) 993.2
ax(e)-grinders' 502
Ayala's 756.89
Ayerza's (pulmonary artery sclerosis with pulmonary hypertension) 416.0
Azorean (of the nervous system) 334.8
Babington's (familial hemorrhagic telangiectasia) 448.0
back bone NEC 733.90
bacterial NEC 040.89
zoonotic NEC 027.9
specified type NEC 027.8
Baehr-Schiffrin (thrombotic thrombocytopenic purpura) 446.6
Baelz's (cheilitis glandularis apostematosa) 528.5
Baerensprung's (eczema marginatum) 110.3
Balfour's (chloroma) 205.3 ☑
balloon (*see also* Effect, adverse, high altitude) 993.2
Baló's 341.1
Bamberger (-Marie) (hypertrophic pulmonary osteoarthropathy) 731.2
Bang's (Brucella abortus) 023.1
Bannister's 995.1
Banti's (with cirrhosis) (with portal hypertension) — *see* Cirrhosis, liver

Disease, diseased — *see also* Syndrome — *continued*
Barcoo (*see also* Ulcer, skin) 707.9
barium lung 503
Barlow (-Möller) (infantile scurvy) 267
barometer makers' 985.0
Barraquer (-Simons) (progressive lipodystrophy) 272.6
basal ganglia 333.90
degenerative NEC 333.0
specified NEC 333.89
Basedow's (exophthalmic goiter) 242.0 ☑
basement membrane NEC 583.89
with
pulmonary hemorrhage (Goodpasture's syndrome) 446.21 [583.81]
Bateman's 078.0
purpura (senile) 287.2
Batten's 330.1 [362.71]
Batten-Mayou (retina) 330.1 [362.71]
Batten-Steinert 359.21
Battey 031.0
Baumgarten-Cruveilhier (cirrhosis of liver) 571.5
bauxite-workers' 503
Bayle's (dementia paralytica) 094.1
Bazin's (primary) (*see also* Tuberculosis) 017.1 ☑
Beard's (neurasthenia) 300.5
Beau's (*see also* Degeneration, myocardial) 429.1
Bechterew's (ankylosing spondylitis) 720.0
Becker's
idiopathic mural endomyocardial disease 425.4
myotonia congenita, recessive form 359.22
Begbie's (exophthalmic goiter) 242.0 ☑
Behr's 362.50
Beigel's (white piedra) 111.2
Bekhterev's (ankylosing spondylitis) 720.0
Bell's (*see also* Psychosis, affective) 296.0 ☑
Bennett's (leukemia) 208.9 ☑
Benson's 379.22
Bergeron's (hysteroepilepsy) 300.11
Berlin's 921.3
Bernard-Soulier (thrombopathy) 287.1
Bernhardt (-Roth) 355.1
beryllium 503
Besnier-Boeck (-Schaumann) (sarcoidosis) 135
Best's 362.76
Beurmann's (sporotrichosis) 117.1
Bielschowsky (-Jansky) 330.1
Biermer's (pernicious anemia) 281.0
Biett's (discoid lupus erythematosus) 695.4
bile duct (*see also* Disease, biliary) 576.9
biliary (duct) (tract) 576.9
with calculus, choledocholithiasis, or stones — *see* Choledocholithiasis
Billroth's (meningocele) (*see also* Spina bifida) 741.9 ☑
Binswanger's 290.12
Bird's (oxaluria) 271.8
bird fanciers' 495.2
black lung 500
bladder 596.9
specified NEC 596.89
bleeder's 286.0
Bloch-Sulzberger (incontinentia pigmenti) 757.33
Blocq's (astasia-abasia) 307.9
blood (-forming organs) 289.9
specified NEC 289.89
vessel 459.9
Bloodgood's 610.1
Blount's (tibia vara) 732.4
blue 746.9
Bodechtel-Guttmann (subacute sclerosing panencephalitis) 046.2
Boeck's (sarcoidosis) 135
bone 733.90
fibrocystic NEC 733.29
jaw 526.2
marrow 289.9

Disease, diseased — *see also* Syndrome — *continued*

bone — *continued*
Paget's (osteitis deformans) 731.0
specified type NEC 733.99
von Recklinghausen's (osteitis fibrosa cystica) 252.01
Bonfils' — *see* Disease, Hodgkin's
Borna 062.9
Bornholm (epidemic pleurodynia) 074.1
Bostock's (*see also* Fever, hay) 477.9
Bouchard's (myopathic dilatation of the stomach) 536.1
Bouillaud's (rheumatic heart disease) 391.9
Bourneville (-Brissaud) (tuberous sclerosis) 759.5
Bouveret (-Hoffmann) (paroxysmal tachycardia) 427.2
bowel 569.9
functional 564.9
psychogenic 306.4
Bowen's (M8081/2) — *see* Neoplasm, skin, in situ
Bozzolo's (multiple myeloma) (M9730/3) 203.0 ☑
Bradley's (epidemic vomiting) 078.82
Brailsford's 732.3
radius, head 732.3
tarsal, scaphoid 732.5
Brailsford-Morquio (mucopolysaccharidosis IV) 277.5
brain 348.9
Alzheimer's 331.0
with dementia — *see* Alzheimer's, dementia
arterial, artery 437.9
arteriosclerotic 437.0
congenital 742.9
degenerative — *see* Degeneration, brain
inflammatory (*see also* Encephalitis)
late effect — *see* category 326
organic 348.9
arteriosclerotic 437.0
parasitic NEC 123.9
Pick's 331.11
with dementia
with behavioral disturbance 331.11 *[294.11]*
without behavioral disturbance 331.11 *[294.10]*
senile 331.2
braziers' 985.8
breast 611.9
cystic (chronic) 610.1
fibrocystic 610.1
inflammatory 611.0
Paget's (M8540/3) 174.0
puerperal, postpartum NEC 676.3 ☑
specified NEC 611.89
Breda's (*see also* Yaws) 102.9
Breisky's (kraurosis vulvae) 624.09
Bretonneau's (diphtheritic malignant angina) 032.0
Bright's (*see also* Nephritis) 583.9
arteriosclerotic (*see also* Hypertension, kidney) 403.90
Brill's (recrudescent typhus) 081.1
flea-borne 081.0
louse-borne 081.1
Brill-Symmers (follicular lymphoma) (M9690/3) 202.0 ☑
Brill-Zinsser (recrudescent typhus) 081.1
Brinton's (leather bottle stomach) (M8142/3) 151.9
Brion-Kayser (*see also* Fever, paratyphoid) 002.9
broad
beta 272.2
ligament, noninflammatory 620.9
specified NEC 620.8
Brocq's 691.8
meaning
atopic (diffuse) neurodermatitis 691.8
dermatitis herpetiformis 694.0
lichen simplex chronicus 698.3

Disease, diseased — *see also* Syndrome — *continued*

Brocq's — *continued*
meaning — *continued*
parapsoriasis 696.2
prurigo 698.2
Brocq-Duhring (dermatitis herpetiformis) 694.0
Brodie's (joint) (*see also* Osteomyelitis) 730.1 ☑
bronchi 519.19
bronchopulmonary 519.19
bronze (Addison's) 255.41
tuberculous (*see also* Tuberculosis) 017.6 ☑
Brown-Séquard 344.89
Bruck's 733.99
Bruck-de Lange (Amsterdam dwarf, intellectual disabilities, and brachycephaly) 759.89
Bruhl's (splenic anemia with fever) 285.8
Bruton's (X-linked agammaglobulinemia) 279.04
buccal cavity 528.9
Buchanan's (juvenile osteochondrosis, iliac crest) 732.1
Buchman's (osteochondrosis juvenile) 732.1
Budgerigar-Fanciers' 495.2
Büdinger-Ludloff-Läwen 717.89
Buerger's (thromboangiitis obliterans) 443.1
Bürger-Grütz (essential familial hyperlipemia) 272.3
Burns' (lower ulna) 732.3
bursa 727.9
Bury's (erythema elevatum diutinum) 695.89
Buschke's 710.1
Busquet's (*see also* Osteomyelitis) 730.1 ☑
Busse-Buschke (cryptococcosis) 117.5
C₂ (*see also* Alcoholism) 303.9 ☑
Caffey's (infantile cortical hyperostosis) 756.59
caisson 993.3
calculous 592.9
California 114.0
Calvé (-Perthes) (osteochondrosis, femoral capital) 732.1
Camurati-Engelmann (diaphyseal sclerosis) 756.59
Canavan's 330.0
capillaries 448.9
Carapata 087.1
cardiac — *see* Disease, heart
cardiopulmonary, chronic 416.9
cardiorenal (arteriosclerotic) (hepatic) (hypertensive) (vascular) (*see also* Hypertension, cardiorenal) 404.90
cardiovascular (arteriosclerotic) 429.2
congenital 746.9
hypertensive (*see also* Hypertension, heart) 402.90
benign 402.10
malignant 402.00
renal (*see also* Hypertension, cardiorenal) 404.90
syphilitic (asymptomatic) 093.9
carotid gland 259.8
Carrión's (Bartonellosis) 088.0
cartilage NEC 733.90
specified NEC 733.99
Castellani's 104.8
cat-scratch 078.3
Cavare's (familial periodic paralysis) 359.3
Cazenave's (pemphigus) 694.4
cecum 569.9
celiac (adult) 579.0
infantile 579.0
cellular tissue NEC 709.9
central core 359.0
cerebellar, cerebellum — *see* Disease, brain
cerebral (*see also* Disease, brain) 348.9
arterial, artery 437.9
degenerative — *see* Degeneration, brain
cerebrospinal 349.9
cerebrovascular NEC 437.9
acute 436
embolic — *see* Embolism, brain

Disease, diseased — *see also* Syndrome — *continued*

cerebrovascular — *continued*
acute — *continued*
late effect — *see* Late effect(s) (of) cerebrovascular disease
puerperal, postpartum, childbirth 674.0 ☑
thrombotic — *see* Thrombosis, brain
arteriosclerotic 437.0
embolic — *see* Embolism, brain
ischemic, generalized NEC 437.1
late effect — *see* Late effect(s) (of) cerebrovascular disease
occlusive 437.1
puerperal, postpartum, childbirth 674.0 ☑
specified type NEC 437.8
thrombotic — *see* Thrombosis, brain
ceroid storage 272.7
cervix (uteri)
inflammatory 616.0
noninflammatory 622.9
specified NEC 622.8
Chabert's 022.9
Chagas' (*see also* Trypanosomiasis, American) 086.2
Chandler's (osteochondritis dissecans, hip) 732.7
Charcôt-Marie-Tooth 356.1
Charcôt's (joint) 094.0 *[713.5]*
spinal cord 094.0
Charlouis' (*see also* Yaws) 102.9
Cheadle (-Möller) (-Barlow) (infantile scurvy) 267
Chédiak-Steinbrinck (-Higashi) (congenital gigantism of peroxidase granules) 288.2
cheek, inner 528.9
chest 519.9
Chiari's (hepatic vein thrombosis) 453.0
Chicago (North American blastomycosis) 116.0
chignon (white piedra) 111.2
chigoe, chigo (jigger) 134.1
childhood granulomatous 288.1
Chinese liver fluke 121.1
chlamydial NEC 078.88
cholecystic (*see also* Disease, gallbladder) 575.9
choroid 363.9
degenerative (*see also* Degeneration, choroid) 363.40
hereditary (*see also* Dystrophy, choroid) 363.50
specified type NEC 363.8
Christian's (chronic histiocytosis X) 277.89
Christian-Weber (nodular nonsuppurative panniculitis) 729.30
Christmas 286.1
ciliary body 364.9
specified NEC 364.89
circulatory (system) NEC 459.9
chronic, maternal, affecting fetus or newborn 760.3
specified NEC 459.89
syphilitic 093.9
congenital 090.5
Civatte's (poikiloderma) 709.09
climacteric 627.2
male 608.89
coagulation factor deficiency (congenital) (*see also* Defect, coagulation) 286.9
Coats' 362.12
coccidioidal pulmonary 114.5
acute 114.0
chronic 114.4
primary 114.0
residual 114.4
Cockayne's (microcephaly and dwarfism) 759.89
Cogan's 370.52
cold
agglutinin 283.0
or hemoglobinuria 283.0

Disease, diseased — *see also* Syndrome — *continued*

cold — *continued*
agglutinin — *continued*
or hemoglobinuria — *continued*
paroxysmal (cold) (nocturnal) 283.2
hemagglutinin (chronic) 283.0
collagen NEC 710.9
nonvascular 710.9
specified NEC 710.8
vascular (allergic) (*see also* Angiitis, hypersensitivity) 446.20
colon 569.9
functional 564.9
congenital 751.3
ischemic 557.1
combined system (of spinal cord) 266.2 *[336.2]*
with anemia (pernicious) 281.0 *[336.2]*
compressed air 993.3
Concato's (pericardial polyserositis) 423.2
peritoneal 568.82
pleural — *see* Pleurisy
congenital NEC 799.89
conjunctiva 372.9
chlamydial 077.98
specified NEC 077.8
specified type NEC 372.89
viral 077.99
specified NEC 077.8
connective tissue, diffuse (*see also* Disease, collagen) 710.9
Conor and Bruch's (boutonneuse fever) 082.1
Conradi (-Hünermann) 756.59
Cooley's (erythroblastic anemia) 282.44
Cooper's 610.1
Corbus' 607.1
cork-handlers' 495.3
cornea (*see also* Keratopathy) 371.9
coronary (*see also* Ischemia, heart) 414.9
congenital 746.85
ostial, syphilitic 093.20
aortic 093.22
mitral 093.21
pulmonary 093.24
tricuspid 093.23
Corrigan's — *see* Insufficiency, aortic
Cotugno's 724.3
Coxsackie (virus) NEC 074.8
cranial nerve NEC 352.9
Creutzfeldt-Jakob (CJD) 046.19
with dementia
with behavioral disturbance 046.19 *[294.11]*
without behavioral disturbance 046.19 *[294.10]*
familial 046.19
iatrogenic 046.19
specified NEC 046.19
sporadic 046.19
variant (vCJD) 046.11
with dementia
with behavioral disturbance 046.11 *[294.11]*
without behavioral disturbance 046.11 *[294.10]*
Crigler-Najjar (congenital hyperbilirubinemia) 277.4
Crocq's (acrocyanosis) 443.89
Crohn's (intestine) (*see also* Enteritis, regional) 555.9
Crouzon's (craniofacial dysostosis) 756.0
Cruchet's (encephalitis lethargica) 049.8
Cruveilhier's 335.21
Cruz-Chagas (*see also* Trypanosomiasis, American) 086.2
crystal deposition (*see also* Arthritis, due to, crystals) 712.9 ☑
Csillag's (lichen sclerosus et atrophicus) 701.0
Curschmann's 359.21
Cushing's (pituitary basophilism) 255.0
cystic
breast (chronic) 610.1

Disease, diseased — *see also* Syndrome — *continued*

cystic — *continued*
kidney, congenital (*see also* Cystic, disease, kidney) 753.10
liver, congenital 751.62
lung 518.89
congenital 748.4
pancreas 577.2
congenital 751.7
renal, congenital (*see also* Cystic, disease, kidney) 753.10
semilunar cartilage 717.5
cysticercus 123.1
cystine storage (with renal sclerosis) 270.0
cytomegalic inclusion (generalized) 078.5
with
pneumonia 078.5 [484.1]
congenital 771.1
Daae (-Finsen) (epidemic pleurodynia) 074.1
dancing 297.8
Danielssen's (anesthetic leprosy) 030.1
Darier's (congenital) (keratosis follicularis) 757.39
erythema annulare centrifugum 695.0
vitamin A deficiency 264.8
Darling's (histoplasmosis) (*see also* Histoplasmosis, American) 115.00
Davies' 425.0
de Beurmann-Gougerot (sporotrichosis) 117.1
Débove's (splenomegaly) 789.2
deer fly (*see also* Tularemia) 021.9
deficiency 269.9
degenerative (*see also* Degeneration)
disc — *see* Degeneration, intervertebral disc
Degos' 447.8
Déjérine (-Sottas) 356.0
Déleage's 359.89
demyelinating, demyelinizating (brain stem) (central nervous system) 341.9
multiple sclerosis 340
specified NEC 341.8
de Quervain's (tendon sheath) 727.04
thyroid (subacute granulomatous thyroiditis) 245.1
Dercum's (adiposis dolorosa) 272.8
Deutschländer's — *see* Fracture, foot
Devergie's (pityriasis rubra pilaris) 696.4
Devic's 341.0
diaphorase deficiency 289.7
diaphragm 519.4
diarrheal, infectious 009.2
diatomaceous earth 502
Diaz's (osteochondrosis astragalus) 732.5
digestive system 569.9
Di Guglielmo's (erythemic myelosis) (M9841/3) 207.0 ☑
Dimitri-Sturge-Weber (encephalocutaneous angiomatosis) 759.6
disc, degenerative — *see* Degeneration, intervertebral disc
discogenic (*see also* Disease, intervertebral disc) 722.90
diverticular — *see* Diverticula
Down's (mongolism) 758.0
Dubini's (electric chorea) 049.8
Dubois' (thymus gland) 090.5
Duchenne's 094.0
locomotor ataxia 094.0
muscular dystrophy 359.1
paralysis 335.22
pseudohypertrophy, muscles 359.1
Duchenne-Griesinger 359.1
ductless glands 259.9
Duhring's (dermatitis herpetiformis) 694.0
Dukes (-Filatov) 057.8
duodenum NEC 537.9
specified NEC 537.89
Duplay's 726.2
Dupré's (meningism) 781.6
Dupuytren's (muscle contracture) 728.6
Durand-Nicolas-Favre (climatic bubo) 099.1
Duroziez's (congenital mitral stenosis) 746.5
Dutton's (trypanosomiasis) 086.9

Disease, diseased — *see also* Syndrome — *continued*

Eales' 362.18
ear (chronic) (inner) NEC 388.9
middle 385.9
adhesive (*see also* Adhesions, middle ear) 385.10
specified NEC 385.89
Eberth's (typhoid fever) 002.0
Ebstein's
heart 746.2
meaning diabetes 250.4 ☑ [581.81]
due to secondary diabetes 249.4 ☑ [581.81]
Echinococcus (*see also* Echinococcus) 122.9
ECHO virus NEC 078.89
Economo's (encephalitis lethargica) 049.8
Eddowes' (brittle bones and blue sclera) 756.51
Edsall's 992.2
Eichstedt's (pityriasis versicolor) 111.0
Ellis-van Creveld (chondroectodermal dysplasia) 756.55
endocardium — *see* Endocarditis
endocrine glands or system NEC 259.9
specified NEC 259.8
endomyocardial, idiopathic mural 425.2
Engelmann's (diaphyseal sclerosis) 756.59
Engel-von Recklinghausen (osteitis fibrosa cystica) 252.01
English (rickets) 268.0
Engman's (infectious eczematoid dermatitis) 690.8
enteroviral, enterovirus NEC 078.89
central nervous system NEC 048
epidemic NEC 136.9
epididymis 608.9
epigastric, functional 536.9
psychogenic 306.4
Erb (-Landouzy) 359.1
Erb-Goldflam 358.00
Erdheim-Chester (ECD) 277.89
Erichsen's (railway spine) 300.16
esophagus 530.9
functional 530.5
psychogenic 306.4
Eulenburg's (congenital paramyotonia) 359.29
Eustachian tube 381.9
Evans' (thrombocytopenic purpura) 287.32
external auditory canal 380.9
extrapyramidal NEC 333.90
eye 379.90
anterior chamber 364.9
inflammatory NEC 364.3
muscle 378.9
eyeball 360.9
eyelid 374.9
eyeworm of Africa 125.2
Fabry's (angiokeratoma corporis diffusum) 272.7
facial nerve (seventh) 351.9
newborn 767.5
Fahr-Volhard (malignant nephrosclerosis) 403.00
fallopian tube, noninflammatory 620.9
specified NEC 620.8
familial periodic 277.31
paralysis 359.3
Fanconi's (congenital pancytopenia) 284.09
Farber's (disseminated lipogranulomatosis) 272.8
fascia 728.9
inflammatory 728.9
Fauchard's (periodontitis) 523.40
Favre-Durand-Nicolas (climatic bubo) 099.1
Favre-Racouchot (elastoidosis cutanea nodularis) 701.8
Fede's 529.0
Feer's 985.0
Felix's (juvenile osteochondrosis, hip) 732.1
Fenwick's (gastric atrophy) 537.89
Fernels' (aortic aneurysm) 441.9
fibrocaseous, of lung (*see also* Tuberculosis, pulmonary) 011.9 ☑
fibrocystic (*see also* Fibrocystic, disease)

Disease, diseased — *see also* Syndrome — *continued*

fibrocystic (*see also* Fibrocystic, disease) — *continued*
newborn 277.01
Fiedler's (leptospiral jaundice) 100.0
fifth 057.0
Filatoff's (infectious mononucleosis) 075
Filatov's (infectious mononucleosis) 075
file-cutters' 984.9
specified type of lead — *see* Table of Drugs and Chemicals
filterable virus NEC 078.89
fish skin 757.1
acquired 701.1
Flajani (-Basedow) (exophthalmic goiter) 242.0 ☑
Flatau-Schilder 341.1
flax-dressers' 504
Fleischner's 732.3
flint 502
fluke — *see* Infestation, fluke
Følling's (phenylketonuria) 270.1
foot and mouth 078.4
foot process 581.3
Forbes' (glycogenosis III) 271.0
Fordyce's (ectopic sebaceous glands) (mouth) 750.26
Fordyce-Fox (apocrine miliaria) 705.82
Fothergill's
meaning scarlatina anginosa 034.1
neuralgia (*see also* Neuralgia, trigeminal) 350.1
Fournier's 608.83
female 616.89
fourth 057.8
Fox (-Fordyce) (apocrine miliaria) 705.82
Francis' (*see also* Tularemia) 021.9
Franklin's (heavy chain) 273.2
Frei's (climatic bubo) 099.1
Freiberg's (flattening metatarsal) 732.5
Friedländer's (endarteritis obliterans) — *see* Arteriosclerosis
Friedreich's
combined systemic or ataxia 334.0
facial hemihypertrophy 756.0
myoclonia 333.2
Fröhlich's (adiposogenital dystrophy) 253.8
Frommel's 676.6 ☑
frontal sinus (chronic) 473.1
acute 461.1
Fuller's earth 502
fungus, fungous NEC 117.9
Gaisböck's (polycythemia hypertonica) 289.0
gallbladder 575.9
congenital 751.60
Gamna's (sideriotic splenomegaly) 289.51
Gamstorp's (adynamia episodica hereditaria) 359.3
Gandy-Nanta (sideriotic splenomegaly) 289.51
Gannister (occupational) 502
Garré's (*see also* Osteomyelitis) 730.1 ☑
gastric (*see also* Disease, stomach) 537.9
gastroesophageal reflux (GERD) 530.81
gastrointestinal (tract) 569.9
amyloid 277.39
functional 536.9
psychogenic 306.4
Gaucher's (adult) (cerebroside lipidosis) (infantile) 272.7
Gayet's (superior hemorrhagic polioencephalitis) 265.1
Gee (-Herter) (-Heubner) (-Thaysen) (nontropical sprue) 579.0
generalized neoplastic (M8000/6) 199.0
genital organs NEC
female 629.9
specified NEC 629.89
male 608.9
Gerhardt's (erythromelalgia) 443.82
Gerlier's (epidemic vertigo) 078.81
Gibert's (pityriasis rosea) 696.3
Gibney's (perispondylitis) 720.9
Gierke's (glycogenosis I) 271.0

Disease, diseased — *see also* Syndrome — *continued*

Gilbert's (familial nonhemolytic jaundice) 277.4
Gilchrist's (North American blastomycosis) 116.0
Gilford (-Hutchinson) (progeria) 259.8
Gilles de la Tourette's (motor-verbal tic) 307.23
Giovannini's 117.9
gland (lymph) 289.9
Glanzmann's (hereditary hemorrhagic thrombasthenia) 287.1
glassblowers' 527.1
Glénard's (enteroptosis) 569.89
Glisson's (*see also* Rickets) 268.0
glomerular
membranous, idiopathic 581.1
minimal change 581.3
glycogen storage (Andersen's) (Cori types 1-7) (Forbes') (McArdle-Schmid-Pearson) (Pompe's) (types I-VII) 271.0
cardiac 271.0 [425.7]
generalized 271.0
glucose–6–phosphatase deficiency 271.0
heart 271.0 [425.7]
hepatorenal 271.0
liver and kidneys 271.0
myocardium 271.0 [425.7]
von Gierke's (glycogenosis I) 271.0
Goldflam-Erb 358.00
Goldscheider's (epidermolysis bullosa) 757.39
Goldstein's (familial hemorrhagic telangiectasia) 448.0
gonococcal NEC 098.0
Goodall's (epidemic vomiting) 078.82
Gordon's (exudative enteropathy) 579.8
Gougerot's (trisymptomatic) 709.1
Gougerot-Carteaud (confluent reticulate papillomatosis) 701.8
Gougerot-Hailey-Hailey (benign familial chronic pemphigus) 757.39
graft-versus-host 279.50
acute 279.51
on chronic 279.53
chronic 279.52
grain-handlers' 495.8
Grancher's (splenopneumonia) — *see* Pneumonia
granulomatous (childhood) (chronic) 288.1
graphite lung 503
Graves' (exophthalmic goiter) 242.0 ☑
Greenfield's 330.0
green monkey 078.89
Griesinger's (*see also* Ancylostomiasis) 126.9
grinders' 502
Grisel's 723.5
Gruby's (tinea tonsurans) 110.0
Guertin's (electric chorea) 049.8
Guillain-Barré 357.0
Guinon's (motor-verbal tic) 307.23
Gull's (thyroid atrophy with myxedema) 244.8
Gull and Sutton's — *see* Hypertension, kidney
gum NEC 523.9
Günther's (congenital erythropoietic porphyria) 277.1
gynecological 629.9
specified NEC 629.89
H 270.0
Haas' 732.3
Habermann's (acute parapsoriasis varioliformis) 696.2
Haff 985.1
Hageman (congenital factor XII deficiency) (*see also* Defect, congenital) 286.3
Haglund's (osteochondrosis os tibiale externum) 732.5
Hagner's (hypertrophic pulmonary osteoarthropathy) 731.2
Hailey-Hailey (benign familial chronic pemphigus) 757.39
hair (follicles) NEC 704.9

Disease, diseased — see also Syndrome — continued

hypophysis — continued
hypofunction 253.2
Iceland (epidemic neuromyasthenia) 049.8
I cell 272.7
ill-defined 799.89
immunologic NEC 279.9
immunoproliferative 203.8 ☑
inclusion 078.5
salivary gland 078.5
infancy, early NEC 779.9
infective NEC 136.9
inguinal gland 289.9
internal semilunar cartilage, cystic 717.5
intervertebral disc 722.90
with myelopathy 722.70
cervical, cervicothoracic 722.91
with myelopathy 722.71
lumbar, lumbosacral 722.93
with myelopathy 722.73
thoracic, thoracolumbar 722.92
with myelopathy 722.72
intestine 569.9
functional 564.9
congenital 751.3
psychogenic 306.4
lardaceous 277.39
organic 569.9
protozoal NEC 007.9
iris 364.9
specified NEC 364.89
iron
metabolism (see also Hemochromatosis) 275.09
storage (see also Hemochromatosis) 275.03
Isambert's (see also Tuberculosis, larynx) 012.3 ☑
Iselin's (osteochondrosis, fifth metatarsal) 732.5
island (scrub typhus) 081.2
itai-itai 985.5
Jadassohn's (maculopapular erythroderma) 696.2
Jadassohn-Pellizari's (anetoderma) 701.3
Jakob-Creutzfeldt (CJD) 046.19
with dementia
with behavioral disturbance 046.19 [294.11]
without behavioral disturbance 046.19 [294.10]
familial 046.19
iatrogenic 046.19
specified NEC 046.19
sporadic 046.19
variant (vCJD) 046.11
with dementia
with behavioral disturbance 046.11 [294.11]
without behavioral disturbance 046.11 [294.10]
Jaksch (-Luzet) (pseudoleukemia infantum) 285.8
Janet's 300.89
Jansky-Bielschowsky 330.1
jaw NEC 526.9
fibrocystic 526.2
Jensen's 363.05
Jeune's (asphyxiating thoracic dystrophy) 756.4
jigger 134.1
Johnson-Stevens (erythema multiforme exudativum) 695.13
joint NEC 719.9 ☑
ankle 719.97
Charcôt 094.0 [713.5]
degenerative (see also Osteoarthrosis) 715.9 ☑
multiple 715.09
spine (see also Spondylosis) 721.90
elbow 719.92
foot 719.97
hand 719.94
hip 719.95

Disease, diseased — see also Syndrome — continued

joint — continued
hypertrophic (chronic) (degenerative) (see also Osteoarthrosis) 715.9 ☑
spine (see also Spondylosis) 721.90
knee 719.96
Luschka 721.90
multiple sites 719.99
pelvic region 719.95
sacroiliac 724.6
shoulder (region) 719.91
specified site NEC 719.98
spine NEC 724.9
pseudarthrosis following fusion 733.82
sacroiliac 724.6
wrist 719.93
Jourdain's (acute gingivitis) 523.00
Jüngling's (sarcoidosis) 135
Kahler (-Bozzolo) (multiple myeloma) (M9730/3) 203.0 ☑
Kalischer's 759.6
Kaposi's 757.33
lichen ruber 697.8
acuminatus 696.4
moniliformis 697.8
xeroderma pigmentosum 757.33
Kaschin-Beck (endemic polyarthritis) 716.00
ankle 716.07
arm 716.02
lower (and wrist) 716.03
upper (and elbow) 716.02
foot (and ankle) 716.07
forearm (and wrist) 716.03
hand 716.04
leg 716.06
lower 716.06
upper 716.05
multiple sites 716.09
pelvic region (hip) (thigh) 716.05
shoulder region 716.01
specified site NEC 716.08
Katayama 120.2
Kawasaki 446.1
Kedani (scrub typhus) 081.2
kidney (functional) (pelvis) (see also Disease, renal) 593.9
chronic 585.9
requiring chronic dialysis 585.6
stage
I 585.1
II (mild) 585.2
III (moderate) 585.3
IV (severe) 585.4
V 585.5
cystic (congenital) 753.10
multiple 753.19
single 753.11
specified NEC 753.19
fibrocystic (congenital) 753.19
in gout 274.10
polycystic (congenital) 753.12
adult type (APKD) 753.13
autosomal dominant 753.13
autosomal recessive 753.14
childhood type (CPKD) 753.14
infantile type 753.14
Kienböck's (carpal lunate) (wrist) 732.3
Kimmelstiel (-Wilson) (intercapillary glomerulosclerosis) 250.4 ☑ [581.81]
due to secondary diabetes 249.4 ☑ [581.81]
Kinnier Wilson's (hepatolenticular degeneration) 275.1
kissing 075
Kleb's (see also Nephritis) 583.9
Klinger's 446.4
Klippel's 723.8
Klippel-Feil (brevicollis) 756.16
knight's 911.1
Köbner's (epidermolysis bullosa) 757.39
Koenig-Wichmann (pemphigus) 694.4
Köhler's
first (osteoarthrosis juvenilis) 732.5

Disease, diseased — see also Syndrome — continued

Köhler's — continued
second (Freiberg's infraction, metatarsal head) 732.5
patellar 732.4
tarsal navicular (bone) (osteoarthrosis juvenilis) 732.5
Köhler-Freiberg (infraction, metatarsal head) 732.5
Köhler-Mouchet (osteoarthrosis juvenilis) 732.5
Köhler-Pellegrini-Stieda (calcification, knee joint) 726.62
Kok 759.89
König's (osteochondritis dissecans) 732.7
Korsakoff's (nonalcoholic) 294.0
alcoholic 291.1
Kostmann's (infantile genetic agranulocytosis) 288.01
Krabbe's 330.0
Kraepelin-Morel (see also Schizophrenia) 295.9 ☑
Kraft-Weber-Dimitri 759.6
Kufs' 330.1
Kugelberg-Welander 335.11
Kuhnt-Junius 362.52
Kümmell's (-Verneuil) (spondylitis) 721.7
Kundrat's (lymphosarcoma) 200.1 ☑
kuru 046.0
Kussmaul (-Meier) (polyarteritis nodosa) 446.0
Kyasanur Forest 065.2
Kyrle's (hyperkeratosis follicularis in cutem penetrans) 701.1
labia
inflammatory 616.10
noninflammatory 624.9
specified NEC 624.8
labyrinth, ear 386.8
lacrimal system (apparatus) (passages) 375.9
gland 375.00
specified NEC 375.89
Lafora's 333.2
Lagleyze-von Hippel (retinocerebral angiomatosis) 759.6
Lancereaux-Mathieu (leptospiral jaundice) 100.0
Landry's 357.0
Lane's 569.89
lardaceous (any site) 277.39
Larrey-Weil (leptospiral jaundice) 100.0
Larsen (-Johansson) (juvenile osteopathia patellae) 732.4
larynx 478.70
Lasègue's (persecution mania) 297.9
Leber's 377.16
Lederer's (acquired infectious hemolytic anemia) 283.19
Legg's (capital femoral osteochondrosis) 732.1
Legg-Calvé-Perthes (capital femoral osteochondrosis) 732.1
Legg-Calvé-Waldenström (femoral capital osteochondrosis) 732.1
Legg-Perthes (femoral capital osteochondrosis) 732.1
Legionnaires' 482.84
Leigh's 330.8
Leiner's (exfoliative dermatitis) 695.89
Leloir's (lupus erythematosus) 695.4
Lenegre's 426.0
lens (eye) 379.39
Leriche's (osteoporosis, posttraumatic) 733.7
Letterer-Siwe (acute histiocytosis X) (M9722/3) 202.5 ☑
Lev's (acquired complete heart block) 426.0
Lewandowski's (see also Tuberculosis) 017.0 ☑
Lewandowski-Lutz (epidermodysplasia verruciformis) 078.19
Lewy body 331.82
with dementia
with behavioral disturbance 331.82 [294.11]

Disease, diseased — see also Syndrome — continued

Lewy body — continued
with dementia — continued
without behavioral disturbance 331.82 [294.10]
Leyden's (periodic vomiting) 536.2
Libman-Sacks (verrucous endocarditis) 710.0 [424.91]
Lichtheim's (subacute combined sclerosis with pernicious anemia) 281.0 [336.2]
ligament 728.9
light chain 203.0 ☑
Lightwood's (renal tubular acidosis) 588.89
Lignac's (cystinosis) 270.0
Lindau's (retinocerebral angiomatosis) 759.6
Lindau-von Hippel (angiomatosis retinocerebellosa) 759.6
lipidosis 272.7
lipoid storage NEC 272.7
Lipschütz's 616.50
lip NEC 528.5
Little's — see Palsy, cerebral
liver 573.9
alcoholic 571.3
acute 571.1
chronic 571.3
chronic 571.9
alcoholic 571.3
cystic, congenital 751.62
drug-induced 573.3
due to
chemicals 573.3
fluorinated agents 573.3
hypersensitivity drugs 573.3
isoniazids 573.3
end stage NEC 572.8
due to hepatitis — see Hepatitis
fibrocystic (congenital) 751.62
glycogen storage 271.0
organic 573.9
polycystic (congenital) 751.62
Lobo's (keloid blastomycosis) 116.2
Lobstein's (brittle bones and blue sclera) 756.51
locomotor system 334.9
Lorain's (pituitary dwarfism) 253.3
Lou Gehrig's 335.20
Lucas-Championnière (fibrinous bronchitis) 466.0
Ludwig's (submaxillary cellulitis) 528.3
luetic — see Syphilis
lumbosacral region 724.6
lung NEC 518.89
black 500
congenital 748.60
cystic 518.89
congenital 748.4
fibroid (chronic) (see also Fibrosis, lung) 515
fluke 121.2
oriental 121.2
in
amyloidosis 277.39 [517.8]
polymyositis 710.4 [517.8]
sarcoidosis 135 [517.8]
Sjögren's syndrome 710.2 [517.8]
syphilis 095.1
systemic lupus erythematosus 710.0 [517.8]
systemic sclerosis 710.1 [517.2]
interstitial (chronic) 515
acute 136.3
respiratory bronchiolitis 516.34
nonspecific, chronic 496
obstructive (chronic) (COPD) 496
with
acute
bronchitis 491.22
exacerbation NEC 491.21
alveolitis, allergic (see also Alveolitis, allergic) 495.9
asthma (chronic) (obstructive) 493.2 ☑
bronchiectasis 494.0
with acute exacerbation 494.1

▼ Subterms under main terms may continue to next column or page

Disease, diseased — *see also* Syndrome — *continued*
lung — *continued*
obstructive — *continued*
with — *continued*
bronchitis (chronic) 491.20
with
acute bronchitis 491.22
exacerbation (acute) 491.21
decompensated 491.21
with exacerbation 491.21
emphysema NEC 492.8
diffuse (with fibrosis) 496
of childhood, specific NEC 516.69
polycystic 518.89
asthma (chronic) (obstructive) 493.2 ✓
congenital 748.4
purulent (cavitary) 513.0
restrictive 518.89
rheumatoid 714.81
diffuse interstitial 714.81
specified NEC 518.89
Lutembacher's (atrial septal defect with mitral stenosis) 745.5
Lutz-Miescher (elastosis perforans serpiginosa) 701.1
Lutz-Splendore-de Almeida (Brazilian blastomycosis) 116.1
Lyell's (toxic epidermal necrolysis) 695.15
due to drug
correct substance properly administered 695.15
overdose or wrong substance given or taken 977.9
specific drug — *see* Table of Drugs and Chemicals
Lyme 088.81
lymphatic (gland) (system) 289.9
channel (noninfective) 457.9
vessel (noninfective) 457.9
specified NEC 457.8
lymphoproliferative (chronic) (M9970/1) 238.79
X linked 759.89
Machado-Joseph 334.8
Madelung's (lipomatosis) 272.8
Madura (actinomycotic) 039.9
mycotic 117.4
Magitot's 526.4
Majocchi's (purpura annularis telangiectodes) 709.1
malarial (*see also* Malaria) 084.6
Malassez's (cystic) 608.89
Malibu 919.8
infected 919.9
malignant (M8000/3) (*see also* Neoplasm, by site, malignant)
previous, affecting management of pregnancy V23.89
Manson's 120.1
maple bark 495.6
maple syrup (urine) 270.3
Marburg (virus) 078.89
Marchiafava (-Bignami) 341.8
Marfan's 090.49
congenital syphilis 090.49
meaning Marfan's syndrome 759.82
Marie-Bamberger (hypertrophic pulmonary osteoarthropathy) (secondary) 731.2
primary or idiopathic (acropachyderma) 757.39
pulmonary (hypertrophic osteoarthropathy) 731.2
Marie-Strümpell (ankylosing spondylitis) 720.0
Marion's (bladder neck obstruction) 596.0
Marsh's (exophthalmic goiter) 242.0 ✓
Martin's 715.27
mast cell 757.33
systemic (M9741/3) 202.6 ✓
mastoid (*see also* Mastoiditis) 383.9
process 385.9
maternal, unrelated to pregnancy NEC, affecting fetus or newborn 760.9

Disease, diseased — *see also* Syndrome — *continued*
Mathieu's (leptospiral jaundice) 100.0
Mauclaire's 732.3
Mauriac's (erythema nodosum syphiliticum) 091.3
Maxcy's 081.0
McArdle (-Schmid-Pearson) (glycogenosis V) 271.0
mediastinum NEC 519.3
Medin's (*see also* Poliomyelitis) 045.9 ✓
Mediterranean 282.40
with hemoglobinopathy 282.49
medullary center (idiopathic) (respiratory) 348.89
Meige's (chronic hereditary edema) 757.0
Meleda 757.39
Ménétrier's (hypertrophic gastritis) 535.2 ✓
Ménière's (active) 386.00
cochlear 386.02
cochleovestibular 386.01
inactive 386.04
in remission 386.04
vestibular 386.03
meningeal — *see* Meningitis
mental (*see also* Psychosis) 298.9
Merzbacher-Pelizaeus 330.0
mesenchymal 710.9
mesenteric embolic 557.0
metabolic NEC 277.9
metal polishers' 502
metastatic — *see* Metastasis
Mibelli's 757.39
microdrepanocytic 282.41
microvascular — code to condition
microvillus
atrophy 751.5
inclusion (MVD) 751.5
Miescher's 709.3
Mikulicz's (dryness of mouth, absent or decreased lacrimation) 527.1
Milkman (-Looser) (osteomalacia with pseudofractures) 268.2
Miller's (osteomalacia) 268.2
Mills' 335.29
Milroy's (chronic hereditary edema) 757.0
Minamata 985.0
Minor's 336.1
Minot's (hemorrhagic disease, newborn) 776.0
Minot-von Willebrand-Jürgens (angiohemophilia) 286.4
Mitchell's (erythromelalgia) 443.82
mitral — *see* Endocarditis, mitral
Mljet (mal de Meleda) 757.39
Möbius', Moebius' 346.2 ✓
Moeller's 267
Möller (-Barlow) (infantile scurvy) 267
Mönckeberg's (*see also* Arteriosclerosis, extremities) 440.20
Mondor's (thrombophlebitis of breast) 451.89
Monge's 993.2
Morel-Kraepelin (*see also* Schizophrenia) 295.9 ✓
Morgagni's (syndrome) (hyperostosis frontalis interna) 733.3
Morgagni-Adams-Stokes (syncope with heart block) 426.9
Morquio (-Brailsford) (-Ullrich) (mucopolysaccharidosis IV) 277.5
Morton's (with metatarsalgia) 355.6
Morvan's 336.0
motor neuron (bulbar) (mixed type) 335.20
Mouchet's (juvenile osteochondrosis, foot) 732.5
mouth 528.9
Moyamoya 437.5
Mucha's (acute parapsoriasis varioliformis) 696.2
mu-chain 273.2
mucolipidosis (I) (II) (III) 272.7
Münchmeyer's (exostosis luxurians) 728.11
Murri's (intermittent hemoglobinuria) 283.2
muscle 359.9
inflammatory 728.9

Disease, diseased — *see also* Syndrome — *continued*
muscle — *continued*
ocular 378.9
musculoskeletal system 729.90
mushroom workers' 495.5
Mya's (congenital dilation, colon) 751.3
mycotic 117.9
myeloproliferative (chronic) (M9960/1) 238.79
myocardium, myocardial (*see also* Degeneration, myocardial) 429.1
hypertensive (*see also* Hypertension, heart 402.90
primary (idiopathic) 425.4
myoneural 358.9
Naegeli's 287.1
nail 703.9
specified type NEC 703.8
Nairobi sheep 066.1
nasal 478.19
cavity NEC 478.19
sinus (chronic) — *see* Sinusitis
navel (newborn) NEC 779.89
delayed separation of umbilical cord 779.83
nemaline body 359.0
neoplastic, generalized (M8000/6) 199.0
nerve — *see* Disorder, nerve
nervous system (central) 349.9
autonomic, peripheral (*see also* Neuropathy, peripheral, autonomic) 337.9
congenital 742.9
inflammatory — *see* Encephalitis
parasympathetic (*see also* Neuropathy, peripheral, autonomic) 337.9
peripheral NEC 355.9
prion NEC 046.79
specified NEC 349.89
sympathetic (*see also* Neuropathy, peripheral, autonomic) 337.9
vegetative (*see also* Neuropathy, peripheral, autonomic) 337.9
Nettleship's (urticaria pigmentosa) 757.33
Neumann's (pemphigus vegetans) 694.4
neurologic (central) NEC (*see also* Disease, nervous system) 349.9
peripheral NEC 355.9
neuromuscular system NEC 358.9
Newcastle 077.8
Nicolas (-Durand) — Favre (climatic bubo) 099.1
Niemann-Pick (lipid histiocytosis) 272.7
nipple 611.9
Paget's (M8540/3) 174.0
Nishimoto (-Takeuchi) 437.5
nonarthropod-borne NEC 078.89
central nervous system NEC 049.9
enterovirus NEC 078.89
nonautoimmune hemolytic NEC 283.10
Nonne-Milroy-Meige (chronic hereditary edema) 757.0
Norrie's (congenital progressive oculoacousticocerebral degeneration) 743.8
nose 478.19
nucleus pulposus — *see* Disease, intervertebral disc
nutritional 269.9
maternal, affecting fetus or newborn 760.4
oasthouse, urine 270.2
obliterative vascular 447.1
Odelberg's (juvenile osteochondrosis) 732.1
Oguchi's (retina) 368.61
Ohara's (*see also* Tularemia) 021.9
Ollier's (chondrodysplasia) 756.4
Opitz's (congestive splenomegaly) 289.51
Oppenheim's 358.8
Oppenheim-Urbach (necrobiosis lipoidica diabeticorum) 250.8 ✓ *[709.3]*
due to secondary diabetes 249.8 ✓ *[709.3]*
optic nerve NEC 377.49
orbit 376.9
specified NEC 376.89
Oriental liver fluke 121.1

Disease, diseased — *see also* Syndrome — *continued*
Oriental lung fluke 121.2
Ormond's 593.4
Osgood-Schlatter 732.4
Osgood's tibia (tubercle) 732.4
Osler (-Vaquez) (polycythemia vera) (M9950/1) 238.4
Osler-Rendu (familial hemorrhagic telangiectasia) 448.0
osteofibrocystic 252.01
Otto's 715.35
outer ear 380.9
ovary (noninflammatory) NEC 620.9
cystic 620.2
polycystic 256.4
specified NEC 620.8
Owren's (congenital) (*see also* Defect, coagulation) 286.3
Paas' 756.59
Paget's (osteitis deformans) 731.0
with infiltrating duct carcinoma of the breast (M8541/3) — *see* Neoplasm, breast, malignant
bone 731.0
osteosarcoma in (M9184/3) — *see* Neoplasm, bone, malignant
breast (M8540/3) 174.0
extramammary (M8542/3) (*see also* Neoplasm, skin, malignant)
anus 154.3
skin 173.59
malignant (M8540/3)
breast 174.0
specified site NEC (M8542/3) — *see* Neoplasm, skin, malignant
unspecified site 174.0
mammary (M8540/3) 174.0
nipple (M8540/3) 174.0
palate (soft) 528.9
Paltauf-Sternberg 201.9 ✓
pancreas 577.9
cystic 577.2
congenital 751.7
fibrocystic 277.00
Panner's 732.3
capitellum humeri 732.3
head of humerus 732.3
tarsal navicular (bone) (osteochondrosis) 732.5
panvalvular — *see* Endocarditis, mitral
parametrium 629.9
parasitic NEC 136.9
cerebral NEC 123.9
intestinal NEC 129
mouth 112.0
skin NEC 134.9
specified type — *see* Infestation
tongue 112.0
parathyroid (gland) 252.9
specified NEC 252.8
Parkinson's 332.0
parodontal 523.9
Parrot's (syphilitic osteochondritis) 090.0
Parry's (exophthalmic goiter) 242.0 ✓
Parson's (exophthalmic goiter) 242.0 ✓
Pavy's 593.6
Paxton's (white piedra) 111.2
Payr's (splenic flexure syndrome) 569.89
pearl-workers' (chronic osteomyelitis) (*see also* Osteomyelitis) 730.1 ✓
Pel-Ebstein — *see* Disease, Hodgkin's
Pelizaeus-Merzbacher 330.0
with dementia
with behavioral disturbance 330.0 *[294.11]*
without behavioral disturbance 330.0 *[294.10]*
Pellegrini-Stieda (calcification, knee joint) 726.62
pelvis, pelvic
female NEC 629.9
specified NEC 629.89
gonococcal (acute) 098.19
chronic or duration of 2 months or over 098.39

✓ **Additional Digit Required** — Refer to the Tabular List for Digit Selection

▽ **Subterms under main terms may continue to next column or page**

Disease, diseased — *see also* Syndrome — *continued*
pelvis, pelvic — *continued*
infection (*see also* Disease, pelvis, inflammatory) 614.9
inflammatory (female) (PID) 614.9
with
abortion — *see* Abortion, by type, with sepsis
ectopic pregnancy (*see also* categories 633.0–633.9) 639.0
molar pregnancy (*see also* categories 630–632) 639.0
acute 614.3
chronic 614.4
complicating pregnancy 646.6 ☑
affecting fetus or newborn 760.8
following
abortion 639.0
ectopic or molar pregnancy 639.0
peritonitis (acute) 614.5
chronic NEC 614.7
puerperal, postpartum, childbirth 670.8 ☑
specified NEC 614.8
organ, female NEC 629.9
specified NEC 629.89
peritoneum, female NEC 629.9
specified NEC 629.89
penis 607.9
inflammatory 607.2
peptic NEC 536.9
acid 536.8
periapical tissues NEC 522.9
pericardium 423.9
specified type NEC 423.8
perineum
female
inflammatory 616.9
specified NEC 616.89
noninflammatory 624.9
specified NEC 624.8
male (inflammatory) 682.2
periodic (familial) (Reimann's) NEC 277.31
paralysis 359.3
periodontal NEC 523.9
specified NEC 523.8
periosteum 733.90
peripheral
arterial 443.9
autonomic nervous system (*see also* Neuropathy, autonomic) 337.9
nerve NEC (*see also* Neuropathy) 356.9
multiple — *see* Polyneuropathy
vascular 443.9
specified type NEC 443.89
peritoneum 568.9
pelvic, female 629.9
specified NEC 629.89
Perrin-Ferraton (snapping hip) 719.65
persistent mucosal (middle ear) (with posterior or superior marginal perforation of ear drum) 382.2
Perthes' (capital femoral osteochondrosis) 732.1
Petit's (*see also* Hernia, lumbar) 553.8
Peutz-Jeghers 759.6
Peyronie's 607.85
Pfeiffer's (infectious mononucleosis) 075
pharynx 478.20
Phocas' 610.1
photochromogenic (acid-fast bacilli) (pulmonary) 031.0
nonpulmonary 031.9
Pick's
brain 331.11
with dementia
with behavioral disturbance 331.11 [294.11]
without behavioral disturbance 331.11 [294.10]
cerebral atrophy 331.11
with dementia
with behavioral disturbance 331.11 [294.11]

Disease, diseased — *see also* Syndrome — *continued*
Pick's — *continued*
cerebral atrophy — *continued*
with dementia — *continued*
without behavioral disturbance 331.11 [294.10]
lipid histiocytosis 272.7
liver (pericardial pseudocirrhosis of liver) 423.2
pericardium (pericardial pseudocirrhosis of liver) 423.2
polyserositis (pericardial pseudocirrhosis of liver) 423.2
Pierson's (osteochondrosis) 732.1
pigeon fanciers' or breeders' 495.2
pineal gland 259.8
pink 985.0
Pinkus' (lichen nitidus) 697.1
pinworm 127.4
pituitary (gland) 253.9
hyperfunction 253.1
hypofunction 253.2
pituitary snuff-takers' 495.8
placenta
affecting fetus or newborn 762.2
complicating pregnancy or childbirth 656.7 ☑
pleura (cavity) (*see also* Pleurisy) 511.0
Plummer's (toxic nodular goiter) 242.3 ☑
pneumatic
drill 994.9
hammer 994.9
policeman's 729.2
Pollitzer's (hidradenitis suppurativa) 705.83
polycystic (congenital) 759.89
congenital 748.4
kidney or renal 753.12
adult type (APKD) 753.13
autosomal dominant 753.13
autosomal recessive 753.14
childhood type (CPKD) 753.14
infantile type 753.14
liver or hepatic 751.62
lung or pulmonary 518.89
ovary, ovaries 256.4
spleen 759.0
polyethylene 996.45
Pompe's (glycogenosis II) 271.0
Poncet's (tuberculous rheumatism) (*see also* Tuberculosis) 015.9 ☑
Posada-Wernicke 114.9
Potain's (pulmonary edema) 514
Pott's (*see also* Tuberculosis) 015.0 ☑ [730.88]
osteomyelitis 015.0 ☑ [730.88]
paraplegia 015.0 ☑ [730.88]
spinal curvature 015.0 ☑ [737.43]
spondylitis 015.0 ☑ [720.81]
Potter's 753.0
Poulet's 714.2
pregnancy NEC (*see also* Pregnancy) 646.9 ☑
Preiser's (osteoporosis) 733.09
Pringle's (tuberous sclerosis) 759.5
Profichet's 729.90
prostate 602.9
specified type NEC 602.8
protozoal NEC 136.8
intestine, intestinal NEC 007.9
pseudo-Hurler's (mucolipidosis III) 272.7
psychiatric (*see also* Psychosis) 298.9
psychotic (*see also* Psychosis) 298.9
Puente's (simple glandular cheilitis) 528.5
puerperal NEC (*see also* Puerperal) 674.9 ☑
pulmonary (*see also* Disease, lung)
amyloid 277.39 [517.8]
artery 417.9
circulation, circulatory 417.9
specified NEC 417.8
diffuse obstructive (chronic) 496
with
acute bronchitis 491.22
asthma (chronic) (obstructive) 493.2 ☑
exacerbation NEC (acute) 491.21

Disease, diseased — *see also* Syndrome — *continued*
pulmonary (*see also* Disease, lung) — *continued*
heart (chronic) 416.9
specified NEC 416.8
hypertensive (vascular) 416.0
cardiovascular 416.0
obstructive diffuse (chronic) 496
with
acute bronchitis 491.22
asthma (chronic) (obstructive) 493.2 ☑
bronchitis (chronic) 491.20
with
exacerbation (acute) 491.21
acute 491.22
exacerbation NEC (acute) 491.21
decompensated 491.21
with exacerbation 491.21
valve (*see also* Endocarditis, pulmonary) 424.3
pulp (dental) NEC 522.9
pulseless 446.7
Putnam's (subacute combined sclerosis with pernicious anemia) 281.0 [336.2]
Pyle (-Cohn) (craniometaphyseal dysplasia) 756.89
pyramidal tract 333.90
Quervain's
tendon sheath 727.04
thyroid (subacute granulomatous thyroiditis) 245.1
Quincke's — *see* Edema, angioneurotic
Quinquaud (acne decalvans) 704.09
rag sorters' 022.1
Raynaud's (paroxysmal digital cyanosis) 443.0
reactive airway — *see* Asthma
Recklinghausen's (M9540/1) 237.71
bone (osteitis fibrosa cystica) 252.01
Recklinghausen-Applebaum (hemochromatosis) (*see also* Hemochromatosis) 275.03
Reclus' (cystic) 610.1
rectum NEC 569.49
Refsum's (heredopathia atactica polyneuritiformis) 356.3
Reichmann's (gastrosuccorrhea) 536.8
Reimann's (periodic) 277.31
Reiter's 099.3
renal (functional) (pelvis) (*see also* Disease, kidney) 593.9
with
edema (*see also* Nephrosis) 581.9
exudative nephritis 583.89
lesion of interstitial nephritis 583.89
stated generalized cause — *see* Nephritis
acute 593.9
basement membrane NEC 583.89
with
pulmonary hemorrhage (Goodpasture's syndrome) 446.21 [583.81]
chronic (*see also* Disease, kidney, chronic) 585.9
complicating pregnancy or puerperium NEC 646.2 ☑
with hypertension — *see* Toxemia, of pregnancy
affecting fetus or newborn 760.1
cystic, congenital (*see also* Cystic, disease, kidney) 753.10
diabetic 250.4 ☑ [583.81]
due to secondary diabetes 249.4 ☑ [581.81]
due to
amyloidosis 277.39 [583.81]
diabetes mellitus 250.4 ☑ [583.81]
due to secondary diabetes 249.4 ☑ [581.81]
systemic lupus erythematosis 710.0 [583.81]

Disease, diseased — *see also* Syndrome — *continued*
renal (*see also* Disease, kidney) — *continued*
end-stage 585.6
exudative 583.89
fibrocystic (congenital) 753.19
gonococcal 098.19 [583.81]
gouty 274.10
hypertensive (*see also* Hypertension, kidney) 403.90
immune complex NEC 583.89
interstitial (diffuse) (focal) 583.89
lupus 710.0 [583.81]
maternal, affecting fetus or newborn 760.1
hypertensive 760.0
phosphate-losing (tubular) 588.0
polycystic (congenital) 753.12
adult type (APKD) 753.13
autosomal dominant 753.13
autosomal recessive 753.14
childhood type (CPKD) 753.14
infantile type 753.14
specified lesion or cause NEC (*see also* Glomerulonephritis) 583.89
subacute 581.9
syphilitic 095.4
tuberculous (*see also* Tuberculosis) 016.0 ☑ [583.81]
tubular (*see also* Nephrosis, tubular) 584.5
Rendu-Osler-Weber (familial hemorrhagic telangiectasia) 448.0
renovascular (arteriosclerotic) (*see also* Hypertension, kidney) 403.90
respiratory (tract) 519.9
acute or subacute (upper) NEC 465.9
due to fumes or vapors 506.3
multiple sites NEC 465.8
noninfectious 478.9
streptococcal 034.0
chronic 519.9
arising in the perinatal period 770.7
due to fumes or vapors 506.4
due to
aspiration of liquids or solids 508.9
external agents 508.9
specified NEC 508.8
fumes or vapors 506.9
acute or subacute NEC 506.3
chronic 506.4
fetus or newborn NEC 770.9
obstructive 496
smoke inhalation 508.2
specified type NEC 519.8
upper (acute) (infectious) NEC 465.9
multiple sites NEC 465.8
noninfectious NEC 478.9
streptococcal 034.0
retina, retinal NEC 362.9
Batten's or Batten-Mayou 330.1 [362.71]
degeneration 362.89
vascular lesion 362.17
rheumatic (*see also* Arthritis) 716.8 ☑
heart — *see* Disease, heart, rheumatic
rheumatoid (heart) — *see* Arthritis, rheumatoid
rickettsial NEC 083.9
specified type NEC 083.8
Riedel's (ligneous thyroiditis) 245.3
Riga (-Fede) (cachectic aphthae) 529.0
Riggs' (compound periodontitis) 523.40
Ritter's 695.81
Rivalta's (cervicofacial actinomycosis) 039.3
Robles' (onchocerciasis) 125.3 [360.13]
Roger's (congenital interventricular septal defect) 745.4
Rokitansky's (*see also* Necrosis, liver) 570
Romberg's 349.89
Rosenthal's (factor XI deficiency) 286.2
Rossbach's (hyperchlorhydria) 536.8
psychogenic 306.4
Roth (-Bernhardt) 355.1
Runeberg's (progressive pernicious anemia) 281.0

☑ Additional Digit Required — Refer to the Tabular List for Digit Selection

▽ Subterms under main terms may continue to next column or page

Disease, diseased — *see also* Syndrome — *continued*

Rust's (tuberculous spondylitis) (*see also* Tuberculosis) 015.0 ☑ *[720.81]*
Rustitskii's (multiple myeloma) (M9730/3) 203.0 ☑
Ruysch's (Hirschsprung's disease) 751.3
Sachs (-Tay) 330.1
sacroiliac NEC 724.6
salivary gland or duct NEC 527.9
  inclusion 078.5
    streptococcal 034.0
    virus 078.5
Sander's (paranoia) 297.1
Sandhoff's 330.1
sandworm 126.9
Savill's (epidemic exfoliative dermatitis) 695.89
Schamberg's (progressive pigmentary dermatosis) 709.09
Schaumann's (sarcoidosis) 135
Schenck's (sporotrichosis) 117.1
Scheuermann's (osteochondrosis) 732.0
Schilder (-Flatau) 341.1
Schimmelbusch's 610.1
Schlatter-Osgood 732.4
Schlatter's tibia (tubercle) 732.4
Schmorl's 722.30
  cervical 722.39
  lumbar, lumbosacral 722.32
  specified region NEC 722.39
  thoracic, thoracolumbar 722.31
Scholz's 330.0
Schönlein (-Henoch) (purpura rheumatica) 287.0
Schottmüller's (*see also* Fever, paratyphoid) 002.9
Schüller-Christian (chronic histiocytosis X) 277.89
Schultz's (agranulocytosis) 288.09
Schwalbe-Ziehen-Oppenheimer 333.6
Schwartz-Jampel 359.23
Schweninger-Buzzi (macular atrophy) 701.3
sclera 379.19
scrofulous (*see also* Tuberculosis) 017.2 ☑
scrotum 608.9
sebaceous glands NEC 706.9
Secretan's (posttraumatic edema) 782.3
semilunar cartilage, cystic 717.5
seminal vesicle 608.9
Senear-Usher (pemphigus erythematosus) 694.4
serum NEC 999.59
Sever's (osteochondrosis calcaneum) 732.5
sexually transmitted — *see* Disease, venereal
Sézary's (reticulosis) (M9701/3) 202.2 ☑
Shaver's (bauxite pneumoconiosis) 503
Sheehan's (postpartum pituitary necrosis) 253.2
shimamushi (scrub typhus) 081.2
shipyard 077.1
sickle cell 282.60
  with
    crisis 282.62
    Hb-S disease 282.61
    other abnormal hemoglobin (Hb-D) (Hb-E) (Hb-G) (Hb-J) (Hb-K) (Hb-O) (Hb-P) (high fetal gene) (without crisis) 282.68
      with crisis 282.69
  elliptocytosis 282.60
  Hb-C (without crisis) 282.63
    with
      crisis 282.64
      vaso-occlusive pain 282.64
  Hb-S 282.61
    with
      crisis 282.62
      Hb-C (without crisis) 282.63
        with
          crisis 282.64
          vaso-occlusive pain 282.64

Disease, diseased — *see also* Syndrome — *continued*

sickle cell — *continued*
  Hb-S — *continued*
    with — *continued*
      other abnormal hemoglobin (Hb-D) (Hb-E) (Hb-G) (Hb-J) (Hb-K) (Hb-O) (Hb-P) (high fetal gene) (without crisis) 282.68
        with crisis 282.69
    spherocytosis 282.60
    thalassemia (without crisis) 282.41
      with
        crisis 282.42
        vaso-occlusive pain 282.42
Siegal-Cattan-Mamou (periodic) 277.31
silo fillers' 506.9
Simian B 054.3
Simmonds' (pituitary cachexia) 253.2
Simons' (progressive lipodystrophy) 272.6
Sinding-Larsen (juvenile osteopathia patellae) 732.4
sinus (*see also* Sinusitis)
  brain 437.9
  specified NEC 478.19
Sirkari's 085.0
sixth (*see also* Exanthem subitum) 058.10
Sjögren (-Gougerot) 710.2
  with lung involvement 710.2 *[517.8]*
Skevas-Zerfus 989.5
skin NEC 709.9
  due to metabolic disorder 277.9
  specified type NEC 709.8
sleeping (*see also* Narcolepsy) 347.00
  meaning sleeping sickness (*see also* Trypanosomiasis) 086.5
small vessel 443.9
Smith-Strang (oasthouse urine) 270.2
Sneddon-Wilkinson (subcorneal pustular dermatosis) 694.1
South African creeping 133.8
Spencer's (epidemic vomiting) 078.82
Spielmeyer-Stock 330.1
Spielmeyer-Vogt 330.1
spine, spinal 733.90
  combined system (*see also* Degeneration, combined) 266.2 *[336.2]*
    with pernicious anemia 281.0 *[336.2]*
  cord NEC 336.9
    congenital 742.9
  demyelinating NEC 341.8
  joint (*see also* Disease, joint, spine) 724.9
    tuberculous 015.0 ☑ *[730.8]* ☑
  spinocerebellar 334.9
    specified NEC 334.8
spleen (organic) (postinfectional) 289.50
  amyloid 277.39
  lardaceous 277.39
  polycystic 759.0
  specified NEC 289.59
sponge divers' 989.5
Stanton's (melioidosis) 025
Stargardt's 362.75
Startle 759.89
Steinert's 359.21
Sternberg's — *see* Disease, Hodgkin's
Stevens-Johnson (erythema multiforme exudativum) 695.13
Sticker's (erythema infectiosum) 057.0
Stieda's (calcification, knee joint) 726.62
Still's (juvenile rheumatoid arthritis) 714.30
  adult onset 714.2
Stiller's (asthenia) 780.79
Stokes' (exophthalmic goiter) 242.0 ☑
Stokes-Adams (syncope with heart block) 426.9
Stokvis (-Talma) (enterogenous cyanosis) 289.7
stomach NEC (organic) 537.9
  functional 536.9
    psychogenic 306.4
  lardaceous 277.39
stonemasons' 502

Disease, diseased — *see also* Syndrome — *continued*

storage
  glycogen (*see also* Disease, glycogen storage) 271.0
  lipid 272.7
  mucopolysaccharide 277.5
striatopallidal system 333.90
  specified NEC 333.89
Strümpell-Marie (ankylosing spondylitis) 720.0
Stuart's (congenital factor X deficiency) (*see also* Defect, coagulation) 286.3
Stuart-Prower (congenital factor X deficiency) (*see also* Defect, coagulation) 286.3
Sturge (-Weber) (-Dimitri) (encephalocutaneous angiomatosis) 759.6
Stuttgart 100.89
Sudeck's 733.7
supporting structures of teeth NEC 525.9
suprarenal (gland) (capsule) 255.9
  hyperfunction 255.3
  hypofunction 255.41
Sutton's 709.09
Sutton and Gull's — *see* Hypertension, kidney
sweat glands NEC 705.9
  specified type NEC 705.89
sweating 078.2
Sweeley-Klionsky 272.7
Swift (-Feer) 985.0
swimming pool (bacillus) 031.1
swineherd's 100.89
Sylvest's (epidemic pleurodynia) 074.1
Symmers (follicular lymphoma) (M9690/3) 202.0 ☑
sympathetic nervous system (*see also* Neuropathy, peripheral, autonomic) 337.9
synovium 727.9
syphilitic — *see* Syphilis
systemic tissue mast cell (M9741/3) 202.6 ☑
Taenzer's 757.4
Takayasu's (pulseless) 446.7
Talma's 728.85
Tangier (familial high-density lipoprotein deficiency) 272.5
Tarral-Besnier (pityriasis rubra pilaris) 696.4
Taylor's 701.8
Tay-Sachs 330.1
tear duct 375.69
teeth, tooth 525.9
  hard tissues 521.9
    specified NEC 521.89
  pulp NEC 522.9
tendon 727.9
  inflammatory NEC 727.9
terminal vessel 443.9
testis 608.9
Thaysen-Gee (nontropical sprue) 579.0
Thomsen's 359.22
Thomson's (congenital poikiloderma) 757.33
Thornwaldt's, Tornwaldt's (pharyngeal bursitis) 478.29
throat 478.20
  septic 034.0
thromboembolic (*see also* Embolism) 444.9
thymus (gland) 254.9
  specified NEC 254.8
thyroid (gland) NEC 246.9
  heart (*see also* Hyperthyroidism) 242.9 ☑ *[425.7]*
  lardaceous 277.39
  specified NEC 246.8
Tietze's 733.6
Tommaselli's
  correct substance properly administered 599.70
  overdose or wrong substance given or taken 961.4
tongue 529.9
tonsils, tonsillar (and adenoids) (chronic) 474.9
  specified NEC 474.8
tooth, teeth 525.9

Disease, diseased — *see also* Syndrome — *continued*

tooth, teeth — *continued*
  hard tissues 521.9
    specified NEC 521.89
  pulp NEC 522.9
Tornwaldt's (pharyngeal bursitis) 478.29
Tourette's 307.23
trachea 519.19
tricuspid — *see* Endocarditis, tricuspid
triglyceride-storage, type I, II, III 272.7
triple vessel (coronary arteries) — *see* Arteriosclerosis, coronary
trisymptomatic, Gougerot's 709.1
trophoblastic (*see also* Hydatidiform mole) 630
  previous, affecting management of pregnancy V23.1
tsutsugamushi (scrub typhus) 081.2
tube (fallopian), noninflammatory 620.9
  specified NEC 620.8
tuberculous NEC (*see also* Tuberculosis) 011.9 ☑
tubo-ovarian
  inflammatory (*see also* Salpingo-oophoritis) 614.2
  noninflammatory 620.9
  specified NEC 620.8
tubotympanic, chronic (with anterior perforation of ear drum) 382.1
tympanum 385.9
Uhl's 746.84
umbilicus (newborn) NEC 779.89
  delayed separation 779.83
Underwood's (sclerema neonatorum) 778.1
undiagnosed 799.9
Unna's (seborrheic dermatitis) 690.18
unstable hemoglobin hemolytic 282.7
Unverricht (-Lundborg) 345.1 ☑
Urbach-Oppenheim (necrobiosis lipoidica diabeticorum) 250.8 ☑ *[709.3]*
  due to secondary diabetes 249.8 ☑ *[709.3]*
Urbach-Wiethe (lipoid proteinosis) 272.8
ureter 593.9
urethra 599.9
  specified type NEC 599.84
urinary (tract) 599.9
  bladder 596.9
    specified NEC 596.89
  maternal, affecting fetus or newborn 760.1
Usher-Senear (pemphigus erythematosus) 694.4
uterus (organic) 621.9
  infective (*see also* Endometritis) 615.9
  inflammatory (*see also* Endometritis) 615.9
  noninflammatory 621.9
    specified type NEC 621.8
uveal tract
  anterior 364.9
  posterior 363.9
vagabonds' 132.1
vagina, vaginal
  inflammatory 616.10
  noninflammatory 623.9
    specified NEC 623.8
Valsuani's (progressive pernicious anemia, puerperal) 648.2 ☑
  complicating pregnancy or puerperium 648.2 ☑
valve, valvular — *see also* Endocarditis
  congenital NEC (*see also* Anomaly, heart, valve) 746.9
  pulmonary 746.00
    specified type NEC 746.89
van Bogaert-Nijssen (-Peiffer) 330.0
van Creveld-von Gierke (glycogenosis I) 271.0
van den Bergh's (enterogenous cyanosis) 289.7
van Neck's (juvenile osteochondrosis) 732.1
Vaquez (-Osler) (polycythemia vera) (M9950/1) 238.4
vascular 459.9

Disease, diseased — *see also* Syndrome — *continued*

vascular — *continued*

arteriosclerotic — *see* Arteriosclerosis

hypertensive — *see* Hypertension

obliterative 447.1

peripheral 443.9

occlusive 459.9

peripheral (occlusive) 443.9

in (due to) (with) diabetes mellitus 250.7 ☑ [443.81]

in (due to) (with) secondary diabetes 249.7 ☑ [443.81]

specified type NEC 443.89

vas deferens 608.9

vasomotor 443.9

vasospastic 443.9

vein 459.9

venereal 099.9

chlamydial NEC 099.50

anus 099.52

bladder 099.53

cervix 099.53

epididymis 099.54

genitourinary NEC 099.55

lower 099.53

specified NEC 099.54

pelvic inflammatory disease 099.54

perihepatic 099.56

peritoneum 099.56

pharynx 099.51

rectum 099.52

specified site NEC 099.59

testis 099.54

vagina 099.53

vulva 099.53

complicating pregnancy, childbirth, or puerperium 647.2 ☑

fifth 099.1

sixth 099.1

specified nature or type NEC 099.8

chlamydial — *see* Disease, venereal, chlamydial

Verneuil's (syphilitic bursitis) 095.7

Verse's (calcinosis intervertebralis) 275.49 [722.90]

vertebra, vertebral NEC 733.90

disc — *see* Disease, Intervertebral disc

vibration NEC 994.9

Vidal's (lichen simplex chronicus) 698.3

Vincent's (trench mouth) 101

Virchow's 733.99

virus (filterable) NEC 078.89

arbovirus NEC 066.9

arthropod-borne NEC 066.9

central nervous system NEC 049.9

specified type NEC 049.8

complicating pregnancy, childbirth, or puerperium 647.6 ☑

contact (with) V01.79

varicella V01.71

exposure to V01.79

varicella V01.71

Marburg 078.89

maternal

with fetal damage affecting management of pregnancy 655.3 ☑

nonarthropod-borne NEC 078.89

central nervous system NEC 049.9

specified NEC 049.8

vaccination, prophylactic (against) V04.89

vitreous 379.29

vocal cords NEC 478.5

Vogt's (Cecile) 333.71

Vogt-Spielmeyer 330.1

Volhard-Fahr (malignant nephrosclerosis) 403.00

Volkmann's

acquired 958.6

von Bechterew's (ankylosing spondylitis) 720.0

von Economo's (encephalitis lethargica) 049.8

von Eulenburg's (congenital paramyotonia) 359.29

Disease, diseased — *see also* Syndrome — *continued*

von Gierke's (glycogenosis I) 271.0

von Graefe's 378.72

von Hippel's (retinocerebral angiomatosis) 759.6

von Hippel-Lindau (angiomatosis retinocerebellosa) 759.6

von Jaksch's (pseudoleukemia infantum) 285.8

von Recklinghausen's (M9540/1) 237.71

bone (osteitis fibrosa cystica) 252.01

von Recklinghausen-Applebaum (hemochromatosis) (*see also* Hemochromatosis) 275.03

von Willebrand (-Jürgens) (angiohemophilia) 286.4

von Zambusch's (lichen sclerosus et atrophicus) 701.0

Voorhoeve's (dyschondroplasia) 756.4

Vrolik's (osteogenesis imperfecta) 756.51

vulva

inflammatory 616.10

noninflammatory 624.9

specified NEC 624.8

Wagner's (colloid milium) 709.3

Waldenström's (osteochondrosis capital femoral) 732.1

Wallgren's (obstruction of splenic vein with collateral circulation) 459.89

Wardrop's (with lymphangitis) 681.9

finger 681.02

toe 681.11

Wassilieff's (leptospiral jaundice) 100.0

wasting NEC 799.4

due to malnutrition 261

paralysis 335.21

Waterhouse-Friderichsen 036.3

waxy (any site) 277.39

Weber-Christian (nodular nonsuppurative panniculitis) 729.30

Wegner's (syphilitic osteochondritis) 090.0

Weil's (leptospiral jaundice) 100.0

of lung 100.0

Weir Mitchell's (erythromelalgia) 443.82

Werdnig-Hoffmann 335.0

Werlhof's (*see also* Purpura, thrombocytopenic) 287.39

Wermer's 258.01

Werner's (progeria adultorum) 259.8

Werner-His (trench fever) 083.1

Werner-Schultz (agranulocytosis) 288.09

Wernicke's (superior hemorrhagic polioencephalitis) 265.1

Wernicke-Posadas 114.9

Whipple's (intestinal lipodystrophy) 040.2

whipworm 127.3

white

White's (congenital) (keratosis follicularis) 757.39

blood cell 288.9

specified NEC 288.8

spot 701.0

Whitmore's (melioidosis) 025

Widal-Abrami (acquired hemolytic jaundice) 283.9

Wilkie's 557.1

Wilkinson-Sneddon (subcorneal pustular dermatosis) 694.1

Willis' (diabetes mellitus) (*see also* Diabetes) 250.0 ☑

due to secondary diabetes 249.0 ☑

Wilson's (hepatolenticular degeneration) 275.1

Wilson-Brocq (dermatitis exfoliativa) 695.89

winter vomiting 078.82

Wise's 696.2

Wohlfart-Kugelberg-Welander 335.11

Woillez's (acute idiopathic pulmonary congestion) 518.52

Wolman's (primary familial xanthomatosis) 272.7

wool-sorters' 022.1

Zagari's (xerostomia) 527.7

Zahorsky's (exanthem subitum) 058.10

Ziehen-Oppenheim 333.6

Disease, diseased — *see also* Syndrome — *continued*

zoonotic, bacterial NEC 027.9

specified type NEC 027.8

Disfigurement (due to scar) 709.2

head V48.6

limb V49.4

neck V48.7

trunk V48.7

Disgerminoma — *see* Dysgerminoma

Disinsertion, retina 361.04

Disintegration, complete, of the body 799.89

traumatic 869.1

Disk kidney 753.3

Dislocatable hip, congenital — *see also* Dislocation, hip, congenital 754.30

Dislocation (articulation) (closed) (displacement) (simple) (subluxation) 839.8

Note — "Closed" includes simple, complete, partial, uncomplicated, and unspecified dislocation.

"Open" includes dislocation specified as infected or compound and dislocation with foreign body.

"Chronic," "habitual," "old," or "recurrent" dislocations should be coded as indicated under the entry "Dislocation, recurrent," and "pathological" as indicated under the entry "Dislocation, pathological."

For late effect of dislocation see Late, effect, dislocation.

---

with fracture — *see* Fracture, by site

acromioclavicular (joint) (closed) 831.04

open 831.14

anatomical site (closed)

specified NEC 839.69

open 839.79

unspecified or ill-defined 839.8

open 839.9

ankle (scaphoid bone) (closed) 837.0

open 837.1

arm (closed) 839.8

open 839.9

astragalus (closed) 837.0

open 837.1

atlanto-axial (closed) 839.01

open 839.11

atlas (closed) 839.01

open 839.11

axis (closed) 839.02

open 839.12

back (closed) 839.8

open 839.9

Bell-Daly 723.8

breast bone (closed) 839.61

open 839.71

capsule, joint — *see* Dislocation, by site

carpal (bone) — *see* Dislocation, wrist

carpometacarpal (joint) (closed) 833.04

open 833.14

cartilage (joint) (*see also* Dislocation, by site)

knee — *see* Tear, meniscus

cervical, cervicodorsal, or cervicothoracic (spine) (vertebra) — *see* Dislocation, vertebra, cervical

chiropractic (*see also* Lesion, nonallopathic) 739.9

chondrocostal — *see* Dislocation, costochondral

chronic — *see* Dislocation, recurrent

clavicle (closed) 831.04

open 831.14

coccyx (closed) 839.41

open 839.51

collar bone (closed) 831.04

open 831.14

compound (open) NEC 839.9

congenital NEC 755.8

hip (*see also* Dislocation, hip, congenital) 754.30

lens 743.37

rib 756.3

sacroiliac 755.69

Dislocation — *continued*

congenital — *continued*

spine NEC 756.19

vertebra 756.19

coracoid (closed) 831.09

open 831.19

costal cartilage (closed) 839.69

open 839.79

costochondral (closed) 839.69

open 839.79

cricoarytenoid articulation (closed) 839.69

open 839.79

cricothyroid (cartilage) articulation (closed) 839.69

open 839.79

dorsal vertebrae (closed) 839.21

open 839.31

ear ossicle 385.23

elbow (closed) 832.00

anterior (closed) 832.01

open 832.11

congenital 754.89

divergent (closed) 832.09

open 832.19

lateral (closed) 832.04

open 832.14

medial (closed) 832.03

open 832.13

posterior (closed) 832.02

open 832.12

recurrent 718.32

specified type NEC 832.09

open 832.19

eye 360.81

lateral 376.36

eyeball 360.81

lateral 376.36

femur

distal end (closed) 836.50

anterior 836.52

open 836.62

lateral 836.54

open 836.64

medial 836.53

open 836.63

open 836.60

posterior 836.51

open 836.61

proximal end (closed) 835.00

anterior (pubic) 835.03

open 835.13

obturator 835.02

open 835.12

open 835.10

posterior 835.01

open 835.11

fibula

distal end (closed) 837.0

open 837.1

proximal end (closed) 836.59

open 836.69

finger(s) (phalanx) (thumb) (closed) 834.00

interphalangeal (joint) 834.02

open 834.12

metacarpal (bone), distal end 834.01

open 834.11

metacarpophalangeal (joint) 834.01

open 834.11

open 834.10

recurrent 718.34

foot (closed) 838.00

open 838.10

recurrent 718.37

forearm (closed) 839.8

open 839.9

fracture — *see* Fracture, by site

glenoid (closed) 831.09

open 831.19

habitual — *see* Dislocation, recurrent

hand (closed) 839.8

open 839.9

hip (closed) 835.00

anterior 835.03

obturator 835.02

open 835.12

☑ **Additional Digit Required** — Refer to the Tabular List for Digit Selection   ▽ **Subterms under main terms may continue to next column or page**

2014 ICD-9-CM   **135**

Dislocation — Dislocation

Dislocation — *continued*
  hip — *continued*
    anterior — *continued*
      open 835.13
    congenital (unilateral) 754.30
      with subluxation of other hip 754.35
      bilateral 754.31
    developmental 718.75
    open 835.10
    posterior 835.01
      open 835.11
    recurrent 718.35
  humerus (closed) 831.00
    distal end (*see also* Dislocation, elbow) 832.00
    open 831.10
    proximal end (closed) 831.00
      anterior (subclavicular) (subcoracoid) (subglenoid) (closed) 831.01
        open 831.11
      inferior (closed) 831.03
        open 831.13
      open 831.10
      posterior (closed) 831.02
        open 831.12
  implant — *see* Complications, mechanical
  incus 385.23
  infracoracoid (closed) 831.01
    open 831.11
  innominate (pubic junction) (sacral junction) (closed) 839.69
    acetabulum (*see also* Dislocation, hip) 835.00
    open 839.79
  interphalangeal (joint)
    finger or hand (closed) 834.02
      open 834.12
    foot or toe (closed) 838.06
      open 838.16
  jaw (cartilage) (meniscus) (closed) 830.0
    open 830.1
    recurrent 524.69
  joint NEC (closed) 839.8
    developmental 718.7 ☑
    open 839.9
    pathological — *see* Dislocation, pathological
    recurrent — *see* Dislocation, recurrent
  knee (closed) 836.50
    anterior 836.51
      open 836.61
    congenital (with genu recurvatum) 754.41
    habitual 718.36
    lateral 836.54
      open 836.64
    medial 836.53
      open 836.63
    old 718.36
    open 836.60
    posterior 836.52
      open 836.62
    recurrent 718.36
    rotatory 836.59
      open 836.69
  lacrimal gland 375.16
  leg (closed) 839.8
    open 839.9
  lens (crystalline) (complete) (partial) 379.32
    anterior 379.33
    congenital 743.37
    ocular implant 996.53
    posterior 379.34
    traumatic 921.3
  ligament — *see* Dislocation, by site
  lumbar (vertebrae) (closed) 839.20
    open 839.30
  lumbosacral (vertebrae) (closed) 839.20
    congenital 756.19
    open 839.30
  mandible (closed) 830.0
    open 830.1
  maxilla (inferior) (closed) 830.0
    open 830.1
  meniscus (knee) (*see also* Tear, meniscus)
    other sites — *see* Dislocation, by site

Dislocation — *continued*
  metacarpal (bone)
    distal end (closed) 834.01
      open 834.11
    proximal end (closed) 833.05
      open 833.15
  metacarpophalangeal (joint) (closed) 834.01
    open 834.11
  metatarsal (bone) (closed) 838.04
    open 838.14
  metatarsophalangeal (joint) (closed) 838.05
    open 838.15
  midcarpal (joint) (closed) 833.03
    open 833.13
  midtarsal (joint) (closed) 838.02
    open 838.12
  Monteggia's — *see* Dislocation, hip
  multiple locations (except fingers only or toes only) (closed) 839.8
    open 839.9
  navicular (bone) foot (closed) 837.0
    open 837.1
  neck (*see also* Dislocation, vertebra, cervical) 839.00
  Nélaton's — *see* Dislocation, ankle
  nontraumatic (joint) — *see* Dislocation, pathological
  nose (closed) 839.69
    open 839.79
  not recurrent, not current injury — *see* Dislocation, pathological
  occiput from atlas (closed) 839.01
    open 839.11
  old — *see* Dislocation, recurrent
  open (compound) NEC 839.9
  ossicle, ear 385.23
  paralytic (flaccid) (spastic) — *see* Dislocation, pathological
  patella (closed) 836.3
    congenital 755.64
    open 836.4
  pathological NEC 718.20
    ankle 718.27
    elbow 718.22
    foot 718.27
    hand 718.24
    hip 718.25
    knee 718.26
    lumbosacral joint 724.6
    multiple sites 718.29
    pelvic region 718.25
    sacroiliac 724.6
    shoulder (region) 718.21
    specified site NEC 718.28
    spine 724.8
      sacroiliac 724.6
    wrist 718.23
  pelvis (closed) 839.69
    acetabulum (*see also* Dislocation, hip) 835.00
    open 839.79
  phalanx
    foot or toe (closed) 838.09
      open 838.19
    hand or finger (*see also* Dislocation, finger) 834.00
  postpoliomyelitic — *see* Dislocation, pathological
  prosthesis, internal — *see* Complications, mechanical
  radiocarpal (joint) (closed) 833.02
    open 833.12
  radioulnar (joint)
    distal end (closed) 833.01
      open 833.11
    proximal end (*see also* Dislocation, elbow) 832.00
  radius
    distal end (closed) 833.00
      open 833.10
    proximal end (closed) 832.01
      open 832.11
  recurrent (*see also* Derangement, joint, recurrent) 718.3 ☑
    elbow 718.32
    hip 718.35

Dislocation — *continued*
  recurrent (*see also* Derangement, joint, recurrent) — *continued*
    joint NEC 718.38
    knee 718.36
    lumbosacral (joint) 724.6
    patella 718.36
    sacroiliac 724.6
    shoulder 718.31
    temporomandibular 524.69
  rib (cartilage) (closed) 839.69
    congenital 756.3
    open 839.79
  sacrococcygeal (closed) 839.42
    open 839.52
  sacroiliac (joint) (ligament) (closed) 839.42
    congenital 755.69
    open 839.52
    recurrent 724.6
  sacrum (closed) 839.42
    open 839.52
  scaphoid (bone)
    ankle or foot (closed) 837.0
      open 837.1
    wrist (closed) (*see also* Dislocation, wrist) 833.00
      open 833.10
  scapula (closed) 831.09
    open 831.19
  semilunar cartilage, knee — *see* Tear, meniscus
  septal cartilage (nose) (closed) 839.69
    open 839.79
  septum (nasal) (old) 470
  sesamoid bone — *see* Dislocation, by site
  shoulder (blade) (ligament) (closed) 831.00
    anterior (subclavicular) (subcoracoid) (subglenoid) (closed) 831.01
      open 831.11
    chronic 718.31
    inferior 831.03
      open 831.13
    open 831.10
    posterior (closed) 831.02
      open 831.12
    recurrent 718.31
  skull — *see* Injury, intracranial
  Smith's — *see* Dislocation, foot
  spine (articular process) (*see also* Dislocation, vertebra) (closed) 839.40
    atlanto-axial (closed) 839.01
      open 839.11
      recurrent 723.8
    cervical, cervicodorsal, cervicothoracic (closed) (*see also* Dislocation, vertebrae, cervical) 839.00
      open 839.10
      recurrent 723.8
    coccyx 839.41
      open 839.51
    congenital 756.19
    due to birth trauma 767.4
    open 839.50
    recurrent 724.9
    sacroiliac 839.42
      recurrent 724.6
    sacrum (sacrococcygeal) (sacroiliac) 839.42
      open 839.52
  spontaneous — *see* Dislocation, pathological
  sternoclavicular (joint) (closed) 839.61
    open 839.71
  sternum (closed) 839.61
    open 839.71
  subastragalar — *see* Dislocation, foot
  subglenoid (closed) 831.01
    open 831.11
  symphysis
    jaw (closed) 830.0
      open 830.1
    mandibular (closed) 830.0
      open 830.1
    pubis (closed) 839.69
      open 839.79
  tarsal (bone) (joint) 838.01

Dislocation — *continued*
  tarsal — *continued*
    open 838.11
  tarsometatarsal (joint) 838.03
    open 838.13
  temporomandibular (joint) (closed) 830.0
    open 830.1
    recurrent 524.69
  thigh
    distal end (*see also* Dislocation, femur, distal end) 836.50
    proximal end (*see also* Dislocation, hip) 835.00
  thoracic (vertebrae) (closed) 839.21
    open 839.31
  thumb(s) (*see also* Dislocation, finger) 834.00
  thyroid cartilage (closed) 839.69
    open 839.79
  tibia
    distal end (closed) 837.0
      open 837.1
    proximal end (closed) 836.50
      anterior 836.51
        open 836.61
      lateral 836.54
        open 836.64
      medial 836.53
        open 836.63
      open 836.60
      posterior 836.52
        open 836.62
      rotatory 836.59
        open 836.69
  tibiofibular
    distal (closed) 837.0
      open 837.1
    superior (closed) 836.59
      open 836.69
  toe(s) (closed) 838.09
    open 838.19
  trachea (closed) 839.69
    open 839.79
  ulna
    distal end (closed) 833.09
      open 833.19
    proximal end — *see* Dislocation, elbow
  vertebra (articular process) (body) (closed) (traumatic) 839.40
    cervical, cervicodorsal or cervicothoracic (closed) 839.00
      first (atlas) 839.01
        open 839.11
      second (axis) 839.02
        open 839.12
      third 839.03
        open 839.13
      fourth 839.04
        open 839.14
      fifth 839.05
        open 839.15
      sixth 839.06
        open 839.16
      seventh 839.07
        open 839.17
      congenital 756.19
      multiple sites 839.08
        open 839.18
      open 839.10
    congenital 756.19
    dorsal 839.21
      open 839.31
      recurrent 724.9
    lumbar, lumbosacral 839.20
      open 839.30
    non-traumatic — *see* Displacement, intervertebral disc
    open NEC 839.50
    recurrent 724.9
    specified region NEC 839.49
      open 839.59
    thoracic 839.21
      open 839.31
  wrist (carpal bone) (scaphoid) (semilunar) (closed) 833.00
    carpometacarpal (joint) 833.04
      open 833.14

☑ **Additional Digit Required — Refer to the Tabular List for Digit Selection**   ▽ **Subterms under main terms may continue to next column or page**

136   2014 ICD-9-CM

Dislocation — *continued*
　wrist — *continued*
　　metacarpal bone, proximal end 833.05
　　　open 833.15
　　midcarpal (joint) 833.03
　　　open 833.13
　　open 833.10
　　radiocarpal (joint) 833.02
　　　open 833.12
　　radioulnar (joint) 833.01
　　　open 833.11
　　recurrent 718.33
　　specified site NEC 833.09
　　　open 833.19
　xiphoid cartilage (closed) 839.61
　　open 839.71
Dislodgement
　artificial skin graft 996.55
　decellularized allodermis graft 996.55
Disobedience, hostile (covert) (overt) — *see also* Disturbance, conduct 312.0 ☑
Disorder — *see also* Disease
　academic underachievement, childhood and adolescence 313.83
　accommodation 367.51
　　drug-induced 367.89
　　toxic 367.89
　adjustment (*see also* Reaction, adjustment) 309.9
　　with
　　　anxiety 309.24
　　　anxiety and depressed mood 309.28
　　　depressed mood 309.0
　　　disturbance of conduct 309.3
　　　disturbance of emotions and conduct 309.4
　adrenal (capsule) (cortex) (gland) 255.9
　　specified type NEC 255.8
　adrenogenital 255.2
　affective (*see also* Psychosis, affective) 296.90
　　atypical 296.81
　aggressive, unsocialized (*see also* Disturbance, conduct) 312.0 ☑
　alcohol, alcoholic (*see also* Alcohol) 291.9
　　induced mood 291.89
　allergic — *see* Allergy
　amino acid (metabolic) (*see also* Disturbance, metabolism, amino acid) 270.9
　　albinism 270.2
　　alkaptonuria 270.2
　　argininosuccinicaciduria 270.6
　　beta-amino-isobutyricaciduria 277.2
　　cystathioninuria 270.4
　　cystinosis 270.0
　　cystinuria 270.0
　　glycinuria 270.0
　　homocystinuria 270.4
　　imidazole 270.5
　　maple syrup (urine) disease 270.3
　　neonatal, transitory 775.89
　　oasthouse urine disease 270.2
　　ochronosis 270.2
　　phenylketonuria 270.1
　　phenylpyruvic oligophrenia 270.1
　　purine NEC 277.2
　　pyrimidine NEC 277.2
　　renal transport NEC 270.0
　　specified type NEC 270.8
　　transport NEC 270.0
　　　renal 270.0
　　xanthinuria 277.2
　amnestic (*see also* Amnestic syndrome) 294.8
　　alcohol-induced persisting 291.1
　　drug-induced persisting 292.83
　　in conditions classified elsewhere 294.0
　anaerobic glycolysis with anemia 282.3
　anxiety (*see also* Anxiety) 300.00
　　due to or associated with physical condition 293.84
　arteriole 447.9
　　specified type NEC 447.8
　artery 447.9
　　specified type NEC 447.8

Disorder — *see also* Disease — *continued*
　articulation — *see* Disorder, joint
　Asperger's 299.8 ☑
　attachment of infancy or early childhood 313.89
　attention deficit 314.00
　　with hyperactivity 314.01
　　predominantly
　　　combined hyperactive/inattentive 314.01
　　　hyperactive/impulsive 314.01
　　　inattentive 314.00
　　residual type 314.8
　auditory processing disorder 388.45
　　acquired 388.45
　　developmental 315.32
　autistic 299.0 ☑
　autoimmune NEC 279.49
　　hemolytic (cold type) (warm type) 283.0
　　parathyroid 252.1
　　thyroid 245.2
　avoidant, childhood or adolescence 313.21
　balance
　　acid-base 276.9
　　　mixed (with hypercapnia) 276.4
　　electrolyte 276.9
　　fluid 276.9
　behavior NEC (*see also* Disturbance, conduct) 312.9
　　disruptive 312.9
　bilirubin excretion 277.4
　bipolar (affective) (alternating) 296.80

Note — Use the following fifth-digit subclassification with categories 296.0–296.6:

0　*unspecifed*

1　*mild*

2　*moderate*

3　*severe, without mention of psychotic behavior*

4　*severe, specified as with psychotic behavior*

5　*in partial or unspecified remission*

6　*in full remission*

---

　　atypical 296.7
　　currently
　　　depressed 296.5 ☑
　　　hypomanic 296.4 ☑
　　　manic 296.4 ☑
　　mixed 296.6 ☑
　　specified type NEC 296.89
　　type I 296.7
　　　most recent episode (or current)
　　　　depressed 296.5 ☑
　　　　hypomanic 296.4 ☑
　　　　manic 296.4 ☑
　　　　mixed 296.6 ☑
　　　　unspecified 296.7
　　　single manic episode 296.0 ☑
　　type II (recurrent major depressive episodes with hypomania) 296.89
　bladder 596.9
　　functional NEC 596.59
　　specified NEC 596.89
　bleeding 286.9
　bone NEC 733.90
　　specified NEC 733.99
　brachial plexus 353.0
　branched-chain amino-acid degradation 270.3
　breast 611.9
　　puerperal, postpartum 676.3 ☑
　　specified NEC 611.89
　Briquet's 300.81
　bursa 727.9
　　shoulder region 726.10
　carbohydrate metabolism, congenital 271.9
　cardiac, functional 427.9
　　postoperative 997.1
　　psychogenic 306.2
　cardiovascular, psychogenic 306.2
　cartilage NEC 733.90

Disorder — *see also* Disease — *continued*
　cartilage — *continued*
　　articular 718.00
　　　ankle 718.07
　　　elbow 718.02
　　　foot 718.07
　　　hand 718.04
　　　hip 718.05
　　　knee 717.9
　　　multiple sites 718.09
　　　pelvic region 718.05
　　　shoulder region 718.01
　　　specified
　　　　site NEC 718.08
　　　　type NEC 733.99
　　　wrist 718.03
　catatonic — *see* Catatonia
　central auditory processing 315.32
　　acquired 388.45
　　developmental 315.32
　cervical region NEC 723.9
　cervical root (nerve) NEC 353.2
　character NEC (*see also* Disorder, personality) 301.9
　ciliary body 364.9
　　specified NEC 364.89
　coagulation (factor) (*see also* Defect, coagulation) 286.9
　　factor VIII (congenital) (functional) 286.0
　　factor IX (congenital) (functional) 286.1
　　neonatal, transitory 776.3
　coccyx 724.70
　　specified NEC 724.79
　cognitive 294.9
　colon 569.9
　　functional 564.9
　　　congenital 751.3
　communication 307.9
　conduct (*see also* Disturbance, conduct) 312.9
　　adjustment reaction 309.3
　　adolescent onset type 312.82
　　childhood onset type 312.81
　　compulsive 312.30
　　　specified type NEC 312.39
　　hyperkinetic 314.2
　　onset unspecified 312.89
　　socialized (type) 312.20
　　　aggressive 312.23
　　　unaggressive 312.21
　　specified NEC 312.89
　conduction, heart 426.9
　　specified NEC 426.89
　conflict
　　sexual orientation 302.0
　congenital
　　glycosylation (CDG) 271.8
　convulsive (secondary) (*see also* Convulsions) 780.39
　　due to injury at birth 767.0
　　idiopathic 780.39
　coordination 781.3
　cornea NEC 371.89
　　due to contact lens 371.82
　corticosteroid metabolism NEC 255.2
　cranial nerve — *see* Disorder, nerve, cranial
　cyclothymic 301.13
　degradation, branched-chain amino acid 270.3
　delusional 297.1
　dentition 520.6
　depersonalization 300.6
　depressive NEC 311
　　atypical 296.82
　　major (*see also* Psychosis, affective) 296.2 ☑
　　　recurrent episode 296.3 ☑
　　　single episode 296.2 ☑
　development, specific 315.9
　　associated with hyperkinesia 314.1
　　coordination 315.4
　　language 315.31
　　　and speech due to hearing loss 315.34
　　learning 315.2
　　　arithmetical 315.1

Disorder — *see also* Disease — *continued*
　development, specific — *continued*
　　learning — *continued*
　　　reading 315.00
　　mixed 315.5
　　motor coordination 315.4
　　specified type NEC 315.8
　　speech 315.39
　　　and language due to hearing loss 315.34
　diaphragm 519.4
　digestive 536.9
　　fetus or newborn 777.9
　　　specified NEC 777.8
　　psychogenic 306.4
　disintegrative, childhood 299.1 ☑
　dissociative 300.15
　　identity 300.14
　　nocturnal 307.47
　　drug-related 292.9
　dysmorphic body 300.7
　dysthymic 300.4
　ear 388.9
　　degenerative NEC 388.00
　　external 380.9
　　　specified 380.89
　　pinna 380.30
　　specified type NEC 388.8
　　vascular NEC 388.00
　eating NEC 307.50
　electrolyte NEC 276.9
　　with
　　　abortion — *see* Abortion, by type, with metabolic disorder
　　　ectopic pregnancy (*see also* categories 633.0–633.9) 639.4
　　　molar pregnancy (*see also* categories 630–632) 639.4
　　acidosis 276.2
　　　metabolic 276.2
　　　respiratory 276.2
　　alkalosis 276.3
　　　metabolic 276.3
　　　respiratory 276.3
　　following
　　　abortion 639.4
　　　ectopic or molar pregnancy 639.4
　　neonatal, transitory NEC 775.5
　emancipation as adjustment reaction 309.22
　emotional (*see also* Disorder, mental, nonpsychotic) V40.9
　endocrine 259.9
　　specified type NEC 259.8
　esophagus 530.9
　　functional 530.5
　　psychogenic 306.4
　explosive
　　intermittent 312.34
　　isolated 312.35
　expressive language 315.31
　eye 379.90
　　globe — *see* Disorder, globe
　　ill-defined NEC 379.99
　　limited duction NEC 378.63
　　specified NEC 379.8
　eyelid 374.9
　　degenerative 374.50
　　sensory 374.44
　　specified type NEC 374.89
　　vascular 374.85
　factitious (with combined psychological and physical signs and symptoms) (with predominantly physical signs and symptoms) 300.19
　　with predominantly psychological signs and symptoms 300.16
　factor, coagulation (*see also* Defect, coagulation) 286.9
　　IX (congenital) (funcitonal) 286.1
　　VIII (congenital) (functional) 286.0
　fascia 728.9
　fatty acid oxidation 277.85
　feeding — *see* Feeding
　female sexual arousal 302.72
　fluency 315.35
　　adult onset 307.0

Dislocation — Disorder

☑ **Additional Digit Required — Refer to the Tabular List for Digit Selection**　　　　　　　▽ **Subterms under main terms may continue to next column or page**

2014 ICD-9-CM　　　　　　　　　　　　　　　　　　　　　　　　　　　　　　　　　　　　　　**137**

Disorder — Disorder

Disorder — *see also* Disease — *continued*
  fluency — *continued*
    childhood onset 315.35
      due to late effect of cerebrovascular accident 438.14
      in conditions classified elsewhere 784.52
  fluid NEC 276.9
  gastric (functional) 536.9
    motility 536.8
    psychogenic 306.4
    secretion 536.8
  gastrointestinal (functional) NEC 536.9
    newborn (neonatal) 777.9
      specified NEC 777.8
    psychogenic 306.4
  gender (child) 302.6
    adult 302.85
  gender identity (childhood) 302.6
    adolescents 302.85
    adults (-life) 302.85
  genitourinary system, psychogenic 306.50
  globe 360.9
    degenerative 360.20
      specified NEC 360.29
    specified type NEC 360.89
  hearing (*see also* Deafness)
    conductive type (air) (*see also* Deafness, conductive) 389.00
    mixed conductive and sensorineural 389.20
      bilateral 389.22
      unilateral 389.21
    nerve
      bilateral 389.12
      unilateral 389.13
    perceptive (*see also* Deafness, perceptive) 389.10
    sensorineural type NEC (*see also* Deafness, sensorineural 389.10
  heart action 427.9
    postoperative 997.1
  hematological, transient neonatal 776.9
    specified type NEC 776.8
  hematopoietic organs 289.9
  hemorrhagic NEC 287.9
    due to intrinsic circulating anticoagulants, antibodies, or inhibitors 286.59
      with
        acquired hemophilia 286.52
        antiphospholipid antibody 286.53
    specified type NEC 287.8
  hemostasis (*see also* Defect, coagulation) 286.9
  homosexual conflict 302.0
  hypomanic (chronic) 301.11
  identity
    childhood and adolescence 313.82
      gender 302.6
  immune mechanism (immunity) 279.9
    single complement (C1-C9) 279.8
    specified type NEC 279.8
  impulse control (*see also* Disturbance, conduct, compulsive) 312.30
  infant sialic acid storage 271.8
  integument, fetus or newborn 778.9
    specified type NEC 778.8
  interactional psychotic (childhood) (*see also* Psychosis, childhood) 299.1 ☑
  intermittent explosive 312.34
  intervertebral disc 722.90
    cervical, cervicothoracic 722.91
    lumbar, lumbosacral 722.93
    thoracic, thoracolumbar 722.92
  intestinal 569.9
    functional NEC 564.9
      congenital 751.3
      postoperative 564.4
    psychogenic 306.4
  introverted, of childhood and adolescence 313.22
  involuntary emotional expression (IEED) 310.81
  iris 364.9
    specified NEC 364.89
  iron, metabolism 275.09

Disorder — *see also* Disease — *continued*
  iron, metabolism — *continued*
    specified type NEC 275.09
  isolated explosive 312.35
  joint NEC 719.90
    ankle 719.97
    elbow 719.92
    foot 719.97
    hand 719.94
    hip 719.95
    knee 719.96
    multiple sites 719.99
    pelvic region 719.95
    psychogenic 306.0
    shoulder (region) 719.91
    specified site NEC 719.98
    temporomandibular 524.60
      sounds on opening or closing 524.64
      specified NEC 524.69
    wrist 719.93
  kidney 593.9
    functional 588.9
      specified NEC 588.89
  labyrinth, labyrinthine 386.9
    specified type NEC 386.8
  lactation 676.9 ☑
  language (developmental) (expressive) 315.31
    mixed receptive-expressive 315.32
  learning 315.9
  ligament 728.9
  ligamentous attachments, peripheral (*see also* Enthesopathy)
    spine 720.1
  limb NEC 729.90
    psychogenic 306.0
  lipid
    metabolism, congenital 272.9
    storage 272.7
  lipoprotein deficiency (familial) 272.5
  low back NEC 724.9
    psychogenic 306.0
  lumbosacral
    plexus 353.1
    root (nerve) NEC 353.4
  lymphoproliferative (chronic) NEC (M9970/1) 238.79
    post-transplant (PTLD) 238.77
  major depressive (*see also* Psychosis, affective) 296.2 ☑
    recurrent episode 296.3 ☑
    single episode 296.2 ☑
  male erectile 607.84
    nonorganic origin 302.72
  manic (*see also* Psychosis, affective) 296.0 ☑
    atypical 296.81
  mathematics 315.1
  meniscus NEC (*see also* Disorder, cartilage, articular) 718.0 ☑
  menopausal 627.9
    specified NEC 627.8
  menstrual 626.9
    psychogenic 306.52
    specified NEC 626.8
  mental (nonpsychotic) 300.9
    affecting management of pregnancy, childbirth, or puerperium 648.4 ☑
    drug-induced 292.9
      hallucinogen persisting perception 292.89
      specified type NEC 292.89
    due to or associated with
      alcoholism 291.9
      drug consumption NEC 292.9
        specified type NEC 292.89
      physical condition NEC 293.9
    induced by drug 292.9
      specified type NEC 292.89
    neurotic (*see also* Neurosis) 300.9
    of infancy, childhood or adolescence 313.9
    persistent
      other
        due to conditions classified elsewhere 294.8

Disorder — *see also* Disease — *continued*
  mental — *continued*
    persistent — *continued*
      unspecified
        due to conditions classified elsewhere 294.9
    presenile 310.1
      psychotic NEC 290.10
    previous, affecting management of pregnancy V23.89
    psychoneurotic (*see also* Neurosis) 300.9
    psychotic (*see also* Psychosis) 298.9
      brief 298.8
      senile 290.20
    specific, following organic brain damage 310.9
      cognitive or personality change of other type 310.1
      frontal lobe syndrome 310.0
      postconcussional syndrome 310.2
      specified type NEC 310.89
    transient
      in conditions classified elsewhere 293.9
  metabolism NEC 277.9
    with
      abortion — *see* Abortion, by type, with metabolic disorder
      ectopic pregnancy (*see also* categories 633.0–633.9) 639.4
      molar pregnancy (*see also* categories 630–632) 639.4
    alkaptonuria 270.2
    amino acid (*see also* Disorder, amino acid) 270.9
      specified type NEC 270.8
    ammonia 270.6
    arginine 270.6
    argininosuccinic acid 270.6
    basal 794.7
    bilirubin 277.4
    calcium 275.40
    carbohydrate 271.9
      specified type NEC 271.8
    cholesterol 272.9
    citrulline 270.6
    copper 275.1
    corticosteroid 255.2
    cystine storage 270.0
    cystinuria 270.0
    fat 272.9
    fatty acid oxidation 277.85
    following
      abortion 639.4
      ectopic or molar pregnancy 639.4
    fructosemia 271.2
    fructosuria 271.2
    fucosidosis 271.8
    galactose-1-phosphate uridyl transferase 271.1
    glutamine 270.7
    glycine 270.7
    glycogen storage NEC 271.0
      hepatorenal 271.0
    hemochromatosis (*see also* Hemochromatosis) 275.03
    in labor and delivery 669.0 ☑
    iron 275.09
    lactose 271.3
    lipid 272.9
      specified type NEC 272.8
      storage 272.7
    lipoprotein (*see also* Hyperlipemia deficiency (familial)) 272.5
    lysine 270.7
    magnesium 275.2
    mannosidosis 271.8
    mineral 275.9
      specified type NEC 275.8
    mitochondrial 277.87
    mucopolysaccharide 277.5
    nitrogen 270.9
    ornithine 270.6
    oxalosis 271.8
    pentosuria 271.8
    phenylketonuria 270.1

Disorder — *see also* Disease — *continued*
  metabolism — *continued*
    phosphate 275.3
    phosphorous 275.3
    plasma protein 273.9
      specified type NEC 273.8
    porphyrin 277.1
    purine 277.2
    pyrimidine 277.2
    serine 270.7
    sodium 276.9
    specified type NEC 277.89
    steroid 255.2
    threonine 270.7
    urea cycle 270.6
    xylose 271.8
  micturition NEC 788.69
    psychogenic 306.53
  misery and unhappiness, of childhood and adolescence 313.1
  mitochondrial metabolism 277.87
  mitral valve 424.0
  mood (*see also* Disorder, bipolar) 296.90
    alcohol-induced 291.89
    episodic 296.90
      specified NEC 296.99
    in conditions classified elsewhere 293.83
  motor tic 307.20
    chronic 307.22
    transient (childhood) 307.21
  movement NEC 333.90
    hysterical 300.11
    medication-induced 333.90
    periodic limb 327.51
    sleep related, unspecified 780.58
      other organic 327.59
    specified type NEC 333.99
    stereotypic 307.3
  mucopolysaccharide 277.5
  muscle 728.9
    psychogenic 306.0
    specified type NEC 728.3
  muscular attachments, peripheral (*see also* Enthesopathy)
    spine 720.1
  musculoskeletal system NEC 729.90
    psychogenic 306.0
  myeloproliferative (chronic) NEC (M9960/1) 238.79
  myoneural 358.9
    due to lead 358.2
    specified type NEC 358.8
    toxic 358.2
  myotonic 359.29
  neck region NEC 723.9
  nerve 349.9
    abducens NEC 378.54
    accessory 352.4
    acoustic 388.5
    auditory 388.5
    auriculotemporal 350.8
    axillary 353.0
    cerebral — *see* Disorder, nerve, cranial
    cranial 352.9
      first 352.0
      second 377.49
      third
        partial 378.51
        total 378.52
      fourth 378.53
      fifth 350.9
      sixth 378.54
      seventh NEC 351.9
      eighth 388.5
      ninth 352.2
      tenth 352.3
      eleventh 352.4
      twelfth 352.5
      multiple 352.6
    entrapment — *see* Neuropathy, entrapment
    facial 351.9
      specified NEC 351.8
    femoral 355.2
    glossopharyngeal NEC 352.2
    hypoglossal 352.5

☑ **Additional Digit Required — Refer to the Tabular List for Digit Selection**   ▽ Subterms under main terms may continue to next column or page

138   **2014 ICD-9-CM**

☑ **Additional Digit Required** — Refer to the Tabular List for Digit Selection   ▽ **Subterms under main terms may continue to next column or page**

2014 ICD-9-CM   **139**

Disorder — Disorder

Disorder — *see also* Disease — *continued*
skin — *continued*
　　psychogenic (allergic) (eczematous) (pruritic) 306.3
　　specified type NEC 709.8
　　vascular 709.1
sleep 780.50
　　with apnea — *see* Apnea, sleep
　　alcohol induced 291.82
　　arousal 307.46
　　　　confusional 327.41
　　circadian rhythm 327.30
　　　　advanced sleep phase type 327.32
　　　　alcohol induced 291.82
　　　　delayed sleep phase type 327.31
　　　　drug induced 292.85
　　　　free running type 327.34
　　　　in conditions classified elsewhere 327.37
　　　　irregular sleep-wake type 327.33
　　　　jet lag type 327.35
　　　　other 327.39
　　　　shift work type 327.36
　　drug induced 292.85
　　initiation or maintenance (*see also* Insomnia) 780.52
　　　　nonorganic origin (transient) 307.41
　　　　　　persistent 307.42
　　nonorganic origin 307.40
　　　　specified type NEC 307.49
　　organic specified type NEC 327.8
　　periodic limb movement 327.51
　　specified NEC 780.59
　　wake
　　　　cycle — *see* Disorder, sleep, circadian rhythm
　　　　schedule — *see* Disorer, sleep, circadian rhythm
social, of childhood and adolescence 313.22
soft tissue 729.90
　　specified type NEC 729.99
somatization 300.81
somatoform (atypical) (undifferentiated) 300.82
　　severe 300.81
　　specified type NEC 300.89
speech NEC 784.59
　　nonorganic origin 307.9
spine NEC 724.9
　　ligamentous or muscular attachments, peripheral 720.1
steroid metabolism NEC 255.2
stomach (functional) (*see also* Disorder, gastric) 536.9
　　psychogenic 306.4
storage, iron 275.09
stress (*see also* Reaction, stress, acute) 308.3
　　posttraumatic
　　　　acute 309.81
　　　　brief 309.81
　　　　chronic 309.81
substitution 300.11
suspected — *see* Observation
synovium 727.9
temperature regulation, fetus or newborn 778.4
temporomandibular joint NEC 524.60
　　sounds on opening or closing 524.64
　　specified NEC 524.69
tendon 727.9
　　shoulder region 726.10
thoracic root (nerve) NEC 353.3
thyrocalcitonin secretion 246.0
thyroid (gland) NEC 246.9
　　specified type NEC 246.8
tic 307.20
　　chronic (motor or vocal) 307.22
　　motor-verbal 307.23
　　organic origin 333.1
　　transient (of childhood) 307.21
tooth NEC 525.9
　　development NEC 520.9
　　　　specified type NEC 520.8
　　eruption 520.6
　　specified type NEC 525.8
Tourette's 307.23

Disorder — *see also* Disease — *continued*
transport, carbohydrate 271.9
　　specified type NEC 271.8
tubular, phosphate-losing 588.0
tympanic membrane 384.9
unaggressive, unsocialized (*see also* Disturbance, conduct) 312.1 ☑
undersocialized, unsocialized (*see also* Disturbance, conduct)
　　aggressive (type) 312.0 ☑
　　unaggressive (type) 312.1 ☑
vision, visual NEC 368.9
　　binocular NEC 368.30
　　cortex 377.73
　　　　associated with
　　　　　　inflammatory disorders 377.73
　　　　　　neoplasms 377.71
　　　　　　vascular disorders 377.72
　　pathway NEC 377.63
　　　　associated with
　　　　　　inflammatory disorders 377.63
　　　　　　neoplasms 377.61
　　　　　　vascular disorders 377.62
vocal tic
　　chronic 307.22
wakefulness (*see also* Hypersomnia) 780.54
　　nonorganic origin (transient) 307.43
　　　　persistent 307.44
written expression 315.2
Disorganized globe 360.29
Displacement, displaced

> *Note* — *For acquired displacement of bones, cartilage, joints, tendons, due to injury, see also Dislocation.*
>
> *Displacements at ages under one year should be considered congenital, provided there is no indication the condition was acquired after birth.*

　　acquired traumatic of bone, cartilage, joint, tendon NEC (without fracture) (*see also* Dislocation) 839.8
　　　　with fracture — *see* Fracture, by site
　　adrenal gland (congenital) 759.1
　　alveolus and teeth, vertical 524.75
　　appendix, retrocecal (congenital) 751.5
　　auricle (congenital) 744.29
　　bladder (acquired) 596.89
　　　　congenital 753.8
　　brachial plexus (congenital) 742.8
　　brain stem, caudal 742.4
　　canaliculus lacrimalis 743.65
　　cardia, through esophageal hiatus 750.6
　　cerebellum, caudal 742.4
　　cervix — *see* Displacement, uterus
　　colon (congenital) 751.4
　　device, implant, or graft — *see* Complications, mechanical
　　epithelium
　　　　columnar of cervix 622.10
　　　　cuboidal, beyond limits of external os (uterus) 752.49
　　esophageal mucosa into cardia of stomach, congenital 750.4
　　esophagus (acquired) 530.89
　　　　congenital 750.4
　　eyeball (acquired) (old) 376.36
　　　　congenital 743.8
　　　　current injury 871.3
　　　　lateral 376.36
　　fallopian tube (acquired) 620.4
　　　　congenital 752.19
　　　　opening (congenital) 752.19
　　gallbladder (congenital) 751.69
　　gastric mucosa 750.7
　　　　into
　　　　　　duodenum 750.7
　　　　　　esophagus 750.7
　　　　　　Meckel's diverticulum, congenital 750.7
　　globe (acquired) (lateral) (old) 376.36
　　　　current injury 871.3
　　graft
　　　　artificial skin graft 996.55
　　　　decellularized allodermis graft 996.55
　　heart (congenital) 746.87

Displacement, displaced — *continued*
heart — *continued*
　　acquired 429.89
　　hymen (congenital) (upward) 752.49
　　internal prosthesis NEC — *see* Complications, mechanical
　　intervertebral disc (with neuritis, radiculitis, sciatica, or other pain) 722.2
　　　　with myelopathy 722.70
　　　　cervical, cervicodorsal, cervicothoracic 722.0
　　　　　　with myelopathy 722.71
　　　　　　due to major trauma — *see* Dislocation, vertebra, cervical
　　　　due to trauma — *see* Dislocation, vertebra
　　　　lumbar, lumbosacral 722.10
　　　　　　with myelopathy 722.73
　　　　　　due to major trauma — *see* Dislocation, vertebra, lumbar
　　　　thoracic, thoracolumbar 722.11
　　　　　　with myelopathy 722.72
　　　　　　due to major trauma — *see* Dislocation, vertebra, thoracic
intrauterine device 996.32
kidney (acquired) 593.0
　　congenital 753.3
lacrimal apparatus or duct (congenital) 743.65
macula (congenital) 743.55
Meckel's diverticulum (congenital) 751.0
nail (congenital) 757.5
　　acquired 703.8
opening of Wharton's duct in mouth 750.26
organ or site, congenital NEC — *see* Malposition, congenital
ovary (acquired) 620.4
　　congenital 752.0
　　free in peritoneal cavity (congenital) 752.0
　　into hernial sac 620.4
oviduct (acquired) 620.4
　　congenital 752.19
parathyroid (gland) 252.8
parotid gland (congenital) 750.26
punctum lacrimale (congenital) 743.65
sacroiliac (congenital) (joint) 755.69
　　current injury — *see* Dislocation, sacroiliac
　　old 724.6
spine (congenital) 756.19
spleen, congenital 759.0
stomach (congenital) 750.7
　　acquired 537.89
subglenoid (closed) 831.01
sublingual duct (congenital) 750.26
teeth, tooth 524.30
　　horizontal 524.33
　　vertical 524.34
tongue (congenital) (downward) 750.19
trachea (congenital) 748.3
ureter or ureteric opening or orifice (congenital) 753.4
uterine opening of oviducts or fallopian tubes 752.19
uterus, uterine (*see also* Malposition, uterus) 621.6
　　congenital 752.39
ventricular septum 746.89
　　with rudimentary ventricle 746.89
xyphoid bone (process) 738.3
Disproportion 653.9 ☑
affecting fetus or newborn 763.1
breast, reconstructed 612.1
　　between native and reconstructed 612.1
caused by
　　conjoined twins 678.1 ☑
　　contraction, pelvis (general) 653.1 ☑
　　　　inlet 653.2 ☑
　　　　midpelvic 653.8 ☑
　　　　midplane 653.8 ☑
　　　　outlet 653.3 ☑
　　fetal
　　　　ascites 653.7 ☑
　　　　hydrocephalus 653.6 ☑
　　　　hydrops 653.7 ☑

Disproportion — *continued*
caused by — *continued*
　　fetal — *continued*
　　　　meningomyelocele 653.7 ☑
　　　　sacral teratoma 653.7 ☑
　　　　tumor 653.7 ☑
　　hydrocephalic fetus 653.6 ☑
　　pelvis, pelvic, abnormality (bony) NEC 653.0 ☑
　　unusually large fetus 653.5 ☑
causing obstructed labor 660.1 ☑
cephalopelvic, normally formed fetus 653.4 ☑
　　causing obstructed labor 660.1 ☑
fetal NEC 653.5 ☑
　　causing obstructed labor 660.1 ☑
fetopelvic, normally formed fetus 653.4 ☑
　　causing obstructed labor 660.1 ☑
mixed maternal and fetal origin, normally formed fetus 653.4 ☑
pelvis, pelvic (bony) NEC 653.1 ☑
　　causing obstructed labor 660.1 ☑
specified type NEC 653.8 ☑
Disruption
cesarean wound 674.1 ☑
family V61.09
　　due to
　　　　child in
　　　　　　care of non-parental family member V61.06
　　　　　　foster care V61.06
　　　　　　welfare custody V61.05
　　　　death of family member V61.07
　　　　divorce V61.03
　　　　estrangement V61.09
　　　　　　parent-child V61.04
　　　　extended absence of family member NEC V61.08
　　　　family member
　　　　　　on military deployment V61.01
　　　　　　return from military deployment V61.02
　　　　legal separation V61.03
gastrointestinal anastomosis 997.49
ligament(s) (*see also* Sprain)
　　knee
　　　　current injury — *see* Dislocation, knee
　　　　old 717.89
　　　　　　capsular 717.85
　　　　　　collateral (medial) 717.82
　　　　　　　　lateral 717.81
　　　　　　cruciate (posterior) 717.84
　　　　　　　　anterior 717.83
　　　　　　specified site NEC 717.85
marital V61.10
　　involving
　　　　divorce V61.03
　　　　estrangement V61.09
operation wound (external) (*see also* Dehiscence) 998.32
　　internal 998.31
organ transplant, anastomosis site — *see* Complications, transplant, organ, by site
ossicles, ossicular chain 385.23
　　traumatic — *see* Fracture, skull, base
parenchyma
　　liver (hepatic) — *see* Laceration, liver, major
　　spleen — *see* Laceration, spleen, parenchyma, massive
phase-shift, of 24-hour sleep-wake cycle, unspecified 780.55
　　nonorganic origin 307.45
sleep-wake cycle (24-hour), unspecified 780.55
　　circadian rhythm 327.33
　　nonorganic origin 307.45
suture line (external) (*see also* Dehiscence) 998.32
　　internal 998.31
wound 998.30
　　cesarean operation 674.1 ☑
　　episiotomy 674.2 ☑
　　operation (surgical) 998.32

☑ Additional Digit Required — Refer to the Tabular List for Digit Selection　　　　　　　　　▽ Subterms under main terms may continue to next column or page

140　　2014 ICD-9-CM

Disruption — *continued*
  wound — *continued*
    operation — *continued*
      cesarean 674.1 ☑
      internal 998.31
    perineal (obstetric) 674.2 ☑
    uterine 674.1 ☑
Disruptio uteri — *see also* Rupture, uterus
  complicating delivery — *see* Delivery, complicated, rupture, uterus
Dissatisfaction with
  employment V62.29
  school environment V62.3
Dissecting — *see* condition
Dissection
  aorta 441.00
    abdominal 441.02
    thoracic 441.01
    thoracoabdominal 441.03
  artery, arterial
    carotid 443.21
    coronary 414.12
    iliac 443.22
    renal 443.23
    specified NEC 443.29
    vertebral 443.24
  vascular 459.9
  wound — *see* Wound, open, by site
Disseminated — *see* condition
Dissociated personality NEC 300.15
Dissociation
  auriculoventricular or atrioventricular (any degree) (AV) 426.89
    with heart block 426.0
  interference 426.89
  isorhythmic 426.89
  rhythm
    atrioventricular (AV) 426.89
    interference 426.89
Dissociative
  identity disorder 300.14
  reaction NEC 300.15
Dissolution, vertebra — *see also* Osteoporosis 733.00
Distention
  abdomen (gaseous) 787.3
  bladder 596.89
  cecum 569.89
  colon 569.89
  gallbladder 575.8
  gaseous (abdomen) 787.3
  intestine 569.89
  kidney 593.89
  liver 573.9
  seminal vesicle 608.89
  stomach 536.8
    acute 536.1
    psychogenic 306.4
  ureter 593.5
  uterus 621.8
Distichia, distichiasis (eyelid) 743.63
Distoma hepaticum infestation 121.3
Distomiasis 121.9
  bile passages 121.3
    due to Clonorchis sinensis 121.1
  hemic 120.9
  hepatic (liver) 121.3
    due to Clonorchis sinensis (clonorchiasis) 121.1
  intestinal 121.4
  liver 121.3
    due to Clonorchis sinensis 121.1
  lung 121.2
  pulmonary 121.2
Distomolar (fourth molar) 520.1
  causing crowding 524.31
Disto-occlusion (division I) (division II) 524.22
Distortion (congenital)
  adrenal (gland) 759.1
  ankle (joint) 755.69
  anus 751.5
  aorta 747.29
  appendix 751.5
  arm 755.59
  artery (peripheral) NEC (*see also* Distortion, peripheral vascular system) 747.60

Distortion — *continued*
  artery (*see also* Distortion, peripheral vascular system) — *continued*
    cerebral 747.81
    coronary 746.85
    pulmonary 747.39
    retinal 743.58
    umbilical 747.5
  auditory canal 744.29
    causing impairment of hearing 744.02
  bile duct or passage 751.69
  bladder 753.8
  brain 742.4
  bronchus 748.3
  cecum 751.5
  cervix (uteri) 752.49
  chest (wall) 756.3
  clavicle 755.51
  clitoris 752.49
  coccyx 756.19
  colon 751.5
  common duct 751.69
  cornea 743.41
  cricoid cartilage 748.3
  cystic duct 751.69
  duodenum 751.5
  ear 744.29
    auricle 744.29
      causing impairment of hearing 744.02
    causing impairment of hearing 744.09
    external 744.29
      causing impairment of hearing 744.02
    inner 744.05
    middle, except ossicles 744.03
      ossicles 744.04
    ossicles 744.04
  endocrine (gland) NEC 759.2
  epiglottis 748.3
  Eustachian tube 744.24
  eye 743.8
    adnexa 743.69
  face bone(s) 756.0
  fallopian tube 752.19
  femur 755.69
  fibula 755.69
  finger(s) 755.59
  foot 755.67
  gallbladder 751.69
  genitalia, genital organ(s)
    female 752.89
      external 752.49
      internal NEC 752.89
    male 752.89
      penis 752.69
  glottis 748.3
  gyri 742.4
  hand bone(s) 755.59
  heart (auricle) (ventricle) 746.89
    valve (cusp) 746.89
  hepatic duct 751.69
  humerus 755.59
  hymen 752.49
  ileum 751.5
  intestine (large) (small) 751.5
    with anomalous adhesions, fixation or malrotation 751.4
  jaw NEC 524.89
  jejunum 751.5
  kidney 753.3
  knee (joint) 755.64
  labium (majus) (minus) 752.49
  larynx 748.3
  leg 755.69
  lens 743.36
  liver 751.69
  lumbar spine 756.19
    with disproportion (fetopelvic) 653.0 ☑
      affecting fetus or newborn 763.1
      causing obstructed labor 660.1 ☑
  lumbosacral (joint) (region) 756.19
  lung (fissures) (lobe) 748.69
  nerve 742.8
  nose 748.1

Distortion — *continued*
  organ
    of Corti 744.05
    of site not listed — *see* Anomaly, specified type NEC
  ossicles, ear 744.04
  ovary 752.0
  oviduct 752.19
  pancreas 751.7
  parathyroid (gland) 759.2
  patella 755.64
  peripheral vascular system NEC 747.60
    gastrointestinal 747.61
    lower limb 747.64
    renal 747.62
    spinal 747.82
    upper limb 747.63
  pituitary (gland) 759.2
  radius 755.59
  rectum 751.5
  rib 756.3
  sacroiliac joint 755.69
  sacrum 756.19
  scapula 755.59
  shoulder girdle 755.59
  site not listed — *see* Anomaly, specified type NEC
  skull bone(s) 756.0
    with
      anencephalus 740.0
      encephalocele 742.0
      hydrocephalus 742.3
        with spina bifida (*see also* Spina bifida) 741.0 ☑
      microcephalus 742.1
  spinal cord 742.59
  spine 756.19
  spleen 759.0
  sternum 756.3
  thorax (wall) 756.3
  thymus (gland) 759.2
  thyroid (gland) 759.2
    cartilage 748.3
  tibia 755.69
  toe(s) 755.66
  tongue 750.19
  trachea (cartilage) 748.3
  ulna 755.59
  ureter 753.4
    causing obstruction 753.20
  urethra 753.8
    causing obstruction 753.6
  uterus 752.39
  vagina 752.49
  vein (peripheral) NEC (*see also* Distortion, peripheral vascular system) 747.60
    great 747.49
    portal 747.49
    pulmonary 747.49
  vena cava (inferior) (superior) 747.49
  vertebra 756.19
  visual NEC 368.15
    shape or size 368.14
  vulva 752.49
  wrist (bones) (joint) 755.59
Distress
  abdomen 789.0 ☑
  colon 564.9
  emotional V40.9
  epigastric 789.0 ☑
  fetal (syndrome) 768.4
    affecting management of pregnancy or childbirth 656.8 ☑
    liveborn infant 768.4
    first noted
      before onset of labor 768.2
      during labor and delivery 768.3
    stillborn infant (death before onset of labor) 768.0
    death during labor 768.1
  gastrointestinal (functional) 536.9
    psychogenic 306.4
  intestinal (functional) NEC 564.9
    psychogenic 306.4
  intrauterine — *see* Distress, fetal
  leg 729.5

Distress — *continued*
  maternal 669.0 ☑
  mental V40.9
  respiratory 786.09
    acute (adult) 518.82
    adult syndrome (following trauma and surgery) 518.52
      specified NEC 518.82
    fetus or newborn 770.89
    syndrome (idiopathic) (newborn) 769
  stomach 536.9
    psychogenic 306.4
Distribution vessel, atypical NEC 747.60
  coronary artery 746.85
  spinal 747.82
Districhiasis 704.2
Disturbance — *see also* Disease
  absorption NEC 579.9
    calcium 269.3
    carbohydrate 579.8
    fat 579.8
    protein 579.8
    specified type NEC 579.8
    vitamin (*see also* Deficiency, vitamin) 269.2
  acid-base equilibrium 276.9
  activity and attention, simple, with hyperkinesis 314.01
  amino acid (metabolic) (*see also* Disorder, amino acid) 270.9
    imidazole 270.5
    maple syrup (urine) disease 270.3
    transport 270.0
  assimilation, food 579.9
  attention, simple 314.00
    with hyperactivity 314.01
  auditory, nerve, except deafness 388.5
  behavior (*see also* Disturbance, conduct) 312.9
  blood clotting (hypoproteinemia) (mechanism) (*see also* Defect, coagulation) 286.9
  central nervous system NEC 349.9
  cerebral nerve NEC 352.9
  circulatory 459.9
  conduct 312.9

> *Note* — Use the following fifth-digit subclassification with categories 312.0–312.2:
>
> 0   unspecified
>
> 1   mild
>
> 2   moderate
>
> 3   severe

  adjustment reaction 309.3
  adolescent onset type 312.82
  childhood onset type 312.81
  compulsive 312.30
    intermittent explosive disorder 312.34
    isolated explosive disorder 312.35
    kleptomania 312.32
    pathological gambling 312.31
    pyromania 312.33
  hyperkinetic 314.2
  intermittent explosive 312.34
  isolated explosive 312.35
  mixed with emotions 312.4
  socialized (type) 312.20
    aggressive 312.23
    unaggressive 312.21
  specified type NEC 312.89
  undersocialized, unsocialized
    aggressive (type) 312.0 ☑
    unaggressive (type) 312.1 ☑
  coordination 781.3
  cranial nerve NEC 352.9
  deep sensibility — *see* Disturbance, sensation
  digestive 536.9
    psychogenic 306.4
  electrolyte — *see* Imbalance, electrolyte
  emotions specific to childhood or adolescence 313.9

Disturbance — see also Disease — continued

emotions specific to childhood or adolescence — continued
  with
    academic underachievement 313.83
    anxiety and fearfulness 313.0
    elective mutism 313.23
    identity disorder 313.82
    jealousy 313.3
    misery and unhappiness 313.1
    oppositional defiant disorder 313.81
    overanxiousness 313.0
    sensitivity 313.21
    shyness 313.21
    social withdrawal 313.22
    withdrawal reaction 313.22
  involving relationship problems 313.3
  mixed 313.89
  specified type NEC 313.89
endocrine (gland) 259.9
  neonatal, transitory 775.9
    specified NEC 775.89
equilibrium 780.4
feeding (elderly) (infant) 783.3
  newborn 779.31
  nonorganic origin NEC 307.59
  psychogenic NEC 307.59
fructose metabolism 271.2
gait 781.2
  hysterical 300.11
gastric (functional) 536.9
  motility 536.8
  psychogenic 306.4
  secretion 536.8
gastrointestinal (functional) 536.9
  psychogenic 306.4
habit, child 307.9
hearing, except deafness 388.40
heart, functional (conditions classifiable to 426, 427, 428)
  due to presence of (cardiac) prosthesis 429.4
  postoperative (immediate) 997.1
    long-term effect of cardiac surgery 429.4
  psychogenic 306.2
hormone 259.9
innervation uterus, sympathetic, parasympathetic 621.8
keratinization NEC
  gingiva 523.10
  lip 528.5
  oral (mucosa) (soft tissue) 528.79
    residual ridge mucosa
      excessive 528.72
      minimal 528.71
  tongue 528.79
labyrinth, labyrinthine (vestibule) 386.9
learning, specific NEC 315.2
memory (see also Amnesia) 780.93
  mild, following organic brain damage 310.89
mental (see also Disorder, mental) 300.9
  associated with diseases classified elsewhere 316
metabolism (acquired) (congenital) (see also Disorder, metabolism) 277.9
  with
    abortion — see Abortion, by type, with metabolic disorder
    ectopic pregnancy (see also categories 633.0–633.9) 639.4
    molar pregnancy (see also categories 630–632) 639.4
  amino acid (see also Disorder, amino acid) 270.9
    aromatic NEC 270.2
    branched-chain 270.3
    specified type NEC 270.8
    straight-chain NEC 270.7
    sulfur-bearing 270.4
    transport 270.0
  ammonia 270.6
  arginine 270.6
  argininosuccinic acid 270.6

Disturbance — see also Disease — continued

metabolism (see also Disorder, metabolism) — continued
  carbohydrate NEC 271.9
  cholesterol 272.9
  citrulline 270.6
  cystathionine 270.4
  fat 272.9
  following
    abortion 639.4
    ectopic or molar pregnancy 639.4
  general 277.9
    carbohydrate 271.9
    iron 275.09
    phosphate 275.3
    sodium 276.9
  glutamine 270.7
  glycine 270.7
  histidine 270.5
  homocystine 270.4
  in labor or delivery 669.0 ☑
  iron 275.09
  isoleucine 270.3
  leucine 270.3
  lipoid 272.9
    specified type NEC 272.8
  lysine 270.7
  methionine 270.4
  neonatal, transitory 775.9
    specified type NEC 775.89
  nitrogen 788.99
  ornithine 270.6
  phosphate 275.3
  phosphatides 272.7
  serine 270.7
  sodium NEC 276.9
  threonine 270.7
  tryptophan 270.2
  tyrosine 270.2
  urea cycle 270.6
  valine 270.3
motor 796.1
nervous functional 799.21
neuromuscular mechanism (eye) due to syphilis 094.84
nutritional 269.9
  nail 703.8
ocular motion 378.87
  psychogenic 306.7
oculogyric 378.87
  psychogenic 306.7
oculomotor NEC 378.87
  psychogenic 306.7
olfactory nerve 781.1
optic nerve NEC 377.49
oral epithelium, including tongue 528.79
  residual ridge mucosa
    excessive 528.72
    minimal 528.71
personality (pattern) (trait) (see also Disorder, personality) 301.9
  following organic brain damage 310.1
polyglandular 258.9
psychomotor 307.9
pupillary 379.49
reflex 796.1
rhythm, heart 427.9
  postoperative (immediate) 997.1
    long-term effect of cardiac surgery 429.4
  psychogenic 306.2
salivary secretion 527.7
sensation (cold) (heat) (localization) (tactile discrimination localization) (texture) (vibratory) NEC 782.0
  hysterical 300.11
  skin 782.0
  smell 781.1
  taste 781.1
sensory (see also Disturbance, sensation) 782.0
  innervation 782.0
situational (transient) (see also Reaction, adjustment) 309.9
  acute 308.3

Disturbance — see also Disease — continued

sleep 780.50
  with apnea — see Apnea, sleep
  initiation or maintenance (see also Insomnia) 780.52
    nonorganic origin 307.41
  nonorganic origin 307.40
    specified type NEC 307.49
  specified NEC 780.59
    nonorganic origin 307.49
  wakefulness (see also Hypersomnia) 780.54
    nonorganic origin 307.43
sociopathic 301.7
speech NEC 784.59
  developmental 315.39
    associated with hyperkinesis 314.1
  secondary to organic lesion 784.59
stomach (functional) (see also Disturbance, gastric) 536.9
sympathetic (nerve) (see also Neuropathy, peripheral, autonomic) 337.9
temperature sense 782.0
  hysterical 300.11
tooth
  eruption 520.6
  formation 520.4
  structure, hereditary NEC 520.5
touch (see also Disturbance, sensation) 782.0
vascular 459.9
  arteriosclerotic — see Arteriosclerosis
vasomotor 443.9
vasospastic 443.9
vestibular labyrinth 386.9
vision, visual NEC 368.9
  psychophysical 368.16
  specified NEC 368.8
  subjective 368.10
voice and resonance 784.40
wakefulness (initiation or maintenance) (see also Hypersomnia) 780.54
  nonorganic origin 307.43

Disulfiduria, beta-mercaptolactate-cysteine 270.0

Disuse atrophy, bone 733.7

Ditthomska syndrome 307.81

Diuresis 788.42

Divers'
palsy or paralysis 993.3
squeeze 993.3

Diverticula, diverticulosis, diverticulum (acute) (multiple) (perforated) (ruptured) 562.10
with diverticulitis 562.11
aorta (Kommerell's) 747.21
appendix (noninflammatory) 543.9
bladder (acquired) (sphincter) 596.3
  congenital 753.8
broad ligament 620.8
bronchus (congenital) 748.3
  acquired 494.0
    with acute exacerbation 494.1
calyx, calyceal (kidney) 593.89
cardia (stomach) 537.1
cecum 562.10
  with
    diverticulitis 562.11
      with hemorrhage 562.13
    hemorrhage 562.12
  congenital 751.5
colon (acquired) 562.10
  with
    diverticulitis 562.11
      with hemorrhage 562.13
    hemorrhage 562.12
  congenital 751.5
duodenum 562.00
  with
    diverticulitis 562.01
      with hemorrhage 562.03
    hemorrhage 562.02
  congenital 751.5
epiphrenic (esophagus) 530.6
esophagus (congenital) 750.4
  acquired 530.6

Diverticula, diverticulosis, diverticulum — continued

esophagus — continued
  epiphrenic 530.6
  pulsion 530.6
  traction 530.6
  Zenker's 530.6
Eustachian tube 381.89
fallopian tube 620.8
gallbladder (congenital) 751.69
gastric 537.1
heart (congenital) 746.89
ileum 562.00
  with
    diverticulitis 562.01
      with hemorrhage 562.03
    hemorrhage 562.02
intestine (large) 562.10
  with
    diverticulitis 562.11
      with hemorrhage 562.13
    hemorrhage 562.12
  congenital 751.5
  small 562.00
    with
      diverticulitis 562.01
        with hemorrhage 562.03
      hemorrhage 562.02
    congenital 751.5
jejunum 562.00
  with
    diverticulitis 562.01
      with hemorrhage 562.03
    hemorrhage 562.02
kidney (calyx) (pelvis) 593.89
  with calculus 592.0
Kommerell's 747.21
laryngeal ventricle (congenital) 748.3
Meckel's (displaced) (hypertrophic) 751.0
midthoracic 530.6
organ or site, congenital NEC — see Distortion
pericardium (congenital) (cyst) 746.89
  acquired (true) 423.8
pharyngoesophageal (pulsion) 530.6
pharynx (congenital) 750.27
pulsion (esophagus) 530.6
rectosigmoid 562.10
  with
    diverticulitis 562.11
      with hemorrhage 562.13
    hemorrhage 562.12
  congenital 751.5
rectum 562.10
  with
    diverticulitis 562.11
      with hemorrhage 562.13
    hemorrhage 562.12
renal (calyces) (pelvis) 593.89
  with calculus 592.0
Rokitansky's 530.6
seminal vesicle 608.0
sigmoid 562.10
  with
    diverticulitis 562.11
      with hemorrhage 562.13
    hemorrhage 562.12
  congenital 751.5
small intestine 562.00
  with
    diverticulitis 562.01
      with hemorrhage 562.03
    hemorrhage 562.02
stomach (cardia) (juxtacardia) (juxtapyloric) (acquired) 537.1
  congenital 750.7
subdiaphragmatic 530.6
trachea (congenital) 748.3
  acquired 519.19
traction (esophagus) 530.6
ureter (acquired) 593.89
  congenital 753.4
ureterovesical orifice 593.89
urethra (acquired) 599.2
  congenital 753.8
ventricle, left (congenital) 746.89

Diverticula, diverticulosis, diverticulum — *continued*
  vesical (urinary) 596.3
    congenital 753.8
  Zenker's (esophagus) 530.6
Diverticulitis (acute) — *see also* Diverticula 562.11
  with hemorrhage 562.13
  bladder (urinary) 596.3
  cecum (perforated) 562.11
    with hemorrhage 562.13
  colon (perforated) 562.11
    with hemorrhage 562.13
  duodenum 562.01
    with hemorrhage 562.03
  esophagus 530.6
  ileum (perforated) 562.01
    with hemorrhage 562.03
  intestine (large) (perforated) 562.11
    with hemorrhage 562.13
    small 562.01
      with hemorrhage 562.03
  jejunum (perforated) 562.01
    with hemorrhage 562.03
  Meckel's (perforated) 751.0
  pharyngoesophageal 530.6
  rectosigmoid (perforated) 562.11
    with hemorrhage 562.13
  rectum 562.11
    with hemorrhage 562.13
  sigmoid (old) (perforated) 562.11
    with hemorrhage 562.13
  small intestine (perforated) 562.01
    with hemorrhage 562.03
  vesical (urinary) 596.3
Diverticulosis — *see* Diverticula
Division
  cervix uteri 622.8
    external os into two openings by frenum 752.44
  external (cervical) into two openings by frenum 752.44
  glans penis 752.69
  hymen 752.49
  labia minora (congenital) 752.49
  ligament (partial or complete) (current) (*see also* Sprain, by site)
    with open wound — *see* Wound, open, by site
  muscle (partial or complete) (current) (*see also* Sprain, by site)
    with open wound — *see* Wound, open, by site
  nerve — *see* Injury, nerve, by site
  penis glans 752.69
  spinal cord — *see* Injury, spinal, by site
  vein 459.9
    traumatic — *see* Injury, vascular, by site
Divorce V61.03
Dix-Hallpike neurolabyrinthitis 386.12
Dizziness 780.4
  hysterical 300.11
  psychogenic 306.9
Doan-Wiseman syndrome (primary splenic neutropenia) 289.53
Dog bite — *see* Wound, open, by site
Döhle body-panmyelopathic syndrome 288.2
Döhle-Heller aortitis 093.1
Dolichocephaly, dolichocephalus 754.0
Dolichocolon 751.5
Dolichostenomelia 759.82
Donohue's syndrome (leprechaunism) 259.8
Donor
  blood V59.01
    other blood components V59.09
    stem cells V59.02
    whole blood V59.01
  bone V59.2
    marrow V59.3
  cornea V59.5
  egg (oocyte) (ovum) V59.70
    over age 35 V59.73
      anonymous recipient V59.73
      designated recipient V59.74
    under age 35 V59.71

Donor — *continued*
  egg — *continued*
    under age 35 — *continued*
      anonymous recipient V59.71
      designated recipient V59.72
  heart V59.8
  kidney V59.4
  liver V59.6
  lung V59.8
  lymphocyte V59.8
  organ V59.9
    specified NEC V59.8
  potential, examination of V70.8
  skin V59.1
  specified organ or tissue NEC V59.8
  sperm V59.8
  stem cells V59.02
  tissue V59.9
    specified type NEC V59.8
Donovanosis (granuloma venereum) 099.2
DOPS (diffuse obstructive pulmonary syndrome) 496
Double
  albumin 273.8
  aortic arch 747.21
  auditory canal 744.29
  auricle (heart) 746.82
  bladder 753.8
  external (cervical) os 752.44
  kidney with double pelvis (renal) 753.3
  larynx 748.3
  meatus urinarius 753.8
  organ or site NEC — *see* Accessory
  orifice
    heart valve NEC 746.89
      pulmonary 746.09
  outlet, right ventricle 745.11
  pelvis (renal) with double ureter 753.4
  penis 752.69
  tongue 750.13
  ureter (one or both sides) 753.4
    with double pelvis (renal) 753.4
  urethra 753.8
  urinary meatus 753.8
  uterus (any degree) 752.2
    with doubling of cervix and vagina 752.2
    in pregnancy or childbirth 654.0 ☑
      affecting fetus or newborn 763.89
  vagina 752.47
    with doubling of cervix and uterus 752.2
  vision 368.2
  vocal cords 748.3
  vulva 752.49
  whammy (syndrome) 360.81
Douglas' pouch, cul-de-sac — *see* condition
Down's disease or syndrome (mongolism) 758.0
Down-growth, epithelial (anterior chamber) 364.61
DPD (dihydropyrimidine dehydrogenase deficiency) 277.6
Dracontiasis 125.7
Dracunculiasis 125.7
Dracunculosis 125.7
Drainage
  abscess (spontaneous) — *see* Abscess
  anomalous pulmonary veins to hepatic veins or right atrium 747.41
  stump (amputation) (surgical) 997.62
  suprapubic, bladder 596.89
Dream state, hysterical 300.13
Drepanocytic anemia — *see also* Disease, sickle cell 282.60
Dresbach's syndrome (elliptocytosis) 282.1
Dreschlera (infection) 118
  hawaiiensis 117.8
Dressler's syndrome (postmyocardial infarction) 411.0
Dribbling (post-void) 788.35
Drift, ulnar 736.09
Drinking (alcohol) — *see also* Alcoholism
  excessive, to excess NEC (*see also* Abuse, drugs, nondependent) 305.0 ☑
    bouts, periodic 305.0 ☑
    continual 303.9 ☑
    episodic 305.0 ☑

Drinking (alcohol) — *see also* Alcoholism — *continued*
  excessive, to excess (*see also* Abuse, drugs, nondependent) — *continued*
    habitual 303.9 ☑
    periodic 305.0 ☑
Drip, postnasal (chronic) 784.91
  due to
    allergic rhinitis — *see* Rhinitis, allergic
    common cold 460
    gastroesophageal reflux — *see* Reflux, gastroesophageal
    nasopharyngitis — *see* Nasopharyngitis
    other known condition — code to condition
    sinusitis — *see* Sinusitis
Drivers' license examination V70.3
Droop
  Cooper's 611.81
  facial 781.94
Drop
  finger 736.29
  foot 736.79
  hematocrit (precipitous) 790.01
  hemoglobin 790.01
  toe 735.8
  wrist 736.05
Dropped
  dead 798.1
  heart beats 426.6
Dropsy, dropsical — *see also* Edema 782.3
  abdomen 789.59
  amnion (*see also* Hydramnios) 657.0 ☑
  brain — *see* Hydrocephalus
  cardiac (*see also* Failure, heart) 428.0
  cardiorenal (*see also* Hypertension, cardiorenal) 404.90
  chest 511.9
  fetus or newborn 778.0
    due to isoimmunization 773.3
  gangrenous (*see also* Gangrene) 785.4
  heart (*see also* Failure, heart) 428.0
  hepatic — *see* Cirrhosis, liver
  infantile — *see* Hydrops, fetalis
  kidney (*see also* Nephrosis) 581.9
  liver — *see* Cirrhosis, liver
  lung 514
  malarial (*see also* Malaria) 084.9
  neonatorum — *see* Hydrops, fetalis
  nephritic 581.9
  newborn — *see* Hydrops, fetalis
  nutritional 269.9
  ovary 620.8
  pericardium (*see also* Pericarditis) 423.9
  renal (*see also* Nephrosis) 581.9
  uremic — *see* Uremia
Drowned, drowning (near) 994.1
  lung 518.52
Drowsiness 780.09
Drug — *see also* condition
  addiction (*see also* listing under Dependence) 304.9 ☑
  adverse effect, correct substance properly administered 995.20
  allergy 995.27
  dependence (*see also* listing under Dependence) 304.9 ☑
  habit (*see also* listing under Dependence) 304.9 ☑
  hypersensitivity 995.27
  induced
    circadian rhythm sleep disorder 292.85
    hypersomnia 292.85
    insomnia 292.85
    mental disorder 292.9
      anxiety 292.89
      mood 292.84
      sexual 292.89
      sleep 292.85
      specified type 292.89
    parasomnia 292.85
    persisting
      amnestic disorder 292.83
      dementia 292.82

Drug — *see also* condition — *continued*
  induced — *continued*
    psychotic disorder
      with
        delusions 292.11
        hallucinations 292.12
      sleep disorder 292.85
  intoxication 292.89
  overdose — *see* Table of Drugs and Chemicals
  poisoning — *see* Table of Drugs and Chemicals
  therapy (maintenance) status NEC
    chemotherapy, antineoplastic V58.11
    immunotherapy, antineoplastic V58.12
    long-term (current) (prophylactic) use V58.69
      antibiotics V58.62
      anticoagulants V58.61
      anti-inflammatories, non-steroidal (NSAID) V58.64
      antiplatelets V58.63
      antithrombotics V58.63
      aspirin V58.66
      bisphosphonates V58.68
      high-risk medications NEC V58.69
      insulin V58.67
      methadone for pain control V58.69
      opiate analgesic V58.69
      steroids V58.65
    methadone 304.00
  wrong substance given or taken in error — *see* Table of Drugs and Chemicals
Drunkenness — *see also* Abuse, drugs, nondependent 305.0 ☑
  acute in alcoholism (*see also* Alcoholism) 303.0 ☑
  chronic (*see also* Alcoholism) 303.9 ☑
  pathologic 291.4
  simple (acute) 305.0 ☑
    in alcoholism 303.0 ☑
  sleep 307.47
Drusen
  optic disc or papilla 377.21
  retina (colloid) (hyaloid degeneration) 362.57
    hereditary 362.77
Drusenfieber 075
Dry, dryness — *see also* condition
  eye 375.15
    syndrome 375.15
  larynx 478.79
  mouth 527.7
  nose 478.19
  skin syndrome 701.1
  socket (teeth) 526.5
  throat 478.29
DSAP (disseminated superficial actinic porokeratosis) 692.75
DSTR (delayed serologic transfusion reaction)
  due to or resulting from
    incompatibility
      ABO 999.69
      non-ABO antigen (minor) (Duffy) (Kell) (Kidd) (Lewis) (M) (N) (P) (S) 999.79
      Rh antigen (C) (c) (D) (E) (e) 999.74
Duane's retraction syndrome 378.71
Duane-Stilling-Türk syndrome (ocular retraction syndrome) 378.71
Dubini's disease (electric chorea) 049.8
Dubin-Johnson disease or syndrome 277.4
Dubois' abscess or disease 090.5
Duchenne's
  disease 094.0
    locomotor ataxia 094.0
    muscular dystrophy 359.1
    pseudohypertrophy, muscles 359.1
  paralysis 335.22
  syndrome 335.22
Duchenne-Aran myelopathic, muscular atrophy (nonprogressive) (progressive) 335.21
Duchenne-Griesinger disease 359.1
Ducrey's
  bacillus 099.0

☑ **Additional Digit Required** — Refer to the Tabular List for Digit Selection   ▽ **Subterms under main terms may continue to next column or page**

2014 ICD-9-CM   **143**

Index

Ducrey's — Dysfunction

Ducrey's — *continued*
chancre 099.0
disease (chancroid) 099.0
Duct, ductus — *see* condition
Duengero 061
Duhring's disease (dermatitis herpetiformis) 694.0
Dukes (-Filatov) disease 057.8
Dullness
cardiac (decreased) (increased) 785.3
Dumb ague — *see also* Malaria 084.6
Dumbness — *see also* Aphasia 784.3
Dumdum fever 085.0
Dumping syndrome (postgastrectomy) 564.2
nonsurgical 536.8
Duodenitis (nonspecific) (peptic) 535.60
with hemorrhage 535.61
due to
Strongyloides stercoralis 127.2
Duodenocholangitis 575.8
Duodenum, duodenal — *see* condition
Duplay's disease, periarthritis, or syndrome 726.2
Duplex — *see also* Accessory
kidney 753.3
placenta — *see* Placenta, abnormal
uterus 752.2
Duplication — *see also* Accessory
anus 751.5
aortic arch 747.21
appendix 751.5
biliary duct (any) 751.69
bladder 753.8
cecum 751.5
and appendix 751.5
cervical, cervix 752.44
clitoris 752.49
cystic duct 751.69
digestive organs 751.8
duodenum 751.5
esophagus 750.4
fallopian tube 752.19
frontonasal process 756.0
gallbladder 751.69
ileum 751.5
intestine (large) (small) 751.5
jejunum 751.5
kidney 753.3
liver 751.69
nose 748.1
pancreas 751.7
penis 752.69
respiratory organs NEC 748.9
salivary duct 750.22
spinal cord (incomplete) 742.51
stomach 750.7
ureter 753.4
vagina 752.47
vas deferens 752.89
vocal cords 748.3
Dupré's disease or syndrome (meningism) 781.6
Dupuytren's
contraction 728.6
disease (muscle contracture) 728.6
fracture (closed) 824.4
ankle (closed) 824.4
open 824.5
fibula (closed) 824.4
open 824.5
open 824.5
radius (closed) 813.42
open 813.52
muscle contracture 728.6
Durand-Nicolas-Favre disease (climatic bubo) 099.1
Durotomy, incidental (inadvertent) — *see also* Tear, dural 349.31
Duroziez's disease (congenital mitral stenosis) 746.5
Dust
conjunctivitis 372.05
reticulation (occupational) 504
Dutton's
disease (trypanosomiasis) 086.9
relapsing fever (West African) 087.1

Dwarf, dwarfism 259.4
with infantilism (hypophyseal) 253.3
achondroplastic 756.4
Amsterdam 759.89
bird-headed 759.89
congenital 259.4
constitutional 259.4
hypophyseal 253.3
infantile 259.4
Levi type 253.3
Lorain-Levi (pituitary) 253.3
Lorain type (pituitary) 253.3
metatropic 756.4
nephrotic-glycosuric, with hypophos-phatemic rickets 270.0
nutritional 263.2
ovarian 758.6
pancreatic 577.8
pituitary 253.3
polydystrophic 277.5
primordial 253.3
psychosocial 259.4
renal 588.0
with hypertension — *see* Hypertension, kidney
Russell's (uterine dwarfism and craniofacial dysostosis) 759.89
Dyke-Young anemia or syndrome (acquired macrocytic hemolytic anemia) (secondary) (symptomatic) 283.9
Dynia abnormality — *see also* Defect, coagulation 286.9
Dysacousis 388.40
Dysadrenocortism 255.9
hyperfunction 255.3
hypofunction 255.41
Dysarthria 784.51
due to late effect of cerebrovascular disease (*see also* Late effect(s) (of) cerebrovascular disease) 438.13
Dysautonomia — *see also* Neuropathy, peripheral, autonomic 337.9
familial 742.8
Dysbarism 993.3
Dysbasia 719.7
angiosclerotica intermittens 443.9
due to atherosclerosis 440.21
hysterical 300.11
lordotica (progressiva) 333.6
nonorganic origin 307.9
psychogenic 307.9
Dysbetalipoproteinemia (familial) 272.2
Dyscalculia 315.1
Dyschezia — *see also* Constipation 564.00
Dyschondroplasia (with hemangiomata) 756.4
Voorhoeve's 756.4
Dyschondrosteosis 756.59
Dyschromia 709.00
Dyscollagenosis 710.9
Dyscoria 743.41
Dyscraniopyophalangy 759.89
Dyscrasia
blood 289.9
with antepartum hemorrhage 641.3 ☑
hemorrhage, subungual 287.8
puerperal, postpartum 666.3 ☑
ovary 256.8
plasma cell 273.9
pluriglandular 258.9
polyglandular 258.9
Dysdiadochokinesia 781.3
Dysectasia, vesical neck 596.89
Dysendocrinism 259.9
Dysentery, dysenteric (bilious) (catarrhal) (diarrhea) (epidemic) (gangrenous) (hemorrhagic) (infectious) (sporadic) (tropical) (ulcerative) 009.0
abscess, liver (*see also* Abscess, amebic) 006.3
amebic (*see also* Amebiasis) 006.9
with abscess — *see* Abscess, amebic
acute 006.0
carrier (suspected) of V02.2
chronic 006.1
arthritis (*see also* Arthritis, due to, dysentery) 009.0 *[711.3]* ☑

Dysentery, dysenteric — *continued*
arthritis (*see also* Arthritis, due to, dysentery) — *continued*
bacillary 004.9 *[711.3]* ☑
asylum 004.9
bacillary 004.9
arthritis 004.9 *[711.3]* ☑
Boyd 004.2
Flexner 004.1
Schmitz (-Stutzer) 004.0
Shiga 004.0
Shigella 004.9
group A 004.0
group B 004.1
group C 004.2
group D 004.3
specified type NEC 004.8
Sonne 004.3
specified type NEC 004.8
bacterium 004.9
balantidial 007.0
Balantidium coli 007.0
Boyd's 004.2
Chilomastix 007.8
Chinese 004.9
choleriform 001.1
coccidial 007.2
Dientamoeba fragilis 007.8
due to specified organism NEC — *see* Enteritis, due to, by organism
Embadomonas 007.8
Endolimax nana — *see* Dysentery, amebic
Entamoba, entamebic — *see* Dysentery, amebic
Flexner's 004.1
Flexner-Boyd 004.2
giardial 007.1
Giardia lamblia 007.1
Hiss-Russell 004.1
lamblia 007.1
leishmanial 085.0
malarial (*see also* Malaria) 084.6
metazoal 127.9
Monilia 112.89
protozoal NEC 007.9
Russell's 004.8
salmonella 003.0
schistosomal 120.1
Schmitz (-Stutzer) 004.0
Shiga 004.0
Shigella NEC (*see also* Dysentery, bacillary) 004.9
boydii 004.2
dysenteriae 004.0
Schmitz 004.0
Shiga 004.0
flexneri 004.1
group A 004.0
group B 004.1
group C 004.2
group D 004.3
Schmitz 004.0
Shiga 004.0
Sonnei 004.3
Sonne 004.3
strongyloidiasis 127.2
trichomonal 007.3
tuberculous (*see also* Tuberculosis) 014.8 ☑
viral (*see also* Enteritis, viral) 008.8
Dysequilibrium 780.4
Dysesthesia 782.0
hysterical 300.11
Dysfibrinogenemia (congenital) — *see also* Defect, coagulation 286.3
Dysfunction
adrenal (cortical) 255.9
hyperfunction 255.3
hypofunction 255.41
associated with sleep stages or arousal from sleep 780.56
nonorganic origin 307.47
bladder NEC 596.59
bleeding, uterus 626.8
brain, minimal (*see also* Hyperkinesia) 314.9
cerebral 348.30
colon 564.9

Dysfunction — *continued*
colon — *continued*
psychogenic 306.4
colostomy or enterostomy 569.62
cystic duct 575.8
diastolic 429.9
with heart failure — *see* Failure, heart
due to
cardiomyopathy — *see* Cardiomyopathy
hypertension — *see* Hypertension, heart
endocrine NEC 259.9
endometrium 621.8
enteric stoma 569.62
enterostomy 569.62
erectile 607.84
nonorganic origin 302.72
esophagostomy 530.87
Eustachian tube 381.81
gallbladder 575.8
gastrointestinal 536.9
gland, glandular NEC 259.9
heart 427.9
postoperative (immediate) 997.1
long-term effect of cardiac surgery 429.4
hemoglobin 289.89
hepatic 573.9
hepatocellular NEC 573.9
hypophysis 253.9
hyperfunction 253.1
hypofunction 253.2
posterior lobe 253.6
hypofunction 253.5
kidney (*see also* Disease, renal) 593.9
labyrinthine 386.50
specified NEC 386.58
liver 573.9
constitutional 277.4
minimal brain (child) (*see also* Hyperkinesia) 314.9
ovary, ovarian 256.9
hyperfunction 256.1
estrogen 256.0
hypofunction 256.39
postablative 256.2
postablative 256.2
specified NEC 256.8
papillary muscle 429.81
with myocardial infarction 410.8 ☑
parathyroid 252.8
hyperfunction 252.00
hypofunction 252.1
pineal gland 259.8
pituitary (gland) 253.9
hyperfunction 253.1
hypofunction 253.2
posterior 253.6
hypofunction 253.5
placental — *see* Placenta, insufficiency
platelets (blood) 287.1
polyglandular 258.9
specified NEC 258.8
psychosexual 302.70
with
dyspareunia (functional) (psychogenic) 302.76
frigidity 302.72
impotence 302.72
inhibition
orgasm
female 302.73
male 302.74
sexual
desire 302.71
excitement 302.72
premature ejaculation 302.75
sexual aversion 302.79
specified disorder NEC 302.79
vaginismus 306.51
pylorus 537.9
rectum 564.9
psychogenic 306.4
segmental (*see also* Dysfunction, somatic) 739.9

☑ **Additional Digit Required — Refer to the Tabular List for Digit Selection**

◄ **Subterms under main terms may continue to next column or page**

Dysfunction — continued
  senile 797
  sexual 302.70
  sinoatrial node 427.81
  somatic 739.9
    abdomen 739.9
    acromioclavicular 739.7
    cervical 739.1
    cervicothoracic 739.1
    costochondral 739.8
    costovertebral 739.8
    extremities
      lower 739.6
      upper 739.7
    head 739.0
    hip 739.5
    lumbar, lumbosacral 739.3
    occipitocervical 739.0
    pelvic 739.5
    pubic 739.5
    rib cage 739.8
    sacral 739.4
    sacrococcygeal 739.4
    sacroiliac 739.4
    specified site NEC 739.9
    sternochondral 739.8
    sternoclavicular 739.7
    temporomandibular 739.0
    thoracic, thoracolumbar 739.2
  stomach 536.9
    psychogenic 306.4
  suprarenal 255.9
    hyperfunction 255.3
    hypofunction 255.41
  symbolic NEC 784.60
    specified type NEC 784.69
  systolic 429.9
    with heart failure — see Failure, heart
  temporomandibular (joint) (joint-pain-syn-
      drome) NEC 524.60
    sounds on opening or closing 524.64
    specified NEC 524.69
  testicular 257.9
    hyperfunction 257.0
    hypofunction 257.2
    specified type NEC 257.8
  thymus 254.9
  thyroid 246.9
    complicating pregnancy, childbirth, or
        puerperium 648.1 ☑
    hyperfunction — see Hyperthyroidism
    hypofunction — see Hypothyroidism
  uterus, complicating delivery 661.9 ☑
    affecting fetus or newborn 763.7
    hypertonic 661.4 ☑
    hypotonic 661.2 ☑
      primary 661.0 ☑
      secondary 661.1 ☑
  velopharyngeal (acquired) 528.9
    congenital 750.29
  ventricular 429.9
    with congestive heart failure (see also
        Failure, heart) 428.0
    due to
      cardiomyopathy — see Cardiomyopa-
          thy
      hypertension — see Hypertension,
          heart
    left, reversible following sudden emo-
        tional stress 429.83
  vesicourethral NEC 596.59
  vestibular 386.50
    specified type NEC 386.58
Dysgammaglobulinemia 279.06
Dysgenesis
  gonadal (due to chromosomal anomaly)
      758.6
    pure 752.7
  kidney(s) 753.0
  ovarian 758.6
  renal 753.0
  reticular 279.2
  seminiferous tubules 758.6
  tidal platelet 287.31

Dysgerminoma (M9060/3)
  specified site — see Neoplasm, by site, ma-
      lignant
  unspecified site
    female 183.0
    male 186.9
Dysgeusia 781.1
Dysgraphia 781.3
Dyshidrosis 705.81
Dysidrosis 705.81
Dysinsulinism 251.8
Dyskaryotic cervical smear 795.09
Dyskeratosis — see also Keratosis 701.1
  bullosa hereditaria 757.39
  cervix 622.10
  congenital 757.39
  follicularis 757.39
    vitamin A deficiency 264.8
  gingiva 523.8
  oral soft tissue NEC 528.79
  tongue 528.79
  uterus NEC 621.8
Dyskinesia 781.3
  biliary 575.8
  esophagus 530.5
  hysterical 300.11
  intestinal 564.89
  neuroleptic-induced tardive 333.85
  nonorganic origin 307.9
  orofacial 333.82
    due to drugs 333.85
  psychogenic 307.9
  subacute, due to drugs 333.85
  tardive (oral) 333.85
Dyslalia 784.59
  developmental 315.39
Dyslexia 784.61
  developmental 315.02
  secondary to organic lesion 784.61
Dyslipidemia 272.4
Dysmaturity — see also Immaturity 765.1 ☑
  lung 770.4
  pulmonary 770.4
Dysmenorrhea (essential) (exfoliative) (func-
    tional) (intrinsic) (membranous) (prima-
    ry) (secondary) 625.3
  psychogenic 306.52
Dysmetabolic syndrome X 277.7
Dysmetria 781.3
**Dysmorodystrophia mesodermalis congeni-
    ta** 759.82
Dysnomia 784.3
Dysorexia 783.0
  hysterical 300.11
Dysostosis
  cleidocranial, cleidocranialis 755.59
  craniofacial 756.0
  Fairbank's (idiopathic familial generalized
      osteophytosis) 756.50
  mandibularis 756.0
  mandibulofacial, incomplete 756.0
  multiplex 277.5
  orodigitofacial 759.89
Dyspareunia (female) 625.0
  male 608.89
  psychogenic 302.76
Dyspepsia (allergic) (congenital) (fermentative)
    (flatulent) (functional) (gastric) (gastroin-
    testinal) (neurogenic) (occupational)
    (reflex) 536.8
  acid 536.8
  atonic 536.3
    psychogenic 306.4
  diarrhea 787.91
    psychogenic 306.4
  intestinal 564.89
    psychogenic 306.4
  nervous 306.4
  neurotic 306.4
  psychogenic 306.4
Dysphagia 787.20
  cervical 787.29
  functional 300.11
  hysterical 300.11
  nervous 300.11
  neurogenic 787.29

Dysphagia — continued
  oral phase 787.21
  oropharyngeal phase 787.22
  pharyngeal phase 787.23
  pharyngoesophageal phase 787.24
  psychogenic 306.4
  sideropenic 280.8
  spastica 530.5
  specified NEC 787.29
Dysphagocytosis, congenital 288.1
Dysphasia 784.59
Dysphonia 784.42
  clericorum 784.49
  functional 300.11
  hysterical 300.11
  psychogenic 306.1
  spastica 478.79
Dyspigmentation — see also Pigmentation
  eyelid (acquired) 374.52
Dyspituitarism 253.9
  hyperfunction 253.1
  hypofunction 253.2
  posterior lobe 253.6
Dysplasia — see also Anomaly
  alveolar capillary, with vein misalignment
      516.64
  anus 569.44
    intraepithelial neoplasia I (AIN I) (histo-
        logically confirmed) 569.44
    intraepithelial neoplasia II (AIN II) (histo-
        logically confirmed) 569.44
    intraepithelial neoplasia III (AIN III) 230.6
      anal canal 230.5
    mild (histologically confirmed) 569.44
    moderate (histologically confirmed)
        569.44
    severe 230.6
      anal canal 230.5
  artery
    fibromuscular NEC 447.8
      carotid 447.8
      renal 447.3
  bladder 596.89
  bone (fibrous) NEC 733.29
    diaphyseal, progressive 756.59
    jaw 526.89
    monostotic 733.29
    polyostotic 756.54
    solitary 733.29
  brain 742.9
  bronchopulmonary, fetus or newborn 770.7
  cervix (uteri) 622.10
    cervical intraepithelial neoplasia I (CIN
        I) 622.11
    cervical intraepithelial neoplasia II (CIN
        II) 622.12
    cervical intraepithelial neoplasia III (CIN
        III) 233.1
    CIN I 622.11
    CIN II 622.12
    CIN III 233.1
    mild 622.11
    moderate 622.12
    severe 233.1
  chondroectodermal 756.55
  chondromatose 756.4
  colon 211.3
  craniocarpotarsal 759.89
  craniometaphyseal 756.89
  dentinal 520.5
  diaphyseal, progressive 756.59
  ectodermal (anhidrotic) (Bason) (Clouston's)
      (congenital) (Feinmesser) (heredi-
      tary) (hidrotic) (Marshall) (Robin-
      son's) 757.31
  epiphysealis 756.9
    multiplex 756.56
    punctata 756.59
  epiphysis 756.9
    multiple 756.56
  epithelial
    epiglottis 478.79
    uterine cervix 622.10
  erythroid NEC 289.89
  eye (see also Microphthalmos) 743.10
  familial metaphyseal 756.89

Dysplasia — see also Anomaly —
    continued
  fibromuscular, artery NEC 447.8
    carotid 447.8
    renal 447.3
  fibrous
    bone NEC 733.29
    diaphyseal, progressive 756.59
    jaw 526.89
    monostotic 733.29
    polyostotic 756.54
    solitary 733.29
  high-grade, focal — see Neoplasm, by site,
      benign
  hip (congenital) 755.63
    with dislocation (see also Dislocation,
        hip, congenital) 754.30
  hypohidrotic ectodermal 757.31
  joint 755.8
  kidney 753.15
  leg 755.69
  linguofacialis 759.89
  lung 748.5
  macular 743.55
  mammary (benign) (gland) 610.9
    cystic 610.1
    specified type NEC 610.8
  metaphyseal 756.9
    familial 756.89
  monostotic fibrous 733.29
  muscle 756.89
  myeloid NEC 289.89
  nervous system (general) 742.9
  neuroectodermal 759.6
  oculoauriculovertebral 756.0
  oculodentodigital 759.89
  olfactogenital 253.4
  osteo-onycho-arthro (hereditary) 756.89
  periosteum 733.99
  polyostotic fibrous 756.54
  progressive diaphyseal 756.59
  prostate 602.3
    intraepithelial neoplasia I [PIN I] 602.3
    intraepithelial neoplasia II [PIN II] 602.3
    intraepithelial neoplasia III [PIN III] 233.4
  renal 753.15
  renofacialis 753.0
  retinal NEC 743.56
  retrolental (see also Retinopathy of prema-
      turity) 362.21
  skin 709.8
  spinal cord 742.9
  thymic, with immunodeficiency 279.2
  vagina 623.0
    mild 623.0
    moderate 623.0
    severe 233.31
  vocal cord 478.5
  vulva 624.8
    intraepithelial neoplasia I (VIN I) 624.01
    intraepithelial neoplasia II (VIN II) 624.02
    intraepithelial neoplasia III (VIN III)
        233.32
    mild 624.01
    moderate 624.02
    severe 233.32
    VIN I 624.01
    VIN II 624.02
    VIN III 233.32
Dyspnea (nocturnal) (paroxysmal) 786.09
  asthmatic (bronchial) (see also Asthma)
      493.9 ☑
    with bronchitis (see also Asthma)
        493.9 ☑
      chronic 493.2 ☑
  cardiac (see also Failure, ventricular, left)
      428.1
  cardiac (see also Failure, ventricular, left)
      428.1
  functional 300.11
  hyperventilation 786.01
  hysterical 300.11
  Monday morning 504
  newborn 770.89
  psychogenic 306.1
  uremic — see Uremia

☑ **Additional Digit Required — Refer to the Tabular List for Digit Selection**   ▽ **Subterms under main terms may continue to next column or page**

Index

Dyspraxia — Ectopic, ectopia

Dyspraxia 781.3
  syndrome 315.4
Dysproteinemia 273.8
  transient with copper deficiency 281.4
Dysprothrombinemia (constitutional) — see
  also Defect, coagulation 286.3
Dysreflexia, autonomic 337.3
Dysrhythmia
  cardiac 427.9
    postoperative (immediate) 997.1
      long-term effect of cardiac surgery
        429.4
    specified type NEC 427.89
  cerebral or cortical 348.30
Dyssecretosis, mucoserous 710.2
**Dyssocial reaction, without manifest psychi-
    atric disorder**
  adolescent V71.02
  adult V71.01
  child V71.02
Dyssomnia NEC 780.56
  nonorganic origin 307.47
Dyssplenism 289.4
Dyssynergia
  biliary (see also Disease, biliary) 576.8
  cerebellaris myoclonica 334.2
  detrusor sphincter (bladder) 596.55
  ventricular 429.89
Dystasia, hereditary areflexic 334.3
Dysthymia 300.4
Dysthymic disorder 300.4
Dysthyroidism 246.9
Dystocia 660.9 ☑
  affecting fetus or newborn 763.1
  cervical 661.2 ☑
    affecting fetus or newborn 763.7
  contraction ring 661.4 ☑
    affecting fetus or newborn 763.7
  fetal 660.9 ☑
    abnormal size 653.5 ☑
    affecting fetus or newborn 763.1
    deformity 653.7 ☑
  maternal 660.9 ☑
    affecting fetus or newborn 763.1
  positional 660.0 ☑
    affecting fetus or newborn 763.1
  shoulder (girdle) 660.4 ☑
    affecting fetus or newborn 763.1
  uterine NEC 661.4 ☑
    affecting fetus or newborn 763.7
Dystonia
  acute
    due to drugs 333.72
      neuroleptic-induced acute 333.72
  deformans progressiva 333.6
  lenticularis 333.6
  musculorum deformans 333.6
  torsion (idiopathic) 333.6
    acquired 333.79
    fragments (of) 333.89
    genetic 333.6
    symptomatic 333.79
Dystonic
  movements 781.0
Dystopia kidney 753.3
Dystrophia myotonica 359.2 ☑
Dystrophy, dystrophia 783.9
  adiposogenital 253.8
  asphyxiating thoracic 756.4
  Becker's type 359.22
  brevicollis 756.16
  Bruch's membrane 362.77
  cervical (sympathetic) NEC 337.09
  chondro-osseus with punctate epiphyseal
    dysplasia 756.59
  choroid (hereditary) 363.50
    central (areolar) (partial) 363.53
      total (gyrate) 363.54
    circinate 363.53
    circumpapillary (partial) 363.51
      total 363.52
    diffuse
      partial 363.56
      total 363.57
    generalized
      partial 363.56

Dystrophy, dystrophia — continued
  choroid — continued
    generalized — continued
      total 363.57
    gyrate
      central 363.54
      generalized 363.57
    helicoid 363.52
    peripapillary — see Dystrophy, choroid,
      circumpapillary
    serpiginous 363.54
  cornea (hereditary) 371.50
    anterior NEC 371.52
    Cogan's 371.52
    combined 371.57
    crystalline 371.56
    endothelial (Fuchs') 371.57
    epithelial 371.50
      juvenile 371.51
      microscopic cystic 371.52
    granular 371.53
    lattice 371.54
    macular 371.55
    marginal (Terrien's) 371.48
    Meesman's 371.51
    microscopic cystic (epithelial) 371.52
    nodular, Salzmann's 371.46
    polymorphous 371.58
    posterior NEC 371.58
    ring-like 371.52
    Salzmann's nodular 371.46
    stromal NEC 371.56
  dermatochondrocorneal 371.50
  Duchenne's 359.1
  due to malnutrition 263.9
  Erb's 359.1
  familial
    hyperplastic periosteal 756.59
    osseous 277.5
  foveal 362.77
  Fuchs', cornea 371.57
  Gowers' muscular 359.1
  hair 704.2
  hereditary, progressive muscular 359.1
  hypogenital, with diabetic tendency 759.81
  Landouzy-Déjérine 359.1
  Leyden-Möbius 359.1
  mesodermalis congenita 759.82
  muscular 359.1
    congenital (hereditary) 359.0
      myotonic 359.22
    distal 359.1
    Duchenne's 359.1
    Erb's 359.1
    fascioscapulohumeral 359.1
    Gowers' 359.1
    hereditary (progressive) 359.1
    Landouzy-Déjérine 359.1
    limb-girdle 359.1
    myotonic 359.21
    progressive (hereditary) 359.1
      Charcôt-Marie-Tooth 356.1
    pseudohypertrophic (infantile) 359.1
  myocardium, myocardial (see also Degener-
    ation, myocardial) 429.1
  myotonic 359.21
  myotonica 359.21
  nail 703.8
    congenital 757.5
  neurovascular (traumatic) (see also Neuropa-
    thy, peripheral, autonomic) 337.9
  nutritional 263.9
  ocular 359.1
  oculocerebrorenal 270.8
  oculopharyngeal 359.1
  ovarian 620.8
  papillary (and pigmentary) 701.1
  pelvicrural atrophic 359.1
  pigmentary (see also Acanthosis) 701.2
  pituitary (gland) 253.8
  polyglandular 258.8
  posttraumatic sympathetic — see Dystro-
    phy, sympathetic
  progressive ophthalmoplegic 359.1
  reflex neuromuscular — see Dystrophy,
    sympathetic

Dystrophy, dystrophia — continued
  retina, retinal (hereditary) 362.70
    albipunctate 362.74
    Bruch's membrane 362.77
    cone, progressive 362.75
    hyaline 362.77
    in
      Bassen-Kornzweig syndrome
        272.5 [362.72]
      cerebroretinal lipidosis 330.1 [362.71]
      Refsum's disease 356.3 [362.72]
      systemic lipidosis 272.7 [362.71]
    juvenile (Stargardt's) 362.75
    pigmentary 362.74
    pigment epithelium 362.76
    progressive cone (-rod) 362.75
    pseudoinflammatory foveal 362.77
    rod, progressive 362.75
    sensory 362.75
    vitelliform 362.76
  Salzmann's nodular 371.46
  scapuloperoneal 359.1
  skin NEC 709.9
  sympathetic (posttraumatic) (reflex) 337.20
    lower limb 337.22
    specified site NEC 337.29
    upper limb 337.21
  tapetoretinal NEC 362.74
  thoracic asphyxiating 756.4
  unguium 703.8
    congenital 757.5
  vitreoretinal (primary) 362.73
    secondary 362.66
  vulva 624.09
Dysuria 788.1
  psychogenic 306.53

E

Eagle-Barrett syndrome 756.71
Eales' disease (syndrome) 362.18
Ear — see also condition
  ache 388.70
    otogenic 388.71
    referred 388.72
  lop 744.29
  piercing V50.3
  swimmers' acute 380.12
  tank 380.12
  tropical 111.8 [380.15]
  wax 380.4
Earache 388.70
  otogenic 388.71
  referred 388.72
Early satiety 780.94
Eaton-Lambert syndrome — see also Syn-
    drome, Lambert-Eaton 358.30
Eberth's disease (typhoid fever) 002.0
Ebstein's
  anomaly or syndrome (downward displace-
    ment, tricuspid valve into right ven-
    tricle) 746.2
  disease (diabetes) 250.4 ☑ [581.81]
    due to secondary diabetes
      249.4 ☑ [581.81]
Eccentro-osteochondrodysplasia 277.5
Ecchondroma (M9210/0) — see Neoplasm,
    bone, benign
Ecchondrosis (M9210/1) 238.0
Ecchordosis physaliphora 756.0
Ecchymosis (multiple) 459.89
  conjunctiva 372.72
  eye (traumatic) 921.0
  eyelids (traumatic) 921.1
  newborn 772.6
  spontaneous 782.7
  traumatic — see Contusion
ECD (Erdheim-Chester disease) 277.89
Echinococciasis — see Echinococcus
Echinococcosis — see Echinococcus
Echinococcus (infection) 122.9
  granulosus 122.4
    liver 122.0
    lung 122.1
    orbit 122.3 [376.13]
    specified site NEC 122.3
    thyroid 122.2

Echinococcus — continued
  liver NEC 122.8
    granulosus 122.0
    multilocularis 122.5
  lung NEC 122.9
    granulosus 122.1
    multilocularis 122.6
  multilocularis 122.7
    liver 122.5
    specified site NEC 122.6
  orbit 122.9 [376.13]
    granulosus 122.3 [376.13]
    multilocularis 122.6 [376.13]
  specified site NEC 122.9
    granulosus 122.3
    multilocularis 122.6 [376.13]
  thyroid NEC 122.9
    granulosus 122.2
    multilocularis 122.6
Echinorhynchiasis 127.7
Echinostomiasis 121.8
Echolalia 784.69
ECHO virus infection NEC 079.1
Eclampsia, eclamptic (coma) (convulsions)
    (delirium) 780.39
  female, child-bearing age NEC — see
    Eclampsia, pregnancy
  gravidarum — see Eclampsia, pregnancy
  male 780.39
  not associated with pregnancy or childbirth
    780.39
  pregnancy, childbirth, or puerperium
    642.6 ☑
    with pre-existing hypertension 642.7 ☑
    affecting fetus or newborn 760.0
  uremic 586
Eclipse blindness (total) 363.31
Economic circumstance affecting care V60.9
  specified type NEC V60.89
Economo's disease (encephalitis lethargica)
    049.8
Ectasia, ectasis
  annuloaortic 424.1
  aorta (see also Ectasia, aortic) 447.70
    with aneurysm 441.9
      ruptured 441.5
  aortic 447.70
    with aneurysm 441.9
    abdominal 447.72
    thoracic 447.71
    thoracoabdominal 447.73
  breast 610.4
  capillary 448.9
  cornea (marginal) (postinfectional) 371.71
  duct (mammary) 610.4
  gastric antral vascular (GAVE) 537.82
    with hemorrhage 537.83
    without hemorrhage 537.82
  kidney 593.89
  mammary duct (gland) 610.4
  papillary 448.9
  renal 593.89
  salivary gland (duct) 527.8
  scar, cornea 371.71
  sclera 379.11
Ecthyma 686.8
  contagiosum 051.2
  gangrenosum 686.09
  infectiosum 051.2
Ectocardia 746.87
Ectodermal dysplasia, congenital 757.31
Ectodermosis erosiva pluriorificialis 695.19
Ectopic, ectopia (congenital) 759.89
  abdominal viscera 751.8
    due to defect in anterior abdominal wall
      756.79
  ACTH syndrome 255.0
  adrenal gland 759.1
  anus 751.5
  auricular beats 427.61
  beats 427.60
  bladder 753.5
  bone and cartilage in lung 748.69
  brain 742.4
  breast tissue 757.6
  cardiac 746.87

☑ **Additional Digit Required — Refer to the Tabular List for Digit Selection**   ▽ **Subterms under main terms may continue to next column or page**

146   2014 ICD-9-CM

Ectopic, ectopia — *continued*
cerebral 742.4
cordis 746.87
endometrium 617.9
gallbladder 751.69
gastric mucosa 750.7
gestation — *see* Pregnancy, ectopic
heart 746.87
hormone secretion NEC 259.3
hyperparathyroidism 259.3
kidney (crossed) (intrathoracic) (pelvis)
753.3
in pregnancy or childbirth 654.4 ☑
causing obstructed labor 660.2 ☑
lens 743.37
lentis 743.37
mole — *see* Pregnancy, ectopic
organ or site NEC — *see* Malposition, congenital
ovary 752.0
pancreas, pancreatic tissue 751.7
pregnancy — *see* Pregnancy, ectopic
pupil 364.75
renal 753.3
sebaceous glands of mouth 750.26
secretion
ACTH 255.0
adrenal hormone 259.3
adrenalin 259.3
adrenocorticotropin 255.0
antidiuretic hormone (ADH) 259.3
epinephrine 259.3
hormone NEC 259.3
norepinephrine 259.3
pituitary (posterior) 259.3
spleen 759.0
testis 752.51
thyroid 759.2
ureter 753.4
ventricular beats 427.69
vesicae 753.5
Ectrodactyly 755.4
finger (*see also* Absence, finger, congenital)
755.29
toe (*see also* Absence, toe, congenital)
755.39
Ectromelia 755.4
lower limb 755.30
upper limb 755.20
Ectropion 374.10
anus 569.49
cervix 622.0
with mention of cervicitis 616.0
cicatricial 374.14
congenital 743.62
eyelid 374.10
cicatricial 374.14
congenital 743.62
mechanical 374.12
paralytic 374.12
senile 374.11
spastic 374.13
iris (pigment epithelium) 364.54
lip (congenital) 750.26
acquired 528.5
mechanical 374.12
paralytic 374.12
rectum 569.49
senile 374.11
spastic 374.13
urethra 599.84
uvea 364.54
Eczema (acute) (allergic) (chronic) (erythematous) (fissum) (occupational) (rubrum)
(squamous) 692.9
asteatotic 706.8
atopic 691.8
contact NEC 692.9
dermatitis NEC 692.9
due to specified cause — *see* Dermatitis,
due to
dyshidrotic 705.81
external ear 380.22
flexural 691.8
gouty 274.89
herpeticum 054.0

Eczema — *continued*
hypertrophicum 701.8
hypostatic — *see* Varicose, vein
impetiginous 684
infantile (acute) (chronic) (due to any substance) (intertriginous) (seborrheic)
690.12
intertriginous NEC 692.9
infantile 690.12
intrinsic 691.8
lichenified NEC 692.9
marginatum 110.3
nummular 692.9
pustular 686.8
seborrheic 690.18
infantile 690.12
solare 692.72
stasis (lower extremity) 454.1
ulcerated 454.2
vaccination, vaccinatum 999.0
varicose (lower extremity) — *see* Varicose,
vein
verrucosum callosum 698.3
Eczematoid, exudative 691.8
Eddowes' syndrome (brittle bones and blue
sclera) 756.51
Edema, edematous 782.3
with nephritis (*see also* Nephrosis) 581.9
allergic 995.1
angioneurotic (allergic) (any site) (with urticaria) 995.1
hereditary 277.6
angiospastic 443.9
Berlin's (traumatic) 921.3
brain (cytotoxic) (vasogenic) 348.5
due to birth injury 767.8
fetus or newborn 767.8
cardiac (*see also* Failure, heart) 428.0
cardiovascular (*see also* Failure, heart) 428.0
cerebral — *see* Edema, brain
cerebrospinal vessel — *see* Edema, brain
cervix (acute) (uteri) 622.8
puerperal, postpartum 674.8 ☑
chronic hereditary 757.0
circumscribed, acute 995.1
hereditary 277.6
complicating pregnancy (gestational)
646.1 ☑
with hypertension — *see* Toxemia, of
pregnancy
conjunctiva 372.73
connective tissue 782.3
cornea 371.20
due to contact lenses 371.24
idiopathic 371.21
secondary 371.22
cystoid macular 362.53
due to
lymphatic obstruction — *see* Edema,
lymphatic
salt retention 276.0
epiglottis — *see* Edema, glottis
essential, acute 995.1
hereditary 277.6
extremities, lower — *see* Edema, legs
eyelid NEC 374.82
familial, hereditary (legs) 757.0
famine 262
fetus or newborn 778.5
genital organs
female 629.89
male 608.86
gestational 646.1 ☑
with hypertension — *see* Toxemia, of
pregnancy
glottis, glottic, glottides (obstructive) (passive) 478.6
allergic 995.1
hereditary 277.6
due to external agent — *see* Condition,
respiratory, acute, due to specified agent
heart (*see also* Failure, heart) 428.0
newborn 779.89
heat 992.7
hereditary (legs) 757.0

Edema, edematous — *continued*
inanition 262
infectious 782.3
intracranial 348.5
due to injury at birth 767.8
iris 364.89
joint (*see also* Effusion, joint) 719.0 ☑
larynx (*see also* Edema, glottis) 478.6
legs 782.3
due to venous obstruction 459.2
hereditary 757.0
localized 782.3
due to venous obstruction 459.2
lower extremity 459.2
lower extremities — *see* Edema, legs
lung 514
acute 518.4
with heart disease or failure (*see also*
Failure, ventricular, left) 428.1
congestive 428.0
chemical (due to fumes or vapors)
506.1
due to
external agent(s) NEC 508.9
specified NEC 508.8
fumes and vapors (chemical) (inhalation) 506.1
radiation 508.0
chemical (acute) 506.1
chronic 506.4
chronic 514
chemical (due to fumes or vapors)
506.4
due to
external agent(s) NEC 508.9
specified NEC 508.8
fumes or vapors (chemical) (inhalation) 506.4
radiation 508.1
due to
external agent 508.9
specified NEC 508.8
high altitude 993.2
near drowning 994.1
postoperative 518.4
terminal 514
lymphatic 457.1
due to mastectomy operation 457.0
macula 362.83
cystoid 362.53
diabetic 250.5 ☑ *[362.07]*
due to secondary diabetes
249.5 ☑ *[362.07]*
malignant (*see also* Gangrene, gas) 040.0
Milroy's 757.0
nasopharynx 478.25
neonatorum 778.5
nutritional (newborn) 262
with dyspigmentation, skin and hair 260
optic disc or nerve — *see* Papilledema
orbit 376.33
circulatory 459.89
palate (soft) (hard) 528.9
pancreas 577.8
penis 607.83
periodic 995.1
hereditary 277.6
pharynx 478.25
pitting 782.3
pulmonary — *see* Edema, lung
Quincke's 995.1
hereditary 277.6
renal (*see also* Nephrosis) 581.9
retina (localized) (macular) (peripheral)
362.83
cystoid 362.53
diabetic 250.5 ☑ *[362.07]*
due to secondary diabetes
249.5 ☑ *[362.07]*
salt 276.0
scrotum 608.86
seminal vesicle 608.86
spermatic cord 608.86
spinal cord 336.1
starvation 262
stasis (*see also* Hypertension, venous) 459.30

Edema, edematous — *continued*
subconjunctival 372.73
subglottic (*see also* Edema, glottis) 478.6
supraglottic (*see also* Edema, glottis) 478.6
testis 608.86
toxic NEC 782.3
traumatic NEC 782.3
tunica vaginalis 608.86
vas deferens 608.86
vocal cord — *see* Edema, glottis
vulva (acute) 624.8
Edentia (complete) (partial) — *see also* Absence, tooth 520.0
acquired (*see also* Edentulism) 525.40
due to
caries 525.13
extraction 525.10
periodontal disease 525.12
specified NEC 525.19
trauma 525.11
causing malocclusion 524.30
congenital (deficiency of tooth buds) 520.0
Edentulism 525.40
complete 525.40
class I 525.41
class II 525.42
class III 525.43
class IV 525.44
partial 525.50
class I 525.51
class II 525.52
class III 525.53
class IV 525.54
Edsall's disease 992.2
Educational handicap V62.3
Edwards' syndrome 758.2
Effect, adverse NEC
abnormal gravitational (G) forces or states
994.9
air pressure — *see* Effect, adverse, atmospheric pressure
altitude (high) — *see* Effect, adverse, high
altitude
anesthetic
in labor and delivery NEC 668.9 ☑
affecting fetus or newborn 763.5
antitoxin — *see* Complications, vaccination
atmospheric pressure 993.9
due to explosion 993.4
high 993.3
low — *see* Effect, adverse, high altitude
specified effect NEC 993.8
biological, correct substance properly administered (*see also* Effect, adverse, drug)
995.20
blood (derivatives) (serum) (transfusion) —
see Complications, transfusion
chemical substance NEC 989.9
specified — *see* Table of Drugs and
Chemicals
cobalt, radioactive (*see also* Effect, adverse,
radioactive substance) 990
cold (temperature) (weather) 991.9
chilblains 991.5
frostbite — *see* Frostbite
specified effect NEC 991.8
drugs and medicinals 995.20
correct substance properly administered
995.20
overdose or wrong substance given or
taken 977.9 ·
specified drug — *see* Table of Drugs
and Chemicals
electric current (shock) 994.8
burn — *see* Burn, by site
electricity (electrocution) (shock) 994.8
burn — *see* Burn, by site
exertion (excessive) 994.5
exposure 994.9
exhaustion 994.4
external cause NEC 994.9
fallout (radioactive) NEC 990
fluoroscopy NEC 990

☑ **Additional Digit Required — Refer to the Tabular List for Digit Selection**

▽ **Subterms under main terms may continue to next column or page**

Effect, adverse — *continued*
  foodstuffs
    anaphylactic reaction or shock due to
      food NEC — *see* Anaphylactic re-
      action or shock, due to food
    noxious 988.9
      specified type NEC (*see also* Poison-
        ing, by name of noxious food-
        stuff) 988.8
  gases, fumes, or vapors — *see* Table of
    Drugs and Chemicals
  glue (airplane) sniffing 304.6 ☑
  heat — *see* Heat
  high altitude NEC 993.2
    anoxia 993.2
    on
      ears 993.0
      sinuses 993.1
    polycythemia 289.0
  hot weather — *see* Heat
  hunger 994.2
  immersion, foot 991.4
  immunization — *see* Complications, vacci-
    nation
  immunological agents — *see* Complications,
    vaccination
  implantation (removable) of isotope or radi-
    um NEC 990
  infrared (radiation) (rays) NEC 990
    burn — *see* Burn, by site
    dermatitis or eczema 692.82
  infusion — *see* Complications, infusion
  ingestion or injection of isotope (therapeu-
    tic) NEC 990
  irradiation NEC (*see also* Effect, adverse, ra-
    diation) 990
  isotope (radioactive) NEC 990
  lack of care (child) (infant) (newborn) 995.52
    adult 995.84
  lightning 994.0
    burn — *see* Burn, by site
  Lirugin — *see* Complications, vaccination
  medicinal substance, correct, properly ad-
    ministered (*see also* Effect, adverse,
    drugs) 995.20
  mesothorium NEC 990
  motion 994.6
  noise, inner ear 388.10
  other drug, medicinal and biological sub-
    stance 995.29
  overheated places — *see* Heat
  polonium NEC 990
  psychosocial, of work environment V62.1
  radiation (diagnostic) (fallout) (infrared)
    (natural source) (therapeutic) (tracer)
    (ultraviolet) (x-ray) NEC 990
    with pulmonary manifestations
      acute 508.0
      chronic 508.1
    dermatitis or eczema 692.82
      due to sun NEC (*see also* Dermatitis,
        due to, sun) 692.70
    fibrosis of lungs 508.1
    maternal with suspected damage to fe-
      tus affecting management of
      pregnancy 655.6 ☑
    pneumonitis 508.0
  radioactive substance NEC 990
    dermatitis or eczema 692.82
  radioactivity NEC 990
  radiotherapy NEC 990
    dermatitis or eczema 692.82
  radium NEC 990
  reduced temperature 991.9
    frostbite — *see* Frostbite
    immersion, foot (hand) 991.4
    specified effect NEC 991.8
  roentgenography NEC 990
  roentgenoscopy NEC 990
  roentgen rays NEC 990
  serum (prophylactic) (therapeutic) NEC
    999.59
  specified NEC 995.89
    external cause NEC 994.9
  strangulation 994.7
  submersion 994.1

Effect, adverse — *continued*
  teletherapy NEC 990
  thirst 994.3
  transfusion — *see* Complications, transfu-
    sion
  ultraviolet (radiation) (rays) NEC 990
    burn (*see also* Burn, by site)
      from sun (*see also* Sunburn) 692.71
    dermatitis or eczema 692.82
      due to sun NEC (*see also* Dermatitis,
        due to, sun) 692.70
  uranium NEC 990
  vaccine (any) — *see* Complications, vaccina-
    tion
  weightlessness 994.9
  whole blood (*see also* Complications, trans-
    fusion)
    overdose or wrong substance given (*see*
      also Table of Drugs and Chemi-
      cals) 964.7
  working environment V62.1
  x-rays NEC 990
    dermatitis or eczema 692.82
Effect, remote
  of cancer — *see* condition
Effects, late — *see* Late, effect (of)
Effluvium, telogen 704.02
Effort
  intolerance 306.2
  syndrome (aviators) (psychogenic) 306.2
Effusion
  amniotic fluid (*see also* Rupture, mem-
    branes, premature) 658.1 ☑
  brain (serous) 348.5
  bronchial (*see also* Bronchitis) 490
  cerebral 348.5
  cerebrospinal (*see also* Meningitis) 322.9
    vessel 348.5
  chest — *see* Effusion, pleura
  intracranial 348.5
  joint 719.00
    ankle 719.07
    elbow 719.02
    foot 719.07
    hand 719.04
    hip 719.05
    knee 719.06
    multiple sites 719.09
    pelvic region 719.05
    shoulder (region) 719.01
    specified site NEC 719.08
    wrist 719.03
  meninges (*see also* Meningitis) 322.9
  pericardium, pericardial (*see also* Pericardi-
    tis) 423.9
    acute 420.90
  peritoneal (chronic) 568.82
  pleura, pleurisy, pleuritic, pleuropericardial
    511.9
    bacterial, nontuberculous 511.1
    fetus or newborn 511.9
    malignant 511.81
    nontuberculous 511.9
      bacterial 511.1
    pneumococcal 511.1
    staphylococcal 511.1
    streptococcal 511.1
    traumatic 862.29
      with open wound 862.39
    tuberculous (*see also* Tuberculosis,
      pleura) 012.0 ☑
      primary progressive 010.1 ☑
  pulmonary — *see* Effusion, pleura
  spinal (*see also* Meningitis) 322.9
  thorax, thoracic — *see* Effusion, pleura
Egg (oocyte) (ovum)
  donor V59.70
    over age 35 V59.73
      anonymous recipient V59.73
      designated recipient V59.74
    under age 35 V59.71
      anonymous recipient V59.71
      designated recipient V59.72
Eggshell nails 703.8
  congenital 757.5

Ego-dystonic
  homosexuality 302.0
  lesbianism 302.0
  sexual orientation 302.0
Egyptian splenomegaly 120.1
Ehlers-Danlos syndrome 756.83
Ehrlichiosis 082.40
  chaffeensis 082.41
  specified type NEC 082.49
Eichstedt's disease (pityriasis versicolor) 111.0
EIN (endometrial intraepithelial neoplasia)
  621.35
Eisenmenger's complex or syndrome (ventricular septal defect) 745.4
Ejaculation, semen
  painful 608.89
    psychogenic 306.59
  premature 302.75
  retrograde 608.87
Ekbom syndrome (restless legs) 333.94
Ekman's syndrome (brittle bones and blue
  sclera) 756.51
Elastic skin 756.83
  acquired 701.8
Elastofibroma (M8820/0) — *see* Neoplasm,
  connective tissue, benign
Elastoidosis
  cutanea nodularis 701.8
  cutis cystica et comedonica 701.8
Elastoma 757.39
  juvenile 757.39
  Miescher's (elastosis perforans serpiginosa)
    701.1
Elastomyofibrosis 425.3
Elastosis 701.8
  atrophicans 701.8
  perforans serpiginosa 701.1
  reactive perforating 701.1
  senilis 701.8
  solar (actinic) 692.74
Elbow — *see* condition
Electric
  current, electricity, effects (concussion) (fa-
    tal) (nonfatal) (shock) 994.8
    burn — *see* Burn, by site
  feet (foot) syndrome 266.2
  shock from electroshock gun (taser) 994.8
Electrocution 994.8
Electrolyte imbalance 276.9
  with
    abortion — *see* Abortion, by type, with
      metabolic disorder
    ectopic pregnancy (*see also* categories
      633.0–633.9) 639.4
    hyperemesis gravidarum (before 22
      completed weeks gestation)
      643.1 ☑
    molar pregnancy (*see also* categories
      630–632) 639.4
  following
    abortion 639.4
    ectopic or molar pregnancy 639.4
Elephantiasis (nonfilarial) 457.1
  arabicum (*see also* Infestation, filarial) 125.9
  congenita hereditaria 757.0
  congenital (any site) 757.0
  due to
    Brugia (malayi) 125.1
    mastectomy operation 457.0
    Wuchereria (bancrofti) 125.0
      malayi 125.1
  eyelid 374.83
  filarial (*see also* Infestation, filarial) 125.9
  filariensis (*see also* Infestation, filarial) 125.9
  gingival 523.8
  glandular 457.1
  graecorum 030.9
  lymphangiectatic 457.1
  lymphatic vessel 457.1
    due to mastectomy operation 457.0
  neuromatosa 237.71
  postmastectomy 457.0
  scrotum 457.1
  streptococcal 457.1
  surgical 997.99
    postmastectomy 457.0

Elephantiasis — *continued*
  telangiectodes 457.1
  vulva (nonfilarial) 624.8
Elephant man syndrome 237.71
Elevated — *see* Elevation
  findings on laboratory examination — *see*
    Findings, abnormal, without diagno-
    sis (examination) (laboratory test)
  GFR (glomerular filtration rate) — *see* Find-
    ings, abnormal, without diagnosis
    (examination) (laboratory test)
Elevation
  17-ketosteroids 791.9
  acid phosphatase 790.5
  alkaline phosphatase 790.5
  amylase 790.5
  antibody titers 795.79
  basal metabolic rate (BMR) 794.7
  blood pressure (*see also* Hypertension) 401.9
    reading (incidental) (isolated) (nonspe-
      cific), no diagnosis of hyperten-
      sion 796.2
  blood sugar 790.29
  body temperature (of unknown origin) (*see*
    also Pyrexia) 780.60
  cancer antigen 125 [CA 125] 795.82
  carcinoembryonic antigen [CEA] 795.81
  cholesterol 272.0
    with high triglycerides 272.2
  conjugate, eye 378.81
  C-reactive protein (CRP) 790.95
  CRP (C-reactive protein) 790.95
  diaphragm, congenital 756.6
  GFR (glomerular filtration rate) — *see* Find-
    ings, abnormal, without diagnosis
    (examination) (laboratory test)
  glucose
    fasting 790.21
    tolerance test 790.22
  immunoglobulin level 795.79
  indolacetic acid 791.9
  lactic acid dehydrogenase (LDH) level 790.4
  leukocytes 288.60
  lipase 790.5
  lipoprotein a level 272.8
  liver function test (LFT) 790.6
    alkaline phosphatase 790.5
    aminotransferase 790.4
    bilirubin 782.4
    hepatic enzyme NEC 790.5
    lactate dehydrogenase 790.4
  lymphocytes 288.61
  prostate specific antigen (PSA) 790.93
  renin 790.99
    in hypertension (*see also* Hypertension,
      renovascular) 405.91
  Rh titer (*see also* Complications, transfusion)
    999.70
  scapula, congenital 755.52
  sedimentation rate 790.1
  SGOT 790.4
  SGPT 790.4
  transaminase 790.4
  triglycerides 272.1
    with high cholesterol 272.2
  vanillylmandelic acid 791.9
  venous pressure 459.89
  VMA 791.9
  white blood cell count 288.60
    specified NEC 288.69
Elliptocytosis (congenital) (hereditary) 282.1
  Hb-C (disease) 282.7
  hemoglobin disease 282.7
  sickle-cell (disease) 282.60
  trait 282.5
Ellison-Zollinger syndrome (gastric hypersecretion with pancreatic islet cell tumor) 251.5
Ellis-van Creveld disease or syndrome
  (chondroectodermal dysplasia) 756.55
Elongation, elongated (congenital) — *see also*
  Distortion
  bone 756.9
  cervix (uteri) 752.49
    acquired 622.6
    hypertrophic 622.6

☑ **Additional Digit Required — Refer to the Tabular List for Digit Selection**   ▽ **Subterms under main terms may continue to next column or page**

148   **2014 ICD-9-CM**

Elongation, elongated — see also Distortion — continued
    colon 751.5
    common bile duct 751.69
    cystic duct 751.69
    frenulum, penis 752.69
    labia minora, acquired 624.8
    ligamentum patellae 756.89
    petiolus (epiglottidis) 748.3
    styloid bone (process) 733.99
    tooth, teeth 520.2
    uvula 750.26
        acquired 528.9
Elschnig bodies or pearls 366.51
El Tor cholera 001.1
Emaciation (due to malnutrition) 261
Emancipation disorder 309.22
Embadomoniasis 007.8
Embarrassment heart, cardiac — see Disease, heart
Embedded
    fragment (status) — see Foreign body, retained
    splinter (status) — see Foreign body, retained
    tooth, teeth 520.6
        root only 525.3
Embolic — see condition
Embolism 444.9
    with
        abortion — see Abortion, by type, with embolism
        ectopic pregnancy (see also categories 633.0–633.9) 639.6
        molar pregnancy (see also categories 630–632) 639.6
    air (any site) 958.0
        with
            abortion — see Abortion, by type, with embolism
            ectopic pregnancy (see also categories 633.0–633.9) 639.6
            molar pregnancy (see also categories 630–632) 639.6
        due to implanted device — see Complications, due to (presence of) any device, implant, or graft classified to 996.0–996.5 NEC
        following
            abortion 639.6
            ectopic or molar pregnancy 639.6
            infusion, perfusion, or transfusion 999.1
        in pregnancy, childbirth, or puerperium 673.0 ☑
        traumatic 958.0
    amniotic fluid (pulmonary) 673.1 ☑
        with
            abortion — see Abortion, by type, with embolism
            ectopic pregnancy (see also categories 633.0–633.9) 639.6
            molar pregnancy (see also categories 630–632) 639.6
        following
            abortion 639.6
            ectopic or molar pregnancy 639.6
    aorta, aortic 444.1
        abdominal 444.09
            saddle 444.01
        bifurcation 444.09
        saddle 444.01
        thoracic 444.1
    artery 444.9
        auditory, internal 433.8 ☑
        basilar (see also Occlusion, artery, basilar) 433.0 ☑
        bladder 444.89
        carotid (common) (internal) (see also Occlusion, artery, carotid) 433.1 ☑
        cerebellar (anterior inferior) (posterior inferior) (superior) 433.8 ☑
        cerebral (see also Embolism, brain) 434.1 ☑
        choroidal (anterior) 433.8 ☑

Embolism — continued
    artery — continued
        communicating posterior 433.8 ☑
        coronary (see also Infarct, myocardium) 410.9 ☑
            without myocardial infarction 411.81
        extremity 444.22
            lower 444.22
            upper 444.21
        hypophyseal 433.8 ☑
        mesenteric (with gangrene) 557.0
        ophthalmic (see also Occlusion, retina) 362.30
        peripheral 444.22
        pontine 433.8 ☑
        precerebral NEC — see Occlusion, artery, precerebral
        pulmonary — see Embolism, pulmonary
        pyemic 449
            pulmonary 415.12
        renal 593.81
        retinal (see also Occlusion, retina) 362.30
        septic 449
            pulmonary 415.12
        specified site NEC 444.89
        vertebral (see also Occlusion, artery, vertebral) 433.2 ☑
    auditory, internal 433.8 ☑
    basilar (artery) (see also Occlusion, artery, basilar) 433.0 ☑
    birth, mother — see Embolism, obstetrical
    blood-clot
        with
            abortion — see Abortion, by type, with embolism
            ectopic pregnancy (see also categories 633.0–633.9) 639.6
            molar pregnancy (see also categories 630–632) 639.6
        following
            abortion 639.6
            ectopic or molar pregnancy 639.6
        in pregnancy, childbirth, or puerperium 673.2 ☑
    brain 434.1 ☑
        with
            abortion — see Abortion, by type, with embolism
            ectopic pregnancy (see also categories 633.0–633.9) 639.6
            molar pregnancy (see also categories 630–632) 639.6
        following
            abortion 639.6
            ectopic or molar pregnancy 639.6
        late effect — see Late effect(s) (of) cerebrovascular disease
        puerperal, postpartum, childbirth 674.0 ☑
    capillary 448.9
    cardiac (see also Infarct, myocardium) 410.9 ☑
    carotid (artery) (common) (internal) (see also Occlusion, artery, carotid) 433.1 ☑
    cavernous sinus (venous) — see Embolism, intracranial venous sinus
    cerebral (see also Embolism, brain) 434.1 ☑
    cholesterol — see Atheroembolism
    choroidal (anterior) (artery) 433.8 ☑
    coronary (artery or vein) (systemic) (see also Infarct, myocardium) 410.9 ☑
        without myocardial infarction 411.81
    due to (presence of) any device, implant, or graft classifiable to 996.0–996.5 — see Complications, due to (presence of) any device, implant, or graft classified to 996.0–996.5 NEC
    encephalomalacia (see also Embolism, brain) 434.1 ☑
    extremities 444.22
        lower 444.22
        upper 444.21
    eye 362.30
    fat (cerebral) (pulmonary) (systemic) 958.1

Embolism — continued
    fat — continued
        with
            abortion — see Abortion, by type, with embolism
            ectopic pregnancy (see also categories 633.0–633.9) 639.6
            molar pregnancy (see also categories 630–632) 639.6
        complicating delivery or puerperium 673.8 ☑
        following
            abortion 639.6
            ectopic or molar pregnancy 639.6
        in pregnancy, childbirth, or the puerperium 673.8 ☑
    femoral (artery) 444.22
        vein 453.6
            deep 453.41
    following
        abortion 639.6
        ectopic or molar pregnancy 639.6
        infusion, perfusion, or transfusion
            air 999.1
            thrombus 999.2
    heart (fatty) (see also Infarct, myocardium) 410.9 ☑
    hepatic (vein) 453.0
    iliac (artery) 444.81
    iliofemoral 444.81
    in pregnancy, childbirth, or puerperium (pulmonary) — see Embolism, obstetrical
    intestine (artery) (vein) (with gangrene) 557.0
    intracranial (see also Embolism, brain) 434.1 ☑
        venous sinus (any) 325
            late effect — see category 326
            nonpyogenic 437.6
                in pregnancy or puerperium 671.5 ☑
    kidney (artery) 593.81
    lateral sinus (venous) — see Embolism, intracranial venous sinus
    longitudinal sinus (venous) — see Embolism, intracranial venous sinus
    lower extremity 444.22
    lung (massive) — see Embolism, pulmonary
    meninges (see also Embolism, brain) 434.1 ☑
    mesenteric (artery) (with gangrene) 557.0
    multiple NEC 444.9
    obstetrical (pulmonary) 673.2 ☑
        air 673.0 ☑
        amniotic fluid (pulmonary) 673.1 ☑
        blood-clot 673.2 ☑
        cardiac 674.8 ☑
        fat 673.8 ☑
        heart 674.8 ☑
        pyemic 673.3 ☑
        septic 673.3 ☑
        specified NEC 674.8 ☑
    ophthalmic (see also Occlusion, retina) 362.30
    paradoxical NEC 444.9
    penis 607.82
    peripheral arteries NEC 444.22
        lower 444.22
        upper 444.21
    pituitary 253.8
    popliteal (artery) 444.22
    portal (vein) 452
    postoperative NEC 997.2
        cerebral 997.02
        mesenteric artery 997.71
        other vessels 997.79
        peripheral vascular 997.2
        pulmonary 415.11
            septic 415.11
        renal artery 997.72
    precerebral artery (see also Occlusion, artery, precerebral) 433.9 ☑
    puerperal — see Embolism, obstetrical
    pulmonary (acute) (artery) (vein) 415.19

Embolism — continued
    pulmonary — continued
        with
            abortion — see Abortion, by type, with embolism
            ectopic pregnancy (see also categories 633.0–633.9) 639.6
            molar pregnancy (see also categories 630–632) 639.6
        chronic 416.2
        following
            abortion 639.6
            ectopic or molar pregnancy 639.6
        healed or old V12.55
        iatrogenic 415.11
        in pregnancy, childbirth, or puerperium — see Embolism, obstetrical
        personal history of V12.55
        postoperative 415.11
        septic 415.12
        pyemic (multiple) (see also Septicemia) 415.12
            with
                abortion — see Abortion, by type, with embolism
                ectopic pregnancy (see also categories 633.0–633.9) 639.6
                molar pregnancy (see also categories 630–632) 639.6
            Aerobacter aerogenes 415.12
            enteric gram-negative bacilli 415.12
            Enterobacter aerogenes 415.12
            Escherichia coli 415.12
            following
                abortion 639.6
                ectopic or molar pregnancy 639.6
            Hemophilus influenzae 415.12
            pneumococcal 415.12
            Proteus vulgaris 415.12
            Pseudomonas (aeruginosa) 415.12
            puerperal, postpartum, childbirth (any organism) 673.3 ☑
            Serratia 415.12
            specified organism NEC 415.12
            staphylococcal 415.12
                aureus 415.12
                specified organism NEC 415.12
            streptococcal 415.12
    renal (artery) 593.81
        vein 453.3
    retina, retinal (see also Occlusion, retina) 362.30
    saddle
        abdominal aorta 444.01
        pulmonary artery 415.13
    septic 415.12
        arterial 449
    septicemic — see Embolism, pyemic
    sinus — see Embolism, intracranial venous sinus
    soap
        with
            abortion — see Abortion, by type, with embolism
            ectopic pregnancy (see also categories 633.0–633.9) 639.6
            molar pregnancy (see also categories 630–632) 639.6
        following
            abortion 639.6
            ectopic or molar pregnancy 639.6
    spinal cord (nonpyogenic) 336.1
        in pregnancy or puerperium 671.5 ☑
        pyogenic origin 324.1
            late effect — see category 326
    spleen, splenic (artery) 444.89
    thrombus (thromboembolism) following infusion, perfusion, or transfusion 999.2
    upper extremity 444.21
    vein 453.9
        with inflammation or phlebitis — see Thrombophlebitis
        antecubital (acute) 453.81
            chronic 453.71
        axillary (acute) 453.84

☑ **Additional Digit Required** — Refer to the Tabular List for Digit Selection   ▽ **Subterms under main terms may continue to next column or page**

2014 ICD-9-CM   149

☑ Additional Digit Required — Refer to the Tabular List for Digit Selection
⏪ Subterms under main terms may continue to next column or page

150

2014 ICD-9-CM

Embolism — Encephalitis

Encephalitis — continued
viral, virus 049.9
  arthropod-borne NEC 064
    mosquito-borne 062.9
      Australian X disease 062.4
      California virus 062.5
      Eastern equine 062.2
      Ilheus virus 062.8
      Japanese (B type) 062.0
      Murray Valley 062.4
      specified type NEC 062.8
      St. Louis 062.3
      type B 062.0
      type C 062.3
      Western equine 062.1
    tick-borne 063.9
      biundulant 063.2
      Central European 063.2
      Czechoslovakian 063.2
      diphasic meningoencephalitis 063.2
      Far Eastern 063.0
      Langat 063.8
      louping ill 063.1
      Powassan 063.8
      Russian spring-summer (taiga) 063.0
      specified type NEC 063.8
    vector unknown 064
    Western equine 062.1
  slow acting NEC 046.8
  specified type NEC 049.8
  vaccination, prophylactic (against) V05.0
von Economo's 049.8
Western equine 062.1
West Nile type 066.41
Encephalocele 742.0
orbit 376.81
Encephalocystocele 742.0
Encephaloduroarteriomyosynangiosis (EDAMS) 437.5
Encephalomalacia (brain) (cerebellar) (cerebral) (cerebrospinal) — see also Softening, brain 348.89
due to
  hemorrhage (see also Hemorrhage, brain) 431
  recurrent spasm of artery 435.9
embolic (cerebral) (see also Embolism, brain) 434.1 ☑
subcorticalis chronicus arteriosclerotica 290.12
thrombotic (see also Thrombosis, brain) 434.0 ☑
Encephalomeningitis — see Meningoencephalitis
Encephalomeningocele 742.0
Encephalomeningomyelitis — see Meningoencephalitis
Encephalomeningopathy — see also Meningoencephalitis 349.9
Encephalomyelitis (chronic) (granulomatous) (myalgic, benign) — see also Encephalitis 323.9
abortive disseminated 049.8
acute disseminated (ADEM) (postinfectious) 136.9 [323.61]
  infectious 136.9 [323.61]
  noninfectious 323.81
  postimmunization 323.51
due to
  cat-scratch disease 078.3 [323.01]
  infectious mononucleosis 075 [323.01]
  ornithosis 073.7 [323.01]
  vaccination (any) 323.51
equine (acute) (infectious) 062.9
  Eastern 062.2
  Venezuelan 066.2
  Western 062.1
funicularis infectiosa 049.8
late effect — see Late, effect, encephalitis
Munch-Peterson's 049.8
postchickenpox 052.0
postimmunization 323.51
postmeasles 055.0
postvaccinal (smallpox) 323.51

Encephalomyelitis — see also Encephalitis — continued
rubella 056.01
specified cause NEC 323.81
syphilitic 094.81
West Nile 066.41
Encephalomyelocele 742.0
Encephalomyelomeningitis — see Meningoencephalitis
Encephalomyeloneuropathy 349.9
Encephalomyelopathy 349.9
subacute necrotizing (infantile) 330.8
Encephalomyeloradiculitis (acute) 357.0
Encephalomyeloradiculoneuritis (acute) 357.0
Encephalomyeloradiculopathy 349.9
Encephalomyocarditis 074.23
Encephalopathia hyperbilirubinemica, newborn 774.7
due to isoimmunization (conditions classifiable to 773.0–773.2) 773.4
Encephalopathy (acute) 348.30
alcoholic 291.2
anoxic — see Damage, brain, anoxic
arteriosclerotic 437.0
  late effect — see Late effect(s) (of) cerebrovascular disease
bilirubin, newborn 774.7
  due to isoimmunization 773.4
congenital 742.9
demyelinating (callosal) 341.8
due to
  birth injury (intracranial) 767.8
  dialysis 294.8
    transient 293.9
  drugs — (see also Table of Drugs and Chemicals) 349.82
  hyperinsulinism — see Hyperinsulinism
  influenza (virus) (see also Influenza) 487.8
  identified
    avian 488.09
    (novel) 2009 H1N1 488.19
  lack of vitamin (see also Deficiency, vitamin) 269.2
  nicotinic acid deficiency 291.2
  serum (nontherapeutic) (therapeutic) 999.59
  syphilis 094.81
  trauma (postconcussional) 310.2
    current (see also Concussion, brain) 850.9
      with skull fracture — see Fracture, skull, by site, with intracranial injury
  vaccination 323.51
hepatic 572.2
hyperbilirubinemic, newborn 774.7
  due to isoimmunization (conditions classifiable to 773.0–773.2) 773.4
hypertensive 437.2
hypoglycemic 251.2
hypoxic (see also Damage, brain, anoxic)
  ischemic (HIE) 768.70
    mild 768.71
    moderate 768.72
    severe 768.73
infantile cystic necrotizing (congenital) 341.8
lead 984.9 [323.71]
leukopolio 330.0
metabolic (see also Delirium) 348.31
  drug induced 349.82
  toxic 349.82
necrotizing
  hemorrhagic (acute) 323.61
  subacute 330.8
other specified type NEC 348.39
pellagrous 265.2
portal-systemic 572.2
postcontusional 310.2
posttraumatic 310.2
saturnine 984.9 [323.71]
septic 348.31
spongiform, subacute (viral) 046.19

Encephalopathy — continued
subacute
  necrotizing 330.8
  spongioform 046.19
  viral, spongiform 046.19
subcortical progressive (Schilder) 341.1
  chronic (Binswanger's) 290.12
toxic 349.82
  metabolic 349.82
traumatic (postconcussional) 310.2
  current (see also Concussion, brain) 850.9
    with skull fracture — see Fracture, skull, by site, with intracranial injury
vitamin B deficiency NEC 266.9
Wernicke's (superior hemorrhagic polioencephalitis) 265.1
Encephalorrhagia — see also Hemorrhage, brain 432.9
healed or old V12.54
late effect — see Late effect(s) (of) cerebrovascular disease
Encephalosis, posttraumatic 310.2
Enchondroma (M9220/0) — see also Neoplasm, bone, benign
multiple, congenital 756.4
Enchondromatosis (cartilaginous) (congenital) (multiple) 756.4
Enchondroses, multiple (cartilaginous) (congenital) 756.4
Encopresis — see also Incontinence, feces 787.60
nonorganic origin 307.7
Encounter for — see also Admission for
administrative purpose only V68.9
  referral of patient without examination or treatment V68.81
  specified purpose NEC V68.89
chemotherapy, (oral) (intravenous), antineoplastic V58.11
determination of fetal viability of pregnancy V23.87
dialysis
  extracorporeal (renal) V56.0
  peritoneal V56.8
disability examination V68.01
end-of-life care V66.7
hospice care V66.7
immunizations (childhood) appropriate for age V20.2
immunotherapy, antineoplastic V58.12
joint prosthesis insertion following prior explantation of joint prosthesis V54.82
palliative care V66.7
paternity testing V70.4
radiotherapy V58.0
respirator [ventilator] dependence
  during
    mechanical failure V46.14
    power failure V46.12
  for weaning V46.13
routine infant and child vision and hearing testing V20.2
school examination V70.3
  following surgery V67.09
screening mammogram NEC V76.12
  for high-risk patient V76.11
terminal care V66.7
weaning from respirator [ventilator] V46.13
Encystment — see Cyst
Endamebiasis — see Amebiasis
Endamoeba — see Amebiasis
Endarteritis (bacterial, subacute) (infective) (septic) 447.6
brain, cerebral or cerebrospinal 437.4
  late effect — see Late effect(s) (of) cerebrovascular disease
coronary (artery) — see Arteriosclerosis, coronary
deformans — see Arteriosclerosis
embolic (see also Embolism) 444.9
obliterans (see also Arteriosclerosis)
  pulmonary 417.8
pulmonary 417.8
retina 362.18

Endarteritis — continued
senile — see Arteriosclerosis
syphilitic 093.89
  brain or cerebral 094.89
  congenital 090.5
  spinal 094.89
tuberculous (see also Tuberculosis) 017.9 ☑
Endemic — see condition
Endocarditis (chronic) (indeterminate) (interstitial) (marantic) (nonbacterial thrombotic) (residual) (sclerotic) (sclerous) (senile) (valvular) 424.90
with
  rheumatic fever (conditions classifiable to 390)
    active — see Endocarditis, acute, rheumatic
    inactive or quiescent (with chorea) 397.9
acute or subacute 421.9
  rheumatic (aortic) (mitral) (pulmonary) (tricuspid) 391.1
    with chorea (acute) (rheumatic) (Sydenham's) 392.0
aortic (heart) (nonrheumatic) (valve) 424.1
  with
    mitral (valve) disease 396.9
      active or acute 391.1
        with chorea (acute) (rheumatic) (Sydenham's) 392.0
    bacterial 421.0
    rheumatic fever (conditions classifiable to 390)
      active — see Endocarditis, acute, rheumatic
      inactive or quiescent (with chorea) 395.9
        with mitral disease 396.9
  acute or subacute 421.9
  arteriosclerotic 424.1
  congenital 746.89
  hypertensive 424.1
  rheumatic (chronic) (inactive) 395.9
    with mitral (valve) disease 396.9
      active or acute 391.1
        with chorea (acute) (rheumatic) (Sydenham's) 392.0
    active or acute 391.1
      with chorea (acute) (rheumatic) (Sydenham's) 392.0
  specified cause, except rheumatic 424.1
  syphilitic 093.22
arteriosclerotic or due to arteriosclerosis 424.99
atypical verrucous (Libman-Sacks) 710.0 [424.91]
bacterial (acute) (any valve) (chronic) (subacute) 421.0
blastomycotic 116.0 [421.1]
candidal 112.81
congenital 425.3
constrictive 421.0
Coxsackie 074.22
due to
  blastomycosis 116.0 [421.1]
  candidiasis 112.81
  Coxsackie (virus) 074.22
  disseminated lupus erythematosus 710.0 [424.91]
  histoplasmosis (see also Histoplasmosis) 115.94
  hypertension (benign) 424.99
  moniliasis 112.81
  prosthetic cardiac valve 996.61
  Q fever 083.0 [421.1]
  serratia marcescens 421.0
  typhoid (fever) 002.0 [421.1]
fetal 425.3
gonococcal 098.84
hypertensive 424.99
infectious or infective (acute) (any valve) (chronic) (subacute) 421.0
lenta (acute) (any valve) (chronic) (subacute) 421.0

☑ **Additional Digit Required** — Refer to the Tabular List for Digit Selection   ▽ **Subterms under main terms may continue to next column or page**

2014 ICD-9-CM   151

Endocarditis — *continued*
  Libman-Sacks 710.0 *[424.91]*
  Loeffler's (parietal fibroplastic) 421.0
  malignant (acute) (any valve) (chronic)
      (subacute) 421.0
  meningococcal 036.42
  mitral (chronic) (double) (fibroid) (heart)
      (inactive) (valve) (with chorea) 394.9
      with
        aortic (valve) disease 396.9
          active or acute 391.1
            with chorea (acute)
                (rheumatic) (Syden-
                ham's) 392.0
          rheumatic fever (conditions classifi-
              able to 390)
            active — *see* Endocarditis, acute,
                rheumatic
            inactive or quiescent (with
                chorea) 394.9
              with aortic valve disease 396.9
        active or acute 391.1
          with chorea (acute) (rheumatic)
              (Sydenham's) 392.0
        bacterial 421.0
      arteriosclerotic 424.0
      congenital 746.89
      hypertensive 424.0
      nonrheumatic 424.0
        acute or subacute 421.9
      syphilitic 093.21
  monilial 112.81
  mycotic (acute) (any valve) (chronic) (suba-
      cute) 421.0
  pneumococcic (acute) (any valve) (chronic)
      (subacute) 421.0
  pulmonary (chronic) (heart) (valve) 424.3
      with
        rheumatic fever (conditions classifi-
            able to 390)
          active — *see* Endocarditis, acute,
              rheumatic
          inactive or quiescent (with
              chorea) 397.1
        acute or subacute 421.9
          rheumatic 391.1
            with chorea (acute) (rheumatic)
                (Sydenham's) 392.0
      arteriosclerotic or due to arteriosclerosis
          424.3
      congenital 746.09
      hypertensive or due to hypertension
          (benign) 424.3
      rheumatic (chronic) (inactive) (with
          chorea) 397.1
        active or acute 391.1
          with chorea (acute) (rheumatic)
              (Sydenham's) 392.0
      syphilitic 093.24
  purulent (acute) (any valve) (chronic) (suba-
      cute) 421.0
  rheumatic (chronic) (inactive) (with chorea)
      397.1
      active or acute (aortic) (mitral) (pul-
          monary) (tricuspid) 391.1
      with chorea (acute) (rheumatic)
          (Sydenham's) 392.0
  septic (acute) (any valve) (chronic) (suba-
      cute) 421.0
  specified cause, except rheumatic 424.99
  streptococcal (acute) (any valve) (chronic)
      (subacute) 421.0
  subacute — *see* Endocarditis, acute
  suppurative (any valve) (acute) (chronic)
      (subacute) 421.0
  syphilitic NEC 093.20
  toxic (*see also* Endocarditis, acute) 421.9
  tricuspid (chronic) (heart) (inactive)
      (rheumatic) (valve) (with chorea)
      397.0
      with
        rheumatic fever (conditions classifi-
            able to 390)
          active — *see* Endocarditis, acute,
              rheumatic

Endocarditis — *continued*
  tricuspid — *continued*
      with — *continued*
        rheumatic fever — *continued*
          inactive or quiescent (with
              chorea) 397.0
      active or acute 391.1
        with chorea (acute) (rheumatic)
            (Sydenham's) 392.0
      arteriosclerotic 424.2
      congenital 746.89
      hypertensive 424.2
      nonrheumatic 424.2
        acute or subacute 421.9
      specified cause, except rheumatic 424.2
      syphilitic 093.23
      tuberculous (*see also* Tuberculosis)
          017.9 ☑ *[424.91]*
  typhoid 002.0 *[421.1]*
  ulcerative (acute) (any valve) (chronic)
      (subacute) 421.0
  vegetative (acute) (any valve) (chronic)
      (subacute) 421.0
  verrucous (acute) (any valve) (chronic)
      (subacute) NEC 710.0 *[424.91]*
      nonbacterial 710.0 *[424.91]*
      nonrheumatic 710.0 *[424.91]*
Endocardium, endocardial — *see also* condi-
    tion
  cushion defect 745.60
      specified type NEC 745.69
Endocervicitis — *see also* Cervicitis 616.0
  due to
      intrauterine (contraceptive) device
          996.65
  gonorrheal (acute) 098.15
      chronic or duration of 2 months or over
          098.35
  hyperplastic 616.0
  syphilitic 095.8
  trichomonal 131.09
  tuberculous (*see also* Tuberculosis) 016.7 ☑
Endocrine — *see* condition
Endocrinopathy, pluriglandular 258.9
Endodontitis 522.0
End-of-life care V66.7
Endomastoiditis — *see also* Mastoiditis 383.9
Endometrioma 617.9
Endometriosis 617.9
  appendix 617.5
  bladder 617.8
  bowel 617.5
  broad ligament 617.3
  cervix 617.0
  colon 617.5
  cul-de-sac (Douglas') 617.3
  exocervix 617.0
  fallopian tube 617.2
  female genital organ NEC 617.8
  gallbladder 617.8
  in scar of skin 617.6
  internal 617.0
  intestine 617.5
  lung 617.8
  myometrium 617.0
  ovary 617.1
  parametrium 617.3
  pelvic peritoneum 617.3
  peritoneal (pelvic) 617.3
  rectovaginal septum 617.4
  rectum 617.5
  round ligament 617.3
  skin 617.6
  specified site NEC 617.8
  stromal (M8931/1) 236.0
  umbilicus 617.8
  uterus 617.0
      internal 617.0
  vagina 617.4
  vulva 617.8
Endometritis (nonspecific) (purulent) (septic)
    (suppurative) 615.9
  with
      abortion — *see* Abortion, by type, with
          sepsis

Endometritis — *continued*
  with — *continued*
      ectopic pregnancy (*see also* categories
          633.0–633.9) 639.0
      molar pregnancy (*see also* categories
          630–632) 639.0
  acute 615.0
  blennorrhagic 098.16
      acute 098.16
      chronic or duration of 2 months or over
          098.36
  cervix, cervical (*see also* Cervicitis) 616.0
      hyperplastic 616.0
  chronic 615.1
  complicating pregnancy 670.1 ☑
      affecting fetus or newborn 760.8
      septic 670.2 ☑
  decidual 615.9
  following
      abortion 639.0
      ectopic or molar pregnancy 639.0
  gonorrheal (acute) 098.16
      chronic or duration of 2 months or over
          098.36
  hyperplastic (*see also* Hyperplasia, en-
      dometrium) 621.30
      cervix 616.0
  polypoid — *see* Endometritis, hyperplastic
  puerperal, postpartum, childbirth 670.1 ☑
      septic 670.2 ☑
  senile (atrophic) 615.9
  subacute 615.0
  tuberculous (*see also* Tuberculosis) 016.7 ☑
Endometrium — *see* condition
Endomyocardiopathy, South African 425.2
Endomyocarditis — *see* Endocarditis
Endomyofibrosis 425.0
Endomyometritis — *see also* Endometritis
    615.9
Endopericarditis — *see* Endocarditis
Endoperineuritis — *see* Disorder, nerve
Endophlebitis — *see also* Phlebitis 451.9
  leg 451.2
      deep (vessels) 451.19
      superficial (vessels) 451.0
  portal (vein) 572.1
  retina 362.18
  specified site NEC 451.89
  syphilitic 093.89
Endophthalmia — *see also* Endophthalmitis
    360.00
  gonorrheal 098.42
Endophthalmitis (globe) (infective)
    (metastatic) (purulent) (subacute) 360.00
  acute 360.01
  bleb associated 379.63
  chronic 360.03
  parasitic 360.13
  phacoanaphylactic 360.19
  specified type NEC 360.19
  sympathetic 360.11
Endosalpingioma (M9111/1) 236.2
Endosalpingiosis 629.89
Endosteitis — *see* Osteomyelitis
Endothelioma, bone (M9260/3) — *see* Neo-
    plasm, bone, malignant
Endotheliosis 287.8
  hemorrhagic infectional 287.8
Endotoxemia — code to condition
Endotoxic shock 785.52
  postoperative 998.02
Endotrachelitis — *see also* Cervicitis 616.0
Enema rash 692.89
Engelmann's disease (diaphyseal sclerosis)
    756.9
**Engel-von Recklinghausen disease or syn-
    drome** (osteitis fibrosa cystica) 252.01
English disease — *see also* Rickets 268.0
Engman's disease (infectious eczematoid
    dermatitis) 690.8
Engorgement
  breast 611.79
      newborn 778.7
      puerperal, postpartum 676.2 ☑
  liver 573.9
  lung 514

Engorgement — *continued*
  pulmonary 514
  retina, venous 362.37
  stomach 536.8
  venous, retina 362.37
Enlargement, enlarged — *see also* Hypertro-
    phy
  abdomen 789.3 ☑
  adenoids 474.12
      and tonsils 474.10
  alveolar process or ridge 525.8
  apertures of diaphragm (congenital) 756.6
  blind spot, visual field 368.42
  gingival 523.8
  heart, cardiac (*see also* Hypertrophy, cardiac)
      429.3
  lacrimal gland, chronic 375.03
  liver (*see also* Hypertrophy, liver) 789.1
  lymph gland or node 785.6
  orbit 376.46
  organ or site, congenital NEC — *see*
      Anomaly, specified type NEC
  parathyroid (gland) 252.01
  pituitary fossa 793.0
  prostate (simple) (soft) 600.00
      with
        other lower urinary tract symptoms
            (LUTS) 600.01
        urinary
            obstruction 600.01
            retention 600.01
  sella turcica 793.0
  spleen (*see also* Splenomegaly) 789.2
      congenital 759.0
  thymus (congenital) (gland) 254.0
  thyroid (gland) (*see also* Goiter) 240.9
  tongue 529.8
  tonsils 474.11
      and adenoids 474.10
  uterus 621.2
Enophthalmos 376.50
  due to
      atrophy of orbital tissue 376.51
      surgery 376.52
      trauma 376.52
Enostosis 526.89
Entamebiasis — *see* Amebiasis
Entamebic — *see* Amebiasis
Entanglement, umbilical cord(s) 663.3 ☑
  with compression 663.2 ☑
  affecting fetus or newborn 762.5
  around neck with compression 663.1 ☑
  twins in monoamniotic sac 663.2 ☑
Enteralgia 789.0 ☑
Enteric — *see* condition
Enteritis (acute) (catarrhal) (choleraic) (chronic)
    (congestive) (diarrheal) (exudative) (fol-
    licular) (hemorrhagic) (infantile) (lienter-
    ic) (noninfectious) (perforative) (phleg-
    monous) (presumed noninfectious)
    (pseudomembranous) 558.9
  adaptive 564.9
  aertrycke infection 003.0
  allergic 558.3
  amebic (*see also* Amebiasis) 006.9
      with abscess — *see* Abscess, amebic
      acute 006.0
          with abscess — *see* Abscess, amebic
          nondysenteric 006.2
      chronic 006.1
          with abscess — *see* Abscess, amebic
          nondysenteric 006.2
      nondysenteric 006.2
  anaerobic (cocci) (gram-negative) (gram-
      positive) (mixed) NEC 008.46
  bacillary NEC 004.9
  bacterial NEC 008.5
      specified NEC 008.49
  Bacteroides (fragilis) (melaninogeniscus)
      (oralis) 008.46
  Butyrivibrio (fibriosolvens) 008.46
  Campylobacter 008.43
  Candida 112.85
  Chilomastix 007.8
  choleriformis 001.1
  chronic 558.9

☑ **Additional Digit Required — Refer to the Tabular List for Digit Selection**   ▽ **Subterms under main terms may continue to next column or page**

152   2014 ICD-9-CM

Enteritis — *continued*
  chronic — *continued*
    ulcerative (*see also* Colitis, ulcerative)
      556.9
  cicatrizing (chronic) 555.0
  Clostridium
    botulinum 005.1
    difficile 008.45
    haemolyticum 008.46
    novyi 008.46
    perfringens (C) (F) 008.46
    specified type NEC 008.46
  coccidial 007.2
  dietetic 558.9
  due to
    achylia gastrica 536.8
    adenovirus 008.62
    Aerobacter aerogenes 008.2
    anaerobes (*see also* Enteritis, anaerobic)
      008.46
    Arizona (bacillus) 008.1
    astrovirus 008.66
    Bacillus coli — *see* Enteritis, E. coli
    bacteria NEC 008.5
      specified NEC 008.49
    Bacteroides (*see also* Enteritis, Bac-
      teroides) 008.46
    Butyrivibrio (fibriosolvens) 008.46
    calicivirus 008.65
    Camplyobacter 008.43
    Clostridium — *see* Enteritis, Clostridium
    Cockle agent 008.64
    Coxsackie (virus) 008.67
    Ditchling agent 008.64
    ECHO virus 008.67
    Enterobacter aerogenes 008.2
    enterococci 008.49
    enterovirus NEC 008.67
    Escherichia coli — *see* Enteritis, E. coli
    Eubacterium 008.46
    Fusobacterium (nucleatum) 008.46
    gram-negative bacteria NEC 008.47
      anaerobic NEC 008.46
    Hawaii agent 008.63
    irritating foods 558.9
    Klebsiella aerogenes 008.47
    Marin County agent 008.66
    Montgomery County agent 008.63
    norovirus 008.63
    Norwalk-like agent 008.63
    Norwalk virus 008.63
    Otofuke agent 008.63
    Paracolobactrum arizonae 008.1
    paracolon bacillus NEC 008.47
      Arizona 008.1
    Paramatta agent 008.64
    Peptococcus 008.46
    Peptostreptococcus 008.46
    Proprionibacterium 008.46
    Proteus (bacillus) (mirabilis) (morganii)
      008.3
    Pseudomonas aeruginosa 008.42
    Rotavirus 008.61
    Sapporo agent 008.63
    small round virus (SRV) NEC 008.64
      featureless NEC 008.63
      structured NEC 008.63
    Snow Mountain (SM) agent 008.63
    specified
      bacteria NEC 008.49
      organism, nonbacterial NEC 008.8
      virus NEC 008.69
    Staphylococcus 008.41
    Streptococcus 008.49
      anaerobic 008.46
    Taunton agent 008.63
    Torovirus 008.69
    Treponema 008.46
    Veillonella 008.46
    virus 008.8
      specified type NEC 008.69
    Wollan (W) agent 008.64
    Yersinia enterocolitica 008.44
  dysentery — *see* Dysentery
  E. coli 008.00
    enterohemorrhagic 008.04

Enteritis — *continued*
  E. coli — *continued*
    enteroinvasive 008.03
    enteropathogenic 008.01
    enterotoxigenic 008.02
    specified type NEC 008.09
  el tor 001.1
  embadomonial 007.8
  eosinophilic 558.41
  epidemic 009.0
  Eubacterium 008.46
  fermentative 558.9
  fulminant 557.0
  Fusobacterium (nucleatum) 008.46
  gangrenous (*see also* Enteritis, due to, by
    organism) 009.0
  giardial 007.1
  gram-negative bacteria NEC 008.47
    anaerobic NEC 008.46
  infectious NEC (*see also* Enteritis, due to, by
    organism) 009.0
    presumed 009.1
  influenzal (*see also* Influenza) 487.8
  ischemic 557.9
    acute 557.0
    chronic 557.1
    due to mesenteric artery insufficiency
      557.1
  membranous 564.9
  mucous 564.9
  myxomembranous 564.9
  necrotic (*see also* Enteritis, due to, by organ-
    ism) 009.0
  necroticans 005.2
  necrotizing of fetus or newborn (*see also*
    Enterocolitis, necrotizing, newborn)
    777.50
  neurogenic 564.9
  newborn 777.8
    necrotizing (*see also* Enterocolitis,
      necrotizing, newborn) 777.50
  parasitic NEC 129
  paratyphoid (fever) (*see also* Fever, paraty-
    phoid) 002.9
  Peptococcus 008.46
  Peptostreptococcus 008.46
  Proprionibacterium 008.46
  protozoal NEC 007.9
  radiation 558.1
  regional (of) 555.9
    intestine
      large (bowel, colon, or rectum) 555.1
        with small intestine 555.2
      small (duodenum, ileum, or jejunum)
        555.0
        with large intestine 555.2
  Salmonella infection 003.0
  salmonellosis 003.0
  segmental (*see also* Enteritis, regional) 555.9
  septic (*see also* Enteritis, due to, by organ-
    ism) 009.0
  Shigella 004.9
  simple 558.9
  spasmodic 564.9
  spastic 564.9
  staphylococcal 008.41
    due to food 005.0
  streptococcal 008.49
    anaerobic 008.46
  toxic 558.2
  Treponema (denticola) (macrodentium)
    008.46
  trichomonal 007.3
  tuberculous (*see also* Tuberculosis) 014.8 ☑
  typhosa 002.0
  ulcerative (chronic) (*see also* Colitis, ulcera-
    tive) 556.9
  Veillonella 008.46
  viral 008.8
    adenovirus 008.62
    enterovirus 008.67
    specified virus NEC 008.69
  Yersinia enterocolitica 008.44
  zymotic 009.0
Enteroarticular syndrome 099.3
Enterobiasis 127.4

Enterobius vermicularis 127.4
Enterocele — *see also* Hernia 553.9
  pelvis, pelvic (acquired) (congenital) 618.6
  vagina, vaginal (acquired) (congenital) 618.6
Enterocolitis — *see also* Enteritis
  fetus or newborn (*see also* Enterocolitis,
    necrotizing, newborn) 777.8
    necrotizing 777.50
  fulminant 557.0
  granulomatous 555.2
  hemorrhagic (acute) 557.0
    chronic 557.1
  necrotizing (acute) (membranous) 557.0
    newborn 777.50
      with
        perforation 777.53
        pneumatosis and perforation
          777.53
        pneumatosis without perforation
          777.52
      without pneumatosis, without perfo-
        ration 777.51
      stage I 777.51
      stage II 777.52
      stage III 777.53
  primary necrotizing (*see also* Enterocolitis,
    necrotizing, newborn) 777.50
  pseudomembranous 008.45
    newborn 008.45
  radiation 558.1
    newborn (*see also* Enterocolitis, necrotiz-
      ing, newborn) 777.50
  ulcerative 556.0
Enterocystoma 751.5
Enterogastritis — *see* Enteritis
Enterogenous cyanosis 289.7
Enterolith, enterolithiasis (impaction) 560.39
  with hernia (*see also* Hernia, by site, with
    obstruction)
    gangrenous — *see* Hernia, by site, with
      gangrene
Enteropathy 569.9
  exudative (of Gordon) 579.8
  gluten 579.0
  hemorrhagic, terminal 557.0
  protein-losing 579.8
Enteroperitonitis — *see also* Peritonitis 567.9
Enteroptosis 569.89
Enterorrhagia 578.9
Enterospasm 564.9
  psychogenic 306.4
Enterostenosis — *see also* Obstruction, intestine 560.9
Enterostomy status V44.4
  with complication 569.60
Enthesopathy 726.90
  ankle and tarsus 726.70
  elbow region 726.30
    specified NEC 726.39
  hip 726.5
  knee 726.60
  peripheral NEC 726.8
  shoulder region 726.10
    adhesive 726.0
  spinal 720.1
  wrist and carpus 726.4
Entrance, air into vein — *see* Embolism, air
Entrapment, nerve — *see* Neuropathy, entrapment
Entropion (eyelid) 374.00
  cicatricial 374.04
  congenital 743.62
  late effect of trachoma (healed) 139.1
  mechanical 374.02
  paralytic 374.02
  senile 374.01
  spastic 374.03
Enucleation of eye (current) (traumatic) 871.3
Enuresis 788.30
  habit disturbance 307.6
  nocturnal 788.36
    psychogenic 307.6
  nonorganic origin 307.6
  psychogenic 307.6
Enzymopathy 277.9
Eosinopenia 288.59

Eosinophilia 288.3
  with
    angiolymphoid hyperplasia (ALHE)
      228.01
  allergic 288.3
  hereditary 288.3
  idiopathic 288.3
  infiltrative 518.3
  Loeffler's 518.3
  myalgia syndrome 710.5
  pulmonary (tropical) 518.3
  secondary 288.3
  tropical 518.3
Eosinophilic — *see also* condition
  fasciitis 728.89
  granuloma (bone) 277.89
  infiltration lung 518.3
Ependymitis (acute) (cerebral) (chronic)
  (granular) — *see also* Meningitis 322.9
Ependymoblastoma (M9392/3)
  specified site — *see* Neoplasm, by site, ma-
    lignant
  unspecified site 191.9
Ependymoma (epithelial) (malignant)
  (M9391/3)
  anaplastic type (M9392/3)
    specified site — *see* Neoplasm, by site,
      malignant
    unspecified site 191.9
  benign (M9391/0)
    specified site — *see* Neoplasm, by site,
      benign
    unspecified site 225.0
  myxopapillary (M9394/1) 237.5
  papillary (M9393/1) 237.5
  specified site — *see* Neoplasm, by site, ma-
    lignant
  unspecified site 191.9
Ependymopathy 349.2
  spinal cord 349.2
Ephelides, ephelis 709.09
Ephemeral fever — *see also* Pyrexia 780.60
Epiblepharon (congenital) 743.62
Epicanthus, epicanthic fold (congenital)
  (eyelid) 743.63
Epicondylitis (elbow) (lateral) 726.32
  medial 726.31
Epicystitis — *see also* Cystitis 595.9
Epidemic — *see* condition
Epidermidalization, cervix — *see* condition
Epidermidization, cervix — *see* condition
Epidermis, epidermal — *see* condition
Epidermization, cervix — *see* condition
Epidermodysplasia verruciformis 078.19
Epidermoid
  cholesteatoma — *see* Cholesteatoma
  inclusion (*see also* Cyst, skin) 706.2
Epidermolysis
  acuta (combustiformis) (toxica) 695.15
  bullosa 757.39
  necroticans combustiformis 695.15
    due to drug
      correct substance properly adminis-
        tered 695.15
      overdose or wrong substance given
        or taken 977.9
      specified drug — *see* Table of
        Drugs and Chemicals
Epidermophytid — *see* Dermatophytosis
Epidermophytosis (infected) — *see* Dermatophytosis
Epidermosis, ear (middle) — *see also*
  Cholesteatoma 385.30
Epididymis — *see* condition
Epididymitis (nonvenereal) 604.90
  with abscess 604.0
  acute 604.99
  blennorrhagic (acute) 098.0
    chronic or duration of 2 months or over
      098.2
  caseous (*see also* Tuberculosis) 016.4 ☑
  chlamydial 099.54
  diphtheritic 032.89 [604.91]
  filarial 125.9 [604.91]
  gonococcal (acute) 098.0

Epididymitis — *continued*
  gonococcal — *continued*
    chronic or duration of 2 months or over 098.2
  recurrent 604.99
  residual 604.99
  syphilitic 095.8 *[604.91]*
  tuberculous (*see also* Tuberculosis) 016.4 ✓
Epididymo-orchitis — *see also* Epididymitis 604.90
  with abscess 604.0
  chlamydial 099.54
  gonococcal (acute) 098.13
    chronic or duration of 2 months or over 098.33
Epidural — *see* condition
Epigastritis — *see also* Gastritis 535.5 ✓
Epigastrium, epigastric — *see* condition
Epigastrocele — *see also* Hernia, epigastric 553.29
Epiglottiditis (acute) 464.30
  with obstruction 464.31
  chronic 476.1
  viral 464.30
    with obstruction 464.31
Epiglottis — *see* condition
Epiglottitis (acute) 464.30
  with obstruction 464.31
  chronic 476.1
  viral 464.30
    with obstruction 464.31
Epignathus 759.4
Epilepsia
  partialis continua (*see also* Epilepsy) 345.7 ✓
  procursiva (*see also* Epilepsy) 345.8 ✓
Epilepsy, epileptic (idiopathic) 345.9 ✓

Note — use the following fifth-digit subclassification with categories 345.0, 345.1, 345.4–345.9:

0 without mention of intractable epilepsy

1 with intractable epilepsy

  pharmacoresistant (pharmacologically resistant)

  poorly controlled

  refractory (medically)

  treatment resistant

  abdominal 345.5 ✓
  absence (attack) 345.0 ✓
  akinetic 345.0 ✓
    psychomotor 345.4 ✓
  automatism 345.4 ✓
  autonomic diencephalic 345.5 ✓
  brain 345.9 ✓
  Bravais-Jacksonian 345.5 ✓
  cerebral 345.9 ✓
  climacteric 345.9 ✓
  clonic 345.1 ✓
  clouded state 345.9 ✓
  coma 345.3
  communicating 345.4 ✓
  complicating pregnancy, childbirth, or the puerperium 649.4 ✓
  congenital 345.9 ✓
  convulsions 345.9 ✓
  cortical (focal) (motor) 345.5 ✓
  cursive (running) 345.8 ✓
  cysticercosis 123.1
  deterioration
    with behavioral disturbance 345.9 ✓ *[294.11]*
    without behavioral disturbance 345.9 ✓ *[294.10]*
  due to syphilis 094.89
  equivalent 345.5 ✓
  fit 345.9 ✓
  focal (motor) 345.5 ✓
  gelastic 345.8 ✓
  generalized 345.9 ✓
    convulsive 345.1 ✓

Epilepsy, epileptic — *continued*
  generalized — *continued*
    flexion 345.1 ✓
    nonconvulsive 345.0 ✓
  grand mal (idiopathic) 345.1 ✓
  Jacksonian (motor) (sensory) 345.5 ✓
  Kojevnikoff's, Kojevnikov's, Kojewnikoff's 345.7 ✓
  laryngeal 786.2
  limbic system 345.4 ✓
  localization related (focal) (partial) and epileptic syndromes
    with
      complex partial seizures 345.4 ✓
      simple partial seizures 345.5 ✓
  major (motor) 345.1 ✓
  minor 345.0 ✓
  mixed (type) 345.9 ✓
  motor partial 345.5 ✓
  musicogenic 345.1 ✓
  myoclonus, myoclonic 345.1 ✓
    progressive (familial) 345.1 ✓
  nonconvulsive, generalized 345.0 ✓
  parasitic NEC 123.9
  partial (focalized) 345.5 ✓
    with
      impairment of consciousness 345.4 ✓
        memory and ideational disturbances 345.4 ✓
      without impairment of consciousness 345.5 ✓
  abdominal type 345.5 ✓
  motor type 345.5 ✓
  psychomotor type 345.4 ✓
  psychosensory type 345.4 ✓
  secondarily generalized 345.4 ✓
  sensory type 345.5 ✓
  somatomotor type 345.5 ✓
  somatosensory type 345.5 ✓
  temporal lobe type 345.4 ✓
  visceral type 345.5 ✓
  visual type 345.5 ✓
  peripheral 345.9 ✓
  petit mal 345.0 ✓
  photokinetic 345.8 ✓
  progressive myoclonic (familial) 345.1 ✓
  psychic equivalent 345.5 ✓
  psychomotor 345.4 ✓
  psychosensory 345.4 ✓
  reflex 345.1 ✓
  seizure 345.9 ✓
  senile 345.9 ✓
  sensory-induced 345.5 ✓
  sleep (*see also* Narcolepsy) 347.00
  somatomotor type 345.5 ✓
  somatosensory 345.5 ✓
  specified type NEC 345.8 ✓
  status (grand mal) 345.3
    focal motor 345.7 ✓
    petit mal 345.2
    psychomotor 345.7 ✓
    temporal lobe 345.7 ✓
  symptomatic 345.9 ✓
  temporal lobe 345.4 ✓
  tonic (-clonic) 345.1 ✓
  traumatic (injury unspecified) 907.0
    injury specified — *see* Late, effect (of) specified injury
  twilight 293.0
  uncinate (gyrus) 345.4 ✓
  Unverricht (-Lundborg) (familial myoclonic) 345.1 ✓
  visceral 345.5 ✓
  visual 345.5 ✓
Epileptiform
  convulsions 780.39
  seizure 780.39
Epiloia 759.5
Epimenorrhea 626.2
Epipharyngitis — *see also* Nasopharyngitis 460
Epiphora 375.20

Epiphora — *continued*
  due to
    excess lacrimation 375.21
    insufficient drainage 375.22
Epiphyseal arrest 733.91
  femoral head 732.2
Epiphyseolysis, epiphysiolysis — *see also* Osteochondrosis 732.9
Epiphysitis — *see also* Osteochondrosis 732.9
  juvenile 732.6
  marginal (Scheuermann's) 732.0
  os calcis 732.5
  syphilitic (congenital) 090.0
  vertebral (Scheuermann's) 732.0
Epiplocele — *see also* Hernia 553.9
Epiploitis — *see also* Peritonitis 567.9
Epiplosarcomphalocele — *see also* Hernia, umbilicus 553.1
Episcleritis 379.00
  gouty 274.89 *[379.09]*
  nodular 379.02
  periodica fugax 379.01
    angioneurotic — *see* Edema, angioneurotic
  specified NEC 379.09
  staphylococcal 379.00
  suppurative 379.00
  syphilitic 095.0
  tuberculous (*see also* Tuberculosis) 017.3 ✓ *[379.09]*
Episode
  brain (*see also* Disease, cerebrovascular, acute) 436
  cerebral (*see also* Disease, cerebrovascular, acute) 436
  depersonalization (in neurotic state) 300.6
  hyporesponsive 780.09
  psychotic (*see also* Psychosis) 298.9
    organic, transient 293.9
  schizophrenic (acute) NEC (*see also* Schizophrenia) 295.4 ✓
Epispadias
  female 753.8
  male 752.62
Episplenitis 289.59
Epistaxis (multiple) 784.7
  hereditary 448.0
  vicarious menstruation 625.8
Epithelioma (malignant) (M8011/3) — *see also* Neoplasm, by site, malignant
  adenoides cysticum (M8100/0) — *see* Neoplasm, skin, benign
  basal cell (M8090/3) — *see* Neoplasm, skin, malignant
  benign (M8011/0) — *see* Neoplasm, by site, benign
  Bowen's (M8081/2) — *see* Neoplasm, skin, in situ
  calcifying (benign) (Malherbe's) (M8110/0) — *see* Neoplasm, skin, benign
  external site — *see* Neoplasm, skin, malignant
  intraepidermal, Jadassohn (M8096/0) — *see* Neoplasm, skin, benign
  squamous cell (M8070/3) — *see* Neoplasm, by site, malignant
Epitheliopathy
  pigment, retina 363.15
  posterior multifocal placoid (acute) 363.15
Epithelium, epithelial — *see* condition
Epituberculosis (allergic) (with atelectasis) — *see also* Tuberculosis 010.8 ✓
Eponychia 757.5
Epstein's
  nephrosis or syndrome (*see also* Nephrosis) 581.9
  pearl (mouth) 528.4
Epstein-Barr infection (viral) 075
  chronic 780.79 *[139.8]*
Epulis (giant cell) (gingiva) 523.8
Equinia 024
Equinovarus (congenital) 754.51
  acquired 736.71
Equivalent
  angina 413.9

Equivalent — *continued*
  convulsive (abdominal) (*see also* Epilepsy) 345.5 ✓
  epileptic (psychic) (*see also* Epilepsy) 345.5 ✓
Erb's
  disease 359.1
  palsy, paralysis (birth) (brachial) (newborn) 767.6
  spinal (spastic) syphilitic 094.89
  pseudohypertrophic muscular dystrophy 359.1
Erb-Goldflam disease or syndrome 358.00
Erb (-Duchenne) paralysis (birth injury) (newborn) 767.6
Erdheim-Chester disease (ECD) 277.89
Erdheim's syndrome (acromegalic macrospondylitis) 253.0
Erection, painful (persistent) 607.3
Ergosterol deficiency (vitamin D) 268.9
  with
    osteomalacia 268.2
    rickets (*see also* Rickets) 268.0
Ergotism (ergotized grain) 988.2
  from ergot used as drug (migraine therapy)
    correct substance properly administered 349.82
    overdose or wrong substance given or taken 975.0
Erichsen's disease (railway spine) 300.16
Erlacher-Blount syndrome (tibia vara) 732.4
Erosio interdigitalis blastomycetica 112.3
Erosion
  arteriosclerotic plaque — *see* Arteriosclerosis, by site
  artery NEC 447.2
    without rupture 447.8
  bone 733.99
  bronchus 519.19
  cartilage (joint) 733.99
  cervix (uteri) (acquired) (chronic) (congenital) 622.0
    with mention of cervicitis 616.0
  cornea (recurrent) (*see also* Keratitis) 371.42
    traumatic 918.1
  dental (idiopathic) (occupational) 521.30
    extending into
      dentine 521.32
      pulp 521.33
    generalized 521.35
    limited to enamel 521.31
    localized 521.34
  duodenum, postpyloric — *see* Ulcer, duodenum
  esophagus 530.89
  gastric 535.4 ✓
  implanted vaginal mesh
    in, into
      pelvic floor muscles 629.31
      surrounding organ(s) or tissue 629.31
  intestine 569.89
  lymphatic vessel 457.8
  pylorus, pyloric (ulcer) 535.4 ✓
  sclera 379.16
  spine, aneurysmal 094.89
  spleen 289.59
  stomach 535.4 ✓
  teeth (idiopathic) (occupational) (*see also* Erosion, dental) 521.30
    due to
      medicine 521.30
      persistent vomiting 521.30
  urethra 599.84
  uterus 621.8
  vaginal prosthetic materials NEC
    in, into
      pelvic floor muscles 629.31
      surrounding organ(s) or tissue 629.31
  vertebra 733.99
Erotomania 302.89
  Clérambault's 297.8
Error
  in diet 269.9
  refractive 367.9
    astigmatism (*see also* Astigmatism) 367.20

✓ **Additional Digit Required** — Refer to the Tabular List for Digit Selection

▽ **Subterms under main terms may continue to next column or page**

Error — *continued*
  refractive — *continued*
    drug-induced 367.89
    hypermetropia 367.0
    hyperopia 367.0
    myopia 367.1
    presbyopia 367.4
    toxic 367.89
Eructation 787.3
  nervous 306.4
  psychogenic 306.4
Eruption
  creeping 126.9
  drug — *see* Dermatitis, due to, drug
  Hutchinson, summer 692.72
  Kaposi's varicelliform 054.0
  napkin (psoriasiform) 691.0
  polymorphous
    light (sun) 692.72
    other source 692.82
  psoriasiform, napkin 691.0
  recalcitrant pustular 694.8
  ringed 695.89
  skin (*see also* Dermatitis) 782.1
    creeping (meaning hookworm) 126.9
    due to
      chemical(s) NEC 692.4
        internal use 693.8
      drug — *see* Dermatitis, due to, drug
      prophylactic inoculation or vaccination against disease — *see* Dermatitis, due to, vaccine
      smallpox vaccination NEC — *see* Dermatitis, due to, vaccine
    erysipeloid 027.1
    feigned 698.4
    Hutchinson, summer 692.72
    Kaposi's, varicelliform 054.0
      vaccinia 999.0
    lichenoid, axilla 698.3
    polymorphous, due to light 692.72
    toxic NEC 695.0
    vesicular 709.8
  teeth, tooth
    accelerated 520.6
    delayed 520.6
    difficult 520.6
    disturbance of 520.6
    in abnormal sequence 520.6
    incomplete 520.6
    late 520.6
    natal 520.6
    neonatal 520.6
    obstructed 520.6
    partial 520.6
    persistent primary 520.6
    premature 520.6
    prenatal 520.6
  vesicular 709.8
Erysipelas (gangrenous) (infantile) (newborn) (phlegmonous) (suppurative) 035
  external ear 035 *[380.13]*
  puerperal, postpartum, childbirth 670.8 ☑
Erysipelatoid (Rosenbach's) 027.1
Erysipeloid (Rosenbach's) 027.1
Erythema, erythematous (generalized) 695.9
  ab igne — *see* Burn, by site, first degree
  annulare (centrifugum) (rheumaticum) 695.0
  arthriticum epidemicum 026.1
  brucellum (*see also* Brucellosis) 023.9
  bullosum 695.19
  caloricum — *see* Burn, by site, first degree
  chronicum migrans 088.81
  circinatum 695.19
  diaper 691.0
  due to
    chemical (contact) NEC 692.4
      internal 693.8
    drug (internal use) 693.0
      contact 692.3
  elevatum diutinum 695.89
  endemic 265.2
  epidemic, arthritic 026.1
  figuratum perstans 695.0
  gluteal 691.0

Erythema, erythematous — *continued*
  gyratum (perstans) (repens) 695.19
  heat — *see* Burn, by site, first degree
  ichthyosiforme congenitum 757.1
  induratum (primary) (scrofulosorum) (*see also* Tuberculosis) 017.1 ☑
    nontuberculous 695.2
  infantum febrile 057.8
  infectional NEC 695.9
  infectiosum 057.0
  inflammation NEC 695.9
  intertrigo 695.89
  iris 695.10
  lupus (discoid) (localized) (*see also* Lupus, erythematosus) 695.4
  marginatum 695.0
    rheumaticum — *see* Fever, rheumatic
  medicamentosum — *see* Dermatitis, due to, drug
  migrans 529.1
    chronicum 088.81
  multiforme 695.10
    bullosum 695.19
    conjunctiva 695.19
    exudativum (Hebra) 695.19
    major 695.12
    minor 695.11
    pemphigoides 694.5
  napkin 691.0
  neonatorum 778.8
  nodosum 695.2
    tuberculous (*see also* Tuberculosis) 017.1 ☑
  nummular, nummulare 695.19
  palmar 695.0
  palmaris hereditarium 695.0
  pernio 991.5
  perstans solare 692.72
  rash, newborn 778.8
  scarlatiniform (exfoliative) (recurrent) 695.0
  simplex marginatum 057.8
  solare (*see also* Sunburn) 692.71
  streptogenes 696.5
  toxic, toxicum NEC 695.0
    newborn 778.8
  tuberculous (primary) (*see also* Tuberculosis) 017.0 ☑
  venenatum 695.0
Erythematosus — *see* condition
Erythematous — *see* condition
Erythermalgia (primary) 443.82
Erythralgia 443.82
Erythrasma 039.0
Erythredema 985.0
  polyneuritica 985.0
  polyneuropathy 985.0
Erythremia (acute) (M9841/3) 207.0 ☑
  chronic (M9842/3) 207.1 ☑
  secondary 289.0
Erythroblastopenia (acquired) 284.89
  congenital 284.01
Erythroblastophthisis 284.01
Erythroblastosis (fetalis) (newborn) 773.2
  due to
    ABO
      antibodies 773.1
      incompatibility, maternal/fetal 773.1
      isoimmunization 773.1
    Rh
      antibodies 773.0
      incompatibility, maternal/fetal 773.0
      isoimmunization 773.0
Erythrocyanosis (crurum) 443.89
Erythrocythemia — *see* Erythremia
Erythrocytopenia 285.9
Erythrocytosis (megalosplenic)
  familial 289.6
  oval, hereditary (*see also* Elliptocytosis) 282.1
  secondary 289.0
  stress 289.0
Erythroderma — *see also* Erythema 695.9
  desquamativa (in infants) 695.89
  exfoliative 695.89
  ichthyosiform, congenital 757.1
  infantum 695.89

Erythroderma — *see also* Erythema — *continued*
  maculopapular 696.2
  neonatorum 778.8
  psoriaticum 696.1
  secondary 695.9
Erythrodysesthesia, palmar plantar (PPE) 693.0
Erythrogenesis imperfecta 284.09
Erythroleukemia (M9840/3) 207.0 ☑
Erythromelalgia 443.82
Erythromelia 701.8
Erythropenia 285.9
Erythrophagocytosis 289.9
Erythrophobia 300.23
Erythroplakia
  oral mucosa 528.79
  tongue 528.79
Erythroplasia (Queyrat) (M8080/2)
  specified site — *see* Neoplasm, skin, in situ
  unspecified site 233.5
Erythropoiesis, idiopathic ineffective 285.0
Escaped beats, heart 427.60
  postoperative 997.1
Escherichia coli (E. coli) — *see* Infection, Escherichia coli
Esoenteritis — *see* Enteritis
Esophagalgia 530.89
Esophagectasis 530.89
  due to cardiospasm 530.0
Esophagismus 530.5
Esophagitis (alkaline) (chemical) (chronic) (infectional) (necrotic) (peptic) (postoperative) (regurgitant) 530.10
  acute 530.12
  candidal 112.84
  eosinophilic 530.13
  reflux 530.11
  specified NEC 530.19
  tuberculous (*see also* Tuberculosis) 017.8 ☑
  ulcerative 530.19
Esophagocele 530.6
Esophagodynia 530.89
Esophagomalacia 530.89
Esophagoptosis 530.89
Esophagospasm 530.5
Esophagostenosis 530.3
Esophagostomiasis 127.7
Esophagostomy
  complication 530.87
    infection 530.86
    malfunctioning 530.87
    mechanical 530.87
Esophagotracheal — *see* condition
Esophagus — *see* condition
Esophoria 378.41
  convergence, excess 378.84
  divergence, insufficiency 378.85
Esotropia (nonaccommodative) 378.00
  accommodative 378.35
  alternating 378.05
    with
      A pattern 378.06
      specified noncomitancy NEC 378.08
      V pattern 378.07
      X pattern 378.08
      Y pattern 378.08
      intermittent 378.22
  intermittent 378.20
    alternating 378.22
    monocular 378.21
  monocular 378.01
    with
      A pattern 378.02
      specified noncomitancy NEC 378.04
      V pattern 378.03
      X pattern 378.04
      Y pattern 378.04
      intermittent 378.21
Espundia 085.5
Essential — *see* condition
Esterapenia 289.89
Esthesioneuroblastoma (M9522/3) 160.0
Esthesioneurocytoma (M9521/3) 160.0
Esthesioneuroepithelioma (M9523/3) 160.0
Esthiomene 099.1

Estivo-autumnal
  fever 084.0
  malaria 084.0
Estrangement V61.09
Estriasis 134.0
Ethanolaminuria 270.8
Ethanolism — *see also* Alcoholism 303.9 ☑
Ether dependence, dependency — *see also* Dependence 304.6 ☑
Etherism — *see also* Dependence 304.6 ☑
Ethmoid, ethmoidal — *see* condition
Ethmoiditis (chronic) (nonpurulent) (purulent) — *see also* Sinusitis, ethmoidal 473.2
  influenzal (*see also* Influenza) 487.1
  Woakes' 471.1
Ethylism — *see also* Alcoholism 303.9 ☑
Eulenburg's disease (congenital paramyotonia) 359.29
Eunuchism 257.2
Eunuchoidism 257.2
  hypogonadotropic 257.2
European blastomycosis 117.5
Eustachian — *see* condition
Euthyroidism 244.9
Euthyroid sick syndrome 790.94
Evaluation
  fetal lung maturity 659.8 ☑
  for suspected condition (*see also* Observation) V71.9
    abuse V71.81
    exposure
      anthrax V71.82
      biologic agent NEC V71.83
      SARS V71.83
    neglect V71.81
    newborn — *see* Observation, suspected, condition, newborn
    specified condition NEC V71.89
  mental health V70.2
    requested by authority V70.1
  nursing care V63.8
  social service V63.8
Evans' syndrome (thrombocytopenic purpura) 287.32
Event, apparent life threatening in newborn and infant (ALTE) 799.82
Eventration
  colon into chest — *see* Hernia, diaphragm
  diaphragm (congenital) 756.6
Eversion
  bladder 596.89
  cervix (uteri) 622.0
    with mention of cervicitis 616.0
  foot NEC 736.79
    congenital 755.67
  lacrimal punctum 375.51
  punctum lacrimale (postinfectional) (senile) 375.51
  ureter (meatus) 593.89
  urethra (meatus) 599.84
  uterus 618.1
    complicating delivery 665.2 ☑
      affecting fetus or newborn 763.89
    puerperal, postpartum 674.8 ☑
Evidence
  of malignancy
    cytologic
      without histologic confirmation
        anus 796.76
        cervix 795.06
        vagina 795.16
Evisceration
  birth injury 767.8
  bowel (congenital) — *see* Hernia, ventral
  congenital (*see also* Hernia, ventral) 553.29
  operative wound 998.32
  traumatic NEC 869.1
    eye 871.3
Evulsion — *see* Avulsion
Ewing's
  angioendothelioma (M9260/3) — *see* Neoplasm, bone, malignant
  sarcoma (M9260/3) — *see* Neoplasm, bone, malignant
  tumor (M9260/3) — *see* Neoplasm, bone, malignant

☑ **Additional Digit Required** — Refer to the Tabular List for Digit Selection   ▽ **Subterms under main terms may continue to next column or page**

2014 ICD-9-CM   155

Exaggerated lumbosacral angle (with imping-ing spine) 756.12
Examination (general) (routine) (of) (for) V70.9
  allergy V72.7
  annual V70.0
  cardiovascular preoperative V72.81
  cervical Papanicolaou smear V76.2
    as a part of routine gynecological exam-ination V72.31
    to confirm findings of recent normal smear following initial abnormal smear V72.32
  child care (routine) V20.2
  clinical research investigation (normal con-trol patient) (participant) V70.7
  dental V72.2
  developmental testing (child) (infant) V20.2
  donor (potential) V70.8
  ear V72.19
  eye V72.0
  following
    accident (motor vehicle) V71.4
    alleged rape or seduction (victim or cul-prit) V71.5
    inflicted injury (victim or culprit) NEC V71.6
    rape or seduction, alleged (victim or culprit) V71.5
    treatment (for) V67.9
      combined V67.6
      fracture V67.4
      involving high-risk medication NEC V67.51
      mental disorder V67.3
      specified condition NEC V67.59
  follow-up (routine) (following) V67.9
    cancer chemotherapy V67.2
    chemotherapy V67.2
    disease NEC V67.59
    high-risk medication NEC V67.51
    injury NEC V67.59
    population survey V70.6
    postpartum V24.2
    psychiatric V67.3
    psychotherapy V67.3
    radiotherapy V67.1
    specified surgery NEC V67.09
    surgery V67.00
    vaginal pap smear V67.01
  gynecological V72.31
    for contraceptive maintenance V25.40
      intrauterine device V25.42
      pill V25.41
      specified method NEC V25.49
  health (of)
    armed forces personnel V70.5
    checkup V70.0
    child, routine V20.2
    defined subpopulation NEC V70.5
    inhabitants of institutions V70.5
    occupational V70.5
    pre-employment screening V70.5
    preschool children V70.5
      for admission to school V70.3
    prisoners V70.5
      for entrance into prison V70.3
    prostitutes V70.5
    refugees V70.5
    school children V70.5
    students V70.5
  hearing V72.19
    following failed hearing screening V72.11
  infant
    8 to 28 days old V20.32
    over 28 days old, routine V20.2
    under 8 days old V20.31
  laboratory V72.60
    ordered as part of a routine general medical examination V72.62
    pre-operative V72.63
    pre-procedural V72.63
    specified NEC V72.69
  lactating mother V24.1
  medical (for) (of) V70.9
    administrative purpose NEC V70.3

Examination — *continued*
  medical — *continued*
    admission to
      old age home V70.3
      prison V70.3
      school V70.3
    adoption V70.3
    armed forces personnel V70.5
    at health care facility V70.0
    camp V70.3
    child, routine V20.2
    clinical research (control) (normal com-parison) (participant) V70.7
    defined subpopulation NEC V70.5
    donor (potential) V70.8
    driving license V70.3
    general V70.9
      routine V70.0
      specified reason NEC V70.8
    immigration V70.3
    inhabitants of institutions V70.5
    insurance certification V70.3
    marriage V70.3
    medicolegal reasons V70.4
    naturalization V70.3
    occupational V70.5
    population survey V70.6
    pre-employment V70.5
    preschool children V70.5
      for admission to school V70.3
    prison V70.3
    prisoners V70.5
      for entrance into prison V70.3
    prostitutes V70.5
    refugees V70.5
    school children V70.5
    specified reason NEC V70.8
    sport competition V70.3
    students V70.5
  medicolegal reason V70.4
  pelvic (annual) (periodic) V72.31
  periodic (annual) (routine) V70.0
  postpartum
    immediately after delivery V24.0
    routine follow-up V24.2
  pregnancy (unconfirmed) (possible) V72.40
    negative result V72.41
    positive result V72.42
  prenatal V22.1
    first pregnancy V22.0
    high-risk pregnancy V23.9
      specified problem NEC V23.89
      to determine fetal viability V23.87
  preoperative V72.84
    cardiovascular V72.81
    respiratory V72.82
    specified NEC V72.83
  preprocedural V72.84
    cardiovascular V72.81
    general physical V72.83
    respiratory V72.82
    specified NEC V72.83
  prior to chemotherapy V72.83
  psychiatric V70.2
    follow-up not needing further care V67.3
    requested by authority V70.1
  radiological NEC V72.5
  respiratory preoperative V72.82
  screening — *see* Screening
  sensitization V72.7
  skin V72.7
    hypersensitivity V72.7
  special V72.9
  specified type or reason NEC V72.85
    preoperative V72.83
      specified NEC V72.83
  teeth V72.2
  vaginal Papanicolaou smear V76.47
    following hysterectomy for malignant condition V67.01
  victim or culprit following
    alleged rape or seduction V71.5
    inflicted injury NEC V71.6
  vision V72.0
  well baby V20.2
Exanthem, exanthema — *see also* Rash 782.1

Exanthem, exanthema — *see also* Rash — *continued*
  Boston 048
  epidemic, with meningitis 048
  lichenoid psoriasiform 696.2
  subitum 058.10
    due to
      human herpesvirus 6 058.11
      human herpesvirus 7 058.12
  viral, virus NEC 057.9
    specified type NEC 057.8
Excess, excessive, excessively
  alcohol level in blood 790.3
  carbohydrate tissue, localized 278.1
  carotene (dietary) 278.3
  cold 991.9
    specified effect NEC 991.8
  convergence 378.84
  crying 780.95
    of
      adolescent 780.95
      adult 780.95
      baby 780.92
      child 780.95
      infant (baby) 780.92
      newborn 780.92
  development, breast 611.1
  diaphoresis (*see also* Hyperhidrosis) 780.8
  distance, interarch 524.28
  divergence 378.85
  drinking (alcohol) NEC (*see also* Abuse, drugs, nondependent) 305.0 ☑
    continual (*see also* Alcoholism) 303.9 ☑
    habitual (*see also* Alcoholism) 303.9 ☑
  eating 783.6
  eyelid fold (congenital) 743.62
  fat 278.02
    in heart (*see also* Degeneration, myocar-dial) 429.1
    tissue, localized 278.1
  foreskin 605
  gas 787.3
  gastrin 251.5
  glucagon 251.4
  heat (*see also* Heat) 992.9
  horizontal
    overjet 524.26
    overlap 524.26
  interarch distance 524.28
  intermaxillary vertical dimension 524.37
  interocclusal distance of teeth 524.37
  large
    colon 564.7
      congenital 751.3
    fetus or infant 766.0
      with obstructed labor 660.1 ☑
        affecting management of pregnancy 656.6 ☑
      causing disproportion 653.5 ☑
    newborn (weight of 4500 grams or more) 766.0
    organ or site, congenital NEC — *see* Anomaly, specified type NEC
  lid fold (congenital) 743.62
  long
    colon 751.5
    organ or site, congenital NEC — *see* Anomaly, specified type NEC
    umbilical cord (entangled)
      affecting fetus or newborn 762.5
      in pregnancy or childbirth 663.3 ☑
        with compression 663.2 ☑
  menstruation 626.2
  number of teeth 520.1
    causing crowding 524.31
  nutrients (dietary) NEC 783.6
  potassium (K) 276.7
  salivation (*see also* Ptyalism) 527.7
  secretion (*see also* Hypersecretion)
    milk 676.6 ☑
    sputum 786.4
    sweat (*see also* Hyperhidrosis) 780.8
  short
    organ or site, congenital NEC — *see* Anomaly, specified type NEC

Excess, excessive, excessively — *continued*
  short — *continued*
    umbilical cord
      affecting fetus or newborn 762.6
      in pregnancy or childbirth 663.4 ☑
  skin NEC 701.9
    eyelid 743.62
      acquired 374.30
  sodium (Na) 276.0
  spacing of teeth 524.32
  sputum 786.4
  sweating (*see also* Hyperhidrosis) 780.8
  tearing (ducts) (eye) (*see also* Epiphora) 375.20
  thirst 783.5
    due to deprivation of water 994.3
  tissue in reconstructed breast 612.0
  tuberosity 524.07
  vitamin
    A (dietary) 278.2
      administered as drug (chronic) (pro-longed excessive intake) 278.2
      reaction to sudden overdose 963.5
    D (dietary) 278.4
      administered as drug (chronic) (pro-longed excessive intake) 278.4
      reaction to sudden overdose 963.5
  weight 278.02
    gain 783.1
      of pregnancy 646.1 ☑
    loss 783.21
Excitability, abnormal, under minor stress 309.29
Excitation
  catatonic (*see also* Schizophrenia) 295.2 ☑
  psychogenic 298.1
  reactive (from emotional stress, psycholog-ical trauma) 298.1
Excitement
  manic (*see also* Psychosis, affective) 296.0 ☑
    recurrent episode 296.1 ☑
    single episode 296.0 ☑
  mental, reactive (from emotional stress, psychological trauma) 298.1
  state, reactive (from emotional stress, psy-chological trauma) 298.1
Excluded pupils 364.76
Excoriation (traumatic) — *see also* Injury, su-perficial, by site 919.8
  neurotic 698.4
Excyclophoria 378.44
Excyclotropia 378.33
Exencephalus, exencephaly 742.0
Exercise
  breathing V57.0
  remedial NEC V57.1
  therapeutic NEC V57.1
Exfoliation
  skin
    due to erythematous condition 695.50
      involving (percent of body surface)
        less than 10 percent 695.50
        10-19 percent 695.51
        20-29 percent 695.52
        30-39 percent 695.53
        40-49 percent 695.54
        50-59 percent 695.55
        60-69 percent 695.56
        70-79 percent 695.57
        80-89 percent 695.58
        90 percent or more 695.59
  teeth
    due to systemic causes 525.0
Exfoliative — *see also* condition
  dermatitis 695.89
Exhaustion, exhaustive (physical NEC) 780.79
  battle (*see also* Reaction, stress, acute) 308.9
  cardiac (*see also* Failure, heart) 428.9
  delirium (*see also* Reaction, stress, acute) 308.9
  due to
    cold 991.8
    excessive exertion 994.5

☑ **Additional Digit Required** — Refer to the Tabular List for Digit Selection   ▽ **Subterms under main terms may continue to next column or page**

156   **2014 ICD-9-CM**

Exhaustion, exhaustive — *continued*
  due to — *continued*
    exposure 994.4
    overexertion 994.5
  fetus or newborn 779.89
  heart (*see also* Failure, heart) 428.9
  heat 992.5
    due to
      salt depletion 992.4
      water depletion 992.3
  manic (*see also* Psychosis, affective) 296.0 ☑
    recurrent episode 296.1 ☑
    single episode 296.0 ☑
  maternal, complicating delivery 669.8 ☑
    affecting fetus or newborn 763.89
  mental 300.5
  myocardium, myocardial (*see also* Failure, heart) 428.9
  nervous 300.5
  old age 797
  postinfectional NEC 780.79
  psychogenic 300.5
  psychosis (*see also* Reaction, stress, acute) 308.9
  senile 797
    dementia 290.0
Exhibitionism (sexual) 302.4
Exomphalos 756.72
Exophoria 378.42
  convergence, insufficiency 378.83
  divergence, excess 378.85
Exophthalmic
  cachexia 242.0 ☑
  goiter 242.0 ☑
  ophthalmoplegia 242.0 ☑ *[376.22]*
Exophthalmos 376.30
  congenital 743.66
  constant 376.31
  endocrine NEC 259.9 *[376.22]*
  hyperthyroidism 242.0 ☑ *[376.21]*
  intermittent NEC 376.34
  malignant 242.0 ☑ *[376.21]*
  pulsating 376.35
    endocrine NEC 259.9 *[376.22]*
  thyrotoxic 242.0 ☑ *[376.21]*
Exostosis 726.91
  cartilaginous (M9210/0) — *see* Neoplasm, bone, benign
  congenital 756.4
  ear canal, external 380.81
  gonococcal 098.89
  hip 726.5
  intracranial 733.3
  jaw (bone) 526.81
  luxurians 728.11
  multiple (cancellous) (congenital) (hereditary) 756.4
  nasal bones 726.91
  orbit, orbital 376.42
  osteocartilaginous (M9210/0) — *see* Neoplasm, bone, benign
  spine 721.8
    with spondylosis — *see* Spondylosis
  syphilitic 095.5
  wrist 726.4
Exotropia 378.10
  alternating 378.15
    with
      A pattern 378.16
      specified noncomitancy NEC 378.18
      V pattern 378.17
      X pattern 378.18
      Y pattern 378.18
    intermittent 378.24
  intermittent 378.20
    alternating 378.24
    monocular 378.23
  monocular 378.11
    with
      A pattern 378.12
      specified noncomitancy NEC 378.14
      V pattern 378.13
      X pattern 378.14
      Y pattern 378.14
    intermittent 378.23

Explanation of
  investigation finding V65.4 ☑
  medication V65.4 ☑
Exposure (suspected) 994.9
  algae bloom V87.32
  cold 991.9
    specified effect NEC 991.8
  effects of 994.9
  exhaustion due to 994.4
  implanted vaginal mesh
    into vagina 629.32
    through vaginal wall 629.32
  to
    AIDS virus V01.79
    anthrax V01.81
    aromatic
      amines V87.11
      dyes V87.19
    arsenic V87.01
    asbestos V15.84
    benzene V87.12
    body fluids (hazardous) V15.85
    cholera V01.0
    chromium compounds V87.09
    communicable disease V01.9
      specified type NEC V01.89
    dyes V87.2
      aromatic V87.19
    Escherichia coli (E. coli) V01.83
    German measles V01.4
    gonorrhea V01.6
    hazardous
      aromatic compounds NEC V87.19
      body fluids V15.85
      chemicals NEC V87.2
      metals V87.09
      substances V87.39
    HIV V01.79
    human immunodeficiency virus V01.79
    lead V15.86
    meningococcus V01.84
    mold V87.31
    nickel dust V87.09
    parasitic disease V01.89
    poliomyelitis V01.2
    polycyclic aromatic hydrocarbons V87.19
    potentially hazardous body fluids V15.85
    rabies V01.5
    rubella V01.4
    SARS-associated coronavirus V01.82
    smallpox V01.3
    syphilis V01.6
    tuberculosis V01.1
    uranium V87.02
    varicella V01.71
    venereal disease V01.6
    viral disease NEC V01.79
      varicella V01.71
    vaginal prosthetic materials NEC
      into vagina 629.32
      through vaginal wall 629.32
Exsanguination, fetal 772.0
Exstrophy
  abdominal content 751.8
  bladder (urinary) 753.5
Extensive — *see* condition
Extra — *see also* Accessory
  rib 756.3
    cervical 756.2
Extraction
  with hook 763.89
  breech NEC 669.6 ☑
    affecting fetus or newborn 763.0
  cataract postsurgical V45.61
  manual NEC 669.8 ☑
    affecting fetus or newborn 763.89
Extrasystole 427.60
  atrial 427.61
  postoperative 997.1
  ventricular 427.69
Extrauterine gestation or pregnancy — *see* Pregnancy, ectopic
Extravasation
  blood 459.0
    lower extremity 459.0
  chemotherapy, vesicant 999.81

Extravasation — *continued*
  chyle into mesentery 457.8
  pelvicalyceal 593.4
  pyelosinus 593.4
  urine 788.8
    from ureter 788.8
  vesicant
    agent NEC 999.82
    chemotherapy 999.81
Extremity — *see* condition
Extrophy — *see* Exstrophy
Extroversion
  bladder 753.5
  uterus 618.1
    complicating delivery 665.2 ☑
      affecting fetus or newborn 763.89
    postpartal (old) 618.1
Extruded tooth 524.34
Extrusion
  alveolus and teeth 524.75
  breast implant (prosthetic) 996.54
  device, implant, or graft — *see* Complications, mechanical
  eye implant (ball) (globe) 996.59
  intervertebral disc — *see* Displacement, intervertebral disc
  lacrimal gland 375.43
  mesh (reinforcing) 996.59
  ocular lens implant 996.53
  prosthetic device NEC — *see* Complications, mechanical
  vitreous 379.26
Exudate, pleura — *see* Effusion, pleura
Exudates, retina 362.82
Exudative — *see* condition
Eye, eyeball, eyelid — *see* condition
Eyestrain 368.13
Eyeworm disease of Africa 125.2

F

Faber's anemia or syndrome (achlorhydric anemia) 280.9
Fabry's disease (angiokeratoma corporis diffusum) 272.7
Face, facial — *see* condition
Facet of cornea 371.44
Faciocephalalgia, autonomic — *see also* Neuropathy, peripheral, autonomic 337.9
Facioscapulohumeral myopathy 359.1
Factitious disorder, illness — *see* Illness, factitious
Factor
  deficiency — *see* Deficiency, factor
  psychic, associated with diseases classified elsewhere 316
  risk — *see* Problem
  V Leiden mutation 289.81
Fahr-Volhard disease (malignant nephrosclerosis) 403.00
Failure, failed
  adenohypophyseal 253.2
  attempted abortion (legal) (*see also* Abortion, failed) 638.9
  bone marrow (anemia) 284.9
    acquired (secondary) 284.89
    congenital 284.09
    idiopathic 284.9
  cardiac (*see also* Failure, heart) 428.9
    newborn 779.89
  cardiorenal (chronic) 428.9
    hypertensive (*see also* Hypertension, cardiorenal) 404.93
  cardiorespiratory 799.1
    specified during or due to a procedure 997.1
      long-term effect of cardiac surgery 429.4
  cardiovascular (chronic) 428.9
  cerebrovascular 437.8
  cervical dilatation in labor 661.0 ☑
    affecting fetus or newborn 763.7
  circulation, circulatory 799.89
    fetus or newborn 779.89
    peripheral 785.50
      postoperative 998.00

Failure, failed — *continued*
  compensation — *see* Disease, heart
  congestive (*see also* Failure, heart) 428.0
  conscious sedation, during procedure 995.24
  coronary (*see also* Insufficiency, coronary) 411.89
  dental implant 525.79
    due to
      infection 525.71
      lack of attached gingiva 525.72
      occlusal trauma (caused by poor prosthetic design) 525.72
      parafunctional habits 525.72
      periodontal infection (peri-implantitis) 525.72
      poor oral hygiene 525.72
      unintentional loading 525.71
    endosseous NEC 525.79
    mechanical 525.73
    osseointegration 525.71
      due to
        complications of systemic disease 525.71
        poor bone quality 525.71
        premature loading 525.71
      iatrogenic 525.71
      prior to intentional prosthetic loading 525.71
    post-osseointegration
      biological 525.72
        iatrogenic 525.72
      due to complications of systemic disease 525.72
      mechanical 525.73
    pre-integration 525.71
    pre-osseointegration 525.71
  dental prosthesis causing loss of dental implant 525.73
  dental restoration
    marginal integrity 525.61
    periodontal anatomical integrity 525.65
  descent of head (at term) 652.5 ☑
    affecting fetus or newborn 763.1
    in labor 660.0 ☑
      affecting fetus or newborn 763.1
  device, implant, or graft — *see* Complications, mechanical
  engagement of head NEC 652.5 ☑
    in labor 660.0 ☑
  extrarenal 788.99
  fetal head to enter pelvic brim 652.5 ☑
    affecting fetus or newborn 763.1
    in labor 660.0 ☑
      affecting fetus or newborn 763.1
  forceps NEC 660.7 ☑
    affecting fetus or newborn 763.1
  fusion (joint) (spinal) 996.49
  growth in childhood 783.43
  heart (acute) (sudden) 428.9
    with
      abortion — *see* Abortion, by type, with specified complication NEC
      acute pulmonary edema (*see also* Failure, ventricular, left) 428.1
        with congestion (*see also* Failure, heart) 428.0
      decompensation (*see also* Failure, heart) 428.0
      dilation — *see* Disease, heart
      ectopic pregnancy (*see also* categories 633.0–633.9) 639.8
      molar pregnancy (*see also* categories 630–632) 639.8
    arteriosclerotic 440.9
    combined left-right sided 428.0
    combined systolic and diastolic 428.40
      acute 428.41
      acute on chronic 428.43
      chronic 428.42
    compensated (*see also* Failure, heart) 428.0

Failure, failed — *continued*
  heart — *continued*
    complicating
      abortion — *see* Abortion, by type, with specified complication NEC
      delivery (cesarean) (instrumental) 669.4 ☑
      ectopic pregnancy (*see also* categories 633.0–633.9) 639.8
      molar pregnancy (*see also* categories 630–632) 639.8
      obstetric anesthesia or sedation 668.1 ☑
      surgery 997.1
    congestive (compensated) (decompensated) (*see also* Failure, heart) 428.0
      with rheumatic fever (conditions classifiable to 390)
        active 391.8
        inactive or quiescent (with chorea) 398.91
      fetus or newborn 779.89
      hypertensive (*see also* Hypertension, heart) 402.91
        with renal disease (*see also* Hypertension, cardiorenal) 404.91
          with renal failure 404.93
        benign 402.11
        malignant 402.01
      rheumatic (chronic) (inactive) (with chorea) 398.91
        active or acute 391.8
          with chorea (Sydenham's) 392.0
    decompensated (*see also* Failure, heart) 428.0
    degenerative (*see also* Degeneration, myocardial) 429.1
    diastolic 428.30
      acute 428.31
      acute on chronic 428.33
      chronic 428.32
    due to presence of (cardiac) prosthesis 429.4
    fetus or newborn 779.89
    following
      abortion 639.8
      cardiac surgery 429.4
      ectopic or molar pregnancy 639.8
    high output NEC 428.9
    hypertensive (*see also* Hypertension, heart) 402.91
      with renal disease (*see also* Hypertension, cardiorenal) 404.91
        with renal failure 404.93
      benign 402.11
      malignant 402.01
    left (ventricular) (*see also* Failure, ventricular, left) 428.1
      with right-sided failure (see also Failure, heart) 428.0
    low output (syndrome) NEC 428.9
    organic — *see* Disease, heart
    postoperative (immediate) 997.1
      long term effect of cardiac surgery 429.4
    rheumatic (chronic) (congestive) (inactive) 398.91
    right (secondary to left heart failure, conditions classifiable to 428.1) (ventricular) (*see also* Failure, heart) 428.0
    senile 797
    specified during or due to a procedure 997.1
      long-term effect of cardiac surgery 429.4
    systolic 428.20
      acute 428.21
      acute on chronic 428.23
      chronic 428.22
    thyrotoxic (*see also* Thyrotoxicosis) 242.9 ☑ *[425.7]*

Failure, failed — *continued*
  heart — *continued*
    valvular — *see* Endocarditis
  hepatic 572.8
    acute 570
    due to a procedure 997.49
  hepatorenal 572.4
  hypertensive heart (*see also* Hypertension, heart) 402.91
    benign 402.11
    malignant 402.01
  induction (of labor) 659.1 ☑
    abortion (legal) (*see also* Abortion, failed) 638.9
    affecting fetus or newborn 763.89
    by oxytocic drugs 659.1 ☑
    instrumental 659.0 ☑
    mechanical 659.0 ☑
    medical 659.1 ☑
    surgical 659.0 ☑
  initial alveolar expansion, newborn 770.4
  involution, thymus (gland) 254.8
  kidney — *see* Failure, renal
  lactation 676.4 ☑
  Leydig's cell, adult 257.2
  liver 572.8
    acute 570
  medullary 799.89
  mitral — *see* Endocarditis, mitral
  moderate sedation, during procedure 995.24
  myocardium, myocardial (*see also* Failure, heart) 428.9
    chronic (*see also* Failure, heart) 428.0
    congestive (*see also* Failure, heart) 428.0
  ovarian (primary) 256.39
    iatrogenic 256.2
    postablative 256.2
    postirradiation 256.2
    postsurgical 256.2
  ovulation 628.0
  prerenal 788.99
  renal (kidney) 586
    with
      abortion — *see* Abortion, by type, with renal failure
      ectopic pregnancy (*see also* categories 633.0–633.9) 639.3
      edema (*see also* Nephrosis) 581.9
      hypertension (*see also* Hypertension, kidney) 403.91
      hypertensive heart disease (conditions classifiable to 402) 404.92
        with heart failure 404.93
        benign 404.12
          with heart failure 404.13
        malignant 404.02
          with heart failure 404.03
      molar pregnancy (*see also* categories 630–632) 639.3
      tubular necrosis (acute) 584.5
    acute 584.9
      with lesion of
        necrosis
          cortical (renal) 584.6
          medullary (renal) (papillary) 584.7
          tubular 584.5
        specified pathology NEC 584.8
    chronic 585.9
      hypertensive or with hypertension (*see also* Hypertension, kidney) 403.91
      due to a procedure 997.5
      following
        abortion 639.3
        crushing 958.5
        ectopic or molar pregnancy 639.3
        labor and delivery (acute) 669.3 ☑
      hypertensive (*see also* Hypertension, kidney) 403.91
      puerperal, postpartum 669.3 ☑
  respiration, respiratory 518.81
    acute 518.81
      following trauma and surgery 518.51

Failure, failed — *continued*
  respiration, respiratory — *continued*
    acute and chronic 518.84
      following trauma and surgery 518.53
    center 348.89
      newborn 770.84
    chronic 518.83
      following trauma and surgery or shock 518.51
      newborn 770.84
    rotation
      cecum 751.4
      colon 751.4
      intestine 751.4
      kidney 753.3
    sedation, during procedure
      conscious 995.24
      moderate 995.24
    segmentation (*see also* Fusion)
      fingers (*see also* Syndactylism, fingers) 755.11
      toes (*see also* Syndactylism, toes) 755.13
    seminiferous tubule, adult 257.2
    senile (general) 797
      with psychosis 290.20
    testis, primary (seminal) 257.2
    to progress 661.2 ☑
    to thrive
      adult 783.7
      child 783.41
      newborn 779.34
    transplant 996.80
      bone marrow 996.85
      organ (immune or nonimmune cause) 996.80
        bone marrow 996.85
        heart 996.83
        intestines 996.87
        kidney 996.81
        liver 996.82
        lung 996.84
        pancreas 996.86
        specified NEC 996.89
      skin 996.52
        artificial 996.55
        decellularized allodermis 996.55
        temporary allograft or pigskin graft — omit code
      stem cell(s) 996.88
        from
          peripheral blood 996.88
          umbilical cord 996.88
    trial of labor NEC 660.6 ☑
      affecting fetus or newborn 763.1
    tubal ligation 998.89
    urinary 586
    vacuum extraction
      abortion — *see* Abortion, failed
      delivery NEC 660.7 ☑
        affecting fetus or newborn 763.1
    vasectomy 998.89
    ventouse NEC 660.7 ☑
      affecting fetus or newborn 763.1
    ventricular (*see also* Failure, heart) 428.9
      left 428.1
        with rheumatic fever (conditions classifiable to 390)
          active 391.8
            with chorea 392.0
          inactive or quiescent (with chorea) 398.91
        hypertensive (*see also* Hypertension, heart) 402.91
          benign 402.11
          malignant 402.01
        rheumatic (chronic) (inactive) (with chorea) 398.91
          active or acute 391.8
            with chorea 392.0
      right (*see also* Failure, heart) 428.0
    vital centers, fetus or newborn 779.89
    weight gain in childhood 783.41
Fainting (fit) (spell) 780.2
Falciform hymen 752.49
Fallen arches 734
Falling, any organ or part — *see* Prolapse

Fall, maternal, affecting fetus or newborn 760.5
Fallopian
  insufflation
    fertility testing V26.21
    following sterilization reversal V26.22
  tube — *see* condition
Fallot's
  pentalogy 745.2
  tetrad or tetralogy 745.2
  triad or trilogy 746.09
Fallout, radioactive (adverse effect) NEC 990
False — *see also* condition
  bundle branch block 426.50
  bursa 727.89
  croup 478.75
  joint 733.82
  labor (pains) 644.1 ☑
  opening, urinary, male 752.69
  passage, urethra (prostatic) 599.4
  positive
    serological test for syphilis 795.6
    Wassermann reaction 795.6
  pregnancy 300.11
Family, familial — *see also* condition
  affected by
    family member
      currently on deployment (military) V61.01
      returned from deployment (military) (current or past conflict) V61.02
  disruption (*see also* Disruption, family) V61.09
  estrangement V61.09
  hemophagocytic
    lymphohistiocytosis 288.4
    reticulosis 288.4
  Li-Fraumeni (syndrome) V84.01
  planning advice V25.09
    natural
      procreative V26.41
      to avoid pregnancy V25.04
  problem V61.9
    specified circumstance NEC V61.8
  retinoblastoma (syndrome) 190.5
Famine 994.2
  edema 262
Fanconi's anemia (congenital pancytopenia) 284.09
Fanconi (-de Toni) (-Debré) syndrome (cystinosis) 270.0
Farber (-Uzman) syndrome or disease (disseminated lipogranulomatosis) 272.8
Farcin 024
Farcy 024
Farmers'
  lung 495.0
  skin 692.74
Farsightedness 367.0
Fascia — *see* condition
Fasciculation 781.0
Fasciculitis optica 377.32
Fasciitis 729.4
  eosinophilic 728.89
  necrotizing 728.86
  nodular 728.79
  perirenal 593.4
  plantar 728.71
  pseudosarcomatous 728.79
  traumatic (old) NEC 728.79
    current — *see* Sprain, by site
Fasciola hepatica infestation 121.3
Fascioliasis 121.3
Fasciolopsiasis (small intestine) 121.4
Fasciolopsis (small intestine) 121.4
Fast pulse 785.0
Fat
  embolism (cerebral) (pulmonary) (systemic) 958.1
    with
      abortion — *see* Abortion, by type, with embolism
      ectopic pregnancy (*see also* categories 633.0–633.9) 639.6

Fat — *continued*
  embolism — *continued*
    with — *continued*
      molar pregnancy (*see also* categories 630–632) 639.6
      complicating delivery or puerperium 673.8 ☑
      following
        abortion 639.6
        ectopic or molar pregnancy 639.6
      in pregnancy, childbirth, or the puerperium 673.8 ☑
  excessive 278.02
    in heart (*see also* Degeneration, myocardial) 429.1
  general 278.02
  hernia, herniation 729.30
    eyelid 374.34
    knee 729.31
    orbit 374.34
    retro-orbital 374.34
    retropatellar 729.31
    specified site NEC 729.39
  indigestion 579.8
  in stool 792.1
  localized (pad) 278.1
    heart (*see also* Degeneration, myocardial) 429.1
    knee 729.31
    retropatellar 729.31
  necrosis (*see also* Fatty, degeneration)
    breast (aseptic) (segmental) 611.3
    mesentery 567.82
    omentum 567.82
    peritoneum 567.82
  pad 278.1
Fatal familial insomnia (FFI) 046.72
Fatal syncope 798.1
Fatigue 780.79
  auditory deafness (*see also* Deafness) 389.9
  chronic, syndrome 780.71
  combat (*see also* Reaction, stress, acute) 308.9
  during pregnancy 646.8 ☑
  general 780.79
    psychogenic 300.5
  heat (transient) 992.6
  muscle 729.89
  myocardium (*see also* Failure, heart) 428.9
  nervous 300.5
  neurosis 300.5
  operational 300.89
  postural 729.89
  posture 729.89
  psychogenic (general) 300.5
  senile 797
  syndrome NEC 300.5
    chronic 780.71
  undue 780.79
  voice 784.49
Fatness 278.02
Fatty — *see also* condition
  apron 278.1
  degeneration (diffuse) (general) NEC 272.8
    localized — *see* Degeneration, by site, fatty
    placenta — *see* Placenta, abnormal
  heart (enlarged) (*see also* Degeneration, myocardial) 429.1
  infiltration (diffuse) (general) (*see also* Degeneration, by site, fatty) 272.8
    heart (enlarged) (*see also* Degeneration, myocardial) 429.1
  liver 571.8
    alcoholic 571.0
  necrosis — *see* Degeneration, fatty
  phanerosis 272.8
Fauces — *see* condition
Fauchard's disease (periodontitis) 523.40
Faucitis 478.29
Faulty — *see also* condition
  position of teeth 524.30
Favism (anemia) 282.2
Favre-Racouchot disease (elastoidosis cutanea nodularis) 701.8
Favus 110.9

Favus — *continued*
  beard 110.0
  capitis 110.0
  corporis 110.5
  eyelid 110.8
  foot 110.4
  hand 110.2
  scalp 110.0
  specified site NEC 110.8
Feared complaint unfounded V65.5
Fear, fearfulness (complex) (reaction) 300.20
  child 313.0
  of
    animals 300.29
    closed spaces 300.29
    crowds 300.29
    eating in public 300.23
    heights 300.29
    open spaces 300.22
      with panic attacks 300.21
    public speaking 300.23
    streets 300.22
      with panic attacks 300.21
    travel 300.22
      with panic attacks 300.21
    washing in public 300.23
  transient 308.0
Febricula (continued) (simple) — *see also* Pyrexia 780.60
Febrile — *see also* Pyrexia 780.60
  convulsion (simple) 780.31
    complex 780.32
    nonhemolytic transfusion reaction (FNHTR) 780.66
  seizure (simple) 780.31
    atypical 780.32
    complex 780.32
    complicated 780.32
Febris — *see also* Fever 780.60
  aestiva (*see also* Fever, hay) 477.9
  flava (*see also* Fever, yellow) 060.9
  melitensis 023.0
  pestis (*see also* Plague) 020.9
  puerperalis 672.0 ☑
  recurrens (*see also* Fever, relapsing) 087.9
    pediculo vestimenti 087.0
  rubra 034.1
  typhoidea 002.0
  typhosa 002.0
Fecal — *see* condition
Fecalith (impaction) 560.32
  with hernia (*see also* Hernia, by site, with obstruction)
    gangrenous — *see* Hernia, by site, with gangrene
  appendix 543.9
  congenital 777.1
Fede's disease 529.0
Feeble-minded 317
Feeble rapid pulse due to shock following injury 958.4
Feeding
  faulty (elderly) (infant) 783.3
    newborn 779.31
  formula check V20.2
  improper (elderly) (infant) 783.3
    newborn 779.31
  problem (elderly) (infant) 783.3
    newborn 779.31
  nonorganic origin 307.59
Feeling of foreign body in throat 784.99
Feer's disease 985.0
Feet — *see* condition
Feigned illness V65.2
Feil-Klippel syndrome (brevicollis) 756.16
Feinmesser's (hidrotic) **ectodermal dysplasia** 757.31
Felix's disease (juvenile osteochondrosis, hip) 732.1
Felon (any digit) (with lymphangitis) 681.01
  herpetic 054.6
Felty's syndrome (rheumatoid arthritis with splenomegaly and leukopenia) 714.1
Feminism in boys 302.6
Feminization, testicular 259.51
  with pseudohermaphroditism, male 259.51

Femoral hernia — *see* Hernia, femoral
Femora vara 736.32
Femur, femoral — *see* condition
Fenestrata placenta — *see* Placenta, abnormal
Fenestration, fenestrated — *see also* Imperfect, closure
  aorta-pulmonary 745.0
  aorticopulmonary 745.0
  aortopulmonary 745.0
  cusps, heart valve NEC 746.89
    pulmonary 746.09
  hymen 752.49
  pulmonic cusps 746.09
Fenwick's disease 537.89
Fermentation (gastric) (gastrointestinal) (stomach) 536.8
  intestine 564.89
    psychogenic 306.4
  psychogenic 306.4
Fernell's disease (aortic aneurysm) 441.9
Fertile eunuch syndrome 257.2
Fertility, meaning multiparity — *see* Multiparity
Fetal
  alcohol syndrome 760.71
  anemia 678.0 ☑
  thrombocytopenia 678.0 ☑
  twin to twin transfusion 678.0 ☑
Fetalis uterus 752.39
Fetid
  breath 784.99
  sweat 705.89
Fetishism 302.81
  transvestic 302.3
Fetomaternal hemorrhage
  affecting management of pregnancy 656.0 ☑
  fetus or newborn 772.0
Fetus, fetal — *see also* condition
  papyraceous 779.89
  type lung tissue 770.4
Fever 780.60
  with chills 780.60
    in malarial regions (*see also* Malaria) 084.6
  abortus NEC 023.9
  aden 061
  African tick-borne 087.1
  American
    mountain tick 066.1
    spotted 082.0
  and ague (*see also* Malaria) 084.6
  aphthous 078.4
  arbovirus hemorrhagic 065.9
  Assam 085.0
  Australian A or Q 083.0
  Bangkok hemorrhagic 065.4
  biliary, Charcôt's intermittent — *see* Choledocholithiasis
  bilious, hemoglobinuric 084.8
  blackwater 084.8
  blister 054.9
  Bonvale Dam 780.79
  boutonneuse 082.1
  brain 323.9
    late effect — *see* category 326
  breakbone 061
  Bullis 082.8
  Bunyamwera 066.3
  Burdwan 085.0
  Bwamba (encephalitis) 066.3
  Cameroon (*see also* Malaria) 084.6
  Canton 081.9
  catarrhal (acute) 460
    chronic 472.0
  cat-scratch 078.3
  cerebral 323.9
    late effect — *see* category 326
  cerebrospinal (meningococcal) (*see also* Meningitis, cerebrospinal) 036.0
  Chagres 084.0
  Chandipura 066.8
  changuinola 066.8
  Charcôt's (biliary) (hepatic) (intermittent) — *see* Choledocholithiasis
  Chikungunya (viral) 066.3

Fever — *continued*
  Chikungunya — *continued*
    hemorrhagic 065.4
  childbed 670.8 ☑
  Chitral 066.0
  Colombo (*see also* Fever, paratyphoid) 002.9
  Colorado tick (virus) 066.1
  congestive
    malarial (*see also* Malaria) 084.6
    remittent (*see also* Malaria) 084.6
  Congo virus 065.0
  continued 780.60
    malarial 084.0
  Corsican (*see also* Malaria) 084.6
  Crimean hemorrhagic 065.0
  Cyprus (*see also* Brucellosis) 023.9
  dandy 061
  deer fly (*see also* Tularemia) 021.9
  dehydration, newborn 778.4
  dengue (virus) 061
    hemorrhagic 065.4
  desert 114.0
  due to heat 992.0
  Dumdum 085.0
  enteric 002.0
  ephemeral (of unknown origin) (*see also* Pyrexia) 780.60
  epidemic, hemorrhagic of the Far East 065.0
  erysipelatous (*see also* Erysipelas) 035
  estivo-autumnal (malarial) 084.0
  etiocholanolone 277.31
  famine (*see also* Fever, relapsing)
    meaning typhus — *see* Typhus
  Far Eastern hemorrhagic 065.0
  five day 083.1
  Fort Bragg 100.89
  gastroenteric 002.0
  gastromalarial (*see also* Malaria) 084.6
  Gibraltar (*see also* Brucellosis) 023.9
  glandular 075
  Guama (viral) 066.3
  Haverhill 026.1
  hay (allergic) (with rhinitis) 477.9
    with
      asthma (bronchial) (*see also* Asthma) 493.0 ☑
    due to
      dander, animal (cat) (dog) 477.2
      dust 477.8
      fowl 477.8
      hair, animal (cat) (dog) 477.2
      pollen, any plant or tree 477.0
      specified allergen other than pollen 477.8
  heat (effects) 992.0
  hematuric, bilious 084.8
  hemoglobinuric (malarial) 084.8
    bilious 084.8
  hemorrhagic (arthropod-borne) NEC 065.9
    with renal syndrome 078.6
    arenaviral 078.7
    Argentine 078.7
    Bangkok 065.4
    Bolivian 078.7
    Central Asian 065.0
    chikungunya 065.4
    Crimean 065.0
    dengue (virus) 065.4
    Ebola 065.8
    epidemic 078.6
      of Far East 065.0
    Far Eastern 065.0
    Junin virus 078.7
    Korean 078.6
    Kyasanur forest 065.2
    Machupo virus 078.7
    mite-borne NEC 065.8
    mosquito-borne 065.4
    Omsk 065.1
    Philippine 065.4
    Russian (Yaroslav) 078.6
    Singapore 065.4
    Southeast Asia 065.4
    Thailand 065.4
    tick-borne NEC 065.3
  hepatic (*see also* Cholecystitis) 575.8

☑ Additional Digit Required — Refer to the Tabular List for Digit Selection   ▽ Subterms under main terms may continue to next column or page

2014 ICD-9-CM   159

Fat — Fever

Fever — *continued*
  hepatic (*see also* Cholecystitis) — *continued*
    intermittent (Charcôt's) — *see* Choledocholithiasis
  herpetic (*see also* Herpes) 054.9
  Hyalomma tick 065.0
  icterohemorrhagic 100.0
  inanition 780.60
    newborn 778.4
  in conditions classified elsewhere 780.61
  infective NEC 136.9
  intermittent (bilious) (*see also* Malaria) 084.6
    hepatic (Charcôt) — *see* Choledocholithiasis
    of unknown origin (*see also* Pyrexia) 780.60
    pernicious 084.0
  iodide
    correct substance properly administered 780.60
    overdose or wrong substance given or taken 975.5
  Japanese river 081.2
  jungle yellow 060.0
  Junin virus, hemorrhagic 078.7
  Katayama 120.2
  Kedani 081.2
  Kenya 082.1
  Korean hemorrhagic 078.6
  Lassa 078.89
  Lone Star 082.8
  lung — *see* Pneumonia
  Machupo virus, hemorrhagic 078.7
  malaria, malarial (*see also* Malaria) 084.6
  Malta (*see also* Brucellosis) 023.9
  Marseilles 082.1
  marsh (*see also* Malaria) 084.6
  Mayaro (viral) 066.3
  Mediterranean (*see also* Brucellosis) 023.9
    familial 277.31
    tick 082.1
  meningeal — *see* Meningitis
  metal fumes NEC 985.8
  Meuse 083.1
  Mexican — *see* Typhus, Mexican
  Mianeh 087.1
  miasmatic (*see also* Malaria) 084.6
  miliary 078.2
  milk, female 672.0 ☑
  mill 504
  mite-borne hemorrhagic 065.8
  Monday 504
  mosquito-borne NEC 066.3
    hemorrhagic NEC 065.4
  mountain 066.1
    meaning
      Rocky Mountain spotted 082.0
      undulant fever (*see also* Brucellosis) 023.9
    tick (American) 066.1
  Mucambo (viral) 066.3
  mud 100.89
  Neapolitan (*see also* Brucellosis) 023.9
  neutropenic 288.00
  newborn (environmentally-induced) 778.4
  nine-mile 083.0
  nonexanthematous tick 066.1
  North Asian tick-borne typhus 082.2
  Omsk hemorrhagic 065.1
  O'nyong-nyong (viral) 066.3
  Oropouche (viral) 066.3
  Oroya 088.0
  paludal (*see also* Malaria) 084.6
  Panama 084.0
  pappataci 066.0
  paratyphoid 002.9
    A 002.1
    B (Schottmüller's) 002.2
    C (Hirschfeld) 002.3
  parrot 073.9
  periodic 277.31
  pernicious, acute 084.0
  persistent (of unknown origin) (*see also* Pyrexia) 780.60
  petechial 036.0

Fever — *continued*
  pharyngoconjunctival 077.2
    adenoviral type 3 077.2
  Philippine hemorrhagic 065.4
  phlebotomus 066.0
  Piry 066.8
  Pixuna (viral) 066.3
  Plasmodium ovale 084.3
  pleural (*see also* Pleurisy) 511.0
  pneumonic — *see* Pneumonia
  polymer fume 987.8
  postimmunization 780.63
  postoperative 780.62
    due to infection 998.59
  posttransfusion 780.66
  postvaccination 780.63
  pretibial 100.89
  puerperal, postpartum 672.0 ☑
  putrid — *see* Septicemia
  pyemic — *see* Septicemia
  Q 083.0
    with pneumonia 083.0 [484.8]
  quadrilateral 083.0
  quartan (malaria) 084.2
  Queensland (coastal) 083.0
    seven-day 100.89
  Quintan (A) 083.1
  quotidian 084.0
  rabbit (*see also* Tularemia) 021.9
  rat-bite 026.9
    due to
      Spirillum minor or minus 026.0
      Spirochaeta morsus muris 026.0
      Streptobacillus moniliformis 026.1
  recurrent — *see* Fever, relapsing
  relapsing 087.9
    Carter's (Asiatic) 087.0
    Dutton's (West African) 087.1
    Koch's 087.9
    louse-borne (epidemic) 087.0
    Novy's (American) 087.1
    Obermeyer's (European) 087.0
    spirillum NEC 087.9
    tick-borne (endemic) 087.1
  remittent (bilious) (congestive) (gastric) (*see also* Malaria) 084.6
  rheumatic (active) (acute) (chronic) (subacute) 390
    with heart involvement 391.9
      carditis 391.9
      endocarditis (aortic) (mitral) (pulmonary) (tricuspid) 391.1
      multiple sites 391.8
      myocarditis 391.2
      pancarditis, acute 391.8
      pericarditis 391.0
      specified type NEC 391.8
      valvulitis 391.1
    cardiac hypertrophy 398.99
    inactive or quiescent
      with cardiac hypertrophy 398.99
      carditis 398.90
      endocarditis 397.9
        aortic (valve) 395.9
          with mitral (valve) disease 396.9
        mitral (valve) 394.9
          with aortic (valve) disease 396.9
        pulmonary (valve) 397.1
        tricuspid (valve) 397.0
      heart conditions (classifiable to 429.3, 429.6, 429.9) 398.99
        failure (congestive) (conditions classifiable to 428.0, 428.9) 398.91
        left ventricular failure (conditions classifiable to 428.1) 398.91
      myocardial degeneration (conditions classifiable to 429.1) 398.0
      myocarditis (conditions classifiable to 429.0) 398.0
      pancarditis 398.99
      pericarditis 393
  Rift Valley (viral) 066.3
  Rocky Mountain spotted 082.0

Fever — *continued*
  rose 477.0
  Ross river (viral) 066.3
  Russian hemorrhagic 078.6
  sandfly 066.0
  San Joaquin (valley) 114.0
  São Paulo 082.0
  scarlet 034.1
  septic — *see* Septicemia
  seven-day 061
    Japan 100.89
    Queensland 100.89
  shin bone 083.1
  Singapore hemorrhagic 065.4
  solar 061
  sore 054.9
  South African tick-bite 087.1
  Southeast Asia hemorrhagic 065.4
  spinal — *see* Meningitis
  spirillary 026.0
  splenic (*see also* Anthrax) 022.9
  spotted (Rocky Mountain) 082.0
    American 082.0
    Brazilian 082.0
    Colombian 082.0
    meaning
      cerebrospinal meningitis 036.0
      typhus 082.9
  spring 309.23
  steroid
    correct substance properly administered 780.60
    overdose or wrong substance given or taken 962.0
  streptobacillary 026.1
  subtertian 084.0
  Sumatran mite 081.2
  sun 061
  swamp 100.89
  sweating 078.2
  swine 003.8
  sylvatic yellow 060.0
  Tahyna 062.5
  tertian — *see* Malaria, tertian
  Thailand hemorrhagic 065.4
  thermic 992.0
  three day 066.0
    with Coxsackie exanthem 074.8
  tick
    American mountain 066.1
    Colorado 066.1
    Kemerovo 066.1
    Mediterranean 082.1
    mountain 066.1
    nonexanthematous 066.1
    Quaranfil 066.1
  tick-bite NEC 066.1
  tick-borne NEC 066.1
    hemorrhagic NEC 065.3
  transitory of newborn 778.4
  trench 083.1
  tsutsugamushi 081.2
  typhogastric 002.0
  typhoid (abortive) (ambulant) (any site) (hemorrhagic) (infection) (intermittent) (malignant) (rheumatic) 002.0
  typhomalarial (*see also* Malaria) 084.6
  typhus — *see* Typhus
  undulant (*see also* Brucellosis) 023.9
  unknown origin (*see also* Pyrexia) 780.60
  uremic — *see* Uremia
  uveoparotid 135
  valley (Coccidioidomycosis) 114.0
  Venezuelan equine 066.2
  Volhynian 083.1
  Wesselsbron (viral) 066.3
  West
    African 084.8
    Nile (viral) 066.40
      with
        cranial nerve disorders 066.42
        encephalitis 066.41
        optic neuritis 066.42
        other complications 066.49
        other neurologic manifestations 066.42

Fever — *continued*
  West — *continued*
    Nile — *continued*
      with — *continued*
        polyradiculitis 066.42
  Whitmore's 025
  Wolhynian 083.1
  worm 128.9
  Yaroslav hemorrhagic 078.6
  yellow 060.9
    jungle 060.0
    sylvatic 060.0
    urban 060.1
    vaccination, prophylactic (against) V04.4
  Zika (viral) 066.3
Fibrillation
  atrial (established) (paroxysmal) 427.31
  auricular (atrial) (established) 427.31
  cardiac (ventricular) 427.41
  coronary (*see also* Infarct, myocardium) 410.9 ☑
  heart (ventricular) 427.41
  muscular 728.9
  postoperative 997.1
  ventricular 427.41
Fibrin
  ball or bodies, pleural (sac) 511.0
  chamber, anterior (eye) (gelatinous exudate) 364.04
Fibrinogenolysis (hemorrhagic) — *see* Fibrinolysis
Fibrinogenopenia (congenital) (hereditary) — *see also* Defect, coagulation 286.3
  acquired 286.6
Fibrinolysis (acquired) (hemorrhagic) (pathologic) 286.6
  with
    abortion — *see* Abortion, by type, with hemorrhage, delayed or excessive
    ectopic pregnancy (*see also* categories 633.0–633.9) 639.1
    molar pregnancy (*see also* categories 630–632) 639.1
  antepartum or intrapartum 641.3 ☑
    affecting fetus or newborn 762.1
  following
    abortion 639.1
    ectopic or molar pregnancy 639.1
  newborn, transient 776.2
  postpartum 666.3 ☑
Fibrinopenia (hereditary) — *see also* Defect, coagulation 286.3
  acquired 286.6
Fibrinopurulent — *see* condition
Fibrinous — *see* condition
Fibroadenoma (M9010/0)
  cellular intracanalicular (M9020/0) 217
  giant (intracanalicular) (M9020/0) 217
  intracanalicular (M9011/0)
    cellular (M9020/0) 217
    giant (M9020/0) 217
    specified site — *see* Neoplasm, by site, benign
    unspecified site 217
  juvenile (M9030/0) 217
  pericanicular (M9012/0)
    specified site — *see* Neoplasm, by site, benign
    unspecified site 217
  phyllodes (M9020/0) 217
  prostate 600.20
    with
      other lower urinary tract symptoms (LUTS) 600.21
      urinary
        obstruction 600.21
        retention 600.21
  specified site — *see* Neoplasm, by site, benign
  unspecified site 217
Fibroadenosis, breast (chronic) (cystic) (diffuse) (periodic) (segmental) 610.2
Fibroangioma (M9160/0) — *see also* Neoplasm, by site, benign

Fibroangioma — *see also* Neoplasm, by site, benign — *continued*
  juvenile (M9160/0)
    specified site — *see* Neoplasm, by site, benign
    unspecified site 210.7
Fibrocellulitis progressiva ossificans 728.11
Fibrochondrosarcoma (M9220/3) — *see* Neoplasm, cartilage, malignant
Fibrocystic
  disease 277.00
    bone NEC 733.29
    breast 610.1
    jaw 526.2
    kidney (congenital) 753.19
    liver 751.62
    lung 518.89
      congenital 748.4
    pancreas 277.00
  kidney (congenital) 753.19
Fibrodysplasia ossificans multiplex (progressiva) 728.11
Fibroelastosis (cordis) (endocardial) (endomyocardial) 425.3
Fibroid (tumor) (M8890/0) — *see also* Neoplasm, connective tissue, benign
  disease, lung (chronic) (*see also* Fibrosis, lung) 515
  heart (disease) (*see also* Myocarditis) 429.0
  induration, lung (chronic) (*see also* Fibrosis, lung) 515
  in pregnancy or childbirth 654.1 ☑
    affecting fetus or newborn 763.89
    causing obstructed labor 660.2 ☑
      affecting fetus or newborn 763.1
  liver — *see* Cirrhosis, liver
  lung (*see also* Fibrosis, lung) 515
  pneumonia (chronic) (*see also* Fibrosis, lung) 515
  uterus (M8890/0) (*see also* Leiomyoma, uterus) 218.9
Fibrolipoma (M8851/0) — *see also* Lipoma, by site 214.9
Fibroliposarcoma (M8850/3) — *see* Neoplasm, connective tissue, malignant
Fibroma (M8810/0) — *see also* Neoplasm, connective tissue, benign
  ameloblastic (M9330/0) 213.1
    upper jaw (bone) 213.0
  bone (nonossifying) 733.99
    ossifying (M9262/0) — *see* Neoplasm, bone, benign
  cementifying (M9274/0) — *see* Neoplasm, bone, benign
  chondromyxoid (M9241/0) — *see* Neoplasm, bone, benign
  desmoplastic (M8823/1) — *see* Neoplasm, connective tissue, uncertain behavior
  facial (M8813/0) — *see* Neoplasm, connective tissue, benign
  invasive (M8821/1) — *see* Neoplasm, connective tissue, uncertain behavior
  molle (M8851/0) (*see also* Lipoma, by site) 214.9
  myxoid (M8811/0) — *see* Neoplasm, connective tissue, benign
  nasopharynx, nasopharyngeal (juvenile) (M9160/0) 210.7
  nonosteogenic (nonossifying) — *see* Dysplasia, fibrous
  odontogenic (M9321/0) 213.1
    upper jaw (bone) 213.0
  ossifying (M9262/0) — *see* Neoplasm, bone, benign
  periosteal (M8812/0) — *see* Neoplasm, bone, benign
  prostate 600.20
    with
      other lower urinary tract symptoms (LUTS) 600.21
      urinary
        obstruction 600.21
        retention 600.21
  soft (M8851/0) (*see also* Lipoma, by site) 214.9
Fibromatosis 728.79

Fibromatosis — *continued*
  abdominal (M8822/1) — *see* Neoplasm, connective tissue, uncertain behavior
  aggressive (M8821/1) — *see* Neoplasm, connective tissue, uncertain behavior
  congenital generalized (CGF) 759.89
  Dupuytren's 728.6
  gingival 523.8
  plantar fascia 728.71
  proliferative 728.79
  pseudosarcomatous (proliferative) (subcutaneous) 728.79
  subcutaneous pseudosarcomatous (proliferative) 728.79
Fibromyalgia 729.1
Fibromyoma (M8890/0) — *see also* Neoplasm, connective tissue, benign
  uterus (corpus) (*see also* Leiomyoma, uterus) 218.9
    in pregnancy or childbirth 654.1 ☑
      affecting fetus or newborn 763.89
      causing obstructed labor 660.2 ☑
        affecting fetus or newborn 763.1
Fibromyositis — *see also* Myositis 729.1
  scapulohumeral 726.2
Fibromyxolipoma (M8852/0) — *see also* Lipoma, by site 214.9
Fibromyxoma (M8811/0) — *see* Neoplasm, connective tissue, benign
Fibromyxosarcoma (M8811/3) — *see* Neoplasm, connective tissue, malignant
Fibro-odontoma, ameloblastic (M9290/0) 213.1
  upper jaw (bone) 213.0
Fibro-osteoma (M9262/0) — *see* Neoplasm, bone, benign
Fibroplasia, retrolental (*see also* Retinopathy of prematurity) 362.21
Fibropurulent — *see* condition
Fibrosarcoma (M8810/3) — *see also* Neoplasm, connective tissue, malignant
  ameloblastic (M9330/3) 170.1
    upper jaw (bone) 170.0
  congenital (M8814/3) — *see* Neoplasm, connective tissue, malignant
  fascial (M8813/3) — *see* Neoplasm, connective tissue, malignant
  infantile (M8814/3) — *see* Neoplasm, connective tissue, malignant
  odontogenic (M9330/3) 170.1
    upper jaw (bone) 170.0
  periosteal (M8812/3) — *see* Neoplasm, bone, malignant
Fibrosclerosis
  breast 610.3
  corpora cavernosa (penis) 607.89
  familial multifocal NEC 710.8
  multifocal (idiopathic) NEC 710.8
  penis (corpora cavernosa) 607.89
Fibrosis, fibrotic
  adrenal (gland) 255.8
  alveolar (diffuse) 516.31
  amnion 658.8 ☑
  anal papillae 569.49
  anus 569.49
  appendix, appendiceal, noninflammatory 543.9
  arteriocapillary — *see* Arteriosclerosis
  bauxite (of lung) 503
  biliary 576.8
    due to Clonorchis sinensis 121.1
  bladder 596.89
    interstitial 595.1
    localized submucosal 595.1
    panmural 595.1
  bone, diffuse 756.59
  breast 610.3
  capillary (*see also* Arteriosclerosis)
    lung (chronic) (*see also* Fibrosis, lung) 515
  cardiac (*see also* Myocarditis) 429.0
  cervix 622.8
  chorion 658.8 ☑
  corpus cavernosum 607.89
  cystic (of pancreas) 277.00

Fibrosis, fibrotic — *continued*
  cystic — *continued*
    with
      manifestations
        gastrointestinal 277.03
        pulmonary 277.02
        specified NEC 277.09
      meconium ileus 277.01
      pulmonary exacerbation 277.02
  due to (presence of) any device, implant, or graft — *see* Complications, due to (presence of) any device, implant, or graft classified to 996.0–996.5 NEC
  ejaculatory duct 608.89
  endocardium (*see also* Endocarditis) 424.90
  endomyocardial (African) 425.0
  epididymis 608.89
  eye muscle 378.62
  graphite (of lung) 503
  heart (*see also* Myocarditis) 429.0
  hepatic (*see also* Cirrhosis, liver)
    due to Clonorchis sinensis 121.1
  hepatolienal — *see* Cirrhosis, liver
  hepatosplenic — *see* Cirrhosis, liver
  infrapatellar fat pad 729.31
  interstitial pulmonary, newborn 770.7
  intrascrotal 608.89
  kidney (*see also* Sclerosis, renal) 587
  liver — *see* Cirrhosis, liver
  lung (atrophic) (capillary) (chronic) (confluent) (massive) (perialveolar) (peribronchial) 515
    with
      anthracosilicosis (occupational) 500
      anthracosis (occupational) 500
      asbestosis (occupational) 501
      bagassosis (occupational) 495.1
      bauxite 503
      berylliosis (occupational) 503
      byssinosis (occupational) 504
      calcicosis (occupational) 502
      chalicosis (occupational) 502
      dust reticulation (occupational) 504
      farmers' lung 495.0
      gannister disease (occupational) 502
      graphite 503
      pneumonoconiosis (occupational) 505
      pneumosiderosis (occupational) 503
      siderosis (occupational) 503
      silicosis (occupational) 502
      tuberculosis (*see also* Tuberculosis) 011.4 ☑
  diffuse (idiopathic) (interstitial) 516.31
  due to
    bauxite 503
    fumes or vapors (chemical) (inhalation) 506.4
    graphite 503
  following radiation 508.1
  postinflammatory 515
  silicotic (massive) (occupational) 502
  tuberculous (*see also* Tuberculosis) 011.4 ☑
  lymphatic gland 289.3
  median bar 600.90
    with
      other lower urinary tract symptoms (LUTS) 600.91
      urinary
        obstruction 600.91
        retention 600.91
  mediastinum (idiopathic) 519.3
  meninges 349.2
  muscle NEC 728.2
    iatrogenic (from injection) 999.9
  myocardium, myocardial (*see also* Myocarditis) 429.0
  oral submucous 528.8
  ovary 620.8
  oviduct 620.8
  pancreas 577.8
    cystic 277.00
      with
        manifestations
          gastrointestinal 277.03

Fibrosis, fibrotic — *continued*
  pancreas — *continued*
    cystic — *continued*
      with — *continued*
        manifestations — *continued*
          pulmonary 277.02
          specified NEC 277.09
        meconium ileus 277.01
        pulmonary exacerbation 277.02
  penis 607.89
  periappendiceal 543.9
  periarticular (*see also* Ankylosis) 718.5 ☑
  pericardium 423.1
  perineum, in pregnancy or childbirth 654.8 ☑
    affecting fetus or newborn 763.89
    causing obstructed labor 660.2 ☑
      affecting fetus or newborn 763.1
  perineural NEC 355.9
    foot 355.6
  periureteral 593.89
  placenta — *see* Placenta, abnormal
  pleura 511.0
  popliteal fat pad 729.31
  preretinal 362.56
  prostate (chronic) 600.90
    with
      other lower urinary tract symptoms (LUTS) 600.91
      urinary
        obstruction 600.91
        retention 600.91
  pulmonary (chronic) (*see also* Fibrosis, lung) 515
    alveolar capillary block 516.8
    idiopathic 516.31
    interstitial
      diffuse (idiopathic) 516.31
      newborn 770.7
  radiation — *see* Effect, adverse, radiation
  rectal sphincter 569.49
  retroperitoneal, idiopathic 593.4
  sclerosing mesenteric (idiopathic) 567.82
  scrotum 608.89
  seminal vesicle 608.89
  senile 797
  skin NEC 709.2
  spermatic cord 608.89
  spleen 289.59
    bilharzial (*see also* Schistosomiasis) 120.9
  subepidermal nodular (M8832/0) — *see* Neoplasm, skin, benign
  submucous NEC 709.2
    oral 528.8
    tongue 528.8
  syncytium — *see* Placenta, abnormal
  testis 608.89
    chronic, due to syphilis 095.8
  thymus (gland) 254.8
  tunica vaginalis 608.89
  ureter 593.89
  urethra 599.84
  uterus (nonneoplastic) 621.8
    bilharzial (*see also* Schistosomiasis) 120.9
    neoplastic (*see also* Leiomyoma, uterus) 218.9
  vagina 623.8
  valve, heart (*see also* Endocarditis) 424.90
  vas deferens 608.89
  vein 459.89
    lower extremities 459.89
  vesical 595.1
Fibrositis (periarticular) (rheumatoid) 729.0
  humeroscapular region 726.2
  nodular, chronic
    Jaccoud's 714.4
    rheumatoid 714.4
  ossificans 728.11
  scapulohumeral 726.2
Fibrothorax 511.0
Fibrotic — *see* Fibrosis
Fibrous — *see* condition
Fibroxanthoma (M8831/0) — *see also* Neoplasm, connective tissue, benign
  atypical (M8831/1) — *see* Neoplasm, connective tissue, uncertain behavior

☑ Additional Digit Required — Refer to the Tabular List for Digit Selection   ▽ Subterms under main terms may continue to next column or page

2014 ICD-9-CM   161

Fibroxanthoma — see also Neoplasm, connective tissue, benign — continued
  malignant (M8831/3) — see Neoplasm, connective tissue, malignant
Fibroxanthosarcoma (M8831/3) — see Neoplasm, connective tissue, malignant
Fiedler's
  disease (leptospiral jaundice) 100.0
  myocarditis or syndrome (acute isolated myocarditis) 422.91
Fiessinger-Leroy (-Reiter) syndrome 099.3
Fiessinger-Rendu syndrome (erythema muliforme exudativum) 695.19
Fifth disease (eruptive) 057.0
  venereal 099.1
Filaria, filarial — see Infestation, filarial
Filariasis — see also Infestation, filarial 125.9
  bancroftian 125.0
  Brug's 125.1
  due to
    bancrofti 125.0
    Brugia (Wuchereria) (malayi) 125.1
    Loa loa 125.2
    malayi 125.1
    organism NEC 125.6
    Wuchereria (bancrofti) 125.0
      malayi 125.1
  Malayan 125.1
  ozzardi 125.5
  specified type NEC 125.6
Filatoff's, Filatov's, Filatow's disease (infectious mononucleosis) 075
File-cutters' disease 984.9
  specified type of lead — see Table of Drugs and Chemicals
Filling defect
  biliary tract 793.3
  bladder 793.5
  duodenum 793.4
  gallbladder 793.3
  gastrointestinal tract 793.4
  intestine 793.4
  kidney 793.5
  stomach 793.4
  ureter 793.4
Filtering bleb, eye (postglaucoma) (status) V45.69
  with complication or rupture 997.99
  postcataract extraction (complication) 997.99
Fimbrial cyst (congenital) 752.11
Fimbriated hymen 752.49
Financial problem affecting care V60.2
Findings, (abnormal), without diagnosis (examination) (laboratory test) 796.4
  17-ketosteroids, elevated 791.9
  acetonuria 791.6
  acid phosphatase 790.5
  albumin-globulin ratio 790.99
  albuminuria 791.0
  alcohol in blood 790.3
  alkaline phosphatase 790.5
  amniotic fluid 792.3
  amylase 790.5
  anisocytosis 790.09
  antenatal screening 796.5
  anthrax, positive 795.31
  antibody titers, elevated 795.79
  anticardiolipin antibody 795.79
  antigen-antibody reaction 795.79
  antiphosphatidylglycerol antibody 795.79
  antiphosphatidylinositol antibody 795.79
  antiphosphatidylserine antibody 795.79
  antiphospholipid antibody 795.79
  bacteriuria 791.9
  ballistocardiogram 794.39
  bicarbonate 276.9
  bile in urine 791.4
  bilirubin 277.4
  bleeding time (prolonged) 790.92
  blood culture, positive 790.7
  blood gas level (arterial) 790.91
  blood sugar level 790.29
    high 790.29
      fasting glucose 790.21

Findings, (abnormal), without diagnosis — continued
  blood sugar level — continued
    high — continued
      glucose tolerance test 790.22
    low 251.2
  calcium 275.40
  cancer antigen 125 [CA 125] 795.82
  carbonate 276.9
  carcinoembryonic antigen [CEA] 795.81
  casts, urine 791.7
  catecholamines 791.9
  cells, urine 791.7
  cerebrospinal fluid (color) (content) (pressure) 792.0
  cervical
    high risk human papillomavirus (HPV) DNA test positive 795.05
    low risk human papillomavirus (HPV) DNA test positive 795.09
    non-atypical endometrial cells 795.09
  chloride 276.9
  cholesterol 272.9
    high 272.0
      with high triglycerides 272.2
  chromosome analysis 795.2
  chyluria 791.1
  circulation time 794.39
  cloudy dialysis effluent 792.5
  cloudy urine 791.9
  coagulation study 790.92
  cobalt, blood 790.6
  color of urine (unusual) NEC 791.9
  copper, blood 790.6
  C-reactive protein (CRP) 790.95
  creatinine clearance 794.4
  crystals, urine 791.9
  culture, positive NEC 795.39
    blood 790.7
    HIV V08
    human immunodeficiency virus V08
    nose 795.39
      Staphylococcus — see Carrier (suspected) of, Staphylococcus
    skin lesion NEC 795.39
    spinal fluid 792.0
    sputum 795.39
    stool 792.1
    throat 795.39
    urine 791.9
    viral
      human immunodeficiency V08
    wound 795.39
  cytology specified site NEC 796.9
  echocardiogram 793.2
  echoencephalogram 794.01
  echogram NEC — see Findings, abnormal, structure
  electrocardiogram (ECG) (EKG) 794.31
  electroencephalogram (EEG) 794.02
  electrolyte level, urinary 791.9
  electromyogram (EMG) 794.17
    ocular 794.14
  electro-oculogram (EOG) 794.12
  electroretinogram (ERG) 794.11
  enzymes, serum NEC 790.5
  fibrinogen titer coagulation study 790.92
  filling defect — see Filling defect
  function study NEC 794.9
    auditory 794.15
    bladder 794.9
    brain 794.00
    cardiac 794.30
    endocrine NEC 794.6
      thyroid 794.5
    kidney 794.4
    liver 794.8
    nervous system
      central 794.00
      peripheral 794.19
    oculomotor 794.14
    pancreas 794.9
    placenta 794.9
    pulmonary 794.2
    retina 794.11
    special senses 794.19

Findings, (abnormal), without diagnosis — continued
  function study — continued
    spleen 794.9
    vestibular 794.16
  gallbladder, nonvisualization 793.3
  glucose 790.29
    elevated
      fasting 790.21
      tolerance test 790.22
  glycosuria 791.5
  heart
    shadow 793.2
    sounds 785.3
  hematinuria 791.2
  hematocrit
    drop (precipitous) 790.01
    elevated 282.7
    low 285.9
  hematologic NEC 790.99
  hematuria 599.70
  hemoglobin
    drop 790.01
    elevated 282.7
    low 285.9
  hemoglobinuria 791.2
  histological NEC 795.4
  hormones 259.9
  immunoglobulins, elevated 795.79
  indolacetic acid, elevated 791.9
  iron 790.6
  karyotype 795.2
  ketonuria 791.6
  lactic acid dehydrogenase (LDH) 790.4
  lead 790.6
  lipase 790.5
  lipids NEC 272.9
  lithium, blood 790.6
  liver function test 790.6
  lung field (shadow) 793.19
    coin lesion 793.11
  magnesium, blood 790.6
  mammogram 793.80
    calcification 793.89
    calculus 793.89
    dense breasts 793.82
    inconclusive 793.82
      due to dense breasts 793.82
    microcalcification 793.81
  mediastinal shift 793.2
  melanin, urine 791.9
  microbiologic NEC 795.39
  mineral, blood NEC 790.6
  myoglobinuria 791.3
  nasal swab, anthrax 795.31
  neonatal screening 796.6
  nitrogen derivatives, blood 790.6
  nonvisualization of gallbladder 793.3
  nose culture, positive 795.39
  odor of urine (unusual) NEC 791.9
  oxygen saturation 790.91
  Papanicolaou (smear) 796.9
    anus 796.70
      with
        atypical squamous cells
          cannot exclude high grade squamous intraepithelial lesion (ASC-H) 796.72
          of undetermined significance (ASC-US) 796.71
        cytologic evidence of malignancy 796.76
        high grade squamous intraepithelial lesion (HGSIL) 796.74
        low grade squamous intraepithelial lesion (LGSIL) 796.73
      glandular 796.70
      specified finding NEC 796.79
    cervix 795.00
      with
        atypical squamous cells
          cannot exclude high grade squamous intraepithelial lesion (ASC-H) 795.02

Findings, (abnormal), without diagnosis — continued
  Papanicolaou — continued
    cervix — continued
      with — continued
        atypical squamous cells — continued
          of undetermined significance (ASC-US) 795.01
        cytologic evidence of malignancy 795.06
        high grade squamous intraepithelial lesion (HGSIL) 795.04
        low grade squamous intraepithelial lesion (LGSIL) 795.03
        non-atypical endometrial cells 795.09
      dyskaryotic 795.09
      non-atypical endometrial cells 795.09
      nonspecific finding NEC 795.09
    other site 796.9
    vagina 795.10
      with
        atypical squamous cells
          cannot exclude high grade squamous intraepithelial lesion (ASC-H) 795.12
          of undetermined significance (ASC-US) 795.11
        cytologic evidence of malignancy 795.16
        high grade squamous intraepithelial lesion (HGSIL) 795.14
        low grade squamous intraepithelial lesion (LGSIL) 795.13
      glandular 795.10
      specified NEC 795.19
  peritoneal fluid 792.9
  phonocardiogram 794.39
  phosphorus 275.3
  pleural fluid 792.9
  pneumoencephalogram 793.0
  PO2-oxygen ratio 790.91
  poikilocytosis 790.09
  potassium
    deficiency 276.8
    excess 276.7
  PPD 795.51
  prostate specific antigen (PSA) 790.93
  protein, serum NEC 790.99
  proteinuria 791.0
  prothrombin time (partial) (prolonged) (PT) (PTT) 790.92
  pyuria 791.9
  radiologic (x-ray) 793.99
    abdomen 793.6
    biliary tract 793.3
    breast 793.89
      abnormal mammogram NOS 793.80
      mammographic
        calcification 793.89
        calculus 793.89
        microcalcification 793.81
    gastrointestinal tract 793.4
    genitourinary organs 793.5
    head 793.0
    image test inconclusive due to excess body fat 793.91
    intrathoracic organs NEC 793.2
    lung 793.19
    musculoskeletal 793.7
    placenta 793.99
    retroperitoneum 793.6
    skin 793.99
    skull 793.0
    subcutaneous tissue 793.99
  red blood cell 790.09
    count 790.09
    morphology 790.09
    sickling 790.09
    volume 790.09
  saliva 792.4
  scan NEC 794.9
    bladder 794.9
    bone 794.9

Findings, (abnormal), without diagnosis — *continued*

scan — *continued*
brain 794.09
kidney 794.4
liver 794.8
lung 794.2
pancreas 794.9
placental 794.9
spleen 794.9
thyroid 794.5
sedimentation rate, elevated 790.1
semen 792.2
serological (for)
human immunodeficiency virus (HIV)
inconclusive 795.71
positive V08
syphilis — *see* Findings, serology for syphilis
serology for syphilis
false positive 795.6
positive 097.1
false 795.6
follow-up of latent syphilis — *see* Syphilis, latent
only finding — *see* Syphilis, latent
serum 790.99
blood NEC 790.99
enzymes NEC 790.5
proteins 790.99
SGOT 790.4
SGPT 790.4
sickling of red blood cells 790.09
skin test, positive 795.79
tuberculin (without active tuberculosis) 795.51
sodium 790.6
deficiency 276.1
excess 276.0
specified NEC 796.9
spermatozoa 792.2
spinal fluid 792.0
culture, positive 792.0
sputum culture, positive 795.39
for acid-fast bacilli 795.39
stool NEC 792.1
bloody 578.1
occult 792.1
color 792.1
culture, positive 792.1
occult blood 792.1
stress test 794.39
structure, body (echogram) (thermogram) (ultrasound) (x-ray) NEC 793.99
abdomen 793.6
breast 793.89
abnormal mammogram 793.80
mammographic
calcification 793.89
calculus 793.89
microcalcification 793.81
gastrointestinal tract 793.4
genitourinary organs 793.5
head 793.0
echogram (ultrasound) 794.01
intrathoracic organs NEC 793.2
lung 793.19
musculoskeletal 793.7
placenta 793.99
retroperitoneum 793.6
skin 793.99
subcutaneous tissue NEC 793.99
synovial fluid 792.9
thermogram — *see* Findings, abnormal, structure
throat culture, positive 795.39
thyroid (function) 794.5
metabolism (rate) 794.5
scan 794.5
uptake 794.5
total proteins 790.99
toxicology (drugs) (heavy metals) 796.0
transaminase (level) 790.4
triglycerides 272.9
high 272.1
with high cholesterol 272.2

Findings, (abnormal), without diagnosis — *continued*

tuberculin skin test (without active tuberculosis) 795.51
tumor markers NEC 795.89
ultrasound (*see also* Findings, abnormal, structure)
cardiogram 793.2
uric acid, blood 790.6
urine, urinary constituents 791.9
acetone 791.6
albumin 791.0
bacteria 791.9
bile 791.4
blood 599.70
casts or cells 791.7
chyle 791.1
culture, positive 791.9
glucose 791.5
hemoglobin 791.2
ketone 791.6
protein 791.0
pus 791.9
sugar 791.5
vaginal
fluid 792.9
high risk human papillomavirus (HPV) DNA test positive 795.15
low risk human papillomavirus (HPV) DNA test positive 795.19
vanillylmandelic acid, elevated 791.9
vectorcardiogram (VCG) 794.39
ventriculogram (cerebral) 793.0
VMA, elevated 791.9
Wassermann reaction
false positive 795.6
positive 097.1
follow-up of latent syphilis — *see* Syphilis, latent
only finding — *see* Syphilis, latent
white blood cell 288.9
count 288.9
elevated 288.60
low 288.50
differential 288.9
morphology 288.9
wound culture 795.39
xerography 793.89
zinc, blood 790.6
Finger — *see* condition
Finnish type nephrosis (congenital) 759.89
Fire, St. Anthony's — *see also* Erysipelas 035
Fish
hook stomach 537.89
meal workers' lung 495.8
Fisher's syndrome 357.0
Fissure, fissured
abdominal wall (congenital) 756.79
anus, anal 565.0
congenital 751.5
buccal cavity 528.9
clitoris (congenital) 752.49
ear, lobule (congenital) 744.29
epiglottis (congenital) 748.3
larynx 478.79
congenital 748.3
lip 528.5
congenital (*see also* Cleft, lip) 749.10
nipple 611.2
puerperal, postpartum 676.1 ☑
palate (congenital) (*see also* Cleft, palate) 749.00
postanal 565.0
rectum 565.0
skin 709.8
streptococcal 686.9
spine (congenital) (*see also* Spina bifida) 741.9 ☑
sternum (congenital) 756.3
tongue (acquired) 529.5
congenital 750.13
Fistula (sinus) 686.9
abdomen (wall) 569.81
bladder 596.2
intestine 569.81
ureter 593.82

Fistula — *continued*

abdomen — *continued*
uterus 619.2
abdominorectal 569.81
abdominosigmoidal 569.81
abdominothoracic 510.0
abdominouterine 619.2
congenital 752.39
abdominovesical 596.2
accessory sinuses (*see also* Sinusitis) 473.9
actinomycotic — *see* Actinomycosis
alveolar
antrum (*see also* Sinusitis, maxillary) 473.0
process 522.7
anorectal 565.1
antrobuccal (*see also* Sinusitis, maxillary) 473.0
antrum (*see also* Sinusitis, maxillary) 473.0
anus, anal (infectional) (recurrent) 565.1
congenital 751.5
tuberculous (*see also* Tuberculosis) 014.8 ☑
aortic sinus 747.29
aortoduodenal 447.2
appendix, appendicular 543.9
arteriovenous (acquired) 447.0
brain 437.3
congenital 747.81
ruptured (*see also* Hemorrhage, subarachnoid) 430
ruptured (*see also* Hemorrhage, subarachnoid) 430
cerebral 437.3
congenital 747.81
congenital (peripheral) 747.60
brain — *see* Fistula, arteriovenous, brain, congenital
coronary 746.85
gastrointestinal 747.61
lower limb 747.64
pulmonary 747.39
renal 747.62
specified site NEC 747.69
upper limb 747.63
coronary 414.19
congenital 746.85
heart 414.19
pulmonary (vessels) 417.0
congenital 747.39
surgically created (for dialysis) V45.11
complication NEC 996.73
atherosclerosis — *see* Arteriosclerosis, extremities
embolism 996.74
infection or inflammation 996.62
mechanical 996.1
occlusion NEC 996.74
thrombus 996.74
traumatic — *see* Injury, blood vessel, by site
artery 447.2
aural 383.81
congenital 744.49
auricle 383.81
congenital 744.49
Bartholin's gland 619.8
bile duct (*see also* Fistula, biliary) 576.4
biliary (duct) (tract) 576.4
congenital 751.69
bladder (neck) (sphincter) 596.2
into seminal vesicle 596.2
bone 733.99
brain 348.89
arteriovenous — *see* Fistula, arteriovenous, brain
branchial (cleft) 744.41
branchiogenous 744.41
breast 611.0
puerperal, postpartum 675.1 ☑
bronchial 510.0
bronchocutaneous, bronchomediastinal, bronchopleural, bronchopleuromediastinal (infective) 510.0
tuberculous (*see also* Tuberculosis) 011.3 ☑

Fistula — *continued*

bronchoesophageal 530.89
congenital 750.3
buccal cavity (infective) 528.3
canal, ear 380.89
carotid-cavernous
congenital 747.81
with hemorrhage 430
traumatic 900.82
with hemorrhage (*see also* Hemorrhage, brain, traumatic) 853.0 ☑
late effect 908.3
cecosigmoidal 569.81
cecum 569.81
cerebrospinal (fluid) 349.81
cervical, lateral (congenital) 744.41
cervicoaural (congenital) 744.49
cervicosigmoidal 619.1
cervicovesical 619.0
cervix 619.8
chest (wall) 510.0
cholecystocolic (*see also* Fistula, gallbladder) 575.5
cholecystocolonic (*see also* Fistula, gallbladder) 575.5
cholecystoduodenal (*see also* Fistula, gallbladder) 575.5
cholecystoenteric (*see also* Fistula, gallbladder) 575.5
cholecystogastric (*see also* Fistula, gallbladder) 575.5
cholecystointestinal (*see also* Fistula, gallbladder) 575.5
choledochoduodenal 576.4
cholocolic (*see also* Fistula, gallbladder) 575.5
coccyx 685.1
with abscess 685.0
colon 569.81
colostomy 569.69
colovaginal (acquired) 619.1
common duct (bile duct) 576.4
congenital, NEC — *see* Anomaly, specified type NEC
cornea, causing hypotony 360.32
coronary, arteriovenous 414.19
congenital 746.85
costal region 510.0
cul-de-sac, Douglas' 619.8
cutaneous 686.9
cystic duct (*see also* Fistula, gallbladder) 575.5
congenital 751.69
cystostomy 596.83
dental 522.7
diaphragm 510.0
bronchovisceral 510.0
pleuroperitoneal 510.0
pulmonoperitoneal 510.0
duodenum 537.4
ear (canal) (external) 380.89
enterocolic 569.81
enterocutaneous 569.81
enteroenteric 569.81
entero-uterine 619.1
congenital 752.39
enterovaginal 619.1
congenital 752.49
enterovesical 596.1
epididymis 608.89
tuberculous (*see also* Tuberculosis) 016.4 ☑
esophagobronchial 530.89
congenital 750.3
esophagocutaneous 530.89
esophagopleurocutaneous 530.89
esophagotracheal 530.84
congenital 750.3
esophagus 530.89
congenital 750.4
ethmoid (*see also* Sinusitis, ethmoidal) 473.2
eyeball (cornea) (sclera) 360.32
eyelid 373.11
fallopian tube (external) 619.2
fecal 569.81

☑ **Additional Digit Required** — Refer to the Tabular List for Digit Selection

⬇ **Subterms under main terms may continue to next column or page**

Fitting — *continued*
  device, unspecified type — *continued*
    prosthetic — *continued*
      specified type NEC V52.8
    special senses V53.09
    substitution
      auditory V53.09
      nervous system V53.09
      visual V53.09
    urinary V53.6
  diaphragm (contraceptive) V25.02
  gastric lap band V53.51
  gastrointestinal appliance and device NEC V53.59
  glasses (reading) V53.1
  growth rod V54.02
  hearing aid V53.2
  ileostomy device V53.5 ☑
  intestinal appliance and device V53.50
  intestinal appliance or device NEC V53.5 ☑
  intrauterine contraceptive device
    insertion V25.11
    removal V25.12
      and reinsertion V25.13
    replacement V25.13
  neuropacemaker (brain) (peripheral nerve) (spinal cord) V53.02
  orthodontic device V53.4
  orthopedic (device) V53.7
    brace V53.7
    cast V53.7
    corset V53.7
    shoes V53.7
  pacemaker (cardiac) V53.31
    brain V53.02
    carotid sinus V53.39
    peripheral nerve V53.02
    spinal cord V53.02
  prosthesis V52.9
    arm (complete) (partial) V52.0
    breast V52.4
      implant exchange (different material) (different size) V52.4
    dental V52.3
    eye V52.2
    leg (complete) (partial) V52.1
    specified type NEC V52.8
  spectacles V53.1
  wheelchair V53.8
Fitz-Hugh and Curtis syndrome 098.86
  due to
    Chlamydia trachomatis 099.56
    Neisseria gonorrhoeae (gonococcal peritonitis) 098.86
Fitz's syndrome (acute hemorrhagic pancreatitis) 577.0
Fixation
  joint — *see* Ankylosis
  larynx 478.79
  pupil 364.76
  stapes 385.22
    deafness (*see also* Deafness, conductive) 389.04
  uterus (acquired) — *see* Malposition, uterus
  vocal cord 478.5
Flaccid — *see also* condition
  foot 736.79
  forearm 736.09
  palate, congenital 750.26
Flail
  chest 807.4
    newborn 767.3
  joint (paralytic) 718.80
    ankle 718.87
    elbow 718.82
    foot 718.87
    hand 718.84
    hip 718.85
    knee 718.86
    multiple sites 718.89
    pelvic region 718.85
    shoulder (region) 718.81
    specified site NEC 718.88
    wrist 718.83
Flajani (-Basedow) syndrome or disease (exophthalmic goiter) 242.0 ☑

Flap, liver 572.8
Flare, anterior chamber (aqueous) (eye) 364.04
Flashback phenomena (drug) (hallucinogenic) 292.89
Flat
  chamber (anterior) (eye) 360.34
  chest, congenital 754.89
  electroencephalogram (EEG) 348.89
  foot (acquired) (fixed type) (painful) (postural) (spastic) 734
    congenital 754.61
      rocker bottom 754.61
      vertical talus 754.61
    rachitic 268.1
    rocker bottom (congenital) 754.61
    vertical talus, congenital 754.61
  organ or site, congenital NEC — *see* Anomaly, specified type NEC
  pelvis 738.6
    with disproportion (fetopelvic) 653.2 ☑
      affecting fetus or newborn 763.1
      causing obstructed labor 660.1 ☑
        affecting fetus or newborn 763.1
    congenital 755.69
Flatau-Schilder disease 341.1
Flattening
  head, femur 736.39
  hip 736.39
  lip (congenital) 744.89
  nose (congenital) 754.0
    acquired 738.0
Flatulence 787.3
Flatus 787.3
  vaginalis 629.89
Flax dressers' disease 504
Flea bite — *see* Injury, superficial, by site
Fleischer (-Kayser) ring (corneal pigmentation) 275.1 *[371.14]*
Fleischner's disease 732.3
Fleshy mole 631.8
Flexibilitas cerea — *see also* Catalepsy 300.11
Flexion
  cervix — *see* Flexion, uterus
  contracture, joint (*see also* Contraction, joint) 718.4 ☑
  deformity, joint (*see also* Contraction, joint) 736.9
    hip, congenital (*see also* Subluxation, congenital, hip) 754.32
  uterus (*see also* Malposition, uterus) 621.6
Flexner's
  bacillus 004.1
  diarrhea (ulcerative) 004.1
  dysentery 004.1
Flexner-Boyd dysentery 004.2
Flexure — *see* condition
Floater, vitreous 379.24
Floating
  cartilage (joint) (*see also* Disorder, cartilage, articular) 718.0 ☑
    knee 717.6
  gallbladder (congenital) 751.69
  kidney 593.0
    congenital 753.3
  liver (congenital) 751.69
  rib 756.3
  spleen 289.59
Flooding 626.2
Floor — *see* condition
Floppy
  infant NEC 781.99
  iris syndrome 364.81
  valve syndrome (mitral) 424.0
Flu — *see also* Influenza
  bird (*see also* Influenza, avian) 488.02
  gastric NEC 008.8
  swine — *see* Influenza (novel) 2009 H1N1
Fluctuating blood pressure 796.4
Fluid
  abdomen 789.59
  chest (*see also* Pleurisy, with effusion) 511.9
  heart (*see also* Failure, heart) 428.0
  joint (*see also* Effusion, joint) 719.0 ☑
  loss (acute) 276.50

Fluid — *continued*
  loss — *continued*
    with
      hypernatremia 276.0
      hyponatremia 276.1
  lung (*see also* Edema, lung)
    encysted 511.89
  peritoneal cavity 789.59
    malignant 789.51
  pleural cavity (*see also* Pleurisy, with effusion) 511.9
  retention 276.69
Flukes NEC — *see also* Infestation, fluke 121.9
  blood NEC (*see also* Infestation, Schistosoma) 120.9
  liver 121.3
Fluor (albus) (vaginalis) 623.5
  trichomonal (Trichomonas vaginalis) 131.00
Fluorosis (dental) (chronic) 520.3
Flushing 782.62
  menopausal 627.2
Flush syndrome 259.2
Flutter
  atrial or auricular 427.32
  heart (ventricular) 427.42
    atrial 427.32
    impure 427.32
    postoperative 997.1
    ventricular 427.42
Flux (bloody) (serosanguineous) 009.0
FNHTR (febrile nonhemolytic transfusion reaction) 780.66
Focal — *see* condition
Fochier's abscess — *see* Abscess, by site
Focus, Assmann's — *see also* Tuberculosis 011.0 ☑
Fogo selvagem 694.4
Foix-Alajouanine syndrome 336.1
Folds, anomalous — *see also* Anomaly, specified type NEC
  Bowman's membrane 371.31
  Descemet's membrane 371.32
  epicanthic 743.63
  heart 746.89
  posterior segment of eye, congenital 743.54
Folie à deux 297.3
Follicle
  cervix (nabothian) (ruptured) 616.0
  graafian, ruptured, with hemorrhage 620.0
  nabothian 616.0
Folliclis (primary) — *see also* Tuberculosis 017.0 ☑
Follicular — *see also* condition
  cyst (atretic) 620.0
Folliculitis 704.8
  abscedens et suffodiens 704.8
  decalvans 704.09
  gonorrheal (acute) 098.0
    chronic or duration of 2 months or more 098.2
  keloid, keloidalis 706.1
  pustular 704.8
  ulerythematosa reticulata 701.8
Folliculosis, conjunctival 372.02
Følling's disease (phenylketonuria) 270.1
Follow-up (examination) (routine) (following) V67.9
  cancer chemotherapy V67.2
  chemotherapy V67.2
  fracture V67.4
  high-risk medication V67.51
  injury NEC V67.59
  postpartum
    immediately after delivery V24.0
    routine V24.2
  psychiatric V67.3
  psychotherapy V67.3
  radiotherapy V67.1
  specified condition NEC V67.59
  specified surgery NEC V67.09
  surgery V67.00
    vaginal pap smear V67.01
  treatment V67.9
    combined NEC V67.6
    fracture V67.4

Follow-up — *continued*
  treatment — *continued*
    involving high-risk medication NEC V67.51
    mental disorder V67.3
    specified NEC V67.59
Fong's syndrome (hereditary osteoonychodysplasia) 756.89
Food
  allergy 693.1
  anaphylactic reaction or shock due to food
  asphyxia (from aspiration or inhalation) (*see also* Asphyxia, food) 933.1
  choked on (*see also* Asphyxia, food) 933.1
  deprivation 994.2
    specified kind of food NEC 269.8
  intoxication (*see also* Poisoning, food) 005.9
  lack of 994.2
  poisoning (*see also* Poisoning, food) 005.9
  refusal or rejection NEC 307.59
  strangulation or suffocation (*see also* Asphyxia, food) 933.1
  toxemia (*see also* Poisoning, food) 005.9
Foot — *see also* condition
  and mouth disease 078.4
  process disease 581.3
Foramen ovale (nonclosure) (patent) (persistent) 745.5
Forbes-Albright syndrome (nonpuerperal amenorrhea and lactation associated with pituitary tumor) 253.1
Forbes'(glycogen storage) disease 271.0
Forced birth or delivery NEC 669.8 ☑
  affecting fetus or newborn NEC 763.89
Forceps
  delivery NEC 669.5 ☑
    affecting fetus or newborn 763.2
Fordyce's disease (ectopic sebaceous glands) (mouth) 750.26
Fordyce-Fox disease (apocrine miliaria) 705.82
Forearm — *see* condition
Foreign body

Note — For foreign body with open wound, or other injury, see Wound, open, or the type of injury specified.

  accidentally left during a procedure 998.4
  anterior chamber (eye) 871.6
    magnetic 871.5
      retained or old 360.51
    retained or old 360.61
  ciliary body (eye) 871.6
    magnetic 871.5
      retained or old 360.52
    retained or old 360.62
  entering through orifice (current) (old)
    accessory sinus 932
    air passage (upper) 933.0
      lower 934.8
    alimentary canal 938
    alveolar process 935.0
    antrum (Highmore) 932
    anus 937
    appendix 936
    asphyxia due to (*see also* Asphyxia, food) 933.1
    auditory canal 931
    auricle 931
    bladder 939.0
    bronchioles 934.8
    bronchus (main) 934.1
    buccal cavity 935.0
    canthus (inner) 930.1
    cecum 936
    cervix (canal) uterine 939.1
    coil, ileocecal 936
    colon 936
    conjunctiva 930.1
    conjunctival sac 930.1
    cornea 930.0
    digestive organ or tract NEC 938
    duodenum 936
    ear (external) 931
    esophagus 935.1
    eye (external) 930.9
      combined sites 930.8

☑ Additional Digit Required — Refer to the Tabular List for Digit Selection   ⏷ Subterms under main terms may continue to next column or page

2014 ICD-9-CM   **165**

Foreign body — *continued*
  entering through orifice — *continued*
    eye — *continued*
      intraocular — *see* Foreign body, by
        site
      specified site NEC 930.8
    eyeball 930.8
      intraocular — *see* Foreign body, in-
        traocular
    eyelid 930.1
      retained or old 374.86
    frontal sinus 932
    gastrointestinal tract 938
    genitourinary tract 939.9
    globe 930.8
      penetrating 871.6
        magnetic 871.5
          retained or old 360.50
        retained or old 360.60
    gum 935.0
    Highmore's antrum 932
    hypopharynx 933.0
    ileocecal coil 936
    ileum 936
    inspiration (of) 933.1
    intestine (large) (small) 936
    lacrimal apparatus, duct, gland, or sac
      930.2
    larynx 933.1
    lung 934.8
    maxillary sinus 932
    mouth 935.0
    nasal sinus 932
    nasopharynx 933.0
    nose (passage) 932
    nostril 932
    oral cavity 935.0
    palate 935.0
    penis 939.3
    pharynx 933.0
    pyriform sinus 933.0
    rectosigmoid 937
      junction 937
    rectum 937
    respiratory tract 934.9
      specified part NEC 934.8
    sclera 930.1
    sinus 932
      accessory 932
      frontal 932
      maxillary 932
      nasal 932
      pyriform 933.0
    small intestine 936
    stomach (hairball) 935.2
    suffocation by (*see also* Asphyxia, food)
      933.1
    swallowed 938
      tongue 933.0
    tear ducts or glands 930.2
    throat 933.0
    tongue 935.0
      swallowed 933.0
    tonsil, tonsillar 933.0
      fossa 933.0
    trachea 934.0
    ureter 939.0
    urethra 939.0
    uterus (any part) 939.1
    vagina 939.2
    vulva 939.2
    wind pipe 934.0
  feeling of, in throat 784.99
  granuloma (old) 728.82
    bone 733.99
    in operative wound (inadvertently left)
      998.4
      due to surgical material intentionally
        left — *see* Complications, due
        to (presence of) any device,
        implant, or graft classified to
        996.0–996.5 NEC
    muscle 728.82
    skin 709.4
    soft tissue 709.4
    subcutaneous tissue 709.4

Foreign body — *continued*
  in
    bone (residual) 733.99
    open wound — *see* Wound, open, by
      site complicated
    soft tissue (residual) 729.6
  inadvertently left in operation wound
    (causing adhesions, obstruction, or
    perforation) 998.4
  ingestion, ingested NEC 938
  inhalation or inspiration (*see also* Asphyxia,
    food) 933.1
  internal organ, not entering through an
    orifice — *see* Injury, internal, by site,
    with open wound
  intraocular (nonmagnetic) 871.6
    combined sites 871.6
      magnetic 871.5
        retained or old 360.59
      retained or old 360.69
    magnetic 871.5
      retained or old 360.50
    retained or old 360.60
    specified site NEC 871.6
      magnetic 871.5
        retained or old 360.59
      retained or old 360.69
  iris (nonmagnetic) 871.6
    magnetic 871.5
      retained or old 360.52
    retained or old 360.62
  lens (nonmagnetic) 871.6
    magnetic 871.5
      retained or old 360.53
    retained or old 360.63
  lid, eye 930.1
  ocular muscle 870.4
    retained or old 376.6
  old or residual
    bone 733.99
    eyelid 374.86
    middle ear 385.83
    muscle 729.6
      ocular 376.6
    retrobulbar 376.6
    skin 729.6
      with granuloma 709.4
    soft tissue 729.6
      with granuloma 709.4
    subcutaneous tissue 729.6
      with granuloma 709.4
  operation wound, left accidentally 998.4
  orbit 870.4
    retained or old 376.6
  posterior wall, eye 871.6
    magnetic 871.5
      retained or old 360.55
    retained or old 360.65
  respiratory tree 934.9
    specified site NEC 934.8
  retained (old) (nonmagnetic) (in) V90.9
    anterior chamber (eye) 360.61
      magnetic 360.51
    ciliary body 360.62
      magnetic 360.52
    eyelid 374.86
    fragment(s)
      acrylics V90.2
      animal quills V90.31
      animal spines V90.31
      cement V90.83
      concrete V90.83
      crystalline V90.83
      depleted
        isotope V90.09
        uranium V90.01
      diethylhexylphthalates V90.2
      glass V90.81
      isocyanate V90.2
      metal V90.10
        magnetic V90.11
        nonmagnetic V90.12
      organic NEC V90.39
      plastic V90.2
      radioactive
        nontherapeutic V90.09

Foreign body — *continued*
  retained — *continued*
    fragment(s) — *continued*
      radioactive — *continued*
        specified NEC V90.09
      stone V90.83
      tooth V90.32
      wood V90.33
    globe 360.60
      magnetic 360.50
    intraocular 360.60
      magnetic 360.50
      specified site NEC 360.69
        magnetic 360.59
    iris 360.62
      magnetic 360.52
    lens 360.63
      magnetic 360.53
    muscle 729.6
    orbit 376.6
    posterior wall of globe 360.65
      magnetic 360.55
    retina 360.65
      magnetic 360.55
    retrobulbar 376.6
    skin 729.6
      with granuloma 709.4
    soft tissue 729.6
      with granuloma 709.4
    specified NEC V90.89
    subcutaneous tissue 729.6
      with granuloma 709.4
    vitreous 360.64
      magnetic 360.54
  retina 871.6
    magnetic 871.5
      retained or old 360.55
    retained or old 360.65
  superficial, without major open wound (*see*
    also Injury, superficial, by site) 919.6
  swallowed NEC 938
  throat, feeling of 784.99
  vitreous (humor) 871.6
    magnetic 871.5
      retained or old 360.54
    retained or old 360.64

Forking, aqueduct of Sylvius 742.3
  with spina bifida (*see also* Spina bifida)
    741.0 ☑
Formation
  bone in scar tissue (skin) 709.3
  connective tissue in vitreous 379.25
  Elschnig pearls (postcataract extraction)
    366.51
  hyaline in cornea 371.49
  sequestrum in bone (due to infection) (*see*
    also Osteomyelitis) 730.1 ☑
  valve
    colon, congenital 751.5
    ureter (congenital) 753.29
Formication 782.0
Fort Bragg fever 100.89
Fossa — *see also* condition
  pyriform — *see* condition
Foster care (status) V60.81
Foster-Kennedy syndrome 377.04
Fothergill's
  disease, meaning scarlatina anginosa 034.1
  neuralgia (*see also* Neuralgia, trigeminal)
    350.1
Foul breath 784.99
Found dead (cause unknown) 798.9
Foundling V20.0
Fournier's disease (idiopathic gangrene)
  608.83
  female 616.89
Fourth
  cranial nerve — *see* condition
  disease 057.8
  molar 520.1
Foville's syndrome 344.89
Fox's
  disease (apocrine miliaria) 705.82
  impetigo (contagiosa) 684
Fox-Fordyce disease (apocrine miliaria) 705.82

Fracture (abduction) (adduction) (avulsion)
  (compression) (crush) (dislocation)
  (oblique) (separation) (closed) 829.0

> *Note — For fracture of any of the fol-*
> *lowing sites with fracture of other bones*
> *— see Fracture, multiple.*
>
> *"Closed" includes the following descrip-*
> *tions of fractures, with or without de-*
> *layed healing, unless they are specified*
> *as open or compound:*
>
> | | |
> |---|---|
> | comminuted | linear |
> | depressed | simple |
> | elevated | slipped epiphysis |
> | fissured | spiral |
> | greenstick | unspecified |
> | impacted | |
>
> *"Open" includes the following descrip-*
> *tions of fractures, with or without de-*
> *layed healing:*
>
> | | |
> |---|---|
> | compound | puncture |
> | infected | with foreign body |
> | missile | |
>
> *For late effect of fracture, see Late, ef-*
> *fect, fracture, by site.*

  with
    internal injuries in same region (condi-
      tions classifiable to 860–869) (*see*
      also Injury, internal, by site)
    pelvic region — *see* Fracture, pelvis
  acetabulum (with visceral injury) (closed)
    808.0
    open 808.1
  acromion (process) (closed) 811.01
    open 811.11
  alveolus (closed) 802.8
    open 802.9
  ankle (malleolus) (closed) 824.8
    bimalleolar (Dupuytren's) (Pott's) 824.4
      open 824.5
    bone 825.21
      open 825.31
    lateral malleolus only (fibular) 824.2
      open 824.3
    medial malleolus only (tibial) 824.0
      open 824.1
    open 824.9
    pathologic 733.16
    talus 825.21
      open 825.31
    trimalleolar 824.6
      open 824.7
  antrum — *see* Fracture, skull, base
  arm (closed) 818.0
    and leg(s) (any bones) 828.0
      open 828.1
    both (any bones) (with rib(s)) (with ster-
      num) 819.0
      open 819.1
    lower 813.80
      open 813.90
    open 818.1
    upper — *see* Fracture, humerus
  astragalus (closed) 825.21
    open 825.31
  atlas — *see* Fracture, vertebra, cervical, first
  axis — *see* Fracture, vertebra, cervical, sec-
    ond
  back — *see* Fracture, vertebra, by site
  Barton's — *see* Fracture, radius, lower end
  basal (skull) — *see* Fracture, skull, base
  Bennett's (closed) 815.01
    open 815.11
  bimalleolar (closed) 824.4
    open 824.5
  bone (closed) NEC 829.0
    birth injury NEC 767.3
    open 829.1
    pathologic NEC (*see also* Fracture,
      pathologic) 733.10

☑ **Additional Digit Required** — Refer to the Tabular List for Digit Selection ▽ **Subterms under main terms may continue to next column or page**

166   **2014 ICD-9-CM**

Fracture — *continued*
- bone — *continued*
  - stress NEC (*see also* Fracture, stress) 733.95
  - boot top — *see* Fracture, fibula
  - boxers' — *see* Fracture, metacarpal bone(s)
  - breast bone — *see* Fracture, sternum
  - bucket handle (semilunar cartilage) — *see* Tear, meniscus
  - buckle — *see* Fracture, torus
  - burst — *see* Fracture, traumatic, by site
  - bursting — *see* Fracture, phalanx, hand, distal
  - calcaneus (closed) 825.0
    - open 825.1
  - capitate (bone) (closed) 814.07
    - open 814.17
  - capitellum (humerus) (closed) 812.49
    - open 812.59
  - carpal bone(s) (wrist NEC) (closed) 814.00
    - open 814.10
    - specified site NEC 814.09
      - open 814.19
  - cartilage, knee (semilunar) — *see* Tear, meniscus
  - cervical — *see* Fracture, vertebra, cervical
  - chauffeur's — *see* Fracture, ulna, lower end
  - chisel — *see* Fracture, radius, upper end
  - chronic — *see* Fracture, pathologic
  - clavicle (interligamentous part) (closed) 810.00
    - acromial end 810.03
      - open 810.13
    - due to birth trauma 767.2
    - open 810.10
    - shaft (middle third) 810.02
      - open 810.12
    - sternal end 810.01
      - open 810.11
  - clayshovelers' — *see* Fracture, vertebra, cervical
  - coccyx (*see also* Fracture, vertebra, coccyx)
    - complicating delivery 665.6 ☑
  - collar bone — *see* Fracture, clavicle
  - Colles' (reversed) (closed) 813.41
    - open 813.51
  - comminuted — *see* Fracture, by site
  - compression (*see also* Fracture, by site)
    - nontraumatic — *see* Fracture, pathologic
  - congenital 756.9
  - coracoid process (closed) 811.02
    - open 811.12
  - coronoid process (ulna) (closed) 813.02
    - mandible (closed) 802.23
      - open 802.33
    - open 813.12
  - corpus cavernosum penis 959.13
  - costochondral junction — *see* Fracture, rib
  - costosternal junction — *see* Fracture, rib
  - cranium — *see* Fracture, skull, by site
  - cricoid cartilage (closed) 807.5
    - open 807.6
  - cuboid (ankle) (closed) 825.23
    - open 825.33
  - cuneiform
    - foot (closed) 825.24
      - open 825.34
    - wrist (closed) 814.03
      - open 814.13
  - dental implant 525.73
  - dental restorative material
    - with loss of material 525.64
    - without loss of material 525.63
  - due to
    - birth injury — *see* Birth injury, fracture
    - gunshot — *see* Fracture, by site, open
    - neoplasm — *see* Fracture, pathologic
    - osteoporosis — *see* Fracture, pathologic
  - Dupuytren's (ankle) (fibula) (closed) 824.4
    - open 824.5
    - radius 813.42
      - open 813.52
  - Duverney's — *see* Fracture, ilium
  - elbow (*see also* Fracture, humerus, lower end)
    - olecranon (process) (closed) 813.01

Fracture — *continued*
- elbow (*see also* Fracture, humerus, lower end) — *continued*
  - olecranon — *continued*
    - open 813.11
  - supracondylar (closed) 812.41
    - open 812.51
  - ethmoid (bone) (sinus) — *see* Fracture, skull, base
  - face bone(s) (closed) NEC 802.8
    - with
      - other bone(s) — *see* Fracture, multiple, skull
      - skull (*see also* Fracture, skull)
        - involving other bones — *see* Fracture, multiple, skull
    - open 802.9
  - fatigue — *see* Fracture, march
  - femur, femoral (closed) 821.00
    - cervicotrochanteric 820.03
      - open 820.13
    - condyles, epicondyles 821.21
      - open 821.31
    - distal end — *see* Fracture, femur, lower end
    - epiphysis (separation)
      - capital 820.01
        - open 820.11
      - head 820.01
        - open 820.11
      - lower 821.22
        - open 821.32
      - trochanteric 820.01
        - open 820.11
      - upper 820.01
        - open 820.11
    - head 820.09
      - open 820.19
    - lower end or extremity (distal end) (closed) 821.20
      - condyles, epicondyles 821.21
        - open 821.31
      - epiphysis (separation) 821.22
        - open 821.32
      - multiple sites 821.29
        - open 821.39
      - specified site NEC 821.29
        - open 821.39
      - supracondylar 821.23
        - open 821.33
      - T-shaped 821.21
        - open 821.31
    - neck (closed) 820.8
      - base (cervicotrochanteric) 820.03
        - open 820.13
      - extracapsular 820.20
        - open 820.30
      - intertrochanteric (section) 820.21
        - open 820.31
      - intracapsular 820.00
        - open 820.10
      - intratrochanteric 820.21
        - open 820.31
      - midcervical 820.02
        - open 820.12
      - open 820.9
      - pathologic 733.14
        - specified part NEC 733.15
      - specified site NEC 820.09
        - open 820.19
      - stress 733.96
      - transcervical 820.02
        - open 820.12
      - transtrochanteric 820.20
        - open 820.30
    - open 821.10
    - pathologic 733.14
      - specified part NEC 733.15
    - peritrochanteric (section) 820.20
      - open 820.30
    - shaft (lower third) (middle third) (upper third) 821.01
      - open 821.11
      - stress 733.97
    - subcapital 820.09

Fracture — *continued*
- femur, femoral — *continued*
  - subcapital — *continued*
    - open 820.19
  - subtrochanteric (region) (section) 820.22
    - open 820.32
  - supracondylar 821.23
    - open 821.33
  - transepiphyseal 820.01
    - open 820.11
  - trochanter (greater) (lesser) (*see also* Fracture, femur, neck, by site) 820.20
    - open 820.30
  - T-shaped, into knee joint 821.21
    - open 821.31
  - upper end 820.8
    - open 820.9
  - fibula (closed) 823.81
    - with tibia 823.82
      - open 823.92
    - distal end 824.8
      - open 824.9
    - epiphysis
      - lower 824.8
        - open 824.9
      - upper — *see* Fracture, fibula, upper end
    - head — *see* Fracture, fibula, upper end
    - involving ankle 824.2
      - open 824.3
    - lower end or extremity 824.8
      - open 824.9
    - malleolus (external) (lateral) 824.2
      - open 824.3
    - open NEC 823.91
    - pathologic 733.16
    - proximal end — *see* Fracture, fibula, upper end
    - shaft 823.21
      - with tibia 823.22
        - open 823.32
      - open 823.31
    - stress 733.93
    - torus 823.41
      - with tibia 823.42
    - upper end or extremity (epiphysis) (head) (proximal end) (styloid) 823.01
      - with tibia 823.02
        - open 823.12
      - open 823.11
  - finger(s), of one hand (closed) (*see also* Fracture, phalanx, hand) 816.00
    - with
      - metacarpal bone(s), of same hand 817.0
        - open 817.1
      - thumb of same hand 816.03
        - open 816.13
    - open 816.10
  - foot, except toe(s) alone (closed) 825.20
    - open 825.30
  - forearm (closed) NEC 813.80
    - lower end (distal end) (lower epiphysis) 813.40
      - open 813.50
    - open 813.90
    - shaft 813.20
      - open 813.30
    - upper end (proximal end) (upper epiphysis) 813.00
      - open 813.10
  - fossa, anterior, middle, or posterior — *see* Fracture, skull, base
  - Fracture (abduction) (adduction) (avulsion) (compression) (crush) (dislocation) (oblique) (separation) (closed) 829.0
  - frontal (bone) (*see also* Fracture, skull, vault)
    - sinus — *see* Fracture, skull, base
  - Galeazzi's — *see* Fracture, radius, lower end
  - glenoid (cavity) (fossa) (scapula) (closed) 811.03
    - open 811.13
  - Gosselin's — *see* Fracture, ankle
  - greenstick — *see* Fracture, by site

Fracture — *continued*
- grenade-throwers' — *see* Fracture, humerus, shaft
- gutter — *see* Fracture, skull, vault
- hamate (closed) 814.08
  - open 814.18
- hand, one (closed) 815.00
  - carpals 814.00
    - open 814.10
    - specified site NEC 814.09
      - open 814.19
  - metacarpals 815.00
    - open 815.10
  - multiple, bones of one hand 817.0
    - open 817.1
  - open 815.10
  - phalanges (*see also* Fracture, phalanx, hand) 816.00
    - open 816.10
- healing
  - aftercare (*see also* Aftercare, fracture) V54.89
  - change of cast V54.89
  - complications — *see* condition
  - convalescence V66.4
  - removal of
    - cast V54.89
    - fixation device
      - external V54.89
      - internal V54.01
- heel bone (closed) 825.0
  - open 825.1
- Hill-Sachs 812.09
- hip (closed) (*see also* Fracture, femur, neck) 820.8
  - open 820.9
  - pathologic 733.14
- humerus (closed) 812.20
  - anatomical neck 812.02
    - open 812.12
  - articular process (*see also* Fracture humerus, condyle(s)) 812.44
    - open 812.54
  - capitellum 812.49
    - open 812.59
  - condyle(s) 812.44
    - lateral (external) 812.42
      - open 812.52
    - medial (internal epicondyle) 812.43
      - open 812.53
    - open 812.54
  - distal end — *see* Fracture, humerus, lower end
  - epiphysis
    - lower (*see also* Fracture, humerus, condyle(s)) 812.44
      - open 812.54
    - upper 812.09
      - open 812.19
  - external condyle 812.42
    - open 812.52
  - great tuberosity 812.03
    - open 812.13
  - head 812.09
    - open 812.19
  - internal epicondyle 812.43
    - open 812.53
  - lesser tuberosity 812.09
    - open 812.19
  - lower end or extremity (distal end) (*see also* Fracture, humerus, by site) 812.40
    - multiple sites NEC 812.49
      - open 812.59
    - open 812.50
    - specified site NEC 812.49
      - open 812.59
  - neck 812.01
    - open 812.11
  - open 812.30
  - pathologic 733.11
  - proximal end — *see* Fracture, humerus, upper end
  - shaft 812.21
    - open 812.31
  - supracondylar 812.41

Fracture — Fracture

☑ **Additional Digit Required** — Refer to the Tabular List for Digit Selection   ▽ **Subterms under main terms may continue to next column or page**

2014 ICD-9-CM   167

Fracture — Fracture

Fracture — *continued*
  humerus — *continued*
    supracondylar — *continued*
      open 812.51
    surgical neck 812.01
      open 812.11
    trochlea 812.49
      open 812.59
    T-shaped 812.44
      open 812.54
    tuberosity — *see* Fracture, humerus, upper end
    upper end or extremity (proximal end) (*see also* Fracture, humerus, by site) 812.00
      open 812.10
      specified site NEC 812.09
        open 812.19
  hyoid bone (closed) 807.5
    open 807.6
  hyperextension — *see* Fracture, radius, lower end
  ilium (with visceral injury) (closed) 808.41
    open 808.51
  impaction, impacted — *see* Fracture, by site
  incus — *see* Fracture, skull, base
  innominate bone (with visceral injury) (closed) 808.49
    open 808.59
  instep, of one foot (closed) 825.20
    with toe(s) of same foot 827.0
      open 827.1
    open 825.30
  insufficiency — *see* Fracture, pathologic, by site
  internal
    ear — *see* Fracture, skull, base
    semilunar cartilage, knee — *see* Tear, meniscus, medial
  intertrochanteric — *see* Fracture, femur, neck, intertrochanteric
  ischium (with visceral injury) (closed) 808.42
    open 808.52
  jaw (bone) (lower) (closed) (*see also* Fracture, mandible) 802.20
    angle 802.25
      open 802.35
    open 802.30
    upper — *see* Fracture, maxilla
  knee
    cap (closed) 822.0
      open 822.1
    cartilage (semilunar) — *see* Tear, meniscus
  labyrinth (osseous) — *see* Fracture, skull, base
  larynx (closed) 807.5
    open 807.6
  late effect — *see* Late, effects (of), fracture
  Le Fort's — *see* Fracture, maxilla
  leg (closed) 827.0
    with rib(s) or sternum 828.0
      open 828.1
    both (any bones) 828.0
      open 828.1
    lower — *see* Fracture, tibia
    open 827.1
    upper — *see* Fracture, femur
  limb
    lower (multiple) (closed) NEC 827.0
      open 827.1
    upper (multiple) (closed) NEC 818.0
      open 818.1
  long bones, due to birth trauma — *see* Birth injury, fracture
  lower end or extremity (anterior lip) (posterior) 824.8
    open 824.9
  lumbar — *see* Fracture, vertebra, lumbar
  lunate bone (closed) 814.02
    open 814.12
  malar bone (closed) 802.4
    open 802.5
  Malgaigne's (closed) 808.43
    open 808.53
  malleolus (closed) 824.8

Fracture — *continued*
  malleolus — *continued*
    bimalleolar 824.4
      open 824.5
    lateral 824.2
      and medial (*see also* Fracture, malleolus, bimalleolar)
        with lip of tibia — *see* Fracture, malleolus, trimalleolar
      open 824.3
    medial (closed) 824.0
      and lateral (*see also* Fracture, malleolus, bimalleolar)
        with lip of tibia — *see* Fracture, malleolus, trimalleolar
      open 824.1
    open 824.9
    trimalleolar (closed) 824.6
      open 824.7
  malleus — *see* Fracture, skull, base
  malunion 733.81
  mandible (closed) 802.20
    angle 802.25
      open 802.35
    body 802.28
      alveolar border 802.27
        open 802.37
      open 802.38
      symphysis 802.26
        open 802.36
    condylar process 802.21
      open 802.31
    coronoid process 802.23
      open 802.33
    multiple sites 802.29
      open 802.39
    open 802.30
    ramus NEC 802.24
      open 802.34
    subcondylar 802.22
      open 802.32
  manubrium — *see* Fracture, sternum
  march 733.95
    femoral neck 733.96
    fibula 733.93
    metatarsals 733.94
    pelvis 733.98
    shaft of femur 733.97
    tibia 733.93
  maxilla, maxillary (superior) (upper jaw) (closed) 802.4
    inferior — *see* Fracture, mandible
    open 802.5
  meniscus, knee — *see* Tear, meniscus
  metacarpus, metacarpal (bone(s)), of one hand (closed) 815.00
    with phalanx, phalanges, hand (finger(s)) (thumb) of same hand 817.0
      open 817.1
    base 815.02
      first metacarpal 815.01
        open 815.11
      open 815.12
      thumb 815.01
        open 815.11
    multiple sites 815.09
      open 815.19
    neck 815.04
      open 815.14
    open 815.10
    shaft 815.03
      open 815.13
  metatarsus, metatarsal (bone(s)), of one foot (closed) 825.25
    with tarsal bone(s) 825.29
      open 825.39
    open 825.35
  Monteggia's (closed) 813.03
    open 813.13
  Moore's — *see* Fracture, radius, lower end
  multangular bone (closed)
    larger 814.05
      open 814.15
    smaller 814.06
      open 814.16

Fracture — *continued*
  multiple (closed) 829.0

> *Note* — *Multiple fractures of sites classifiable to the same three- or four-digit category are coded to that category, except for sites classifiable to 810–818 or 820–827 in different limbs.*
>
> *Multiple fractures of sites classifiable to different fourth-digit subdivisions within the same three-digit category should be dealt with according to coding rules.*
>
> *Multiple fractures of sites classifiable to different three-digit categories (identifiable from the listing under "Fracture"), and of sites classifiable to 810–818 or 820–827 in different limbs should be coded according to the following list, which should be referred to in the following priority order: skull or face bones, pelvis or vertebral column, legs, arms.*

    arm (multiple bones in same arm except in hand alone) (sites classifiable to 810–817 with sites classifiable to a different three-digit category in 810–817 in same arm) (closed) 818.0
      open 818.1
    arms, both or arm(s) with rib(s) or sternum (sites classifiable to 810–818 with sites classifiable to same range of categories in other limb or to 807) (closed) 819.0
      open 819.1
    bones of trunk NEC (closed) 809.0
      open 809.1
    hand, metacarpal bone(s) with phalanx or phalanges of same hand (sites classifiable to 815 with sites classifiable to 816 in same hand) (closed) 817.0
      open 817.1
    leg (multiple bones in same leg) (sites classifiable to 820–826 with sites classifiable to a different three-digit category in that range in same leg) (closed) 827.0
      open 827.1
    legs, both or leg(s) with arm(s), rib(s), or sternum (sites classifiable to 820–827 with sites classifiable to same range of categories in other leg or to 807 or 810–819) (closed) 828.0
      open 828.1
    open 829.1
    pelvis with other bones except skull or face bones (sites classifiable to 808 with sites classifiable to 805–807 or 810–829) (closed) 809.0
      open 809.1

Fracture — *continued*
  multiple — *continued*
    skull, specified or unspecified bones, or face bone(s) with any other bone(s) (sites classifiable to 800–803 with sites classifiable to 805–829) (closed) 804.0 ☑

> *Note* — *Use the following fifth-digit subclassification with categories 800, 801, 803, and 804:*
>
> 0   *unspecified state of consciousness*
>
> 1   *with no loss of consciousness*
>
> 2   *with brief [less than one hour] loss of consciousness*
>
> 3   *with moderate [1–24 hours] loss of consciousness*
>
> 4   *with prolonged [more than 24 hours] loss of consciousness and return to pre-existing conscious level*
>
> 5   *with prolonged [more than 24 hours] loss of consciousness, without return to pre-existing conscious level*
>
> *Use fifth-digit 5 to designate when a patient is unconscious and dies before regaining consciousness, regardless of the duration of the loss of consciousness*
>
> 6   *with loss of consciousness of unspecified duration*
>
> 9   *with concussion, unspecified*

      with
        contusion, cerebral 804.1 ☑
        epidural hemorrhage 804.2 ☑
        extradural hemorrhage 804.2 ☑
        hemorrhage (intracranial) NEC 804.3 ☑
        intracranial injury NEC 804.4 ☑
        laceration, cerebral 804.1 ☑
        subarachnoid hemorrhage 804.2 ☑
        subdural hemorrhage 804.2 ☑
      open 804.5 ☑
        with
          contusion, cerebral 804.6 ☑
          epidural hemorrhage 804.7 ☑
          extradural hemorrhage 804.7 ☑
          hemorrhage (intracranial) NEC 804.8 ☑
          intracranial injury NEC 804.9 ☑
          laceration, cerebral 804.6 ☑
          subarachnoid hemorrhage 804.7 ☑
          subdural hemorrhage 804.7 ☑
    vertebral column with other bones, except skull or face bones (sites classifiable to 805 or 806 with sites classifiable to 807–808 or 810–829) (closed) 809.0
      open 809.1
  nasal (bone(s)) (closed) 802.0
    open 802.1
    sinus — *see* Fracture, skull, base
  navicular
    carpal (wrist) (closed) 814.01
      open 814.11
    tarsal (ankle) (closed) 825.22
      open 825.32
  neck — *see* Fracture, vertebra, cervical
  neural arch — *see* Fracture, vertebra, by site
  nonunion 733.82
  nose, nasal, (bone) (septum) (closed) 802.0
    open 802.1
  occiput — *see* Fracture, skull, base
  odontoid process — *see* Fracture, vertebra, cervical
  olecranon (process) (ulna) (closed) 813.01

Fracture — *continued*
olecranon — *continued*
open 813.11
open 829.1
orbit, orbital (bone) (region) (closed) 802.8
floor (blow-out) 802.6
open 802.7
open 802.9
roof — *see* Fracture, skull, base
specified part NEC 802.8
open 802.9
os
calcis (closed) 825.0
open 825.1
magnum (closed) 814.07
open 814.17
pubis (with visceral injury) (closed) 808.2
open 808.3
triquetrum (closed) 814.03
open 814.13
osseous
auditory meatus — *see* Fracture, skull, base
labyrinth — *see* Fracture, skull, base
ossicles, auditory (incus) (malleus) (stapes) — *see* Fracture, skull, base
osteoporotic — *see* Fracture, pathologic
palate (closed) 802.8
open 802.9
paratrooper — *see* Fracture, tibia, lower end
parietal bone — *see* Fracture, skull, vault
parry — *see* Fracture, Monteggia's
patella (closed) 822.0
open 822.1
pathologic (cause unknown) 733.10
ankle 733.16
femur (neck) 733.14
specified NEC 733.15
fibula 733.16
hip 733.14
humerus 733.11
radius (distal) 733.12
specified site NEC 733.19
tibia 733.16
ulna 733.12
vertebrae (collapse) 733.13
wrist 733.12
pedicle (of vertebral arch) — *see* Fracture, vertebra, by site
pelvis, pelvic (bone(s)) (with visceral injury) (closed) 808.8
multiple
with
disruption of pelvic circle 808.43
open 808.53
disruption of pelvic ring 808.43
open 808.53
without
disruption of pelvic circle 808.44
open 808.54
disruption of pelvic ring 808.44
open 808.54
open 808.9
rim (closed) 808.49
open 808.59
stress 733.98
peritrochanteric (closed) 820.20
open 820.30
phalanx, phalanges, of one
foot (closed) 826.0
with bone(s) of same lower limb 827.0
open 827.1
open 826.1
hand (closed) 816.00
with metacarpal bone(s) of same hand 817.0
open 817.1
distal 816.02
open 816.12
middle 816.01
open 816.11
multiple sites NEC 816.03
open 816.13
open 816.10
proximal 816.01

Fracture — *continued*
phalanx, phalanges, of one — *continued*
hand — *continued*
proximal — *continued*
open 816.11
pisiform (closed) 814.04
open 814.14
pond — *see* Fracture, skull, vault
Pott's (closed) 824.4
open 824.5
prosthetic device, internal — *see* Complications, mechanical
pubis (with visceral injury) (closed) 808.2
open 808.3
Quervain's (closed) 814.01
open 814.11
radius (alone) (closed) 813.81
with ulna NEC 813.83
open 813.93
distal end — *see* Fracture, radius, lower end
epiphysis
lower — *see* Fracture, radius, lower end
upper — *see* Fracture, radius, upper end
head — *see* Fracture, radius, upper end
lower end or extremity (distal end) (lower epiphysis) 813.42
with ulna (lower end) 813.44
open 813.54
open 813.52
torus 813.45
with ulna 813.47
neck — *see* Fracture, radius, upper end
open NEC 813.91
pathologic 733.12
proximal end — *see* Fracture, radius, upper end
shaft (closed) 813.21
with ulna (shaft) 813.23
open 813.33
open 813.31
upper end 813.07
with ulna (upper end) 813.08
open 813.18
epiphysis 813.05
open 813.15
head 813.05
open 813.15
multiple sites 813.07
open 813.17
neck 813.06
open 813.16
open 813.17
specified site NEC 813.07
open 813.17
ramus
inferior or superior (with visceral injury) (closed) 808.2
open 808.3
ischium — *see* Fracture, ischium
mandible 802.24
open 802.34
rib(s) (closed) 807.0 ☑

Note — *Use the following fifth-digit subclassification with categories 807.0–807.1:*

0   *rib(s), unspecified*

1   *one rib*

2   *two ribs*

3   *three ribs*

4   *four ribs*

5   *five ribs*

6   *six ribs*

7   *seven ribs*

8   *eight or more ribs*

9   *multiple ribs, unspecified*

with flail chest (open) 807.4
open 807.1 ☑
root, tooth 873.63

Fracture — *continued*
root, tooth — *continued*
complicated 873.73
sacrum — *see* Fracture, vertebra, sacrum
scaphoid
ankle (closed) 825.22
open 825.32
wrist (closed) 814.01
open 814.11
scapula (closed) 811.00
acromial, acromion (process) 811.01
open 811.11
body 811.09
open 811.19
coracoid process 811.02
open 811.12
glenoid (cavity) (fossa) 811.03
open 811.13
neck 811.03
open 811.13
open 811.10
semilunar
bone, wrist (closed) 814.02
open 814.12
cartilage (interior) (knee) — *see* Tear, meniscus
sesamoid bone — *see* Fracture, by site
Shepherd's (closed) 825.21
open 825.31
shoulder (*see also* Fracture, humerus, upper end)
blade — *see* Fracture, scapula
silverfork — *see* Fracture, radius, lower end
sinus (ethmoid) (frontal) (maxillary) (nasal) (sphenoidal) — *see* Fracture, skull, base
Skillern's — *see* Fracture, radius, shaft
skull (multiple NEC) (with face bones) (closed) 803.0 ☑

Note — *Use the following fifth-digit subclassification with categories 800, 801, 803, and 804:*

0   *unspecified state of consciousness*

1   *with no loss of consciousness*

2   *with brief [less than one hour] loss of consciousness*

3   *with moderate [1-24 hours] loss of consciousness*

4   *with prolonged [more than 24 hours] loss of consciousness and return to pre-existing conscious level*

5   *with prolonged [more than 24 hours] loss of consciousness, without return to pre-existing conscious level*

Use fifth-digit 5 to designate when a patient is unconscious and dies before regaining consciousness, regardless of the duration of the loss of consciousness

6   *with loss of consciousness of unspecified duration*

9   *with concussion, unspecified*

with
contusion, cerebral 803.1 ☑
epidural hemorrhage 803.2 ☑
extradural hemorrhage 803.2 ☑
hemorrhage (intracranial) NEC 803.3 ☑
intracranial injury NEC 803.4 ☑
laceration, cerebral 803.1 ☑
other bones — *see* Fracture, multiple, skull
subarachnoid hemorrhage 803.2 ☑
subdural hemorrhage 803.2 ☑
base (antrum) (ethmoid bone) (fossa) (internal ear) (nasal sinus) (occiput) (sphenoid) (temporal bone) (closed) 801.0 ☑

Fracture — *continued*
skull — *continued*
base — *continued*
with
NULL
contusion, cerebral 801.1 ☑
epidural hemorrhage 801.2 ☑
extradural hemorrhage 801.2 ☑
hemorrhage (intracranial) NEC 801.3 ☑
intracranial injury NEC 801.4 ☑
laceration, cerebral 801.1 ☑
subarachnoid hemorrhage 801.2 ☑
subdural hemorrhage 801.2 ☑
open 801.5 ☑
with
contusion, cerebral 801.6 ☑
epidural hemorrhage 801.7 ☑
extradural hemorrhage 801.7 ☑
hemorrhage (intracranial) NEC 801.8 ☑
intracranial injury NEC 801.9 ☑
laceration, cerebral 801.6 ☑
subarachnoid hemorrhage 801.7 ☑
subdural hemorrhage 801.7 ☑
birth injury 767.3
face bones — *see* Fracture, face bones
open 803.5 ☑
open 801.5 ☑
with
contusion, cerebral 803.6 ☑
epidural hemorrhage 803.7 ☑
extradural hemorrhage 803.7 ☑
hemorrhage (intracranial) NEC 803.8 ☑
intracranial injury NEC 803.9 ☑
laceration, cerebral 803.6 ☑
subarachnoid hemorrhage 803.7 ☑
subdural hemorrhage 803.7 ☑
NULL
NULL
vault (frontal bone) (parietal bone) (vertex) (closed) 800.0 ☑
with
contusion, cerebral 800.1 ☑
epidural hemorrhage 800.2 ☑
extradural hemorrhage 800.2 ☑
hemorrhage (intracranial) NEC 800.3 ☑
intracranial injury NEC 800.4 ☑
laceration, cerebral 800.1 ☑
subarachnoid hemorrhage 800.2 ☑
subdural hemorrhage 800.2 ☑
open 800.5 ☑
with
contusion, cerebral 800.6 ☑
epidural hemorrhage 800.7 ☑
extradural hemorrhage 800.7 ☑
hemorrhage (intracranial) NEC 800.8 ☑
intracranial injury NEC 800.9 ☑
laceration, cerebral 800.6 ☑
subarachnoid hemorrhage 800.7 ☑
subdural hemorrhage 800.7 ☑
Smith's 813.41
open 813.51
sphenoid (bone) (sinus) — *see* Fracture, skull, base
spine (*see also* Fracture, vertebra, by site due to birth trauma) 767.4
spinous process — *see* Fracture, vertebra, by site

Fracture — Fracture

☑ **Additional Digit Required** — Refer to the Tabular List for Digit Selection   ▽ **Subterms under main terms may continue to next column or page**

2014 ICD-9-CM   **169**

Fracture — *continued*
spontaneous — *see* Fracture, pathologic
sprinters' — *see* Fracture, ilium
stapes — *see* Fracture, skull, base
stave (*see also* Fracture, metacarpus, metacarpal bone(s))
spine — *see* Fracture, tibia, upper end
sternum (closed) 807.2
  with flail chest (open) 807.4
  open 807.3
Stieda's — *see* Fracture, femur, lower end
stress 733.95
  femoral neck 733.96
  fibula 733.93
  metatarsals 733.94
  pelvis 733.98
  shaft of femur 733.97
  specified site NEC 733.95
  tibia 733.93
styloid process
  metacarpal (closed) 815.02
    open 815.12
  radius — *see* Fracture, radius, lower end
  temporal bone — *see* Fracture, skull, base
  ulna — *see* Fracture, ulna, lower end
supracondylar, elbow 812.41
  open 812.51
symphysis pubis (with visceral injury) (closed) 808.2
  open 808.3
talus (ankle bone) (closed) 825.21
  open 825.31
tarsus, tarsal bone(s) (with metatarsus) of one foot (closed) NEC 825.29
  open 825.39
temporal bone (styloid) — *see* Fracture, skull, base
tendon — *see* Sprain, by site
thigh — *see* Fracture, femur, shaft
thumb (and finger(s)) of one hand (closed) (*see also* Fracture, phalanx, hand) 816.00
  with metacarpal bone(s) of same hand 817.0
    open 817.1
  metacarpal(s) — *see* Fracture, metacarpus
  open 816.10
thyroid cartilage (closed) 807.5
  open 807.6
tibia (closed) 823.80
  with fibula 823.82
    open 823.92
  condyles — *see* Fracture, tibia, upper end
  distal end 824.8
    open 824.9
  epiphysis
    lower 824.8
      open 824.9
    upper — *see* Fracture, tibia, upper end
  head (involving knee joint) — *see* Fracture, tibia, upper end
  intercondyloid eminence — *see* Fracture, tibia, upper end
  involving ankle 824.0
    open 824.9
  lower end or extremity (anterior lip) (posterior lip) 824.8
    open 824.9
  malleolus (internal) (medial) 824.0
    open 824.1
  open NEC 823.90
  pathologic 733.16
  proximal end — *see* Fracture, tibia, upper end
  shaft 823.20
    with fibula 823.22
      open 823.32
    open 823.30
  spine — *see* Fracture, tibia, upper end
  stress 733.93
  torus 823.40
    with fibula 823.42

Fracture — *continued*
tibia — *continued*
  tuberosity — *see* Fracture, tibia, upper end
  upper end or extremity (condyle) (epiphysis) (head) (spine) (proximal end) (tuberosity) 823.00
    with fibula 823.02
      open 823.12
    open 823.10
toe(s), of one foot (closed) 826.0
  with bone(s) of same lower limb 827.0
    open 827.1
  open 826.1
tooth (root) 873.63
  complicated 873.73
torus
  fibula 823.41
    with tibia 823.42
  humerus 812.49
  radius (alone) 813.45
    with ulna 813.47
  tibia 823.40
    with fibula 823.42
  ulna (alone) 813.46
    with radius 813.47
trachea (closed) 807.5
  open 807.6
transverse process — *see* Fracture, vertebra, by site
trapezium (closed) 814.05
  open 814.15
trapezoid bone (closed) 814.06
  open 814.16
trimalleolar (closed) 824.6
  open 824.7
triquetral (bone) (closed) 814.03
  open 814.13
trochanter (greater) (lesser) (closed) (*see also* Fracture, femur, neck, by site) 820.20
  open 820.30
trunk (bones) (closed) 809.0
  open 809.1
tuberosity (external) — *see* Fracture, by site
ulna (alone) (closed) 813.82
  with radius NEC 813.83
    open 813.93
  coronoid process (closed) 813.02
    open 813.12
  distal end — *see* Fracture, ulna, lower end
  epiphysis
    lower — *see* Fracture, ulna, lower end
    upper — *see* Fracture, ulna, upper end
  head — *see* Fracture, ulna, lower end
  lower end (distal end) (head) (lower epiphysis) (styloid process) 813.43
    with radius (lower end) 813.44
      open 813.54
    open 813.53
  olecranon process (closed) 813.01
    open 813.11
  open NEC 813.92
  pathologic 733.12
  proximal end — *see* Fracture, ulna, upper end
  shaft 813.22
    with radius (shaft) 813.23
      open 813.33
    open 813.32
  styloid process — *see* Fracture, ulna, lower end
  torus 813.46
    with radius 813.47
  transverse — *see* Fracture, ulna, by site
  upper end (epiphysis) 813.04
    with radius (upper end) 813.08
      open 813.18
    multiple sites 813.04
      open 813.14
    open 813.14
    specified site NEC 813.04
      open 813.14

Fracture — *continued*
unciform (closed) 814.08
  open 814.18
vertebra, vertebral (back) (body) (column) (neural arch) (pedicle) (spine) (spinous process) (transverse process) (closed) 805.8
  with
    hematomyelia — *see* Fracture, vertebra, by site, with spinal cord injury
    injury to
      cauda equina — *see* Fracture, vertebra, sacrum, with spinal cord injury
      nerve — *see* Fracture, vertebra, by site, with spinal cord injury
    paralysis — *see* Fracture, vertebra, by site, with spinal cord injury
    paraplegia — *see* Fracture, vertebra, by site, with spinal cord injury
    quadriplegia — *see* Fracture, vertebra, by site, with spinal cord injury
    spinal concussion — *see* Fracture, vertebra, by site, with spinal cord injury
    spinal cord injury (closed) NEC 806.8

Note — Use the following fifth-digit subclassification with categories 806.0–806.3:

C_1–C_4 or unspecified level and D_1–D_6 (T_1–T_6) or unspecified level with

0 unspecified spinal cord injury

1 complete lesion of cord

2 anterior cord syndrome

3 central cord syndrome

4 specified injury NEC

C_5–C_7 level and D_7–D_{12} level with:

5 unspecified spinal cord injury

6 complete lesion of cord

7 anterior cord syndrome

8 central cord syndrome

9 specified injury NEC

      cervical 806.0 ☑
        open 806.1 ☑
      dorsal, dorsolumbar 806.2 ☑
        open 806.3 ☑
      open 806.9
      thoracic, thoracolumbar 806.2 ☑
        open 806.3 ☑
  atlanto-axial — *see* Fracture, vertebra, cervical
  cervical (hangman) (teardrop) (closed) 805.00
    with spinal cord injury — *see* Fracture, vertebra, with spinal cord injury, cervical
    first (atlas) 805.01
      open 805.11
    second (axis) 805.02
      open 805.12
    third 805.03
      open 805.13
    fourth 805.04
      open 805.14
    fifth 805.05
      open 805.15
    sixth 805.06
      open 805.16
    seventh 805.07
      open 805.17
    multiple sites 805.08
      open 805.18
    open 805.10
  chronic 733.13
  coccyx (closed) 805.6

Fracture — *continued*
vertebra, vertebral — *continued*
  coccyx — *continued*
    with spinal cord injury (closed) 806.60
      cauda equina injury 806.62
        complete lesion 806.61
          open 806.71
        open 806.72
      open 806.70
      specified type NEC 806.69
        open 806.79
    open 805.7
  collapsed 733.13
  compression, not due to trauma 733.13
  dorsal (closed) 805.2
    with spinal cord injury — *see* Fracture, vertebra, with spinal cord injury, dorsal
    open 805.3
  dorsolumbar (closed) 805.2
    with spinal cord injury — *see* Fracture, vertebra, with spinal cord injury, dorsal
    open 805.3
  due to osteoporosis 733.13
  fetus or newborn 767.4
  lumbar (closed) 805.4
    with spinal cord injury (closed) 806.4
      open 806.5
    open 805.5
  nontraumatic 733.13
  open NEC 805.9
  pathologic (any site) 733.13
  sacrum (closed) 805.6
    with spinal cord injury 806.60
      cauda equina injury 806.62
        complete lesion 806.61
          open 806.71
        open 806.72
      open 806.70
      specified type NEC 806.69
        open 806.79
    open 805.7
  site unspecified (closed) 805.8
    with spinal cord injury (closed) 806.8
      open 806.9
    open 805.9
  stress (any site) 733.95
  thoracic (closed) 805.2
    with spinal cord injury — *see* Fracture, vertebra, with spinal cord injury, thoracic
    open 805.3
  vertex — *see* Fracture, skull, vault
  vomer (bone) 802.0
    open 802.1
Wagstaffe's — *see* Fracture, ankle
wrist (closed) 814.00
  open 814.10
  pathologic 733.12
xiphoid (process) — *see* Fracture, sternum
zygoma (zygomatic arch) (closed) 802.4
  open 802.5

Fragile X syndrome 759.83
Fragilitas
  crinium 704.2
  hair 704.2
  ossium 756.51
    with blue sclera 756.51
  unguium 703.8
    congenital 757.5
Fragility
  bone 756.51
    with deafness and blue sclera 756.51
  capillary (hereditary) 287.8
  hair 704.2
  nails 703.8
Fragmentation — *see* Fracture, by site
Frailty 797
Frambesia, frambesial (tropica) — *see also* Yaws 102.9
  initial lesion or ulcer 102.0
  primary 102.0
Frambeside
  gummatous 102.4

Frambeside — *continued*
　　of early yaws 102.2
Frambesioma 102.1
Franceschetti's syndrome (mandibulofacial dysostosis) 756.0
Francis' disease — *see also* Tularemia 021.9
Franklin's disease (heavy chain) 273.2
Frank's essential thrombocytopenia — *see also* Purpura, thrombocytopenic 287.39
Fraser's syndrome 759.89
Freckle 709.09
　　malignant melanoma in (M8742/3) — *see* Melanoma
　　melanotic (of Hutchinson) (M8742/2) — *see* Neoplasm, skin, in situ
　　retinal 239.81
Freeman-Sheldon syndrome 759.89
Freezing 991.9
　　specified effect NEC 991.8
Freiberg's
　　disease (osteochondrosis, second metatarsal) 732.5
　　infraction of metatarsal head 732.5
　　osteochondrosis 732.5
Frei's disease (climatic bubo) 099.1
Fremitus, friction, cardiac 785.3
Frenulum linguae 750.0
Frenum
　　external os 752.44
　　tongue 750.0
Frequency (urinary) NEC 788.41
　　micturition 788.41
　　nocturnal 788.43
　　polyuria 788.42
　　psychogenic 306.53
Frey's syndrome (auriculotemporal syndrome) 705.22
Friction
　　burn (*see also* Injury, superficial, by site) 919.0
　　fremitus, cardiac 785.3
　　precordial 785.3
　　sounds, chest 786.7
Friderichsen-Waterhouse syndrome or disease 036.3
Friedländer's
　　B (bacillus) NEC (*see also* condition) 041.3
　　　　sepsis or septicemia 038.49
　　disease (endarteritis obliterans) — *see* Arteriosclerosis
Friedreich's
　　ataxia 334.0
　　combined systemic disease 334.0
　　disease 333.2
　　　　combined systemic 334.0
　　myoclonia 333.2
　　sclerosis (spinal cord) 334.0
Friedrich-Erb-Arnold syndrome (acropachyderma) 757.39
Frigidity 302.72
　　psychic or psychogenic 302.72
Fröhlich's disease or syndrome (adiposogenital dystrophy) 253.8
Froin's syndrome 336.8
Frommel-Chiari syndrome 676.6 ☑
Frommel's disease 676.6 ☑
Frontal — *see also* condition
　　lobe syndrome 310.0
Frostbite 991.3

Frostbite — *continued*
　　face 991.0
　　foot 991.2
　　hand 991.1
　　specified site NEC 991.3
Frotteurism 302.89
Frozen 991.9
　　pelvis 620.8
　　shoulder 726.0
Fructosemia 271.2
Fructosuria (benign) (essential) 271.2
Fuchs'
　　black spot (myopic) 360.21
　　corneal dystrophy (endothelial) 371.57
　　heterochromic cyclitis 364.21
Fucosidosis 271.8
Fugue 780.99
　　dissociative 300.13
　　hysterical (dissociative) 300.13
　　reaction to exceptional stress (transient) 308.1
Fukuhara syndrome 277.87
Fuller Albright's syndrome (osteitis fibrosa disseminata) 756.59
Fuller's earth disease 502
Fulminant, fulminating — *see* condition
Functional — *see* condition
Functioning
　　borderline intellectual V62.89
Fundus — *see also* condition
　　flavimaculatus 362.76
Fungemia 117.9
Fungus, fungous
　　cerebral 348.89
　　disease NEC 117.9
　　infection — *see* Infection, fungus
　　testis (*see also* Tuberculosis)
　　　　016.5 ☑ [608.81]
Funiculitis (acute) 608.4
　　chronic 608.4
　　endemic 608.4
　　gonococcal (acute) 098.14
　　　　chronic or duration of 2 months or over 098.34
　　tuberculous (*see also* Tuberculosis) 016.5 ☑
Funnel
　　breast (acquired) 738.3
　　　　congenital 754.81
　　　　late effect of rickets 268.1
　　chest (acquired) 738.3
　　　　congenital 754.81
　　　　late effect of rickets 268.1
　　pelvis (acquired) 738.6
　　　　with disproportion (fetopelvic) 653.3 ☑
　　　　　　affecting fetus or newborn 763.1
　　　　　　causing obstructed labor 660.1 ☑
　　　　　　　　affecting fetus or newborn 763.1
　　　　congenital 755.69
　　　　tuberculous (*see also* Tuberculosis) 016.9 ☑
FUO — *see also* Pyrexia 780.60
Furfur 690.18
　　microsporon 111.0
Furor, paroxysmal (idiopathic) — *see also* Epilepsy 345.8 ☑
Furriers' lung 495.8
Furrowed tongue 529.5
　　congenital 750.13
Furrowing nail(s) (transverse) 703.8

Furrowing nail(s) — *continued*
　　congenital 757.5
Furuncle 680.9
　　abdominal wall 680.2
　　ankle 680.6
　　anus 680.5
　　arm (any part, above wrist) 680.3
　　auditory canal, external 680.0
　　axilla 680.3
　　back (any part) 680.2
　　breast 680.2
　　buttock 680.5
　　chest wall 680.2
　　corpus cavernosum 607.2
　　ear (any part) 680.0
　　eyelid 373.13
　　face (any part, except eye) 680.0
　　finger (any) 680.4
　　flank 680.2
　　foot (any part) 680.7
　　forearm 680.3
　　gluteal (region) 680.5
　　groin 680.2
　　hand (any part) 680.4
　　head (any part, except face) 680.8
　　heel 680.7
　　hip 680.6
　　kidney (*see also* Abscess, kidney) 590.2
　　knee 680.6
　　labium (majus) (minus) 616.4
　　lacrimal
　　　　gland (*see also* Dacryoadenitis) 375.00
　　　　passages (duct) (sac) (*see also* Dacryocystitis) 375.30
　　leg, any part except foot 680.6
　　malignant 022.0
　　multiple sites 680.9
　　neck 680.1
　　nose (external) (septum) 680.0
　　orbit 376.01
　　partes posteriores 680.5
　　pectoral region 680.2
　　penis 607.2
　　perineum 680.2
　　pinna 680.0
　　scalp (any part) 680.8
　　scrotum 608.4
　　seminal vesicle 608.0
　　shoulder 680.3
　　skin NEC 680.9
　　specified site NEC 680.8
　　spermatic cord 608.4
　　temple (region) 680.0
　　testis 604.90
　　thigh 680.6
　　thumb 680.4
　　toe (any) 680.7
　　trunk 680.2
　　tunica vaginalis 608.4
　　umbilicus 680.2
　　upper arm 680.3
　　vas deferens 608.4
　　vulva 616.4
　　wrist 680.4
Furunculosis — *see also* Furuncle 680.9
　　external auditory meatus 680.0 *[380.13]*
Fusarium (infection) 118
Fusion, fused (congenital)
　　anal (with urogenital canal) 751.5

Fusion, fused — *continued*
　　aorta and pulmonary artery 745.0
　　astragaloscaphoid 755.67
　　atria 745.5
　　atrium and ventricle 745.69
　　auditory canal 744.02
　　auricles, heart 745.5
　　binocular, with defective stereopsis 368.33
　　bone 756.9
　　cervical spine — *see* Fusion, spine
　　choanal 748.0
　　commissure, mitral valve 746.5
　　cranial sutures, premature 756.0
　　cusps, heart valve NEC 746.89
　　　　mitral 746.5
　　　　tricuspid 746.89
　　ear ossicles 744.04
　　fingers (*see also* Syndactylism, fingers) 755.11
　　hymen 752.42
　　hymeno-urethral 599.89
　　　　causing obstructed labor 660.1 ☑
　　　　　　affecting fetus or newborn 763.1
　　joint (acquired) (*see also* Ankylosis)
　　　　congenital 755.8
　　kidneys (incomplete) 753.3
　　labium (majus) (minus) 752.49
　　larynx and trachea 748.3
　　limb 755.8
　　　　lower 755.69
　　　　upper 755.59
　　lobe, lung 748.5
　　lumbosacral (acquired) 724.6
　　　　congenital 756.15
　　　　surgical V45.4
　　nares (anterior) (posterior) 748.0
　　nose, nasal 748.0
　　nostril(s) 748.0
　　organ or site NEC — *see* Anomaly, specified type NEC
　　ossicles 756.9
　　　　auditory 744.04
　　pulmonary valve segment 746.02
　　pulmonic cusps 746.02
　　ribs 756.3
　　sacroiliac (acquired) (joint) 724.6
　　　　congenital 755.69
　　　　surgical V45.4
　　skull, imperfect 756.0
　　spine (acquired) 724.9
　　　　arthrodesis status V45.4
　　　　congenital (vertebra) 756.15
　　　　postoperative status V45.4
　　sublingual duct with submaxillary duct at opening in mouth 750.26
　　talonavicular (bar) 755.67
　　teeth, tooth 520.2
　　testes 752.89
　　toes (*see also* Syndactylism, toes) 755.13
　　trachea and esophagus 750.3
　　twins 759.4
　　urethral-hymenal 599.89
　　vagina 752.49
　　valve cusps — *see* Fusion, cusps, heart valve
　　ventricles, heart 745.4
　　vertebra (arch) — *see* Fusion, spine
　　vulva 752.49
Fusospirillosis (mouth) (tongue) (tonsil) 101
Fussy infant (baby) 780.91

☑ **Additional Digit Required** — Refer to the Tabular List for Digit Selection   ▽ **Subterms under main terms may continue to next column or page**

2014 ICD-9-CM   **171**

G

Gafsa boil 085.1
Gain, weight (abnormal) (excessive) — *see also*
Weight, gain 783.1
Gaisböck's disease or syndrome (polycythemia hypertonica) 289.0
Gait
abnormality 781.2
hysterical 300.11
ataxic 781.2
hysterical 300.11
disturbance 781.2
hysterical 300.11
paralytic 781.2
scissor 781.2
spastic 781.2
staggering 781.2
hysterical 300.11
Galactocele (breast) (infected) 611.5
puerperal, postpartum 676.8 ☑
Galactophoritis 611.0
puerperal, postpartum 675.2 ☑
Galactorrhea 676.6 ☑
not associated with childbirth 611.6
Galactosemia (classic) (congenital) 271.1
Galactosuria 271.1
Galacturia 791.1
bilharziasis 120.0
Galen's vein — *see* condition
Gallbladder — *see also* condition
acute (*see also* Disease, gallbladder) 575.0
Gall duct — *see* condition
Gallop rhythm 427.89
Gallstone (cholemic) (colic) (impacted) — *see
also* Cholelithiasis
causing intestinal obstruction 560.31
Gambling, pathological 312.31
Gammaloidosis 277.39
Gammopathy 273.9
macroglobulinemia 273.3
monoclonal (benign) (essential) (idiopathic)
(with lymphoplasmacytic dyscrasia)
273.1
Gamna's disease (siderotic splenomegaly)
289.51
Gampsodactylia (congenital) 754.71
Gamstorp's disease (adynamia episodica
hereditaria) 359.3
Gandy-Nanta disease (siderotic splenomegaly)
289.51
**Gang activity, without manifest psychiatric
disorder** V71.09
adolescent V71.02
adult V71.01
child V71.02
Gangliocytoma (M9490/0) — *see* Neoplasm,
connective tissue, benign
Ganglioglioma (M9505/1) — *see* Neoplasm,
by site, uncertain behavior
Ganglion 727.43
joint 727.41
of yaws (early) (late) 102.6
periosteal (*see also* Periostitis) 730.3 ☑
tendon sheath (compound) (diffuse) 727.42
tuberculous (*see also* Tuberculosis) 015.9 ☑
Ganglioneuroblastoma (M9490/3) — *see*
Neoplasm, connective tissue, malignant
Ganglioneuroma (M9490/0) — *see also* Neoplasm, connective tissue, benign
malignant (M9490/3) — *see* Neoplasm,
connective tissue, malignant
Ganglioneuromatosis (M9491/0) — *see* Neoplasm, connective tissue, benign
Ganglionitis
fifth nerve (*see also* Neuralgia, trigeminal)
350.1
gasserian 350.1
geniculate 351.1
herpetic 053.11
newborn 767.5
herpes zoster 053.11
herpetic geniculate (Hunt's syndrome)
053.11
Gangliosidosis 330.1
Gangosa 102.5

Gangrene, gangrenous (anemia) (artery)
(cellulitis) (dermatitis) (dry) (infective)
(moist) (pemphigus) (septic) (skin) (stasis) (ulcer) 785.4
with
arteriosclerosis (native artery) 440.24
bypass graft 440.30
autologous vein 440.31
nonautologous biological 440.32
diabetes (mellitus) 250.7 ☑ *[785.4]*
due to secondary diabetes
249.7 ☑ *[785.4]*
abdomen (wall) 785.4
adenitis 683
alveolar 526.5
angina 462
diphtheritic 032.0
anus 569.49
appendices epiploicae — *see* Gangrene,
mesentery
appendix — *see* Appendicitis, acute
arteriosclerotic — *see* Arteriosclerosis, with,
gangrene
auricle 785.4
Bacillus welchii (*see also* Gangrene, gas)
040.0
bile duct (*see also* Cholangitis) 576.8
bladder 595.89
bowel — *see* Gangrene, intestine
cecum — *see* Gangrene, intestine
Clostridium perfringens or welchii (*see also*
Gangrene, gas) 040.0
colon — *see* Gangrene, intestine
connective tissue 785.4
cornea 371.40
corpora cavernosa (infective) 607.2
noninfective 607.89
cutaneous, spreading 785.4
decubital (*see also* Ulcer, pressure)
707.00 *[785.4]*
diabetic (any site) 250.7 ☑ *[785.4]*
due to secondary diabetes
249.7 ☑ *[785.4]*
dropsical 785.4
emphysematous (*see also* Gangrene, gas)
040.0
epidemic (ergotized grain) 988.2
epididymis (infectional) (*see also* Epididymitis) 604.99
erysipelas (*see also* Erysipelas) 035
extremity (lower) (upper) 785.4
gallbladder or duct (*see also* Cholecystitis,
acute) 575.0
gas (bacillus) 040.0
with
abortion — *see* Abortion, by type,
with sepsis
ectopic pregnancy (*see also* categories 633.0–633.9) 639.0
molar pregnancy (*see also* categories
630–632) 639.0
following
abortion 639.0
ectopic or molar pregnancy 639.0
puerperal, postpartum, childbirth
670.8 ☑
glossitis 529.0
gum 523.8
hernia — *see* Hernia, by site, with gangrene
hospital noma 528.1
intestine, intestinal (acute) (hemorrhagic)
(massive) 557.0
with
hernia — *see* Hernia, by site, with
gangrene
mesenteric embolism or infarction
557.0
obstruction (*see also* Obstruction, intestine) 560.9
laryngitis 464.00
with obstruction 464.01
liver 573.8
lung 513.0
spirochetal 104.8
lymphangitis 457.2
Meleney's (cutaneous) 686.09

Gangrene, gangrenous — *continued*
mesentery 557.0
with
embolism or infarction 557.0
intestinal obstruction (*see also* Obstruction, intestine) 560.9
mouth 528.1
noma 528.1
orchitis 604.90
ovary (*see also* Salpingo-oophoritis) 614.2
pancreas 577.0
penis (infectional) 607.2
noninfective 607.89
perineum 785.4
pharynx 462
pneumonia 513.0
Pott's 440.24
presenile 443.1
pulmonary 513.0
pulp, tooth 522.1
quinsy 475
Raynaud's (symmetric gangrene)
443.0 *[785.4]*
rectum 569.49
retropharyngeal 478.24
rupture — *see* Hernia, by site, with gangrene
scrotum 608.4
noninfective 608.83
senile 440.24
septic 034.0
sore throat 462
spermatic cord 608.4
noninfective 608.89
spine 785.4
spirochetal NEC 104.8
spreading cutaneous 785.4
stomach 537.89
stomatitis 528.1
symmetrical 443.0 *[785.4]*
testis (infectional) (*see also* Orchitis) 604.99
noninfective 608.89
throat 462
diphtheritic 032.0
thyroid (gland) 246.8
tonsillitis (acute) 463
tooth (pulp) 522.1
tuberculous NEC (*see also* Tuberculosis)
011.9 ☑
tunica vaginalis 608.4
noninfective 608.89
umbilicus 785.4
uterus (*see also* Endometritis) 615.9
uvulitis 528.3
vas deferens 608.4
noninfective 608.89
vulva (*see also* Vulvitis) 616.10
Gannister disease (occupational) 502
with tuberculosis — *see* Tuberculosis, pulmonary
Ganser's syndrome, hysterical 300.16
Gardner-Diamond syndrome (autoerythrocyte sensitization) 287.2
Gargoylism 277.5
Garré's
disease (*see also* Osteomyelitis) 730.1 ☑
osteitis (sclerosing) (*see also* Osteomyelitis)
730.1 ☑
osteomyelitis (*see also* Osteomyelitis)
730.1 ☑
Garrod's pads, knuckle 728.79
Gartner's duct
cyst 752.41
persistent 752.41
Gas 787.3
asphyxia, asphyxiation, inhalation, poisoning, suffocation NEC 987.9
specified gas — *see* Table of Drugs and
Chemicals
bacillus gangrene or infection — *see* Gas,
gangrene
cyst, mesentery 568.89
excessive 787.3
gangrene 040.0

Gas — *continued*
gangrene — *continued*
with
abortion — *see* Abortion, by type,
with sepsis
ectopic pregnancy (*see also* categories 633.0–633.9) 639.0
molar pregnancy (*see also* categories
630–632) 639.0
following
abortion 639.0
ectopic or molar pregnancy 639.0
puerperal, postpartum, childbirth
670.8 ☑
on stomach 787.3
pains 787.3
Gastradenitis 535.0 ☑
Gastralgia 536.8
psychogenic 307.89
Gastrectasis, gastrectasia 536.1
psychogenic 306.4
Gastric — *see* condition
Gastrinoma (M8153/1)
malignant (M8153/3)
pancreas 157.4
specified site NEC — *see* Neoplasm, by
site, malignant
unspecified site 157.4
specified site — *see* Neoplasm, by site, uncertain behavior
unspecified site 235.5
Gastritis 535.5 ☑

> Note — Use the following fifth-digit
> subclassification for category 535:
>
> 0   without mention of hemorrhage
>
> 1   with hemorrhage

acute 535.0 ☑
alcoholic 535.3 ☑
allergic 535.4 ☑
antral 535.4 ☑
atrophic 535.1 ☑
atrophic-hyperplastic 535.1 ☑
bile-induced 535.4 ☑
catarrhal 535.0 ☑
chronic (atrophic) 535.1 ☑
cirrhotic 535.4 ☑
corrosive (acute) 535.4 ☑
dietetic 535.4 ☑
due to diet deficiency 269.9 *[535.4]* ☑
eosinophilic 535.7 ☑
erosive 535.4 ☑
follicular 535.4 ☑
chronic 535.1 ☑
giant hypertrophic 535.2 ☑
glandular 535.4 ☑
chronic 535.1 ☑
hypertrophic (mucosa) 535.2 ☑
chronic giant 211.1
irritant 535.4 ☑
nervous 306.4
phlegmonous 535.0 ☑
psychogenic 306.4
sclerotic 535.4 ☑
spastic 536.8
subacute 535.0 ☑
superficial 535.4 ☑
suppurative 535.0 ☑
toxic 535.4 ☑
tuberculous (*see also* Tuberculosis) 017.9 ☑
Gastrocarcinoma (M8010/3) 151.9
Gastrocolic — *see* condition
Gastrocolitis — *see* Enteritis
Gastrodisciasis 121.8
Gastroduodenitis — *see also* Gastritis 535.5 ☑
catarrhal 535.0 ☑
infectional 535.0 ☑
virus, viral 008.8
specified type NEC 008.69
Gastrodynia 536.8
Gastroenteritis (acute) (catarrhal) (congestive)
(hemorrhagic) (noninfectious) — *see also*
Enteritis 558.9
aertrycke infection 003.0

Gastroenteritis — *see also* Enteritis — *continued*
  allergic 558.3
  chronic 558.9
    ulcerative (*see also* Colitis, ulcerative) 556.9
  dietetic 558.9
  due to
    antineoplastic chemotherapy 558.9
    food poisoning (*see also* Poisoning, food) 005.9
    radiation 558.1
  eosinophilic 558.41
  epidemic 009.0
  functional 558.9
  infectious (*see also* Enteritis, due to, by organism) 009.0
    presumed 009.1
  salmonella 003.0
  septic (*see also* Enteritis, due to, by organism) 009.0
  toxic 558.2
  tuberculous (*see also* Tuberculosis) 014.8 ☑
  ulcerative (*see also* Colitis, ulcerative) 556.9
  viral NEC 008.8
    specified type NEC 008.69
  zymotic 009.0
Gastroenterocolitis — *see* Enteritis
Gastroenteropathy, protein-losing 579.8
Gastroenteroptosis 569.89
Gastroesophageal laceration-hemorrhage syndrome 530.7
Gastroesophagitis 530.19
Gastrohepatitis — *see also* Gastritis 535.5 ☑
Gastrointestinal — *see* condition
Gastrojejunal — *see* condition
Gastrojejunitis — *see also* Gastritis 535.5 ☑
Gastrojejunocolic — *see* condition
Gastroliths 537.89
Gastromalacia 537.89
Gastroparalysis 536.3
  diabetic 250.6 ☑ [536.3]
    due to secondary diabetes 249.6 ☑ [536.3]
Gastroparesis 536.3
  diabetic 250.6 ☑ [536.3]
    due to secondary diabetes 249.6 ☑ [536.3]
Gastropathy 537.9
  congestive portal 537.89
  erythematous 535.5 ☑
  exudative 579.8
  portal hypertensive 537.89
Gastroptosis 537.5
Gastrorrhagia 578.0
Gastrorrhea 536.8
  psychogenic 306.4
Gastroschisis (congenital) 756.73
  acquired 569.89
Gastrospasm (neurogenic) (reflex) 536.8
  neurotic 306.4
  psychogenic 306.4
Gastrostaxis 578.0
Gastrostenosis 537.89
Gastrostomy
  attention to V55.1
  complication 536.40
    specified type 536.49
  infection 536.41
  malfunctioning 536.42
  status V44.1
Gastrosuccorrhea (continuous) (intermittent) 536.8
  neurotic 306.4
  psychogenic 306.4
Gaucher's
  disease (adult) (cerebroside lipidosis) (infantile) 272.7
  hepatomegaly 272.7
  splenomegaly (cerebroside lipidosis) 272.7
GAVE (gastric antral vascular ectasia) 537.82
  with hemorrhage 537.83
  without hemorrhage 537.82
Gayet's disease (superior hemorrhagic polioencephalitis) 265.1

Gayet-Wernicke's syndrome (superior hemorrhagic polioencephalitis) 265.1
Gee (-Herter) (-Heubner) (-Thaysen) disease or syndrome (nontropical sprue) 579.0
Gélineau's syndrome — *see also* Narcolepsy 347.00
Gemination, teeth 520.2
Gemistocytoma (M9411/3)
  specified site — *see* Neoplasm, by site, malignant
  unspecified site 191.9
General, generalized — *see* condtion
Genetic
  susceptibility to
    MEN (multiple endocrine neoplasia) V84.81
    neoplasia
      multiple endocrine (MEN) V84.81
    neoplasm
      malignant, of
        breast V84.01
        endometrium V84.04
        other V84.09
        ovary V84.02
        prostate V84.03
    specified disease NEC V84.89
Genital — *see* condition
  warts 078.11
Genito-anorectal syndrome 099.1
Genitourinary system — *see* condition
Genu
  congenital 755.64
  extrorsum (acquired) 736.42
    congenital 755.64
    late effects of rickets 268.1
  introrsum (acquired) 736.41
    congenital 755.64
    late effects of rickets 268.1
  rachitic (old) 268.1
  recurvatum (acquired) 736.5
    congenital 754.40
      with dislocation of knee 754.41
    late effects of rickets 268.1
  valgum (acquired) (knock-knee) 736.41
    congenital 755.64
    late effects of rickets 268.1
  varum (acquired) (bowleg) 736.42
    congenital 755.64
    late effect of rickets 268.1
Geographic tongue 529.1
Geophagia 307.52
Geotrichosis 117.9
  intestine 117.9
  lung 117.9
  mouth 117.9
Gephyrophobia 300.29
Gerbode defect 745.4
GERD (gastroesophageal reflux disease) 530.81
Gerhardt's
  disease (erythromelalgia) 443.82
  syndrome (vocal cord paralysis) 478.30
Gerlier's disease (epidemic vertigo) 078.81
German measles 056.9
  exposure to V01.4
Germinoblastoma (diffuse) (M9614/3) 202.8 ☑
  follicular (M9692/3) 202.0 ☑
Germinoma (M9064/3) — *see* Neoplasm, by site, malignant
Gerontoxon 371.41
Gerstmann-Sträussler-Scheinker syndrome (GSS) 046.71
Gerstmann's syndrome (finger agnosia) 784.69
Gestation (period) — *see also* Pregnancy
  ectopic NEC (*see also* Pregnancy, ectopic) 633.90
    with intrauterine pregnancy 633.91
  multiple
    placenta status
      quadruplet
        two or more monoamniotic fetuses V91.22
        two or more monochorionic fetuses V91.21

Gestation — *see also* Pregnancy — *continued*
  multiple — *continued*
    placenta status — *continued*
      quadruplet — *continued*
        unable to determine number of placenta and number of amniotic sacs V91.29
        unspecified number of placenta and unspecified number of amniotic sacs V91.20
      specified (greater than quadruplets) NEC
        two or more monoamniotic fetuses V91.92
        two or more monochorionic fetuses V91.91
        unable to determine number of placenta and number of amniotic sacs V91.99
        unspecified number of placenta and unspecified number of amniotic sacs V91.90
      triplet
        two or more monoamniotic fetuses V91.12
        two or more monochorionic fetuses V91.11
        unable to determine number of placenta and number of amniotic sacs V91.19
        unspecified number of placenta, unspecified number of amniotic sacs V91.10
      twin
        dichorionic/diamniotic (two placentae, two amniotic sacs) V91.03
        monochorionic/diamniotic (one placenta, two amniotic sacs) V91.02
        monochorionic/monoamniotic (one placenta, one amniotic sac) V91.01
        unable to determine number of placenta and number of amniotic sacs V91.09
        unspecified number of placenta, unspecified number of amniotic sacs V91.00
Gestational proteinuria 646.2 ☑
  with hypertension — *see* Toxemia, of pregnancy
Ghon tubercle primary infection — *see also* Tuberculosis 010.0 ☑
Ghost
  teeth 520.4
  vessels, cornea 370.64
Ghoul hand 102.3
Gianotti Crosti syndrome 057.8
  due to known virus — *see* Infection, virus
  due to unknown virus 057.8
Giant
  cell
    epulis 523.8
      peripheral (gingiva) 523.8
    tumor, tendon sheath 727.02
  colon (congenital) 751.3
  esophagus (congenital) 750.4
  kidney 753.3
  urticaria 995.1
    hereditary 277.6
Giardia lamblia infestation 007.1
Giardiasis 007.1
Gibert's disease (pityriasis rosea) 696.3
Gibraltar fever — *see* Brucellosis
Giddiness 780.4
  hysterical 300.11
  psychogenic 306.9
Gierke's disease (glycogenosis I) 271.0
Gigantism (cerebral) (hypophyseal) (pituitary) 253.0
Gilbert's disease or cholemia (familial nonhemolytic jaundice) 277.4
Gilchrist's disease (North American blastomycosis) 116.0

Gilford (-Hutchinson) disease or syndrome (progeria) 259.8
Gilles de la Tourette's disease (motor-verbal tic) 307.23
Gillespie's syndrome (dysplasia oculodentodigitalis) 759.89
Gingivitis 523.10
  acute 523.00
    necrotizing 101
    non-plaque induced 523.01
    plaque induced 523.00
  catarrhal 523.00
  chronic 523.10
    non-plaque induced 523.11
  desquamative 523.10
  expulsiva 523.40
  hyperplastic 523.10
  marginal, simple 523.10
  necrotizing, acute 101
  non-plaque induced 523.11
  pellagrous 265.2
  plaque induced 523.10
  ulcerative 523.10
    acute necrotizing 101
  Vincent's 101
Gingivoglossitis 529.0
Gingivopericementitis 523.40
Gingivosis 523.10
Gingivostomatitis 523.10
  herpetic 054.2
Giovannini's disease 117.9
GISA (glycopeptide intermediate staphylococcus aureus) V09.8 ☑
Glanders 024
Gland, glandular — *see* condition
Glanzmann (-Naegeli) disease or thrombasthenia 287.1
Glassblowers' disease 527.1
Glaucoma (capsular) (inflammatory) (noninflammatory) (primary) 365.9
  with increased episcleral venous pressure 365.82
  absolute 360.42
  acute 365.22
    narrow angle 365.22
    secondary 365.60
  angle closure 365.20
    acute 365.22
    attack 365.22
    chronic 365.23
    crisis 365.22
    intermittent 365.21
    interval 365.21
    primary 365.20
      chronic 365.23
    residual stage 365.24
    subacute 365.21
  angle recession 365.65
  borderline 365.00
  chronic 365.11
    noncongestive 365.11
    open angle 365.11
    simple 365.11
  closed angle — *see* Glaucoma, angle closure
  congenital 743.20
    associated with other eye anomalies 743.22
    simple 743.21
  congestive — *see* Glaucoma, narrow angle
  corticosteroid-induced (glaucomatous stage) 365.31
    residual stage 365.32
  exfoliation 365.52
  hemorrhagic 365.60
  hypersecretion 365.81
  infantile 365.14
    congenital 743.20
      associated with other eye anomalies 743.22
      simple 743.21
  inflammatory 365.62
  in or with
    aniridia 365.42
    Axenfeld's anomaly 365.41
    congenital syndromes NEC 759.89 [365.44]

☑ **Additional Digit Required** — Refer to the Tabular List for Digit Selection   ⬛ **Subterms under main terms may continue to next column or page**

2014 ICD-9-CM   173

Glaucoma — continued
　in or with — continued
　　disorder of lens NEC 365.59
　　inflammation, ocular 365.62
　　iris
　　　anomalies NEC 365.42
　　　atrophy, essential 365.42
　　　bombé 365.61
　　microcornea 365.43
　　neurofibromatosis 237.71 [365.44]
　　ocular
　　　cysts NEC 365.64
　　　disorders NEC 365.60
　　　trauma 365.65
　　　tumors NEC 365.64
　　pupillary block or seclusion 365.61
　　Rieger's anomaly or syndrome 365.41
　　seclusion of pupil 365.61
　　Sturge-Weber (-Dimitri) syndrome
　　　759.6 [365.44]
　　systemic syndrome NEC 365.44
　　tumor of globe 365.64
　　vascular disorders NEC 365.63
　juvenile 365.14
　low tension 365.12
　malignant 365.83
　narrow angle (primary) 365.20
　　acute 365.22
　　chronic 365.23
　　intermittent 365.21
　　interval 365.21
　　residual stage 365.24
　　subacute 365.21
　neovascular 365.63
　newborn 743.20
　　associated with other eye anomalies
　　　743.22
　　simple 743.21
　noncongestive (chronic) 365.11
　nonobstructive (chronic) 365.11
　normal tension 365.12
　obstructive 365.60
　　due to lens changes 365.59
　open angle 365.10
　　with
　　　abnormal optic disc appearance or
　　　　asymmetry 365.01
　　　borderline findings
　　　　high risk 365.05
　　　　intraocular pressure 365.01
　　　　low risk 365.01
　　　cupping of optic discs 365.01
　　　thin central corneal thickness
　　　　(pachymetry) 365.01
　　high risk 365.05
　　low risk 365.01
　　primary 365.11
　　residual stage 365.15
　phacoanaphylactic 365.59
　phacolytic 365.51
　phacomorphic
　　acute 365.22
　　borderline 365.06
　pigmentary 365.13
　pigment dispersion 365.13
　postinfectious 365.60
　pseudoexfoliation 365.52
　secondary NEC 365.60
　　due to
　　　steroids 365.31
　　　surgery 365.60
　simple (chronic) 365.11
　simplex 365.11
　stage
　　advanced 365.73
　　early 365.71
　　end-stage 365.73
　　indeterminate 365.74
　　mild 365.71
　　moderate 365.72
　　severe 365.73
　　unspecified 365.70
　steroid
　　induced 365.31
　　responders 365.03
　suspect 365.00

Glaucoma — continued
　suspect — continued
　　primary angle closure 365.02
　　syphilitic 095.8
　　traumatic NEC 365.65
　　　newborn 767.8
　　uveitic 365.62
　　wide angle (see also Glaucoma, open angle)
　　　365.10
Glaucomatous flecks (subcapsular) 366.31
Glazed tongue 529.4
Gleet 098.2
Glénard's disease or syndrome (enteroptosis)
　569.89
Glinski-Simmonds syndrome (pituitary
　cachexia) 253.2
Glioblastoma (multiforme) (M9440/3)
　with sarcomatous component (M9442/3)
　　specified site — see Neoplasm, by site,
　　　malignant
　　unspecified site 191.9
　giant cell (M9441/3)
　　specified site — see Neoplasm, by site,
　　　malignant
　　unspecified site 191.9
　specified site — see Neoplasm, by site, ma-
　　lignant
　unspecified site 191.9
Glioma (malignant) (M9380/3)
　astrocytic (M9400/3)
　　specified site — see Neoplasm, by site,
　　　malignant
　　unspecified site 191.9
　mixed (M9382/3)
　　specified site — see Neoplasm, by site,
　　　malignant
　　unspecified site 191.9
　nose 748.1
　specified site NEC — see Neoplasm, by site,
　　malignant
　subependymal (M9383/1) 237.5
　unspecified site 191.9
Gliomatosis cerebri (M9381/3) 191.0
Glioneuroma (M9505/1) — see Neoplasm, by
　site, uncertain behavior
Gliosarcoma (M9380/3)
　specified site — see Neoplasm, by site, ma-
　　lignant
　unspecified site 191.9
Gliosis (cerebral) 349.89
　spinal 336.0
Glisson's
　cirrhosis — see Cirrhosis, portal
　disease (see also Rickets) 268.0
Glissonitis 573.3
Globinuria 791.2
Globus 306.4
　hystericus 300.11
Glomangioma (M8712/0) — see also Heman-
　gioma 228.00
Glomangiosarcoma (M8710/3) — see Neo-
　plasm, connective tissue, malignant
Glomerular nephritis — see also Nephritis
　583.9
Glomerulitis — see also Nephritis 583.9
Glomerulonephritis — see also Nephritis 583.9
　with
　　edema (see also Nephrosis) 581.9
　　lesion of
　　　exudative nephritis 583.89
　　　interstitial nephritis (diffuse) (focal)
　　　　583.89
　　　necrotizing glomerulitis 583.4
　　　　acute 580.4
　　　　chronic 582.4
　　　renal necrosis 583.9
　　　　cortical 583.6
　　　　medullary 583.7
　　　specified pathology NEC 583.89
　　　　acute 580.89
　　　　chronic 582.89
　　necrosis, renal 583.9
　　　cortical 583.6
　　　medullary (papillary) 583.7
　　specified pathology or lesion NEC 583.89
　acute 580.9

Glomerulonephritis — see also Nephritis —
　continued
　acute — continued
　　with
　　　exudative nephritis 580.89
　　　interstitial nephritis (diffuse) (focal)
　　　　580.89
　　　necrotizing glomerulitis 580.4
　　　extracapillary with epithelial crescents
　　　　580.4
　　　poststreptococcal 580.0
　　　proliferative (diffuse) 580.0
　　　rapidly progressive 580.4
　　　specified pathology NEC 580.89
　arteriolar (see also Hypertension, kidney)
　　403.90
　arteriosclerotic (see also Hypertension, kid-
　　ney) 403.90
　ascending (see also Pyelitis) 590.80
　basement membrane NEC 583.89
　　with
　　　pulmonary hemorrhage (Goodpas-
　　　　ture's syndrome)
　　　　446.21 [583.81]
　chronic 582.9
　　with
　　　exudative nephritis 582.89
　　　interstitial nephritis (diffuse) (focal)
　　　　582.89
　　　necrotizing glomerulitis 582.4
　　　specified pathology or lesion NEC
　　　　582.89
　　endothelial 582.2
　　extracapillary with epithelial crescents
　　　582.4
　　hypocomplementemic persistent 582.2
　　lobular 582.2
　　membranoproliferative 582.2
　　membranous 582.1
　　　and proliferative (mixed) 582.2
　　　sclerosing 582.1
　　mesangiocapillary 582.2
　　mixed membranous and proliferative
　　　582.2
　　proliferative (diffuse) 582.0
　　rapidly progressive 582.4
　　sclerosing 582.1
　cirrhotic — see Sclerosis, renal
　desquamative — see Nephrosis
　due to or associated with
　　amyloidosis 277.39 [583.81]
　　　with nephrotic syndrome
　　　　277.39 [581.81]
　　　chronic 277.39 [582.81]
　　diabetes mellitus 250.4 ☑ [583.81]
　　　with nephrotic syndrome
　　　　250.4 ☑ [581.81]
　　　due to secondary diabetes
　　　　249.4 ☑ [581.81]
　　　due to secondary diabetes
　　　　249.4 ☑ [581.81]
　　diphtheria 032.89 [580.81]
　　gonococcal infection (acute)
　　　098.19 [583.81]
　　　chronic or duration of 2 months or
　　　　over 098.39 [583.81]
　　infectious hepatitis 070.9 [580.81]
　　malaria (with nephrotic syndrome)
　　　084.9 [581.81]
　　mumps 072.79 [580.81]
　　polyarteritis (nodosa) (with nephrotic
　　　syndrome) 446.0 [581.81]
　　specified pathology NEC 583.89
　　　acute 580.89
　　　chronic 582.89
　　streptotrichosis 039.8 [583.81]
　　subacute bacterial endocarditis
　　　421.0 [580.81]
　　syphilis (late) 095.4
　　　congenital 090.5 [583.81]
　　　early 091.69 [583.81]
　　systemic lupus erythematosus
　　　710.0 [583.81]
　　　with nephrotic syndrome
　　　　710.0 [581.81]
　　　chronic 710.0 [582.81]

Glomerulonephritis — see also Nephritis —
　continued
　due to or associated with — continued
　　tuberculosis (see also Tuberculosis)
　　　016.0 ☑ [583.81]
　　typhoid fever 002.0 [580.81]
　extracapillary with epithelial crescents 583.4
　　acute 580.4
　　chronic 582.4
　exudative 583.89
　　acute 580.89
　　chronic 582.89
　focal (see also Nephritis) 583.9
　　embolic 580.4
　granular 582.89
　granulomatous 582.89
　hydremic (see also Nephrosis) 581.9
　hypocomplementemic persistent 583.2
　　with nephrotic syndrome 581.2
　　chronic 582.2
　immune complex NEC 583.89
　infective (see also Pyelitis) 590.80
　interstitial (diffuse) (focal) 583.89
　　with nephrotic syndrome 581.89
　　acute 580.89
　　chronic 582.89
　latent or quiescent 582.9
　lobular 583.2
　　with nephrotic syndrome 581.2
　　chronic 582.2
　membranoproliferative 583.2
　　with nephrotic syndrome 581.2
　　chronic 582.2
　membranous 583.1
　　with nephrotic syndrome 581.1
　　and proliferative (mixed) 583.2
　　　with nephrotic syndrome 581.2
　　　chronic 582.2
　　chronic 582.1
　　sclerosing 582.1
　　　with nephrotic syndrome 581.1
　mesangiocapillary 583.2
　　with nephrotic syndrome 581.2
　　chronic 582.2
　minimal change 581.3
　mixed membranous and proliferative 583.2
　　with nephrotic syndrome 581.2
　　chronic 582.2
　necrotizing 583.4
　　acute 580.4
　　chronic 582.4
　nephrotic (see also Nephrosis) 581.9
　old — see Glomerulonephritis, chronic
　parenchymatous 581.89
　poststreptococcal 580.0
　proliferative (diffuse) 583.0
　　with nephrotic syndrome 581.0
　　acute 580.0
　　chronic 582.0
　purulent (see also Pyelitis) 590.80
　quiescent — see Nephritis, chronic
　rapidly progressive 583.4
　　acute 580.4
　　chronic 582.4
　sclerosing membranous (chronic) 582.1
　　with nephrotic syndrome 581.1
　septic (see also Pyelitis) 590.80
　specified pathology or lesion NEC 583.89
　　with nephrotic syndrome 581.89
　　acute 580.89
　　chronic 582.89
　suppurative (acute) (disseminated) (see also
　　Pyelitis) 590.80
　toxic — see Nephritis, acute
　tubal, tubular — see Nephrosis, tubular
　type II (Ellis) — see Nephrosis
　vascular — see Hypertension, kidney
Glomerulosclerosis — see also Sclerosis, renal
　587
　focal 582.1
　　with nephrotic syndrome 581.1
　intercapillary (nodular) (with diabetes)
　　250.4 ☑ [581.81]
　　due to secondary diabetes
　　　249.4 ☑ [581.81]
Glossagra 529.6

Glossalgia 529.6
Glossitis 529.0
  areata exfoliativa 529.1
  atrophic 529.4
  benign migratory 529.1
  gangrenous 529.0
  Hunter's 529.4
  median rhomboid 529.2
  Moeller's 529.4
  pellagrous 265.2
Glossocele 529.8
Glossodynia 529.6
  exfoliativa 529.4
Glossoncus 529.8
Glossophytia 529.3
Glossoplegia 529.8
Glossoptosis 529.8
Glossopyrosis 529.6
Glossotrichia 529.3
Glossy skin 701.9
Glottis — see condition
Glottitis — see Glossitis
Glucagonoma (M8152/0)
  malignant (M8152/3)
    pancreas 157.4
    specified site NEC — see Neoplasm, by site, malignant
    unspecified site 157.4
  pancreas 211.7
  specified site NEC — see Neoplasm, by site, benign
  unspecified site 211.7
Glucoglycinuria 270.7
Glue ear syndrome 381.20
Glue sniffing (airplane glue) — see also Dependence 304.6 ☑
Glycinemia (with methylmalonic acidemia) 270.7
Glycinuria (renal) (with ketosis) 270.0
Glycogen
  infiltration (see also Disease, glycogen storage) 271.0
  storage disease (see also Disease, glycogen storage) 271.0
Glycogenosis — see also Disease, glycogen storage 271.0
  cardiac 271.0 [425.7]
  Cori, types I-VII 271.0
  diabetic, secondary 250.8 ☑ [259.8]
    due to secondary diabetes 249.8 ☑ [259.8]
  diffuse (with hepatic cirrhosis) 271.0
  generalized 271.0
  glucose-6-phosphatase deficiency 271.0
  hepatophosphorylase deficiency 271.0
  hepatorenal 271.0
  myophosphorylase deficiency 271.0
  pulmonary interstitial 516.62
Glycopenia 251.2
Glycopeptide
  intermediate staphylococcus aureus (GISA) V09.8 ☑
  resistant
    enterococcus V09.8 ☑
    staphylococcus aureus (GRSA) V09.8 ☑
Glycoprolinuria 270.8
Glycosuria 791.5
  renal 271.4
Gnathostoma (spinigerum) (infection) (infestation) 128.1
  wandering swellings from 128.1
Gnathostomiasis 128.1
Goiter (adolescent) (colloid) (diffuse) (dipping) (due to iodine deficiency) (endemic) (euthyroid) (heart) (hyperplastic) (internal) (intrathoracic) (juvenile) (mixed type) (nonendemic) (parenchymatous) (plunging) (sporadic) (subclavicular) (substernal) 240.9
  with
    hyperthyroidism (recurrent) (see also Goiter, toxic) 242.0 ☑
    thyrotoxicosis (see also Goiter, toxic) 242.0 ☑
  adenomatous (see also Goiter, nodular) 241.9

Goiter — continued
  cancerous (M8000/3) 193
  complicating pregnancy, childbirth, or puerperium 648.1 ☑
  congenital 246.1
  cystic (see also Goiter, nodular) 241.9
  due to enzyme defect in synthesis of thyroid hormone (butane-insoluble iodine) (coupling) (deiodinase) (iodide trapping or organification) (iodotyrosine dehalogenase) (peroxidase) 246.1
  dyshormonogenic 246.1
  exophthalmic (see also Goiter, toxic) 242.0 ☑
  familial (with deaf-mutism) 243
  fibrous 245.3
  lingual 759.2
  lymphadenoid 245.2
  malignant (M8000/3) 193
  multinodular (nontoxic) 241.1
    toxic or with hyperthyroidism (see also Goiter, toxic) 242.2 ☑
  nodular (nontoxic) 241.9
    with
      hyperthyroidism (see also Goiter, toxic) 242.3 ☑
      thyrotoxicosis (see also Goiter, toxic) 242.3 ☑
    endemic 241.9
    exophthalmic (diffuse) (see also Goiter, toxic) 242.0 ☑
    multinodular (nontoxic) 241.1
    sporadic 241.9
    toxic (see also Goiter, toxic) 242.3 ☑
    uninodular (nontoxic) 241.0
  nontoxic (nodular) 241.9
    multinodular 241.1
    uninodular 241.0
  pulsating (see also Goiter, toxic) 242.0 ☑
  simple 240.0
  toxic 242.0 ☑

> *Note* — *Use the following fifth-digit subclassification with category 242:*
>
> 0   *without mention of thyrotoxic crisis or storm*
>
> 1   *with mention of thyrotoxic crisis or storm*

    adenomatous 242.3 ☑
      multinodular 242.2 ☑
      uninodular 242.1 ☑
    multinodular 242.2 ☑
    nodular 242.3 ☑
      multinodular 242.2 ☑
      uninodular 242.1 ☑
    uninodular 242.1 ☑
  uninodular (nontoxic) 241.0
    toxic or with hyperthyroidism (see also Goiter, toxic) 242.1 ☑
Goldberg (-Maxwell) (-Morris) syndrome (testicular feminization) 259.51
Goldblatt's
  hypertension 440.1
  kidney 440.1
Goldenhar's syndrome (oculoauriculovertebral dysplasia) 756.0
Goldflam-Erb disease or syndrome 358.00
Goldscheider's disease (epidermolysis bullosa) 757.39
Goldstein's disease (familial hemorrhagic telangiectasia) 448.0
Golfer's elbow 726.32
Goltz-Gorlin syndrome (dermal hypoplasia) 757.39
Gonadoblastoma (M9073/1)
  specified site — see Neoplasm, by site uncertain behavior
  unspecified site
    female 236.2
    male 236.4
Gonecystitis — see also Vesiculitis 608.0
Gongylonemiasis 125.6
  mouth 125.6
Goniosynechiae 364.73
Gonococcemia 098.89

Gonococcus, gonococcal (disease) (infection) — see also condition 098.0
  anus 098.7
  bursa 098.52
  chronic NEC 098.2
  complicating pregnancy, childbirth, or puerperium 647.1 ☑
    affecting fetus or newborn 760.2
  conjunctiva, conjunctivitis (neonatorum) 098.40
  dermatosis 098.89
  endocardium 098.84
  epididymo-orchitis 098.13
    chronic or duration of 2 months or over 098.33
  eye (newborn) 098.40
  fallopian tube (chronic) 098.37
    acute 098.17
  genitourinary (acute) (organ) (system) (tract) (see also Gonorrhea) 098.0
    lower 098.0
      chronic 098.2
    upper 098.10
      chronic 098.30
  heart NEC 098.85
  joint 098.50
  keratoderma 098.81
  keratosis (blennorrhagica) 098.81
  lymphatic (gland) (node) 098.89
  meninges 098.82
  orchitis (acute) 098.13
    chronic or duration of 2 months or over 098.33
  pelvis (acute) 098.19
    chronic or duration of 2 months or over 098.39
  pericarditis 098.83
  peritonitis 098.86
  pharyngitis 098.6
  pharynx 098.6
  proctitis 098.7
  pyosalpinx (chronic) 098.37
    acute 098.17
  rectum 098.7
  septicemia 098.89
  skin 098.89
  specified site NEC 098.89
  synovitis 098.51
  tendon sheath 098.51
  throat 098.6
  urethra (acute) 098.0
    chronic or duration of 2 months or over 098.2
  vulva (acute) 098.0
    chronic or duration of 2 months or over 098.2
Gonocytoma (M9073/1)
  specified site — see Neoplasm, by site, uncertain behavior
  unspecified site
    female 236.2
    male 236.4
Gonorrhea 098.0
  acute 098.0
  Bartholin's gland (acute) 098.0
    chronic or duration of 2 months or over 098.2
  bladder (acute) 098.11
    chronic or duration of 2 months or over 098.31
  carrier (suspected of) V02.7
  cervix (acute) 098.15
    chronic or duration of 2 months or over 098.35
  chronic 098.2
  complicating pregnancy, childbirth, or puerperium 647.1 ☑
    affecting fetus or newborn 760.2
  conjunctiva, conjunctivitis (neonatorum) 098.40
  contact V01.6
  Cowper's gland (acute) 098.0
    chronic or duration of 2 months or over 098.2
  duration of two months or over 098.2
  exposure to V01.6

Gonorrhea — continued
  fallopian tube (chronic) 098.37
    acute 098.17
  genitourinary (acute) (organ) (system) (tract) 098.0
    chronic 098.2
    duration of two months or over 098.2
  kidney (acute) 098.19
    chronic or duration of 2 months or over 098.39
  ovary (acute) 098.19
    chronic or duration of 2 months or over 098.39
  pelvis (acute) 098.19
    chronic or duration of 2 months or over 098.39
  penis (acute) 098.0
    chronic or duration of 2 months or over 098.2
  prostate (acute) 098.12
    chronic or duration of 2 months or over 098.32
  seminal vesicle (acute) 098.14
    chronic or duration of 2 months or over 098.34
  specified site NEC — see Gonococcus
  spermatic cord (acute) 098.14
    chronic or duration of 2 months or over 098.34
  urethra (acute) 098.0
    chronic or duration of 2 months or over 098.2
  vagina (acute) 098.0
    chronic or duration of 2 months or over 098.2
  vas deferens (acute) 098.14
    chronic or duration of 2 months or over 098.34
  vulva (acute) 098.0
    chronic or duration of 2 months or over 098.2
Goodpasture's syndrome (pneumorenal) 446.21
Good's syndrome 279.06
Gopalan's syndrome (burning feet) 266.2
Gordon's disease (exudative enteropathy) 579.8
Gorlin-Chaudhry-Moss syndrome 759.89
Gougerot-Blum syndrome (pigmented purpuric lichenoid dermatitis) 709.1
Gougerot-Carteaud disease or syndrome (confluent reticulate papillomatosis) 701.8
Gougerot-Hailey-Hailey disease (benign familial chronic pemphigus) 757.39
Gougerot (-Houwer) -Sjögren syndrome (keratoconjunctivitis sicca) 710.2
Gougerot's syndrome (trisymptomatic) 709.1
Gouley's syndrome (constrictive pericarditis) 423.2
Goundou 102.6
Gout, gouty 274.9
  with
    specified manifestations NEC 274.89
    tophi (tophus) 274.03
  acute 274.01
  arthritis 274.00
    acute 274.01
  arthropathy 274.00
    acute 274.01
    chronic (without mention of tophus (tophi)) 274.02
      with tophus (tophi) 274.03
  attack 274.01
  chronic 274.02
    tophaceous 274.03
  degeneration, heart 274.82
  diathesis 274.9
  eczema 274.89
  episcleritis 274.89 [379.09]
  external ear (tophus) 274.81
  flare 274.01
  glomerulonephritis 274.10
  iritis 274.89 [364.11]
  joint 274.00
  kidney 274.10

☑ Additional Digit Required — Refer to the Tabular List for Digit Selection   Subterms under main terms may continue to next column or page

2014 ICD-9-CM   175

Index

Gout, gouty — Gynandrism

Gout, gouty — *continued*
  lead 984.9
    specified type of lead — *see* Table of Drugs and Chemicals
  nephritis 274.10
  neuritis 274.89 *[357.4]*
  phlebitis 274.89 *[451.9]*
  rheumatic 714.0
  saturnine 984.9
    specified type of lead — *see* Table of Drugs and Chemicals
  spondylitis 274.00
  synovitis 274.00
  syphilitic 095.8
  tophi 274.03
    ear 274.81
    heart 274.82
  specified site NEC 274.82
Gowers'
  muscular dystrophy 359.1
  syndrome (vasovagal attack) 780.2
Gowers-Paton-Kennedy syndrome 377.04
Gradenigo's syndrome 383.02
Graft-versus-host disease 279.50
  due to organ transplant NEC — *see* Complications, transplant, organ
Graham Steell's murmur (pulmonic regurgitation) — *see also* Endocarditis, pulmonary 424.3
Grain-handlers' disease or lung 495.8
Grain mite (itch) 133.8
Grand
  mal (idiopathic) (*see also* Epilepsy) 345.1 ☑
    hysteria of Charcôt 300.11
    nonrecurrent or isolated 780.39
  multipara
    affecting management of labor and delivery 659.4 ☑
    status only (not pregnant) V61.5
Granite workers' lung 502
Granular — *see also* condition
  inflammation, pharynx 472.1
  kidney (contracting) (*see also* Sclerosis, renal) 587
  liver — *see* Cirrhosis, liver
  nephritis — *see* Nephritis
Granulation tissue, abnormal — *see also* Granuloma
  abnormal or excessive 701.5
  postmastoidectomy cavity 383.33
  postoperative 701.5
  skin 701.5
Granulocytopenia, granulocytopenic (primary) 288.00
  malignant 288.09
Granulomatosis NEC 686.1
  disciformis chronica et progressiva 709.3
  infantiseptica 771.2
  lipoid 277.89
  lipophagic, intestinal 040.2
  miliary 027.0
  necrotizing, respiratory 446.4
  progressive, septic 288.1
  Wegener's (necrotizing respiratory) 446.4
Granulomatous tissue — *see* Granuloma
Granuloma NEC 686.1
  abdomen (wall) 568.89
    skin (pyogenicum) 686.1
      from residual foreign body 709.4
  annulare 695.89
  anus 569.49
  apical 522.6
  appendix 543.9
  aural 380.23
  beryllium (skin) 709.4
    lung 503
  bone (*see also* Osteomyelitis) 730.1 ☑
    eosinophilic 277.89
    from residual foreign body 733.99
  canaliculus lacrimalis 375.81
  cerebral 348.89
  cholesterin, middle ear 385.82
  coccidioidal (progressive) 114.3
    lung 114.4
    meninges 114.2
    primary (lung) 114.0

Granuloma — *continued*
  colon 569.89
  conjunctiva 372.61
  dental 522.6
  ear, middle (cholesterin) 385.82
    with otitis media — *see* Otitis media
  eosinophilic 277.89
    bone 277.89
    lung 277.89
    oral mucosa 528.9
  exuberant 701.5
  eyelid 374.89
  facial
    lethal midline 446.3
    malignant 446.3
  faciale 701.8
  fissuratum (gum) 523.8
  foot NEC 686.1
  foreign body (in soft tissue) NEC 728.82
    bone 733.99
    in operative wound 998.4
    muscle 728.82
    skin 709.4
    subcutaneous tissue 709.4
  fungoides 202.1 ☑
  gangraenescens 446.3
  giant cell (central) (jaw) (reparative) 526.3
    gingiva 523.8
    peripheral (gingiva) 523.8
  gland (lymph) 289.3
  Hodgkin's (M9661/3) 201.1 ☑
  ileum 569.89
  infectious NEC 136.9
  inguinale (Donovan) 099.2
    venereal 099.2
  intestine 569.89
  iridocyclitis 364.10
  jaw (bone) 526.3
    reparative giant cell 526.3
  kidney (*see also* Infection, kidney) 590.9
  lacrimal sac 375.81
  larynx 478.79
  lethal midline 446.3
  lipid 277.89
  lipoid 277.89
  liver 572.8
  lung (infectious) (*see also* Fibrosis, lung) 515
    coccidioidal 114.4
    eosinophilic 277.89
  lymph gland 289.3
  Majocchi's 110.6
  malignant, face 446.3
  mandible 526.3
  mediastinum 519.3
  midline 446.3
  monilial 112.3
  muscle 728.82
    from residual foreign body 728.82
  nasal sinus (*see also* Sinusitis) 473.9
  operation wound 998.59
    foreign body 998.4
    stitch (external) 998.89
      internal wound 998.89
    talc 998.7
  oral mucosa, eosinophilic or pyogenic 528.9
  orbit, orbital 376.11
  paracoccidioidal 116.1
  penis, venereal 099.2
  periapical 522.6
  peritoneum 568.89
    due to ova of helminths NEC (*see also* Helminthiasis) 128.9
  postmastoidectomy cavity 383.33
  postoperative — *see* Granuloma, operation wound
  prostate 601.8
  pudendi (ulcerating) 099.2
  pudendorum (ulcerative) 099.2
  pulp, internal (tooth) 521.49
  pyogenic, pyogenicum (skin) 686.1
    maxillary alveolar ridge 522.6
    oral mucosa 528.9
  rectum 569.49
  reticulohistiocytic 277.89
  rubrum nasi 705.89
  sarcoid 135

Granuloma — *continued*
  Schistosoma 120.9
  septic (skin) 686.1
  silica (skin) 709.4
  sinus (accessory) (infectional) (nasal) (*see also* Sinusitis) 473.9
  skin (pyogenicum) 686.1
    from foreign body or material 709.4
  sperm 608.89
  spine
    syphilitic (epidural) 094.89
    tuberculous (*see also* Tuberculosis) 015.0 ☑ *[730.88]*
  stitch (postoperative) 998.89
    internal wound 998.89
  suppurative (skin) 686.1
  suture (postoperative) 998.89
    internal wound 998.89
  swimming pool 031.1
  talc 728.82
    in operation wound 998.7
  telangiectaticum (skin) 686.1
  tracheostomy 519.09
  trichophyticum 110.6
  tropicum 102.4
  umbilicus 686.1
    newborn 771.4
  urethra 599.84
  uveitis 364.10
  vagina 099.2
  venereum 099.2
  vocal cords 478.5
  Wegener's (necrotizing respiratory granulomatosis) 446.4
Granulosis rubra nasi 705.89
Graphite fibrosis (of lung) 503
Graphospasm 300.89
  organic 333.84
Grating scapula 733.99
Gravel (urinary) — *see also* Calculus 592.9
Graves' disease (exophthalmic goiter) — *see also* Goiter, toxic 242.0 ☑
Gravis — *see* condition
Grawitz's tumor (hypernephroma) (M8312/3) 189.0
Grayness, hair (premature) 704.3
  congenital 757.4
Gray or grey syndrome (chloramphenicol) (newborn) 779.4
Greenfield's disease 330.0
Green sickness 280.9
Greenstick fracture — *see* Fracture, by site
Greig's syndrome (hypertelorism) 756.0
Grief 309.0
Griesinger's disease — *see also* Ancylostomiasis 126.9
Grinders'
  asthma 502
  lung 502
  phthisis (*see also* Tuberculosis) 011.4 ☑
Grinding, teeth 306.8
Grip
  Dabney's 074.1
  devil's 074.1
Grippe, grippal — *see also* Influenza
  Balkan 083.0
  intestinal (*see also* Influenza) 487.8
  summer 074.8
Grippy cold — *see also* Influenza 487.1
Grisel's disease 723.5
Groin — *see* condition
Grooved
  nails (transverse) 703.8
  tongue 529.5
    congenital 750.13
Ground itch 126.9
Growing pains, children 781.99
Growth (fungoid) (neoplastic) (new) (M8000/1) — *see also* Neoplasm, by site, unspecified nature
  adenoid (vegetative) 474.12
  benign (M8000/0) — *see* Neoplasm, by site, benign
  fetal, poor 764.9 ☑
    affecting management of pregnancy 656.5 ☑

Growth — *see also* Neoplasm, by site, unspecified nature — *continued*
  malignant (M8000/3) — *see* Neoplasm, by site, malignant
  rapid, childhood V21.0
  secondary (M8000/6) — *see* Neoplasm, by site, malignant, secondary
GRSA (glycopeptide resistant staphylococcus aureus) V09.8 ☑
Gruber's hernia — *see* Hernia, Gruber's
Gruby's disease (tinea tonsurans) 110.0
GSS (Gerstmann-Sträussler-Scheinker syndrome) 046.71
G-trisomy 758.0
Guama fever 066.3
Gubler (-Millard) paralysis or syndrome 344.89
Guérin-Stern syndrome (arthrogryposis multiplex congenita) 754.89
Guertin's disease (electric chorea) 049.8
Guillain-Barré disease or syndrome 357.0
Guinea worms (infection) (infestation) 125.7
Guinon's disease (motor-verbal tic) 307.23
Gull and Sutton's disease — *see* Hypertension, kidney
Gull's disease (thyroid atrophy with myxedema) 244.8
Gum — *see* condition
Gumboil 522.7
Gumma (syphilitic) 095.9
  artery 093.89
    cerebral or spinal 094.89
  bone 095.5
    of yaws (late) 102.6
  brain 094.89
  cauda equina 094.89
  central nervous system NEC 094.9
  ciliary body 095.8 *[364.11]*
  congenital 090.5
    testis 090.5
  eyelid 095.8 *[373.5]*
  heart 093.89
  intracranial 094.89
  iris 095.8 *[364.11]*
  kidney 095.4
  larynx 095.8
  leptomeninges 094.2
  liver 095.3
  meninges 094.2
  myocardium 093.82
  nasopharynx 095.8
  neurosyphilitic 094.9
  nose 095.8
  orbit 095.8
  palate (soft) 095.8
  penis 095.8
  pericardium 093.81
  pharynx 095.8
  pituitary 095.8
  scrofulous (see also Tuberculosis) 017.0 ☑
  skin 095.8
  specified site NEC 095.8
  spinal cord 094.89
  tongue 095.8
  tonsil 095.8
  trachea 095.8
  tuberculous (*see also* Tuberculosis) 017.0 ☑
  ulcerative due to yaws 102.4
  ureter 095.8
  yaws 102.4
    bone 102.6
Gunn's syndrome (jaw-winking syndrome) 742.8
Gunshot wound — *see also* Wound, open, by site
  fracture — *see* Fracture, by site, open
  internal organs (abdomen, chest, or pelvis) — *see* Injury, internal, by site, with open wound
  intracranial — *see* Laceration, brain, with open intracranial wound
Günther's disease or syndrome (congenital erythropoietic porphyria) 277.1
Gustatory hallucination 780.1
Gynandrism 752.7

☑ **Additional Digit Required** — Refer to the Tabular List for Digit Selection   ▽ **Subterms under main terms may continue to next column or page**

Gynandroblastoma (M8632/1)
   specified site — see Neoplasm, by site, uncertain behavior
   unspecified site
      female 236.2
      male 236.4
Gynandromorphism 752.7
Gynatresia (congenital) 752.49
Gynecoid pelvis, male 738.6
Gynecological examination V72.31
   for contraceptive maintenance V25.40
Gynecomastia 611.1
Gynephobia 300.29
Gyrate scalp 757.39

H

Haas' disease (osteochondrosis head of humerus) 732.3
Habermann's disease (acute parapsoriasis varioliformis) 696.2
Habit, habituation
   chorea 307.22
   disturbance, child 307.9
   drug (see also Dependence) 304.9 ☑
   laxative (see also Abuse, drugs, nondependent) 305.9 ☑
   spasm 307.20
      chronic 307.22
      transient (of childhood) 307.21
   tic 307.20
      chronic 307.22
      transient (of childhood) 307.21
   use of
      nonprescribed drugs (see also Abuse, drugs, nondependent) 305.9 ☑
      patent medicines (see also Abuse, drugs, nondependent) 305.9 ☑
   vomiting 536.2
Hadfield-Clarke syndrome (pancreatic infantilism) 577.8
Haff disease 985.1
Hageman factor defect, deficiency, or disease — see also Defect, coagulation 286.3
Haglund's disease (osteochondrosis os tibiale externum) 732.5
Haglund-Läwen-Fründ syndrome 717.89
Hagner's disease (hypertrophic pulmonary osteoarthropathy) 731.2
Hag teeth, tooth 524.39
Hailey-Hailey disease (benign familial chronic pemphigus) 757.39
Hair — see also condition
   plucking 307.9
Hairball in stomach 935.2
Hairy black tongue 529.3
Half vertebra 756.14
Halitosis 784.99
Hallermann-Streiff syndrome 756.0
Hallervorden-Spatz disease or syndrome 333.0
Hallopeau's
   acrodermatitis (continua) 696.1
   disease (lichen sclerosis et atrophicus) 701.0
Hallucination (auditory) (gustatory) (olfactory) (tactile) 780.1
   alcohol-induced 291.3
   drug-induced 292.12
   visual 368.16
Hallucinosis 298.9
   alcohol-induced (acute) 291.3
   drug-induced 292.12
Hallus — see Hallux
Hallux 735.9
   limitus 735.8
   malleus (acquired) 735.3
   rigidus (acquired) 735.2
      congenital 755.66
      late effects of rickets 268.1
   valgus (acquired) 735.0
      congenital 755.66
   varus (acquired) 735.1
      congenital 755.66
Halo, visual 368.15
Hamartoblastoma 759.6
Hamartoma 759.6

Hamartoma — continued
   epithelial (gingival), odontogenic, central, or peripheral (M9321/0) 213.1
      upper jaw (bone) 213.0
   vascular 757.32
Hamartosis, hamartoses NEC 759.6
Hamman's disease or syndrome (spontaneous mediastinal emphysema) 518.1
Hamman-Rich syndrome (diffuse interstitial pulmonary fibrosis) 516.33
Hammer toe (acquired) 735.4
   congenital 755.66
   late effects of rickets 268.1
Hand — see condition
Hand-foot syndrome 693.0
Hand-Schüller-Christian disease or syndrome (chronic histiocytosis x) 277.89
Hanging (asphyxia) (strangulation) (suffocation) 994.7
Hangnail (finger) (with lymphangitis) 681.02
Hangover (alcohol) — see also Abuse, drugs, nondependent 305.0 ☑
Hanot-Chauffard (-Troisier) syndrome (bronze diabetes) 275.01
Hanot's cirrhosis or disease — see Cirrhosis, biliary
Hansen's disease (leprosy) 030.9
   benign form 030.1
   malignant form 030.0
Harada's disease or syndrome 363.22
Hard chancre 091.0
Hardening
   artery — see Arteriosclerosis
   brain 348.89
   liver 571.8
Hard firm prostate 600.10
   with
      urinary
         obstruction 600.11
         retention 600.11
Harelip — see also Cleft, lip 749.10
Hare's syndrome (M8010/3) (carcinoma, pulmonary apex) 162.3
Harkavy's syndrome 446.0
Harlequin (fetus) 757.1
   color change syndrome 779.89
Harley's disease (intermittent hemoglobinuria) 283.2
Harris'
   lines 733.91
   syndrome (organic hyperinsulinism) 251.1
Hart's disease or syndrome (pellagra-cerebellar ataxia-renal aminoaciduria) 270.0
Hartmann's pouch (abnormal sacculation of gallbladder neck) 575.8
   of intestine V44.3
      attention to V55.3
Hartnup disease (pellagra-cerebellar ataxia-renal aminoaciduria) 270.0
Harvester lung 495.0
Hashimoto's disease or struma (struma lymphomatosa) 245.2
Hassall-Henle bodies (corneal warts) 371.41
Haut mal — see also Epilepsy 345.1 ☑
Haverhill fever 026.1
Hawaiian wood rose dependence 304.5 ☑
Hawkins' keloid 701.4
Hay
   asthma (see also Asthma) 493.0 ☑
   fever (allergic) (with rhinitis) 477.9
      with asthma (bronchial) (see also Asthma) 493.0 ☑
      allergic, due to grass, pollen, ragweed, or tree 477.0
      conjunctivitis 372.05
      due to
         dander, animal (cat) (dog) 477.2
         dust 477.8
         fowl 477.8
         hair, animal (cat) (dog) 477.2
         pollen 477.0
         specified allergen other than pollen 477.8
Hayem-Faber syndrome (achlorhydric anemia) 280.9

Hayem-Widal syndrome (acquired hemolytic jaundice) 283.9
Haygarth's nodosities 715.04
Hazard-Crile tumor (M8350/3) 193
Hb (abnormal)
   disease — see Disease, hemoglobin
   trait — see Trait
H disease 270.0
Head — see also condition
   banging 307.3
Headache 784.0
   allergic 339.00
   associated with sexual activity 339.82
   cluster 339.00
      chronic 339.02
      episodic 339.01
   daily
      chronic 784.0
      new persistent (NPDH) 339.42
   drug induced 339.3
   due to
      loss, spinal fluid 349.0
      lumbar puncture 349.0
      saddle block 349.0
   emotional 307.81
   histamine 339.00
   hypnic 339.81
   lumbar puncture 349.0
   medication overuse 339.3
   menopausal 627.2
   menstrual 346.4 ☑
   migraine 346.9 ☑
   nasal septum 784.0
   nonorganic origin 307.81
   orgasmic 339.82
   postspinal 349.0
   post-traumatic 339.20
      acute 339.21
      chronic 339.22
   premenstrual 346.4 ☑
   preorgasmic 339.82
   primary
      cough 339.83
      exertional 339.84
      stabbing 339.85
      thunderclap 339.43
   psychogenic 307.81
   psychophysiologic 307.81
   rebound 339.3
   short lasting unilateral neuralgiform with conjunctival injection and tearing (SUNCT) 339.05
   sick 346.9 ☑
   spinal 349.0
      complicating labor and delivery 668.8 ☑
      postpartum 668.8 ☑
   spinal fluid loss 349.0
   syndrome
      cluster 339.00
      complicated NEC 339.44
      periodic in child or adolescent 346.2 ☑
      specified NEC 339.89
   tension 307.81
      type 339.10
         chronic 339.12
         episodic 339.11
   vascular 784.0
      migraine type 346.9 ☑
   vasomotor 346.9 ☑
Health
   advice V65.4 ☑
   audit V70.0
   checkup V70.0
   education V65.4 ☑
   hazard (see also History of) V15.9
      falling V15.88
      specified cause NEC V15.89
   instruction V65.4 ☑
   services provided because (of)
      boarding school residence V60.6
      holiday relief for person providing home care V60.5
      inadequate
         housing V60.1
         resources V60.2
      lack of housing V60.0

Health — continued
   services provided because — continued
      no care available in home V60.4
      person living alone V60.3
      poverty V60.3
      residence in institution V60.6
      specified cause NEC V60.89
      vacation relief for person providing home care V60.5
Healthy
   donor (see also Donor) V59.9
   infant or child
      accompanying sick mother V65.0
      receiving care V20.1
   person
      accompanying sick relative V65.0
      admitted for sterilization V25.2
      receiving prophylactic inoculation or vaccination (see also Vaccination, prophylactic) V05.9
Hearing
   conservation and treatment V72.12
   examination V72.19
      following failed hearing screening V72.11
Heart — see condition
Heartburn 787.1
   psychogenic 306.4
Heat (effects) 992.9
   apoplexy 992.0
   burn (see also Burn, by site)
      from sun (see also Sunburn) 692.71
   collapse 992.1
   cramps 992.2
   dermatitis or eczema 692.89
   edema 992.7
   erythema — see Burn, by site
   excessive 992.9
      specified effect NEC 992.8
   exhaustion 992.5
      anhydrotic 992.3
      due to
         salt (and water) depletion 992.4
         water depletion 992.3
   fatigue (transient) 992.6
   fever 992.0
   hyperpyrexia 992.0
   prickly 705.1
   prostration — see Heat, exhaustion
   pyrexia 992.0
   rash 705.1
   specified effect NEC 992.8
   stroke 992.0
   sunburn (see also Sunburn) 692.71
   syncope 992.1
Heavy-chain disease 273.2
Heavy-for-dates (fetus or infant) 766.1
   4500 grams or more 766.0
   exceptionally 766.0
Hebephrenia, hebephrenic (acute) — see also Schizophrenia 295.1 ☑
   dementia (praecox) (see also Schizophrenia) 295.1 ☑
   schizophrenia (see also Schizophrenia) 295.1 ☑
Heberden's
   disease or nodes 715.04
   syndrome (angina pectoris) 413.9
Hebra's disease
   dermatitis exfoliativa 695.89
   erythema multiforme exudativum 695.19
   pityriasis 695.89
      maculata et circinata 696.3
      rubra 695.89
      pilaris 696.4
   prurigo 698.2
Hebra, nose 040.1
Hedinger's syndrome (malignant carcinoid) 259.2
Heel — see condition
Heerfordt's disease or syndrome (uveoparotitis) 135
Hegglin's anomaly or syndrome 288.2
Heidenhain's disease 290.10
   with dementia 290.10

☑ **Additional Digit Required** — Refer to the Tabular List for Digit Selection   🔻 **Subterms under main terms may continue to next column or page**

2014 ICD-9-CM   **177**

Heilmeyer-Schöner disease (M9842/3) 207.1 ☑

Heine-Medin disease — *see also* Poliomyelitis 045.9 ☑

Heinz-body anemia, congenital 282.7

Heller's disease or syndrome (infantile psychosis) — *see also* Psychosis, childhood 299.1 ☑

H.E.L.L.P 642.5 ☑

Helminthiasis — *see also* Infestation, by specific parasite 128.9
  Ancylostoma (*see also* Ancylostoma) 126.9
  intestinal 127.9
    mixed types (types classifiable to more than one of the categories 120.0–127.7) 127.8
    specified type 127.7
  mixed types (intestinal) (types classifiable to more than one of the categories 120.0–127.7) 127.8
  Necator americanus 126.1
  specified type NEC 128.8
  Trichinella 124

Heloma 700

Hemangioblastoma (M9161/1) — *see also* Neoplasm, connective tissue, uncertain behavior
  malignant (M9161/3) — *see* Neoplasm, connective tissue, malignant

Hemangioblastomatosis, cerebelloretinal 759.6

Hemangioendothelioma (M9130/1) — *see also* Neoplasm, by site, uncertain behavior
  benign (M9130/0) 228.00
  bone (diffuse) (M9130/3) — *see* Neoplasm, bone, malignant
  malignant (M9130/3) — *see* Neoplasm, connective tissue, malignant
  nervous system (M9130/0) 228.09

Hemangioendotheliosarcoma (M9130/3) — *see* Neoplasm, connective tissue, malignant

Hemangiofibroma (M9160/0) — *see* Neoplasm, by site, benign

Hemangiolipoma (M8861/0) — *see* Lipoma

Hemangioma (M9120/0) 228.00
  arteriovenous (M9123/0) — *see* Hemangioma, by site
  brain 228.02
  capillary (M9131/0) — *see* Hemangioma, by site
  cavernous (M9121/0) — *see* Hemangioma, by site
  central nervous system NEC 228.09
  choroid 228.09
  heart 228.09
  infantile (M9131/0) — *see* Hemangioma, by site
  intra-abdominal structures 228.04
  intracranial structures 228.02
  intramuscular (M9132/0) — *see* Hemangioma, by site
  iris 228.09
  juvenile (M9131/0) — *see* Hemangioma, by site
  malignant (M9120/3) — *see* Neoplasm, connective tissue, malignant
  meninges 228.09
    brain 228.02
    spinal cord 228.09
  peritoneum 228.04
  placenta — *see* Placenta, abnormal
  plexiform (M9131/0) — *see* Hemangioma, by site
  racemose (M9123/0) — *see* Hemangioma, by site
  retina 228.03
  retroperitoneal tissue 228.04
  sclerosing (M8832/0) — *see* Neoplasm, skin, benign
  simplex (M9131/0) — *see* Hemangioma, by site
  skin and subcutaneous tissue 228.01
  specified site NEC 228.09
  spinal cord 228.09

Hemangioma — *continued*
  venous (M9122/0) — *see* Hemangioma, by site
  verrucous keratotic (M9142/0) — *see* Hemangioma, by site

Hemangiomatosis (systemic) 757.32
  involving single site — *see* Hemangioma

Hemangiopericytoma (M9150/1) — *see also* Neoplasm, connective tissue, uncertain behavior
  benign (M9150/0) — *see* Neoplasm, connective tissue, benign
  malignant (M9150/3) — *see* Neoplasm, connective tissue, malignant

Hemangiosarcoma (M9120/3) — *see* Neoplasm, connective tissue, malignant

Hemarthrosis (nontraumatic) 719.10
  ankle 719.17
  elbow 719.12
  foot 719.17
  hand 719.14
  hip 719.15
  knee 719.16
  multiple sites 719.19
  pelvic region 719.15
  shoulder (region) 719.11
  specified site NEC 719.18
  traumatic — *see* Sprain, by site
  wrist 719.13

Hematemesis 578.0
  with ulcer — *see* Ulcer, by site, with hemorrhage
  due to S. japonicum 120.2
  Goldstein's (familial hemorrhagic telangiectasia) 448.0
  newborn 772.4
    due to swallowed maternal blood 777.3

Hematidrosis 705.89

Hematinuria — *see also* Hemoglobinuria 791.2
  malarial 084.8
  paroxysmal 283.2

Hematite miners' lung 503

Hematobilia 576.8

Hematocele (congenital) (diffuse) (idiopathic) 608.83
  broad ligament 620.7
  canal of Nuck 629.0
  cord, male 608.83
  fallopian tube 620.8
  female NEC 629.0
  ischiorectal 569.89
  male NEC 608.83
  ovary 629.0
  pelvis, pelvic
    female 629.0
      with ectopic pregnancy (*see also* Pregnancy, ectopic) 633.90
      with intrauterine pregnancy 633.91
    male 608.83
  periuterine 629.0
  retrouterine 629.0
  scrotum 608.83
  spermatic cord (diffuse) 608.83
  testis 608.84
  traumatic — *see* Injury, internal, pelvis
  tunica vaginalis 608.83
  uterine ligament 629.0
  uterus 621.4
  vagina 623.6
  vulva 624.5

Hematocephalus 742.4

Hematochezia — *see also* Melena 578.1

Hematochyluria — *see also* Infestation, filarial 125.9

Hematocolpos 626.8

Hematocornea 371.12

Hematogenous — *see* condition

Hematoma (skin surface intact) (traumatic) — *see also* Contusion

> Note — Hematomas are coded according to origin and the nature and site of the hematoma or the accompanying injury. Hematomas of unspecified origin are coded as injuries of the sites involved, except:
>
> (a) hematomas of genital organs which are coded as diseases of the organ involved unless they complicate pregnancy or delivery
>
> (b) hematomas of the eye which are coded as diseases of the eye.
>
> For late effect of hematoma classifiable to 920–924 see Late, effect, contusion

  with
    crush injury — *see* Crush
    fracture — *see* Fracture, by site
    injury of internal organs (*see also* Injury, internal, by site)
      kidney — *see* Hematoma, kidney traumatic
      liver — *see* Hematoma, liver, traumatic
      spleen — *see* Hematoma, spleen
    nerve injury — *see* Injury, nerve
    open wound — *see* Wound, open, by site
    skin surface intact — *see* Contusion
  abdomen (wall) — *see* Contusion, abdomen
  amnion 658.8 ☑
  aorta, dissecting 441.00
    abdominal 441.02
    thoracic 441.01
    thoracoabdominal 441.03
  aortic intramural — *see* Dissection, aorta
  arterial (complicating trauma) 904.9
    specified site — *see* Injury, blood vessel, by site
  auricle (ear) 380.31
  birth injury 767.8
    skull 767.19
  brain (traumatic) 853.0 ☑

> Note — Use the following fifth-digit subclassification with categories 851–854:
>
> 0   unspecified state of consciousness
>
> 1   with no loss of consciousness
>
> 2   with brief [less than one hour] loss of consciousness
>
> 3   with moderate [1–24 hours] loss of consciousness
>
> 4   with prolonged [more than 24 hours] loss of consciousness and return to pre–existing conscious level
>
> 5   with prolonged [more than 24 hours] loss of consciousness, without return to pre–existing conscious level
>
> Use fifth-digit 5 to designate when a patient is unconscious and dies before regaining consciousness, regardless of the duration of the loss of consciousness
>
> 6   with loss of consciousness of unspecified duration
>
> 9   with concussion, unspecified

    with
      cerebral
        contusion — *see* Contusion, brain
        laceration — *see* Laceration, brain
      open intracranial wound 853.1 ☑
      skull fracture — *see* Fracture, skull, by site
    extradural or epidural 852.4 ☑
      with open intracranial wound 852.5 ☑
      fetus or newborn 767.0

Hematoma — *see also* Contusion — *continued*
  brain — *continued*
    extradural or epidural — *continued*
      nontraumatic 432.0
    fetus or newborn NEC 767.0
    nontraumatic (*see also* Hemorrhage, brain) 431
      epidural or extradural 432.0
      newborn NEC 772.8
      subarachnoid, arachnoid, or meningeal (*see also* Hemorrhage, subarachnoid) 430
      subdural (*see also* Hemorrhage, subdural) 432.1
    subarachnoid, arachnoid, or meningeal 852.0 ☑
      with open intracranial wound 852.1 ☑
      fetus or newborn 772.2
      nontraumatic (*see also* Hemorrhage, subarachnoid) 430
    subdural 852.2 ☑
      with open intracranial wound 852.3 ☑
      fetus or newborn (localized) 767.0
      nontraumatic (*see also* Hemorrhage, subdural) 432.1
  breast (nontraumatic) 611.89
  broad ligament (nontraumatic) 620.7
    complicating delivery 665.7 ☑
    traumatic — *see* Injury, internal, broad ligament
  calcified NEC 959.9
  capitis 920
    due to birth injury 767.19
    newborn 767.19
  cerebral — *see* Hematoma, brain
  cesarean section wound 674.3 ☑
  chorion — *see* Placenta, abnormal
  complicating delivery (perineum) (vulva) 664.5 ☑
    pelvic 665.7 ☑
    vagina 665.7 ☑
  corpus
    cavernosum (nontraumatic) 607.82
    luteum (nontraumatic) (ruptured) 620.1
  dura (mater) — *see* Hematoma, brain, subdural
  epididymis (nontraumatic) 608.83
  epidural (traumatic) (*see also* Hematoma, brain, extradural)
    spinal — *see* Injury, spinal, by site
  episiotomy 674.3 ☑
  external ear 380.31
  extradural (*see also* Hematoma, brain, extradural)
    fetus or newborn 767.0
    nontraumatic 432.0
      fetus or newborn 767.0
  fallopian tube 620.8
  genital organ (nontraumatic)
    female NEC 629.89
    male NEC 608.83
    traumatic (external site) 922.4
      internal — *see* Injury, internal, genital organ
  graafian follicle (ruptured) 620.0
  internal organs (abdomen, chest, or pelvis) (*see also* Injury, internal, by site)
    kidney — *see* Hematoma, kidney, traumatic
    liver — *see* Hematoma, liver, traumatic
    spleen — *see* Hematoma, spleen
  intracranial — *see* Hematoma, brain
  kidney, cystic 593.81
    traumatic 866.01
      with open wound into cavity 866.11
  labia (nontraumatic) 624.5
  lingual (and other parts of neck, scalp, or face, except eye) 920
  liver (subcapsular) 573.8
    birth injury 767.8
    fetus or newborn 767.8
    traumatic NEC 864.01

☑ **Additional Digit Required** — Refer to the Tabular List for Digit Selection   ▽ **Subterms under main terms may continue to next column or page**

178   **2014 ICD-9-CM**

Hematoma — see also Contusion —
continued
liver — continued
traumatic — continued
with
laceration — see Laceration, liver
open wound into cavity 864.11
mediastinum — see Injury, internal, mediastinum
meninges, meningeal (brain) (see also
Hematoma, brain, subarachnoid)
spinal — see Injury, spinal, by site
mesosalpinx (nontraumatic) 620.8
traumatic — see Injury, internal, pelvis
muscle (traumatic) — see Contusion, by site
nontraumatic 729.92
nasal (septum) (and other part(s) of neck,
scalp, or face, except eye) 920
obstetrical surgical wound 674.3 ☑
orbit, orbital (nontraumatic) 376.32
traumatic 921.2
ovary (corpus luteum) (nontraumatic) 620.1
traumatic — see Injury, internal, ovary
pelvis (female) (nontraumatic) 629.89
complicating delivery 665.7 ☑
male 608.83
traumatic (see also Injury, internal, pelvis)
specified organ NEC (see also Injury,
internal, pelvis) 867.6
penis (nontraumatic) 607.82
pericranial (and neck, or face any part, except eye) 920
due to injury at birth 767.19
perineal wound (obstetrical) 674.3 ☑
complicating delivery 664.5 ☑
perirenal, cystic 593.81
pinna 380.31
placenta — see Placenta, abnormal
postoperative 998.12
retroperitoneal (nontraumatic) 568.81
traumatic — see Injury, internal,
retroperitoneum
retropubic, male 568.81
scalp (and neck, or face any part, except eye)
920
fetus or newborn 767.19
scrotum (nontraumatic) 608.83
traumatic 922.4
seminal vesicle (nontraumatic) 608.83
traumatic — see Injury, internal, seminal,
vesicle
soft tissue 729.92
spermatic cord (see also Injury, internal,
spermatic cord)
nontraumatic 608.83
spinal (cord) (meninges) (see also Injury,
spinal, by site)
fetus or newborn 767.4
nontraumatic 336.1
spleen 865.01
with
laceration — see Laceration, spleen
open wound into cavity 865.11
sternocleidomastoid, birth injury 767.8
sternomastoid, birth injury 767.8
subarachnoid (see also Hematoma, brain,
subarachnoid)
fetus or newborn 772.2
nontraumatic (see also Hemorrhage,
subarachnoid) 430
newborn 772.2
subdural (see also Hematoma, brain, subdural)
fetus or newborn (localized) 767.0
nontraumatic (see also Hemorrhage,
subdural) 432.1
subperiosteal (syndrome) 267
traumatic — see Hematoma, by site
superficial, fetus or newborn 772.6
syncytium — see Placenta, abnormal
testis (nontraumatic) 608.83
birth injury 767.8
traumatic 922.4
tunica vaginalis (nontraumatic) 608.83
umbilical cord 663.6 ☑
affecting fetus or newborn 762.6

Hematoma — see also Contusion —
continued
uterine ligament (nontraumatic) 620.7
traumatic — see Injury, internal, pelvis
uterus 621.4
traumatic — see Injury, internal, pelvis
vagina (nontraumatic) (ruptured) 623.6
complicating delivery 665.7 ☑
traumatic 922.4
vas deferens (nontraumatic) 608.83
traumatic — see Injury, internal, vas
deferens
vitreous 379.23
vocal cord 920
vulva (nontraumatic) 624.5
complicating delivery 664.5 ☑
fetus or newborn 767.8
traumatic 922.4
Hematometra 621.4
Hematomyelia 336.1
with fracture of vertebra (see also Fracture,
vertebra, by site, with spinal cord injury) 806.8
fetus or newborn 767.4
Hematomyelitis 323.9
late effect — see category 326
Hematoperitoneum — see also Hemoperitoneum 568.81
Hematopneumothorax — see also Hemothorax 511.89
Hematopoiesis, cyclic 288.02
Hematoporphyria (acquired) (congenital)
277.1
Hematoporphyrinuria (acquired) (congenital)
277.1
Hematorachis, hematorrhachis 336.1
fetus or newborn 767.4
Hematosalpinx 620.8
with
ectopic pregnancy (see also categories
633.0–633.9) 639.2
infectional (see also Salpingo-oophoritis)
614.2
molar pregnancy (see also categories
630–632) 639.2
Hematospermia 608.82
Hematothorax — see also Hemothorax 511.89
Hematotympanum 381.03
Hematuria (benign) (essential) (idiopathic)
599.70
due to S. hematobium 120.0
endemic 120.0
gross 599.71
intermittent 599.70
malarial 084.8
microscopic 599.72
paroxysmal 599.70
sulfonamide
correct substance properly administered
599.70
overdose or wrong substance given or
taken 961.0
tropical (bilharziasis) 120.0
tuberculous (see also Tuberculosis) 016.9 ☑
Hematuric bilious fever 084.8
Hemeralopia 368.10
Hemiabiotrophy 799.89
Hemi-akinesia 781.8
Hemianalgesia — see also Disturbance, sensation 782.0
Hemianencephaly 740.0
Hemianesthesia — see also Disturbance, sensation 782.0
Hemianopia, hemianopsia (altitudinal)
(homonymous) 368.46
binasal 368.47
bitemporal 368.47
heteronymous 368.47
syphilitic 095.8
Hemiasomatognosia 307.9
Hemiathetosis 781.0
Hemiatrophy 799.89
cerebellar 334.8
face 349.89
progressive 349.89
fascia 728.9

Hemiatrophy — continued
leg 728.2
tongue 529.8
Hemiballism (us) 333.5
Hemiblock (cardiac) (heart) (left) 426.2
Hemicardia 746.89
Hemicephalus, hemicephaly 740.0
Hemichorea 333.5
Hemicrania 346.9 ☑
congenital malformation 740.0
continua 339.41
paroxysmal 339.03
chronic 339.04
episodic 339.03
Hemidystrophy — see Hemiatrophy
Hemiectromelia 755.4
Hemihypalgesia — see also Disturbance, sensation 782.0
Hemihypertrophy (congenital) 759.89
cranial 756.0
Hemihypesthesia — see also Disturbance,
sensation 782.0
Hemi-inattention 781.8
Hemimelia 755.4
lower limb 755.30
paraxial (complete) (incomplete) (intercalary) (terminal) 755.32
fibula 755.37
tibia 755.36
transverse (complete) (partial) 755.31
upper limb 755.20
paraxial (complete) (incomplete) (intercalary) (terminal) 755.22
radial 755.26
ulnar 755.27
transverse (complete) (partial) 755.21
Hemiparalysis — see also Hemiplegia 342.9
Hemiparesis — see also Hemiplegia 342.9
Hemiparesthesia — see also Disturbance,
sensation 782.0
Hemiplegia 342.9 ☑
acute (see also Disease, cerebrovascular,
acute) 436
alternans facialis 344.89
apoplectic (see also Disease, cerebrovascular, acute) 436
late effect or residual
affecting
dominant side 438.21
nondominant side 438.22
unspecified side 438.20
arteriosclerotic 437.0
late effect or residual
affecting
dominant side 438.21
nondominant side 438.22
unspecified side 438.20
ascending (spinal) NEC 344.89
attack (see also Disease, cerebrovascular,
acute) 436
brain, cerebral (current episode) 437.8
congenital 343.1
cerebral — see Hemiplegia, brain
congenital (cerebral) (spastic) (spinal) 343.1
conversion neurosis (hysterical) 300.11
cortical — see Hemiplegia, brain
due to
arteriosclerosis 437.0
late effect or residual
affecting
dominant side 438.21
nondominant side 438.22
unspecified side 438.20
cerebrovascular lesion (see also Disease,
cerebrovascular, acute) 436
late effect
affecting
dominant side 438.21
nondominant side 438.22
unspecified side 438.20
embolic (current) (see also Embolism, brain)
434.1 ☑
late effect
affecting
dominant side 438.21
nondominant side 438.22

Hemiplegia — continued
embolic (see also Embolism, brain) — continued
late effect — continued
affecting — continued
unspecified side 438.20
flaccid 342.0 ☑
hypertensive (current episode) 437.8
infantile (postnatal) 343.4
late effect
birth injury, intracranial or spinal 343.4
cerebrovascular lesion — see Late effect(s) (of) cerebrovascular disease
viral encephalitis 139.0
middle alternating NEC 344.89
newborn NEC 767.0
seizure (current episode) (see also Disease,
cerebrovascular, acute) 436
spastic 342.1 ☑
congenital or infantile 343.1
specified NEC 342.8 ☑
thrombotic (current) (see also Thrombosis,
brain) 434.0 ☑
late effect — see Late effect(s) (of) cerebrovascular disease
Hemisection, spinal cord — see Fracture,
vertebra, by site, with spinal cord injury
Hemispasm 781.0
facial 781.0
Hemispatial neglect 781.8
Hemisporosis 117.9
Hemitremor 781.0
Hemivertebra 756.14
Hemobilia 576.8
Hemocholecyst 575.8
Hemochromatosis (acquired) (liver) (myocardium) (secondary) 275.03
with refractory anemia 238.72
diabetic 275.03
due to repeated red blood cell transfusions
275.02
hereditary 275.01
primary idiopathic 275.01
specified NEC 275.03
transfusion associated (red blood cell)
275.02
Hemodialysis V56.0
Hemoglobin — see also condition
abnormal (disease) — see Disease,
hemoglobin
AS genotype 282.5
fetal, hereditary persistence 282.7
H Constant Spring 282.43
H disease 282.43
high-oxygen-affinity 289.0
low NEC 285.9
S (Hb-S), heterozygous 282.5
Hemoglobinemia 283.2
due to blood transfusion NEC 999.89
bone marrow 996.85
paroxysmal 283.2
Hemoglobinopathy (mixed) — see also Disease, hemoglobin 282.7
with thalassemia 282.49
sickle-cell 282.60
with thalassemia (without crisis) 282.41
with
crisis 282.42
vaso-occlusive pain 282.42
Hemoglobinuria, hemoglobinuric 791.2
with anemia, hemolytic, acquired (chronic)
NEC 283.2
cold (agglutinin) (paroxysmal) (with Raynaud's syndrome) 283.2
due to
exertion 283.2
hemolysis (from external causes) NEC
283.2
exercise 283.2
fever (malaria) 084.8
infantile 791.2
intermittent 283.2
malarial 084.8
march 283.2
nocturnal (paroxysmal) 283.2

☑ Additional Digit Required — Refer to the Tabular List for Digit Selection
▽ Subterms under main terms may continue to next column or page
2014 ICD-9-CM
179

Hemoglobinuria, hemoglobinuric —
continued
  paroxysmal (cold) (nocturnal) 283.2
Hemolymphangioma (M9175/0) 228.1
Hemolysis
  fetal — *see* Jaundice, fetus or newborn
  intravascular (disseminated) NEC 286.6
    with
      abortion — *see* Abortion, by type,
        with hemorrhage, delayed or
        excessive
      ectopic pregnancy (*see also* cate-
        gories 633.0–633.9) 639.1
      hemorrhage of pregnancy 641.3 ☑
        affecting fetus or newborn 762.1
      molar pregnancy (*see also* categories
        630–632) 639.1
    acute 283.2
    following
      abortion 639.1
      ectopic or molar pregnancy 639.1
  neonatal — *see* Jaundice, fetus or newborn
  transfusion NEC 999.89
    bone marrow 996.85
Hemolytic — *see also* condition
  anemia — *see* Anemia, hemolytic
  uremic syndrome 283.11
Hemometra 621.4
Hemopericardium (with effusion) 423.0
  newborn 772.8
  traumatic (*see also* Hemothorax, traumatic)
    860.2
    with open wound into thorax 860.3
Hemoperitoneum 568.81
  infectional (*see also* Peritonitis) 567.29
  traumatic — *see* Injury, internal, peritoneum
Hemophagocytic syndrome 288.4
  infection-associated 288.4
Hemophilia (familial) (hereditary) 286.0
  A 286.0
    carrier (asymptomatic) V83.01
      symptomatic V83.02
  acquired 286.52
  autoimmune 286.52
  B (Leyden) 286.1
  C 286.2
  calcipriva (*see also* Fibrinolysis) 286.7
  classical 286.0
  nonfamilial 286.7
  secondary 286.52
  vascular 286.4
Hemophilus influenzae NEC 041.5
  arachnoiditis (basic) (brain) (spinal) 320.0
    late effect — *see* category 326
  bronchopneumonia 482.2
  cerebral ventriculitis 320.0
    late effect — *see* category 326
  cerebrospinal inflammation 320.0
    late effect — *see* category 326
  infection NEC 041.5
  leptomeningitis 320.0
    late effect — *see* category 326
  meningitis (cerebral) (cerebrospinal) (spinal)
    320.0
    late effect — *see* category 326
  meningomyelitis 320.0
    late effect — *see* category 326
  pachymeningitis (adhesive) (fibrous) (hem-
    orrhagic) (hypertrophic) (spinal)
    320.0
    late effect — *see* category 326
  pneumonia (broncho-) 482.2
Hemophthalmos 360.43
Hemopneumothorax — *see also* Hemothorax
  511.89
  traumatic 860.4
    with open wound into thorax 860.5
Hemoptysis 786.30
  due to Paragonimus (westermani) 121.2
  newborn 770.3
  specified NEC 786.39
  tuberculous (*see also* Tuberculosis, pul-
    monary) 011.9 ☑
Hemorrhage, hemorrhagic (nontraumatic)
  459.0
  abdomen 459.0

Hemorrhage, hemorrhagic — *continued*
  accidental (antepartum) 641.2 ☑
    affecting fetus or newborn 762.1
  adenoid 474.8
  adrenal (capsule) (gland) (medulla) 255.41
    newborn 772.5
  after labor — *see* Hemorrhage, postpartum
  alveolar
    lung, newborn 770.3
    process 525.8
  alveolus 525.8
  amputation stump (surgical) 998.11
    secondary, delayed 997.69
  anemia (chronic) 280.0
    acute 285.1
  antepartum — *see* Hemorrhage, pregnancy
  anus (sphincter) 569.3
  apoplexy (stroke) 432.9
  arachnoid — *see* Hemorrhage, subarach-
    noid
  artery NEC 459.0
    brain (*see also* Hemorrhage, brain) 431
    middle meningeal — *see* Hemorrhage,
      subarachnoid
  basilar (ganglion) (*see also* Hemorrhage,
    brain) 431
  bladder 596.89
  blood dyscrasia 289.9
  bowel 578.9
    newborn 772.4
  brain (miliary) (nontraumatic) 431
    with
      birth injury 767.0
    arachnoid — *see* Hemorrhage, subarach-
      noid
    due to
      birth injury 767.0
      rupture of aneurysm (congenital) (*see
        also* Hemorrhage, subarach-
        noid) 430
      mycotic 431
      syphilis 094.89
    epidural or extradural — *see* Hemor-
      rhage, extradural
    fetus or newborn (anoxic) (hypoxic) (due
      to birth trauma) (nontraumatic)
      767.0
      intraventricular 772.10
        grade I 772.11
        grade II 772.12
        grade III 772.13
        grade IV 772.14
    iatrogenic 997.02
    postoperative 997.02
    puerperal, postpartum, childbirth
      674.0 ☑
    stem 431
    subarachnoid, arachnoid, or meningeal
      — *see* Hemorrhage, subarach-
      noid
    subdural — *see* Hemorrhage, subdural

Hemorrhage, hemorrhagic — *continued*
  brain — *continued*
    traumatic NEC 853.0 ☑

> Note — Use the following fifth-digit
> subclassification with categories
> 851–854:
>
> 0 unspecified state of consciousness
>
> 1 with no loss of consciousness
>
> 2 with brief [less than one hour]
>   loss of consciousness
>
> 3 with moderate [1–24 hours] loss
>   of consciousness
>
> 4 with prolonged [more than 24
>   hours] loss of consciousness and
>   return to pre–existing conscious
>   level
>
> 5 with prolonged [more than 24
>   hours] loss of consciousness,
>   without return to pre–existing
>   conscious level
>
> Use fifth-digit 5 to designate when a
> patient is unconscious and dies before
> regaining consciousness, regardless of
> the duration of the loss of consciousness
>
> 6 with loss of consciousness of un-
>   specified duration
>
> 9 with concussion, unspecified

    with
      cerebral
        contusion — *see* Contusion,
          brain
        laceration — *see* Laceration,
          brain
      open intracranial wound 853.1 ☑
      skull fracture — *see* Fracture,
        skull, by site
    extradural or epidural 852.4 ☑
      with open intracranial wound
        852.5 ☑
    subarachnoid 852.0 ☑
      with open intracranial wound
        852.1 ☑
    subdural 852.2 ☑
      with open intracranial wound
        852.3 ☑
  breast 611.79
  bronchial tube — *see* Hemorrhage, lung
  bronchopulmonary — *see* Hemorrhage,
    lung
  bronchus (cause unknown) (*see also* Hemor-
    rhage, lung) 786.30
  bulbar (*see also* Hemorrhage, brain) 431
  bursa 727.89
  capillary 448.9
    primary 287.8
  capsular — *see* Hemorrhage, brain
  cardiovascular 429.89
  cecum 578.9
  cephalic (*see also* Hemorrhage, brain) 431
  cerebellar (*see also* Hemorrhage, brain) 431
  cerebellum (*see also* Hemorrhage, brain) 431
  cerebral (*see also* Hemorrhage, brain) 431
    fetus or newborn (anoxic) (traumatic)
      767.0
  cerebromeningeal (*see also* Hemorrhage,
    brain) 431
  cerebrospinal (*see also* Hemorrhage, brain)
    431
  cerebrovascular accident — *see* Hemor-
    rhage, brain
  cerebrum (*see also* Hemorrhage, brain) 431
  cervix (stump) (uteri) 622.8
  cesarean section wound 674.3 ☑
  chamber, anterior (eye) 364.41
  childbirth — *see* Hemorrhage, complicating,
    delivery
  choroid 363.61
    expulsive 363.62
  ciliary body 364.41
  cochlea 386.8
  colon — *see* Hemorrhage, intestine

Hemorrhage, hemorrhagic — *continued*
  complicating
    delivery 641.9 ☑
      affecting fetus or newborn 762.1
      associated with
        afibrinogenemia 641.3 ☑
          affecting fetus or newborn
          763.89
        coagulation defect 641.3 ☑
          affecting fetus or newborn
          763.89
        hyperfibrinolysis 641.3 ☑
          affecting fetus or newborn
          763.89
        hypofibrinogenemia 641.3 ☑
          affecting fetus or newborn
          763.89
      due to
        low-lying placenta 641.1 ☑
          affecting fetus or newborn
          762.0
        placenta previa 641.1 ☑
          affecting fetus or newborn
          762.0
        premature separation of placenta
          641.2 ☑
          affecting fetus or newborn
          762.1
      retained
        placenta 666.0 ☑
        secundines 666.2 ☑
      trauma 641.8 ☑
        affecting fetus or newborn
          763.89
      uterine leiomyoma 641.8 ☑
        affecting fetus or newborn
          763.89
    surgical procedure 998.11
  complication(s)
    of dental implant placement 525.71
  concealed NEC 459.0
  congenital 772.9
  conjunctiva 372.72
    newborn 772.8
  cord, newborn 772.0
    slipped ligature 772.3
    stump 772.3
  corpus luteum (ruptured) 620.1
  cortical (*see also* Hemorrhage, brain) 431
  cranial 432.9
  cutaneous 782.7
    newborn 772.6
  cystitis — *see* Cystitis
  cyst, pancreas 577.2
  delayed
    with
      abortion — *see* Abortion, by type,
        with hemorrhage, delayed or
        excessive
      ectopic pregnancy (*see also* cate-
        gories 633.0–633.9) 639.1
      molar pregnancy (*see also* categories
        630–632) 639.1
    following
      abortion 639.1
      ectopic or molar pregnancy 639.1
    postpartum 666.2 ☑
  diathesis (familial) 287.9
    newborn 776.0
  disease 287.9
    newborn 776.0
    specified type NEC 287.8
  disorder 287.9
    due to intrinsic circulating anticoagu-
      lants, antibodies, or inhibitors
      286.59
      with
        acquired hemophilia 286.52
        antiphospholipid antibody 286.53
    specified type NEC 287.8
  due to
    any device, implant or graft (presence
      of) classifiable to 996.0–996.5 —
      see Complications, due to (pres-
      ence of) any device, implant, or
      graft classified to 996.0–996.5NEC

☑ **Additional Digit Required** — Refer to the Tabular List for Digit Selection   ▽ **Subterms under main terms may continue to next column or page**

180   2014 ICD-9-CM

Hemorrhage, hemorrhagic — *continued*
  pulmonary (*see also* Hemorrhage, lung)
    786.30
      acute idiopathic in infants (AIPHI) (over
        28 days old) 786.31
      newborn (massive) 770.3
      renal syndrome 446.21
  purpura (primary) (*see also* Purpura, throm-
    bocytopenic) 287.39
  rectum (sphincter) 569.3
  recurring, following initial hemorrhage at
    time of injury 958.2
  renal 593.81
    pulmonary syndrome 446.21
  respiratory tract (*see also* Hemorrhage, lung)
    786.30
  retina, retinal (deep) (superficial) (vessels)
    362.81
    diabetic 250.5 ☑ *[362.01]*
      due to secondary diabetes
        249.5 ☑ *[362.01]*
    due to birth injury 772.8
  retrobulbar 376.89
  retroperitoneal 459.0
  retroplacental (*see also* Placenta, separation)
    641.2 ☑
  scalp 459.0
    due to injury at birth 767.19
  scrotum 608.83
  secondary (nontraumatic) 459.0
    following initial hemorrhage at time of
      injury 958.2
  seminal vesicle 608.83
  skin 782.7
    newborn 772.6
  spermatic cord 608.83
  spinal (cord) 336.1
    aneurysm (ruptured) 336.1
      syphilitic 094.89
    due to birth injury 767.4
    fetus or newborn 767.4
  spleen 289.59
  spontaneous NEC 459.0
    petechial 782.7
  stomach 578.9
    newborn 772.4
    ulcer — *see* Ulcer, stomach, with hemor-
      rhage
  subaponeurotic, newborn 767.11
    massive (birth injury) 767.11
  subarachnoid (nontraumatic) 430
    fetus or newborn (anoxic) (traumatic)
      772.2
    puerperal, postpartum, childbirth
      674.0 ☑
    traumatic — *see* Hemorrhage, brain,
      traumatic, subarachnoid
  subconjunctival 372.72
    due to birth injury 772.8
    newborn 772.8
  subcortical (*see also* Hemorrhage, brain) 431
  subcutaneous 782.7
  subdiaphragmatic 459.0
  subdural (nontraumatic) 432.1
    due to birth injury 767.0
    fetus or newborn (anoxic) (hypoxic) (due
      to birth trauma) 767.0
    puerperal, postpartum, childbirth
      674.0 ☑
    spinal 336.1
    traumatic — *see* Hemorrhage, brain,
      traumatic, subdural
  subgaleal 767.11
  subhyaloid 362.81
  subperiosteal 733.99
  subretinal 362.81
  subtentorial (*see also* Hemorrhage, subdu-
    ral) 432.1
  subungual 703.8
    due to blood dyscrasia 287.8
  suprarenal (capsule) (gland) 255.41
    fetus or newborn 772.5
  tentorium (traumatic) (*see also* Hemorrhage,
    brain, traumatic)
    fetus or newborn 767.0

Hemorrhage, hemorrhagic — *continued*
  tentorium (*see also* Hemorrhage, brain,
    traumatic) — *continued*
    nontraumatic — *see* Hemorrhage, sub-
      dural
  testis 608.83
  thigh 459.0
  third stage 666.0 ☑
  thorax — *see* Hemorrhage, lung
  throat 784.8
  thrombocythemia 238.71
  thymus (gland) 254.8
  thyroid (gland) 246.3
    cyst 246.3
  tongue 529.8
  tonsil 474.8
    postoperative 998.11
  tooth socket (postextraction) 998.11
  trachea — *see* Hemorrhage, lung
  traumatic (*see also* nature of injury)
    brain — *see* Hemorrhage, brain, traumat-
      ic
    recurring or secondary (following initial
      hemorrhage at time of injury)
      958.2
  tuberculous NEC (*see also* Tuberculosis,
    pulmonary) 011.9 ☑
  tunica vaginalis 608.83
  ulcer — *see* Ulcer, by site, with hemorrhage
  umbilicus, umbilical cord 772.0
    after birth, newborn 772.3
    complicating delivery 663.8 ☑
      affecting fetus or newborn 772.0
    slipped ligature 772.3
    stump 772.3
  unavoidable (due to placenta previa)
    641.1 ☑
    affecting fetus or newborn 762.0
  upper extremity 459.0
  urethra (idiopathic) 599.84
  uterus, uterine (abnormal) 626.9
    climacteric 627.0
    complicating delivery — *see* Hemor-
      rhage, complicating, delivery
    due to
      intrauterine contraceptive device
        996.76
      perforating uterus 996.32
    functional or dysfunctional 626.8
    in pregnancy — *see* Hemorrhage, preg-
      nancy
    intermenstrual 626.6
      irregular 626.6
      regular 626.5
    postmenopausal 627.1
    postpartum (*see also* Hemorrhage,
      postpartum) 666.1 ☑
    prepubertal 626.8
    pubertal 626.3
    puerperal (immediate) 666.1 ☑
  vagina 623.8
  vasa previa 663.5 ☑
    affecting fetus or newborn 772.0
  vas deferens 608.83
  ventricular (*see also* Hemorrhage, brain) 431
  vesical 596.89
  viscera 459.0
    newborn 772.8
  vitreous (humor) (intraocular) 379.23
  vocal cord 478.5
  vulva 624.8
Hemorrhoids (anus) (rectum) (without compli-
    cation) 455.6
  bleeding, prolapsed, strangulated, or ulcer-
    ated NEC 455.8
    external 455.5
    internal 455.2
  complicated NEC 455.8
  complicating pregnancy and puerperium
    671.8 ☑
  external 455.3
    with complication NEC 455.5
    bleeding, prolapsed, strangulated, or
      ulcerated 455.5
    thrombosed 455.4
  internal 455.0

Hemorrhoids — *continued*
  internal — *continued*
    with complication NEC 455.2
    bleeding, prolapsed, strangulated, or
      ulcerated 455.2
    thrombosed 455.1
  residual skin tag 455.9
  sentinel pile 455.9
  thrombosed NEC 455.7
    external 455.4
    internal 455.1
Hemosalpinx 620.8
Hemosiderosis 275.09
  dietary 275.09
  pulmonary (idiopathic) 275.09 *[516.1]*
  transfusion NEC 275.02
    bone marrow 996.85
Hemospermia 608.82
Hemothorax 511.89
  bacterial, nontuberculous 511.1
  newborn 772.8
  nontuberculous 511.89
    bacterial 511.1
  pneumococcal 511.1
  postoperative 998.11
  staphylococcal 511.1
  streptococcal 511.1
  traumatic 860.2
    with
      open wound into thorax 860.3
      pneumothorax 860.4
        with open wound into thorax
          860.5
  tuberculous (*see also* Tuberculosis, pleura)
    012.0 ☑
Hemotympanum 385.89
Hench-Rosenberg syndrome (palindromic
    arthritis) — *see also* Rheumatism, palin-
    dromic 719.3 ☑
Henle's warts 371.41
Henoch (-Schönlein)
  disease or syndrome (allergic purpura) 287.0
  purpura (allergic) 287.0
Henpue, henpuye 102.6
Heparin-induced thrombocytopenia (HIT)
    289.84
Heparitinuria 277.5
Hepar lobatum 095.3
Hepatalgia 573.8
Hepatic — *see also* condition
  flexure syndrome 569.89
Hepatitis 573.3
  acute (*see also* Necrosis, liver) 570
    alcoholic 571.1
    infective 070.1
      with hepatic coma 070.0
  alcoholic 571.1
  amebic — *see* Abscess, liver, amebic
  anicteric (acute) — *see* Hepatitis, viral
  antigen-associated (HAA) — *see* Hepatitis,
    viral, type B
  Australian antigen (positive) — *see* Hepati-
    tis, viral, type B
  autoimmune 571.42
  catarrhal (acute) 070.1
    with hepatic coma 070.0
    chronic 571.40
    newborn 070.1
      with hepatic coma 070.0
  chemical 573.3
  cholangiolitic 573.8
  cholestatic 573.8
  chronic 571.40
    active 571.49
      viral — *see* Hepatitis, viral
    aggressive 571.49
    persistent 571.41
    viral — *see* Hepatitis, viral
  cytomegalic inclusion virus 078.5 *[573.1]*
  diffuse 573.3
  "dirty needle" — *see* Hepatitis, viral
  drug-induced 573.3
  due to
    Coxsackie 074.8 *[573.1]*
    cytomegalic inclusion virus 078.5 *[573.1]*
    infectious mononucleosis 075 *[573.1]*

Hepatitis — *continued*
  due to — *continued*
    malaria 084.9 *[573.2]*
    mumps 072.71
    secondary syphilis 091.62
    toxoplasmosis (acquired) 130.5
      congenital (active) 771.2
  epidemic — *see* Hepatitis, viral, type A
  fetus or newborn 774.4
  fibrous (chronic) 571.49
    acute 570
  from injection, inoculation, or transfusion
    (blood) (other substance) (plasma)
    (serum) (onset within 8 months after
    administration) — *see* Hepatitis, viral
  fulminant (viral) (*see also* Hepatitis, viral)
    070.9
    with hepatic coma 070.6
    type A 070.1
      with hepatic coma 070.0
    type B — *see* Hepatitis, viral, type B
  giant cell (neonatal) 774.4
  hemorrhagic 573.8
  history of
    B V12.09
    C V12.09
  homologous serum — *see* Hepatitis, viral
  hypertrophic (chronic) 571.49
    acute 570
  infectious, infective (acute) (chronic) (suba-
    cute) 070.1
    with hepatic coma 070.0
  inoculation — *see* Hepatitis, viral
  interstitial (chronic) 571.49
    acute 570
  lupoid 571.49
  malarial 084.9 *[573.2]*
  malignant (*see also* Necrosis, liver) 570
  neonatal (toxic) 774.4
  newborn 774.4
  parenchymatous (acute) (*see also* Necrosis,
    liver) 570
  peliosis 573.3
  persistent, chronic 571.41
  plasma cell 571.49
  postimmunization — *see* Hepatitis, viral
  postnecrotic 571.49
  posttransfusion — *see* Hepatitis, viral
  recurrent 571.49
  septic 573.3
  serum — *see* Hepatitis, viral
    carrier (suspected of) V02.61
  subacute (*see also* Necrosis, liver) 570
  suppurative (diffuse) 572.0
  syphilitic (late) 095.3
    congenital (early) 090.0 *[573.2]*
    late 090.5 *[573.2]*
    secondary 091.62
  toxic (noninfectious) 573.3
    fetus or newborn 774.4
  tuberculous (*see also* Tuberculosis) 017.9 ☑
  viral (acute) (anicteric) (cholangiolitic)
    (cholestatic) (chronic) (subacute)
    070.9
    with hepatic coma 070.6
    AU-SH type virus — *see* Hepatitis, viral,
      type B
    Australian antigen — *see* Hepatitis, viral,
      type B
    B-antigen — *see* Hepatitis, viral, type B
    Coxsackie 074.8 *[573.1]*
    cytomegalic inclusion 078.5 *[573.1]*
    IH (virus) — *see* Hepatitis, viral, type A
    infectious hepatitis virus — *see* Hepati-
      tis, viral, type A
    serum hepatitis virus — *see* Hepatitis,
      viral, type B
    SH — *see* Hepatitis, viral, type B
    specified type NEC 070.59
      with hepatic coma 070.49
    type A 070.1
      with hepatic coma 070.0
    type B (acute) 070.30
      with
        hepatic coma 070.20
          with hepatitis delta 070.21

☑ **Additional Digit Required** — Refer to the Tabular List for Digit Selection **Subterms under main terms may continue to next column or page**

182 2014 ICD-9-CM

Hepatitis — *continued*
  viral — *continued*
    type B — *continued*
      with — *continued*
        hepatitis delta 070.31
          with hepatic coma 070.21
      carrier status V02.61
      chronic 070.32
        with
          hepatic coma 070.22
            with hepatitis delta 070.23
          hepatitis delta 070.33
            with hepatic coma 070.23
    type C
      acute 070.51
        with hepatic coma 070.41
      carrier status V02.62
      chronic 070.54
        with hepatic coma 070.44
      in remission 070.54
      unspecified 070.70
        with hepatic coma 070.71
    type delta (with hepatitis B carrier state) 070.52
      with
        active hepatitis B disease — *see* Hepatitis, viral, type B
        hepatic coma 070.42
    type E 070.53
      with hepatic coma 070.43
    vaccination and inoculation (prophylactic) V05.3
  Waldenström's (lupoid hepatitis) 571.49
Hepatization, lung (acute) — *see also* Pneumonia, lobar
  chronic (*see also* Fibrosis, lung) 515
Hepatoblastoma (M8970/3) 155.0
Hepatocarcinoma (M8170/3) 155.0
Hepatocholangiocarcinoma (M8180/3) 155.0
Hepatocholangioma, benign (M8180/0) 211.5
Hepatocholangitis 573.8
Hepatocystitis — *see also* Cholecystitis 575.10
Hepatodystrophy 570
Hepatolenticular degeneration 275.1
Hepatolithiasis — *see* Choledocholithiasis
Hepatoma (malignant) (M8170/3) 155.0
  benign (M8170/0) 211.5
  congenital (M8970/3) 155.0
  embryonal (M8970/3) 155.0
Hepatomegalia glycogenica diffusa 271.0
Hepatomegaly — *see also* Hypertrophy, liver 789.1
  congenital 751.69
    syphilitic 090.0
  due to Clonorchis sinensis 121.1
  Gaucher's 272.7
  syphilitic (congenital) 090.0
Hepatoptosis 573.8
Hepatorrhexis 573.8
Hepatosis, toxic 573.8
Hepatosplenomegaly 571.8
  due to S. japonicum 120.2
  hyperlipemic (Bürger-Grutz type) 272.3
Herald patch 696.3
Hereditary — *see* condition
Heredodegeneration 330.9
  macular 362.70
Heredopathia atactica polyneuritiformis 356.3
Heredosyphilis — *see also* Syphilis, congenital 090.9
Hermaphroditism (true) 752.7
  with specified chromosomal anomaly — *see* Anomaly, chromosomes, sex
Hernia, hernial (acquired) (recurrent) 553.9
  with
    gangrene (obstructed) NEC 551.9
    obstruction NEC 552.9
      and gangrene 551.9
  abdomen (wall) — *see* Hernia, ventral
  abdominal, specified site NEC 553.8
    with
      gangrene (obstructed) 551.8
      obstruction 552.8
        and gangrene 551.8
  appendix 553.8

Hernia, hernial — *continued*
  appendix — *continued*
    with
      gangrene (obstructed) 551.8
      obstruction 552.8
        and gangrene 551.8
  bilateral (inguinal) — *see* Hernia, inguinal
  bladder (sphincter)
    congenital (female) (male) 756.71
    female (*see also* Cystocele, female) 618.01
    male 596.89
  brain 348.4
    congenital 742.0
  broad ligament 553.8
  cartilage, vertebral — *see* Displacement, intervertebral disc
  cerebral 348.4
    congenital 742.0
    endaural 742.0
  ciliary body 364.89
    traumatic 871.1
  colic 553.9
    with
      gangrene (obstructed) 551.9
      obstruction 552.9
        and gangrene 551.9
  colon 553.9
    with
      gangrene (obstructed) 551.9
      obstruction 552.9
        and gangrene 551.9
  colostomy (stoma) 569.69
  Cooper's (retroperitoneal) 553.8
    with
      gangrene (obstructed) 551.8
      obstruction 552.8
        and gangrene 551.8
  crural — *see* Hernia, femoral
  cystostomy 596.83
  diaphragm, diaphragmatic 553.3
    with
      gangrene (obstructed) 551.3
      obstruction 552.3
        and gangrene 551.3
    congenital 756.6
    due to gross defect of diaphragm 756.6
    traumatic 862.0
      with open wound into cavity 862.1
  direct (inguinal) — *see* Hernia, inguinal
  disc, intervertebral — *see* Displacement, intervertebral disc
  diverticulum, intestine 553.9
    with
      gangrene (obstructed) 551.9
      obstruction 552.9
        and gangrene 551.9
  double (inguinal) — *see* Hernia, inguinal
  due to adhesion with obstruction 552.9
  duodenojejunal 553.8
    with
      gangrene (obstructed) 551.8
      obstruction 552.8
        and gangrene 551.8
  en glissade — *see* Hernia, inguinal
  enterostomy (stoma) 569.69
  epigastric 553.29
    with
      gangrene (obstruction) 551.29
      obstruction 552.29
        and gangrene 551.29
    recurrent 553.21
      with
        gangrene (obstructed) 551.21
        obstruction 552.21
          and gangrene 551.21
  esophageal hiatus (sliding) 553.3
    with
      gangrene (obstructed) 551.3
      obstruction 552.3
        and gangrene 551.3
    congenital 750.6
  external (inguinal) — *see* Hernia, inguinal
  fallopian tube 620.4
  fascia 728.89
  fat 729.30

Hernia, hernial — *continued*
  fat — *continued*
    eyelid 374.34
    orbital 374.34
    pad 729.30
      eye, eyelid 374.34
      knee 729.31
      orbit 374.34
      popliteal (space) 729.31
      specified site NEC 729.39
  femoral (unilateral) 553.00
    with
      gangrene (obstructed) 551.00
      obstruction 552.00
        with gangrene 551.00
    bilateral 553.02
      gangrenous (obstructed) 551.02
      obstructed 552.02
        with gangrene 551.02
      recurrent 553.03
        gangrenous (obstructed) 551.03
        obstructed 552.03
          with gangrene 551.03
    recurrent (unilateral) 553.01
      bilateral 553.03
        gangrenous (obstructed) 551.03
        obstructed 552.03
          with gangrene 551.01
      gangrenous (obstructed) 551.01
      obstructed 552.01
        with gangrene 551.01
  foramen
    Bochdalek 553.3
      with
        gangrene (obstructed) 551.3
        obstruction 552.3
          and gangrene 551.3
      congenital 756.6
    magnum 348.4
    Morgagni, Morgagnian 553.3
      with
        gangrene 551.3
        obstruction 552.3
          and gangrene 551.3
      congenital 756.6
  funicular (umbilical) 553.1
    with
      gangrene (obstructed) 551.1
      obstruction 552.1
        and gangrene 551.1
    spermatic cord — *see* Hernia, inguinal
  gangrenous — *see* Hernia, by site, with gangrene
  gastrointestinal tract 553.9
    with
      gangrene (obstructed) 551.9
      obstruction 552.9
        and gangrene 551.9
  gluteal — *see* Hernia, femoral
  Gruber's (internal mesogastric) 553.8
    with
      gangrene (obstructed) 551.8
      obstruction 552.8
        and gangrene 551.8
  Hesselbach's 553.8
    with
      gangrene (obstructed) 551.8
      obstruction 552.8
        and gangrene 551.8
  hiatal (esophageal) (sliding) 553.3
    with
      gangrene (obstructed) 551.3
      obstruction 552.3
        and gangrene 551.3
    congenital 750.6
  incarcerated (*see also* Hernia, by site, with obstruction) 552.9
    gangrenous (*see also* Hernia, by site, with gangrene) 551.9
  incisional 553.21
    with
      gangrene (obstructed) 551.21
      obstruction 552.21
        and gangrene 551.21
    lumbar — *see* Hernia, lumbar
    recurrent 553.21

Hernia, hernial — *continued*
  incisional — *continued*
    recurrent — *continued*
      with
        gangrene (obstructed) 551.21
        obstruction 552.21
          and gangrene 551.21
  indirect (inguinal) — *see* Hernia, inguinal
  infantile — *see* Hernia, inguinal
  infrapatellar fat pad 729.31
  inguinal (direct) (double) (encysted) (external) (funicular) (indirect) (infantile) (internal) (interstitial) (oblique) (scrotal) (sliding) 550.9 ☑

> **Note** — *Use the following fifth-digit subclassification with category 550:*
>
> **0** *unilateral or unspecified (not specified as recurrent)*
>
> **1** *unilateral or unspecified, recurrent*
>
> **2** *bilateral (not specified as recurrent)*
>
> **3** *bilateral, recurrent*

    with
      gangrene (obstructed) 550.0 ☑
      obstruction 550.1 ☑
        and gangrene 550.0 ☑
  internal 553.8
    with
      gangrene (obstructed) 551.8
      obstruction 552.8
        and gangrene 551.8
    inguinal — *see* Hernia, inguinal
  interstitial 553.9
    with
      gangrene (obstructed) 551.9
      obstruction 552.9
        and gangrene 551.9
    inguinal — *see* Hernia, inguinal
  intervertebral cartilage or disc — *see* Displacement, intervertebral disc
  intestine, intestinal 553.9
    with
      gangrene (obstructed) 551.9
      obstruction 552.9
        and gangrene 551.9
  intra-abdominal 553.9
    with
      gangrene (obstructed) 551.9
      obstruction 552.9
        and gangrene 551.9
  intraparietal 553.9
    with
      gangrene (obstructed) 551.9
      obstruction 552.9
        and gangrene 551.9
  iris 364.89
    traumatic 871.1
  irreducible (*see also* Hernia, by site, with obstruction) 552.9
    gangrenous (with obstruction) (*see also* Hernia, by site, with gangrene) 551.9
  ischiatic 553.8
    with
      gangrene (obstructed) 551.8
      obstruction 552.8
        and gangrene 551.8
  ischiorectal 553.8
    with
      gangrene (obstructed) 551.8
      obstruction 552.8
        and gangrene 551.8
  lens 379.32
    traumatic 871.1
  linea
    alba — *see* Hernia, epigastric
    semilunaris — *see* Hernia, spigelian
  Littre's (diverticular) 553.9
    with
      gangrene (obstructed) 551.9
      obstruction 552.9
        and gangrene 551.9
  lumbar 553.8

Hernia, hernial — *continued*
  lumbar — *continued*
    with
      gangrene (obstructed) 551.8
      obstruction 552.8
        and gangrene 551.8
    intervertebral disc 722.10
  lung (subcutaneous) 518.89
    congenital 748.69
  mediastinum 519.3
  mesenteric (internal) 553.8
    with
      gangrene (obstructed) 551.8
      obstruction 552.8
        and gangrene 551.8
  mesocolon 553.8
    with
      gangrene (obstructed) 551.8
      obstruction 552.8
        and gangrene 551.8
  muscle (sheath) 728.89
  nucleus pulposus — *see* Displacement, intervertebral disc
  oblique (inguinal) — *see* Hernia, inguinal
  obstructive (*see also* Hernia, by site, with obstruction) 552.9
    gangrenous (with obstruction) (*see also* Hernia, by site, with gangrene) 551.9
  obturator 553.8
    with
      gangrene (obstructed) 551.8
      obstruction 552.8
        and gangrene 551.8
  omental 553.8
    with
      gangrene (obstructed) 551.8
      obstruction 552.8
        and gangrene 551.8
  orbital fat (pad) 374.34
  ovary 620.4
  oviduct 620.4
  paracolostomy (stoma) 569.69
  paraduodenal 553.8
    with
      gangrene (obstructed) 551.8
      obstruction 552.8
        and gangrene 551.8
  paraesophageal 553.3
    with
      gangrene (obstructed) 551.3
      obstruction 552.3
        and gangrene 551.3
    congenital 750.6
  parahiatal 553.3
    with
      gangrene (obstructed) 551.3
      obstruction 552.3
        and gangrene 551.3
  paraumbilical 553.1
    with
      gangrene (obstructed) 551.1
      obstruction 552.1
        and gangrene 551.1
  parietal 553.9
    with
      gangrene (obstructed) 551.9
      obstruction 552.9
        and gangrene 551.9
  perineal 553.8
    with
      gangrene (obstructed) 551.8
      obstruction 552.8
        and gangrene 551.8
  peritoneal sac, lesser 553.8
    with
      gangrene (obstructed) 551.8
      obstruction 552.8
        and gangrene 551.8
  popliteal fat pad 729.31
  postoperative 553.21
    with
      gangrene (obstructed) 551.21
      obstruction 552.21
        and gangrene 551.21
  pregnant uterus 654.4 ☑

Hernia, hernial — *continued*
  prevesical 596.89
  properitoneal 553.8
    with
      gangrene (obstructed) 551.8
      obstruction 552.8
        and gangrene 551.8
  pudendal 553.8
    with
      gangrene (obstructed) 551.8
      obstruction 552.8
        and gangrene 551.8
  rectovaginal 618.6
  retroperitoneal 553.8
    with
      gangrene (obstructed) 551.8
      obstruction 552.8
        and gangrene 551.8
  Richter's (parietal) 553.9
    with
      gangrene (obstructed) 551.9
      obstruction 552.9
        and gangrene 551.9
  Rieux's, Riex's (retrocecal) 553.8
    with
      gangrene (obstructed) 551.8
      obstruction 552.8
        and gangrene 551.8
  sciatic 553.8
    with
      gangrene (obstructed) 551.8
      obstruction 552.8
        and gangrene 551.8
  scrotum, scrotal — *see* Hernia, inguinal
  sliding (inguinal) (*see also* Hernia, inguinal)
    hiatus — *see* Hernia, hiatal
  spigelian 553.29
    with
      gangrene (obstructed) 551.29
      obstruction 552.29
        and gangrene 551.29
  spinal (*see also* Spina bifida) 741.9 ☑
    with hydrocephalus 741.0 ☑
  strangulated (*see also* Hernia, by site, with obstruction) 552.9
    gangrenous (with obstruction) (*see also* Hernia, by site, with gangrene) 551.9
  supraumbilicus (linea alba) — *see* Hernia, epigastric
  tendon 727.9
  testis (nontraumatic) 550.9 ☑
    meaning
      scrotal hernia 550.9 ☑
      symptomatic late syphilis 095.8
  Treitz's (fossa) 553.8
    with
      gangrene (obstructed) 551.8
      obstruction 552.8
        and gangrene 551.8
  tunica
    albuginea 608.89
    vaginalis 752.89
  umbilicus, umbilical 553.1
    with
      gangrene (obstructed) 551.1
      obstruction 552.1
        and gangrene 551.1
  ureter 593.89
    with obstruction 593.4
  uterus 621.8
    pregnant 654.4 ☑
  vaginal (posterior) 618.6
  Velpeau's (femoral) (*see also* Hernia, femoral) 553.00
  ventral 553.20
    with
      gangrene (obstructed) 551.20
      obstruction 552.20
        and gangrene 551.20
    incisional 553.21
    recurrent 553.21
      with
        gangrene (obstructed) 551.21
        obstruction 552.21
          and gangrene 551.21

Hernia, hernial — *continued*
  vesical
    congenital (female) (male) 756.71
    female (*see also* Cystocele, female) 618.01
    male 596.89
  vitreous (into anterior chamber) 379.21
    traumatic 871.1
Herniation — *see also* Hernia
  brain (stem) 348.4
  cerebral 348.4
  gastric mucosa (into duodenal bulb) 537.89
  mediastinum 519.3
  nucleus pulposus — *see* Displacement, intervertebral disc
Herpangina 074.0
Herpes, herpetic 054.9
  auricularis (zoster) 053.71
    simplex 054.73
  blepharitis (zoster) 053.20
    simplex 054.41
  circinate 110.5
  circinatus 110.5
    bullous 694.5
  conjunctiva (simplex) 054.43
    zoster 053.21
  cornea (simplex) 054.43
    disciform (simplex) 054.43
    zoster 053.21
  encephalitis 054.3
  eye (zoster) 053.29
    simplex 054.40
  eyelid (zoster) 053.20
    simplex 054.41
  febrilis 054.9
  fever 054.9
  geniculate ganglionitis 053.11
  genital, genitalis 054.10
    specified site NEC 054.19
  gestationis 646.8 ☑
  gingivostomatitis 054.2
  iridocyclitis (simplex) 054.44
    zoster 053.22
  iris (any site) 695.10
  iritis (simplex) 054.44
  keratitis (simplex) 054.43
    dendritic 054.42
    disciform 054.43
    interstitial 054.43
      zoster 053.21
  keratoconjunctivitis (simplex) 054.43
    zoster 053.21
  labialis 054.9
    meningococcal 036.89
  lip 054.9
  meningitis (simplex) 054.72
    zoster 053.0
  ophthalmicus (zoster) 053.20
    simplex 054.40
  otitis externa (zoster) 053.71
    simplex 054.73
  penis 054.13
  perianal 054.10
  pharyngitis 054.79
  progenitalis 054.10
  scrotum 054.19
  septicemia 054.5
  simplex 054.9
    complicated 054.8
      ophthalmic 054.40
        specified NEC 054.49
      specified NEC 054.79
    congenital 771.2
    external ear 054.73
    keratitis 054.43
      dendritic 054.42
    meningitis 054.72
    myelitis 054.74
    neuritis 054.79
    specified complication NEC 054.79
      ophthalmic 054.49
    visceral 054.71
  stomatitis 054.2
  tonsurans 110.0
    maculosus (of Hebra) 696.3
  visceral 054.71

Herpes, herpetic — *continued*
  vulva 054.12
  vulvovaginitis 054.11
  whitlow 054.6
  zoster 053.9
    auricularis 053.71
    complicated 053.8
      specified NEC 053.79
    conjunctiva 053.21
    cornea 053.21
    ear 053.71
    eye 053.29
    geniculate 053.11
    keratitis 053.21
      interstitial 053.21
    myelitis 053.14
    neuritis 053.10
    ophthalmicus(a) 053.20
    oticus 053.71
    otitis externa 053.71
    specified complication NEC 053.79
    specified site NEC 053.9
  zosteriform, intermediate type 053.9
Herrick's
  anemia (hemoglobin S disease) 282.61
  syndrome (hemoglobin S disease) 282.61
Hers' disease (glycogenosis VI) 271.0
Herter (-Gee) disease or syndrome (nontropical sprue) 579.0
Herter's infantilism (nontropical sprue) 579.0
Herxheimer's disease (diffuse idiopathic cutaneous atrophy) 701.8
Herxheimer's reaction 995.91
Hesitancy, urinary 788.64
Hesselbach's hernia — *see* Hernia, Hesselbach's
Heterochromia (congenital) 743.46
  acquired 364.53
  cataract 366.33
  cyclitis 364.21
  hair 704.3
  iritis 364.21
  retained metallic foreign body 360.62
    magnetic 360.52
  uveitis 364.21
Heterophoria 378.40
  alternating 378.45
  vertical 378.43
Heterophyes, small intestine 121.6
Heterophyiasis 121.6
Heteropsia 368.8
Heterotopia, heterotopic — *see also* Malposition, congenital
  cerebralis 742.4
  pancreas, pancreatic 751.7
  spinalis 742.59
Heterotropia 378.30
  intermittent 378.20
    vertical 378.31
  vertical (constant) (intermittent) 378.31
Heubner's disease 094.89
Heubner-Herter disease or syndrome (nontropical sprue) 579.0
Hexadactylism 755.0 ☑
Heyd's syndrome (hepatorenal) 572.4
HGSIL (high grade squamous intraepithelial lesion) (cytologic finding) (Pap smear finding)
  anus 796.74
  cervix 795.04
    biopsy finding — code to CIN II or CIN III
  vagina 795.14
Hibernoma (M8880/0) — *see* Lipoma
Hiccough 786.8
  epidemic 078.89
  psychogenic 306.1
Hiccup — *see also* Hiccough 786.8
Hicks (-Braxton) contractures 644.1 ☑
Hidden penis 752.65
Hidradenitis (axillaris) (suppurative) 705.83
Hidradenoma (nodular) (M8400/0) — *see also* Neoplasm, skin, benign
  clear cell (M8402/0) — *see* Neoplasm, skin, benign

☑ **Additional Digit Required** — **Refer to the Tabular List for Digit Selection**   ▽ **Subterms under main terms may continue to next column or page**

184   **2014 ICD-9-CM**

Index

Hernia, hernial — Hidradenoma

Hidradenoma — see also Neoplasm, skin, benign — continued
  papillary (M8405/0) — see Neoplasm, skin, benign
Hidrocystoma (M8404/0) — see Neoplasm, skin, benign
HIE (hypoxic-ischemic encephalopathy) 768.70
  mild 768.71
  moderate 768.72
  severe 768.73
High
  A₂ anemia 282.46
  altitude effects 993.2
    anoxia 993.2
    on
      ears 993.0
      sinuses 993.1
    polycythemia 289.0
  arch
    foot 755.67
    palate 750.26
  artery (arterial) tension (see also Hypertension) 401.9
    without diagnosis of hypertension 796.2
  basal metabolic rate (BMR) 794.7
  blood pressure (see also Hypertension) 401.9
    borderline 796.2
    incidental reading (isolated) (nonspecific), no diagnosis of hypertension 796.2
  cholesterol 272.0
    with high triglycerides 272.2
  compliance bladder 596.4
  diaphragm (congenital) 756.6
  frequency deafness (congenital) (regional) 389.8
  head at term 652.5 ☑
    affecting fetus or newborn 763.1
  output failure (cardiac) (see also Failure, heart) 428.9
  oxygen-affinity hemoglobin 289.0
  palate 750.26
  risk
    behavior — see Problem
    family situation V61.9
      specified circumstance NEC V61.8
    human papillomavirus (HPV) DNA test positive
      anal 796.75
      cervical 795.05
      vaginal 795.15
    individual NEC V62.89
    infant NEC V20.1
    patient taking drugs (prescribed) V67.51
      nonprescribed (see also Abuse, drugs, nondependent) 305.9 ☑
    pregnancy V23.9
      inadequate prenatal care V23.7
      inconclusive fetal viability V23.87
      specified problem NEC V23.89
  temperature (of unknown origin) (see also Pyrexia) 780.60
  thoracic rib 756.3
  triglycerides 272.1
    with high cholesterol 272.2
Hildenbrand's disease (typhus) 081.9
Hilger's syndrome 337.09
Hill diarrhea 579.1
Hilliard's lupus — see also Tuberculosis 017.0 ☑
Hilum — see condition
Hip — see condition
Hippel's disease (retinocerebral angiomatosis) 759.6
Hippus 379.49
Hirschfeld's disease (acute diabetes mellitus) — see also Diabetes 250.0 ☑
  due to secondary diabetes 249.0 ☑
Hirschsprung's disease or megacolon (congenital) 751.3
Hirsuties — see also Hypertrichosis 704.1
Hirsutism — see also Hypertrichosis 704.1
Hirudiniasis (external) (internal) 134.2
Hiss-Russell dysentery 004.1
Histamine cephalgia 339.00
Histidinemia 270.5

Histidinuria 270.5
Histiocytic syndromes 288.4
Histiocytoma (M8832/0) — see also Neoplasm, skin, benign
  fibrous (M8830/0) (see also Neoplasm, skin, benign)
    atypical (M8830/1) — see Neoplasm, connective tissue, uncertain behavior
    malignant (M8830/3) — see Neoplasm, connective tissue, malignant
Histiocytosis (acute) (chronic) (subacute) 277.89
  acute differentiated progressive (M9722/3) 202.5 ☑
  adult pulmonary Langerhans cell (PLCH) 516.5
  cholesterol 277.89
  essential 277.89
  lipid, lipoid (essential) 272.7
  lipochrome (familial) 288.1
  malignant (M9720/3) 202.3 ☑
  non-Langerhans cell 277.89
  polyostotic sclerosing 277.89
  X (chronic) 277.89
    acute (progressive) (M9722/3) 202.5 ☑
Histoplasmosis 115.90
  with
    endocarditis 115.94
    meningitis 115.91
    pericarditis 115.93
    pneumonia 115.95
    retinitis 115.92
    specified manifestation NEC 115.99
  African (due to Histoplasma duboisii) 115.10
    with
      endocarditis 115.14
      meningitis 115.11
      pericarditis 115.13
      pneumonia 115.15
      retinitis 115.12
      specified manifestation NEC 115.19
  American (due to Histoplasma capsulatum) 115.00
    with
      endocarditis 115.04
      meningitis 115.01
      pericarditis 115.03
      pneumonia 115.05
      retinitis 115.02
      specified manifestation NEC 115.09
  Darling's — see Histoplasmosis, American
  large form (see also Histoplasmosis, African) 115.10
  lung 115.05
  small form (see also Histoplasmosis, American) 115.00
History (personal) of
  abuse
    emotional V15.42
    neglect V15.42
    physical V15.41
    sexual V15.41
  affective psychosis V11.1
  alcoholism V11.3
    specified as drinking problem (see also Abuse, drugs, nondependent) 305.0 ☑
  allergy to V15.09
    analgesic agent NEC V14.6
    anesthetic NEC V14.4
    antibiotic agent NEC V14.1
      penicillin V14.0
    anti-infective agent NEC V14.3
    arachnid bite V15.06
    diathesis V15.09
    drug V14.9
      specified type NEC V14.8
    eggs V15.03
    food additives V15.05
    insect bite V15.06
    latex V15.07
    medicinal agents V14.9
      specified type NEC V14.8
    milk products V15.02
    narcotic agent NEC V14.5

History of — continued
  allergy to — continued
    nuts V15.05
      peanuts V15.01
    penicillin V14.0
    radiographic dye V15.08
    seafood V15.04
    serum V14.7
    specified food NEC V15.05
    specified nonmedicinal agents NEC V15.09
    spider bite V15.06
    sulfa V14.2
    sulfonamides V14.2
    therapeutic agent NEC V15.09
    vaccine V14.7
  anaphylactic reaction or shock V13.81
  anaphylaxis V13.81
  anemia V12.3
  arrest, sudden cardiac V12.53
  arthritis V13.4
  attack, transient ischemic (TIA) V12.54
  benign neoplasm of brain V12.41
  blood disease V12.3
  calculi, urinary V13.01
  cardiovascular disease V12.50
    myocardial infarction 412
  chemotherapy, antineoplastic V87.41
  child abuse V15.41
  cigarette smoking V15.82
  circulatory system disease V12.50
    myocardial infarction 412
  cleft lip and palate, corrected V13.64
  combat and operational stress reaction V11.4
  congenital malformation (corrected)
    circulatory system V13.65
    digestive system V13.67
    ear V13.64
    eye V13.64
    face V13.64
    genitourinary system V13.62
    heart V13.65
    integument V13.68
    limbs V13.68
    musculoskeletal V13.68
    neck V13.64
    nervous system V13.63
    respiratory system V13.66
    specified type NEC V13.69
  contraception V15.7
  death, sudden, successfully resuscitated V12.53
  deficit
    prolonged reversible ischemic neurologic (PRIND) V12.54
    reversible ischemic neurologic (RIND) V12.54
  diathesis, allergic V15.09
  digestive system disease V12.70
    peptic ulcer V12.71
    polyps, colonic V12.72
    specified NEC V12.79
  disease (of) V13.9
    blood V12.3
    blood-forming organs V12.3
    cardiovascular system V12.50
    circulatory system V12.50
      specified NEC V12.59
    digestive system V12.70
      peptic ulcer V12.71
      polyps, colonic V12.72
      specified NEC V12.79
    infectious V12.00
      malaria V12.03
      methicillin resistant Staphylococcus aureus (MRSA) V12.04
      MRSA (methicillin resistant Staphylococcus aureus) V12.04
      poliomyelitis V12.02
      specified NEC V12.09
      tuberculosis V12.01
    parasitic V12.00
      specified NEC V12.09
    respiratory system V12.60
      pneumonia V12.61

History of — continued
  disease — continued
    respiratory system — continued
      specified NEC V12.69
    skin V13.3
    specified site NEC V13.89
    subcutaneous tissue V13.3
    trophoblastic V13.1
      affecting management of pregnancy V23.1
  disorder (of) V13.9
    endocrine V12.29
      gestational diabetes V12.21
    genital system V13.29
    hematological V12.3
    immunity V12.29
    mental V11.9
      affective type V11.1
      manic-depressive V11.1
      neurosis V11.2
      schizophrenia V11.0
      specified type NEC V11.8
    metabolic V12.29
    musculoskeletal NEC V13.59
    nervous system V12.40
      specified type NEC V12.49
    obstetric V13.29
      affecting management of current pregnancy V23.49
      ectopic pregnancy V23.42
      pre-term labor V23.41
      pre-term labor V13.21
    sense organs V12.40
      specified type NEC V12.49
    specified site NEC V13.89
    urinary system V13.00
      calculi V13.01
      infection V13.02
      nephrotic syndrome V13.03
      specified NEC V13.09
  drug use
    nonprescribed (see also Abuse, drugs, nondependent) 305.9 ☑
    patent (see also Abuse, drugs, non-dependent) 305.9 ☑
  dysplasia
    cervical (conditions classifiable to 622.10-622.12) V13.22
    vaginal (conditions classifiable to 623.0) V13.23
    vulvar (conditions classifiable to 624.01-624.02) V13.24
  effect NEC of external cause V15.89
  embolism V12.51
    pulmonary V12.55
  emotional abuse V15.42
  encephalitis V12.42
  endocrine disorder V12.29
    gestational diabetes V12.21
  estrogen therapy V87.43
  extracorporeal membrane oxygenation (ECMO) V15.87
  failed
    conscious sedation V15.80
    moderate sedation V15.80
  falling V15.88
  family
    allergy V19.6
    anemia V18.2
    arteriosclerosis V17.49
    arthritis V17.7
    asthma V17.5
    blindness V19.0
    blood disorder NEC V18.3
    cardiovascular disease V17.49
    carrier, genetic disease V18.9
    cerebrovascular disease V17.1
    chronic respiratory condition NEC V17.6
    colonic polyps V18.51
    congenital anomalies V19.5
    consanguinity V19.7
    coronary artery disease V17.3
    cystic fibrosis V18.19
    deafness V19.2
    diabetes mellitus V18.0
    digestive disorders V18.59

☑ **Additional Digit Required** — Refer to the Tabular List for Digit Selection   ▽ **Subterms under main terms may continue to next column or page**

2014 ICD-9-CM   185

History of — *continued*
  family — *continued*
    disabilities, intellectual V18.4
    disease or disorder (of)
      allergic V19.6
      blood NEC V18.3
      cardiovascular NEC V17.49
      cerebrovascular V17.1
      colonic polyps V18.51
      coronary artery V17.3
      death, sudden cardiac (SCD) V17.41
      digestive V18.59
      ear NEC V19.3
      endocrine V18.19
        multiple neoplasia (MEN) syndrome V18.11
      eye NEC V19.19
        glaucoma V19.11
      genitourinary NEC V18.7
      glaucoma V19.11
      hypertensive V17.49
      infectious V18.8
      ischemic heart V17.3
      kidney V18.69
        polycystic V18.61
      mental V17.0
      metabolic V18.19
      musculoskeletal NEC V17.89
        osteoporosis V17.81
      neurological NEC V17.2
      parasitic V18.8
      psychiatric condition V17.0
      skin condition V19.4
    ear disorder NEC V19.3
    endocrine disease V18.19
      multiple neoplasia (MEN) syndrome V18.11
    epilepsy V17.2
    eye disorder NEC V19.19
      glaucoma V19.11
    genetic disease carrier V18.9
    genitourinary disease NEC V18.7
    glaucoma V19.11
    glomerulonephritis V18.69
    gout V18.19
    hay fever V17.6
    hearing loss V19.2
    hematopoietic neoplasia V16.7
    Hodgkin's disease V16.7
    Huntington's chorea V17.2
    hydrocephalus V19.5
    hypertension V17.49
    infarction, myocardial V17.3
    infectious disease V18.8
    intellectual disabilities V18.4
    ischemic heart disease V17.3
    kidney disease V18.69
      polycystic V18.61
    leukemia V16.6
    lymphatic malignant neoplasia NEC V16.7
    malignant neoplasm (of) NEC V16.9
      anorectal V16.0
      anus V16.0
      appendix V16.0
      bladder V16.52
      bone V16.8
      brain V16.8
      breast V16.3
        male V16.8
      bronchus V16.1
      cecum V16.0
      cervix V16.49
      colon V16.0
      duodenum V16.0
      esophagus V16.0
      eye V16.8
      gallbladder V16.0
      gastrointestinal tract V16.0
      genital organs V16.40
      hemopoietic NEC V16.7
      ileum V16.0
      ilium V16.8
      intestine NEC V16.0
      intrathoracic organs NEC V16.2
      kidney V16.51

History of — *continued*
  family — *continued*
    malignant neoplasm — *continued*
      larynx V16.2
      liver V16.0
      lung V16.1
      lymphatic NEC V16.7
      ovary V16.41
      oviduct V16.41
      pancreas V16.0
      penis V16.49
      prostate V16.42
      rectum V16.0
      respiratory organs NEC V16.2
      skin V16.8
      specified site NEC V16.8
      stomach V16.0
      testis V16.43
      trachea V16.1
      ureter V16.59
      urethra V16.59
      urinary organs V16.59
      uterus V16.49
      vagina V16.49
      vulva V16.49
    MEN (multiple endocrine neoplasia syndrome) V18.11
    mental retardation — *see* History, family, intellectual disabilities
    metabolic disease NEC V18.19
    mongolism V19.5
    multiple
      endocrine neoplasia (MEN) syndrome V18.11
      myeloma V16.7
    musculoskeletal disease NEC V17.89
      osteoporosis V17.81
    myocardial infarction V17.3
    nephritis V18.69
    nephrosis V18.69
    osteoporosis V17.81
    parasitic disease V18.8
    polycystic kidney disease V18.61
    psychiatric disorder V17.0
    psychosis V17.0
    retinitis pigmentosa V19.19
    schizophrenia V17.0
    skin conditions V19.4
    specified condition NEC V19.8
    stroke (cerebrovascular) V17.1
    sudden cardiac death (SCD) V17.41
    visual loss V19.0
  foreign body fully removed V15.53
  fracture, healed
    pathologic V13.51
    stress V13.52
    traumatic V15.51
  genital system disorder V13.29
    pre-term labor V13.21
  gestational diabetes V12.21
  health hazard V15.9
    falling V15.88
    specified cause NEC V15.89
  hepatitis
    B V12.09
    C V12.09
  Hodgkin's disease V10.72
  hypospadias (corrected) V13.61
  immunity disorder V12.29
  immunosuppression therapy V87.46
  infarction, cerebral, without residual deficits V12.54
  infection
    central nervous system V12.42
    urinary (tract) V13.02
  infectious disease V12.00
    malaria V12.03
    methicillin resistant Staphylococcus aureus (MRSA) V12.04
    MRSA (methicillin resistant Staphylococcus aureus) V12.04
    poliomyelitis V12.02
    specified NEC V12.09
    tuberculosis V12.01
  injury NEC V15.59
    traumatic brain V15.52

History of — *continued*
  insufficient prenatal care V23.7
  in utero procedure
    during pregnancy V15.21
    while a fetus V15.22
  irradiation V15.3
  leukemia V10.60
    lymphoid V10.61
    monocytic V10.63
    myeloid V10.62
    specified type NEC V10.69
  little or no prenatal care V23.7
  low birth weight (*see* Status, low birth weight) V21.30
  lymphosarcoma V10.71
  malaria V12.03
  malignant carcinoid tumor V10.91
  malignant neoplasm (of) V10.90
    accessory sinus V10.22
    adrenal V10.88
    anus V10.06
    bile duct V10.09
    bladder V10.51
    bone V10.81
    brain V10.85
    breast V10.3
    bronchus V10.11
    cervix uteri V10.41
    colon V10.05
    connective tissue NEC V10.89
    corpus uteri V10.42
    digestive system V10.00
      specified part NEC V10.09
    duodenum V10.09
    endocrine gland NEC V10.88
    epididymis V10.48
    esophagus V10.03
    eye V10.84
    fallopian tube V10.44
    female genital organ V10.40
      specified site NEC V10.44
    gallbladder V10.09
    gastrointestinal tract V10.00
    gum V10.02
    hematopoietic NEC V10.79
    hypopharynx V10.02
    ileum V10.09
    intrathoracic organs NEC V10.20
    jejunum V10.09
    kidney V10.52
    large intestine V10.05
    larynx V10.21
    lip V10.02
    liver V10.07
    lung V10.11
    lymphatic NEC V10.79
    lymph glands or nodes NEC V10.79
    male genital organ V10.45
      specified site NEC V10.49
    mediastinum V10.29
    melanoma (of skin) V10.82
    middle ear V10.22
    mouth V10.02
      specified part NEC V10.02
    nasal cavities V10.22
    nasopharynx V10.02
    nervous system NEC V10.86
    nose V10.22
    oropharynx V10.02
    ovary V10.43
    pancreas V10.09
    parathyroid V10.88
    penis V10.49
    pharynx V10.02
    pineal V10.88
    pituitary V10.88
    placenta V10.44
    pleura V10.29
    prostate V10.46
    rectosigmoid junction V10.06
    rectum V10.06
    renal pelvis V10.53
    respiratory organs NEC V10.20
    salivary gland V10.02
    skin V10.83
      melanoma V10.82

History of — *continued*
  malignant neoplasm — *continued*
    small intestine NEC V10.09
    soft tissue NEC V10.89
    specified site NEC V10.89
    stomach V10.04
    testis V10.47
    thymus V10.29
    thyroid V10.87
    tongue V10.01
    trachea V10.12
    ureter V10.59
    urethra V10.59
    urinary organ V10.50
    uterine adnexa V10.44
    uterus V10.42
    vagina V10.44
    vulva V10.44
  malignant neuroendocrine tumor V10.91
  manic-depressive psychosis V11.1
  meningitis V12.42
  mental disorder V11.9
    affective type V11.1
      manic-depressive V11.1
    neurosis V11.2
    schizophrenia V11.0
    specified type NEC V11.8
  Merkel cell carcinoma V10.91
  metabolic disorder V12.29
  methicillin resistant Staphylococcus aureus (MRSA) V12.04
  MRSA (methicillin resistant Staphylococcus aureus) V12.04
  musculoskeletal disorder NEC V13.59
  myocardial infarction 412
  neglect (emotional) V15.42
  nephrotic syndrome V13.03
  nervous system disorder V12.40
    specified type NEC V12.49
  neurosis V11.2
  noncompliance with medical treatment V15.81
  nutritional deficiency V12.1
  obstetric disorder V13.29
    affecting management of current pregnancy V23.49
      ectopic pregnancy V23.42
      pre-term labor V23.41
    pre-term labor V13.21
  parasitic disease V12.00
    specified NEC V12.09
  perinatal problems V13.7
    low birth weight (*see also* Status, low birth weight) V21.30
  physical abuse V15.41
  poisoning V15.6
  poliomyelitis V12.02
  polyps, colonic V12.72
  poor obstetric V13.29
    affecting management of current pregnancy V23.49
      ectopic pregnancy V23.42
      pre-term labor V23.41
    pre-term labor V13.21
  prolonged reversible ischemic neurologic deficit (PRIND) V12.54
  psychiatric disorder V11.9
    affective type V11.1
      manic-depressive V11.1
    neurosis V11.2
    schizophrenia V11.0
    specified type NEC V11.8
  psychological trauma V15.49
    emotional abuse V15.42
    neglect V15.42
    physical abuse V15.41
    rape V15.41
  psychoneurosis V11.2
  radiation therapy V15.3
  rape V15.41
  respiratory system disease V12.60
    pneumonia V12.61
    specified NEC V12.69
  reticulosarcoma V10.71
  return from military deployment V62.22

☑ **Additional Digit Required** — Refer to the Tabular List for Digit Selection   ▽ **Subterms under main terms may continue to next column or page**

186   **2014 ICD-9-CM**

Index — History — History

History of — continued
  reversible ischemic neurologic deficit (RIND)
    V12.54
  schizophrenia V11.0
  skin disease V13.3
  smoking (tobacco) V15.82
  steroid therapy V87.45
    inhaled V87.44
    systemic V87.45
  stroke without residual deficits V12.54
  subcutaneous tissue disease V13.3
  sudden
    cardiac
      arrest V12.53
      death (successfully resuscitated)
        V12.53
  surgery to
    great vessels V15.1
    heart V15.1
    in utero
      during pregnancy V15.21
      while a fetus V15.22
    organs NEC V15.29
  syndrome, nephrotic V13.03
  therapy
    antineoplastic drug V87.41
    drug NEC V87.49
    estrogen V87.43
    immunosuppression V87.46
    monoclonal drug V87.42
    steroid V87.45
      inhaled V87.44
      systemic V87.45
  thrombophlebitis V12.52
  thrombosis V12.51
    pulmonary V12.55
  tobacco use V15.82
  trophoblastic disease V13.1
    affecting management of pregnancy
      V23.1
  tuberculosis V12.01
  ulcer, peptic V12.71
  urinary system disorder V13.00
    calculi V13.01
    infection V13.02
    nephrotic syndrome V13.03
    specified NEC V13.09
His-Werner disease (trench fever) 083.1
HIT (heparin-induced thrombocytopenia)
  289.84
Hives (bold) — see also Urticaria 708.9
HIV infection (disease) (illness) — see Human
  immunodeficiency virus (disease) (illness) (infection)
Hoarseness 784.42
Hobnail liver — see Cirrhosis, portal
Hobo, hoboism V60.0
Hodgkin's
  disease (M9650/3) 201.9 ☑
    lymphocytic
      depletion (M9653/3) 201.7 ☑
        diffuse fibrosis (M9654/3)
          201.7 ☑
        reticular type (M9655/3) 201.7 ☑
      predominance (M9651/3) 201.4 ☑
    lymphocytic-histiocytic predominance
      (M9651/3) 201.4 ☑
    mixed cellularity (M9652/3) 201.6 ☑
    nodular sclerosis (M9656/3) 201.5 ☑
      cellular phase (M9657/3) 201.5 ☑
  granuloma (M9661/3) 201.1 ☑
  lymphogranulomatosis (M9650/3) 201.9 ☑
  lymphoma (M9650/3) 201.9 ☑
  lymphosarcoma (M9650/3) 201.9 ☑
  paragranuloma (M9660/3) 201.0 ☑
  sarcoma (M9662/3) 201.2 ☑
Hodgson's disease (aneurysmal dilatation of
  aorta) 441.9
  ruptured 441.5
Hodi-potsy 111.0
Hoffa (-Kastert) disease or syndrome (liposynovitis prepatellaris) 272.8
Hoffmann-Bouveret syndrome (paroxysmal
  tachycardia) 427.2
Hoffman's syndrome 244.9 [359.5]

Hole
  macula 362.54
  optic disc, crater-like 377.22
  retina (macula) 362.54
  round 361.31
    with detachment 361.01
Holla disease — see also Spherocytosis 282.0
Holländer-Simons syndrome (progressive
  lipodystrophy) 272.6
Hollow foot (congenital) 754.71
  acquired 736.73
Holmes' syndrome (visual disorientation)
  368.16
Holoprosencephaly 742.2
  due to
    trisomy 13 758.1
    trisomy 18 758.2
Holthouse's hernia — see Hernia, inguinal
Homesickness 309.89
Homicidal ideation V62.85
Homocystinemia 270.4
Homocystinuria 270.4
Homologous serum jaundice (prophylactic)
  (therapeutic) — see Hepatitis, viral
Homosexuality — omit code
  ego-dystonic 302.0
  pedophilic 302.2
  problems with 302.0
Homozygous Hb-S disease 282.61
Honeycomb lung 518.89
  congenital 748.4
Hong Kong ear 117.3
HOOD (hereditary osteo-onychodysplasia)
  756.89
Hooded
  clitoris 752.49
  penis 752.69
Hookworm (anemia) (disease) (infestation) —
  see Ancylostomiasis
Hoppe-Goldflam syndrome 358.00
Hordeolum (external) (eyelid) 373.11
  internal 373.12
Horn
  cutaneous 702.8
    cheek 702.8
    eyelid 702.8
    penis 702.8
  iliac 756.89
  nail 703.8
    congenital 757.5
  papillary 700
Horner's
  syndrome (see also Neuropathy, peripheral,
    autonomic) 337.9
    traumatic 954.0
  teeth 520.4
Horseshoe kidney (congenital) 753.3
Horton's
  disease (temporal arteritis) 446.5
  headache or neuralgia 339.00
Hospice care V66.7
Hospitalism (in children) NEC 309.83
Hourglass contraction, contracture
  bladder 596.89
  gallbladder 575.2
    congenital 751.69
  stomach 536.8
    congenital 750.7
    psychogenic 306.4
  uterus 661.4 ☑
    affecting fetus or newborn 763.7
Household circumstance affecting care V60.9
  specified type NEC V60.89
Housemaid's knee 727.2
Housing circumstance affecting care V60.9
  specified type NEC V60.89
HTLV-I infection 079.51
HTLV-II infection 079.52
HTLV-III/LAV (disease) (illness) (infection) —
  see Human immunodeficiency virus
  (disease) (illness) (infection)
HTLV-III (disease) (illness) (infection) — see
  Human immunodeficiency virus (dis-
  ease) (illness) (infection)

HTR (hemolytic transfusion reaction)
  due to or resulting from
    incompatibility
      ABO 999.61
        acute 999.62
        delayed 999.63
      non-ABO antigen (minor) (Duffy)
        (Kell) (Kidd) (Lewis) (M) (N) (P)
        (S) 999.76
        acute 999.77
        delayed 999.78
      Rh antigen (C) (c) (D) (E) (e) 999.71
        acute 999.72
        delayed 999.73
Huchard's disease (continued arterial hypertension) 401.9
Hudson-Ståhli lines 371.11
Huguier's disease (uterine fibroma) 218.9
Human bite (open wound) — see also Wound,
  open, by site
  intact skin surface — see Contusion
Human immunodeficiency virus (disease)
  (illness) 042
  infection V08
    with symptoms, symptomatic 042
Human immunodeficiency virus-2 infection
  079.53
Human immunovirus (disease) (illness) (infection) — see Human immunodeficiency
  virus (disease) (illness) (infection)
Human papillomavirus 079.4
  high risk, DNA test positive
    anal 796.75
    cervical 795.05
    vaginal 795.15
  low risk, DNA test positive
    anal 796.79
    cervical 795.09
    vaginal 795.19
Human parvovirus 079.83
**Human T-cell lymphotrophic virus-I infec-
  tion** 079.51
**Human T-cell lymphotrophic virus-II infec-
  tion** 079.52
Human T-cell lymphotrophic virus-III (disease) (illness) (infection) — see Human
  immunodeficiency virus (disease) (ill-
  ness) (infection)
Humpback (acquired) 737.9
  congenital 756.19
Hum, venous — omit code
Hunchback (acquired) 737.9
  congenital 756.19
Hunger 994.2
  air, psychogenic 306.1
  disease 251.1
Hungry bone syndrome 275.5
Hunner's ulcer — see also Cystitis 595.1
Hunt's
  neuralgia 053.11
  syndrome (herpetic geniculate ganglionitis)
    053.11
    dyssynergia cerebellaris myoclonica
      334.2
Hunter's glossitis 529.4
Hunterian chancre 091.0
Hunter (-Hurler) syndrome (mucopolysaccharidosis II) 277.5
Huntington's
  chorea 333.4
  disease 333.4
Huppert's disease (multiple myeloma)
  (M9730/3) 203.0 ☑
Hurler (-Hunter) disease or syndrome (mu-
  copolysaccharidosis II) 277.5
Hürthle cell
  adenocarcinoma (M8290/3) 193
  adenoma (M8290/0) 226
  carcinoma (M8290/3) 193
  tumor (M8290/0) 226
Hutchinson's
  disease meaning
    angioma serpiginosum 709.1
    cheiropompholyx 705.81
    prurigo estivalis 692.72

Hutchinson's — continued
  disease meaning — continued
    summer eruption, or summer prurigo
      692.72
  incisors 090.5
  melanotic freckle (M8742/2) (see also Neo-
    plasm, skin, in situ)
    malignant melanoma in (M8742/3) —
      see Melanoma
  teeth or incisors (congenital syphilis) 090.5
Hutchinson-Boeck disease or syndrome
  (sarcoidosis) 135
Hutchinson-Gilford disease or syndrome
  (progeria) 259.8
Hyaline
  degeneration (diffuse) (generalized) 728.9
    localized — see Degeneration, by site
  membrane (disease) (lung) (newborn) 769
Hyalinosis cutis et mucosae 272.8
Hyalin plaque, sclera, senile 379.16
Hyalitis (asteroid) 379.22
  syphilitic 095.8
Hydatid
  cyst or tumor (see also Echinococcus)
    fallopian tube 752.11
  mole — see Hydatidiform mole
  Morgagni (congenital) 752.89
    fallopian tube 752.11
Hydatidiform mole (benign) (complicating
  pregnancy) (delivered) (undelivered) 630
  invasive (M9100/1) 236.1
  malignant (M9100/1) 236.1
  previous, affecting management of pregnan-
    cy V23.1
Hydatidosis — see Echinococcus
Hyde's disease (prurigo nodularis) 698.3
Hydradenitis 705.83
Hydradenoma (M8400/0) — see Hidradenoma
Hydralazine lupus or syndrome
  correct substance properly administered
    695.4
  overdose or wrong substance given or taken
    972.6
Hydramnios 657.0 ☑
  affecting fetus or newborn 761.3
Hydrancephaly 742.3
  with spina bifida (see also Spina bifida)
    741.0 ☑
Hydranencephaly 742.3
  with spina bifida (see also Spina bifida)
    741.0 ☑
Hydrargyrism NEC 985.0
Hydrarthrosis — see also Effusion, joint
  719.0 ☑
  gonococcal 098.50
  intermittent (see also Rheumatism, palin-
    dromic) 719.3 ☑
  of yaws (early) (late) 102.6
  syphilitic 095.8
    congenital 090.5
Hydremia 285.9
Hydrencephalocele (congenital) 742.0
Hydrencephalomeningocele (congenital)
  742.0
Hydroa 694.0
  aestivale 692.72
  gestationis 646.8 ☑
  herpetiformis 694.0
  pruriginosa 694.0
  vacciniforme 692.72
Hydroadenitis 705.83
Hydrocalycosis — see also Hydronephrosis 591
  congenital 753.29
Hydrocalyx — see also Hydronephrosis 591
Hydrocele (calcified) (chylous) (idiopathic)
  (infantile) (inguinal canal) (recurrent)
  (senile) (spermatic cord) (testis) (tunica
  vaginalis) 603.9
  canal of Nuck (female) 629.1
    male 603.9
  congenital 778.6
  encysted 603.0
    congenital 778.6
  female NEC 629.89
  infected 603.1
  round ligament 629.89

☑ Additional Digit Required — Refer to the Tabular List for Digit Selection   ▽ Subterms under main terms may continue to next column or page

2014 ICD-9-CM   187

☑ Additional Digit Required — Refer to the Tabular List for Digit Selection   ▽ Subterms under main terms may continue to next column or page

188   2014 ICD-9-CM

Hyperfunction — *continued*
ovary 256.1
estrogen 256.0
pancreas 577.8
parathyroid (gland) 252.00
pituitary (anterior) (gland) (lobe) 253.1
testicular 257.0
Hypergammaglobulinemia 289.89
monoclonal, benign (BMH) 273.1
polyclonal 273.0
Waldenström's 273.0
Hyperglobulinemia 273.8
Hyperglycemia 790.29
maternal
affecting fetus or newborn 775.0
manifest diabetes in infant 775.1
postpancreatectomy (complete) (partial)
251.3
Hyperglyceridemia 272.1
endogenous 272.1
essential 272.1
familial 272.1
hereditary 272.1
mixed 272.3
pure 272.1
Hyperglycinemia 270.7
Hypergonadism
ovarian 256.1
testicular (infantile) (primary) 257.0
Hyperheparinemia — *see also* Circulating, intrinsic anticoagulants 287.5
Hyperhidrosis, hyperidrosis 705.21
axilla 705.21
face 705.21
focal (localized) 705.21
primary 705.21
axilla 705.21
face 705.21
palms 705.21
soles 705.21
secondary 705.22
axilla 705.22
face 705.22
palms 705.22
soles 705.22
generalized 780.8
palms 705.21
psychogenic 306.3
secondary 780.8
soles 705.21
Hyperhistidinemia 270.5
Hyperinsulinism (ectopic) (functional) (organic) NEC 251.1
iatrogenic 251.0
reactive 251.2
spontaneous 251.2
therapeutic misadventure (from administration of insulin) 962.3
Hyperiodemia 276.9
Hyperirritability (cerebral), in newborn 779.1
Hyperkalemia 276.7
Hyperkeratosis — *see also* Keratosis 701.1
cervix 622.2
congenital 757.39
cornea 371.89
due to yaws (early) (late) (palmar or plantar)
102.3
eccentrica 757.39
figurata centrifuga atrophica 757.39
follicularis 757.39
in cutem penetrans 701.1
limbic (cornea) 371.89
palmoplantaris climacterica 701.1
pinta (carate) 103.1
senile (with pruritus) 702.0
tongue 528.79
universalis congenita 757.1
vagina 623.1
vocal cord 478.5
vulva 624.09
Hyperkinesia, hyperkinetic (disease) (reaction) (syndrome) 314.9
with
attention deficit — *see* Disorder, attention deficit
conduct disorder 314.2

Hyperkinesia, hyperkinetic — *continued*
with — *continued*
developmental delay 314.1
simple disturbance of activity and attention 314.01
specified manifestation NEC 314.8
heart (disease) 429.82
of childhood or adolescence NEC 314.9
Hyperlacrimation — *see also* Epiphora 375.20
Hyperlipemia — *see also* Hyperlipidemia 272.4
Hyperlipidemia 272.4
carbohydrate-induced 272.1
combined 272.2
endogenous 272.1
exogenous 272.3
fat-induced 272.3
group
A 272.0
B 272.1
C 272.2
D 272.3
mixed 272.2
specified type NEC 272.4
Hyperlipidosis 272.7
hereditary 272.7
Hyperlipoproteinemia (acquired) (essential)
(familial) (hereditary) (primary) (secondary) 272.4
Fredrickson type
I 272.3
IIa 272.0
IIb 272.2
III 272.2
IV 272.1
V 272.3
low-density-lipoid-type (LDL) 272.0
very-low-density-lipoid-type (VLDL) 272.1
Hyperlucent lung, unilateral 492.8
Hyperluteinization 256.1
Hyperlysinemia 270.7
Hypermagnesemia 275.2
neonatal 775.5
Hypermaturity (fetus or newborn)
post-term infant 766.21
prolonged gestation infant 766.22
Hypermenorrhea 626.2
Hypermetabolism 794.7
Hypermethioninemia 270.4
Hypermetropia (congenital) 367.0
Hypermobility
cecum 564.9
coccyx 724.71
colon 564.9
psychogenic 306.4
ileum 564.89
joint (acquired) 718.80
ankle 718.87
elbow 718.82
foot 718.87
hand 718.84
hip 718.85
knee 718.86
multiple sites 718.89
pelvic region 718.85
shoulder (region) 718.81
specified site NEC 718.88
wrist 718.83
kidney, congenital 753.3
meniscus (knee) 717.5
scapula 718.81
stomach 536.8
psychogenic 306.4
syndrome 728.5
testis, congenital 752.52
urethral 599.81
Hypermotility
gastrointestinal 536.8
intestine 564.9
psychogenic 306.4
stomach 536.8
Hypernasality 784.43
Hypernatremia 276.0
with water depletion 276.0
Hypernephroma (M8312/3) 189.0
Hyperopia 367.0
Hyperorexia 783.6

Hyperornithinemia 270.6
Hyperosmia — *see also* Disturbance, sensation
781.1
Hyperosmolality 276.0
Hyperosteogenesis 733.99
Hyperostosis 733.99
calvarial 733.3
cortical 733.3
infantile 756.59
frontal, internal of skull 733.3
interna frontalis 733.3
monomelic 733.99
skull 733.3
congenital 756.0
vertebral 721.8
with spondylosis — *see* Spondylosis
ankylosing 721.6
Hyperovarianism 256.1
Hyperovarism, hyperovaria 256.1
Hyperoxaluria (primary) 271.8
Hyperoxia 987.8
Hyperparathyroidism 252.00
ectopic 259.3
other 252.08
primary 252.01
secondary (of renal origin) 588.81
non-renal 252.02
tertiary 252.08
Hyperpathia — *see also* Disturbance, sensation
782.0
psychogenic 307.80
Hyperperistalsis 787.4
psychogenic 306.4
Hyperpermeability, capillary 448.9
Hyperphagia 783.6
Hyperphenylalaninemia 270.1
Hyperphoria 378.40
alternating 378.45
Hyperphosphatemia 275.3
Hyperpiesia — *see also* Hypertension 401.9
Hyperpiesis — *see also* Hypertension 401.9
Hyperpigmentation — *see* Pigmentation
Hyperpinealism 259.8
Hyperpipecolatemia 270.7
Hyperpituitarism 253.1
Hyperplasia, hyperplastic
adenoids (lymphoid tissue) 474.12
and tonsils 474.10
adrenal (capsule) (cortex) (gland) 255.8
with
sexual precocity (male) 255.2
virilism, adrenal 255.2
virilization (female) 255.2
congenital 255.2
due to excess ACTH (ectopic) (pituitary)
255.0
medulla 255.8
alpha cells (pancreatic)
with
gastrin excess 251.5
glucagon excess 251.4
angiolymphoid, with eosinophilia (ALHE)
228.01
appendix (lymphoid) 543.0
artery, fibromuscular NEC 447.8
carotid 447.8
renal 447.3
bone 733.99
marrow 289.9
breast (*see also* Hypertrophy, breast) 611.1
ductal 610.8
atypical 610.8
carotid artery 447.8
cementation, cementum (teeth) (tooth)
521.5
cervical gland 785.6
cervix (uteri) 622.10
basal cell 622.10
congenital 752.49
endometrium 622.10
polypoid 622.10
chin 524.05
clitoris, congenital 752.49
dentin 521.5
endocervicitis 616.0

Hyperplasia, hyperplastic — *continued*
endometrium, endometrial (adenomatous)
(atypical) (cystic) (glandular) (polypoid) (uterus) 621.30
with atypia 621.33
without atypia
complex 621.32
simple 621.31
benign 621.34
cervix 622.10
epithelial 709.8
focal, oral, including tongue 528.79
mouth (focal) 528.79
nipple 611.89
skin 709.8
tongue (focal) 528.79
vaginal wall 623.0
erythroid 289.9
fascialis ossificans (progressiva) 728.11
fibromuscular, artery NEC 447.8
carotid 447.8
renal 447.3
genital
female 629.89
male 608.89
gingiva 523.8
glandularis
cystica uteri 621.30
endometrium (uterus) 621.30
interstitialis uteri 621.30
granulocytic 288.69
gum 523.8
hymen, congenital 752.49
islands of Langerhans 251.1
islet cell (pancreatic) 251.9
alpha cells
with excess
gastrin 251.5
glucagon 251.4
beta cells 251.1
juxtaglomerular (complex) (kidney) 593.89
kidney (congenital) 753.3
liver (congenital) 751.69
lymph node (gland) 785.6
lymphoid (diffuse) (nodular) 785.6
appendix 543.0
intestine 569.89
mandibular 524.02
alveolar 524.72
unilateral condylar 526.89
Marchand multiple nodular (liver) — *see*
Cirrhosis, postnecrotic
maxillary 524.01
alveolar 524.71
medulla, adrenal 255.8
myometrium, myometrial 621.2
neuroendocrine cell, of infancy 516.61
nose (lymphoid) (polypoid) 478.19
oral soft tissue (inflammatory) (irritative)
(mucosa) NEC 528.9
gingiva 523.8
tongue 529.8
organ or site, congenital NEC — *see*
Anomaly, specified type NEC
ovary 620.8
palate, papillary 528.9
pancreatic islet cells 251.9
alpha
with excess
gastrin 251.5
glucagon 251.4
beta 251.1
parathyroid (gland) 252.01
persistent, vitreous (primary) 743.51
pharynx (lymphoid) 478.29
prostate 600.90
with
other lower urinary tract symptoms
(LUTS) 600.91
urinary
obstruction 600.91
retention 600.91
adenofibromatous 600.20
with
other lower urinary tract symptoms (LUTS) 600.21

Hyperfunction — Hyperplasia, hyperplastic

Hyperplasia, hyperplastic — *continued*
  prostate — *continued*
    adenofibromatous — *continued*
      with — *continued*
        urinary
          obstruction 600.21
          retention 600.21
    nodular 600.10
      with
        urinary
          obstruction 600.11
          retention 600.11
  renal artery (fibromuscular) 447.3
  reticuloendothelial (cell) 289.9
  salivary gland (any) 527.1
  Schimmelbusch's 610.1
  suprarenal (capsule) (gland) 255.8
  thymus (gland) (persistent) 254.0
  thyroid (*see also* Goiter) 240.9
    primary 242.0 ☑
    secondary 242.2 ☑
  tonsil (lymphoid tissue) 474.11
    and adenoids 474.10
  urethrovaginal 599.89
  uterus, uterine (myometrium) 621.2
    endometrium (*see also* Hyperplasia, endometrium) 621.30
  vitreous (humor), primary persistent 743.51
  vulva 624.3
  zygoma 738.11
Hyperpnea — *see also* Hyperventilation 786.01
Hyperpotassemia 276.7
Hyperprebetalipoproteinemia 272.1
  with chylomicronemia 272.3
  familial 272.1

Hyperprolactinemia 253.1
Hyperprolinemia 270.8
Hyperproteinemia 273.8
Hyperprothrombinemia 289.89
Hyperpselaphesia 782.0
Hyperpyrexia 780.60
  heat (effects of) 992.0
  malarial (*see also* Malaria) 084.6
  malignant, due to anesthetic 995.86
  rheumatic — *see* Fever, rheumatic
  unknown origin (*see also* Pyrexia) 780.60
Hyperreactor, vascular 780.2
Hyperreflexia 796.1
  bladder, autonomic 596.54
    with cauda equina 344.61
  detrusor 344.61
Hypersalivation — *see also* Ptyalism 527.7
Hypersarcosinemia 270.8
Hypersecretion
  ACTH 255.3
  androgens (ovarian) 256.1
  calcitonin 246.0
  corticoadrenal 255.3
  cortisol 255.0
  estrogen 256.0
  gastric 536.8
    psychogenic 306.4
  gastrin 251.5
  glucagon 251.4
  hormone
    ACTH 255.3
    anterior pituitary 253.1
    growth NEC 253.0
    ovarian androgen 256.1
    testicular 257.0

Hypersecretion — *continued*
  hormone — *continued*
    thyroid stimulating 242.8 ☑
  insulin — *see* Hyperinsulinism
  lacrimal glands (*see also* Epiphora) 375.20
  medulloadrenal 255.6
  milk 676.6 ☑
  ovarian androgens 256.1
  pituitary (anterior) 253.1
  salivary gland (any) 527.7
  testicular hormones 257.0
  thyrocalcitonin 246.0
  upper respiratory 478.9
Hypersegmentation, hereditary 288.2
  eosinophils 288.2
  neutrophil nuclei 288.2
Hypersensitive, hypersensitiveness, hypersensitivity — *see also* Allergy
  angiitis 446.20
    specified NEC 446.29
  carotid sinus 337.01
  colon 564.9
    psychogenic 306.4
  DNA (deoxyribonucleic acid) NEC 287.2
  drug (*see also* Allergy, drug) 995.27
  due to correct medical substance properly administered 995.27
  esophagus 530.89
  insect bites — *see* Injury, superficial, by site
  labyrinth 386.58
  pain (*see also* Disturbance, sensation) 782.0
  pneumonitis NEC 495.9
  reaction (*see also* Allergy) 995.3
    upper respiratory tract NEC 478.8
  stomach (allergic) (nonallergic) 536.8

Hypersensitive, hypersensitiveness, hypersensitivity — *see also* Allergy — *continued*
  stomach — *continued*
    psychogenic 306.4
Hypersomatotropism (classic) 253.0
Hypersomnia, unspecified 780.54
  with sleep apnea, unspecified 780.53
  alcohol induced 291.82
  drug induced 292.85
  due to
    medical condition classified elsewhere 327.14
    mental disorder 327.15
  idiopathic
    with long sleep time 327.11
    without long sleep time 327.12
  menstrual related 327.13
  nonorganic origin 307.43
    persistent (primary) 307.44
    transient 307.43
  organic 327.10
    other 327.19
  primary 307.44
  recurrent 327.13
Hypersplenia 289.4
Hypersplenism 289.4
Hypersteatosis 706.3
Hyperstimulation, ovarian 256.1
Hypersuprarenalism 255.3
Hypersusceptibility — *see* Allergy
Hyper-TBG-nemia 246.8
Hypertelorism 756.0
  orbit, orbital 376.41

	Malignant	Benign	Unspecified
Hypertension, hypertensive (arterial) (arteriolar) (crisis) (degeneration) (disease) (essential) (fluctuating) (idiopathic) (intermittent) (labile) (low renin) (orthostatic) (paroxysmal) (primary) (systemic) (uncontrolled) (vascular)	401.0	401.1	401.9
with			
chronic kidney disease			
stage I through stage IV, or unspecified	403.00	403.10	403.90
stage V or end stage renal disese	403.01	403.11	403.91
heart involvement (conditions classifiable to 429.0–429.3, 429.8, 429.9 due to hypertension) (*see also* Hypertension, heart)	402.00	402.10	402.90
with kidney involvement — *see* Hypertension, cardiorenal			
renal (kidney) involvement (only conditions classifiable to 585, 587) (excludes conditions classifiable to 584) (*see also* Hypertension, kidney)	403.00	403.10	403.90
with heart involvement — *see* Hypertension, cardiorenal			
failure (and sclerosis) (*see also* Hypertension, kidney)	403.01	403.11	403.91
sclerosis without failure (*see also* Hypertension, kidney)	403.00	403.10	403.90
accelerated (*see also* Hypertension, by type, malignant))	401.0	—	—
antepartum — *see* Hypertension, complicating pregnancy, childbirth, or the puerperium			
borderline	—	—	796.2
cardiorenal (disease)	404.00	404.10	404.90
with			
chronic kidney disease			
stage I through stage IV, or unspecified	404.00	404.10	404.90
and heart failure	404.01	404.11	404.91
stage V or end stage renal disease	404.02	404.12	404.92
and heart failure	404.03	404.13	404.93
heart failure	404.01	404.11	404.91
and chronic kidney disease	404.01	404.11	404.91
stage I through stage IV or unspecified	404.01	404.11	404.91
stave V or end stage renal disease	404.03	404.13	404.93
cardiovascular disease (arteriosclerotic) (sclerotic)	402.00	402.10	402.90
with			
heart failure	402.01	402.11	402.91
renal involvement (conditions classifiable to 403) (*see also* Hypertension, cardiorenal)	404.00	404.10	404.90
cardiovascular renal (disease) (sclerosis) (*see also* Hypertension, cardiorenal)	404.00	404.10	404.90
cerebrovascular disease NEC	437.2	—	—
complicating pregnancy, childbirth, or the puerperium	642.2	642.0	642.9
with			
albuminuria (and edema) (mild)	—	—	642.4
severe	—	—	642.5
chronic kidney disesae	642.2	—	—
and heart disease	642.2	—	—
edema (mild)	—	—	642.4
severe	—	—	642.5
heart disease	642.2	—	—
and chronic kidney disease	642.2	—	—
renal disease	642.2	—	—
and heart disease	642.2	—	—
chronic	642.2	642.0	—
with pre-eclampsia or eclampsia	642.7	—	—
fetus or newborn	760.0	—	—
essential	—	642.0	—
with pre-eclampsia or eclampsia	—	642.7	—
fetus or newborn	760.0	—	—
fetus or newborn	760.0	—	—
gestational	—	—	642.3
pre-existing	642.2	642.0	—
with pre-eclampsia or eclampsia	642.7	—	—
fetus or newborn	760.0	—	—
secondary to renal disease	642.1	—	—
with pre-eclampsia or eclampsia	642.7	—	—
fetus or newborn	760.0	—	—
transient	—	—	642.3
due to			
aldosteronism, primary	405.09	405.19	405.99
brain tumor	405.09	405.19	405.99
bulbar poliomyelitis	405.09	405.19	405.99
calculus			
kidney	405.09	405.19	405.99

	Malignant	Benign	Unspecified
Hypertension, hypertensive — *continued*			
due to — *continued*			
calculus — *continued*			
ureter	405.09	405.19	405.99
coarctation, aorta	405.09	405.19	405.99
Cushing's disease	405.09	405.19	405.99
glomerulosclerosis (*see also* Hypertension, kidney)	403.00	403.10	403.90
periarteritis nodosa	405.09	405.19	405.99
pheochromocytoma	405.09	405.19	405.99
polycystic kidney(s)	405.09	405.19	405.99
polycythemia	405.09	405.19	405.99
porphyria	405.09	405.19	405.99
pyelonephritis	405.09	405.19	405.99
renal (artery)			
aneurysm	405.01	405.11	405.91
anomaly	405.01	405.11	405.91
embolism	405.01	405.11	405.91
fibromuscular hyperplasia	405.01	405.11	405.91
occlusion	405.01	405.11	405.91
stenosis	405.01	405.11	405.91
thrombosis	405.01	405.11	405.91
encephalopathy	437.2	—	—
gestational (transient) NEC	—	—	642.3
Goldblatt's	440.1	—	—
heart (disease) (conditions classifiable to 429.0–429.3, 429.8, 429.9 due to hypertension)	402.00	402.10	402.90
with heart failure	402.01	402.11	402.91
hypertensive kidney disease (conditions classifiable to 403) (*see also* Hypertension, cardiorenal)	404.00	404.10	404.90
renal sclerosis (*see also* Hypertension, cardiorenal)	404.00	404.10	404.90
intracranial, benign	—	348.2	—
intraocular	—	—	365.04
kidney	403.00	403.10	403.90
with			
chronic kidney disease			
stage I through stage IV, or unspecified	403.00	403.10	403.90
stage V or end stage renal disese	403.01	403.11	403.91
heart involvement (conditions classifiable to 429.0–429.3, 429.8, 429.9 due to hypertension) (*see also* Hypertension, cardiorenal)	404.00	404.10	404.90
hypertensive heart (disease) (conditions classifiable to 402) (*see also* Hypertension, cardiorenal)	404.00	404.10	404.90
lesser circulation	—	—	416.0
necrotizing	401.0	—	—
ocular	—	—	365.04
pancreatic duct — code to underlying condition			
with			
chronic pancreatitis	—	—	577.1
portal (due to chronic liver disease)	—	—	572.3
postoperative	—	—	997.91
psychogenic	—	—	306.2
puerperal, postpartum — *see* Hypertension, complicating pregnancy, childbirth, or the puerperium			
pulmonary (artery) (secondary)	—	—	416.8
with			
cor pulmonale (chronic)	—	—	416.8
acute	—	—	415.0
right heart ventricular strain/failure	—	—	416.8
acute	—	—	415.0
idiopathic	—	—	416.0
primary	—	—	416.0
of newborn	—	—	747.83
secondary	—	—	416.8
renal (disease) (*see also* Hypertension, kidney)	403.00	403.10	403.90
renovascular NEC	405.01	405.11	405.91
secondary NEC	405.09	405.19	405.99
due to			
aldosteronism, primary	405.09	405.19	405.99
brain tumor	405.09	405.19	405.99
bulbar poliomyelitis	405.09	405.19	405.99
calculus			
kidney	405.09	405.19	405.99
ureter	405.09	405.19	405.99
coarctation, aorta	405.09	405.19	405.99
Cushing's disease	405.09	405.19	405.99
glomerulosclerosis (*see also* Hypertension, kidney)	403.00	403.10	403.90

	Malignant	Benign	Unspecified
Hypertension, hypertensive — *continued*			
secondary — *continued*			
due to — *continued*			
periarteritis nodosa	405.09	405.19	405.99
pheochromocytoma	405.09	405.19	405.99
polycystic kidney(s)	405.09	405.19	405.99
polycythemia	405.09	405.19	405.99
porphyria	405.09	405.19	405.99
pyelonephritis	405.09	405.19	405.99
renal (artery)			
aneurysm	405.01	405.11	405.91
anomaly	405.01	405.11	405.91
embolism	405.01	405.11	405.91
fibromuscular hyperplasia	405.01	405.11	405.91
occlusion	405.01	405.11	405.91
stenosis	405.01	405.11	405.91
thrombosis	405.01	405.11	405.91
transient	—	—	796.2
of pregnancy	—	—	642.3
vascular degeneration	401.0	401.1	401.9
venous, chronic (asymptomatic) (idiopathic)	—	—	459.30
with			
complication, NEC	—	—	459.39
inflammation	—	—	459.32
with ulcer	—	—	459.33
ulcer	—	—	459.31
with inflammation	—	—	459.33
due to			
deep vein thrombosis (*see also* Syndrome, postphlebetic)	—	—	459.10

Hypertensive urgency — *see* Hypertension
Hyperthecosis, ovary 256.8
Hyperthermia (of unknown origin) — *see also* Pyrexia 780.60
  malignant (due to anesthesia) 995.86
  newborn 778.4
Hyperthymergasia — *see also* Psychosis, affective 296.0 ☑
  reactive (from emotional stress, psychological trauma) 298.1
  recurrent episode 296.1 ☑
  single episode 296.0 ☑
Hyperthymism 254.8
Hyperthyroid (recurrent) — *see* Hyperthyroidism
Hyperthyroidism (latent) (preadult) (recurrent) (without goiter) 242.9 ☑

> *Note* — Use the following fifth-digit subclassification with category 242:
>
> 0 *without mention of thyrotoxic crisis or storm*
>
> 1 *with mention of thyrotoxic crisis or storm*

  with
    goiter (diffuse) 242.0 ☑
      adenomatous 242.3 ☑
        multinodular 242.2 ☑
        uninodular 242.1 ☑
      nodular 242.3 ☑
        multinodular 242.2 ☑
        uninodular 242.1 ☑
    thyroid nodule 242.1 ☑
  complicating pregnancy, childbirth, or puerperium 648.1 ☑
  neonatal (transient) 775.3
Hypertonia — *see* Hypertonicity
Hypertonicity
  bladder 596.51
  fetus or newborn 779.89
  gastrointestinal (tract) 536.8
  infancy 779.89
    due to electrolyte imbalance 779.89
  muscle 728.85
  stomach 536.8
    psychogenic 306.4
  uterus, uterine (contractions) 661.4 ☑
    affecting fetus or newborn 763.7
Hypertony — *see* Hypertonicity
Hypertransaminemia 790.4
Hypertrichosis 704.1
  congenital 757.4
  eyelid 374.54
  lanuginosa 757.4
    acquired 704.1
Hypertriglyceridemia, essential 272.1
Hypertrophy, hypertrophic
  adenoids (infectional) 474.12
    and tonsils (faucial) (infective) (lingual) (lymphoid) 474.10
  adrenal 255.8
  alveolar process or ridge 525.8
  anal papillae 569.49
  apocrine gland 705.82
  artery NEC 447.8
    carotid 447.8
    congenital (peripheral) NEC 747.60
      gastrointestinal 747.61
      lower limb 747.64
      renal 747.62
      specified NEC 747.69
      spinal 747.82
      upper limb 747.63
    renal 447.3
  arthritis (chronic) (*see also* Osteoarthrosis) 715.9 ☑
    spine (*see also* Spondylosis) 721.90
  arytenoid 478.79
  asymmetrical (heart) 429.9
  auricular — *see* Hypertrophy, cardiac
  Bartholin's gland 624.8
  bile duct 576.8
  bladder (sphincter) (trigone) 596.89
  blind spot, visual field 368.42
  bone 733.99

Hypertrophy, hypertrophic — *continued*
  brain 348.89
  breast 611.1
    cystic 610.1
    fetus or newborn 778.7
    fibrocystic 610.1
    massive pubertal 611.1
    puerperal, postpartum 676.3 ☑
    senile (parenchymatous) 611.1
  cardiac (chronic) (idiopathic) 429.3
    with
      rheumatic fever (conditions classifiable to 390)
        active 391.8
          with chorea 392.0
        inactive or quiescent (with chorea) 398.99
    congenital NEC 746.89
    fatty (*see also* Degeneration, myocardial) 429.1
    hypertensive (*see also* Hypertension, heart) 402.90
    rheumatic (with chorea) 398.99
      active or acute 391.8
        with chorea 392.0
    valve (*see also* Endocarditis) 424.90
      congenital NEC 746.89
  cartilage 733.99
  cecum 569.89
  cervix (uteri) 622.6
    congenital 752.49
    elongation 622.6
  clitoris (cirrhotic) 624.2
    congenital 752.49
  colon 569.89
    congenital 751.3
  conjunctiva, lymphoid 372.73
  cornea 371.89
  corpora cavernosa 607.89
  duodenum 537.89
  endometrium (uterus) (*see also* Hyperplasia, endometrium) 621.30
    cervix 622.6
  epididymis 608.89
  esophageal hiatus (congenital) 756.6
    with hernia — *see* Hernia, diaphragm
  eyelid 374.30
  falx, skull 733.99
  fat pad 729.30
    infrapatellar 729.31
    knee 729.31
    orbital 374.34
    popliteal 729.31
    prepatellar 729.31
    retropatellar 729.31
    specified site NEC 729.39
  foot (congenital) 755.67
  frenum, frenulum (tongue) 529.8
    linguae 529.8
    lip 528.5
  gallbladder or cystic duct 575.8
  gastric mucosa 535.2 ☑
  gingiva 523.8
  gland, glandular (general) NEC 785.6
  gum (mucous membrane) 523.8
  heart (idiopathic) (*see also* Hypertrophy, cardiac)
    valve (*see also* Endocarditis)
      congenital NEC 746.89
  hemifacial 754.0
  hepatic — *see* Hypertrophy, liver
  hiatus (esophageal) 756.6
  hilus gland 785.6
  hymen, congenital 752.49
  ileum 569.89
  infrapatellar fat pad 729.31
  intestine 569.89
  jejunum 569.89
  kidney (compensatory) 593.1
    congenital 753.3
  labial frenulum 528.5
  labium (majus) (minus) 624.3
  lacrimal gland, chronic 375.03
  ligament 728.9
    spinal 724.8
  linguae frenulum 529.8

Hypertrophy, hypertrophic — *continued*
  lingual tonsil (infectional) 474.11
  lip (frenum) 528.5
    congenital 744.81
  liver 789.1
    acute 573.8
    cirrhotic — *see* Cirrhosis, liver
    congenital 751.69
    fatty — *see* Fatty, liver
  lymph gland 785.6
    tuberculous — *see* Tuberculosis, lymph gland
  mammary gland — *see* Hypertrophy, breast
  maxillary frenulum 528.5
  Meckel's diverticulum (congenital) 751.0
  medial meniscus, acquired 717.3
  median bar 600.90
    with
      other lower urinary tract symptoms (LUTS) 600.91
      urinary
        obstruction 600.91
        retention 600.91
  mediastinum 519.3
  meibomian gland 373.2
  meniscus, knee, congenital 755.64
  metatarsal head 733.99
  metatarsus 733.99
  mouth 528.9
  mucous membrane
    alveolar process 523.8
    nose 478.19
    turbinate (nasal) 478.0
  muscle 728.9
  muscular coat, artery NEC 447.8
    carotid 447.8
    renal 447.3
  myocardium (*see also* Hypertrophy, cardiac) 429.3
    idiopathic 425.18
  myometrium 621.2
  nail 703.8
    congenital 757.5
  nasal 478.19
    alae 478.19
    bone 738.0
    cartilage 478.19
    mucous membrane (septum) 478.19
    sinus (*see also* Sinusitis) 473.9
    turbinate 478.0
  nasopharynx, lymphoid (infectional) (tissue) (wall) 478.29
  neck, uterus 622.6
  nipple 611.1
  normal aperture diaphragm (congenital) 756.6
  nose (*see also* Hypertrophy, nasal) 478.19
  orbit 376.46
  organ or site, congenital NEC — *see* Anomaly, specified type NEC
  osteoarthropathy (pulmonary) 731.2
  ovary 620.8
  palate (hard) 526.89
    soft 528.9
  pancreas (congenital) 751.7
  papillae
    anal 569.49
    tongue 529.3
  parathyroid (gland) 252.01
  parotid gland 527.1
  penis 607.89
  phallus 607.89
    female (clitoris) 624.2
  pharyngeal tonsil 474.12
  pharyngitis 472.1
  pharynx 478.29
    lymphoid (infectional) (tissue) (wall) 478.29
  pituitary (fossa) (gland) 253.8
  popliteal fat pad 729.31
  preauricular (lymph) gland (Hampstead) 785.6
  prepuce (congenital) 605
    female 624.2
  prostate (asymptomatic) (early) (recurrent) 600.90

Hypertrophy, hypertrophic — *continued*
  prostate — *continued*
    with
      other lower urinary tract symptoms (LUTS) 600.91
      urinary
        obstruction 600.91
        retention 600.91
    adenofibromatous 600.20
      with
        other lower urinary tract symptoms (LUTS) 600.21
        urinary
          obstruction 600.21
          retention 600.21
    benign 600.00
      with
        other lower urinary tract symptoms (LUTS) 600.01
        urinary
          obstruction 600.01
          retention 600.01
    congenital 752.89
  pseudoedematous hypodermal 757.0
  pseudomuscular 359.1
  pylorus (muscle) (sphincter) 537.0
    congenital 750.5
    infantile 750.5
  rectal sphincter 569.49
  rectum 569.49
  renal 593.1
  rhinitis (turbinate) 472.0
  salivary duct or gland 527.1
    congenital 750.26
  scaphoid (tarsal) 733.99
  scar 701.4
  scrotum 608.89
  sella turcica 253.8
  seminal vesicle 608.89
  sigmoid 569.89
  skin condition NEC 701.9
  spermatic cord 608.89
  spinal ligament 724.8
  spleen — *see* Splenomegaly
  spondylitis (spine) (*see also* Spondylosis) 721.90
  stomach 537.89
  subaortic stenosis (idiopathic) 425.11
  sublingual gland 527.1
    congenital 750.26
  submaxillary gland 527.1
  suprarenal (gland) 255.8
  tendon 727.9
  testis 608.89
    congenital 752.89
  thymic, thymus (congenital) (gland) 254.0
  thyroid (gland) (*see also* Goiter) 240.9
    primary 242.0 ☑
    secondary 242.2 ☑
  toe (congenital) 755.65
    acquired 735.8
  tongue 529.8
    congenital 750.15
    frenum 529.8
    papillae (foliate) 529.3
  tonsil (faucial) (infective) (lingual) (lymphoid) 474.11
    with
      adenoiditis 474.01
      tonsillitis 474.00
        and adenoiditis 474.02
    and adenoids 474.10
  tunica vaginalis 608.89
  turbinate (mucous membrane) 478.0
  ureter 593.89
  urethra 599.84
  uterus 621.2
    puerperal, postpartum 674.8 ☑
  uvula 528.9
  vagina 623.8
  vas deferens 608.89
  vein 459.89
  ventricle, ventricular (heart) (left) (right) (*see also* Hypertrophy, cardiac)
    congenital 746.89

☑ **Additional Digit Required** — Refer to the Tabular List for Digit Selection   🔖 **Subterms under main terms may continue to next column or page**

2014 ICD-9-CM

193

Hypertrophy, hypertrophic — *continued*
  ventricle, ventricular (*see also* Hypertrophy, cardiac) — *continued*
    due to hypertension (left) (right) (*see also* Hypertension, heart) 402.90
      benign 402.10
      malignant 402.00
    right with ventricular septal defect, pulmonary stenosis or atresia, and dextraposition of aorta 745.2
  verumontanum 599.89
  vesical 596.89
  vocal cord 478.5
  vulva 624.3
    stasis (nonfilarial) 624.3
Hypertropia (intermittent) (periodic) 378.31
Hypertyrosinemia 270.2
Hyperuricemia 790.6
Hypervalinemia 270.3
Hyperventilation (tetany) 786.01
  hysterical 300.11
  psychogenic 306.1
  syndrome 306.1
Hyperviscidosis 277.00
Hyperviscosity (of serum) (syndrome) NEC 273.3
  polycythemic 289.0
  sclerocythemic 282.8
Hypervitaminosis (dietary) NEC 278.8
  A (dietary) 278.2
  D (dietary) 278.4
  from excessive administration or use of vitamin preparations (chronic) 278.8
    reaction to sudden overdose 963.5
  vitamin A 278.2
    reaction to sudden overdose 963.5
  vitamin D 278.4
    reaction to sudden overdose 963.5
  vitamin K
    correct substance properly administered 278.8
    overdose or wrong substance given or taken 964.3
Hypervolemia 276.69
Hypesthesia — *see also* Disturbance, sensation 782.0
  cornea 371.81
Hyphema (anterior chamber) (ciliary body) (iris) 364.41
  traumatic 921.3
Hyphemia — *see* Hyphema
Hypoacidity, gastric 536.8
  psychogenic 306.4
Hypoactive labyrinth (function) — *see* Hypofunction, labyrinth
Hypoadrenalism 255.41
  tuberculous (*see also* Tuberculosis) 017.6 ☑
Hypoadrenocorticism 255.41
  pituitary 253.4
Hypoalbuminemia 273.8
Hypoaldosteronism 255.42
Hypoalphalipoproteinemia 272.5
Hypobarism 993.2
Hypobaropathy 993.2
Hypobetalipoproteinemia (familial) 272.5
Hypocalcemia 275.41
  cow's milk 775.4
  dietary 269.3
  neonatal 775.4
  phosphate-loading 775.4
Hypocalcification, teeth 520.4
Hypochloremia 276.9
Hypochlorhydria 536.8
  neurotic 306.4
  psychogenic 306.4
Hypocholesteremia 272.5
Hypochondria (reaction) 300.7
Hypochondriac 300.7
Hypochondriasis 300.7
Hypochromasia blood cells 280.9
Hypochromic anemia 280.9
  due to blood loss (chronic) 280.0
    acute 285.1
  microcytic 280.9
Hypocoagulability — *see also* Defect, coagulation 286.9

Hypocomplementemia 279.8
Hypocythemia (progressive) 284.9
Hypodontia — *see also* Anodontia 520.0
Hypoeosinophilia 288.59
Hypoesthesia — *see also* Disturbance, sensation 782.0
  cornea 371.81
  tactile 782.0
Hypoestrinism 256.39
Hypoestrogenism 256.39
Hypoferremia 280.9
  due to blood loss (chronic) 280.0
Hypofertility
  female 628.9
  male 606.1
Hypofibrinogenemia 286.3
  acquired 286.6
  congenital 286.3
Hypofunction
  adrenal (gland) 255.41
    cortex 255.41
    medulla 255.5
    specified NEC 255.5
  cerebral 331.9
  corticoadrenal NEC 255.41
  intestinal 564.89
  labyrinth (unilateral) 386.53
    with loss of labyrinthine reactivity 386.55
    bilateral 386.54
      with loss of labyrinthine reactivity 386.56
  Leydig cell 257.2
  ovary 256.39
    postablative 256.2
  pituitary (anterior) (gland) (lobe) 253.2
    posterior 253.5
  testicular 257.2
    iatrogenic 257.1
    postablative 257.1
    postirradiation 257.1
    postsurgical 257.1
Hypogammaglobulinemia 279.00
  acquired primary 279.06
  non-sex-linked, congenital 279.06
  sporadic 279.06
  transient of infancy 279.09
Hypogenitalism (congenital) (female) (male) 752.89
  penis 752.69
Hypoglycemia (spontaneous) 251.2
  coma 251.0
    diabetic 250.3 ☑
      due to secondary diabetes 249.3 ☑
  diabetic 250.8 ☑
    due to secondary diabetes 249.8 ☑
  due to insulin 251.0
    therapeutic misadventure 962.3
  familial (idiopathic) 251.2
  following gastrointestinal surgery 579.3
  infantile (idiopathic) 251.2
  in infant of diabetic mother 775.0
  leucine-induced 270.3
  neonatal 775.6
  reactive 251.2
  specified NEC 251.1
Hypoglycemic shock 251.0
  diabetic 250.8 ☑
    due to secondary diabetes 249.8 ☑
  due to insulin 251.0
  functional (syndrome) 251.1
Hypogonadism
  female 256.39
  gonadotrophic (isolated) 253.4
  hypogonadotropic (isolated) (with anosmia) 253.4
  isolated 253.4
  male 257.2
    hereditary familial (Reifenstein's syndrome) 259.52
  ovarian (primary) 256.39
  pituitary (secondary) 253.4
  testicular (primary) (secondary) 257.2
Hypohidrosis 705.0
Hypohidrotic ectodermal dysplasia 757.31
Hypoidrosis 705.0
Hypoinsulinemia, postsurgical 251.3

Hypoinsulinemia, postsurgical — *continued*
  postpancreatectomy (complete) (partial) 251.3
Hypokalemia 276.8
Hypokinesia 780.99
Hypoleukia splenica 289.4
Hypoleukocytosis 288.50
Hypolipidemia 272.5
Hypolipoproteinemia 272.5
Hypomagnesemia 275.2
  neonatal 775.4
Hypomania, hypomanic reaction — *see also* Psychosis, affective 296.0 ☑
  recurrent episode 296.1 ☑
  single episode 296.0 ☑
Hypomastia (congenital) 611.82
Hypomenorrhea 626.1
Hypometabolism 783.9
Hypomotility
  gastrointestinal tract 536.8
    psychogenic 306.4
  intestine 564.89
    psychogenic 306.4
  stomach 536.8
    psychogenic 306.4
Hyponasality 784.44
Hyponatremia 276.1
Hypo-ovarianism 256.39
Hypo-ovarism 256.39
Hypoparathyroidism (idiopathic) (surgically induced) 252.1
  neonatal 775.4
Hypoperfusion (in)
  newborn 779.89
Hypopharyngitis 462
Hypophoria 378.40
Hypophosphatasia 275.3
Hypophosphatemia (acquired) (congenital) (familial) 275.3
  renal 275.3
Hypophyseal, hypophysis — *see also* condition
  dwarfism 253.3
  gigantism 253.0
  syndrome 253.8
Hypophyseothalamic syndrome 253.8
Hypopiesis — *see* Hypotension
Hypopigmentation 709.00
  eyelid 374.53
Hypopinealism 259.8
Hypopituitarism (juvenile) (syndrome) 253.2
  due to
    hormone therapy 253.7
    hypophysectomy 253.7
    radiotherapy 253.7
  postablative 253.7
  postpartum hemorrhage 253.2
Hypoplasia, hypoplasis 759.89
  adrenal (gland) 759.1
  alimentary tract 751.8
    lower 751.2
    upper 750.8
  angiolymphoid, with eosinophilia (ALHE) 228.01
  anus, anal (canal) 751.2
  aorta 747.22
  aortic
    arch (tubular) 747.10
    orifice or valve with hypoplasia of ascending aorta and defective development of left ventricle (with mitral valve atresia) 746.7
  appendix 751.2
  areola 757.6
  arm (*see also* Absence, arm, congenital) 755.20
  artery (congenital) (peripheral) 747.60
    brain 747.81
    cerebral 747.81
    coronary 746.85
    gastrointestinal 747.61
    lower limb 747.64
    pulmonary 747.31
    renal 747.62
    retinal 743.58

Hypoplasia, hypoplasis — *continued*
  artery — *continued*
    specified NEC 747.69
    spinal 747.82
    umbilical 747.5
    upper limb 747.63
  auditory canal 744.29
    causing impairment of hearing 744.02
  biliary duct (common) or passage 751.61
  bladder 753.8
  bone NEC 756.9
    face 756.0
    malar 756.0
    mandible 524.04
      alveolar 524.74
    marrow 284.9
      acquired (secondary) 284.89
      congenital 284.09
      idiopathic 284.9
    maxilla 524.03
      alveolar 524.73
    skull (*see also* Hypoplasia, skull) 756.0
  brain 742.1
    gyri 742.2
    specified part 742.2
  breast (areola) 611.82
  bronchus (tree) 748.3
  cardiac 746.89
    valve — *see* Hypoplasia, heart, valve
    vein 746.89
  carpus (*see also* Absence, carpal, congenital) 755.28
  cartilaginous 756.9
  cecum 751.2
  cementum 520.4
    hereditary 520.5
  cephalic 742.1
  cerebellum 742.2
  cervix (uteri) 752.43
  chin 524.06
  clavicle 755.51
  coccyx 756.19
  colon 751.2
  corpus callosum 742.2
  cricoid cartilage 748.3
  dermal, focal (Goltz) 757.39
  digestive organ(s) or tract NEC 751.8
    lower 751.2
    upper 750.8
  ear 744.29
    auricle 744.23
    lobe 744.29
    middle, except ossicles 744.03
      ossicles 744.04
    ossicles 744.04
  enamel of teeth (neonatal) (postnatal) (prenatal) 520.4
    hereditary 520.5
  endocrine (gland) NEC 759.2
  endometrium 621.8
  epididymis 752.89
  epiglottis 748.3
  erythroid, congenital 284.01
  erythropoietic, chronic acquired 284.81
  esophagus 750.3
  Eustachian tube 744.24
  eye (*see also* Microphthalmos) 743.10
    lid 743.62
  face 744.89
    bone(s) 756.0
  fallopian tube 752.19
  femur (*see also* Absence, femur, congenital) 755.34
  fibula (*see also* Absence, fibula, congenital) 755.37
  finger (*see also* Absence, finger, congenital) 755.29
  focal dermal 757.39
  foot 755.31
  gallbladder 751.69
  genitalia, genital organ(s)
    female 752.89
      external 752.49
      internal NEC 752.89
    in adiposogenital dystrophy 253.8
    male 752.89

Hypoplasia, hypoplasis — *continued*
genitalia, genital organ(s) — *continued*
male — *continued*
penis 752.69
glottis 748.3
hair 757.4
hand 755.21
heart 746.89
left (complex) (syndrome) 746.7
valve NEC 746.89
pulmonary 746.01
humerus (*see also* Absence, humerus, congenital) 755.24
hymen 752.49
intestine (small) 751.1
large 751.2
iris 743.46
jaw 524.09
kidney(s) 753.0
labium (majus) (minus) 752.49
labyrinth, membranous 744.05
lacrimal duct (apparatus) 743.65
larynx 748.3
leg (*see also* Absence, limb, congenital, lower) 755.30
limb 755.4
lower (*see also* Absence, limb, congenital, lower) 755.30
upper (*see also* Absence, limb, congenital, upper) 755.20
liver 751.69
lung (lobe) 748.5
mammary (areolar) 611.82
mandibular 524.04
alveolar 524.74
unilateral condylar 526.89
maxillary 524.03
alveolar 524.73
medullary 284.9
megakaryocytic 287.30
metacarpus (*see also* Absence, metacarpal, congenital) 755.28
metatarsus (*see also* Absence, metatarsal, congenital) 755.38
muscle 756.89
eye 743.69
myocardium (congenital) (Uhl's anomaly) 746.84
nail(s) 757.5
nasolacrimal duct 743.65
nervous system NEC 742.8
neural 742.8
nose, nasal 748.1
ophthalmic (*see also* Microphthalmos) 743.10
optic nerve 377.43
organ
of Corti 744.05
or site NEC — *see* Anomaly, by site
osseous meatus (ear) 744.03
ovary 752.0
oviduct 752.19
pancreas 751.7
parathyroid (gland) 759.2
parotid gland 750.26
patella 755.64
pelvis, pelvic girdle 755.69
penis 752.69
peripheral vascular system (congenital) NEC 747.60
gastrointestinal 747.61
lower limb 747.64
renal 747.62
specified NEC 747.69
spinal 747.82
upper limb 747.63
pituitary (gland) 759.2
pulmonary 748.5

Hypoplasia, hypoplasis — *continued*
pulmonary — *continued*
arteriovenous 747.32
artery 747.31
valve 746.01
punctum lacrimale 743.65
radioulnar (*see also* Absence, radius, congenital, with ulna) 755.25
radius (*see also* Absence, radius, congenital) 755.26
rectum 751.2
respiratory system NEC 748.9
rib 756.3
sacrum 756.19
scapula 755.59
shoulder girdle 755.59
skin 757.39
skull (bone) 756.0
with
anencephalus 740.0
encephalocele 742.0
hydrocephalus 742.3
with spina bifida (*see also* Spina bifida) 741.0 ☑
microcephalus 742.1
spinal (cord) (ventral horn cell) 742.59
vessel 747.82
spine 756.19
spleen 759.0
sternum 756.3
tarsus (*see also* Absence, tarsal, congenital) 755.38
testis, testicle 752.89
thymus (gland) 279.11
thyroid (gland) 243
cartilage 748.3
tibiofibular (*see also* Absence, tibia, congenital, with fibula) 755.35
toe (*see also* Absence, toe, congenital) 755.39
tongue 750.16
trachea (cartilage) (rings) 748.3
Turner's (tooth) 520.4
ulna (*see also* Absence, ulna, congenital) 755.27
umbilical artery 747.5
ureter 753.29
uterus 752.32
vagina 752.45
vascular (peripheral) NEC (*see also* Hypoplasia, peripheral vascular system) 747.60
brain 747.81
vein(s) (peripheral) NEC (*see also* Hypoplasia, peripheral vascular system) 747.60
brain 747.81
cardiac 746.89
great 747.49
portal 747.49
pulmonary 747.49
vena cava (inferior) (superior) 747.49
vertebra 756.19
vulva 752.49
zonule (ciliary) 743.39
zygoma 738.12
Hypopotassemia 276.8
Hypoproaccelerinemia — *see also* Defect, coagulation 286.3
Hypoproconvertinemia (congenital) — *see also* Defect, coagulation 286.3
Hypoproteinemia (essential) (hypermetabolic) (idiopathic) 273.8
Hypoproteinosis 260
Hypoprothrombinemia (congenital) (hereditary) (idiopathic) — *see also* Defect, coagulation 286.3
acquired 286.7
newborn 776.3

Hypopselaphesia 782.0
Hypopyon (anterior chamber) (eye) 364.05
iritis 364.05
ulcer (cornea) 370.04
Hypopyrexia 780.99
Hyporeflex 796.1
Hyporeninemia, extreme 790.99
in primary aldosteronism 255.10
Hyporesponsive episode 780.09
Hyposecretion
ACTH 253.4
ovary 256.39
postablative 256.2
salivary gland (any) 527.7
Hyposegmentation of neutrophils, hereditary 288.2
Hyposiderinemia 280.9
Hyposmolality 276.1
syndrome 276.1
Hyposomatotropism 253.3
Hyposomnia, unspecified — *see also* Insomnia 780.52
with sleep apnea, unspecified 780.51
Hypospadias (male) 752.61
female 753.8
Hypospermatogenesis 606.1
Hyposphagma 372.72
Hyposplenism 289.59
Hypostasis, pulmonary 514
Hypostatic — *see* condition
Hyposthenuria 593.89
Hyposuprarenalism 255.41
Hypo-TBG-nemia 246.8
Hypotension (arterial) (constitutional) 458.9
chronic 458.1
iatrogenic 458.29
maternal, syndrome (following labor and delivery) 669.2 ☑
of hemodialysis 458.21
orthostatic (chronic) 458.0
dysautonomic-dyskinetic syndrome 333.0
permanent idiopathic 458.1
postoperative 458.29
postural 458.0
specified type NEC 458.8
transient 796.3
Hypothermia (accidental) 991.6
anesthetic 995.89
associated with low environmental temperature 991.6
newborn NEC 778.3
not associated with low environmental temperature 780.65
Hypothymergasia — *see also* Psychosis, affective 296.2 ☑
recurrent episode 296.3 ☑
single episode 296.2 ☑
Hypothyroidism (acquired) 244.9
complicating pregnancy, childbirth, or puerperium 648.1 ☑
congenital 243
due to
ablation 244.1
radioactive iodine 244.1
surgical 244.0
iodine (administration) (ingestion) 244.2
radioactive 244.1
irradiation therapy 244.1
p-aminosalicylic acid (PAS) 244.3
phenylbutazone 244.3
resorcinol 244.3
specified cause NEC 244.8
surgery 244.0
goitrous (sporadic) 246.1
iatrogenic NEC 244.3
iodine 244.2

Hypothyroidism — *continued*
pituitary 244.8
postablative NEC 244.1
postsurgical 244.0
primary 244.9
secondary NEC 244.8
specified cause NEC 244.8
sporadic goitrous 246.1
Hypotonia, hypotonicity, hypotony 781.3
benign congenital 358.8
bladder 596.4
congenital 779.89
benign 358.8
eye 360.30
due to
fistula 360.32
ocular disorder NEC 360.33
following loss of aqueous or vitreous 360.33
primary 360.31
infantile muscular (benign) 359.0
muscle 728.9
uterus, uterine (contractions) — *see* Inertia, uterus
Hypotrichosis 704.09
congenital 757.4
lid (congenital) 757.4
acquired 374.55
postinfectional NEC 704.09
Hypotropia 378.32
Hypoventilation 786.09
congenital central alveolar syndrome 327.25
idiopathic sleep related nonobstructive alveolar 327.24
obesity 278.03
sleep related, in conditions classifiable elsewhere 327.26
Hypovitaminosis — *see also* Deficiency, vitamin 269.2
Hypovolemia 276.52
surgical shock 998.09
traumatic (shock) 958.4
Hypoxemia — *see also* Anoxia 799.02
sleep related, in conditions classifiable elsewhere 327.26
Hypoxia — *see also* Anoxia 799.02
cerebral 348.1
during or resulting from a procedure 997.01
newborn 770.88
mild or moderate 768.6
severe 768.5
fetal, affecting newborn 770.88
intrauterine — *see* Distress, fetal
myocardial (*see also* Insufficiency, coronary) 411.89
arteriosclerotic — *see* Arteriosclerosis, coronary
newborn 770.88
sleep related 327.24
Hypoxic-ischemic encephalopathy (HIE) 768.70
mild 768.71
moderate 768.72
severe 768.73
Hypsarrhythmia — *see also* Epilepsy 345.6 ☑
Hysteralgia, pregnant uterus 646.8 ☑
Hysteria, hysterical 300.10
anxiety 300.20
Charcôt's gland 300.11
conversion (any manifestation) 300.11
dissociative type NEC 300.15
psychosis, acute 298.1
Hysteroepilepsy 300.11
Hysterotomy, affecting fetus or newborn 763.89

I

Iatrogenic syndrome of excess cortisol 255.0
IBM (inclusion body myositis) 359.71
Iceland disease (epidemic neuromyasthenia) 049.8
Ichthyosis (congenita) 757.1
  acquired 701.1
  fetalis gravior 757.1
  follicularis 757.1
  hystrix 757.39
  lamellar 757.1
  lingual 528.6
  palmaris and plantaris 757.39
  simplex 757.1
  vera 757.1
  vulgaris 757.1
Ichthyotoxism 988.0
  bacterial (*see also* Poisoning, food) 005.9
Icteroanemia, hemolytic (acquired) 283.9
  congenital (*see also* Spherocytosis) 282.0
Icterus — *see also* Jaundice 782.4
  catarrhal — *see* Icterus, infectious
  conjunctiva 782.4
    newborn 774.6
  epidemic — *see* Icterus, infectious
  febrilis — *see* Icterus, infectious
  fetus or newborn — *see* Jaundice, fetus or newborn
  gravis (*see also* Necrosis, liver) 570
    complicating pregnancy 646.7 ☑
      affecting fetus or newborn 760.8
    fetus or newborn NEC 773.0
    obstetrical 646.7 ☑
      affecting fetus or newborn 760.8
  hematogenous (acquired) 283.9
  hemolytic (acquired) 283.9
    congenital (*see also* Spherocytosis) 282.0
  hemorrhagic (acute) 100.0
    leptospiral 100.0
    newborn 776.0
    spirochetal 100.0
  infectious 070.1
    with hepatic coma 070.0
    leptospiral 100.0
    spirochetal 100.0
  intermittens juvenilis 277.4
  malignant (*see also* Necrosis, liver) 570
  neonatorum (*see also* Jaundice, fetus or newborn) 774.6
  pernicious (*see also* Necrosis, liver) 570
  spirochetal 100.0
Ictus solaris, solis 992.0
Ideation
  homicidal V62.85
  suicidal V62.84
Identity disorder 313.82
  dissociative 300.14
  gender role (child) 302.6
    adult 302.85
  psychosexual (child) 302.6
    adult 302.85
Idioglossia 307.9
Idiopathic — *see* condition
Idiosyncrasy — *see also* Allergy 995.3
  drug, medicinal substance, and biological — *see* Allergy, drug
Idiot, idiocy (congenital) 318.2
  amaurotic (Bielschowsky) (-Jansky) (family) (infantile) (late) (juvenile) (late) (Vogt-Spielmeyer) 330.1
  microcephalic 742.1
  Mongolian 758.0
  oxycephalic 756.0
Id reaction (due to bacteria) 692.89
IEED (involuntary emotional expression disorder) 310.81
IFIS (intraoperative floppy iris syndrome) 364.81
IgE asthma 493.0 ☑
Ileitis (chronic) — *see also* Enteritis 558.9
  infectious 009.0
  noninfectious 558.9
  regional (ulcerative) 555.0
    with large intestine 555.2
  segmental 555.0

Ileitis — *see also* Enteritis — *continued*
  segmental — *continued*
    with large intestine 555.2
  terminal (ulcerative) 555.0
    with large intestine 555.2
Ileocolitis — *see also* Enteritis 558.9
  infectious 009.0
  regional 555.2
  ulcerative 556.1
Ileostomy status V44.2
  with complication 569.60
Ileotyphus 002.0
Ileum — *see* condition
Ileus (adynamic) (bowel) (colon) (inhibitory) (intestine) (neurogenic) (paralytic) 560.1
  arteriomesenteric duodenal 537.2
  due to gallstone (in intestine) 560.31
  duodenal, chronic 537.2
  following gastrointestinal surgery 997.49
  gallstone 560.31
  mechanical (*see also* Obstruction, intestine) 560.9
  meconium 777.1
    due to cystic fibrosis 277.01
  myxedema 564.89
  postoperative 997.49
  transitory, newborn 777.4
Iliac — *see* condition
Iliotibial band friction syndrome 728.89
Illegitimacy V61.6
Ill, louping 063.1
Illness — *see also* Disease
  factitious 300.19
    with
      combined psychological and physical signs and symptoms 300.19
      predominantly
        physical signs and symptoms 300.19
        psychological symptoms 300.16
  chronic (with physical symptoms) 301.51
  heart — *see* Disease, heart
  manic-depressive (*see also* Psychosis, affective) 296.80
  mental (*see also* Disorder, mental) 300.9
Imbalance 781.2
  autonomic (*see also* Neuropathy, peripheral, autonomic) 337.9
  electrolyte 276.9
    with
      abortion — *see* Abortion, by type, with metabolic disorder
      ectopic pregnancy (*see also* categories 633.0–633.9) 639.4
      hyperemesis gravidarum (before 22 completed weeks gestation) 643.1 ☑
      molar pregnancy (*see also* categories 630–632) 639.4
    following
      abortion 639.4
      ectopic or molar pregnancy 639.4
    neonatal, transitory NEC 775.5
  endocrine 259.9
  eye muscle NEC 378.9
    heterophoria — *see* Heterophoria
  glomerulotubular NEC 593.89
  hormone 259.9
  hysterical (*see also* Hysteria) 300.10
  labyrinth NEC 386.50
  posture 729.90
  sympathetic (*see also* Neuropathy, peripheral, autonomic) 337.9
Imbecile, imbecility 318.0
  moral 301.7
  old age 290.9
  senile 290.9
  specified IQ — *see* IQ
  unspecified IQ 318.0
Imbedding, intrauterine device 996.32
Imbibition, cholesterol (gallbladder) 575.6
Imerslund (-Gräsbeck) syndrome (anemia due to familial selective vitamin B_{12} malabsorption) 281.1
Iminoacidopathy 270.8
Iminoglycinuria, familial 270.8

Immature — *see also* Immaturity
  personality 301.89
Immaturity 765.1 ☑
  extreme 765.0 ☑
  fetus or infant light-for-dates — *see* Light-for-dates
  lung, fetus or newborn 770.4
  organ or site NEC — *see* Hypoplasia
  pulmonary, fetus or newborn 770.4
  reaction 301.89
  sexual (female) (male) 259.0
Immersion 994.1
  foot 991.4
  hand 991.4
Immobile, immobility
  complete
    due to severe physical disability or frailty 780.72
  intestine 564.89
  joint — *see* Ankylosis
  syndrome (paraplegic) 728.3
Immunization
  ABO
    affecting management of pregnancy 656.2 ☑
    fetus or newborn 773.1
  complication — *see* Complications, vaccination
  Rh factor
    affecting management of pregnancy 656.1 ☑
    fetus or newborn 773.0
    from transfusion (*see also* Complications, transfusion) 999.70
Immunodeficiency 279.3
  with
    adenosine-deaminase deficiency 279.2
    defect, predominant
      B-cell 279.00
      T-cell 279.10
    hyperimmunoglobulinemia 279.2
    lymphopenia, hereditary 279.2
    thrombocytopenia and eczema 279.12
    thymic
      aplasia 279.2
      dysplasia 279.2
  autosomal recessive, Swiss-type 279.2
  common variable 279.06
  severe combined (SCID) 279.2
  to Rh factor
    affecting management of pregnancy 656.1 ☑
    fetus or newborn 773.0
  X-linked, with increased IgM 279.05
Immunotherapy, prophylactic V07.2
  antineoplastic V58.12
Impaction, impacted
  bowel, colon, rectum 560.30
    with hernia (*see also* Hernia, by site, with obstruction)
      gangrenous — *see* Hernia, by site, with gangrene
    by
      calculus 560.32
      gallstone 560.31
    fecal 560.32
    specified type NEC 560.32
  calculus — *see* Calculus
  cerumen (ear) (external) 380.4
  cuspid 520.6
  dental 520.6
  fecal, feces 560.32
    with hernia (*see also* Hernia, by site, with obstruction)
      gangrenous — *see* Hernia, by site, with gangrene
  fracture — *see* Fracture, by site
  gallbladder — *see* Cholelithiasis
  gallstone(s) — *see* Cholelithiasis
    in intestine (any part) 560.31
  intestine(s) 560.30
    with hernia (*see also* Hernia, by site, with obstruction)
      gangrenous — *see* Hernia, by site, with gangrene

Impaction, impacted — *continued*
  intestine(s) — *continued*
    by
      calculus 560.32
      gallstone 560.31
    fecal 560.32
    specified type NEC 560.32
  intrauterine device (IUD) 996.32
  molar 520.6
  shoulder 660.4 ☑
    affecting fetus or newborn 763.1
  tooth, teeth 520.6
  turbinate 733.99
Impaired, impairment (function)
  arm V49.1
    movement, involving
      musculoskeletal system V49.1
      nervous system V49.2
  auditory discrimination 388.43
  back V48.3
  body (entire) V49.89
  cognitive, mild, so stated 331.83
  combined visual hearing V49.85
  dual sensory V49.85
  glucose
    fasting 790.21
    tolerance test (oral) 790.22
  hearing (*see also* Deafness) 389.9
    combined with visual impairment V49.85
  heart — *see* Disease, heart
  kidney (*see also* Disease, renal) 593.9
    disorder resulting from 588.9
      specified NEC 588.89
  leg V49.1
    movement, involving
      musculoskeletal system V49.1
      nervous system V49.2
  limb V49.1
    movement, involving
      musculoskeletal system V49.1
      nervous system V49.2
  liver 573.8
  mastication 524.9
  mild cognitive, so stated 331.83
  mobility
    ear ossicles NEC 385.22
    incostapedial joint 385.22
    malleus 385.21
  myocardium, myocardial (*see also* Insufficiency, myocardial) 428.0
  neuromusculoskeletal NEC V49.89
    back V48.3
    head V48.2
    limb V49.2
    neck V48.3
    spine V48.3
    trunk V48.3
  rectal sphincter 787.99
  renal (*see also* Disease, renal) 593.9
    disorder resulting from 588.9
      specified NEC 588.89
  spine V48.3
  vision NEC 369.9
    both eyes NEC 369.3
      combined with hearing impairment V49.85
      moderate 369.74
        both eyes 369.25
          with impairment of lesser eye (specified as)
            blind, not further specified 369.15
            low vision, not further specified 369.23
            near-total 369.17
            profound 369.18
            severe 369.24
            total 369.16
      one eye 369.74
        with vision of other eye (specified as)
          near-normal 369.75
          normal 369.76
      near-total 369.64
        both eyes 369.04

Impaired, impairment — *continued*
  vision — *continued*
    near-total — *continued*
      both eyes — *continued*
        with impairment of lesser eye
            (specified as)
          blind, not further specified
              369.02
          total 369.03
        one eye 369.64
          with vision of other eye (specified
              as)
            near normal 369.65
            normal 369.66
      one eye 369.60
        with low vision of other eye 369.10
      profound 369.67
        both eyes 369.08
          with impairment of lesser eye
              (specified as)
            blind, not further specified
                369.05
            near-total 369.07
            total 369.06
        one eye 369.67
          with vision of other eye (specified
              as)
            near-normal 369.68
            normal 369.69
      severe 369.71
        both eyes 369.22
          with impairment of lesser eye
              (specified as)
            blind, not further specified
                369.11
            low vision, not further speci-
                fied 369.21
            near-total 369.13
            profound 369.14
            total 369.12
        one eye 369.71
          with vision of other eye (specified
              as)
            near-normal 369.72
            normal 369.73
      total
        both eyes 369.01
        one eye 369.61
          with vision of other eye (specified
              as)
            near-normal 369.62
            normal 369.63
Impaludism — *see* Malaria
Impediment, speech NEC 784.59
  psychogenic 307.9
  secondary to organic lesion 784.59
Impending
  cerebrovascular accident or attack 435.9
  coronary syndrome 411.1
  delirium tremens 291.0
  myocardial infarction 411.1
Imperception, auditory (acquired) (congeni-
    tal) 389.9
Imperfect
  aeration, lung (newborn) 770.5
  closure (congenital)
    alimentary tract NEC 751.8
      lower 751.5
      upper 750.8
    atrioventricular ostium 745.69
    atrium (secundum) 745.5
      primum 745.61
    branchial cleft or sinus 744.41
    choroid 743.59
    cricoid cartilage 748.3
    cusps, heart valve NEC 746.89
      pulmonary 746.09
    ductus
      arteriosus 747.0
      Botalli 747.0
    ear drum 744.29
      causing impairment of hearing
          744.03
    endocardial cushion 745.60
    epiglottis 748.3

Imperfect — *continued*
  closure — *continued*
    esophagus with communication to
        bronchus or trachea 750.3
    Eustachian valve 746.89
    eyelid 743.62
    face, facial (*see also* Cleft, lip) 749.10
    foramen
      Botalli 745.5
      ovale 745.5
    genitalia, genital organ(s) or system
      female 752.89
        external 752.49
        internal NEC 752.89
        uterus 752.39
      male 752.89
        penis 752.69
    glottis 748.3
    heart valve (cusps) NEC 746.89
    interatrial ostium or septum 745.5
    interauricular ostium or septum 745.5
    interventricular ostium or septum 745.4
    iris 743.46
    kidney 753.3
    larynx 748.3
    lens 743.36
    lip (*see also* Cleft, lip) 749.10
    nasal septum or sinus 748.1
    nose 748.1
    omphalomesenteric duct 751.0
    optic nerve entry 743.57
    organ or site NEC — *see* Anomaly, spec-
        ified type, by site
    ostium
      interatrial 745.5
      interauricular 745.5
      interventricular 745.4
    palate (*see also* Cleft, palate) 749.00
    preauricular sinus 744.46
    retina 743.56
    roof of orbit 742.0
    sclera 743.47
    septum
      aortic 745.0
      aorticopulmonary 745.0
      atrial (secundum) 745.5
        primum 745.61
      between aorta and pulmonary artery
          745.0
      heart 745.9
      interatrial (secundum) 745.5
        primum 745.61
      interauricular (secundum) 745.5
        primum 745.61
      interventricular 745.4
        with pulmonary stenosis or atre-
            sia, dextraposition of aor-
            ta, and hypertrophy of
            right ventricle 745.2
          in tetralogy of Fallot 745.2
      nasal 748.1
      ventricular 745.4
        with pulmonary stenosis or atre-
            sia, dextraposition of aor-
            ta, and hypertrophy of
            right ventricle 745.2
          in tetralogy of Fallot 745.2
    skull 756.0
      with
        anencephalus 740.0
        encephalocele 742.0
        hydrocephalus 742.3
          with spina bifida (*see also*
              Spina bifida) 741.0 ☑
        microcephalus 742.1
    spine (with meningocele) (*see also* Spina
        bifida) 741.90
    thyroid cartilage 748.3
    trachea 748.3
    tympanic membrane 744.29
      causing impairment of hearing
          744.03
    uterus (with communication to bladder,
        intestine, or rectum) 752.39
    uvula 749.02

Imperfect — *continued*
  closure — *continued*
    uvula — *continued*
      with cleft lip (*see also* Cleft, palate,
          with cleft lip) 749.20
      vitelline duct 751.0
    development — *see* Anomaly, by site
    erection 607.84
    fusion — *see* Imperfect, closure
    inflation lung (newborn) 770.5
    intestinal canal 751.5
    poise 729.90
    rotation — *see* Malrotation
    septum, ventricular 745.4
Imperfectly descended testis 752.51
Imperforate (congenital) — *see also* Atresia
  anus 751.2
  bile duct 751.61
  cervix (uteri) 752.49
  esophagus 750.3
  hymen 752.42
  intestine (small) 751.1
    large 751.2
  jejunum 751.1
  pharynx 750.29
  rectum 751.2
  salivary duct 750.23
  urethra 753.6
  urinary meatus 753.6
  vagina 752.49
Impervious (congenital) — *see also* Atresia
  anus 751.2
  bile duct 751.61
  esophagus 750.3
  intestine (small) 751.1
    large 751.5
  rectum 751.2
  urethra 753.6
Impetiginization of other dermatoses 684
Impetigo (any organism) (any site) (bullous)
    (circinate) (contagiosa) (neonatorum)
    (simplex) 684
  Bockhart's (superficial folliculitis) 704.8
  external ear 684 *[380.13]*
  eyelid 684 *[373.5]*
  Fox's (contagiosa) 684
  furfuracea 696.5
  herpetiformis 694.3
    nonobstetrical 694.3
  staphylococcal infection 684
  ulcerative 686.8
  vulgaris 684
Impingement, soft tissue between teeth
    524.89
  anterior 524.81
  posterior 524.82
Implantation
  anomalous (*see also* Anomaly, specified
      type, by site)
    ureter 753.4
  cyst
    external area or site (skin) NEC 709.8
    iris 364.61
    vagina 623.8
    vulva 624.8
  dermoid (cyst)
    external area or site (skin) NEC 709.8
    iris 364.61
    vagina 623.8
    vulva 624.8
  placenta, low or marginal — *see* Placenta
      previa
Implant, endometrial 617.9
Impotence (sexual) 607.84
  organic origin NEC 607.84
  psychogenic 302.72
Impoverished blood 285.9
Impression, basilar 756.0
Imprisonment V62.5
Improper
  development, infant 764.9 ☑
Improperly tied umbilical cord (causing
    hemorrhage) 772.3
Impulses, obsessional 300.3
Impulsive 799.23
  neurosis 300.3

Impulsiveness 799.23
Inaction, kidney — *see also* Disease, renal
    593.9
Inactive — *see* condition
Inadequate, inadequacy
  aesthetics of dental restoration 525.67
  biologic 301.6
  cardiac and renal — *see* Hypertension, car-
      diorenal
  constitutional 301.6
  development
    child 783.40
    fetus 764.9 ☑
      affecting management of pregnancy
          656.5 ☑
    genitalia
      after puberty NEC 259.0
      congenital — *see* Hypoplasia, geni-
          talia
    lungs 748.5
    organ or site NEC — *see* Hypoplasia, by
        site
  dietary 269.9
  distance, interarch 524.28
  education V62.3
  environment
    economic problem V60.2
    household condition NEC V60.1
    poverty V60.2
    unemployment V62.0
  functional 301.6
  household care, due to
    family member
      handicapped or ill V60.4
      temporarily away from home V60.4
        on vacation V60.5
    technical defects in home V60.1
    temporary absence from home of person
        rendering care V60.4
  housing (heating) (space) V60.1
  interarch distance 524.28
  material resources V60.2
  mental (*see also* Disability, intellectual) 319
  nervous system 799.29
  personality 301.6
  prenatal care in current pregnancy V23.7
  pulmonary
    function 786.09
      newborn 770.89
    ventilation, newborn 770.89
  respiration 786.09
    newborn 770.89
  sample
    cytology
      anal 796.78
      cervical 795.08
      vaginal 795.18
  social 301.6
Inanition 263.9
  with edema 262
  due to
    deprivation of food 994.2
    malnutrition 263.9
  fever 780.60
Inappropriate
  change in quantitative human chorionic
      gonadotropin (hCG) in early pregnan-
      cy 631.0
  level of quantitative human chorionic go-
      nadotropin (hCG) for gestational age
      in early pregnancy 631.0
  secretion
    ACTH 255.0
    antidiuretic hormone (ADH) (excessive)
        253.6
    deficiency 253.5
    ectopic hormone NEC 259.3
    pituitary (posterior) 253.6
Inattention after or at birth 995.52
Inborn errors of metabolism — *see* Disorder,
    metabolism
Incarceration, incarcerated
  bubonocele (*see also* Hernia, inguinal, with
      obstruction)
    gangrenous — *see* Hernia, inguinal, with
        gangrene

☑ Additional Digit Required — Refer to the Tabular List for Digit Selection

▽ Subterms under main terms may continue to next column or page

Incarceration, incarcerated — *continued*
　colon (by hernia) (*see also* Hernia, by site
　　with obstruction)
　　gangrenous — *see* Hernia, by site, with
　　　gangrene
　enterocele 552.9
　　gangrenous 551.9
　epigastrocele 552.29
　　gangrenous 551.29
　epiplocele 552.9
　　gangrenous 551.9
　exomphalos 552.1
　　gangrenous 551.1
　fallopian tube 620.8
　hernia (*see also* Hernia, by site, with obstruc-
　　tion)
　　gangrenous — *see* Hernia, by site, with
　　　gangrene
　iris, in wound 871.1
　lens, in wound 871.1
　merocele (*see also* Hernia, femoral, with
　　obstruction) 552.00
　omentum (by hernia) (*see also* Hernia, by
　　site, with obstruction)
　　gangrenous — *see* Hernia, by site, with
　　　gangrene
　omphalocele 756.72
　rupture (meaning hernia) (*see also* Hernia,
　　by site, with obstruction) 552.9
　　gangrenous (*see also* Hernia, by site, with
　　　gangrene) 551.9
　sarcoepiplocele 552.9
　　gangrenous 551.9
　sarcoepiplomphalocele 552.1
　　with gangrene 551.1
　uterus 621.8
　　gravid 654.3 ☑
　　　causing obstructed labor 660.2 ☑
　　　affecting fetus or newborn 763.1
Incident, cerebrovascular — *see also* Disease,
　cerebrovascular, acute 436
Incineration (entire body) (from fire, conflagra-
　tion, electricity, or lightning) — *see* Burn,
　multiple, specified sites
Incised wound
　external — *see* Wound, open, by site
　internal organs (abdomen, chest, or pelvis)
　　— *see* Injury, internal, by site, with
　　open wound
Incision, incisional
　hernia — *see* Hernia, incisional
　surgical, complication — *see* Complications,
　　surgical procedures
　traumatic
　　external — *see* Wound, open, by site
　　internal organs (abdomen, chest, or
　　　pelvis) — *see* Injury, internal, by
　　　site, with open wound
Inclusion
　azurophilic leukocytic 288.2
　blennorrhea (neonatal) (newborn) 771.6
　cyst — *see* Cyst, skin
　gallbladder in liver (congenital) 751.69
Incompatibility
　ABO
　　affecting management of pregnancy
　　　656.2 ☑
　　fetus or newborn 773.1
　　infusion or transfusion reaction (*see also*
　　　Complications, transfusion)
　　　999.60
　blood (group) (Duffy) (E) (K(ell)) (Kidd)
　　(Lewis) (M) (N) (P) (S) NEC
　　affecting management of pregnancy
　　　656.2 ☑
　　fetus or newborn 773.2
　　infusion or transfusion reaction (*see also*
　　　Complications, transfusion)
　　　999.75
　contour of existing restoration of tooth
　　with oral health 525.65
　marital V61.10
　　involving
　　　divorce V61.03
　　　estrangement V61.09

Incompatibility — *continued*
　non-ABO (*see also* Complications, transfu-
　　sion) 999.75
　Rh (antigen) (C) (c) (D) (E) (e) (blood group)
　　(factor)
　　affecting management of pregnancy
　　　656.1 ☑
　　fetus or newborn 773.0
　　infusion or transfusion reaction (*see also*
　　　Complications, transfusion)
　　　999.70
　Rhesus — *see* Incompatibility, Rh
Incompetency, incompetence, incompetent
　annular
　　aortic (valve) (*see also* Insufficiency, aor-
　　　tic) 424.1
　　mitral (valve) (*see also* Insufficiency, mi-
　　　tral) 424.0
　　pulmonary valve (heart) (*see also* Endo-
　　　carditis, pulmonary) 424.3
　aortic (valve) (*see also* Insufficiency, aortic)
　　424.1
　　syphilitic 093.22
　cardiac (orifice) 530.0
　　valve — *see* Endocarditis
　cervix, cervical (os) 622.5
　　in pregnancy 654.5 ☑
　　　affecting fetus or newborn 761.0
　chronotropic 426.89
　　with
　　　autonomic dysfunction 337.9
　　　ischemic heart disease 414.9
　　　left ventricular dysfunction 429.89
　　　sinus node dysfunction 427.81
　esophagogastric (junction) (sphincter) 530.0
　heart valve, congenital 746.89
　mitral (valve) — *see* Insufficiency, mitral
　papillary muscle (heart) 429.81
　pelvic fundus
　　pubocervical tissue 618.81
　　rectovaginal tissue 618.82
　pulmonary valve (heart) (*see also* Endocardi-
　　tis, pulmonary) 424.3
　　congenital 746.09
　tricuspid (annular) (rheumatic) (valve) (*see
　　also* Endocarditis, tricuspid) 397.0
　valvular — *see* Endocarditis
　vein, venous (saphenous) (varicose) (*see also*
　　Varicose, vein) 454.9
　velopharyngeal (closure)
　　acquired 528.9
　　congenital 750.29
Incomplete — *see also* condition
　bladder emptying 788.21
　defecation 787.61
　expansion lungs (newborn) 770.5
　gestation (liveborn) — *see* Immaturity
　rotation — *see* Malrotation
Inconclusive
　image test due to excess body fat 793.91
　mammogram, mammography 793.82
　　due to dense breasts 793.82
Incontinence 788.30
　without sensory awareness 788.34
　anal sphincter 787.60
　continuous leakage 788.37
　feces, fecal 787.60
　　due to hysteria 300.11
　　nonorganic origin 307.7
　hysterical 300.11
　mixed (male) (female) (urge and stress)
　　788.33
　overflow 788.38
　paradoxical 788.39
　rectal 787.60
　specified NEC 788.39
　stress (female) 625.6
　　male NEC 788.32
　urethral sphincter 599.84
　urge 788.31
　　and stress (male) (female) 788.33
　urine 788.30
　　active 788.30
　　due to
　　　cognitive impairment 788.91
　　　immobility 788.91

Incontinence — *continued*
　urine — *continued*
　　due to — *continued*
　　　severe physical disability 788.91
　　functional 788.91
　　male 788.30
　　　stress 788.32
　　　and urge 788.33
　　neurogenic 788.39
　　nonorganic origin 307.6
　　stress (female) 625.6
　　　male NEC 788.32
　　urge 788.31
　　　and stress 788.33
Incontinentia pigmenti 757.33
Incoordinate
　uterus (action) (contractions) 661.4 ☑
　　affecting fetus or newborn 763.7
Incoordination
　esophageal-pharyngeal (newborn) 787.24
　muscular 781.3
　papillary muscle 429.81
Increase, increased
　abnormal, in development 783.9
　androgens (ovarian) 256.1
　anticoagulants (antithrombin) (anti-II) (anti-
　　VIIIa) (anti-IXa) (anti-XIa) (prothrom-
　　bin) (*see also* Anticoagulants 286.59
　　anti-IIa 287.8
　　anti-Xa 287.8
　　extrinsic 287.8
　　postpartum 666.3 ☑
　cold sense (*see also* Disturbance, sensation)
　　782.0
　estrogen 256.0
　function
　　adrenal (cortex) 255.3
　　　medulla 255.6
　　pituitary (anterior) (gland) (lobe) 253.1
　　　posterior 253.6
　heat sense (*see also* Disturbance, sensation)
　　782.0
　intracranial pressure 781.99
　　injury at birth 767.8
　light reflex of retina 362.13
　permeability, capillary 448.9
　pressure
　　intracranial 781.99
　　　injury at birth 767.8
　　intraocular 365.00
　pulsations 785.9
　pulse pressure 785.9
　sphericity, lens 743.36
　splenic activity 289.4
　venous pressure 459.89
　　portal 572.3
Incrustation, cornea, lead or zinc 930.0
Incyclophoria 378.44
Incyclotropia 378.33
Indeterminate sex 752.7
India rubber skin 756.83
Indicanuria 270.2
Indigestion (bilious) (functional) 536.8
　acid 536.8
　catarrhal 536.8
　due to decomposed food NEC 005.9
　fat 579.8
　nervous 306.4
　psychogenic 306.4
Indirect — *see* condition
Indolent bubo NEC 099.8
Induced
　abortion — *see* Abortion, induced
　birth, affecting fetus or newborn 763.89
　delivery — *see* Delivery
　labor — *see* Delivery
Induration, indurated
　brain 348.89
　breast (fibrous) 611.79
　　puerperal, postpartum 676.3 ☑
　broad ligament 620.8
　chancre 091.0
　　anus 091.1
　　congenital 090.0
　　extragenital NEC 091.2
　corpora cavernosa (penis) (plastic) 607.89

Induration, indurated — *continued*
　liver (chronic) 573.8
　　acute 573.8
　lung (black) (brown) (chronic) (fibroid) (*see
　　also* Fibrosis, lung) 515
　　essential brown 275.09 [516.1]
　penile 607.89
　phlebitic — *see* Phlebitis
　skin 782.8
　stomach 537.89
Induratio penis plastica 607.89
Industrial — *see* condition
Inebriety — *see also* Abuse, drugs, nondepen-
　dent 305.0 ☑
Inefficiency
　kidney (*see also* Disease, renal) 593.9
　thyroid (acquired) (gland) 244.9
Inelasticity, skin 782.8
Inequality, leg (acquired) (length) 736.81
　congenital 755.30
Inertia
　bladder 596.4
　　neurogenic 596.54
　　　with cauda equina syndrome 344.61
　stomach 536.8
　　psychogenic 306.4
　uterus, uterine 661.2 ☑
　　affecting fetus or newborn 763.7
　　primary 661.0 ☑
　　secondary 661.1 ☑
　vesical 596.4
　　neurogenic 596.54
　　　with cauda equina 344.61
Infant — *see also* condition
　excessive crying of 780.92
　fussy (baby) 780.91
　held for adoption V68.89
　newborn — *see* Newborn
　post-term (gestation period over 40 com-
　　pleted weeks to 42 completed
　　weeks) 766.21
　prolonged gestation of (period over 42
　　completed weeks) 766.22
　syndrome of diabetic mother 775.0
"Infant Hercules" syndrome 255.2
Infantile — *see also* condition
　genitalia, genitals 259.0
　　in pregnancy or childbirth NEC 654.4 ☑
　　　affecting fetus or newborn 763.89
　　　causing obstructed labor 660.2 ☑
　　　　affecting fetus or newborn 763.1
　heart 746.9
　kidney 753.3
　lack of care 995.52
　macula degeneration 362.75
　melanodontia 521.05
　os, uterus (*see also* Infantile, genitalia) 259.0
　pelvis 738.6
　　with disproportion (fetopelvic) 653.1 ☑
　　　affecting fetus or newborn 763.1
　　　causing obstructed labor 660.1 ☑
　　　　affecting fetus or newborn 763.1
　penis 259.0
　testis 257.2
　uterus (*see also* Infantile, genitalia) 259.0
　vulva 752.49
Infantilism 259.9
　with dwarfism (hypophyseal) 253.3
　Brissaud's (infantile myxedema) 244.9
　celiac 579.0
　Herter's (nontropical sprue) 579.0
　hypophyseal 253.3
　hypothalamic (with obesity) 253.8
　idiopathic 259.9
　intestinal 579.0
　pancreatic 577.8
　pituitary 253.3
　renal 588.0
　sexual (with obesity) 259.0
Infants, healthy liveborn — *see* Newborn
Infarct, infarction
　adrenal (capsule) (gland) 255.41
　amnion 658.8 ☑
　anterior (with contiguous portion of intra-
　　ventricular septum) NEC (*see also* In-
　　farct, myocardium) 410.1 ☑

☑ **Additional Digit Required** — Refer to the Tabular List for Digit Selection　　　　　　　▽ **Subterms under main terms may continue to next column or page**

198　　**2014 ICD-9-CM**

Index to Diseases
Infection, infected, infective
Index
Infarct, infarction — Infection, infected, infective

Infarct, infarction — *continued*
appendices epiploicae 557.0
bowel 557.0
brain (stem) 434.91
embolic (*see also* Embolism, brain) 434.11
healed or old without residuals V12.54
iatrogenic 997.02
lacunar 434.91
late effect — *see* Late effect(s) (of) cerebrovascular disease
postoperative 997.02
puerperal, postpartum, childbirth 674.0 ☑
thrombotic (*see also* Thrombosis, brain) 434.01
breast 611.89
Brewer's (kidney) 593.81
cardiac (*see also* Infarct, myocardium) 410.9 ☑
cerebellar (*see also* Infarct, brain) 434.91
embolic (*see also* Embolism, brain) 434.11
cerebral (*see also* Infarct, brain) 434.91
aborted 434.91
embolic (*see also* Embolism, brain) 434.11
thrombotic (*see also* Infarct, brain) 434.01
chorion 658.8 ☑
colon (acute) (agnogenic) (embolic) (hemorrhagic) (nonocclusive) (nonthrombotic) (occlusive) (segmental) (thrombotic) (with gangrene) 557.0
coronary artery (*see also* Infarct, myocardium) 410.9 ☑
cortical 434.91
embolic (*see also* Embolism) 444.9
fallopian tube 620.8
gallbladder 575.8
heart (*see also* Infarct, myocardium) 410.9 ☑
hepatic 573.4
hypophysis (anterior lobe) 253.8
impending (myocardium) 411.1
intestine (acute) (agnogenic) (embolic) (hemorrhagic) (nonocclusive) (nonthrombotic) (occlusive) (thrombotic) (with gangrene) 557.0
kidney 593.81
lacunar 434.91
liver 573.4
lung (embolic) (thrombotic) 415.19
with
abortion — *see* Abortion, by type, with, embolism
ectopic pregnancy (*see also* categories 633.0–633.9) 639.6
molar pregnancy (*see also* categories 630–632) 639.6
following
abortion 639.6
ectopic or molar pregnancy 639.6
iatrogenic 415.11
in pregnancy, childbirth, or puerperium — *see* Embolism, obstetrical
postoperative 415.11
septic 415.12
lymph node or vessel 457.8
medullary (brain) — *see* Infarct, brain
meibomian gland (eyelid) 374.85
mesentery, mesenteric (embolic) (thrombotic) (with gangrene) 557.0
midbrain — *see* Infarct, brain
myocardium, myocardial (acute or with a stated duration of 8 weeks or less) (with hypertension) 410.9 ☑

Note — Use the following fifth-digit subclassification with category 410:

0   episode unspecified

1   initial episode

2   subsequent episode without recurrence

Infarct, infarction — *continued*
myocardium, myocardial — *continued*
with symptoms after 8 weeks from date of infarction 414.8
anterior (wall) (with contiguous portion of intraventricular septum) NEC 410.1 ☑
anteroapical (with contiguous portion of intraventricular septum) 410.1 ☑
anterolateral (wall) 410.0 ☑
anteroseptal (with contiguous portion of intraventricular septum) 410.1 ☑
apical-lateral 410.5 ☑
atrial 410.8 ☑
basal-lateral 410.5 ☑
chronic (with symptoms after 8 weeks from date of infarction) 414.8
diagnosed on ECG, but presenting no symptoms 412
diaphragmatic wall (with contiguous portion of intraventricular septum) 410.4 ☑
healed or old, currently presenting no symptoms 412
high lateral 410.5 ☑
impending 411.1
inferior (wall) (with contiguous portion of intraventricular septum) 410.4 ☑
inferolateral (wall) 410.2 ☑
inferoposterior wall 410.3 ☑
intraoperative 997.1
lateral wall 410.5 ☑
non-Q wave 410.7 ☑
non-ST elevation (NSTEMI)
nontransmural 410.7 ☑
papillary muscle 410.8 ☑
past (diagnosed on ECG or other special investigation, but currently presenting no symptoms) 412
with symptoms NEC 414.8
posterior (strictly) (true) (wall) 410.6 ☑
posterobasal 410.6 ☑
posteroinferior 410.3 ☑
posterolateral 410.5 ☑
postprocedural 997.1
previous, currently presenting no symptoms 412
Q wave (*see also* Infarct, myo-cardium, by site) 410.9 ☑
septal 410.8 ☑
specified site NEC 410.8 ☑
ST elevation (STEMI) 410.9 ☑
anterior (wall) 410.1 ☑
anterolateral (wall) 410.0 ☑
inferior (wall) 410.4 ☑
inferolateral (wall) 410.2 ☑
inferoposterior wall 410.3 ☑
lateral wall 410.5 ☑
posterior (strictly) (true) (wall) 410.6 ☑
specified site NEC 410.8 ☑
subendocardial 410.7 ☑
syphilitic 093.82
non-ST elevation myocardial infarction (NSTEMI) 410.7 ☑
nontransmural 410.7 ☑
omentum 557.0
ovary 620.8
pancreas 577.8
papillary muscle (*see also* Infarct, myocardium) 410.8 ☑
parathyroid gland 252.8
pituitary (gland) 253.8
placenta (complicating pregnancy) 656.7 ☑
affecting fetus or newborn 762.2
pontine — *see* Infarct, brain
posterior NEC (*see also* Infarct, myocardium) 410.6 ☑
prostate 602.8
pulmonary (artery) (hemorrhagic) (vein) 415.19

Infarct, infarction — *continued*
pulmonary — *continued*
with
abortion — *see* Abortion, by type, with embolism
ectopic pregnancy (*see also* categories 633.0–633.9) 639.6
molar pregnancy (*see also* categories 630–632) 639.6
following
abortion 639.6
ectopic or molar pregnancy 639.6
iatrogenic 415.11
in pregnancy, childbirth, or puerperium — *see* Embolism, obstetrical
postoperative 415.11
septic 415.12
renal 593.81
embolic or thrombotic 593.81
retina, retinal 362.84
with occlusion — *see* Occlusion, retina
spinal (acute) (cord) (embolic) (nonembolic) 336.1
spleen 289.59
embolic or thrombotic 444.89
subchorionic — *see* Infarct, placenta
subendocardial (*see also* Infarct, myocardium) 410.7 ☑
suprarenal (capsule) (gland) 255.41
syncytium — *see* Infarct, placenta
testis 608.83
thrombotic (*see also* Thrombosis) 453.9
artery, arterial — *see* Embolism
thyroid (gland) 246.3
ventricle (heart) (*see also* Infarct, myocardium) 410.9 ☑
Infecting — *see* condition
Infection, infected, infective (opportunistic) 136.9
with
influenza viruses occurring in pigs or other animals — *see* Influenza, due to identified, novel influenza A virus
lymphangitis — *see* Lymphangitis
abortion — *see* Abortion, by type, with, sepsis
abscess (skin) — *see* Abscess, by site
Absidia 117.7
acanthamoeba 136.21
Acanthocheilonema (perstans) 125.4
streptocerca 125.6
accessory sinus (chronic) (*see also* Sinusitis) 473.9
Achorion — *see* Dermatophytosis
Acremonium falciforme 117.4
acromioclavicular (joint) 711.91
actinobacillus
lignieresii 027.8
mallei 024
muris 026.1
actinomadura — *see* Actinomycosis
Actinomyces (israelii) (*see also* Actinomycosis)
muris-ratti 026.1
Actinomycetales (actinomadura) (Actinomyces) (Nocardia) (Streptomyces) — *see* Actinomycosis
actinomycotic NEC (*see also* Actinomycosis) 039.9
adenoid (chronic) 474.01
acute 463
and tonsil (chronic) 474.02
acute or subacute 463
adenovirus NEC 079.0
in diseases classified elsewhere — *see* category 079 ☑
unspecified nature or site 079.0
Aerobacter aerogenes NEC 041.85
enteritis 008.2
aerogenes capsulatus (*see also* Gangrene, gas) 040.0
aertrycke (*see also* Infection, Salmonella) 003.9
ajellomyces dermatitidis 116.0

Infection, infected, infective — *continued*
alimentary canal NEC (*see also* Enteritis, due to, by organism) 009.0
Allescheria boydii 117.6
Alternaria 118
alveolus, alveolar (process) (pulpal origin) 522.4
ameba, amebic (histolytica) (*see also* Amebiasis) 006.9
acute 006.0
chronic 006.1
free-living 136.29
hartmanni 007.8
specified
site NEC 006.8
type NEC 007.8
amniotic fluid or cavity 658.4 ☑
affecting fetus or newborn 762.7
anaerobes (cocci) (gram-negative) (gram-positive) (mixed) NEC 041.84
anal canal 569.49
Ancylostoma braziliense 126.2
Angiostrongylus cantonensis 128.8
anisakiasis 127.1
Anisakis larva 127.1
anthrax (*see also* Anthrax) 022.9
antrum (chronic) (*see also* Sinusitis, maxillary) 473.0
anus (papillae) (sphincter) 569.49
arbor virus NEC 066.9
arbovirus NEC 066.9
argentophil-rod 027.0
Ascaris lumbricoides 127.0
ascomycetes 117.4
Aspergillus (flavus) (fumigatus) (terreus) 117.3
atypical
acid-fast (bacilli) (*see also* Mycobacterium, atypical) 031.9
mycobacteria (*see also* Mycobacterium, atypical) 031.9
auditory meatus (circumscribed) (diffuse) (external) (*see also* Otitis, externa) 380.10
auricle (ear) (*see also* Otitis, externa) 380.10
axillary gland 683
Babesiasis 088.82
Babesiosis 088.82
Bacillus NEC 041.89
abortus 023.1
anthracis (*see also* Anthrax) 022.9
cereus (food poisoning) 005.89
coli — *see* Infection, Escherichia coli
coliform NEC 041.85
Ducrey's (any location) 099.0
Flexner's 004.1
Friedländer's NEC 041.3
fusiformis 101
gas (gangrene) (*see also* Gangrene, gas) 040.0
mallei 024
melitensis 023.0
paratyphoid, paratyphosus 002.9
A 002.1
B 002.2
C 002.3
Schmorl's 040.3
Shiga 004.0
suipestifer (*see also* Infection, Salmonella) 003.9
swimming pool 031.1
typhosa 002.0
welchii (*see also* Gangrene, gas) 040.0
Whitmore's 025
bacterial NEC 041.9
specified NEC 041.89
anaerobic NEC 041.84
gram-negative NEC 041.85
anaerobic NEC 041.84
Bacterium
paratyphosum 002.9
A 002.1
B 002.2
C 002.3
typhosum 002.0

☑ Additional Digit Required — Refer to the Tabular List for Digit Selection
▽ Subterms under main terms may continue to next column or page
2014 ICD-9-CM
199

Infection, infected, infective — *continued*

Bacteroides (fragilis) (melaninogenicus) (oralis) NEC 041.82
balantidium coli 007.0
Bartholin's gland 616.89
Basidiobolus 117.7
Bedsonia 079.98
   specified NEC 079.88
bile duct 576.1
bladder (*see also* Cystitis) 595.9
Blastomyces, blastomycotic 116.0
   brasiliensis 116.1
   dermatitidis 116.0
   European 117.5
   loboi 116.2
   North American 116.0
   South American 116.1
bleb
   postprocedural 379.60
      stage 1 379.61
      stage 2 379.62
      stage 3 379.63
blood stream (*see also* Septicemia)
   catheter-related (CRBSI) 999.31
   central line-associated (CLABSI) 999.32
   due to central venous catheter 999.32
bone 730.9 ☑
   specified — *see* Osteomyelitis
Bordetella 033.9
   bronchiseptica 033.8
   parapertussis 033.1
   pertussis 033.0
Borrelia
   bergdorfi 088.81
   vincentii (mouth) (pharynx) (tonsil) 101
bovine stomatitis 059.11
brain (*see also* Encephalitis) 323.9
   late effect — *see* category 326
   membranes (*see also* Meningitis) 322.9
   septic 324.0
      late effect — *see* category 326
      meninges (*see also* Meningitis) 320.9
branchial cyst 744.42
breast 611.0
   puerperal, postpartum 675.2 ☑
      with nipple 675.9 ☑
         specified type NEC 675.8 ☑
      nonpurulent 675.2 ☑
      purulent 675.1 ☑
bronchus (*see also* Bronchitis) 490
   fungus NEC 117.9
Brucella 023.9
   abortus 023.1
   canis 023.3
   melitensis 023.0
   mixed 023.8
   suis 023.2
Brugia (Wuchereria) malayi 125.1
bursa — *see* Bursitis
buttocks (skin) 686.9
Candida (albicans) (tropicalis) (*see also* Candidiasis) 112.9
   congenital 771.7
Candiru 136.8
Capillaria
   hepatica 128.8
   philippinensis 127.5
cartilage 733.99
catheter-related bloodstream (CRBSI) 999.31
cat liver fluke 121.0
cellulitis — *see* Cellulitis, by site
central line-associated 999.31
   bloodstream 999.32
Cephalosporum falciforme 117.4
Cercomonas hominis (intestinal) 007.3
cerebrospinal (*see also* Meningitis) 322.9
   late effect — *see* category 326
cervical gland 683
cervix (*see also* Cervicitis) 616.0
cesarean section wound 674.3 ☑
Chilomastix (intestinal) 007.8
Chlamydia 079.98
   specified NEC 079.88
cholera (*see also* Cholera) 001.9
chorionic plate 658.8 ☑

Infection, infected, infective — *continued*

Cladosporium
   bantianum 117.8
   carrionii 117.2
   mansoni 111.1
   trichoides 117.8
   wernecki 111.1
Clonorchis (sinensis) (liver) 121.1
Clostridium (haemolyticum) (novyi) NEC 041.84
   botulinum 005.1
   histolyticum (*see also* Gangrene, gas) 040.0
   oedematiens (*see also* Gangrene, gas) 040.0
   perfringens 041.83
      due to food 005.2
   septicum (*see also* Gangrene, gas) 040.0
   sordellii (*see also* Gangrene, gas) 040.0
   welchii (*see also* Gangrene, gas) 040.0
      due to food 005.2
Coccidioides (immitis) (*see also* Coccidioidomycosis) 114.9
coccus NEC 041.89
colon (*see also* Enteritis, due to, by organism) 009.0
   bacillus — *see* Infection, Escherichia coli
colostomy or enterostomy 569.61
common duct 576.1
complicating pregnancy, childbirth, or puerperium NEC 647.9 ☑
   affecting fetus or newborn 760.2
Condiobolus 117.7
congenital NEC 771.89
   Candida albicans 771.7
   chronic 771.2
   cytomegalovirus 771.1
   hepatitis, viral 771.2
   herpes simplex 771.2
   listeriosis 771.2
   malaria 771.2
   poliomyelitis 771.2
   rubella 771.0
   toxoplasmosis 771.2
   tuberculosis 771.2
   urinary (tract) 771.82
   vaccinia 771.2
coronavirus 079.89
   SARS-associated 079.82
corpus luteum (*see also* Salpingo-oophoritis) 614.2
Corynebacterium diphtheriae — *see* Diphtheria
cotia virus 059.8
Coxsackie (*see also* Coxsackie) 079.2
   endocardium 074.22
   heart NEC 074.20
   in diseases classified elsewhere — *see* category 079 ☑
   meninges 047.0
   myocardium 074.23
   pericardium 074.21
   pharynx 074.0
   specified disease NEC 074.8
   unspecified nature or site 079.2
Cryptococcus neoformans 117.5
Cryptosporidia 007.4
Cunninghamella 117.7
cyst — *see* Cyst
Cysticercus cellulosae 123.1
cystostomy 596.83
cytomegalovirus 078.5
   congenital 771.1
dental (pulpal origin) 522.4
deuteromycetes 117.4
Dicrocoelium dendriticum 121.8
Dipetalonema (perstans) 125.4
   streptocerca 125.6
diphtherial — *see* Diphtheria
Diphyllobothrium (adult) (latum) (pacificum) 123.4
   larval 123.5
Diplogonoporus (grandis) 123.8
Dipylidium (caninum) 123.8
Dirofilaria 125.6
dog tapeworm 123.8

Infection, infected, infective — *continued*

Dracunculus medinensis 125.7
Dreschlera 118
   hawaiiensis 117.8
Ducrey's bacillus (any site) 099.0
due to or resulting from
   central venous catheter (*see also* Complications, due to, catheter, central venous) 999.31
      bloodstream 999.32
      localized 999.33
   device, implant, or graft (any) (presence of) — *see* Complications, infection and inflammation, due to (presence of) any device, implant, or graft classified to 996.0–996.5 NEC
   injection, inoculation, infusion, transfusion, or vaccination (prophylactic) (therapeutic) 999.39
      blood and blood products
         acute 999.34
   injury NEC — *see* Wound, open, by site, complicated
   surgery 998.59
   duodenum 535.6 ☑
ear (*see also* Otitis)
   external (*see also* Otitis, externa) 380.10
   inner (*see also* Labyrinthitis) 386.30
   middle — *see* Otitis, media
Eaton's agent NEC 041.81
Eberthella typhosa 002.0
Ebola 078.89
echinococcosis 122.9
Echinococcus (*see also* Echinococcus) 122.9
Echinostoma 121.8
ECHO virus 079.1
   in diseases classified elsewhere — *see* category 079 ☑
   unspecified nature or site 079.1
Ehrlichiosis 082.40
   chaffeensis 082.41
   specified type NEC 082.49
Endamoeba — *see* Infection, ameba
endocardium (*see also* Endocarditis) 421.0
endocervix (*see also* Cervicitis) 616.0
Entamoeba — *see* Infection, ameba
enteric (*see also* Enteritis, due to, by organism) 009.0
Enterobacter aerogenes NEC 041.85
Enterobacter sakazakii 041.85
Enterobius vermicularis 127.4
enterococcus NEC 041.04
enterovirus NEC 079.89
   central nervous system NEC 048
   enteritis 008.67
   meningitis 047.9
Entomophthora 117.7
Epidermophyton — *see* Dermatophytosis
epidermophytosis — *see* Dermatophytosis
episiotomy 674.3 ☑
Epstein-Barr virus 075
   chronic 780.79 *[139.8]*
erysipeloid 027.1
Erysipelothrix (insidiosa) (rhusiopathiae) 027.1
erythema infectiosum 057.0
Escherichia coli (E. coli) 041.49
   enteritis — *see* Enteritis, E. coli
   generalized 038.42
   intestinal — *see* Enteritis, E. coli
   non-Shiga toxin-producing 041.49
   Shiga toxin-producing (STEC) 041.43
      with
         unspecified O group 041.43
         non-O157 (with known O group) 041.43
      O157 (with confirmation of Shiga toxin when H antigen is unknown, or is not H7) 041.41
      O157:H7 with or without confirmation of Shiga toxin-production 041.41
      O157:H- (nonmotile) with confirmation of Shiga toxin 041.41
   specified NEC 041.42

Infection, infected, infective — *continued*

esophagostomy 530.86
ethmoidal (chronic) (sinus) (*see also* Sinusitis, ethmoidal) 473.2
Eubacterium 041.84
Eustachian tube (ear) 381.50
   acute 381.51
   chronic 381.52
exanthema subitum (*see also* Exanthem subitum) 058.10
exit site 999.33
external auditory canal (meatus) (*see also* Otitis, externa) 380.10
eyelid 373.9
   specified NEC 373.8
eye NEC 360.00
fallopian tube (*see also* Salpingo-oophoritis) 614.2
fascia 728.89
Fasciola
   gigantica 121.3
   hepatica 121.3
Fasciolopsis (buski) 121.4
fetus (intra-amniotic) — *see* Infection, congenital
filarial — *see* Infestation, filarial
finger (skin) 686.9
   abscess (with lymphangitis) 681.00
      pulp 681.01
   cellulitis (with lymphangitis) 681.00
   distal closed space (with lymphangitis) 681.00
   nail 681.02
      fungus 110.1
fish tapeworm 123.4
   larval 123.5
flagellate, intestinal 007.9
fluke — *see* Infestation, fluke
focal
   teeth (pulpal origin) 522.4
   tonsils 474.00
      and adenoids 474.02
Fonsecaea
   compactum 117.2
   pedrosoi 117.2
food (*see also* Poisoning, food) 005.9
foot (skin) 686.9
   fungus 110.4
Francisella tularensis (*see also* Tularemia) 021.9
frontal sinus (chronic) (*see also* Sinusitis, frontal) 473.1
fungus NEC 117.9
   beard 110.0
   body 110.5
   dermatiaceous NEC 117.8
   foot 110.4
   groin 110.3
   hand 110.2
   nail 110.1
   pathogenic to compromised host only 118
   perianal (area) 110.3
   scalp 110.0
   scrotum 110.8
   skin 111.9
      foot 110.4
      hand 110.2
   toenails 110.1
   trachea 117.9
Fusarium 118
Fusobacterium 041.84
gallbladder (*see also* Cholecystitis, acute) 575.0
Gardnerella vaginalis 041.89
gas bacillus (*see also* Gas, gangrene) 040.0
gastric (*see also* Gastritis) 535.5 ☑
Gastrodiscoides hominis 121.8
gastroenteric (*see also* Enteritis, due to, by organism) 009.0
gastrointestinal (*see also* Enteritis, due to, by organism) 009.0
gastrostomy 536.41
generalized NEC (*see also* Septicemia) 038.9
genital organ or tract NEC
   female 614.9

Infection, infected, infective — *continued*
genital organ or tract — *continued*
female — *continued*
with
abortion — *see* Abortion, by type, with sepsis
ectopic pregnancy (*see also* categories 633.0–633.9) 639.0
molar pregnancy (*see also* categories 630–632) 639.0
complicating pregnancy 646.6 ☑
affecting fetus or newborn 760.8
following
abortion 639.0
ectopic or molar pregnancy 639.0
puerperal, postpartum, childbirth 670.8 ☑
minor or localized 646.6 ☑
affecting fetus or newborn 760.8
male 608.4
genitourinary tract NEC 599.0
Ghon tubercle, primary (*see also* Tuberculosis) 010.0 ☑
Giardia lamblia 007.1
gingival (chronic) 523.10
acute 523.00
Vincent's 101
glanders 024
Glenosporopsis amazonica 116.2
Gnathostoma spinigerum 128.1
Gongylonema 125.6
gonococcal NEC (*see also* Gonococcus) 098.0
gram-negative bacilli NEC 041.85
anaerobic 041.84
guinea worm 125.7
gum (*see also* Infection, gingival) 523.10
Hantavirus 079.81
heart 429.89
Helicobacter pylori [H. pylori] 041.86
helminths NEC 128.9
intestinal 127.9
mixed (types classifiable to more than one category in 120.0–127.7) 127.8
specified type NEC 127.7
specified type NEC 128.8
Hemophilus influenzae NEC 041.5
generalized 038.41
herpes (simplex) (*see also* Herpes, simplex) 054.9
congenital 771.2
zoster (*see also* Herpes, zoster) 053.9
eye NEC 053.29
Heterophyes heterophyes 121.6
Histoplasma (*see also* Histoplasmosis) 115.90
capsulatum (*see also* Histoplasmosis, American) 115.00
duboisii (*see also* Histoplasmosis, African) 115.10
HIV V08
with symptoms, symptomatic 042
hookworm (*see also* Ancylostomiasis) 126.9
human herpesvirus 6 058.81
human herpesvirus 7 058.82
human herpesvirus 8 058.89
human herpesvirus NEC 058.89
human immunodeficiency virus V08
with symptoms, symptomatic 042
human papillomavirus 079.4
hydrocele 603.1
hydronephrosis 591
Hymenolepis 123.6
hypopharynx 478.29
inguinal glands 683
due to soft chancre 099.0
insertion site 999.33
intestine, intestinal (*see also* Enteritis, due to, by organism) 009.0
intrauterine (*see also* Endometritis) 615.9
complicating delivery 646.6 ☑
isospora belli or hominis 007.2
Japanese B encephalitis 062.0
jaw (bone) (acute) (chronic) (lower) (subacute) (upper) 526.4
joint — *see* Arthritis, infectious or infective

Infection, infected, infective — *continued*
Kaposi's sarcoma-associated herpesvirus 058.89
kidney (cortex) (hematogenous) 590.9
with
abortion — *see* Abortion, by type, with urinary tract infection
calculus 592.0
ectopic pregnancy (*see also* categories 633.0–633.9) 639.8
molar pregnancy (*see also* categories 630–632) 639.8
complicating pregnancy or puerperium 646.6 ☑
affecting fetus or newborn 760.1
following
abortion 639.8
ectopic or molar pregnancy 639.8
pelvis and ureter 590.3
Klebsiella pneumoniae NEC 041.3
knee (skin) NEC 686.9
joint — *see* Arthritis, infectious
Koch's (*see also* Tuberculosis, pulmonary) 011.9 ☑
labia (majora) (minora) (*see also* Vulvitis) 616.10
lacrimal
gland (*see also* Dacryoadenitis) 375.00
passages (duct) (sac) (*see also* Dacryocystitis) 375.30
larynx NEC 478.79
leg (skin) NEC 686.9
Leishmania (*see also* Leishmaniasis) 085.9
braziliensis 085.5
donovani 085.0
ethiopica 085.3
furunculosa 085.1
infantum 085.0
mexicana 085.4
tropica (minor) 085.1
major 085.2
Leptosphaeria senegalensis 117.4
leptospira (*see also* Leptospirosis) 100.9
Australis 100.89
Bataviae 100.89
pyrogenes 100.89
specified type NEC 100.89
leptospirochetal NEC (*see also* Leptospirosis) 100.9
Leptothrix — *see* Actinomycosis
Listeria monocytogenes (listeriosis) 027.0
congenital 771.2
liver fluke — *see* Infestation, fluke, liver
Loa loa 125.2
eyelid 125.2 [373.6]
Loboa loboi 116.2
local, skin (staphylococcal) (streptococcal) NEC 686.9
abscess — *see* Abscess, by site
cellulitis — *see* Cellulitis, by site
ulcer (*see also* Ulcer, skin) 707.9
Loefflerella
mallei 024
whitmori 025
lung 518.89
atypical Mycobacterium 031.0
tuberculous (*see also* Tuberculosis, pulmonary) 011.9 ☑
basilar 518.89
chronic 518.89
fungus NEC 117.9
spirochetal 104.8
virus — *see* Pneumonia, virus
lymph gland (axillary) (cervical) (inguinal) 683
mesenteric 289.2
lymphoid tissue, base of tongue or posterior pharynx, NEC 474.00
madurella
grisea 117.4
mycetomii 117.4
major
with
abortion — *see* Abortion, by type, with sepsis

Infection, infected, infective — *continued*
major — *continued*
with — *continued*
ectopic pregnancy (*see also* categories 633.0–633.9) 639.0
molar pregnancy (*see also* categories 630–632) 639.0
following
abortion 639.0
ectopic or molar pregnancy 639.0
puerperal, postpartum, childbirth 670.0 ☑
Malassezia furfur 111.0
Malleomyces
mallei 024
pseudomallei 025
mammary gland 611.0
puerperal, postpartum 675.2 ☑
Mansonella (ozzardi) 125.5
mastoid (suppurative) — *see* Mastoiditis
maxilla, maxillary 526.4
sinus (chronic) (*see also* Sinusitis, maxillary) 473.0
mediastinum 519.2
medina 125.7
meibomian
cyst 373.12
gland 373.12
melioidosis 025
meninges (*see also* Meningitis) 320.9
meningococcal (*see also* condition) 036.9
brain 036.1
cerebrospinal 036.0
endocardium 036.42
generalized 036.2
meninges 036.0
meningococcemia 036.2
specified site NEC 036.89
mesenteric lymph nodes or glands NEC 289.2
Metagonimus 121.5
metatarsophalangeal 711.97
methicillin
resistant Staphylococcus aureus (MRSA) 041.12
susceptible Staphylococcus aureus (MSSA) 041.11
microorganism resistant to drugs — *see* Resistance (to), drugs by microorganisms
Microsporidia 136.8
microsporum, microsporic — *see* Dermatophytosis
Mima polymorpha NEC 041.85
mixed flora NEC 041.89
Monilia (*see also* Candidiasis) 112.9
neonatal 771.7
monkeypox 059.01
Monosporium apiospermum 117.6
mouth (focus) NEC 528.9
parasitic 136.9
MRSA (methicillin resistant Staphylococcus aureus) 041.12
MSSA (methicillin susceptible Staphylococcus aureus) 041.11
Mucor 117.7
muscle NEC 728.89
mycelium NEC 117.9
mycetoma
actinomycotic NEC (*see also* Actinomycosis) 039.9
mycotic NEC 117.4
Mycobacterium, mycobacterial (*see also* Mycobacterium) 031.9
Mycoplasma NEC 041.81
mycotic NEC 117.9
pathogenic to compromised host only 118
skin NEC 111.9
systemic 117.9
myocardium NEC 422.90
nail (chronic) (with lymphangitis) 681.9
finger 681.02
fungus 110.1
ingrowing 703.0
toe 681.11

Infection, infected, infective — *continued*
nail — *continued*
toe — *continued*
fungus 110.1
nasal sinus (chronic) (*see also* Sinusitis) 473.9
nasopharynx (chronic) 478.29
acute 460
navel 686.9
newborn 771.4
Neisserian — *see* Gonococcus
Neotestudina rosatii 117.4
newborn, generalized 771.89
nipple 611.0
puerperal, postpartum 675.0 ☑
with breast 675.9 ☑
specified type NEC 675.8 ☑
Nocardia — *see* Actinomycosis
nose 478.19
nostril 478.19
obstetrical surgical wound 674.3 ☑
Oesophagostomum (apiostomum) 127.7
Oestrus ovis 134.0
Oidium albicans (*see also* Candidiasis) 112.9
Onchocerca (volvulus) 125.3
eye 125.3 [360.13]
eyelid 125.3 [373.6]
operation wound 998.59
Opisthorchis (felineus) (tenuicollis) (viverrini) 121.0
orbit 376.00
chronic 376.10
orthopoxvirus 059.00
specified NEC 059.09
ovary (*see also* Salpingo-oophoritis) 614.2
Oxyuris vermicularis 127.4
pancreas 577.0
Paracoccidioides brasiliensis 116.1
Paragonimus (westermani) 121.2
parainfluenza virus 079.89
parameningococcus NEC 036.9
with meningitis 036.0
parapoxvirus 059.10
specified NEC 059.19
parasitic NEC 136.9
paratyphoid 002.9
type A 002.1
type B 002.2
type C 002.3
paraurethral ducts 597.89
parotid gland 527.2
Pasteurella NEC 027.2
multocida (cat-bite) (dog-bite) 027.2
pestis (*see also* Plague) 020.9
pseudotuberculosis 027.2
septica (cat-bite) (dog-bite) 027.2
tularensis (*see also* Tularemia) 021.9
pelvic, female (*see also* Disease, pelvis, inflammatory) 614.9
penis (glans) (retention) NEC 607.2
herpetic 054.13
Peptococcus 041.84
Peptostreptococcus 041.84
periapical (pulpal origin) 522.4
peridental 523.30
perineal wound (obstetrical) 674.3 ☑
periodontal 523.31
periorbital 376.00
chronic 376.10
perirectal 569.49
perirenal (*see also* Infection, kidney) 590.9
peritoneal (*see also* Peritonitis) 567.9
periureteral 593.89
periurethral 597.89
Petriellidium boydii 117.6
pharynx 478.29
Coxsackie virus 074.0
phlegmonous 462
posterior, lymphoid 474.00
Phialophora
gougerotii 117.8
jeanselmei 117.8
verrucosa 117.2
Piedraia hortai 111.3
pinna, acute 380.11
pinta 103.9
intermediate 103.1

☑ **Additional Digit Required** — Refer to the Tabular List for Digit Selection   🔽 **Subterms under main terms may continue to next column or page**

2014 ICD-9-CM   201

Infection, infected, infective — *continued*

pinta — *continued*
    late 103.2
    mixed 103.3
    primary 103.0
pinworm 127.4
pityrosporum furfur 111.0
pleuropneumonia-like organisms NEC (PPLO) 041.81
pneumococcal NEC 041.2
    generalized (purulent) 038.2
Pneumococcus NEC 041.2
port 999.33
postoperative wound 998.59
posttraumatic NEC 958.3
postvaccinal 999.39
poxvirus 059.9
    specified NEC 059.8
prepuce NEC 607.1
Proprionibacterium 041.84
prostate (capsule) (*see also* Prostatitis) 601.9
Proteus (mirabilis) (morganii) (vulgaris) NEC 041.6
    enteritis 008.3
protozoal NEC 136.8
    intestinal NEC 007.9
Pseudomonas NEC 041.7
    mallei 024
    pneumonia 482.1
    pseudomallei 025
psittacosis 073.9
puerperal, postpartum (major) 670.0 ☑
    minor 646.6 ☑
pulmonary — *see* Infection, lung
purulent — *see* Abscess
putrid, generalized — *see* Septicemia
pyemic — *see* Septicemia
Pyrenochaeta romeroi 117.4
Q fever 083.0
rabies 071
rectum (sphincter) 569.49
renal (*see also* Infection, kidney) 590.9
    pelvis and ureter 590.3
reservoir 999.33
resistant to drugs — *see* Resistance (to), drugs by microorganisms
respiratory 519.8
    chronic 519.8
    influenzal (acute) (upper) (*see also* Influenza) 487.1
    lung 518.89
    rhinovirus 460
    syncytial virus 079.6
    upper (acute) (infectious) NEC 465.9
        with flu, grippe, or influenza (*see also* Influenza) 487.1
        influenzal (*see also* Influenza) 487.1
        multiple sites NEC 465.8
        streptococcal 034.0
        viral NEC 465.9
respiratory syncytial virus (RSV) 079.6
resulting from presence of shunt or other internal prosthetic device — *see* Complications, infection and inflammation, due to (presence of) any device, implant, or graft classified to 996.0–996.5 NEC
retroperitoneal 567.39
retrovirus 079.50
    human immunodeficiency virus type 2 (HIV2) 079.53
    human T-cell lymphotrophic virus type I (HTLV-I) 079.51
    human T-cell lymphotrophic virus type II (HTLV-II) 079.52
    specified NEC 079.59
Rhinocladium 117.1
Rhinosporidium — *see* beri 117.0
rhinovirus
    in diseases classified elsewhere — *see* category 079 ☑
    unspecified nature or site 079.3
Rhizopus 117.7
rickettsial 083.9
rickettsialpox 083.2
rubella (*see also* Rubella) 056.9

Infection, infected, infective — *continued*

rubella (*see also* Rubella) — *continued*
    congenital 771.0
Saccharomyces (*see also* Candidiasis) 112.9
Saksenaea 117.7
salivary duct or gland (any) 527.2
Salmonella (aertrycke) (callinarum) (choleraesuis) (enteritidis) (suipestifer) (typhimurium) 003.9
    with
        arthritis 003.23
        gastroenteritis 003.0
        localized infection 003.20
            specified type NEC 003.29
        meningitis 003.21
        osteomyelitis 003.24
        pneumonia 003.22
        septicemia 003.1
        specified manifestation NEC 003.8
    due to food (poisoning) (any serotype) (*see also* Poisoning, food, due to, Salmonella)
    hirschfeldii 002.3
    localized 003.20
        specified type NEC 003.29
    paratyphi 002.9
        A 002.1
        B 002.2
        C 002.3
    schottmuelleri 002.2
    specified type NEC 003.8
    typhi 002.0
    typhosa 002.0
saprophytic 136.8
Sarcocystis, lindemanni 136.5
SARS-associated coronavirus 079.82
scabies 133.0
Schistosoma — *see* Infestation, Schistosoma
Schmorl's bacillus 040.3
scratch or other superficial injury — *see* Injury, superficial, by site
scrotum (acute) NEC 608.4
sealpox 059.12
secondary, burn or open wound (dislocation) (fracture) 958.3
seminal vesicle (*see also* Vesiculitis) 608.0
septic
    generalized — *see* Septicemia
    localized, skin (*see also* Abscess) 682.9
septicemic — *see* Septicemia
seroma 998.51
Serratia (marcescens) 041.85
    generalized 038.44
sheep liver fluke 121.3
Shigella 004.9
    boydii 004.2
    dysenteriae 004.0
    flexneri 004.1
    group
        A 004.0
        B 004.1
        C 004.2
        D 004.3
    Schmitz (-Stutzer) 004.0
    schmitzii 004.0
    Shiga 004.0
    sonnei 004.3
    specified type NEC 004.8
Sin Nombre virus 079.81
sinus (*see also* Sinusitis) 473.9
    pilonidal 685.1
        with abscess 685.0
    skin NEC 686.9
Skene's duct or gland (*see also* Urethritis) 597.89
skin (local) (staphylococcal) (streptococcal) NEC 686.9
    abscess — *see* Abscess, by site
    cellulitis — *see* Cellulitis, by site
    due to fungus 111.9
        specified type NEC 111.8
    mycotic 111.9
        specified type NEC 111.8
    ulcer (*see also* Ulcer, skin) 707.9
slow virus 046.9
    specified condition NEC 046.8

Infection, infected, infective — *continued*

Sparganum (mansoni) (proliferum) 123.5
spermatic cord NEC 608.4
sphenoidal (chronic) (sinus) (*see also* Sinusitis, sphenoidal) 473.3
Spherophorus necrophorus 040.3
spinal cord NEC (*see also* Encephalitis) 323.9
    abscess 324.1
    late effect — *see* category 326
    late effect — *see* category 326
    meninges — *see* Meningitis
    streptococcal 320.2
Spirillum
    minus or minor 026.0
    morsus muris 026.0
    obermeieri 087.0
spirochetal NEC 104.9
    lung 104.8
    specified nature or site NEC 104.8
spleen 289.59
Sporothrix schenckii 117.1
Sporotrichum (schenckii) 117.1
Sporozoa 136.8
staphylococcal NEC 041.10
    aureus 041.11
        methicillin
            resistant (MRSA) 041.12
            susceptible (MSSA) 041.11
    food poisoning 005.0
    generalized (purulent) 038.10
        aureus 038.11
            methicillin
                resistant 038.12
                susceptible 038.11
        specified organism NEC 038.19
    pneumonia 482.40
        aureus 482.41
            methicillin
                resistant (MRSA) 482.42
                susceptible (MSSA) 482.41
        MRSA (methicillin resistant Staphylococcus aureus) 482.42
        MSSA (methicillin susceptible Staphylococcus aureus) 482.41
        specified type NEC 482.49
    septicemia 038.10
        aureus 038.11
            methicillin
                resistant (MRSA) 038.12
                susceptible (MSSA) 038.11
        MRSA (methicillin resistant Staphylococcus aureus) 038.12
        MSSA (methicillin susceptible Staphylococcus aureus) 038.11
        specified organism NEC 038.19
    specified NEC 041.19
steatoma 706.2
Stellantchasmus falcatus 121.6
Streptobacillus moniliformis 026.1
streptococcal NEC 041.00
    generalized (purulent) 038.0
    Group
        A 041.01
        B 041.02
        C 041.03
        D [enterococcus] 041.04
        G 041.05
    pneumonia — *see* Pneumonia, streptococcal
    septicemia 038.0
    sore throat 034.0
    specified NEC 041.09
Streptomyces — *see* Actinomycosis
streptotrichosis — *see* Actinomycosis
Strongyloides (stercoralis) 127.2
stump (amputation) (posttraumatic) (surgical) 997.62
    traumatic — *see* Amputation, traumatic, by site, complicated
subcutaneous tissue, local NEC 686.9
submaxillary region 528.9
suipestifer (*see also* Infection, Salmonella) 003.9
swimming pool bacillus 031.1

Infection, infected, infective — *continued*

syphilitic — *see* Syphilis
systemic — *see* Septicemia
Taenia — *see* Infestation, Taenia
Taeniarhynchus saginatus 123.2
tanapox 059.21
tapeworm — *see* Infestation, tapeworm
tendon (sheath) 727.89
Ternidens diminutus 127.7
testis (*see also* Orchitis) 604.90
thigh (skin) 686.9
threadworm 127.4
throat 478.29
    pneumococcal 462
    staphylococcal 462
    streptococcal 034.0
    viral NEC (*see also* Pharyngitis) 462
thumb (skin) 686.9
    abscess (with lymphangitis) 681.00
        pulp 681.01
    cellulitis (with lymphangitis) 681.00
    nail 681.02
thyroglossal duct 529.8
toe (skin) 686.9
    abscess (with lymphangitis) 681.10
    cellulitis (with lymphangitis) 681.10
    nail 681.11
        fungus 110.1
tongue NEC 529.0
    parasitic 112.0
tonsil (faucial) (lingual) (pharyngeal) 474.00
    acute or subacute 463
    and adenoid 474.02
    tag 474.00
tooth, teeth 522.4
    periapical (pulpal origin) 522.4
    peridental 523.30
    periodontal 523.31
    pulp 522.0
    socket 526.5
TORCH — *see* Infection, congenital NEC without active infection 760.2
Torula histolytica 117.5
Toxocara (cani) (cati) (felis) 128.0
Toxoplasma gondii (*see also* Toxoplasmosis) 130.9
trachea, chronic 491.8
    fungus 117.9
traumatic NEC 958.3
trematode NEC 121.9
trench fever 083.1
Treponema
    denticola 041.84
    macrodenticum 041.84
    pallidum (*see also* Syphilis) 097.9
Trichinella (spiralis) 124
Trichomonas 131.9
    bladder 131.09
    cervix 131.09
    hominis 007.3
    intestine 007.3
    prostate 131.03
    specified site NEC 131.8
    urethra 131.02
    urogenitalis 131.00
    vagina 131.01
    vulva 131.01
Trichophyton, trichophytid — *see* Dermatophytosis
Trichosporon (beigelii) cutaneum 111.2
Trichostrongylus 127.6
Trichuris (trichiuria) 127.3
Trombicula (irritans) 133.8
Trypanosoma (*see also* Trypanosomiasis) 086.9
    cruzi 086.2
tubal (*see also* Salpingo-oophoritis) 614.2
tuberculous NEC (*see also* Tuberculosis) 011.9 ☑
tubo-ovarian (*see also* Salpingo-oophoritis) 614.2
tunica vaginalis 608.4
tunnel 999.33
tympanic membrane — *see* Myringitis
typhoid (abortive) (ambulant) (bacillus) 002.0

Subterms under main terms may continue to next column or page

Infection, infected, infective — *continued*
  typhus 081.9
    flea-borne (endemic) 081.0
    louse-borne (epidemic) 080
    mite-borne 081.2
    recrudescent 081.1
    tick-borne 082.9
      African 082.1
      North Asian 082.2
  umbilicus (septic) 686.9
    newborn NEC 771.4
  ureter 593.89
  urethra (*see also* Urethritis) 597.80
  urinary (tract) NEC 599.0
    with
      abortion — *see* Abortion, by type, with urinary tract infection
      ectopic pregnancy (*see also* categories 633.0–633.9) 639.8
      molar pregnancy (*see also* categories 630–632) 639.8
    candidal 112.2
    complicating pregnancy, childbirth, or puerperium 646.6 ☑
      affecting fetus or newborn 760.1
      asymptomatic 646.5 ☑
        affecting fetus or newborn 760.1
    diplococcal (acute) 098.0
      chronic 098.2
    due to Trichomonas (vaginalis) 131.00
    following
      abortion 639.8
      ectopic or molar pregnancy 639.8
    gonococcal (acute) 098.0
      chronic or duration of 2 months or over 098.2
    newborn 771.82
    trichomonal 131.00
    tuberculous (*see also* Tuberculosis) 016.3 ☑
  uterus, uterine (*see also* Endometritis) 615.9
  utriculus masculinus NEC 597.89
  vaccination 999.39
  vagina (granulation tissue) (wall) (*see also* Vaginitis) 616.10
  varicella 052.9
  varicose veins — *see* Varicose, veins
  variola 050.9
    major 050.0
    minor 050.1
  vas deferens NEC 608.4
  Veillonella 041.84
  verumontanum 597.89
  vesical (*see also* Cystitis) 595.9
  Vibrio
    cholerae 001.0
      El Tor 001.1
    parahaemolyticus (food poisoning) 005.4
    vulnificus 041.85
  Vincent's (gums) (mouth) (tonsil) 101
  vaccination 999.39
  virus, viral 079.99
    adenovirus
      in diseases classified elsewhere — *see* category 079 ☑
      unspecified nature or site 079.0
    central nervous system NEC 049.9
      enterovirus 048
        meningitis 047.9
          specified type NEC 047.8
      slow virus 046.9
      specified condition NEC 046.8
    chest 519.8
    conjunctivitis 077.99
      specified type NEC 077.8
    coronavirus 079.89
      SARS-associated 079.82
    Coxsackie (*see also* Infection, Coxsackie) 079.2
    Ebola 065.8
    ECHO
      in diseases classified elsewhere — *see* category 079 ☑
      unspecified nature or site 079.1

Infection, infected, infective — *continued*
  virus, viral — *continued*
    encephalitis 049.9
      arthropod-borne NEC 064
      tick-borne 063.9
        specified type NEC 063.8
    enteritis NEC (*see also* Enteritis, viral) 008.8
    exanthem NEC 057.9
    Hantavirus 079.81
    human papilloma 079.4
    in diseases classified elsewhere — *see* category 079 ☑
    intestine (*see also* Enteritis, viral) 008.8
    lung — *see* Pneumonia, viral
    respiratory syncytial (RSV) 079.6
    retrovirus 079.50
    rhinovirus
      in diseases classified elsewhere — *see* category 079 ☑
      unspecified nature or site 079.3
    salivary gland disease 078.5
    slow 046.9
      specified condition NEC 046.8
    specified type NEC 079.89
      in diseases classified elsewhere — *see* category 079 ☑
    unspecified nature or site 079.99
    warts 078.10
      specified NEC 078.19
    yaba monkey tumor 059.22
  vulva (*see also* Vulvitis) 616.10
  whipworm 127.3
  Whitmore's bacillus 025
  wound (local) (posttraumatic) NEC 958.3
    with
      dislocation — *see* Dislocation, by site, open
      fracture — *see* Fracture, by site, open
      open wound — *see* Wound, open, by site, complicated
    postoperative 998.59
    surgical 998.59
  Wuchereria 125.0
    bancrofti 125.0
    malayi 125.1
  yaba monkey tumor virus 059.22
  yatapoxvirus 059.20
  yaws — *see* Yaws
  yeast (*see also* Candidiasis) 112.9
  yellow fever (*see also* Fever, yellow) 060.9
  Yersinia pestis (*see also* Plague) 020.9
  Zeis' gland 373.12
  zoonotic bacterial NEC 027.9
  Zopfia senegalensis 117.4
Infective, infectious — *see* condition
Inferiority complex 301.9
  constitutional psychopathic 301.9
Infertility
  female 628.9
    age related 628.8
    associated with
      adhesions, peritubal 614.6 *[628.2]*
      anomaly
        cervical mucus 628.4
        congenital
          cervix 628.4
          fallopian tube 628.2
          uterus 628.3
          vagina 628.4
      anovulation 628.0
      dysmucorrhea 628.4
      endometritis, tuberculous (*see also* Tuberculosis) 016.7 ☑ *[628.3]*
      Stein-Leventhal syndrome 256.4 *[628.0]*
    due to
      adiposogenital dystrophy 253.8 *[628.1]*
      anterior pituitary disorder NEC 253.4 *[628.1]*
        hyperfunction 253.1 *[628.1]*
      cervical anomaly 628.4
      fallopian tube anomaly 628.2
      ovarian failure 256.39 *[628.0]*

Infertility — *continued*
  female — *continued*
    due to — *continued*
      Stein-Leventhal syndrome 256.4 *[628.0]*
      uterine anomaly 628.3
      vaginal anomaly 628.4
    nonimplantation 628.3
    origin
      cervical 628.4
      pituitary-hypothalamus NEC 253.8 *[628.1]*
        anterior pituitary NEC 253.4 *[628.1]*
        hyperfunction NEC 253.1 *[628.1]*
        dwarfism 253.3 *[628.1]*
        panhypopituitarism 253.2 *[628.1]*
      specified NEC 628.8
      tubal (block) (occlusion) (stenosis) 628.2
        adhesions 614.6 *[628.2]*
      uterine 628.3
      vaginal 628.4
    previous, requiring supervision of pregnancy V23.0
  male 606.9
    absolute 606.0
    due to
      azoospermia 606.0
      drug therapy 606.8
      extratesticular cause NEC 606.8
      germinal cell
        aplasia 606.0
        desquamation 606.1
      hypospermatogenesis 606.1
      infection 606.8
      obstruction, afferent ducts 606.8
      oligospermia 606.1
      radiation 606.8
      spermatogenic arrest (complete) 606.0
        incomplete 606.1
      systemic disease 606.8
Infestation 134.9
  Acanthocheilonema (perstans) 125.4
    streptocerca 125.6
  Acariasis 133.9
    demodex folliculorum 133.8
    Sarcoptes scabiei 133.0
    trombiculae 133.8
  Agamofilaria streptocerca 125.6
  Ancylostoma, Ankylostoma 126.9
    americanum 126.1
    braziliense 126.2
    canium 126.8
    ceylanicum 126.3
    duodenale 126.0
    new world 126.1
    old world 126.0
  Angiostrongylus cantonensis 128.8
  anisakiasis 127.1
  Anisakis larva 127.1
  arthropod NEC 134.1
  Ascaris lumbricoides 127.0
  Bacillus fusiformis 101
  Balantidium coli 007.0
  beef tapeworm 123.2
  Bothriocephalus (latus) 123.4
    larval 123.5
  broad tapeworm 123.4
    larval 123.5
  Brugia malayi 125.1
  Candiru 136.8
  Capillaria
    hepatica 128.8
    philippinensis 127.5
  cat liver fluke 121.0
  Cercomonas hominis (intestinal) 007.3
  cestodes 123.9
    specified type NEC 123.8
  chigger 133.8
  chigoe 134.1
  Chilomastix 007.8
  Clonorchis (sinensis) (liver) 121.1
  coccidia 007.2

Infestation — *continued*
  complicating pregnancy, childbirth, or puerperium 647.9 ☑
    affecting fetus or newborn 760.8
  Cysticercus cellulosae 123.1
  Demodex folliculorum 133.8
  Dermatobia (hominis) 134.0
  Dibothriocephalus (latus) 123.4
    larval 123.5
  Dicrocoelium dendriticum 121.8
  Diphyllobothrium (adult) (intestinal) (latum) (pacificum) 123.4
    larval 123.5
  Diplogonoporus (grandis) 123.8
  Dipylidium (caninum) 123.8
  Distoma hepaticum 121.3
  dog tapeworm 123.8
  Dracunculus medinensis 125.7
  dragon worm 125.7
  dwarf tapeworm 123.6
  Echinococcus (*see also* Echinococcus) 122.9
  Echinostoma ilocanum 121.8
  Embadomonas 007.8
  Endamoeba (histolytica) — *see* Infection, ameba
  Entamoeba (histolytica) — *see* Infection, ameba
  Enterobius vermicularis 127.4
  Epidermophyton — *see* Dermatophytosis
  eyeworm 125.2
  Fasciola
    gigantica 121.3
    hepatica 121.3
  Fasciolopsis (buski) (small intestine) 121.4
  blood NEC (*see also* Schistosomiasis) 120.9
  cat liver 121.0
  filarial 125.9
    due to
      Acanthocheilonema (perstans) 125.4
        streptocerca 125.6
      Brugia (Wuchereria) malayi 125.1
      Dracunculus medinensis 125.7
      guinea worms 125.7
      Mansonella (ozzardi) 125.5
      Onchocerca volvulus 125.3
        eye 125.3 *[360.13]*
        eyelid 125.3 *[373.6]*
      Wuchereria (bancrofti) 125.0
        malayi 125.1
    specified type NEC 125.6
  fish tapeworm 123.4
    larval 123.5
  fluke 121.9
    intestinal (giant) 121.4
    liver (sheep) 121.3
      cat 121.0
      Chinese 121.1
      clonorchiasis 121.1
      fascioliasis 121.3
      Oriental 121.1
    lung (oriental) 121.2
    sheep liver 121.3
  fly larva 134.0
  Gasterophilus (intestinalis) 134.0
  Gastrodiscoides hominis 121.8
  Giardia lamblia 007.1
  Gnathostoma (spinigerum) 128.1
  Gongylonema 125.6
  guinea worm 125.7
  helminth NEC 128.9
    intestinal 127.9
      mixed (types classifiable to more than one category in 120.0–127.7) 127.8
      specified type NEC 127.7
    specified type NEC 128.8
  Heterophyes heterophyes (small intestine) 121.6
  hookworm (*see also* Infestation, ancylostoma) 126.9
  Hymenolepis (diminuta) (nana) 123.6
  intestinal NEC 129
  leeches (aquatic) (land) 134.2
  Leishmania — *see* Leishmaniasis

☑ **Additional Digit Required** — Refer to the Tabular List for Digit Selection   ⬙ **Subterms under main terms may continue to next column or page**

2014 ICD-9-CM   203

Infestation — *continued*
  lice (*see also* Infestation, pediculus) 132.9
  Linguatulidae, linguatula (pentastoma)
      (serrata) 134.1
  Loa loa 125.2
    eyelid 125.2 *[373.6]*
  louse (*see also* Infestation, pediculus) 132.9
    body 132.1
    head 132.0
    pubic 132.2
  maggots 134.0
  Mansonella (ozzardi) 125.5
  medina 125.7
  Metagonimus yokogawai (small intestine)
      121.5
  Microfilaria streptocerca 125.3
    eye 125.3 *[360.13]*
    eyelid 125.3 *[373.6]*
  Microsporon furfur 111.0
  microsporum — *see* Dermatophytosis
  mites 133.9
    scabic 133.0
    specified type NEC 133.8
  monilia (albicans) (*see also* Candidiasis)
      112.9
    vagina 112.1
    vulva 112.1
  mouth 112.0
  Necator americanus 126.1
  nematode (intestinal) 127.9
    Ancylostoma (*see also* Ancylostoma)
        126.9
    Ascaris lumbricoides 127.0
    conjunctiva NEC 128.9
    Dioctophyma 128.8
    Enterobius vermicularis 127.4
    Gnathostoma spinigerum 128.1
    Oesophagostomum (apiostomum) 127.7
    Physaloptera 127.4
    specified type NEC 127.7
    Strongyloides stercoralis 127.2
    Ternidens diminutus 127.7
    Trichinella spiralis 124
    Trichostrongylus 127.6
    Trichuris (trichiuria) 127.3
  Oesophagostomum (apiostomum) 127.7
  Oestrus ovis 134.0
  Onchocerca (volvulus) 125.3
    eye 125.3 *[360.13]*
    eyelid 125.3 *[373.6]*
  Opisthorchis (felineus) (tenuicollis) (viverrini) 121.0
  Oxyuris vermicularis 127.4
  Paragonimus (westermani) 121.2
  parasite, parasitic NEC 136.9
    eyelid 134.9 *[373.6]*
    intestinal 129
    mouth 112.0
    orbit 376.13
    skin 134.9
    tongue 112.0
  pediculus 132.9
    capitis (humanus) (any site) 132.0
    corporis (humanus) (any site) 132.1
    eyelid 132.0 *[373.6]*
    mixed (classifiable to more than one
        category in 132.0–132.2) 132.3
    pubis (any site) 132.2
  phthirus (pubis) (any site) 132.2
    with any infestation classifiable to 132.0,
        132.1 and 132.3
  pinworm 127.4
  pork tapeworm (adult) 123.0
  protozoal NEC 136.8
  pubic louse 132.2
  rat tapeworm 123.6
  red bug 133.8
  roundworm (large) NEC 127.0
  sand flea 134.1
  saprophytic NEC 136.8
  Sarcoptes scabiei 133.0
  scabies 133.0
  Schistosoma 120.9
    bovis 120.8
    cercariae 120.3
    hematobium 120.0

Infestation — *continued*
  Schistosoma — *continued*
    intercalatum 120.8
    japonicum 120.2
    mansoni 120.1
    mattheii 120.8
    specified
      site — *see* Schistosomiasis
      type NEC 120.8
    spindale 120.8
  screw worms 134.0
  skin NEC 134.9
  Sparganum (mansoni) (proliferum) 123.5
    larval 123.5
  specified type NEC 134.8
  Spirometra larvae 123.5
  Sporozoa NEC 136.8
  Stellantchasmus falcatus 121.6
  Strongyloides 127.2
  Strongylus (gibsoni) 127.7
  Taenia 123.3
    diminuta 123.6
    Echinococcus (*see also* Echinococcus)
        122.9
    mediocanellata 123.2
    nana 123.6
    saginata (mediocanellata) 123.2
    solium (intestinal form) 123.0
      larval form 123.1
  Taeniarhynchus saginatus 123.2
  tapeworm 123.9
    beef 123.2
    broad 123.4
      larval 123.5
    dog 123.8
    dwarf 123.6
    fish 123.4
      larval 123.5
    pork 123.0
    rat 123.6
  Ternidens diminutus 127.7
  Tetranychus molestissimus 133.8
  threadworm 127.4
  tongue 112.0
  Toxocara (cani) (cati) (felis) 128.0
  trematode(s) NEC 121.9
  Trichina spiralis 124
  Trichinella spiralis 124
  Trichocephalus 127.3
  Trichomonas 131.9
    bladder 131.09
    cervix 131.09
    intestine 007.3
    prostate 131.03
    specified site NEC 131.8
    urethra (female) (male) 131.02
    urogenital 131.00
    vagina 131.01
    vulva 131.01
  Trichophyton — *see* Dermatophytosis
  Trichostrongylus instabilis 127.6
  Trichuris (trichiuria) 127.3
  Trombicula (irritans) 133.8
  Trypanosoma — *see* Trypanosomiasis
  Tunga penetrans 134.1
  Uncinaria americana 126.1
  whipworm 127.3
  worms NEC 128.9
    intestinal 127.9
  Wuchereria 125.0
    bancrofti 125.0
    malayi 125.1

Infiltrate, infiltration
  with an iron compound 275.09
  amyloid (any site) (generalized) 277.39
  calcareous (muscle) NEC 275.49
    localized — *see* Degeneration, by site
  calcium salt (muscle) 275.49
  chemotherapy, vesicant 999.81
  corneal (*see also* Edema, cornea) 371.20
  eyelid 373.9
  fatty (diffuse) (generalized) 272.8
    localized — *see* Degeneration, by site,
        fatty
  glycogen, glycogenic (*see also* Disease,
      glycogen storage) 271.0

Infiltrate, infiltration — *continued*
  heart, cardiac
    fatty (*see also* Degeneration, myocardial)
        429.1
    glycogenic 271.0 *[425.7]*
  inflammatory in vitreous 379.29
  kidney (*see also* Disease, renal) 593.9
  leukemic (M9800/3) — *see* Leukemia
  liver 573.8
    fatty — *see* Fatty, liver
    glycogen (*see also* Disease, glycogen
        storage) 271.0
  lung (*see also* Infiltrate, pulmonary) 793.19
    eosinophilic 518.3
    x-ray finding only 793.19
  lymphatic (*see also* Leukemia, lymphatic)
      204.9 ☑
    gland, pigmentary 289.3
  muscle, fatty 728.9
  myelogenous (*see also* Leukemia, myeloid)
      205.9 ☑
  myocardium, myocardial
    fatty (*see also* Degeneration, myocardial)
        429.1
    glycogenic 271.0 *[425.7]*
  pulmonary 793.19
    with
      eosinophilia 518.3
      pneumonia — *see* Pneumonia, by
          type
    x-ray finding only 793.19
  Ranke's primary (*see also* Tuberculosis)
      010.0 ☑
  skin, lymphocytic (benign) 709.8
  thymus (gland) (fatty) 254.8
  urine 788.8
  vesicant
    agent NEC 999.82
    chemotherapy 999.81
  vitreous humor 379.29

Infirmity 799.89
  senile 797

Inflammation, inflamed, inflammatory (with
    exudation)
  abducens (nerve) 378.54
  accessory sinus (chronic) (*see also* Sinusitis)
      473.9
  adrenal (gland) 255.8
  alimentary canal — *see* Enteritis
  alveoli (teeth) 526.5
    scorbutic 267
  amnion — *see* Amnionitis
  anal canal 569.49
  antrum (chronic) (*see also* Sinusitis, maxillary) 473.0
  anus 569.49
  appendix (*see also* Appendicitis) 541
  arachnoid — *see* Meningitis
  areola 611.0
    puerperal, postpartum 675.0 ☑
  areolar tissue NEC 686.9
  artery — *see* Arteritis
  auditory meatus (external) (*see also* Otitis,
      externa) 380.10
  Bartholin's gland 616.89
  bile duct or passage 576.1
  bladder (*see also* Cystitis) 595.9
  bleb
    postprocedural 379.60
      stage 1 379.61
      stage 2 379.62
      stage 3 379.63
  bone — *see* Osteomyelitis
  bowel (*see also* Enteritis) 558.9
  brain (*see also* Encephalitis) 323.9
    late effect — *see* category 326
    membrane — *see* Meningitis
  breast 611.0
    puerperal, postpartum 675.2 ☑
  broad ligament (*see also* Disease, pelvis, inflammatory) 614.4
    acute 614.3
  bronchus — *see* Bronchitis
  bursa — *see* Bursitis
  capsule
    liver 573.3

Inflammation, inflamed, inflammatory —
    continued
  capsule — *continued*
    spleen 289.59
  catarrhal (*see also* Catarrh) 460
    vagina 616.10
  cecum (*see also* Appendicitis) 541
  cerebral (*see also* Encephalitis) 323.9
    late effect — *see* category 326
    membrane — *see* Meningitis
  cerebrospinal (*see also* Meningitis) 322.9
    late effect — *see* category 326
    meningococcal 036.0
    tuberculous (*see also* Tuberculosis)
        013.6 ☑
  cervix (uteri) (*see also* Cervicitis) 616.0
  chest 519.9
  choroid NEC (*see also* Choroiditis) 363.20
  cicatrix (tissue) — *see* Cicatrix
  colon (*see also* Enteritis) 558.9
    granulomatous 555.1
    newborn 558.9
  connective tissue (diffuse) NEC 728.9
  cornea (*see also* Keratitis) 370.9
    with ulcer (*see also* Ulcer, cornea) 370.00
  corpora cavernosa (penis) 607.2
  cranial nerve — *see* Disorder, nerve, cranial
  diarrhea — *see* Diarrhea
  disc (intervertebral) (space) 722.90
    cervical, cervicothoracic 722.91
    lumbar, lumbosacral 722.93
    thoracic, thoracolumbar 722.92
  Douglas' cul-de-sac or pouch (chronic) (*see
      also* Disease, pelvis, inflammatory)
      614.4
    acute 614.3
  due to (presence of) any device, implant, or
      graft classifiable to 996.0–996.5 —
      see Complications, infection and inflammation, due to (presence of) any
      device, implant, or graft classified to
      996.0–996.5 NEC
  duodenum 535.6 ☑
  dura mater — *see* Meningitis
  ear (*see also* Otitis)
    external (*see also* Otitis, externa) 380.10
    inner (*see also* Labyrinthitis) 386.30
    middle — *see* Otitis media
  esophagus 530.10
  ethmoidal (chronic) (sinus) (*see also* Sinusitis, ethmoidal) 473.2
  Eustachian tube (catarrhal) 381.50
    acute 381.51
    chronic 381.52
  extrarectal 569.49
  eye 379.99
  eyelid 373.9
    specified NEC 373.8
  fallopian tube (*see also* Salpingo-oophoritis)
      614.2
  fascia 728.9
  fetal membranes (acute) 658.4 ☑
    affecting fetus or newborn 762.7
  follicular, pharynx 472.1
  frontal (chronic) (sinus) (*see also* Sinusitis,
      frontal) 473.1
  gallbladder (*see also* Cholecystitis, acute)
      575.0
  gall duct (*see also* Cholecystitis) 575.10
  gastrointestinal (*see also* Enteritis) 558.9
  genital organ (diffuse) (internal)
    female 614.9
      with
        abortion — *see* Abortion, by type,
            with sepsis
        ectopic pregnancy (*see also* categories 633.0–633.9) 639.0
        molar pregnancy (*see also* categories 630–632) 639.0
      complicating pregnancy, childbirth,
          or puerperium 646.6 ☑
        affecting fetus or newborn 760.8
      following
        abortion 639.0
        ectopic or molar pregnancy 639.0
    male 608.4

☑ **Additional Digit Required** — Refer to the Tabular List for Digit Selection ⬧ **Subterms under main terms may continue to next column or page**

204   **2014 ICD-9-CM**

Inflammation, inflamed, inflammatory — *continued*
  gland (lymph) (*see also* Lymphadenitis) 289.3
  glottis (*see also* Laryngitis) 464.00
    with obstruction 464.01
  granular, pharynx 472.1
  gum 523.10
  heart (*see also* Carditis) 429.89
  hepatic duct 576.8
  hernial sac — *see* Hernia, by site
  ileum (*see also* Enteritis) 558.9
    terminal or regional 555.0
      with large intestine 555.2
  intervertebral disc 722.90
    cervical, cervicothoracic 722.91
    lumbar, lumbosacral 722.93
    thoracic, thoracolumbar 722.92
  intestine (*see also* Enteritis) 558.9
  jaw (acute) (bone) (chronic) (lower) (suppurative) (upper) 526.4
  jejunum — *see* Enteritis
  joint NEC (*see also* Arthritis) 716.9 ☑
    sacroiliac 720.2
  kidney (*see also* Nephritis) 583.9
  knee (joint) 716.66
    tuberculous (active) (*see also* Tuberculosis) 015.2 ☑
  labium (majus) (minus) (*see also* Vulvitis) 616.10
  lacrimal
    gland (*see also* Dacryoadenitis) 375.00
    passages (duct) (sac) (*see also* Dacryocystitis) 375.30
  larynx (*see also* Laryngitis) 464.00
    with obstruction 464.01
    diphtheritic 032.3
  leg NEC 686.9
  lip 528.5
  liver (capsule) (*see also* Hepatitis) 573.3
    acute 570
    chronic 571.40
    suppurative 572.0
  lung (acute) (*see also* Pneumonia) 486
    chronic (interstitial) 518.89
  lymphatic vessel (*see also* Lymphangitis) 457.2
  lymph node or gland (*see also* Lymphadenitis) 289.3
  mammary gland 611.0
    puerperal, postpartum 675.2 ☑
  maxilla, maxillary 526.4
    sinus (chronic) (*see also* Sinusitis, maxillary) 473.0
  membranes of brain or spinal cord — *see* Meningitis
  meninges — *see* Meningitis
  mouth 528.00
  muscle 728.9
  myocardium (*see also* Myocarditis) 429.0
  nasal sinus (chronic) (*see also* Sinusitis) 473.9
  nasopharynx — *see* Nasopharyngitis
  navel 686.9
    newborn NEC 771.4
  nerve NEC 729.2
  nipple 611.0
    puerperal, postpartum 675.0 ☑
  nose 478.19
    suppurative 472.0
  oculomotor nerve 378.51
  optic nerve 377.30
  orbit (chronic) 376.10
    acute 376.00
    chronic 376.10
  ovary (*see also* Salpingo-oophoritis) 614.2
  oviduct (*see also* Salpingo-oophoritis) 614.2
  pancreas — *see* Pancreatitis
  parametrium (chronic) (*see also* Disease, pelvis, inflammatory) 614.4
    acute 614.3
  parotid region 686.9
    gland 527.2
  pelvis, female (*see also* Disease, pelvis, inflammatory) 614.9
  penis (corpora cavernosa) 607.2
  perianal 569.49

Inflammation, inflamed, inflammatory — *continued*
  pericardium (*see also* Pericarditis) 423.9
  perineum (female) (male) 686.9
  perirectal 569.49
  peritoneum (*see also* Peritonitis) 567.9
  periuterine (*see also* Disease, pelvis, inflammatory) 614.9
  perivesical (*see also* Cystitis) 595.9
  petrous bone (*see also* Petrositis) 383.20
  pharynx (*see also* Pharyngitis) 462
    follicular 472.1
    granular 472.1
  pia mater — *see* Meningitis
  pleura — *see* Pleurisy
  postmastoidectomy cavity 383.30
    chronic 383.33
  pouch, internal ileoanal 569.71
  prostate (*see also* Prostatitis) 601.9
  rectosigmoid — *see* Rectosigmoiditis
  rectum (*see also* Proctitis) 569.49
  respiratory, upper (*see also* Infection, respiratory, upper) 465.9
    chronic, due to external agent — *see* Condition, respiratory, chronic, due to, external agent
    due to
      fumes or vapors (chemical) (inhalation) 506.2
      radiation 508.1
  retina (*see also* Retinitis) 363.20
  retrocecal (*see also* Appendicitis) 541
  retroperitoneal (*see also* Peritonitis) 567.9
  salivary duct or gland (any) (suppurative) 527.2
  scorbutic, alveoli, teeth 267
  scrotum 608.4
  sigmoid — *see* Enteritis
  sinus (*see also* Sinusitis) 473.9
  Skene's duct or gland (*see also* Urethritis) 597.89
  skin 686.9
  spermatic cord 608.4
  sphenoidal (sinus) (*see also* Sinusitis, sphenoidal) 473.3
  spinal
    cord (*see also* Encephalitis) 323.9
      late effect — *see* category 326
    membrane — *see* Meningitis
    nerve — *see* Disorder, nerve
  spine (*see also* Spondylitis) 720.9
  spleen (capsule) 289.59
  stomach — *see* Gastritis
  stricture, rectum 569.49
  subcutaneous tissue NEC 686.9
  suprarenal (gland) 255.8
  synovial (fringe) (membrane) — *see* Bursitis
  tendon (sheath) NEC 726.90
  testis (*see also* Orchitis) 604.90
  thigh 686.9
  throat (*see also* Sore throat) 462
  thymus (gland) 254.8
  thyroid (gland) (*see also* Thyroiditis) 245.9
  tongue 529.0
  tonsil — *see* Tonsillitis
  trachea — *see* Tracheitis
  trochlear nerve 378.53
  tubal (*see also* Salpingo-oophoritis) 614.2
  tuberculous NEC (*see also* Tuberculosis) 011.9 ☑
  tubo-ovarian (*see also* Salpingo-oophoritis) 614.2
  tunica vaginalis 608.4
  tympanic membrane — *see* Myringitis
  umbilicus, umbilical 686.9
    newborn NEC 771.4
  uterine ligament (*see also* Disease, pelvis, inflammatory) 614.4
    acute 614.3
  uterus (catarrhal) (*see also* Endometritis) 615.9
  uveal tract (anterior) (*see also* Iridocyclitis) 364.3
    posterior — *see* Chorioretinitis
    sympathetic 360.11
  vagina (*see also* Vaginitis) 616.10

Inflammation, inflamed, inflammatory — *continued*
  vas deferens 608.4
  vein (*see also* Phlebitis) 451.9
    thrombotic 451.9
      cerebral (*see also* Thrombosis, brain) 434.0 ☑
      leg 451.2
        deep (vessels) NEC 451.19
        superficial (vessels) 451.0
      lower extremity 451.2
        deep (vessels) NEC 451.19
        superficial (vessels) 451.0
  vocal cord 478.5
  vulva (*see also* Vulvitis) 616.10

Inflation, lung imperfect (newborn) 770.5

Influenza, influenzal 487.1
  with
    bronchitis 487.1
    bronchopneumonia 487.0
    cold (any type) 487.1
    digestive manifestations 487.8
    hemoptysis 487.1
    involvement of
      gastrointestinal tract 487.8
      nervous system 487.8
    laryngitis 487.1
    manifestations NEC 487.8
      respiratory 487.1
        pneumonia 487.0
    pharyngitis 487.1
    pneumonia (any form classifiable to 480–483, 485–486) 487.0
    respiratory manifestations NEC 487.1
    sinusitis 487.1
    sore throat 487.1
    tonsillitis 487.1
    tracheitis 487.1
    upper respiratory infection (acute) 487.1
  abdominal 487.8
  A/H5N1 (*see also* Influenza, avian) 488.02
  Asian 487.1
  avian 488.02
    with involvement of gastrointestinal tract 488.09
    bronchopneumonia 488.01
    laryngitis 488.02
    manifestations NEC 488.09
      respiratory 488.02
    pharyngitis 488.02
    pneumonia (any form classifiable to 480-483, 485-486) 488.01
    respiratory infection (acute) (upper) 488.02
  bronchial 487.1
  bronchopneumonia 487.0
  catarrhal 487.1
  due to identified
    animal origin influenza virus — *see* Influenza, due to identified, novel influenza A virus
    avian influenza virus 488.02
      with
        manifestations NEC 488.09
          respiratory 488.02
        pneumonia (any form classifiable to 480-483, 485-486) 488.01
    (novel 2009) H1N1 influenza virus 488.12
      with
        manifestations NEC 488.19
          respiratory 488.12
        pneumonia 488.11
    novel influenza A virus 488.82
      with
        encephalopathy 488.89
        involvement of gastrointestinal tract 488.89
        laryngitis 488.82
        manifestations NEC 488.89
          respiratory (acute) (upper) 488.82
        pharyngitis 488.82
        pneumonia 488.81
  epidemic 487.1
  gastric 487.8

Influenza, influenzal — *continued*
  intestinal 487.8
  laryngitis 487.1
  maternal affecting fetus or newborn 760.2
    manifest influenza in infant 771.2
  (novel) 2009 H1N1 488.12
    with involvement of gastrointestinal tract 488.19
    bronchopneumonia 488.11
    laryngitis 488.12
    manifestations NEC 488.19
      respiratory 488.12
    pharyngitis 488.12
    pneumonia (any form classifiable to 480-483, 485-486) 488.11
    respiratory infection (acute) (upper) 488.12
  novel A/H1N1 (*see also* Influenza, (novel) 2009 H1N1) 488.12
  novel influenza A viruses not previously found in humans — *see* Influenza, due to identified, novel influenza A virus
  pharyngitis 487.1
  pneumonia (any form) 487.0
  respiratory (upper) 487.1
  specified NEC 487.1
  stomach 487.8
  vaccination, prophylactic (against) V04.81

Influenza-like disease — *see also* Influenza 487.1

Infraction, Freiberg's (metatarsal head) 732.5

Infraeruption, teeth 524.34

Infusion complication, misadventure, or reaction — *see* Complication, infusion

Ingestion
  chemical — *see* Table of Drugs and Chemicals
  drug or medicinal substance
    overdose or wrong substance given or taken 977.9
      specified drug — *see* Table of Drugs and Chemicals
  foreign body NEC (*see also* Foreign body) 938

Ingrowing
  hair 704.8
  nail (finger) (toe) (infected) 703.0

Inguinal — *see also* condition
  testis 752.51

Inhalation
  carbon monoxide 986
  flame
    lung 947.1
    mouth 947.0
  food or foreign body (*see also* Asphyxia, food or foreign body) 933.1
  gas, fumes, or vapor (noxious) 987.9
    specified agent — *see* Table of Drugs and Chemicals
  liquid or vomitus (*see also* Asphyxia, food or foreign body) 933.1
  lower respiratory tract NEC 934.9
  meconium (fetus or newborn) 770.11
    with respiratory symptoms 770.12
  mucus (*see also* Asphyxia, mucus) 933.1
  oil (causing suffocation) (*see also* Asphyxia, food or foreign body) 933.1
  pneumonia — *see* Pneumonia, aspiration
  smoke 508.2
  steam 987.9
  stomach contents or secretions (*see also* Asphyxia, food or foreign body) 933.1
    in labor and delivery 668.0 ☑

Inhibition, inhibited
  academic as adjustment reaction 309.23
  orgasm
    female 302.73
    male 302.74
  sexual
    desire 302.71
    excitement 302.72
  work as adjustment reaction 309.23

Inhibitor
  autoimmune, to clotting factors 286.52

☑ **Additional Digit Required** — Refer to the Tabular List for Digit Selection   ▽ **Subterms under main terms may continue to next column or page**

Inhibitor — *continued*
  systemic lupus erythematosus (presence of) 795.79
    with
      hemorrhagic disorder 286.53
      hypercoagulable state 289.81
Iniencephalus, iniencephaly 740.2
Injected eye 372.74
Injury 959.9

> *Note — For abrasion, insect bite (non-venomous), blister, or scratch, see Injury, superficial.*
>
> *For laceration, traumatic rupture, tear, or penetrating wound of internal organs, such as heart, lung, liver, kidney, pelvic organs, whether or not accompanied by open wound in the same region, see Injury, internal.*
>
> *For nerve injury, see Injury, nerve.*
>
> *For late effect of injuries classifiable to 850–854, 860–869, 900–919, 950–959, see Late, effect, injury, by type.*

  abdomen, abdominal (viscera) (*see also* Injury, internal, abdomen)
    muscle or wall 959.12
  acoustic, resulting in deafness 951.5
  adenoid 959.09
  adrenal (gland) — *see* Injury, internal, adrenal
  alveolar (process) 959.09
  ankle (and foot) (and knee) (and leg, except thigh) 959.7
  anterior chamber, eye 921.3
  anus 959.19
  aorta (thoracic) 901.0
    abdominal 902.0
  appendix — *see* Injury, internal, appendix
  arm, upper (and shoulder) 959.2
  artery (complicating trauma) (*see also* Injury, blood vessel, by site) 904.9
    cerebral or meningeal (*see also* Hemorrhage, brain, traumatic, subarachnoid) 852.0 ☑
  auditory canal (external) (meatus) 959.09
  auricle, auris, ear 959.09
  axilla 959.2
  back 959.19
  bile duct — *see* Injury, internal, bile duct
  birth (*see also* Birth, injury)
    canal NEC, complicating delivery 665.9 ☑
  bladder (sphincter) — *see* Injury, internal, bladder
  blast (air) (hydraulic) (immersion) (underwater) NEC 869.0
    with open wound into cavity NEC 869.1
    abdomen or thorax — *see* Injury, internal, by site
    brain — *see* Concussion, brain
    ear (acoustic nerve trauma) 951.5
      with perforation of tympanic membrane — *see* Wound, open, ear, drum
  blood vessel NEC 904.9
    abdomen 902.9
      multiple 902.87
      specified NEC 902.89
    aorta (thoracic) 901.0
      abdominal 902.0
    arm NEC 903.9
    axillary 903.00
      artery 903.01
      vein 903.02
    azygos vein 901.89
    basilic vein 903.1
    brachial (artery) (vein) 903.1
    bronchial 901.89
    carotid artery 900.00
      common 900.01
      external 900.02
      internal 900.03
    celiac artery 902.20
      specified branch NEC 902.24
    cephalic vein (arm) 903.1

Injury — *continued*
  blood vessel — *continued*
    colica dextra 902.26
    cystic
      artery 902.24
      vein 902.39
    deep plantar 904.6
    digital (artery) (vein) 903.5
    due to accidental puncture or laceration during procedure 998.2
    extremity
      lower 904.8
        multiple 904.7
        specified NEC 904.7
      upper 903.9
        multiple 903.8
        specified NEC 903.8
    femoral
      artery (superficial) 904.1
        above profunda origin 904.0
        common 904.0
      vein 904.2
    gastric
      artery 902.21
      vein 902.39
    head 900.9
      intracranial — *see* Injury, intracranial
      multiple 900.82
      specified NEC 900.89
    hemiazygos vein 901.89
    hepatic
      artery 902.22
      vein 902.11
    hypogastric 902.59
      artery 902.51
      vein 902.52
    ileocolic
      artery 902.26
      vein 902.31
    iliac 902.50
      artery 902.53
      specified branch NEC 902.59
      vein 902.54
    innominate
      artery 901.1
      vein 901.3
    intercostal (artery) (vein) 901.81
    jugular vein (external) 900.81
      internal 900.1
    leg NEC 904.8
    mammary (artery) (vein) 901.82
    mesenteric
      artery 902.20
        inferior 902.27
        specified branch NEC 902.29
        superior (trunk) 902.25
          branches, primary 902.26
      vein 902.39
        inferior 902.32
        superior (and primary subdivisions) 902.31
    neck 900.9
      multiple 900.82
      specified NEC 900.89
    ovarian 902.89
      artery 902.81
      vein 902.82
    palmar artery 903.4
    pelvis 902.9
      multiple 902.87
      specified NEC 902.89
    plantar (deep) (artery) (vein) 904.6
    popliteal 904.40
      artery 904.41
      vein 904.42
    portal 902.33
    pulmonary 901.40
      artery 901.41
      vein 901.42
    radial (artery) (vein) 903.2
    renal 902.40
      artery 902.41
      specified NEC 902.49
      vein 902.42
    saphenous
      artery 904.7

Injury — *continued*
  blood vessel — *continued*
    saphenous — *continued*
      vein (greater) (lesser) 904.3
    splenic
      artery 902.23
      vein 902.34
    subclavian
      artery 901.1
      vein 901.3
    suprarenal 902.49
    thoracic 901.9
      multiple 901.83
      specified NEC 901.89
    tibial 904.50
      artery 904.50
        anterior 904.51
        posterior 904.53
      vein 904.50
        anterior 904.52
        posterior 904.54
    ulnar (artery) (vein) 903.3
    uterine 902.59
      artery 902.55
      vein 902.56
    vena cava
      inferior 902.10
        specified branches NEC 902.19
      superior 901.2
  brachial plexus 953.4
    newborn 767.6
  brain (traumatic) NEC (*see also* Injury, intracranial) 854.0 ☑
    due to fracture of skull — *see* Fracture, skull, by site
  breast 959.19
  broad ligament — *see* Injury, internal, broad ligament
  bronchus, bronchi — *see* Injury, internal, bronchus
  brow 959.09
  buttock 959.19
  canthus, eye 921.1
  cathode ray 990
  cauda equina 952.4
    with fracture, vertebra — *see* Fracture, vertebra, sacrum
  cavernous sinus (*see also* Injury, intracranial) 854.0 ☑
  cecum — *see* Injury, internal, cecum
  celiac ganglion or plexus 954.1
  cerebellum (*see also* Injury, intracranial) 854.0 ☑
  cervix (uteri) — *see* Injury, internal, cervix
  cheek 959.09
  chest (*see also* Injury, internal, chest)
    wall 959.11
  childbirth (*see also* Birth, injury)
    maternal NEC 665.9 ☑
  chin 959.09
  choroid (eye) 921.3
  clitoris 959.14
  coccyx 959.19
    complicating delivery 665.6 ☑
  colon — *see* Injury, internal, colon
  common duct — *see* Injury, internal, common duct
  conjunctiva 921.1
    superficial 918.2
  cord
    spermatic — *see* Injury, internal, spermatic cord
    spinal — *see* Injury, spinal, by site
  cornea 921.3
    abrasion 918.1
    due to contact lens 371.82
    penetrating — *see* Injury, eyeball, penetrating
    superficial 918.1
      due to contact lens 371.82
  cortex (cerebral) (*see also* Injury, intracranial) 854.0 ☑
    visual 950.3
  costal region 959.11
  costochondral 959.11

Injury — *continued*
  cranial
    bones — *see* Fracture, skull, by site
    cavity (*see also* Injury, intracranial) 854.0 ☑
    nerve — *see* Injury, nerve, cranial
  crushing — *see* Crush
  cutaneous sensory nerve
    lower limb 956.4
    upper limb 955.5
  deep tissue — *see* Contusion, by site
    meaning pressure ulcer 707.25
  delivery (*see also* Birth, injury)
    maternal NEC 665.9 ☑
  Descemet's membrane — *see* Injury, eyeball, penetrating
  diaphragm — *see* Injury, internal, diaphragm
  diffuse axonal — *see* Injury, intracranial
  duodenum — *see* Injury, internal, duodenum
  ear (auricle) (canal) (drum) (external) 959.09
  elbow (and forearm) (and wrist) 959.3
  epididymis 959.14
  epigastric region 959.12
  epiglottis 959.09
  epiphyseal, current — *see* Fracture, by site
  esophagus — *see* Injury, internal, esophagus
  Eustachian tube 959.09
  extremity (lower) (upper) NEC 959.8
  eye 921.9
    penetrating eyeball — *see* Injury, eyeball, penetrating
    superficial 918.9
  eyeball 921.3
    penetrating 871.7
      with
        partial loss (of intraocular tissue) 871.2
        prolapse or exposure (of intraocular tissue) 871.1
      without prolapse 871.0
      foreign body (nonmagnetic) 871.6
        magnetic 871.5
    superficial 918.9
  eyebrow 959.09
  eyelid(s) 921.1
    laceration — *see* Laceration, eyelid
    superficial 918.0
  face (and neck) 959.09
  fallopian tube — *see* Injury, internal, fallopian tube
  finger(s) (nail) 959.5
  flank 959.19
  foot (and ankle) (and knee) (and leg, except thigh) 959.7
  forceps NEC 767.9
    scalp 767.19
  forearm (and elbow) (and wrist) 959.3
  forehead 959.09
  gallbladder — *see* Injury, internal, gallbladder
  gasserian ganglion 951.2
  gastrointestinal tract — *see* Injury, internal, gastrointestinal tract
  genital organ(s)
    with
      abortion — *see* Abortion, by type, with, damage to pelvic organs
      ectopic pregnancy (*see also* categories 633.0–633.9) 639.2
      molar pregnancy (*see also* categories 630–632) 639.2
    external 959.14
      fracture of corpus cavernosum penis 959.13
    following
      abortion 639.2
      ectopic or molar pregnancy 639.2
    internal — *see* Injury, internal, genital organs
    obstetrical trauma NEC 665.9 ☑
      affecting fetus or newborn 763.89
  gland
    lacrimal 921.1

Injury — *continued*
 gland — *continued*
  lacrimal — *continued*
   laceration 870.8
  parathyroid 959.09
  salivary 959.09
  thyroid 959.09
 globe (eye) (*see also* Injury, eyeball) 921.3
 grease gun — *see* Wound, open, by site,
  complicated
 groin 959.19
 gum 959.09
 hand(s) (except fingers) 959.4
 head NEC 959.01
  with
   loss of consciousness 850.5
   skull fracture — *see* Fracture, skull,
    by site
 heart — *see* Injury, internal, heart
 heel 959.7
 hip (and thigh) 959.6
 hymen 959.14
 hyperextension (cervical) (vertebra) 847.0
 ileum — *see* Injury, internal, ileum
 iliac region 959.19
 infrared rays NEC 990
 instrumental (during surgery) 998.2
  birth injury — *see* Birth, injury
  nonsurgical (*see also* Injury, by site) 959.9
  obstetrical 665.9 ☑
   affecting fetus or newborn 763.89
   bladder 665.5 ☑
   cervix 665.3 ☑
   high vaginal 665.4 ☑
   perineal NEC 664.9 ☑
   urethra 665.5 ☑
   uterus 665.5 ☑
 internal 869.0

> Note — For injury of internal organ(s) by foreign body entering through a natural orifice (e.g., inhaled, ingested, or swallowed) — see Foreign body, entering through orifice.
>
> For internal injury of any of the following sites with internal injury of any other of the sites — see Injury, internal, multiple.

  with
   fracture
    pelvis — *see* Fracture, pelvis
    specified site, except pelvis — *see*
     Injury, internal, by site
   open wound into cavity 869.1
  abdomen, abdominal (viscera) NEC
   868.00
   with
    fracture, pelvis — *see* Fracture,
     pelvis
    open wound into cavity
     868.10
    specified site NEC 868.09
     with open wound into cavity
      868.19
  adrenal (gland) 868.01
   with open wound into cavity 868.11
  aorta (thoracic) 901.0
   abdominal 902.0
  appendix 863.85
   with open wound into cavity 863.95
  bile duct 868.02
   with open wound into cavity 868.12
  bladder (sphincter) 867.0
   with
    abortion — *see* Abortion, by type,
     with damage to pelvic organs
    ectopic pregnancy (*see also* categories 633.0–633.9) 639.2
    molar pregnancy (*see also* categories 630–632) 639.2
    open wound into cavity 867.1
   following
    abortion 639.2
    ectopic or molar pregnancy 639.2
   obstetrical trauma 665.5 ☑

Injury — *continued*
 internal — *continued*
  bladder — *continued*
   obstetrical trauma — *continued*
    affecting fetus or newborn 763.89
  blood vessel — *see* Injury, blood vessel,
   by site
  broad ligament 867.6
   with open wound into cavity 867.7
  bronchus, bronchi 862.21
   with open wound into cavity 862.31
  cecum 863.89
   with open wound into cavity 863.99
  cervix (uteri) 867.4
   with
    abortion — *see* Abortion, by type,
     with damage to pelvic organs
    ectopic pregnancy (*see also* categories 633.0–633.9) 639.2
    molar pregnancy (*see also* categories 630–632) 639.2
    open wound into cavity 867.5
   following
    abortion 639.2
    ectopic or molar pregnancy 639.2
   obstetrical trauma 665.3 ☑
    affecting fetus or newborn 763.89
  chest (*see also* Injury, internal, intrathoracic organs) 862.8
   with open wound into cavity 862.9
  colon 863.40
   with
    open wound into cavity 863.50
    rectum 863.46
     with open wound into cavity
      863.56
   ascending (right) 863.41
    with open wound into cavity
     863.51
   descending (left) 863.43
    with open wound into cavity
     863.53
   multiple sites 863.46
    with open wound into cavity
     863.56
   sigmoid 863.44
    with open wound into cavity
     863.54
   specified site NEC 863.49
    with open wound into cavity
     863.59
   transverse 863.42
    with open wound into cavity
     863.52
  common duct 868.02
   with open wound into cavity 868.12
  complicating delivery 665.9 ☑
   affecting fetus or newborn 763.89
  diaphragm 862.0
   with open wound into cavity 862.1
  duodenum 863.21
   with open wound into cavity 863.31
  esophagus (intrathoracic) 862.22
   with open wound into cavity 862.32
   cervical region 874.4
    complicated 874.5
  fallopian tube 867.6
   with open wound into cavity 867.7
  gallbladder 868.02
   with open wound into cavity 868.12
  gastrointestinal tract NEC 863.80
   with open wound into cavity 863.90
  genital organ NEC 867.6
   with open wound into cavity 867.7
  heart 861.00
   with open wound into thorax 861.10
  ileum 863.29
   with open wound into cavity 863.39
  intestine NEC 863.89
   with open wound into cavity 863.99
   large NEC 863.40
    with open wound into cavity
     863.50
   small NEC 863.20

Injury — *continued*
 internal — *continued*
  intestine — *continued*
   small — *continued*
    with open wound into cavity
     863.30
  intra-abdominal (organ) 868.00
   with open wound into cavity 868.10
   multiple sites 868.09
    with open wound into cavity
     868.19
   specified site NEC 868.09
    with open wound into cavity
     868.19
  intrathoracic organs (multiple) 862.8
   with open wound into cavity 862.9
   diaphragm (only) — *see* Injury, internal, diaphragm
   heart (only) — *see* Injury, internal, heart
   lung (only) — *see* Injury, internal, lung
   specified site NEC 862.29
    with open wound into cavity
     862.39
  intrauterine (*see also* Injury, internal, uterus) 867.4
   with open wound into cavity 867.5
  jejunum 863.29
   with open wound into cavity 863.39
  kidney (subcapsular) 866.00
   with
    disruption of parenchyma (complete) 866.03
     with open wound into cavity
      866.13
    hematoma (without rupture of capsule) 866.01
     with open wound into cavity
      866.11
    laceration 866.02
     with open wound into cavity
      866.12
   open wound into cavity 866.10
  liver 864.00
   with
    contusion 864.01
     with open wound into cavity
      864.11
    hematoma 864.01
     with open wound into cavity
      864.11
    laceration 864.05
     with open wound into cavity
      864.15
    major (disruption of hepatic parenchyma) 864.04
     with open wound into cavity 864.14
    minor (capsule only) 864.02
     with open wound into cavity 864.12
    moderate (involving parenchyma) 864.03
     with open wound into cavity 864.13
    multiple 864.04
    stellate 864.04
     with open wound into cavity 864.14
   open wound into cavity 864.10
  lung 861.20
   with open wound into thorax 861.30
   aspiration 507.0
   hemopneumothorax — *see* Hemopneumothorax, traumatic
   hemothorax — *see* Hemothorax, traumatic
   pneumohemothorax — *see* Pneumohemothorax, traumatic
   pneumothorax — *see* Pneumothorax, traumatic
   transfusion related, acute (TRALI) 518.7
  mediastinum 862.29
   with open wound into cavity 862.39

Injury — *continued*
 internal — *continued*
  mesentery 863.89
   with open wound into cavity 863.99
  mesosalpinx 867.6
   with open wound into cavity 867.7
  multiple 869.0

> Note — Multiple internal injuries of sites classifiable to the same three- or four-digit category should be classified to that category.
>
> Multiple injuries classifiable to different fourth-digit subdivisions of 861 (heart and lung injuries) should be dealt with according to coding rules.

   internal
    with open wound into cavity 869.1
   intra-abdominal organ (sites classifiable to 863–868)
    with
     intrathoracic organ(s) (sites classifiable to 861–862) 869.0
      with open wound into cavity 869.1
     other intra-abdominal organ(s) (sites classifiable to 863–868, except where classifiable to the same three-digit category) 868.09
      with open wound into cavity 868.19
   intrathoracic organ (sites classifiable to 861–862)
    with
     intra-abdominal organ(s) (sites classifiable to 863–868) 869.0
      with open wound into cavity 869.1
     other intrathoracic organ(s) (sites classifiable to 861–862, except where classifiable to the same three-digit category) 862.8
      with open wound into cavity 862.9
  myocardium — *see* Injury, internal, heart
  ovary 867.6
   with open wound into cavity 867.7
  pancreas (multiple sites) 863.84
   with open wound into cavity 863.94
   body 863.82
    with open wound into cavity
     863.92
   head 863.81
    with open wound into cavity
     863.91
   tail 863.83
    with open wound into cavity
     863.93
  pelvis, pelvic (organs) (viscera) 867.8
   with
    fracture, pelvis — *see* Fracture, pelvis
    open wound into cavity 867.9
   specified site NEC 867.6
    with open wound into cavity
     867.7
  peritoneum 868.03
   with open wound into cavity 868.13
  pleura 862.29
   with open wound into cavity 862.39
  prostate 867.6
   with open wound into cavity 867.7
  rectum 863.45
   with
    colon 863.46
     with open wound into cavity
      863.56
    open wound into cavity 863.55
  retroperitoneum 868.04

☑ Additional Digit Required — Refer to the Tabular List for Digit Selection   ⚑ Subterms under main terms may continue to next column or page

2014 ICD-9-CM   207

Injury — continued
  internal — *continued*
    retroperitoneum — *continued*
      with open wound into cavity 868.14
    round ligament 867.6
      with open wound into cavity 867.7
    seminal vesicle 867.6
      with open wound into cavity 867.7
    spermatic cord 867.6
      with open wound into cavity 867.7
      scrotal — *see* Wound, open, spermatic cord
    spleen 865.00
      with
        disruption of parenchyma (massive) 865.04
          with open wound into cavity 865.14
        hematoma (without rupture of capsule) 865.01
          with open wound into cavity 865.11
        open wound into cavity 865.10
        tear, capsular 865.02
          with open wound into cavity 865.12
        extending into parenchyma 865.03
          with open wound into cavity 865.13
    stomach 863.0
      with open wound into cavity 863.1
    suprarenal gland (multiple) 868.01
      with open wound into cavity 868.11
    thorax, thoracic (cavity) (organs) (multiple) (*see also* Injury, internal, intrathoracic organs) 862.8
      with open wound into cavity 862.9
    thymus (gland) 862.29
      with open wound into cavity 862.39
    trachea (intrathoracic) 862.29
      with open wound into cavity 862.39
      cervical region (*see also* Wound, open, trachea) 874.02
    ureter 867.2
      with open wound into cavity 867.3
    urethra (sphincter) 867.0
      with
        abortion — *see* Abortion, by type, with damage to pelvic organs
        ectopic pregnancy (*see also* categories 633.0–633.9) 639.2
        molar pregnancy (*see also* categories 630–632) 639.2
        open wound into cavity 867.1
      following
        abortion 639.2
        ectopic or molar pregnancy 639.2
      obstetrical trauma 665.5 ☑
        affecting fetus or newborn 763.89
    uterus 867.4
      with
        abortion — *see* Abortion, by type, with damage to pelvic organs
        ectopic pregnancy (*see also* categories 633.0–633.9) 639.2
        molar pregnancy (*see also* categories 630–632) 639.2
        open wound into cavity 867.5
      following
        abortion 639.2
        ectopic or molar pregnancy 639.2
      obstetrical trauma NEC 665.5 ☑
        affecting fetus or newborn 763.89
    vas deferens 867.6
      with open wound into cavity 867.7
    vesical (sphincter) 867.0
      with open wound into cavity 867.1
    viscera (abdominal) (*see also* Injury, internal, multiple) 868.00
      with
        fracture, pelvis — *see* Fracture, pelvis
        open wound into cavity 868.10

Injury — continued
  internal — *continued*
    viscera (*see also* Injury, internal, multiple) — *continued*
      thoracic NEC (*see also* Injury, internal, intrathoracic organs) 862.8
        with open wound into cavity 862.9
    interscapular region 959.19
    intervertebral disc 959.19
    intestine — *see* Injury, internal, intestine
    intra-abdominal (organs) NEC — *see* Injury, internal, intra-abdominal
    intracranial (traumatic) 854.0 ☑

Note — *Use the following fifth-digit subclassification with categories 851–854:*

0   unspecified state of consciousness

1   with no loss of consciousness

2   with brief [less than one hour] loss of consciousness

3   with moderate [1–24 hours] loss of consciousness

4   with prolonged [more than 24 hours] loss of consciousness and return to pre–existing conscious level

5   with prolonged [more than 24 hours] loss of consciousness, without return to pre–existing conscious level

Use fifth-digit 5 to designate when a patient is unconscious and dies before regaining consciousness, regardless of the duration of the loss of consciousness

6   with loss of consciousness of unspecified duration

9   with concussion, unspecified

    with
      open intracranial wound 854.1 ☑
      skull fracture — *see* Fracture, skull, by site
    contusion 851.8 ☑
      with open intracranial wound 851.9 ☑
      brain stem 851.4 ☑
        with open intracranial wound 851.5 ☑
      cerebellum 851.4 ☑
        with open intracranial wound 851.5 ☑
      cortex (cerebral) 851.0 ☑
        with open intracranial wound 851.2 ☑
    hematoma — *see* Injury, intracranial, hemorrhage
    hemorrhage 853.0 ☑
      with
        laceration — *see* Injury, intracranial, laceration
        open intracranial wound 853.1 ☑
      extradural 852.4 ☑
        with open intracranial wound 852.5 ☑
      subarachnoid 852.0 ☑
        with open intracranial wound 852.1 ☑
      subdural 852.2 ☑
        with open intracranial wound 852.3 ☑
    laceration 851.8 ☑
      with open intracranial wound 851.9 ☑
      brain stem 851.6 ☑
        with open intracranial wound 851.7 ☑
      cerebellum 851.6 ☑
        with open intracranial wound 851.7 ☑
      cortex (cerebral) 851.2 ☑

Injury — continued
  intracranial — *continued*
    laceration — *continued*
      cortex — *continued*
        with open intracranial wound 851.3 ☑
    intraocular — *see* Injury, eyeball, penetrating
    intrathoracic organs (multiple) — *see* Injury, internal, intrathoracic organs
    intrauterine — *see* Injury, internal, intrauterine
    iris 921.3
      penetrating — *see* Injury, eyeball, penetrating
    jaw 959.09
    jejunum — *see* Injury, internal, jejunum
    joint NEC 959.9
      old or residual 718.80
        ankle 718.87
        elbow 718.82
        foot 718.87
        hand 718.84
        hip 718.85
        knee 718.86
        multiple sites 718.89
        pelvic region 718.85
        shoulder (region) 718.81
        specified site NEC 718.88
        wrist 718.83
    kidney — *see* Injury, internal, kidney
      acute (nontraumatic) 584.9
    knee (and ankle) (and foot) (and leg, except thigh) 959.7
    labium (majus) (minus) 959.14
    labyrinth, ear 959.09
    lacrimal apparatus, gland, or sac 921.1
      laceration 870.8
    larynx 959.09
    late effect — *see* Late, effects (of), injury
    leg, except thigh (and ankle) (and foot) (and knee) 959.7
      upper or thigh 959.6
    lens, eye 921.3
      penetrating — *see* Injury, eyeball, penetrating
    lid, eye — *see* Injury, eyelid
    lip 959.09
    liver — *see* Injury, internal, liver
    lobe, parietal — *see* Injury, intracranial
    lumbar (region) 959.19
      plexus 953.5
    lumbosacral (region) 959.19
      plexus 953.5
    lung — *see* Injury, internal, lung
    malar region 959.09
    mastoid region 959.09
    maternal, during pregnancy, affecting fetus or newborn 760.5
    maxilla 959.09
    mediastinum — *see* Injury, internal, mediastinum
    membrane
      brain (*see also* Injury, intracranial) 854.0 ☑
      tympanic 959.09
    meningeal artery — *see* Hemorrhage, brain, traumatic, subarachnoid
    meninges (cerebral) — *see* Injury, intracranial
    mesenteric
      artery — *see* Injury, blood vessel, mesenteric, artery
      plexus, inferior 954.1
      vein — *see* Injury, blood vessel, mesenteric, vein
    mesentery — *see* Injury, internal, mesentery
    mesosalpinx — *see* Injury, internal, mesosalpinx
    middle ear 959.09
    midthoracic region 959.11
    mouth 959.09
    multiple (sites not classifiable to the same four-digit category in 959.0–959.7) 959.8
      internal 869.0

Injury — continued
  multiple — *continued*
    internal — *continued*
      with open wound into cavity 869.1
    musculocutaneous nerve 955.4
    nail
      finger 959.5
      toe 959.7
    nasal (septum) (sinus) 959.09
    nasopharynx 959.09
    neck (and face) 959.09
    nerve 957.9
      abducens 951.3
      abducent 951.3
      accessory 951.6
      acoustic 951.5
      ankle and foot 956.9
      anterior crural, femoral 956.1
      arm (*see also* Injury, nerve, upper limb) 955.9
      auditory 951.5
      axillary 955.0
      brachial plexus 953.4
      cervical sympathetic 954.0
      cranial 951.9
        first or olfactory 951.8
        second or optic 950.0
        third or oculomotor 951.0
        fourth or trochlear 951.1
        fifth or trigeminal 951.2
        sixth or abducens 951.3
        seventh or facial 951.4
        eighth, acoustic, or auditory 951.5
        ninth or glossopharyngeal 951.8
        tenth, pneumogastric, or vagus 951.8
        eleventh or accessory 951.6
        twelfth or hypoglossal 951.7
        newborn 767.7
      cutaneous sensory
        lower limb 956.4
        upper limb 955.5
      digital (finger) 955.6
        toe 956.5
      facial 951.4
        newborn 767.5
      femoral 956.1
      finger 955.9
      foot and ankle 956.9
      forearm 955.9
      glossopharyngeal 951.8
      hand and wrist 955.9
      head and neck, superficial 957.0
      hypoglossal 951.7
      involving several parts of body 957.8
      leg (*see also* Injury, nerve, lower limb) 956.9
      lower limb 956.9
        multiple 956.8
        specified site NEC 956.5
      lumbar plexus 953.5
      lumbosacral plexus 953.5
      median 955.1
        forearm 955.1
        wrist and hand 955.1
      multiple (in several parts of body) (sites not classifiable to the same three-digit category) 957.8
      musculocutaneous 955.4
      musculospiral 955.3
        upper arm 955.3
      oculomotor 951.0
      olfactory 951.8
      optic 950.0
      pelvic girdle 956.9
        multiple sites 956.8
        specified site NEC 956.5
      peripheral 957.9
        multiple (in several regions) (sites not classifiable to the same three-digit category) 957.8
        specified site NEC 957.1
      peroneal 956.3
        ankle and foot 956.3
        lower leg 956.3
      plantar 956.5
      plexus 957.9

Injury — *continued*
  nerve — *continued*
    plexus — *continued*
      celiac 954.1
      mesenteric, inferior 954.1
      spinal 953.9
        brachial 953.4
        lumbosacral 953.5
        multiple sites 953.8
      sympathetic NEC 954.1
    pneumogastric 951.8
    radial 955.3
      wrist and hand 955.3
    sacral plexus 953.5
    sciatic 956.0
      thigh 956.0
    shoulder girdle 955.9
      multiple 955.8
      specified site NEC 955.7
    specified site NEC 957.1
    spinal 953.9
      plexus — *see* Injury, nerve, plexus, spinal
      root 953.9
        cervical 953.0
        dorsal 953.1
        lumbar 953.2
        multiple sites 953.8
        sacral 953.3
    splanchnic 954.1
    sympathetic NEC 954.1
      cervical 954.0
    thigh 956.9
    tibial 956.5
      ankle and foot 956.2
      lower leg 956.5
      posterior 956.2
    toe 956.9
    trigeminal 951.2
    trochlear 951.1
    trunk, excluding shoulder and pelvic girdles 954.9
      specified site NEC 954.8
      sympathetic NEC 954.1
    ulnar 955.2
      forearm 955.2
      wrist (and hand) 955.2
    upper limb 955.9
      multiple 955.8
      specified site NEC 955.7
    vagus 951.8
    wrist and hand 955.9
  nervous system, diffuse 957.8
  nose (septum) 959.09
  obstetrical NEC 665.9 ☑
    affecting fetus or newborn 763.89
  occipital (region) (scalp) 959.09
    lobe (*see also* Injury, intracranial) 854.0 ☑
  optic 950.9
    chiasm 950.1
    cortex 950.3
    nerve 950.0
    pathways 950.2
  orbit, orbital (region) 921.2
    penetrating 870.3
      with foreign body 870.4
  ovary — *see* Injury, internal, ovary
  paint-gun — *see* Wound, open, by site, complicated
  palate (soft) 959.09
  pancreas — *see* Injury, internal, pancreas
  parathyroid (gland) 959.09
  parietal (region) (scalp) 959.09
    lobe — *see* Injury, intracranial
  pelvic
    floor 959.19
      complicating delivery 664.1 ☑
        affecting fetus or newborn 763.89
    joint or ligament, complicating delivery 665.6 ☑
      affecting fetus or newborn 763.89
    organs (*see also* Injury, internal, pelvis)

Injury — *continued*
  pelvic — *continued*
    organs (*see also* Injury, internal, pelvis) — *continued*
      with
        abortion — *see* Abortion, by type, with damage to pelvic organs
        ectopic pregnancy (*see also* categories 633.0–633.9) 639.2
        molar pregnancy (*see also* categories 633.0–633.9) 639.2
      following
        abortion 639.2
        ectopic or molar pregnancy 639.2
      obstetrical trauma 665.5 ☑
        affecting fetus or newborn 763.89
  pelvis 959.19
  penis 959.14
    fracture of corpus cavernosum 959.13
  perineum 959.14
  peritoneum — *see* Injury, internal, peritoneum
  periurethral tissue
    with
      abortion — *see* Abortion, by type, with damage to pelvic organs
      ectopic pregnancy (*see also* categories 633.0–633.9) 639.2
      molar pregnancy (*see also* categories 630–632) 639.2
    complicating delivery 664.8 ☑
      affecting fetus or newborn 763.89
    following
      abortion 639.2
      ectopic or molar pregnancy 639.2
  phalanges
    foot 959.7
    hand 959.5
  pharynx 959.09
  pleura — *see* Injury, internal, pleura
  popliteal space 959.7
  post-cardiac surgery (syndrome) 429.4
  prepuce 959.14
  prostate — *see* Injury, internal, prostate
  pubic region 959.19
  pudenda 959.14
  radiation NEC 990
  radioactive substance or radium NEC 990
  rectovaginal septum 959.14
  rectum — *see* Injury, internal, rectum
  retina 921.3
    penetrating — *see* Injury, eyeball, penetrating
  retroperitoneal — *see* Injury, internal, retroperitoneum
  roentgen rays NEC 990
  round ligament — *see* Injury, internal, round ligament
  sacral (region) 959.19
    plexus 953.5
  sacroiliac ligament NEC 959.19
  sacrum 959.19
  salivary ducts or glands 959.09
  scalp 959.09
    due to birth trauma 767.19
    fetus or newborn 767.19
  scapular region 959.2
  sclera 921.3
    penetrating — *see* Injury, eyeball, penetrating
    superficial 918.2
  scrotum 959.14
  seminal vesicle — *see* Injury, internal, seminal vesicle
  shoulder (and upper arm) 959.2
  sinus
    cavernous (*see also* Injury, intracranial) 854.0 ☑
    nasal 959.09
  skeleton NEC, birth injury 767.3
  skin NEC 959.9
  skull — *see* Fracture, skull, by site
  soft tissue (of external sites) (severe) — *see* Wound, open, by site
  specified site NEC 959.8

Injury — *continued*
  spermatic cord — *see* Injury, internal, spermatic cord
  spinal (cord) 952.9
    with fracture, vertebra — *see* Fracture, vertebra, by site, with spinal cord injury
    cervical (C_1-C_4) 952.00
      with
        anterior cord syndrome 952.02
        central cord syndrome 952.03
        complete lesion of cord 952.01
        incomplete lesion NEC 952.04
        posterior cord syndrome 952.04
    C_5-C_7 level 952.05
      with
        anterior cord syndrome 952.07
        central cord syndrome 952.08
        complete lesion of cord 952.06
        incomplete lesion NEC 952.09
        posterior cord syndrome 952.09
      specified type NEC 952.09
    specified type NEC 952.04
    dorsal (D_1-D_6) (T_1-T_6) (thoracic) 952.10
      with
        anterior cord syndrome 952.12
        central cord syndrome 952.13
        complete lesion of cord 952.11
        incomplete lesion NEC 952.14
        posterior cord syndrome 952.14
    D_7-D_{12} level (T_7-T_{12}) 952.15
      with
        anterior cord syndrome 952.17
        central cord syndrome 952.18
        complete lesion of cord 952.16
        incomplete lesion NEC 952.19
        posterior cord syndrome 952.19
      specified type NEC 952.19
    specified type NEC 952.14
    lumbar 952.2
    multiple sites 952.8
    nerve (root) NEC — *see* Injury, nerve, spinal, root
    plexus 953.9
      brachial 953.4
      lumbosacral 953.5
      multiple sites 953.8
    sacral 952.3
    thoracic (*see also* Injury, spinal, dorsal) 952.10
  spleen — *see* Injury, internal, spleen
  stellate ganglion 954.1
  sternal region 959.11
  stomach — *see* Injury, internal, stomach
  subconjunctival 921.1
  subcutaneous 959.9
  subdural — *see* Injury, intracranial
  submaxillary region 959.09
  submental region 959.09
  subungual
    fingers 959.5
    toes 959.7

Injury — *continued*
  superficial 919 ☑

> Note — Use the following fourth-digit subdivisions with categories 910–919:
>
> 0   Abrasion or friction burn without mention of infection
>
> 1   Abrasion or friction burn, infected
>
> 2   Blister without mention of infection
>
> 3   Blister, infected
>
> 4   Insect bite, nonvenomous, without mention of infection
>
> 5   Insect bite, nonvenomous, infected
>
> 6   Superficial foreign body (splinter) without major open wound and without mention of infection
>
> 7   Superficial foreign body (splinter) without major open wound, infected
>
> 8   Other and unspecified superficial injury without mention of infection
>
> 9   Other and unspecified superficial injury, infected
>
> *For late effects of superficial injury, see category 906.2.*

    abdomen, abdominal (muscle) (wall) (and other part(s) of trunk) 911 ☑
    ankle (and hip, knee, leg, or thigh) 916 ☑
    anus (and other part(s) of trunk) 911 ☑
    arm 913 ☑
      upper (and shoulder) 912 ☑
    auditory canal (external) (meatus) (and other part(s) of face, neck, or scalp, except eye) 910 ☑
    axilla (and upper arm) 912 ☑
    back (and other part(s) of trunk) 911 ☑
    breast (and other part(s) of trunk) 911 ☑
    brow (and other part(s) of face, neck, or scalp, except eye) 910 ☑
    buttock (and other part(s) of trunk) 911 ☑
    canthus, eye 918.0
    cheek(s) (and other part(s) of face, neck, or scalp, except eye) 910 ☑
    chest wall (and other part(s) of trunk) 911 ☑
    chin (and other part(s) of face, neck, or scalp, except eye) 910 ☑
    clitoris (and other part(s) of trunk) 911 ☑
    conjunctiva 918.2
    cornea 918.1
      due to contact lens 371.82
    costal region (and other part(s) of trunk) 911 ☑
    ear(s) (auricle) (canal) (drum) (external) (and other part(s) of face, neck, or scalp, except eye) 910 ☑
    elbow (and forearm) (and wrist) 913 ☑
    epididymis (and other part(s) of trunk) 911 ☑
    epigastric region (and other part(s) of trunk) 911 ☑
    epiglottis (and other part(s) of face, neck, or scalp, except eye) 910 ☑
    eyelid(s) (and periocular area) 918.0
    eye(s) (and adnexa) NEC 918.9
    face (any part(s), except eye) (and neck or scalp) 910 ☑
    finger(s) (nail) (any) 915 ☑
    flank (and other part(s) of trunk) 911 ☑
    foot (phalanges) (and toe(s)) 917 ☑
    forearm (and elbow) (and wrist) 913 ☑
    forehead (and other part(s) of face, neck, or scalp, except eye) 910 ☑
    globe (eye) 918.9

☑ **Additional Digit Required** — Refer to the Tabular List for Digit Selection   ▼ **Subterms under main terms may continue to next column or page**

2014 ICD-9-CM   **209**

Injury — *continued*
  superficial — *continued*
    groin (and other part) of trunk) 911 ☑
    gum(s) (and other part(s) of face, neck, or scalp, except eye) 910 ☑
    hand(s) (except fingers alone) 914 ☑
    head (and other part(s) of face, neck, or scalp, except eye) 910 ☑
    heel (and foot or toe) 917 ☑
    hip (and ankle, knee, leg, or thigh) 916 ☑
    iliac region (and other part(s) of trunk) 911 ☑
    interscapular region (and other part(s) of trunk) 911 ☑
    iris 918.9
    knee (and ankle, hip, leg, or thigh) 916 ☑
    labium (majus) (minus) (and other part(s) of trunk) 911 ☑
    lacrimal (apparatus) (gland) (sac) 918.0
    leg (lower) (upper) (and ankle, hip, knee, or thigh) 916 ☑
    lip(s) (and other part(s) of face, neck, or scalp, except eye) 910 ☑
    lower extremity (except foot) 916 ☑
    lumbar region (and other part(s) of trunk) 911 ☑
    malar region (and other part(s) of face, neck, or scalp, except eye) 910 ☑
    mastoid region (and other part(s) of face, neck, or scalp, except eye) 910 ☑
    midthoracic region (and other part(s) of trunk) 911 ☑
    mouth (and other part(s) of face, neck, or scalp, except eye) 910 ☑
    multiple sites (not classifiable to the same three-digit category) 919 ☑
    nasal (septum) (and other part(s) of face, neck, or scalp, except eye) 910 ☑
    neck (and face or scalp, any part(s), except eye) 910 ☑
    nose (septum) (and other part(s) of face, neck, or scalp, except eye) 910 ☑
    occipital region (and other part(s) of face, neck, or scalp, except eye) 910 ☑
    orbital region 918.0
    palate (soft) (and other part(s) of face, neck, or scalp, except eye) 910 ☑
    parietal region (and other part(s) of face, neck, or scalp, except eye) 910 ☑
    penis (and other part(s) of trunk) 911 ☑
    perineum (and other part(s) of trunk) 911 ☑
    periocular area 918.0
    pharynx (and other part(s) of face, neck, or scalp, except eye) 910 ☑
    popliteal space (and ankle, hip, leg, or thigh) 916 ☑
    prepuce (and other part(s) of trunk) 911 ☑
    pubic region (and other part(s) of trunk) 911 ☑
    pudenda (and other part(s) of trunk) 911 ☑
    sacral region (and other part(s) of trunk) 911 ☑
    salivary (ducts) (glands) (and other part(s) of face, neck, or scalp, except eye) 910 ☑
    scalp (and other part(s) of face or neck, except eye) 910 ☑
    scapular region (and upper arm) 912 ☑
    sclera 918.2
    scrotum (and other part(s) of trunk) 911 ☑
    shoulder (and upper arm) 912 ☑
    skin NEC 919 ☑
    specified site(s) NEC 919 ☑
    sternal region (and other part(s) of trunk) 911 ☑
    subconjunctival 918.2
    subcutaneous NEC 919 ☑

Injury — *continued*
  superficial — *continued*
    submaxillary region (and other part(s) of face, neck, or scalp, except eye) 910 ☑
    submental region (and other part(s) of face, neck, or scalp, except eye) 910 ☑
    supraclavicular fossa (and other part(s) of face, neck, or scalp, except eye) 910 ☑
    supraorbital 918.0
    temple (and other part(s) of face, neck, or scalp, except eye) 910 ☑
    temporal region (and other part(s) of face, neck, or scalp, except eye) 910 ☑
    testis (and other part(s) of trunk) 911 ☑
    thigh (and ankle, hip, knee, or leg) 916 ☑
    thorax, thoracic (external) (and other part(s) of trunk) 911 ☑
    throat (and other part(s) of face, neck, or scalp, except eye) 910 ☑
    thumb(s) (nail) 915 ☑
    toe(s) (nail) (subungual) (and foot) 917 ☑
    tongue (and other part(s) of face, neck, or scalp, except eye) 910 ☑
    tooth, teeth (*see also* Abrasion, dental) 521.20
    trunk (any part(s)) 911 ☑
    tunica vaginalis 959.14
    tympanum, tympanic membrane (and other part(s) of face, neck, or scalp, except eye) 910 ☑
    upper extremity NEC 913 ☑
    uvula (and other part(s) of face, neck, or scalp, except eye) 910 ☑
    vagina (and other part(s) of trunk) 911 ☑
    vulva (and other part(s) of trunk) 911 ☑
    wrist (and elbow) (and forearm) 913 ☑
  supraclavicular fossa 959.19
  supraorbital 959.09
  surgical complication (external or internal site) 998.2
  symphysis pubis 959.19
    complicating delivery 665.6 ☑
      affecting fetus or newborn 763.89
  temple 959.09
  temporal region 959.09
  testis 959.14
  thigh (and hip) 959.6
  thorax, thoracic (external) 959.11
    cavity — *see* Injury, internal, thorax
    internal — *see* Injury, internal, intrathoracic organs
  throat 959.09
  thumb(s) (nail) 959.5
  thymus — *see* Injury, internal, thymus
  thyroid (gland) 959.09
  toe (nail) (any) 959.7
  tongue 959.09
  tonsil 959.09
  tooth NEC 873.63
    complicated 873.73
  trachea — *see* Injury, internal, trachea
  trunk 959.19
  tunica vaginalis 959.14
  tympanum, tympanic membrane 959.09
  ultraviolet rays NEC 990
  ureter — *see* Injury, internal, ureter
  urethra (sphincter) — *see* Injury, internal, urethra
  uterus — *see* Injury, internal, uterus
  uvula 959.09
  vagina 959.14
  vascular — *see* Injury, blood vessel
  vas deferens — *see* Injury, internal, vas deferens
  vein (*see also* Injury, blood vessel, by site) 904.9
  vena cava
    inferior 902.10
    superior 901.2

Injury — *continued*
  vesical (sphincter) — *see* Injury, internal, vesical
  viscera (abdominal) — *see* Injury, internal, viscera
    with fracture, pelvis — *see* Fracture, pelvis
  visual 950.9
    cortex 950.3
  vitreous (humor) 871.2
  vulva 959.14
  whiplash (cervical spine) 847.0
  wringer — *see* Crush, by site
  wrist (and elbow) (and forearm) 959.3
  x-ray NEC 990
Inoculation — *see also* Vaccination
  complication or reaction — *see* Complication, vaccination
INPH (idiopathic normal pressure hydrocephalus) 331.5
Insanity, insane — *see also* Psychosis 298.9
  adolescent (*see also* Schizophrenia) 295.9 ☑
  alternating (*see also* Psychosis, affective, circular) 296.7
  confusional 298.9
    acute 293.0
    subacute 293.1
  delusional 298.9
  paralysis, general 094.1
    progressive 094.1
  paresis, general 094.1
  senile 290.20
Insect
  bite — *see* Injury, superficial, by site
  venomous, poisoning by 989.5
Insemination, artificial V26.1
Insensitivity
  adrenocorticotropin hormone (ACTH) 255.41
  androgen 259.50
    complete 259.51
    partial 259.52
Insertion
  cord (umbilical) lateral or velamentous 663.8 ☑
    affecting fetus or newborn 762.6
  intrauterine contraceptive device V25.11
  placenta, vicious — *see* Placenta, previa
  subdermal implantable contraceptive V25.5
  velamentous, umbilical cord 663.8 ☑
    affecting fetus or newborn 762.6
Insolation 992.0
  meaning sunstroke 992.0
Insomnia, unspecified 780.52
  with sleep apnea, unspecified 780.51
  adjustment 307.41
  alcohol induced 291.82
  behavioral, of childhood V69.5
  drug induced 292.85
  due to
    medical condition classified elsewhere 327.01
    mental disorder 327.02
  fatal familial (FFI) 046.72
  idiopathic 307.42
  nonorganic origin 307.41
    persistent (primary) 307.42
    transient 307.41
  organic 327.00
    other 327.09
  paradoxical 307.42
  primary 307.42
  psychophysiological 307.42
  subjective complaint 307.49
Inspiration
  food or foreign body (*see also* Asphyxia, food or foreign body) 933.1
  mucus (*see also* Asphyxia, mucus) 933.1
Inspissated bile syndrome, newborn 774.4
Instability
  detrusor 596.59
  emotional (excessive) 301.3
  joint (posttraumatic) 718.80
    ankle 718.87
    elbow 718.82
    foot 718.87

Instability — *continued*
  joint — *continued*
    hand 718.84
    hip 718.85
    knee 718.86
    lumbosacral 724.6
    multiple sites 718.89
    pelvic region 718.85
    sacroiliac 724.6
    shoulder (region) 718.81
    specified site NEC 718.88
    wrist 718.83
  lumbosacral 724.6
  nervous 301.89
  personality (emotional) 301.59
  thyroid, paroxysmal 242.9 ☑
  urethral 599.83
  vasomotor 780.2
Insufficiency, insufficient
  accommodation 367.4
  adrenal (gland) (acute) (chronic) 255.41
    medulla 255.5
    primary 255.41
    specified site NEC 255.5
  adrenocortical 255.41
  anterior (occlusal) guidance 524.54
  anus 569.49
  aortic (valve) 424.1
    with
      mitral (valve) disease 396.1
        insufficiency, incompetence, or regurgitation 396.3
        stenosis or obstruction 396.1
      stenosis or obstruction 424.1
        with mitral (valve) disease 396.8
    congenital 746.4
    rheumatic 395.1
      with
        mitral (valve) disease 396.1
          insufficiency, incompetence, or regurgitation 396.3
          stenosis or obstruction 396.1
        stenosis or obstruction 395.2
          with mitral (valve) disease 396.8
    specified cause NEC 424.1
    syphilitic 093.22
  arterial 447.1
    basilar artery 435.0
    carotid artery 435.8
    cerebral 437.1
    coronary (acute or subacute) 411.89
    mesenteric 557.1
    peripheral 443.9
    precerebral 435.9
    vertebral artery 435.1
    vertebrobasilar 435.3
  arteriovenous 459.9
  basilar artery 435.0
  biliary 575.8
  cardiac (*see also* Insufficiency, myocardial) 428.0
    complicating surgery 997.1
    due to presence of (cardiac) prosthesis 429.4
    postoperative 997.1
      long-term effect of cardiac surgery 429.4
    specified during or due to a procedure 997.1
      long-term effect of cardiac surgery 429.4
  cardiorenal (*see also* Hypertension, cardiorenal) 404.90
  cardiovascular (*see also* Disease, cardiovascular) 429.2
    renal (*see also* Hypertension, cardiorenal) 404.90
  carotid artery 435.8
  cerebral (vascular) 437.9
  cerebrovascular 437.9
    with transient focal neurological signs and symptoms 435.9
    acute 437.1
      with transient focal neurological signs and symptoms 435.9

☑ **Additional Digit Required** — Refer to the Tabular List for Digit Selection ⬇ **Subterms under main terms may continue to next column or page**

210 **2014 ICD-9-CM**

Insufficiency, insufficient — *continued*
circulatory NEC 459.9
  fetus or newborn 779.89
convergence 378.83
coronary (acute or subacute) 411.89
  chronic or with a stated duration of over 8 weeks 414.8
corticoadrenal 255.41
dietary 269.9
divergence 378.85
food 994.2
gastroesophageal 530.89
gonadal
  ovary 256.39
  testis 257.2
gonadotropic hormone secretion 253.4
heart (*see also* Insufficiency, myocardial)
  fetus or newborn 779.89
  valve (*see also* Endocarditis) 424.90
    congenital NEC 746.89
hepatic 573.8
idiopathic autonomic 333.0
interocclusal distance of teeth (ridge) 524.36
kidney
  acute 593.9
  chronic 585.9
labyrinth, labyrinthine (function) 386.53
  bilateral 386.54
  unilateral 386.53
lacrimal 375.15
liver 573.8
lung (acute) (*see also* Insufficiency, pulmonary) 518.82
  following trauma and surgery 518.52
  newborn 770.89
mental (congenital) (*see also* Disability, intellectual) 319
mesenteric 557.1
mitral (valve) 424.0
  with
    aortic (valve) disease 396.3
      insufficiency, incompetence, or regurgitation 396.3
      stenosis or obstruction 396.2
    obstruction or stenosis 394.2
      with aortic valve disease 396.8
  congenital 746.6
  rheumatic 394.1
    with
      aortic (valve) disease 396.3
        insufficiency, incompetence, or regurgitation 396.3
        stenosis or obstruction 396.2
      obstruction or stenosis 394.2
        with aortic valve disease 396.8
      active or acute 391.1
        with chorea, rheumatic (Sydenham's) 392.0
  specified cause, except rheumatic 424.0
muscle
  heart — *see* Insufficiency, myocardial
  ocular (*see also* Strabismus) 378.9
myocardial, myocardium (with arteriosclerosis) 428.0
  with rheumatic fever (conditions classifiable to 390)
    active, acute, or subacute 391.2
      with chorea 392.0
    inactive or quiescent (with chorea) 398.0
  congenital 746.89
  due to presence of (cardiac) prosthesis 429.4
  fetus or newborn 779.89
  following cardiac surgery 429.4
  hypertensive (*see also* Hypertension, heart) 402.91
    benign 402.11
    malignant 402.01
  postoperative 997.1
    long-term effect of cardiac surgery 429.4
  rheumatic 398.0
    active, acute, or subacute 391.2
      with chorea (Sydenham's) 392.0
  syphilitic 093.82

Insufficiency, insufficient — *continued*
nourishment 994.2
organic 799.89
ovary 256.39
  postablative 256.2
pancreatic 577.8
parathyroid (gland) 252.1
peripheral vascular (arterial) 443.9
pituitary (anterior) 253.2
  posterior 253.5
placental — *see* Placenta, insufficiency
platelets 287.5
prenatal care in current pregnancy V23.7
progressive pluriglandular 258.9
pseudocholinesterase 289.89
pulmonary (acute) 518.82
  following
    shock 518.52
    surgery 518.52
    trauma 518.52
  newborn 770.89
  valve (*see also* Endocarditis, pulmonary) 424.3
    congenital 746.09
pyloric 537.0
renal 593.9
  acute 593.9
  chronic 585.9
  due to a procedure 997.5
respiratory 786.09
  acute 518.82
    following trauma and surgery 518.52
  newborn 770.89
rotation — *see* Malrotation
suprarenal 255.41
  medulla 255.5
tarso-orbital fascia, congenital 743.66
tear film 375.15
testis 257.2
thyroid (gland) (acquired) (*see also* Hypothyroidism)
  congenital 243
tricuspid (*see also* Endocarditis, tricuspid) 397.0
  congenital 746.89
  syphilitic 093.23
urethral sphincter 599.84
valve, valvular (heart) (*see also* Endocarditis) 424.90
vascular 459.9
  intestine NEC 557.9
  mesenteric 557.1
  peripheral 443.9
  renal (*see also* Hypertension, kidney) 403.90
velopharyngeal
  acquired 528.9
  congenital 750.29
venous (peripheral) 459.81
ventricular — *see* Insufficiency, myocardial
vertebral artery 435.1
vertebrobasilar artery 435.3
weight gain during pregnancy 646.8 ☑
zinc 269.3

Insufflation
fallopian
  fertility testing V26.21
  following sterilization reversal V26.22
meconium 770.11
  with respiratory symptoms 770.12

Insular — *see* condition

Insulinoma (M8151/0)
malignant (M8151/3)
  pancreas 157.4
  specified site — *see* Neoplasm, by site, malignant
  unspecified site 157.4
pancreas 211.7
specified site — *see* Neoplasm, by site, benign
unspecified site 211.7

Insuloma — *see* Insulinoma

Insult
brain 437.9
  acute 436
cerebral 437.9

Insult — *continued*
cerebral — *continued*
  acute 436
cerebrovascular 437.9
  acute 436
vascular NEC 437.9
  acute 436

Insurance examination (certification) V70.3

Intemperance — *see also* Alcoholism 303.9 ☑

Interception of pregnancy (menstrual extraction) V25.3

Interference
balancing side 524.56
non-working side 524.56

Intermenstrual
bleeding 626.6
  irregular 626.6
  regular 626.5
hemorrhage 626.6
  irregular 626.6
  regular 626.5
pain(s) 625.2

Intermittent — *see* condition

Internal — *see* condition

Interproximal wear 521.10

Interrogation
cardiac defibrillator (automatic) (implantable) V53.32
cardiac pacemaker V53.31
cardiac (event) (loop) recorder V53.39
infusion pump (implanted) (intrathecal) V53.09
neurostimulator V53.02

Interruption
aortic arch 747.11
bundle of His 426.50
fallopian tube (for sterilization) V25.2
phase-shift, sleep cycle 307.45
repeated REM-sleep 307.48
sleep
  due to perceived environmental disturbances 307.48
  phase-shift, of 24-hour sleep-wake cycle 307.45
  repeated REM-sleep type 307.48
vas deferens (for sterilization) V25.2

Intersexuality 752.7

Interstitial — *see* condition

Intertrigo 695.89
  labialis 528.5

Intervertebral disc — *see* condition

Intestine, intestinal — *see also* condition
flu 487.8

Intolerance
carbohydrate NEC 579.8
cardiovascular exercise, with pain (at rest) (with less than ordinary activity) (with ordinary activity) V47.2
cold 780.99
dissacharide (hereditary) 271.3
drug
  correct substance properly administered 995.27
  wrong substance given or taken in error 977.9
  specified drug — *see* Table of Drugs and Chemicals
effort 306.2
fat NEC 579.8
foods NEC 579.8
fructose (hereditary) 271.2
glucose (-galactose) (congenital) 271.3
gluten 579.0
lactose (hereditary) (infantile) 271.3
lysine (congenital) 270.7
milk NEC 579.8
protein (familial) 270.7
starch NEC 579.8
sucrose (-isomaltose) (congenital) 271.3

Intoxicated NEC — *see also* Alcoholism 305.0 ☑

Intoxication
acid 276.2
acute
  alcoholic 305.0 ☑
    with alcoholism 303.0 ☑

Intoxication — *continued*
acute — *continued*
  alcoholic — *continued*
    hangover effects 305.0 ☑
  caffeine 305.9 ☑
  hallucinogenic (*see also* Abuse, drugs, nondependent) 305.3 ☑
alcohol (acute) 305.0 ☑
  with alcoholism 303.0 ☑
  hangover effects 305.0 ☑
  idiosyncratic 291.4
  pathological 291.4
alimentary canal 558.2
ammonia (hepatic) 572.2
caffeine 305.9 ☑
chemical (*see also* Table of Drugs and Chemicals)
  via placenta or breast milk 760.70
    alcohol 760.71
    anticonvulsants
    antifungals
    anti-infective agents 760.74
    antimetabolics
    cocaine 760.75
    "crack" 760.75
    hallucinogenic agents NEC 760.73
    medicinal agents NEC 760.79
    narcotics 760.72
    obstetric anesthetic or analgesic drug 763.5
    specified agent NEC 760.79
    suspected, affecting management of pregnancy 655.5 ☑
cocaine, through placenta or breast milk 760.75
delirium
  alcohol 291.0
  drug 292.81
drug 292.89
  with delirium 292.81
  correct substance properly administered (*see also* Allergy, drug) 995.27
  newborn 779.4
  obstetric anesthetic or sedation 668.9 ☑
    affecting fetus or newborn 763.5
  overdose or wrong substance given or taken — *see* Table of Drugs and Chemicals
  pathologic 292.2
  specific to newborn 779.4
  via placenta or breast milk 760.70
    alcohol 760.71
    anticonvulsants 760.77
    antifungals 760.74
    anti-infective agents 760.74
    antimetabolics 760.78
    cocaine 760.75
    "crack" 760.75
    hallucinogenic agents 760.73
    medicinal agents NEC 760.79
    narcotics 760.72
    obstetric anesthetic or analgesic drug 763.5
    specified agent NEC 760.79
    suspected, affecting management of pregnancy 655.5 ☑
enteric — *see* Intoxication, intestinal
fetus or newborn, via placenta or breast milk 760.70
  alcohol 760.71
  anticonvulsants 760.77
  antifungals 760.74
  anti-infective agents 760.74
  antimetabolics 760.78
  cocaine 760.75
  "crack" 760.75
  hallucinogenic agents 760.73
  medicinal agents NEC 760.79
  narcotics 760.72
  obstetric anesthetic or analgesic drug 763.5
  specified agent NEC 760.79
  suspected, affecting management of pregnancy 655.5 ☑
food — *see* Poisoning, food
gastrointestinal 558.2

☑ Additional Digit Required — Refer to the Tabular List for Digit Selection   ⩔ Subterms under main terms may continue to next column or page

Intoxication — *continued*
  hallucinogenic (acute) 305.3 ☑
  hepatocerebral 572.2
  idiosyncratic alcohol 291.4
  intestinal 569.89
    due to putrefaction of food 005.9
  methyl alcohol (*see also* Alcoholism) 305.0 ☑
    with alcoholism 303.0 ☑
  non-foodborne due to toxins of Clostridium botulinum [C. botulinum] — *see* Botulism
  pathologic 291.4
    drug 292.2
  potassium (K) 276.7
  septic
    with
      abortion — *see* Abortion, by type, with sepsis
      ectopic pregnancy (*see also* categories 633.0–633.9) 639.0
      molar pregnancy (*see also* categories 630–632) 639.0
    during labor 659.3 ☑
    following
      abortion 639.0
      ectopic or molar pregnancy 639.0
    generalized — *see* Septicemia
    puerperal, postpartum, childbirth 670.2 ☑
  serum (prophylactic) (therapeutic) 999.59
  uremic — *see* Uremia
  water 276.69
Intracranial — *see* condition
Intrahepatic gallbladder 751.69
Intraligamentous — *see also* condition
  pregnancy — *see* Pregnancy, cornual
Intraocular — *see also* condition
  sepsis 360.00
Intrathoracic — *see also* condition
  kidney 753.3
  stomach — *see* Hernia, diaphragm
Intrauterine contraceptive device
  checking V25.42
  insertion V25.11
  in situ V45.51
  management V25.42
  prescription V25.02
    repeat V25.42
  reinsertion V25.13
  removal V25.12
    and reinsertion V25.13
  replacement V25.13
Intraventricular — *see* condition
Intrinsic deformity — *see* Deformity
Intruded tooth 524.34
Intrusion, repetitive, of sleep (due to environmental disturbances) (with atypical polysomnographic features) 307.48
Intumescent, lens (eye) NEC 366.9
  senile 366.12
Intussusception (colon) (enteric) (intestine) (rectum) 560.0
  appendix 543.9
  congenital 751.5
  fallopian tube 620.8
  ileocecal 560.0
  ileocolic 560.0
  ureter (with obstruction) 593.4
Invagination
  basilar 756.0
  colon or intestine 560.0
Invalid (since birth) 799.89
Invalidism (chronic) 799.89
Inversion
  albumin-globulin (A-G) ratio 273.8
  bladder 596.89
  cecum (*see also* Intussusception) 560.0
  cervix 622.8
  nipple 611.79
    congenital 757.6
    puerperal, postpartum 676.3 ☑
  optic papilla 743.57
  organ or site, congenital NEC — *see* Anomaly, specified type NEC
  sleep rhythm 327.39

Inversion — *continued*
  sleep rhythm — *continued*
    nonorganic origin 307.45
  testis (congenital) 752.51
  uterus (postinfectional) (postpartal, old) 621.7
    chronic 621.7
    complicating delivery 665.2 ☑
      affecting fetus or newborn 763.89
  vagina — *see* Prolapse, vagina
Investigation
  allergens V72.7
  clinical research (control) (normal comparison) (participant) V70.7
Inviability — *see* Immaturity
Involuntary movement, abnormal 781.0
Involution, involutional — *see also* condition
  breast, cystic or fibrocystic 610.1
  depression (*see also* Psychosis, affective) 296.2 ☑
    recurrent episode 296.3 ☑
    single episode 296.2 ☑
  melancholia (*see also* Psychosis, affective) 296.2 ☑
    recurrent episode 296.3 ☑
    single episode 296.2 ☑
  ovary, senile 620.3
  paranoid state (reaction) 297.2
  paraphrenia (climacteric) (menopause) 297.2
  psychosis 298.8
  thymus failure 254.8
IQ
  under 20 318.2
  20-34 318.1
  35-49 318.0
  50-70 317
IRDS 769
Irideremia 743.45
Iridis rubeosis 364.42
  diabetic 250.5 ☑ [364.42]
    due to secondary diabetes 249.5 ☑ [364.42]
Iridochoroiditis (panuveitis) 360.12
Iridocyclitis NEC 364.3
  acute 364.00
    primary 364.01
    recurrent 364.02
  chronic 364.10
    in
      lepromatous leprosy 030.0 [364.11]
      sarcoidosis 135 [364.11]
      tuberculosis (*see also* Tuberculosis) 017.3 ☑ [364.11]
  due to allergy 364.04
  endogenous 364.01
  gonococcal 098.41
  granulomatous 364.10
  herpetic (simplex) 054.44
    zoster 053.22
  hypopyon 364.05
  lens induced 364.23
  nongranulomatous 364.00
  primary 364.01
  recurrent 364.02
  rheumatic 364.10
  secondary 364.04
    infectious 364.03
    noninfectious 364.04
  subacute 364.00
    primary 364.01
    recurrent 364.02
  sympathetic 360.11
  syphilitic (secondary) 091.52
  tuberculous (chronic) (*see also* Tuberculosis) 017.3 ☑ [364.11]
Iridocyclochoroiditis (panuveitis) 360.12
Iridodialysis 364.76
Iridodonesis 364.89
Iridoplegia (complete) (partial) (reflex) 379.49
Iridoschisis 364.52
IRIS (Immune Reconstitution Inflammatory Syndrome) 995.90
Iris — *see* condition
Iritis 364.3
  acute 364.00

Iritis — *continued*
  acute — *continued*
    primary 364.01
    recurrent 364.02
  chronic 364.10
    in
      sarcoidosis 135 [364.11]
      tuberculosis (*see also* Tuberculosis) 017.3 ☑ [364.11]
  diabetic 250.5 ☑ [364.42]
    due to secondary diabetes 249.5 ☑ [364.42]
  due to
    allergy 364.04
    herpes simplex 054.44
    leprosy 030.0 [364.11]
  endogenous 364.01
  gonococcal 098.41
  gouty 274.89 [364.11]
  granulomatous 364.10
  hypopyon 364.05
  lens induced 364.23
  nongranulomatous 364.00
  papulosa 095.8 [364.11]
  primary 364.01
  recurrent 364.02
  rheumatic 364.10
  secondary 364.04
    infectious 364.03
    noninfectious 364.04
  subacute 364.00
    primary 364.01
    recurrent 364.02
  sympathetic 360.11
  syphilitic (secondary) 091.52
    congenital 090.0 [364.11]
    late 095.8 [364.11]
  tuberculous (*see also* Tuberculosis) 017.3 ☑ [364.11]
  uratic 274.89 [364.11]
Iron
  deficiency anemia 280.9
  metabolism disease 275.09
  storage disease 275.09
Iron-miners' lung 503
Irradiated enamel (tooth, teeth) 521.89
Irradiation
  burn — *see* Burn, by site
  effects, adverse 990
Irreducible, irreducibility — *see* condition
Irregular, irregularity
  action, heart 427.9
  alveolar process 525.8
  bleeding NEC 626.4
  breathing 786.09
  colon 569.89
  contour
    acquired 371.70
    of cornea 743.41
      acquired 371.70
    reconstructed breast 612.0
  dentin in pulp 522.3
  eye movements NEC 379.59
  menstruation (cause unknown) 626.4
  periods 626.4
  prostate 602.9
  pupil 364.75
  respiratory 786.09
  septum (nasal) 470
  shape, organ or site, congenital NEC — *see* Distortion
  sleep-wake rhythm (non-24-hour) 327.39
    nonorganic origin 307.45
  vertebra 733.99
Irritability 799.22
  bladder 596.89
    neurogenic 596.54
      with cauda equina syndrome 344.61
  bowel (syndrome) 564.1
  bronchial (*see also* Bronchitis) 490
  cerebral, newborn 779.1
  colon 564.1
    psychogenic 306.4
  duodenum 564.89
  heart (psychogenic) 306.2
  ileum 564.89

Irritability — *continued*
  jejunum 564.89
  myocardium 306.2
  nervousness 799.21
  rectum 564.89
  stomach 536.9
    psychogenic 306.4
  sympathetic (nervous system) (*see also* Neuropathy, peripheral, autonomic) 337.9
  urethra 599.84
  ventricular (heart) (psychogenic) 306.2
Irritable — *see also* Irritability 799.22
Irritation
  anus 569.49
  axillary nerve 353.0
  bladder 596.89
  brachial plexus 353.0
  brain (traumatic) (*see also* Injury, intracranial) 854.0 ☑
    nontraumatic — *see* Encephalitis
  bronchial (*see also* Bronchitis) 490
  cerebral (traumatic) (*see also* Injury, intracranial) 854.0 ☑
    nontraumatic — *see* Encephalitis
  cervical plexus 353.2
  cervix (*see also* Cervicitis) 616.0
  choroid, sympathetic 360.11
  cranial nerve — *see* Disorder, nerve, cranial
  digestive tract 536.9
    psychogenic 306.4
  gastric 536.9
    psychogenic 306.4
  gastrointestinal (tract) 536.9
    functional 536.9
    psychogenic 306.4
  globe, sympathetic 360.11
  intestinal (bowel) 564.9
  labyrinth 386.50
  lumbosacral plexus 353.1
  meninges (traumatic) (*see also* Injury, intracranial) 854.0 ☑
    nontraumatic — *see* Meningitis
  myocardium 306.2
  nerve — *see* Disorder, nerve
  nervous 799.21
  nose 478.19
  penis 607.89
  perineum 709.9
  peripheral
    autonomic nervous system (*see also* Neuropathy, peripheral, autonomic) 337.9
    nerve — *see* Disorder, nerve
  peritoneum (*see also* Peritonitis) 567.9
  pharynx 478.29
  plantar nerve 355.6
  spinal (cord) (traumatic) (*see also* Injury, spinal, by site)
    nerve (*see also* Disorder, nerve)
      root NEC 724.9
      traumatic — *see* Injury, nerve, spinal
    nontraumatic — *see* Myelitis
  stomach 536.9
    psychogenic 306.4
  sympathetic nerve NEC (*see also* Neuropathy, peripheral, autonomic) 337.9
  ulnar nerve 354.2
  vagina 623.9
Isambert's disease 012.3 ☑
Ischemia, ischemic 459.9
  basilar artery (with transient neurologic deficit) 435.0
  bone NEC 733.40
  bowel (transient) 557.9
    acute 557.0
    chronic 557.1
    due to mesenteric artery insufficiency 557.1
  brain (*see also* Ischemia, cerebral)
    recurrent focal 435.9
  cardiac (*see also* Ischemia, heart) 414.9
  cardiomyopathy 414.8
  carotid artery (with transient neurologic deficit) 435.8
  cerebral (chronic) (generalized) 437.1

☑ **Additional Digit Required** — Refer to the Tabular List for Digit Selection

▽ **Subterms under main terms may continue to next column or page**

Ischemia, ischemic — *continued*
  cerebral — *continued*
    arteriosclerotic 437.0
    intermittent (with transient neurologic
        deficit) 435.9
    newborn 779.2
    puerperal, postpartum, childbirth
        674.0 ☑
    recurrent focal (with transient neurologic
        deficit) 435.9
    transient (with transient neurologic
        deficit) 435.9
  colon 557.9
    acute 557.0
    chronic 557.1
    due to mesenteric artery insufficiency
        557.1
  coronary (chronic) (*see also* Ischemia, heart)
        414.9
  demand 411.89
  heart (chronic or with a stated duration of
        over 8 weeks) 414.9
    acute or with a stated duration of 8
        weeks or less (*see also* Infarct,
        myocardium) 410.9 ☑
        without myocardial infarction 411.89
        with coronary (artery) occlusion
            411.81
    subacute 411.89
  intestine (transient) 557.9
    acute 557.0
    chronic 557.1
    due to mesenteric artery insufficiency
        557.1
  kidney 593.81
  labyrinth 386.50

Ischemia, ischemic — *continued*
  muscles, leg 728.89
  myocardium, myocardial (chronic or with a
        stated duration of over 8 weeks)
        414.8
    acute (*see also* Infarct, myocardium)
        410.9 ☑
        without myocardial infarction 411.89
        with coronary (artery) occlusion
            411.81
  renal 593.81
  retina, retinal 362.84
  small bowel 557.9
    acute 557.0
    chronic 557.1
    due to mesenteric artery insufficiency
        557.1
  spinal cord 336.1
  subendocardial (*see also* Insufficiency,
        coronary) 411.89
  supply (*see also* Angina) 414.9
  vertebral artery (with transient neurologic
        deficit) 435.1
Ischialgia — *see also* Sciatica 724.3
Ischiopagus 759.4
Ischium, ischial — *see* condition
Ischomenia 626.8
Ischuria 788.5
Iselin's disease or osteochondrosis 732.5
Islands of
  parotid tissue in
    lymph nodes 750.26
    neck structures 750.26
  submaxillary glands in
    fascia 750.26
    lymph nodes 750.26

Islands of — *continued*
  submaxillary glands in — *continued*
    neck muscles 750.26
Islet cell tumor, pancreas (M8150/0) 211.7
Isoimmunization NEC — *see also* Incompati-
        bility 656.2 ☑
  anti-E 656.2 ☑
  fetus or newborn 773.2
    ABO blood groups 773.1
    Rhesus (Rh) factor 773.0
Isolation V07.0
  social V62.4
Isosporosis 007.2
Issue
  medical certificate NEC V68.09
    cause of death V68.09
    disability examination V68.01
    fitness V68.09
    incapacity V68.09
  repeat prescription NEC V68.1
    appliance V68.1
    contraceptive V25.40
      device NEC V25.49
        intrauterine V25.42
        specified type NEC V25.49
      pill V25.41
    glasses V68.1
    medicinal substance V68.1
Itch — *see also* Pruritus 698.9
  bakers' 692.89
  barbers' 110.0
  bricklayers' 692.89
  cheese 133.8
  clam diggers' 120.3
  coolie 126.9
  copra 133.8

Itch — *see also* Pruritus — *continued*
  Cuban 050.1
  dew 126.9
  dhobie 110.3
  eye 379.99
  filarial (*see also* Infestation, filarial) 125.9
  grain 133.8
  grocers' 133.8
  ground 126.9
  harvest 133.8
  jock 110.3
  Malabar 110.9
    beard 110.0
    foot 110.4
    scalp 110.0
  meaning scabies 133.0
  Norwegian 133.0
  perianal 698.0
  poultrymen's 133.8
  sarcoptic 133.0
  scrub 134.1
  seven year V61.10
    meaning scabies 133.0
  straw 133.8
  swimmers' 120.3
  washerwoman's 692.4
  water 120.3
  winter 698.8
Itsenko-Cushing syndrome (pituitary ba-
        sophilism) 255.0
Ivemark's syndrome (asplenia with congenital
        heart disease) 759.0
Ivory bones 756.52
Ixodes 134.8
Ixodiasis 134.8

☑ Additional Digit Required — Refer to the Tabular List for Digit Selection   ▽ Subterms under main terms may continue to next column or page

2014 ICD-9-CM   213

J

Jaccoud's nodular fibrositis, chronic (Jaccoud's syndrome) 714.4
Jackson's
  membrane 751.4
  paralysis or syndrome 344.89
  veil 751.4
Jacksonian
  epilepsy (*see also* Epilepsy) 345.5 ☑
  seizures (focal) (*see also* Epilepsy) 345.5 ☑
Jacob's ulcer (M8090/3) — *see* Neoplasm, skin, malignant, by site
Jacquet's dermatitis (diaper dermatitis) 691.0
Jadassohn's
  blue nevus (M8780/0) — *see* Neoplasm, skin, benign
  disease (maculopapular erythroderma) 696.2
  intraepidermal epithelioma (M8096/0) — *see* Neoplasm, skin, benign
Jadassohn-Lewandowski syndrome (pachyonychia congenita) 757.5
Jadassohn-Pellizari's disease (anetoderma) 701.3
Jadassohn-Tièche nevus (M8780/0) — *see* Neoplasm, skin, benign
Jaffe-Lichtenstein (-Uehlinger) syndrome 252.01
Jahnke's syndrome (encephalocutaneous angiomatosis) 759.6
Jakob-Creutzfeldt disease (CJD) (syndrome) 046.19
  with dementia
    with behavioral disturbance 046.19 [294.11]
    without behavioral disturbance 046.19 [294.10]
  familial 046.19
  iatrogenic 046.19
  specified NEC 046.19
  sporadic 046.19
  variant (vCJD) 046.11
    with dementia
      with behavioral disturbance 046.11 [294.11]
      without behavioral disturbance 046.11 [294.10]
Jaksch (-Luzet) disease or syndrome (pseudoleukemia infantum) 285.8
Jamaican
  neuropathy 349.82
  paraplegic tropical ataxic-spastic syndrome 349.82
Janet's disease (psychasthenia) 300.89
Janiceps 759.4
Jansky-Bielschowsky amaurotic familial idiocy 330.1
Japanese
  B type encephalitis 062.0
  river fever 081.2
  seven-day fever 100.89
Jaundice (yellow) 782.4
  acholuric (familial) (splenomegalic) (*see also* Spherocytosis) 282.0
    acquired 283.9
  breast milk 774.39
  catarrhal (acute) 070.1
    with hepatic coma 070.0
    chronic 571.9
    epidemic — *see* Jaundice, epidemic
  cholestatic (benign) 782.4
  chronic idiopathic 277.4
  epidemic (catarrhal) 070.1
    with hepatic coma 070.0
    leptospiral 100.0
    spirochetal 100.0
  febrile (acute) 070.1
    with hepatic coma 070.0
    leptospiral 100.0
    spirochetal 100.0
  fetus or newborn 774.6
    due to or associated with
      ABO
        absence or deficiency of enzyme system for bilirubin conjugation (congenital) 774.39

Jaundice — *continued*
  fetus or newborn — *continued*
    due to or associated with — *continued*
      antibodies 773.1
      blood group incompatibility NEC 773.2
      breast milk inhibitors to conjugation 774.39
        associated with preterm delivery 774.2
      bruising 774.1
      Crigler-Najjar syndrome 277.4 [774.31]
      delayed conjugation 774.30
        associated with preterm delivery 774.2
        development 774.39
      drugs or toxins transmitted from mother 774.1
      G-6-PD deficiency 282.2 [774.0]
      galactosemia 271.1 [774.5]
      Gilbert's syndrome 277.4 [774.31]
      hepatocellular damage 774.4
      hereditary hemolytic anemia (*see also* Anemia, hemolytic) 282.9 [774.0]
      hypothyroidism, congenital 243 [774.31]
      incompatibility, maternal/fetal 773.1
      incompatibility, maternal/fetal NEC 773.2
      infection 774.1
      inspissated bile syndrome 774.4
      isoimmunization 773.1
      isoimmunization NEC 773.2
      mucoviscidosis 277.01 [774.5]
      obliteration of bile duct, congenital 751.61 [774.5]
      polycythemia 774.1
      preterm delivery 774.2
      red cell defect 282.9 [774.0]
      Rh
        antibodies 773.0
        incompatibility, maternal/fetal 773.0
        isoimmunization 773.0
      spherocytosis (congenital) 282.0 [774.0]
      swallowed maternal blood 774.1
    physiological NEC 774.6
  from injection, inoculation, infusion, or transfusion (blood) (plasma) (serum) (other substance) (onset within 8 months after administration) — *see* Hepatitis, viral
  Gilbert's (familial nonhemolytic) 277.4
  hematogenous 283.9
  hemolytic (acquired) 283.9
    congenital (*see also* Spherocytosis) 282.0
  hemorrhagic (acute) 100.0
    leptospiral 100.0
    newborn 776.0
    spirochetal 100.0
  hepatocellular 573.8
  homologous (serum) — *see* Hepatitis, viral
  idiopathic, chronic 277.4
  infectious (acute) (subacute) 070.1
    with hepatic coma 070.0
    leptospiral 100.0
    spirochetal 100.0
  leptospiral 100.0
  malignant (*see also* Necrosis, liver) 570
  newborn (physiological) (*see also* Jaundice, fetus or newborn) 774.6
  nonhemolytic, congenital familial (Gilbert's) 277.4
  nuclear, newborn (*see also* Kernicterus of newborn) 774.7
  obstructive NEC (*see also* Obstruction, biliary) 576.8
  postimmunization — *see* Hepatitis, viral
  posttransfusion — *see* Hepatitis, viral
  regurgitation (*see also* Obstruction, biliary) 576.8

Jaundice — *continued*
  serum (homologous) (prophylactic) (therapeutic) — *see* Hepatitis, viral
  spirochetal (hemorrhagic) 100.0
  symptomatic 782.4
    newborn 774.6
Jaw — *see* condition
Jaw-blinking 374.43
  congenital 742.8
Jaw-winking phenomenon or syndrome 742.8
Jealousy
  alcoholic 291.5
  childhood 313.3
  sibling 313.3
Jejunitis — *see also* Enteritis 558.9
Jejunostomy status V44.4
Jejunum, jejunal — *see* condition
Jensen's disease 363.05
Jericho boil 085.1
Jerks, myoclonic 333.2
Jervell-Lange-Nielsen syndrome 426.82
Jeune's disease or syndrome (asphyxiating thoracic dystrophy) 756.4
Jigger disease 134.1
Job's syndrome (chronic granulomatous disease) 288.1
Jod-Basedow phenomenon 242.8 ☑
Johnson-Stevens disease (erythema multiforme exudativum) 695.13
Joint — *see also* condition
  Charcôt's 094.0 [713.5]
  false 733.82
  flail — *see* Flail, joint
  mice — *see* Loose, body, joint, by site
  sinus to bone 730.9 ☑
  von Gies' 095.8
Jordan's anomaly or syndrome 288.2
Josephs-Diamond-Blackfan anemia (congenital hypoplastic) 284.01
Joubert syndrome 759.89
Jumpers' knee 727.2
Jungle yellow fever 060.0
Jüngling's disease (sarcoidosis) 135
Junin virus hemorrhagic fever 078.7
Juvenile — *see also* condition
  delinquent 312.9
    group (*see also* Disturbance, conduct) 312.2 ☑
  neurotic 312.4

K

Kabuki syndrome 759.89
Kahler (-Bozzolo) disease (multiple myeloma) (M9730/3) 203.0 ☑
Kakergasia 300.9
Kakke 265.0
Kala-azar (Indian) (infantile) (Mediterranean) (Sudanese) 085.0
Kalischer's syndrome (encephalocutaneous angiomatosis) 759.6
Kallmann's syndrome (hypogonadotropic hypogonadism with anosmia) 253.4
Kanner's syndrome (autism) — *see also* Psychosis, childhood 299.0 ☑
Kaolinosis 502
Kaposi's
  disease 757.33
    lichen ruber 696.4
      acuminatus 696.4
      moniliformis 697.8
    xeroderma pigmentosum 757.33
  sarcoma (M9140/3) 176.9
    adipose tissue 176.1
    aponeurosis 176.1
    artery 176.1
    associated herpesvirus infection 058.89
    blood vessel 176.1
    bursa 176.1
    connective tissue 176.1
    external genitalia 176.8
    fascia 176.1
    fatty tissue 176.1
    fibrous tissue 176.1
    gastrointestinal tract NEC 176.3
    ligament 176.1

Kaposi's — *continued*
  sarcoma — *continued*
    lung 176.4
    lymph
      gland(s) 176.5
      node(s) 176.5
    lymphatic(s) NEC 176.1
    muscle (skeletal) 176.1
    oral cavity NEC 176.8
    palate 176.2
    scrotum 176.8
    skin 176.0
    soft tissue 176.1
    specified site NEC 176.8
    subcutaneous tissue 176.1
    synovia 176.1
    tendon (sheath) 176.1
    vein 176.1
    vessel 176.1
    viscera NEC 176.9
    vulva 176.8
  varicelliform eruption 054.0
    vaccinia 999.0
Kartagener's syndrome or triad (sinusitis, bronchiectasis, situs inversus) 759.3
Kasabach-Merritt syndrome (capillary hemangioma associated with thrombocytopenic purpura) 287.39
Kaschin-Beck disease (endemic polyarthritis) — *see* Disease, Kaschin-Beck
Kast's syndrome (dyschondroplasia with hemangiomas) 756.4
Katatonia — *see* Catatonia
Katayama disease or fever 120.2
Kathisophobia 781.0
Kawasaki disease 446.1
Kayser-Fleischer ring (cornea) (pseudosclerosis) 275.1 [371.14]
Kaznelson's syndrome (congenital hypoplastic anemia) 284.01
Kearns-Sayre syndrome 277.87
Kedani fever 081.2
Kelis 701.4
Kelly (-Patterson) syndrome (sideropenic dysphagia) 280.8
Keloid, cheloid 701.4
  Addison's (morphea) 701.0
  cornea 371.00
  Hawkins' 701.4
  scar 701.4
Keloma 701.4
Kenya fever 082.1
Keratectasia 371.71
  congenital 743.41
Keratinization NEC
  alveolar ridge mucosa
    excessive 528.72
    minimal 528.71
Keratitis (nodular) (nonulcerative) (simple) (zonular) NEC 370.9
  with ulceration (*see also* Ulcer, cornea) 370.00
  actinic 370.24
  arborescens 054.42
  areolar 370.22
  bullosa 370.8
  deep — *see* Keratitis, interstitial
  dendritic(a) 054.42
  desiccation 370.34
  diffuse interstitial 370.52
  disciform(is) 054.43
    varicella 052.7 [370.44]
  epithelialis vernalis 372.13 [370.32]
  exposure 370.34
  filamentary 370.23
  gonococcal (congenital) (prenatal) 098.43
  herpes, herpetic (simplex) NEC 054.43
    zoster 053.21
  hypopyon 370.04
  in
    chickenpox 052.7 [370.44]
    exanthema (*see also* Exanthem) 057.9 [370.44]
    paravaccinia (*see also* Paravaccinia) 051.9 [370.44]

☑ **Additional Digit Required — Refer to the Tabular List for Digit Selection**   ▽ **Subterms under main terms may continue to next column or page**

Kyphosis, kyphotic — *continued*
  due to or associated with — *continued*
    osteitis
      deformans 731.0 *[737.41]*
      fibrosa cystica 252.01 *[737.41]*
    osteoporosis (*see also* Osteoporosis)
      733.0 ☑ *[737.41]*
    poliomyelitis (*see also* Poliomyelitis)
      138 *[737.41]*
    radiation 737.11
    tuberculosis (*see also* Tuberculosis)
      015.0 ☑ *[737.41]*
  Kümmell's 721.7
  late effect of rickets 268.1 *[737.41]*
  Morquio-Brailsford type (spinal)
    277.5 *[737.41]*
  pelvis 738.6
  postlaminectomy 737.12
  specified cause NEC 737.19
  syphilitic, congenital 090.5 *[737.41]*
  tuberculous (*see also* Tuberculosis)
    015.0 ☑ *[737.41]*
Kyrle's disease (hyperkeratosis follicularis in
  cutem penetrans) 701.1

L

Labia, labium — *see* condition
Labiated hymen 752.49
Labile
  blood pressure 796.2
  emotions, emotionality 301.3
  vasomotor system 443.9
Lability, emotional 799.24
Labioglossal paralysis 335.22
Labium leporinum — *see also* Cleft, lip 749.10
Labor — *see also* Delivery
  with complications — *see* Delivery, compli-
    cated
  abnormal NEC 661.9 ☑
    affecting fetus or newborn 763.7
  arrested active phase 661.1 ☑
    affecting fetus or newborn 763.7
  desultory 661.2 ☑
    affecting fetus or newborn 763.7
  dyscoordinate 661.4 ☑
    affecting fetus or newborn 763.7
  early onset (22-36 weeks gestation)
    644.2 ☑
  failed
    induction 659.1 ☑
      mechanical 659.0 ☑
      medical 659.1 ☑
      surgical 659.0 ☑
    trial (vaginal delivery) 660.6 ☑
  false 644.1 ☑
  forced or induced, affecting fetus or new-
    born 763.89
  hypertonic 661.4 ☑
    affecting fetus or newborn 763.7
  hypotonic 661.2 ☑
    affecting fetus or newborn 763.7
    primary 661.0 ☑
      affecting fetus or newborn 763.7
    secondary 661.1 ☑
      affecting fetus or newborn 763.7
  incoordinate 661.4 ☑
    affecting fetus or newborn 763.7
  irregular 661.2 ☑
    affecting fetus or newborn 763.7
  long — *see* Labor, prolonged
  missed (at or near term) 656.4 ☑
  obstructed NEC 660.9 ☑
    affecting fetus or newborn 763.1
    due to female genital mutilation
      660.8 ☑
    specified cause NEC 660.8 ☑
      affecting fetus or newborn 763.1
  pains, spurious 644.1 ☑
  precipitate 661.3 ☑
    affecting fetus or newborn 763.6
  premature 644.2 ☑
    threatened 644.0 ☑
  prolonged or protracted 662.1 ☑
    first stage 662.0 ☑
      affecting fetus or newborn 763.89

Labor — *see also* Delivery — *continued*
  prolonged or protracted — *continued*
    second stage 662.2 ☑
      affecting fetus or newborn 763.89
    affecting fetus or newborn 763.89
  threatened NEC 644.1 ☑
  undelivered 644.1 ☑
Labored breathing — *see also* Hyperventilation 786.09
Labyrinthitis (inner ear) (destructive) (latent)
  386.30
  circumscribed 386.32
  diffuse 386.31
  focal 386.32
  purulent 386.33
  serous 386.31
  suppurative 386.33
  syphilitic 095.8
  toxic 386.34
  viral 386.35
Laceration — *see also* Wound, open, by site
  accidental, complicating surgery 998.2
  Achilles tendon 845.09
    with open wound 892.2
  anus (sphincter) 879.6
    with
      abortion — *see* Abortion, by type,
        with damage to pelvic organs
      ectopic pregnancy (*see also* cate-
        gories 633.0–633.9) 639.2
      molar pregnancy (*see also* categories
        630–632) 639.2
    complicated 879.7
    complicating delivery (healed) (old)
      654.8 ☑
      with laceration of anal or rectal mu-
        cosa 664.3 ☑
      not associated with third-degree
        perineal laceration 664.6 ☑
    following
      abortion 639.2
      ectopic or molar pregnancy 639.2
    nontraumatic, nonpuerperal (healed)
      (old) 569.43
  bladder (urinary)
    with
      abortion — *see* Abortion, by type,
        with damage to pelvic organs
      ectopic pregnancy (*see also* cate-
        gories 633.0–633.9) 639.2
      molar pregnancy (*see also* categories
        630–632) 639.2
    following
      abortion 639.2
      ectopic or molar pregnancy 639.2
    obstetrical trauma 665.5 ☑
  blood vessel — *see* Injury, blood vessel, by
    site
  bowel
    with
      abortion — *see* Abortion, by type,
        with damage to pelvic organs
      ectopic pregnancy (*see also* cate-
        gories 633.0–633.9) 639.2
      molar pregnancy (*see also* categories
        630–632) 639.2
    following
      abortion 639.2
      ectopic or molar pregnancy 639.2
    obstetrical trauma 665.5 ☑

Laceration — *see also* Wound, open, by site —
  continued
  brain (cerebral) (membrane) (with hemor-
    rhage) 851.8 ☑

> Note — Use the following fifth-digit
> subclassification with categories
> 851–854:
>
> 0 unspecified state of consciousness
>
> 1 with no loss of consciousness
>
> 2 with brief [less than one hour]
>   loss of consciousness
>
> 3 with moderate [1–24 hours] loss
>   of consciousness
>
> 4 with prolonged [more than 24
>   hours] loss of consciousness and
>   return to pre–existing conscious
>   level
>
> 5 with prolonged [more than 24
>   hours] loss of consciousness,
>   without return to pre–existing
>   conscious level
>
> Use fifth-digit 5 to designate when a
> patient is unconscious and dies before
> regaining consciousness, regardless of
> the duration of the loss of consciousness
>
> 6 with loss of consciousness of un-
>   specified duration
>
> 9 with concussion, unspecified

      with
        open intracranial wound 851.9 ☑
        skull fracture — *see* Fracture, skull,
          by site
      cerebellum 851.6 ☑
        with open intracranial wound
          851.7 ☑
      cortex 851.2 ☑
        with open intracranial wound
          851.3 ☑
      during birth 767.0
      stem 851.6 ☑
        with open intracranial wound
          851.7 ☑
    broad ligament
      with
        abortion — *see* Abortion, by type,
          with damage to pelvic organs
        ectopic pregnancy (*see also* cate-
          gories 633.0–633.9) 639.2
        molar pregnancy (*see also* categories
          630–632) 639.2
      following
        abortion 639.2
        ectopic or molar pregnancy 639.2
      nontraumatic 620.6
      obstetrical trauma 665.6 ☑
      syndrome (nontraumatic) 620.6
    capsule, joint — *see* Sprain, by site
    cardiac — *see* Laceration, heart
    causing eversion of cervix uteri (old) 622.0
    central, complicating delivery 664.4 ☑
    cerebellum — *see* Laceration, brain, cerebel-
      lum
    cerebral (*see also* Laceration, brain)
      during birth 767.0
    cervix (uteri)
      with
        abortion — *see* Abortion, by type,
          with damage to pelvic organs
        ectopic pregnancy (*see also* cate-
          gories 633.0–633.9) 639.2
        molar pregnancy (*see also* categories
          630–632) 639.2
      following
        abortion 639.2
        ectopic or molar pregnancy 639.2
      nonpuerperal, nontraumatic 622.3
      obstetrical trauma (current) 665.3 ☑
      old (postpartal) 622.3
      traumatic — *see* Injury, internal, cervix
    chordae heart 429.5
    complicated 879.9

Laceration — *see also* Wound, open, by site —
  continued
  cornea — *see* Laceration, eyeball
    superficial 918.1
  cortex (cerebral) — *see* Laceration, brain,
    cortex
  esophagus 530.89
  eye(s) — *see* Laceration, ocular
  eyeball NEC 871.4
    with prolapse or exposure of intraocular
      tissue 871.1
    penetrating — *see* Penetrating wound,
      eyeball
    specified as without prolapse of intraoc-
      ular tissue 871.0
  eyelid NEC 870.8
    full thickness 870.1
      involving lacrimal passages 870.2
    skin (and periocular area) 870.0
      penetrating — *see* Penetrating
        wound, orbit
  fourchette
    with
      abortion — *see* Abortion, by type,
        with damage to pelvic organs
      ectopic pregnancy (*see also* cate-
        gories 633.0–633.9) 639.2
      molar pregnancy (*see also* categories
        630–632) 639.2
    complicating delivery 664.0 ☑
    following
      abortion 639.2
      ectopic or molar pregnancy 639.2
  heart (without penetration of heart cham-
    bers) 861.02
    with
      open wound into thorax 861.12
      penetration of heart chambers
        861.03
        with open wound into thorax
          861.13
  hernial sac — *see* Hernia, by site
  internal organ (abdomen) (chest) (pelvis)
    NEC — *see* Injury, internal, by site
    NEC — *see* Injury, internal, by site
  kidney (parenchyma) 866.02
    with
      complete disruption of parenchyma
        (rupture) 866.03
        with open wound into cavity
          866.13
      open wound into cavity 866.12
  labia
    complicating delivery 664.0 ☑
  ligament (*see also* Sprain, by site)
    with open wound — *see* Wound, open,
      by site
  liver 864.05
    with open wound into cavity 864.15
    major (disruption of hepatic parenchy-
      ma) 864.04
      with open wound into cavity 864.14
    minor (capsule only) 864.02
      with open wound into cavity 864.12
    moderate (involving parenchyma with-
      out major disruption) 864.03
      with open wound into cavity 864.13
    multiple 864.04
      with open wound into cavity
        864.14
    stellate 864.04
      with open wound into cavity 864.14
  lung 861.22
    with open wound into thorax 861.32
  meninges — *see* Laceration, brain
  meniscus (knee) (*see also* Tear, meniscus)
    836.2
    old 717.5
    site other than knee (*see also* Sprain, by
      site)
      old NEC (*see also* Disorder, cartilage,
        articular) 718.0 ☑
  muscle (*see also* Sprain, by site)
    with open wound — *see* Wound, open,
      by site
  myocardium — *see* Laceration, heart

☑ **Additional Digit Required** — Refer to the Tabular List for Digit Selection   ▼ **Subterms under main terms may continue to next column or page**

216   **2014 ICD-9-CM**

Laceration — *see also* Wound, open, by site — *continued*
nerve — *see* Injury, nerve, by site
ocular NEC (*see also* Laceration, eyeball) 871.4
  adnexa NEC 870.8
    penetrating 870.3
      with foreign body 870.4
orbit (eye) 870.8
  penetrating 870.3
    with foreign body 870.4
pelvic
  floor (muscles)
    with
      abortion — *see* Abortion, by type, with damage to pelvic organs
      ectopic pregnancy (*see also* categories 633.0–633.9) 639.2
      molar pregnancy (*see also* categories 630–632) 639.2
    complicating delivery 664.1 ☑
    following
      abortion 639.2
      ectopic or molar pregnancy 639.2
    nonpuerperal 618.7
    old (postpartal) 618.7
  organ NEC
    with
      abortion — *see* Abortion, by type, with damage to pelvic organs
      ectopic pregnancy (*see also* categories 633.0–633.9) 639.2
      molar pregnancy (*see also* categories 630–632) 639.2
    complicating delivery 665.5 ☑
      affecting fetus or newborn 763.89
    following
      abortion 639.2
      ectopic or molar pregnancy 639.2
      obstetrical trauma 665.5 ☑
perineum, perineal (old) (postpartal) 618.7
  with
    abortion — *see* Abortion, by type, with damage to pelvic floor
    ectopic pregnancy (*see also* categories 633.0–633.9) 639.2
    molar pregnancy (*see also* categories 630–632) 639.2
  complicating delivery 664.4 ☑
    first degree 664.0 ☑
    second degree 664.1 ☑
    third degree 664.2 ☑
    fourth degree 664.3 ☑
    anal sphincter (healed) (old) 654.8 ☑
      not associated with third-degree perineal laceration 664.6 ☑
      sphincter (anal) (healed) (old) 654.8 ☑
        not associated with third-degree perineal laceration 664.6 ☑
    central 664.4 ☑
    involving
      anal sphincter 664.2 ☑
      fourchette 664.0 ☑
      hymen 664.0 ☑
      labia 664.0 ☑
      pelvic floor 664.1 ☑
      perineal muscles 664.1 ☑
      rectovaginal septum 664.2 ☑
        with anal mucosa 664.3 ☑
      skin 664.0 ☑
      sphincter (anal) 664.2 ☑
        with anal mucosa 664.3 ☑
      vagina 664.0 ☑
      vaginal muscles 664.1 ☑
      vulva 664.0 ☑
    secondary 674.2 ☑
  following
    abortion 639.2
    ectopic or molar pregnancy 639.2
  male 879.6

Laceration — *see also* Wound, open, by site — *continued*
perineum, perineal — *continued*
  male — *continued*
    complicated 879.7
  muscles, complicating delivery 664.1 ☑
  nonpuerperal, current injury 879.6
    complicated 879.7
  secondary (postpartal) 674.2 ☑
peritoneum
  with
    abortion — *see* Abortion, by type, with damage to pelvic organs
    ectopic pregnancy (*see also* categories 633.0–633.9) 639.2
    molar pregnancy (*see also* categories 630–632) 639.2
  following
    abortion 639.2
    ectopic or molar pregnancy 639.2
  obstetrical trauma 665.5 ☑
periurethral tissue
  with
    abortion — *see* Abortion, by type, with damage to pelvic organs
    ectopic pregnancy (*see also* categories 633.0–633.9) 639.2
    molar pregnancy (*see also* categories 630–632) 639.2
  following
    abortion 639.2
    ectopic or molar pregnancy 639.2
  obstetrical trauma 664.8 ☑
rectovaginal (septum)
  with
    abortion — *see* Abortion, by type, with damage to pelvic organs
    ectopic pregnancy (*see also* categories 633.0–633.9) 639.2
    molar pregnancy (*see also* categories 630–632) 639.2
  complicating delivery 665.4 ☑
    with perineum 664.2 ☑
      involving anal or rectal mucosa 664.3 ☑
  following
    abortion 639.2
    ectopic or molar pregnancy 639.2
  nonpuerperal 623.4
  old (postpartal) 623.4
spinal cord (meninges) (*see also* Injury, spinal, by site)
  due to injury at birth 767.4
  fetus or newborn 767.4
spleen 865.09
  with
    disruption of parenchyma (massive) 865.04
      with open wound into cavity 865.14
    open wound into cavity 865.19
  capsule (without disruption of parenchyma) 865.02
    with open wound into cavity 865.12
  parenchyma 865.03
    with open wound into cavity 865.13
    massive disruption (rupture) 865.04
      with open wound into cavity 865.14
tendon 848.9
  with open wound — *see* Wound, open, by site
  Achilles 845.09
    with open wound 892.2
  lower limb NEC 844.9
    with open wound NEC 894.2
  upper limb NEC 840.9
    with open wound NEC 884.2
tentorium cerebelli — *see* Laceration, brain, cerebellum
tongue 873.64
  complicated 873.74
urethra
  with
    abortion — *see* Abortion, by type, with damage to pelvic organs

Laceration — *see also* Wound, open, by site — *continued*
urethra — *continued*
  with — *continued*
    ectopic pregnancy (*see also* categories 633.0–633.9) 639.2
    molar pregnancy (*see also* categories 630–632) 639.2
  following
    abortion 639.2
    ectopic or molar pregnancy 639.2
  nonpuerperal, nontraumatic 599.84
  obstetrical trauma 665.5 ☑
uterus
  with
    abortion — *see* Abortion, by type, with damage to pelvic organs
    ectopic pregnancy (*see also* categories 633.0–633.9) 639.2
    molar pregnancy (*see also* categories 630–632) 639.2
  following
    abortion 639.2
    ectopic or molar pregnancy 639.2
  nonpuerperal, nontraumatic 621.8
  obstetrical trauma NEC 665.5 ☑
  old (postpartal) 621.8
vagina
  with
    abortion — *see* Abortion, by type, with damage to pelvic organs
    ectopic pregnancy (*see also* categories 633.0–633.9) 639.2
    molar pregnancy (*see also* categories 630–632) 639.2
    perineal involvement, complicating delivery 664.0 ☑
  complicating delivery 665.4 ☑
    first degree 664.0 ☑
    second degree 664.1 ☑
    third degree 664.2 ☑
    fourth degree 664.3 ☑
    high 665.4 ☑
    muscles 664.1 ☑
    sulcus 665.4 ☑
    wall 665.4 ☑
  following
    abortion 639.2
    ectopic or molar pregnancy 639.2
  nonpuerperal, nontraumatic 623.4
  old (postpartal) 623.4
valve, heart — *see* Endocarditis
vulva
  with
    abortion — *see* Abortion, by type, with damage to pelvic organs
    ectopic pregnancy (*see also* categories 633.0–633.9) 639.2
    molar pregnancy (*see also* categories 630–632) 639.2
  complicating delivery 664.0 ☑
  following
    abortion 639.2
    ectopic or molar pregnancy 639.2
  nonpuerperal, nontraumatic 624.4
  old (postpartal) 624.4
Lachrymal — *see* condition
Lachrymonasal duct — *see* condition
Lack of
adequate intermaxillary vertical dimension 524.36
appetite (*see also* Anorexia) 783.0
care
  in home V60.4
  of adult 995.84
  of infant (at or after birth) 995.52
coordination 781.3
development (*see also* Hypoplasia)
  physiological in childhood 783.40
education V62.3
energy 780.79
financial resources V60.2
food 994.2
  in environment V60.89
growth in childhood 783.43
heating V60.1

Lack of — *continued*
housing (permanent) (temporary) V60.0
  adequate V60.1
material resources V60.2
medical attention 799.89
memory (*see also* Amnesia) 780.93
  mild, following organic brain damage 310.89
ovulation 628.0
person able to render necessary care V60.4
physical exercise V69.0
physiologic development in childhood 783.40
posterior occlusal support 524.57
prenatal care in current pregnancy V23.7
shelter V60.0
sleep V69.4
water 994.3
Lacrimal — *see* condition
Lacrimation, abnormal — *see also* Epiphora 375.20
Lacrimonasal duct — *see* condition
Lactation, lactating (breast) (puerperal) (postpartum)
defective 676.4 ☑
disorder 676.9 ☑
  specified type NEC 676.8 ☑
excessive 676.6 ☑
failed 676.4 ☑
mastitis NEC 675.2 ☑
mother (care and/or examination) V24.1
nonpuerperal 611.6
suppressed 676.5 ☑
Lacticemia 271.3
excessive 276.2
Lactosuria 271.3
Lacunar skull 756.0
Laennec's cirrhosis (alcoholic) 571.2
nonalcoholic 571.5
Lafora's disease 333.2
Lagleyze-von Hippel disease (retinocerebral angiomatosis) 759.6
Lag, lid (nervous) 374.41
Lagophthalmos (eyelid) (nervous) 374.20
cicatricial 374.23
keratitis (*see also* Keratitis) 370.34
mechanical 374.22
paralytic 374.21
La grippe — *see* Influenza
Lahore sore 085.1
Lakes, venous (cerebral) 437.8
Laki-Lorand factor deficiency — *see also* Defect, coagulation 286.3
Lalling 307.9
Lambliasis 007.1
Lame back 724.5
Lancereaux's diabetes (diabetes mellitus with marked emaciation) 250.8 ☑ *[261]*
due to secondary diabetes 249.8 ☑ *[261]*
Landau-Kleffner syndrome 345.8 ☑
Landouzy-Déjérine dystrophy (fascioscapulohumeral atrophy) 359.1
Landry's disease or paralysis 357.0
Landry-Guillain-Barré syndrome 357.0
Lane's
band 751.4
disease 569.89
kink (*see also* Obstruction, intestine) 560.9
Langdon Down's syndrome (mongolism) 758.0
Language abolition 784.69
Lanugo (persistent) 757.4
Laparoscopic surgical procedure converted to open procedure V64.41
Lardaceous
degeneration (any site) 277.39
disease 277.39
kidney 277.39 *[583.81]*
liver 277.39
Large
baby (regardless of gestational age) 766.1
  exceptionally (weight of 4500 grams or more) 766.0
  of diabetic mother 775.0
ear 744.22
fetus (*see also* Oversize, fetus)

☑ **Additional Digit Required — Refer to the Tabular List for Digit Selection**   ▽ **Subterms under main terms may continue to next column or page**

2014 ICD-9-CM   **217**

Laceration — Large

Large — continued
  fetus (see also Oversize, fetus) — continued
    causing disproportion 653.5 ☑
      with obstructed labor 660.1 ☑
    for dates
      fetus or newborn (regardless of gestational age) 766.1
      affecting management of pregnancy 656.6 ☑
      exceptionally (weight of 4500 grams or more) 766.0
    physiological cup 743.57
    stature 783.9
    waxy liver 277.39
    white kidney — see Nephrosis
Larsen-Johansson disease (juvenile osteopathia patellae) 732.4
Larsen's syndrome (flattened facies and multiple congenital dislocations) 755.8
Larva migrans
  cutaneous NEC 126.9
    ancylostoma 126.9
  of Diptera in vitreous 128.0
  visceral NEC 128.0
Laryngeal — see also condition 786.2
  syncope 786.2
Laryngismus (acute) (infectious) (stridulous) 478.75
  congenital 748.3
  diphtheritic 032.3
Laryngitis (acute) (edematous) (fibrinous) (gangrenous) (infective) (infiltrative) (malignant) (membranous) (phlegmonous) (pneumococcal) (pseudomembranous) (septic) (subglottic) (suppurative) (ulcerative) (viral) 464.00
  with
    influenza, flu, or grippe (see also Influenza) 487.1
    obstruction 464.01
    tracheitis (see also Laryngotracheitis) 464.20
      with obstruction 464.21
      acute 464.20
        with obstruction 464.21
      chronic 476.1
  atrophic 476.0
  Borrelia vincentii 101
  catarrhal 476.0
  chronic 476.0
    with tracheitis (chronic) 476.1
    due to external agent — see Condition, respiratory, chronic, due to
  diphtheritic (membranous) 032.3
  due to external agent — see Inflammation, respiratory, upper, due to
  Hemophilus influenzae 464.00
    with obstruction 464.01
  H. influenzae 464.00
    with obstruction 464.01
  hypertrophic 476.0
  influenzal (see also Influenza) 487.1
  pachydermic 478.79
  sicca 476.0
  spasmodic 478.75
    acute 464.00
      with obstruction 464.01
  streptococcal 034.0
  stridulous 478.75
  syphilitic 095.8
    congenital 090.5
  tuberculous (see also Tuberculosis, larynx) 012.3 ☑
  Vincent's 101
Laryngocele (congenital) (ventricular) 748.3
Laryngofissure 478.79
  congenital 748.3
Laryngomalacia (congenital) 748.3
Laryngopharyngitis (acute) 465.0
  chronic 478.9
    due to external agent — see Condition, respiratory, chronic, due to
  due to external agent — see Inflammation, respiratory, upper, due to
  septic 034.0

Laryngoplegia — see also Paralysis, vocal cord 478.30
Laryngoptosis 478.79
Laryngospasm 478.75
  due to external agent — see Condition, respiratory, acute, due to
Laryngostenosis 478.74
  congenital 748.3
Laryngotracheitis (acute) (infectional) (viral) — see also Laryngitis 464.20
  with obstruction 464.21
  atrophic 476.1
  Borrelia vincenti 101
  catarrhal 476.1
  chronic 476.1
    due to external agent — see Condition, respiratory, chronic, due to
  diphtheritic (membranous) 032.3
  due to external agent — see Inflammation, respiratory, upper, due to
  H. influenzae 464.20
    with obstruction 464.21
  hypertrophic 476.1
  influenzal (see also Influenza) 487.1
  pachydermic 478.75
  sicca 476.1
  spasmodic 478.75
    acute 464.20
      with obstruction 464.21
  streptococcal 034.0
  stridulous 478.75
  syphilitic 095.8
    congenital 090.5
  tuberculous (see also Tuberculosis, larynx) 012.3 ☑
  Vincent's 101
Laryngotracheobronchitis — see also Bronchitis 490
  acute 466.0
  chronic 491.8
  viral 466.0
Laryngotracheobronchopneumonitis — see Pneumonia, broncho-
Larynx, laryngeal — see condition
Lasègue's disease (persecution mania) 297.9
Lassa fever 078.89
Lassitude — see also Weakness 780.79
Late — see also condition
  effect(s) (of) (see also condition)
    abscess
      intracranial or intraspinal (conditions classifiable to 324) — see category 326
    adverse effect of drug, medicinal or biological substance 909.5
    allergic reaction 909.9
    amputation
      postoperative (late) 997.60
      traumatic (injury classifiable to 885–887 and 895–897) 905.9
    burn (injury classifiable to 948–949) 906.9
      extremities NEC (injury classifiable to 943 or 945) 906.7
      hand or wrist (injury classifiable to 944) 906.6
      eye (injury classifiable to 940) 906.5
      face, head, and neck (injury classifiable to 941) 906.5
      specified site NEC (injury classifiable to 942 and 946–947) 906.8
    cerebrovascular disease (conditions classifiable to 430–437) 438.9
      with
        alterations of sensations 438.6
        aphasia 438.11
        apraxia 438.81
        ataxia 438.84
        cognitive deficits 438.0
        disturbances of vision 438.7
        dysarthria 438.13
        dysphagia 438.82
        dysphasia 438.12
        facial droop 438.83
        facial weakness 438.83
        fluency disorder 438.14

Late — see also condition — continued
  effect(s) (see also condition) — continued
    cerebrovascular disease — continued
      with — continued
        hemiplegia/hemiparesis affecting
          dominant side 438.21
          nondominant side 438.22
          unspecified side 438.20
        monoplegia of lower limb affecting
          dominant side 438.41
          nondominant side 438.42
          unspecified side 438.40
        monoplegia of upper limb affecting
          dominant side 438.31
          nondominant side 438.32
          unspecified side 438.30
        paralytic syndrome NEC affecting
          bilateral 438.53
          dominant side 438.51
          nondominant side 438.52
          unspecified side 438.50
        speech and language deficit 438.10
          specified type NEC 438.19
        stuttering 438.14
        vertigo 438.85
      specified type NEC 438.89
    childbirth complication(s) 677
    complication(s) of
      childbirth 677
      delivery 677
      pregnancy 677
      puerperium 677
      surgical and medical care (conditions classifiable to 996–999) 909.3
      trauma (conditions classifiable to 958) 908.6
    contusion (injury classifiable to 920–924) 906.3
    crushing (injury classifiable to 925–929) 906.4
    delivery complication(s) 677
    dislocation (injury classifiable to 830–839) 905.6
    encephalitis or encephalomyelitis (conditions classifiable to 323) — see category 326
      in infectious diseases 139.8
      viral (conditions classifiable to 049.8, 049.9, 062–064) 139.0
    external cause NEC (conditions classifiable to 995) 909.9
      certain conditions classifiable to categories 991–994 909.4
    foreign body in orifice (injury classifiable to 930–939) 908.5
    fracture (multiple) (injury classifiable to 828–829) 905.5
    extremity
      lower (injury classifiable to 821–827) 905.4
      neck of femur (injury classifiable to 820) 905.3
      upper (injury classifiable to 810–819) 905.2
    face and skull (injury classifiable to 800–804) 905.0
    skull and face (injury classifiable to 800–804) 905.0
    spine and trunk (injury classifiable to 805 and 807–809) 905.1
      with spinal cord lesion (injury classifiable to 806) 907.2
    infection
      pyogenic, intracranial — see category 326
    infectious diseases (conditions classifiable to 001–136) NEC 139.8
    injury (injury classifiable to 959) 908.9

Late — see also condition — continued
  effect(s) (see also condition) — continued
    injury — continued
      blood vessel 908.3
        abdomen and pelvis (injury classifiable to 902) 908.4
        extremity (injury classifiable to 903–904) 908.3
        head and neck (injury classifiable to 900) 908.3
        intracranial (injury classifiable to 850–854) 907.0
          with skull fracture 905.0
        thorax (injury classifiable to 901) 908.4
      internal organ NEC (injury classifiable to 867 and 869) 908.2
        abdomen (injury classifiable to 863–866 and 868) 908.1
        thorax (injury classifiable to 860–862) 908.0
      intracranial (injury classifiable to 850–854) 907.0
        with skull fracture (injury classifiable to 800–801 and 803–804) 905.0
      nerve NEC (injury classifiable to 957) 907.9
        cranial (injury classifiable to 950–951) 907.1
        peripheral NEC (injury classifiable to 957) 907.9
          lower limb and pelvic girdle (injury classifiable to 956) 907.5
          upper limb and shoulder girdle (injury classifiable to 955) 907.4
        roots and plexus(es), spinal (injury classifiable to 953) 907.3
        trunk (injury classifiable to 954) 907.3
      spinal
        cord (injury classifiable to 806 and 952) 907.2
        nerve root(s) and plexus(es) (injury classifiable to 953) 907.3
      superficial (injury classifiable to 910–919) 906.2
      tendon (tendon injury classifiable to 840–848, 880–884 with .2, and 890–894 with .2) 905.8
    meningitis
      bacterial (conditions classifiable to 320) — see category 326
      unspecified cause (conditions classifiable to 322) — see category 326
    myelitis (see also Late, effect(s) (of), encephalitis) — see category 326
    parasitic diseases (conditions classifiable to 001–136 NEC) 139.8
    phlebitis or thrombophlebitis of intracranial venous sinuses (conditions classifiable to 325) — see category 326
    poisoning due to drug, medicinal or biological substance (conditions classifiable to 960–979) 909.0
    poliomyelitis, acute (conditions classifiable to 045) 138
    pregnancy complication(s) 677
    puerperal complication(s) 677
    radiation (conditions classifiable to 990) 909.2
    rickets 268.1
    sprain and strain without mention of tendon injury (injury classifiable to 840–848, except tendon injury) 905.7
      tendon involvement 905.8

Late — *see also* condition — *continued*
effect(s) (*see also* condition) — *continued*
  toxic effect of
    drug, medicinal or biological substance (conditions classifiable to 960–979) 909.0
    nonmedical substance (conditions classifiable to 980–989) 909.1
  trachoma (conditions classifiable to 076) 139.1
  tuberculosis 137.0
    bones and joints (conditions classifiable to 015) 137.3
    central nervous system (conditions classifiable to 013) 137.1
    genitourinary (conditions classifiable to 016) 137.2
    pulmonary (conditions classifiable to 010–012) 137.0
    specified organs NEC (conditions classifiable to 014, 017–018) 137.4
    viral encephalitis (conditions classifiable to 049.8, 049.9, 062–064) 139.0
  wound, open
    extremity (injury classifiable to 880–884 and 890–894, except .2) 906.1
      tendon (injury classifiable to 880–884 with .2 and 890–894 with .2) 905.8
    head, neck, and trunk (injury classifiable to 870–879) 906.0
infant
  post-term (gestation period over 40 completed weeks to 42 completed weeks) 766.21
  prolonged gestation (period over 42 completed weeks) 766.22
Latent — *see* condition
Lateral — *see* condition
Laterocession — *see* Lateroversion
Lateroflexion — *see* Lateroversion
Lateroversion
  cervix — *see* Lateroversion, uterus
  uterus, uterine (cervix) (postinfectional) (postpartal, old) 621.6
    congenital 752.39
    in pregnancy or childbirth 654.4 ☑
      affecting fetus or newborn 763.89
Lathyrism 988.2
Launois-Bensaude's lipomatosis 272.8
Launois-Cléret syndrome (adiposogenital dystrophy) 253.8
Launois' syndrome (pituitary gigantism) 253.0
Laurence-Moon-Biedl syndrome (obesity, polydactyly, and intellectual disabilities) 759.89
LAV (disease) (illness) (infection) — *see* Human immunodeficiency virus (disease) (illness) (infection)
LAV/HTLV-III (disease) (illness) (infection) — *see* Human immunodeficiency virus (disease) (illness) (infection)
Lawford's syndrome (encephalocutaneous angiomatosis) 759.6
Laxative habit — *see also* Abuse, drugs, nondependent 305.9 ☑
Lax, laxity — *see also* Relaxation
  ligament 728.4
  skin (acquired) 701.8
    congenital 756.83
Lazy leukocyte syndrome 288.09
LCAD (long chain/very long chain acyl CoA dehydrogenase deficiency, VLCAD) 277.85
LCHAD (long chain 3-hydroxyacyl CoA dehydrogenase deficiency) 277.85
Lead — *see also* condition
  exposure (suspected) to V15.86
  incrustation of cornea 371.15
  poisoning 984.9
    specified type of lead — *see* Table of Drugs and Chemicals
Lead miners' lung 503

Leakage
  amniotic fluid 658.1 ☑
    with delayed delivery 658.2 ☑
    affecting fetus or newborn 761.1
  bile from drainage tube (T tube) 997.49
  blood (microscopic), fetal, into maternal circulation 656.0 ☑
    affecting management of pregnancy or puerperium 656.0 ☑
  device, implant, or graft — *see* Complications, mechanical
  spinal fluid at lumbar puncture site 997.09
  urine, continuous 788.37
Leaky heart — *see* Endocarditis
Learning defect, specific NEC (strephosymbolia) 315.2
Leather bottle stomach (M8142/3) 151.9
Leber's
  congenital amaurosis 362.76
  optic atrophy (hereditary) 377.16
Lederer's anemia or disease (acquired infectious hemolytic anemia) 283.19
Lederer-Brill syndrome (acquired infectious hemolytic anemia) 283.19
Leeches (aquatic) (land) 134.2
Left-sided neglect 781.8
Leg — *see* condition
Legal investigation V62.5
Legg (-Calvé) -Perthes disease or syndrome (osteochondrosis, femoral capital) 732.1
Legionnaires' disease 482.84
Leigh's disease 330.8
Leiner's disease (exfoliative dermatitis) 695.89
Leiofibromyoma (M8890/0) — *see also* Leiomyoma
  uterus (cervix) (corpus) (*see also* Leiomyoma, uterus) 218.9
Leiomyoblastoma (M8891/1) — *see* Neoplasm, connective tissue, uncertain behavior
Leiomyofibroma (M8890/0) — *see also* Neoplasm, connective tissue, benign
  uterus (cervix) (corpus) (*see also* Leiomyoma, uterus) 218.9
Leiomyoma (M8890/0) — *see also* Neoplasm, connective tissue, benign
  bizarre (M8893/0) — *see* Neoplasm, connective tissue, benign
  cellular (M8892/1) — *see* Neoplasm, connective tissue, uncertain behavior
  epithelioid (M8891/1) — *see* Neoplasm, connective tissue, uncertain behavior
  prostate (polypoid) 600.20
    with
      other lower urinary tract symptoms (LUTS) 600.21
      urinary
        obstruction 600.21
        retention 600.21
  uterus (cervix) (corpus) 218.9
    interstitial 218.1
    intramural 218.1
    submucous 218.0
    subperitoneal 218.2
    subserous 218.2
  vascular (M8894/0) — *see* Neoplasm, connective tissue, benign
Leiomyomatosis (intravascular) (M8890/1) — *see* Neoplasm, connective tissue, uncertain behavior
Leiomyosarcoma (M8890/3) — *see also* Neoplasm, connective tissue, malignant
  epithelioid (M8891/3) — *see* Neoplasm, connective tissue, malignant
Leishmaniasis 085.9
  American 085.5
    cutaneous 085.4
    mucocutaneous 085.5
  Asian desert 085.2
  Brazilian 085.5
  cutaneous 085.9
    acute necrotizing 085.2
    American 085.4
    Asian desert 085.2
    diffuse 085.3
    dry form 085.1

Leishmaniasis — *continued*
  cutaneous — *continued*
    Ethiopian 085.3
    eyelid 085.5 [373.6]
    late 085.1
    lepromatous 085.3
    recurrent 085.1
    rural 085.2
    ulcerating 085.1
    urban 085.1
    wet form 085.2
    zoonotic form 085.2
  dermal (*see also* Leishmaniasis, cutaneous)
    post kala-azar 085.0
  eyelid 085.5 [373.6]
  infantile 085.0
  Mediterranean 085.0
  mucocutaneous (American) 085.5
  naso-oral 085.5
  nasopharyngeal 085.5
  Old World 085.1
  tegumentaria diffusa 085.4
  vaccination, prophylactic (against) V05.2
  visceral (Indian) 085.0
Leishmanoid, dermal — *see also* Leishmaniasis, cutaneous
  post kala-azar 085.0
Leloir's disease 695.4
Lemiere syndrome 451.89
Lenegre's disease 426.0
Lengthening, leg 736.81
Lennox-Gastaut syndrome 345.0 ☑
  with tonic seizures 345.1 ☑
Lennox's syndrome — *see also* Epilepsy 345.0 ☑
Lens — *see* condition
Lenticonus (anterior) (posterior) (congenital) 743.36
Lenticular degeneration, progressive 275.1
Lentiglobus (posterior) (congenital) 743.36
Lentigo (congenital) 709.09
  juvenile 709.09
  Maligna (M8742/2) (*see also* Neoplasm, skin, in situ)
    melanoma (M8742/3) — *see* Melanoma
  senile 709.09
Leonine leprosy 030.0
Leontiasis
  ossium 733.3
  syphilitic 095.8
    congenital 090.5
Léopold-Lévi's syndrome (paroxysmal thyroid instability) 242.9 ☑
Lepore hemoglobin syndrome 282.45
Lepothrix 039.0
Lepra 030.9
  Willan's 696.1
Leprechaunism 259.8
Lepromatous leprosy 030.0
Leprosy 030.9
  anesthetic 030.1
  beriberi 030.1
  borderline (group B) (infiltrated) (neuritic) 030.3
  cornea (*see also* Leprosy, by type) 030.9 [371.89]
  dimorphous (group B) (infiltrated) (lepromatous) (neuritic) (tuberculoid) 030.3
  eyelid 030.0 [373.4]
  indeterminate (group I) (macular) (neuritic) (uncharacteristic) 030.2
  leonine 030.0
  lepromatous (diffuse) (infiltrated) (macular) (neuritic) (nodular) (type L) 030.0
  macular (early) (neuritic) (simple) 030.2
  maculoanesthetic 030.1
  mixed 030.0
  neuro 030.1
  nodular 030.0
  primary neuritic 030.3
  specified type or group NEC 030.8
  tubercular 030.1
  tuberculoid (macular) (maculoanesthetic) (major) (minor) (neuritic) (type T) 030.1
Leptocytosis, hereditary 282.40

Leptomeningitis (chronic) (circumscribed) (hemorrhagic) (nonsuppurative) — *see also* Meningitis 322.9
  aseptic 047.9
    adenovirus 049.1
    Coxsackie virus 047.0
    ECHO virus 047.1
    enterovirus 047.9
    lymphocytic choriomeningitis 049.0
  epidemic 036.0
  late effect — *see* category 326
  meningococcal 036.0
  pneumococcal 320.1
  syphilitic 094.2
  tuberculous (*see also* Tuberculosis, meninges) 013.0 ☑
Leptomeningopathy — *see also* Meningitis 322.9
Leptospiral — *see* condition
Leptospirochetal — *see* condition
Leptospirosis 100.9
  autumnalis 100.89
  canicula 100.89
  grippotyphosa 100.89
  hebdomidis 100.89
  icterohemorrhagica 100.0
  nanukayami 100.89
  pomona 100.89
  Weil's disease 100.0
Leptothricosis — *see* Actinomycosis
Leptothrix infestation — *see* Actinomycosis
Leptotricosis — *see* Actinomycosis
Leptus dermatitis 133.8
Leriche's syndrome (aortic bifurcation occlusion) 444.09
Léris pleonosteosis 756.89
Léri-Weill syndrome 756.59
Lermoyez's syndrome — *see also* Disease, Ménière's 386.00
Lesbianism — *omit code*
  ego-dystonic 302.0
  problems with 302.0
Lesch-Nyhan syndrome (hypoxanthineguanine-phosphoribosyltransferase deficiency) 277.2
Lesion(s)
  abducens nerve 378.54
  alveolar process 525.8
  anorectal 569.49
  aortic (valve) — *see* Endocarditis, aortic
  auditory nerve 388.5
  basal ganglion 333.90
  bile duct (*see also* Disease, biliary) 576.8
  bladder 596.9
  bone 733.90
  brachial plexus 353.0
  brain 348.89
    congenital 742.9
    vascular (*see also* Lesion, cerebrovascular) 437.9
      degenerative 437.1
      healed or old without residuals V12.54
      hypertensive 437.2
      late effect — *see* Late effect(s) (of) cerebrovascular disease
  buccal 528.9
  calcified — *see* Calcification
  canthus 373.9
  carate — *see* Pinta, lesions
  cardia 537.89
  cardiac — *see also* Disease, heart
    congenital 746.9
    valvular — *see* Endocarditis
  cauda equina 344.60
    with neurogenic bladder 344.61
  cecum 569.89
  cerebral — *see* Lesion, brain
  cerebrovascular (*see also* Disease, cerebrovascular NEC) 437.9
    degenerative 437.1
      healed or old without residuals V12.54
    hypertensive 437.2
    specified type NEC 437.8
  cervical root (nerve) NEC 353.2

Lesion(s) — *continued*
  chiasmal 377.54
    associated with
      inflammatory disorders 377.54
      neoplasm NEC 377.52
        pituitary 377.51
      pituitary disorders 377.51
      vascular disorders 377.53
  chorda tympani 351.8
  coin, lung 793.11
  colon 569.89
  congenital — *see* Anomaly
  conjunctiva 372.9
  coronary artery (*see also* Ischemia, heart) 414.9
  cranial nerve 352.9
    first 352.0
    second 377.49
    third
      partial 378.51
      total 378.52
    fourth 378.53
    fifth 350.9
    sixth 378.54
    seventh 351.9
    eighth 388.5
    ninth 352.2
    tenth 352.3
    eleventh 352.4
    twelfth 352.5
  cystic — *see* Cyst
  degenerative — *see* Degeneration
  dermal (skin) 709.9
  Dieulafoy (hemorrhagic)
    of
      duodenum 537.84
      intestine 569.86
      stomach 537.84
  duodenum 537.89
    with obstruction 537.3
  eyelid 373.9
  gasserian ganglion 350.8
  gastric 537.89
  gastroduodenal 537.89
  gastrointestinal 569.89
  glossopharyngeal nerve 352.2
  heart (organic) (*see also* Disease, heart)
    vascular — *see* Disease, cardiovascular
  helix (ear) 709.9
  high grade myelodysplastic syndrome 238.73
  hyperchromic, due to pinta (carate) 103.1
  hyperkeratotic (*see also* Hyperkeratosis) 701.1
  hypoglossal nerve 352.5
  hypopharynx 478.29
  hypothalamic 253.9
  ileocecal coil 569.89
  ileum 569.89
  iliohypogastric nerve 355.79
  ilioinguinal nerve 355.79
  in continuity — *see* Injury, nerve, by site
  inflammatory — *see* Inflammation
  intestine 569.89
  intracerebral — *see* Lesion, brain
  intrachiasmal (optic) (*see also* Lesion, chiasmal) 377.54
  intracranial, space-occupying NEC 784.2
  joint 719.90
    ankle 719.97
    elbow 719.92
    foot 719.97
    hand 719.94
    hip 719.95
    knee 719.96
    multiple sites 719.99
    pelvic region 719.95
    sacroiliac (old) 724.6
    shoulder (region) 719.91
    specified site NEC 719.98
    wrist 719.93
  keratotic (*see also* Keratosis) 701.1
  kidney (*see also* Disease, renal) 593.9
  laryngeal nerve (recurrent) 352.3
  leonine 030.0
  lip 528.5

Lesion(s) — *continued*
  liver 573.8
  low grade myelodysplastic syndrome 238.72
  lumbosacral
    plexus 353.1
    root (nerve) NEC 353.4
  lung 518.89
    coin 793.11
  maxillary sinus 473.0
  mitral — *see* Endocarditis, mitral
  Morel Lavallée — *see* Hematoma, by site
  motor cortex 348.89
  nerve (*see also* Disorder, nerve) 355.9
  nervous system 349.9
    congenital 742.9
  nonallopathic NEC 739.9
    in region (of)
      abdomen 739.9
      acromioclavicular 739.7
      cervical, cervicothoracic 739.1
      costochondral 739.8
      costovertebral 739.8
      extremity
        lower 739.6
        upper 739.7
      head 739.0
      hip 739.5
      lower extremity 739.6
      lumbar, lumbosacral 739.3
      occipitocervical 739.0
      pelvic 739.5
      pubic 739.5
      rib cage 739.8
      sacral, sacrococcygeal, sacroiliac 739.4
      sternochondral 739.8
      sternoclavicular 739.7
      thoracic, thoracolumbar 739.2
      upper extremity 739.7
  nose (internal) 478.19
  obstructive — *see* Obstruction
  obturator nerve 355.79
  occlusive
    artery — *see* Embolism, artery
  organ or site NEC — *see* Disease, by site
  osteolytic 733.90
  paramacular, of retina 363.32
  peptic 537.89
  periodontal, due to traumatic occlusion 523.8
  perirectal 569.49
  peritoneum (granulomatous) 568.89
  pigmented (skin) 709.00
  pinta — *see* Pinta, lesions
  polypoid — *see* Polyp
  prechiasmal (optic) (*see also* Lesion, chiasmal) 377.54
  primary (*see also* Syphilis, primary)
    carate 103.0
    pinta 103.0
    yaws 102.0
  pulmonary 518.89
    valve (*see also* Endocarditis, pulmonary) 424.3
  pylorus 537.89
  radiation NEC 990
  radium NEC 990
  rectosigmoid 569.89
  retina, retinal (*see also* Retinopathy)
    vascular 362.17
  retroperitoneal 568.89
  romanus 720.1
  sacroiliac (joint) 724.6
  salivary gland 527.8
    benign lymphoepithelial 527.8
  saphenous nerve 355.79
  secondary — *see* Syphilis, secondary
  sigmoid 569.89
  sinus (accessory) (nasal) (*see also* Sinusitis) 473.9
  skin 709.9
    suppurative 686.00
  SLAP (superior glenoid labrum) 840.7
  space-occupying, intracranial NEC 784.2
  spinal cord 336.9
    congenital 742.9

Lesion(s) — *continued*
  spinal cord — *continued*
    traumatic (complete) (incomplete) (transverse) (*see also* Injury, spinal, by site)
      with
        broken
          back — *see* Fracture, vertebra, by site, with spinal cord injury
          neck — *see* Fracture, vertebra, cervical, with spinal cord injury
        fracture, vertebra — *see* Fracture, vertebra, by site, with spinal cord injury
  spleen 289.50
  stomach 537.89
  superior glenoid labrum (SLAP) 840.7
  syphilitic — *see* Syphilis
  tertiary — *see* Syphilis, tertiary
  thoracic root (nerve) 353.3
  tonsillar fossa 474.9
  tooth, teeth 525.8
    white spot 521.01
  traumatic NEC (*see also* nature and site of injury) 959.9
  tricuspid (valve) — *see* Endocarditis, tricuspid
  trigeminal nerve 350.9
  ulcerated or ulcerative — *see* Ulcer
  uterus NEC 621.9
  vagina 623.8
  vagus nerve 352.3
  valvular — *see* Endocarditis
  vascular 459.9
    affecting central nervous system (*see also* Lesion, cerebrovascular) 437.9
    following trauma (*see also* Injury, blood vessel, by site) 904.9
    retina 362.17
    traumatic — *see* Injury, blood vessel, by site
    umbilical cord 663.6 ☑
      affecting fetus or newborn 762.6
  visual
    cortex NEC (*see also* Disorder, visual, cortex) 377.73
    pathway NEC (*see also* Disorder, visual, pathway) 377.63
  warty — *see* Verruca
  white spot, on teeth 521.01
  x-ray NEC 990
Lethargic — *see* condition
Lethargy 780.79
Letterer-Siwe disease (acute histiocytosis X) (M9722/3) 202.5 ☑
Leucinosis 270.3
Leucocoria 360.44
Leucosarcoma (M9850/3) 207.8 ☑
Leukasmus 270.2
Leukemia, leukemic (congenital) (M9800/3) 208.9 ☑

> *Note – Use the following fifth-digit subclassification for categories 203–208:*
>
> **0**   *without mention of having achieved remission*
>
>   *failed remission*
>
> **1**   *with remission*
>
> **2**   *in relapse*

  acute NEC (M9801/3) 208.0 ☑
  aleukemic NEC (M9804/3) 208.8 ☑
    granulocytic (M9864/3) 205.8 ☑
  basophilic (M9870/3) 205.1 ☑
  blast (cell) (M9801/3) 208.0 ☑
  blastic (M9801/3) 208.0 ☑
    granulocytic (M9861/3) 205.0 ☑
  chronic NEC (M9803/3) 208.1 ☑
  compound (M9810/3) 207.8 ☑
  eosinophilic (M9880/3) 205.1 ☑
  giant cell (M9910/3) 207.2 ☑
  granulocytic (M9860/3) 205.9 ☑
    acute (M9861/3) 205.0 ☑

Leukemia, leukemic — *continued*
  granulocytic — *continued*
    aleukemic (M9864/3) 205.8 ☑
    blastic (M9861/3) 205.0 ☑
    chronic (M9863/3) 205.1 ☑
    subacute (M9862/3) 205.2 ☑
    subleukemic (M9864/3) 205.8 ☑
  hairy cell (M9940/3) 202.4 ☑
  hemoblastic (M9801/3) 208.0 ☑
  histiocytic (M9890/3) 206.9 ☑
  lymphatic (M9820/3) 204.9 ☑
    acute (M9821/3) 204.0 ☑
    aleukemic (M9824/3) 204.8 ☑
    chronic (M9823/3) 204.1 ☑
    subacute (M9822/3) 204.2 ☑
    subleukemic (M9824/3) 204.8 ☑
  lymphoblastic (M9821/3) 204.0 ☑
  lymphocytic (M9820/3) 204.9 ☑
    acute (M9821/3) 204.0 ☑
    aleukemic (M9824/3) 204.8 ☑
    chronic (M9823/3) 204.1 ☑
    granular
      large T-cell 204.8 ☑
    subacute (M9822/3) 204.2 ☑
    subleukemic (M9824/3) 204.8 ☑
  lymphogenous (M9820/3) — *see* Leukemia, lymphoid
  lymphoid (M9820/3) 204.9 ☑
    acute (M9821/3) 204.0 ☑
    aleukemic (M9824/3) 204.8 ☑
    blastic (M9821/3) 204.0 ☑
    chronic (M9823/3) 204.1 ☑
    subacute (M9822/3) 204.2 ☑
    subleukemic (M9824/3) 204.8 ☑
  lymphosarcoma cell (M9850/3) 207.8 ☑
  mast cell (M9900/3) 207.8 ☑
  megakaryocytic (M9910/3) 207.2 ☑
  megakaryocytoid (M9910/3) 207.2 ☑
  mixed (cell) (M9810/3) 207.8 ☑
  monoblastic (M9891/3) 206.0 ☑
  monocytic (Schilling-type) (M9890/3) 206.9 ☑
    acute (M9891/3) 206.0 ☑
    aleukemic (M9894/3) 206.8 ☑
    chronic (M9893/3) 206.1 ☑
    Naegeli-type (M9863/3) 205.1 ☑
    subacute (M9892/3) 206.2 ☑
    subleukemic (M9894/3) 206.8 ☑
  monocytoid (M9890/3) 206.9 ☑
    acute (M9891/3) 206.0 ☑
    aleukemic (M9894/3) 206.8 ☑
    chronic (M9893/3) 206.1 ☑
    myelogenous (M9863/3) 205.1 ☑
    subacute (M9892/3) 206.2 ☑
    subleukemic (M9894/3) 206.8 ☑
  monomyelocytic (M9860/3) — *see* Leukemia, myelomonocytic
  myeloblastic (M9861/3) 205.0 ☑
  myelocytic (M9863/3) 205.1 ☑
    acute (M9861/3) 205.0 ☑
  myelogenous (M9860/3) 205.9 ☑
    acute (M9861/3) 205.0 ☑
    aleukemic (M9864/3) 205.8 ☑
    chronic (M9863/3) 205.1 ☑
    monocytoid (M9863/3) 205.1 ☑
    subacute (M9862/3) 205.2 ☑
    subleukemic (M9864) 205.8 ☑
  myeloid (M9860/3) 205.9 ☑
    acute (M9861/3) 205.0 ☑
    aleukemic (M9864/3) 205.8 ☑
    chronic (M9863/3) 205.1 ☑
    subacute (M9862/3) 205.2 ☑
    subleukemic (M9864/3) 205.8 ☑
  myelomonocytic (M9860/3) 205.9 ☑
    acute (M9861/3) 205.0 ☑
    chronic (M9863/3) 205.1 ☑
  Naegeli-type monocytic (M9863/3) 205.1 ☑
  neutrophilic (M9865/3) 205.1 ☑
  plasma cell (M9830/3) 203.1 ☑
  plasmacytic (M9830/3) 203.1 ☑
  prolymphocytic (M9825/3) — *see* Leukemia, lymphoid
  promyelocytic, acute (M9866/3) 205.0 ☑

☑ **Additional Digit Required — Refer to the Tabular List for Digit Selection**   ▽ **Subterms under main terms may continue to next column or page**

220   **2014 ICD-9-CM**

Leukemia, leukemic — Lipomatosis

☑ Additional Digit Required — Refer to the Tabular List for Digit Selection   ▽ Subterms under main terms may continue to next column or page

2014 ICD-9-CM   221

Lipomatosis — continued
   Launois-Bensaude's 272.8
Lipomyohemangioma (M8860/0)
   specified site — see Neoplasm, connective
      tissue, benign
   unspecified site 223.0
Lipomyoma (M8860/0)
   specified site — see Neoplasm, connective
      tissue, benign
   unspecified site 223.0
Lipomyxoma (M8852/0) — see Lipoma, by site
Lipomyxosarcoma (M8852/3) — see Neoplasm, connective tissue, malignant
Lipophagocytosis 289.89
Lipoproteinemia (alpha) 272.4
   broad-beta 272.2
   floating-beta 272.2
   hyper-pre-beta 272.1
Lipoproteinosis (Rössle-Urbach-Wiethe) 272.8
Liposarcoma (M8850/3) — see also Neoplasm,
   connective tissue, malignant
   differentiated type (M8851/3) — see Neo-
      plasm, connective tissue, malignant
   embryonal (M8852/3) — see Neoplasm,
      connective tissue, malignant
   mixed type (M8855/3) — see Neoplasm,
      connective tissue, malignant
   myxoid (M8852/3) — see Neoplasm, connec-
      tive tissue, malignant
   pleomorphic (M8854/3) — see Neoplasm,
      connective tissue, malignant
   round cell (M8853/3) — see Neoplasm,
      connective tissue, malignant
   well differentiated type (M8851/3) — see
      Neoplasm, connective tissue, malig-
Liposynovitis prepatellaris 272.8
Lipping
   cervix 622.0
   spine (see also Spondylosis) 721.90
   vertebra (see also Spondylosis) 721.90
Lip pits (mucus), congenital 750.25
Lipschütz disease or ulcer 616.50
Lipuria 791.1
   bilharziasis 120.0
Liquefaction, vitreous humor 379.21
Lisping 307.9
Lissauer's paralysis 094.1
Lissencephalia, lissencephaly 742.2
Listerellose 027.0
Listeriose 027.0
Listeriosis 027.0
   congenital 771.2
   fetal 771.2
   suspected fetal damage affecting manage-
      ment of pregnancy 655.4 ☑
Listlessness 780.79
Lithemia 790.6
Lithiasis — see also Calculus
   hepatic (duct) — see Choledocholithiasis
   urinary 592.9
Lithopedion 779.9
   affecting management of pregnancy
      656.8 ☑
Lithosis (occupational) 502
   with tuberculosis — see Tuberculosis, pul-
      monary
Lithuria 791.9
Litigation V62.5
Little
   league elbow 718.82
   stroke syndrome 435.9
Little's disease — see Palsy, cerebral
Littre's
   gland — see condition
   hernia — see Hernia, Littre's
Littritis — see also Urethritis 597.89
Livedo 782.61
   annularis 782.61
   racemose 782.61
   reticularis 782.61
Live flesh 781.0
Liver — see also condition
   donor V59.6
Livida, asphyxia
   newborn 768.6

Living
   alone V60.3
      with handicapped person V60.4
Lloyd's syndrome 258.1
Loa loa 125.2
Loasis 125.2
Lobe, lobar — see condition
Lobo's disease or blastomycosis 116.2
Lobomycosis 116.2
Lobotomy syndrome 310.0
Lobstein's disease (brittle bones and blue
   sclera) 756.51
Lobster-claw hand 755.58
Lobulation (congenital) — see also Anomaly,
   specified type NEC, by site
   kidney, fetal 753.3
   liver, abnormal 751.69
   spleen 759.0
Lobule, lobular — see condition
Local, localized — see condition
Locked bowel or intestine — see also Obstruc-
   tion, intestine 560.9
Locked-in state 344.81
Locked twins 660.5 ☑
   affecting fetus or newborn 763.1
Locking
   joint (see also Derangement, joint) 718.90
   knee 717.9
Lockjaw — see also Tetanus 037
Locomotor ataxia (progressive) 094.0
Löffler's
   endocarditis 421.0
   eosinophilia or syndrome 518.3
   pneumonia 518.3
   syndrome (eosinophilic pneumonitis) 518.3
Löfgren's syndrome (sarcoidosis) 135
Loiasis 125.2
   eyelid 125.2 [373.6]
Loneliness V62.89
Lone star fever 082.8
Longitudinal stripes or grooves, nails 703.8
   congenital 757.5
Long labor 662.1 ☑
   affecting fetus or newborn 763.89
   first stage 662.0 ☑
   second stage 662.2 ☑
Long-term (current) (prophylactic) **drug use**
   V58.69
   antibiotics V58.62
   anticoagulants V58.61
   anti-inflammatories, non-steroidal (NSAID)
      V58.64
   antiplatelets/antithrombotics V58.63
   aspirin V58.66
   bisphosphonates V58.68
   high-risk medications NEC V58.69
   insulin V58.67
   methadone for pain control V58.69
   opiate analgesic V58.69
   pain killers V58.69
      anti-inflammatories, non-steroidal
         (NSAID) V58.64
      aspirin V58.66
   steroids V58.65
   tamoxifen V07.51
Loop
   intestine (see also Volvulus) 560.2
   intrascleral nerve 379.29
   vascular on papilla (optic) 743.57
Loose — see also condition
   body
      in tendon sheath 727.82
      joint 718.10
         ankle 718.17
         elbow 718.12
         foot 718.17
         hand 718.14
         hip 718.15
         knee 717.6
         multiple sites 718.19
         pelvic region 718.15
         prosthetic implant — see Complica-
            tions, mechanical
         shoulder (region) 718.11
         specified site NEC 718.18
         wrist 718.13

Loose — see also condition — continued
   cartilage (joint) (see also Loose, body, joint)
      718.1 ☑
      knee 717.6
   facet (vertebral) 724.9
   prosthetic implant — see Complications,
      mechanical
   sesamoid, joint (see also Loose, body, joint)
      718.1 ☑
   tooth, teeth 525.8
Loosening epiphysis 732.9
Looser (-Debray)-Milkman syndrome (osteomalacia with pseudofractures) 268.2
Lop ear (deformity) 744.29
Lorain's disease or syndrome (pituitary
   dwarfism) 253.3
Lorain-Levi syndrome (pituitary dwarfism)
   253.3
Lordosis (acquired) (postural) 737.20
   congenital 754.2
   due to or associated with
      Charcôt-Marie-Tooth disease
         356.1 [737.42]
      mucopolysaccharidosis 277.5 [737.42]
      neurofibromatosis 237.71 [737.42]
      osteitis
         deformans 731.0 [737.42]
         fibrosa cystica 252.01 [737.42]
      osteoporosis (see also Osteoporosis)
         733.00 [737.42]
      poliomyelitis (see also Poliomyelitis)
         138 [737.42]
      tuberculosis (see also Tuberculosis)
         015.0 ☑ [737.42]
   late effect of rickets 268.1 [737.42]
   postlaminectomy 737.21
   postsurgical NEC 737.22
   rachitic 268.1 [737.42]
   specified NEC 737.29
   tuberculous (see also Tuberculosis)
      015.0 ☑ [737.42]
Loss
   appetite 783.0
      hysterical 300.11
      nonorganic origin 307.59
      psychogenic 307.59
   blood — see Hemorrhage
   central vision 368.41
   consciousness 780.09
      transient 780.2
   control, sphincter, rectum 787.60
      nonorganic origin 307.7
   ear ossicle, partial 385.24
   elasticity, skin 782.8
   extremity or member, traumatic, current —
      see Amputation, traumatic
   fluid (acute) 276.50
      with
         hypernatremia 276.0
         hyponatremia 276.1
      fetus or newborn 775.5
   hair 704.00
   hearing (see also Deafness)
      central 389.14
      conductive (air) 389.00
         with sensorineural hearing loss
            389.20
            bilateral 389.22
            unilateral 389.21
         bilateral 389.06
         combined types 389.08
         external ear 389.01
         inner ear 389.04
         middle ear 389.03
         multiple types 389.08
         tympanic membrane 389.02
         unilateral 389.05
      mixed conductive and sensorineural
         389.2
         bilateral 389.22
         unilateral 389.21
      mixed type 389.20
         bilateral 389.22
         unilateral 389.21
      nerve
         bilateral 389.12

Loss — continued
   hearing (see also Deafness) — continued
      nerve — continued
         unilateral 389.13
      neural
         bilateral 389.12
         unilateral 389.13
      noise-induced 388.12
      perceptive NEC (see also Loss, hearing,
         sensorineural) 389.10
      sensorineural 389.10
         with conductive hearing loss 389.20
            bilateral 389.22
            unilateral 389.21
         asymmetrical 389.16
         bilateral 389.18
         central 389.14
         neural 389.12
           bilateral 389.12
           unilateral 389.13
         sensory
           bilateral 389.11
           unilateral 389.17
         unilateral 389.15
      sensory
         bilateral 389.11
         unilateral 389.17
      specified type NEC 389.8
      sudden NEC 388.2
   height 781.91
   labyrinthine reactivity (unilateral) 386.55
      bilateral 386.56
   memory (see also Amnesia) 780.93
      mild, following organic brain damage
         310.89
   mind (see also Psychosis) 298.9
   occlusal vertical dimension 524.37
   organ or part — see Absence, by site, ac-
      quired
   recurrent pregnancy — see Pregnancy,
      management affected by, abortion,
      habitual
   sensation 782.0
   sense of
      smell (see also Disturbance, sensation)
         781.1
      taste (see also Disturbance, sensation)
         781.1
      touch (see also Disturbance, sensation)
         781.1
   sight (acquired) (complete) (congenital) —
      see Blindness
   spinal fluid
      headache 349.0
   substance of
      bone (see also Osteoporosis) 733.00
      cartilage 733.99
      ear 380.32
      vitreous (humor) 379.26
   tooth, teeth
      acquired 525.10
         due to
            caries 525.13
            extraction 525.10
            periodontal disease 525.12
            specified NEC 525.19
            trauma 525.11
   vision, visual (see also Blindness) 369.9
      both eyes (see also Blindness, both eyes)
         369.3
      complete (see also Blindness, both eyes)
         369.00
      one eye 369.8
      sudden 368.11
      transient 368.12
   vitreous 379.26
   voice (see also Aphonia) 784.41
   weight (cause unknown) 783.21
Lou Gehrig's disease 335.20
Louis-Bar syndrome (ataxia-telangiectasia)
   334.8
Louping ill 063.1
Lousiness — see Lice
Low
   back syndrome 724.2
   basal metabolic rate (BMR) 794.7

☑ **Additional Digit Required** — Refer to the Tabular List for Digit Selection   ⬇ **Subterms under main terms may continue to next column or page**

Low — continued
- birthweight 765.1 ☑
  - extreme (less than 1000 grams) 765.0 ☑
  - for gestational age 764.0 ☑
  - status (see also Status, low birth weight) V21.30
- bladder compliance 596.52
- blood pressure (see also Hypotension) 458.9
  - reading (incidental) (isolated) (nonspecific) 796.3
- cardiac reserve — see Disease, heart
- compliance bladder 596.52
- frequency deafness — see Disorder, hearing
- function (see also Hypofunction)
  - kidney (see also Disease, renal) 593.9
  - liver 573.9
- hemoglobin 285.9
- implantation, placenta — see Placenta, previa
- insertion, placenta — see Placenta, previa
- lying
  - kidney 593.0
  - organ or site, congenital — see Malposition, congenital
  - placenta — see Placenta, previa
- output syndrome (cardiac) (see also Failure, heart) 428.9
- platelets (blood) (see also Thrombocytopenia) 287.5
- reserve, kidney (see also Disease, renal) 593.9
- risk
  - human papillomavirus (HPA) DNA test positive
    - anal 796.79
    - cervical 795.09
    - vaginal 795.19
- salt syndrome 593.9
- tension glaucoma 365.12
- vision 369.9
  - both eyes 369.20
  - one eye 369.70

Lower extremity — see condition
Lowe (-Terrey-MacLachlan) syndrome (oculocerebrorenal dystrophy) 270.8
Lown (-Ganong) -Levine syndrome (short P-R interval, normal QRS complex, and paroxysmal supraventricular tachycardia) 426.81
LSD reaction — see also Abuse, drugs, nondependent 305.3 ☑
L-shaped kidney 753.3
Lucas-Championnière disease (fibrinous bronchitis) 466.0
Lucey-Driscoll syndrome (jaundice due to delayed conjugation) 774.30
Ludwig's
- angina 528.3
- disease (submaxillary cellulitis) 528.3
Lues (venerea), **luetic** — see Syphilis
Luetscher's syndrome (dehydration) 276.51
Lumbago 724.2
- due to displacement, intervertebral disc 722.10
Lumbalgia 724.2
- due to displacement, intervertebral disc 722.10
Lumbar — see condition
Lumbarization, vertebra 756.15
Lumbermen's itch 133.8
Lump — see also Mass
- abdominal 789.3 ☑
- breast 611.72
- chest 786.6
- epigastric 789.3 ☑
- head 784.2
- kidney 753.3
- liver 789.1
- lung 786.6
- mediastinal 786.6
- neck 784.2
- nose or sinus 784.2
- pelvic 789.3 ☑
- skin 782.2
- substernal 786.6
- throat 784.2

Lump — see also Mass — continued
- umbilicus 789.3 ☑
Lunacy — see also Psychosis 298.9
Lunatomalacia 732.3
Lung — see also condition
- donor V59.8
- drug addict's 417.8
- mainliners' 417.8
- vanishing 492.0
Lupoid (miliary) **of Boeck** 135
Lupus 710.0
- anticoagulant 795.79
  - with
    - hemorrhagic disorder 286.53
    - hypercoagulable state 289.81
- Cazenave's (erythematosus) 695.4
- discoid (local) 695.4
- disseminated 710.0
- erythematodes (discoid) (local) 695.4
- erythematosus (discoid) (local) 695.4
  - disseminated 710.0
  - eyelid 373.34
  - systemic 710.0
    - with
      - encephalitis 710.0 [323.81]
      - lung involvement 710.0 [517.8]
      - inhibitor (presence of) 795.79
        - with hypercoagulable state 289.81
- exedens 017.0 ☑
- eyelid (see also Tuberculosis)
  - 017.0 ☑ [373.4]
- Hilliard's 017.0 ☑
- hydralazine
  - correct substance properly administered 695.4
  - overdose or wrong substance given or taken 972.6
- miliaris disseminatus faciei 017.0 ☑
- nephritis 710.0 [583.81]
  - acute 710.0 [580.81]
  - chronic 710.0 [582.81]
- nontuberculous, not disseminated 695.4
- pernio (Besnier) 135
- tuberculous (see also Tuberculosis) 017.0 ☑
  - eyelid (see also Tuberculosis)
    - 017.0 ☑ [373.4]
- vulgaris 017.0 ☑
Luschka's joint disease 721.90
Luteinoma (M8610/0) 220
Lutembacher's disease or syndrome (atrial septal defect with mitral stenosis) 745.5
Luteoma (M8610/0) 220
Lutz-Miescher disease (elastosis perforans serpiginosa) 701.1
Lutz-Splendore-de Almeida disease (Brazilian blastomycosis) 116.1
Luxatio
- bulbi due to birth injury 767.8
- coxae congenita (see also Dislocation, hip, congenital) 754.30
- erecta — see Dislocation, shoulder
- imperfecta — see Sprain, by site
- perinealis — see Dislocation, hip
Luxation — see also Dislocation, by site
- eyeball 360.81
  - due to birth injury 767.8
  - lateral 376.36
- genital organs (external) NEC — see Wound, open, genital organs
- globe (eye) 360.81
  - lateral 376.36
- lacrimal gland (postinfectional) 375.16
- lens (old) (partial) 379.32
  - congenital 743.37
    - syphilitic 090.49 [379.32]
  - Marfan's disease 090.49
  - spontaneous 379.32
- penis — see Wound, open, penis
- scrotum — see Wound, open, scrotum
- testis — see Wound, open, testis
L-xyloketosuria 271.8
Lycanthropy — see also Psychosis 298.9
Lyell's disease or syndrome (toxic epidermal necrolysis) 695.15

Lyell's disease or syndrome — continued
- due to drug
  - correct substance properly administered 695.15
  - overdose or wrong substance given or taken 977.9
  - specified drug — see Table of Drugs and Chemicals
Lyme disease 088.81
Lymph
- gland or node — see condition
- scrotum (see also Infestation, filarial) 125.9
Lymphadenitis 289.3
- with
  - abortion — see Abortion, by type, with sepsis
  - ectopic pregnancy (see also categories 633.0–633.9) 639.0
  - molar pregnancy (see also categories 630–632) 639.0
- acute 683
  - mesenteric 289.2
- any site, except mesenteric 289.3
  - acute 683
  - chronic 289.1
  - mesenteric (acute) (chronic) (nonspecific) (subacute) 289.2
  - subacute 289.1
    - mesenteric 289.2
- breast, puerperal, postpartum 675.2 ☑
- chancroidal (congenital) 099.0
- chronic 289.1
  - mesenteric 289.2
- dermatopathic 695.89
- due to
  - anthracosis (occupational) 500
  - Brugia (Wuchereria) malayi 125.1
  - diphtheria (toxin) 032.89
  - lymphogranuloma venereum 099.1
  - Wuchereria bancrofti 125.0
- following
  - abortion 639.0
  - ectopic or molar pregnancy 639.0
- generalized 289.3
- gonorrheal 098.89
- granulomatous 289.1
- infectional 683
- mesenteric (acute) (chronic) (nonspecific) (subacute) 289.2
  - due to Bacillus typhi 002.0
  - tuberculous (see also Tuberculosis) 014.8 ☑
- mycobacterial 031.8
- purulent 683
- pyogenic 683
- regional 078.3
- septic 683
- streptococcal 683
- subacute, unspecified site 289.1
- suppurative 683
- syphilitic (early) (secondary) 091.4
  - late 095.8
- tuberculous — see Tuberculosis, lymph gland
- venereal 099.1
Lymphadenoid goiter 245.2
Lymphadenopathy (general) 785.6
- due to toxoplasmosis (acquired) 130.7
  - congenital (active) 771.2
Lymphadenopathy-associated virus (disease) (illness) (infection) — see Human immunodeficiency virus (disease) (illness) (infection)
Lymphadenosis 785.6
- acute 075
Lymphangiectasis 457.1
- conjunctiva 372.89
- postinfectional 457.1
- scrotum 457.1
Lymphangiectatic elephantiasis, nonfilarial 457.1
Lymphangioendothelioma (M9170/0) 228.1
- malignant (M9170/3) — see Neoplasm, connective tissue, malignant
Lymphangioleiomyomatosis 516.4
Lymphangioma (M9170/0) 228.1

Lymphangioma — continued
- capillary (M9171/0) 228.1
- cavernous (M9172/0) 228.1
- cystic (M9173/0) 228.1
- malignant (M9170/3) — see Neoplasm, connective tissue, malignant
Lymphangiomyoma (M9174/0) 228.1
Lymphangiomyomatosis 516.4
Lymphangiosarcoma (M9170/3) — see Neoplasm, connective tissue, malignant
Lymphangitis 457.2
- with
  - abortion — see Abortion, by type, with sepsis
  - abscess — see Abscess, by site
  - cellulitis — see Abscess, by site
  - ectopic pregnancy (see also categories 633.0–633.9) 639.0
  - molar pregnancy (see also categories 630–632) 639.0
- acute (with abscess or cellulitis) 682.9
  - specified site — see Abscess, by site
- breast, puerperal, postpartum 675.2 ☑
- chancroidal 099.0
- chronic (any site) 457.2
- due to
  - Brugia (Wuchereria) malayi 125.1
  - Wuchereria bancrofti 125.0
- following
  - abortion 639.0
  - ectopic or molar pregnancy 639.0
- gangrenous 457.2
- penis
  - acute 607.2
  - gonococcal (acute) 098.0
    - chronic or duration of 2 months or more 098.2
- puerperal, postpartum, childbirth 670.8 ☑
- strumous, tuberculous (see also Tuberculosis) 017.2 ☑
- subacute (any site) 457.2
- tuberculous — see Tuberculosis, lymph gland
Lymphatic (vessel) — see condition
Lymphatism 254.8
- scrofulous (see also Tuberculosis) 017.2 ☑
Lymphectasia 457.1
Lymphedema — see also Elephantiasis 457.1
- acquired (chronic) 457.1
- chronic hereditary 757.0
- congenital 757.0
- idiopathic hereditary 757.0
- praecox 457.1
- secondary 457.1
- surgical NEC 997.99
  - postmastectomy (syndrome) 457.0
Lymph-hemangioma (M9120/0) — see Hemangioma, by site
Lymphoblastic — see condition
Lymphoblastoma (diffuse) (M9630/3) 200.1 ☑
- giant follicular (M9690/3) 202.0 ☑
- macrofollicular (M9690/3) 202.0 ☑
Lymphoblastosis, acute benign 075
Lymphocele 457.8
Lymphocythemia 288.51
Lymphocytic — see also condition
- chorioencephalitis (acute) (serous) 049.0
- choriomeningitis (acute) (serous) 049.0
Lymphocytoma (diffuse) (malignant) (M9620/3) 200.1 ☑
Lymphocytomatosis (M9620/3) 200.1 ☑
Lymphocytopenia 288.51
Lymphocytosis (symptomatic) 288.61
- infectious (acute) 078.89
Lymphoepithelioma (M8082/3) — see Neoplasm, by site, malignant
Lymphogranuloma (malignant) (M9650/3) 201.9 ☑
- inguinale 099.1
- venereal (any site) 099.1
  - with stricture of rectum 099.1
- venereum 099.1
Lymphogranulomatosis (malignant) (M9650/3) 201.9 ☑
- benign (Boeck's sarcoid) (Schaumann's) 135
- Hodgkin's (M9650/3) 201.9 ☑

Lymphohistiocytosis, familial hemophago-cytic 288.4
Lymphoid — *see* condition
Lympholeukoblastoma (M9850/3) 207.8 ☑
Lympholeukosarcoma (M9850/3) 207.8 ☑
Lymphoma (malignant) (M9590/3) 202.8 ☑

Note — *Use the following fifth-digit subclassification with categories 200–202:*

0   *unspecified site, extranodal and solid organ sites*

1   *lymph nodes of head, face, and neck*

2   *intrathoracic lymph nodes*

3   *intra–abdominal lymph nodes*

4   *lymph nodes of axilla and upper limb*

5   *lymph nodes of inguinal region and lower limb*

6   *intrapelvic lymph nodes*

7   *spleen*

8   *lymph nodes of multiple sites*

benign (M9590/0) — *see* Neoplasm, by site, benign
Burkitt's type (lymphoblastic) (undifferentiated) (M9750/3) 200.2 ☑
Castleman's (mediastinal lymph node hyperplasia) 785.6
centroblastic-centrocytic
   diffuse (M9614/3) 202.8 ☑
   follicular (M9692/3) 202.0 ☑
centroblastic type (diffuse) (M9632/3) 202.8 ☑
   follicular (M9697/3) 202.0 ☑
centrocytic (M9622/3) 202.8 ☑
compound (M9613/3) 200.8 ☑
convoluted cell type (lymphoblastic) (M9602/3) 202.8 ☑
diffuse NEC (M9590/3) 202.8 ☑
   large B cell 202.8 ☑
follicular (giant) (M9690/3) 202.0 ☑
   center cell (diffuse) (M9615/3) 202.8 ☑
   cleaved (diffuse) (M9623/3) 202.8 ☑
     follicular (M9695/3) 202.0 ☑
   non-cleaved (diffuse) (M9633/3) 202.8 ☑
     follicular (M9698/3) 202.0 ☑
   centroblastic-centrocytic (M9692/3) 202.0 ☑
   centroblastic type (M9697/3) 202.0 ☑
   large cell 202.0 ☑
   lymphocytic
     intermediate differentiation (M9694/3) 202.0 ☑
     poorly differentiated (M9696/3) 202.0 ☑
   mixed (cell type) (lymphocytic-histiocytic) (small cell and large cell) (M9691/3) 202.0 ☑
germinocytic (M9622/3) 202.8 ☑
giant, follicular or follicle (M9690/3) 202.0 ☑
histiocytic (diffuse) (M9640/3) 200.0 ☑
   nodular (M9642/3) 200.0 ☑
   pleomorphic cell type (M9641/3) 200.0 ☑
Hodgkin's (M9650/3) (*see also* Disease, Hodgkin's) 201.9 ☑
immunoblastic (type) (M9612/3) 200.8 ☑
large cell (M9640/3) 200.7 ☑
   anaplastic 200.6 ☑
   nodular (M9642/3) 202.0 ☑
   pleomorphic cell type (M9641/3) 200.0 ☑
lymphoblastic (diffuse) (M9630/3) 200.1 ☑
   Burkitt's type (M9750/3) 200.2 ☑
   convoluted cell type (M9602/3) 202.8 ☑
lymphocytic (cell type) (diffuse) (M9620/3) 200.1 ☑

Lymphoma — *continued*
lymphocytic — *continued*
   with plasmacytoid differentiation, diffuse (M9611/3) 200.8 ☑
   intermediate differentiation (diffuse) (M9621/3) 200.1 ☑
     follicular (M9694/3) 202.0 ☑
     nodular (M9694/3) 202.0 ☑
   nodular (M9690/3) 202.0 ☑
   poorly differentiated (diffuse) (M9630/3) 200.1 ☑
     follicular (M9696/3) 202.0 ☑
     nodular (M9696/3) 202.0 ☑
   well differentiated (diffuse) (M9620/3) 200.1 ☑
     follicular (M9693/3) 202.0 ☑
     nodular (M9693/3) 202.0 ☑
lymphocytic-histiocytic, mixed (diffuse) (M9613/3) 200.8 ☑
   follicular (M9691/3) 202.0 ☑
   nodular (M9691/3) 202.0 ☑
lymphoplasmacytoid type (M9611/3) 200.8 ☑
lymphosarcoma type (M9610/3) 200.1 ☑
macrofollicular (M9690/3) 202.0 ☑
mantle cell 200.4 ☑
marginal zone 200.3 ☑
   extranodal B-cell 200.3 ☑
   nodal B-cell 200.3 ☑
   splenic B-cell 200.3 ☑
mixed cell type (diffuse) (M9613/3) 200.8 ☑
   follicular (M9691/3) 202.0 ☑
   nodular (M9691/3) 202.0 ☑
nodular (M9690/3) 202.0 ☑
   histiocytic (M9642/3) 200.0 ☑
   lymphocytic (M9690/3) 202.0 ☑
     intermediate differentiation (M9694/3) 202.0 ☑
     poorly differentiated (M9696/3) 202.0 ☑
   mixed (cell type) (lymphocytic-histiocytic) (small cell and large cell) (M9691/3) 202.0 ☑
non-Hodgkin's type NEC (M9591/3) 202.8 ☑
peripheral T-cell 202.7 ☑
primary central nervous system 200.5 ☑
reticulum cell (type) (M9640/3) 200.0 ☑
small cell and large cell, mixed (diffuse) (M9613/3) 200.8 ☑
   follicular (M9691/3) 202.0 ☑
   nodular (M9691/3) 202.0 ☑
stem cell (type) (M9601/3) 202.8 ☑
T-cell 202.1 ☑
   peripheral 202.7 ☑
undifferentiated (cell type) (non-Burkitt's) (M9600/3) 202.8 ☑
   Burkitt's type (M9750/3) 200.2 ☑
Lymphomatosis (M9590/3) — *see also* Lymphoma
granulomatous 099.1
Lymphopathia
venereum 099.1
veneris 099.1
Lymphopenia 288.51
familial 279.2
Lymphoreticulosis, benign (of inoculation) 078.3
Lymphorrhea 457.8
Lymphosarcoma (M9610/3) 200.1 ☑
diffuse (M9610/3) 200.1 ☑
   with plasmacytoid differentiation (M9611/3) 200.8 ☑
   lymphoplasmacytic (M9611/3) 200.8 ☑
follicular (giant) (M9690/3) 202.0 ☑
   lymphoblastic (M9696/3) 202.0 ☑
   lymphocytic, intermediate differentiation (M9694/3) 202.0 ☑
   mixed cell type (M9691/3) 202.0 ☑
giant follicular (M9690/3) 202.0 ☑
Hodgkin's (M9650/3) 201.9 ☑
immunoblastic (M9612/3) 200.8 ☑
lymphoblastic (diffuse) (M9630/3) 200.1 ☑
   follicular (M9696/3) 202.0 ☑
   nodular (M9696/3) 202.0 ☑

Lymphosarcoma — *continued*
lymphocytic (diffuse) (M9620/3) 200.1 ☑
   intermediate differentiation (diffuse) (M9621/3) 200.1 ☑
     follicular (M9694/3) 202.0 ☑
     nodular (M9694/3) 202.0 ☑
mixed cell type (diffuse) (M9613/3) 200.8 ☑
   follicular (M9691/3) 202.0 ☑
   nodular (M9691/3) 202.0 ☑
nodular (M9690/3) 202.0 ☑
   lymphoblastic (M9696/3) 202.0 ☑
   lymphocytic, intermediate differentiation (M9694/3) 202.0 ☑
   mixed cell type (M9691/3) 202.0 ☑
prolymphocytic (M9631/3) 200.1 ☑
reticulum cell (M9640/3) 200.0 ☑
Lymphostasis 457.8
Lypemania — *see also* Melancholia 296.2 ☑
Lyssa 071

M

Macacus ear 744.29
Maceration
fetus (cause not stated) 779.9
wet feet, tropical (syndrome) 991.4
Machado-Joseph disease 334.8
Machupo virus hemorrhagic fever 078.7
Macleod's syndrome (abnormal transradiancy, one lung) 492.8
Macrocephalia, macrocephaly 756.0
Macrocheilia (congenital) 744.81
Macrochilia (congenital) 744.81
Macrocolon (congenital) 751.3
Macrocornea 743.41
associated with buphthalmos 743.22
Macrocytic — *see* condition
Macrocytosis 289.89
Macrodactylia, macrodactylism (fingers) (thumbs) 755.57
toes 755.65
Macrodontia 520.2
Macroencephaly 742.4
Macrogenia 524.05
Macrogenitosomia (female) (male) (praecox) 255.2
Macrogingivae 523.8
Macroglobulinemia (essential) (idiopathic) (monoclonal) (primary) (syndrome) (Waldenström's) 273.3
Macroglossia (congenital) 750.15
acquired 529.8
Macrognathia, macrognathism (congenital) 524.00
mandibular 524.02
   alveolar 524.72
maxillary 524.01
   alveolar 524.71
Macrogyria (congenital) 742.4
Macrohydrocephalus — *see also* Hydrocephalus 331.4
Macromastia — *see also* Hypertrophy, breast 611.1
Macrophage activation syndrome 288.4
Macropsia 368.14
Macrosigmoid 564.7
congenital 751.3
Macrospondylitis, acromegalic 253.0
Macrostomia (congenital) 744.83
Macrotia (external ear) (congenital) 744.22
Macula
cornea, corneal
   congenital 743.43
     interfering with vision 743.42
   interfering with central vision 371.03
   not interfering with central vision 371.02
degeneration (*see also* Degeneration, macula) 362.50
hereditary (*see also* Dystrophy, retina) 362.70
edema, cystoid 362.53
Maculae ceruleae 132.1
Macules and papules 709.8
Maculopathy, toxic 362.55
Madarosis 374.55

Madelung's
deformity (radius) 755.54
disease (lipomatosis) 272.8
lipomatosis 272.8
Madness — *see also* Psychosis 298.9
myxedema (acute) 293.0
   subacute 293.1
Madura
disease (actinomycotic) 039.9
   mycotic 117.4
foot (actinomycotic) 039.4
   mycotic 117.4
Maduromycosis (actinomycotic) 039.9
mycotic 117.4
Maffucci's syndrome (dyschondroplasia with hemangiomas) 756.4
Magenblase syndrome 306.4
Main en griffe (acquired) 736.06
congenital 755.59
Maintenance
chemotherapy regimen or treatment V58.11
dialysis regimen or treatment
   extracorporeal (renal) V56.0
   peritoneal V56.8
   renal V56.0
drug therapy or regimen
   chemotherapy, antineoplastic V58.11
   immunotherapy, antineoplastic V58.12
external fixation NEC V54.89
methadone 304.00
radiotherapy V58.0
traction NEC V54.89
Majocchi's
disease (purpura annularis telangiectodes) 709.1
granuloma 110.6
Major — *see* condition
Mal
cerebral (idiopathic) (*see also* Epilepsy) 345.9 ☑
comital (*see also* Epilepsy) 345.9 ☑
de los pintos (*see also* Pinta) 103.9
de Meleda 757.39
de mer 994.6
lie — *see* Presentation, fetal
perforant (*see also* Ulcer, lower extremity) 707.15
Malabar itch 110.9
beard 110.0
foot 110.4
scalp 110.0
Malabsorption 579.9
calcium 579.8
carbohydrate 579.8
disaccharide 271.3
drug-induced 579.8
due to bacterial overgrowth 579.8
fat 579.8
folate, congenital 281.2
galactose 271.1
glucose-galactose (congenital) 271.3
intestinal 579.9
isomaltose 271.3
lactose (hereditary) 271.3
methionine 270.4
monosaccharide 271.8
postgastrectomy 579.3
postsurgical 579.3
protein 579.8
sucrose (-isomaltose) (congenital) 271.3
syndrome 579.9
   postgastrectomy 579.3
   postsurgical 579.3
Malacia, bone 268.2
juvenile (*see also* Rickets) 268.0
Kienböck's (juvenile) (lunate) (wrist) 732.3
   adult 732.8
Malacoplakia
bladder 596.89
colon 569.89
pelvis (kidney) 593.89
ureter 593.89
urethra 599.84
Malacosteon 268.2
juvenile (*see also* Rickets) 268.0
Maladaptation — *see* Maladjustment

☑ **Additional Digit Required** — **Refer to the Tabular List for Digit Selection**   ▽ **Subterms under main terms may continue to next column or page**

Maladie de Roger 745.4
Maladjustment
  conjugal V61.10
    involving
      divorce V61.03
      estrangement V61.09
  educational V62.3
  family V61.9
    specified circumstance NEC V61.8
  marital V61.10
    involving
      divorce V61.03
      estrangement V61.09
  occupational V62.29
    current military deployment status
      V62.21
  simple, adult (see also Reaction, adjustment)
    309.9
  situational acute (see also Reaction, adjust-
    ment) 309.9
  social V62.4
Malaise 780.79
Malakoplakia — see Malacoplakia
Malaria, malarial (fever) 084.6
  algid 084.9
  any type, with
    algid malaria 084.9
    blackwater fever 084.8
    fever
      blackwater 084.8
      hemoglobinuric (bilious) 084.8
    hemoglobinuria, malarial 084.8
    hepatitis 084.9 [573.2]
    nephrosis 084.9 [581.81]
    pernicious complication NEC 084.9
      cardiac 084.9
      cerebral 084.9
  cardiac 084.9
  carrier (suspected) of V02.9
  cerebral 084.9
  complicating pregnancy, childbirth, or
    puerperium 647.4 ✓
  congenital 771.2
  congestion, congestive 084.6
    brain 084.9
  continued 084.0
  estivo-autumnal 084.0
  falciparum (malignant tertian) 084.0
  hematinuria 084.8
  hematuria 084.8
  hemoglobinuria 084.8
  hemorrhagic 084.6
  induced (therapeutically) 084.7
    accidental — see Malaria, by type
  liver 084.9 [573.2]
  malariae (quartan) 084.2
  malignant (tertian) 084.0
  mixed infections 084.5
  monkey 084.4
  ovale 084.3
  pernicious, acute 084.0
  Plasmodium, P.
    falciparum 084.0
    malariae 084.2
    ovale 084.3
    vivax 084.1
  quartan 084.2
  quotidian 084.0
  recurrent 084.6
    induced (therapeutically) 084.7
      accidental — see Malaria, by type
  remittent 084.6
  specified types NEC 084.4
  spleen 084.6
  subtertian 084.0
  tertian (benign) 084.1
    malignant 084.0
  tropical 084.0
  typhoid 084.6
  vivax (benign tertian) 084.1
Malassez's disease (testicular cyst) 608.89
Malassimilation 579.9
Maldescent, testis 752.51
Maldevelopment — see also Anomaly, by site
  brain 742.9
  colon 751.5

Maldevelopment — see also Anomaly, by site
  — continued
  hip (joint) 755.63
    congenital dislocation (see also Disloca-
      tion, hip, congenital) 754.30
  mastoid process 756.0
  middle ear, except ossicles 744.03
    ossicles 744.04
  newborn (not malformation) 764.9 ✓
  ossicles, ear 744.04
  spine 756.10
  toe 755.66
Male type pelvis 755.69
  with disproportion (fetopelvic) 653.2 ✓
    affecting fetus or newborn 763.1
    causing obstructed labor 660.1 ✓
      affecting fetus or newborn 763.1
Malformation (congenital) — see also
  Anomaly
  arteriovenous
    pulmonary 747.32
  bone 756.9
  bursa 756.9
  Chiari
    type I 348.4
    type II (see also Spina bifida) 741.0 ✓
    type III 742.0
    type IV 742.2
  circulatory system NEC 747.9
    specified type NEC 747.89
  cochlea 744.05
  digestive system NEC 751.9
    lower 751.5
    specified type NEC 751.8
    upper 750.9
  eye 743.9
  gum 750.9
  heart NEC 746.9
    specified type NEC 746.89
    valve 746.9
  internal ear 744.05
  joint NEC 755.9
    specified type NEC 755.8
  Mondini's (congenital) (malformation,
    cochlea) 744.05
  muscle 756.9
  nervous system (central) 742.9
  pelvic organs or tissues
    in pregnancy or childbirth 654.9 ✓
      affecting fetus or newborn 763.89
      causing obstructed labor 660.2 ✓
        affecting fetus or newborn 763.1
  placenta (see also Placenta, abnormal)
    656.7 ✓
  respiratory organs 748.9
    specified type NEC 748.8
  Rieger's 743.44
  sense organs NEC 742.9
    specified type NEC 742.8
  skin 757.9
    specified type NEC 757.8
  spinal cord 742.9
  teeth, tooth NEC 520.9
  tendon 756.9
  throat 750.9
  umbilical cord (complicating delivery)
    663.9 ✓
    affecting fetus or newborn 762.6
  umbilicus 759.9
  urinary system NEC 753.9
    specified type NEC 753.8
  venous — see Anomaly, vein
Malfunction — see also Dysfunction
  arterial graft 996.1
  cardiac pacemaker 996.01
  catheter device — see Complications, me-
    chanical, catheter
  colostomy 569.62
    valve 569.62
  cystostomy 596.82
    infection 596.81
    mechanical 596.82
    specified complication NEC 596.83
  device, implant, or graft NEC — see Compli-
    cations, mechanical
  enteric stoma 569.62

Malfunction — see also Dysfunction —
  continued
  enterostomy 569.62
  esophagostomy 530.87
  gastroenteric 536.8
  gastrostomy 536.42
  ileostomy
    valve 569.62
  nephrostomy 997.5
  pacemaker — see Complications, mechani-
    cal, pacemaker
  prosthetic device, internal — see Complica-
    tions, mechanical
  tracheostomy 519.02
  valve
    colostomy 569.62
    ileostomy 569.62
  vascular graft or shunt 996.1
Malgaigne's fracture (closed) 808.43
  open 808.53
Malherbe's
  calcifying epithelioma (M8110/0) — see
    Neoplasm, skin, benign
  tumor (M8110/0) — see Neoplasm, skin,
    benign
Malibu disease 919.8
  infected 919.9
Malignancy (M8000/3) — see Neoplasm, by
  site, malignant
Malignant — see condition
Malingerer, malingering V65.2
Mallet, finger (acquired) 736.1
  congenital 755.59
  late effect of rickets 268.1
Malleus 024
Mallory's bodies 034.1
Mallory-Weiss syndrome 530.7
Malnutrition (calorie) 263.9
  complicating pregnancy 648.9 ✓
  degree
    first 263.1
    second 263.0
    third 262
    mild (protein) 263.1
    moderate (protein) 263.0
    severe 261
      protein-calorie 262
  fetus 764.2 ✓
    "light-for-dates" 764.1 ✓
  following gastrointestinal surgery 579.3
  intrauterine or fetal 764.2 ✓
    fetus or infant "light-for-dates" 764.1 ✓
  lack of care, or neglect (child) (infant) 995.52
    adult 995.84
  malignant 260
  mild (protein) 263.1
  moderate (protein) 263.0
  protein 260
  protein-calorie 263.9
    mild 263.1
    moderate 263.0
    severe 262
    specified type NEC 263.8
  severe 261
    protein-calorie NEC 262
Malocclusion (teeth) 524.4
  angle's class I 524.21
  angle's class II 524.22
  angle's class III 524.23
  due to
    abnormal swallowing 524.59
    accessory teeth (causing crowding)
      524.31
    dentofacial abnormality NEC 524.89
    impacted teeth (causing crowding) 520.6
    missing teeth 524.30
    mouth breathing 524.59
    sleep postures 524.59
    supernumerary teeth (causing crowding)
      524.31
    thumb sucking 524.59
    tongue, lip, or finger habits 524.59
    temporomandibular (joint) 524.69
Malposition
  cardiac apex (congenital) 746.87
  cervix — see Malposition, uterus

Malposition — continued
  congenital
    adrenal (gland) 759.1
    alimentary tract 751.8
      lower 751.5
      upper 750.8
    aorta 747.21
    appendix 751.5
    arterial trunk 747.29
    artery (peripheral) NEC (see also Malposi-
      tion, congenital, peripheral vascu-
      lar system) 747.60
      coronary 746.85
      pulmonary 747.39
    auditory canal 744.29
      causing impairment of hearing
        744.02
    auricle (ear) 744.29
      causing impairment of hearing
        744.02
    cervical 744.43
    biliary duct or passage 751.69
    bladder (mucosa) 753.8
      exteriorized or extroverted 753.5
    brachial plexus 742.8
    brain tissue 742.4
    breast 757.6
    bronchus 748.3
    cardiac apex 746.87
    cecum 751.5
    clavicle 755.51
    colon 751.5
    digestive organ or tract NEC 751.8
      lower 751.5
      upper 750.8
    ear (auricle) (external) 744.29
      ossicles 744.04
    endocrine (gland) NEC 759.2
    epiglottis 748.3
    Eustachian tube 744.24
    eye 743.8
    facial features 744.89
    fallopian tube 752.19
    finger(s) 755.59
      supernumerary 755.01
    foot 755.67
    gallbladder 751.69
    gastrointestinal tract 751.8
    genitalia, genital organ(s) or tract
      female 752.89
        external 752.49
        internal NEC 752.89
      male 752.89
        penis 752.69
        scrotal transposition 752.81
    glottis 748.3
    hand 755.59
    heart 746.87
      dextrocardia 746.87
        with complete transposition of
          viscera 759.3
    hepatic duct 751.69
    hip (joint) (see also Dislocation, hip,
      congenital) 754.30
    intestine (large) (small) 751.5
      with anomalous adhesions, fixation,
        or malrotation 751.4
    joint NEC 755.8
    kidney 753.3
    larynx 748.3
    limb 755.8
      lower 755.69
      upper 755.59
    liver 751.69
    lung (lobe) 748.69
    nail(s) 757.5
    nerve 742.8
    nervous system NEC 742.8
    nose, nasal (septum) 748.1
    organ or site NEC — see Anomaly, spec-
      ified type NEC, by site
    ovary 752.0
    pancreas 751.7
    parathyroid (gland) 759.2
    patella 755.64
    peripheral vascular system 747.60

Malposition — *continued*
  congenital — *continued*
    peripheral vascular system — *continued*
      gastrointestinal 747.61
      lower limb 747.64
      renal 747.62
      specified NEC 747.69
      spinal 747.82
      upper limb 747.63
    pituitary (gland) 759.2
    respiratory organ or system NEC 748.9
    rib (cage) 756.3
      supernumerary in cervical region 756.2
    scapula 755.59
    shoulder 755.59
    spinal cord 742.59
    spine 756.19
    spleen 759.0
    sternum 756.3
    stomach 750.7
    symphysis pubis 755.69
    testis (undescended) 752.51
    thymus (gland) 759.2
    thyroid (gland) (tissue) 759.2
      cartilage 748.3
    toe(s) 755.66
      supernumerary 755.02
    tongue 750.19
    trachea 748.3
    uterus 752.39
    vein(s) (peripheral) NEC (*see also* Malposition, congenital, peripheral vascular system) 747.60
      great 747.49
      portal 747.49
      pulmonary 747.49
    vena cava (inferior) (superior) 747.49
  device, implant, or graft — *see* Complications, mechanical
  fetus NEC (*see also* Presentation, fetal) 652.9 ☑
    with successful version 652.1 ☑
    affecting fetus or newborn 763.1
    before labor, affecting fetus or newborn 761.7
    causing obstructed labor 660.0 ☑
    in multiple gestation (one fetus or more) 652.6 ☑
      with locking 660.5 ☑
      causing obstructed labor 660.0 ☑
  gallbladder (*see also* Disease, gallbladder) 575.8
  gastrointestinal tract 569.89
    congenital 751.8
  heart (*see also* Malposition, congenital, heart) 746.87
  intestine 569.89
    congenital 751.5
  pelvic organs or tissues
    in pregnancy or childbirth 654.4 ☑
      affecting fetus or newborn 763.89
      causing obstructed labor 660.2 ☑
        affecting fetus or newborn 763.1
  placenta — *see* Placenta, previa
  stomach 537.89
    congenital 750.7
  tooth, teeth 524.30
    with impaction 520.6
  uterus (acquired) (acute) (adherent) (any degree) (asymptomatic) (postinfectional) (postpartal) (old) 621.6
    anteflexion or anteversion (*see also* Anteversion, uterus) 621.6
    congenital 752.39
    flexion 621.6
      lateral (*see also* Lateroversion, uterus) 621.6
    in pregnancy or childbirth 654.4 ☑
      affecting fetus or newborn 763.89
      causing obstructed labor 660.2 ☑
        affecting fetus or newborn 763.1
    inversion 621.6
    lateral (flexion) (version) (*see also* Lateroversion, uterus) 621.6

Malposition — *continued*
  uterus — *continued*
    lateroflexion (*see also* Lateroversion, uterus) 621.6
    lateroversion (*see also* Lateroversion, uterus) 621.6
    retroflexion or retroversion (*see also* Retroversion, uterus) 621.6
Malposture 729.90
Malpresentation, fetus — *see also* Presentation, fetal 652.9 ☑
Malrotation
  cecum 751.4
  colon 751.4
  intestine 751.4
  kidney 753.3
MALT (mucosa associated lymphoid tissue) 200.3 ☑
Malta fever — *see also* Brucellosis 023.9
Maltosuria 271.3
Maltreatment (of)
  adult 995.80
    emotional 995.82
    multiple forms 995.85
    neglect (nutritional) 995.84
    physical 995.81
    psychological 995.82
    sexual 995.83
  child 995.50
    emotional 995.51
    multiple forms 995.59
    neglect (nutritional) 995.52
    physical 995.54
      shaken infant syndrome 995.55
    psychological 995.51
    sexual 995.53
  spouse (*see also* Maltreatment, adult) 995.80
Malt workers' lung 495.4
Malum coxae senilis 715.25
Malunion, fracture 733.81
Mammillitis — *see also* Mastitis 611.0
  puerperal, postpartum 675.2 ☑
Mammitis — *see also* Mastitis 611.0
  puerperal, postpartum 675.2 ☑
Mammographic
  calcification 793.89
  calculus 793.89
  microcalcification 793.81
Mammoplasia 611.1
Management
  contraceptive V25.9
    specified type NEC V25.8
  procreative V26.9
    specified type NEC V26.89
Mangled NEC — *see also* nature and site of injury 959.9
Mania (monopolar) — *see also* Psychosis, affective 296.0 ☑
  alcoholic (acute) (chronic) 291.9
  Bell's — *see* Mania, chronic
  chronic 296.0 ☑
    recurrent episode 296.1 ☑
    single episode 296.0 ☑
  compulsive 300.3
  delirious (acute) 296.0 ☑
    recurrent episode 296.1 ☑
    single episode 296.0 ☑
  epileptic (*see also* Epilepsy) 345.4 ☑
  hysterical 300.10
  inhibited 296.89
  puerperal (after delivery) 296.0 ☑
    recurrent episode 296.1 ☑
    single episode 296.0 ☑
  recurrent episode 296.1 ☑
  senile 290.8
  single episode 296.0 ☑
  stupor 296.89
  stuporous 296.89
  unproductive 296.89
Manic-depressive insanity, psychosis, reaction, or syndrome — *see also* Psychosis, affective 296.80
  circular (alternating) 296.7
    currently
      depressed 296.5 ☑
      episode unspecified 296.7

Manic-depressive insanity, psychosis, reaction, or syndrome — *see also* Psychosis, affective — *continued*
  circular — *continued*
    currently — *continued*
      hypomanic, previously depressed 296.4 ☑
      manic 296.4 ☑
      mixed 296.6 ☑
  depressed (type), depressive 296.2 ☑
    atypical 296.82
    recurrent episode 296.3 ☑
    single episode 296.2 ☑
  hypomanic 296.0 ☑
    recurrent episode 296.1 ☑
    single episode 296.0 ☑
  manic 296.0 ☑
    atypical 296.81
    recurrent episode 296.1 ☑
    single episode 296.0 ☑
  mixed NEC 296.89
  perplexed 296.89
  stuporous 296.89
Manifestations, rheumatoid
  lungs 714.81
  pannus — *see* Arthritis, rheumatoid
  subcutaneous nodules — *see* Arthritis, rheumatoid
Mankowsky's syndrome (familial dysplastic osteopathy) 731.2
Mannoheptulosuria 271.8
Mannosidosis 271.8
Manson's
  disease (schistosomiasis) 120.1
  pyosis (pemphigus contagiosus) 684
  schistosomiasis 120.1
Mansonellosis 125.5
Manual — *see* condition
Maple bark disease 495.6
Maple bark-strippers' lung 495.6
Maple syrup (urine) disease or syndrome 270.3
Marable's syndrome (celiac artery compression) 447.4
Marasmus 261
  brain 331.9
  due to malnutrition 261
  intestinal 569.89
  nutritional 261
  senile 797
  tuberculous NEC (*see also* Tuberculosis) 011.9 ☑
Marble
  bones 756.52
  skin 782.61
Marburg disease (virus) 078.89
March
  foot 733.94
  hemoglobinuria 283.2
Marchand multiple nodular hyperplasia (liver) 571.5
Marchesani (-Weill) syndrome (brachymorphism and ectopia lentis) 759.89
Marchiafava (-Bignami) disease or syndrome 341.8
Marchiafava-Micheli syndrome (paroxysmal nocturnal hemoglobinuria) 283.2
Marcus Gunn's syndrome (jaw-winking syndrome) 742.8
Marfan's
  congenital syphilis 090.49
  disease 090.49
  syndrome (arachnodactyly) 759.82
    meaning congenital syphilis 090.49
      with luxation of lens 090.49 [379.32]
Marginal
  implantation, placenta — *see* Placenta, previa
  placenta — *see* Placenta, previa
  sinus (hemorrhage) (rupture) 641.2 ☑
    affecting fetus or newborn 762.1
Marie's
  cerebellar ataxia 334.2
  syndrome (acromegaly) 253.0

Marie-Bamberger disease or syndrome (hypertrophic) (pulmonary) (secondary) 731.2
  idiopathic (acropachyderma) 757.39
  primary (acropachyderma) 757.39
Marie-Charcôt-Tooth neuropathic atrophy, muscle 356.1
Marie-Strümpell arthritis or disease (ankylosing spondylitis) 720.0
Marihuana, marijuana
  abuse (*see also* Abuse, drugs, nondependent) 305.2 ☑
  dependence (*see also* Dependence) 304.3 ☑
Marion's disease (bladder neck obstruction) 596.0
Marital conflict V61.10
Mark
  port wine 757.32
  raspberry 757.32
  strawberry 757.32
  stretch 701.3
  tattoo 709.09
Maroteaux-Lamy syndrome (mucopolysaccharidosis VI) 277.5
Marriage license examination V70.3
Marrow (bone)
  arrest 284.9
  megakaryocytic 287.30
  poor function 289.9
Marseilles fever 082.1
Marshall's (hidrotic) **ectodermal dysplasia** 757.31
Marsh's disease (exophthalmic goiter) 242.0 ☑
Marsh fever — *see also* Malaria 084.6
Martin-Albright syndrome (pseudohypoparathyroidism) 275.49
Martin's disease 715.27
Martorell-Fabre syndrome (pulseless disease) 446.7
Masculinization, female, with adrenal hyperplasia 255.2
Masculinovoblastoma (M8670/0) 220
Masochism 302.83
Masons' lung 502
Mass
  abdominal 789.3 ☑
  anus 787.99
  bone 733.90
  breast 611.72
  cheek 784.2
  chest 786.6
  cystic — *see* Cyst
  ear 388.8
  epigastric 789.3 ☑
  eye 379.92
  female genital organ 625.8
  gum 784.2
  head 784.2
  intracranial 784.2
  joint 719.60
    ankle 719.67
    elbow 719.62
    foot 719.67
    hand 719.64
    hip 719.65
    knee 719.66
    multiple sites 719.69
    pelvic region 719.65
    shoulder (region) 719.61
    specified site NEC 719.68
    wrist 719.63
  kidney (*see also* Disease, kidney) 593.9
  lung 786.6
  lymph node 785.6
  malignant (M8000/3) — *see* Neoplasm, by site, malignant
  mediastinal 786.6
  mouth 784.2
  muscle (limb) 729.89
  neck 784.2
  nose or sinus 784.2
  palate 784.2
  pelvis, pelvic 789.3 ☑
  penis 607.89
  perineum 625.8

Mass — *continued*
  rectum 787.99
  scrotum 608.89
  skin 782.2
  specified organ NEC — *see* Disease of specified organ or site
  splenic 789.2
  substernal 786.6
    thyroid (*see also* Goiter) 240.9
  superficial (localized) 782.2
  testes 608.89
  throat 784.2
  tongue 784.2
  umbilicus 789.3 ☑
  uterus 625.8
  vagina 625.8
  vulva 625.8
Massive — *see* condition
Mastalgia 611.71
  psychogenic 307.89
Mast cell
  disease 757.33
    systemic (M9741/3) 202.6 ☑
  leukemia (M9900/3) 207.8 ☑
  sarcoma (M9740/3) 202.6 ☑
  tumor (M9740/1) 238.5
    malignant (M9740/3) 202.6 ☑
Masters-Allen syndrome 620.6
Mastitis (acute) (adolescent) (diffuse) (interstitial) (lobular) (nonpuerperal) (nonsuppurative) (parenchymatous) (phlegmonous) (simple) (subacute) (suppurative) 611.0
  chronic (cystic) (fibrocystic) 610.1
  cystic 610.1
    Schimmelbusch's type 610.1
  fibrocystic 610.1
  infective 611.0
  lactational 675.2 ☑
  lymphangitis 611.0
  neonatal (noninfective) 778.7
    infective 771.5
  periductal 610.4
  plasma cell 610.4
  puerperalis 675.2 ☑
  puerperal, postpartum, (interstitial) (nonpurulent) (parenchymatous) 675.2 ☑
    purulent 675.1 ☑
    stagnation 676.2 ☑
  retromammary 611.0
    puerperal, postpartum 675.1 ☑
  submammary 611.0
    puerperal, postpartum 675.1 ☑
Mastocytoma (M9740/1) 238.5
  malignant (M9740/3) 202.6 ☑
Mastocytosis 757.33
  malignant (M9741/3) 202.6 ☑
  systemic (M9741/3) 202.6 ☑
Mastodynia 611.71
  psychogenic 307.89
Mastoid — *see* condition
Mastoidalgia — *see also* Otalgia 388.70
Mastoiditis (coalescent) (hemorrhagic) (pneumococcal) (streptococcal) (suppurative) 383.9
  acute or subacute 383.00
    with
      Gradenigo's syndrome 383.02
      petrositis 383.02
      specified complication NEC 383.02
      subperiosteal abscess 383.01
  chronic (necrotic) (recurrent) 383.1
  tuberculous (*see also* Tuberculosis) 015.6 ☑
Mastopathy, mastopathia 611.9
  chronica cystica 610.1
  diffuse cystic 610.1
  estrogenic 611.89
  ovarian origin 611.89
Mastoplasia 611.1
Masturbation 307.9
Maternal condition, affecting fetus or newborn
  acute yellow atrophy of liver 760.8
  albuminuria 760.1
  anesthesia or analgesia 763.5
  blood loss 762.1

Maternal condition, affecting fetus or newborn — *continued*
  chorioamnionitis 762.7
  circulatory disease, chronic (conditions classifiable to 390–459, 745–747) 760.3
  congenital heart disease (conditions classifiable to 745–746) 760.3
  cortical necrosis of kidney 760.1
  death 761.6
  diabetes mellitus 775.0
    manifest diabetes in the infant 775.1
  disease NEC 760.9
    circulatory system, chronic (conditions classifiable to 390–459, 745–747) 760.3
    genitourinary system (conditions classifiable to 580–599) 760.1
    respiratory (conditions classifiable to 490–519, 748) 760.3
  eclampsia 760.0
  hemorrhage NEC 762.1
  hepatitis acute, malignant, or subacute 760.8
  hyperemesis (gravidarum) 761.8
  hypertension (arising during pregnancy) (conditions classifiable to 642) 760.0
  infection
    disease classifiable to 001-136 ☑, 760.2
    genital tract NEC 760.8
    urinary tract 760.1
  influenza 760.2
    manifest influenza in the infant 771.2
  injury (conditions classifiable to 800–996) 760.5
  malaria 760.2
    manifest malaria in infant or fetus 771.2
  malnutrition 760.4
  necrosis of liver 760.8
  nephritis (conditions classifiable to 580–583) 760.1
  nephrosis (conditions classifiable to 581) 760.1
  noxious substance transmitted via breast milk or placenta 760.70
    alcohol 760.71
    anticonvulsants 760.77
    antifungals 760.74
    anti-infective agents 760.74
    antimetabolics 760.78
    cocaine 760.75
    "crack" 760.75
    diethylstilbestrol [DES] 760.76
    hallucinogenic agents 760.73
    medicinal agents NEC 760.79
    narcotics 760.72
    obstetric anesthetic or analgesic drug 760.72
    specified agent NEC 760.79
  nutritional disorder (conditions classifiable to 260–269) 760.4
  operation unrelated to current delivery (*see also* Newborn, affected by) 760.64
  pre-eclampsia 760.0
  pyelitis or pyelonephritis, arising during pregnancy (conditions classifiable to 590) 760.1
  renal disease or failure 760.1
  respiratory disease, chronic (conditions classifiable to 490–519, 748) 760.3
  rheumatic heart disease (chronic) (conditions classifiable to 393–398) 760.3
  rubella (conditions classifiable to 056) 760.2
    manifest rubella in the infant or fetus 771.0
  surgery unrelated to current delivery (*see also* Newborn, affected by) 760.64
    to uterus or pelvic organs 760.64
  syphilis (conditions classifiable to 090–097) 760.2
    manifest syphilis in the infant or fetus 090.0
  thrombophlebitis 760.3
  toxemia (of pregnancy) 760.0
    pre-eclamptic 760.0

Maternal condition, affecting fetus or newborn — *continued*
  toxoplasmosis (conditions classifiable to 130) 760.2
    manifest toxoplasmosis in the infant or fetus 771.2
  transmission of chemical substance through the placenta 760.70
    alcohol 760.71
    anticonvulsants 760.77
    antifungals 760.74
    anti-infective 760.74
    antimetabolics 760.78
    cocaine 760.75
    "crack" 760.75
    diethylstilbestrol [DES] 760.76
    hallucinogenic agents 760.73
    narcotics 760.72
    specified substance NEC 760.79
  uremia 760.1
  urinary tract conditions (conditions classifiable to 580–599) 760.1
  vomiting (pernicious) (persistent) (vicious) 761.8
Maternity — *see* Delivery
Matheiu's disease (leptospiral jaundice) 100.0
Mauclaire's disease or osteochondrosis 732.3
Maxcy's disease 081.0
Maxilla, maxillary — *see* condition
May (-Hegglin) anomaly or syndrome 288.2
Mayaro fever 066.3
Mazoplasia 610.8
MBD (minimal brain dysfunction), child — *see also* Hyperkinesia 314.9
MCAD (medium chain acyl CoA dehydrogenase deficiency) 277.85
McArdle (-Schmid-Pearson) disease or syndrome (glycogenosis V) 271.0
McCune-Albright syndrome (osteitis fibrosa disseminata) 756.59
MCLS (mucocutaneous lymph node syndrome) 446.1
McQuarrie's syndrome (idiopathic familial hypoglycemia) 251.2
Measles (black) (hemorrhagic) (suppressed) 055.9
  with
    encephalitis 055.0
    keratitis 055.71
    keratoconjunctivitis 055.71
    otitis media 055.2
    pneumonia 055.1
  complication 055.8
    specified type NEC 055.79
  encephalitis 055.0
  French 056.9
  German 056.9
  keratitis 055.71
  keratoconjunctivitis 055.71
  liberty 056.9
  otitis media 055.2
  pneumonia 055.1
  specified complications NEC 055.79
  vaccination, prophylactic (against) V04.2
Meatitis, urethral — *see also* Urethritis 597.89
Meat poisoning — *see* Poisoning, food
Meatus, meatal — *see* condition
Meat-wrappers' asthma 506.9
Meckel's
  diverticulitis 751.0
  diverticulum (displaced) (hypertrophic) 751.0
Meconium
  aspiration 770.11
    with
      pneumonia 770.12
      pneumonitis 770.12
      respiratory symptoms 770.12
    below vocal cords 770.11
      with respiratory symptoms 770.12
  syndrome 770.12
  delayed passage in newborn 777.1
  ileus 777.1
    due to cystic fibrosis 277.01
  in liquor 792.3
    noted during delivery 656.8 ☑

Meconium — *continued*
  insufflation 770.11
    with respiratory symptoms 770.12
  obstruction
    fetus or newborn 777.1
      in mucoviscidosis 277.01
  passage of 792.3
    noted during delivery 763.84
  peritonitis 777.6
  plug syndrome (newborn) NEC 777.1
  staining 779.84
Median — *see also* condition
  arcuate ligament syndrome 447.4
  bar (prostate) 600.90
    with
      other lower urinary tract symptoms (LUTS) 600.91
      urinary
        obstruction 600.91
        retention 600.91
  rhomboid glossitis 529.2
  vesical orifice 600.90
    with
      other lower urinary tract symptoms (LUTS) 600.91
      urinary
        obstruction 600.91
        retention 600.91
Mediastinal shift 793.2
Mediastinitis (acute) (chronic) 519.2
  actinomycotic 039.8
  syphilitic 095.8
  tuberculous (*see also* Tuberculosis) 012.8 ☑
Mediastinopericarditis — *see also* Pericarditis 423.9
  acute 420.90
  chronic 423.8
    rheumatic 393
  rheumatic, chronic 393
Mediastinum, mediastinal — *see* condition
Medical services provided for — *see* Health, services provided because (of)
Medicine poisoning (by overdose) (wrong substance given or taken in error) 977.9
  specified drug or substance — *see* Table of Drugs and Chemicals
Medin's disease (poliomyelitis) 045.9 ☑
Mediterranean
  anemia 282.40
    with other hemoglobinopathy 282.49
  disease or syndrome (hemopathic) 282.40
    with other hemoglobinopathy 282.49
  fever (*see also* Brucellosis) 023.9
    familial 277.31
  kala-azar 085.0
  leishmaniasis 085.0
  tick fever 082.1
Medulla — *see* condition
Medullary
  cystic kidney 753.16
  sponge kidney 753.17
Medullated fibers
  optic (nerve) 743.57
  retina 362.85
Medulloblastoma (M9470/3)
  desmoplastic (M9471/3) 191.6
  specified site — *see* Neoplasm, by site, malignant
  unspecified site 191.6
Medulloepithelioma (M9501/3) — *see also* Neoplasm, by site, malignant
  teratoid (M9502/3) — *see* Neoplasm, by site, malignant
Medullomyoblastoma (M9472/3)
  specified site — *see* Neoplasm, by site, malignant
  unspecified site 191.6
Meekeren-Ehlers-Danlos syndrome 756.83
Megacaryocytic — *see* condition
Megacolon (acquired) (functional) (not Hirschsprung's disease) 564.7
  aganglionic 751.3
  congenital, congenitum 751.3
  Hirschsprung's (disease) 751.3
  psychogenic 306.4
  toxic (*see also* Colitis, ulcerative) 556.9

☑ **Additional Digit Required** — Refer to the Tabular List for Digit Selection   ⬇ **Subterms under main terms may continue to next column or page**

2014 ICD-9-CM   227

Mass — Megacolon

Megaduodenum 537.3
Megaesophagus (functional) 530.0
  congenital 750.4
Megakaryocytic — *see* condition
Megalencephaly 742.4
Megalerythema (epidermicum) (infectiosum) 057.0
Megalia, cutis et ossium 757.39
Megaloappendix 751.5
Megalocephalus, megalocephaly NEC 756.0
Megalocornea 743.41
  associated with buphthalmos 743.22
Megalocytic anemia 281.9
Megalodactylia (fingers) (thumbs) 755.57
  toes 755.65
Megaloduodenum 751.5
Megaloesophagus (functional) 530.0
  congenital 750.4
Megalogastria (congenital) 750.7
Megalomania 307.9
Megalophthalmos 743.8
Megalopsia 368.14
Megalosplenia — *see also* Splenomegaly 789.2
Megaloureter 593.89
  congenital 753.22
Megarectum 569.49
Megasigmoid 564.7
  congenital 751.3
Megaureter 593.89
  congenital 753.22
Megrim 346.9 ☑
Meibomian
  cyst 373.2
    infected 373.12
  gland — *see* condition
  infarct (eyelid) 374.85
  stye 373.11
Meibomitis 373.12
Meige
  -Milroy disease (chronic hereditary edema) 757.0
  syndrome (blepharospasm-oromandibular dystonia) 333.82
Melalgia, nutritional 266.2
Melancholia — *see also* Psychosis, affective 296.90
  climacteric 296.2 ☑
    recurrent episode 296.3 ☑
    single episode 296.2 ☑
  hypochondriac 300.7
  intermittent 296.2 ☑
    recurrent episode 296.3 ☑
    single episode 296.2 ☑
  involutional 296.2 ☑
    recurrent episode 296.3 ☑
    single episode 296.2 ☑
  menopausal 296.2 ☑
    recurrent episode 296.3 ☑
    single episode 296.2 ☑
  puerperal 296.2 ☑
  reactive (from emotional stress, psychological trauma) 298.0
  recurrent 296.3 ☑
  senile 290.21
  stuporous 296.2 ☑
    recurrent episode 296.3 ☑
    single episode 296.2 ☑
Melanemia 275.09
Melanoameloblastoma (M9363/0) — *see* Neoplasm, bone, benign
Melanoblastoma (M8720/3) — *see* Melanoma
Melanoblastosis
  Block-Sulzberger 757.33
  cutis linearis sive systematisata 757.33
Melanocarcinoma (M8720/3) — *see* Melanoma
Melanocytoma, eyeball (M8726/0) 224.0
Melanocytosis, neurocutaneous 757.33
Melanoderma, melanodermia 709.09
  Addison's (primary adrenal insufficiency) 255.41
Melanodontia, infantile 521.05
Melanodontoclasia 521.05
Melanoepithelioma (M8720/3) — *see* Melanoma

Melanoma (malignant) (M8720/3) 172.9

Note — Except where otherwise indicated, the morphological varieties of melanoma in the list below should be coded by site as for "Melanoma (malignant)". Internal sites should be coded to malignant neoplasm of those sites.

  abdominal wall 172.5
  ala nasi 172.3
  amelanotic (M8730/3) — *see* Melanoma, by site
  ankle 172.7
  anus, anal 154.3
    canal 154.2
  arm 172.6
  auditory canal (external) 172.2
  auricle (ear) 172.2
  auricular canal (external) 172.2
  axilla 172.5
  axillary fold 172.5
  back 172.5
  balloon cell (M8722/3) — *see* Melanoma, by site
  benign (M8720/0) — *see* Neoplasm, skin, benign
  breast (female) (male) 172.5
  brow 172.3
  buttock 172.5
  canthus (eye) 172.1
  cheek (external) 172.3
  chest wall 172.5
  chin 172.3
  choroid 190.6
  conjunctiva 190.3
  ear (external) 172.2
  epithelioid cell (M8771/3) (*see also* Melanoma, by site)
    and spindle cell, mixed (M8775/3) — *see* Melanoma, by site
  external meatus (ear) 172.2
  eye 190.9
  eyebrow 172.3
  eyelid (lower) (upper) 172.1
  face NEC 172.3
  female genital organ (external) NEC 184.4
  finger 172.6
  flank 172.5
  foot 172.7
  forearm 172.6
  forehead 172.3
  foreskin 187.1
  gluteal region 172.5
  groin 172.5
  hand 172.6
  heel 172.7
  helix 172.2
  hip 172.7
  in
    giant pigmented nevus (M8761/3) — *see* Melanoma, by site
    Hutchinson's melanotic freckle (M8742/3) — *see* Melanoma, by site
    junctional nevus (M8740/3) — *see* Melanoma, by site
    precancerous melanosis (M8741/3) — *see* Melanoma, by site
  in situ — *see* Melanoma, by site
    skin 172.9
  interscapular region 172.5
  iris 190.0
  jaw 172.3
  juvenile (M8770/0) — *see* Neoplasm, skin, benign
  knee 172.7
  labium
    majus 184.1
    minus 184.2
  lacrimal gland 190.2
  leg 172.7
  lip (lower) (upper) 172.0
  liver 197.7
  lower limb NEC 172.7
  male genital organ (external) NEC 187.9
  meatus, acoustic (external) 172.2
  meibomian gland 172.1

Melanoma — *continued*
  metastatic
    of or from specified site — *see* Melanoma, by site
    site not of skin — *see* Neoplasm, by site, malignant, secondary
    to specified site — *see* Neoplasm, by site, malignant, secondary
    unspecified site 172.9
  nail 172.9
    finger 172.6
    toe 172.7
  neck 172.4
  nodular (M8721/3) — *see* Melanoma, by site
  nose, external 172.3
  orbit 190.1
  penis 187.4
  perianal skin 172.5
  perineum 172.5
  pinna 172.2
  popliteal (fossa) (space) 172.7
  prepuce 187.1
  pubes 172.5
  pudendum 184.4
  retina 190.5
  scalp 172.4
  scrotum 187.7
  septum nasal (skin) 172.3
  shoulder 172.6
  skin NEC 172.8
    in situ 172.9
  spindle cell (M8772/3) (*see also* Melanoma, by site)
    type A (M8773/3) 190.0
    type B (M8774/3) 190.0
  submammary fold 172.5
  superficial spreading (M8743/3) — *see* Melanoma, by site
  temple 172.3
  thigh 172.7
  toe 172.7
  trunk NEC 172.5
  umbilicus 172.5
  upper limb NEC 172.6
  vagina vault 184.0
  vulva 184.4
Melanoplakia 528.9
Melanosarcoma (M8720/3) — *see also* Melanoma
  epithelioid cell (M8771/3) — *see* Melanoma
Melanosis 709.09
  addisonian (primary adrenal insufficiency) 255.41
    tuberculous (*see also* Tuberculosis) 017.6 ☑
  adrenal 255.41
  colon 569.89
  conjunctiva 372.55
    congenital 743.49
  corii degenerativa 757.33
  cornea (presenile) (senile) 371.12
    congenital 743.43
      interfering with vision 743.42
  eye 372.55
    congenital 743.49
  jute spinners' 709.09
  lenticularis progressiva 757.33
  liver 573.8
  precancerous (M8741/2) (*see also* Neoplasm, skin, in situ)
    malignant melanoma in (M8741/3) — *see* Melanoma
  prenatal 743.43
    interfering with vision 743.42
  Riehl's 709.09
  sclera 379.19
    congenital 743.47
  suprarenal 255.41
  tar 709.09
  toxic 709.09
Melanuria 791.9
Melasma 709.09
  adrenal (gland) 255.41
  suprarenal (gland) 255.41

MELAS syndrome (mitochondrial encephalopathy, lactic acidosis and stroke-like episodes) 277.87
Melena 578.1
  due to
    swallowed maternal blood 777.3
    ulcer — *see* Ulcer, by site, with hemorrhage
  newborn 772.4
    due to swallowed maternal blood 777.3
Meleney's
  gangrene (cutaneous) 686.09
  ulcer (chronic undermining) 686.09
Melioidosis 025
Melitensis, febris 023.0
Melitococcosis 023.0
Melkersson (-Rosenthal) syndrome 351.8
Mellitus, diabetes — *see* Diabetes
Melorheostosis (bone) (leri) 733.99
Meloschisis 744.83
Melotia 744.29
Membrana
  capsularis lentis posterior 743.39
  epipapillaris 743.57
Membranacea placenta — *see* Placenta, abnormal
Membranaceous uterus 621.8
Membrane, membranous — *see also* condition
  folds, congenital — *see* Web
  Jackson's 751.4
  over face (causing asphyxia), fetus or newborn 768.9
  premature rupture — *see* Rupture, membranes, premature
  pupillary 364.74
    persistent 743.46
  retained (complicating delivery) (with hemorrhage) 666.2 ☑
    without hemorrhage 667.1 ☑
  secondary (eye) 366.50
  unruptured (causing asphyxia) 768.9
  vitreous humor 379.25
Membranitis, fetal 658.4 ☑
  affecting fetus or newborn 762.7
Memory disturbance, loss or lack — *see also* Amnesia 780.93
  mild, following organic brain damage 310.89
MEN (multiple endocrine neoplasia) (syndromes)
  type I 258.01
  type IIA 258.02
  type IIB 258.03
Menadione (vitamin K) **deficiency** 269.0
Menarche, precocious 259.1
Mendacity, pathologic 301.7
Mendelson's syndrome (resulting from a procedure) 997.32
  obstetric 668.0 ☑
Mende's syndrome (ptosis-epicanthus) 270.2
Ménétrier's disease or syndrome (hypertrophic gastritis) 535.2 ☑
Ménière's disease, syndrome, or vertigo 386.00
  cochlear 386.02
  cochleovestibular 386.01
  inactive 386.04
  in remission 386.04
  vestibular 386.03
Meninges, meningeal — *see* condition
Meningioma (M9530/0) — *see also* Neoplasm, meninges, benign
  angioblastic (M9535/0) — *see* Neoplasm, meninges, benign
  angiomatous (M9534/0) — *see* Neoplasm, meninges, benign
  endotheliomatous (M9531/0) — *see* Neoplasm, meninges, benign
  fibroblastic (M9532/0) — *see* Neoplasm, meninges, benign
  fibrous (M9532/0) — *see* Neoplasm, meninges, benign
  hemangioblastic (M9535/0) — *see* Neoplasm, meninges, benign

Meningioma — see also Neoplasm, meninges, benign — continued
  hemangiopericytic (M9536/0) — see Neoplasm, meninges, benign
  malignant (M9530/3) — see Neoplasm, meninges, malignant
  meningiothelial (M9531/0) — see Neoplasm, meninges, benign
  meningotheliomatous (M9531/0) — see Neoplasm, meninges, benign
  mixed (M9537/0) — see Neoplasm, meninges, benign
  multiple (M9530/1) 237.6
  papillary (M9538/1) 237.6
  psammomatous (M9533/0) — see Neoplasm, meninges, benign
  syncytial (M9531/0) — see Neoplasm, meninges, benign
  transitional (M9537/0) — see Neoplasm, meninges, benign
Meningiomatosis (diffuse) (M9530/1) 237.6
Meningism — see also Meningismus 781.6
Meningismus (infectional) (pneumococcal) 781.6
  due to serum or vaccine 997.09 *[321.8]*
  influenzal NEC (see also Influenza) 487.8
Meningitis (basal) (basic) (basilar) (brain) (cerebral) (cervical) (congestive) (diffuse) (hemorrhagic) (infantile) (membranous) (metastatic) (nonspecific) (pontine) (progressive) (simple) (spinal) (subacute) (sympathetica) (toxic) 322.9
  abacterial NEC (see also Meningitis, aseptic) 047.9
  actinomycotic 039.8 *[320.7]*
  adenoviral 049.1
  Aerobacter aerogenes 320.82
  anaerobes (cocci) (gram-negative) (gram-positive) (mixed) (NEC) 320.81
  arbovirus NEC 066.9 *[321.2]*
    specified type NEC 066.8 *[321.2]*
  aseptic (acute) NEC 047.9
    adenovirus 049.1
    Coxsackie virus 047.0
    due to
      adenovirus 049.1
      Coxsackie virus 047.0
      ECHO virus 047.1
      enterovirus 047.9
      mumps 072.1
      poliovirus (see also Poliomyelitis) 045.2 ☑ *[321.2]*
    ECHO virus 047.1
    herpes (simplex) virus 054.72
      zoster 053.0
    leptospiral 100.81
    lymphocytic choriomeningitis 049.0
    noninfective 322.0
  Bacillus pyocyaneus 320.89
  bacterial NEC 320.9
    anaerobic 320.81
    gram-negative 320.82
      anaerobic 320.81
  Bacteroides (fragilis) (oralis) (melaninogenicus) 320.81
  cancerous (M8000/6) 198.4
  candidal 112.83
  carcinomatous (M8010/6) 198.4
  caseous (see also Tuberculosis, meninges) 013.0 ☑
  cerebrospinal (acute) (chronic) (diplococcal) (endemic) (epidemic) (fulminant) (infectious) (malignant) (meningococcal) (sporadic) 036.0
    carrier (suspected) of V02.59
  chronic NEC 322.2
  clear cerebrospinal fluid NEC 322.0
  Clostridium (haemolyticum) (novyi) NEC 320.81
  coccidioidomycosis 114.2
  Coxsackie virus 047.0
  cryptococcal 117.5 *[321.0]*
  diplococcal 036.0
    gram-negative 036.0
    gram-positive 320.1

Meningitis — continued
Diplococcus pneumoniae 320.1
due to
  actinomycosis 039.8 *[320.7]*
  adenovirus 049.1
  coccidiomycosis 114.2
  enterovirus 047.9
    specified NEC 047.8
  histoplasmosis (see also Histoplasmosis) 115.91
  Listerosis 027.0 *[320.7]*
  Lyme disease 088.81 *[320.7]*
  moniliasis 112.83
  mumps 072.1
  neurosyphilis 094.2
  nonbacterial organisms NEC 321.8
  oidiomycosis 112.83
  poliovirus (see also Poliomyelitis) 045.2 ☑ *[321.2]*
  preventive immunization, inoculation, or vaccination 997.09 *[321.8]*
  sarcoidosis 135 *[321.4]*
  sporotrichosis 117.1 *[321.1]*
  syphilis 094.2
    acute 091.81
    congenital 090.42
    secondary 091.81
  trypanosomiasis (see also Trypanosomiasis) 086.9 *[321.3]*
  whooping cough 033.9 *[320.7]*
ECHO virus 047.1
E. coli 320.82
endothelial-leukocytic, benign, recurrent 047.9
Enterobacter aerogenes 320.82
enteroviral 047.9
  specified type NEC 047.8
enterovirus 047.9
  specified NEC 047.8
eosinophilic 322.1
epidemic NEC 036.0
Escherichia coli (E. coli) 320.82
Eubacterium 320.81
fibrinopurulent NEC 320.9
  specified type NEC 320.89
Friedländer (bacillus) 320.82
fungal NEC 117.9 *[321.1]*
Fusobacterium 320.81
gonococcal 098.82
gram-negative bacteria NEC 320.82
  anaerobic 320.81
  cocci 036.0
    specified NEC 320.82
gram-negative cocci NEC 036.0
  specified NEC 320.82
gram-positive cocci NEC 320.9
herpes (simplex) virus 054.72
  zoster 053.0
H. influenzae 320.0
infectious NEC 320.9
influenzal 320.0
Klebsiella pneumoniae 320.82
late effect — see Late, effect, meningitis
leptospiral (aseptic) 100.81
Listerella (monocytogenes) 027.0 *[320.7]*
Listeria monocytogenes 027.0 *[320.7]*
lymphocytic (acute) (benign) (serous) 049.0
  choriomeningitis virus 049.0
meningococcal (chronic) 036.0
Mima polymorpha 320.82
Mollaret's 047.9
monilial 112.83
mumps (virus) 072.1
mycotic NEC 117.9 *[321.1]*
Neisseria 036.0
neurosyphilis 094.2
nonbacterial NEC (see also Meningitis, aseptic) 047.9
nonpyogenic NEC 322.0
oidiomycosis 112.83
ossificans 349.2
Peptococcus 320.81
Peptostreptococcus 320.81
pneumococcal 320.1
poliovirus (see also Poliomyelitis) 045.2 ☑ *[321.2]*

Meningitis — continued
Proprionibacterium 320.81
Proteus morganii 320.82
Pseudomonas (aeruginosa) (pyocyaneus) 320.82
purulent NEC 320.9
  specified organism NEC 320.89
pyogenic NEC 320.9
  specified organism NEC 320.89
Salmonella 003.21
septic NEC 320.9
  specified organism NEC 320.89
serosa circumscripta NEC 322.0
serous NEC (see also Meningitis, aseptic) 047.9
  lymphocytic 049.0
  syndrome 348.2
Serratia (marcescens) 320.82
specified organism NEC 320.89
sporadic cerebrospinal 036.0
sporotrichosis 117.1 *[321.1]*
staphylococcal 320.3
sterile 997.09
streptococcal (acute) 320.2
suppurative 320.9
  specified organism NEC 320.89
syphilitic 094.2
  acute 091.81
  congenital 090.42
  secondary 091.81
torula 117.5 *[321.0]*
traumatic (complication of injury) 958.8
Treponema (denticola) (macrodenticum) 320.81
trypanosomiasis 086.1 *[321.3]*
tuberculous (see also Tuberculosis, meninges) 013.0 ☑
typhoid 002.0 *[320.7]*
Veillonella 320.81
Vibrio vulnificus 320.82
viral, virus NEC (see also Meningitis, aseptic) 047.9
Wallgren's (see also Meningitis, aseptic) 047.9
Meningocele (congenital) (spinal) — see also Spina bifida 741.9 ☑
  acquired (traumatic) 349.2
  cerebral 742.0
  cranial 742.0
Meningocerebritis — see Meningoencephalitis
Meningococcemia (acute) (chronic) 036.2
Meningococcus, meningococcal — see also condition 036.9
  adrenalitis, hemorrhagic 036.3
  carditis 036.40
  carrier (suspected) of V02.59
  cerebrospinal fever 036.0
  encephalitis 036.1
  endocarditis 036.42
  exposure to V01.84
  infection NEC 036.9
  meningitis (cerebrospinal) 036.0
  myocarditis 036.43
  optic neuritis 036.81
  pericarditis 036.41
  septicemia (chronic) 036.2
Meningoencephalitis — see also Encephalitis 323.9
acute NEC 048
bacterial, purulent, pyogenic, or septic — see Meningitis
chronic NEC 094.1
diffuse NEC 094.1
diphasic 063.2
due to
  actinomycosis 039.8 *[320.7]*
  blastomycosis NEC (see also Blastomycosis) 116.0 *[323.41]*
  free-living amebae 136.29
  Listeria monocytogenes 027.0 *[320.7]*
  Lyme disease 088.81 *[320.7]*
  mumps 072.2
  Naegleria (amebae) (gruberi) (organisms) 136.29
  rubella 056.01

Meningoencephalitis — see also Encephalitis — continued
due to — continued
  sporotrichosis 117.1 *[321.1]*
  toxoplasmosis (acquired) 130.0
    congenital (active) 771.2 *[323.41]*
  Trypanosoma 086.1 *[323.2]*
epidemic 036.0
herpes 054.3
herpetic 054.3
H. influenzae 320.0
infectious (acute) 048
influenzal 320.0
late effect — see category 326
Listeria monocytogenes 027.0 *[320.7]*
lymphocytic (serous) 049.0
mumps 072.2
parasitic NEC 123.9 *[323.41]*
pneumococcal 320.1
primary amebic 136.29
rubella 056.01
serous 048
  lymphocytic 049.0
specific 094.2
staphylococcal 320.3
streptococcal 320.2
syphilitic 094.2
toxic NEC 989.9 *[323.71]*
  due to
    carbon tetrachloride (vapor) 987.8 *[323.71]*
    hydroxyquinoline derivatives poisoning 961.3 *[323.71]*
    lead 984.9 *[323.71]*
    mercury 985.0 *[323.71]*
    thallium 985.8 *[323.71]*
toxoplasmosis (acquired) 130.0
trypanosomic 086.1 *[323.2]*
tuberculous (see also Tuberculosis, meninges) 013.0 ☑
virus NEC 048
Meningoencephalocele 742.0
syphilitic 094.89
congenital 090.49
Meningoencephalomyelitis — see also Meningoencephalitis 323.9
acute NEC 048
  disseminated (postinfectious) 136.9 *[323.61]*
    postimmunization or postvaccination 323.51
due to
  actinomycosis 039.8 *[320.7]*
  torula 117.5 *[323.41]*
  toxoplasma or toxoplasmosis (acquired) 130.0
    congenital (active) 771.2 *[323.41]*
late effect — see category 326
Meningoencephalomyelopathy — see also Meningoencephalomyelitis 349.9
Meningoencephalopathy — see also Meningoencephalitis 348.39
Meningoencephalopoliomyelitis — see also Poliomyelitis, bulbar 045.0 ☑
  late effect 138
Meningomyelitis — see also Meningoencephalitis 323.9
blastomycotic NEC (see also Blastomycosis) 116.0 *[323.41]*
due to
  actinomycosis 039.8 *[320.7]*
  blastomycosis (see also Blastomycosis) 116.0 *[323.41]*
  Meningococcus 036.0
  sporotrichosis 117.1 *[323.41]*
  torula 117.5 *[323.41]*
late effect — see category 326
lethargic 049.8
meningococcal 036.0
syphilitic 094.2
tuberculous (see also Tuberculosis, meninges) 013.0 ☑
Meningomyelocele — see also Spina bifida 741.9 ☑
syphilitic 094.89

Meningomyeloneuritis — *see* Meningoencephalitis
Meningoradiculitis — *see* Meningitis
Meningovascular — *see* condition
Meniscocytosis 282.60
Menkes' syndrome — *see* Syndrome, Menkes'
Menolipsis 626.0
Menometrorrhagia 626.2
Menopause, menopausal (symptoms) (syndrome) 627.2
  arthritis (any site) NEC 716.3 ☑
  artificial 627.4
  bleeding 627.0
  crisis 627.2
  depression (*see also* Psychosis, affective) 296.2 ☑
    agitated 296.2 ☑
      recurrent episode 296.3 ☑
      single episode 296.2 ☑
    psychotic 296.2 ☑
      recurrent episode 296.3 ☑
      single episode 296.2 ☑
    recurrent episode 296.3 ☑
    single episode 296.2 ☑
    melancholia (*see also* Psychosis, affective) 296.2 ☑
      recurrent episode 296.3 ☑
      single episode 296.2 ☑
  paranoid state 297.2
  paraphrenia 297.2
  postsurgical 627.4
  premature 256.31
    postirradiation 256.2
    postsurgical 256.2
  psychoneurosis 627.2
  psychosis NEC 298.8
  surgical 627.4
  toxic polyarthritis NEC 716.39
Menorrhagia (primary) 626.2
  climacteric 627.0
  menopausal 627.0
  postclimacteric 627.1
  postmenopausal 627.1
  preclimacteric 627.0
  premenopausal 627.0
  puberty (menses retained) 626.3
Menorrhalgia 625.3
Menoschesis 626.8
Menostaxis 626.2
Menses, retention 626.8
Menstrual — *see also* Menstruation
  cycle, irregular 626.4
  disorders NEC 626.9
  extraction V25.3
  fluid, retained 626.8
  molimen 625.4
  period, normal V65.5
  regulation V25.3
Menstruation
  absent 626.0
  anovulatory 628.0
  delayed 626.8
  difficult 625.3
  disorder 626.9
    psychogenic 306.52
    specified NEC 626.8
  during pregnancy 640.8 ☑
  excessive 626.2
  frequent 626.2
  infrequent 626.1
  irregular 626.4
  latent 626.8
  membranous 626.8
  painful (primary) (secondary) 625.3
    psychogenic 306.52
  passage of clots 626.2
  precocious 259.1
  protracted 626.8
  retained 626.8
  retrograde 626.8
  scanty 626.1
  suppression 626.8
  vicarious (nasal) 625.8
Mentagra — *see also* Sycosis 704.8
Mental — *see also* condition

Mental — *see also* condition — *continued*
  deficiency (*see also* Disability, intellectual) 319
  deterioration (*see also* Psychosis) 298.9
  disorder (*see also* Disorder, mental) 300.9
  exhaustion 300.5
  insufficiency (congenital) (*see also* Disability, intellectual) 319
  observation without need for further medical care NEC V71.09
  retardation —*see* Disability, intellectual
  subnormality (*see also* Disability, intellectual) 319
    mild 317
    moderate 318.0
    profound 318.2
    severe 318.1
  upset (*see also* Disorder, mental) 300.9
Meralgia paresthetica 355.1
Mercurial — *see* condition
Mercurialism NEC 985.0
Merergasia 300.9
Merkel cell tumor — *see* Carcinoma, Merkel cell
Merocele — *see also* Hernia, femoral 553.00
Meromelia 755.4
  lower limb 755.30
    intercalary 755.32
      femur 755.34
        tibiofibular (complete) (incomplete) 755.33
      fibula 755.37
      metatarsal(s) 755.38
      tarsal(s) 755.38
      tibia 755.36
      tibiofibular 755.35
    terminal (complete) (partial) (transverse) 755.31
    longitudinal 755.32
      metatarsal(s) 755.38
      phalange(s) 755.39
      tarsal(s) 755.38
    transverse 755.31
  upper limb 755.20
    intercalary 755.22
      carpal(s) 755.28
      humeral 755.24
        radioulnar (complete) (incomplete) 755.23
      metacarpal(s) 755.28
      phalange(s) 755.29
      radial 755.26
      radioulnar 755.25
      ulnar 755.27
    terminal (complete) (partial) (transverse) 755.21
    longitudinal 755.22
      carpal(s) 755.28
      metacarpal(s) 755.28
      phalange(s) 755.29
    transverse 755.21
Merosmia 781.1
MERRF syndrome (myoclonus with epilepsy and with ragged red fibers) 277.87
Merycism — *see also* Vomiting
  psychogenic 307.53
Merzbacher-Pelizaeus disease 330.0
Mesaortitis — *see* Aortitis
Mesarteritis — *see* Arteritis
Mesencephalitis — *see also* Encephalitis 323.9
  late effect — *see* category 326
Mesenchymoma (M8990/1) — *see also* Neoplasm, connective tissue, uncertain behavior
  benign (M8990/0) — *see* Neoplasm, connective tissue, benign
  malignant (M8990/3) — *see* Neoplasm, connective tissue, malignant
Mesenteritis
  retractile 567.82
  sclerosing 567.82
Mesentery, mesenteric — *see* condition
Mesiodens, mesiodentes 520.1
  causing crowding 524.31
Mesio-occlusion 524.23
Mesocardia (with asplenia) 746.87

Mesocolon — *see* condition
Mesonephroma (malignant) (M9110/3) — *see also* Neoplasm, by site, malignant
  benign (M9110/0) — *see* Neoplasm, by site, benign
Mesophlebitis — *see* Phlebitis
Mesostromal dysgenesis 743.51
Mesothelioma (malignant) (M9050/3) — *see also* Neoplasm, by site, malignant
  benign (M9050/0) — *see* Neoplasm, by site, benign
  biphasic type (M9053/3) (*see also* Neoplasm, by site, malignant)
    benign (M9053/0) — *see* Neoplasm, by site, benign
  epithelioid (M9052/3) (*see also* Neoplasm, by site, malignant)
    benign (M9052/0) — *see* Neoplasm, by site, benign
  fibrous (M9051/3) (*see also* Neoplasm, by site, malignant)
    benign (M9051/0) — *see* Neoplasm, by site, benign
Metabolic syndrome 277.7
Metabolism disorder 277.9
  specified type NEC 277.89
Metagonimiasis 121.5
Metagonimus infestation (small intestine) 121.5
Metal
  pigmentation (skin) 709.00
  polishers' disease 502
Metalliferous miners' lung 503
Metamorphopsia 368.14
Metaplasia
  bone, in skin 709.3
  breast 611.89
  cervix — *omit code*
  endometrium (squamous) 621.8
  esophagus 530.85
  intestinal, of gastric mucosa 537.89
  kidney (pelvis) (squamous) (*see also* Disease, renal) 593.89
  myelogenous 289.89
  myeloid 289.89
    agnogenic 238.76
    megakaryocytic 238.76
  spleen 289.59
  squamous cell
    amnion 658.8 ☑
    bladder 596.89
    cervix — *see* condition
    trachea 519.19
    tracheobronchial tree 519.19
    uterus 621.8
      cervix — *see* condition
Metastasis, metastatic
  abscess — *see* Abscess
  calcification 275.40
  cancer, neoplasm, or disease
    from specified site (M8000/3) — *see* Neoplasm, by site, malignant
    to specified site (M8000/6) — *see* Neoplasm, by site, secondary
  deposits (in) (M8000/6) — *see* Neoplasm, by site, secondary
  mesentery, of neuroendocrine tumor 209.74
  pneumonia 038.8 *[484.8]*
  spread (to) (M8000/6) — *see* Neoplasm, by site, secondary
Metatarsalgia 726.70
  anterior 355.6
  due to Freiberg's disease 732.5
  Morton's 355.6
Metatarsus, metatarsal — *see also* condition
  abductus valgus (congenital) 754.60
  adductus varus (congenital) 754.53
  primus varus 754.52
  valgus (adductus) (congenital) 754.60
  varus (abductus) (congenital) 754.53
    primus 754.52
Methadone use 304.00
Methemoglobinemia 289.7
  acquired (with sulfhemoglobinemia) 289.7
  congenital 289.7
  enzymatic 289.7

Methemoglobinemia — *continued*
  Hb-M disease 289.7
  hereditary 289.7
  toxic 289.7
Methemoglobinuria — *see also* Hemoglobinuria 791.2
Methicillin
  resistant staphyloccocus aureus (MRSA) 041.12
    colonization V02.54
    personal history of V12.04
  susceptible staphylococcus aureus (MSSA) 041.11
    colonization V02.53
Methioninemia 270.4
Metritis (catarrhal) (septic) (suppurative) — *see also* Endometritis 615.9
  blennorrhagic 098.16
    chronic or duration of 2 months or over 098.36
  cervical (*see also* Cervicitis) 616.0
  gonococcal 098.16
    chronic or duration of 2 months or over 098.36
  hemorrhagic 626.8
  puerperal, postpartum, childbirth 670.1 ☑
    septic 670.2 ☑
  tuberculous (*see also* Tuberculosis) 016.7 ☑
Metropathia hemorrhagica 626.8
Metroperitonitis — *see also* Peritonitis, pelvic, female 614.5
Metrorrhagia 626.6
  arising during pregnancy — *see* Hemorrhage, pregnancy
  postpartum NEC 666.2 ☑
  primary 626.6
  psychogenic 306.59
  puerperal 666.2 ☑
Metrorrhexis — *see* Rupture, uterus
Metrosalpingitis — *see also* Salpingo-oophoritis 614.2
Metrostaxis 626.6
Metrovaginitis — *see also* Endometritis 615.9
  gonococcal (acute) 098.16
    chronic or duration of 2 months or over 098.36
Mexican fever — *see* Typhus, Mexican
Meyenburg-Altherr-Uehlinger syndrome 733.99
Meyer-Schwickerath and Weyers syndrome (dysplasia oculodentodigitalis) 759.89
Meynert's amentia (nonalcoholic) 294.0
  alcoholic 291.1
Mibelli's disease 757.39
Mice, joint — *see also* Loose, body, joint 718.1 ☑
  knee 717.6
Micheli-Rietti syndrome (thalassemia minor) 282.46
Michotte's syndrome 721.5
Micrencephalon, micrencephaly 742.1
Microalbuminuria 791.0
Microaneurysm, retina 362.14
  diabetic 250.5 ☑ *[362.01]*
    due to secondary diabetes 249.5 ☑ *[362.01]*
Microangiopathy 443.9
  diabetic (peripheral) 250.7 ☑ *[443.81]*
    due to secondary diabetes 249.7 ☑ *[443.81]*
    retinal 250.5 ☑ *[362.01]*
      due to secondary diabetes 249.5 ☑ *[362.01]*
  peripheral 443.9
    diabetic 250.7 ☑ *[443.81]*
      due to secondary diabetes 249.7 ☑ *[443.81]*
  retinal 362.18
    diabetic 250.5 ☑ *[362.01]*
      due to secondary diabetes 249.5 ☑ *[362.01]*
  thrombotic 446.6
    Moschcowitz's (thrombotic thrombocytopenic purpura) 446.6
Microcalcification, mammographic 793.81

Microcephalus, microcephalic, microcephaly 742.1
due to toxoplasmosis (congenital) 771.2
Microcheilia 744.82
Microcolon (congenital) 751.5
Microcornea (congenital) 743.41
Microcytic — see condition
Microdeletions NEC 758.33
Microdontia 520.2
Microdrepanocytosis (thalassemia-Hb-S disease) 282.41
with sickle cell crisis 282.42
Microembolism
atherothrombotic — see Atheroembolism
retina 362.33
Microencephalon 742.1
Microfilaria streptocerca infestation 125.3
Microgastria (congenital) 750.7
Microgenia 524.06
Microgenitalia (congenital) 752.89
penis 752.64
Microglioma (M9710/3)
specified site — see Neoplasm, by site, malignant
unspecified site 191.9
Microglossia (congenital) 750.16
Micrognathia, micrognathism (congenital) 524.00
mandibular 524.04
alveolar 524.74
maxillary 524.03
alveolar 524.73
Microgyria (congenital) 742.2
Microinfarct, heart — see also Insufficiency, coronary 411.89
Microlithiasis, alveolar, pulmonary 516.2
Micromastia 611.82
Micromyelia (congenital) 742.59
Micropenis 752.64
Microphakia (congenital) 743.36
Microphthalmia (congenital) — see also Microphthalmos 743.10
Microphthalmos (congenital) 743.10
associated with eye and adnexal anomalies NEC 743.12
due to toxoplasmosis (congenital) 771.2
isolated 743.11
simple 743.11
syndrome 759.89
Micropsia 368.14
Microsporidiosis 136.8
Microsporon furfur infestation 111.0
Microsporosis — see also Dermatophytosis 110.9
nigra 111.1
Microstomia (congenital) 744.84
Microthelia 757.6
Microthromboembolism — see Embolism
Microtia (congenital) (external ear) 744.23
Microtropia 378.34
Microvillus inclusion disease (MVD) 751.5
Micturition
disorder NEC 788.69
psychogenic 306.53
frequency 788.41
psychogenic 306.53
nocturnal 788.43
painful 788.1
psychogenic 306.53
Middle
ear — see condition
lobe (right) syndrome 518.0
Midplane — see condition
Miescher's disease 709.3
cheilitis 351.8
granulomatosis disciformis 709.3
Miescher-Leder syndrome or granulomatosis 709.3
Mieten's syndrome 759.89

Migraine (idiopathic) 346.9 ☑

Note — The following fifth digit subclassification is for use with category 346:

0   without mention of intractable migraine without mention of status migrainosus

without mention of refractory migraine without mention of status migrainosus

1   with intractable migraine, so stated, without mention of status migrainosus

with refractory migraine, so stated, without mention of status migrainosus

2   without mention of intractable migraine with status migrainosus

without mention of refractory migraine with status migrainosus

3   with intractable migraine, so stated, with status migrainosus

with refractory migraine, so stated, with status migrainosus

with aura (acute-onset) (without headache) (prolonged) (typical) 346.0 ☑
without aura 346.1 ☑
chronic 346.7 ☑
transformed 346.7 ☑
abdominal (syndrome) 346.2 ☑
allergic (histamine) 346.2 ☑
atypical 346.8 ☑
basilar 346.0 ☑
chronic without aura 346.7 ☑
classic(al) 346.0 ☑
common 346.1 ☑
complicated 346.0 ☑
hemiplegic 346.3 ☑
familial 346.3 ☑
sporadic 346.3 ☑
lower-half 339.00
menstrual 346.4 ☑
menstrually related 346.4 ☑
ophthalmic 346.8 ☑
ophthalmoplegic 346.2 ☑
premenstrual 346.4 ☑
pure menstrual 346.4 ☑
retinal 346.0 ☑
specified form NEC 346.8 ☑
transformed without aura 346.7 ☑
variant 346.2 ☑
Migrant, social V60.0
Migratory, migrating — see also condition
person V60.0
testis, congenital 752.52
Mikulicz's disease or syndrome (dryness of mouth, absent or decreased lacrimation) 527.1
Milian atrophia blanche 701.3
Miliaria (crystallina) (rubra) (tropicalis) 705.1
apocrine 705.82
Miliary — see condition
Milium — see also Cyst, sebaceous 706.2
colloid 709.3
eyelid 374.84
Milk
crust 690.11
excess secretion 676.6 ☑
fever, female 672.0 ☑
poisoning 988.8
retention 676.2 ☑
sickness 988.8
spots 423.1
Milkers' nodes 051.1
Milk-leg (deep vessels) 671.4 ☑
complicating pregnancy 671.3 ☑
nonpuerperal 451.19
puerperal, postpartum, childbirth 671.4 ☑
Milkman (-Looser) disease or syndrome (osteomalacia with pseudofractures) 268.2

Milky urine — see also Chyluria 791.1
Millar's asthma (laryngismus stridulus) 478.75
Millard-Gubler-Foville paralysis 344.89
Millard-Gubler paralysis or syndrome 344.89
Miller-Dieker syndrome 758.33
Miller's disease (osteomalacia) 268.2
Miller Fisher's syndrome 357.0
Milles' syndrome (encephalocutaneous angiomatosis) 759.6
Mills' disease 335.29
Millstone makers' asthma or lung 502
Milroy's disease (chronic hereditary edema) 757.0
Miners' — see also condition
asthma 500
elbow 727.2
knee 727.2
lung 500
nystagmus 300.89
phthisis (see also Tuberculosis) 011.4 ☑
tuberculosis (see also Tuberculosis) 011.4 ☑
Minkowski-Chauffard syndrome — see also Spherocytosis 282.0
Minor — see condition
Minor's disease 336.1
Minot's disease (hemorrhagic disease, newborn) 776.0
Minot-von Willebrand (-Jürgens) disease or syndrome (angiohemophilia) 286.4
Minus (and plus) hand (intrinsic) 736.09
Miosis (persistent) (pupil) 379.42
Mirizzi's syndrome (hepatic duct stenosis) — see also Obstruction, biliary 576.2
with calculus, cholelithiasis, or stones — see Choledocholithiasis
Mirror writing 315.09
secondary to organic lesion 784.69
Misadventure (prophylactic) (therapeutic) — see also Complications 999.9
administration of insulin 962.3
infusion — see Complications, infusion
local applications (of fomentations, plasters, etc.) 999.9
burn or scald — see Burn, by site
medical care (early) (late) NEC 999.9
adverse effect of drugs or chemicals — see Table of Drugs and Chemicals
burn or scald — see Burn, by site
radiation NEC 990
radiotherapy NEC 990
surgical procedure (early) (late) — see Complications, surgical procedure
transfusion — see Complications, transfusion
vaccination or other immunological procedure — see Complications, vaccination
Misanthropy 301.7
Miscarriage — see Abortion, spontaneous
Mischief, malicious, child — see also Disturbance, conduct 312.0 ☑
Misdirection
aqueous 365.83
Mismanagement, feeding 783.3
Misplaced, misplacement
kidney (see also Disease, renal) 593.0
congenital 753.3
organ or site, congenital NEC — see Malposition, congenital
Missed
abortion 632
delivery (at or near term) 656.4 ☑
labor (at or near term) 656.4 ☑
Misshapen reconstructed breast 612.0
Missing — see also Absence
teeth (acquired) 525.10
congenital (see also Anodontia) 520.0
due to
caries 525.13
extraction 525.10
periodontal disease 525.12
specified NEC 525.19
trauma 525.11
vertebrae (congenital) 756.13
Misuse of drugs NEC — see also Abuse, drug, nondependent 305.9 ☑

Mitchell's disease (erythromelalgia) 443.82
Mite(s)
diarrhea 133.8
grain (itch) 133.8
hair follicle (itch) 133.8
in sputum 133.8
Mitochondrial encephalopathy, lactic acidosis and stroke-like episodes (MELAS syndrome) 277.87
Mitochondrial neurogastrointestinal encephalopathy syndrome (MNGIE) 277.87
Mitral — see condition
Mittelschmerz 625.2
Mixed — see condition
Mljet disease (mal de Meleda) 757.39
Mobile, mobility
cecum 751.4
coccyx 733.99
excessive — see Hypermobility
gallbladder 751.69
kidney 593.0
congenital 753.3
organ or site, congenital NEC — see Malposition, congenital
spleen 289.59
Mobitz heart block (atrioventricular) 426.10
type I (Wenckebach's) 426.13
type II 426.12
Möbius'
disease 346.2 ☑
syndrome
congenital oculofacial paralysis 352.6
ophthalmoplegic migraine 346.2 ☑
Moeller(-Barlow) disease (infantile scurvy) 267
glossitis 529.4
Mohr's syndrome (types I and II) 759.89
Mola destruens (M9100/1) 236.1
Molarization, premolars 520.2
Molar pregnancy 631.8
hydatidiform (delivered) (undelivered) 630
Molding, head (during birth) — omit code
Mold(s) in vitreous 117.9
Mole (pigmented) (M8720/0) — see also Neoplasm, skin, benign
blood 631.8
Breus' 631.8
cancerous (M8720/3) — see Melanoma
carneous 631.8
destructive (M9100/1) 236.1
ectopic — see Pregnancy, ectopic
fleshy 631.8
hemorrhagic 631.8
hydatid, hydatidiform (benign) (complicating pregnancy) (delivered) (undelivered) (see also Hydatidiform mole) 630
invasive (M9100/1) 236.1
malignant (M9100/1) 236.1
previous, affecting management of pregnancy V23.1
invasive (hydatidiform) (M9100/1) 236.1
malignant
meaning
malignant hydatidiform mole (M9100/1) 236.1
melanoma (M8720/3) — see Melanoma
nonpigmented (M8730/0) — see Neoplasm, skin, benign
pregnancy NEC 631.8
skin (M8720/0) — see Neoplasm, skin, benign
stone 631.8
tubal — see Pregnancy, tubal
vesicular (see also Hydatidiform mole) 630
Molimen, molimina (menstrual) 625.4
Mollaret's meningitis 047.9
Mollities (cerebellar) (cerebral) 437.8
ossium 268.2
Molluscum
contagiosum 078.0
epitheliale 078.0
fibrosum (M8851/0) — see Lipoma, by site
pendulum (M8851/0) — see Lipoma, by site

☑ Additional Digit Required — Refer to the Tabular List for Digit Selection   ▽ Subterms under main terms may continue to next column or page

2014 ICD-9-CM

231

Mönckeberg's arteriosclerosis, degeneration, disease, or sclerosis — see also Arteriosclerosis, extremities 440.20
Monday fever 504
Monday morning dyspnea or asthma 504
Mondini's malformation (cochlea) 744.05
Mondor's disease (thrombophlebitis of breast) 451.89
Mongolian, mongolianism, mongolism, mongoloid 758.0
  spot 757.33
Monilethrix (congenital) 757.4
Monilia infestation — see Candidiasis
Moniliasis — see also Candidiasis
  neonatal 771.7
  vulvovaginitis 112.1
Monkeypox 059.01
Monoarthritis 716.60
  ankle 716.67
  arm 716.62
    lower (and wrist) 716.63
    upper (and elbow) 716.62
  foot (and ankle) 716.67
  forearm (and wrist) 716.63
  hand 716.64
  leg 716.66
    lower 716.66
    upper 716.65
  pelvic region (hip) (thigh) 716.65
  shoulder (region) 716.61
  specified site NEC 716.68
Monoblastic — see condition
Monochromatism (cone) (rod) 368.54
Monocytic — see condition
Monocytopenia 288.59
Monocytosis (symptomatic) 288.63
Monofixation syndrome 378.34
Monomania — see also Psychosis 298.9
Mononeuritis 355.9
  cranial nerve — see Disorder, nerve, cranial
  femoral nerve 355.2
  lateral
    cutaneous nerve of thigh 355.1
    popliteal nerve 355.3
  lower limb 355.8
    specified nerve NEC 355.79
  medial popliteal nerve 355.4
  median nerve 354.1
  multiplex 354.5
  plantar nerve 355.6
  posterior tibial nerve 355.5
  radial nerve 354.3
  sciatic nerve 355.0
  ulnar nerve 354.2
  upper limb 354.9
    specified nerve NEC 354.8
  vestibular 388.5
Mononeuropathy — see also Mononeuritis 355.9
  diabetic NEC 250.6 ☑ [355.9]
    due to secondary diabetes 249.6 ☑ [355.9]
    lower limb 250.6 ☑ [355.8]
      due to secondary diabetes 249.6 ☑ [355.8]
    upper limb 250.6 ☑ [354.9]
      due to secondary diabetes 249.6 ☑ [354.9]
  iliohypogastric nerve 355.79
  ilioinguinal nerve 355.79
  obturator nerve 355.79
  saphenous nerve 355.79
Mononucleosis, infectious 075
  with hepatitis 075 [573.1]
Monoplegia 344.5
  brain (current episode) (see also Paralysis, brain) 437.8
    fetus or newborn 767.8
  cerebral (current episode) (see also Paralysis, brain) 437.8
  congenital or infantile (cerebral) (spastic) (spinal) 343.3
  embolic (current) (see also Embolism, brain) 434.1 ☑
    late effect — see Late effect(s) (of) cerebrovascular disease

Monoplegia — continued
  infantile (cerebral) (spastic) (spinal) 343.3
  lower limb 344.30
    affecting
      dominant side 344.31
      nondominant side 344.32
    due to late effect of cerebrovascular accident — see Late effect(s) (of) cerebrovascular accident
    newborn 767.8
    psychogenic 306.0
      specified as conversion reaction 300.11
    thrombotic (current) (see also Thrombosis, brain) 434.0 ☑
      late effect — see Late effect(s) (of) cerebrovascular disease
  transient 781.4
  upper limb 344.40
    affecting
      dominant side 344.41
      nondominant side 344.42
    due to late effect of cerebrovascular accident — see Late effect(s) (of) cerebrovascular accident
Monorchism, monorchidism 752.89
Monteggia's fracture (closed) 813.03
  open 813.13
Mood swings
  brief compensatory 296.99
  rebound 296.99
Mooren's ulcer (cornea) 370.07
Moore's syndrome — see also Epilepsy 345.5 ☑
Mooser bodies 081.0
Mooser-Neill reaction 081.0
Moral
  deficiency 301.7
  imbecility 301.7
Morax-Axenfeld conjunctivitis 372.03
Morbilli — see also Measles 055.9
Morbus
  anglicus, anglorum 268.0
  Beigel 111.2
  caducus (see also Epilepsy) 345.9 ☑
  caeruleus 746.89
  celiacus 579.0
  comitialis (see also Epilepsy) 345.9 ☑
  cordis (see also Disease, heart)
    valvulorum — see Endocarditis
  coxae 719.95
    tuberculous (see also Tuberculosis) 015.1 ☑
  hemorrhagicus neonatorum 776.0
  maculosus neonatorum 772.6
  renum 593.0
  senilis (see also Osteoarthrosis) 715.9 ☑
Morel-Kraepelin disease — see also Schizophrenia 295.9 ☑
Morel-Moore syndrome (hyperostosis frontalis interna) 733.3
Morel-Morgagni syndrome (hyperostosis frontalis interna) 733.3
Morgagni
  cyst, organ, hydatid, or appendage 752.89
    fallopian tube 752.11
  disease or syndrome (hyperostosis frontalis interna) 733.3
Morgagni-Adams-Stokes syndrome (syncope with heart block) 426.9
Morgagni-Stewart-Morel syndrome (hyperostosis frontalis interna) 733.3
Moria — see also Psychosis 298.9
Morning sickness 643.0 ☑
Moron 317
Morphea (guttate) (linear) 701.0
Morphine dependence — see also Dependence 304.0 ☑
Morphinism — see also Dependence 304.0 ☑
Morphinomania — see also Dependence 304.0 ☑
Morphoea 701.0
Morquio (-Brailsford) (-Ullrich) disease or syndrome (mucopolysaccharidosis IV) 277.5
  kyphosis 277.5

Morris syndrome (testicular feminization) 259.51
Morsus humanus (open wound) — see also Wound, open, by site
  skin surface intact — see Contusion
Mortification (dry) (moist) — see also Gangrene 785.4
Morton's
  disease 355.6
  foot 355.6
  metatarsalgia (syndrome) 355.6
  neuralgia 355.6
  neuroma 355.6
  syndrome (metatarsalgia) (neuralgia) 355.6
  toe 355.6
Morvan's disease 336.0
Mosaicism, mosaic (chromosomal) 758.9
  autosomal 758.5
  sex 758.81
Moschcowitz's syndrome (thrombotic thrombocytopenic purpura) 446.6
Mother yaw 102.0
Motion sickness (from travel, any vehicle) (from roundabouts or swings) 994.6
Mottled teeth (enamel) (endemic) (nonendemic) 520.3
Mottling enamel (endemic) (nonendemic) (teeth) 520.3
Mouchet's disease 732.5
Mould(s) (in vitreous) 117.9
Moulders'
  bronchitis 502
  tuberculosis (see also Tuberculosis) 011.4 ☑
Mounier-Kuhn syndrome 748.3
  with
    acute exacerbation 494.1
    bronchiectasis 494.0
      with (acute) exacerbation 494.1
  acquired 519.19
    with bronchiectasis 494.0
      with (acute) exacerbation 494.1
Mountain
  fever — see Fever, mountain
  sickness 993.2
    with polycythemia, acquired 289.0
    acute 289.0
  tick fever 066.1
Mouse, joint — see also Loose, body, joint 718.1 ☑
  knee 717.6
Mouth — see condition
Movable
  coccyx 724.71
  kidney (see also Disease, renal) 593.0
    congenital 753.3
  organ or site, congenital NEC — see Malposition, congenital
  spleen 289.59
Movement
  abnormal (dystonic) (involuntary) 781.0
  decreased fetal 655.7 ☑
  paradoxical facial 374.43
Moya Moya disease 437.5
Mozart's ear 744.29
MRSA (methicillin-resistant staphylococcus aureus) 041.12
  colonization V02.54
  personal history of V12.04
MSSA (methicillin susceptible staphylococcus aureus) 041.11
  colonization V02.53
Mucha's disease (acute parapsoriasis varioliformis) 696.2
Mucha-Haberman syndrome (acute parapsoriasis varioliformis) 696.2
Mu-chain disease 273.2
Mucinosis (cutaneous) (papular) 701.8
Mucocele
  appendix 543.9
  buccal cavity 528.9
  gallbladder (see also Disease, gallbladder) 575.3
  lacrimal sac 375.43
  orbit (eye) 376.81
  salivary gland (any) 527.6
  sinus (accessory) (nasal) 478.19

Mucocele — continued
  turbinate (bone) (middle) (nasal) 478.19
  uterus 621.8
Mucocutaneous lymph node syndrome (acute) (febrile) (infantile) 446.1
Mucoenteritis 564.9
Mucolipidosis I, II, III 272.7
Mucopolysaccharidosis (types 1-6) 277.5
  cardiopathy 277.5 [425.7]
Mucormycosis (lung) 117.7
Mucosa associated lymphoid tissue (MALT) 200.3 ☑
Mucositis — see also Inflammation, by site 528.00
  cervix (ulcerative) 616.81
  due to
    antineoplastic therapy (ulcerative) 528.01
    other drugs (ulcerative) 528.02
    specified NEC 528.09
  gastrointestinal (ulcerative) 538
  nasal (ulcerative) 478.11
  necroticans agranulocytica (see also Agranulocytosis) 288.09
  ulcerative 528.00
  vagina (ulcerative) 616.81
  vulva (ulcerative) 616.81
Mucous — see also condition
  patches (syphilitic) 091.3
    congenital 090.0
Mucoviscidosis 277.00
  with meconium obstruction 277.01
Mucus
  asphyxia or suffocation (see also Asphyxia, mucus) 933.1
    newborn 770.18
  in stool 792.1
  plug (see also Asphyxia, mucus) 933.1
    aspiration, of newborn 770.17
    tracheobronchial 519.19
      newborn 770.18
Muguet 112.0
Mulberry molars 090.5
Müllerian mixed tumor (M8950/3) — see Neoplasm, by site, malignant
Multicystic kidney 753.19
Multilobed placenta — see Placenta, abnormal
Multinodular prostate 600.10
  with
    urinary
      obstruction 600.11
      retention 600.11
Multiparity V61.5
  affecting
    fetus or newborn 763.89
    management of
      labor and delivery 659.4 ☑
      pregnancy V23.3
  requiring contraceptive management (see also Contraception) V25.9
Multipartita placenta — see Placenta, abnormal
Multiple, multiplex — see also condition
  birth
    affecting fetus or newborn 761.5
    healthy liveborn — see Newborn, multiple
  digits (congenital) 755.00
    fingers 755.01
    toes 755.02
  organ or site NEC — see Accessory
  personality 300.14
  renal arteries 747.62
Mumps 072.9
  with complication 072.8
    specified type NEC 072.79
  encephalitis 072.2
  hepatitis 072.71
  meningitis (aseptic) 072.1
  meningoencephalitis 072.2
  oophoritis 072.79
  orchitis 072.0
  pancreatitis 072.3
  polyneuropathy 072.72
  vaccination, prophylactic (against) V04.6

Mumu — see also Infestation, filarial 125.9
Münchausen syndrome 301.51
Münchmeyer's disease or syndrome (exostosis luxurians) 728.11
Mural — see condition
Murmur (cardiac) (heart) (nonorganic) (organic) 785.2
  abdominal 787.5
  aortic (valve) (see also Endocarditis, aortic) 424.1
  benign — omit code
  cardiorespiratory 785.2
  diastolic — see condition
  Flint (see also Endocarditis, aortic) 424.1
  functional — omit code
  Graham Steell (pulmonic regurgitation) (see also Endocarditis, pulmonary) 424.3
  innocent — omit code
  insignificant — omit code
  midsystolic 785.2
  mitral (valve) — see Stenosis, mitral
  physiologic — see condition
  presystolic, mitral — see Insufficiency, mitral
  pulmonic (valve) (see also Endocarditis, pulmonary) 424.3
  Still's (vibratory) — omit code
  systolic (valvular) — see condition
  tricuspid (valve) — see Endocarditis, tricuspid
  undiagnosed 785.2
  valvular — see condition
  vibratory — omit code
Murri's disease (intermittent hemoglobinuria) 283.2
Muscae volitantes 379.24
Muscle, muscular — see condition
Musculoneuralgia 729.1
Mushrooming hip 718.95
Mushroom workers' (pickers') lung 495.5
Mutation(s)
  factor V Leiden 289.81
  prothrombin gene 289.81
  surfactant, of lung 516.63
Mutism — see also Aphasia 784.3
  akinetic 784.3
  deaf (acquired) (congenital) 389.7
  hysterical 300.11
  selective (elective) 313.23
    adjustment reaction 309.83
MVD (microvillus inclusion disease) 751.5
MVID (microvillus inclusion disease) 751.5
Myà's disease (congenital dilation, colon) 751.3
Myalgia (intercostal) 729.1
  eosinophilia syndrome 710.5
  epidemic 074.1
    cervical 078.89
  psychogenic 307.89
  traumatic NEC 959.9
Myasthenia 358.00
  cordis — see Failure, heart
  gravis 358.00
    with exacerbation (acute) 358.01
    in crisis 358.01
    neonatal 775.2
    pseudoparalytica 358.00
  stomach 536.8
    psychogenic 306.4
  syndrome
    in
      botulism 005.1 [358.1]
      diabetes mellitus 250.6 ☑ [358.1]
        due to secondary diabetes 249.6 ☑ [358.1]
      hypothyroidism (see also Hypothyroidism) 244.9 [358.1]
      malignant neoplasm NEC 199.1 [358.1]
      pernicious anemia 281.0 [358.1]
      thyrotoxicosis (see also Thyrotoxicosis) 242.9 ☑ [358.1]
Myasthenic 728.87
Mycelium infection NEC 117.9
Mycetismus 988.1
Mycetoma (actinomycotic) 039.9
  bone 039.8

Mycetoma — continued
  bone — continued
    mycotic 117.4
  foot 039.4
    mycotic 117.4
  madurae 039.9
    mycotic 117.4
  maduromycotic 039.9
    mycotic 117.4
  mycotic 117.4
  nocardial 039.9
Mycobacteriosis — see Mycobacterium
Mycobacterium, mycobacterial (infection) 031.9
  acid-fast (bacilli) 031.9
  anonymous (see also Mycobacterium, atypical) 031.9
  atypical (acid-fast bacilli) 031.9
    cutaneous 031.1
    pulmonary 031.0
      tuberculous (see also Tuberculosis, pulmonary) 011.9 ☑
    specified site NEC 031.8
  avium 031.0
    intracellulare complex bacteremia (MAC) 031.2
  balnei 031.1
  Battey 031.0
  cutaneous 031.1
  disseminated 031.2
    avium-intracellulare complex (DMAC) 031.2
  fortuitum 031.0
  intracellulare (battey bacillus) 031.0
  kakerifu 031.8
  kansasii 031.0
  kasongo 031.8
  leprae — see Leprosy
  luciflavum 031.0
  marinum 031.1
  pulmonary 031.0
    tuberculous (see also Tuberculosis, pulmonary) 011.9 ☑
  scrofulaceum 031.1
  tuberculosis (human, bovine) (see also Tuberculosis)
    avian type 031.0
  ulcerans 031.1
  xenopi 031.0
Mycosis, mycotic 117.9
  cutaneous NEC 111.9
  ear 111.8 [380.15]
  fungoides (M9700/3) 202.1 ☑
  mouth 112.0
  pharynx 117.9
  skin NEC 111.9
  stomatitis 112.0
  systemic NEC 117.9
  tonsil 117.9
  vagina, vaginitis 112.1
Mydriasis (persistent) (pupil) 379.43
Myelatelia 742.59
Myelinoclasis, perivascular, acute (postinfectious) NEC 136.9 [323.61]
  postimmunization or postvaccinal 323.51
Myelinosis, central pontine 341.8
Myelitis (ascending) (cerebellar) (childhood) (chronic) (descending) (diffuse) (disseminated) (pressure) (progressive) (spinal cord) (subacute) — see also Encephalitis 323.9
  acute (transverse) 341.20
    idiopathic 341.22
    in conditions classified elsewhere 341.21
  due to
    other infection classified elsewhere 136.9 [323.42]
    specified cause NEC 323.82
    vaccination (any) 323.52
    viral diseases classified elsewhere 323.02
  herpes simplex 054.74
  herpes zoster 053.14
  late effect — see category 326
  optic neuritis in 341.0
  postchickenpox 052.2
  postimmunization 323.52

Myelitis — see also Encephalitis — continued
  postinfectious 136.9 [323.63]
  postvaccinal 323.52
  postvaricella 052.2
  syphilitic (transverse) 094.89
  toxic 989.9 [323.72]
  transverse 323.82
    acute 341.20
      idiopathic 341.22
      in conditions classified elsewhere 341.21
    idiopathic 341.22
    tuberculous (see also Tuberculosis) 013.6 ☑
    virus 049.9
Myeloblastic — see condition
Myelocele — see also Spina bifida 741.9 ☑
  with hydrocephalus 741.0 ☑
Myelocystocele — see also Spina bifida 741.9 ☑
Myelocytic — see condition
Myelocytoma 205.1 ☑
Myelodysplasia (spinal cord) 742.59
  meaning myelodysplastic syndrome — see Syndrome, myelodysplastic
Myeloencephalitis — see Encephalitis
Myelofibrosis 289.83
  with myeloid metaplasia 238.76
  idiopathic (chronic) 238.76
  megakaryocytic 238.79
  primary 238.76
  secondary 289.83
Myelogenous — see condition
Myeloid — see condition
Myelokathexis 288.09
Myeloleukodystrophy 330.0
Myelolipoma (M8870/0) — see Neoplasm, by site, benign
Myeloma (multiple) (plasma cell) (plasmacytic) (M9730/3) 203.0 ☑
  monostotic (M9731/1) 238.6
  solitary (M9731/1) 238.6
Myelomalacia 336.8
Myelomata, multiple (M9730/3) 203.0 ☑
Myelomatosis (M9730/3) 203.0 ☑
Myelomeningitis — see Meningoencephalitis
Myelomeningocele (spinal cord) — see also Spina bifida 741.9 ☑
  fetal, causing fetopelvic disproportion 653.7 ☑
Myelo-osteo-musculodysplasia hereditaria 756.89
Myelopathic — see condition
Myelopathy (spinal cord) 336.9
  cervical 721.1
  diabetic 250.6 ☑ [336.3]
    due to secondary diabetes 249.6 ☑ [336.3]
  drug-induced 336.8
  due to or with
    carbon tetrachloride 987.8 [323.72]
    degeneration or displacement, intervertebral disc 722.70
      cervical, cervicothoracic 722.71
      lumbar, lumbosacral 722.73
      thoracic, thoracolumbar 722.72
    hydroxyquinoline derivatives 961.3 [323.72]
    infection — see Encephalitis
    intervertebral disc disorder 722.70
      cervical, cervicothoracic 722.71
      lumbar, lumbosacral 722.73
      thoracic, thoracolumbar 722.72
    lead 984.9 [323.72]
    mercury 985.0 [323.72]
    neoplastic disease (see also Neoplasm, by site) 239.9 [336.3]
    pernicious anemia 281.0 [336.3]
    spondylosis 721.91
      cervical 721.1
      lumbar, lumbosacral 721.42
      thoracic 721.41
    thallium 985.8 [323.72]
  lumbar, lumbosacral 721.42
  necrotic (subacute) 336.1
  radiation-induced 336.8

Myelopathy — continued
  spondylogenic NEC 721.91
    cervical 721.1
    lumbar, lumbosacral 721.42
    thoracic 721.41
  thoracic 721.41
  toxic NEC 989.9 [323.72]
  transverse (see also Myelitis) 323.82
  vascular 336.1
Myelophthisis 284.2
Myeloproliferative disease (M9960/1) 238.79
Myeloradiculitis — see also Polyneuropathy 357.0
Myeloradiculodysplasia (spinal) 742.59
Myelosarcoma (M9930/3) 205.3 ☑
Myelosclerosis 289.89
  with myeloid metaplasia (M9961/1) 238.76
  disseminated, of nervous system 340
  megakaryocytic (M9961/1) 238.79
Myelosis (M9860/3) — see also Leukemia, myeloid 205.9 ☑
  acute (M9861/3) 205.0 ☑
  aleukemic (M9864/3) 205.8 ☑
  chronic (M9863/3) 205.1 ☑
  erythremic (M9840/3) 207.0 ☑
    acute (M9841/3) 207.0 ☑
  megakaryocytic (M9920/3) 207.2 ☑
  nonleukemic (chronic) 288.8
  subacute (M9862/3) 205.2 ☑
Myesthenia — see Myasthenia
Myiasis (cavernous) 134.0
  orbit 134.0 [376.13]
Myoadenoma, prostate 600.20
  with
    other lower urinary tract symptoms (LUTS) 600.21
    urinary
      obstruction 600.21
      retention 600.21
Myoblastoma
  granular cell (M9580/0) (see also Neoplasm, connective tissue, benign)
    malignant (M9580/3) — see Neoplasm, connective tissue, malignant
  tongue (M9580/0) 210.1
Myocardial — see condition
Myocardiopathy (congestive) (constrictive) (familial) (idiopathic) (infiltrative) (obstructive) (primary) (restrictive) (sporadic) 425.4
  alcoholic 425.5
  amyloid 277.39 [425.7]
  beriberi 265.0 [425.7]
  cobalt-beer 425.5
  due to
    amyloidosis 277.39 [425.7]
    beriberi 265.0 [425.7]
    cardiac glycogenosis 271.0 [425.7]
    Chagas' disease 086.0
    Friedreich's ataxia 334.0 [425.8]
    influenza (see also Influenza) 487.8 [425.8]
    mucopolysaccharidosis 277.5 [425.7]
    myotonia atrophica 359.21 [425.8]
    progressive muscular dystrophy 359.1 [425.8]
    sarcoidosis 135 [425.8]
  glycogen storage 271.0 [425.7]
  hypertrophic 425.18
    nonobstructive 425.18
    obstructive 425.11
  metabolic NEC 277.9 [425.7]
  nutritional 269.9 [425.7]
  obscure (African) 425.2
  peripartum 674.5 ☑
  postpartum 674.5 ☑
  secondary 425.9
  thyrotoxic (see also Thyrotoxicosis) 242.9 ☑ [425.7]
  toxic NEC 425.9
Myocarditis (fibroid) (interstitial) (old) (progressive) (senile) (with arteriosclerosis) 429.0
  with
    rheumatic fever (conditions classifiable to 390) 398.0

☑ Additional Digit Required — Refer to the Tabular List for Digit Selection   ⬙ Subterms under main terms may continue to next column or page

2014 ICD-9-CM   233

Myocarditis — continued
  with — continued
    rheumatic fever — continued
      active (see also Myocarditis, acute, rheumatic) 391.2
      inactive or quiescent (with chorea) 398.0
  active (nonrheumatic) 422.90
    rheumatic 391.2
      with chorea (acute) (rheumatic) (Sydenham's) 392.0
  acute or subacute (interstitial) 422.90
    due to Streptococcus (beta-hemolytic) 391.2
    idiopathic 422.91
    rheumatic 391.2
      with chorea (acute) (rheumatic) (Sydenham's) 392.0
    specified type NEC 422.99
  aseptic of newborn 074.23
  bacterial (acute) 422.92
  chagasic 086.0
  chronic (interstitial) 429.0
  congenital 746.89
  constrictive 425.4
  Coxsackie (virus) 074.23
  diphtheritic 032.82
  due to or in
    Coxsackie (virus) 074.23
    diphtheria 032.82
    epidemic louse-borne typhus 080 [422.0]
    influenza (see also Influenza) 487.8 [422.0]
    Lyme disease 088.81 [422.0]
    scarlet fever 034.1 [422.0]
    toxoplasmosis (acquired) 130.3
    tuberculosis (see also Tuberculosis) 017.9 ☑ [422.0]
    typhoid 002.0 [422.0]
    typhus NEC 081.9 [422.0]
  eosinophilic 422.91
  epidemic of newborn 074.23
  Fiedler's (acute) (isolated) (subacute) 422.91
  giant cell (acute) (subacute) 422.91
  gonococcal 098.85
  granulomatous (idiopathic) (isolated) (non-specific) 422.91
  hypertensive (see also Hypertension, heart) 402.90
  idiopathic 422.91
    granulomatous 422.91
  infective 422.92
  influenzal (see also Influenza) 487.8 [422.0]
  isolated (diffuse) (granulomatous) 422.91
  malignant 422.99
  meningococcal 036.43
  nonrheumatic, active 422.90
  parenchymatous 422.90
  pneumococcal (acute) (subacute) 422.92
  rheumatic (chronic) (inactive) (with chorea) 398.0
    active or acute 391.2
      with chorea (acute) (rheumatic) (Sydenham's) 392.0
  septic 422.92
  specific (giant cell) (productive) 422.91
  staphylococcal (acute) (subacute) 422.92
  suppurative 422.92
  syphilitic (chronic) 093.82
  toxic 422.93
    rheumatic (see also Myocarditis, acute rheumatic) 391.2
  tuberculous (see also Tuberculosis) 017.9 ☑ [422.0]
  typhoid 002.0 [422.0]
  valvular — see Endocarditis
  viral, except Coxsackie 422.91
    Coxsackie 074.23
    of newborn (Coxsackie) 074.23
Myocardium, myocardial — see condition
Myocardosis — see also Cardiomyopathy 425.4
Myoclonia (essential) 333.2
  epileptica 345.1 ☑
  Friedrich's 333.2
  massive 333.2

Myoclonic
  epilepsy, familial (progressive) 345.1 ☑
  jerks 333.2
Myoclonus (familial essential) (multifocal) (simplex) 333.2
  with epilepsy and with ragged red fibers (MERRF syndrome) 277.87
  facial 351.8
  massive (infantile) 333.2
  palatal 333.2
  pharyngeal 333.2
Myocytolysis 429.1
Myodiastasis 728.84
Myoendocarditis — see also Endocarditis
  acute or subacute 421.9
Myoepithelioma (M8982/0) — see Neoplasm, by site, benign
Myofascitis (acute) 729.1
  low back 724.2
Myofibroma (M8890/0) — see also Neoplasm, connective tissue, benign
  uterus (cervix) (corpus) (see also Leiomyoma) 218.9
Myofibromatosis
  infantile 759.89
Myofibrosis 728.2
  heart (see also Myocarditis) 429.0
  humeroscapular region 726.2
  scapulohumeral 726.2
Myofibrositis — see also Myositis 729.1
  scapulohumeral 726.2
Myogelosis (occupational) 728.89
Myoglobinuria 791.3
Myoglobulinuria, primary 791.3
Myokymia — see also Myoclonus
  facial 351.8
Myolipoma (M8860/0)
  specified site — see Neoplasm, connective tissue, benign
  unspecified site 223.0
Myoma (M8895/0) — see also Neoplasm, connective tissue, benign
  cervix (stump) (uterus) (see also Leiomyoma) 218.9
  malignant (M8895/3) — see Neoplasm, connective tissue, malignant
  prostate 600.20
    with
      other lower urinary tract symptoms (LUTS) 600.21
    urinary
      obstruction 600.21
      retention 600.21
  uterus (cervix) (corpus) (see also Leiomyoma) 218.9
  in pregnancy or childbirth 654.1 ☑
    affecting fetus or newborn 763.89
    causing obstructed labor 660.2 ☑
      affecting fetus or newborn 763.1
Myomalacia 728.9
  cordis, heart (see also Degeneration, myocardial) 429.1
Myometritis — see also Endometritis 615.9
Myometrium — see condition
Myonecrosis, clostridial 040.0
Myopathy 359.9
  alcoholic 359.4
  amyloid 277.39 [359.6]
  benign, congenital 359.0
  central core 359.0
  centronuclear 359.0
  congenital (benign) 359.0
  critical illness 359.81
  distal 359.1
  due to drugs 359.4
  endocrine 259.9 [359.5]
    specified type NEC 259.8 [359.5]
  extraocular muscles 376.82
  facioscapulohumeral 359.1
  in
    Addison's disease 255.41 [359.5]
    amyloidosis 277.39 [359.6]
    cretinism 243 [359.5]
    Cushing's syndrome 255.0 [359.5]
    disseminated lupus erythematosus 710.0 [359.6]

Myopathy — continued
  in — continued
    giant cell arteritis 446.5 [359.6]
    hyperadrenocorticism NEC 255.3 [359.5]
    hyperparathyroidism 252.01 [359.5]
    hypopituitarism 253.2 [359.5]
    hypothyroidism (see also Hypothyroidism) 244.9 [359.5]
    malignant neoplasm NEC (M8000/3) 199.1 [359.6]
    myxedema (see also Myxedema) 244.9 [359.5]
    polyarteritis nodosa 446.0 [359.6]
    rheumatoid arthritis 714.0 [359.6]
    sarcoidosis 135 [359.6]
    scleroderma 710.1 [359.6]
    Sjögren's disease 710.2 [359.6]
    thyrotoxicosis (see also Thyrotoxicosis) 242.9 ☑ [359.5]
  inflammatory 359.79
    immune NEC 359.79
    specified NEC 359.79
  intensive care (ICU) 359.81
  limb-girdle 359.1
  myotubular 359.0
  necrotizing, acute 359.81
  nemaline 359.0
  ocular 359.1
  oculopharyngeal 359.1
  of critical illness 359.81
  primary 359.89
  progressive NEC 359.89
  proximal myotonic (PROMM) 359.21
  quadriplegic, acute 359.81
  rod body 359.0
  scapulohumeral 359.1
  specified type NEC 359.89
  toxic 359.4
Myopericarditis — see also Pericarditis 423.9
Myopia (axial) (congenital) (increased curvature or refraction, nucleus of lens) 367.1
  degenerative, malignant 360.21
  malignant 360.21
  progressive high (degenerative) 360.21
Myosarcoma (M8895/3) — see Neoplasm, connective tissue, malignant
Myosis (persistent) 379.42
  stromal (endolymphatic) (M8931/1) 236.0
Myositis 729.1
  clostridial 040.0
  due to posture 729.1
  epidemic 074.1
  fibrosa or fibrous (chronic) 728.2
    Volkmann's (complicating trauma) 958.6
  inclusion body (IBM) 359.71
  infective 728.0
  interstitial 728.81
  multiple — see Polymyositis
  occupational 729.1
  orbital, chronic 376.12
  ossificans 728.12
    circumscribed 728.12
    progressive 728.11
    traumatic 728.12
  progressive fibrosing 728.11
  purulent 728.0
  rheumatic 729.1
  rheumatoid 729.1
  suppurative 728.0
  syphilitic 095.6
  traumatic (old) 729.1
Myospasia impulsiva 307.23
Myotonia (acquisita) (intermittens) 728.85
  atrophica 359.21
  congenita 359.22
    acetazolamide responsive 359.22
    dominant form 359.22
    recessive form 359.22
  drug-induced 359.24
  dystrophica 359.21
  fluctuans 359.29
  levior 359.22
  permanens 359.29
Myotonic pupil 379.46
Myriapodiasis 134.1

Myringitis
  with otitis media — see Otitis media
  acute 384.00
    specified type NEC 384.09
  bullosa hemorrhagica 384.01
  bullous 384.01
  chronic 384.1
Mysophobia 300.29
Mytilotoxism 988.0
Myxadenitis labialis 528.5
Myxedema (adult) (idiocy) (infantile) (juvenile) (thyroid gland) — see also Hypothyroidism 244.9
  circumscribed 242.9 ☑
  congenital 243
  cutis 701.8
  localized (pretibial) 242.9 ☑
  madness (acute) 293.0
    subacute 293.1
  papular 701.8
  pituitary 244.8
  postpartum 674.8 ☑
  pretibial 242.9 ☑
  primary 244.9
Myxochondrosarcoma (M9220/3) — see Neoplasm, cartilage, malignant
Myxofibroma (M8811/0) — see also Neoplasm, connective tissue, benign
  odontogenic (M9320/0) 213.1
    upper jaw (bone) 213.0
Myxofibrosarcoma (M8811/3) — see Neoplasm, connective tissue, malignant
Myxolipoma (M8852/0) — see also Lipoma, by site 214.9
Myxoliposarcoma (M8852/3) — see Neoplasm, connective tissue, malignant
Myxoma (M8840/0) — see also Neoplasm, connective tissue, benign
  odontogenic (M9320/0) 213.1
    upper jaw (bone) 213.0
Myxosarcoma (M8840/3) — see Neoplasm, connective tissue, malignant

N

Naegeli's
  disease (hereditary hemorrhagic thrombasthenia) 287.1
  leukemia, monocytic (M9863/3) 205.1 ☑
  syndrome (incontinentia pigmenti) 757.33
Naffziger's syndrome 353.0
Naga sore — see also Ulcer, skin 707.9
Nägele's pelvis 738.6
  with disproportion (fetopelvic) 653.0 ☑
    affecting fetus or newborn 763.1
    causing obstructed labor 660.1 ☑
      affecting fetus or newborn 763.1
Nager-de Reynier syndrome (dysostosis mandibularis) 756.0
Nail — see also condition
  biting 307.9
  patella syndrome (hereditary osteoonychodysplasia) 756.89
Nanism, nanosomia — see also Dwarfism 259.4
  hypophyseal 253.3
  pituitary 253.3
  renis, renalis 588.0
Nanukayami 100.89
Napkin rash 691.0
Narcissism 301.81
Narcolepsy 347.00
  with cataplexy 347.01
  in conditions classified elsewhere 347.10
    with cataplexy 347.11
Narcosis
  carbon dioxide (respiratory) 786.09
  due to drug
    correct substance properly administered 780.09
    overdose or wrong substance given or taken 977.9
      specified drug — see Table of Drugs and Chemicals
Narcotism (chronic) — see also Dependence 304.9 ☑

Narcotism (chronic) — see also Dependence — continued
acute
correct substance properly administered 349.82
overdose or wrong substance given or taken 967.8
specified drug — see Table of Drugs and Chemicals
NARP (ataxia and retinitis pigmentosa) 277.87
Narrow
anterior chamber angle 365.02
pelvis (inlet) (outlet) — see Contraction, pelvis
Narrowing
artery NEC 447.1
auditory, internal 433.8 ☑
basilar 433.0 ☑
with other precerebral artery 433.3 ☑
bilateral 433.3 ☑
carotid 433.1 ☑
with other precerebral artery 433.3 ☑
bilateral 433.3 ☑
cerebellar 433.8 ☑
choroidal 433.8 ☑
communicating posterior 433.8 ☑
coronary (see also Arteriosclerosis, coronary)
congenital 746.85
due to syphilis 090.5
hypophyseal 433.8 ☑
pontine 433.8 ☑
precerebral NEC 433.9 ☑
multiple or bilateral 433.3 ☑
specified NEC 433.8 ☑
vertebral 433.2 ☑
with other precerebral artery 433.3 ☑
bilateral 433.3 ☑
auditory canal (external) (see also Stricture, ear canal, acquired) 380.50
cerebral arteries 437.0
cicatricial — see Cicatrix
congenital — see Anomaly, congenital
coronary artery — see Narrowing, artery, coronary
ear, middle 385.22
Eustachian tube (see also Obstruction, Eustachian tube) 381.60
eyelid 374.46
congenital 743.62
intervertebral disc or space NEC — see Degeneration, intervertebral disc
joint space, hip 719.85
larynx 478.74
lids 374.46
congenital 743.62
mesenteric artery (with gangrene) 557.0
palate 524.89
palpebral fissure 374.46
retinal artery 362.13
ureter 593.3
urethra (see also Stricture, urethra) 598.9
Narrowness, abnormal, eyelid 743.62
Nasal — see condition
Nasolacrimal — see condition
Nasopharyngeal — see also condition
bursa 478.29
pituitary gland 759.2
torticollis 723.5
Nasopharyngitis (acute) (infective) (subacute) 460
chronic 472.2
due to external agent — see Condition, respiratory, chronic, due to
due to external agent — see Condition, respiratory, due to
septic 034.0
streptococcal 034.0
suppurative (chronic) 472.2
ulcerative (chronic) 472.2
Nasopharynx, nasopharyngeal — see condition
Natal tooth, teeth 520.6

Nausea — see also Vomiting 787.02
with vomiting 787.01
epidemic 078.82
gravidarum — see Hyperemesis, gravidarum
marina 994.6
Navel — see condition
Neapolitan fever — see also Brucellosis 023.9
Near drowning 994.1
Nearsightedness 367.1
Near-syncope 780.2
Nebécourt's syndrome 253.3
Nebula, cornea (eye) 371.01
congenital 743.43
interfering with vision 743.42
Necator americanus infestation 126.1
Necatoriasis 126.1
Neck — see condition
Necrencephalus — see also Softening, brain 437.8
Necrobacillosis 040.3
Necrobiosis 799.89
brain or cerebral (see also Softening, brain) 437.8
lipoidica 709.3
diabeticorum 250.8 ☑ [709.3]
due to secondary diabetes 249.8 ☑ [709.3]
Necrodermolysis 695.15
Necrolysis, toxic epidermal 695.15
due to drug
correct substance properly administered 695.15
overdose or wrong substance given or taken 977.9
specified drug — see Table of Drugs and Chemicals
Stevens-Johnson syndrome overlap (SJS-TEN overlap syndrome) 695.14
Necrophilia 302.89
Necrosis, necrotic
adrenal (capsule) (gland) 255.8
antrum, nasal sinus 478.19
aorta (hyaline) (see also Aneurysm, aorta) 441.9
cystic medial 441.00
abdominal 441.02
thoracic 441.01
thoracoabdominal 441.03
ruptured 441.5
arteritis 446.0
artery 447.5
aseptic, bone 733.40
femur (head) (neck) 733.42
medial condyle 733.43
humoral head 733.41
jaw 733.45
medial femoral condyle 733.43
specific site NEC 733.49
talus 733.44
avascular, bone NEC (see also Necrosis, aseptic, bone) 733.40
bladder (aseptic) (sphincter) 596.89
bone (see also Osteomyelitis) 730.1 ☑
acute 730.0 ☑
aseptic or avascular 733.40
femur (head) (neck) 733.42
medial condyle 733.43
humoral head 733.41
jaw 733.45
medial femoral condyle 733.43
specified site NEC 733.49
talus 733.44
ethmoid 478.19
ischemic 733.40
jaw 526.4
asceptic 733.45
marrow 289.89
Paget's (osteitis deformans) 731.0
tuberculous — see Tuberculosis, bone
brain (softening) (see also Softening, brain) 437.8
breast (aseptic) (fat) (segmental) 611.3
bronchus, bronchi 519.19
central nervous system NEC (see also Softening, brain) 437.8
cerebellar (see also Softening, brain) 437.8

Necrosis, necrotic — continued
cerebral (softening) (see also Softening, brain) 437.8
cerebrospinal (softening) (see also Softening, brain) 437.8
colon 557.0
cornea (see also Keratitis) 371.40
cortical, kidney 583.6
cystic medial (aorta) 441.00
abdominal 441.02
thoracic 441.01
thoracoabdominal 441.03
dental 521.09
pulp 522.1
due to swallowing corrosive substance — see Burn, by site
ear (ossicle) 385.24
esophagus 530.89
ethmoid (bone) 478.19
eyelid 374.50
fat, fatty (generalized) (see also Degeneration, fatty) 272.8
abdominal wall 567.82
breast (aseptic) (segmental) 611.3
intestine 569.89
localized — see Degeneration, by site, fatty
mesentery 567.82
omentum 567.82
pancreas 577.8
peritoneum 567.82
skin (subcutaneous) 709.3
newborn 778.1
femur (aseptic) (avascular) 733.42
head 733.42
medial condyle 733.43
neck 733.42
gallbladder (see also Cholecystitis, acute) 575.0
gangrenous 785.4
gastric 537.89
glottis 478.79
heart (myocardium) — see Infarct, myocardium
hepatic (see also Necrosis, liver) 570
hip (aseptic) (avascular) 733.42
intestine (acute) (hemorrhagic) (massive) 557.0
ischemic 785.4
jaw 526.4
asceptic 733.45
kidney (bilateral) 583.9
acute 584.9
cortical 583.6
acute 584.6
with
abortion — see Abortion, by type, with renal failure
ectopic pregnancy (see also categories 633.0–633.9) 639.3
molar pregnancy (see also categories 630–632) 639.3
complicating pregnancy 646.2 ☑
affecting fetus or newborn 760.1
following labor and delivery 669.3 ☑
medullary (papillary) (see also Pyelitis) 590.80
in
acute renal failure 584.7
nephritis, nephropathy 583.7
papillary (see also Pyelitis) 590.80
in
acute renal failure 584.7
nephritis, nephropathy 583.7
tubular 584.5
with
abortion — see Abortion, by type, with renal failure
ectopic pregnancy (see also categories 633.0–633.9) 639.3
molar pregnancy (see also categories 630–632) 639.3

Necrosis, necrotic — continued
kidney — continued
tubular — continued
complicating
abortion 639.3
ectopic or molar pregnancy 639.3
pregnancy 646.2 ☑
affecting fetus or newborn 760.1
following labor and delivery 669.3 ☑
traumatic 958.5
larynx 478.79
liver (acute) (congenital) (diffuse) (massive) (subacute) 570
with
abortion — see Abortion, by type, with specified complication NEC
ectopic pregnancy (see also categories 633.0–633.9) 639.8
molar pregnancy (see also categories 630–632) 639.8
complicating pregnancy 646.7 ☑
affecting fetus or newborn 760.8
following
abortion 639.8
ectopic or molar pregnancy 639.8
obstetrical 646.7 ☑
postabortal 639.8
puerperal, postpartum 674.8 ☑
toxic 573.3
lung 513.0
lymphatic gland 683
mammary gland 611.3
mastoid (chronic) 383.1
mesentery 557.0
fat 567.82
mitral valve — see Insufficiency, mitral
myocardium, myocardial — see Infarct, myocardium
nose (septum) 478.19
omentum 557.0
with mesenteric infarction 557.0
fat 567.82
orbit, orbital 376.10
ossicles, ear (aseptic) 385.24
ovary (see also Salpingo-oophoritis) 614.2
pancreas (aseptic) (duct) (fat) 577.8
acute 577.0
infective 577.0
papillary, kidney (see also Pyelitis) 590.80
perineum 624.8
peritoneum 557.0
with mesenteric infarction 557.0
fat 567.82
pharynx 462
in granulocytopenia 288.09
phosphorus 983.9
pituitary (gland) (postpartum) (Sheehan) 253.2
placenta (see also Placenta, abnormal) 656.7 ☑
pneumonia 513.0
pulmonary 513.0
pulp (dental) 522.1
pylorus 537.89
radiation — see Necrosis, by site
radium — see Necrosis, by site
renal — see Necrosis, kidney
sclera 379.19
scrotum 608.89
skin or subcutaneous tissue 709.8
due to burn — see Burn, by site
gangrenous 785.4
spine, spinal (column) 730.18
acute 730.18
cord 336.1
spleen 289.59
stomach 537.89
stomatitis 528.1
subcutaneous fat 709.3
fetus or newborn 778.1
subendocardial — see Infarct, myocardium
suprarenal (capsule) (gland) 255.8
teeth, tooth 521.09
testis 608.89

☑ Additional Digit Required — Refer to the Tabular List for Digit Selection
Subterms under main terms may continue to next column or page
2014 ICD-9-CM
235
Narcotism (chronic) — Necrosis, necrotic
Index

Necrosis, necrotic — *continued*
   thymus (gland) 254.8
   tonsil 474.8
   trachea 519.19
   tuberculous NEC — *see* Tuberculosis
   tubular (acute) (anoxic) (toxic) 584.5
      due to a procedure 997.5
   umbilical cord, affecting fetus or newborn
         762.6
   vagina 623.8
   vertebra (lumbar) 730.18
      acute 730.18
      tuberculous (*see also* Tuberculosis)
            015.0 ☑ [730.8] ☑
   vesical (aseptic) (bladder) 596.89
   vulva 624.8

Necrosis, necrotic — *continued*
   x-ray — *see* Necrosis, by site
Necrospermia 606.0
Necrotizing angiitis 446.0
Negativism 301.7
Neglect (child) (newborn) NEC 995.52
   adult 995.84
   after or at birth 995.52
   hemispatial 781.8
   left-sided 781.8
   sensory 781.8
   visuospatial 781.8
Negri bodies 071
Neill-Dingwall syndrome (microcephaly and
      dwarfism) 759.89
Neisserian infection NEC — *see* Gonococcus

Nematodiasis NEC — *see also* Infestation, Ne-
      matode 127.9
   ancylostoma (*see also* Ancylostomiasis)
         126.9
Neoformans cryptococcus infection 117.5
Neonatal — *see also* condition
   abstinence syndrome 779.5
   adrenoleukodystrophy 277.86
   teeth, tooth 520.6
Neonatorum — *see* condition
Neoplasia
   anal intraepithelial I (AIN I) (histologically
      confirmed) 569.44
   anal intraepithelial II (AIN II) (histologically
      confirmed) 569.44
   anal intraepithelial III (AIN III) 230.6

Neoplasia — *continued*
   anal intraepithelial III — *continued*
      anal canal 230.5
   endometrial intraepithelial (EIN) 621.35
   multiple endocrine (MEN)
      type I 258.01
      type IIA 258.02
      type IIB 258.03
   vaginal intraepithelial I (VAIN I) 623.0
   vaginal intraepithelial II (VAIN II) 623.0
   vaginal intraepithelial III (VAIN III) 233.31
   vulvular intraepithelial I (VIN I) 624.01
   vulvular intraepithelial II (VIN II) 624.02
   vulvular intraepithelial III (VIN III) 233.32

☑ **Additional Digit Required — Refer to the Tabular List for Digit Selection**

▽ **Subterms under main terms may continue to next column or page**

	Malignant			Benign	Uncertain Behavior	Unspecified
	Primary	Secondary	Ca in situ			
Neoplasm, neoplastic	199.1	—	234.9	229.9	238.9	239.9

Notes — 1. The list below gives the code numbers for neoplasms by anatomical site. For each site there are six possible code numbers according to whether the neoplasm in question is malignant, benign, in situ, of uncertain behavior, or of unspecified nature. The description of the neoplasm will often indicate which of the six columns is appropriate; e.g., malignant melanoma of skin, benign fibroadenoma of breast, carcinoma in situ of cervix uteri.

Where such descriptors are not present, the remainder of the Index should be consulted where guidance is given to the appropriate column for each morphological (histological) variety listed; e.g., Mesonephroma — see Neoplasm, malignant; Embryoma — see also Neoplasm, uncertain behavior; Disease, Bowen's — see Neoplasm, skin, in situ. However, the guidance in the Index can be overridden if one of the descriptors mentioned above is present; e.g., malignant adenoma of colon is coded to 153.9 and not to 211.3 as the adjective "malignant" overrides the Index entry "Adenoma — see also Neoplasm, benign."

2. Sites marked with the sign * (e.g., face NEC*) should be classified to malignant neoplasm of skin of these sites if the variety of neoplasm is a squamous cell carcinoma or an epidermoid carcinoma, and to benign neoplasm of skin of these sites if the variety of neoplasm is a papilloma (any type).

	Primary	Secondary	Ca in situ	Benign	Uncertain Behavior	Unspecified
abdomen, abdominal	195.2	198.89	234.8	229.8	238.8	239.89
cavity	195.2	198.89	234.8	229.8	238.8	239.89
organ	195.2	198.89	234.8	229.8	238.8	239.89
viscera	195.2	198.89	234.8	229.8	238.8	239.89
wall	173.50	198.2	232.5	216.5	238.2	239.2
basal cell carcinoma	173.51	—	—	—	—	—
connective tissue	171.5	198.89	—	215.5	238.1	239.2
specified type NEC	173.59	—	—	—	—	—
squamous cell carcinoma	173.52	—	—	—	—	—
abdominopelvic	195.8	198.89	234.8	229.8	238.8	239.89
accessory sinus — see Neoplasm, sinus						
acoustic nerve	192.0	198.4	—	225.1	237.9	239.7
acromion (process)	170.4	198.5	—	213.4	238.0	239.2
adenoid (pharynx) (tissue)	147.1	198.89	230.0	210.7	235.1	239.0
adipose tissue (see also Neoplasm, connective tissue)	171.9	198.89	—	215.9	238.1	239.2
adnexa (uterine)	183.9	198.82	233.39	221.8	236.3	239.5
adrenal (cortex) (gland) (medulla)	194.0	198.7	234.8	227.0	237.2	239.7
ala nasi (external)	173.30	198.2	232.3	216.3	238.2	239.2
alimentary canal or tract NEC	159.9	197.8	230.9	211.9	235.5	239.0
alveolar	143.9	198.89	230.0	210.4	235.1	239.0
mucosa	143.9	198.89	230.0	210.4	235.1	239.0
lower	143.1	198.89	230.0	210.4	235.1	239.0
upper	143.0	198.89	230.0	210.4	235.1	239.0
ridge or process	170.1	198.5	—	213.1	238.0	239.2
carcinoma	143.9	—	—	—	—	—
lower	143.1	—	—	—	—	—
upper	143.0	—	—	—	—	—
lower	170.1	198.5	—	213.1	238.0	239.2
mucosa	143.9	198.89	230.0	210.4	235.1	239.0
lower	143.1	198.89	230.0	210.4	235.1	239.0
upper	143.0	198.89	230.0	210.4	235.1	239.0
upper	170.0	198.5	—	213.0	238.0	239.2
sulcus	145.1	198.89	230.0	210.4	235.1	239.0
alveolus	143.9	198.89	230.0	210.4	235.1	239.0
lower	143.1	198.89	230.0	210.4	235.1	239.0
upper	143.0	198.89	230.0	210.4	235.1	239.0
ampulla of Vater	156.2	197.8	230.8	211.5	235.3	239.0
ankle NEC*	195.5	198.89	232.7	229.8	238.8	239.89
anorectum, anorectal (junction)	154.8	197.5	230.7	211.4	235.2	239.0
antecubital fossa or space*	195.4	198.89	232.6	229.8	238.8	239.89

	Primary	Secondary	Ca in situ	Benign	Uncertain Behavior	Unspecified
Neoplasm, neoplastic — *continued*						
antrum (Highmore) (maxillary)	160.2	197.3	231.8	212.0	235.9	239.1
pyloric	151.2	197.8	230.2	211.1	235.2	239.0
tympanicum	160.1	197.3	231.8	212.0	235.9	239.1
anus, anal	154.3	197.5	230.6	211.4	235.5	239.0
canal	154.2	197.5	230.5	211.4	235.5	239.0
contiguous sites with rectosigmoid junction or rectum	154.8	—	—	—	—	—
margin (see also Neoplasm, anus, skin)	173.50	198.2	232.5	216.6	238.2	239.2
skin	173.50	198.2	232.5	216.5	238.2	239.2
basal cell carcinoma	173.51	—	—	—	—	—
specified type NEC	173.59	—	—	—	—	—
squamous cell carcinoma	173.52	—	—	—	—	—
sphincter	154.2	197.5	230.5	211.4	235.5	239.0
aorta (thoracic)	171.4	198.89	—	215.4	238.1	239.2
abdominal	171.5	198.89	—	215.5	238.1	239.2
aortic body	194.6	198.89	—	227.6	237.3	239.7
aponeurosis	171.9	198.89	—	215.9	238.1	239.2
palmar	171.2	198.89	—	215.2	238.1	239.2
plantar	171.3	198.89	—	215.3	238.1	239.2
appendix	153.5	197.5	230.3	211.3	235.2	239.0
arachnoid (cerebral)	192.1	198.4	—	225.2	237.6	239.7
spinal	192.3	198.4	—	225.4	237.6	239.7
areola (female)	174.0	198.81	233.0	217	238.3	239.3
male	175.0	198.81	233.0	217	238.3	239.3
arm NEC*	195.4	198.89	232.6	229.8	238.8	239.89
artery — see Neoplasm, connective tissue						
aryepiglottic fold	148.2	198.89	230.0	210.8	235.1	239.0
hypopharyngeal aspect	148.2	198.89	230.0	210.8	235.1	239.0
laryngeal aspect	161.1	197.3	231.0	212.1	235.6	239.1
marginal zone	148.2	198.89	230.0	210.8	235.1	239.0
arytenoid (cartilage)	161.3	197.3	231.0	212.1	235.6	239.1
fold — see Neoplasm, aryepiglottic						
associated with transplanted organ	199.2	—	—	—	—	—
atlas	170.2	198.5	—	213.2	238.0	239.2
atrium, cardiac	164.1	198.89	—	212.7	238.8	239.89
auditory						
canal (external) (skin) (see also Neoplasm, skin, ear)	173.20	198.2	232.2	216.2	238.2	239.2
internal	160.1	197.3	231.8	212.0	235.9	239.1
nerve	192.0	198.4	—	225.1	237.9	239.7
tube	160.1	197.3	231.8	212.0	235.9	239.1
Eustachian	160.1	197.3	231.8	212.0	235.9	239.1
opening	147.2	198.89	230.0	210.7	235.1	239.0
auricle, ear see also Neoplasm, skin, ear)	173.20	198.2	232.2	216.2	238.2	239.2
cartilage	171.0	198.89	—	215.0	238.1	239.2
auricular canal (external) (see also Neoplasm, skin, ear)	173.20	198.2	232.2	216.2	238.2	239.2
internal	160.1	197.3	231.8	212.0	235.9	239.1
autonomic nerve or nervous system NEC	171.9	198.89	—	215.9	238.1	239.2
axilla, axillary	195.1	198.89	234.8	229.8	238.8	239.89
fold (see also Neoplasm, skin, trunk)	173.50	198.2	232.5	216.5	238.2	239.2

	Malignant					
	Primary	Secondary	Ca in situ	Benign	Uncertain Behavior	Unspecified
Neoplasm, neoplastic— *continued*						
back NEC*	195.8	198.89	232.5	229.8	238.8	239.89
Bartholin's gland	184.1	198.82	233.32	221.2	236.3	239.5
basal ganglia	191.0	198.3	—	225.0	237.5	239.6
basis pedunculi	191.7	198.3	—	225.0	237.5	239.6
bile or biliary (tract)	156.9	197.8	230.8	211.5	235.3	239.0
canaliculi (biliferi) (intrahepatic)	155.1	197.8	230.8	211.5	235.3	239.0
canals, interlobular	155.1	197.8	230.8	211.5	235.3	239.0
contiguous sites	156.8	—	—	—	—	—
duct or passage (common) (cystic) (extrahepatic)	156.1	197.8	230.8	211.5	235.3	239.0
contiguous sites with gallbladder	156.8	—	—	—	—	—
interlobular	155.1	197.8	230.8	211.5	235.3	239.0
intrahepatic	155.1	197.8	230.8	211.5	235.3	239.0
and extrahepatic	156.9	197.8	230.8	211.5	235.3	239.0
bladder (urinary)	188.9	198.1	233.7	223.3	236.7	239.4
contiguous sites	188.8	—	—	—	—	—
dome	188.1	198.1	233.7	223.3	236.7	239.4
neck	188.5	198.1	233.7	223.3	236.7	239.4
orifice	188.9	198.1	233.7	223.3	236.7	239.4
ureteric	188.6	198.1	233.7	223.3	236.7	239.4
urethral	188.5	198.1	233.7	223.3	236.7	239.4
sphincter	188.8	198.1	233.7	223.3	236.7	239.4
trigone	188.0	198.1	233.7	223.3	236.7	239.4
urachus	188.7	—	233.7	223.3	236.7	239.4
wall	188.9	198.1	233.7	223.3	236.7	239.4
anterior	188.3	198.1	233.7	223.3	236.7	239.4
lateral	188.2	198.1	233.7	223.3	236.7	239.4
posterior	188.4	198.1	233.7	223.3	236.7	239.4
blood vessel — *see* Neoplasm, connective tissue						
bone (periosteum)	170.9	198.5	—	213.9	238.0	239.2

> Note — Carcinomas and adenocarcinomas, of any type other than intraosseous or odontogenic, of the sites listed under "Neoplasm, bone" should be considered as constituting metastatic spread from an unspecified primary site and coded to 198.5 for morbidity coding.

	Primary	Secondary	Ca in situ	Benign	Uncertain Behavior	Unspecified
acetabulum	170.6	198.5	—	213.6	238.0	239.2
acromion (process)	170.4	198.5	—	213.4	238.0	239.2
ankle	170.8	198.5	—	213.8	238.0	239.2
arm NEC	170.4	198.5	—	213.4	238.0	239.2
astragalus	170.8	198.5	—	213.8	238.0	239.2
atlas	170.2	198.5	—	213.2	238.0	239.2
axis	170.2	198.5	—	213.2	238.0	239.2
back NEC	170.2	198.5	—	213.2	238.0	239.2
calcaneus	170.8	198.5	—	213.8	238.0	239.2
calvarium	170.0	198.5	—	213.0	238.0	239.2
carpus (any)	170.5	198.5	—	213.5	238.0	239.2
cartilage NEC	170.9	198.5	—	213.9	238.0	239.2
clavicle	170.3	198.5	—	213.3	238.0	239.2
clivus	170.0	198.5	—	213.0	238.0	239.2
coccygeal vertebra	170.6	198.5	—	213.6	238.0	239.2
coccyx	170.6	198.5	—	213.6	238.0	239.2
costal cartilage	170.3	198.5	—	213.3	238.0	239.2
costovertebral joint	170.3	198.5	—	213.3	238.0	239.2
cranial	170.0	198.5	—	213.0	238.0	239.2
cuboid	170.8	198.5	—	213.8	238.0	239.2
cuneiform	170.9	198.5	—	213.9	238.0	239.2
ankle	170.8	198.5	—	213.8	238.0	239.2
wrist	170.5	198.5	—	213.5	238.0	239.2
digital	170.9	198.5	—	213.9	238.0	239.2
finger	170.5	198.5	—	213.5	238.0	239.2
toe	170.8	198.5	—	213.8	238.0	239.2

	Malignant					
	Primary	Secondary	Ca in situ	Benign	Uncertain Behavior	Unspecified
Neoplasm, neoplastic— *continued*						
bone — *continued*						
elbow	170.4	198.5	—	213.4	238.0	239.2
ethmoid (labyrinth)	170.0	198.5	—	213.0	238.0	239.2
face	170.0	198.5	—	213.0	238.0	239.2
lower jaw	170.1	198.5	—	213.1	238.0	239.2
femur (any part)	170.7	198.5	—	213.7	238.0	239.2
fibula (any part)	170.7	198.5	—	213.7	238.0	239.2
finger (any)	170.5	198.5	—	213.5	238.0	239.2
foot	170.8	198.5	—	213.8	238.0	239.2
forearm	170.4	198.5	—	213.4	238.0	239.2
frontal	170.0	198.5	—	213.0	238.0	239.2
hand	170.5	198.5	—	213.5	238.0	239.2
heel	170.8	198.5	—	213.8	238.0	239.2
hip	170.6	198.5	—	213.6	238.0	239.2
humerus (any part)	170.4	198.5	—	213.4	238.0	239.2
hyoid	170.0	198.5	—	213.0	238.0	239.2
ilium	170.6	198.5	—	213.6	238.0	239.2
innominate	170.6	198.5	—	213.6	238.0	239.2
intervertebral cartilage or disc	170.2	198.5	—	213.2	238.0	239.2
ischium	170.6	198.5	—	213.6	238.0	239.2
jaw (lower)	170.1	198.5	—	213.1	238.0	239.2
upper	170.0	198.5	—	213.0	238.0	239.2
knee	170.7	198.5	—	213.7	238.0	239.2
leg NEC	170.7	198.5	—	213.7	238.0	239.2
limb NEC	170.9	198.5	—	213.9	238.0	239.2
lower (long bones)	170.7	198.5	—	213.7	238.0	239.2
short bones	170.8	198.5	—	213.8	238.0	239.2
upper (long bones)	170.4	198.5	—	213.4	238.0	239.2
short bones	170.5	198.5	—	213.5	238.0	239.2
long	170.9	198.5	—	213.9	238.0	239.2
lower limbs NEC	170.7	198.5	—	213.7	238.0	239.2
upper limbs NEC	170.4	198.5	—	213.4	238.0	239.2
malar	170.0	198.5	—	213.0	238.0	239.2
mandible	170.1	198.5	—	213.1	238.0	239.2
marrow NEC	202.9	198.5	—	—	—	238.79
mastoid	170.0	198.5	—	213.0	238.0	239.2
maxilla, maxillary (superior)	170.0	198.5	—	213.0	238.0	239.2
inferior	170.1	198.5	—	213.1	238.0	239.2
metacarpus (any)	170.5	198.5	—	213.5	238.0	239.2
metatarsus (any)	170.8	198.5	—	213.8	238.0	239.2
navicular (ankle)	170.8	198.5	—	213.8	238.0	239.2
hand	170.5	198.5	—	213.5	238.0	239.2
nose, nasal	170.0	198.5	—	213.0	238.0	239.2
occipital	170.0	198.5	—	213.0	238.0	239.2
orbit	170.0	198.5	—	213.0	238.0	239.2
parietal	170.0	198.5	—	213.0	238.0	239.2
patella	170.8	198.5	—	213.8	238.0	239.2
pelvic	170.6	198.5	—	213.6	238.0	239.2
phalanges	170.9	198.5	—	213.9	238.0	239.2
foot	170.8	198.5	—	213.8	238.0	239.2
hand	170.5	198.5	—	213.5	238.0	239.2
pubic	170.6	198.5	—	213.6	238.0	239.2
radius (any part)	170.4	198.5	—	213.4	238.0	239.2
rib	170.3	198.5	—	213.3	238.0	239.2
sacral vertebra	170.6	198.5	—	213.6	238.0	239.2
sacrum	170.6	198.5	—	213.6	238.0	239.2
scaphoid (of hand)	170.5	198.5	—	213.5	238.0	239.2
of ankle	170.8	198.5	—	213.8	238.0	239.2
scapula (any part)	170.4	198.5	—	213.4	238.0	239.2
sella turcica	170.0	198.5	—	213.0	238.0	239.2
short	170.9	198.5	—	213.9	238.0	239.2
lower limb	170.8	198.5	—	213.8	238.0	239.2

☑ Additional Digit Required — Refer to the Tabular List for Digit Selection   ▽ Subterms under main terms may continue to next column or page

238   2014 ICD-9-CM

	Malignant			Benign	Uncertain Behavior	Unspecified
	Primary	Secondary	Ca in situ			

Neoplasm, neoplastic —
continued
  bone — *continued*
    short — *continued*

	Primary	Secondary	Ca in situ	Benign	Uncertain Behavior	Unspecified
upper limb	170.5	198.5	—	213.5	238.0	239.2
shoulder	170.4	198.5	—	213.4	238.0	239.2
skeleton, skeletal NEC	170.9	198.5	—	213.9	238.0	239.2
skull	170.0	198.5	—	213.0	238.0	239.2
sphenoid	170.0	198.5	—	213.0	238.0	239.2
spine, spinal (column)	170.2	198.5	—	213.2	238.0	239.2
coccyx	170.6	198.5	—	213.6	238.0	239.2
sacrum	170.6	198.5	—	213.6	238.0	239.2
sternum	170.3	198.5	—	213.3	238.0	239.2
tarsus (any)	170.8	198.5	—	213.8	238.0	239.2
temporal	170.0	198.5	—	213.0	238.0	239.2
thumb	170.5	198.5	—	213.5	238.0	239.2
tibia (any part)	170.7	198.5	—	213.7	238.0	239.2
toe (any)	170.8	198.5	—	213.8	238.0	239.2
trapezium	170.5	198.5	—	213.5	238.0	239.2
trapezoid	170.5	198.5	—	213.5	238.0	239.2
turbinate	170.0	198.5	—	213.0	238.0	239.2
ulna (any part)	170.4	198.5	—	213.4	238.0	239.2
unciform	170.5	198.5	—	213.5	238.0	239.2
vertebra (column)	170.2	198.5	—	213.2	238.0	239.2
coccyx	170.6	198.5	—	213.6	238.0	239.2
sacrum	170.6	198.5	—	213.6	238.0	239.2
vomer	170.0	198.5	—	213.0	238.0	239.2
wrist	170.5	198.5	—	213.5	238.0	239.2
xiphoid process	170.3	198.5	—	213.3	238.0	239.2
zygomatic	170.0	198.5	—	213.0	238.0	239.2
book-leaf (mouth)	145.8	198.89	230.0	210.4	235.1	239.0
bowel — *see* Neoplasm, intestine						
brachial plexus	171.2	198.89	—	215.2	238.1	239.2
brain NEC	191.9	198.3	—	225.0	237.5	239.6
basal ganglia	191.0	198.3	—	225.0	237.5	239.6
cerebellopontine angle	191.6	198.3	—	225.0	237.5	239.6
cerebellum NOS	191.6	198.3	—	225.0	237.5	239.6
cerebrum	191.0	198.3	—	225.0	237.5	239.6
choroid plexus	191.5	198.3	—	225.0	237.5	239.6
contiguous sites	191.8	—	—	—	—	—
corpus callosum	191.8	198.3	—	225.0	237.5	239.6
corpus striatum	191.0	198.3	—	225.0	237.5	239.6
cortex (cerebral)	191.0	198.3	—	225.0	237.5	239.6
frontal lobe	191.1	198.3	—	225.0	237.5	239.6
globus pallidus	191.0	198.3	—	225.0	237.5	239.6
hippocampus	191.2	198.3	—	225.0	237.5	239.6
hypothalamus	191.0	198.3	—	225.0	237.5	239.6
internal capsule	191.0	198.3	—	225.0	237.5	239.6
medulla oblongata	191.7	198.3	—	225.0	237.5	239.6
meninges	192.1	198.4	—	225.2	237.6	239.7
midbrain	191.7	198.3	—	225.0	237.5	239.6
occipital lobe	191.4	198.3	—	225.0	237.5	239.6
parietal lobe	191.3	198.3	—	225.0	237.5	239.6
peduncle	191.7	198.3	—	225.0	237.5	239.6
pons	191.7	198.3	—	225.0	237.5	239.6
stem	191.7	198.3	—	225.0	237.5	239.6
tapetum	191.8	198.3	—	225.0	237.5	239.6
temporal lobe	191.2	198.3	—	225.0	237.5	239.6
thalamus	191.0	198.3	—	225.0	237.5	239.6
uncus	191.2	198.3	—	225.0	237.5	239.6
ventricle (floor)	191.5	198.3	—	225.0	237.5	239.6
branchial (cleft) (vestiges)	146.8	198.89	230.0	210.6	235.1	239.0
breast (connective tissue) (female) (glandular tissue) (soft parts)	174.9	198.81	233.0	217	238.3	239.3
areola	174.0	198.81	233.0	217	238.3	239.3
male	175.0	198.81	233.0	217	238.3	239.3
axillary tail	174.6	198.81	233.0	217	238.3	239.3

Neoplasm, neoplastic —
continued
  breast — *continued*

	Primary	Secondary	Ca in situ	Benign	Uncertain Behavior	Unspecified
central portion	174.1	198.81	233.0	217	238.3	239.3
contiguous sites	174.8	—	—	—	—	—
ectopic sites	174.8	198.81	233.0	217	238.3	239.3
inner	174.8	198.81	233.0	217	238.3	239.3
lower	174.8	198.81	233.0	217	238.3	239.3
lower-inner quadrant	174.3	198.81	233.0	217	238.3	239.3
lower-outer quadrant	174.5	198.81	233.0	217	238.3	239.3
male	175.9	198.81	233.0	217	238.3	239.3
areola	175.0	198.81	233.0	217	238.3	239.3
ectopic tissue	175.9	198.81	233.0	217	238.3	239.3
nipple	175.0	198.81	233.0	217	238.3	239.3
mastectomy site (skin) (*see also* Neoplasm, mastectomy site)	173.50	198.2	—	—	—	—
specified as breast tissue	174.8	198.81	—	—	—	—
midline	174.8	198.81	233.0	217	238.3	239.3
nipple	174.0	198.81	233.0	217	238.3	239.3
male	175.0	198.81	233.0	217	238.3	239.3
outer	174.8	198.81	233.0	217	238.3	239.3
skin (*see also* Neoplasm, mastectomy site)	173.50	198.2	232.5	216.5	238.2	239.2
tail (axillary)	174.6	198.81	233.0	217	238.3	239.3
upper	174.8	198.81	233.0	217	238.3	239.3
upper-inner quadrant	174.2	198.81	233.0	217	238.3	239.3
upper-outer quadrant	174.4	198.81	233.0	217	238.3	239.3
broad ligament	183.3	198.82	233.39	221.0	236.3	239.5
bronchiogenic, bronchogenic (lung)	162.9	197.0	231.2	212.3	235.7	239.1
bronchiole	162.9	197.0	231.2	212.3	235.7	239.1
bronchus	162.9	197.0	231.2	212.3	235.7	239.1
carina	162.2	197.0	231.2	212.3	235.7	239.1
contiguous sites with lung or trachea	162.8	—	—	—	—	—
lower lobe of lung	162.5	197.0	231.2	212.3	235.7	239.1
main	162.2	197.0	231.2	212.3	235.7	239.1
middle lobe of lung	162.4	197.0	231.2	212.3	235.7	239.1
upper lobe of lung	162.3	197.0	231.2	212.3	235.7	239.1
brow	173.30	198.2	232.3	216.3	238.2	239.2
basal cell carcinoma	173.31	—	—	—	—	—
specified type NEC	173.39	—	—	—	—	—
squamous cell carcinoma	173.32	—	—	—	—	—
buccal (cavity)	145.9	198.89	230.0	210.4	235.1	239.0
commissure	145.0	198.89	230.0	210.4	235.1	239.0
groove (lower) (upper)	145.1	198.89	230.0	210.4	235.1	239.0
mucosa	145.0	198.89	230.0	210.4	235.1	239.0
sulcus (lower) (upper)	145.1	198.89	230.0	210.4	235.1	239.0
bulbourethral gland	189.3	198.1	233.9	223.81	236.99	239.5
bursa — *see* Neoplasm, connective tissue						
buttock NEC*	195.3	198.89	232.5	229.8	238.8	239.89
calf*	195.5	198.89	232.7	229.8	238.8	239.89
calvarium	170.0	198.5	—	213.0	238.0	239.2
calyx, renal	189.1	198.0	233.9	223.1	236.91	239.5
canal anal	154.2	197.5	230.5	211.4	235.5	239.0

	Malignant					
	Primary	Secondary	Ca in situ	Benign	Uncertain Behavior	Unspecified
Neoplasm, neoplastic — *continued*						
canal — *continued*						
auditory (external) (see also Neoplasm, skin, ear)	173.20	198.2	232.2	216.2	238.2	239.2
auricular (external) (see also Neoplasm, skin, ear)	173.20	198.2	232.2	216.2	238.2	239.2
canaliculi, biliary (biliferi) (intrahepatic)	155.1	197.8	230.8	211.5	235.3	239.0
canthus (eye) (inner) (outer)	173.10	198.2	232.1	216.1	238.2	239.2
basal cell carcinoma	173.11	—	—	—	—	—
specified type NEC	173.19					
squamous cell carcinoma	173.12	—	—	—	—	—
capillary — *see* Neoplasm, connective tissue						
caput coli	153.4	197.5	230.3	211.3	235.2	239.0
cardia (gastric)	151.0	197.8	230.2	211.1	235.2	239.0
cardiac orifice (stomach)	151.0	197.8	230.2	211.1	235.2	239.0
cardio-esophageal junction	151.0	197.8	230.2	211.1	235.2	239.0
cardio-esophagus	151.0	197.8	230.2	211.1	235.2	239.0
carina (bronchus)	162.2	197.0	231.2	212.3	235.7	239.1
carotid (artery)	171.0	198.89	—	215.0	238.1	239.2
body	194.5	198.89	—	227.5	237.3	239.7
carpus (any bone)	170.5	198.5	—	213.5	238.0	239.2
cartilage (articular) (joint) NEC (see also Neoplasm, bone)	170.9	198.5	—	213.9	238.0	239.2
arytenoid	161.3	197.3	231.0	212.1	235.6	239.1
auricular	171.0	198.89	—	215.0	238.1	239.2
bronchi	162.2	197.3	—	212.3	235.7	239.1
connective tissue — *see* Neoplasm, connective tissue						
costal	170.3	198.5	—	213.3	238.0	239.2
cricoid	161.3	197.3	231.0	212.1	235.6	239.1
cuneiform	161.3	197.3	231.0	212.1	235.6	239.1
ear (external)	171.0	198.89	—	215.0	238.1	239.2
ensiform	170.3	198.5	—	213.3	238.0	239.2
epiglottis	161.1	197.3	231.0	212.1	235.6	239.1
anterior surface	146.4	198.89	230.0	210.6	235.1	239.0
eyelid	171.0	198.89	—	215.0	238.1	239.2
intervertebral	170.2	198.5	—	213.2	238.0	239.2
larynx, laryngeal	161.3	197.3	231.0	212.1	235.6	239.1
nose, nasal	160.0	197.3	231.8	212.0	235.9	239.1
pinna	171.0	198.89	—	215.0	238.1	239.2
rib	170.3	198.5	—	213.3	238.0	239.2
semilunar (knee)	170.7	198.5	—	213.7	238.0	239.2
thyroid	161.3	197.3	231.0	212.1	235.6	239.1
trachea	162.0	197.3	231.1	212.2	235.7	239.1
cauda equina	192.2	198.3	—	225.3	237.5	239.7
cavity						
buccal	145.9	198.89	230.0	210.4	235.1	239.0
nasal	160.0	197.3	231.8	212.0	235.9	239.1
oral	145.9	198.89	230.0	210.4	235.1	239.0
peritoneal	158.9	197.6	—	211.8	235.4	239.0
tympanic	160.1	197.3	231.8	212.0	235.9	239.1
cecum	153.4	197.5	230.3	211.3	235.2	239.0
central nervous system — *see* Neoplasm, nervous system						
white matter	191.0	198.3	—	225.0	237.5	239.6
Neoplasm, neoplastic — *continued*						
cerebellopontine (angle)	191.6	198.3	—	225.0	237.5	239.6
cerebellum, cerebellar	191.6	198.3	—	225.0	237.5	239.6
cerebrum, cerebral (cortex) (hemisphere) (white matter)	191.0	198.3	—	225.0	237.5	239.6
meninges	192.1	198.4	—	225.2	237.6	239.7
peduncle	191.7	198.3	—	225.0	237.5	239.6
ventricle (any)	191.5	198.3	—	225.0	237.5	239.6
cervical region	195.0	198.89	234.8	229.8	238.8	239.89
cervix (cervical) (uteri) (uterus)	180.9	198.82	233.1	219.0	236.0	239.5
canal	180.0	198.82	233.1	219.0	236.0	239.5
contiguous sites	180.8	—	—	—	—	—
endocervix (canal) (gland)	180.0	198.82	233.1	219.0	236.0	239.5
exocervix	180.1	198.82	233.1	219.0	236.0	239.5
external os	180.1	198.82	233.1	219.0	236.0	239.5
internal os	180.0	198.82	233.1	219.0	236.0	239.5
nabothian gland	180.0	198.82	233.1	219.0	236.0	239.5
squamocolumnar junction	180.8	198.82	233.1	219.0	236.0	239.5
stump	180.8	198.82	233.1	219.0	236.0	239.5
cheek	195.0	198.89	234.8	229.8	238.8	239.89
external	173.30	198.2	232.3	216.3	238.2	239.2
basal cell carcinoma	173.31	—	—	—	—	—
specified type NEC	173.39	—		—	—	—
squamous cell carcinoma	173.32	—	—	—	—	—
inner aspect	145.0	198.89	230.0	210.4	235.1	239.0
internal	145.0	198.89	230.0	210.4	235.1	239.0
mucosa	145.0	198.89	230.0	210.4	235.1	239.0
chest (wall) NEC	195.1	198.89	234.8	229.8	238.8	239.89
chiasma opticum	192.0	198.4	—	225.1	237.9	239.7
chin	173.30	198.2	232.3	216.3	238.2	239.2
basal cell carcinoma	173.31	—	—	—	—	—
specified type NEC	173.39	—		—	—	—
squamous cell carcinoma	173.32	—	—	—	—	—
choana	147.3	198.89	230.0	210.7	235.1	239.0
cholangiole	155.1	197.8	230.8	211.5	235.3	239.0
choledochal duct	156.1	197.8	230.8	211.5	235.3	239.0
choroid	190.6	198.4	234.0	224.6	238.8	239.81
plexus	191.5	198.3	—	225.0	237.5	239.6
ciliary body	190.0	198.4	234.0	224.0	238.8	239.89
clavicle	170.3	198.5	—	213.3	238.0	239.2
clitoris	184.3	198.82	233.32	221.2	236.3	239.5
clivus	170.0	198.5	—	213.0	238.0	239.2
cloacogenic zone	154.8	197.5	230.7	211.4	235.5	239.0
coccygeal body or glomus	194.6	198.89	—	227.6	237.3	239.7
vertebra	170.6	198.5	—	213.6	238.0	239.2
coccyx	170.6	198.5	—	213.6	238.0	239.2
colon — *see also* Neoplasm, intestine, large	153.9	197.5	230.3	211.3	235.2	239.0
with rectum	154.0	197.5	230.4	211.4	235.2	239.0
columnella (see also Neoplasm, skin, face)	173.30	198.2	232.3	216.3	238.2	239.2
column, spinal — *see* Neoplasm, spine						
commissure						
labial, lip	140.6	198.89	230.0	210.4	235.1	239.0
laryngeal	161.0	197.3	231.0	212.1	235.6	239.1
common (bile) duct	156.1	197.8	230.8	211.5	235.3	239.0

☑ Additional Digit Required — Refer to the Tabular List for Digit Selection   ▽ Subterms under main terms may continue to next column or page

240   2014 ICD-9-CM

Neoplasm, neoplastic —	Malignant Primary	Malignant Secondary	Malignant Ca in situ	Benign	Uncertain Behavior	Unspecified
continued						
concha (see also Neoplasm, skin, ear)	173.20	198.2	232.2	216.2	238.2	239.2
nose	160.0	197.3	231.8	212.0	235.9	239.1
conjunctiva	190.3	198.4	234.0	224.3	238.8	239.89
connective tissue NEC	171.9	198.89	—	215.9	238.1	239.2

Note — For neoplasms of connective tissue (blood vessel, bursa, fascia, ligament, muscle, peripheral nerves, sympathetic and parasympathetic nerves and ganglia, synovia, tendon, etc.) or of morphological types that indicate connective tissue, code according to the list under "Neoplasm, connective tissue"; for sites that do not appear in this list, code to neoplasm of that site; e.g.,

liposarcoma, shoulder 171.2

leiomyosarcoma, stomach 151.9

neurofibroma, chest wall 215.4

Morphological types that indicate connective tissue appear in the proper place in the alphabetic index with the instruction "see Neoplasm, connective tissue…"

	Primary	Secondary	Ca in situ	Benign	Uncertain Behavior	Unspecified
abdomen	171.5	198.89	—	215.5	238.1	239.2
abdominal wall	171.5	198.89	—	215.5	238.1	239.2
ankle	171.3	198.89	—	215.3	238.1	239.2
antecubital fossa or space	171.2	198.89	—	215.2	238.1	239.2
arm	171.2	198.89	—	215.2	238.1	239.2
auricle (ear)	171.0	198.89	—	215.0	238.1	239.2
axilla	171.4	198.89	—	215.4	238.1	239.2
back	171.7	198.89	—	215.7	238.1	239.2
breast (female) (see also Neoplasm, breast)	174.9	198.81	233.0	217	238.3	239.3
male	175.9	198.81	233.0	217	238.3	239.3
buttock	171.6	198.89	—	215.6	238.1	239.2
calf	171.3	198.89	—	215.3	238.1	239.2
cervical region	171.0	198.89	—	215.0	238.1	239.2
cheek	171.0	198.89	—	215.0	238.1	239.2
chest (wall)	171.4	198.89	—	215.4	238.1	239.2
chin	171.0	198.89	—	215.0	238.1	239.2
contiguous sites	171.8	—	—	—	—	—
diaphragm	171.4	198.89	—	215.4	238.1	239.2
ear (external)	171.0	198.89	—	215.0	238.1	239.2
elbow	171.2	198.89	—	215.2	238.1	239.2
extrarectal	171.6	198.89	—	215.6	238.1	239.2
extremity	171.8	198.89	—	215.8	238.1	239.2
lower	171.3	198.89	—	215.3	238.1	239.2
upper	171.2	198.89	—	215.2	238.1	239.2
eyelid	171.0	198.89	—	215.0	238.1	239.2
face	171.0	198.89	—	215.0	238.1	239.2
finger	171.2	198.89	—	215.2	238.1	239.2
flank	171.7	198.89	—	215.7	238.1	239.2
foot	171.3	198.89	—	215.3	238.1	239.2
forearm	171.2	198.89	—	215.2	238.1	239.2
forehead	171.0	198.89	—	215.0	238.1	239.2
gastric	171.5	198.89	—	215.5	238.1	—
gastrointestinal	171.5	198.89	—	215.5	238.1	—
gluteal region	171.6	198.89	—	215.6	238.1	239.2
great vessels NEC	171.4	198.89	—	215.4	238.1	239.2
groin	171.6	198.89	—	215.6	238.1	239.2
hand	171.2	198.89	—	215.2	238.1	239.2
head	171.0	198.89	—	215.0	238.1	239.2
heel	171.3	198.89	—	215.3	238.1	239.2
hip	171.3	198.89	—	215.3	238.1	239.2
hypochondrium	171.5	198.89	—	215.5	238.1	239.2
iliopsoas muscle	171.6	198.89	—	215.5	238.1	239.2
infraclavicular region	171.4	198.89	—	215.4	238.1	239.2
inguinal (canal) (region)	171.6	198.89	—	215.6	238.1	239.2
intestine	171.5	198.89	—	215.5	238.1	—
intrathoracic	171.4	198.89	—	215.4	238.1	239.2
ischorectal fossa	171.6	198.89	—	215.6	238.1	239.2
jaw	143.9	198.89	230.0	210.4	235.1	239.0

Neoplasm, neoplastic — continued / connective tissue — continued	Primary	Secondary	Ca in situ	Benign	Uncertain Behavior	Unspecified
knee	171.3	198.89	—	215.3	238.1	239.2
leg	171.3	198.89	—	215.3	238.1	239.2
limb NEC	171.9	198.89	—	215.8	238.1	239.2
lower	171.3	198.89	—	215.3	238.1	239.2
upper	171.2	198.89	—	215.2	238.1	239.2
nates	171.6	198.89	—	215.6	238.1	239.2
neck	171.0	198.89	—	215.0	238.1	239.2
orbit	190.1	198.4	234.0	224.1	238.8	239.89
pararectal	171.6	198.89	—	215.6	238.1	239.2
para-urethral	171.6	198.89	—	215.6	238.1	239.2
paravaginal	171.6	198.89	—	215.6	238.1	239.2
pelvis (floor)	171.6	198.89	—	215.6	238.1	239.2
pelvo-abdominal	171.8	198.89	—	215.8	238.1	239.2
perineum	171.6	198.89	—	215.6	238.1	239.2
perirectal (tissue)	171.6	198.89	—	215.6	238.1	239.2
periurethral (tissue)	171.6	198.89	—	215.6	238.1	239.2
popliteal fossa or space	171.3	198.89	—	215.3	238.1	239.2
presacral	171.6	198.89	—	215.6	238.1	239.2
psoas muscle	171.5	198.89	—	215.5	238.1	239.2
pterygoid fossa	171.0	198.89	—	215.0	238.1	239.2
rectovaginal septum or wall	171.6	198.89	—	215.6	238.1	239.2
rectovesical	171.6	198.89	—	215.6	238.1	239.2
retroperitoneum	158.0	197.6	—	211.8	235.4	239.0
sacrococcygeal region	171.6	198.89	—	215.6	238.1	239.2
scalp	171.0	198.89	—	215.0	238.1	239.2
scapular region	171.4	198.89	—	215.4	238.1	239.2
shoulder	171.2	198.89	—	215.2	238.1	239.2
skin (dermis) NEC	173.90	198.2	232.9	216.9	238.2	239.2
stomach	171.5	198.89	—	215.5	238.1	—
submental	171.0	198.89	—	215.0	238.1	239.2
supraclavicular region	171.0	198.89	—	215.0	238.1	239.2
temple	171.0	198.89	—	215.0	238.1	239.2
temporal region	171.0	198.89	—	215.0	238.1	239.2
thigh	171.3	198.89	—	215.3	238.1	239.2
thoracic (duct) (wall)	171.4	198.89	—	215.4	238.1	239.2
thorax	171.4	198.89	—	215.4	238.1	239.2
thumb	171.2	198.89	—	215.2	238.1	239.2
toe	171.3	198.89	—	215.3	238.1	239.2
trunk	171.7	198.89	—	215.7	238.1	239.2
umbilicus	171.5	198.89	—	215.5	238.1	239.2
vesicorectal	171.6	198.89	—	215.6	238.1	239.2
wrist	171.2	198.89	—	215.2	238.1	239.2
conus medullaris	192.2	198.3	—	225.3	237.5	239.7
cord (true) (vocal)	161.0	197.3	231.0	212.1	235.6	239.1
false	161.1	197.3	231.0	212.1	235.6	239.1
spermatic	187.6	198.82	233.6	222.8	236.6	239.5
spinal (cervical) (lumbar) (thoracic)	192.2	198.3	—	225.3	237.5	239.7
cornea (limbus)	190.4	198.4	234.0	224.4	238.8	239.89
corpus						
albicans	183.0	198.6	233.39	220	236.2	239.5
callosum, brain	191.8	198.3	—	225.0	237.5	239.6
cavernosum	187.3	198.82	233.5	222.1	236.6	239.5
gastric	151.4	197.8	230.2	211.1	235.2	239.0
penis	187.3	198.82	233.5	222.1	236.6	239.5
striatum, cerebrum	191.0	198.3	—	225.0	237.5	239.6
uteri	182.0	198.82	233.2	219.1	236.0	239.5
isthmus	182.1	198.82	233.2	219.1	236.0	239.5
cortex						
adrenal	194.0	198.7	234.8	227.0	237.2	239.7
cerebral	191.0	198.3	—	225.0	237.5	239.6
costal cartilage	170.3	198.5	—	213.3	238.0	239.2

☑ Additional Digit Required — Refer to the Tabular List for Digit Selection   ▽ Subterms under main terms may continue to next column or page

2014 ICD-9-CM   241

	Malignant			Benign	Uncertain Behavior	Unspecified
	Primary	Secondary	Ca in situ			
Neoplasm, neoplastic — *continued*						
costovertebral joint	170.3	198.5	—	213.3	238.0	239.2
Cowper's gland	189.3	198.1	233.9	223.81	236.99	239.5
cranial (fossa, any)	191.9	198.3	—	225.0	237.5	239.6
meninges	192.1	198.4	—	225.2	237.6	239.7
nerve (any)	192.0	198.4	—	225.1	237.9	239.7
craniobuccal pouch	194.3	198.89	234.8	227.3	237.0	239.7
craniopharyngeal (duct) (pouch)	194.3	198.89	234.8	227.3	237.0	239.7
cricoid	148.0	198.89	230.0	210.8	235.1	239.0
cartilage	161.3	197.3	231.0	212.1	235.6	239.1
cricopharynx	148.0	198.89	230.0	210.8	235.1	239.0
crypt of Morgagni	154.8	197.5	230.7	211.4	235.2	239.0
crystalline lens	190.0	198.4	234.0	224.0	238.8	239.89
cul-de-sac (Douglas')	158.8	197.6	—	211.8	235.4	239.0
cuneiform cartilage	161.3	197.3	231.0	212.1	235.6	239.1
cutaneous — *see* Neoplasm, skin						
cutis — *see* Neoplasm, skin						
cystic (bile) duct (common)	156.1	197.8	230.8	211.5	235.3	239.0
dermis — *see* Neoplasm, skin						
diaphragm	171.4	198.89	—	215.4	238.1	239.2
digestive organs, system, tube, or tract NEC	159.9	197.8	230.9	211.9	235.5	239.0
contiguous sites with peritoneum	159.8	—	—	—	—	—
disc, intervertebral	170.2	198.5	—	213.2	238.0	239.2
disease, generalized	199.0	—	234.9	229.9	238.9	—
disseminated	199.0	—	234.9	229.9	238.9	—
Douglas' cul-de-sac or pouch	158.8	197.6	—	211.8	235.4	239.0
duodenojejunal junction	152.8	197.4	230.7	211.2	235.2	239.0
duodenum	152.0	197.4	230.7	211.2	235.2	239.0
dura (cranial) (mater)	192.1	198.4	—	225.2	237.6	239.7
cerebral	192.1	198.4	—	225.2	237.6	239.7
spinal	192.3	198.4	—	225.4	237.6	239.7
ear (external) (*see also* Neoplasm, ear, skin)	173.20	198.2	232.2	216.2	238.2	239.2
auricle or auris (*see also* Neoplasm, ear, skin)	173.20	198.2	232.2	216.2	238.2	239.2
canal, external (*see also* Neoplasm, ear, skin)	173.20	198.2	232.2	216.2	238.2	239.2
cartilage	171.0	198.89	—	215.0	238.1	239.2
external meatus (*see also* Neoplasm, ear, skin)	173.20	198.2	232.2	216.2	238.2	239.2
inner	160.1	197.3	231.8	212.0	235.9	239.89
lobule (*see also* Neoplasm, ear, skin)	173.20	198.2	232.2	216.2	238.2	239.2
middle	160.1	197.3	231.8	212.0	235.9	239.89
contiguous sites with accessory sinuses or nasal cavities	160.8	—	—	—	—	—
skin	173.20	198.2	232.2	216.2	238.2	239.2
basal cell carcinoma	173.21	—	—	—	—	—
specified type NEC	173.29	—	—	—	—	—
squamous cell carcinoma	173.22	—	—	—	—	—
earlobe	173.20	198.2	232.2	216.2	238.2	239.2
Neoplasm, neoplastic — *continued*						
earlobe — *continued* basal cell carcinoma	173.21	—	—	—	—	—
specified type NEC	173.29	—	—	—	—	—
squamous cell carcinoma	173.22	—	—	—	—	—
ejaculatory duct	187.8	198.82	233.6	222.8	236.6	239.5
elbow NEC*	195.4	198.89	232.6	229.8	238.8	239.89
endocardium	164.1	198.89	—	212.7	238.8	239.89
endocervix (canal) (gland)	180.0	198.82	233.1	219.0	236.0	239.5
endocrine gland NEC	194.9	198.89	—	227.9	237.4	239.7
pluriglandular NEC	194.8	198.89	234.8	227.8	237.4	239.7
endometrium (gland) (stroma)	182.0	198.82	233.2	219.1	236.0	239.5
ensiform cartilage	170.3	198.5	—	213.3	238.0	239.2
enteric — *see* Neoplasm, intestine						
ependyma (brain)	191.5	198.3	—	225.0	237.5	239.6
epicardium	164.1	198.89	—	212.7	238.8	239.89
epididymis	187.5	198.82	233.6	222.3	236.6	239.5
epidural	192.9	198.4	—	225.9	237.9	239.7
epiglottis	161.1	197.3	231.0	212.1	235.6	239.1
anterior aspect or surface	146.4	198.89	230.0	210.6	235.1	239.0
cartilage	161.3	197.3	231.0	212.1	235.6	239.1
free border (margin)	146.4	198.89	230.0	210.6	235.1	239.0
junctional region	146.5	198.89	230.0	210.6	235.1	239.0
posterior (laryngeal) surface	161.1	197.3	231.0	212.1	235.6	239.1
suprahyoid portion	161.1	197.3	231.0	212.1	235.6	239.1
esophagogastric junction	151.0	197.8	230.2	211.1	235.2	239.0
esophagus	150.9	197.8	230.1	211.0	235.5	239.0
abdominal	150.2	197.8	230.1	211.0	235.5	239.0
cervical	150.0	197.8	230.1	211.0	235.5	239.0
contiguous sites	150.8	—	—	—	—	—
distal (third)	150.5	197.8	230.1	211.0	235.5	239.0
lower (third)	150.5	197.8	230.1	211.0	235.5	239.0
middle (third)	150.4	197.8	230.1	211.0	235.5	239.0
proximal (third)	150.3	197.8	230.1	211.0	235.5	239.0
specified part NEC	150.8	197.8	230.1	211.0	235.5	239.0
thoracic	150.1	197.8	230.1	211.0	235.5	239.0
upper (third)	150.3	197.8	230.1	211.0	235.5	239.0
ethmoid (sinus)	160.3	197.3	231.8	212.0	235.9	239.1
bone or labyrinth	170.0	198.5	—	213.0	238.0	239.2
Eustachian tube	160.1	197.3	231.8	212.0	235.9	239.1
exocervix	180.1	198.82	233.1	219.0	236.0	239.5
external meatus (ear) (*see also* Neoplasm, skin, ear)	173.20	198.2	232.2	216.2	238.2	239.2
os, cervix uteri	180.1	198.82	233.1	219.0	236.0	239.5
extradural	192.9	198.4	—	225.9	237.9	239.7
extrahepatic (bile) duct	156.1	197.8	230.8	211.5	235.3	239.0
contiguous sites with gallbladder	156.8	—	—	—	—	—
extraocular muscle	190.1	198.4	234.0	224.1	238.8	239.89
extrarectal	195.3	198.89	234.8	229.8	238.8	239.89
extremity*	195.8	198.89	232.8	229.8	238.8	239.89
lower*	195.5	198.89	232.7	229.8	238.8	239.89
upper*	195.4	198.89	232.6	229.8	238.8	239.89
eyeball	190.0	198.4	234.0	224.0	238.8	239.89
eyebrow	173.30	198.2	232.3	216.3	238.2	239.2

☑ **Additional Digit Required — Refer to the Tabular List for Digit Selection**

▽ **Subterms under main terms may continue to next column or page**

	Malignant			Benign	Uncertain Behavior	Unspecified
	Primary	Secondary	Ca in situ			

Neoplasm, neoplastic — continued

	Primary	Secondary	Ca in situ	Benign	Uncertain Behavior	Unspecified
eyebrow — *continued*						
basal cell carcinoma	173.31	—	—	—	—	—
specified type NEC	173.39	—	—	—	—	—
squamous cell carcinoma	173.32	—	—	—	—	—
eyelid (lower) (skin) (upper)	173.10	198.2	232.1	216.1	238.2	239.2
basal cell carcinoma	173.11	—	—	—	—	—
cartilage	171.0	198.89	—	215.0	238.1	239.2
specified type NEC	173.19	—	—	—	—	—
squamous cell carcinoma	173.12	—	—	—	—	—
eye NEC	190.9	198.4	234.0	224.9	238.8	239.89
contiguous sites	190.8	—	—	—	—	—
specified sites NEC	190.8	198.4	234.0	224.8	238.8	239.89
face NEC*	195.0	198.89	232.3	229.8	238.8	239.89
fallopian tube (accessory)	183.2	198.82	233.39	221.0	236.3	239.5
falx (cerebelli) (cerebri)	192.1	198.4		225.2	237.6	239.7
fascia (*see also* Neoplasm, connective tissue)						
palmar	171.2	198.89	—	215.2	238.1	239.2
plantar	171.3	198.89	—	215.3	238.1	239.2
fatty tissue — *see* Neoplasm, connective tissue						
fauces, faucial NEC	146.9	198.89	230.0	210.6	235.1	239.0
pillars	146.2	198.89	230.0	210.6	235.1	239.0
tonsil	146.0	198.89	230.0	210.5	235.1	239.0
femur (any part)	170.7	198.5	—	213.7	238.0	239.2
fetal membrane	181	198.82	233.2	219.8	236.1	239.5
fibrous tissue — *see* Neoplasm, connective tissue						
fibula (any part)	170.7	198.5	—	213.7	238.0	239.2
filum terminale	192.2	198.3	—	225.3	237.5	239.7
finger NEC*	195.4	198.89	232.6	229.8	238.8	239.89
flank NEC*	195.8	198.89	232.5	229.8	238.8	239.89
follicle, nabothian	180.0	198.82	233.1	219.0	236.0	239.5
foot NEC*	195.5	198.89	232.7	229.8	238.8	239.89
forearm NEC*	195.4	198.89	232.6	229.8	238.8	239.89
forehead (skin)	173.30	198.2	232.3	216.3	238.2	239.2
basal cell carcinoma	173.31	—	—	—	—	—
specified type NEC	173.39	—	—	—	—	—
squamous cell carcinoma	173.32	—	—	—	—	—
foreskin	187.1	198.82	233.5	222.1	236.6	239.5
fornix						
pharyngeal	147.3	198.89	230.0	210.7	235.1	239.0
vagina	184.0	198.82	233.31	221.1	236.3	239.5
fossa (of)						
anterior (cranial)	191.9	198.3	—	225.0	237.5	239.6
cranial	191.9	198.3	—	225.0	237.5	239.6
ischiorectal	195.3	198.89	234.8	229.8	238.8	239.89
middle (cranial)	191.9	198.3	—	225.0	237.5	239.6
pituitary	194.3	198.89	234.8	227.3	237.0	239.7
posterior (cranial)	191.9	198.3	—	225.0	237.5	239.6
pterygoid	171.0	198.89	—	215.0	238.1	239.2
pyriform	148.1	198.89	230.0	210.8	235.1	239.0
Rosenmüller	147.2	198.89	230.0	210.7	235.1	239.0
tonsillar	146.1	198.89	230.0	210.6	235.1	239.0
fourchette	184.4	198.82	233.32	221.2	236.3	239.5
frenulum						
labii — *see* Neoplasm, lip, internal						

Neoplasm, neoplastic — continued

	Primary	Secondary	Ca in situ	Benign	Uncertain Behavior	Unspecified
frenulum — *continued*						
linguae	141.3	198.89	230.0	210.1	235.1	239.0
frontal						
bone	170.0	198.5	—	213.0	238.0	239.2
lobe, brain	191.1	198.3	—	225.0	237.5	239.6
meninges	192.1	198.4	—	225.2	237.6	239.7
pole	191.1	198.3	—	225.0	237.5	239.6
sinus	160.4	197.3	231.8	212.0	235.9	239.1
fundus						
stomach	151.3	197.8	230.2	211.1	235.2	239.0
uterus	182.0	198.82	233.2	219.1	236.0	239.5
gallbladder	156.0	197.8	230.8	211.5	235.3	239.0
contiguous sites with extrahepatic bile ducts	156.8	—	—	—	—	—
gall duct (extrahepatic)	156.1	197.8	230.8	211.5	235.3	239.0
intrahepatic	155.1	197.8	230.8	211.5	235.3	239.0
ganglia (*see also* Neoplasm, connective tissue)	171.9	198.89	—	215.9	238.1	239.2
basal	191.0	198.3	—	225.0	237.5	239.6
ganglion (*see also* Neoplasm, connective tissue)	171.9	198.89	—	215.9	238.1	239.2
cranial nerve	192.0	198.4	—	225.1	237.9	239.7
Gartner's duct	184.0	198.82	233.31	221.1	236.3	239.5
gastric — *see* Neoplasm, stomach						
gastrocolic	159.8	197.8	230.9	211.9	235.5	239.0
gastroesophageal junction	151.0	197.8	230.2	211.1	235.2	239.0
gastrointestinal (tract) NEC	159.9	197.8	230.9	211.9	235.5	239.0
generalized	199.0	—	234.9	229.9	238.9	—
genital organ or tract						
female NEC	184.9	198.82	233.39	221.9	236.3	239.5
contiguous sites	184.8	—	—	—	—	—
specified site NEC	184.8	198.82	233.39	221.8	236.3	239.5
male NEC	187.9	198.82	233.6	222.9	236.6	239.5
contiguous sites	187.8	—	—	—	—	—
specified site NEC	187.8	198.82	233.6	222.8	236.6	239.5
genitourinary tract						
female	184.9	198.82	233.39	221.9	236.3	239.5
male	187.9	198.82	233.6	222.9	236.6	239.5
gingiva (alveolar) (marginal)	143.9	198.89	230.0	210.4	235.1	239.0
lower	143.1	198.89	230.0	210.4	235.1	239.0
mandibular	143.1	198.89	230.0	210.4	235.1	239.0
maxillary	143.0	198.89	230.0	210.4	235.1	239.0
upper	143.0	198.89	230.0	210.4	235.1	239.0
gland, glandular (lymphatic) (system) (*see also* Neoplasm, lymph gland)						
endocrine NEC	194.9	198.89		227.9	237.4	239.7
salivary — *see* Neoplasm, salivary, gland						
glans penis	187.2	198.82	233.5	222.1	236.6	239.5
globus pallidus	191.0	198.3	—	225.0	237.5	239.6
glomus						
coccygeal	194.6	198.89	—	227.6	237.3	239.7
jugularis	194.6	198.89	—	227.6	237.3	239.7
glosso-epiglottic fold(s)	146.4	198.89	230.0	210.6	235.1	239.0
glossopalatine fold	146.2	198.89	230.0	210.6	235.1	239.0
glossopharyngeal sulcus	146.1	198.89	230.0	210.6	235.1	239.0

	Malignant					
	Primary	Secondary	Ca in situ	Benign	Uncertain Behavior	Unspecified
Neoplasm, neoplastic— *continued*						
glottis	161.0	197.3	231.0	212.1	235.6	239.1
gluteal region*	195.3	198.89	232.5	229.8	238.8	239.89
great vessels NEC	171.4	198.89	—	215.4	238.1	239.2
groin NEC	195.3	198.89	232.5	229.8	238.8	239.89
gum	143.9	198.89	230.0	210.4	235.1	239.0
contiguous sites	143.8	—	—	—	—	—
lower	143.1	198.89	230.0	210.4	235.1	239.0
upper	143.0	198.89	230.0	210.4	235.1	239.0
hand NEC*	195.4	198.89	232.6	229.8	238.8	239.89
head NEC*	195.0	198.89	232.4	229.8	238.8	239.89
heart	164.1	198.89	—	212.7	238.8	239.89
contiguous sites with mediastinum or thymus	164.8	—	—	—	—	—
heel NEC*	195.5	198.89	232.7	229.8	238.8	239.89
helix (*see also* Neoplasm, skin, ear)	173.20	198.2	232.2	216.2	238.2	239.2
hematopoietic, hemopoietic tissue NEC	202.8	198.89	—	—	—	238.79
hemisphere, cerebral	191.0	198.3	—	225.0	237.5	239.6
hemorrhoidal zone	154.2	197.5	230.5	211.4	235.5	239.0
hepatic	155.2	197.7	230.8	211.5	235.3	239.0
duct (bile)	156.1	197.8	230.8	211.5	235.3	239.0
flexure (colon)	153.0	197.5	230.3	211.3	235.2	239.0
primary	155.0	—	—	—	—	—
hilus of lung	162.2	197.0	231.2	212.3	235.7	239.1
hippocampus, brain	191.2	198.3	—	225.0	237.5	239.6
hip NEC*	195.5	198.89	232.7	229.8	238.8	239.89
humerus (any part)	170.4	198.5	—	213.4	238.0	239.2
hymen	184.0	198.82	233.31	221.1	236.3	239.5
hypopharynx, hypopharyngeal NEC	148.9	198.89	230.0	210.8	235.1	239.0
contiguous sites	148.8	—	—	—	—	—
postcricoid region	148.0	198.89	230.0	210.8	235.1	239.0
posterior wall	148.3	198.89	230.0	210.8	235.1	239.0
pyriform fossa (sinus)	148.1	198.89	230.0	210.8	235.1	239.0
specified site NEC	148.8	198.89	230.0	210.8	235.1	239.0
wall	148.9	198.89	230.0	210.8	235.1	239.0
posterior	148.3	198.89	230.0	210.8	235.1	239.0
hypophysis	194.3	198.89	234.8	227.3	237.0	239.7
hypothalamus	191.0	198.3	—	225.0	237.5	239.6
ileocecum, ileocecal (coil) (junction) (valve)	153.4	197.5	230.3	211.3	235.2	239.0
ileum	152.2	197.4	230.7	211.2	235.2	239.0
ilium	170.6	198.5	—	213.6	238.0	239.2
immunoproliferative NEC	203.8	—	—	—	—	—
infraclavicular (region)*	195.1	198.89	232.5	229.8	238.8	239.89
inguinal (region)*	195.3	198.89	232.5	229.8	238.8	239.89
insula	191.0	198.3	—	225.0	237.5	239.6
insular tissue (pancreas)	157.4	197.8	230.9	211.7	235.5	239.0
brain	191.0	198.3	—	225.0	237.5	239.6
interarytenoid fold	148.2	198.89	230.0	210.8	235.1	239.0
hypopharyngeal aspect	148.2	198.89	230.0	210.8	235.1	239.0
laryngeal aspect	161.1	197.3	231.0	212.1	235.6	239.1
marginal zone	148.2	198.89	230.0	210.8	235.1	239.0
interdental papillae	143.9	198.89	230.0	210.4	235.1	239.0
lower	143.1	198.89	230.0	210.4	235.1	239.0
upper	143.0	198.89	230.0	210.4	235.1	239.0
internal capsule	191.0	198.3	—	225.0	237.5	239.6
os (cervix)	180.0	198.82	233.1	219.0	236.0	239.5
Neoplasm, neoplastic— *continued*						
intervertebral cartilage or disc	170.2	198.5	—	213.2	238.0	239.2
intestine, intestinal	159.0	197.8	230.7	211.9	235.2	239.0
large	153.9	197.5	230.3	211.3	235.2	239.0
appendix	153.5	197.5	230.3	211.3	235.2	239.0
caput coli	153.4	197.5	230.3	211.3	235.2	239.0
cecum	153.4	197.5	230.3	211.3	235.2	239.0
colon	153.9	197.5	230.3	211.3	235.2	239.0
and rectum	154.0	197.5	230.4	211.4	235.2	239.0
ascending	153.6	197.5	230.3	211.3	235.2	239.0
caput	153.4	197.5	230.3	211.3	235.2	239.0
contiguous sites	153.8	—	—	—	—	—
descending	153.2	197.5	230.3	211.3	235.2	239.0
distal	153.2	197.5	230.3	211.3	235.2	239.0
left	153.2	197.5	230.3	211.3	235.2	239.0
pelvic	153.3	197.5	230.3	211.3	235.2	239.0
right	153.6	197.5	230.3	211.3	235.2	239.0
sigmoid (flexure)	153.3	197.5	230.3	211.3	235.2	239.0
transverse	153.1	197.5	230.3	211.3	235.2	239.0
contiguous sites	153.8	—	—	—	—	—
hepatic flexure	153.0	197.5	230.3	211.3	235.2	239.0
ileocecum, ileocecal (coil) (valve)	153.4	197.5	230.3	211.3	235.2	239.0
sigmoid flexure (lower) (upper)	153.3	197.5	230.3	211.3	235.2	239.0
splenic flexure	153.7	197.5	230.3	211.3	235.2	239.0
small	152.9	197.4	230.7	211.2	235.2	239.0
contiguous sites	152.8	—	—	—	—	—
duodenum	152.0	197.4	230.7	211.2	235.2	239.0
ileum	152.2	197.4	230.7	211.2	235.2	239.0
jejunum	152.1	197.4	230.7	211.2	235.2	239.0
tract NEC	159.0	197.8	230.7	211.9	235.2	239.0
intra-abdominal	195.2	198.89	234.8	229.8	238.8	239.89
intracranial NEC	191.9	198.3	—	225.0	237.5	239.6
intrahepatic (bile) duct	155.1	197.8	230.8	211.5	235.3	239.0
intraocular	190.0	198.4	234.0	224.0	238.8	239.89
intraorbital	190.1	198.4	234.0	224.1	238.8	239.89
intrasellar	194.3	198.89	234.8	227.3	237.0	239.7
intrathoracic (cavity) (organs NEC)	195.1	198.89	234.8	229.8	238.8	239.89
contiguous sites with respiratory organs	165.8	—	—	—	—	—
iris	190.0	198.4	234.0	224.0	238.8	239.89
ischiorectal (fossa)	195.3	198.89	234.8	229.8	238.8	239.89
ischium	170.6	198.5	—	213.6	238.0	239.2
island of Reil	191.0	198.3	—	225.0	237.5	239.6
islands or islets of Langerhans	157.4	197.8	230.9	211.7	235.5	239.0
isthmus uteri	182.1	198.82	233.2	219.1	236.0	239.5
jaw	195.0	198.89	234.8	229.8	238.8	239.89
bone	170.1	198.5	—	213.1	238.0	239.2
carcinoma	143.9	—	—	—	—	—
lower	143.1	—	—	—	—	—
upper	143.0	—	—	—	—	—
lower	170.1	198.5	—	213.1	238.0	239.2
upper	170.0	198.5	—	213.0	238.0	239.2
carcinoma (any type) (lower) (upper)	195.0	—	—	—	—	—
skin (*see also* Neoplasm, skin, face)	173.30	198.2	232.3	216.3	238.2	239.2
soft tissues	143.9	198.89	230.0	210.4	235.1	239.0
lower	143.1	198.89	230.0	210.4	235.1	239.0
upper	143.0	198.89	230.0	210.4	235.1	239.0
jejunum	152.1	197.4	230.7	211.2	235.2	239.0

☑ **Additional Digit Required — Refer to the Tabular List for Digit Selection**

▽ **Subterms under main terms may continue to next column or page**

Neoplasm, joint — Neoplasm, lobe

Neoplasm, neoplastic—continued	Primary	Secondary	Ca in situ	Benign	Uncertain Behavior	Unspecified
joint NEC (see also Neoplasm, bone)	170.9	198.5	—	213.9	238.0	239.2
acromioclavicular	170.4	198.5	—	213.4	238.0	239.2
bursa or synovial membrane — see Neoplasm, connective tissue						
costovertebral	170.3	198.5	—	213.3	238.0	239.2
sternocostal	170.3	198.5	—	213.3	238.0	239.2
temporomandibular	170.1	198.5	—	213.1	238.0	239.2
junction						
anorectal	154.8	197.5	230.7	211.4	235.5	239.0
cardioesophageal	151.0	197.8	230.2	211.1	235.2	239.0
esophagogastric	151.0	197.8	230.2	211.1	235.2	239.0
gastroesophageal	151.0	197.8	230.2	211.1	235.2	239.0
hard and soft palate	145.5	198.89	230.0	210.4	235.1	239.0
ileocecal	153.4	197.5	230.3	211.3	235.2	239.0
pelvirectal	154.0	197.5	230.4	211.4	235.2	239.0
pelviureteric	189.1	198.0	233.9	223.1	236.91	239.5
rectosigmoid	154.0	197.5	230.4	211.4	235.2	239.0
squamocolumnar, of cervix	180.8	198.82	233.1	219.0	236.0	239.5
kidney (parenchyma)	189.0	198.0	233.9	223.0	236.91	239.5
calyx	189.1	198.0	233.9	223.1	236.91	239.5
hilus	189.1	198.0	233.9	223.1	236.91	239.5
pelvis	189.1	198.0	233.9	223.1	236.91	239.5
knee NEC*	195.5	198.89	232.7	229.8	238.8	239.89
labia (skin)	184.4	198.82	233.32	221.2	236.3	239.5
majora	184.1	198.82	233.32	221.2	236.3	239.5
minora	184.2	198.82	233.32	221.2	236.3	239.5
labial (see also Neoplasm, lip)						
sulcus (lower) (upper)	145.1	198.89	230.0	210.4	235.1	239.0
labium (skin)	184.4	198.82	233.32	221.2	236.3	239.5
majus	184.1	198.82	233.32	221.2	236.3	239.5
minus	184.2	198.82	233.32	221.2	236.3	239.5
lacrimal						
canaliculi	190.7	198.4	234.0	224.7	238.8	239.89
duct (nasal)	190.7	198.4	234.0	224.7	238.8	239.89
gland	190.2	198.4	234.0	224.2	238.8	239.89
punctum	190.7	198.4	234.0	224.7	238.8	239.89
sac	190.7	198.4	234.0	224.7	238.8	239.89
Langerhans, islands or islets	157.4	197.8	230.9	211.7	235.5	239.0
laryngopharynx	148.9	198.89	230.0	210.8	235.1	239.0
larynx, laryngeal						
NEC	161.9	197.3	231.0	212.1	235.6	239.1
aryepiglottic fold	161.1	197.3	231.0	212.1	235.6	239.1
cartilage (arytenoid) (cricoid) (cuneiform) (thyroid)	161.3	197.3	231.0	212.1	235.6	239.1
commissure (anterior) (posterior)	161.0	197.3	231.0	212.1	235.6	239.1
contiguous sites	161.8	—	—	—	—	—
extrinsic NEC	161.1	197.3	231.0	212.1	235.6	239.1
meaning hypopharynx	148.9	198.89	230.0	210.8	235.1	239.0
interarytenoid fold	161.1	197.3	231.0	212.1	235.6	239.1
intrinsic	161.0	197.3	231.0	212.1	235.6	239.1
ventricular band	161.1	197.3	231.0	212.1	235.6	239.1
leg NEC*	195.5	198.89	232.7	229.8	238.8	239.89
lens, crystalline	190.0	198.4	234.0	224.0	238.8	239.89
lid (lower) (upper)	173.10	198.2	232.1	216.1	238.2	239.2
basal cell carcinoma	173.11	—	—	—	—	—
specified type NEC	173.19	—	—	—	—	—
squamous cell carcinoma	173.12	—	—	—	—	—

Neoplasm, neoplastic—continued	Primary	Secondary	Ca in situ	Benign	Uncertain Behavior	Unspecified
ligament (see also Neoplasm, connective tissue)						
broad	183.3	198.82	233.39	221.0	236.3	239.5
Mackenrodt's	183.8	198.82	233.39	221.8	236.3	239.5
non-uterine — see Neoplasm, connective tissue						
round	183.5	198.82	—	221.0	236.3	239.5
sacro-uterine	183.4	198.82	—	221.0	236.3	239.5
uterine	183.4	198.82	—	221.0	236.3	239.5
utero-ovarian	183.8	198.82	233.39	221.8	236.3	239.5
uterosacral	183.4	198.82	—	221.0	236.3	239.5
limb*	195.8	198.89	232.8	229.8	238.8	239.89
lower*	195.5	198.89	232.7	229.8	238.8	239.89
upper*	195.4	198.89	232.6	229.8	238.8	239.89
limbus of cornea	190.4	198.4	234.0	224.4	238.8	239.89
lingual NEC (see also Neoplasm, tongue)	141.9	198.89	230.0	210.1	235.1	239.0
lingula, lung	162.3	197.0	231.2	212.3	235.7	239.1
lip (external) (lipstick area) (vermillion border)	140.9	198.89	230.0	210.0	235.1	239.0
buccal aspect — see Neoplasm, lip, internal						
commissure	140.6	198.89	230.0	210.4	235.1	239.0
contiguous sites	140.8	—	—	—	—	—
with oral cavity or pharynx	149.8	—	—	—	—	—
frenulum — see Neoplasm, lip, internal						
inner aspect — see Neoplasm, lip, internal						
internal (buccal) (frenulum) (mucosa) (oral)	140.5	198.89	230.0	210.0	235.1	239.0
lower	140.4	198.89	230.0	210.0	235.1	239.0
upper	140.3	198.89	230.0	210.0	235.1	239.0
lower	140.1	198.89	230.0	210.0	235.1	239.0
internal (buccal) (frenulum) (mucosa) (oral)	140.4	198.89	230.0	210.0	235.1	239.0
mucosa — see Neoplasm, lip, internal						
oral aspect — see Neoplasm, lip, internal						
skin (commissure) (lower) (upper)	173.00	198.2	232.0	216.0	238.2	239.2
basal cell carcinoma	173.01	—	—	—	—	—
specified type NEC	173.09	—	—	—	—	—
squamous cell carcinoma	173.02	—	—	—	—	—
upper	140.0	198.89	230.0	210.0	235.1	239.0
internal (buccal) (frenulum) (mucosa) (oral)	140.3	198.89	230.0	210.0	235.1	239.0
liver	155.2	197.7	230.8	211.5	235.3	239.0
primary	155.0	—	—	—	—	—
lobe						
azygos	162.3	197.0	231.2	212.3	235.7	239.1
frontal	191.1	198.3	—	225.0	237.5	239.6
lower	162.5	197.0	231.2	212.3	235.7	239.1
middle	162.4	197.0	231.2	212.3	235.7	239.1
occipital	191.4	198.3	—	225.0	237.5	239.6

☑ Additional Digit Required — Refer to the Tabular List for Digit Selection

▽ Subterms under main terms may continue to next column or page

Neoplasm, neoplastic—	Malignant			Benign	Uncertain Behavior	Unspecified
	Primary	Secondary	Ca in situ			
continued						
lobe — *continued*						
parietal	191.3	198.3	—	225.0	237.5	239.6
temporal	191.2	198.3	—	225.0	237.5	239.6
upper	162.3	197.0	231.2	212.3	235.7	239.1
lumbosacral plexus	171.6	198.4	—	215.6	238.1	239.2
lung	162.9	197.0	231.2	212.3	235.7	239.1
azygos lobe	162.3	197.0	231.2	212.3	235.7	239.1
carina	162.2	197.0	231.2	212.3	235.7	239.1
contiguous sites with bronchus or trachea	162.8	—	—	—	—	—
hilus	162.2	197.0	231.2	212.3	235.7	239.1
lingula	162.3	197.0	231.2	212.3	235.7	239.1
lobe NEC	162.9	197.0	231.2	212.3	235.7	239.1
lower lobe	162.5	197.0	231.2	212.3	235.7	239.1
main bronchus	162.2	197.0	231.2	212.3	235.7	239.1
middle lobe	162.4	197.0	231.2	212.3	235.7	239.1
upper lobe	162.3	197.0	231.2	212.3	235.7	239.1
lymph, lymphatic channel NEC (*see also* Neoplasm, connective tissue)	171.9	198.89	—	215.9	238.1	239.2
gland						
(secondary)	—	196.9	—	229.0	238.8	239.89
abdominal	—	196.2	—	229.0	238.8	239.89
aortic	—	196.2	—	229.0	238.8	239.89
arm	—	196.3	—	229.0	238.8	239.89
auricular (anterior) (posterior)	—	196.0	—	229.0	238.8	239.89
axilla, axillary	—	196.3	—	229.0	238.8	239.89
brachial	—	196.3	—	229.0	238.8	239.89
bronchial	—	196.1	—	229.0	238.8	239.89
bronchopulmonary	—	196.1	—	229.0	238.8	239.89
celiac	—	196.2	—	229.0	238.8	239.89
cervical	—	196.0	—	229.0	238.8	239.89
cervicofacial	—	196.0	—	229.0	238.8	239.89
Cloquet	—	196.5	—	229.0	238.8	239.89
colic	—	196.2	—	229.0	238.8	239.89
common duct	—	196.2	—	229.0	238.8	239.89
cubital	—	196.3	—	229.0	238.8	239.89
diaphragmatic	—	196.1	—	229.0	238.8	239.89
epigastric, inferior	—	196.6	—	229.0	238.8	239.89
epitrochlear	—	196.3	—	229.0	238.8	239.89
esophageal	—	196.1	—	229.0	238.8	239.89
face	—	196.0	—	229.0	238.8	239.89
femoral	—	196.5	—	229.0	238.8	239.89
gastric	—	196.2	—	229.0	238.8	239.89
groin	—	196.5	—	229.0	238.8	239.89
head	—	196.0	—	229.0	238.8	239.89
hepatic	—	196.2	—	229.0	238.8	239.89
hilar (pulmonary)	—	196.1	—	229.0	238.8	239.89
splenic	—	196.2	—	229.0	238.8	239.89
hypogastric	—	196.6	—	229.0	238.8	239.89
ileocolic	—	196.2	—	229.0	238.8	239.89
iliac	—	196.6	—	229.0	238.8	239.89
infraclavicular	—	196.3	—	229.0	238.8	239.89
inguina, inguinal	—	196.5	—	229.0	238.8	239.89
innominate	—	196.1	—	229.0	238.8	239.89
intercostal	—	196.1	—	229.0	238.8	239.89
intestinal	—	196.2	—	229.0	238.8	239.89
intra-abdominal	—	196.2	—	229.0	238.8	239.89
intrapelvic	—	196.6	—	229.0	238.8	239.89
intrathoracic	—	196.1	—	229.0	238.8	239.9
jugular	—	196.0	—	229.0	238.8	239.89
leg	—	196.5	—	229.0	238.8	239.89
limb						
lower	—	196.5	—	229.0	238.8	239.9
upper	—	196.3	—	229.0	238.8	239.89
lower limb	—	196.5	—	229.0	238.8	239.9
lumbar	—	196.2	—	229.0	238.8	239.89

Neoplasm, neoplastic—	Malignant			Benign	Uncertain Behavior	Unspecified
	Primary	Secondary	Ca in situ			
continued						
lymph, lymphatic — *continued*						
gland — *continued*						
mandibular	—	196.0	—	229.0	238.8	239.89
mediastinal	—	196.1	—	229.0	238.8	239.89
mesenteric (inferior) (superior)	—	196.2	—	229.0	238.8	239.89
midcolic	—	196.2	—	229.0	238.8	239.89
multiple sites in categories 196.0–196.6	—	196.8	—	229.0	238.8	239.89
neck	—	196.0	—	229.0	238.8	239.89
obturator	—	196.6	—	229.0	238.8	239.89
occipital	—	196.0	—	229.0	238.8	239.89
pancreatic	—	196.2	—	229.0	238.8	239.89
para-aortic	—	196.2	—	229.0	238.8	239.89
paracervical	—	196.6	—	229.0	238.8	239.89
parametrial	—	196.6	—	229.0	238.8	239.89
parasternal	—	196.1	—	229.0	238.8	239.89
parotid	—	196.0	—	229.0	238.8	239.89
pectoral	—	196.3	—	229.0	238.8	239.89
pelvic	—	196.6	—	229.0	238.8	239.89
peri-aortic	—	196.2	—	229.0	238.8	239.89
peripancreatic	—	196.2	—	229.0	238.8	239.89
popliteal	—	196.5	—	229.0	238.8	239.89
porta hepatis	—	196.2	—	229.0	238.8	239.89
portal	—	196.2	—	229.0	238.8	239.89
preauricular	—	196.0	—	229.0	238.8	239.89
prelaryngeal	—	196.0	—	229.0	238.8	239.89
presymphysial	—	196.6	—	229.0	238.8	239.89
pretracheal	—	196.0	—	229.0	238.8	239.89
primary (any site) NEC	202.9	—	—	—	—	—
pulmonary (hiler)	—	196.1	—	229.0	238.8	239.89
pyloric	—	196.2	—	229.0	238.8	239.89
retroperitoneal	—	196.2	—	229.0	238.8	239.89
retropharyngeal	—	196.0	—	229.0	238.8	239.89
Rosenmüller's	—	196.5	—	229.0	238.8	239.89
sacral	—	196.6	—	229.0	238.8	239.89
scalene	—	196.0	—	229.0	238.8	239.89
site NEC	—	196.9	—	229.0	238.8	239.89
splenic (hilar)	—	196.2	—	229.0	238.8	239.89
subclavicular	—	196.3	—	229.0	238.8	239.89
subinguinal	—	196.5	—	229.0	238.8	239.89
sublingual	—	196.0	—	229.0	238.8	239.89
submandibular	—	196.0	—	229.0	238.8	239.89
submaxillary	—	196.0	—	229.0	238.8	239.89
submental	—	196.0	—	229.0	238.8	239.89
subscapular	—	196.3	—	229.0	238.8	239.89
supraclavicular	—	196.0	—	229.0	238.8	239.89
thoracic	—	196.1	—	229.0	238.8	239.89
tibial	—	196.5	—	229.0	238.8	239.89
tracheal	—	196.1	—	229.0	238.8	239.89
tracheobronchial	—	196.1	—	229.0	238.8	239.89
upper limb	—	196.3	—	229.0	238.8	239.89
Virchow's	—	196.0	—	229.0	238.8	239.89
node (*see also* Neoplasm, lymph gland)						
primary NEC	202.9	—	—	—	—	—
vessel (*see also* Neoplasm, connective tissue)	171.9	198.89	—	215.9	238.1	239.2
Mackenrodt's ligament	183.8	198.82	233.39	221.8	236.3	239.5
malar	170.0	198.5	—	213.0	238.0	239.2
region — *see* Neoplasm, cheek						
mammary gland — *see* Neoplasm, breast						
mandible	170.1	198.5	—	213.1	238.0	239.2
alveolar						

☑ **Additional Digit Required — Refer to the Tabular List for Digit Selection**

▽ **Subterms under main terms may continue to next column or page**

Neoplasm, neoplastic — continued

	Malignant					
	Primary	Secondary	Ca in situ	Benign	Uncertain Behavior	Unspecified
mandible — *continued*						
alveolar — *continued*						
mucosa	143.1	198.89	230.0	210.4	235.1	239.0
mucose	143.1	198.89	230.0	210.4	235.1	239.0
ridge or process	170.1	198.5	—	213.1	238.0	239.2
carcinoma	143.1	—	—	—	—	—
carcinoma	143.1	—	—	—	—	—
marrow (bone) NEC	202.9	198.5	—	—	—	238.79
mastectomy site (skin)	173.50	198.2	—			
basal cell carcinoma	173.51	—	—			
specified as breast tissue	174.8	198.81				
specified type NEC	173.59	—	—			
squamous cell carcinoma	173.52	—	—			
mastoid (air cells) (antrum) (cavity)	160.1	197.3	231.8	212.0	235.9	239.1
bone or process	170.0	198.5	—	213.0	238.0	239.2
maxilla, maxillary (superior)	170.0	198.5	—	213.0	238.0	239.2
alveolar						
mucosa	143.0	198.89	230.0	210.4	235.1	239.0
ridge or process	170.0	198.5	—	213.0	238.0	239.2
carcinoma	143.0	—	—	—	—	—
antrum	160.2	197.3	231.8	212.0	235.9	239.1
carcinoma	143.0	—	—	—	—	—
inferior — *see* Neoplasm, mandible						
sinus	160.2	197.3	231.8	212.0	235.9	239.1
meatus						
external (ear) (*see also* Neoplasm, skin, ear)	173.20	198.2	232.2	216.2	238.2	239.2
Meckel's diverticulum	152.3	197.4	230.7	211.2	235.2	239.0
mediastinum, mediastinal	164.9	197.1	—	212.5	235.8	239.89
anterior	164.2	197.1	—	212.5	235.8	239.89
contiguous sites with heart and thymus	164.8	—	—	—	—	—
posterior	164.3	197.1	—	212.5	235.8	239.89
medulla						
adrenal	194.0	198.7	234.8	227.0	237.2	239.7
oblongata	191.7	198.3	—	225.0	237.5	239.6
meibomian gland	173.10	198.2	232.1	216.1	238.2	239.2
basal cell carcinoma	173.11	—	—	—	—	—
specified type NEC	173.19	—	—	—	—	—
squamous cell carcinoma	173.12	—	—	—	—	—
meninges (brain) (cerebral) (cranial) (intracranial)	192.1	198.4		225.0	237.6	239.7
spinal (cord)	192.3	198.4	—	225.4	237.6	239.7
meniscus, knee joint (lateral) (medial)	170.7	198.5	—	213.7	238.0	239.2
mesentery, mesenteric	158.8	197.6	—	211.8	235.4	239.0
mesoappendix	158.8	197.6	—	211.8	235.4	239.0
mesocolon	158.8	197.6	—	211.8	235.4	239.0
mesopharynx — *see* Neoplasm, oropharynx						
mesosalpinx	183.3	198.82	233.39	221.0	236.3	239.5
mesovarium	183.3	198.82	233.39	221.0	236.3	239.5

Neoplasm, neoplastic — continued

	Malignant					
	Primary	Secondary	Ca in situ	Benign	Uncertain Behavior	Unspecified
metacarpus (any bone)	170.5	198.5	—	213.5	238.0	239.2
metastatic NEC (*see also* Neoplasm, by site, secondary)	—	199.1	—	—	—	—
metatarsus (any bone)	170.8	198.5	—	213.8	238.0	239.2
midbrain	191.7	198.3	—	225.0	237.5	239.6
milk duct — *see* Neoplasm, breast						
mons						
pubis	184.4	198.82	233.32	221.2	236.3	239.5
veneris	184.4	198.82	233.32	221.2	236.3	239.5
motor tract	192.9	198.4	—	225.9	237.9	239.7
brain	191.9	198.3	—	225.0	237.5	239.6
spinal	192.2	198.3	—	225.3	237.5	239.7
mouth	145.9	198.89	230.0	210.4	235.1	239.0
contiguous sites	145.8	—	—	—	—	—
floor	144.9	198.89	230.0	210.3	235.1	239.0
anterior portion	144.0	198.89	230.0	210.3	235.1	239.0
contiguous sites	144.8	—	—	—	—	—
lateral portion	144.1	198.89	230.0	210.3	235.1	239.0
roof	145.5	198.89	230.0	210.4	235.1	239.0
specified part NEC	145.8	198.89	230.0	210.4	235.1	239.0
vestibule	145.1	198.89	230.0	210.4	235.1	239.0
mucosa						
alveolar (ridge or process)	143.9	198.89	230.0	210.4	235.1	239.0
lower	143.1	198.89	230.0	210.4	235.1	239.0
upper	143.0	198.89	230.0	210.4	235.1	239.0
buccal	145.0	198.89	230.0	210.4	235.1	239.0
cheek	145.0	198.89	230.0	210.4	235.1	239.0
lip — *see* Neoplasm, lip, internal						
nasal	160.0	197.3	231.8	212.0	235.9	239.1
oral	145.0	198.89	230.0	210.4	235.1	239.0
Müllerian duct						
female	184.8	198.82	233.39	221.8	236.3	239.5
male	187.8	198.82	233.6	222.8	236.6	239.5
multiple sites NEC	199.0	—	234.9	229.9	238.9	—
muscle (*see also* Neoplasm, connective tissue)						
extraocular	190.1	198.4	234.0	224.1	238.8	239.89
myocardium	164.1	198.89	—	212.7	238.8	239.89
myometrium	182.0	198.82	233.2	219.1	236.0	239.5
myopericardium	164.1	198.89	—	212.7	238.8	239.89
nabothian gland (follicle)	180.0	198.82	233.1	219.0	236.0	239.5
nail	173.90	198.2	232.9	216.9	238.2	239.2
finger (*see also* Neoplasm, skin, limb, upper)	173.60	198.2	232.6	216.6	238.2	239.2
toe (*see also* Neoplasm, skin, limb, lower)	173.70	198.2	232.7	216.7	238.2	239.2
nares, naris (anterior) (posterior)	160.0	197.3	231.8	212.0	235.9	239.1
nasal — *see* Neoplasm, nose						
nasolabial groove (*see also* Neoplasm, skin, face)	173.30	198.2	232.3	216.3	238.2	239.2
nasolacrimal duct	190.7	198.4	234.0	224.7	238.8	239.89
nasopharynx, nasopharyngeal	147.9	198.89	230.0	210.7	235.1	239.0
contiguous sites	147.8	—	—	—	—	—
floor	147.3	198.89	230.0	210.7	235.1	239.0
roof	147.0	198.89	230.0	210.7	235.1	239.0
specified site NEC	147.8	198.89	230.0	210.7	235.1	239.0
wall	147.9	198.89	230.0	210.7	235.1	239.0

☑ Additional Digit Required — Refer to the Tabular List for Digit Selection   ▽ Subterms under main terms may continue to next column or page

2014 ICD-9-CM   247

	Malignant			Benign	Uncertain Behavior	Unspecified
	Primary	Secondary	Ca in situ			
Neoplasm, neoplastic — *continued*						
nasopharynx, nasopharyngeal — *continued*						
wall — *continued*						
anterior	147.3	198.89	230.0	210.7	235.1	239.0
lateral	147.2	198.89	230.0	210.7	235.1	239.0
posterior	147.1	198.89	230.0	210.7	235.1	239.0
superior	147.0	198.89	230.0	210.7	235.1	239.0
nates (*see also* Neoplasm, skin, trunk)	173.50	198.2	232.5	216.5	238.2	239.2
neck NEC*	195.0	198.89	234.8	229.8	238.8	239.89
skin	173.40	198.2	232.4	216.4	238.2	239.2
basal cell carcinoma	173.41	—	—	—	—	—
specified type NEC	173.49	—	—	—	—	—
squamous cell carcinoma	173.42	—	—	—	—	—
nerve (autonomic) (ganglion) (parasympathetic) (peripheral) (sympathetic) (*see also* Neoplasm, connective tissue)						
abducens	192.0	198.4	—	225.1	237.9	239.7
accessory (spinal)	192.0	198.4	—	225.1	237.9	239.7
acoustic	192.0	198.4	—	225.1	237.9	239.7
auditory	192.0	198.4	—	225.1	237.9	239.7
brachial	171.2	198.89	—	215.2	238.1	239.2
cranial (any)	192.0	198.4	—	225.1	237.9	239.7
facial	192.0	198.4	—	225.1	237.9	239.7
femoral	171.3	198.89	—	215.3	238.1	239.2
glossopharyngeal	192.0	198.4	—	225.1	237.9	239.7
hypoglossal	192.0	198.4	—	225.1	237.9	239.7
intercostal	171.4	198.89	—	215.4	238.1	239.2
lumbar	171.7	198.89	—	215.7	238.1	239.2
median	171.2	198.89	—	215.2	238.1	239.2
obturator	171.3	198.89	—	215.3	238.1	239.2
oculomotor	192.0	198.4	—	225.1	237.9	239.7
olfactory	192.0	198.4	—	225.1	237.9	239.7
optic	192.0	198.4	—	225.1	237.9	239.7
peripheral NEC	171.9	198.89	—	215.9	238.1	239.2
radial	171.2	198.89	—	215.2	238.1	239.2
sacral	171.6	198.89	—	215.6	238.1	239.2
sciatic	171.3	198.89	—	215.3	238.1	239.2
spinal NEC	171.9	198.89	—	215.9	238.1	239.2
trigeminal	192.0	198.4	—	225.1	237.9	239.7
trochlear	192.0	198.4	—	225.1	237.9	239.7
ulnar	171.2	198.89	—	215.2	238.1	239.2
vagus	192.0	198.4	—	225.1	237.9	239.7
nervous system (central) NEC	192.9	198.4	—	225.9	237.9	239.7
autonomic NEC	171.9	198.89	—	215.9	238.1	239.2
brain (*see also* Neoplasm, brain)						
membrane or meninges	192.1	198.4	—	225.2	237.6	239.7
contiguous sites	192.8	—	—	—	—	—
parasympathetic NEC	171.9	198.89	—	215.9	238.1	239.2
sympathetic NEC	171.9	198.89	—	215.9	238.1	239.2
nipple (female)	174.0	198.81	233.0	217	238.3	239.3
male	175.0	198.81	233.0	217	238.3	239.3
nose, nasal	195.0	198.89	234.8	229.8	238.8	239.89
ala (external) (*see also* Neoplasm, nose, skin)	173.30	198.2	232.3	216.3	238.2	239.2
bone	170.0	198.5	—	213.0	238.0	239.2
cartilage	160.0	197.3	231.8	212.0	235.9	239.1
cavity	160.0	197.3	231.8	212.0	235.9	239.1
contiguous sites with accessory	160.8	—	—	—	—	—

	Malignant			Benign	Uncertain Behavior	Unspecified
	Primary	Secondary	Ca in situ			
Neoplasm, neoplastic — *continued*						
nose, nasal — *continued*						
cavity — *continued*						
contiguous sites with accessory sinuses or middle ear — *continued*						
sinuses or middle ear						
choana	147.3	198.89	230.0	210.7	235.1	239.0
external (skin) (*see also* Neoplasm, nose, skin)	173.30	198.2	232.3	216.3	238.2	239.2
fossa	160.0	197.3	231.8	212.0	235.9	239.1
internal	160.0	197.3	231.8	212.0	235.9	239.1
mucosa	160.0	197.3	231.8	212.0	235.9	239.1
septum	160.0	197.3	231.8	212.0	235.9	239.1
posterior margin	147.3	198.89	230.0	210.7	235.1	239.0
sinus — *see* Neoplasm, sinus						
skin	173.30	198.2	232.3	216.3	238.2	239.2
basal cell carcinoma	173.31	—	—	—	—	—
specified type NEC	173.39	—	—	—	—	—
squamous cell carcinoma	173.32	—	—	—	—	—
turbinate (mucosa)	160.0	197.3	231.8	212.0	235.9	239.1
bone	170.0	198.5	—	213.0	238.0	239.2
vestibule	160.0	197.3	231.8	212.0	235.9	239.1
nostril	160.0	197.3	231.8	212.0	235.9	239.1
nucleus pulposus	170.2	198.5	—	213.2	238.0	239.2
occipital bone	170.0	198.5	—	213.0	238.0	239.2
lobe or pole, brain	191.4	198.3	—	225.0	237.5	239.6
odontogenic — *see* Neoplasm, jaw bone						
oesophagus — *see* Neoplasm, esophagus						
olfactory nerve or bulb	192.0	198.4	—	225.1	237.9	239.7
olive (brain)	191.7	198.3	—	225.0	237.5	239.6
omentum	158.8	197.6	—	211.8	235.4	239.0
operculum (brain)	191.0	198.3	—	225.0	237.5	239.6
optic nerve, chiasm, or tract	192.0	198.4	—	225.1	237.9	239.7
oral (cavity)	145.9	198.89	230.0	210.4	235.1	239.0
contiguous sites with lip or pharynx	149.8	—	—	—	—	—
ill-defined	149.9	198.89	230.0	210.4	235.1	239.0
mucosa	145.9	198.89	230.0	210.4	235.1	239.0
orbit	190.1	198.4	234.0	224.1	238.8	239.89
bone	170.0	198.5	—	213.0	238.0	239.2
eye	190.1	198.4	234.0	224.1	238.8	239.89
soft parts	190.1	198.4	234.0	224.1	238.8	239.89
organ of Zuckerkandl	194.6	198.89	—	227.6	237.3	239.7
oropharynx	146.9	198.89	230.0	210.6	235.1	239.0
branchial cleft (vestige)	146.8	198.89	230.0	210.6	235.1	239.0
contiguous sites	146.8	—	—	—	—	—
junctional region	146.5	198.89	230.0	210.6	235.1	239.0
lateral wall	146.6	198.89	230.0	210.6	235.1	239.0
pillars of fauces	146.2	198.89	230.0	210.6	235.1	239.0
posterior wall	146.7	198.89	230.0	210.6	235.1	239.0
specified part NEC	146.8	198.89	230.0	210.6	235.1	239.0
vallecula	146.3	198.89	230.0	210.6	235.1	239.0
os external	180.1	198.82	233.1	219.0	236.0	239.5

	Malignant			Benign	Uncertain Behavior	Unspecified
	Primary	Secondary	Ca in situ			

Neoplasm, neoplastic — continued

os — continued

	Primary	Secondary	Ca in situ	Benign	Uncertain Behavior	Unspecified
internal	180.0	198.82	233.1	219.0	236.0	239.5
ovary	183.0	198.6	233.39	220	236.2	239.5
oviduct	183.2	198.82	233.39	221.0	236.3	239.5
palate	145.5	198.89	230.0	210.4	235.1	239.0
hard	145.2	198.89	230.0	210.4	235.1	239.0
junction of hard and soft palate	145.5	198.89	230.0	210.4	235.1	239.0
soft	145.3	198.89	230.0	210.4	235.1	239.0
nasopharyngeal surface	147.3	198.89	230.0	210.7	235.1	239.0
posterior surface	147.3	198.89	230.0	210.7	235.1	239.0
superior surface	147.3	198.89	230.0	210.7	235.1	239.0
palatoglossal arch	146.2	198.89	230.0	210.6	235.1	239.0
palatopharyngeal arch	146.2	198.89	230.0	210.6	235.1	239.0
pallium	191.0	198.3	—	225.0	237.5	239.6
palpebra	173.10	198.2	232.1	216.1	238.2	239.2
basal cell carcinoma	173.11	—	—	—	—	—
specified type NEC	173.19	—	—	—	—	—
squamous cell carcinoma	173.12	—	—	—	—	—
pancreas	157.9	197.8	230.9	211.6	235.5	239.0
body	157.1	197.8	230.9	211.6	235.5	239.0
contiguous sites	157.8	—	—	—	—	—
duct (of Santorini) (of Wirsung)	157.3	197.8	230.9	211.6	235.5	239.0
ectopic tissue	157.8	197.8	230.9	211.6	235.5	239.0
head	157.0	197.8	230.9	211.6	235.5	239.0
islet cells	157.4	197.8	230.9	211.7	235.5	239.0
neck	157.8	197.8	230.9	211.6	235.5	239.0
tail	157.2	197.8	230.9	211.6	235.5	239.0
para-aortic body	194.6	198.89	—	227.6	237.3	239.7
paraganglion NEC	194.6	198.89	—	227.6	237.3	239.7
parametrium	183.4	198.82	—	221.0	236.3	239.5
paranephric	158.0	197.6	—	211.8	235.4	239.0
pararectal	195.3	198.89	—	229.8	238.8	239.89
parasagittal (region)	195.0	198.89	234.8	229.8	238.8	239.89
parasellar	192.9	198.4	—	225.9	237.9	239.7
parathyroid (gland)	194.1	198.89	234.8	227.1	237.4	239.7
paraurethral	195.3	198.89	—	229.8	238.8	239.89
gland	189.4	198.1	233.9	223.89	236.99	239.5
paravaginal	195.3	198.89	—	229.8	238.8	239.89
parenchyma, kidney	189.0	198.0	233.9	223.0	236.91	239.5
parietal						
bone	170.0	198.5	—	213.0	238.0	239.2
lobe, brain	191.3	198.3	—	225.0	237.5	239.6
paroophoron	183.3	198.82	233.39	221.0	236.3	239.5
parotid (duct) (gland)	142.0	198.89	230.0	210.2	235.0	239.0
parovarium	183.3	198.82	233.39	221.0	236.3	239.5
patella	170.8	198.5	—	213.8	238.0	239.2
peduncle, cerebral	191.7	198.3	—	225.0	237.5	239.6
pelvirectal junction	154.0	197.5	230.4	211.4	235.2	239.0
pelvis, pelvic	195.3	198.89	234.8	229.8	238.8	239.89
bone	170.6	198.5	—	213.6	238.0	239.2
floor	195.3	198.89	234.8	229.8	238.8	239.89
renal	189.1	198.0	233.9	223.1	236.91	239.5
viscera	195.3	198.89	234.8	229.8	238.8	239.89
wall	195.3	198.89	234.8	229.8	238.8	239.89
pelvo-abdominal	195.8	198.89	234.8	229.8	238.8	239.89
penis	187.4	198.82	233.5	222.1	236.6	239.5
body	187.3	198.82	233.5	222.1	236.6	239.5
corpus (cavernosum)	187.3	198.82	233.5	222.1	236.6	239.5
glans	187.2	198.82	233.5	222.1	236.6	239.5
skin NEC	187.4	198.82	233.5	222.1	236.6	239.5
periadrenal (tissue)	158.0	197.6	—	211.8	235.4	239.0

Neoplasm, neoplastic — continued

	Primary	Secondary	Ca in situ	Benign	Uncertain Behavior	Unspecified
perianal (skin) (see also Neoplasm, skin, anus)	173.50	198.2	232.5	216.5	238.2	239.2
pericardium	164.1	198.89	—	212.7	238.8	239.89
perinephric	158.0	197.6	—	211.8	235.4	239.0
perineum	195.3	198.89	234.8	229.8	238.8	239.89
periodontal tissue NEC	143.9	198.89	230.0	210.4	235.1	239.0
periosteum — see Neoplasm, bone						
peripancreatic	158.0	197.6	—	211.8	235.4	239.0
peripheral nerve NEC	171.9	198.89	—	215.9	238.1	239.2
perirectal (tissue)	195.3	198.89	—	229.8	238.8	239.89
perirenal (tissue)	158.0	197.6	—	211.8	235.4	239.0
peritoneum, peritoneal (cavity)	158.9	197.6	—	211.8	235.4	239.0
contiguous sites	158.8	—	—	—	—	—
with digestive organs	159.8	—	—	—	—	—
parietal	158.8	197.6	—	211.8	235.4	239.0
pelvic	158.8	197.6	—	211.8	235.4	239.0
specified part NEC	158.8	197.6	—	211.8	235.4	239.0
peritonsillar (tissue)	195.3	198.89	234.8	229.8	238.8	239.89
periurethral tissue	195.3	198.89	—	229.8	238.8	239.89
phalanges	170.9	198.5	—	213.9	238.0	239.2
foot	170.8	198.5	—	213.8	238.0	239.2
hand	170.5	198.5	—	213.5	238.0	239.2
pharynx, pharyngeal	149.0	198.89	230.0	210.9	235.1	239.0
bursa	147.1	198.89	230.0	210.7	235.1	239.0
fornix	147.3	198.89	230.0	210.7	235.1	239.0
recess	147.2	198.89	230.0	210.7	235.1	239.0
region	149.0	198.89	230.0	210.9	235.1	239.0
tonsil	147.1	198.89	230.0	210.7	235.1	239.0
wall (lateral) (posterior)	149.0	198.89	230.0	210.9	235.1	239.0
pia mater (cerebral) (cranial)	192.1	198.4	—	225.2	237.6	239.7
spinal	192.3	198.4	—	225.4	237.6	239.7
pillars of fauces	146.2	198.89	230.0	210.6	235.1	239.0
pineal (body) (gland)	194.4	198.89	234.8	227.4	237.1	239.7
pinna (ear) NEC (see also Neoplasm, skin, ear)	173.20	198.2	232.2	216.2	238.2	239.2
cartilage	171.0	198.89	—	215.0	238.1	239.2
piriform fossa or sinus	148.1	198.89	230.0	210.8	235.1	239.0
pituitary (body) (fossa) (gland) (lobe)	194.3	198.89	234.8	227.3	237.0	239.7
placenta	181	198.82	233.2	219.8	236.1	239.5
pleura, pleural (cavity)	163.9	197.2	—	212.4	235.8	239.1
contiguous sites	163.8	—	—	—	—	—
parietal	163.0	197.2	—	212.4	235.8	239.1
visceral	163.1	197.2	—	212.4	235.8	239.1
plexus						
brachial	171.2	198.89	—	215.2	238.1	239.2
cervical	171.0	198.89	—	215.0	238.1	239.2
choroid	191.5	198.3	—	225.0	237.5	239.6
lumbosacral	171.6	198.89	—	215.6	238.1	239.2
sacral	171.6	198.89	—	215.6	238.1	239.2
pluri-endocrine	194.8	198.89	234.8	227.8	237.4	239.7
pole						
frontal	191.1	198.3	—	225.0	237.5	239.6
occipital	191.4	198.3	—	225.0	237.5	239.6
pons (varolii)	191.7	198.3	—	225.0	237.5	239.6
popliteal fossa or space*	195.5	198.89	234.8	229.8	238.8	239.89
postcricoid (region)	148.0	198.89	230.0	210.8	235.1	239.0

☑ **Additional Digit Required — Refer to the Tabular List for Digit Selection**

▽ **Subterms under main terms may continue to next column or page**

Neoplasm, neoplastic— continued	Malignant			Benign	Uncertain Behavior	Unspecified
	Primary	Secondary	Ca in situ			
posterior fossa (cranial)	191.9	198.3	—	225.0	237.5	239.6
postnasal space	147.9	198.89	230.0	210.7	235.1	239.0
prepuce	187.1	198.82	233.5	222.1	236.6	239.5
prepylorus	151.1	197.8	230.2	211.1	235.2	239.0
presacral (region)	195.3	198.89	—	229.8	238.8	239.89
prostate (gland)	185	198.82	233.4	222.2	236.5	239.5
utricle	189.3	198.1	233.9	223.81	236.99	239.5
pterygoid fossa	171.0	198.89	—	215.0	238.1	239.2
pubic bone	170.6	198.5	—	213.6	238.0	239.2
pudenda, pudendum (female)	184.4	198.82	233.32	221.2	236.3	239.5
pulmonary	162.9	197.0	231.2	212.3	235.7	239.1
putamen	191.0	198.3	—	225.0	237.5	239.6
pyloric						
antrum	151.2	197.8	230.2	211.1	235.2	239.0
canal	151.1	197.8	230.2	211.1	235.2	239.0
pylorus	151.1	197.8	230.2	211.1	235.2	239.0
pyramid (brain)	191.7	198.3	—	225.0	237.5	239.6
pyriform fossa or sinus	148.1	198.89	230.0	210.8	235.1	239.0
radius (any part)	170.4	198.5	—	213.4	238.0	239.2
Rathke's pouch	194.3	198.89	234.8	227.3	237.0	239.7
rectosigmoid (colon) (junction)	154.0	197.5	230.4	211.4	235.2	239.0
contiguous sites with anus or rectum	154.8	—	—	—	—	—
rectouterine pouch	158.8	197.6	—	211.8	235.4	239.0
rectovaginal septum or wall	195.3	198.89	234.8	229.8	238.8	239.89
rectovesical septum	195.3	198.89	234.8	229.8	238.8	239.89
rectum (ampulla)	154.1	197.5	230.4	211.4	235.2	239.0
and colon	154.0	197.5	230.4	211.4	235.2	239.0
contiguous sites with anus or rectosigmoid junction	154.8	—	—	—	—	—
renal	189.0	198.0	233.9	223.0	236.91	239.5
calyx	189.1	198.0	233.9	223.1	236.91	239.5
hilus	189.1	198.0	233.9	223.1	236.91	239.5
parenchyma	189.0	198.0	233.9	223.0	236.91	239.5
pelvis	189.1	198.0	233.9	223.1	236.91	239.5
respiratory						
organs or system NEC	165.9	197.3	231.9	212.9	235.9	239.1
contiguous sites with intrathoracic organs	165.8	—	—	—	—	—
specified sites NEC	165.8	197.3	231.8	212.8	235.9	239.1
tract NEC	165.9	197.3	231.9	212.9	235.9	239.1
upper	165.0	197.3	231.9	212.9	235.9	239.1
retina	190.5	198.4	234.0	224.5	238.8	239.81
retrobulbar	190.1	198.4	—	224.1	238.8	239.89
retrocecal	158.0	197.6	—	211.8	235.4	239.0
retromolar (area) (triangle) (trigone)	145.6	198.89	230.0	210.4	235.1	239.0
retro-orbital	195.0	198.89	234.8	229.8	238.8	239.89
retroperitoneal (space) (tissue)	158.0	197.6	—	211.8	235.4	239.0
contiguous sites	158.8	—	—	—	—	—
retroperitoneum	158.0	197.6	—	211.8	235.4	239.0
contiguous sites	158.8	—	—	—	—	—
retropharyngeal	149.0	198.89	230.0	210.9	235.1	239.0
retrovesical (septum)	195.3	198.89	234.8	229.8	238.8	239.89
rhinencephalon	191.0	198.3	—	225.0	237.5	239.6
rib	170.3	198.5	—	213.3	238.0	239.2
Rosenmüller's fossa	147.2	198.89	230.0	210.7	235.1	239.0
round ligament	183.5	198.82	—	221.0	236.3	239.5

Neoplasm, neoplastic— continued	Malignant			Benign	Uncertain Behavior	Unspecified
	Primary	Secondary	Ca in situ			
sacrococcyx, sacrococcygeal	170.6	198.5	—	213.6	238.0	239.2
region	195.3	198.89	234.8	229.8	238.8	239.89
sacrouterine ligament	183.4	198.82	—	221.0	236.3	239.5
sacrum, sacral (vertebra)	170.6	198.5	—	213.6	238.0	239.2
salivary gland or duct (major)	142.9	198.89	230.0	210.2	235.0	239.0
contiguous sites	142.8	—	—	—	—	—
minor NEC	145.9	198.89	230.0	210.4	235.1	239.0
parotid	142.0	198.89	230.0	210.2	235.0	239.0
pluriglandular	142.8	198.89	—	210.2	235.0	239.0
sublingual	142.2	198.89	230.0	210.2	235.0	239.0
submandibular	142.1	198.89	230.0	210.2	235.0	239.0
submaxillary	142.1	198.89	230.0	210.2	235.0	239.0
salpinx (uterine)	183.2	198.82	233.39	221.0	236.3	239.5
Santorini's duct	157.3	197.8	230.9	211.6	235.5	239.0
scalp	173.40	198.2	232.4	216.4	238.2	239.2
basal cell carcinoma	173.41	—	—	—	—	—
specified type NEC	173.49	—	—	—	—	—
squamous cell carcinoma	173.42	—	—	—	—	—
scapula (any part)	170.4	198.5	—	213.4	238.0	239.2
scapular region	195.1	198.89	234.8	229.8	238.8	239.89
scar NEC (see also Neoplasm, skin)	173.90	198.2	232.9	216.9	238.2	239.2
sciatic nerve	171.3	198.89	—	215.3	238.1	239.2
sclera	190.0	198.4	234.0	224.0	238.8	239.89
scrotum (skin)	187.7	198.82	—	222.4	236.6	239.5
sebaceous gland — see Neoplasm, skin						
sella turcica	194.3	198.89	234.8	227.3	237.0	239.7
bone	170.0	198.5	—	213.0	238.0	239.2
semilunar cartilage (knee)	170.7	198.5	—	213.7	238.0	239.2
seminal vesicle	187.8	198.82	233.6	222.8	236.6	239.5
septum						
nasal	160.0	197.3	231.8	212.0	235.9	239.1
posterior margin	147.3	198.89	230.0	210.7	235.1	239.0
rectovaginal	195.3	198.89	234.8	229.8	238.8	239.89
rectovesical	195.3	198.89	234.8	229.8	238.8	239.89
urethrovaginal	184.9	198.82	233.39	221.9	236.3	239.5
vesicovaginal	184.9	198.82	233.39	221.9	236.3	239.5
shoulder NEC*	195.4	198.89	232.6	229.8	238.8	239.89
sigmoid flexure (lower) (upper)	153.3	197.5	230.3	211.3	235.2	239.0
sinus (accessory)	160.9	197.3	231.8	212.0	235.9	239.1
bone (any)	170.0	198.5	—	213.0	238.0	239.2
contiguous sites with middle ear or nasal cavities	160.8	—	—	—	—	—
ethmoidal	160.3	197.3	231.8	212.0	235.9	239.1
frontal	160.4	197.3	231.8	212.0	235.9	239.1
maxillary	160.2	197.3	231.8	212.0	235.9	239.1
nasal, paranasal NEC	160.9	197.3	231.8	212.0	235.9	239.1
pyriform	148.1	198.89	230.0	210.8	235.1	239.0
sphenoidal	160.5	197.3	231.8	212.0	235.9	239.1
skeleton, skeletal NEC	170.9	198.5	—	213.9	238.0	239.2
Skene's gland	189.4	198.1	233.9	223.89	236.99	239.5
skin NOS	173.90	198.2	232.9	216.9	238.2	239.2
abdominal wall	173.50	198.2	232.5	216.5	238.2	239.2
basal cell carcinoma	173.51	—	—	—	—	—
specified type NEC	173.59	—	—	—	—	—
squamous cell carcinoma	173.52	—	—	—	—	—

☑ Additional Digit Required — Refer to the Tabular List for Digit Selection   ⬇ Subterms under main terms may continue to next column or page

250   2014 ICD-9-CM

Neoplasm, neoplastic — continued
skin — continued

	Malignant			Benign	Uncertain Behavior	Unspecified
	Primary	Secondary	Ca in situ			
ala nasi (see also Neoplasm, skin, face)	173.30	198.2	232.3	216.3	238.2	239.2
ankle (see also Neoplasm, skin, limb, lower)	173.70	198.2	232.7	216.7	238.2	239.2
antecubital space (see also Neoplasm, skin, limb, upper)	173.60	198.2	232.6	216.6	238.2	239.2
anus	173.50	198.2	232.5	216.5	238.2	239.2
basal cell carcinoma	173.51	—	—	—	—	—
specified type NEC	173.59	—	—	—	—	—
squamous cell carcinoma	173.52	—	—	—	—	—
arm (see also Neoplasm, skin, limb, upper)	173.60	198.2	232.6	216.6	238.2	239.2
auditory canal (external) (see also Neoplasm, skin, ear)	173.20	198.2	232.2	216.2	238.2	239.2
auricle (ear) (see also Neoplasm, skin, ear)	173.20	198.2	232.2	216.2	238.2	239.2
auricular canal (external) (see also Neoplasm, skin, ear)	173.20	198.2	232.2	216.2	238.2	239.2
axilla, axillary fold (see also Neoplasm, skin, trunk)	173.50	198.2	232.5	216.5	238.2	239.2
back	173.50	198.2	232.5	216.5	238.2	239.2
basal cell carcinoma	173.51	—	—	—	—	—
specified type NEC	173.59	—	—	—	—	—
squamous cell carcinoma	173.52	—	—	—	—	—
basal cell carcinoma, unspecified site	173.91	—	—	—	—	—
breast (see also Neoplasm, skin, trunk)	173.50	198.2	232.5	216.5	238.2	239.2
brow (see also Neoplasm, skin, face)	173.30	198.2	232.3	216.3	238.2	239.2
buttock (see also Neoplasm, skin, trunk)	173.50	198.2	232.5	216.5	238.2	239.2
calf (see also Neoplasm, skin, limb, lower)	173.70	198.2	232.7	216.7	238.2	239.2
canthus (eye) (inner) (outer)	173.10	198.2	232.1	216.1	238.2	239.2
basal cell carcinoma	173.11	—	—	—	—	—
specified type NEC	173.19	—	—	—	—	—
squamous cell carcinoma	173.12	—	—	—	—	—
cervical region (see also Neoplasm, skin, neck)	173.40	198.2	232.4	216.4	238.2	239.2
cheek (external) (see also Neoplasm, skin, face)	173.30	198.2	232.3	216.3	238.2	239.2
chest (wall) (see also Neoplasm, skin, trunk)	173.50	198.2	232.5	216.5	238.2	239.2
chin (see also Neoplasm, skin, face)	173.30	198.2	232.3	216.3	238.2	239.2

Neoplasm, neoplastic — continued
skin — continued

	Malignant			Benign	Uncertain Behavior	Unspecified
	Primary	Secondary	Ca in situ			
clavicular area (see also Neoplasm, skin, trunk)	173.50	198.2	232.5	216.5	238.2	239.2
clitoris	—	198.82	233.32	221.2	236.3	239.5
columnella (see also Neoplasm, skin, face)	173.30	198.2	232.3	216.3	238.2	239.2
concha (see also Neoplasm, skin, ear)	173.20	198.2	232.2	216.2	238.2	239.2
contiguous sites	173.80	—	—	—	—	—
basal cell carcinoma	173.81	—	—	—	—	—
specified type NEC	173.89	—	—	—	—	—
squamous cell carcinoma	173.82	—	—	—	—	—
ear (external)	173.20	198.2	232.2	216.2	238.2	239.2
basal cell carcinoma	173.21	—	—	—	—	—
specified type NEC	173.29	—	—	—	—	—
squamous cell carcinoma	173.22	—	—	—	—	—
elbow (see also Neoplasm, skin, limb, upper)	173.60	198.2	232.6	216.6	238.2	239.2
eyebrow (see also Neoplasm, skin, face)	173.30	198.2	232.3	216.3	238.2	239.2
eyelid	173.10	198.2	232.1	—	238.2	239.2
basal cell carcinoma	173.11	—	—	—	—	—
specified type NEC	173.19	—	—	—	—	—
squamous cell carcinoma	173.12	—	—	—	—	—
face NEC	173.30	198.2	232.3	216.3	238.2	239.2
basal cell carcinoma	173.31	—	—	—	—	—
specified type NEC	173.39	—	—	—	—	—
squamous cell carcinoma	173.32	—	—	—	—	—
female genital organs (external)	184.4	198.82	233.30	221.2	236.3	239.5
clitoris	184.3	198.82	233.32	221.2	236.3	239.5
labium NEC	184.4	198.82	233.32	221.2	236.3	239.5
majus	184.1	198.82	233.32	221.2	236.3	239.5
minus	184.2	198.82	233.32	221.2	236.3	239.5
pudendum	184.4	198.82	233.32	221.2	236.3	239.5
vulva	184.4	198.82	233.32	221.2	236.3	239.5
finger (see also Neoplasm, skin, limb, upper)	173.60	198.2	232.6	216.6	238.2	239.2
flank (see also Neoplasm, skin, trunk)	173.50	198.2	232.5	216.5	238.2	239.2
foot (see also Neoplasm, skin, limb, lower)	173.70	198.2	232.7	216.7	238.2	239.2
forearm (see also Neoplasm, skin, limb, upper)	173.60	198.2	232.6	216.6	238.2	239.2
forehead (see also Neoplasm, skin, face)	173.30	198.2	232.3	216.3	238.2	239.2
glabella (see also Neoplasm, skin, face)	173.30	198.2	232.3	216.3	238.2	239.2
gluteal region (see also Neoplasm, skin, trunk)	173.50	198.2	232.5	216.5	238.2	239.2
groin (see also Neoplasm, skin, trunk)	173.50	198.2	232.5	216.5	238.2	239.2

☑ Additional Digit Required — Refer to the Tabular List for Digit Selection

▽ Subterms under main terms may continue to next column or page

	Malignant					
	Primary	Secondary	Ca in situ	Benign	Uncertain Behavior	Unspecified
Neoplasm, neoplastic— continued						
skin — continued						
hand (see also Neoplasm, skin, limb, upper)	173.60	198.2	232.6	216.6	238.2	239.2
head NEC (see also Neoplasm, skin, scalp)	173.40	198.2	232.4	216.4	238.2	239.2
heel (see also Neoplasm, skin, limb, lower)	173.70	198.2	232.7	216.7	238.2	239.2
helix (see also Neoplasm, skin, ear)	173.20	198.2	—	216.2	238.2	239.2
hip	173.70	198.2	232.7	216.7	238.2	239.2
basal cell carcinoma	173.71	—	—	—	—	—
specified type NEC	173.79	—	—	—	—	—
squamous cell carcinoma	173.72	—	—	—	—	—
infraclavicular region (see also Neoplasm, skin, trunk)	173.50	198.2	232.5	216.5	238.2	239.2
inguinal region (see also Neoplasm, skin, trunk)	173.50	198.2	232.5	216.5	238.2	239.2
jaw (see also Neoplasm, skin, face)	173.30	198.2	232.3	216.3	238.2	239.2
knee (see also Neoplasm, skin, limb, lower)	173.70	198.2	232.7	216.7	238.2	239.2
labia						
majora	184.1	198.82	233.32	221.2	236.3	239.5
minora	184.2	198.82	233.32	221.2	236.3	239.5
leg (see also Neoplasm, skin, limb, lower)	173.70	198.2	232.7	216.7	238.2	239.2
lid (lower) (upper)	173.10	198.2	232.1	216.1	238.2	239.2
basal cell carcinoma	173.11	—	—	—	—	—
specified type NEC	173.19	—	—	—	—	—
squamous cell carcinoma	173.12	—	—	—	—	—
limb NEC	173.90	198.2	232.9	216.9	238.2	239.5
lower	173.70	198.2	232.7	216.7	238.2	239.2
basal cell carcinoma	173.71	—	—	—	—	—
specified type NEC	173.79	—	—	—	—	—
squamous cell carcinoma	173.72	—	—	—	—	—
upper	173.60	198.2	232.6	216.6	238.2	239.2
basal cell carcinoma	173.61	—	—	—	—	—
specified type NEC	173.69	—	—	—	—	—
squamous cell carcinoma	173.62	—	—	—	—	—
lip (lower) (upper)	173.00	198.2	232.0	216.0	238.2	239.2
basal cell carcinoma	173.01	—	—	—	—	—
specified type NEC	173.09	—	—	—	—	—
squamous cell carcinoma	173.02	—	—	—	—	—
male genital organs	187.9	198.82	233.6	222.9	236.6	239.5
penis	187.4	198.82	233.5	222.1	236.6	239.5
prepuce	187.1	198.82	233.5	222.1	236.6	239.5
scrotum	187.7	198.82	233.6	222.4	236.6	239.5

	Malignant					
	Primary	Secondary	Ca in situ	Benign	Uncertain Behavior	Unspecified
Neoplasm, neoplastic— continued						
skin — continued						
mastectomy site (see also Neoplasm, skin, trunk)	173.50	198.2	—	—	—	—
specified as breast tissue	174.8	198.81	—	—	—	—
meatus, acoustic (external) (see also Neoplasm, skin, ear)	173.20	198.2	232.2	216.2	238.2	239.2
nates (see also Neoplasm, skin, trunk)	173.50	198.2	232.5	216.5	238.2	239.0
neck	173.40	198.2	232.4	216.4	238.2	239.2
basal cell carcinoma	173.41	—	—	—	—	—
specified type NEC	173.49	—	—	—	—	—
squamous cell carcinoma	173.42	—	—	—	—	—
nose (external) (see also Neoplasm, skin, face)	173.30	198.2	232.3	216.3	238.2	239.2
palm (see also Neoplasm, skin, limb, upper)	173.60	198.2	232.6	216.6	238.2	239.2
palpebra	173.10	198.2	232.1	216.1	238.2	239.2
basal cell carcinoma	173.11	—	—	—	—	—
specified type NEC	173.19	—	—	—	—	—
squamous cell carcinoma	173.12	—	—	—	—	—
penis NEC	187.4	198.82	233.5	222.1	236.6	239.5
perianal (see also Neoplasm, skin, anus)	173.50	198.2	232.5	216.5	238.2	239.2
perineum (see also Neoplasm, skin, anus)	173.50	198.2	232.5	216.5	238.2	239.2
pinna (see also Neoplasm, skin, ear)	173.20	198.2	232.2	216.2	238.2	239.2
plantar (see also Neoplasm, skin, limb, lower)	173.70	198.2	232.7	216.7	238.2	239.2
popliteal fossa or space (see also Neoplasm, skin, limb, lower)	173.70	198.2	232.7	216.7	238.2	239.2
prepuce	187.1	198.82	233.5	222.1	236.6	239.5
pubes (see also Neoplasm, skin, trunk)	173.50	198.2	232.5	216.5	238.2	239.2
sacrococcygeal region (see also Neoplasm, skin, trunk)	173.50	198.2	232.5	216.5	238.2	239.2
scalp	173.40	198.2	232.4	216.4	238.2	239.2
basal cell carcinoma	173.41	—	—	—	—	—
specified type NEC	173.49	—	—	—	—	—
squamous cell carcinoma	173.42	—	—	—	—	—
scapular region (see also Neoplasm, skin, trunk)	173.50	198.2	232.5	216.5	238.2	239.2
scrotum	187.7	198.82	233.6	222.4	236.6	239.5
shoulder	173.60	198.2	232.6	216.6	238.2	239.2
basal cell carcinoma	173.61	—	—	—	—	—
specified type NEC	173.69	—	—	—	—	—
squamous cell carcinoma	173.62	—	—	—	—	—

☑ **Additional Digit Required — Refer to the Tabular List for Digit Selection**

▽ **Subterms under main terms may continue to next column or page**

Neoplasm, neoplastic — continued	Malignant Primary	Malignant Secondary	Malignant Ca in situ	Benign	Uncertain Behavior	Unspecified
skin — continued						
sole (foot) (see also Neoplasm, skin, limb, lower)	173.70	198.2	232.7	216.7	238.2	239.2
specified sites NEC	173.80	198.2	232.8	216.8	—	239.2
basal cell carcinoma	173.81	—	—	—	—	—
specified type NEC	173.89	—	—	—	—	—
squamous cell carcinoma	173.82	—	—	—	—	—
specified type NEC, unspecified site	173.99	—	—	—	—	—
squamous cell carcinoma, unspecified site	173.92	—	—	—	—	—
submammary fold (see also Neoplasm, skin, trunk)	173.50	198.2	232.5	216.5	238.2	239.2
supraclavicular region (see also Neoplasm, skin, neck)	173.40	198.2	232.4	216.4	238.2	239.2
temple (see also Neoplasm, skin, face)	173.30	198.2	232.3	216.3	238.2	239.2
thigh (see also Neoplasm, skin, limb, lower)	173.70	198.2	232.7	216.7	238.2	239.2
thoracic wall (see also Neoplasm, skin, trunk)	173.50	198.2	232.5	216.5	238.2	239.2
thumb (see also Neoplasm, skin, limb, upper)	173.60	198.2	232.6	216.6	238.2	239.2
toe (see also Neoplasm, skin, limb, lower)	173.70	198.2	232.7	216.7	238.2	239.2
tragus (see also Neoplasm, skin, ear)	173.20	198.2	232.2	216.2	238.2	239.2
trunk	173.50	198.2	232.5	216.5	238.2	239.2
basal cell carcinoma	173.51	—	—	—	—	—
specified type NEC	173.59	—	—	—	—	—
squamous cell carcinoma	173.52	—	—	—	—	—
umbilicus (see also Neoplasm, skin, trunk)	173.50	198.2	232.5	216.5	238.2	239.2
vulva	184.4	198.82	233.32	221.2	236.3	239.5
wrist (see also Neoplasm, skin, limb, upper)	173.60	198.2	232.6	216.6	238.2	239.2
skull	170.0	198.5	—	213.0	238.0	239.2
soft parts or tissues — see Neoplasm, connective tissue						
specified site — see Neoplasm, skin						
specified site NEC	195.8	198.89	234.8	229.8	238.8	239.89
spermatic cord	187.6	198.82	233.6	222.8	236.6	239.5
sphenoid	160.5	197.3	231.8	212.0	235.9	239.1
bone	170.0	198.5	—	213.0	238.0	239.2
sinus	160.5	197.3	231.8	212.0	235.9	239.1
sphincter anal	154.2	197.5	230.5	211.4	235.5	239.0
of Oddi	156.1	197.8	230.8	211.5	235.3	239.0
spine, spinal (column)	170.2	198.5	—	213.2	238.0	239.2
bulb	191.7	198.3	—	225.0	237.5	239.6
coccyx	170.6	198.5	—	213.6	238.0	239.2

Neoplasm, neoplastic — continued	Malignant Primary	Malignant Secondary	Malignant Ca in situ	Benign	Uncertain Behavior	Unspecified
spine, spinal — continued						
cord (cervical) (lumbar) (sacral) (thoracic)	192.2	198.3	—	225.3	237.5	239.7
dura mater	192.3	198.4	—	225.4	237.6	239.7
lumbosacral	170.2	198.5	—	213.2	238.0	239.2
membrane	192.3	198.4	—	225.4	237.6	239.7
meninges	192.3	198.4	—	225.4	237.6	239.7
nerve (root)	171.9	198.89	—	215.9	238.1	239.2
pia mater	192.3	198.4	—	225.4	237.6	239.7
root	171.9	198.89	—	215.9	238.1	239.2
sacrum	170.6	198.5	—	213.6	238.0	239.2
spleen, splenic NEC	159.1	197.8	230.9	211.9	235.5	239.0
flexure (colon)	153.7	197.5	230.3	211.3	235.2	239.0
stem, brain	191.7	198.3	—	225.0	237.5	239.6
Stensen's duct	142.0	198.89	230.0	210.2	235.0	239.0
sternum	170.3	198.5	—	213.3	238.0	239.2
stomach	151.9	197.8	230.2	211.1	235.2	239.0
antrum (pyloric)	151.2	197.8	230.2	211.1	235.2	239.0
body	151.4	197.8	230.2	211.1	235.2	239.0
cardia	151.0	197.8	230.2	211.1	235.2	239.0
cardiac orifice	151.0	197.8	230.2	211.1	235.2	239.0
contiguous sites	151.8	—	—	—	—	—
corpus	151.4	197.8	230.2	211.1	235.2	239.0
fundus	151.3	197.8	230.2	211.1	235.2	239.0
greater curvature NEC	151.6	197.8	230.2	211.1	235.2	239.0
lesser curvature NEC	151.5	197.8	230.2	211.1	235.2	239.0
prepylorus	151.1	197.8	230.2	211.1	235.2	239.0
pylorus	151.1	197.8	230.2	211.1	235.2	239.0
wall NEC	151.9	197.8	230.2	211.1	235.2	239.0
anterior NEC	151.8	197.8	230.2	211.1	235.2	239.0
posterior NEC	151.8	197.8	230.2	211.1	235.2	239.0
stroma, endometrial	182.0	198.82	233.2	219.1	236.0	239.5
stump, cervical	180.8	198.82	233.1	219.0	236.0	239.5
subcutaneous (nodule) (tissue) NEC — see Neoplasm, connective tissue						
subdural	192.1	198.4	—	225.2	237.6	239.7
subglottis, subglottic	161.2	197.3	231.0	212.1	235.6	239.1
sublingual	144.9	198.89	230.0	210.3	235.1	239.0
gland or duct	142.2	198.89	230.0	210.2	235.0	239.0
submandibular gland	142.1	198.89	230.0	210.2	235.0	239.0
submaxillary gland or duct	142.1	198.89	230.0	210.2	235.0	239.0
submental	195.0	198.89	234.8	229.8	238.8	239.89
subpleural	162.9	197.0	—	212.3	235.7	239.1
substernal	164.2	197.1	—	212.5	235.8	239.89
sudoriferous, sudoriparous gland, site unspecified	173.90	198.2	232.9	216.9	238.2	239.2
specified site — see Neoplasm, skin						
supraclavicular region	195.0	198.89	234.8	229.8	238.8	239.89
supraglottis	161.1	197.3	231.0	212.1	235.6	239.1
suprarenal (capsule) (cortex) (gland) (medulla)	194.0	198.7	234.8	227.0	237.2	239.7
suprasellar (region)	191.9	198.3	—	225.0	237.5	239.6
sweat gland (apocrine) (eccrine), site unspecified	173.90	198.2	232.9	216.9	238.2	239.2
sympathetic nerve or nervous system NEC	171.9	198.89	—	215.9	238.1	239.2

Neoplasm, neoplastic— *continued*	Malignant			Benign	Uncertain Behavior	Unspecified
	Primary	Secondary	Ca in situ			
symphysis pubis	170.6	198.5	—	213.6	238.0	239.2
synovial membrane — *see* Neoplasm, connective tissue						
tapetum, brain	191.8	198.3	—	225.0	237.5	239.6
tarsus (any bone)	170.8	198.5	—	213.8	238.0	239.2
temple (skin) (*see also* Neoplasm, skin, face)	173.30	198.2	232.3	216.3	238.2	239.2
temporal						
bone	170.0	198.5	—	213.0	238.0	239.2
lobe or pole	191.2	198.3	—	225.0	237.5	239.6
region	195.0	198.89	234.8	229.8	238.8	239.89
skin (*see also* Neoplasm, skin, face)	173.30	198.2	232.3	216.3	238.2	239.2
tendon (sheath) — *see* Neoplasm, connective tissue						
tentorium (cerebelli)	192.1	198.4	—	225.2	237.6	239.7
testis, testes (descended) (scrotal)	186.9	198.82	233.6	222.0	236.4	239.5
ectopic	186.0	198.82	233.6	222.0	236.4	239.5
retained	186.0	198.82	233.6	222.0	236.4	239.5
undescended	186.0	198.82	233.6	222.0	236.4	239.5
thalamus	191.0	198.3	—	225.0	237.5	239.6
thigh NEC*	195.5	198.89	234.8	229.8	238.8	239.89
thorax, thoracic (cavity) (organs NEC)	195.1	198.89	234.8	229.8	238.8	239.89
duct	171.4	198.89	—	215.4	238.1	239.2
wall NEC	195.1	198.89	234.8	229.8	238.8	239.89
throat	149.0	198.89	230.0	210.9	235.1	239.0
thumb NEC*	195.4	198.89	232.6	229.8	238.8	239.89
thymus (gland)	164.0	198.89	—	212.6	235.8	239.89
contiguous sites with heart and mediastinum	164.8	—	—	—	—	—
thyroglossal duct	193	198.89	234.8	226	237.4	239.7
thyroid (gland)	193	198.89	234.8	226	237.4	239.7
cartilage	161.3	197.3	231.0	212.1	235.6	239.1
tibia (any part)	170.7	198.5	—	213.7	238.0	239.2
toe NEC*	195.5	198.89	232.7	229.8	238.8	239.89
tongue	141.9	198.89	230.0	210.1	235.1	239.0
anterior (two-thirds) NEC	141.4	198.89	230.0	210.1	235.1	239.0
dorsal surface	141.1	198.89	230.0	210.1	235.1	239.0
ventral surface	141.3	198.89	230.0	210.1	235.1	239.0
base (dorsal surface)	141.0	198.89	230.0	210.1	235.1	239.0
border (lateral)	141.2	198.89	230.0	210.1	235.1	239.0
contiguous sites	141.8	—	—	—	—	—
dorsal surface NEC	141.1	198.89	230.0	210.1	235.1	239.0
fixed part NEC	141.0	198.89	230.0	210.1	235.1	239.0
foreamen cecum	141.1	198.89	230.0	210.1	235.1	239.0
frenulum linguae	141.3	198.89	230.0	210.1	235.1	239.0
junctional zone	141.5	198.89	230.0	210.1	235.1	239.0
margin (lateral)	141.2	198.89	230.0	210.1	235.1	239.0
midline NEC	141.1	198.89	230.0	210.1	235.1	239.0
mobile part NEC	141.4	198.89	230.0	210.1	235.1	239.0
posterior (third)	141.0	198.89	230.0	210.1	235.1	239.0
root	141.0	198.89	230.0	210.1	235.1	239.0
surface (dorsal)	141.1	198.89	230.0	210.1	235.1	239.0
base	141.0	198.89	230.0	210.1	235.1	239.0
ventral	141.3	198.89	230.0	210.1	235.1	239.0
tip	141.2	198.89	230.0	210.1	235.1	239.0
tonsil	141.6	198.89	230.0	210.1	235.1	239.0
tonsil	146.0	198.89	230.0	210.5	235.1	239.0
fauces, faucial	146.0	198.89	230.0	210.5	235.1	239.0
lingual	141.6	198.89	230.0	210.1	235.1	239.0
palatine	146.0	198.89	230.0	210.5	235.1	239.0
pharyngeal	147.1	198.89	230.0	210.7	235.1	239.0

Neoplasm, neoplastic— *continued*	Malignant			Benign	Uncertain Behavior	Unspecified
	Primary	Secondary	Ca in situ			
tonsil — *continued*						
pillar (anterior) (posterior)	146.2	198.89	230.0	210.6	235.1	239.0
tonsillar fossa	146.1	198.89	230.0	210.6	235.1	239.0
tooth socket NEC	143.9	198.89	230.0	210.4	235.1	239.0
trachea (cartilage) (mucosa)	162.0	197.3	231.1	212.2	235.7	239.1
contiguous sites with bronchus or lung	162.8	—	—	—	—	—
tracheobronchial	162.8	197.3	231.1	212.2	235.7	239.1
contiguous sites with lung	162.8	—	—	—	—	—
tragus (*see also* Neoplasm, skin, ear)	173.20	198.2	232.2	216.2	238.2	239.2
trunk NEC*	195.8	198.89	232.5	229.8	238.8	239.89
tubo-ovarian	183.8	198.82	233.39	221.8	236.3	239.5
tunica vaginalis	187.8	198.82	233.6	222.8	236.6	239.5
turbinate (bone)	170.0	198.5	—	213.0	238.0	239.2
nasal	160.0	197.3	231.8	212.0	235.9	239.1
tympanic cavity	160.1	197.3	231.8	212.0	235.9	239.1
ulna (any part)	170.4	198.5	—	213.4	238.0	239.2
umbilicus, umbilical (*see also* Neoplasm, skin, trunk)	173.50	198.2	232.5	216.5	238.2	239.2
uncus, brain	191.2	198.3	—	225.0	237.5	239.6
unknown site or unspecified	199.1	199.1	234.9	229.9	238.9	239.9
urachus	188.7	198.1	233.7	223.3	236.7	239.4
ureter-bladder (junction)	188.6	198.1	233.7	223.3	236.7	239.4
ureter, ureteral	189.2	198.1	233.9	223.2	236.91	239.5
orifice (bladder)	188.6	198.1	233.7	223.3	236.7	239.4
urethra, urethral (gland)	189.3	198.1	233.9	223.81	236.99	239.5
orifice, internal	188.5	198.1	233.7	223.3	236.7	239.4
urethrovaginal (septum)	184.9	198.82	233.39	221.9	236.3	239.5
urinary organ or system NEC	189.9	198.1	233.9	223.9	236.99	239.5
bladder — *see* Neoplasm, bladder						
contiguous sites	189.8	—	—	—	—	—
specified sites NEC	189.8	198.1	233.9	223.89	236.99	239.5
utero-ovarian	183.8	198.82	233.39	221.8	236.3	239.5
ligament	183.3	198.82	—	221.0	236.3	239.5
uterosacral ligament	183.4	198.82	—	221.0	236.3	239.5
uterus, uteri, uterine	179	198.82	233.2	219.9	236.0	239.5
adnexa NEC	183.9	198.82	233.39	221.8	236.3	239.5
contiguous sites	183.8	—	—	—	—	—
body	182.0	198.82	233.2	219.1	236.0	239.5
contiguous sites	182.8	—	—	—	—	—
cervix	180.9	198.82	233.1	219	236.0	239.5
cornu	182.0	198.82	233.2	219.1	236.0	239.5
corpus	182.0	198.82	233.2	219.1	236.0	239.5
endocervix (canal) (gland)	180.0	198.82	233.1	219.0	236.0	239.5
endometrium	182.0	198.82	233.2	219.1	236.0	239.5
exocervix	180.1	198.82	233.1	219.0	236.0	239.5
external os	180.1	198.82	233.1	219.0	236.0	239.5
fundus	182.0	198.82	233.2	219.1	236.0	239.5
internal os	180.0	198.82	233.1	219.0	236.0	239.5
isthmus	182.1	198.82	233.2	219.1	236.0	239.5
ligament	183.4	198.82	—	221.0	236.3	239.5
broad	183.3	198.82	233.39	221.0	236.3	239.5
round	183.5	198.82	—	221.0	236.3	239.5
lower segment	182.1	198.82	233.2	219.1	236.0	239.5
myometrium	182.0	198.82	233.2	219.1	236.0	239.5

☑ Additional Digit Required — Refer to the Tabular List for Digit Selection　　　　　　　▽ Subterms under main terms may continue to next column or page

254　　　　　　　　　　　　　　　　　　　　　　　　　　　　　　　　　　　　　　　2014 ICD-9-CM

	Malignant					
	Primary	Secondary	Ca in situ	Benign	Uncertain Behavior	Unspecified
Neoplasm, neoplastic — *continued*						
uterus, uteri, uterine — *continued*						
squamocolumnar junction	180.8	198.82	233.1	219.0	236.0	239.5
tube	183.2	198.82	233.39	221.0	236.3	239.5
utricle, prostatic	189.3	198.1	233.9	223.81	236.99	239.5
uveal tract	190.0	198.4	234.0	224.0	238.8	239.89
uvula	145.4	198.89	230.0	210.4	235.1	239.0
vagina, vaginal (fornix) (vault) (wall)	184.0	198.82	233.31	221.1	236.3	239.5
vaginovesical	184.9	198.82	233.39	221.9	236.3	239.5
septum	184.9	198.82	233.39	221.9	236.3	239.5
vallecula (epiglottis)	146.3	198.89	230.0	210.6	235.1	239.0
vascular — *see* Neoplasm, connective tissue						
vas deferens	187.6	198.82	233.6	222.8	236.6	239.5
Vater's ampulla	156.2	197.8	230.8	211.5	235.3	239.0
vein, venous — *see* Neoplasm, connective tissue						
vena cava (abdominal) (inferior)	171.5	198.89	—	215.5	238.1	239.2
superior	171.4	198.89	—	215.4	238.1	239.2
ventricle (cerebral) (floor) (fourth) (lateral) (third)	191.5	198.3	—	225.0	237.5	239.6
cardiac (left) (right)	164.1	198.89	—	212.7	238.8	239.89
ventricular band of larynx	161.1	197.3	231.0	212.1	235.6	239.1
ventriculus — see Neoplasm, stomach						
vermillion border — *see* Neoplasm, lip						
vermis, cerebellum	191.6	198.3	—	225.0	237.5	239.6
vertebra (column)	170.2	198.5	—	213.2	238.0	239.2
coccyx	170.6	198.5	—	213.6	238.0	239.2
sacrum	170.6	198.5	—	213.6	238.0	239.2
vesical — *see* Neoplasm, bladder						
vesicle, seminal	187.8	198.82	233.6	222.8	236.6	239.5
vesicocervical tissue	184.9	198.82	233.39	221.9	236.3	239.5
vesicorectal	195.3	198.89	234.8	229.8	238.8	239.89
vesicovaginal	184.9	198.82	233.39	221.9	236.3	239.5
septum	184.9	198.82	233.39	221.9	236.3	239.5
vessel (blood) — *see* Neoplasm, connective tissue						
vestibular gland, greater	184.1	198.82	233.32	221.2	236.3	239.5
vestibule						
mouth	145.1	198.89	230.0	210.4	235.1	239.0
nose	160.0	197.3	231.8	212.0	235.9	239.1
Virchow's gland	—	196.0	—	229.0	238.8	239.89
viscera NEC	195.8	198.89	234.8	229.8	238.8	239.89
vocal cords (true)	161.0	197.3	231.0	212.1	235.6	239.1
false	161.1	197.3	231.0	212.1	235.6	239.1
vomer	170.0	198.5	—	213.0	238.0	239.2
vulva	184.4	198.82	233.32	221.2	236.3	239.5
vulvovaginal gland	184.4	198.82	233.32	221.2	236.3	239.5
Waldeyer's ring	149.1	198.89	230.0	210.9	235.1	239.0
Wharton's duct	142.1	198.89	230.0	210.2	235.0	239.0
white matter (central) (cerebral)	191.0	198.3	—	225.0	237.5	239.6
windpipe	162.0	197.3	231.1	212.2	235.7	239.1
Wirsung's duct	157.3	197.8	230.9	211.6	235.5	239.0
wolffian (body) (duct) female	184.8	198.82	233.39	221.8	236.3	239.5
male	187.8	198.82	233.6	222.8	236.6	239.5
womb — *see* Neoplasm, uterus						

	Malignant					
	Primary	Secondary	Ca in situ	Benign	Uncertain Behavior	Unspecified
Neoplasm, neoplastic — *continued*						
wrist NEC*	195.4	198.89	232.6	229.8	238.8	239.89
xiphoid process	170.3	198.5	—	213.3	238.0	239.2
Zuckerkandl's organ	194.6	198.89	—	227.6	237.3	239.7

☑ Additional Digit Required — Refer to the Tabular List for Digit Selection

▽ Subterms under main terms may continue to next column or page

Neovascularization
- choroid 362.16
- ciliary body 364.42
- cornea 370.60
  - deep 370.63
  - localized 370.61
- iris 364.42
- retina 362.16
- subretinal 362.16

Nephralgia 788.0

Nephritis, nephritic (albuminuric) (azotemic) (congenital) (degenerative) (diffuse) (disseminated) (epithelial) (familial) (focal) (granulomatous) (hemorrhagic) (infantile) (nonsuppurative, excretory) (uremic) 583.9
- with
  - edema — see Nephrosis
  - lesion of
    - glomerulonephritis
      - hypocomplementemic persistent 583.2
        - with nephrotic syndrome 581.2
        - chronic 582.2
      - lobular 583.2
        - with nephrotic syndrome 581.2
        - chronic 582.2
      - membranoproliferative 583.2
        - with nephrotic syndrome 581.2
        - chronic 582.2
      - membranous 583.1
        - with nephrotic syndrome 581.1
        - chronic 582.1
      - mesangiocapillary 583.2
        - with nephrotic syndrome 581.2
        - chronic 582.2
      - mixed membranous and proliferative 583.2
        - with nephrotic syndrome 581.2
        - chronic 582.2
      - proliferative (diffuse) 583.0
        - with nephrotic syndrome 581.0
        - acute 580.0
        - chronic 582.0
      - rapidly progressive 583.4
        - acute 580.4
        - chronic 582.4
    - interstitial nephritis (diffuse) (focal) 583.89
      - with nephrotic syndrome 581.89
      - acute 580.89
      - chronic 582.89
    - necrotizing glomerulitis 583.4
      - acute 580.4
      - chronic 582.4
    - renal necrosis 583.9
      - cortical 583.6
      - medullary 583.7
    - specified pathology NEC 583.89
      - with nephrotic syndrome 581.89
      - acute 580.89
      - chronic 582.89
- necrosis, renal 583.9
  - cortical 583.6
  - medullary (papillary) 583.7
- nephrotic syndrome (see also Nephrosis) 581.9
- papillary necrosis 583.7
- specified pathology NEC 583.89
- acute 580.9
  - extracapillary with epithelial crescents 580.4
  - hypertensive (see also Hypertension, kidney) 403.90
  - necrotizing 580.4
  - poststreptococcal 580.0
  - proliferative (diffuse) 580.0
  - rapidly progressive 580.4
  - specified pathology NEC 580.89

Nephritis, nephritic — continued
- amyloid 277.39 [583.81]
  - chronic 277.39 [582.81]
- arteriolar (see also Hypertension, kidney) 403.90
- arteriosclerotic (see also Hypertension, kidney) 403.90
- ascending (see also Pyelitis) 590.80
- atrophic 582.9
- basement membrane NEC 583.89
  - with
    - pulmonary hemorrhage (Goodpasture's syndrome) 446.21 [583.81]
- calculous, calculus 592.0
- cardiac (see also Hypertension, kidney) 403.90
- cardiovascular (see also Hypertension, kidney) 403.90
- chronic 582.9
  - arteriosclerotic (see also Hypertension, kidney) 403.90
  - hypertensive (see also Hypertension, kidney) 403.90
- cirrhotic (see also Sclerosis, renal) 587
- complicating pregnancy, childbirth, or puerperium 646.2 ☑
  - with hypertension 642.1 ☑
    - affecting fetus or newborn 760.0
  - affecting fetus or newborn 760.1
- croupous 580.9
- desquamative — see Nephrosis
- due to
  - amyloidosis 277.39 [583.81]
    - chronic 277.39 [582.81]
  - arteriosclerosis (see also Hypertension, kidney) 403.90
  - diabetes mellitus 250.4 ☑ [583.81]
    - with nephrotic syndrome 250.4 ☑ [581.81]
    - due to secondary diabetes 249.4 ☑ [583.81]
    - due to secondary diabetes 249.4 ☑ [583.81]
  - diphtheria 032.89 [580.81]
  - gonococcal infection (acute) 098.19 [583.81]
    - chronic or duration of 2 months or over 098.39 [583.81]
  - gout 274.10
  - infectious hepatitis 070.9 [580.81]
  - mumps 072.79 [580.81]
  - specified kidney pathology NEC 583.89
    - acute 580.89
    - chronic 582.89
  - streptotrichosis 039.8 [583.81]
  - subacute bacterial endocarditis 421.0 [580.81]
  - systemic lupus erythematosus 710.0 [583.81]
    - chronic 710.0 [582.81]
  - typhoid fever 002.0 [580.81]
- endothelial 582.2
- end stage (chronic) (terminal) NEC 585.6
- epimembranous 581.1
- exudative 583.89
  - with nephrotic syndrome 581.89
  - acute 580.89
  - chronic 582.89
- gonococcal (acute) 098.19 [583.81]
  - chronic or duration of 2 months or over 098.39 [583.81]
- gouty 274.10
- hereditary (Alport's syndrome) 759.89
- hydremic — see Nephrosis
- hypertensive (see also Hypertension, kidney) 403.90
- hypocomplementemic persistent 583.2
  - with nephrotic syndrome 581.2
  - chronic 582.2
- immune complex NEC 583.89
- infective (see also Pyelitis) 590.80
- interstitial (diffuse) (focal) 583.89
  - with nephrotic syndrome 581.89
  - acute 580.89
  - chronic 582.89

Nephritis, nephritic — continued
- latent or quiescent — see Nephritis, chronic
- lead 984.9
  - specified type of lead — see Table of Drugs and Chemicals
- lobular 583.2
  - with nephrotic syndrome 581.2
  - chronic 582.2
- lupus 710.0 [583.81]
  - acute 710.0 [580.81]
  - chronic 710.0 [582.81]
- membranoproliferative 583.2
  - with nephrotic syndrome 581.2
  - chronic 582.2
- membranous 583.1
  - with nephrotic syndrome 581.1
  - chronic 582.1
- mesangiocapillary 583.2
  - with nephrotic syndrome 581.2
  - chronic 582.2
- minimal change 581.3
- mixed membranous and proliferative 583.2
  - with nephrotic syndrome 581.2
  - chronic 582.2
- necrotic, necrotizing 583.4
  - acute 580.4
  - chronic 582.4
- nephrotic — see Nephrosis
- old — see Nephritis, chronic
- parenchymatous 581.89
- polycystic 753.12
  - adult type (APKD) 753.13
  - autosomal dominant 753.13
  - autosomal recessive 753.14
  - childhood type (CPKD) 753.14
  - infantile type 753.14
- poststreptococcal 580.0
- pregnancy — see Nephritis, complicating pregnancy
- proliferative 583.0
  - with nephrotic syndrome 581.0
  - acute 580.0
  - chronic 582.0
- purulent (see also Pyelitis) 590.80
- rapidly progressive 583.4
  - acute 580.4
  - chronic 582.4
- salt-losing or salt-wasting (see also Disease, renal) 593.9
- saturnine 584.9
  - specified type of lead — see Table of Drugs and Chemicals
- septic (see also Pyelitis) 590.80
- specified pathology NEC 583.89
  - acute 580.89
  - chronic 582.89
- staphylococcal (see also Pyelitis) 590.80
- streptotrichosis 039.8 [583.81]
- subacute (see also Nephrosis) 581.9
- suppurative (see also Pyelitis) 590.80
- syphilitic (late) 095.4
  - congenital 090.5 [583.81]
  - early 091.69 [583.81]
- terminal (chronic) (end-stage) NEC 585.6
- toxic — see Nephritis, acute
- tubal, tubular — see Nephrosis, tubular
- tuberculous (see also Tuberculosis) 016.0 ☑ [583.81]
- type II (Ellis) — see Nephrosis
- vascular — see Hypertension, kidney
- war 580.9

Nephroblastoma (M8960/3) 189.0
- epithelial (M8961/3) 189.0
- mesenchymal (M8962/3) 189.0

Nephrocalcinosis 275.49

Nephrocystitis, pustular — see also Pyelitis 590.80

Nephrolithiasis (congenital) (pelvis) (recurrent) 592.0
- uric acid 274.11

Nephroma (M8960/3) 189.0
- mesoblastic (M8960/1) 236.9 ☑

Nephronephritis — see also Nephrosis 581.9

Nephronopthisis 753.16

Nephropathy — see also Nephritis 583.9

Nephropathy — see also Nephritis — continued
- with
  - exudative nephritis 583.89
  - interstitial nephritis (diffuse) (focal) 583.89
  - medullary necrosis 583.7
  - necrosis 583.9
    - cortical 583.6
    - medullary or papillary 583.7
  - papillary necrosis 583.7
  - specified lesion or cause NEC 583.89
- analgesic 583.89
  - with medullary necrosis, acute 584.7
- arteriolar (see also Hypertension, kidney) 403.90
- arteriosclerotic (see also Hypertension, kidney) 403.90
- complicating pregnancy 646.2 ☑
- diabetic 250.4 ☑ [583.81]
  - due to secondary diabetes 249.4 ☑ [583.81]
- gouty 274.10
  - specified type NEC 274.19
- hereditary amyloid 277.31
- hypercalcemic 588.89
- hypertensive (see also Hypertension, kidney) 403.90
- hypokalemic (vacuolar) 588.89
- IgA 583.9
- obstructive 593.89
  - congenital 753.20
- phenacetin 584.7
- phosphate-losing 588.0
- potassium depletion 588.89
- proliferative (see also Nephritis, proliferative) 583.0
- protein-losing 588.89
- salt-losing or salt-wasting (see also Disease, renal) 593.9
- sickle-cell (see also Disease, sickle-cell) 282.60 [583.81]
- toxic 584.5
- vasomotor 584.5
- water-losing 588.89

Nephroptosis — see also Disease, renal 593.0
- congenital (displaced) 753.3

Nephropyosis — see also Abscess, kidney 590.2

Nephrorrhagia 593.81

Nephrosclerosis (arteriolar) (arteriosclerotic) (chronic) (hyaline) — see also Hypertension, kidney 403.90
- gouty 274.10
- hyperplastic (arteriolar) (see also Hypertension, kidney) 403.90
- senile (see also Sclerosis, renal) 587

Nephrosis, nephrotic (Epstein's) (syndrome) 581.9
- with
  - lesion of
    - focal glomerulosclerosis 581.1
    - glomerulonephritis
      - endothelial 581.2
      - hypocomplementemic persistent 581.2
      - lobular 581.2
      - membranoproliferative 581.2
      - membranous 581.1
      - mesangiocapillary 581.2
      - minimal change 581.3
      - mixed membranous and proliferative 581.2
      - proliferative 581.0
      - segmental hyalinosis 581.1
    - specified pathology NEC 581.89
- acute — see Nephrosis, tubular
- anoxic — see Nephrosis, tubular
- arteriosclerotic (see also Hypertension, kidney) 403.90
- chemical — see Nephrosis, tubular
- cholemic 572.4
- complicating pregnancy, childbirth, or puerperium — see Nephritis, complicating pregnancy
- diabetic 250.4 ☑ [581.81]

Nephrosis, nephrotic — *continued*
  diabetic — *continued*
    due to secondary diabetes
      249.4 ☑ *[581.81]*
  Finnish type (congenital) 759.89
  hemoglobinuric — *see* Nephrosis, tubular
  in
    amyloidosis 277.39 *[581.81]*
    diabetes mellitus 250.4 ☑ *[581.81]*
      due to secondary diabetes
        249.4 ☑ *[581.81]*
    epidemic hemorrhagic fever 078.6
    malaria 084.9 *[581.81]*
    polyarteritis 446.0 *[581.81]*
    systemic lupus erythematosus
      710.0 *[581.81]*
  ischemic — *see* Nephrosis, tubular
  lipoid 581.3
  lower nephron — *see* Nephrosis, tubular
  lupoid 710.0 *[581.81]*
  lupus 710.0 *[581.81]*
  malarial 084.9 *[581.81]*
  minimal change 581.3
  necrotizing — *see* Nephrosis, tubular
  osmotic (sucrose) 588.89
  polyarteritic 446.0 *[581.81]*
  radiation 581.9
  specified lesion or cause NEC 581.89
  syphilitic 095.4
  toxic — *see* Nephrosis, tubular
  tubular (acute) 584.5
    due to a procedure 997.5
    radiation 581.9
Nephrosonephritis hemorrhagic (endemic)
  078.6
Nephrostomy status V44.6
  with complication 997.5
Nerve — *see* condition
Nerves 799.21
Nervous — *see also* condition 799.21
  breakdown 300.9
  heart 306.2
  stomach 306.4
  tension 799.21
Nervousness 799.21
Nesidioblastoma (M8150/0)
  pancreas 211.7
  specified site NEC — *see* Neoplasm, by site,
    benign
  unspecified site 211.7
Netherton's syndrome (ichthyosiform erythroderma) 757.1
Nettle rash 708.8
Nettleship's disease (urticaria pigmentosa)
  757.33
Neumann's disease (pemphigus vegetans)
  694.4
Neuralgia, neuralgic (acute) — *see also* Neuritis 729.2
  accessory (nerve) 352.4
  acoustic (nerve) 388.5
  ankle 355.8
  anterior crural 355.8
  anus 787.99
  arm 723.4
  auditory (nerve) 388.5
  axilla 353.0
  bladder 788.1
  brachial 723.4
  brain — *see* Disorder, nerve, cranial
  broad ligament 625.9
  cerebral — *see* Disorder, nerve, cranial
  ciliary 339.00
  cranial nerve (*see also* Disorder, nerve, cra-
    nial)
    fifth or trigeminal (*see also* Neuralgia,
      trigeminal) 350.1
  ear 388.71
    middle 352.1
  facial 351.8
  finger 354.9
  flank 355.8
  foot 355.8
  forearm 354.9
  Fothergill's (*see also* Neuralgia, trigeminal)
    350.1

Neuralgia, neuralgic — *see also* Neuritis
  — *continued*
  Fothergill's (*see also* Neuralgia, trigeminal)
    — *continued*
    postherpetic 053.12
  glossopharyngeal (nerve) 352.1
  groin 355.8
  hand 354.9
  heel 355.8
  Horton's 339.00
  Hunt's 053.11
  hypoglossal (nerve) 352.5
  iliac region 355.8
  infraorbital (*see also* Neuralgia, trigeminal)
    350.1
  inguinal 355.8
  intercostal (nerve) 353.8
    postherpetic 053.19
  jaw 352.1
  kidney 788.0
  knee 355.8
  loin 355.8
  malarial (*see also* Malaria) 084.6
  mastoid 385.89
  maxilla 352.1
  median thenar 354.1
  metatarsal 355.6
  middle ear 352.1
  migrainous 339.00
  Morton's 355.6
  nerve, cranial — *see* Disorder, nerve, cranial
  nose 352.0
  occipital 723.8
  olfactory (nerve) 352.0
  ophthalmic 377.30
    postherpetic 053.19
  optic (nerve) 377.30
  penis 607.9
  perineum 355.8
  pleura 511.0
  postherpetic NEC 053.19
    geniculate ganglion 053.11
    ophthalmic 053.19
    trifacial 053.12
    trigeminal 053.12
  pubic region 355.8
  radial (nerve) 723.4
  rectum 787.99
  sacroiliac joint 724.3
  sciatic (nerve) 724.3
  scrotum 608.9
  seminal vesicle 608.9
  shoulder 354.9
  Sluder's 337.09
  specified nerve NEC — *see* Disorder, nerve
  spermatic cord 608.9
  sphenopalatine (ganglion) 337.09
  subscapular (nerve) 723.4
  suprascapular (nerve) 723.4
  testis 608.89
  thenar (median) 354.1
  thigh 355.8
  tongue 352.5
  trifacial (nerve) (*see also* Neuralgia, trigemi-
    nal) 350.1
  trigeminal (nerve) 350.1
    postherpetic 053.12
  tympanic plexus 388.71
  ulnar (nerve) 723.4
  vagus (nerve) 352.3
  wrist 354.9
  writers' 300.89
    organic 333.84
Neurapraxia — *see* Injury, nerve, by site
Neurasthenia 300.5
  cardiac 306.2
  gastric 306.4
  heart 306.2
  postfebrile 780.79
  postviral 780.79
Neurilemmoma (M9560/0) — *see also* Neoplasm, connective tissue, benign
  acoustic (nerve) 225.1
  malignant (M9560/3) (*see also* Neoplasm,
    connective tissue, malignant)
    acoustic (nerve) 192.0

Neurilemmosarcoma (M9560/3) — *see* Neoplasm, connective tissue, malignant
Neurilemoma — *see* Neurilemmoma
Neurinoma (M9560/0) — *see* Neurilemmoma
Neurinomatosis (M9560/1) — *see also* Neoplasm, connective tissue, uncertain behavior
  centralis 759.5
Neuritis — *see also* Neuralgia 729.2
  abducens (nerve) 378.54
  accessory (nerve) 352.4
  acoustic (nerve) 388.5
    syphilitic 094.86
  alcoholic 357.5
    with psychosis 291.1
  amyloid, any site 277.39 *[357.4]*
  anterior crural 355.8
  arising during pregnancy 646.4 ☑
  arm 723.4
  ascending 355.2
  auditory (nerve) 388.5
  brachial (nerve) NEC 723.4
    due to displacement, intervertebral disc
      722.0
  cervical 723.4
  chest (wall) 353.8
  costal region 353.8
  cranial nerve (*see also* Disorder, nerve, cra-
    nial)
    first or olfactory 352.0
    second or optic 377.30
    third or oculomotor 378.52
    fourth or trochlear 378.53
    fifth or trigeminal (*see also* Neuralgia,
      trigeminal) 350.1
    sixth or abducens 378.54
    seventh or facial 351.8
      newborn 767.5
    eighth or acoustic 388.5
    ninth or glossopharyngeal 352.1
    tenth or vagus 352.3
    eleventh or accessory 352.4
    twelfth or hypoglossal 352.5
  Déjérine-Sottas 356.0
  diabetic 250.6 ☑ *[357.2]*
    due to secondary diabetes
      249.6 ☑ *[357.2]*
  diphtheritic 032.89 *[357.4]*
  due to
    beriberi 265.0 *[357.4]*
    displacement, prolapse, protrusion, or
      rupture of intervertebral disc
      722.2
      cervical 722.0
      lumbar, lumbosacral 722.10
      thoracic, thoracolumbar 722.11
    herniation, nucleus pulposus 722.2
      cervical 722.0
      lumbar, lumbosacral 722.10
      thoracic, thoracolumbar 722.11
  endemic 265.0 *[357.4]*
  facial (nerve) 351.8
    newborn 767.5
  general — *see* Polyneuropathy
  geniculate ganglion 351.1
    due to herpes 053.11
  glossopharyngeal (nerve) 352.1
  gouty 274.89 *[357.4]*
  hypoglossal (nerve) 352.5
  ilioinguinal (nerve) 355.8
  in diseases classified elsewhere — *see*
    Polyneuropathy, in
  infectious (multiple) 357.0
  intercostal (nerve) 353.8
  interstitial hypertrophic progressive NEC
    356.9
  leg 355.8
  lumbosacral NEC 724.4
  median (nerve) 354.1
    thenar 354.1
  multiple (acute) (infective) 356.9
    endemic 265.0 *[357.4]*
  multiplex endemica 265.0 *[357.4]*
  nerve root (*see also* Radiculitis) 729.2
  oculomotor (nerve) 378.52
  olfactory (nerve) 352.0

Neuritis — *see also* Neuralgia — *continued*
  optic (nerve) 377.30
    in myelitis 341.0
    meningococcal 036.81
  pelvic 355.8
  peripheral (nerve) (*see also* Neuropathy,
    peripheral)
    complicating pregnancy or puerperium
      646.4 ☑
    specified nerve NEC — *see* Mononeuritis
  pneumogastric (nerve) 352.3
  postchickenpox 052.7
  postherpetic 053.19
  progressive hypertrophic interstitial NEC
    356.9
  puerperal, postpartum 646.4 ☑
  radial (nerve) 723.4
  retrobulbar 377.32
    syphilitic 094.85
  rheumatic (chronic) 729.2
  sacral region 355.8
  sciatic (nerve) 724.3
    due to displacement of intervertebral
      disc 722.10
  serum 999.59
  specified nerve NEC — *see* Disorder, nerve
  spinal (nerve) 355.9
    root (*see also* Radiculitis) 729.2
  subscapular (nerve) 723.4
  suprascapular (nerve) 723.4
  syphilitic 095.8
  thenar (median) 354.1
  thoracic NEC 724.4
  toxic NEC 357.7
  trochlear (nerve) 378.53
  ulnar (nerve) 723.4
  vagus (nerve) 352.3
Neuroangiomatosis, encephalofacial 759.6
Neuroastrocytoma (M9505/1) — *see* Neoplasm, by site, uncertain behavior
Neuro-avitaminosis 269.2
Neuroblastoma (M9500/3)
  olfactory (M9522/3) 160.0
  specified site — *see* Neoplasm, by site, ma-
    lignant
  unspecified site 194.0
Neurochorioretinitis — *see also* Chorioretinitis
  363.20
Neurocirculatory asthenia 306.2
Neurocytoma (M9506/0) — *see* Neoplasm, by
  site, benign
Neurodermatitis (circumscribed) (circumscripta) (local) 698.3
  atopic 691.8
  diffuse (Brocq) 691.8
  disseminated 691.8
  nodulosa 698.3
Neuroencephalomyelopathy, optic 341.0
Neuroendocrine tumor — *see* Tumor, neuroendocrine
Neuroepithelioma (M9503/3) — *see also*
  Neoplasm, by site, malignant
  olfactory (M9521/3) 160.0
Neurofibroma (M9540/0) — *see also* Neoplasm, connective tissue, benign
  melanotic (M9541/0) — *see* Neoplasm,
    connective tissue, benign
  multiple (M9540/1) 237.70
    type 1 237.71
    type 2 237.72
  plexiform (M9550/0) — *see* Neoplasm,
    connective tissue, benign
Neurofibromatosis (multiple) (M9540/1)
  237.70
  acoustic 237.72
  malignant (M9540/3) — *see* Neoplasm,
    connective tissue, malignant
  Schwannomatosis 237.73
  specified type NEC 237.79
  type 1 237.71
  type 2 237.72
  von Recklinghausen's 237.71
Neurofibrosarcoma (M9540/3) — *see* Neoplasm, connective tissue, malignant
Neurogenic — *see also* condition

☑ **Additional Digit Required** — Refer to the Tabular List for Digit Selection   ▽ **Subterms under main terms may continue to next column or page**

Index

Neurogenic — *see also* condition — *continued*
  bladder (atonic) (automatic) (autonomic) (flaccid) (hypertonic) (hypotonic) (inertia) (infranuclear) (irritable) (motor) (nonreflex) (nuclear) (paralysis) (reflex) (sensory) (spastic) (supranuclear) (uninhibited) 596.54
    with cauda equina syndrome 344.61
  bowel 564.81
  heart 306.2
Neuroglioma (M9505/1) — *see* Neoplasm, by site, uncertain behavior
Neurolabyrinthitis (of Dix and Hallpike) 386.12
Neurolathyrism 988.2
Neuroleprosy 030.1
Neuroleptic malignant syndrome 333.92
Neurolipomatosis 272.8
Neuroma (M9570/0) — *see also* Neoplasm, connective tissue, benign
  acoustic (nerve) (M9560/0) 225.1
  amputation (traumatic) (*see also* Injury, nerve, by site)
    surgical complication (late) 997.61
  appendix 211.3
  auditory nerve 225.1
  digital 355.6
    toe 355.6
  interdigital (toe) 355.6
  intermetatarsal 355.6
  Morton's 355.6
  multiple 237.70
    type 1 237.71
    type 2 237.72
  nonneoplastic 355.9
    arm NEC 354.9
    leg NEC 355.8
    lower extremity NEC 355.8
    specified site NEC — *see* Mononeuritis, by site
    upper extremity NEC 354.9
  optic (nerve) 225.1
  plantar 355.6
  plexiform (M9550/0) — *see* Neoplasm, connective tissue, benign
  surgical (nonneoplastic) 355.9
    arm NEC 354.9
    leg NEC 355.8
    lower extremity NEC 355.8
    upper extremity NEC 354.9
  traumatic (*see also* Injury, nerve, by site)
    old — *see* Neuroma, nonneoplastic
Neuromyalgia 729.1
Neuromyasthenia (epidemic) 049.8
Neuromyelitis 341.8
  ascending 357.0
  optica 341.0
Neuromyopathy NEC 358.9
Neuromyositis 729.1
Neuronevus (M8725/0) — *see* Neoplasm, skin, benign
Neuronitis 357.0
  ascending (acute) 355.2
  vestibular 386.12
Neuroparalytic — *see* condition
Neuropathy, neuropathic — *see also* Disorder, nerve 355.9
  acute motor 357.82
  alcoholic 357.5
    with psychosis 291.1
  arm NEC 354.9
  ataxia and retinitis pigmentosa (NARP syndrome) 277.87
  autonomic (peripheral) — *see* Neuropathy, peripheral, autonomic
  axillary nerve 353.0
  brachial plexus 353.0
  cervical plexus 353.2
  chronic
    progressive segmentally demyelinating 357.89
    relapsing demyelinating 357.89
  congenital sensory 356.2
  Déjérine-Sottas 356.0
  diabetic 250.6 ☑ *[357.2]*
    autonomic (peripheral) 250.6 ☑ *[337.1]*

Neuropathy, neuropathic — *see also* Disorder, nerve — *continued*
  diabetic — *continued*
    due to secondary diabetes 249.6 ☑ *[357.2]*
    autonomic (peripheral) 249.6 ☑ *[337.1]*
  entrapment 355.9
    iliohypogastric nerve 355.79
    ilioinguinal nerve 355.79
    lateral cutaneous nerve of thigh 355.1
    median nerve 354.0
    obturator nerve 355.79
    peroneal nerve 355.3
    posterior tibial nerve 355.5
    saphenous nerve 355.79
    ulnar nerve 354.2
  facial nerve 351.9
  hereditary 356.9
    peripheral 356.0
    sensory (radicular) 356.2
  hypertrophic
    Charcôt-Marie-Tooth 356.1
    Déjérine-Sottas 356.0
    interstitial 356.9
    Refsum 356.3
  intercostal nerve 354.8
  ischemic — *see* Disorder, nerve
  Jamaican (ginger) 357.7
  leg NEC 355.8
  lower extremity NEC 355.8
  lumbar plexus 353.1
  median nerve 354.1
  motor
    acute 357.82
  multiple (acute) (chronic) (*see also* Polyneuropathy) 356.9
  optic 377.39
    ischemic 377.41
    nutritional 377.33
    toxic 377.34
  peripheral (nerve) (*see also* Polyneuropathy) 356.9
    arm NEC 354.9
    autonomic 337.9
      amyloid 277.39 *[337.1]*
      idiopathic 337.00
      in
        amyloidosis 277.39 *[337.1]*
        diabetes (mellitus) 250.6 ☑ *[337.1]*
          due to secondary diabetes 249.6 ☑ *[337.1]*
        diseases classified elsewhere 337.1
        gout 274.89 *[337.1]*
        hyperthyroidism 242.9 ☑ *[337.1]*
      due to
        antitetanus serum 357.6
        arsenic 357.7
        drugs 357.6
        lead 357.7
        organophosphate compounds 357.7
        toxic agent NEC 357.7
      hereditary 356.0
      idiopathic 356.9
        progressive 356.4
        specified type NEC 356.8
      in diseases classified elsewhere — *see* Polyneuropathy, in
    leg NEC 355.8
    lower extremity NEC 355.8
    upper extremity NEC 354.9
  plantar nerves 355.6
  progressive
    hypertrophic interstitial 356.9
    inflammatory 357.89
  radicular NEC 729.2
    brachial 723.4
    cervical NEC 723.4
    hereditary sensory 356.2
    lumbar 724.4
    lumbosacral 724.4
    thoracic NEC 724.4
  sacral plexus 353.1
  sciatic 355.0

Neuropathy, neuropathic — *see also* Disorder, nerve — *continued*
  spinal nerve NEC 355.9
    root (*see also* Radiculitis) 729.2
  toxic 357.7
  trigeminal sensory 350.8
  ulnar nerve 354.2
  upper extremity NEC 354.9
  uremic 585.9 *[357.4]*
  vitamin B$_{12}$ 266.2 *[357.4]*
    with anemia (pernicious) 281.0 *[357.4]*
      due to dietary deficiency 281.1 *[357.4]*
Neurophthisis — *see also* Disorder, nerve
  diabetic 250.6 ☑ *[357.2]*
    due to secondary diabetes 249.6 ☑ *[357.2]*
  peripheral 356.9
Neuropraxia — *see* Injury, nerve
Neuroretinitis 363.05
  syphilitic 094.85
Neurosarcoma (M9540/3) — *see* Neoplasm, connective tissue, malignant
Neurosclerosis — *see* Disorder, nerve
Neurosis, neurotic 300.9
  accident 300.16
  anancastic, anankastic 300.3
  anxiety (state) 300.00
    generalized 300.02
    panic type 300.01
  asthenic 300.5
  bladder 306.53
  cardiac (reflex) 306.2
  cardiovascular 306.2
  climacteric, unspecified type 627.2
  colon 306.4
  compensation 300.16
  compulsive, compulsion 300.3
  conversion 300.11
  craft 300.89
  cutaneous 306.3
  depersonalization 300.6
  depressive (reaction) (type) 300.4
  endocrine 306.6
  environmental 300.89
  fatigue 300.5
  functional (*see also* Disorder, psychosomatic) 306.9
  gastric 306.4
  gastrointestinal 306.4
  genitourinary 306.50
  heart 306.2
  hypochondriacal 300.7
  hysterical 300.10
    conversion type 300.11
    dissociative type 300.15
  impulsive 300.3
  incoordination 306.0
    larynx 306.1
    vocal cord 306.1
  intestine 306.4
  larynx 306.1
    hysterical 300.11
    sensory 306.1
  menopause, unspecified type 627.2
  mixed NEC 300.89
  musculoskeletal 306.0
  obsessional 300.3
    phobia 300.3
  obsessive-compulsive 300.3
  occupational 300.89
  ocular 306.7
  oral (*see also* Disorder, fluency) 315.35
  organ (*see also* Disorder, psychosomatic) 306.9
  pharynx 306.1
  phobic 300.20
  posttraumatic (acute) (situational) 309.81
    chronic 309.81
  psychasthenic (type) 300.89
  railroad 300.16
  rectum 306.4
  respiratory 306.1
  rumination 306.4
  senile 300.89
  sexual 302.70

Neurosis, neurotic — *continued*
  situational 300.89
  specified type NEC 300.89
  state 300.9
    with depersonalization episode 300.6
  stomach 306.4
  vasomotor 306.2
  visceral 306.4
  war 300.16
Neurospongioblastosis diffusa 759.5
Neurosyphilis (arrested) (early) (inactive) (late) (latent) (recurrent) 094.9
  with ataxia (cerebellar) (locomotor) (spastic) (spinal) 094.0
  acute meningitis 094.2
  aneurysm 094.89
  arachnoid (adhesive) 094.2
  arteritis (any artery) 094.89
  asymptomatic 094.3
  congenital 090.40
  dura (mater) 094.89
  general paresis 094.1
  gumma 094.9
  hemorrhagic 094.9
  juvenile (asymptomatic) (meningeal) 090.40
  leptomeninges (aseptic) 094.2
  meningeal 094.2
  meninges (adhesive) 094.2
  meningovascular (diffuse) 094.2
  optic atrophy 094.84
  parenchymatous (degenerative) 094.1
  paresis (*see also* Paresis, general) 094.1
  paretic (*see also* Paresis, general) 094.1
  relapse 094.9
  remission in (sustained) 094.9
  serological 094.3
  specified nature or site NEC 094.89
  tabes (dorsalis) 094.0
    juvenile 090.40
  tabetic 094.0
    juvenile 090.40
  taboparesis 094.1
    juvenile 090.40
  thrombosis 094.89
  vascular 094.89
Neurotic — *see also* Neurosis 300.9
  excoriation 698.4
    psychogenic 306.3
Neurotmesis — *see* Injury, nerve, by site
Neurotoxemia — *see* Toxemia
Neutro-occlusion 524.21
Neutropenia, neutropenic (idiopathic) (pernicious) (primary) 288.00
  chronic 288.09
    hypoplastic 288.09
  congenital (nontransient) 288.01
  cyclic 288.02
  drug induced 288.03
  due to infection 288.04
  fever 288.00
  genetic 288.01
  immune 288.09
  infantile 288.01
  malignant 288.09
  neonatal, transitory (isoimmune) (maternal transfer) 776.7
  periodic 288.02
  splenic 289.53
  splenomegaly 289.53
  toxic 288.09
Neutrophilia, hereditary giant 288.2
Nevocarcinoma (M8720/3) — *see* Melanoma
Nevus (M8720/0) — *see also* Neoplasm, skin, benign

> *Note* — Except where otherwise indicated, varieties of nevus in the list below that are followed by a morphology code number (M----/0) should be coded by site as for "Neoplasm, skin, benign."

  acanthotic 702.8
  achromic (M8730/0)
  amelanotic (M8730/0)
  anemic, anemicus 709.09
  angiomatous (M9120/0) (*see also* Hemangioma) 228.00
  araneus 448.1

Neurogenic — Nevus

Nevus — see also Neoplasm, skin, benign — continued
avasculosus 709.09
balloon cell (M8722/0)
bathing trunk (M8761/1) 238.2
blue (M8780/0)
cellular (M8790/0)
giant (M8790/0)
Jadassohn's (M8780/0)
malignant (M8780/3) — see Melanoma
capillary (M9131/0) (see also Hemangioma) 228.00
cavernous (M9121/0) (see also Hemangioma) 228.00
cellular (M8720/0)
blue (M8790/0)
comedonicus 757.33
compound (M8760/0)
conjunctiva (M8720/0) 224.3
dermal (M8750/0)
and epidermal (M8760/0)
epithelioid cell (and spindle cell) (M8770/0)
flammeus 757.32
osteohypertrophic 759.89
hairy (M8720/0)
halo (M8723/0)
hemangiomatous (M9120/0) (see also Hemangioma) 228.00
intradermal (M8750/0)
intraepidermal (M8740/0)
involuting (M8724/0)
Jadassohn's (blue) (M8780/0)
junction, junctional (M8740/0)
malignant melanoma in (M8740/3) — see Melanoma
juvenile (M8770/0)
lymphatic (M9170/0) 228.1
magnocellular (M8726/0)
specified site — see Neoplasm, by site, benign
unspecified site 224.0
malignant (M8720/3) — see Melanoma
meaning hemangioma (M9120/0) (see also Hemangioma) 228.00
melanotic (pigmented) (M8720/0)
multiplex 759.5
nonneoplastic 448.1
nonpigmented (M8730/0)
nonvascular (M8720/0)
oral mucosa, white sponge 750.26
osteohypertrophic, flammeus 759.89
papillaris (M8720/0)
papillomatosus (M8720/0)
pigmented (M8720/0)
giant (M8761/1) (see also Neoplasm, skin, uncertain behavior)
malignant melanoma in (M8761/3) — see Melanoma
systematicus 757.33
pilosus (M8720/0)
port wine 757.32
sanguineous 757.32
sebaceous (senile) 702.8
senile 448.1
spider 448.1
spindle cell (and epithelioid cell) (M8770/0)
stellar 448.1
strawberry 757.32
syringocystadenomatous papilliferous (M8406/0)
unius lateris 757.33
Unna's 757.32
vascular 757.32
verrucous 757.33
white sponge (oral mucosa) 750.26
Newborn (infant) (liveborn)
abstinence syndrome 779.5
affected by
amniocentesis 760.61
maternal abuse of drugs (gestational) (via placenta) (via breast milk) (see also Noxious, substances transmitted through placenta or breast milk (affecting fetus or newborn)) 760.70
methamphetamine(s) 760.72

Newborn — continued
affected by — continued
procedure
amniocentesis 760.61
in utero NEC 760.62
surgical on mother
during pregnancy NEC 760.63
previous not associated with pregnancy 760.64
apnea 770.81
obstructive 770.82
specified NEC 770.82
breast buds 779.89
cardiomyopathy 425.4
congenital 425.3
convulsion 779.0
electrolyte imbalance NEC (transitory) 775.5
fever (environmentally-induced) 778.4
gestation
24 completed weeks 765.22
25-26 completed weeks 765.23
27-28 completed weeks 765.24
29-30 completed weeks 765.25
31-32 completed weeks 765.26
33-34 completed weeks 765.27
35-36 completed weeks 765.28
37 or more completed weeks 765.29
less than 24 completed weeks 765.21
unspecified completed weeks 765.20
infection 771.89
candida 771.7
mastitis 771.5
specified NEC 771.89
urinary tract 771.82
mastitis 771.5
multiple NEC
born in hospital (without mention of cesarean delivery or section) V37.00
with cesarean delivery or section V37.01
born outside hospital
hospitalized V37.1
not hospitalized V37.2
mates all liveborn
born in hospital (without mention of cesarean delivery or section) V34.00
with cesarean delivery or section V34.01
born outside hospital
hospitalized V34.1
not hospitalized V34.2
mates all stillborn
born in hospital (without mention of cesarean delivery or section) V35.00
with cesarean delivery or section V35.01
born outside hospital
hospitalized V35.1
not hospitalized V35.2
mates liveborn and stillborn
born in hospital (without mention of cesarean delivery or section) V36.00
with cesarean delivery or section V36.01
born outside hospital
hospitalized V36.1
not hospitalized V36.2
omphalitis 771.4
seizure 779.0
sepsis 771.81
single
born in hospital (without mention of cesarean delivery or section) V30.00
with cesarean delivery or section V30.01
born outside hospital
hospitalized V30.1
not hospitalized V30.2
specified condition NEC 779.89

Newborn — continued
twin NEC
born in hospital (without mention of cesarean delivery or section) V33.00
with cesarean delivery or section V33.01
born outside hospital
hospitalized V33.1
not hospitalized V33.2
mate liveborn
born in hospital V31.0 ☑
born outside hospital
hospitalized V31.1
not hospitalized V31.2
mate stillborn
born in hospital V32.0 ☑
born outside hospital
hospitalized V32.1
not hospitalized V32.2
unspecified as to single or multiple birth
born in hospital (without mention of cesarean delivery or section) V39.00
with cesarean delivery or section V39.01
born outside hospital
hospitalized V39.1
not hospitalized V39.2
weight check V20.32
Newcastle's conjunctivitis or disease 077.8
Nezelof's syndrome (pure alymphocytosis) 279.13
Niacin (amide) **deficiency** 265.2
Nicolas-Durand-Favre disease (climatic bubo) 099.1
Nicolas-Favre disease (climatic bubo) 099.1
Nicotinic acid (amide) **deficiency** 265.2
Niemann-Pick disease (lipid histiocytosis) (splenomegaly) 272.7
Night
blindness (see also Blindness, night) 368.60
congenital 368.61
vitamin A deficiency 264.5
cramps 729.82
sweats 780.8
terrors, child 307.46
Nightmare 307.47
REM-sleep type 307.47
Nipple — see condition
Nisbet's chancre 099.0
Nishimoto (-Takeuchi) disease 437.5
Nitritoid crisis or reaction — see Crisis, nitritoid
Nitrogen retention, extrarenal 788.99
Nitrosohemoglobinemia 289.89
Njovera 104.0
No
diagnosis 799.9
disease (found) V71.9
room at the inn V65.0
Nocardiasis — see Nocardiosis
Nocardiosis 039.9
with pneumonia 039.1
lung 039.1
specified type NEC 039.8
Nocturia 788.43
psychogenic 306.53
Nocturnal — see also condition
dyspnea (paroxysmal) 786.09
emissions 608.89
enuresis 788.36
psychogenic 307.6
frequency (micturition) 788.43
psychogenic 306.53
Nodal rhythm disorder 427.89
Nodding of head 781.0
Node(s) — see also Nodule(s)
Heberden's 715.04
larynx 478.79
lymph — see condition
milkers' 051.1
Osler's 421.0
rheumatic 729.89
Schmorl's 722.30
lumbar, lumbosacral 722.32

Node(s) — see also Nodule(s) — continued
Schmorl's — continued
specified region NEC 722.39
thoracic, thoracolumbar 722.31
singers' 478.5
skin NEC 782.2
tuberculous — see Tuberculosis, lymph gland
vocal cords 478.5
Nodosities, Haygarth's 715.04
Nodule(s), nodular
actinomycotic (see also Actinomycosis) 039.9
arthritic — see Arthritis, nodosa
breast 793.89
cutaneous 782.2
Haygarth's 715.04
inflammatory — see Inflammation
juxta-articular 102.7
syphilitic 095.7
yaws 102.7
larynx 478.79
lung
emphysematous 492.8
solitary 793.11
milkers' 051.1
prostate 600.10
with
urinary
obstruction 600.11
retention 600.11
pulmonary, solitary (subsegmental branch of the bronchial tree) 793.11
multiple 793.19
retrocardiac 785.9
rheumatic 729.89
rheumatoid — see Arthritis, rheumatoid
scrotum (inflammatory) 608.4
singers' 478.5
skin NEC 782.2
solitary, lung 793.11
emphysematous 492.8
subcutaneous 782.2
thyroid (gland) (nontoxic) (uninodular) 241.0
with
hyperthyroidism 242.1 ☑
thyrotoxicosis 242.1 ☑
toxic or with hyperthyroidism 242.1 ☑
vocal cords 478.5
Noma (gangrenous) (hospital) (infective) 528.1
auricle (see also Gangrene) 785.4
mouth 528.1
pudendi (see also Vulvitis) 616.10
vulvae (see also Vulvitis) 616.10
Nomadism V60.0
Non-adherence
artificial skin graft 996.55
decellularized allodermis graft 996.55
Non-autoimmune hemolytic anemia NEC 283.10
Nonclosure — see also Imperfect, closure
ductus
arteriosus 747.0
Botalli 747.0
Eustachian valve 746.89
foramen
Botalli 745.5
ovale 745.5
Noncompliance with medical treatment V15.81
renal dialysis V45.12
Nondescent (congenital) — see also Malposition, congenital
cecum 751.4
colon 751.4
testis 752.51
Nondevelopment
brain 742.1
specified part 742.2
heart 746.89
organ or site, congenital NEC — see Hypoplasia
Nonengagement
head NEC 652.5 ☑
in labor 660.1 ☑
affecting fetus or newborn 763.1

☑ **Additional Digit Required** — Refer to the Tabular List for Digit Selection

▽ **Subterms under main terms may continue to next column or page**

Nonexanthematous tick fever 066.1
Nonexpansion, lung (newborn) NEC 770.4
Nonfunctioning
 cystic duct (*see also* Disease, gallbladder) 575.8
 gallbladder (*see also* Disease, gallbladder) 575.8
 kidney (*see also* Disease, renal) 593.9
 labyrinth 386.58
Nonhealing
 stump (surgical) 997.69
 wound, surgical 998.83
Nonimplantation of ovum, causing infertility 628.3
Noninsufflation, fallopian tube 628.2
Nonne-Milroy-Meige syndrome (chronic hereditary edema) 757.0
Nonovulation 628.0
Nonpatent fallopian tube 628.2
Nonpneumatization, lung NEC 770.4
Nonreflex bladder 596.54
 with cauda equina 344.61
Nonretention of food — *see* Vomiting
Nonrotation — *see* Malrotation
Nonsecretion, urine — *see also* Anuria 788.5
 newborn 753.3
Nonunion
 fracture 733.82
 organ or site, congenital NEC — *see* Imperfect, closure
 symphysis pubis, congenital 755.69
 top sacrum, congenital 756.19
Nonviability 765.0 ☑
Nonvisualization, gallbladder 793.3
Nonvitalized tooth 522.9
Non-working side interference 524.56
Normal
 delivery — *see* category 650
 menses V65.5
 state (feared complaint unfounded) V65.5
Normoblastosis 289.89

Normocytic anemia (infectional) 285.9
 due to blood loss (chronic) 280.0
 acute 285.1
Norrie's disease (congenital) (progressive oculoacousticocerebral degeneration) 743.8
North American blastomycosis 116.0
Norwegian itch 133.0
Nosebleed 784.7
Nose, nasal — *see* condition
Nosomania 298.9
Nosophobia 300.29
Nostalgia 309.89
Notched lip, congenital — *see also* Cleft, lip 749.10
Notching nose, congenital (tip) 748.1
Notch of iris 743.46
Nothnagel's
 syndrome 378.52
 vasomotor acroparesthesia 443.89
Novy's relapsing fever (American) 087.1
Noxious
 foodstuffs, poisoning by
  fish 988.0
  fungi 988.1
  mushrooms 988.1
  plants (food) 988.2
  shellfish 988.0
  specified type NEC 988.8
  toadstool 988.1
 substances transmitted through placenta or breast milk (affecting fetus or newborn) 760.70
  acetretin 760.78
  alcohol 760.71
  aminopterin 760.78
  antiandrogens 760.79
  anticonvulsant 760.77
  antifungal 760.74
  anti-infective agents 760.74
  antimetabolic 760.78

Noxious — *continued*
 substances transmitted through placenta or breast milk — *continued*
  atorvastatin 760.78
  carbamazepine 760.77
  cocaine 760.75
  "crack" 760.75
  diethylstilbestrol (DES) 760.76
  divalproex sodium 760.77
  endocrine disrupting chemicals 760.79
  estrogens 760.79
  etretinate 760.78
  fluconazole 760.74
  fluvastatin 760.78
  hallucinogenic agents NEC 760.73
  hormones 760.79
  lithium 760.79
  lovastatin 760.78
  medicinal agents NEC 760.79
  methotrexate 760.78
  misoprostil 760.79
  narcotics 760.72
  obstetric anesthetic or analgesic 763.5
  phenobarbital 760.77
  phenytoin 760.77
  pravastatin 760.78
  progestins 760.79
  retinoic acid 760.78
  simvastatin 760.78
  solvents 760.79
  specified agent NEC 760.79
  statins 760.78
  suspected, affecting management of pregnancy 655.5 ☑
  tetracycline 760.74
  thalidomide 760.79
  trimethadione 760.77
  valproate 760.77
  valproic acid 760.77
  vitamin A 760.78
NPDH (new persistent daily headache) 339.42

Nuchal hitch (arm) 652.8 ☑
Nucleus pulposus — *see* condition
Numbness 782.0
Nuns' knee 727.2
Nursemaid's
 elbow 832.2
 shoulder 831.0 ☑
Nutmeg liver 573.8
Nutrition, deficient or insufficient (particular kind of food) 269.9
 due to
  insufficient food 994.2
  lack of
   care (child) (infant) 995.52
    adult 995.84
   food 994.2
Nyctalopia — *see also* Blindness, night 368.60
 vitamin A deficiency 264.5
Nycturia 788.43
 psychogenic 306.53
Nymphomania 302.89
Nystagmus 379.50
 associated with vestibular system disorders 379.54
 benign paroxysmal positional 386.11
 central positional 386.2
 congenital 379.51
 deprivation 379.53
 dissociated 379.55
 latent 379.52
 miners' 300.89
 positional
  benign paroxysmal 386.11
  central 386.2
 specified NEC 379.56
 vestibular 379.54
 visual deprivation 379.53

O

Oasthouse urine disease 270.2
Obermeyer's relapsing fever (European) 087.0
Obesity (constitutional) (exogenous) (familial) (nutritional) (simple) 278.00
　adrenal 255.8
　complicating pregnancy, childbirth, or puerperium 649.1 ☑
　due to hyperalimentation 278.00
　endocrine NEC 259.9
　endogenous 259.9
　Fröhlich's (adiposogenital dystrophy) 253.8
　glandular NEC 259.9
　hypothyroid (*see also* Hypothyroidism) 244.9
　hypoventilation syndrome 278.03
　morbid 278.01
　of pregnancy 649.1 ☑
　pituitary 253.8
　severe 278.01
　thyroid (*see also* Hypothyroidism) 244.9
Oblique — *see also* condition
　lie before labor, affecting fetus or newborn 761.7
Obliquity, pelvis 738.6
Obliteration
　abdominal aorta 446.7
　appendix (lumen) 543.9
　artery 447.1
　ascending aorta 446.7
　bile ducts 576.8
　　with calculus, choledocholithiasis, or stones — *see* Choledocholithiasis
　　congenital 751.61
　　jaundice from 751.61 [774.5]
　common duct 576.8
　　with calculus, choledocholithiasis, or stones — *see* Choledocholithiasis
　　congenital 751.61
　cystic duct 575.8
　　with calculus, choledocholithiasis, or stones — *see* Choledocholithiasis
　disease, arteriolar 447.1
　endometrium 621.8
　eye, anterior chamber 360.34
　fallopian tube 628.2
　lymphatic vessel 457.1
　　postmastectomy 457.0
　organ or site, congenital NEC — *see* Atresia
　placental blood vessels — *see* Placenta, abnormal
　supra-aortic branches 446.7
　ureter 593.89
　urethra 599.84
　vein 459.9
　vestibule (oral) 525.8
Observation (for) V71.9
　without need for further medical care V71.9
　accident NEC V71.4
　　at work V71.3
　criminal assault V71.6
　deleterious agent ingestion V71.89
　disease V71.9
　　cardiovascular V71.7
　　heart V71.7
　　mental V71.09
　　specified condition NEC V71.89
　foreign body ingestion V71.89
　growth and development variations V21.8
　injuries (accidental) V71.4
　　inflicted NEC V71.6
　　　during alleged rape or seduction V71.5
　malignant neoplasm, suspected V71.1
　postpartum
　　immediately after delivery V24.0
　　routine follow-up V24.2
　pregnancy
　　high-risk V23.9
　　　inconclusive fetal viability V23.87
　　　specified problem NEC V23.89
　　normal (without complication) V22.1
　　　with nonobstetric complication V22.2
　　　first V22.0
　rape or seduction, alleged V71.5
　　injury during V71.5

Observation — *continued*
　suicide attempt, alleged V71.89
　suspected (undiagnosed) (unproven)
　　abuse V71.81
　　cardiovascular disease V71.7
　　child or wife battering victim V71.6
　　concussion (cerebral) V71.6
　　condition NEC V71.89
　　　infant — *see* Observation, suspected, condition, newborn
　　　maternal and fetal
　　　　amniotic cavity and membrane problem V89.01
　　　　cervical shortening V89.05
　　　　fetal anomaly V89.03
　　　　fetal growth problem V89.04
　　　　oligohydramnios V89.01
　　　　other specified problem NEC V89.09
　　　　placental problem V89.02
　　　　polyhydramnios V89.01
　　　newborn V29.9
　　　　cardiovascular disease V29.8
　　　　congenital anomaly V29.8
　　　　genetic V29.3
　　　　infectious V29.0
　　　　ingestion foreign object V29.8
　　　　injury V29.8
　　　　metabolic V29.3
　　　　neoplasm V29.8
　　　　neurological V29.1
　　　　poison, poisoning V29.8
　　　　respiratory V29.2
　　　　specified NEC V29.8
　　exposure
　　　anthrax V71.82
　　　biologic agent NEC V71.83
　　　SARS V71.83
　　infectious disease not requiring isolation V71.89
　　malignant neoplasm V71.1
　　mental disorder V71.09
　　neglect V71.81
　　neoplasm
　　　benign V71.89
　　　malignant V71.1
　　specified condition NEC V71.89
　　tuberculosis V71.2
　tuberculosis, suspected V71.2
Obsession, obsessional 300.3
　ideas and mental images 300.3
　impulses 300.3
　neurosis 300.3
　phobia 300.3
　psychasthenia 300.3
　ruminations 300.3
　state 300.3
　syndrome 300.3
Obsessive-compulsive 300.3
　neurosis 300.3
　personality 301.4
　reaction 300.3
Obstetrical trauma NEC (complicating delivery) 665.9 ☑
　with
　　abortion — *see* Abortion, by type, with damage to pelvic organs
　　ectopic pregnancy (*see also* categories 633.0–633.9) 639.2
　　molar pregnancy (*see also* categories 630–632) 639.2
　affecting fetus or newborn 763.89
　following
　　abortion 639.2
　　ectopic or molar pregnancy 639.2
Obstipation — *see also* Constipation 564.00
　psychogenic 306.4
Obstruction, obstructed, obstructive
　airway NEC 519.8
　　with
　　　allergic alveolitis NEC 495.9
　　　asthma NEC (*see also* Asthma) 493.9 ☑
　　　bronchiectasis 494.0
　　　　with acute exacerbation 494.1

Obstruction, obstructed, obstructive — *continued*
　airway — *continued*
　　with — *continued*
　　　bronchitis (chronic) (*see also* Bronchitis, with, obstruction) 491.20
　　　emphysema NEC 492.8
　　chronic 496
　　　with
　　　　allergic alveolitis NEC 495.5
　　　　asthma NEC (*see also* Asthma) 493.2 ☑
　　　　bronchiectasis 494.0
　　　　　with acute exacerbation 494.1
　　　　bronchitis (chronic) (*see also* Bronchitis, with, obstruction) 491.20
　　　　emphysema NEC 492.8
　　　due to
　　　　bronchospasm 519.11
　　　　foreign body 934.9
　　　　inhalation of fumes or vapors 506.9
　　　　laryngospasm 478.75
　alimentary canal (*see also* Obstruction, intestine) 560.9
　ampulla of Vater 576.2
　　with calculus, cholelithiasis, or stones — *see* Choledocholithiasis
　aortic (heart) (valve) (*see also* Stenosis, aortic) 424.1
　　rheumatic (*see also* Stenosis, aortic, rheumatic) 395.0
　aortoiliac 444.09
　aqueduct of Sylvius 331.4
　　congenital 742.3
　　　with spina bifida (*see also* Spina bifida) 741.0 ☑
　Arnold-Chiari (*see also* Spina bifida) 741.0 ☑
　artery (*see also* Embolism, artery) 444.9
　　basilar (complete) (partial) (*see also* Occlusion, artery, basilar) 433.0 ☑
　　carotid (complete) (partial) (*see also* Occlusion, artery, carotid) 433.1 ☑
　　precerebral — *see* Occlusion, artery, precerebral NEC
　　retinal (central) (*see also* Occlusion, retina) 362.30
　　vertebral (complete) (partial) (*see also* Occlusion, artery, vertebral) 433.2 ☑
　asthma (chronic) (with obstructive pulmonary disease) 493.2 ☑
　band (intestinal) 560.81
　bile duct or passage (*see also* Obstruction, biliary) 576.2
　　congenital 751.61
　　　jaundice from 751.61 [774.5]
　biliary (duct) (tract) 576.2
　　with calculus 574.51
　　　with cholecystitis (chronic) 574.41
　　　　acute 574.31
　　congenital 751.61
　　　jaundice from 751.61 [774.5]
　　gallbladder 575.2
　　　with calculus 574.21
　　　　with cholecystitis (chronic) 574.11
　　　　　acute 574.01
　bladder neck (acquired) 596.0
　　congenital 753.6
　bowel (*see also* Obstruction, intestine) 560.9
　bronchus 519.19
　canal, ear (*see also* Stricture, ear canal, acquired) 380.50
　cardia 537.89
　caval veins (inferior) (superior) 459.2
　cecum (*see also* Obstruction, intestine) 560.9
　circulatory 459.9
　colon (*see also* Obstruction, intestine) 560.9
　　sympathicotonic 560.89
　common duct (*see also* Obstruction, biliary) 576.2
　　congenital 751.61
　coronary (artery) (heart) (*see also* Arteriosclerosis, coronary)
　　acute (*see also* Infarct, myocardium) 410.9 ☑

Obstruction, obstructed, obstructive — *continued*
　coronary (*see also* Arteriosclerosis, coronary) — *continued*
　　acute (*see also* Infarct, myocardium) — *continued*
　　　without myocardial infarction 411.81
　cystic duct (*see also* Obstruction, gallbladder) 575.2
　　congenital 751.61
　device, implant, or graft — *see* Complications, due to (presence of) any device, implant, or graft classified to 996.0–996.5 NEC
　due to foreign body accidentally left in operation wound 998.4
　duodenum 537.3
　　congenital 751.1
　　due to
　　　compression NEC 537.3
　　　cyst 537.3
　　　intrinsic lesion or disease NEC 537.3
　　　scarring 537.3
　　　torsion 537.3
　　　ulcer 532.91
　　　volvulus 537.3
　ejaculatory duct 608.89
　endocardium 424.90
　　arteriosclerotic 424.99
　　specified cause, except rheumatic 424.99
　esophagus 530.3
　eustachian tube (complete) (partial) 381.60
　　cartilaginous
　　　extrinsic 381.63
　　　intrinsic 381.62
　　due to
　　　cholesteatoma 381.61
　　　osseous lesion NEC 381.61
　　　polyp 381.61
　　　osseous 381.61
　fallopian tube (bilateral) 628.2
　fecal 560.32
　　with hernia (*see also* Hernia, by site, with obstruction)
　　gangrenous — *see* Hernia, by site, with gangrene
　foramen of Monro (congenital) 742.3
　　with spina bifida (*see also* Spina bifida) 741.0 ☑
　foreign body — *see* Foreign body
　gallbladder 575.2
　　with calculus, cholelithiasis, or stones 574.21
　　　with cholecystitis (chronic) 574.11
　　　　acute 574.01
　　congenital 751.69
　　　jaundice from 751.69 [774.5]
　gastric outlet 537.0
　gastrointestinal (*see also* Obstruction, intestine) 560.9
　glottis 478.79
　hepatic 573.8
　　duct (*see also* Obstruction, biliary) 576.2
　　　congenital 751.61
　icterus (*see also* Obstruction, biliary) 576.8
　　congenital 751.61
　ileocecal coil (*see also* Obstruction, intestine) 560.9
　ileum (*see also* Obstruction, intestine) 560.9
　iliofemoral (artery) 444.81
　internal anastomosis — *see* Complications, mechanical, graft
　intestine (mechanical) (neurogenic) (paroxysmal) (postinfectional) (reflex) 560.9
　　with
　　　adhesions (intestinal) (peritoneal) 560.81
　　　hernia (*see also* Hernia, by site, with obstruction)
　　　　gangrenous — *see* Hernia, by site, with gangrene
　　adynamic (*see also* Ileus) 560.1
　　by gallstone 560.31
　　congenital or infantile (small) 751.1
　　　large 751.2

Obstruction, obstructed, obstructive —
continued
intestine — *continued*
  due to
    Ascaris lumbricoides 127.0
    mural thickening 560.89
    procedure 997.49
      involving urinary tract 997.5
  impaction 560.32
  infantile — *see* Obstruction, intestine, congenital
  newborn
    due to
      fecaliths 777.1
      inspissated milk 777.2
      meconium (plug) 777.1
        in mucoviscidosis 277.01
    transitory 777.4
  specified cause NEC 560.89
  transitory, newborn 777.4
  volvulus 560.2
  intracardiac ball valve prosthesis 996.02
jaundice (*see also* Obstruction, biliary) 576.8
  congenital 751.61
jejunum (*see also* Obstruction, intestine) 560.9
kidney 593.89
labor 660.9 ☑
  affecting fetus or newborn 763.1
  by
    bony pelvis (conditions classifiable to 653.0–653.9) 660.1 ☑
    deep transverse arrest 660.3 ☑
    impacted shoulder 660.4 ☑
    locked twins 660.5 ☑
    malposition (fetus) (conditions classifiable to 652.0–652.9) 660.0 ☑
      head during labor 660.3 ☑
    persistent occipitoposterior position 660.3 ☑
    soft tissue, pelvic (conditions classifiable to 654.0–654.9) 660.2 ☑
lacrimal
  canaliculi 375.53
  congenital 743.65
  punctum 375.52
  sac 375.54
lacrimonasal duct 375.56
  congenital 743.65
  neonatal 375.55
lacteal, with steatorrhea 579.2
laryngitis (*see also* Laryngitis) 464.01
larynx 478.79
  congenital 748.3
liver 573.8
  cirrhotic (*see also* Cirrhosis, liver) 571.5
lung 518.89
  with
    asthma — *see* Asthma
    bronchitis (chronic) 491.20
    emphysema NEC 492.8
  airway, chronic 496
  chronic NEC 496
    with
      asthma (chronic) (obstructive) 493.2 ☑
    disease, chronic 496
      with
        asthma (chronic) (obstructive) 493.2 ☑
    emphysematous 492.8
lymphatic 457.1
meconium
  fetus or newborn 777.1
    in mucoviscidosis 277.01
  newborn due to fecaliths 777.1
mediastinum 519.3
mitral (rheumatic) — *see* Stenosis, mitral
nasal 478.19
  duct 375.56
    neonatal 375.55
  sinus — *see* Sinusitis
nasolacrimal duct 375.56
  congenital 743.65
  neonatal 375.55

Obstruction, obstructed, obstructive —
continued
nasopharynx 478.29
nose 478.19
organ or site, congenital NEC — *see* Atresia
pancreatic duct 577.8
parotid gland 527.8
pelviureteral junction (*see also* Obstruction, ureter) 593.4
pharynx 478.29
portal (circulation) (vein) 452
prostate 600.90
  with
    other lower urinary tract symptoms (LUTS) 600.91
    urinary
      obstruction 600.91
      retention 600.91
  valve (urinary) 596.0
pulmonary
  valve (heart) (*see also* Endocarditis, pulmonary) 424.3
  vein, isolated 747.49
pyemic — *see* Septicemia
pylorus (acquired) 537.0
  congenital 750.5
  infantile 750.5
rectosigmoid (*see also* Obstruction, intestine) 560.9
rectum 569.49
renal 593.89
respiratory 519.8
  chronic 496
retinal (artery) (vein) (central) (*see also* Occlusion, retina) 362.30
salivary duct (any) 527.8
  with calculus 527.5
sigmoid (*see also* Obstruction, intestine) 560.9
sinus (accessory) (nasal) (*see also* Sinusitis) 473.9
Stensen's duct 527.8
stomach 537.89
  acute 536.1
  congenital 750.7
submaxillary gland 527.8
  with calculus 527.5
thoracic duct 457.1
thrombotic — *see* Thrombosis
tooth eruption 520.6
trachea 519.19
tracheostomy airway 519.09
tricuspid — *see* Endocarditis, tricuspid
upper respiratory, congenital 748.8
ureter (functional) 593.4
  congenital 753.20
  due to calculus 592.1
ureteropelvic junction, congenital 753.21
ureterovesical junction, congenital 753.22
urethra 599.60
  congenital 753.6
urinary (moderate) 599.60
  organ or tract (lower) 599.60
    due to
      benign prostatic hypertrophy (BPH) - see category 600
    specified NEC 599.69
      due to
        benign prostatic hypertrophy (BPH) — see category 600
  prostatic valve 596.0
uropathy 599.60
uterus 621.8
vagina 623.2
valvular — *see* Endocarditis
vascular graft or shunt 996.1
  atherosclerosis — *see* Arteriosclerosis, coronary
  embolism 996.74
  occlusion NEC 996.74
  thrombus 996.74
vein, venous 459.2
  caval (inferior) (superior) 459.2
  thrombotic — *see* Thrombosis
vena cava (inferior) (superior) 459.2

Obstruction, obstructed, obstructive —
continued
ventricular shunt 996.2
vesical 596.0
vesicourethral orifice 596.0
vessel NEC 459.9
Obturator — *see* condition
Occlusal
  plane deviation 524.76
  wear, teeth 521.10
Occlusion
anus 569.49
  congenital 751.2
  infantile 751.2
aortoiliac (chronic) 444.09
aqueduct of Sylvius 331.4
  congenital 742.3
    with spina bifida (*see also* Spina bifida) 741.0 ☑
arteries of extremities, lower 444.22
  without thrombus or embolus (*see also* Arteriosclerosis, extremities) 440.20
  due to stricture or stenosis 447.1
  upper 444.21
    without thrombus or embolus (*see also* Arteriosclerosis, extremities) 440.20
    due to stricture or stenosis 447.1
artery NEC (*see also* Embolism, artery) 444.9
  auditory, internal 433.8 ☑
  basilar 433.0 ☑
    with other precerebral artery 433.3 ☑
    bilateral 433.3 ☑
  brain or cerebral (*see also* Infarct, brain) 434.9 ☑
  carotid 433.1 ☑
    with other precerebral artery 433.3 ☑
    bilateral 433.3 ☑
  cerebellar (anterior inferior) (posterior inferior) (superior) 433.8 ☑
  cerebral (*see also* Infarct, brain) 434.9 ☑
  choroidal (anterior) 433.8 ☑
  chronic total
    coronary 414.2
    extremity(ies) 440.4
  communicating posterior 433.8 ☑
  complete
    coronary 414.2
    extremity(ies) 440.4
  coronary (thrombotic) (*see also* Infarct, myocardium) 410.9 ☑
    acute 410.9 ☑
      without myocardial infarction 411.81
    chronic total 414.2
    complete 414.2
    healed or old 412
    total 414.2
  extremity(ies)
    chronic total 440.4
    complete 440.4
    total 440.4
  hypophyseal 433.8 ☑
  iliac (artery) 444.81
  mesenteric (embolic) (thrombotic) (with gangrene) 557.0
  pontine 433.8 ☑
  precerebral NEC 433.9 ☑
    late effect — *see* Late effect(s) (of) cerebrovascular disease
    multiple or bilateral 433.3 ☑
    puerperal, postpartum, childbirth 674.0 ☑
    specified NEC 433.8 ☑
  renal 593.81
  retinal — *see* Occlusion, retina, artery
  spinal 433.8 ☑
  vertebral 433.2 ☑
    with other precerebral artery 433.3 ☑
    bilateral 433.3 ☑

Occlusion — *continued*
  basilar (artery) — *see* Occlusion, artery, basilar
  bile duct (any) (*see also* Obstruction, biliary) 576.2
  bowel (*see also* Obstruction, intestine) 560.9
  brain (artery) (vascular) (*see also* Infarct, brain) 434.9 ☑
  breast (duct) 611.89
  carotid (artery) (common) (internal) — *see* Occlusion, artery, carotid
  cerebellar (anterior inferior) (artery) (posterior inferior) (superior) 433.8 ☑
  cerebral (artery) (*see also* Infarct, brain) 434.9 ☑
  cerebrovascular (*see also* Infarct, brain) 434.9 ☑
    diffuse 437.0
  cervical canal (*see also* Stricture, cervix) 622.4
    by falciparum malaria 084.0
  cervix (uteri) (*see also* Stricture, cervix) 622.4
  choanal 748.0
  choroidal (artery) 433.8 ☑
  colon (*see also* Obstruction, intestine) 560.9
  communicating posterior artery 433.8 ☑
  coronary (artery) (thrombotic) (*see also* Infarct, myocardium) 410.9 ☑
    without myocardial infarction 411.81
    acute 410.9 ☑
      without myocardial infarction 411.81
    healed or old 412
  cystic duct (*see also* Obstruction, gallbladder) 575.2
    congenital 751.69
  disto
    division I 524.22
    division II 524.22
  embolic — *see* Embolism
  fallopian tube 628.2
    congenital 752.19
  gallbladder (*see also* Obstruction, gallbladder) 575.2
    congenital 751.69
      jaundice from 751.69 [774.5]
  gingiva, traumatic 523.8
  hymen 623.3
    congenital 752.42
  hypophyseal (artery) 433.8 ☑
  iliac artery 444.81
  intestine (*see also* Obstruction, intestine) 560.9
  kidney 593.89
  lacrimal apparatus — *see* Stenosis, lacrimal
  lung 518.89
  lymph or lymphatic channel 457.1
  mammary duct 611.89
  mesenteric artery (embolic) (thrombotic) (with gangrene) 557.0
  nose 478.1 ☑
    congenital 748.0
  organ or site, congenital NEC — *see* Atresia
  oviduct 628.2
    congenital 752.19
  periodontal, traumatic 523.8
  peripheral arteries (lower extremity) 444.22
    without thrombus or embolus (*see also* Arteriosclerosis, extremities) 440.20
    due to stricture or stenosis 447.1
    upper extremity 444.21
      without thrombus or embolus (*see also* Arteriosclerosis, extremities) 440.20
      due to stricture or stenosis 447.1
  pontine (artery) 433.8 ☑
  posterior lingual, of mandibular teeth 524.29
  precerebral artery — *see* Occlusion, artery, precerebral NEC
  puncta lacrimalia 375.52
  pupil 364.74
  pylorus (*see also* Stricture, pylorus) 537.0
  renal artery 593.81
  retina, retinal (vascular) 362.30
    artery, arterial 362.30

Occlusion — *continued*
  retina, retinal — *continued*
    artery, arterial — *continued*
      branch 362.32
      central (total) 362.31
      partial 362.33
      transient 362.34
      tributary 362.32
    vein 362.30
      branch 362.36
      central (total) 362.35
      incipient 362.37
      partial 362.37
      tributary 362.36
  spinal artery 433.8 ☑
  stent
    coronary 996.72
  teeth (mandibular) (posterior lingual) 524.29
  thoracic duct 457.1
  tubal 628.2
  ureter (complete) (partial) 593.4
    congenital 753.29
  urethra (*see also* Stricture, urethra) 598.9
    congenital 753.6
  uterus 621.8
  vagina 623.2
  vascular NEC 459.9
  vein — *see* Thrombosis
  vena cava
    inferior 453.2
    superior (acute) 453.87
      chronic 453.77
  ventricle (brain) NEC 331.4
  vertebral (artery) — *see* Occlusion, artery, vertebral
  vessel (blood) NEC 459.9
  vulva 624.8
Occlusio pupillae 364.74
Occupational
  problems NEC V62.29
  therapy V57.21
Ochlophobia 300.29
Ochronosis (alkaptonuric) (congenital) (endogenous) 270.0
  with chloasma of eyelid 270.2
Ocular muscle — *see also* condition
  myopathy 359.1
  torticollis 781.93
Oculoauriculovertebral dysplasia 756.0
Oculogyric
  crisis or disturbance 378.87
    psychogenic 306.7
Oculomotor syndrome 378.81
Oddi's sphincter spasm 576.5
Odelberg's disease (juvenile osteochondrosis) 732.1
Odontalgia 525.9
Odontoameloblastoma (M9311/0) 213.1
  upper jaw (bone) 213.0
Odontoclasia 521.05
Odontoclasis 873.63
  complicated 873.73
Odontodysplasia, regional 520.4
Odontogenesis imperfecta 520.5
Odontoma (M9280/0) 213.1
  ameloblastic (M9311/0) 213.1
    upper jaw (bone) 213.0
  calcified (M9280/0) 213.1
    upper jaw (bone) 213.0
  complex (M9282/0) 213.1
    upper jaw (bone) 213.0
  compound (M9281/0) 213.1
    upper jaw (bone) 213.0
  fibroameloblastic (M9290/0) 213.1
    upper jaw (bone) 213.0
  follicular 526.0
  upper jaw (bone) 213.0
Odontomyelitis (closed) (open) 522.0
Odontonecrosis 521.09
Odontorrhagia 525.8
Odontosarcoma, ameloblastic (M9290/3) 170.1
  upper jaw (bone) 170.0
Odynophagia 787.20
Oesophagostomiasis 127.7
Oesophagostomum infestation 127.7

Oestriasis 134.0
Ogilvie's syndrome (sympathicotonic colon obstruction) 560.89
Oguchi's disease (retina) 368.61
Ohara's disease — *see also* Tularemia 021.9
Oidiomycosis — *see also* Candidiasis 112.9
Oidiomycotic meningitis 112.83
Oidium albicans infection — *see also* Candidiasis 112.9
Old age 797
  dementia (of) 290.0
Olfactory — *see* condition
Oligemia 285.9
Oligergasia — *see also* Disability, intellectual 319
Oligoamnios 658.0 ☑
  affecting fetus or newborn 761.2
Oligoastrocytoma, mixed (M9382/3)
  specified site — *see* Neoplasm, by site, malignant
  unspecified site 191.9
Oligocythemia 285.9
Oligodendroblastoma (M9460/3)
  specified site — *see* Neoplasm, by site, malignant
  unspecified site 191.9
Oligodendroglioma (M9450/3)
  anaplastic type (M9451/3)
    specified site — *see* Neoplasm, by site, malignant
    unspecified site 191.9
  specified site — *see* Neoplasm, by site, malignant
  unspecified site 191.9
Oligodendroma — *see* Oligodendroglioma
Oligodontia — *see also* Anodontia 520.0
Oligoencephalon 742.1
Oligohydramnios 658.0 ☑
  affecting fetus or newborn 761.2
  due to premature rupture of membranes 658.1 ☑
    affecting fetus or newborn 761.2
Oligohydrosis 705.0
Oligomenorrhea 626.1
Oligophrenia — *see also* Disability, intellectual 319
  phenylpyruvic 270.1
Oligospermia 606.1
Oligotrichia 704.09
  congenita 757.4
Oliguria 788.5
  with
    abortion — *see* Abortion, by type, with renal failure
    ectopic pregnancy (*see also* categories 633.0–633.9) 639.3
    molar pregnancy (*see also* categories 630–632) 639.3
  complicating
    abortion 639.3
    ectopic or molar pregnancy 639.3
    pregnancy 646.2 ☑
      with hypertension — *see* Toxemia, of pregnancy
    due to a procedure 997.5
    following labor and delivery 669.3 ☑
    heart or cardiac — *see* Failure, heart
    puerperal, postpartum 669.3 ☑
    specified due to a procedure 997.5
Ollier's disease (chondrodysplasia) 756.4
Omentitis — *see also* Peritonitis 567.9
Omentocele — *see also* Hernia, omental 553.8
Omentum, omental — *see* condition
Omphalitis (congenital) (newborn) 771.4
  not of newborn 686.9
    tetanus 771.3
Omphalocele 756.72
Omphalomesenteric duct, persistent 751.0
Omphalorrhagia, newborn 772.3
Omsk hemorrhagic fever 065.1
Onanism 307.9
Onchocerciasis 125.3
  eye 125.3 [360.13]
Onchocercosis 125.3
Oncocytoma (M8290/0) — *see* Neoplasm, by site, benign

Ondine's curse 348.89
Oneirophrenia — *see also* Schizophrenia 295.4 ☑
Onychauxis 703.8
  congenital 757.5
Onychia (with lymphangitis) 681.9
  dermatophytic 110.1
  finger 681.02
  toe 681.11
Onychitis (with lymphangitis) 681.9
  finger 681.02
  toe 681.11
Onychocryptosis 703.0
Onychodystrophy 703.8
  congenital 757.5
Onychogryphosis 703.8
Onychogryposis 703.8
Onycholysis 703.8
Onychomadesis 703.8
Onychomalacia 703.8
Onychomycosis 110.1
  finger 110.1
  toe 110.1
Onycho-osteodysplasia 756.89
Onychophagy 307.9
Onychoptosis 703.8
Onychorrhexis 703.8
  congenital 757.5
Onychoschizia 703.8
Onychotrophia — *see also* Atrophy, nail 703.8
O'nyong-nyong fever 066.3
Onyxis (finger) (toe) 703.0
Onyxitis (with lymphangitis) 681.9
  finger 681.02
  toe 681.11
Oocyte (egg) (ovum)
  donor V59.70
    over age 35 V59.73
      anonymous recipient V59.73
      designated recipient V59.74
    under age 35 V59.71
      anonymous recipient V59.71
      designated recipient V59.72
Oophoritis (cystic) (infectional) (interstitial) — *see also* Salpingo-oophoritis 614.2
  complicating pregnancy 646.6 ☑
  fetal (acute) 752.0
  gonococcal (acute) 098.19
    chronic or duration of 2 months or over 098.39
  tuberculous (*see also* Tuberculosis) 016.6 ☑
Opacity, opacities
  cornea 371.00
    central 371.03
    congenital 743.43
      interfering with vision 743.42
    degenerative (*see also* Degeneration, cornea) 371.40
    hereditary (*see also* Dystrophy, cornea) 371.50
    inflammatory (*see also* Keratitis) 370.9
    late effect of trachoma (healed) 139.1
    minor 371.01
    peripheral 371.02
  enamel (fluoride) (nonfluoride) (teeth) 520.3
  lens (*see also* Cataract) 366.9
  snowball 379.22
  vitreous (humor) 379.24
    congenital 743.51
Opalescent dentin (hereditary) 520.5
Open, opening
  abnormal, organ or site, congenital — *see* Imperfect, closure
  angle
    with
      borderline findings
        high risk 365.05
        intraocular pressure 365.01
        low risk 365.01
      cupping of discs 365.01
      high risk 365.05
      low risk 365.01
    bite
      anterior 524.24
      posterior 524.25
    false — *see* Imperfect, closure

Open, opening — *continued*
  margin on tooth restoration 525.61
    restoration margins 525.61
  wound — *see* Wound, open, by site
Operation
  causing mutilation of fetus 763.89
  destructive, on live fetus, to facilitate birth 763.89
  for delivery, fetus or newborn 763.89
  maternal, unrelated to current delivery, affecting fetus or newborn (*see also* Newborn, affected by) 760.64
Operational fatigue 300.89
Operative — *see* condition
Operculitis (chronic) 523.40
  acute 523.30
Operculum, retina 361.32
  with detachment 361.01
Ophiasis 704.01
Ophthalmia — *see also* Conjunctivitis 372.30
  actinic rays 370.24
  allergic (acute) 372.05
    chronic 372.14
  blennorrhagic (neonatorum) 098.40
  catarrhal 372.03
  diphtheritic 032.81
  Egyptian 076.1
  electric, electrica 370.24
  gonococcal (neonatorum) 098.40
  metastatic 360.11
  migraine 346.8 ☑
  neonatorum, newborn 771.6
    gonococcal 098.40
  nodosa 360.14
  phlyctenular 370.31
    with ulcer (*see also* Ulcer, cornea) 370.00
  sympathetic 360.11
Ophthalmitis — *see* Ophthalmia
Ophthalmocele (congenital) 743.66
Ophthalmoneuromyelitis 341.0
Ophthalmopathy, infiltrative with thyrotoxicosis 242.0 ☑
Ophthalmoplegia — *see also* Strabismus 378.9
  anterior internuclear 378.86
  ataxia-areflexia syndrome 357.0
  bilateral 378.9
  diabetic 250.5 ☑ [378.86]
    due to secondary diabetes 249.5 ☑ [378.86]
  exophthalmic 242.0 ☑ [376.22]
  external 378.55
    progressive 378.72
    total 378.56
  internal (complete) (total) 367.52
  internuclear 378.86
  migraine 346.2 ☑
  painful 378.55
  Parinaud's 378.81
  progressive external 378.72
  supranuclear, progressive 333.0
  total (external) 378.56
    internal 367.52
  unilateral 378.9
Opisthognathism 524.00
Opisthorchiasis (felineus) (tenuicollis) (viverrini) 121.0
Opisthotonos, opisthotonus 781.0
Opitz's disease (congestive splenomegaly) 289.51
Opiumism — *see also* Dependence 304.0 ☑
Opsoclonia 379.59
Optic nerve — *see* condition
Orbit — *see* condition
Orchioblastoma (M9071/3) 186.9
Orchitis (nonspecific) (septic) 604.90
  with abscess 604.0
  blennorrhagic (acute) 098.13
    chronic or duration of 2 months or over 098.33
  diphtheritic 032.89 [604.91]
  filarial 125.9 [604.91]

☑ **Additional Digit Required** — Refer to the Tabular List for Digit Selection   ▼ **Subterms under main terms may continue to next column or page**

2014 ICD-9-CM   **263**

Orchitis — *continued*
 gangrenous 604.99
 gonococcal (acute) 098.13
  chronic or duration of 2 months or over
   098.33
 mumps 072.0
 parotidea 072.0
 suppurative 604.99
 syphilitic 095.8 [604.91]
 tuberculous (*see also* Tuberculosis)
  016.5 ☑ [608.81]
Orf 051.2
Organic — *see also* condition
 heart — *see* Disease, heart
 insufficiency 799.89
Oriental
 bilharziasis 120.2
 schistosomiasis 120.2
 sore 085.1
Orientation
 ego-dystonic sexual 302.0
Orifice — *see* condition
Origin, both great vessels from right ventricle 745.11
Ormond's disease or syndrome 593.4
Ornithosis 073.9
 with
  complication 073.8
   specified NEC 073.7
  pneumonia 073.0
  pneumonitis (lobular) 073.0
Orodigitofacial dysostosis 759.89
Oropouche fever 066.3
Orotaciduria, oroticaciduria (congenital)
  (hereditary) (pyrimidine deficiency)
  281.4
Oroya fever 088.0
Orthodontics V58.5
 adjustment V53.4
 aftercare V58.5
 fitting V53.4
Orthopnea 786.02
Orthoptic training V57.4
Osgood-Schlatter
 disease 732.4
 osteochondrosis 732.4
Osler's
 disease (M9950/1) (polycythemia vera)
  238.4
 nodes 421.0
Osler-Rendu disease (familial hemorrhagic
  telangiectasia) 448.0
Osler-Vaquez disease (M9950/1) (polycythemia vera) 238.4
Osler-Weber-Rendu syndrome (familial
  hemorrhagic telangiectasia) 448.0
Osmidrosis 705.89
Osseous — *see* condition
Ossification
 artery — *see* Arteriosclerosis
 auricle (ear) 380.39
 bronchus 519.19
 cardiac (*see also* Degeneration, myocardial)
  429.1
 cartilage (senile) 733.99
 coronary (artery) — *see* Arteriosclerosis,
  coronary
 diaphragm 728.10
 ear 380.39
  middle (*see also* Otosclerosis) 387.9
 falx cerebri 349.2
 fascia 728.10
 fontanel
  defective or delayed 756.0
  premature 756.0
 heart (*see also* Degeneration, myocardial)
  429.1
  valve — *see* Endocarditis
 larynx 478.79
 ligament
  posterior longitudinal 724.8
   cervical 723.7
 meninges (cerebral) 349.2
  spinal 336.8
 multiple, eccentric centers 733.99
 muscle 728.10

Ossification — *continued*
 muscle — *continued*
  heterotopic, postoperative 728.13
 myocardium, myocardial (*see also* Degeneration, myocardial) 429.1
 penis 607.81
 periarticular 728.89
 sclera 379.16
 tendon 727.82
 trachea 519.19
 tympanic membrane (*see also* Tympanosclerosis) 385.00
 vitreous (humor) 360.44
Osteitis — *see also* Osteomyelitis 730.2 ☑
 acute 730.0 ☑
 alveolar 526.5
 chronic 730.1 ☑
 condensans (ilii) 733.5
 deformans (Paget's) 731.0
  due to or associated with malignant
   neoplasm (*see also* Neoplasm,
   bone, malignant) 170.9 [731.1]
 due to yaws 102.6
 fibrosa NEC 733.29
  cystica (generalisata) 252.01
  disseminata 756.59
  osteoplastica 252.01
 fragilitans 756.51
 Garré's (sclerosing) 730.1 ☑
 infectious (acute) (subacute) 730.0 ☑
  chronic or old 730.1 ☑
 jaw (acute) (chronic) (lower) (neonatal)
  (suppurative) (upper) 526.4
 parathyroid 252.01
 petrous bone (*see also* Petrositis) 383.20
 pubis 733.5
 sclerotic, nonsuppurative 730.1 ☑
 syphilitic 095.5
 tuberculosa
  cystica (of Jüngling) 135
  multiplex cystoides 135
Osteoarthritica spondylitis (spine) — *see also*
  Spondylosis 721.90
Osteoarthritis — *see also* Osteoarthrosis
  715.9 ☑
 distal interphalangeal 715.9 ☑
 hyperplastic 731.2
 interspinalis (*see also* Spondylosis) 721.90
 spine, spinal NEC (*see also* Spondylosis)
  721.90
Osteoarthropathy — *see also* Osteoarthrosis
  715.9 ☑
 chronic idiopathic hypertrophic 757.39
 familial idiopathic 757.39
 hypertrophic pulmonary 731.2
  secondary 731.2
 idiopathic hypertrophic 757.39
 primary hypertrophic 731.2
 pulmonary hypertrophic 731.2
 secondary hypertrophic 731.2
Osteoarthrosis (degenerative) (hypertrophic)
  (rheumatoid) 715.9 ☑

Note — Use the following fifth-digit
subclassification with category 715:

0 site unspecified
1 shoulder region
2 upper arm
3 forearm
4 hand
5 pelvic region and thigh
6 lower leg
7 ankle and foot
8 other specified sites except spine
9 multiple sites

 Deformans alkaptonurica 270.2
 generalized 715.09
 juvenilis (Köhler's) 732.5
 localized 715.3 ☑
  idiopathic 715.1 ☑
  primary 715.1 ☑

Osteoarthrosis — *continued*
 localized — *continued*
  secondary 715.2 ☑
 multiple sites, not specified as generalized
  715.89
 polyarticular 715.09
 spine (*see also* Spondylosis) 721.90
 temporomandibular joint 524.69
Osteoblastoma (M9200/0) — *see* Neoplasm,
  bone, benign
Osteochondritis — *see also* Osteochondrosis
  732.9
 dissecans 732.7
  hip 732.7
 ischiopubica 732.1
 multiple 756.59
 syphilitic (congenital) 090.0
Osteochondrodermodysplasia 756.59
Osteochondrodystrophy 277.5
 deformans 277.5
 familial 277.5
 fetalis 756.4
Osteochondrolysis 732.7
Osteochondroma (M9210/0) — *see also* Neoplasm, bone, benign
 multiple, congenital 756.4
Osteochondromatosis (M9210/1) 238.0
 synovial 727.82
Osteochondromyxosarcoma (M9180/3) —
  see Neoplasm, bone, malignant
Osteochondropathy NEC 732.9
Osteochondrosarcoma (M9180/3) — *see*
  Neoplasm, bone, malignant
Osteochondrosis 732.9
 acetabulum 732.1
 adult spine 732.8
 astragalus 732.5
 Blount's 732.4
 Buchanan's (juvenile osteochondrosis of iliac crest) 732.1
 Buchman's (juvenile osteochondrosis) 732.1
 Burns' 732.3
 calcaneus 732.5
 capitular epiphysis (femur) 732.1
 carpal
  lunate (wrist) 732.3
  scaphoid 732.3
 coxae juvenilis 732.1
 deformans juvenilis (coxae) (hip) 732.1
  Scheuermann's 732.0
  spine 732.0
  tibia 732.4
  vertebra 732.0
 Diaz's (astragalus) 732.5
 dissecans (knee) (shoulder) 732.7
 femoral capital epiphysis 732.1
 femur (head) (juvenile) 732.1
 foot (juvenile) 732.5
 Freiberg's (disease) (second metatarsal)
  732.5
 Haas' 732.3
 Haglund's (os tibiale externum) 732.5
 hand (juvenile) 732.3
 head of
  femur 732.1
  humerus (juvenile) 732.3
 hip (juvenile) 732.1
 humerus (juvenile) 732.3
 iliac crest (juvenile) 732.1
 ilium (juvenile) 732.1
 ischiopubic synchondrosis 732.1
 Iselin's (osteochondrosis fifth metatarsal)
  732.5
 juvenile, juvenilis 732.6
  arm 732.3
   capital femoral epiphysis 732.1
   capitellum humeri 732.3
   capitular epiphysis 732.1
   carpal scaphoid 732.3
   clavicle, sternal epiphysis 732.6
   coxae 732.1
   deformans 732.1
   foot 732.5
   hand 732.3
   hip and pelvis 732.1
   lower extremity, except foot 732.4

Osteochondrosis — *continued*
 juvenile, juvenilis — *continued*
   lunate, wrist 732.3
   medial cuneiform bone 732.5
   metatarsal (head) 732.5
   metatarsophalangeal 732.5
   navicular, ankle 732.5
   patella 732.4
   primary patellar center (of Köhler) 732.4
   specified site NEC 732.6
   spine 732.0
   tarsal scaphoid 732.5
   tibia (epiphysis) (tuberosity) 732.4
   upper extremity 732.3
   vertebra (body) (Calvé) 732.0
    epiphyseal plates (of Scheuermann)
     732.0
 Kienböck's (disease) 732.3
 Köhler's (disease) (navicular, ankle) 732.5
  patellar 732.4
  tarsal navicular 732.5
 Legg-Calvé-Perthes (disease) 732.1
 lower extremity (juvenile) 732.4
 lunate bone 732.3
 Mauclaire's 732.3
 metacarpal heads (of Mauclaire) 732.3
 metatarsal (fifth) (head) (second) 732.5
 navicular, ankle 732.5
 os calcis 732.5
 Osgood-Schlatter 732.4
 os tibiale externum 732.5
 Panner's 732.3
 patella (juvenile) 732.4
 patellar center
  primary (of Köhler) 732.4
  secondary (of Sinding-Larsen) 732.4
 pelvis (juvenile) 732.1
 Pierson's 732.1
 radial head (juvenile) 732.3
 Scheuermann's 732.0
 Sever's (calcaneum) 732.5
 Sinding-Larsen (secondary patellar center)
  732.4
 spine (juvenile) 732.0
  adult 732.8
 symphysis pubis (of Pierson) (juvenile) 732.1
 syphilitic (congenital) 090.0
 tarsal (navicular) (scaphoid) 732.5
 tibia (proximal) (tubercle) 732.4
 tuberculous — *see* Tuberculosis, bone
 ulna 732.3
 upper extremity (juvenile) 732.3
 van Neck's (juvenile osteochondrosis) 732.1
 vertebral (juvenile) 732.0
  adult 732.8
Osteoclastoma (M9250/1) 238.0
 malignant (M9250/3) — *see* Neoplasm,
  bone, malignant
Osteocopic pain 733.90
Osteodynia 733.90
Osteodystrophy
 azotemic 588.0
 chronica deformans hypertrophica 731.0
 congenital 756.50
  specified type NEC 756.59
 deformans 731.0
 fibrosa localisata 731.0
 parathyroid 252.01
 renal 588.0
Osteofibroma (M9262/0) — *see* Neoplasm,
  bone, benign
Osteofibrosarcoma (M9182/3) — *see* Neoplasm, bone, malignant
Osteogenesis imperfecta 756.51
Osteogenic — *see* condition
Osteoma (M9180/0) — *see also* Neoplasm,
  bone, benign
 osteoid (M9191/0) (*see also* Neoplasm, bone,
  benign)
  giant (M9200/0) — *see* Neoplasm, bone,
   benign
Osteomalacia 268.2
 chronica deformans hypertrophica 731.0
 due to vitamin D deficiency 268.2
 infantile (*see also* Rickets) 268.0
 juvenile (*see also* Rickets) 268.0

Osteomalacia — *continued*
- oncogenic 275.8
- pelvis 268.2
- vitamin D-resistant 275.3

Osteomalacic bone 268.2
Osteomalacosis 268.2
Osteomyelitis (general) (infective) (localized) (neonatal) (purulent) (pyogenic) (septic) (staphylococcal) (streptococcal) (suppurative) (with periostitis) 730.2 ☑

> *Note — Use the following fifth-digit subclassification with category 730:*
>
> 0   *site unspecified*
> 1   *shoulder region*
> 2   *upper arm*
> 3   *forearm*
> 4   *hand*
> 5   *pelvic region and thigh*
> 6   *lower leg*
> 7   *ankle and foot*
> 8   *other specified sites*
> 9   *multiple sites*

- acute or subacute 730.0 ☑
- chronic or old 730.1 ☑
- due to or associated with
  - diabetes mellitus 250.8 ☑ *[731.8]*
    - due to secondary diabetes 249.8 ☑ *[731.8]*
  - tuberculosis (*see also* Tuberculosis, bone) 015.9 ☑ *[730.8]* ☑
    - limb bones 015.5 ☑ *[730.8]* ☑
    - specified bones NEC 015.7 ☑ *[730.8]* ☑
    - spine 015.0 ☑ *[730.8]* ☑
  - typhoid 002.0 *[730.8]* ☑
- Garré's 730.1 ☑
- jaw (acute) (chronic) (lower) (neonatal) (suppurative) (upper) 526.4
- nonsuppurating 730.1 ☑
- orbital 376.03
- petrous bone (*see also* Petrositis) 383.20
- Salmonella 003.24
- sclerosing, nonsuppurative 730.1 ☑
- sicca 730.1 ☑
- syphilitic 095.5
  - congenital 090.0 *[730.8]* ☑
- tuberculous — *see* Tuberculosis, bone
- typhoid 002.0 *[730.8]* ☑

Osteomyelofibrosis 289.89
Osteomyelosclerosis 289.89
Osteonecrosis 733.40
- meaning osteomyelitis 730.1 ☑

Osteo-onycho-arthro dysplasia 756.89
Osteo-onychodysplasia, hereditary 756.89
Osteopathia
- condensans disseminata 756.53
- hyperostotica multiplex infantilis 756.59
- hypertrophica toxica 731.2
- striata 756.4

Osteopathy resulting from poliomyelitis — *see also* Poliomyelitis 045.9 ☑ *[730.7]* ☑
- familial dysplastic 731.2

Osteopecilia 756.53
Osteopenia 733.90
- borderline 733.90

Osteoperiostitis — *see also* Osteomyelitis 730.2 ☑
- ossificans toxica 731.2
- toxica ossificans 731.2

Osteopetrosis (familial) 756.52
Osteophyte — *see* Exostosis
Osteophytosis — *see* Exostosis
Osteopoikilosis 756.53
Osteoporosis (generalized) 733.00
- circumscripta 731.0
- disuse 733.03
- drug-induced 733.09
- idiopathic 733.02
- postmenopausal 733.01
- posttraumatic 733.7

Osteoporosis — *continued*
- screening V82.81
- senile 733.01
- specified type NEC 733.09

Osteoporosis-osteomalacia syndrome 268.2
Osteopsathyrosis 756.51
Osteoradionecrosis, jaw 526.89
Osteosarcoma (M9180/3) — *see also* Neoplasm, bone, malignant
- chondroblastic (M9181/3) — *see* Neoplasm, bone, malignant
- fibroblastic (M9182/3) — *see* Neoplasm, bone, malignant
- in Paget's disease of bone (M9184/3) — *see* Neoplasm, bone, malignant
- juxtacortical (M9190/3) — *see* Neoplasm, bone, malignant
- parosteal (M9190/3) — *see* Neoplasm, bone, malignant
- telangiectatic (M9183/3) — *see* Neoplasm, bone, malignant

Osteosclerosis 756.52
- fragilis (generalisata) 756.52

Osteosclerotic anemia 289.89
Osteosis
- acromegaloid 757.39
- cutis 709.3
- parathyroid 252.01
- renal fibrocystic 588.0

Österreicher-Turner syndrome 756.89
Ostium
- atrioventriculare commune 745.69
- primum (arteriosum) (defect) (persistent) 745.61
- secundum (arteriosum) (defect) (patent) (persistent) 745.5

Ostrum-Furst syndrome 756.59
Os, uterus — *see* condition
Otalgia 388.70
- otogenic 388.71
- referred 388.72

Othematoma 380.31
Otitic hydrocephalus 348.2
Otitis 382.9
- with effusion 381.4
  - purulent 382.4
  - secretory 381.4
  - serous 381.4
  - suppurative 382.4
- acute 382.9
- adhesive (*see also* Adhesions, middle ear) 385.10
- chronic 382.9
  - with effusion 381.3
  - mucoid, mucous (simple) 381.20
  - purulent 382.3
  - secretory 381.3
  - serous 381.10
  - suppurative 382.3
- diffuse parasitic 136.8
- externa (acute) (diffuse) (hemorrhagica) 380.10
  - actinic 380.22
  - candidal 112.82
  - chemical 380.22
  - chronic 380.23
    - mycotic — *see* Otitis, externa, mycotic
    - specified type NEC 380.23
  - circumscribed 380.10
  - contact 380.22
  - due to
    - erysipelas 035 *[380.13]*
    - impetigo 684 *[380.13]*
    - seborrheic dermatitis 690.10 *[380.13]*
  - eczematoid 380.22
  - furuncular 680.0 *[380.13]*
  - infective 380.10
    - chronic 380.16
  - malignant 380.14
  - mycotic (chronic) 380.15
    - due to
      - aspergillosis 117.3 *[380.15]*
      - moniliasis 112.82
      - otomycosis 111.8 *[380.15]*
  - reactive 380.22

Otitis — *continued*
- externa — *continued*
  - specified type NEC 380.22
  - tropical 111.8 *[380.15]*
- insidiosa (*see also* Otosclerosis) 387.9
- interna (*see also* Labyrinthitis) 386.30
- media (hemorrhagic) (staphylococcal) (streptococcal) 382.9
  - acute 382.9
    - with effusion 381.00
    - allergic 381.04
      - mucoid 381.05
      - sanguineous 381.06
      - serous 381.04
    - catarrhal 381.00
    - exudative 381.00
    - mucoid 381.02
      - allergic 381.05
    - necrotizing 382.00
      - with spontaneous rupture of ear drum 382.01
      - in
        - influenza (*see also* Influenza) 487.8 *[382.02]*
        - measles 055.2
        - scarlet fever 034.1 *[382.02]*
    - nonsuppurative 381.00
    - purulent 382.00
      - with spontaneous rupture of ear drum 382.01
    - sanguineous 381.03
      - allergic 381.06
    - secretory 381.01
    - seromucinous 381.02
    - serous 381.01
      - allergic 381.04
    - suppurative 382.00
      - with spontaneous rupture of ear drum 382.01
      - due to
        - influenza (*see also* Influenza) 487.8 *[382.02]*
        - scarlet fever 034.1 *[382.02]*
    - transudative 381.00
  - adhesive (*see also* Adhesions, middle ear) 385.10
  - allergic 381.4
    - acute 381.04
      - mucoid 381.05
      - sanguineous 381.06
      - serous 381.04
    - chronic 381.3
  - catarrhal 381.4
    - acute 381.00
    - chronic (simple) 381.10
  - chronic 382.9
    - with effusion 381.3
    - adhesive (*see also* Adhesions, middle ear) 385.10
    - allergic 381.3
    - atticoantral, suppurative (with posterior or superior marginal perforation of ear drum) 382.2
    - benign suppurative (with anterior perforation of ear drum) 382.1
    - catarrhal 381.10
    - exudative 381.3
    - mucinous 381.20
    - mucoid, mucous (simple) 381.20
    - mucosanguineous 381.29
    - nonsuppurative 381.3
    - purulent 382.3
    - secretory 381.3
    - seromucinous 381.3
    - serosanguineous 381.19
    - serous (simple) 381.10
    - suppurative 382.3
      - atticoantral (with posterior or superior marginal perforation of ear drum) 382.2
      - benign (with anterior perforation of ear drum) 382.1
      - tuberculous (*see also* Tuberculosis) 017.4 ☑
    - tubotympanic 382.1
    - transudative 381.3

Otitis — *continued*
- media — *continued*
  - exudative 381.4
    - acute 381.00
    - chronic 381.3
  - fibrotic (*see also* Adhesions, middle ear) 385.10
  - mucoid, mucous 381.4
    - acute 381.02
    - chronic (simple) 381.20
  - mucosanguineous, chronic 381.29
  - nonsuppurative 381.4
    - acute 381.00
    - chronic 381.3
  - postmeasles 055.2
  - purulent 382.4
    - acute 382.00
      - with spontaneous rupture of ear drum 382.01
    - chronic 382.3
  - sanguineous, acute 381.03
    - allergic 381.06
  - secretory 381.4
    - acute or subacute 381.01
    - chronic 381.3
  - seromucinous 381.4
    - acute or subacute 381.02
    - chronic 381.3
  - serosanguineous, chronic 381.19
  - serous 381.4
    - acute or subacute 381.01
    - chronic (simple) 381.10
  - subacute — *see* Otitis, media, acute
  - suppurative 382.4
    - acute 382.00
      - with spontaneous rupture of ear drum 382.01
    - chronic 382.3
      - atticoantral 382.2
      - benign 382.1
      - tuberculous (*see also* Tuberculosis) 017.4 ☑
      - tubotympanic 382.1
  - transudative 381.4
    - acute 381.00
    - chronic 381.3
  - tuberculous (*see also* Tuberculosis) 017.4 ☑
- postmeasles 055.2

Otoconia 386.8
Otolith syndrome 386.19
Otomycosis 111.8 *[380.15]*
- in
  - aspergillosis 117.3 *[380.15]*
  - moniliasis 112.82

Otopathy 388.9
Otoporosis — *see also* Otosclerosis 387.9
Otorrhagia 388.69
- traumatic — *see* nature of injury

Otorrhea 388.60
- blood 388.69
- cerebrospinal (fluid) 388.61

Otosclerosis (general) 387.9
- cochlear (endosteal) 387.2
- involving
  - otic capsule 387.2
  - oval window
    - nonobliterative 387.0
    - obliterative 387.1
  - round window 387.2
- nonobliterative 387.0
- obliterative 387.1
- specified type NEC 387.8

Otospongiosis — *see also* Otosclerosis 387.9
Otto's disease or pelvis 715.35
Outburst, aggressive — *see also* Disturbance, conduct 312.0 ☑
- in children or adolescents 313.9

Outcome of delivery
- multiple birth NEC V27.9
  - all liveborn V27.5
  - all stillborn V27.7
  - some liveborn V27.6
  - unspecified V27.9
- single V27.9
  - liveborn V27.0

☑ **Additional Digit Required — Refer to the Tabular List for Digit Selection**   ▼ **Subterms under main terms may continue to next column or page**

2014 ICD-9-CM   265

Outcome of delivery — *continued*
  single — *continued*
    stillborn V27.1
  twins V27.9
    both liveborn V27.2
    both stillborn V27.4
    one liveborn, one stillborn V27.3
Outlet — *see also* condition
  syndrome (thoracic) 353.0
Outstanding ears (bilateral) 744.29
Ovalocytosis (congenital) (hereditary) — *see also* Elliptocytosis 282.1
Ovarian — *see also* condition
  pregnancy — *see* Pregnancy, ovarian
  remnant syndrome 620.8
  vein syndrome 593.4
Ovaritis (cystic) — *see also* Salpingo-oophoritis 614.2
Ovary, ovarian — *see* condition
Overactive — *see also* Hyperfunction
  bladder 596.51
  eye muscle (*see also* Strabismus) 378.9
  hypothalamus 253.8
  thyroid (*see also* Thyrotoxicosis) 242.9 ☑
Overactivity, child 314.01
Overbite (deep) (excessive) (horizontal) (vertical) 524.29
Overbreathing — *see also* Hyperventilation 786.01
Overconscientious personality 301.4
Overdevelopment — *see also* Hypertrophy
  breast (female) (male) 611.1
  nasal bones 738.0
  prostate, congenital 752.89
Overdistention — *see* Distention
Overdose overdosage (drug) 977.9
  specified drug or substance — *see* Table of Drugs and Chemicals
Overeating 783.6
  nonorganic origin 307.51
Overexertion (effects) (exhaustion) 994.5
Overexposure (effects) 994.9
  exhaustion 994.4
Overfeeding — *see also* Overeating 783.6
Overfill, endodontic 526.62
Overgrowth, bone NEC 733.99
Overhanging
  tooth restoration 525.62
  unrepairable, dental restorative materials 525.62
Overheated (effects) (places) — *see* Heat
Overinhibited child 313.0
Overjet 524.29
  excessive horizontal 524.26
Overlaid, overlying (suffocation) 994.7
Overlap
  excessive horizontal 524.26
Overlapping toe (acquired) 735.8
  congenital (fifth toe) 755.66
Overload
  fluid 276.69
    due to transfusion (blood) (blood components) 276.61
  iron, due to repeated red blood cell transfusions 275.02
  potassium (K) 276.7
  sodium (Na) 276.0
  transfusion associated circulatory (TACO) 276.61
Overnutrition — *see also* Hyperalimentation 783.6
Overproduction — *see also* Hypersecretion
  ACTH 255.3
  cortisol 255.0
  growth hormone 253.0
  thyroid-stimulating hormone (TSH) 242.8 ☑
Overriding
  aorta 747.21
  finger (acquired) 736.29
    congenital 755.59
  toe (acquired) 735.8
    congenital 755.66
Oversize
  fetus (weight of 4500 grams or more) 766.0
    affecting management of pregnancy 656.6 ☑

Oversize — *continued*
  fetus — *continued*
    causing disproportion 653.5 ☑
    with obstructed labor 660.1 ☑
    affecting fetus or newborn 763.1
Overstimulation, ovarian 256.1
Overstrained 780.79
  heart — *see* Hypertrophy, cardiac
Overweight — *see also* Obesity 278.02
Overwork 780.79
Oviduct — *see* condition
Ovotestis 752.7
Ovulation (cycle)
  failure or lack of 628.0
  pain 625.2
Ovum
  blighted 631.8
  donor V59.70
    over age 35 V59.73
      anonymous recipient V59.73
      designated recipient V59.74
    under age 35 V59.71
      anonymous recipient V59.71
      designated recipient V59.72
  dropsical 631.8
  pathologic 631.8
Owren's disease or syndrome (parahemophilia) — *see also* Defect, coagulation 286.3
Oxalosis 271.8
Oxaluria 271.8
Ox heart — *see* Hypertrophy, cardiac
OX syndrome 758.6
Oxycephaly, oxycephalic 756.0
  syphilitic, congenital 090.0
Oxyuriasis 127.4
Oxyuris vermicularis (infestation) 127.4
Ozena 472.0

P

Pacemaker syndrome 429.4
Pachyderma, pachydermia 701.8
  laryngis 478.5
  laryngitis 478.79
  larynx (verrucosa) 478.79
Pachydermatitis 701.8
Pachydermatocele (congenital) 757.39
  acquired 701.8
Pachydermatosis 701.8
Pachydermoperiostitis
  secondary 731.2
Pachydermoperiostosis
  primary idiopathic 757.39
  secondary 731.2
Pachymeningitis (adhesive) (basal) (brain) (cerebral) (cervical) (chronic) (circumscribed) (external) (fibrous) (hemorrhagic) (hypertrophic) (internal) (purulent) (spinal) (suppurative) — *see also* Meningitis 322.9
  gonococcal 098.82
Pachyonychia (congenital) 757.5
  acquired 703.8
Pachyperiosteodermia
  primary or idiopathic 757.39
  secondary 731.2
Pachyperiostosis
  primary or idiopathic 757.39
  secondary 731.2
Pacinian tumor (M9507/0) — *see* Neoplasm, skin, benign
Pads, knuckle or Garrod's 728.79
Paget's disease (osteitis deformans) 731.0
  with infiltrating duct carcinoma of the breast (M8541/3) — *see* Neoplasm, breast, malignant
  bone 731.0
    osteosarcoma in (M9184/3) — *see* Neoplasm, bone, malignant
  breast (M8540/3) 174.0
  extramammary (M8542/3) (*see also* Neoplasm, skin, malignant)
    anus 154.3
    skin 173.59
  malignant (M8540/3)
    breast 174.0

Paget's disease — *continued*
  malignant — *continued*
    specified site NEC (M8542/3) — *see* Neoplasm, skin, malignant
    unspecified site 174.0
  mammary (M8540/3) 174.0
  necrosis of bone 731.0
  nipple (M8540/3) 174.0
  osteitis deformans 731.0
Paget-Schroetter syndrome (intermittent venous claudication) 453.89
Pain(s) (*see also* Painful) 780.96
  abdominal 789.0 ☑
  acute 338.19
    due to trauma 338.11
    postoperative 338.18
      post-thoracotomy 338.12
  adnexa (uteri) 625.9
  alimentary, due to vascular insufficiency 557.9
  anginoid (*see also* Pain, precordial) 786.51
  anus 569.42
  arch 729.5
  arm 729.5
  axillary 729.5
  back (postural) 724.5
    low 724.2
    psychogenic 307.89
  bile duct 576.9
  bladder 788.99
  bone 733.90
  breast 611.71
    psychogenic 307.89
  broad ligament 625.9
  cancer associated 338.3
  cartilage NEC 733.90
  cecum 789.0 ☑
  cervicobrachial 723.3
  chest (central) 786.50
    atypical 786.59
    midsternal 786.51
    musculoskeletal 786.59
    noncardiac 786.59
    substernal 786.51
    wall (anterior) 786.52
  chronic 338.29
    associated with significant psychosocial dysfunction 338.4
    due to trauma 338.21
    postoperative 338.28
      post-thoracotomy 338.22
    syndrome 338.4
  coccyx 724.79
  colon 789.0 ☑
  common duct 576.9
  coronary — *see* Angina
  costochondral 786.52
  diaphragm 786.52
  due to (presence of) any device, implant, or graft classifiable to 996.0–996.5 — *see* Complications, due to (presence of) any device, implant, or graft classified to 996.0–996.5 NEC
    malignancy (primary) (secondary) 338.3
  ear (*see also* Otalgia) 388.70
  epigastric, epigastrium 789.06
  extremity (lower) (upper) 729.5
  eye 379.91
  face, facial 784.0
    atypical 350.2
    nerve 351.8
  false (labor) 644.1 ☑
  female genital organ NEC 625.9
    psychogenic 307.89
  finger 729.5
  flank 789.0 ☑
  foot 729.5
  gallbladder 575.9
  gas (intestinal) 787.3
  gastric 536.8
  generalized 780.96
  genital organ
    female 625.9
    male 608.9
    psychogenic 307.89
  groin 789.0 ☑

Pain(s) (*see also* Painful) — *continued*
  growing 781.99
  hand 729.5
  head (*see also* Headache) 784.0
  heart (see also Pain, precordial) 786.51
  infraorbital (*see also* Neuralgia, trigeminal) 350.1
  intermenstrual 625.2
  jaw 784.92
  joint 719.40
    ankle 719.47
    elbow 719.42
    foot 719.47
    hand 719.44
    hip 719.45
    knee 719.46
    multiple sites 719.49
    pelvic region 719.45
    psychogenic 307.89
    shoulder (region) 719.41
    specified site NEC 719.48
    wrist 719.43
  kidney 788.0
  labor, false or spurious 644.1 ☑
  laryngeal 784.1
  leg 729.5
  limb 729.5
  low back 724.2
  lumbar region 724.2
  mandible, mandibular 784.92
  mastoid (*see also* Otalgia) 388.70
  maxilla 784.92
  menstrual 625.3
  metacarpophalangeal (joint) 719.44
  metatarsophalangeal (joint) 719.47
  mouth 528.9
  muscle 729.1
    intercostal 786.59
  musculoskeletal (see also Pain, by site) 729.1
  nasal 478.19
  nasopharynx 478.29
  neck NEC 723.1
    psychogenic 307.89
  neoplasm related (acute) (chronic) 338.3
  nerve NEC 729.2
  neuromuscular 729.1
  nose 478.19
  ocular 379.91
  ophthalmic 379.91
  orbital region 379.91
  osteocopic 733.90
  ovary 625.9
    psychogenic 307.89
  over heart (*see also* Pain, precordial) 786.51
  ovulation 625.2
  pelvic (female) 625.9
    male NEC 789.0 ☑
      psychogenic 307.89
    psychogenic 307.89
  penis 607.9
    psychogenic 307.89
  pericardial (*see also* Pain, precordial) 786.51
  perineum
    female 625.9
    male 608.9
  pharynx 478.29
  pleura, pleural, pleuritic 786.52
  postoperative 338.18
    acute 338.18
    chronic 338.28
  post-thoracotomy 338.12
    acute 338.12
    chronic 338.22
  preauricular 388.70
  precordial (region) 786.51
    psychogenic 307.89
  premenstrual 625.4
  psychogenic 307.80
    cardiovascular system 307.89
    gastrointestinal system 307.89
    genitourinary system 307.89
    heart 307.89
    musculoskeletal system 307.89
    respiratory system 307.89
    skin 306.3
  radicular (spinal) (*see also* Radiculitis) 729.2

Pain(s) (see also Painful) — continued
rectum 569.42
respiration 786.52
retrosternal 786.51
rheumatic NEC 729.0
  muscular 729.1
rib 786.50
root (spinal) (see also Radiculitis) 729.2
round ligament (stretch) 625.9
sacroiliac 724.6
sciatic 724.3
scrotum 608.9
  psychogenic 307.89
seminal vesicle 608.9
sinus 478.19
skin 782.0
spermatic cord 608.9
spinal root (see also Radiculitis) 729.2
stomach 536.8
  psychogenic 307.89
substernal 786.51
testis 608.9
  psychogenic 307.89
thoracic spine 724.1
  with radicular and visceral pain 724.4
throat 784.1
tibia 733.90
toe 729.5
tongue 529.6
tooth 525.9
total hip replacement 996.77
total knee replacement 996.77
trigeminal (see also Neuralgia, trigeminal) 350.1
tumor associated 338.3
umbilicus 789.05
ureter 788.0
urinary (organ) (system) 788.0
uterus 625.9
  psychogenic 307.89
vagina 625.9
vertebrogenic (syndrome) 724.5
vesical 788.99
vulva 625.9
xiphoid 733.90
Painful — see also Pain
arc syndrome 726.19
coitus
  female 625.0
  male 608.89
  psychogenic 302.76
ejaculation (semen) 608.89
  psychogenic 302.79
erection 607.3
feet syndrome 266.2
menstruation 625.3
  psychogenic 306.52
micturition 788.1
ophthalmoplegia 378.55
respiration 786.52
scar NEC 709.2
urination 788.1
wire sutures 998.89
Painters' colic 984.9
specified type of lead — see Table of Drugs and Chemicals
Palate — see condition
Palatoplegia 528.9
Palatoschisis — see also Cleft, palate 749.00
Palilalia 784.69
Palindromic arthritis — see also Rheumatism, palindromic 719.3 ☑
Palliative care V66.7
Pallor 782.61
temporal, optic disc 377.15
Palmar — see also condition
fascia — see condition
Palpable
cecum 569.89
kidney 593.89
liver 573.9
lymph nodes 785.6
ovary 620.8
prostate 602.9
spleen (see also Splenomegaly) 789.2
uterus 625.8

Palpitation (heart) 785.1
psychogenic 306.2
Palsy — see also Paralysis 344.9
atrophic diffuse 335.20
Bell's 351.0
  newborn 767.5
birth 767.7
brachial plexus 353.0
  fetus or newborn 767.6
brain (see also Palsy, cerebral)
  noncongenital or noninfantile 344.89
    late effect — see Late effect(s) (of) cerebrovascular disease
  syphilitic 094.89
    congenital 090.49
bulbar (chronic) (progressive) 335.22
  pseudo NEC 335.23
  supranuclear NEC 344.8 ☑
cerebral (congenital) (infantile) (spastic) 343.9
  athetoid 333.71
  diplegic 343.0
    late effect — see Late effect(s) (of) cerebrovascular disease
  hemiplegic 343.1
  monoplegic 343.3
  noncongenital or noninfantile 437.8
    late effect — see Late effect(s) (of) cerebrovascular disease
  paraplegic 343.0
  quadriplegic 343.2
  spastic, not congenital or infantile 344.89
  syphilitic 094.89
    congenital 090.49
  tetraplegic 343.2
cranial nerve (see also Disorder, nerve, cranial)
  multiple 352.6
creeping 335.21
divers' 993.3
Erb's (birth injury) 767.6
facial 351.0
  newborn 767.5
glossopharyngeal 352.2
Klumpke (-Déjérine) 767.6
lead 984.9
  specified type of lead — see Table of Drugs and Chemicals
median nerve (tardy) 354.0
peroneal nerve (acute) (tardy) 355.3
progressive supranuclear 333.0
pseudobulbar NEC 335.23
radial nerve (acute) 354.3
seventh nerve 351.0
  newborn 767.5
shaking (see also Parkinsonism) 332.0
spastic (cerebral) (spinal) 343.9
  hemiplegic 343.1
specified nerve NEC — see Disorder, nerve
supranuclear NEC 356.8
  progressive 333.0
ulnar nerve (tardy) 354.2
wasting 335.21
Paltauf-Sternberg disease 201.9 ☑
Paludism — see Malaria
Panama fever 084.0
Panaris (with lymphangitis) 681.9
finger 681.02
toe 681.11
Panaritium (with lymphangitis) 681.9
finger 681.02
toe 681.11
Panarteritis (nodosa) 446.0
brain or cerebral 437.4
Pancake heart 793.2
with cor pulmonale (chronic) 416.9
Pancarditis (acute) (chronic) 429.89
with
  rheumatic
    fever (active) (acute) (chronic) (subacute) 391.8
      inactive or quiescent 398.99
  rheumatic, acute 391.8
    chronic or inactive 398.99

Pancoast's syndrome or tumor (carcinoma, pulmonary apex) (M8010/3) 162.3
Pancoast-Tobias syndrome (M8010/3) (carcinoma, pulmonary apex) 162.3
Pancolitis 556.6
Pancreas, pancreatic — see condition
Pancreatitis 577.0
acute (edematous) (hemorrhagic) (recurrent) 577.0
annular 577.0
apoplectic 577.0
calcereous 577.0
chronic (infectious) 577.1
  recurrent 577.1
cystic 577.2
fibrous 577.8
gangrenous 577.0
hemorrhagic (acute) 577.0
interstitial (chronic) 577.1
  acute 577.0
malignant 577.0
mumps 072.3
painless 577.1
recurrent 577.1
relapsing 577.1
subacute 577.0
suppurative 577.0
syphilitic 095.8
Pancreatolithiasis 577.8
Pancytolysis 289.9
Pancytopenia (acquired) 284.19
with
  malformations 284.09
  myelodysplastic syndrome — see Syndrome, myelodysplastic
congenital 284.09
due to
  antineoplastic chemotherapy 284.11
  drug, specified NEC 284.12
specified NEC 284.19
Panencephalitis — see also Encephalitis
subacute, sclerosing 046.2
Panhematopenia 284.81
congenital 284.09
constitutional 284.09
splenic, primary 289.4
Panhemocytopenia 284.81
congenital 284.09
constitutional 284.09
Panhypogonadism 257.2
Panhypopituitarism 253.2
prepubertal 253.3
Panic (attack) (state) 300.01
reaction to exceptional stress (transient) 308.0
Panmyelopathy, familial constitutional 284.09
Panmyelophthisis 284.2
acquired (secondary) 284.81
congenital 284.2
idiopathic 284.9
Panmyelosis (acute) (M9951/1) 238.79
Panner's disease 732.3
capitellum humeri 732.3
head of humerus 732.3
tarsal navicular (bone) (osteochondrosis) 732.5
Panneuritis endemica 265.0 [357.4]
Panniculitis 729.30
back 724.8
knee 729.31
mesenteric 567.82
neck 723.6
nodular, nonsuppurative 729.30
sacral 724.8
specified site NEC 729.39
Panniculus adiposus (abdominal) 278.1
Pannus (corneal) 370.62
abdominal (symptomatic) 278.1
allergic eczematous 370.62
degenerativus 370.62
keratic 370.62
rheumatoid — see Arthritis, rheumatoid
trachomatosus, trachomatous (active) 076.1 [370.62]
  late effect 139.1

Panophthalmitis 360.02
Panotitis — see Otitis media
Pansinusitis (chronic) (hyperplastic) (nonpurulent) 473.8
acute 461.8
due to fungus NEC 117.9
tuberculous (see also Tuberculosis) 012.8 ☑
Panuveitis 360.12
sympathetic 360.11
Panvalvular disease — see Endocarditis, mitral
Papageienkrankheit 073.9
Papanicolaou smear
anus 796.70
  with
    atypical squamous cells
      cannot exclude high grade squamous intraepithelial lesion (ASC-H) 796.72
      of undetermined significance (ASC-US) 796.71
    cytologic evidence of malignancy 796.76
    high grade squamous intraepithelial lesion (HGSIL) 796.74
    low grade squamous intraepithelial lesion (LGSIL) 796.73
  glandular 796.70
  specified finding NEC 796.79
  unsatisfactory cytology 796.78
cervix (screening test) V76.2
  as part of gynecological examination V72.31
  for suspected malignant neoplasm V76.2
  no disease found V71.1
  inadequate cytology sample 795.08
  nonspecific abnormal finding 795.00
    with
      atypical squamous cells
        cannot exclude high grade squamous intraepithelial lesion (ASC-H) 795.02
        of undetermined significance (ASC-US) 795.01
      cytologic evidence of malignancy 795.06
      high grade squamous intraepithelial lesion (HGSIL) 795.04
      low grade squamous intraepithelial lesion (LGSIL) 795.03
      nonspecific finding NEC 795.09
  to confirm findings of recent normal smear following initial abnormal smear V72.32
  satisfactory smear but lacking transformation zone 795.07
  unsatisfactory cervical cytology 795.08
other specified site (see also Screening, malignant neoplasm)
  for suspected malignant neoplasm (see also Screening, malignant neoplasm)
  no disease found V71.1
  nonspecific abnormal finding 796.9
vagina V76.47
  with
    atypical squamous cells
      cannot exclude high grade squamous intraepithelial lesion (ASC-H) 795.12
      of undetermined significance (ASC-US) 795.11
    cytologic evidence of malignancy 795.16
    high grade squamous intraepithelial lesion (HGSIL) 795.14
    low grade squamous intraepithelial lesion (LGSIL) 795.13
  abnormal NEC 795.19
  following hysterectomy for malignant condition V67.01
  inadequate cytology sample 795.18
  unsatisfactory cytology 795.18
Papilledema 377.00
associated with
  decreased ocular pressure 377.02

☑ **Additional Digit Required** — Refer to the Tabular List for Digit Selection   ▽ **Subterms under main terms may continue to next column or page**

Papilledema — *continued*
  associated with — *continued*
    increased intracranial pressure 377.01
      retinal disorder 377.03
  choked disc 377.00
  infectional 377.00
Papillitis 377.31
  anus 569.49
  chronic lingual 529.4
  necrotizing, kidney 584.7
  optic 377.31
  rectum 569.49
  renal, necrotizing 584.7
  tongue 529.0
Papilloma (M8050/0) — *see also* Neoplasm, by site, benign

> *Note* — *Except where otherwise indicated, the morphological varieties of papilloma in the list below should be coded by site as for "Neoplasm, benign."*

  acuminatum (female) (male) 078.11
  bladder (urinary) (transitional cell) (M8120/1) 236.7
    benign (M8120/0) 223.3
  choroid plexus (M9390/0) 225.0
    anaplastic type (M9390/3) 191.5
    malignant (M9390/3) 191.5
  ductal (M8503/0)
  dyskeratotic (M8052/0)
  epidermoid (M8052/0)
  hyperkeratotic (M8052/0)
  intracystic (M8504/0)
  intraductal (M8503/0)
  inverted (M8053/0)
  keratotic (M8052/0)
  parakeratotic (M8052/0)
  pinta (primary) 103.0
  renal pelvis (transitional cell) (M8120/1) 236.99
    benign (M8120/0) 223.1
  Schneiderian (M8121/0)
    specified site — *see* Neoplasm, by site, benign
    unspecified site 212.0
  serous surface (M8461/0)
    borderline malignancy (M8461/1)
      specified site — *see* Neoplasm, by site, uncertain behavior
      unspecified site 236.2
    specified site — *see* Neoplasm, by site, benign
    unspecified site 220
  squamous (cell) (M8052/0)
  transitional (cell) (M8120/0)
    bladder (urinary) (M8120/1) 236.7
    inverted type (M8121/1) — *see* Neoplasm, by site, uncertain behavior
    renal pelvis (M8120/1) 236.91
    ureter (M8120/1) 236.91
  ureter (transitional cell) (M8120/1) 236.91
    benign (M8120/0) 223.2
  urothelial (M8120/1) — *see* Neoplasm, by site, uncertain behavior
  verrucous (M8051/0)
  villous (M8261/1) — *see* Neoplasm, by site, uncertain behavior
  yaws, plantar or palmar 102.1
Papillomata, multiple, of yaws 102.1
Papillomatosis (M8060/0) — *see also* Neoplasm, by site, benign
  confluent and reticulate 701.8
  cutaneous 701.8
  ductal, breast 610.1
  Gougerot-Carteaud (confluent reticulate) 701.8
  intraductal (diffuse) (M8505/0) — *see* Neoplasm, by site, benign
  subareolar duct (M8506/0) 217
Papillon-Léage and Psaume syndrome (orodigitofacial dysostosis) 759.89
Papule 709.8
  carate (primary) 103.0
  fibrous, of nose (M8724/0) 216.3
  pinta (primary) 103.0
Papulosis
  lymphomatoid 709.8

Papulosis — *continued*
  malignant 447.8
Papyraceous fetus 779.89
  complicating pregnancy 646.0 ☑
Paracephalus 759.7
Parachute mitral valve 746.5
Paracoccidioidomycosis 116.1
  mucocutaneous-lymphangitic 116.1
  pulmonary 116.1
  visceral 116.1
Paracoccidiomycosis — *see* Paracoccidioidomycosis
Paracusis 388.40
Paradentosis 523.5
Paradoxical facial movements 374.43
Paraffinoma 999.9
Paraganglioma (M8680/1)
  adrenal (M8700/0) 227.0
    malignant (M8700/3) 194.0
  aortic body (M8691/1) 237.3
    malignant (M8691/3) 194.6
  carotid body (M8692/1) 237.3
    malignant (M8692/3) 194.5
  chromaffin (M8700/0) (*see also* Neoplasm, by site, benign)
    malignant (M8700/3) — *see* Neoplasm, by site, malignant
  extra-adrenal (M8693/1)
    malignant (M8693/3)
      specified site — *see* Neoplasm, by site, malignant
      unspecified site 194.6
    specified site — *see* Neoplasm, by site, uncertain behavior
    unspecified site 237.3
  glomus jugulare (M8690/1) 237.3
    malignant (M8690/3) 194.6
  jugular (M8690/1) 237.3
    malignant (M8680/3)
      specified site — *see* Neoplasm, by site, malignant
      unspecified site 194.6
  nonchromaffin (M8693/1)
    malignant (M8693/3)
      specified site — *see* Neoplasm, by site, malignant
      unspecified site 194.6
    specified site — *see* Neoplasm, by site, uncertain behavior
    unspecified site 237.3
  parasympathetic (M8682/1)
    specified site — *see* Neoplasm, by site, uncertain behavior
    unspecified site 237.3
  specified site — *see* Neoplasm, by site, uncertain behavior
  sympathetic (M8681/1)
    specified site — *see* Neoplasm, by site, uncertain behavior
    unspecified site 237.3
  unspecified site 237.3
Parageusia 781.1
  psychogenic 306.7
Paragonimiasis 121.2
Paragranuloma, Hodgkin's (M9660/3) 201.0 ☑
Parahemophilia — *see also* Defect, coagulation 286.3
Parakeratosis 690.8
  psoriasiformis 696.2
  variegata 696.2
Paralysis, paralytic (complete) (incomplete) 344.9
  with
    broken
      back — *see* Fracture, vertebra, by site, with spinal cord injury
      neck — *see* Fracture, vertebra, cervical, with spinal cord injury
    fracture, vertebra — *see* Fracture, vertebra, by site, with spinal cord injury
    syphilis 094.89
  abdomen and back muscles 355.9
  abdominal muscles 355.9
  abducens (nerve) 378.54

Paralysis, paralytic — *continued*
  abductor 355.9
    lower extremity 355.8
    upper extremity 354.9
  accessory nerve 352.4
  accommodation 367.51
    hysterical 300.11
  acoustic nerve 388.5
  agitans 332.0
    arteriosclerotic 332.0
  alternating 344.89
    oculomotor 344.89
  amyotrophic 335.20
  ankle 355.8
  anterior serratus 355.9
  anus (sphincter) 569.49
  apoplectic (current episode) (*see also* Disease, cerebrovascular, acute) 436
    late effect — *see* Late effect(s) (of) cerebrovascular disease
  arm 344.40
    affecting
      dominant side 344.41
      nondominant side 344.42
    both 344.2
    hysterical 300.11
    late effect — *see* Late effect(s) (of) cerebrovascular disease
    psychogenic 306.0
    transient 781.4
    traumatic NEC (*see also* Injury, nerve, upper limb) 955.9
  arteriosclerotic (current episode) 437.0
    late effect — *see* Late effect(s) (of) cerebrovascular disease
  ascending (spinal), acute 357.0
  associated, nuclear 344.89
  asthenic bulbar 358.00
  ataxic NEC 334.9
    general 094.1
  athetoid 333.71
  atrophic 356.9
    infantile, acute (*see also* Poliomyelitis, with paralysis) 045.1 ☑
    muscle NEC 355.9
    progressive 335.21
    spinal (acute) (*see also* Poliomyelitis, with paralysis) 045.1 ☑
  attack (*see also* Disease, cerebrovascular, acute) 436
  axillary 353.0
  Babinski-Nageotte's 344.89
  Bell's 351.0
    newborn 767.5
  Benedikt's 344.89
  birth (injury) 767.7
    brain 767.0
    intracranial 767.0
    spinal cord 767.4
  bladder (sphincter) 596.53
    neurogenic 596.54
      with cauda equina syndrome 344.61
    puerperal, postpartum, childbirth 665.5 ☑
    sensory 596.54
      with cauda equina 344.61
    spastic 596.54
      with cauda equina 344.61
  bowel, colon, or intestine (*see also* Ileus) 560.1
  brachial plexus 353.0
    due to birth injury 767.6
    newborn 767.6
  brain
    congenital — *see* Palsy, cerebral
    current episode 437.8
    diplegia 344.2
    hemiplegia 342.9 ☑
      late effect — *see* Late effect(s) (of) cerebrovascular disease
    infantile — *see* Palsy, cerebral
    late effect — *see* Late effect(s) (of) cerebrovascular disease
    monoplegia (*see also* Monoplegia)
      late effect — *see* Late effect(s) (of) cerebrovascular disease

Paralysis, paralytic — *continued*
  brain — *continued*
    paraplegia 344.1
    quadriplegia — *see* Quadriplegia
    syphilitic, congenital 090.49
    triplegia 344.89
  bronchi 519.19
  Brown-Séquard's 344.89
  bulbar (chronic) (progressive) 335.22
    infantile (*see also* Poliomyelitis, bulbar) 045.0 ☑
    poliomyelitic (*see also* Poliomyelitis, bulbar) 045.0 ☑
    pseudo 335.23
    supranuclear 344.89
  bulbospinal 358.00
  cardiac (*see also* Failure, heart) 428.9
  cerebral
    current episode 437.8
    spastic, infantile — *see* Palsy, cerebral
  cerebrocerebellar 437.8
    diplegic infantile 343.0
  cervical
    plexus 353.2
    sympathetic NEC 337.09
  Céstan-Chenais 344.89
  Charcôt-Marie-Tooth type 356.1
  childhood — *see* Palsy, cerebral
  Clark's 343.9
  colon (*see also* Ileus) 560.1
  compressed air 993.3
  compression
    arm NEC 354.9
    cerebral — *see* Paralysis, brain
    leg NEC 355.8
    lower extremity NEC 355.8
    upper extremity NEC 354.9
  congenital (cerebral) (spastic) (spinal) — *see* Palsy, cerebral
  conjugate movement (of eye) 378.81
    cortical (nuclear) (supranuclear) 378.81
  convergence 378.83
  cordis (*see also* Failure, heart) 428.9
  cortical (*see also* Paralysis, brain) 437.8
  cranial or cerebral nerve (*see also* Disorder, nerve, cranial) 352.9
  creeping 335.21
  crossed leg 344.89
  crutch 953.4
  deglutition 784.99
    hysterical 300.11
  dementia 094.1
  descending (spinal) NEC 335.9
  diaphragm (flaccid) 519.4
    due to accidental section of phrenic nerve during procedure 998.2
  digestive organs NEC 564.89
  diplegic — *see* Diplegia
  divergence (nuclear) 378.85
  divers' 993.3
  Duchenne's 335.22
  due to intracranial or spinal birth injury — *see* Palsy, cerebral
  embolic (current episode) (*see also* Embolism, brain) 434.1 ☑
    late effect — *see* Late effect(s) (of) cerebrovascular disease
  enteric (*see also* Ileus) 560.1
    with hernia — *see* Hernia, by site, with obstruction
  Erb (-Duchenne) (birth) (newborn) 767.6
  Erb's syphilitic spastic spinal 094.89
  esophagus 530.89
  essential, infancy (*see also* Poliomyelitis) 045.9 ☑
  extremity
    lower — *see* Paralysis, leg
    spastic (hereditary) 343.3
      noncongenital or noninfantile 344.1
    transient (cause unknown) 781.4
    upper — *see* Paralysis, arm
  eye muscle (extrinsic) 378.55
    intrinsic 367.51
  facial (nerve) 351.0
    birth injury 767.5
    congenital 767.5

☑ **Additional Digit Required** — Refer to the Tabular List for Digit Selection   ▽ **Subterms under main terms may continue to next column or page**

268   **2014 ICD-9-CM**

Paralysis, paralytic — Paralysis, paralytic

☑ **Additional Digit Required** — Refer to the Tabular List for Digit Selection   ▽ **Subterms under main terms may continue to next column or page**

☑ **Additional Digit Required** — Refer to the Tabular List for Digit Selection   ▽ **Subterms under main terms may continue to next column or page**

Pathology (of) — *see also* Disease
periradicular, associated with previous en-
dodontic treatment 526.69
Patterned motor discharge, idiopathic —
see also Epilepsy 345.5 ☑
Patulous — *see also* Patent
anus 569.49
Eustachian tube 381.7
Pause, sinoatrial 427.81
Pavor nocturnus 307.46
Pavy's disease 593.6
Paxton's disease (white piedra) 111.2
Payr's disease or syndrome (splenic flexure
syndrome) 569.89
PBA (pseudobulbar affect) 310.81
Pearls
Elschnig 366.51
enamel 520.2
Pearl-workers' disease (chronic osteomyelitis)
— *see also* Osteomyelitis 730.1 ☑
Pectenitis 569.49
Pectenosis 569.49
Pectoral — *see* condition
Pectus
carinatum (congenital) 754.82
acquired 738.3
rachitic (*see also* Rickets) 268.0
excavatum (congenital) 754.81
acquired 738.3
rachitic (*see also* Rickets) 268.0
recurvatum (congenital) 754.81
acquired 738.3
Pedatrophia 261
Pederosis 302.2
Pediculosis (infestation) 132.9
capitis (head louse) (any site) 132.0
corporis (body louse) (any site) 132.1
eyelid 132.0 *[373.6]*
mixed (classifiable to more than one category in 132.0–132.2) 132.3
pubis (pubic louse) (any site) 132.2
vestimenti 132.1
vulvae 132.2
Pediculus (infestation) — *see* Pediculosis
Pedophilia 302.2
Peg-shaped teeth 520.2
Pelade 704.01
Pel's crisis 094.0
Pel-Ebstein disease — *see* Disease, Hodgkin's
Pelger-Huët anomaly or syndrome (hereditary hyposegmentation) 288.2
Peliosis (rheumatica) 287.0
Pelizaeus-Merzbacher
disease 330.0
sclerosis, diffuse cerebral 330.0
Pellagra (alcoholic or with alcoholism) 265.2
with polyneuropathy 265.2 *[357.4]*
Pellagra-cerebellar-ataxia-renal
aminoaciduria syndrome 270.0
Pellegrini's disease (calcification, knee joint)
726.62
Pellegrini (-Stieda) disease or syndrome
(calcification, knee joint) 726.62
Pellizzi's syndrome (pineal) 259.8
Pelvic — *see also* condition
congestion-fibrosis syndrome 625.5
kidney 753.3
Pelvioectasis 591
Pelviolithiasis 592.0
Pelviperitonitis
female (*see also* Peritonitis, pelvic, female)
614.5
male (*see also* Peritonitis) 567.21
Pelvis, pelvic — *see also* condition or type
infantile 738.6
Nägele's 738.6
obliquity 738.6
Robert's 755.69
Pemphigoid 694.5
benign, mucous membrane 694.60
with ocular involvement 694.61
bullous 694.5
cicatricial 694.60
with ocular involvement 694.61
juvenile 694.2
Pemphigus 694.4

Pemphigus — *continued*
benign 694.5
chronic familial 757.39
Brazilian 694.4
circinatus 694.0
congenital, traumatic 757.39
conjunctiva 694.61
contagiosus 684
erythematodes 694.4
erythematosus 694.4
foliaceus 694.4
frambesiodes 694.4
gangrenous (*see also* Gangrene) 785.4
malignant 694.4
neonatorum, newborn 684
ocular 694.61
papillaris 694.4
seborrheic 694.4
South American 694.4
syphilitic (congenital) 090.0
vegetans 694.4
vulgaris 694.4
wildfire 694.4
Pendred's syndrome (familial goiter with deaf-
mutism) 243
Pendulous
abdomen 701.9
in pregnancy or childbirth 654.4 ☑
affecting fetus or newborn 763.89
breast 611.89
Penetrating wound — *see also* Wound, open,
by site
with internal injury — *see* Injury, internal,
by site, with open wound
eyeball 871.7
with foreign body (nonmagnetic) 871.6
magnetic 871.5
ocular (*see also* Penetrating wound, eyeball)
871.7
adnexa 870.3
with foreign body 870.4
orbit 870.3
with foreign body 870.4
Penetration, pregnant uterus by instrument
with
abortion — *see* Abortion, by type, with
damage to pelvic organs
ectopic pregnancy (*see also* categories
633.0–633.9) 639.2
molar pregnancy (*see also* categories
630–632) 639.2
complication of delivery 665.1 ☑
affecting fetus or newborn 763.89
following
abortion 639.2
ectopic or molar pregnancy 639.2
Penfield's syndrome — *see also* Epilepsy
345.5 ☑
Penicilliosis of lung 117.3
Penis — *see* condition
Penitis 607.2
Pentalogy (of Fallot) 745.2
Penta X syndrome 758.81
Pentosuria (benign) (essential) 271.8
Peptic acid disease 536.8
Peregrinating patient V65.2
Perforated — *see* Perforation
Perforation, perforative (nontraumatic)
antrum (*see also* Sinusitis, maxillary) 473.0
appendix 540.0
with peritoneal abscess 540.1
atrial septum, multiple 745.5
attic, ear 384.22
healed 384.81
bile duct, except cystic (*see also* Disease,
biliary) 576.3
cystic 575.4
bladder (urinary) 596.6
with
abortion — *see* Abortion, by type,
with damage to pelvic organs
ectopic pregnancy (*see also* categories 633.0–633.9) 639.2
molar pregnancy (*see also* categories
630–632) 639.2

Perforation, perforative — *continued*
bladder — *continued*
following
abortion 639.2
ectopic or molar pregnancy 639.2
obstetrical trauma 665.5 ☑
bowel 569.83
with
abortion — *see* Abortion, by type,
with damage to pelvic organs
ectopic pregnancy (*see also* categories 633.0–633.9) 639.2
molar pregnancy (*see also* categories
630–632) 639.2
fetus or newborn 777.6
following
abortion 639.2
ectopic or molar pregnancy 639.2
obstetrical trauma 665.5 ☑
broad ligament
with
abortion — *see* Abortion, by type,
with damage to pelvic organs
ectopic pregnancy (*see also* categories 633.0–633.9) 639.2
molar pregnancy (*see also* categories
630–632) 639.2
following
abortion 639.2
ectopic or molar pregnancy 639.2
obstetrical trauma 665.6 ☑
by
device, implant, or graft — *see* Complications, mechanical
foreign body left accidentally in operation wound 998.4
instrument (any) during a procedure,
accidental 998.2
cecum 540.0
with peritoneal abscess 540.1
cervix (uteri) (*see also* Injury, internal, cervix)
with
abortion — *see* Abortion, by type,
with damage to pelvic organs
ectopic pregnancy (*see also* categories 633.0–633.9) 639.2
molar pregnancy (*see also* categories
630–632) 639.2
following
abortion 639.2
ectopic or molar pregnancy 639.2
obstetrical trauma 665.3 ☑
colon 569.83
common duct (bile) 576.3
cornea (*see also* Ulcer, cornea) 370.00
due to ulceration 370.06
cystic duct 575.4
diverticulum (*see also* Diverticula) 562.10
small intestine 562.00
duodenum, duodenal (ulcer) — *see* Ulcer,
duodenum, with perforation
ear drum — *see* Perforation, tympanum
enteritis — *see* Enteritis
esophagus 530.4
ethmoidal sinus (*see also* Sinusitis, ethmoidal) 473.2
foreign body (external site) (*see also* Wound,
open, by site, complicated)
internal site, by ingested object — *see*
Foreign body
frontal sinus (*see also* Sinusitis, frontal) 473.1
gallbladder or duct (*see also* Disease, gallbladder) 575.4
gastric (ulcer) — *see* Ulcer, stomach, with
perforation
heart valve — *see* Endocarditis
ileum (*see also* Perforation, intestine) 569.83
instrumental
external — *see* Wound, open, by site
pregnant uterus, complicating delivery
665.9 ☑
surgical (accidental) (blood vessel)
(nerve) (organ) 998.2
intestine 569.83

Perforation, perforative — *continued*
intestine — *continued*
with
abortion — *see* Abortion, by type,
with damage to pelvic organs
ectopic pregnancy (*see also* categories 633.0–633.9) 639.2
molar pregnancy (*see also* categories
630–632) 639.2
fetus or newborn 777.6
obstetrical trauma 665.5 ☑
ulcerative NEC 569.83
jejunum, jejunal 569.83
ulcer — *see* Ulcer, gastrojejunal, with
perforation
mastoid (antrum) (cell) 383.89
maxillary sinus (*see also* Sinusitis, maxillary)
473.0
membrana tympani — *see* Perforation,
tympanum
nasal
septum 478.19
congenital 748.1
syphilitic 095.8
sinus (*see also* Sinusitis) 473.9
congenital 748.1
palate (hard) 526.89
soft 528.9
syphilitic 095.8
syphilitic 095.8
palatine vault 526.89
syphilitic 095.8
congenital 090.5
pelvic
floor
with
abortion — *see* Abortion, by type,
with damage to pelvic or-
gans
ectopic pregnancy (*see also* categories 633.0–633.9) 639.2
molar pregnancy (*see also* categories 630–632) 639.2
obstetrical trauma 664.1 ☑
organ
with
abortion — *see* Abortion, by type,
with damage to pelvic or-
gans
ectopic pregnancy (*see also* categories 633.0–633.9) 639.2
molar pregnancy (*see also* categories 630–632) 639.2
following
abortion 639.2
ectopic or molar pregnancy 639.2
obstetrical trauma 665.5 ☑
perineum — *see* Laceration, perineum
periurethral tissue
with
abortion — *see* Abortion, by type,
with damage to pelvic organs
ectopic pregnancy (*see also* categories 630–632) 639.2
molar pregnancy (*see also* categories
630–632) 639.2
pharynx 478.29
pylorus, pyloric (ulcer) — *see* Ulcer, stomach, with perforation
rectum 569.49
root canal space 526.61
sigmoid 569.83
sinus (accessory) (chronic) (nasal) (*see also*
Sinusitis) 473.9
sphenoidal sinus (*see also* Sinusitis, sphenoidal) 473.3
stomach (due to ulcer) — *see* Ulcer, stomach, with perforation
surgical (accidental) (by instrument) (blood
vessel) (nerve) (organ) 998.2
traumatic
external — *see* Wound, open, by site
eye (*see also* Penetrating wound, ocular)
871.7
internal organ — *see* Injury, internal, by
site

☑ **Additional Digit Required** — Refer to the Tabular List for Digit Selection

▽ **Subterms under main terms may continue to next column or page**

Perforation, perforative — *continued*
  tympanum (membrane) (persistent posttraumatic) (postinflammatory) 384.20
    with
        otitis media — *see* Otitis media
    attic 384.22
    central 384.21
    healed 384.81
    marginal NEC 384.23
    multiple 384.24
    pars flaccida 384.22
    total 384.25
    traumatic — *see* Wound, open, ear, drum
  typhoid, gastrointestinal 002.0
  ulcer — *see* Ulcer, by site, with perforation
  ureter 593.89
  urethra
    with
        abortion — *see* Abortion, by type, with damage to pelvic organs
        ectopic pregnancy (*see also* categories 633.0–633.9) 639.2
        molar pregnancy (*see also* categories 630–632) 639.2
    following
        abortion 639.2
        ectopic or molar pregnancy 639.2
    obstetrical trauma 665.5 ☑
  uterus (*see also* Injury, internal, uterus)
    with
        abortion — *see* Abortion, by type, with damage to pelvic organs
        ectopic pregnancy (*see also* categories 633.0–633.9) 639.2
        molar pregnancy (*see also* categories 630–632) 639.2
    by intrauterine contraceptive device 996.32
    following
        abortion 639.2
        ectopic or molar pregnancy 639.2
    obstetrical trauma — *see* Injury, internal, uterus, obstetrical trauma
  uvula 528.9
    syphilitic 095.8
  vagina — *see* Laceration, vagina
  viscus NEC 799.89
    traumatic 868.00
        with open wound into cavity 868.10
Periadenitis mucosa necrotica recurrens 528.2
Periangiitis 446.0
Periantritis 535.4 ☑
Periappendicitis (acute) — *see also* Appendicitis 541
Periarteritis (disseminated) (infectious) (necrotizing) (nodosa) 446.0
Periarthritis (joint) 726.90
  Duplay's 726.2
  gonococcal 098.50
  humeroscapularis 726.2
  scapulohumeral 726.2
  shoulder 726.2
  wrist 726.4
Periarthrosis (angioneural) — *see* Periarthritis
Peribronchitis 491.9
  tuberculous (*see also* Tuberculosis) 011.3 ☑
Pericapsulitis, adhesive (shoulder) 726.0
Pericarditis (granular) (with decompensation) (with effusion) 423.9
  with
      rheumatic fever (conditions classifiable to 390)
          active (*see also* Pericarditis, rheumatic) 391.0
          inactive or quiescent 393
  actinomycotic 039.8 *[420.0]*
  acute (nonrheumatic) 420.90
      with chorea (acute) (rheumatic) (Sydenham's) 392.0
      bacterial 420.99
      benign 420.91
      hemorrhagic 420.90
      idiopathic 420.91
      infective 420.90

Pericarditis — *continued*
  acute — *continued*
      nonspecific 420.91
      rheumatic 391.0
          with chorea (acute) (rheumatic) (Sydenham's) 392.0
      sicca 420.90
      viral 420.91
  adhesive or adherent (external) (internal) 423.1
      acute — *see* Pericarditis, acute
      rheumatic (external) (internal) 393
  amebic 006.8 *[420.0]*
  bacterial (acute) (subacute) (with serous or seropurulent effusion) 420.99
  calcareous 423.2
  cholesterol (chronic) 423.8
      acute 420.90
  chronic (nonrheumatic) 423.8
      rheumatic 393
  constrictive 423.2
  Coxsackie 074.21
  due to
      actinomycosis 039.8 *[420.0]*
      amebiasis 006.8 *[420.0]*
      Coxsackie (virus) 074.21
      histoplasmosis (*see also* Histoplasmosis) 115.93
      nocardiosis 039.8 *[420.0]*
      tuberculosis (*see also* Tuberculosis) 017.9 ☑ *[420.0]*
  fibrinocaseous (*see also* Tuberculosis) 017.9 ☑ *[420.0]*
  fibrinopurulent 420.99
  fibrinous — *see* Pericarditis, rheumatic
  fibropurulent 420.99
  fibrous 423.1
  gonococcal 098.83
  hemorrhagic 423.0
  idiopathic (acute) 420.91
  infective (acute) 420.90
  meningococcal 036.41
  neoplastic (chronic) 423.8
      acute 420.90
  nonspecific 420.91
  obliterans, obliterating 423.1
  plastic 423.1
  pneumococcal (acute) 420.99
  postinfarction 411.0
  purulent (acute) 420.99
  rheumatic (active) (acute) (with effusion) (with pneumonia) 391.0
      with chorea (acute) (rheumatic) (Sydenham's) 392.0
      chronic or inactive (with chorea) 393
  septic (acute) 420.99
  serofibrinous — *see* Pericarditis, rheumatic
  staphylococcal (acute) 420.99
  streptococcal (acute) 420.99
  suppurative (acute) 420.99
  syphilitic 093.81
  tuberculous (acute) (chronic) (*see also* Tuberculosis) 017.9 ☑ *[420.0]*
  uremic 585.9 *[420.0]*
  viral (acute) 420.91
Pericardium, pericardial — *see* condition
Pericellulitis — *see also* Cellulitis 682.9
Pericementitis 523.40
  acute 523.30
  chronic (suppurative) 523.40
Pericholecystitis — *see also* Cholecystitis 575.10
Perichondritis
  auricle 380.00
      acute 380.01
      chronic 380.02
  bronchus 491.9
  ear (external) 380.00
      acute 380.01
      chronic 380.02
  larynx 478.71
      syphilitic 095.8
      typhoid 002.0 *[478.71]*
  nose 478.19
  pinna 380.00
      acute 380.01

Perichondritis — *continued*
  pinna — *continued*
      chronic 380.02
  trachea 478.9
Periclasia 523.5
Pericolitis 569.89
Pericoronitis (chronic) 523.40
  acute 523.33
Pericystitis — *see also* Cystitis 595.9
Pericytoma (M9150/1) — *see also* Neoplasm, connective tissue, uncertain behavior
  benign (M9150/0) — *see* Neoplasm, connective tissue, benign
  malignant (M9150/3) — *see* Neoplasm, connective tissue, malignant
Peridacryocystitis, acute 375.32
Peridiverticulitis — *see also* Diverticulitis 562.11
Periduodenitis 535.6 ☑
Periendocarditis — *see also* Endocarditis 424.90
  acute or subacute 421.9
Periepididymitis — *see also* Epididymitis 604.90
Perifolliculitis (abscedens) 704.8
  capitis, abscedens et suffodiens 704.8
  dissecting, scalp 704.8
  scalp 704.8
  superficial pustular 704.8
Perigastritis (acute) 535.0 ☑
Perigastrojejunitis (acute) 535.0 ☑
Perihepatitis (acute) 573.3
  chlamydial 099.56
  gonococcal 098.86
Peri-ileitis (subacute) 569.89
Perilabyrinthitis (acute) — *see* Labyrinthitis
Perimeningitis — *see* Meningitis
Perimetritis — *see also* Endometritis 615.9
Perimetrosalpingitis — *see also* Salpingo-oophoritis 614.2
Perineocele 618.05
Perinephric — *see* condition
Perinephritic — *see* condition
Perinephritis — *see also* Infection, kidney 590.9
  purulent (*see also* Abscess, kidney) 590.2
Perineum, perineal — *see* condition
Perineuritis NEC 729.2
Periodic — *see also* condition
  disease (familial) 277.31
  edema 995.1
      hereditary 277.6
  fever 277.31
  headache syndromes in child or adolescent 346.2 ☑
  limb movement disorder 327.51
  paralysis (familial) 359.3
  peritonitis 277.31
  polyserositis 277.31
  somnolence (*see also* Narcolepsy) 347.00
Periodontal
  cyst 522.8
  pocket 523.8
Periodontitis (chronic) (complex) (compound) (simplex) 523.40
  acute 523.33
  aggressive 523.30
      generalized 523.32
      localized 523.31
  apical 522.6
      acute (pulpal origin) 522.4
  generalized 523.42
  localized 523.41
Periodontoclasia 523.5
Periodontosis 523.5
Periods — *see also* Menstruation
  heavy 626.2
  irregular 626.4
Perionychia (with lymphangitis) 681.9
  finger 681.02
  toe 681.11
Perioophoritis — *see also* Salpingo-oophoritis 614.2
Periorchitis — *see also* Orchitis 604.90
Periosteum, periosteal — *see* condition

Periostitis (circumscribed) (diffuse) (infective) 730.3 ☑

Note — Use the following fifth-digit subclassification with category 730:

0	*site unspecified*
1	*shoulder region*
2	*upper arm*
3	*forearm*
4	*hand*
5	*pelvic region and thigh*
6	*lower leg*
7	*ankle and foot*
8	*other specified sites*
9	*multiple sites*

  with osteomyelitis (*see also* Osteomyelitis) 730.2 ☑
      acute or subacute 730.0 ☑
      chronic or old 730.1 ☑
  albuminosa, albuminosus 730.3 ☑
  alveolar 526.5
  alveolodental 526.5
  dental 526.5
  gonorrheal 098.89
  hyperplastica, generalized 731.2
  jaw (lower) (upper) 526.4
  monomelic 733.99
  orbital 376.02
  syphilitic 095.5
      congenital 090.0 *[730.8]* ☑
      secondary 091.61
  tuberculous (*see also* Tuberculosis, bone) 015.9 ☑ *[730.8]* ☑
  yaws (early) (hypertrophic) (late) 102.6
Periostosis — *see also* Periostitis 730.3 ☑
  with osteomyelitis (*see also* Osteomyelitis) 730.2 ☑
      acute or subacute 730.0 ☑
      chronic or old 730.1 ☑
  hyperplastic 756.59
Peripartum cardiomyopathy 674.5 ☑
Periphlebitis — *see also* Phlebitis 451.9
  lower extremity 451.2
      deep (vessels) 451.19
      superficial (vessels) 451.0
  portal 572.1
  retina 362.18
  superficial (vessels) 451.0
  tuberculous (*see also* Tuberculosis) 017.9 ☑
      retina 017.3 ☑ *[362.18]*
Peripneumonia — *see* Pneumonia
Periproctitis 569.49
Periprostatitis — *see also* Prostatitis 601.9
Perirectal — *see* condition
Perirenal — *see* condition
Perisalpingitis — *see also* Salpingo-oophoritis 614.2
Perisigmoiditis 569.89
Perisplenitis (infectional) 289.59
Perispondylitis — *see* Spondylitis
Peristalsis reversed or visible 787.4
Peritendinitis — *see also* Tenosynovitis 726.90
  adhesive (shoulder) 726.0
Perithelioma (M9150/1) — *see* Pericytoma
Peritoneum, peritoneal — *see also* condition
  equilibration test V56.32
Peritonitis (acute) (adhesive) (fibrinous) (hemorrhagic) (idiopathic) (localized) (perforative) (primary) (with adhesions) (with effusion) 567.9
  with or following
      abortion — *see* Abortion, by type, with sepsis
      abscess 567.21
      appendicitis 540.0
          with peritoneal abscess 540.1
      ectopic pregnancy (*see also* categories 633.0–633.9) 639.0
      molar pregnancy (*see also* categories 630–632) 639.0
  aseptic 998.7

☑ **Additional Digit Required** — Refer to the Tabular List for Digit Selection   ▽ **Subterms under main terms may continue to next column or page**

272   **2014 ICD-9-CM**

Peritonitis — continued
  bacterial 567.29
    spontaneous 567.23
  bile, biliary 567.81
  chemical 998.7
  chlamydial 099.56
  chronic proliferative 567.89
  congenital NEC 777.6
  diaphragmatic 567.22
  diffuse NEC 567.29
  diphtheritic 032.83
  disseminated NEC 567.29
  due to
    bile 567.81
    foreign
      body or object accidentally left during a procedure (instrument) (sponge) (swab) 998.4
      substance accidentally left during a procedure (chemical) (powder) (talc) 998.7
    talc 998.7
    urine 567.89
  fibrinopurulent 567.29
  fibrinous 567.29
  fibrocaseous (see also Tuberculosis) 014.0 ☑
  fibropurulent 567.29
  general, generalized (acute) 567.21
  gonococcal 098.86
  in infective disease NEC 136.9 [567.0]
  meconium (newborn) 777.6
  pancreatic 577.8
  paroxysmal, benign 277.31
  pelvic
    female (acute) 614.5
      chronic NEC 614.7
        with adhesions 614.6
      puerperal, postpartum, childbirth 670.8 ☑
    male (acute) 567.21
  periodic (familial) 277.31
  phlegmonous 567.29
  pneumococcal 567.1
  postabortal 639.0
  proliferative, chronic 567.89
  puerperal, postpartum, childbirth 670.8 ☑
  purulent 567.29
  septic 567.29
  spontaneous bacterial 567.23
  staphylococcal 567.29
  streptococcal 567.29
  subdiaphragmatic 567.29
  subphrenic 567.29
  suppurative 567.29
  syphilitic 095.2
    congenital 090.0 [567.0]
  talc 998.7
  tuberculous (see also Tuberculosis) 014.0 ☑
  urine 567.89
Peritonsillar — see condition
Peritonsillitis 475
Perityphlitis — see also Appendicitis 541
Periureteritis 593.89
Periurethral — see condition
Periurethritis (gangrenous) 597.89
Periuterine — see condition
Perivaginitis — see also Vaginitis 616.10
Perivasculitis, retinal 362.18
Perivasitis (chronic) 608.4
Periventricular leukomalacia 779.7
Perivesiculitis (seminal) — see also Vesiculitis 608.0
Perlèche 686.8
  due to
    moniliasis 112.0
    riboflavin deficiency 266.0
Pernicious — see condition
Pernio, perniosis 991.5
Persecution
  delusion 297.9
  social V62.4
Perseveration (tonic) 784.69
Persistence, persistent (congenital) 759.89
  anal membrane 751.2
  arteria stapedia 744.04
  atrioventricular canal 745.69

Persistence, persistent — continued
  bloody ejaculate 792.2
  branchial cleft 744.41
  bulbus cordis in left ventricle 745.8
  canal of Cloquet 743.51
  capsule (opaque) 743.51
  cilioretinal artery or vein 743.51
  cloaca 751.5
  communication — see Fistula, congenital
  convolutions
    aortic arch 747.21
    fallopian tube 752.19
    oviduct 752.19
    uterine tube 752.19
  double aortic arch 747.21
  ductus
    arteriosus 747.0
    Botalli 747.0
  fetal
    circulation 747.83
    form of cervix (uteri) 752.49
    hemoglobin (hereditary) ("Swiss variety") 282.7
    pulmonary hypertension 747.83
  foramen
    Botalli 745.5
    ovale 745.5
  Gartner's duct 752.41
  hemoglobin, fetal (hereditary) (HPFH) 282.7
  hyaloid
    artery (generally incomplete) 743.51
    system 743.51
  hymen (tag)
    in pregnancy or childbirth 654.8 ☑
      causing obstructed labor 660.2 ☑
  lanugo 757.4
  left
    posterior cardinal vein 747.49
    root with right arch of aorta 747.21
    superior vena cava 747.49
  Meckel's diverticulum 751.0
  mesonephric duct 752.89
    fallopian tube 752.11
  mucosal disease (middle ear) (with posterior or superior marginal perforation of ear drum) 382.2
  nail(s), anomalous 757.5
  occiput, anterior or posterior 660.3 ☑
    fetus or newborn 763.1
  omphalomesenteric duct 751.0
  organ or site NEC — see Anomaly, specified type NEC
  ostium
    atrioventriculare commune 745.69
    primum 745.61
    secundum 745.5
  ovarian rests in fallopian tube 752.19
  pancreatic tissue in intestinal tract 751.5
  primary (deciduous)
    teeth 520.6
    vitreous hyperplasia 743.51
  pulmonary hypertension 747.83
  pupillary membrane 743.46
    iris 743.46
  Rhesus (Rh) titer (see also Complications, transfusion) 999.70
  right aortic arch 747.21
  sinus
    urogenitalis 752.89
    venosus with imperfect incorporation in right auricle 747.49
  thymus (gland) 254.8
    hyperplasia 254.0
  thyroglossal duct 759.2
  thyrolingual duct 759.2
  truncus arteriosus or communis 745.0
  tunica vasculosa lentis 743.39
  umbilical sinus 753.7
  urachus 753.7
  vegetative state 780.03
  vitelline duct 751.0
  wolffian duct 752.89
Person (with)
  admitted for clinical research, as participant or control subject V70.7

Person — continued
  affected by
    family member
      currently on deployment (military) V61.01
      returned from deployment (military) (current or past conflict) V61.02
  awaiting admission to adequate facility elsewhere V63.2
  undergoing social agency investigation V63.8
  concern (normal) about sick person in family V61.49
  consulting on behalf of another V65.19
    pediatric
      pre-adoption visit for adoptive parents V65.11
      pre-birth visit for expectant parents V65.11
  currently deployed in theater or in support of military war, peacekeeping and humanitarian operations V62.21
  feared
    complaint in whom no diagnosis was made V65.5
    condition not demonstrated V65.5
  feigning illness V65.2
  healthy, accompanying sick person V65.0
  history of military war, peacekeeping and humanitarian deployment (current or past conflict) V62.22
  living (in)
    without
      adequate
        financial resources V60.2
        housing (heating) (space) V60.1
      housing (permanent) (temporary) V60.0
      material resources V60.2
      person able to render necessary care V60.4
      shelter V60.0
    alone V60.3
    boarding school V60.6
    residence remote from hospital or medical care facility V63.0
    residential institution V60.6
  medical services in home not available V63.1
  on waiting list V63.2
    undergoing social agency investigation V63.8
  sick or handicapped in family V61.49
  "worried well" V65.5
Personality
  affective 301.10
  aggressive 301.3
  amoral 301.7
  anancastic, anankastic 301.4
  antisocial 301.7
  asocial 301.7
  asthenic 301.6
  avoidant 301.82
  borderline 301.83
  change 310.1
  compulsive 301.4
  cycloid 301.13
  cyclothymic 301.13
  dependent 301.6
  depressive (chronic) 301.12
  disorder, disturbance NEC 301.9
    with
      antisocial disturbance 301.7
      pattern disturbance NEC 301.9
      sociopathic disturbance 301.7
      trait disturbance 301.9
  dual 300.14
  dyssocial 301.7
  eccentric 301.89
    "haltlose" type 301.89
  emotionally unstable 301.59
  epileptoid 301.3
  explosive 301.3
  fanatic 301.0
  histrionic 301.50
  hyperthymic 301.11

Personality — continued
  hypomanic 301.11
  hypothymic 301.12
  hysterical 301.50
  immature 301.89
  inadequate 301.6
  labile 301.59
  masochistic 301.89
  morally defective 301.7
  multiple 300.14
  narcissistic 301.81
  obsessional 301.4
  obsessive-compulsive 301.4
  overconscientious 301.4
  paranoid 301.0
  passive (-dependent) 301.6
  passive-aggressive 301.84
  pathologic NEC 301.9
  pattern defect or disturbance 301.9
  pseudosocial 301.7
  psychoinfantile 301.59
  psychoneurotic NEC 301.89
  psychopathic 301.9
    with
      amoral trend 301.7
      antisocial trend 301.7
      asocial trend 301.7
      pathologic sexuality (see also Deviation, sexual) 302.9
    mixed types 301.9
  schizoid 301.20
  type A 301.4
  unstable (emotional) 301.59
Perthes' disease (capital femoral osteochondrosis) 732.1
Pertussis — see also Whooping cough 033.9
  vaccination, prophylactic (against) V03.6
Peruvian wart 088.0
Perversion, perverted
  appetite 307.52
    hysterical 300.11
  function
    pineal gland 259.8
    pituitary gland 253.9
      anterior lobe
        deficient 253.2
        excessive 253.1
      posterior lobe 253.6
    placenta — see Placenta, abnormal
  sense of smell or taste 781.1
    psychogenic 306.7
  sexual (see also Deviation, sexual) 302.9
Pervious, congenital — see also Imperfect, closure
  ductus arteriosus 747.0
Pes (congenital) — see also Talipes 754.70
  abductus (congenital) 754.60
    acquired 736.79
  acquired NEC 736.79
    planus 734
  adductus (congenital) 754.79
    acquired 736.79
  cavus 754.71
    acquired 736.73
  planovalgus (congenital) 754.69
    acquired 736.79
  planus (acquired) (any degree) 734
    congenital 754.61
    rachitic 268.1
  valgus (congenital) 754.61
    acquired 736.79
  varus (congenital) 754.50
    acquired 736.79
Pest — see also Plague 020.9
Pestis — see also Plague 020.9
  bubonica 020.0
  fulminans 020.0
  minor 020.8
  pneumonica — see Plague, pneumonic
Petechial
  fever 036.0
  typhus 081.9
Petechia, petechiae 782.7
  fetus or newborn 772.6
Petges-Cléjat or Petges-Clégat syndrome (poikilodermatomyositis) 710.3

Petit's
- disease (*see also* Hernia, lumbar) 553.8
Petit mal (idiopathic) — *see also* Epilepsy 345.0 ☑
  status 345.2
Petrellidosis 117.6
Petrositis 383.20
  acute 383.21
  chronic 383.22
Peutz-Jeghers disease or syndrome 759.6
Peyronie's disease 607.85
Pfeiffer's disease 075
Phacentocele 379.32
  traumatic 921.3
Phacoanaphylaxis 360.19
Phacocele (old) 379.32
  traumatic 921.3
Phaehyphomycosis 117.8
Phagedena (dry) (moist) — *see also* Gangrene 785.4
  arteriosclerotic 440.24
  geometric 686.09
  penis 607.89
  senile 440.2 ☑ *[785.4]*
  sloughing 785.4
  tropical (*see also* Ulcer, skin) 707.9
  vulva 616.50
Phagedenic — *see also* condition
  abscess (*see also* Abscess)
    chancroid 099.0
  bubo NEC 099.8
  chancre 099.0
  ulcer (tropical) (*see also* Ulcer, skin) 707.9
Phagomania 307.52
Phakoma 362.89
Phantom limb (syndrome) 353.6
Pharyngeal — *see also* condition
  arch remnant 744.41
  pouch syndrome 279.11
Pharyngitis (acute) (catarrhal) (gangrenous) (infective) (malignant) (membranous) (phlegmonous) (pneumococcal) (pseudomembranous) (simple) (staphylococcal) (subacute) (suppurative) (ulcerative) (viral) 462
  with influenza, flu, or grippe (*see also* Influenza) 487.1
  aphthous 074.0
  atrophic 472.1
  chlamydial 099.51
  chronic 472.1
  Coxsackie virus 074.0
  diphtheritic (membranous) 032.0
  follicular 472.1
  fusospirochetal 101
  gonococcal 098.6
  granular (chronic) 472.1
  herpetic 054.79
  hypertrophic 472.1
  infectional, chronic 472.1
  influenzal (*see also* Influenza) 487.1
  lymphonodular, acute 074.8
  septic 034.0
  streptococcal 034.0
  tuberculous (*see also* Tuberculosis) 012.8 ☑
  vesicular 074.0
Pharyngoconjunctival fever 077.2
Pharyngoconjunctivitis, viral 077.2
Pharyngolaryngitis (acute) 465.0
  chronic 478.9
  septic 034.0
Pharyngoplegia 478.29
Pharyngotonsillitis 465.8
  tuberculous 012.8 ☑
Pharyngotracheitis (acute) 465.8
  chronic 478.9
Pharynx, pharyngeal — *see* condition
Phase of life problem NEC V62.89
Phenomenon
  Arthus' 995.21
  flashback (drug) 292.89
  jaw-winking 742.8
  Jod-Basedow 242.8 ☑
  L. E. cell 710.0
  lupus erythematosus cell 710.0

Phenomenon — *continued*
  Pelger-Huët (hereditary hyposegmentation) 288.2
  Raynaud's (paroxysmal digital cyanosis) (secondary) 443.0
  Reilly's (*see also* Neuropathy, peripheral, autonomic) 337.9
  vasomotor 780.2
  vasospastic 443.9
  vasovagal 780.2
  Wenckebach's, heart block (second degree) 426.13
Phenylketonuria (PKU) 270.1
Phenylpyruvicaciduria 270.1
Pheochromoblastoma (M8700/3)
  specified site — *see* Neoplasm, by site, malignant
  unspecified site 194.0
Pheochromocytoma (M8700/0)
  malignant (M8700/3)
    specified site — *see* Neoplasm, by site, malignant
    unspecified site 194.0
  specified site — *see* Neoplasm, by site, benign
  unspecified site 227.0
Phimosis (congenital) 605
  chancroidal 099.0
  due to infection 605
Phlebectasia — *see also* Varicose, vein 454.9
  congenital NEC 747.60
  esophagus (*see also* Varix, esophagus) 456.1
    with hemorrhage (*see also* Varix, esophagus, bleeding) 456.0
Phlebitis (infective) (pyemic) (septic) (suppurative) 451.9
  antecubital vein 451.82
  arm NEC 451.84
    axillary vein 451.89
    basilic vein 451.82
    deep 451.83
    superficial 451.82
  axillary vein 451.89
  basilic vein 451.82
  blue 451.9
  brachial vein 451.83
  breast, superficial 451.89
  cavernous (venous) sinus — *see* Phlebitis, intracranial sinus
  cephalic vein 451.82
  cerebral (venous) sinus — *see* Phlebitis, intracranial sinus
  chest wall, superficial 451.89
  complicating pregnancy or puerperium 671.2 ☑
    affecting fetus or newborn 760.3
  cranial (venous) sinus — *see* Phlebitis, intracranial sinus
  deep (vessels) 451.19
    femoral vein 451.11
    specified vessel NEC 451.19
  due to implanted device — *see* Complications, due to (presence of) any device, implant, or graft classified to 996.0–996.5 NEC
  during or resulting from a procedure 997.2
  femoral vein (deep) (superficial) 451.11
  femoropopliteal 451.19
  following infusion, perfusion, or transfusion 999.2
  gouty 274.89 *[451.9]*
  hepatic veins 451.89
  iliac vein 451.81
  iliofemoral 451.11
  intracranial sinus (any) (venous) 325
    late effect — *see* category 326
    nonpyogenic 437.6
      in pregnancy or puerperium 671.5 ☑
  jugular vein 451.89
  lateral (venous) sinus — *see* Phlebitis, intracranial sinus
  leg 451.2
    deep (vessels) 451.19
      femoral vein 451.11
      specified vessel NEC 451.19
    superficial (vessels) 451.0

Phlebitis — *continued*
  leg — *continued*
    superficial — *continued*
      femoral vein 451.11
  longitudinal sinus — *see* Phlebitis, intracranial sinus
  lower extremity 451.2
    deep (vessels) 451.19
      femoral vein 451.11
      specified vessel NEC 451.19
    migrans, migrating (superficial) 453.1
    superficial (vessels) 451.0
      femoral vein 451.11
  pelvic
    with
      abortion — *see* Abortion, by type, with sepsis
      ectopic pregnancy (*see also* categories 633.0–633.9) 639.0
      molar pregnancy (*see also* categories 630–632) 639.0
    following
      abortion 639.0
      ectopic or molar pregnancy 639.0
    puerperal, postpartum 671.4 ☑
  popliteal vein 451.19
  portal (vein) 572.1
  postoperative 997.2
  pregnancy 671.2 ☑
    deep 671.3 ☑
    specified type NEC 671.5 ☑
    superficial 671.2 ☑
  puerperal, postpartum, childbirth 671.2 ☑
    deep 671.3 ☑
    lower extremities 671.2 ☑
    pelvis 671.4 ☑
    specified site NEC 671.5 ☑
    superficial 671.2 ☑
  radial vein 451.83
  retina 362.18
  saphenous (great) (long) 451.0
    accessory or small 451.0
  sinus (meninges) — *see* Phlebitis, intracranial sinus
  specified site NEC 451.89
  subclavian vein 451.89
  syphilitic 093.89
  tibial vein 451.19
  ulcer, ulcerative 451.9
    leg 451.2
      deep (vessels) 451.19
        femoral vein 451.11
        specified vessel NEC 451.19
      superficial (vessels) 451.0
        femoral vein 451.11
    lower extremity 451.2
      deep (vessels) 451.19
        femoral vein 451.11
        specified vessel NEC 451.19
      superficial (vessels) 451.0
  ulnar vein 451.83
  umbilicus 451.89
  upper extremity (*see also* Phlebitis, arm)
    deep (veins) 451.83
      brachial vein 451.83
      radial vein 451.83
      ulnar vein 451.83
    superficial (veins) 451.82
      antecubital vein 451.82
      basilica vein 451.82
      cephalic vein 451.82
  uterus (septic) (*see also* Endometritis) 615.9
  varicose (leg) (lower extremity) (*see also* Varicose, vein) 454.1
Phlebofibrosis 459.89
Phleboliths 459.89
Phlebosclerosis 459.89
Phlebothrombosis — *see* Thrombosis
Phlebotomus fever 066.0
Phlegmasia
  alba dolens (deep vessels) 451.19
    complicating pregnancy 671.3 ☑
    nonpuerperal 451.19
    puerperal, postpartum, childbirth 671.4 ☑
  cerulea dolens 451.19

Phlegm, choked on 933.1
Phlegmon — *see also* Abscess 682.9
  erysipelatous (*see also* Erysipelas) 035
  iliac 682.2
    fossa 540.1
  throat 478.29
Phlegmonous — *see* condition
Phlyctenulosis (allergic) (keratoconjunctivitis) (nontuberculous) 370.31
  cornea 370.31
    with ulcer (*see also* Ulcer, cornea) 370.00
  tuberculous (*see also* Tuberculosis) 017.3 ☑ *[370.31]*
Phobia, phobic (reaction) 300.20
  animal 300.29
  isolated NEC 300.29
  obsessional 300.3
  simple NEC 300.29
  social 300.23
  specified NEC 300.29
  state 300.20
Phocas' disease 610.1
Phocomelia 755.4
  lower limb 755.32
    complete 755.33
    distal 755.35
    proximal 755.34
  upper limb 755.22
    complete 755.23
    distal 755.25
    proximal 755.24
Phoria — *see also* Heterophoria 378.40
Phosphate-losing tubular disorder 588.0
Phosphatemia 275.3
Phosphaturia 275.3
Photoallergic response 692.72
Photocoproporphyria 277.1
Photodermatitis (sun) 692.72
  light other than sun 692.82
Photokeratitis 370.24
Photo-ophthalmia 370.24
Photophobia 368.13
Photopsia 368.15
Photoretinitis 363.31
Photoretinopathy 363.31
Photosensitiveness (sun) 692.72
  light other than sun 692.82
Photosensitization (skin) (sun) 692.72
  light other than sun 692.82
Phototoxic response 692.72
Phrenitis 323.9
Phrynoderma 264.8
Phthiriasis (pubis) (any site) 132.2
  with any infestation classifiable to 132.0, 132.1, 132.3
Phthirus infestation — *see* Phthiriasis
Phthisis — *see also* Tuberculosis 011.9 ☑
  bulbi (infectional) 360.41
  colliers' 011.4 ☑
  cornea 371.05
  eyeball (due to infection) 360.41
  millstone makers' 011.4 ☑
  miners' 011.4 ☑
  potters' 011.4 ☑
  sandblasters' 011.4 ☑
  stonemasons' 011.4 ☑
Phycomycosis 117.7
Physalopteriasis 127.7
Physical therapy NEC V57.1
  breathing exercises V57.0
Physiological cup, optic papilla
  borderline, glaucoma suspect 365.00
  enlarged 377.14
  glaucomatous 377.14
Phytobezoar 938
  intestine 936
  stomach 935.2
Pian — *see also* Yaws 102.9
Pianoma 102.1
Piarhemia, piarrhemia — *see also* Hyperlipemia 272.4
  bilharziasis 120.9
Pica 307.52
  hysterical 300.11
Pick's
  cerebral atrophy 331.11

☑ **Additional Digit Required** — **Refer to the Tabular List for Digit Selection**   ▽ **Subterms under main terms may continue to next column or page**

274   **2014 ICD-9-CM**

Pick's — *continued*
  cerebral atrophy — *continued*
    with dementia
      with behavioral disturbance
        331.11 *[294.11]*
      without behavioral disturbance
        331.11 *[294.10]*
  disease
    brain 331.11
      dementia in
        with behavioral disturbance
          331.11 *[294.11]*
        without behavioral disturbance
          331.11 *[294.10]*
    lipid histiocytosis 272.7
    liver (pericardial pseudocirrhosis of liver) 423.2
    pericardium (pericardial pseudocirrhosis of liver) 423.2
    polyserositis (pericardial pseudocirrhosis of liver) 423.2
  syndrome
    heart (pericardial pseudocirrhosis of liver) 423.2
    liver (pericardial pseudocirrhosis of liver) 423.2
  tubular adenoma (M8640/0)
    specified site — *see* Neoplasm, by site, benign
    unspecified site
      female 220
      male 222.0
Pick-Herxheimer syndrome (diffuse idiopathic cutaneous atrophy) 701.8
Pick-Niemann disease (lipid histiocytosis) 272.7
Pickwickian syndrome (cardiopulmonary obesity) 278.03
Piebaldism, classic 709.09
Piedra 111.2
  beard 111.2
    black 111.3
    white 111.2
  black 111.3
  scalp 111.3
    black 111.3
    white 111.2
  white 111.2
Pierre Marie-Bamberger syndrome (hypertrophic pulmonary osteoarthropathy) 731.2
Pierre Marie's syndrome (pulmonary hypertrophic osteoarthropathy) 731.2
Pierre Mauriac's syndrome (diabetes-dwarfism-obesity) 258.1
Pierre Robin deformity or syndrome (congenital) 756.0
Pierson's disease or osteochondrosis 732.1
Pigeon
  breast or chest (acquired) 738.3
    congenital 754.82
    rachitic (*see also* Rickets) 268.0
  breeders' disease or lung 495.2
  fanciers' disease or lung 495.2
  toe 735.8
Pigmentation (abnormal) 709.00
  anomaly 709.00
    congenital 757.33
    specified NEC 709.09
  conjunctiva 372.55
  cornea 371.10
    anterior 371.11
    posterior 371.13
    stromal 371.12
  lids (congenital) 757.33
    acquired 374.52
  limbus corneae 371.10
  metals 709.00
  optic papilla, congenital 743.57
  retina (congenital) (grouped) (nevoid) 743.53
    acquired 362.74
  scrotum, congenital 757.33
Piles — *see* Hemorrhoids
Pili
  annulati or torti (congenital) 757.4

Pili — *continued*
  incarnati 704.8
Pill roller hand (intrinsic) 736.09
Pilomatrixoma (M8110/0) — *see* Neoplasm, skin, benign
Pilonidal — *see* condition
Pimple 709.8
PIN I (prostatic intraepithelial neoplasia I) 602.3
PIN II (prostatic intraepithelial neoplasia II) 602.3
PIN III (prostatic intraepithelial neoplasia III) 233.4
Pinched nerve — *see* Neuropathy, entrapment
Pineal body or gland — *see* condition
Pinealoblastoma (M9362/3) 194.4
Pinealoma (M9360/1) 237.1
  malignant (M9360/3) 194.4
Pineoblastoma (M9362/3) 194.4
Pineocytoma (M9361/1) 237.1
Pinguecula 372.51
Pingueculitis 372.34
Pinhole meatus — *see also* Stricture, urethra 598.9
Pink
  disease 985.0
  eye 372.03
  puffer 492.8
Pinkus' disease (lichen nitidus) 697.1
Pinpoint
  meatus (*see also* Stricture, urethra) 598.9
  os uteri (*see also* Stricture, cervix) 622.4
Pinselhaare (congenital) 757.4
Pinta 103.9
  cardiovascular lesions 103.2
  chancre (primary) 103.0
  erythematous plaques 103.1
  hyperchromic lesions 103.1
  hyperkeratosis 103.1
  lesions 103.9
    cardiovascular 103.2
    hyperchromic 103.1
    intermediate 103.1
    late 103.2
    mixed 103.3
    primary 103.0
    skin (achromic) (cicatricial) (dyschromic) 103.2
      hyperchromic 103.1
      mixed (achromic and hyperchromic) 103.3
  papule (primary) 103.0
  skin lesions (achromic) (cicatricial) (dyschromic) 103.2
    hyperchromic 103.1
    mixed (achromic and hyperchromic) 103.3
  vitiligo 103.2
Pintid 103.0
Pinworms (disease) (infection) (infestation) 127.4
Piry fever 066.8
Pistol wound — *see* Gunshot wound
Pitchers' elbow 718.82
Pithecoid pelvis 755.69
  with disproportion (fetopelvic) 653.2 ☑
    affecting fetus or newborn 763.1
    causing obstructed labor 660.1 ☑
Pithiatism 300.11
Pit, lip (mucus), **congenital** 750.25
Pitted — *see also* Pitting
  teeth 520.4
Pitting (edema) — *see also* Edema 782.3
  lip 782.3
  nail 703.8
    congenital 757.5
Pituitary gland — *see* condition
Pituitary snuff-takers' disease 495.8
Pityriasis 696.5
  alba 696.5
  capitis 690.11
  circinata (et maculata) 696.3
  Hebra's (exfoliative dermatitis) 695.89
  lichenoides et varioliformis 696.2
  maculata (et circinata) 696.3
  nigra 111.1
  pilaris 757.39

Pityriasis — *continued*
  pilaris — *continued*
    acquired 701.1
    Hebra's 696.4
  rosea 696.3
  rotunda 696.3
  rubra (Hebra) 695.89
    pilaris 696.4
  sicca 690.18
  simplex 690.18
  specified type NEC 696.5
  streptogenes 696.5
  versicolor 111.0
    scrotal 111.0
Placenta, placental
  ablatio 641.2 ☑
    affecting fetus or newborn 762.1
  abnormal, abnormality 656.7 ☑
    with hemorrhage 641.8 ☑
      affecting fetus or newborn 762.1
    affecting fetus or newborn 762.2
  abruptio 641.2 ☑
    affecting fetus or newborn 762.1
  accessory lobe — *see* Placenta, abnormal
  accreta (without hemorrhage) 667.0 ☑
    with hemorrhage 666.0 ☑
  adherent (without hemorrhage) 667.0 ☑
    with hemorrhage 666.0 ☑
  apoplexy — *see* Placenta, separation
  battledore — *see* Placenta, abnormal
  bilobate — *see* Placenta, abnormal
  bipartita — *see* Placenta, abnormal
  carneous mole 631.8
  centralis — *see* Placenta, previa
  circumvallata — *see* Placenta, abnormal
  cyst (amniotic) — *see* Placenta, abnormal
  deficiency — *see* Placenta, insufficiency
  degeneration — *see* Placenta, insufficiency
  detachment (partial) (premature) (with hemorrhage) 641.2 ☑
    affecting fetus or newborn 762.1
  dimidiata — *see* Placenta, abnormal
  disease 656.7 ☑
    affecting fetus or newborn 762.2
  duplex — *see* Placenta, abnormal
  dysfunction — *see* Placenta, insufficiency
  fenestrata — *see* Placenta, abnormal
  fibrosis — *see* Placenta, abnormal
  fleshy mole 631.8
  hematoma — *see* Placenta, abnormal
  hemorrhage NEC — *see* Placenta, separation
  hormone disturbance or malfunction — *see* Placenta, abnormal
  hyperplasia — *see* Placenta, abnormal
  increta (without hemorrhage) 667.0 ☑
    with hemorrhage 666.0 ☑
  infarction 656.7 ☑
    affecting fetus or newborn 762.2
  insertion, vicious — *see* Placenta, previa
  insufficiency
    affecting
      fetus or newborn 762.2
      management of pregnancy 656.5 ☑
  lateral — *see* Placenta, previa
  low implantation or insertion — *see* Placenta, previa
  low-lying — *see* Placenta, previa
  malformation — *see* Placenta, abnormal
  malposition — *see* Placenta, previa
  marginalis, marginata — *see* Placenta, previa
  marginal sinus (hemorrhage) (rupture) 641.2 ☑
    affecting fetus or newborn 762.1
  membranacea — *see* Placenta, abnormal
  multilobed — *see* Placenta, abnormal
  multipartita — *see* Placenta, abnormal
  necrosis — *see* Placenta, abnormal
  percreta (without hemorrhage) 667.0 ☑
    with hemorrhage 666.0 ☑
  polyp 674.4 ☑
  previa (central) (centralis) (complete) (lateral) (marginal) (marginalis) (partial) (partialis) (total) (with hemorrhage) 641.1 ☑

Placenta, placental — *continued*
  previa — *continued*
    without hemorrhage (before labor and delivery) (during pregnancy) 641.0 ☑
      affecting fetus or newborn 762.0
      noted
        before labor, without hemorrhage (with cesarean delivery) 641.0 ☑
        during pregnancy (without hemorrhage) 641.0 ☑
  retention (with hemorrhage) 666.0 ☑
    without hemorrhage 667.0 ☑
    fragments, complicating puerperium (delayed hemorrhage) 666.2 ☑
      without hemorrhage 667.1 ☑
    postpartum, puerperal 666.2 ☑
  separation (normally implanted) (partial) (premature) (with hemorrhage) 641.2 ☑
    affecting fetus or newborn 762.1
  septuplex — *see* Placenta, abnormal
  small — *see* Placenta, insufficiency
  softening (premature) — *see* Placenta, abnormal
  spuria — *see* Placenta, abnormal
  succenturiata — *see* Placenta, abnormal
  syphilitic 095.8
  transfusion syndromes 762.3
  transmission of chemical substance — *see* Absorption, chemical, through placenta
  trapped (with hemorrhage) 666.0 ☑
    without hemorrhage 667.0 ☑
  trilobate — *see* Placenta, abnormal
  tripartita — *see* Placenta, abnormal
  triplex — *see* Placenta, abnormal
  varicose vessel — *see* Placenta, abnormal
  vicious insertion — *see* Placenta, previa
Placentitis
  affecting fetus or newborn 762.7
  complicating pregnancy 658.4 ☑
Plagiocephaly (skull) 754.0
Plague 020.9
  abortive 020.8
  ambulatory 020.8
  bubonic 020.0
  cellulocutaneous 020.1
  lymphatic gland 020.0
  pneumonic 020.5
    primary 020.3
    secondary 020.4
  pulmonary — *see* Plague, pneumonic
  pulmonic — *see* Plague, pneumonic
  septicemic 020.2
  tonsillar 020.9
    septicemic 020.2
  vaccination, prophylactic (against) V03.3
Planning, family V25.09
  contraception V25.9
  natural
    procreative V26.41
    to avoid pregnancy V25.04
  procreation V26.49
    natural V26.41
Plaque
  artery, arterial — *see* Arteriosclerosis
  calcareous — *see* Calcification
  Hollenhorst's (retinal) 362.33
  tongue 528.6
Plasma cell myeloma 203.0 ☑
Plasmacytoma, plasmocytoma (solitary) (M9731/1) 238.6
  benign (M9731/0) — *see* Neoplasm, by site, benign
  malignant (M9731/3) 203.8 ☑
Plasmacytopenia 288.59
Plasmacytosis 288.64
Plaster ulcer — *see also* Ulcer, pressure 707.00
Plateau iris syndrome (without glaucoma) 364.82
  with glaucoma 365.23
Platybasia 756.0
Platyonychia (congenital) 757.5
  acquired 703.8

☑ **Additional Digit Required** — **Refer to the Tabular List for Digit Selection**   ▽ **Subterms under main terms may continue to next column or page**

2014 ICD-9-CM   **275**

Pick's — Platyonychia

Platypelloid pelvis 738.6
- with disproportion (fetopelvic) 653.2 ☑
  - affecting fetus or newborn 763.1
  - causing obstructed labor 660.1 ☑
    - affecting fetus or newborn 763.1
- congenital 755.69

Platyspondylia 756.19

Plethora 782.62
- newborn 776.4

Pleuralgia 786.52

Pleura, pleural — *see* condition

Pleurisy (acute) (adhesive) (chronic) (costal) (diaphragmatic) (double) (dry) (fetid) (fibrinous) (fibrous) (interlobar) (latent) (lung) (old) (plastic) (primary) (residual) (sicca) (sterile) (subacute) (unresolved) (with adherent pleura) 511.0
- with
  - effusion (without mention of cause) 511.9
    - bacterial, nontuberculous 511.1
    - nontuberculous NEC 511.9
      - bacterial 511.1
    - pneumococcal 511.1
    - specified type NEC 511.89
    - staphylococcal 511.1
    - streptococcal 511.1
    - tuberculous (*see also* Tuberculosis, pleura) 012.0 ☑
      - primary, progressive 010.1 ☑
  - influenza, flu, or grippe (*see also* Influenza) 487.1
  - tuberculosis — *see* Pleurisy, tuberculous
- encysted 511.89
- exudative (*see also* Pleurisy, with effusion) 511.9
  - bacterial, nontuberculous 511.1
- fibrinopurulent 510.9
  - with fistula 510.0
- fibropurulent 510.9
  - with fistula 510.0
- hemorrhagic 511.89
- influenzal (*see also* Influenza) 487.1
- pneumococcal 511.0
  - with effusion 511.1
- purulent 510.9
  - with fistula 510.0
- septic 510.9
  - with fistula 510.0
- serofibrinous (*see also* Pleurisy, with effusion) 511.9
  - bacterial, nontuberculous 511.1
- seropurulent 510.9
  - with fistula 510.0
- serous (*see also* Pleurisy, with effusion) 511.9
  - bacterial, nontuberculous 511.1
- staphylococcal 511.0
  - with effusion 511.1
- streptococcal 511.0
  - with effusion 511.1
- suppurative 510.9
  - with fistula 510.0
- traumatic (post) (current) 862.29
  - with open wound into cavity 862.39
- tuberculous (with effusion) (*see also* Tuberculosis, pleura) 012.0 ☑
  - primary, progressive 010.1 ☑

Pleuritis sicca — *see* Pleurisy

Pleurobronchopneumonia — *see also* Pneumonia, broncho- 485

Pleurodynia 786.52
- epidemic 074.1
- viral 074.1

Pleurohepatitis 573.8

Pleuropericarditis — *see also* Pericarditis 423.9
- acute 420.90

Pleuropneumonia (acute) (bilateral) (double) (septic) — *see also* Pneumonia 486
- chronic (*see also* Fibrosis, lung) 515

Pleurorrhea — *see also* Hydrothorax 511.89

Plexitis, brachial 353.0

Plica
- knee 727.83
- polonica 132.0
- syndrome 727.83
- tonsil 474.8

Plicae dysphonia ventricularis 784.49

Plicated tongue 529.5
- congenital 750.13

Plug
- bronchus NEC 519.19
- meconium (newborn) NEC 777.1
- mucus — *see* Mucus, plug

Plumbism 984.9
- specified type of lead — *see* Table of Drugs and Chemicals

Plummer's disease (toxic nodular goiter) 242.3 ☑

Plummer-Vinson syndrome (sideropenic dysphagia) 280.8

Pluricarential syndrome of infancy 260

Plurideficiency syndrome of infancy 260

Plus (and minus) hand (intrinsic) 736.09

PMDD (premenstrual dysphoric disorder) 625.4

PMS 625.4

Pneumathemia — *see* Air, embolism, by type

Pneumatic drill or hammer disease 994.9

Pneumatocele (lung) 518.89
- intracranial 348.89
- tension 492.0

Pneumatosis
- cystoides intestinalis 569.89
- peritonei 568.89
- pulmonum 492.8

Pneumaturia 599.84

Pneumoblastoma (M8981/3) — *see* Neoplasm, lung, malignant

Pneumocephalus 348.89

Pneumococcemia 038.2

Pneumococcus, pneumococcal — *see* condition

Pneumoconiosis (due to) (inhalation of) 505
- aluminum 503
- asbestos 501
- bagasse 495.1
- bauxite 503
- beryllium 503
- carbon electrode makers' 503
- coal
  - miners' (simple) 500
  - workers' (simple) 500
- cotton dust 504
- diatomite fibrosis 502
- dust NEC 504
  - inorganic 503
  - lime 502
  - marble 502
  - organic NEC 504
- fumes or vapors (from silo) 506.9
- graphite 503
- hard metal 503
- mica 502
- moldy hay 495.0
- rheumatoid 714.81
- silicate NEC 502
- silica NEC 502
  - and carbon 500
- talc 502

Pneumocystis carinii pneumonia 136.3

Pneumocystis jiroveci pneumonia 136.3

Pneumocystosis 136.3
- with pneumonia 136.3

Pneumoenteritis 025

Pneumohemopericardium — *see also* Pericarditis 423.9

Pneumohemothorax — *see also* Hemothorax 511.89
- traumatic 860.4
  - with open wound into thorax 860.5

Pneumohydropericardium — *see also* Pericarditis 423.9

Pneumohydrothorax — *see also* Hydrothorax 511.89

Pneumomediastinum 518.1
- congenital 770.2
- fetus or newborn 770.2

Pneumomycosis 117.9

Pneumonia (acute) (Alpenstich) (benign) (bilateral) (brain) (cerebral) (circumscribed) (congestive) (creeping) (delayed resolution) (double) (epidemic) (fever) (flash) (fulminant) (fungoid) (granulomatous) (hemorrhagic) (incipient) (infantile) (infectious) (infiltration) (insular) (intermittent) (latent) (lobe) (migratory) (newborn) (organized) (overwhelming) (primary) (progressive) (pseudolobar) (purulent) (resolved) (secondary) (senile) (septic) (suppurative) (terminal) (true) (unresolved) (vesicular) 486
- with influenza, flu, or grippe 487.0
  - due to
    - identified (virus)
      - avian 488.01
      - (novel) 2009 H1N1 488.11
    - novel influenza A 488.81
- adenoviral 480.0
- adynamic 514
- alba 090.0
- allergic 518.3
- alveolar — *see* Pneumonia, lobar
- anaerobes 482.81
- anthrax 022.1 [484.5]
- apex, apical — *see* Pneumonia, lobar
- ascaris 127.0 [484.8]
- aspiration 507.0
  - due to
    - aspiration of microorganisms
      - bacterial 482.9
        - specified type NEC 482.89
      - specified organism NEC 483.8
        - bacterial NEC 482.89
      - viral 480.9
        - specified type NEC 480.8
    - food (regurgitated) 507.0
    - gastric secretions 507.0
    - milk 507.0
    - oils, essences 507.1
    - solids, liquids NEC 507.8
    - vomitus 507.0
  - fetal 770.18
    - due to
      - blood 770.16
      - clear amniotic fluid 770.14
      - meconium 770.12
      - postnatal stomach contents 770.86
    - newborn 770.18
      - due to
        - blood 770.16
        - clear amniotic fluid 770.14
        - meconium 770.12
        - postnatal stomach contents 770.86
- asthenic 514
- atypical (disseminated) (focal) (primary) 486
  - with influenza (*see also* Influenza) 487.0
- bacillus 482.9
  - specified type NEC 482.89
- bacterial 482.9
  - specified type NEC 482.89
- Bacteroides (fragilis) (oralis) (melaninogenicus) 482.81
- basal, basic, basilar — *see* Pneumonia, by type
- bronchiolitis obliterans organized (BOOP) 516.8
- broncho-, bronchial (confluent) (croupous) (diffuse) (disseminated) (hemorrhagic) (involving lobes) (lobar) (terminal) 485
  - with influenza 487.0
    - due to
      - identified (virus)
        - avian 488.01
        - (novel) 2009 H1N1 488.11
      - novel influenza A 488.81
  - allergic 518.3
  - aspiration (*see also* Pneumonia, aspiration) 507.0
  - bacterial 482.9
    - specified type NEC 482.89
  - capillary 466.19

Pneumonia — *continued*
- broncho-, bronchial — *continued*
  - capillary — *continued*
    - with bronchospasm or obstruction 466.19
  - chronic (*see also* Fibrosis, lung) 515
  - congenital (infective) 770.0
  - diplococcal 481
  - Eaton's agent 483.0
  - Escherichia coli (E. coli) 482.82
  - Friedländer's bacillus 482.0
  - Hemophilus influenzae 482.2
  - hiberno-vernal 083.0 [484.8]
  - hypostatic 514
  - influenzal (*see also* Influenza) 487.0
  - inhalation (*see also* Pneumonia, aspiration) 507.0
    - due to fumes or vapors (chemical) 506.0
  - Klebsiella 482.0
  - lipid 507.8
    - endogenous 516.8
  - Mycoplasma (pneumoniae) 483.0
  - ornithosis 073.0
  - pleuropneumonia-like organisms (PPLO) 483.0
  - pneumococcal 481
  - Proteus 482.83
  - Pseudomonas 482.1
  - specified organism NEC 483.8
    - bacterial NEC 482.89
  - staphylococcal 482.40
    - aureus 482.41
      - methicillin
        - resistant (MRSA) 482.42
        - susceptible (MSSA) 482.41
    - specified type NEC 482.49
  - streptococcal — *see* Pneumonia, streptococcal
  - typhoid 002.0 [484.8]
  - viral, virus (*see also* Pneumonia, viral) 480.9
- Butyrivibrio (fibriosolvens) 482.81
- Candida 112.4
- capillary 466.19
  - with bronchospasm or obstruction 466.19
- caseous (*see also* Tuberculosis) 011.6 ☑
- catarrhal — *see* Pneumonia, broncho-
- central — *see* Pneumonia, lobar
- Chlamydia, chlamydial 483.1
  - pneumoniae 483.1
  - psittaci 073.0
  - specified type NEC 483.1
  - trachomatis 483.1
- cholesterol 516.8
- chronic (*see also* Fibrosis, lung) 515
- cirrhotic (chronic) (*see also* Fibrosis, lung) 515
- Clostridium (haemolyticum) (novyi) NEC 482.81
- confluent — *see* Pneumonia, broncho-
- congenital (infective) 770.0
  - aspiration 770.18
- croupous — *see* Pneumonia, lobar
- cryptogenic organizing 516.36
- cytomegalic inclusion 078.5 [484.1]
- deglutition (*see also* Pneumonia, aspiration) 507.0
- desquamative interstitial 516.37
- diffuse — *see* Pneumonia, broncho-
- diplococcal, diplococcus (broncho-) (lobar) 481
- disseminated (focal) — *see* Pneumonia, broncho-
- due to
  - adenovirus 480.0
  - anaerobes 482.81
  - Bacterium anitratum 482.83
  - Chlamydia, chlamydial 483.1
    - pneumoniae 483.1
    - psittaci 073.0
    - specified type NEC 483.1
    - trachomatis 483.1
  - coccidioidomycosis 114.0
  - Diplococcus (pneumoniae) 481

☑ **Additional Digit Required** — Refer to the Tabular List for Digit Selection   ▽ **Subterms under main terms may continue to next column or page**

276   **2014 ICD-9-CM**

Pneumonia — continued
  due to — continued
    Eaton's agent 483.0
    Escherichia coli (E. coli) 482.82
    Friedländer's bacillus 482.0
    fumes or vapors (chemical) (inhalation) 506.0
    fungus NEC 117.9 [484.7]
      coccidioidomycosis 114.0
    Hemophilus influenzae (H. influenzae) 482.2
    Herellea 482.83
    influenza (see also Influenza) 487.0
    Klebsiella pneumoniae 482.0
    Mycoplasma (pneumoniae) 483.0
    parainfluenza virus 480.2
    pleuropneumonia-like organism (PPLO) 483.0
    Pneumococcus 481
    Pneumocystis carinii 136.3
    Pneumocystis jiroveci 136.3
    Proteus 482.83
    Pseudomonas 482.1
    respiratory syncytial virus 480.1
    rickettsia 083.9 [484.8]
    SARS-associated coronavirus 480.3
    specified
      bacteria NEC 482.89
      organism NEC 483.8
      virus NEC 480.8
    Staphylococcus 482.40
      aureus 482.41
        methicillin
          resistant (MRSA) 482.42
          susceptible (MSSA) 482.41
      specified type NEC 482.49
    Streptococcus (see also Pneumonia, streptococcal)
      pneumoniae 481
    virus (see also Pneumonia, viral) 480.9
      SARS-associated coronavirus 480.3
  Eaton's agent 483.0
  embolic, embolism — (see Embolism, pulmonary)
  eosinophilic 518.3
  Escherichia coli (E. coli) 482.82
  Eubacterium 482.81
  fibrinous — see Pneumonia, lobar
  fibroid (chronic) (see also Fibrosis, lung) 515
  fibrous (see also Fibrosis, lung) 515
  Friedländer's bacillus 482.0
  Fusobacterium (nucleatum) 482.81
  gangrenous 513.0
  giant cell (see also Pneumonia, viral) 480.9
  gram-negative bacteria NEC 482.83
    anaerobic 482.81
  grippal (see also Influenza) 487.0
  Hemophilus influenzae (bronchial) (lobar) 482.2
  hypostatic (broncho-) (lobar) 514
  in
    actinomycosis 039.1
    anthrax 022.1 [484.5]
    aspergillosis 117.3 [484.6]
    candidiasis 112.4
    coccidioidomycosis 114.0
    cytomegalic inclusion disease 078.5 [484.1]
    histoplasmosis (see also Histoplasmosis) 115.95
    infectious disease NEC 136.9 [484.8]
    measles 055.1
    mycosis, systemic NEC 117.9 [484.7]
    nocardiasis, nocardiosis 039.1
    ornithosis 073.0
    pneumocystosis 136.3
    psittacosis 073.0
    Q fever 083.0 [484.8]
    salmonellosis 003.22
    toxoplasmosis 130.4
    tularemia 021.2
    typhoid (fever) 002.0 [484.8]
    varicella 052.1
    whooping cough (see also Whooping cough) 033.9 [484.3]
  infective, acquired prenatally 770.0

Pneumonia — continued
  influenzal (broncho) (lobar) (virus) (see also Influenza) 487.0
  inhalation (see also Pneumonia, aspiration) 507.0
    fumes or vapors (chemical) 506.0
  interstitial 516.8
    with influenzal (see also Influenza) 487.0
    acute
      due to Pneumocystis (carinii) (jiroveci) 136.3
      meaning:
        acute interstitial pneumonitis 516.33
        atypical pneumonia — see Pneumonia, atypical
        bacterial pneumonia — see Pneumonia, bacterial
    chronic (see also Fibrosis, lung) 515
    desquamative 516.37
    hypostatic 514
    idiopathic 516.30
      lymphoid 516.35
    lipoid 507.1
    lymphoid (due to known underlying cause) 516.8
    non-specific (due to known underlying cause) 516.8
    organizing (due to known underlying cause) 516.8
    plasma cell 136.3
    Pseudomonas 482.1
  intrauterine (infective) 770.0
    aspiration 770.18
      blood 770.16
      clear amniotic fluid 770.14
      meconium 770.12
      postnatal stomach contents 770.86
  Klebsiella pneumoniae 482.0
  Legionnaires' 482.84
  lipid, lipoid (exogenous) (interstitial) 507.1
    endogenous 516.8
  lobar (diplococcal) (disseminated) (double) (interstitial) (pneumococcal, any type) 481
    with influenza (see also Influenza) 487.0
    bacterial 482.9
      specified type NEC 482.89
    chronic (see also Fibrosis, lung) 515
    Escherichia coli (E. coli) 482.82
    Friedländer's bacillus 482.0
    Hemophilus influenzae (H. influenzae) 482.2
    hypostatic 514
    influenzal (see also Influenza) 487.0
    Klebsiella 482.0
    ornithosis 073.0
    Proteus 482.83
    Pseudomonas 482.1
    psittacosis 073.0
    specified organism NEC 483.8
      bacterial NEC 482.89
    staphylococcal 482.40
      aureus 482.41
        methicillin
          resistant (MRSA) 482.42
          susceptible (MSSA) 482.41
      specified type NEC 482.49
    streptococcal — see Pneumonia, streptococcal
    viral, virus (see also Pneumonia, viral) 480.9
  lobular (confluent) — see Pneumonia, broncho-
  Löffler's 518.3
  massive — see Pneumonia, lobar
  meconium aspiration 770.12
  metastatic NEC 038.8 [484.8]
  methicillin resistant Staphylococcus aureus (MRSA) 482.42
  methicillin susceptible Staphylococcus aureus (MSSA) 482.41
  MRSA (methicillin resistant Staphylococcus aureus) 482.42
  MSSA (methicillin susceptible Staphylococcus aureus) 482.41

Pneumonia — continued
  multilobar — see Pneumonia, by type
  Mycoplasma (pneumoniae) 483.0
  necrotic 513.0
  nitrogen dioxide 506.9
  orthostatic 514
  parainfluenza virus 480.2
  parenchymatous (see also Fibrosis, lung) 515
  passive 514
  patchy — see Pneumonia, broncho-
  Peptococcus 482.81
  Peptostreptococcus 482.81
  plasma cell 136.3
  pleurolobar — see Pneumonia, lobar
  pleuropneumonia-like organism (PPLO) 483.0
  pneumococcal (broncho) (lobar) 481
  Pneumocystis (carinii) (jiroveci) 136.3
  postinfectional NEC 136.9 [484.8]
  postmeasles 055.1
  postoperative 997.39
    aspiration 997.32
  primary atypical 486
  Proprionibacterium 482.81
  Proteus 482.83
  Pseudomonas 482.1
  psittacosis 073.0
  radiation 508.0
  respiratory syncytial virus 480.1
  resulting from a procedure 997.39
    aspiration 997.32
  rheumatic 390 [517.1]
  Salmonella 003.22
  SARS-associated coronavirus 480.3
  segmented, segmental — see Pneumonia, broncho-
  Serratia (marcescens) 482.83
  specified
    bacteria NEC 482.89
    organism NEC 483.8
    virus NEC 480.8
  spirochetal 104.8 [484.8]
  staphylococcal (broncho) (lobar) 482.40
    aureus 482.41
      methicillin
        resistant 482.42
        susceptible (MSSA) 482.41
    specified type NEC 482.49
  static, stasis 514
  streptococcal (broncho) (lobar) NEC 482.30
    Group
      A 482.31
      B 482.32
      specified NEC 482.39
    pneumoniae 481
    specified type NEC 482.39
  Streptococcus pneumoniae 481
  traumatic (complication) (early) (secondary) 958.8
  tuberculous (any) (see also Tuberculosis) 011.6 ☑
  tularemic 021.2
  TWAR agent 483.1
  varicella 052.1
  Veillonella 482.81
  ventilator associated 997.31
  viral, virus (broncho) (interstitial) (lobar) 480.9
    with influenza, flu, or grippe (see also Influenza) 487.0
    adenoviral 480.0
    parainfluenza 480.2
    respiratory syncytial 480.1
    SARS-associated coronavirus 480.3
    specified type NEC 480.8
  white (congenital) 090.0
Pneumonic — see condition
Pneumonitis (acute) (primary) — see also Pneumonia 486
  allergic 495.9
    specified type NEC 495.8
  aspiration 507.0
    due to fumes or gases 506.0
    fetal 770.18
      due to
        blood 770.16

Pneumonitis — see also Pneumonia — continued
  aspiration — continued
    fetal — continued
      due to — continued
        clear amniotic fluid 770.14
        meconium 770.12
        postnatal stomach contents 770.86
    newborn 770.18
      due to
        blood 770.16
        clear amniotic fluid 770.14
        meconium 770.12
        postnatal stomach contents 770.86
    obstetric 668.0 ☑
  chemical 506.0
    due to fumes or gases 506.0
    resulting from a procedure 997.32
  cholesterol 516.8
  chronic (see also Fibrosis, lung) 515
  congenital rubella 771.0
  crack 506.0
  due to
    crack (cocaine) 506.0
    fumes or vapors 506.0
    inhalation
      food (regurgitated), milk, vomitus 507.0
      oils, essences 507.1
      saliva 507.0
      solids, liquids NEC 507.8
    toxoplasmosis (acquired) 130.4
      congenital (active) 771.2 [484.8]
  eosinophilic 518.3
  fetal aspiration 770.18
    due to
      blood 770.16
      clear amniotic fluid 770.14
      meconium 770.12
      postnatal stomach contents 770.86
  hypersensitivity 495.9
  interstitial (chronic) (see also Fibrosis, lung) 515
    acute 516.33
    idiopathic
      lymphocytic 516.35
      non-specific 516.32
    lymphoid 516.8
  lymphoid, interstitial 516.8
  meconium aspiration 770.12
  postanesthetic
    correct substance properly administered 507.0
    obstetric 668.0 ☑
    overdose or wrong substance given 968.4
      specified anesthetic — see Table of Drugs and Chemicals
  postoperative 997.3 ☑
    aspiration 997.32
    obstetric 668.0 ☑
  radiation 508.0
  rubella, congenital 771.0
  "ventilation" 495.7
  ventilator associated 997.31
  wood-dust 495.8
Pneumonoconiosis — see Pneumoconiosis
Pneumoparotid 527.8
Pneumopathy NEC 518.89
  alveolar 516.9
    specified NEC 516.8
  due to dust NEC 504
  parietoalveolar 516.9
    specified condition NEC 516.8
Pneumopericarditis — see also Pericarditis 423.9
  acute 420.90
Pneumopericardium — see also Pericarditis
  congenital 770.2
  fetus or newborn 770.2
  traumatic (post) (see also Pneumothorax, traumatic) 860.0
    with open wound into thorax 860.1
Pneumoperitoneum 568.89

☑ **Additional Digit Required — Refer to the Tabular List for Digit Selection**   ▽ **Subterms under main terms may continue to next column or page**

2014 ICD-9-CM   **277**

Pneumoperitoneum — *continued*
  fetus or newborn 770.2
Pneumophagia (psychogenic) 306.4
Pneumopleurisy, pneumopleuritis — *see also* Pneumonia 486
Pneumopyopericardium 420.99
Pneumopyothorax — *see also* Pyopneumothorax 510.9
  with fistula 510.0
Pneumorrhagia 786.30
  newborn 770.3
  tuberculous (*see also* Tuberculosis, pulmonary) 011.9 ☑
Pneumosiderosis (occupational) 503
Pneumothorax 512.89
  acute 512.89
  chronic 512.83
  congenital 770.2
  due to operative injury of chest wall or lung 512.1
    accidental puncture or laceration 512.1
  fetus or newborn 770.2
  iatrogenic 512.1
  postoperative 512.1
  specified type NEC 512.89
  spontaneous 512.89
    fetus or newborn 770.2
    primary 512.81
    secondary 512.82
    tension 512.0
  sucking 512.89
    iatrogenic 512.1
    postoperative 512.1
  tense valvular, infectional 512.0
  tension 512.0
    iatrogenic 512.1
    postoperative 512.1
    spontaneous 512.0
  traumatic 860.0
    with
      hemothorax 860.4
        with open wound into thorax 860.5
      open wound into thorax 860.1
  tuberculous (*see also* Tuberculosis) 011.7 ☑
Pocket(s)
  endocardial (*see also* Endocarditis) 424.90
  periodontal 523.8
Podagra 274.01
Podencephalus 759.89
Poikilocytosis 790.09
Poikiloderma 709.09
  Civatte's 709.09
  congenital 757.33
  vasculare atrophicans 696.2
Poikilodermatomyositis 710.3
Pointed ear 744.29
Poise imperfect 729.90
Poisoned — *see* Poisoning
Poisoning (acute) — *see also* Table of Drugs and Chemicals
  Bacillus, B.
    aertrycke (*see also* Infection, Salmonella) 003.9
    botulinus 005.1
    cholerae (suis) (*see also* Infection, Salmonella) 003.9
    paratyphosus (*see also* Infection, Salmonella) 003.9
    suipestifer (*see also* Infection, Salmonella) 003.9
  bacterial toxins NEC 005.9
  berries, noxious 988.2
  blood (general) — *see* Septicemia
  botulism 005.1
  bread, moldy, mouldy — *see* Poisoning, food
  Ciguatera 988.0
  damaged meat — *see* Poisoning, food
  death-cap (Amanita phalloides) (Amanita verna) 988.1
  decomposed food — *see* Poisoning, food
  diseased food — *see* Poisoning, food
  drug — *see* Table of Drugs and Chemicals
  epidemic, fish, meat, or other food — *see* Poisoning, food

Poisoning — *see also* Table of Drugs and Chemicals — *continued*
  fava bean 282.2
  fish (bacterial) (*see also* Poisoning, food)
    noxious 988.0
  food (acute) (bacterial) (diseased) (infected) NEC 005.9
    due to
      bacillus
        aertrycke (*see also* Poisoning, food, due to Salmonella) 003.9
        botulinus 005.1
        cereus 005.89
        choleraesuis (*see also* Poisoning, food, due to Salmonella) 003.9
        paratyphosus (*see also* Poisoning, food, due to Salmonella) 003.9
        suipestifer (*see also* Poisoning, food, due to Salmonella) 003.9
      Clostridium 005.3
        botulinum 005.1
        perfringens 005.2
        welchii 005.2
      Salmonella (aertrycke) (callinarum) (choleraesuis) (enteritidis) (paratyphi) (suipestifer) 003.9
        with
          gastroenteritis 003.0
          localized infection(s) (*see also* Infection, Salmonella) 003.20
          septicemia 003.1
          specified manifestation NEC 003.8
      specified bacterium NEC 005.89
      Staphylococcus 005.0
      Streptococcus 005.89
      Vibrio parahaemolyticus 005.4
      Vibrio vulnificus 005.81
    noxious or naturally toxic 988.0
      berries 988.2
      fish 988.0
      mushroom 988.1
      plants NEC 988.2
  ice cream — *see* Poisoning, food
  ichthyotoxism (bacterial) 005.9
  kreotoxism, food 005.9
  malarial — *see* Malaria
  meat — *see* Poisoning, food
  mushroom (noxious) 988.1
  mussel (*see also* Poisoning, food)
    noxious 988.0
  noxious foodstuffs (*see also* Poisoning, food, noxious) 988.9
    specified type NEC 988.8
  plants, noxious 988.2
  pork (*see also* Poisoning, food)
    specified NEC 988.8
    Trichinosis 124
  ptomaine — *see* Poisoning, food
  putrefaction, food — *see* Poisoning, food
  radiation 508.0
  Salmonella (*see also* Infection, Salmonella) 003.9
  sausage (*see also* Poisoning, food)
    Trichinosis 124
  saxitoxin 988.0
  shellfish (*see also* Poisoning, food)
    noxious (amnesic) (azaspiracid) (diarrheic) (neurotoxic) (paralytic) 988.0
  Staphylococcus, food 005.0
  toxic, from disease NEC 799.89
  truffles — *see* Poisoning, food
  uremic — *see* Uremia
  uric acid 274.9
  water 276.69
Poison ivy, oak, sumac or other plant dermatitis 692.6
Poker spine 720.0
Policeman's disease 729.2
Polioencephalitis (acute) (bulbar) — *see also* Poliomyelitis, bulbar 045.0 ☑

Polioencephalitis — *see also* Poliomyelitis, bulbar — *continued*
  inferior 335.22
  influenzal (*see also* Influenza) 487.8
  superior hemorrhagic (acute) (Wernicke's) 265.1
  Wernicke's (superior hemorrhagic) 265.1
Polioencephalomyelitis (acute) (anterior) (bulbar) — *see also* Polioencephalitis 045.0 ☑
Polioencephalopathy, superior hemorrhagic 265.1
  with
    beriberi 265.0
    pellagra 265.2
Poliomeningoencephalitis — *see* Meningoencephalitis
Poliomyelitis (acute) (anterior) (epidemic) 045.9 ☑

Note — Use the following fifth-digit subclassification with category 045:

0   poliovirus, unspecified type

1   poliovirus, type I

2   poliovirus, type II

3   poliovirus, type III

  with
    paralysis 045.1 ☑
      bulbar 045.0 ☑
  abortive 045.2 ☑
  ascending 045.9 ☑
    progressive 045.9 ☑
  bulbar 045.0 ☑
  cerebral 045.0 ☑
  chronic 335.21
  congenital 771.2
  contact V01.2
  deformities 138
  exposure to V01.2
  late effect 138
  nonepidemic 045.9 ☑
  nonparalytic 045.2 ☑
  old with deformity 138
  posterior, acute 053.19
  residual 138
  sequelae 138
  spinal, acute 045.9 ☑
  syphilitic (chronic) 094.89
  vaccination, prophylactic (against) V04.0
Poliosis (eyebrow) (eyelashes) 704.3
  circumscripta (congenital) 757.4
    acquired 704.3
  congenital 757.4
Pollakiuria 788.41
  psychogenic 306.53
Pollinosis 477.0
Pollitzer's disease (hidradenitis suppurativa) 705.83
Polyadenitis — *see also* Adenitis 289.3
  malignant 020.0
Polyalgia 729.99
Polyangiitis (essential) 446.0
Polyarteritis (nodosa) (renal) 446.0
Polyarthralgia 719.49
  psychogenic 306.0
Polyarthritis, polyarthropathy NEC 716.59
  due to or associated with other specified conditions — *see* Arthritis, due to or associated with
  endemic (*see also* Disease, Kaschin-Beck) 716.0 ☑
  inflammatory 714.9
    specified type NEC 714.89
  juvenile (chronic) 714.30
    acute 714.31
  migratory — *see* Fever, rheumatic
  rheumatic 714.0
    fever, acute — *see* Fever, rheumatic
Polycarential syndrome of infancy 260
Polychondritis (atrophic) (chronic) (relapsing) 733.99
Polycoria 743.46
Polycystic (congenital) (disease) 759.89

Polycystic — *continued*
  degeneration, kidney — *see* Polycystic, kidney
  kidney (congenital) 753.12
    adult type (APKD) 753.13
    autosomal dominant 753.13
    autosomal recessive 753.14
    childhood type (CPKD) 753.14
    infantile type 753.14
  liver 751.62
  lung 518.89
    congenital 748.4
  ovary, ovaries 256.4
  spleen 759.0
Polycythemia (primary) (rubra) (vera) (M9950/1) 238.4
  acquired 289.0
  benign 289.0
    familial 289.6
  due to
    donor twin 776.4
    fall in plasma volume 289.0
    high altitude 289.0
    maternal-fetal transfusion 776.4
    stress 289.0
  emotional 289.0
  erythropoietin 289.0
  familial (benign) 289.6
  Gaisböck's (hypertonica) 289.0
  high altitude 289.0
  hypertonica 289.0
  hypoxemic 289.0
  neonatorum 776.4
  nephrogenous 289.0
  relative 289.0
  secondary 289.0
  spurious 289.0
  stress 289.0
Polycytosis cryptogenica 289.0
Polydactylism, polydactyly 755.00
  fingers 755.01
  toes 755.02
Polydipsia 783.5
Polydystrophic oligophrenia 277.5
Polyembryoma (M9072/3) — *see* Neoplasm, by site, malignant
Polygalactia 676.6 ☑
Polyglandular
  deficiency 258.9
  dyscrasia 258.9
  dysfunction 258.9
  syndrome 258.8
Polyhydramnios — *see also* Hydramnios 657.0 ☑
Polymastia 757.6
Polymenorrhea 626.2
Polymicrogyria 742.2
Polymyalgia 725
  arteritica 446.5
  rheumatica 725
Polymyositis (acute) (chronic) (hemorrhagic) 710.4
  with involvement of
    lung 710.4 [517.8]
    skin 710.3
  ossificans (generalisata) (progressiva) 728.19
  Wagner's (dermatomyositis) 710.3
Polyneuritis, polyneuritic — *see also* Polyneuropathy 356.9
  alcoholic 357.5
    with psychosis 291.1
  cranialis 352.6
  demyelinating, chronic inflammatory (CIDP) 357.81
  diabetic 250.6 ☑ [357.2]
    due to secondary diabetes 249.6 ☑ [357.2]
  due to lack of vitamin NEC 269.2 [357.4]
  endemic 265.0 [357.4]
  erythredema 985.0
  febrile 357.0
  hereditary ataxic 356.3
  idiopathic, acute 357.0
  infective (acute) 357.0
  nutritional 269.9 [357.4]
  postinfectious 357.0

Polyneuropathy (peripheral) 356.9
  alcoholic 357.5
  amyloid 277.39 *[357.4]*
  arsenical 357.7
  critical illness 357.82
  demyelinating, chronic inflammatory (CIDP) 357.81
  diabetic 250.6 ☑ *[357.2]*
    due to secondary diabetes 249.6 ☑ *[357.2]*
  due to
    antitetanus serum 357.6
    arsenic 357.7
    drug or medicinal substance 357.6
      correct substance properly administered 357.6
      overdose or wrong substance given or taken 977.9
        specified drug — *see* Table of Drugs and Chemicals
    lack of vitamin NEC 269.2 *[357.4]*
    lead 357.7
    organophosphate compounds 357.7
    pellagra 265.2 *[357.4]*
    porphyria 277.1 *[357.4]*
    serum 357.6
    toxic agent NEC 357.7
  hereditary 356.0
  idiopathic 356.9
    progressive 356.4
  in
    amyloidosis 277.39 *[357.4]*
    avitaminosis 269.2 *[357.4]*
      specified NEC 269.1 *[357.4]*
    beriberi 265.0 *[357.4]*
    collagen vascular disease NEC 710.9 *[357.1]*
    deficiency
      B-complex NEC 266.2 *[357.4]*
      vitamin B 266.1 *[357.4]*
      vitamin B6 266.9 *[357.4]*
    diabetes 250.6 ☑ *[357.2]*
      due to secondary diabetes 249.6 ☑ *[357.2]*
    diphtheria (*see also* Diphtheria) 032.89 *[357.4]*
    disseminated lupus erythematosus 710.0 *[357.1]*
    herpes zoster 053.13
    hypoglycemia 251.2 *[357.4]*
    malignant neoplasm (M8000/3) NEC 199.1 *[357.3]*
    mumps 072.72
    pellagra 265.2 *[357.4]*
    polyarteritis nodosa 446.0 *[357.1]*
    porphyria 277.1 *[357.4]*
    rheumatoid arthritis 714.0 *[357.1]*
    sarcoidosis 135 *[357.4]*
    uremia 585.9 *[357.4]*
  lead 357.7
  nutritional 269.9 *[357.4]*
    specified NEC 269.8 *[357.4]*
  postherpetic 053.13
  progressive 356.4
  sensory (hereditary) 356.2
  specified NEC 356.8
Polyonychia 757.5
Polyopia 368.2
  refractive 368.15
Polyorchism, polyorchidism (three testes) 752.89
Polyorrhymenitis (peritoneal) — *see also* Polyserositis 568.82
  pericardial 423.2
Polyostotic fibrous dysplasia 756.54
Polyotia 744.1
Polyphagia 783.6
Polypoid — *see* condition
Polyposis — *see also* Polyp
  coli (adenomatous) (M8220/0) 211.3
    adenocarcinoma in (M8220/3) 153.9
    carcinoma in (M8220/3) 153.9
  familial (M8220/0) 211.3
  intestinal (adenomatous) (M8220/0) 211.3
  multiple (M8221/0) — *see* Neoplasm, by site, benign

Polyp, polypus

Note — Polyps of organs or sites that do not appear in the list below should be coded to the residual category for diseases of the organ or site concerned.

  accessory sinus 471.8
  adenoid tissue 471.0
  adenomatous (M8210/0) (*see also* Neoplasm, by site, benign)
    adenocarcinoma in (M8210/3) — *see* Neoplasm, by site, malignant
    carcinoma in (M8210/3) — *see* Neoplasm, by site, malignant
    multiple (M8221/0) — *see* Neoplasm, by site, benign
  antrum 471.8
  anus, anal (canal) (nonadenomatous) 569.0
    adenomatous 211.4
  Bartholin's gland 624.6
  bladder (M8120/1) 236.7
  broad ligament 620.8
  cervix (uteri) 622.7
    adenomatous 219.0
    in pregnancy or childbirth 654.6 ☑
      affecting fetus or newborn 763.89
      causing obstructed labor 660.2 ☑
    mucous 622.7
    nonneoplastic 622.7
  choanal 471.0
  cholesterol 575.6
  clitoris 624.6
  colon (M8210/0) (*see also* Polyp, adenomatous) 211.3
  corpus uteri 621.0
  dental 522.0
  ear (middle) 385.30
  endometrium 621.0
  ethmoidal (sinus) 471.8
  fallopian tube 620.8
  female genital organs NEC 624.8
  frontal (sinus) 471.8
  gallbladder 575.6
  gingiva 523.8
  gum 523.8
  labia 624.6
  larynx (mucous) 478.4
  malignant (M8000/3) — *see* Neoplasm, by site, malignant
  maxillary (sinus) 471.8
  middle ear 385.30
  myometrium 621.0
  nares
    anterior 471.9
    posterior 471.0
  nasal (mucous) 471.9
    cavity 471.0
    septum 471.9
  nasopharyngeal 471.0
  neoplastic (M8210/0) — *see* Neoplasm, by site, benign
  nose (mucous) 471.9
  oviduct 620.8
  paratubal 620.8
  pharynx 478.29
    congenital 750.29
  placenta, placental 674.4 ☑
  prostate 600.20
    with
      other lower urinary tract symptoms (LUTS) 600.21
      urinary
        obstruction 600.21
        retention 600.21
  pudenda 624.6
  pulp (dental) 522.0
  rectosigmoid 211.4
  rectum (nonadenomatous) 569.0
    adenomatous 211.4
  septum (nasal) 471.9
  sinus (accessory) (ethmoidal) (frontal) (maxillary) (sphenoidal) 471.8
  sphenoidal (sinus) 471.8
  stomach (M8210/0) 211.1
  tube, fallopian 620.8
  turbinate, mucous membrane 471.8
  ureter 593.89

Polyp, polypus — *continued*
  urethra 599.3
  uterine
    ligament 620.8
    tube 620.8
  uterus (body) (corpus) (mucous) 621.0
    in pregnancy or childbirth 654.1 ☑
      affecting fetus or newborn 763.89
      causing obstructed labor 660.2 ☑
  vagina 623.7
  vocal cord (mucous) 478.4
  vulva 624.6
Polyradiculitis (acute) 357.0
Polyradiculoneuropathy (acute) (segmentally demyelinating) 357.0
Polysarcia 278.00
Polyserositis (peritoneal) 568.82
  due to pericarditis 423.2
  paroxysmal (familial) 277.31
  pericardial 423.2
  periodic (familial) 277.31
  pleural — *see* Pleurisy
  recurrent 277.31
  tuberculous (*see also* Tuberculosis, polyserositis) 018.9 ☑
Polysialia 527.7
Polysplenia syndrome 759.0
Polythelia 757.6
Polytrichia — *see also* Hypertrichosis 704.1
Polyunguia (congenital) 757.5
  acquired 703.8
Polyuria 788.42
Pompe's disease (glycogenosis II) 271.0
Pompholyx 705.81
Poncet's disease (tuberculous rheumatism) — *see also* Tuberculosis 015.9 ☑
Pond fracture — *see* Fracture, skull, vault
Ponos 085.0
Pons, pontine — *see* condition
Poor
  aesthetics of existing restoration of tooth 525.67
  contractions, labor 661.2 ☑
    affecting fetus or newborn 763.7
  fetal growth NEC 764.9 ☑
    affecting management of pregnancy 656.5 ☑
  incorporation
    artificial skin graft 996.55
    decellularized allodermis graft 996.55
  obstetrical history V13.29
    affecting management of current pregnancy V23.49
      ectopic pregnancy V23.42
      pre-term labor V23.41
    pre-term labor V13.21
  sucking reflex (newborn) 796.1
  vision NEC 369.9
Poradenitis, nostras 099.1
Porencephaly (congenital) (developmental) (true) 742.4
  acquired 348.0
  nondevelopmental 348.0
  traumatic (post) 310.2
Porocephaliasis 134.1
Porokeratosis 757.39
  disseminated superficial actinic (DSAP) 692.75
Poroma, eccrine (M8402/0) — *see* Neoplasm, skin, benign
Porphyria (acute) (congenital) (constitutional) (erythropoietic) (familial) (hepatica) (idiopathic) (idiosyncratic) (intermittent) (latent) (mixed hepatic) (photosensitive) (South African genetic) (Swedish) 277.1
  acquired 277.1
  cutaneatarda
    hereditaria 277.1
    symptomatica 277.1
  due to drugs
    correct substance properly administered 277.1
    overdose or wrong substance given or taken 977.9
      specified drug — *see* Table of Drugs and Chemicals

Porphyria — *continued*
  secondary 277.1
  toxic NEC 277.1
  variegata 277.1
Porphyrinuria (acquired) (congenital) (secondary) 277.1
Porphyruria (acquired) (congenital) 277.1
Portal — *see* condition
Port wine nevus or mark 757.32
Posadas-Wernicke disease 114.9
Position
  fetus, abnormal (*see also* Presentation, fetal) 652.9 ☑
  teeth, faulty (*see also* Anomaly, position tooth) 524.30
Positive
  culture (nonspecific) 795.39
    AIDS virus V08
    blood 790.7
    HIV V08
    human immunodeficiency virus V08
    nose 795.39
      Staphylococcus — *see* Carrier (suspected) of, Staphylococcus
    skin lesion NEC 795.39
    spinal fluid 792.0
    sputum 795.39
    stool 792.1
    throat 795.39
    urine 791.9
    wound 795.39
  findings, anthrax 795.31
  HIV V08
  human immunodeficiency virus (HIV) V08
  PPD 795.51
  serology
    AIDS virus V08
      inconclusive 795.71
    HIV V08
      inconclusive 795.71
    human immunodeficiency virus (HIV) V08
      inconclusive 795.71
    syphilis 097.1
      with signs or symptoms — *see* Syphilis, by site and stage
      false 795.6
  skin test 795.7 ☑
    tuberculin (without active tuberculosis) 795.51
  VDRL 097.1
    with signs or symptoms — *see* Syphilis, by site and stage
    false 795.6
  Wassermann reaction 097.1
    false 795.6
Postcardiotomy syndrome 429.4
Postcaval ureter 753.4
Postcholecystectomy syndrome 576.0
Postclimacteric bleeding 627.1
Postcommissurotomy syndrome 429.4
Postconcussional syndrome 310.2
Postcontusional syndrome 310.2
Postcricoid region — *see* condition
Post-dates (pregnancy) — *see* Pregnancy
Postencephalitic — *see also* condition
  syndrome 310.89
Posterior — *see* condition
Posterolateral sclerosis (spinal cord) — *see* Degeneration, combined
Postexanthematous — *see* condition
Postfebrile — *see* condition
Postgastrectomy dumping syndrome 564.2
Posthemiplegic chorea 344.89
Posthemorrhagic anemia (chronic) 280.0
  acute 285.1
  newborn 776.5
Posthepatitis syndrome 780.79
Postherpetic neuralgia (intercostal) (syndrome) (zoster) 053.19
  geniculate ganglion 053.11
  ophthalmica 053.19
  trigeminal 053.12
Posthitis 607.1
Postimmunization complication or reaction — *see* Complications, vaccination

---

Postinfectious — *see* condition
Postinfluenzal syndrome 780.79
Postlaminectomy syndrome 722.80
  cervical, cervicothoracic 722.81
  kyphosis 737.12
  lumbar, lumbosacral 722.83
  thoracic, thoracolumbar 722.82
Postleukotomy syndrome 310.0
Postlobectomy syndrome 310.0
Postmastectomy lymphedema (syndrome) 457.0
Postmaturity, postmature (fetus or newborn) (gestation period over 42 completed weeks) 766.22
  affecting management of pregnancy
    post-term pregnancy 645.1 ☑
    prolonged pregnancy 645.2 ☑
  syndrome 766.22
Postmeasles — *see also* condition
  complication 055.8
    specified NEC 055.79
Postmenopausal
  endometrium (atrophic) 627.8
    suppurative (see also Endometritis) 615.9
  hormone replacement therapy V07.4
  status (age related) (natural) V49.81
Postnasal drip 784.91
Postnatal — *see* condition
Postoperative — *see also* condition
  confusion state 293.9
  psychosis 293.9
  status NEC (*see also* Status (post)) V45.89
Postpancreatectomy hyperglycemia 251.3
Postpartum — *see also* condition
  anemia 648.2 ☑
  cardiomyopathy 674.5 ☑
  observation
    immediately after delivery V24.0
    routine follow-up V24.2
Postperfusion syndrome NEC 999.89
  bone marrow 996.85
Postpoliomyelitic — *see* condition
Postsurgery status NEC — *see also* Status (post V45.89
Post-term (pregnancy) 645.1 ☑
  infant (gestation period over 40 completed weeks to 42 completed weeks) 766.21
Post-transplant lymphoproliferative disorder (PTLD) 238.77
Posttraumatic — *see* condition
Posttraumatic brain syndrome, nonpsychotic 310.2
Post-traumatic stress disorder (PTSD) 309.81
Postures, hysterical 300.11
Postvaccinal reaction or complication — *see* Complications, vaccination
Postvagotomy syndrome 564.2
Postvalvulotomy syndrome 429.4
Postvasectomy sperm count V25.8
Potain's disease (pulmonary edema) 514
Potain's syndrome (gastrectasis with dyspepsia) 536.1
Pott's
  curvature (spinal) (*see also* Tuberculosis) 015.0 ☑ *[737.43]*
  disease or paraplegia (*see also* Tuberculosis) 015.0 ☑ *[730.88]*
  fracture (closed) 824.4
    open 824.5
  gangrene 440.24
  osteomyelitis (*see also* Tuberculosis) 015.0 ☑ *[730.88]*
  spinal curvature (*see also* Tuberculosis) 015.0 ☑ *[737.43]*
  tumor, puffy (*see also* Osteomyelitis) 730.2 ☑
Potter's
  asthma 502
  disease 753.0
  facies 754.0
  lung 502
  syndrome (with renal agenesis) 753.0

Pouch
  bronchus 748.3
  Douglas' — *see* condition
  esophagus, esophageal (congenital) 750.4
    acquired 530.6
  gastric 537.1
  Hartmann's (abnormal sacculation of gallbladder neck) 575.8
    of intestine V44.3
      attention to V55.3
  pharynx, pharyngeal (congenital) 750.27
Pouchitis 569.71
Poulet's disease 714.2
Poultrymen's itch 133.8
Poverty V60.2
PPE (palmar plantar erythrodysesthesia) 693.0
Prader-Labhart-Willi-Fanconi syndrome (hypogenital dystrophy with diabetic tendency) 759.81
Prader-Willi syndrome (hypogenital dystrophy with diabetic tendency) 759.81
Preachers' voice 784.49
Pre-AIDS — *see* Human immunodeficiency virus (disease) (illness) (infection)
Preauricular appendage 744.1
Prebetalipoproteinemia (acquired) (essential) (familial) (hereditary) (primary) (secondary) 272.1
  with chylomicronemia 272.3
Precipitate labor 661.3 ☑
  affecting fetus or newborn 763.6
Preclimacteric bleeding 627.0
  menorrhagia 627.0
Precocious
  adrenarche 259.1
  menarche 259.1
  menstruation 259.1
  pubarche 259.1
  puberty NEC 259.1
  sexual development NEC 259.1
  thelarche 259.1
Precocity, sexual (constitutional) (cryptogenic) (female) (idiopathic) (male) NEC 259.1
  with adrenal hyperplasia 255.2
Precordial pain 786.51
  psychogenic 307.89
Predeciduous teeth 520.2
Prediabetes, prediabetic 790.29
  complicating pregnancy, childbirth, or puerperium 648.8 ☑
  fetus or newborn 775.89
Predislocation status of hip, at birth — *see also* Subluxation, congenital, hip 754.32
Preeclampsia (mild) 642.4 ☑
  with pre-existing hypertension 642.7 ☑
  affecting fetus or newborn 760.0
  severe 642.5 ☑
  superimposed on pre-existing hypertensive disease 642.7 ☑
Preeruptive color change, teeth, tooth 520.8
Preexcitation 426.7
  atrioventricular conduction 426.7
  ventricular 426.7
Preglaucoma 365.00
Pregnancy (single) (uterine) (without sickness) V22.2

Note — Use the following fifth-digit subclassification with categories 640–649, 651–679:

0 unspecified as to episode of care

1 delivered, with or without mention of antepartum condition

2 delivered, with mention of postpartum complication

3 antepartum condition or complication

4 postpartum condition or complication

  abdominal (ectopic) 633.00
    with intrauterine pregnancy 633.01
    affecting fetus or newborn 761.4
  abnormal NEC 646.9 ☑
  ampullar — *see* Pregnancy, tubal

Pregnancy — *continued*
  biochemical 631.0
  broad ligament — *see* Pregnancy, cornual
  cervical — *see* Pregnancy, cornual
  chemical 631.0
  combined (extrauterine and intrauterine) — *see* Pregnancy, cornual
  complicated (by) 646.9 ☑
    abnormal, abnormality NEC 646.9 ☑
      cervix 654.6 ☑
      cord (umbilical) 663.9 ☑
      glucose tolerance (conditions classifiable to 790.21–790.29) 648.8 ☑
      pelvic organs or tissues NEC 654.9 ☑
      pelvis (bony) 653.0 ☑
      perineum or vulva 654.8 ☑
      placenta, placental (vessel) 656.7 ☑
      position
        cervix 654.4 ☑
        placenta 641.1 ☑
          without hemorrhage 641.0 ☑
        uterus 654.4 ☑
      size, fetus 653.5 ☑
      uterus (congenital) 654.0 ☑
    abscess or cellulitis
      bladder 646.6 ☑
      genitourinary tract (conditions classifiable to 590, 595, 597, 599.0, 614.0–614.5, 614.7–614.9, 615) 646.6 ☑
      kidney 646.6 ☑
      urinary tract NEC 646.6 ☑
    adhesion, pelvic peritoneal 648.9 ☑
    air embolism 673.0 ☑
    albuminuria 646.2 ☑
      with hypertension — *see* Toxemia, of pregnancy
    amnionitis 658.4 ☑
    amniotic fluid embolism 673.1 ☑
    anemia (conditions classifiable to 280–285) 648.2 ☑
    appendicitis 648.9 ☑
    atrophy, yellow (acute) (liver) (subacute) 646.7 ☑
    bacilluria, asymptomatic 646.5 ☑
    bacteriuria, asymptomatic 646.5 ☑
    bariatric surgery status 649.2 ☑
    bicornis or bicornuate uterus 654.0 ☑
    biliary problems 646.8 ☑
    bone and joint disorders (conditions classifiable to 720–724 or conditions affecting lower limbs classifiable to 711–719, 725–738) 648.7 ☑
    breech presentation (buttocks) (complete) (frank) 652.2 ☑
      with successful version 652.1 ☑
    cardiovascular disease (conditions classifiable to 390–398, 410–429) 648.6 ☑
      congenital (conditions classifiable to 745–747) 648.5 ☑
    cerebrovascular disorders (conditions classifiable to 430–434, 436–437) 674.0 ☑
    cervicitis (conditions classifiable to 616.0) 646.6 ☑
    chloasma (gravidarum) 646.8 ☑
    cholelithiasis 646.8 ☑
    cholestasis 646.7 ☑
    chorea (gravidarum) — *see* Eclampsia, pregnancy
    coagulation defect 649.3 ☑
    conjoined twins 678.1 ☑
    contraction, pelvis (general) 653.1 ☑
      inlet 653.2 ☑
      outlet 653.3 ☑
    convulsions (eclamptic) (uremic) 642.6 ☑
      with pre-existing hypertension 642.7 ☑

Pregnancy — *continued*
  complicated — *continued*
    current disease or condition (nonobstetric)
      abnormal glucose tolerance 648.8 ☑
      anemia 648.2 ☑
      biliary tract 646.7 ☑
      bone and joint (lower limb) 648.7 ☑
      cardiovascular 648.6 ☑
        congenital 648.5 ☑
      cerebrovascular 674.0 ☑
      diabetes (conditions classifiable to 249 and 250) 648.0 ☑
      drug dependence 648.3 ☑
      female genital mutilation 648.9 ☑
      genital organ or tract 646.6 ☑
      gonorrheal 647.1 ☑
      hypertensive 642.2 ☑
        chronic kidney 642.2 ☑
        renal 642.1 ☑
      infectious 647.9 ☑
        specified type NEC 647.8 ☑
      liver 646.7 ☑
      malarial 647.4 ☑
      nutritional deficiency 648.9 ☑
      parasitic NEC 647.8 ☑
      periodontal disease 648.9 ☑
      renal 646.2 ☑
        hypertensive 642.1 ☑
      rubella 647.5 ☑
      specified condition NEC 648.9 ☑
      syphilitic 647.0 ☑
      thyroid 648.1 ☑
      tuberculous 647.3 ☑
      urinary 646.6 ☑
      venereal 647.2 ☑
      viral NEC 647.6 ☑
    cystitis 646.6 ☑
    cystocele 654.4 ☑
    death of fetus (near term) 656.4 ☑
      early pregnancy (before 22 completed weeks gestation) 632
    deciduitis 646.6 ☑
    decreased fetal movements 655.7 ☑
    diabetes (mellitus) (conditions classifiable to 249 and 250) 648.0 ☑
    disorders of liver and biliary tract 646.7 ☑
    displacement, uterus NEC 654.4 ☑
    disproportion — *see* Disproportion
    double uterus 654.0 ☑
    drug dependence (conditions classifiable to 304) 648.3 ☑
    dysplasia, cervix 654.6 ☑
    early onset of delivery (spontaneous) 644.2 ☑
    eclampsia, eclamptic (coma) (convulsions) (delirium) (nephritis) (uremia) 642.6 ☑
      with pre-existing hypertension 642.7 ☑
    edema 646.1 ☑
      with hypertension — *see* Toxemia, of pregnancy
    effusion, amniotic fluid 658.1 ☑
      delayed delivery following 658.2 ☑
    embolism
      air 673.0 ☑
      amniotic fluid 673.1 ☑
      blood-clot 673.2 ☑
      cerebral 674.0 ☑
      pulmonary NEC 673.2 ☑
      pyemic 673.3 ☑
      septic 673.3 ☑
    emesis (gravidarum) — *see* Pregnancy, complicated, vomiting
    endometritis (conditions classifiable to 615.0–615.9) 670.1 ☑
      decidual 646.6 ☑
    epilepsy 649.4 ☑
    excessive weight gain NEC 646.1 ☑
    face presentation 652.4 ☑
    failure, fetal head to enter pelvic brim 652.5 ☑

☑ **Additional Digit Required** — Refer to the Tabular List for Digit Selection   ▽ **Subterms under main terms may continue to next column or page**

280   **2014 ICD-9-CM**

Pregnancy — *continued*
  complicated — *continued*
    false labor (pains) 644.1 ☑
    fatigue 646.8 ☑
    fatty metamorphosis of liver 646.7 ☑
    female genital mutilation 648.9 ☑
    fetal
      anemia 678.0 ☑
      complications from in utero proce-
        dure 679.1 ☑
      conjoined twins 678.1 ☑
      death (near term) 656.4 ☑
        early (before 22 completed weeks
          gestation) 632
      deformity 653.7 ☑
      distress 656.8 ☑
      hematologic conditions 678.0 ☑
      reduction of multiple fetuses reduced
        to single fetus 651.7 ☑
      thrombocytopenia 678.0 ☑
      twin to twin transfusion 678.0 ☑
    fibroid (tumor) (uterus) 654.1 ☑
    footling presentation 652.8 ☑
      with successful version 652.1 ☑
    gallbladder disease 646.8 ☑
    gastric banding status 649.2 ☑
    gastric bypass status for obesity
      649.2 ☑
    genital herpes (asymptomatic) (history
      of) (inactive) 647.6 ☑
    goiter 648.1 ☑
    gonococcal infection (conditions classifi-
      able to 098) 647.1 ☑
    gonorrhea (conditions classifiable to
      098) 647.1 ☑
    hemorrhage 641.9 ☑
      accidental 641.2 ☑
      before 22 completed weeks gesta-
        tion NEC 640.9 ☑
      cerebrovascular 674.0 ☑
      due to
        afibrinogenemia or other coagu-
          lation defect (conditions
          classifiable to 286.0–286.9)
          641.3 ☑
        leiomyoma, uterine 641.8 ☑
        marginal sinus (rupture) 641.2 ☑
        premature separation, placenta
          641.2 ☑
        trauma 641.8 ☑
      early (before 22 completed weeks
        gestation) 640.9 ☑
      threatened abortion 640.0 ☑
      unavoidable 641.1 ☑
    hepatitis (acute) (malignant) (subacute)
      646.7 ☑
      viral 647.6 ☑
    herniation of uterus 654.4 ☑
    high head at term 652.5 ☑
    hydatidiform mole (delivered) (undeliv-
      ered) 630
    hydramnios 657.0 ☑
    hydrocephalic fetus 653.6 ☑
    hydrops amnii 657.0 ☑
    hydrorrhea 658.1 ☑
    hyperemesis (gravidarum) — *see* Hyper-
      emesis, gravidarum
    hypertension — *see* Hypertension,
      complicating pregnancy
    hypertensive
      chronic kidney disease 642.2 ☑
      heart and chronic kidney disease
        642.2 ☑
      heart and renal disease 642.2 ☑
      heart disease 642.2 ☑
      renal disease 642.2 ☑
    hypertensive heart and chronic kidney
      disease 642.2 ☑
    hyperthyroidism 648.1 ☑
    hypothyroidism 648.1 ☑
    hysteralgia 646.8 ☑
    icterus gravis 646.7 ☑
    incarceration, uterus 654.3 ☑
    incompetent cervix (os) 654.5 ☑
    infection 647.9 ☑

Pregnancy — *continued*
  complicated — *continued*
    infection — *continued*
      amniotic fluid 658.4 ☑
      bladder 646.6 ☑
      genital organ (conditions classifiable
        to 614.0–614.5, 614.7–614.9,
        615) 646.6 ☑
      kidney (conditions classifiable to
        590.0–590.9) 646.6 ☑
      urinary (tract) 646.6 ☑
        asymptomatic 646.5 ☑
    infective and parasitic diseases NEC
      647.8 ☑
    inflammation
      bladder 646.6 ☑
      genital organ (conditions classifiable
        to 614.0–614.5, 614.7–614.9,
        615) 646.6 ☑
      urinary tract NEC 646.6 ☑
    insufficient weight gain 646.8 ☑
    insulin resistance 648.8 ☑
    intrauterine fetal death (near term) NEC
      656.4 ☑
      early (before 22 completed weeks'
        gestation) 632
    malaria (conditions classifiable to 084)
      647.4 ☑
    malformation, uterus (congenital)
      654.0 ☑
    malnutrition (conditions classifiable to
      260–269) 648.9 ☑
    malposition
      fetus — *see* Pregnancy, complicated,
        malpresentation
      uterus or cervix 654.4 ☑
    malpresentation 652.9 ☑
      with successful version 652.1 ☑
      in multiple gestation 652.6 ☑
      specified type NEC 652.8 ☑
    marginal sinus hemorrhage or rupture
      641.2 ☑
    maternal complications from in utero
      procedure 679.0 ☑
    maternal drug abuse 648.4 ☑
    maternal obesity syndrome 646.1 ☑
    menstruation 640.8 ☑
    mental disorders (conditions classifiable
      to 290–303, 305.0, 305.2-305.9,
      306–316, 317–319) 648.4 ☑
    mentum presentation 652.4 ☑
    missed
      abortion 632
      delivery (at or near term) 656.4 ☑
      labor (at or near term) 656.4 ☑
    necrosis
      genital organ or tract (conditions
        classifiable to 614.0–614.5,
        614.7–614.9, 615) 646.6 ☑
      liver (conditions classifiable to 570)
        646.7 ☑
      renal, cortical 646.2 ☑
    nephritis or nephrosis (conditions classi-
      fiable to 580–589) 646.2 ☑
      with hypertension 642.1 ☑
    nephropathy NEC 646.2 ☑
    neuritis (peripheral) 646.4 ☑
    nutritional deficiency (conditions classi-
      fiable to 260–269) 648.9 ☑
    obesity 649.1 ☑
      surgery status 649.2 ☑
    oblique lie or presentation 652.3 ☑
      with successful version 652.1 ☑
    obstetrical trauma NEC 665.9 ☑
    oligohydramnios NEC 658.0 ☑
    onset of contractions before 37 weeks
      644.0 ☑
    oversize fetus 653.5 ☑
    papyraceous fetus 646.0 ☑
    patent cervix 654.5 ☑
    pelvic inflammatory disease (conditions
      classifiable to 614.0–614.5,
      614.7–614.9, 615) 646.6 ☑
    pelvic peritoneal adhesion 648.9 ☑

Pregnancy — *continued*
  complicated — *continued*
    placenta, placental
      abnormality 656.7 ☑
      abruptio or ablatio 641.2 ☑
      detachment 641.2 ☑
      disease 656.7 ☑
      infarct 656.7 ☑
      low implantation 641.1 ☑
        without hemorrhage 641.0 ☑
      malformation 656.7 ☑
      malposition 641.1 ☑
        without hemorrhage 641.0 ☑
      marginal sinus hemorrhage 641.2 ☑
      previa 641.1 ☑
        without hemorrhage 641.0 ☑
      separation (premature) (undelivered)
        641.2 ☑
    placentitis 658.4 ☑
    pneumonia 648.9 ☑
    polyhydramnios 657.0 ☑
    postmaturity
      post-term 645.1 ☑
      prolonged 645.2 ☑
    prediabetes 648.8 ☑
    pre-eclampsia (mild) 642.4 ☑
      severe 642.5 ☑
      superimposed on pre-existing hyper-
        tensive disease 642.7 ☑
    premature rupture of membranes
      658.1 ☑
      with delayed delivery 658.2 ☑
    previous
      ectopic pregnancy V23.42
      infertility V23.0
      in utero procedure during previous
        pregnancy V23.86
      nonobstetric condition V23.89
      poor obstetrical history V23.49
      premature delivery V23.41
      trophoblastic disease (conditions
        classifiable to 630) V23.1
    prolapse, uterus 654.4 ☑
    proteinuria (gestational) 646.2 ☑
      with hypertension — *see* Toxemia,
        of pregnancy
    pruritus (neurogenic) 646.8 ☑
    psychosis or psychoneurosis 648.4 ☑
    ptyalism 646.8 ☑
    pyelitis (conditions classifiable to
      590.0–590.9) 646.6 ☑
    renal disease or failure NEC 646.2 ☑
      with secondary hypertension
        642.1 ☑
      hypertensive 642.2 ☑
    retention, retained dead ovum 631.8
    retroversion, uterus 654.3 ☑
    Rh immunization, incompatibility, or
      sensitization 656.1 ☑
    rubella (conditions classifiable to 056)
      647.5 ☑
    rupture
      amnion (premature) 658.1 ☑
        with delayed delivery 658.2 ☑
      marginal sinus (hemorrhage)
        641.2 ☑
      membranes (premature) 658.1 ☑
        with delayed delivery 658.2 ☑
      uterus (before onset of labor)
        665.0 ☑
    salivation (excessive) 646.8 ☑
    salpingo–oophoritis (conditions classifi-
      able to 614.0–614.2) 646.6 ☑
    septicemia (conditions classifiable to
      038.0–038.9) 647.8 ☑
      postpartum 670.2 ☑
      puerperal 670.2 ☑
    smoking 649.0 ☑
    spasms, uterus (abnormal) 646.8 ☑
    specified condition NEC 646.8 ☑
    spotting 649.5 ☑
    spurious labor pains 644.1 ☑
    status post
      bariatric surgery 649.2 ☑

Pregnancy — *continued*
  complicated — *continued*
    status post — *continued*
      gastric banding 649.2 ☑
      gastric bypass for obesity 649.2 ☑
      obesity surgery 649.2 ☑
    superfecundation 651.9 ☑
    superfetation 651.9 ☑
    syphilis (conditions classifiable to
      090–097) 647.0 ☑
    threatened
      abortion 640.0 ☑
      premature delivery 644.2 ☑
      premature labor 644.0 ☑
    thrombophlebitis (superficial) 671.2 ☑
      deep 671.3 ☑
      septic 670.3 ☑
    thrombosis 671.2 ☑
      venous (superficial) 671.2 ☑
        deep 671.3 ☑
    thyroid dysfunction (conditions classifi-
      able to 240–246) 648.1 ☑
    thyroiditis 648.1 ☑
    thyrotoxicosis 648.1 ☑
    tobacco use disorder 649.0 ☑
    torsion of uterus 654.4 ☑
    toxemia — *see* Toxemia, of pregnancy
    transverse lie or presentation 652.3 ☑
      with successful version 652.1 ☑
    trauma 648.9 ☑
      obstetrical 665.9 ☑
    tuberculosis (conditions classifiable to
      010–018) 647.3 ☑
    tumor
      cervix 654.6 ☑
      ovary 654.4 ☑
      pelvic organs or tissue NEC 654.4 ☑
      uterus (body) 654.1 ☑
        cervix 654.6 ☑
      vagina 654.7 ☑
      vulva 654.8 ☑
    unstable lie 652.0 ☑
    uremia — *see* Pregnancy, complicated,
      renal disease
    urethritis 646.6 ☑
    vaginitis or vulvitis (conditions classifi-
      able to 616.1) 646.6 ☑
    varicose
      placental vessels 656.7 ☑
      veins (legs) 671.0 ☑
        perineum 671.1 ☑
        vulva 671.1 ☑
    varicosity, labia or vulva 671.1 ☑
    venereal disease NEC (conditions classi-
      fiable to 099) 647.2 ☑
    venous complication 671.9 ☑
    viral disease NEC (conditions classifiable
      to 042, 050–055, 057–079,
      795.05, 795.15, 796.75) 647.6 ☑
    vomiting (incoercible) (pernicious) (per-
      sistent) (uncontrollable) (vicious)
      643.9 ☑
      due to organic disease or other cause
        643.8 ☑
      early — *see* Hyperemesis, gravi-
        darum
      late (after 22 completed weeks gesta-
        tion) 643.2 ☑
    young maternal age 659.8 ☑
  complications NEC 646.9 ☑
  cornual 633.80
    with intrauterine pregnancy 633.81
    affecting fetus or newborn 761.4
  death, maternal NEC 646.9 ☑
  delivered — *see* Delivery
  ectopic (ruptured) NEC 633.90
    with intrauterine pregnancy 633.91
    abdominal — *see* Pregnancy, abdominal
    affecting fetus or newborn 761.4
    combined (extrauterine and intrauter-
      ine) — *see* Pregnancy, cornual
    ovarian — *see* Pregnancy, ovarian
    specified type NEC 633.80
      with intrauterine pregnancy 633.81

☑ Additional Digit Required — Refer to the Tabular List for Digit Selection   ▽ Subterms under main terms may continue to next column or page

Pregnancy — continued
  ectopic — continued
    specified type — continued
      affecting fetus or newborn 761.4
    tubal — see Pregnancy, tubal
  examination, pregnancy
    negative result V72.41
    not confirmed V72.40
    positive result V72.42
  extrauterine — see Pregnancy, ectopic
  fallopian — see Pregnancy, tubal
  false 300.11
    labor (pains) 644.1 ☑
  fatigue 646.8 ☑
  illegitimate V61.6
  incidental finding V22.2
  in double uterus 654.0 ☑
  interstitial — see Pregnancy, cornual
  intraligamentous — see Pregnancy, cornual
  intramural — see Pregnancy, cornual
  intraperitoneal — see Pregnancy, abdominal
  isthmian — see Pregnancy, tubal
  management affected by
    abnormal, abnormality
      fetus (suspected) 655.9 ☑
        specified NEC 655.8 ☑
      placenta 656.7 ☑
    advanced maternal age NEC 659.6 ☑
      multigravida 659.6 ☑
      primigravida 659.5 ☑
    antibodies (maternal)
      anti-c 656.1 ☑
      anti-d 656.1 ☑
      anti-e 656.1 ☑
      blood group (ABO) 656.2 ☑
        Rh(esus) 656.1 ☑
    appendicitis 648.9 ☑
    bariatric surgery status 649.2 ☑
    coagulation defect 649.3 ☑
    elderly multigravida 659.6 ☑
    elderly primigravida 659.5 ☑
    epilepsy 649.4 ☑
    fetal (suspected)
      abnormality 655.9 ☑
        abdominal 655.8 ☑
        acid-base balance 656.8 ☑
        cardiovascular 655.8 ☑
        facial 655.8 ☑
        gastrointestinal 655.8 ☑
        gentourinary 655.8 ☑
        heart rate or rhythm 659.7 ☑
        limb 655.8 ☑
        specified NEC 655.8 ☑
      acidemia 656.3 ☑
      anencephaly 655.0 ☑
      aneuploidy 655.1 ☑
      bradycardia 659.7 ☑
      central nervous system malformation 655.0 ☑
      chromosomal abnormalities (conditions classifiable to 758.0–758.9) 655.1 ☑
      damage from
        drugs 655.5 ☑
          obstetric, anesthetic, or sedative 655.5 ☑
        environmental toxins 655.8 ☑
        intrauterine contraceptive device 655.8 ☑
        maternal
          alcohol addiction 655.4 ☑
          disease NEC 655.4 ☑
          drug use 655.5 ☑
          listeriosis 655.4 ☑
          rubella 655.3 ☑
          toxoplasmosis 655.4 ☑
          viral infection 655.3 ☑
        radiation 655.6 ☑
      death (near term) 656.4 ☑
        early (before 22 completed weeks' gestation) 632
      distress 656.8 ☑
      excessive growth 656.6 ☑

Pregnancy — continued
  management affected by — continued
    fetal — continued
      fetal-maternal hemorrhage 656.0 ☑
      growth retardation 656.5 ☑
      hereditary disease 655.2 ☑
      hereditary disease in family (possibly) affecting fetus 655.2 ☑
      hydrocephalus 655.0 ☑
      incompatibility, blood groups (ABO) 656.2 ☑
      intrauterine death 656.4 ☑
      poor growth 656.5 ☑
      Rh(esus) 656.1 ☑
      spina bifida (with myelomeningocele) 655.0 ☑
    gastric banding status 649.2 ☑
    gastric bypass status for obesity 649.2 ☑
    insufficient prenatal care V23.7
    insulin resistance 648.8 ☑
    intrauterine death 656.4 ☑
    isoimmunization (ABO) 656.2 ☑
      Rh(esus) 656.1 ☑
    large-for-dates fetus 656.6 ☑
    light-for-dates fetus 656.5 ☑
    meconium in liquor 656.8 ☑
    mental disorder (conditions classifiable to 290–303, 305.0, 305.2–305.9, 306–316, 317–319) 648.4 ☑
    multiparity (grand) 659.4 ☑
    obesity 649.1 ☑
      surgery status 649.2 ☑
    poor obstetric history V23.49
      pre-term labor V23.41
    postmaturity
      post-term 645.1 ☑
      prolonged 645.2 ☑
    post-term pregnancy 645.1 ☑
    previous
      abortion V23.2
        habitual 646.3 ☑
      cesarean delivery 654.2 ☑
      difficult delivery V23.49
      ectopic pregnancy V23.42
      forceps delivery V23.49
      habitual abortions 646.3 ☑
      hemorrhage, antepartum or postpartum V23.49
      hydatidiform mole V23.1
      infertility V23.0
      in utero procedure during previous pregnancy V23.86
      malignancy NEC V23.89
      nonobstetrical conditions V23.8 ☑
      premature delivery V23.41
      recurrent pregnancy loss 646.3 ☑
      trophoblastic disease (conditions in 630) V23.1
      vesicular mole V23.1
    prolonged pregnancy 645.2 ☑
    recurrent pregnancy loss 646.3 ☑
    small-for-dates fetus 656.5 ☑
    smoking 649.0 ☑
    spotting 649.5 ☑
    suspected conditions not found
      amniotic cavity and membrane problem V89.01
      cervical shortening V89.05
      fetal anomaly V89.03
      fetal growth problem V89.04
      oligohydramnios V89.01
      other specified problem NEC V89.09
      placental problem V89.02
      polyhydramnios V89.01
    tobacco use disorder 649.0 ☑
    venous complication 671.9 ☑
    young maternal age 659.8 ☑
  maternal death NEC 646.9 ☑
  mesometric (mural) — see Pregnancy, cornual
  molar 631.8
    hydatidiform (see also Hydatidiform mole) 630
      previous, affecting management of pregnancy V23.1

Pregnancy — continued
  molar — continued
    previous, affecting management of pregnancy V23.49
  multiple NEC 651.9 ☑
    with fetal loss and retention of one or more fetus(es) 651.6 ☑
    affecting fetus or newborn 761.5
    following (elective) fetal reduction 651.7 ☑
    specified type NEC 651.8 ☑
      with fetal loss and retention of one or more fetus(es) 651.6 ☑
      following (elective) fetal reduction 651.7 ☑
  mural — see Pregnancy, cornual
  observation NEC V22.1
    first pregnancy V22.0
    high-risk V23.9
      inconclusive fetal viability V23.87
      specified problem NEC V23.89
  ovarian 633.20
    with intrauterine pregnancy 633.21
    affecting fetus or newborn 761.4
  possible, not (yet) confirmed V72.40
  postmature
    post-term 645.1 ☑
    prolonged 645.2 ☑
  post-term 645.1 ☑
  prenatal care only V22.1
    first pregnancy V22.0
    high-risk V23.9
      inconclusive fetal viability V23.87
      specified problem NEC V23.89
  prolonged 645.2 ☑
  quadruplet NEC 651.2 ☑
    with fetal loss and retention of one or more fetus(es) 651.5 ☑
    affecting fetus or newborn 761.5
    following (elective) fetal reduction 651.7 ☑
  quintuplet NEC 651.8 ☑
    with fetal loss and retention of one or more fetus(es) 651.6 ☑
    affecting fetus or newborn 761.5
    following (elective) fetal reduction 651.7 ☑
  resulting from
    assisted reproductive technology V23.85
    in vitro fertilization V23.85
  sextuplet NEC 651.8 ☑
    with fetal loss and retention of one or more fetus(es) 651.6 ☑
    affecting fetus or newborn 761.5
    following (elective) fetal reduction 651.7 ☑
  spurious 300.11
  superfecundation NEC 651.9 ☑
    with fetal loss and retention of one or more fetus(es) 651.6 ☑
    following (elective) fetal reduction 651.7 ☑
  superfetation NEC 651.9 ☑
    with fetal loss and retention of one or more fetus(es) 651.6 ☑
    following (elective) fetal reduction 651.7 ☑
  supervision (of) (for) (see also Pregnancy, management affected by)
    elderly
      multigravida V23.82
      primigravida V23.81
    high-risk V23.9
      inconclusive fetal viability V23.87
      insufficient prenatal care V23.7
      specified problem NEC V23.89
    inconclusive fetal viability V23.87
    multiparity V23.3
    normal NEC V22.1
      first V22.0
    poor
      obstetric history V23.49
        ectopic pregnancy V23.42
        pre-term labor V23.41
      reproductive history V23.5

Pregnancy — continued
  supervision (see also Pregnancy, management affected by) — continued
    previous
      abortion V23.2
      hydatidiform mole V23.1
      infertility V23.0
      neonatal death V23.5
      stillbirth V23.5
      trophoblastic disease V23.1
      vesicular mole V23.1
    specified problem NEC V23.89
    young
      multigravida V23.84
      primigravida V23.83
  triplet NEC 651.1 ☑
    with fetal loss and retention of one or more fetus(es) 651.4 ☑
    affecting fetus or newborn 761.5
    following (elective) fetal reduction 651.7 ☑
  tubal (with rupture) 633.10
    with intrauterine pregnancy 633.11
    affecting fetus or newborn 761.4
  twin NEC 651.0 ☑
    with fetal loss and retention of one fetus 651.3 ☑
    affecting fetus or newborn 761.5
    conjoined 678.1 ☑
    following (elective) fetal reduction 651.7 ☑
  unconfirmed V72.40
  undelivered (no other diagnosis) V22.2
    with false labor 644.1 ☑
    high-risk V23.9
      specified problem NEC V23.89
  unwanted NEC V61.7
Pregnant uterus — see condition
Preiser's disease (osteoporosis) 733.09
Prekwashiorkor 260
Preleukemia 238.75
Preluxation of hip, congenital — see also Subluxation, congenital, hip 754.32
Premature — see also condition
  beats (nodal) 427.60
    atrial 427.61
    auricular 427.61
    postoperative 997.1
    specified type NEC 427.69
    supraventricular 427.61
    ventricular 427.69
  birth NEC 765.1 ☑
  closure
    cranial suture 756.0
    fontanel 756.0
    foramen ovale 745.8
  contractions 427.60
    atrial 427.61
    auricular 427.61
    auriculoventricular 427.61
    heart (extrasystole) 427.60
    junctional 427.60
    nodal 427.60
    postoperative 997.1
    ventricular 427.69
  ejaculation 302.75
  infant NEC 765.1 ☑
    excessive 765.0 ☑
    light-for-dates — see Light-for-dates
  labor 644.2 ☑
    threatened 644.0 ☑
  lungs 770.4
  menopause 256.31
  puberty 259.1
  rupture of membranes or amnion 658.1 ☑
    affecting fetus or newborn 761.1
    delayed delivery following 658.2 ☑
  senility (syndrome) 259.8
  separation, placenta (partial) — see Placenta, separation
  ventricular systole 427.69
Prematurity NEC 765.1 ☑
  extreme 765.0 ☑
Premenstrual syndrome 625.4
Premenstrual tension 625.4
Premolarization, cuspids 520.2

Premyeloma 273.1
Prenatal
care, normal pregnancy V22.1
first V22.0
death, cause unknown — *see* Death, fetus
screening — *see* Antenatal, screening
teeth 520.6
Prepartum — *see* condition
Preponderance, left or right ventricular
429.3
Prepuce — *see* condition
PRES (posterior reversible encephalopathy syndrome) 348.39
Presbycardia 797
hypertensive (*see also* Hypertension, heart) 402.90
Presbycusis 388.01
Presbyesophagus 530.89
Presbyophrenia 310.1
Presbyopia 367.4
Prescription of contraceptives NEC V25.02
diaphragm V25.02
oral (pill) V25.01
emergency V25.03
postcoital V25.03
repeat V25.41
repeat V25.40
oral (pill) V25.41
Presenile — *see also* condition
aging 259.8
dementia (*see also* Dementia, presenile) 290.10
Presenility 259.8
Presentation, fetal
abnormal 652.9 ☑
with successful version 652.1 ☑
before labor, affecting fetus or newborn 761.7
causing obstructed labor 660.0 ☑
affecting fetus or newborn, any, except breech 763.1
in multiple gestation (one or more) 652.6 ☑
specified NEC 652.8 ☑
arm 652.7 ☑
causing obstructed labor 660.0 ☑
breech (buttocks) (complete) (frank) 652.2 ☑
with successful version 652.1 ☑
before labor, affecting fetus or newborn 761.7
before labor, affecting fetus or newborn 761.7
brow 652.4 ☑
causing obstructed labor 660.0 ☑
buttocks 652.2 ☑
chin 652.4 ☑
complete 652.2 ☑
compound 652.8 ☑
cord 663.0 ☑
extended head 652.4 ☑
face 652.4 ☑
to pubes 652.8 ☑
footling 652.8 ☑
frank 652.2 ☑
hand, leg, or foot NEC 652.8 ☑
incomplete 652.8 ☑
mentum 652.4 ☑
multiple gestation (one fetus or more) 652.6 ☑
oblique 652.3 ☑
with successful version 652.1 ☑
shoulder 652.8 ☑
affecting fetus or newborn 763.1
transverse 652.3 ☑
with successful version 652.1 ☑
umbilical cord 663.0 ☑
unstable 652.0 ☑
Prespondylolisthesis (congenital) (lumbosacral) 756.11
Pressure
area, skin ulcer (*see also* Ulcer, pressure) 707.00
atrophy, spine 733.99
birth, fetus or newborn NEC 767.9

Pressure — *continued*
brachial plexus 353.0
brain 348.4
injury at birth 767.0
cerebral — *see* Pressure, brain
chest 786.59
cone, tentorial 348.4
injury at birth 767.0
funis — *see* Compression, umbilical cord
hyposystolic (*see also* Hypotension) 458.9
increased
intracranial 781.99
due to
benign intracranial hypertension 348.2
hydrocephalus — *see* hydrocephalus
injury at birth 767.8
intraocular 365.00
lumbosacral plexus 353.1
mediastinum 519.3
necrosis (chronic) (skin) (*see also* Decubitus) 707.00
nerve — *see* Compression, nerve
paralysis (*see also* Neuropathy, entrapment) 355.9
pre-ulcer skin changes limited to persistent focal erythema (*see also* Ulcer, pressure) 707.21
sore (chronic) (*see also* Ulcer, pressure) 707.00
spinal cord 336.9
ulcer (chronic) (*see also* Ulcer, pressure) 707.00
umbilical cord — *see* Compression, umbilical cord
venous, increased 459.89
Pre-syncope 780.2
Preterm infant NEC 765.1 ☑
extreme 765.0 ☑
Priapism (penis) 607.3
Prickling sensation — *see also* Disturbance, sensation 782.0
Prickly heat 705.1
Primary — *see also* condition
angle closure suspect 365.02
Primigravida, elderly
affecting
fetus or newborn 763.89
management of pregnancy, labor, and delivery 659.5 ☑
Primipara, old
affecting
fetus or newborn 763.89
management of pregnancy, labor, and delivery 659.5 ☑
Primula dermatitis 692.6
Primus varus (bilateral) (metatarsus) 754.52
PRIND (prolonged reversible ischemic neurologic deficit) 434.91
history of (personal) V12.54
Pringle's disease (tuberous sclerosis) 759.5
Prinzmetal's angina 413.1
Prinzmetal-Massumi syndrome (anterior chest wall) 786.52
Prizefighter ear 738.7
Problem (with) V49.9
academic V62.3
acculturation V62.4
adopted child V61.24
aged
in-law V61.3
parent V61.3
person NEC V61.8
alcoholism in family V61.41
anger reaction (*see also* Disturbance, conduct) 312.0 ☑
behavioral V40.9
specified NEC V40.39
behavior, child 312.9
betting V69.3
biological child V61.23
cardiorespiratory NEC V47.2
career choice V62.29
care of sick or handicapped person in family or household V61.49

Problem — *continued*
communication V40.1
conscience regarding medical care V62.6
delinquency (juvenile) 312.9
diet, inappropriate V69.1
digestive NEC V47.3
ear NEC V41.3
eating habits, inappropriate V69.1
economic V60.2
affecting care V60.9
specified type NEC V60.89
educational V62.3
enuresis, child 307.6
exercise, lack of V69.0
eye NEC V41.1
family V61.9
specified circumstance NEC V61.8
fear reaction, child 313.0
feeding (elderly) (infant) 783.3
newborn 779.31
nonorganic 307.59
fetal, affecting management of pregnancy 656.9 ☑
specified type NEC 656.8 ☑
financial V60.2
foster child V61.25
functional V41.9
specified type NEC V41.8
gambling V69.3
genital NEC V47.5
head V48.9
deficiency V48.0
disfigurement V48.6
mechanical V48.2
motor V48.2
movement of V48.2
sensory V48.4
specified condition NEC V48.8
hearing V41.2
high-risk sexual behavior V69.2
identity 313.82
influencing health status NEC V49.89
internal organ NEC V47.9
deficiency V47.0
mechanical or motor V47.1
interpersonal NEC V62.81
jealousy, child 313.3
learning V40.0
legal V62.5
life circumstance NEC V62.89
lifestyle V69.9
specified NEC V69.8
limb V49.9
deficiency V49.0
disfigurement V49.4
mechanical V49.1
motor V49.2
movement, involving
musculoskeletal system V49.1
nervous system V49.2
sensory V49.3
specified condition NEC V49.5
litigation V62.5
living alone V60.3
loneliness NEC V62.89
marital V61.10
involving
divorce V61.03
estrangement V61.09
psychosexual disorder 302.9
sexual function V41.7
relationship V61.10
mastication V41.6
medical care, within family V61.49
mental V40.9
specified NEC V40.2
mental hygiene, adult V40.9
multiparity V61.5
nail biting, child 307.9
neck V48.9
deficiency V48.1
disfigurement V48.7
mechanical V48.3
motor V48.3
movement V48.3
sensory V48.5

Problem — *continued*
neck — *continued*
specified condition NEC V48.8
neurological NEC 781.99
none (feared complaint unfounded) V65.5
occupational V62.29
parent-child V61.20
adopted child V61.24
biological child V61.23
foster child V61.25
relationship V61.20
partner V61.10
relationship V61.10
personality (*see also* Disorder, personality) 301.9
personal NEC V62.89
interpersonal conflict NEC V62.81
phase of life V62.89
placenta, affecting management of pregnancy 656.9 ☑
specified type NEC 656.8 ☑
poverty V60.2
presence of sick or handicapped person in family or household V61.49
psychiatric 300.9
psychosocial V62.9
specified type NEC V62.89
relational NEC V62.81
relationship, childhood 313.3
religious or spiritual belief
other than medical care V62.89
regarding medical care V62.6
self-damaging behavior V69.8
sexual
behavior, high-risk V69.2
function NEC V41.7
sibling
relational V61.8
relationship V61.8
sight V41.0
sleep disorder, child 307.40
sleep, lack of V69.4
smell V41.5
speech V40.1
spite reaction, child (*see also* Disturbance, conduct) 312.0 ☑
spoiled child reaction (*see also* Disturbance, conduct) 312.1 ☑
substance abuse in family V61.42
swallowing V41.6
tantrum, child (*see also* Disturbance, conduct) 312.1 ☑
taste V41.5
thumb sucking, child 307.9
tic (child) 307.21
trunk V48.9
deficiency V48.1
disfigurement V48.7
mechanical V48.3
motor V48.3
movement V48.3
sensory V48.5
specified condition NEC V48.8
unemployment V62.0
urinary NEC V47.4
voice production V41.4
Procedure (surgical) **not done** NEC V64.3
because of
contraindication V64.1
patient's decision V64.2
for reasons of conscience or religion V62.6
specified reason NEC V64.3
Procidentia
anus (sphincter) 569.1
rectum (sphincter) 569.1
stomach 537.89
uteri 618.1
Proctalgia 569.42
fugax 564.6
spasmodic 564.6
psychogenic 307.89
Proctitis 569.49
amebic 006.8
chlamydial 099.52
gonococcal 098.7

☑ **Additional Digit Required** — Refer to the Tabular List for Digit Selection

▽ **Subterms under main terms may continue to next column or page**

Proctitis — *continued*
 granulomatous 555.1
 idiopathic 556.2
  with ulcerative sigmoiditis 556.3
 tuberculous (*see also* Tuberculosis) 014.8 ☑
 ulcerative (chronic) (nonspecific) 556.2
  with ulcerative sigmoiditis 556.3
Proctocele
 female (without uterine prolapse) 618.04
  with uterine prolapse 618.4
   complete 618.3
   incomplete 618.2
 male 569.49
Proctocolitis, idiopathic 556.2
 with ulcerative sigmoiditis 556.3
Proctoptosis 569.1
Proctosigmoiditis 569.89
 ulcerative (chronic) 556.3
Proctospasm 564.6
 psychogenic 306.4
Prodromal-AIDS — *see* Human immunodeficiency virus (disease) (illness) (infection)
Profichet's disease or syndrome 729.90
Progeria (adultorum) (syndrome) 259.8
Prognathism (mandibular) (maxillary) 524.10
Progonoma (melanotic) (M9363/0) — *see* Neoplasm, by site, benign
Progressive — *see* condition
Prolapse, prolapsed
 anus, anal (canal) (sphincter) 569.1
 arm or hand, complicating delivery 652.7 ☑
  causing obstructed labor 660.0 ☑
   affecting fetus or newborn 763.1
  fetus or newborn 763.1
 bladder (acquired) (mucosa) (sphincter)
  congenital (female) (male) 756.71
  female (*see also* Cystocele, female) 618.01
  male 596.89
 breast implant (prosthetic) 996.54
 cecostomy 569.69
 cecum 569.89
 cervix, cervical (hypertrophied) 618.1
  anterior lip, obstructing labor 660.2 ☑
   affecting fetus or newborn 763.1
  congenital 752.49
  postpartal (old) 618.1
  stump 618.84
 ciliary body 871.1
 colon (pedunculated) 569.89
 colostomy 569.69
 conjunctiva 372.73
 cord — *see* Prolapse, umbilical cord
 cystostomy 596.83
 disc (intervertebral) — *see* Displacement, intervertebral disc
 duodenum 537.89
 eye implant (orbital) 996.59
  lens (ocular) 996.53
 fallopian tube 620.4
 fetal extremity, complicating delivery 652.8 ☑
  causing obstructed labor 660.0 ☑
  fetus or newborn 763.1
 funis — *see* Prolapse, umbilical cord
 gastric (mucosa) 537.89
 genital, female 618.9
  specified NEC 618.89
 globe 360.81
 ileostomy bud 569.69
 intervertebral disc — *see* Displacement, intervertebral disc
 intestine (small) 569.89
 iris 364.89
  traumatic 871.1
 kidney (*see also* Disease, renal) 593.0
  congenital 753.3
 laryngeal muscles or ventricle 478.79
 leg, complicating delivery 652.8 ☑
  causing obstructed labor 660.0 ☑
  fetus or newborn 763.1
 liver 573.8
 meatus urinarius 599.5
 mitral valve 424.0
 ocular lens implant 996.53

Prolapse, prolapsed — *continued*
 organ or site, congenital NEC — *see* Malposition, congenital
 ovary 620.4
 pelvic (floor), female 618.89
 perineum, female 618.89
 pregnant uterus 654.4 ☑
 rectum (mucosa) (sphincter) 569.1
  due to Trichuris trichiuria 127.3
 spleen 289.59
 stomach 537.89
 umbilical cord
  affecting fetus or newborn 762.4
  complicating delivery 663.0 ☑
 ureter 593.89
  with obstruction 593.4
 ureterovesical orifice 593.89
 urethra (acquired) (infected) (mucosa) 599.5
  congenital 753.8
 uterovaginal 618.4
  complete 618.3
  incomplete 618.2
  specified NEC 618.89
 uterus (first degree) (second degree) (third degree) (complete) (without vaginal wall prolapse) 618.1
  with mention of vaginal wall prolapse — *see* Prolapse, uterovaginal
  congenital 752.39
  in pregnancy or childbirth 654.4 ☑
   affecting fetus or newborn 763.1
   causing obstructed labor 660.2 ☑
    affecting fetus or newborn 763.1
  postpartal (old) 618.1
 uveal 871.1
 vagina (anterior) (posterior) (vault) (wall) (without uterine prolapse) 618.00
  with uterine prolapse 618.4
   complete 618.3
   incomplete 618.2
  paravaginal 618.02
  posthysterectomy 618.5
  specified NEC 618.09
 vitreous (humor) 379.26
  traumatic 871.1
 womb — *see* Prolapse, uterus
Prolapsus, female 618.9
Proliferative — *see* condition
Prolinemia 270.8
Prolinuria 270.8
Prolonged, prolongation
 bleeding time (*see also* Defect, coagulation) 790.92
  "idiopathic" (in von Willebrand's disease) 286.4
 coagulation time (*see also* Defect, coagulation) 790.92
 gestation syndrome 766.22
 labor 662.1 ☑
  affecting fetus or newborn 763.89
  first stage 662.0 ☑
  second stage 662.2 ☑
 pregnancy 645.2 ☑
 PR interval 426.11
 prothrombin time (*see also* Defect, coagulation) 790.92
 QT interval 794.31
  syndrome 426.82
 rupture of membranes (24 hours or more prior to onset of labor) 658.2 ☑
 uterine contractions in labor 661.4 ☑
  affecting fetus or newborn 763.7
Prominauris 744.29
Prominence
 auricle (ear) (congenital) 744.29
  acquired 380.32
 ischial spine or sacral promontory
  with disproportion (fetopelvic) 653.3 ☑
   affecting fetus or newborn 763.1
   causing obstructed labor 660.1 ☑
    affecting fetus or newborn 763.1
 nose (congenital) 748.1
  acquired 738.0
PROMM (proximal myotonic myotonia) 359.21
Pronation
 ankle 736.79

Pronation — *continued*
 foot 736.79
  congenital 755.67
Prophylactic
 administration of
  antibiotics, long-term V58.62
   short-term — *omit code*
  antitoxin, any V07.2
  antivenin V07.2
  chemotherapeutic agent NEC V07.39
   fluoride V07.31
  diphtheria antitoxin V07.2
  drug V07.39
  exemestar (Aromasin) V07.52
  gamma globulin V07.2
  immune sera (gamma globulin) V07.2
  RhoGAM V07.2
  tetanus antitoxin V07.2
 chemotherapy NEC V07.39
  fluoride V07.31
 hormone replacement (postmenopausal) V07.4
 immunotherapy V07.2
 measure V07.9
  specified type NEC V07.8
 medication V07.39
 postmenopausal hormone replacement V07.4
 sterilization V25.2
Proptosis (ocular) — *see also* Exophthalmos 376.30
 thyroid 242.0 ☑
Propulsion
 eyeball 360.81
Prosecution, anxiety concerning V62.5
Prosopagnosia 368.16
Prostate, prostatic — *see* condition
Prostatism 600.90
 with
  other lower urinary tract symptoms (LUTS) 600.91
  urinary
   obstruction 600.91
   retention 600.91
Prostatitis (congestive) (suppurative) 601.9
 acute 601.0
 cavitary 601.8
 chlamydial 099.54
 chronic 601.1
 diverticular 601.8
 due to Trichomonas (vaginalis) 131.03
 fibrous 600.90
  with
   other lower urinary tract symptoms (LUTS) 600.91
   urinary
    obstruction 600.91
    retention 600.91
 gonococcal (acute) 098.12
  chronic or duration of 2 months or over 098.32
 granulomatous 601.8
 hypertrophic 600.00
  with
   other lower urinary tract symptoms (LUTS) 600.01
   urinary
    obstruction 600.01
    retention 600.01
 specified type NEC 601.8
 subacute 601.1
 trichomonal 131.03
 tuberculous (*see also* Tuberculosis) 016.5 ☑ [601.4]
Prostatocystitis 601.3
Prostatorrhea 602.8
Prostatoseminovesiculitis, trichomonal 131.03
Prostration 780.79
 heat 992.5
  anhydrotic 992.3
  due to
   salt (and water) depletion 992.4
   water depletion 992.3
 nervous 300.5
 newborn 779.89

Prostration — *continued*
 senile 797
Protanomaly 368.51
Protanopia (anomalous trichromat) (complete) (incomplete) 368.51
Protection (against) (from) — *see* Prophylactic
Protein
 deficiency 260
 malnutrition 260
 sickness (prophylactic) (therapeutic) 999.59
Proteinemia 790.99
Proteinosis
 alveolar, lung or pulmonary 516.0
 lipid 272.8
 lipoid (of Urbach) 272.8
Proteinuria — *see also* Albuminuria 791.0
 Bence-Jones NEC 791.0
 gestational 646.2 ☑
  with hypertension — *see* Toxemia, of pregnancy
 orthostatic 593.6
 postural 593.6
Proteolysis, pathologic 286.6
Protocoproporphyria 277.1
Protoporphyria (erythrohepatic) (erythropoietic) 277.1
Protrusio acetabuli 718.65
Protrusion
 acetabulum (into pelvis) 718.65
 device, implant, or graft — *see* Complications, mechanical
 ear, congenital 744.29
 intervertebral disc — *see* Displacement, intervertebral disc
 nucleus pulposus — *see* Displacement, intervertebral disc
Proud flesh 701.5
Prune belly (syndrome) 756.71
Prurigo (ferox) (gravis) (Hebra's) (hebrae) (mitis) (simplex) 698.2
 agria 698.3
 asthma syndrome 691.8
 Besnier's (atopic dermatitis) (infantile eczema) 691.8
 eczematodes allergicum 691.8
 estivalis (Hutchinson's) 692.72
 Hutchinson's 692.72
 nodularis 698.3
 psychogenic 306.3
Pruritus, pruritic 698.9
 ani 698.0
  psychogenic 306.3
 conditions NEC 698.9
  psychogenic 306.3
 due to Onchocerca volvulus 125.3
 ear 698.9
 essential 698.9
 genital organ(s) 698.1
  psychogenic 306.3
 gravidarum 646.8 ☑
 hiemalis 698.8
 neurogenic (any site) 306.3
 perianal 698.0
 psychogenic (any site) 306.3
 scrotum 698.1
  psychogenic 306.3
 senile, senilis 698.8
 Trichomonas 131.9
 vulva, vulvae 698.1
  psychogenic 306.3
Psammocarcinoma (M8140/3) — *see* Neoplasm, by site, malignant
Pseudarthrosis, pseudoarthrosis (bone) 733.82
 joint following fusion V45.4
Pseudoacanthosis
 nigricans 701.8
Pseudoaneurysm — *see* Aneurysm
Pseudoangina (pectoris) — *see* Angina
Pseudoangioma 452
Pseudo-Argyll-Robertson pupil 379.45
Pseudoarteriosus 747.89
Pseudoarthrosis — *see* Pseudarthrosis
Pseudoataxia 799.89
Pseudobulbar affect (PBA) 310.81
Pseudobursa 727.89

☑ **Additional Digit Required** — Refer to the Tabular List for Digit Selection   ▽ **Subterms under main terms may continue to next column or page**

284   **2014 ICD-9-CM**

Pseudocholera 025
Pseudochromidrosis 705.89
Pseudocirrhosis, liver, pericardial 423.2
Pseudocoarctation 747.21
Pseudocowpox 051.1
Pseudocoxalgia 732.1
Pseudocroup 478.75
Pseudocyesis 300.11
Pseudocyst
    lung 518.89
    pancreas 577.2
    retina 361.19
Pseudodementia 300.16
Pseudoelephantiasis neuroarthritica 757.0
Pseudoemphysema 518.89
Pseudoencephalitis
    superior (acute) hemorrhagic 265.1
Pseudoerosion cervix, congenital 752.49
Pseudoexfoliation, lens capsule 366.11
Pseudofracture (idiopathic) (multiple) (spontaneous) (symmetrical) 268.2
Pseudoglanders 025
Pseudoglioma 360.44
Pseudogout — see Chondrocalcinosis
Pseudohallucination 780.1
Pseudohemianesthesia 782.0
Pseudohemophilia (Bernuth's) (hereditary) (typeB) 286.4
    type A 287.8
    vascular 287.8
Pseudohermaphroditism 752.7
    with chromosomal anomaly — see Anomaly, chromosomal
    adrenal 255.2
    female (without adrenocortical disorder) 752.7
        with adrenocortical disorder 255.2
        adrenal 255.2
    male (without gonadal disorder) 752.7
        with
            adrenocortical disorder 255.2
            cleft scrotum 752.7
            feminizing testis 259.51
            gonadal disorder 257.9
            adrenal 255.2
Pseudohole, macula 362.54
Pseudo-Hurler's disease (mucolipidosis III) 272.7
Pseudohydrocephalus 348.2
Pseudohypertrophic muscular dystrophy (Erb's) 359.1
Pseudohypertrophy, muscle 359.1
Pseudohypoparathyroidism 275.49
Pseudoinfluenza — see also Influenza 487.1
Pseudoinsomnia 307.49
Pseudoleukemia 288.8
    infantile 285.8
Pseudomembranous — see condition
Pseudomeningocele (cerebral) (infective) 349.2
    postprocedural 997.01
    spinal 349.2
Pseudomenstruation 626.8
Pseudomucinous
    cyst (ovary) (M8470/0) 220
    peritoneum 568.89
Pseudomyeloma 273.1
Pseudomyxoma peritonei (M8480/6) 197.6
Pseudoneuritis optic (nerve) 377.24
    papilla 377.24
        congenital 743.57
Pseudoneuroma — see Injury, nerve, by site
Pseudo-obstruction
    intestine (chronic) (idiopathic) (intermittent secondary) (primary) 564.89
        acute 560.89
Pseudopapilledema 377.24
Pseudoparalysis
    arm or leg 781.4
    atonic, congenital 358.8
Pseudopelade 704.09
Pseudophakia V43.1
Pseudopolycythemia 289.0
Pseudopolyposis, colon 556.4
Pseudoporencephaly 348.0
Pseudopseudohypoparathyroidism 275.49

Pseudopsychosis 300.16
Pseudopterygium 372.52
Pseudoptosis (eyelid) 374.34
Pseudorabies 078.89
Pseudoretinitis, pigmentosa 362.65
Pseudorickets 588.0
    senile (Pozzi's) 731.0
Pseudorubella 057.8
Pseudoscarlatina 057.8
Pseudosclerema 778.1
Pseudosclerosis (brain)
    Jakob's 046.19
    of Westphal (-Strümpell) (hepatolenticular degeneration) 275.1
    spastic 046.19
        with dementia
            with behavioral disturbance 046.19 *[294.11]*
            without behavioral disturbance 046.19 *[294.10]*
Pseudoseizure 780.39
    non-psychiatric 780.39
    psychiatric 300.11
Pseudotabes 799.89
    diabetic 250.6 ☑ *[337.1]*
        due to secondary diabetes 249.6 ☑ *[337.1]*
Pseudotetanus — see also Convulsions 780.39
Pseudotetany 781.7
    hysterical 300.11
Pseudothalassemia 285.0
Pseudotrichinosis 710.3
Pseudotruncus arteriosus 747.29
Pseudotuberculosis, pasteurella (infection) 027.2
Pseudotumor
    cerebri 348.2
    orbit (inflammatory) 376.11
Pseudo-Turner's syndrome 759.89
Pseudoxanthoma elasticum 757.39
Psilosis (sprue) (tropical) 579.1
    Monilia 112.89
    nontropical 579.0
    not sprue 704.00
Psittacosis 073.9
Psoitis 728.89
Psora NEC 696.1
Psoriasis 696.1
    any type, except arthropathic 696.1
    arthritic, arthropathic 696.0
    buccal 528.6
    flexural 696.1
    follicularis 696.1
    guttate 696.1
    inverse 696.1
    mouth 528.6
    nummularis 696.1
    psychogenic 316 *[696.1]*
    punctata 696.1
    pustular 696.1
    rupioides 696.1
    vulgaris 696.1
Psorospermiasis 136.4
Psorospermosis 136.4
    follicularis (vegetans) 757.39
Psychalgia 307.80
Psychasthenia 300.89
    compulsive 300.3
    mixed compulsive states 300.3
    obsession 300.3
Psychiatric disorder or problem NEC 300.9
Psychogenic — see also condition
    factors associated with physical conditions 316
Psychoneurosis, psychoneurotic — see also Neurosis 300.9
    anxiety (state) 300.00
    climacteric 627.2
    compensation 300.16
    compulsion 300.3
    conversion hysteria 300.11
    depersonalization 300.6
    depressive type 300.4
    dissociative hysteria 300.15
    hypochondriacal 300.7
    hysteria 300.10

Psychoneurosis, psychoneurotic — see also Neurosis — continued
    hysteria — continued
        conversion type 300.11
        dissociative type 300.15
    mixed NEC 300.89
    neurasthenic 300.5
    obsessional 300.3
    obsessive-compulsive 300.3
    occupational 300.89
    personality NEC 301.89
    phobia 300.20
    senile NEC 300.89
Psychopathic — see also condition
    constitution, posttraumatic 310.2
        with psychosis 293.9
    personality 301.9
        amoral trends 301.7
        antisocial trends 301.7
        asocial trends 301.7
        mixed types 301.7
    state 301.9
Psychopathy, sexual — see also Deviation, sexual 302.9
Psychophysiologic, psychophysiological condition — see Reaction, psychophysiologic
Psychose passionelle 297.8
Psychosexual identity disorder 302.6
    adult-life 302.85
    childhood 302.6
Psychosis 298.9
    acute hysterical 298.1
    affecting management of pregnancy, childbirth, or puerperium 648.4 ☑
    affective (see also Disorder, mood) 296.90

> Note — Use the following fifth-digit subclassification with categories 296.0–296.6:
>
> 0   unspecified
>
> 1   mild
>
> 2   moderate
>
> 3   severe, without mention of psychotic behavior
>
> 4   severe, specified as with psychotic behavior
>
> 5   in partial or unspecified remission
>
> 6   in full remission

    drug-induced 292.84
    due to or associated with physical condition 293.83
    involutional 293.83
        recurrent episode 296.3 ☑
        single episode 296.2 ☑
    manic-depressive 296.80
        circular (alternating) 296.7
            currently depressed 296.5 ☑
            currently manic 296.4 ☑
        depressed type 296.2 ☑
            atypical 296.82
            recurrent episode 296.3 ☑
            single episode 296.2 ☑
        manic 296.0 ☑
            atypical 296.81
            recurrent episode 296.1 ☑
            single episode 296.0 ☑
        mixed type NEC 296.89
        specified type NEC 296.89
    senile 290.21
    specified type NEC 296.99
    alcoholic 291.9
        with
            anxiety 291.89
            delirium tremens 291.0
            delusions 291.5
            dementia 291.2
            hallucinosis 291.3
            jealousy 291.5
            mood disturbance 291.89
            paranoia 291.5
            persisting amnesia 291.1
            sexual dysfunction 291.89

Psychosis — continued
    alcoholic — continued
        with — continued
            sleep disturbance 291.89
        amnestic confabulatory 291.1
        delirium tremens 291.0
        hallucinosis 291.3
        Korsakoff's, Korsakov's, Korsakow's 291.1
        paranoid type 291.5
        pathological intoxication 291.4
        polyneuritic 291.1
        specified type NEC 291.89
    alternating (see also Psychosis, manic-depressive, circular) 296.7
    anergastic (see also Psychosis, organic) 294.9
    arteriosclerotic 290.40
        with
            acute confusional state 290.41
            delirium 290.41
            delusions 290.42
            depressed mood 290.43
        depressed type 290.43
        paranoid type 290.42
        simple type 290.40
        uncomplicated 290.40
    atypical 298.9
        depressive 296.82
        manic 296.81
    borderline (schizophrenia) (see also Schizophrenia) 295.5 ☑
        of childhood (see also Psychosis, childhood) 299.8 ☑
        prepubertal 299.8 ☑
    brief reactive 298.8
    childhood, with origin specific to 299.9 ☑

> Note — Use the following fifth-digit subclassification with category 299:
>
> 0   current or active state
>
> 1   residual state

        atypical 299.8 ☑
        specified type NEC 299.8 ☑
    circular (see also Psychosis, manic-depressive, circular) 296.7
    climacteric (see also Psychosis, involutional) 298.8
    confusional 298.9
        acute 293.0
        reactive 298.2
        subacute 293.1
    depressive (see also Psychosis, affective) 296.2 ☑
        atypical 296.82
        involutional 296.2 ☑
            with hypomania (bipolar II) 296.89
            recurrent episode 296.3 ☑
            single episode 296.2 ☑
        psychogenic 298.0
        reactive (emotional stress) (psychological trauma) 298.0
        recurrent episode 296.3 ☑
            with hypomania (bipolar II) 296.89
        single episode 296.2 ☑
    disintegrative, childhood (see also Psychosis, childhood) 299.1 ☑
    drug 292.9
        with
            affective syndrome 292.84
            amnestic syndrome 292.83
            anxiety 292.89
            delirium 292.81
                 withdrawal 292.0
            delusions 292.11
            dementia 292.82
            depressive state 292.84
            hallucinations 292.12
            hallucinosis 292.12
            mood disorder 292.84
            mood disturbance 292.84
            organic personality syndrome NEC 292.89
            sexual dysfunction 292.89
            sleep disturbance 292.89
            withdrawal syndrome (and delirium) 292.0

☑ **Additional Digit Required** — Refer to the Tabular List for Digit Selection   ▽ **Subterms under main terms may continue to next column or page**

Psychosis — continued
  drug — continued
    affective syndrome 292.84
    delusions 292.11
    hallucinatory state 292.12
    hallucinosis 292.12
    paranoid state 292.11
    specified type NEC 292.89
    withdrawal syndrome (and delirium) 292.0
  due to or associated with physical condition (see also Psychosis, organic) 293.9
  epileptic NEC 293.9
  excitation (psychogenic) (reactive) 298.1
  exhaustive (see also Reaction, stress, acute) 308.9
  hypomanic (see also Psychosis, affective) 296.0 ☑
    recurrent episode 296.1 ☑
    single episode 296.0 ☑
  hysterical 298.8
    acute 298.1
  in
    conditions classified elsewhere
      with
        delusions 293.81
        hallucinations 293.82
    pregnancy, childbirth, or puerperium 648.4 ☑
  incipient 298.8
    schizophrenic (see also Schizophrenia) 295.5 ☑
  induced 297.3
  infantile (see also Psychosis, childhood) 299.0 ☑
  infective 293.9
    acute 293.0
    subacute 293.1
  interactional (childhood) (see also Psychosis, childhood) 299.1 ☑
  involutional 298.8
    depressive (see also Psychosis, affective) 296.2 ☑
      recurrent episode 296.3 ☑
      single episode 296.2 ☑
    melancholic 296.2 ☑
      recurrent episode 296.3 ☑
      single episode 296.2 ☑
    paranoid state 297.2
    paraphrenia 297.2
  Korsakoff's, Korakov's, Korsakow's (nonalcoholic) 294.0
    alcoholic 291.1
  mania (phase) (see also Psychosis, affective) 296.0 ☑
    recurrent episode 296.1 ☑
    single episode 296.0 ☑
  manic (see also Psychosis, affective) 296.0 ☑
    atypical 296.81
    recurrent episode 296.1 ☑
    single episode 296.0 ☑
  manic-depressive 296.80
    circular 296.7
      currently
        depressed 296.5 ☑
        manic 296.4 ☑
        mixed 296.6 ☑
    depressive 296.2 ☑
      recurrent episode 296.3 ☑
        with hypomania (bipolar II) 296.89
      single episode 296.2 ☑
    hypomanic 296.0 ☑
      recurrent episode 296.1 ☑
      single episode 296.0 ☑
    manic 296.0 ☑
      atypical 296.81
      recurrent episode 296.1 ☑
      single episode 296.0 ☑
    mixed NEC 296.89
    perplexed 296.89
    stuporous 296.89
  menopausal (see also Psychosis, involutional) 298.8

Psychosis — continued
  mixed schizophrenic and affective (see also Schizophrenia) 295.7 ☑
  multi-infarct (cerebrovascular) (see also Psychosis, arteriosclerotic) 290.40
  organic NEC 294.9
    due to or associated with
      addiction
        alcohol (see also Psychosis, alcoholic) 291.9
        drug (see also Psychosis, drug) 292.9
      alcohol intoxication, acute (see also Psychosis, alcoholic) 291.9
      alcoholism (see also Psychosis, alcoholic) 291.9
      arteriosclerosis (cerebral) (see also Psychosis, arteriosclerotic) 290.40
      cerebrovascular disease
        acute (psychosis) 293.0
        arteriosclerotic (see also Psychosis, arteriosclerotic) 290.40
      childbirth — see Psychosis, puerperal
      dependence
        alcohol (see also Psychosis, alcoholic) 291.9
        drug 292.9
      disease
        alcoholic liver (see also Psychosis, alcoholic) 291.9
        brain
          arteriosclerotic (see also Psychosis, arteriosclerotic) 290.40
          cerebrovascular
            acute (psychosis) 293.0
            arteriosclerotic (see also Psychosis, arteriosclerotic) 290.40
        endocrine or metabolic 293.9
          acute (psychosis) 293.0
          subacute (psychosis) 293.1
        Jakob-Creutzfeldt 046.19
          with behavioral disturbance 046.19 [294.11]
          without behavioral disturbance 046.19 [294.10]
          familial 046.19
          iatrogenic 046.19
          specified NEC 046.19
          sporadic 046.19
          variant 046.11
            with dementia
              with behavioral disturbance 046.11 [294.11]
              without behavioral disturbance 046.11 [294.10]
        liver, alcoholic (see also Psychosis, alcoholic) 291.9
      disorder
        cerebrovascular
          acute (psychosis) 293.0
        endocrine or metabolic 293.9
          acute (psychosis) 293.0
          subacute (psychosis) 293.1
      epilepsy
        with behavioral disturbance 345.9 ☑ [294.11]
        without behavioral disturbance 345.9 ☑ [294.10]
        transient (acute) 293.0
      Huntington's chorea
        with behavioral disturbance 333.4 [294.11]
        without behavioral disturbance 333.4 [294.10]
      infection
        brain 293.9
          acute (psychosis) 293.0
          chronic 294.8
          subacute (psychosis) 293.1
        intracranial NEC 293.9

Psychosis — continued
  organic — continued
    due to or associated with — continued
      infection — continued
        intracranial — continued
          acute (psychosis) 293.0
          chronic 294.8
          subacute (psychosis) 293.1
      intoxication
        alcoholic (acute) (see also Psychosis, alcoholic) 291.9
        pathological 291.4
        drug (see also Psychosis, drug) 292.9
      ischemia
        cerebrovascular (generalized) (see also Psychosis, arteriosclerotic) 290.40
      Jakob-Creutzfeldt disease (syndrome) 046.19
        with behavioral disturbance 046.19 [294.11]
        without behavioral disturbance 046.19 [294.10]
        variant 046.11
          with dementia
            with behavioral disturbance 046.11 [294.11]
            without behavioral disturbance 046.11 [294.10]
      multiple sclerosis
        with behavioral disturbance 340 [294.11]
        without behavioral disturbance 340 [294.10]
      physical condition NEC 293.9
        with
          delusions 293.81
          hallucinations 293.82
      presenility 290.10
      puerperium — see Psychosis, puerperal
      sclerosis, multiple
        with behavioral disturbance 340 [294.11]
        without behavioral disturbance 340 [294.10]
      senility 290.20
      status epilepticus
        with behavioral disturbance 345.3 [294.11]
        without behavioral disturbance 345.3 [294.10]
      trauma
        brain (birth) (from electrical current) (surgical) 293.9
        acute (psychosis) 293.0
        chronic 294.8
        subacute (psychosis) 293.1
      unspecified physical condition 293.9
        with
          delusion 293.81
          hallucinations 293.82
    infective 293.9
      acute (psychosis) 293.0
      subacute 293.1
    posttraumatic 293.9
      acute 293.0
      subacute 293.1
    specified type NEC 294.8
    transient 293.9
      with
        anxiety 293.84
        delusions 293.81
        depression 293.83
        hallucinations 293.82
      depressive type 293.83
      hallucinatory type 293.82
      paranoid type 293.81
      specified type NEC 293.89
  paranoic 297.1
  paranoid (chronic) 297.9

Psychosis — continued
  paranoid — continued
    alcoholic 291.5
    chronic 297.1
    climacteric 297.2
    involutional 297.2
    menopausal 297.2
    protracted reactive 298.4
    psychogenic 298.4
      acute 298.3
    schizophrenic (see also Schizophrenia) 295.3 ☑
    senile 290.20
    paroxysmal 298.9
    senile 290.20
  polyneuritic, alcoholic 291.1
  postoperative 293.9
  postpartum — see Psychosis, puerperal
  prepsychotic (see also Schizophrenia) 295.5 ☑
  presbyophrenic (type) 290.8
  presenile (see also Dementia, presenile) 290.10
  prison 300.16
  psychogenic 298.8
    depressive 298.0
    paranoid 298.4
      acute 298.3
  puerperal
    specified type — see categories 295-298 ☑
    unspecified type 293.89
      acute 293.0
      chronic 293.89
      subacute 293.1
  reactive (emotional stress) (psychological trauma) 298.8
    brief 298.8
    confusion 298.2
    depressive 298.0
    excitation 298.1
  schizo-affective (depressed) (excited) (see also Schizophrenia) 295.7 ☑
  schizophrenia, schizophrenic (see also Schizophrenia) 295.9 ☑
    borderline type 295.5 ☑
      of childhood (see also Psychosis, childhood) 299.8 ☑
    catatonic (excited) (withdrawn) 295.2 ☑
    childhood type (see also Psychosis, childhood) 299.9 ☑
    hebephrenic 295.1 ☑
    incipient 295.5 ☑
    latent 295.5 ☑
    paranoid 295.3 ☑
    prepsychotic 295.5 ☑
    prodromal 295.5 ☑
    pseudoneurotic 295.5 ☑
    pseudopsychopathic 295.5 ☑
    schizophreniform 295.4 ☑
    simple 295.0 ☑
    undifferentiated type 295.9 ☑
  schizophreniform 295.4 ☑
  senile NEC 290.20
    with
      delusional features 290.20
      depressive features 290.21
    depressed type 290.21
    paranoid type 290.20
    simple deterioration 290.20
    specified type — see categories 295-298 ☑
  shared 297.3
  situational (reactive) 298.8
  symbiotic (childhood) (see also Psychosis, childhood) 299.1 ☑
  toxic (acute) 293.9
Psychotic — see also condition 298.9
  episode 298.9
    due to or associated with physical conditions (see also Psychosis, organic) 293.9
Pterygium (eye) 372.40
  central 372.43
  colli 744.5

☑ **Additional Digit Required** — Refer to the Tabular List for Digit Selection

▼ **Subterms under main terms may continue to next column or page**

Pterygium — *continued*
  double 372.44
  peripheral (stationary) 372.41
    progressive 372.42
  recurrent 372.45
Ptilosis 374.55
PTLD (post-transplant lymphoproliferative disorder) 238.77
Ptomaine (poisoning) — *see also* Poisoning, food 005.9
Ptosis (adiposa) 374.30
  breast 611.81
  cecum 569.89
  colon 569.89
  congenital (eyelid) 743.61
    specified site NEC — *see* Anomaly, specified type NEC
  epicanthus syndrome 270.2
  eyelid 374.30
    congenital 743.61
    mechanical 374.33
    myogenic 374.32
    paralytic 374.31
  gastric 537.5
  intestine 569.89
  kidney (*see also* Disease, renal) 593.0
    congenital 753.3
  liver 573.8
  renal (*see also* Disease, renal) 593.0
    congenital 753.3
  splanchnic 569.89
  spleen 289.59
  stomach 537.5
  viscera 569.89
PTP (posttransfusion purpura) 287.41
PTSD (Post-traumatic stress disorder) 309.81
Ptyalism 527.7
  hysterical 300.11
  periodic 527.2
  pregnancy 646.8 ✓
  psychogenic 306.4
Ptyalolithiasis 527.5
Pubalgia 848.8
Pubarche, precocious 259.1
Pubertas praecox 259.1
Puberty V21.1
  abnormal 259.9
  bleeding 626.3
  delayed 259.0
  precocious (constitutional) (cryptogenic) (idiopathic) NEC 259.1
    due to
      adrenal
        cortical hyperfunction 255.2
        hyperplasia 255.2
      cortical hyperfunction 255.2
      ovarian hyperfunction 256.1
        estrogen 256.0
      pineal tumor 259.8
      testicular hyperfunction 257.0
  premature 259.1
    due to
      adrenal cortical hyperfunction 255.2
      pineal tumor 259.8
      pituitary (anterior) hyperfunction 253.1
Puckering, macula 362.56
Pudenda, pudendum — *see* condition
Puente's disease (simple glandular cheilitis) 528.5
Puerperal
  abscess
    areola 675.1 ✓
    Bartholin's gland 646.6 ✓
    breast 675.1 ✓
    cervix (uteri) 670.8 ✓
    fallopian tube 670.8 ✓
    genital organ 670.8 ✓
    kidney 646.6 ✓
    mammary 675.1 ✓
    mesosalpinx 670.8 ✓
    nabothian 646.6 ✓
    nipple 675.0 ✓
    ovary, ovarian 670.8 ✓
    oviduct 670.8 ✓
    parametric 670.8 ✓

Puerperal — *continued*
  abscess — *continued*
    para-uterine 670.8 ✓
    pelvic 670.8 ✓
    perimetric 670.8 ✓
    periuterine 670.8 ✓
    retro-uterine 670.8 ✓
    subareolar 675.1 ✓
    suprapelvic 670.8 ✓
    tubal (ruptured) 670.8 ✓
    tubo-ovarian 670.8 ✓
    urinary tract NEC 646.6 ✓
    uterine, uterus 670.8 ✓
    vagina (wall) 646.6 ✓
    vaginorectal 646.6 ✓
    vulvovaginal gland 646.6 ✓
  accident 674.9 ✓
  adnexitis 670.8 ✓
  afibrinogenemia, or other coagulation defect 666.3 ✓
  albuminuria (acute) (subacute) 646.2 ✓
    pre-eclamptic 642.4 ✓
  anemia (conditions classifiable to 280–285) 648.2 ✓
  anuria 669.3 ✓
  apoplexy 674.0 ✓
  asymptomatic bacteriuria 646.5 ✓
  atrophy, breast 676.3 ✓
  blood dyscrasia 666.3 ✓
  caked breast 676.2 ✓
  cardiomyopathy 674.5 ✓
  cellulitis — *see* Puerperal, abscess
  cerebrovascular disorder (conditions classifiable to 430–434, 436–437) 674.0 ✓
  cervicitis (conditions classifiable to 616.0) 646.6 ✓
  coagulopathy (any) 666.3 ✓
  complications 674.9 ✓
    specified type NEC 674.8 ✓
  convulsions (eclamptic) (uremic) 642.6 ✓
    with pre-existing hypertension 642.7 ✓
  cracked nipple 676.1 ✓
  cystitis 646.6 ✓
  cystopyelitis 646.6 ✓
  deciduitis (acute) 670.8 ✓
  delirium NEC 293.9
  diabetes (mellitus) (conditions classifiable to 249 and 250) 648.0 ✓
  disease 674.9 ✓
    breast NEC 676.3 ✓
    cerebrovascular (acute) 674.0 ✓
    nonobstetric NEC (*see also* Pregnancy, complicated, current disease or condition) 648.9 ✓
    pelvis inflammatory 670.8 ✓
    renal NEC 646.2 ✓
    tubo-ovarian 670.8 ✓
    Valsuani's (progressive pernicious anemia) 648.2 ✓
  disorder
    lactation 676.9 ✓
      specified type NEC 676.8 ✓
    nonobstetric NEC (*see also* Pregnancy, complicated, current disease or condition) 648.9 ✓
  disruption
    cesarean wound 674.1 ✓
    episiotomy wound 674.2 ✓
    perineal laceration wound 674.2 ✓
  drug dependence (conditions classifiable to 304) 648.3 ✓
  eclampsia 642.6 ✓
    with pre-existing hypertension 642.7 ✓
  embolism (pulmonary) 673.2 ✓
    air 673.0 ✓
    amniotic fluid 673.1 ✓
    blood-clot 673.2 ✓
    brain or cerebral 674.0 ✓
    cardiac 674.8 ✓
    fat 673.8 ✓
    intracranial sinus (venous) 671.5 ✓
    pyemic 673.3 ✓
    septic 673.3 ✓
    spinal cord 671.5 ✓

Puerperal — *continued*
  endometritis (conditions classifiable to 615.0–615.9) 670.1 ✓
  endophlebitis — *see* Puerperal, phlebitis
  endotrachelitis 646.6 ✓
  engorgement, breasts 676.2 ✓
  erysipelas 670.8 ✓
  failure
    lactation 676.4 ✓
    renal, acute 669.3 ✓
  fever 672 ✓
    meaning pyrexia (of unknown origin) 672.0 ✓
    meaning sepsis 670.2 ✓
  fissure, nipple 676.1 ✓
  fistula
    breast 675.1 ✓
    mammary gland 675.1 ✓
    nipple 675.0 ✓
  galactophoritis 675.2 ✓
  galactorrhea 676.6 ✓
  gangrene
    gas 670.8 ✓
      with sepsis 670.2 ✓
    uterus 670.8 ✓
  gonorrhea (conditions classifiable to 098) 647.1 ✓
  hematoma, subdural 674.0 ✓
  hematosalpinx, infectional 670.8 ✓
  hemiplegia, cerebral 674.0 ✓
  hemorrhage 666.1 ✓
    brain 674.0 ✓
    bulbar 674.0 ✓
    cerebellar 674.0 ✓
    cerebral 674.0 ✓
    cortical 674.0 ✓
    delayed (after 24 hours) (uterine) 666.2 ✓
    extradural 674.0 ✓
    internal capsule 674.0 ✓
    intracranial 674.0 ✓
    intrapontine 674.0 ✓
    meningeal 674.0 ✓
    pontine 674.0 ✓
    subarachnoid 674.0 ✓
    subcortical 674.0 ✓
    subdural 674.0 ✓
    uterine, delayed 666.2 ✓
    ventricular 674.0 ✓
  hemorrhoids 671.8 ✓
  hepatorenal syndrome 674.8 ✓
  hypertrophy
    breast 676.3 ✓
    mammary gland 676.3 ✓
  induration breast (fibrous) 676.3 ✓
  infarction
    lung — *see* Puerperal, embolism
    pulmonary — *see* Puerperal, embolism
  infection
    Bartholin's gland 646.6 ✓
    breast 675.2 ✓
      with nipple 675.9 ✓
        specified type NEC 675.8 ✓
    cervix 646.6 ✓
    endocervix 646.6 ✓
    fallopian tube 670.8 ✓
    generalized 670.0 ✓
    genital tract (major) 670.0 ✓
      minor or localized 646.6 ✓
    kidney (bacillus coli) 646.6 ✓
    mammary gland 675.2 ✓
      with nipple 675.9 ✓
        specified type NEC 675.8 ✓
    nipple 675.0 ✓
      with breast 675.9 ✓
        specified type NEC 675.8 ✓
    ovary 670.8 ✓
    pelvic 670.8 ✓
    peritoneum 670.8 ✓
    renal 646.6 ✓
    tubo-ovarian 670.8 ✓
    urinary (tract) NEC 646.6 ✓
      asymptomatic 646.5 ✓

Puerperal — *continued*
  infection — *continued*
    uterus, uterine 670.8 ✓
    vagina 646.6 ✓
  inflammation (*see also* Puerperal, infection)
    areola 675.1 ✓
    Bartholin's gland 646.6 ✓
    breast 675.2 ✓
    broad ligament 670.8 ✓
    cervix (uteri) 646.6 ✓
    fallopian tube 670.8 ✓
    genital organs 670.8 ✓
      localized 646.6 ✓
    mammary gland 675.2 ✓
    nipple 675.0 ✓
    ovary 670.8 ✓
    oviduct 670.8 ✓
    pelvis 670.8 ✓
    periuterine 670.8 ✓
    tubal 670.8 ✓
    vagina 646.6 ✓
    vein — *see* Puerperal, phlebitis
  inversion, nipple 676.3 ✓
  ischemia, cerebral 674.0 ✓
  lymphangitis 670.8 ✓
    breast 675.2 ✓
  malaria (conditions classifiable to 084) 647.4 ✓
  malnutrition 648.9 ✓
  mammillitis 675.0 ✓
  mammitis 675.2 ✓
  mania 296.0 ✓
    recurrent episode 296.1 ✓
    single episode 296.0 ✓
  mastitis 675.2 ✓
    purulent 675.1 ✓
    retromammary 675.1 ✓
    submammary 675.1 ✓
  melancholia 296.2 ✓
    recurrent episode 296.3 ✓
    single episode 296.2 ✓
  mental disorder (conditions classifiable to 290–303, 305.0, 305.2–305.9, 306–316, 317–319) 648.4 ✓
  metritis (suppurative) 670.1 ✓
    septic 670.2 ✓
  metroperitonitis 670.8 ✓
  metrorrhagia 666.2 ✓
  metrosalpingitis 670.8 ✓
  metrovaginitis 670.8 ✓
  milk leg 671.4 ✓
  monoplegia, cerebral 674.0 ✓
  necrosis
    kidney, tubular 669.3 ✓
    liver (acute) (subacute) (conditions classifiable to 570) 674.8 ✓
    ovary 670.8 ✓
    renal cortex 669.3 ✓
  nephritis or nephrosis (conditions classifiable to 580–589) 646.2 ✓
    with hypertension 642.1 ✓
  nutritional deficiency (conditions classifiable to 260–269) 648.9 ✓
  occlusion, precerebral artery 674.0 ✓
  oliguria 669.3 ✓
  oophoritis 670.8 ✓
  ovaritis 670.8 ✓
  paralysis
    bladder (sphincter) 665.5 ✓
    cerebral 674.0 ✓
  paralytic stroke 674.0 ✓
  parametritis 670.8 ✓
  paravaginitis 646.6 ✓
  pelviperitonitis 670.8 ✓
  perimetritis 670.8 ✓
  perimetrosalpingitis 670.8 ✓
  perinephritis 646.6 ✓
  perioophoritis 670.8 ✓
  periphlebitis — *see* Puerperal, phlebitis
  perisalpingitis 670.8 ✓
  peritoneal infection 670.8 ✓
  peritonitis (pelvic) 670.8 ✓
  perivaginitis 646.6 ✓

☑ **Additional Digit Required — Refer to the Tabular List for Digit Selection**   ▽ **Subterms under main terms may continue to next column or page**

2014 ICD-9-CM   287

Puerperal — *continued*
phlebitis 671.2 ☑
deep 671.4 ☑
intracranial sinus (venous) 671.5 ☑
pelvic 671.4 ☑
specified site NEC 671.5 ☑
superficial 671.2 ☑
phlegmasia alba dolens 671.4 ☑
placental polyp 674.4 ☑
pneumonia, embolic — *see* Puerperal, embolism
prediabetes 648.8 ☑
pre-eclampsia (mild) 642.4 ☑
with pre-existing hypertension 642.7 ☑
severe 642.5 ☑
psychosis, unspecified (*see also* Psychosis, puerperal) 293.89
pyelitis 646.6 ☑
pyelocystitis 646.6 ☑
pyelohydronephrosis 646.6 ☑
pyelonephritis 646.6 ☑
pyelonephrosis 646.6 ☑
pyemia 670.2 ☑
pyocystitis 646.6 ☑
pyometra 670.8 ☑
pyonephritis 646.6 ☑
pyonephrosis 646.6 ☑
pyo-oophoritis 670.8 ☑
pyosalpingitis 670.8 ☑
pyosalpinx 670.8 ☑
pyrexia (of unknown origin) 672.0 ☑
renal
disease NEC 646.2 ☑
failure, acute 669.3 ☑
retention
decidua (fragments) (with delayed hemorrhage) 666.2 ☑
without hemorrhage 667.1 ☑
placenta (fragments) (with delayed hemorrhage) 666.2 ☑
without hemorrhage 667.1 ☑
secundines (fragments) (with delayed hemorrhage) 666.2 ☑
without hemorrhage 667.1 ☑
retracted nipple 676.0 ☑
rubella (conditions classifiable to 056) 647.5 ☑
salpingitis 670.8 ☑
salpingo-oophoritis 670.8 ☑
salpingo-ovaritis 670.8 ☑
salpingoperitonitis 670.8 ☑
sapremia 670.2 ☑
secondary perineal tear 674.2 ☑
sepsis (pelvic) 670.2 ☑
septicemia 670.2 ☑
subinvolution (uterus) 674.8 ☑
sudden death (cause unknown) 674.9 ☑
suppuration — *see* Puerperal, abscess
syphilis (conditions classifiable to 090–097) 647.0 ☑
tetanus 670.8 ☑
thelitis 675.0 ☑
thrombocytopenia 666.3 ☑
thrombophlebitis (superficial) 671.2 ☑
deep 671.4 ☑
pelvic 671.4 ☑
septic 670.3 ☑
specified site NEC 671.5 ☑
thrombosis (venous) — *see* Thrombosis, puerperal
thyroid dysfunction (conditions classifiable to 240–246) 648.1 ☑
toxemia (*see also* Toxemia, of pregnancy) 642.4 ☑
eclamptic 642.6 ☑
with pre-existing hypertension 642.7 ☑
pre-eclamptic (mild) 642.4 ☑
with
convulsions 642.6 ☑
pre-existing hypertension 642.7 ☑
severe 642.5 ☑

Puerperal — *continued*
tuberculosis (conditions classifiable to 010–018) 647.3 ☑
uremia 669.3 ☑
vaginitis (conditions classifiable to 616.1) 646.6 ☑
varicose veins (legs) 671.0 ☑
vulva or perineum 671.1 ☑
venous complication 671.9 ☑
vulvitis (conditions classifiable to 616.1) 646.6 ☑
vulvovaginitis (conditions classifiable to 616.1) 646.6 ☑
white leg 671.4 ☑
Pulled muscle — *see* Sprain, by site
Pulmolithiasis 518.89
Pulmonary — *see* condition
Pulmonitis (unknown etiology) 486
Pulpitis (acute) (anachoretic) (chronic) (hyperplastic) (putrescent) (suppurative) (ulcerative) 522.0
Pulpless tooth 522.9
Pulse
alternating 427.89
psychogenic 306.2
bigeminal 427.89
fast 785.0
feeble, rapid, due to shock following injury 958.4
rapid 785.0
slow 427.89
strong 785.9
trigeminal 427.89
water-hammer (*see also* Insufficiency, aortic) 424.1
weak 785.9
Pulseless disease 446.7
Pulsus
alternans or trigeminy 427.89
psychogenic 306.2
Punch drunk 310.2
Puncta lacrimalia occlusion 375.52
Punctiform hymen 752.49
Puncture (traumatic) — *see also* Wound, open, by site
accidental, complicating surgery 998.2
bladder, nontraumatic 596.6
by
device, implant, or graft — *see* Complications, mechanical
foreign body
internal organs (*see also* Injury, internal, by site)
by ingested object — *see* Foreign body
left accidentally in operation wound 998.4
instrument (any) during a procedure, accidental 998.2
internal organs, abdomen, chest, or pelvis — *see* Injury, internal, by site
kidney, nontraumatic 593.89
Pupil — *see* condition
Pupillary membrane 364.74
persistent 743.46
Pupillotonia 379.46
pseudotabetic 379.46
Purpura 287.2
abdominal 287.0
allergic 287.0
anaphylactoid 287.0
annularis telangiectodes 709.1
arthritic 287.0
autoerythrocyte sensitization 287.2
autoimmune 287.0
bacterial 287.0
Bateman's (senile) 287.2
capillary fragility (hereditary) (idiopathic) 287.8
cryoglobulinemic 273.2
devil's pinches 287.2
fibrinolytic (*see also* Fibrinolysis) 286.6
fulminans, fulminous 286.6
gangrenous 287.0
hemorrhagic (*see also* Purpura, thrombocytopenic) 287.39

Purpura — *continued*
hemorrhagic (*see also* Purpura, thrombocytopenic) — *continued*
nodular 272.7
nonthrombocytopenic 287.0
thrombocytopenic 287.39
Henoch's (purpura nervosa) 287.0
Henoch-Schönlein (allergic) 287.0
hypergammaglobulinemic (benign primary) (Waldenström's) 273.0
idiopathic 287.31
nonthrombocytopenic 287.0
thrombocytopenic 287.31
immune thrombocytopenic 287.31
infectious 287.0
malignant 287.0
neonatorum 772.6
nervosa 287.0
newborn NEC 772.6
nonthrombocytopenic 287.2
hemorrhagic 287.0
idiopathic 287.0
nonthrombopenic 287.2
peliosis rheumatica 287.0
pigmentaria, progressiva 709.09
posttransfusion (PTP) 287.41
from whole blood (fresh) or blood products 287.41
primary 287.0
primitive 287.0
red cell membrane sensitivity 287.2
rheumatica 287.0
Schönlein (-Henoch) (allergic) 287.0
scorbutic 267
senile 287.2
simplex 287.2
symptomatica 287.0
telangiectasia annularis 709.1
thrombocytopenic (*see also* Thrombocytopenia) 287.30
congenital 287.33
essential 287.30
hereditary 287.31
idiopathic 287.31
immune 287.31
neonatal, transitory (*see also* Thrombocytopenia, neonatal transitory) 776.1
primary 287.30
puerperal, postpartum 666.3 ☑
thrombotic 446.6
thrombohemolytic (*see also* Fibrinolysis) 286.6
thrombopenic (*see also* Thrombocytopenia) 287.30
congenital 287.33
essential 287.30
thrombotic 446.6
thrombocytic 446.6
thrombocytopenic 446.6
toxic 287.0
variolosa 050.0
vascular 287.0
visceral symptoms 287.0
Werlhof's (*see also* Purpura, thrombocytopenic) 287.39
Purpuric spots 782.7
Purulent — *see* condition
Pus
absorption, general — *see* Septicemia
in
stool 792.1
urine 791.9
tube (rupture) (*see also* Salpingo-oophoritis) 614.2
Pustular rash 782.1
Pustule 686.9
malignant 022.0
nonmalignant 686.9
Putnam-Dana syndrome (subacute combined sclerosis with pernicious anemia) 281.0 *[336.2]*
Putnam's disease (subacute combined sclerosis with pernicious anemia) 281.0 *[336.2]*
Putrefaction, intestinal 569.89
Putrescent pulp (dental) 522.1

Pyarthritis — *see* Pyarthrosis
Pyarthrosis — *see also* Arthritis, pyogenic 711.0 ☑
tuberculous — *see* Tuberculosis, joint
Pycnoepilepsy, pycnolepsy (idiopathic) — *see also* Epilepsy 345.0 ☑
Pyelectasia 593.89
Pyelectasis 593.89
Pyelitis (congenital) (uremic) 590.80
with
abortion — *see* Abortion, by type, with specified complication NEC
contracted kidney 590.00
ectopic pregnancy (*see also* categories 633.0–633.9) 639.8
molar pregnancy (*see also* categories 630–632) 639.8
acute 590.10
with renal medullary necrosis 590.11
chronic 590.00
with
renal medullary necrosis 590.01
complicating pregnancy, childbirth, or puerperium 646.6 ☑
affecting fetus or newborn 760.1
cystica 590.3
following
abortion 639.8
ectopic or molar pregnancy 639.8
gonococcal 098.19
chronic or duration of 2 months or over 098.39
tuberculous (*see also* Tuberculosis) 016.0 ☑ *[590.81]*
Pyelocaliectasis 593.89
Pyelocystitis — *see also* Pyelitis 590.80
Pyelohydronephrosis 591
Pyelonephritis — *see also* Pyelitis 590.80
acute 590.10
with renal medullary necrosis 590.11
chronic 590.00
syphilitic (late) 095.4
tuberculous (*see also* Tuberculosis) 016.0 ☑ *[590.81]*
Pyelonephrosis — *see also* Pyelitis 590.80
chronic 590.00
Pyelophlebitis 451.89
Pyelo-ureteritis cystica 590.3
Pyemia, pyemic (purulent) — *see* Septicemia 038.9
abscess — *see* Abscess
arthritis (*see also* Arthritis, pyogenic) 711.0 ☑
Bacillus coli 038.42
embolism (*see also* Septicemia) 415.12
fever 038.9
infection 038.9
joint (*see also* Arthritis, pyogenic) 711.0 ☑
liver 572.1
meningococcal 036.2
newborn 771.81
phlebitis — *see* Phlebitis
pneumococcal 038.2
portal 572.1
postvaccinal 999.39
puerperal 670.2 ☑
specified organism NEC 038.8
staphylococcal 038.10
aureus 038.11
methicillin
resistant 038.12
susceptible 038.11
specified organism NEC 038.19
streptococcal 038.0
tuberculous — *see* Tuberculosis, miliary
Pygopagus 759.4
Pykno-epilepsy, pyknolepsy (idiopathic) — *see also* Epilepsy 345.0 ☑
Pyle (-Cohn) disease (craniometaphyseal dysplasia) 756.89
Pylephlebitis (suppurative) 572.1
Pylethrombophlebitis 572.1
Pylethrombosis 572.1
Pyloritis — *see also* Gastritis 535.5 ☑
Pylorospasm (reflex) 537.81
congenital or infantile 750.5

☑ **Additional Digit Required** — Refer to the Tabular List for Digit Selection

▽ **Subterms under main terms may continue to next column or page**

Pylorospasm — *continued*
neurotic 306.4
newborn 750.5
psychogenic 306.4
Pylorus, pyloric — *see* condition
Pyoarthrosis — *see* Pyarthrosis
Pyocele
mastoid 383.00
sinus (accessory) (nasal) (*see also* Sinusitis) 473.9
turbinate (bone) 473.9
urethra (*see also* Urethritis) 597.0
Pyococcal dermatitis 686.00
Pyococcide, skin 686.00
Pyocolpos — *see also* Vaginitis 616.10
Pyocyaneus dermatitis 686.09
Pyocystitis — *see also* Cystitis 595.9
Pyoderma, pyodermia 686.00
gangrenosum 686.01
specified type NEC 686.09
vegetans 686.8
Pyodermatitis 686.00
vegetans 686.8
Pyogenic — *see* condition
Pyohemia — *see* Septicemia
Pyohydronephrosis — *see also* Pyelitis 590.80
Pyometra 615.9
Pyometritis — *see also* Endometritis 615.9
Pyometrium — *see also* Endometritis 615.9
Pyomyositis 728.0
ossificans 728.19
tropical (bungpagga) 040.81
Pyonephritis — *see also* Pyelitis 590.80
chronic 590.00
Pyonephrosis (congenital) — *see also* Pyelitis 590.80
acute 590.10
Pyo-oophoritis — *see also* Salpingo-oophoritis 614.2
Pyo-ovarium — *see also* Salpingo-oophoritis 614.2
Pyopericarditis 420.99
Pyopericardium 420.99
Pyophlebitis — *see* Phlebitis
Pyopneumopericardium 420.99
Pyopneumothorax (infectional) 510.9
with fistula 510.0
subdiaphragmatic (*see also* Peritonitis) 567.29
subphrenic (*see also* Peritonitis) 567.29
tuberculous (*see also* Tuberculosis, pleura) 012.0 ☑
Pyorrhea (alveolar) (alveolaris) 523.40
degenerative 523.5
Pyosalpingitis — *see also* Salpingo-oophoritis 614.2
Pyosalpinx — *see also* Salpingo-oophoritis 614.2
Pyosepticemia — *see* Septicemia
Pyosis
Corlett's (impetigo) 684
Manson's (pemphigus contagiosus) 684
Pyothorax 510.9
with fistula 510.0
tuberculous (*see also* Tuberculosis, pleura) 012.0 ☑
Pyoureter 593.89
tuberculous (*see also* Tuberculosis) 016.2 ☑
Pyramidopallidonigral syndrome 332.0
Pyrexia (of unknown origin) (P.U.O.) 780.60
atmospheric 992.0
during labor 659.2 ☑
environmentally-induced newborn 778.4
heat 992.0
newborn, environmentally-induced 778.4
puerperal 672.0 ☑
Pyroglobulinemia 273.8
Pyromania 312.33
Pyrosis 787.1
Pyrroloporphyria 277.1
Pyuria (bacterial) 791.9

Q

Q fever 083.0
with pneumonia 083.0 [484.8]
Quadricuspid aortic valve 746.89

Quadrilateral fever 083.0
Quadriparesis — *see* Quadriplegia
meaning muscle weakness 728.87
Quadriplegia 344.00
with fracture, vertebra (process) — *see* Fracture, vertebra, cervical, with spinal cord injury
brain (current episode) 437.8
C1-C4
complete 344.01
incomplete 344.02
C5-C7
complete 344.03
incomplete 344.04
cerebral (current episode) 437.8
congenital or infantile (cerebral) (spastic) (spinal) 343.2
cortical 437.8
embolic (current episode) (*see also* Embolism, brain) 434.1 ☑
functional 780.72
infantile (cerebral) (spastic) (spinal) 343.2
newborn NEC 767.0
specified NEC 344.00
thrombotic (current episode) (*see also* Thrombosis, brain) 434.0 ☑
traumatic — *see* Injury, spinal, cervical
Quadruplet
affected by maternal complications of pregnancy 761.5
healthy liveborn — *see* Newborn, multiple
pregnancy (complicating delivery) NEC 651.8 ☑
with fetal loss and retention of one or more fetus(es) 651.5 ☑
following (elective) fetal reduction 651.7 ☑
Quarrelsomeness 301.3
Quartan
fever 084.2
malaria (fever) 084.2
Queensland fever 083.0
coastal 083.0
seven-day 100.89
Quervain's disease 727.04
thyroid (subacute granulomatous thyroiditis) 245.1
Queyrat's erythroplasia (M8080/2)
specified site — *see* Neoplasm, skin, in situ
unspecified site 233.5
Quincke's disease or edema — *see* Edema, angioneurotic
Quinquaud's disease (acne decalvans) 704.09
Quinsy (gangrenous) 475
Quintan fever 083.1
Quintuplet
affected by maternal complications of pregnancy 761.5
healthy liveborn — *see* Newborn, multiple
pregnancy (complicating delivery) NEC 651.2 ☑
with fetal loss and retention of one or more fetus(es) 651.6 ☑
following (elective) fetal reduction 651.7 ☑
Quotidian
fever 084.0
malaria (fever) 084.0

R

Rabbia 071
Rabbit fever — *see also* Tularemia 021.9
Rabies 071
contact V01.5
exposure to V01.5
inoculation V04.5
reaction — *see* Complications, vaccination
vaccination, prophylactic (against) V04.5
Rachischisis — *see also* Spina bifida 741.9 ☑
Rachitic — *see also* condition
deformities of spine 268.1
pelvis 268.1
with disproportion (fetopelvic) 653.2 ☑
affecting fetus or newborn 763.1

Rachitic — *see also* condition — *continued*
pelvis — *continued*
with disproportion — *continued*
causing obstructed labor 660.1 ☑
affecting fetus or newborn 763.1
Rachitis, rachitism — *see also* Rickets
acute 268.0
fetalis 756.4
renalis 588.0
tarda 268.0
Racket nail 757.5
Radial nerve — *see* condition
Radiation effects or sickness — *see also* Effect, adverse, radiation
cataract 366.46
dermatitis 692.82
sunburn (*see also* Sunburn) 692.71
Radiculitis (pressure) (vertebrogenic) 729.2
accessory nerve 723.4
anterior crural 724.4
arm 723.4
brachial 723.4
cervical NEC 723.4
due to displacement of intervertebral disc — *see* Neuritis, due to, displacement intervertebral disc
leg 724.4
lumbar NEC 724.4
lumbosacral 724.4
rheumatic 729.2
syphilitic 094.89
thoracic (with visceral pain) 724.4
Radiculomyelitis 357.0
toxic, due to
Clostridium tetani 037
Corynebacterium diphtheriae 032.89
Radiculopathy — *see also* Radiculitis 729.2
Radioactive substances, adverse effect — *see* Effect, adverse, radioactive substance
Radiodermal burns (acute) (chronic) (occupational) — *see* Burn, by site
Radiodermatitis 692.82
Radionecrosis — *see* Effect, adverse, radiation
Radiotherapy session V58.0
Radium, adverse effect — *see* Effect, adverse, radioactive substance
Raeder-Harbitz syndrome (pulseless disease) 446.7
Rage — *see also* Disturbance, conduct 312.0 ☑
meaning rabies 071
Rag sorters' disease 022.1
Raillietiniasis 123.8
Railroad neurosis 300.16
Railway spine 300.16
Raised — *see* Elevation
Raiva 071
Rake teeth, tooth 524.39
Rales 786.7
Ramifying renal pelvis 753.3
Ramsay Hunt syndrome (herpetic geniculate ganglionitis) 053.11
meaning dyssynergia cerebellaris myoclonica 334.2
Ranke's primary infiltration — *see also* Tuberculosis 010.0 ☑
Ranula 527.6
congenital 750.26
Rape
adult 995.83
alleged, observation or examination V71.5
child 995.53
Rapid
feeble pulse, due to shock, following injury 958.4
heart (beat) 785.0
psychogenic 306.2
respiration 786.06
psychogenic 306.1
second stage (delivery) 661.3 ☑
affecting fetus or newborn 763.6
time-zone change syndrome 327.35
Rarefaction, bone 733.99
Rash 782.1
canker 034.1
diaper 691.0
drug (internal use) 693.0

Rash — *continued*
drug — *continued*
contact 692.3
ECHO 9 virus 078.89
enema 692.89
food (*see also* Allergy, food) 693.1
heat 705.1
napkin 691.0
nettle 708.8
pustular 782.1
rose 782.1
epidemic 056.9
of infants 057.8
scarlet 034.1
serum (prophylactic) (therapeutic) 999.59
toxic 782.1
wandering tongue 529.1
Rasmussen's aneurysm — *see also* Tuberculosis 011.2 ☑
Rat-bite fever 026.9
due to Streptobacillus moniliformis 026.1
spirochetal (morsus muris) 026.0
Rathke's pouch tumor (M9350/1) 237.0
Raymond (-Céstan) syndrome 433.8 ☑
Raynaud's
disease or syndrome (paroxysmal digital cyanosis) 443.0
gangrene (symmetric) 443.0 [785.4]
phenomenon (paroxysmal digital cyanosis) (secondary) 443.0
RDS 769
Reaction
acute situational maladjustment (*see also* Reaction, adjustment) 309.9
adaptation (*see also* Reaction, adjustment) 309.9
adjustment 309.9
with
anxious mood 309.24
with depressed mood 309.28
conduct disturbance 309.3
combined with disturbance of emotions 309.4
depressed mood 309.0
brief 309.0
with anxious mood 309.28
prolonged 309.1
elective mutism 309.83
mixed emotions and conduct 309.4
mutism, elective 309.83
physical symptoms 309.82
predominant disturbance (of)
conduct 309.3
emotions NEC 309.29
mixed 309.28
mixed, emotions and conduct 309.4
specified type NEC 309.89
specific academic or work inhibition 309.23
withdrawal 309.83
depressive 309.0
with conduct disturbance 309.4
brief 309.0
prolonged 309.1
specified type NEC 309.89
adverse food NEC 995.7
affective (*see also* Psychosis, affective) 296.90
specified type NEC 296.99
aggressive 301.3
unsocialized (*see also* Disturbance, conduct) 312.0 ☑
allergic (*see also* Allergy) 995.3
drug, medicinal substance, and biological — *see* Allergy, drug
due to correct medical substance properly administered 995.27
food — *see* Allergy, food
serum 999.59
anaphylactic — *see* Anaphylactic reaction
anesthesia — *see* Anesthesia, complication
anger 312.0 ☑
antisocial 301.7
antitoxin (prophylactic) (therapeutic) — *see* Complications, vaccination

Pylorospasm — Reaction

Reaction — *continued*
- anxiety 300.00
- Arthus 995.21
- asthenic 300.5
- compulsive 300.3
- conversion (anesthetic) (autonomic) (hyperkinetic) (mixed paralytic) (paresthetic) 300.11
- deoxyribonuclease (DNA) (DNase) hypersensitivity NEC 287.2
- depressive 300.4
    - acute 309.0
    - affective (*see also* Psychosis, affective) 296.2 ☑
        - recurrent episode 296.3 ☑
        - single episode 296.2 ☑
    - brief 309.0
    - manic (*see also* Psychosis, affective) 296.80
    - neurotic 300.4
    - psychoneurotic 300.4
    - psychotic 298.0
- dissociative 300.15
- drug NEC (*see also* Table of Drugs and Chemicals) 995.20
    - allergic (*see also* Allergy, drug) 995.27
    - correct substance properly administered 995.20
    - obstetric anesthetic or analgesic NEC 668.9 ☑
        - affecting fetus or newborn 763.5
        - specified drug — *see* Table of Drugs and Chemicals
    - overdose or poisoning 977.9
        - specified drug — *see* Table of Drugs and Chemicals
    - specific to newborn 779.4
    - transmitted via placenta or breast milk — *see* Absorption, drug, through placenta
    - withdrawal NEC 292.0
        - infant of dependent mother 779.5
    - wrong substance given or taken in error 977.9
        - specified drug — *see* Table of Drugs and Chemicals
- dyssocial 301.7
- dystonic, acute, due to drugs 333.72
- erysipeloid 027.1
- fear 300.20
    - child 313.0
- fluid loss, cerebrospinal 349.0
- food (*see also* Allergy, food)
    - adverse NEC 995.7
    - anaphylactic shock — *see* Anaphylactic reaction or shock, due to, food
- foreign
    - body NEC 728.82
        - in operative wound (inadvertently left) 998.4
            - due to surgical material intentionally left — *see* Complications, due to (presence of) any device, implant, or graft classified to 996.0–996.5 NEC
        - substance accidentally left during a procedure (chemical) (powder) (talc) 998.7
        - body or object (instrument) (sponge) (swab) 998.4
- graft-versus-host (GVH) 279.50
- grief (acute) (brief) 309.0
    - prolonged 309.1
- gross stress (*see also* Reaction, stress, acute) 308.9
- group delinquent (*see also* Disturbance, conduct) 312.2 ☑
- Herxheimer's 995.91
- hyperkinetic (*see also* Hyperkinesia) 314.9
- hypochondriacal 300.7
- hypoglycemic, due to insulin 251.0
    - therapeutic misadventure 962.3
- hypomanic (*see also* Psychosis, affective) 296.0 ☑
    - recurrent episode 296.1 ☑

Reaction — *continued*
- hypomanic (*see also* Psychosis, affective) — *continued*
    - single episode 296.0 ☑
- hysterical 300.10
    - conversion type 300.11
    - dissociative 300.15
- id (bacterial cause) 692.89
- immaturity NEC 301.89
    - aggressive 301.3
    - emotional instability 301.59
- immunization — *see* Complications, vaccination
- incompatibility
    - blood group (*see also* Complications, transfusion) 999.80
        - ABO (due to transfusion of blood or blood products) (*see also* Complications, transfusion) 999.60
        - minor blood group 999.89
        - non-ABO — *see also* Complications, transfusion 999.75
        - Rh antigen (C) (c) (D) (E) (e) (factor) (infusion) (transfusion) (*see also* Complications, transfusion) 999.70
- inflammatory — *see* Infection
- infusion — *see* Complications, infusion
- inoculation (immune serum) — *see* Complications, vaccination
- insulin 995.23
- involutional
    - paranoid 297.2
    - psychotic (*see also* Psychosis, affective, depressive) 296.2 ☑
- leukemoid (basophilic) (lymphocytic) (monocytic) (myelocytic) (neutrophilic) 288.62
- LSD (*see also* Abuse, drugs, nondependent) 305.3 ☑
- lumbar puncture 349.0
- manic-depressive (*see also* Psychosis, affective) 296.80
    - depressed 296.2 ☑
        - recurrent episode 296.3 ☑
        - single episode 296.2 ☑
    - hypomanic 296.0 ☑
- neurasthenic 300.5
- neurogenic (*see also* Neurosis) 300.9
- neurotic-depressive 300.4
- neurotic NEC 300.9
- nitritoid — *see* Crisis, nitritoid
- nonspecific
    - to
        - cell mediated immunity measurement of gamma interferon antigen response without active tuberculosis 795.52
        - QuantiFERON-TB test (QFT) without active tuberculosis 795.52
        - tuberculin test (*see also* Reaction, tuberculin skin test) 795.51
- obsessive compulsive 300.3
- organic 293.9
    - acute 293.0
    - subacute 293.1
- overanxious, child or adolescent 313.0
- paranoid (chronic) 297.9
    - acute 298.3
    - climacteric 297.2
    - involutional 297.2
    - menopausal 297.2
    - senile 290.20
    - simple 297.0
- passive
    - aggressive 301.84
    - dependency 301.6
- personality (*see also* Disorder, personality) 301.9
- phobic 300.20
- postradiation — *see* Effect, adverse, radiation
- psychogenic NEC 300.9
- psychoneurotic (*see also* Neurosis) 300.9
    - anxiety 300.00
    - compulsive 300.3

Reaction — *continued*
- psychoneurotic (*see also* Neurosis) — *continued*
    - conversion 300.11
    - depersonalization 300.6
    - depressive 300.4
    - dissociative 300.15
    - hypochondriacal 300.7
    - hysterical 300.10
        - conversion type 300.11
        - dissociative type 300.15
    - neurasthenic 300.5
    - obsessive 300.3
    - obsessive-compulsive 300.3
    - phobic 300.20
    - tension state 300.9
- psychophysiologic NEC (*see also* Disorder, psychosomatic) 306.9
    - cardiovascular 306.2
    - digestive 306.4
    - endocrine 306.6
    - gastrointestinal 306.4
    - genitourinary 306.50
    - heart 306.2
    - hemic 306.8
    - intestinal (large) (small) 306.4
    - laryngeal 306.1
    - lymphatic 306.8
    - musculoskeletal 306.0
    - pharyngeal 306.1
    - respiratory 306.1
    - skin 306.3
    - special sense organs 306.7
- psychosomatic (*see also* Disorder, psychosomatic) 306.9
- psychotic (*see also* Psychosis) 298.9
    - depressive 298.0
    - due to or associated with physical condition (*see also* Psychosis, organic) 293.9
    - involutional (*see also* Psychosis, affective) 296.2 ☑
        - recurrent episode 296.3 ☑
        - single episode 296.2 ☑
- pupillary (myotonic) (tonic) 379.46
- radiation — *see* Effect, adverse, radiation
- runaway (*see also* Disturbance, conduct)
    - socialized 312.2 ☑
    - undersocialized, unsocialized 312.1 ☑
- scarlet fever toxin — *see* Complications, vaccination
- schizophrenic (*see also* Schizophrenia) 295.9 ☑
    - latent 295.5 ☑
- serological for syphilis — *see* Serology for syphilis
- serum (prophylactic) (therapeutic) 999.59
    - anaphylactic 999.49
    - due to
        - administration of blood and blood products 999.51
            - anaphylactic 999.41
        - vaccination 999.52
            - anaphylactic 999.41
    - immediate 999.49
- situational (*see also* Reaction, adjustment) 309.9
    - acute, to stress 308.3
    - adjustment (*see also* Reaction, adjustment) 309.9
- somatization (*see also* Disorder, psychosomatic) 306.9
- spinal puncture 349.0
- spite, child (*see also* Disturbance, conduct) 312.0 ☑
- stress, acute 308.9
    - with predominant disturbance (of)
        - consciousness 308.1
        - emotions 308.0
        - mixed 308.4
        - psychomotor 308.2
        - specified type NEC 308.3
    - bone or cartilage — *see* Fracture, stress
- surgical procedure — *see* Complications, surgical procedure

Reaction — *continued*
- tetanus antitoxin — *see* Complications, vaccination
- toxin-antitoxin — *see* Complications, vaccination
- transfusion (blood) (bone marrow) (lymphocytes) (allergic) (*see also* Complications, transfusion) 999.80
- tuberculin skin test, nonspecific (without active tuberculosis) 795.51
    - positive (without active tuberculosis) 795.51
- ultraviolet — *see* Effect, adverse, ultraviolet
- undersocialized, unsocialized (*see also* Disturbance, conduct)
    - aggressive (type) 312.0 ☑
    - unaggressive (type) 312.1 ☑
- vaccination (any) — *see* Complications, vaccination
- white graft (skin) 996.52
- withdrawing, child or adolescent 313.22
- x-ray — *see* Effect, adverse, x-rays

Reactive depression — *see also* Reaction, depressive 300.4
- neurotic 300.4
- psychoneurotic 300.4
- psychotic 298.0

Rebound tenderness 789.6 ☑
Recalcitrant patient V15.81
Recanalization, thrombus — *see* Thrombosis
Recession, receding
- chamber angle (eye) 364.77
- chin 524.06
- gingival (postinfective) (postoperative) 523.20
    - generalized 523.25
    - localized 523.24
    - minimal 523.21
    - moderate 523.22
    - severe 523.23

Recklinghausen-Applebaum disease (hemochromatosis) 275.03
Recklinghausen's disease (M9540/1) 237.71
- bones (osteitis fibrosa cystica) 252.01
Reclus' disease (cystic) 610.1
Recrudescent typhus (fever) 081.1
Recruitment, auditory 388.44
Rectalgia 569.42
Rectitis 569.49
Rectocele
- female (without uterine prolapse) 618.04
    - with uterine prolapse 618.4
        - complete 618.3
        - incomplete 618.2
    - in pregnancy or childbirth 654.4 ☑
        - causing obstructed labor 660.2 ☑
            - affecting fetus or newborn 763.1
- male 569.49
- vagina, vaginal (outlet) 618.04
Rectosigmoiditis 569.89
- ulcerative (chronic) 556.3
Rectosigmoid junction — *see* condition
Rectourethral — *see* condition
Rectovaginal — *see* condition
Rectovesical — *see* condition
Rectum, rectal — *see* condition
Recurrent — *see* condition
- pregnancy loss — *see* Pregnancy, management affected by, abortion, habitual
Red bugs 133.8
Red cedar asthma 495.8
Redness
- conjunctiva 379.93
- eye 379.93
- nose 478.19
Reduced ventilatory or vital capacity 794.2
Reduction
- function
    - kidney (*see also* Disease, renal) 593.9
    - liver 573.8
- ventilatory capacity 794.2
- vital capacity 794.2
Redundant, redundancy
- abdomen 701.9
- anus 751.5
- cardia 537.89

Redundant, redundancy — *continued*
  clitoris 624.2
  colon (congenital) 751.5
  foreskin (congenital) 605
  intestine 751.5
  labia 624.3
  organ or site, congenital NEC — *see* Accessory
  panniculus (abdominal) 278.1
  prepuce (congenital) 605
  pylorus 537.89
  rectum 751.5
  scrotum 608.89
  sigmoid 751.5
  skin (of face) 701.9
    eyelids 374.30
  stomach 537.89
  uvula 528.9
  vagina 623.8
Reduplication — *see* Duplication
Referral
  adoption (agency) V68.89
  nursing care V63.8
  patient without examination or treatment V68.81
  social services V63.8
Reflex — *see also* condition
  blink, deficient 374.45
  hyperactive gag 478.29
  neurogenic bladder NEC 596.54
    atonic 596.54
    with cauda equina syndrome 344.61
  vasoconstriction 443.9
  vasovagal 780.2
Reflux 530.81
  acid 530.81
  esophageal 530.81
    with esophagitis 530.11
  esophagitis 530.11
  gastroesophageal 530.81
  mitral — *see* Insufficiency, mitral
  ureteral — *see* Reflux, vesicoureteral
  vesicoureteral 593.70
    with
      reflux nephropathy 593.73
        bilateral 593.72
        unilateral 593.71
Reformed gallbladder 576.0
Reforming, artificial openings — *see also* Attention to, artificial, opening V55.9
Refractive error — *see also* Error, refractive 367.9
Refsum's disease or syndrome (heredopathia atactica polyneuritiformis) 356.3
Refusal of
  food 307.59
    hysterical 300.11
  treatment because of, due to
    patient's decision NEC V64.2
    reason of conscience or religion V62.6
Regaud
  tumor (M8082/3) — *see* Neoplasm, nasopharynx, malignant
  type carcinoma (M8082/3) — *see* Neoplasm, nasopharynx, malignant
Regional — *see* condition
Regulation feeding (elderly) (infant) 783.3
  newborn 779.31
Regurgitated
  food, choked on 933.1
  stomach contents, choked on 933.1
Regurgitation 787.03
  aortic (valve) (*see also* Insufficiency, aortic) 424.1
    congenital 746.4
    syphilitic 093.22
  food (*see also* Vomiting)
    with reswallowing — *see* Rumination
    newborn 779.33
  gastric contents — *see* Vomiting
  heart — *see* Endocarditis
  mitral (valve) (*see also* Insufficiency, mitral)
    congenital 746.6
  myocardial — *see* Endocarditis
  pulmonary (heart) (valve) (*see also* Endocarditis, pulmonary) 424.3

Regurgitation — *continued*
  stomach — *see* Vomiting
  tricuspid — *see* Endocarditis, tricuspid
  valve, valvular — *see* Endocarditis
  vesicoureteral — *see* Reflux, vesicoureteral
Rehabilitation V57.9
  multiple types V57.89
  occupational V57.21
  specified type NEC V57.89
  speech (-language) V57.3
  vocational V57.22
Reichmann's disease or syndrome (gastrosuccorrhea) 536.8
Reifenstein's syndrome (hereditary familial hypogonadism, male) 259.52
Reilly's syndrome or phenomenon — *see also* Neuropathy, peripheral, autonomic 337.9
Reimann's periodic disease 277.31
Reinsertion, contraceptive device V25.42
  intrauterine V25.13
Reiter's disease, syndrome, or urethritis 099.3 *[711.1]* ☑
Rejection
  food, hysterical 300.11
  transplant 996.80
    bone marrow 996.85
    corneal 996.51
    organ (immune or nonimmune cause) 996.80
      bone marrow 996.85
      heart 996.83
      intestines 996.87
      kidney 996.81
      liver 996.82
      lung 996.84
      pancreas 996.86
      specified NEC 996.89
    skin 996.52
      artificial 996.55
      decellularized allodermis 996.55
    stem cells(s) 996.88
      from
        peripheral blood 996.88
        umbilical cord 996.88
Relapsing fever 087.9
  Carter's (Asiatic) 087.0
  Dutton's (West African) 087.1
  Koch's 087.9
  louse-borne (epidemic) 087.0
  Novy's (American) 087.1
  Obermeyer's (European) 087.0
  Spirillum 087.9
  tick-borne (endemic) 087.1
Relaxation
  anus (sphincter) 569.49
    due to hysteria 300.11
  arch (foot) 734
    congenital 754.61
  back ligaments 728.4
  bladder (sphincter) 596.59
  cardio-esophageal 530.89
  cervix (*see also* Incompetency, cervix) 622.5
  diaphragm 519.4
  inguinal rings — *see* Hernia, inguinal
  joint (capsule) (ligament) (paralytic) (*see also* Derangement, joint) 718.90
    congenital 755.8
  lumbosacral joint 724.6
  pelvic floor 618.89
  pelvis 618.89
  perineum 618.89
  posture 729.90
  rectum (sphincter) 569.49
  sacroiliac (joint) 724.6
  scrotum 608.89
  urethra (sphincter) 599.84
  uterus (outlet) 618.89
  vagina (outlet) 618.89
  vesical 596.59
Remains
  canal of Cloquet 743.51
  capsule (opaque) 743.51
Remittent fever (malarial) 084.6
Remnant
  canal of Cloquet 743.51

Remnant — *continued*
  capsule (opaque) 743.51
  cervix, cervical stump (acquired) (postoperative) 622.8
  cystic duct, postcholecystectomy 576.0
  fingernail 703.8
    congenital 757.5
  meniscus, knee 717.5
  thyroglossal duct 759.2
  tonsil 474.8
    infected 474.00
  urachus 753.7
Remote effect of cancer — *see* condition
Removal (of)
  catheter (urinary) (indwelling) V53.6
    from artificial opening — *see* Attention to, artificial, opening
    non-vascular V58.82
    vascular V58.81
  cerebral ventricle (communicating) shunt V53.01
  device (*see also* Fitting (of))
    contraceptive V25.12
      with reinsertion V25.13
    fixation
      external V54.89
      internal V54.01
    traction V54.89
  drains V58.49
  dressing
    wound V58.30
      nonsurgical V58.30
      surgical V58.31
  ileostomy V55.2
  Kirschner wire V54.89
  nonvascular catheter V58.82
  pin V54.01
  plaster cast V54.89
  plate (fracture) V54.01
  rod V54.01
  screw V54.01
  splint, external V54.89
  staples V58.32
  subdermal implantable contraceptive V25.43
  sutures V58.32
  traction device, external V54.89
  vascular catheter V58.81
  wound packing V58.30
    nonsurgical V58.30
    surgical V58.31
Ren
  arcuatus 753.3
  mobile, mobilis (*see also* Disease, renal) 593.0
    congenital 753.3
  unguliformis 753.3
Renal — *see also* condition
  glomerulohyalinosis-diabetic syndrome 250.4 ☑ *[581.81]*
    due to secondary diabetes 249.4 ☑ *[581.81]*
Rendu-Osler-Weber disease or syndrome (familial hemorrhagic telangiectasia) 448.0
Reninoma (M8361/1) 236.91
Rénon-Delille syndrome 253.8
Repair
  pelvic floor, previous, in pregnancy or childbirth 654.4 ☑
    affecting fetus or newborn 763.89
  scarred tissue V51.8
Replacement by artificial or mechanical device or prosthesis of — *see also* Fitting (of
  artificial skin V43.83
  bladder V43.5
  blood vessel V43.4
  breast V43.82
  eye globe V43.0
  heart
    with
      assist device V43.21
      fully implantable artificial heart V43.22
    valve V43.3

Replacement by artificial or mechanical device or prosthesis of — *see also* Fitting (of — *continued*
  intestine V43.89
  joint V43.60
    ankle V43.66
    elbow V43.62
    finger V43.69
    hip (partial) (total) V43.64
    knee V43.65
    shoulder V43.61
    specified NEC V43.69
    wrist V43.63
  kidney V43.89
  larynx V43.81
  lens V43.1
  limb(s) V43.7
  liver V43.89
  lung V43.89
  organ NEC V43.89
  pancreas V43.89
  skin (artificial) V43.83
  tissue NEC V43.89
Reprogramming
  cardiac pacemaker V53.31
Request for expert evidence V68.2
Reserve, decreased or low
  cardiac — *see* Disease, heart
  kidney (*see also* Disease, renal) 593.9
Residual — *see also* condition
  bladder 596.89
  foreign body — *see* Retention, foreign body
  state, schizophrenic (*see also* Schizophrenia) 295.6 ☑
  urine 788.69
Resistance, resistant (to)
  activated protein C 289.81

> *Note* — use the following subclassification for categories V09.5, V09.7, V09.8, V09.9:
>
> 0 *without mention of resistance to multiple drugs*
>
> 1 *with resistance to multiple drugs*
>
>   V09.5 *quinolones and fluoroquinolones*
>
>   V09.7 *antimycobacterial agents*
>
>   V09.8 *specified drugs NEC*
>
>   V09.9 *unspecified drugs*

  drugs by microorganisms V09.9 ☑
    Amikacin V09.4
    aminoglycosides V09.4
    Amodiaquine V09.5 ☑
    Amoxicillin V09.0
    Ampicillin V09.0
    antimycobacterial agents V09.7 ☑
    Azithromycin V09.2
    Azlocillin V09.0
    Aztreonam V09.1
    Bacampicillin V09.0
    Bacitracin V09.8 ☑
    Benznidazole V09.8 ☑
    B-lactam antibiotics V09.1
    Capreomycin V09.7 ☑
    Carbenicillin V09.0
    Cefaclor V09.1
    Cefadroxil V09.1
    Cefamandole V09.1
    Cefatetan V09.1
    Cefazolin V09.1
    Cefixime V09.1
    Cefonicid V09.1
    Cefoperazone V09.1
    Ceforanide V09.1
    Cefotaxime V09.1
    Cefoxitin V09.1
    Ceftazidime V09.1
    Ceftizoxime V09.1
    Ceftriaxone V09.1
    Cefuroxime V09.1
    Cephalexin V09.1
    Cephaloglycin V09.1
    Cephaloridine V09.1

☑ **Additional Digit Required** — Refer to the Tabular List for Digit Selection   ▽ **Subterms under main terms may continue to next column or page**

2014 ICD-9-CM

291

Resistance, resistant — *continued*
   drugs by microorganisms — *continued*
      Cephalosporins V09.1
      Cephalothin V09.1
      Cephapirin V09.1
      Cephradine V09.1
      Chloramphenicol V09.8 ☑
      Chloraquine V09.5 ☑
      Chlorguanide V09.8 ☑
      Chlorproguanil V09.8 ☑
      Chlortetracycline V09.3
      Cinoxacin V09.5 ☑
      Ciprofloxacin V09.5 ☑
      Clarithromycin V09.2
      Clindamycin V09.8 ☑
      Clioquinol V09.5 ☑
      Clofazimine V09.7 ☑
      Cloxacillin V09.0
      Cyclacillin V09.0
      Cycloserine V09.7 ☑
      Dapsone [DZ] V09.7 ☑
      Demeclocycline V09.3
      Dicloxacillin V09.0
      Doxycycline V09.3
      Enoxacin V09.5 ☑
      Erythromycin V09.2
      Ethambutol [EMB] V09.7 ☑
      Ethionamide [ETA] V09.7 ☑
      fluoroquinolones V09.5 ☑
      Gentamicin V09.4
      Halofantrine V09.8 ☑
      Imipenem V09.1
      Iodoquinol V09.5 ☑
      Isoniazid [INH] V09.7 ☑
      Kanamycin V09.4
      macrolides V09.2
      Mafenide V09.6
      MDRO (multiple drug resistant organisms) NOS V09.91
      Mefloquine V09.8 ☑
      Melasoprol V09.8 ☑
      Methacycline V09.3
      Methenamine V09.8 ☑
      Methicillin — *see* Infection, Methicillin V09.0
      Metronidazole V09.8 ☑
      Mezlocillin V09.0
      Minocycline V09.3
      multiple drug resistant organisms NOS V09.91
      Nafcillin V09.0
      Nalidixic acid V09.5 ☑
      Natamycin V09.2
      Neomycin V09.4
      Netilmicin V09.4
      Nimorazole V09.8 ☑
      Nitrofurantoin V09.8 ☑
      Nitrofurtimox V09.8 ☑
      Norfloxacin V09.5 ☑
      Nystatin V09.2
      Ofloxacin V09.5 ☑
      Oleandomycin V09.2
      Oxacillin V09.0
      Oxytetracycline V09.3
      Para-amino salicylic acid [PAS] V09.7 ☑
      Paromomycin V09.4
      Penicillin (G) (V) (VK) V09.0
      penicillins V09.0
      Pentamidine V09.8 ☑
      Piperacillin V09.0
      Primaquine V09.5 ☑
      Proguanil V09.8 ☑
      Pyrazinamide [PZA] V09.7 ☑
      Pyrimethamine/Sulfalene V09.8 ☑
      Pyrimethamine/Sulfodoxine V09.8 ☑
      Quinacrine V09.5 ☑
      Quinidine V09.8 ☑
      Quinine V09.8 ☑
      quinolones V09.5 ☑
      Rifabutin V09.7 ☑
      Rifampin [RIF] V09.7 ☑
      Rifamycin V09.7 ☑
      Rolitetracycline V09.3
      specified drugs NEC V09.8 ☑
      Spectinomycin V09.8 ☑

Resistance, resistant — *continued*
   drugs by microorganisms — *continued*
      Spiramycin V09.2
      Streptomycin [SM] V09.4
      Sulfacetamide V09.6
      Sulfacytine V09.6
      Sulfadiazine V09.6
      Sulfadoxine V09.6
      Sulfamethoxazole V09.6
      Sulfapyridine V09.6
      Sulfasalizine V09.6
      Sulfasoxazole V09.6
      sulfonamides V09.6
      Sulfoxone V09.7 ☑
      tetracycline V09.3
      tetracyclines V09.3
      Thiamphenicol V09.8 ☑
      Ticarcillin V09.0
      Tinidazole V09.8 ☑
      Tobramycin V09.4
      Triamphenicol V09.8 ☑
      Trimethoprim V09.8 ☑
      Vancomycin V09.8 ☑
   insulin 277.7
      complicating pregnancy 648.8 ☑
   thyroid hormone 246.8
Resorption
   biliary 576.8
      purulent or putrid (*see also* Cholecystitis) 576.8
   dental (roots) 521.40
      alveoli 525.8
      pathological
         external 521.42
         internal 521.41
         specified NEC 521.49
   septic — *see* Septicemia
   teeth (roots) 521.40
      pathological
         external 521.42
         internal 521.41
         specified NEC 521.49
Respiration
   asymmetrical 786.09
   bronchial 786.09
   Cheyne-Stokes (periodic respiration) 786.04
   decreased, due to shock following injury 958.4
   disorder of 786.00
      psychogenic 306.1
      specified NEC 786.09
   failure 518.81
      acute 518.81
         following trauma and surgery 518.51
      acute and chronic 518.84
         following trauma and surgery 518.53
      chronic 518.83
         following trauma and surgery 518.51
      newborn 770.84
   insufficiency 786.09
      acute 518.82
      newborn NEC 770.89
   Kussmaul (air hunger) 786.09
   painful 786.52
   periodic 786.09
      high altitude 327.22
   poor 786.09
      newborn NEC 770.89
   sighing 786.7
      psychogenic 306.1
   wheezing 786.07
Respiratory — *see also* condition
   distress 786.09
      acute 518.82
      fetus or newborn NEC 770.89
      syndrome (newborn) 769
         adult (following trauma and surgery) 518.52
            specified NEC 518.82
   failure 518.81
      acute 518.81
         following trauma and surgery 518.51
      acute and chronic 518.84
         following trauma and surgery 518.53
      chronic 518.83
         following trauma and surgery 518.51

Respiratory syncytial virus (RSV) 079.6
   bronchiolitis 466.11
   pneumonia 480.1
   vaccination, prophylactic (against) V04.82
Response
   photoallergic 692.72
   phototoxic 692.72
Restless legs syndrome (RLS) 333.94
Restlessness 799.29
Restoration of organ continuity from previous sterilization (tuboplasty) (vasoplasty) V26.0
Rest, rests
   mesonephric duct 752.89
      fallopian tube 752.11
   ovarian, in fallopian tubes 752.19
   wolffian duct 752.89
Restriction of housing space V60.1
Restzustand, schizophrenic — *see also* Schizophrenia 295.6 ☑
Retained — *see* Retention
Retardation
   development, developmental, specific (*see also* Disorder, development, specific) 315.9
      learning, specific 315.2
         arithmetical 315.1
         language (skills) 315.31
            expressive 315.31
            mixed receptive-expressive 315.32
         mathematics 315.1
         reading 315.00
            phonological 315.39
         written expression 315.2
      motor 315.4
   endochondral bone growth 733.91
   growth (physical) in childhood 783.43
      due to malnutrition 263.2
      fetal (intrauterine) 764.9 ☑
         affecting management of pregnancy 656.5 ☑
   intrauterine growth 764.9 ☑
      affecting management of pregnancy 656.5 ☑
   mental — *see* Disability, intellectual
   motor, specific 315.4
   physical 783.43
      child 783.43
      due to malnutrition 263.2
      fetus (intrauterine) 764.9 ☑
         affecting management of pregnancy 656.5 ☑
   psychomotor NEC 307.9
   reading 315.00
Retching — *see* Vomiting
Retention, retained
   bladder (*see also* Retention, urine) 788.20
      psychogenic 306.53
   carbon dioxide 276.2
   cholelithiasis, following cholecystectomy 997.41
   cyst — *see* Cyst
   dead
      fetus (after 22 completed weeks gestation) 656.4 ☑
         early fetal death (before 22 completed weeks gestation) 632
      ovum 631.8
   decidua (following delivery) (fragments) (with hemorrhage) 666.2 ☑
      without hemorrhage 667.1 ☑
   deciduous tooth 520.6
   dental root 525.3
   fecal (*see also* Constipation) 564.00
   fluid 276.69
   foreign body (*see also* Foreign body, retained)
      bone 733.99
      current trauma — *see* Foreign body, by site or type
      middle ear 385.83
      muscle 729.6
      soft tissue NEC 729.6
   gallstones, following cholecystectomy 997.41

Retention, retained — *continued*
   gastric 536.8
   membranes (following delivery) (with hemorrhage) 666.2 ☑
      with abortion — *see* Abortion, by type
      without hemorrhage 667.1 ☑
   menses 626.8
   milk (puerperal) 676.2 ☑
   nitrogen, extrarenal 788.99
   placenta (total) (with hemorrhage) 666.0 ☑
      with abortion — *see* Abortion, by type
      without hemorrhage 667.0 ☑
      portions or fragments 666.2 ☑
         without hemorrhage 667.1 ☑
   products of conception
      early pregnancy (fetal death before 22 completed weeks gestation) 632
      following
         abortion — *see* Abortion, by type
         delivery 666.2 ☑
            with hemorrhage 666.2 ☑
            without hemorrhage 667.1 ☑
   secundines (following delivery) (with hemorrhage) 666.2 ☑
      with abortion — *see* Abortion, by type
      without hemorrhage 667.1 ☑
      complicating puerperium (delayed hemorrhage) 666.2 ☑
   smegma, clitoris 624.8
   urine NEC 788.20
      bladder, incomplete emptying 788.21
      due to
         benign prostatic hypertrophy (BPH) — see category 600
      due to
         benign prostatic hypertrophy (BPH) — see category 600
      psychogenic 306.53
      specified NEC 788.29
   water (in tissue) (*see also* Edema) 782.3
Reticulation, dust (occupational) 504
Reticulocytosis NEC 790.99
Reticuloendotheliosis
   acute infantile (M9722/3) 202.5 ☑
   leukemic (M9940/3) 202.4 ☑
   malignant (M9720/3) 202.3 ☑
   nonlipid (M9722/3) 202.5 ☑
Reticulohistiocytoma (giant cell) 277.89
Reticulohistiocytosis, multicentric 272.8
Reticulolymphosarcoma (diffuse) (M9613/3) 200.8 ☑
   follicular (M9691/3) 202.0 ☑
   nodular (M9691/3) 202.0 ☑
Reticulosarcoma (M9640/3) 200.0 ☑
   nodular (M9642/3) 200.0 ☑
   pleomorphic cell type (M9641/3) 200.0 ☑
Reticulosis (skin)
   acute of infancy (M9722/3) 202.5 ☑
   familial hemophagocytic 288.4
   histiocytic medullary (M9721/3) 202.3 ☑
   lipomelanotic 695.89
   malignant (M9720/3) 202.3 ☑
   Sézary's (M9701/3) 202.2 ☑
Retina, retinal — *see* condition
Retinitis — *see also* Chorioretinitis 363.20
   albuminurica 585.9 [363.10]
   arteriosclerotic 440.8 [362.13]
   central angiospastic 362.41
   Coat's 362.12
   diabetic 250.5 ☑ [362.01]
      due to secondary diabetes 249.5 ☑ [362.01]
   disciformis 362.52
   disseminated 363.10
      metastatic 363.14
      neurosyphilitic 094.83
      pigment epitheliopathy 363.15
   exudative 362.12
   focal 363.00
      in histoplasmosis 115.92
         capsulatum 115.02
         duboisii 115.12
      juxtapapillary 363.05
      macular 363.06
      paramacular 363.06

Retinitis — see also Chorioretinitis —
   continued
  focal — continued
    peripheral 363.08
    posterior pole NEC 363.07
  gravidarum 646.8 ☑
  hemorrhagica externa 362.12
  juxtapapillary (Jensen's) 363.05
  luetic — see Retinitis, syphilitic
  metastatic 363.14
  pigmentosa 362.74
  proliferans 362.29
  proliferating 362.29
  punctata albescens 362.76
  renal 585.9 [363.13]
  syphilitic (secondary) 091.51
    congenital 090.0 [363.13]
    early 091.51
    late 095.8 [363.13]
  syphilitica, central, recurrent 095.8 [363.13]
  tuberculous (see also Tuberculous)
    017.3 ☑ [363.13]
Retinoblastoma (M9510/3) 190.5
  differentiated type (M9511/3) 190.5
  undifferentiated type (M9512/3) 190.5
Retinochoroiditis — see also Chorioretinitis
  363.20
  central angiospastic 362.41
  disseminated 363.10
    metastatic 363.14
    neurosyphilitic 094.83
    pigment epitheliopathy 363.15
    syphilitic 094.83
  due to toxoplasmosis (acquired) (focal)
    130.2
  focal 363.00
    in histoplasmosis 115.92
      capsulatum 115.02
      duboisii 115.12
    juxtapapillary (Jensen's) 363.05
    macular 363.06
    paramacular 363.06
    peripheral 363.08
    posterior pole NEC 363.07
  juxtapapillaris 363.05
  syphilitic (disseminated) 094.83
Retinopathy (background) 362.10
  arteriosclerotic 440.8 [362.13]
  atherosclerotic 440.8 [362.13]
  central serous 362.41
  circinate 362.10
  Coat's 362.12
  diabetic 250.5 ☑ [362.01]
    due to secondary diabetes
      249.5 ☑ [362.01]
    nonproliferative 250.5 ☑ [362.03]
      due to secondary diabetes
        249.5 ☑ [362.03]
      mild 250.5 ☑ [362.04]
        due to secondary diabetes
          249.5 ☑ [362.04]
      moderate 250.5 ☑ [362.05]
        due to secondary diabetes
          249.5 ☑ [362.05]
      severe 250.5 ☑ [362.06]
        due to secondary diabetes
          249.5 ☑ [362.06]
    proliferative 250.5 ☑ [362.02]
      due to secondary diabetes
        249.5 ☑ [362.02]
  exudative 362.12
  hypertensive 362.11
  nonproliferative
    diabetic 250.5 ☑ [362.03]
      due to secondary diabetes
        249.5 ☑ [362.03]
      mild 250.5 ☑ [362.04]
        due to secondary diabetes
          249.5 ☑ [362.04]
      moderate 250.5 ☑ [362.05]
        due to secondary diabetes
          249.5 ☑ [362.05]
      severe 250.5 ☑ [362.06]
        due to secondary diabetes
          249.5 ☑ [362.06]
  of prematurity 362.20

Retinopathy — continued
  of prematurity — continued
    cicatricial 362.21
    stage
      0 362.22
      1 362.23
      2 362.24
      3 362.25
      4 362.26
      5 362.27
  pigmentary, congenital 362.74
  proliferative 362.29
    diabetic 250.5 ☑ [362.02]
      due to secondary diabetes
        249.5 ☑ [362.02]
    sickle-cell 282.60 [362.29]
  solar 363.31
Retinoschisis 361.10
  bullous 361.12
  congenital 743.56
  flat 361.11
  juvenile 362.73
Retractile testis 752.52
Retraction
  cervix — see Retraction, uterus
  drum (membrane) 384.82
  eyelid 374.41
  finger 736.29
  head 781.0
  lid 374.41
  lung 518.89
  mediastinum 519.3
  nipple 611.79
    congenital 757.6
    puerperal, postpartum 676.0 ☑
  palmar fascia 728.6
  pleura (see also Pleurisy) 511.0
  ring, uterus (Bandl's) (pathological) 661.4 ☑
    affecting fetus or newborn 763.7
  sternum (congenital) 756.3
    acquired 738.3
    during respiration 786.9
  substernal 738.3
  supraclavicular 738.8
  syndrome (Duane's) 378.71
  uterus 621.6
  valve (heart) — see Endocarditis
Retrobulbar — see condition
Retrocaval ureter 753.4
Retrocecal — see also condition
  appendix (congenital) 751.5
Retrocession — see Retroversion
Retrodisplacement — see Retroversion
Retroflection, retroflexion — see Retrover-
  sion
Retrognathia, retrognathism (mandibular)
  (maxillary) 524.10
Retrograde
  ejaculation 608.87
  menstruation 626.8
Retroiliac ureter 753.4
Retroperineal — see condition
Retroperitoneal — see condition
Retroperitonitis 567.39
Retropharyngeal — see condition
Retroplacental — see condition
Retroposition — see Retroversion
Retroprosthetic membrane 996.51
Retrosternal thyroid (congenital) 759.2
Retroversion, retroverted
  cervix — see Retroversion, uterus
  female NEC (see also Retroversion, uterus)
    621.6
  iris 364.70
  testis (congenital) 752.51
  uterus, uterine (acquired) (acute) (adherent)
    (any degree) (asymptomatic) (cervix)
    (postinfectional) (postpartal, old)
    621.6
    congenital 752.39
    in pregnancy or childbirth 654.3 ☑
      affecting fetus or newborn 763.89
      causing obstructed labor 660.2 ☑
        affecting fetus or newborn 763.1
Retrusion, premaxilla (developmental) 524.04
Rett's syndrome 330.8

Reverse, reversed
  peristalsis 787.4
Reye-Sheehan syndrome (postpartum pituitary necrosis) 253.2
Reye's syndrome 331.81
Rhabdomyolysis (idiopathic) 728.88
Rhabdomyoma (M8900/0) — see also Neoplasm, connective tissue, benign
  adult (M8904/0) — see Neoplasm, connec-
    tive tissue, benign
  fetal (M8903/0) — see Neoplasm, connec-
    tive tissue, benign
  glycogenic (M8904/0) — see Neoplasm,
    connective tissue, benign
Rhabdomyosarcoma (M8900/3) — see also
  Neoplasm, connective tissue, malignant
  alveolar (M8920/3) — see Neoplasm, con-
    nective tissue, malignant
  embryonal (M8910/3) — see Neoplasm,
    connective tissue, malignant
  mixed type (M8902/3) — see Neoplasm,
    connective tissue, malignant
  pleomorphic (M8901/3) — see Neoplasm,
    connective tissue, malignant
Rhabdosarcoma (M8900/3) — see Rhabdomyosarcoma
Rh antigen (C) (c) (D) (E) (e) (factor)
  hemolytic disease 773.0
  incompatibility, immunization, or sensitiza-
    tion
    affecting management of pregnancy
      656.1 ☑
    fetus or newborn 773.0
    transfusion reaction (see also Complica-
      tions, transfusion) 999.70
  negative mother, affecting fetus or newborn
    773.0
  titer elevated (see also Complications,
    transfusion) 999.70
  transfusion reaction (see also Complications,
    transfusion) 999.70
Rhesus (factor) (Rh) incompatibility — see Rh,
  incompatibility
Rheumaticosis — see Rheumatism
Rheumatism, rheumatic (acute NEC) 729.0
  adherent pericardium 393
  arthritis
    acute or subacute — see Fever,
      rheumatic
    chronic 714.0
      spine 720.0
  articular (chronic) NEC (see also Arthritis)
    716.9 ☑
    acute or subacute — see Fever,
      rheumatic
  back 724.9
  blennorrhagic 098.59
  carditis — see Disease, heart, rheumatic
  cerebral — see Fever, rheumatic
  chorea (acute) — see Chorea, rheumatic
  chronic NEC 729.0
  coronary arteritis 391.9
    chronic 398.99
  degeneration, myocardium (see also Degen-
    eration, myocardium, with rheumatic
    fever) 398.0
  desert 114.0
  febrile — see Fever, rheumatic
  fever — see Fever, rheumatic
  gonococcal 098.59
  gout 714.0
  heart
    disease (see also Disease, heart,
      rheumatic) 398.90
    failure (chronic) (congestive) (inactive)
      398.91
    hemopericardium — see Rheumatic, peri-
      carditis
    hydropericardium — see Rheumatic, peri-
      carditis
    inflammatory (acute) (chronic) (subacute)
      — see Fever, rheumatic
  intercostal 729.1
    meaning Tietze's disease 733.6
  joint (chronic) NEC (see also Arthritis)
    716.9 ☑

Rheumatism, rheumatic — continued
  joint (see also Arthritis) — continued
    acute — see Fever, rheumatic
  mediastinopericarditis — see Rheumatic,
    pericarditis
  muscular 729.0
  myocardial degeneration (see also Degener-
    ation, myocardium, with rheumatic
    fever) 398.0
  myocarditis (chronic) (inactive) (with
    chorea) 398.0
    active or acute 391.2
      with chorea (acute) (rheumatic)
        (Sydenham's) 392.0
  myositis 729.1
  neck 724.9
  neuralgic 729.0
  neuritis (acute) (chronic) 729.2
  neuromuscular 729.0
  nodose — see Arthritis, nodosa
  nonarticular 729.0
  palindromic 719.30
    ankle 719.37
    elbow 719.32
    foot 719.37
    hand 719.34
    hip 719.35
    knee 719.36
    multiple sites 719.39
    pelvic region 719.35
    shoulder (region) 719.31
    specified site NEC 719.38
    wrist 719.33
  pancarditis, acute 391.8
    with chorea (acute) (rheumatic) (Syden-
      ham's) 392.0
    chronic or inactive 398.99
  pericarditis (active) (acute) (with effusion)
    (with pneumonia) 391.0
    with chorea (acute) (rheumatic) (Syden-
      ham's) 392.0
    chronic or inactive 393
  pericardium — see Rheumatic, pericarditis
  pleuropericarditis — see Rheumatic, peri-
    carditis
  pneumonia 390 [517.1]
  pneumonitis 390 [517.1]
  pneumopericarditis — see Rheumatic,
    pericarditis
  polyarthritis
    acute or subacute — see Fever,
      rheumatic
    chronic 714.0
  polyarticular NEC (see also Arthritis) 716.9 ☑
  psychogenic 306.0
  radiculitis 729.2
  sciatic 724.3
  septic — see Fever, rheumatic
  spine 724.9
  subacute NEC 729.0
  torticollis 723.5
  tuberculous NEC (see also Tuberculosis)
    015.9 ☑
  typhoid fever 002.0
Rheumatoid — see also condition
  lungs 714.81
Rhinitis (atrophic) (catarrhal) (chronic)
  (croupous) (fibrinous) (hyperplastic)
  (hypertrophic) (membranous) (purulent)
  (suppurative) (ulcerative) 472.0
  with
    hay fever (see also Fever, hay) 477.9
      with asthma (bronchial) 493.0 ☑
    sore throat — see Nasopharyngitis
  acute 460
  allergic (nonseasonal) (seasonal) (see also
    Fever, hay) 477.9
    with asthma (see also Asthma) 493.0 ☑
    due to food 477.1
  granulomatous 472.0
  infective 460
  obstructive 472.0
  pneumococcal 460
  syphilitic 095.8
    congenital 090.0
  tuberculous (see also Tuberculosis) 012.8 ☑

☑ **Additional Digit Required** — Refer to the Tabular List for Digit Selection   ▽ **Subterms under main terms may continue to next column or page**

2014 ICD-9-CM

293

Rhinitis — *continued*
  vasomotor (*see also* Fever, hay) 477.9
Rhinoantritis (chronic) 473.0
  acute 461.0
Rhinodacryolith 375.57
Rhinolalia (aperta) (clausa) (open) 784.43
Rhinolith 478.19
  nasal sinus (*see also* Sinusitis) 473.9
Rhinomegaly 478.19
Rhinopharyngitis (acute) (subacute) — *see also* Nasopharyngitis 460
  chronic 472.2
  destructive ulcerating 102.5
  mutilans 102.5
Rhinophyma 695.3
Rhinorrhea 478.19
  cerebrospinal (fluid) 349.81
  paroxysmal (*see also* Fever, hay) 477.9
  spasmodic (*see also* Fever, hay) 477.9
Rhinosalpingitis 381.50
  acute 381.51
  chronic 381.52
Rhinoscleroma 040.1
Rhinosporidiosis 117.0
Rhinovirus infection 079.3
Rhizomelic chrondrodysplasia punctata 277.86
Rhizomelique, pseudopolyarthritic 446.5
Rhoads and Bomford anemia (refractory) 238.72
Rhus
  diversiloba dermatitis 692.6
  radicans dermatitis 692.6
  toxicodendron dermatitis 692.6
  venenata dermatitis 692.6
  verniciflua dermatitis 692.6
Rhythm
  atrioventricular nodal 427.89
  disorder 427.9
    coronary sinus 427.89
    ectopic 427.89
    nodal 427.89
  escape 427.89
  heart, abnormal 427.9
    fetus or newborn — *see* Abnormal, heart rate
  idioventricular 426.89
    accelerated 427.89
  nodal 427.89
  sleep, inversion 327.39
    nonorganic origin 307.45
Rhytidosis facialis 701.8
Rib — *see also* condition
  cervical 756.2
Riboflavin deficiency 266.0
Rice bodies — *see also* Loose, body, joint 718.1 ☑
  knee 717.6
Richter's hernia — *see* Hernia, Richter's
Ricinism 988.2
Rickets (active) (acute) (adolescent) (adult) (chest wall) (congenital) (current) (infantile) (intestinal) 268.0
  celiac 579.0
  fetal 756.4
  hemorrhagic 267
  hypophosphatemic with nephrotic-glycosuric dwarfism 270.0
  kidney 588.0
  late effect 268.1
  renal 588.0
  scurvy 267
  vitamin D-resistant 275.3
Rickettsial disease 083.9
  specified type NEC 083.8
Rickettsialpox 083.2
Rickettsiosis NEC 083.9
  specified type NEC 083.8
  tick-borne 082.9
    specified type NEC 082.8
  vesicular 083.2
Ricord's chancre 091.0
Riddoch's syndrome (visual disorientation) 368.16
Rider's
  bone 733.99

Rider's — *continued*
  chancre 091.0
Ridge, alveolus — *see also* condition
  edentulous
    atrophy 525.20
      mandible 525.20
        minimal 525.21
        moderate 525.22
        severe 525.23
      maxilla 525.20
        minimal 525.24
        moderate 525.25
        severe 525.26
    flabby 525.20
Ridged ear 744.29
Riedel's
  disease (ligneous thyroiditis) 245.3
  lobe, liver 751.69
  struma (ligneous thyroiditis) 245.3
  thyroiditis (ligneous) 245.3
Rieger's anomaly or syndrome (mesodermal dysgenesis, anterior ocular segment) 743.44
Riehl's melanosis 709.09
Rietti-Greppi-Micheli anemia or syndrome 282.46
Rieux's hernia — *see* Hernia, Rieux's
Rift Valley fever 066.3
Riga's disease (cachectic aphthae) 529.0
Riga-Fede disease (cachectic aphthae) 529.0
Riggs' disease (compound periodontitis) 523.40
Right middle lobe syndrome 518.0
Rigid, rigidity — *see also* condition
  abdominal 789.4 ☑
  articular, multiple congenital 754.89
  back 724.8
  cervix uteri
    in pregnancy or childbirth 654.6 ☑
      affecting fetus or newborn 763.89
      causing obstructed labor 660.2 ☑
        affecting fetus or newborn 763.1
  hymen (acquired) (congenital) 623.3
  nuchal 781.6
  pelvic floor
    in pregnancy or childbirth 654.4 ☑
      affecting fetus or newborn 763.89
      causing obstructed labor 660.2 ☑
        affecting fetus or newborn 763.1
  perineum or vulva
    in pregnancy or childbirth 654.8 ☑
      affecting fetus or newborn 763.89
      causing obstructed labor 660.2 ☑
        affecting fetus or newborn 763.1
  spine 724.8
  vagina
    in pregnancy or childbirth 654.7 ☑
      affecting fetus or newborn 763.89
      causing obstructed labor 660.2 ☑
        affecting fetus or newborn 763.1
Rigors 780.99
Riley-Day syndrome (familial dysautonomia) 742.8
RIND (reversible ischemic neurological deficit) 434.91
  history of (personal) V12.54
Ring(s)
  aorta 747.21
  Bandl's, complicating delivery 661.4 ☑
    affecting fetus or newborn 763.7
  contraction, complicating delivery 661.4 ☑
    affecting fetus or newborn 763.7
  esophageal (congenital) 750.3
  Fleischer (-Kayser) (cornea) 275.1 [371.14]
  hymenal, tight (acquired) (congenital) 623.3
  Kayser-Fleischer (cornea) 275.1 [371.14]
  retraction, uterus, pathological 661.4 ☑
    affecting fetus or newborn 763.7
  Schatzki's (esophagus) (congenital) (lower) 750.3
    acquired 530.3
  Soemmering's 366.51
  trachea, abnormal 748.3
  vascular (congenital) 747.21
  Vossius' 921.3
    late effect 366.21

Ringed hair (congenital) 757.4
Ringing in the ear — *see also* Tinnitus 388.30
Ringworm 110.9
  beard 110.0
  body 110.5
  Burmese 110.9
  corporeal 110.5
  foot 110.4
  groin 110.3
  hand 110.2
  honeycomb 110.0
  nails 110.1
  perianal (area) 110.3
  scalp 110.0
  specified site NEC 110.8
  Tokelau 110.5
Rise, venous pressure 459.89
Risk
  factor — *see* Problem
  falling V15.88
  suicidal 300.9
Ritter's disease (dermatitis exfoliativa neonatorum) 695.81
Rivalry, sibling 313.3
Rivalta's disease (cervicofacial actinomycosis) 039.3
River blindness 125.3 [360.13]
Robert's pelvis 755.69
  with disproportion (fetopelvic) 653.0 ☑
    affecting fetus or newborn 763.1
    causing obstructed labor 660.1 ☑
      affecting fetus or newborn 763.1
Robinson's (hidrotic) **ectodermal dysplasia** 757.31
Robin's syndrome 756.0
Robles' disease (onchocerciasis) 125.3 [360.13]
Rochalimea — *see* Rickettsial disease
Rocky Mountain fever (spotted) 082.0
Rodent ulcer (M8090/3) — *see also* Neoplasm, skin, malignant
  cornea 370.07
Roentgen ray, adverse effect — *see* Effect, adverse, x-ray
Roetheln 056.9
Roger's disease (congenital interventricular septal defect) 745.4
Rokitansky's
  disease (*see also* Necrosis, liver) 570
  tumor 620.2
Rokitansky-Aschoff sinuses (mucosal outpouching of gallbladder) — *see also* Disease, gallbladder 575.8
Rokitansky-Kuster-Hauser syndrome (congenital absence vagina) 752.45
Rollet's chancre (syphilitic) 091.0
Rolling of head 781.0
Romano-Ward syndrome (prolonged QT interval syndrome) 426.82
Romanus lesion 720.1
Romberg's disease or syndrome 349.89
Roof, mouth — *see* condition
Rosacea 695.3
  acne 695.3
  keratitis 695.3 [370.49]
Rosary, rachitic 268.0
Rose
  cold 477.0
  fever 477.0
  rash 782.1
    epidemic 056.9
    of infants 057.8
Rosenbach's erysipelatoid or erysipeloid 027.1
Rosen-Castleman-Liebow syndrome (pulmonary proteinosis) 516.0
Rosenthal's disease (factor XI deficiency) 286.2
Roseola 057.8
  infantum, infantilis (*see also* Exanthem subitum) 058.10
Rossbach's disease (hyperchlorhydria) 536.8
  psychogenic 306.4
Rössle-Urbach-Wiethe lipoproteinosis 272.8
Ross river fever 066.3
Rostan's asthma (cardiac) — *see also* Failure, ventricular, left 428.1

Rot
  Barcoo (*see also* Ulcer, skin) 707.9
  knife-grinders' (*see also* Tuberculosis) 011.4 ☑
Rotation
  anomalous, incomplete or insufficient — *see* Malrotation
  cecum (congenital) 751.4
  colon (congenital) 751.4
  manual, affecting fetus or newborn 763.89
  spine, incomplete or insufficient 737.8
  tooth, teeth 524.35
  vertebra, incomplete or insufficient 737.8
Rot-Bernhardt disease 355.1
Röteln 056.9
Roth-Bernhardt disease or syndrome 355.1
Roth's disease or meralgia 355.1
Rothmund (-Thomson) syndrome 757.33
Rotor's disease or syndrome (idiopathic hyperbilirubinemia) 277.4
Rotundum ulcus — *see* Ulcer, stomach
Round
  back (with wedging of vertebrae) 737.10
    late effect of rickets 268.1
  hole, retina 361.31
    with detachment 361.01
  ulcer (stomach) — *see* Ulcer, stomach
  worms (infestation) (large) NEC 127.0
Roussy-Lévy syndrome 334.3
Routine postpartum follow-up V24.2
Roy (-Jutras) syndrome (acropachyderma) 757.39
Rubella (German measles) 056.9
  complicating pregnancy, childbirth, or puerperium 647.5 ☑
  complication 056.8
    neurological 056.00
      encephalomyelitis 056.01
      specified type NEC 056.09
    specified type NEC 056.79
  congenital 771.0
  contact V01.4
  exposure to V01.4
  maternal
    with suspected fetal damage affecting management of pregnancy 655.3 ☑
    affecting fetus or newborn 760.2
      manifest rubella in infant 771.0
  specified complications NEC 056.79
  vaccination, prophylactic (against) V04.3
Rubeola (measles) — *see also* Measles 055.9
  complicated 055.8
  meaning rubella (*see also* Rubella) 056.9
  scarlatinosis 057.8
Rubeosis iridis 364.42
  diabetica 250.5 ☑ [364.42]
    due to secondary diabetes 249.5 ☑ [364.42]
Rubinstein-Taybi's syndrome (brachydactylia, short stature and intellectual disabilities) 759.89
Rudimentary (congenital) — *see also* Agenesis
  arm 755.22
  bone 756.9
  cervix uteri 752.43
  eye (*see also* Microphthalmos) 743.10
  fallopian tube 752.19
  leg 755.32
  lobule of ear 744.21
  patella 755.64
  respiratory organs in thoracopagus 759.4
  tracheal bronchus 748.3
  uterine horn 752.39
  uterus 752.39
    in male 752.7
    solid or with cavity 752.39
  vagina 752.45
Rud's syndrome (mental deficiency, epilepsy, and infantilism) 759.89
Ruiter-Pompen (-Wyers) syndrome (angiokeratoma corporis diffusum) 272.7
Ruled out condition — *see also* Observation, suspected V71.9
Rumination — *see also* Vomiting
  disorder 307.53

☑ Additional Digit Required — Refer to the Tabular List for Digit Selection   Subterms under main terms may continue to next column or page

Rumination — *see also* Vomiting — *continued*
 neurotic 300.3
 obsessional 300.3
 psychogenic 307.53
Runaway reaction — *see also* Disturbance, conduct
 socialized 312.2 ☑
 undersocialized, unsocialized 312.1 ☑
Runeberg's disease (progressive pernicious anemia) 281.0
Runge's syndrome (postmaturity) 766.22
Runny nose 784.99
Rupia 091.3
 congenital 090.0
 tertiary 095.9
Rupture, ruptured 553.9
 abdominal viscera NEC 799.89
  obstetrical trauma 665.5 ☑
 abscess (spontaneous) — *see* Abscess, by site
 amnion — *see* Rupture, membranes
 aneurysm — *see* Aneurysm
 anus (sphincter) — *see* Laceration, anus
 aorta, aortic 441.5
  abdominal 441.3
  arch 441.1
  ascending 441.1
  descending 441.5
   abdominal 441.3
   thoracic 441.1
  syphilitic 093.0
  thoracoabdominal 441.6
  thorax, thoracic 441.1
  transverse 441.1
  traumatic (thoracic) 901.0
   abdominal 902.0
  valve or cusp (*see also* Endocarditis, aortic) 424.1
 appendix (with peritonitis) 540.0
  with peritoneal abscess 540.1
  traumatic — *see* Injury, internal, gastrointestinal tract
 arteriovenous fistula, brain (congenital) 430
 artery 447.2
  brain (*see also* Hemorrhage, brain) 431
  coronary (*see also* Infarct, myocardium) 410.9 ☑
  heart (*see also* Infarct, myocardium) 410.9 ☑
  pulmonary 417.8
  traumatic (complication) (*see also* Injury, blood vessel, by site) 904.9
 bile duct, except cystic (*see also* Disease, biliary) 576.3
  cystic 575.4
  traumatic — *see* Injury, internal, intra-abdominal
 bladder (sphincter) 596.6
  with
   abortion — *see* Abortion, by type, with damage to pelvic organs
   ectopic pregnancy (*see also* categories 633.0–633.9) 639.2
   molar pregnancy (*see also* categories 630–632) 639.2
  following
   abortion 639.2
   ectopic or molar pregnancy 639.2
  nontraumatic 596.6
  obstetrical trauma 665.5 ☑
  spontaneous 596.6
  traumatic — *see* Injury, internal, bladder
 blood vessel (*see also* Hemorrhage) 459.0
  brain (*see also* Hemorrhage, brain) 431
  heart (*see also* Infarct, myocardium) 410.9 ☑
  traumatic (complication) (*see also* Injury, blood vessel, by site) 904.9
 bone — *see* Fracture, by site
 bowel 569.89
  traumatic — *see* Injury, internal, intestine
 Bowman's membrane 371.31

Rupture, ruptured — *continued*
 brain
  aneurysm (congenital) (*see also* Hemorrhage, subarachnoid) 430
   late effect — *see* Late effect(s) (of) cerebrovascular disease
  syphilitic 094.87
  hemorrhagic (*see also* Hemorrhage, brain) 431
  injury at birth 767.0
  syphilitic 094.89
 capillaries 448.9
 cardiac (*see also* Infarct, myocardium) 410.9 ☑
 cartilage (articular) (current) (*see also* Sprain, by site)
  knee — *see* Tear, meniscus
  semilunar — *see* Tear, meniscus
 cecum (with peritonitis) 540.0
  with peritoneal abscess 540.1
  traumatic 863.89
   with open wound into cavity 863.99
 cerebral aneurysm (congenital) (*see also* Hemorrhage, subarachnoid) 430
  late effect — *see* Late effect(s) (of) cerebrovascular disease
 cervix (uteri)
  with
   abortion — *see* Abortion, by type, with damage to pelvic organs
   ectopic pregnancy (*see also* categories 633.0–633.9) 639.2
   molar pregnancy (*see also* categories 630–632) 639.2
  following
   abortion 639.2
   ectopic or molar pregnancy 639.2
  obstetrical trauma 665.3 ☑
  traumatic — *see* Injury, internal, cervix
 chordae tendineae 429.5
 choroid (direct) (indirect) (traumatic) 363.63
 circle of Willis (*see also* Hemorrhage, subarachnoid) 430
  late effect — *see* Late effect(s) (of) cerebrovascular disease
 colon 569.89
  traumatic — *see* Injury, internal, colon
 cornea (traumatic) (*see also* Rupture, eye)
  due to ulcer 370.00
 coronary (artery) (thrombotic) (*see also* Infarct, myocardium) 410.9 ☑
 corpus luteum (infected) (ovary) 620.1
 cyst — *see* Cyst
 cystic duct (*see also* Disease, gallbladder) 575.4
 Descemet's membrane 371.33
  traumatic — *see* Rupture, eye
 diaphragm (*see also* Hernia, diaphragm)
  traumatic — *see* Injury, internal, diaphragm
 diverticulum
  bladder 596.3
  intestine (large) (*see also* Diverticula) 562.10
   small 562.00
 duodenal stump 537.89
 duodenum (ulcer) — *see* Ulcer, duodenum, with perforation
 ear drum (*see also* Perforation, tympanum) 384.20
  with otitis media — *see* Otitis media
  traumatic — *see* Wound, open, ear
 esophagus 530.4
  traumatic 862.22
   with open wound into cavity 862.32
   cervical region — *see* Wound, open, esophagus
 eye (without prolapse of intraocular tissue) 871.0
  with
   exposure of intraocular tissue 871.1
   partial loss of intraocular tissue 871.2
   prolapse of intraocular tissue 871.1
  due to burn 940.5
 fallopian tube 620.8

Rupture, ruptured — *continued*
 fallopian tube — *continued*
  due to pregnancy — *see* Pregnancy, tubal
  traumatic — *see* Injury, internal, fallopian tube
 fontanel 767.3
 free wall (ventricle) (*see also* Infarct, myocardium) 410.9 ☑
 gallbladder or duct (*see also* Disease, gallbladder) 575.4
  traumatic — *see* Injury, internal, gallbladder
 gastric (*see also* Rupture, stomach) 537.89
  vessel 459.0
 globe (eye) (traumatic) — *see* Rupture, eye
 graafian follicle (hematoma) 620.0
 heart (auricle) (ventricle) (*see also* Infarct, myocardium) 410.9 ☑
  infectional 422.90
  traumatic — *see* Rupture, myocardium, traumatic
 hymen 623.8
 internal
  organ, traumatic (*see also* Injury, internal, by site)
   heart — *see* Rupture, myocardium, traumatic
   kidney — *see* Rupture, kidney
   liver — *see* Rupture, liver
   spleen — *see* Rupture, spleen, traumatic
  semilunar cartilage — *see* Tear, meniscus
  intervertebral disc — *see* Displacement, intervertebral disc
   traumatic (current) — *see* Dislocation, vertebra
 intestine 569.89
  traumatic — *see* Injury, internal, intestine
 intracranial, birth injury 767.0
 iris 364.76
  traumatic — *see* Rupture, eye
 joint capsule — *see* Sprain, by site
 kidney (traumatic) 866.03
  with open wound into cavity 866.13
  due to birth injury 767.8
  nontraumatic 593.89
 lacrimal apparatus (traumatic) 870.2
 lens (traumatic) 366.20
 ligament (*see also* Sprain, by site)
  with open wound — *see* Wound, open, by site
  old (*see also* Disorder, cartilage, articular) 718.0 ☑
 liver (traumatic) 864.04
  with open wound into cavity 864.14
  due to birth injury 767.8
  nontraumatic 573.8
 lymphatic (node) (vessel) 457.8
 marginal sinus (placental) (with hemorrhage) 641.2 ☑
  affecting fetus or newborn 762.1
 meaning hernia — *see* Hernia
 membrana tympani (*see also* Perforation, tympanum) 384.20
  with otitis media — *see* Otitis media
  traumatic — *see* Wound, open, ear
 membranes (spontaneous)
  artificial
   delayed delivery following 658.3 ☑
    affecting fetus or newborn 761.1
   fetus or newborn 761.1
  delayed delivery following 658.2 ☑
   affecting fetus or newborn 761.1
  premature (less than 24 hours prior to onset of labor) 658.1 ☑
   affecting fetus or newborn 761.1
   delayed delivery following 658.2 ☑
    affecting fetus or newborn 761.1
 meningeal artery (*see also* Hemorrhage, subarachnoid) 430
  late effect — *see* Late effect(s) (of) cerebrovascular disease
 meniscus (knee) (*see also* Tear, meniscus)

Rupture, ruptured — *continued*
 meniscus (*see also* Tear, meniscus) — *continued*
  old (*see also* Derangement, meniscus) 717.5
  site other than knee — *see* Disorder, cartilage, articular
  site other than knee — *see* Sprain, by site
 mesentery 568.89
  traumatic — *see* Injury, internal, mesentery
 mitral — *see* Insufficiency, mitral
 muscle (traumatic) NEC (*see also* Sprain, by site)
  with open wound — *see* Wound, open, by site
  nontraumatic 728.83
 musculotendinous cuff (nontraumatic) (shoulder) 840.4
 mycotic aneurysm, causing cerebral hemorrhage (*see also* Hemorrhage, subarachnoid) 430
  late effect — *see* Late effect(s) (of) cerebrovascular disease
 myocardium, myocardial (*see also* Infarct, myocardium) 410.9 ☑
  traumatic 861.03
   with open wound into thorax 861.13
 nontraumatic (meaning hernia) (*see also* Hernia, by site) 553.9
 obstructed (*see also* Hernia, by site, with obstruction) 552.9
  gangrenous (*see also* Hernia, by site, with gangrene) 551.9
 operation wound (*see also* Dehiscence) 998.32
  internal 998.31
 ovary, ovarian 620.8
  corpus luteum 620.1
  follicle (graafian) 620.0
 oviduct 620.8
  due to pregnancy — *see* Pregnancy, tubal
 pancreas 577.8
  traumatic — *see* Injury, internal, pancreas
 papillary muscle (ventricular) 429.6
 pelvic
  floor, complicating delivery 664.1 ☑
  organ NEC — *see* Injury, pelvic, organs
 penis (traumatic) — *see* Wound, open, penis
 perineum 624.8
  during delivery (*see also* Laceration, perineum, complicating delivery) 664.4 ☑
 pharynx (nontraumatic) (spontaneous) 478.29
 pregnant uterus (before onset of labor) 665.0 ☑
 prostate (traumatic) — *see* Injury, internal, prostate
 pulmonary
  artery 417.8
  valve (heart) (*see also* Endocarditis, pulmonary) 424.3
  vein 417.8
  vessel 417.8
 pupil, sphincter 364.75
 pus tube (*see also* Salpingo-oophoritis) 614.2
 pyosalpinx (*see also* Salpingo-oophoritis) 614.2
 rectum 569.49
  traumatic — *see* Injury, internal, rectum
 retina, retinal (traumatic) (without detachment) 361.30
  with detachment (*see also* Detachment, retina, with retinal defect) 361.00
 rotator cuff (capsule) (traumatic) 840.4
  nontraumatic (complete) 727.61
   partial 726.13
 sclera 871.0
 semilunar cartilage, knee (*see also* Tear, meniscus) 836.2

☑ Additional Digit Required — Refer to the Tabular List for Digit Selection   ▽ Subterms under main terms may continue to next column or page

Rupture, ruptured — *continued*
semilunar cartilage, knee (*see also* Tear, meniscus) — *continued*
old (*see also* Derangement, meniscus) 717.5
septum (cardiac) 410.8 ☑
sigmoid 569.89
traumatic — *see* Injury, internal, colon, sigmoid
sinus of Valsalva 747.29
spinal cord (*see also* Injury, spinal, by site)
due to injury at birth 767.4
fetus or newborn 767.4
syphilitic 094.89
traumatic (*see also* Injury, spinal, by site)
with fracture — *see* Fracture, vertebra, by site, with spinal cord injury
spleen 289.59
congenital 767.8
due to injury at birth 767.8
malarial 084.9
nontraumatic 289.59
spontaneous 289.59
traumatic 865.04
with open wound into cavity 865.14
splenic vein 459.0
stomach 537.89
due to injury at birth 767.8
traumatic — *see* Injury, internal, stomach
ulcer — *see* Ulcer, stomach, with perforation
synovium 727.50
specified site NEC 727.59
tendon (traumatic) (*see also* Sprain, by site)
with open wound — *see* Wound, open, by site
Achilles 845.09
nontraumatic 727.67
ankle 845.09
nontraumatic 727.68
biceps (long bead) 840.8
nontraumatic 727.62
foot 845.10
interphalangeal (joint) 845.13

Rupture, ruptured — *continued*
tendon (*see also* Sprain, by site) — *continued*
foot — *continued*
metatarsophalangeal (joint) 845.12
nontraumatic 727.68
specified site NEC 845.19
tarsometatarsal (joint) 845.11
hand 842.10
carpometacarpal (joint) 842.11
interphalangeal (joint) 842.13
metacarpophalangeal (joint) 842.12
nontraumatic 727.63
extensors 727.63
flexors 727.64
specified site NEC 842.19
nontraumatic 727.60
specified site NEC 727.69
patellar 844.8
nontraumatic 727.66
quadriceps 844.8
nontraumatic 727.65
rotator cuff (capsule) 840.4
nontraumatic (complete) 727.61
partial 726.13
wrist 842.00
carpal (joint) 842.01
nontraumatic 727.63
extensors 727.63
flexors 727.64
radiocarpal (joint) (ligament) 842.02
radioulnar (joint), distal 842.09
specified site NEC 842.09
testis (traumatic) 878.2
complicated 878.3
due to syphilis 095.8
thoracic duct 457.8
tonsil 474.8
traumatic
with open wound — *see* Wound, open, by site
aorta — *see* Rupture, aorta, traumatic
ear drum — *see* Wound, open, ear, drum
external site — *see* Wound, open, by site
eye 871.2
globe (eye) — *see* Wound, open, eyeball

Rupture, ruptured — *continued*
traumatic — *continued*
internal organ (abdomen, chest, or pelvis) (*see also* Injury, internal, by site)
heart — *see* Rupture, myocardium, traumatic
kidney — *see* Rupture, kidney
liver — *see* Rupture, liver
spleen — *see* Rupture, spleen, traumatic
ligament, muscle, or tendon (*see also* Sprain, by site)
with open wound — *see* Wound, open, by site
meaning hernia — *see* Hernia
tricuspid (heart) (valve) — *see* Endocarditis, tricuspid
tube, tubal 620.8
abscess (*see also* Salpingo-oophoritis) 614.2
due to pregnancy — *see* Pregnancy, tubal
tympanum, tympanic (membrane) (*see also* Perforation, tympanum) 384.20
with otitis media — *see* Otitis media
traumatic — *see* Wound, open, ear, drum
umbilical cord 663.8 ☑
fetus or newborn 772.0
ureter (traumatic) (*see also* Injury, internal, ureter) 867.2
nontraumatic 593.89
urethra 599.84
with
abortion — *see* Abortion, by type, with damage to pelvic organs
ectopic pregnancy (*see also* categories 633.0–633.9) 639.2
molar pregnancy (*see also* categories 630–632) 639.2
following
abortion 639.2
ectopic or molar pregnancy 639.2
obstetrical trauma 665.5 ☑
traumatic — *see* Injury, internal urethra

Rupture, ruptured — *continued*
uterosacral ligament 620.8
uterus (traumatic) (*see also* Injury, internal uterus)
affecting fetus or newborn 763.89
during labor 665.1 ☑
nonpuerperal, nontraumatic 621.8
nontraumatic 621.8
pregnant (during labor) 665.1 ☑
before labor 665.0 ☑
vagina 878.6
complicated 878.7
complicating delivery — *see* Laceration, vagina, complicating delivery
valve, valvular (heart) — *see* Endocarditis
varicose vein — *see* Varicose, vein
varix — *see* Varix
vena cava 459.0
ventricle (free wall) (left) (*see also* Infarct, myocardium) 410.9 ☑
vesical (urinary) 596.6
traumatic — *see* Injury, internal, bladder
vessel (blood) 459.0
pulmonary 417.8
viscus 799.89
vulva 878.4
complicated 878.5
complicating delivery 664.0 ☑
Russell's dwarf (uterine dwarfism and craniofacial dysostosis) 759.89
Russell's dysentery 004.8
Russell (-Silver) syndrome (congenital hemihypertrophy and short stature) 759.89
Russian spring-summer type encephalitis 063.0
Rust's disease (tuberculous spondylitis) 015.0 ☑ *[720.81]*
Rustitskii's disease (multiple myeloma) (M9730/3) 203.0 ☑
Ruysch's disease (Hirschsprung's disease) 751.3
Rytand-Lipsitch syndrome (complete atrioventricular block) 426.0

S

Saber
shin 090.5
tibia 090.5
Saccharomyces infection — *see also* Candidiasis 112.9
Saccharopinuria 270.7
Saccular — *see* condition
Sacculation
aorta (nonsyphilitic) (*see also* Aneurysm, aorta) 441.9
ruptured 441.5
syphilitic 093.0
bladder 596.3
colon 569.89
intralaryngeal (congenital) (ventricular) 748.3
larynx (congenital) (ventricular) 748.3
organ or site, congenital — *see* Distortion
pregnant uterus, complicating delivery 654.4 ☑
affecting fetus or newborn 763.1
causing obstructed labor 660.2 ☑
affecting fetus or newborn 763.1
rectosigmoid 569.89
sigmoid 569.89
ureter 593.89
urethra 599.2
vesical 596.3
Sachs (-Tay) disease (amaurotic familial idiocy) 330.1
Sacks-Libman disease 710.0 [424.91]
Sac, lacrimal — *see* condition
Sacralgia 724.6
Sacralization
fifth lumbar vertebra 756.15
incomplete (vertebra) 756.15
Sacrodynia 724.6
Sacroiliac joint — *see* condition
Sacroiliitis NEC 720.2
Sacrum — *see* condition
Saddle
back 737.8
embolus
abdominal aorta 444.01
pulmonary artery 415.13
injury — code to condition
nose 738.0
congenital 754.0
due to syphilis 090.5
Sadism (sexual) 302.84
Saemisch's ulcer 370.04
Saenger's syndrome 379.46
Sago spleen 277.39
Sailors' skin 692.74
Saint
Anthony's fire (*see also* Erysipelas) 035
Guy's dance — *see* Chorea
Louis-type encephalitis 062.3
triad (*see also* Hernia, diaphragm) 553.3
Vitus' dance — *see* Chorea
Salicylism
correct substance properly administered 535.4 ☑
overdose or wrong substance given or taken 965.1
Salivary duct or gland — *see also* condition
virus disease 078.5
Salivation (excessive) — *see also* Ptyalism 527.7
Salmonella (aertrycke) (choleraesuis) (enteritidis) (gallinarum) (suipestifer) (typhimurium) — *see also* Infection, Salmonella 003.9
arthritis 003.23
carrier (suspected) of V02.3
meningitis 003.21
osteomyelitis 003.24
pneumonia 003.22
septicemia 003.1
typhosa 002.0
carrier (suspected) of V02.1
Salmonellosis 003.0
with pneumonia 003.22

Salpingitis (catarrhal) (fallopian tube) (nodular) (pseudofollicular) (purulent) (septic) — *see also* Salpingo-oophoritis 614.2
ear 381.50
acute 381.51
chronic 381.52
Eustachian (tube) 381.50
acute 381.51
chronic 381.52
follicularis 614.1
gonococcal (chronic) 098.37
acute 098.17
interstitial, chronic 614.1
isthmica nodosa 614.1
old — *see* Salpingo-oophoritis, chronic
puerperal, postpartum, childbirth 670.8 ☑
specific (chronic) 098.37
acute 098.17
tuberculous (acute) (chronic) (*see also* Tuberculosis) 016.6 ☑
venereal (chronic) 098.37
acute 098.17
Salpingocele 620.4
Salpingo-oophoritis (catarrhal) (purulent) (ruptured) (septic) (suppurative) 614.2
acute 614.0
with
abortion — *see* Abortion, by type, with sepsis
ectopic pregnancy (*see also* categories 633.0–633.9) 639.0
molar pregnancy (*see also* categories 630–632) 639.0
following
abortion 639.0
ectopic or molar pregnancy 639.0
gonococcal 098.17
puerperal, postpartum, childbirth 670.8 ☑
tuberculous (*see also* Tuberculosis) 016.6 ☑
chronic 614.1
gonococcal 098.37
tuberculous (*see also* Tuberculosis) 016.6 ☑
complicating pregnancy 646.6 ☑
affecting fetus or newborn 760.8
gonococcal (chronic) 098.37
acute 098.17
old — *see* Salpingo-oophoritis, chronic
puerperal 670.8 ☑
specific — *see* Salpingo-oophoritis, gonococcal
subacute (*see also* Salpingo-oophoritis, acute) 614.0
tuberculous (acute) (chronic) (*see also* Tuberculosis) 016.6 ☑
venereal — *see* Salpingo-oophoritis, gonococcal
Salpingo-ovaritis — *see also* Salpingo-oophoritis 614.2
Salpingoperitonitis — *see also* Salpingo-oophoritis 614.2
Salt-losing
nephritis (*see also* Disease, renal) 593.9
syndrome (*see also* Disease, renal) 593.9
Salt-rheum — *see also* Eczema 692.9
Salzmann's nodular dystrophy 371.46
Sampling
chorionic villus V28.89
Sampson's cyst or tumor 617.1
Sandblasters'
asthma 502
lung 502
Sander's disease (paranoia) 297.1
Sandfly fever 066.0
Sandhoff's disease 330.1
Sanfilippo's syndrome (mucopolysaccharidosis III) 277.5
Sanger-Brown's ataxia 334.2
San Joaquin Valley fever 114.0
Sao Paulo fever or typhus 082.0
Saponification, mesenteric 567.89
Sapremia — *see* Septicemia
Sarcocele (benign)
syphilitic 095.8

Sarcocele — *continued*
syphilitic — *continued*
congenital 090.5
Sarcoepiplocele — *see also* Hernia 553.9
Sarcoepiplomphalocele — *see also* Hernia, umbilicus 553.1
Sarcoid (any site) 135
with lung involvement 135 [517.8]
Boeck's 135
Darier-Roussy 135
Spiegler-Fendt 686.8
Sarcoidosis 135
cardiac 135 [425.8]
lung 135 [517.8]
Sarcoma (M8800/3) — *see also* Neoplasm, connective tissue, malignant
alveolar soft part (M9581/3) — *see* Neoplasm, connective tissue, malignant
ameloblastic (M9330/3) 170.1
upper jaw (bone) 170.0
botryoid (M8910/3) — *see* Neoplasm, connective tissue, malignant
botryoides (M8910/3) — *see* Neoplasm, connective tissue, malignant
cerebellar (M9480/3) 191.6
circumscribed (arachnoidal) (M9471/3) 191.6
circumscribed (arachnoidal) cerebellar (M9471/3) 191.6
clear cell, of tendons and aponeuroses (M9044/3) — *see* Neoplasm, connective tissue, malignant
embryonal (M8991/3) — *see* Neoplasm, connective tissue, malignant
endometrial (stromal) (M8930/3) 182.0
isthmus 182.1
endothelial (M9130/3) (*see also* Neoplasm, connective tissue, malignant)
bone (M9260/3) — *see* Neoplasm, bone, malignant
epithelioid cell (M8804/3) — *see* Neoplasm, connective tissue, malignant
Ewing's (M9260/3) — *see* Neoplasm, bone, malignant
follicular dendritic cell 202.9 ☑
germinoblastic (diffuse) (M9632/3) 202.8 ☑
follicular (M9697/3) 202.0 ☑
giant cell (M8802/3) (*see also* Neoplasm, connective tissue, malignant)
bone (M9250/3) — *see* Neoplasm, bone, malignant
glomoid (M8710/3) — *see* Neoplasm, connective tissue, malignant
granulocytic (M9930/3) 205.3 ☑
hemangioendothelial (M9130/3) — *see* Neoplasm, connective tissue, malignant
hemorrhagic, multiple (M9140/3) — *see* Kaposi's, sarcoma
Hodgkin's (M9662/3) 201.2 ☑
immunoblastic (M9612/3) 200.8 ☑
interdigitating dendritic cell 202.9 ☑
Kaposi's (M9140/3) — *see* Kaposi's, sarcoma
Kupffer cell (M9124/3) 155.0
Langerhans cell 202.9 ☑
leptomeningeal (M9530/3) — *see* Neoplasm, meninges, malignant
lymphangioendothelial (M9170/3) — *see* Neoplasm, connective tissue, malignant
lymphoblastic (M9630/3) 200.1 ☑
lymphocytic (M9620/3) 200.1 ☑
mast cell (M9740/3) 202.6 ☑
melanotic (M8720/3) — *see* Melanoma
meningeal (M9530/3) — *see* Neoplasm, meninges, malignant
meningothelial (M9530/3) — *see* Neoplasm, meninges, malignant
mesenchymal (M8800/3) (*see also* Neoplasm, connective tissue, malignant)
mixed (M8990/3) — *see* Neoplasm, connective tissue, malignant
mesothelial (M9050/3) — *see* Neoplasm, by site, malignant

Sarcoma — *see also* Neoplasm, connective tissue, malignant — *continued*
monstrocellular (M9481/3)
specified site — *see* Neoplasm, by site, malignant
unspecified site 191.9
myeloid (M9930/3) 205.3 ☑
neurogenic (M9540/3) — *see* Neoplasm, connective tissue, malignant
odontogenic (M9270/3) 170.1
upper jaw (bone) 170.0
osteoblastic (M9180/3) — *see* Neoplasm, bone, malignant
osteogenic (M9180/3) (*see also* Neoplasm, bone, malignant)
juxtacortical (M9190/3) — *see* Neoplasm, bone, malignant
periosteal (M9190/3) — *see* Neoplasm, bone, malignant
periosteal (M8812/3) (*see also* Neoplasm, bone, malignant)
osteogenic (M9190/3) — *see* Neoplasm, bone, malignant
plasma cell (M9731/3) 203.8 ☑
pleomorphic cell (M8802/3) — *see* Neoplasm, connective tissue, malignant
reticuloendothelial (M9720/3) 202.3 ☑
reticulum cell (M9640/3) 200.0 ☑
nodular (M9642/3) 200.0 ☑
pleomorphic cell type (M9641/3) 200.0 ☑
round cell (M8803/3) — *see* Neoplasm, connective tissue, malignant
small cell (M8803/3) — *see* Neoplasm, connective tissue, malignant
spindle cell (M8801/3) — *see* Neoplasm, connective tissue, malignant
stromal (endometrial) (M8930/3) 182.0
isthmus 182.1
synovial (M9040/3) (*see also* Neoplasm, connective tissue, malignant)
biphasic type (M9043/3) — *see* Neoplasm, connective tissue, malignant
epithelioid cell type (M9042/3) — *see* Neoplasm, connective tissue, malignant
spindle cell type (M9041/3) — *see* Neoplasm, connective tissue, malignant
Sarcomatosis
meningeal (M9539/3) — *see* Neoplasm, meninges, malignant
specified site NEC (M8800/3) — *see* Neoplasm, connective tissue, malignant
unspecified site (M8800/6) 171.9
Sarcosinemia 270.8
Sarcosporidiosis 136.5
Satiety, early 780.94
Satisfactory smear but lacking transformation zone
anal 796.77
cervical 795.07
Saturnine — *see* condition
Saturnism 984.9
specified type of lead — *see* Table of Drugs and Chemicals
Satyriasis 302.89
Sauriasis — *see* Ichthyosis
Sauriderma 757.39
Sauriosis — *see* Ichthyosis
Savill's disease (epidemic exfoliative dermatitis) 695.89
SBE (subacute bacterial endocarditis) 421.0
Scabies (any site) 133.0
Scabs 782.8
Scaglietti-Dagnini syndrome (acromegalic macrospondylitis) 253.0
Scald, scalded — *see* Burn, by site
skin syndrome 695.81
Scalenus anticus (anterior) syndrome 353.0
Scales 782.8
Scalp — *see* condition
Scaphocephaly 756.0
Scaphoiditis, tarsal 732.5
Scapulalgia 733.90

☑ **Additional Digit Required** — Refer to the Tabular List for Digit Selection   ⚐ **Subterms under main terms may continue to next column or page**

2014 ICD-9-CM   297

Scapulohumeral myopathy 359.1
Scarabiasis 134.1
Scarlatina 034.1
  anginosa 034.1
  maligna 034.1
  myocarditis, acute 034.1 *[422.0]*
    old (*see also* Myocarditis) 429.0
  otitis media 034.1 *[382.02]*
  ulcerosa 034.1
Scarlatinella 057.8
Scarlet fever (albuminuria) (angina) (convulsions) (lesions of lid) (rash) 034.1
Scar, scarring — *see also* Cicatrix 709.2
  adherent 709.2
  atrophic 709.2
  cervix
    in pregnancy or childbirth 654.6 ☑
      affecting fetus or newborn 763.89
      causing obstructed labor 660.2 ☑
        affecting fetus or newborn 763.1
  cheloid 701.4
  chorioretinal 363.30
    disseminated 363.35
    macular 363.32
    peripheral 363.34
    posterior pole NEC 363.33
  choroid (*see also* Scar, chorioretinal) 363.30
  compression, pericardial 423.9
  congenital 757.39
  conjunctiva 372.64
  cornea 371.00
    xerophthalmic 264.6
  due to previous cesarean delivery, complicating pregnancy or childbirth 654.2 ☑
    affecting fetus or newborn 763.89
  duodenal (bulb) (cap) 537.3
  hypertrophic 701.4
  keloid 701.4
  labia 624.4
  lung (base) 518.89
  macula 363.32
    disseminated 363.35
    peripheral 363.34
  muscle 728.89
  myocardium, myocardial 412
  painful 709.2
  papillary muscle 429.81
  posterior pole NEC 363.33
    macular — *see* Scar, macula
  postnecrotic (hepatic) (liver) 571.9
  psychic V15.49
  retina (*see also* Scar, chorioretinal) 363.30
  trachea 478.9
  uterus 621.8
    in pregnancy or childbirth NEC 654.9 ☑
      affecting fetus or newborn 763.89
      due to previous cesarean delivery 654.2 ☑
  vulva 624.4
Schamberg's disease, dermatitis, or dermatosis (progressive pigmentary dermatosis) 709.09
Schatzki's ring (esophagus) (lower) (congenital) 750.3
  acquired 530.3
Schaufenster krankheit 413.9
Schaumann's
  benign lymphogranulomatosis 135
  disease (sarcoidosis) 135
  syndrome (sarcoidosis) 135
Scheie's syndrome (mucopolysaccharidosis IS) 277.5
Schenck's disease (sporotrichosis) 117.1
Scheuermann's disease or osteochondrosis 732.0
Scheuthauer-Marie-Sainton syndrome (cleidocranialis dysostosis) 755.59
Schilder (-Flatau) disease 341.1
Schilling-type monocytic leukemia (M9890/3) 206.9 ☑
Schimmelbusch's disease, cystic mastitis, or hyperplasia 610.1
Schirmer's syndrome (encephalocutaneous angiomatosis) 759.6
Schistocelia 756.79

Schistoglossia 750.13
Schistosoma infestation — *see* Infestation, Schistosoma
Schistosomiasis 120.9
  Asiatic 120.2
  bladder 120.0
  chestermani 120.8
  colon 120.1
  cutaneous 120.3
  due to
    S. hematobium 120.0
    S. japonicum 120.2
    S. mansoni 120.1
    S. mattheii 120.8
  eastern 120.2
  genitourinary tract 120.0
  intestinal 120.1
  lung 120.2
  Manson's (intestinal) 120.1
  Oriental 120.2
  pulmonary 120.2
  specified type NEC 120.8
  vesical 120.0
Schizencephaly 742.4
Schizo-affective psychosis — *see also* Schizophrenia 295.7 ☑
Schizodontia 520.2
Schizoid personality 301.20
  introverted 301.21
  schizotypal 301.22
Schizophrenia, schizophrenic (reaction) 295.9 ☑

Note — *Use the following fifth-digit subclassification with category 295:*

0   *unspecified*

1   *subchronic*

2   *chronic*

3   *subchronic with acute exacerbation*

4   *chronic with acute exacerbation*

5   *in remission*

  acute (attack) NEC 295.8 ☑
    episode 295.4 ☑
  atypical form 295.8 ☑
  borderline 295.5 ☑
  catalepsy 295.2 ☑
  catatonic (type) (acute) (excited) (withdrawn) 295.2 ☑
  childhood (type) (*see also* Psychosis, childhood) 299.9 ☑
  chronic NEC 295.6 ☑
  coenesthesiopathic 295.8 ☑
  cyclic (type) 295.7 ☑
  disorganized (type) 295.1 ☑
  flexibilitas cerea 295.2 ☑
  hebephrenic (type) (acute) 295.1 ☑
  incipient 295.5 ☑
  latent 295.5 ☑
  paranoid (type) (acute) 295.3 ☑
  paraphrenic (acute) 295.3 ☑
  prepsychotic 295.5 ☑
  primary (acute) 295.0 ☑
  prodromal 295.5 ☑
  pseudoneurotic 295.5 ☑
  pseudopsychopathic 295.5 ☑
  reaction 295.9 ☑
  residual type (state) 295.6 ☑
  restzustand 295.6 ☑
  schizo-affective (type) (depressed) (excited) 295.7 ☑
  schizophreniform type 295.4 ☑
  simple (type) (acute) 295.0 ☑
  simplex (acute) 295.0 ☑
  specified type NEC 295.8 ☑
  syndrome of childhood NEC (*see also* Psychosis, childhood) 299.9 ☑
  undifferentiated type 295.9 ☑
    acute 295.8 ☑
    chronic 295.6 ☑
Schizothymia 301.20
  introverted 301.21

Schizothymia — *continued*
  schizotypal 301.22
Schlafkrankheit 086.5
Schlatter-Osgood disease (osteochondrosis, tibial tubercle) 732.4
Schlatter's tibia (osteochondrosis) 732.4
Schloffer's tumor — *see also* Peritonitis 567.29
Schmidt's syndrome
  sphallo-pharyngo-laryngeal hemiplegia 352.6
  thyroid-adrenocortical insufficiency 258.1
  vagoaccessory 352.6
Schmincke
  carcinoma (M8082/3) — *see* Neoplasm, nasopharynx, malignant
  tumor (M8082/3) — *see* Neoplasm, nasopharynx, malignant
Schmitz (-Stutzer) dysentery 004.0
Schmorl's disease or nodes 722.30
  lumbar, lumbosacral 722.32
  specified region NEC 722.39
  thoracic, thoracolumbar 722.31
Schneiderian
  carcinoma (M8121/3)
    specified site — *see* Neoplasm, by site, malignant
    unspecified site 160.0
  papilloma (M8121/0)
    specified site — *see* Neoplasm, by site, benign
    unspecified site 212.0
Schneider's syndrome 047.9
Schnitzler syndrome 273.1
Schoffer's tumor — *see also* Peritonitis 567.29
Scholte's syndrome (malignant carcinoid) 259.2
Scholz's disease 330.0
Scholz (-Bielschowsky-Henneberg) syndrome 330.0
Schönlein (-Henoch) disease (primary) (purpura) (rheumatic) 287.0
School examination V70.3
  following surgery V67.09
Schottmüller's disease — *see also* Fever, paratyphoid 002.9
Schroeder's syndrome (endocrine-hypertensive) 255.3
Schüller-Christian disease or syndrome (chronic histiocytosis X) 277.89
Schultz's disease or syndrome (agranulocytosis) 288.09
Schultze's acroparesthesia, simple 443.89
Schwalbe-Ziehen-Oppenheimer disease 333.6
Schwannoma (M9560/0) — *see also* Neoplasm, connective tissue, benign
  malignant (M9560/3) — *see* Neoplasm, connective tissue, malignant
Schwannomatosis 237.73
Schwartz-Bartter syndrome (inappropriate secretion of antidiuretic hormone) 253.6
Schwartz (-Jampel) syndrome 359.23
Schweninger-Buzzi disease (macular atrophy) 701.3
Sciatic — *see* condition
Sciatica (infectional) 724.3
  due to
    displacement of intervertebral disc 722.10
    herniation, nucleus pulposus 722.10
  wallet 724.3
Scimitar syndrome (anomalous venous drainage, right lung to inferior vena cava) 747.49
Sclera — *see* condition
Sclerectasia 379.11
Scleredema
  adultorum 710.1
  Buschke's 710.1
  newborn 778.1
Sclerema
  adiposum (newborn) 778.1
  adultorum 710.1
  edematosum (newborn) 778.1
  neonatorum 778.1
  newborn 778.1

Scleriasis — *see* Scleroderma
Scleritis 379.00
  with corneal involvement 379.05
  anterior (annular) (localized) 379.03
  brawny 379.06
  granulomatous 379.09
  posterior 379.07
  specified NEC 379.09
  suppurative 379.09
  syphilitic 095.0
  tuberculous (nodular) (*see also* Tuberculosis) 017.3 ☑ *[379.09]*
Sclerochoroiditis — *see also* Scleritis 379.00
Scleroconjunctivitis — *see also* Scleritis 379.00
Sclerocystic ovary (syndrome) 256.4
Sclerodactylia 701.0
Scleroderma, sclerodermia (acrosclerotic) (diffuse) (generalized) (progressive) (pulmonary) 710.1
  circumscribed 701.0
  linear 701.0
  localized (linear) 701.0
  newborn 778.1
Sclerokeratitis 379.05
  meaning sclerosing keratitis 370.54
  tuberculous (*see also* Tuberculosis) 017.3 ☑ *[379.09]*
Scleromalacia
  multiple 731.0
  perforans 379.04
Scleroma, trachea 040.1
Scleromyxedema 701.8
Scleroperikeratitis 379.05
Sclerose en plaques 340
Sclerosis, sclerotic
  adrenal (gland) 255.8
  Alzheimer's 331.0
    with dementia — *see* Alzheimer's, dementia
  amyotrophic (lateral) 335.20
  annularis fibrosi
    aortic 424.1
    mitral 424.0
  aorta, aortic 440.0
    valve (*see also* Endocarditis, aortic) 424.1
  artery, arterial, arteriolar, arteriovascular — *see* Arteriosclerosis
  ascending multiple 340
  Baló's (concentric) 341.1
  basilar — *see* Sclerosis, brain
  bone (localized) NEC 733.99
  brain (general) (lobular) 348.89
    Alzheimer's — *see* Alzheimer's, dementia
    artery, arterial 437.0
    atrophic lobar 331.0
      with dementia
        with behavioral disturbance 331.0 *[294.11]*
        without behavioral disturbance 331.0 *[294.10]*
    diffuse 341.1
      familial (chronic) (infantile) 330.0
      infantile (chronic) (familial) 330.0
      Pelizaeus-Merzbacher type 330.0
    disseminated 340
    hereditary 334.2
    hippocampal 348.81
    infantile (degenerative) (diffuse) 330.0
    insular 340
    Krabbe's 330.0
    mesial temporal 348.81
    miliary 340
    multiple 340
    Pelizaeus-Merzbacher 330.0
    progressive familial 330.0
    senile 437.0
    temporal 348.81
      mesial 348.81
    tuberous 759.5
  bulbar, progressive 340
  bundle of His 426.50
    left 426.3
    right 426.4
  cardiac — *see* Arteriosclerosis, coronary

☑ **Additional Digit Required** — Refer to the Tabular List for Digit Selection

▽ **Subterms under main terms may continue to next column or page**

Sclerosis, sclerotic — *continued*
  cardiorenal (*see also* Hypertension, cardiorenal) 404.90
  cardiovascular (*see also* Disease, cardiovascular) 429.2
    renal (*see also* Hypertension, cardiorenal) 404.90
  centrolobar, familial 330.0
  cerebellar — *see* Sclerosis, brain
  cerebral — *see* Sclerosis, brain
  cerebrospinal 340
    disseminated 340
    multiple 340
  cerebrovascular 437.0
  choroid 363.40
    diffuse 363.56
  combined (spinal cord) (*see also* Degeneration, combined)
    multiple 340
  concentric, Baló's 341.1
  cornea 370.54
  coronary (artery) — *see* Arteriosclerosis, coronary
  corpus cavernosum
    female 624.8
    male 607.89
  Dewitzky's
    aortic 424.1
    mitral 424.0
  diffuse NEC 341.1
  disease, heart — *see* Arteriosclerosis, coronary
  disseminated 340
  dorsal 340
  dorsolateral (spinal cord) — *see* Degeneration, combined
  endometrium 621.8
  extrapyramidal 333.90
  eye, nuclear (senile) 366.16
  Friedreich's (spinal cord) 334.0
  funicular (spermatic cord) 608.89
  gastritis 535.4 ☑
  general (vascular) — *see* Arteriosclerosis
  gland (lymphatic) 457.8
  hepatic 571.9
  hereditary
    cerebellar 334.2
    spinal 334.0
  hippocampal 348.81
  idiopathic cortical (Garré's) (*see also* Osteomyelitis) 730.1 ☑
  ilium, piriform 733.5
  insular 340
    pancreas 251.8
  Islands of Langerhans 251.8
  kidney — *see* Sclerosis, renal
  larynx 478.79
  lateral 335.24
    amyotrophic 335.20
    descending 335.24
    primary 335.24
    spinal 335.24
  liver 571.9
  lobar, atrophic (of brain) 331.0
    with dementia
      with behavioral disturbance 331.0 [294.11]
      without behavioral disturbance 331.0 [294.10]
  lung (*see also* Fibrosis, lung) 515
  mastoid 383.1
  mesial temporal 348.81
  mitral — *see* Endocarditis, mitral
  Mönckeberg's (medial) (*see also* Arteriosclerosis, extremities) 440.20
  multiple (brain stem) (cerebral) (generalized) (spinal cord) 340
  myocardium, myocardial — *see* Arteriosclerosis, coronary
  nuclear (senile), eye 366.16
  ovary 620.8
  pancreas 577.8
  penis 607.89
  peripheral arteries (*see also* Arteriosclerosis, extremities) 440.20
  plaques 340

Sclerosis, sclerotic — *continued*
  pluriglandular 258.8
  polyglandular 258.8
  posterior (spinal cord) (syphilitic) 094.0
  posterolateral (spinal cord) — *see* Degeneration, combined
  prepuce 607.89
  primary lateral 335.24
  progressive systemic 710.1
  pulmonary (*see also* Fibrosis, lung) 515
    artery 416.0
    valve (heart) (*see also* Endocarditis, pulmonary) 424.3
  renal 587
    with
      cystine storage disease 270.0
      hypertension (*see also* Hypertension, kidney) 403.90
      hypertensive heart disease (conditions classifiable to 402) (*see also* Hypertension, cardiorenal) 404.90
      arteriolar (hyaline) (*see also* Hypertension, kidney) 403.90
      hyperplastic (*see also* Hypertension, kidney) 403.90
  retina (senile) (vascular) 362.17
  rheumatic
    aortic valve 395.9
    mitral valve 394.9
  Schilder's 341.1
  senile — *see* Arteriosclerosis
  spinal (cord) (general) (progressive) (transverse) 336.8
    ascending 357.0
    combined (*see also* Degeneration, combined)
      multiple 340
      syphilitic 094.89
    disseminated 340
    dorsolateral — *see* Degeneration, combined
    hereditary (Friedreich's) (mixed form) 334.0
    lateral (amyotrophic) 335.24
    multiple 340
    posterior (syphilitic) 094.0
  stomach 537.89
  subendocardial, congenital 425.3
  systemic (progressive) 710.1
    with lung involvement 710.1 [517.2]
  temporal 348.81
    mesial 348.81
  tricuspid (heart) (valve) — *see* Endocarditis, tricuspid
  tuberous (brain) 759.5
  tympanic membrane (*see also* Tympanosclerosis) 385.00
  valve, valvular (heart) — *see* Endocarditis
  vascular — *see* Arteriosclerosis
  vein 459.89
Sclerotenonitis 379.07
Sclerotitis — *see also* Scleritis 379.00
  syphilitic 095.0
  tuberculous (*see also* Tuberculosis) 017.3 ☑ [379.09]
Scoliosis (acquired) (postural) 737.30
  congenital 754.2
  due to or associated with
    Charcôt-Marie-Tooth disease 356.1 [737.43]
    mucopolysaccharidosis 277.5 [737.43]
    neurofibromatosis 237.71 [737.43]
    osteitis
      deformans 731.0 [737.43]
      fibrosa cystica 252.01 [737.43]
    osteoporosis (*see also* Osteoporosis) 733.00 [737.43]
    poliomyelitis 138 [737.43]
    radiation 737.33
    tuberculosis (*see also* Tuberculosis) 015.0 ☑ [737.43]
  idiopathic 737.30
    infantile
      progressive 737.32
      resolving 737.31

Scoliosis — *continued*
  paralytic 737.39
  rachitic 268.1
  sciatic 724.3
  specified NEC 737.39
  thoracogenic 737.34
  tuberculous (*see also* Tuberculosis) 015.0 ☑ [737.43]
Scoliotic pelvis 738.6
  with disproportion (fetopelvic) 653.0 ☑
    affecting fetus or newborn 763.1
    causing obstructed labor 660.1 ☑
      affecting fetus or newborn 763.1
Scorbutus, scorbutic 267
  anemia 281.8
Scotoma (ring) 368.44
  arcuate 368.43
  Bjerrum 368.43
  blind spot area 368.42
  central 368.41
  centrocecal 368.41
  paracecal 368.42
  paracentral 368.41
  scintillating 368.12
  Seidel 368.43
Scratch — *see* Injury, superficial, by site
Scratchy throat 784.99
Screening (for) V82.9
  alcoholism V79.1
  anemia, deficiency NEC V78.1
    iron V78.0
  anomaly, congenital V82.89
  antenatal, of mother V28.9
    alphafetoprotein levels, raised V28.1
    based on amniocentesis V28.2
      chromosomal anomalies V28.0
      raised alphafetoprotein levels V28.1
    fetal growth retardation using ultrasonics V28.4
      ultrasonics V28.4
    genomic V28.89
    isoimmunization V28.5
    malformations using ultrasonics V28.3
    proteomic V28.89
    raised alphafetoprotein levels V28.1
    risk
      pre-term labor V28.82
    specified condition NEC V28.89
    Streptococcus B V28.6
  arterial hypertension V81.1
  arthropod-borne viral disease NEC V73.5
  asymptomatic bacteriuria V81.5
  bacterial
    and spirochetal sexually transmitted diseases V74.5
    conjunctivitis V74.4
    disease V74.9
      sexually transmitted V74.5
      specified condition NEC V74.8
  bacteriuria, asymptomatic V81.5
  blood disorder NEC V78.9
    specified type NEC V78.8
  bronchitis, chronic V81.3
  brucellosis V74.8
  cancer — *see* Screening, malignant neoplasm
  cardiovascular disease NEC V81.2
  cataract V80.2
  Chagas' disease V75.3
  chemical poisoning V82.5
  cholera V74.0
  cholesterol level V77.91
  chromosomal
    anomalies
      by amniocentesis, antenatal V28.0
      maternal postnatal V82.4
    athletes V70.3
  colonoscopy V76.51
  condition
    cardiovascular NEC V81.2
    eye NEC V80.2
    genitourinary NEC V81.6
    neurological NEC V80.09
    respiratory NEC V81.4
    skin V82.0
    specified NEC V82.89

Screening — *continued*
  congenital
    anomaly V82.89
      eye V80.2
    dislocation of hip V82.3
    eye condition or disease V80.2
  conjunctivitis, bacterial V74.4
  contamination NEC (*see also* Poisoning) V82.5
  coronary artery disease V81.0
  cystic fibrosis V77.6
  deficiency anemia NEC V78.1
    iron V78.0
  dengue fever V73.5
  depression V79.0
  developmental handicap V79.9
    in early childhood V79.3
    specified type NEC V79.8
  diabetes mellitus V77.1
  diphtheria V74.3
  disease or disorder V82.9
    bacterial V74.9
      specified NEC V74.8
    blood V78.9
      specified type NEC V78.8
    blood-forming organ V78.9
      specified type NEC V78.8
    cardiovascular NEC V81.2
      hypertensive V81.1
      ischemic V81.0
    Chagas' V75.3
    chlamydial V73.98
      specified NEC V73.88
    ear NEC V80.3
    endocrine NEC V77.99
    eye NEC V80.2
    genitourinary NEC V81.6
    heart NEC V81.2
      hypertensive V81.1
      ischemic V81.0
    HPV (human papillomavirus) V73.81
    human papillomavirus V73.81
    immunity NEC V77.99
    infectious NEC V75.9
    lipoid NEC V77.91
    mental V79.9
      specified type NEC V79.8
    metabolic NEC V77.99
      inborn NEC V77.7
    neurological NEC V80.09
    nutritional NEC V77.99
    rheumatic NEC V82.2
    rickettsial V75.0
    sexually transmitted V74.5
      bacterial V74.5
      spirochetal V74.5
    sickle-cell V78.2
      trait V78.2
    specified type NEC V82.89
    thyroid V77.0
    vascular NEC V81.2
      ischemic V81.0
    venereal V74.5
    viral V73.99
      arthropod-borne NEC V73.5
      specified type NEC V73.89
  dislocation of hip, congenital V82.3
  drugs in athletes V70.3
  elevated titer V82.9
  emphysema (chronic) V81.3
  encephalitis, viral (mosquito or tick borne) V73.5
  endocrine disorder NEC V77.99
  eye disorder NEC V80.2
    congenital V80.2
  fever
    dengue V73.5
    hemorrhagic V73.5
    yellow V73.4
  filariasis V75.6
  galactosemia V77.4
  genetic V82.79
    disease carrier status V82.71
  genitourinary condition NEC V81.6
  glaucoma V80.1
  gonorrhea V74.5

☑ **Additional Digit Required** — Refer to the Tabular List for Digit Selection   🔻 **Subterms under main terms may continue to next column or page**

Screening — continued
  gout V77.5
  Hansen's disease V74.2
  heart disease NEC V81.2
    hypertensive V81.1
    ischemic V81.0
  heavy metal poisoning V82.5
  helminthiasis, intestinal V75.7
  hematopoietic malignancy V76.89
  hemoglobinopathies NEC V78.3
  hemorrhagic fever V73.5
  Hodgkin's disease V76.89
  hormones in athletes V70.3
  HPV (human papillomavirus) V73.81
  human papillomavirus (HPV) V73.81
  hypercholesterolemia V77.91
  hyperlipidemia V77.91
  hypertension V81.1
  immunity disorder NEC V77.99
  inborn errors of metabolism NEC V77.7
  infection
    bacterial V74.9
      specified type NEC V74.8
    mycotic V75.4
    parasitic NEC V75.8
  infectious disease V75.9
    specified type NEC V75.8
  ingestion of radioactive substance V82.5
  intellectual disabilities V79.2
  intestinal helminthiasis V75.7
  iron deficiency anemia V78.0
  ischemic heart disease V81.0
  lead poisoning V82.5
  leishmaniasis V75.2
  leprosy V74.2
  leptospirosis V74.8
  leukemia V76.89
  lipoid disorder NEC V77.91
  lymphoma V76.89
  malaria V75.1
  malignant neoplasm (of) V76.9
    bladder V76.3
    blood V76.89
    breast V76.10
      mammogram NEC V76.12
        for high-risk patient V76.11
      specified type NEC V76.19
    cervix V76.2
    colon V76.51
    colorectal V76.51
    hematopoietic system V76.89
    intestine V76.50
      colon V76.51
      small V76.52
    lung V76.0
    lymph (glands) V76.89
    nervous system V76.81
    oral cavity V76.42
    other specified neoplasm NEC V76.89
    ovary V76.46
    prostate V76.44
    rectum V76.41
    respiratory organs V76.0
    skin V76.43
    specified sites NEC V76.49
    testis V76.45
    vagina V76.47
      following hysterectomy for malig-
        nant condition V67.01
  malnutrition V77.2
  mammogram NEC V76.12
    for high-risk patient V76.11
  maternal postnatal chromosomal anomalies
    V82.4
  measles V73.2
  mental
    disorder V79.9
      specified type NEC V79.8
    retardation — see Screening, intellectual
      disabilities
  metabolic disorder NEC V77.99
  metabolic errors, inborn V77.7
  mucoviscidosis V77.6
  multiphasic V82.6
  mycosis V75.4
  mycotic infection V75.4

Screening — continued
  nephropathy V81.5
  neurological condition NEC V80.09
  nutritional disorder V77.99
  obesity V77.8
  osteoporosis V82.81
  parasitic infection NEC V75.8
  phenylketonuria V77.3
  plague V74.8
  poisoning
    chemical NEC V82.5
    contaminated water supply V82.5
      heavy metal V82.5
  poliomyelitis V73.0
  postnatal chromosomal anomalies, mater-
    nal V82.4
  prenatal — see Screening, antenatal
  pulmonary tuberculosis V74.1
  radiation exposure V82.5
  renal disease V81.5
  respiratory condition NEC V81.4
  rheumatic disorder NEC V82.2
  rheumatoid arthritis V82.1
  rickettsial disease V75.0
  rubella V73.3
  schistosomiasis V75.5
  senile macular lesions of eye V80.2
  sexually transmitted diseases V74.5
    bacterial V74.5
    spirochetal V74.5
  sickle-cell anemia, disease, or trait V78.2
  skin condition V82.0
  sleeping sickness V75.3
  smallpox V73.1
  special V82.9
    specified condition NEC V82.89
  specified type NEC V82.89
  spirochetal disease V74.9
    sexually transmitted V74.5
    specified type NEC V74.8
  stimulants in athletes V70.3
  syphilis V74.5
  tetanus V74.8
  thyroid disorder V77.0
  trachoma V73.6
  traumatic brain injury V80.01
  trypanosomiasis V75.3
  tuberculosis, pulmonary V74.1
  venereal disease V74.5
  viral encephalitis
    mosquito-borne V73.5
    tick-borne V73.5
  whooping cough V74.8
  worms, intestinal V75.7
  yaws V74.6
  yellow fever V73.4
Scrofula — see also Tuberculosis 017.2 ☑
Scrofulide (primary) — see also Tuberculosis
    017.0 ☑
Scrofuloderma, scrofulodermia (any site)
    (primary) — see also Tuberculosis
    017.0 ☑
Scrofulosis (universal) — see also Tuberculosis
    017.2 ☑
Scrofulosis lichen (primary) — see also Tuber-
    culosis 017.0 ☑
Scrofulous — see condition
Scrotal tongue 529.5
  congenital 750.13
Scrotum — see condition
Scurvy (gum) (infantile) (rickets) (scorbutic) 267
Sea-blue histiocyte syndrome 272.7
Seabright-Bantam syndrome (pseudohy-
    poparathyroidism) 275.49
Sealpox 059.12
Seasickness 994.6
Seatworm 127.4
Sebaceous
  cyst (see also Cyst, sebaceous) 706.2
  gland disease NEC 706.9
Sebocystomatosis 706.2
Seborrhea, seborrheic 706.3
  adiposa 706.3
  capitis 690.11
  congestiva 695.4
  corporis 706.3

Seborrhea, seborrheic — continued
  dermatitis 690.10
    infantile 690.12
  diathesis in infants 695.89
  eczema 690.18
    infantile 690.12
  keratosis 702.19
    inflamed 702.11
  nigricans 705.89
  sicca 690.18
  wart 702.19
    inflamed 702.11
Seckel's syndrome 759.89
Seclusion pupil 364.74
Seclusiveness, child 313.22
Secondary — see also condition
  neoplasm — see Neoplasm, by site, malig-
    nant, secondary
Secretan's disease or syndrome (posttraumat-
    ic edema) 782.3
Secretion
  antidiuretic hormone, inappropriate (syn-
    drome) 253.6
  catecholamine, by pheochromocytoma
    255.6
  hormone
    antidiuretic, inappropriate (syndrome)
      253.6
    by
      carcinoid tumor 259.2
      pheochromocytoma 255.6
    ectopic NEC 259.3
  urinary
    excessive 788.42
    suppression 788.5
Section
  cesarean
    affecting fetus or newborn 763.4
    post mortem, affecting fetus or newborn
      761.6
    previous, in pregnancy or childbirth
      654.2 ☑
      affecting fetus or newborn 763.89
  nerve, traumatic — see Injury, nerve, by site
Seeligmann's syndrome (ichthyosis congeni-
    ta) 757.1
Segmentation, incomplete (congenital) —
    see also Fusion
  bone NEC 756.9
  lumbosacral (joint) 756.15
  vertebra 756.15
    lumbosacral 756.15
Seizure(s) 780.39
  akinetic (idiopathic) (see also Epilepsy)
    345.0 ☑
    psychomotor 345.4 ☑
  apoplexy, apoplectic (see also Disease,
    cerebrovascular, acute) 436
  atonic (see also Epilepsy) 345.0 ☑
  autonomic 300.11
  brain or cerebral (see also Disease, cere-
    brovascular, acute) 436
  convulsive (see also Convulsions) 780.39
  cortical (focal) (motor) (see also Epilepsy)
    345.5 ☑
  disorder (see also Epilepsy) 345.9 ☑
    due to stroke 438.89
  epilepsy, epileptic (cryptogenic) (see also
    Epilepsy) 345.9 ☑
  epileptiform, epileptoid 780.39
    focal (see also Epilepsy) 345.5 ☑
  febrile (simple) 780.31
    with status epilepticus 345.3
    atypical 780.32
    complex 780.32
    complicated 780.32
  heart — see Disease, heart
  hysterical 300.11
  Jacksonian (focal) (see also Epilepsy)
    345.5 ☑
    motor type 345.5 ☑
    sensory type 345.5 ☑
  migraine triggered 346.0 ☑
  newborn 779.0
  paralysis (see also Disease, cerebrovascular,
    acute) 436

Seizure(s) — continued
  posttraumatic 780.33
  recurrent 345.8 ☑
    epileptic — see Epilepsy
  repetitive 780.39
    epileptic — see Epilepsy
  salaam (see also Epilepsy) 345.6 ☑
  uncinate (see also Epilepsy) 345.4 ☑
Self-mutilation 300.9
Semicoma 780.09
Semiconsciousness 780.09
Seminal
  vesicle — see condition
  vesiculitis (see also Vesiculitis) 608.0
Seminoma (M9061/3)
  anaplastic type (M9062/3)
    specified site — see Neoplasm, by site,
      malignant
    unspecified site 186.9
  specified site — see Neoplasm, by site, ma-
    lignant
  spermatocytic (M9063/3)
    specified site — see Neoplasm, by site,
      malignant
    unspecified site 186.9
  unspecified site 186.9
Semliki Forest encephalitis 062.8
Senear-Usher disease or syndrome (pemphi-
    gus erythematosus) 694.4
Senecio jacobae dermatitis 692.6
Senectus 797
Senescence 797
Senile — see also condition 797
  cervix (atrophic) 622.8
  degenerative atrophy, skin 701.3
  endometrium (atrophic) 621.8
  fallopian tube (atrophic) 620.3
  heart (failure) 797
  lung 492.8
  ovary (atrophic) 620.3
  syndrome 259.8
  vagina, vaginitis (atrophic) 627.3
  wart 702.0
Senility 797
  with
    acute confusional state 290.3
    delirium 290.3
    mental changes 290.9
    psychosis NEC (see also Psychosis, senile)
      290.20
  premature (syndrome) 259.8
Sensation
  burning (see also Disturbance, sensation)
    782.0
    tongue 529.6
  choking 784.99
  loss of (see also Disturbance, sensation)
    782.0
  prickling (see also Disturbance, sensation)
    782.0
  tingling (see also Disturbance, sensation)
    782.0
Sense loss (touch) — see also Disturbance,
    sensation 782.0
  smell 781.1
  taste 781.1
Sensibility disturbance NEC (cortical) (deep)
    (vibratory) — see also Disturbance, sen-
    sation 782.0
Sensitive dentine 521.89
Sensitiver Beziehungswahn 297.8
Sensitivity, sensitization — see also Allergy
  autoerythrocyte 287.2
  carotid sinus 337.01
  child (excessive) 313.21
  cold, autoimmune 283.0
  methemoglobin 289.7
  suxamethonium 289.89
  tuberculin, without clinical or radiological
    symptoms 795.51
Sensory
  extinction 781.8
  neglect 781.8
Separation
  acromioclavicular — see Dislocation,
    acromioclavicular

Separation — *continued*
anxiety, abnormal 309.21
apophysis, traumatic — *see* Fracture, by site
choroid 363.70
  hemorrhagic 363.72
  serous 363.71
costochondral (simple) (traumatic) — *see* Dislocation, costochondral
delayed
  umbilical cord 779.83
epiphysis, epiphyseal
  nontraumatic 732.9
   upper femoral 732.2
  traumatic — *see* Fracture, by site
fracture — *see* Fracture, by site
infundibulum cardiac from right ventricle by a partition 746.83
joint (current) (traumatic) — *see* Dislocation, by site
placenta (normally implanted) — *see* Placenta, separation
pubic bone, obstetrical trauma 665.6 ☑
retina, retinal (*see also* Detachment, retina) 361.9
  layers 362.40
   sensory (*see also* Retinoschisis) 361.10
  pigment epithelium (exudative) 362.42
   hemorrhagic 362.43
sternoclavicular (traumatic) — *see* Dislocation, sternoclavicular
symphysis pubis, obstetrical trauma 665.6 ☑
tracheal ring, incomplete (congenital) 748.3
Sepsis (generalized) 995.91
with
  abortion — *see* Abortion, by type, with sepsis
  acute organ dysfunction 995.92
  ectopic pregnancy (*see also* categories 633.0–633.9) 639.0
  molar pregnancy (*see also* categories 630–632) 639.0
  multiple organ dysfunction (MOD) 995.92
buccal 528.3
complicating labor 659.3 ☑
dental (pulpal origin) 522.4
female genital organ NEC 614.9
fetus (intrauterine) 771.81
following
  abortion 639.0
  ectopic or molar pregnancy 639.0
  infusion, perfusion, or transfusion 999.39
Friedländer's 038.49
intra-abdominal 567.22
intraocular 360.00
localized — code to specific localized infection
  in operation wound 998.59
  skin (*see also* Abscess) 682.9
malleus 024
nadir 038.9
newborn (organism unspecified) NEC 771.81
oral 528.3
puerperal, postpartum, childbirth (pelvic) 670.2 ☑
resulting from infusion, injection, transfusion, or vaccination 999.39
severe 995.92
skin, localized (*see also* Abscess) 682.9
umbilical (newborn) (organism unspecified) 771.89
  tetanus 771.3
urinary 599.0
  meaning sepsis 995.91
  meaning urinary tract infection 599.0
Septate — *see also* Septum
Septic — *see also* condition
adenoids 474.01
  and tonsils 474.02
arm (with lymphangitis) 682.3
embolus — *see* Embolism
finger (with lymphangitis) 681.00
foot (with lymphangitis) 682.7
gallbladder (*see also* Cholecystitis) 575.8

Septic — *see also* condition — *continued*
hand (with lymphangitis) 682.4
joint (*see also* Arthritis, septic) 711.0 ☑
kidney (*see also* Infection, kidney) 590.9
leg (with lymphangitis) 682.6
mouth 528.3
nail 681.9
  finger 681.02
  toe 681.11
shock (endotoxic) 785.52
  postoperative 998.02
sore (*see also* Abscess) 682.9
  throat 034.0
   milk-borne 034.0
   streptococcal 034.0
spleen (acute) 289.59
teeth (pulpal origin) 522.4
throat 034.0
thrombus — *see* Thrombosis
toe (with lymphangitis) 681.10
tonsils 474.00
  and adenoids 474.02
umbilical cord (newborn) (organism unspecified) 771.89
uterus (*see also* Endometritis) 615.9
Septicemia, septicemic (generalized) (suppurative) 038.9
with
  abortion — *see* Abortion, by type, with sepsis
  ectopic pregnancy (*see also* categories 633.0–633.9) 639.0
  molar pregnancy (*see also* categories 630–632) 639.0
Aerobacter aerogenes 038.49
anaerobic 038.3
anthrax 022.3
Bacillus coli 038.42
Bacteroides 038.3
Clostridium 038.3
complicating labor 659.3 ☑
cryptogenic 038.9
enteric gram-negative bacilli 038.40
Enterobacter aerogenes 038.49
Erysipelothrix (insidiosa) (rhusiopathiae) 027.1
Escherichia coli 038.42
following
  abortion 639.0
  ectopic or molar pregnancy 639.0
  infusion, injection, transfusion, or vaccination 999.39
Friedländer's (bacillus) 038.49
gangrenous 038.9
gonococcal 098.89
gram-negative (organism) 038.40
  anaerobic 038.3
Hemophilus influenzae 038.41
herpes (simplex) 054.5
herpetic 054.5
Listeria monocytogenes 027.0
meningeal — *see* Meningitis
meningococcal (chronic) (fulminating) 036.2
methicillin
  resistant Staphylococcus aureus (MRSA) 038.12
  susceptible Staphylococcus aureus (MSSA) 038.11
MRSA (methicillin resistant Staphylococcus aureus) 038.12
MSSA (methicillin susceptible Staphylococcus aureus) 038.11
navel, newborn (organism unspecified) 771.89
newborn (organism unspecified) 771.81
plague 020.2
pneumococcal 038.2
postabortal 639.0
postoperative 998.59
Proteus vulgaris 038.49
Pseudomonas (aeruginosa) 038.43
puerperal, postpartum 670.2 ☑
Salmonella (aertrycke) (callinarum) (choleraesuis) (enteritidis) (suipestifer) 003.1
Serratia 038.44
Shigella (*see also* Dysentery, bacillary) 004.9

Septicemia, septicemic — *continued*
specified organism NEC 038.8
staphylococcal 038.10
  aureus 038.11
   methicillin
    resistant (MRSA) 038.12
    susceptible (MSSA) 038.11
  specified organism NEC 038.19
streptococcal (anaerobic) 038.0
Streptococcus pneumoniae 038.2
suipestifer 003.1
umbilicus, newborn (organism unspecified) 771.89
viral 079.99
Yersinia enterocolitica 038.49
Septum, septate (congenital) — *see also* Anomaly, specified type NEC
anal 751.2
aqueduct of Sylvius 742.3
  with spina bifida (*see also* Spina bifida) 741.0 ☑
hymen 752.49
uterus (complete) (partial) 752.35
vagina
  in pregnancy or childbirth 654.7 ☑
   affecting fetus or newborn 763.89
   causing obstructed labor 660.2 ☑
    affecting fetus or newborn 763.1
  longitudinal (with or without obstruction) 752.47
  transverse 752.46
Sequestration
lung (congenital) (extralobar) (intralobar) 748.5
orbit 376.10
pulmonary artery (congenital) 747.39
splenic 289.52
Sequestrum
bone (*see also* Osteomyelitis) 730.1 ☑
  jaw 526.4
dental 525.8
jaw bone 526.4
sinus (accessory) (nasal) (*see also* Sinusitis) 473.9
  maxillary 473.0
Sequoiosis asthma 495.8
Serology for syphilis
doubtful
  with signs or symptoms — *see* Syphilis, by site and stage
  follow-up of latent syphilis — *see* Syphilis, latent
false positive 795.6
negative, with signs or symptoms — *see* Syphilis, by site and stage
positive 097.1
  with signs or symptoms — *see* Syphilis, by site and stage
  false 795.6
  follow-up of latent syphilis — *see* Syphilis, latent
  only finding — *see* Syphilis, latent
reactivated 097.1
Seroma (postoperative) (non-infected) 998.13
infected 998.51
post-traumatic 729.91
Seropurulent — *see* condition
Serositis, multiple 569.89
pericardial 423.2
peritoneal 568.82
pleural — *see* Pleurisy
Serotonin syndrome 333.99
Serous — *see* condition
Sertoli cell
adenoma (M8640/0)
  specified site — *see* Neoplasm, by site, benign
  unspecified site
   female 220
   male 222.0
carcinoma (M8640/3)
  specified site — *see* Neoplasm, by site, malignant
  unspecified site 186.9
syndrome (germinal aplasia) 606.0

Sertoli cell — *continued*
tumor (M8640/0)
  with lipid storage (M8641/0)
   specified site — *see* Neoplasm, by site, benign
   unspecified site
    female 220
    male 222.0
  specified site — *see* Neoplasm, by site, benign
  unspecified site
   female 220
   male 222.0
Sertoli-Leydig cell tumor (M8631/0)
specified site — *see* Neoplasm, by site, benign
unspecified site
  female 220
  male 222.0
Serum
allergy, allergic reaction 999.59
  shock 999.49
arthritis 999.59 [713.6]
complication or reaction NEC 999.59
disease NEC 999.59
hepatitis 070.3 ☑
intoxication 999.59
jaundice (homologous) — *see* Hepatitis, viral, type B
neuritis 999.59
poisoning NEC 999.59
rash NEC 999.59
reaction NEC 999.59
sickness NEC 999.59
Sesamoiditis 733.99
Seven-day fever 061
of
  Japan 100.89
  Queensland 100.89
Sever's disease or osteochondrosis (calcaneum) 732.5
Sex chromosome mosaics 758.81
Sex reassignment surgery status (*see also* Trans-sexualism) 302.50
Sextuplet
affected by maternal complications of pregnancy 761.5
healthy liveborn — *see* Newborn, multiple
pregnancy (complicating delivery) NEC 651.8 ☑
  with fetal loss and retention of one or more fetus(es) 651.6 ☑
  following (elective) fetal reduction 651.7 ☑
Sexual
anesthesia 302.72
deviation (*see also* Deviation, sexual) 302.9
disorder (*see also* Deviation, sexual) 302.9
frigidity (female) 302.72
function, disorder of (psychogenic) 302.70
  specified type NEC 302.79
immaturity (female) (male) 259.0
impotence 607.84
  organic origin NEC 607.84
  psychogenic 302.72
precocity (constitutional) (cryptogenic) (female) (idiopathic) (male) NEC 259.1
  with adrenal hyperplasia 255.2
sadism 302.84
Sexuality, pathological — *see also* Deviation, sexual 302.9
Sézary's disease, reticulosis, or syndrome (M9701/3) 202.2 ☑
Shadow, lung 793.19
Shaken infant syndrome 995.55
Shaking
head (tremor) 781.0
palsy or paralysis (*see also* Parkinsonism) 332.0
Shallowness, acetabulum 736.39
Shaver's disease or syndrome (bauxite pneumoconiosis) 503
Shearing
artificial skin graft 996.55
decellularized allodermis graft 996.55
Sheath (tendon) — *see* condition

☑ **Additional Digit Required** — Refer to the Tabular List for Digit Selection   ▽ **Subterms under main terms may continue to next column or page**

2014 ICD-9-CM   **301**

Shedding
nail 703.8
teeth, premature, primary (deciduous) 520.6
Sheehan's disease or syndrome (postpartum pituitary necrosis) 253.2
Shelf, rectal 569.49
Shell
shock (current) (see also Reaction, stress, acute) 308.9
lasting state 300.16
teeth 520.5
Shield kidney 753.3
Shifting
pacemaker 427.89
sleep-work schedule (affecting sleep) 327.36
Shift, mediastinal 793.2
Shiga's
bacillus 004.0
dysentery 004.0
Shigella (dysentery) — see also Dysentery, bacillary 004.9
carrier (suspected) of V02.3
Shigellosis — see also Dysentery, bacillary 004.9
Shingles — see also Herpes, zoster 053.9
eye NEC 053.29
Shin splints 844.9
Shipyard eye or disease 077.1
Shirodkar suture, in pregnancy 654.5 ☑
Shock 785.50
with
abortion — see Abortion, by type, with shock
ectopic pregnancy (see also categories 633.0–633.9) 639.5
molar pregnancy (see also categories 630–632) 639.5
allergic — see Anaphylactic reaction or shock
anaclitic 309.21
anaphylactic — see also Anaphylactic reaction or shock
due to administration of blood and blood products 999.41
anaphylactoid — see Anaphylactic reaction or shock
anesthetic
correct substance properly administered 995.4
overdose or wrong substance given 968.4
specified anesthetic — see Table of Drugs and Chemicals
birth, fetus or newborn NEC 779.89
cardiogenic 785.51
chemical substance — see Table of Drugs and Chemicals
circulatory 785.59
complicating
abortion — see Abortion, by type, with shock
ectopic pregnancy (see also categories 633.0–633.9) 639.5
labor and delivery 669.1 ☑
molar pregnancy (see also categories 630–632) 639.5
culture 309.29
due to
drug 995.0
correct substance properly administered 995.0
overdose or wrong substance given or taken 977.9
specified drug — see Table of Drugs and Chemicals
food — see Anaphylactic shock, due to, food
during labor and delivery 669.1 ☑
electric 994.8
from electroshock gun (taser) 994.8
endotoxic 785.52
due to surgical procedure 998.02
postoperative 998.02
following
abortion 639.5
ectopic or molar pregnancy 639.5

Shock — continued
following — continued
injury (immediate) (delayed) 958.4
labor and delivery 669.1 ☑
gram-negative 785.52
postoperative 998.02
hematogenic 785.59
hemorrhagic
due to
disease 785.59
surgery (intraoperative) (postoperative) 998.09
trauma 958.4
hypovolemic NEC 785.59
surgical 998.09
traumatic 958.4
insulin 251.0
therapeutic misadventure 962.3
kidney 584.5
traumatic (following crushing) 958.5
lightning 994.0
lung 518.82
related to trauma and surgery 518.52
nervous (see also Reaction, stress, acute) 308.9
obstetric 669.1 ☑
with
abortion — see Abortion, by type, with shock
ectopic pregnancy (see also categories 633.0–633.9) 639.5
molar pregnancy (see also categories 630–632) 639.5
following
abortion 639.5
ectopic or molar pregnancy 639.5
paralysis, paralytic (see also Disease, cerebrovascular, acute) 436
late effect — see Late effect(s) (of) cerebrovascular disease
pleural (surgical) 998.09
due to trauma 958.4
postoperative 998.00
with
abortion — see Abortion, by type, with shock
ectopic pregnancy (see also categories 633.0–633.9) 639.5
molar pregnancy (see also categories 630–632) 639.5
cardiogenic 998.01
following
abortion 639.5
ectopic or molar pregnancy 639.5
hypovolemic 998.09
septic (endotoxic) (gram-negative) 998.02
specified NEC 998.09
psychic (see also Reaction, stress, acute) 308.9
past history (of) V15.49
psychogenic (see also Reaction, stress, acute) 308.9
septic 785.52
with
abortion — see Abortion, by type, with shock
ectopic pregnancy (see also categories 633.0–633.9) 639.5
molar pregnancy (see also categories 630–632) 639.5
due to
surgical procedure 998.02
transfusion NEC 999.89
bone marrow 996.85
following
abortion 639.5
ectopic or molar pregnancy 639.5
surgical procedure 998.02
transfusion NEC 999.89
bone marrow 996.85
postoperative 998.02
spinal (see also Injury, spinal, by site)
with spinal bone injury — see Fracture, vertebra, by site, with spinal cord injury

Shock — continued
surgical 998.00
therapeutic misadventure NEC (see also Complications) 998.89
thyroxin 962.7
toxic 040.82
transfusion — see Complications, transfusion
traumatic (immediate) (delayed) 958.4
Shoemakers' chest 738.3
Short, shortening, shortness
Achilles tendon (acquired) 727.81
arm 736.89
congenital 755.20
back 737.9
bowel syndrome 579.3
breath 786.05
cervical, cervix 649.7 ☑
gravid uterus 649.7 ☑
non-gravid uterus 622.5
acquired 622.5
congenital 752.49
chain acyl CoA dehydrogenase deficiency (SCAD) 277.85
common bile duct, congenital 751.69
cord (umbilical) 663.4 ☑
affecting fetus or newborn 762.6
cystic duct, congenital 751.69
esophagus (congenital) 750.4
femur (acquired) 736.81
congenital 755.34
frenulum linguae 750.0
frenum, lingual 750.0
hamstrings 727.81
hip (acquired) 736.39
congenital 755.63
leg (acquired) 736.81
congenital 755.30
metatarsus (congenital) 754.79
acquired 736.79
organ or site, congenital NEC — see Distortion
palate (congenital) 750.26
P-R interval syndrome 426.81
radius (acquired) 736.09
congenital 755.26
round ligament 629.89
sleeper 307.49
stature, constitutional (hereditary) (idiopathic) 783.43
tendon 727.81
Achilles (acquired) 727.81
congenital 754.79
congenital 756.89
thigh (acquired) 736.81
congenital 755.34
tibialis anticus 727.81
umbilical cord 663.4 ☑
affecting fetus or newborn 762.6
urethra 599.84
uvula (congenital) 750.26
vagina 623.8
Shortsightedness 367.1
Shoshin (acute fulminating beriberi) 265.0
Shoulder — see condition
Shovel-shaped incisors 520.2
Shower, thromboembolic — see Embolism
Shunt (status)
aortocoronary bypass V45.81
arterial-venous (dialysis) V45.11
arteriovenous, pulmonary (acquired) 417.0
congenital 747.39
traumatic (complication) 901.40
cerebral ventricle (communicating) in situ V45.2
coronary artery bypass V45.81
surgical, prosthetic, with complications — see Complications, shunt
vascular NEC V45.89
Shutdown
renal 586
with
abortion — see Abortion, by type, with renal failure
ectopic pregnancy (see also categories 633.0–633.9) 639.3

Shutdown — continued
renal — continued
with — continued
molar pregnancy (see also categories 630–632) 639.3
complicating
abortion 639.3
ectopic or molar pregnancy 639.3
following labor and delivery 669.3 ☑
Shwachman's syndrome 288.02
Shy-Drager syndrome (orthostatic hypotension with multisystem degeneration) 333.0
Sialadenitis (any gland) (chronic) (suppurative) 527.2
epidemic — see Mumps
Sialadenosis, periodic 527.2
Sialaporia 527.7
Sialectasia 527.8
Sialitis 527.2
Sialoadenitis — see also Sialadenitis 527.2
Sialoangitis 527.2
Sialodochitis (fibrinosa) 527.2
Sialodocholithiasis 527.5
Sialolithiasis 527.5
Sialorrhea — see also Ptyalism 527.7
periodic 527.2
Sialosis 527.8
rheumatic 710.2
Siamese twin 759.4
complicating pregnancy 678.1 ☑
Sicard's syndrome 352.6
Sicca syndrome (keratoconjunctivitis) 710.2
Sick 799.9
cilia syndrome 759.89
or handicapped person in family V61.49
Sickle-cell
anemia (see also Disease, sickle-cell) 282.60
disease (see also Disease, sickle-cell) 282.60
hemoglobin
C disease (without crisis) 282.63
with
crisis 282.64
vaso-occlusive pain 282.64
D disease (without crisis) 282.68
with crisis 282.69
E disease (without crisis) 282.68
with crisis 282.69
thalassemia (without crisis) 282.41
with
crisis 282.42
vaso-occlusive pain 282.42
trait 282.5
Sicklemia — see also Disease, sickle-cell 282.60
trait 282.5
Sickness
air (travel) 994.6
airplane 994.6
alpine 993.2
altitude 993.2
Andes 993.2
aviators' 993.2
balloon 993.2
car 994.6
compressed air 993.3
decompression 993.3
green 280.9
harvest 100.89
milk 988.8
morning 643.0 ☑
motion 994.6
mountain 993.2
acute 289.0
protein (see also Complications, vaccination) 999.59
radiation NEC 990
roundabout (motion) 994.6
sea 994.6
serum NEC 999.59
sleeping (African) 086.5
by Trypanosoma 086.5
gambiense 086.3
rhodesiense 086.4
Gambian 086.3
late effect 139.8
Rhodesian 086.4

Sickness — *continued*
 sweating 078.2
 swing (motion) 994.6
 train (railway) (travel) 994.6
 travel (any vehicle) 994.6
Sick sinus syndrome 427.81
Sideropenia — *see also* Anemia, iron deficiency 280.9
Siderosis (lung) (occupational) 503
 central nervous system (CNS) 437.8
 cornea 371.15
 eye (bulbi) (vitreous) 360.23
 lens 360.23
Siegal-Cattan-Mamou disease (periodic) 277.31
Siemens' syndrome
 ectodermal dysplasia 757.31
 keratosis follicularis spinulosa (decalvans) 757.39
Sighing respiration 786.7
Sigmoid
 flexure — *see* condition
 kidney 753.3
Sigmoiditis — *see* Enteritis
Silfverskiöld's syndrome 756.50
Silicosis, silicotic (complicated) (occupational) (simple) 502
 fibrosis, lung (confluent) (massive) (occupational) 502
 non-nodular 503
 pulmonum 502
Silicotuberculosis — *see also* Tuberculosis 011.4 ☑
Silo fillers' disease 506.9
Silver's syndrome (congenital hemihypertrophy and short stature) 759.89
Silver wire arteries, retina 362.13
Silvestroni-Bianco syndrome (thalassemia minima) 282.49
Simian crease 757.2
Simmonds' cachexia or disease (pituitary cachexia) 253.2
Simons' disease or syndrome (progressive lipodystrophy) 272.6
Simple, simplex — *see* condition
Sinding-Larsen disease (juvenile osteopathia patellae) 732.4
Singapore hemorrhagic fever 065.4
Singers' node or nodule 478.5
Single
 atrium 745.69
 coronary artery 746.85
 umbilical artery 747.5
 ventricle 745.3
Singultus 786.8
 epidemicus 078.89
Sinus — *see also* Fistula
 abdominal 569.81
 arrest 426.6
 arrhythmia 427.89
 bradycardia 427.89
  chronic 427.81
 branchial cleft (external) (internal) 744.41
 coccygeal (infected) 685.1
  with abscess 685.0
 dental 522.7
 dermal (congenital) 685.1
  with abscess 685.0
 draining — *see* Fistula
 infected, skin NEC 686.9
 marginal, ruptured or bleeding 641.2 ☑
  affecting fetus or newborn 762.1
 pause 426.6
 pericranii 742.0
 pilonidal (infected) (rectum) 685.1
  with abscess 685.0
 preauricular 744.46
 rectovaginal 619.1
 sacrococcygeal (dermoid) (infected) 685.1
  with abscess 685.0
 skin
  infected NEC 686.9
  noninfected — *see* Ulcer, skin
 tachycardia 427.89
 tarsi syndrome 726.79
 testis 608.89

Sinus — *see also* Fistula — *continued*
 tract (postinfectional) — *see* Fistula
 urachus 753.7
Sinuses, Rokitansky-Aschoff — *see also* Disease, gallbladder 575.8
Sinusitis (accessory) (nasal) (hyperplastic) (nonpurulent) (purulent) (chronic) 473.9
 with influenza, flu, or grippe (*see also* Influenza) 487.1
 acute 461.9
  ethmoidal 461.2
  frontal 461.1
  maxillary 461.0
  specified type NEC 461.8
  sphenoidal 461.3
 allergic (*see also* Fever, hay) 477.9
 antrum — *see* Sinusitis, maxillary
 due to
  fungus, any sinus 117.9
  high altitude 993.1
 ethmoidal 473.2
  acute 461.2
 frontal 473.1
  acute 461.1
 influenzal (*see also* Influenza) 487.1
 maxillary 473.0
  acute 461.0
 specified site NEC 473.8
 sphenoidal 473.3
  acute 461.3
 syphilitic, any sinus 095.8
 tuberculous, any sinus (*see also* Tuberculosis) 012.8 ☑
Sinusitis-bronchiectasis-situs inversus (syndrome) (triad) 759.3
Sioloangitis 527.2
Sipple's syndrome (medullary thyroid carcinoma-pheochromocytoma) 258.02
Sirenomelia 759.89
Siriasis 992.0
Sirkari's disease 085.0
SIRS (systemic inflammatory response syndrome) 995.90
 due to
  infectious process 995.91
   with acute organ dysfunction 995.92
  non-infectious process 995.93
   with acute organ dysfunction 995.94
Siti 104.0
Sitophobia 300.29
Situational
 disturbance (transient) (*see also* Reaction, adjustment) 309.9
  acute 308.3
 maladjustment, acute (*see also* Reaction, adjustment) 309.9
 reaction (*see also* Reaction, adjustment) 309.9
  acute 308.3
Situation, psychiatric 300.9
Situs inversus or transversus 759.3
 abdominalis 759.3
 thoracis 759.3
Sixth disease
 due to
  human herpesvirus 6 058.11
  human herpesvirus 7 058.12
Sjögren-Larsson syndrome (ichthyosis congenita) 757.1
Sjögren (-Gougerot) syndrome or disease (keratoconjunctivitis sicca) 710.2
 with lung involvement 710.2 *[517.8]*
SJS-TEN (Stevens-Johnson syndrome - toxic epidermal necrolysis overlap syndrome) 695.14
Skeletal — *see* condition
Skene's gland — *see* condition
Skenitis — *see also* Urethritis 597.89
 gonorrheal (acute) 098.0
  chronic or duration of 2 months or over 098.2
Skerljevo 104.0
Skevas-Zerfus disease 989.5
Skin — *see also* condition
 donor V59.1
 hidebound 710.9

SLAP lesion (superior glenoid labrum) 840.7
Slate-dressers' lung 502
Slate-miners' lung 502
Sleep
 deprivation V69.4
 disorder 780.50
  with apnea — *see* Apnea, sleep
  child 307.40
  movement, unspecified 780.58
  nonorganic origin 307.40
   specified type NEC 307.49
 disturbance 780.50
  with apnea — *see* Apnea, sleep
  nonorganic origin 307.40
   specified type NEC 307.49
 drunkenness 307.47
 movement disorder, unspecified 780.58
 paroxysmal (*see also* Narcolepsy) 347.00
 related movement disorder, unspecified 780.58
 rhythm inversion 327.39
  nonorganic origin 307.45
 walking 307.46
  hysterical 300.13
Sleeping sickness 086.5
 late effect 139.8
Sleeplessness — *see also* Insomnia 780.52
 menopausal 627.2
 nonorganic origin 307.41
Slipped, slipping
 epiphysis (postinfectional) 732.9
  traumatic (old) 732.9
  current — *see* Fracture, by site
  upper femoral (nontraumatic) 732.2
 intervertebral disc — *see* Displacement, intervertebral disc
 ligature, umbilical 772.3
 patella 717.89
 rib 733.99
 sacroiliac joint 724.6
 tendon 727.9
 ulnar nerve, nontraumatic 354.2
 vertebra NEC (*see also* Spondylolisthesis) 756.12
Slocumb's syndrome 255.3
Sloughing (multiple) (skin) 686.9
 abscess — *see* Abscess, by site
 appendix 543.9
 bladder 596.89
 fascia 728.9
 graft — *see* Complications, graft
 phagedena (*see also* Gangrene) 785.4
 reattached extremity (*see also* Complications, reattached extremity) 996.90
 rectum 569.49
 scrotum 608.89
 tendon 727.9
 transplanted organ (*see also* Rejection, transplant, organ, by site) 996.80
 ulcer (*see also* Ulcer, skin) 707.9
Slow
 feeding newborn 779.31
 fetal, growth NEC 764.9 ☑
  affecting management of pregnancy 656.5 ☑
Slowing
 heart 427.89
 urinary stream 788.62
Sluder's neuralgia or syndrome 337.09
Slurred, slurring, speech 784.59
Small-for-dates — *see also* Light-for-dates 764.0 ☑
 affecting management of pregnancy 656.5 ☑
Smallpox 050.9
 contact V01.3
 exposure to V01.3
 hemorrhagic (pustular) 050.0
 malignant 050.0
 modified 050.2
 vaccination
  complications — *see* Complications, vaccination
  prophylactic (against) V04.1
Small, smallness
 cardiac reserve — *see* Disease, heart

Small, smallness — *continued*
 for dates
  fetus or newborn 764.0 ☑
   with malnutrition 764.1 ☑
   affecting management of pregnancy 656.5 ☑
  infant, term 764.0 ☑
   with malnutrition 764.1 ☑
   affecting management of pregnancy 656.5 ☑
 introitus, vagina 623.3
 kidney, unknown cause 589.9
  bilateral 589.1
  unilateral 589.0
 ovary 620.8
 pelvis
  with disproportion (fetopelvic) 653.1 ☑
   affecting fetus or newborn 763.1
  causing obstructed labor 660.1 ☑
   affecting fetus or newborn 763.1
 placenta — *see* Placenta, insufficiency
 uterus 621.8
 white kidney 582.9
Smearing, fecal 787.62
Smith's fracture (separation) (closed) 813.41
 open 813.51
Smith-Lemli Opitz syndrome (cerebrohepatorenal syndrome) 759.89
Smith-Magenis syndrome 758.33
Smith-Strang disease (oasthouse urine) 270.2
Smokers'
 bronchitis 491.0
 cough 491.0
 syndrome (*see also* Abuse, drugs, nondependent) 305.1
 throat 472.1
 tongue 528.6
Smoking complicating pregnancy, childbirth, or the puerperium 649.0 ☑
Smothering spells 786.09
Snaggle teeth, tooth 524.39
Snapping
 finger 727.05
 hip 719.65
 jaw 524.69
  temporomandibular joint sounds on opening or closing 524.64
 knee 717.9
 thumb 727.05
Sneddon-Wilkinson disease or syndrome (subcorneal pustular dermatosis) 694.1
Sneezing 784.99
 intractable 478.19
Sniffing
 cocaine (*see also* Dependence) 304.2 ☑
 ether (*see also* Dependence) 304.6 ☑
 glue (airplane) (*see also* Dependence) 304.6 ☑
Snoring 786.09
Snow blindness 370.24
Snuffles (nonsyphilitic) 460
 syphilitic (infant) 090.0
Social migrant V60.0
Sodoku 026.0
Soemmering's ring 366.51
Soft — *see also* condition
 enlarged prostate 600.00
  with
   other lower urinary tract symptoms (LUTS) 600.01
   urinary
    obstruction 600.01
    retention 600.01
 nails 703.8
Softening
 bone 268.2
 brain (necrotic) (progressive) 348.89
  arteriosclerotic 437.0
  congenital 742.4
  due to cerebrovascular accident 438.89
  embolic (*see also* Embolism, brain) 434.1 ☑
  hemorrhagic (*see also* Hemorrhage, brain) 431
  occlusive 434.9 ☑

☑ **Additional Digit Required** — **Refer to the Tabular List for Digit Selection**   ▽ **Subterms under main terms may continue to next column or page**

Softening — *continued*
  brain — *continued*
    thrombotic (*see also* Thrombosis, brain) 434.0 ☑
  cartilage 733.92
  cerebellar — *see* Softening, brain
  cerebral — *see* Softening, brain
  cerebrospinal — *see* Softening, brain
  myocardial, heart (*see also* Degeneration, myocardial) 429.1
  nails 703.8
  spinal cord 336.8
  stomach 537.89
Soiling, fecal 787.62
Solar fever 061
Soldier's
  heart 306.2
  patches 423.1
Solitary
  cyst
    bone 733.21
    kidney 593.2
  kidney (congenital) 753.0
  tubercle, brain (*see also* Tuberculosis, brain) 013.2 ☑
  ulcer, bladder 596.89
Somatization reaction, somatic reaction — *see also* Disorder, psychosomatic 306.9
  disorder 300.81
Somatoform disorder 300.82
  atypical 300.82
  severe 300.81
  undifferentiated 300.82
Somnambulism 307.46
  hysterical 300.13
Somnolence 780.09
  nonorganic origin 307.43
  periodic 349.89
Sonne dysentery 004.3
Soor 112.0
Sore
  Delhi 085.1
  desert (*see also* Ulcer, skin) 707.9
  eye 379.99
  Lahore 085.1
  mouth 528.9
    canker 528.2
    due to dentures 528.9
  muscle 729.1
  Naga (*see also* Ulcer, skin) 707.9
  oriental 085.1
  pressure (*see also* Ulcer, pressure) 707.00
    with gangrene (*see also* Ulcer, pressure) 707.00 [785.4]
  skin NEC 709.9
  soft 099.0
  throat 462
    with influenza, flu, or grippe (*see also* Influenza) 487.1
    acute 462
    chronic 472.1
    clergyman's 784.49
    coxsackie (virus) 074.0
    diphtheritic 032.0
    epidemic 034.0
    gangrenous 462
    herpetic 054.79
    influenzal (*see also* Influenza) 487.1
    malignant 462
    purulent 462
    putrid 462
    septic 034.0
    streptococcal (ulcerative) 034.0
    ulcerated 462
    viral NEC 462
      Coxsackie 074.0
  tropical (*see also* Ulcer, skin) 707.9
  veldt (*see also* Ulcer, skin) 707.9
Sotos' syndrome (cerebral gigantism) 253.0
Sounds
  friction, pleural 786.7
  succussion, chest 786.7
  temporomandibular joint
    on opening or closing 524.64
South African cardiomyopathy syndrome 425.2

South American
  blastomycosis 116.1
  trypanosomiasis — *see* Trypanosomiasis
Southeast Asian hemorrhagic fever 065.4
Spacing, teeth, abnormal 524.30
  excessive 524.32
Spade-like hand (congenital) 754.89
Spading nail 703.8
  congenital 757.5
Spanemia 285.9
Spanish collar 605
Sparganosis 123.5
Spasmodic — *see* condition
Spasmophilia — *see also* Tetany 781.7
Spasm, spastic, spasticity — *see also* condition 781.0
  accommodation 367.53
  ampulla of Vater (*see also* Disease, gallbladder) 576.8
  anus, ani (sphincter) (reflex) 564.6
    psychogenic 306.4
  artery NEC 443.9
    basilar 435.0
    carotid 435.8
    cerebral 435.9
      specified artery NEC 435.8
    retinal (*see also* Occlusion, retinal, artery) 362.30
    vertebral 435.1
    vertebrobasilar 435.3
  Bell's 351.0
  bladder (sphincter, external or internal) 596.89
  bowel 564.9
    psychogenic 306.4
  bronchus, bronchiole 519.11
  cardia 530.0
  cardiac — *see* Angina
  carpopedal (*see also* Tetany) 781.7
  cecum 564.9
    psychogenic 306.4
  cerebral (arteries) (vascular) 435.9
    specified artery NEC 435.8
  cerebrovascular 435.9
  cervix, complicating delivery 661.4 ☑
    affecting fetus or newborn 763.7
  ciliary body (of accommodation) 367.53
  colon 564.1
    psychogenic 306.4
  common duct (*see also* Disease, biliary) 576.8
  compulsive 307.22
  conjugate 378.82
  convergence 378.84
  coronary (artery) — *see* Angina
  diaphragm (reflex) 786.8
    psychogenic 306.1
  duodenum, duodenal (bulb) 564.89
  esophagus (diffuse) 530.5
    psychogenic 306.4
  facial 351.8
  fallopian tube 620.8
  gait 781.2
  gastrointestinal (tract) 536.8
    psychogenic 306.4
  glottis 478.75
    hysterical 300.11
    psychogenic 306.1
      specified as conversion reaction 300.11
    reflex through recurrent laryngeal nerve 478.75
  habit 307.20
    chronic 307.22
    transient (of childhood) 307.21
  heart — *see* Angina
  hourglass — *see* Contraction, hourglass
  hysterical 300.11
  infantile (*see also* Epilepsy) 345.6 ☑
  internal oblique, eye 378.51
  intestinal 564.9
    psychogenic 306.4
  larynx, laryngeal 478.75
    hysterical 300.11
    psychogenic 306.1

Spasm, spastic, spasticity — *see also* condition — *continued*
  larynx, laryngeal — *continued*
    psychogenic — *continued*
      specified as conversion reaction 300.11
    levator palpebrae superioris 333.81
    lightning (*see also* Epilepsy) 345.6 ☑
    mobile 781.0
    muscle 728.85
      back 724.8
      psychogenic 306.0
    nerve, trigeminal 350.1
    nervous 306.0
    nodding 307.3
      infantile (*see also* Epilepsy) 345.6 ☑
    occupational 300.89
    oculogyric 378.87
    ophthalmic artery 362.30
    orbicularis 781.0
    perineal 625.8
    peroneo-extensor (*see also* Flat, foot) 734
    pharynx (reflex) 478.29
      hysterical 300.11
      psychogenic 306.1
        specified as conversion reaction 300.11
    pregnant uterus, complicating delivery 661.4 ☑
    psychogenic 306.0
    pylorus 537.81
      adult hypertrophic 537.0
      congenital or infantile 750.5
      psychogenic 306.4
    rectum (sphincter) 564.6
      psychogenic 306.4
    retinal artery NEC (*see also* Occlusion, retina, artery) 362.30
    sacroiliac 724.6
    salaam (infantile) (*see also* Epilepsy) 345.6 ☑
    saltatory 781.0
    sigmoid 564.9
      psychogenic 306.4
    sphincter of Oddi (*see also* Disease, gallbladder) 576.5
    stomach 536.8
      neurotic 306.4
    throat 478.29
      hysterical 300.11
      psychogenic 306.1
        specified as conversion reaction 300.11
    tic 307.20
      chronic 307.22
      transient (of childhood) 307.21
    tongue 529.8
    torsion 333.6
    trigeminal nerve 350.1
      postherpetic 053.12
    ureter 593.89
    urethra (sphincter) 599.84
    uterus 625.8
      complicating labor 661.4 ☑
        affecting fetus or newborn 763.7
    vagina 625.1
      psychogenic 306.51
    vascular NEC 443.9
    vasomotor NEC 443.9
    vein NEC 459.89
    vesical (sphincter, external or internal) 596.89
    viscera 789.0 ☑
Spasmus nutans 307.3
Spastic — *see also* Spasm
  child 343.9
Spasticity — *see also* Spasm
  cerebral, child 343.9
Speakers' throat 784.49
Specific, specified — *see* condition
Speech
  defect, disorder, disturbance, impediment NEC 784.59
    psychogenic 307.9
  (language) therapy V57.3
Spells 780.39

Spells — *continued*
  breath-holding 786.9
Spencer's disease (epidemic vomiting) 078.82
Spens' syndrome (syncope with heart block) 426.9
Spermatic cord — *see* condition
Spermatocele 608.1
  congenital 752.89
Spermatocystitis 608.4
Spermatocytoma (M9063/3)
  specified site — *see* Neoplasm, by site, malignant
  unspecified site 186.9
Spermatorrhea 608.89
Sperm counts
  fertility testing V26.21
  following sterilization reversal V26.22
  postvasectomy V25.8
Sphacelus — *see also* Gangrene 785.4
Sphenoidal — *see* condition
Sphenoiditis (chronic) — *see also* Sinusitis, sphenoidal 473.3
Sphenopalatine ganglion neuralgia 337.09
Sphericity, increased, lens 743.36
Spherocytosis (congenital) (familial) (hereditary) 282.0
  hemoglobin disease 282.7
  sickle-cell (disease) 282.60
Spherophakia 743.36
Sphincter — *see* condition
Sphincteritis, sphincter of Oddi — *see also* Cholecystitis 576.8
Sphingolipidosis 272.7
Sphingolipodystrophy 272.7
Sphingomyelinosis 272.7
Spicule tooth 520.2
Spider
  finger 755.59
  nevus 448.1
  vascular 448.1
Spiegler-Fendt sarcoid 686.8
Spielmeyer-Stock disease 330.1
Spielmeyer-Vogt disease 330.1
Spina bifida (aperta) 741.9 ☑

> *Note — Use the following fifth-digit subclassification with category 741:*
>
> 0   unspecified region
>
> 1   cervical region
>
> 2   dorsal [thoracic} region
>
> 3   lumbar region

  with hydrocephalus 741.0 ☑
    fetal (suspected), affecting management of pregnancy 655.0 ☑
  occulta 756.17
Spindle, Krukenberg's 371.13
Spine, spinal — *see* condition
Spiradenoma (eccrine) (M8403/0) — *see* Neoplasm, skin, benign
Spirillosis NEC — *see also* Fever, relapsing 087.9
Spirillum minus 026.0
Spirillum obermeieri infection 087.0
Spirochetal — *see* condition
Spirochetosis 104.9
  arthritic, arthritica 104.9 [711.8] ☑
  bronchopulmonary 104.8
  icterohemorrhagica 100.0
  lung 104.8
Spitting blood — *see also* Hemoptysis 786.30
Splanchnomegaly 569.89
Splanchnoptosis 569.89
Spleen, splenic — *see also* condition
  agenesis 759.0
  flexure syndrome 569.89
  neutropenia syndrome 289.53
  sequestration syndrome 289.52
Splenectasis — *see also* Splenomegaly 789.2
Splenitis (interstitial) (malignant) (nonspecific) 289.59
  malarial (*see also* Malaria) 084.6
  tuberculous (*see also* Tuberculosis) 017.7 ☑
Splenocele 289.59
Splenomegalia — *see* Splenomegaly
Splenomegalic — *see* condition

Splenomegaly 789.2
  Bengal 789.2
  cirrhotic 289.51
  congenital 759.0
  congestive, chronic 289.51
  cryptogenic 789.2
  Egyptian 120.1
  Gaucher's (cerebroside lipidosis) 272.7
  idiopathic 789.2
  malarial (see also Malaria) 084.6
  neutropenic 289.53
  Niemann-Pick (lipid histiocytosis) 272.7
  siderotic 289.51
  syphilitic 095.8
    congenital 090.0
  tropical (Bengal) (idiopathic) 789.2
Splenopathy 289.50
Splenopneumonia — see Pneumonia
Splenoptosis 289.59
Splinter — see Injury, superficial, by site
Split, splitting
  heart sounds 427.89
  lip, congenital (see also Cleft, lip) 749.10
  nails 703.8
  urinary stream 788.61
Spoiled child reaction — see also Disturbance,
    conduct 312.1 ☑
Spondylarthritis — see also Spondylosis
    721.90
Spondylarthrosis — see also Spondylosis
    721.90
Spondylitis 720.9
  ankylopoietica 720.0
  ankylosing (chronic) 720.0
  atrophic 720.9
    ligamentous 720.9
  chronic (traumatic) (see also Spondylosis)
    721.90
  deformans (chronic) (see also Spondylosis)
    721.90
  gonococcal 098.53
  gouty 274.00
  hypertrophic (see also Spondylosis) 721.90
  infectious NEC 720.9
  juvenile (adolescent) 720.0
  Kümmell's 721.7
  Marie-Strümpell (ankylosing) 720.0
  muscularis 720.9
  ossificans ligamentosa 721.6
  osteoarthritica (see also Spondylosis) 721.90
  posttraumatic 721.7
  proliferative 720.0
  rheumatoid 720.0
  rhizomelica 720.0
  sacroiliac NEC 720.2
  senescent (see also Spondylosis) 721.90
  senile (see also Spondylosis) 721.90
  static (see also Spondylosis) 721.90
  traumatic (chronic) (see also Spondylosis)
    721.90
  tuberculous (see also Tuberculosis)
    015.0 ☑ [720.81]
  typhosa 002.0 [720.81]
Spondyloarthrosis — see also Spondylosis
    721.90
Spondylolisthesis (congenital) (lumbosacral)
    756.12
  with disproportion (fetopelvic) 653.3 ☑
    affecting fetus or newborn 763.1
    causing obstructed labor 660.1 ☑
      affecting fetus or newborn 763.1
  acquired 738.4
  degenerative 738.4
  traumatic 738.4
    acute (lumbar) — see Fracture, vertebra,
      lumbar
    site other than lumbosacral — see
      Fracture, vertebra, by site
Spondylolysis (congenital) 756.11
  acquired 738.4
  cervical 756.19
  lumbosacral region 756.11
    with disproportion (fetopelvic) 653.3 ☑
      affecting fetus or newborn 763.1
      causing obstructed labor 660.1 ☑
        affecting fetus or newborn 763.1

Spondylopathy
  inflammatory 720.9
    specified type NEC 720.89
  traumatic 721.7
Spondylose rhizomelique 720.0
Spondylosis 721.90
  with
    disproportion 653.3 ☑
      affecting fetus or newborn 763.1
      causing obstructed labor 660.1 ☑
        affecting fetus or newborn 763.1
    myelopathy NEC 721.91
  cervical, cervicodorsal 721.0
    with myelopathy 721.1
  inflammatory 720.9
  lumbar, lumbosacral 721.3
    with myelopathy 721.42
  sacral 721.3
    with myelopathy 721.42
  thoracic 721.2
    with myelopathy 721.41
  traumatic 721.7
Sponge
  divers' disease 989.5
  inadvertently left in operation wound 998.4
  kidney (medullary) 753.17
Spongioblastoma (M9422/3)
  multiforme (M9440/3)
    specified site — see Neoplasm, by site,
      malignant
    unspecified site 191.9
  polare (M9423/3)
    specified site — see Neoplasm, by site,
      malignant
    unspecified site 191.9
  primitive polar (M9443/3)
    specified site — see Neoplasm, by site,
      malignant
    unspecified site 191.9
  specified site — see Neoplasm, by site, ma-
    lignant
  unspecified site 191.9
Spongiocytoma (M9400/3)
  specified site — see Neoplasm, by site, ma-
    lignant
  unspecified site 191.9
Spongioneuroblastoma (M9504/3) — see
    Neoplasm, by site, malignant
Spontaneous — see also condition
  fracture — see Fracture, pathologic
Spoon nail 703.8
  congenital 757.5
Sporadic — see condition
Sporotrichosis (bones) (cutaneous) (dissemi-
    nated) (epidermal) (lymphatic) (lympho-
    cutaneous) (mucous membranes) (pul-
    monary) (skeletal) (visceral) 117.1
Sporotrichum schenckii infection 117.1
Spots, spotting
  atrophic (skin) 701.3
  Bitôt's (in the young child) 264.1
  café au lait 709.09
  cayenne pepper 448.1
  complicating pregnancy 649.5 ☑
  cotton wool (retina) 362.83
  de Morgan's (senile angiomas) 448.1
  Fúchs' black (myopic) 360.21
  intermenstrual
    irregular 626.6
    regular 626.5
  interpalpebral 372.53
  Koplik's 055.9
  liver 709.09
  Mongolian (pigmented) 757.33
  of pregnancy 649.5 ☑
  purpuric 782.7
  ruby 448.1
Spotted fever — see Fever, spotted
Sprain, strain (joint) (ligament) (muscle) (ten-
    don) 848.9
  abdominal wall (muscle) 848.8
  Achilles tendon 845.09
  acromioclavicular 840.0
  ankle 845.00
    and foot 845.00
  anterior longitudinal, cervical 847.0

Sprain, strain — continued
  arm 840.9
    upper 840.9
      and shoulder 840.9
  astragalus 845.00
  atlanto-axial 847.0
  atlanto-occipital 847.0
  atlas 847.0
  axis 847.0
  back (see also Sprain, spine) 847.9
  breast bone 848.40
  broad ligament — see Injury, internal, broad
    ligament
  calcaneofibular 845.02
  carpal 842.01
  carpometacarpal 842.11
  cartilage
    costal, without mention of injury to
      sternum 848.3
      involving sternum 848.42
    ear 848.8
    knee 844.9
      with current tear (see also Tear,
        meniscus) 836.2
    semilunar (knee) 844.8
      with current tear (see also Tear,
        meniscus) 836.2
    septal, nose 848.0
    thyroid region 848.2
    xiphoid 848.49
  cervical, cervicodorsal, cervicothoracic 847.0
  chondrocostal, without mention of injury
    to sternum 848.3
    involving sternum 848.42
  chondrosternal 848.42
  chronic (joint) — see Derangement, joint
  clavicle 840.9
  coccyx 847.4
  collar bone 840.9
  collateral, knee (medial) (tibial) 844.1
    lateral (fibular) 844.0
    recurrent or old 717.89
      lateral 717.81
      medial 717.82
  coracoacromial 840.8
  coracoclavicular 840.1
  coracohumeral 840.2
  coracoid (process) 840.9
  coronary, knee 844.8
  costal cartilage, without mention of injury
    to sternum 848.3
    involving sternum 848.42
  cricoarytenoid articulation 848.2
  cricothyroid articulation 848.2
  cruciate
    knee 844.2
    old 717.89
      anterior 717.83
      posterior 717.84
  deltoid
    ankle 845.01
    shoulder 840.8
  dorsal (spine) 847.1
  ear cartilage 848.8
  elbow 841.9
    and forearm 841.9
    specified site NEC 841.8
  femur (proximal end) 843.9
    distal end 844.9
  fibula (proximal end) 844.9
    distal end 845.00
  fibulocalcaneal 845.02
  finger(s) 842.10
  foot 845.10
    and ankle 845.00
  forearm 841.9
    and elbow 841.9
    specified site NEC 841.8
  glenoid (shoulder) (see also SLAP lesion)
    840.8
  hand 842.10
  hip 843.9
    and thigh 843.9
  humerus (proximal end) 840.9
    distal end 841.9
  iliofemoral 843.0

Sprain, strain — continued
  infraspinatus 840.3
  innominate
    acetabulum 843.9
    pubic junction 848.5
    sacral junction 846.1
  internal
    collateral, ankle 845.01
    semilunar cartilage 844.8
      with current tear (see also Tear,
        meniscus) 836.2
      old 717.5
  interphalangeal
    finger 842.13
    toe 845.13
  ischiocapsular 843.1
  jaw (cartilage) (meniscus) 848.1
    old 524.69
  knee 844.9
    and leg 844.9
    old 717.5
      collateral
        lateral 717.81
        medial 717.82
      cruciate
        anterior 717.83
        posterior 717.84
  late effect — see Late, effects (of), sprain
  lateral collateral, knee 844.0
    old 717.81
  leg 844.9
    and knee 844.9
  ligamentum teres femoris 843.8
  low back 846.9
  lumbar (spine) 847.2
  lumbosacral 846.0
    chronic or old 724.6
  mandible 848.1
    old 524.69
  maxilla 848.1
  medial collateral, knee 844.1
    old 717.82
  meniscus
    jaw 848.1
      old 524.69
    knee 844.8
      with current tear (see also Tear,
        meniscus) 836.2
      old 717.5
    mandible 848.1
      old 524.69
    specified site NEC 848.8
  metacarpal 842.10
    distal 842.12
    proximal 842.11
  metacarpophalangeal 842.12
  metatarsal 845.10
  metatarsophalangeal 845.12
  midcarpal 842.19
  midtarsal 845.19
  multiple sites, except fingers alone or toes
    alone 848.8
  neck 847.0
  nose (septal cartilage) 848.0
  occiput from atlas 847.0
  old — see Derangement, joint
  orbicular, hip 843.8
  patella(r) 844.8
    old 717.89
  pelvis 848.5
  phalanx
    finger 842.10
    toe 845.10
  radiocarpal 842.02
  radiohumeral 841.2
  radioulnar 841.9
    distal 842.09
  radius, radial (proximal end) 841.9
    and ulna 841.9
      distal 842.09
    collateral 841.0
    distal end 842.00
  recurrent — see Sprain, by site
  rib (cage), without mention of injury to
    sternum 848.3
    involving sternum 848.42

☑ Additional Digit Required — Refer to the Tabular List for Digit Selection ▽ Subterms under main terms may continue to next column or page

Sprain, strain — continued
  rotator cuff (capsule) 840.4
  round ligament (see also Injury, internal, round ligament)
    femur 843.8
  sacral (spine) 847.3
  sacrococcygeal 847.3
  sacroiliac (region) 846.9
    chronic or old 724.6
    ligament 846.1
    specified site NEC 846.8
  sacrospinatus 846.2
  sacrospinous 846.2
  sacrotuberous 846.3
  scaphoid bone, ankle 845.00
  scapula(r) 840.9
  semilunar cartilage (knee) 844.8
    with current tear (see also Tear, meniscus) 836.2
    old 717.5
  septal cartilage (nose) 848.0
  shoulder 840.9
    and arm, upper 840.9
    blade 840.9
  specified site NEC 848.8
  spine 847.9
    cervical 847.0
    coccyx 847.4
    dorsal 847.1
    lumbar 847.2
    lumbosacral 846.0
      chronic or old 724.6
    sacral 847.3
    sacroiliac (see also Sprain, sacroiliac) 846.9
      chronic or old 724.6
    thoracic 847.1
  sternoclavicular 848.41
  sternum 848.40
  subglenoid (see also SLAP lesion) 840.8
  subscapularis 840.5
  supraspinatus 840.6
  symphysis
    jaw 848.1
      old 524.69
    mandibular 848.1
      old 524.69
    pubis 848.5
  talofibular 845.09
  tarsal 845.10
  tarsometatarsal 845.11
  temporomandibular 848.1
    old 524.69
  teres
    ligamentum femoris 843.8
    major or minor 840.8
  thigh (proximal end) 843.9
    and hip 843.9
    distal end 844.9
  thoracic (spine) 847.1
  thorax 848.8
  thumb 842.10
  thyroid cartilage or region 848.2
  tibia (proximal end) 844.9
    distal end 845.00
  tibiofibular
    distal 845.03
    superior 844.3
  toe(s) 845.10
  trachea 848.8
  trapezoid 840.8
  ulna, ulnar (proximal end) 841.9
    collateral 841.1
    distal end 842.00
  ulnohumeral 841.3
  vertebrae (see also Sprain, spine) 847.9
    cervical, cervicodorsal, cervicothoracic 847.0
  wrist (cuneiform) (scaphoid) (semilunar) 842.00
  xiphoid cartilage 848.49
Sprengel's deformity (congenital) 755.52
Spring fever 309.23
Sprue 579.1
  celiac 579.0
  idiopathic 579.0

Sprue — continued
  meaning thrush 112.0
  nontropical 579.0
  tropical 579.1
Spur — see also Exostosis
  bone 726.91
    calcaneal 726.73
  calcaneal 726.73
  iliac crest 726.5
  nose (septum) 478.19
    bone 726.91
  septal 478.19
Spuria placenta — see Placenta, abnormal
Spurway's syndrome (brittle bones and blue sclera) 756.51
Sputum, abnormal (amount) (color) (excessive) (odor) (purulent) 786.4
  bloody 786.30
Squamous — see also condition
  cell metaplasia
    bladder 596.89
    cervix — see condition
  epithelium in
    cervical canal (congenital) 752.49
    uterine mucosa (congenital) 752.39
  metaplasia
    bladder 596.89
    cervix — see condition
Squashed nose 738.0
  congenital 754.0
Squeeze, divers' 993.3
Squint — see also Strabismus 378.9
  accommodative (see also Esotropia) 378.00
  concomitant (see also Heterotropia) 378.30
Stab — see also Wound, open, by site
  internal organs — see Injury, internal, by site, with open wound
Staggering gait 781.2
  hysterical 300.11
Staghorn calculus 592.0
Stain, staining
  meconium 779.84
  port wine 757.32
  tooth, teeth (hard tissues) 521.7
    due to
      accretions 523.6
      deposits (betel) (black) (green) (materia alba) (orange) (tobacco) 523.6
      metals (copper) (silver) 521.7
      nicotine 523.6
      pulpal bleeding 521.7
      tobacco 523.6
Stälh's
  ear 744.29
  pigment line (cornea) 371.11
Stälhi's pigment lines (cornea) 371.11
Stammering — see also Disorder, fluency 315.35
Standstill
  atrial 426.6
  auricular 426.6
  cardiac (see also Arrest, cardiac) 427.5
  sinoatrial 426.6
  sinus 426.6
  ventricular (see also Arrest, cardiac) 427.5
Stannosis 503
Stanton's disease (melioidosis) 025
Staphylitis (acute) (catarrhal) (chronic) (gangrenous) (membranous) (suppurative) (ulcerative) 528.3
Staphylococcemia 038.10
  aureus 038.11
  specified organism NEC 038.19
Staphylococcus, staphylococcal — see condition
Staphyloderma (skin) 686.00
Staphyloma 379.11
  anterior, localized 379.14
  ciliary 379.11
  cornea 371.73
  equatorial 379.13
  posterior 379.12
  posticum 379.12
  ring 379.15
  sclera NEC 379.11

Starch eating 307.52
Stargardt's disease 362.75
Starvation (inanition) (due to lack of food) 994.2
  edema 262
  voluntary NEC 307.1
Stasis
  bile (duct) (see also Disease, biliary) 576.8
  bronchus (see also Bronchitis) 490
  cardiac (see also Failure, heart) 428.0
  cecum 564.89
  colon 564.89
  dermatitis (see also Varix, with stasis dermatitis) 454.1
  duodenal 536.8
  eczema (see also Varix, with stasis dermatitis) 454.1
  edema (see also Hypertension, venous) 459.30
  foot 991.4
  gastric 536.3
  ileocecal coil 564.89
  ileum 564.89
  intestinal 564.89
  jejunum 564.89
  kidney 586
  liver 571.9
    cirrhotic — see Cirrhosis, liver
  lymphatic 457.8
  pneumonia 514
  portal 571.9
  pulmonary 514
  rectal 564.89
  renal 586
    tubular 584.5
  stomach 536.3
  ulcer
    with varicose veins 454.0
    without varicose veins 459.81
  urine NEC (see also Retention, urine) 788.20
  venous 459.81
State
  affective and paranoid, mixed, organic psychotic 294.8
  agitated 307.9
    acute reaction to stress 308.2
  anxiety (neurotic) (see also Anxiety) 300.00
    specified type NEC 300.09
  apprehension (see also Anxiety) 300.00
    specified type NEC 300.09
  climacteric, female 627.2
    following induced menopause 627.4
  clouded
    epileptic (see also Epilepsy) 345.9 ☑
    paroxysmal (idiopathic) (see also Epilepsy) 345.9 ☑
  compulsive (mixed) (with obsession) 300.3
  confusional 298.9
    acute 293.0
      with
        arteriosclerotic dementia 290.41
        presenile brain disease 290.11
        senility 290.3
      alcoholic 291.0
      drug-induced 292.81
    epileptic 293.0
    postoperative 293.9
    reactive (emotional stress) (psychological trauma) 298.2
    subacute 293.1
  constitutional psychopathic 301.9
  convulsive (see also Convulsions) 780.39
  depressive NEC 311
    induced by drug 292.84
    neurotic 300.4
  dissociative 300.15
  hallucinatory 780.1
    induced by drug 292.12
  hypercoagulable (primary) 289.81
    secondary 289.82
  hyperdynamic beta-adrenergic circulatory 429.82
  locked-in 344.81
  menopausal 627.2
    artificial 627.4
    following induced menopause 627.4

State — continued
  neurotic NEC 300.9
    with depersonalization episode 300.6
  obsessional 300.3
  oneiroid (see also Schizophrenia) 295.4 ☑
  panic 300.01
  paranoid 297.9
    alcohol-induced 291.5
    arteriosclerotic 290.42
    climacteric 297.2
    drug-induced 292.11
    in
      presenile brain disease 290.12
      senile brain disease 290.20
    involutional 297.2
    menopausal 297.2
    senile 290.20
    simple 297.0
  postleukotomy 310.0
  pregnant (see also Pregnancy) V22.2
  psychogenic, twilight 298.2
  psychotic, organic (see also Psychosis, organic) 294.9
    mixed paranoid and affective 294.8
    senile or presenile NEC 290.9
    transient NEC 293.9
      with
        anxiety 293.84
        delusions 293.81
        depression 293.83
        hallucinations 293.82
  residual schizophrenic (see also Schizophrenia) 295.6 ☑
  tension (see also Anxiety) 300.9
  transient organic psychotic 293.9
    anxiety type 293.84
    depressive type 293.83
    hallucinatory type 293.83
    paranoid type 293.81
    specified type NEC 293.89
  twilight
    epileptic 293.0
    psychogenic 298.2
  vegetative (persistent) 780.03
Status (post)
  absence
    epileptic (see also Epilepsy) 345.2 ☑
    of organ, acquired (postsurgical) — see Absence, by site, acquired
  administration of tPA(rtPA) in a different institution within the last 24 hours prior to admission to facility V45.88
  anastomosis of intestine (for bypass) V45.3
  anginosus 413.9
  angioplasty, percutaneous transluminal coronary V45.82
  ankle prosthesis V43.66
  aortocoronary bypass or shunt V45.81
  arthrodesis V45.4
  artificially induced condition NEC V45.89
  artificial opening (of) V44.9
    gastrointestinal tract NEC V44.4
    specified site NEC V44.8
    urinary tract NEC V44.6
    vagina V44.7
  aspirator V46.0
  asthmaticus (see also Asthma) 493.9 ☑
  awaiting organ transplant V49.83
  bariatric surgery V45.86
    complicating pregnancy, childbirth, or the puerperium 649.2 ☑
  bed confinement V49.84
  breast
    correction V43.82
    implant removal V45.83
    reconstruction V43.82
  cardiac
    device (in situ) V45.00
      carotid sinus V45.09
        fitting or adjustment V53.39
      defibrillator, automatic implantable (with synchronous cardiac pacemaker) V45.02
      pacemaker V45.01
        fitting or adjustment V53.31
  carotid sinus stimulator V45.09

☑ **Additional Digit Required** — Refer to the Tabular List for Digit Selection   ▽ **Subterms under main terms may continue to next column or page**

306   **2014 ICD-9-CM**

Status — *continued*
cataract extraction V45.61
chemotherapy V66.2
   current V58.69
circumcision, female 629.20
clitorectomy (female genital mutilation type I) 629.21
   with excision of labia minora (female genital mutilation type II) 629.22
colonization — *see* Carrier (suspected) of
colostomy V44.3
contraceptive device V45.59
   intrauterine V45.51
   subdermal V45.52
convulsivus idiopathicus (*see also* Epilepsy) 345.3
coronary artery bypass or shunt V45.81
cutting
   female genital 629.20
      specified NEC 629.29
      type I 629.21
      type II 629.22
      type III 629.23
      type IV 629.29
cystostomy V44.50
   appendico-vesicostomy V44.52
   cutaneous-vesicostomy V44.51
   specified type NEC V44.59
defibrillator, automatic implantable cardiac (with synchronous cardiac pacemaker) V45.02
delinquent immunization V15.83
dental crowns V45.84
dental fillings V45.84
dental restoration V45.84
dental sealant V49.82
dialysis (hemo) (peritoneal) V45.11
donor V59.9
do not resuscitate V49.86
drug therapy or regimen V67.59
   high-risk medication NEC V67.51
elbow prosthesis V43.62
embedded
   fragment — *see* Foreign body, retained
   splinter — *see* Foreign body, retained
enterostomy V44.4
epileptic, epilepticus (absence) (grand mal) (*see also* Epilepsy) 345.3
   focal motor 345.7 ☑
   partial 345.7 ☑
   petit mal 345.2
   psychomotor 345.7 ☑
   temporal lobe 345.7 ☑
estrogen receptor
   negative [ER-] V86.1
   positive [ER+] V86.0
explantation of joint prosthesis NEC V88.29
   hip V88.21
   knee V88.22
eye (adnexa) surgery V45.69
female genital
   cutting 629.20
      specified NEC 629.29
      type I 629.21
      type II 629.22
      type III 629.23
      type IV 629.29
   mutilation 629.20
      type I 629.21
      type II 629.22
      type III 629.23
      type IV 629.29
filtering bleb (eye) (postglaucoma) V45.69
   with rupture or complication 997.99
   postcataract extraction (complication) 997.99
finger joint prosthesis V43.69
foster care V60.81
gastric
   banding V45.86
      complicating pregnancy, childbirth, or the puerperium 649.2 ☑
   bypass for obesity V45.86
      complicating pregnancy, childbirth, or the puerperium 649.2 ☑
gastrostomy V44.1

Status — *continued*
grand mal 345.3
heart valve prosthesis V43.3
hemodialysis V45.11
hip prosthesis (joint) (partial) (total) V43.64
   explantation V88.21
hysterectomy V88.01
   partial with remaining cervical stump V88.02
   total V88.01
ileostomy V44.2
infibulation (female genital mutilation type III) 629.23
insulin pump V45.85
intestinal bypass V45.3
intrauterine contraceptive device V45.51
jejunostomy V44.4
joint prosthesis NEC V43.69
   explantation V88.29
knee joint prosthesis V43.65
   explantation V88.22
lacunaris 437.8
lacunosis 437.8
lapsed immunization schedule V15.83
low birth weight V21.30
   less than 500 grams V21.31
   1000–1499 grams V21.33
   1500–1999 grams V21.34
   2000–2500 grams V21.35
   500–999 grams V21.32
lymphaticus 254.8
malignant neoplasm, ablated or excised — *see* History, malignant neoplasm
marmoratus 333.79
military deployment V62.22
mutilation, female 629.20
   type I 629.21
   type II 629.22
   type III 629.23
   type IV 629.29
nephrostomy V44.6
neuropacemaker NEC V45.89
   brain V45.89
   carotid sinus V45.09
   neurologic NEC V45.89
obesity surgery V45.86
   complicating pregnancy, childbirth, or the puerperium 649.2 ☑
organ replacement
   by artificial or mechanical device or prosthesis of
      artery V43.4
      artificial skin V43.83
      bladder V43.5
      blood vessel V43.4
      breast V43.82
      eye globe V43.0
      heart
         assist device V43.21
         fully implantable artificial heart V43.22
         valve V43.3
      intestine V43.89
      joint V43.60
         ankle V43.66
         elbow V43.62
         finger V43.69
         hip (partial) (total) V43.64
         knee V43.65
         shoulder V43.61
         specified NEC V43.69
         wrist V43.63
      kidney V43.89
      larynx V43.81
      lens V43.1
      limb(s) V43.7
      liver V43.89
      lung V43.89
      organ NEC V43.89
      pancreas V43.89
      skin (artificial) V43.83
      tissue NEC V43.89
      vein V43.4
   by organ transplant (heterologous) (homologous) — *see* Status, transplant

Status — *continued*
pacemaker
   brain V45.89
   cardiac V45.01
   carotid sinus V45.09
   neurologic NEC V45.89
   specified site NEC V45.89
percutaneous transluminal coronary angioplasty V45.82
peritoneal dialysis V45.11
petit mal 345.2
physical restraints V49.87
postcommotio cerebri 310.2
postmenopausal (age related) (natural) V49.81
postoperative NEC V45.89
postpartum NEC V24.2
   care immediately following delivery V24.0
   routine follow-up V24.2
postsurgical NEC V45.89
renal dialysis V45.11
   noncompliance V45.12
respirator [ventilator] V46.11
   encounter
      during
         mechanical failure V46.14
         power failure V46.12
      for weaning V46.13
retained foreign body — *see* Foreign body, retained
reversed jejunal transposition (for bypass) V45.3
sex reassignment surgery (*see also* Transsexualism) 302.50
shoulder prosthesis V43.61
shunt
   aortocoronary bypass V45.81
   arteriovenous (for dialysis) V45.11
   cerebrospinal fluid V45.2
   vascular NEC V45.89
      aortocoronary (bypass) V45.81
   ventricular (communicating) (for drainage) V45.2
sterilization
   tubal ligation V26.51
   vasectomy V26.52
subdermal contraceptive device V45.52
thymicolymphaticus 254.8
thymicus 254.8
thymolymphaticus 254.8
tooth extraction 525.10
tracheostomy V44.0
transplant
   blood vessel V42.89
   bone V42.4
      marrow V42.81
   cornea V42.5
   heart V42.1
      valve V42.2
   intestine V42.84
   kidney V42.0
   liver V42.7
   lung V42.6
   organ V42.9
      removal (due to complication, failure, rejection or infection) V45.87
      specified site NEC V42.89
   pancreas V42.83
   peripheral stem cells V42.82
   skin V42.3
   stem cells, peripheral V42.82
   tissue V42.9
      specified type NEC V42.89
   vessel, blood V42.89
tubal ligation V26.51
underimmunization V15.83
ureterostomy V44.6
urethrostomy V44.6
vagina, artificial V44.7
vascular shunt NEC V45.89
   aortocoronary (bypass) V45.81
vasectomy V26.52
ventilator [respirator] V46.11

Status — *continued*
ventilator [respirator] — *continued*
   encounter
      during
         mechanical failure V46.14
         power failure V46.12
      for weaning V46.13
   wheelchair confinement V46.3
   wrist prosthesis V43.63
Stave fracture — *see* Fracture, metacarpus, metacarpal bone(s)
Steal
subclavian artery 435.2
vertebral artery 435.1
Stealing, solitary, child problem — *see also* Disturbance, conduct 312.1 ☑
Steam burn — *see* Burn, by site
Steatocystoma multiplex 706.2
Steatoma (infected) 706.2
eyelid (cystic) 374.84
infected 373.13
Steatorrhea (chronic) 579.8
with lacteal obstruction 579.2
idiopathic 579.0
   adult 579.0
   infantile 579.0
pancreatic 579.4
primary 579.0
secondary 579.8
specified cause NEC 579.8
tropical 579.1
Steatosis 272.8
heart (*see also* Degeneration, myocardial) 429.1
kidney 593.89
liver 571.8
Steele-Richardson (-Olszewski) Syndrome 333.0
Steinbrocker's syndrome — *see also* Neuropathy, peripheral, autonomic 337.9
Steinert's disease 359.21
Stein-Leventhal syndrome (polycystic ovary) 256.4
Stein's syndrome (polycystic ovary) 256.4
STEMI (ST elevation myocardial infarction — *see also* — Infarct, myocardium, ST elevation 410.9 ☑
Stenocardia — *see also* Angina 413.9
Stenocephaly 756.0
Stenosis (cicatricial) — *see also* Stricture
ampulla of Vater 576.2
   with calculus, cholelithiasis, or stones — *see* Choledocholithiasis
anus, anal (canal) (sphincter) 569.2
   congenital 751.2
aorta (ascending) 747.22
   arch 747.10
   arteriosclerotic 440.0
   calcified 440.0
aortic (valve) 424.1
   with
      mitral (valve)
         insufficiency or incompetence 396.2
         stenosis or obstruction 396.0
   atypical 396.0
   congenital 746.3
   rheumatic 395.0
      with
         insufficiency, incompetency or regurgitation 395.2
         with mitral (valve) disease 396.8
      mitral (valve)
         disease (stenosis) 396.0
         insufficiency or incompetence 396.2
         stenosis or obstruction 396.0
   specified cause, except rheumatic 424.1
   syphilitic 093.22
aqueduct of Sylvius (congenital) 742.3
   with spina bifida (*see also* Spina bifida) 741.0 ☑
   acquired 331.4
artery NEC (*see also* Arteriosclerosis) 447.1
   basilar — *see* Narrowing, artery, basilar

Stenosis — see also Stricture — continued
artery (see also Arteriosclerosis) — continued
  carotid (common) (internal) — see Narrowing, artery, carotid
  celiac 447.4
  cerebral 437.0
    due to
      embolism (see also Embolism, brain) 434.1 ☑
      thrombus (see also Thrombosis, brain) 434.0 ☑
  extremities 440.20
  precerebral — see Narrowing, artery, precerebral
  pulmonary (congenital) 747.31
    acquired 417.8
  renal 440.1
  vertebral — see Narrowing, artery, vertebral
bile duct or biliary passage (see also Obstruction, biliary) 576.2
  congenital 751.61
bladder neck (acquired) 596.0
  congenital 753.6
brain 348.89
bronchus 519.19
  syphilitic 095.8
cardia (stomach) 537.89
  congenital 750.7
cardiovascular (see also Disease, cardiovascular) 429.2
carotid artery — see Narrowing, artery, carotid
cervix, cervical (canal) 622.4
  congenital 752.49
  in pregnancy or childbirth 654.6 ☑
    affecting fetus or newborn 763.89
    causing obstructed labor 660.2 ☑
      affecting fetus or newborn 763.1
colon (see also Obstruction, intestine) 560.9
  congenital 751.2
colostomy 569.62
common bile duct (see also Obstruction, biliary) 576.2
  congenital 751.61
coronary (artery) — see Arteriosclerosis, coronary
cystic duct (see also Obstruction, gallbladder) 575.2
  congenital 751.61
due to (presence of) any device, implant, or graft classifiable to 996.0–996.5 — see Complications, due to (presence of) any device, implant, or graft classified to 996.0–996.5 NEC
duodenum 537.3
  congenital 751.1
ejaculatory duct NEC 608.89
endocervical os — see Stenosis, cervix
enterostomy 569.62
esophagostomy 530.87
esophagus 530.3
  congenital 750.3
  syphilitic 095.8
    congenital 090.5
external ear canal 380.50
  secondary to
    inflammation 380.53
    surgery 380.52
    trauma 380.51
gallbladder (see also Obstruction, gallbladder) 575.2
glottis 478.74
heart valve (acquired) (see also Endocarditis)
  congenital NEC 746.89
    aortic 746.3
    mitral 746.5
    pulmonary 746.02
    tricuspid 746.1
hepatic duct (see also Obstruction, biliary) 576.2
hymen 623.3
hypertrophic subaortic (idiopathic) 425.11
infundibulum cardiac 746.83

Stenosis — see also Stricture — continued
intestine (see also Obstruction, intestine) 560.9
  congenital (small) 751.1
    large 751.2
lacrimal
  canaliculi 375.53
  duct 375.56
    congenital 743.65
  punctum 375.52
    congenital 743.65
  sac 375.54
    congenital 743.65
lacrimonasal duct 375.56
  congenital 743.65
  neonatal 375.55
larynx 478.74
  congenital 748.3
  syphilitic 095.8
    congenital 090.5
mitral (valve) (chronic) (inactive) 394.0
  with
    aortic (valve)
      disease (insufficiency) 396.1
      insufficiency or incompetence 396.1
      stenosis or obstruction 396.0
    incompetency, insufficiency or regurgitation 394.2
      with aortic valve disease 396.8
  active or acute 391.1
    with chorea (acute) (rheumatic) (Sydenham's) 392.0
  congenital 746.5
  specified cause, except rheumatic 424.0
  syphilitic 093.21
myocardium, myocardial (see also Degeneration, myocardial) 429.1
  hypertrophic subaortic (idiopathic) 425.11
nares (anterior) (posterior) 478.19
  congenital 748.0
nasal duct 375.56
  congenital 743.65
nasolacrimal duct 375.56
  congenital 743.65
  neonatal 375.55
organ or site, congenital NEC — see Atresia
papilla of Vater 576.2
  with calculus, cholelithiasis, or stones — see Choledocholithiasis
pulmonary (artery) (congenital) 747.31
  with ventricular septal defect, dextraposition of aorta and hypertrophy of right ventricle 745.2
  acquired 417.8
  infundibular 746.83
  in tetralogy of Fallot 745.2
  subvalvular 746.83
  valve (see also Endocarditis, pulmonary) 424.3
    congenital 746.02
  vein 747.49
    acquired 417.8
  vessel NEC 417.8
pulmonic (congenital) 746.02
  infundibular 746.83
  subvalvular 746.83
pylorus (hypertrophic) 537.0
  adult 537.0
  congenital 750.5
  infantile 750.5
rectum (sphincter) (see also Stricture, rectum) 569.2
renal artery 440.1
salivary duct (any) 527.8
sphincter of Oddi (see also Obstruction, biliary) 576.2
spinal 724.00
  cervical 723.0
  lumbar, lumbosacral (without neurogenic claudication) 724.02
    with neurogenic claudication 724.03
  nerve (root) NEC 724.9
  specified region NEC 724.09
  thoracic, thoracolumbar 724.01

Stenosis — see also Stricture — continued
stomach, hourglass 537.6
subaortic 746.81
  hypertrophic (idiopathic) 425.11
supra (valvular)-aortic 747.22
trachea 519.19
  congenital 748.3
  syphilitic 095.8
  tuberculous (see also Tuberculosis) 012.8 ☑
tracheostomy 519.02
tricuspid (valve) (see also Endocarditis, tricuspid) 397.0
  congenital 746.1
  nonrheumatic 424.2
tubal 628.2
ureter (see also Stricture, ureter) 593.3
  congenital 753.29
urethra (see also Stricture, urethra) 598.9
vagina 623.2
  congenital 752.49
  in pregnancy or childbirth 654.7 ☑
    affecting fetus or newborn 763.89
    causing obstructed labor 660.2 ☑
      affecting fetus or newborn 763.1
valve (cardiac) (heart) (see also Endocarditis) 424.90
  congenital NEC 746.89
    aortic 746.3
    mitral 746.5
    pulmonary 746.02
    tricuspid 746.1
    urethra 753.6
valvular (see also Endocarditis) 424.90
  congenital NEC 746.89
    urethra 753.6
vascular graft or shunt 996.1
  atherosclerosis — see Arteriosclerosis, extremities
  embolism 996.74
  occlusion NEC 996.74
  thrombus 996.74
vena cava (inferior) (superior) 459.2
  congenital 747.49
ventricular shunt 996.2
vulva 624.8

Stent jail 996.72
Stercolith — see also Fecalith 560.32
  appendix 543.9
Stercoraceous, stercoral ulcer 569.82
  anus or rectum 569.41
Stereopsis, defective
  with fusion 368.33
  without fusion 368.32
Stereotypes NEC 307.3
Sterility
  female — see Infertility, female
  male (see also Infertility, male) 606.9
Sterilization, admission for V25.2
  status
    tubal ligation V26.51
    vasectomy V26.52
Sternalgia — see also Angina 413.9
Sternopagus 759.4
Sternum bifidum 756.3
Sternutation 784.99
Steroid
  effects (adverse) (iatrogenic)
    cushingoid
      correct substance properly administered 255.0
      overdose or wrong substance given or taken 962.0
    diabetes — see Diabetes, secondary
      correct substance properly administered 251.8
      overdose or wrong substance given or taken 962.0
    due to
      correct substance properly administered 255.8
      overdose or wrong substance given or taken 962.0
    fever
      correct substance properly administered 780.60

Steroid — continued
  effects — continued
    fever — continued
      overdose or wrong substance given or taken 962.0
    withdrawal
      correct substance properly administered 255.41
      overdose or wrong substance given or taken 962.0
  responder 365.03
Stevens-Johnson disease or syndrome (erythema multiforme exudativum) 695.13
  toxic epidermal necrolysis overlap (SJS-TEN overlap syndrome) 695.14
Stewart-Morel syndrome (hyperostosis frontalis interna) 733.3
Sticker's disease (erythema infectiosum) 057.0
Stickler syndrome 759.89
Sticky eye 372.03
Stieda's disease (calcification, knee joint) 726.62
Stiff
  back 724.8
  neck (see also Torticollis) 723.5
Stiff-baby 759.89
Stiff-man syndrome 333.91
Stiffness, joint NEC 719.50
  ankle 719.57
  back 724.8
  elbow 719.52
  finger 719.54
  hip 719.55
  knee 719.56
  multiple sites 719.59
  sacroiliac 724.6
  shoulder 719.51
  specified site NEC 719.58
  spine 724.9
  surgical fusion V45.4
  wrist 719.53
Stigmata, congenital syphilis 090.5
Stillbirth, stillborn NEC 779.9
Still's disease or syndrome 714.30
  adult onset 714.2
Stiller's disease (asthenia) 780.79
Still-Felty syndrome (rheumatoid arthritis with splenomegaly and leukopenia) 714.1
Stilling-Türk-Duane syndrome (ocular retraction syndrome) 378.71
Stimulation, ovary 256.1
Sting (animal) (bee) (fish) (insect) (jellyfish) (Portuguese man-o-war) (wasp) (venomous) 989.5
  anaphylactic shock or reaction 989.5
  plant 692.6
Stippled epiphyses 756.59
Stitch
  abscess 998.59
  burst (in external operation wound) (see also Dehiscence) 998.32
    internal 998.31
  in back 724.5
Stojano's (subcostal) **syndrome** 098.86
Stokes-Adams syndrome (syncope with heart block) 426.9
Stokes' disease (exophthalmic goiter) 242.0 ☑
Stokvis' (-Talma) disease (enterogenous cyanosis) 289.7
Stomach — see condition
Stoma malfunction
  colostomy 569.62
  cystostomy 596.82
    infection 596.81
    mechanical 596.82
    specified complication NEC 596.83
  enterostomy 569.62
  esophagostomy 530.87
  gastrostomy 536.42
  ileostomy 569.62
  nephrostomy 997.5
  tracheostomy 519.02
  ureterostomy 997.5
Stomatitis 528.00
  angular 528.5

☑ Additional Digit Required — Refer to the Tabular List for Digit Selection
Subterms under main terms may continue to next column or page

308

2014 ICD-9-CM

Stomatitis — *continued*
  angular — *continued*
    due to dietary or vitamin deficiency 266.2
  aphthous 528.2
  bovine 059.11
  candidal 112.0
  catarrhal 528.00
  denture 528.9
  diphtheritic (membranous) 032.0
  due to
    dietary deficiency 266.0
    thrush 112.0
    vitamin deficiency 266.0
  epidemic 078.4
  epizootic 078.4
  follicular 528.00
  gangrenous 528.1
  herpetic 054.2
  herpetiformis 528.2
  malignant 528.00
  membranous acute 528.00
  monilial 112.0
  mycotic 112.0
  necrotic 528.1
    ulcerative 101
  necrotizing ulcerative 101
  parasitic 112.0
  septic 528.00
  specified NEC 528.09
  spirochetal 101
  suppurative (acute) 528.00
  ulcerative 528.00
    necrotizing 101
  ulceromembranous 101
  vesicular 528.00
    with exanthem 074.3
  Vincent's 101
Stomatocytosis 282.8
Stomatomycosis 112.0
Stomatorrhagia 528.9
Stone(s) — *see also* Calculus
  bladder 594.1
    diverticulum 594.0
  cystine 270.0
  heart syndrome (*see also* Failure, ventricular, left) 428.1
  kidney 592.0
  prostate 602.0
  pulp (dental) 522.2
  renal 592.0
  salivary duct or gland (any) 527.5
  ureter 592.1
  urethra (impacted) 594.2
  urinary (duct) (impacted) (passage) 592.9
    bladder 594.1
      diverticulum 594.0
    lower tract NEC 594.9
    specified site 594.8
  xanthine 277.2
Stonecutters' lung 502
  tuberculous (*see also* Tuberculosis) 011.4 ☑
Stonemasons'
  asthma, disease, or lung 502
    tuberculous (*see also* Tuberculosis) 011.4 ☑
  phthisis (*see also* Tuberculosis) 011.4 ☑
Stoppage
  bowel (*see also* Obstruction, intestine) 560.9
  heart (*see also* Arrest, cardiac) 427.5
  intestine (*see also* Obstruction, intestine) 560.9
  urine NEC (*see also* Retention, urine) 788.20
Storm, thyroid (apathetic) — *see also* Thyrotoxicosis 242.9 ☑
Strabismus (alternating) (congenital) (nonparalytic) 378.9
  concomitant (*see also* Heterotropia) 378.30
    convergent (*see also* Esotropia) 378.00
    divergent (*see also* Exotropia) 378.10
  convergent (*see also* Esotropia) 378.00
  divergent (*see also* Exotropia) 378.10
  due to adhesions, scars — *see* Strabismus, mechanical
  in neuromuscular disorder NEC 378.73
    intermittent 378.20

Strabismus — *continued*
  in neuromuscular disorder — *continued*
    intermittent — *continued*
      vertical 378.31
  latent 378.40
    convergent (esophoria) 378.41
    divergent (exophoria) 378.42
    vertical 378.43
  mechanical 378.60
    due to
      Brown's tendon sheath syndrome 378.61
      specified musculofascial disorder NEC 378.62
  paralytic 378.50
    third or oculomotor nerve (partial) 378.51
      total 378.52
    fourth or trochlear nerve 378.53
    sixth or abducens nerve 378.54
  specified type NEC 378.73
  vertical (hypertropia) 378.31
Strain — *see also* Sprain, by site
  eye NEC 368.13
  heart — *see* Disease, heart
  meaning gonorrhea — *see* Gonorrhea
  on urination 788.65
  physical NEC V62.89
  postural 729.90
  psychological NEC V62.89
Strands
  conjunctiva 372.62
  vitreous humor 379.25
Strangulation, strangulated 994.7
  appendix 543.9
  asphyxiation or suffocation by 994.7
  bladder neck 596.0
  bowel — *see* Strangulation, intestine
  colon — *see* Strangulation, intestine
  cord (umbilical) — *see* Compression, umbilical cord
  due to birth injury 767.8
  food or foreign body (*see also* Asphyxia, food) 933.1
  hemorrhoids 455.8
    external 455.5
    internal 455.2
  hernia (*see also* Hernia, by site, with obstruction)
    gangrenous — *see* Hernia, by site, with gangrene
  intestine (large) (small) 560.2
    with hernia (*see also* Hernia, by site, with obstruction)
      gangrenous — *see* Hernia, by site, with gangrene
    congenital (small) 751.1
    large 751.2
  mesentery 560.2
  mucus (*see also* Asphyxia, mucus) 933.1
    newborn 770.18
  omentum 560.2
  organ or site, congenital NEC — *see* Atresia
  ovary 620.8
    due to hernia 620.4
  penis 607.89
    foreign body 939.3
  rupture (*see also* Hernia, by site, with obstruction) 552.9
    gangrenous (*see also* Hernia, by site, with gangrene) 551.9
  stomach, due to hernia (*see also* Hernia, by site, with obstruction) 552.9
    with gangrene (*see also* Hernia, by site, with gangrene) 551.9
  umbilical cord — *see* Compression, umbilical cord
  vesicourethral orifice 596.0
Strangury 788.1
Strawberry
  gallbladder (*see also* Disease, gallbladder) 575.6
  mark 757.32
  tongue (red) (white) 529.3
Straw itch 133.8
Streak, ovarian 752.0

Strephosymbolia 315.01
  secondary to organic lesion 784.69
Streptobacillary fever 026.1
Streptobacillus moniliformis 026.1
Streptococcemia 038.0
Streptococcicosis — *see* Infection, streptococcal
Streptococcus, streptococcal — *see* condition
Streptoderma 686.00
Streptomycosis — *see* Actinomycosis
Streptothricosis — *see* Actinomycosis
Streptothrix — *see* Actinomycosis
Streptotrichosis — *see* Actinomycosis
Stress 308.9
  fracture — *see* Fracture, stress
  polycythemia 289.0
  reaction (gross) (*see also* Reaction, stress, acute) 308.9
Stretching, nerve — *see* Injury, nerve, by site
Striae (albicantes) (atrophicae) (cutis distensae) (distensae) 701.3
Striations of nails 703.8
Stricture — *see also* Stenosis 799.89
  ampulla of Vater 576.2
    with calculus, cholelithiasis, or stones — *see* Choledocholithiasis
  anus (sphincter) 569.2
    congenital 751.2
    infantile 751.2
  aorta (ascending) 747.22
    arch 747.10
    arteriosclerotic 440.0
    calcified 440.0
  aortic (valve) (*see also* Stenosis, aortic) 424.1
    congenital 746.3
  aqueduct of Sylvius (congenital) 742.3
    with spina bifida (*see also* Spina bifida) 741.0 ☑
    acquired 331.4
  artery 447.1
    basilar — *see* Narrowing, artery, basilar
    carotid (common) (internal) — *see* Narrowing, artery, carotid
    celiac 447.4
    cerebral 437.0
      congenital 747.81
      due to
        embolism (*see also* Embolism, brain) 434.1 ☑
        thrombus (*see also* Thrombosis, brain) 434.0 ☑
    congenital (peripheral) 747.60
      cerebral 747.81
      coronary 746.85
      gastrointestinal 747.61
      lower limb 747.64
      renal 747.62
      retinal 743.58
      specified NEC 747.69
      spinal 747.82
      umbilical 747.5
      upper limb 747.63
    coronary — *see* Arteriosclerosis, coronary
      congenital 746.85
    precerebral — *see* Narrowing, artery, precerebral NEC
    pulmonary (congenital) 747.31
      acquired 417.8
    renal 440.1
    vertebral — *see* Narrowing, artery, vertebral
  auditory canal (congenital) (external) 744.02
    acquired (*see also* Stricture, ear canal, acquired) 380.50
  bile duct or passage (any) (postoperative) (*see also* Obstruction, biliary) 576.2
    congenital 751.61
  bladder 596.89
    congenital 753.6
    neck 596.0
      congenital 753.6
  bowel (*see also* Obstruction, intestine) 560.9
  brain 348.89
  bronchus 519.19
    syphilitic 095.8

Stricture — *see also* Stenosis — *continued*
  cardia (stomach) 537.89
    congenital 750.7
  cardiac (*see also* Disease, heart)
    orifice (stomach) 537.89
  cardiovascular (*see also* Disease, cardiovascular) 429.2
  carotid artery — *see* Narrowing, artery, carotid
  cecum (*see also* Obstruction, intestine) 560.9
  cervix, cervical (canal) 622.4
    congenital 752.49
    in pregnancy or childbirth 654.6 ☑
      affecting fetus or newborn 763.89
      causing obstructed labor 660.2 ☑
        affecting fetus or newborn 763.1
  colon (*see also* Obstruction, intestine) 560.9
    congenital 751.2
  colostomy 569.62
  common bile duct (*see also* Obstruction, biliary) 576.2
    congenital 751.61
  coronary (artery) — *see* Arteriosclerosis, coronary
    congenital 746.85
  cystic duct (*see also* Obstruction, gallbladder) 575.2
    congenital 751.61
  cystostomy 596.83
  digestive organs NEC, congenital 751.8
  duodenum 537.3
    congenital 751.1
  ear canal (external) (congenital) 744.02
    acquired 380.50
      secondary to
        inflammation 380.53
        surgery 380.52
        trauma 380.51
  ejaculatory duct 608.85
  enterostomy 569.62
  esophagostomy 530.87
  esophagus (corrosive) (peptic) 530.3
    congenital 750.3
    syphilitic 095.8
      congenital 090.5
  eustachian tube (*see also* Obstruction, Eustachian tube) 381.60
    congenital 744.24
  fallopian tube 628.2
    gonococcal (chronic) 098.37
      acute 098.17
    tuberculous (*see also* Tuberculosis) 016.6 ☑
  gallbladder (*see also* Obstruction, gallbladder) 575.2
    congenital 751.69
  glottis 478.74
  heart (*see also* Disease, heart)
    congenital NEC 746.89
    valve (*see also* Endocarditis)
      congenital NEC 746.89
        aortic 746.3
        mitral 746.5
        pulmonary 746.02
        tricuspid 746.1
  hepatic duct (*see also* Obstruction, biliary) 576.2
  hourglass, of stomach 537.6
  hymen 623.3
  hypopharynx 478.29
  intestine (*see also* Obstruction, intestine) 560.9
    congenital (small) 751.1
      large 751.2
    ischemic 557.1
  lacrimal
    canaliculi 375.53
      congenital 743.65
    punctum 375.52
      congenital 743.65
    sac 375.54
      congenital 743.65
  lacrimonasal duct 375.56
    congenital 743.65
    neonatal 375.55
  larynx 478.79

Stomatitis — Stricture

☑ Additional Digit Required — Refer to the Tabular List for Digit Selection   ▽ Subterms under main terms may continue to next column or page

2014 ICD-9-CM   309

Stricture — *see also* Stenosis — *continued*
larynx — *continued*
  congenital 748.3
  syphilitic 095.8
    congenital 090.5
lung 518.89
meatus
  ear (congenital) 744.02
    acquired (*see also* Stricture, ear canal,
      acquired) 380.50
  osseous (congenital) (ear) 744.03
    acquired (*see also* Stricture, ear canal,
      acquired) 380.50
  urinarius (*see also* Stricture, urethra)
    598.9
    congenital 753.6
mitral (valve) (*see also* Stenosis, mitral) 394.0
  congenital 746.5
  specified cause, except rheumatic 424.0
myocardium, myocardial (*see also* Degeneration, myocardial) 429.1
  hypertrophic subaortic (idiopathic)
    425.11
nares (anterior) (posterior) 478.19
  congenital 748.0
nasal duct 375.56
  congenital 743.65
  neonatal 375.55
nasolacrimal duct 375.56
  congenital 743.65
  neonatal 375.55
nasopharynx 478.29
  syphilitic 095.8
nephrostomy 997.5
nose 478.19
  congenital 748.0
nostril (anterior) (posterior) 478.19
  congenital 748.0
organ or site, congenital NEC — *see* Atresia
osseous meatus (congenital) (ear) 744.03
  acquired (*see also* Stricture, ear canal,
    acquired) 380.50
os uteri (*see also* Stricture, cervix) 622.4
oviduct — *see* Stricture, fallopian tube
pelviureteric junction 593.3
pharynx (dilation) 478.29
prostate 602.8
pulmonary, pulmonic
  artery (congenital) 747.31
    acquired 417.8
    noncongenital 417.8
  infundibulum (congenital) 746.83
  valve (*see also* Endocarditis, pulmonary)
    424.3
    congenital 746.02
  vein (congenital) 747.49
    acquired 417.8
  vessel NEC 417.8
punctum lacrimale 375.52
  congenital 743.65
pylorus (hypertrophic) 537.0
  adult 537.0
  congenital 750.5
  infantile 750.5
rectosigmoid 569.89
rectum (sphincter) 569.2
  congenital 751.2
  due to
    chemical burn 947.3
    irradiation 569.2
    lymphogranuloma venereum 099.1
  gonococcal 098.7
  inflammatory 099.1
  syphilitic 095.8
  tuberculous (*see also* Tuberculosis)
    014.8 ☑
renal artery 440.1
salivary duct or gland (any) 527.8
sigmoid (flexure) (*see also* Obstruction, intestine) 560.9
spermatic cord 608.85
stoma (following) (of)
  colostomy 569.62
  cystostomy 596.83
  enterostomy 569.62
  esophagostomy 530.87

Stricture — *see also* Stenosis — *continued*
stoma — *continued*
  gastrostomy 536.42
  ileostomy 569.62
  nephrostomy 997.5
  tracheostomy 519.02
  ureterostomy 997.5
stomach 537.89
  congenital 750.7
  hourglass 537.6
subaortic 746.81
  hypertrophic (acquired) (idiopathic)
    425.11
subglottic 478.74
syphilitic NEC 095.8
tendon (sheath) 727.81
trachea 519.19
  congenital 748.3
  syphilitic 095.8
  tuberculous (*see also* Tuberculosis)
    012.8 ☑
tracheostomy 519.02
tricuspid (valve) (*see also* Endocarditis, tricuspid) 397.0
  congenital 746.1
  nonrheumatic 424.2
tunica vaginalis 608.85
ureter (postoperative) 593.3
  congenital 753.29
  tuberculous (*see also* Tuberculosis)
    016.2 ☑
ureteropelvic junction 593.3
  congenital 753.21
ureterovesical orifice 593.3
  congenital 753.22
urethra (anterior) (meatal) (organic) (posterior) (spasmodic) 598.9
  associated with schistosomiasis (*see also*
    Schistosomiasis) 120.9 [598.01]
  congenital (valvular) 753.6
  due to
    infection 598.00
      syphilis 095.8 [598.01]
    trauma 598.1
  gonococcal 098.2 [598.01]
  gonorrheal 098.2 [598.01]
  infective 598.00
  late effect of injury 598.1
  postcatheterization 598.2
  postobstetric 598.1
  postoperative 598.2
  specified cause NEC 598.8
  syphilitic 095.8 [598.01]
  traumatic 598.1
  valvular, congenital 753.6
urinary meatus (*see also* Stricture, urethra)
  598.9
  congenital 753.6
uterus, uterine 621.5
  os (external) (internal) — *see* Stricture,
    cervix
vagina (outlet) 623.2
  congenital 752.49
valve (cardiac) (heart) (*see also* Endocarditis)
  424.90
  congenital (cardiac) (heart) NEC 746.89
    aortic 746.3
    mitral 746.5
    pulmonary 746.02
    tricuspid 746.1
    urethra 753.6
valvular (*see also* Endocarditis) 424.90
vascular graft or shunt 996.1
  atherosclerosis — *see* Arteriosclerosis,
    extremities
  embolism 996.74
  occlusion NEC 996.74
  thrombus 996.74
vas deferens 608.85
  congenital 752.89
vein 459.2
vena cava (inferior) (superior) NEC 459.2
  congenital 747.49
ventricular shunt 996.2
vesicourethral orifice 596.0
  congenital 753.6

Stricture — *see also* Stenosis — *continued*
  vulva (acquired) 624.8
Stridor 786.1
  congenital (larynx) 748.3
Stridulous — *see* condition
Strippling of nails 703.8
Stroke 434.91
  apoplectic (*see also* Disease, cerebrovascular, acute) 436
  brain — *see* Infarct, brain
  embolic 434.11
  epileptic — *see* Epilepsy
  healed or old V12.54
  heart — *see* Disease, heart
  heat 992.0
  hemorrhagic — *see* Hemorrhage, brain
  iatrogenic 997.02
  in evolution 434.91
  ischemic 434.91
  late effect — *see* Late effect(s) (of) cerebrovascular disease
  lightning 994.0
  paralytic — *see* Infarct, brain
  postoperative 997.02
  progressive 435.9
  thrombotic 434.01
Stromatosis, endometrial (M8931/1) 236.0
Strong pulse 785.9
Strongyloides stercoralis infestation 127.2
Strongyloidiasis 127.2
Strongyloidosis 127.2
Strongylus (gibsoni) infestation 127.7
Strophulus (newborn) 779.89
  pruriginosus 698.2
Struck by lightning 994.0
Struma — *see also* Goiter 240.9
  fibrosa 245.3
  Hashimoto (struma lymphomatosa) 245.2
  lymphomatosa 245.2
  nodosa (simplex) 241.9
    endemic 241.9
    multinodular 241.1
    sporadic 241.9
    toxic or with hyperthyroidism 242.3 ☑
      multinodular 242.2 ☑
      uninodular 242.1 ☑
    toxicosa 242.3 ☑
      multinodular 242.2 ☑
      uninodular 242.1 ☑
    uninodular 241.0
  ovarii (M9090/0) 220
    and carcinoid (M9091/1) 236.2
    malignant (M9090/3) 183.0
  Riedel's (ligneous thyroiditis) 245.3
  scrofulous (*see also* Tuberculosis) 017.2 ☑
  tuberculous (*see also* Tuberculosis) 017.2 ☑
    abscess 017.2 ☑
    adenitis 017.2 ☑
    lymphangitis 017.2 ☑
    ulcer 017.2 ☑
Strumipriva cachexia — *see also* Hypothyroidism 244.9
Strümpell-Marie disease or spine (ankylosing spondylitis) 720.0
Strümpell-Westphal pseudosclerosis (hepatolenticular degeneration) 275.1
Stuart's disease (congenital factor X deficiency) — *see also* Defect, coagulation 286.3
Stuart-Prower factor deficiency (congenital factor X deficiency) — *see also* Defect, coagulation 286.3
Students' elbow 727.2
Stuffy nose 478.19
Stump — *see also* Amputation
  cervix, cervical (healed) 622.8
Stupor 780.09
  catatonic (*see also* Schizophrenia) 295.2 ☑
  circular (*see also* Psychosis, manic-depressive, circular) 296.7
  manic 296.89
  manic-depressive (*see also* Psychosis, affective) 296.89
  mental (anergic) (delusional) 298.9
  psychogenic 298.8
  reaction to exceptional stress (transient)
    308.2

Stupor — *continued*
  traumatic NEC (*see also* Injury, intracranial)
    with spinal (cord)
      lesion — *see* Injury, spinal, by site
      shock — *see* Injury, spinal, by site
Sturge (-Weber) (-Dimitri) disease or syndrome (encephalocutaneous angiomatosis) 759.6
Sturge-Kalischer-Weber syndrome (encephalocutaneous angiomatosis) 759.6
Stuttering 315.35
  adult onset 307.0
  childhood onset 315.35
  due to late effect of cerebrovascular disease
    (*see also* Late effect(s) (of) cerebrovascular disease) 438.14
  in conditions classified elsewhere 784.52
Sty, stye 373.11
  external 373.11
  internal 373.12
  meibomian 373.12
Subacidity, gastric 536.8
  psychogenic 306.4
Subacute — *see* condition
Subarachnoid — *see* condition
Subclavian steal syndrome 435.2
Subcortical — *see* condition
Subcostal syndrome 098.86
  nerve compression 354.8
Subcutaneous, subcuticular — *see* condition
Subdelirium 293.1
Subdural — *see* condition
Subendocardium — *see* condition
Subependymoma (M9383/1) 237.5
Suberosis 495.3
Subglossitis — *see* Glossitis
Subhemophilia 286.0
Subinvolution (uterus) 621.1
  breast (postlactational) (postpartum) 611.89
  chronic 621.1
  puerperal, postpartum 674.8 ☑
Sublingual — *see* condition
Sublinguitis 527.2
Subluxation — *see also* Dislocation, by site
  congenital NEC (*see also* Malposition, congenital)
    hip (unilateral) 754.32
      with dislocation of other hip 754.35
      bilateral 754.33
    joint
      lower limb 755.69
      shoulder 755.59
      upper limb 755.59
    lower limb (joint) 755.69
    shoulder (joint) 755.59
    upper limb (joint) 755.59
  lens 379.32
    anterior 379.33
    posterior 379.34
  radial head 832.2
  rotary, cervical region of spine — *see* Fracture, vertebra, cervical
Submaxillary — *see* condition
Submersion (fatal) (nonfatal) 994.1
Submissiveness (undue), in child 313.0
Submucous — *see* condition
Subnormal, subnormality
  accommodation (*see also* Disorder, accommodation) 367.9
  mental (*see also* Disability, intellectual) 319
    mild 317
    moderate 318.0
    profound 318.2
    severe 318.1
  temperature (accidental) 991.6
    not associated with low environmental temperature 780.99
Subphrenic — *see* condition
Subscapular nerve — *see* condition
Subseptus uterus 752.35
Subsiding appendicitis 542
Substance abuse in family V61.42
Substernal thyroid — *see also* Goiter 240.9
  congenital 759.2
Substitution disorder 300.11
Subtentorial — *see* condition

☑ **Additional Digit Required — Refer to the Tabular List for Digit Selection**　　　　🔻 **Subterms under main terms may continue to next column or page**

310

2014 ICD-9-CM

Subtertian
- fever 084.0
- malaria (fever) 084.0

Subthyroidism (acquired) — *see also* Hypothyroidism 244.9
- congenital 243

Succenturiata placenta — *see* Placenta, abnormal

Succussion sounds, chest 786.7

Sucking thumb, child 307.9

Sudamen 705.1

Sudamina 705.1

Sudanese kala-azar 085.0

Sudden
- death, cause unknown (less than 24 hours) 798.1
  - cardiac (SCD)
    - family history of V17.41
    - personal history of, successfully resuscitated V12.53
  - during childbirth 669.9 ☑
  - infant 798.0
  - puerperal, postpartum 674.9 ☑
- hearing loss NEC 388.2
- heart failure (*see also* Failure, heart) 428.9
- infant death syndrome 798.0

Sudeck's atrophy, disease, or syndrome 733.7

SUDS (sudden unexplained death) 798.2

Suffocation — *see also* Asphyxia 799.01
- by
  - bed clothes 994.7
  - bunny bag 994.7
  - cave-in 994.7
  - constriction 994.7
  - drowning 994.1
  - inhalation
    - food or foreign body (*see also* Asphyxia, food or foreign body) 933.1
    - oil or gasoline (*see also* Asphyxia, food or foreign body) 933.1
  - overlying 994.7
  - plastic bag 994.7
  - pressure 994.7
  - strangulation 994.7
- during birth 768.1
- mechanical 994.7

Sugar
- blood
  - high 790.29
  - low 251.2
- in urine 791.5

Suicide, suicidal (attempted)
- by poisoning — *see* Table of Drugs and Chemicals
- ideation V62.84
- risk 300.9
- tendencies 300.9
- trauma NEC (*see also* nature and site of injury) 959.9

Suipestifer infection — *see also* Infection, Salmonella 003.9

Sulfatidosis 330.0

Sulfhemoglobinemia, sulphemoglobinemia (acquired) (congenital) 289.7

Sumatran mite fever 081.2

Summer — *see* condition

Sunburn 692.71
- first degree 692.71
- second degree 692.76
- third degree 692.77
- dermatitis 692.71
- due to
  - other ultraviolet radiation 692.82
  - tanning bed 692.82

SUNCT (short lasting unilateral neuralgiform headache with conjunctival injection and tearing) 339.05

Sunken
- acetabulum 718.85
- fontanels 756.0

Sunstroke 992.0

Superfecundation 651.9 ☑
- with fetal loss and retention of one or more fetus(es) 651.6 ☑
- following (elective) fetal reduction 651.7 ☑

Superfetation 651.9 ☑
- with fetal loss and retention of one or more fetus(es) 651.6 ☑
- following (elective) fetal reduction 651.7 ☑

Superinvolution uterus 621.8

Supernumerary (congenital)
- aortic cusps 746.89
- auditory ossicles 744.04
- bone 756.9
- breast 757.6
- carpal bones 755.56
- cusps, heart valve NEC 746.89
  - mitral 746.5
  - pulmonary 746.09
- digit(s) 755.00
  - finger 755.01
  - toe 755.02
- ear (lobule) 744.1
- fallopian tube 752.19
- finger 755.01
- hymen 752.49
- kidney 753.3
- lacrimal glands 743.64
- lacrimonasal duct 743.65
- lobule (ear) 744.1
- mitral cusps 746.5
- muscle 756.82
- nipples 757.6
- organ or site NEC — *see* Accessory
- ossicles, auditory 744.04
- ovary 752.0
- oviduct 752.19
- pulmonic cusps 746.09
- rib 756.3
  - cervical or first 756.2
    - syndrome 756.2
- roots (of teeth) 520.2
- spinal vertebra 756.19
- spleen 759.0
- tarsal bones 755.67
- teeth 520.1
  - causing crowding 524.31
- testis 752.89
- thumb 755.01
- toe 755.02
- uterus 752.2
- vagina 752.49
- vertebra 756.19

Supervision (of)
- contraceptive method previously prescribed V25.40
  - intrauterine device V25.42
  - oral contraceptive (pill) V25.41
  - specified type NEC V25.49
  - subdermal implantable contraceptive V25.43
- dietary (for) V65.3
  - allergy (food) V65.3
  - colitis V65.3
  - diabetes mellitus V65.3
  - food allergy intolerance V65.3
  - gastritis V65.3
  - hypercholesterolemia V65.3
  - hypoglycemia V65.3
  - intolerance (food) V65.3
  - obesity V65.3
  - specified NEC V65.3
- lactation V24.1
- newborn health
  - 8 to 28 days old V20.32
  - under 8 days old V20.31
- pregnancy — *see* Pregnancy, supervision of

Supplemental teeth 520.1
- causing crowding 524.31

Suppression
- binocular vision 368.31
- lactation 676.5 ☑
- menstruation 626.8
- ovarian secretion 256.39
- renal 586
- urinary secretion 788.5
- urine 788.5

Suppuration, suppurative — *see also* condition

Suppuration, suppurative — *see also* condition — *continued*
- accessory sinus (chronic) (*see also* Sinusitis) 473.9
- adrenal gland 255.8
- antrum (chronic) (*see also* Sinusitis, maxillary) 473.0
- bladder (*see also* Cystitis) 595.89
- bowel 569.89
- brain 324.0
  - late effect 326
- breast 611.0
  - puerperal, postpartum 675.1 ☑
- dental periosteum 526.5
- diffuse (skin) 686.00
- ear (middle) (*see also* Otitis media) 382.4
  - external (*see also* Otitis, externa) 380.10
  - internal 386.33
- ethmoidal (sinus) (chronic) (*see also* Sinusitis, ethmoidal) 473.2
- fallopian tube (*see also* Salpingo-oophoritis) 614.2
- frontal (sinus) (chronic) (*see also* Sinusitis, frontal) 473.1
- gallbladder (*see also* Cholecystitis, acute) 575.0
- gum 523.30
- hernial sac — *see* Hernia, by site
- intestine 569.89
- joint (*see also* Arthritis, suppurative) 711.0 ☑
- labyrinthine 386.33
- lung 513.0
- mammary gland 611.0
  - puerperal, postpartum 675.1 ☑
- maxilla, maxillary 526.4
  - sinus (chronic) (*see also* Sinusitis, maxillary) 473.0
- muscle 728.0
- nasal sinus (chronic) (*see also* Sinusitis) 473.9
- pancreas 577.0
- parotid gland 527.2
- pelvis, pelvic
  - female (*see also* Disease, pelvis, inflammatory) 614.4
    - acute 614.3
  - male (*see also* Peritonitis) 567.21
- pericranial (*see also* Osteomyelitis) 730.2 ☑
- salivary duct or gland (any) 527.2
- sinus (nasal) (*see also* Sinusitis) 473.9
- sphenoidal (sinus) (chronic) (*see also* Sinusitis, sphenoidal) 473.3
- thymus (gland) 254.1
- thyroid (gland) 245.0
- tonsil 474.8
- uterus (*see also* Endometritis) 615.9
- vagina 616.10
- wound (*see also* Wound, open, by site, complicated)
  - dislocation — *see* Dislocation, by site, compound
  - fracture — *see* Fracture, by site, open
  - scratch or other superficial injury — *see* Injury, superficial, by site

Supraeruption, teeth 524.34

Supraglottitis 464.50
- with obstruction 464.51

Suprapubic drainage 596.89

Suprarenal (gland) — *see* condition

Suprascapular nerve — *see* condition

Suprasellar — *see* condition

Supraspinatus syndrome 726.10

Surfer knots 919.8
- infected 919.9

Surgery
- cosmetic NEC V50.1
  - breast reconstruction following mastectomy V51.0
  - following healed injury or operation V51.8
  - hair transplant V50.0
- elective V50.9
  - breast
    - augmentation or reduction V50.1
    - reconstruction following mastectomy V51.0

Surgery — *continued*
- elective — *continued*
  - circumcision, ritual or routine (in absence of medical indication) V50.2
  - cosmetic NEC V50.1
  - ear piercing V50.3
  - face-lift V50.1
  - following healed injury or operation V51.8
  - hair transplant V50.0
- not done because of
  - contraindication V64.1
  - patient's decision V64.2
  - specified reason NEC V64.3
- plastic
  - breast
    - augmentation or reduction V50.1
    - reconstruction following mastectomy V51.0
  - cosmetic V50.1
  - face-lift V50.1
  - following healed injury or operation V51.8
  - repair of scarred tissue (following healed injury or operation) V51.8
  - specified type NEC V50.8
- previous, in pregnancy or childbirth
  - cervix 654.6 ☑
    - affecting fetus or newborn (*see also* Newborn, affected by) 760.63
    - causing obstructed labor 660.2 ☑
      - affecting fetus or newborn 763.1
  - pelvic soft tissues NEC 654.9 ☑
    - affecting fetus or newborn (*see also* Newborn, affected by) 760.63
    - causing obstructed labor 660.2 ☑
      - affecting fetus or newborn 763.1
  - perineum or vulva 654.8 ☑
  - uterus NEC 654.9 ☑
    - affecting fetus or newborn (*see also* Newborn, affected by) 760.63
    - causing obstructed labor 660.2 ☑
      - affecting fetus or newborn 763.1
    - due to previous cesarean delivery 654.2 ☑
  - vagina 654.7 ☑

Surgical
- abortion — *see* Abortion, legal
- emphysema 998.81
- kidney (*see also* Pyelitis) 590.80
- operation NEC 799.9
- procedures, complication or misadventure — *see* Complications, surgical procedure
- shock 998.00

Survey
- fetal anatomic V28.81

Susceptibility
- genetic
  - to
    - MEN (multiple endocrine neoplasia) V84.81
    - neoplasia
      - multiple endocrine (MEN) V84.81
    - neoplasm
      - malignant, of
        - breast V84.01
        - endometrium V84.04
        - other V84.09
        - ovary V84.02
        - prostate V84.03
      - specified disease V84.89

Suspected condition, ruled out — *see also* Observation, suspected V71.9
- specified condition NEC V71.89

Suspended uterus, in pregnancy or childbirth 654.4 ☑
- affecting fetus or newborn 763.89
- causing obstructed labor 660.2 ☑
  - affecting fetus or newborn 763.1

Sutton and Gull's disease (arteriolar nephrosclerosis) — *see also* Hypertension, kidney 403.90

Sutton's disease 709.09

☑ **Additional Digit Required** — **Refer to the Tabular List for Digit Selection**   ▽ **Subterms under main terms may continue to next column or page**

2014 ICD-9-CM   311

Suture
burst (in external operation wound) (*see also* Dehiscence) 998.32
internal 998.31
inadvertently left in operation wound 998.4
removal V58.32
Shirodkar, in pregnancy (with or without cervical incompetence) 654.5 ✓
Swab inadvertently left in operation wound 998.4
Swallowed, swallowing
difficulty (*see also* Dysphagia) 787.20
foreign body NEC (*see also* Foreign body) 938
Swamp fever 100.89
Swan neck hand (intrinsic) 736.09
Sweat(s), sweating
disease or sickness 078.2
excessive (*see also* Hyperhidrosis) 780.8
fetid 705.89
fever 078.2
gland disease 705.9
specified type NEC 705.89
miliary 078.2
night 780.8
Sweeley-Klionsky disease (angiokeratoma corporis diffusum) 272.7
Sweet's syndrome (acute febrile neutrophilic dermatosis) 695.89
Swelling 782.3
abdominal (not referable to specific organ) 789.3 ✓
adrenal gland, cloudy 255.8
ankle 719.07
anus 787.99
arm 729.81
breast 611.72
Calabar 125.2
cervical gland 785.6
cheek 784.2
chest 786.6
ear 388.8
epigastric 789.3 ✓
extremity (lower) (upper) 729.81
eye 379.92
female genital organ 625.8
finger 729.81
foot 729.81
glands 785.6
gum 784.2
hand 729.81
head 784.2
inflammatory — *see* Inflammation
joint (*see also* Effusion, joint) 719.0 ✓
tuberculous — *see* Tuberculosis, joint
kidney, cloudy 593.89
leg 729.81
limb 729.81
liver 573.8
lung 786.6
lymph nodes 785.6
mediastinal 786.6
mouth 784.2
muscle (limb) 729.81
neck 784.2
nose or sinus 784.2
palate 784.2
pelvis 789.3 ✓
penis 607.83
perineum 625.8
rectum 787.99
scrotum 608.86
skin 782.2
splenic (*see also* Splenomegaly) 789.2
substernal 786.6
superficial, localized (skin) 782.2
testicle 608.86
throat 784.2
toe 729.81
tongue 784.2
tubular (*see also* Disease, renal) 593.9
umbilicus 789.3 ✓
uterus 625.8
vagina 625.8
vulva 625.8

Swelling — *continued*
wandering, due to Gnathostoma (spinigerum) 128.1
white — *see* Tuberculosis, arthritis
Swift's disease 985.0
Swimmers'
ear (acute) 380.12
itch 120.3
Swimming in the head 780.4
Swollen — *see also* Swelling
glands 785.6
Swyer-James syndrome (unilateral hyperlucent lung) 492.8
Swyer's syndrome (XY pure gonadal dysgenesis) 752.7
Sycosis 704.8
barbae (not parasitic) 704.8
contagiosa 110.0
lupoid 704.8
mycotic 110.0
parasitic 110.0
vulgaris 704.8
Sydenham's chorea — *see* Chorea, Sydenham's
Sylvatic yellow fever 060.0
Sylvest's disease (epidemic pleurodynia) 074.1
Symblepharon 372.63
congenital 743.62
Symonds' syndrome 348.2
Sympathetic — *see* condition
Sympatheticotonia — *see also* Neuropathy, peripheral, autonomic 337.9
Sympathicoblastoma (M9500/3)
specified site — *see* Neoplasm, by site, malignant
unspecified site 194.0
Sympathicogonioma (M9500/3) — *see* Sympathicoblastoma
Sympathoblastoma (M9500/3) — *see* Sympathicoblastoma
Sympathogonioma (M9500/3) — *see* Sympathicoblastoma
Symphalangy — *see also* Syndactylism 755.10
Symptoms, specified (general) NEC 780.99
abdomen NEC 789.9
bone NEC 733.90
breast NEC 611.79
cardiac NEC 785.9
cardiovascular NEC 785.9
chest NEC 786.9
cognition 799.59
development NEC 783.9
digestive system NEC 787.99
emotional state NEC 799.29
eye NEC 379.99
gastrointestinal tract NEC 787.99
genital organs NEC
female 625.9
male 608.9
head and neck NEC 784.99
heart NEC 785.9
jaw 784.92
joint NEC 719.60
ankle 719.67
elbow 719.62
foot 719.67
hand 719.64
hip 719.65
knee 719.66
multiple sites 719.69
pelvic region 719.65
shoulder (region) 719.61
specified site NEC 719.68
temporomandibular 524.69
wrist 719.63
larynx NEC 784.99
limbs NEC 729.89
lymphatic system NEC 785.9
maxilla 784.92
menopausal 627.2
metabolism NEC 783.9
mouth NEC 528.9
muscle NEC 728.9
musculoskeletal NEC 781.99
limbs NEC 729.89
nervous system NEC 781.99

Symptoms, specified — *continued*
neurotic NEC 300.9
nutrition, metabolism, and development NEC 783.9
pelvis NEC 789.9
female 625.9
peritoneum NEC 789.9
respiratory system NEC 786.9
skin and integument NEC 782.9
subcutaneous tissue NEC 782.9
throat NEC 784.99
tonsil NEC 784.99
urinary system NEC 788.99
vascular NEC 785.9
Sympus 759.89
Synarthrosis 719.80
ankle 719.87
elbow 719.82
foot 719.87
hand 719.84
hip 719.85
knee 719.86
multiple sites 719.89
pelvic region 719.85
shoulder (region) 719.81
specified site NEC 719.88
wrist 719.83
Syncephalus 759.4
Synchondrosis 756.9
abnormal (congenital) 756.9
ischiopubic (van Neck's) 732.1
Synchysis (senile) (vitreous humor) 379.21
scintillans 379.22
Syncope (near) (pre-) 780.2
anginosa 413.9
bradycardia 427.89
cardiac 780.2
carotid sinus 337.01
complicating delivery 669.2 ✓
due to lumbar puncture 349.0
fatal 798.1
heart 780.2
heat 992.1
laryngeal 786.2
tussive 786.2
vasoconstriction 780.2
vasodepressor 780.2
vasomotor 780.2
vasovagal 780.2
Syncytial infarct — *see* Placenta, abnormal
Syndactylism, syndactyly (multiple sites) 755.10
fingers (without fusion of bone) 755.11
with fusion of bone 755.12
toes (without fusion of bone) 755.13
with fusion of bone 755.14
Syndrome — *see also* Disease
with 5q deletion 238.74
5q minus 238.74
abdominal
acute 789.0 ✓
migraine 346.2 ✓
muscle deficiency 756.79
Abercrombie's (amyloid degeneration) 277.39
abnormal innervation 374.43
abstinence
alcohol 291.81
drug 292.0
neonatal 779.5
Abt-Letterer-Siwe (acute histiocytosis X) (M9722/3) 202.5 ✓
Achard-Thiers (adrenogenital) 255.2
acid pulmonary aspiration 997.39
obstetric (Mendelson's) 668.0 ✓
acquired immune deficiency 042
acquired immunodeficiency 042
acrocephalosyndactylism 755.55
acute abdominal 789.0 ✓
acute chest 517.3
acute coronary 411.1
Adair-Dighton (brittle bones and blue sclera, deafness) 756.51
Adams-Stokes (-Morgagni) (syncope with heart block) 426.9
Addisonian 255.41

Syndrome — *see also* Disease — *continued*
Adie (-Holmes) (pupil) 379.46
adiposogenital 253.8
adrenal
hemorrhage 036.3
meningococcic 036.3
adrenocortical 255.3
adrenogenital (acquired) (congenital) 255.2
feminizing 255.2
iatrogenic 760.79
virilism (acquired) (congenital) 255.2
affective organic NEC 293.89
drug-induced 292.84
afferent loop NEC 537.89
African macroglobulinemia 273.3
Ahumada-Del Castillo (nonpuerperal galactorrhea and amenorrhea) 253.1
air blast concussion — *see* Injury, internal, by site
Alagille 759.89
Albright (-Martin) (pseudohypoparathyroidism) 275.49
Albright-McCune-Sternberg (osteitis fibrosa disseminata) 756.59
alcohol withdrawal 291.81
Alder's (leukocyte granulation anomaly) 288.2
Aldrich (-Wiskott) (eczema-thrombocytopenia) 279.12
Alibert-Bazin (mycosis fungoides) (M9700/3) 202.1 ✓
Alice in Wonderland 293.89
alien hand 781.8
Allen-Masters 620.6
Alligator baby (ichthyosis congenita) 757.1
Alport's (hereditary hematuria-nephropathy-deafness) 759.89
Alvarez (transient cerebral ischemia) 435.9
alveolar capillary block 516.8
Alzheimer's 331.0
with dementia — *see* Alzheimer's, dementia
amnestic (confabulatory) 294.0
alcohol-induced persisting 291.1
drug-induced 292.83
posttraumatic 294.0
amotivational 292.89
amyostatic 275.1
amyotrophic lateral sclerosis 335.20
androgen insensitivity 259.51
partial 259.52
Angelman 759.89
angina (*see also* Angina) 413.9
ankyloglossia superior 750.0
anterior
chest wall 786.52
compartment (tibial) 958.8
spinal artery 433.8 ✓
compression 721.1
tibial (compartment) 958.8
antibody deficiency 279.00
agammaglobulinemic 279.00
congenital 279.04
hypogammaglobulinemic 279.00
anticardiolipin antibody 289.81
antimongolism 758.39
antiphospholipid antibody 289.81
Anton (-Babinski) (hemiasomatognosia) 307.9
anxiety (*see also* Anxiety) 300.00
organic 293.84
aortic
arch 446.7
bifurcation (occlusion) 444.09
ring 747.21
Apert's (acrocephalosyndactyly) 755.55
Apert-Gallais (adrenogenital) 255.2
aphasia-apraxia-alexia 784.69
apical ballooning 429.83
"approximate answers" 300.16
arcuate ligament (-celiac axis) 447.4
arcus aortae 446.7
arc welders' 370.24
argentaffin, argintaffinoma 259.2
Argonz-Del Castillo (nonpuerperal galactorrhea and amenorrhea) 253.1

✓ **Additional Digit Required** — Refer to the Tabular List for Digit Selection   ▽ **Subterms under main terms may continue to next column or page**

312   2014 ICD-9-CM

Syndrome — *see also* Disease — *continued*
  Argyll Robertson's (syphilitic) 094.89
    nonsyphilitic 379.45
  Armenian 277.31
  arm-shoulder (*see also* Neuropathy, peripheral, autonomic) 337.9
  Arnold-Chiari (*see also* Spina bifida) 741.0 ☑
    type I 348.4
    type II 741.0 ☑
    type III 742.0
    type IV 742.2
  Arrillaga-Ayerza (pulmonary artery sclerosis with pulmonary hypertension) 416.0
  arteriomesenteric duodenum occlusion 537.89
  arteriovenous steal 996.73
  arteritis, young female (obliterative brachiocephalic) 446.7
  aseptic meningitis — *see* Meningitis, aseptic
  Asherman's 621.5
  Asperger's 299.8 ☑
  asphyctic (*see also* Anxiety) 300.00
  aspiration, of newborn (massive) 770.18
    meconium 770.12
  ataxia-telangiectasia 334.8
  Audry's (acropachyderma) 757.39
  auriculotemporal 350.8
  autoimmune lymphoproliferative (ALPS) 279.41
  autosomal (*see also* Abnormal, autosomes NEC)
    deletion 758.39
      5p 758.31
      22q11.2 758.32
  Avellis' 344.89
  Axenfeld's 743.44
  Ayerza (-Arrillaga) (pulmonary artery sclerosis with pulmonary hypertension) 416.0
  Baader's (erythema multiforme exudativum) 695.19
  Baastrup's 721.5
  Babinski (-Vaquez) (cardiovascular syphilis) 093.89
  Babinski-Fröhlich (adiposogenital dystrophy) 253.8
  Babinski-Nageotte 344.89
  Bagratuni's (temporal arteritis) 446.5
  Bakwin-Krida (craniometaphyseal dysplasia) 756.89
  Balint's (psychic paralysis of visual disorientation) 368.16
  Ballantyne (-Runge) (postmaturity) 766.22
  ballooning posterior leaflet 424.0
  Banti's — *see* Cirrhosis, liver
  Bardet-Biedl (obesity, polydactyly, and intellectual disabiilties) 759.89
  Bard-Pic's (carcinoma, head of pancreas) 157.0
  Barlow's (mitral valve prolapse) 424.0
  Barlow (-Möller) (infantile scurvy) 267
  Baron Munchausen's 301.51
  Barré-Guillain 357.0
  Barré-Liéou (posterior cervical sympathetic) 723.2
  Barrett's (chronic peptic ulcer of esophagus) 530.85
  Bársony-Polgár (corkscrew esophagus) 530.5
  Bársony-Teschendorf (corkscrew esophagus) 530.5
  Barth 759.89
  Bartter's (secondary hyperaldosteronism with juxtaglomerular hyperplasia) 255.13
  basal cell nevus 759.89
  Basedow's (exophthalmic goiter) 242.0 ☑
  basilar artery 435.0
  basofrontal 377.04
  Bassen-Kornzweig (abetalipoproteinemia) 272.5
  Batten-Steinert 359.21
  battered
    adult 995.81
    baby or child 995.54
    spouse 995.81

Syndrome — *see also* Disease — *continued*
  Baumgarten-Cruveilhier (cirrhosis of liver) 571.5
  Beals 759.82
  Bearn-Kunkel (-Slater) (lupoid hepatitis) 571.49
  Beau's (*see also* Degeneration, myocardial) 429.1
  Bechterew-Strümpell-Marie (ankylosing spondylitis) 720.0
  Beck's (anterior spinal artery occlusion) 433.8 ☑
  Beckwith (-Wiedemann) 759.89
  Behçet's 136.1
  Bekhterev-Strümpell-Marie (ankylosing spondylitis) 720.0
  Benedikt's 344.89
  Béquez César (-Steinbrinck-Chédiak-Higashi) (congenital gigantism of peroxidase granules) 288.2
  Bernard-Horner (*see also* Neuropathy, peripheral, autonomic) 337.9
  Bernard-Sergent (acute adrenocortical insufficiency) 255.41
  Bernhardt-Roth 355.1
  Bernheim's (*see also* Failure, heart) 428.0
  Bertolotti's (sacralization of fifth lumbar vertebra) 756.15
  Besnier-Boeck-Schaumann (sarcoidosis) 135
  Bianchi's (aphasia-apraxia-alexia syndrome) 784.69
  Biedl-Bardet (obesity, polydactyly, and intellectual disabilities) 759.89
  Biemond's (obesity, polydactyly, and intellectual disabilities) 759.89
  big spleen 289.4
  bilateral polycystic ovarian 256.4
  Bing-Horton's 339.00
  Biörck (-Thorson) (malignant carcinoid) 259.2
  Birt-Hogg-Dube 759.89
  Blackfan-Diamond (congenital hypoplastic anemia) 284.01
  black lung 500
  black widow spider bite 989.5
  bladder neck (*see also* Incontinence, urine) 788.30
  blast (concussion) — *see* Blast, injury
  blind loop (postoperative) 579.2
  Bloch-Siemens (incontinentia pigmenti) 757.33
  Bloch-Sulzberger (incontinentia pigmenti) 757.33
  Bloom (-Machacek) (-Torre) 757.39
  Blount-Barber (tibia vara) 732.4
  blue
    bloater 491.20
      with
        acute bronchitis 491.22
          exacerbation (acute) 491.21
    diaper 270.0
    drum 381.02
    sclera 756.51
    toe 445.02
  Boder-Sedgwick (ataxia-telangiectasia) 334.8
  Boerhaave's (spontaneous esophageal rupture) 530.4
  Bonnevie-Ullrich 758.6
  Bonnier's 386.19
  Borjeson-Forssman-Lehmann 759.89
  Bouillaud's (rheumatic heart disease) 391.9
  Bourneville (-Pringle) (tuberous sclerosis) 759.5
  Bouveret (-Hoffmann) (paroxysmal tachycardia) 427.2
  brachial plexus 353.0
  Brachman-de Lange (Amsterdam dwarf, intellectual disabilities, and brachycephaly) 759.89
  bradycardia-tachycardia 427.81
  Brailsford-Morquio (dystrophy) (mucopolysaccharidosis IV) 277.5
  brain (acute) (chronic) (nonpsychotic) (organic) (with behavioral reaction) (with neurotic reaction) 310.9

Syndrome — *see also* Disease — *continued*
  brain — *continued*
    with
      presenile brain disease (*see also* Dementia, presenile) 290.10
      psychosis, psychotic reaction (*see also* Psychosis, organic) 294.9
    chronic alcoholic 291.2
    congenital (*see also* Disability, intellectual) 319
    postcontusional 310.2
    posttraumatic
      nonpsychotic 310.2
      psychotic 293.9
        acute 293.0
        chronic (*see also* Psychosis, organic) 294.8
        subacute 293.1
    psycho-organic (*see also* Syndrome, psycho-organic) 310.9
    psychotic (*see also* Psychosis, organic) 294.9
    senile (*see also* Dementia, senile) 290.0
  branchial arch 744.41
  Brandt's (acrodermatitis enteropathica) 686.8
  Brennemann's 289.2
  Briquet's 300.81
  Brissaud-Meige (infantile myxedema) 244.9
  broad ligament laceration 620.6
  Brock's (atelectasis due to enlarged lymph nodes) 518.0
  broken heart 429.83
  Brown-Séquard 344.89
  brown spot 756.59
  Brown's tendon sheath 378.61
  Brugada 746.89
  Brugsch's (acropachyderma) 757.39
  bubbly lung 770.7
  Buchem's (hyperostosis corticalis) 733.3
  Budd-Chiari (hepatic vein thrombosis) 453.0
  Büdinger-Ludloff-Läwen 717.89
  bulbar 335.22
    lateral (*see also* Disease, cerebrovascular, acute) 436
  Bullis fever 082.8
  bundle of Kent (anomalous atrioventricular excitation) 426.7
  Bürger-Grütz (essential familial hyperlipemia) 272.3
  Burke's (pancreatic insufficiency and chronic neutropenia) 577.8
  Burnett's (milk-alkali) 275.42
  Burnier's (hypophyseal dwarfism) 253.3
  burning feet 266.2
  Bywaters' 958.5
  Caffey's (infantile cortical hyperostosis) 756.59
  Calvé-Legg-Perthes (osteochondrosis, femoral capital) 732.1
  Caplan (-Colinet) syndrome 714.81
  capsular thrombosis (*see also* Thrombosis, brain) 434.0 ☑
  carbohydrate-deficient glycoprotein (CDGS) 271.8
  carcinogenic thrombophlebitis 453.1
  carcinoid 259.2
  cardiac asthma (*see also* Failure, ventricular, left) 428.1
  cardiacos negros 416.0
  cardiofaciocutaneous 759.89
  cardiopulmonary obesity 278.03
  cardiorenal (*see also* Hypertension, cardiorenal) 404.90
  cardiorespiratory distress (idiopathic), newborn 769
  cardiovascular renal (*see also* Hypertension, cardiorenal) 404.90
  cardiovasorenal 272.7
  Carini's (ichthyosis congenita) 757.1
  carotid
    artery (internal) 435.8
    body or sinus 337.01
  carpal tunnel 354.0
  Carpenter's 759.89

Syndrome — *see also* Disease — *continued*
  Cassidy (-Scholte) (malignant carcinoid) 259.2
  cat-cry 758.31
  cauda equina 344.60
  causalgia 355.9
    lower limb 355.71
    upper limb 354.4
  cavernous sinus 437.6
  celiac 579.0
    artery compression 447.4
    axis 447.4
  central pain 338.0
  cerebellomedullary malformation (*see also* Spina bifida) 741.0 ☑
  cerebral gigantism 253.0
  cerebrohepatorenal 759.89
  cervical (root) (spine) NEC 723.8
    disc 722.71
    posterior, sympathetic 723.2
    rib 353.0
    sympathetic paralysis 337.09
    traumatic (acute) NEC 847.0
  cervicobrachial (diffuse) 723.3
  cervicocranial 723.2
  cervicodorsal outlet 353.2
  Céstan's 344.89
  Céstan (-Raymond) 433.8 ☑
  Céstan-Chenais 344.89
  chancriform 114.1
  Charcôt's (intermittent claudication) 443.9
    angina cruris 443.9
    due to atherosclerosis 440.21
  Charcôt-Marie-Tooth 356.1
  Charcôt-Weiss-Baker 337.01
  CHARGE association 759.89
  Cheadle (-Möller) (-Barlow) (infantile scurvy) 267
  Chédiak-Higashi (-Steinbrinck) (congenital gigantism of peroxidase granules) 288.2
  chest wall 786.52
  Chiari's (hepatic vein thrombosis) 453.0
  Chiari-Frommel 676.6 ☑
  chiasmatic 368.41
  Chilaiditi's (subphrenic displacement, colon) 751.4
  chondroectodermal dysplasia 756.55
  chorea-athetosis-agitans 275.1
  Christian's (chronic histiocytosis X) 277.89
  chromosome 4 short arm deletion 758.39
  chronic pain 338.4
  Churg-Strauss 446.4
  Clarke-Hadfield (pancreatic infantilism) 577.8
  Claude's 352.6
  Claude Bernard-Horner (*see also* Neuropathy, peripheral, autonomic) 337.9
  Clérambault's
    automatism 348.89
    erotomania 297.8
  Clifford's (postmaturity) 766.22
  climacteric 627.2
  Clouston's (hidrotic ectodermal dysplasia) 757.31
  clumsiness 315.4
  Cockayne's (microencephaly and dwarfism) 759.89
  Cockayne-Weber (epidermolysis bullosa) 757.39
  Coffin-Lowry 759.89
  Cogan's (nonsyphilitic interstitial keratitis) 370.52
  cold injury (newborn) 778.2
  Collet (-Sicard) 352.6
  combined immunity deficiency 279.2
  compartment(al) (anterior) (deep) (posterior) 958.8
    nontraumatic
      abdomen 729.73
      arm 729.71
      buttock 729.72
      fingers 729.71
      foot 729.72
      forearm 729.71
      hand 729.71

☑ Additional Digit Required — Refer to the Tabular List for Digit Selection   ▽ Subterms under main terms may continue to next column or page

2014 ICD-9-CM   313

Syndrome — see also Disease — continued

compartment — continued

nontraumatic — continued

hip 729.72

leg 729.72

lower extremity 729.72

shoulder 729.71

specified site NEC 729.79

thigh 729.72

toes 729.72

upper extremity 729.71

wrist 729.71

post-surgical (see also Syndrome, compartment, non-traumatic) 998.89

traumatic 958.90

abdomen 958.93

arm 958.91

buttock 958.92

fingers 958.91

foot 958.92

forearm 958.91

hand 958.91

hip 958.92

leg 958.92

lower extremity 958.92

shoulder 958.91

specified site NEC 958.99

thigh 958.92

tibial 958.92

toes 958.92

upper extremity 958.91

wrist 958.91

complex regional pain — see also Dystrophy, sympathetic

type I — see Dystrophy, sympathetic (posttraumatic) (reflex)

type II — see Causalgia

compression 958.5

cauda equina 344.60

with neurogenic bladder 344.61

concussion 310.2

congenital

affecting more than one system 759.7

specified type NEC 759.89

congenital central alveolar hypoventilation 327.25

facial diplegia 352.6

muscular hypertrophy-cerebral 759.89

congestion-fibrosis (pelvic) 625.5

conjunctivourethrosynovial 099.3

Conn (-Louis) (primary aldosteronism) 255.12

Conradi (-Hünermann) (chondrodysplasia calcificans congenita) 756.59

conus medullaris 336.8

Cooke-Apert-Gallais (adrenogenital) 255.2

Cornelia de Lange's (Amsterdam dwarf, intellectual disabilities, and brachycephaly) 759.8 ☑

coronary insufficiency or intermediate 411.1

cor pulmonale 416.9

corticosexual 255.2

Costen's (complex) 524.60

costochondral junction 733.6

costoclavicular 353.0

costovertebral 253.0

Cotard's (paranoia) 297.1

Cowden 759.6

craniovertebral 723.2

Creutzfeldt-Jakob 046.19

with dementia

with behavioral disturbance 046.19 [294.11]

without behavioral disturbance 046.19 [294.10]

variant 046.11

with dementia

with behavioral disturbance 046.11 [294.11]

without behavioral disturbance 046.11 [294.10]

crib death 798.0

cricopharyngeal 787.20

cri-du-chat 758.31

Crigler-Najjar (congenital hyperbilirubinemia) 277.4

Syndrome — see also Disease — continued

crocodile tears 351.8

Cronkhite-Canada 211.3

croup 464.4

CRST (cutaneous systemic sclerosis) 710.1

crush 958.5

crushed lung (see also Injury, internal, lung) 861.20

Cruveilhier-Baumgarten (cirrhosis of liver) 571.5

cubital tunnel 354.2

Cuiffini-Pancoast (M8010/3) (carcinoma, pulmonary apex) 162.3

Curschmann (-Batten) (-Steinert) 359.21

Cushing's (iatrogenic) (idiopathic) (pituitary basophilism) (pituitary-dependent) 255.0

overdose or wrong substance given or taken 962.0

Cyriax's (slipping rib) 733.99

cystic duct stump 576.0

Da Costa's (neurocirculatory asthenia) 306.2

Dameshek's (erythroblastic anemia) 282.49

Dana-Putnam (subacute combined sclerosis with pernicious anemia) 281.0 [336.2]

Danbolt (-Closs) (acrodermatitis enteropathica) 686.8

Dandy-Walker (atresia, foramen of Magendie) 742.3

with spina bifida (see also Spina bifida) 741.0 ☑

Danlos' 756.83

Davies-Colley (slipping rib) 733.99

dead fetus 641.3 ☑

defeminization 255.2

defibrination (see also Fibrinolysis) 286.6

Degos' 447.8

Deiters' nucleus 386.19

Déjérine-Roussy 338.0

Déjérine-Thomas 333.0

de Lange's (Amsterdam dwarf, intellectual disabilities, and brachycephaly) (Cornelia) 759.89

Del Castillo's (germinal aplasia) 606.0

deletion chromosomes 758.39

delusional

induced by drug 292.11

dementia-aphonia, of childhood (see also Psychosis, childhood) 299.1 ☑

demyelinating NEC 341.9

denial visual hallucination 307.9

depersonalization 300.6

de Quervain's 259.51

Dercum's (adiposis dolorosa) 272.8

de Toni-Fanconi (-Debré) (cystinosis) 270.0

diabetes-dwarfism-obesity (juvenile) 258.1

diabetes mellitus-hypertension-nephrosis 250.4 ☑ [581.81]

due to secondary diabetes 249.4 ☑ [581.81]

diabetes mellitus in newborn infant 775.1

diabetes-nephrosis 250.4 ☑ [581.81]

due to secondary diabetes 249.4 ☑ [581.81]

diabetic amyotrophy 250.6 ☑ [353.5]

due to secondary diabetes 249.6 ☑ [353.5]

Diamond-Blackfan (congenital hypoplastic anemia) 284.01

Diamond-Gardener (autoerythrocyte sensitization) 287.2

DIC (diffuse or disseminated intravascular coagulopathy) (see also Fibrinolysis) 286.6

diencephalohypophyseal NEC 253.8

diffuse cervicobrachial 723.3

diffuse obstructive pulmonary 496

DiGeorge's (thymic hypoplasia) 279.11

Dighton's 756.51

Di Guglielmo's (erythremic myelosis) (M9841/3) 207.0 ☑

disequilibrium 276.9

disseminated platelet thrombosis 446.6

Ditthomska 307.81

Doan-Wiseman (primary splenic neutropenia) 289.53

Syndrome — see also Disease — continued

Döhle body-panmyelopathic 288.2

Donohue's (leprechaunism) 259.8

dorsolateral medullary (see also Disease, cerebrovascular, acute) 436

double athetosis 333.71

double whammy 360.81

Down's (mongolism) 758.0

Dresbach's (elliptocytosis) 282.1

Dressler's (postmyocardial infarction) 411.0

hemoglobinuria 283.2

postcardiotomy 429.4

drug withdrawal, infant, of dependent mother 779.5

dry skin 701.1

eye 375.15

DSAP (disseminated superficial actinic porokeratosis) 692.75

Duane's (retraction) 378.71

Duane-Stilling-Türk (ocular retraction syndrome) 378.71

Dubin-Johnson (constitutional hyperbilirubinemia) 277.4

Dubin-Sprinz (constitutional hyperbilirubinemia) 277.4

Duchenne's 335.22

due to abnormality

autosomal NEC (see also Abnormal, autosomes NEC) 758.5

13 758.1

18 758.2

21 or 22 758.0

D1 758.1

E3 758.2

G 758.0

chromosomal 758.89

sex 758.81

dumping 564.2

nonsurgical 536.8

Duplay's 726.2

Dupré's (meningism) 781.6

Dyke-Young (acquired macrocytic hemolytic anemia) 283.9

dyspraxia 315.4

dystocia, dystrophy 654.9 ☑

Eagle-Barret 756.71

Eales' 362.18

Eaton-Lambert (see also Syndrome, Lambert-Eaton) 358.30

Ebstein's (downward displacement, tricuspid valve into right ventricle) 746.2

ectopic ACTH secretion 255.0

eczema-thrombocytopenia 279.12

Eddowes' (brittle bones and blue sclera) 756.51

Edwards' 758.2

efferent loop 537.89

effort (aviators') (psychogenic) 306.2

Ehlers-Danlos 756.83

Eisenmenger's (ventricular septal defect) 745.4

Ekbom's (restless legs) 333.94

Ekman's (brittle bones and blue sclera) 756.51

electric feet 266.2

Elephant man 237.71

Ellison-Zollinger (gastric hypersecretion with pancreatic islet cell tumor) 251.5

Ellis-van Creveld (chondroectodermal dysplasia) 756.55

embryonic fixation 270.2

empty sella (turcica) 253.8

endocrine-hypertensive 255.3

Engel-von Recklinghausen (osteitis fibrosa cystica) 252.01

enteroarticular 099.3

entrapment — see Neuropathy, entrapment

eosinophilia myalgia 710.5

epidemic vomiting 078.82

Epstein's — see Nephrosis

Erb (-Oppenheim)-Goldflam 358.00

Erdheim's (acromegalic macrospondylitis) 253.0

Erdheim-Chester 277.89

Erlacher-Blount (tibia vara) 732.4

erythrocyte fragmentation 283.19

Syndrome — see also Disease — continued

euthyroid sick 790.94

Evans' (thrombocytopenic purpura) 287.32

excess cortisol, iatrogenic 255.0

exhaustion 300.5

extrapyramidal 333.90

eyelid-malar-mandible 756.0

eye retraction 378.71

Faber's (achlorhydric anemia) 280.9

Fabry (-Anderson) (angiokeratoma corporis diffusum) 272.7

facet 724.8

Fallot's 745.2

falx (see also Hemorrhage, brain) 431

familial eczema-thrombocytopenia 279.12

Fanconi's (anemia) (congenital pancytopenia) 284.09

Fanconi (-de Toni) (-Debré) (cystinosis) 270.0

Farber (-Uzman) (disseminated lipogranulomatosis) 272.8

fatigue NEC 300.5

chronic 780.71

faulty bowel habit (idiopathic megacolon) 564.7

FDH (focal dermal hypoplasia) 757.39

fecal reservoir 560.39

Feil-Klippel (brevicollis) 756.16

Felty's (rheumatoid arthritis with splenomegaly and leukopenia) 714.1

fertile eunuch 257.2

fetal alcohol 760.71

late effect 760.71

fibrillation-flutter 427.32

fibrositis (periarticular) 729.0

Fiedler's (acute isolated myocarditis) 422.91

Fiessinger-Leroy (-Reiter) 099.3

Fiessinger-Rendu (erythema multiforme exudativum) 695.19

first arch 756.0

Fisher's 357.0

fish odor 270.8

Fitz's (acute hemorrhagic pancreatitis) 577.0

Fitz-Hugh and Curtis 098.86

due to

Chlamydia trachomatis 099.56

Neisseria gonorrhoeae (gonococcal peritonitis) 098.86

Flajani (-Basedow) (exophthalmic goiter) 242.0 ☑

flat back

acquired 737.29

postprocedural 738.5

floppy

infant 781.99

iris 364.81

valve (mitral) 424.0

flush 259.2

Foix-Alajouanine 336.1

Fong's (hereditary osteo-onychodysplasia) 756.89

foramen magnum 348.4

Forbes-Albright (nonpuerperal amenorrhea and lactation associated with pituitary tumor) 253.1

Foster-Kennedy 377.04

Foville's (peduncular) 344.89

fragile X 759.83

Franceschetti's (mandibulofacial dysostosis) 756.0

Fraser's 759.89

Freeman-Sheldon 759.89

Frey's (auriculotemporal) 705.22

Friderichsen-Waterhouse 036.3

Friedrich-Erb-Arnold (acropachyderma) 757.39

Fröhlich's (adiposogenital dystrophy) 253.8

Froin's 336.8

Frommel-Chiari 676.6 ☑

frontal lobe 310.0

Fukuhara 277.87

Fuller Albright's (osteitis fibrosa disseminata) 756.59

functional

bowel 564.9

prepubertal castrate 752.89

☑ Additional Digit Required — Refer to the Tabular List for Digit Selection   ▽ Subterms under main terms may continue to next column or page

314

2014 ICD-9-CM

Syndrome — *see also* Disease — *continued*

Gaisböck's (polycythemia hypertonica) 289.0
ganglion (basal, brain) 333.90
geniculi 351.1
Ganser's, hysterical 300.16
Gardner-Diamond (autoerythrocyte sensitization) 287.2
gastroesophageal junction 530.0
gastroesophageal laceration-hemorrhage 530.7
gastrojejunal loop obstruction 537.89
Gayet-Wernicke's (superior hemorrhagic polioencephalitis) 265.1
Gee-Herter-Heubner (nontropical sprue) 579.0
Gélineau's (*see also* Narcolepsy) 347.00
genito-anorectal 099.1
Gerhardt's (vocal cord paralysis) 478.30
Gerstmann's (finger agnosia) 784.69
Gerstmann-Sträussler-Scheinker (GSS) 046.71
Gianotti Crosti 057.8
due to known virus — *see* Infection, virus
due to unknown virus 057.8
Gilbert's 277.4
Gilford (-Hutchinson) (progeria) 259.8
Gilles de la Tourette's 307.23
Gillespie's (dysplasia oculodentodigitalis) 759.89
Glénard's (enteroptosis) 569.89
Glinski-Simmonds (pituitary cachexia) 253.2
glucuronyl transferase 277.4
glue ear 381.20
Goldberg (-Maxwell) (-Morris) (testicular feminization) 259.51
Goldenhar's (oculoauriculovertebral dysplasia) 756.0
Goldflam-Erb 358.00
Goltz-Gorlin (dermal hypoplasia) 757.39
Good's 279.06
Goodpasture's (pneumorenal) 446.21
Gopalan's (burning feet) 266.2
Gorlin's 759.89
Gorlin-Chaudhry-Moss 759.89
Gougerot-Blum (pigmented purpuric lichenoid dermatitis) 709.1
Gougerot-Carteaud (confluent reticulate papillomatosis) 701.8
Gougerot (-Houwer)-Sjögren (keratoconjunctivitis sicca) 710.2
Gouley's (constrictive pericarditis) 423.2
Gowers' (vasovagal attack) 780.2
Gowers-Paton-Kennedy 377.04
Gradenigo's 383.02
gray or grey (chloramphenicol) (newborn) 779.2
Greig's (hypertelorism) 756.0
GSS (Gerstmann-Sträussler-Scheinker) 046.71
Gubler-Millard 344.89
Guérin-Stern (arthrogryposis multiplex congenita) 754.89
Guillain-Barré (-Strohl) 357.0
Gunn's (jaw-winking syndrome) 742.8
Günther's (congenital erythropoietic porphyria) 277.1
gustatory sweating 350.8
H₃O 759.81
Hadfield-Clarke (pancreatic infantilism) 577.8
Haglund-Läwen-Fründ 717.89
hairless women 257.8
hair tourniquet (*see also* Injury, superficial, by site)
finger 915.8
infected 915.9
penis 911.8
infected 911.9
toe 917.8
infected 917.9
Hallermann-Streiff 756.0
Hallervorden-Spatz 333.0
Hamman's (spontaneous mediastinal emphysema) 518.1

Syndrome — *see also* Disease — *continued*

Hamman-Rich (diffuse interstitial pulmonary fibrosis) 516.33
hand-foot 693.0
Hand-Schüller-Christian (chronic histiocytosis X) 277.89
Hanot-Chauffard (-Troisier) (bronze diabetes) 275.01
Harada's 363.22
Hare's (M8010/3) (carcinoma, pulmonary apex) 162.3
Harkavy's 446.0
harlequin color change 779.89
Harris' (organic hyperinsulinism) 251.1
Hart's (pellagra-cerebellar ataxia-renal aminoaciduria) 270.0
Hayem-Faber (achlorhydric anemia) 280.9
Hayem-Widal (acquired hemolytic jaundice) 283.9
headache — *see* Headache, syndrome
Heberden's (angina pectoris) 413.9
Hedinger's (malignant carcinoid) 259.2
Hegglin's 288.2
Heller's (infantile psychosis) (*see also* Psychosis, childhood) 299.1 ☑
H.E.L.L.P 642.5 ☑
hemolytic-uremic (adult) (child) 283.11
hemophagocytic 288.4
infection-associated 288.4
Hench-Rosenberg (palindromic arthritis) (*see also* Rheumatism, palindromic) 719.3 ☑
Henoch-Schönlein (allergic purpura) 287.0
hepatic flexure 569.89
hepatopulmonary 573.5
hepatorenal 572.4
due to a procedure 997.49
following delivery 674.8 ☑
hepatourologic 572.4
Herrick's (hemoglobin S disease) 282.61
Herter (-Gee) (nontropical sprue) 579.0
Heubner-Herter (nontropical sprue) 579.0
Heyd's (hepatorenal) 572.4
HHHO 759.81
high grade myelodysplastic 238.73
with 5q deletion 238.73
Hilger's 337.09
histiocytic 288.4
Hoffa (-Kastert) (liposynovitis prepatellaris) 272.8
Hoffmann's 244.9 [359.5]
Hoffmann-Bouveret (paroxysmal tachycardia) 427.2
Hoffmann-Werdnig 335.0
Holländer-Simons (progressive lipodystrophy) 272.6
Holmes' (visual disorientation) 368.16
Holmes-Adie 379.46
Hoppe-Goldflam 358.00
Horner's (*see also* Neuropathy, peripheral, autonomic) 337.9
traumatic — *see* Injury, nerve, cervical sympathetic
hospital addiction 301.51
hungry bone 275.5
Hunt's (herpetic geniculate ganglionitis) 053.11
dyssynergia cerebellaris myoclonica 334.2
Hunter (-Hurler) (mucopolysaccharidosis II) 277.5
hunterian glossitis 529.4
Hurler (-Hunter) (mucopolysaccharidosis II) 277.5
Hutchinson-Boeck (sarcoidosis) 135
Hutchinson-Gilford (progeria) 259.8
Hutchinson's incisors or teeth 090.5
hydralazine
correct substance properly administered 695.4
overdose or wrong substance given or taken 972.6
hydraulic concussion (abdomen) (*see also* Injury, internal, abdomen) 868.00
hyperabduction 447.8
hyperactive bowel 564.9

Syndrome — *see also* Disease — *continued*

hyperaldosteronism with hypokalemic alkalosis (Bartter's) 255.13
hypercalcemic 275.42
hypercoagulation NEC 289.89
hypereosinophilic (idiopathic) 288.3
hyperkalemic 276.7
hyperkinetic (*see also* Hyperkinesia)
heart 429.82
hyperlipemia-hemolytic anemia-icterus 571.1
hypermobility 728.5
hypernatremia 276.0
hyperosmolarity 276.0
hyperperfusion 997.01
hypersomnia-bulimia 349.89
hypersplenic 289.4
hypersympathetic (*see also* Neuropathy, peripheral, autonomic) 337.9
hypertransfusion, newborn 776.4
hyperventilation, psychogenic 306.1
hyperviscosity (of serum) NEC 273.3
polycythemic 289.0
sclerothymic 282.8
hypoglycemic (familial) (neonatal) 251.2
functional 251.1
hypokalemic 276.8
hypophyseal 253.8
hypophyseothalamic 253.8
hypopituitarism 253.2
hypoplastic left heart 746.7
hypopotassemia 276.8
hyposmolality 276.1
hypotension, maternal 669.2 ☑
hypothenar hammer 443.89
hypotonia-hypomentia-hypogonadism-obesity 759.81
ICF (intravascular coagulation-fibrinolysis) (*see also* Fibrinolysis) 286.6
idiopathic cardiorespiratory distress, newborn 769
idiopathic nephrotic (infantile) 581.9
iliotibial band 728.89
Imerslund (-Gräsbeck) (anemia due to familial selective vitamin B₁₂ malabsorption) 281.1
immobility (paraplegic) 728.3
immune reconstitution inflammatory (IRIS) 995.90
immunity deficiency, combined 279.2
impending coronary 411.1
impingement
shoulder 726.2
vertebral bodies 724.4
inappropriate secretion of antidiuretic hormone (ADH) 253.6
incomplete
mandibulofacial 756.0
infant
death, sudden (SIDS) 798.0
Hercules 255.2
of diabetic mother 775.0
shaken 995.55
infantilism 253.3
inferior vena cava 459.2
influenza-like (*see also* Influenza) 487.1
inspissated bile, newborn 774.4
insufficient sleep 307.44
intermediate coronary (artery) 411.1
internal carotid artery (*see also* Occlusion, artery, carotid) 433.1 ☑
interspinous ligament 724.8
intestinal
carcinoid 259.2
gas 787.3
knot 560.2
intraoperative floppy iris (IFIS) 364.81
intravascular
coagulation-fibrinolysis (ICF) (*see also* Fibrinolysis) 286.6
coagulopathy (*see also* Fibrinolysis) 286.6
inverted Marfan's 759.89
IRDS (idiopathic respiratory distress, newborn) 769
irritable
bowel 564.1

Syndrome — *see also* Disease — *continued*

irritable — *continued*
heart 306.2
weakness 300.5
ischemic bowel (transient) 557.9
chronic 557.1
due to mesenteric artery insufficiency 557.1
Itsenko-Cushing (pituitary basophilism) 255.0
IVC (intravascular coagulopathy) (*see also* Fibrinolysis) 286.6
Ivemark's (asplenia with congenital heart disease) 759.0
Jaccoud's 714.4
Jackson's 344.89
Jadassohn-Lewandowski (pachyonchia congenita) 757.5
Jaffe-Lichtenstein (-Uehlinger) 252.01
Jahnke's (encephalocutaneous angiomatosis) 759.6
Jakob-Creutzfeldt 046.19
with dementia
with behavioral disturbance 046.19 [294.11]
without behavioral disturbance 046.19 [294.10]
variant 046.11
with dementia
with behavioral disturbance 046.11 [294.11]
without behavioral disturbance 046.11 [294.10]
Jaksch's (pseudoleukemia infantum) 285.8
Jaksch-Hayem (-Luzet) (pseudoleukemia infantum) 285.8
jaw-winking 742.8
jejunal 564.2
Jervell-Lange-Nielsen 426.82
jet lag 327.35
Jeune's (asphyxiating thoracic dystrophy of newborn) 756.4
Job's (chronic granulomatous disease) 288.1
Jordan's 288.2
Joseph-Diamond-Blackfan (congenital hypoplastic anemia) 284.01
Joubert 759.89
jugular foramen 352.6
Kabuki 759.89
Kahler's (multiple myeloma) (M9730/3) 203.0 ☑
Kalischer's (encephalocutaneous angiomatosis) 759.6
Kallmann's (hypogonadotropic hypogonadism with anosmia) 253.4
Kanner's (autism) (*see also* Psychosis, childhood) 299.0 ☑
Kartagener's (sinusitis, bronchiectasis, situs inversus) 759.3
Kasabach-Merritt (capillary hemangioma associated with thrombocytopenic purpura) 287.39
Kast's (dyschondroplasia with hemangiomas) 756.4
Kaznelson's (congenital hypoplastic anemia) 284.01
Kearns-Sayre 277.87
Kelly's (sideropenic dysphagia) 280.8
Kimmelstiel-Wilson (intercapillary glomerulosclerosis) 250.4 ☑ [581.81]
due to secondary diabetes 249.4 ☑ [581.81]
Klauder's (erythema multiforme exudativum) 695.19
Kleine-Levin 327.35
Klein-Waardenburg (ptosis-epicanthus) 270.2
Klinefelter's 758.7
Klippel-Feil (brevicollis) 756.16
Klippel-Trenaunay 759.89
Klumpke (-Déjérine) (injury to brachial plexus at birth) 767.6
Klüver-Bucy (-Terzian) 310.0
Köhler-Pellegrini-Stieda (calcification, knee joint) 726.62
König's 564.89

Index

Syndrome — Syndrome

☑ **Additional Digit Required** — Refer to the Tabular List for Digit Selection   ▽ **Subterms under main terms may continue to next column or page**

2014 ICD-9-CM   317

Syndrome — *see also* Disease — *continued*

Rud's (mental deficiency, epilepsy, and infantilism) 759.89
Ruiter-Pompen (-Wyers) (angiokeratoma
corporis diffusum) 272.7
Runge's (postmaturity) 766.22
Russell (-Silver) (congenital hemihypertrophy and short stature) 759.89
Rytand-Lipsitch (complete atrioventricular
block) 426.0
sacralization-scoliosis-sciatica 756.15
sacroiliac 724.6
Saenger's 379.46
salt
depletion (*see also* Disease, renal) 593.9
due to heat NEC 992.8
causing heat exhaustion or prostration 992.4
low (*see also* Disease, renal) 593.9
salt-losing (*see also* Disease, renal) 593.9
Sanfilippo's (mucopolysaccharidosis III)
277.5
Scaglietti-Dagnini (acromegalic
macrospondylitis) 253.0
scalded skin 695.81
scalenus anticus (anterior) 353.0
scapulocostal 354.8
scapuloperoneal 359.1
scapulovertebral 723.4
Schaumann's (sarcoidosis) 135
Scheie's (mucopolysaccharidosis IS) 277.5
Scheuthauer-Marie-Sainton (cleidocranialis
dysostosis) 755.59
Schirmer's (encephalocutaneous angiomatosis) 759.6
schizophrenic, of childhood NEC (*see also*
Psychosis, childhood) 299.9 ☑
Schmidt's
sphallo-pharyngo-laryngeal hemiplegia
352.6
thyroid-adrenocortical insufficiency
258.1
vagoaccessory 352.6
Schneider's 047.9
Schnitzler 273.1
Scholte's (malignant carcinoid) 259.2
Scholz (-Bielschowsky-Henneberg) 330.0
Schroeder's (endocrine-hypertensive) 255.3
Schüller-Christian (chronic histiocytosis X)
277.89
Schultz's (agranulocytosis) 288.09
Schwartz (-Jampel) 359.23
Schwartz-Bartter (inappropriate secretion
of antidiuretic hormone) 253.6
Scimitar (anomalous venous drainage, right
lung to inferior vena cava) 747.49
sclerocystic ovary 256.4
sea-blue histiocyte 272.7
Seabright-Bantam (pseudohypoparathy-
roidism) 275.49
Seckel's 759.89
Secretan's (posttraumatic edema) 782.3
secretoinhibitor (keratoconjunctivitis sicca)
710.2
Seeligmann's (ichthyosis congenita) 757.1
Senear-Usher (pemphigus erythematosus)
694.4
senilism 259.8
seroconversion, retroviral (acute) V08
serotonin 333.99
serous meningitis 348.2
Sertoli cell (germinal aplasia) 606.0
sex chromosome mosaic 758.81
Sézary's (reticulosis) (M9701/3) 202.2 ☑
shaken infant 995.55
Shaver's (bauxite pneumoconiosis) 503
Sheehan's (postpartum pituitary necrosis)
253.2
shock (traumatic) 958.4
kidney 584.5
following crush injury 958.5
lung 518.82
related to trauma and surgery 518.52
neurogenic 308.9
psychic 308.9
Shone's 746.84

Syndrome — *see also* Disease — *continued*

short
bowel 579.3
P-R interval 426.81
shoulder-arm (*see also* Neuropathy, peripheral, autonomic) 337.9
shoulder-girdle 723.4
shoulder-hand (*see also* Neuropathy, peripheral, autonomic) 337.9
Shwachman's 288.02
Shy-Drager (orthostatic hypotension with
multisystem degeneration) 333.0
Sicard's 352.6
sicca (keratoconjunctivitis) 710.2
sick
cell 276.1
cilia 759.89
sinus 427.81
sideropenic 280.8
Siemens'
ectodermal dysplasia 757.31
keratosis follicularis spinulosa (decalvans) 757.39
Silfverskiöld's (osteochondrodystrophy, extremities) 756.50
Silver's (congenital hemihypertrophy and
short stature) 759.89
Silvestroni-Bianco (thalassemia minima)
282.46
Simons' (progressive lipodystrophy) 272.6
sinusitis-bronchiectasis-situs inversus 759.3
sinus tarsi 726.79
Sipple's (medullary thyroid carcinoma-
pheochromocytoma) 258.02
Sjögren (-Gougerot) (keratoconjunctivitis
sicca) 710.2
with lung involvement 710.2 [517.8]
Sjögren-Larsson (ichthyosis congenita)
757.1
SJS-TEN (Stevens-Johnson syndrome - toxic
epidermal necrolysis overlap) 695.14
Slocumb's 255.3
Sluder's 337.09
Smith-Lemli-Opitz (cerebrohepatorenal
syndrome) 759.89
Smith-Magenis 758.33
smokers' 305.1
Sneddon-Wilkinson (subcorneal pustular
dermatosis) 694.1
Sotos' (cerebral gigantism) 253.0
South African cardiomyopathy 425.2
spasmodic
upward movement, eye(s) 378.82
winking 307.20
Spens' (syncope with heart block) 426.9
spherophakia-brachymorphia 759.89
spinal cord injury (*see also* Injury, spinal, by
site)
with fracture, vertebra — *see* Fracture,
vertebra, by site, with spinal cord
injury
cervical — *see* Injury, spinal, cervical
fluid malabsorption (acquired) 331.3
splenic
agenesis 759.0
flexure 569.89
neutropenia 289.53
sequestration 289.52
Spurway's (brittle bones and blue sclera)
756.51
staphylococcal scalded skin 695.81
Stein's (polycystic ovary) 256.4
Steinbrocker's (*see also* Neuropathy, peripheral, autonomic) 337.9
Stein-Leventhal (polycystic ovary) 256.4
Stevens-Johnson (erythema multiforme
exudativum) 695.13
toxic epidermal necrolysis overlap (SJS-
TEN overlap syndrome) 695.14
Stewart-Morel (hyperostosis frontalis interna) 733.3
Stickler 759.89
stiff-baby 759.89
stiff-man 333.91
Still's (juvenile rheumatoid arthritis) 714.30

Syndrome — *see also* Disease — *continued*

Still-Felty (rheumatoid arthritis with
splenomegaly and leukopenia) 714.1
Stilling-Türk-Duane (ocular retraction syndrome) 378.71
Stojano's (subcostal) 098.86
Stokes (-Adams) (syncope with heart block)
426.9
Stokvis-Talma (enterogenous cyanosis)
289.7
stone heart (*see also* Failure, ventricular, left)
428.1
straight-back 756.19
stroke (*see also* Disease, cerebrovascular,
acute) 436
little 435.9
Sturge-Kalischer-Weber (encephalotrigeminal angiomatosis) 759.6
Sturge-Weber (-Dimitri) (encephalocutaneous angiomatosis) 759.6
subclavian-carotid obstruction (chronic)
446.7
subclavian steal 435.2
subcoracoid-pectoralis minor 447.8
subcostal 098.86
nerve compression 354.8
subperiosteal hematoma 267
subphrenic interposition 751.4
sudden infant death (SIDS) 798.0
Sudeck's 733.7
Sudeck-Leriche 733.7
superior
cerebellar artery (*see also* Disease, cerebrovascular, acute) 436
mesenteric artery 557.1
pulmonary sulcus (tumor) (M8010/3)
162.3
semi-circular canal dehiscence 386.8
vena cava 459.2
suprarenal cortical 255.3
supraspinatus 726.10
Susac 348.39
swallowed blood 777.3
sweat retention 705.1
Sweet's (acute febrile neutrophilic dermatosis) 695.89
Swyer's (XY pure gonadal dysgenesis) 752.7
Swyer-James (unilateral hyperlucent lung)
492.8
Symonds' 348.2
sympathetic
cervical paralysis 337.09
pelvic 625.5
syndactylic oxycephaly 755.55
syphilitic-cardiovascular 093.89
systemic
fibrosclerosing 710.8
inflammatory response (SIRS) 995.90
due to
infectious process 995.91
with acute organ dysfunction
995.92
non-infectious process 995.93
with acute organ dysfunction
995.94
systolic click (-murmur) 785.2
Tabagism 305.1
tachycardia-bradycardia 427.81
Takayasu (-Onishi) (pulseless disease) 446.7
Takotsubo 429.83
Tapia's 352.6
tarsal tunnel 355.5
Taussig-Bing (transposition, aorta and
overriding pulmonary artery) 745.11
Taybi's (otopalatodigital) 759.89
Taylor's 625.5
teething 520.7
tegmental 344.89
telangiectasis-pigmentation-cataract 757.33
temporal 383.02
lobectomy behavior 310.0
temporomandibular joint-pain-dysfunction
[TMJ] NEC 524.60
specified NEC 524.69
Terry's (*see also* Retinopathy of prematurity)
362.21

Syndrome — *see also* Disease — *continued*

testicular feminization 259.51
testis, nonvirilizing 257.8
tethered (spinal) cord 742.59
thalamic 338.0
Thibierge-Weissenbach (cutaneous systemic
sclerosis) 710.1
Thiele 724.6
thoracic outlet (compression) 353.0
thoracogenous rheumatic (hypertrophic
pulmonary osteoarthropathy) 731.2
Thorn's (*see also* Disease, renal) 593.9
Thorson-Biörck (malignant carcinoid) 259.2
thrombopenia-hemangioma 287.39
thyroid-adrenocortical insufficiency 258.1
Tietze's 733.6
time-zone (rapid) 327.35
Tobias' (carcinoma, pulmonary apex)
(M8010/3) 162.3
toilet seat 926.0
Tolosa-Hunt 378.55
Toni-Fanconi (cystinosis) 270.0
Touraine's (hereditary osteo-onychodysplasia) 756.89
Touraine-Solente-Golé (acropachyderma)
757.39
toxic
oil 710.5
shock 040.82
transfusion
fetal-maternal 772.0
twin
donor (infant) 772.0
recipient (infant) 776.4
transient left ventricular apical ballooning
429.83
Treacher Collins' (incomplete mandibulofacial dysostosis) 756.0
trigeminal plate 259.8
triple X female 758.81
trisomy NEC 758.5
13 or D$_1$ 758.1
16-18 or E 758.2
18 or E$_3$ 758.2
20 758.5
21 or G (mongolism) 758.0
22 or G (mongolism) 758.0
G 758.0
Troisier-Hanot-Chauffard (bronze diabetes)
275.01
tropical wet feet 991.4
Trousseau's (thrombophlebitis migrans visceral cancer) 453.1
tumor lysis (following antineoplastic drug
therapy) (spontaneous) 277.88
Türk's (ocular retraction syndrome) 378.71
Turner's 758.6
Turner-Varny 758.6
Twiddler's (due to)
automatic implantable defibrillator
996.04
pacemaker 996.01
twin-to-twin transfusion 762.3
recipient twin 776.4
Uehlinger's (acropachyderma) 757.39
Ullrich (-Bonnevie) (-Turner) 758.6
Ullrich-Feichtiger 759.89
underwater blast injury (abdominal) (*see
also* Injury, internal, abdomen)
868.00
universal joint, cervix 620.6
Unverricht (-Lundborg) 345.1 ☑
Unverricht-Wagner (dermatomyositis) 710.3
upward gaze 378.81
Urbach-Oppenheim (necrobiosis lipoidica
diabeticorum) 250.8 ☑ [709.3]
due to secondary diabetes
249.8 ☑ [709.3]
Urbach-Wiethe (lipoid proteinosis) 272.8
uremia, chronic 585.9
urethral 597.81
urethro-oculoarticular 099.3
urethro-oculosynovial 099.3
urohepatic 572.4
uveocutaneous 364.24
uveomeningeal, uveomeningitis 363.22

Syndrome — *see also* Disease — *continued*
vagohypoglossal 352.6
vagovagal 780.2
van Buchem's (hyperostosis corticalis) 733.3
van der Hoeve's (brittle bones and blue sclera, deafness) 756.51
van der Hoeve-Halbertsma-Waardenburg (ptosis-epicanthus) 270.2
van der Hoeve-Waardenburg-Gualdi (ptosis-epicanthus) 270.2
vanishing twin 651.33
van Neck-Odelberg (juvenile osteochondrosis) 732.1
vascular splanchnic 557.0
vasomotor 443.9
vasovagal 780.2
VATER 759.89
Velo-cardio-facial 758.32
vena cava (inferior) (superior) (obstruction) 459.2
Verbiest's (claudicatio intermittens spinalis) 435.1
Vernet's 352.6
vertebral
    artery 435.1
        compression 721.1
        lumbar 724.4
        steal 435.1
vertebrogenic (pain) 724.5
vertiginous NEC 386.9
video display tube 723.8
Villaret's 352.6
Vinson-Plummer (sideropenic dysphagia) 280.8
virilizing adrenocortical hyperplasia, congenital 255.2
virus, viral 079.99
visceral larval migrans 128.0
visual disorientation 368.16
vitamin B$_6$ deficiency 266.1
vitreous touch 997.99
Vogt's (corpus striatum) 333.71
Vogt-Koyanagi 364.24
Volkmann's 958.6
von Bechterew-Strümpell (ankylosing spondylitis) 720.0
von Graefe's 378.72
von Hippel-Lindau (angiomatosis retinocerebellosa) 759.6
von Schroetter's (intermittent venous claudication) 453.89
von Willebrand (-Jürgens) (angiohemophilia) 286.4
Waardenburg-Klein (ptosis epicanthus) 270.2
Wagner (-Unverricht) (dermatomyositis) 710.3
Waldenström's (macroglobulinemia) 273.3
Waldenström-Kjellberg (sideropenic dysphagia) 280.8
Wallenberg's (posterior inferior cerebellar artery) (*see also* Disease, cerebrovascular, acute) 436
Waterhouse (-Friderichsen) 036.3
water retention 276.69
Weber's 344.89
Weber-Christian (nodular nonsuppurative panniculitis) 729.30
Weber-Cockayne (epidermolysis bullosa) 757.39
Weber-Dimitri (encephalocutaneous angiomatosis) 759.6
Weber-Gubler 344.89
Weber-Leyden 344.89
Weber-Osler (familial hemorrhagic telangiectasia) 448.0
Wegener's (necrotizing respiratory granulomatosis) 446.4
Weill-Marchesani (brachymorphism and ectopia lentis) 759.89
Weingarten's (tropical eosinophilia) 518.3
Weiss-Baker (carotid sinus syncope) 337.01
Weissenbach-Thibierge (cutaneous systemic sclerosis) 710.1
Werdnig-Hoffmann 335.0

Syndrome — *see also* Disease — *continued*
Werlhof-Wichmann (*see also* Purpura, thrombocytopenic) 287.39
Wermer's (polyendocrine adenomatosis) 258.01
Werner's (progeria adultorum) 259.8
Wernicke's (nonalcoholic) (superior hemorrhagic polioencephalitis) 265.1
Wernicke-Korsakoff (nonalcoholic) 294.0
    alcoholic 291.1
Westphal-Strümpell (hepatolenticular degeneration) 275.1
wet
    brain (alcoholic) 303.9 ☑
    feet (maceration) (tropical) 991.4
    lung
        adult 518.52
        newborn 770.6
whiplash 847.0
Whipple's (intestinal lipodystrophy) 040.2
"whistling face" (craniocarpotarsal dystrophy) 759.89
Widal (-Abrami) (acquired hemolytic jaundice) 283.9
Wilkie's 557.1
Wilkinson-Sneddon (subcorneal pustular dermatosis) 694.1
Willan-Plumbe (psoriasis) 696.1
Willebrand (-Jürgens) (angiohemophilia) 286.4
Willi-Prader (hypogenital dystrophy with diabetic tendency) 759.81
Wilson's (hepatolenticular degeneration) 275.1
Wilson-Mikity 770.7
Wiskott-Aldrich (eczema-thrombocytopenia) 279.12
withdrawal
    alcohol 291.81
    drug 292.0
        infant of dependent mother 779.5
Woakes' (ethmoiditis) 471.1
Wolff-Parkinson-White (anomalous atrioventricular excitation) 426.7
Wright's (hyperabduction) 447.8
X
    cardiac 413.9
    dysmetabolic 277.7
xiphoidalgia 733.99
XO 758.6
XXX 758.81
XXXXY 758.81
XXY 758.7
yellow vernix (placental dysfunction) 762.2
Zahorsky's 074.0
Zellweger 277.86
Zieve's (jaundice, hyperlipemia and hemolytic anemia) 571.1
Zollinger-Ellison (gastric hypersecretion with pancreatic islet cell tumor) 251.5
Zuelzer-Ogden (nutritional megaloblastic anemia) 281.2
Synechia (iris) (pupil) 364.70
    anterior 364.72
        peripheral 364.73
    intrauterine (traumatic) 621.5
    posterior 364.71
    vulvae, congenital 752.49
Synesthesia — *see also* Disturbance, sensation 782.0
Synodontia 520.2
Synophthalmus 759.89
Synorchidism 752.89
Synorchism 752.89
Synostosis (congenital) 756.59
    astragaloscaphoid 755.67
    radioulnar 755.53
    talonavicular (bar) 755.67
    tarsal 755.67
Synovial — *see* condition
Synovioma (M9040/3) — *see also* Neoplasm, connective tissue, malignant
    benign (M9040/0) — *see* Neoplasm, connective tissue, benign
Synoviosarcoma (M9040/3) — *see* Neoplasm, connective tissue, malignant

Synovitis (*see also* Tenosynovitis) 727.00
    chronic crepitant, wrist 727.2
    due to crystals — *see* Arthritis, due to crystals
    gonococcal 098.51
    gouty 274.00
    specified NEC 727.09
    syphilitic 095.7
        congenital 090.0
    traumatic, current — *see* Sprain, by site
    tuberculous — *see* Tuberculosis, synovitis
    villonodular 719.20
        ankle 719.27
        elbow 719.22
        foot 719.27
        hand 719.24
        hip 719.25
        knee 719.26
        multiple sites 719.29
        pelvic region 719.25
        shoulder (region) 719.21
        specified site NEC 719.28
        wrist 719.23
Syphilide 091.3
    congenital 090.0
    newborn 090.0
    tubercular 095.8
        congenital 090.0
Syphilis, syphilitic (acquired) 097.9
    with lung involvement 095.1
    abdomen (late) 095.2
    acoustic nerve 094.86
    adenopathy (secondary) 091.4
    adrenal (gland) 095.8
        with cortical hypofunction 095.8
    age under 2 years NEC (*see also* Syphilis, congenital) 090.9
        acquired 097.9
    alopecia (secondary) 091.82
    anemia 095.8
    aneurysm (artery) (ruptured) 093.89
        aorta 093.0
        central nervous system 094.89
        congenital 090.5
    anus 095.8
        primary 091.1
        secondary 091.3
    aorta, aortic (arch) (abdominal) (insufficiency) (pulmonary) (regurgitation) (stenosis) (thoracic) 093.89
        aneurysm 093.0
    arachnoid (adhesive) 094.2
    artery 093.89
        cerebral 094.89
        spinal 094.89
    arthropathy (neurogenic) (tabetic) 094.0 *[713.5]*
    asymptomatic — *see* Syphilis, latent
    ataxia, locomotor (progressive) 094.0
    atrophoderma maculatum 091.3
    auricular fibrillation 093.89
    Bell's palsy 094.89
    bladder 095.8
    bone 095.5
        secondary 091.61
    brain 094.89
    breast 095.8
    bronchus 095.8
    bubo 091.0
    bulbar palsy 094.89
    bursa (late) 095.7
    cardiac decompensation 093.89
    cardiovascular (early) (late) (primary) (secondary) (tertiary) 093.89
        specified type and site NEC 093.89
    causing death under 2 years of age (*see also* Syphilis, congenital) 090.9
        stated to be acquired NEC 097.9
    central nervous system (any site) (early) (late) (latent) (primary) (recurrent) (relapse) (secondary) (tertiary) 094.9
        with
            ataxia 094.0
            paralysis, general 094.1
                juvenile 090.40
            paresis (general) 094.1

Syphilis, syphilitic — *continued*
    central nervous system — *continued*
        with — *continued*
            paresis — *continued*
                juvenile 090.40
                tabes (dorsalis) 094.0
                    juvenile 090.40
                taboparesis 094.1
                    juvenile 090.40
            aneurysm (ruptured) 094.87
                congenital 090.40
                juvenile 090.40
            remission in (sustained) 094.9
            serology doubtful, negative, or positive 094.9
            specified nature or site NEC 094.89
            vascular 094.89
        cerebral 094.89
            meningovascular 094.2
            nerves 094.89
            sclerosis 094.89
            thrombosis 094.89
        cerebrospinal 094.89
            tabetic 094.0
        cerebrovascular 094.89
    cervix 095.8
    chancre (multiple) 091.0
        extragenital 091.2
        Rollet's 091.2
    Charcôt's joint 094.0 *[713.5]*
    choked disc 094.89 *[377.00]*
    chorioretinitis 091.51
        congenital 090.0 *[363.13]*
        late 094.83
    choroiditis 091.51
        congenital 090.0 *[363.13]*
        late 094.83
        prenatal 090.0 *[363.13]*
    choroidoretinitis (secondary) 091.51
        congenital 090.0 *[363.13]*
        late 094.83
    ciliary body (secondary) 091.52
        late 095.8 *[364.11]*
    colon (late) 095.8
    combined sclerosis 094.89
    complicating pregnancy, childbirth or puerperium 647.0 ☑
        affecting fetus or newborn 760.2
    condyloma (latum) 091.3
    congenital 090.9
        with
            encephalitis 090.41
            paresis (general) 090.40
            tabes (dorsalis) 090.40
            taboparesis 090.40
        chorioretinitis, choroiditis 090.0 *[363.13]*
        early or less than 2 years after birth NEC 090.2
            with manifestations 090.0
            latent (without manifestations) 090.1
                negative spinal fluid test 090.1
                serology, positive 090.1
            symptomatic 090.0
            interstitial keratitis 090.3
            juvenile neurosyphilis 090.40
        late or 2 years or more after birth NEC 090.7
            chorioretinitis, choroiditis 090.5 *[363.13]*
            interstitial keratitis 090.3
            juvenile neurosyphilis NEC 090.40
            latent (without manifestations) 090.6
                negative spinal fluid test 090.6
                serology, positive 090.6
            symptomatic or with manifestations NEC 090.5
                interstitial keratitis 090.3
        conjugal 097.9
            tabes 094.0
        conjunctiva 095.8 *[372.10]*
        contact V01.6
        cord, bladder 094.0
        cornea, late 095.8 *[370.59]*
        coronary (artery) 093.89
            sclerosis 093.89
        coryza 095.8

☑ **Additional Digit Required — Refer to the Tabular List for Digit Selection**   ▽ **Subterms under main terms may continue to next column or page**

2014 ICD-9-CM   **319**

Syphilis, syphilitic — *continued*
  coryza — *continued*
    congenital 090.0
  cranial nerve 094.89
  cutaneous — *see* Syphilis, skin
  dacryocystitis 095.8
  degeneration, spinal cord 094.89
  d'emblée 095.8
  dementia 094.1
    paralytica 094.1
      juvenilis 090.40
  destruction of bone 095.5
  dilatation, aorta 093.0
  due to blood transfusion 097.9
  dura mater 094.89
  ear 095.8
    inner 095.8
      nerve (eighth) 094.86
      neurorecurrence 094.86
  early NEC 091.0
    cardiovascular 093.9
    central nervous system 094.9
      paresis 094.1
      tabes 094.0
    latent (without manifestations) (less
      than 2 years after infection) 092.9
    negative spinal fluid test 092.9
    serological relapse following treat-
      ment 092.0
    serology positive 092.9
    paresis 094.1
    relapse (treated, untreated) 091.7
    skin 091.3
    symptomatic NEC 091.89
      extragenital chancre 091.2
      primary, except extragenital chancre
        091.0
      secondary (*see also* Syphilis, sec-
        ondary) 091.3
        relapse (treated, untreated) 091.7
    tabes 094.0
    ulcer 091.3
  eighth nerve 094.86
  endemic, nonvenereal 104.0
  endocarditis 093.20
    aortic 093.22
    mitral 093.21
    pulmonary 093.24
    tricuspid 093.23
  epididymis (late) 095.8
  epiglottis 095.8
  epiphysitis (congenital) 090.0
  esophagus 095.8
  Eustachian tube 095.8
  exposure to V01.6
  eye 095.8 *[363.13]*
    neuromuscular mechanism 094.85
  eyelid 095.8 *[373.5]*
    with gumma 095.8 *[373.5]*
    ptosis 094.89
  fallopian tube 095.8
  fracture 095.5
  gallbladder (late) 095.8
  gastric 095.8
    crisis 094.0
    polyposis 095.8
  general 097.9
    paralysis 094.1
      juvenile 090.40
  genital (primary) 091.0
  glaucoma 095.8
  gumma (late) NEC 095.9
    cardiovascular system 093.9
    central nervous system 094.9
    congenital 090.5
    heart or artery 093.89
  heart 093.89
    block 093.89
    decompensation 093.89
    disease 093.89
    failure 093.89
    valve (*see also* Syphilis, endocarditis)
      093.20
  hemianesthesia 094.89
  hemianopsia 095.8
  hemiparesis 094.89

Syphilis, syphilitic — *continued*
  hemiplegia 094.89
  hepatic artery 093.89
  hepatitis 095.3
  hepatomegaly 095.3
    congenital 090.0
  hereditaria tarda (*see also* Syphilis, congeni-
    tal, late) 090.7
  hereditary (*see also* Syphilis, congenital)
    090.9
    interstitial keratitis 090.3
  Hutchinson's teeth 090.5
  hyalitis 095.8
  inactive — *see* Syphilis, latent
  infantum NEC (*see also* Syphilis, congenital)
    090.9
  inherited — *see* Syphilis, congenital
  internal ear 095.8
  intestine (late) 095.8
  iris, iritis (secondary) 091.52
    late 095.8 *[364.11]*
  joint (late) 095.8
  keratitis (congenital) (early) (interstitial)
    (late) (parenchymatous) (punctata
    profunda) 090.3
  kidney 095.4
  lacrimal apparatus 095.8
  laryngeal paralysis 095.8
  larynx 095.8
  late 097.0
    cardiovascular 093.9
    central nervous system 094.9
    latent or 2 years or more after infection
      (without manifestations) 096
      negative spinal fluid test 096
      serology positive 096
    paresis 094.1
    specified site NEC 095.8
    symptomatic or with symptoms 095.9
    tabes 094.0
  latent 097.1
    central nervous system 094.9
    date of infection unspecified 097.1
    early or less than 2 years after infection
      092.9
    late or 2 years or more after infection 096
    serology
      doubtful
        follow-up of latent syphilis 097.1
        central nervous system 094.9
        date of infection unspecified
          097.1
        early or less than 2 years after
          infection 092.9
        late or 2 years or more after
          infection 096
      positive, only finding 097.1
        date of infection unspecified
          097.1
        early or less than 2 years after in-
          fection 097.1
        late or 2 years or more after infec-
          tion 097.1
  lens 095.8
  leukoderma 091.3
    late 095.8
  lienis 095.8
  lip 091.3
    chancre 091.2
    late 095.8
    primary 091.2
  Lissauer's paralysis 094.1
  liver 095.3
    secondary 091.62
  locomotor ataxia 094.0
  lung 095.1
  lymphadenitis (secondary) 091.4
  lymph gland (early) (secondary) 091.4
    late 095.8
  macular atrophy of skin 091.3
    striated 095.8
  maternal, affecting fetus or newborn 760.2
    manifest syphilis in newborn — *see*
      Syphilis, congenital
  mediastinum (late) 095.8

Syphilis, syphilitic — *continued*
  meninges (adhesive) (basilar) (brain) (spinal
    cord) 094.2
  meningitis 094.2
    acute 091.81
    congenital 090.42
  meningoencephalitis 094.2
  meningovascular 094.2
    congenital 090.49
  mesarteritis 093.89
    brain 094.89
    spine 094.89
  middle ear 095.8
  mitral stenosis 093.21
  monoplegia 094.89
  mouth (secondary) 091.3
    late 095.8
  mucocutaneous 091.3
    late 095.8
  mucous
    membrane 091.3
      late 095.8
    patches 091.3
      congenital 090.0
  mulberry molars 090.5
  muscle 095.6
  myocardium 093.82
  myositis 095.6
  nasal sinus 095.8
  neonatorum NEC (*see also* Syphilis, congen-
    ital) 090.9
  nerve palsy (any cranial nerve) 094.89
  nervous system, central 094.9
  neuritis 095.8
    acoustic nerve 094.86
  neurorecidive of retina 094.83
  neuroretinitis 094.83
  newborn (*see also* Syphilis, congenital) 090.9
  nodular superficial 095.8
  nonvenereal, endemic 104.0
  nose 095.8
    saddle back deformity 090.5
    septum 095.8
      perforated 095.8
  occlusive arterial disease 093.89
  ophthalmic 095.8 *[363.13]*
  ophthalmoplegia 094.89
  optic nerve (atrophy) (neuritis) (papilla)
    094.84
  orbit (late) 095.8
  orchitis 095.8
  organic 097.9
  osseous (late) 095.5
  osteochondritis (congenital) 090.0
  osteoporosis 095.5
  ovary 095.8
  oviduct 095.8
  palate 095.8
    gumma 095.8
    perforated 090.5
  pancreas (late) 095.8
  pancreatitis 095.8
  paralysis 094.89
    general 094.1
    juvenile 090.40
  paraplegia 094.89
  paresis (general) 094.1
    juvenile 090.40
  paresthesia 094.89
  Parkinson's disease or syndrome 094.82
  paroxysmal tachycardia 093.89
  pemphigus (congenital) 090.0
  penis 091.0
    chancre 091.0
    late 095.8
  pericardium 093.81
  perichondritis, larynx 095.8
  periosteum 095.5
    congenital 090.0
    early 091.61
    secondary 091.61
  peripheral nerve 095.8
  petrous bone (late) 095.5
  pharynx 095.8
    secondary 091.3
  pituitary (gland) 095.8

Syphilis, syphilitic — *continued*
  placenta 095.8
  pleura (late) 095.8
  pneumonia, white 090.0
  pontine (lesion) 094.89
  portal vein 093.89
  primary NEC 091.2
    anal 091.1
    and secondary (*see also* Syphilis, sec-
      ondary) 091.9
    cardiovascular 093.9
    central nervous system 094.9
    extragenital chancre NEC 091.2
    fingers 091.2
    genital 091.0
    lip 091.2
    specified site NEC 091.2
    tonsils 091.2
  prostate 095.8
  psychosis (intracranial gumma) 094.89
  ptosis (eyelid) 094.89
  pulmonary (late) 095.1
    artery 093.89
  pulmonum 095.1
  pyelonephritis 095.4
  recently acquired, symptomatic NEC 091.89
  rectum 095.8
  respiratory tract 095.8
  retina
    late 094.83
    neurorecidive 094.83
  retrobulbar neuritis 094.85
  salpingitis 095.8
  sclera (late) 095.0
  sclerosis
    cerebral 094.89
    coronary 093.89
    multiple 094.89
    subacute 094.89
  scotoma (central) 095.8
  scrotum 095.8
  secondary (and primary) 091.9
    adenopathy 091.4
    anus 091.3
    bone 091.61
    cardiovascular 093.9
    central nervous system 094.9
    chorioretinitis, choroiditis 091.51
    hepatitis 091.62
    liver 091.62
    lymphadenitis 091.4
    meningitis, acute 091.81
    mouth 091.3
    mucous membranes 091.3
    periosteum 091.61
    periostitis 091.61
    pharynx 091.3
    relapse (treated) (untreated) 091.7
    skin 091.3
    specified form NEC 091.89
    tonsil 091.3
    ulcer 091.3
    viscera 091.69
    vulva 091.3
  seminal vesicle (late) 095.8
  seronegative
    with signs or symptoms — *see* Syphilis,
      by site or stage
  seropositive
    with signs or symptoms — *see* Syphilis,
      by site and stage
    follow-up of latent syphilis — *see*
      Syphilis, latent
    only finding — *see* Syphilis, latent
  seventh nerve (paralysis) 094.89
  sinus 095.8
  sinusitis 095.8
  skeletal system 095.5
  skin (early) (secondary) (with ulceration)
    091.3
    late or tertiary 095.8
  small intestine 095.8
  spastic spinal paralysis 094.0
  spermatic cord (late) 095.8
  spinal (cord) 094.89

☑ **Additional Digit Required** — **Refer to the Tabular List for Digit Selection**

▽ **Subterms under main terms may continue to next column or page**

Syphilis, syphilitic — *continued*
  spinal — *continued*
    with
      paresis 094.1
      tabes 094.0
  spleen 095.8
  splenomegaly 095.8
  spondylitis 095.5
  staphyloma 095.8
  stigmata (congenital) 090.5
  stomach 095.8
  synovium (late) 095.7
  tabes dorsalis (early) (late) 094.0
    juvenile 090.40
  tabetic type 094.0
    juvenile 090.40
  taboparesis 094.1
    juvenile 090.40
  tachycardia 093.89
  tendon (late) 095.7
  tertiary 097.0
    with symptoms 095.8
    cardiovascular 093.9
    central nervous system 094.9
    multiple NEC 095.8
    specified site NEC 095.8
  testis 095.8
  thorax 095.8
  throat 095.8
  thymus (gland) 095.8
  thyroid (late) 095.8
  tongue 095.8
  tonsil (lingual) 095.8
    primary 091.2
    secondary 091.3
  trachea 095.8
  tricuspid valve 093.23
  tumor, brain 094.89
  tunica vaginalis (late) 095.8
  ulcer (any site) (early) (secondary) 091.3
    late 095.9
    perforating 095.9
      foot 094.0
  urethra (stricture) 095.8
  urogenital 095.8
  uterus 095.8
  uveal tract (secondary) 091.50
    late 095.8 *[363.13]*
  uveitis (secondary) 091.50
    late 095.8 *[363.13]*
  uvula (late) 095.8
    perforated 095.8
  vagina 091.0
    late 095.8
  valvulitis NEC 093.20
  vascular 093.89
    brain or cerebral 094.89
  vein 093.89
    cerebral 094.89
  ventriculi 095.8
  vesicae urinariae 095.8
  viscera (abdominal) 095.2
    secondary 091.69
  vitreous (hemorrhage) (opacities) 095.8
  vulva 091.0
    late 095.8
    secondary 091.3
Syphiloma 095.9
  cardiovascular system 093.9
  central nervous system 094.9
  circulatory system 093.9
  congenital 090.5
Syphilophobia 300.29
Syringadenoma (M8400/0) — *see also* Neoplasm, skin, benign
  papillary (M8406/0) — *see* Neoplasm, skin, benign
Syringobulbia 336.0
Syringocarcinoma (M8400/3) — *see* Neoplasm, skin, malignant
Syringocystadenoma (M8400/0) — *see also* Neoplasm, skin, benign
  papillary (M8406/0) — *see* Neoplasm, skin, benign
Syringocystoma (M8407/0) — *see* Neoplasm, skin, benign

Syringoma (M8407/0) — *see also* Neoplasm, skin, benign
  chondroid (M8940/0) — *see* Neoplasm, by site, benign
Syringomyelia 336.0
Syringomyelitis 323.9
  late effect — *see* category 326
Syringomyelocele — *see also* Spina bifida 741.9 ☑
Syringopontia 336.0
System, systemic — *see also* condition
  disease, combined — *see* Degeneration, combined
  fibrosclerosing syndrome 710.8
  inflammatory response syndrome (SIRS) 995.90
    due to
      infectious process 995.91
        with acute organ dysfunction 995.92
      non-infectious process 995.93
        with acute organ dysfunction 995.94
  lupus erythematosus 710.0
    inhibitor 795.79

T

Tab — *see* Tag
Tabacism 989.84
Tabacosis 989.84
Tabardillo 080
  flea-borne 081.0
  louse-borne 080
Tabes, tabetic
  with
    central nervous system syphilis 094.0
    Charcôt's joint 094.0 *[713.5]*
    cord bladder 094.0
    crisis, viscera (any) 094.0
    paralysis, general 094.1
    paresis (general) 094.1
    perforating ulcer 094.0
  arthropathy 094.0 *[713.5]*
  bladder 094.0
  bone 094.0
  cerebrospinal 094.0
  congenital 090.40
  conjugal 094.0
  dorsalis 094.0
    neurosyphilis 094.0
  early 094.0
  juvenile 090.40
  latent 094.0
  mesenterica (*see also* Tuberculosis) 014.8 ☑
  paralysis insane, general 094.1
  peripheral (nonsyphilitic) 799.89
  spasmodic 094.0
    not dorsal or dorsalis 343.9
  syphilis (cerebrospinal) 094.0
Taboparalysis 094.1
Taboparesis (remission) 094.1
  with
    Charcôt's joint 094.1 *[713.5]*
    cord bladder 094.1
    perforating ulcer 094.1
  juvenile 090.40
Tache noir 923.20
Tachyalimentation 579.3
Tachyarrhythmia, tachyrhythmia — *see also* Tachycardia
  paroxysmal with sinus bradycardia 427.81
Tachycardia 785.0
  atrial 427.89
  auricular 427.89
  AV nodal re-entry (re-entrant) 427.89
  junctional ectopic 427.0
  newborn 779.82
  nodal 427.89
    nonparoxysmal atrioventricular 426.89
  nonparoxysmal atrioventricular (nodal) 426.89
  nonsustained 427.2
  paroxysmal 427.2
    with sinus bradycardia 427.81
    atrial (PAT) 427.0
      psychogenic 316 *[427.0]*

Tachycardia — *continued*
  paroxysmal — *continued*
    atrioventricular (AV) 427.0
      psychogenic 316 *[427.0]*
    essential 427.2
    junctional 427.0
    nodal 427.0
    psychogenic 316 *[427.2]*
      atrial 316 *[427.0]*
      supraventricular 316 *[427.0]*
      ventricular 316 *[427.1]*
    supraventricular 427.0
      psychogenic 316 *[427.0]*
    ventricular 427.1
      psychogenic 316 *[427.1]*
  postoperative 997.1
  psychogenic 306.2
  sick sinus 427.81
  sinoauricular 427.89
  sinus 427.89
  supraventricular 427.89
  sustained 427.2
    supraventricular 427.0
    ventricular 427.1
  ventricular (paroxysmal) 427.1
    psychogenic 316 *[427.1]*
Tachygastria 536.8
Tachypnea 786.06
  hysterical 300.11
  newborn (idiopathic) (transitory) 770.6
  psychogenic 306.1
  transitory, of newborn 770.6
TACO (transfusion associated circulatory overload) 276.61
Taenia (infection) (infestation) — *see also* Infestation, taenia 123.3
  diminuta 123.6
  echinococcal infestation (*see also* Echinococcus) 122.9
  nana 123.6
  saginata infestation 123.2
  solium (intestinal form) 123.0
    larval form 123.1
Taeniasis (intestine) — *see also* Infestation, taenia 123.3
  saginata 123.2
  solium 123.0
Taenzer's disease 757.4
Tag (hypertrophied skin) (infected) 701.9
  adenoid 474.8
  anus 455.9
  endocardial (*see also* Endocarditis) 424.90
  hemorrhoidal 455.9
  hymen 623.8
  perineal 624.8
  preauricular 744.1
  rectum 455.9
  sentinel 455.9
  skin 701.9
    accessory 757.39
    anus 455.9
    congenital 757.39
    preauricular 744.1
    rectum 455.9
  tonsil 474.8
  urethra, urethral 599.84
  vulva 624.8
Tahyna fever 062.5
Takayasu (-Onishi) disease or syndrome (pulseless disease) 446.7
Takotsubo syndrome 429.83
Talc granuloma 728.82
  in operation wound 998.7
Talcosis 502
Talipes (congenital) 754.70
  acquired NEC 736.79
    planus 734
  asymmetric 754.79
    acquired 736.79
  calcaneovalgus 754.62
    acquired 736.76
  calcaneovarus 754.59
    acquired 736.76
  calcaneus 754.79
    acquired 736.76
  cavovarus 754.59

Talipes — *continued*
  cavovarus — *continued*
    acquired 736.75
  cavus 754.71
    acquired 736.73
  equinovalgus 754.69
    acquired 736.72
  equinovarus 754.51
    acquired 736.71
  equinus 754.79
    acquired, NEC 736.72
  percavus 754.71
    acquired 736.73
  planovalgus 754.69
    acquired 736.79
  planus (acquired) (any degree) 734
    congenital 754.61
    due to rickets 268.1
  valgus 754.60
    acquired 736.79
  varus 754.50
    acquired 736.79
Talma's disease 728.85
Talon noir 924.20
  hand 923.20
  heel 924.20
  toe 924.3
Tamponade heart (Rose's) — *see also* Pericarditis 423.3
Tanapox 059.21
Tangier disease (familial high-density lipoprotein deficiency) 272.5
Tank ear 380.12
Tantrum (childhood) — *see also* Disturbance, conduct 312.1 ☑
Tapeworm (infection) (infestation) — *see also* Infestation, tapeworm 123.9
Tapia's syndrome 352.6
Tarantism 297.8
Target-oval cell anemia 285.8
  with thalassemia — *see* Thalassemia
Tarlov's cyst 355.9
Tarral-Besnier disease (pityriasis rubra pilaris) 696.4
Tarsalgia 729.2
Tarsal tunnel syndrome 355.5
Tarsitis (eyelid) 373.00
  syphilitic 095.8 *[373.00]*
  tuberculous (*see also* Tuberculosis) 017.0 ☑ *[373.4]*
Tartar (teeth) 523.6
Tattoo (mark) 709.09
Taurodontism 520.2
Taussig-Bing defect, heart, or syndrome (transposition, aorta and overriding pulmonary artery) 745.11
Taybi's syndrome (otopalatodigital) 759.89
Tay's choroiditis 363.41
Taylor's
  disease (diffuse idiopathic cutaneous atrophy) 701.8
  syndrome 625.5
Tay-Sachs
  amaurotic familial idiocy 330.1
  disease 330.1
TBI (traumatic brain injury) — *see also* Injury, intracranial 854.0 ☑
  with skull fracture — *see* Fracture, skull, by site
Tear stone 375.57
Tear, torn (traumatic) — *see also* Wound, open, by site
  annular fibrosis 722.51
  anus, anal (sphincter) 863.89
    with open wound in cavity 863.99
    complicating delivery (healed) (old) 654.8 ☑
      with mucosa 664.3 ☑
      not associated with third-degree perineal laceration 664.6 ☑
    nontraumatic, nonpuerperal (healed) (old) 569.43
  articular cartilage, old (*see also* Disorder, cartilage, articular) 718.0 ☑

☑ **Additional Digit Required** — Refer to the Tabular List for Digit Selection
🔻 **Subterms under main terms may continue to next column or page**
2014 ICD-9-CM
321

Index

Tear, torn — Teratoma

Tear, torn — *see also* Wound, open, by site — *continued*
  bladder
    with
      abortion — *see* Abortion, by type, with damage to pelvic organs
      ectopic pregnancy (*see also* categories 633.0–633.9) 639.2
      molar pregnancy (*see also* categories 630–632) 639.2
    following
      abortion 639.2
      ectopic or molar pregnancy 639.2
    obstetrical trauma 665.5 ☑
  bowel
    with
      abortion — *see* Abortion, by type, with damage to pelvic organs
      ectopic pregnancy (*see also* categories 633.0–633.9) 639.2
      molar pregnancy (*see also* categories 630–632) 639.2
    following
      abortion 639.2
      ectopic or molar pregnancy 639.2
    obstetrical trauma 665.5 ☑
  broad ligament
    with
      abortion — *see* Abortion, by type, with damage to pelvic organs
      ectopic pregnancy (*see also* categories 633.0–633.9) 639.2
      molar pregnancy (*see also* categories 630–632) 639.2
    following
      abortion 639.2
      ectopic or molar pregnancy 639.2
    obstetrical trauma 665.6 ☑
  bucket handle (knee) (meniscus) — *see* Tear, meniscus
  capsule
    joint — *see* Sprain, by site
    spleen — *see* Laceration, spleen, capsule
  cartilage (*see also* Sprain, by site)
    articular, old (*see also* Disorder, cartilage, articular) 718.0 ☑
    knee — *see* Tear, meniscus
    semilunar (knee) (current injury) — *see* Tear, meniscus
  cervix
    with
      abortion — *see* Abortion, by type, with damage to pelvic organs
      ectopic pregnancy (*see also* categories 633.0–633.9) 639.2
      molar pregnancy (*see also* categories 630–632) 639.2
    following
      abortion 639.2
      ectopic or molar pregnancy 639.2
    obstetrical trauma (current) 665.3 ☑
    old 622.3
  dural 349.31
    accidental puncture or laceration during a procedure 349.31
    incidental (inadvertent) 349.31
    nontraumatic NEC 349.39
  internal organ (abdomen, chest, or pelvis) — *see* Injury, internal, by site
  ligament (*see also* Sprain, by site)
    with open wound — *see* Wound, open by site
  meniscus (knee) (current injury) 836.2
    bucket handle 836.0
      old 717.0
    lateral 836.1
      anterior horn 836.1
        old 717.42
      bucket handle 836.1
        old 717.41
      old 717.40
      posterior horn 836.1
        old 717.43
      specified site NEC 836.1
        old 717.49
    medial 836.0

Tear, torn — *see also* Wound, open, by site — *continued*
  meniscus — *continued*
    medial — *continued*
      anterior horn 836.0
        old 717.1
      bucket handle 836.0
        old 717.0
      posterior horn 836.0
        old 717.2
    old NEC 717.5
    site other than knee — *see* Sprain, by site
  muscle (*see also* Sprain, by site)
    with open wound — *see* Wound, open by site
  pelvic
    floor, complicating delivery 664.1 ☑
    organ NEC
      with
        abortion — *see* Abortion, by type, with damage to pelvic organs
        ectopic pregnancy (*see also* categories 633.0–633.9) 639.2
        molar pregnancy (*see also* categories 630–632) 639.2
      following
        abortion 639.2
        ectopic or molar pregnancy 639.2
      obstetrical trauma 665.5 ☑
  perineum (*see also* Laceration, perineum)
    obstetrical trauma 665.5 ☑
  periurethral tissue
    with
      abortion — *see* Abortion, by type, with damage to pelvic organs
      ectopic pregnancy (*see also* categories 633.0–633.9) 639.2
      molar pregnancy (*see also* categories 630–632) 639.2
    following
      abortion 639.2
      ectopic or molar pregnancy 639.2
    obstetrical trauma 664.8 ☑
  rectovaginal septum — *see* Laceration, rectovaginal septum
  retina, retinal (recent) (with detachment) 361.00
    without detachment 361.30
    dialysis (juvenile) (with detachment) 361.04
    giant (with detachment) 361.03
    horseshoe (without detachment) 361.32
    multiple (with detachment) 361.02
      without detachment 361.33
    old
      delimited (partial) 361.06
      partial 361.06
      total or subtotal 361.07
    partial (without detachment)
      giant 361.03
      multiple defects 361.02
      old (delimited) 361.06
      single defect 361.01
    round hole (without detachment) 361.31
    single defect (with detachment) 361.01
    total or subtotal (recent) 361.05
      old 361.07
  rotator cuff (traumatic) 840.4
    current injury 840.4
    degenerative 726.10
    nontraumatic (complete) 727.61
    partial 726.13
  semilunar cartilage, knee (*see also* Tear, meniscus) 836.2
    old 717.5
  tendon (*see also* Sprain, by site)
    with open wound — *see* Wound, open by site
  tentorial, at birth 767.0
  umbilical cord
    affecting fetus or newborn 772.0
    complicating delivery 663.8 ☑

Tear, torn — *see also* Wound, open, by site — *continued*
  urethra
    with
      abortion — *see* Abortion, by type, with damage to pelvic organs
      ectopic pregnancy (*see also* categories 633.0–633.9) 639.2
      molar pregnancy (*see also* categories 630–632) 639.2
    following
      abortion 639.2
      ectopic or molar pregnancy 639.2
    obstetrical trauma 665.5 ☑
  uterus — *see* Injury, internal, uterus
  vagina — *see* Laceration, vagina
  vessel, from catheter 998.2
  vulva, complicating delivery 664.0 ☑
Teething 520.7
  syndrome 520.7
Teeth, tooth — *see also* condition
  grinding 306.8
  prenatal 520.6
Tegmental syndrome 344.89
Telangiectasia, telangiectasis (verrucous) 448.9
  ataxic (cerebellar) 334.8
  familial 448.0
  hemorrhagic, hereditary (congenital) (senile) 448.0
  hereditary hemorrhagic 448.0
  retina 362.15
  spider 448.1
Telecanthus (congenital) 743.63
Telescoped bowel or intestine — *see also* Intussusception 560.0
Teletherapy, adverse effect NEC 990
Telogen effluvium 704.02
Temperature
  body, high (of unknown origin) (*see also* Pyrexia) 780.60
  cold, trauma from 991.9
    newborn 778.2
    specified effect NEC 991.8
  high
    body (of unknown origin) (*see also* Pyrexia) 780.60
    trauma from — *see* Heat
Temper tantrum (childhood) — *see also* Disturbance, conduct 312.1 ☑
Temple — *see* condition
Temporal — *see also* condition
  lobe syndrome 310.0
Temporomandibular joint-pain-dysfunction syndrome 524.60
Temporosphenoidal — *see* condition
Tendency
  bleeding (*see also* Defect, coagulation) 286.9
  homosexual, ego-dystonic 302.0
  paranoid 301.0
  suicide 300.9
Tenderness
  abdominal (generalized) (localized) 789.6 ☑
  rebound 789.6 ☑
  skin 782.0
Tendinitis, tendonitis — *see also* Tenosynovitis 726.90
  Achilles 726.71
  adhesive 726.90
    shoulder 726.0
  calcific 727.82
    shoulder 726.11
  gluteal 726.5
  patellar 726.64
  peroneal 726.79
  pes anserinus 726.61
  psoas 726.5
  tibialis (anterior) (posterior) 726.72
  trochanteric 726.5
Tendon — *see* condition
Tendosynovitis — *see* Tenosynovitis
Tendovaginitis — *see* Tenosynovitis
Tenesmus 787.99
  rectal 787.99
  vesical 788.99
Tenia — *see* Taenia

Teniasis — *see* Taeniasis
Tennis elbow 726.32
Tenonitis — *see also* Tenosynovitis
  eye (capsule) 376.04
Tenontosynovitis — *see* Tenosynovitis
Tenontothecitis — *see* Tenosynovitis
Tenophyte 727.9
Tenosynovitis (*see also* Synovitis) 727.00
  adhesive 726.90
    shoulder 726.0
  ankle 727.06
  bicipital (calcifying) 726.12
  buttock 727.09
  due to crystals — *see* Arthritis, due to crystals
  elbow 727.09
  finger 727.05
  foot 727.06
  gonococcal 098.51
  hand 727.05
  hip 727.09
  knee 727.09
  radial styloid 727.04
  shoulder 726.10
    adhesive 726.0
  specified NEC 727.09
  spine 720.1
  supraspinatus 726.10
  toe 727.06
  tuberculous — *see* Tuberculosis, tenosynovitis
  wrist 727.05
Tenovaginitis — *see* Tenosynovitis
Tension
  arterial, high (*see also* Hypertension) 401.9
    without diagnosis of hypertension 796.2
  headache 307.81
  intraocular (elevated) 365.00
  nervous 799.21
  ocular (elevated) 365.00
  pneumothorax 512.0
    iatrogenic 512.1
    postoperative 512.1
    spontaneous 512.0
  premenstrual 625.4
  state 300.9
Tentorium — *see* condition
Teratencephalus 759.89
Teratism 759.7
Teratoblastoma (malignant) (M9080/3) — *see* Neoplasm, by site, malignant
Teratocarcinoma (M9081/3) — *see also* Neoplasm, by site, malignant
  liver 155.0
Teratoma (solid) (M9080/1) — *see also* Neoplasm, by site, uncertain behavior
  adult (cystic) (M9080/0) — *see* Neoplasm, by site, benign
  and embryonal carcinoma, mixed (M9081/3) — *see* Neoplasm, by site, malignant
  benign (M9080/0) — *see* Neoplasm, by site, benign
  combined with choriocarcinoma (M9101/3) — *see* Neoplasm, by site, malignant
  cystic (adult) (M9080/0) — *see* Neoplasm, by site, benign
  differentiated type (M9080/0) — *see* Neoplasm, by site, benign
  embryonal (M9080/3) (*see also* Neoplasm, by site, malignant)
    liver 155.0
  fetal
    sacral, causing fetopelvic disproportion 653.7 ☑
  immature (M9080/3) — *see* Neoplasm, by site, malignant
  liver (M9080/3) 155.0
    adult, benign, cystic, differentiated type or mature (M9080/0) 211.5
  malignant (M9080/3) (*see also* Neoplasm, by site, malignant)
    anaplastic type (M9082/3) — *see* Neoplasm, by site, malignant
    intermediate type (M9083/3) — *see* Neoplasm, by site, malignant
    liver (M9080/3) 155.0

☑ Additional Digit Required — Refer to the Tabular List for Digit Selection
▼ Subterms under main terms may continue to next column or page
322
2014 ICD-9-CM

Teratoma — *see also* Neoplasm, by site, uncertain behavior — *continued*
  malignant (*see also* Neoplasm, by site, malignant) — *continued*
    trophoblastic (M9102/3)
      specified site — *see* Neoplasm, by site, malignant
      unspecified site 186.9
    undifferentiated type (M9082/3) — *see* Neoplasm, by site, malignant
    mature (M9080/0) — *see* Neoplasm, by site, benign
      malignant (M9080/3) — *see* Neoplasm, by site, malignant
    ovary (M9080/0) 220
      embryonal, immature, or malignant (M9080/3) 183.0
    suprasellar (M9080/3) — *see* Neoplasm, by site, malignant
    testis (M9080/3) 186.9
      adult, benign, cystic, differentiated type or mature (M9080/0) 222.0
      undescended 186.0
Terminal care V66.7
Termination
  anomalous (*see also* Malposition, congenital)
    portal vein 747.49
    right pulmonary vein 747.42
  pregnancy (legal) (therapeutic) — *see* Abortion, legal 635.9 ☑
    fetus NEC 779.6
    illegal (*see also* Abortion, illegal) 636.9 ☑
Ternidens diminutus infestation 127.7
Terrors, night (child) 307.46
Terry's syndrome (*see also* Retinopathy of prematurity) 362.21
Tertiary — *see* condition
Tessellated fundus, retina (tigroid) 362.89
Test(s)
  adequacy
    hemodialysis V56.31
    peritoneal dialysis V56.32
  AIDS virus V72.69
  allergen V72.7
  bacterial disease NEC (*see also* Screening, by name of disease) V74.9
  basal metabolic rate V72.69
  blood
    alcohol V70.4
    drug V70.4
      for therapeutic drug monitoring V58.83
      for routine general physical examination V72.62
      prior to treatment or procedure V72.63
      typing V72.86
        Rh typing V72.86
  developmental, infant or child V20.2
  Dick V74.8
  fertility V26.21
  genetic
    female V26.32
    for genetic disease carrier status
      female V26.31
      male V26.34
    male V26.39
  hearing V72.19
    following failed hearing screening V72.11
    routine, for infant and child V20.2
  HIV V72.69
  human immunodeficiency virus V72.69
  immunity status V72.61
  Kveim V82.89
  laboratory V72.60
    for medicolegal reason V70.4
    ordered as part of a routine general medical examination V72.62
    pre-operative V72.63
    pre-procedural V72.63
    specified NEC V72.69
  male partner of female with recurrent pregnancy loss V26.35
  Mantoux (for tuberculosis) V74.1

Test(s) — *continued*
  mycotic organism V75.4
  nuchal translucency V28.89
  parasitic agent NEC V75.8
  paternity V70.4
  peritoneal equilibration V56.32
  pregnancy
    negative result V72.41
    positive result V72.42
      first pregnancy V72.42
    unconfirmed V72.40
  preoperative V72.84
    cardiovascular V72.81
    respiratory V72.82
    specified NEC V72.83
  procreative management NEC V26.29
    genetic disease carrier status
      female V26.31
      male V26.34
  Rh typing V72.86
  sarcoidosis V82.89
  Schick V74.3
  Schultz-Charlton V74.8
  skin, diagnostic
    allergy V72.7
    bacterial agent NEC (*see also* Screening, by name of disease) V74.9
    Dick V74.8
    hypersensitivity V72.7
    Kveim V82.89
    Mantoux V74.1
    mycotic organism V75.4
    parasitic agent NEC V75.8
    sarcoidosis V82.89
    Schick V74.3
    Schultz-Charlton V74.8
    tuberculin V74.1
  specified type NEC V72.85
  tuberculin V74.1
  vision V72.0
    routine, for infant and child V20.2
  Wassermann
    positive (*see also* Serology for syphilis, positive) 097.1
    false 795.6
Testicle, testicular, testis — *see also* condition
  feminization (syndrome) 259.51
Tetanus, tetanic (cephalic) (convulsions) 037
  with
    abortion — *see* Abortion, by type, with sepsis
    ectopic pregnancy (*see also* categories 633.0–633.9) 639.0
    molar pregnancy (*see also* categories 630–632 639.0
  following
    abortion 639.0
    ectopic or molar pregnancy 639.0
  inoculation V03.7
    reaction (due to serum) — *see* Complications, vaccination
  neonatorum 771.3
  puerperal, postpartum, childbirth 670.8 ☑
Tetany, tetanic 781.7
  alkalosis 276.3
  associated with rickets 268.0
  convulsions 781.7
    hysterical 300.11
  functional (hysterical) 300.11
  hyperkinetic 781.7
    hysterical 300.11
  hyperpnea 786.01
    hysterical 300.11
    psychogenic 306.1
  hyperventilation 786.01
    hysterical 300.11
    psychogenic 306.1
  hypocalcemic, neonatal 775.4
  hysterical 300.11
  neonatal 775.4
  parathyroid (gland) 252.1
  parathyroprival 252.1
  postoperative 252.1
  postthyroidectomy 252.1
  pseudotetany 781.7
    hysterical 300.11

Tetany, tetanic — *continued*
  psychogenic 306.1
    specified as conversion reaction 300.11
Tetralogy of Fallot 745.2
Tetraplegia — *see* Quadriplegia
Thailand hemorrhagic fever 065.4
Thalassanemia 282.40
Thalassemia (disease) 282.40
  with other hemoglobinopathy 282.49
  alpha (major) (severe) (triple gene defect) 282.43
    silent carrier 282.46
  beta (homozygous) (major) (severe) 282.44
  delta-beta (homozygous) 282.45
  dominant 282.49
  Hb-S (without crisis) 282.41
    with
      crisis 282.42
      vaso-occlusive pain 282.42
  hemoglobin
    C (Hb-C) 282.49
    D (Hb-D) 282.49
    E (Hb-E) 282.49
    E-beta 282.47
    H (Hb-H) 282.49
    I (Hb-I) 282.49
  high fetal gene (*see also* Thalassemia) 282.40
  high fetal hemoglobin (*see also* Thalassemia) 282.40
  intermedia 282.44
  major 282.44
  minor (alpha) (beta) 282.46
  mixed 282.49
  sickle-cell (without crisis) 282.41
    with
      crisis 282.42
      vaso-occlusive pain 282.42
  specified NEC 282.49
  trait (alpha) (beta) (delta-beta) 282.46
Thalassemic variants 282.49
Thaysen-Gee disease (nontropical sprue) 579.0
Thecoma (M8600/0) 220
  malignant (M8600/3) 183.0
Thelarche, precocious 259.1
Thelitis 611.0
  puerperal, postpartum 675.0 ☑
Therapeutic — *see* condition
Therapy V57.9
  blood transfusion, without reported diagnosis V58.2
  breathing V57.0
  chemotherapy, antineoplastic V58.11
    fluoride V07.31
    prophylactic NEC V07.39
  dialysis (intermittent) (treatment)
    extracorporeal V56.0
    peritoneal V56.8
    renal V56.0
    specified type NEC V56.8
  exercise NEC V57.1
    breathing V57.0
  extracorporeal dialysis (renal) V56.0
  fluoride prophylaxis V07.31
  hemodialysis V56.0
  hormone replacement (postmenopausal) V07.4
  immunotherapy antineoplastic V58.12
  long term oxygen therapy V46.2
  occupational V57.21
  orthoptic V57.4
  orthotic V57.81
  peritoneal dialysis V56.8
  physical NEC V57.1
  postmenopausal hormone replacement V07.4
  radiation V58.0
  speech (-language) V57.3
  vocational V57.22
Thermalgesia 782.0
Thermalgia 782.0
Thermanalgesia 782.0
Thermanesthesia 782.0
Thermic — *see* condition
Thermography (abnormal) 793.99
  breast 793.89

Thermoplegia 992.0
Thesaurismosis
  amyloid 277.39
  bilirubin 277.4
  calcium 275.40
  cystine 270.0
  glycogen (*see also* Disease, glycogen storage) 271.0
  kerasin 272.7
  lipoid 272.7
  melanin 255.41
  phosphatide 272.7
  urate 274.9
Thiaminic deficiency 265.1
  with beriberi 265.0
Thibierge-Weissenbach syndrome (cutaneous systemic sclerosis) 710.1
Thickened endometrium 793.5
Thickening
  bone 733.99
    extremity 733.99
  breast 611.79
  hymen 623.3
  larynx 478.79
  nail 703.8
    congenital 757.5
  periosteal 733.99
  pleura (*see also* Pleurisy) 511.0
  skin 782.8
  subepiglottic 478.79
  tongue 529.8
  valve, heart — *see* Endocarditis
Thiele syndrome 724.6
Thigh — *see* condition
Thinning vertebra — *see also* Osteoporosis 733.00
Thirst, excessive 783.5
  due to deprivation of water 994.3
Thomsen's disease 359.22
Thomson's disease (congenital poikiloderma) 757.33
Thoracic — *see also* condition
  kidney 753.3
  outlet syndrome 353.0
  stomach — *see* Hernia, diaphragm
Thoracogastroschisis (congenital) 759.89
Thoracopagus 759.4
Thoracoschisis 756.3
Thoracoscopic surgical procedure converted to open procedure V64.42
Thorax — *see* condition
Thorn's syndrome — *see also* Disease, renal 593.9
Thornwaldt's, Tornwaldt's
  bursitis (pharyngeal) 478.29
  cyst 478.26
  disease (pharyngeal bursitis) 478.29
Thorson-Biörck syndrome (malignant carcinoid) 259.2
Threadworm (infection) (infestation) 127.4
Threatened
  abortion or miscarriage 640.0 ☑
    with subsequent abortion (*see also* Abortion, spontaneous) 634.9 ☑
    affecting fetus 762.1
  labor 644.1 ☑
    affecting fetus or newborn 761.8
    premature 644.0 ☑
  miscarriage 640.0 ☑
    affecting fetus 762.1
  premature
    delivery 644.2 ☑
      affecting fetus or newborn 761.8
    labor 644.0 ☑
      before 22 completed weeks gestation 640.0 ☑
Three-day fever 066.0
Threshers' lung 495.0
Thrix annulata (congenital) 757.4
Throat — *see* condition
Thrombasthenia (Glanzmann's) (hemorrhagic) (hereditary) 287.1
Thromboangiitis 443.1
  obliterans (general) 443.1
    cerebral 437.1

☑ Additional Digit Required — Refer to the Tabular List for Digit Selection   ▽ Subterms under main terms may continue to next column or page

2014 ICD-9-CM   323

Teratoma — Thromboangiitis

Thromboangiitis — *continued*
  obliterans — *continued*
    vessels
      brain 437.1
      spinal cord 437.1
Thromboarteritis — *see* Arteritis
Thromboasthenia (Glanzmann's) (hemorrhagic) (hereditary) 287.1
Thrombocytasthenia (Glanzmann's) 287.1
Thrombocythemia (primary) (M9962/1) 238.71
  essential 238.71
  hemorrhagic 238.71
  idiopathic (hemorrhagic) (M9962/1) 238.71
Thrombocytopathy (dystrophic) (granulopenic) 287.1
Thrombocytopenia, thrombocytopenic 287.5
  with
    absent radii (TAR) syndrome 287.33
    giant hemangioma 287.39
  amegakaryocytic, congenital 287.33
  congenital 287.33
  cyclic 287.39
  dilutional 287.49
  due to
    drugs 287.49
    extracorporeal circulation of blood 287.49
    massive blood transfusion 287.49
    platelet alloimmunization 287.49
  essential 287.30
  fetal 678.0 ☑
  heparin-induced (HIT) 289.84
  hereditary 287.3
  Kasabach-Merritt 287.39
  neonatal, transitory 776.1
    due to
      exchange transfusion 776.1
      idiopathic maternal thrombocytopenia 776.1
      isoimmunization 776.1
  primary 287.30
  puerperal, postpartum 666.3 ☑
  purpura (*see also* Purpura, thrombocytopenic) 287.30
    thrombotic 446.6
  secondary NEC 287.49
  sex-linked 287.39
Thrombocytosis 238.71
  essential 238.71
  primary 238.71
Thromboembolism — *see* Embolism
Thrombopathy (Bernard-Soulier) 287.1
  constitutional 286.4
  Willebrand-Jürgens (angiohemophilia) 286.4
Thrombopenia — *see also* Thrombocytopenia 287.5
Thrombophlebitis 451.9
  antecubital vein 451.82
  antepartum (superficial) 671.2 ☑
    affecting fetus or newborn 760.3
    deep 671.3 ☑
  arm 451.89
    deep 451.83
    superficial 451.82
  breast, superficial 451.89
  cavernous (venous) sinus — *see* Thrombophlebitis, intracranial venous sinus
  cephalic vein 451.82
  cerebral (sinus) (vein) 325
    late effect — *see* category 326
    nonpyogenic 437.6
      in pregnancy or puerperium 671.5 ☑
      late effect — *see* Late effect(s) (of) cerebrovascular disease
  due to implanted device — *see* Complications, due to (presence of) any device, implant or graft classified to 996.0–996.5 NEC
  during or resulting from a procedure NEC 997.2
  femoral 451.11
  femoropopliteal 451.19
  following infusion, perfusion, or transfusion 999.2
  hepatic (vein) 451.89
  idiopathic, recurrent 453.1

Thrombophlebitis — *continued*
  iliac vein 451.81
  iliofemoral 451.11
  intracranial venous sinus (any) 325
    late effect — *see* category 326
    nonpyogenic 437.6
      in pregnancy or puerperium 671.5 ☑
      late effect — *see* Late effect(s) (of) cerebrovascular disease
  jugular vein 451.89
  lateral (venous) sinus — *see* Thrombophlebitis, intracranial venous sinus
  leg 451.2
    deep (vessels) 451.19
      femoral vein 451.11
      specified vessel NEC 451.19
    superficial (vessels) 451.0
      femoral vein 451.11
  longitudinal (venous) sinus — *see* Thrombophlebitis, intracranial venous sinus
  lower extremity 451.2
    deep (vessels) 451.19
      femoral vein 451.11
      specified vessel NEC 451.19
    superficial (vessels) 451.0
  migrans, migrating 453.1
  pelvic
    with
      abortion — *see* Abortion, by type, with sepsis
      ectopic pregnancy (*see also* categories 633.0–633.9) 639.0
      molar pregnancy (*see also* categories 630–632) 639.0
    following
      abortion 639.0
      ectopic or molar pregnancy 639.0
    puerperal 671.4 ☑
  popliteal vein 451.19
  portal (vein) 572.1
  postoperative 997.2
  pregnancy (superficial) 671.2 ☑
    affecting fetus or newborn 760.3
    deep 671.3 ☑
  puerperal, postpartum, childbirth (extremities) (superficial) 671.2 ☑
    deep 671.4 ☑
    pelvic 671.4 ☑
    septic 670.3 ☑
    specified site NEC 671.5 ☑
  radial vein 451.83
  saphenous (greater) (lesser) 451.0
  sinus (intracranial) — *see* Thrombophlebitis, intracranial venous sinus
    specified site NEC 451.89
  tibial vein 451.19
Thrombosis, thrombotic (marantic) (multiple) (progressive) (vein) (vessel) 453.9
  with childbirth or during the puerperium — *see* Thrombosis, puerperal, postpartum
  antepartum — *see* Thrombosis, pregnancy
  aorta, aortic 444.1
    abdominal 444.09
      saddle 444.01
    bifurcation 444.09
    saddle 444.01
    terminal 444.09
    thoracic 444.1
    valve — *see* Endocarditis, aortic
  apoplexy (*see also* Thrombosis, brain) 434.0 ☑
    late effect — *see* Late effect(s) (of) cerebrovascular disease
  appendix, septic — *see* Appendicitis, acute
  arteriolar-capillary platelet, disseminated 446.6
  artery, arteries (postinfectional) 444.9
    auditory, internal 433.8 ☑
    basilar (*see also* Occlusion, artery, basilar) 433.0 ☑
    carotid (common) (internal) (*see also* Occlusion, artery, carotid) 433.1 ☑
      with other precerebral artery 433.3 ☑

Thrombosis, thrombotic — *continued*
  artery, arteries — *continued*
    cerebellar (anterior inferior) (posterior inferior) (superior) 433.8 ☑
    cerebral (*see also* Thrombosis, brain) 434.0 ☑
    choroidal (anterior) 433.8 ☑
    communicating posterior 433.8 ☑
    coronary (*see also* Infarct, myocardium) 410.9 ☑
      without myocardial infarction 411.81
      due to syphilis 093.89
      healed or specified as old 412
    extremities 444.22
      lower 444.22
      upper 444.21
    femoral 444.22
    hepatic 444.89
    hypophyseal 433.8 ☑
    meningeal, anterior or posterior 433.8 ☑
    mesenteric (with gangrene) 557.0
    ophthalmic (*see also* Occlusion, retina) 362.30
    pontine 433.8 ☑
    popliteal 444.22
    precerebral — *see* Occlusion, artery, precerebral NEC
    pulmonary 415.19
      iatrogenic 415.11
      personal history of V12.55
      postoperative 415.11
      septic 415.12
    renal 593.81
    retinal (*see also* Occlusion, retina) 362.30
    specified site NEC 444.89
    spinal, anterior or posterior 433.8 ☑
    traumatic (complication) (early) (*see also* Injury, blood vessel, by site) 904.9
    vertebral (*see also* Occlusion, artery, vertebral) 433.2 ☑
      with other precerebral artery 433.3 ☑
  atrial (endocardial) 424.90
    without endocarditis 429.89
    due to syphilis 093.89
  auricular (*see also* Infarct, myocardium) 410.9 ☑
  axillary (acute) (vein) 453.84
    chronic 453.74
    personal history of V12.51
  basilar (artery) (*see also* Occlusion, artery, basilar) 433.0 ☑
  bland NEC 453.9
  brain (artery) (stem) 434.0 ☑
    due to syphilis 094.89
    iatrogenic 997.02
    late effect — *see* Late effect(s) (of) cerebrovascular disease
    postoperative 997.02
    puerperal, postpartum, childbirth 674.0 ☑
    sinus (*see also* Thrombosis, intracranial venous sinus) 325
  capillary 448.9
    arteriolar, generalized 446.6
  cardiac (*see also* Infarct, myocardium) 410.9 ☑
    due to syphilis 093.89
    healed or specified as old 412
    valve — *see* Endocarditis
  carotid (artery) (common) (internal) (*see also* Occlusion, artery, carotid) 433.1 ☑
    with other precerebral artery 433.3 ☑
  cavernous sinus (venous) — *see* Thrombosis, intracranial venous sinus
  cerebellar artery (anterior inferior) (posterior inferior) (superior) 433.8 ☑
    late effect — *see* Late effect(s) (of) cerebrovascular disease
  cerebral (arteries) (*see also* Thrombosis, brain) 434.0 ☑
    late effect — *see* Late effect(s) (of) cerebrovascular disese
  coronary (artery) (*see also* Infarct, myocardium) 410.9 ☑

Thrombosis, thrombotic — *continued*
  coronary (*see also* Infarct, myocardium) — *continued*
    without myocardial infarction 411.81
    due to syphilis 093.89
    healed or specified as old 412
  corpus cavernosum 607.82
  cortical (*see also* Thrombosis, brain) 434.0 ☑
  due to (presence of) any device, implant, or graft classifiable to 996.0–996.5 — *see* Complications, due to (presence of) any device, implant, or graft classified to 996.0–996.5 NEC
  effort 453.89
  endocardial — *see* Infarct, myocardium
  eye (*see also* Occlusion, retina) 362.30
  femoral (vein) 453.6
    with inflammation or phlebitis 451.11
    artery 444.22
    deep 453.41
    personal history of V12.51
  genital organ, male 608.83
  heart (chamber) (*see also* Infarct, myocardium) 410.9 ☑
  hepatic (vein) 453.0
    artery 444.89
    infectional or septic 572.1
  iliac (acute) (vein) 453.41
    with inflammation or phlebitis 451.81
    artery (common) (external) (internal) 444.81
    chronic 453.51
    personal history of V12.51
  inflammation, vein — *see* Thrombophlebitis
  internal carotid artery (*see also* Occlusion, artery, carotid) 433.1 ☑
    with other precerebral artery 433.3 ☑
  intestine (with gangrene) 557.0
  intracranial (*see also* Thrombosis, brain) 434.0 ☑
    venous sinus (any) 325
      nonpyogenic origin 437.6
        in pregnancy or puerperium 671.5 ☑
  intramural (*see also* Infarct, myocardium) 410.9 ☑
    without
      cardiac condition 429.89
      coronary artery disease 429.89
      myocardial infarction 429.89
    healed or specified as old 412
  jugular (bulb)
    external (acute) 453.89
      chronic 453.79
    internal (acute) 453.86
      chronic 453.76
  kidney 593.81
    artery 593.81
  lateral sinus (venous) — *see* Thrombosis, intracranial venous sinus
  leg (*see also* Thrombosis, lower extremity) 453.6
    with inflammation or phlebitis — *see* Thrombophlebitis
    deep (vessels) 453.40
      acute 453.40
        lower distal 453.42
        upper (proximal) 453.41
      chronic 453.50
        lower (distal) 453.52
        upper (proximal) 453.51
      lower (distal) 453.42
      upper (proximal) 453.41
    personal history of V12.51
    superficial (vessels) 453.6
  liver (venous) 453.0
    artery 444.89
    infectional or septic 572.1
    portal vein 452
  longitudinal sinus (venous) — *see* Thrombosis, intracranial venous sinus
  lower extremity (superficial) 453.6
    deep vessels 453.40
      acute 453.40
        calf 453.42
        distal (lower leg) 453.42

☑ **Additional Digit Required** — **Refer to the Tabular List for Digit Selection**

▽ **Subterms under main terms may continue to next column or page**

Thrombosis, thrombotic — *continued*
  lower extremity — *continued*
    deep vessels — *continued*
      acute — *continued*
        femoral 453.41
        iliac 453.41
        lower leg 453.42
        peroneal 453.42
        popliteal 453.41
        proximal (upper leg) 453.41
        thigh 453.41
        tibial 453.42
      chronic 453.50
        calf 453.52
        distal (lower leg) 453.52
        femoral 453.51
        iliac 453.51
        lower leg 453.52
        peroneal 453.52
        popliteal 453.51
        proximal (upper leg) 453.51
        thigh 453.51
        tibial 453.52
    personal history of V12.51
    saphenous (greater) (lesser) 453.6
    superficial 453.6
  lung 415.19
    iatrogenic 415.11
    personal history of V12.55
    postoperative 415.11
    septic 415.12
  marantic, dural sinus 437.6
  meninges (brain) (see also Thrombosis, brain) 434.0 ☑
  mesenteric (artery) (with gangrene) 557.0
    vein (inferior) (superior) 557.0
  mitral — see Insufficiency, mitral
  mural (heart chamber) (see also Infarct, myocardium) 410.9 ☑
    without
      cardiac condition 429.89
      coronary artery disease 429.89
      myocardial infarction 429.89
    due to syphilis 093.89
    following myocardial infarction 429.79
    healed or specified as old 412
  omentum (with gangrene) 557.0
  ophthalmic (artery) (see also Occlusion, retina) 362.30
  pampiniform plexus (male) 608.83
    female 620.8
  parietal (see also Infarct, myocardium) 410.9 ☑
  penis, penile 607.82
  peripheral arteries 444.22
    lower 444.22
    upper 444.21
  platelet 446.6
  portal 452
    due to syphilis 093.89
    infectional or septic 572.1
  precerebral artery (see also Occlusion, artery, precerebral NEC)
  pregnancy 671.2 ☑
    deep (vein) 671.3 ☑
    superficial (vein) 671.2 ☑
  puerperal, postpartum, childbirth 671.2 ☑
    brain (artery) 674.0 ☑
      venous 671.5 ☑
    cardiac 674.8 ☑
    cerebral (artery) 674.0 ☑
      venous 671.5 ☑
    deep (vein) 671.4 ☑
    intracranial sinus (nonpyogenic) (venous) 671.5 ☑
    pelvic 671.4 ☑
    pulmonary (artery) 673.2 ☑
    specified site NEC 671.5 ☑
    superficial 671.2 ☑
  pulmonary (artery) (vein) 415.19
    iatrogenic 415.11
    personal history of V12.55
    postoperative 415.11
    septic 415.12
  renal (artery) 593.81
    vein 453.3

Thrombosis, thrombotic — *continued*
  resulting from presence of shunt or other internal prosthetic device — see Complications, due to (presence of) any device, implant, or graft classified to 996.0–996.5 NEC
  retina, retinal (artery) 362.30
    arterial branch 362.32
    central 362.31
    partial 362.33
    vein
      central 362.35
      tributary (branch) 362.36
  saphenous vein (greater) (lesser) 453.6
  scrotum 608.83
  seminal vesicle 608.83
  sigmoid (venous) sinus — see Thrombosis, intracranial venous sinus 325
  silent NEC 453.9
  sinus, intracranial (venous) (any) (see also Thrombosis, intracranial venous sinus) 325
  softening, brain (see also Thrombosis, brain) 434.0 ☑
  specified site NEC (acute) 453.89
    chronic 453.79
  spermatic cord 608.83
  spinal cord 336.1
    due to syphilis 094.89
    in pregnancy or puerperium 671.5 ☑
    pyogenic origin 324.1
      late effect — see category 326
  spleen, splenic 289.59
    artery 444.89
  testis 608.83
  traumatic (complication) (early) (see also Injury, blood vessel, by site) 904.9
  tricuspid — see Endocarditis, tricuspid
  tumor — see Neoplasm, by site
  tunica vaginalis 608.83
  umbilical cord (vessels) 663.6 ☑
    affecting fetus or newborn 762.6
  upper extremity (acute) 453.83
    chronic 453.73
      deep 453.72
      superficial 453.71
    deep 453.82
    superficial 453.81
  vas deferens 608.83
  vein
    antecubital (acute) 453.81
      chronic 453.71
    axillary (acute) 453.84
      chronic 453.74
    basilic (acute) 453.81
      chronic 453.71
    brachial (acute) 453.82
      chronic 453.72
    brachiocephalic (innominate) (acute) 453.87
      chronic 453.77
    cephalic (acute) 453.81
      chronic 453.71
    deep 453.40
      personal history of V12.51
    internal jugular (acute) 453.86
      chronic 453.76
    lower extremity — see Thrombosis, lower extremity
    personal history of V12.51
    radial (acute) 453.82
      chronic 453.72
    saphenous (greater) (lesser) 453.6
    specified site NEC (acute) 453.89
      chronic 453.79
    subclavian (acute) 453.85
      chronic 453.75
    superior vena cava (acute) 453.87
      chronic 453.77
    thoracic (acute) 453.87
      chronic 453.77
    ulnar (acute) 453.82
      chronic 453.72
    upper extremity — see Thrombosis, upper extremity

Thrombosis, thrombotic — *continued*
  vena cava
    inferior 453.2
    personal history of V12.51
    superior (acute) 453.87
      chronic 453.77
Thrombus — *see* Thrombosis
Thrush 112.0
  newborn 771.7
Thumb — *see also* condition
  gamekeeper's 842.12
  sucking (child problem) 307.9
Thygeson's superficial punctate keratitis 370.21
Thymergasia — *see also* Psychosis, affective 296.80
Thymitis 254.8
Thymoma (benign) (M8580/0) 212.6
  malignant (M8580/3) 164.0
Thymus, thymic (gland) — *see* condition
Thyrocele — *see also* Goiter 240.9
Thyroglossal — *see also* condition
  cyst 759.2
  duct, persistent 759.2
Thyroid (body) (gland) — *see also* condition
  hormone resistance 246.8
  lingual 759.2
Thyroiditis 245.9
  acute (pyogenic) (suppurative) 245.0
    nonsuppurative 245.0
  autoimmune 245.2
  chronic (nonspecific) (sclerosing) 245.8
    fibrous 245.3
    lymphadenoid 245.2
    lymphocytic 245.2
    lymphoid 245.2
  complicating pregnancy, childbirth, or puerperium 648.1 ☑
  de Quervain's (subacute granulomatous) 245.1
  fibrous (chronic) 245.3
  giant (cell) (follicular) 245.1
  granulomatous (de Quervain's) (subacute) 245.1
  Hashimoto's (struma lymphomatosa) 245.2
  iatrogenic 245.4
  invasive (fibrous) 245.3
  ligneous 245.3
  lymphocytic (chronic) 245.2
  lymphoid 245.2
  lymphomatous 245.2
  pseudotuberculous 245.1
  pyogenic 245.0
  radiation 245.4
  Riedel's (ligneous) 245.3
  subacute 245.1
  suppurative 245.0
  tuberculous (see also Tuberculosis) 017.5 ☑
  viral 245.1
  woody 245.3
Thyrolingual duct, persistent 759.2
Thyromegaly 240.9
Thyrotoxic
  crisis or storm (see also Thyrotoxicosis) 242.9 ☑
  heart failure (see also Thyrotoxicosis) 242.9 ☑ [425.7]
Thyrotoxicosis 242.9 ☑

Note — *Use the following fifth-digit subclassification with category 242:*

0   *without mention of thyrotoxic crisis or storm*

1   *with mention of thyrotoxic crisis or storm*

  with
    goiter (diffuse) 242.0 ☑
      adenomatous 242.3 ☑
        multinodular 242.2 ☑
        uninodular 242.1 ☑
      nodular 242.3 ☑
        multinodular 242.2 ☑
        uninodular 242.1 ☑
    infiltrative
      dermopathy 242.0 ☑

Thyrotoxicosis — *continued*
  with — *continued*
    infiltrative — *continued*
      ophthalmopathy 242.0 ☑
    thyroid acropachy 242.0 ☑
  complicating pregnancy, childbirth, or puerperium 648.1 ☑
  due to
    ectopic thyroid nodule 242.4 ☑
    ingestion of (excessive) thyroid material 242.8 ☑
    specified cause NEC 242.8 ☑
  factitia 242.8 ☑
  heart 242.9 ☑ [425.7]
  neonatal (transient) 775.3
TIA (transient ischemic attack) 435.9
  with transient neurologic deficit 435.9
  late effect — see Late effect(s) (of) cerebrovascular disease
Tibia vara 732.4
Tic 307.20
  breathing 307.20
  child problem 307.21
  compulsive 307.22
  convulsive 307.20
  degenerative (generalized) (localized) 333.3
    facial 351.8
  douloureux (see also Neuralgia, trigeminal) 350.1
    atypical 350.2
  habit 307.20
    chronic (motor or vocal) 307.22
    transient (of childhood) 307.21
  lid 307.20
    transient (of childhood) 307.21
  motor-verbal 307.23
  occupational 300.89
  orbicularis 307.20
    transient (of childhood) 307.21
  organic origin 333.3
  postchoreic — see Chorea
  psychogenic 307.20
    compulsive 307.22
  salaam 781.0
  spasm 307.20
    chronic (motor or vocal) 307.22
    transient (of childhood) 307.21
Tick-bite fever NEC 066.1
  African 087.1
  Colorado (virus) 066.1
  Rocky Mountain 082.0
Tick (-borne) fever NEC 066.1
  American mountain 066.1
  Colorado 066.1
  hemorrhagic NEC 065.3
    Crimean 065.0
    Kyasanur Forest 065.2
    Omsk 065.1
  mountain 066.1
  nonxanthematous 066.1
Tick paralysis 989.5
Tics and spasms, compulsive 307.22
Tietze's disease or syndrome 733.6
Tight, tightness
  anus 564.89
  chest 786.59
  fascia (lata) 728.9
  foreskin (congenital) 605
  hymen 623.3
  introitus (acquired) (congenital) 623.3
  rectal sphincter 564.89
  tendon 727.81
    Achilles (heel) 727.81
  urethral sphincter 598.9
Tilting vertebra 737.9
Timidity, child 313.21
Tinea (intersecta) (tarsi) 110.9
  amiantacea 110.0
  asbestina 110.0
  barbae 110.0
  beard 110.0
  black dot 110.0
  blanca 111.2
  capitis 110.0
  corporis 110.5
  cruris 110.3

☑ **Additional Digit Required** — Refer to the Tabular List for Digit Selection   ▽ **Subterms under main terms may continue to next column or page**

2014 ICD-9-CM   **325**

Tinea — *continued*
  decalvans 704.09
  flava 111.0
  foot 110.4
  furfuracea 111.0
  imbricata (Tokelau) 110.5
  lepothrix 039.0
  manuum 110.2
  microsporic (*see also* Dermatophytosis)
      110.9
  nigra 111.1
  nodosa 111.2
  pedis 110.4
  scalp 110.0
  specified site NEC 110.8
  sycosis 110.0
  tonsurans 110.0
  trichophytic (*see also* Dermatophytosis)
      110.9
  unguium 110.1
  versicolor 111.0
Tingling sensation — *see also* Disturbance,
      sensation 782.0
Tin-miners' lung 503
Tinnitus (aurium) 388.30
  audible 388.32
  objective 388.32
  subjective 388.31
Tipped, teeth 524.33
Tipping
  pelvis 738.6
      with disproportion (fetopelvic) 653.0 ☑
          affecting fetus or newborn 763.1
          causing obstructed labor 660.1 ☑
              affecting fetus or newborn 763.1
  teeth 524.33
Tiredness 780.79
Tissue — *see* condition
Tobacco
  abuse (affecting health) NEC (*see also* Abuse,
      drugs, nondependent) 305.1
  heart 989.84
  use disorder complicating pregnancy,
      childbirth, or the puerperium
      649.0 ☑
Tobias' syndrome (carcinoma, pulmonary
      apex) (M8010/3) 162.3
Tocopherol deficiency 269.1
Todd's
  cirrhosis — *see* Cirrhosis, biliary
  paralysis (postepileptic transitory paralysis)
      344.89
Toe — *see* condition
Toilet, artificial opening — *see also* Attention
      to, artificial, opening V55.9
Tokelau ringworm 110.5
Tollwut 071
Tolosa-Hunt syndrome 378.55
Tommaselli's disease
  correct substance properly administered
      599.70
  overdose or wrong substance given or taken
      961.4
Tongue — *see also* condition
  worms 134.1
Tongue tie 750.0
Tonic pupil 379.46
Toni-Fanconi syndrome (cystinosis) 270.0
Tonsil — *see* condition
Tonsillitis (acute) (catarrhal) (croupous) (follic-
      ular) (gangrenous) (infective) (lacunar)
      (lingual) (malignant) (membranous)
      (phlegmonous) (pneumococcal) (pseu-
      domembranous) (purulent) (septic)
      (staphylococcal) (subacute) (suppura-
      tive) (toxic) (ulcerative) (vesicular) (viral)
      463
  with influenza, flu, or grippe (*see also* Influen-
      za) 487.1
  chronic 474.00
  diphtheritic (membranous) 032.0
  hypertrophic 474.00
  influenzal (*see also* Influenza) 487.1
  parenchymatous 475
  streptococcal 034.0
  tuberculous (*see also* Tuberculosis) 012.8 ☑

Tonsillitis — *continued*
  Vincent's 101
Tonsillopharyngitis 465.8
Toothache 525.9
Tooth, teeth — *see* condition
Topagnosis 782.0
Tophi (gouty) 274.03
  ear 274.81
  heart 274.82
  specified site NEC 274.82
TORCH infection — *see also* Infection, congen-
      ital 760.2
Torn — *see* Tear, torn
Tornwaldt's bursitis (disease) (pharyngeal
      bursitis) 478.29
  cyst 478.26
Torpid liver 573.9
Torsion
  accessory tube 620.5
  adnexa (female) 620.5
  aorta (congenital) 747.29
      acquired 447.1
  appendix
      epididymis 608.24
      testis 608.23
  bile duct 576.8
      with calculus, choledocholithiasis or
          stones — *see* Choledocholithiasis
      congenital 751.69
  bowel, colon, or intestine 560.2
  cervix — *see* Malposition, uterus
  duodenum 537.3
  dystonia — *see* Dystonia, torsion
  epididymis 608.24
      appendix 608.24
  fallopian tube 620.5
  gallbladder (*see also* Disease, gallbladder)
      575.8
      congenital 751.69
  gastric 537.89
  hydatid of Morgagni (female) 620.5
  kidney (pedicle) 593.89
  Meckel's diverticulum (congenital) 751.0
  mesentery 560.2
  omentum 560.2
  organ or site, congenital NEC — *see*
      Anomaly, specified type NEC
  ovary (pedicle) 620.5
      congenital 752.0
  oviduct 620.5
  penis 607.89
      congenital 752.69
  renal 593.89
  spasm — *see* Dystonia, torsion
  spermatic cord 608.22
      extravaginal 608.21
      intravaginal 608.22
  spleen 289.59
  testicle, testis 608.20
      appendix 608.23
  tibia 736.89
  umbilical cord — *see* Compression, umbili-
      cal cord
  uterus (*see also* Malposition, uterus) 621.6
Torticollis (intermittent) (spastic) 723.5
  congenital 754.1
      sternomastoid 754.1
  due to birth injury 767.8
  hysterical 300.11
  ocular 781.93
  psychogenic 306.0
      specified as conversion reaction 300.11
  rheumatic 723.5
  rheumatoid 714.0
  spasmodic 333.83
  traumatic, current NEC 847.0
Tortuous
  artery 447.1
  fallopian tube 752.19
  organ or site, congenital NEC — *see* Distor-
      tion
  renal vessel (congenital) 747.62
  retina vessel (congenital) 743.58
      acquired 362.17
  ureter 593.4
  urethra 599.84

Tortuous — *continued*
  vein — *see* Varicose, vein
Torula, torular (infection) 117.5
  histolytica 117.5
  lung 117.5
Torulosis 117.5
Torus
  fracture
      fibula 823.41
          with tibia 823.42
      humerus 812.49
      radius (alone) 813.45
          with ulna 813.47
      tibia 823.40
          with fibula 823.42
      ulna (alone) 813.46
          with radius 813.47
  mandibularis 526.81
  palatinus 526.81
Touch, vitreous 997.99
Touraine-Solente-Golé syndrome
      (acropachyderma) 757.39
Touraine's syndrome (hereditary osteo-ony-
      chodysplasia) 756.89
Tourette's disease (motor-verbal tic) 307.23
Tower skull 756.0
  with exophthalmos 756.0
Toxemia 799.89
  with
      abortion — *see* Abortion, by type, with
          toxemia
      bacterial — *see* Septicemia
  biliary (*see also* Disease, biliary) 576.8
  burn — *see* Burn, by site
  congenital NEC 779.89
  eclamptic 642.6 ☑
      with pre-existing hypertension 642.7 ☑
  erysipelatous (*see also* Erysipelas) 035
  fatigue 799.89
  fetus or newborn NEC 779.89
  food (*see also* Poisoning, food) 005.9
  gastric 537.89
  gastrointestinal 558.2
  intestinal 558.2
  kidney (*see also* Disease, renal) 593.9
  lung 518.89
  malarial NEC (*see also* Malaria) 084.6
  maternal (of pregnancy), affecting fetus or
      newborn 760.0
  myocardial — *see* Myocarditis, toxic
  of pregnancy (mild) (pre-eclamptic)
      642.4 ☑
      with
          convulsions 642.6 ☑
          pre-existing hypertension 642.7 ☑
      affecting fetus or newborn 760.0
      severe 642.5 ☑
  pre-eclamptic — *see* Toxemia, of pregnancy
  puerperal, postpartum — *see* Toxemia, of
      pregnancy
  pulmonary 518.89
  renal (*see also* Disease, renal) 593.9
  septic (*see also* Septicemia) 038.9
  small intestine 558.2
  staphylococcal 038.10
      aureus 038.11
      due to food 005.0
      specified organism NEC 038.19
  stasis 799.89
  stomach 537.89
  uremic (*see also* Uremia) 586
  urinary 586
Toxemica cerebropathia psychica (nonalco-
      holic) 294.0
  alcoholic 291.1
Toxic (poisoning) — *see also* condition
  from drug or poison — *see* Table of Drugs
      and Chemicals
  oil syndrome 710.5
  shock syndrome 040.82
  thyroid (gland) (*see also* Thyrotoxicosis)
      242.9 ☑
Toxicemia — *see* Toxemia
Toxicity
  dilantin
      asymptomatic 796.0

Toxicity — *continued*
  dilantin — *continued*
      symptomatic — *see* Table of Drugs and
          Chemicals
  drug
      asymptomatic 796.0
      symptomatic — *see* Table of Drugs and
          Chemicals
  fava bean 282.2
  from drug or poison
      asymptomatic 796.0
      symptomatic — *see* Table of Drugs and
          Chemicals
Toxicosis — *see also* Toxemia 799.89
  capillary, hemorrhagic 287.0
Toxinfection 799.89
  gastrointestinal 558.2
Toxocariasis 128.0
Toxoplasma infection, generalized 130.9
Toxoplasmosis (acquired) 130.9
  with pneumonia 130.4
  congenital, active 771.2
  disseminated (multisystemic) 130.8
  maternal
      with suspected damage to fetus affect-
          ing management of pregnancy
          655.4 ☑
      affecting fetus or newborn 760.2
      manifest toxoplasmosis in fetus or
          newborn 771.2
  multiple sites 130.8
  multisystemic disseminated 130.8
  specified site NEC 130.7
Trabeculation, bladder 596.89
Trachea — *see* condition
Tracheitis (acute) (catarrhal) (infantile) (mem-
      branous) (plastic) (pneumococcal) (sep-
      tic) (suppurative) (viral) 464.10
  with
      bronchitis 490
          acute or subacute 466.0
          chronic 491.8
          tuberculosis — *see* Tuberculosis,
              pulmonary
      laryngitis (acute) 464.20
          with obstruction 464.21
          chronic 476.1
          tuberculous (*see also* Tuberculosis,
              larynx) 012.3 ☑
      obstruction 464.11
  chronic 491.8
      with
          bronchitis (chronic) 491.8
          laryngitis (chronic) 476.1
          due to external agent — *see* Condition,
              respiratory, chronic, due to
  diphtheritic (membranous) 032.3
  due to external agent — *see* Inflamma-
      tion, respiratory, upper, due to
  edematous 464.11
  influenzal (*see also* Influenza) 487.1
  streptococcal 034.0
  syphilitic 095.8
  tuberculous (*see also* Tuberculosis) 012.8 ☑
Trachelitis (nonvenereal) — *see also* Cervicitis
      616.0
  trichomonal 131.09
Tracheobronchial — *see* condition
Tracheobronchitis — *see also* Bronchitis 490
  acute or subacute 466.0
      with bronchospasm or obstruction 466.0
  chronic 491.8
  influenzal (*see also* Influenza) 487.1
  senile 491.8
Tracheobronchomegaly (congenital) 748.3
  with bronchiectasis 494.0
      with (acute) exacerbation 494.1
  acquired 519.19
      with bronchiectasis 494.0
          with (acute) exacerbation 494.1
Tracheobronchopneumonitis — *see* Pneumo-
      nia, broncho
Tracheocele (external) (internal) 519.19
  congenital 748.3
Tracheomalacia 519.19
  congenital 748.3

Tracheopharyngitis (acute) 465.8
  chronic 478.9
    due to external agent — *see* Condition, respiratory, chronic, due to
    due to external agent — *see* Inflammation, respiratory, upper, due to
Tracheostenosis 519.19
  congenital 748.3
Tracheostomy
  attention to V55.0
  complication 519.00
  granuloma 519.09
  hemorrhage 519.09
  infection 519.01
  malfunctioning 519.02
  obstruction 519.09
  sepsis 519.01
  status V44.0
  stenosis 519.02
Trachoma, trachomatous 076.9
  active (stage) 076.1
  contraction of conjunctiva 076.1
  dubium 076.0
  healed or late effect 139.1
  initial (stage) 076.0
  Türck's (chronic catarrhal laryngitis) 476.0
Trachyphonia 784.49
Traction, vitreomacular 379.27
Training
  insulin pump V65.46
  orthoptic V57.4
  orthotic V57.81
Train sickness 994.6
Trait
  hemoglobin
    abnormal NEC 282.7
      with thalassemia 282.46
    C (*see also* Disease, hemoglobin, C) 282.7
      with elliptocytosis 282.7
    S (Hb-S) 282.5
    Lepore 282.49
    with other abnormal hemoglobin NEC 282.49
  paranoid 301.0
  sickle-cell 282.5
    with
      elliptocytosis 282.5
      spherocytosis 282.5
    thalassemia (alpha) (beta) (delta-beta) 282.46
Traits, paranoid 301.0
Tramp V60.0
Trance 780.09
  hysterical 300.13
Transaminasemia 790.4
Transfusion, blood
  without reported diagnosis V58.2
  donor V59.01
    stem cells V59.02
  fetal twin to twin 678.0 ☑
  incompatible (*see also* Complications, transfusion) 999.80
    ABO (*see also* Complications, transfusion) 999.60
    minor blood group 999.89
    non-ABO (*see also* Complications, transfusion) 999.75
    Rh (antigen) (C) (c) (D) (E) (e) (*see also* Complications, transfusion) 999.70
  reaction or complication — *see* Complications, transfusion
  related acute lung injury (TRALI) 518.7
  syndrome
    fetomaternal 772.0
    twin-to-twin
      blood loss (donor twin) 772.0
      recipient twin 776.4
  twin to twin fetal 678.0 ☑
Transient — *see also* condition
  alteration of awareness 780.02
  blindness 368.12
  deafness (ischemic) 388.02
  global amnesia 437.7
  hyperglycemia (post-procedural) 790.29
  hypoglycemia (post-procedural) 251.2

Transient — *see also* condition — *continued*
  person (homeless) NEC V60.0
Transitional, lumbosacral joint of vertebra 756.19
Translocation
  autosomes NEC 758.5
    13-15 758.1
    16-18 758.2
    21 or 22 758.0
    balanced in normal individual 758.4
    D₁ 758.1
    E₃ 758.2
    G 758.0
  balanced autosomal in normal individual 758.4
  chromosomes NEC 758.89
  Down's syndrome 758.0
Translucency, iris 364.53
Transmission of chemical substances through the placenta (affecting fetus or newborn) 760.70
  alcohol 760.71
  anticonvulsants 760.77
  antifungals 760.74
  anti-infective agents 760.74
  antimetabolics 760.78
  cocaine 760.75
  "crack" 760.75
  diethylstilbestrol [DES] 760.76
  hallucinogenic agents 760.73
  medicinal agents NEC 760.79
  narcotics 760.72
  obstetric anesthetic or analgesic drug 763.5
  specified agent NEC 760.79
  suspected, affecting management of pregnancy 655.5 ☑
Transplant(ed)
  bone V42.4
    marrow V42.81
  complication (*see also* Complications, due to (presence of) any device, implant, or graft classified to 996.0–996.5 NEC)
    bone marrow 996.85
    corneal graft NEC 996.79
      infection or inflammation 996.69
      reaction 996.51
      rejection 996.51
    organ (failure) (immune or nonimmune cause) (infection) (rejection) 996.80
      bone marrow 996.85
      heart 996.83
      intestines 996.87
      kidney 996.81
      liver 996.82
      lung 996.84
      pancreas 996.86
      specified NEC 996.89
    previously removed due to complication, failure, rejection or infection V45.87
    removal status V45.87
    skin NEC 996.79
      infection or inflammation 996.69
      rejection 996.51
        artificial 996.55
        decellularized allodermis 996.55
    stem cell(s) 996.88
      from
        peripheral blood 996.88
        umbilical cord 996.88
  cornea V42.5
  hair V50.0
  heart V42.1
    valve V42.2
  intestine V42.84
  kidney V42.0
  liver V42.7
  lung V42.6
  organ V42.9
    specified NEC V42.89
  pancreas V42.83
  peripheral stem cells V42.82
  skin V42.3

Transplant(ed) — *continued*
  stem cells, peripheral V42.82
  tissue V42.9
    specified NEC V42.89
Transplants, ovarian, endometrial 617.1
Transposed — *see* Transposition
Transposition (congenital) — *see also* Malposition, congenital
  abdominal viscera 759.3
  aorta (dextra) 745.11
  appendix 751.5
  arterial trunk 745.10
  colon 751.5
  great vessels (complete) 745.10
    both originating from right ventricle 745.11
    corrected 745.12
    double outlet right ventricle 745.11
    incomplete 745.11
    partial 745.11
    specified type NEC 745.19
  heart 746.87
    with complete transposition of viscera 759.3
  intestine (large) (small) 751.5
  pulmonary veins 747.49
  reversed jejunal (for bypass) (status) V45.3
  scrotal 752.81
  stomach 750.7
    with general transposition of viscera 759.3
  teeth, tooth 524.30
  vessels (complete) 745.10
    partial 745.11
  viscera (abdominal) (thoracic) 759.3
Trans-sexualism 302.50
  with
    asexual history 302.51
    heterosexual history 302.53
    homosexual history 302.52
Transverse — *see also* condition
  arrest (deep), in labor 660.3 ☑
    affecting fetus or newborn 763.1
  lie 652.3 ☑
    before labor, affecting fetus or newborn 761.7
    causing obstructed labor 660.0 ☑
      affecting fetus or newborn 763.1
    during labor, affecting fetus or newborn 763.1
Transvestism, transvestitism (transvestic fetishism) 302.3
Trapped placenta (with hemorrhage) 666.0 ☑
  without hemorrhage 667.0 ☑
Traumatic — *see also* condition
  brain injury (TBI) (*see also* Injury, intracranial) 854.0 ☑
    with skull fracture — *see* Fracture, skull, by site
Trauma, traumatism — *see also* Injury, by site 959.9
  birth — *see* Birth, injury NEC
  causing hemorrhage of pregnancy or delivery 641.8 ☑
  complicating
    abortion — *see* Abortion, by type, with damage to pelvic organs
    ectopic pregnancy (*see also* categories 633.0–633.9) 639.2
    molar pregnancy (*see also* categories 630–632) 639.2
  during delivery NEC 665.9 ☑
  following
    abortion 639.2
    ectopic or molar pregnancy 639.2
  maternal, during pregnancy, affecting fetus or newborn 760.5
  neuroma — *see* Injury, nerve, by site
  previous major, affecting management of pregnancy, childbirth, or puerperium V23.89
  psychic (current) (*see also* Reaction, adjustment)
    previous (history) V15.49
  psychologic, previous (affecting health) V15.49

Trauma, traumatism — *see also* Injury, by site — *continued*
  transient paralysis — *see* Injury, nerve, by site
Treacher Collins' syndrome (incomplete facial dysostosis) 756.0
Treitz's hernia — *see* Hernia, Treitz's
Trematode infestation NEC 121.9
Trematodiasis NEC 121.9
Trembles 988.8
Trembling paralysis — *see also* Parkinsonism 332.0
Tremor 781.0
  essential (benign) 333.1
  familial 333.1
  flapping (liver) 572.8
  hereditary 333.1
  hysterical 300.11
  intention 333.1
  medication-induced postural 333.1
  mercurial 985.0
  muscle 728.85
  Parkinson's (*see also* Parkinsonism) 332.0
  psychogenic 306.0
    specified as conversion reaction 300.11
  senilis 797
  specified type NEC 333.1
Trench
  fever 083.1
  foot 991.4
  mouth 101
  nephritis — *see* Nephritis, acute
Treponema pallidum infection — *see also* Syphilis 097.9
Treponematosis 102.9
  due to
    T. pallidum — *see* Syphilis
    T. pertenue (yaws) (*see also* Yaws) 102.9
Triad
  Kartagener's 759.3
  Reiter's (complete) (incomplete) 099.3
  Saint's (*see also* Hernia, diaphragm) 553.3
Trichiasis 704.2
  cicatricial 704.2
  eyelid 374.05
    with entropion (*see also* Entropion) 374.00
Trichinella spiralis (infection) (infestation) 124
Trichinelliasis 124
Trichinellosis 124
Trichiniasis 124
Trichinosis 124
Trichobezoar 938
  intestine 936
  stomach 935.2
Trichocephaliasis 127.3
Trichocephalosis 127.3
Trichocephalus infestation 127.3
Trichoclasis 704.2
Trichoepithelioma (M8100/0) — *see also* Neoplasm, skin, benign
  breast 217
  genital organ NEC — *see* Neoplasm, by site, benign
  malignant (M8100/3) — *see* Neoplasm, skin, malignant
Trichofolliculoma (M8101/0) — *see* Neoplasm, skin, benign
Tricholemmoma (M8102/0) — *see* Neoplasm, skin, benign
Trichomatosis 704.2
Trichomoniasis 131.9
  bladder 131.09
  cervix 131.09
  intestinal 007.3
  prostate 131.03
  seminal vesicle 131.09
  specified site NEC 131.8
  urethra 131.02
  urogenitalis 131.00
  vagina 131.01
  vulva 131.01
  vulvovaginal 131.01
Trichomycosis 039.0
  axillaris 039.0
  nodosa 111.2

☑ **Additional Digit Required** — Refer to the Tabular List for Digit Selection

▽ **Subterms under main terms may continue to next column or page**

Trichomycosis — *continued*
  nodularis 111.2
  rubra 039.0
Trichonocardiosis (axillaris) (palmellina) 039.0
Trichonodosis 704.2
Trichophytide — *see* Dermatophytosis
Trichophytid, trichophyton infection — *see also* Dermatophytosis 110.9
Trichophytobezoar 938
  intestine 936
  stomach 935.2
Trichophytosis — *see* Dermatophytosis
Trichoptilosis 704.2
Trichorrhexis (nodosa) 704.2
Trichosporosis nodosa 111.2
Trichostasis spinulosa (congenital) 757.4
Trichostrongyliasis (small intestine) 127.6
Trichostrongylosis 127.6
Trichostrongylus (instabilis) infection 127.6
Trichotillomania 312.39
Trichromat, anomalous (congenital) 368.59
Trichromatopsia, anomalous (congenital) 368.59
Trichuriasis 127.3
Trichuris trichiuria (any site) (infection) (infestation) 127.3
Tricuspid (valve) — *see* condition
Trifid — *see also* Accessory
  kidney (pelvis) 753.3
  tongue 750.13
Trigeminal neuralgia — *see also* Neuralgia, trigeminal 350.1
Trigeminoencephaloangiomatosis 759.6
Trigeminy 427.89
  postoperative 997.1
Trigger finger (acquired) 727.03
  congenital 756.89
Trigonitis (bladder) (chronic) (pseudomembranous) 595.3
  tuberculous (*see also* Tuberculosis) 016.1 ☑
Trigonocephaly 756.0
Trihexosidosis 272.7
Trilobate placenta — *see* Placenta, abnormal
Trilocular heart 745.8
Trimethylaminuria 270.8
Tripartita placenta — *see* Placenta, abnormal
Triple — *see also* Accessory
  kidneys 753.3
  uteri 752.2
  X female 758.81
Triplegia 344.89
  congenital or infantile 343.8
Triplet
  affected by maternal complications of pregnancy 761.5
  healthy liveborn — *see* Newborn, multiple
  pregnancy (complicating delivery) NEC 651.1 ☑
    with fetal loss and retention of one or more fetus(es) 651.4 ☑
    following (elective) fetal reduction 651.7 ☑
Triplex placenta — *see* Placenta, abnormal
Triplication — *see* Accessory
Trismus 781.0
  neonatorum 771.3
  newborn 771.3
Trisomy (syndrome) NEC 758.5
  13 (partial) 758.1
  16-18 758.2
  18 (partial) 758.2
  21 (partial) 758.0
  22 758.0
  autosomes NEC 758.5
  D$_1$ 758.1
  E$_3$ 758.2
  G (group) 758.0
  group D$_1$ 758.1
  group E 758.2
  group G 758.0
Tritanomaly 368.53
Tritanopia 368.53
Troisier-Hanot-Chauffard syndrome (bronze diabetes) 275.01
Trombidiosis 133.8
Trophedema (hereditary) 757.0

Trophedema — *continued*
  congenital 757.0
Trophoblastic disease — *see also* Hydatidiform mole 630
  previous, affecting management of pregnancy V23.1
Tropholymphedema 757.0
Trophoneurosis NEC 356.9
  arm NEC 354.9
  disseminated 710.1
  facial 349.89
  leg NEC 355.8
  lower extremity NEC 355.8
  upper extremity NEC 354.9
Tropical — *see also* condition
  maceration feet (syndrome) 991.4
  wet foot (syndrome) 991.4
Trouble — *see also* Disease
  bowel 569.9
  heart — *see* Disease, heart
  intestine 569.9
  kidney (*see also* Disease, renal) 593.9
  nervous 799.21
  sinus (*see also* Sinusitis) 473.9
Trousseau's syndrome (thrombophlebitis migrans) 453.1
Truancy, childhood — *see also* Disturbance, conduct
  socialized 312.2 ☑
  undersocialized, unsocialized 312.1 ☑
Truncus
  arteriosus (persistent) 745.0
  common 745.0
  communis 745.0
Trunk — *see* condition
Trychophytide — *see* Dermatophytosis
Trypanosoma infestation — *see* Trypanosomiasis
Trypanosomiasis 086.9
  with meningoencephalitis 086.9 [323.2]
  African 086.5
    due to Trypanosoma 086.5
      gambiense 086.3
      rhodesiense 086.4
  American 086.2
    with
      heart involvement 086.0
      other organ involvement 086.1
    without mention of organ involvement 086.2
  Brazilian — *see* Trypanosomiasis, American
  Chagas' — *see* Trypanosomiasis, American
  due to Trypanosoma
    cruzi — *see* Trypanosomiasis, American
    gambiense 086.3
    rhodesiense 086.4
  gambiensis, Gambian 086.3
  North American — *see* Trypanosomiasis, American
  rhodesiensis, Rhodesian 086.4
  South American — *see* Trypanosomiasis, American
T-shaped incisors 520.2
Tsutsugamushi fever 081.2
Tubercle — *see also* Tuberculosis
  brain, solitary 013.2 ☑
  Darwin's 744.29
  epithelioid noncaseating 135
  Ghon, primary infection 010.0 ☑
Tuberculid, tuberculide (indurating) (lichenoid) (miliary) (papulonecrotic) (primary) (skin) (subcutaneous) — *see also* Tuberculosis 017.0 ☑
Tuberculoma — *see also* Tuberculosis
  brain (any part) 013.2 ☑
  meninges (cerebral) (spinal) 013.1 ☑
  spinal cord 013.4 ☑

Tuberculosis, tubercular, tuberculous (calcification) (calcified) (caseous) (chromogenic acid-fast bacilli) (congenital) (degeneration) (disease) (fibrocaseous) (fistula) (gangrene) (interstitial) (isolated circumscribed lesions) (necrosis) (parenchymatous) (ulcerative) 011.9 ☑

> *Note* — *Use the following fifth-digit subclassification with categories 010–018:*
>
> 0   *unspecified*
>
> 1   *bacteriological or histological examination not done*
>
> 2   *bacteriological or histological examination unknown (at present)*
>
> 3   *tubercle bacilli found (in sputum) by microscopy*
>
> 4   *tubercle bacilli not found (in sputum) by microscopy, but found by bacterial culture*
>
> 5   *tubercle bacilli not found by bacteriological examination, but tuberculosis confirmed histologically*
>
> 6   *tubercle bacilli not found by bacteriological or histological examination, but tuberculosis confirmed by other methods [inoculation of animals]*
>
> *For tuberculous conditions specified as late effects or sequelae, see category 137.*

  abdomen 014.8 ☑
    lymph gland 014.8 ☑
  abscess 011.9 ☑
    arm 017.9 ☑
    bone (*see also* Osteomyelitis, due to, tuberculosis) 015.9 ☑ [730.8]
      hip 015.1 ☑ [730.85]
      knee 015.2 ☑ [730.86]
      sacrum 015.0 ☑ [730.88]
      specified site NEC 015.7 ☑ [730.88]
      spinal 015.0 ☑ [730.88]
      vertebra 015.0 ☑ [730.88]
    brain 013.3 ☑
    breast 017.9 ☑
    Cowper's gland 016.5 ☑
    dura (mater) 013.8 ☑
      brain 013.3 ☑
      spinal cord 013.5 ☑
    epidural 013.8 ☑
      brain 013.3 ☑
      spinal cord 013.5 ☑
    frontal sinus — *see* Tuberculosis, sinus
    genital organs NEC 016.9 ☑
      female 016.7 ☑
      male 016.5 ☑
    genitourinary NEC 016.9 ☑
    gland (lymphatic) — *see* Tuberculosis, lymph gland
    hip 015.1 ☑
    iliopsoas 015.0 ☑ [730.88]
    intestine 014.8 ☑
    ischiorectal 014.8 ☑
    joint 015.9 ☑
      hip 015.1 ☑
      knee 015.2 ☑
      specified joint NEC 015.8 ☑
      vertebral 015.0 ☑ [730.88]
    kidney 016.0 ☑ [590.81]
    knee 015.2 ☑
    lumbar 015.0 ☑ [730.88]
    lung 011.2 ☑
      primary, progressive 010.8 ☑
    meninges (cerebral) (spinal) 013.0 ☑
    pelvic 016.9 ☑
      female 016.7 ☑
      male 016.5 ☑
    perianal 014.8 ☑
      fistula 014.8 ☑
    perinephritic 016.0 ☑ [590.81]

Tuberculosis, tubercular, tuberculous — *continued*
  abscess — *continued*
    perineum 017.9 ☑
    perirectal 014.8 ☑
    psoas 015.0 ☑ [730.88]
    rectum 014.8 ☑
    retropharyngeal 012.8 ☑
    sacrum 015.0 ☑ [730.88]
    scrofulous 017.2 ☑
    scrotum 016.5 ☑
    skin 017.0 ☑
      primary 017.0 ☑
    spinal cord 013.5 ☑
    spine or vertebra (column) 015.0 ☑ [730.88]
    strumous 017.2 ☑
    subdiaphragmatic 014.8 ☑
    testis 016.5 ☑
    thigh 017.9 ☑
    urinary 016.3 ☑
      kidney 016.0 ☑ [590.81]
    uterus 016.7 ☑
  accessory sinus — *see* Tuberculosis, sinus
  Addison's disease 017.6 ☑
  adenitis (*see also* Tuberculosis, lymph gland) 017.2 ☑
  adenoids 012.8 ☑
  adenopathy (*see also* Tuberculosis, lymph gland) 017.2 ☑
    tracheobronchial 012.1 ☑
      primary progressive 010.8 ☑
  adherent pericardium 017.9 ☑ [420.0]
  adnexa (uteri) 016.7 ☑
  adrenal (capsule) (gland) 017.6 ☑
  air passage NEC 012.8 ☑
  alimentary canal 014.8 ☑
  anemia 017.9 ☑
  ankle (joint) 015.8 ☑
    bone 015.5 ☑ [730.87]
  anus 014.8 ☑
  apex (*see also* Tuberculosis, pulmonary) 011.9 ☑
  apical (*see also* Tuberculosis, pulmonary) 011.9 ☑
  appendicitis 014.8 ☑
  appendix 014.8 ☑
  arachnoid 013.0 ☑
  artery 017.9 ☑
  arthritis (chronic) (synovial) 015.9 ☑ [711.40]
    ankle 015.8 ☑ [730.87]
    hip 015.1 ☑ [711.45]
    knee 015.2 ☑ [711.46]
    specified site NEC 015.8 ☑ [711.48]
    spine or vertebra (column) 015.0 ☑ [720.81]
    wrist 015.8 ☑ [730.83]
  articular — *see* Tuberculosis, joint
  ascites 014.0 ☑
  asthma (*see also* Tuberculosis, pulmonary) 011.9 ☑
  axilla, axillary 017.2 ☑
    gland 017.2 ☑
  bilateral (*see also* Tuberculosis, pulmonary) 011.9 ☑
  bladder 016.1 ☑
  bone (*see also* Osteomyelitis, due to, tuberculosis) 015.9 ☑ [730.8] ☑
    hip 015.1 ☑ [730.85]
    knee 015.2 ☑ [730.86]
    limb NEC 015.5 ☑ [730.88]
    sacrum 015.0 ☑ [730.88]
    specified site NEC 015.7 ☑ [730.88]
    spinal or vertebral column 015.0 ☑ [730.88]
  bowel 014.8 ☑
    miliary 018.9 ☑
  brain 013.2 ☑
  breast 017.9 ☑
  broad ligament 016.7 ☑
  bronchi, bronchial, bronchus 011.3 ☑
    ectasia, ectasis 011.5 ☑
    fistula 011.3 ☑

☑ **Additional Digit Required** — Refer to the Tabular List for Digit Selection   ▽ **Subterms under main terms may continue to next column or page**

328   2014 ICD-9-CM

Tuberculosis, tubercular, tuberculous — *continued*

bronchi, bronchial, bronchus — *continued*
  fistula — *continued*
    primary, progressive 010.8 ☑
    gland 012.1 ☑
      primary, progressive 010.8 ☑
    isolated 012.2 ☑
    lymph gland or node 012.1 ☑
      primary, progressive 010.8 ☑
bronchiectasis 011.5 ☑
bronchitis 011.3 ☑
bronchopleural 012.0 ☑
bronchopneumonia, bronchopneumonic 011.6 ☑
bronchorrhagia 011.3 ☑
bronchotracheal 011.3 ☑
  isolated 012.2 ☑
bronchus — *see* Tuberculosis, bronchi
bronze disease (Addison's) 017.6 ☑
buccal cavity 017.9 ☑
bulbourethral gland 016.5 ☑
bursa (*see also* Tuberculosis, joint) 015.9 ☑
cachexia NEC (*see also* Tuberculosis, pulmonary) 011.9 ☑
cardiomyopathy 017.9 ☑ *[425.8]*
caries (*see also* Tuberculosis, bone) 015.9 ☑ *[730.8]*
cartilage (*see also* Tuberculosis, bone) 015.9 ☑ *[730.8]*
  intervertebral 015.0 ☑ *[730.88]*
catarrhal (*see also* Tuberculosis, pulmonary) 011.9 ☑
cecum 014.8 ☑
cellular tissue (primary) 017.0 ☑
cellulitis (primary) 017.0 ☑
central nervous system 013.9 ☑
  specified site NEC 013.8 ☑
cerebellum (current) 013.2 ☑
cerebral (current) 013.2 ☑
  meninges 013.0 ☑
cerebrospinal 013.6 ☑
  meninges 013.0 ☑
cerebrum (current) 013.2 ☑
cervical 017.2 ☑
  gland 017.2 ☑
  lymph nodes 017.2 ☑
cervicitis (uteri) 016.7 ☑
cervix 016.7 ☑
chest (*see also* Tuberculosis, pulmonary) 011.9 ☑
childhood type or first infection 010.0 ☑
choroid 017.3 ☑ *[363.13]*
choroiditis 017.3 ☑ *[363.13]*
ciliary body 017.3 ☑ *[364.11]*
colitis 014.8 ☑
colliers' 011.4 ☑
colliquativa (primary) 017.0 ☑
colon 014.8 ☑
  ulceration 014.8 ☑
complex, primary 010.0 ☑
complicating pregnancy, childbirth, or puerperium 647.3 ☑
  affecting fetus or newborn 760.2
congenital 771.2
conjunctiva 017.3 ☑ *[370.31]*
connective tissue 017.9 ☑
  bone — *see* Tuberculosis, bone
contact V01.1
converter (tuberculin skin test) (without disease) 795.51
cornea (ulcer) 017.3 ☑ *[370.31]*
Cowper's gland 016.5 ☑
coxae 015.1 ☑ *[730.85]*
coxalgia 015.1 ☑ *[730.85]*
cul-de-sac of Douglas 014.8 ☑
curvature, spine 015.0 ☑ *[737.40]*
cutis (colliquativa) (primary) 017.0 ☑
cystitis 016.1 ☑
cyst, ovary 016.6 ☑
dacryocystitis 017.3 ☑ *[375.32]*
dactylitis 015.5 ☑
diarrhea 014.8 ☑

diffuse (*see also* Tuberculosis, miliary) 018.9 ☑
  lung — *see* Tuberculosis, pulmonary
  meninges 013.0 ☑
digestive tract 014.8 ☑
disseminated (*see also* Tuberculosis, miliary) 018.9 ☑
  meninges 013.0 ☑
duodenum 014.8 ☑
dura (mater) 013.9 ☑
  abscess 013.8 ☑
    cerebral 013.3 ☑
    spinal 013.5 ☑
dysentery 014.8 ☑
ear (inner) (middle) 017.4 ☑
  bone 015.6 ☑
  external (primary) 017.0 ☑
  skin (primary) 017.0 ☑
elbow 015.8 ☑
emphysema — *see* Tuberculosis, pulmonary
empyema 012.0 ☑
encephalitis 013.6 ☑
endarteritis 017.9 ☑
endocarditis (any valve) 017.9 ☑ *[424.91]*
endocardium (any valve) 017.9 ☑ *[424.91]*
endocrine glands NEC 017.9 ☑
endometrium 016.7 ☑
enteric, enterica 014.8 ☑
enteritis 014.8 ☑
enterocolitis 014.8 ☑
epididymis 016.4 ☑
epididymitis 016.4 ☑
epidural abscess 013.8 ☑
  brain 013.3 ☑
  spinal cord 013.5 ☑
epiglottis 012.3 ☑
episcleritis 017.3 ☑ *[379.00]*
erythema (induratum) (nodosum) (primary) 017.1 ☑
esophagus 017.8 ☑
Eustachian tube 017.4 ☑
exposure to V01.1
exudative 012.0 ☑
  primary, progressive 010.1 ☑
eye 017.3 ☑
eyelid (primary) 017.0 ☑
  lupus 017.0 ☑ *[373.4]*
fallopian tube 016.6 ☑
fascia 017.9 ☑
fauces 012.8 ☑
finger 017.9 ☑
first infection 010.0 ☑
fistula, perirectal 014.8 ☑
Florida 011.6 ☑
foot 017.9 ☑
funnel pelvis 137.3
gallbladder 017.9 ☑
galloping (*see also* Tuberculosis, pulmonary) 011.9 ☑
ganglionic 015.9 ☑
gastritis 017.9 ☑
gastrocolic fistula 014.8 ☑
gastroenteritis 014.8 ☑
gastrointestinal tract 014.8 ☑
general, generalized 018.9 ☑
  acute 018.0 ☑
  chronic 018.8 ☑
genital organs NEC 016.9 ☑
  female 016.7 ☑
  male 016.5 ☑
genitourinary NEC 016.9 ☑
genu 015.2 ☑
glandulae suprarenalis 017.6 ☑
glandular, general 017.2 ☑
glottis 012.3 ☑
grinders' 011.4 ☑
groin 017.2 ☑
gum 017.9 ☑
hand 017.9 ☑
heart 017.9 ☑ *[425.8]*
hematogenous — *see* Tuberculosis, miliary

hemoptysis (*see also* Tuberculosis, pulmonary) 011.9 ☑
hemorrhage NEC (*see also* Tuberculosis, pulmonary) 011.9 ☑
hemothorax 012.0 ☑
hepatitis 017.9 ☑
hilar lymph nodes 012.1 ☑
  primary, progressive 010.8 ☑
hip (disease) (joint) 015.1 ☑
  bone 015.1 ☑ *[730.85]*
hydrocephalus 013.8 ☑
hydropneumothorax 012.0 ☑
hydrothorax 012.0 ☑
hypoadrenalism 017.6 ☑
hypopharynx 012.8 ☑
ileocecal (hyperplastic) 014.8 ☑
ileocolitis 014.8 ☑
ileum 014.8 ☑
iliac spine (superior) 015.0 ☑ *[730.88]*
incipient NEC (*see also* Tuberculosis, pulmonary) 011.9 ☑
indurativa (primary) 017.1 ☑
infantile 010.0 ☑
infection NEC 011.9 ☑
  without clinical manifestation 010.0 ☑
infraclavicular gland 017.2 ☑
inguinal gland 017.2 ☑
inguinalis 017.2 ☑
intestine (any part) 014.8 ☑
iris 017.3 ☑ *[364.11]*
iritis 017.3 ☑ *[364.11]*
ischiorectal 014.8 ☑
jaw 015.7 ☑ *[730.88]*
jejunum 014.8 ☑
joint 015.9 ☑
  hip 015.1 ☑
  knee 015.2 ☑
  specified site NEC 015.8 ☑
  vertebral 015.0 ☑ *[730.88]*
keratitis 017.3 ☑ *[370.31]*
  interstitial 017.3 ☑ *[370.59]*
keratoconjunctivitis 017.3 ☑ *[370.31]*
kidney 016.0 ☑
knee (joint) 015.2 ☑
kyphoscoliosis 015.0 ☑ *[737.43]*
kyphosis 015.0 ☑ *[737.41]*
lacrimal apparatus, gland 017.3 ☑
laryngitis 012.3 ☑
larynx 012.3 ☑
latent 795.51
leptomeninges, leptomeningitis (cerebral) (spinal) 013.0 ☑
lichenoides (primary) 017.0 ☑
linguae 017.9 ☑
lip 017.9 ☑
liver 017.9 ☑
lordosis 015.0 ☑ *[737.42]*
lung — *see* Tuberculosis, pulmonary
luposa 017.0 ☑
  eyelid 017.0 ☑ *[373.4]*
lymphadenitis — *see* Tuberculosis, lymph gland
lymphangitis — *see* Tuberculosis, lymph gland
lymphatic (gland) (vessel) — *see* Tuberculosis, lymph gland
lymph gland or node (peripheral) 017.2 ☑
  abdomen 014.8 ☑
  bronchial 012.1 ☑
    primary, progressive 010.8 ☑
  cervical 017.2 ☑
  hilar 012.1 ☑
    primary, progressive 010.8 ☑
  intrathoracic 012.1 ☑
    primary, progressive 010.8 ☑
  mediastinal 012.1 ☑
    primary, progressive 010.8 ☑
  mesenteric 014.8 ☑
  peripheral 017.2 ☑
  retroperitoneal 014.8 ☑
  tracheobronchial 012.1 ☑

lymph gland or node — *continued*
  tracheobronchial — *continued*
    primary, progressive 010.8 ☑
malignant NEC (*see also* Tuberculosis, pulmonary) 011.9 ☑
mammary gland 017.9 ☑
marasmus NEC (*see also* Tuberculosis, pulmonary) 011.9 ☑
mastoiditis 015.6 ☑
maternal, affecting fetus or newborn 760.2
mediastinal (lymph) gland or node 012.1 ☑
  primary, progressive 010.8 ☑
mediastinitis 012.8 ☑
  primary, progressive 010.8 ☑
mediastinopericarditis 017.9 ☑ *[420.0]*
mediastinum 012.8 ☑
  primary, progressive 010.8 ☑
medulla 013.9 ☑
  brain 013.2 ☑
  spinal cord 013.4 ☑
melanosis, Addisonian 017.6 ☑
membrane, brain 013.0 ☑
meninges (cerebral) (spinal) 013.0 ☑
meningitis (basilar) (brain) (cerebral) (cerebrospinal) (spinal) 013.0 ☑
meningoencephalitis 013.0 ☑
mesentery, mesenteric 014.8 ☑
  lymph gland or node 014.8 ☑
miliary (any site) 018.9 ☑
  acute 018.0 ☑
  chronic 018.8 ☑
  specified type NEC 018.8 ☑
millstone makers' 011.4 ☑
miners' 011.4 ☑
moulders' 011.4 ☑
mouth 017.9 ☑
multiple 018.9 ☑
  acute 018.0 ☑
  chronic 018.8 ☑
muscle 017.9 ☑
myelitis 013.6 ☑
myocarditis 017.9 ☑ *[422.0]*
myocardium 017.9 ☑ *[422.0]*
nasal (passage) (sinus) 012.8 ☑
nasopharynx 012.8 ☑
neck gland 017.2 ☑
nephritis 016.0 ☑ *[583.81]*
nerve 017.9 ☑
nose (septum) 012.8 ☑
ocular 017.3 ☑
old NEC 137.0
  without residuals V12.01
omentum 014.8 ☑
oophoritis (acute) (chronic) 016.6 ☑
optic 017.3 ☑ *[377.39]*
  nerve trunk 017.3 ☑ *[377.39]*
  papilla, papillae 017.3 ☑ *[377.39]*
orbit 017.3 ☑
orchitis 016.5 ☑ *[608.81]*
organ, specified NEC 017.9 ☑
orificialis (primary) 017.0 ☑
osseous (*see also* Tuberculosis, bone) 015.9 ☑ *[730.8]*
osteitis (*see also* Tuberculosis, bone) 015.9 ☑ *[730.8]*
osteomyelitis (*see also* Tuberculosis, bone) 015.9 ☑ *[730.8]*
otitis (media) 017.4 ☑
ovaritis (acute) (chronic) 016.6 ☑
ovary (acute) (chronic) 016.6 ☑
oviducts (acute) (chronic) 016.6 ☑
pachymeningitis 013.0 ☑
palate (soft) 017.9 ☑
pancreas 017.9 ☑
papulonecrotic (primary) 017.0 ☑
parathyroid glands 017.9 ☑
paronychia (primary) 017.0 ☑
parotid gland or region 017.9 ☑
pelvic organ NEC 016.9 ☑
  female 016.7 ☑
  male 016.5 ☑

☑ **Additional Digit Required** — Refer to the Tabular List for Digit Selection
▽ Subterms under main terms may continue to next column or page
2014 ICD-9-CM
329

Tuberculosis, tubercular, tuberculous —
continued

pelvis (bony) 015.7 ☑ *[730.85]*
penis 016.5 ☑
peribronchitis 011.3 ☑
pericarditis 017.9 ☑ *[420.0]*
pericardium 017.9 ☑ *[420.0]*
perichondritis, larynx 012.3 ☑
perineum 017.9 ☑
periostitis (*see also* Tuberculosis, bone)
    015.9 ☑ *[730.8]*
periphlebitis 017.9 ☑
    eye vessel 017.3 ☑ *[362.18]*
    retina 017.3 ☑ *[362.18]*
perirectal fistula 014.8 ☑
peritoneal gland 014.8 ☑
peritoneum 014.0 ☑
peritonitis 014.0 ☑
pernicious NEC (*see also* Tuberculosis, pul-
    monary) 011.9 ☑
pharyngitis 012.8 ☑
pharynx 012.8 ☑
phlyctenulosis (conjunctiva)
    017.3 ☑ *[370.31]*
phthisis NEC (*see also* Tuberculosis, pul-
    monary) 011.9 ☑
pituitary gland 017.9 ☑
placenta 016.7 ☑
pleura, pleural, pleurisy, pleuritis (fibrinous)
    (obliterative) (purulent) (simple
    plastic) (with effusion) 012.0 ☑
    primary, progressive 010.1 ☑
pneumonia, pneumonic 011.6 ☑
pneumothorax 011.7 ☑
polyserositis 018.9 ☑
    acute 018.0 ☑
    chronic 018.8 ☑
potters' 011.4 ☑
prepuce 016.5 ☑
primary 010.9 ☑
    complex 010.0 ☑
    complicated 010.8 ☑
        with pleurisy or effusion 010.1 ☑
    progressive 010.8 ☑
        with pleurisy or effusion 010.1 ☑
    skin 017.0 ☑
proctitis 014.8 ☑
prostate 016.5 ☑ *[601.4]*
prostatitis 016.5 ☑ *[601.4]*
pulmonaris (*see also* Tuberculosis, pul-
    monary) 011.9 ☑
pulmonary (artery) (incipient) (malignant)
    (multiple round foci) (pernicious)
    (reinfection stage) 011.9 ☑
    cavitated or with cavitation 011.2 ☑
        primary, progressive 010.8 ☑
    childhood type or first infection 010.0 ☑
    chromogenic acid-fast bacilli 795.39
    fibrosis or fibrotic 011.4 ☑
    infiltrative 011.0 ☑
        primary, progressive 010.9 ☑
    nodular 011.1 ☑
    specified NEC 011.8 ☑
    sputum positive only 795.39
    status following surgical collapse of lung
        NEC 011.9 ☑
pyelitis 016.0 ☑ *[590.81]*
pyelonephritis 016.0 ☑ *[590.81]*
pyemia — *see* Tuberculosis, miliary
pyonephrosis 016.0 ☑
pyopneumothorax 012.0 ☑
pyothorax 012.0 ☑
rectum (with abscess) 014.8 ☑
    fistula 014.8 ☑
reinfection stage (*see also* Tuberculosis,
    pulmonary) 011.9 ☑
renal 016.0 ☑
renis 016.0 ☑
reproductive organ 016.7 ☑
respiratory NEC (*see also* Tuberculosis, pul-
    monary) 011.9 ☑
    specified site NEC 012.8 ☑
retina 017.3 ☑ *[363.13]*

Tuberculosis, tubercular, tuberculous —
continued

retroperitoneal (lymph gland or node)
    014.8 ☑
    gland 014.8 ☑
retropharyngeal abscess 012.8 ☑
rheumatism 015.9 ☑
rhinitis 012.8 ☑
sacroiliac (joint) 015.8 ☑
sacrum 015.0 ☑ *[730.88]*
salivary gland 017.9 ☑
salpingitis (acute) (chronic) 016.6 ☑
sandblasters' 011.4 ☑
sclera 017.3 ☑ *[379.09]*
scoliosis 015.0 ☑ *[737.43]*
scrofulous 017.2 ☑
scrotum 016.5 ☑
seminal tract or vesicle 016.5 ☑ *[608.81]*
senile NEC (*see also* Tuberculosis, pul-
    monary) 011.9 ☑
septic NEC (*see also* Tuberculosis, miliary)
    018.9 ☑
shoulder 015.8 ☑
    blade 015.7 ☑ *[730.8]*
sigmoid 014.8 ☑
sinus (accessory) (nasal) 012.8 ☑
    bone 015.7 ☑ *[730.88]*
    epididymis 016.4 ☑
skeletal NEC (*see also* Osteomyelitis, due to
    tuberculosis) 015.9 ☑ *[730.8]*
skin (any site) (primary) 017.0 ☑
small intestine 014.8 ☑
soft palate 017.9 ☑
spermatic cord 016.5 ☑
spinal
    column 015.0 ☑ *[730.88]*
    cord 013.4 ☑
    disease 015.0 ☑ *[730.88]*
    medulla 013.4 ☑
    membrane 013.0 ☑
    meninges 013.0 ☑
spine 015.0 ☑ *[730.88]*
spleen 017.7 ☑
splenitis 017.7 ☑
spondylitis 015.0 ☑ *[720.81]*
spontaneous pneumothorax — *see* Tuber-
    culosis, pulmonary
sternoclavicular joint 015.8 ☑
stomach 017.9 ☑
stonemasons' 011.4 ☑
struma 017.2 ☑
subcutaneous tissue (cellular) (primary)
    017.0 ☑
subcutis (primary) 017.0 ☑
subdeltoid bursa 017.9 ☑
submaxillary 017.9 ☑
    region 017.9 ☑
supraclavicular gland 017.2 ☑
suprarenal (capsule) (gland) 017.6 ☑
swelling, joint (*see also* Tuberculosis, joint)
    015.9 ☑
symphysis pubis 015.7 ☑ *[730.88]*
synovitis 015.9 ☑ *[727.01]*
    hip 015.1 ☑ *[727.01]*
    knee 015.2 ☑ *[727.01]*
    specified site NEC 015.8 ☑ *[727.01]*
    spine or vertebra 015.0 ☑ *[727.01]*
systemic — *see* Tuberculosis, miliary
tarsitis (eyelid) 017.0 ☑ *[373.4]*
    ankle (bone) 015.5 ☑ *[730.87]*
tendon (sheath) — *see* Tuberculosis,
    tenosynovitis
tenosynovitis 015.9 ☑ *[727.01]*
    hip 015.1 ☑ *[727.01]*
    knee 015.2 ☑ *[727.01]*
    specified site NEC 015.8 ☑ *[727.01]*
    spine or vertebra 015.0 ☑ *[727.01]*
testis 016.5 ☑ *[608.81]*
throat 012.8 ☑
thymus gland 017.9 ☑
thyroid gland 017.5 ☑
toe 017.9 ☑
tongue 017.9 ☑

Tuberculosis, tubercular, tuberculous —
continued

tonsil (lingual) 012.8 ☑
tonsillitis 012.8 ☑
trachea, tracheal 012.8 ☑
    gland 012.1 ☑
        primary, progressive 010.8 ☑
    isolated 012.2 ☑
tracheobronchial 011.3 ☑
    glandular 012.1 ☑
        primary, progressive 010.8 ☑
    isolated 012.2 ☑
    lymph gland or node 012.1 ☑
        primary, progressive 010.8 ☑
tubal 016.6 ☑
tunica vaginalis 016.5 ☑
typhlitis 014.8 ☑
ulcer (primary) (skin) 017.0 ☑
    bowel or intestine 014.8 ☑
    specified site NEC — *see* Tuberculosis,
        by site
    unspecified site — *see* Tuberculosis, pul-
        monary
ureter 016.2 ☑
urethra, urethral 016.3 ☑
urinary organ or tract 016.3 ☑
    kidney 016.0 ☑
uterus 016.7 ☑
uveal tract 017.3 ☑ *[363.13]*
uvula 017.9 ☑
vaccination, prophylactic (against) V03.2
vagina 016.7 ☑
vas deferens 016.5 ☑
vein 017.9 ☑
verruca (primary) 017.0 ☑
verrucosa (cutis) (primary) 017.0 ☑
vertebra (column) 015.0 ☑ *[730.88]*
vesiculitis 016.5 ☑ *[608.81]*
viscera NEC 014.8 ☑
vulva 016.7 ☑ *[616.51]*
wrist (joint) 015.8 ☑
    bone 015.5 ☑ *[730.83]*

Tuberculum
auriculae 744.29
occlusal 520.2
paramolare 520.2
Tuberosity
jaw, excessive 524.07
maxillary, entire 524.07
Tuberous sclerosis (brain) 759.5
Tube, tubal, tubular — *see also* condition
ligation, admission for V25.2
Tubo-ovarian — *see* condition
Tuboplasty, after previous sterilization V26.0
Tubotympanitis 381.10
Tularemia 021.9
    with
        conjunctivitis 021.3
        pneumonia 021.2
    bronchopneumonic 021.2
    conjunctivitis 021.3
    cryptogenic 021.1
    disseminated 021.8
    enteric 021.1
    generalized 021.8
    glandular 021.8
    intestinal 021.1
    oculoglandular 021.3
    ophthalmic 021.3
    pneumonia 021.2
    pulmonary 021.2
    specified NEC 021.8
    typhoidal 021.1
    ulceroglandular 021.0
    vaccination, prophylactic (against) V03.4
Tularensis conjunctivitis 021.3
Tumefaction — *see also* Swelling
    liver (*see also* Hypertrophy, liver) 789.1
Tumor (M8000/1) — *see also* Neoplasm, by site,
    unspecified nature
Abrikossov's (M9580/0) (*see also* Neoplasm,
    connective tissue, benign)
    malignant (M9580/3) — *see* Neoplasm,
        connective tissue, malignant

Tumor — *see also* Neoplasm, by site,
    unspecified nature — *continued*
acinar cell (M8550/1) — *see* Neoplasm, by
    site, uncertain behavior
acinic cell (M8550/1) — *see* Neoplasm, by
    site, uncertain behavior
adenomatoid (M9054/0) (*see also* Neoplasm,
    by site, benign)
    odontogenic (M9300/0) 213.1
        upper jaw (bone) 213.0
adnexal (skin) (M8390/0) — *see* Neoplasm,
    skin, benign
adrenal
    cortical (benign) (M8370/0) 227.0
        malignant (M8370/3) 194.0
    rest (M8671/0) — *see* Neoplasm, by site,
        benign
alpha cell (M8152/0)
    malignant (M8152/3)
        pancreas 157.4
        specified site NEC — *see* Neoplasm,
            by site, malignant
        unspecified site 157.4
    pancreas 211.7
    specified site NEC — *see* Neoplasm, by
        site, benign
    unspecified site 211.7
aneurysmal (*see also* Aneurysm) 442.9
aortic body (M8691/1) 237.3
    malignant (M8691/3) 194.6
argentaffin (M8241/1) — *see* Neoplasm, by
    site, uncertain behavior
basal cell (M8090/1) (*see also* Neoplasm,
    skin, uncertain behavior)
benign (M8000/0) — *see* Neoplasm, by site,
    benign
beta cell (M8151/0)
    malignant (M8151/3)
        pancreas 157.4
        specified site — *see* Neoplasm, by
            site, malignant
        unspecified site 157.4
    pancreas 211.7
    specified site NEC — *see* Neoplasm, by
        site, benign
    unspecified site 211.7
blood — *see* Hematoma
Brenner (M9000/0) 220
    borderline malignancy (M9000/1) 236.2
    malignant (M9000/3) 183.0
    proliferating (M9000/1) 236.2
Brooke's (M8100/0) — *see* Neoplasm, skin,
    benign
brown fat (M8880/0) — *see* Lipoma, by site
Burkitt's (M9750/3) 200.2 ☑
calcifying epithelial odontogenic (M9340/0)
    213.1
    upper jaw (bone) 213.0
carcinoid (M8240/1) 209.60
    benign 209.60
        appendix 209.51
        ascending colon 209.53
        bronchus 209.61
        cecum 209.52
        colon 209.50
        descending colon 209.55
        duodenum 209.41
        foregut 209.65
        hindgut 209.67
        ileum 209.43
        jejunum 209.42
        kidney 209.64
        large intestine 209.50
        lung 209.61
        midgut 209.66
        rectum 209.57
        sigmoid colon 209.56
        small intestine 209.40
        specified NEC 209.69
        stomach 209.63
        thymus 209.62
        transverse colon 209.54
    malignant (of) 209.20
        appendix 209.11
        ascending colon 209.13
        bronchus 209.21

Tumor — *see also* Neoplasm, by site, unspecified nature — *continued*
carcinoid — *continued*
  malignant — *continued*
    cecum 209.12
    colon 209.10
    descending colon 209.15
    duodenum 209.01
    foregut 209.25
    hindgut 209.27
    ileum 209.03
    jejunum 209.02
    kidney 209.24
    large intestine 209.10
    lung 209.21
    midgut 209.26
    rectum 209.17
    sigmoid colon 209.16
    small intestine 209.00
    specified NEC 209.29
    stomach 209.23
    thymus 209.22
    transverse colon 209.14
  secondary — *see* Tumor, neuroendocrine, secondary
carotid body (M8692/1) 237.3
  malignant (M8692/3) 194.5
Castleman's (mediastinal lymph node hyperplasia) 785.6
cells (M8001/1) (*see also* Neoplasm, by site, unspecified nature)
  benign (M8001/0) — *see* Neoplasm, by site, benign
  malignant (M8001/3) — *see* Neoplasm, by site, malignant
  uncertain whether benign or malignant (M8001/1) — *see* Neoplasm, by site, uncertain nature
cervix
  in pregnancy or childbirth 654.6 ☑
    affecting fetus or newborn 763.89
    causing obstructed labor 660.2 ☑
      affecting fetus or newborn 763.1
chondromatous giant cell (M9230/0) — *see* Neoplasm, bone, benign
chromaffin (M8700/0) (*see also* Neoplasm, by site, benign)
  malignant (M8700/3) — *see* Neoplasm, by site, malignant
Cock's peculiar 706.2
Codman's (benign chondroblastoma) (M9230/0) — *see* Neoplasm, bone, benign
dentigerous, mixed (M9282/0) 213.1
  upper jaw (bone) 213.0
dermoid (M9084/0) — *see* Neoplasm, by site, benign
  with malignant transformation (M9084/3) 183.0
desmoid (extra-abdominal) (M8821/1) (*see also* Neoplasm, connective tissue, uncertain behavior)
  abdominal (M8822/1) — *see* Neoplasm, connective tissue, uncertain behavior
embryonal (mixed) (M9080/1) (*see also* Neoplasm, by site, uncertain behavior)
  liver (M9080/3) 155.0
endodermal sinus (M9071/3)
  specified site — *see* Neoplasm, by site, malignant
  unspecified site
    female 183.0
    male 186.9
epithelial
  benign (M8010/0) — *see* Neoplasm, by site, benign
  malignant (M8010/3) — *see* Neoplasm, by site, malignant
Ewing's (M9260/3) — *see* Neoplasm, bone, malignant
fatty — *see* Lipoma
fetal, causing disproportion 653.7 ☑
  causing obstructed labor 660.1 ☑
fibroid (M8890/0) — *see* Leiomyoma

Tumor — *see also* Neoplasm, by site, unspecified nature — *continued*
G cell (M8153/1)
  malignant (M8153/3)
    pancreas 157.4
    specified site NEC — *see* Neoplasm, by site, malignant
    unspecified site 157.4
  specified site — *see* Neoplasm, by site, uncertain behavior
  unspecified site 235.5
giant cell (type) (M8003/1) (*see also* Neoplasm, by site, unspecified nature)
  bone (M9250/1) 238.0
    malignant (M9250/3) — *see* Neoplasm, bone, malignant
  chondromatous (M9230/0) — *see* Neoplasm, bone, benign
  malignant (M8003/3) — *see* Neoplasm, by site, malignant
  peripheral (gingiva) 523.8
  soft parts (M9251/1) (*see also* Neoplasm, connective tissue, uncertain behavior)
    malignant (M9251/3) — *see* Neoplasm, connective tissue, malignant
  tendon sheath 727.02
glomus (M8711/0) (*see also* Hemangioma, by site)
  jugulare (M8690/1) 237.3
    malignant (M8690/3) 194.6
gonadal stromal (M8590/1) — *see* Neoplasm, by site, uncertain behavior
granular cell (M9580/0) (*see also* Neoplasm, connective tissue, benign)
  malignant (M9580/3) — *see* Neoplasm, connective tissue, malignant
granulosa cell (M8620/1) 236.2
  malignant (M8620/3) 183.0
granulosa cell-theca cell (M8621/1) 236.2
  malignant (M8621/3) 183.0
Grawitz's (hypernephroma) (M8312/3) 189.0
hazard-crile (M8350/3) 193
hemorrhoidal — *see* Hemorrhoids
hilar cell (M8660/0) 220
Hürthle cell (benign) (M8290/0) 226
  malignant (M8290/3) 193
hydatid (*see also* Echinococcus) 122.9
hypernephroid (M8311/1) (*see also* Neoplasm, by site, uncertain behavior)
interstitial cell (M8650/1) (*see also* Neoplasm, by site, uncertain behavior)
  benign (M8650/0) — *see* Neoplasm, by site, benign
  malignant (M8650/3) — *see* Neoplasm, by site, malignant
islet cell (M8150/0)
  malignant (M8150/3)
    pancreas 157.4
    specified site — *see* Neoplasm, by site, malignant
    unspecified site 157.4
  pancreas 211.7
  specified site NEC — *see* Neoplasm, by site, benign
  unspecified site 211.7
juxtaglomerular (M8361/1) 236.91
Krukenberg's (M8490/6) 198.6
Leydig cell (M8650/1)
  benign (M8650/0)
    specified site — *see* Neoplasm, by site, benign
    unspecified site
      female 220
      male 222.0
  malignant (M8650/3)
    specified site — *see* Neoplasm, by site, malignant
    unspecified site
      female 183.0
      male 186.9
  specified site — *see* Neoplasm, by site, uncertain behavior
  unspecified site
    female 236.2

Tumor — *see also* Neoplasm, by site, unspecified nature — *continued*
Leydig cell — *continued*
  unspecified site — *continued*
    male 236.4
lipid cell, ovary (M8670/0) 220
lipoid cell, ovary (M8670/0) 220
lymphomatous, benign (M9590/0) (*see also* Neoplasm, by site, benign)
lysis syndrome (following antineoplastic drug therapy) (spontaneous) 277.88
Malherbe's (M8110/0) — *see* Neoplasm, skin, benign
malignant (M8000/3) (*see also* Neoplasm, by site, malignant)
  fusiform cell (type) (M8004/3) — *see* Neoplasm, by site, malignant
  giant cell (type) (M8003/3) — *see* Neoplasm, by site, malignant
  mixed NEC (M8940/3) — *see* Neoplasm, by site, malignant
  small cell (type) (M8002/3) — *see* Neoplasm, by site, malignant
  spindle cell (type) (M8004/3) — *see* Neoplasm, by site, malignant
mast cell (M9740/1) 238.5
  malignant (M9740/3) 202.6 ☑
melanotic, neuroectodermal (M9363/0) — *see* Neoplasm, by site, benign
Merkel cell — *see* Carcinoma, Merkel cell
mesenchymal
  malignant (M8800/3) — *see* Neoplasm, connective tissue, malignant
  mixed (M8990/1) — *see* Neoplasm, connective tissue, uncertain behavior
mesodermal, mixed (M8951/3) — *see* Neoplasm, by site, malignant
  liver 155.0
mesonephric (M9110/1) (*see also* Neoplasm, by site, uncertain behavior)
  malignant (M9110/3) — *see* Neoplasm, by site, malignant
metastatic
  from specified site (M8000/3) — *see* Neoplasm, by site, malignant
  to specified site (M8000/6) — *see* Neoplasm, by site, malignant, secondary
mixed NEC (M8940/0) (*see also* Neoplasm, by site, benign)
  malignant (M8940/3) — *see* Neoplasm, by site, malignant
mucocarcinoid, malignant (M8243/3) — *see* Neoplasm, by site, malignant
mucoepidermoid (M8430/1) — *see* Neoplasm, by site, uncertain behavior
Müllerian, mixed (M8950/3) — *see* Neoplasm, by site, malignant
myoepithelial (M8982/0) — *see* Neoplasm, by site, benign
neuroendocrine 209.60
  malignant poorly differentiated 209.30
  secondary 209.70
    bone 209.73
    distant lymph nodes 209.71
    liver 209.72
    peritoneum 209.74
    site specified NEC 209.79
neurogenic olfactory (M9520/3) 160.0
nonencapsulated sclerosing (M8350/3) 193
odontogenic (M9270/1) 238.0
  adenomatoid (M9300/0) 213.1
    upper jaw (bone) 213.0
  benign (M9270/0) 213.1
    upper jaw (bone) 213.0
  calcifying epithelial (M9340/0) 213.1
    upper jaw (bone) 213.0
  malignant (M9270/3) 170.1
    upper jaw (bone) 170.0
  squamous (M9312/0) 213.1
    upper jaw (bone) 213.0
ovarian stromal (M8590/1) 236.2
ovary
  in pregnancy or childbirth 654.4 ☑
    affecting fetus or newborn 763.89

Tumor — *see also* Neoplasm, by site, unspecified nature — *continued*
ovary — *continued*
  in pregnancy or childbirth — *continued*
    causing obstructed labor 660.2 ☑
      affecting fetus or newborn 763.1
pacinian (M9507/0) — *see* Neoplasm, skin, benign
Pancoast's (M8010/3) 162.3
papillary — *see* Papilloma
pelvic, in pregnancy or childbirth 654.9 ☑
  affecting fetus or newborn 763.89
  causing obstructed labor 660.2 ☑
    affecting fetus or newborn 763.1
phantom 300.11
plasma cell (M9731/1) 238.6
  benign (M9731/0) — *see* Neoplasm, by site, benign
  malignant (M9731/3) 203.8 ☑
polyvesicular vitelline (M9071/3)
  specified site — *see* Neoplasm, by site, malignant
  unspecified site
    female 183.0
    male 186.9
Pott's puffy (*see also* Osteomyelitis) 730.2 ☑
Rathke's pouch (M9350/1) 237.0
regaud's (M8082/3) — *see* Neoplasm, nasopharynx, malignant
rete cell (M8140/0) 222.0
retinal anlage (M9363/0) — *see* Neoplasm, by site, benign
Rokitansky's 620.2
salivary gland type, mixed (M8940/0) (*see also* Neoplasm, by site, benign)
  malignant (M8940/3) — *see* Neoplasm, by site, malignant
Sampson's 617.1
Schloffer's (*see also* Peritonitis) 567.29
Schmincke (M8082/3) — *see* Neoplasm, nasopharynx, malignant
sebaceous (*see also* Cyst, sebaceous) 706.2
secondary (M8000/6) — *see* Neoplasm, by site, secondary
  carcinoid — *see* Tumor, neuroendocrine, secondary
  neuroendocrine — *see* Tumor, neuroendocrine, secondary
Sertoli cell (M8640/0)
  with lipid storage (M8641/0)
    specified site — *see* Neoplasm, by site, benign
    unspecified site
      female 220
      male 222.0
  specified site — *see* Neoplasm, by site, benign
  unspecified site
    female 220
    male 222.0
Sertoli-Leydig cell (M8631/0)
  specified site — *see* Neoplasm, by site, benign
  unspecified site
    female 220
    male 222.0
sex cord (-stromal) (M8590/1) — *see* Neoplasm, by site, uncertain behavior
skin appendage (M8390/0) — *see* Neoplasm, skin, benign
soft tissue
  benign (M8800/0) — *see* Neoplasm, connective tissue, benign
  malignant (M8800/3) — *see* Neoplasm, connective tissue, malignant
sternomastoid 754.1
stromal
  abdomen
    benign 215.5
    malignant NEC 171.5
    uncertain behavior 238.1
  digestive system 238.1
    benign 215.5
    malignant NEC 171.5
    uncertain behavior 238.1

Tumor — see also Neoplasm, by site, unspecified nature — continued
  stromal — continued
    endometrium (endometrial) 236.0
    gastric 238.1
      benign 215.5
      malignant 151.9
      uncertain behavior 238.1
    gastrointestinal 238.1
      benign 215.5
      malignant NEC 171.5
      uncertain behavior 238.1
    intestine (small) 238.1
      benign 215.5
      malignant 152.9
      uncertain behavior 238.1
    stomach 238.1
      benign 215.5
      malignant 151.9
      uncertain behavior 238.1
  superior sulcus (lung) (pulmonary) (syndrome) (M8010/3) 162.3
  suprasulcus (M8010/3) 162.3
  sweat gland (M8400/1) (see also Neoplasm, skin, uncertain behavior)
    benign (M8400/0) — see Neoplasm, skin, benign
    malignant (M8400/3) — see Neoplasm, skin, malignant
  syphilitic brain 094.89
    congenital 090.49
  testicular stromal (M8590/1) 236.4
  theca cell (M8600/0) 220
  theca cell-granulosa cell (M8621/1) 236.2
  theca-lutein (M8610/0) 220
  turban (M8200/0) 216.4
  uterus
    in pregnancy or childbirth 654.1 ☑
      affecting fetus or newborn 763.89
      causing obstructed labor 660.2 ☑
        affecting fetus or newborn 763.1
  vagina
    in pregnancy or childbirth 654.7 ☑
      affecting fetus or newborn 763.89
      causing obstructed labor 660.2 ☑
        affecting fetus or newborn 763.1
  varicose (see also Varicose, vein) 454.9
  von Recklinghausen's (M9540/1) 237.71
  vulva
    in pregnancy or childbirth 654.8 ☑
      affecting fetus or newborn 763.89
      causing obstructed labor 660.2 ☑
        affecting fetus or newborn 763.1
  Warthin's (salivary gland) (M8561/0) 210.2
  white (see also Tuberculosis, arthritis)
  White-Darier 757.39
  Wilms' (nephroblastoma) (M8960/3) 189.0
  yolk sac (M9071/3)
    specified site — see Neoplasm, by site, malignant
    unspecified site
      female 183.0
      male 186.9
Tumorlet (M8040/1) — see Neoplasm, by site, uncertain behavior
Tungiasis 134.1
Tunica vasculosa lentis 743.39
Tunnel vision 368.45
Turban tumor (M8200/0) 216.4
Türck's trachoma (chronic catarrhal laryngitis) 476.0
Türk's syndrome (ocular retraction syndrome) 378.71
Turner's
  hypoplasia (tooth) 520.4
  syndrome 758.6
  tooth 520.4
Turner-Kieser syndrome (hereditary osteo-onychodysplasia) 756.89
Turner-Varny syndrome 758.6
Turricephaly 756.0
Tussis convulsiva — see also Whooping cough 033.9
Twiddler's syndrome (due to)
  automatic implantable defibrillator 996.04
  pacemaker 996.01

Twin
  affected by maternal complications of pregnancy 761.5
  conjoined 759.4
    fetal 678.1 ☑
  healthy liveborn — see Newborn, twin
  pregnancy (complicating delivery) NEC 651.0 ☑
    with fetal loss and retention of one fetus 651.3 ☑
    conjoined 678.1 ☑
    following (elective) fetal reduction 651.7 ☑
Twinning, teeth 520.2
Twist, twisted
  bowel, colon, or intestine 560.2
  hair (congenital) 757.4
  mesentery 560.2
  omentum 560.2
  organ or site, congenital NEC — see Anomaly, specified type NEC
  ovarian pedicle 620.5
    congenital 752.0
  umbilical cord — see Compression, umbilical cord
Twitch 781.0
Tylosis 700
  buccalis 528.6
  gingiva 523.8
  linguae 528.6
  palmaris et plantaris 757.39
Tympanism 787.3
Tympanites (abdominal) (intestine) 787.3
Tympanitis — see Myringitis
Tympanosclerosis 385.00
  involving
    combined sites NEC 385.09
      with tympanic membrane 385.03
    tympanic membrane 385.01
      with ossicles 385.02
        and middle ear 385.03
Tympanum — see condition
Tympany
  abdomen 787.3
  chest 786.7
Typhlitis — see also Appendicitis 541
Typhoenteritis 002.0
Typhogastric fever 002.0
Typhoid (abortive) (ambulant) (any site) (fever) (hemorrhagic) (infection) (intermittent) (malignant) (rheumatic) 002.0
  with pneumonia 002.0 [484.8]
  abdominal 002.0
  carrier (suspected) of V02.1
  cholecystitis (current) 002.0
  clinical (Widal and blood test negative) 002.0
  endocarditis 002.0 [421.1]
  inoculation reaction — see Complications, vaccination
  meningitis 002.0 [320.7]
  mesenteric lymph nodes 002.0
  myocarditis 002.0 [422.0]
  osteomyelitis (see also Osteomyelitis, due to, typhoid) 002.0 [730.8] ☑
  perichondritis, larynx 002.0 [478.71]
  pneumonia 002.0 [484.8]
  spine 002.0 [720.81]
  ulcer (perforating) 002.0
  vaccination, prophylactic (against) V03.1
  Widal negative 002.0
Typhomalaria (fever) — see also Malaria 084.6
Typhomania 002.0
Typhoperitonitis 002.0
Typhus (fever) 081.9
  abdominal, abdominalis 002.0
  African tick 082.1
  amarillic (see also Fever, Yellow) 060.9
  brain 081.9
  cerebral 081.9
  classical 080
  endemic (flea-borne) 081.0
  epidemic (louse-borne) 080
  exanthematicus SAI 080
    brillii SAI 081.1
    Mexicanus SAI 081.0

Typhus — continued
  exanthematicus SAI — continued
    pediculo vestimenti causa 080
    typhus murinus 081.0
  exanthematic NEC 080
  flea-borne 081.0
  Indian tick 082.1
  Kenya tick 082.1
  louse-borne 080
  Mexican 081.0
    flea-borne 081.0
    louse-borne 080
    tabardillo 080
  mite-borne 081.2
  murine 081.0
  North Asian tick-borne 082.2
  petechial 081.9
  Queensland tick 082.3
  rat 081.0
  recrudescent 081.1
  recurrent (see also Fever, relapsing) 087.9
  São Paulo 082.0
  scrub (China) (India) (Malaya) (New Guinea) 081.2
  shop (of Malaya) 081.0
  Siberian tick 082.2
  tick-borne NEC 082.9
  tropical 081.2
  vaccination, prophylactic (against) V05.8
Tyrosinemia 270.2
  neonatal 775.89
Tyrosinosis (Medes) (Sakai) 270.2
Tyrosinuria 270.2
Tyrosyluria 270.2

U

Uehlinger's syndrome (acropachyderma) 757.39
Uhl's anomaly or disease (hypoplasia of myocardium, right ventricle) 746.84
Ulcerosa scarlatina 034.1
Ulcer, ulcerated, ulcerating, ulceration, ulcerative 707.9
  with gangrene 707.9 [785.4]
  abdomen (wall) (see also Ulcer, skin) 707.8
  ala, nose 478.19
  alveolar process 526.5
  amebic (intestine) 006.9
    skin 006.6
  anastomotic — see Ulcer, gastrojejunal
  anorectal 569.41
  antral — see Ulcer, stomach
  anus (sphincter) (solitary) 569.41
    varicose — see Varicose, ulcer, anus
  aorta — see Aneuysm
  aphthous (oral) (recurrent) 528.2
    genital organ(s)
      female 616.50
      male 608.89
    mouth 528.2
  arm (see also Ulcer, skin) 707.8
  arteriosclerotic plaque — see Arteriosclerosis, by site
  artery NEC 447.2
    without rupture 447.8
  atrophic NEC — see Ulcer, skin
  Barrett's (chronic peptic ulcer of esophagus) 530.85
  bile duct 576.8
  bladder (solitary) (sphincter) 596.89
    bilharzial (see also Schistosomiasis) 120.9 [595.4]
    submucosal (see also Cystitis) 595.1
    tuberculous (see also Tuberculosis) 016.1 ☑
  bleeding NEC — see Ulcer, peptic, with hemorrhage
  bone 730.9 ☑
  bowel (see also Ulcer, intestine) 569.82
  breast 611.0
  bronchitis 491.8
  bronchus 519.19
  buccal (cavity) (traumatic) 528.9
  burn (acute) — see Ulcer, duodenum
  Buruli 031.1
  buttock (see also Ulcer, skin) 707.8

Ulcer, ulcerated, ulcerating, ulceration, ulcerative — continued
  buttock (see also Ulcer, skin) — continued
    decubitus (see also Ulcer, pressure) 707.00
  cancerous (M8000/3) — see Neoplasm, by site, malignant
  cardia — see Ulcer, stomach
  cardio-esophageal (peptic) 530.20
    with bleeding 530.21
  cecum (see also Ulcer, intestine) 569.82
  cervix (uteri) (trophic) 622.0
    with mention of cervicitis 616.0
  chancroidal 099.0
  chest (wall) (see also Ulcer, skin) 707.8
  Chiclero 085.4
  chin (pyogenic) (see also Ulcer, skin) 707.8
  chronic (cause unknown) (see also Ulcer, skin)
    penis 607.89
  Cochin-China 085.1
  colitis — see Colitis, ulcerative
  colon (see also Ulcer, intestine) 569.82
  conjunctiva (acute) (postinfectional) 372.00
  cornea (infectional) 370.00
    with perforation 370.06
    annular 370.02
    catarrhal 370.01
    central 370.03
    dendritic 054.42
    marginal 370.01
    mycotic 370.05
    phlyctenular, tuberculous (see also Tuberculosis) 017.3 ☑ [370.31]
    ring 370.02
    rodent 370.07
    serpent, serpiginous 370.04
    superficial marginal 370.01
    tuberculous (see also Tuberculosis) 017.3 ☑ [370.31]
  corpus cavernosum (chronic) 607.89
  crural — see Ulcer, lower extremity
  Curling's — see Ulcer, duodenum
  Cushing's — see Ulcer, peptic
  cystitis (interstitial) 595.1
  decubitus (unspecified site) (see also Ulcer, pressure) 707.00
    with gangrene 707.00 [785.4]
    ankle 707.06
    back
      lower 707.03
      upper 707.02
    buttock 707.05
    coccyx 707.03
    elbow 707.01
    head 707.09
    heel 707.07
    hip 707.04
    other site 707.09
    sacrum 707.03
    shoulder blades 707.02
  dendritic 054.42
  diabetes, diabetic (mellitus) 250.8 ☑ [707.9]
    due to secondary diabetes 249.8 ☑ [707.9]
    lower limb 250.8 ☑ [707.10]
      ankle 250.8 ☑ [707.13]
        due to secondary diabetes 249.8 ☑ [707.13]
      calf 250.8 ☑ [707.12]
        due to secondary diabetes 249.8 ☑ [707.12]
      due to secondary diabetes 249.8 ☑ [707.10]
      foot 250.8 ☑ [707.15]
        due to secondary diabetes 249.8 ☑ [707.15]
      heel 250.8 ☑ [707.14]
        due to secondary diabetes 249.8 ☑ [707.14]
      knee 250.8 ☑ [707.19]
        due to secondary diabetes 249.8 ☑ [707.19]
      specified site NEC 250.8 ☑ [707.19]

Ulcer, ulcerated, ulcerating, ulceration, ulcerative — *continued*
  diabetes, diabetic — *continued*
    lower limb — *continued*
      specified site — *continued*
        due to secondary diabetes
          249.8 ☑ [707.19]
        thigh 250.8 ☑ [707.11]
          due to secondary diabetes
            249.8 ☑ [707.11]
        toes 250.8 ☑ [707.15]
          due to secondary diabetes
            249.8 ☑ [707.15]
      specified site NEC 250.8 ☑ [707.8]
        due to secondary diabetes
          249.8 ☑ [707.8]
  Dieulafoy — *see* Lesion, Dieulafoy
  due to
    infection NEC — *see* Ulcer, skin
    radiation, radium — *see* Ulcer, by site
    trophic disturbance (any region) — *see* Ulcer, skin
    x-ray — *see* Ulcer, by site
  duodenum, duodenal (eroded) (peptic) 532.9 ☑

Note — Use the following fifth-digit subclassification with categories 531–534:

0   without mention of obstruction

1   with obstruction

    with
      hemorrhage (chronic) 532.4 ☑
        and perforation 532.6 ☑
      perforation (chronic) 532.5 ☑
        and hemorrhage 532.6 ☑
    acute 532.3 ☑
      with
        hemorrhage 532.0 ☑
          and perforation 532.2 ☑
        perforation 532.1 ☑
          and hemorrhage 532.2 ☑
    bleeding (recurrent) — *see* Ulcer, duodenum, with hemorrhage
    chronic 532.7 ☑
      with
        hemorrhage 532.4 ☑
          and perforation 532.6 ☑
        perforation 532.5 ☑
          and hemorrhage 532.6 ☑
    penetrating — *see* Ulcer, duodenum, with perforation
    perforating — *see* Ulcer, duodenum, with perforation
  dysenteric NEC 009.0
  elusive 595.1
  endocarditis (any valve) (acute) (chronic) (subacute) 421.0
  enteritis — *see* Colitis, ulcerative
  enterocolitis 556.0
  epiglottis 478.79
  esophagus (peptic) 530.20
    with bleeding 530.21
    due to ingestion
      aspirin 530.20
      chemicals 530.20
      medicinal agents 530.20
    fungal 530.20
    infectional 530.20
    varicose (*see also* Varix, esophagus) 456.1
      bleeding (*see also* Varix, esophagus, bleeding) 456.0
  eyelid (region) 373.01
  eye NEC 360.00
    dendritic 054.42
  face (*see also* Ulcer, skin) 707.8
  fauces 478.29
  Fenwick (-Hunner) (solitary) (*see also* Cystitis) 595.1
  fistulous NEC — *see* Ulcer, skin
  foot (indolent) (*see also* Ulcer, lower extremity) 707.15
    perforating 707.15
      leprous 030.1
      syphilitic 094.0

Ulcer, ulcerated, ulcerating, ulceration, ulcerative — *continued*
  foot (*see also* Ulcer, lower extremity) — *continued*
    trophic 707.15
    varicose 454.0
      inflamed or infected 454.2
  frambesial, initial or primary 102.0
  gallbladder or duct 575.8
  gall duct 576.8
  gangrenous (*see also* Gangrene) 785.4
  gastric — *see* Ulcer, stomach
  gastrocolic — *see* Ulcer, gastrojejunal
  gastroduodenal — *see* Ulcer, peptic
  gastroesophageal — *see* Ulcer, stomach
  gastrohepatic — *see* Ulcer, stomach
  gastrointestinal — *see* Ulcer, gastrojejunal
  gastrojejunal (eroded) (peptic) 534.9 ☑

Note — Use the following fifth-digit subclassification with categories 531–534:

0   without mention of obstruction

1   with obstruction

    with
      hemorrhage (chronic) 534.4 ☑
        and perforation 534.6 ☑
      perforation 534.5 ☑
        and hemorrhage 534.6 ☑
    acute 534.3 ☑
      with
        hemorrhage 534.0 ☑
          and perforation 534.2 ☑
        perforation 534.1 ☑
          and hemorrhage 534.2 ☑
    bleeding (recurrent) — *see* Ulcer, gastrojejunal, with hemorrhage
    chronic 534.7 ☑
      with
        hemorrhage 534.4 ☑
          and perforation 534.6 ☑
        perforation 534.5 ☑
          and hemorrhage 534.6 ☑
    penetrating — *see* Ulcer, gastrojejunal, with perforation
    perforating — *see* Ulcer, gastrojejunal, with perforation
  gastrojejunocolic — *see* Ulcer, gastrojejunal
  genital organ
    female 629.89
    male 608.89
  gingiva 523.8
  gingivitis 523.10
  glottis 478.79
  granuloma of pudenda 099.2
  groin (*see also* Ulcer, skin) 707.8
  gum 523.8
  gumma, due to yaws 102.4
  hand (*see also* Ulcer, skin) 707.8
  hard palate 528.9
  heel (*see also* Ulcer, lower extremity) 707.14
    decubitus (*see also* Ulcer, pressure) 707.07
  hemorrhoids 455.8
    external 455.5
    internal 455.2
  hip (*see also* Ulcer, skin) 707.8
    decubitus (*see also* Ulcer, pressure) 707.04
  Hunner's 595.1
  hypopharynx 478.29
  hypopyon (chronic) (subacute) 370.04
  hypostaticum — *see* Ulcer, varicose
  ileocolitis 556.1
  ileum (*see also* Ulcer, intestine) 569.82
  intestine, intestinal 569.82
    with perforation 569.83
    amebic 006.9
    duodenal — *see* Ulcer, duodenum
    granulocytopenic (with hemorrhage) 288.09
    marginal 569.82
    perforating 569.83
    small, primary 569.82
    stercoraceous 569.82

Ulcer, ulcerated, ulcerating, ulceration, ulcerative — *continued*
  intestine, intestinal — *continued*
    stercoral 569.82
    tuberculous (*see also* Tuberculosis) 014.8 ☑
    typhoid (fever) 002.0
    varicose 456.8
  ischemic 707.9
    lower extremity (*see also* Ulcer, lower extremity) 707.10
      ankle 707.13
      calf 707.12
      foot 707.15
      heel 707.14
      knee 707.19
      specified site NEC 707.19
      thigh 707.11
      toes 707.15
  jejunum, jejunal — *see* Ulcer, gastrojejunal
  keratitis (*see also* Ulcer, cornea) 370.00
  knee — *see* Ulcer, lower extremity
  labium (majus) (minus) 616.50
  laryngitis (*see also* Laryngitis) 464.00
    with obstruction 464.01
  larynx (aphthous) (contact) 478.79
    diphtheritic 032.3
  leg — *see* Ulcer, lower extremity
  lip 528.5
  Lipschütz's 616.50
  lower extremity (atrophic) (chronic) (neurogenic) (perforating) (pyogenic) (trophic) (tropical) 707.10
    with gangrene (*see also* Ulcer, lower extremity) 707.10 [785.4]
      arteriosclerotic 440.24
    ankle 707.13
      arteriosclerotic 440.23
        with gangrene 440.24
    calf 707.12
    decubitus (*see also* Ulcer, pressure) 707.00
      with gangrene 707.00 [785.4]
      ankle 707.06
      buttock 707.05
      heel 707.07
      hip 707.04
    foot 707.15
    heel 707.14
    knee 707.19
    specified site NEC 707.19
    thigh 707.11
    toes 707.15
    varicose 454.0
      inflamed or infected 454.2
  luetic — *see* Ulcer, syphilitic
  lung 518.89
    tuberculous (*see also* Tuberculosis) 011.2 ☑
  malignant (M8000/3) — *see* Neoplasm, by site, malignant
  marginal NEC — *see* Ulcer, gastrojejunal
  meatus (urinarius) 597.89
  Meckel's diverticulum 751.0
  Meleney's (chronic undermining) 686.09
  Mooren's (cornea) 370.07
  mouth (traumatic) 528.9
  mycobacterial (skin) 031.1
  nasopharynx 478.29
  navel cord (newborn) 771.4
  neck (*see also* Ulcer, skin) 707.8
    uterus 622.0
  neurogenic NEC — *see* Ulcer, skin
  nose, nasal (infectional) (passage) 478.19
    septum 478.19
      varicose 456.8
    skin — *see* Ulcer, skin
    spirochetal NEC 104.8
  oral mucosa (traumatic) 528.9
  palate (soft) 528.9
  penetrating NEC — *see* Ulcer, peptic, with perforation
  penis (chronic) 607.89

Ulcer, ulcerated, ulcerating, ulceration, ulcerative — *continued*
  peptic (site unspecified) 533.9 ☑

Note — Use the following fifth-digit subclassification with categories 531–534:

0   without mention of obstruction

1   with obstruction

    with
      hemorrhage 533.4 ☑
        and perforation 533.6 ☑
      perforation (chronic) 533.5 ☑
        and hemorrhage 533.6 ☑
    acute 533.3 ☑
      with
        hemorrhage 533.0 ☑
          and perforation 533.2 ☑
        perforation 533.1 ☑
          and hemorrhage 533.2 ☑
    bleeding (recurrent) — *see* Ulcer, peptic, with hemorrhage
    chronic 533.7 ☑
      with
        hemorrhage 533.4 ☑
          and perforation 533.6 ☑
        perforation 533.5 ☑
          and hemorrhage 533.6 ☑
    penetrating — *see* Ulcer, peptic, with perforation
    perforating NEC (*see also* Ulcer, peptic, with perforation) 533.5 ☑
  skin 707.9
  perineum (*see also* Ulcer, skin) 707.8
  peritonsillar 474.8
  phagedenic (tropical) NEC — *see* Ulcer, skin
  pharynx 478.29
  phlebitis — *see* Phlebitis
  plaster (*see also* Ulcer, pressure) 707.00
  popliteal space — *see* Ulcer, lower extremity
  postpyloric — *see* Ulcer, duodenum
  prepuce 607.89
  prepyloric — *see* Ulcer, stomach
  pressure 707.00
    with
      abrasion, blister, partial thickness skin loss involving epidermis and/or dermis 707.22
      full thickness skin loss involving damage or necrosis of subcutaneous tissue 707.23
      gangrene 707.00 [785.4]
      necrosis of soft tissue through to underlying muscle, tendon, or bone 707.24
    ankle 707.06
    back
      lower 707.03
      upper 707.02
    buttock 707.05
    coccyx 707.03
    elbow 707.01
    head 707.09
    healed — omit code
    healing — code to Ulcer, pressure, by stage
    heel 707.07
    hip 707.04
    other site 707.09
    sacrum 707.03
    shoulder blades 707.02
    stage
      I (healing) 707.21
      II (healing) 707.22
      III (healing) 707.23
      IV (healing) 707.24
      unspecified (healing) 707.20
    unstageable 707.25
  primary of intestine 569.82
    with perforation 569.83
  proctitis 556.2
    with ulcerative sigmoiditis 556.3
  prostate 601.8
  pseudopeptic — *see* Ulcer, peptic
  pyloric — *see* Ulcer, stomach

☑ **Additional Digit Required** — Refer to the Tabular List for Digit Selection   ▽ **Subterms under main terms may continue to next column or page**

2014 ICD-9-CM   333

Ulcer, ulcerated, ulcerating, ulceration, ulcerative — *continued*
rectosigmoid 569.82
  with perforation 569.83
rectum (sphincter) (solitary) 569.41
  stercoraceous, stercoral 569.41
  varicose — *see* Varicose, ulcer, anus
retina (*see also* Chorioretinitis) 363.20
rodent (M8090/3) (*see also* Neoplasm, skin, malignant)
  cornea 370.07
round — *see* Ulcer, stomach
sacrum (region) (*see also* Ulcer, skin) 707.8
Saemisch's 370.04
scalp (*see also* Ulcer, skin) 707.8
sclera 379.09
scrofulous (*see also* Tuberculosis) 017.2 ☑
scrotum 608.89
  tuberculous (*see also* Tuberculosis) 016.5 ☑
  varicose 456.4
seminal vesicle 608.89
sigmoid 569.82
  with perforation 569.83
skin (atrophic) (chronic) (neurogenic) (non-healing) (perforating) (pyogenic) (trophic) 707.9
  with gangrene 707.9 *[785.4]*
  amebic 006.6
  decubitus (*see also* Ulcer, pressure) 707.00
    with gangrene 707.00 *[785.4]*
  in granulocytopenia 288.09
  lower extremity (*see also* Ulcer, lower extremity) 707.10
    with gangrene 707.10 *[785.4]*
      arteriosclerotic 440.24
    ankle 707.13
    arteriosclerotic 440.23
      with gangrene 440.24
    calf 707.12
    foot 707.15
    heel 707.14
    knee 707.19
    specified site NEC 707.19
    thigh 707.11
    toes 707.15
  mycobacterial 031.1
  syphilitic (early) (secondary) 091.3
  tuberculous (primary) (*see also* Tuberculosis) 017.0 ☑
  varicose — *see* Ulcer, varicose
sloughing NEC — *see* Ulcer, skin
soft palate 528.9
solitary, anus or rectum (sphincter) 569.41
sore throat 462
  streptococcal 034.0
spermatic cord 608.89
spine (tuberculous) 015.0 ☑ *[730.88]*
stasis (leg) (venous) 454.0
  with varicose veins 454.0
  without varicose veins 459.81
  inflamed or infected 454.2
stercoral, stercoraceous 569.82
  with perforation 569.83
  anus or rectum 569.41
stoma, stomal — *see* Ulcer, gastrojejunal
stomach (eroded) (peptic) (round) 531.9 ☑

Note — Use the following fifth-digit subclassification with categories 531–534:

0 *without mention of obstruction*

1 *with obstruction*

  with
    hemorrhage 531.4 ☑
      and perforation 531.6 ☑
    perforation (chronic) 531.5 ☑
      and hemorrhage 531.6 ☑
  acute 531.3 ☑
    with
      hemorrhage 531.0 ☑
        and perforation 531.2 ☑
      perforation 531.1 ☑
        and hemorrhage 531.2 ☑

Ulcer, ulcerated, ulcerating, ulceration, ulcerative — *continued*
stomach — *continued*
  bleeding (recurrent) — *see* Ulcer, stomach, with hemorrhage
  chronic 531.7 ☑
    with
      hemorrhage 531.4 ☑
        and perforation 531.6 ☑
      perforation 531.5 ☑
        and hemorrhage 531.6 ☑
  penetrating — *see* Ulcer, stomach, with perforation
  perforating — *see* Ulcer, stomach, with perforation
stomatitis 528.00
stress — *see* Ulcer, peptic
strumous (tuberculous) (*see also* Tuberculosis) 017.2 ☑
submental (*see also* Ulcer, skin) 707.8
submucosal, bladder 595.1
syphilitic (any site) (early) (secondary) 091.3
  late 095.9
    perforating 095.9
      foot 094.0
testis 608.89
thigh — *see* Ulcer, lower extremity
throat 478.29
  diphtheritic 032.0
toe — *see* Ulcer, lower extremity
tongue (traumatic) 529.0
tonsil 474.8
  diphtheritic 032.0
trachea 519.19
trophic — *see* Ulcer, skin
tropical NEC (*see also* Ulcer, skin) 707.9
tuberculous — *see* Tuberculosis, ulcer
tunica vaginalis 608.89
turbinate 730.9 ☑
typhoid (fever) 002.0
  perforating 002.0
umbilicus (newborn) 771.4
unspecified site NEC — *see* Ulcer, skin
urethra (meatus) (*see also* Urethritis) 597.89
uterus 621.8
  cervix 622.0
    with mention of cervicitis 616.0
  neck 622.0
    with mention of cervicitis 616.0
vagina 616.89
valve, heart 421.0
varicose (lower extremity, any part) 454.0
  anus — *see* Varicose, ulcer, anus
  broad ligament 456.5
  esophagus (*see also* Varix, esophagus) 456.1
    bleeding (*see also* Varix, esophagus, bleeding) 456.0
  inflamed or infected 454.2
  nasal septum 456.8
  perineum 456.6
  rectum — *see* Varicose, ulcer, anus
  scrotum 456.4
  specified site NEC 456.8
  sublingual 456.3
  vulva 456.6
vas deferens 608.89
vesical (*see also* Ulcer, bladder) 596.89
vulva (acute) (infectional) 616.50
  Behçet's syndrome 136.1 *[616.51]*
  herpetic 054.12
  tuberculous 016.7 ☑ *[616.51]*
vulvobuccal, recurring 616.50
x-ray — *see* Ulcer, by site
yaws 102.4
Ulcus — *see also* Ulcer
cutis tuberculosum (*see also* Tuberculosis) 017.0 ☑
duodeni — *see* Ulcer, duodenum
durum 091.0
  extragenital 091.2
gastrojejunale — *see* Ulcer, gastrojejunal
hypostaticum — *see* Ulcer, varicose
molle (cutis) (skin) 099.0
serpens corneae (pneumococcal) 370.04
ventriculi — *see* Ulcer, stomach

Ulegyria 742.4
Ulerythema
  acneiforma 701.8
  centrifugum 695.4
  ophryogenes 757.4
Ullrich-Feichtiger syndrome 759.89
Ullrich (-Bonnevie) (-Turner) syndrome 758.6
Ulnar — *see* condition
Ulorrhagia 523.8
Ulorrhea 523.8
Umbilicus, umbilical — *see also* condition
  cord necrosis, affecting fetus or newborn 762.6
Unacceptable
  existing dental restoration
    contours 525.65
    morphology 525.65
Unavailability of medical facilities (at) V63.9
  due to
    investigation by social service agency V63.8
    lack of services at home V63.1
    remoteness from facility V63.0
    waiting list V63.2
  home V63.1
  outpatient clinic V63.0
  specified reason NEC V63.8
Uncinaria americana infestation 126.1
Uncinariasis — *see also* Ancylostomiasis 126.9
Unconscious, unconsciousness 780.09
Underdevelopment — *see also* Undeveloped
  sexual 259.0
Underfill, endodontic 526.63
Undernourishment 269.9
Undernutrition 269.9
Under observation — *see* Observation
Underweight 783.22
  for gestational age — *see* Light-for-dates
Underwood's disease (sclerema neonatorum) 778.1
Undescended — *see also* Malposition, congenital
  cecum 751.4
  colon 751.4
  testis 752.51
Undetermined diagnosis or cause 799.9
Undeveloped, undevelopment — *see also* Hypoplasia
  brain (congenital) 742.1
  cerebral (congenital) 742.1
  fetus or newborn 764.9 ☑
  heart 746.89
  lung 748.5
  testis 257.2
  uterus 259.0
Undiagnosed (disease) 799.9
Undulant fever — *see also* Brucellosis 023.9
Unemployment, anxiety concerning V62.0
Unequal leg (acquired) (length) 736.81
  congenital 755.30
Unerupted teeth, tooth 520.6
Unextracted dental root 525.3
Unguis incarnatus 703.0
Unicornis uterus 752.33
Unicornuate uterus (with or without a separate uterine horn) 752.33
Unicorporeus uterus 752.39
Uniformis uterus 752.39
Unilateral — *see also* condition
  development, breast 611.89
  organ or site, congenital NEC — *see* Agenesis
  vagina 752.49
Unilateralis uterus 752.39
Unilocular heart 745.8
Uninhibited bladder 596.54
  with cauda equina syndrome 344.61
  neurogenic — *see also* Neurogenic, bladder 596.54
Union, abnormal — *see also* Fusion
  divided tendon 727.89
  larynx and trachea 748.3
Universal
  joint, cervix 620.6
  mesentery 751.4

Unknown
  cause of death 799.9
  diagnosis 799.9
Unna's disease (seborrheic dermatitis) 690.10
Unresponsiveness, adrenocorticotropin (ACTH) 255.41
Unsatisfactory
  cytology smear
    anal 796.78
    cervical 795.08
    vaginal 795.18
  restoration, tooth (existing) 525.60
    specified NEC 525.69
Unsoundness of mind — *see also* Psychosis 298.9
Unspecified cause of death 799.9
Unstable
  back NEC 724.9
  colon 569.89
  joint — *see* Instability, joint
  lie 652.0 ☑
    affecting fetus or newborn (before labor) 761.7
      causing obstructed labor 660.0 ☑
        affecting fetus or newborn 763.1
  lumbosacral joint (congenital) 756.19
    acquired 724.6
  sacroiliac 724.6
  spine NEC 724.9
Untruthfulness, child problem — *see also* Disturbance, conduct 312.0 ☑
Unverricht (-Lundborg) disease, syndrome, or epilepsy 345.1 ☑
Unverricht-Wagner syndrome (dermatomyositis) 710.3
Upper respiratory — *see* condition
Upset
  gastric 536.8
    psychogenic 306.4
  gastrointestinal 536.8
    psychogenic 306.4
    virus (*see also* Enteritis, viral) 008.8
  intestinal (large) (small) 564.9
    psychogenic 306.4
  menstruation 626.9
  mental 300.9
  stomach 536.8
    psychogenic 306.4
Urachus — *see also* condition
  patent 753.7
  persistent 753.7
Uratic arthritis 274.00
Urbach's lipoid proteinosis 272.8
Urbach-Oppenheim disease or syndrome (necrobiosis lipoidica diabeticorum) 250.8 ☑ *[709.3]*
  due to secondary diabetes 249.8 ☑ *[709.3]*
Urbach-Wiethe disease or syndrome (lipoid proteinosis) 272.8
Urban yellow fever 060.1
Urea, blood, high — *see* Uremia
Uremia, uremic (absorption) (amaurosis) (amblyopia) (aphasia) (apoplexy) (coma) (delirium) (dementia) (dropsy) (dyspnea) (fever) (intoxication) (mania) (paralysis) (poisoning) (toxemia) (vomiting) 586
  with
    abortion — *see* Abortion, by type, with renal failure
    ectopic pregnancy (*see also* categories 633.0–633.9) 639.3
    hypertension (*see also* Hypertension, kidney) 403.91
    molar pregnancy (*see also* categories 630–632) 639.3
  chronic 585.9
  complicating
    abortion 639.3
    ectopic or molar pregnancy 639.3
    hypertension (*see also* Hypertension, kidney) 403.91
    labor and delivery 669.3 ☑
  congenital 779.89
  extrarenal 788.99
  hypertensive (chronic) (*see also* Hypertension, kidney) 403.91

Uremia, uremic — *continued*
   maternal NEC, affecting fetus or newborn 760.1
   neuropathy 585.9 *[357.4]*
   pericarditis 585.9 *[420.0]*
   prerenal 788.99
   pyelitic (*see also* Pyelitis) 590.80
Ureteralgia 788.0
Ureterectasis 593.89
Ureteritis 593.89
   cystica 590.3
   due to calculus 592.1
   gonococcal (acute) 098.19
     chronic or duration of 2 months or over 098.39
   nonspecific 593.89
Ureterocele (acquired) 593.89
   congenital 753.23
Ureterolith 592.1
Ureterolithiasis 592.1
Ureterostomy status V44.6
   with complication 997.5
Ureter, ureteral — *see* condition
Urethralgia 788.99
Urethra, urethral — *see* condition
Urethritis (abacterial) (acute) (allergic) (anterior) (chronic) (nonvenereal) (posterior) (recurrent) (simple) (subacute) (ulcerative) (undifferentiated) 597.80
   diplococcal (acute) 098.0
     chronic or duration of 2 months or over 098.2
   due to Trichomonas (vaginalis) 131.02
   gonococcal (acute) 098.0
     chronic or duration of 2 months or over 098.2
   nongonococcal (sexually transmitted) 099.40
     Chlamydia trachomatis 099.41
     Reiter's 099.3
     specified organism NEC 099.49
   nonspecific (sexually transmitted) (*see also* Urethritis, nongonococcal) 099.40
   not sexually transmitted 597.80
   Reiter's 099.3
   trichomonal or due to Trichomonas (vaginalis) 131.02
   tuberculous (*see also* Tuberculosis) 016.3 ☑
   venereal NEC (*see also* Urethritis, nongonococcal) 099.40
Urethrocele
   female 618.03
     with uterine prolapse 618.4
       complete 618.3
       incomplete 618.2
   male 599.5
Urethrolithiasis 594.2
Urethro-oculoarticular syndrome 099.3
Urethro-oculosynovial syndrome 099.3
Urethrorectal — *see* condition
Urethrorrhagia 599.84
Urethrorrhea 788.7
Urethrostomy status V44.6
   with complication 997.5

Urethrotrigonitis 595.3
Urethrovaginal — *see* condition
Urgency
   fecal 787.63
   hypertensive — *see* Hypertension
Urhidrosis, uridrosis 705.89
Uric acid
   diathesis 274.9
   in blood 790.6
Uricacidemia 790.6
Uricemia 790.6
Uricosuria 791.9
Urination
   frequent 788.41
   painful 788.1
   urgency 788.63
Urinemia — *see* Uremia
Urine, urinary — *see also* condition
   abnormality NEC 788.69
   blood in (*see also* Hematuria) 599.70
   discharge, excessive 788.42
   enuresis 788.30
     nonorganic origin 307.6
   extravasation 788.8
   frequency 788.41
   hesitancy 788.64
   incontinence 788.30
     active 788.30
     female 788.30
       stress 625.6
         and urge 788.33
     male 788.30
       stress 788.32
         and urge 788.33
     mixed (stress and urge) 788.33
     neurogenic 788.39
     nonorganic origin 307.6
     overflow 788.38
     stress (female) 625.6
       male NEC 788.32
   intermittent stream 788.61
   pus in 791.9
   retention or stasis NEC 788.20
     bladder, incomplete emptying 788.21
     psychogenic 306.53
     specified NEC 788.29
   secretion
     deficient 788.5
     excessive 788.42
     frequency 788.41
   strain 788.65
   stream
     intermittent 788.61
     slowing 788.62
     splitting 788.61
     weak 788.62
   urgency 788.63
Urinoma NEC 599.9
   bladder 596.89
   kidney 593.89
   renal 593.89
   ureter 593.89
   urethra 599.84
Uroarthritis, infectious 099.3

Urodialysis 788.5
Urolithiasis 592.9
Uronephrosis 593.89
Uropathy 599.9
   obstructive 599.60
Urosepsis 599.0
   meaning sepsis 995.91
   meaning urinary tract infection 599.0
Urticaria 708.9
   with angioneurotic edema 995.1
     hereditary 277.6
   allergic 708.0
   cholinergic 708.5
   chronic 708.8
   cold, familial 708.2
   dermatographic 708.3
   due to
     cold or heat 708.2
     drugs 708.0
     food 708.0
     inhalants 708.0
     plants 708.8
     serum 999.59
   factitial 708.3
   giant 995.1
     hereditary 277.6
   gigantea 995.1
     hereditary 277.6
   idiopathic 708.1
   larynx 995.1
     hereditary 277.6
   neonatorum 778.8
   nonallergic 708.1
   papulosa (Hebra) 698.2
   perstans hemorrhagica 757.39
   pigmentosa 757.33
   recurrent periodic 708.8
   serum 999.59
   solare 692.72
   specified type NEC 708.8
   thermal (cold) (heat) 708.2
   vibratory 708.4
Urticarioides acarodermatitis 133.9
Use of
   agents affecting estrogen receptors and estrogen levels NEC V07.59
   anastrozole (Arimidex) V07.52
   aromatase inhibitors V07.52
   estrogen receptor downregulators V07.59
   exemestane (Aromasin) V07.52
   fulvestrant (Faslodex) V07.59
   gonadotropin-releasing hormone (GnRH) agonist V07.59
   goserelin acetate (Zoladex) V07.59
   letrozole (Femara) V07.52
   leuprolide acetate (leuprorelin) (Lupron) V07.59
   megestrol acetate (Megace) V07.59
   methadone 304.00
   nonprescribed drugs (*see also* Abuse, drugs, nondependent) 305.9 ☑
   patent medicines (*see also* Abuse, drugs, nondependent) 305.9 ☑
   raloxifene (Evista) V07.51

Use of — *continued*
   selective estrogen receptor modulators (SERMs) V07.51
   tamoxifen (Nolvadex) V07.51
   toremifene (Fareston) V07.51
Usher-Senear disease (pemphigus erythematosus) 694.4
Uta 085.5
Uterine size-date discrepancy 649.6 ☑
Uteromegaly 621.2
Uterovaginal — *see* condition
Uterovesical — *see* condition
Uterus — *see also* condition
   with only one functioning horn 752.33
Utriculitis (utriculus prostaticus) 597.89
Uveal — *see* condition
Uveitis (anterior) — *see also* Iridocyclitis 364.3
   acute or subacute 364.00
     due to or associated with
       gonococcal infection 098.41
       herpes (simplex) 054.44
         zoster 053.22
     primary 364.01
     recurrent 364.02
     secondary (noninfectious) 364.04
       infectious 364.03
   allergic 360.11
   chronic 364.10
     due to or associated with
       sarcoidosis 135 *[364.11]*
       tuberculosis (*see also* Tuberculosis) 017.3 ☑ *[364.11]*
   due to
     operation 360.11
     toxoplasmosis (acquired) 130.2
       congenital (active) 771.2
   granulomatous 364.10
   heterochromic 364.21
   lens-induced 364.23
   nongranulomatous 364.00
   posterior 363.20
     disseminated — *see* Chorioretinitis, disseminated
     focal — *see* Chorioretinitis, focal
   recurrent 364.02
   sympathetic 360.11
   syphilitic (secondary) 091.50
     congenital 090.0 *[363.13]*
     late 095.8 *[363.13]*
   tuberculous (*see also* Tuberculosis) 017.3 ☑ *[364.11]*
Uveoencephalitis 363.22
Uveokeratitis — *see also* Iridocyclitis 364.3
Uveoparotid fever 135
Uveoparotitis 135
Uvula — *see* condition
Uvulitis (acute) (catarrhal) (chronic) (gangrenous) (membranous) (suppurative) (ulcerative) 528.3

☑ Additional Digit Required — Refer to the Tabular List for Digit Selection
▽ Subterms under main terms may continue to next column or page
2014 ICD-9-CM
335

V

Vaccination
complication or reaction — see Complications, vaccination
delayed V64.00
not carried out V64.00
  because of
    acute illness V64.01
    allergy to vaccine or component V64.04
    caregiver refusal V64.05
    chronic illness V64.02
    guardian refusal V64.05
    immune compromised state V64.03
    parent refusal V64.05
    patient had disease being vaccinated against V64.08
    patient refusal V64.06
    reason NEC V64.09
    religious reasons V64.07
prophylactic (against) V05.9
  arthropod-borne viral
    disease NEC V05.1
    encephalitis V05.0
  chickenpox V05.4
  cholera (alone) V03.0
    with typhoid-paratyphoid (cholera + TAB) V06.0
  common cold V04.7
  diphtheria (alone) V03.5
    with
      poliomyelitis (DTP+ polio) V06.3
      tetanus V06.5
        pertussis combined (DTP) (DTaP) V06.1
        typhoid-paratyphoid (DTP + TAB) V06.2
  disease (single) NEC V05.9
    bacterial NEC V03.9
      specified type NEC V03.89
    combination NEC V06.9
      specified type NEC V06.8
    specified type NEC V05.8
  encephalitis, viral, arthropod-borne V05.0
  Hemophilus influenzae, type B [Hib] V03.81
  hepatitis, viral V05.3
  influenza V04.81
    with
      Streptococcus pneumoniae [pneumococcus] V06.6
  leishmaniasis V05.2
  measles (alone) V04.2
    with mumps-rubella (MMR) V06.4
  mumps (alone) V04.6
    with measles and rubella (MMR) V06.4
  pertussis alone V03.6
  plague V03.3
  poliomyelitis V04.0
    with diphtheria-tetanus-pertussis (DTP + polio) V06.3
  rabies V04.5
  respiratory syncytial virus (RSV) V04.82
  rubella (alone) V04.3
    with measles and mumps (MMR) V06.4
  smallpox V04.1
  Streptococcus pneumoniae [pneumococcus] V03.82
    with
      influenza V06.6
  tetanus toxoid (alone) V03.7
    with diphtheria [Td] [DT] V06.5
      with
        pertussis (DTP) (DTaP) V06.1
          with poliomyelitis (DTP+polio) V06.3
  tuberculosis (BCG) V03.2
  tularemia V03.4
  typhoid-paratyphoid (TAB) (alone) V03.1
    with diphtheria-tetanus-pertussis (TAB + DTP) V06.2
  varicella V05.4

Vaccination — continued
prophylactic — continued
  viral
    disease NEC V04.89
    encephalitis, arthropod-borne V05.0
    hepatitis V05.3
    yellow fever V04.4
Vaccinia (generalized) 999.0
without vaccination 051.02
congenital 771.2
conjunctiva 999.39
eyelids 999.0 [373.5]
localized 999.39
nose 999.39
not from vaccination 051.02
  eyelid 051.02 [373.5]
sine vaccinatione 051.02
Vacuum
extraction of fetus or newborn 763.3
in sinus (accessory) (nasal) (see also Sinusitis) 473.9
Vagabond V60.0
Vagabondage V60.0
Vagabonds' disease 132.1
Vaginalitis (tunica) 608.4
Vagina, vaginal — see also condition
high risk human papillomavirus (HPV) DNA test positive 795.15
low risk human papillomavirus (HPV) DNA test positive 795.19
Vaginismus (reflex) 625.1
functional 306.51
hysterical 300.11
psychogenic 306.51
Vaginitis (acute) (chronic) (circumscribed) (diffuse) (emphysematous) (Hemophilus vaginalis) (nonspecific) (nonvenereal) (ulcerative) 616.10
  with
    abortion — see Abortion, by type, with sepsis
    ectopic pregnancy (see also categories 633.0–633.9) 639.0
    molar pregnancy (see also categories 630–632) 639.0
  adhesive, congenital 752.49
  atrophic, postmenopausal 627.3
  bacterial 616.10
  blennorrhagic (acute) 098.0
    chronic or duration of 2 months or over 098.2
  candidal 112.1
  chlamydial 099.53
  complicating pregnancy or puerperium 646.6 ☑
    affecting fetus or newborn 760.8
  congenital (adhesive) 752.49
  due to
    C. albicans 112.1
    Trichomonas (vaginalis) 131.01
  following
    abortion 639.0
    ectopic or molar pregnancy 639.0
  gonococcal (acute) 098.0
    chronic or duration of 2 months or over 098.2
  granuloma 099.2
  Monilia 112.1
  mycotic 112.1
  pinworm 127.4 [616.11]
  postirradiation 616.10
  postmenopausal atrophic 627.3
  senile (atrophic) 627.3
  syphilitic (early) 091.0
    late 095.8
  trichomonal 131.01
  tuberculous (see also Tuberculosis) 016.7 ☑
  venereal NEC 099.8
Vaginosis — see Vaginitis
Vagotonia 352.3
Vagrancy V60.0
VAIN I (vaginal intraepithelial neoplasia I) 623.0
VAIN II (vaginal intraepithelial neoplasia II) 623.0
VAIN III (vaginal intraepithelial neoplasia III) 233.31

Vallecula — see condition
Valley fever 114.0
Valsuani's disease (progressive pernicious anemia, puerperal) 648.2 ☑
Valve, valvular (formation) — see also condition
cerebral ventricle (communicating) in situ V45.2
cervix, internal os 752.49
colon 751.5
congenital NEC — see Atresia
formation, congenital NEC — see Atresia
heart defect — see Anomaly, heart, valve
ureter 753.29
  pelvic junction 753.21
  vesical orifice 753.22
urethra 753.6
Valvulitis (chronic) — see also Endocarditis 424.90
rheumatic (chronic) (inactive) (with chorea) 397.9
  active or acute (aortic) (mitral) (pulmonary) (tricuspid) 391.1
syphilitic NEC 093.20
  aortic 093.22
  mitral 093.21
  pulmonary 093.24
  tricuspid 093.23
Valvulopathy — see Endocarditis
van Bogaert-Nijssen (-Peiffer) disease 330.0
van Bogaert's leukoencephalitis (sclerosing) (subacute) 046.2
van Buchem's syndrome (hyperostosis corticalis) 733.3
Vancomycin (glycopeptide)
intermediate staphylococcus aureus (VISA/GISA) V09.8 ☑
resistant
  enterococcus (VRE) V09.8 ☑
  staphylococcus aureus (VRSA/GRSA) V09.8 ☑
van Creveld-von Gierke disease (glycogenosis I) 271.0
van den Bergh's disease (enterogenous cyanosis) 289.7
van der Hoeve-Halbertsma-Waardenburg syndrome (ptosis-epicanthus) 270.2
van der Hoeve-Waardenburg-Gualdi syndrome (ptosis epicanthus) 270.2
van der Hoeve's syndrome (brittle bones and blue sclera, deafness) 756.51
Vanillism 692.89
Vanishing lung 492.0
Vanishing twin 651.33
van Neck (-Odelberg) disease or syndrome (juvenile osteochondrosis) 732.1
Vapor asphyxia or suffocation NEC 987.9
specified agent — see Table of Drugs and Chemicals
Vaquez's disease (M9950/1) 238.4
Vaquez-Osler disease (polycythemia vera) (M9950/1) 238.4
Variance, lethal ball, prosthetic heart valve 996.02
Variants, thalassemic 282.49
Variations in hair color 704.3
Varicella 052.9
with
  complication 052.8
    specified NEC 052.7
  pneumonia 052.1
  vaccination and inoculation (prophylactic) V05.4
exposure to V01.71
vaccination and inoculation (against) (prophylactic) V05.4
Varices — see Varix
Varicocele (scrotum) (thrombosed) 456.4
ovary 456.5
perineum 456.6
spermatic cord (ulcerated) 456.4
Varicose
aneurysm (ruptured) (see also Aneurysm) 442.9
dermatitis (lower extremity) — see Varicose, vein, inflamed or infected

Varicose — continued
eczema — see Varicose, vein
phlebitis — see Varicose, vein, inflamed or infected
placental vessel — see Placenta, abnormal
tumor — see Varicose, vein
ulcer (lower extremity, any part) 454.0
  anus 455.8
    external 455.5
    internal 455.2
  esophagus (see also Varix, esophagus) 456.1
    bleeding (see also Varix, esophagus, bleeding) 456.0
    inflamed or infected 454.2
  nasal septum 456.8
  perineum 456.6
  rectum — see Varicose, ulcer, anus
  scrotum 456.4
  specified site NEC 456.8
vein (lower extremity) (ruptured) (see also Varix) 454.9
  with
    complications NEC 454.8
    edema 454.8
    inflammation or infection 454.1
      ulcerated 454.2
    pain 454.8
    stasis dermatitis 454.1
      with ulcer 454.2
    swelling 454.8
    ulcer 454.0
      inflamed or infected 454.2
  anus — see Hemorrhoids
  broad ligament 456.5
  congenital (peripheral) 747.60
    gastrointestinal 747.61
    lower limb 747.64
    renal 747.62
    specified NEC 747.69
    upper limb 747.63
  esophagus (ulcerated) (see also Varix, esophagus) 456.1
    bleeding (see also Varix, esophagus, bleeding) 456.0
  inflamed or infected 454.1
    with ulcer 454.2
  in pregnancy or puerperium 671.0 ☑
    vulva or perineum 671.1 ☑
  nasal septum (with ulcer) 456.8
  pelvis 456.5
  perineum 456.6
    in pregnancy, childbirth, or puerperium 671.1 ☑
  rectum — see Hemorrhoids
  scrotum (ulcerated) 456.4
  specified site NEC 456.8
  sublingual 456.3
  ulcerated 454.0
    inflamed or infected 454.2
  umbilical cord, affecting fetus or newborn 762.6
  urethra 456.8
  vulva 456.6
    in pregnancy, childbirth, or puerperium 671.1 ☑
vessel (see also Varix)
  placenta — see Placenta, abnormal
Varicosis, varicosities, varicosity — see also Varix 454.9
Variola 050.9
hemorrhagic (pustular) 050.0
major 050.0
minor 050.1
modified 050.2
Varioloid 050.2
Variolosa, purpura 050.0
Varix (lower extremity) (ruptured) 454.9
with
  complications NEC 454.8
  edema 454.8
  inflammation or infection 454.1
    with ulcer 454.2
  pain 454.8
  stasis dermatitis 454.1
    with ulcer 454.2

Varix — *continued*
  with — *continued*
    swelling 454.8
    ulcer 454.0
      with inflammation or infection 454.2
  aneurysmal (*see also* Aneurysm) 442.9
  anus — *see* Hemorrhoids
  arteriovenous (congenital) (peripheral) NEC 747.60
    gastrointestinal 747.61
    lower limb 747.64
    renal 747.62
    specified NEC 747.69
    spinal 747.82
    upper limb 747.63
  bladder 456.5
  broad ligament 456.5
  congenital (peripheral) 747.60
  esophagus (ulcerated) 456.1
    bleeding 456.0
      in
        cirrhosis of liver 571.5 *[456.20]*
        portal hypertension 572.3 *[456.20]*
    congenital 747.69
      in
        cirrhosis of liver 571.5 *[456.21]*
          with bleeding 571.5 *[456.20]*
        portal hypertension 572.3 *[456.21]*
          with bleeding 572.3 *[456.20]*
  gastric 456.8
  inflamed or infected 454.1
    ulcerated 454.2
  in pregnancy or puerperium 671.0 ☑
    perineum 671.1 ☑
    vulva 671.1 ☑
  labia (majora) 456.6
  orbit 456.8
    congenital 747.69
  ovary 456.5
  papillary 448.1
  pelvis 456.5
  perineum 456.6
    in pregnancy or puerperium 671.1 ☑
  pharynx 456.8
  placenta — *see* Placenta, abnormal
  prostate 456.8
  rectum — *see* Hemorrhoids
  renal papilla 456.8
  retina 362.17
  scrotum (ulcerated) 456.4
  sigmoid colon 456.8
  specified site NEC 456.8
  spinal (cord) (vessels) 456.8
  spleen, splenic (vein) (with phlebolith) 456.8
  sublingual 456.3
  ulcerated 454.0
    inflamed or infected 454.2
  umbilical cord, affecting fetus or newborn 762.6
  uterine ligament 456.5
  vocal cord 456.8
  vulva 456.6
    in pregnancy, childbirth, or puerperium 671.1 ☑
Vasa previa 663.5 ☑
  affecting fetus or newborn 762.6
  hemorrhage from, affecting fetus or newborn 772.0
Vascular — *see also* condition
  loop on papilla (optic) 743.57
  sheathing, retina 362.13
  spasm 443.9
  spider 448.1
Vascularity, pulmonary, congenital 747.39
Vascularization
  choroid 362.16
  cornea 370.60
    deep 370.63
    localized 370.61
  retina 362.16
  subretinal 362.16
Vasculitis 447.6
  allergic 287.0
  cryoglobulinemic 273.2

Vasculitis — *continued*
  disseminated 447.6
  kidney 447.8
  leukocytoclastic 446.29
  nodular 695.2
  retinal 362.18
  rheumatic — *see* Fever, rheumatic
Vasculopathy
  cardiac allograft 996.83
Vas deferens — *see* condition
Vas deferentitis 608.4
Vasectomy, admission for V25.2
Vasitis 608.4
  nodosa 608.4
  scrotum 608.4
  spermatic cord 608.4
  testis 608.4
  tuberculous (*see also* Tuberculosis) 016.5 ☑
  tunica vaginalis 608.4
  vas deferens 608.4
Vasodilation 443.9
Vasomotor — *see* condition
Vasoplasty, after previous sterilization V26.0
Vasoplegia, splanchnic — *see also* Neuropathy, peripheral, autonomic 337.9
Vasospasm 443.9
  cerebral (artery) 435.9
    with transient neurologic deficit 435.9
  coronary 413.1
  nerve
    arm NEC 354.9
    autonomic 337.9
    brachial plexus 353.0
    cervical plexus 353.2
    leg NEC 355.8
    lower extremity NEC 355.8
    peripheral NEC 355.9
    spinal NEC 355.9
    sympathetic 337.9
    upper extremity NEC 354.9
  peripheral NEC 443.9
  retina (artery) (*see also* Occlusion, retinal, artery) 362.30
Vasospastic — *see* condition
Vasovagal attack (paroxysmal) 780.2
  psychogenic 306.2
Vater's ampulla — *see* condition
VATER syndrome 759.89
vCJD (variant Creutzfeldt-Jakob disease) 046.11
Vegetation, vegetative
  adenoid (nasal fossa) 474.2
  consciousness (persistent) 780.03
  endocarditis (acute) (any valve) (chronic) (subacute) 421.0
  heart (mycotic) (valve) 421.0
  state (persistent) 780.03
Veil
  Jackson's 751.4
  over face (causing asphyxia) 768.9
Vein, venous — *see* condition
Veldt sore — *see also* Ulcer, skin 707.9
Velo-cardio-facial syndrome 758.32
Velpeau's hernia — *see* Hernia, femoral
Venereal
  balanitis NEC 099.8
  bubo 099.1
  disease 099.9
    specified nature or type NEC 099.8
  granuloma inguinale 099.2
  lymphogranuloma (Durand-Nicolas-Favre), any site 099.1
  salpingitis 098.37
  urethritis (*see also* Urethritis, nongonococcal) 099.40
  vaginitis NEC 099.8
  warts 078.11
Vengefulness, in child — *see also* Disturbance, conduct 312.0 ☑
Venofibrosis 459.89
Venom, venomous
  bite or sting (animal or insect) 989.5
  poisoning 989.5
Venous — *see* condition
Ventouse delivery NEC 669.5 ☑
  affecting fetus or newborn 763.3
Ventral — *see* condition

Ventricle, ventricular — *see also* condition
  escape 427.69
  standstill (*see also* Arrest, cardiac) 427.5
Ventriculitis, cerebral — *see also* Meningitis 322.9
Ventriculostomy status V45.2
Verbiest's syndrome (claudicatio intermittens spinalis) 435.1
Vernet's syndrome 352.6
Verneuil's disease (syphilitic bursitis) 095.7
Verruca (filiformis) 078.10
  acuminata (any site) 078.11
  necrogenica (primary) (*see also* Tuberculosis) 017.0 ☑
  peruana 088.0
  peruviana 088.0
  plana (juvenilis) 078.19
  plantaris 078.12
  seborrheica 702.19
    inflamed 702.11
  senilis 702.0
  tuberculosa (primary) (*see also* Tuberculosis) 017.0 ☑
  venereal 078.11
  viral 078.10
    specified NEC 078.19
  vulgaris 078.10
Verrucosities — *see also* Verruca 078.10
Verrucous endocarditis (acute) (any valve) (chronic) (subacute) 710.0 *[424.91]*
  nonbacterial 710.0 *[424.91]*
Verruga
  peruana 088.0
  peruviana 088.0
Verse's disease (calcinosis intervertebralis) 275.49 *[722.90]*
Version
  before labor, affecting fetus or newborn 761.7
  cephalic (correcting previous malposition) 652.1 ☑
    affecting fetus or newborn 763.1
  cervix — *see* Version, uterus
  uterus (postinfectional) (postpartal, old) (*see also* Malposition, uterus) 621.6
    forward — *see* Anteversion, uterus
    lateral — *see* Lateroversion, uterus
Vertebra, vertebral — *see* condition
Vertigo 780.4
  auditory 386.19
  aural 386.19
  benign paroxysmal positional 386.11
  central origin 386.2
  cerebral 386.2
  Dix and Hallpike (epidemic) 386.12
  endemic paralytic 078.81
  epidemic 078.81
    Dix and Hallpike 386.12
    Gerlier's 078.81
    Pedersen's 386.12
    vestibular neuronitis 386.12
  epileptic — *see* Epilepsy
  Gerlier's (epidemic) 078.81
  hysterical 300.11
  labyrinthine 386.10
  laryngeal 786.2
  malignant positional 386.2
  Ménière's (*see also* Disease, Ménière's) 386.00
  menopausal 627.2
  otogenic 386.19
  paralytic 078.81
  paroxysmal positional, benign 386.11
  Pedersen's (epidemic) 386.12
  peripheral 386.10
    specified type NEC 386.19
  positional
    benign paroxysmal 386.11
    malignant 386.2
Verumontanitis (chronic) — *see also* Urethritis 597.89
Vesania — *see also* Psychosis 298.9
Vesical — *see* condition
Vesicle
  cutaneous 709.8
  seminal — *see* condition

Vesicle — *continued*
  skin 709.8
Vesicocolic — *see* condition
Vesicoperineal — *see* condition
Vesicorectal — *see* condition
Vesicourethrorectal — *see* condition
Vesicovaginal — *see* condition
Vesicular — *see* condition
Vesiculitis (seminal) 608.0
  amebic 006.8
  gonorrheal (acute) 098.14
    chronic or duration of 2 months or over 098.34
  trichomonal 131.09
  tuberculous (*see also* Tuberculosis) 016.5 ☑ *[608.81]*
Vestibulitis (ear) — *see also* Labyrinthitis 386.30
  nose (external) 478.19
  vulvar 625.71
Vestibulopathy, acute peripheral (recurrent) 386.12
Vestige, vestigial — *see also* Persistence
  branchial 744.41
  structures in vitreous 743.51
Vibriosis NEC 027.9
Vidal's disease (lichen simplex chronicus) 698.3
Video display tube syndrome 723.8
Vienna-type encephalitis 049.8
Villaret's syndrome 352.6
Villous — *see* condition
VIN I (vulvar intraepithelial neoplasia I) 624.01
VIN II (vulvar intraepithelial neoplasia II) 624.02
VIN III (vulvar intraepithelial neoplasia III) 233.32
Vincent's
  angina 101
  bronchitis 101
  disease 101
  gingivitis 101
  infection (any site) 101
  laryngitis 101
  stomatitis 101
  tonsillitis 101
Vinson-Plummer syndrome (sideropenic dysphagia) 280.8
Viosterol deficiency — *see also* Deficiency, calciferol 268.9
Virchow's disease 733.99
Viremia 790.8
Virilism (adrenal) (female) NEC 255.2
  with
    3-beta-hydroxysteroid dehydrogenase defect 255.2
    11-hydroxylase defect 255.2
    21-hydroxylase defect 255.2
    adrenal
      hyperplasia 255.2
      insufficiency (congenital) 255.2
    cortical hyperfunction 255.2
Virilization (female) (suprarenal) — *see also* Virilism 255.2
  isosexual 256.4
Virulent bubo 099.0
Virus, viral — *see also* condition
  infection NEC (*see also* Infection, viral) 079.99
  septicemia 079.99
  yaba monkey tumor 059.22
VISA (vancomycin intermediate staphylococcus aureus) V09.8 ☑
Viscera, visceral — *see* condition
Visceroptosis 569.89
Visible peristalsis 787.4
Vision, visual
  binocular, suppression 368.31
  blurred, blurring 368.8
    hysterical 300.11
  defect, defective (*see also* Impaired, vision) 369.9
  disorientation (syndrome) 368.16
  disturbance NEC (*see also* Disturbance, vision) 368.9
    hysterical 300.11
  examination V72.0

☑ **Additional Digit Required** — Refer to the Tabular List for Digit Selection   ▽ Subterms under main terms may continue to next column or page

2014 ICD-9-CM 337

Vision, visual — *continued*
  field, limitation 368.40
  fusion, with defective steropsis 368.33
  hallucinations 368.16
  halos 368.16
  loss 369.9
    both eyes (*see also* Blindness, both eyes) 369.3
    complete (*see also* Blindness, both eyes) 369.00
    one eye 369.8
    sudden 368.16
  low (both eyes) 369.20
    one eye (other eye normal) (*see also* Impaired, vision) 369.70
      blindness, other eye 369.10
  perception, simultaneous without fusion 368.32
  tunnel 368.45
Vitality, lack or want of 780.79
  newborn 779.89
Vitamin deficiency NEC — *see also* Deficiency, vitamin 269.2
Vitelline duct, persistent 751.0
Vitiligo 709.01
  due to pinta (carate) 103.2
  eyelid 374.53
  vulva 624.8
Vitium cordis — *see* Disease, heart
Vitreous — *see also* condition
  touch syndrome 997.99
VLCAD (long chain/very long chain acyl CoA dehydrogenase deficiency, LCAD) 277.85
Vocal cord — *see* condition
Vocational rehabilitation V57.22
Vogt's (Cecile) disease or syndrome 333.7 ☑
Vogt-Koyanagi syndrome 364.24
Vogt-Spielmeyer disease (amaurotic familial idiocy) 330.1
Voice
  change (*see also* Dysphonia) 784.49
  loss (*see also* Aphonia) 784.41
Volhard-Fahr disease (malignant nephrosclerosis) 403.00
Volhynian fever 083.1
Volkmann's ischemic contracture or paralysis (complicating trauma) 958.6
Voluntary starvation 307.1
Volvulus (bowel) (colon) (intestine) 560.2
  with
    hernia (*see also* Hernia, by site, with obstruction)
      gangrenous — *see* Hernia, by site, with gangrene
    perforation 560.2
  congenital 751.5
  duodenum 537.3
  fallopian tube 620.5
  oviduct 620.5
  stomach (due to absence of gastrocolic ligament) 537.89
Vomiting 787.03
  with nausea 787.01
  allergic 535.4 ☑
  asphyxia 933.1
  bilious (cause unknown) 787.04
    following gastrointestinal surgery 564.3
    newborn 779.32
  blood (*see also* Hematemesis) 578.0
  causing asphyxia, choking, or suffocation (*see also* Asphyxia, food) 933.1
  cyclical 536.2
    associated with migraine 346.2 ☑
    psychogenic 306.4
  epidemic 078.82
  fecal matter 569.87
  following gastrointestinal surgery 564.3
  functional 536.8
    psychogenic 306.4
  habit 536.2
  hysterical 300.11
  nervous 306.4
  neurotic 306.4
  newborn 779.33
    bilious 779.32
  of or complicating pregnancy 643.9 ☑

Vomiting — *continued*
  of or complicating pregnancy — *continued*
    due to
      organic disease 643.8 ☑
      specific cause NEC 643.8 ☑
    early — *see* Hyperemesis, gravidarum
    late (after 22 completed weeks of gestation) 643.2 ☑
  pernicious or persistent 536.2
    complicating pregnancy — *see* Hyperemesis, gravidarum
    psychogenic 306.4
  physiological 787.03
    bilious 787.04
  psychic 306.4
  psychogenic 307.54
  stercoral 569.89
  uncontrollable 536.2
    psychogenic 306.4
  uremic — *see* Uremia
  winter 078.82
von Bechterew (-Strumpell) disease or syndrome (ankylosing spondylitis) 720.0
von Bezold's abscess 383.01
von Economo's disease (encephalitis lethargica) 049.8
von Eulenburg's disease (congenital paramyotonia) 359.29
von Gierke's disease (glycogenosis I) 271.0
von Gies' joint 095.8
von Graefe's disease or syndrome 378.72
von Hippel (-Lindau) disease or syndrome (retinocerebral angiomatosis) 759.6
von Jaksch's anemia or disease (pseudoleukemia infantum) 285.8
von Recklinghausen-Applebaum disease (hemochromatosis) — *see also* Hemochromatosis 275.03
von Recklinghausen's
  disease or syndrome (nerves) (skin) (M9540/1) 237.71
  bones (osteitis fibrosa cystica) 252.01
  tumor (M9540/1) 237.71
von Schroetter's syndrome (intermittent venous claudication) 453.89
von Willebrand (-Jürgens) disease or syndrome (angiohemophilia) 286.4
von Zambusch's disease (lichen sclerosus et atrophicus) 701.0
Voorhoeve's disease or dyschondroplasia 756.4
Vossius' ring 921.3
  late effect 366.21
Voyeurism 302.82
VRE (vancomycin resistant enterococcus) V09.8 ☑
Vrolik's disease (osteogenesis imperfecta) 756.51
VRSA (vancomycin resistant staphylococcus aureus) V09.8 ☑
Vulva — *see* condition
Vulvismus 625.1
Vulvitis (acute) (allergic) (chronic) (gangrenous) (hypertrophic) (intertriginous) 616.10
  with
    abortion — *see* Abortion, by type, with sepsis
    ectopic pregnancy (*see also* categories 633.0–633.9) 639.0
    molar pregnancy (*see also* categories 630–632) 639.0
  adhesive, congenital 752.49
  blennorrhagic (acute) 098.0
    chronic or duration of 2 months or over 098.2
  chlamydial 099.53
  complicating pregnancy or puerperium 646.6 ☑
  due to Ducrey's bacillus 099.0
  following
    abortion 639.0
    ectopic or molar pregnancy 639.0
  gonococcal (acute) 098.0

Vulvitis — *continued*
  gonococcal — *continued*
    chronic or duration of 2 months or over 098.2
  herpetic 054.11
  leukoplakic 624.09
  monilial 112.1
  puerperal, postpartum, childbirth 646.6 ☑
  syphilitic (early) 091.0
    late 095.8
  trichomonal 131.01
Vulvodynia 625.70
  specified NEC 625.79
Vulvorectal — *see* condition
Vulvovaginitis — *see also* Vulvitis 616.10
  amebic 006.8
  chlamydial 099.53
  gonococcal (acute) 098.0
    chronic or duration of 2 months or over 098.2
  herpetic 054.11
  monilial 112.1
  trichomonal (Trichomonas vaginalis) 131.01

W

Waardenburg-Klein syndrome (ptosis-epicanthus) 270.2
Waardenburg's syndrome 756.89
  meaning ptosis-epicanthus 270.2
Wagner's disease (colloid milium) 709.3
Wagner (-Unverricht) syndrome (dermatomyositis) 710.3
Waiting list, person on V63.2
  undergoing social agency investigation V63.8
Wakefulness disorder — *see also* Hypersomnia 780.54
  nonorganic origin 307.43
Waldenström's
  disease (osteochondrosis, capital femoral) 732.1
  hepatitis (lupoid hepatitis) 571.49
  hypergammaglobulinemia 273.0
  macroglobulinemia 273.3
  purpura, hypergammaglobulinemic 273.0
  syndrome (macroglobulinemia) 273.3
Waldenström-Kjellberg syndrome (sideropenic dysphagia) 280.8
Walking
  difficulty 719.7
    psychogenic 307.9
  sleep 307.46
    hysterical 300.13
Wall, abdominal — *see* condition
Wallenberg's syndrome (posterior inferior cerebellar artery) — *see also* Disease, cerebrovascular, acute 436
Wallgren's
  disease (obstruction of splenic vein with collateral circulation) 459.89
  meningitis (*see also* Meningitis, aseptic) 047.9
Wandering
  acetabulum 736.39
  gallbladder 751.69
  in diseases classified elsewhere V40.31
  kidney, congenital 753.3
  organ or site, congenital NEC — *see* Malposition, congenital
  pacemaker (atrial) (heart) 427.89
  spleen 289.59
Wardrop's disease (with lymphangitis) 681.9
  finger 681.02
  toe 681.11
War neurosis 300.16
Wart (digitate) (filiform) (infectious) (viral) 078.10
  common 078.19
  external genital organs (venereal) 078.11
  fig 078.19
  flat 078.19
  genital 078.11
  Hassall-Henle's (of cornea) 371.41
  Henle's (of cornea) 371.41
  juvenile 078.19
  moist 078.10

Wart — *continued*
  Peruvian 088.0
  plantar 078.12
  prosector (*see also* Tuberculosis) 017.0 ☑
  seborrheic 702.19
    inflamed 702.11
  senile 702.0
  specified NEC 078.19
  syphilitic 091.3
  tuberculous (*see also* Tuberculosis) 017.0 ☑
  venereal (female) (male) 078.11
Warthin's tumor (salivary gland) (M8561/0) 210.2
Washerwoman's itch 692.4
Wassilieff's disease (leptospiral jaundice) 100.0
Wasting
  disease 799.4
    due to malnutrition 261
  extreme (due to malnutrition) 261
  muscular NEC 728.2
  palsy, paralysis 335.21
  pelvic muscle 618.83
Water
  clefts 366.12
  deprivation of 994.3
  in joint (*see also* Effusion, joint) 719.0 ☑
  intoxication 276.69
  itch 120.3
  lack of 994.3
  loading 276.69
  on
    brain — *see* Hydrocephalus
    chest 511.89
  poisoning 276.69
Waterbrash 787.1
Water-hammer pulse — *see also* Insufficiency, aortic 424.1
Waterhouse (-Friderichsen) disease or syndrome 036.3
Water-losing nephritis 588.89
Watermelon stomach 537.82
  with hemorrhage 537.83
  without hemorrhage 537.82
Wax in ear 380.4
Waxy
  degeneration, any site 277.39
  disease 277.39
  kidney 277.39 [583.81]
  liver (large) 277.39
  spleen 277.39
Weak, weakness (generalized) 780.79
  arches (acquired) 734
    congenital 754.61
  bladder sphincter 596.59
  congenital 779.89
  eye muscle — *see* Strabismus
  facial 781.94
  foot (double) — *see* Weak, arches
  heart, cardiac (*see also* Failure, heart) 428.9
    congenital 746.9
  mind 317
  muscle (generalized) 728.87
  myocardium (*see also* Failure, heart) 428.9
  newborn 779.89
  pelvic fundus
    pubocervical tissue 618.81
    rectovaginal tissue 618.82
  pulse 785.9
  senile 797
  urinary stream 788.62
  valvular — *see* Endocarditis
Wear, worn, tooth, teeth (approximal) (hard tissues) (interproximal) (occlusal) — *see also* Attrition, teeth 521.10
Weather, weathered
  effects of
    cold NEC 991.9
      specified effect NEC 991.8
    hot (*see also* Heat) 992.9
    skin 692.74
Weber-Christian disease or syndrome (nodular nonsuppurative panniculitis) 729.30
Weber-Cockayne syndrome (epidermolysis bullosa) 757.39

☑ Additional Digit Required — Refer to the Tabular List for Digit Selection   ▽ Subterms under main terms may continue to next column or page

338   2014 ICD-9-CM

☑ **Additional Digit Required** — Refer to the Tabular List for Digit Selection   ▽ **Subterms under main terms may continue to next column or page**

2014 ICD-9-CM   **339**

Wound, open — *continued*

Descemet's membrane (*see also* Wound, open, intraocular) 871.9

digit(s)
foot 893.0
with tendon involvement 893.2
complicated 893.1
hand 883.0
with tendon involvement 883.2
complicated 883.1

drumhead, ear 872.61
complicated 872.71

ear 872.8
canal 872.02
complicated 872.12
complicated 872.9
drum 872.61
complicated 872.71
external 872.00
complicated 872.10
multiple sites 872.69
complicated 872.79
ossicles (incus) (malleus) (stapes) 872.62
complicated 872.72
specified part NEC 872.69
complicated 872.79

elbow 881.01
with tendon involvement 881.21
complicated 881.11

epididymis 878.2
complicated 878.3

epigastric region 879.2
complicated 879.3

epiglottis 874.01
complicated 874.11

esophagus (cervical) 874.4
complicated 874.5
thoracic — *see* Injury, internal, esophagus

Eustachian tube 872.63
complicated 872.73

extremity
lower (multiple) NEC 894.0
with tendon involvement 894.2
complicated 894.1
upper (multiple) NEC 884.0
with tendon involvement 884.2
complicated 884.1

eye(s) (globe) — *see* Wound, open, intraocular

eyeball NEC 871.9
laceration (*see also* Laceration, eyeball) 871.4
penetrating (*see also* Penetrating wound, eyeball) 871.7

eyebrow 873.42
complicated 873.52

eyelid NEC 870.8
laceration — *see* Laceration, eyelid

face 873.40
complicated 873.50
multiple sites 873.49
complicated 873.59
specified part NEC 873.49
complicated 873.59

fallopian tube — *see* Injury, internal, fallopian tube

finger(s) (nail) (subungual) 883.0
with tendon involvement 883.2
complicated 883.1

flank 879.4
complicated 879.5

foot (any part except toe(s) alone) 892.0
with tendon involvement 892.2
complicated 892.1

forearm 881.00
with tendon involvement 881.20
complicated 881.10

forehead 873.42
complicated 873.52

genital organs (external) NEC 878.8
complicated 878.9
internal — *see* Injury, internal, by site

globe (eye) (*see also* Wound, open, eyeball) 871.9

groin 879.4

Wound, open — *continued*

groin — *continued*
complicated 879.5

gum(s) 873.62
complicated 873.72

hand (except finger(s) alone) 882.0
with tendon involvement 882.2
complicated 882.1

head NEC 873.8
with intracranial injury — *see* Injury, intracranial
due to or associated with skull fracture — *see* Fracture, skull
complicated 873.9
scalp — *see* Wound, open, scalp

heel 892.0
with tendon involvement 892.2
complicated 892.1

high-velocity (grease gun) — *see* Wound, open, complicated, by site

hip 890.0
with tendon involvement 890.2
complicated 890.1

hymen 878.6
complicated 878.7

hypochondrium 879.4
complicated 879.5

hypogastric region 879.2
complicated 879.3

iliac (region) 879.4
complicated 879.5

incidental to
dislocation — *see* Dislocation, open, by site
fracture — *see* Fracture, open, by site
intracranial injury — *see* Injury, intracranial, with open intracranial wound
nerve injury — *see* Injury, nerve, by site

inguinal region 879.4
complicated 879.5

instep 892.0
with tendon involvement 892.2
complicated 892.1

interscapular region 876.0
complicated 876.1

intracranial — *see* Injury, intracranial, with open intracranial wound

intraocular 871.9
with
partial loss (of intraocular tissue) 871.2
prolapse or exposure (of intraocular tissue) 871.1
without prolapse (of intraocular tissue) 871.0
laceration (*see also* Laceration, eyeball) 871.4
penetrating 871.7
with foreign body (nonmagnetic) 871.6
magnetic 871.5

iris (*see also* Wound, open, eyeball) 871.9

jaw (fracture not involved) 873.44
with fracture — *see* Fracture, jaw
complicated 873.54

knee 891.0
with tendon involvement 891.2
complicated 891.1

labium (majus) (minus) 878.4
complicated 878.5

lacrimal apparatus, gland, or sac 870.8
with laceration of eyelid 870.2

larynx 874.01
with trachea 874.00
complicated 874.10
complicated 874.11

leg (multiple) 891.0
with tendon involvement 891.2
complicated 891.1
lower 891.0
with tendon involvement 891.2
complicated 891.1
thigh 890.0
with tendon involvement 890.2
complicated 890.1

Wound, open — *continued*

leg — *continued*
upper 890.0
with tendon involvement 890.2
complicated 890.1

lens (eye) (alone) (*see also* Cataract, traumatic) 366.20
with involvement of other eye structures — *see* Wound, open, eyeball

limb
lower (multiple) NEC 894.0
with tendon involvement 894.2
complicated 894.1
upper (multiple) NEC 884.0
with tendon involvement 884.2
complicated 884.1

lip 873.43
complicated 873.53

loin 876.0
complicated 876.1

lumbar region 876.0
complicated 876.1

malar region 873.41
complicated 873.51

mastoid region 873.49
complicated 873.59

mediastinum — *see* Injury, internal, mediastinum

midthoracic region 875.0
complicated 875.1

mouth 873.60
complicated 873.70
floor 873.64
complicated 873.74
multiple sites 873.69
complicated 873.79
specified site NEC 873.69
complicated 873.79

multiple, unspecified site(s) 879.8

> *Note — Multiple open wounds of sites classifiable to the same four-digit category should be classified to that category unless they are in different limbs.*
>
> *Multiple open wounds of sites classifiable to different four-digit categories, or to different limbs, should be coded separately.*

complicated 879.9
lower limb(s) (one or both) (sites classifiable to more than one three-digit category in 890 to 893) 894.0
with tendon involvement 894.2
complicated 894.1
upper limb(s) (one or both) (sites classifiable to more than one three-digit category in 880 to 883) 884.0
with tendon involvement 884.2
complicated 884.1

muscle — *see* Sprain, by site

nail
finger(s) 883.0
complicated 883.1
thumb 883.0
complicated 883.1
toe(s) 893.0
complicated 893.1

nape (neck) 874.8
complicated 874.9
specified part NEC 874.8
complicated 874.9

nasal (*see also* Wound, open, nose)
cavity 873.22
complicated 873.32
septum 873.21
complicated 873.31
sinuses 873.23
complicated 873.33

nasopharynx 873.22
complicated 873.32

neck 874.8
complicated 874.9
nape 874.8
complicated 874.9
specified part NEC 874.8

Wound, open — *continued*

neck — *continued*
specified part — *continued*
complicated 874.9

nerve — *see* Injury, nerve, by site

non-healing surgical 998.83

nose 873.20
complicated 873.30
multiple sites 873.29
complicated 873.39
septum 873.21
complicated 873.31
sinuses 873.23
complicated 873.33

occipital region — *see* Wound, open, scalp

ocular NEC 871.9
adnexa 870.9
specified region NEC 870.8
laceration (*see also* Laceration, ocular) 871.4
muscle (extraocular) 870.3
with foreign body 870.4
eyelid 870.1
intraocular — *see* Wound, open, eyeball
penetrating (*see also* Penetrating wound, ocular) 871.7

orbit 870.8
penetrating 870.3
with foreign body 870.4

orbital region 870.9

ovary — *see* Injury, internal, pelvic organs

palate 873.65
complicated 873.75

palm 882.0
with tendon involvement 882.2
complicated 882.1

parathyroid (gland) 874.2
complicated 874.3

parietal region — *see* Wound, open, scalp

pelvic floor or region 879.6
complicated 879.7

penis 878.0
complicated 878.1

perineum 879.6
complicated 879.7

periocular area 870.8
laceration of skin 870.0

pharynx 874.4
complicated 874.5

pinna 872.01
complicated 872.11

popliteal space 891.0
with tendon involvement 891.2
complicated 891.1

prepuce 878.0
complicated 878.1

pubic region 879.2
complicated 879.3

pudenda 878.8
complicated 878.9

rectovaginal septum 878.8
complicated 878.9

sacral region 877.0
complicated 877.1

sacroiliac region 877.0
complicated 877.1

salivary (ducts) (glands) 873.69
complicated 873.79

scalp 873.0
complicated 873.1

scalpel, fetus or newborn 767.8

scapular region 880.01
with tendon involvement 880.21
complicated 880.11
involving other sites of upper arm 880.09
with tendon involvement 880.29
complicated 880.19

sclera (*see also* Wound, open, intraocular) 871.9

scrotum 878.2
complicated 878.3

seminal vesicle — *see* Injury, internal, pelvic organs

shin 891.0
with tendon involvement 891.2

☑ **Additional Digit Required** — Refer to the Tabular List for Digit Selection   ▽ **Subterms under main terms may continue to next column or page**

340   **2014 ICD-9-CM**

Wound, open — continued
  shin — continued
    complicated 891.1
  shoulder 880.00
    with tendon involvement 880.20
    complicated 880.10
    involving other sites of upper arm 880.09
      with tendon involvement 880.29
      complicated 880.19
  skin NEC 879.8
    complicated 879.9
  skull (see also Injury, intracranial, with open
    intracranial wound)
    with skull fracture — see Fracture, skull
  spermatic cord (scrotal) 878.2
    complicated 878.3
    pelvic region — see Injury, internal,
      spermatic cord
  spinal cord — see Injury, spinal
  sternal region 875.0
    complicated 875.1
  subconjunctival — see Wound, open, in-
    traocular
  subcutaneous NEC 879.8
    complicated 879.9
  submaxillary region 873.44
    complicated 873.54
  submental region 873.44
    complicated 873.54
  subungual
    finger(s) (thumb) — see Wound, open,
      finger
    toe(s) — see Wound, open, toe
  supraclavicular region 874.8
    complicated 874.9
  supraorbital 873.42
    complicated 873.52
  surgical, non-healing 998.83
  temple 873.49
    complicated 873.59
  temporal region 873.49
    complicated 873.59
  testis 878.2
    complicated 878.3
  thigh 890.0
    with tendon involvement 890.2
    complicated 890.1
  thorax, thoracic (external) 875.0
    routined 875.1
  throat 874.8
    complicated 874.9
  thumb (nail) (subungual) 883.0
    with tendon involvement 883.2
    complicated 883.1
  thyroid (gland) 874.2
    complicated 874.3
  toe(s) (nail) (subungual) 893.0
    with tendon involvement 893.2
    complicated 893.1
  tongue 873.64
    complicated 873.74
  tonsil — see Wound, open, neck
  trachea (cervical region) 874.02
    with larynx 874.00
      complicated 874.10
    complicated 874.12
    intrathoracic — see Injury, internal, tra-
      chea
  trunk (multiple) NEC 879.6
    complicated 879.7
    specified site NEC 879.6
      complicated 879.7

Wound, open — continued
  tunica vaginalis 878.2
    complicated 878.3
  tympanic membrane 872.61
    complicated 872.71
  tympanum 872.61
    complicated 872.71
  umbilical region 879.2
    complicated 879.3
  ureter — see Injury, internal, ureter
  urethra — see Injury, internal, urethra
  uterus — see Injury, internal, uterus
  uvula 873.69
    complicated 873.79
  vagina 878.6
    complicated 878.7
  vas deferens — see Injury, internal, vas def-
    erens
  vitreous (humor) 871.2
  vulva 878.4
    complicated 878.5
  wrist 881.02
    with tendon involvement 881.22
    complicated 881.12
Wright's syndrome (hyperabduction) 447.8
  pneumonia 390 [517.1]
Wringer injury — see Crush injury, by site
Wrinkling of skin 701.8
Wrist — see also condition
  drop (acquired) 736.05
Wrong drug (given in error) NEC 977.9
  specified drug or substance — see Table of
    Drugs and Chemicals
Wry neck — see also Torticollis
  congenital 754.1
Wuchereria infestation 125.0
  bancrofti 125.0
  Brugia malayi 125.1
  malayi 125.1
Wuchereriasis 125.0
Wuchereriosis 125.0
Wuchernde struma langhans (M8332/3) 193

X

Xanthelasma 272.2
  eyelid 272.2 [374.51]
  palpebrarum 272.2 [374.51]
Xanthelasmatosis (essential) 272.2
Xanthelasmoidea 757.33
Xanthine stones 277.2
Xanthinuria 277.2
Xanthofibroma (M8831/0) — see Neoplasm,
  connective tissue, benign
Xanthoma(s), xanthomatosis 272.2
  with
    hyperlipoproteinemia
      type I 272.3
      type III 272.2
      type IV 272.1
      type V 272.3
  bone 272.7
  craniohypophyseal 277.89
  cutaneotendinous 272.7
  diabeticorum 250.8 ☑ [272.2]
    due to secondary diabetes
      249.8 ☑ [272.2]
  disseminatum 272.7
  eruptive 272.2
  eyelid 272.2 [374.51]
  familial 272.7
  hereditary 272.7

Xanthoma(s), xanthomatosis —
  continued
  hypercholesterinemic 272.0
  hypercholesterolemic 272.0
  hyperlipemic 272.4
  hyperlipidemic 272.4
  infantile 272.7
  joint 272.7
  juvenile 272.7
  multiple 272.7
  multiplex 272.7
  primary familial 272.7
  tendon (sheath) 272.7
  tuberosum 272.2
  tuberous 272.2
  tubo-eruptive 272.2
Xanthosis 709.09
  surgical 998.81
Xenophobia 300.29
Xeroderma (congenital) 757.39
  acquired 701.1
    eyelid 373.33
  eyelid 373.33
  pigmentosum 757.33
  vitamin A deficiency 264.8
Xerophthalmia 372.53
  vitamin A deficiency 264.7
Xerosis
  conjunctiva 372.53
    with Bitôt's spot 372.53
      vitamin A deficiency 264.1
    vitamin A deficiency 264.0
  cornea 371.40
    with corneal ulceration 370.00
      vitamin A deficiency 264.3
    vitamin A deficiency 264.2
  cutis 706.8
  skin 706.8
Xerostomia 527.7
Xiphodynia 733.90
Xiphoidalgia 733.90
Xiphoiditis 733.99
Xiphopagus 759.4
XO syndrome 758.6
X-ray
  effects, adverse, NEC 990
  of chest
    for suspected tuberculosis V71.2
    routine V72.5
XXX syndrome 758.81
XXXXY syndrome 758.81
XXY syndrome 758.7
Xyloketosuria 271.8
Xylosuria 271.8
Xylulosuria 271.8
XYY syndrome 758.81

Y

Yaba monkey tumor virus 059.22
Yawning 786.09
  psychogenic 306.1
Yaws 102.9
  bone or joint lesions 102.6
  butter 102.1
  chancre 102.0
  cutaneous, less than five years after infec-
    tion 102.2
  early (cutaneous) (macular) (maculopapular)
    (micropapular) (papular) 102.2
    frambeside 102.2
    skin lesions NEC 102.2

Yaws — continued
  eyelid 102.9 [373.4]
  ganglion 102.6
  gangosis, gangosa 102.5
  gumma, gummata 102.4
    bone 102.6
  gummatous
    frambeside 102.4
    osteitis 102.6
    periostitis 102.6
  hydrarthrosis 102.6
  hyperkeratosis (early) (late) (palmar) (plan-
    tar) 102.3
  initial lesions 102.0
  joint lesions 102.6
  juxta-articular nodules 102.7
  late nodular (ulcerated) 102.4
  latent (without clinical manifestations) (with
    positive serology) 102.8
  mother 102.0
  mucosal 102.7
  multiple papillomata 102.1
  nodular, late (ulcerated) 102.4
  osteitis 102.6
  papilloma, papillomata (palmar) (plantar)
    102.1
  periostitis (hypertrophic) 102.6
  ulcers 102.4
  wet crab 102.1
Yeast infection — see also Candidiasis 112.9
Yellow
  atrophy (liver) 570
    chronic 571.8
    resulting from administration of blood,
      plasma, serum, or other biological
      substance (within 8 months of
      administration) — see Hepatitis,
      viral
  fever — see Fever, yellow
  jack (see also Fever, yellow) 060.9
  jaundice (see also Jaundice) 782.4
  vernix syndrome 762.2
Yersinia septica 027.8

Z

Zagari's disease (xerostomia) 527.7
Zahorsky's disease (exanthema subitum) (see
  also Exanthem subitum) 058.10
  syndrome (herpangina) 074.0
Zellweger syndrome 277.86
Zenker's diverticulum (esophagus) 530.6
Ziehen-Oppenheim disease 333.6
Zieve's syndrome (jaundice, hyperlipemia,
  and hemolytic anemia) 571.1
Zika fever 066.3
Zollinger-Ellison syndrome (gastric hyper-
  secretion with pancreatic islet cell tu-
  mor) 251.5
Zona — see also Herpes, zoster 053.9
Zoophilia (erotica) 302.1
Zoophobia 300.29
Zoster (herpes) — see also Herpes, zoster 053.9
Zuelzer (-Ogden) anemia or syndrome (nu-
  tritional megaloblastic anemia) 281.2
Zygodactyly — see also Syndactylism 755.10
Zygomycosis 117.7
Zymotic — see condition

☑ **Additional Digit Required — Refer to the Tabular List for Digit Selection**
▽ **Subterms under main terms may continue to next column or page**

2014 ICD-9-CM   **341**

SECTION 2

Alphabetic Index to Poisoning and External Causes of Adverse Effects of Drugs and Other Chemical Substances

TABLE OF DRUGS AND CHEMICALS

This table contains a classification of drugs and other chemical substances to identify poisoning states and external causes of adverse effects.

Each of the listed substances in the table is assigned a code according to the poisoning classification (960-989). These codes are used when there is a statement of poisoning, overdose, wrong substance given or taken, or intoxication.

The table also contains a listing of external causes of adverse effects. An adverse effect is a pathologic manifestation due to ingestion or exposure to drugs or other chemical substances (e.g., dermatitis, hypersensitivity reaction, aspirin gastritis). The adverse effect is to be identified by the appropriate code found in Section 1, Index to Diseases and Injuries. An external cause code can then be used to identify the circumstances involved. The table headings pertaining to external causes are defined below:

Accidental poisoning (E850-E869) — accidental overdose of drug, wrong substance given or taken, drug taken inadvertently, accidents in the usage of drugs and biologicals in medical and surgical procedures, and to show external causes of poisonings classifiable to 980-989.

Therapeutic use (E930-E949) — a correct substance properly administered in therapeutic or prophylactic dosage as the external cause of adverse effects.

Suicide attempt (E950-E952) — instances in which self-inflicted injuries or poisonings are involved.

Assault (E961-E962) — injury or poisoning inflicted by another person with the intent to injure or kill.

Undetermined (E980-E982) — to be used when the intent of the poisoning or injury cannot be determined whether it was intentional or accidental.

The American Hospital Formulary Service list numbers are included in the table to help classify new drugs not identified in the table by name. The AHFS list numbers are keyed to the continually revised American Hospital Formulary Service (AHFS).* These listings are found in the table under the main term **Drug**.

Excluded from the table are radium and other radioactive substances. The classification of adverse effects and complications pertaining to these substances will be found in Section 1, Index to Diseases and Injuries, and Section 3, Index to External Causes of Injuries.

Although certain substances are indexed with one or more subentries, the majority are listed according to one use or state. It is recognized that many substances may be used in various ways, in medicine and in industry, and may cause adverse effects whatever the state of the agent (solid, liquid, or fumes arising from a liquid). In cases in which the reported data indicates a use or state not in the table, or which is clearly different from the one listed, an attempt should be made to classify the substance in the form which most nearly expresses the reported facts.

*American Hospital Formulary Service, 2 vol. (Washington, D.C.: American Society of Hospital Pharmacists, 1959-)

	Poisoning	Accident	Therapeutic Use	Suicide Attempt	Assault	Undetermined
1-propanol	980.3	E860.4	—	E950.9	E962.1	E980.9
2-propanol	980.2	E860.3	—	E950.9	E962.1	E980.9
2, 4-D (dichlorophenoxyacetic acid)	989.4	E863.5	—	E950.6	E962.1	E980.7
2, 4-toluene diisocyanate	983.0	E864.0	—	E950.7	E962.1	E980.6
2, 4, 5-T (trichlorophenoxyacetic acid)	989.2	E863.5	—	E950.6	E962.1	E980.7
14-hydroxydihydromorphinone	965.09	E850.2	E935.2	E950.0	E962.0	E980.0
ABOB	961.7	E857	E931.7	E950.4	E962.0	E980.4
Abrus (seed)	988.2	E865.3	—	E950.9	E962.1	E980.9
Absinthe	980.0	E860.1	—	E950.9	E962.1	E980.9
beverage	980.0	E860.0	—	E950.9	E962.1	E980.9
Acenocoumarin, acenocoumarol	964.2	E858.2	E934.2	E950.4	E962.0	E980.4
Acepromazine	969.1	E853.0	E939.1	E950.3	E962.0	E980.3
Acetal	982.8	E862.4	—	E950.9	E962.1	E980.9
Acetaldehyde (vapor)	987.8	E869.8	—	E952.8	E962.2	E982.8
liquid	989.89	E866.8	—	E950.9	E962.1	E980.9
Acetaminophen	965.4	E850.4	E935.4	E950.0	E962.0	E980.0
Acetaminosalol	965.1	E850.3	E935.3	E950.0	E962.0	E980.0
Acetanilid(e)	965.4	E850.4	E935.4	E950.0	E962.0	E980.0
Acetarsol, acetarsone	961.1	E857	E931.1	E950.4	E962.0	E980.4
Acetazolamide	974.2	E858.5	E944.2	E950.4	E962.0	E980.4
Acetic						
acid	983.1	E864.1	—	E950.7	E962.1	E980.6
with sodium acetate (ointment)	976.3	E858.7	E946.3	E950.4	E962.0	E980.4
irrigating solution	974.5	E858.5	E944.5	E950.4	E962.0	E980.4
lotion	976.2	E858.7	E946.2	E950.4	E962.0	E980.4
anhydride	983.1	E864.1	—	E950.7	E962.1	E980.6
ether (vapor)	982.8	E862.4	—	E950.9	E962.1	E980.9
Acetohexamide	962.3	E858.0	E932.3	E950.4	E962.0	E980.4
Acetomenaphthone	964.3	E858.2	E934.3	E950.4	E962.0	E980.4
Acetomorphine	965.01	E850.0	E935.0	E950.0	E962.0	E980.0
Acetone (oils) (vapor)	982.8	E862.4	—	E950.9	E962.1	E980.9
Acetophenazine						
(maleate)	969.1	E853.0	E939.1	E950.3	E962.0	E980.3
Acetophenetidin	965.4	E850.4	E935.4	E950.0	E962.0	E980.0
Acetophenone	982.8	E862.4	—	E950.9	E962.1	E980.9
Acetorphine	965.09	E850.2	E935.2	E950.0	E962.0	E980.0
Acetosulfone (sodium)	961.8	E857	E931.8	E950.4	E962.0	E980.4
Acetrizoate (sodium)	977.8	E858.8	E947.8	E950.4	E962.0	E980.4
Acetylcarbromal	967.3	E852.2	E937.3	E950.2	E962.0	E980.2
Acetylcholine (chloride)	971.0	E855.3	E941.0	E950.4	E962.0	E980.4
Acetylcysteine	975.5	E858.6	E945.5	E950.4	E962.0	E980.4
Acetyldigitoxin	972.1	E858.3	E942.1	E950.4	E962.0	E980.4
Acetyldihydrocodeine	965.09	E850.2	E935.2	E950.0	E962.0	E980.0
Acetyldihydrocodeinone	965.09	E850.2	E935.2	E950.0	E962.0	E980.0
Acetylene (gas) (industrial)	987.1	E868.1	—	E951.8	E962.2	E981.8
incomplete combustion of — see Carbon monoxide, fuel, utility						
tetrachloride (vapor)	982.3	E862.4	—	E950.9	E962.1	E980.9
Acetyliodosalicylic acid	965.1	E850.3	E935.3	E950.0	E962.0	E980.0
Acetylphenylhydrazine	965.8	E850.8	E935.8	E950.0	E962.0	E980.0
Acetylsalicylic acid	965.1	E850.3	E935.3	E950.0	E962.0	E980.0
Achromycin	960.4	E856	E930.4	E950.4	E962.0	E980.4
ophthalmic preparation	976.5	E858.7	E946.5	E950.4	E962.0	E980.4
topical NEC	976.0	E858.7	E946.0	E950.4	E962.0	E980.4
Acidifying agents	963.2	E858.1	E933.2	E950.4	E962.0	E980.4
Acids (corrosive) NEC	983.1	E864.1	—	E950.7	E962.1	E980.6
Aconite (wild)	988.2	E865.4	—	E950.9	E962.1	E980.9
Aconitine (liniment)	976.8	E858.7	E946.8	E950.4	E962.0	E980.4
Aconitum ferox	988.2	E865.4	—	E950.9	E962.1	E980.9
Acridine	983.0	E864.0	—	E950.7	E962.1	E980.6
vapor	987.8	E869.8	—	E952.8	E962.2	E982.8
Acriflavine	961.9	E857	E931.9	E950.4	E962.0	E980.4
Acrisorcin	976.0	E858.7	E946.0	E950.4	E962.0	E980.4
Acrolein (gas)	987.8	E869.8	—	E952.8	E962.2	E982.8
liquid	989.89	E866.8	—	E950.9	E962.1	E980.9
Actaea spicata	988.2	E865.4	—	E950.9	E962.1	E980.9
Acterol	961.5	E857	E931.5	E950.4	E962.0	E980.4
ACTH	962.4	E858.0	E932.4	E950.4	E962.0	E980.4
Acthar	962.4	E858.0	E932.4	E950.4	E962.0	E980.4
Actinomycin (C) (D)	960.7	E856	E930.7	E950.4	E962.0	E980.4
Adalin (acetyl)	967.3	E852.2	E937.3	E950.2	E962.0	E980.2
Adenosine (phosphate)	977.8	E858.8	E947.8	E950.4	E962.0	E980.4
ADH	962.5	E858.0	E932.5	E950.4	E962.0	E980.4
Adhesives	989.89	E866.6	—	E950.9	E962.1	E980.9

	Poisoning	Accident	Therapeutic Use	Suicide Attempt	Assault	Undetermined
Adicillin	960.0	E856	E930.0	E950.4	E962.0	E980.4
Adiphenine	975.1	E855.6	E945.1	E950.4	E962.0	E980.4
Adjunct, pharmaceutical	977.4	E858.8	E947.4	E950.4	E962.0	E980.4
Adrenal (extract, cortex or medulla) (glucocorticoids) (hormones) (mineralocorticoids)	962.0	E858.0	E932.0	E950.4	E962.0	E980.4
ENT agent	976.6	E858.7	E946.6	E950.4	E962.0	E980.4
ophthalmic preparation	976.5	E858.7	E946.5	E950.4	E962.0	E980.4
topical NEC	976.0	E858.7	E946.0	E950.4	E962.0	E980.4
Adrenalin	971.2	E855.5	E941.2	E950.4	E962.0	E980.4
Adrenergic blocking agents	971.3	E855.6	E941.3	E950.4	E962.0	E980.4
Adrenergics	971.2	E855.5	E941.2	E950.4	E962.0	E980.4
Adrenochrome (derivatives)	972.8	E858.3	E942.8	E950.4	E962.0	E980.4
Adrenocorticotropic hormone	962.4	E858.0	E932.4	E950.4	E962.0	E980.4
Adrenocorticotropin	962.4	E858.0	E932.4	E950.4	E962.0	E980.4
Adriamycin	960.7	E856	E930.7	E950.4	E962.0	E980.4
Aerosol spray — see Sprays						
Aerosporin	960.8	E856	E930.8	E950.4	E962.0	E980.4
ENT agent	976.6	E858.7	E946.6	E950.4	E962.0	E980.4
ophthalmic preparation	976.5	E858.7	E946.5	E950.4	E962.0	E980.4
topical NEC	976.0	E858.7	E946.0	E950.4	E962.0	E980.4
Aethusa cynapium	988.2	E865.4	—	E950.9	E962.1	E980.9
Afghanistan black	969.6	E854.1	E939.6	E950.3	E962.0	E980.3
Aflatoxin	989.7	E865.9	—	E950.9	E962.1	E980.9
African boxwood	988.2	E865.4	—	E950.9	E962.1	E980.9
Agar (-agar)	973.3	E858.4	E943.3	E950.4	E962.0	E980.4
Agricultural agent NEC	989.89	E863.9	—	E950.6	E962.1	E980.7
Agrypnal	967.0	E851	E937.0	E950.1	E962.0	E980.1
Air contaminant(s), source or type not specified	987.9	E869.9	—	E952.9	E962.2	E982.9
specified type — see specific substance						
Akee	988.2	E865.4	—	E950.9	E962.1	E980.9
Akrinol	976.0	E858.7	E946.0	E950.4	E962.0	E980.4
Alantolactone	961.6	E857	E931.6	E950.4	E962.0	E980.4
Albamycin	960.8	E856	E930.8	E950.4	E962.0	E980.4
Albumin (normal human serum)	964.7	E858.2	E934.7	E950.4	E962.0	E980.4
Albuterol	975.7	E858.6	E945.7	E950.4	E962.0	E980.4
Alcohol	980.9	E860.9	—	E950.9	E962.1	E980.9
absolute	980.0	E860.1	—	E950.9	E962.1	E980.9
beverage	980.0	E860.0	E947.8	E950.9	E962.1	E980.9
amyl	980.3	E860.4	—	E950.9	E962.1	E980.9
antifreeze	980.1	E860.2	—	E950.9	E962.1	E980.9
butyl	980.3	E860.4	—	E950.9	E962.1	E980.9
dehydrated	980.0	E860.1	—	E950.9	E962.1	E980.9
beverage	980.0	E860.0	E947.8	E950.9	E962.1	E980.9
denatured	980.0	E860.1	—	E950.9	E962.1	E980.9
deterrents	977.3	E858.8	E947.3	E950.4	E962.0	E980.4
diagnostic (gastric function)	977.8	E858.8	E947.8	E950.4	E962.0	E980.4
ethyl	980.0	E860.1	—	E950.9	E962.1	E980.9
beverage	980.0	E860.0	E947.8	E950.9	E962.1	E980.9
grain	980.0	E860.1	—	E950.9	E962.1	E980.9
beverage	980.0	E860.0	E947.8	E950.9	E962.1	E980.9
industrial	980.9	E860.9	—	E950.9	E962.1	E980.9
isopropyl	980.2	E860.3	—	E950.9	E962.1	E980.9
methyl	980.1	E860.2	—	E950.9	E962.1	E980.9
preparation for consumption	980.0	E860.0	E947.8	E950.9	E962.1	E980.9
propyl	980.3	E860.4	—	E950.9	E962.1	E980.9
secondary	980.2	E860.3	—	E950.9	E962.1	E980.9
radiator	980.1	E860.2	—	E950.9	E962.1	E980.9
rubbing	980.2	E860.3	—	E950.9	E962.1	E980.9
specified type NEC	980.8	E860.8	—	E950.9	E962.1	E980.9
surgical	980.9	E860.9	—	E950.9	E962.1	E980.9
vapor (from any type of alcohol)	987.8	E869.8	—	E952.8	E962.2	E982.8
wood	980.1	E860.2	—	E950.9	E962.1	E980.9
Alcuronium chloride	975.2	E858.6	E945.2	E950.4	E962.0	E980.4
Aldactone	974.4	E858.5	E944.4	E950.4	E962.0	E980.4
Aldicarb	989.3	E863.2	—	E950.6	E962.1	E980.7
Aldomet	972.6	E858.3	E942.6	E950.4	E962.0	E980.4
Aldosterone	962.0	E858.0	E932.0	E950.4	E962.0	E980.4
Aldrin (dust)	989.2	E863.0	—	E950.6	E962.1	E980.7
Algeldrate	973.0	E858.4	E943.0	E950.4	E962.0	E980.4
Alidase	963.4	E858.1	E933.4	E950.4	E962.0	E980.4
Aliphatic thiocyanates	989.0	E866.8	—	E950.9	E962.1	E980.9

External Cause (E-Code) — Left column

Substance	Poisoning	Accident	Therapeutic Use	Suicide Attempt	Assault	Undetermined
Alkaline antiseptic solution (aromatic)	976.6	E858.7	E946.6	E950.4	E962.0	E980.4
Alkalinizing agents (medicinal)	963.3	E858.1	E933.3	E950.4	E962.0	E980.4
Alkalis, caustic	983.2	E864.2	—	E950.7	E962.1	E980.6
Alkalizing agents (medicinal)	963.3	E858.1	E933.3	E950.4	E962.0	E980.4
Alka-seltzer	965.1	E850.3	E935.3	E950.0	E962.0	E980.0
Alkavervir	972.6	E858.3	E942.6	E950.4	E962.0	E980.4
Allegron	969.05	E854.0	E939.0	E950.3	E962.0	E980.3
Alleve — Naproxen						
Allobarbital, allobarbitone	967.0	E851	E937.0	E950.1	E962.0	E980.1
Allopurinol	974.7	E858.5	E944.7	E950.4	E962.0	E980.4
Allylestrenol	962.2	E858.0	E932.2	E950.4	E962.0	E980.4
Allylisopropylacetylurea	967.8	E852.8	E937.8	E950.2	E962.0	E980.2
Allylisopropylmalonylurea	967.0	E851	E937.0	E950.1	E962.0	E980.1
Allyltribromide	967.3	E852.2	E937.3	E950.2	E962.0	E980.2
Aloe, aloes, aloin	973.1	E858.4	E943.1	E950.4	E962.0	E980.4
Alosetron	973.8	E858.4	E943.8	E950.4	E962.0	E980.4
Aloxidone	966.0	E855.0	E936.0	E950.4	E962.0	E980.4
Aloxiprin	965.1	E850.3	E935.3	E950.0	E962.0	E980.0
Alpha-1 blockers	971.3	E855.6	E941.3	E950.4	E962.0	E980.4
Alpha amylase	963.4	E858.1	E933.4	E950.4	E962.0	E980.4
Alphaprodine (hydrochloride)	965.09	E850.2	E935.2	E950.0	E962.0	E980.0
Alpha tocopherol	963.5	E858.1	E933.5	E950.4	E962.0	E980.4
Alseroxylon	972.6	E858.3	E942.6	E950.4	E962.0	E980.4
Alum (ammonium) (potassium)	983.2	E864.2	—	E950.7	E962.1	E980.6
medicinal (astringent) NEC	976.2	E858.7	E946.2	E950.4	E962.0	E980.4
Aluminium, aluminum (gel) (hydroxide)	973.0	E858.4	E943.0	E950.4	E962.0	E980.4
acetate solution	976.2	E858.7	E946.2	E950.4	E962.0	E980.4
aspirin	965.1	E850.3	E935.3	E950.0	E962.0	E980.0
carbonate	973.0	E858.4	E943.0	E950.4	E962.0	E980.4
glycinate	973.0	E858.4	E943.0	E950.4	E962.0	E980.4
nicotinate	972.2	E858.3	E942.2	E950.4	E962.0	E980.4
ointment (surgical) (topical)	976.3	E858.7	E946.3	E950.4	E962.0	E980.4
phosphate	973.0	E858.4	E943.0	E950.4	E962.0	E980.4
subacetate	976.2	E858.7	E946.2	E950.4	E962.0	E980.4
topical NEC	976.3	E858.7	E946.3	E950.4	E962.0	E980.4
Alurate	967.0	E851	E937.0	E950.1	E962.0	E980.1
Alverine (citrate)	975.1	E858.6	E945.1	E950.4	E962.0	E980.4
Alvodine	965.09	E850.2	E935.2	E950.0	E962.0	E980.0
Amanita phalloides	988.1	E865.5	—	E950.9	E962.1	E980.9
Amantadine (hydrochloride)	966.4	E855.0	E936.4	E950.4	E962.0	E980.4
Ambazone	961.9	E857	E931.9	E950.4	E962.0	E980.4
Ambenonium	971.0	E855.3	E941.0	E950.4	E962.0	E980.4
Ambutonium bromide	971.1	E855.4	E941.1	E950.4	E962.0	E980.4
Ametazole	977.8	E858.8	E947.8	E950.4	E962.0	E980.4
Amethocaine (infiltration) (topical)	968.5	E855.2	E938.5	E950.4	E962.0	E980.4
nerve block (peripheral) (plexus)	968.6	E855.2	E938.6	E950.4	E962.0	E980.4
spinal	968.7	E855.2	E938.7	E950.4	E962.0	E980.4
Amethopterin	963.1	E858.1	E933.1	E950.4	E962.0	E980.4
Amfepramone	977.0	E858.8	E947.0	E950.4	E962.0	E980.4
Amidon	965.02	E850.1	E935.1	E950.0	E962.0	E980.0
Amidopyrine	965.5	E850.5	E935.5	E950.0	E962.0	E980.0
Aminacrine	976.0	E858.7	E946.0	E950.4	E962.0	E980.4
Aminitrozole	961.5	E857	E931.5	E950.4	E962.0	E980.4
Aminoacetic acid	974.5	E858.5	E944.5	E950.4	E962.0	E980.4
Amino acids	974.5	E858.5	E944.5	E950.4	E962.0	E980.4
Aminocaproic acid	964.4	E858.2	E934.4	E950.4	E962.0	E980.4
Aminoethylisothiourium	963.8	E858.1	E933.8	E950.4	E962.0	E980.4
Aminoglutethimide	966.3	E855.0	E936.3	E950.4	E962.0	E980.4
Aminometradine	974.3	E858.5	E944.3	E950.4	E962.0	E980.4
Aminopentamide	971.1	E855.4	E941.1	E950.4	E962.0	E980.4
Aminophenazone	965.5	E850.5	E935.5	E950.0	E962.0	E980.0
Aminophenol	983.0	E864.0	—	E950.7	E962.1	E980.6
Aminophenylpyridone	969.5	E853.8	E939.5	E950.3	E962.0	E980.3
Aminophyllin	975.7	E858.6	E945.7	E950.4	E962.0	E980.4
Aminopterin	963.1	E858.1	E933.1	E950.4	E962.0	E980.4
Aminopyrine	965.5	E850.5	E935.5	E950.0	E962.0	E980.0
Aminosalicylic acid	961.8	E857	E931.8	E950.4	E962.0	E980.4
Amiphenazole	970.1	E854.3	E940.1	E950.4	E962.0	E980.4
Amiquinsin	972.6	E858.3	E942.6	E950.4	E962.0	E980.4

External Cause (E-Code) — Right column

Substance	Poisoning	Accident	Therapeutic Use	Suicide Attempt	Assault	Undetermined
Amisometradine	974.3	E858.5	E944.3	E950.4	E962.0	E980.4
Amitriptyline	969.05	E854.0	E939.0	E950.3	E962.0	E980.3
Ammonia (fumes) (gas) (vapor)	987.8	E869.8	—	E952.8	E962.2	E982.8
liquid (household) NEC	983.2	E861.4	—	E950.7	E962.1	E980.6
spirit, aromatic	970.89	E854.3	E940.8	E950.4	E962.0	E980.4
Ammoniated mercury	976.0	E858.7	E946.0	E950.4	E962.0	E980.4
Ammonium carbonate	983.2	E864.2	—	E950.7	E962.1	E980.6
chloride (acidifying agent)	963.2	E858.1	E933.2	E950.4	E962.0	E980.4
expectorant	975.5	E858.6	E945.5	E950.4	E962.0	E980.4
compounds (household) NEC	983.2	E861.4	—	E950.7	E962.1	E980.6
fumes (any usage)	987.8	E869.8	—	E952.8	E962.2	E982.8
industrial	983.2	E864.2	—	E950.7	E962.1	E980.6
ichthyosulfonate	976.4	E858.7	E946.4	E950.4	E962.0	E980.4
mandelate	961.9	E857	E931.9	E950.4	E962.0	E980.4
Amobarbital	967.0	E851	E937.0	E950.1	E962.0	E980.1
Amodiaquin(e)	961.4	E857	E931.4	E950.4	E962.0	E980.4
Amopyroquin(e)	961.4	E857	E931.4	E950.4	E962.0	E980.4
Amphenidone	969.5	E853.8	E939.5	E950.3	E962.0	E980.3
Amphetamine	969.72	E854.2	E939.7	E950.3	E962.0	E980.3
Amphomycin	960.8	E856	E930.8	E950.4	E962.0	E980.4
Amphotericin B	960.1	E856	E930.1	E950.4	E962.0	E980.4
topical	976.0	E858.7	E946.0	E950.4	E962.0	E980.4
Ampicillin	960.0	E856	E930.0	E950.4	E962.0	E980.4
Amprotropine	971.1	E855.4	E941.1	E950.4	E962.0	E980.4
Amygdalin	977.8	E858.8	E947.8	E950.4	E962.0	E980.4
Amyl acetate (vapor)	982.8	E862.4	—	E950.9	E962.1	E980.9
alcohol	980.3	E860.4	—	E950.9	E962.1	E980.9
nitrite (medicinal)	972.4	E858.3	E942.4	E950.4	E962.0	E980.4
Amylase (alpha)	963.4	E858.1	E933.4	E950.4	E962.0	E980.4
Amylene hydrate	980.8	E860.8	—	E950.9	E962.1	E980.9
Amylobarbitone	967.0	E851	E937.0	E950.1	E962.0	E980.1
Amylocaine	968.9	E855.2	E938.9	E950.4	E962.0	E980.4
infiltration (subcutaneous)	968.5	E855.2	E938.5	E950.4	E962.0	E980.4
nerve block (peripheral) (plexus)	968.6	E855.2	E938.6	E950.4	E962.0	E980.4
spinal	968.7	E855.2	E938.7	E950.4	E962.0	E980.4
topical (surface)	968.5	E855.2	E938.5	E950.4	E962.0	E980.4
Amytal (sodium)	967.0	E851	E937.0	E950.1	E962.0	E980.1
Analeptics	970.0	E854.3	E940.0	E950.4	E962.0	E980.4
Analgesics	965.9	E850.9	E935.9	E950.0	E962.0	E980.0
aromatic NEC	965.4	E850.4	E935.4	E950.0	E962.0	E980.0
non-narcotic NEC	965.7	E850.7	E935.7	E950.0	E962.0	E980.0
specified NEC	965.8	E850.8	E935.8	E950.0	E962.0	E980.0
Anamirta cocculus	988.2	E865.3	—	E950.9	E962.1	E980.9
Ancillin	960.0	E856	E930.0	E950.4	E962.0	E980.4
Androgens (anabolic congeners)	962.1	E858.0	E932.1	E950.4	E962.0	E980.4
Androstalone	962.1	E858.0	E932.1	E950.4	E962.0	E980.4
Androsterone	962.1	E858.0	E932.1	E950.4	E962.0	E980.4
Anemone pulsatilla	988.2	E865.4	—	E950.9	E962.1	E980.9
Anesthesia, anesthetic (general) NEC	968.4	E855.1	E938.4	E950.4	E962.0	E980.4
block (nerve) (plexus)	968.6	E855.2	E938.6	E950.4	E962.0	E980.4
gaseous NEC	968.2	E855.1	E938.2	E950.4	E962.0	E980.4
halogenated hydrocarbon derivatives NEC	968.2	E855.1	E938.2	E950.4	E962.0	E980.4
infiltration (intradermal) (subcutaneous) (submucosal)	968.5	E855.2	E938.5	E950.4	E962.0	E980.4
intravenous	968.3	E855.1	E938.3	E950.4	E962.0	E980.4
local NEC	968.9	E855.2	E938.9	E950.4	E962.0	E980.4
nerve blocking (peripheral) (plexus)	968.6	E855.2	E938.6	E950.4	E962.0	E980.4
rectal NEC	968.3	E855.1	E938.3	E950.4	E962.0	E980.4
spinal	968.7	E855.2	E938.7	E950.4	E962.0	E980.4
surface	968.5	E855.2	E938.5	E950.4	E962.0	E980.4
topical	968.5	E855.2	E938.5	E950.4	E962.0	E980.4
Aneurine	963.5	E858.1	E933.5	E950.4	E962.0	E980.4
Anginine — see Glyceryl trinitrate						
Angio-Conray	977.8	E858.8	E947.8	E950.4	E962.0	E980.4
Angiotensin	971.2	E855.5	E941.2	E950.4	E962.0	E980.4
Anhydrohydroxyprogesterone	962.2	E858.0	E932.2	E950.4	E962.0	E980.4
Anhydron	974.3	E858.5	E944.3	E950.4	E962.0	E980.4
Anileridine	965.09	E850.2	E935.2	E950.0	E962.0	E980.0

	External Cause (E-Code)					
	Poisoning	Accident	Therapeutic Use	Suicide Attempt	Assault	Undetermined
Aniline (dye) (liquid)	983.0	E864.0	—	E950.7	E962.1	E980.6
analgesic	965.4	E850.4	E935.4	E950.0	E962.0	E980.0
derivatives, therapeutic NEC	965.4	E850.4	E935.4	E950.0	E962.0	E980.0
vapor	987.8	E869.8	—	E952.8	E962.2	E982.8
Aniscoropine	971.1	E855.4	E941.1	E950.4	E962.0	E980.4
Anisindione	964.2	E858.2	E934.2	E950.4	E962.0	E980.4
Anorexic agents	977.0	E858.8	E947.0	E950.4	E962.0	E980.4
Ant (bite) (sting)	—	E905.5	—	E950.9	E962.1	E980.9
Antabuse	977.3	E858.8	E947.3	E950.4	E962.0	E980.4
Antacids	973.0	E858.4	E943.0	E950.4	E962.0	E980.4
Antazoline	963.0	E858.1	E933.0	E950.4	E962.0	E980.4
Anthralin	976.4	E858.7	E946.4	E950.4	E962.0	E980.4
Anthramycin	960.7	E856	E930.7	E950.4	E962.0	E980.4
Antiadrenergics	971.3	E855.6	E941.3	E950.4	E962.0	E980.4
Antiallergic agents	963.0	E858.1	E933.0	E950.4	E962.0	E980.4
Antianemic agents NEC	964.1	E858.2	E934.1	E950.4	E962.0	E980.4
Antiaris toxicaria	988.2	E865.4	—	E950.9	E962.1	E980.9
Antiarteriosclerotic agents	972.2	E858.3	E942.2	E950.4	E962.0	E980.4
Antiasthmatics	975.7	E858.6	E945.7	E950.4	E962.0	E980.4
Antibiotics	960.9	E856	E930.9	E950.4	E962.0	E980.4
antifungal	960.1	E856	E930.1	E950.4	E962.0	E980.4
antimycobacterial	960.6	E856	E930.6	E950.4	E962.0	E980.4
antineoplastic	960.7	E856	E930.7	E950.4	E962.0	E980.4
cephalosporin (group)	960.5	E856	E930.5	E950.4	E962.0	E980.4
chloramphenicol (group)	960.2	E856	E930.2	E950.4	E962.0	E980.4
macrolides	960.3	E856	E930.3	E950.4	E962.0	E980.4
specified NEC	960.8	E856	E930.8	E950.4	E962.0	E980.4
tetracycline (group)	960.4	E856	E930.4	E950.4	E962.0	E980.4
Anticancer agents NEC	963.1	E858.1	E933.1	E950.4	E962.0	E980.4
antibiotics	960.7	E856	E930.7	E950.4	E962.0	E980.4
Anticholinergics	971.1	E855.4	E941.1	E950.4	E962.0	E980.4
Anticholinesterase (organophosphorus) (reversible)	971.0	E855.3	E941.0	E950.4	E962.0	E980.4
Anticoagulants	964.2	E858.2	E934.2	E950.4	E962.0	E980.4
antagonists	964.5	E858.2	E934.5	E950.4	E962.0	E980.4
Anti-common cold agents NEC	975.6	E858.6	E945.6	E950.4	E962.0	E980.4
Anticonvulsants NEC	966.3	E855.0	E936.3	E950.4	E962.0	E980.4
Antidepressants	969.00	E854.0	E939.0	E950.3	E962.0	E980.3
monoamine oxidase inhibitors (MAOI)	969.01	E854.0	E939.0	E950.3	E962.0	E980.3
specified type NEC	969.09	E854.0	E939.0	E950.3	E962.0	E980.3
SSNRI (selective serotonin and norepinephrine reuptake inhibitors)	969.02	E854.0	E939.0	E950.3	E962.0	E980.3
SSRI (selective serotonin reuptake inhibitors)	969.03	E854.0	E939.0	E950.3	E962.0	E980.3
tetracyclic	969.04	E854.0	E939.0	E950.3	E962.0	E980.3
tricyclic	969.05	E854.0	E939.0	E950.3	E962.0	E980.3
Antidiabetic agents	962.3	E858.0	E932.3	E950.4	E962.0	E980.4
Antidiarrheal agents	973.5	E858.4	E943.5	E950.4	E962.0	E980.4
Antidiuretic hormone	962.5	E858.0	E932.5	E950.4	E962.0	E980.4
Antidotes NEC	977.2	E858.8	E947.2	E950.4	E962.0	E980.4
Antiemetic agents	963.0	E858.1	E933.0	E950.4	E962.0	E980.4
Antiepilepsy agent NEC	966.3	E855.0	E936.3	E950.4	E962.0	E980.4
Antifertility pills	962.2	E858.0	E932.2	E950.4	E962.0	E980.4
Antiflatulents	973.8	E858.4	E943.8	E950.4	E962.0	E980.4
Antifreeze	989.89	E866.8	—	E950.9	E962.1	E980.9
alcohol	980.1	E860.2	—	E950.9	E962.1	E980.9
ethylene glycol	982.8	E862.4	—	E950.9	E962.1	E980.9
Antifungals (nonmedicinal) (sprays)	989.4	E863.6	—	E950.6	E962.1	E980.7
medicinal NEC	961.9	E857	E931.9	E950.4	E962.0	E980.4
antibiotic	960.1	E856	E930.1	E950.4	E962.0	E980.4
topical	976.0	E858.7	E946.0	E950.4	E962.0	E980.4
Antigastric secretion agents	973.0	E858.4	E943.0	E950.4	E962.0	E980.4
Antihelmintics	961.6	E857	E931.6	E950.4	E962.0	E980.4
Antihemophilic factor (human)	964.7	E858.2	E934.7	E950.4	E962.0	E980.4
Antihistamine	963.0	E858.1	E933.0	E950.4	E962.0	E980.4
Antihypertensive agents NEC	972.6	E858.3	E942.6	E950.4	E962.0	E980.4
Anti-infectives NEC	961.9	E857	E931.9	E950.4	E962.0	E980.4
antibiotics	960.9	E856	E930.9	E950.4	E962.0	E980.4
specified NEC	960.8	E856	E930.8	E950.4	E962.0	E980.4
antihelmintic	961.6	E857	E931.6	E950.4	E962.0	E980.4
antimalarial	961.4	E857	E931.4	E950.4	E962.0	E980.4
antimycobacterial NEC	961.8	E857	E931.8	E950.4	E962.0	E980.4
Anti-infectives — *continued*						
antimycobacterial — *continued*						
antibiotics	960.6	E856	E930.6	E950.4	E962.0	E980.4
antiprotozoal NEC	961.5	E857	E931.5	E950.4	E962.0	—
blood	961.4	E857	E931.4	E950.4	E962.0	E980.4
antiviral	961.7	E857	E931.7	E950.4	E962.0	E980.4
arsenical	961.1	E857	E931.1	E950.4	E962.0	E980.4
ENT agents	976.6	E858.7	E946.6	E950.4	E962.0	E980.4
heavy metals NEC	961.2	E857	E931.2	E950.4	E962.0	E980.4
local	976.0	E858.7	E946.0	E950.4	E962.0	E980.4
ophthalmic preparation	976.5	E858.7	E946.5	E950.4	E962.0	E980.4
topical NEC	976.0	E858.7	E946.0	E950.4	E962.0	E980.4
Anti-inflammatory agents (topical)	976.0	E858.7	E946.0	E950.4	E962.0	E980.4
Antiknock (tetraethyl lead)	984.1	E862.1	—	E950.9	—	E980.9
Antilipemics	972.2	E858.3	E942.2	E950.4	E962.0	E980.4
Antimalarials	961.4	E857	E931.4	E950.4	E962.0	E980.4
Antimony (compounds) (vapor) NEC	985.4	E866.2	—	E950.9	E962.1	E980.9
anti-infectives	961.2	E857	E931.2	E950.4	E962.0	E980.4
pesticides (vapor)	985.4	E863.4	—	E950.6	E962.2	E980.7
potassium tartrate	961.2	E857	E931.2	E950.4	E962.0	E980.4
tartrated	961.2	E857	E931.2	E950.4	E962.0	E980.4
Antimuscarinic agents	971.1	E855.4	E941.1	E950.4	E962.0	E980.4
Antimycobacterials NEC	961.8	E857	E931.8	E950.4	E962.0	E980.4
antibiotics	960.6	E856	E930.6	E950.4	E962.0	E980.4
Antineoplastic agents	963.1	E858.1	E933.1	E950.4	E962.0	E980.4
antibiotics	960.7	E856	E930.7	E950.4	E962.0	E980.4
Anti-Parkinsonism agents	966.4	E855.0	E936.4	E950.4	E962.0	E980.4
Antiphlogistics	965.69	E850.6	E935.6	E950.0	E962.0	E980.0
Antiprotozoals NEC	961.5	E857	E931.5	E950.4	E962.0	E980.4
blood	961.4	E857	E931.4	E950.4	E962.0	E980.4
Antipruritics (local)	976.1	E858.7	E946.1	E950.4	E962.0	E980.4
Antipsychotic agents NEC	969.3	E853.8	E939.3	E950.3	E962.0	E980.3
Antipyretics	965.9	E850.9	E935.9	E950.0	E962.0	E980.0
specified NEC	965.8	E850.8	E935.8	E950.0	E962.0	E980.0
Antipyrine	965.5	E850.5	E935.5	E950.0	E962.0	E980.0
Antirabies serum (equine)	979.9	E858.8	E949.9	E950.4	E962.0	E980.4
Antirheumatics	965.69	E850.6	E935.6	E950.0	E962.0	E980.0
Antiseborrheics	976.4	E858.7	E946.4	E950.4	E962.0	E980.4
Antiseptics (external) (medicinal)	976.0	E858.7	E946.0	E950.4	E962.0	E980.4
Antistine	963.0	E858.1	E933.0	E950.4	E962.0	E980.4
Antithyroid agents	962.8	E858.0	E932.8	E950.4	E962.0	E980.4
Antitoxin, any	979.9	E858.8	E949.9	E950.4	E962.0	E980.4
Antituberculars	961.8	E857	E931.8	E950.4	E962.0	E980.4
antibiotics	960.6	E856	E930.6	E950.4	E962.0	E980.4
Antitussives	975.4	E858.6	E945.4	E950.4	E962.0	E980.4
Antivaricose agents (sclerosing)	972.7	E858.3	E942.7	E950.4	E962.0	E980.4
Antivenin (crotaline) (spider-bite)	979.9	E858.8	E949.9	E950.4	E962.0	E980.4
Antivert	963.0	E858.1	E933.0	E950.4	E962.0	E980.4
Antivirals NEC	961.7	E857	E931.7	E950.4	E962.0	E980.4
Ant poisons — *see* Pesticides						
Antrol	989.4	E863.4	—	E950.6	E962.1	E980.7
fungicide	989.4	E863.6	—	E950.6	E962.1	E980.7
Apomorphine hydrochloride (emetic)	973.6	E858.4	E943.6	E950.4	E962.0	E980.4
Appetite depressants, central	977.0	E858.8	E947.0	E950.4	E962.0	E980.4
Apresoline	972.6	E858.3	E942.6	E950.4	E962.0	E980.4
Aprobarbital, aprobarbitone	967.0	E851	E937.0	E950.1	E962.0	E980.1
Apronalide	967.8	E852.8	E937.8	E950.2	E962.0	E980.2
Aqua fortis	983.1	E864.1	—	E950.7	E962.1	E980.6
Arachis oil (topical)	976.3	E858.7	E946.3	E950.4	E962.0	E980.4
cathartic	973.2	E858.4	E943.2	E950.4	E962.0	E980.4
Aralen	961.4	E857	E931.4	E950.4	E962.0	E980.4
Arginine salts	974.5	E858.5	E944.5	E950.4	E962.0	E980.4
Argyrol	976.0	E858.7	E946.0	E950.4	E962.0	E980.4
ENT agent	976.6	E858.7	E946.6	E950.4	E962.0	E980.4
ophthalmic preparation	976.5	E858.7	E946.5	E950.4	E962.0	E980.4
Aristocort	962.0	E858.0	E932.0	E950.4	E962.0	E980.4
ENT agent	976.6	E858.7	E946.6	E950.4	E962.0	E980.4
ophthalmic preparation	976.5	E858.7	E946.5	E950.4	E962.0	E980.4
topical NEC	976.0	E858.7	E946.0	E950.4	E962.0	E980.4

Aniline — Aristocort

Nontherapeutic use substance

⬇ Subterms under main terms may continue to next column or page

	Poisoning	Accident	Therapeutic Use	Suicide Attempt	Assault	Undetermined
Aromatics, corrosive	983.0	E864.0	—	E950.7	E962.1	E980.6
disinfectants	983.0	E861.4	—	E950.7	E962.1	E980.6
Arsenate of lead (insecticide)	985.1	E863.4	—	E950.8	E962.1	E980.8
herbicide	985.1	E863.5	—	E950.8	E962.1	E980.8
Arsenic, arsenicals (compounds) (dust) (fumes) (vapor) NEC	985.1	E866.3	—	E950.8	E962.1	E980.8
anti-infectives	961.1	E857	E931.1	E950.4	E962.0	E980.4
pesticide (dust) (fumes)	985.1	E863.4	—	E950.8	E962.1	E980.8
Arsine (gas)	985.1	E866.3	—	E950.8	E962.1	E980.8
Arsphenamine (silver)	961.1	E857	E931.1	E950.4	E962.0	E980.4
Arsthinol	961.1	E857	E931.1	E950.4	E962.0	E980.4
Artane	971.1	E855.4	E941.1	E950.4	E962.0	E980.4
Arthropod (venomous) NEC	989.5	E905.5	—	E950.9	E962.1	E980.9
Asbestos	989.81	E866.8	—	E950.9	E962.1	E980.9
Ascaridole	961.6	E857	E931.6	E950.4	E962.0	E980.4
Ascorbic acid	963.5	E858.1	E933.5	E950.4	E962.0	E980.4
Asiaticoside	976.0	E858.7	E946.0	E950.4	E962.0	E980.4
Aspidium (oleoresin)	961.6	E857	E931.6	E950.4	E962.0	E980.4
Aspirin	965.1	E850.3	E935.3	E950.0	E962.0	E980.0
Astringents (local)	976.2	E858.7	E946.2	E950.4	E962.0	E980.4
Atabrine	961.3	E857	E931.3	E950.4	E962.0	E980.4
Ataractics	969.5	E853.8	E939.5	E950.3	E962.0	E980.3
Atonia drug, intestinal	973.3	E858.4	E943.3	E950.4	E962.0	E980.4
Atophan	974.7	E858.5	E944.7	E950.4	E962.0	E980.4
Atropine	971.1	E855.4	E941.1	E950.4	E962.0	E980.4
Attapulgite	973.5	E858.4	E943.5	E950.4	E962.0	E980.4
Attenuvax	979.4	E858.8	E949.4	E950.4	E962.0	E980.4
Aureomycin	960.4	E856	E930.4	E950.4	E962.0	E980.4
ophthalmic preparation	976.5	E858.7	E946.5	E950.4	E962.0	E980.4
topical NEC	976.0	E858.7	E946.0	E950.4	E962.0	E980.4
Aurothioglucose	965.69	E850.6	E935.6	E950.0	E962.0	E980.0
Aurothioglycanide	965.69	E850.6	E935.6	E950.0	E962.0	E980.0
Aurothiomalate	965.69	E850.6	E935.6	E950.0	E962.0	E980.0
Automobile fuel	981	E862.1	—	E950.9	E962.1	E980.9
Autonomic nervous system agents NEC	971.9	E855.9	E941.9	E950.4	E962.0	E980.4
Avlosulfon	961.8	E857	E931.8	E950.4	E962.0	E980.4
Avomine	967.8	E852.8	E937.8	E950.2	E962.0	E980.2
Azacyclonol	969.5	E853.8	E939.5	E950.3	E962.0	E980.3
Azapetine	971.3	E855.6	E941.3	E950.4	E962.0	E980.4
Azaribine	963.1	E858.1	E933.1	E950.4	E962.0	E980.4
Azaserine	960.7	E856	E930.7	E950.4	E962.0	E980.4
Azathioprine	963.1	E858.1	E933.1	E950.4	E962.0	E980.4
Azosulfamide	961.0	E857	E931.0	E950.4	E962.0	E980.4
Azulfidine	961.0	E857	E931.0	E950.4	E962.0	E980.4
Azuresin	977.8	E858.8	E947.8	E950.4	E962.0	E980.4
Bacimycin	976.0	E858.7	E946.0	E950.4	E962.0	E980.4
ophthalmic preparation	976.5	E858.7	E946.5	E950.4	E962.0	E980.4
Bacitracin	960.8	E856	E930.8	E950.4	E962.0	E980.4
ENT agent	976.6	E858.7	E946.6	E950.4	E962.0	E980.4
ophthalmic preparation	976.5	E858.7	E946.5	E950.4	E962.0	E980.4
topical NEC	976.0	E858.7	E946.0	E950.4	E962.0	E980.4
Baking soda	963.3	E858.1	E933.3	E950.4	E962.0	E980.4
BAL	963.8	E858.1	E933.8	E950.4	E962.0	E980.4
Bamethan (sulfate)	972.5	E858.3	E942.5	E950.4	E962.0	E980.4
Bamipine	963.0	E858.1	E933.0	E950.4	E962.0	E980.4
Baneberry	988.2	E865.4	—	E950.9	E962.1	E980.9
Banewort	988.2	E865.4	—	E950.9	E962.1	E980.9
Barbenyl	967.0	E851	E937.0	E950.1	E962.0	E980.1
Barbital, barbitone	967.0	E851	E937.0	E950.1	E962.0	E980.1
Barbiturates, barbituric acid	967.0	E851	E937.0	E950.1	E962.0	E980.1
anesthetic (intravenous)	968.3	E855.1	E938.3	E950.4	E962.0	E980.4
Barium (carbonate) (chloride) (sulfate)	985.8	E866.4	—	E950.9	E962.1	E980.9
diagnostic agent	977.8	E858.8	E947.8	E950.4	E962.0	E980.4
pesticide	985.8	E863.4	—	E950.6	E962.1	E980.7
rodenticide	985.8	E863.7	—	E950.6	E962.1	E980.7
Barrier cream	976.3	E858.7	E946.3	E950.4	E962.0	E980.4
Battery acid or fluid	983.1	E864.1	—	E950.7	E962.1	E980.6
Bay rum	980.8	E860.8	—	E950.9	E962.1	E980.9
BCG vaccine	978.0	E858.8	E948.0	E950.4	E962.0	E980.4
Bearsfoot	988.2	E865.4	—	E950.9	E962.1	E980.9
Beclamide	966.3	E855.0	E936.3	E950.4	E962.0	E980.4
Bee (sting) (venom)	989.5	E905.3	—	E950.9	E962.1	E980.9
Belladonna (alkaloids)	971.1	E855.4	E941.1	E950.4	E962.0	E980.4
Bemegride	970.0	E854.3	E940.0	E950.4	E962.0	E980.4
Benactyzine	969.8	E855.8	E939.8	E950.3	E962.0	E980.3
Benadryl	963.0	E858.1	E933.0	E950.4	E962.0	E980.4

	Poisoning	Accident	Therapeutic Use	Suicide Attempt	Assault	Undetermined
Bendrofluazide	974.3	E858.5	E944.3	E950.4	E962.0	E980.4
Bendroflumethiazide	974.3	E858.5	E944.3	E950.4	E962.0	E980.4
Benemid	974.7	E858.5	E944.7	E950.4	E962.0	E980.4
Benethamine penicillin G	960.0	E856	E930.0	E950.4	E962.0	E980.4
Benisone	976.0	E858.7	E946.0	E950.4	E962.0	E980.4
Benoquin	976.8	E858.7	E946.8	E950.4	E962.0	E980.4
Benoxinate	968.5	E855.2	E938.5	E950.4	E962.0	E980.4
Bentonite	976.3	E858.7	E946.3	E950.4	E962.0	E980.4
Benzalkonium (chloride)	976.0	E858.7	E946.0	E950.4	E962.0	E980.4
ophthalmic preparation	976.5	E858.7	E946.5	E950.4	E962.0	E980.4
Benzamidosalicylate (calcium)	961.8	E857	E931.8	E950.4	E962.0	E980.4
Benzathine penicillin	960.0	E856	E930.0	E950.4	E962.0	E980.4
Benzcarbimine	963.1	E858.1	E933.1	E950.4	E962.0	E980.4
Benzedrex	971.2	E855.5	E941.2	E950.4	E962.0	E980.4
Benzedrine (amphetamine)	969.72	E854.2	E939.7	E950.3	E962.0	E980.3
Benzene (acetyl) (dimethyl) (methyl) (solvent) (vapor)	982.0	E862.4	—	E950.9	E962.1	E980.9
hexachloride (gamma) (insecticide) (vapor)	989.2	E863.0	—	E950.6	E962.1	E980.7
Benzethonium	976.0	E858.7	E946.0	E950.4	E962.0	E980.4
Benzhexol (chloride)	966.4	E855.0	E936.4	E950.4	E962.0	E980.4
Benzilonium	971.1	E855.4	E941.1	E950.4	E962.0	E980.4
Benzin(e) — *see* Ligroin						
Benziodarone	972.4	E858.3	E942.4	E950.4	E962.0	E980.4
Benzocaine	968.5	E855.2	E938.5	E950.4	E962.0	E980.4
Benzodiapin	969.4	E853.2	E939.4	E950.3	E962.0	E980.3
Benzodiazepines (tranquilizers) NEC	969.4	E853.2	E939.4	E950.3	E962.0	E980.3
Benzoic acid (with salicylic acid) (anti-infective)	976.0	E858.7	E946.0	E950.4	E962.0	E980.4
Benzoin	976.3	E858.7	E946.3	E950.4	E962.0	E980.4
Benzol (vapor)	982.0	E862.4	—	E950.9	E962.1	E980.9
Benzomorphan	965.09	E850.2	E935.2	E950.0	E962.0	E980.0
Benzonatate	975.4	E858.6	E945.4	E950.4	E962.0	E980.4
Benzothiadiazides	974.3	E858.5	E944.3	E950.4	E962.0	E980.4
Benzoylpas	961.8	E857	E931.8	E950.4	E962.0	E980.4
Benzperidol	969.5	E853.8	E939.5	E950.3	E962.0	E980.3
Benzphetamine	977.0	E858.8	E947.0	E950.4	E962.0	E980.4
Benzpyrinium	971.0	E855.3	E941.0	E950.4	E962.0	E980.4
Benzquinamide	963.0	E858.1	E933.0	E950.4	E962.0	E980.4
Benzthiazide	974.3	E858.5	E944.3	E950.4	E962.0	E980.4
Benztropine	971.1	E855.4	E941.1	E950.4	E962.0	E980.4
Benzyl						
acetate	982.8	E862.4	—	E950.9	E962.1	E980.9
benzoate (anti-infective)	976.0	E858.7	E946.0	E950.4	E962.0	E980.4
morphine	965.09	E850.2	E935.2	E950.0	E962.0	E980.0
penicillin	960.0	E856	E930.0	E950.4	E962.0	E980.4
Bephenium hydroxynapthoate	961.6	E857	E931.6	E950.4	E962.0	E980.4
Bergamot oil	989.89	E866.8	—	E950.9	E962.1	E980.9
Berries, poisonous	988.2	E865.3	—	E950.9	E962.1	E980.9
Beryllium (compounds) (fumes)	985.3	E866.4	—	E950.9	E962.1	E980.9
Beta-carotene	976.3	E858.7	E946.3	E950.4	E962.0	E980.4
Beta-Chlor	967.1	E852.0	E937.1	E950.2	E962.0	E980.2
Betamethasone	962.0	E858.0	E932.0	E950.4	E962.0	E980.4
topical	976.0	E858.7	E946.0	E950.4	E962.0	E980.4
Betazole	977.8	E858.8	E947.8	E950.4	E962.0	E980.4
Bethanechol	971.0	E855.3	E941.0	E950.4	E962.0	E980.4
Bethanidine	972.6	E858.3	E942.6	E950.4	E962.0	E980.4
Betula oil	976.3	E858.7	E946.3	E950.4	E962.0	E980.4
Bhang	969.6	E854.1	E939.6	E950.3	E962.0	E980.3
Bialamicol	961.5	E857	E931.5	E950.4	E962.0	E980.4
Bichloride of mercury — *see* Mercury, chloride						
Bichromates (calcium) (crystals) (potassium) (sodium)	983.9	E864.3	—	E950.7	E962.1	E980.6
fumes	987.8	E869.8	—	E952.8	E962.2	E982.8
Biguanide derivatives, oral	962.3	E858.0	E932.3	E950.4	E962.0	E980.4
Biligrafin	977.8	E858.8	E947.8	E950.4	E962.0	E980.4
Bilopaque	977.8	E858.8	E947.8	E950.4	E962.0	E980.4
Bioflavonoids	972.8	E858.3	E942.8	E950.4	E962.0	E980.4
Biological substance NEC	979.9	E858.8	E949.9	E950.4	E962.0	E980.4
Biperiden	966.4	E855.0	E936.4	E950.4	E962.0	E980.4
Bisacodyl	973.1	E858.4	E943.1	E950.4	E962.0	E980.4
Bishydroxycoumarin	964.2	E858.2	E934.2	E950.4	E962.0	E980.4

Nontherapeutic use substance

▼ Subterms under main terms may continue to next column or page

	Poisoning	Accident	Therapeutic Use	Suicide Attempt	Assault	Undeter-mined
Bismarsen	961.1	E857	E931.1	E950.4	E962.0	E980.4
Bismuth (compounds)						
NEC	985.8	E866.4	—	E950.9	E962.1	E980.9
anti-infectives	961.2	E857	E931.2	E950.4	E962.0	E980.4
subcarbonate	973.5	E858.4	E943.5	E950.4	E962.0	E980.4
sulfarsphenamine	961.1	E857	E931.1	E950.4	E962.0	E980.4
Bisphosphonates						
intravenous	963.1	E858.1	E933.7	E950.4	E962.0	E980.4
oral	963.1	E858.1	E933.6	E950.4	E962.0	E980.4
Bithionol	961.6	E857	E931.6	E950.4	E962.0	E980.4
Bitter almond oil	989.0	E866.8	—	E950.9	E962.1	E980.9
Bittersweet	988.2	E865.4	—	E950.9	E962.1	E930.9
Black						
flag	989.4	E863.4	—	E950.6	E962.1	E980.7
henbane	988.2	E865.4	—	E950.9	E962.1	E980.9
leaf (40)	989.4	E863.4	—	E950.6	E962.1	E980.7
widow spider (bite)	989.5	E905.1	—	E950.9	E962.1	E980.9
antivenin	979.9	E858.8	E949.9	E950.4	E962.0	E980.4
Blast furnace gas (carbon monoxide from)	986	E868.8	—	E952.1	E962.2	E982.1
Bleaching solutions	983.9	E864.3	—	E950.7	E962.1	E980.6
Bleach NEC	983.9	E864.3	—	E950.7	E962.1	E980.6
Bleomycin (sulfate)	960.7	E856	E930.7	E950.4	E962.0	E980.4
Blockain	968.9	E855.2	E938.9	E950.4	E962.0	E980.4
infiltration (subcuta-neous)	968.5	E855.2	E938.5	E950.4	E962.0	E980.4
nerve block (peripheral) (plexus)	968.6	E855.2	E938.6	E950.4	E962.0	E980.4
topical (surface)	968.5	E855.2	E938.5	E950.4	E962.0	E980.4
Blood (derivatives) (natural) (plasma) (whole)	964.7	E858.2	E934.7	E950.4	E962.0	E980.4
affecting agent	964.9	E858.2	E934.9	E950.4	E962.0	E980.4
specified NEC	964.8	E858.2	E934.8	E950.4	E962.0	E980.4
substitute (macromolecu-lar)	964.8	E858.2	E934.8	E950.4	E962.0	E980.4
Blue velvet	965.09	E850.2	E935.2	E950.0	E962.0	E980.0
Bone meal	989.89	E866.5	—	E950.9	E962.1	E980.9
Bonine	963.0	E858.1	E933.0	E950.4	E962.0	E980.4
Boracic acid	976.0	E858.7	E946.0	E950.4	E962.0	E980.4
ENT agent	976.6	E858.7	E946.6	E950.4	E962.0	E980.4
ophthalmic preparation	976.5	E858.7	E946.5	E950.4	E962.0	E980.4
Borate (cleanser) (sodi-um)	989.6	E861.3	—	E950.9	E962.1	E980.9
Borax (cleanser)	989.6	E861.3	—	E950.9	E962.1	E980.9
Boric acid	976.0	E858.7	E946.0	E950.4	E962.0	E980.4
ENT agent	976.6	E858.7	E946.6	E950.4	E962.0	E980.4
ophthalmic preparation	976.5	E858.7	E946.5	E950.4	E962.0	E980.4
Boron hydride NEC	989.89	E866.8	—	E950.9	E962.1	E980.9
fumes or gas	987.8	E869.8	—	E952.8	E962.2	E982.8
Botox	975.3	E858.6	E945.3	E950.4	E962.0	E980.4
Brake fluid vapor	987.8	E869.8	—	E952.8	E962.2	E982.8
Brass (compounds) (fumes)	985.8	E866.4	—	E950.9	E962.1	E980.9
Brasso	981	E861.3	—	E950.9	E962.1	E980.9
Bretylium (tosylate)	972.6	E858.3	E942.6	E950.4	E962.0	E980.4
Brevital (sodium)	968.3	E855.1	E938.3	E950.4	E962.0	E980.4
British antilewisite	963.8	E858.1	E933.8	E950.4	E962.0	E980.4
Bromal (hydrate)	967.3	E852.2	E937.3	E950.2	E962.0	E980.2
Bromelains	963.4	E858.1	E933.4	E950.4	E962.0	E980.4
Bromides NEC	967.3	E852.2	E937.3	E950.2	E962.0	E980.2
Bromine (vapor)	987.8	E869.8	—	E952.8	E962.2	E982.8
compounds (medicinal)	967.3	E852.2	E937.3	E950.2	E962.0	E980.2
Bromisovalum	967.3	E852.2	E937.3	E950.2	E962.0	E980.2
Bromobenzyl cyanide	987.5	E869.3	—	E952.8	E962.2	E982.8
Bromodiphenhydramine	963.0	E858.1	E933.0	E950.4	E962.0	E980.4
Bromoform	967.3	E852.2	E937.3	E950.2	E962.0	E980.2
Bromophenol blue reagent	977.8	E858.8	E947.8	E950.4	E962.0	E980.4
Bromosalicylhydroxamic acid	961.8	E857	E931.8	E950.4	E962.0	E980.4
Bromo-seltzer	965.4	E850.4	E935.4	E950.0	E962.0	E980.0
Brompheniramine	963.0	E858.1	E933.0	E950.4	E962.0	E980.4
Bromural	967.3	E852.2	E937.3	E950.2	E962.0	E980.2
Brown spider (bite) (ven-om)	989.5	E905.1	—	E950.9	E962.1	E980.9
Brucia	988.2	E865.3	—	E950.9	E962.1	E980.9
Brucine	989.1	E863.7	—	E950.6	E962.1	E980.7
Brunswick green — *see* Copper						
Bruten — *see* Ibuprofen						
Bryonia (alba) (dioica)	988.2	E865.4	—	E950.9	E962.1	E980.9
Buclizine	969.5	E853.8	E939.5	E950.3	E962.0	E980.3

	Poisoning	Accident	Therapeutic Use	Suicide Attempt	Assault	Undeter-mined
Bufferin	965.1	E850.3	E935.3	E950.0	E962.0	E980.0
Bufotenine	969.6	E854.1	E939.6	E950.3	E962.0	E980.3
Buphenine	971.2	E855.5	E941.2	E950.4	E962.0	E980.4
Bupivacaine	968.9	E855.2	E938.9	E950.4	E962.0	E980.4
infiltration (subcuta-neous)	968.5	E855.2	E938.5	E950.4	E962.0	E980.4
nerve block (peripheral) (plexus)	968.6	E855.2	E938.6	E950.4	E962.0	E980.4
Busulfan	963.1	E858.1	E933.1	E950.4	E962.0	E980.4
Butabarbital (sodium)	967.0	E851	E937.0	E950.1	E962.0	E980.1
Butabarbitone	967.0	E851	E937.0	E950.1	E962.0	E980.1
Butabarpal	967.0	E851	E937.0	E950.1	E962.0	E980.1
Butacaine	968.5	E855.2	E938.5	E950.4	E962.0	E980.4
Butallylonal	967.0	E851	E937.0	E950.1	E962.0	E980.1
Butane (distributed in mobile container)	987.0	E868.0	—	E951.1	E962.2	E981.1
distributed through pipes	987.0	E867	—	E951.0	E962.2	E981.0
incomplete combustion of — *see* Carbon monoxide, butane						
Butanol	980.3	E860.4	—	E950.9	E962.1	E980.9
Butanone	982.8	E862.4	—	E950.9	E962.1	E980.9
Butaperazine	969.1	E853.0	E939.1	E950.3	E962.0	E980.3
Butazolidin	965.5	E850.5	E935.5	E950.0	E962.0	E980.0
Butethal	967.0	E851	E937.0	E950.1	E962.0	E980.1
Butethamate	971.1	E855.4	E941.1	E950.4	E962.0	E980.4
Buthalitone (sodium)	968.3	E855.1	E938.3	E950.4	E962.0	E980.4
Butisol (sodium)	967.0	E851	E937.0	E950.1	E962.0	E980.1
Butobarbital, butobarbi-tone	967.0	E851	E937.0	E950.1	E962.0	E980.1
Butriptyline	969.05	E854.0	E939.0	E950.3	E962.0	E980.3
Buttercups	988.2	E865.4	—	E950.9	E962.1	E980.9
Butter of antimony — *see* Antimony						
Butyl						
acetate (secondary)	982.8	E862.4	—	E950.9	E962.1	E980.9
alcohol	980.3	E860.4	—	E950.9	E962.1	E980.9
carbinol	980.8	E860.8	—	E950.9	E962.1	E980.9
carbitol	982.8	E862.4	—	E950.9	E962.1	E980.9
cellosolve	982.8	E862.4	—	E950.9	E962.1	E980.9
chloral (hydrate)	967.1	E852.0	E937.1	E950.2	E962.0	E980.2
formate	982.8	E862.4	—	E950.9	E962.1	E980.9
scopolammonium bro-mide	971.1	E855.4	E941.1	E950.4	E962.0	E980.4
Butyn	968.5	E855.2	E938.5	E950.4	E962.0	E980.4
Butyrophenone (-based tran-quilizers)	969.2	E853.1	E939.2	E950.3	E962.0	E980.3
Cacodyl, cacodylic acid — *see* Arsenic						
Cactinomycin	960.7	E856	E930.7	E950.4	E962.0	E980.4
Cade oil	976.4	E858.7	E946.4	E950.4	E962.0	E980.4
Cadmium (chloride) (com-pounds) (dust) (fumes) (ox-ide)	985.5	E866.4	—	E950.9	E962.1	E980.9
sulfide (medicinal) NEC	976.4	E858.7	E946.4	E950.4	E962.0	E980.4
Caffeine	969.71	E854.2	E939.7	E950.3	E962.0	E980.3
Calabar bean	988.2	E865.4	—	E950.9	E962.1	E980.9
Caladium seguinium	988.2	E865.4	—	E950.9	E962.1	E980.9
Calamine (liniment) (lo-tion)	976.3	E858.7	E946.3	E950.4	E962.0	E980.4
Calciferol	963.5	E858.1	E933.5	E950.4	E962.0	E980.4
Calcium (salts) NEC	974.5	E858.5	E944.5	E950.4	E962.0	E980.4
acetylsalicylate	965.1	E850.3	E935.3	E950.0	E962.0	E980.0
benzamidosalicylate	961.8	E857	E931.8	E950.4	E962.0	E980.4
carbaspirin	965.1	E850.3	E935.3	E950.0	E962.0	E980.0
carbimide (citrated)	977.3	E858.8	E947.3	E950.4	E962.0	E980.4
carbonate (antacid)	973.0	E858.4	E943.0	E950.4	E962.0	E980.4
cyanide (citrated)	977.3	E858.8	E947.3	E950.4	E962.0	E980.4
dioctyl sulfosuccinate	973.2	E858.4	E943.2	E950.4	E962.0	E980.4
disodium edathamil	963.8	E858.1	E933.8	E950.4	E962.0	E980.4
disodium edetate	963.8	E858.1	E933.8	E950.4	E962.0	E980.4
EDTA	963.8	E858.1	E933.8	E950.4	E962.0	E980.4
hydrate, hydroxide	983.2	E864.2	—	E950.7	E962.1	E980.6
mandelate	961.9	E857	E931.9	E950.4	E962.0	E980.4
oxide	983.2	E864.2	—	E950.7	E962.1	E980.6
Calomel — *see* Mercury, chloride						
Caloric agents NEC	974.5	E858.5	E944.5	E950.4	E962.0	E980.4
Calusterone	963.1	E858.1	E933.1	E950.4	E962.0	E980.4
Camoquin	961.4	E857	E931.4	E950.4	E962.0	E980.4
Camphor (oil)	976.1	E858.7	E946.1	E950.4	E962.0	E980.4

Nontherapeutic use substance

� Subterms under main terms may continue to next column or page

Index

Candeptin — Central nervous system

Substance	Poisoning	Accident	Therapeutic Use	Suicide Attempt	Assault	Undetermined
Candeptin	976.0	E858.7	E946.0	E950.4	E962.0	E980.4
Candicidin	976.0	E858.7	E946.0	E950.4	E962.0	E980.4
Cannabinols	969.6	E854.1	E939.6	E950.3	E962.0	E980.3
Cannabis (derivatives) (indica) (sativa)	969.6	E854.1	E939.6	E950.3	E962.0	E980.3
Canned heat	980.1	E860.2	—	E950.9	E962.1	E980.9
Cantharides, cantharidin, cantharis	976.8	E858.7	E946.8	E950.4	E962.0	E980.4
Capillary agents	972.8	E858.3	E942.8	E950.4	E962.0	E980.4
Capreomycin	960.6	E856	E930.6	E950.4	E962.0	E980.4
Captodiame, captodiamine	969.5	E853.8	E939.5	E950.3	E962.0	E980.3
Caramiphen (hydrochloride)	971.1	E855.4	E941.1	E950.4	E962.0	E980.4
Carbachol	971.0	E855.3	E941.0	E950.4	E962.0	E980.4
Carbacrylamine resins	974.5	E858.5	E944.5	E950.4	E962.0	E980.4
Carbamate (sedative)	967.8	E852.8	E937.8	E950.2	E962.0	E980.2
herbicide	989.3	E863.5	—	E950.6	E962.1	E980.7
insecticide	989.3	E863.2	—	E950.6	E962.1	E980.7
Carbamazepine	966.3	E855.0	E936.3	E950.4	E962.0	E980.4
Carbamic esters	967.8	E852.8	E937.8	E950.2	E962.0	E980.2
Carbamide	974.4	E858.5	E944.4	E950.4	E962.0	E980.4
topical	976.8	E858.7	E946.8	E950.4	E962.0	E980.4
Carbamylcholine chloride	971.0	E855.3	E941.0	E950.4	E962.0	E980.4
Carbarsone	961.1	E857	E931.1	E950.4	E962.0	E980.4
Carbaryl	989.3	E863.2	—	E950.6	E962.1	E980.7
Carbaspirin	965.1	E850.3	E935.3	E950.0	E962.0	E980.0
Carbazochrome	972.8	E858.3	E942.8	E950.4	E962.0	E980.4
Carbenicillin	960.0	E856	E930.0	E950.4	E962.0	E980.4
Carbenoxolone	973.8	E858.4	E943.8	E950.4	E962.0	E980.4
Carbetapentane	975.4	E858.6	E945.4	E950.4	E962.0	E980.4
Carbimazole	962.8	E858.0	E932.8	E950.4	E962.0	E980.4
Carbinol	980.1	E860.2	—	E950.9	E962.1	E980.9
Carbinoxamine	963.0	E858.1	E933.0	E950.4	E962.0	E980.4
Carbitol	982.8	E862.4	—	E950.9	E962.1	E980.9
Carbocaine	968.9	E855.2	E938.9	E950.4	E962.0	E980.4
infiltration (subcutaneous)	968.5	E855.2	E938.5	E950.4	E962.0	E980.4
nerve block (peripheral) (plexus)	968.6	E855.2	E938.6	E950.4	E962.0	E980.4
topical (surface)	968.5	E855.2	E938.5	E950.4	E962.0	E980.4
Carbol-fuchsin solution	976.0	E858.7	E946.0	E950.4	E962.0	E980.4
Carbolic acid — see also Phenol	983.0	E864.0	—	E950.7	E962.1	E980.6
Carbomycin	960.8	E856	E930.8	E950.4	E962.0	E980.4
Carbon						
bisulfide (liquid) (vapor)	982.2	E862.4	—	E950.9	E962.1	E980.9
dioxide (gas)	987.8	E869.8	—	E952.8	E962.2	E982.8
disulfide (liquid) (vapor)	982.2	E862.4	—	E950.9	E962.1	E980.9
monoxide (from incomplete combustion of) (in)						
NEC	986	E868.9	—	E952.1	E962.2	E982.1
blast furnace gas	986	E868.8	—	E952.1	E962.2	E982.1
butane (distributed in mobile container)	986	E868.0	—	E951.1	E962.2	E981.1
distributed through pipes	986	E867	—	E951.0	E962.2	E981.0
charcoal fumes	986	E868.3	—	E952.1	E962.2	E982.1
coal						
gas (piped)	986	E867	—	E951.0	E962.2	E981.0
solid (in domestic stoves, fireplaces)	986	E868.3	—	E952.1	E962.2	E982.1
coke (in domestic stoves, fireplaces)	986	E868.3	—	E952.1	E962.2	E982.1
exhaust gas (motor) not in transit	986	E868.2	—	E952.0	E962.2	E982.0
combustion engine, any not in watercraft	986	E868.2	—	E952.0	E962.2	E982.0
farm tractor, not in transit	986	E868.2	—	E952.0	E962.2	E982.0
gas engine	986	E868.2	—	E952.0	E962.2	E982.0
motor pump	986	E868.2	—	E952.0	E962.2	E982.0
motor vehicle, not in transit	986	E868.2	—	E952.0	E962.2	E982.0
fuel (in domestic use)	986	E868.3	—	E952.1	E962.2	E982.1
gas (piped)	986	E867	—	E951.0	E962.2	E981.0
in mobile container	986	E868.0	—	E951.1	E962.2	E981.1
utility	986	E868.1	—	E951.8	E962.2	E981.1
in mobile container	986	E868.0	—	E951.1	E962.2	E981.1
piped (natural)	986	E867	—	E951.0	E962.2	E981.0
illuminating gas	986	E868.1	—	E951.8	E962.2	E981.8
Carbon — continued						
monoxide — continued						
industrial fuels or gases, any	986	E868.8	—	E952.1	E962.2	E982.1
kerosene (in domestic stoves, fireplaces)	986	E868.3	—	E952.1	E962.2	E982.1
kiln gas or vapor	986	E868.8	—	E952.1	E962.2	E982.1
motor exhaust gas, not in transit	986	E868.2	—	E952.0	E962.2	E982.0
piped gas (manufactured) (natural)	986	E867	—	E951.0	E962.2	E981.0
producer gas	986	E868.8	—	E952.1	E962.2	E982.1
propane (distributed in mobile container)	986	E868.0	—	E951.1	E962.2	E981.1
distributed through pipes	986	E867	—	E951.0	E962.2	E981.0
specified source NEC	986	E868.8	—	E952.1	E962.2	E982.1
stove gas	986	E868.1	—	E951.8	E962.2	E981.8
piped	986	E867	—	E951.0	E962.2	E981.0
utility gas	986	E868.1	—	E951.8	E962.2	E981.8
piped	986	E867	—	E951.0	E962.2	E981.0
water gas	986	E868.1	—	E951.8	E962.2	E981.8
wood (in domestic stoves, fireplaces)	986	E868.3	—	E952.1	E962.2	E982.1
tetrachloride (vapor) NEC	987.8	E869.8	—	E952.8	E962.2	E982.8
liquid (cleansing agent)						
NEC	982.1	E861.3	—	E950.9	E962.1	E980.9
solvent	982.1	E862.4	—	E950.9	E962.1	E980.9
Carbonic acid (gas)	987.8	E869.8	—	E952.8	E962.2	E982.8
anhydrase inhibitors	974.2	E858.5	E944.2	E950.4	E962.0	E980.4
Carbowax	976.3	E858.7	E946.3	E950.4	E962.0	E980.4
Carbrital	967.0	E851	E937.0	E950.1	E962.0	E980.1
Carbromal (derivatives)	967.3	E852.2	E937.3	E950.2	E962.0	E980.2
Cardiac						
depressants	972.0	E858.3	E942.0	E950.4	E962.0	E980.4
rhythm regulators	972.0	E858.3	E942.0	E950.4	E962.0	E980.4
Cardiografin	977.8	E858.8	E947.8	E950.4	E962.0	E980.4
Cardio-green	977.8	E858.8	E947.8	E950.4	E962.0	E980.4
Cardiotonic glycosides	972.1	E858.3	E942.1	E950.4	E962.0	E980.4
Cardiovascular agents						
NEC	972.9	E858.3	E942.9	E950.4	E962.0	E980.4
Cardrase	974.2	E858.5	E944.2	E950.4	E962.0	E980.4
Carfusin	976.0	E858.7	E946.0	E950.4	E962.0	E980.4
Carisoprodol	968.0	E855.1	E938.0	E950.4	E962.0	E980.4
Carmustine	963.1	E858.1	E933.1	E950.4	E962.0	E980.4
Carotene	963.5	E858.1	E933.5	E950.4	E962.0	E980.4
Carphenazine (maleate)	969.1	E853.0	E939.1	E950.3	E962.0	E980.3
Carter's Little Pills	973.1	E858.4	E943.1	E950.4	E962.0	E980.4
Cascara (sagrada)	973.1	E858.4	E943.1	E950.4	E962.0	E980.4
Cassava	988.2	E865.4	—	E950.9	E962.1	E980.9
Castellani's paint	976.0	E858.7	E946.0	E950.4	E962.0	E980.4
Castor						
bean	988.2	E865.3	—	E950.9	E962.1	E980.9
oil	973.1	E858.4	E943.1	E950.4	E962.0	E980.4
Caterpillar (sting)	989.5	E905.5	—	E950.9	E962.1	E980.9
Catha (edulis)	970.89	E854.3	E940.8	E950.4	E962.0	E980.4
Cathartics NEC	973.3	E858.4	E943.3	E950.4	E962.0	E980.4
contact	973.1	E858.4	E943.1	E950.4	E962.0	E980.4
emollient	973.2	E858.4	E943.2	E950.4	E962.0	E980.4
intestinal irritants	973.1	E858.4	E943.1	E950.4	E962.0	E980.4
saline	973.3	E858.4	E943.3	E950.4	E962.0	E980.4
Cathomycin	960.8	E856	E930.8	E950.4	E962.0	E980.4
Caustic(s)	983.9	E864.4	—	E950.7	E962.1	E980.6
alkali	983.2	E864.2	—	E950.7	E962.1	E980.6
hydroxide	983.2	E864.2	—	E950.7	E962.1	E980.6
potash	983.2	E864.2	—	E950.7	E962.1	E980.6
soda	983.2	E864.2	—	E950.7	E962.1	E980.6
specified NEC	983.9	E864.3	—	E950.7	E962.1	E980.6
Ceepryn	976.0	E858.7	E946.0	E950.4	E962.0	E980.4
ENT agent	976.6	E858.7	E946.6	E950.4	E962.0	E980.4
lozenges	976.6	E858.7	E946.6	E950.4	E962.0	E980.4
Celestone	962.0	E858.0	E932.0	E950.4	E962.0	E980.4
topical	976.0	E858.7	E946.0	E950.4	E962.0	E980.4
Cellosolve	982.8	E862.4	—	E950.9	E962.1	E980.9
Cell stimulants and proliferants	976.8	E858.7	E946.8	E950.4	E962.0	E980.4
Cellulose derivatives, cathartic	973.3	E858.4	E943.3	E950.4	E962.0	E980.4
nitrates (topical)	976.3	E858.7	E946.3	E950.4	E962.0	E980.4
Centipede (bite)	989.5	E905.4	—	E950.9	E962.1	E980.9
Central nervous system						
depressants	968.4	E855.1	E938.4	E950.4	E962.0	E980.4

Nontherapeutic use substance

▽ Subterms under main terms may continue to next column or page

	Poisoning	Accident	Therapeutic Use	Suicide Attempt	Assault	Undetermined
Central nervous system — *continued*						
depressants — continued						
anesthetic (general)						
NEC	968.4	E855.1	E938.4	E950.4	E962.0	E980.4
gases NEC	968.2	E855.1	E938.2	E950.4	E962.0	E980.4
intravenous	968.3	E855.1	E938.3	E950.4	E962.0	E980.4
barbiturates	967.0	E851	E937.0	E950.1	E962.0	E980.1
bromides	967.3	E852.2	E937.3	E950.2	E962.0	E980.2
cannabis sativa	969.6	E854.1	E939.6	E950.3	E962.0	E980.3
chloral hydrate	967.1	E852.0	E937.1	E950.2	E962.0	E980.2
hallucinogenics	969.6	E854.1	E939.6	E950.3	E962.0	E980.3
hypnotics	967.9	E852.9	E937.9	E950.2	E962.0	E980.2
specified NEC	967.8	E852.8	E937.8	E950.2	E962.0	E980.2
muscle relaxants	968.0	E855.1	E938.0	E950.4	E962.0	E980.4
paraldehyde	967.2	E852.1	E937.2	E950.2	E962.0	E980.2
sedatives	967.9	E852.9	E937.9	E950.2	E962.0	E980.2
mixed NEC	967.6	E852.5	E937.6	E950.2	E962.0	E980.2
specified NEC	967.8	E852.8	E937.8	E950.2	E962.0	E980.2
muscle-tone depressants	968.0	E855.1	E938.0	E950.4	E962.0	E980.4
stimulants	970.9	E854.3	E940.9	E950.4	E962.0	E980.4
amphetamines	969.72	E854.2	E939.7	E950.3	E962.0	E980.3
analeptics	970.0	E854.3	E940.0	E950.4	E962.0	E980.4
antidepressants	969.00	E854.0	E939.0	E950.3	E962.0	E980.3
opiate antagonists	970.1	E854.3	E940.0	E950.4	E962.0	E980.4
specified NEC	970.89	E854.3	E940.8	E950.4	E962.0	E980.4
Cephalexin	960.5	E856	E930.5	E950.4	E962.0	E980.4
Cephaloglycin	960.5	E856	E930.5	E950.4	E962.0	E980.4
Cephaloridine	960.5	E856	E930.5	E950.4	E962.0	E980.4
Cephalosporins NEC	960.5	E856	E930.5	E950.4	E962.0	E980.4
N (adicillin)	960.0	E856	E930.0	E950.4	E962.0	E980.4
Cephalothin (sodium)	960.5	E856	E930.5	E950.4	E962.0	E980.4
Cerbera (odallam)	988.2	E865.4	—	E950.9	E962.1	E980.9
Cerberin	972.1	E858.3	E942.1	E950.4	E962.0	E980.4
Cerebral stimulants	970.9	E854.3	E940.9	E950.4	E962.0	E980.4
psychotherapeutic	969.79	E854.2	E939.7	E950.3	E962.0	E980.3
specified NEC	970.89	E854.3	E940.8	E950.4	E962.0	E980.4
Cetalkonium (chloride)	976.0	E858.7	E946.0	E950.4	E962.0	E980.4
Cetoxime	963.0	E858.1	E933.0	E950.4	E962.0	E980.4
Cetrimide	976.2	E858.7	E946.2	E950.4	E962.0	E980.4
Cetylpyridinium	976.0	E858.7	E946.0	E950.4	E962.0	E980.4
ENT agent	976.6	E858.7	E946.6	E950.4	E962.0	E980.4
lozenges	976.6	E858.7	E946.6	E950.4	E962.0	E980.4
Cevadilla — *see* Sabadilla						
Cevitamic acid	963.5	E858.1	E933.5	E950.4	E962.0	E980.4
Chalk, precipitated	973.0	E858.4	E943.0	E950.4	E962.0	E980.4
Charcoal						
fumes (carbon monox-ide)	986	E868.3	—	E952.1	E962.2	E982.1
industrial	986	E868.8	—	E952.1	E962.2	E982.1
medicinal (activated)	973.0	E858.4	E943.0	E950.4	E962.0	E980.4
Chelating agents NEC	977.2	E858.8	E947.2	E950.4	E962.0	E980.4
Chelidonium majus	988.2	E865.4	—	E950.9	E962.1	E980.9
Chemical substance	989.9	E866.9	—	E950.9	E962.1	E980.9
specified NEC	989.89	E866.8	—	E950.9	E962.1	E980.9
Chemotherapy, antineoplastic	963.1	E858.1	E933.1	E950.4	E962.0	E980.4
Chenopodium (oil)	961.6	E857	E931.6	E950.4	E962.0	E980.4
Cherry laurel	988.2	E865.4	—	E950.9	E962.1	E980.9
Chiniofon	961.3	E857	E931.3	E950.4	E962.0	E980.4
Chlophedianol	975.4	E858.6	E945.4	E950.4	E962.0	E980.4
Chloral (betaine) (formamide) (hydrate)	967.1	E852.0	E937.1	E950.2	E962.0	E980.2
Chloralamide	967.1	E852.0	E937.1	E950.2	E962.0	E980.2
Chlorambucil	963.1	E858.1	E933.1	E950.4	E962.0	E980.4
Chloramphenicol	960.2	E856	E930.2	E950.4	E962.0	E980.4
ENT agent	976.6	E858.7	E946.6	E950.4	E962.0	E980.4
ophthalmic preparation	976.5	E858.7	E946.5	E950.4	E962.0	E980.4
topical NEC	976.0	E858.7	E946.0	E950.4	E962.0	E980.4
Chlorate(s) (potassium) (sodium) NEC	983.9	E864.3	—	E950.7	E962.1	E980.6
herbicides	989.4	E863.5	—	E950.6	E962.1	E980.7
Chlorcyclizine	963.0	E858.1	E933.0	E950.4	E962.0	E980.4
Chlordan(e) (dust)	989.2	E863.0	—	E950.6	E962.1	E980.7
Chlordantoin	976.0	E858.7	E946.0	E950.4	E962.0	E980.4
Chlordiazepoxide	969.4	E853.2	E939.4	E950.3	E962.0	E980.3
Chloresium	976.8	E858.7	E946.8	E950.4	E962.0	E980.4
Chlorethiazol	967.1	E852.0	E937.1	E950.2	E962.0	E980.2
Chlorethyl — *see* Ethyl, chloride						
Chloretone	967.1	E852.0	E937.1	E950.2	E962.0	E980.2
Chlorex	982.3	E862.4	—	E950.9	E962.1	E980.9

	Poisoning	Accident	Therapeutic Use	Suicide Attempt	Assault	Undetermined
Chlorhexadol	967.1	E852.0	E937.1	E950.2	E962.0	E980.2
Chlorhexidine (hydrochloride)	976.0	E858.7	E946.0	E950.4	E962.0	E980.4
Chlorhydroxyquinolin	976.0	E858.7	E946.0	E950.4	E962.0	E980.4
Chloride of lime (bleach)	983.9	E864.3	—	E950.7	E962.1	E980.6
Chlorinated						
camphene	989.2	E863.0	—	E950.6	E962.1	E980.7
diphenyl	989.89	E866.8	—	E950.9	E962.1	E980.9
hydrocarbons NEC	989.2	E863.0	—	E950.6	E962.1	E980.7
solvent	982.3	E862.4	—	E950.9	E962.1	E980.9
lime (bleach)	983.9	E864.3	—	E950.7	E962.1	E980.6
naphthalene — see Naphthalene						
pesticides NEC	989.2	E863.0	—	E950.6	E962.1	E980.7
soda — see Sodium, hypochlorite						
Chlorine (fumes) (gas)	987.6	E869.8	—	E952.8	E962.2	E982.8
bleach	983.9	E864.3	—	E950.7	E962.1	E980.6
compounds NEC	983.9	E864.3	—	E950.7	E962.1	E980.6
disinfectant	983.9	E861.4	—	E950.7	E962.1	E980.6
releasing agents NEC	983.9	E864.3	—	E950.7	E962.1	E980.6
Chlorisondamine	972.3	E858.3	E942.3	E950.4	E962.0	E980.4
Chlormadinone	962.2	E858.0	E932.2	E950.4	E962.0	E980.4
Chlormerodrin	974.0	E858.5	E944.0	E950.4	E962.0	E980.4
Chlormethiazole	967.1	E852.0	E937.1	E950.2	E962.0	E980.2
Chlormethylenecycline	960.4	E856	E930.4	E950.4	E962.0	E980.4
Chlormezanone	969.5	E853.8	E939.5	E950.3	E962.0	E980.3
Chloroacetophenone	987.5	E869.3	—	E952.8	E962.2	E982.8
Chloroaniline	983.0	E864.0	—	E950.7	E962.1	E980.6
Chlorobenzene, chlorobenzol	982.0	E862.4	—	E950.9	E962.1	E980.9
Chlorobutanol	967.1	E852.0	E937.1	E950.2	E962.0	E980.2
Chlorodinitrobenzene	983.0	E864.0	—	E950.7	E962.1	E980.6
dust or vapor	987.8	E869.8	—	E952.8	E962.2	E982.8
Chloroethane — see Ethyl, chloride						
Chloroform (fumes) (vapor)	987.8	E869.8	—	E952.8	E962.2	E982.8
anesthetic (gas)	968.2	E855.1	E938.2	E950.4	E962.0	E980.4
liquid NEC	968.4	E855.1	E938.4	E950.4	E962.0	E980.4
solvent	982.3	E862.4	—	E950.9	E962.1	E980.9
Chloroguanide	961.4	E857	E931.4	E950.4	E962.0	E980.4
Chloromycetin	960.2	E856	E930.2	E950.4	E962.0	E980.4
ENT agent	976.6	E858.7	E946.6	E950.4	E962.0	E980.4
ophthalmic preparation	976.5	E858.7	E946.5	E950.4	E962.0	E980.4
otic solution	976.6	E858.7	E946.6	E950.4	E962.0	E980.4
topical NEC	976.0	E858.7	E946.0	E950.4	E962.0	E980.4
Chloronitrobenzene	983.0	E864.0	—	E950.7	E962.1	E980.6
dust or vapor	987.8	E869.8	—	E952.8	E962.2	E982.8
Chlorophenol	983.0	E864.0	—	E950.7	E962.1	E980.6
Chlorophenothane	989.2	E863.0	—	E950.6	E962.1	E980.7
Chlorophyll (derivatives)	976.8	E858.7	E946.8	E950.4	E962.0	E980.4
Chloropicrin (fumes)	987.8	E869.8	—	E952.8	E962.2	E982.8
fumigant	989.4	E863.8	—	E950.6	E962.1	E980.7
fungicide	989.4	E863.6	—	E950.6	E962.1	E980.7
pesticide (fumes)	989.4	E863.4	—	E950.6	E962.1	E980.7
Chloroprocaine	968.9	E855.2	E938.9	E950.4	E962.0	E980.4
infiltration (subcutaneous)	968.5	E855.2	E938.5	E950.4	E962.0	E980.4
nerve block (peripheral) (plexus)	968.6	E855.2	E938.6	E950.4	E962.0	E980.4
Chloroptic	976.5	E858.7	E946.5	E950.4	E962.0	E980.4
Chloropurine	963.1	E858.1	E933.1	E950.4	E962.0	E980.4
Chloroquine (hydrochloride) (phosphate)	961.4	E857	E931.4	E950.4	E962.0	E980.4
Chlorothen	963.0	E858.1	E933.0	E950.4	E962.0	E980.4
Chlorothiazide	974.3	E858.5	E944.3	E950.4	E962.0	E980.4
Chlorotrianisene	962.2	E858.0	E932.2	E950.4	E962.0	E980.4
Chlorovinyldichloroarsine	985.1	E866.3	—	E950.8	E962.1	E980.8
Chloroxylenol	976.0	E858.7	E946.0	E950.4	E962.0	E980.4
Chlorphenesin (carbamate)	968.0	E855.1	E938.0	E950.4	E962.0	E980.4
topical (antifungal)	976.0	E858.7	E946.0	E950.4	E962.0	E980.4
Chlorpheniramine	963.0	E858.1	E933.0	E950.4	E962.0	E980.4
Chlorphenoxamine	966.4	E855.0	E936.4	E950.4	E962.0	E980.4
Chlorphentermine	977.0	E858.8	E947.0	E950.4	E962.0	E980.4
Chlorproguanil	961.4	E857	E931.4	E950.4	E962.0	E980.4
Chlorpromazine	969.1	E853.0	E939.1	E950.3	E962.0	E980.3
Chlorpropamide	962.3	E858.0	E932.3	E950.4	E962.0	E980.4
Chlorprothixene	969.3	E853.8	E939.3	E950.3	E962.0	E980.3
Chlorquinaldol	976.0	E858.7	E946.0	E950.4	E962.0	E980.4

Nontherapeutic use substance

Subterms under main terms may continue to next column or page

	Poisoning	Accident	Therapeutic Use	Suicide Attempt	Assault	Undetermined
External Cause (E-Code)						
Chlortetracycline	960.4	E856	E930.4	E950.4	E962.0	E980.4
Chlorthalidone	974.4	E858.5	E944.4	E950.4	E962.0	E980.4
Chlortrianisene	962.2	E858.0	E932.2	E950.4	E962.0	E980.4
Chlor-Trimeton	963.0	E858.1	E933.0	E950.4	E962.0	E980.4
Chlorzoxazone	968.0	E855.1	E938.0	E950.4	E962.0	E980.4
Choke damp	987.8	E869.8	—	E952.8	E962.2	E982.8
Cholebrine	977.8	E858.8	E947.8	E950.4	E962.0	E980.4
Cholera vaccine	978.2	E858.8	E948.2	E950.4	E962.0	E980.4
Cholesterol-lowering agents	972.2	E858.3	E942.2	E950.4	E962.0	E980.4
Cholestyramine (resin)	972.2	E858.3	E942.2	E950.4	E962.0	E980.4
Cholic acid	973.4	E858.4	E943.4	E950.4	E962.0	E980.4
Choline						
dihydrogen citrate	977.1	E858.8	E947.1	E950.4	E962.0	E980.4
salicylate	965.1	E850.3	E935.3	E950.0	E962.0	E980.0
theophyllinate	974.1	E858.5	E944.1	E950.4	E962.0	E980.4
Cholinergics	971.0	E855.3	E941.0	E950.4	E962.0	E980.4
Cholografin	977.8	E858.8	E947.8	E950.4	E962.0	E980.4
Chorionic gonadotropin	962.4	E858.0	E932.4	E950.4	E962.0	E980.4
Chromates	983.9	E864.3	—	E950.7	E962.1	E980.6
dust or mist	987.8	E869.8	—	E952.8	E962.2	E982.8
lead	984.0	E866.0	—	E950.9	E962.1	E980.9
paint	984.0	E861.5	—	E950.9	E962.1	E980.9
Chromic acid	983.9	E864.3	—	E950.7	E962.1	E980.6
dust or mist	987.8	E869.8	—	E952.8	E962.2	E982.8
Chromium	985.6	E866.4	—	E950.9	E962.1	E980.9
compounds — see Chromates						
Chromonar	972.4	E858.3	E942.4	E950.4	E962.0	E980.4
Chromyl chloride	983.9	E864.3	—	E950.7	E962.1	E980.6
Chrysarobin (ointment)	976.4	E858.7	E946.4	E950.4	E962.0	E980.4
Chrysazin	973.1	E858.4	E943.1	E950.4	E962.0	E980.4
Chymar	963.4	E858.1	E933.4	E950.4	E962.0	E980.4
ophthalmic preparation	976.5	E858.7	E946.5	E950.4	E962.0	E980.4
Chymotrypsin	963.4	E858.1	E933.4	E950.4	E962.0	E980.4
ophthalmic preparation	976.5	E858.7	E946.5	E950.4	E962.0	E980.4
Cicuta maculata or virosa	988.2	E865.4	—	E950.9	E962.1	E980.9
Cigarette lighter fluid	981	E862.1	—	E950.9	E962.1	E980.9
Cinchocaine (spinal)	968.7	E855.2	E938.7	E950.4	E962.0	E980.4
topical (surface)	968.5	E855.2	E938.5	E950.4	E962.0	E980.4
Cinchona	961.4	E857	E931.4	E950.4	E962.0	E980.4
Cinchonine alkaloids	961.4	E857	E931.4	E950.4	E962.0	E980.4
Cinchophen	974.7	E858.5	E944.7	E950.4	E962.0	E980.4
Cinnarizine	963.0	E858.1	E933.0	E950.4	E962.0	E980.4
Citanest	968.9	E855.2	E938.9	E950.4	E962.0	E980.4
infiltration (subcutaneous)	968.5	E855.2	E938.5	E950.4	E962.0	E980.4
nerve block (peripheral) (plexus)	968.6	E855.2	E938.6	E950.4	E962.0	E980.4
Citric acid	989.89	E866.8	—	E950.9	E962.1	E980.9
Citrovorum factor	964.1	E858.2	E934.1	E950.4	E962.0	E980.4
Claviceps purpurea	988.2	E865.4	—	E950.9	E962.1	E980.9
Cleaner, cleansing agent, type not specified	989.89	E861.9	—	E950.9	E962.1	E980.9
of paint or varnish	982.8	E862.9	—	E950.9	E962.1	E980.9
specified type NEC	989.89	E861.3	—	E950.9	E962.1	E980.9
Clematis vitalba	988.2	E865.4	—	E950.9	E962.1	E980.9
Clemizole	963.0	E858.1	E933.0	E950.4	E962.0	E980.4
penicillin	960.0	E856	E930.0	E950.4	E962.0	E980.4
Clidinium	971.1	E855.4	E941.1	E950.4	E962.0	E980.4
Clindamycin	960.8	E856	E930.8	E950.4	E962.0	E980.4
Cliradon	965.09	E850.2	E935.2	E950.0	E962.0	E980.0
Clocortolone	962.0	E858.0	E932.0	E950.4	E962.0	E980.4
Clofedanol	975.4	E858.6	E945.4	E950.4	E962.0	E980.4
Clofibrate	972.2	E858.3	E942.2	E950.4	E962.0	E980.4
Clomethiazole	967.1	E852.0	E937.1	E950.2	E962.0	E980.2
Clomiphene	977.8	E858.8	E947.8	E950.4	E962.0	E980.4
Clonazepam	969.4	E853.2	E939.4	E950.3	E962.0	E980.3
Clonidine	972.6	E858.3	E942.6	E950.4	E962.0	E980.4
Clopamide	974.3	E858.5	E944.3	E950.4	E962.0	E980.4
Clorazepate	969.4	E853.2	E939.4	E950.3	E962.0	E980.3
Clorexolone	974.4	E858.5	E944.4	E950.4	E962.0	E980.4
Clorox (bleach)	983.9	E864.3	—	E950.7	E962.1	E980.6
Clortermine	977.0	E858.8	E947.0	E950.4	E962.0	E980.4
Clotrimazole	976.0	E858.7	E946.0	E950.4	E962.0	E980.4
Cloxacillin NEC	960.0	E856	E930.0	E950.4	E962.0	E980.4
Coagulants NEC	964.5	E858.2	E934.5	E950.4	E962.0	E980.4
Coal (carbon monoxide from) — see also Carbon, monoxide, coal						
oil — see Kerosene						

	Poisoning	Accident	Therapeutic Use	Suicide Attempt	Assault	Undetermined
External Cause (E-Code)						
Coal — see also Carbon, monoxide, coal — continued						
tar NEC	983.0	E864.0	—	E950.7	E962.1	E980.6
fumes	987.8	E869.8	—	E952.8	E962.2	E982.8
medicinal (ointment)	976.4	E858.7	E946.4	E950.4	E962.0	E980.4
analgesics NEC	965.5	E850.5	E935.5	E950.0	E962.0	E980.0
naphtha (solvent)	981	E862.0	—	E950.9	E962.1	E980.9
Cobalt (fumes) (industrial)	985.8	E866.4	—	E950.9	E962.1	E980.9
Cobra (venom)	989.5	E905.0	—	E950.9	E962.1	E980.9
Coca (leaf)	970.81	E854.3	E940.8	E950.4	E962.0	E980.4
Cocaine (hydrochloride) (salt)	970.81	E854.3	E940.8	E950.4	E962.0	E980.4
topical anesthetic	968.5	E855.2	E938.5	E950.4	E962.0	E980.4
Coccidioidin	977.8	E858.8	E947.8	E950.4	E962.0	E980.4
Cocculus indicus	988.2	E865.3	—	E950.9	E962.1	E980.9
Cochineal	989.89	E866.8	—	E950.9	E962.1	E980.9
medicinal products	977.4	E858.8	E947.4	E950.4	E962.0	E980.4
Codeine	965.09	E850.2	E935.2	E950.0	E962.0	E980.0
Coffee	989.89	E866.8	—	E950.9	E962.1	E980.9
Cogentin	971.1	E855.4	E941.1	E950.4	E962.0	E980.4
Coke fumes or gas (carbon monoxide)	986	E868.3	—	E952.1	E962.2	E982.1
industrial use	986	E868.8	—	E952.1	E962.2	E982.1
Colace	973.2	E858.4	E943.2	E950.4	E962.0	E980.4
Colchicine	974.7	E858.5	E944.7	E950.4	E962.0	E980.4
Colchicum	988.2	E865.3	—	E950.9	E962.1	E980.9
Cold cream	976.3	E858.7	E946.3	E950.4	E962.0	E980.4
Colestipol	972.2	E858.3	E942.2	E950.4	E962.0	E980.4
Colistimethate	960.8	E856	E930.8	E950.4	E962.0	E980.4
Colistin	960.8	E856	E930.8	E950.4	E962.0	E980.4
Collagen	977.8	E866.8	E947.8	E950.9	E962.1	E980.9
Collagenase	976.8	E858.7	E946.8	E950.4	E962.0	E980.4
Collodion (flexible)	976.3	E858.7	E946.3	E950.4	E962.0	E980.4
Colocynth	973.1	E858.4	E943.1	E950.4	E962.0	E980.4
Coloring matter — see Dye(s)						
Combustion gas — see Carbon, monoxide						
Compazine	969.1	E853.0	E939.1	E950.3	E962.0	E980.3
Compound						
42 (warfarin)	989.4	E863.7	—	E950.6	E962.1	E980.7
269 (endrin)	989.2	E863.0	—	E950.6	E962.1	E980.7
497 (dieldrin)	989.2	E863.0	—	E950.6	E962.1	E980.7
1080 (sodium fluoroacetate)	989.4	E863.7	—	E950.6	E962.1	E980.7
3422 (parathion)	989.3	E863.1	—	E950.6	E962.1	E980.7
3911 (phorate)	989.3	E863.1	—	E950.6	E962.1	E980.7
3956 (toxaphene)	989.2	E863.0	—	E950.6	E962.1	E980.7
4049 (malathion)	989.3	E863.1	—	E950.6	E962.1	E980.7
4124 (dicapthon)	989.4	E863.4	—	E950.6	E962.1	E980.7
E (cortisone)	962.0	E858.0	E932.0	E950.4	E962.0	E980.4
F (hydrocortisone)	962.0	E858.0	E932.0	E950.4	E962.0	E980.4
Congo red	977.8	E858.8	E947.8	E950.4	E962.0	E980.4
Coniine, conine	965.7	E850.7	E935.7	E950.0	E962.0	E980.0
Conium (maculatum)	988.2	E865.4	—	E950.9	E962.1	E980.9
Conjugated estrogens (equine)	962.2	E858.0	E932.2	E950.4	E962.0	E980.4
Contac	975.6	E858.6	E945.6	E950.4	E962.0	E980.4
Contact lens solution	976.5	E858.7	E946.5	E950.4	E962.0	E980.4
Contraceptives (oral)	962.2	E858.0	E932.2	E950.4	E962.0	E980.4
vaginal	976.8	E858.7	E946.8	E950.4	E962.0	E980.4
Contrast media (roentgenographic)	977.8	E858.8	E947.8	E950.4	E962.0	E980.4
Convallaria majalis	988.2	E865.4	—	E950.9	E962.1	E980.9
Copperhead snake (bite) (venom)	989.5	E905.0	—	E950.9	E962.1	E980.9
Copper (dust) (fumes) (salts) NEC	985.8	E866.4	—	E950.9	E962.1	E980.9
arsenate, arsenite	985.1	E866.3	—	E950.8	E962.1	E980.8
insecticide	985.1	E863.4	—	E950.8	E962.1	E980.8
emetic	973.6	E858.4	E943.6	E950.4	E962.0	E980.4
fungicide	985.8	E863.6	—	E950.6	E962.1	E980.7
insecticide	985.8	E863.4	—	E950.6	E962.1	E980.7
oleate	976.0	E858.7	E946.0	E950.4	E962.0	E980.4
sulfate	983.9	E864.3	—	E950.7	E962.1	E980.6
cupric	973.6	E858.4	E943.6	E950.4	E962.0	E980.4
cuprous	983.9	E864.3	—	E950.7	E962.1	E980.6
fungicide	983.9	E863.6	—	E950.7	E962.1	E980.6
Coral (sting)	989.5	E905.6	—	E950.9	E962.1	E980.9
snake (bite) (venom)	989.5	E905.0	—	E950.9	E962.1	E980.9
Cordran	976.0	E858.7	E946.0	E950.4	E962.0	E980.4
Corn cures	976.4	E858.7	E946.4	E950.4	E962.0	E980.4
Cornhusker's lotion	976.3	E858.7	E946.3	E950.4	E962.0	E980.4

Nontherapeutic use substance

☞ Subterms under main terms may continue to next column or page

	Poisoning	External Cause (E-Code)				
		Accident	Therapeutic Use	Suicide Attempt	Assault	Undetermined
Corn starch	976.3	E858.7	E946.3	E950.4	E962.0	E980.4
Corrosive	983.9	E864.4	—	E950.7	E962.1	E980.6
acids NEC	983.1	E864.1	—	E950.7	E962.1	E980.6
aromatics	983.0	E864.0	—	E950.7	E962.1	E980.6
disinfectant	983.0	E861.4	—	E950.7	E962.1	E980.6
fumes NEC	987.9	E869.9	—	E952.9	E962.2	E982.9
specified NEC	983.9	E864.3	—	E950.7	E962.1	E980.6
sublimate — see Mercury, chloride						
Cortate	962.0	E858.0	E932.0	E950.4	E962.0	E980.4
Cort-Dome	962.0	E858.0	E932.0	E950.4	E962.0	E980.4
ENT agent	976.6	E858.7	E946.6	E950.4	E962.0	E980.4
ophthalmic preparation	976.5	E858.7	E946.5	E950.4	E962.0	E980.4
topical NEC	976.0	E858.7	E946.0	E950.4	E962.0	E980.4
Cortef	962.0	E858.0	E932.0	E950.4	E962.0	E980.4
ENT agent	976.6	E858.7	E946.6	E950.4	E962.0	E980.4
ophthalmic preparation	976.5	E858.7	E946.5	E950.4	E962.0	E980.4
topical NEC	976.0	E858.7	E946.0	E950.4	E962.0	E980.4
Corticosteroids (fluorinated)	962.0	E858.0	E932.0	E950.4	E962.0	E980.4
ENT agent	976.6	E858.7	E946.6	E950.4	E962.0	E980.4
ophthalmic preparation	976.5	E858.7	E946.5	E950.4	E962.0	E980.4
topical NEC	976.0	E858.7	E946.0	E950.4	E962.0	E980.4
Corticotropin	962.4	E858.0	E932.4	E950.4	E962.0	E980.4
Cortisol	962.0	E858.0	E932.0	E950.4	E962.0	E980.4
ENT agent	976.6	E858.7	E946.6	E950.4	E962.0	E980.4
ophthalmic preparation	976.5	E858.7	E946.5	E950.4	E962.0	E980.4
topical NEC	976.0	E858.7	E946.0	E950.4	E962.0	E980.4
Cortisone derivatives (acetate)	962.0	E858.0	E932.0	E950.4	E962.0	E980.4
ENT agent	976.6	E858.7	E946.6	E950.4	E962.0	E980.4
ophthalmic preparation	976.5	E858.7	E946.5	E950.4	E962.0	E980.4
topical NEC	976.0	E858.7	E946.0	E950.4	E962.0	E980.4
Cortogen	962.0	E858.0	E932.0	E950.4	E962.0	E980.4
ENT agent	976.6	E858.7	E946.6	E950.4	E962.0	E980.4
ophthalmic preparation	976.5	E858.7	E946.5	E950.4	E962.0	E980.4
Cortone	962.0	E858.0	E932.0	E950.4	E962.0	E980.4
ENT agent	976.6	E858.7	E946.6	E950.4	E962.0	E980.4
ophthalmic preparation	976.5	E858.7	E946.5	E950.4	E962.0	E980.4
Cortril	962.0	E858.0	E932.0	E950.4	E962.0	E980.4
ENT agent	976.6	E858.7	E946.6	E950.4	E962.0	E980.4
ophthalmic preparation	976.5	E858.7	E946.5	E950.4	E962.0	E980.4
topical NEC	976.0	E858.7	E946.0	E950.4	E962.0	E980.4
Cosmetics	989.89	E866.7	—	E950.9	E962.1	E980.9
Cosyntropin	977.8	E858.8	E947.8	E950.4	E962.0	E980.4
Cotarnine	964.5	E858.2	E934.5	E950.4	E962.0	E980.4
Cottonseed oil	976.3	E858.7	E946.3	E950.4	E962.0	E980.4
Cough mixtures (antitussives)	975.4	E858.6	E945.4	E950.4	E962.0	E980.4
containing opiates	965.09	E850.2	E935.2	E950.0	E962.0	E980.0
expectorants	975.5	E858.6	E945.5	E950.4	E962.0	E980.4
Coumadin	964.2	E858.2	E934.2	E950.4	E962.0	E980.4
rodenticide	989.4	E863.7	—	E950.6	E962.1	E980.7
Coumarin	964.2	E858.2	E934.2	E950.4	E962.0	E980.4
Coumetarol	964.2	E858.2	E934.2	E950.4	E962.0	E980.4
Cowbane	988.2	E865.4	—	E950.9	E962.1	E980.9
Cozyme	963.5	E858.1	E933.5	E950.4	E962.0	E980.4
Crack	970.81	E854.3	E940.8	E950.4	E962.0	E980.4
Creolin	983.0	E864.0	—	E950.7	E962.1	E980.6
disinfectant	983.0	E861.4	—	E950.7	E962.1	E980.6
Creosol (compound)	983.0	E864.0	—	E950.7	E962.1	E980.6
Creosote (beechwood) (coal tar)	983.0	E864.0	—	E950.7	E962.1	E980.6
medicinal (expectorant)	975.5	E858.6	E945.5	E950.4	E962.0	E980.4
syrup	975.5	E858.6	E945.5	E950.4	E962.0	E980.4
Cresol	983.0	E864.0	—	E950.7	E962.1	E980.6
disinfectant	983.0	E861.4	—	E950.7	E962.1	E980.6
Cresylic acid	983.0	E864.0	—	E950.7	E962.1	E980.6
Cropropamide	965.7	E850.7	E935.7	E950.0	E962.0	E980.0
with crotethamide	970.0	E854.3	E940.0	E950.4	E962.0	E980.4
Crotamiton	976.0	E858.7	E946.0	E950.4	E962.0	E980.4
Crotethamide	965.7	E850.7	E935.7	E950.0	E962.0	E980.0
with cropropamide	970.0	E854.3	E940.0	E950.4	E962.0	E980.4
Croton (oil)	973.1	E858.4	E943.1	E950.4	E962.0	E980.4
chloral	967.1	E852.0	E937.1	E950.2	E962.0	E980.2
Crude oil	981	E862.1	—	E950.9	E962.1	E980.9
Cryogenine	965.8	E850.8	E935.8	E950.0	E962.0	E980.0
Cryolite (pesticide)	989.4	E863.4	—	E950.6	E962.1	E980.7
Cryptenamine	972.6	E858.3	E942.6	E950.4	E962.0	E980.4
Crystal violet	976.0	E858.7	E946.0	E950.4	E962.0	E980.4
Cuckoopint	988.2	E865.4	—	E950.9	E962.1	E980.9
Cumetharol	964.2	E858.2	E934.2	E950.4	E962.0	E980.4
Cupric sulfate	973.6	E858.4	E943.6	E950.4	E962.0	E980.4
Cuprous sulfate	983.9	E864.3	—	E950.7	E962.1	E980.6
Curare, curarine	975.2	E858.6	E945.2	E950.4	E962.0	E980.4
Cyanic acid — see Cyanide(s)						
Cyanide(s) (compounds) (hydrogen) (potassium) (sodium) NEC	989.0	E866.8	—	E950.9	E962.1	E980.9
dust or gas (inhalation) NEC	987.7	E869.8	—	E952.8	E962.2	E982.8
fumigant	989.0	E863.8	—	E950.6	E962.1	E980.7
mercuric — see Mercury						
pesticide (dust) (fumes)	989.0	E863.4	—	E950.6	E962.1	E980.7
Cyanocobalamin	964.1	E858.2	E934.1	E950.4	E962.0	E980.4
Cyanogen (chloride) (gas) NEC	987.8	E869.8	—	E952.8	E962.2	E982.8
Cyclaine	968.5	E855.2	E938.5	E950.4	E962.0	E980.4
Cyclamen europaeum	988.2	E865.4	—	E950.9	E962.1	E980.9
Cyclandelate	972.5	E858.3	E942.5	E950.4	E962.0	E980.4
Cyclazocine	965.09	E850.2	E935.2	E950.0	E962.0	E980.0
Cyclizine	963.0	E858.1	E933.0	E950.4	E962.0	E980.4
Cyclobarbital, cyclobarbitone	967.0	E851	E937.0	E950.1	E962.0	E980.1
Cycloguanil	961.4	E857	E931.4	E950.4	E962.0	E980.4
Cyclohexane	982.0	E862.4	—	E950.9	E962.1	E980.9
Cyclohexanol	980.8	E860.8	—	E950.9	E962.1	E980.9
Cyclohexanone	982.8	E862.4	—	E950.9	E962.1	E980.9
Cyclomethycaine	968.5	E855.2	E938.5	E950.4	E962.0	E980.4
Cyclopentamine	971.2	E855.5	E941.2	E950.4	E962.0	E980.4
Cyclopenthiazide	974.3	E858.5	E944.3	E950.4	E962.0	E980.4
Cyclopentolate	971.1	E855.4	E941.1	E950.4	E962.0	E980.4
Cyclophosphamide	963.1	E858.1	E933.1	E950.4	E962.0	E980.4
Cyclopropane	968.2	E855.1	E938.2	E950.4	E962.0	E980.4
Cycloserine	960.6	E856	E930.6	E950.4	E962.0	E980.4
Cyclothiazide	974.3	E858.5	E944.3	E950.4	E962.0	E980.4
Cycrimine	966.4	E855.0	E936.4	E950.4	E962.0	E980.4
Cymarin	972.1	E858.3	E942.1	E950.4	E962.0	E980.4
Cyproheptadine	963.0	E858.1	E933.0	E950.4	E962.0	E980.4
Cyprolidol	969.09	E854.0	E939.0	E950.3	E962.0	E980.3
Cytarabine	963.1	E858.1	E933.1	E950.4	E962.0	E980.4
Cytisus						
laburnum	988.2	E865.4	—	E950.9	E962.1	E980.9
scoparius	988.2	E865.4	—	E950.9	E962.1	E980.9
Cytomel	962.7	E858.0	E932.7	E950.4	E962.0	E980.4
Cytosine (antineoplastic)	963.1	E858.1	E933.1	E950.4	E962.0	E980.4
Cytoxan	963.1	E858.1	E933.1	E950.4	E962.0	E980.4
Dacarbazine	963.1	E858.1	E933.1	E950.4	E962.0	E980.4
Dactinomycin	960.7	E856	E930.7	E950.4	E962.0	E980.4
DADPS	961.8	E857	E931.8	E950.4	E962.0	E980.4
Dakin's solution (external)	976.0	E858.7	E946.0	E950.4	E962.0	E980.4
Dalmane	969.4	E853.2	E939.4	E950.3	E962.0	E980.3
DAM	977.2	E858.8	E947.2	E950.4	E962.0	E980.4
Danilone	964.2	E858.2	E934.2	E950.4	E962.0	E980.4
Danthron	973.1	E858.4	E943.1	E950.4	E962.0	E980.4
Dantrolene	975.2	E858.6	E945.2	E950.4	E962.0	E980.4
Daphne (gnidium) (mezereum)	988.2	E865.4	—	E950.9	E962.1	E980.9
berry	988.2	E865.3	—	E950.9	E962.1	E980.9
Dapsone	961.8	E857	E931.8	E950.4	E962.0	E980.4
Daraprim	961.4	E857	E931.4	E950.4	E962.0	E980.4
Darnel	988.2	E865.3	—	E950.9	E962.1	E980.9
Darvon	965.8	E850.8	E935.8	E950.0	E962.0	E980.0
Daunorubicin	960.7	E856	E930.7	E950.4	E962.0	E980.4
DBI	962.3	E858.0	E932.3	E950.4	E962.0	E980.4
D-Con (rodenticide)	989.4	E863.7	—	E950.6	E962.1	E980.7
DDS	961.8	E857	E931.8	E950.4	E962.0	E980.4
DDT	989.2	E863.0	—	E950.6	E962.1	E980.7
Deadly nightshade	988.2	E865.4	—	E950.9	E962.1	E980.9
berry	988.2	E865.3	—	E950.9	E962.1	E980.9
Deanol	969.79	E854.2	E939.7	E950.3	E962.0	E980.3
Debrisoquine	972.6	E858.3	E942.6	E950.4	E962.0	E980.4
Decaborane	989.89	E866.8	—	E950.9	E962.1	E980.9
fumes	987.8	E869.8	—	E952.8	E962.2	E982.8
Decadron	962.0	E858.0	E932.0	E950.4	E962.0	E980.4
ENT agent	976.6	E858.7	E946.6	E950.4	E962.0	E980.4
ophthalmic preparation	976.5	E858.7	E946.5	E950.4	E962.0	E980.4
topical NEC	976.0	E858.7	E946.0	E950.4	E962.0	E980.4
Decahydronaphthalene	982.0	E862.4	—	E950.9	E962.1	E980.9
Decalin	982.0	E862.4	—	E950.9	E962.1	E980.9
Decamethonium	975.2	E858.6	E945.2	E950.4	E962.0	E980.4
Decholin	973.4	E858.4	E943.4	E950.4	E962.0	E980.4
sodium (diagnostic)	977.8	E858.8	E947.8	E950.4	E962.0	E980.4

Nontherapeutic use substance

⚕ Subterms under main terms may continue to next column or page

	Poisoning	Accident	Therapeutic Use	Suicide Attempt	Assault	Undetermined
Declomycin	960.4	E856	E930.4	E950.4	E962.0	E980.4
Deferoxamine	963.8	E858.1	E933.8	E950.4	E962.0	E980.4
Dehydrocholic acid	973.4	E858.4	E943.4	E950.4	E962.0	E980.4
Dekalin	982.0	E862.4	—	E950.9	E962.1	E980.9
Delalutin	962.2	E858.0	E932.2	E950.4	E962.0	E980.4
Delphinium	988.2	E865.3	—	E950.9	E962.1	E980.9
Deltasone	962.0	E858.0	E932.0	E950.4	E962.0	E980.4
Deltra	962.0	E858.0	E932.0	E950.4	E962.0	E980.4
Delvinal	967.0	E851	E937.0	E950.1	E962.0	E980.1
Demecarium (bromide)	971.0	E855.3	E941.0	E950.4	E962.0	E980.4
Demeclocycline	960.4	E856	E930.4	E950.4	E962.0	E980.4
Demecolcine	963.1	E858.1	E933.1	E950.4	E962.0	E980.4
Demelanizing agents	976.8	E858.7	E946.8	E950.4	E962.0	E980.4
Demerol	965.09	E850.2	E935.2	E950.0	E962.0	E980.0
Demethylchlortetracy-cline	960.4	E856	E930.4	E950.4	E962.0	E980.4
Demethyltetracycline	960.4	E856	E930.4	E950.4	E962.0	E980.4
Demeton	989.3	E863.1	—	E950.6	E962.1	E980.7
Demulcents	976.3	E858.7	E946.3	E950.4	E962.0	E980.4
Demulen	962.2	E858.0	E932.2	E950.4	E962.0	E980.4
Denatured alcohol	980.0	E860.1	—	E950.9	E962.1	E980.9
Dendrid	976.5	E858.7	E946.5	E950.4	E962.0	E980.4
Dental agents, topical	976.7	E858.7	E946.7	E950.4	E962.0	E980.4
Deodorant spray (feminine hygiene)	976.8	E858.7	E946.8	E950.4	E962.0	E980.4
Deoxyribonuclease	963.4	E858.1	E933.4	E950.4	E962.0	E980.4
Depressants						
appetite, central	977.0	E858.8	E947.0	E950.4	E962.0	E980.4
cardiac	972.0	E858.3	E942.0	E950.4	E962.0	E980.4
central nervous system (anes-thetic)	968.4	E855.1	E938.4	E950.4	E962.0	E980.4
psychotherapeutic	969.5	E853.9	E939.5	E950.3	E962.0	E980.3
Dequalinium	976.0	E858.7	E946.0	E950.4	E962.0	E980.4
Dermolate	976.2	E858.7	E946.2	E950.4	E962.0	E980.4
DES	962.2	E858.0	E932.2	E950.4	E962.0	E980.4
Desenex	976.0	E858.7	E946.0	E950.4	E962.0	E980.4
Deserpidine	972.6	E858.3	E942.6	E950.4	E962.0	E980.4
Desipramine	969.05	E854.0	E939.0	E950.3	E962.0	E980.3
Deslanoside	972.1	E858.3	E942.1	E950.4	E962.0	E980.4
Desocodeine	965.09	E850.2	E935.2	E950.0	E962.0	E980.0
Desomorphine	965.09	E850.2	E935.2	E950.0	E962.0	E980.0
Desonide	976.0	E858.7	E946.0	E950.4	E962.0	E980.4
Desoxycorticosterone derivatives	962.0	E858.0	E932.0	E950.4	E962.0	E980.4
Desoxyephedrine	969.72	E854.2	E939.7	E950.3	E962.0	E980.3
DET	969.6	E854.1	E939.6	E950.3	E962.0	E980.3
Detergents (ingested) (synthetic)	989.6	E861.0	—	E950.9	E962.1	E980.9
ENT agent	976.6	E858.7	E946.6	E950.4	E962.0	E980.4
external medication	976.2	E858.7	E946.2	E950.4	E962.0	E980.4
ophthalmic preparation	976.5	E858.7	E946.5	E950.4	E962.0	E980.4
topical NEC	976.0	E858.7	E946.0	E950.4	E962.0	E980.4
Deterrent, alcohol	977.3	E858.8	E947.3	E950.4	E962.0	E980.4
Detrothyronine	962.7	E858.0	E932.7	E950.4	E962.0	E980.4
Dettol (external medication)	976.0	E858.7	E946.0	E950.4	E962.0	E980.4
Dexamethasone	962.0	E858.0	E932.0	E950.4	E962.0	E980.4
Dexamphetamine	969.72	E854.2	E939.7	E950.3	E962.0	E980.3
Dexedrine	969.72	E854.2	E939.7	E950.3	E962.0	E980.3
Dexpanthenol	963.5	E858.1	E933.5	E950.4	E962.0	E980.4
Dextran	964.8	E858.2	E934.8	E950.4	E962.0	E980.4
Dextriferron	964.0	E858.2	E934.0	E950.4	E962.0	E980.4
Dextroamphetamine	969.72	E854.2	E939.7	E950.3	E962.0	E980.3
Dextro calcium pantothenate	963.5	E858.1	E933.5	E950.4	E962.0	E980.4
Dextromethorphan	975.4	E858.6	E945.4	E950.4	E962.0	E980.4
Dextromoramide	965.09	E850.2	E935.2	E950.0	E962.0	E980.0
Dextro pantothenyl alcohol	963.5	E858.1	E933.5	E950.4	E962.0	E980.4
topical	976.8	E858.7	E946.8	E950.4	E962.0	E980.4
Dextropropoxyphene (hydrochloride)	965.8	E850.8	E935.8	E950.0	E962.0	E980.0
Dextrorphan	965.09	E850.2	E935.2	E950.0	E962.0	E980.0
Dextrose NEC	974.5	E858.5	E944.5	E950.4	E962.0	E980.4
Dextrothyroxin	962.7	E858.0	E932.7	E950.4	E962.0	E980.4
DFP	971.0	E855.3	E941.0	E950.4	E962.0	E980.4
DHE-45	972.9	E858.3	E942.9	E950.4	E962.0	E980.4
Diabinese	962.3	E858.0	E932.3	E950.4	E962.0	E980.4
Diacetyl monoxime	977.2	E858.8	E947.2	E950.4	E962.0	E980.4
Diacetylmorphine	965.01	E850.0	E935.0	E950.0	E962.0	E980.0
Diagnostic agents	977.8	E858.8	E947.8	E950.4	E962.0	E980.4
Dial (soap)	976.2	E858.7	E946.2	E950.4	E962.0	E980.4

	Poisoning	Accident	Therapeutic Use	Suicide Attempt	Assault	Undetermined
Dial — *continued*						
sedative	967.0	E851	E937.0	E950.1	E962.0	E980.1
Diallylbarbituric acid	967.0	E851	E937.0	E950.1	E962.0	E980.1
Diaminodiphenylsulfone	961.8	E857	E931.8	E950.4	E962.0	E980.4
Diamorphine	965.01	E850.0	E935.0	E950.0	E962.0	E980.0
Diamox	974.2	E858.5	E944.2	E950.4	E962.0	E980.4
Diamthazole	976.0	E858.7	E946.0	E950.4	E962.0	E980.4
Diaphenylsulfone	961.8	E857	E931.8	E950.4	E962.0	E980.4
Diasone (sodium)	961.8	E857	E931.8	E950.4	E962.0	E980.4
Diazepam	969.4	E853.2	E939.4	E950.3	E962.0	E980.3
Diazinon	989.3	E863.1	—	E950.6	E962.1	E980.7
Diazomethane (gas)	987.8	E869.8	—	E952.8	E962.2	E982.8
Diazoxide	972.5	E858.3	E942.5	E950.4	E962.0	E980.4
Dibenamine	971.3	E855.6	E941.3	E950.4	E962.0	E980.4
Dibenzheptropine	963.0	E858.1	E933.0	E950.4	E962.0	E980.4
Dibenzyline	971.3	E855.6	E941.3	E950.4	E962.0	E980.4
Diborane (gas)	987.8	E869.8	—	E952.8	E962.2	E982.8
Dibromomannitol	963.1	E858.1	E933.1	E950.4	E962.0	E980.4
Dibucaine (spinal)	968.7	E855.2	E938.7	E950.4	E962.0	E980.4
topical (surface)	968.5	E855.2	E938.5	E950.4	E962.0	E980.4
Dibunate sodium	975.4	E858.6	E945.4	E950.4	E962.0	E980.4
Dibutoline	971.1	E855.4	E941.1	E950.4	E962.0	E980.4
Dicapthon	989.4	E863.4	—	E950.6	E962.1	E980.7
Dichloralphenazone	967.1	E852.0	E937.1	E950.2	E962.0	E980.2
Dichlorodifluo-romethane	987.4	E869.2	—	E952.8	E962.2	E982.8
Dichloroethane	982.3	E862.4	—	E950.9	E962.1	E980.9
Dichloroethylene	982.3	E862.4	—	E950.9	E962.1	E980.9
Dichloroethyl sulfide	987.8	E869.8	—	E952.8	E962.2	E982.8
Dichlorohydrin	982.3	E862.4	—	E950.9	E962.1	E980.9
Dichloromethane (solvent) (vapor)	982.3	E862.4	—	E950.9	E962.1	E980.9
Dichlorophen(e)	961.6	E857	E931.6	E950.4	E962.0	E980.4
Dichlorphenamide	974.2	E858.5	E944.2	E950.4	E962.0	E980.4
Dichlorvos	989.3	E863.1	—	E950.6	E962.1	E980.7
Diclofenac sodium	965.69	E850.6	E935.6	E950.0	E962.0	E980.0
Dicoumarin, dicumarol	964.2	E858.2	E934.2	E950.4	E962.0	E980.4
Dicyanogen (gas)	987.8	E869.8	—	E952.8	E962.2	E982.8
Dicyclomine	971.1	E855.4	E941.1	E950.4	E962.0	E980.4
Dieldrin (vapor)	989.2	E863.0	—	E950.6	E962.1	E980.7
Dienestrol	962.2	E858.0	E932.2	E950.4	E962.0	E980.4
Dietetics	977.0	E858.8	E947.0	E950.4	E962.0	E980.4
Diethazine	966.4	E855.0	E936.4	E950.4	E962.0	E980.4
Diethyl						
barbituric acid	967.0	E851	E937.0	E950.1	E962.0	E980.1
carbamazine	961.6	E857	E931.6	E950.4	E962.0	E980.4
carbinol	980.8	E860.8	—	E950.9	E962.1	E980.9
carbonate	982.8	E862.4	—	E950.9	E962.1	E980.9
dioxide	982.8	E862.4	—	E950.9	E962.1	E980.9
ether (vapor) — see Ether(s)						
glycol (monoacetate) (monoethyl ether)	982.8	E862.4	—	E950.9	E962.1	E980.9
propion	977.0	E858.8	E947.0	E950.4	E962.0	E980.4
stilbestrol	962.2	E858.0	E932.2	E950.4	E962.0	E980.4
Diethylene						
dioxide	982.8	E862.4	—	E950.9	E962.1	E980.9
glycol (monoacetate) (monoethyl ether)	982.8	E862.4	—	E950.9	E962.1	E980.9
Diethylsulfone-diethyl-methane	967.8	E852.8	E937.8	E950.2	E962.0	E980.2
Difencloxazine	965.09	E850.2	E935.2	E950.0	E962.0	E980.0
Diffusin	963.4	E858.1	E933.4	E950.4	E962.0	E980.4
Diflos	971.0	E855.3	E941.0	E950.4	E962.0	E980.4
Digestants	973.4	E858.4	E943.4	E950.4	E962.0	E980.4
Digitalin(e)	972.1	E858.3	E942.1	E950.4	E962.0	E980.4
Digitalis glycosides	972.1	E858.3	E942.1	E950.4	E962.0	E980.4
Digitoxin	972.1	E858.3	E942.1	E950.4	E962.0	E980.4
Digoxin	972.1	E858.3	E942.1	E950.4	E962.0	E980.4
Dihydrocodeine	965.09	E850.2	E935.2	E950.0	E962.0	E980.0
Dihydrocodeinone	965.09	E850.2	E935.2	E950.0	E962.0	E980.0
Dihydroergocristine	972.9	E858.3	E942.9	E950.4	E962.0	E980.4
Dihydroergotamine	972.9	E858.3	E942.9	E950.4	E962.0	E980.4
Dihydroergotoxine	972.9	E858.3	E942.9	E950.4	E962.0	E980.4
Dihydrohydroxy-codeinone	965.09	E850.2	E935.2	E950.0	E962.0	E980.0
Dihydrohydroxymorphi-none	965.09	E850.2	E935.2	E950.0	E962.0	E980.0
Dihydroisocodeine	965.09	E850.2	E935.2	E950.0	E962.0	E980.0
Dihydromorphine	965.09	E850.2	E935.2	E950.0	E962.0	E980.0
Dihydromorphinone	965.09	E850.2	E935.2	E950.0	E962.0	E980.0
Dihydrostreptomycin	960.6	E856	E930.6	E950.4	E962.0	E980.4
Dihydrotachysterol	962.6	E858.0	E932.6	E950.4	E962.0	E980.4

	External Cause (E-Code)					
	Poisoning	Accident	Therapeutic Use	Suicide Attempt	Assault	Undetermined
Dihydroxyanthraquinone	973.1	E858.4	E943.1	E950.4	E962.0	E980.4
Dihydroxycodeinone	965.09	E850.2	E935.2	E950.0	E962.0	E980.0
Diiodohydroxyquin	961.3	E857	E931.3	E950.4	E962.0	E980.4
topical	976.0	E858.7	E946.0	E950.4	E962.0	E980.4
Diiodohydroxyquinoline	961.3	E857	E931.3	E950.4	E962.0	E980.4
Dilantin	966.1	E855.0	E936.1	E950.4	E962.0	E980.4
Dilaudid	965.09	E850.2	E935.2	E950.0	E962.0	E980.0
Diloxanide	961.5	E857	E931.5	E950.4	E962.0	E980.4
Dimefline	970.0	E854.3	E940.0	E950.4	E962.0	E980.4
Dimenhydrinate	963.0	E858.1	E933.0	E950.4	E962.0	E980.4
Dimercaprol	963.8	E858.1	E933.8	E950.4	E962.0	E980.4
Dimercaptopropanol	963.8	E858.1	E933.8	E950.4	E962.0	E980.4
Dimetane	963.0	E858.1	E933.0	E950.4	E962.0	E980.4
Dimethicone	976.3	E858.7	E946.3	E950.4	E962.0	E980.4
Dimethindene	963.0	E858.1	E933.0	E950.4	E962.0	E980.4
Dimethisoquin	968.5	E855.2	E938.5	E950.4	E962.0	E980.4
Dimethisterone	962.2	E858.0	E932.2	E950.4	E962.0	E980.4
Dimethoxanate	975.4	E858.6	E945.4	E950.4	E962.0	E980.4
Dimethyl						
arsine, arsinic acid — see Arsenic						
carbinol	980.2	E860.3	—	E950.9	E962.1	E980.9
diguanide	962.3	E858.0	E932.3	E950.4	E962.0	E980.4
ketone	982.8	E862.4	—	E950.9	E962.1	E980.9
vapor	987.8	E869.8	—	E952.8	E962.2	E982.8
meperidine	965.09	E850.2	E935.2	E950.0	E962.0	E980.0
parathion	989.3	E863.1	—	E950.6	E962.1	E980.7
polysiloxane	973.8	E858.4	E943.8	E950.4	E962.0	E980.4
sulfate (fumes)	987.8	E869.8	—	E952.8	E962.2	E982.8
liquid	983.9	E864.3	—	E950.7	E962.1	E980.6
sulfoxide NEC	982.8	E862.4	—	E950.9	E962.1	E980.9
medicinal	976.4	E858.7	E946.4	E950.4	E962.0	E980.4
triptamine	969.6	E854.1	E939.6	E950.3	E962.0	E980.3
tubocurarine	975.2	E858.6	E945.2	E950.4	E962.0	E980.4
Dindevan	964.2	E858.2	E934.2	E950.4	E962.0	E980.4
Dinitrobenzene	983.0	E864.0	—	E950.7	E962.1	E980.6
vapor	987.8	E869.8	—	E952.8	E962.2	E982.8
Dinitro (-ortho-) cresol (herbicide) (spray)	989.4	E863.5	—	E950.6	E962.1	E980.7
insecticide	989.4	E863.4	—	E950.6	E962.1	E980.7
Dinitro-orthocresol (herbicide) (cide)	989.4	E863.5	—	E950.6	E962.1	E980.7
insecticide	989.4	E863.4	—	E950.6	E962.1	E980.7
Dinitrophenol (herbicide) (spray)	989.4	E863.5	—	E950.6	E962.1	E980.7
insecticide	989.4	E863.4	—	E950.6	E962.1	E980.7
Dinoprost	975.0	E858.6	E945.0	E950.4	E962.0	E980.4
Dioctyl sulfosuccinate (calcium) (sodium)	973.2	E858.4	E943.2	E950.4	E962.0	E980.4
Diodoquin	961.3	E857	E931.3	E950.4	E962.0	E980.4
Dione derivatives NEC	966.3	E855.0	E936.3	E950.4	E962.0	E980.4
Dionin	965.09	E850.2	E935.2	E950.0	E962.0	E980.0
Dioxane	982.8	E862.4	—	E950.9	E962.1	E980.9
Dioxin — see Herbicide						
Dioxyline	972.5	E858.3	E942.5	E950.4	E962.0	E980.4
Dipentene	982.8	E862.4	—	E950.9	E962.1	E980.9
Diphemanil	971.1	E855.4	E941.1	E950.4	E962.0	E980.4
Diphenadione	964.2	E858.2	E934.2	E950.4	E962.0	E980.4
Diphenhydramine	963.0	E858.1	E933.0	E950.4	E962.0	E980.4
Diphenidol	963.0	E858.1	E933.0	E950.4	E962.0	E980.4
Diphenoxylate	973.5	E858.4	E943.5	E950.4	E962.0	E980.4
Diphenylchloroarsine	985.1	E866.3	—	E950.8	E962.1	E980.8
Diphenylhydantoin (sodium)	966.1	E855.0	E936.1	E950.4	E962.0	E980.4
Diphenylpyraline	963.0	E858.1	E933.0	E950.4	E962.0	E980.4
Diphtheria						
antitoxin	979.9	E858.8	E949.9	E950.4	E962.0	E980.4
toxoid	978.5	E858.8	E948.5	E950.4	E962.0	E980.4
with tetanus toxoid	978.9	E858.8	E948.9	E950.4	E962.0	E980.4
with pertussis component	978.6	E858.8	E948.6	E950.4	E962.0	E980.4
vaccine	978.5	E858.8	E948.5	E950.4	E962.0	E980.4
Dipipanone	965.09	E850.2	E935.2	E950.0	E962.0	E980.0
Diplovax	979.5	E858.8	E949.5	E950.4	E962.0	E980.4
Diprophylline	975.1	E858.6	E945.1	E950.4	E962.0	E980.4
Dipyridamole	972.4	E858.3	E942.4	E950.4	E962.0	E980.4
Dipyrone	965.5	E850.5	E935.5	E950.0	E962.0	E980.0
Diquat	989.4	E863.5	—	E950.6	E962.1	E980.7
Disinfectant NEC	983.9	E861.4	—	E950.7	E962.1	E980.6
alkaline	983.2	E861.4	—	E950.7	E962.1	E980.6
aromatic	983.0	E861.4	—	E950.7	E962.1	E980.6

	External Cause (E-Code)					
	Poisoning	Accident	Therapeutic Use	Suicide Attempt	Assault	Undetermined
Disipal	966.4	E855.0	E936.4	E950.4	E962.0	E980.4
Disodium edetate	963.8	E858.1	E933.8	E950.4	E962.0	E980.4
Disulfamide	974.4	E858.5	E944.4	E950.4	E962.0	E980.4
Disulfanilamide	961.0	E857	E931.0	E950.4	E962.0	E980.4
Disulfiram	977.3	E858.8	E947.3	E950.4	E962.0	E980.4
Dithiazanine	961.6	E857	E931.6	E950.4	E962.0	E980.4
Dithioglycerol	963.8	E858.1	E933.8	E950.4	E962.0	E980.4
Dithranol	976.4	E858.7	E946.4	E950.4	E962.0	E980.4
Diucardin	974.3	E858.5	E944.3	E950.4	E962.0	E980.4
Diupres	974.3	E858.5	E944.3	E950.4	E962.0	E980.4
Diuretics NEC	974.4	E858.5	E944.4	E950.4	E962.0	E980.4
carbonic acid anhydrase inhibitors	974.2	E858.5	E944.2	E950.4	E962.0	E980.4
mercurial	974.0	E858.5	E944.0	E950.4	E962.0	E980.4
osmotic	974.4	E858.5	E944.4	E950.4	E962.0	E980.4
purine derivatives	974.1	E858.5	E944.1	E950.4	E962.0	E980.4
saluretic	974.3	E858.5	E944.3	E950.4	E962.0	E980.4
Diuril	974.3	E858.5	E944.3	E950.4	E962.0	E980.4
Divinyl ether	968.2	E855.1	E938.2	E950.4	E962.0	E980.4
D-lysergic acid diethylamide	969.6	E854.1	E939.6	E950.3	E962.0	E980.3
DMCT	960.4	E856	E930.4	E950.4	E962.0	E980.4
DMSO	982.8	E862.4	—	E950.9	E962.1	E980.9
DMT	969.6	E854.1	E939.6	E950.3	E962.0	E980.3
DNOC	989.4	E863.5	—	E950.6	E962.1	E980.7
DOCA	962.0	E858.0	E932.0	E950.4	E962.0	E980.4
Dolophine	965.02	E850.1	E935.1	E950.0	E962.0	E980.0
Doloxene	965.8	E850.8	E935.8	E950.0	E962.0	E980.0
DOM	969.6	E854.1	E939.6	E950.3	E962.0	E980.3
Domestic gas — see Gas, utility						
Domiphen (bromide) (lozenges)	976.6	E858.7	E946.6	E950.4	E962.0	E980.4
Dopa (levo)	966.4	E855.0	E936.4	E950.4	E962.0	E980.4
Dopamine	971.2	E855.5	E941.2	E950.4	E962.0	E980.4
Doriden	967.5	E852.4	E937.5	E950.2	E962.0	E980.2
Dormiral	967.0	E851	E937.0	E950.1	E962.0	E980.1
Dormison	967.8	E852.8	E937.8	E950.2	E962.0	E980.2
Dornase	963.4	E858.1	E933.4	E950.4	E962.0	E980.4
Dorsacaine	968.5	E855.2	E938.5	E950.4	E962.0	E980.4
Dothiepin hydrochloride	969.05	E854.0	E939.0	E950.3	E962.0	E980.3
Doxapram	970.0	E854.3	E940.0	E950.4	E962.0	E980.4
Doxepin	969.05	E854.0	E939.0	E950.3	E962.0	E980.3
Doxorubicin	960.7	E856	E930.7	E950.4	E962.0	E980.4
Doxycycline	960.4	E856	E930.4	E950.4	E962.0	E980.4
Doxylamine	963.0	E858.1	E933.0	E950.4	E962.0	E980.4
Dramamine	963.0	E858.1	E933.0	E950.4	E962.0	E980.4
Drano (drain cleaner)	983.2	E864.2	—	E950.7	E962.1	E980.6
Dromoran	965.09	E850.2	E935.2	E950.0	E962.0	E980.0
Dromostanolone	962.1	E858.0	E932.1	E950.4	E962.0	E980.4
Droperidol	969.2	E853.1	E939.2	E950.3	E962.0	E980.3
Drotrecogin alfa	964.2	E858.2	E934.2	E950.4	E962.0	E980.4
Drug	977.9	E858.9	E947.9	E950.5	E962.0	E980.5
AHFS List						
4:00 antihistamine drugs	963.0	E858.1	E933.0	E950.4	E962.0	E980.4
8:04 amebacides	961.5	E857	E931.5	E950.4	E962.0	E980.4
arsenical anti-infectives	961.1	E857	E931.1	E950.4	E962.0	E980.4
quinoline derivatives	961.3	E857	E931.3	E950.4	E962.0	E980.4
8:08 anthelmintics	961.6	E857	E931.6	E950.4	E962.0	E980.4
quinoline derivatives	961.3	E857	E931.3	E950.4	E962.0	E980.4
8:12.04 antifungal antibiotics	960.1	E856	E930.1	E950.4	E962.0	E980.4
8:12.06 cephalosporins	960.5	E856	E930.5	E950.4	E962.0	E980.4
8:12.08 chloramphenicol	960.2	E856	E930.2	E950.4	E962.0	E980.4
8:12.12 erythromycins	960.3	E856	E930.3	E950.4	E962.0	E980.4
8:12.16 penicillins	960.0	E856	E930.0	E950.4	E962.0	E980.4
8:12.20 streptomycins	960.6	E856	E930.6	E950.4	E962.0	E980.4
8:12.24 tetracyclines	960.4	E856	E930.4	E950.4	E962.0	E980.4
8:12.28 other antibiotics	960.8	E856	E930.8	E950.4	E962.0	E980.4
antimycobacterial	960.6	E856	E930.6	E950.4	E962.0	E980.4
macrolides	960.3	E856	E930.3	E950.4	E962.0	E980.4
8:16 antituberculars	961.8	E857	E931.8	E950.4	E962.0	E980.4
antibiotics	960.6	E856	E930.6	E950.4	E962.0	E980.4
8:18 antivirals	961.7	E857	E931.7	E950.4	E962.0	E980.4
8:20 plasmodicides (antimalarials)	961.4	E857	E931.4	E950.4	E962.0	E980.4
8:24 sulfonamides	961.0	E857	E931.0	E950.4	E962.0	E980.4
8:26 sulfones	961.8	E857	E931.8	E950.4	E962.0	E980.4
8:28 treponemicides	961.2	E857	E931.2	E950.4	E962.0	E980.4
8:32 trichomonacides	961.5	E857	E931.5	E950.4	E962.0	E980.4
nitrofuran derivatives	961.9	E857	E931.9	E950.4	E962.0	E980.4
quinoline derivatives	961.3	E857	E931.3	E950.4	E962.0	E980.4

Nontherapeutic use substance

Subterms under main terms may continue to next column or page

Drug — continued	Poisoning	Accident	Therapeutic Use	Suicide Attempt	Assault	Undetermined
8:36 urinary germicides	961.9	E857	E931.9	E950.4	E962.0	E980.4
quinoline derivatives	961.3	E857	E931.3	E950.4	E962.0	E980.4
8:40 other anti-infectives	961.9	E857	E931.9	E950.4	E962.0	E980.4
10:00 antineoplastic agents	963.1	E858.1	E933.1	E950.4	E962.0	E980.4
antibiotics	960.7	E856	E930.7	E950.4	E962.0	E980.4
progestogens	962.2	E858.0	E932.2	E950.4	E962.0	E980.4
12:04 parasympathomimetic (cholinergic) agents	971.0	E855.3	E941.0	E950.4	E962.0	E980.4
12:08 parasympatholytic (cholinergic-blocking) agents	971.1	E855.4	E941.1	E950.4	E962.0	E980.4
12:12 Sympathomimetic (adrenergic) agents	971.2	E855.5	E941.2	E950.4	E962.0	E980.4
12:16 sympatholytic (adrenergic-blocking) agents	971.3	E855.6	E941.3	E950.4	E962.0	E980.4
12:20 skeletal muscle relaxants						
central nervous system muscle-tone depressants	968.0	E855.1	E938.0	E950.4	E962.0	E980.4
myoneural blocking agents	975.2	E858.6	E945.2	E950.4	E962.0	E980.4
16:00 blood derivatives	964.7	E858.2	E934.7	E950.4	E962.0	E980.4
20:04.04 iron preparations	964.0	E858.2	E934.0	E950.4	E962.0	E980.4
20:04.08 liver and stomach preparations	964.1	E858.2	E934.1	E950.4	E962.0	E980.4
20:04 antianemia drugs	964.1	E858.2	E934.1	E950.4	E962.0	E980.4
20:12.04 anticoagulants	964.2	E858.2	E934.2	E950.4	E962.0	E980.4
20:12.08 antiheparin agents	964.5	E858.2	E934.5	E950.4	E962.0	E980.4
20:12.12 coagulants	964.5	E858.2	E934.5	E950.4	E962.0	E980.4
20:12.16 hemostatics NEC	964.5	E858.2	E934.5	E950.4	E962.0	E980.4
capillary active drugs	972.8	E858.3	E942.8	E950.4	E962.0	E980.4
24:04 cardiac drugs	972.9	E858.3	E942.9	E950.4	E962.0	E980.4
cardiotonic agents	972.1	E858.3	E942.1	E950.4	E962.0	E980.4
rhythm regulators	972.0	E858.3	E942.0	E950.4	E962.0	E980.4
24:06 antilipemic agents	972.2	E858.3	E942.2	E950.4	E962.0	E980.4
thyroid derivatives	962.7	E858.0	E932.7	E950.4	E962.0	E980.4
24:08 hypotensive agents	972.6	E858.3	E942.6	E950.4	E962.0	E980.4
adrenergic blocking agents	971.3	E855.6	E941.3	E950.4	E962.0	E980.4
ganglion blocking agents	972.3	E858.3	E942.3	E950.4	E962.0	E980.4
vasodilators	972.5	E858.3	E942.5	E950.4	E962.0	E980.4
24:12 vasodilating agents NEC	972.5	E858.3	E942.5	E950.4	E962.0	E980.4
coronary	972.4	E858.3	E942.4	E950.4	E962.0	E980.4
nicotinic acid derivatives	972.2	E858.3	E942.2	E950.4	E962.0	E980.4
24:16 sclerosing agents	972.7	E858.3	E942.7	E950.4	E962.0	E980.4
28:04 general anesthetics	968.4	E855.1	E938.4	E950.4	E962.0	E980.4
gaseous anesthetics	968.2	E855.1	E938.2	E950.4	E962.0	E980.4
halothane	968.1	E855.1	E938.1	E950.4	E962.0	E980.4
intravenous anesthetics	968.3	E855.1	E938.3	E950.4	E962.0	E980.4
28:08 analgesics and antipyretics	965.9	E850.9	E935.9	E950.0	E962.0	E980.0
antirheumatics	965.69	E850.6	E935.6	E950.0	E962.0	E980.0
aromatic analgesics	965.4	E850.4	E935.4	E950.0	E962.0	E980.0
non-narcotic NEC	965.7	E850.7	E935.7	E950.0	E962.0	E980.0
opium alkaloids	965.00	E850.2	E935.2	E950.0	E962.0	E980.0
heroin	965.01	E850.0	E935.0	E950.0	E962.0	E980.0
methadone	965.02	E850.1	E935.1	E950.0	E962.0	E980.0
specified type NEC	965.09	E850.2	E935.2	E950.0	E962.0	E980.0
pyrazole derivatives	965.5	E850.5	E935.5	E950.0	E962.0	E980.0
salicylates	965.1	E850.3	E935.3	E950.0	E962.0	E980.0
specified NEC	965.8	E850.8	E935.8	E950.0	E962.0	E980.0
28:10 narcotic antagonists	970.1	E854.3	E940.1	E950.4	E962.0	E980.4
28:12 anticonvulsants	966.3	E855.0	E936.3	E950.4	E962.0	E980.4
barbiturates	967.0	E851	E937.0	E950.1	E962.0	E980.1
benzodiazepine-based tranquilizers	969.4	E853.2	E939.4	E950.3	E962.0	E980.3
bromides	967.3	E852.2	E937.3	E950.2	E962.0	E980.2
hydantoin derivatives	966.1	E855.0	E936.1	E950.4	E962.0	E980.4
oxazolidine (derivatives)	966.0	E855.0	E936.0	E950.4	E962.0	E980.4
succinimides	966.2	E855.0	E936.2	E950.4	E962.0	E980.4

Drug — continued	Poisoning	Accident	Therapeutic Use	Suicide Attempt	Assault	Undetermined
28:16.04 antidepressants	969.00	E854.0	E939.0	E950.3	E962.0	E980.3
28:16.08 tranquilizers	969.5	E853.9	E939.5	E950.3	E962.0	E980.3
benzodiazepine-based	969.4	E853.2	E939.4	E950.3	E962.0	E980.3
butyrophenone-based	969.2	E853.1	E939.2	E950.3	E962.0	E980.3
major NEC	969.3	E853.8	E939.3	E950.3	E962.0	E980.3
phenothiazine-based	969.1	E853.0	E939.1	E950.3	E962.0	E980.3
28:16.12 other psychotherapeutic agents	969.8	E855.8	E939.8	E950.3	E962.0	E980.3
28:20 respiratory and cerebral stimulants	970.9	E854.3	E940.9	E950.4	E962.0	E980.4
analeptics	970.0	E854.3	E940.0	E950.4	E962.0	E980.4
anorexigenic agents	977.0	E858.8	E947.0	E950.4	E962.0	E980.4
psychostimulants	969.70	E854.2	E939.7	E950.3	E962.0	E980.3
specified NEC	970.89	E854.3	E940.8	E950.4	E962.0	E980.4
28:24 sedatives and hypnotics	967.9	E852.9	E937.9	E950.2	E962.0	E980.2
barbiturates	967.0	E851	E937.0	E950.1	E962.0	E980.1
benzodiazepine-based tranquilizers	969.4	E853.2	E939.4	E950.3	E962.0	E980.3
chloral hydrate (group)	967.1	E852.0	E937.1	E950.2	E962.0	E980.2
glutethamide group	967.5	E852.4	E937.5	E950.2	E962.0	E980.2
intravenous anesthetics	968.3	E855.1	E938.3	E950.4	E962.0	E980.4
methaqualone (compounds)	967.4	E852.3	E937.4	E950.2	E962.0	E980.2
paraldehyde	967.2	E852.1	E937.2	E950.2	E962.0	E980.2
phenothiazine-based tranquilizers	969.1	E853.0	E939.1	E950.3	E962.0	E980.3
specified NEC	967.8	E852.8	E937.8	E950.2	E962.0	E980.2
thiobarbiturates	968.3	E855.1	E938.3	E950.4	E962.0	E980.4
tranquilizer NEC	969.5	E853.9	E939.5	E950.3	E962.0	E980.3
36:04 to 36:88 diagnostic agents	977.8	E858.8	E947.8	E950.4	E962.0	E980.4
40:00 electrolyte, caloric, and water balance agents NEC	974.5	E858.5	E944.5	E950.4	E962.0	E980.4
40:04 acidifying agents	963.2	E858.1	E933.2	E950.4	E962.0	E980.4
40:08 alkalinizing agents	963.3	E858.1	E933.3	E950.4	E962.0	E980.4
40:10 ammonia detoxicants	974.5	E858.5	E944.5	E950.4	E962.0	E980.4
40:12 replacement solutions	974.5	E858.5	E944.5	E950.4	E962.0	E980.4
plasma expanders	964.8	E858.2	E934.8	E950.4	E962.0	E980.4
40:16 sodium-removing resins	974.5	E858.5	E944.5	E950.4	E962.0	E980.4
40:18 potassium-removing resins	974.5	E858.5	E944.5	E950.4	E962.0	E980.4
40:20 caloric agents	974.5	E858.5	E944.5	E950.4	E962.0	E980.4
40:24 salt and sugar substitutes	974.5	E858.5	E944.5	E950.4	E962.0	E980.4
40:28 diuretics NEC	974.4	E858.5	E944.4	E950.4	E962.0	E980.4
carbonic acid anhydrase inhibitors	974.2	E858.5	E944.2	E950.4	E962.0	E980.4
mercurials	974.0	E858.5	E944.0	E950.4	E962.0	E980.4
purine derivatives	974.1	E858.5	E944.1	E950.4	E962.0	E980.4
saluretics	974.3	E858.5	E944.3	E950.4	E962.0	E980.4
thiazides	974.3	E858.5	E944.3	E950.4	E962.0	E980.4
40:36 irrigating solutions	974.5	E858.5	E944.5	E950.4	E962.0	E980.4
40:40 uricosuric agents	974.7	E858.5	E944.7	E950.4	E962.0	E980.4
44:00 enzymes	963.4	E858.1	E933.4	E950.4	E962.0	E980.4
fibrinolysis-affecting agents	964.4	E858.2	E934.4	E950.4	E962.0	E980.4
gastric agents	973.4	E858.4	E943.4	E950.4	E962.0	E980.4
48:00 expectorants and cough preparations						
antihistamine agents	963.0	E858.1	E933.0	E950.4	E962.0	E980.4
antitussives	975.4	E858.6	E945.4	E950.4	E962.0	E980.4
codeine derivatives	965.09	E850.2	E935.2	E950.0	E962.0	E980.0
expectorants	975.5	E858.6	E945.5	E950.4	E962.0	E980.4
narcotic agents NEC	965.09	E850.2	E935.2	E950.0	E962.0	E980.0
52:04.04 antibiotics (EENT)						
ENT agent	976.6	E858.7	E946.6	E950.4	E962.0	E980.4
ophthalmic preparation	976.5	E858.7	E946.5	E950.4	E962.0	E980.4
52:04.06 antivirals (EENT)						
ENT agent	976.6	E858.7	E946.6	E950.4	E962.0	E980.4
ophthalmic preparation	976.5	E858.7	E946.5	E950.4	E962.0	E980.4
52:04.08 sulfonamides (EENT)						
ENT agent	976.6	E858.7	E946.6	E950.4	E962.0	E980.4
ophthalmic preparation	976.5	E858.7	E946.5	E950.4	E962.0	E980.4
52:04.12 miscellaneous anti-infectives (EENT)						
ENT agent	976.6	E858.7	E946.6	E950.4	E962.0	E980.4

▼ **Nontherapeutic use substance**

▼ **Subterms under main terms may continue to next column or page**

Drug — continued	Poisoning	Accident	Therapeutic Use	Suicide Attempt	Assault	Undetermined
52:04.12 miscellaneous anti-infectives — continued						
ophthalmic preparation	976.5	E858.7	E946.5	E950.4	E962.0	E980.4
52:04 anti-infectives (EENT)						
ENT agent	976.6	E858.7	E946.6	E950.4	E962.0	E980.4
ophthalmic preparation	976.5	E858.7	E946.5	E950.4	E962.0	E980.4
52:08 anti-inflammatory agents (EENT)						
ENT agent	976.6	E858.7	E946.6	E950.4	E962.0	E980.4
ophthalmic preparation	976.5	E858.7	E946.5	E950.4	E962.0	E980.4
52:10 carbonic anhydrase inhibitors	974.2	E858.5	E944.2	E950.4	E962.0	E980.4
52:12 contact lens solutions	976.5	E858.7	E946.5	E950.4	E962.0	E980.4
52:16 local anesthetics (EENT)	968.5	E855.2	E938.5	E950.4	E962.0	E980.4
52:20 miotics	971.0	E855.3	E941.0	E950.4	E962.0	E980.4
52:24 mydriatics						
adrenergics	971.2	E855.5	E941.2	E950.4	E962.0	E980.4
anticholinergics	971.1	E855.4	E941.1	E950.4	E962.0	E980.4
antimuscarinics	971.1	E855.4	E941.1	E950.4	E962.0	E980.4
parasympatholytics	971.1	E855.4	E941.1	E950.4	E962.0	E980.4
spasmolytics	971.1	E855.4	E941.1	E950.4	E962.0	E980.4
sympathomimetics	971.2	E855.5	E941.2	E950.4	E962.0	E980.4
52:28 mouth washes and gargles	976.6	E858.7	E946.6	E950.4	E962.0	E980.4
52:32 vasoconstrictors (EENT)	971.2	E855.5	E941.2	E950.4	E962.0	E980.4
52:36 unclassified agents (EENT)						
ENT agent	976.6	E858.7	E946.6	E950.4	E962.0	E980.4
ophthalmic preparation	976.5	E858.7	E946.5	E950.4	E962.0	E980.4
56:04 antacids and adsorbents	973.0	E858.4	E943.0	E950.4	E962.0	E980.4
56:08 antidiarrhea agents	973.5	E858.4	E943.5	E950.4	E962.0	E980.4
56:10 antiflatulents	973.8	E858.4	E943.8	E950.4	E962.0	E980.4
56:12 cathartics NEC	973.3	E858.4	E943.3	E950.4	E962.0	E980.4
emollients	973.2	E858.4	E943.2	E950.4	E962.0	E980.4
irritants	973.1	E858.4	E943.1	E950.4	E962.0	E980.4
56:16 digestants	973.4	E858.4	E943.4	E950.4	E962.0	E980.4
56:20 emetics and antiemetics						
antiemetics	963.0	E858.1	E933.0	E950.4	E962.0	E980.4
emetics	973.6	E858.4	E943.6	E950.4	E962.0	E980.4
56:24 lipotropic agents	977.1	E858.8	E947.1	E950.4	E962.0	E980.4
56:40 miscellaneous G.I. drugs	973.8	E858.4	E943.8	E950.4	E962.0	E980.4
60:00 gold compounds	965.69	E850.6	E935.6	E950.0	E962.0	E980.0
64:00 heavy metal antagonists	963.8	E858.1	E933.8	E950.4	E962.0	E980.4
68:04 adrenals	962.0	E858.0	E932.0	E950.4	E962.0	E980.4
68:08 androgens	962.1	E858.0	E932.1	E950.4	E962.0	E980.4
68:12 contraceptives, oral	962.2	E858.0	E932.2	E950.4	E962.0	E980.4
68:16 estrogens	962.2	E858.0	E932.2	E950.4	E962.0	E980.4
68:18 gonadotropins	962.4	E858.0	E932.4	E950.4	E962.0	E980.4
68:20.08 insulins	962.3	E858.0	E932.3	E950.4	E962.0	E980.4
68:20 insulins and antidiabetic agents	962.3	E858.0	E932.3	E950.4	E962.0	E980.4
68:24 parathyroid	962.6	E858.0	E932.6	E950.4	E962.0	E980.4
68:28 pituitary (posterior)	962.5	E858.0	E932.5	E950.4	E962.0	E980.4
anterior	962.4	E858.0	E932.4	E950.4	E962.0	E980.4
68:32 progestogens	962.2	E858.0	E932.2	E950.4	E962.0	E980.4
68:34 other corpus luteum hormones NEC	962.2	E858.0	E932.2	E950.4	E962.0	E980.4
68:36 thyroid and antithyroid						
antithyroid	962.8	E858.0	E932.8	E950.4	E962.0	E980.4
thyroid (derivatives)	962.7	E858.0	E932.7	E950.4	E962.0	E980.4
72:00 local anesthetics						
NEC	968.9	E855.2	E938.9	E950.4	E962.0	E980.4
infiltration (intradermal) (subcutaneous) (submucosal)	968.5	E855.2	E938.5	E950.4	E962.0	E980.4
nerve blocking (peripheral) (plexus) (regional)	968.6	E855.2	E938.6	E950.4	E962.0	E980.4
spinal	968.7	E855.2	E938.7	E950.4	E962.0	E980.4
topical (surface)	968.5	E855.2	E938.5	E950.4	E962.0	E980.4
76:00 oxytocics	975.0	E858.6	E945.0	E950.4	E962.0	E980.4
78:00 radioactive agents	990	—	—	—	—	—
80:04 serums NEC	979.9	E858.8	E949.9	E950.4	E962.0	E980.4

Drug — continued	Poisoning	Accident	Therapeutic Use	Suicide Attempt	Assault	Undetermined
80:04 serums — continued						
immune gamma globulin (human)	964.6	E858.2	E934.6	E950.4	E962.0	E980.4
80:08 toxoids NEC	978.8	E858.8	E948.8	E950.4	E962.0	E980.4
diphtheria	978.5	E858.8	E948.5	E950.4	E962.0	E980.4
and diphtheria	978.9	E858.8	E948.9	E950.4	E962.0	E980.4
with pertussis component	978.6	E858.8	E948.6	E950.4	E962.0	E980.4
and tetanus	978.9	E858.8	E948.9	E950.4	E962.0	E980.4
with pertussis component	978.6	E858.8	E948.6	E950.4	E962.0	E980.4
tetanus	978.4	E858.8	E948.4	E950.4	E962.0	E980.4
80:12 vaccines	979.9	E858.8	E949.9	E950.4	E962.0	E980.4
bacterial NEC	978.8	E858.8	E948.8	E950.4	E962.0	E980.4
with						
other bacterial components	978.9	E858.8	E948.9	E950.4	E962.0	E980.4
pertussis component	978.6	E858.8	E948.6	E950.4	E962.0	E980.4
viral and rickettsial components	979.7	E858.8	E949.7	E950.4	E962.0	E980.4
rickettsial NEC	979.6	E858.8	E949.6	E950.4	E962.0	E980.4
with						
bacterial component	979.7	E858.8	E949.7	E950.4	E962.0	E980.4
pertussis component	978.6	E858.8	E948.6	E950.4	E962.0	E980.4
viral component	979.7	E858.8	E949.7	E950.4	E962.0	E980.4
viral NEC	979.6	E858.8	E949.6	E950.4	E962.0	E980.4
with						
bacterial component	979.7	E858.8	E949.7	E950.4	E962.0	E980.4
pertussis component	978.6	E858.8	E948.6	E950.4	E962.0	E980.4
rickettsial component	979.7	E858.8	E949.7	E950.4	E962.0	E980.4
84:04.04 antibiotics (skin and mucous membrane)	976.0	E858.7	E946.0	E950.4	E962.0	E980.4
84:04.08 fungicides (skin and mucous membrane)	976.0	E858.7	E946.0	E950.4	E962.0	E980.4
84:04.12 scabicides and pediculicides (skin and mucous membrane)	976.0	E858.7	E946.0	E950.4	E962.0	E980.4
84:04.16 miscellaneous local anti-infectives (skin and mucous membrane)	976.0	E858.7	E946.0	E950.4	E962.0	E980.4
84:06 anti-inflammatory agents (skin and mucous membrane)	976.0	E858.7	E946.0	E950.4	E962.0	E980.4
84:08 antipruritics and local anesthetics						
antipruritics	976.1	E858.7	E946.1	E950.4	E962.0	E980.4
local anesthetics	968.5	E855.2	E938.5	E950.4	E962.0	E980.4
84:12 astringents	976.2	E858.7	E946.2	E950.4	E962.0	E980.4
84:16 cell stimulants and proliferants	976.8	E858.7	E946.8	E950.4	E962.0	E980.4
84:20 detergents	976.2	E858.7	E946.2	E950.4	E962.0	E980.4
84:24 emollients, demulcents, and protectants	976.3	E858.7	E946.3	E950.4	E962.0	E980.4
84:28 keratolytic agents	976.4	E858.7	E946.4	E950.4	E962.0	E980.4
84:32 keratoplastic agents	976.4	E858.7	E946.4	E950.4	E962.0	E980.4
84:36 miscellaneous agents (skin and mucous membrane)	976.8	E858.7	E946.8	E950.4	E962.0	E980.4
86:00 spasmolytic agents	975.1	E858.6	E945.1	E950.4	E962.0	E980.4
antiasthmatics	975.7	E858.6	E945.7	E950.4	E962.0	E980.4
papaverine	972.5	E858.3	E942.5	E950.4	E962.0	E980.4
theophylline	974.1	E858.5	E944.1	E950.4	E962.0	E980.4
88:04 vitamin A	963.5	E858.1	E933.5	E950.4	E962.0	E980.4
88:08 vitamin B complex	963.5	E858.1	E933.5	E950.4	E962.0	E980.4
hematopoietic vitamin	964.1	E858.2	E934.1	E950.4	E962.0	E980.4
nicotinic acid derivatives	972.2	E858.3	E942.2	E950.4	E962.0	E980.4
88:12 vitamin C	963.5	E858.1	E933.5	E950.4	E962.0	E980.4
88:16 vitamin D	963.5	E858.1	E933.5	E950.4	E962.0	E980.4
88:20 vitamin E	963.5	E858.1	E933.5	E950.4	E962.0	E980.4
88:24 vitamin K activity	964.3	E858.2	E934.3	E950.4	E962.0	E980.4
88:28 multivitamin preparations	963.5	E858.1	E933.5	E950.4	E962.0	E980.4

		External Cause (E-Code)						**External Cause (E-Code)**			
	Poisoning	Accident	Therapeutic Use	Suicide Attempt	Assault	Undeter-mined	Poisoning	Accident	Therapeutic Use	Suicide Attempt	Assault	Undeter-mined

Drug — continued							Ethacrynic acid	974.4	E858.5	E944.4	E950.4	E962.0	E980.4
92:00 unclassified therapeutic							Ethambutol	961.8	E857	E931.8	E950.4	E962.0	E980.4
agents	977.8	E858.8	E947.8	E950.4	E962.0	E980.4	Ethamide	974.2	E858.5	E944.2	E950.4	E962.0	E980.4
specified NEC	977.8	E858.8	E947.8	E950.4	E962.0	E980.4	Ethamivan	970.0	E854.3	E940.0	E950.4	E962.0	E980.4
Duboisine	971.1	E855.4	E941.1	E950.4	E962.0	E980.4	Ethamsylate	964.5	E858.2	E934.5	E950.4	E962.0	E980.4
Dulcolax	973.1	E858.4	E943.1	E950.4	E962.0	E980.4	Ethanol	980.0	E860.1	—	E950.9	E962.1	E980.9
Duponol (C) (EP)	976.2	E858.7	E946.2	E950.4	E962.0	E980.4	beverage	980.0	E860.0	—	E950.9	E962.1	E980.9
Durabolin	962.1	E858.0	E932.1	E950.4	E962.0	E980.4	Ethchlorvynol	967.8	E852.8	E937.8	E950.2	E962.0	E980.2
Dyclone	968.5	E855.2	E938.5	E950.4	E962.0	E980.4	Ethebenecid	974.7	E858.5	E944.7	E950.4	E962.0	E980.4
Dyclonine	968.5	E855.2	E938.5	E950.4	E962.0	E980.4	Ether(s) (diethyl) (ethyl) (va-						
Dydrogesterone	962.2	E858.0	E932.2	E950.4	E962.0	E980.4	por)	987.8	E869.8	—	E952.8	E962.2	E982.8
Dyes NEC	989.89	E866.8	—	E950.9	E962.1	E980.9	anesthetic	968.2	E855.1	E938.2	E950.4	E962.0	E980.4
diagnostic agents	977.8	E858.8	E947.8	E950.4	E962.0	E980.4	petroleum — see Ligroin						
pharmaceutical NEC	977.4	E858.8	E947.4	E950.4	E962.0	E980.4	solvent	982.8	E862.4	—	E950.9	E962.1	E980.9
Dyfols	971.0	E855.3	E941.0	E950.4	E962.0	E980.4	Ethidine chloride (vapor)	987.8	E869.8	—	E952.8	E962.2	E982.8
Dymelor	962.3	E858.0	E932.3	E950.4	E962.0	E980.4	liquid (solvent)	982.3	E862.4	—	E950.9	E962.1	E980.9
Dynamite	989.89	E866.8	—	E950.9	E962.1	E980.9	Ethinamate	967.8	E852.8	E937.8	E950.2	E962.0	E980.2
fumes	987.8	E869.8	—	E952.8	E962.2	E982.8	Ethinylestradiol	962.2	E858.0	E932.2	E950.4	E962.0	E980.4
Dyphylline	975.1	E858.6	E945.1	E950.4	E962.0	E980.4	Ethionamide	961.8	E857	E931.8	E950.4	E962.0	E980.4
Ear preparations	976.6	E858.7	E946.6	E950.4	E962.0	E980.4	Ethisterone	962.2	E858.0	E932.2	E950.4	E962.0	E980.4
Echothiopate, ecoth-							Ethobral	967.0	E851	E937.0	E950.1	E962.0	E980.1
iopate	971.0	E855.3	E941.0	E950.4	E962.0	E980.4	Ethocaine (infiltration) (topi-						
Ecstasy	969.72	E854.2	E939.7	E950.3	E962.0	E980.3	cal)	968.5	E855.2	E938.5	E950.4	E962.0	E980.4
Ectylurea	967.8	E852.8	E937.8	E950.2	E962.0	E980.2	nerve block (peripheral)						
Edathamil disodium	963.8	E858.1	E933.8	E950.4	E962.0	E980.4	(plexus)	968.6	E855.2	E938.6	E950.4	E962.0	E980.4
Edecrin	974.4	E858.5	E944.4	E950.4	E962.0	E980.4	spinal	968.7	E855.2	E938.7	E950.4	E962.0	E980.4
Edetate, disodium (calci-							Ethoheptazine (citrate)	965.7	E850.7	E935.7	E950.0	E962.0	E980.0
um)	963.8	E858.1	E933.8	E950.4	E962.0	E980.4	Ethopropazine	966.4	E855.0	E936.4	E950.4	E962.0	E980.4
Edrophonium	971.0	E855.3	E941.0	E950.4	E962.0	E980.4	Ethosuximide	966.2	E855.0	E936.2	E950.4	E962.0	E980.4
Elase	976.8	E858.7	E946.8	E950.4	E962.0	E980.4	Ethotoin	966.1	E855.0	E936.1	E950.4	E962.0	E980.4
Elaterium	973.1	E858.4	E943.1	E950.4	E962.0	E980.4	Ethoxazene	961.9	E857	E931.9	E950.4	E962.0	E980.4
Elder	988.2	E865.4	—	E950.9	E962.1	E980.9	Ethoxzolamide	974.2	E858.5	E944.2	E950.4	E962.0	E980.4
berry (unripe)	988.2	E865.3	—	E950.9	E962.1	E980.9	Ethyl						
Electrolytes NEC	974.5	E858.5	E944.5	E950.4	E962.0	E980.4	acetate (vapor)	982.8	E862.4	—	E950.9	E962.1	E980.9
Electrolytic agent NEC	974.5	E858.5	E944.5	E950.4	E962.0	E980.4	alcohol	980.0	E860.1	—	E950.9	E962.1	E980.9
Embramine	963.0	E858.1	E933.0	E950.4	E962.0	E980.4	beverage	980.0	E860.0	—	E950.9	E962.1	E980.9
Emetics	973.6	E858.4	E943.6	E950.4	E962.0	E980.4	aldehyde (vapor)	987.8	E869.8	—	E952.8	E962.2	E982.8
Emetine (hydrochloride)	961.5	E857	E931.5	E950.4	E962.0	E980.4	liquid	989.89	E866.8	—	E950.9	E962.1	E980.9
Emollients	976.3	E858.7	E946.3	E950.4	E962.0	E980.4	aminobenzoate	968.5	E855.2	E938.5	E950.4	E962.0	E980.4
Emylcamate	969.5	E853.8	E939.5	E950.3	E962.0	E980.3	biscoumacetate	964.2	E858.2	E934.2	E950.4	E962.0	E980.4
Encyprate	969.09	E854.0	E939.0	E950.3	E962.0	E980.3	bromide (anesthetic)	968.2	E855.1	E938.2	E950.4	E962.0	E980.4
Endocaine	968.5	E855.2	E938.5	E950.4	E962.0	E980.4	carbamate (antineoplas-						
Endrin	989.2	E863.0	—	E950.6	E962.1	E980.7	tic)	963.1	E858.1	E933.1	E950.4	E962.0	E980.4
Enflurane	968.2	E855.1	E938.2	E950.4	E962.0	E980.4	carbinol	980.3	E860.4	—	E950.9	E962.1	E980.9
Enovid	962.2	E858.0	E932.2	E950.4	E962.0	E980.4	chaulmoograte	961.8	E857	E931.8	E950.4	E962.0	E980.4
ENT preparations (anti-infec-							chloride (vapor)	987.8	E869.8	—	E952.8	E962.2	E982.8
tives)	976.6	E858.7	E946.6	E950.4	E962.0	E980.4	anesthetic (local)	968.5	E855.2	E938.5	E950.4	E962.0	E980.4
Enzodase	963.4	E858.1	E933.4	E950.4	E962.0	E980.4	inhaled	968.2	E855.1	E938.2	E950.4	E962.0	E980.4
Enzymes NEC	963.4	E858.1	E933.4	E950.4	E962.0	E980.4	solvent	982.3	E862.4	—	E950.9	E962.1	E980.9
Epanutin	966.1	E855.0	E936.1	E950.4	E962.0	E980.4	estranol	962.1	E858.0	E932.1	E950.4	E962.0	E980.4
Ephedra (tincture)	971.2	E855.5	E941.2	E950.4	E962.0	E980.4	ether — see Ether(s)						
Ephedrine	971.2	E855.5	E941.2	E950.4	E962.0	E980.4	formate (solvent) NEC	982.8	E862.4	—	E950.9	E962.1	E980.9
Epiestriol	962.2	E858.0	E932.2	E950.4	E962.0	E980.4	iodoacetate	987.5	E869.3	—	E952.8	E962.2	E982.8
Epilim — see Sodium val-							lactate (solvent) NEC	982.8	E862.4	—	E950.9	E962.1	E980.9
proate							methylcarbinol	980.8	E860.8	—	E950.9	E962.1	E980.9
Epinephrine	971.2	E855.5	E941.2	E950.4	E962.0	E980.4	morphine	965.09	E850.2	E935.2	E950.0	E962.0	E980.0
Epsom salt	973.3	E858.4	E943.3	E950.4	E962.0	E980.4	Ethylene (gas)	987.1	E869.8	—	E952.8	E962.2	E982.8
Equanil	969.5	E853.8	E939.5	E950.3	E962.0	E980.3	anesthetic (general)	968.2	E855.1	E938.2	E950.4	E962.0	E980.4
Equisetum (diuretic)	974.4	E858.5	E944.4	E950.4	E962.0	E980.4	chlorohydrin (vapor)	982.3	E862.4	—	E950.9	E962.1	E980.9
Ergometrine	975.0	E858.6	E945.0	E950.4	E962.0	E980.4	dichloride (vapor)	982.3	E862.4	—	E950.9	E962.1	E980.9
Ergonovine	975.0	E858.6	E945.0	E950.4	E962.0	E980.4	glycol(s) (any) (vapor)	982.8	E862.4	—	E950.9	E962.1	E980.9
Ergotamine (tartrate) (for mi-							Ethylidene						
graine) NEC	972.9	E858.3	E942.9	E950.4	E962.0	E980.4	chloride NEC	982.3	E862.4	—	E950.9	E962.1	E980.9
Ergotrate	975.0	E858.6	E945.0	E950.4	E962.0	E980.4	diethyl ether	982.8	E862.4	—	E950.9	E962.1	E980.9
Ergot NEC	988.2	E865.4	—	E950.9	E962.1	E980.9	Ethynodiol	962.2	E858.0	E932.2	E950.4	E962.0	E980.4
medicinal (alkaloids)	975.0	E858.6	E945.0	E950.4	E962.0	E980.4	Etidocaine	968.9	E855.2	E938.9	E950.4	E962.0	E980.4
Erythrityl tetranitrate	972.4	E858.3	E942.4	E950.4	E962.0	E980.4	infiltration (subcuta-						
Erythrol tetranitrate	972.4	E858.3	E942.4	E950.4	E962.0	E980.4	neous)	968.5	E855.2	E938.5	E950.4	E962.0	E980.4
Erythromycin	960.3	E856	E930.3	E950.4	E962.0	E980.4	nerve (peripheral)						
ophthalmic preparation	976.5	E858.7	E946.5	E950.4	E962.0	E980.4	(plexus)	968.6	E855.2	E938.6	E950.4	E962.0	E980.4
topical NEC	976.0	E858.7	E946.0	E950.4	E962.0	E980.4	Etilfen	967.0	E851	E937.0	E950.1	E962.0	E980.1
Eserine	971.0	E855.3	E941.0	E950.4	E962.0	E980.4	Etomide	965.7	E850.7	E935.7	E950.0	E962.0	E980.0
Eskabarb	967.0	E851	E937.0	E950.1	E962.0	E980.1	Etorphine	965.09	E850.2	E935.2	E950.0	E962.0	E980.0
Eskalith	969.8	E855.8	E939.8	E950.3	E962.0	E980.3	Etoval	967.0	E851	E937.0	E950.1	E962.0	E980.1
Estradiol (cypionate) (dipropi-							Etryptamine	969.01	E854.0	E939.0	E950.3	E962.0	E980.3
onate) (valerate)	962.2	E858.0	E932.2	E950.4	E962.0	E980.4	Eucaine	968.5	E855.2	E938.5	E950.4	E962.0	E980.4
Estriol	962.2	E858.0	E932.2	E950.4	E962.0	E980.4	Eucalyptus (oil) NEC	975.5	E858.6	E945.5	E950.4	E962.0	E980.4
Estrogens (with progesto-							Eucatropine	971.1	E855.4	E941.1	E950.4	E962.0	E980.4
gens)	962.2	E858.0	E932.2	E950.4	E962.0	E980.4	Eucodal	965.09	E850.2	E935.2	E950.0	E962.0	E980.0
Estrone	962.2	E858.0	E932.2	E950.4	E962.0	E980.4	Euneryl	967.0	E851	E937.0	E950.1	E962.0	E980.1
Etafedrine	971.2	E855.5	E941.2	E950.4	E962.0	E980.4	Euphthalmine	971.1	E855.4	E941.1	E950.4	E962.0	E980.4
Ethacrynate sodium	974.4	E858.5	E944.4	E950.4	E962.0	E980.4	Eurax	976.0	E858.7	E946.0	E950.4	E962.0	E980.4

	Poisoning	Accident	Therapeutic Use	Suicide Attempt	Assault	Undetermined
Euresol	976.4	E858.7	E946.4	E950.4	E962.0	E980.4
Euthroid	962.7	E858.0	E932.7	E950.4	E962.0	E980.4
Evans blue	977.8	E858.8	E947.8	E950.4	E962.0	E980.4
Evipal	967.0	E851	E937.0	E950.1	E962.0	E980.1
sodium	968.3	E855.1	E938.3	E950.4	E962.0	E980.4
Evipan	967.0	E851	E937.0	E950.1	E962.0	E980.1
sodium	968.3	E855.1	E938.3	E950.4	E962.0	E980.4
Exalgin	965.4	E850.4	E935.4	E950.0	E962.0	E980.0
Excipients, pharmaceutical	977.4	E858.8	E947.4	E950.4	E962.0	E980.4
Exhaust gas — see Carbon, monoxide						
Ex-Lax (phenolphthalein)	973.1	E858.4	E943.1	E950.4	E962.0	E980.4
Expectorants	975.5	E858.6	E945.5	E950.4	E962.0	E980.4
External medications (skin)						
(mucous membrane)	976.9	E858.7	E946.9	E950.4	E962.0	E980.4
dental agent	976.7	E858.7	E946.7	E950.4	E962.0	E980.4
ENT agent	976.6	E858.7	E946.6	E950.4	E962.0	E980.4
ophthalmic preparation	976.5	E858.7	E946.5	E950.4	E962.0	E980.4
specified NEC	976.8	E858.7	E946.8	E950.4	E962.0	E980.4
Eye agents (anti-infective)	976.5	E858.7	E946.5	E950.4	E962.0	E980.4
Factor IX complex (human)	964.5	E858.2	E934.5	E950.4	E962.0	E980.4
Fecal softeners	973.2	E858.4	E943.2	E950.4	E962.0	E980.4
Fenbutrazate	977.0	E858.8	E947.0	E950.4	E962.0	E980.4
Fencamfamin	970.89	E854.3	E940.8	E950.4	E962.0	E980.4
Fenfluramine	977.0	E858.8	E947.0	E950.4	E962.0	E980.4
Fenoprofen	965.61	E850.6	E935.6	E950.0	E962.0	E980.0
Fentanyl	965.09	E850.2	E935.2	E950.0	E962.0	E980.0
Fentazin	969.1	E853.0	E939.1	E950.3	E962.0	E980.3
Fenticlor, fentichlor	976.0	E858.7	E946.0	E950.4	E962.0	E980.4
Fer de lance (bite) (venom)	989.5	E905.0	—	E950.9	E962.1	E980.9
Ferric — see Iron						
Ferrocholinate	964.0	E858.2	E934.0	E950.4	E962.0	E980.4
Ferrous fumerate, gluconate, lactate, salt NEC, sulfate (medicinal)	964.0	E858.2	E934.0	E950.4	E962.0	E980.4
Ferrum — see Iron						
Fertilizers NEC	989.89	E866.5	—	E950.9	E962.1	E980.9
with herbicide mixture	989.4	E863.5	—	E950.6	E962.1	E980.7
Fibrinogen (human)	964.7	E858.2	E934.7	E950.4	E962.0	E980.4
Fibrinolysin	964.4	E858.2	E934.4	E950.4	E962.0	E980.4
Fibrinolysis-affecting agents	964.4	E858.2	E934.4	E950.4	E962.0	E980.4
Filix mas	961.6	E857	E931.6	E950.4	E962.0	E980.4
Fiorinal	965.1	E850.3	E935.3	E950.0	E962.0	E980.0
Fire damp	987.1	E869.8	—	E952.8	E962.2	E982.8
Fish, nonbacterial or noxious	988.0	E865.2	—	E950.9	E962.1	E980.9
shell	988.0	E865.1	—	E950.9	E962.1	E980.9
Flagyl	961.5	E857	E931.5	E950.4	E962.0	E980.4
Flavoxate	975.1	E858.6	E945.1	E950.4	E962.0	E980.4
Flaxedil	975.2	E858.6	E945.2	E950.4	E962.0	E980.4
Flaxseed (medicinal)	976.3	E858.7	E946.3	E950.4	E962.0	E980.4
Flomax	971.3	E855.6	E941.3	E950.4	E962.0	E980.4
Florantyrone	973.4	E858.4	E943.4	E950.4	E962.0	E980.4
Floraquin	961.3	E857	E931.3	E950.4	E962.0	E980.4
Florinef	962.0	E858.0	E932.0	E950.4	E962.0	E980.4
ENT agent	976.6	E858.7	E946.6	E950.4	E962.0	E980.4
ophthalmic preparation	976.5	E858.7	E946.5	E950.4	E962.0	E980.4
topical NEC	976.0	E858.7	E946.0	E950.4	E962.0	E980.4
Flowers of sulfur	976.4	E858.7	E946.4	E950.4	E962.0	E980.4
Floxuridine	963.1	E858.1	E933.1	E950.4	E962.0	E980.4
Flucytosine	961.9	E857	E931.9	E950.4	E962.0	E980.4
Fludrocortisone	962.0	E858.0	E932.0	E950.4	E962.0	E980.4
ENT agent	976.6	E858.7	E946.6	E950.4	E962.0	E980.4
ophthalmic preparation	976.5	E858.7	E946.5	E950.4	E962.0	E980.4
topical NEC	976.0	E858.7	E946.0	E950.4	E962.0	E980.4
Flumethasone	976.0	E858.7	E946.0	E950.4	E962.0	E980.4
Flumethiazide	974.3	E858.5	E944.3	E950.4	E962.0	E980.4
Flumidin	961.7	E857	E931.7	E950.4	E962.0	E980.4
Flunitrazepam	969.4	E853.2	E939.4	E950.3	E962.0	E980.3
Fluocinolone	976.0	E858.7	E946.0	E950.4	E962.0	E980.4
Fluocortolone	962.0	E858.0	E932.0	E950.4	E962.0	E980.4
Fluohydrocortisone	962.0	E858.0	E932.0	E950.4	E962.0	E980.4
ENT agent	976.6	E858.7	E946.6	E950.4	E962.0	E980.4
ophthalmic preparation	976.5	E858.7	E946.5	E950.4	E962.0	E980.4
topical NEC	976.0	E858.7	E946.0	E950.4	E962.0	E980.4
Fluonid	976.0	E858.7	E946.0	E950.4	E962.0	E980.4
Fluopromazine	969.1	E853.0	E939.1	E950.3	E962.0	E980.3

	Poisoning	Accident	Therapeutic Use	Suicide Attempt	Assault	Undetermined
Fluoracetate	989.4	E863.7	—	E950.6	E962.1	E980.7
Fluorescein (sodium)	977.8	E858.8	E947.8	E950.4	E962.0	E980.4
Fluoride(s) (pesticides) (sodium) NEC	989.4	E863.4	—	E950.6	E962.1	E980.7
hydrogen — see Hydrofluoric acid						
medicinal	976.7	E858.7	E946.7	E950.4	E962.0	E980.4
not pesticide NEC	983.9	E864.4	—	E950.7	E962.1	E980.6
stannous	976.7	E858.7	E946.7	E950.4	E962.0	E980.4
Fluorinated corticosteroids	962.0	E858.0	E932.0	E950.4	E962.0	E980.4
Fluorine (compounds) (gas)	987.8	E869.8	—	E952.8	E962.2	E982.8
salt — see Fluoride(s)						
Fluoristan	976.7	E858.7	E946.7	E950.4	E962.0	E980.4
Fluoroacetate	989.4	E863.7	—	E950.6	E962.1	E980.7
Fluorodeoxyuridine	963.1	E858.1	E933.1	E950.4	E962.0	E980.4
Fluorometholone (topical) NEC	976.0	E858.7	E946.0	E950.4	E962.0	E980.4
ophthalmic preparation	976.5	E858.7	E946.5	E950.4	E962.0	E980.4
Fluorouracil	963.1	E858.1	E933.1	E950.4	E962.0	E980.4
Fluothane	968.1	E855.1	E938.1	E950.4	E962.0	E980.4
Fluoxetine hydrochloride	969.03	E854.0	E939.0	E950.3	E962.0	E980.3
Fluoxymesterone	962.1	E858.0	E932.1	E950.4	E962.0	E980.4
Fluphenazine	969.1	E853.0	E939.1	E950.3	E962.0	E980.3
Fluprednisolone	962.0	E858.0	E932.0	E950.4	E962.0	E980.4
Flurandrenolide	976.0	E858.7	E946.0	E950.4	E962.0	E980.4
Flurazepam (hydrochloride)	969.4	E853.2	E939.4	E950.3	E962.0	E980.3
Flurbiprofen	965.61	E850.6	E935.6	E950.0	E962.0	E980.0
Flurobate	976.0	E858.7	E946.0	E950.4	E962.0	E980.4
Flurothyl	969.8	E855.8	E939.8	E950.3	E962.0	E980.3
Fluroxene	968.2	E855.1	E938.2	E950.4	E962.0	E980.4
Folacin	964.1	E858.2	E934.1	E950.4	E962.0	E980.4
Folic acid	964.1	E858.2	E934.1	E950.4	E962.0	E980.4
Follicle stimulating hormone	962.4	E858.0	E932.4	E950.4	E962.0	E980.4
Food, foodstuffs, nonbacterial or noxious	988.9	E865.9	—	E950.9	E962.1	E980.9
berries, seeds	988.2	E865.3	—	E950.9	E962.1	E980.9
fish	988.0	E865.2	—	E950.9	E962.1	E980.9
mushrooms	988.1	E865.5	—	E950.9	E962.1	E980.9
plants	988.2	E865.9	—	E950.9	E962.1	E980.9
specified type NEC	988.2	E865.4	—	E950.9	E962.1	E980.9
shellfish	988.0	E865.1	—	E950.9	E962.1	E980.9
specified NEC	988.8	E865.8	—	E950.9	E962.1	E980.9
Fool's parsley	988.2	E865.4	—	E950.9	E962.1	E980.9
Formaldehyde (solution)	989.89	E861.4	—	E950.9	E962.1	E980.9
fungicide	989.4	E863.6	—	E950.6	E962.1	E980.7
gas or vapor	987.8	E869.8	—	E952.8	E962.2	E982.8
Formalin	989.89	E861.4	—	E950.9	E962.1	E980.9
fungicide	989.4	E863.6	—	E950.6	E962.1	E980.7
vapor	987.8	E869.8	—	E952.8	E962.2	E982.8
Formic acid	983.1	E864.1	—	E950.7	E962.1	E980.6
automobile	981	E862.1	—	E950.9	E962.1	E980.9
exhaust gas, not in transit	986	E868.2	—	E952.0	E962.2	E982.0
vapor NEC	987.1	E869.8	—	E952.8	E962.2	E982.8
gas (domestic use) (see also Carbon, monoxide, fuel)						
utility	987.1	E868.1	—	E951.8	E962.2	E981.8
incomplete combustion of — see Carbon, monoxide, fuel, utility						
in mobile container	987.0	E868.0	—	E951.1	E962.2	E981.1
piped (natural)	987.1	E867	—	E951.0	E962.2	E981.0
industrial, incomplete combustion	986	E868.3	—	E952.1	E962.2	E982.1
vapor	987.8	E869.8	—	E952.8	E962.2	E982.8
Fowler's solution	985.1	E866.3	—	E950.8	E962.1	E980.8
Foxglove	988.2	E865.4	—	E950.9	E962.1	E980.9
Fox green	977.8	E858.8	E947.8	E950.4	E962.0	E980.4
Framycetin	960.8	E856	E930.8	E950.4	E962.0	E980.4
Frangula (extract)	973.1	E858.4	E943.1	E950.4	E962.0	E980.4
Frei antigen	977.8	E858.8	E947.8	E950.4	E962.0	E980.4
Freons	987.4	E869.2	—	E952.8	E962.2	E982.8
Fructose	974.5	E858.5	E944.5	E950.4	E962.0	E980.4
Frusemide	974.4	E858.5	E944.4	E950.4	E962.0	E980.4
FSH	962.4	E858.0	E932.4	E950.4	E962.0	E980.4
Fuel						
Fugillin	960.8	E856	E930.8	E950.4	E962.0	E980.4

▽ Subterms under main terms may continue to next column or page

	External Cause (E-Code)					
	Poisoning	Accident	Therapeutic Use	Suicide Attempt	Assault	Undeter-mined
Fulminate of mercury	985.0	E866.1	—	E950.9	E962.1	E980.9
Fulvicin	960.1	E856	E930.1	E950.4	E962.0	E980.4
Fumadil	960.8	E856	E930.8	E950.4	E962.0	E980.4
Fumagillin	960.8	E856	E930.8	E950.4	E962.0	E980.4
Fumes (from)	987.9	E869.9	—	E952.9	E962.2	E982.9
carbon monoxide — see Carbon, monoxide						
charcoal (domestic use)	986	E868.3	—	E952.1	E962.2	E982.1
chloroform — see Chloroform						
coke (in domestic stoves, fireplaces)	986	E868.3	—	E952.1	E962.2	E982.1
corrosive NEC	987.8	E869.8	—	E952.8	E962.2	E982.8
ether — see Ether(s)						
freons	987.4	E869.2	—	E952.8	E962.2	E982.8
hydrocarbons	987.1	E869.8	—	E952.8	E962.2	E982.8
petroleum (liquefied)	987.0	E868.0	—	E951.1	E962.2	E981.1
distributed through pipes (pure or mixed with air)	987.0	E867		E951.0	E962.2	E981.0
lead — see Lead						
metals — see specified metal						
nitrogen dioxide	987.2	E869.0	—	E952.8	E962.2	E982.8
pesticides — see Pesticides						
petroleum (liquefied)	987.0	E868.0	—	E951.1	E962.2	E981.1
distributed through pipes (pure or mixed with air)	987.0	E867		E951.0	E962.2	E981.0
polyester	987.8	E869.8	—	E952.8	E962.2	E982.8
specified, source other (see also substance specified)	987.8	E869.8	—	E952.8	E962.2	E982.8
sulfur dioxide	987.3	E869.1	—	E952.8	E962.2	E982.8
Fumigants	989.4	E863.8	—	E950.6	E962.1	E980.7
Fungicides — see also Antifungals	989.4	E863.6	—	E950.6	E962.1	E980.7
Fungi, noxious, used as food	988.1	E865.5	—	E950.9	E962.1	E980.9
Fungizone	960.1	E856	E930.1	E950.4	E962.0	E980.4
topical	976.0	E858.7	E946.0	E950.4	E962.0	E980.4
Furacin	976.0	E858.7	E946.0	E950.4	E962.0	E980.4
Furadantin	961.9	E857	E931.9	E950.4	E962.0	E980.4
Furazolidone	961.9	E857	E931.9	E950.4	E962.0	E980.4
Furnace (coal burning) (domestic), gas from	986	E868.3	—	E952.1	E962.2	E982.1
industrial	986	E868.8	—	E952.1	E962.2	E982.1
Furniture polish	989.89	E861.2	—	E950.9	E962.1	E980.9
Furosemide	974.4	E858.5	E944.4	E950.4	E962.0	E980.4
Furoxone	961.9	E857	E931.9	E950.4	E962.0	E980.4
Fusel oil (amyl) (butyl) (propyl)	980.3	E860.4	—	E950.9	E962.1	E980.9
Fusidic acid	960.8	E856	E930.8	E950.4	E962.0	E980.4
Gallamine	975.2	E858.6	E945.2	E950.4	E962.0	E980.4
Gallotannic acid	976.2	E858.7	E946.2	E950.4	E962.0	E980.4
Gamboge	973.1	E858.4	E943.1	E950.4	E962.0	E980.4
Gamimune	964.6	E858.2	E934.6	E950.4	E962.0	E980.4
Gamma-benzene hexachloride (vapor)	989.2	E863.0	—	E950.6	E962.1	E980.7
Gamma globulin	964.6	E858.2	E934.6	E950.4	E962.0	E980.4
Gamma hydroxy butyrate (GHB)	968.4	E855.1	E938.4	E950.4	E962.0	E980.4
Gamulin	964.6	E858.2	E934.6	E950.4	E962.0	E980.4
Ganglionic blocking agents	972.3	E858.3	E942.3	E950.4	E962.0	E980.4
Ganja	969.6	E854.1	E939.6	E950.3	E962.0	E980.3
Garamycin	960.8	E856	E930.8	E950.4	E962.0	E980.4
ophthalmic preparation	976.5	E858.7	E946.5	E950.4	E962.0	E980.4
topical NEC	976.0	E858.7	E946.0	E950.4	E962.0	E980.4
Gardenal	967.0	E851	E937.0	E950.1	E962.0	E980.1
Gardepanyl	967.0	E851	E937.0	E950.1	E962.0	E980.1
Gas	987.9	E869.9	—	E952.9	E962.2	E982.9
acetylene	987.1	E868.1	—	E951.8	E962.2	E981.8
incomplete combustion of — see Carbon, monoxide, fuel, utility						
air contaminants, source or type not specified	987.9	E869.9	—	E952.9	E962.2	E982.9
anesthetic (general) NEC	968.2	E855.1	E938.2	E950.4	E962.0	E980.4
blast furnace	986	E868.8	—	E952.1	E962.2	E982.1
butane — see Butane						
carbon monoxide — see Carbon, monoxide						

Gas — continued	Poisoning	Accident	Therapeutic Use	Suicide Attempt	Assault	Undeter-mined
chlorine	987.6	E869.8	—	E952.8	E962.2	E982.8
coal — see Carbon, monoxide, coal						
cyanide	987.7	E869.8	—	E952.8	E962.2	E982.8
dicyanogen	987.8	E869.8	—	E952.8	E962.2	E982.8
domestic — see Gas, utility						
exhaust — see Carbon, monoxide, exhaust gas						
from wood- or coal-burning stove or fireplace	986	E868.3	—	E952.1	E962.2	E982.1
fuel (domestic use) (see also Carbon, monoxide, fuel)						
industrial use	986	E868.8	—	E952.1	E962.2	E982.1
utility	987.1	E868.1	—	E951.8	E962.2	E981.8
incomplete combustion of — see Carbon, monoxide, fuel, utility						
in mobile container	987.0	E868.0	—	E951.1	E962.2	E981.1
piped (natural)	987.1	E867	—	E951.0	E962.2	E981.0
garage	986	E868.2	—	E952.0	E962.2	E982.0
hydrocarbon NEC	987.1	E869.8	—	E952.8	E962.2	E982.8
incomplete combustion of — see Carbon, monoxide, fuel, utility						
liquefied (mobile container)	987.0	E868.0	—	E951.1	E962.2	E981.1
piped	987.0	E867	—	E951.0	E962.2	E981.0
hydrocyanic acid	987.7	E869.8	—	E952.8	E962.2	E982.8
illuminating — see Gas, utility						
incomplete combustion, any — see Carbon, monoxide						
kiln	986	E868.8	—	E952.1	E962.2	E982.1
lacrimogenic	987.5	E869.3	—	E952.8	E962.2	E982.8
marsh	987.1	E869.8	—	E952.8	E962.2	E982.8
motor exhaust, not in transit	986	E868.8	—	E952.1	E962.2	E982.1
mustard — see Mustard, gas						
natural	987.1	E867	—	E951.0	E962.2	E981.0
nerve (war)	987.9	E869.9	—	E952.9	E962.2	E982.9
oils	981	E862.1	—	E950.9	E962.1	E980.9
petroleum (liquefied) (distributed in mobile containers)	987.0	E868.0	—	E951.1	E962.2	E981.1
piped (pure or mixed with air)	987.0	E867	—	E951.1	E962.2	E981.1
piped (manufactured) (natural) NEC	987.1	E867	—	E951.0	E962.2	E981.0
producer	986	E868.8	—	E952.1	E962.2	E982.1
propane — see Propane						
refrigerant (freon)	987.4	E869.2	—	E952.8	E962.2	E982.8
not freon	987.9	E869.9	—	E952.9	E962.2	E982.9
sewer	987.8	E869.8	—	E952.8	E962.2	E982.8
specified source NEC (see also substance specified)	987.8	E869.8	—	E952.8	E962.2	E982.8
stove — see Gas, utility						
tear	987.5	E869.3	—	E952.8	E962.2	E982.8
utility (for cooking, heating, or lighting) (piped) NEC	987.1	E868.1	—	E951.8	E962.2	E981.8
incomplete combustion of — see Carbon, monoxide, fuel, utility						
in mobile container	987.0	E868.0	—	E951.1	E962.2	E981.1
piped (natural)	987.1	E867	—	E951.0	E962.2	E981.0
water	987.1	E868.1	—	E951.8	E962.2	E981.8
incomplete combustion of — see Carbon, monoxide, fuel, utility						
Gaseous substance — see Gas						
Gasoline, gasolene	981	E862.1	—	E950.9	E962.1	E980.9
vapor	987.1	E869.8	—	E952.8	E962.2	E982.8
Gastric enzymes	973.4	E858.4	E943.4	E950.4	E962.0	E980.4
Gastrografin	977.8	E858.8	E947.8	E950.4	E962.0	E980.4
Gastrointestinal agents	973.9	E858.4	E943.9	E950.4	E962.0	E980.4
specified NEC	973.8	E858.4	E943.8	E950.4	E962.0	E980.4
Gaultheria procumbens	988.2	E865.4	—	E950.9	E962.1	E980.9
Gelatin (intravenous)	964.8	E858.2	E934.8	E950.4	E962.0	E980.4
absorbable (sponge)	964.5	E858.2	E934.5	E950.4	E962.0	E980.4
Gelfilm	976.8	E858.7	E946.8	E950.4	E962.0	E980.4
Gelfoam	964.5	E858.2	E934.5	E950.4	E962.0	E980.4

	External Cause (E-Code)					
	Poisoning	Accident	Therapeutic Use	Suicide Attempt	Assault	Undetermined
Gelsemine	970.89	E854.3	E940.8	E950.4	E962.0	E980.4
Gelsemium (semper-virens)	988.2	E865.4	—	E950.9	E962.1	E980.9
Gemonil	967.0	E851	E937.0	E950.1	E962.0	E980.1
Gentamicin	960.8	E856	E930.8	E950.4	E962.0	E980.4
ophthalmic preparation	976.5	E858.7	E946.5	E950.4	E962.0	E980.4
topical NEC	976.0	E858.7	E946.0	E950.4	E962.0	E980.4
Gentian violet	976.0	E858.7	E946.0	E950.4	E962.0	E980.4
Gexane	976.0	E858.7	E946.0	E950.4	E962.0	E980.4
Gila monster (venom)	989.5	E905.0	—	E950.9	E962.1	E980.9
Ginger, Jamaica	989.89	E866.8	—	E950.9	E962.1	E980.9
Gitalin	972.1	E858.3	E942.1	E950.4	E962.0	E980.4
Gitoxin	972.1	E858.3	E942.1	E950.4	E962.0	E980.4
Glandular extract (medicinal) NEC	977.9	E858.9	E947.9	E950.5	E962.0	E980.5
Glaucarubin	961.5	E857	E931.5	E950.4	E962.0	E980.4
Globin zinc insulin	962.3	E858.0	E932.3	E950.4	E962.0	E980.4
Glucagon	962.3	E858.0	E932.3	E950.4	E962.0	E980.4
Glucochloral	967.1	E852.0	E937.1	E950.2	E962.0	E980.2
Glucocorticoids	962.0	E858.0	E932.0	E950.4	E962.0	E980.4
Glucose	974.5	E858.5	E944.5	E950.4	E962.0	E980.4
oxidase reagent	977.8	E858.8	E947.8	E950.4	E962.0	E980.4
Glucosulfone sodium	961.8	E857	E931.8	E950.4	E962.0	E980.4
Glue(s)	989.89	E866.6	—	E950.9	E962.1	E980.9
Glutamic acid (hydrochloride)	973.4	E858.4	E943.4	E950.4	E962.0	E980.4
Glutaraldehyde	989.89	E861.4	—	E950.9	E962.1	E980.9
Glutathione	963.8	E858.1	E933.8	E950.4	E962.0	E980.4
Glutethimide (group)	967.5	E852.4	E937.5	E950.2	E962.0	E980.2
Glycerin (lotion)	976.3	E858.7	E946.3	E950.4	E962.0	E980.4
Glycerol (topical)	976.3	E858.7	E946.3	E950.4	E962.0	E980.4
Glyceryl						
guaiacolate	975.5	E858.6	E945.5	E950.4	E962.0	E980.4
triacetate (topical)	976.0	E858.7	E946.0	E950.4	E962.0	E980.4
trinitrate	972.4	E858.3	E942.4	E950.4	E962.0	E980.4
Glycine	974.5	E858.5	E944.5	E950.4	E962.0	E980.4
Glycobiarsol	961.1	E857	E931.1	E950.4	E962.0	E980.4
Glycols (ether)	982.8	E862.4	—	E950.9	E962.1	E980.9
Glycopyrrolate	971.1	E855.4	E941.1	E950.4	E962.0	E980.4
Glymidine	962.3	E858.0	E932.3	E950.4	E962.0	E980.4
Gold (compounds) (salts)	965.69	E850.6	E935.6	E950.0	E962.0	E980.0
Golden sulfide of antimony	985.4	E866.2	—	E950.9	E962.1	E980.9
Goldylocks	988.2	E865.4	—	E950.9	E962.1	E980.9
Gonadal tissue extract	962.9	E858.0	E932.9	E950.4	E962.0	E980.4
female	962.2	E858.0	E932.2	E950.4	E962.0	E980.4
male	962.1	E858.0	E932.1	E950.4	E962.0	E980.4
Gonadotropin	962.4	E858.0	E932.4	E950.4	E962.0	E980.4
Grain alcohol	980.0	E860.1	—	E950.9	E962.1	E980.9
beverage	980.0	E860.0	—	E950.9	E962.1	E980.9
Gramicidin	960.8	E856	E930.8	E950.4	E962.0	E980.4
Gratiola officinalis	988.2	E865.4	—	E950.9	E962.1	E980.9
Grease	989.89	E866.8	—	E950.9	E962.1	E980.9
Green hellebore	988.2	E865.4	—	E950.9	E962.1	E980.9
Green soap	976.2	E858.7	E946.2	E950.4	E962.0	E980.4
Grifulvin	960.1	E856	E930.1	E950.4	E962.0	E980.4
Griseofulvin	960.1	E856	E930.1	E950.4	E962.0	E980.4
Growth hormone	962.4	E858.0	E932.4	E950.4	E962.0	E980.4
Guaiacol	975.5	E858.6	E945.5	E950.4	E962.0	E980.4
Guaiac reagent	977.8	E858.8	E947.8	E950.4	E962.0	E980.4
Guaifenesin	975.5	E858.6	E945.5	E950.4	E962.0	E980.4
Guaiphenesin	975.5	E858.6	E945.5	E950.4	E962.0	E980.4
Guanatol	961.4	E857	E931.4	E950.4	E962.0	E980.4
Guanethidine	972.6	E858.3	E942.6	E950.4	E962.0	E980.4
Guano	989.89	E866.5	—	E950.9	E962.1	E980.9
Guanochlor	972.6	E858.3	E942.6	E950.4	E962.0	E980.4
Guanoctine	972.6	E858.3	E942.6	E950.4	E962.0	E980.4
Guanoxan	972.6	E858.3	E942.6	E950.4	E962.0	E980.4
Hair treatment agent NEC	976.4	E858.7	E946.4	E950.4	E962.0	E980.4
Halcinonide	976.0	E858.7	E946.0	E950.4	E962.0	E980.4
Halethazole	976.0	E858.7	E946.0	E950.4	E962.0	E980.4
Hallucinogens	969.6	E854.1	E939.6	E950.3	E962.0	E980.3
Haloperidol	969.2	E853.1	E939.2	E950.3	E962.0	E980.3
Haloprogin	976.0	E858.7	E946.0	E950.4	E962.0	E980.4
Halotex	976.0	E858.7	E946.0	E950.4	E962.0	E980.4
Halothane	968.1	E855.1	E938.1	E950.4	E962.0	E980.4
Halquinols	976.0	E858.7	E946.0	E950.4	E962.0	E980.4
Hand sanitizer	976.0	E858.7	E946.0	E950.4	E962.0	E980.4
Harmonyl	972.6	E858.3	E942.6	E950.4	E962.0	E980.4
Hartmann's solution	974.5	E858.5	E944.5	E950.4	E962.0	E980.4
Hashish	969.6	E854.1	E939.6	E950.3	E962.0	E980.3
Hawaiian wood rose seeds	969.6	E854.1	E939.6	E950.3	E962.0	E980.3
Headache cures, drugs, powders NEC	977.9	E858.9	E947.9	E950.5	E962.0	E980.9
Heavenly Blue (morning glory)	969.6	E854.1	E939.6	E950.3	E962.0	E980.3
Heavy metal antagonists	963.8	E858.1	E933.8	E950.4	E962.0	E980.4
anti-infectives	961.2	E857	E931.2	E950.4	E962.0	E980.4
Hedaquinium	976.0	E858.7	E946.0	E950.4	E962.0	E980.4
Hedge hyssop	988.2	E865.4	—	E950.9	E962.1	E980.9
Heet	976.8	E858.7	E946.8	E950.4	E962.0	E980.4
Helenin	961.6	E857	E931.6	E950.4	E962.0	E980.4
Hellebore (black) (green) (white)	988.2	E865.4	—	E950.9	E962.1	E980.9
Hemlock	988.2	E865.4	—	E950.9	E962.1	E980.9
Hemostatics	964.5	E858.2	E934.5	E950.4	E962.0	E980.4
capillary active drugs	972.8	E858.3	E942.8	E950.4	E962.0	E980.4
Henbane	988.2	E865.4	—	E950.9	E962.1	E980.9
Heparin (sodium)	964.2	E858.2	E934.2	E950.4	E962.0	E980.4
Heptabarbital, heptabarbitone	967.0	E851	E937.0	E950.1	E962.0	E980.1
Heptachlor	989.2	E863.0	—	E950.6	E962.1	E980.7
Heptalgin	965.09	E850.2	E935.2	E950.0	E962.0	E980.0
Herbicides	989.4	E863.5	—	E950.6	E962.1	E980.7
Heroin	965.01	E850.0	E935.0	E950.0	E962.0	E980.0
Herplex	976.5	E858.7	E946.5	E950.4	E962.0	E980.4
HES	964.8	E858.2	E934.8	E950.4	E962.0	E980.4
Hetastarch	964.8	E858.2	E934.8	E950.4	E962.0	E980.4
Hexachlorocyclohexane	989.2	E863.0	—	E950.6	E962.1	E980.7
Hexachlorophene	976.2	E858.7	E946.2	E950.4	E962.0	E980.4
Hexadimethrine (bromide)	964.5	E858.2	E934.5	E950.4	E962.0	E980.4
Hexafluorenium	975.2	E858.6	E945.2	E950.4	E962.0	E980.4
Hexa-germ	976.2	E858.7	E946.2	E950.4	E962.0	E980.4
Hexahydrophenol	980.8	E860.8	—	E950.9	E962.1	E980.9
Hexalin	980.8	E860.8	—	E950.9	E962.1	E980.9
Hexamethonium	972.3	E858.3	E942.3	E950.4	E962.0	E980.4
Hexamethyleneamine	961.9	E857	E931.9	E950.4	E962.0	E980.4
Hexamine	961.9	E857	E931.9	E950.4	E962.0	E980.4
Hexanone	982.8	E862.4	—	E950.9	E962.1	E980.9
Hexapropymate	967.8	E852.8	E937.8	E950.2	E962.0	E980.2
Hexestrol	962.2	E858.0	E932.2	E950.4	E962.0	E980.4
Hexethal (sodium)	967.0	E851	E937.0	E950.1	E962.0	E980.1
Hexetidine	976.0	E858.7	E946.0	E950.4	E962.0	E980.4
Hexobarbital, hexobarbitone	967.0	E851	E937.0	E950.1	E962.0	E980.1
sodium (anesthetic)	968.3	E855.1	E938.3	E950.4	E962.0	E980.4
soluble	968.3	E855.1	E938.3	E950.4	E962.0	E980.4
Hexocyclium	971.1	E855.4	E941.1	E950.4	E962.0	E980.4
Hexoestrol	962.2	E858.0	E932.2	E950.4	E962.0	E980.4
Hexone	982.8	E862.4	—	E950.9	E962.1	E980.9
Hexylcaine	968.5	E855.2	E938.5	E950.4	E962.0	E980.4
Hexylresorcinol	961.6	E857	E931.6	E950.4	E962.0	E980.4
Hinkle's pills	973.1	E858.4	E943.1	E950.4	E962.0	E980.4
Histalog	977.8	E858.8	E947.8	E950.4	E962.0	E980.4
Histamine (phosphate)	972.5	E858.3	E942.5	E950.4	E962.0	E980.4
Histoplasmin	977.8	E858.8	E947.8	E950.4	E962.0	E980.4
Holly berries	988.2	E865.3	—	E950.9	E962.1	E980.9
Homatropine	971.1	E855.4	E941.1	E950.4	E962.0	E980.4
Homo-tet	964.6	E858.2	E934.6	E950.4	E962.0	E980.4
Hormones (synthetic substitute) NEC	962.9	E858.0	E932.9	E950.4	E962.0	E980.4
adrenal cortical steroids	962.0	E858.0	E932.0	E950.4	E962.0	E980.4
antidiabetic agents	962.3	E858.0	E932.3	E950.4	E962.0	E980.4
follicle stimulating	962.4	E858.0	E932.4	E950.4	E962.0	E980.4
gonadotropic	962.4	E858.0	E932.4	E950.4	E962.0	E980.4
growth	962.4	E858.0	E932.4	E950.4	E962.0	E980.4
ovarian (substitutes)	962.2	E858.0	E932.2	E950.4	E962.0	E980.4
parathyroid (derivatives)	962.6	E858.0	E932.6	E950.4	E962.0	E980.4
pituitary (posterior)	962.5	E858.0	E932.5	E950.4	E962.0	E980.4
anterior	962.4	E858.0	E932.4	E950.4	E962.0	E980.4
thyroid (derivative)	962.7	E858.0	E932.7	E950.4	E962.0	E980.4
Hornet (sting)	989.5	E905.3	—	E950.9	E962.1	E980.9
Horticulture agent NEC	989.4	E863.9	—	E950.6	E962.1	E980.7
Hyaluronidase	963.4	E858.1	E933.4	E950.4	E962.0	E980.4
Hyazyme	963.4	E858.1	E933.4	E950.4	E962.0	E980.4
Hycodan	965.09	E850.2	E935.2	E950.0	E962.0	E980.0
Hydantoin derivatives	966.1	E855.0	E936.1	E950.4	E962.0	E980.4
Hydeltra	962.0	E858.0	E932.0	E950.4	E962.0	E980.4
Hydergine	971.3	E855.6	E941.3	E950.4	E962.0	E980.4
Hydrabamine penicillin	960.0	E856	E930.0	E950.4	E962.0	E980.4

Nontherapeutic use substance

☞ Subterms under main terms may continue to next column or page

	External Cause (E-Code)					
	Poisoning	Accident	Therapeutic Use	Suicide Attempt	Assault	Undetermined
Hydralazine, hydrallazine	972.6	E858.3	E942.6	E950.4	E962.0	E980.4
Hydrargaphen	976.0	E858.7	E946.0	E950.4	E962.0	E980.4
Hydrazine	983.9	E864.3	—	E950.7	E962.1	E980.6
Hydriodic acid	975.5	E858.6	E945.5	E950.4	E962.0	E980.4
Hydrocarbon gas	987.1	E869.8	—	E952.8	E962.2	E982.8
incomplete combustion of — see Carbon, monoxide, fuel, utility						
liquefied (mobile container)	987.0	E868.0	—	E951.1	E962.2	E981.1
piped (natural)	987.0	E867	—	E951.0	E962.2	E981.0
Hydrochloric acid (liquid)	983.1	E864.1	—	E950.7	E962.1	E980.6
medicinal	973.4	E858.4	E943.4	E950.4	E962.0	E980.4
vapor	987.8	E869.8	—	E952.8	E962.2	E982.8
Hydrochlorothiazide	974.3	E858.5	E944.3	E950.4	E962.0	E980.4
Hydrocodone	965.09	E850.2	E935.2	E950.0	E962.0	E980.0
Hydrocortisone	962.0	E858.0	E932.0	E950.4	E962.0	E980.4
ENT agent	976.6	E858.7	E946.6	E950.4	E962.0	E980.4
ophthalmic preparation	976.5	E858.7	E946.5	E950.4	E962.0	E980.4
topical NEC	976.0	E858.7	E946.0	E950.4	E962.0	E980.4
Hydrocortone	962.0	E858.0	E932.0	E950.4	E962.0	E980.4
ENT agent	976.6	E858.7	E946.6	E950.4	E962.0	E980.4
ophthalmic preparation	976.5	E858.7	E946.5	E950.4	E962.0	E980.4
topical NEC	976.0	E858.7	E946.0	E950.4	E962.0	E980.4
Hydrocyanic acid — see Cyanide(s)						
Hydroflumethiazide	974.3	E858.5	E944.3	E950.4	E962.0	E980.4
Hydrofluoric acid (liquid)	983.1	E864.1	—	E950.7	E962.1	E980.6
vapor	987.8	E869.8	—	E952.8	E962.2	E982.8
Hydrogen	987.8	E869.8	—	E952.8	E962.2	E982.8
arsenide	985.1	E866.3	—	E950.8	E962.1	E980.8
arseniureted	985.1	E866.3	—	E950.8	E962.1	E980.8
cyanide (salts)	989.0	E866.8	—	E950.9	E962.1	E980.9
gas	987.7	E869.8	—	E952.8	E962.2	E982.8
fluoride (liquid)	983.1	E864.1	—	E950.7	E962.1	E980.6
vapor	987.8	E869.8	—	E952.8	E962.2	E982.8
peroxide (solution)	976.6	E858.7	E946.6	E950.4	E962.0	E980.4
phosphureted	987.8	E869.8	—	E952.8	E962.2	E982.8
sulfide (gas)	987.8	E869.8	—	E952.8	E962.2	E982.8
arseniureted	985.1	E866.3	—	E950.8	E962.1	E980.8
sulfureted	987.8	E869.8	—	E952.8	E962.2	E982.8
Hydromorphinol	965.09	E850.2	E935.2	E950.0	E962.0	E980.0
Hydromorphinone	965.09	E850.2	E935.2	E950.0	E962.0	E980.0
Hydromorphone	965.09	E850.2	E935.2	E950.0	E962.0	E980.0
Hydromox	974.3	E858.5	E944.3	E950.4	E962.0	E980.4
Hydrophilic lotion	976.3	E858.7	E946.3	E950.4	E962.0	E980.4
Hydroquinone	983.0	E864.0	—	E950.7	E962.1	E980.6
vapor	987.8	E869.8	—	E952.8	E962.2	E982.8
Hydrosulfuric acid (gas)	987.8	E869.8	—	E952.8	E962.2	E982.8
Hydrous wool fat (lotion)	976.3	E858.7	E946.3	E950.4	E962.0	E980.4
Hydroxide, caustic	983.2	E864.2	—	E950.7	E962.1	E980.6
Hydroxocobalamin	964.1	E858.2	E934.1	E950.4	E962.0	E980.4
Hydroxyamphetamine	971.2	E855.5	E941.2	E950.4	E962.0	E980.4
Hydroxychloroquine	961.4	E857	E931.4	E950.4	E962.0	E980.4
Hydroxydihydrocodeinone	965.09	E850.2	E935.2	E950.0	E962.0	E980.0
Hydroxyethyl starch	964.8	E858.2	E934.8	E950.4	E962.0	E980.4
Hydroxyphenamate	969.5	E853.8	E939.5	E950.3	E962.0	E980.3
Hydroxyphenylbutazone	965.5	E850.5	E935.5	E950.0	E962.0	E980.0
Hydroxyprogesterone	962.2	E858.0	E932.2	E950.4	E962.0	E980.4
Hydroxyquinoline derivatives	961.3	E857	E931.3	E950.4	E962.0	E980.4
Hydroxystilbamidine	961.5	E857	E931.5	E950.4	E962.0	E980.4
Hydroxyurea	963.1	E858.1	E933.1	E950.4	E962.0	E980.4
Hydroxyzine	969.5	E853.8	E939.5	E950.3	E962.0	E980.3
Hyoscine (hydrobromide)	971.1	E855.4	E941.1	E950.4	E962.0	E980.4
Hyoscyamine	971.1	E855.4	E941.1	E950.4	E962.0	E980.4
Hyoscyamus (albus) (niger)	988.2	E865.4	—	E950.9	E962.1	E980.9
Hypaque	977.8	E858.8	E947.8	E950.4	E962.0	E980.4
Hypertussis	964.6	E858.2	E934.6	E950.4	E962.0	E980.4
Hypnotics NEC	967.9	E852.9	E937.9	E950.2	E962.0	E980.2
Hypochlorites — see Sodium, hypochlorite						
Hypotensive agents NEC	972.6	E858.3	E942.6	E950.4	E962.0	E980.4
Ibufenac	965.69	E850.6	E935.6	E950.0	E962.0	E980.0
Ibuprofen	965.61	E850.6	E935.6	E950.0	E962.0	E980.0
ICG	977.8	E858.8	E947.8	E950.4	E962.0	E980.4
Ichthammol	976.4	E858.7	E946.4	E950.4	E962.0	E980.4
Ichthyol	976.4	E858.7	E946.4	E950.4	E962.0	E980.4
Idoxuridine	976.5	E858.7	E946.5	E950.4	E962.0	E980.4

	External Cause (E-Code)					
	Poisoning	Accident	Therapeutic Use	Suicide Attempt	Assault	Undetermined
IDU	976.5	E858.7	E946.5	E950.4	E962.0	E980.4
Iletin	962.3	E858.0	E932.3	E950.4	E962.0	E980.4
Ilex	988.2	E865.4	—	E950.9	E962.1	E980.9
Illuminating gas — see Gas, utility						
Ilopan	963.5	E858.1	E933.5	E950.4	E962.0	E980.4
Ilotycin	960.3	E856	E930.3	E950.4	E962.0	E980.4
ophthalmic preparation	976.5	E858.7	E946.5	E950.4	E962.0	E980.4
topical NEC	976.0	E858.7	E946.0	E950.4	E962.0	E980.4
Imipramine	969.05	E854.0	E939.0	E950.3	E962.0	E980.3
Immu-G	964.6	E858.2	E934.6	E950.4	E962.0	E980.4
Immuglobin	964.6	E858.2	E934.6	E950.4	E962.0	E980.4
Immune serum globulin	964.6	E858.2	E934.6	E950.4	E962.0	E980.4
Immunosuppressive agents	963.1	E858.1	E933.1	E950.4	E962.0	E980.4
Immu-tetanus	964.6	E858.2	E934.6	E950.4	E962.0	E980.4
Indandione (derivatives)	964.2	E858.2	E934.2	E950.4	E962.0	E980.4
Inderal	972.0	E858.3	E942.0	E950.4	E962.0	E980.4
Indian						
hemp	969.6	E854.1	E939.6	E950.3	E962.0	E980.3
tobacco	988.2	E865.4	—	E950.9	E962.1	E980.9
Indigo carmine	977.8	E858.8	E947.8	E950.4	E962.0	E980.4
Indocin	965.69	E850.6	E935.6	E950.0	E962.0	E980.0
Indocyanine green	977.8	E858.8	E947.8	E950.4	E962.0	E980.4
Indomethacin	965.69	E850.6	E935.6	E950.0	E962.0	E980.0
Industrial						
alcohol	980.9	E860.9	—	E950.9	E962.1	E980.9
fumes	987.8	E869.8	—	E952.8	E962.2	E982.8
solvents (fumes) (vapors)	982.8	E862.9	—	E950.9	E962.1	E980.9
Influenza vaccine	979.6	E858.8	E949.6	E950.4	E962.0	E982.8
Ingested substances NEC	989.9	E866.9	—	E950.9	E962.1	E980.9
INH (isoniazid)	961.8	E857	E931.8	E950.4	E962.0	E980.4
Inhalation, gas (noxious) — see Gas						
Ink	989.89	E866.8	—	E950.9	E962.1	E980.9
Innovar	967.6	E852.5	E937.6	E950.2	E962.0	E980.2
Inositol niacinate	972.2	E858.3	E942.2	E950.4	E962.0	E980.4
Inproquone	963.1	E858.1	E933.1	E950.4	E962.0	E980.4
Insecticides — see also Pesticides	989.4	E863.4	—	E950.6	E962.1	E980.7
chlorinated	989.2	E863.0	—	E950.6	E962.1	E980.7
mixtures	989.4	E863.3	—	E950.6	E962.1	E980.7
organochlorine (compounds)	989.2	E863.0	—	E950.6	E962.1	E980.7
organophosphorus (compounds)	989.3	E863.1	—	E950.6	E962.1	E980.7
Insect (sting), venomous	989.5	E905.5	—	E950.9	E962.1	E980.9
Insular tissue extract	962.3	E858.0	E932.3	E950.4	E962.0	E980.4
Insulin (amorphous) (globin) (isophane) (Lente) (NPH) (protamine) (Semilente) (Ultralente) (zinc)	962.3	E858.0	E932.3	E950.4	E962.0	E980.4
Intranarcon	968.3	E855.1	E938.3	E950.4	E962.0	E980.4
Inulin	977.8	E858.8	E947.8	E950.4	E962.0	E980.4
Invert sugar	974.5	E858.5	E944.5	E950.4	E962.0	E980.4
Inza — see Naproxen						
Iodide NEC — see also Iodine						
dine	976.0	E858.7	E946.0	E950.4	E962.0	E980.4
mercury (ointment)	976.0	E858.7	E946.0	E950.4	E962.0	E980.4
methylate	976.0	E858.7	E946.0	E950.4	E962.0	E980.4
potassium (expectorant) NEC	975.5	E858.6	E945.5	E950.4	E962.0	E980.4
Iodinated glycerol	975.5	E858.6	E945.5	E950.4	E962.0	E980.4
Iodine (antiseptic, external) (tincture) NEC	976.0	E858.7	E946.0	E950.4	E962.0	E980.4
diagnostic	977.8	E858.8	E947.8	E950.4	E962.0	E980.4
for thyroid conditions (antithyroid)	962.8	E858.0	E932.8	E950.4	E962.0	E980.4
vapor	987.8	E869.8	—	E952.8	E962.2	E982.8
Iodized oil	977.8	E858.8	E947.8	E950.4	E962.0	E980.4
Iodobismitol	961.2	E857	E931.2	E950.4	E962.0	E980.4
Iodochlorhydroxyquin	961.3	E857	E931.3	E950.4	E962.0	E980.4
topical	976.0	E858.7	E946.0	E950.4	E962.0	E980.4
Iodoform	976.0	E858.7	E946.0	E950.4	E962.0	E980.4
Iodopanoic acid	977.8	E858.8	E947.8	E950.4	E962.0	E980.4
Iodophthalein	977.8	E858.8	E947.8	E950.4	E962.0	E980.4
Ion exchange resins	974.5	E858.5	E944.5	E950.4	E962.0	E980.4
Iopanoic acid	977.8	E858.8	E947.8	E950.4	E962.0	E980.4
Iophendylate	977.8	E858.8	E947.8	E950.4	E962.0	E980.4
Iothiouracil	962.8	E858.0	E932.8	E950.4	E962.0	E980.4
Ipecac	973.6	E858.4	E943.6	E950.4	E962.0	E980.4
Ipecacuanha	973.6	E858.4	E943.6	E950.4	E962.0	E980.4

	Poisoning	Accident	Therapeutic Use	Suicide Attempt	Assault	Undetermined
Ipodate	977.8	E858.8	E947.8	E950.4	E962.0	E980.4
Ipral	967.0	E851	E937.0	E950.1	E962.0	E980.1
Ipratropium	975.1	E858.6	E945.1	E950.4	E962.0	E980.4
Iproniazid	969.01	E854.0	E939.0	E950.3	E962.0	E980.3
Iron (compounds) (medicinal)						
(preparations)	964.0	E858.2	E934.0	E950.4	E962.0	E980.4
dextran	964.0	E858.2	E934.0	E950.4	E962.0	E980.4
nonmedicinal (dust) (fumes) NEC	985.8	E866.4	—	E950.9	E962.1	E980.9
Irritant drug	977.9	E858.9	E947.9	E950.5	E962.0	E980.5
Ismelin	972.6	E858.3	E942.6	E950.4	E962.0	E980.4
Isoamyl nitrite	972.4	E858.3	E942.4	E950.4	E962.0	E980.4
Isobutyl acetate	982.8	E862.4	—	E950.9	E962.1	E980.9
Isocarboxazid	969.01	E854.0	E939.0	E950.3	E962.0	E980.3
Isoephedrine	971.2	E855.5	E941.2	E950.4	E962.0	E980.4
Isoetharine	971.2	E855.5	E941.2	E950.4	E962.0	E980.4
Isofluorophate	971.0	E855.3	E941.0	E950.4	E962.0	E980.4
Isoniazid (INH)	961.8	E857	E931.8	E950.4	E962.0	E980.4
Isopentaquine	961.4	E857	E931.4	E950.4	E962.0	E980.4
Isophane insulin	962.3	E858.0	E932.3	E950.4	E962.0	E980.4
Isopregnenone	962.2	E858.0	E932.2	E950.4	E962.0	E980.4
Isoprenaline	971.2	E855.5	E941.2	E950.4	E962.0	E980.4
Isopropamide	971.1	E855.4	E941.1	E950.4	E962.0	E980.4
Isopropanol	980.2	E860.3	—	E950.9	E962.1	E980.9
topical (germicide)	976.0	E858.7	E946.0	E950.4	E962.0	E980.4
Isopropyl						
acetate	982.8	E862.4	—	E950.9	E962.1	E980.9
alcohol	980.2	E860.3	—	E950.9	E962.1	E980.9
topical (germicide)	976.0	E858.7	E946.0	E950.4	E962.0	E980.4
ether	982.8	E862.4	—	E950.9	E962.1	E980.9
Isoproterenol	971.2	E855.5	E941.2	E950.4	E962.0	E980.4
Isosorbide dinitrate	972.4	E858.3	E942.4	E950.4	E962.0	E980.4
Isothipendyl	963.0	E858.1	E933.0	E950.4	E962.0	E980.4
Isoxazolyl penicillin	960.0	E856	E930.0	E950.4	E962.0	E980.4
Isoxsuprine hydrochloride	972.5	E858.3	E942.5	E950.4	E962.0	E980.4
l-thyroxine sodium	962.7	E858.0	E932.7	E950.4	E962.0	E980.4
Jaborandi (pilocarpus) (extract)	971.0	E855.3	E941.0	E950.4	E962.0	E980.4
Jalap	973.1	E858.4	E943.1	E950.4	E962.0	E980.4
Jamaica						
dogwood (bark)	965.7	E850.7	E935.7	E950.0	E962.0	E980.0
ginger	989.89	E866.8	—	E950.9	E962.1	E980.9
Jatropha	988.2	E865.4	—	E950.9	E962.1	E980.9
curcas	988.2	E865.3	—	E950.9	E962.1	E980.9
Jectofer	964.0	E858.2	E934.0	E950.4	E962.0	E980.4
Jellyfish (sting)	989.5	E905.6	—	E950.9	E962.1	E980.9
Jequirity (bean)	988.2	E865.3	—	E950.9	E962.1	E980.9
Jimson weed	988.2	E865.4	—	E950.9	E962.1	E980.9
seeds	988.2	E865.3	—	E950.9	E962.1	E980.9
Juniper tar (oil) (ointment)	976.4	E858.7	E946.4	E950.4	E962.0	E980.4
Kallikrein	972.5	E858.3	E942.5	E950.4	E962.0	E980.4
Kanamycin	960.6	E856	E930.6	E950.4	E962.0	E980.4
Kantrex	960.6	E856	E930.6	E950.4	E962.0	E980.4
Kaolin	973.5	E858.4	E943.5	E950.4	E962.0	E980.4
Karaya (gum)	973.3	E858.4	E943.3	E950.4	E962.0	E980.4
Kemithal	968.3	E855.1	E938.3	E950.4	E962.0	E980.4
Kenacort	962.0	E858.0	E932.0	E950.4	E962.0	E980.4
Keratolytics	976.4	E858.7	E946.4	E950.4	E962.0	E980.4
Keratoplastics	976.4	E858.7	E946.4	E950.4	E962.0	E980.4
Kerosene, kerosine (fuel) (solvent) NEC	981	E862.1	—	E950.9	E962.1	E980.9
insecticide	981	E863.4	—	E950.6	E962.1	E980.7
vapor	987.1	E869.8	—	E952.8	E962.2	E982.8
Ketamine	968.3	E855.1	E938.3	E950.4	E962.0	E980.4
Ketobemidone	965.09	E850.2	E935.2	E950.0	E962.0	E980.0
Ketols	982.8	E862.4	—	E950.9	E962.1	E980.9
Ketone oils	982.8	E862.4	—	E950.9	E962.1	E980.9
Ketoprofen	965.61	E850.6	E935.6	E950.0	E962.0	E980.0
Kiln gas or vapor (carbon monoxide)	986	E868.8	—	E952.1	E962.2	E982.1
Konsyl	973.3	E858.4	E943.3	E950.4	E962.0	E980.4
Kosam seed	988.2	E865.3	—	E950.9	E962.1	E980.9
Krait (venom)	989.5	E905.0	—	E950.9	E962.1	E980.9
Kwell (insecticide)	989.2	E863.0	—	E950.6	E962.1	E980.7
anti-infective (topical)	976.0	E858.7	E946.0	E950.4	E962.0	E980.4
Laburnum (flowers) (seeds)	988.2	E865.4	—	E950.9	E962.1	E980.9
leaves	988.2	E865.4	—	E950.9	E962.1	E980.9
Lacquers	989.89	E861.6	—	E950.9	E962.1	E980.9
Lacrimogenic gas	987.5	E869.3	—	E952.8	E962.2	E982.8

	Poisoning	Accident	Therapeutic Use	Suicide Attempt	Assault	Undetermined
Lactic acid	983.1	E864.1	—	E950.7	E962.1	E980.6
Lactobacillus acidophilus	973.5	E858.4	E943.5	E950.4	E962.0	E980.4
Lactoflavin	963.5	E858.1	E933.5	E950.4	E962.0	E980.4
Lactuca (virosa) (extract)	967.8	E852.8	E937.8	E950.2	E962.0	E980.2
Lactucarium	967.8	E852.8	E937.8	E950.2	E962.0	E980.2
Laevulose	974.5	E858.5	E944.5	E950.4	E962.0	E980.4
Lanatoside (C)	972.1	E858.3	E942.1	E950.4	E962.0	E980.4
Lanolin (lotion)	976.3	E858.7	E946.3	E950.4	E962.0	E980.4
Largactil	969.1	E853.0	E939.1	E950.3	E962.0	E980.3
Larkspur	988.2	E865.3	—	E950.9	E962.1	E980.9
Laroxyl	969.05	E854.0	E939.0	E950.3	E962.0	E980.3
Lasix	974.4	E858.5	E944.4	E950.4	E962.0	E980.4
Latex	989.82	E866.8	—	E950.9	E962.1	E980.9
Lathyrus (seed)	988.2	E865.3	—	E950.9	E962.1	E980.9
Laudanum	965.09	E850.2	E935.2	E950.0	E962.0	E980.0
Laudexium	975.2	E858.6	E945.2	E950.4	E962.0	E980.4
Laurel, black or cherry	988.2	E865.4	—	E950.9	E962.1	E980.9
Laurolinium	976.0	E858.7	E946.0	E950.4	E962.0	E980.4
Lauryl sulfoacetate	976.2	E858.7	E946.2	E950.4	E962.0	E980.4
Laxatives NEC	973.3	E858.4	E943.3	E950.4	E962.0	E980.4
emollient	973.2	E858.4	E943.2	E950.4	E962.0	E980.4
L-dopa	966.4	E855.0	E936.4	E950.4	E962.0	E980.4
Lead (dust) (fumes) (vapor)						
NEC	984.9	E866.0	—	E950.9	E962.1	E980.9
acetate (dust)	984.1	E866.0	—	E950.9	E962.1	E980.9
anti-infectives	961.2	E857	E931.2	E950.4	E962.0	E980.4
antiknock compound (tetraethyl)	984.1	E862.1	—	E950.9	E962.1	E980.9
arsenate, arsenite (dust) (insecticide) (vapor)	985.1	E863.4	—	E950.8	E962.1	E980.8
herbicide	985.1	E863.5	—	E950.8	E962.1	E980.8
carbonate	984.0	E866.0	—	E950.9	E962.1	E980.9
paint	984.0	E861.5	—	E950.9	E962.1	E980.9
chromate	984.0	E866.0	—	E950.9	E962.1	E980.9
paint	984.0	E861.5	—	E950.9	E962.1	E980.9
dioxide	984.0	E866.0	—	E950.9	E962.1	E980.9
inorganic (compound)	984.0	E866.0	—	E950.9	E962.1	E980.9
paint	984.0	E861.5	—	E950.9	E962.1	E980.9
iodide	984.0	E866.0	—	E950.9	E962.1	E980.9
pigment (paint)	984.0	E861.5	—	E950.9	E962.1	E980.9
monoxide (dust)	984.0	E866.0	—	E950.9	E962.1	E980.9
paint	984.0	E861.5	—	E950.9	E962.1	E980.9
organic	984.1	E866.0	—	E950.9	E962.1	E980.9
oxide	984.0	E866.0	—	E950.9	E962.1	E980.9
paint	984.0	E861.5	—	E950.9	E962.1	E980.9
paint	984.0	E861.5	—	E950.9	E962.1	E980.9
salts	984.0	E866.0	—	E950.9	E962.1	E980.9
specified compound NEC	984.8	E866.0	—	E950.9	E962.1	E980.9
tetra-ethyl	984.1	E862.1	—	E950.9	E962.1	E980.9
Lebanese red	969.6	E854.1	E939.6	E950.3	E962.0	E980.3
Lente Iletin (insulin)	962.3	E858.0	E932.3	E950.4	E962.0	E980.4
Leptazol	970.0	E854.3	E940.0	E950.4	E962.0	E980.4
Leritine	965.09	E850.2	E935.2	E950.0	E962.0	E980.0
Letter	962.7	E858.0	E932.7	E950.4	E962.0	E980.4
Lettuce opium	967.8	E852.8	E937.8	E950.2	E962.0	E980.2
Leucovorin (factor)	964.1	E858.2	E934.1	E950.4	E962.0	E980.4
Leukeran	963.1	E858.1	E933.1	E950.4	E962.0	E980.4
Levalbuterol	975.7	E858.6	E945.7	E950.4	E962.0	E980.4
Levallorphan	970.1	E854.3	E940.1	E950.4	E962.0	E980.4
Levanil	967.8	E852.8	E937.8	E950.2	E962.0	E980.2
Levarterenol	971.2	E855.5	E941.2	E950.4	E962.0	E980.4
Levodopa	966.4	E855.0	E936.4	E950.4	E962.0	E980.4
Levo-dromoran	965.09	E850.2	E935.2	E950.0	E962.0	E980.0
Levoid	962.7	E858.0	E932.7	E950.4	E962.0	E980.4
Levo-iso-methadone	965.02	E850.1	E935.1	E950.0	E962.0	E980.0
Levomepromazine	967.8	E852.8	E937.8	E950.2	E962.0	E980.2
Levoprome	967.8	E852.8	E937.8	E950.2	E962.0	E980.2
Levopropoxyphene	975.4	E858.6	E945.4	E950.4	E962.0	E980.4
Levorphan, levophanol	965.09	E850.2	E935.2	E950.0	E962.0	E980.0
Levothyroxine (sodium)	962.7	E858.0	E932.7	E950.4	E962.0	E980.4
Levsin	971.1	E855.4	E941.1	E950.4	E962.0	E980.4
Levulose	974.5	E858.5	E944.5	E950.4	E962.0	E980.4
Lewisite (gas)	985.1	E866.3	—	E950.8	E962.1	E980.8
Librium	969.4	E853.2	E939.4	E950.3	E962.0	E980.3
Lidex	976.0	E858.7	E946.0	E950.4	E962.0	E980.4
Lidocaine (infiltration) (topical)	968.5	E855.2	E938.5	E950.4	E962.0	E980.4
nerve block (peripheral) (plexus)	968.6	E855.2	E938.6	E950.4	E962.0	E980.4
spinal	968.7	E855.2	E938.7	E950.4	E962.0	E980.4
Lighter fluid	981	E862.1	—	E950.9	E962.1	E980.9

▽ Subterms under main terms may continue to next column or page

	Poisoning	Accident	Therapeutic Use	Suicide Attempt	Assault	Undetermined
External Cause (E-Code)						
Lignocaine (infiltration) (topical)	968.5	E855.2	E938.5	E950.4	E962.0	E980.4
nerve block (peripheral) (plexus)	968.6	E855.2	E938.6	E950.4	E962.0	E980.4
spinal	968.7	E855.2	E938.7	E950.4	E962.0	E980.4
Ligroin(e) (solvent)	981	E862.0	—	E950.9	E962.1	E980.9
vapor	987.1	E869.8	—	E952.8	E962.2	E982.8
Ligustrum vulgare	988.2	E865.3	—	E950.9	E962.1	E980.9
Lily of the valley	988.2	E865.4	—	E950.9	E962.1	E980.9
Lime (chloride)	983.2	E864.2	—	E950.7	E962.1	E980.6
solution, sulferated	976.4	E858.7	E946.4	E950.4	E962.0	E980.4
Limonene	982.8	E862.4	—	E950.9	E962.1	E980.9
Lincomycin	960.8	E856	E930.8	E950.4	E962.0	E980.4
Lindane (insecticide) (vapor)	989.2	E863.0	—	E950.6	E962.1	E980.7
anti-infective (topical)	976.0	E858.7	E946.0	E950.4	E962.0	E980.4
Liniments NEC	976.9	E858.7	E946.9	E950.4	E962.0	E980.4
Linoleic acid	972.2	E858.3	E942.2	E950.4	E962.0	E980.4
Liothyronine	962.7	E858.0	E932.7	E950.4	E962.0	E980.4
Liotrix	962.7	E858.0	E932.7	E950.4	E962.0	E980.4
Lipancreatin	973.4	E858.4	E943.4	E950.4	E962.0	E980.4
Lipo-Lutin	962.2	E858.0	E932.2	E950.4	E962.0	E980.4
Lipotropic agents	977.1	E858.8	E947.1	E950.4	E962.0	E980.4
Liquefied petroleum gases	987.0	E868.0	—	E951.1	E962.2	E981.1
piped (pure or mixed with air)	987.0	E867	—	E951.0	E962.2	E981.0
Liquid petrolatum	973.2	E858.4	E943.2	E950.4	E962.0	E980.4
substance	989.9	E866.9	—	E950.9	E962.1	E980.9
specified NEC	989.89	E866.8	—	E950.9	E962.1	E980.9
Lirugen	979.4	E858.8	E949.4	E950.4	E962.0	E980.4
Lithane	969.8	E855.8	E939.8	E950.3	E962.0	E980.3
Lithium	985.8	E866.4	—	E950.9	E962.1	E980.9
carbonate	969.8	E855.8	E939.8	E950.3	E962.0	E980.3
Lithonate	969.8	E855.8	E939.8	E950.3	E962.0	E980.3
Liver (extract) (injection) (preparations)	964.1	E858.2	E934.1	E950.4	E962.0	E980.4
Lizard (bite) (venom)	989.5	E905.0	—	E950.9	E962.1	E980.9
LMD	964.8	E858.2	E934.8	E950.4	E962.0	E980.4
Lobelia	988.2	E865.4	—	E950.9	E962.1	E980.9
Lobeline	970.0	E854.3	E940.0	E950.4	E962.0	E980.4
Locorten	976.0	E858.7	E946.0	E950.4	E962.0	E980.4
Lolium temulentum	988.2	E865.3	—	E950.9	E962.1	E980.9
Lomotil	973.5	E858.4	E943.5	E950.4	E962.0	E980.4
Lomustine	963.1	E858.1	E933.1	E950.4	E962.0	E980.4
Lophophora williamsii	969.6	E854.1	E939.6	E950.3	E962.0	E980.3
Lorazepam	969.4	E853.2	E939.4	E950.3	E962.0	E980.3
Lotions NEC	976.9	E858.7	E946.9	E950.4	E962.0	E980.4
Lotronex	973.8	E858.4	E943.8	E950.4	E962.0	E980.4
Lotusate	967.0	E851	E937.0	E950.1	E962.0	E980.1
Lowila	976.2	E858.7	E946.2	E950.4	E962.0	E980.4
Loxapine	969.3	E853.8	E939.3	E950.3	E962.0	E980.3
Lozenges (throat)	976.6	E858.7	E946.6	E950.4	E962.0	E980.4
LSD (25)	969.6	E854.1	E939.6	E950.3	E962.0	E980.3
L-Tryptophan — see amino acid						
Lubricating oil NEC	981	E862.2	—	E950.9	E962.1	E980.9
Lucanthone	961.6	E857	E931.6	E950.4	E962.0	E980.4
Luminal	967.0	E851	E937.0	E950.1	E962.0	E980.1
Lung irritant (gas) NEC	987.9	E869.9	—	E952.9	E962.2	E982.9
Lutocylol	962.2	E858.0	E932.2	E950.4	E962.0	E980.4
Lutromone	962.2	E858.0	E932.2	E950.4	E962.0	E980.4
Lututrin	975.0	E858.6	E945.0	E950.4	E962.0	E980.4
Lye (concentrated)	983.2	E864.2	—	E950.7	E962.1	E980.6
Lygranum (skin test)	977.8	E858.8	E947.8	E950.4	E962.0	E980.4
Lymecycline	960.4	E856	E930.4	E950.4	E962.0	E980.4
Lymphogranuloma venereum antigen	977.8	E858.8	E947.8	E950.4	E962.0	E980.4
Lynestrenol	962.2	E858.0	E932.2	E950.4	E962.0	E980.4
Lyovac Sodium Edecrin	974.4	E858.5	E944.4	E950.4	E962.0	E980.4
Lypressin	962.5	E858.0	E932.5	E950.4	E962.0	E980.4
Lysergic acid (amide) (diethylamide)	969.6	E854.1	E939.6	E950.3	E962.0	E980.3
Lysergide	969.6	E854.1	E939.6	E950.3	E962.0	E980.3
Lysine vasopressin	962.5	E858.0	E932.5	E950.4	E962.0	E980.4
Lysol	983.0	E864.0	—	E950.7	E962.1	E980.6
Lytta (vitatta)	976.8	E858.7	E946.8	E950.4	E962.0	E980.4
Mace	987.5	E869.3	—	E952.8	E962.2	E982.8
Macrolides (antibiotics)	960.3	E856	E930.3	E950.4	E962.0	E980.4
Mafenide	976.0	E858.7	E946.0	E950.4	E962.0	E980.4
Magaldrate	973.0	E858.4	E943.0	E950.4	E962.0	E980.4
Magic mushroom	969.6	E854.1	E939.6	E950.3	E962.0	E980.3

	Poisoning	Accident	Therapeutic Use	Suicide Attempt	Assault	Undetermined
External Cause (E-Code)						
Magnamycin	960.8	E856	E930.8	E950.4	E962.0	E980.4
Magnesia magma	973.0	E858.4	E943.0	E950.4	E962.0	E980.4
Magnesium (compounds) (fumes) NEC	985.8	E866.4	—	E950.9	E962.1	E980.9
antacid	973.0	E858.4	E943.0	E950.4	E962.0	E980.4
carbonate	973.0	E858.4	E943.0	E950.4	E962.0	E980.4
cathartic	973.3	E858.4	E943.3	E950.4	E962.0	E980.4
citrate	973.3	E858.4	E943.3	E950.4	E962.0	E980.4
hydroxide	973.0	E858.4	E943.0	E950.4	E962.0	E980.4
oxide	973.0	E858.4	E943.0	E950.4	E962.0	E980.4
sulfate (oral)	973.3	E858.4	E943.3	E950.4	E962.0	E980.4
intravenous	966.3	E855.0	E936.3	E950.4	E962.0	E980.4
trisilicate	973.0	E858.4	E943.0	E950.4	E962.0	E980.4
Malathion (insecticide)	989.3	E863.1	—	E950.6	E962.1	E980.7
Male fern (oleoresin)	961.6	E857	E931.6	E950.4	E962.0	E980.4
Mandelic acid	961.9	E857	E931.9	E950.4	E962.0	E980.4
Manganese compounds (fumes) NEC	985.2	E866.4	—	E950.9	E962.1	E980.9
Mannitol (diuretic) (medicinal) NEC	974.4	E858.5	E944.4	E950.4	E962.0	E980.4
hexanitrate	972.4	E858.3	E942.4	E950.4	E962.0	E980.4
mustard	963.1	E858.1	E933.1	E950.4	E962.0	E980.4
Mannomustine	963.1	E858.1	E933.1	E950.4	E962.0	E980.4
MAO inhibitors	969.01	E854.0	E939.0	E950.3	E962.0	E980.3
Mapharsen	961.1	E857	E931.1	E950.4	E962.0	E980.4
Marcaine	968.9	E855.2	E938.9	E950.4	E962.0	E980.4
infiltration (subcutaneous)	968.5	E855.2	E938.5	E950.4	E962.0	E980.4
nerve block (peripheral) (plexus)	968.6	E855.2	E938.6	E950.4	E962.0	E980.4
Marezine	963.0	E858.1	E933.0	E950.4	E962.0	E980.4
Marihuana, marijuana (derivatives)	969.6	E854.1	E939.6	E950.3	E962.0	E980.3
Marine animals or plants (sting)	989.5	E905.6	—	E950.9	E962.1	E980.9
Marplan	969.01	E854.0	E939.0	E950.3	E962.0	E980.3
Marsh gas	987.1	E869.8	—	E952.8	E962.2	E982.8
Marsilid	969.01	E854.0	E939.0	E950.3	E962.0	E980.3
Matulane	963.1	E858.1	E933.1	E950.4	E962.0	E980.4
Mazindol	977.0	E858.8	E947.0	E950.4	E962.0	E980.4
MDMA	969.72	E854.2	E939.7	E950.3	E962.0	E980.3
Meadow saffron	988.2	E865.3	—	E950.9	E962.1	E980.9
Measles vaccine	979.4	E858.8	E949.4	E950.4	E962.0	E980.4
Meat, noxious or nonbacterial	988.8	E865.0	—	E950.9	E962.1	E980.9
Mebanazine	969.01	E854.0	E939.0	E950.3	E962.0	E980.3
Mebaral	967.0	E851	E937.0	E950.1	E962.0	E980.1
Mebendazole	961.6	E857	E931.6	E950.4	E962.0	E980.4
Mebeverine	975.1	E858.6	E945.1	E950.4	E962.0	E980.4
Mebhydroline	963.0	E858.1	E933.0	E950.4	E962.0	E980.4
Mebrophenhydramine	963.0	E858.1	E933.0	E950.4	E962.0	E980.4
Mebutamate	969.5	E853.8	E939.5	E950.3	E962.0	E980.3
Mecamylamine (chloride)	972.3	E858.3	E942.3	E950.4	E962.0	E980.4
Mechlorethamine hydrochloride	963.1	E858.1	E933.1	E950.4	E962.0	E980.4
Meclizene (hydrochloride)	963.0	E858.1	E933.0	E950.4	E962.0	E980.4
Meclofenoxate	970.0	E854.3	E940.0	E950.4	E962.0	E980.4
Meclozine (hydrochloride)	963.0	E858.1	E933.0	E950.4	E962.0	E980.4
Medazepam	969.4	E853.2	E939.4	E950.3	E962.0	E980.3
Medicine, medicinal substance	977.9	E858.9	E947.9	E950.5	E962.0	E980.5
specified NEC	977.8	E858.8	E947.8	E950.4	E962.0	E980.4
Medinal	967.0	E851	E937.0	E950.1	E962.0	E980.1
Medomin	967.0	E851	E937.0	E950.1	E962.0	E980.1
Medroxyprogesterone	962.2	E858.0	E932.2	E950.4	E962.0	E980.4
Medrysone	976.5	E858.7	E946.5	E950.4	E962.0	E980.4
Mefenamic acid	965.7	E850.7	E935.7	E950.0	E962.0	E980.0
Megahallucinogen	969.6	E854.1	E939.6	E950.3	E962.0	E980.3
Megestrol	962.2	E858.0	E932.2	E950.4	E962.0	E980.4
Meglumine	977.8	E858.8	E947.8	E950.4	E962.0	E980.4
Meladinin	976.3	E858.7	E946.3	E950.4	E962.0	E980.4
Melanizing agents	976.3	E858.7	E946.3	E950.4	E962.0	E980.4
Melarsoprol	961.1	E857	E931.1	E950.4	E962.0	E980.4
Melia azedarach	988.2	E865.3	—	E950.9	E962.1	E980.9
Mellaril	969.1	E853.0	E939.1	E950.3	E962.0	E980.3
Meloxine	976.3	E858.7	E946.3	E950.4	E962.0	E980.4
Melphalan	963.1	E858.1	E933.1	E950.4	E962.0	E980.4
Menadiol sodium diphosphate	964.3	E858.2	E934.3	E950.4	E962.0	E980.4
Menadione (sodium bisulfite)	964.3	E858.2	E934.3	E950.4	E962.0	E980.4
Menaphthone	964.3	E858.2	E934.3	E950.4	E962.0	E980.4

	Poisoning	Accident	Therapeutic Use	Suicide Attempt	Assault	Undetermined
Meningococcal vaccine	978.8	E858.8	E948.8	E950.4	E962.0	E980.4
Menningovax-C	978.8	E858.8	E948.8	E950.4	E962.0	E980.4
Menotropins	962.4	E858.0	E932.4	E950.4	E962.0	E980.4
Menthol NEC	976.1	E858.7	E946.1	E950.4	E962.0	E980.4
Mepacrine	961.3	E857	E931.3	E950.4	E962.0	E980.4
Meparfynol	967.8	E852.8	E937.8	E950.2	E962.0	E980.2
Mepazine	969.1	E853.0	E939.1	E950.3	E962.0	E980.3
Mepenzolate	971.1	E855.4	E941.1	E950.4	E962.0	E980.4
Meperidine	965.09	E850.2	E935.2	E950.0	E962.0	E980.0
Mephenamin(e)	966.4	E855.0	E936.4	E950.4	E962.0	E980.4
Mephenesin (carbamate)	968.0	E855.1	E938.0	E950.4	E962.0	E980.4
Mephenoxalone	969.5	E853.8	E939.5	E950.3	E962.0	E980.3
Mephentermine	971.2	E855.5	E941.2	E950.4	E962.0	E980.4
Mephenytoin	966.1	E855.0	E936.1	E950.4	E962.0	E980.4
Mephobarbital	967.0	E851	E937.0	E950.1	E962.0	E980.1
Mepiperphenidol	971.1	E855.4	E941.1	E950.4	E962.0	E980.4
Mepivacaine	968.9	E855.2	E938.9	E950.4	E962.0	E980.4
infiltration (subcutaneous)	968.5	E855.2	E938.5	E950.4	E962.0	E980.4
nerve block (peripheral) (plexus)	968.6	E855.2	E938.6	E950.4	E962.0	E980.4
topical (surface)	968.5	E855.2	E938.5	E950.4	E962.0	E980.4
Meprednisone	962.0	E858.0	E932.0	E950.4	E962.0	E980.4
Meprobam	969.5	E853.8	E939.5	E950.3	E962.0	E980.3
Meprobamate	969.5	E853.8	E939.5	E950.3	E962.0	E980.3
Mepyramine (maleate)	963.0	E858.1	E933.0	E950.4	E962.0	E980.4
Meralluride	974.0	E858.5	E944.0	E950.4	E962.0	E980.4
Merbaphen	974.0	E858.5	E944.0	E950.4	E962.0	E980.4
Merbromin	976.0	E858.7	E946.0	E950.4	E962.0	E980.4
Mercaptomerin	974.0	E858.5	E944.0	E950.4	E962.0	E980.4
Mercaptopurine	963.1	E858.1	E933.1	E950.4	E962.0	E980.4
Mercumatilin	974.0	E858.5	E944.0	E950.4	E962.0	E980.4
Mercuramide	974.0	E858.5	E944.0	E950.4	E962.0	E980.4
Mercuranin	976.0	E858.7	E946.0	E950.4	E962.0	E980.4
Mercurochrome	976.0	E858.7	E946.0	E950.4	E962.0	E980.4
Mercury, mercuric, mercurous (compounds) (cyanide) (fumes) (nonmedicinal) (vapor) NEC	985.0	E866.1	—	E950.9	E962.1	E980.9
ammoniated	976.0	E858.7	E946.0	E950.4	E962.0	E980.4
anti-infective	961.2	E857	E931.2	E950.4	E962.0	E980.4
topical	976.0	E858.7	E946.0	E950.4	E962.0	E980.4
chloride (antiseptic) NEC	976.0	E858.7	E946.0	E950.4	E962.0	E980.4
fungicide	985.0	E863.6	—	E950.6	E962.1	E980.7
diuretic compounds	974.0	E858.5	E944.0	E950.4	E962.0	E980.4
fungicide	985.0	E863.6	—	E950.6	E962.1	E980.7
organic (fungicide)	985.0	E863.6	—	E950.6	E962.1	E980.7
Merethoxylline	974.0	E858.5	E944.0	E950.4	E962.0	E980.4
Mersalyl	974.0	E858.5	E944.0	E950.4	E962.0	E980.4
Merthiolate (topical)	976.0	E858.7	E946.0	E950.4	E962.0	E980.4
ophthalmic preparation	976.5	E858.7	E946.5	E950.4	E962.0	E980.4
Meruvax	979.4	E858.8	E949.4	E950.4	E962.0	E980.4
Mescal buttons	969.6	E854.1	E939.6	E950.3	E962.0	E980.3
Mescaline (salts)	969.6	E854.1	E939.6	E950.3	E962.0	E980.3
Mesoridazine besylate	969.1	E853.0	E939.1	E950.3	E962.0	E980.3
Mestanolone	962.1	E858.0	E932.1	E950.4	E962.0	E980.4
Mestranol	962.2	E858.0	E932.2	E950.4	E962.0	E980.4
Metacresylacetate	976.0	E858.7	E946.0	E950.4	E962.0	E980.4
Metaldehyde (snail killer) NEC	989.4	E863.4	—	E950.6	E962.1	E980.7
Metals (heavy) (nonmedicinal) NEC	985.9	E866.4	—	E950.9	E962.1	E980.9
dust, fumes, or vapor NEC	985.9	E866.4	—	E950.9	E962.1	E980.9
light NEC	985.9	E866.4	—	E950.9	E962.1	E980.9
dust, fumes, or vapor NEC	985.9	E866.4	—	E950.9	E962.1	E980.9
pesticides (dust) (vapor)	985.9	E863.4	—	E950.6	E962.1	E980.7
Metamucil	973.3	E858.4	E943.3	E950.4	E962.0	E980.4
Metaphen	976.0	E858.7	E946.0	E950.4	E962.0	E980.4
Metaproterenol	975.1	E858.6	E945.1	E950.4	E962.0	E980.4
Metaraminol	972.8	E858.3	E942.8	E950.4	E962.0	E980.4
Metaxalone	968.0	E855.1	E938.0	E950.4	E962.0	E980.4
Metformin	962.3	E858.0	E932.3	E950.4	E962.0	E980.4
Methacycline	960.4	E856	E930.4	E950.4	E962.0	E980.4
Methadone	965.02	E850.1	E935.1	E950.0	E962.0	E980.0
Methallenestril	962.2	E858.0	E932.2	E950.4	E962.0	E980.4
Methamphetamine	969.72	E854.2	E939.7	E950.3	E962.0	E980.3
Methandienone	962.1	E858.0	E932.1	E950.4	E962.0	E980.4
Methandriol	962.1	E858.0	E932.1	E950.4	E962.0	E980.4
Methandrostenolone	962.1	E858.0	E932.1	E950.4	E962.0	E980.4
Methane gas	987.1	E869.8	—	E952.8	E962.2	E982.8
Methanol	980.1	E860.2	—	E950.9	E962.1	E980.9
vapor	987.8	E869.8	—	E952.8	E962.2	E982.8
Methantheline	971.1	E855.4	E941.1	E950.4	E962.0	E980.4
Methaphenilene	963.0	E858.1	E933.0	E950.4	E962.0	E980.4
Methapyrilene	963.0	E858.1	E933.0	E950.4	E962.0	E980.4
Methaqualone (compounds)	967.4	E852.3	E937.4	E950.2	E962.0	E980.2
Metharbital, metharbitone	967.0	E851	E937.0	E950.1	E962.0	E980.1
Methazolamide	974.2	E858.5	E944.2	E950.4	E962.0	E980.4
Methdilazine	963.0	E858.1	E933.0	E950.4	E962.0	E980.4
Methedrine	969.72	E854.2	E939.7	E950.3	E962.0	E980.3
Methenamine (mandelate)	961.9	E857	E931.9	E950.4	E962.0	E980.4
Methenolone	962.1	E858.0	E932.1	E950.4	E962.0	E980.4
Methergine	975.0	E858.6	E945.0	E950.4	E962.0	E980.4
Methiacil	962.8	E858.0	E932.8	E950.4	E962.0	E980.4
Methicillin (sodium)	960.0	E856	E930.0	E950.4	E962.0	E980.4
Methimazole	962.8	E858.0	E932.8	E950.4	E962.0	E980.4
Methionine	977.1	E858.8	E947.1	E950.4	E962.0	E980.4
Methisazone	961.7	E857	E931.7	E950.4	E962.0	E980.4
Methitural	967.0	E851	E937.0	E950.1	E962.0	E980.1
Methixene	971.1	E855.4	E941.1	E950.4	E962.0	E980.4
Methobarbital, methobarbitone	967.0	E851	E937.0	E950.1	E962.0	E980.1
Methocarbamol	968.0	E855.1	E938.0	E950.4	E962.0	E980.4
Methohexital, methohexitone (sodium)	968.3	E855.1	E938.3	E950.4	E962.0	E980.4
Methoin	966.1	E855.0	E936.1	E950.4	E962.0	E980.4
Methopholine	965.7	E850.7	E935.7	E950.0	E962.0	E980.0
Methorate	975.4	E858.6	E945.4	E950.4	E962.0	E980.4
Methoserpidine	972.6	E858.3	E942.6	E950.4	E962.0	E980.4
Methotrexate	963.1	E858.1	E933.1	E950.4	E962.0	E980.4
Methotrimeprazine	967.8	E852.8	E937.8	E950.2	E962.0	E980.2
Methoxa-Dome	976.3	E858.7	E946.3	E950.4	E962.0	E980.4
Methoxamine	971.2	E855.5	E941.2	E950.4	E962.0	E980.4
Methoxsalen	976.3	E858.7	E946.3	E950.4	E962.0	E980.4
Methoxybenzyl penicillin	960.0	E856	E930.0	E950.4	E962.0	E980.4
Methoxychlor	989.2	E863.0	—	E950.6	E962.1	E980.7
Methoxyflurane	968.2	E855.1	E938.2	E950.4	E962.0	E980.4
Methoxyphenamine	971.2	E855.5	E941.2	E950.4	E962.0	E980.4
Methoxypromazine	969.1	E853.0	E939.1	E950.3	E962.0	E980.3
Methoxypsoralen	976.3	E858.7	E946.3	E950.4	E962.0	E980.4
Methscopolamine (bromide)	971.1	E855.4	E941.1	E950.4	E962.0	E980.4
Methsuximide	966.2	E855.0	E936.2	E950.4	E962.0	E980.4
Methyclothiazide	974.3	E858.5	E944.3	E950.4	E962.0	E980.4
Methyl						
acetate	982.8	E862.4	—	E950.9	E962.1	E980.9
acetone	982.8	E862.4	—	E950.9	E962.1	E980.9
alcohol	980.1	E860.2	—	E950.9	E962.1	E980.9
amphetamine	969.72	E854.2	E939.7	E950.3	E962.0	E980.3
androstanolone	962.1	E858.0	E932.1	E950.4	E962.0	E980.4
atropine	971.1	E855.4	E941.1	E950.4	E962.0	E980.4
benzene	982.0	E862.4	—	E950.9	E962.1	E980.9
bromide (gas)	987.8	E869.8	—	E952.8	E962.2	E982.8
fumigant	987.8	E863.8	—	E950.6	E962.2	E980.7
butanol	980.8	E860.8	—	E950.9	E962.1	E980.9
carbinol	980.1	E860.2	—	E950.9	E962.1	E980.9
cellosolve	982.8	E862.4	—	E950.9	E962.1	E980.9
cellulose	973.3	E858.4	E943.3	E950.4	E962.0	E980.4
chloride (gas)	987.8	E869.8	—	E952.8	E962.2	E982.8
cyclohexane	982.8	E862.4	—	E950.9	E962.1	E980.9
cyclohexanone	982.8	E862.4	—	E950.9	E962.1	E980.9
dihydromorphinone	965.09	E850.2	E935.2	E950.0	E962.0	E980.0
ergometrine	975.0	E858.6	E945.0	E950.4	E962.0	E980.4
ergonovine	975.0	E858.6	E945.0	E950.4	E962.0	E980.4
ethyl ketone	982.8	E862.4	—	E950.9	E962.1	E980.9
hydrazine	983.9	E864.3	—	E950.7	E962.1	E980.6
isobutyl ketone	982.8	E862.4	—	E950.9	E962.1	E980.9
morphine NEC	965.09	E850.2	E935.2	E950.0	E962.0	E980.0
parafynol	967.8	E852.8	E937.8	E950.2	E962.0	E980.2
parathion	989.3	E863.1	—	E950.6	E962.1	E980.7
pentynol NEC	967.8	E852.8	E937.8	E950.2	E962.0	E980.2
peridol	969.2	E853.1	E939.2	E950.3	E962.0	E980.3
phenidate	969.73	E854.2	E939.7	E950.3	E962.0	E980.3
prednisolone	962.0	E858.0	E932.0	E950.4	E962.0	E980.4
ENT agent	976.6	E858.7	E946.6	E950.4	E962.0	E980.4
ophthalmic preparation	976.5	E858.7	E946.5	E950.4	E962.0	E980.4
topical NEC	976.0	E858.7	E946.0	E950.4	E962.0	E980.4
propylcarbinol	980.8	E860.8	—	E950.9	E962.1	E980.9

Methyl — continued

	Poisoning	Accident	Therapeutic Use	Suicide Attempt	Assault	Undetermined
External Cause (E-Code)						
rosaniline NEC	976.0	E858.7	E946.0	E950.4	E962.0	E980.4
salicylate NEC	976.3	E858.7	E946.3	E950.4	E962.0	E980.4
sulfate (fumes)	987.8	E869.8	—	E952.8	E962.2	E982.8
liquid	983.9	E864.3	—	E950.7	E962.1	E980.6
sulfonal	967.8	E852.8	E937.8	E950.2	E962.0	E980.2
testosterone	962.1	E858.0	E932.1	E950.4	E962.0	E980.4
thiouracil	962.8	E858.0	E932.8	E950.4	E962.0	E980.4
Methylated spirit	980.0	E860.1	—	E950.9	E962.1	E980.9
Methyldopa	972.6	E858.3	E942.6	E950.4	E962.0	E980.4
Methylene						
blue	961.9	E857	E931.9	E950.4	E962.0	E980.4
chloride or dichloride (solvent) NEC	982.3	E862.4	—	E950.9	E962.1	E980.9
Methylhexabital	967.0	E851	E937.0	E950.1	E962.0	E980.1
Methylparaben (ophthalmic)	976.5	E858.7	E946.5	E950.4	E962.0	E980.4
Methyprylon	967.5	E852.4	E937.5	E950.2	E962.0	E980.2
Methysergide	971.3	E855.6	E941.3	E950.4	E962.0	E980.4
Metoclopramide	963.0	E858.1	E933.0	E950.4	E962.0	E980.4
Metofoline	965.7	E850.7	E935.7	E950.0	E962.0	E980.0
Metopon	965.09	E850.2	E935.2	E950.0	E962.0	E980.0
Metronidazole	961.5	E857	E931.5	E950.4	E962.0	E980.4
Metycaine	968.9	E855.2	E938.9	E950.4	E962.0	E980.4
infiltration (subcutaneous)	968.5	E855.2	E938.5	E950.4	E962.0	E980.4
nerve block (peripheral) (plexus)	968.6	E855.2	E938.6	E950.4	E962.0	E980.4
topical (surface)	968.5	E855.2	E938.5	E950.4	E962.0	E980.4
Metyrapone	977.8	E858.8	E947.8	E950.4	E962.0	E980.4
Mevinphos	989.3	E863.1	—	E950.6	E962.1	E980.7
Mezereon (berries)	988.2	E865.3	—	E950.9	E962.1	E980.9
Micatin	976.0	E858.7	E946.0	E950.4	E962.0	E980.4
Miconazole	976.0	E858.7	E946.0	E950.4	E962.0	E980.4
Midol	965.1	E850.3	E935.3	E950.0	E962.0	E980.0
Mifepristone	962.9	E858.0	E932.9	E950.4	E962.0	E980.4
Milk of magnesia	973.0	E858.4	E943.0	E950.4	E962.0	E980.4
Millipede (tropical) (venomous)	989.5	E905.4	—	E950.9	E962.1	E980.9
Miltown	969.5	E853.8	E939.5	E950.3	E962.0	E980.3
Mineral						
oil (medicinal)	973.2	E858.4	E943.2	E950.4	E962.0	E980.4
nonmedicinal	981	E862.1	—	E950.9	E962.1	E980.9
topical	976.3	E858.7	E946.3	E950.4	E962.0	E980.4
salts NEC	974.6	E858.5	E944.6	E950.4	E962.0	E980.4
spirits	981	E862.0	—	E950.9	E962.1	E980.9
Minocycline	960.4	E856	E930.4	E950.4	E962.0	E980.4
Mithramycin (antineoplastic)	960.7	E856	E930.7	E950.4	E962.0	E980.4
Mitobronitol	963.1	E858.1	E933.1	E950.4	E962.0	E980.4
Mitomycin (antineoplastic)	960.7	E856	E930.7	E950.4	E962.0	E980.4
Mitotane	963.1	E858.1	E933.1	E950.4	E962.0	E980.4
Moderil	972.6	E858.3	E942.6	E950.4	E962.0	E980.4
Mogadon — see Nitrazepam						
Molindone	969.3	E853.8	E939.3	E950.3	E962.0	E980.3
Monistat	976.0	E858.7	E946.0	E950.4	E962.0	E980.4
Monkshood	988.2	E865.4	—	E950.9	E962.1	E980.9
Monoamine oxidase inhibitors	969.01	E854.0	E939.0	E950.3	E962.0	E980.3
Monochlorobenzene	982.0	E862.4	—	E950.9	E962.1	E980.9
Monosodium glutamate	989.89	E866.8	—	E950.9	E962.1	E980.9
Monoxide, carbon — see Carbon, monoxide						
Moperone	969.2	E853.1	E939.2	E950.3	E962.0	E980.3
Morning glory seeds	969.6	E854.1	E939.6	E950.3	E962.0	E980.3
Moroxydine (hydrochloride)	961.7	E857	E931.7	E950.4	E962.0	E980.4
Morphazinamide	961.8	E857	E931.8	E950.4	E962.0	E980.4
Morphinans	965.09	E850.2	E935.2	E950.0	E962.0	E980.0
Morphine NEC	965.09	E850.2	E935.2	E950.0	E962.0	E980.0
antagonists	970.1	E854.3	E940.1	E950.4	E962.0	E980.4
Morpholinylethylmorphine	965.09	E850.2	E935.2	E950.0	E962.0	E980.0
Morrhuate sodium	972.7	E858.3	E942.7	E950.4	E962.0	E980.4
Moth balls — see also Pesticides	989.4	E863.4	—	E950.6	E962.1	E980.7
naphthalene	983.0	E863.4	—	E950.7	E962.1	E980.6
Motor exhaust gas — see Carbon, monoxide, exhaust gas						
Mouth wash	976.6	E858.7	E946.6	E950.4	E962.0	E980.4

	Poisoning	Accident	Therapeutic Use	Suicide Attempt	Assault	Undetermined
External Cause (E-Code)						
Mucolytic agent	975.5	E858.6	E945.5	E950.4	E962.0	E980.4
Mucomyst	975.5	E858.6	E945.5	E950.4	E962.0	E980.4
Mucous membrane agents						
(external)	976.9	E858.7	E946.9	E950.4	E962.0	E980.4
specified NEC	976.8	E858.7	E946.8	E950.4	E962.0	E980.4
Mumps						
immune globulin (human)	964.6	E858.2	E934.6	E950.4	E962.0	E980.4
skin test antigen	977.8	E858.8	E947.8	E950.4	E962.0	E980.4
vaccine	979.6	E858.8	E949.6	E950.4	E962.0	E980.4
Mumpsvax	979.6	E858.8	E949.6	E950.4	E962.0	E980.4
Muriatic acid — see Hydrochloric acid						
Muscarine	971.0	E855.3	E941.0	E950.4	E962.0	E980.4
Muscle affecting agents						
NEC	975.3	E858.6	E945.3	E950.4	E962.0	E980.4
oxytocic	975.0	E858.6	E945.0	E950.4	E962.0	E980.4
relaxants	975.3	E858.6	E945.3	E950.4	E962.0	E980.4
central nervous system	968.0	E855.1	E938.0	E950.4	E962.0	E980.4
skeletal	975.2	E858.6	E945.2	E950.4	E962.0	E980.4
smooth	975.1	E858.6	E945.1	E950.4	E962.0	E980.4
Mushrooms, noxious	988.1	E865.5	—	E950.9	E962.1	E980.9
Mussel, noxious	988.0	E865.1	—	E950.9	E962.1	E980.9
Mustard (emetic)	973.6	E858.4	E943.6	E950.4	E962.0	E980.4
gas	987.8	E869.8	—	E952.8	E962.2	E982.8
nitrogen	963.1	E858.1	E933.1	E950.4	E962.0	E980.4
Mustine	963.1	E858.1	E933.1	E950.4	E962.0	E980.4
M-vac	979.4	E858.8	E949.4	E950.4	E962.0	E980.4
Mycifradin	960.8	E856	E930.8	E950.4	E962.0	E980.4
topical	976.0	E858.7	E946.0	E950.4	E962.0	E980.4
Mycitracin	960.8	E856	E930.8	E950.4	E962.0	E980.4
ophthalmic preparation	976.5	E858.7	E946.5	E950.4	E962.0	E980.4
Mycostatin	960.1	E856	E930.1	E950.4	E962.0	E980.4
topical	976.0	E858.7	E946.0	E950.4	E962.0	E980.4
Mydriacyl	971.1	E855.4	E941.1	E950.4	E962.0	E980.4
Myelobromal	963.1	E858.1	E933.1	E950.4	E962.0	E980.4
Myleran	963.1	E858.1	E933.1	E950.4	E962.0	E980.4
Myochrysin(e)	965.69	E850.6	E935.6	E950.0	E962.0	E980.0
Myoneural blocking agents	975.2	E858.6	E945.2	E950.4	E962.0	E980.4
Myristica fragrans	988.2	E865.3	—	E950.9	E962.1	E980.9
Myristicin	988.2	E865.3	—	E950.9	E962.1	E980.9
Mysoline	966.3	E855.0	E936.3	E950.4	E962.0	E980.4
Nafcillin (sodium)	960.0	E856	E930.0	E950.4	E962.0	E980.4
Nail polish remover	982.8	E862.4	—	E950.9	E962.1	E908.9
Nalidixic acid	961.9	E857	E931.9	E950.4	E962.0	E980.4
Nalorphine	970.1	E854.3	E940.1	E950.4	E962.0	E980.4
Naloxone	970.1	E854.3	E940.1	E950.4	E962.0	E980.4
Nandrolone (decanoate) (phenproprionate)	962.1	E858.0	E932.1	E950.4	E962.0	E980.4
Naphazoline	971.2	E855.5	E941.2	E950.4	E962.0	E980.4
Naphtha (painter's) (petroleum)	981	E862.0	—	E950.9	E962.1	E980.9
solvent	981	E862.0	—	E950.9	E962.1	E980.9
vapor	987.1	E869.8	—	E952.8	E962.2	E982.8
Naphthalene (chlorinated)	983.0	E864.0	—	E950.7	E962.1	E980.6
insecticide or moth repellent	983.0	E863.4	—	E950.7	E962.1	E980.6
vapor	987.8	E869.8	—	E952.8	E962.2	E982.8
Naphthol	983.0	E864.0	—	E950.7	E962.1	E980.6
Naphthylamine	983.0	E864.0	—	E950.7	E962.1	E980.6
Naprosyn — see Naproxen						
Naproxen	965.61	E850.6	E935.6	E950.0	E962.0	E980.0
Narcotic (drug)	967.9	E852.9	E937.9	E950.2	E962.0	E980.2
analgesic NEC	965.8	E850.8	E935.8	E950.0	E962.0	E980.0
antagonist	970.1	E854.3	E940.1	E950.4	E962.0	E980.4
specified NEC	967.8	E852.8	E937.8	E950.2	E962.0	E980.2
Narcotine	975.4	E858.6	E945.4	E950.4	E962.0	E980.4
Nardil	969.01	E854.0	E939.0	E950.3	E962.0	E980.3
Natrium cyanide — see Cyanide(s)						
Natural						
blood (product)	964.7	E858.2	E934.7	E950.4	E962.0	E980.4
gas (piped)	987.1	E867	—	E951.0	E962.2	E981.0
incomplete combustion	986	E867	—	E951.0	E962.2	E981.0
Nealbarbital, nealbarbitone	967.0	E851	E937.0	E950.1	E962.0	E980.1
Nectadon	975.4	E858.6	E945.4	E950.4	E962.0	E980.4
Nematocyst (sting)	989.5	E905.6	—	E950.9	E962.1	E980.9
Nembutal	967.0	E851	E937.0	E950.1	E962.0	E980.1
Neoarsphenamine	961.1	E857	E931.1	E950.4	E962.0	E980.4

	Poisoning	Accident	Therapeutic Use	Suicide Attempt	Assault	Undetermined
Neocinchophen	974.7	E858.5	E944.7	E950.4	E962.0	E980.4
Neomycin	960.8	E856	E930.8	E950.4	E962.0	E980.4
ENT agent	976.6	E858.7	E946.6	E950.4	E962.0	E980.4
ophthalmic preparation	976.5	E858.7	E946.5	E950.4	E962.0	E980.4
topical NEC	976.0	E858.7	E946.0	E950.4	E962.0	E980.4
Neonal	967.0	E851	E937.0	E950.1	E962.0	E980.1
Neoprontosil	961.0	E857	E931.0	E950.4	E962.0	E980.4
Neosalvarsan	961.1	E857	E931.1	E950.4	E962.0	E980.4
Neosilversalvarsan	961.1	E857	E931.1	E950.4	E962.0	E980.4
Neosporin	960.8	E856	E930.8	E950.4	E962.0	E980.4
ENT agent	976.6	E858.7	E946.6	E950.4	E962.0	E980.4
opthalmic preparation	976.5	E858.7	E946.5	E950.4	E962.0	E980.4
topical NEC	976.0	E858.7	E946.0	E950.4	E962.0	E980.4
Neostigmine	971.0	E855.3	E941.0	E950.4	E962.0	E980.4
Neraval	967.0	E851	E937.0	E950.1	E962.0	E980.1
Neravan	967.0	E851	E937.0	E950.1	E962.0	E980.1
Nerium oleander	988.2	E865.4	—	E950.9	E962.1	E980.9
Nerve gases (war)	987.9	E869.9	—	E952.9	E962.2	E982.9
Nesacaine	968.9	E855.2	E938.9	E950.4	E962.0	E980.4
infiltration (subcutaneous)	968.5	E855.2	E938.5	E950.4	E962.0	E980.4
nerve block (peripheral) (plexus)	968.6	E855.2	E938.6	E950.4	E962.0	E980.4
Neurobarb	967.0	E851	E937.0	E950.1	E962.0	E980.1
Neuroleptics NEC	969.3	E853.8	E939.3	E950.3	E962.0	E980.3
Neuroprotective agent	977.8	E858.8	E947.8	E950.4	E962.0	E980.4
Neutral spirits	980.0	E860.1	—	E950.9	E962.1	E980.9
beverage	980.0	E860.0	—	E950.9	E962.1	E980.9
Niacin, niacinamide	972.2	E858.3	E942.2	E950.4	E962.0	E980.4
Nialamide	969.01	E854.0	E939.0	E950.3	E962.0	E980.3
Nickle (carbonyl) (compounds) (fumes) (tetracarbonyl) (vapor)	985.8	E866.4	—	E950.9	E962.1	E980.9
Niclosamide	961.6	E857	E931.6	E950.4	E962.0	E980.4
Nicomorphine	965.09	E850.2	E935.2	E950.0	E962.0	E980.0
Nicotinamide	972.2	E858.3	E942.2	E950.4	E962.0	E980.4
Nicotine (insecticide) (spray) (sulfate) NEC	989.4	E863.4	—	E950.6	E962.1	E980.7
not insecticide	989.89	E866.8	—	E950.9	E962.1	E980.9
Nicotinic acid (derivatives)	972.2	E858.3	E942.2	E950.4	E962.0	E980.4
Nicotinyl alcohol	972.2	E858.3	E942.2	E950.4	E962.0	E980.4
Nicoumalone	964.2	E858.2	E934.2	E950.4	E962.0	E980.4
Nifenazone	965.5	E850.5	E935.5	E950.0	E962.0	E980.0
Nifuraldezone	961.9	E857	E931.9	E950.4	E962.0	E980.4
Nightshade (deadly)	988.2	E865.4	—	E950.9	E962.1	E980.9
Nikethamide	970.0	E854.3	E940.0	E950.4	E962.0	E980.4
Nilstat	960.1	E856	E930.1	E950.4	E962.0	E980.4
topical	976.0	E858.7	E946.0	E950.4	E962.0	E980.4
Nimodipine	977.8	E858.8	E947.8	E950.4	E962.0	E980.4
Niridazole	961.6	E857	E931.6	E950.4	E962.0	E980.4
Nisentil	965.09	E850.2	E935.2	E950.0	E962.0	E980.0
Nitrates	972.4	E858.3	E942.4	E950.4	E962.0	E980.4
Nitrazepam	969.4	E853.2	E939.4	E950.3	E962.0	E980.3
Nitric						
acid (liquid)	983.1	E864.1	—	E950.7	E962.1	E980.6
vapor	987.8	E869.8	—	E952.8	E962.2	E982.8
oxide (gas)	987.2	E869.0	—	E952.8	E962.2	E982.8
Nitrite, amyl (medicinal) (vapor)	972.4	E858.3	E942.4	E950.4	E962.0	E980.4
Nitroaniline	983.0	E864.0	—	E950.7	E962.1	E980.6
vapor	987.8	E869.8	—	E952.8	E962.2	E982.8
Nitrobenzene, nitrobenzol	983.0	E864.0	—	E950.7	E962.1	E980.6
vapor	987.8	E869.8	—	E952.8	E962.2	E982.8
Nitrocellulose	976.3	E858.7	E946.3	E950.4	E962.0	E980.4
Nitrofuran derivatives	961.9	E857	E931.9	E950.4	E962.0	E980.4
Nitrofurantoin	961.9	E857	E931.9	E950.4	E962.0	E980.4
Nitrofurazone	976.0	E858.7	E946.0	E950.4	E962.0	E980.4
Nitrogen (dioxide) (gas) (oxide)	987.2	E869.0	—	E952.8	E962.2	E982.8
mustard (antineoplastic)	963.1	E858.1	E933.1	E950.4	E962.0	E980.4
nonmedicinal	989.89	E866.8	—	E950.9	E962.1	E980.9
fumes	987.8	E869.8	—	E952.8	E962.2	E982.8
Nitroglycerin, nitroglycerol (medicinal)	972.4	E858.3	E942.4	E950.4	E962.0	E980.4
Nitrohydrochloric acid	983.1	E864.1	—	E950.7	E962.1	E980.6
Nitromersol	976.0	E858.7	E946.0	E950.4	E962.0	E980.4
Nitronaphthalene	983.0	E864.0	—	E950.7	E962.1	E980.6
Nitrophenol	983.0	E864.0	—	E950.7	E962.2	E980.6
Nitrothiazol	961.6	E857	E931.6	E950.4	E962.0	E980.4
Nitrotoluene, nitrotoluol	983.0	E864.0	—	E950.7	E962.1	E980.6
Nitrotoluene, nitrotoluol — continued						
vapor	987.8	E869.8	—	E952.8	E962.2	E982.8
Nitrous	968.2	E855.1	E938.2	E950.4	E962.0	E980.4
acid (liquid)	983.1	E864.1	—	E950.7	E962.1	E980.6
fumes	987.2	E869.0	—	E952.8	E962.2	E982.8
oxide (anesthetic) NEC	968.2	E855.1	E938.2	E950.4	E962.0	E980.4
Nitrozone	976.0	E858.7	E946.0	E950.4	E962.0	E980.4
Noctec	967.1	E852.0	E937.1	E950.2	E962.0	E980.2
Noludar	967.5	E852.4	E937.5	E950.2	E962.0	E980.2
Noptil	967.0	E851	E937.0	E950.1	E962.0	E980.1
Noradrenalin	971.2	E855.5	E941.2	E950.4	E962.0	E980.4
Noramidopyrine	965.5	E850.5	E935.5	E950.0	E962.0	E980.0
Norepinephrine	971.2	E855.5	E941.2	E950.4	E962.0	E980.4
Norethandrolone	962.1	E858.0	E932.1	E950.4	E962.0	E980.4
Norethindrone	962.2	E858.0	E932.2	E950.4	E962.0	E980.4
Norethisterone	962.2	E858.0	E932.2	E950.4	E962.0	E980.4
Norethynodrel	962.2	E858.0	E932.2	E950.4	E962.0	E980.4
Norlestrin	962.2	E858.0	E932.2	E950.4	E962.0	E980.4
Norlutin	962.2	E858.0	E932.2	E950.4	E962.0	E980.4
Normison — see Benzodiazepines						
Normorphine	965.09	E850.2	E935.2	E950.0	E962.0	E980.0
Nortriptyline	969.05	E854.0	E939.0	E950.3	E962.0	E980.3
Noscapine	975.4	E858.6	E945.4	E950.4	E962.0	E980.4
Nose preparations	976.6	E858.7	E946.6	E950.4	E962.0	E980.4
Novobiocin	960.8	E856	E930.8	E950.4	E962.0	E980.4
Novocain (infiltration) (topical)	968.5	E855.2	E938.5	E950.4	E962.0	E980.4
nerve block (peripheral) (plexus)	968.6	E855.2	E938.6	E950.4	E962.0	E980.4
spinal	968.7	E855.2	E938.7	E950.4	E962.0	E980.4
Noxythiolin	961.9	E857	E931.9	E950.4	E962.0	E980.4
NPH Iletin (insulin)	962.3	E858.0	E932.3	E950.4	E962.0	E980.4
Numorphan	965.09	E850.2	E935.2	E950.0	E962.0	E980.0
Nunol	967.0	E851	E937.0	E950.1	E962.0	E980.1
Nupercaine (spinal anesthetic)	968.7	E855.2	E938.7	E950.4	E962.0	E980.4
topical (surface)	968.5	E855.2	E938.5	E950.4	E962.0	E980.4
Nutmeg oil (liniment)	976.3	E858.7	E946.3	E950.4	E962.0	E980.4
Nux vomica	989.1	E863.7	—	E950.6	E962.1	E980.7
Nydrazid	961.8	E857	E931.8	E950.4	E962.0	E980.4
Nylidrin	971.2	E855.5	E941.2	E950.4	E962.0	E980.4
Nystatin	960.1	E856	E930.1	E950.4	E962.0	E980.4
topical	976.0	E858.7	E946.0	E950.4	E962.0	E980.4
Nytol	963.0	E858.1	E933.0	E950.4	E962.0	E980.4
Oblivion	967.8	E852.8	E937.8	E950.2	E962.0	E980.2
Octyl nitrite	972.4	E858.3	E942.4	E950.4	E962.0	E980.4
Oestradiol (cypionate) (dipropionate) (valerate)	962.2	E858.0	E932.2	E950.4	E962.0	E980.4
Oestriol	962.2	E858.0	E932.2	E950.4	E962.0	E980.4
Oestrone	962.2	E858.0	E932.2	E950.4	E962.0	E980.4
Oil (of) NEC	989.89	E866.8	—	E950.9	E962.1	E980.9
bitter almond	989.0	E866.8	—	E950.9	E962.1	E980.9
camphor	976.1	E858.7	E946.1	E950.4	E962.0	E980.4
colors	989.89	E861.6	—	E950.9	E962.1	E980.9
fumes	987.8	E869.8	—	E952.8	E962.2	E982.8
lubricating	981	E862.2	—	E950.9	E962.1	E980.9
specified source, other — see substance specified						
vitriol (liquid)	983.1	E864.1	—	E950.7	E962.1	E980.6
fumes	987.8	E869.8	—	E952.8	E962.2	E982.8
wintergreen (bitter) NEC	976.3	E858.7	E946.3	E950.4	E962.0	E980.4
Ointments NEC	976.9	E858.7	E946.9	E950.4	E962.0	E980.4
Oleander	988.2	E865.4	—	E950.9	E962.1	E980.9
Oleandomycin	960.3	E856	E930.3	E950.4	E962.0	E980.4
Oleovitamin A	963.5	E858.1	E933.5	E950.4	E962.0	E980.4
Oleum ricini	973.1	E858.4	E943.1	E950.4	E962.0	E980.4
Olive oil (medicinal) NEC	973.2	E858.4	E943.2	E950.4	E962.0	E980.4
OMPA	989.3	E863.1	—	E950.6	E962.1	E980.7
Oncovin	963.1	E858.1	E933.1	E950.4	E962.0	E980.4
Ophthaine	968.5	E855.2	E938.5	E950.4	E962.0	E980.4
Ophthetic	968.5	E855.2	E938.5	E950.4	E962.0	E980.4
Opiates, opioids, opium NEC	965.00	E850.2	E935.2	E950.0	E962.0	E980.0
antagonists	970.1	E854.3	E940.1	E950.4	E962.0	E980.4
Oracon	962.2	E858.0	E932.2	E950.4	E962.0	E980.4
Oragrafin	977.8	E858.8	E947.8	E950.4	E962.0	E980.4
Oral contraceptives	962.2	E858.0	E932.2	E950.4	E962.0	E980.4
Orciprenaline	975.1	E858.6	E945.1	E950.4	E962.0	E980.4
Organidin	975.5	E858.6	E945.5	E950.4	E962.0	E980.4
Organophosphates	989.3	E863.1	—	E950.6	E962.1	E980.7

Substance	Poisoning	Accident	Therapeutic Use	Suicide Attempt	Assault	Undetermined
Orimune	979.5	E858.8	E949.5	E950.4	E962.0	E980.4
Orinase	962.3	E858.0	E932.3	E950.4	E962.0	E980.4
Orphenadrine	966.4	E855.0	E936.4	E950.4	E962.0	E980.4
Ortal (sodium)	967.0	E851	E937.0	E950.1	E962.0	E980.1
Orthoboric acid	976.0	E858.7	E946.0	E950.4	E962.0	E980.4
ENT agent	976.6	E858.7	E946.6	E950.4	E962.0	E980.4
ophthalmic preparation	976.5	E858.7	E946.5	E950.4	E962.0	E980.4
Orthocaine	968.5	E855.2	E938.5	E950.4	E962.0	E980.4
Ortho-Novum	962.2	E858.0	E932.2	E950.4	E962.0	E980.4
Orthotolidine (reagent)	977.8	E858.8	E947.8	E950.4	E962.0	E980.4
Osmic acid (liquid)	983.1	E864.1	—	E950.7	E962.1	E980.6
fumes	987.8	E869.8	—	E952.8	E962.2	E982.8
Osmotic diuretics	974.4	E858.5	E944.4	E950.4	E962.0	E980.4
Ouabain	972.1	E858.3	E942.1	E950.4	E962.0	E980.4
Ovarian hormones (synthetic substitutes)	962.2	E858.0	E932.2	E950.4	E962.0	E980.4
Ovral	962.2	E858.0	E932.2	E950.4	E962.0	E980.4
Ovulation suppressants	962.2	E858.0	E932.2	E950.4	E962.0	E980.4
Ovulen	962.2	E858.0	E932.2	E950.4	E962.0	E980.4
Oxacillin (sodium)	960.0	E856	E930.0	E950.4	E962.0	E980.4
Oxalic acid	983.1	E864.1	—	E950.7	E962.1	E980.6
Oxanamide	969.5	E853.8	E939.5	E950.3	E962.0	E980.3
Oxandrolone	962.1	E858.0	E932.1	E950.4	E962.0	E980.4
Oxaprozin	965.61	E850.6	E935.6	E950.0	E962.0	E980.0
Oxazepam	969.4	E853.2	E939.4	E950.3	E962.0	E980.3
Oxazolidine derivatives	966.0	E855.0	E936.0	E950.4	E962.0	E980.4
Ox bile extract	973.4	E858.4	E943.4	E950.4	E962.0	E980.4
Oxedrine	971.2	E855.5	E941.2	E950.4	E962.0	E980.4
Oxeladin	975.4	E858.6	E945.4	E950.4	E962.0	E980.4
Oxethazaine NEC	968.5	E855.2	E938.5	E950.4	E962.0	E980.4
Oxidizing agents NEC	983.9	E864.3	—	E950.7	E962.1	E980.6
Oxolinic acid	961.3	E857	E931.3	E950.4	E962.0	E980.4
Oxophenarsine	961.1	E857	E931.1	E950.4	E962.0	E980.4
Oxsoralen	976.3	E858.7	E946.3	E950.4	E962.0	E980.4
Oxtriphylline	975.7	E858.6	E945.7	E950.4	E962.0	E980.4
Oxybuprocaine	968.5	E855.2	E938.5	E950.4	E962.0	E980.4
Oxybutynin	975.1	E858.6	E945.1	E950.4	E962.0	E980.4
Oxycodone	965.09	E850.2	E935.2	E950.0	E962.0	E980.0
Oxygen	987.8	E869.8	—	E952.8	E962.2	E982.8
Oxylone	976.0	E858.7	E946.0	E950.4	E962.0	E980.4
ophthalmic preparation	976.5	E858.7	E946.5	E950.4	E962.0	E980.4
Oxymesterone	962.1	E858.0	E932.1	E950.4	E962.0	E980.4
Oxymetazoline	971.2	E855.5	E941.2	E950.4	E962.0	E980.4
Oxymetholone	962.1	E858.0	E932.1	E950.4	E962.0	E980.4
Oxymorphone	965.09	E850.2	E935.2	E950.0	E962.0	E980.0
Oxypertine	969.09	E854.0	E939.0	E950.3	E962.0	E980.3
Oxyphenbutazone	965.5	E850.5	E935.5	E950.0	E962.0	E980.0
Oxyphencyclimine	971.1	E855.4	E941.1	E950.4	E962.0	E980.4
Oxyphenisatin	973.1	E858.4	E943.1	E950.4	E962.0	E980.4
Oxyphenonium	971.1	E855.4	E941.1	E950.4	E962.0	E980.4
Oxyquinoline	961.3	E857	E931.3	E950.4	E962.0	E980.4
Oxytetracycline	960.4	E856	E930.4	E950.4	E962.0	E980.4
Oxytocics	975.0	E858.6	E945.0	E950.4	E962.0	E980.4
Oxytocin	975.0	E858.6	E945.0	E950.4	E962.0	E980.4
Ozone	987.8	E869.8	—	E952.8	E962.2	E982.8
PABA	976.3	E858.7	E946.3	E950.4	E962.0	E980.4
Packed red cells	964.7	E858.2	E934.7	E950.4	E962.0	E980.4
Paint NEC	989.89	E861.6	—	E950.9	E962.1	E980.9
cleaner	982.8	E862.9	—	E950.9	E962.1	E980.9
fumes NEC	987.8	E869.8	—	E952.8	E962.1	E982.8
lead (fumes)	984.0	E861.5	—	E950.9	E962.1	E980.9
solvent NEC	982.8	E862.9	—	E950.9	E962.1	E980.9
stripper	982.8	E862.9	—	E950.9	E962.1	E980.9
Palfium	965.09	E850.2	E935.2	E950.0	E962.0	E980.0
Palivizumab	979.9	E858.8	E949.6	E950.4	E962.0	E980.4
Paludrine	961.4	E857	E931.4	E950.4	E962.0	E980.4
PAM	977.2	E855.8	E947.2	E950.4	E962.0	E980.4
Pamaquine (naphthoate)	961.4	E857	E931.4	E950.4	E962.0	E980.4
Pamprin	965.1	E850.3	E935.3	E950.0	E962.0	E980.0
Panadol	965.4	E850.4	E935.4	E950.0	E962.0	E980.0
Pancreatic dornase (mucolytic)	963.4	E858.1	E933.4	E950.4	E962.0	E980.4
Pancreatin	973.4	E858.4	E943.4	E950.4	E962.0	E980.4
Pancrelipase	973.4	E858.4	E943.4	E950.4	E962.0	E980.4
Pangamic acid	963.5	E858.1	E933.5	E950.4	E962.0	E980.4
Panthenol	963.5	E858.1	E933.5	E950.4	E962.0	E980.4
topical	976.8	E858.7	E946.8	E950.4	E962.0	E980.4
Pantopaque	977.8	E858.8	E947.8	E950.4	E962.0	E980.4
Pantopon	965.00	E850.2	E935.2	E950.0	E962.0	E980.0
Pantothenic acid	963.5	E858.1	E933.5	E950.4	E962.0	E980.4
Panwarfin	964.2	E858.2	E934.2	E950.4	E962.0	E980.4
Papain	973.4	E858.4	E943.4	E950.4	E962.0	E980.4
Papaverine	972.5	E858.3	E942.5	E950.4	E962.0	E980.4
Para-aminobenzoic acid	976.3	E858.7	E946.3	E950.4	E962.0	E980.4
Para-aminophenol derivatives	965.4	E850.4	E935.4	E950.0	E962.0	E980.0
Para-aminosalicylic acid (derivatives)	961.8	E857	E931.8	E950.4	E962.0	E980.4
Paracetaldehyde (medicinal)	967.2	E852.1	E937.2	E950.2	E962.0	E980.2
Paracetamol	965.4	E850.4	E935.4	E950.0	E962.0	E980.0
Paracodin	965.09	E850.2	E935.2	E950.0	E962.0	E980.0
Paradione	966.0	E855.0	E936.0	E950.4	E962.0	E980.4
Paraffin(s) (wax)	981	E862.3	—	E950.9	E962.1	E980.9
liquid (medicinal)	973.2	E858.4	E943.2	E950.4	E962.0	E980.4
nonmedicinal (oil)	981	E962.1	—	E950.9	—	E980.9
Paraldehyde (medicinal)	967.2	E852.1	E937.2	E950.2	E962.0	E980.2
Paramethadione	966.0	E855.0	E936.0	E950.4	E962.0	E980.4
Paramethasone	962.0	E858.0	E932.0	E950.4	E962.0	E980.4
Paraquat	989.4	E863.5	—	E950.6	E962.1	E980.7
Parasympatholytics	971.1	E855.4	E941.1	E950.4	E962.0	E980.4
Parasympathomimetics	971.0	E855.3	E941.0	E950.4	E962.0	E980.4
Parathion	989.3	E863.1	—	E950.6	E962.1	E980.7
Parathormone	962.6	E858.0	E932.6	E950.4	E962.0	E980.4
Parathyroid (derivatives)	962.6	E858.0	E932.6	E950.4	E962.0	E980.4
Paratyphoid vaccine	978.1	E858.8	E948.1	E950.4	E962.0	E980.4
Paredrine	971.2	E855.5	E941.2	E950.4	E962.0	E980.4
Paregoric	965.00	E850.2	E935.2	E950.0	E962.0	E980.0
Pargyline	972.3	E858.3	E942.3	E950.4	E962.0	E980.4
Paris green	985.1	E866.3	—	E950.8	E962.1	E980.8
insecticide	985.1	E863.4	—	E950.8	E962.1	E980.8
Parnate	969.01	E854.0	E939.0	E950.3	E962.0	E980.3
Paromomycin	960.8	E856	E930.8	E950.4	E962.0	E980.4
Paroxypropione	963.1	E858.1	E933.1	E950.4	E962.0	E980.4
Parzone	965.09	E850.2	E935.2	E950.0	E962.0	E980.0
PAS	961.8	E857	E931.8	E950.4	E962.0	E980.4
PCBs	981	E862.3	—	E950.9	E962.1	E980.9
PCP (pentachlorophenol)	989.4	E863.6	—	E950.6	E962.1	E980.7
herbicide	989.4	E863.5	—	E950.6	E962.1	E980.7
insecticide	989.4	E863.4	—	E950.6	E962.1	E980.7
phencyclidine	968.3	E855.1	E938.3	E950.4	E962.0	E980.4
Peach kernel oil (emulsion)	973.2	E858.4	E943.2	E950.4	E962.0	E980.4
Peanut oil (emulsion) NEC	973.2	E858.4	E943.2	E950.4	E962.0	E980.4
topical	976.3	E858.7	E946.3	E950.4	E962.0	E980.4
Pearly Gates (morning glory seeds)	969.6	E854.1	E939.6	E950.3	E962.0	E980.3
Pecazine	969.1	E853.0	E939.1	E950.3	E962.0	E980.3
Pecilocin	960.1	E856	E930.1	E950.4	E962.0	E980.4
Pectin (with kaolin) NEC	973.5	E858.4	E943.5	E950.4	E962.0	E980.4
Pelletierine tannate	961.6	E857	E931.6	E950.4	E962.0	E980.4
Pemoline	969.79	E854.2	E939.7	E950.3	E962.0	E980.3
Pempidine	972.3	E858.3	E942.3	E950.4	E962.0	E980.4
Penamecillin	960.0	E856	E930.0	E950.4	E962.0	E980.4
Penethamate hydriodide	960.0	E856	E930.0	E950.4	E962.0	E980.4
Penicillamine	963.8	E858.1	E933.8	E950.4	E962.0	E980.4
Penicillin (any type)	960.0	E856	E930.0	E950.4	E962.0	E980.4
Penicillinase	963.4	E858.1	E933.4	E950.4	E962.0	E980.4
Pentachlorophenol (fungicide)	989.4	E863.6	—	E950.6	E962.1	E980.7
herbicide	989.4	E863.5	—	E950.6	E962.1	E980.7
insecticide	989.4	E863.4	—	E950.6	E962.1	E980.7
Pentaerythritol	972.4	E858.3	E942.4	E950.4	E962.0	E980.4
chloral	967.1	E852.0	E937.1	E950.2	E962.0	E980.2
tetranitrate NEC	972.4	E858.3	E942.4	E950.4	E962.0	E980.4
Pentagastrin	977.8	E858.8	E947.8	E950.4	E962.0	E980.4
Pentalin	982.3	E862.4	—	E950.9	E962.1	E980.9
Pentamethonium (bromide)	972.3	E858.3	E942.3	E950.4	E962.0	E980.4
Pentamidine	961.5	E857	E931.5	E950.4	E962.0	E980.4
Pentanol	980.8	E860.8	—	E950.9	E962.1	E980.9
Pentaquine	961.4	E857	E931.4	E950.4	E962.0	E980.4
Pentazocine	965.8	E850.8	E935.8	E950.0	E962.0	E980.0
Penthienate	971.1	E855.4	E941.1	E950.4	E962.0	E980.4
Pentobarbital, pentobarbitone (sodium)	967.0	E851	E937.0	E950.1	E962.0	E980.1
Pentolinium (tartrate)	972.3	E858.3	E942.3	E950.4	E962.0	E980.4
Pentothal	968.3	E855.1	E938.3	E950.4	E962.0	E980.4
Pentylenetetrazol	970.0	E854.3	E940.0	E950.4	E962.0	E980.4
Pentylsalicylamide	961.8	E857	E931.8	E950.4	E962.0	E980.4
Pepsin	973.4	E858.4	E943.4	E950.4	E962.0	E980.4
Peptavlon	977.8	E858.8	E947.8	E950.4	E962.0	E980.4
Percaine (spinal)	968.7	E855.2	E938.7	E950.4	E962.0	E980.4

External Cause (E-Code)

	Poisoning	Accident	Therapeutic Use	Suicide Attempt	Assault	Undetermined
Percaine — *continued*						
topical (surface)	968.5	E855.2	E938.5	E950.4	E962.0	E980.4
Perchloroethylene (vapor)	982.3	E862.4	—	E950.9	E962.1	E980.9
medicinal	961.6	E857	E931.6	E950.4	E962.0	E980.4
Percodan	965.09	E850.2	E935.2	E950.0	E962.0	E980.0
Percogesic	965.09	E850.2	E935.2	E950.0	E962.0	E980.0
Percorten	962.0	E858.0	E932.0	E950.4	E962.0	E980.4
Pergonal	962.4	E858.0	E932.4	E950.4	E962.0	E980.4
Perhexiline	972.4	E858.3	E942.4	E950.4	E962.0	E980.4
Periactin	963.0	E858.1	E933.0	E950.4	E962.0	E980.4
Periclor	967.1	E852.0	E937.1	E950.2	E962.0	E980.2
Pericyazine	969.1	E853.0	E939.1	E950.3	E962.0	E980.3
Peritrate	972.4	E858.3	E942.4	E950.4	E962.0	E980.4
Permanganates NEC	983.9	E864.3	—	E950.7	E962.1	E980.6
potassium (topical)	976.0	E858.7	E946.0	E950.4	E962.0	E980.4
Pernocton	967.0	E851	E937.0	E950.1	E962.0	E980.1
Pernoston	967.0	E851	E937.0	E950.1	E962.0	E980.1
Peronin(e)	965.09	E850.2	E935.2	E950.0	E962.0	E980.0
Perphenazine	969.1	E853.0	E939.1	E950.3	E962.0	E980.3
Pertofrane	969.05	E854.0	E939.0	E950.3	E962.0	E980.3
Pertussis						
immune serum (human)	964.6	E858.2	E934.6	E950.4	E962.0	E980.4
vaccine (with diphtheria toxoid) (with tetanus toxoid)	978.6	E858.8	E948.6	E950.4	E962.0	E980.4
Peruvian balsam	976.8	E858.7	E946.8	E950.4	E962.0	E980.4
Pesticides (dust) (fumes) (vapor)	989.4	E863.4	—	E950.6	E962.1	E980.7
arsenic	985.1	E863.4	—	E950.8	E962.1	E980.8
chlorinated	989.2	E863.0	—	E950.6	E962.1	E980.7
cyanide	989.0	E863.4	—	E950.6	E962.1	E980.7
kerosene	981	E863.4	—	E950.6	E962.1	E980.7
mixture (of compounds)	989.4	E863.3	—	E950.6	E962.1	E980.7
naphthalene	983.0	E863.4	—	E950.7	E962.1	E980.6
organochlorine (compounds)	989.2	E863.0	—	E950.6	E962.1	E980.7
petroleum (distillate) (products) NEC	981	E863.4	—	E950.6	E962.1	E980.7
specified ingredient NEC	989.4	E863.4	—	E950.6	E962.1	E980.7
strychnine	989.1	E863.4	—	E950.6	E962.1	E980.7
thallium	985.8	E863.7	—	E950.6	E962.1	E980.7
Pethidine (hydrochloride)	965.09	E850.2	E935.2	E950.0	E962.0	E980.0
Petrichloral	967.1	E852.0	E937.1	E950.2	E962.0	E980.2
Petrol	981	E862.1		E950.9	E962.1	E980.9
vapor	987.1	E869.8		E952.8	E962.2	E982.8
Petrolatum (jelly) (ointment)	976.3	E858.7	E946.3	E950.4	E962.0	E980.4
hydrophilic	976.3	E858.7	E946.3	E950.4	E962.0	E980.4
liquid	973.2	E858.4	E943.2	E950.4	E962.0	E980.4
topical	976.3	E858.7	E946.3	E950.4	E962.0	E980.4
nonmedicinal	981	E862.1		E950.9	E962.1	E980.9
Petroleum (cleaners) (fuels) (products) NEC	981	E862.1		E950.9	E962.1	E980.9
benzin(e) — see Ligroin						
ether — see Ligroin						
jelly — see Petrolatum						
naphtha — see Ligroin						
pesticide	981	E863.4	—	E950.6	E962.1	E980.7
solids	981	E862.3	—	E950.9	E962.1	E980.9
solvents	981	E862.0	—	E950.9	E962.1	E980.9
vapor	987.1	E869.8	—	E952.8	E962.2	E982.8
Peyote	969.6	E854.1	E939.6	E950.3	E962.0	E980.3
Phanodorm, phanodorn	967.0	E851	E937.0	E950.1	E962.0	E980.1
Phanquinone, phanquone	961.5	E857	E931.5	E950.4	E962.0	E980.4
Pharmaceutical excipient or adjunct	977.4	E858.8	E947.4	E950.4	E962.0	E980.4
Phenacemide	966.3	E855.0	E936.3	E950.4	E962.0	E980.4
Phenacetin	965.4	E850.4	E935.4	E950.0	E962.0	E980.0
Phenadoxone	965.09	E850.2	E935.2	E950.0	E962.0	E980.0
Phenaglycodol	969.5	E853.8	E939.5	E950.3	E962.0	E980.3
Phenantoin	966.1	E855.0	E936.1	E950.4	E962.0	E980.4
Phenaphthazine reagent	977.8	E858.8	E947.8	E950.4	E962.0	E980.4
Phenazocine	965.09	E850.2	E935.2	E950.0	E962.0	E980.0
Phenazone	965.5	E850.5	E935.5	E950.0	E962.0	E980.0
Phenazopyridine	976.1	E858.7	E946.1	E950.4	E962.0	E980.4
Phenbenicillin	960.0	E856	E930.0	E950.4	E962.0	E980.4
Phenbutrazate	977.0	E858.8	E947.0	E950.4	E962.0	E980.4
Phencyclidine	968.3	E855.1	E938.3	E950.4	E962.0	E980.4
Phendimetrazine	977.0	E858.8	E947.0	E950.4	E962.0	E980.4
Phenelzine	969.01	E854.0	E939.0	E950.3	E962.0	E980.3
Phenergan	967.8	E852.8	E937.8	E950.2	E962.0	E980.2
Phenethicillin (potassium)	960.0	E856	E930.0	E950.4	E962.0	E980.4
Phenetsal	965.1	E850.3	E935.3	E950.0	E962.0	E980.0
Pheneturide	966.3	E855.0	E936.3	E950.4	E962.0	E980.4
Phenformin	962.3	E858.0	E932.3	E950.4	E962.0	E980.4
Phenglutarimide	971.1	E855.4	E941.1	E950.4	E962.0	E980.4
Phenicarbazide	965.8	E850.8	E935.8	E950.0	E962.0	E980.0
Phenindamine (tartrate)	963.0	E858.1	E933.0	E950.4	E962.0	E980.4
Phenindione	964.2	E858.2	E934.2	E950.4	E962.0	E980.4
Pheniprazine	969.01	E854.0	E939.0	E950.3	E962.0	E980.3
Pheniramine (maleate)	963.0	E858.1	E933.0	E950.4	E962.0	E980.4
Phenmetrazine	977.0	E858.8	E947.0	E950.4	E962.0	E980.4
Phenobal	967.0	E851	E937.0	E950.1	E962.0	E980.1
Phenobarbital	967.0	E851	E937.0	E950.1	E962.0	E980.1
Phenobarbitone	967.0	E851	E937.0	E950.1	E962.0	E980.1
Phenoctide	976.0	E858.7	E946.0	E950.4	E962.0	E980.4
Phenolphthalein	973.1	E858.4	E943.1	E950.4	E962.0	E980.4
Phenolsulfonphthalein	977.8	E858.8	E947.8	E950.4	E962.0	E980.4
Phenol (derivatives) NEC	983.0	E864.0	—	E950.7	E962.1	E980.6
disinfectant	983.0	E864.0	—	E950.7	E962.1	E980.6
pesticide	989.4	E863.4	—	E950.6	E962.1	E980.7
red	977.8	E858.8	E947.8	E950.4	E962.0	E980.4
Phenomorphan	965.09	E850.2	E935.2	E950.0	E962.0	E980.0
Phenonyl	967.0	E851	E937.0	E950.1	E962.0	E980.1
Phenoperidine	965.09	E850.2	E935.2	E950.0	E962.0	E980.0
Phenoquin	974.7	E858.5	E944.7	E950.4	E962.0	E980.4
Phenothiazines (tranquilizers) NEC	969.1	E853.0	E939.1	E950.3	E962.0	E980.3
insecticide	989.3	E863.4	—	E950.6	E962.1	E980.7
Phenoxybenzamine	971.3	E855.6	E941.3	E950.4	E962.0	E980.4
Phenoxymethyl penicillin	960.0	E856	E930.0	E950.4	E962.0	E980.4
Phenprocoumon	964.2	E858.2	E934.2	E950.4	E962.0	E980.4
Phensuximide	966.2	E855.0	E936.2	E950.4	E962.0	E980.4
Phentermine	977.0	E858.8	E947.0	E950.4	E962.0	E980.4
Phentolamine	971.3	E855.6	E941.3	E950.4	E962.0	E980.4
Phenyl						
butazone	965.5	E850.5	E935.5	E950.0	E962.0	E980.0
enediamine	983.0	E864.0	—	E950.7	E962.1	E980.6
hydrazine	983.0	E864.0	—	E950.7	E962.1	E980.6
antineoplastic	963.1	E858.1	E933.1	E950.4	E962.0	E980.4
mercuric compounds — see Mercury						
salicylate	976.3	E858.7	E946.3	E950.4	E962.0	E980.4
Phenylephrine	971.2	E855.5	E941.2	E950.4	E962.0	E980.4
Phenylethylbiguanide	962.3	E858.0	E932.3	E950.4	E962.0	E980.4
Phenylpropanolamine	971.2	E855.5	E941.2	E950.4	E962.0	E980.4
Phenylsulfthion	989.3	E863.1	—	E950.6	E962.1	E980.7
Phenyramidol, phenyramidon	965.7	E850.7	E935.7	E950.0	E962.0	E980.0
Phenytoin	966.1	E855.0	E936.1	E950.4	E962.0	E980.4
pHisoHex	976.2	E858.7	E946.2	E950.4	E962.0	E980.4
Pholcodine	965.09	E850.2	E935.2	E950.0	E962.0	E980.0
Phorate	989.3	E863.1	—	E950.6	E962.1	E980.7
Phosdrin	989.3	E863.1	—	E950.6	E962.1	E980.7
Phosgene (gas)	987.8	E869.8	—	E952.8	E962.2	E982.8
Phosphate (tricresyl)	989.89	E866.8	—	E950.9	E962.1	E980.9
organic	989.3	E863.1	—	E950.6	E962.1	E980.7
solvent	982.8	E862.4	—	E950.9	E926.1	E980.9
Phosphine	987.8	E869.8	—	E952.8	E962.2	E982.8
fumigant	987.8	E863.8	—	E950.6	E962.2	E980.7
Phospholine	971.0	E855.3	E941.0	E950.4	E962.0	E980.4
Phosphoric acid	983.1	E864.1	—	E950.7	E962.1	E980.6
Phosphorus (compounds) NEC	983.9	E864.3	—	E950.7	E962.1	E980.6
rodenticide	983.9	E863.7	—	E950.7	E962.1	E980.6
Phthalimidoglutarimide	967.8	E852.8	E937.8	E950.2	E962.0	E980.2
Phthalylsulfathiazole	961.0	E857	E931.0	E950.4	E962.0	E980.4
Phylloquinone	964.3	E858.2	E934.3	E950.4	E962.0	E980.4
Physeptone	965.02	E850.1	E935.1	E950.0	E962.0	E980.0
Physostigma venenosum	988.2	E865.4	—	E950.9	E962.1	E980.9
Physostigmine	971.0	E855.3	E941.0	E950.4	E962.0	E980.4
Phytolacca decandra	988.2	E865.4	—	E950.9	E962.1	E980.9
Phytomenadione	964.3	E858.2	E934.3	E950.4	E962.0	E980.4
Phytonadione	964.3	E858.2	E934.3	E950.4	E962.0	E980.4
Picric (acid)	983.0	E864.0	—	E950.7	E962.1	E980.6
Picrotoxin	970.0	E854.3	E940.0	E950.4	E962.0	E980.4
Pilocarpine	971.0	E855.3	E941.0	E950.4	E962.0	E980.4
Pilocarpus (jaborandi) extract	971.0	E855.3	E941.0	E950.4	E962.0	E980.4

	Poisoning	Accident	Therapeutic Use	Suicide Attempt	Assault	Undetermined
Pimaricin	960.1	E856	E930.1	E950.4	E962.0	E980.4
Piminodine	965.09	E850.2	E935.2	E950.0	E962.0	E980.0
Pine oil, pinesol (disinfectant)	983.9	E861.4	—	E950.7	E962.1	E980.6
Pinkroot	961.6	E857	E931.6	E950.4	E962.0	E980.4
Pipadone	965.09	E850.2	E935.2	E950.0	E962.0	E980.0
Pipamazine	963.0	E858.1	E933.0	E950.4	E962.0	E980.4
Pipazethate	975.4	E858.6	E945.4	E950.4	E962.0	E980.4
Pipenzolate	971.1	E855.4	E941.1	E950.4	E962.0	E980.4
Piperacetazine	969.1	E853.0	E939.1	E950.3	E962.0	E980.3
Piperazine NEC	961.6	E857	E931.6	E950.4	E962.0	E980.4
estrone sulfate	962.2	E858.0	E932.2	E950.4	E962.0	E980.4
Piper cubeba	988.2	E865.4	—	E950.9	E962.1	E980.9
Piperidione	975.4	E858.6	E945.4	E950.4	E962.0	E980.4
Piperidolate	971.1	E855.4	E941.1	E950.4	E962.0	E980.4
Piperocaine	968.9	E855.2	E938.9	E950.4	E962.0	E980.4
infiltration (subcutaneous)	968.5	E855.2	E938.5	E950.4	E962.0	E980.4
nerve block (peripheral) (plexus)	968.6	E855.2	E938.6	E950.4	E962.0	E980.4
topical (surface)	968.5	E855.2	E938.5	E950.4	E962.0	E980.4
Pipobroman	963.1	E858.1	E933.1	E950.4	E962.0	E980.4
Pipradrol	970.89	E854.3	E940.8	E950.4	E962.0	E980.4
Piscidia (bark) (erythrina)	965.7	E850.7	E935.7	E950.0	E962.0	E980.0
Pitch	983.0	E864.0	—	E950.7	E962.1	E980.6
Pitkin's solution	968.7	E855.2	E938.7	E950.4	E962.0	E980.4
Pitocin	975.0	E858.6	E945.0	E950.4	E962.0	E980.4
Pitressin (tannate)	962.5	E858.0	E932.5	E950.4	E962.0	E980.4
Pituitary extracts (posterior)	962.5	E858.0	E932.5	E950.4	E962.0	E980.4
anterior	962.4	E858.0	E932.4	E950.4	E962.0	E980.4
Pituitrin	962.5	E858.0	E932.5	E950.4	E962.0	E980.4
Placental extract	962.9	E858.0	E932.9	E950.4	E962.0	E980.4
Placidyl	967.8	E852.8	E937.8	E950.2	E962.0	E980.2
Plague vaccine	978.3	E858.8	E948.3	E950.4	E962.0	E980.4
Plant foods or fertilizers NEC	989.89	E866.5	—	E950.9	E962.1	E980.9
mixed with herbicides	989.4	E863.5	—	E950.6	E962.1	E980.7
Plants, noxious, used as food	988.2	E865.9	—	E950.9	E962.1	E980.9
berries and seeds	988.2	E865.3	—	E950.9	E962.1	E980.9
specified type NEC	988.2	E865.4	—	E950.9	E962.1	E980.9
Plasma (blood)	964.7	E858.2	E934.7	E950.4	E962.0	E980.4
expanders	964.8	E858.2	E934.8	E950.4	E962.0	E980.4
Plasmanate	964.7	E858.2	E934.7	E950.4	E962.0	E980.4
Plegicil	969.1	E853.0	E939.1	E950.3	E962.0	E980.3
Podophyllin	976.4	E858.7	E946.4	E950.4	E962.0	E980.4
Podophyllum resin	976.4	E858.7	E946.4	E950.4	E962.0	E980.4
Poisonous berries	988.2	E865.3	—	E950.9	E962.1	E980.9
Poison NEC	989.9	E866.9	—	E950.9	E962.1	E980.9
Pokeweed (any part)	988.2	E865.4	—	E950.9	E962.1	E980.9
Poldine	971.1	E855.4	E941.1	E950.4	E962.0	E980.4
Poliomyelitis vaccine	979.5	E858.8	E949.5	E950.4	E962.0	E980.4
Poliovirus vaccine	979.5	E858.8	E949.5	E950.4	E962.0	E980.4
Polish (car) (floor) (furniture) (metal) (silver)	989.89	E861.2	—	E950.9	E962.1	E980.9
abrasive	989.89	E861.3	—	E950.9	E962.1	E980.9
porcelain	989.89	E861.3	—	E950.9	E962.1	E980.9
Poloxalkol	973.2	E858.4	E943.2	E950.4	E962.0	E980.4
Polyaminostyrene resins	974.5	E858.5	E944.5	E950.4	E962.0	E980.4
Polychlorinated biphenyl — see PCBs						
Polycycline	960.4	E856	E930.4	E950.4	E962.0	E980.4
Polyester resin hardener	982.8	E862.4	—	E950.9	E962.1	E980.9
fumes	987.8	E869.8	—	E952.8	E962.2	E982.8
Polyestradiol (phosphate)	962.2	E858.0	E932.2	E950.4	E962.0	E980.4
Polyethanolamine alkyl sulfate	976.2	E858.7	E946.2	E950.4	E962.0	E980.4
Polyethylene glycol	976.3	E858.7	E946.3	E950.4	E962.0	E980.4
Polyferose	964.0	E858.2	E934.0	E950.4	E962.0	E980.4
Polymyxin B	960.8	E856	E930.8	E950.4	E962.0	E980.4
ENT agent	976.6	E858.7	E946.6	E950.4	E962.0	E980.4
ophthalmic preparation	976.5	E858.7	E946.5	E950.4	E962.0	E980.4
topical NEC	976.0	E858.7	E946.0	E950.4	E962.0	E980.4
Polynoxylin(e)	976.0	E858.7	E946.0	E950.4	E962.0	E980.4
Polyoxymethyleneurea	976.0	E858.7	E946.0	E950.4	E962.0	E980.4
Polytetrafluoroethylene (inhaled)	987.8	E869.8	—	E952.8	E962.2	E982.8
Polythiazide	974.3	E858.5	E944.3	E950.4	E962.0	E980.4
Polyvinylpyrrolidone	964.8	E858.2	E934.8	E950.4	E962.0	E980.4
Pontocaine (hydrochloride) (infiltration) (topical)	968.5	E855.2	E938.5	E950.4	E962.0	E980.4
nerve block (peripheral) (plexus)	968.6	E855.2	E938.6	E950.4	E962.0	E980.4
spinal	968.7	E855.2	E938.7	E950.4	E962.0	E980.4
Pot	969.6	E854.1	E939.6	E950.3	E962.0	E980.3
Potash (caustic)	983.2	E864.2	—	E950.7	E962.1	E980.6
Potassic saline injection (lactated)	974.5	E858.5	E944.5	E950.4	E962.0	E980.4
Potassium (salts) NEC	974.5	E858.5	E944.5	E950.4	E962.0	E980.4
aminosalicylate	961.8	E857	E931.8	E950.4	E962.0	E980.4
arsenite (solution)	985.1	E866.3	—	E950.8	E962.1	E980.8
bichromate	983.9	E864.3	—	E950.7	E962.1	E980.6
bisulfate	983.9	E864.3	—	E950.7	E962.1	E980.6
bromide (medicinal) NEC	967.3	E852.2	E937.3	E950.2	E962.0	E980.2
carbonate	983.2	E864.2	—	E950.7	E962.1	E980.6
chlorate NEC	983.9	E864.3	—	E950.7	E962.1	E980.6
cyanide — see Cyanide						
hydroxide	983.2	E864.2	—	E950.7	E962.1	E980.6
iodide (expectorant) NEC	975.5	E858.6	E945.5	E950.4	E962.0	E980.4
nitrate	989.89	E866.8	—	E950.9	E962.1	E980.9
oxalate	983.9	E864.3	—	E950.7	E962.1	E980.6
perchlorate NEC	977.8	E858.8	E947.8	E950.4	E962.0	E980.4
antithyroid	962.8	E858.0	E932.8	E950.4	E962.0	E980.4
permanganate	976.0	E858.7	E946.0	E950.4	E962.0	E980.4
nonmedicinal	983.9	E864.3	—	E950.7	E962.1	E980.6
Povidone-iodine (anti-infective) NEC	976.0	E858.7	E946.0	E950.4	E962.0	E980.4
Practolol	972.0	E858.3	E942.0	E950.4	E962.0	E980.4
Pralidoxime (chloride)	977.2	E858.8	E947.2	E950.4	E962.0	E980.4
Pramoxine	968.5	E855.2	E938.5	E950.4	E962.0	E980.4
Prazosin	972.6	E858.3	E942.6	E950.4	E962.0	E980.4
Prednisolone	962.0	E858.0	E932.0	E950.4	E962.0	E980.4
ENT agent	976.6	E858.7	E946.6	E950.4	E962.0	E980.4
ophthalmic preparation	976.5	E858.7	E946.5	E950.4	E962.0	E980.4
topical NEC	976.0	E858.7	E946.0	E950.4	E962.0	E980.4
Prednisone	962.0	E858.0	E932.0	E950.4	E962.0	E980.4
Pregnanediol	962.2	E858.0	E932.2	E950.4	E962.0	E980.4
Pregneninolone	962.2	E858.0	E932.2	E950.4	E962.0	E980.4
Preludin	977.0	E858.8	E947.0	E950.4	E962.0	E980.4
Premarin	962.2	E858.0	E932.2	E950.4	E962.0	E980.4
Prenylamine	972.4	E858.3	E942.4	E950.4	E962.0	E980.4
Preparation H	976.8	E858.7	E946.8	E950.4	E962.0	E980.4
Preservatives	989.89	E866.8	—	E950.9	E962.1	E980.9
Pride of China	988.2	E865.3	—	E950.9	E962.1	E980.9
Prilocaine	968.9	E855.2	E938.9	E950.4	E962.0	E980.4
infiltration (subcutaneous)	968.5	E855.2	E938.5	E950.4	E962.0	E980.4
nerve block (peripheral) (plexus)	968.6	E855.2	E938.6	E950.4	E962.0	E980.4
Primaquine	961.4	E857	E931.4	E950.4	E962.0	E980.4
Primidone	966.3	E855.0	E936.3	E950.4	E962.0	E980.4
Primula (veris)	988.2	E865.4	—	E950.9	E962.1	E980.9
Prinadol	965.09	E850.2	E935.2	E950.0	E962.0	E980.0
Priscol, Priscoline	971.3	E855.6	E941.3	E950.4	E962.0	E980.4
Privet	988.2	E865.4	—	E950.9	E962.1	E980.9
Privine	971.2	E855.5	E941.2	E950.4	E962.0	E980.4
Pro-Banthine	971.1	E855.4	E941.1	E950.4	E962.0	E980.4
Probarbital	967.0	E851	E937.0	E950.1	E962.0	E980.1
Probenecid	974.7	E858.5	E944.7	E950.4	E962.0	E980.4
Procainamide (hydrochloride)	972.0	E858.3	E942.0	E950.4	E962.0	E980.4
Procaine (hydrochloride) (infiltration) (topical)	968.5	E855.2	E938.5	E950.4	E962.0	E980.4
nerve block (peripheral) (plexus)	968.6	E855.2	E938.6	E950.4	E962.0	E980.4
penicillin G	960.0	E856	E930.0	E950.4	E962.0	E980.4
spinal	968.7	E855.2	E938.7	E950.4	E962.0	E980.4
Procalmidol	969.5	E853.8	E939.5	E950.3	E962.0	E980.3
Procarbazine	963.1	E858.1	E933.1	E950.4	E962.0	E980.4
Prochlorperazine	969.1	E853.0	E939.1	E950.3	E962.0	E980.3
Procyclidine	966.4	E855.0	E936.4	E950.4	E962.0	E980.4
Producer gas	986	E868.8	—	E952.1	E962.2	E982.1
Profenamine	966.4	E855.0	E936.4	E950.4	E962.0	E980.4
Profenil	975.1	E858.6	E945.1	E950.4	E962.0	E980.4
Progesterones	962.2	E858.0	E932.2	E950.4	E962.0	E980.4
Progestin	962.2	E858.0	E932.2	E950.4	E962.0	E980.4
Progestogens (with estrogens)	962.2	E858.0	E932.2	E950.4	E962.0	E980.4
Progesterone	962.2	E858.0	E932.2	E950.4	E962.0	E980.4
Proguanil	961.4	E857	E931.4	E950.4	E962.0	E980.4
Prolactin	962.4	E858.0	E932.4	E950.4	E962.0	E980.4

	Poisoning	Accident	Therapeutic Use	Suicide Attempt	Assault	Undetermined
External Cause (E-Code)						
Proloid	962.7	E858.0	E932.7	E950.4	E962.0	E980.4
Proluton	962.2	E858.0	E932.2	E950.4	E962.0	E980.4
Promacetin	961.8	E857	E931.8	E950.4	E962.0	E980.4
Promazine	969.1	E853.0	E939.1	E950.3	E962.0	E980.3
Promedol	965.09	E850.2	E935.2	E950.0	E962.0	E980.0
Promethazine	967.8	E852.8	E937.8	E950.2	E962.0	E980.2
Promin	961.8	E857	E931.8	E950.4	E962.0	E980.4
Pronestyl (hydrochloride)	972.0	E858.3	E942.0	E950.4	E962.0	E980.4
Pronetalol, pronethalol	972.0	E858.3	E942.0	E950.4	E962.0	E980.4
Prontosil	961.0	E857	E931.0	E950.4	E962.0	E980.4
Propamidine isethionate	961.5	E857	E931.5	E950.4	E962.0	E980.4
Propanal (medicinal)	967.8	E852.8	E937.8	E950.2	E962.0	E980.2
Propane (gas) (distributed in mobile container)	987.0	E868.0	—	E951.1	E962.2	E981.1
distributed through pipes	987.0	E867	—	E951.0	E962.2	E981.0
incomplete combustion of — see Carbon monoxide, Propane						
Propanidid	968.3	E855.1	E938.3	E950.4	E962.0	E980.4
Propanol	980.3	E860.4	—	E950.9	E962.1	E980.9
Propantheline	971.1	E855.4	E941.1	E950.4	E962.0	E980.4
Proparacaine	968.5	E855.2	E938.5	E950.4	E962.0	E980.4
Propatyl nitrate	972.4	E858.3	E942.4	E950.4	E962.0	E980.4
Propicillin	960.0	E856	E930.0	E950.4	E962.0	E980.4
Propiolactone (vapor)	987.8	E869.8	—	E952.8	E962.2	E982.8
Propiomazine	967.8	E852.8	E937.8	E950.2	E962.0	E980.2
Propionaldehyde (medicinal)	967.8	E852.8	E937.8	E950.2	E962.0	E980.2
Propionate compound	976.0	E858.7	E946.0	E950.4	E962.0	E980.4
Propion gel	976.0	E858.7	E946.0	E950.4	E962.0	E980.4
Propitocaine	968.9	E855.2	E938.9	E950.4	E962.0	E980.4
infiltration (subcutaneous)	968.5	E855.2	E938.5	E950.4	E962.0	E980.4
nerve block (peripheral) (plexus)	968.6	E855.2	E938.6	E950.4	E962.0	E980.4
Propoxur	989.3	E863.2	—	E950.6	E962.1	E980.7
Propoxycaine	968.9	E855.2	E938.9	E950.4	E962.0	E980.4
infiltration (subcutaneous)	968.5	E855.2	E938.5	E950.4	E962.0	E980.4
nerve block (peripheral) (plexus)	968.6	E855.2	E938.6	E950.4	E962.0	E980.4
topical (surface)	968.5	E855.2	E938.5	E950.4	E962.0	E980.4
Propoxyphene (hydrochloride)	965.8	E850.8	E935.8	E950.0	E962.0	E980.0
Propranolol	972.0	E858.3	E942.0	E950.4	E962.0	E980.4
Propyl						
alcohol	980.3	E860.4	—	E950.9	E962.1	E980.9
carbinol	980.3	E860.4	—	E950.9	E962.1	E980.9
hexadrine	971.2	E855.5	E941.2	E950.4	E962.0	E980.4
iodone	977.8	E858.8	E947.8	E950.4	E962.0	E980.4
thiouracil	962.8	E858.0	E932.8	E950.4	E962.0	E980.4
Propylene	987.1	E869.8	—	E952.8	E962.2	E982.8
Propylparaben (ophthalmic)	976.5	E858.7	E946.5	E950.4	E962.0	E980.4
Proscillaridin	972.1	E858.3	E942.1	E950.4	E962.0	E980.4
Prostaglandins	975.0	E858.6	E945.0	E950.4	E962.0	E980.4
Prostigmin	971.0	E855.3	E941.0	E950.4	E962.0	E980.4
Protamine (sulfate)	964.5	E858.2	E934.5	E950.4	E962.0	E980.4
zinc insulin	962.3	E858.0	E932.3	E950.4	E962.0	E980.4
Protectants (topical)	976.3	E858.7	E946.3	E950.4	E962.0	E980.4
Protein hydrolysate	974.5	E858.5	E944.5	E950.4	E962.0	E980.4
Prothiaden — see Dothiepin hydrochloride						
Prothionamide	961.8	E857	E931.8	E950.4	E962.0	E980.4
Prothipendyl	969.5	E853.8	E939.5	E950.3	E962.0	E980.3
Protokylol	971.2	E855.5	E941.2	E950.4	E962.0	E980.4
Protopam	977.2	E858.8	E947.2	E950.4	E962.0	E980.4
Protoveratrine(s) (A) (B)	972.6	E858.3	E942.6	E950.4	E962.0	E980.4
Protriptyline	969.05	E854.0	E939.0	E950.3	E962.0	E980.3
Provera	962.2	E858.0	E932.2	E950.4	E962.0	E980.4
Provitamin A	963.5	E858.1	E933.5	E950.4	E962.0	E980.4
Proxymetacaine	968.5	E855.2	E938.5	E950.4	E962.0	E980.4
Proxyphylline	975.1	E858.6	E945.1	E950.4	E962.0	E980.4
Prozac — see Fluoxetine hydrochloride						
Prunus						
laurocerasus	988.2	E865.4	—	E950.9	E962.1	E980.9
virginiana	988.2	E865.4	—	E950.9	E962.1	E980.9
Prussic acid	989.0	E866.8	—	E950.9	E962.1	E980.9
vapor	987.7	E869.8	—	E952.8	E962.2	E982.8
Pseudoephedrine	971.2	E855.5	E941.2	E950.4	E962.0	E980.4

	Poisoning	Accident	Therapeutic Use	Suicide Attempt	Assault	Undetermined
External Cause (E-Code)						
Psilocin	969.6	E854.1	E939.6	E950.3	E962.0	E980.3
Psilocybin	969.6	E854.1	E939.6	E950.3	E962.0	E980.3
PSP	977.8	E858.8	E947.8	E950.4	E962.0	E980.4
Psychedelic agents	969.6	E854.1	E939.6	E950.3	E962.0	E980.3
Psychodysleptics	969.6	E854.1	E939.6	E950.3	E962.0	E980.3
Psychostimulants	969.70	E854.2	E939.7	E950.3	E962.0	E980.3
Psychotherapeutic agents	969.9	E855.9	E939.9	E950.3	E962.0	E980.3
antidepressants	969.00	E854.0	E939.0	E950.3	E962.0	E980.3
specified NEC	969.8	E855.8	E939.8	E950.3	E962.0	E980.3
tranquilizers NEC	969.5	E853.9	E939.5	E950.3	E962.0	E980.3
Psychotomimetic agents	969.6	E854.1	E939.6	E950.3	E962.0	E980.3
Psychotropic agents	969.9	E854.8	E939.9	E950.3	E962.0	E980.3
specified NEC	969.8	E854.8	E939.8	E950.3	E962.0	E980.3
Psyllium	973.3	E858.4	E943.3	E950.4	E962.0	E980.4
Pteroylglutamic acid	964.1	E858.2	E934.1	E950.4	E962.0	E980.4
Pteroyltriglutamate	963.1	E858.1	E933.1	E950.4	E962.0	E980.4
PTFE	987.8	E869.8	—	E952.8	E962.2	E982.8
Pulsatilla	988.2	E865.4	—	E950.9	E962.1	E980.9
Purex (bleach)	983.9	E864.3	—	E950.7	E962.1	E980.6
Purine diuretics	974.1	E858.5	E944.1	E950.4	E962.0	E980.4
Purinethol	963.1	E858.1	E933.1	E950.4	E962.0	E980.4
PVP	964.8	E858.2	E934.8	E950.4	E962.0	E980.4
Pyrabital	965.7	E850.7	E935.7	E950.0	E962.0	E980.0
Pyramidon	965.5	E850.5	E935.5	E950.0	E962.0	E980.0
Pyrantel (pamoate)	961.6	E857	E931.6	E950.4	E962.0	E980.4
Pyrathiazine	963.0	E858.1	E933.0	E950.4	E962.0	E980.4
Pyrazinamide	961.8	E857	E931.8	E950.4	E962.0	E980.4
Pyrazinoic acid (amide)	961.8	E857	E931.8	E950.4	E962.0	E980.4
Pyrazole (derivatives)	965.5	E850.5	E935.5	E950.0	E962.0	E980.0
Pyrazolone (analgesics)	965.5	E850.5	E935.5	E950.0	E962.0	E980.0
Pyrethrins, pyrethrum	989.4	E863.4	—	E950.6	E962.1	E980.7
Pyribenzamine	963.0	E858.1	E933.0	E950.4	E962.0	E980.4
Pyridine (liquid) (vapor)	982.0	E862.4	—	E950.9	E962.1	E980.9
aldoxime chloride	977.2	E858.8	E947.2	E950.4	E962.0	E980.4
Pyridium	976.1	E858.7	E946.1	E950.4	E962.0	E980.4
Pyridostigmine	971.0	E855.3	E941.0	E950.4	E962.0	E980.4
Pyridoxine	963.5	E858.1	E933.5	E950.4	E962.0	E980.4
Pyrilamine	963.0	E858.1	E933.0	E950.4	E962.0	E980.4
Pyrimethamine	961.4	E857	E931.4	E950.4	E962.0	E980.4
Pyrogallic acid	983.0	E864.0	—	E950.7	E962.1	E980.6
Pyroxylin	976.3	E858.7	E946.3	E950.4	E962.0	E980.4
Pyrrobutamine	963.0	E858.1	E933.0	E950.4	E962.0	E980.4
Pyrrocitine	968.5	E855.2	E938.5	E950.4	E962.0	E980.4
Pyrvinium (pamoate)	961.6	E857	E931.6	E950.4	E962.0	E980.4
PZI	962.3	E858.0	E932.3	E950.4	E962.0	E980.4
Quaalude	967.4	E852.3	E937.4	E950.2	E962.0	E980.2
Quaternary ammonium derivatives	971.1	E855.4	E941.1	E950.4	E962.0	E980.4
Quicklime	983.2	E864.2	—	E950.7	E962.1	E980.6
Quinacrine	961.3	E857	E931.3	E950.4	E962.0	E980.4
Quinaglute	972.0	E858.3	E942.0	E950.4	E962.0	E980.4
Quinalbarbitone	967.0	E851	E937.0	E950.1	E962.0	E980.1
Quinestradiol	962.2	E858.0	E932.2	E950.4	E962.0	E980.4
Quinethazone	974.3	E858.5	E944.3	E950.4	E962.0	E980.4
Quinidine (gluconate) (polygalacturonate) (salts) (sulfate)	972.0	E858.3	E942.0	E950.4	E962.0	E980.4
Quinine	961.4	E857	E931.4	E950.4	E962.0	E980.4
Quiniobine	961.3	E857	E931.3	E950.4	E962.0	E980.4
Quinolines	961.3	E857	E931.3	E950.4	E962.0	E980.4
Quotane	968.5	E855.2	E938.5	E950.4	E962.0	E980.4
Rabies						
immune globulin (human)	964.6	E858.2	E934.6	E950.4	E962.0	E980.4
vaccine	979.1	E858.8	E949.1	E950.4	E962.0	E980.4
Racemoramide	965.09	E850.2	E935.2	E950.0	E962.0	E980.0
Racemorphan	965.09	E850.2	E935.2	E950.0	E962.0	E980.0
Radiator alcohol	980.1	E860.2	—	E950.9	E962.1	E980.9
Radio-opaque (drugs) (materials)	977.8	E858.8	E947.8	E950.4	E962.0	E980.4
Ranunculus	988.2	E865.4	—	E950.9	E962.1	E980.9
Rat poison	989.4	E863.7	—	E950.6	E962.1	E980.7
Rattlesnake (venom)	989.5	E905.0	—	E950.9	E962.1	E980.9
Raudixin	972.6	E858.3	E942.6	E950.4	E962.0	E980.4
Rautensin	972.6	E858.3	E942.6	E950.4	E962.0	E980.4
Rautina	972.6	E858.3	E942.6	E950.4	E962.0	E980.4
Rautotal	972.6	E858.3	E942.6	E950.4	E962.0	E980.4
Rauwiloid	972.6	E858.3	E942.6	E950.4	E962.0	E980.4
Rauwoldin	972.6	E858.3	E942.6	E950.4	E962.0	E980.4
Rauwolfia (alkaloids)	972.6	E858.3	E942.6	E950.4	E962.0	E980.4
Realgar	985.1	E866.3	—	E950.8	E962.1	E980.8

Subterms under main terms may continue to next column or page

	Poisoning	Accident	Therapeutic Use	Suicide Attempt	Assault	Undetermined
Red cells, packed	964.7	E858.2	E934.7	E950.4	E962.0	E980.4
Reducing agents, industrial NEC	983.9	E864.3	—	E950.7	E962.1	E980.6
Refrigerant gas (freon)	987.4	E869.2	—	E952.8	E962.2	E982.8
central nervous system	968.0	E855.1	E938.0	E950.4	E962.0	E980.4
not freon	987.9	E869.9	—	E952.9	E962.2	E982.9
Regroton	974.4	E858.5	E944.4	E950.4	E962.0	E980.4
Rela	968.0	E855.1	E938.0	E950.4	E962.0	E980.4
Relaxants, skeletal muscle (autonomic)	975.2	E858.6	E945.2	E950.4	E962.0	E980.4
Renese	974.3	E858.5	E944.3	E950.4	E962.0	E980.4
Renografin	977.8	E858.8	E947.8	E950.4	E962.0	E980.4
Replacement solutions	974.5	E858.5	E944.5	E950.4	E962.0	E980.4
Rescinnamine	972.6	E858.3	E942.6	E950.4	E962.0	E980.4
Reserpine	972.6	E858.3	E942.6	E950.4	E962.0	E980.4
Resorcin, resorcinol	976.4	E858.7	E946.4	E950.4	E962.0	E980.4
Respaire	975.5	E858.6	E945.5	E950.4	E962.0	E980.4
Respiratory agents NEC	975.8	E858.6	E945.8	E950.4	E962.0	E980.4
Retinoic acid	976.8	E858.7	E946.8	E950.4	E962.0	E980.4
Retinol	963.5	E858.1	E933.5	E950.4	E962.0	E980.4
Rh (D) immune globulin (human)	964.6	E858.2	E934.6	E950.4	E962.0	E980.4
Rhodine	965.1	E850.3	E935.3	E950.0	E962.0	E980.0
RhoGAM	964.6	E858.2	E934.6	E950.4	E962.0	E980.4
Riboflavin	963.5	E858.1	E933.5	E950.4	E962.0	E980.4
Ricin	989.89	E866.8	—	E950.9	E962.1	E980.9
Ricinus communis	988.2	E865.3	—	E950.9	E962.1	E980.9
Rickettsial vaccine NEC	979.6	E858.8	E949.6	E950.4	E962.0	E980.4
with viral and bacterial vaccine	979.7	E858.8	E949.7	E950.4	E962.0	E980.4
Rifampin	960.6	E856	E930.6	E950.4	E962.0	E980.4
Rimifon	961.8	E857	E931.8	E950.4	E962.0	E980.4
Ringer's injection (lactated)	974.5	E858.5	E944.5	E950.4	E962.0	E980.4
Ristocetin	960.8	E856	E930.8	E950.4	E962.0	E980.4
Ritalin	969.73	E854.2	E939.7	E950.3	E962.0	E980.3
Roach killers — *see* Pesticides						
Rocky Mountain spotted fever vaccine	979.6	E858.8	E949.6	E950.4	E962.0	E980.4
Rodenticides	989.4	E863.7	—	E950.6	E962.1	E980.7
Rohypnol	969.4	E853.2	E939.4	E950.3	E962.0	E980.3
Rolaids	973.0	E858.4	E943.0	E950.4	E962.0	E980.4
Rolitetracycline	960.4	E856	E930.4	E950.4	E962.0	E980.4
Romilar	975.4	E858.6	E945.4	E950.4	E962.0	E980.4
Rose water ointment	976.3	E858.7	E946.3	E950.4	E962.0	E980.4
Rosuvastatin calcium	972.1	E858.3	E942.2	E950.4	E962.0	E980.4
Rotenone	989.4	E863.7	—	E950.6	E962.1	E980.7
Rotoxamine	963.0	E858.1	E933.0	E950.4	E962.0	E980.4
Rough-on-rats	989.4	E863.7	—	E950.6	E962.1	E980.7
RU486	962.9	E858.0	E932.9	E950.4	E962.0	E980.4
Rubbing alcohol	980.2	E860.3	—	E950.9	E962.1	E980.9
Rubella virus vaccine	979.4	E858.8	E949.4	E950.4	E962.0	E980.4
Rubelogen	979.4	E858.8	E949.4	E950.4	E962.0	E980.4
Rubeovax	979.4	E858.8	E949.4	E950.4	E962.0	E980.4
Rubidomycin	960.7	E856	E930.7	E950.4	E962.0	E980.4
Rue	988.2	E865.4	—	E950.9	E962.1	E980.9
Ruta	988.2	E865.4	—	E950.9	E962.1	E980.9
Sabadilla (medicinal)	976.0	E858.7	E946.0	E950.4	E962.0	E980.4
pesticide	989.4	E863.4	—	E950.6	E962.1	E980.7
Sabin oral vaccine	979.5	E858.8	E949.5	E950.4	E962.0	E980.4
Saccharated iron oxide	964.0	E858.2	E934.0	E950.4	E962.0	E980.4
Saccharin	974.5	E858.5	E944.5	E950.4	E962.0	E980.4
Safflower oil	972.2	E858.3	E942.2	E950.4	E962.0	E980.4
Salbutamol sulfate	975.7	E858.6	E945.7	E950.4	E962.0	E980.4
Salicylamide	965.1	E850.3	E935.3	E950.0	E962.0	E980.0
Salicylate(s)	965.1	E850.3	E935.3	E950.0	E962.0	E980.0
methyl	976.3	E858.7	E946.3	E950.4	E962.0	E980.4
theobromine calcium	974.1	E858.5	E944.1	E950.4	E962.0	E980.4
Salicylazosulfapyridine	961.0	E857	E931.0	E950.4	E962.0	E980.4
Salicylhydroxamic acid	976.0	E858.7	E946.0	E950.4	E962.0	E980.4
Salicylic acid (keratolytic) NEC	976.4	E858.7	E946.4	E950.4	E962.0	E980.4
congeners	965.1	E850.3	E935.3	E950.0	E962.0	E980.0
salts	965.1	E850.3	E935.3	E950.0	E962.0	E980.0
Saliniazid	961.8	E857	E931.8	E950.4	E962.0	E980.4
Salol	976.3	E858.7	E946.3	E950.4	E962.0	E980.4
Salt (substitute) NEC	974.5	E858.5	E944.5	E950.4	E962.0	E980.4
Saluretics	974.3	E858.5	E944.3	E950.4	E962.0	E980.4
Saluron	974.3	E858.5	E944.3	E950.4	E962.0	E980.4
Salvarsan 606 (neosilver) (silver)	961.1	E857	E931.1	E950.4	E962.0	E980.4
Sambucus canadensis	988.2	E865.4	—	E950.9	E962.1	E980.9
Sambucus canadensis — *continued*						
berry	988.2	E865.3	—	E950.9	E962.1	E980.9
Sandril	972.6	E858.3	E942.6	E950.4	E962.0	E980.4
Sanguinaria canadensis	988.2	E865.4	—	E950.9	E962.1	E980.9
Saniflush (cleaner)	983.9	E861.3	—	E950.7	E962.1	E980.6
Santonin	961.6	E857	E931.6	E950.4	E962.0	E980.4
Santyl	976.8	E858.7	E946.8	E950.4	E962.0	E980.4
Sarkomycin	960.7	E856	E930.7	E950.4	E962.0	E980.4
Saroten	969.05	E854.0	E939.0	E950.3	E962.0	E980.3
Saturnine — *see* Lead						
Savin (oil)	976.4	E858.7	E946.4	E950.4	E962.0	E980.4
Scammony	973.1	E858.4	E943.1	E950.4	E962.0	E980.4
Scarlet red	976.8	E858.7	E946.8	E950.4	E962.0	E980.4
Scheele's green	985.1	E866.3	—	E950.8	E962.1	E980.8
insecticide	985.1	E863.4	—	E950.8	E962.1	E980.8
Schradan	989.3	E863.1	—	E950.6	E962.1	E980.7
Schweinfurt(h) green	985.1	E866.3	—	E950.8	E962.1	E980.8
insecticide	985.1	E863.4	—	E950.8	E962.1	E980.8
Scilla — *see* Squill						
Sclerosing agents	972.7	E858.3	E942.7	E950.4	E962.0	E980.4
Scopolamine	971.1	E855.4	E941.1	E950.4	E962.0	E980.4
Scouring powder	989.89	E861.3	—	E950.9	E962.1	E980.9
Sea						
anemone (sting)	989.5	E905.6	—	E950.9	E962.1	E980.9
cucumber (sting)	989.5	E905.6	—	E950.9	E962.1	E980.9
snake (bite) (venom)	989.5	E905.0	—	E950.9	E962.1	E980.9
urchin spine (puncture)	989.5	E905.6	—	E950.9	E962.1	E980.9
Secbutabarbital	967.0	E851	E937.0	E950.1	E962.0	E980.1
Secbutabarbitone	967.0	E851	E937.0	E950.1	E962.0	E980.1
Secobarbital	967.0	E851	E937.0	E950.1	E962.0	E980.1
Seconal	967.0	E851	E937.0	E950.1	E962.0	E980.1
Secretin	977.8	E858.8	E947.8	E950.4	E962.0	E980.4
Sedatives, nonbarbiturate	967.9	E852.9	E937.9	E950.2	E962.0	E980.2
specified NEC	967.8	E852.8	E937.8	E950.2	E962.0	E980.2
Sedormid	967.8	E852.8	E937.8	E950.2	E962.0	E980.2
Seed (plant)	988.2	E865.3	—	E950.9	E962.1	E980.9
disinfectant or dressing	989.89	E866.5	—	E950.9	E962.1	E980.9
Selective serotonin and norepinephrine reuptake inhibitors (SSNRI)	969.02	E854.0	E939.0	E950.3	E962.0	E980.3
Selective serotonin reuptake inhibitors (SSRI)	969.03	E854.0	E939.0	E950.3	E962.0	E980.3
Selenium (fumes) NEC	985.8	E866.4	—	E950.9	E962.1	E980.9
disulfide or sulfide	976.4	E858.7	E946.4	E950.4	E962.0	E980.4
Selsun	976.4	E858.7	E946.4	E950.4	E962.0	E980.4
Senna	973.1	E858.4	E943.1	E950.4	E962.0	E980.4
Septisol	976.2	E858.7	E946.2	E950.4	E962.0	E980.4
Serax	969.4	E853.2	E939.4	E950.3	E962.0	E980.3
Serenesil	967.8	E852.8	E937.8	E950.2	E962.0	E980.2
Serenium (hydrochloride)	961.9	E857	E931.9	E950.4	E962.0	E980.4
Serepax — *see* Oxazepam						
Sernyl	968.3	E855.1	E938.3	E950.4	E962.0	E980.4
Serotonin	977.8	E858.8	E947.8	E950.4	E962.0	E980.4
Serpasil	972.6	E858.3	E942.6	E950.4	E962.0	E980.4
Sewer gas	987.8	E869.8	—	E952.8	E962.2	E982.8
Shampoo	989.6	E861.0	—	E950.9	E962.1	E980.9
Shellfish, nonbacterial or noxious	988.0	E865.1	—	E950.9	E962.1	E980.9
Silicones NEC	989.83	E866.8	E947.8	E950.9	E962.1	E980.9
Silvadene	976.0	E858.7	E946.0	E950.4	E962.0	E980.4
Silver (compound) (medicinal) NEC	976.0	E858.7	E946.0	E950.4	E962.0	E980.4
anti-infectives	976.0	E858.7	E946.0	E950.4	E962.0	E980.4
arsphenamine	961.1	E857	E931.1	E950.4	E962.0	E980.4
nitrate	976.0	E858.7	E946.0	E950.4	E962.0	E980.4
ophthalmic preparation	976.5	E858.7	E946.5	E950.4	E962.0	E980.4
toughened (keratolytic)	976.4	E858.7	E946.4	E950.4	E962.0	E980.4
nonmedicinal (dust)	985.8	E866.4	—	E950.9	E962.1	E980.9
protein (mild) (strong)	976.0	E858.7	E946.0	E950.4	E962.0	E980.4
salvarsan	961.1	E857	E931.1	E950.4	E962.0	E980.4
Simethicone	973.8	E858.4	E943.8	E950.4	E962.0	E980.4
Sinequan	969.05	E854.0	E939.0	E950.3	E962.0	E980.3
Singoserp	972.6	E858.3	E942.6	E950.4	E962.0	E980.4
Sintrom	964.2	E858.2	E934.2	E950.4	E962.0	E980.4
Sitosterols	972.2	E858.3	E942.2	E950.4	E962.0	E980.4
Skeletal muscle relaxants	975.2	E858.6	E945.2	E950.4	E962.0	E980.4
Skin						
agents (external)	976.9	E858.7	E946.9	E950.4	E962.0	E980.4
specified NEC	976.8	E858.7	E946.8	E950.4	E962.0	E980.4

	Poisoning	Accident	Therapeutic Use	Suicide Attempt	Assault	Undetermined
Skin — *continued*						
test antigen	977.8	E858.8	E947.8	E950.4	E962.0	E980.4
Sleep-eze	963.0	E858.1	E933.0	E950.4	E962.0	E980.4
Sleeping draught (drug) (pill) (tablet)	967.9	E852.9	E937.9	E950.2	E962.0	E980.2
Smallpox vaccine	979.0	E858.8	E949.0	E950.4	E962.0	E980.4
Smelter fumes NEC	985.9	E866.4	—	E950.9	E962.1	E980.9
Smog	987.3	E869.1	—	E952.8	E962.2	E982.8
Smoke NEC	987.9	E869.9	—	E952.9	E962.2	E982.9
Smooth muscle relaxant	975.1	E858.6	E945.1	E950.4	E962.0	E980.4
Snail killer	989.4	E863.4	—	E950.6	E962.1	E980.7
Snake (bite) (venom)	989.5	E905.0	—	E950.9	E962.1	E980.9
Snuff	989.89	E866.8	—	E950.9	E962.1	E980.9
Soap (powder) (product)	989.6	E861.1	—	E950.9	E962.1	E980.9
bicarb	963.3	E858.1	E933.3	E950.4	E962.0	E980.4
chlorinated — see Sodium, hypochlorite						
medicinal, soft	976.2	E858.7	E946.2	E950.4	E962.0	E980.4
Soda (caustic)	983.2	E864.2	—	E950.7	E962.1	E980.6
Sodium						
acetosulfone	961.8	E857	E931.8	E950.4	E962.0	E980.4
acetrizoate	977.8	E858.8	E947.8	E950.4	E962.0	E980.4
amytal	967.0	E851	E937.0	E950.1	E962.0	E980.1
arsenate — see Arsenic						
bicarbonate	963.3	E858.1	E933.3	E950.4	E962.0	E980.4
bichromate	983.9	E864.3	—	E950.7	E962.1	E980.6
biphosphate	963.2	E858.1	E933.2	E950.4	E962.0	E980.4
bisulfate	983.9	E864.3	—	E950.7	E962.1	E980.6
borate (cleanser)	989.6	E861.3	—	E950.9	E962.1	E980.9
bromide NEC	967.3	E852.2	E937.3	E950.2	E962.0	E980.2
cacodylate (nonmedicinal) NEC	978.8	E858.8	E948.8	E950.4	E962.0	E980.4
anti-infective	961.1	E857	E931.1	E950.4	E962.0	E980.4
herbicide	989.4	E863.5	—	E950.6	E962.1	E980.7
calcium edetate	963.8	E858.1	E933.8	E950.4	E962.0	E980.4
carbonate NEC	983.2	E864.2	—	E950.7	E962.1	E980.6
chlorate NEC	983.9	E864.3	—	E950.7	E962.1	E980.6
herbicide	983.9	E863.5	—	E950.7	E962.1	E980.6
chloride NEC	974.5	E858.5	E944.5	E950.4	E962.0	E980.4
chromate	983.9	E864.3	—	E950.7	E962.1	E980.6
citrate	963.3	E858.1	E933.3	E950.4	E962.0	E980.4
cyanide — see Cyanide(s)						
cyclamate	974.5	E858.5	E944.5	E950.4	E962.0	E980.4
diatrizoate	977.8	E858.8	E947.8	E950.4	E962.0	E980.4
dibunate	975.4	E858.6	E945.4	E950.4	E962.0	E980.4
dioctyl sulfosuccinate	973.2	E858.4	E943.2	E950.4	E962.0	E980.4
edetate	963.8	E858.1	E933.8	E950.4	E962.0	E980.4
ethacrynate	974.4	E858.5	E944.4	E950.4	E962.0	E980.4
fluoracetate (dust) (rodenticide)	989.4	E863.7	—	E950.6	E962.1	E980.7
fluoride — see Fluoride(s)						
free salt	974.5	E858.5	E944.5	E950.4	E962.0	E980.4
glucosulfone	961.8	E857	E931.8	E950.4	E962.0	E980.4
hydroxide	983.2	E864.2	—	E950.7	E962.1	E980.6
hypochlorite (bleach) NEC	983.9	E864.3	—	E950.7	E962.1	E980.6
disinfectant	983.9	E861.4	—	E950.7	E962.1	E980.6
medicinal (anti-infective) (external)	976.0	E858.7	E946.0	E950.4	E962.0	E980.4
vapor	987.8	E869.8	—	E952.8	E962.2	E982.8
hyposulfite	976.0	E858.7	E946.0	E950.4	E962.0	E980.4
indigotindisulfonate	977.8	E858.8	E947.8	E950.4	E962.0	E980.4
iodide	977.8	E858.8	E947.8	E950.4	E962.0	E980.4
iothalamate	977.8	E858.8	E947.8	E950.4	E962.0	E980.4
iron edetate	964.0	E858.2	E934.0	E950.4	E962.0	E980.4
lactate	963.3	E858.1	E933.3	E950.4	E962.0	E980.4
lauryl sulfate	976.2	E858.7	E946.2	E950.4	E962.0	E980.4
L-triiodothyronine	962.7	E858.0	E932.7	E950.4	E962.0	E980.4
metrizoate	977.8	E858.8	E947.8	E950.4	E962.0	E980.4
monofluoracetate (dust) (rodenticide)	989.4	E863.7	—	E950.6	E962.1	E980.7
morrhuate	972.7	E858.3	E942.7	E950.4	E962.0	E980.4
nafcillin	960.0	E856	E930.0	E950.4	E962.0	E980.4
nitrate (oxidizing agent)	983.9	E864.3	—	E950.7	E962.1	E980.6
nitrite (medicinal)	972.4	E858.3	E942.4	E950.4	E962.0	E980.4
nitroferricyanide	972.6	E858.3	E942.6	E950.4	E962.0	E980.4
nitroprusside	972.6	E858.3	E942.6	E950.4	E962.0	E980.4
para-aminohippurate	977.8	E858.8	E947.8	E950.4	E962.0	E980.4
perborate (nonmedicinal) NEC	989.89	E866.8	—	E950.9	E962.1	E980.9
medicinal	976.6	E858.7	E946.6	E950.4	E962.0	E980.4
soap	989.6	E861.1	—	E950.9	E962.1	E980.9
Sodium — *continued*						
percarbonate — see Sodium, perborate						
phosphate	973.3	E858.4	E943.3	E950.4	E962.0	E980.4
polystyrene sulfonate	974.5	E858.5	E944.5	E950.4	E962.0	E980.4
propionate	976.0	E858.7	E946.0	E950.4	E962.0	E980.4
psylliate	972.7	E858.3	E942.7	E950.4	E962.0	E980.4
removing resins	974.5	E858.5	E944.5	E950.4	E962.0	E980.4
salicylate	965.1	E850.3	E935.3	E950.0	E962.0	E980.0
sulfate	973.3	E858.4	E943.3	E950.4	E962.0	E980.4
sulfoxone	961.8	E857	E931.8	E950.4	E962.0	E980.4
tetradecyl sulfate	972.7	E858.3	E942.7	E950.4	E962.0	E980.4
thiopental	968.3	E855.1	E938.3	E950.4	E962.0	E980.4
thiosalicylate	965.1	E850.3	E935.3	E950.0	E962.0	E980.0
thiosulfate	976.0	E858.7	E946.0	E950.4	E962.0	E980.4
tolbutamide	977.8	E858.8	E947.8	E950.4	E962.0	E980.4
tyropanoate	977.8	E858.8	E947.8	E950.4	E962.0	E980.4
valproate	966.3	E855.0	E936.3	E950.4	E962.0	E980.4
Solanine	977.8	E858.8	E947.8	E950.4	E962.0	E980.4
Solanum dulcamara	988.2	E865.4	—	E950.9	E962.1	E980.9
Solapsone	961.8	E857	E931.8	E950.4	E962.0	E980.4
Solasulfone	961.8	E857	E931.8	E950.4	E962.0	E980.4
Soldering fluid	983.1	E864.1	—	E950.7	E962.1	E980.6
Solid substance	989.9	E866.9	—	E950.9	E962.1	E980.9
specified NEC	989.9	E866.8	—	E950.9	E962.1	E980.9
Solvents, industrial	982.8	E862.9	—	E950.9	E962.1	E980.9
naphtha	981	E862.0	—	E950.9	E962.1	E980.9
petroleum	981	E862.0	—	E950.9	E962.1	E980.9
specified NEC	982.8	E862.4	—	E950.9	E962.1	E980.9
Soma	968.0	E855.1	E938.0	E950.4	E962.0	E980.4
Somatotropin	962.4	E858.0	E932.4	E950.4	E962.0	E980.4
Sominex	963.0	E858.1	E933.0	E950.4	E962.0	E980.4
Somnos	967.1	E852.0	E937.1	E950.2	E962.0	E980.2
Somonal	967.0	E851	E937.0	E950.1	E962.0	E980.1
Soneryl	967.0	E851	E937.0	E950.1	E962.0	E980.1
Soothing syrup	977.9	E858.9	E947.9	E950.5	E962.0	E980.5
Sopor	967.4	E852.3	E937.4	E950.2	E962.0	E980.2
Soporific drug	967.9	E852.9	E937.9	E950.2	E962.0	E980.2
specified type NEC	967.8	E852.8	E937.8	E950.2	E962.0	E980.2
Sorbitol NEC	977.4	E858.8	E947.4	E950.4	E962.0	E980.4
Sotradecol	972.7	E858.3	E942.7	E950.4	E962.0	E980.4
Spacoline	975.1	E858.6	E945.1	E950.4	E962.0	E980.4
Spanish fly	976.8	E858.7	E946.8	E950.4	E962.0	E980.4
Sparine	969.1	E853.0	E939.1	E950.3	E962.0	E980.3
Sparteine	975.0	E858.6	E945.0	E950.4	E962.0	E980.4
Spasmolytics	975.1	E858.6	E945.1	E950.4	E962.0	E980.4
anticholinergics	971.1	E855.4	E941.1	E950.4	E962.0	E980.4
Spectinomycin	960.8	E856	E930.8	E950.4	E962.0	E980.4
Speed	969.72	E854.2	E939.7	E950.3	E962.0	E980.3
Spermicides	976.8	E858.7	E946.8	E950.4	E962.0	E980.4
Spider (bite) (venom)	989.5	E905.1	—	E950.9	E962.1	E980.9
antivenin	979.9	E858.8	E949.9	E950.4	E962.0	E980.4
Spigelia (root)	961.6	E857	E931.6	E950.4	E962.0	E980.4
Spiperone	969.2	E853.1	E939.2	E950.3	E962.0	E980.3
Spiramycin	960.3	E856	E930.3	E950.4	E962.0	E980.4
Spirilene	969.5	E853.8	E939.5	E950.3	E962.0	E980.3
Spirit(s) (neutral) NEC	980.0	E860.1	—	E950.9	E962.1	E980.9
beverage	980.0	E860.0	—	E950.9	E962.1	E980.9
industrial	980.9	E860.9	—	E950.9	E962.1	E980.9
mineral	981	E862.0	—	E950.9	E962.1	E980.9
of salt — see Hydrochloric acid						
surgical	980.9	E860.9	—	E950.9	E962.1	E980.9
Spironolactone	974.4	E858.5	E944.4	E950.4	E962.0	E980.4
Sponge, absorbable (gelatin)	964.5	E858.2	E934.5	E950.4	E962.0	E980.4
Sporostacin	976.0	E858.7	E946.0	E950.4	E962.0	E980.4
Sprays (aerosol)	989.89	E866.8	—	E950.9	E962.1	E980.9
cosmetic	989.89	E866.7	—	E950.9	E962.1	E980.9
medicinal NEC	977.9	E858.9	E947.9	E950.5	E962.0	E980.5
pesticides — see Pesticides						
specified content — see substance specified						
Spurge flax	988.2	E865.4	—	E950.9	E962.1	E980.9
Spurges	988.2	E865.4	—	E950.9	E962.1	E980.9
Squill (expectorant) NEC	975.5	E858.6	E945.5	E950.4	E962.0	E980.4
rat poison	989.4	E863.7	—	E950.6	E962.1	E980.7
Squirting cucumber (cathartic)	973.1	E858.4	E943.1	E950.4	E962.0	E980.4
SSNRI (selective serotonin and norepinephrine reuptake inhibitors)	969.02	E854.0	E939.0	E950.3	E962.0	E980.3

▨ Nontherapeutic use substance

✶ Subterms under main terms may continue to next column or page

	External Cause (E-Code)					
	Poisoning	Accident	Therapeutic Use	Suicide Attempt	Assault	Undetermined
SSRI (selective serotonin reuptake inhibitors)	969.03	E854.0	E939.0	E950.3	E962.0	E980.3
Stains	989.89	E866.8	—	E950.9	E962.1	E980.9
Stannous — see also Tin						
fluoride	976.7	E858.7	E946.7	E950.4	E962.0	E980.4
Stanolone	962.1	E858.0	E932.1	E950.4	E962.0	E980.4
Stanozolol	962.1	E858.0	E932.1	E950.4	E962.0	E980.4
Staphisagria or stavesacre (pediculicide)	976.0	E858.7	E946.0	E950.4	E962.0	E980.4
Stelazine	969.1	E853.0	E939.1	E950.3	E962.0	E980.3
Stemetil	969.1	E853.0	E939.1	E950.3	E962.0	E980.3
Sterculia (cathartic) (gum)	973.3	E858.4	E943.3	E950.4	E962.0	E980.4
Sternutator gas	987.8	E869.8	—	E952.8	E962.2	E982.8
Steroids NEC	962.0	E858.0	E932.0	E950.4	E962.0	E980.4
ENT agent	976.6	E858.7	E946.6	E950.4	E962.0	E980.4
ophthalmic preparation	976.5	E858.7	E946.5	E950.4	E962.0	E980.4
topical NEC	976.0	E858.7	E946.0	E950.4	E962.0	E980.4
Stibine	985.8	E866.4	—	E950.9	E962.1	E980.9
Stibophen	961.2	E857	E931.2	E950.4	E962.0	E980.4
Stilbamide, stilbamidine	961.5	E857	E931.5	E950.4	E962.0	E980.4
Stilbestrol	962.2	E858.0	E932.2	E950.4	E962.0	E980.4
Stimulants (central nervous system)	970.9	E854.3	E940.9	E950.4	E962.0	E980.4
analeptics	970.0	E854.3	E940.0	E950.4	E962.0	E980.4
opiate antagonist	970.1	E854.3	E940.1	E950.4	E962.0	E980.4
psychotherapeutic NEC	969.09	E854.0	E939.0	E950.3	E962.0	E980.3
specified NEC	970.89	E854.3	E940.8	E950.4	E962.0	E980.4
Storage batteries (acid) (cells)	983.1	E864.1	—	E950.7	E962.1	E980.6
Stovaine	968.9	E855.2	E938.9	E950.4	E962.0	E980.4
infiltration (subcutaneous)	968.5	E855.2	E938.5	E950.4	E962.0	E980.4
nerve block (peripheral) (plexus)	968.6	E855.2	E938.6	E950.4	E962.0	E980.4
spinal	968.7	E855.2	E938.7	E950.4	E962.0	E980.4
topical (surface)	968.5	E855.2	E938.5	E950.4	E962.0	E980.4
Stovarsal	961.1	E857	E931.1	E950.4	E962.0	E980.4
Stove gas — see Gas, utility						
Stoxil	976.5	E858.7	E946.5	E950.4	E962.0	E980.4
STP	969.6	E854.1	E939.6	E950.3	E962.0	E980.3
Stramonium (medicinal) NEC	971.1	E855.4	E941.1	E950.4	E962.0	E980.4
natural state	988.2	E865.4	—	E950.9	E962.1	E980.9
Streptodornase	964.4	E858.2	E934.4	E950.4	E962.0	E980.4
Streptoduocin	960.6	E856	E930.6	E950.4	E962.0	E980.4
Streptokinase	964.4	E858.2	E934.4	E950.4	E962.0	E980.4
Streptomycin	960.6	E856	E930.6	E950.4	E962.0	E980.4
Streptozocin	960.7	E856	E930.7	E950.4	E962.0	E980.4
Stripper (paint) (solvent)	982.8	E862.9	—	E950.9	E962.1	E980.9
Strobane	989.2	E863.0	—	E950.6	E962.1	E980.7
Strophanthin	972.1	E858.3	E942.1	E950.4	E962.0	E980.4
Strophanthus hispidus or kombe	988.2	E865.4	—	E950.9	E962.1	E980.9
Strychnine (rodenticide) (salts)	989.1	E863.7	—	E950.6	E962.1	E980.7
medicinal NEC	970.89	E854.3	E940.8	E950.4	E962.0	E980.4
Strychnos (ignatii) — see Strychnine						
Styramate	968.0	E855.1	E938.0	E950.4	E962.0	E980.4
Styrene	983.0	E864.0	—	E950.7	E962.1	E980.6
Succinimide (anticonvulsant)	966.2	E855.0	E936.2	E950.4	E962.0	E980.4
mercuric — see Mercury						
Succinylcholine	975.2	E858.6	E945.2	E950.4	E962.0	E980.4
Succinylsulfathiazole	961.0	E857	E931.0	E950.4	E962.0	E980.4
Sucrose	974.5	E858.5	E944.5	E950.4	E962.0	E980.4
Sulfacetamide	961.0	E857	E931.0	E950.4	E962.0	E980.4
ophthalmic preparation	976.5	E858.7	E946.5	E950.4	E962.0	E980.4
Sulfachlorpyridazine	961.0	E857	E931.0	E950.4	E962.0	E980.4
Sulfacytine	961.0	E857	E931.0	E950.4	E962.0	E980.4
Sulfadiazine	961.0	E857	E931.0	E950.4	E962.0	E980.4
silver (topical)	976.0	E858.7	E946.0	E950.4	E962.0	E980.4
Sulfadimethoxine	961.0	E857	E931.0	E950.4	E962.0	E980.4
Sulfadimidine	961.0	E857	E931.0	E950.4	E962.0	E980.4
Sulfaethidole	961.0	E857	E931.0	E950.4	E962.0	E980.4
Sulfafurazole	961.0	E857	E931.0	E950.4	E962.0	E980.4
Sulfaguanidine	961.0	E857	E931.0	E950.4	E962.0	E980.4
Sulfamerazine	961.0	E857	E931.0	E950.4	E962.0	E980.4
Sulfameter	961.0	E857	E931.0	E950.4	E962.0	E980.4
Sulfamethizole	961.0	E857	E931.0	E950.4	E962.0	E980.4
Sulfamethoxazole	961.0	E857	E931.0	E950.4	E962.0	E980.4
Sulfamethoxydiazine	961.0	E857	E931.0	E950.4	E962.0	E980.4

	External Cause (E-Code)					
	Poisoning	Accident	Therapeutic Use	Suicide Attempt	Assault	Undetermined
Sulfamethoxypyridazine	961.0	E857	E931.0	E950.4	E962.0	E980.4
Sulfamethylthiazole	961.0	E857	E931.0	E950.4	E962.0	E980.4
Sulfamylon	976.0	E858.7	E946.0	E950.4	E962.0	E980.4
Sulfan blue (diagnostic dye)	977.8	E858.8	E947.8	E950.4	E962.0	E980.4
Sulfanilamide	961.0	E857	E931.0	E950.4	E962.0	E980.4
Sulfanilylguanidine	961.0	E857	E931.0	E950.4	E962.0	E980.4
Sulfaphenazole	961.0	E857	E931.0	E950.4	E962.0	E980.4
Sulfaphenylthiazole	961.0	E857	E931.0	E950.4	E962.0	E980.4
Sulfaproxyline	961.0	E857	E931.0	E950.4	E962.0	E980.4
Sulfapyridine	961.0	E857	E931.0	E950.4	E962.0	E980.4
Sulfapyrimidine	961.0	E857	E931.0	E950.4	E962.0	E980.4
Sulfarsphenamine	961.1	E857	E931.1	E950.4	E962.0	E980.4
Sulfasalazine	961.0	E857	E931.0	E950.4	E962.0	E980.4
Sulfasomizole	961.0	E857	E931.0	E950.4	E962.0	E980.4
Sulfasuxidine	961.0	E857	E931.0	E950.4	E962.0	E980.4
Sulfinpyrazone	974.7	E858.5	E944.7	E950.4	E962.0	E980.4
Sulfisoxazole	961.0	E857	E931.0	E950.4	E962.0	E980.4
ophthalmic preparation	976.5	E858.7	E946.5	E950.4	E962.0	E980.4
Sulfomyxin	960.8	E856	E930.8	E950.4	E962.0	E980.4
Sulfonal	967.8	E852.8	E937.8	E950.2	E962.0	E980.2
Sulfonamides (mixtures)	961.0	E857	E931.0	E950.4	E962.0	E980.4
Sulfones	961.8	E857	E931.8	E950.4	E962.0	E980.4
Sulfonethylmethane	967.8	E852.8	E937.8	E950.2	E962.0	E980.2
Sulfonmethane	967.8	E852.8	E937.8	E950.2	E962.0	E980.2
Sulfonphthal, sulfonphthol	977.8	E858.8	E947.8	E950.4	E962.0	E980.4
Sulfonylurea derivatives, oral	962.3	E858.0	E932.3	E950.4	E962.0	E980.4
Sulfoxone	961.8	E857	E931.8	E950.4	E962.0	E980.4
Sulfur, sulfureted, sulfuric, sulfurous, sulfuryl (compounds) NEC	989.89	E866.8	—	E950.9	E962.1	E980.9
acid	983.1	E864.1	—	E950.7	E962.1	E980.6
dioxide	987.3	E869.1	—	E952.8	E962.2	E982.8
ether — see Ether(s)						
hydrogen	987.8	E869.8	—	E952.8	E962.2	E982.8
medicinal (keratolytic) (ointment) NEC	976.4	E858.7	E946.4	E950.4	E962.0	E980.4
pesticide (vapor)	989.4	E863.4	—	E950.6	E962.1	E980.7
vapor NEC	987.8	E869.8	—	E952.8	E962.2	E982.8
Sulkowitch's reagent	977.8	E858.8	E947.8	E950.4	E962.0	E980.4
Sulphadione	961.8	E857	E931.8	E950.4	E962.0	E980.4
Sulph — see also Sulf-						
Sulthiame, sultiame	966.3	E855.0	E936.3	E950.4	E962.0	E980.4
Superinone	975.5	E858.6	E945.5	E950.4	E962.0	E980.4
Suramin	961.5	E857	E931.5	E950.4	E962.0	E980.4
Surfacaine	968.5	E855.2	E938.5	E950.4	E962.0	E980.4
Surital	968.3	E855.1	E938.3	E950.4	E962.0	E980.4
Sutilains	976.8	E858.7	E946.8	E950.4	E962.0	E980.4
Suxamethonium (bromide) (chloride) (iodide)	975.2	E858.6	E945.2	E950.4	E962.0	E980.4
Suxethonium (bromide)	975.2	E858.6	E945.2	E950.4	E962.0	E980.4
Sweet oil (birch)	976.3	E858.7	E946.3	E950.4	E962.0	E980.4
Sym-dichloroethyl ether	982.3	E862.4	—	E950.9	E962.1	E980.9
Sympatholytics	971.3	E855.6	E941.3	E950.4	E962.0	E980.4
Sympathomimetics	971.2	E855.5	E941.2	E950.4	E962.0	E980.4
Synagis	979.6	E858.8	E949.6	E950.4	E962.0	E980.4
Synalar	976.0	E858.7	E946.0	E950.4	E962.0	E980.4
Synthroid	962.7	E858.0	E932.7	E950.4	E962.0	E980.4
Syntocinon	975.0	E858.6	E945.0	E950.4	E962.0	—
Syrosingopine	972.6	E858.3	E942.6	E950.4	E962.0	E980.4
Systemic agents (primarily)	963.9	E858.1	E933.9	E950.4	E962.0	E980.4
specified NEC	963.8	E858.1	E933.8	E950.4	E962.0	E980.4
Tablets — see also specified substance	977.9	E858.9	E947.9	E950.5	E962.0	E980.5
Tace	962.2	E858.0	E932.2	E950.4	E962.0	E980.4
Tacrine	971.0	E855.3	E941.0	E950.4	E962.0	E980.4
Talbutal	967.0	E851	E937.0	E950.1	E962.0	E980.1
Talc	976.3	E858.7	E946.3	E950.4	E962.0	E980.4
Talcum	976.3	E858.7	E946.3	E950.4	E962.0	E980.4
Tamsulosin	971.3	E855.6	E941.3	E950.4	E962.0	E980.4
Tandearil, tanderil	965.5	E850.5	E935.5	E950.0	E962.0	E980.0
Tannic acid	983.1	E864.1	—	E950.7	E962.1	E980.6
medicinal (astringent)	976.2	E858.7	E946.2	E950.4	E962.0	E980.4
Tannin — see Tannic acid						
Tansy	988.2	E865.4	—	E950.9	E962.1	E980.9
TAO	960.3	E856	E930.3	E950.4	E962.0	E980.4
Tapazole	962.8	E858.0	E932.8	E950.4	E962.0	E980.4
Taractan	969.3	E853.8	E939.3	E950.3	E962.0	E980.3
Tarantula (venomous)	989.5	E905.1	—	E950.9	E962.1	E980.9

Substance		External Cause (E-Code)				
	Poisoning	Accident	Therapeutic Use	Suicide Attempt	Assault	Undetermined
Tartar emetic (anti-infective)	961.2	E857	E931.2	E950.4	E962.0	E980.4
Tartaric acid	983.1	E864.1	—	E950.7	E962.1	E980.6
Tartrated antimony (anti-infective)	961.2	E857	E931.2	E950.4	E962.0	E980.4
Tar NEC	983.0	E864.0	—	E950.7	E962.1	E980.6
camphor — see Naphthalene						
fumes	987.8	E869.8	—	E952.8	E962.2	E982.8
TCA — see Trichloroacetic acid						
TDI	983.0	E864.0	—	E950.7	E962.1	E980.6
vapor	987.8	E869.8	—	E952.8	E962.2	E982.8
Tear gas	987.5	E869.3	—	E952.8	E962.2	E982.8
Teclothiazide	974.3	E858.5	E944.3	E950.4	E962.0	E980.4
Tegretol	966.3	E855.0	E936.3	E950.4	E962.0	E980.4
Telepaque	977.8	E858.8	E947.8	E950.4	E962.0	E980.4
Tellurium	985.8	E866.4	—	E950.9	E962.1	E980.9
fumes	985.8	E866.4	—	E950.9	E962.1	E980.9
TEM	963.1	E858.1	E933.1	E950.4	E962.0	E980.4
Temazepan — see Benzodiazepines						
TEPA	963.1	E858.1	E933.1	E950.4	E962.0	E980.4
TEPP	989.3	E863.1	—	E950.6	E962.1	E980.7
Terbutaline	971.2	E855.5	E941.2	E950.4	E962.0	E980.4
Teroxalene	961.6	E857	E931.6	E950.4	E962.0	E980.4
Terpin hydrate	975.5	E858.6	E945.5	E950.4	E962.0	E980.4
Terramycin	960.4	E856	E930.4	E950.4	E962.0	E980.4
Tessalon	975.4	E858.6	E945.4	E950.4	E962.0	E980.4
Testosterone	962.1	E858.0	E932.1	E950.4	E962.0	E980.4
Tetanus (vaccine)	978.4	E858.8	E948.4	E950.4	E962.0	E980.4
antitoxin	979.9	E858.8	E949.9	E950.4	E962.0	E980.4
immune globulin (human)	964.6	E858.2	E934.6	E950.4	E962.0	E980.4
toxoid	978.4	E858.8	E948.4	E950.4	E962.0	E980.4
with diphtheria toxoid	978.9	E858.8	E948.9	E950.4	E962.0	E980.4
with pertussis	978.6	E858.8	E948.6	E950.4	E962.0	E980.4
Tetrabenazine	969.5	E853.8	E939.5	E950.3	E962.0	E980.3
Tetracaine (infiltration) (topical)	968.5	E855.2	E938.5	E950.4	E962.0	E980.4
nerve block (peripheral) (plexus)	968.6	E855.2	E938.6	E950.4	E962.0	E980.4
spinal	968.7	E855.2	E938.7	E950.4	E962.0	E980.4
Tetrachlorethylene — see Tetrachloroethylene						
Tetrachlormethiazide	974.3	E858.5	E944.3	E950.4	E962.0	E980.4
Tetrachloroethane (liquid) (vapor)	982.3	E862.4	—	E950.9	E962.1	E980.9
paint or varnish	982.3	E861.6	—	E950.9	E962.1	E980.9
Tetrachloroethylene (liquid) (vapor)	982.3	E862.4	—	E950.9	E962.1	E980.9
medicinal	961.6	E857	E931.6	E950.4	E962.0	E980.4
Tetrachloromethane — see Carbon, tetrachloride						
Tetracycline	960.4	E856	E930.4	E950.4	E962.0	E980.4
ophthalmic preparation	976.5	E858.7	E946.5	E950.4	E962.0	E980.4
topical NEC	976.0	E858.7	E946.0	E950.4	E962.0	E980.4
Tetraethylammonium chloride	972.3	E858.3	E942.3	E950.4	E962.0	E980.4
Tetraethyl lead (antiknock compound)	984.1	E862.1	—	E950.9	E962.1	E980.9
Tetraethyl pyrophosphate	989.3	E863.1	—	E950.6	E962.1	E980.7
Tetraethylthiuram disulfide	977.3	E858.8	E947.3	E950.4	E962.0	E980.4
Tetrahydroaminoacridine	971.0	E855.3	E941.0	E950.4	E962.0	E980.4
Tetrahydrocannabinol	969.6	E854.1	E939.6	E950.3	E962.0	E980.3
Tetrahydronaphthalene	982.0	E862.4	—	E950.9	E962.1	E980.9
Tetrahydrozoline	971.2	E855.5	E941.2	E950.4	E962.0	E980.4
Tetralin	982.0	E862.4	—	E950.9	E962.1	E980.9
Tetramethylthiuram (disulfide) NEC	989.4	E863.6	—	E950.6	E962.1	E980.7
medicinal	976.2	E858.7	E946.2	E950.4	E962.0	E980.4
Tetronal	967.8	E852.8	E937.8	E950.2	E962.0	E980.2
Tetryl	983.0	E864.0	—	E950.7	E962.1	E980.6
Thalidomide	967.8	E852.8	E937.8	E950.2	E962.0	E980.2
Thallium (compounds) (dust) NEC	985.8	E866.4	—	E950.9	E962.1	E980.9
pesticide (rodenticide)	985.8	E863.7	—	E950.6	E962.1	E980.7
THC	969.6	E854.1	E939.6	E950.3	E962.0	E980.3
Thebacon	965.09	E850.2	E935.2	E950.0	E962.0	E980.0
Thebaine	965.09	E850.2	E935.2	E950.0	E962.0	E980.0
Theobromine (calcium salicylate)	974.1	E858.5	E944.1	E950.4	E962.0	E980.4
Theophylline (diuretic)	974.1	E858.5	E944.1	E950.4	E962.0	E980.4
ethylenediamine	975.7	E858.6	E945.7	E950.4	E962.0	E980.4
Thiabendazole	961.6	E857	E931.6	E950.4	E962.0	E980.4
Thialbarbital, thialbarbitone	968.3	E855.1	E938.3	E950.4	E962.0	E980.4
Thiamine	963.5	E858.1	E933.5	E950.4	E962.0	E980.4
Thiamylal (sodium)	968.3	E855.1	E938.3	E950.4	E962.0	E980.4
Thiazesim	969.09	E854.0	E939.0	E950.3	E962.0	E980.3
Thiazides (diuretics)	974.3	E858.5	E944.3	E950.4	E962.0	E980.4
Thiethylperazine	963.0	E858.1	E933.0	E950.4	E962.0	E980.4
Thimerosal (topical)	976.0	E858.7	E946.0	E950.4	E962.0	E980.4
ophthalmic preparation	976.5	E858.7	E946.5	E950.4	E962.0	E980.4
Thioacetazone	961.8	E857	E931.8	E950.4	E962.0	E980.4
Thiobarbiturates	968.3	E855.1	E938.3	E950.4	E962.0	E980.4
Thiobismol	961.2	E857	E931.2	E950.4	E962.0	E980.4
Thiocarbamide	962.8	E858.0	E932.8	E950.4	E962.0	E980.4
Thiocarbarsone	961.1	E857	E931.1	E950.4	E962.0	E980.4
Thiocarlide	961.8	E857	E931.8	E950.4	E962.0	E980.4
Thioguanine	963.1	E858.1	E933.1	E950.4	E962.0	E980.4
Thiomercaptomerin	974.0	E858.5	E944.0	E950.4	E962.0	E980.4
Thiomerin	974.0	E858.5	E944.0	E950.4	E962.0	E980.4
Thiopental, thiopentone (sodium)	968.3	E855.1	E938.3	E950.4	E962.0	E980.4
Thiopropazate	969.1	E853.0	E939.1	E950.3	E962.0	E980.3
Thioproperazine	969.1	E853.0	E939.1	E950.3	E962.0	E980.3
Thioridazine	969.1	E853.0	E939.1	E950.3	E962.0	E980.3
Thio-TEPA, thiotepa	963.1	E858.1	E933.1	E950.4	E962.0	E980.4
Thiothixene	969.3	E853.8	E939.3	E950.3	E962.0	E980.4
Thiouracil	962.8	E858.0	E932.8	E950.4	E962.0	E980.4
Thiourea	962.8	E858.0	E932.8	E950.4	E962.0	E980.4
Thiphenamil	971.1	E855.4	E941.1	E950.4	E962.0	E980.4
Thiram NEC	989.4	E863.6	—	E950.6	E962.1	E980.7
medicinal	976.2	E858.7	E946.2	E950.4	E962.0	E980.4
Thonzylamine	963.0	E858.1	E933.0	E950.4	E962.0	E980.4
Thorazine	969.1	E853.0	E939.1	E950.3	E962.0	E980.3
Thornapple	988.2	E865.4	—	E950.9	E962.1	E980.9
Throat preparation (lozenges) NEC	976.6	E858.7	E946.6	E950.4	E962.0	E980.4
Thrombin	964.5	E858.2	E934.5	E950.4	E962.0	E980.4
Thrombolysin	964.4	E858.2	E934.4	E950.4	E962.0	E980.4
Thymol	983.0	E864.0	—	E950.7	E962.1	E980.6
Thymus extract	962.9	E858.0	E932.9	E950.4	E962.0	E980.4
Thyroglobulin	962.7	E858.0	E932.7	E950.4	E962.0	E980.4
Thyroid (derivatives) (extract)	962.7	E858.0	E932.7	E950.4	E962.0	E980.4
Thyrolar	962.7	E858.0	E932.7	E950.4	E962.0	E980.4
Thyrothrophin, thyrotropin	977.8	E858.8	E947.8	E950.4	E962.0	E980.4
Thyroxin(e)	962.7	E858.0	E932.7	E950.4	E962.0	E980.4
Tigan	963.0	E858.1	E933.0	E950.4	E962.0	E980.4
Tigloidine	968.0	E855.1	E938.0	E950.4	E962.0	E980.4
Tinactin	976.0	E858.7	E946.0	E950.4	E962.0	E980.4
Tincture, iodine — see Iodine						
Tindal	969.1	E853.0	E939.1	E950.3	E962.0	E980.3
Tin (chloride) (dust) (oxide) NEC	985.8	E866.4	—	E950.9	E962.1	E980.9
anti-infectives	961.2	E857	E931.2	E950.4	E962.0	E980.4
Titanium (compounds) (vapor)	985.8	E866.4	—	E950.9	E962.1	E980.9
ointment	976.3	E858.7	E946.3	E950.4	E962.0	E980.4
Titroid	962.7	E858.0	E932.7	E950.4	E962.0	E980.4
TMTD — see Tetramethylthiuram disulfide						
TNT	989.89	E866.8	—	E950.9	E962.1	E980.9
fumes	987.8	E869.8	—	E952.8	E962.2	E982.8
Toadstool	988.1	E865.5	—	E950.9	E962.1	E980.9
Tobacco NEC	989.84	E866.8	—	E950.9	E962.1	E980.9
Indian	988.2	E865.4	—	E950.9	E962.1	E980.9
smoke, second-hand	987.8	E869.4	—	—	—	—
Tocopherol	963.5	E858.1	E933.5	E950.4	E962.0	E980.4
Tocosamine	975.0	E858.6	E945.0	E950.4	E962.0	E980.4
Tofranil	969.05	E854.0	E939.0	E950.3	E962.0	E980.3
Toilet deodorizer	989.89	E866.8	—	E950.9	E962.1	E980.9
Tolazamide	962.3	E858.0	E932.3	E950.4	E962.0	E980.4
Tolazoline	971.3	E855.6	E941.3	E950.4	E962.0	E980.4
Tolbutamide	962.3	E858.0	E932.3	E950.4	E962.0	E980.4
sodium	977.8	E858.8	E947.8	E950.4	E962.0	E980.4
Tolmetin	965.69	E850.6	E935.6	E950.0	E962.0	E980.0
Tolnaftate	976.0	E858.7	E946.0	E950.4	E962.0	E980.4
Tolpropamine	976.1	E858.7	E946.1	E950.4	E962.0	E980.4

	Poisoning	Accident	Therapeutic Use	Suicide Attempt	Assault	Undetermined
Tolserol	968.0	E855.1	E938.0	E950.4	E962.0	E980.4
Toluene (liquid) (vapor)	982.0	E862.4	—	E950.9	E962.1	E980.9
diisocyanate	983.0	E864.0	—	E950.7	E962.1	E980.6
Toluidine	983.0	E864.0	—	E950.7	E962.1	E980.6
vapor	987.8	E869.8	—	E952.8	E962.2	E982.8
Toluol (liquid) (vapor)	982.0	E862.4	—	E950.9	E962.1	E980.9
Tolylene-2, 4-diiso-cyanate	983.0	E864.0	—	E950.7	E962.1	E980.6
Tonics, cardiac	972.1	E858.3	E942.1	E950.4	E962.0	E980.4
Toxaphene (dust) (spray)	989.2	E863.0	—	E950.6	E962.1	E980.7
Toxoids NEC	978.8	E858.8	E948.8	E950.4	E962.0	E980.4
Tractor fuel NEC	981	E862.1	—	E950.9	E962.1	E980.9
Tragacanth	973.3	E858.4	E943.3	E950.4	E962.0	E980.4
Tramazoline	971.2	E855.5	E941.2	E950.4	E962.0	E980.4
Tranquilizers	969.5	E853.9	E939.5	E950.3	E962.0	E980.3
benzodiazepine-based	969.4	E853.2	E939.4	E950.3	E962.0	E980.3
butyrophenone-based	969.2	E853.1	E939.2	E950.3	E962.0	E980.3
major NEC	969.3	E853.8	E939.3	E950.3	E962.0	E980.3
phenothiazine-based	969.1	E853.0	E939.1	E950.3	E962.0	E980.3
specified NEC	969.5	E853.8	E939.5	E950.3	E962.0	E980.3
Trantoin	961.9	E857	E931.9	E950.4	E962.0	E980.4
Tranxene	969.4	E853.2	E939.4	E950.3	E962.0	E980.3
Tranylcypromine (sulfate)	969.01	E854.0	E939.0	E950.3	E962.0	E980.3
Trasentine	975.1	E858.6	E945.1	E950.4	E962.0	E980.4
Travert	974.5	E858.5	E944.5	E950.4	E962.0	E980.4
Trecator	961.8	E857	E931.8	E950.4	E962.0	E980.4
Tretinoin	976.8	E858.7	E946.8	E950.4	E962.0	E980.4
Triacetin	976.0	E858.7	E946.0	E950.4	E962.0	E980.4
Triacetyloleandomycin	960.3	E856	E930.3	E950.4	E962.0	E980.4
Triamcinolone	962.0	E858.0	E932.0	E950.4	E962.0	E980.4
ENT agent	976.6	E858.7	E946.6	E950.4	E962.0	E980.4
medicinal (keratolytic)	976.4	E858.7	E946.4	E950.4	E962.0	E980.4
ophthalmic preparation	976.5	E858.7	E946.5	E950.4	E962.0	E980.4
topical NEC	976.0	E858.7	E946.0	E950.4	E962.0	E980.4
Triamterene	974.4	E858.5	E944.4	E950.4	E962.0	E980.4
Triaziquone	963.1	E858.1	E933.1	E950.4	E962.0	E980.4
Tribromacetaldehyde	967.3	E852.2	E937.3	E950.2	E962.0	E980.2
Tribromoethanol	968.2	E855.1	E938.2	E950.4	E962.0	E980.4
Tribromomethane	967.3	E852.2	E937.3	E950.2	E962.0	E980.2
Trichlorethane	982.3	E862.4	—	E950.9	E962.1	E980.9
Trichlormethiazide	974.3	E858.5	E944.3	E950.4	E962.0	E980.4
Trichloroacetic acid	983.1	E864.1	—	E950.7	E962.1	E980.6
Trichloroethanol	967.1	E852.0	E937.1	E950.2	E962.0	E980.2
Trichloroethylene (liquid) (vapor)	982.3	E862.4	—	E950.9	E962.1	E980.9
anesthetic (gas)	968.2	E855.1	E938.2	E950.4	E962.0	E980.4
Trichloroethyl phosphate	967.1	E852.0	E937.1	E950.2	E962.0	E980.2
Trichlorofluoromethane NEC	987.4	E869.2	—	E952.8	E962.2	E982.8
Trichlorotriethylamine	963.1	E858.1	E933.1	E950.4	E962.0	E980.4
Trichomonacides NEC	961.5	E857	E931.5	E950.4	E962.0	E980.4
Trichomycin	960.1	E856	E930.1	E950.4	E962.0	E980.4
Triclofos	967.1	E852.0	E937.1	E950.2	E962.0	E980.2
Tricresyl phosphate	989.89	E866.8	—	E950.9	E962.1	E980.9
solvent	982.8	E862.4	—	E950.9	E962.1	E980.9
Tricyclamol	966.4	E855.0	E936.4	E950.4	E962.0	E980.4
Tridesilon	976.0	E858.7	E946.0	E950.4	E962.0	E980.4
Tridihexethyl	971.1	E855.4	E941.1	E950.4	E962.0	E980.4
Tridione	966.0	E855.0	E936.0	E950.4	E962.0	E980.4
Triethanolamine NEC	983.2	E864.2	—	E950.7	E962.1	E980.6
detergent	983.2	E861.0	—	E950.7	E962.1	E980.6
trinitrate	972.4	E858.3	E942.4	E950.4	E962.0	E980.4
Triethanomelamine	963.1	E858.1	E933.1	E950.4	E962.0	E980.4
Triethylene melamine	963.1	E858.1	E933.1	E950.4	E962.0	E980.4
Triethylenephosphoramide	963.1	E858.1	E933.1	E950.4	E962.0	E980.4
Triethylenethiophosphoramide	963.1	E858.1	E933.1	E950.4	E962.0	E980.4
Trifluoperazine	969.1	E853.0	E939.1	E950.3	E962.0	E980.3
Trifluperidol	969.2	E853.1	E939.2	E950.3	E962.0	E980.3
Triflupromazine	969.1	E853.0	E939.1	E950.3	E962.0	E980.3
Trihexyphenidyl	971.1	E855.4	E941.1	E950.4	E962.0	E980.4
Triiodothyronine	962.7	E858.0	E932.7	E950.4	E962.0	E980.4
Trilene	968.2	E855.1	E938.2	E950.4	E962.0	E980.4
Trimeprazine	963.0	E858.1	E933.0	E950.4	E962.0	E980.4
Trimetazidine	972.4	E858.3	E942.4	E950.4	E962.0	E980.4
Trimethadione	966.0	E855.0	E936.0	E950.4	E962.0	E980.4
Trimethaphan	972.3	E858.3	E942.3	E950.4	E962.0	E980.4
Trimethidinium	972.3	E858.3	E942.3	E950.4	E962.0	E980.4
Trimethobenzamide	963.0	E858.1	E933.0	E950.4	E962.0	E980.4
Trimethylcarbinol	980.8	E860.8	—	E950.9	E962.1	E980.9
Trimethylpsoralen	976.3	E858.7	E946.3	E950.4	E962.0	E980.4
Trimeton	963.0	E858.1	E933.0	E950.4	E962.0	E980.4
Trimipramine	969.05	E854.0	E939.0	E950.3	E962.0	E980.3
Trimustine	963.1	E858.1	E933.1	E950.4	E962.0	E980.4
Trinitrin	972.4	E858.3	E942.4	E950.4	E962.0	E980.4
Trinitrophenol	983.0	E864.0	—	E950.7	E962.1	E980.6
Trinitrotoluene	989.89	E866.8	—	E950.9	E962.1	E980.9
fumes	987.8	E869.8	—	E952.8	E962.2	E982.8
Trional	967.8	E852.8	E937.8	E950.2	E962.0	E980.2
Trioxide of arsenic — *see* Arsenic						
Trioxsalen	976.3	E858.7	E946.3	E950.4	E962.0	E980.4
Tripelennamine	963.0	E858.1	E933.0	E950.4	E962.0	E980.4
Triperidol	969.2	E853.1	E939.2	E950.3	E962.0	E980.3
Triprolidine	963.0	E858.1	E933.0	E950.4	E962.0	E980.4
Trisoralen	976.3	E858.7	E946.3	E950.4	E962.0	E980.4
Troleandomycin	960.3	E856	E930.3	E950.4	E962.0	E980.4
Trolnitrate (phosphate)	972.4	E858.3	E942.4	E950.4	E962.0	E980.4
Trometamol	963.3	E858.1	E933.3	E950.4	E962.0	E980.4
Tromethamine	963.3	E858.1	E933.3	E950.4	E962.0	E980.4
Tronothane	968.5	E855.2	E938.5	E950.4	E962.0	E980.4
Tropicamide	971.1	E855.4	E941.1	E950.4	E962.0	E980.4
Troxidone	966.0	E855.0	E936.0	E950.4	E962.0	E980.4
Tryparsamide	961.1	E857	E931.1	E950.4	E962.0	E980.4
Trypsin	963.4	E858.1	E933.4	E950.4	E962.0	E980.4
Tryptizol	969.05	E854.0	E939.0	E950.3	E962.0	E980.3
Tuaminoheptane	971.2	E855.5	E941.2	E950.4	E962.0	E980.4
Tuberculin (old)	977.8	E858.8	E947.8	E950.4	E962.0	E980.4
Tubocurare	975.2	E858.6	E945.2	E950.4	E962.0	E980.4
Tubocurarine	975.2	E858.6	E945.2	E950.4	E962.0	E980.4
Turkish green	969.6	E854.1	E939.6	E950.3	E962.0	E980.3
Turpentine (spirits of) (liquid) (vapor)	982.8	E862.4	—	E950.9	E962.1	E980.9
Tybamate	969.5	E853.8	E939.5	E950.3	E962.0	E980.3
Tyloxapol	975.5	E858.6	E945.5	E950.4	E962.0	E980.4
Tymazoline	971.2	E855.5	E941.2	E950.4	E962.0	E980.4
Typhoid vaccine	978.1	E858.8	E948.1	E950.4	E962.0	E980.4
Typhus vaccine	979.2	E858.8	E949.2	E950.4	E962.0	E980.4
Tyrothricin	976.0	E858.7	E946.0	E950.4	E962.0	E980.4
ENT agent	976.6	E858.7	E946.6	E950.4	E962.0	E980.4
ophthalmic preparation	976.5	E858.7	E946.5	E950.4	E962.0	E980.4
Undecenoic acid	976.0	E858.7	E946.0	E950.4	E962.0	E980.4
Undecylenic acid	976.0	E858.7	E946.0	E950.4	E962.0	E980.4
Unna's boot	976.3	E858.7	E946.3	E950.4	E962.0	E980.4
Uracil mustard	963.1	E858.1	E933.1	E950.4	E962.0	E980.4
Uramustine	963.1	E858.1	E933.1	E950.4	E962.0	E980.4
Urari	975.2	E858.6	E945.2	E950.4	E962.0	E980.4
Urea	974.4	E858.5	E944.4	E950.4	E962.0	E980.4
topical	976.8	E858.7	E946.8	E950.4	E962.0	E980.4
Urethan(e) (antineoplastic)	963.1	E858.1	E933.1	E950.4	E962.0	E980.4
Urginea (maritima) (scilla) — *see* Squill						
Uric acid metabolism agents NEC	974.7	E858.5	E944.7	E950.4	E962.0	E980.4
Urokinase	964.4	E858.2	E934.4	E950.4	E962.0	E980.4
Urokon	977.8	E858.8	E947.8	E950.4	E962.0	E980.4
Urotropin	961.9	E857	E931.9	E950.4	E962.0	E980.4
Urtica	988.2	E865.4	—	E950.9	E962.1	E980.9
Utility gas — *see* Gas, utility						
Vaccine NEC	979.9	E858.8	E949.9	E950.4	E962.0	E980.4
bacterial NEC	978.8	E858.8	E948.8	E950.4	E962.0	E980.4
with other bacterial component	978.9	E858.8	E948.9	E950.4	E962.0	E980.4
pertussis component	978.6	E858.8	E948.6	E950.4	E962.0	E980.4
viral-rickettsial component	979.7	E858.8	E949.7	E950.4	E962.0	E980.4
mixed NEC	978.9	E858.8	E948.9	E950.4	E962.0	E980.4
BCG	978.0	E858.8	E948.0	E950.4	E962.0	E980.4
cholera	978.2	E858.8	E948.2	E950.4	E962.0	E980.4
diphtheria	978.5	E858.8	E948.5	E950.4	E962.0	E980.4
influenza	979.6	E858.8	E949.6	E950.4	E962.0	E980.4
measles	979.4	E858.8	E949.4	E950.4	E962.0	E980.4
meningococcal	978.8	E858.8	E948.8	E950.4	E962.0	E980.4
mumps	979.6	E858.8	E949.6	E950.4	E962.0	E980.4
paratyphoid	978.1	E858.8	E948.1	E950.4	E962.0	E980.4
pertussis (with diphtheria toxoid) (with tetanus toxoid)	978.6	E858.8	E948.6	E950.4	E962.0	E980.4
plague	978.3	E858.8	E948.3	E950.4	E962.0	E980.4

	Poisoning	Accident	Therapeutic Use	Suicide Attempt	Assault	Undetermined
Vaccine — *continued*						
poliomyelitis	979.5	E858.8	E949.5	E950.4	E962.0	E980.4
poliovirus	979.5	E858.8	E949.5	E950.4	E962.0	E980.4
rabies	979.1	E858.8	E949.1	E950.4	E962.0	E980.4
respiratory syncytial virus	979.6	E858.8	E949.6	E950.4	E962.0	E980.4
rickettsial NEC	979.6	E858.8	E949.6	E950.4	E962.0	E980.4
with						
bacterial component	979.7	E858.8	E949.7	E950.4	E962.0	E980.4
pertussis component	978.6	E858.8	E948.6	E950.4	E962.0	E980.4
viral component	979.7	E858.8	E949.7	E950.4	E962.0	E980.4
Rocky mountain spotted fever	979.6	E858.8	E949.6	E950.4	E962.0	E980.4
rotavirus	979.6	E858.8	E949.6	E950.4	E962.0	E980.4
rubella virus	979.4	E858.8	E949.4	E950.4	E962.0	E980.4
sabin oral	979.5	E858.8	E949.5	E950.4	E962.0	E980.4
smallpox	979.0	E858.8	E949.0	E950.4	E962.0	E980.4
tetanus	978.4	E858.8	E948.4	E950.4	E962.0	E980.4
typhoid	978.1	E858.8	E948.1	E950.4	E962.0	E980.4
typhus	979.2	E858.8	E949.2	E950.4	E962.0	E980.4
viral NEC	979.6	E858.8	E949.6	E950.4	E962.0	E980.4
with						
bacterial component	979.7	E858.8	E949.7	E950.4	E962.0	E980.4
pertussis component	978.6	E858.8	E948.6	E950.4	E962.0	E980.4
rickettsial component	979.7	E858.8	E949.7	E950.4	E962.0	E980.4
yellow fever	979.3	E858.8	E949.3	E950.4	E962.0	E980.4
Vaccinia immune globulin (human)	964.6	E858.2	E934.6	E950.4	E962.0	E980.4
Vaginal contraceptives	976.8	E858.7	E946.8	E950.4	E962.0	E980.4
Valethamate	971.1	E855.4	E941.1	E950.4	E962.0	E980.4
Valisone	976.0	E858.7	E946.0	E950.4	E962.0	E980.4
Valium	969.4	E853.2	E939.4	E950.3	E962.0	E980.3
Valmid	967.8	E852.8	E937.8	E950.2	E962.0	E980.2
Vanadium	985.8	E866.4	—	E950.9	E962.1	E980.9
Vancomycin	960.8	E856	E930.8	E950.4	E962.0	E980.4
Vapor — *see also* Gas	987.9	E869.9		E952.9	E962.2	E982.9
kiln (carbon monoxide)	986	E868.8	—	E952.1	E962.2	E982.1
lead — *see* Lead						
specified source NEC (*see also* specific substance)	987.8	E869.8	—	E952.8	E962.2	E982.8
Varidase	964.4	E858.2	E934.4	E950.4	E962.0	E980.4
Varnish	989.89	E861.6		E950.9	E962.1	E980.9
cleaner	982.8	E862.9		E950.9	E962.1	E980.9
Vaseline	976.3	E858.7	E946.3	E950.4	E962.0	E980.4
Vasodilan	972.5	E858.3	E942.5	E950.4	E962.0	E980.4
Vasodilators NEC	972.5	E858.3	E942.5	E950.4	E962.0	E980.4
coronary	972.4	E858.3	E942.4	E950.4	E962.0	E980.4
Vasopressin	962.5	E858.0	E932.5	E950.4	E962.0	E980.4
Vasopressor drugs	962.5	E858.0	E932.5	E950.4	E962.0	E980.4
Venom, venomous (bite) (sting)	989.5	E905.9	—	E950.9	E962.1	E980.9
arthropod NEC	989.5	E905.5	—	E950.9	E962.1	E980.9
bee	989.5	E905.3	—	E950.9	E962.1	E980.9
centipede	989.5	E905.4	—	E950.9	E962.1	E980.9
hornet	989.5	E905.3	—	E950.9	E962.1	E980.9
lizard	989.5	E905.0	—	E950.9	E962.1	E980.9
marine animals or plants	989.5	E905.6	—	E950.9	E962.1	E980.9
millipede (tropical)	989.5	E905.4	—	E950.9	E962.1	E980.9
plant NEC	989.5	E905.7	—	E950.9	E962.1	E980.9
marine	989.5	E905.6	—	E950.9	E962.1	E980.9
scorpion	989.5	E905.2	—	E950.9	E962.1	E980.9
snake	989.5	E905.0	—	E950.9	E962.1	E980.9
specified NEC	989.5	E905.8	—	E950.9	E962.1	E980.9
spider	989.5	E905.1	—	E950.9	E962.1	E980.9
wasp	989.5	E905.3	—	E950.9	E962.1	E980.9
Ventolin — *see* Salbutamol sulfate						
Veramon	967.0	E851	E937.0	E950.1	E962.0	E980.1
Veratrum						
album	988.2	E865.4	—	E950.9	E962.1	E980.9
alkaloids	972.6	E858.3	E942.6	E950.4	E962.0	E980.4
viride	988.2	E865.4	—	E950.9	E962.1	E980.9
Verdigris — *see also* Copper	985.8	E866.4	—	E950.9	E962.1	E980.9
Veronal	967.0	E851	E937.0	E950.1	E962.0	E980.1
Veroxil	961.6	E857	E931.6	E950.4	E962.0	E980.4
Versidyne	965.7	E850.7	E935.7	E950.0	E962.0	E980.0
Viagra	972.5	E858.3	E942.5	E950.4	E962.0	E980.4
Vienna						
green	985.1	E866.3	—	E950.8	E962.1	E980.8
insecticide	985.1	E863.4	—	E950.6	E962.1	E980.7
red	989.89	E866.8	—	E950.9	E962.1	E980.9
pharmaceutical dye	977.4	E858.8	E947.4	E950.4	E962.0	E980.4

	Poisoning	Accident	Therapeutic Use	Suicide Attempt	Assault	Undetermined
Vinbarbital, vinbarbitone	967.0	E851	E937.0	E950.1	E962.0	E980.1
Vinblastine	963.1	E858.1	E933.1	E950.4	E962.0	E980.4
Vincristine	963.1	E858.1	E933.1	E950.4	E962.0	E980.4
Vinesthene, vinethene	968.2	E855.1	E938.2	E950.4	E962.0	E980.4
Vinyl						
bital	967.0	E851	E937.0	E950.1	E962.0	E980.1
ether	968.2	E855.1	E938.2	E950.4	E962.0	E980.4
Vioform	961.3	E857	E931.3	E950.4	E962.0	E980.4
topical	976.0	E858.7	E946.0	E950.4	E962.0	E980.4
Viomycin	960.6	E856	E930.6	E950.4	E962.0	E980.4
Viosterol	963.5	E858.1	E933.5	E950.4	E962.0	E980.4
Viper (venom)	989.5	E905.0	—	E950.9	E962.1	E980.9
Viprynium (embonate)	961.6	E857	E931.6	E950.4	E962.0	E980.4
Virugon	961.7	E857	E931.7	E950.4	E962.0	E980.4
Visine	976.5	E858.7	E946.5	E950.4	E962.0	E980.4
Vitamins NEC	963.5	E858.1	E933.5	E950.4	E962.0	E980.4
B_{12}	964.1	E858.2	E934.1	E950.4	E962.0	E980.4
hematopoietic	964.1	E858.2	E934.1	E950.4	E962.0	E980.4
K	964.3	E858.2	E934.3	E950.4	E962.0	E980.4
Vleminckx's solution	976.4	E858.7	E946.4	E950.4	E962.0	E980.4
Voltaren — *see* Diclofenac sodium						
Warfarin (potassium) (sodium)	964.2	E858.2	E934.2	E950.4	E962.0	E980.4
rodenticide	989.4	E863.7	—	E950.6	E962.1	E980.7
Wasp (sting)	989.5	E905.3	—	E950.9	E962.1	E980.9
Water						
balance agents NEC	974.5	E858.5	E944.5	E950.4	E962.0	E980.4
gas	987.1	E868.1	—	E951.8	E962.2	E981.8
incomplete combustion of — *see* Carbon, monoxide, fuel, utility						
hemlock	988.2	E865.4	—	E950.9	E962.1	E980.9
moccasin (venom)	989.5	E905.0	—	E950.9	E962.1	E980.9
Wax (paraffin) (petroleum)	981	E862.3	—	E950.9	E962.1	E980.9
automobile	989.89	E861.2	—	E950.9	E962.1	E980.9
floor	981	E862.0	—	E950.9	E962.1	E980.9
Weed killers NEC	989.4	E863.5	—	E950.6	E962.1	E980.7
Welldorm	967.1	E852.0	E937.1	E950.2	E962.0	E980.2
White						
arsenic — *see* Arsenic						
hellebore	988.2	E865.4	—	E950.9	E962.1	E980.9
lotion (keratolytic)	976.4	E858.7	E946.4	E950.4	E962.0	E980.4
spirit	981	E862.0	—	E950.9	E962.1	E980.9
Whitewashes	989.89	E861.6	—	E950.9	E962.1	E980.9
Whole blood	964.7	E858.2	E934.7	E950.4	E962.0	E980.4
Wild						
black cherry	988.2	E865.4	—	E950.9	E962.1	E980.9
poisonous plants NEC	988.2	E865.4	—	E950.9	E962.1	E980.9
Window cleaning fluid	989.89	E861.3	—	E950.9	E962.1	E980.9
Wintergreen (oil)	976.3	E858.7	E946.3	E950.4	E962.0	E980.4
Witch hazel	976.2	E858.7	E946.2	E950.4	E962.0	E980.4
Wood						
alcohol	980.1	E860.2	—	E950.9	E962.1	E980.9
spirit	980.1	E860.2	—	E950.9	E962.1	E980.9
Woorali	975.2	E858.6	E945.2	E950.4	E962.0	E980.4
Wormseed, American	961.6	E857	E931.6	E950.4	E962.0	E980.4
Xanthine diuretics	974.1	E858.5	E944.1	E950.4	E962.0	E980.4
Xanthocillin	960.0	E856	E930.0	E950.4	E962.0	E980.4
Xanthotoxin	976.3	E858.7	E946.3	E950.4	E962.0	E980.4
Xigris	964.2	E858.2	E934.2	E950.4	E962.0	E980.4
Xylene (liquid) (vapor)	982.0	E862.4	—	E950.9	E962.1	E980.9
Xylocaine (infiltration) (topical)	968.5	E855.2	E938.5	E950.4	E962.0	E980.4
nerve block (peripheral) (plexus)	968.6	E855.2	E938.6	E950.4	E962.0	E980.4
spinal	968.7	E855.2	E938.7	E950.4	E962.0	E980.4
Xylol (liquid) (vapor)	982.0	E862.4	—	E950.9	E962.1	E980.9
Xylometazoline	971.2	E855.5	E941.2	E950.4	E962.0	E980.4
Yellow						
fever vaccine	979.3	E858.8	E949.3	E950.4	E962.0	E980.4
jasmine	988.2	E865.4	—	E950.9	E962.1	E980.9
Yew	988.2	E865.4	—	E950.9	E962.1	E980.9
Zactane	965.7	E850.7	E935.7	E950.0	E962.0	E980.0
Zaroxolyn	974.3	E858.5	E944.3	E950.4	E962.0	E980.4
Zephiran (topical)	976.0	E858.7	E946.0	E950.4	E962.0	E980.4
ophthalmic preparation	976.5	E858.7	E946.5	E950.4	E962.0	E980.4
Zerone	980.1	E860.2	—	E950.9	E962.1	E980.9
Zinc (compounds) (fumes) (salts) (vapor) NEC	985.8	E866.4	—	E950.9	E962.1	E980.9
anti-infectives	976.0	E858.7	E946.0	E950.4	E962.0	E980.4

	Poisoning	External Cause (E-Code)				
		Accident	Therapeutic Use	Suicide Attempt	Assault	Undeter-mined
Zinc — continued						
antivaricose	972.7	E858.3	E942.7	E950.4	E962.0	E980.4
bacitracin	976.0	E858.7	E946.0	E950.4	E962.0	E980.4
chloride	976.2	E858.7	E946.2	E950.4	E962.0	E980.4
gelatin	976.3	E858.7	E946.3	E950.4	E962.0	E980.4
oxide	976.3	E858.7	E946.3	E950.4	E962.0	E980.4
peroxide	976.0	E858.7	E946.0	E950.4	E962.0	E980.4
pesticides	985.8	E863.4	—	E950.6	E962.1	E980.7
phosphide (rodenticide)	985.8	E863.7	—	E950.6	E962.1	E980.7
stearate	976.3	E858.7	E946.3	E950.4	E962.0	E980.4
sulfate (antivaricose)	972.7	E858.3	E942.7	E950.4	E962.0	E980.4
ENT agent	976.6	E858.7	E946.6	E950.4	E962.0	E980.4
ophthalmic solution	976.5	E858.7	E946.5	E950.4	E962.0	E980.4
topical NEC	976.0	E858.7	E946.0	E950.4	E962.0	E980.4
undecylenate	976.0	E858.7	E946.0	E950.4	E962.0	E980.4
Zovant	964.2	E858.2	E934.2	E950.4	E962.0	E980.4
Zoxazolamine	968.0	E855.1	E938.0	E950.4	E962.0	E980.4
Zygadenus (venenosus)	988.2	E865.4	—	E950.9	E962.1	E980.9
Zyprexa	969.3	E853.8	E939.3	E950.3	E962.0	E980.3

SECTION 3

Alphabetic Index to External Causes of Injury and Poisoning (E Code)

This section contains the index to the codes which classify environmental events, circumstances, and other conditions as the cause of injury and other adverse effects. Where a code from the section Supplementary Classification of External Causes of Injury and Poisoning (E800-E999) is applicable, it is intended that the E code shall be used in addition to a code from the main body of the classification, Chapters 1 to 17.

The alphabetic index to the E codes is organized by main terms which describe the accident, circumstance, event, or specific agent which caused the injury or other adverse effect.

Note — Transport accidents (E800-E848) include accidents involving:

- *aircraft and spacecraft (E840-E845)*
- *watercraft (E830-E838)*
- *motor vehicle (E810-E825)*
- *railway (E800-E807)*
- *other road vehicles (E826-E829)*

For definitions and examples related to transport accidents — see Volume 1 code categories E800-E848.

The fourth-digit subdivisions for use with categories E800-E848 to identify the injured person are found at the end of this section.

For identifying the place in which an accident or poisoning occurred (circumstances classifiable to categories E850-E869 and E880-E928) — see the listing in this section under "Accident, occurring."

See the Table of Drugs and Chemicals (Section 2 of this volume) for identifying the specific agent involved in drug overdose or a wrong substance given or taken in error, and for intoxication or poisoning by a drug or other chemical substance.

The specific adverse effect, reaction, or localized toxic effect to a correct drug or substance properly administered in therapeutic or prophylactic dosage should be classified according to the nature of the adverse effect (e.g., allergy, dermatitis, tachycardia) listed in Section 1 of this volume.

☑ **Additional Digit Required — Refer to the Tabular List for Digit Selection** ▽ **Subterms under main terms may continue to next column or page**

2014 ICD-9-CM 377

Abandonment — Accident (to)

A

Abandonment
causing exposure to weather conditions —
  see Exposure
child, with intent to injure or kill E968.4
helpless person, infant, newborn E904.0
  with intent to injure or kill E968.4
Abortion, criminal, injury to child E968.8
Abuse (alleged) (suspected)
  adult
    by
      child E967.4
      ex-partner E967.3
      ex-spouse E967.3
      father E967.0
      grandchild E967.7
      grandparent E967.6
      mother E967.2
      non-related caregiver E967.8
      other relative E967.7
      other specified person E967.1
      partner E967.3
      sibling E967.5
      spouse E967.3
      stepfather E967.0
      stepmother E967.2
      unspecified person E967.9
  child
    by
      boyfriend of parent or guardian
        E967.0
      child E967.4
      father E967.0
      female partner of parent or guardian
        E967.2
      girlfriend of parent or guardian
        E967.2
      grandchild E967.7
      grandparent E967.6
      male partner of parent or guardian
        E967.0
      mother E967.2
      non-related caregiver E967.8
      other relative E967.7
      other specified person(s) E967.1
      sibling E967.5
      stepfather E967.0
      stepmother E967.2
      unspecified person E967.9
Accident (to) E928.9
  aircraft (in transit) (powered) E841 ☑
    at landing, take-off E840 ☑
    due to, caused by cataclysm — *see* cate-
      gories E908 ☑, E909 ☑
    late effect of E929.1
    unpowered (*see also* Collision, aircraft,
      unpowered) E842 ☑
    while alighting, boarding E843 ☑
  amphibious vehicle
    on
      land — *see* Accident, motor vehicle
      water — *see* Accident, watercraft
  animal-drawn vehicle NEC E827 ☑
  animal, ridden NEC E828 ☑
  balloon (*see also* Collision, aircraft, unpow-
    ered) E842 ☑
  caused by, due to
    abrasive wheel (metalworking) E919.3
    animal NEC E906.9
      being ridden (in sport or transport)
        E828 ☑
    avalanche NEC E909.2
    band saw E919.4
    bench saw E919.4
    bore, earth-drilling or mining (land)
      (seabed) E919.1
    bulldozer E919.7
    cataclysmic
      earth surface movement or eruption
        E909.9
      storm E908.9
    chain
      hoist E919.2
        agricultural operations E919.0
        mining operations E919.1

Accident (to) — *continued*
  caused by, due to — *continued*
    chain — *continued*
      saw E920.1
      circular saw E919.4
      cold (excessive) (*see also* Cold, exposure
        to) E901.9
      combine E919.0
      conflagration — *see* Conflagration
      corrosive liquid, substance NEC E924.1
      cotton gin E919.8
      crane E919.2
        agricultural operations E919.0
        mining operations E919.1
      cutting or piercing instrument (*see also*
        Cut) E920.9
      dairy equipment E919.8
      derrick E919.2
        agricultural operations E919.0
        mining operations E919.1
      drill E920.1
        earth (land) (seabed) E919.1
        hand (powered) E920.1
          not powered E920.4
        metalworking E919.3
        woodworking E919.4
      earth(-)
        drilling machine E919.1
        moving machine E919.7
        scraping machine E919.7
      electric
        current (*see also* Electric shock)
          E925.9
        motor (*see also* Accident, machine,
          by type of machine)
          current (of) — *see* Electric shock
      elevator (building) (grain) E919.2
        agricultural operations E919.0
        mining operations E919.1
      environmental factors NEC E928.9
      excavating machine E919.7
      explosive material (*see also* Explosion)
        E923.9
      farm machine E919.0
      firearm missile — *see* Shooting
      fire, flames (*see also* Fire)
        conflagration — *see* Conflagration
      forging (metalworking) machine E919.3
      forklift (truck) E919.2
        agricultural operations E919.0
        mining operations E919.1
      gas turbine E919.5
      harvester E919.0
      hay derrick, mower, or rake E919.0
      heat (excessive) (*see also* Heat) E900.9
      hoist (*see also* Accident, caused by, due
        to, lift) E919.2
        chain — *see* Accident, caused by, due
          to, chain
        shaft E919.1
      hot
        liquid E924.0
          caustic or corrosive E924.1
        object (not producing fire or flames)
          E924.8
        substance E924.9
          caustic or corrosive E924.1
          liquid (metal) NEC E924.0
          specified type NEC E924.8
      human bite E928.3
      ignition — *see* Ignition
      internal combustion engine E919.5
      landslide NEC E909.2
      lathe (metalworking) E919.3
        turnings E920.8
        woodworking E919.4
      lift, lifting (appliances) E919.2
        agricultural operations E919.0
        mining operations E919.1
        shaft E919.1
      lightning NEC E907
      machine, machinery (*see also* Accident,
        machine)
        drilling, metal E919.3
        manufacturing, for manufacture of
          beverages E919.8

Accident (to) — *continued*
  caused by, due to — *continued*
    machine, machinery (*see also* Accident,
      machine) — *continued*
      manufacturing, for manufacture of
        — *continued*
        clothing E919.8
        foodstuffs E919.8
        paper E919.8
        textiles E919.8
      milling, metal E919.3
      moulding E919.4
      power press, metal E919.3
      printing E919.8
      rolling mill, metal E919.3
      sawing, metal E919.3
      specified type NEC E919.8
      spinning E919.8
      weaving E919.8
    natural factor NEC E928.9
    overhead plane E919.4
    plane E920.4
      overhead E919.4
    powered
      hand tool NEC E920.1
      saw E919.4
        hand E920.1
    printing machine E919.8
    pulley (block) E919.2
      agricultural operations E919.0
      mining operations E919.1
      transmission E919.6
    radial saw E919.4
    radiation — *see* Radiation
    reaper E919.0
    road scraper E919.7
      when in transport under its own
        power — *see* categories
        E810-E825 ☑
    roller coaster E919.8
    sander E919.4
    saw E920.4
      band E919.4
      bench E919.4
      chain E920.1
      circular E919.4
      hand E920.4
        powered, except hand E919.4
      radial E919.4
    sawing machine, metal E919.3
    shaft
      hoist E919.1
      lift E919.1
      transmission E919.6
    shears E920.4
      hand E920.1
        powered E920.1
      mechanical E919.3
    shovel E920.4
      steam E919.7
    spinning machine E919.8
    steam (*see also* Burning, steam)
      engine E919.5
      shovel E919.7
    thresher E919.0
    thunderbolt NEC E907
    tractor E919.0
      when in transport under its own
        power — *see* categories
        E810-E825 ☑
    transmission belt, cable, chain, gear,
      pinion, pulley, shaft E919.6
    turbine (gas) (water driven) E919.5
    under-cutter E919.1
    weaving machine E919.8
    winch E919.2
      agricultural operations E919.0
      mining operations E919.1
  diving E883.0
    with insufficient air supply E913.2
  glider (hang) (*see also* Collision, aircraft, un-
    powered) E842 ☑
  hovercraft
    on
      land — *see* Accident, motor vehicle

Accident (to) — *continued*
  hovercraft — *continued*
    on — *continued*
      water — *see* Accident, watercraft
  ice yacht (*see also* Accident, vehicle NEC)
    E848
  in
    medical, surgical procedure
      as, or due to misadventure — *see*
        Misadventure
      causing an abnormal reaction or later
        complication without men-
        tion of misadventure — *see*
        Reaction, abnormal
  kite carrying a person (*see also* Collision, in-
    volving aircraft, unpowered) E842 ☑
  land yacht (*see also* Accident, vehicle NEC)
    E848
  late effect of — *see* Late effect
  launching pad E845 ☑
  machine, machinery (*see also* Accident,
    caused by, due to, by specific type of
    machine) E919.9
    agricultural including animal-powered
      E919.0
    earth-drilling E919.1
    earth moving or scraping E919.7
    excavating E919.7
    involving transport under own power
      on highway or transport vehicle
      — *see* categories
      E810-E825 ☑, E840-E845 ☑
    lifting (appliances) E919.2
    metalworking E919.3
    mining E919.1
    prime movers, except electric motors
      E919.5
      electric motors — *see* Accident, ma-
        chine, by specific type of ma-
        chine
    recreational E919.8
    specified type NEC E919.8
    transmission E919.6
    watercraft (deck) (engine room) (galley)
      (laundry) (loading) E836 ☑
    woodworking or forming E919.4
  motor vehicle (on public highway) (traffic)
    E819 ☑
    due to cataclysm — *see* categories
      E908 ☑, E909 ☑
    involving
      collision (*see also* Collision, motor
        vehicle) E812 ☑
      nontraffic, not on public highway — *see*
        categories E820-E825 ☑
      not involving collision — *see* categories
        E816-E819 ☑
  nonmotor vehicle NEC E829 ☑
    nonroad — *see* Accident, vehicle NEC
    road, except pedal cycle, animal-drawn
      vehicle, or animal being ridden
      E829 ☑
  nonroad vehicle NEC — *see* Accident, vehi-
    cle NEC
  not elsewhere classifiable involving
    cable car (not on rails) E847
      on rails E829 ☑
    coal car in mine E846
    hand truck — *see* Accident, vehicle NEC
    logging car E846
    sled(ge), meaning snow or ice vehicle
      E848
    tram, mine or quarry E846
    truck
      mine or quarry E846
      self-propelled, industrial E846
      station baggage E846
    tub, mine or quarry E846
    vehicle NEC E848
      snow and ice E848
      used only on industrial premises
        E846
    wheelbarrow E848
  occurring (at) (in)
    apartment E849.0
    baseball field, diamond E849.4

☑ **Additional Digit Required** — **Refer to the Tabular List for Digit Selection**   🖙 **Subterms under main terms may continue to next column or page**

2014 ICD-9-CM   379

Accident (to) — Activity

Activity — continued

- personal — continued
  - hygiene NEC E013.8
  - showering E013.0
  - physical
    - games generally associated with school recess, summer camp and children E007.8
    - training NEC E009.9
  - piano playing E018.0
  - pilates E010.3
  - platform diving E002.1
  - playing musical instrument
    - brass instrument E018.3
    - drum E018.1
    - musical keyboard (electronic) E018.0
    - percussion instrument NEC E018.1
    - piano E018.0
    - string instrument E018.2
    - wind instrument E018.3
  - property maintenance NEC E016.9
  - pruning (garden and lawn) E016.1
  - pull-ups E010.1
  - push-ups E010.1
  - racquetball E008.2
  - rafting (in calm and turbulent water) E002.5
  - raking (leaves) E016.0
  - rappelling E004.1
  - refereeing a sports activity E029.0
  - residential relocation E013.5
  - rhythmic
    - gymnastics E005.2
    - movement NEC E005.9
  - riding
    - horseback E006.1
    - roller coaster E017.0
  - rock climbing E004.0
  - roller coaster riding E017.0
  - roller skating (inline) E006.0
  - rough housing and horseplay E029.2
  - rowing (in calm and turbulent water) E002.5
  - rugby E007.2
  - running E001.1
  - SCUBA diving E002.4
  - sewing E012.1
  - shoveling E016.0
    - dirt E016.0
    - snow E016.0
  - showering (personal) E013.0
  - sit-ups E010.1
  - skateboarding E006.0
  - skating (ice) E003.0
    - roller E006.0
  - skiing (alpine) (downhill) E003.2
    - cross country E003.3
    - nordic E003.3
  - sledding (snow) E003.2
  - smoking and grilling food E015.1
  - snorkeling E002.4
  - snow NEC E003.9
    - boarding E003.2
    - shoveling E016.0
    - sledding E003.2
    - tubing E003.2
  - soccer E007.5
  - softball E007.3
  - specified NEC E029.9
  - spectator at an event E029.1
  - sports played as a team or group NEC E007.9
  - sports played individually NEC E006.9
  - sports NEC E008.9
  - springboard diving E002.1
  - squash E008.2
  - stationary bike E009.0
  - step (stepping) exercise (class) E009.2
  - stepper machine E009.0
  - stove E015.2
  - string instrument playing E018.2
  - surfing E002.7
  - swimming E002.0
  - tackle football E007.0
  - tap dancing E005.0
  - tennis E008.2
  - tobogganing E003.2
  - touch football E007.1
  - track and field events (non-running) E006.6

Activity — continued

- track and field events — continued
  - running E001.1
  - trampoline E005.3
  - treadmill E009.0
  - trimming shrubs E016.1
  - tubing (in calm and turbulent water) E002.5
    - snow E003.2
  - ultimate frisbee E008.3
  - underwater diving E002.4
  - unpacking in moving to a new residence E013.5
  - use of stove, oven and microwave oven E015.2
  - vacuuming E013.2
  - volleyball (beach) (court) E007.7
  - wake boarding E002.6
  - walking (on level or elevated terrain) E001.0
    - an animal E019.0
  - walking an animal E019.0
  - wall climbing E004.0
  - warm up and cool down exercises E009.1
  - water NEC E002.9
    - aerobics E002.3
    - craft NEC E002.9
    - exercise E002.3
    - polo E002.2
    - skiing E002.6
    - sliding E002.8
    - survival training and testing E002.9
  - weeding (garden and lawn) E016.1
  - wind instrument playing E018.3
  - windsurfing E002.7
  - wrestling E008.1
  - yoga E005.1

Activity status E000.9

- child assisting in compensated work of other family member E000.8
- civilian
  - done for
    - financial or other compensation E000.0
    - pay or income E000.0
- family member assisting in compensated work of other family member E000.8
- for income E000.0
- hobby or leisure E000.8
- military E000.1
  - off duty E000.8
- off duty military E000.8
- recreation E000.8
- specified NEC E000.8
- sport not for income E000.8
- student E000.8
- volunteer E000.2

Aeroneurosis E902.1

Aero-otitis media — see Effects of, air pressure

Aerosinusitis — see Effects of, air pressure

After-effect, late — see Late effect

Air

- blast
  - in
    - terrorism E979.2
    - war operations E993.9
- embolism (traumatic) NEC E928.9
  - in
    - infusion or transfusion E874.1
    - perfusion E874.2
  - sickness E903

Alpine sickness E902.0

Altitude sickness — see Effects of, air pressure

Anaphylactic shock, anaphylaxis — see also Table of Drugs and Chemicals E947.9

- due to bite or sting (venomous) — see Bite, venomous

Andes disease E902.0

Apoplexy

- heat — see Heat

Arachnidism E905.1

Arson E968.0

Asphyxia, asphyxiation

- by
  - chemical
    - in
      - terrorism E979.7

Asphyxia, asphyxiation — continued

- by — continued
  - chemical — continued
    - in — continued
      - war operations E997.2
    - explosion — see Explosion
    - food (bone) (regurgitated food) (seed) E911
    - foreign object, except food E912
    - fumes
      - in
        - terrorism (chemical weapons) E979.7
        - war operations E997.2
    - gas (see also Table of Drugs and Chemicals)
      - in
        - terrorism E979.7
        - war operations E997.2
      - legal
        - execution E978
        - intervention (tear) E972
      - tear E972
    - mechanical means (see also Suffocation) E913.9
  - from
    - conflagration — see Conflagration
    - fire (see also Fire) E899
      - in
        - terrorism E979.3
        - war operations E990.9
    - ignition — see Ignition

Aspiration

- foreign body — see Foreign body, aspiration
- mucus, not of newborn (with asphyxia, obstruction respiratory passage, suffocation) E912
- phlegm (with asphyxia, obstruction respiratory passage, suffocation) E912
- vomitus (with asphyxia, obstruction respiratory passage, suffocation) (see also Foreign body, aspiration, food) E911

Assassination (attempt) — see also Assault E968.9

Assault (homicidal) (by) (in) E968.9

- acid E961
  - swallowed E962.1
- air gun E968.6
- BB gun E968.6
- bite NEC E968.8
  - of human being E968.7
- bomb ((placed in) car or house) E965.8
  - antipersonnel E965.5
  - letter E965.7
  - petrol E965.6
- brawl (hand) (fists) (foot) E960.0
- burning, burns (by fire) E968.0
  - acid E961
    - swallowed E962.1
  - caustic, corrosive substance E961
    - swallowed E962.1
  - chemical from swallowing caustic, corrosive substance NEC E962.1
  - hot liquid E968.3
  - scalding E968.3
  - vitriol E961
    - swallowed E962.1
- caustic, corrosive substance E961
  - swallowed E962.1
- cut, any part of body E966
- dagger E966
- drowning E964
- explosive(s) E965.9
  - bomb (see also Assault, bomb) E965.8
  - dynamite E965.8
- fight (hand) (fists) (foot) E960.0
  - with weapon E968.9
    - blunt or thrown E968.2
    - cutting or piercing E966
    - firearm — see Shooting, homicide
- fire E968.0
- firearm(s) — see Shooting, homicide
- garrotting E963
- gunshot (wound) — see Shooting, homicide
- hanging E963
- injury NEC E968.9

Assault — continued

- knife E966
- late effect of E969
- ligature E963
- poisoning E962.9
  - drugs or medicinals E962.0
  - gas(es) or vapors, except drugs and medicinals E962.2
  - solid or liquid substances, except drugs and medicinals E962.1
- puncture, any part of body E966
- pushing
  - before moving object, train, vehicle E968.5
  - from high place E968.1
- rape E960.1
- scalding E968.3
- shooting — see Shooting, homicide
- sodomy E960.1
- stab, any part of body E966
- strangulation E963
- submersion E964
- suffocation E963
- transport vehicle E968.5
- violence NEC E968.9
- vitriol E961
  - swallowed E962.1
- weapon E968.9
  - blunt or thrown E968.2
  - cutting or piercing E966
  - firearm — see Shooting, homicide
- wound E968.9
  - cutting E966
  - gunshot — see Shooting, homicide
  - knife E966
  - piercing E966
  - puncture E966
  - stab E966

Attack by animal NEC E906.9

Avalanche E909.2

- falling on or hitting
  - motor vehicle (in motion) (on public highway) E909.2
  - railway train E909.2

Aviators' disease E902.1

B

Barotitis, barodontalgia, barosinusitis, barotrauma (otitic) (sinus) — see Effects of, air pressure

Battered

- baby or child (syndrome) — see Abuse, child; category E967 ✓
- person other than baby or child — see Assault

Bayonet wound — see also Cut, by bayonet E920.3

- in
  - legal intervention E974
  - terrorism E979.8
  - war operations E995.2

Bean in nose E912

Bed set on fire NEC E898.0

Beheading (by guillotine)

- homicide E966
- legal execution E978

Bending, injury

- due to
  - repetitive movement E927.3
  - sudden strenuous movement E927.0

Bends E902.0

Bite

- animal NEC E906.5
  - other specified (except arthropod) E906.3
  - venomous NEC E905.9
- arthropod (nonvenomous) NEC E906.4
  - venomous — see Sting
- black widow spider E905.1
- cat E906.3
- centipede E905.4
- cobra E905.0
- copperhead snake E905.0
- coral snake E905.0
- dog E906.0
- fer de lance E905.0

Bite — *continued*
  gila monster E905.0
  human being
    accidental E928.3
    assault E968.7
  insect (nonvenomous) E906.4
    venomous — *see* Sting
  krait E905.0
  late effect of — *see* Late effect
  lizard E906.2
    venomous E905.0
  mamba E905.0
  marine animal
    nonvenomous E906.3
      snake E906.2
    venomous E905.6
      snake E905.0
  millipede E906.4
    venomous E905.4
  moray eel E906.3
  rat E906.1
  rattlesnake E905.0
  rodent, except rat E906.3
  serpent — *see* Bite, snake
  shark E906.3
  snake (venomous) E905.0
    nonvenomous E906.2
    sea E905.0
  spider E905.1
    nonvenomous E906.4
  tarantula (venomous) E905.1
  venomous NEC E905.9
    by specific animal — *see category*
      E905 ☑
  viper E905.0
  water moccasin E905.0
Blast (air)
  from nuclear explosion E996 ☑
  in
    terrorism E979.2
      from nuclear explosion E979.5
      underwater E979.0
    war operations E993.9
      from nuclear explosion — *see* War
        operations, injury due to, nu-
        clear weapons
      underwater E992.9
Blizzard E908.3
Blow E928.9
  by law-enforcing agent, police (on duty)
    E975
    with blunt object (baton) (nightstick)
      (stave) (truncheon) E973
Blowing up — *see also* Explosion E923.9
Brawl (hand) (fists) (foot) E960.0
Breakage (accidental)
  cable of cable car not on rails E847
  ladder (causing fall) E881.0
  part (any) of
    animal-drawn vehicle E827 ☑
    ladder (causing fall) E881.0
    motor vehicle
      in motion (on public highway)
        E818 ☑
        not on public highway E825 ☑
    nonmotor road vehicle, except animal-
      drawn vehicle or pedal cycle
      E829 ☑
    off-road type motor vehicle (not on
      public highway) NEC E821 ☑
      on public highway E818 ☑
    pedal cycle E826 ☑
    scaffolding (causing fall) E881.1
    snow vehicle, motor-driven (not on
      public highway) E820 ☑
      on public highway E818 ☑
    vehicle NEC — *see* Accident, vehicle
Broken
  glass
    fall on E888.0
    injury by E920.8
  power line (causing electric shock) E925.1
Bumping against, into (accidentally)
  object (moving) E917.9
    caused by crowd E917.1
      with subsequent fall E917.6

Bumping against, into — *continued*
  object — *continued*
    furniture E917.3
      with subsequent fall E917.7
    in
      running water E917.2
      sports E917.0
        with subsequent fall E917.5
    stationary E917.4
      with subsequent fall E917.8
  person(s) E917.9
    with fall E886.9
      in sports E886.0
    as, or caused by, a crowd E917.1
      with subsequent fall E917.6
    in sports E917.0
      with fall E886.0
Burning, burns (accidental) (by) (from) (on)
  E899
  acid (any kind) E924.1
    swallowed — *see* Table of Drugs and
      Chemicals
  airgun E928.7
  bedclothes (*see also* Fire, specified NEC)
    E898.0
  blowlamp (*see also* Fire, specified NEC)
    E898.1
  blowtorch (*see also* Fire, specified NEC)
    E898.1
  boat, ship, watercraft — *see* categories
    E830 ☑, E831 ☑, E837 ☑
  bonfire (controlled) E897
    uncontrolled E892
  candle (*see also* Fire, specified NEC) E898.1
  caustic liquid, substance E924.1
    swallowed — *see* Table of Drugs and
      Chemicals
  chemical E924.1
    from swallowing caustic, corrosive sub-
      stance — *see* Table of Drugs and
      Chemicals
    in
      terrorism E979.7
      war operations E997.2
  cigar(s) or cigarette(s) (*see also* Fire, speci-
    fied NEC) E898.1
  clothes, clothing, nightdress — *see* Ignition,
    clothes
    with conflagration — *see* Conflagration
  conflagration — *see* Conflagration
  corrosive liquid, substance E924.1
    swallowed — *see* Table of Drugs and
      Chemicals
  electric current (*see also* Electric shock)
    E925.9
  firearm E928.7
  fire, flames (*see also* Fire) E899
  flare, Verey pistol E922.8
  heat
    from appliance (electrical) E924.8
    in local application, or packing during
      medical or surgical procedure
      E873.5
  homicide (attempt) (*see also* Assault, burn-
    ing) E968.0
  hot
    liquid E924.0
      caustic or corrosive E924.1
    object (not producing fire or flames)
      E924.8
    substance E924.9
      caustic or corrosive E924.1
      liquid (metal) NEC E924.0
      specified type NEC E924.8
    tap water E924.2
  ignition (*see also* Ignition)
    clothes, clothing, nightdress (*see also*
      Ignition, clothes)
      with conflagration — *see* Conflagra-
        tion
    highly inflammable material (benzine)
      (fat) (gasoline) (kerosene) (paraf-
      fin) (petrol) E894
  in
    terrorism E979.3
      from nuclear explosion E979.5

Burning, burns — *continued*
  in — *continued*
    terrorism — *continued*
      petrol bomb E979.3
    war operations (from fire-producing de-
      vice or conventional weapon)
      E990.9
      from nuclear explosion (*see also* War
        operations, injury due to, nu-
        clear weapons) E996.2
      incendiary bomb E990.0
      petrol bomb E990.0
  inflicted by other person
    stated as
      homicidal, intentional (*see also* As-
        sault, burning) E968.0
      undetermined whether accidental or
        intentional (*see also* Burn,
        stated as undetermined
        whether accidental or inten-
        tional) E988.1
  internal, from swallowed caustic, corrosive
    liquid, substance — *see* Table of
    Drugs and Chemicals
  lamp (*see also* Fire, specified NEC) E898.1
  late effect of NEC E929.4
  lighter (cigar) (cigarette) (*see also* Fire,
    specified NEC) E898.1
  lightning E907
  liquid (boiling) (hot) (molten) E924.0
    caustic, corrosive (external) E924.1
      swallowed — *see* Table of Drugs and
        Chemicals
  local application of externally applied sub-
    stance in medical or surgical care
    E873.5
  machinery — *see* Accident, machine
  matches (*see also* Fire, specified NEC) E898.1
  medicament, externally applied E873.5
  metal, molten E924.0
  object (hot) E924.8
    producing fire or flames — *see* Fire
  oven (electric) (gas) E924.8
  pipe (smoking) (*see also* Fire, specified NEC)
    E898.1
  radiation — *see* Radiation
  railway engine, locomotive, train (*see also*
    Explosion, railway engine) E803 ☑
  self-inflicted (unspecified whether acciden-
    tal or intentional) E988.1
    caustic or corrosive substance NEC
      E988.7
    stated as intentional, purposeful E958.1
      caustic or corrosive substance NEC
        E958.7
    stated as undetermined whether accidental
      or intentional E988.1
      caustic or corrosive substance NEC
        E988.7
  steam E924.0
    pipe E924.8
  substance (hot) E924.9
    boiling or molten E924.0
    caustic, corrosive (external) E924.1
      swallowed — *see* Table of Drugs and
        Chemicals
  suicidal (attempt) NEC E958.1
    caustic substance E958.7
    late effect of E959
  tanning bed E926.2
  therapeutic misadventure
    overdose of radiation E873.2
  torch, welding (*see also* Fire, specified NEC)
    E898.1
  trash fire (*see also* Burning, bonfire) E897
  vapor E924.0
  vitriol E924.1
  x-rays E926.3
    in medical, surgical procedure — *see*
      Misadventure, failure, in dosage,
      radiation
Butted by animal E906.8

C

Cachexia, lead or saturnine E866.0

Cachexia, lead or saturnine — *continued*
  from pesticide NEC (*see also* Table of Drugs
    and Chemicals) E863.4
Caisson disease E902.2
Capital punishment (any means) E978
Car sickness E903
Casualty (not due to war) NEC E928.9
  terrorism E979.8
  war (*see also* War operations) E995.9
Cat
  bite E906.3
  scratch E906.8
Cataclysmic (any injury)
  earth surface movement or eruption E909.9
    specified type NEC E909.8
  storm or flood resulting from storm E908.9
    specified type NEC E908.8
Catching fire — *see* Ignition
Caught
  between
    objects (moving) (stationary and mov-
      ing) E918
      and machinery — *see* Accident, ma-
        chine
  by cable car, not on rails E847
  in
    machinery (moving parts of) — *see*, Ac-
      cident, machine
    object E918
Cave-in (causing asphyxia, suffocation (by
  pressure)) — *see also* Suffocation, due
  to, cave-in E913.3
  with injury other than asphyxia or suffoca-
    tion E916
    with asphyxia or suffocation (*see also*
      Suffocation, due to, cave-in)
      E913.3
  struck or crushed by E916
    with asphyxia or suffocation (*see also*
      Suffocation, due to, cave-in)
      E913.3
Change(s) in air pressure — *see also* Effects
  of, air pressure
  sudden, in aircraft (ascent) (descent) (caus-
    ing aeroneurosis or aviators' disease)
    E902.1
Chilblains E901.0
  due to manmade conditions E901.1
Choking (on) (any object except food or vomitus) E912
  apple E911
  bone E911
  food, any type (regurgitated) E911
  mucus or phlegm E912
  seed E911
Civil insurrection — *see* War operations
Cloudburst E908.8
Cold, exposure to (accidental) (excessive)
  (extreme) (place) E901.9
  causing chilblains or immersion foot E901.0
  due to
    manmade conditions E901.1
    specified cause NEC E901.8
    weather (conditions) E901.0
  late effect of NEC E929.5
  self-inflicted (undetermined whether acci-
    dental or intentional) E988.3
    suicidal E958.3
  suicide E958.3
Colic, lead, painter's, or saturnine — *see*
  category E866 ☑
Collapse
  building E916
    burning (uncontrolled fire) E891.8
      in terrorism E979.3
      private E890.8
  dam E909.3
  due to heat — *see* Heat
  machinery — *see* Accident, machine or ve-
    hicle
  man-made structure E909.3
  postoperative NEC E878.9
  structure
    burning (uncontrolled fire) NEC E891.8
      in terrorism E979.3

Collision — Collision

Collision (accidental)

Note — In the case of collisions between different types of vehicles, persons and objects, priority in classification is in the following order:

  Aircraft

  Watercraft

  Motor vehicle

  Railway vehicle

  Pedal cycle

  Animal-drawn vehicle

  Animal being ridden

  Streetcar or other nonmotor road vehicle

  Other vehicle

  Pedestrian or person using pedestrian conveyance

  Object (except where falling from or set in motion by vehicle etc. listed above)

In the listing below, the combinations are listed only under the vehicle etc. having priority. For definitions, see Supplementary Classification of External Causes of Injury and Poisoning (E800-E999).

aircraft (with object or vehicle) (fixed) (movable) (moving) E841 ☑
  with
    person (while landing, taking off) (without accident to aircraft) E844 ☑
    powered (in transit) (with unpowered aircraft) E841 ☑
      while landing, taking off E840 ☑
    unpowered E842 ☑
      while landing, taking off E840 ☑
animal being ridden (in sport or transport) E828 ☑
  and
    animal (being ridden) (herded) (unattended) E828 ☑
    nonmotor road vehicle, except pedal cycle or animal-drawn vehicle E828 ☑
    object (fallen) (fixed) (movable) (moving) not falling from or set in motion by vehicle of higher priority E828 ☑
    pedestrian (conveyance or vehicle) E828 ☑
animal-drawn vehicle E827 ☑
  and
    animal (being ridden) (herded) (unattended) E827 ☑
    nonmotor road vehicle, except pedal cycle E827 ☑
    object (fallen) (fixed) (movable) (moving) not falling from or set in motion by vehicle of higher priority E827 ☑
    pedestrian (conveyance or vehicle) E827 ☑
    streetcar E827 ☑
motor vehicle (on public highway) (traffic accident) E812 ☑
  after leaving, running off, public highway (without antecedent collision) (without re-entry) E816 ☑
    with antecedent collision on public highway — see categories E810-E815 ☑
    with re-entrance collision with another motor vehicle E811 ☑
  and
    abutment (bridge) (overpass) E815 ☑
    animal (herded) (unattended) E815 ☑

Collision — continued
  motor vehicle — continued
    and — continued
      animal — continued
        carrying person, property E813 ☑
      animal-drawn vehicle E813 ☑
      another motor vehicle (abandoned) (disabled) (parked) (stalled) (stopped) E812 ☑
        with, involving re-entrance (on same roadway) (across median strip) E811 ☑
      any object, person, or vehicle off the public highway resulting from a noncollision motor vehicle nontraffic accident E816 ☑
      avalanche, fallen or not moving E815 ☑
        falling E909.2
      boundary fence E815 ☑
      culvert E815 ☑
      fallen
        stone E815 ☑
        tree E815 ☑
      guard post or guard rail E815 ☑
      inter-highway divider E815 ☑
      landslide, fallen or not moving E815 ☑
        moving E909 ☑
      machinery (road) E815 ☑
      nonmotor road vehicle NEC E813 ☑
      object (any object, person, or vehicle off the public highway resulting from a noncollision motor vehicle nontraffic accident) E815 ☑
        off, normally not on, public highway resulting from a noncollision motor vehicle traffic accident E816 ☑
      pedal cycle E813 ☑
      pedestrian (conveyance) E814 ☑
      person (using pedestrian conveyance) E814 ☑
      post or pole (lamp) (light) (signal) (telephone) (utility) E815 ☑
      railway rolling stock, train, vehicle E810 ☑
      safety island E815 ☑
      street car E813 ☑
      traffic signal, sign, or marker (temporary) E815 ☑
      tree E815 ☑
      tricycle E813 ☑
      wall of cut made for road E815 ☑
    due to cataclysm — see categories E908 ☑, E909 ☑
    not on public highway, nontraffic accident E822 ☑
      and
        animal (carrying person, property) (herded) (unattended) E822 ☑
        animal-drawn vehicle E822 ☑
        another motor vehicle (moving), except off-road motor vehicle E822 ☑
          stationary E823 ☑
        avalanche, fallen, not moving E823 ☑
          moving E909.2
        landslide, fallen, not moving E823 ☑
          moving E909.2
        nonmotor vehicle (moving) E822 ☑
          stationary E823 ☑
        object (fallen) (normally) (fixed) (movable but not in motion) (stationary) E823 ☑
          moving, except when falling from, set in motion by, aircraft or cataclysm E822 ☑
        pedal cycle (moving) E822 ☑

Collision — continued
  motor vehicle — continued
    not on public highway, nontraffic accident — continued
      and — continued
        pedal cycle — continued
          stationary E823 ☑
        pedestrian (conveyance) E822 ☑
        person (using pedestrian conveyance) E822 ☑
        railway rolling stock, train, vehicle (moving) E822 ☑
          stationary E823 ☑
        road vehicle (any) (moving) E822 ☑
          stationary E823 ☑
        tricycle (moving) E822 ☑
          stationary E823 ☑
    off-road type motor vehicle (not on public highway) E821 ☑
      and
        animal (being ridden) (-drawn vehicle) E821 ☑
        another off-road motor vehicle, except snow vehicle E821 ☑
        other motor vehicle, not on public highway E821 ☑
        other object or vehicle NEC, fixed or movable, not set in motion by aircraft, motor vehicle on highway, or snow vehicle, motor driven E821 ☑
        pedal cycle E821 ☑
        pedestrian (conveyance) E821 ☑
        railway train E821 ☑
      on public highway — see Collision, motor vehicle
  pedal cycle E826 ☑
    and
      animal (carrying person, property) (herded) (unherded) E826 ☑
      animal-drawn vehicle E826 ☑
      another pedal cycle E826 ☑
      nonmotor road vehicle E826 ☑
      object (fallen) (fixed) (movable) (moving) not falling from or set in motion by aircraft, motor vehicle, or railway train NEC E826 ☑
      pedestrian (conveyance) E826 ☑
      person (using pedestrian conveyance) E826 ☑
      street car E826 ☑
  pedestrian(s) (conveyance) E917.9
    with fall E886.9
    in sports E886.0
    and
      crowd, human stampede E917.1
        with subsequent fall E917.6
      furniture E917.3
        with subsequent fall E917.7
      machinery — see Accident, machine
      object (fallen) (moving) not falling from NEC, fixed or set in motion by any vehicle classifiable to E800-E848 ☑, E917.9
        with subsequent fall E917.6
        caused by a crowd E917.1
          with subsequent fall E917.6
        furniture E917.3
          with subsequent fall E917.7
      in
        running water E917.2
          with drowning or submersion — see Submersion
        sports E917.0
          with subsequent fall E917.5
        stationary E917.4
          with subsequent fall E917.8
      vehicle, nonmotor, nonroad E848
    in
      running water E917.2

Collision — continued
  pedestrian(s) — continued
    in — continued
      running water — continued
        with drowning or submersion — see Submersion
      sports E917.0
        with fall E886.0
    person(s) (using pedestrian conveyance) (see also Collision, pedestrian) E917.9
  railway (rolling stock) (train) (vehicle) (with subsequent) derailment, explosion, fall or fire) E800 ☑
    with antecedent derailment E802 ☑
    and
      animal (carrying person) (herded) (unattended) E801 ☑
      another railway train or vehicle E800 ☑
      buffers E801 ☑
      fallen tree on railway E801 ☑
      farm machinery, nonmotor (in transport) (stationary) E801 ☑
      gates E801 ☑
      nonmotor vehicle E801 ☑
      object (fallen) (fixed) (movable) (moving) not falling from, set in motion by, aircraft or motor vehicle NEC E801 ☑
      pedal cycle E801 ☑
      pedestrian (conveyance) E805 ☑
      person (using pedestrian conveyance) E805 ☑
      platform E801 ☑
      rock on railway E801 ☑
      street car E801 ☑
    snow vehicle, motor-driven (not on public highway) E820 ☑
      and
        animal (being ridden) (-drawn vehicle) E820 ☑
        another off-road motor vehicle E820 ☑
        other motor vehicle, not on public highway E820 ☑
        other object or vehicle NEC, fixed or movable, not set in motion by aircraft or motor vehicle on highway E820 ☑
        pedal cycle E820 ☑
        pedestrian (conveyance) E820 ☑
        railway train E820 ☑
      on public highway — see Collision, motor vehicle
    street car(s) E829 ☑
      and
        animal, herded, not being ridden, unattended E829 ☑
        nonmotor road vehicle NEC E829 ☑
        object (fallen) (fixed) (movable) (moving) not falling from or set in motion by aircraft, animal-drawn vehicle, animal being ridden, motor vehicle, pedal cycle, or railway train E829 ☑
        pedestrian (conveyance) E829 ☑
        person (using pedestrian conveyance) E829 ☑
  vehicle
    animal-drawn — see Collision, animal-drawn vehicle
    motor — see Collision, motor vehicle
    nonmotor
      nonroad E848
        and
          another nonmotor, nonroad vehicle E848

Collision — *continued*
  vehicle — *continued*
    nonmotor — *continued*
      nonroad — *continued*
        and — *continued*
          object (fallen) (fixed) (movable) (moving) not falling from or set in motion by aircraft, animal-drawn vehicle, animal being ridden, motor vehicle, nonmotor road vehicle, pedal cycle, railway train, or streetcar E848
      road, except animal being ridden, animal-drawn vehicle, or pedal cycle E829 ☑
      and
        animal, herded, not being ridden, unattended E829 ☑
        another nonmotor road vehicle, except animal being ridden, animal-drawn vehicle, or pedal cycle E829 ☑
        object (fallen) (fixed) (movable) (moving) not falling from or set in motion by, aircraft, animal-drawn vehicle, animal being ridden, motor vehicle, pedal cycle, or railway train E829 ☑
        pedestrian (conveyance) E829 ☑
        person (using pedestrian conveyance) E829 ☑
        vehicle, nonmotor, nonroad E829 ☑
  watercraft E838 ☑
    and
      person swimming or water skiing E838 ☑
    causing
      drowning, submersion E830 ☑
      injury except drowning, submersion E831 ☑

Combustion, spontaneous — *see* Ignition
Complication of medical or surgical procedure or treatment
  as an abnormal reaction — *see* Reaction, abnormal
  delayed, without mention of misadventure — *see* Reaction, abnormal
  due to misadventure — *see* Misadventure
Compression
  divers' squeeze E902.2
  trachea by
    food E911
    foreign body, except food E912
Conflagration
  building or structure, except private dwelling (barn) (church) (convalescent or residential home) (factory) (farm outbuilding) (hospital) (hotel) (institution) (educational) (domitory) (residential) (school) (shop) (store) (theater) E891.9
  with or causing (injury due to)
    accident or injury NEC E891.9
      specified circumstance NEC E891.8
    burns, burning E891.3
    carbon monoxide E891.2
    fumes E891.2
      polyvinylchloride (PVC) or similar material E891.1
    smoke E891.2
  causing explosion E891.0
  in terrorism E979.3
  not in building or structure E892

Conflagration — *continued*
  private dwelling (apartment) (boarding house) (camping place) (caravan) (farmhouse) (home (private)) (house) (lodging house) (private garage) (rooming house) (tenement) E890.9
  with or causing (injury due to)
    accident or injury NEC E890.9
      specified circumstance NEC E890.8
    burns, burning E890.3
    carbon monoxide E890.2
    fumes E890.2
      polyvinylchloride (PVC) or similar material E890.1
    smoke E890.2
  causing explosion E890.0
Constriction, external
  caused by
    hair E928.4
    other object E928.5
Contact with
  dry ice E901.1
  liquid air, hydrogen, nitrogen E901.1
Cramp(s)
  Heat — *see* Heat
  swimmers (*see also* category E910) E910.2
    not in recreation or sport E910.3
Cranking (car) (truck) (bus) (engine), injury by E917.9
Crash
  aircraft (in transit) (powered) E841 ☑
    at landing, take-off E840 ☑
    in
      terrorism E979.1
      war operations E994.9
    on runway NEC E840 ☑
    stated as
      homicidal E968.8
      suicidal E958.6
      undetermined whether accidental or intentional E988.6
    unpowered E842 ☑
  glider E842 ☑
  motor vehicle (*see also* Accident, motor vehicle)
    homicidal E968.5
    suicidal E958.5
    undetermined whether accidental or intentional E988.5
Crushed (accidentally) E928.9
  between
    boat(s), ship(s), watercraft (and dock or pier) (without accident to watercraft) E838 ☑
    after accident to, or collision, watercraft E831 ☑
    objects (moving) (stationary and moving) E918
  by
    avalanche NEC E909.2
    boat, ship, watercraft after accident to, collision, watercraft E831 ☑
    cave-in E916
      with asphyxiation or suffocation (*see also* Suffocation, due to, cave-in) E913.3
    crowd, human stampede E917.1
    falling
      aircraft (*see also* Accident, aircraft) E841 ☑
      in
        terrorism E979.1
        war operations E994.8
      earth, material E916
        with asphyxiation or suffocation (*see also* Suffocation, due to, cave-in) E913.3
      object E916
        on ship, watercraft E838 ☑
        while loading, unloading watercraft E838 ☑
    firearm E928.7
    landslide NEC E909.2
    lifeboat after abandoning ship E831 ☑
    machinery — *see* Accident, machine

Crushed — *continued*
  by — *continued*
    railway rolling stock, train, vehicle (part of) E805 ☑
    slide trigger mechanism, scope or other part of gun E928.7
    street car E829 ☑
    vehicle NEC — *see* Accident, vehicle NEC
  in
    machinery — *see* Accident, machine
    object E918
    transport accident — *see* categories E800-E848 ☑
  late effect of NEC E929.9
Cut, cutting (any part of body) (accidental) E920.9
  by
    arrow E920.8
    axe E920.4
    bayonet (*see also* Bayonet wound) E920.3
      in war operations E995.2
    blender E920.2
    broken glass E920.8
      following fall E888.0
    can opener E920.4
      powered E920.2
    chisel E920.4
    circular saw E919.4
    cutting or piercing instrument (*see also* category) E920 ☑
      following fall E888.0
      late effect of E929.8
    dagger E920.3
    dart E920.8
    drill — *see* Accident, caused by drill
    edge of stiff paper E920.8
    electric
      beater E920.2
      fan E920.2
      knife E920.2
      mixer E920.2
    firearm component E928.7
    fork E920.4
    garden fork E920.4
    hand saw or tool (not powered) E920.4
      powered E920.1
    hedge clipper E920.4
      powered E920.1
    hoe E920.4
    ice pick E920.4
    knife E920.3
      electric E920.2
      in war operations E995.2
    lathe turnings E920.8
    lawn mower E920.4
      powered E920.0
      riding E919.8
    machine — *see* Accident, machine
    meat
      grinder E919.8
      slicer E919.8
    nails E920.8
    needle E920.4
      hypodermic E920.5
    object, edged, pointed, sharp — *see* category E920 ☑
      following fall E888.0
    paper cutter E920.4
    piercing instrument (*see also* category) E920 ☑
      late effect of E929.8
    pitchfork E920.4
    powered
      can opener E920.2
      garden cultivator E920.1
        riding E919.8
      hand saw E920.1
      hand tool NEC E920.1
      hedge clipper E920.1
      household appliance or implement E920.2
      lawn mower (hand) E920.0
        riding E919.8
      rivet gun E920.1
      staple gun E920.1

Cut, cutting — *continued*
  by — *continued*
    rake E920.4
    saw
      circular E919.4
      hand E920.4
    scissors E920.4
    screwdriver E920.4
    sewing machine (electric) (powered) E920.2
      not powered E920.4
    shears E920.4
    shovel E920.4
    slide trigger mechanism, scope or other part of gun E928.7
    spade E920.4
    splinters E920.8
    sword E920.3
      in war operations E995.2
    tin can lid E920.8
    wood slivers E920.8
  homicide (attempt) E966
  inflicted by other person
    stated as
      intentional, homicidal E966
      undetermined whether accidental or intentional E986
  late effect of NEC E929.8
  legal
    execution E978
    intervention E974
  self-inflicted (unspecified whether accidental or intentional) E986
    stated as intentional, purposeful E956
    stated as undetermined whether accidental or intentional E986
  suicidal (attempt) E956
  terrorism E979.8
  war operations E995.2
Cyclone E908.1

D

Death due to injury occurring one year or more previous — *see* Late effect
Decapitation (accidental circumstances) NEC E928.9
  homicidal E966
  legal execution (by guillotine) E978
Deprivation — *see also* Privation
  homicidal intent E968.4
Derailment (accidental)
  railway (rolling stock) (train) (vehicle) (with subsequent collision) E802 ☑
    with
      collision (antecedent) (*see also* Collision, railway) E800 ☑
      explosion (subsequent) (without antecedent collision) E802 ☑
        antecedent collision E803 ☑
      fall (without collision (antecedent)) E802 ☑
      fire (without collision (antecedent)) E802 ☑
  street car E829 ☑
Descent
  parachute (voluntary) (without accident to aircraft) E844 ☑
    due to accident to aircraft — *see* categories E840-E842 ☑
Desertion
  child, with intent to injure or kill E968.4
  helpless person, infant, newborn E904.0
    with intent to injure or kill E968.4
Destitution — *see* Privation
Dirty bomb (*see also* War operations, injury due to, nuclear weapons) E996.9
Disability, late effect or sequela of injury — *see* Late effect
Disease
  Andes E902.0
  aviators' E902.1
  caisson E902.2
  range E902.0
Divers' disease, palsy, paralysis, squeeze E902.0

Dog bite E906.0
Dragged by
cable car (not on rails) E847
  on rails E829 ☑
motor vehicle (on highway) E814 ☑
  not on highway, nontraffic accident E825 ☑
street car E829 ☑
Drinking poison (accidental) — *see* Table of Drugs and Chemicals
Drowning — *see* Submersion
Dust in eye E914

E

Earth falling (on) (with asphyxia or suffocation (by pressure)) — *see also* Suffocation, due to, cave-in E913.3
as, or due to, a cataclysm (involving any transport vehicle) — *see* categories E908 ☑, E909 ☑
not due to cataclysmic action E913.3
  motor vehicle (in motion) (on public highway) E813 ☑
    not on public highway E825 ☑
  nonmotor road vehicle NEC E829 ☑
  pedal cycle E826 ☑
  railway rolling stock, train, vehicle E806 ☑
  street car E829 ☑
  struck or crushed by E916
    with asphyxiation or suffocation E913.3
    with injury other than asphyxia, suffocation E916
Earthquake (any injury) E909.0
Effect(s) (adverse) of
air pressure E902.9
  at high altitude E902.9
    in aircraft E902.1
    residence or prolonged visit (causing conditions classifiable to E902.0) E902.0
  due to
    diving E902.2
    specified cause NEC E902.8
  in aircraft E902.1
cold, excessive (exposure to) (*see also* Cold, exposure to) E901.9
heat (excessive) (*see also* Heat) E900.9
hot
  place — *see* Heat
  weather E900.0
insulation — *see* Heat
late — *see* Late effect of
motion E903
nuclear explosion or weapon
  in
    terrorism E979.5
    war operations (*see also* War operations, injury due to, nuclear weapons) E996.9
radiation — *see* Radiation
terrorism, secondary E979.9
travel E903
Electric shock, electrocution (accidental) (from exposed wire, faulty appliance, high voltage cable, live rail, open socket) (by) (in) E925.9
appliance or wiring
  domestic E925.0
  factory E925.2
  farm (building) E925.8
  house E925.0
  home E925.0
  industrial (conductor) (control apparatus) (transformer) E925.2
  outdoors E925.8
  public building E925.8
  residential institution E925.8
  school E925.8
  specified place NEC E925.8
caused by other person
  stated as
    intentional, homicidal E968.8

Electric shock, electrocution — *continued*
caused by other person — *continued*
  stated as — *continued*
    undetermined whether accidental or intentional E988.4
electric power generating plant, distribution station E925.1
electroshock gun (taser) (stun gun) E925.8
  caused by other person E968.8
    legal intervention E975
    stated as accidental E925.8
    stated as intentional E968.8
  due to legal intervention E975
  stated as intentional self-harm (suicidal attempt) E958.4
  stated as undetermined whether accidental or intentional E988.4
  suicide (attempt) E958.4
homicidal (attempt) E968.8
legal execution E978
lightning E907
machinery E925.9
  domestic E925.0
  factory E925.2
  farm E925.8
  home E925.0
misadventure in medical or surgical procedure
  in electroshock therapy E873.4
self-inflicted (undetermined whether accidental or intentional) E988.4
  stated as intentional E958.4
  stated as undetermined whether accidental or intentional E988.4
  suicidal (attempt) E958.4
transmission line E925.1
Electrocution — *see* Electric shock
Embolism
air (traumatic) NEC — *see* Air, embolism
Encephalitis
lead or saturnine E866.0
  from pesticide NEC E863.4
Entanglement
in
  bedclothes, causing suffocation E913.0
  wheel of pedal cycle E826 ☑
Entry of foreign body, material, any — *see* Foreign body
Execution, legal (any method) E978
Exertion, excessive physical, from prolonged activity E927.2
Exhaustion
cold — *see* Cold, exposure to
due to excessive exertion E927.2
heat — *see* Heat
Explosion (accidental) (in) (of) (on) E923.9
acetylene E923.2
aerosol can E921.8
aircraft (in transit) (powered) E841 ☑
  at landing, take-off E840 ☑
  in
    terrorism E979.1
    war operations
      from
        enemy fire or explosive(s) (device placed on aircraft) E994.0
        own onboard explosives E994.1
  unpowered E842 ☑
air tank (compressed) (in machinery) E921.1
anesthetic gas in operating theatre E923.2
automobile tire NEC E921.8
  causing transport accident — *see* categories E810-E825 ☑
blasting (cap) (materials) E923.1
boiler (machinery), not on transport vehicle E921.0
  steamship — *see* Explosion, watercraft
bomb E923.8
  in
    terrorism E979.2
    war operations E993.8
      after cessation of hostilities E998.1

Explosion — *continued*
bomb — *continued*
  in — *continued*
    war operations — *continued*
      atom, hydrogen or nuclear (*see also* War operations, injury due to, nuclear weapons) E996.9
      injury by fragments from E991.9
        antipersonnel bomb E991.3
butane E923.2
caused by
  other person
    stated as
      intentional, homicidal — *see* Assault, explosive
      undetermined whether accidental or homicidal E985.5
coal gas E923.2
detonator E923.1
dynamite E923.1
explosive (material) NEC E923.9
  gas(es) E923.2
  missile E923.8
    in
      terrorism E979.2
      war operations E993.1
        injury by fragments from E991.9
        antipersonnel bomb E991.3
  used in blasting operations E923.1
fire-damp E923.2
fireworks E923.0
gas E923.2
  cylinder (in machinery) E921.1
  pressure tank (in machinery) E921.1
gasoline (fumes) (tank) not in moving motor vehicle E923.2
grain store (military) (munitions) E923.8
grenade E923.8
  in
    terrorism E979.2
    war operations E993.8
      injury by fragments from E991.4
homicide (attempt) — *see* Assault, explosive
hot water heater, tank (in machinery) E921.0
in mine (of explosive gases) NEC E923.2
late effect of NEC E929.8
machinery (*see also* Accident, machine)
  pressure vessel — *see* Explosion, pressure vessel
methane E923.2
missile E923.8
  in
    terrorism E979.2
    war operations E993.1
      injury by fragments from E991.4
motor vehicle (part of)
  in motion (on public highway) E818 ☑
    not on public highway E825 ☑
munitions (dump) (factory) E923.8
  in
    terrorism E979.2
    war operations E993.9
of mine E923.8
  in
    terrorism
      at sea or in harbor E979.0
      land E979.2
      marine E979.0
    war operations
      after cessation of hostilities E998.0
      at sea or in harbor E992.2
      land E993.8
        after cessation of hostilities E998.0
        injury by fragments from E991.4
      marine E992.2
own weapons
  in
    terrorism (*see also* Suicide) E979.2
    war operations E993.7
      injury by fragments from E991.9

Explosion — *continued*
own weapons — *continued*
  in — *continued*
    war operations — *continued*
      injury by fragments from — *continued*
        antipersonnel bomb E991.3
pressure
  cooker E921.8
  gas tank (in machinery) E921.1
  vessel (in machinery) E921.9
    on transport vehicle — *see* categories E800-E848 ☑
    specified type NEC E921.8
propane E923.2
railway engine, locomotive, train (boiler) (with subsequent collision, derailment, fall) E803 ☑
  with
    collision (antecedent) (*see also* Collision, railway) E800 ☑
    derailment (antecedent) E802 ☑
    fire (without antecedent collision or derailment) E803 ☑
secondary fire resulting from — *see* Fire
self-inflicted (unspecified whether accidental or intentional) E985.5
  stated as intentional, purposeful E955.5
shell (artillery) E923.8
  in
    terrorism E979.2
    war operations E993.2
      injury by fragments from E991.4
stated as undetermined whether caused accidentally or purposely inflicted E985.5
steam or water lines (in machinery) E921.0
suicide (attempted) E955.5
terrorism — *see* Terrorism, explosion
torpedo E923.8
  in
    terrorism E979.0
    war operations E992.0
transport accident — *see* categories E800-E848 ☑
war operations — *see* War operations, explosion
watercraft (boiler) E837 ☑
  causing drowning, submersion (after jumping from watercraft) E830 ☑
Exposure (weather) (conditions) (rain) (wind) E904.3
with homicidal intent E968.4
environmental
  to
    algae bloom E928.6
    blue-green algae bloom E928.6
    brown tide E928.6
    cyanobacteria bloom E928.6
    Florida red tide E928.6
    harmful alage
      and toxins E928.6
      bloom E928.6
    pfiesteria piscicida E928.6
    red tide E928.6
excessive E904.3
  cold (*see also* Cold, exposure to) E901.9
    self-inflicted — *see* Cold, exposure to, self-inflicted
  heat (*see also* Heat) E900.9
helpless person, infant, newborn due to abandonment or neglect E904.0
noise E928.1
prolonged in deep-freeze unit or refrigerator E901.1
radiation — *see* Radiation
resulting from transport accident — *see* categories E800-E848 ☑
smoke from, due to
  fire — *see* Fire
  tobacco, second-hand E869.4
vibration E928.2
External cause status E000.9
child assisting in compensated work of other family member E000.8

External cause status — *continued*
  civilian
    done for
      financial or other compensation
        E000.0
      pay or income E000.0
    family member assisting in compensated
      work of other family member E000.8
    for income E000.0
    hobby or leisure E000.8
    military E000.1
      off duty E000.8
    off duty military E000.8
    recreation E000.8
    specified NEC E000.8
    sport not for income E000.8
    student E000.8
    volunteer E000.2

F

Fallen on by
  animal (horse) (not being ridden) E906.8
    being ridden (in sport or transport)
      E828 ☑
Fall, falling (accidental) E888.9
  building E916
    burning E891.8
      private E890.8
  down
    escalator E880.0
    ladder E881.0
      in boat, ship, watercraft E833 ☑
    staircase E880.9
    stairs, steps — *see* Fall, from, stairs
  earth (with asphyxia or suffocation (by
    pressure)) (*see also* Earth, falling)
    E913.3
  from, off
    aircraft (at landing, take-off) (in-transit)
      (while alighting, boarding)
      E843 ☑
      resulting from accident to aircraft —
        see categories E840-E842 ☑
    animal (in sport or transport) E828 ☑
    animal-drawn vehicle E827 ☑
    balcony E882
    bed E884.4
    bicycle E826 ☑
    boat, ship, watercraft (into water)
      E832 ☑
      after accident to, collision, fire on
        E830 ☑
        and subsequently struck by (part
          of) boat E831 ☑
      and subsequently struck by (part of)
        while alighting, boat E831 ☑
      burning, crushed, sinking E830 ☑
        and subsequently struck by (part
          of) boat E831 ☑
    bridge E882
    building E882
      burning (uncontrolled fire) E891.8
        in terrorism E979.3
      private E890.8
    bunk in boat, ship, watercraft E834 ☑
      due to accident to watercraft
        E831 ☑
    cable car (not on rails) E847
      on rails E829 ☑
    car — *see* Fall from motor vehicle
    chair E884.2
    cliff E884.1
    commode E884.6
    curb (sidewalk) E880.1
    elevation aboard ship E834 ☑
      due to accident to ship E831 ☑
    embankment E884.9
    escalator E880.0
    fire escape E882
    flagpole E882
    furniture NEC E884.5
    gangplank (into water) (*see also* Fall,
      from, boat) E832 ☑
      to deck, dock E834 ☑
    hammock on ship E834 ☑

Fall, falling — *continued*
  from, off — *continued*
    hammock on ship — *continued*
      due to accident to watercraft
        E831 ☑
    haystack E884.9
    heelies E885.1
    high place NEC E884.9
      stated as undetermined whether ac-
        cidental or intentional — *see*
        Jumping, from, high place
    horse (in sport or transport) E828 ☑
    in-line skates E885.1
    ladder E881.0
      in boat, ship, watercraft E833 ☑
      due to accident to watercraft
        E831 ☑
    machinery (*see also* Accident, machine)
      not in operation E884.9
    motorized
      mobility scooter E884.3
      wheelchair E884.3
    motor vehicle (in motion) (on public
      highway) E818 ☑
      not on public highway E825 ☑
        stationary, except while alighting,
          boarding, entering, leav-
          ing E884.9
        while alighting, boarding, enter-
          ing, leaving E824 ☑
      stationary, except while alighting,
        boarding, entering, leaving
        E884.9
      while alighting, boarding, entering,
        leaving, except off-road type
        motor vehicle E817 ☑
      off-road type — *see* Fall, from,
        off-road type motor vehi-
        cle
    nonmotor road vehicle (while alighting,
      boarding) NEC E829 ☑
      stationary, except while alighting,
        boarding, entering, leaving
        E884.9
    off road type motor vehicle (not on
      public highway) NEC E821 ☑
      on public highway E818 ☑
        while alighting, boarding, enter-
          ing, leaving E817 ☑
      snow vehicle — *see* Fall from snow
        vehicle, motor-driven
    one
      deck to another on ship E834 ☑
        due to accident to ship E831 ☑
      level to another NEC E884.9
        boat, ship, or watercraft E834 ☑
        due to accident to watercraft
          E831 ☑
    pedal cycle E826 ☑
    playground equipment E884.0
    railway rolling stock, train, vehicle (while
      alighting, boarding) E804 ☑
      with
        collision (*see also* Collision, rail-
          way) E800 ☑
        derailment (*see also* Derailment,
          railway) E802 ☑
        explosion (*see also* Explosion,
          railway engine) E803 ☑
    rigging (aboard ship) E834 ☑
      due to accident to watercraft
        E831 ☑
    roller skates E885.1
    scaffolding E881.1
    scooter (nonmotorized) E885.0
      motorized mobility E884.3
    sidewalk (curb) E880.1
      moving E885.9
    skateboard E885.2
    skis E885.3
    snowboard E885.4
    snow vehicle, motor-driven (not on
      public highway) E820 ☑
      on public highway E818 ☑

Fall, falling — *continued*
  from, off — *continued*
    snow vehicle, motor-driven — *contin-
      ued*
      on public highway — *continued*
        while alighting, boarding, enter-
          ing, leaving E817 ☑
    stairs, steps E880.9
      boat, ship, watercraft E833 ☑
        due to accident to watercraft
          E831 ☑
      motor bus, motor vehicle — *see* Fall,
        from, motor vehicle, while
        alighting, boarding
      street car E829 ☑
    stationary vehicle NEC E884.9
    stepladder E881.0
    street car (while boarding, alighting)
      E829 ☑
      stationary, except while boarding or
        alighting E884.9
    structure NEC E882
      burning (uncontrolled fire) E891.8
        in terrorism E979.3
    table E884.9
    toilet E884.6
    tower E882
    tree E884.9
    turret E882
    vehicle NEC (*see also* Accident, vehicle
      NEC)
      stationary E884.9
    viaduct E882
    wall E882
    wheelchair (electric) (motorized) E884.3
    wheelies E885.1
    window E882
  in, on
    aircraft (at landing, take-off) (in-transit)
      E843 ☑
      resulting from accident to aircraft —
        see categories E840-E842 ☑
    boat, ship, watercraft E835 ☑
      due to accident to watercraft
        E831 ☑
      one level to another NEC E834 ☑
      on ladder, stairs E833 ☑
    cutting or piercing instrument or ma-
      chine E888.0
    deck (of boat, ship, watercraft) E835 ☑
      due to accident to watercraft
        E831 ☑
    escalator E880.0
    gangplank E835 ☑
    glass, broken E888.0
    knife E888.0
    ladder E881.0
      in boat, ship, watercraft E833 ☑
      due to accident to watercraft
        E831 ☑
    object
      edged, pointed or sharp E888.0
      other E888.1
    pitchfork E888.0
    railway rolling stock, train, vehicle (while
      alighting, boarding) E804 ☑
      with
        collision (*see also* Collision, rail-
          way) E800 ☑
        derailment (*see also* Derailment,
          railway) E802 ☑
        explosion (see also Explosion,
          railway engine) E803 ☑
    scaffolding E881.1
    scissors E888.0
    staircase, stairs, steps (*see also* Fall, from,
      stairs) E880.9
    street car E829 ☑
    water transport (*see also* Fall, in, boat)
      E835 ☑
  into
    cavity E883.9
    dock E883.9
      from boat, ship, watercraft (*see also*
        Fall, from, boat) E832 ☑

Fall, falling — *continued*
  into — *continued*
    hold (of ship) E834 ☑
      due to accident to watercraft
        E831 ☑
    hole E883.9
    manhole E883.2
    moving part of machinery — *see* Acci-
      dent, machine
    opening in surface NEC E883.9
    pit E883.9
    quarry E883.9
    shaft E883.9
    storm drain E883.2
    tank E883.9
    water (with drowning or submersion)
      E910.9
    well E883.1
  late effect of NEC E929.3
  object (*see also* Hit by, object, falling) E916
  other E888.8
  over
    animal E885.9
    cliff E884.1
    embankment E884.9
    small object E885.9
  overboard (*see also* Fall, from, boat) E832 ☑
  resulting in striking against object E888.1
    sharp E888.0
  rock E916
  same level NEC E888.9
    aircraft (any kind) E843 ☑
      resulting from accident to aircraft —
        see categories E840-E842 ☑
    boat, ship, watercraft E835 ☑
      due to accident to, collision, water-
        craft E831 ☑
    from
      collision, pushing, shoving, by or
        with other person(s) E886.9
        as, or caused by, a crowd E917.6
        in sports E886.0
      in-line skates E885.1
      roller skates E885.1
      scooter (nonmotorized) E885.0
      skateboard E885.2
      slipping stumbling, tripping E885
      snowboard E885.4
  snowslide E916
    as avalanche E909.2
  stone E916
  through
    hatch (on ship) E834 ☑
      due to accident to watercraft
        E831 ☑
    roof E882
    window E882
  timber E916
  while alighting from, boarding, entering,
    leaving
    aircraft (any kind) E843 ☑
    motor bus, motor vehicle — *see* Fall,
      from, motor vehicle, while
      alighting, boarding
    nonmotor road vehicle NEC E829 ☑
    railway train E804 ☑
    street car E829 ☑
Fell or jumped from high place, so stated —
  see Jumping, from, high place
Felo-de-se — *see also* Suicide E958.9
Fever
  heat — *see* Heat
  thermic — *see* Heat
Fight (hand) (fist) (foot) — *see also* Assault,
  fight E960.9
Fire (accidental) (caused by great heat from
  appliance (electrical), hot object or hot
  substance) (secondary, resulting from
  explosion) E899
  conflagration — *see* Conflagration
  controlled, normal (in brazier, fireplace,
    furnace, or stove) (charcoal) (coal)
    (coke) (electric) (gas) (wood)
    bonfire E897
    brazier, not in building or structure E897

☑ **Additional Digit Required** — Refer to the Tabular List for Digit Selection   ▽ **Subterms under main terms may continue to next column or page**

2014 ICD-9-CM   **385**

Fire, hot object or hot substance — *continued*

controlled, normal — *continued*

in building or structure, except private dwelling (barn) (church) (convalescent or residential home) (factory) (farm outbuilding) (hospital) (hotel) (institution (educational) (dormitory) (residential) (private garage) (school) (shop) (store) (theatre) E896

in private dwelling (apartment) (boarding house) (camping place) (caravan) (farmhouse) (home (private)) (house) (lodging house) (rooming house) (tenement) E895

not in building or structure E897

trash E897

forest (uncontrolled) E892

grass (uncontrolled) E892

hay (uncontrolled) E892

homicide (attempt) E968.0

late effect of E969

in, of, on, starting in E892

aircraft (in transit) (powered) E841 ✓

at landing, take-off E840 ✓

stationary E892

unpowered (balloon) (glider) E842 ✓

balloon E842 ✓

boat, ship, watercraft — *see* categories E830 ✓, E831 ✓, E837 ✓

building or structure, except private dwelling (barn) (church) (convalescent or residential home) (factory) (farm outbuilding) (hospital) (hotel) (institution (educational) (dormitory) (residential) (school) (shop) (store) (theatre) (*see also* Conflagration, building or structure, except private dwelling) E891.9

forest (uncontrolled) E892

glider E842 ✓

grass (uncontrolled) E892

hay (uncontrolled) E892

lumber (uncontrolled) E892

machinery — *see* Accident, machine

mine (uncontrolled) E892

motor vehicle (in motion) (on public highway) E818 ✓

not on public highway E825 ✓

stationary E892

prairie (uncontrolled) E892

private dwelling (apartment) (boarding house) (camping place) (caravan) (farmhouse) (home (private)) (house) (lodging house) (private garage) (rooming house) (tenement) (*see also* Conflagration, private dwelling) E890.9

railway rolling stock, train, vehicle (*see also* Explosion, railway engine) E803 ✓

stationary E892

room NEC E898.1

street car (in motion) E829 ✓

stationary E892

terrorism (by fire-producing device) E979.3

fittings or furniture (burning building) (uncontrolled fire) E979.3

from nuclear explosion E979.5

transport vehicle, stationary NEC E892

tunnel (uncontrolled) E892

war operations (by fire-producing device or conventional weapon) E990.9

from nuclear explosion (*see also* War operations, injury due to, nuclear weapons) E996.2

incendiary bomb E990.0

petrol bomb E990.0

late effect of NEC E929.4

lumber (uncontrolled) E892

mine (uncontrolled) E892

prairie (uncontrolled) E892

Fire, hot object or hot substance — *continued*

self-inflicted (unspecified whether accidental or intentional) E988.1

stated as intentional, purposeful E958.1

specified NEC E898.1

with

conflagration — *see* Conflagration

ignition (of)

clothing — *see* Ignition, clothes

highly inflammable material (benzine) (fat) (gasoline) (kerosene) (paraffin) (petrol) E894

started by other person

stated as

with intent to injure or kill E968.0

undetermined whether or not with intent to injure or kill E988.1

suicide (attempted) E958.1

late effect of E959

tunnel (uncontrolled) E892

Fireball effects from nuclear explosion

in

terrorism E979.5

war operations (*see also* War operations, injury due to, nuclear weapons) E996.2

Fireworks (explosion) E923.0

Flash burns from explosion — *see also* Explosion E923.9

Flood (any injury) (resulting from storm) E908.2

caused by collapse of dam or manmade structure E909.3

Forced landing (aircraft) E840 ✓

Foreign body, object or material (entrance into) (accidental)

air passage (causing injury) E915

with asphyxia, obstruction, suffocation E912

food or vomitus E911

nose (with asphyxia, obstruction, suffocation) E912

causing injury without asphyxia, obstruction, suffocation E915

alimentary canal (causing injury) (with obstruction) E915

with asphyxia, obstruction respiratory passage, suffocation E912

food E911

mouth E915

with asphyxia, obstruction, suffocation E912

food E911

pharynx E915

with asphyxia, obstruction, suffocation E912

food E911

aspiration (with asphyxia, obstruction respiratory passage, suffocation) E912

causing injury without asphyxia, obstruction respiratory passage, suffocation E915

food (regurgitated) (vomited) E911

causing injury without asphyxia, obstruction respiratory passage, suffocation E915

mucus (not of newborn) E912

phlegm E912

bladder (causing injury or obstruction) E915

bronchus, bronchi — *see* Foreign body, air passages

conjunctival sac E914

digestive system — *see* Foreign body, alimentary canal

ear (causing injury or obstruction) E915

esophagus (causing injury or obstruction) (*see also* Foreign body, alimentary canal) E915

eye (any part) E914

eyelid E914

hairball (stomach) (with obstruction) E915

ingestion — *see* Foreign body, alimentary canal

inhalation — *see* Foreign body, aspiration

Foreign body, object or material — *continued*

intestine (causing injury or obstruction) E915

iris E914

lacrimal apparatus E914

larynx — *see* Foreign body, air passage

late effect of NEC E929.8

lung — *see* Foreign body, air passage

mouth — *see* Foreign body, alimentary canal, mouth

nasal passage — *see* Foreign body, air passage, nose

nose — *see* Foreign body, air passage, nose

ocular muscle E914

operation wound (left in) — *see* Misadventure, foreign object

orbit E914

pharynx — *see* Foreign body, alimentary canal, pharynx

rectum (causing injury or obstruction) E915

stomach (hairball) (causing injury or obstruction) E915

tear ducts or glands E914

trachea — *see* Foreign body, air passage

urethra (causing injury or obstruction) E915

vagina (causing injury or obstruction) E915

Found dead, injured

from exposure (to) — *see* Exposure

on

public highway E819 ✓

railway right of way E807 ✓

Fracture (circumstances unknown or unspecified) E887

due to specified external means — *see* manner of accident

late effect of NEC E929.3

occurring in water transport NEC E835 ✓

Freezing — *see* Cold, exposure to

Frostbite E901.0

due to manmade conditions E901.1

Frozen — *see* Cold, exposure to

G

Garrotting, homicidal (attempted) E963

Gored E906.8

Gunshot wound — *see also* Shooting E922.9

H

Hailstones, injury by E904.3

Hairball (stomach) (with obstruction) E915

Hanged himself — *see also* Hanging, self-inflicted E983.0

Hang gliding E842 ✓

Hanging (accidental) E913.8

caused by other person

in accidental circumstances E913.8

stated as

intentional, homicidal E963

undetermined whether accidental or intentional E983.0

homicide (attempt) E963

in bed or cradle E913.0

legal execution E978

self-inflicted (unspecified whether accidental or intentional) E983.0

in accidental circumstances E913.8

stated as intentional, purposeful E953.0

stated as undetermined whether accidental or intentional E983.0

suicidal (attempt) E953.0

Heat (apoplexy) (collapse) (cramps) (effects of) (excessive) (exhaustion) (fever) (prostration) (stroke) E900.9

due to

manmade conditions (as listed in E900.1, except boat, ship, watercraft) E900.1

weather (conditions) E900.0

from

electric heating apparatus causing burning E924.8

nuclear explosion

in

terrorism E979.5

Heat — *continued*

from — *continued*

nuclear explosion — *continued*

in — *continued*

war operations (*see also* War operations, injury due to, nuclear weapons) E996.2

generated in, boiler, engine, evaporator, fire room of boat, ship, watercraft E838 ✓

inappropriate in local application or packing in medical or surgical procedure E873.5

late effect of NEC E989

Hemorrhage

delayed following medical or surgical treatment without mention of misadventure — *see* Reaction, abnormal

during medical or surgical treatment as misadventure — *see* Misadventure, cut

High

altitude, effects E902.9

level of radioactivity, effects — *see* Radiation

pressure effects (*see also* Effects of, air pressure)

from rapid descent in water (causing caisson or divers' disease, palsy, or paralysis) E902.2

temperature, effects — *see* Heat

Hit, hitting (accidental) by

aircraft (propeller) (without accident to aircraft) E844 ✓

unpowered E842 ✓

avalanche E909.2

being thrown against object in or part of motor vehicle (in motion) (on public highway) E818 ✓

not on public highway E825 ✓

nonmotor road vehicle NEC E829 ✓

street car E829 ✓

boat, ship, watercraft

after fall from watercraft E838 ✓

damaged, involved in accident E831 ✓

while swimming, water skiing E838 ✓

bullet (*see also* Shooting) E922.9

from air gun E922.4

in

terrorism E979.4

war operations E991.2

rubber E991.0

flare, Verey pistol (*see also* Shooting) E922.8

hailstones E904.3

landslide E909.2

law-enforcing agent (on duty) E975

with blunt object (baton) (night stick) (stave) (truncheon) E973

machine — *see* Accident, machine

missile

firearm (*see also* Shooting) E922.9

in

terrorism — *see* Terrorism, missile

war operations — *see* War operations, missile

motor vehicle (on public highway) (traffic accident) E814 ✓

not on public highway, nontraffic accident E822 ✓

nonmotor road vehicle NEC E829 ✓

object

falling E916

from, in, on

aircraft E844 ✓

due to accident to aircraft — *see* categories E840-E842 ✓

unpowered E842 ✓

boat, ship, watercraft E838 ✓

due to accident to watercraft E831 ✓

building E916

burning (uncontrolled fire) E891.8

in terrorism E979.3

Hit, hitting by — continued
object — continued
  falling — continued
    from, in, on — continued
      building — continued
        burning — continued
          private E890.8
        cataclysmic
          earth surface movement or
            eruption E909.9
          storm E908.9
        cave-in E916
          with asphyxiation or suffoca-
            tion (see also Suffoca-
            tion, due to, cave-in)
            E913.3
        earthquake E909.0
        motor vehicle (in motion) (on
          public highway) E818 ☑
          not on public highway
            E825 ☑
          stationary E916
        nonmotor road vehicle NEC
          E829 ☑
        pedal cycle E826 ☑
        railway rolling stock, train, vehicle
          E806 ☑
        street car E829 ☑
        structure, burning NEC E891.8
        vehicle, stationary E916
  moving NEC — see Striking against, ob-
    ject
  projected NEC — see Striking against,
    object
  set in motion by
    compressed air or gas, spring, strik-
      ing, throwing — see Striking
      against, object
    explosion — see Explosion
  thrown into, on, or towards
    motor vehicle (in motion) (on public
      highway) E818 ☑
      not on public highway E825 ☑
      nonmotor road vehicle NEC E829 ☑
      pedal cycle E826 ☑
      street car E829 ☑
  off-road type motor vehicle (not on public
    highway) E821 ☑
  on public highway E814 ☑
  other person(s) E917.9
    with blunt or thrown object E917.9
      in sports E917.0
        with subsequent fall E917.5
      intentionally, homicidal E968.2
    as, or caused by, a crowd E917.1
      with subsequent fall E917.6
      in sports E917.0
  pedal cycle E826 ☑
  police (on duty) E975
    with blunt object (baton) (nightstick)
      (stave) (truncheon) E973
  railway, rolling stock, train, vehicle (part of)
    E805 ☑
  shot — see Shooting
  snow vehicle, motor-driven (not on public
    highway) E820 ☑
    on public highway E814 ☑
  street car E829 ☑
  vehicle NEC — see Accident, vehicle NEC
Homicide, homicidal (attempt) (justifiable) —
  see also Assault E968.9
Hot
liquid, object, substance, accident caused
  by (see also Accident, caused by, hot,
  by type of substance)
  late effect of E929.8
place, effects — see Heat
weather, effects E900.0
Humidity, causing problem E904.3
Hunger E904.1
resulting from
  abandonment or neglect E904.0
  transport accident — see categories
    E800-E848 ☑
Hurricane (any injury) E908.0

Hypobarism, hypobaropathy — see Effects
  of, air pressure
Hypothermia — see Cold, exposure to

I

Ictus
caloris — see Heat
solaris E900.0
Ignition (accidental)
anesthetic gas in operating theatre E923.2
bedclothes
  with
    conflagration — see Conflagration
    ignition (of)
      clothing — see Ignition, clothes
      highly inflammable material
        (benzine) (fat) (gasoline)
        (kerosene) (paraffin)
        (petrol) E894
benzine E894
clothes, clothing (from controlled fire) (in
  building) E893.9
  with conflagration — see Conflagration
  from
    bonfire E893.2
    highly inflammable material E894
    sources or material as listed in E893.8
    trash fire E893.2
    uncontrolled fire — see Conflagra-
      tion
  in
    private dwelling E893.0
    specified building or structure, ex-
      cept private dwelling E893.1
    not in building or structure E893.2
explosive material — see Explosion
fat E894
gasoline E894
kerosene E894
material
  explosive — see Explosion
  highly inflammable E894
    with conflagration — see Conflagra-
      tion
    with explosion E923.2
nightdress — see Ignition, clothes
paraffin E894
petrol E894
Immersion — see Submersion
Implantation of quills of porcupine E906.8
Inanition (from) E904.9
hunger — see Lack of, food
resulting from homicidal intent E968.4
thirst — see Lack of, water
Inattention after, at birth E904.0
homicidal, infanticidal intent E968.4
Infanticide — see also Assault
Ingestion
foreign body (causing injury) (with obstruction) — see Foreign body, alimentary
  canal
poisonous substance NEC — see Table of
  Drugs and Chemicals
Inhalation
excessively cold substance, manmade
  E901.1
foreign body — see Foreign body, aspiration
liquid air, hydrogen, nitrogen E901.1
mucus, not of newborn (with asphyxia, obstruction respiratory passage, suffocation) E912
phlegm (with asphyxia, obstruction respiratory passage, suffocation) E912
poisonous gas — see Table of Drugs and
  Chemicals
smoke from, due to
  fire — see Fire
tobacco, second-hand E869.4
vomitus (with asphyxia, obstruction respiratory passage, suffocation) E911
Injury, injured (accidental(ly)) NEC E928.9
by, caused by, from
  air rifle (BB gun) E922.4
  animal (not being ridden) NEC E906.9
    being ridden (in sport or transport)
      E828 ☑

Injury, injured — continued
by, caused by, from — continued
  assault (see also Assault) E968.9
  avalanche E909.2
  bayonet (see also Bayonet wound)
    E920.3
  being thrown against some part of, or
    object in
    motor vehicle (in motion) (on public
      highway) E818 ☑
      not on public highway E825 ☑
    nonmotor road vehicle NEC E829 ☑
    off-road motor vehicle NEC E821 ☑
    railway train E806 ☑
    snow vehicle, motor-driven E820 ☑
    street car E829 ☑
  bending
    due to
      repetitive movement E927.3
      sudden strenuous movement
        E927.0
  bite, human E928.3
  broken glass E920.8
  bullet — see Shooting
  cave-in (see also Suffocation, due to,
    cave-in) E913.3
    without asphyxiation or suffocation
      E916
    earth surface movement or eruption
      E909.9
    storm E908.9
  cloudburst E908.8
  component of firearm or air gun E928.7
  cutting or piercing instrument (see also
    Cut) E920.9
  cyclone E908.1
  earthquake E909.0
  earth surface movement or eruption
    E909.9
  electric current (see also Electric shock)
    E925.9
  explosion (see also Explosion) E923.9
    of gun part E928.7
  fire — see Fire
  flare, Verey pistol E922.8
  flood E908.2
  foreign body — see Foreign body
  gun recoil E928.7
  hailstones E904.3
  hurricane E908.0
  landslide E909.2
  law-enforcing agent, police, in course of
    legal intervention — see Legal
    intervention
  lightning E907
  live rail or live wire — see Electric shock
  machinery (see also Accident, machine)
    aircraft, without accident to aircraft
      E844 ☑
    boat, ship, watercraft (deck) (engine
      room) (galley) (laundry)
      (loading) E836 ☑
  mechanism of firearm or air gun E928.7
  missile
    explosive E923.8
    firearm — see Shooting
    in
      terrorism — see Terrorism, mis-
        sile
      war operations — see War opera-
        tions, missile
  moving part of motor vehicle (in motion)
    (on public highway) E818 ☑
    not on public highway, nontraffic
      accident E825 ☑
    while alighting, boarding, entering,
      leaving — see Fall, from, mo-
      tor vehicle, while alighting,
      boarding
  nail E920.8
  needle (sewing) E920.4
    hypodermic E920.5
  noise E928.1

Injury, injured — continued
by, caused by, from — continued
  object
    fallen on
      motor vehicle (in motion) (on
        public highway) E818 ☑
      not on public highway
        E825 ☑
    falling — see Hit by, object, falling
  paintball gun E922.5
  radiation — see Radiation
  railway rolling stock, train, vehicle (part
    of) E805 ☑
    door or window E806 ☑
  recoil of firearm E928.7
  rotating propeller, aircraft E844 ☑
  rough landing of off-road type motor
    vehicle (after leaving ground or
    rough terrain) E821 ☑
  snow vehicle E820 ☑
  saber (see also Wound, saber) E920.3
  shot — see Shooting
  sound waves E928.1
  splinter or sliver, wood E920.8
  straining
    due to
      repetitive movement E927.3
      sudden strenuous movement
        E927.0
  street car (door) E829 ☑
  suicide (attempt) E958.9
  sword E920.3
  terrorism — see Terrorism
  third rail — see Electric shock
  thunderbolt E907
  tidal wave E909.4
    caused by storm E908.0
  tornado E908.1
  torrential rain E908.2
  twisting
    due to
      repetitive movement E927.3
      sudden strenuous movement
        E927.0
  vehicle NEC — see Accident, vehicle NEC
  vibration E928.2
  volcanic eruption E909.1
  weapon burst, in war operations E993.9
  weightlessness (in spacecraft, real or
    simulated) E928.0
  wood splinter or sliver E920.8
due to
  civil insurrection — see War operations
    occurring after cessation of hostilities
      E998.9
  terrorism — see Terrorism
  war operations — see War operations
    occurring after cessation of hostilities
      E998.9
  weapon of mass destruction [WMD]
    E997.3
homicidal (see also Assault) E968.9
inflicted (by)
  in course of arrest (attempted), suppres-
    sion of disturbance, maintenance
    of order, by law enforcing agents
    — see Legal intervention
  law-enforcing agent (on duty) — see
    Legal intervention
  other person
    stated as
      accidental E928.9
      homicidal, intentional — see As-
        sault
      undetermined whether acciden-
        tal or intentional — see
        Injury, stated as undeter-
        mined
  police (on duty) — see Legal interven-
    tion
in, on
  civil insurrection — see War operations
  fight E960.0
  parachute descent (voluntary) (without
    accident to aircraft) E844 ☑

Injury, injured — *continued*
  in, on — *continued*
    parachute descent — *continued*
      with accident to aircraft — *see* categories E840-E842 ☑
    public highway E819 ☑
    railway right of way E807 ☑
    terrorism — *see* Terrorism
    war operations — *see* War operations
  late effect of E929.9
  purposely (inflicted) by other person(s) — *see* Assault
  self-inflicted (unspecified whether accidental or intentional) E988.9
    stated as
      accidental E928.9
      intentionally, purposely E958.9
  specified cause NEC E928.8
  stated as
    hanging E983.0
    knife E986
    late effect of E989
    puncture (any part of body) E986
    shooting — *see* Shooting, stated as undetermined whether accidental or intentional
    specified means NEC E988.8
    stab (any part of body) E986
    strangulation — *see* Suffocation, stated as undetermined whether accidental or intentional
    submersion E984
    suffocation — *see* Suffocation, stated as undetermined whether accidental or intentional
  undetermined whether accidentally or purposely inflicted (by) E988.9
    cut (any part of body) E986
    cutting or piercing instrument (classifiable to E920) E986
    drowning E984
    explosive(s) (missile) E985.5
    falling from high place E987.9
      manmade structure, except residential E987.1
    natural site E987.2
    residential premises E987.0
  to child due to criminal abortion E968.8
Insufficient nourishment — *see* Lack of, food
  homicidal intent E968.4
Insulation, effects — *see* Heat
Interruption of respiration by
  food lodged in esophagus E911
  foreign body, except food, in esophagus E912
Intervention, legal — *see* Legal intervention
Intoxication, drug or poison — *see* Table of Drugs and Chemicals
Irradiation — *see* Radiation

J

Jammed (accidentally)
  between objects (moving) (stationary and moving) E918
  in object E918
Jumped or fell from high place, so stated — *see* Jumping, from, high place, stated as in undetermined circumstances
Jumping
  before train, vehicle or other moving object (unspecified whether accidental or intentional) E988.0
    stated as
      intentional, purposeful E958.0
      suicidal (attempt) E958.0
  from
    aircraft
      by parachute (voluntarily) (without accident to aircraft) E844 ☑
      due to accident to aircraft — *see* categories E840-E842 ☑
    boat, ship, watercraft (into water)
      after accident to, fire on, watercraft E830 ☑

Jumping — *continued*
  from — *continued*
    boat, ship, watercraft — *continued*
      after accident to, fire on, watercraft — *continued*
        and subsequently struck by (part of) boat E831 ☑
      burning, crushed, sinking E830 ☑
        and subsequently struck by (part of) boat E831 ☑
      voluntarily, without accident (to boat) with injury other than drowning or submersion E883.0
    building (*see also* Jumping, from, high place)
    burning (uncontrolled fire) E891.8
      in terrorism E979.3
      private E890.8
    cable car (not on rails) E847
      on rails E829 ☑
    high place
      in accidental circumstances or in sport — *see* categories E880-E884 ☑
      stated as
        with intent to injure self E957.9
          man-made structures NEC E957.1
          natural sites E957.2
          residential premises E957.0
        in undetermined circumstances E987.9
          man-made structures NEC E987.1
          natural sites E987.2
          residential premises E987.0
        suicidal (attempt) E957.9
          man-made structures NEC E957.1
          natural sites E957.1
          residential premises E957.0
    motor vehicle (in motion) (on public highway) — *see* Fall, from, motor vehicle
    nonmotor road vehicle NEC E829 ☑
    street car E829 ☑
    structure (*see also* Jumping, from, high place)
      burning NEC (uncontrolled fire) E891.8
      in terrorism E979.3
  into water
    with injury other than drowning or submersion E883.0
    drowning or submersion — *see* Submersion
  from, off, watercraft — *see* Jumping, from, boat
Justifiable homicide — *see* Assault

K

Kicked by
  animal E906.8
  person(s) (accidentally) E917.9
    with intent to injure or kill E960.0
    as, or caused by a crowd E917.1
      with subsequent fall E917.6
    in fight E960.0
    in sports E917.0
      with subsequent fall E917.5
Kicking against
  object (moving) E917.9
    in sports E917.0
      with subsequent fall E917.5
    stationary E917.4
      with subsequent fall E917.8
  person — *see* Striking against, person
Killed, killing (accidentally) NEC — *see also* Injury E928.9
  in
    action — *see* War operations
    brawl, fight (hand) (fists) (foot) E960.0
      by weapon (*see also* Assault)
        cutting, piercing E966
        firearm — *see* Shooting, homicide

Killed, killing — *see also* Injury — *continued*
  self
    stated as
      accident E928.9
      suicide — *see* Suicide
    unspecified whether accidental or suicidal E988.9
Knocked down (accidentally) (by) NEC E928.9
  animal (not being ridden) E906.8
    being ridden (in sport or transport) E828 ☑
  blast from explosion (*see also* Explosion) E923.9
  crowd, human stampede E917.6
  late effect of — *see* Late effect
  person (accidentally) E917.9
    in brawl, fight E960.0
    in sports E917.5
  transport vehicle — *see* vehicle involved under Hit by
  while boxing E917.5

L

Laceration NEC E928.9
Lack of
  air (refrigerator or closed place), suffocation by E913.2
  care (helpless person) (infant) (newborn) E904.0
    homicidal intent E968.4
  food except as result of transport accident E904.1
    helpless person, infant, newborn due to abandonment or neglect E904.0
  water except as result of transport accident E904.2
    helpless person, infant, newborn due to abandonment or neglect E904.0
Landslide E909.2
  falling on, hitting
    motor vehicle (any) (in motion) (on or off public highway) E909.2
    railway rolling stock, train, vehicle E909.2
Late effect of
  accident NEC (accident classifiable to E928.9) E929.9
    specified NEC (accident classifiable to E910–E928.8) E929.8
  assault E969
  fall, accidental (accident classifiable to E880–E888) E929.3
  fire, accident caused by (accident classifiable to E890–E899) E929.4
  homicide, attempt (any means) E969
  injury due to terrorism E999.1
  injury undetermined whether accidentally or purposely inflicted (injury classifiable to E980–E988) E989
  legal intervention (injury classifiable to E970–E976) E977
  medical or surgical procedure, test or therapy
    as, or resulting in, or from
      abnormal or delayed reaction or complication — *see* Reaction, abnormal
      misadventure — *see* Misadventure
  motor vehicle accident (accident classifiable to E810–E825) E929.0
  natural or environmental factor, accident due to (accident classifiable to E900–E909) E929.5
  poisoning, accidental (accident classifiable to E850–E858, E860–E869) E929.2
  suicide, attempt (any means) E959
  transport accident NEC (accident classifiable to E800–E807, E826–E838, E840–E848) E929.1
  war operations, injury due to (injury classifiable to E990–E998) E999.0
Launching pad accident E845 ☑
Legal
  execution, any method E978
  intervention (by) (injury from) E976
    baton E973

Legal — *continued*
  intervention — *continued*
    bayonet E974
    blow E975
    blunt object (baton) (nightstick) (stave) (truncheon) E973
    cutting or piercing instrument E974
    dynamite E971
    execution, any method E973
    explosive(s) (shell) E971
    firearm(s) E970
    gas (asphyxiation) (poisoning) (tear) E972
    grenade E971
    late effect of E977
    machine gun E970
    manhandling E975
    mortar bomb E971
    nightstick E973
    revolver E970
    rifle E970
    specified means NEC E975
    stabbing E974
    stave E973
    truncheon E973
Lifting, injury
  due to
    repetitive movement E927.3
    sudden strenuous movement E927.0
Lightning (shock) (stroke) (struck by) E907
Liquid (noncorrosive) in eye E914
  corrosive E924.1
Loss of control
  motor vehicle (on public highway) (without antecedent collision) E816 ☑
    with
      antecedent collision on public highway — *see* Collision, motor vehicle
      involving any object, person or vehicle not on public highway E816 ☑
    not on public highway, nontraffic accident E825 ☑
      with antecedent collision — *see* Collision, motor vehicle, not on public highway
    on public highway — *see* Collision, motor vehicle
    off-road type motor vehicle (not on public highway) E821 ☑
      on public highway — *see* Loss of control, motor vehicle
    snow vehicle, motor-driven (not on public highway) E820 ☑
      on public highway — *see* Loss of control, motor vehicle
Lost at sea E832 ☑
  with accident to watercraft E830 ☑
  in war operations E995.8
Low
  pressure, effects — *see* Effects of, air pressure
  temperature, effects — *see* Cold, exposure to
Lying before train, vehicle or other moving object (unspecified whether accidental or intentional) E988.0
  stated as intentional, purposeful, suicidal (attempt) E958.0
Lynching — *see also* Assault E968.9

M

Malfunction, atomic power plant in water transport E838 ☑
Mangled (accidentally) NEC E928.9
Manhandling (in brawl, fight) E960.0
  legal intervention E975
Manslaughter (nonaccidental) — *see* Assault
Marble in nose E912
Mauled by animal E906.8
Medical procedure, complication of
  delayed or as an abnormal reaction without mention of misadventure — *see* Reaction, abnormal

Medical procedure, complication of — *continued*
    due to or as a result of misadventure — *see* Misadventure
Melting of fittings and furniture in burning
    in terrorism E979.3
Minamata disease E865.2
Misadventure(s) to patient(s) during surgical or medical care E876.9
    contaminated blood, fluid, drug or biological substance (presence of agents and toxins as listed in E875) E875.9
      administered (by) NEC E875.9
        infusion E875.0
        injection E875.1
        specified means NEC E875.2
        transfusion E875.0
        vaccination E875.1
    cut, cutting, puncture, perforation or hemorrhage (accidental) (inadvertent) (inappropriate) (during) E870.9
      aspiration of fluid or tissue (by puncture or catheterization, except heart) E870.5
      biopsy E870.8
        needle (aspirating) E870.5
      blood sampling E870.5
      catheterization E870.5
        heart E870.6
      dialysis (kidney) E870.2
      endoscopic examination E870.4
      enema E870.7
      infusion E870.1
      injection E870.3
      lumbar puncture E870.5
      needle biopsy E870.5
      paracentesis, abdominal E870.5
      perfusion E870.2
      specified procedure NEC E870.8
      surgical operation E870.0
      thoracentesis E870.5
      transfusion E870.1
      vaccination E870.1
    excessive amount of blood or other fluid during transfusion or infusion E873.0
    failure
      in dosage E873.9
        electroshock therapy E873.4
        inappropriate temperature (too hot or too cold) in local application and packing E873.5
        infusion
          excessive amount of fluid E873.0
          incorrect dilution of fluid E873.1
        insulin-shock therapy E873.4
        nonadministration of necessary drug or medicinal E873.6
        overdose (*see also* Overdose)
          radiation, in therapy E873.2
        radiation
          inadvertent exposure of patient (receiving radiation for test or therapy) E873.3
          not receiving radiation for test or therapy — *see* Radiation
          overdose E873.2
        specified procedure NEC E873.8
        transfusion
          excessive amount of blood E873.0
      mechanical, of instrument or apparatus (during procedure) E874.9
        aspiration of fluid or tissue (by puncture or catheterization, except of heart) E874.4
        biopsy E874.8
          needle (aspirating) E874.4
        blood sampling E874.4
        catheterization E874.4
          heart E874.5
        dialysis (kidney) E874.2
        endoscopic examination E874.3
        enema E874.8
        infusion E874.1
        injection E874.8
        lumbar puncture E874.4

Misadventure(s) to patient(s) during surgical or medical care — *continued*
    failure — *continued*
      mechanical, of instrument or apparatus — *continued*
        needle biopsy E874.4
        paracentesis, abdominal E874.4
        perfusion E874.2
        specified procedure NEC E874.8
        surgical operation E874.0
        thoracentesis E874.4
        transfusion E874.1
        vaccination E874.8
      sterile precautions (during procedure) E872.9
        aspiration of fluid or tissue (by puncture or catheterization, except heart) E872.5
        biopsy E872.8
          needle (aspirating) E872.5
        blood sampling E872.5
        catheterization E872.5
          heart E872.6
        dialysis (kidney) E872.2
        endoscopic examination E872.4
        enema E872.8
        infusion E872.1
        injection E872.3
        lumbar puncture E872.5
        needle biopsy E872.5
        paracentesis, abdominal E872.5
        perfusion E872.2
        removal of catheter or packing E872.5
        specified procedure NEC E872.8
        surgical operation E872.0
        thoracentesis E872.5
        transfusion E872.1
        vaccination E872.3
      suture or ligature during surgical procedure E876.2
      to introduce or to remove tube or instrument E876.4
        foreign object left in body — *see* Misadventure, foreign object
    foreign object left in body (during procedure) E871.9
      aspiration of fluid or tissue (by puncture or catheterization, except heart) E871.5
      biopsy E871.8
        needle (aspirating) E871.5
      blood sampling E871.5
      catheterization E871.5
        heart E871.6
      dialysis (kidney) E871.2
      endoscopic examination E871.4
      enema E871.8
      infusion E871.1
      injection E871.3
      lumbar puncture E871.5
      needle biopsy E871.5
      paracentesis, abdominal E871.5
      perfusion E871.2
      removal of catheter or packing E871.7
      specified procedure NEC E871.8
      surgical operation E871.0
      thoracentesis E871.5
      transfusion E871.1
      vaccination E871.3
    hemorrhage — *see* Misadventure, cut
    inadvertent exposure of patient to radiation (being received for test or therapy) E873.3
    inappropriate
      temperature (too hot or too cold) in local application or packing E873.5
    infusion (*see also* Misadventure, by specific type, infusion)
      excessive amount of fluid E873.0
      incorrect dilution of fluid E873.1
      wrong fluid E876.1
    mismatched blood in transfusion E876.0
    nonadministration of necessary drug or medicinal E873.6
    overdose (*see also* Overdose)

Misadventure(s) to patient(s) during surgical or medical care — *continued*
    overdose (*see also* Overdose) — *continued*
      radiation, in therapy E873.2
    perforation — *see* Misadventure, cut
    performance of correct operation (procedure) on wrong
      body part E876.7
      side E876.7
      site E876.7
    performance of operation (procedure)
      intended for another patient E876.6
      on patient not scheduled for surgery E876.6
      on wrong patient E876.6
    performance of wrong operation on correct patient E876.5
    puncture — *see* Misadventure, cut
    specified type NEC E876.8
      failure
        suture or ligature during surgical operation E876.2
        to introduce or to remove tube or instrument E876.4
          foreign object left in body E871.9
      infusion of wrong fluid E876.1
      performance of inappropriate operation E876.5
      transfusion of mismatched blood E876.0
      wrong
        fluid in infusion E876.1
        placement of endotracheal tube during anesthetic procedure E876.3
    transfusion (*see also* Misadventure, by specific type, transfusion)
      excessive amount of blood E873.0
      mismatched blood E876.0
    wrong
      device implanted into correct surgical site E876.5
      drug given in error — *see* Table of Drugs and Chemicals
      fluid in infusion E876.1
      placement of endotracheal tube during anesthetic procedure E876.3
      procedure (operation) performed on the correct patient E876.5
Motion (effects) E903
    sickness E903
Mountain sickness E902.0
Mucus aspiration or inhalation, not of newborn (with asphyxia, obstruction respiratory passage, suffocation) E912
Mudslide of cataclysmic nature E909.2
Murder (attempt) — *see also* Assault E968.9

N

Nail, injury by E920.8
Needlestick (sewing needle) E920.4
    hypodermic E920.5
Neglect — *see also* Privation
    criminal E968.4
    homicidal intent E968.4
Noise (causing injury) (pollution) E928.1
Nuclear weapon — *see also* War operations, injury due to, nuclear weapons E996.9

O

Object
    falling
      from, in, on, hitting
        aircraft E844 ☑
          due to accident to aircraft — *see* categories E840-E842 ☑
        machinery (*see also* Accident, machine)
          not in operation E916
        motor vehicle (in motion) (on public highway) E818 ☑
        nonmotor road vehicle NEC E829 ☑
          not on public highway E825 ☑
        pedal cycle E826 ☑

Object — *continued*
    falling — *continued*
      from, in, on, hitting — *continued*
        motor vehicle — *continued*
          person E916
          railway rolling stock, train, vehicle E806 ☑
          stationary E916
          street car E829 ☑
          watercraft E838 ☑
            due to accident to watercraft E831 ☑
      set in motion by
        accidental explosion of pressure vessel — *see* category E921 ☑
        firearm — *see* category E922 ☑
        machine(ry) — *see* Accident, machine
        transport vehicle — *see* categories E800-E848 ☑
      thrown from, in, on, towards
        aircraft E844 ☑
        cable car (not on rails) E847
          on rails E829 ☑
        motor vehicle (in motion) (on public highway) E818 ☑
          not on public highway E825 ☑
        nonmotor road vehicle NEC E829 ☑
        pedal cycle E826 ☑
        street car E829 ☑
        vehicle NEC — *see* Accident, vehicle NEC
Obstruction
    air passages, larynx, respiratory passages by
        external means NEC — *see* Suffocation
        food, any type (regurgitated) (vomited) E911
        material or object, except food E912
        mucus E912
        phlegm E912
        vomitus E911
    digestive tract, except mouth or pharynx by
        food, any type E915
        foreign body (any) E915
    esophagus
      without asphyxia or obstruction of respiratory passage E915
      food E911
      foreign body, except food E912
    mouth or pharynx by
        food, any type E911
        material or object, except food E912
    respiration — *see* Obstruction, air passages
Oil in eye E914
Overdose
    anesthetic (drug) — *see* Table of Drugs and Chemicals
    drug — *see* Table of Drugs and Chemicals
Overexertion E927.9
    from
      lifting
        repetitive movement E927.3
        sudden strenuous movement E927.0
      maintaining prolonged positions E927.1
        holding E927.1
        sitting E927.1
        standing E927.1
      prolonged static position E927.1
      pulling
        repetitive movement E927.3
        sudden strenuous movement E927.0
      pushing
        repetitive movement E927.3
        sudden strenuous movement E927.0
      specified NEC E927.8
      sudden strenuous movement E927.0
Overexposure (accidental) (to)
    cold (*see also* Cold, exposure to) E901.9
      due to manmade conditions E901.1
    heat (*see also* Heat) E900.9
    radiation — *see* Radiation
    radioactivity — *see* Radiation
    sun, except sunburn E900.0
    weather — *see* Exposure

☑ **Additional Digit Required** — Refer to the Tabular List for Digit Selection   ▽ **Subterms under main terms may continue to next column or page**

2014 ICD-9-CM   **389**

Overexposure — *continued*
  wind — *see* Exposure
Overheated — *see also* Heat E900.9
Overlaid E913.0
Overturning (accidental)
  animal-drawn vehicle E827 ☑
  boat, ship, watercraft
    causing
      drowning, submersion E830 ☑
      injury except drowning, submersion E831 ☑
    machinery — *see* Accident, machine
  motor vehicle (*see also* Loss of control, motor vehicle) E816 ☑
    with antecedent collision on public highway — *see* Collision, motor vehicle
    not on public highway, nontraffic accident E825 ☑
      with antecedent collision — *see* Collision, motor vehicle, not on public highway
  nonmotor road vehicle NEC E829 ☑
  off-road type motor vehicle — *see* Loss of control, off-road type motor vehicle
  pedal cycle E826 ☑
  railway rolling stock, train, vehicle (*see also* Derailment, railway) E802 ☑
  street car E829 ☑
  vehicle NEC — *see* Accident, vehicle NEC

P

Palsy, divers' E902.2
Parachuting (voluntary) (without accident to aircraft) E844 ☑
  due to accident to aircraft — *see* categories E840-E842 ☑
Paralysis
  divers' E902.2
  lead or saturnine E866.0
    from pesticide NEC E863.4
Pecked by bird E906.8
Performance of correct operation (procedure) **on wrong**
  body part E876.7
  side E876.7
  site E876.7
Performance of operation (procedure)
  intended for another patient E876.6
  on patient not scheduled for surgery E876.6
  on wrong patient E876.6
Performance of wrong operation on correct patient E876.5
Phlegm aspiration or inhalation (with asphyxia, obstruction respiratory passage, suffocation) E912
Piercing — *see also* Cut E920.9
  by slide trigger mechanism, scope or other part of gun E928.7
Pinched
  between objects (moving) (stationary and moving) E918
  by slide trigger mechanism, scope or other part of gun E928.7
  in object E918
Pinned under
  machine(ry) — *see* Accident, machine
Place of occurrence of accident — *see* Accident (to), occurring (at) (in)
Plumbism E866.0
  from insecticide NEC E863.4
Poisoning (accidental) (by) — *see also* Table of Drugs and Chemicals
  carbon monoxide
    generated by
      aircraft in transit E844 ☑
      motor vehicle
        in motion (on public highway) E818 ☑
        not on public highway E825 ☑
      watercraft (in transit) (not in transit) E838 ☑

Poisoning — *see also* Table of Drugs and Chemicals — *continued*
  caused by injection of poisons or toxins into or through skin by plant thorns, spines, or other mechanism E905.7
    marine or sea plants E905.6
  fumes or smoke due to
    conflagration — *see* Conflagration
    explosion or fire — *see* Fire
    ignition — *see* Ignition
  gas
    in legal intervention E972
    legal execution, by E978
    on watercraft E838 ☑
    used as anesthetic — *see* Table of Drugs and Chemicals
  in
    terrorism (chemical weapons) E979.7
    war operations E997.2
      execution E978
      intervention
        by gas E972
  late effect of — *see* Late effect
  legal
Pressure, external, causing asphyxia, suffocation — *see also* Suffocation E913.9
Privation E904.9
  food (*see also* Lack of, food) E904.1
  helpless person, infant, newborn due to abandonment or neglect E904.0
  late effect of NEC E929.5
  resulting from transport accident — *see* categories E800-E848 ☑
  water (*see also* Lack of, water) E904.2
Projected objects, striking against or struck by — *see* Striking against, object
Prolonged stay in
  high altitude (causing conditions as listed in E902.0) E902.0
  weightless environment E928.0
Prostration
  heat — *see* Heat
Pulling, injury
  due to
    repetitive movement E927.3
    sudden strenuous movement E927.0
Puncture, puncturing — *see also* Cut E920.9
  by
    plant thorns or spines E920.8
      toxic reaction E905.7
        marine or sea plants E905.6
    sea-urchin spine E905.6
Pushing (injury in) (overexertion)
  by other person(s) (accidental) E917.9
    with fall E886.9
    in sports E886.0
    as, or caused by, a crowd, human stampede E917.1
      with subsequent fall E917.6
    before moving vehicle or object
      stated as
        intentional, homicidal E968.5
        undetermined whether accidental or intentional E988.8
    from
      high place
        in accidental circum-stances — *see* categories E880-E884 ☑
        stated as
          intentional, homicidal E968.1
          undetermined whether accidental or intentional E987.9
          man-made structure, except residential E987.1
          natural site E987.2
          residential E987.0
      motor vehicle (*see also* Fall, from, motor vehicle) E818 ☑
        stated as
          intentional, homicidal E968.5
          undetermined whether accidental or intentional E988.8

Pushing — *continued*
  by other person(s) — *continued*
    in sports E917.0
      with fall E886.0
  due to
    repetitive movement E927.3
    sudden strenuous movement E927.0

R

Radiation (exposure to) E926.9
  abnormal reaction to medical test or therapy E879.2
  arc lamps E926.2
  atomic power plant (malfunction) NEC E926.9
    in water transport E838 ☑
  electromagnetic, ionizing E926.3
  gamma rays E926.3
  in
    terrorism (from or following nuclear explosion) (direct) (secondary) E979.5
      laser E979.8
    war operations (*see also* War operations, injury due to, nuclear weapons) E996.3
      laser(s) E997.0
      water transport E838 ☑
  inadvertent exposure of patient (receiving test or therapy) E873.3
  infrared (heaters and lamps) E926.1
    excessive heat E900.1
  ionized, ionizing (particles, artificially accelerated) E926.8
    electromagnetic E926.3
  isotopes, radioactive — *see* Radiation, radioactive isotopes
  laser(s) E926.4
    in
      terrorism E979.8
      war operations E997.0
    misadventure in medical care — *see* Misadventure, failure, in dosage, radiation
  late effect of NEC E929.8
    excessive heat from — *see* Heat
  light sources (visible) (ultraviolet) E926.2
  misadventure in medical or surgical procedure — *see* Misadventure, failure, in dosage, radiation
  overdose (in medical or surgical procedure) E873.2
  radar E926.0
  radioactive isotopes E926.5
    atomic power plant malfunction E926.5
      in water transport E838 ☑
    misadventure in medical or surgical treatment — *see* Misadventure, failure, in dosage, radiation
  radiobiologicals — *see* Radiation, radioactive isotopes
  radiofrequency E926.0
  radiopharmaceuticals — *see* Radiation, radioactive isotopes
  radium NEC E926.9
  sun E926.2
    excessive heat from E900.0
  tanning bed E926.2
  welding arc or torch E926.2
    excessive heat from E900.1
  x-rays (hard) (soft) E926.3
    misadventure in medical or surgical treatment — *see* Misadventure, failure, in dosage, radiation
Rape E960.1
Reaction, abnormal to or following (medical or surgical procedure) E879.9
  amputation (of limbs) E878.5
  anastomosis (arteriovenous) (blood vessel) (gastrojejunal) (skin) (tendon) (natural, artificial material, tissue) E878.2
    external stoma, creation of E878.3
  aspiration (of fluid) E879.4
    tissue E879.8
  biopsy E879.8

Reaction, abnormal to or following — *continued*
  blood
    sampling E879.7
    transfusion
      procedure E879.8
    bypass — *see* Reaction, abnormal, anastomosis
  catheterization
    cardiac E879.0
    urinary E879.6
  colostomy E878.3
  cystostomy E878.3
  dialysis (kidney) E879.1
  drugs or biologicals — *see* Table of Drugs and Chemicals
  duodenostomy E878.3
  electroshock therapy E879.3
  formation of external stoma E878.3
  gastrostomy E878.3
  graft — *see* Reaction, abnormal, anastomosis
  hypothermia E879.8
  implant, implantation (of)
    artificial
      internal device (cardiac pacemaker) (electrodes in brain) (heart valve prosthesis) (orthopedic) E878.1
      material or tissue (for anastomosis or bypass) E878.2
        with creation of external stoma E878.3
    natural tissues (for anastomosis or bypass) E878.2
      with creation of external stoma E878.3
    as transplantion — *see* Reaction, abnormal, transplant
  infusion
    procedure E879.8
  injection
    procedure E879.8
    specific type of procedure) E879.9
  insertion of gastric or duodenal sound E879.5
  insulin-shock therapy E879.3
  lumbar puncture E879.4
  perfusion E879.1
  procedures other than surgical operation (*see also* Reaction, abnormal, by specified procedure NEC E879.8
  radiological procedure or therapy E879.2
  removal of organ (partial) (total) NEC E878.6
    with
      anastomosis, bypass or graft E878.2
      formation of external stoma E878.3
      implant of artificial internal device E878.1
      transplant(ation)
        partial organ E878.4
        whole organ E878.0
  sampling
    blood E879.7
    fluid NEC E879.4
    tissue E879.8
  shock therapy E879.3
  surgical operation (*see also* Reaction, abnormal, by specified type of operation) E878.9
    restorative NEC E878.4
      with
        anastomosis, bypass or graft E878.2
        fomation of external stoma E878.3
        implant(ation) — *see* Reaction, abnormal, implant
        transplant(ation) — *see* Reaction, abnormal, transplant
  specified operation NEC E878.8
  thoracentesis E879.4
  transfusion
    procedure E879.8
  transplant, transplantation (heart) (kidney) (liver) E878.0

Reaction, abnormal to or following — *continued*
  transplant, transplantation — *continued*
    partial organ E878.4
    ureterostomy E878.3
  vaccination E879.8
Reduction in
  atmospheric pressure (*see also* Effects of, air pressure)
    while surfacing from
      deep water diving causing caisson or divers' disease, palsy or paralysis E902.2
      underground E902.8
Repetitive movements NEC E927.8
Residual (effect) — *see* Late effect
Rock falling on or hitting (accidentally)
  motor vehicle (in motion) (on public highway) E818 ☑
    not on public highway E825 ☑
  nonmotor road vehicle NEC E829 ☑
  pedal cycle E826 ☑
  person E916
  railway rolling stock, train, vehicle E806 ☑
Running off, away
  animal (being ridden) (in sport or transport) E828 ☑
    not being ridden E906.8
  animal-drawn vehicle E827 ☑
  rails, railway (*see also* Derailment) E802 ☑
  roadway
    motor vehicle (without antecedent collision) E816 ☑
      with
        antecedent collision — *see* Collision motor vehicle
        subsequent collision
          involving any object, person or vehicle not on public highway E816 ☑
          on public highway E811 ☑
      nontraffic accident E825 ☑
        with antecedent collision — *see* Collision, motor vehicle, not on public highway
    nonmotor road vehicle NEC E829 ☑
    pedal cycle E826 ☑
Run over (accidentally) (by)
  animal (not being ridden) E906.8
    being ridden (in sport or transport) E828 ☑
  animal-drawn vehicle E827 ☑
  machinery — *see* Accident, machine
  motor vehicle (on public highway) — *see* Hit by, motor vehicle
  nonmotor road vehicle NEC E829 ☑
  railway train E805 ☑
  street car E829 ☑
  vehicle NEC E848

S

Saturnism E866.0
  from insecticide NEC E863.4
Scald, scalding (accidental) (by) (from) (in) E924.0
  acid — *see* Scald, caustic
  boiling tap water E924.2
  caustic or corrosive liquid, substance E924.1
    swallowed — *see* Table of Drugs and Chemicals
  homicide (attempt) — *see* Assault, burning
  inflicted by other person
    stated as
      intentional or homicidal E968.3
      undetermined whether accidental or intentional E988.2
  late effect of NEC E929.8
  liquid (boiling) (hot) E924.0
  local application of externally applied substance in medical or surgical care E873.5
  molten metal E924.0
  self-inflicted (unspecified whether accidental or intentional) E988.2
    stated as intentional, purposeful E958.2

Scald, scalding — *continued*
  stated as undetermined whether accidental or intentional E988.2
    steam E924.0
    tap water (boiling) E924.2
    transport accident — *see* categories E800-E848 ☑
    vapor E924.0
Scratch, cat E906.8
Sea
  sickness E903
Self-mutilation — *see* Suicide
Sequelae (of)
  in
    terrorism E999.1
    war operations E999.0
Shock
  anaphylactic (*see also* Table of Drugs and Chemicals) E947.9
    due to
      bite (venomous) — *see* Bite, venomous NEC
      sting — *see* Sting
  electric (*see also* Electric shock) E925.9
    from electric appliance or current (*see also* Electric shock) E925.9
Shooting, shot (accidental(ly)) E922.9
  air gun E922.4
  BB gun E922.4
  hand gun (pistol) (revolver) E922.0
  himself (*see also* Shooting, self-inflicted) E985.4
    hand gun (pistol) (revolver) E985.0
    military firearm, except hand gun E985.3
      hand gun (pistol) (revolver) E985.0
    rifle (hunting) E985.2
      military E985.3
    shotgun (automatic) E985.1
    specified firearm NEC E985.4
    Verey pistol E985.4
  homicide (attempt) E965.4
    air gun E968.6
    BB gun E968.6
    hand gun (pistol) (revolver) E965.0
    military firearm, except hand gun E965.3
      hand gun (pistol) (revolver) E965.0
    paintball gun E965.4
    rifle (hunting) E965.2
      military E965.3
    shotgun (automatic) E965.1
    specified firearm NEC E965.4
    Verey pistol E965.4
  in
    terrorism — *see* Terrorism, shooting
    war operations — *see* War operations, shooting
  inflicted by other person
    in accidental circumstances E922.9
      hand gun (pistol) (revolver) E922.0
      military firearm, except hand gun E922.3
        hand gun (pistol) (revolver) E922.0
      rifle (hunting) E922.2
        military E922.3
      shotgun (automatic) E922.1
      specified firearm NEC E922.8
      Verey pistol E922.8
    stated as
      intentional, homicidal E965.4
        hand gun (pistol) (revolver) E965.0
        military firearm, except hand gun E965.3
          hand gun (pistol) (revolver) E965.0
        paintball gun E965.4
        rifle (hunting) E965.2
          military E965.3
        shotgun (automatic) E965.1
        specified firearm E965.4
        Verey pistol E965.4
      undetermined whether accidental or intentional E985.4
        air gun E985.6
        BB gun E985.6

Shooting, shot — *continued*
  inflicted by other person — *continued*
    stated as — *continued*
      undetermined whether accidental or intentional — *continued*
        hand gun (pistol) (revolver) E985.0
        military firearm, except hand gun E985.3
          hand gun (pistol) (revolver) E985.0
        paintball gun E985.7
        rifle (hunting) E985.2
        shotgun (automatic) E985.1
        specified firearm NEC E985.4
        Verey pistol E985.4
  legal
    execution E978
    intervention E970
  military firearm, except hand gun E922.3
    hand gun (pistol) (revolver) E922.0
  paintball gun E922.5
  rifle (hunting) E922.2
    military E922.3
  self-inflicted (unspecified whether accidental or intentional) E985.4
    air gun E985.6
    BB gun E985.6
    hand gun (pistol) (revolver) E985.0
    military firearm, except hand gun E985.3
      hand gun (pistol) (revolver) E985.0
    paintball gun E985.7
    rifle (hunting) E985.2
      military E985.3
    shotgun (automatic) E985.1
    specified firearm NEC E985.4
    stated as
      accidental E922.9
        hand gun (pistol) (revolver) E922.0
        military firearm, except hand gun E922.3
          hand gun (pistol) (revolver) E922.0
        paintball gun E922.5
        rifle (hunting) E922.2
          military E922.3
        shotgun (automatic) E922.1
        specified firearm NEC E922.8
        Verey pistol E922.8
      intentional, purposeful E955.4
        hand gun (pistol) (revolver) E955.0
        military firearm, except hand gun E955.3
          hand gun (pistol) (revolver) E955.0
        paintball gun E955.7
        rifle (hunting) E955.2
          military E955.3
        shotgun (automatic) E955.1
        specified firearm NEC E955.4
        Verey pistol E955.4
  shotgun (automatic) E922.1
  specified firearm NEC E922.8
  stated as undetermined whether accidental or intentional E985.4
    hand gun (pistol) (revolver) E985.0
    military firearm, except hand gun E985.3
      hand gun (pistol) (revolver) E985.0
    paintball gun E985.7
    rifle (hunting) E985.2
      military E985.3
    shotgun (automatic) E985.1
    specified firearm NEC E985.4
    Verey pistol E985.4
  suicidal (attempt) E955.4
    air gun E955.6
    BB gun E955.6
    hand gun (pistol) (revolver) E955.0
    military firearm, except hand gun E955.3
      hand gun (pistol) (revolver) E955.0
    paintball gun E955.7
    rifle (hunting) E955.2
      military E955.3
    shotgun (automatic) E955.1

Shooting, shot — *continued*
  suicidal — *continued*
    specified firearm NEC E955.4
    Verey pistol E955.4
  Verey pistol E922.8
Shoving (accidentally) by other person — *see also* Pushing by other person E917.9
Sickness
  air E903
  alpine E902.0
  car E903
  motion E903
  mountain E902.0
  sea E903
  travel E903
Sinking (accidental)
  boat, ship, watercraft (causing drowning, submersion) E830 ☑
    causing injury except drowning, submersion E831 ☑
Siriasis E900.0
Skydiving E844 ☑
Slashed wrists — *see also* Cut, self-inflicted E986
Slipping (accidental)
  on
    deck (of boat, ship, watercraft) (icy) (oily) (wet) E835 ☑
    ice E885.9
    ladder of ship E833 ☑
      due to accident to watercraft E831 ☑
    mud E885.9
    oil E885.9
    snow E885.9
    stairs of ship E833 ☑
      due to accident to watercraft E831 ☑
    surface
      slippery E885 ☑
      wet E885 ☑
Sliver, wood, injury by E920.8
Smothering, smothered — *see also* Suffocation E913.9
Smouldering building or structure in terrorism E979.3
Sodomy (assault) E960.1
Solid substance in eye (any part) or adnexa E914
Sound waves (causing injury) E928.1
Splinter, injury by E920.8
Stab, stabbing E966
  accidental — *see* Cut
Starvation E904.1
  helpless person, infant, newborn — *see* Lack of food
  homicidal intent E968.4
  late effect of NEC E929.5
  resulting from accident connected with transport — *see* categories E800-E848 ☑
Stepped on
  by
    animal (not being ridden) E906.8
      being ridden (in sport or transport) E828 ☑
    crowd E917.1
    person E917.9
      in sports E917.0
  in sports E917.0
Stepping on
  object (moving) E917.9
    in sports E917.0
      with subsequent fall E917.5
    stationary E917.4
      with subsequent fall E917.8
  person E917.9
    as, or caused by a crowd E917.1
      with subsequent fall E917.6
    in sports E917.0
Sting E905.9
  ant E905.5
  bee E905.3
  caterpillar E905.5
  coral E905.6
  hornet E905.3

☑ **Additional Digit Required — Refer to the Tabular List for Digit Selection**   ▽ **Subterms under main terms may continue to next column or page**

2014 ICD-9-CM   **391**

Sting — continued
insect NEC E905.5
jellyfish E905.6
marine animal or plant E905.6
nematocysts E905.6
scorpion E905.2
sea anemone E905.6
sea cucumber E905.6
wasp E905.3
yellow jacket E905.3
Storm E908.9
specified type NEC E908.8
Straining, injury
due to
repetitive movement E927.3
sudden strenuous movement E927.0
Strangling — see Suffocation
Strangulation — see Suffocation
Strenuous movements (in recreational or other activities) NEC E927.8
Striking against
bottom (when jumping or diving into water) E883.0
object (moving) E917.9
caused by crowd E917.1
with subsequent fall E917.6
furniture E917.3
with subsequent fall E917.7
in
running water E917.2
with drowning or submersion — see Submersion
sports E917.0
with subsequent fall E917.5
stationary E917.4
with subsequent fall E917.8
person(s) E917.9
with fall E886.9
in sports E886.0
as, or caused by, a crowd E917.1
with subsequent fall E917.6
in sports E917.0
with fall E886.0
Stroke
heat — see Heat
lightning E907
Struck by — see also Hit by
bullet
in
terrorism E979.4
war operations E991.2
rubber E991.0
lightning E907
missile
in terrorism — see Terrorism, missile
object
falling
from, in, on
building
burning (uncontrolled fire) in terrorism E979.3
thunderbolt E907
Stumbling over animal, carpet, curb, rug or (small) object (with fall) E885.9
without fall — see Striking against, object
Submersion (accidental) E910.8
boat, ship, watercraft (causing drowning, submersion) E830 ☑
causing injury except drowning, submersion E831 ☑
by other person
in accidental circumstances — see category E910 ☑
intentional, homicidal E964
stated as undetermined whether accidental or intentional E984
due to
accident
machinery — see Accident, machine
to boat, ship, watercraft E830 ☑
transport — see categories E800-E848 ☑
avalanche E909.2
cataclysmic
earth surface movement or eruption E909.9

Submersion (accidental) — continued
due to — continued
cataclysmic — continued
storm E908.9
cloudburst E908.8
cyclone E908.1
fall
from
boat, ship, watercraft (not involved in accident) E832 ☑
burning, crushed E830 ☑
involved in accident, collision E830 ☑
gangplank (into water) E832 ☑
overboard NEC E832 ☑
flood E908.2
hurricane E908.0
jumping into water E910.8
from boat, ship, watercraft
burning, crushed, sinking E830 ☑
involved in accident, collision E830 ☑
not involved in accident, for swim E910.2
in recreational activity (without diving equipment) E910.2
with or using diving equipment E910.1
to rescue another person E910.3
homicide (attempt) E964
in
bathtub E910.4
specified activity, not sport, transport or recreational E910.3
sport or recreational activity (without diving equipment) E910.2
with or using diving equipment E910.1
water skiing E910.0
swimming pool NEC E910.8
terrorism E979.8
war operations E995.4
intentional E995.3
water transport E832 ☑
due to accident to boat, ship, watercraft E830 ☑
landslide E909.2
overturning boat, ship, watercraft E909.2
sinking boat, ship, watercraft E909.2
submersion boat, ship, watercraft E909.2
tidal wave E909.4
caused by storm E908.0
torrential rain E908.2
late effect of NEC E929.8
quenching tank E910.8
self-inflicted (unspecified whether accidental or intentional) E984
in accidental circumstances — see category E910 ☑
stated as intentional, purposeful E954
stated as undetermined whether accidental or intentional E984
suicidal (attempted) E954
while
attempting rescue of another person E910.3
engaged in
fishing, not from boat E910.2
hunting, not from boat E910.2
ice skating E910.2
pearl diving E910.3
placing fishing nets E910.3
playing in water E910.2
scuba diving E910.1
nonrecreational E910.3
skin diving E910.1
snorkel diving E910.2
spear fishing underwater E910.1
surfboarding E910.2
swimming (swimming pool) E910.2
wading (in water) E910.2
water skiing E910.0
Sucked
into
jet (aircraft) E844 ☑

Suffocation (accidental) (by external means) (by pressure) (mechanical) E913.9
caused by other person
in accidental circumstances — see category E913 ☑
stated as
intentional, homicidal E963
undetermined whether accidental or intentional E983.9
by, in
hanging E983.0
plastic bag E983.1
specified means NEC E983.8
due to, by
avalanche E909.2
bedclothes E913.0
bib E913.0
blanket E913.0
cave-in E913.3
caused by cataclysmic earth surface movement or eruption E909.9
conflagration — see Conflagration
explosion — see Explosion
falling earth, other substance E913.3
fire — see Fire
food, any type (ingestion) (inhalation) (regurgitated) (vomited) E911
foreign body, except food (ingestion) (inhalation) E912
ignition — see Ignition
landslide E909.2
machine(ry) — see Accident, machine
material, object except food entering by nose or mouth, ingested, inhaled E912
mucus (aspiration) (inhalation), not of newborn E912
phlegm (aspiration) (inhalation) E912
pillow E913.0
plastic bag — see Suffocation, in, plastic bag
sheet (plastic) E913.0
specified means NEC E913.8
vomitus (aspiration) (inhalation) E911
homicidal (attempt) E963
in war operations E995.3
in
airtight enclosed place E913.2
baby carriage E913.0
bed E913.0
closed place E913.2
cot, cradle E913.0
perambulator E913.0
plastic bag (in accidental circumstances) E913.1
homicidal, purposely inflicted by other person E963
self-inflicted (unspecified whether accidental or intentional) E983.1
in accidental circumstances E913.1
intentional, suicidal E953.1
stated as undetermined whether accidentally or purposely inflicted E983.1
suicidal, purposely self-inflicted E953.1
refrigerator E913.2
war operations E995.3
self-inflicted (see also Suffocation, stated as undetermined whether accidental or intentional) E953.9
in accidental circumstances — see category E913 ☑
stated as intentional, purposeful — see Suicide, suffocation
stated as undetermined whether accidental or intentional E983.9
by, in
hanging E983.0
plastic bag E983.1
specified means NEC E983.8
suicidal — see Suicide, suffocation
Suicide, suicidal (attempted) (by) E958.9
burning, burns E958.1

Suicide, suicidal — continued
caustic substance E958.7
poisoning E950.7
swallowed E950.7
cold, extreme E958.3
cut (any part of body) E956
cutting or piercing instrument (classifiable to E920) E956
drowning E954
electrocution E958.4
explosive(s) (classifiable to E923) E955.5
fire E958.1
firearm (classifiable to E922) — see Shooting, suicidal
hanging E953.0
jumping
before moving object, train, vehicle E958.0
from high place — see Jumping, from, high place, stated as, suicidal
knife E956
late effect of E959
motor vehicle, crashing of E958.5
poisoning — see Table of Drugs and Chemicals
puncture (any part of body) E956
scald E958.2
shooting — see Shooting, suicidal
specified means NEC E958.8
stab (any part of body) E956
strangulation — see Suicide, suffocation
submersion E954
suffocation E953.9
by, in
hanging E953.0
plastic bag E953.1
specified means NEC E953.8
wound NEC E958.9
Sunburn E926.2
Sunstroke E900.0
Supersonic waves (causing injury) E928.1
Surgical procedure, complication of
delayed or as an abnormal reaction without mention of misadventure — see Reaction, abnormal
due to or as a result of misadventure — see Misadventure
Swallowed, swallowing
foreign body — see Foreign body, alimentary canal
poison — see Table of Drugs and Chemicals
substance
caustic — see Table of Drugs and Chemicals
corrosive — see Table of Drugs and Chemicals
poisonous — see Table of Drugs and Chemicals
Swimmers cramp — see also category E910 E910.2
not in recreation or sport E910.3
Syndrome, battered
baby or child — see Abuse, child
wife — see Assault

T

Tackle in sport E886.0
Terrorism (injury) (by) (in) E979.8
air blast E979.2
aircraft burned, destroyed, exploded, shot down E979.1
used as a weapon E979.1
anthrax E979.6
asphyxia from
chemical (weapons) E979.7
fire, conflagration (caused by fire-producing device) E979.3
from nuclear explosion E979.5
gas or fumes E979.7
bayonet E979.8
biological agents E979.6
blast (air) (effects) E979.2
from nuclear explosion E979.5
underwater E979.0
bomb (antipersonnel) (mortar) (explosion) (fragments) E979.2

☑ Additional Digit Required — Refer to the Tabular List for Digit Selection

▽ Subterms under main terms may continue to next column or page

Terrorism — *continued*
  bullet(s) (from carbine, machine gun, pistol, rifle, shotgun) E979.4
  burn from
    chemical E979.7
    fire, conflagration (caused by fire-producing device) E979.3
      from nuclear explosion E979.5
    gas E979.7
  burning aircraft E979.1
  chemical E979.7
  cholera E979.6
  conflagration E979.3
  crushed by falling aircraft E979.1
  depth-charge E979.0
  destruction of aircraft E979.1
  disability, as sequelae one year or more after injury E999.1
  drowning E979.8
  effect
    of nuclear weapon (direct) (secondary) E979.5
    secondary NEC E979.9
    sequelae E999.1
  explosion (artillery shell) (breech-block) (cannon block) E979.2
    aircraft E979.1
    bomb (antipersonnel) (mortar) E979.2
      nuclear (atom) (hydrogen) E979.5
    depth-charge E979.0
    grenade E979.2
    injury by fragments from E979.2
    land-mine E979.2
    marine weapon E979.0
    mine (land) E979.2
      at sea or in harbor E979.0
      marine E979.0
    missile (explosive) NEC E979.2
    munitions (dump) (factory) E979.2
    nuclear (weapon) E979.5
      other direct and secondary effects of E979.5
    sea-based artillery shell E979.0
    torpedo E979.0
  exposure to ionizing radiation from nuclear explosion E979.5
  falling aircraft E979.1
  firearms E979.4
  fireball effects from nuclear explosion E979.5
  fire or fire-producing device E979.3
  fragments from artillery shell, bomb NEC, grenade, guided missile, land-mine, rocket, shell, shrapnel E979.2
  gas or fumes E979.7
  grenade (explosion) (fragments) E979.2
  guided missile (explosion) (fragments) E979.2
    nuclear E979.5
  heat from nuclear explosion E979.5
  hot substances E979.3
  hydrogen cyanide E979.7
  land-mine (explosion) (fragments) E979.2
  laser(s) E979.8
  late effect of E999.1
  lewisite E979.7
  lung irritant (chemical) (fumes) (gas) E979.7
  marine mine E979.0
  mine E979.2
    at sea E979.0
    in harbor E979.0
    land (explosion) (fragments) E979.2
    marine E979.0
  missile (explosion) (fragments) (guided) E979.2
    marine E979.0
    nuclear weapons E979.5
  mortar bomb (explosion) (fragments) E979.2
  mustard gas E979.7
  nerve gas E979.7
  nuclear weapons E979.5
  pellets (shotgun) E979.4
  petrol bomb E979.3
  phosgene E979.7
  piercing object E979.8
  poisoning (chemical) (fumes) (gas) E979.7

Terrorism — *continued*
  radiation, ionizing from nuclear explosion E979.5
  rocket (explosion) (fragments) E979.2
  saber, sabre E979.8
  sarin E979.7
  screening smoke E979.7
  sequelae effect (of) E999.1
  shell (aircraft) (artillery) (cannon) (land-based) (explosion) (fragments) E979.2
    sea-based E979.0
  shooting E979.4
    bullet(s) E979.4
    pellet(s) (rifle) (shotgun) E979.4
  shrapnel E979.2
  smallpox E979.7
  stabbing object(s) E979.8
  submersion E979.8
  torpedo E979.0
  underwater blast E979.0
  vesicant (chemical) (fumes) (gas) E979.7
  weapon burst E979.2
Thermic fever E900.9
Thermoplegia E900.9
Thirst — *see also* Lack of water
  resulting from accident connected with transport — *see* categories E800-E848 ☑
Thrown (accidently)
  against object in or part of vehicle
    by motion of vehicle
      aircraft E844 ☑
      boat, ship, watercraft E838 ☑
      motor vehicle (on public highway) E818 ☑
        not on public highway E825 ☑
        off-road type (not on public highway) E821 ☑
          on public highway E818 ☑
        snow vehicle E820 ☑
          on public highway E818 ☑
      nonmotor road vehicle NEC E829 ☑
      railway rolling stock, train, vehicle E806 ☑
      street car E829 ☑
  from
    animal (being ridden) (in sport or transport) E828 ☑
    high place, homicide (attempt) E968.1
    machinery — *see* Accident, machine
    vehicle NEC — *see* Accident, vehicle NEC
  off — *see* Thrown, from
  overboard (by motion of boat, ship, watercraft) E832 ☑
    by accident to boat, ship, watercraft E830 ☑
Thunderbolt NEC E907
Tidal wave (any injury) E909.4
  caused by storm E908.0
Took
  overdose of drug — *see* Table of Drugs and Chemicals
  poison — *see* Table of Drugs and Chemicals
Tornado (any injury) E908.1
Torrential rain (any injury) E908.2
Traffic accident NEC E819 ☑
Trampled by animal E906.8
  being ridden (in sport or transport) E828 ☑
Trapped (accidently)
  between
    objects (moving) (stationary and moving) E918
  by
    door of
      elevator E918
      motor vehicle (on public highway) (while alighting, boarding) — *see* Fall, from, motor vehicle, while alighting
      railway train (underground) E806 ☑
      street car E829 ☑
      subway train E806 ☑
  in object E918

Trauma
  cumulative
    from
      repetitive
        impact E927.4
        motion or movements E927.3
      sudden from strenuous movement E927.0
Travel (effects) E903
  sickness E903
Tree
  falling on or hitting E916
    motor vehicle (in motion) (on public highway) E818 ☑
      not on public highway E825 ☑
    nonmotor road vehicle NEC E829 ☑
    pedal cycle E826 ☑
    person E916
    railway rolling stock, train, vehicle E806 ☑
    street car E829 ☑
Trench foot E901.0
Tripping over animal, carpet, curb, rug, or small object (with fall) E885 ☑
  without fall — *see* Striking against, object
Tsunami E909.4
Twisting, injury
  due to
    repetitive movement E927.3
    sudden strenuous movement E927.0

V

Violence, nonaccidental — *see also* Assault E968.9
Volcanic eruption (any injury) E909.1
Vomitus in air passages (with asphyxia, obstruction or suffocation) E911

W

War operations (during hostilities) (injury) (by) (in) E995.9
  after cessation of hostilities, injury due to E998.9
  air blast E993.9
  aircraft burned, destroyed, exploded, shot down E994 ☑
  asphyxia from
    chemical E997.2
    fire, conflagration (caused by fire producing device or conventional weapon) E990.9
      from nuclear explosion (*see also* War operations, injury due to, nuclear weapons) E996.8
    incendiary bomb E990.0
    petrol bomb E990.0
    fumes E997.2
    gas E997.2
  baton (nightstick) E995.1
  battle wound NEC E995.8
  bayonet E995.2
  biological warfare agents E997.1
  blast (air) (effects) E993.9
    from nuclear explosion — *see* War operations, injury due to, nuclear weapons
    underwater E992.9
  bomb (mortar) (explosion) E993.2
    after cessation of hostilities E998.1
    fragments, injury by E991.4
      antipersonnel E991.3
  bullet(s) (from carbine, machine gun, pistol, rifle, shotgun) E991.2
    rubber E991.0
  burn from
    chemical E997.2
    fire, conflagration (caused by fire-producing device or conventional weapon) E990.9
    from
      conventional weapon E990.3
      flamethrower E990.1
      incendiary bomb E990.0
      incendiary bullet E990.2
      nuclear explosion E996.2
    petrol bomb E990.0

War operations — *continued*
  burn from — *continued*
    gas E997.2
  burning aircraft E994.3
  chemical E997.2
  chlorine E997.2
  conventional warfare, specified form NEC E995.8
  crushing by falling aircraft E994.8
  depth charge E992.1
  destruction of aircraft E994.9
  detonation of own munitions (ammunition) (artillery) (mortars), unintentional E993.6
  disability as sequela one year or more after injury E999.9
  discharge of own munitions launch device (autocannons) (automatic grenade launchers) (missile launchers) (small arms), unintentional E993.7
  drowning E995.4
  effect nuclear weapon (*see also* War operations, injury due to, nuclear weapons) E996.9
  explosion (breech block) (cannon shell) E993.9
    after cessation of hostilities
      bomb placed in war E998.1
      mine placed in war E998.0
    aircraft E994.1
      due to
        enemy fire or explosives E994.0
        own onboard explosives E994.1
    artillery shell E993.2
    bomb (mortar) E993.2
      aerial E993.0
      atom (*see also* War operations, injury due to, nuclear weapons) E996.9
      hydrogen (*see also* War operations, injury due to, nuclear weapons) E996.9
      injury by fragments from E991.4
        antipersonnel E991.3
      nuclear (*see also* War operations, injury due to, nuclear weapons) E996.9
    depth charge E992.1
    injury by fragments from E991.4
      antipersonnel E991.3
    marine weapon NEC E992.8
    mine
      at sea or in harbor E992.2
      land E993.8
        injury by fragments from E991.4
      marine E992.2
    missile, guided E993.1
    mortar E993.2
    munitions (accidental) (being used in war) (dump) (factory) E993.9
      own E993.7
        ammunition (artillery) (mortars) E993.6
        launch device (autocannons) (automatic grenade launchers) (missile launchers) (small arms) E993.7
    nuclear (weapon) (*see also* War operations, injury due to, nuclear weapons) E996.9
    own weapons (accidental) E993.7
      injury by fragments from E991.9
        antipersonnel E991.3
    sea-based artillery shell E992.3
    specified NEC E993.8
    torpedo E992.0
  exposure to ionizing radiation from nuclear explosion (*see also* War operations, injury due to, nuclear weapons) E996.3
  falling aircraft E994.8
  fireball effects from nuclear explosion E996.2
  fire or fire-producing device E990.9
    flamethrower E990.1

☑ **Additional Digit Required — Refer to the Tabular List for Digit Selection**   ◪ **Subterms under main terms may continue to next column or page**

2014 ICD-9-CM   393

War operations — *continued*
  fire or fire-producing device — *continued*
    incendiary bomb E990.0
    incendiary bullet E990.2
    indirectly caused from conventional weapon E990.3
    petrol bomb E990.0
  fragments from
    antipersonnel bomb E991.3
    artillery shell E991.4
    bomb NEC E991.4
    grenade E991.4
    guided missile E991.4
    land mine E991.4
    rocket E991.4
    shell E991.4
    shrapnel E991.9
  fumes E997.2
  gas E997.2
  grenade (explosion) E993.8
    fragments, injury by E991.4
  guided missile (explosion) E993.1
    fragments, injury by E991.4
    nuclear (*see also* War operations, injury due to, nuclear weapons) E996.9
  heat from nuclear explosion E996.2
  injury due to
    aerial bomb E993.0
    air blast E993.9
    aircraft shot down E994.0
    artillery shell E993.2
    blast E993.9
      wave E993.9
      wind E993.9
    bomb E993.8
    but occurring after cessation of hostilities
      explosion of bombs E998.1
      explosion of mines E998.0
      specified NEC E998.8
    conventional warfare E995.9
      specified form NEC E995.8
    depth charge E992.1
    destruction of aircraft E994.9
      due to
        air to air missile E994.0
        collision with other aircraft E994.2
        enemy fire or explosives E994.0
        on board explosion (explosives) E994.1
        on board fire E994.3
        rocket propelled grenade [RPG] E994.0
        small arms fire E994.0
        surface to air missile E994.0
      specified NEC E994.8
    dirty bomb (*see also* War operations, injury due to, nuclear weapons) E996.9
    drowning E995.4
    explosion (direct pressure) (indirect pressure) (due to) E993.9
      depth charge E992.1
      improvised explosive device [IED]
        person borne E993.3
        roadside E993.5
        specified NEC E993.5
        transport vehicle (air) (land) (water) borne E993.4

War operations — *continued*
  injury due to — *continued*
    explosion — *continued*
      improvised explosive device [IED] — *continued*
        vehicle (air) (land) (water) borne E993.4
      marine mines (in harbor) (at sea) E992.2
      marine weapons E992.9
        specified NEC E992.8
      sea based artillery shell E992.3
      specified NEC E993.8
      torpedo E992.0
      unintentional (of own)
        autocannons E993.7
        automatic grenade launchers E993.7
        launch device discharge E993.7
        missile launchers E993.7
        munitions detonation (ammunition) (artillery) (mortars) E993.6
        small arms E993.7
    fragments (from) E991.9
      artillery E991.8
      artillery shells E991.4
      autocannons E991.8
      automatic grenade launchers [AGL] E991.8
      bombs E991.4
        antipersonnel E991.3
      detonation of unexploded ordnance [UXO] E991.4
      grenade E991.4
      guided missile E991.4
      improvised explosive device [IED]
        person borne E991.5
        roadside E991.7
        specified NEC E991.7
        transport vehicle (air) (land) (water) borne E991.6
        vehicle (air) (land) (water) borne E991.6
      land mine E991.4
      missile launchers E991.8
      mortars E991.8
      munitions (artillery shells) (bombs) (grenades) (rockets) (shells) E991.4
      rockets E991.4
      shells E991.4
      small arms E991.8
      specified NEC E991.9
      weapons (artillery) (autocannons) (mortars) (small arms) E991.8
    grenade E993.8
    guided missile E993.1
    hand to hand combat, unarmed E995.4
    improvised explosive device [IED]
      person borne E993.3
      roadside E993.5
      specified NEC E993.5
      transport vehicle (air) (land) (water) borne E993.4
      vehicle (air) (land) (water) borne E993.4
    inability to surface or obtain air E995.4
    land mine E993.8
    marine mines (in harbor) (at sea) E992.2
    marine weapons E992.9

War operations — *continued*
  injury due to — *continued*
    marine weapons — *continued*
      specified NEC E992.8
    mortar E993.2
    nuclear weapons E996.9
      beta burns E996.3
      blast debris E996.1
      blast pressure E996.0
      burns due to thermal radiation E996.2
      direct blast effect E996.0
      fallout exposure E996.3
      fireball effect E996.2
      flash burns E996.2
      heat effect E996.2
      indirect blast effect E996.1
      nuclear radiation effects E996.3
      radiation exposure (acute) E996.3
      radiation sickness E996.3
      secondary effects E996.3
      specified effects NEC E996.8
      thermal radiation effect E996.2
    piercing object E995.2
    restriction of airway, intentional E995.3
    sea based artillery shell E992.3
    shrapnel E991.9
    stave E995.1
    strangulation E995.3
    strike by blunt object (baton) (nightstick) (stave) E995.1
    submersion (accidental) (unintentional) E995.4
      intentional E995.3
    suffocation E995.3
      accidental E995.4
    torpedo E992.0
    underwater blast E992.9
    weapon of mass destruction [WMD] E997.3
  knife E995.2
  lacrimator (gas) (chemical) E997.2
  land mine (explosion) E993.8
    after cessation of hostilities E998.0
    fragments, injury by E991.4
  laser(s) E997.0
  late effect of E999.0
  lewisite E997.2
  lung irritant (chemical) (fumes) (gas) E997.2
  marine mine E992.2
  mine
    after cessation of hostilities E998.0
    at sea E992.2
    in harbor E992.2
    land (explosion) E993.8
      fragments, injury by E991.4
    marine E992.2
  missile (guided) (explosion) E993.1
    fragments, injury by E991.4
    marine E992.8
    nuclear (*see also* War operations, injury due to, nuclear weapons) E996.9
  mortar bomb (explosion) E993.2
    fragments, injury by E991.4
  mustard gas E997.2
  nerve gas E997.2
  phosgene E997.2
  piercing object E995.2
  poisoning (chemical) (fumes) (gas) E997.2

War operations — *continued*
  radiation, ionizing from nuclear explosion (*see also* War operations, injury due to, nuclear weapons) E996.3
  rocket (explosion) E993.8
    fragments, injury by E991.4
  saber, sabre E995.2
  screening smoke E997.8
  shell (aircraft) (artillery) (cannon) (land based) (explosion) E993.2
    fragments, injury by E991.4
    sea-based E992.3
  shooting E991.2
    after cessation of hostilities E998.8
    bullet(s) E991.2
      rubber E991.0
    pellet(s) (rifle) E991.1
    shrapnel E991.9
    submersion E995 ☑
    torpedo E992 ☑
  stave E995.2
  strike by blunt object (baton) (nightstick) (stave) E995.1
  submersion E995.4
    intentional E995.3
  sword E995.2
  torpedo E992.0
  unconventional warfare, except by nuclear weapon E997.9
    biological (warfare) E997.1
    gas, fumes, chemicals E997.2
    laser(s) E997.0
    specified type NEC E997.8
  underwater blast E992.9
  vesicant (chemical) (fumes) (gas) E997.2
  weapon burst E993.9
Washed
  away by flood — *see* Flood
  away by tidal wave — *see* Tidal wave
  off road by storm (transport vehicle) E908.9
  overboard E832 ☑
Weapon of mass destruction [WMD] E997.3
Weather exposure — *see also* Exposure
  cold E901.0
  hot E900.0
Weightlessness (causing injury) (effects of) (in spacecraft, real or simulated) E928.0
Wound (accidental) NEC — *see also* Injury E928.9
  battle (*see also* War operations) E995.9
  bayonet E920.3
    in
      legal intervention E974
      war operations E995.2
  gunshot — *see* Shooting
  incised — *see* Cut
  saber, sabre E920.3
    in war operations E995.2
Wrong
  body part, performance of correct operation (procedure) on E876.7
  device implanted into correct surgical site E876.5
  patient, performance of operation (procedure) on E876.6
  procedure (operation) performed on correct patient E876.5
  side, performance of correct operation (procedure) on E876.7
  site, performance of correct operation (procedure) on E876.7

☑ Additional Digit Required — Refer to the Tabular List for Digit Selection   ▽ Subterms under main terms may continue to next column or page

394   2014 ICD-9-CM

Railway Accidents (E800-E807)

The following fourth-digit subdivisions are for use with categories E800-E807 to identify the injured person:

.0 **Railway employee**
Any person who by virtue of his employment in connection with a railway, whether by the railway company or not, is at increased risk of involvement in a railway accident, such as:
catering staff on train
postal staff on train
driver
railway fireman
guard
shunter
porter
sleeping car attendant

.1 **Passenger on railway**
Any authorized person traveling on a train, except a railway employee
EXCLUDES intending passenger waiting at station (.8)
unauthorized rider on railway vehicle (.8)

.2 **Pedestrian** See definition (r), E-Codes-2

.3 **Pedal cyclist** See definition (p), E-Codes-2

.8 **Other specified person** Intending passenger waiting at station
Unauthorized rider on railway vehicle

.9 **Unspecified person**

Motor Vehicle Traffic and Nontraffic Accidents (E810-E825)

The following fourth-digit subdivisions are for use with categories E810-E819 and E820-E825 to identify the injured person:

.0 **Driver of motor vehicle other than motorcycle** See definition (1), E-Codes-2

.1 **Passenger in motor vehicle other than motorcycle** See definition (1), E-Codes-2

.2 **Motorcyclist** See definition (1), E-Codes-2

.3 **Passenger on motorcycle** See definition (1), E-Codes-2

.4 **Occupant of streetcar**

.5 **Rider of animal; occupant of animal-drawn vehicle**

.6 **Pedal cyclist** See definition (p), E-Codes-2

.7 **Pedestrian** See definition (r), E-Codes-2

.8 **Other specified person**
Occupant of vehicle other than above
Person in railway train involved in accident
Unauthorized rider of motor vehicle

.9 **Unspecified person**

Other Road Vehicle Accidents (E826-E829)
(animal-drawn vehicle, streetcar, pedal cycle, and other nonmotor road vehicle accidents)

The following fourth-digit subdivisions are for use with categories E826-E829 to identify the injured person:

.0 **Pedestrian** See definition (r), E-Codes-2

.1 **Pedal cyclist** (does not apply to codes E827, E828, E829) See definition (p), E-Codes-2

.2 **Rider of animal** (does not apply to code E829)

.3 **Occupant of animal-drawn vehicle (does not apply to codes E828, E829)**

.4 **Occupant of streetcar**

.8 **Other specified person**

.9 **Unspecified person**

Water Transport Accidents (E830-E838)

The following fourth-digit subdivisions are for use with categories E830-E838 to identify the injured person:

.0 **Occupant of small boat, unpowered**

.1 **Occupant of small boat, powered** See definition (t), E-Codes-2
EXCLUDES water skier (.4)

.2 **Occupant of other watercraft — crew**
Persons:
engaged in operation of watercraft
providing passenger services [cabin attendants, ship's physician, catering personnel]
working on ship during voyage in other capacity [musician in band, operators of shops and beauty parlors]

.3 **Occupant of other watercraft — other than crew**
Passenger
Occupant of lifeboat, other than crew, after abandoning ship

.4 **Water skier**

.5 **Swimmer**

.6 **Dockers, stevedores**
Longshoreman employed on the dock in loading and unloading ships

.8 **Other specified person**
Immigration and custom officials on board ship
Persons:
accompanying passenger or member of crew visiting boat
Pilot (guiding ship into port)

.9 **Unspecified person**

Air and Space Transport Accidents (E840-E845)

The following fourth-digit subdivisions are for use with categories E840-E845 to identify the injured person:

.0 **Occupant of spacecraft**
Crew
Passenger (civilian)(military)
Troops
in military aircraft [air force] [army] [national guard] [navy]

.1 **Occupant of military aircraft, any**
EXCLUDES occupants of aircraft operated under jurisdiction of police departments (.5) parachutist (.7)

.2 **Crew of commercial aircraft (powered) in surface to surface transport**

.3 **Other occupant of commercial aircraft (powered) in surface to surface transport**
Flight personnel:
not part of crew
on familiarization flight
Passenger on aircraft

.4 **Occupant of commercial aircraft (powered) in surface to air transport**
Occupant [crew] [passenger] of aircraft (powered) engaged in activities, such as:
air drops of emergency supplies
air drops of parachutists, except from military craft
crop dusting
lowering of construction material [bridge or telephone pole]
sky writing

.5 **Occupant of other powered aircraft**
Occupant [crew] [passenger] of aircraft (powered) engaged in activities, such as:
aerial spraying (crops)(fire retardants)
aerobatic flying
aircraft racing
rescue operation
storm surveillance
traffic suveillance
Occupant of private plane NOS

.6 **Occupant of unpowered aircraft, except parachutist**
Occupant of aircraft classifiable to E842

.7 **Parachutist (military)(other)**
Person making voluntary descent
person making descent after accident to aircraft (.1-.6)

.8 **Ground crew, airline employee**
Persons employed at airfields (civil)(military) or launching pads, not occupants of aircraft

.9 **Other person**

☑ Additional Digit Required — Refer to the Tabular List for Digit Selection
2014 ICD-9-CM
▽ Subterms under main terms may continue to next column or page
395

Chapter 1: Infections and Parasitic Diseases (001–139)

Coding Guidance

Communicable diseases as well as diseases of unknown origin but possibly due to infectious organisms are found in this chapter. Infections confined to a specific body system are classified to chapters covering the specific body site. Congenitally acquired infections, postoperative infections, and infections complicating pregnancy and delivery are classified elsewhere. An additional code from the "Infectious and Parasitic Disease" chapter may be used in combination with the codes from other chapters to further describe the nature of the infection.

Infective organisms classified to categories 001–139 include arthropods, bacteria, chlamydia, fungi, helminths, mycoplasms, protozoans, rickettsias, and viruses. This chapter classifies infectious and parasitic diseases by anatomic site, by type of infectious organism or parasite, as well as by a combination of site and type of organism.

Steps to coding infection:

1. Locate the main term "Infection" in the alphabetic index.
2. Locate the subterm for the causal organism.
3. The subterm for the organism takes precedence over the more general subterms such as acute or chronic.
4. When the index directs the user to another chapter to code the infection, an additional code from the "Infectious and Parasitic Disease" chapter is generally required to further describe the nature of the infection.
5. The coder may also search the alphabetic index under the main term for the condition.
6. Locate the code in the tabular list and read all "includes" and "excludes" notes for the category to verify code assignments.

Intestinal Infectious Diseases (001–009)

This subchapter includes diseases specific to the intestines caused by infectious organisms and parasites (except for helminthiases, which are classified to subcategories 120.0–129). Some of the main categories in this subchapter include cholera, typhoid, salmonella, shigellosis, food poisoning, amebiasis, Escherichia coli (E. coli), septicemia and enteritis.

Important notes for coding this subsection:

- Determine whether the infection is acute or chronic.
- Determine from documentation in the medical record positive identification of the organism.
- Note the site of infection, whether localized or generalized.
- Note extraintestinal complications due to the infection.

Tuberculosis (010–018)

Infectious diseases caused primarily by the acid fast bacilli *Mycobacterium tuberculosis*, but also *M. bovis, M. africanum, M. leprae* and other variants are included in this subchapter. Infection occurs almost exclusively through the respiratory system by inhalation of the tubercule bacilli released by an infected host. The disease spreads from the primary lesion in the lung to other parts of the body. Tuberculosis is first coded according to site or type.

Other Bacterial Diseases (030–041)

Leprosy, diphtheria, whooping cough, scarlet fever, streptococcal sore throat, meningitis, tetanus, septicemia, actinomycotic infections, and gas gangrene are grouped as other bacterial diseases in this subchapter.

Methicillin-resistant *Staphylococcus aureus* (MRSA) is a variant form of the bacterium that is resistant to traditional beta lactam class of antibiotics such as penicillin, methicillin, and cephalosporins. Sometimes referred to as a "superbug," MRSA is a major cause of hospital-acquired infections as well as community-acquired infections. Community-acquired MRSA infections (CA-MRSA) are generally not life-threatening. Skin, and soft tissue infections are spread through direct contact. The term methicillin-susceptible *Staphylococcus aureus* (MSSA) identifies certain strains of *Staphylococcus aureus* that are penicillin-resistant yet susceptible or treatable with methicillin.

Note that category 041 is provided to identify the bacterial agent in diseases classified elsewhere, or of an unspecified nature or site. For example an E. coli infection of an unspecified site of the urinary tract is coded first to urinary tract infection 599.0. The instructional note under this subcategory directs the use of an additional code to identify the organism, in this case *E. coli*. The complete code assignment is 599.0 and 041.4.

Septicemia (038)

Septicemia is a systemic infection associated with the presence and persistence of microorganisms and their toxins in the blood. Since it is a systemic disease, site-specific or organ-specific sepsis is not coded as septicemia.

Certain forms of septicemia are more appropriately classified elsewhere. Search the alphabetic index under the main term "Septicemia" for subterms that identify particular forms of septicemia. Septicemia, not otherwise specified, is reported with code 038.9. When reporting the diagnosis of sepsis, however, the instructional note at subcategory 995.9 directs the coder to sequence the underlying cause of the infection first. The default code assigned for the underlying infection is 038.9 Unspecified septicemia. Systemic inflammatory response syndrome (SIRS) generally is a systemic response to infection, trauma/burns, or other insult (such as cancer). The term 'sepsis' generally refers to SIRS due to infection. Severe sepsis is sepsis with associated acute organ dysfunction.

Coding of SIRS, sepsis and severe sepsis requires a minimum of 2 codes: a code for the underlying cause (such as infection or trauma) and a code from subcategory 995.9 Systemic inflammatory response syndrome (SIRS). The code for the underlying cause must be sequenced before the code from subcategory 995.9 Systemic inflammatory response syndrome (SIRS). For sepsis, if the causal organism is not documented, assign code 038.9, Unspecified septicemia. Severe sepsis requires additional code(s) for the associated acute organ dysfunction(s).

If sepsis or severe sepsis is present on admission, and meets the definition of principal diagnosis, the systemic infection code (e.g., 038.xx, 112.5, etc) should be assigned as the principal diagnosis, followed by code 995.91 Sepsis, or 995.92 Severe sepsis, as required by the sequencing rules. When sepsis or severe sepsis develops during the encounter (not present on admission), the systemic infection code and code 995.91 or 995.92 should be assigned as secondary diagnoses.

Septic shock is a form of organ dysfunction, and circulatory failure, associated with systemic inflammatory response syndrome (SIRS) due to infectious process which cannot occur in the absence of severe sepsis. Septic shock can be stated as severe sepsis with shock. Note: severe sepsis with shock involves persistent hypotension with systolic blood pressure < 90 mmHg, or a 40 mmHg drop in previous blood pressure, with no response to adequate fluid resuscitation. As a result, reduced myocardial performance occurs, or heart failure is an inherent characteristic of severe sepsis. Therefore, heart failure is inclusive in the code 785.52 and should not be listed separately.

For all cases of septic shock, the code for the systemic infection should be sequenced first, followed by codes 995.92 and 785.52. Any additional codes for other acute organ dysfunctions should also be assigned. Septic shock cannot be assigned as a principal diagnosis.

If sepsis or severe sepsis is documented as associated with a noninfectious condition, such as a burn or serious injury, the code for the noninfectious condition should be sequenced first, followed by the code for the systemic infection and either code 995.91 Sepsis, or 995.92 Severe sepsis. Additional codes for any associated acute organ dysfunction(s) should also be assigned for cases of severe sepsis. If the sepsis or severe sepsis meets the definition of principal diagnosis, the systemic infection and sepsis codes should be sequenced before the noninfectious condition. When both the associated noninfectious condition and the sepsis or severe sepsis meet the definition of principal diagnosis, either code may be assigned as the principal diagnosis. However, only one code from subcategory 995.9 should be assigned.

Methicillin-Resistant Staphylococcus Aureus (MRSA) Conditions (041.2)

When a patient is diagnosed with an infection that is due to methicillin-resistant *Staphylococcus aureus* (MRSA), and that infection has a combination code that includes the causal organism assign the appropriate code for the condition (e.g., code 038.12, Methicillin-resistant Staphylococcus aureus septicemia or code 482.42, Methicillin-resistant pneumonia due to Staphylococcus aureus). Do not assign code 041.12, Methicillin-resistant Staphylococcus aureus, as an additional code because the code includes the type of infection and the MRSA organism. Do not assign a code from subcategory V09.0, Infection with microorganisms resistant to penicillins, as an additional diagnosis.

When there is documentation of a current infection (e.g., wound infection, stitch abscess, urinary tract infection) due to MRSA and that infection does not have a combination code that includes the causal organism, select the appropriate code to identify the condition along with code 041.12, Methicillin-resistant Staphylococcus aureus, for the MRSA infection.

The condition or state of being colonized means that MSSA or MSRA is present on or in the body without necessarily causing illness. Assign code V02.54, Carrier or suspected carrier, Methicillin-resistant Staphylococcus aureus, for patients documented as having MRSA colonization or V02.53, Carrier or suspected carrier, Methicillin-susceptible Staphylococcus aureus, for a patient documented as having MSSA colonization.

If a patient is documentd as having both MRSA colonization and infection during a hospital admission, code V02.54, Carrier or suspected carrier, Methicillin-resistant Staphylococcus aureus, and the code for the MRSA infection may both be assigned.

Other Specified Botulism (040.4)

Botulism, an uncommon but serious neuromuscular poisoning caused by the toxin Clostridium botulinum, occurs in three forms. Food-borne botulism is a result of ingesting foods containing the botulism toxin and is reported with code 005.1. Wound botulism (040.42), caused by a toxin produced from a wound infected with Clostridium botulinum, is frequently the result of a traumatic injury or a deep puncture wound. Often caused by abscess formation due to self-injected illegal drugs, its manifestations include neurological symptoms with onset typically two weeks following the initial wound or trauma. To report wound botulism or botulism classifiable to code 040.42, use an additional code to identify the complicated wound, by site.

Infant botulism (040.41) is a result of consuming the spores of the botulinum bacteria and occurs most often in infants less than six months of age. The spores colonize in the large intestine, frequently resulting in constipation and progressing to neuromuscular paralysis. All forms of botulism can be fatal, with life-threatening impairment of respiratory function being one of the greatest complications.

Human Immunodeficiency Virus Infection (042)

Human immunodeficiency virus (HIV) disease is coded to category 042. Code 042 is reported when the medical record documentations states: AIDS, acquired immune deficiency syndrome, acquired immunodeficiency syndrome, AIDS-like syndrome, AIDS-like disease, AIDS-related complex (ARC), AIDS-related conditions, Pre-AIDS, Prodromal-AIDS, and HIV disease. Manifestations of AIDS and HIV infection are often numerous and all should be coded.

Category 042 is assigned only when the physician states a positive diagnosis. Code 042 is sequenced first when a patient is seen for an HIV infection or complication due to the presence of the HIV infection. Additional codes identify associated complications.

Code 042 is not sequenced first if the patient is seen for a condition unrelated to HIV infection. Rather, 042 is assigned as a secondary diagnosis. For example, a patient is seen for a fractured wrist, the fracture is sequenced first and the code for HIV is sequenced second.

An asymptomatic patient with a positive HIV test result is assigned V08 Asymptomatic human immunodeficiency virus [HIV] infection status. As an asymptomatic patient develops HIV related symptoms assign code 042 for subsequent visits.

Patients with nonspecific serologic evidence of HIV infection but with inconclusive HIV test results are assigned code 795.71 Nonspecific serologic evidence of human immunodeficiency virus [HIV].

A patient concerned about HIV status is reported by code V73.89 Screening for other specified viral disease.

Slow Virus Infections and Prion Diseases of Central Nervous System (046)

Prion diseases or transmissible spongiform encephalopathies (TSE) are a family of rare progressive neurodegenerative disorders that affect both humans and animals. They are distinguished by long incubation periods, characteristic spongiform changes associated with neuronal loss, and a failure to induce inflammatory response. The causative agent of TSEs is believed to be a prion, an abnormal, transmissible agent that is able to induce abnormal folding of normal cellular prion proteins in the brain, leading to brain damage and the characteristic signs and symptoms of the disease.

Other Human Herpesviruses (058)

Human herpesviruses type 6 (HHV-6) and HHV-7 infect the majority of individuals primarily during childhood and are associated with various clinical manifestations such as fever, rash, and seizures. Immunocompromised hosts, such as transplant recipients or those with AIDS, are at increased risk for symptomatic primary disease or reactivation disease.

Code category 058 reports specific herpesviruses not specifically classifiable elsewhere to type. Herpesvirus infections that are classifiable elsewhere in chapter 1 include cytomegalovirus/HHV-5 (078.5), Epstein-Barr/HHV-4 (075), and other forms of human herpesviruses (categories 052–054).

Arthropod-borne Viral Diseases (060–066)

This section includes the viral diseases transmitted by arthropods, that phylum of exoskeletal organisms having paired and jointed legs.

Notable among these diseases is West Nile virus. Report code 066.41 if diagnosed with encephalitis, code 066.42 for other neurologic manifestations, code 066.49 for other complications, and code 066.40 if the West Nile virus is unspecified.

Other Diseases Due to Viruses and Chlamydiae (070–079)

Viral hepatitis, rabies, mumps, infectious mononucleosis, trachoma, viral warts, cat-scratch fever, cytomegaloviral disease (CMV), respiratory syncitial virus (RSV), and coxsackie viral infections are included in this section.

Viral hepatitis is classified according to virus type A, B, C, or E. Secondly, viral hepatitis is classified according to hepatic coma. For example, viral hepatitis B with hepatic coma is assigned 070.20 and viral hepatitis B without mention of hepatic coma is coded 070.30

A fifth-digit assignment for viral hepatitis B identifies the presence of hepatitis D (hepatitis delta) as well as whether the condition is acute or chronic. Hepatitis D occurs simultaneously or after an infection of hepatitis B and may increase the severity of the disease.

Verrucae (warts) are classified according to site and type. Code 078.10 is assigned for verruca vulgaris, or the common wart of the hands and fingers. This is also the default code assignment for verruca NOS. Warts specified as "condyloma" or "genital" are coded to 078.11 Condyloma acuminatum. Verruca plantaris, verruca of the sole of the feet, is assigned code 078.12. Verruca plana, flat wart of the face, neck, hands, wrists, and back is assigned code 078.19.

Parvovirus B19 (079.83), the only parvovirus that causes disease in humans, may be referred to as human parvovirus. Parvovirus B19 infection may manifest with anemia or neurological symptoms. When polyneuropathy is associated with parvovirus B19, reporting the condition requires mandatory manifestation/etiology dual coding, whereby codes 079.83 Parvovirus B19 and 711.5x Arthropathy associated with other viral diseases are reported.

Syphilis and Other Venereal Diseases (090–099)

Syphilis is classified by type, early or late, and whether symptomatic, latent, or unspecified. Syphilis affecting the cardiovascular or nervous system is classified separately.

Venereal disease is classified by type, whether acute or chronic, and by site of complication. For example, acute gonococcal infection of the bladder is coded 098.11. Chronic gonococcal infection of the seminal vesicles is coded 098.34.

Mycoses (110–118)

Diseases caused by a fungus are found in this section of the classification system, excluding Actinomycotic infections, which are coded to category 039. Additional coding is necessary to identify manifestations of the disease. For example, systemic cryptococcosis with meningitis is coded 117.5 and 321.0

Helminthiases (120–129)

Helminths are parasitic worms that cause a number of diseases including schistomsomiasis (120.x), hydatid disease (122.x), tapeworm infection (123.x), trichinosis (124.x), roundworm infection (127.0), and pinworm infection (127.4).

Late Effects of Infectious and Parasitic Diseases (137–139)

Late effects of tuberculosis (137), acute poliomyelitis (138), and other infectious and parasitic diseases (139) are classified to this section. Since the infection is no longer present, a code from one of these three categories is assigned in conjunction with the residual condition code. For example, focal glomerulosclerosis from past episode of tuberculosis of the kidney is coded 582.1 and 137.2.

1. INFECTIOUS AND PARASITIC DISEASES (001-139)

Note: Categories for "late effects" of infectious and parasitic diseases are to be found at 137-139.

INCLUDES diseases generally recognized as communicable or transmissible as well as a few diseases of unknown but possibly infectious origin

EXCLUDES acute respiratory infections (460-466)
carrier or suspected carrier of infectious organism (V02.0-V02.9)
certain localized infections
influenza (487.0-487.8, 488.01-488.19)

INTESTINAL INFECTIOUS DISEASES (001-009)

EXCLUDES helminthiases (120.0-129)

√4ᵗʰ **001 Cholera**
DEF: An acute infectious enteritis caused by a potent enterotoxin produced by *Vibrio cholerae*; changes the permeability of the mucosa of the intestines and leads to diarrhea and dehydration.

001.0 Due to Vibrio cholerae

001.1 Due to Vibrio cholerae el tor

001.9 Cholera, unspecified

√4ᵗʰ **002 Typhoid and paratyphoid fevers**
DEF: Typhoid fever: an acute generalized illness caused by *Salmonella typhi*; clinical features are fever, headache, abdominal pain, cough, toxemia, leukopenia, abnormal pulse, rose spots on the skin, bacteremia, hyperplasia of intestinal lymph nodes, mesenteric lymphadenopathy, and Peyer's patches in the intestines.
DEF: Paratyphoid fever: a prolonged febrile illness, caused by salmonella serotypes other than *S. typhi*, especially *S. enteritidis* serotypes paratyphi A and B and *S. choleraesuis*.

002.0 Typhoid fever
Typhoid (fever) (infection) [any site]

002.1 Paratyphoid fever A

002.2 Paratyphoid fever B

002.3 Paratyphoid fever C

002.9 Paratyphoid fever, unspecified

√4ᵗʰ **003 Other salmonella infections**
INCLUDES infection or food poisoning by Salmonella [any serotype]
DEF: Infections caused by a genus of gram-negative, anaerobic bacteria of the family *Enterobacteriaceae*; major symptoms are enteric fevers, acute gastroenteritis and septicemia.

003.0 Salmonella gastroenteritis
Salmonellosis

003.1 Salmonella septicemia

√5ᵗʰ **003.2 Localized salmonella infections**

003.20 Localized salmonella infection, unspecified

003.21 Salmonella meningitis

003.22 Salmonella pneumonia

003.23 Salmonella arthritis

003.24 Salmonella osteomyelitis

003.29 Other

003.8 Other specified salmonella infections

003.9 Salmonella infection, unspecified

√4ᵗʰ **004 Shigellosis**
INCLUDES bacillary dysentery
DEF: Acute infectious dysentery caused by the genus *Shigella*, of the family *Enterobacteriaceae*; affecting the colon causing blood-stained stools, tenesmus, abdominal cramps and fever.

004.0 Shigella dysenteriae
Infection by group A Shigella (Schmitz) (Shiga)

004.1 Shigella flexneri
Infection by group B Shigella

004.2 Shigella boydii
Infection by group C Shigella

004.3 Shigella sonnei
Infection by group D Shigella

004.8 Other specified Shigella infections

004.9 Shigellosis, unspecified

√4ᵗʰ **005 Other food poisoning (bacterial)**
EXCLUDES salmonella infections (003.0-003.9)
toxic effect of:
food contaminants (989.7)
noxious foodstuffs (988.0-988.9)
DEF: Enteritis caused by ingesting contaminated foods and characterized by diarrhea, abdominal pain, vomiting; symptoms may be mild or life threatening.

005.0 Staphylococcal food poisoning
Staphylococcal toxemia specified as due to food

005.1 Botulism food poisoning
Botulism NOS
Food poisoning due to Clostridium botulinum
EXCLUDES infant botulism (040.41)
wound botulism (040.42)

005.2 Food poisoning due to Clostridium perfringens [C. welchii]
Enteritis necroticans

005.3 Food poisoning due to other Clostridia

005.4 Food poisoning due to Vibrio parahaemolyticus

√5ᵗʰ **005.8 Other bacterial food poisoning**
EXCLUDES salmonella food poisoning (003.0-003.9)

005.81 Food poisoning due to Vibrio vulnificus

005.89 Other bacterial food poisoning
Food poisoning due to Bacillus cereus

005.9 Food poisoning, unspecified

√4ᵗʰ **006 Amebiasis**
INCLUDES infection due to Entamoeba histolytica
EXCLUDES amebiasis due to organisms other than Entamoeba histolytica (007.8)
DEF: Infection of the large intestine caused by *Entamoeba histolytica*; usually asymptomatic but symptoms may range from mild diarrhea to profound life-threatening dysentery. Extraintestinal complications include hepatic abscess, which may rupture, causing life-threatening infections.

006.0 Acute amebic dysentery without mention of abscess
Acute amebiasis
DEF: Sudden, severe *Entamoeba histolytica* infection causing bloody stools.

006.1 Chronic intestinal amebiasis without mention of abscess
Chronic:
amebiasis
amebic dysentery

006.2 Amebic nondysenteric colitis
DEF: *Entamoeba histolytica* infection with inflamed colon but no dysentery.

006.3 Amebic liver abscess
Hepatic amebiasis

006.4 Amebic lung abscess
Amebic abscess of lung (and liver)

006.5 Amebic brain abscess
Amebic abscess of brain (and liver) (and lung)

006.6 Amebic skin ulceration
Cutaneous amebiasis

006.8 Amebic infection of other sites
Amebic: Ameboma
appendicitis
balanitis
EXCLUDES specific infections by free-living amebae (136.21-136.29)

006.9 Amebiasis, unspecified
Amebiasis NOS

Infectious and Parasitic Diseases

007–009.1

✓4ᵗʰ **007 Other protozoal intestinal diseases**
> INCLUDES   protozoal:
> > colitis
> > diarrhea
> > dysentery

007.0 Balantidiasis
> Infection by Balantidium coli

007.1 Giardiasis
> Infection by Giardia lamblia
> Lambliasis

007.2 Coccidiosis
> Infection by Isospora belli and Isospora hominis
> Isosporiasis

007.3 Intestinal trichomoniasis
> DEF: Colitis, diarrhea, or dysentery caused by the protozoa *Trichomonas*.

007.4 Cryptosporidiosis
> DEF: An intestinal infection by protozoan parasites causing intractable diarrhea in patients with AIDS and other immunosuppressed individuals.

007.5 Cyclosporiasis
> DEF: An infection of the small intestine by the protozoal organism, *Cyclospora cayetanesis*, spread to humans through ingestion of contaminated water or food. Symptoms include watery diarrhea, loss of appetite, increased gas, stomach cramps, nausea, vomiting, muscle aches, low grade fever, and fatigue.

007.8 Other specified protozoal intestinal diseases
> Amebiasis due to organisms other than Entamoeba histolytica

007.9 Unspecified protozoal intestinal disease
> Flagellate diarrhea
> Protozoal dysentery NOS

✓4ᵗʰ **008 Intestinal infections due to other organisms**
> INCLUDES   any condition classifiable to 009.0-009.3 with mention of the responsible organisms
> EXCLUDES   *food poisoning by these organisms (005.0-005.9)*

✓5ᵗʰ **008.0 Escherichia coli [E. coli]**

008.00 E. coli, unspecified
> E. coli enteritis NOS

008.01 Enteropathogenic E. coli
> DEF: *E. coli* causing inflammation of intestines.

008.02 Enterotoxigenic E. coli
> DEF: A toxic reaction to *E. coli* of the intestinal mucosa, causing voluminous watery secretions.

008.03 Enteroinvasive E. coli
> DEF: *E. coli* infection penetrating intestinal mucosa.

008.04 Enterohemorrhagic E. coli
> DEF: *E. coli* infection penetrating the intestinal mucosa, producing microscopic ulceration and bleeding.

008.09 Other intestinal E. coli infections

008.1 Arizona group of paracolon bacilli

008.2 Aerobacter aerogenes
> Enterobacter aeogenes

008.3 Proteus (mirabilis) (morganii)

✓5ᵗʰ **008.4 Other specified bacteria**

008.41 Staphylococcus
> Staphylococcal enterocolitis

008.42 Pseudomonas

008.43 Campylobacter

008.44 Yersinia enterocolitica

008.45 Clostridium difficile
> Pseudomembranous colitis
> DEF: An overgrowth of a species of bacterium that is a part of the normal colon flora in human infants and sometimes in adults; produces a toxin that causes pseudomembranous enterocolitis; typically is seen in patients undergoing antibiotic therapy.

008.46 Other anaerobes
> Anaerobic enteritis NOS
> Bacteroides (fragilis)
> Gram-negative anaerobes

008.47 Other gram-negative bacteria
> Gram-negative enteritis NOS
> EXCLUDES   *gram-negative anaerobes (008.46)*

008.49 Other

008.5 Bacterial enteritis, unspecified

✓5ᵗʰ **008.6 Enteritis due to specified virus**

008.61 Rotavirus

008.62 Adenovirus

008.63 Norwalk virus
> Norovirus
> Norwalk-like agent

008.64 Other small round viruses [SRVs]
> Small round virus NOS

008.65 Calicivirus
> DEF: Enteritis due to a subgroup of *Picornaviruses*.

008.66 Astrovirus

008.67 Enterovirus NEC
> Coxsackie virus
> Echovirus
> EXCLUDES   *poliovirus (045.0-045.9)*

008.69 Other viral enteritis
> Torovirus

008.8 Other organism, not elsewhere classified
> Viral:
> > enteritis NOS
> > gastroenteritis
> EXCLUDES   *influenza with involvement of gastrointestinal tract (487.8, 488.09, 488.19)*

✓4ᵗʰ **009 Ill-defined intestinal infections**
> EXCLUDES   *diarrheal disease or intestinal infection due to specified organism (001.0-008.8)*
> > *diarrhea following gastrointestinal surgery (564.4)*
> > *intestinal malabsorption (579.0-579.9)*
> > *ischemic enteritis (557.0-557.9)*
> > *other noninfectious gastroenteritis and colitis (558.1-558.9)*
> > *regional enteritis (555.0-555.9)*
> > *ulcerative colitis (556)*

009.0 Infectious colitis, enteritis, and gastroenteritis
> Colitis ⎤
> Enteritis ⎬ septic
> Gastroenteritis ⎦
> Dysentery:
> > NOS
> > catarrhal
> > hemorrhagic
> DEF: Colitis: An inflammation of mucous membranes of the colon.
> DEF: Enteritis: An inflammation of mucous membranes of the small intestine.
> DEF: Gastroenteritis: An inflammation of mucous membranes of stomach and intestines.

009.1 Colitis, enteritis, and gastroenteritis of presumed infectious origin
> EXCLUDES   *colitis NOS (558.9)*
> > *enteritis NOS (558.9)*
> > *gastroenteritis NOS (558.9)*

009.2 Infectious diarrhea
Diarrhea:
dysenteric
epidemic
Infectious diarrheal disease NOS

009.3 Diarrhea of presumed infectious origin
EXCLUDES   *diarrhea NOS (787.91)*

TUBERCULOSIS (010-018)

INCLUDES   infection by Mycobacterium tuberculosis (human) (bovine)

EXCLUDES   *congenital tuberculosis (771.2)*
late effects of tuberculosis (137.0-137.4)

The following fifth-digit subclassification is for use with categories 010-018:
0 **unspecified**
1 **bacteriological or histological examination not done**
2 **bacteriological or histological examination unknown (at present)**
3 **tubercle bacilli found (in sputum) by microscopy**
4 **tubercle bacilli not found (in sputum) by microscopy, but found by bacterial culture**
5 **tubercle bacilli not found by bacteriological examination, but tuberculosis confirmed histologically**
6 **tubercle bacilli not found by bacteriological or histological examination but tuberculosis confirmed by other methods [inoculation of animals]**

DEF: An infection by Mycobacterium tuberculosis causing the formation of small, rounded nodules, called tubercles, that can disseminate throughout the body via lymph and blood vessels. Localized tuberculosis is most often seen in the lungs.

√4ᵗʰ **010 Primary tuberculous infection**
DEF: Tuberculosis of the lungs occurring when the patient is first infected.

√5ᵗʰ **010.0 Primary tuberculous infection**
[0-6]   EXCLUDES   *nonspecific reaction to test for tuberculosis without active tuberculosis (795.51-795.52)*
positive PPD (795.51)
positive tuberculin skin test without active tuberculosis (795.51)
DEF: Hilar or paratracheal lymph node enlargement in pulmonary tuberculosis.

√5ᵗʰ **010.1 Tuberculous pleurisy in primary progressive**
[0-6]   **tuberculosis**
DEF: Inflammation and exudation in the lining of the tubercular lung.

√5ᵗʰ **010.8 Other primary progressive tuberculosis**
[0-6]   EXCLUDES   *tuberculous erythema nodosum (017.1)*

√5ᵗʰ **010.9 Primary tuberculous infection, unspecified**
[0-6]

√4ᵗʰ **011 Pulmonary tuberculosis**
Use additional code to identify any associated silicosis (502)

√5ᵗʰ **011.0 Tuberculosis of lung, infiltrative**
[0-6]

√5ᵗʰ **011.1 Tuberculosis of lung, nodular**
[0-6]

√5ᵗʰ **011.2 Tuberculosis of lung with cavitation**
[0-6]

√5ᵗʰ **011.3 Tuberculosis of bronchus**
[0-6]   EXCLUDES   *isolated bronchial tuberculosis (012.2)*

√5ᵗʰ **011.4 Tuberculous fibrosis of lung**
[0-6]

√5ᵗʰ **011.5 Tuberculous bronchiectasis**
[0-6]

√5ᵗʰ **011.6 Tuberculous pneumonia [any form]**
[0-6]   **DEF:** Inflammatory pulmonary reaction to tuberculous cells.

√5ᵗʰ **011.7 Tuberculous pneumothorax**
[0-6]   **DEF:** Spontaneous rupture of damaged tuberculous pulmonary tissue.

√5ᵗʰ **011.8 Other specified pulmonary tuberculosis**
[0-6]

√5ᵗʰ **011.9 Pulmonary tuberculosis, unspecified**
[0-6]   Respiratory tuberculosis NOS
Tuberculosis of lung NOS

√4ᵗʰ **012 Other respiratory tuberculosis**
EXCLUDES   *respiratory tuberculosis, unspecified (011.9)*

√5ᵗʰ **012.0 Tuberculous pleurisy**
[0-6]   Tuberculosis of pleura
Tuberculous empyema
Tuberculous hydrothorax
EXCLUDES   *pleurisy with effusion without mention of cause (511.9)*
tuberculous pleurisy in primary progressive tuberculosis (010.1)
DEF: Inflammation and exudation in the lining of the tubercular lung.

√5ᵗʰ **012.1 Tuberculosis of intrathoracic lymph nodes**
[0-6]   Tuberculosis of lymph nodes:
hilar
mediastinal
tracheobronchial
Tuberculous tracheobronchial adenopathy
EXCLUDES   *that specified as primary (010.0-010.9)*

√5ᵗʰ **012.2 Isolated tracheal or bronchial tuberculosis**
[0-6]

√5ᵗʰ **012.3 Tuberculous laryngitis**
[0-6]   Tuberculosis of glottis

√5ᵗʰ **012.8 Other specified respiratory tuberculosis**
[0-6]   Tuberculosis of:
mediastinum
nasopharynx
nose (septum)
sinus [any nasal]

√4ᵗʰ **013 Tuberculosis of meninges and central nervous system**

√5ᵗʰ **013.0 Tuberculous meningitis**
[0-6]   Tuberculosis of meninges (cerebral) (spinal)
Tuberculous:
leptomeningitis
meningoencephalitis
EXCLUDES   *tuberculoma of meninges (013.1)*

√5ᵗʰ **013.1 Tuberculoma of meninges**
[0-6]

√5ᵗʰ **013.2 Tuberculoma of brain**
[0-6]   Tuberculosis of brain (current disease)

√5ᵗʰ **013.3 Tuberculous abscess of brain**
[0-6]

√5ᵗʰ **013.4 Tuberculoma of spinal cord**
[0-6]

√5ᵗʰ **013.5 Tuberculous abscess of spinal cord**
[0-6]

√5ᵗʰ **013.6 Tuberculous encephalitis or myelitis**
[0-6]

√5ᵗʰ **013.8 Other specified tuberculosis of central**
[0-6]   **nervous system**

√5ᵗʰ **013.9 Unspecified tuberculosis of central**
[0-6]   **nervous system**
Tuberculosis of central nervous system NOS

√4ᵗʰ **014 Tuberculosis of intestines, peritoneum, and mesenteric glands**

√5ᵗʰ **014.0 Tuberculous peritonitis**
[0-6]   Tuberculous ascites
DEF: Tuberculous inflammation of the membrane lining the abdomen.

Infectious and Parasitic Diseases

014.8–017.9

√5ᵗʰ **014.8 Other**
[0-6]   Tuberculosis (of):
                    anus
                    intestine (large) (small)
                    mesenteric glands
                    rectum
                    retroperitoneal (lymph nodes)
               Tuberculous enteritis

√4ᵗʰ **015 Tuberculosis of bones and joints**
          Use additional code to identify manifestation, as:
          tuberculous:
               arthropathy (711.4)
               necrosis of bone (730.8)
               osteitis (730.8)
               osteomyelitis (730.8)
               synovitis (727.01)
               tenosynovitis (727.01)

√5ᵗʰ **015.0 Vertebral column**
[0-6]   Pott's disease
               Use additional code to identify manifestation, as:
                    curvature of spine [Pott's] (737.4)
                    kyphosis (737.4)
                    spondylitis (720.81)

√5ᵗʰ **015.1 Hip**
[0-6]

√5ᵗʰ **015.2 Knee**
[0-6]

√5ᵗʰ **015.5 Limb bones**
[0-6]   Tuberculous dactylitis

√5ᵗʰ **015.6 Mastoid**
[0-6]   Tuberculous mastoiditis

√5ᵗʰ **015.7 Other specified bone**
[0-6]

√5ᵗʰ **015.8 Other specified joint**
[0-6]

√5ᵗʰ **015.9 Tuberculosis of unspecified bones and joints**
[0-6]

√4ᵗʰ **016 Tuberculosis of genitourinary system**

√5ᵗʰ **016.0 Kidney**
[0-6]   Renal tuberculosis
               Use additional code to identify manifestation, as:
               tuberculous:
                    nephropathy (583.81)
                    pyelitis (590.81)
                    pyelonephritis (590.81)

√5ᵗʰ **016.1 Bladder**
[0-6]

√5ᵗʰ **016.2 Ureter**
[0-6]

√5ᵗʰ **016.3 Other urinary organs**
[0-6]

√5ᵗʰ **016.4 Epididymis**
[0-6]

√5ᵗʰ **016.5 Other male genital organs**
[0-6]   Use additional code to identify manifestation, as:
               tuberculosis of:
                    prostate (601.4)
                    seminal vesicle (608.81)
                    testis (608.81)

√5ᵗʰ **016.6 Tuberculous oophoritis and salpingitis**
[0-6]

√5ᵗʰ **016.7 Other female genital organs**
[0-6]   Tuberculous:
                    cervicitis
                    endometritis

√5ᵗʰ **016.9 Genitourinary tuberculosis, unspecified**
[0-6]

√4ᵗʰ **017 Tuberculosis of other organs**

√5ᵗʰ **017.0 Skin and subcutaneous cellular tissue**
[0-6]   Lupus: Tuberculosis:
               exedens   colliquativa
               vulgaris   cutis
          Scrofuloderma   lichenoides
                                          papulonecrotica
                                          verrucosa cutis
          EXCLUDES *lupus erythematosus (695.4)*
                         disseminated (710.0)
                    lupus NOS (710.0)
                    nonspecific reaction to test for tuberculosis
                         without active tuberculosis
                         (795.51-795.52)
                    positive PPD (795.51)
                    positive tuberculin skin test without active
                         tuberculosis (795.51)

√5ᵗʰ **017.1 Erythema nodosum with hypersensitivity**
[0-6]   **reaction in tuberculosis**
          Bazin's disease
          Erythema:
               induratum
               nodosum, tuberculous
          Tuberculosis indurativa
          EXCLUDES *erythema nodosum NOS (695.2)*

          DEF: Tender, inflammatory, bilateral nodules appearing on
          the shins and thought to be an allergic reaction to
          tuberculotoxin.

√5ᵗʰ **017.2 Peripheral lymph nodes**
[0-6]   Scrofula
          Scrofulous abscess
          Tuberculous adenitis
          EXCLUDES *tuberculosis of lymph nodes:*
                    bronchial and mediastinal (012.1)
                    mesenteric and retroperitoneal (014.8)
                    tuberculous tracheobronchial adenopathy
                         (012.1)

          DEF: Scrofula: Old name for tuberculous cervical
          lymphadenitis.

√5ᵗʰ **017.3 Eye**
[0-6]   Use additional code to identify manifestation, as:
          tuberculous:
               chorioretinitis, disseminated (363.13)
               episcleritis (379.09)
               interstitial keratitis (370.59)
               iridocyclitis, chronic (364.11)
               keratoconjunctivitis (phlyctenular) (370.31)

√5ᵗʰ **017.4 Ear**
[0-6]   Tuberculosis of ear
          Tuberculous otitis media
          EXCLUDES *tuberculous mastoiditis (015.6)*

√5ᵗʰ **017.5 Thyroid gland**
[0-6]

√5ᵗʰ **017.6 Adrenal glands**
[0-6]   Addison's disease, tuberculous

√5ᵗʰ **017.7 Spleen**
[0-6]

√5ᵗʰ **017.8 Esophagus**
[0-6]

√5ᵗʰ **017.9 Other specified organs**
[0-6]   Use additional code to identify manifestation, as:
          tuberculosis of:
               endocardium [any valve] (424.91)
               myocardium (422.0)
               pericardium (420.0)

018 Miliary tuberculosis
> **INCLUDES** tuberculosis:
>> disseminated
>> generalized
>> miliary, whether of a single specified site, multiple sites, or unspecified site
>> polyserositis

DEF: A form of tuberculosis caused by caseous material carried through the bloodstream planting seedlike tubercles in various body organs.

018.0 Acute miliary tuberculosis
[0-6]

018.8 Other specified miliary tuberculosis
[0-6]

018.9 Miliary tuberculosis, unspecified
[0-6]

ZOONOTIC BACTERIAL DISEASES (020-027)

020 Plague
> **INCLUDES** infection by Yersinia [Pasteurella] pestis

020.0 Bubonic
DEF: Most common acute and severe form of plague characterized by lymphadenopathy (buboes), chills, fever and headache.

020.1 Cellulocutaneous
DEF: Plague characterized by inflammation and necrosis of skin.

020.2 Septicemic
DEF: Plague characterized by massive infection in the bloodstream.

020.3 Primary pneumonic
DEF: Plague characterized by massive pulmonary infection.

020.4 Secondary pneumonic
DEF: Lung infection as a secondary complication of plague.

020.5 Pneumonic, unspecified

020.8 Other specified types of plague
Abortive plague   Pestis minor
Ambulatory plague

020.9 Plague, unspecified

021 Tularemia
> **INCLUDES** deerfly fever
>> infection by Francisella [Pasteurella] tularensis
>> rabbit fever

DEF: A febrile disease transmitted by the bites of deer flies, fleas and ticks, by inhalations of aerosolized *F. tularensis* or by ingestion of contaminated food or water; patients quickly develop fever, chills, weakness, headache, backache and malaise.

021.0 Ulceroglandular tularemia
DEF: Lesions occur at the site *Francisella tularensis* organism enters body, usually the fingers or hands.

021.1 Enteric tularemia
Tularemia:
> cryptogenic
> intestinal
> typhoidal

021.2 Pulmonary tularemia
Bronchopneumonic tularemia

021.3 Oculoglandular tularemia
DEF: Painful conjunctival infection by *Francisella tularensis* organism with possible corneal, preauricular lymph, or lacrimal involvement.

021.8 Other specified tularemia
Tularemia:
> generalized or disseminated
> glandular

021.9 Unspecified tularemia

022 Anthrax
DEF: An bacterial disease usually transmitted by contact with infected animals or their discharges; primary routes of inoculation are cutaneous, gastrointestinal and inhalation.

022.0 Cutaneous anthrax
Malignant pustule

022.1 Pulmonary anthrax
Respiratory anthrax
Wool-sorters' disease

022.2 Gastrointestinal anthrax

022.3 Anthrax septicemia

022.8 Other specified manifestations of anthrax

022.9 Anthrax, unspecified

023 Brucellosis
> **INCLUDES** fever:
>> Malta
>> Mediterranean
>> undulant

DEF: An infectious disease caused by gram-negative, aerobic coccobacilli organisms transmitted to humans through contact with infected tissue or dairy products; fever, sweating, weakness, and aching are symptoms.

023.0 Brucella melitensis
DEF: Infection from direct or indirect contact with infected sheep or goats.

023.1 Brucella abortus
DEF: Infection from direct or indirect contact with infected cattle.

023.2 Brucella suis
DEF: Infection from direct or indirect contact with infected swine.

023.3 Brucella canis
DEF: Infection from direct or indirect contact with infected dogs.

023.8 Other brucellosis
Infection by more than one organism

023.9 Brucellosis, unspecified

024 Glanders
Infection by:
> actinobacillus mallei
> malleomyces mallei
> pseudomonas mallei
Farcy
Malleus
DEF: Equine infection causing mucosal inflammation and skin ulcers in humans.

025 Melioidosis
Infection by:
> malleomyces pseudomallei
> pseudomonas pseudomallei
> whitmore's bacillus
Pseudoglanders
DEF: Rare infection caused by *Pseudomonas pseudomallei*; clinical symptoms range from localized infection to fatal septicemia.

026 Rat-bite fever

026.0 Spirillary fever
Rat-bite fever due to Spirillum minor [S. minus]
Sodoku

026.1 Streptobacillary fever
Epidemic arthritic erythema
Haverhill fever
Rat-bite fever due to Streptobacillus moniliformis

026.9 Unspecified rat-bite fever

027 Other zoonotic bacterial diseases

027.0 Listeriosis
Infection
Septicemia } by Listeria monocytogenes

Use additional code to identify manifestation, as meningitis (320.7)
> **EXCLUDES** *congenital listeriosis (771.2)*

Infectious and Parasitic Diseases

027.1–036.0

027.1   Erysipelothrix infection
Erysipeloid (of Rosenbach)

Infection } by Erysipelothrix insidiosa [E.
Septicemia }   rhusiopathiae]

DEF: Usually associated with handling of fish, meat, or poultry; symptoms range from localized inflammation to septicemia.

027.2   Pasteurellosis
Pasteurella pseudotuberculosis infection

Mesenteric adenitis   }
Septic infection (cat   } by Pasteurella multocida
    bite) (dog bite)   }   [P. septica]

EXCLUDES   infection by:
Francisella [Pasteurella] tularensis (021.0-021.9)
Yersinia [Pasteurella] pestis (020.0-020.9)

DEF: Swelling, abscesses, or septicemia from *Pasteurella multocida*, commonly transmitted to humans by a dog or cat scratch.

027.8   Other specified zoonotic bacterial diseases

027.9   Unspecified zoonotic bacterial disease

OTHER BACTERIAL DISEASES (030-041)

EXCLUDES   bacterial venereal diseases (098.0-099.9)
bartonellosis (088.0)

✓4th   **030   Leprosy**
INCLUDES   Hansen's disease
infection by Mycobacterium leprae

030.0   Lepromatous [type L]
Lepromatous leprosy (macular) (diffuse) (infiltrated) (nodular) (neuritic)

DEF: Infectious, disseminated leprosy bacilli with lesions and deformities.

030.1   Tuberculoid [type T]
Tuberculoid leprosy (macular) (maculoanesthetic) (major) (minor) (neuritic)

DEF: Relatively benign, self-limiting leprosy with neuralgia and scales.

030.2   Indeterminate [group I]
Indeterminate [uncharacteristic] leprosy (macular) (neuritic)

DEF: Uncharacteristic leprosy, frequently an early manifestation.

030.3   Borderline [group B]
Borderline or dimorphous leprosy (infiltrated) (neuritic)

DEF: Transitional form of leprosy, neither lepromatous nor tuberculoid.

030.8   Other specified leprosy

030.9   Leprosy, unspecified

✓4th   **031   Diseases due to other mycobacteria**

031.0   Pulmonary
Battey disease
Infection by Mycobacterium:
avium
intracellulare [Battey bacillus]
kansasii

031.1   Cutaneous
Buruli ulcer
Infection by Mycobacterium:
marinum [M. balnei]
ulcerans

031.2   Disseminated
Disseminated mycobacterium avium-intracellulare complex (DMAC)
Mycobacterium avium-intracellulare complex (MAC) bacteremia

DEF: Disseminated mycobacterium avium-intracellulare complex (DMAC): A serious systemic form of MAC commonly observed in patients in the late course of AIDS.

DEF: Mycobacterium avium-intracellulare complex (MAC) bacterium: Human pulmonary disease, lymphadenitis in children and systemic disease in immunocompromised individuals caused by a slow growing, gram-positive, aerobic organism.

031.8   Other specified mycobacterial diseases

031.9   Unspecified diseases due to mycobacteria
Atypical mycobacterium infection NOS

✓4th   **032   Diphtheria**
INCLUDES   infection by Corynebacterium diphtheriae

032.0   Faucial diphtheria
Membranous angina, diphtheritic
DEF: Diphtheria of the throat.

032.1   Nasopharyngeal diphtheria

032.2   Anterior nasal diphtheria

032.3   Laryngeal diphtheria
Laryngotracheitis, diphtheritic

✓5th   **032.8   Other specified diphtheria**

032.81   Conjunctival diphtheria
Pseudomembranous diphtheritic conjunctivitis

032.82   Diphtheritic myocarditis

032.83   Diphtheritic peritonitis

032.84   Diphtheritic cystitis

032.85   Cutaneous diphtheria

032.89   Other

032.9   Diphtheria, unspecified

✓4th   **033   Whooping cough**
INCLUDES   pertussis
Use additional code to identify any associated pneumonia (484.3)
DEF: An acute, highly contagious respiratory tract infection caused by *Bordetella pertussis* and *B. bronchiseptica*; characteristic paroxysmal cough.

033.0   Bordetella pertussis [B. pertussis]

033.1   Bordetella parapertussis [B. parapertussis]

033.8   Whooping cough due to other specified organism
Bordetella bronchiseptica [B. bronchiseptica]

033.9   Whooping cough, unspecified organism

✓4th   **034   Streptococcal sore throat and scarlet fever**

034.0   Streptococcal sore throat

Septic: Streptococcal:
angina   angina
sore throat   laryngitis
                     pharyngitis
                     tonsillitis

034.1   Scarlet fever
Scarlatina
EXCLUDES   parascarlatina (057.8)
DEF: Streptococcal infection and fever with red rash spreading from trunk.

035   Erysipelas
EXCLUDES   postpartum or puerperal erysipelas (670.8)
DEF: An acute superficial cellulitis involving the dermal lymphatics; it is often caused by group A streptococci.

✓4th   **036   Meningococcal infection**

036.0   Meningococcal meningitis
Cerebrospinal fever (meningococcal)
Meningitis:
cerebrospinal
epidemic

036.1   **Meningococcal encephalitis**

036.2   **Meningococcemia**
       Meningococcal septicemia

036.3   **Waterhouse-Friderichsen syndrome, meningococcal**
       Meningococcal hemorrhagic adrenalitis
       Meningococcic adrenal syndrome
       Waterhouse-Friderichsen syndrome NOS

√5ᵗʰ **036.4**   **Meningococcal carditis**

     036.40   **Meningococcal carditis, unspecified**

     036.41   **Meningococcal pericarditis**
          DEF: Meningococcal infection of the outer membrane of the heart.

     036.42   **Meningococcal endocarditis**
          DEF: Meningococcal infection of the membranes lining the cavities of the heart.

     036.43   **Meningococcal myocarditis**
          DEF: Meningococcal infection of the muscle of the heart.

√5ᵗʰ **036.8**   **Other specified meningococcal infections**

     036.81   **Meningococcal optic neuritis**

     036.82   **Meningococcal arthropathy**

     036.89   **Other**

036.9   **Meningococcal infection, unspecified**
       Meningococcal infection NOS

037   **Tetanus**
     EXCLUDES   *tetanus:*
          complicating:
             abortion (634-638 with .0, 639.0)
             ectopic or molar pregnancy (639.0)
          neonatorum (771.3)
          puerperal (670.8)
     DEF: An acute, often fatal, infectious disease caused by the anaerobic, spore-forming bacillus *Clostridium tetani*; the bacillus enters the body through a contaminated wound, burns, surgical wounds, or cutaneous ulcers. Symptoms: lockjaw, spasms, seizures, and paralysis.

√4ᵗʰ **038**   **Septicemia**
     Use additional code for systemic inflammatory response syndrome (SIRS) (995.91-995.92)
     EXCLUDES   *bacteremia (790.7)*
          during labor (659.3)
          following ectopic or molar pregnancy (639.0)
          following infusion, injection, transfusion, or vaccination (999.3)
          postpartum, puerperal (670)
          septicemia (sepsis) of newborn (771.81)
          that complicating abortion (634-638 with .0, 639.0)
     DEF: A systemic disease associated with the presence and persistence of pathogenic microorganisms or their toxins in the blood.

038.0   **Streptococcal septicemia**

√5ᵗʰ **038.1**   **Staphylococcal septicemia**

     038.10   **Staphylococcal septicemia, unspecified**

     038.11   **Methicillin susceptible Staphylococcus aureus septicemia**
          MSSA septicemia
          Staphylococcus aureus septicemia NOS

     038.12   **Methicillin resistant Staphylococcus aureus septicemia**

     038.19   **Other staphylococcal septicemia**

038.2   **Pneumococcal septicemia [Streptococcus pneumoniae septicemia]**

038.3   **Septicemia due to anaerobes**
       Septicemia due to bacteroides
     EXCLUDES   *gas gangrene (040.0)*
          that due to anaerobic streptococci (038.0)
     DEF: Infection of blood by microorganisms that thrive without oxygen.

√5ᵗʰ **038.4**   **Septicemia due to other gram-negative organisms**
     DEF: Infection of blood by microorganisms categorized as gram-negative by Gram's method of staining for identification of bacteria.

     038.40   **Gram-negative organism, unspecified**
          Gram-negative septicemia NOS

     038.41   **Hemophilus influenzae [H. influenzae]**

     038.42   **Escherichia coli [E. coli]**

     038.43   **Pseudomonas**

     038.44   **Serratia**

     038.49   **Other**

038.8   **Other specified septicemias**
     EXCLUDES   *septicemia (due to):*
          anthrax (022.3)
          gonococcal (098.89)
          herpetic (054.5)
          meningococcal (036.2)
          septicemic plague (020.2)

038.9   **Unspecified septicemia**
       Septicemia NOS
     EXCLUDES   *bacteremia NOS (790.7)*

√4ᵗʰ **039**   **Actinomycotic infections**
     INCLUDES   actinomycotic mycetoma
          infection by Actinomycetales, such as species of Actinomyces, Actinomadura, Nocardia, Streptomyces
          maduromycosis (actinomycotic)
          schizomycetoma (actinomycotic)
     DEF: Inflammatory lesions and abscesses at site of infection by *Actinomyces israelii*.

039.0   **Cutaneous**
       Erythrasma
       Trichomycosis axillaris

039.1   **Pulmonary**
       Thoracic actinomycosis

039.2   **Abdominal**

039.3   **Cervicofacial**

039.4   **Madura foot**
     EXCLUDES   *madura foot due to mycotic infection (117.4)*

039.8   **Of other specified sites**

039.9   **Of unspecified site**
       Actinomycosis NOS
       Maduromycosis NOS
       Nocardiosis NOS

√4ᵗʰ **040**   **Other bacterial diseases**
     EXCLUDES   *bacteremia NOS (790.7)*
          bacterial infection NOS (041.9)

040.0   **Gas gangrene**
       Gas bacillus infection or gangrene
       Infection by Clostridium:
          histolyticum
          oedematiens
          perfringens [welchii]
          septicum
          sordellii
       Malignant edema
       Myonecrosis, clostridial
       Myositis, clostridial

040.1   **Rhinoscleroma**
     DEF: Growths on the nose and nasopharynx caused by *Klebsiella rhinoscleromatis*.

040.2   **Whipple's disease**
       Intestinal lipodystrophy

040.3   **Necrobacillosis**
     DEF: Infection with *Fusobacterium necrophorum* causing abscess or necrosis.

Infectious and Parasitic Diseases

040.4–042

√5ᵗʰ **040.4 Other specified botulism**
Non-foodborne intoxication due to toxins of Clostridium botulinum [C. botulinum]
> **EXCLUDES** *botulism NOS (005.1)*
> *food poisoning due to toxins of Clostridium botulinum (005.1)*

040.41 Infant botulism
DEF: Colonization of *Clostridium botulinum* spores in the large intestine; release of neurotoxins results in constipation; may progress to neuromuscular paralysis; affects infants of less than six months.

040.42 Wound botulism
Non-foodborne botulism NOS
Use additional code to identify complicated open wound

√5ᵗʰ **040.8 Other specified bacterial diseases**
040.81 Tropical pyomyositis

040.82 Toxic shock syndrome
Use additional code to identify the organism
DEF: Syndrome caused by staphylococcal exotoxin that may rapidly progress to severe and intractable shock; symptoms include sunburn-like rash with peeling of skin on palms and soles, sudden onset high fever, vomiting, diarrhea, myalgia, and hypotension.

040.89 Other

√4ᵗʰ **041 Bacterial infection in conditions classified elsewhere and of unspecified site**
Note: This category is provided to be used as an additional code to identify the bacterial agent in diseases classified elsewhere. This category will also be used to classify bacterial infections of unspecified nature or site.
> **EXCLUDES** *septicemia (038.0-038.9)*

√5ᵗʰ **041.0 Streptococcus**
041.00 Streptococcus, unspecified
041.01 Group A
041.02 Group B
041.03 Group C
041.04 Group D [Enterococcus]
041.05 Group G
041.09 Other Streptococcus

√5ᵗʰ **041.1 Staphylococcus**
041.10 Staphylococcus, unspecified
041.11 Methicillin susceptible Staphylococcus aureus
MSSA
Staphylococcus aureus NOS
041.12 Methicillin resistant Staphylococcus aureus
Methicillin-resistant staphylococcus aureus (MRSA)
041.19 Other Staphylococcus

041.2 Pneumococcus

041.3 Klebsiella pneumoniae

√5ᵗʰ **041.4 Escherichia coli [E. coli]**
041.41 Shiga toxin-producing Escherichia coli [E. coli] (STEC) O157
E. coli O157:H- (nonmotile) with confirmation of Shiga toxin
E. coli O157 with confirmation of Shiga toxin when H antigen is unknown, or is not H7
O157:H7 Escherichia coli [E.coli] with or without confirmation of Shiga toxin-production
Shiga toxin-producing Escherichia coli [E.coli] O157:H7 with or without confirmation of Shiga toxin-production
STEC O157:H7 with or without confirmation of Shiga toxin-production

041.42 Other specified Shiga toxin-producing Escherichia coli [E. coli] (STEC)
Non-O157 Shiga toxin-producing Escherichia coli [E.coli]
Non-O157 Shiga toxin-producing Escherichia coli [E.coli] with known O group

041.43 Shiga toxin-producing Escherichia coli [E. coli] (STEC), unspecified
Shiga toxin-producing Escherichia coli [E. coli] with unspecified O group
STEC NOS

041.49 Other and unspecified Escherichia coli [E. coli]
Escherichia coli [E. coli] NOS
Non-Shiga toxin-producing E. Coli

041.5 Hemophilus influenzae [H. influenzae]

041.6 Proteus (mirabilis) (morganii)

041.7 Pseudomonas

√5ᵗʰ **041.8 Other specified bacterial infections**
041.81 Mycoplasma
Eaton's agent
Pleuropneumonia-like organisms [PPLO]

041.82 Bacteroides fragilis
DEF: Anaerobic gram-negative bacilli of the gastrointestinal tract; frequently implicated in intra-abdominal infection; commonly resistant to antibiotics.

041.83 Clostridium perfringens

041.84 Other anaerobes
Gram-negative anaerobes
> **EXCLUDES** *Helicobacter pylori (041.86)*

041.85 Other gram-negative organisms
Aerobacter aerogenes
Gram-negative bacteria NOS
Mima polymorpha
Serratia
> **EXCLUDES** *gram-negative anaerobes (041.84)*

041.86 Helicobacter pylori [H. pylori]

041.89 Other specified bacteria

041.9 Bacterial infection, unspecified

HUMAN IMMUNODEFICIENCY VIRUS (HIV) INFECTION (042)

042 Human immunodeficiency virus [HIV] disease
Acquired immune deficiency syndrome
Acquired immunodeficiency syndrome
AIDS
AIDS-like syndrome
AIDS-related complex
ARC
HIV infection, symptomatic
Use additional code(s) to identify all manifestations of HIV
Use additional code to identify HIV-2 infection (079.53)
> **EXCLUDES** *asymptomatic HIV infection status (V08)*
> *exposure to HIV virus (V01.79)*
> *nonspecific serologic evidence of HIV (795.71)*

POLIOMYELITIS AND OTHER NON-ARTHROPOD-BORNE VIRAL DISEASES AND PRION DISEASES OF CENTRAL NERVOUS SYSTEM (045-049)

√4ᵗʰ **045 Acute poliomyelitis**

> EXCLUDES   *late effects of acute poliomyelitis (138)*

> The following fifth-digit subclassification is for use with category 045:
> **0 poliovirus, unspecified type**
> **1 poliovirus type I**
> **2 poliovirus type II**
> **3 poliovirus type III**

√5ᵗʰ **045.0 Acute paralytic poliomyelitis specified as bulbar**
[0-3] Infantile paralysis (acute)   ⎫
Poliomyelitis (acute) (anterior)   ⎬ specified as bulbar
Polioencephalitis (acute) (bulbar)
Polioencephalomyelitis (acute) (anterior) (bulbar)
DEF: Acute paralytic infection occurring where the brain merges with the spinal cord; affecting breathing, swallowing, and heart rate.

√5ᵗʰ **045.1 Acute poliomyelitis with other paralysis**
[0-3] Paralysis:
acute atrophic, spinal
infantile, paralytic
Poliomyelitis (acute)   ⎫
anterior   ⎬ with paralysis except
epidemic   ⎭ bulbar
DEF: Paralytic infection affecting peripheral or spinal nerves.

√5ᵗʰ **045.2 Acute nonparalytic poliomyelitis**
[0-3] Poliomyelitis (acute)   ⎫
anterior   ⎬ specified as nonparalytic
epidemic   ⎭
DEF: Nonparalytic infection causing pain, stiffness, and paresthesias.

√5ᵗʰ **045.9 Acute poliomyelitis, unspecified**
[0-3] Infantile paralysis   ⎫
Poliomyelitis (acute)   ⎬ unspecified whether paralytic
anterior   ⎬ or nonparalytic
epidemic   ⎭

√4ᵗʰ **046 Slow virus infections and prion diseases of central nervous system**

046.0 Kuru
DEF: A chronic, progressive, fatal nervous system disorder; clinical symptoms include cerebellar ataxia, trembling, spasticity and progressive dementia.

√5ᵗʰ **046.1 Jakob-Creutzfeldt disease**
Use additional code to identify dementia:
with behavioral disturbance (294.11)
without behavioral disturbance (294.10)

046.11 Variant Creutzfeldt-Jakob disease
vCJD

046.19 Other and unspecified Creutzfeldt-Jakob disease
CJD
Familial Creutzfeldt-Jakob disease
Iatrogenic Creutzfeldt-Jakob disease
Jakob-Creutzfeldt disease, unspecified
Sporadic Creutzfeldt-Jakob disease
Subacute spongiform encephalopathy
> EXCLUDES   *variant Creutzfeldt-Jakob disease (vCJD) (046.11)*
DEF: Communicable, progressive spongiform encephalopathy thought to be caused by an infectious particle known as a "prion" (proteinaceous infection particle); a progressive, fatal disease manifested principally by mental deterioration.

046.2 Subacute sclerosing panencephalitis
Dawson's inclusion body encephalitis
Van Bogaert's sclerosing leukoencephalitis
DEF: Progressive viral infection causing cerebral dysfunction, blindness, dementia, and death (SSPE).

046.3 Progressive multifocal leukoencephalopathy
Multifocal leukoencephalopathy NOS
DEF: Infection affecting cerebral cortex in patients with weakened immune systems.

√5ᵗʰ **046.7 Other specified prion diseases of central nervous system**
> EXCLUDES   *Creutzfeldt-Jakob disease (046.11-046.19)*
> *Jakob-Creutzfeldt disease (046.11-046.19)*
> *kuru (046.0)*
> *variant Creutzfeldt-Jakob disease (vCJD) (046.11)*

046.71 Gerstmann-Sträussler-Scheinker syndrome
GSS syndrome

046.72 Fatal familial insomnia
FFI

046.79 Other and unspecified prion disease of central nervous system

046.8 Other specified slow virus infection of central nervous system

046.9 Unspecified slow virus infection of central nervous system

√4ᵗʰ **047 Meningitis due to enterovirus**
> INCLUDES   meningitis:
> abacterial
> aseptic
> viral
> EXCLUDES   *meningitis due to:*
> *adenovirus (049.1)*
> *arthropod-borne virus (060.0-066.9)*
> *leptospira (100.81)*
> *virus of:*
> *herpes simplex (054.72)*
> *herpes zoster (053.0)*
> *lymphocytic choriomeningitis (049.0)*
> *mumps (072.1)*
> *poliomyelitis (045.0-045.9)*
> *any other infection specifically classified elsewhere*

047.0 Coxsackie virus

047.1 ECHO virus
Meningo-eruptive syndrome

047.8 Other specified viral meningitis

047.9 Unspecified viral meningitis
Viral meningitis NOS

048 Other enterovirus diseases of central nervous system
Boston exanthem

√4ᵗʰ **049 Other non-arthropod-borne viral diseases of central nervous system**
> EXCLUDES   *late effects of viral encephalitis (139.0)*

049.0 Lymphocytic choriomeningitis
Lymphocytic:
meningitis (serous) (benign)
meningoencephalitis (serous) (benign)

049.1 Meningitis due to adenovirus
DEF: Inflammation of lining of brain caused by Arenaviruses and usually occurring in adults in fall and winter months.

049.8 Other specified non-arthropod-borne viral diseases of central nervous system
Encephalitis: Encephalitis:
acute: lethargica
inclusion body   Rio Bravo
necrotizing   von Economo's disease
epidemic
> EXCLUDES   *human herpesvirus 6 encephalitis (058.21)*
> *other human herpesvirus encephalitis (058.29)*

049.9 Unspecified non-arthropod-borne viral diseases of central nervous system
Viral encephalitis NOS

VIRAL DISEASES GENERALLY ACCOMPANIED BY EXANTHEM (050-059)

EXCLUDES   arthropod-borne viral diseases (060.0-066.9)
           Boston exanthem (048)

√4ᵗʰ **050 Smallpox**

050.0 Variola major

| Hemorrhagic (pustular) | Malignant smallpox |
| smallpox | Purpura variolosa |

DEF: Form of smallpox known for its high mortality; exists only in laboratories.

050.1 Alastrim

Variola minor

DEF: Mild form of smallpox known for its low mortality rate.

050.2 Modified smallpox

Varioloid

DEF: Mild form occurring in patients with history of infection or vaccination.

050.9 Smallpox, unspecified

√4ᵗʰ **051 Cowpox and paravaccinia**

√5ᵗʰ **051.0 Cowpox and vaccinia not from vaccination**

051.01 Cowpox

DEF: A disease contracted by milking infected cows; vesicles usually appear on the fingers, hands and adjacent areas and usually disappear without scarring; other symptoms: local edema, lymphangitis, and regional lymphadenitis with or without fever.

051.02 Vaccinia not from vaccination

EXCLUDES   vaccinia (generalized) (from vaccination) (999.0)

051.1 Pseudocowpox

Milkers' node

DEF: Hand lesions and mild fever in dairy workers caused by exposure to paravaccinia.

051.2 Contagious pustular dermatitis

Ecthyma contagiosum
Orf

DEF: Skin eruptions caused by exposure to poxvirus-infected sheep or goats.

051.9 Paravaccinia, unspecified

√4ᵗʰ **052 Chickenpox**

DEF: Contagious infection by Varicella-zoster virus causing rash with pustules and fever.

052.0 Postvaricella encephalitis

Postchickenpox encephalitis

052.1 Varicella (hemorrhagic) pneumonitis

052.2 Postvaricella myelitis

Postchickenpox myelitis

052.7 With other specified complications

052.8 With unspecified complication

052.9 Varicella without mention of complication

Chickenpox NOS
Varicella NOS

√4ᵗʰ **053 Herpes zoster**

INCLUDES   shingles
           zona

DEF: Self-limiting infection by Varicella-zoster virus causing unilateral eruptions and neuralgia along affected nerves.

053.0 With meningitis

DEF: Varicella-zoster virus infection causing inflammation of the lining of the brain and/or spinal cord.

√5ᵗʰ **053.1 With other nervous system complications**

053.10 With unspecified nervous system complication

053.11 Geniculate herpes zoster

Herpetic geniculate ganglionitis

DEF: Unilateral eruptions and neuralgia along the facial nerve geniculum affecting face and outer and middle ear.

053.12 Postherpetic trigeminal neuralgia

DEF: Severe oral or nasal pain following a herpes zoster infection.

053.13 Postherpetic polyneuropathy

DEF: Multiple areas of pain following a herpes zoster infection.

053.14 Herpes zoster myelitis

053.19 Other

√5ᵗʰ **053.2 With ophthalmic complications**

053.20 Herpes zoster dermatitis of eyelid

Herpes zoster ophthalmicus

053.21 Herpes zoster keratoconjunctivitis

053.22 Herpes zoster iridocyclitis

053.29 Other

√5ᵗʰ **053.7 With other specified complications**

053.71 Otitis externa due to herpes zoster

053.79 Other

053.8 With unspecified complication

053.9 Herpes zoster without mention of complication

Herpes zoster NOS

√4ᵗʰ **054 Herpes simplex**

EXCLUDES   congenital herpes simplex (771.2)

054.0 Eczema herpeticum

Kaposi's varicelliform eruption

DEF: Herpes simplex virus invading site of preexisting skin inflammation.

√5ᵗʰ **054.1 Genital herpes**

054.10 Genital herpes, unspecified

Herpes progenitalis

054.11 Herpetic vulvovaginitis

054.12 Herpetic ulceration of vulva

054.13 Herpetic infection of penis

054.19 Other

054.2 Herpetic gingivostomatitis

054.3 Herpetic meningoencephalitis

Herpes encephalitis
Simian B disease

EXCLUDES   human herpesvirus 6 encephalitis (058.21)
           other human herpesvirus encephalitis (058.29)

DEF: Inflammation of the brain and its lining, caused by infection of herpes simplex 1 in adults and simplex 2 in newborns.

√5ᵗʰ **054.4 With ophthalmic complications**

054.40 With unspecified ophthalmic complication

054.41 Herpes simplex dermatitis of eyelid

054.42 Dendritic keratitis

054.43 Herpes simplex disciform keratitis

054.44 Herpes simplex iridocyclitis

054.49 Other

054.5 Herpetic septicemia

054.6 Herpetic whitlow

Herpetic felon

DEF: A primary infection of the terminal segment of a finger by herpes simplex; intense itching and pain start the disease, vesicles form, and tissue ultimately is destroyed.

√5ᵗʰ **054.7 With other specified complications**

054.71 Visceral herpes simplex

054.72 Herpes simplex meningitis

    054.73   **Herpes simplex otitis externa**

    054.74   **Herpes simplex myelitis**

    054.79   **Other**

  054.8   **With unspecified complication**

  054.9   **Herpes simplex without mention of complication**

✓4th **055**   **Measles**

    INCLUDES   morbilli

              rubeola

  055.0   **Postmeasles encephalitis**

  055.1   **Postmeasles pneumonia**

  055.2   **Postmeasles otitis media**

✓5th   **055.7**   **With other specified complications**

    055.71   **Measles keratoconjunctivitis**

           Measles keratitis

    055.79   **Other**

  055.8   **With unspecified complication**

  055.9   **Measles without mention of complication**

✓4th **056**   **Rubella**

    INCLUDES   German measles

    EXCLUDES   *congenital rubella (771.0)*

    DEF: Acute but usually benign togavirus infection causing fever, sore throat, and rash; associated with complications to fetus as a result of maternal infection.

✓5th   **056.0**   **With neurological complications**

    056.00   **With unspecified neurological complication**

    056.01   **Encephalomyelitis due to rubella**

           Encephalitis   ⎫

           Meningoencephalitis ⎬ due to rubella

    056.09   **Other**

✓5th   **056.7**   **With other specified complications**

    056.71   **Arthritis due to rubella**

    056.79   **Other**

  056.8   **With unspecified complications**

  056.9   **Rubella without mention of complication**

✓4th **057**   **Other viral exanthemata**

    DEF: Skin eruptions or rashes and fever caused by viruses, including poxviruses.

  057.0   **Erythema infectiosum [fifth disease]**

    DEF: A moderately contagious, benign, epidemic disease, usually seen in children, of probable viral etiology; a red macular rash appears on face and may spread to the limbs and trunk.

  057.8   **Other specified viral exanthemata**

     Dukes (-Filatow) disease   Parascarlatina

     Fourth disease   Pseudoscarlatina

    EXCLUDES   *exanthema subitum [sixth disease]*

            (058.10-058.12)

            roseola infantum (058.10-058.12)

  057.9   **Viral exanthem, unspecified**

✓4th **058**   **Other human herpesvirus**

    EXCLUDES   *congenital herpes (771.2)*

            cytomegalovirus (078.5)

            Epstein-Barr virus (075)

            herpes NOS (054.0-054.9)

            herpes simplex (054.0-054.9)

            herpes zoster (053.0-053.9)

            human herpesvirus NOS (054.0-054.9)

            human herpesvirus 1 (054.0-054.9)

            human herpesvirus 2 (054.0-054.9)

            human herpesvirus 3 (052.0-053.9)

            human herpesvirus 4 (075)

            human herpesvirus 5 (078.5)

            varicella (052.0-052.9)

            varicella-zoster virus (052.0-053.9)

✓5th   **058.1**   **Roseola infantum**

     Exanthema subitum [sixth disease]

    058.10   **Roseola infantum, unspecified**

           Exanthema subitum [sixth disease], unspecified

    058.11   **Roseola infantum due to human herpesvirus 6**

           Exanthema subitum [sixth disease] due to human herpesvirus 6

    058.12   **Roseola infantum due to human herpesvirus 7**

           Exanthema subitum [sixth disease] due to human herpesvirus 7

✓5th   **058.2**   **Other human herpesvirus encephalitis**

    EXCLUDES   *herpes encephalitis NOS (054.3)*

            herpes simplex encephalitis (054.3)

            human herpesvirus encephalitis NOS (054.3)

            simian B herpesvirus encephalitis (054.3)

    058.21   **Human herpesvirus 6 encephalitis**

    058.29   **Other human herpesvirus encephalitis**

           Human herpesvirus 7 encephalitis

✓5th   **058.8**   **Other human herpesvirus infections**

    058.81   **Human herpesvirus 6 infection**

    058.82   **Human herpesvirus 7 infection**

    058.89   **Other human herpesvirus infection**

           Human herpesvirus 8 infection

           Kaposi's sarcoma-associated herpesvirus infection

✓4th **059**   **Other poxvirus infections**

    EXCLUDES   *contagious pustular dermatitis (051.2)*

            cowpox (051.01)

            ecthyma contagiosum (051.2)

            milker's nodule (051.1)

            orf (051.2)

            paravaccinia NOS (051.9)

            pseudocowpox (051.1)

            smallpox (050.0-050.9)

            vaccinia (generalized) (from vaccination) (999.0)

            vaccinia not from vaccination (051.02)

✓5th   **059.0**   **Other orthopoxvirus infections**

    059.00   **Orthopoxvirus infection, unspecified**

    059.01   **Monkeypox**

    059.09   **Other orthopoxvirus infection**

✓5th   **059.1**   **Other parapoxvirus infections**

    059.10   **Parapoxvirus infection, unspecified**

    059.11   **Bovine stomatitis**

    059.12   **Sealpox**

    059.19   **Other parapoxvirus infections**

✓5th   **059.2**   **Yatapoxvirus infections**

    059.20   **Yatapoxvirus infection, unspecified**

    059.21   **Tanapox**

    059.22   **Yaba monkey tumor virus**

  059.8   **Other poxvirus infections**

  059.9   **Poxvirus infections, unspecified**

ARTHROPOD-BORNE VIRAL DISEASES (060-066)

     Use additional code to identify any associated meningitis (321.2)

    EXCLUDES   *late effects of viral encephalitis (139.0)*

✓4th **060**   **Yellow fever**

    DEF: Fever and jaundice from infection by mosquito-borne virus of genus *Flavivirus*.

  060.0   **Sylvatic**

     Yellow fever: Yellow fever:

       jungle   sylvan

    DEF: Yellow fever transmitted from animal to man, via mosquito.

  060.1   **Urban**

    DEF: Yellow fever transmitted from man to man, via mosquito.

  060.9   **Yellow fever, unspecified**

Infectious and Parasitic Diseases

061–066.9

061 Dengue
Breakbone fever
EXCLUDES *hemorrhagic fever caused by dengue virus (065.4)*
DEF: Acute, self-limiting infection by mosquito-borne virus characterized by fever and generalized aches.

☑4ᵗʰ **062 Mosquito-borne viral encephalitis**

062.0 Japanese encephalitis
Japanese B encephalitis
DEF: *Flavivirus* causing inflammation of the brain, with a wide range of clinical manifestations.

062.1 Western equine encephalitis
DEF: Alphavirus WEE infection causing inflammation of the brain, found in areas west of the Mississippi; transmitted horse to mosquito to man.

062.2 Eastern equine encephalitis
EXCLUDES *Venezuelan equine encephalitis (066.2)*
DEF: Alphavirus EEE causing inflammation of the brain and spinal cord, found from Canada to South America and Mexico; transmitted horse to mosquito to man.

062.3 St. Louis encephalitis
DEF: Epidemic form caused by *Flavivirus* and transmitted by mosquito, and characterized by fever, difficulty in speech, and headache.

062.4 Australian encephalitis
Australian arboencephalitis
Australian X disease
Murray Valley encephalitis
DEF: *Flavivirus* causing inflammation of the brain, occurring in Australia and New Guinea.

062.5 California virus encephalitis
Encephalitis: Tahyna fever
   California
   La Crosse
DEF: Bunyamwere virus causing inflammation of the brain.

062.8 Other specified mosquito-borne viral encephalitis
Encephalitis by Ilheus virus
EXCLUDES *West Nile virus (066.40-066.49)*

062.9 Mosquito-borne viral encephalitis, unspecified

☑4ᵗʰ **063 Tick-borne viral encephalitis**
INCLUDES diphasic meningoencephalitis

063.0 Russian spring-summer [taiga] encephalitis

063.1 Louping ill
DEF: Inflammation of brain caused by virus transmitted sheep to tick to man; incidence usually limited to British Isles.

063.2 Central European encephalitis
DEF: Inflammation of brain caused by virus transmitted by tick; limited to central Europe and presenting with two distinct phases.

063.8 Other specified tick-borne viral encephalitis
Langat encephalitis   Powassan encephalitis

063.9 Tick-borne viral encephalitis, unspecified

064 Viral encephalitis transmitted by other and unspecified arthropods
Arthropod-borne viral encephalitis, vector unknown
Negishi virus encephalitis
EXCLUDES *viral encephalitis NOS (049.9)*

☑4ᵗʰ **065 Arthropod-borne hemorrhagic fever**

065.0 Crimean hemorrhagic fever [CHF Congo virus]
Central Asian hemorrhagic fever

065.1 Omsk hemorrhagic fever

065.2 Kyasanur Forest disease

065.3 Other tick-borne hemorrhagic fever

065.4 Mosquito-borne hemorrhagic fever
Chikungunya hemorrhagic fever
Dengue hemorrhagic fever
EXCLUDES *Chikungunya fever (066.3)*
dengue (061)
yellow fever (060.0-060.9)

065.8 Other specified arthropod-borne hemorrhagic fever
Mite-borne hemorrhagic fever

065.9 Arthropod-borne hemorrhagic fever, unspecified
Arbovirus hemorrhagic fever NOS

☑4ᵗʰ **066 Other arthropod-borne viral diseases**

066.0 Phlebotomus fever
Changuinola fever
Sandfly fever
DEF: Sandfly-borne viral infection occurring in Asia, Mideast and South America.

066.1 Tick-borne fever
Nairobi sheep disease
Tick fever:
   American mountain
   Colorado
   Kemerovo
   Quaranfil

066.2 Venezuelan equine fever
Venezuelan equine encephalitis
DEF: Alphavirus VEE infection causing inflammation of the brain, usually limited to South America, Mexico, and Florida; transmitted horse to mosquito to man.

066.3 Other mosquito-borne fever
Fever (viral):   Fever (viral):
   Bunyamwera   Oropouche
   Bwamba   Pixuna
   Chikungunya   Rift valley
   Guama   Ross river
   Mayaro   Wesselsbron
   Mucambo   Zika
   O'Nyong-Nyong
EXCLUDES *dengue (061)*
yellow fever (060.0-060.9)

☑5ᵗʰ **066.4 West Nile fever**
DEF: Mosquito-borne fever causing fatal inflammation of the brain, the lining of the brain, or of the lining of the brain and spinal cord.

066.40 West Nile fever, unspecified
West Nile fever NOS
West Nile fever without complications
West Nile virus NOS

066.41 West Nile fever with encephalitis
West Nile encephalitis
West Nile encephalomyelitis

066.42 West Nile fever with other neurologic manifestation
Use additional code to specify the neurologic manifestation

066.49 West Nile fever with other complications
Use additional code to specify the other conditions

066.8 Other specified arthropod-borne viral diseases
Chandipura fever
Piry fever

066.9 Arthropod-borne viral disease, unspecified
Arbovirus infection NOS

OTHER DISEASES DUE TO VIRUSES AND CHLAMYDIAE (070-079)

√4th **070 Viral hepatitis**

INCLUDES viral hepatitis (acute) (chronic)
EXCLUDES *cytomegalic inclusion virus hepatitis (078.5)*

The following fifth-digit subclassification is for use with categories 070.2 and 070.3:
  0 **acute or unspecified, without mention of hepatitis delta**
  1 **acute or unspecified, with hepatitis delta**
  2 **chronic, without mention of hepatitis delta**
  3 **chronic, with hepatitis delta**

DEF: Hepatitis A: HAV infection is self-limiting with flulike symptoms; transmission, fecal-oral.
DEF: Hepatitis B: HBV infection can be chronic and systemic; transmission, bodily fluids.
DEF: Hepatitis C: HCV infection can be chronic and systemic; transmission, blood transfusion and unidentified agents.
DEF: Hepatitis D (delta): HDV occurs only in the presence of hepatitis B virus.
DEF: Hepatitis E: HEV is epidemic form; transmission and nature under investigation.

070.0 Viral hepatitis A with hepatic coma

070.1 Viral hepatitis A without mention of hepatic coma
    Infectious hepatitis

√5th **070.2 Viral hepatitis B with hepatic coma**
    [0-3]

√5th **070.3 Viral hepatitis B without mention of hepatic coma**
    [0-3]   Serum hepatitis

√5th **070.4 Other specified viral hepatitis with hepatic coma**

    070.41 Acute hepatitis C with hepatic coma

    070.42 Hepatitis delta without mention of active hepatitis B disease with hepatic coma
        Hepatitis delta with hepatitis B carrier state

    070.43 Hepatitis E with hepatic coma

    070.44 Chronic hepatitis C with hepatic coma

    070.49 Other specified viral hepatitis with hepatic coma

√5th **070.5 Other specified viral hepatitis without mention of hepatic coma**

    070.51 Acute hepatitis C without mention of hepatic coma

    070.52 Hepatitis delta without mention of active hepatitis B disease or hepatic coma

    070.53 Hepatitis E without mention of hepatic coma

    070.54 Chronic hepatitis C without mention of hepatic coma

    070.59 Other specified viral hepatitis without mention of hepatic coma

070.6 Unspecified viral hepatitis with hepatic coma
    EXCLUDES *unspecified viral hepatitis C with hepatic coma (070.71)*

√5th **070.7 Unspecified viral hepatitis C**

    070.70 Unspecified viral hepatitis C without hepatic coma
        Unspecified viral hepatitis C NOS

    070.71 Unspecified viral hepatitis C with hepatic coma

070.9 Unspecified viral hepatitis without mention of hepatic coma
    Viral hepatitis NOS
    EXCLUDES *unspecified viral hepatitis C without hepatic coma (070.70)*

071 Rabies
    Hydrophobia
    Lyssa
    DEF: Acute infectious disease of the CNS caused by a rhabdovirus; usually spread by bites by infected animals; progresses from fever, restlessness, and extreme excitability, to hydrophobia, seizures, confusion and death.

√4th **072 Mumps**
    DEF: Acute infectious disease caused by paramyxovirus; usually seen in children less than 15 years of age; salivary glands are typically enlarged, involves other organs, such as testes, pancreas and meninges.

    072.0 Mumps orchitis

    072.1 Mumps meningitis

    072.2 Mumps encephalitis
        Mumps meningoencephalitis

    072.3 Mumps pancreatitis

√5th **072.7 Mumps with other specified complications**

    072.71 Mumps hepatitis

    072.72 Mumps polyneuropathy

    072.79 Other

    072.8 Mumps with unspecified complication

    072.9 Mumps without mention of complication
        Epidemic parotitis
        Infectious parotitis

√4th **073 Ornithosis**
    INCLUDES parrot fever
            psittacosis
    DEF: *Chlamydia psittaci* infection often transmitted from birds to humans.

    073.0 With pneumonia
        Lobular pneumonitis due to ornithosis

    073.7 With other specified complications

    073.8 With unspecified complication

    073.9 Ornithosis, unspecified

√4th **074 Specific diseases due to Coxsackie virus**
    EXCLUDES *Coxsackie virus:*
            infection NOS (079.2)
            meningitis (047.0)

    074.0 Herpangina
        Vesicular pharyngitis
        DEF: Acute infectious coxsackie virus infection causing throat lesions, fever, and vomiting; generally affects children in summer.

    074.1 Epidemic pleurodynia
        Bornholm disease   Epidemic:
        Devil's grip   myalgia
                                      myositis
        DEF: Paroxysmal pain in chest, accompanied by fever and usually limited to children and young adults; caused by coxsackie virus.

√5th **074.2 Coxsackie carditis**

    074.20 Coxsackie carditis, unspecified

    074.21 Coxsackie pericarditis
        DEF: Coxsackie infection of the outer lining of the heart.

    074.22 Coxsackie endocarditis
        DEF: Coxsackie infection within the heart's cavities.

    074.23 Coxsackie myocarditis
        Aseptic myocarditis of newborn
        DEF: Coxsackie infection of the muscle of the heart.

    074.3 Hand, foot, and mouth disease
        Vesicular stomatitis and exanthem
        DEF: Mild coxsackie infection causing lesions on hands, feet and oral mucosa, most commonly seen in preschool children.

Infectious and Parasitic Diseases

074.8–079.1

074.8   **Other specified diseases due to Coxsackie virus**
Acute lymphonodular pharyngitis

075   **Infectious mononucleosis**
Glandular fever   Pfeiffer's disease
Monocytic angina

DEF: Acute infection by Epstein-Barr virus causing fever, sore throat, enlarged lymph glands and spleen, and fatigue; usually seen in teens and young adults.

√4ᵗʰ **076**   **Trachoma**
EXCLUDES   *late effect of trachoma (139.1)*

DEF: A chronic infectious disease of the cornea and conjunctiva caused by a strain of the bacteria *Chlamydia trachomatis*; the infection can cause photophobia, pain, excessive tearing and sometimes blindness.

076.0   **Initial stage**
Trachoma dubium

076.1   **Active stage**
Granular conjunctivitis (trachomatous)
Trachomatous:
    follicular conjunctivitis
    pannus

076.9   **Trachoma, unspecified**
Trachoma NOS

√4ᵗʰ **077**   **Other diseases of conjunctiva due to viruses and Chlamydiae**
EXCLUDES   *ophthalmic complications of viral diseases classified elsewhere*

077.0   **Inclusion conjunctivitis**
Paratrachoma   Swimming pool conjunctivitis
EXCLUDES   *inclusion blennorrhea (neonatal) (771.6)*

DEF: Pus in conjunctiva caused by *Chlamydiae trachomatis*.

077.1   **Epidemic keratoconjunctivitis**
Shipyard eye

DEF: Highly contagious corneal or conjunctival infection caused by adenovirus type 8; symptoms include inflammation and corneal infiltrates.

077.2   **Pharyngoconjunctival fever**
Viral pharyngoconjunctivitis

077.3   **Other adenoviral conjunctivitis**
Acute adenoviral follicular conjunctivitis

077.4   **Epidemic hemorrhagic conjunctivitis**
Apollo:
    conjunctivitis
    disease
Conjunctivitis due to enterovirus type 70
Hemorrhagic conjunctivitis (acute) (epidemic)

077.8   **Other viral conjunctivitis**
Newcastle conjunctivitis

√5ᵗʰ **077.9**   **Unspecified diseases of conjunctiva due to viruses and Chlamydiae**

077.98   **Due to Chlamydiae**

077.99   **Due to viruses**
Viral conjunctivitis NOS

√4ᵗʰ **078**   **Other diseases due to viruses and Chlamydiae**
EXCLUDES   *viral infection NOS (079.0-079.9)*
                viremia NOS (790.8)

078.0   **Molluscum contagiosum**
DEF: Benign poxvirus infection causing small bumps on the skin or conjunctiva; transmitted by close contact.

√5ᵗʰ **078.1**   **Viral warts**
Viral warts due to human papilloma virus

DEF: A keratotic papilloma of the epidermis caused by the human papilloma virus; the superficial vegetative lesions last for varying durations and eventually regress spontaneously.

078.10   **Viral warts, unspecified**
Verruca:
    Vulgaris
Warts (infectious)

078.11   **Condyloma acuminatum**
Condyloma NOS
Genital warts NOS

DEF: Clusters of mucosa or epidermal lesions on external genitalia; viral infection is sexually transmitted.

078.12   **Plantar wart**
Verruca plantaris

078.19   **Other specified viral warts**
Common wartx   Veruca planna
Flat wart

078.2   **Sweating fever**
Miliary fever
Sweating disease

DEF: A viral infection characterized by profuse sweating; various papular, vesicular and other eruptions cause the blockage of sweat glands.

078.3   **Cat-scratch disease**
Benign lymphoreticulosis (of inoculation)
Cat-scratch fever

078.4   **Foot and mouth disease**
Aphthous fever   Epizootic:
Epizootic: stomatitis
    aphthae

DEF: Ulcers on oral mucosa, legs, and feet after exposure to infected animal.

078.5   **Cytomegaloviral disease**
Cytomegalic inclusion disease
Salivary gland virus disease
Use additional code to identify manifestation, as:
    cytomegalic inclusion virus:
       hepatitis (573.1)
       pneumonia (484.1)
EXCLUDES   *congenital cytomegalovirus infection (771.1)*

DEF: A herpesvirus associated with serious disease morbidity including fever, leukopenia, pneumonia, retinitis, hepatitis and organ transplant; often leads to hepatomegaly, splenomegaly and thrombocytopenia; a common post-transplant complication.

078.6   **Hemorrhagic nephrosonephritis**
Hemorrhagic fever: Hemorrhagic fever:
    epidemic   Russian
    Korean   with renal syndrome

DEF: Viral infection causing kidney dysfunction and bleeding disorders.

078.7   **Arenaviral hemorrhagic fever**
Hemorrhagic fever: Hemorrhagic fever:
    Argentine   Junin virus
    Bolivian   Machupo virus

√5ᵗʰ **078.8**   **Other specified diseases due to viruses and Chlamydiae**
EXCLUDES   *epidemic diarrhea (009.2)*
                lymphogranuloma venereum (099.1)

078.81   **Epidemic vertigo**

078.82   **Epidemic vomiting syndrome**
Winter vomiting disease

078.88   **Other specified diseases due to Chlamydiae**

078.89   **Other specified diseases due to viruses**
Epidemic cervical myalgia
Marburg disease

√4ᵗʰ **079**   **Viral and chlamydial infection in conditions classified elsewhere and of unspecified site**
Note: This category is provided to be used as an additional code to identify the viral agent in diseases classifiable elsewhere. This category will also be used to classify virus infection of unspecified nature or site.

079.0   **Adenovirus**

079.1   **ECHO virus**
DEF: An "orphan" enteric RNA virus, certain serotypes of which are associated with human disease, especially aseptic meningitis.

079.2 Coxsackie virus

DEF: A heterogenous group of viruses associated with aseptic meningitis, myocarditis, pericarditis, and acute onset juvenile diabetes.

079.3 Rhinovirus

DEF: Rhinoviruses affect primarily the upper respiratory tract. Over 100 distinct types infect humans.

079.4 Human papillomavirus

DEF: Viral infection caused by the genus *Papillomavirus* causing cutaneous and genital warts, including verruca vulgaris and condyloma acuminatum; certain types are associated with cervical dysplasia, cancer and other genital malignancies.

√5ᵗʰ **079.5 Retrovirus**

EXCLUDES   human immunodeficiency virus, type 1 [HIV-1] (042)
human T-cell lymphotrophic virus, type III [HTLV-III] (042)
lymphadenopathy-associated virus [LAV] (042)

DEF: A large group of RNA viruses that carry reverse transcriptase and include the leukoviruses and lentiviruses.

079.50 Retrovirus, unspecified

079.51 Human T-cell lymphotrophic virus, type I [HTLV-I]

079.52 Human T-cell lymphotrophic virus, type II [HTLV-II]

079.53 Human immunodeficiency virus, type 2 [HIV-2]

079.59 Other specified retrovirus

079.6 Respiratory syncytial virus [RSV]

DEF: The major respiratory pathogen of young children, causing severe bronchitis and bronchopneumonia, and minor infection in adults.

√5ᵗʰ **079.8 Other specified viral and chlamydial infections**

079.81 Hantavirus

DEF: An infection caused by the Muerto Canyon virus whose primary rodent reservoir is the deer mouse Peromyscus maniculatus; commonly characterized by fever, myalgias, headache, cough.

079.82 SARS-associated coronavirus

DEF: A life-threatening respiratory disease, severe acute respiratory syndrome (SARS); etiology coronavirus; presenting symptoms may range from mild to severe forms of flu-like conditions; fever, chills, cough, headache, myalgia; diagnosis of SARS is based upon clinical, laboratory, and epidemiological criteria.

079.83 Parvovirus B19

Human parvovirus   Parvovirus NOS

EXCLUDES   erythema infectiosum [fifth disease] (057.0)

DEF: The only known parvovirus to cause disease in humans; manifestation is erythema infectiosum; also associated with polyarthropathy, chronic anemia, red cell aplasia, and fetal hydrops.

079.88 Other specified chlamydial infection

079.89 Other specified viral infection

√5ᵗʰ **079.9 Unspecified viral and chlamydial infections**

EXCLUDES   viremia NOS (790.8)

079.98 Unspecified chlamydial infection

Chlamydial infections NOS

079.99 Unspecified viral infection

Viral infections NOS

RICKETTSIOSES AND OTHER ARTHROPOD-BORNE DISEASES (080-088)

EXCLUDES   arthropod-borne viral diseases (060.0-066.9)

080 Louse-borne [epidemic] typhus

Typhus (fever):   Typhus (fever):
classical   exanthematic NOS
epidemic   louse-borne

DEF: *Rickettsia prowazekii*; causes severe headache, rash, high fever.

√4ᵗʰ **081 Other typhus**

081.0 Murine [endemic] typhus

Typhus (fever):   Typhus (fever):
endemic   flea-borne

DEF: Milder typhus caused by *Rickettsia typhi (mooseri)*; transmitted by rat flea.

081.1 Brill's disease

Brill-Zinsser disease   Recrudescent typhus (fever)

081.2 Scrub typhus

Japanese river fever   Mite-borne typhus
Kedani fever   Tsutsugamushi

DEF: Typhus caused by *Rickettsia tsutsugamushi* transmitted by chigger.

081.9 Typhus, unspecified

Typhus (fever) NOS

√4ᵗʰ **082 Tick-borne rickettsioses**

082.0 Spotted fevers

Rocky mountain spotted fever
Sao Paulo fever

082.1 Boutonneuse fever

African tick typhus   Marseilles fever
India tick typhus   Mediterranean tick fever
Kenya tick typhus

082.2 North Asian tick fever

Siberian tick typhus

082.3 Queensland tick typhus

√5ᵗʰ **082.4 Ehrlichiosis**

082.40 Ehrlichiosis, unspecified

082.41 Ehrlichiosis chaffeensis [E. chaffeensis]

DEF: A febrile illness caused by bacterial infection, also called human monocytic ehrlichiosis (HME). Causal organism is *Ehrlichia chaffeensis*, transmitted by the Lone Star tick. Symptoms include fever, chills, myalgia, nausea, vomiting, diarrhea, confusion, and severe headache occurring one week after a tick bite. Clinical findings are lymphadenopathy, rash, thrombocytopenia, leukopenia, and abnormal liver function tests.

082.49 Other ehrlichiosis

082.8 Other specified tick-borne rickettsioses

Lone star fever

082.9 Tick-borne rickettsiosis, unspecified

Tick-borne typhus NOS

√4ᵗʰ **083 Other rickettsioses**

083.0 Q fever

DEF: Infection of *Coxiella burnettii* usually acquired through airborne organisms.

083.1 Trench fever

Quintan fever   Wolhynian fever

083.2 Rickettsialpox

Vesicular rickettsiosis

DEF: Infection of *Rickettsia akari* usually acquired through a mite bite.

083.8 Other specified rickettsioses

083.9 Rickettsiosis, unspecified

084 Malaria

Note: Subcategories 084.0-084.6 exclude the listed conditions with mention of pernicious complications (084.8-084.9).

EXCLUDES congenital malaria (771.2)

DEF: Mosquito-borne disease causing high fever and prostration and cataloged by species of *Plasmodium*: *P. falciparum*, *P. malariae*, *P. ovale*, and *P. vivax*.

084.0 Falciparum malaria [malignant tertian]
Malaria (fever):
by Plasmodium falciparum
subtertian

084.1 Vivax malaria [benign tertian]
Malaria (fever) by Plasmodium vivax

084.2 Quartan malaria
Malaria (fever) by Plasmodium malariae
Malariae malaria

084.3 Ovale malaria
Malaria (fever) by Plasmodium ovale

084.4 Other malaria
Monkey malaria

084.5 Mixed malaria
Malaria (fever) by more than one parasite

084.6 Malaria, unspecified
Malaria (fever) NOS

084.7 Induced malaria
Therapeutically induced malaria
EXCLUDES accidental infection from syringe, blood transfusion, etc. (084.0-084.6, above, according to parasite species) transmission from mother to child during delivery (771.2)

084.8 Blackwater fever
Hemoglobinuric:
fever (bilious)
malaria
Malarial hemoglobinuria
DEF: Severe hemic and renal complication of *Plasmodium falciparum* infection.

084.9 Other pernicious complications of malaria
Algid malaria
Cerebral malaria
Use additional code to identify complication, as:
malarial:
hepatitis (573.2)
nephrosis (581.81)

085 Leishmaniasis

085.0 Visceral [kala-azar]
Dumdum fever
Infection by Leishmania:
donovani
infantum
Leishmaniasis:
dermal, post-kala-azar
Mediterranean
visceral (Indian)

085.1 Cutaneous, urban
Aleppo boil
Baghdad boil
Delhi boil
Infection by Leishmania tropica (minor)
Leishmaniasis, cutaneous:
dry form
late
recurrent
ulcerating
Oriental sore

085.2 Cutaneous, Asian desert
Infection by Leishmania tropica major
Leishmaniasis, cutaneous:
acute necrotizing
rural
wet form
zoonotic form

085.3 Cutaneous, Ethiopian
Infection by Leishmania ethiopica
Leishmaniasis, cutaneous:
diffuse
lepromatous

085.4 Cutaneous, American
Chiclero ulcer
Infection by Leishmania mexicana
Leishmaniasis tegumentaria diffusa

085.5 Mucocutaneous (American)
Espundia
Infection by Leishmania braziliensis
Uta

085.9 Leishmaniasis, unspecified

086 Trypanosomiasis
Use additional code to identify manifestations, as:
trypanosomiasis:
encephalitis (323.2)
meningitis (321.3)

086.0 Chagas' disease with heart involvement
American trypanosomiasis
Infection by Trypanosoma cruzi } with heart involvement
Any condition classifiable to 086.2 with heart involvement

086.1 Chagas' disease with other organ involvement
American trypanosomiasis
Infection by Trypanosoma cruzi } with involvement of organ other than heart
Any condition classifiable to 086.2 with involvement of organ other than heart

086.2 Chagas' disease without mention of organ involvement
American trypanosomiasis
Infection by Trypanosoma cruzi

086.3 Gambian trypanosomiasis
Gambian sleeping sickness
Infection by Trypanosoma gambiense

086.4 Rhodesian trypanosomiasis
Infection by Trypanosoma rhodesiense
Rhodesian sleeping sickness

086.5 African trypanosomiasis, unspecified
Sleeping sickness NOS

086.9 Trypanosomiasis, unspecified

087 Relapsing fever
INCLUDES recurrent fever
DEF: Infection of *Borrelia*; symptoms are episodic and include fever and arthralgia.

087.0 Louse-borne

087.1 Tick-borne

087.9 Relapsing fever, unspecified

088 Other arthropod-borne diseases

088.0 Bartonellosis
Carrión's disease
Oroya fever
Verruga peruana

088.8 Other specified arthropod-borne diseases

088.81 Lyme disease
Erythema chronicum migrans
DEF: A recurrent multisystem disorder caused by the spirochete *Borrelia burgdorferi* with the carrier being the tick; begins with lesions of erythema chronicum migrans; followed by arthritis of the large joints, myalgia, malaise, and neurological and cardiac manifestations.

088.82 Babesiosis
Babesiasis
DEF: A tick-borne disease caused by infection of *Babesia*, characterized by fever, malaise, listlessness, severe anemia and hemoglobinuria.

088.89   Other

088.9   Arthropod-borne disease, unspecified

SYPHILIS AND OTHER VENEREAL DISEASES (090-099)

> EXCLUDES   nonvenereal endemic syphilis (104.0)
>   urogenital trichomoniasis (131.0)

√4th **090   Congenital syphilis**

DEF: Infection by spirochete *Treponema pallidum* acquired in utero from the infected mother.

090.0   Early congenital syphilis, symptomatic

Congenital syphilitic:	Congenital syphilitic:
choroiditis	splenomegaly
coryza (chronic)	Syphilitic (congenital):
hepatomegaly	epiphysitis
mucous patches	osteochondritis
periostitis	pemphigus

Any congenital syphilitic condition specified as early or manifest less than two years after birth

090.1   Early congenital syphilis, latent

Congenital syphilis without clinical manifestations, with positive serological reaction and negative spinal fluid test, less than two years after birth

090.2   Early congenital syphilis, unspecified

Congenital syphilis NOS, less than two years after birth

090.3   Syphilitic interstitial keratitis

Syphilitic keratitis:
   parenchymatous
   punctata profunda

> EXCLUDES   interstitial keratitis NOS (370.50)

√5th **090.4   Juvenile neurosyphilis**

Use additional code to identify any associated mental disorder

DEF: *Treponema pallidum* infection involving the nervous system.

090.40   Juvenile neurosyphilis, unspecified

Congenital neurosyphilis
Dementia paralytica juvenilis
Juvenile:
   general paresis
   tabes
   taboparesis

090.41   Congenital syphilitic encephalitis

DEF: Congenital *Treponema pallidum* infection involving the brain.

090.42   Congenital syphilitic meningitis

DEF: Congenital *Treponema pallidum* infection involving the lining of the brain and/or spinal cord.

090.49   Other

090.5   Other late congenital syphilis, symptomatic

Gumma due to congenital syphilis
Hutchinson's teeth
Syphilitic saddle nose
Any congenital syphilitic condition specified as late or manifest two years or more after birth

090.6   Late congenital syphilis, latent

Congenital syphilis without clinical manifestations, with positive serological reaction and negative spinal fluid test, two years or more after birth

090.7   Late congenital syphilis, unspecified

Congenital syphilis NOS, two years or more after birth

090.9   Congenital syphilis, unspecified

√4th **091   Early syphilis, symptomatic**

> EXCLUDES   early cardiovascular syphilis (093.0-093.9)
>   early neurosyphilis (094.0-094.9)

091.0   Genital syphilis (primary)

Genital chancre

DEF: Genital lesion at the site of initial infection by *Treponema pallidum*.

091.1   Primary anal syphilis

DEF: Anal lesion at the site of initial infection by *Treponema pallidum*.

091.2   Other primary syphilis

Primary syphilis of:
   breast
   fingers
   lip
   tonsils

DEF: Lesion at the site of initial infection by *Treponema pallidum*.

091.3   Secondary syphilis of skin or mucous membranes

Condyloma latum
Secondary syphilis of:
   anus
   mouth
   pharynx
   skin
   tonsils
   vulva

DEF: Transitory or chronic lesions following initial syphilis infection.

091.4   Adenopathy due to secondary syphilis

Syphilitic adenopathy (secondary)
Syphilitic lymphadenitis (secondary)

√5th **091.5   Uveitis due to secondary syphilis**

091.50   Syphilitic uveitis, unspecified

091.51   Syphilitic chorioretinitis (secondary)

DEF: Inflammation of choroid and retina as a secondary infection.

091.52   Syphilitic iridocyclitis (secondary)

DEF: Inflammation of iris and ciliary body as a secondary infection.

√5th **091.6   Secondary syphilis of viscera and bone**

091.61   Secondary syphilitic periostitis

DEF: Inflammation of outer layers of bone as a secondary infection.

091.62   Secondary syphilitic hepatitis

Secondary syphilis of liver

091.69   Other viscera

091.7   Secondary syphilis, relapse

Secondary syphilis, relapse (treated) (untreated)

DEF: Return of symptoms of syphilis following asymptomatic period.

√5th **091.8   Other forms of secondary syphilis**

091.81   Acute syphilitic meningitis (secondary)

DEF: Sudden, severe inflammation of the lining of the brain and/or spinal cord as a secondary infection.

091.82   Syphilitic alopecia

DEF: Hair loss following initial syphilis infection.

091.89   Other

091.9   Unspecified secondary syphilis

√4th **092   Early syphilis, latent**

> INCLUDES   syphilis (acquired) without clinical manifestations, with positive serological reaction and negative spinal fluid test, less than two years after infection

092.0   Early syphilis, latent, serological relapse after treatment

092.9   Early syphilis, latent, unspecified

√4th **093   Cardiovascular syphilis**

093.0   Aneurysm of aorta, specified as syphilitic

Dilatation of aorta, specified as syphilitic

093.1   Syphilitic aortitis

DEF: Inflammation of the aorta – the main artery leading from the heart.

093.2 Syphilitic endocarditis
> **DEF:** Inflammation of the tissues lining the cavities of the heart.

093.20 Valve, unspecified
> Syphilitic ostial coronary disease

093.21 Mitral valve

093.22 Aortic valve
> Syphilitic aortic incompetence or stenosis

093.23 Tricuspid valve

093.24 Pulmonary valve

093.8 Other specified cardiovascular syphilis

093.81 Syphilitic pericarditis
> **DEF:** Inflammation of the outer lining of the heart.

093.82 Syphilitic myocarditis
> **DEF:** Inflammation of the muscle of the heart.

093.89 Other

093.9 Cardiovascular syphilis, unspecified

094 Neurosyphilis
> Use additional code to identify any associated mental disorder

094.0 Tabes dorsalis
> Locomotor ataxia (progressive)
> Posterior spinal sclerosis (syphilitic)
> Tabetic neurosyphilis
> Use additional code to identify manifestation, as:
> neurogenic arthropathy [Charcot's joint disease] (713.5)
> **DEF:** Progressive degeneration of nerves associated with long-term syphilis; causing pain, wasting away, incontinence, and ataxia.

094.1 General paresis
> Dementia paralytica
> General paralysis (of the insane) (progressive)
> Paretic neurosyphilis
> Taboparesis
> **DEF:** Degeneration of brain associated with long-term syphilis, causing loss of brain function, progressive dementia, and paralysis.

094.2 Syphilitic meningitis
> Meningovascular syphilis
> **EXCLUDES** acute syphilitic meningitis (secondary) (091.81)
> **DEF:** Inflammation of the lining of the brain and/or spinal cord.

094.3 Asymptomatic neurosyphilis

094.8 Other specified neurosyphilis

094.81 Syphilitic encephalitis

094.82 Syphilitic Parkinsonism
> **DEF:** Decreased motor function, tremors, and muscular rigidity.

094.83 Syphilitic disseminated retinochoroiditis
> **DEF:** Inflammation of retina and choroid due to neurosyphilis.

094.84 Syphilitic optic atrophy
> **DEF:** Degeneration of the eye and its nerves due to neurosyphilis.

094.85 Syphilitic retrobulbar neuritis
> **DEF:** Inflammation of the posterior optic nerve due to neurosyphilis.

094.86 Syphilitic acoustic neuritis
> **DEF:** Inflammation of acoustic nerve due to neurosyphilis.

094.87 Syphilitic ruptured cerebral aneurysm

094.89 Other

094.9 Neurosyphilis, unspecified
> Gumma (syphilitic)
> Syphilis (early) (late)   } of central nervous system
> Syphiloma   NOS

095 Other forms of late syphilis, with symptoms
> **INCLUDES** gumma (syphilitic)
> syphilis, late, tertiary, or unspecified stage

095.0 Syphilitic episcleritis

095.1 Syphilis of lung

095.2 Syphilitic peritonitis

095.3 Syphilis of liver

095.4 Syphilis of kidney

095.5 Syphilis of bone

095.6 Syphilis of muscle
> Syphilitic myositis

095.7 Syphilis of synovium, tendon, and bursa
> Syphilitic:
> bursitis
> synovitis

095.8 Other specified forms of late symptomatic syphilis
> **EXCLUDES** cardiovascular syphilis (093.0-093.9)
> neurosyphilis (094.0-094.9)

095.9 Late symptomatic syphilis, unspecified

096 Late syphilis, latent
> Syphilis (acquired) without clinical manifestations, with positive serological reaction and negative spinal fluid test, two years or more after infection

097 Other and unspecified syphilis

097.0 Late syphilis, unspecified

097.1 Latent syphilis, unspecified
> Positive serological reaction for syphilis

097.9 Syphilis, unspecified
> Syphilis (acquired) NOS
> **EXCLUDES** syphilis NOS causing death under two years of age (090.9)

098 Gonococcal infections
> **DEF:** Neisseria gonorrhoeae infection generally acquired in utero or in sexual congress.

098.0 Acute, of lower genitourinary tract
> Gonococcal: Gonorrhea (acute):
> Bartholinitis (acute)   NOS
> urethritis (acute)   genitourinary (tract) NOS
> vulvovaginitis (acute)

098.1 Acute, of upper genitourinary tract

098.10 Gonococcal infection (acute) of upper genitourinary tract, site unspecified

098.11 Gonococcal cystitis (acute) upper
> Gonorrhea (acute) of bladder

098.12 Gonococcal prostatitis (acute)

098.13 Gonococcal epididymo-orchitis (acute)
> Gonococcal orchitis (acute)
> **DEF:** Acute inflammation of the testes.

098.14 Gonococcal seminal vesiculitis (acute)
> Gonorrhea (acute) of seminal vesicle

098.15 Gonococcal cervicitis (acute)
> Gonorrhea (acute) of cervix

098.16 Gonococcal endometritis (acute)
> Gonorrhea (acute) of uterus

098.17 Gonococcal salpingitis, specified as acute
> **DEF:** Acute inflammation of the fallopian tubes.

098.19 Other

098.2 Chronic, of lower genitourinary tract
> Gonoccocal:
> Bartholinitis
> urethritis   } specified as chronic or with
> vulvovaginitis   duration of two
> Gonorrhea: months or more
> NOS
> genitourinary (tract)
> Any condition classifiable to 098.0 specified as chronic or with duration of two months or more

√5ᵗʰ **098.3 Chronic, of upper genitourinary tract**

     INCLUDES   any condition classifiable to 098.1 stated as chronic or with a duration of two months or more

098.30 Chronic gonococcal infection of upper genitourinary tract, site unspecified

098.31 Gonococcal cystitis, chronic
Gonorrhea of bladder, chronic
Any condition classifiable to 098.11, specified as chronic

098.32 Gonococcal prostatitis, chronic
Any condition classifiable to 098.12, specified as chronic

098.33 Gonococcal epididymo-orchitis, chronic
Chronic gonococcal orchitis
Any condition classifiable to 098.13, specified as chronic
DEF: Chronic inflammation of the testes.

098.34 Gonococcal seminal vesiculitis, chronic
Gonorrhea of seminal vesicle, chronic
Any condition classifiable to 098.14, specified as chronic

098.35 Gonococcal cervicitis, chronic
Gonorrhea of cervix, chronic
Any condition classifiable to 098.15, specified as chronic

098.36 Gonococcal endometritis, chronic
Any condition classifiable to 098.16, specified as chronic
DEF: Chronic inflammation of the uterus.

098.37 Gonococcal salpingitis (chronic)
DEF: Chronic inflammation of the fallopian tubes.

098.39 Other

√5ᵗʰ **098.4 Gonococcal infection of eye**

098.40 Gonococcal conjunctivitis (neonatorum)
Gonococcal ophthalmia (neonatorum)
DEF: Infection of conjunctiva present at birth.

098.41 Gonococcal iridocyclitis
DEF: Inflammation and infection of iris and ciliary body.

098.42 Gonococcal endophthalmia
DEF: Inflammation and infection of contents of eyeball.

098.43 Gonococcal keratitis
DEF: Inflammation and infection of the cornea.

098.49 Other

√5ᵗʰ **098.5 Gonococcal infection of joint**

098.50 Gonococcal arthritis
Gonococcal infection of joint NOS

098.51 Gonococcal synovitis and tenosynovitis

098.52 Gonococcal bursitis
DEF: Inflammation of the sac-like cavities in a joint.

098.53 Gonococcal spondylitis

098.59 Other
Gonococcal rheumatism

098.6 Gonococcal infection of pharynx

098.7 Gonococcal infection of anus and rectum
Gonococcal proctitis

√5ᵗʰ **098.8 Gonococcal infection of other specified sites**

098.81 Gonococcal keratosis (blennorrhagica)
DEF: Pustular skin lesions caused by *Neisseria gonorrhoeae*.

098.82 Gonococcal meningitis
DEF: Inflammation of lining of brain and/or spinal cord.

098.83 Gonococcal pericarditis
DEF: Inflammation of the outer lining of the heart.

098.84 Gonococcal endocarditis
DEF: Inflammation of tissues lining the cavities of heart.

098.85 Other gonococcal heart disease

098.86 Gonococcal peritonitis
DEF: Inflammation of the membrane lining the abdomen.

098.89 Other
Gonococcemia

√4ᵗʰ **099 Other venereal diseases**

099.0 Chancroid
Bubo (inguinal):
  chancroidal
  due to Hemophilus ducreyi
Chancre:
  Ducrey's
  simple
  soft
Ulcus molle (cutis)(skin)
DEF: A sexually transmitted disease caused by *Haemophilus ducreyi*; identified by a painful primary ulcer at the site of inoculation (usually external genitalia) with related lymphadenitis.

099.1 Lymphogranuloma venereum
Climatic or tropical bubo
(Durand-) Nicolas-Favre disease
Esthiomene
Lymphogranuloma inguinale
DEF: Sexually transmitted infection of *Chlamydia trachomatis* causing skin lesions.

099.2 Granuloma inguinale
Donovanosis
Granuloma pudendi (ulcerating)
Granuloma venereum
Pudendal ulcer
DEF: Chronic, sexually transmitted infection of *Calymmatobacterium granulomatis* causing progressive, anogenital skin ulcers.

099.3 Reiter's disease
Reactive arthritis
Reiter's syndrome
Use additional code for associated:
  arthropathy (711.1)
  conjunctivitis (372.33)
DEF: A symptom complex of unknown etiology consisting of urethritis, conjunctivitis, arthritis and myocutaneous lesions; occurs most commonly in young men and patients with HIV. Also a form of reactive arthritis.

√5ᵗʰ **099.4 Other nongonococcal urethritis [NGU]**

099.40 Unspecified
Nonspecific urethritis

099.41 Chlamydia trachomatis

099.49 Other specified organism

√5ᵗʰ **099.5 Other venereal diseases due to Chlamydia trachomatis**
   EXCLUDES   *Chlamydia trachomatis infection of conjunctiva (076.0-076.9, 077.0, 077.9) Lymphogranuloma venereum (099.1)*
DEF: Venereal diseases caused by *Chlamydia trachomatis* at other sites besides the urethra (e.g., pharynx, anus and rectum, conjunctiva and peritoneum).

099.50 Unspecified site

099.51 Pharynx

099.52 Anus and rectum

099.53 Lower genitourinary sites
Use additional code to specify site of infection, such as:
bladder (595.4)
cervix (616.0)
vagina and vulva (616.11)
EXCLUDES urethra (099.41)

099.54 Other genitourinary sites
Use additional code to specify site of infection, such as:
pelvic inflammatory disease NOS (614.9)
testis and epididymis (604.91)

099.55 Unspecified genitourinary site

099.56 Peritoneum
Perihepatitis

099.59 Other specified site

099.8 Other specified venereal diseases

099.9 Venereal disease, unspecified

OTHER SPIROCHETAL DISEASES (100-104)

☑4ᵗʰ **100 Leptospirosis**
DEF: A blood infection of any spirochete of the genus *Leptospire*; transmitted to humans by exposure to contaminated animal tissues or water. Patients present with flulike symptoms, characteristic muscle aches involving the thighs and low back.

100.0 Leptospirosis icterohemorrhagica
Leptospiral or spirochetal jaundice (hemorrhagic)
Weil's disease

☑5ᵗʰ **100.8 Other specified leptospiral infections**

100.81 Leptospiral meningitis (aseptic)

100.89 Other

Fever:	Infection by Leptospira:
Fort Bragg	australis
pretibial	bataviae
swamp	pyrogenes

100.9 Leptospirosis, unspecified

101 Vincent's angina
Acute necrotizing ulcerative:
gingivitis
stomatitis
Fusospirochetal pharyngitis
Spirochetal stomatitis
Trench mouth
Vincent's:
gingivitis
infection [any site]
DEF: Painful ulceration with edema and hypermic patches of the oropharyngeal and throat membranes; it is caused by spreading of acute ulcerative gingivitis.

☑4ᵗʰ **102 Yaws**
INCLUDES frambesia
pian
DEF: An infectious, endemic, tropical disease caused by *Treponema pertenue*; usually affects persons 15 years old or younger; a primary cutaneous lesion develops, then a granulomatous skin eruption, and occasionally lesions that destroy skin and bone.

102.0 Initial lesions

Chancre of yaws	Initial frambesial ulcer
Frambesia, initial or primary	Mother yaw

102.1 Multiple papillomata and wet crab yaws
Butter yaws
Frambesioma
Pianoma
Plantar or palmar papilloma of yaws

102.2 Other early skin lesions
Cutaneous yaws, less than five years after infection
Early yaws (cutaneous) (macular) (papular) (maculopapular) (micropapular)
Frambeside of early yaws

102.3 Hyperkeratosis
Ghoul hand
Hyperkeratosis, palmar or plantar (early) (late) due to yaws
Worm-eaten soles
DEF: Overgrowth of skin of palm or bottoms of feet, due to yaws.

102.4 Gummata and ulcers
Gummatous frambeside
Nodular late yaws (ulcerated)
DEF: Rubbery lesions and areas of dead skin caused by yaws.

102.5 Gangosa
Rhinopharyngitis mutilans
DEF: Massive, mutilating lesions of the nose and oral cavity caused by yaws.

102.6 Bone and joint lesions
Goundou
Gumma, bone } of yaws (late)
Gummatous osteitis or periostitis

Hydrarthrosis
Osteitis } of yaws (early) (late)
Periostitis (hypertrophic)

102.7 Other manifestations
Juxta-articular nodules of yaws
Mucosal yaws

102.8 Latent yaws
Yaws without clinical manifestations, with positive serology

102.9 Yaws, unspecified

☑4ᵗʰ **103 Pinta**
DEF: A chronic form of treponematosis, endemic in areas of tropical America; it is identified by the presence of red, violet, blue, coffee-colored or white spots on the skin.

103.0 Primary lesions
Chancre (primary)
Papule (primary) } of pinta [carate]
Pintid

103.1 Intermediate lesions
Erythematous plaques
Hyperchronic lesions } of pinta [carate]
Hyperkeratosis

103.2 Late lesions
Cardiovascular lesions
Skin lesions:
achromic
cicatricial } of pinta [carate]
dyschromic
Vitiligo

103.3 Mixed lesions
Achromic and hyperchromic skin lesions of pinta [carate]

103.9 Pinta, unspecified

☑4ᵗʰ **104 Other spirochetal infection**

104.0 Nonvenereal endemic syphilis
Bejel
Njovera
DEF: *Treponema pallidum, T. pertenue,* or *T. caroteum* infection transmitted non-sexually, causing lesions on mucosa and skin.

104.8 Other specified spirochetal infections
EXCLUDES relapsing fever (087.0-087.9)
syphilis (090.0-097.9)

104.9 Spirochetal infection, unspecified

MYCOSES (110-118)

Use additional code to identify manifestation as:
arthropathy (711.6)
meningitis (321.0-321.1)
otitis externa (380.15)

> EXCLUDES *infection by Actinomycetales, such as species of Actinomyces, Actinomadura, Nocardia, Streptomyces (039.0-039.9)*

✓4ᵗʰ **110 Dermatophytosis**

> INCLUDES infection by species of Epidermophyton, Microsporum, and Trichophyton
> tinea, any type except those in 111

DEF: Superficial infection of the skin caused by a parasitic fungus.

110.0 Of scalp and beard
Kerion
Sycosis, mycotic
Trichophytic tinea [black dot tinea], scalp

110.1 Of nail
Dermatophytic onychia
Onychomycosis
Tinea unguium

110.2 Of hand
Tinea manuum

110.3 Of groin and perianal area
Dhobie itch
Eczema marginatum
Tinea cruris

110.4 Of foot
Athlete's foot
Tinea pedis

110.5 Of the body
Herpes circinatus
Tinea imbricata [Tokelau]

110.6 Deep seated dermatophytosis
Granuloma trichophyticum
Majocchi's granuloma

110.8 Of other specified sites

110.9 Of unspecified site
Favus NOS
Microsporic tinea NOS
Ringworm NOS

✓4ᵗʰ **111 Dermatomycosis, other and unspecified**

111.0 Pityriasis versicolor
Infection by Malassezia [Pityrosporum] furfur
Tinea flava
Tinea versicolor

111.1 Tinea nigra
Infection by Cladosporium species
Keratomycosis nigricans
Microsporosis nigra
Pityriasis nigra
Tinea palmaris nigra

111.2 Tinea blanca
Infection by Trichosporon (beigelii) cutaneum
White piedra

111.3 Black piedra
Infection by Piedraia hortai

111.8 Other specified dermatomycoses

111.9 Dermatomycosis, unspecified

✓4ᵗʰ **112 Candidiasis**

> INCLUDES infection by Candida species
> moniliasis

> EXCLUDES *neonatal monilial infection (771.7)*

DEF: Fungal infection caused by *Candida*; usually seen in mucous membranes or skin.

112.0 Of mouth
Thrush (oral)

112.1 Of vulva and vagina
Candidal vulvovaginitis
Monilial vulvovaginitis

112.2 Of other urogenital sites
Candidal balanitis

112.3 Of skin and nails
Candidal intertrigo
Candidal onychia
Candidal perionyxis [paronychia]

112.4 Of lung
Candidal pneumonia

112.5 Disseminated
Systemic candidiasis

✓5ᵗʰ **112.8 Of other specified sites**

112.81 Candidal endocarditis

112.82 Candidal otitis externa
Otomycosis in moniliasis

112.83 Candidal meningitis

112.84 Candidal esophagitis

112.85 Candidal enteritis

112.89 Other

112.9 Of unspecified site

✓4ᵗʰ **114 Coccidioidomycosis**

> INCLUDES infection by Coccidioides (immitis)
> Posada-Wernicke disease

DEF: A fungal disease caused by inhalation of dust particles containing arthrospores of *Coccidiodes immitis*; a self-limited respiratory infection; the primary form is known as San Joaquin fever, desert fever or valley fever.

114.0 Primary coccidioidomycosis (pulmonary)
Acute pulmonary coccidioidomycosis
Coccidioidomycotic pneumonitis
Desert rheumatism
Pulmonary coccidioidomycosis
San Joaquin Valley fever
DEF: Acute, self-limiting *Coccidioides immitis* infection of the lung.

114.1 Primary extrapulmonary coccidioidomycosis
Chancriform syndrome
Primary cutaneous coccidioidomycosis
DEF: Acute, self-limiting *Coccidioides immitis* infection in nonpulmonary site.

114.2 Coccidioidal meningitis
DEF: *Coccidioides immitis* infection of the lining of the brain and/or spinal cord.

114.3 Other forms of progressive coccidioidomycosis
Coccidioidal granuloma
Disseminated coccidioidomycosis

114.4 Chronic pulmonary coccidioidomycosis

114.5 Pulmonary coccidioidomycosis, unspecified

114.9 Coccidioidomycosis, unspecified

Infectious and Parasitic Diseases

115–121.0

√4ᵗʰ **115 Histoplasmosis**

The following fifth-digit subclassification is for use with category 115:

0 without mention of manifestation
1 meningitis
2 retinitis
3 pericarditis
4 endocarditis
5 pneumonia
9 other

√5ᵗʰ **115.0 Infection by Histoplasma capsulatum**
[0-5, 9]   American histoplasmosis
Darling's disease
Reticuloendothelial cytomycosis
Small form histoplasmosis
DEF: Infection resulting from inhalation of fungal spores, causing acute pneumonia, an influenza-like illness, or a disseminated disease of the reticuloendothelial system. In immunocompromised patients it can reactivate, affecting lungs, meninges, heart, peritoneum and adrenals.

√5ᵗʰ **115.1 Infection by Histoplasma duboisii**
[0-5, 9]   African histoplasmosis
Large form histoplasmosis

√5ᵗʰ **115.9 Histoplasmosis, unspecified**
[0-5, 9]   Histoplasmosis NOS

√4ᵗʰ **116 Blastomycotic infection**

116.0 Blastomycosis
Blastomycotic dermatitis
Chicago disease
Cutaneous blastomycosis
Disseminated blastomycosis
Gilchrist's disease
Infection by Blastomyces [Ajellomyces] dermatitidis
North American blastomycosis
Primary pulmonary blastomycosis

116.1 Paracoccidioidomycosis
Brazilian blastomycosis
Infection by Paracoccidioides [Blastomyces] brasiliensis
Lutz-Splendore-Almeida disease
Mucocutaneous-lymphangitic paracoccidioidomycosis
Pulmonary paracoccidioidomycosis
South American blastomycosis
Visceral paracoccidioidomycosis

116.2 Lobomycosis
Infections by Loboa [Blastomyces] loboi
Keloidal blastomycosis
Lobo's disease

√4ᵗʰ **117 Other mycoses**

117.0 Rhinosporidiosis
Infection by Rhinosporidium seeberi

117.1 Sporotrichosis
Cutaneous sporotrichosis
Disseminated sporotrichosis
Infection by Sporothrix [Sporotrichum] schenckii
Lymphocutaneous sporotrichosis
Pulmonary sporotrichosis
Sporotrichosis of the bones

117.2 Chromoblastomycosis
Chromomycosis
Infection by Cladosporidium carrionii, Fonsecaea compactum, Fonsecaea pedrosoi, Phialophora verrucosa

117.3 Aspergillosis
Infection by Aspergillus species, mainly A. fumigatus, A. flavus group, A. terreus group

117.4 Mycotic mycetomas
Infection by various genera and species of Ascomycetes and Deuteromycetes, such as Acremonium [Cephalosporium] falciforme, Neotestudina rosatii, Madurella grisea, Madurella mycetomii, Pyrenochaeta romeroi, Zopfia [Leptosphaeria] senegalensis
Madura foot, mycotic
Maduromycosis, mycotic
EXCLUDES actinomycotic mycetomas (039.0-039.9)

117.5 Cryptococcosis
Busse-Buschke's disease
European cryptococcosis
Infection by Cryptococcus neoformans
Pulmonary cryptococcosis
Systemic cryptococcosis
Torula

117.6 Allescheriosis [Petriellidosis]
Infections by Allescheria [Petriellidium] boydii [Monosporium apiospermum]
EXCLUDES mycotic mycetoma (117.4)

117.7 Zygomycosis [Phycomycosis or Mucormycosis]
Infection by species of Absidia, Basidiobolus, Conidiobolus, Cunninghamella, Entomophthora, Mucor, Rhizopus, Saksenaea

117.8 Infection by dematiacious fungi, [Phaehyphomycosis]
Infection by dematiacious fungi, such as Cladosporium trichoides [bantianum], Dreschlera hawaiiensis, Phialophora gougerotii, Phialophora jeanselmi

117.9 Other and unspecified mycoses

√4ᵗʰ **118 Opportunistic mycoses**
Infection of skin, subcutaneous tissues, and/or organs by a wide variety of fungi generally considered to be pathogenic to compromised hosts only (e.g., infection by species of Alternaria, Dreschlera, Fusarium)
Use additional code to identify manifestation, such as: keratitis (370.8)

HELMINTHIASES (120-129)

√4ᵗʰ **120 Schistosomiasis [bilharziasis]**
DEF: Infection caused by *Schistosoma*, a genus of flukes or trematode parasites.

120.0 Schistosoma haematobium
Vesical schistosomiasis NOS

120.1 Schistosoma mansoni
Intestinal schistosomiasis NOS

120.2 Schistosoma japonicum
Asiatic schistosomiasis NOS
Katayama disease or fever

120.3 Cutaneous
Cercarial dermatitis
Infection by cercariae of Schistosoma
Schistosome dermatitis
Swimmers' itch

120.8 Other specified schistosomiasis
Infection by Schistosoma:
bovis
intercalatum
mattheii
spindale
Schistosomiasis chestermani

120.9 Schistosomiasis, unspecified
Blood flukes NOS
Hemic distomiasis

√4ᵗʰ **121 Other trematode infections**

121.0 Opisthorchiasis
Infection by:
cat liver fluke
Opisthorchis (felineus) (tenuicollis) (viverrini)

121.1 **Clonorchiasis**
Biliary cirrhosis due to clonorchiasis
Chinese liver fluke disease
Hepatic distomiasis due to Clonorchis sinensis
Oriental liver fluke disease

121.2 **Paragonimiasis**
Infection by Paragonimus
Lung fluke disease (oriental)
Pulmonary distomiasis

121.3 **Fascioliasis**
Infection by Fasciola:
gigantica
hepatica
Liver flukes NOS
Sheep liver fluke infection

121.4 **Fasciolopsiasis**
Infection by Fasciolopsis (buski)
Intestinal distomiasis

121.5 **Metagonimiasis**
Infection by Metagonimus yokogawai

121.6 **Heterophyiasis**
Infection by:
Heterophyes heterophyes
Stellantchasmus falcatus

121.8 **Other specified trematode infections**
Infection by:
Dicrocoelium dendriticum
Echinostoma ilocanum
Gastrodiscoides hominis

121.9 **Trematode infection, unspecified**
Distomiasis NOS
Fluke disease NOS

✓4ᵗʰ 122 **Echinococcosis**
INCLUDES   echinococciasis
hydatid disease
hydatidosis
DEF: Infection caused by larval forms of tapeworms of the genus *Echinococcus.*

122.0 **Echinococcus granulosus infection of liver**

122.1 **Echinococcus granulosus infection of lung**

122.2 **Echinococcus granulosus infection of thyroid**

122.3 **Echinococcus granulosus infection, other**

122.4 **Echinococcus granulosus infection, unspecified**

122.5 **Echinococcus multilocularis infection of liver**

122.6 **Echinococcus multilocularis infection, other**

122.7 **Echinococcus multilocularis infection, unspecified**

122.8 **Echinococcosis, unspecified, of liver**

122.9 **Echinococcosis, other and unspecified**

✓4ᵗʰ 123 **Other cestode infection**

123.0 **Taenia solium infection, intestinal form**
Pork tapeworm (adult) (infection)

123.1 **Cysticercosis**
Cysticerciasis
Infection by Cysticercus cellulosae [larval form of Taenia solium]

123.2 **Taenia saginata infection**
Beef tapeworm (infection)
Infection by Taeniarhynchus saginatus

123.3 **Taeniasis, unspecified**

123.4 **Diphyllobothriasis, intestinal**
Diphyllobothrium (adult) (latum) (pacificum) infection
Fish tapeworm (infection)

123.5 **Sparganosis [larval diphyllobothriasis]**
Infection by:
Diphyllobothrium larvae
Sparganum (mansoni) (proliferum)
Spirometra larvae

123.6 **Hymenolepiasis**
Dwarf tapeworm (infection)
Hymenolepis (diminuta) (nana) infection
Rat tapeworm (infection)

123.8 **Other specified cestode infection**
Diplogonoporus (grandis) ⎫
Dipylidium (caninum)   ⎬ infection
Dog tapeworm (infection)   ⎭

123.9 **Cestode infection, unspecified**
Tapeworm (infection) NOS

124 **Trichinosis**
Trichinella spiralis infection
Trichinellosis
Trichiniasis
DEF: Infection by *Trichinella spiralis,* the smallest of the parasitic nematodes.

✓4ᵗʰ 125 **Filarial infection and dracontiasis**

125.0 **Bancroftian filariasis**
Chyluria   ⎫
Elephantiasis   ⎪
Infection   ⎬ due to Wuchereria bancrofti
Lymphadenitis   ⎪
Lymphangitis   ⎭
Wuchereriasis

125.1 **Malayan filariasis**
Brugia filariasis ⎫
Chyluria   ⎪
Elephantiasis   ⎪
Infection   ⎬ due to Wuchereria bancrofti
Lymphadenitis   ⎪
Lymphangitis   ⎭

125.2 **Loiasis**
Eyeworm disease of Africa
Loa loa infection

125.3 **Onchocerciasis**
Onchocerca volvulus infection
Onchocercosis

125.4 **Dipetalonemiasis**
Infection by:
Acanthocheilonema perstans
Dipetalonema perstans

125.5 **Mansonella ozzardi infection**
Filariasis ozzardi

125.6 **Other specified filariasis**
Dirofilaria infection
Infection by:
Acanthocheilonema streptocerca
Dipetalonema streptocerca

125.7 **Dracontiasis**
Guinea-worm infection
Infection by Dracunculus medinensis

125.9 **Unspecified filariasis**

✓4ᵗʰ 126 **Ancylostomiasis and necatoriasis**
INCLUDES   cutaneous larva migrans due to Ancylostoma
hookworm (disease) (infection)
uncinariasis

126.0 **Ancylostoma duodenale**

126.1 **Necator americanus**

126.2 **Ancylostoma braziliense**

126.3 **Ancylostoma ceylanicum**

126.8 **Other specified Ancylostoma**

126.9 **Ancylostomiasis and necatoriasis, unspecified**
Creeping eruption NOS
Cutaneous larva migrans NOS

✓4ᵗʰ 127 **Other intestinal helminthiases**

127.0 **Ascariasis**
Ascaridiasis
Infection by Ascaris lumbricoides
Roundworm infection

127.1 Anisakiasis
Infection by Anisakis larva

127.2 Strongyloidiasis
Infection by Strongyloides stercoralis
EXCLUDES trichostrongyliasis (127.6)

127.3 Trichuriasis
Infection by Trichuris trichiuria
Trichocephaliasis
Whipworm (disease) (infection)

127.4 Enterobiasis
Infection by Enterobius vermicularis
Oxyuriasis
Oxyuris vermicularis infection
Pinworm (disease) (infection)
Threadworm infection

127.5 Capillariasis
Infection by Capillaria philippinensis
EXCLUDES infection by Capillaria hepatica (128.8)

127.6 Trichostrongyliasis
Infection by Trichostrongylus species

127.7 Other specified intestinal helminthiasis
Infection by:
Oesophagostomum apiostomum and related species
Ternidens diminutus
other specified intestinal helminth
Physalopteriasis

127.8 Mixed intestinal helminthiasis
Infection by intestinal helminths classified to more than one of the categories 120.0-127.7
Mixed helminthiasis NOS

127.9 Intestinal helminthiasis, unspecified

√4th **128 Other and unspecified helminthiases**

128.0 Toxocariasis
Larva migrans visceralis
Toxocara (canis) (cati) infection
Visceral larva migrans syndrome

128.1 Gnathostomiasis
Infection by Gnathostoma spinigerum and related species

128.8 Other specified helminthiasis
Infection by:
Angiostrongylus cantonensis
Capillaria hepatica
other specified helminth

128.9 Helminth infection, unspecified
Helminthiasis NOS
Worms NOS

129 Intestinal parasitism, unspecified

OTHER INFECTIOUS AND PARASITIC DISEASES (130–136)

√4th **130 Toxoplasmosis**
INCLUDES infection by toxoplasma gondii
toxoplasmosis (acquired)
EXCLUDES congenital toxoplasmosis (771.2)

130.0 Meningoencephalitis due to toxoplasmosis
Encephalitis due to acquired toxoplasmosis

130.1 Conjunctivitis due to toxoplasmosis

130.2 Chorioretinitis due to toxoplasmosis
Focal retinochoroiditis due to acquired toxoplasmosis

130.3 Myocarditis due to toxoplasmosis

130.4 Pneumonitis due to toxoplasmosis

130.5 Hepatitis due to toxoplasmosis

130.7 Toxoplasmosis of other specified sites

130.8 Multisystemic disseminated toxoplasmosis
Toxoplasmosis of multiple sites

130.9 Toxoplasmosis, unspecified

√4th **131 Trichomoniasis**
INCLUDES infection due to Trichomonas (vaginalis)

√5th **131.0 Urogenital trichomoniasis**

131.00 Urogenital trichomoniasis, unspecified
Fluor (vaginalis) | trichomonal or due to
Leukorrhea | Trichomonas
(vaginalis) | (vaginalis)
DEF: Trichomonas vaginalis infection of reproductive and urinary organs, transmitted through coitus.

131.01 Trichomonal vulvovaginitis
Vaginitis, trichomonal or due to Trichomonas (vaginalis)
DEF: Trichomonas vaginalis infection of vulva and vagina; often asymptomatic, transmitted through coitus.

131.02 Trichomonal urethritis
DEF: Trichomonas vaginalis infection of the urethra.

131.03 Trichomonal prostatitis
DEF: Trichomonas vaginalis infection of the prostate.

131.09 Other

131.8 Other specified sites
EXCLUDES intestinal (007.3)

131.9 Trichomoniasis, unspecified

√4th **132 Pediculosis and phthirus infestation**

132.0 Pediculus capitis [head louse]

132.1 Pediculus corporis [body louse]

132.2 Phthirus pubis [pubic louse]
Pediculus pubis

132.3 Mixed infestation
Infestation classifiable to more than one of the categories 132.0-132.2

132.9 Pediculosis, unspecified

√4th **133 Acariasis**

133.0 Scabies
Infestation by Sarcoptes scabiei
Norwegian scabies
Sarcoptic itch

133.8 Other acariasis
Chiggers
Infestation by:
Demodex folliculorum
Trombicula

133.9 Acariasis, unspecified
Infestation by mites NOS

√4th **134 Other infestation**

134.0 Myiasis
Infestation by:
Dermatobia (hominis)
fly larvae
Gasterophilus (intestinalis)
maggots
Oestrus ovis

134.1 Other arthropod infestation
Infestation by:
chigoe
sand flea
Tunga penetrans
Jigger disease
Scarabiasis
Tungiasis

134.2 Hirudiniasis
Hirudiniasis (external) (internal)
Leeches (aquatic) (land)

134.8 Other specified infestations

134.9　Infestation, unspecified
　　　Infestation (skin) NOS
　　　Skin parasites NOS

135　Sarcoidosis
　　Besnier-Boeck-Schaumann disease
　　Lupoid (miliary) of Boeck
　　Lupus pernio (Besnier)
　　Lymphogranulomatosis, benign (Schaumann's)
　　Sarcoid (any site):
　　　NOS
　　　Boeck
　　　Darier-Roussy
　　Uveoparotid fever
　　DEF: A chronic, granulomatous reticulosis (abnormal increase in cells), affecting any organ or tissue; acute form has high rate of remission; chronic form is progressive.

✓4ᵗʰ 136　Other and unspecified infectious and parasitic diseases

136.0　Ainhum
　　　Dactylolysis spontanea
　　　DEF: A disease affecting the toes, especially the fifth digit, and the fingers, mostly seen in black adult males; characterized by a linear constriction around the affected digit leading to spontaneous amputation of the distal part of the digit.

136.1　Behçet's syndrome
　　　DEF: A chronic inflammatory disorder of unknown etiology involving the small blood vessels; characterized by recurrent aphthous ulceration of the oral and pharyngeal mucous membranes and the genitalia, skin lesions, severe uveitis, retinal vascularitis and optic atrophy.

✓5ᵗʰ 136.2　Specific infections by free-living amebae

136.21　Specific infection due to acanthamoeba
　　　　　Use additional code to identify manifestation, such as:
　　　　　　keratitis (370.8)

136.29　Other specific infections by free-living amebae
　　　　　Meningoencephalitis due to Naegleria

136.3　Pneumocystosis
　　　Pneumonia due to Pneumocystis carinii
　　　Pneumonia due to Pneumocystis jiroveci
　　　DEF: *Pneumocystis carinii* fungus causing pneumonia in immunocompromised patients; a leading cause of death among AIDS patients.

136.4　Psorospermiasis

136.5　Sarcosporidiosis
　　　Infection by Sarcocystis lindemanni
　　　DEF: *Sarcocystis* infection causing muscle cysts of intestinal inflammation.

136.8　Other specified infectious and parasitic diseases
　　　Candiru infestation

136.9　Unspecified infectious and parasitic diseases
　　　Infectious disease NOS
　　　Parasitic disease NOS

LATE EFFECTS OF INFECTIOUS AND PARASITIC DISEASES (137-139)

✓4ᵗʰ 137　Late effects of tuberculosis
　　Note: This category is to be used to indicate conditions classifiable to 010-018 as the cause of late effects, which are themselves classified elsewhere. The "late effects" include those specified as such, as sequelae, or as due to old or inactive tuberculosis, without evidence of active disease.

137.0　Late effects of respiratory or unspecified tuberculosis

137.1　Late effects of central nervous system tuberculosis

137.2　Late effects of genitourinary tuberculosis

137.3　Late effects of tuberculosis of bones and joints

137.4　Late effects of tuberculosis of other specified organs

138　Late effects of acute poliomyelitis
　　Note: This category is to be used to indicate conditions classifiable to 045 as the cause of late effects, which are themselves classified elsewhere. The "late effects" include conditions specified as such, or as sequelae, or as due to old or inactive poliomyelitis, without evidence of active disease.

✓4ᵗʰ 139　Late effects of other infectious and parasitic diseases
　　Note: This category is to be used to indicate conditions classifiable to categories 001-009, 020-041, 046-136 as the cause of late effects, which are themselves classified elsewhere. The "late effects" include conditions specified as such; they also include sequela of diseases classifiable to the above categories if there is evidence that the disease itself is no longer present.

139.0　Late effects of viral encephalitis
　　　Late effects of conditions classifiable to 049.8-049.9, 062-064

139.1　Late effects of trachoma
　　　Late effects of conditions classifiable to 076

139.8　Late effects of other and unspecified infectious and parasitic diseases

Chapter 2: Neoplasms (140–239)

Coding Guidance

Code neoplasms by behavior and site. According to the most widely accepted definition, a neoplasm is an abnormal mass of tissue, the growth of which exceeds and is uncoordinated with that of the normal tissues and persists in the same excessive manner after cessation of the stimulus that evoked the change.

For ICD-9-CM classification purposes, neoplasms are described in the following four ways:

- Behavior - malignant, benign, uncertain, and unspecified
- Malignant neoplasms are further differentiated into three types. Primary neoplasm identifies the originating site of the tumor. Secondary neoplasm identifies the site to which a primary tumor has metastasized. And carcinoma in situ identifies tumors that are confined to their point of origin and have not invaded surrounding tissue.
- Site - anatomic location of the neoplasm and is used as a subdivision for each of the four types of behaviors
- Functional activity - effects certain neoplasms have on tissues that are functionally active
- Morphology - classification of neoplasms according to tissue type or cell origin

The morphology of a neoplasm is reported using M codes, which are provided as a separate code listing in ICD-9-CM, Appendix A. Morphology codes are usually reported only by the hospital health information management (HIM) department to the national cancer registry. Home Health agencies do not report the morphology of neoplasms to the payers or registry.

Metastatic (secondary) neoplasms are classified to categories 196–198.

Benign neoplasms, classified to categories 210–229, are tumors in which the dividing cells adhere to each other, with the resulting neoplastic mass remaining as a circumscribed lesion.

Uncertain behavior is the term used to describe neoplasms whose behavior cannot be determined at the time of discovery and continued study is necessary to accurately classify the neoplasm by behavior.

Unspecified behavior is assigned when the medical documentation does not specify the behavior of the neoplasm.

The major groups of malignant neoplasms are carcinomas, sarcomas, and mixed tissue tumors. Examples of the mixed tissue tumors are tumors of the kidney, ovary, and testes.

Steps in coding neoplasms using the alphabetic index and neoplasm table:

- Locate the main term for the morphologic type in the alphabetic index.
- Review the subterm entries.
- Look for cross-references and site.
- If the site is not listed as a subterm refer to the neoplasm table according to the cross-reference.
- Locate the anatomical site in the table that lists sites alphabetically.
- Select the appropriate behavior type for the neoplasm.
- Select the appropriate code and verify the code in the tabular list.

Example:

Primary hepatic cell carcinoma.

Using the alphabetic index: Under the main term "Carcinoma" in the alphabetic index locate the subterm hepatic cell. The index directs the coder to the code 155.0. The tabular verifies that code 155.0 includes hepatocellular carcinoma specified as primary. Note that the morphology code indicates this is a primary site malignancy.

Carcinoma (M8010/3)—see also Neoplasm, by site, malignant
    hepatic cell (M8170/3) 155.0
    hepatocellular (M8170/3) 155.0 and bile duct, mixed
        (M8180/3) 155.0

Using the Neoplasm Table

To locate the code for primary hepatic cell carcinoma using the table, search the table for the main entry of anatomic site. In this case hepatic cell carcinoma is neoplasm of the liver. Locate the main term "liver" in the table. The entry contains the subterm "primary." Since the diagnostic statement and the behavior code for primary hepatic cell (liver) carcinoma indicate that this neoplasm is of a primary malignant nature, the coder uses the code listed under the table heading "Malignant." Again the code choice is 155.0.

Coding Metastatic Neoplasms

For neoplasms that have multiple metastatic sites, code all as secondary and code the primary site if indicated.

Example:

Metastatic neoplasm of the lung and brain from the oropharynx. The oropharynx is the primary site (146.8) and the lung (197.0) and brain (198.3) are secondary sites.

When either the primary or the secondary site is not indicated or documented, code 199.1 Malignant neoplasm without specification of site, is assigned. For neoplasms that have multiple metastatic sites and no primary site indicated, code all as secondary and code the primary site to 199.1.

In those cases where the neoplasm is a single metastatic site and the morphologic type is indicated, the coder first locates the morphologic term in the alphabetic index either as a separate entry or under the main term "Carcinoma."

For example, metastatic hepatic cell carcinoma of the stomach is coded 155.0 and 197.8. The user is directed by the index under the main term "Carcinoma" to code hepatic cell carcinoma 155.0 Malignant neoplasm, liver, primary. The secondary site is the stomach and is coded as 197.8. Do not assign the unspecified code 199.1 when the morphologic type indicates a primary site.

If the morphology does not indicate a primary site and the neoplasm is identified as a single metastatic site, assign code 199.1, indicating the unspecified primary site. In addition, assign a code identifying the single specified metastatic site.

For patients who are in remission or are no longer considered to have a malignant neoplasm, personal history of malignant neoplasm codes V10.00–V10.9, should be updated.

Malignant Neoplasms of Solid Tumor Type (140–199)

Solid tumors have the capacity to spread to adjacent (direct extension metastasis) or distant sites in the body (embolic metastasis). The method of spreading is not reflected in the code assignment, only the fact that there has been metastasis. When there has been direct extension and the site of origin cannot be determined (i.e., the neoplasm exists over two adjacent [contiguous] sites), ICD-9-CM classifies that neoplasm as other specified site, fourth digit of 8.

Code 199.2 reports malignant neoplasm associated with a transplanted organ. Organ recipients are routinely placed on immunosuppressive drugs to prevent rejection of the transplanted organ, but this immunosuppression also renders them vulnerable to infection and disease, including malignancy. Additionally, a transplanted organ may contain malignant cells that were undetected prior to transplant. Multiple transplant operations may be a result of transplanted organ failure, rejection, or other complications such as neoplasm. Instructional notes are included with code 199.2 Malignant neoplasm associated with transplanted organ to "code first complication of transplanted organ (996.80–996.89)" and "use additional code for specific malignancy site." Multiple codes are required and are reported in a specific sequence.

Malignant Neoplasms of Lymphatic and Hematopoietic Tissue (200–208)

Malignant neoplasms of the lymphatic and hematopoietic tissues are considered primary neoplasms and are not considered to spread to secondary sites. The malignant cells circulate to other areas but these are not considered secondary sites.

Some of the types of neoplasms included in this section are lymphosarcomas, Hodgkin's disease, lymphomas, malignant histocytosis, multiple myeloma, myeloid leukemia, acute leukemia and chronic leukemia.

Fifth-digit subclassification used with categories 200–202 specifies the lymph node involvement with the disease. It is acceptable to assign two different fourth-digit codes from the same three-digit category. For example, a patient diagnosed with T-cell lymphoma and Sezary syndrome is assigned both 202.2x Sezary syndrome, and 202.1x Mycosis fungoides.

Relapse, or recurrence, of leukemia occurs when the disease returns either during therapy or after being successfully treated (remission). Relapse during or soon after the completion of treatment is generally considered less favorable than relapse after remission has been achieved. Interventions and treatments may vary from induction (primary) therapy, and may be more aggressive in nature. Due to the increased risks associated with treating leukemia that relapsed prior to achieving remission, the fifth-digit definitions to the hematopoietic neoplasm code categories 203–208 facilitate tracking disease progression of relapse with or without having achieved remission.

Sequencing guidelines governing code assignment for cases involving neoplasms depends on focus of the treatment. If treatment is directed to the primary site, code the primary malignancy first. If treatment is directed toward the secondary site only, code the secondary neoplasm as principal diagnosis. When a patient is admitted only for chemotherapy or radiotherapy, assign code V58.0 or V58.1 [V58.11], respectively, with the malignancy coded as a secondary diagnosis. For treatment directed toward a complication of therapy, code the complication as primary and the malignancy as a secondary code.

Neuroendocrine Tumors (209)

Carcinoid tumors are a specific type of slow-growing malignant neoplasms originating in the cells of the neuroendocrine system. Although the terms "carcinoid" and "neuroendocrine" may be used interchangeably in the clinical environment to describe specific types of neoplasm, carcinoid tumor is one type of neuroendocrine neoplasm. Neuroendocrine cells produce and secrete regulatory hormones. Tumors comprised of these cells are consequently capable of producing hormonal syndromes (e.g., carcinoid syndrome), in which the normal hormonal balance required to support body system functions is adversely affected. Symptoms caused by neuroendocrine tumors arise from the abnormal secretion of hormones due to the presence of neoplastic growth and its affected tissues. As a result, many of these tumors are associated with a diverse range of characteristic hormonal syndromes such as multiple endocrine neoplasia syndromes, classifiable to subcategory 258.0 and carcinoid syndrome (259.2). Carcinoid syndrome (259.2) is the most common systemic syndrome associated with carcinoid tumors. Carcinoid syndrome causes patients to have flushing, diarrhea, and heart disease. It is caused by an abnormally high concentration of serotonin secretion. Carcinoid tumors occur most commonly in the respiratory and gastrointestinal tract, and usually originate in hormone-producing cells in the linings of these organs. They can also occur in the pancreas, testes, ovaries, or lungs. Gastrointestinal carcinoid tumors are classified according to the presumed embryonic site of origin: the foregut (bronchi and stomach), the midgut (small intestine and appendix), and the hindgut (colon and rectum). Carcinoid tumors have different expected outcomes than more common neoplasms, and require different treatments. For example, an adenocarcinoma may be treated with cytotoxic chemotherapy, while a neuroendocrine tumor is likely to be more responsive to hormonal therapies due to the nature of the neoplasm.

Benign Neoplasms (210–229)

Benign neoplasms, classified to categories 210–229, are tumors in which the dividing cells adhere to each other, with the resulting neoplastic mass remaining as a circumscribed lesion. These tumor cells, which are not cancerous, do not metastasize or invade adjacent structures.

Carcinoma In Situ (230–234)

Carcinoma in situ are neoplasms that have the potential for spreading to surrounding tissue but remain limited and have not extended beyond the basement membrane of the epithelial tissue. Other common terms used to describe carcinoma in situ are noninfiltrating, noninvasive, intraepithelial, or preinvasive carcinoma. Neoplasms classified to this section of ICD-9-CM include carcinoma of the digestive tract, respiratory system, skin, breast, and genitourinary system.

For example, in situ carcinoma of the breast, lower outer quadrant is coded 233.0. Coders may use either the neoplasm table or the Index to locate this code. In the Index under the main term "Carcinoma" locate the subterm "in situ (M8010/2)—see also Neoplasm, by site, in situ." This indicates that the coder should refer to the neoplasm table under "Breast, in situ."

Certain severe dysplasias are classified as carcinoma in situ. Dysplastic tissue may be described as an alteration of cellular organization, size, and shape. These alterations may progress to cancerous conditions. Dysplasia and carcinoma in situ are definitive diagnoses based upon histological examination of biopsied tissue. For example, vaginal intraepithelial neoplasia (VAIN III) is reported with code 233.31 Carcinoma in situ of other and unspecified female genital organs, vagina, while vulvar intraepithelial neoplasia (VIN III) is reported with code 233.32 Carcinoma in situ of other and unspecified female genital organs, vulva.

Neoplasms of Uncertain Behavior (235–238)

Neoplasms of uncertain behavior consist of cells in an intermediate stage that require further testing to determine subsequent behavior. These neoplasms are classified to category codes 235–238. Codes from this column should only be used when "uncertain behavior" appears on the pathology report. Note: Uncertain behavior is a histomorphological determination, as distinguished from "unspecified," which indicates lack of documentation to support a more specific code assignment. Do not confuse "uncertain behavior" with "unspecified." The two terms are not interchangeable.

Post-transplant lymphoproliferative disorder (PTLD) (238.77) is a disease of uncontrolled proliferation or production of B cell lymphocytes, often following infection with the Epstein-Barr virus for post-transplant patients. The clinical presentation of PTLD varies. The patient may present asymptomatically or with localized or systemic symptoms such as one or more nodal or extranodal tumors. Systemic presentations may range from an unexplained infectious syndrome or mononucleosis-like illness with or without lymphadenopathy to a disseminated sepsis syndrome. Symptoms of PTLD are related to the site of tumor growth. For example, gastrointestinal tumors can cause abdominal pain with hemorrhage and perforation, resulting in peritonitis. Diagnosis may be confirmed with histopathological changes on biopsy. After cessation of immunosuppressive drug therapy, PTLD may regress spontaneously.

Code 238.77 includes an instructional note to "code first complications of transplant (996.80–996.89)." Therefore, PTLD is reported as a secondary diagnosis, with the appropriate subcategory 996.8 as the first-listed diagnosis.

Neoplasms of Unspecified Nature (239)

Category 239 classifies by site neoplasms of unspecified morphology or behavior. This means the medical record contains no further information to more accurately code the condition. Neoplasm of unspecified nature indicates a lack of specific information in the documentation while neoplasm of uncertain behavior refers to incomplete assessment of the neoplasm. Other terms often documented in records with no further information include neoplasm, new growth, tumor, or growth.

Coding and Sequencing Complications of Malignancy or Antineoplastic Therapy

When the encounter is for management of an anemia associated with the malignancy and the care is directed only toward the anemia, the appropriate anemia code (such as code 285.22, Anemia in neoplastic disease) is designated as the principal diagnosis and is followed by the appropriate code(s) for the malignancy. Code 285.22 may also be used as a secondary code if the patient suffers from anemia and is being treated for the malignancy.

When the encounter is for management of an anemia due to chemotherapy, immunotherapy, or radiotherapy and the care is directed only toward the anemia, the anemia is sequenced first. The appropriate neoplasm code should be assigned as an additional code.

Code 285.22 Anemia in neoplastic disease, and code 285.3 Antineoplastic chemotherapy induced anemia, may both be assigned if anemia in neoplastic disease and anemia due to antineoplastic chemotherapy are both documented.

When the encounter is for management of dehydration due to the malignancy or the therapy, or a combination of both, and only the dehydration is being treated (intravenous rehydration), the dehydration is sequenced first, followed by the code(s) for the malignancy.

When the encounter is for treatment of a complication resulting from a surgical procedure, designate the complication as the principal or first-listed diagnosis.

2. NEOPLASMS (140-239)

Notes:

1. Content

   This chapter contains the following broad groups:

   140-195   Malignant neoplasms, stated or presumed to be primary, of specified sites, except of lymphatic and hematopoietic tissue

   196-198   Malignant neoplasms, stated or presumed to be secondary, of specified sites

   199   Malignant neoplasms, without specification of site

   200-208   Malignant neoplasms, stated or presumed to be primary, of lymphatic and hematopoietic tissue

   209   Neuroendocrine tumors

   210-229   Benign neoplasms

   230-234   Carcinoma in situ

   235-238   Neoplasms of uncertain behavior [see Note, above category 235]

   239   Neoplasms of unspecified nature

2. Functional activity

   All neoplasms are classified in this chapter, whether or not functionally active. An additional code from Chapter 3 may be used to identify such functional activity associated with any neoplasm, e.g.:

   > catecholamine-producing malignant pheochromocytoma of adrenal:
   >
   > > code 194.0, additional code 255.6
   >
   > basophil adenoma of pituitary with Cushing's syndrome:
   >
   > > code 227.3, additional code 255.0

3. Morphology [Histology]

   For those wishing to identify the histological type of neoplasms, a comprehensive coded nomenclature, which comprises the morphology rubrics of the ICD-Oncology, is given in Appendix A.

4. Malignant neoplasms overlapping site boundaries

   Categories 140-195 are for the classification of primary malignant neoplasms according to their point of origin. A malignant neoplasm that overlaps two or more subcategories within a three-digit rubric and whose point of origin cannot be determined should be classified to the subcategory .8 "Other."

   For example, "carcinoma involving tip and ventral surface of tongue" should be assigned to 141.8. On the other hand, "carcinoma of tip of tongue, extending to involve the ventral surface" should be coded to 141.2, as the point of origin, the tip, is known. Three subcategories (149.8, 159.8, 165.8) have been provided for malignant neoplasms that overlap the boundaries of three-digit rubrics within certain systems.

   Overlapping malignant neoplasms that cannot be classified as indicated above should be assigned to the appropriate subdivision of category 195 (Malignant neoplasm of other and ill-defined sites).

   > **DEF:** An abnormal growth; morphology determines behavior, i.e., whether it will remain intact (benign) or spread to adjacent tissue (malignant). The term mass is not synonymous with neoplasm, as it is often used to describe cysts and thickenings such as those occurring with hematoma or infection.

MALIGNANT NEOPLASM OF LIP, ORAL CAVITY, AND PHARYNX (140-149)

> EXCLUDES   carcinoma in situ (230.0)

✓4ᵗʰ **140 Malignant neoplasm of lip**

> EXCLUDES   malignant melanoma of skin of lip (172.0)
> malignant neoplasm of skin of lip (173.00-173.09)

140.0 Upper lip, vermilion border

Upper lip:
NOS
external
lipstick area

140.1 Lower lip, vermilion border

Lower lip:
NOS
external
lipstick area

Lip

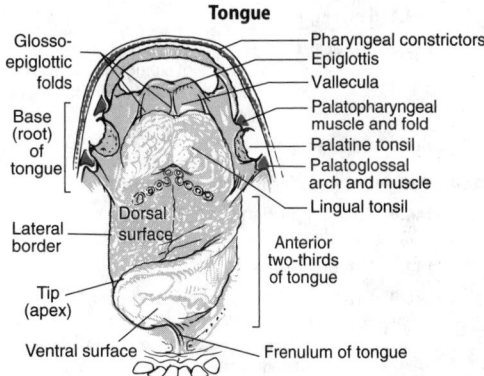

140.3 Upper lip, inner aspect

Upper lip:
buccal aspect
frenulum
mucosa
oral aspect

140.4 Lower lip, inner aspect

Lower lip:
buccal aspect
frenulum
mucosa
oral aspect

140.5 Lip, unspecified, inner aspect

Lip, not specified whether upper or lower:
buccal aspect
frenulum
mucosa
oral aspect

140.6 Commissure of lip

Labial commissure

140.8 Other sites of lip

Malignant neoplasm of contiguous or overlapping sites of lip whose point of origin cannot be determined

140.9 Lip, unspecified, vermilion border

Lip, not specified as upper or lower:
NOS
external
lipstick area

✓4ᵗʰ **141 Malignant neoplasm of tongue**

141.0 Base of tongue

Dorsal surface of base of tongue
Fixed part of tongue NOS

141.1 Dorsal surface of tongue

Anterior two-thirds of tongue, dorsal surface
Dorsal tongue NOS
Midline of tongue

> EXCLUDES   *dorsal surface of base of tongue (141.0)*

141.2 Tip and lateral border of tongue

Tongue

Main Salivary Glands

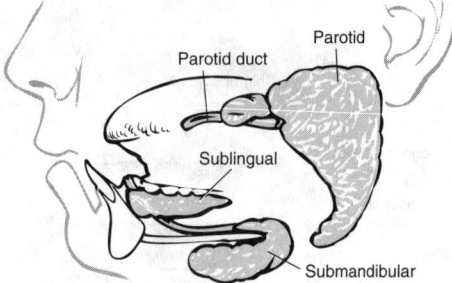

141.3 Ventral surface of tongue
Anterior two-thirds of tongue, ventral surface
Frenulum linguae

141.4 Anterior two-thirds of tongue, part unspecified
Mobile part of tongue NOS

141.5 Junctional zone
Border of tongue at junction of fixed and mobile parts at insertion of anterior tonsillar pillar

141.6 Lingual tonsil

141.8 Other sites of tongue
Malignant neoplasm of contiguous or overlapping sites of tongue whose point of origin cannot be determined

141.9 Tongue, unspecified
Tongue NOS

√4ᵗʰ 142 Malignant neoplasm of major salivary glands
INCLUDES salivary ducts
EXCLUDES *malignant neoplasm of minor salivary glands:*
NOS (145.9)
buccal mucosa (145.0)
soft palate (145.3)
tongue (141.0-141.9)
tonsil, palatine (146.0)

142.0 Parotid gland

142.1 Submandibular gland
Submaxillary gland

142.2 Sublingual gland

142.8 Other major salivary glands
Malignant neoplasm of contiguous or overlapping sites of salivary glands and ducts whose point of origin cannot be determined

142.9 Salivary gland, unspecified
Salivary gland (major) NOS

√4ᵗʰ 143 Malignant neoplasm of gum
INCLUDES alveolar (ridge) mucosa
gingiva (alveolar) (marginal)
interdental papillae
EXCLUDES *malignant odontogenic neoplasms (170.0-170.1)*

143.0 Upper gum

143.1 Lower gum

143.8 Other sites of gum
Malignant neoplasm of contiguous or overlapping sites of gum whose point of origin cannot be determined

143.9 Gum, unspecified

√4ᵗʰ 144 Malignant neoplasm of floor of mouth

144.0 Anterior portion
Anterior to the premolar-canine junction

144.1 Lateral portion

144.8 Other sites of floor of mouth
Malignant neoplasm of contiguous or overlapping sites of floor of mouth whose point of origin cannot be determined

144.9 Floor of mouth, part unspecified

Mouth

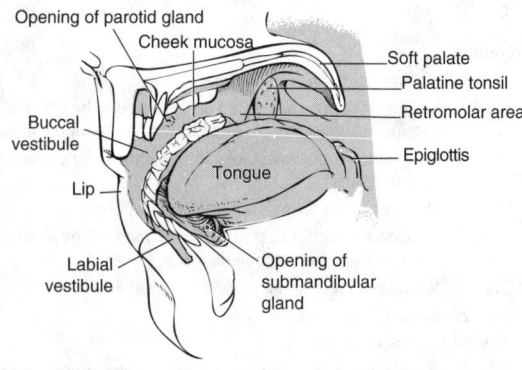

√4ᵗʰ 145 Malignant neoplasm of other and unspecified parts of mouth
EXCLUDES *mucosa of lips (140.0-140.9)*

145.0 Cheek mucosa
Buccal mucosa
Cheek, inner aspect

145.1 Vestibule of mouth
Buccal sulcus (upper) (lower)
Labial sulcus (upper) (lower)

145.2 Hard palate

145.3 Soft palate
EXCLUDES *nasopharyngeal [posterior] [superior] surface of soft palate (147.3)*

145.4 Uvula

145.5 Palate, unspecified
Junction of hard and soft palate
Roof of mouth

145.6 Retromolar area

145.8 Other specified parts of mouth
Malignant neoplasm of contiguous or overlapping sites of mouth whose point of origin cannot be determined

145.9 Mouth, unspecified
Buccal cavity NOS
Minor salivary gland, unspecified site
Oral cavity NOS

√4ᵗʰ 146 Malignant neoplasm of oropharynx

146.0 Tonsil
Tonsil:
NOS
faucial
palatine
EXCLUDES *lingual tonsil (141.6)*
pharyngeal tonsil (147.1)

146.1 Tonsillar fossa

Oropharynx

Nasopharynx

Hypopharynx

146.2 Tonsillar pillars (anterior) (posterior)
Faucial pillar   Palatoglossal arch
Glossopalatine fold   Palatopharyngeal arch

146.3 Vallecula
Anterior and medial surface of the pharyngoepiglottic fold

146.4 Anterior aspect of epiglottis
Epiglottis, free border [margin]
Glossoepiglottic fold(s)
EXCLUDES   *epiglottis:*
     NOS (161.1)
     suprahyoid portion (161.1)

146.5 Junctional region
Junction of the free margin of the epiglottis, the aryepiglottic fold, and the pharyngoepiglottic fold

146.6 Lateral wall of oropharynx

146.7 Posterior wall of oropharynx

146.8 Other specified sites of oropharynx
Branchial cleft
Malignant neoplasm of contiguous or overlapping sites of oropharynx whose point of origin cannot be determined

146.9 Oropharynx, unspecified

✓4ᵗʰ **147 Malignant neoplasm of nasopharynx**

147.0 Superior wall
Roof of nasopharynx

147.1 Posterior wall
Adenoid
Pharyngeal tonsil

147.2 Lateral wall
Fossa of Rosenmüller
Opening of auditory tube
Pharyngeal recess

147.3 Anterior wall
Floor of nasopharynx
Nasopharyngeal [posterior] [superior] surface of soft palate
Posterior margin of nasal septum and choanae

147.8 Other specified sites of nasopharynx
Malignant neoplasm of contiguous or overlapping sites of nasopharynx whose point of origin cannot be determined

147.9 Nasopharynx, unspecified
Nasopharyngeal wall NOS

✓4ᵗʰ **148 Malignant neoplasm of hypopharynx**

148.0 Postcricoid region

148.1 Pyriform sinus
Pyriform fossa

148.2 Aryepiglottic fold, hypopharyngeal aspect
Aryepiglottic fold or interarytenoid fold:
    NOS
    marginal zone
EXCLUDES   *aryepiglottic fold or interarytenoid fold, laryngeal aspect (161.1)*

148.3 Posterior hypopharyngeal wall

148.8 Other specified sites of hypopharynx
Malignant neoplasm of contiguous or overlapping sites of hypopharynx whose point of origin cannot be determined

148.9 Hypopharynx, unspecified
Hypopharyngeal wall NOS
Hypopharynx NOS

✓4ᵗʰ **149 Malignant neoplasm of other and ill-defined sites within the lip, oral cavity, and pharynx**

149.0 Pharynx, unspecified

149.1 Waldeyer's ring

149.8 Other
Malignant neoplasms of lip, oral cavity, and pharynx whose point of origin cannot be assigned to any one of the categories 140-148
EXCLUDES   *"book leaf" neoplasm [ventral surface of tongue and floor of mouth] (145.8)*

149.9 Ill-defined

MALIGNANT NEOPLASM OF DIGESTIVE ORGANS AND PERITONEUM (150-159)
EXCLUDES   *carcinoma in situ (230.1-230.9)*

✓4ᵗʰ **150 Malignant neoplasm of esophagus**

150.0 Cervical esophagus

150.1 Thoracic esophagus

150.2 Abdominal esophagus
EXCLUDES   *adenocarcinoma (151.0)*
     cardio-esophageal junction (151.0)

150.3 Upper third of esophagus
Proximal third of esophagus

150.4 Middle third of esophagus

150.5 Lower third of esophagus
Distal third of esophagus
EXCLUDES   *adenocarcinoma (151.0)*
     cardio-esophageal junction (151.0)

150.8 Other specified part
Malignant neoplasm of contiguous or overlapping sites of esophagus whose point of origin cannot be determined

150.9 Esophagus, unspecified

✓4ᵗʰ **151 Malignant neoplasm of stomach**
EXCLUDES   *benign carcinoid tumor of stomach (209.63)*
     malignant carcinoid tumor of stomach (209.23)

151.0 Cardia
Cardiac orifice
Cardio-esophageal junction
EXCLUDES   *squamous cell carcinoma (150.2, 150.5)*

151.1 Pylorus
Prepylorus
Pyloric canal

151.2 Pyloric antrum
Antrum of stomach NOS

151.3 Fundus of stomach

151.4 Body of stomach

151.5 Lesser curvature, unspecified
Lesser curvature, not classifiable to 151.1-151.4

151.6 Greater curvature, unspecified
Greater curvature, not classifiable to 151.0-151.4

151.8 Other specified sites of stomach
Anterior wall, not classifiable to 151.0-151.4
Posterior wall, not classifiable to 151.0-151.4
Malignant neoplasm of contiguous or overlapping sites of stomach whose point of origin cannot be determined

151.9 Stomach, unspecified
Carcinoma ventriculi
Gastric cancer

✓4ᵗʰ **152 Malignant neoplasm of small intestine, including duodenum**
EXCLUDES   *benign carcinoid tumor of small intestine and duodenum (209.40-209.43)*
malignant carcinoid tumor of small intestine and duodenum (209.00-209.03)

152.0 Duodenum

152.1 Jejunum

152.2 Ileum
EXCLUDES   *ileocecal valve (153.4)*

152.3 Meckel's diverticulum

152.8 Other specified sites of small intestine
Duodenojejunal junction
Malignant neoplasm of contiguous or overlapping sites of small intestine whose point of origin cannot be determined

152.9 Small intestine, unspecified

✓4ᵗʰ **153 Malignant neoplasm of colon**
EXCLUDES   *benign carcinoid tumor of colon (209.50-209.56)*
malignant carcinoid tumor of colon (209.10-209.16)

153.0 Hepatic flexure

153.1 Transverse colon

153.2 Descending colon
Left colon

153.3 Sigmoid colon
Sigmoid (flexure)
EXCLUDES   *rectosigmoid junction (154.0)*

153.4 Cecum
Ileocecal valve

153.5 Appendix

153.6 Ascending colon
Right colon

153.7 Splenic flexure

153.8 Other specified sites of large intestine
Malignant neoplasm of contiguous or overlapping sites of colon whose point of origin cannot be determined
EXCLUDES   *ileocecal valve (153.4)*
rectosigmoid junction (154.0)

153.9 Colon, unspecified
Large intestine NOS

✓4ᵗʰ **154 Malignant neoplasm of rectum, rectosigmoid junction, and anus**
EXCLUDES   *benign carcinoid tumor of rectum (209.57)*
malignant carcinoid tumor of rectum (209.17)

154.0 Rectosigmoid junction
Colon with rectum
Rectosigmoid (colon)

154.1 Rectum
Rectal ampulla

154.2 Anal canal
Anal sphincter
EXCLUDES   *malignant melanoma of skin of anus (172.5)*
malignant neoplasm of skin of anus (173.50-173.59)

154.3 Anus, unspecified
EXCLUDES   *malignant melanoma of:*
anus:
margin (172.5)
skin (172.5)
perianal skin (172.5)
malignant neoplasm of:
anus:
margin (173.50-173.59)
skin (173.50-173.59)
perianal skin (173.50-173.59)

154.8 Other
Anorectum
Cloacogenic zone
Malignant neoplasm of contiguous or overlapping sites of rectum, rectosigmoid junction, and anus whose point of origin cannot be determined

✓4ᵗʰ **155 Malignant neoplasm of liver and intrahepatic bile ducts**

155.0 Liver, primary
Carcinoma:
liver, specified as primary
hepatocellular
liver cell
Hepatoblastoma

155.1 Intrahepatic bile ducts
Canaliculi biliferi   Intrahepatic:
Interlobular: biliary passages
  bile ducts   canaliculi
  biliary canals   gall duct
EXCLUDES   *hepatic duct (156.1)*

155.2 Liver, not specified as primary or secondary

✓4ᵗʰ **156 Malignant neoplasm of gallbladder and extrahepatic bile ducts**

156.0 Gallbladder

156.1 Extrahepatic bile ducts
Biliary duct or passage NOS
Common bile duct
Cystic duct
Hepatic duct
Sphincter of Oddi

Colon

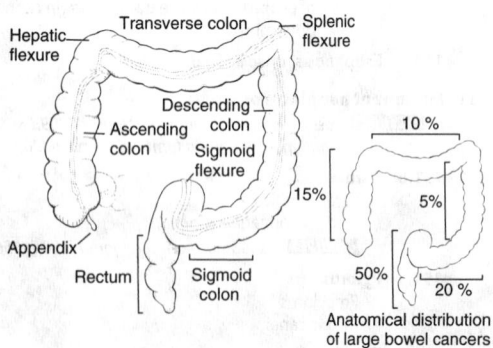

Anatomical distribution of large bowel cancers

Retroperitoneum and Peritoneum

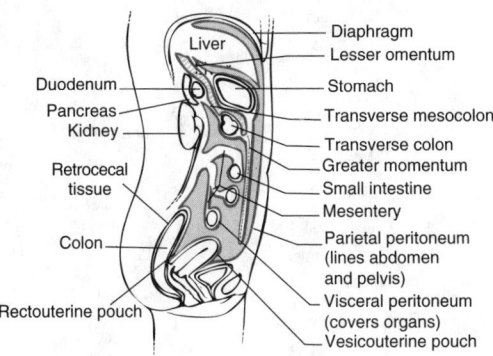

156.2 Ampulla of Vater
> **DEF:** Malignant neoplasm in the area of dilation at the juncture of the common bile and pancreatic ducts near the opening into the lumen of the duodenum.

156.8 Other specified sites of gallbladder and extrahepatic bile ducts
> Malignant neoplasm of contiguous or overlapping sites of gallbladder and extrahepatic bile ducts whose point of origin cannot be determined

156.9 Biliary tract, part unspecified
> Malignant neoplasm involving both intrahepatic and extrahepatic bile ducts

✓4ᵗʰ 157 Malignant neoplasm of pancreas

157.0 Head of pancreas

157.1 Body of pancreas

157.2 Tail of pancreas

157.3 Pancreatic duct
> Duct of:
> Santorini
> Wirsung

157.4 Islets of Langerhans
> Islets of Langerhans, any part of pancreas
> Use additional code to identify any functional activity
> **DEF:** Malignant neoplasm within the structures of the pancreas that produce insulin, somatostatin and glucagon.

157.8 Other specified sites of pancreas
> Ectopic pancreatic tissue
> Malignant neoplasm of contiguous or overlapping sites of pancreas whose point of origin cannot be determined

157.9 Pancreas, part unspecified

✓4ᵗʰ 158 Malignant neoplasm of retroperitoneum and peritoneum

158.0 Retroperitoneum
> Periadrenal tissue   Perirenal tissue
> Perinephric tissue   Retrocecal tissue

158.8 Specified parts of peritoneum
> Cul-de-sac (of Douglas)
> Malignant neoplasm of contiguous or overlapping sites of retroperitoneum and peritoneum whose point of origin cannot be determined
> Mesentery
> Mesocolon
> Omentum
> Peritoneum:
> parietal
> pelvic
> Rectouterine pouch

158.9 Peritoneum, unspecified

✓4ᵗʰ 159 Malignant neoplasm of other and ill-defined sites within the digestive organs and peritoneum

159.0 Intestinal tract, part unspecified
> Intestine NOS

159.1 Spleen, not elsewhere classified
> Angiosarcoma ⎱ of spleen
> Fibrosarcoma ⎰
> **EXCLUDES**   Hodgkin's disease (201.0-201.9)
> lymphosarcoma (200.1)
> reticulosarcoma (200.0)

159.8 Other sites of digestive system and intra-abdominal organs
> Malignant neoplasm of digestive organs and peritoneum whose point of origin cannot be assigned to any one of the categories 150-158
> **EXCLUDES**   anus and rectum (154.8)
> cardio-esophageal junction (151.0)
> colon and rectum (154.0)

159.9 Ill-defined
> Alimentary canal or tract NOS
> Gastrointestinal tract NOS
> **EXCLUDES**   abdominal NOS (195.2)
> intra-abdominal NOS (195.2)

NEOPLASM OF RESPIRATORY AND INTRATHORACIC ORGANS (160-165)

> **EXCLUDES**   carcinoma in situ (231.0-231.9)

✓4ᵗʰ 160 Malignant neoplasm of nasal cavities, middle ear, and accessory sinuses

160.0 Nasal cavities
> Cartilage of nose   Septum of nose
> Conchae, nasal   Vestibule of nose
> Internal nose
> **EXCLUDES**   malignant melanoma of skin of nose (172.3)
> malignant neoplasm of skin of nose (173.30-173.39)
> nasal bone (170.0)
> nose NOS (195.0)
> olfactory bulb (192.0)
> posterior margin of septum and choanae (147.3)
> turbinates (170.0)

160.1 Auditory tube, middle ear, and mastoid air cells
> Antrum tympanicum
> Eustachian tube
> Tympanic cavity
> **EXCLUDES**   bone of ear (meatus) (170.0)
> cartilage of ear (171.0)
> malignant melanoma of:
> auditory canal (external) (172.2)
> ear (external) (skin) (172.2)
> malignant neoplasm of:
> auditory canal (external) (173.20-173.29)
> ear (external) (skin) (173.20-173.29)

160.2 Maxillary sinus
> Antrum (Highmore) (maxillary)

160.3 Ethmoidal sinus

160.4 Frontal sinus

160.5 Sphenoidal sinus

160.8 Other
> Malignant neoplasm of contiguous or overlapping sites of nasal cavities, middle ear, and accessory sinuses whose point of origin cannot be determined

160.9 Accessory sinus, unspecified

✓4ᵗʰ 161 Malignant neoplasm of larynx

161.0 Glottis
> Intrinsic larynx
> Laryngeal commissure (anterior) (posterior)
> True vocal cord
> Vocal cord NOS

161.1 Supraglottis
Aryepiglottic fold or interarytenoid fold, laryngeal aspect
Epiglottis (suprahyoid portion) NOS
Extrinsic larynx
False vocal cords
Posterior (laryngeal) surface of epiglottis
Ventricular bands
> EXCLUDES *anterior aspect of epiglottis (146.4)*
> *aryepiglottic fold or interarytenoid fold:*
> *NOS (148.2)*
> *hypopharyngeal aspect (148.2)*
> *marginal zone (148.2)*

161.2 Subglottis

161.3 Laryngeal cartilages
Cartilage:
  arytenoid
  cricoid
  cuneiform
  thyroid

161.8 Other specified sites of larynx
Malignant neoplasm of contiguous or overlapping sites of larynx whose point of origin cannot be determined

161.9 Larynx, unspecified

√4ᵗʰ **162 Malignant neoplasm of trachea, bronchus, and lung**
> EXCLUDES *benign carcinoid tumor of bronchus (209.61)*
> *malignant carcinoid tumor of bronchus (209.21)*

162.0 Trachea
Cartilage
Mucosa } of trachea

162.2 Main bronchus
Carina
Hilus of lung

162.3 Upper lobe, bronchus or lung

162.4 Middle lobe, bronchus or lung

162.5 Lower lobe, bronchus or lung

162.8 Other parts of bronchus or lung
Malignant neoplasm of contiguous or overlapping sites of bronchus or lung whose point of origin cannot be determined

162.9 Bronchus and lung, unspecified

√4ᵗʰ **163 Malignant neoplasm of pleura**

163.0 Parietal pleura

163.1 Visceral pleura

163.8 Other specified sites of pleura
Malignant neoplasm of contiguous or overlapping sites of pleura whose point of origin cannot be determined

163.9 Pleura, unspecified

√4ᵗʰ **164 Malignant neoplasm of thymus, heart, and mediastinum**

164.0 Thymus
> EXCLUDES *benign carcinoid tumor of the thymus (209.62)*
> *malignant carcinoid tumor of the thymus (209.22)*

164.1 Heart
Endocardium
Epicardium
Myocardium
Pericardium
> EXCLUDES *great vessels (171.4)*

164.2 Anterior mediastinum

164.3 Posterior mediastinum

164.8 Other
Malignant neoplasm of contiguous or overlapping sites of thymus, heart, and mediastinum whose point of origin cannot be determined

164.9 Mediastinum, part unspecified

Skull

√4ᵗʰ **165 Malignant neoplasm of other and ill-defined sites within the respiratory system and intrathoracic organs**

165.0 Upper respiratory tract, part unspecified

165.8 Other
Malignant neoplasm of respiratory and intrathoracic organs whose point of origin cannot be assigned to any one of the categories 160-164

165.9 Ill-defined sites within the respiratory system
Respiratory tract NOS
> EXCLUDES *intrathoracic NOS (195.1)*
> *thoracic NOS (195.1)*

MALIGNANT NEOPLASM OF BONE, CONNECTIVE TISSUE, SKIN, AND BREAST (170-176)
> EXCLUDES *carcinoma in situ:*
> *breast (233.0)*
> *skin (232.0-232.9)*

√4ᵗʰ **170 Malignant neoplasm of bone and articular cartilage**
> INCLUDES cartilage (articular) (joint)
> periosteum
> EXCLUDES *bone marrow NOS (202.9)*
> *cartilage:*
> *ear (171.0)*
> *eyelid (171.0)*
> *larynx (161.3)*
> *nose (160.0)*
> *synovia (171.0-171.9)*

170.0 Bones of skull and face, except mandible

Bone:	Bone:
ethmoid	sphenoid
frontal	temporal
malar	zygomatic
nasal	Maxilla (superior)
occipital	Turbinate
orbital	Upper jaw bone
parietal	Vomer

> EXCLUDES *carcinoma, any type except intraosseous or odontogenic:*
> *maxilla, maxillary (sinus) (160.2)*
> *upper jaw bone (143.0)*
> *jaw bone (lower) (170.1)*

170.1 Mandible
Inferior maxilla
Jaw bone NOS
Lower jaw bone
> EXCLUDES *carcinoma, any type except intraosseous or odontogenic:*
> *jaw bone NOS (143.9)*
> *lower (143.1)*
> *upper jaw bone (170.0)*

170.2 Vertebral column, excluding sacrum and coccyx
Spinal column
Spine
Vertebra
> EXCLUDES *sacrum and coccyx (170.6)*

170.3   Ribs, sternum, and clavicle
Costal cartilage
Costovertebral joint
Xiphoid process

170.4   Scapula and long bones of upper limb
Acromion
Bones NOS of upper limb
Humerus
Radius
Ulna

170.5   Short bones of upper limb

Carpal	Scaphoid (of hand)
Cuneiform, wrist	Semilunar or lunate
Metacarpal	Trapezium
Navicular, of hand	Trapezoid
Phalanges of hand	Unciform
Pisiform	

170.6   Pelvic bones, sacrum, and coccyx
Coccygeal vertebra
Ilium
Ischium
Pubic bone
Sacral vertebra

170.7   Long bones of lower limb
Bones NOS of lower limb
Femur
Fibula
Tibia

170.8   Short bones of lower limb

Astragalus [talus]	Navicular (of ankle)
Calcaneus	Patella
Cuboid	Phalanges of foot
Cuneiform, ankle	Tarsal
Metatarsal	

170.9   Bone and articular cartilage, site unspecified

√4ᵗʰ **171   Malignant neoplasm of connective and other soft tissue**

INCLUDES   blood vessel
bursa
fascia
fat
ligament, except uterine
muscle
peripheral, sympathetic, and parasympathetic
    nerves and ganglia
synovia
tendon (sheath)

EXCLUDES   *cartilage (of):*
    articular (170.0-170.9)
    larynx (161.3)
    nose (160.0)
connective tissue:
    breast (174.0-175.9)
    internal organs–code to malignant neoplasm of the
        site [e.g., leiomyosarcoma of stomach, 151.9]
heart (164.1)
uterine ligament (183.4)

171.0   Head, face, and neck
Cartilage of:
    ear
    eyelid

171.2   Upper limb, including shoulder
Arm
Finger
Forearm
Hand

171.3   Lower limb, including hip
Foot
Leg
Popliteal space
Thigh
Toe

171.4   Thorax
Axilla
Diaphragm
Great vessels
EXCLUDES   *heart (164.1)*
    mediastinum (164.2-164.9)
    thymus (164.0)

171.5   Abdomen
Abdominal wall
Hypochondrium
EXCLUDES   *peritoneum (158.8)*
    retroperitoneum (158.0)

171.6   Pelvis
Buttock
Groin
Inguinal region
Perineum
EXCLUDES   *pelvic peritoneum (158.8)*
    retroperitoneum (158.0)
    uterine ligament, any (183.3-183.5)

171.7   Trunk, unspecified
Back NOS
Flank NOS

171.8   Other specified sites of connective and other soft tissue
Malignant neoplasm of contiguous or overlapping sites
    of connective tissue whose point of origin cannot
    be determined

171.9   Connective and other soft tissue, site unspecified

√4ᵗʰ **172   Malignant melanoma of skin**

INCLUDES   melanocarcinoma
melanoma (skin) NOS
melanoma in situ of skin

EXCLUDES   *skin of genital organs (184.0-184.9, 187.1-187.9)*
    sites other than skin–code to malignant neoplasm of
        the site

DEF: Malignant neoplasm of melanocytes; most common in skin,
may involve oral cavity, esophagus, anal canal, vagina,
leptomeninges, or conjunctiva.

172.0   Lip
EXCLUDES   *vermilion border of lip (140.0-140.1, 140.9)*

172.1   Eyelid, including canthus

172.2   Ear and external auditory canal
Auricle (ear)
Auricular canal, external
External [acoustic] meatus
Pinna

172.3   Other and unspecified parts of face
Cheek (external)
Chin
Eyebrow
Forehead
Nose, external
Temple

172.4   Scalp and neck

172.5   Trunk, except scrotum

Axilla	Perianal skin
Breast	Perineum
Buttock	Umbilicus
Groin	

EXCLUDES   *anal canal (154.2)*
    anus NOS (154.3)
    scrotum (187.7)

172.6   Upper limb, including shoulder

Arm	Forearm
Finger	Hand

172.7   Lower limb, including hip

Ankle	Leg
Foot	Popliteal area
Heel	Thigh
Knee	Toe

172.8   **Other specified sites of skin**
Malignant melanoma of contiguous or overlapping sites of skin whose point of origin cannot be determined

172.9   **Melanoma of skin, site unspecified**

√4ᵗʰ **173**   **Other and unspecified malignant neoplasm of skin**

[INCLUDES]   malignant neoplasm of:
    sebaceous glands
    sudoriferous, sudoriparous glands
    sweat glands

[EXCLUDES]   *Kaposi's sarcoma (176.0-176.9)*
malignant melanoma of skin (172.0-172.9)
Merkel cell carcinoma of skin (209.31-209.36)
skin of genital organs (184.0-184.9, 187.1-187.9)

√5ᵗʰ **173.0**   **Other and unspecified malignant neoplasm of skin of lip**

[EXCLUDES]   *vermilion border of lip (140.0-140.1, 140.9)*

173.00   **Unspecified malignant neoplasm of skin of lip**

173.01   **Basal cell carcinoma of skin of lip**

173.02   **Squamous cell carcinoma of skin of lip**

173.09   **Other specified malignant neoplasm of skin of lip**

√5ᵗʰ **173.1**   **Other and unspecified malignant neoplasm of skin of eyelid, including canthus**

[EXCLUDES]   *cartilage of eyelid (171.0)*

173.10   **Unspecified malignant neoplasm of eyelid, including canthus**

173.11   **Basal cell carcinoma of eyelid, including canthus**

173.12   **Squamous cell carcinoma of eyelid, including canthus**

173.19   **Other specified malignant neoplasm of eyelid, including canthus**

√5ᵗʰ **173.2**   **Other and unspecified malignant neoplasm of skin of ear and external auditory canal**
Auricle (ear)
Auricular canal, external
External meatus
Pinna

[EXCLUDES]   *cartilage of ear (171.0)*

173.20   **Unspecified malignant neoplasm of skin of ear and external auditory canal**

173.21   **Basal cell carcinoma of skin of ear and external auditory canal**

173.22   **Squamous cell carcinoma of skin of ear and external auditory canal**

173.29   **Other specified malignant neoplasm of skin of ear and external auditory canal**

√5ᵗʰ **173.3**   **Other and unspecified malignant neoplasm of skin of other and unspecified parts of face**
Cheek, external   Forehead
Chin   Nose, external
Eyebrow   Temple

173.30   **Unspecified malignant neoplasm of skin of other and unspecified parts of face**

173.31   **Basal cell carcinoma of skin of other and unspecified parts of face**

173.32   **Squamous cell carcinoma of skin of other and unspecified parts of face**

173.39   **Other specified malignant neoplasm of skin of other and unspecified parts of face**

√5ᵗʰ **173.4**   **Other and unspecified malignant neoplasm of scalp and skin of neck**

173.40   **Unspecified malignant neoplasm of scalp and skin of neck**

173.41   **Basal cell carcinoma of scalp and skin of neck**

173.42   **Squamous cell carcinoma of scalp and skin of neck**

173.49   **Other specified malignant neoplasm of scalp and skin of neck**

√5ᵗʰ **173.5**   **Other and unspecified malignant neoplasm of skin of trunk, except scrotum**
Axillary fold   Skin of:
Perianal skin   buttock
Skin of: chest wall
   abdominal wall   groin
   anus   perineum
   back   Umbilicus
   breast

[EXCLUDES]   *anal canal (154.2)*
anus NOS (154.3)
skin of scrotum (187.7)

173.50   **Unspecified malignant neoplasm of skin of trunk, except scrotum**

173.51   **Basal cell carcinoma of skin of trunk, except scrotum**

173.52   **Squamous cell carcinoma of skin of trunk, except scrotum**

173.59   **Other specified malignant neoplasm of skin of trunk, except scrotum**

√5ᵗʰ **173.6**   **Other and unspecified malignant neoplasm of skin of upper limb, including shoulder**
Arm   Forearm
Finger   Hand

173.60   **Unspecified malignant neoplasm of skin of upper limb, including shoulder**

173.61   **Basal cell carcinoma of skin of upper limb, including shoulder**

173.62   **Squamous cell carcinoma of skin of upper limb, including shoulder**

173.69   **Other specified malignant neoplasm of skin of upper limb, including shoulder**

√5ᵗʰ **173.7**   **Other and unspecified malignant neoplasm of skin of lower limb, including hip**
Ankle   Leg
Foot   Popliteal area
Heel   Thigh
Knee   Toe

173.70   **Unspecified malignant neoplasm of skin of lower limb, including hip**

173.71   **Basal cell carcinoma of skin of lower limb, including hip**

173.72   **Squamous cell carcinoma of skin of lower limb, including hip**

173.79   **Other specified malignant neoplasm of skin of lower limb, including hip**

√5ᵗʰ **173.8**   **Other and unspecified malignant neoplasm of other specified sites of skin**
Malignant neoplasm of contiguous or overlapping sites of skin whose point of origin cannot be determined

173.80   **Unspecified malignant neoplasm of other specified sites of skin**

173.81   **Basal cell carcinoma of other specified sites of skin**

173.82   **Squamous cell carcinoma of other specified sites of skin**

173.89   **Other specified malignant neoplasm of other specified sites of skin**

√5ᵗʰ **173.9**   **Other and unspecified malignant neoplasm of skin, site unspecified**

173.90   **Unspecified malignant neoplasm of skin, site unspecified**
Malignant neoplasm of skin NOS

173.91   **Basal cell carcinoma of skin, site unspecified**

173.92   **Squamous cell carcinoma of skin, site unspecified**

173.99   **Other specified malignant neoplasm of skin, site unspecified**

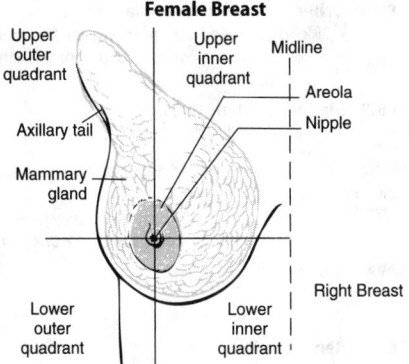

Female Breast

Upper outer quadrant

Upper inner quadrant

Midline

Areola

Nipple

Axillary tail

Mammary gland

Right Breast

Lower outer quadrant

Lower inner quadrant

✓4ᵗʰ **174 Malignant neoplasm of female breast**

INCLUDES breast (female)
connective tissue
soft parts
Paget's disease of:
  breast
  nipple

Use additional code to identify estrogen receptor status (V86.0, V86.1)

EXCLUDES *malignant melanoma of skin of breast (172.5)*
malignant neoplasm of skin of breast (173.50-173.59)

174.0 Nipple and areola

174.1 Central portion

174.2 Upper-inner quadrant

174.3 Lower-inner quadrant

174.4 Upper-outer quadrant

174.5 Lower-outer quadrant

174.6 Axillary tail

174.8 Other specified sites of female breast
Ectopic sites
Inner breast
Lower breast
Midline of breast
Outer breast
Upper breast
Malignant neoplasm of contiguous or overlapping sites of breast whose point of origin cannot be determined

174.9 Breast (female), unspecified

✓4ᵗʰ **175 Malignant neoplasm of male breast**
Use additional code to identify estrogen receptor status (V86.0, V86.1)

EXCLUDES *malignant melanoma of skin of breast (172.5)*
malignant neoplasm of skin of breast (173.50-173.59)

175.0 Nipple and areola

175.9 Other and unspecified sites of male breast
Ectopic breast tissue, male

✓4ᵗʰ **176 Kaposi's sarcoma**

176.0 Skin

176.1 Soft tissue
Blood vessel
Connective tissue
Fascia
Ligament
Lymphatic(s) NEC
Muscle
EXCLUDES *lymph glands and nodes (176.5)*

176.2 Palate

176.3 Gastrointestinal sites

176.4 Lung

176.5 Lymph nodes

176.8 Other specified sites
Oral cavity NEC

176.9 Unspecified
Viscera NOS

MALIGNANT NEOPLASM OF GENITOURINARY ORGANS (179-189)
EXCLUDES *carcinoma in situ (233.1-233.9)*

179 Malignant neoplasm of uterus, part unspecified

✓4ᵗʰ **180 Malignant neoplasm of cervix uteri**
INCLUDES invasive malignancy [carcinoma]
EXCLUDES *carcinoma in situ (233.1)*

180.0 Endocervix
Cervical canal NOS
Endocervical canal
Endocervical gland

180.1 Exocervix

180.8 Other specified sites of cervix
Cervical stump
Squamocolumnar junction of cervix
Malignant neoplasm of contiguous or overlapping sites of cervix uteri whose point of origin cannot be determined

180.9 Cervix uteri, unspecified

181 Malignant neoplasm of placenta
Choriocarcinoma NOS
Chorioepithelioma NOS
EXCLUDES *chorioadenoma (destruens) (236.1)*
hydatidiform mole (630)
  malignant (236.1)
invasive mole (236.1)
male choriocarcinoma NOS (186.0-186.9)

✓4ᵗʰ **182 Malignant neoplasm of body of uterus**
EXCLUDES *carcinoma in situ (233.2)*

182.0 Corpus uteri, except isthmus
Cornu
Endometrium
Fundus
Myometrium

182.1 Isthmus
Lower uterine segment

182.8 Other specified sites of body of uterus
Malignant neoplasm of contiguous or overlapping sites of body of uterus whose point of origin cannot be determined
EXCLUDES *uterus NOS (179)*

✓4ᵗʰ **183 Malignant neoplasm of ovary and other uterine adnexa**
EXCLUDES *Douglas' cul-de-sac (158.8)*

183.0 Ovary
Use additional code to identify any functional activity

183.2 Fallopian tube
Oviduct
Uterine tube

183.3 Broad ligament
Mesovarium
Parovarian region

183.4 Parametrium
Uterine ligament NOS
Uterosacral ligament

183.5 Round ligament

183.8 Other specified sites of uterine adnexa
Tubo-ovarian
Utero-ovarian
Malignant neoplasm of contiguous or overlapping sites of ovary and other uterine adnexa whose point of origin cannot be determined

183.9 Uterine adnexa, unspecified

174–183.9

✓4ᵗʰ 184 Malignant neoplasm of other and unspecified female genital organs
>   *EXCLUDES*   *carcinoma in situ (233.30-233.39)*

184.0 Vagina
> Gartner's duct
> Vaginal vault

184.1 Labia majora
> Greater vestibular [Bartholin's] gland

184.2 Labia minora

184.3 Clitoris

184.4 Vulva, unspecified
> External female genitalia NOS
> Pudendum

184.8 Other specified sites of female genital organs
> Malignant neoplasm of contiguous or overlapping sites of female genital organs whose point of origin cannot be determined

184.9 Female genital organ, site unspecified
> Female genitourinary tract NOS

185 Malignant neoplasm of prostate
>   *EXCLUDES*   *seminal vesicles (187.8)*

✓4ᵗʰ 186 Malignant neoplasm of testis
> Use additional code to identify any functional activity

186.0 Undescended testis
> Ectopic testis
> Retained testis

186.9 Other and unspecified testis
> Testis:
>> NOS
>> descended
>> scrotal

✓4ᵗʰ 187 Malignant neoplasm of penis and other male genital organs

187.1 Prepuce
> Foreskin

187.2 Glans penis

187.3 Body of penis
> Corpus cavernosum

187.4 Penis, part unspecified
> Skin of penis NOS

187.5 Epididymis

187.6 Spermatic cord
> Vas deferens

187.7 Scrotum
> Skin of scrotum

187.8 Other specified sites of male genital organs
> Seminal vesicle
> Tunica vaginalis
> Malignant neoplasm of contiguous or overlapping sites of penis and other male genital organs whose point of origin cannot be determined

187.9 Male genital organ, site unspecified
> Male genital organ or tract NOS

✓4ᵗʰ 188 Malignant neoplasm of bladder
>   *EXCLUDES*   *carcinoma in situ (233.7)*

188.0 Trigone of urinary bladder

188.1 Dome of urinary bladder

188.2 Lateral wall of urinary bladder

188.3 Anterior wall of urinary bladder

188.4 Posterior wall of urinary bladder

188.5 Bladder neck
> Internal urethral orifice

188.6 Ureteric orifice

188.7 Urachus

188.8 Other specified sites of bladder
> Malignant neoplasm of contiguous or overlapping sites of bladder whose point of origin cannot be determined

188.9 Bladder, part unspecified
> Bladder wall NOS

✓4ᵗʰ 189 Malignant neoplasm of kidney and other and unspecified urinary organs
>   *EXCLUDES*   *benign carcinoid tumor of kidney (209.64)*
>   *malignant carcinoid tumor of kidney (209.24)*

189.0 Kidney, except pelvis
> Kidney NOS
> Kidney parenchyma

189.1 Renal pelvis
> Renal calyces
> Ureteropelvic junction

189.2 Ureter
>   *EXCLUDES*   *ureteric orifice of bladder (188.6)*

189.3 Urethra
>   *EXCLUDES*   *urethral orifice of bladder (188.5)*

189.4 Paraurethral glands

189.8 Other specified sites of urinary organs
> Malignant neoplasm of contiguous or overlapping sites of kidney and other urinary organs whose point of origin cannot be determined

189.9 Urinary organ, site unspecified
> Urinary system NOS

MALIGNANT NEOPLASM OF OTHER AND UNSPECIFIED SITES (190-199)
>   *EXCLUDES*   *carcinoma in situ (234.0-234.9)*

✓4ᵗʰ 190 Malignant neoplasm of eye
>   *EXCLUDES*   *carcinoma in situ (234.0)*
>   *dark area on retina and choroid (239.81)*
>   *cartilage (171.0)*
>   *malignant melanoma of eyelid (skin) (172.1)*
>   *malignant neoplasm of eyelid (skin) (173.10-173.19)*
>   *optic nerve (192.0)*
>   *orbital bone (170.0)*
>   *retinal freckle (239.81)*

190.0 Eyeball, except conjunctiva, cornea, retina, and choroid
> Ciliary body   Sclera
> Crystalline lens   Uveal tract
> Iris

190.1 Orbit
> Connective tissue of orbit
> Extraocular muscle
> Retrobulbar
>   *EXCLUDES*   *bone of orbit (170.0)*

190.2 Lacrimal gland

190.3 Conjunctiva

190.4 Cornea

190.5 Retina

190.6 Choroid

190.7 Lacrimal duct
> Lacrimal sac
> Nasolacrimal duct

190.8 Other specified sites of eye
> Malignant neoplasm of contiguous or overlapping sites of eye whose point of origin cannot be determined

190.9 Eye, part unspecified

✓4ᵗʰ 191 Malignant neoplasm of brain
>   *EXCLUDES*   *cranial nerves (192.0)*
>   *retrobulbar area (190.1)*

191.0 Cerebrum, except lobes and ventricles
> Basal ganglia   Globus pallidus
> Cerebral cortex   Hypothalamus
> Corpus striatum   Thalamus

Brain and Meninges

Fourth ventricle · Cerebrum · Corpus callosum · Thalamus · Hypothalamus · Hypophysis · Pons · Cerebellum · Medulla oblongata

Midsagittal Section (between hemispheres)

191.1 Frontal lobe

191.2 Temporal lobe
    Hippocampus   Uncus

191.3 Parietal lobe

191.4 Occipital lobe

191.5 Ventricles
    Choroid plexus   Floor of ventricle

191.6 Cerebellum NOS
    Cerebellopontine angle

191.7 Brain stem
    Cerebral peduncle
    Medulla oblongata
    Midbrain
    Pons

191.8 Other parts of brain
    Corpus callosum
    Tapetum
    Malignant neoplasm of contiguous or overlapping sites of brain whose point of origin cannot be determined

191.9 Brain, unspecified
    Cranial fossa NOS

✓4ᵗʰ **192 Malignant neoplasm of other and unspecified parts of nervous system**
    EXCLUDES *peripheral, sympathetic, and parasympathetic nerves and ganglia (171.0-171.9)*

192.0 Cranial nerves
    Olfactory bulb

192.1 Cerebral meninges
    Dura (mater)   Meninges NOS
    Falx (cerebelli) (cerebri)   Tentorium

192.2 Spinal cord
    Cauda equina

192.3 Spinal meninges

192.8 Other specified sites of nervous system
    Malignant neoplasm of contiguous or overlapping sites of other parts of nervous system whose point of origin cannot be determined

192.9 Nervous system, part unspecified
    Nervous system (central) NOS
    EXCLUDES *meninges NOS (192.1)*

193 Malignant neoplasm of thyroid gland
    Thyroglossal duct
    Use additional code to identify any functional activity

✓4ᵗʰ **194 Malignant neoplasm of other endocrine glands and related structures**
    EXCLUDES *islets of Langerhans (157.4)*
        neuroendocrine tumors (209.00-209.69)
        ovary (183.0)
        testis (186.0-186.9)
        thymus (164.0)

194.0 Adrenal gland
    Adrenal cortex   Suprarenal gland
    Adrenal medulla

194.1 Parathyroid gland

194.3 Pituitary gland and craniopharyngeal duct
    Craniobuccal pouch   Rathke's pouch
    Hypophysis   Sella turcica

194.4 Pineal gland

194.5 Carotid body

194.6 Aortic body and other paraganglia
    Coccygeal body
    Glomus jugulare
    Para-aortic body

194.8 Other
    Pluriglandular involvement NOS
    Note: If the sites of multiple involvements are known, they should be coded separately.

194.9 Endocrine gland, site unspecified

✓4ᵗʰ **195 Malignant neoplasm of other and ill-defined sites**
    INCLUDES malignant neoplasms of contiguous sites, not elsewhere classified, whose point of origin cannot be determined
    EXCLUDES *malignant neoplasm:*
        lymphatic and hematopoietic tissue (200.0-208.9)
        secondary sites (196.0-198.8)
        unspecified site (199.0-199.1)

195.0 Head, face, and neck
    Cheek NOS   Nose NOS
    Jaw NOS   Supraclavicular region NOS

195.1 Thorax
    Axilla
    Chest (wall) NOS
    Intrathoracic NOS

195.2 Abdomen
    Intra-abdominal NOS

195.3 Pelvis
    Groin
    Inguinal region NOS
    Presacral region
    Sacrococcygeal region
    Sites overlapping systems within pelvis, as:
        rectovaginal (septum)
        rectovesical (septum)

195.4 Upper limb

195.5 Lower limb

195.8 Other specified sites
    Back NOS
    Flank NOS
    Trunk NOS

✓4ᵗʰ **196 Secondary and unspecified malignant neoplasm of lymph nodes**
    EXCLUDES *any malignant neoplasm of lymph nodes, specified as primary (200.0-202.9)*
        Hodgkin's disease (201.0-201.9)
        lymphosarcoma (200.1)
        other forms of lymphoma (202.0-202.9)
        reticulosarcoma (200.0)
        secondary neuroendocrine tumor of (distant) lymph nodes (209.71)

196.0 Lymph nodes of head, face, and neck
    Cervical   Scalene
    Cervicofacial   Supraclavicular

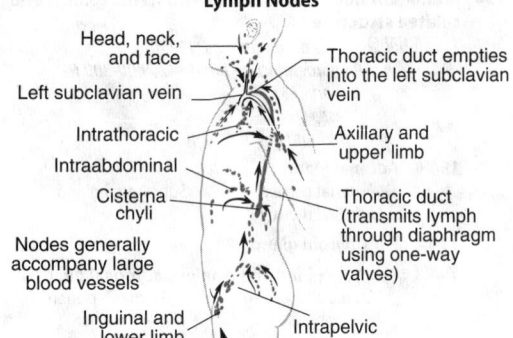

Lymph Nodes

Head, neck, and face
Thoracic duct empties into the left subclavian vein
Left subclavian vein
Intrathoracic
Axillary and upper limb
Intraabdominal
Cisterna chyli
Thoracic duct (transmits lymph through diaphragm using one-way valves)
Nodes generally accompany large blood vessels
Inguinal and lower limb
Intrapelvic

196.1 Intrathoracic lymph nodes
Bronchopulmonary   Mediastinal
Intercostal   Tracheobronchial

196.2 Intra-abdominal lymph nodes
Intestinal
Mesenteric
Retroperitoneal

196.3 Lymph nodes of axilla and upper limb
Brachial   Infraclavicular
Epitrochlear   Pectoral

196.5 Lymph nodes of inguinal region and lower limb
Femoral   Popliteal
Groin   Tibial

196.6 Intrapelvic lymph nodes
Hypogastric   Obturator
Iliac   Parametrial

196.8 Lymph nodes of multiple sites

196.9 Site unspecified
Lymph nodes NOS

√4ᵗʰ **197 Secondary malignant neoplasm of respiratory and digestive systems**
EXCLUDES *lymph node metastasis (196.0-196.9)*
secondary neuroendocrine tumor of liver (209.72)
secondary neuroendocrine tumor of respiratory organs (209.79)

197.0 Lung
Bronchus

197.1 Mediastinum

197.2 Pleura

197.3 Other respiratory organs
Trachea

197.4 Small intestine, including duodenum

197.5 Large intestine and rectum

197.6 Retroperitoneum and peritoneum

197.7 Liver, specified as secondary

197.8 Other digestive organs and spleen

√4ᵗʰ **198 Secondary malignant neoplasm of other specified sites**
EXCLUDES *lymph node metastasis (196.0-196.9)*
secondary neuroendocrine tumor of other specified sites (209.79)

198.0 Kidney

198.1 Other urinary organs

198.2 Skin
Skin of breast

198.3 Brain and spinal cord

198.4 Other parts of nervous system
Meninges (cerebral) (spinal)

198.5 Bone and bone marrow

198.6 Ovary

198.7 Adrenal gland
Suprarenal gland

√5ᵗʰ **198.8 Other specified sites**
198.81 Breast
EXCLUDES *skin of breast (198.2)*
198.82 Genital organs
198.89 Other
EXCLUDES *retroperitoneal lymph nodes (196.2)*

√4ᵗʰ **199 Malignant neoplasm without specification of site**
EXCLUDES *malignant carcinoid tumor of unknown primary site (209.20)*
malignant (poorly differentiated) neuroendocrine carcinoma, any site (209.30)
malignant (poorly differentiated) neuroendocrine tumor, any site (209.30)
neuroendocrine carcinoma (high grade), any site (209.30)

199.0 Disseminated
Carcinomatosis
Generalized: } unspecified site (primary)
    cancer   (secondary)
    malignancy
Multiple cancer

199.1 Other
Cancer   } unspecified site (primary)
Carcinoma   (secondary)
Malignancy

199.2 Malignant neoplasm associated with transplanted organ
Code first complication of transplanted organ (996.80-996.89)
Use additional code for specific malignancy

MALIGNANT NEOPLASM OF LYMPHATIC AND HEMATOPOIETIC TISSUE (200-208)

EXCLUDES *autoimmune lymphoproliferative syndrome (279.41)*
secondary and unspecified neoplasm of lymph nodes (196.0-196.9)
secondary neoplasm of:
    bone marrow (198.5)
    spleen (197.8)

The following fifth-digit subclassification is for use with categories 200-202:
    0 unspecified site, extranodal and solid organ sites
    1 lymph nodes of head, face, and neck
    2 intrathoracic lymph nodes
    3 intra-abdominal lymph nodes
    4 lymph nodes of axilla and upper limb
    5 lymph nodes of inguinal region and lower limb
    6 intrapelvic lymph nodes
    7 spleen
    8 lymph nodes of multiple sites

√4ᵗʰ **200 Lymphosarcoma and reticulosarcoma and other specified malignant tumors of lymphatic tissue**

√5ᵗʰ **200.0 Reticulosarcoma**
[0-8]   Lymphoma (malignant):   Reticulum cell sarcoma:
            histiocytic (diffuse):   NOS
                nodular   pleomorphic cell type
                pleomorphic cell type
            reticulum cell type

DEF: Malignant lymphoma of primarily histolytic cells; commonly originates in reticuloendothelium of lymph nodes.

√5ᵗʰ **200.1 Lymphosarcoma**
[0-8]
    Lymphoblastoma (diffuse)
    Lymphoma (malignant):
        lymphoblastic (diffuse)
        lymphocytic (cell type) (diffuse)
        lymphosarcoma type
        prolymphocytic
    Lymphosarcoma:
        NOS
        diffuse NOS
        lymphoblastic (diffuse)
        lymphocytic (diffuse)
        prolymphocytic

> **EXCLUDES** *lymphosarcoma:*
>   *follicular or nodular (202.0)*
>   *mixed cell type (200.8)*
>   *lymphosarcoma cell leukemia (207.8)*

DEF: Malignant lymphoma created from anaplastic lymphoid cells resembling lymphocytes or lymphoblasts.

√5ᵗʰ **200.2 Burkitt's tumor or lymphoma**
[0-8]
    Malignant lymphoma, Burkitt's type

DEF: Large osteolytic lesion most common in jaw or as abdominal mass; usually found in central Africa but reported elsewhere.

√5ᵗʰ **200.3 Marginal zone lymphoma**
[0-8]
    Extranodal marginal zone B-cell lymphoma
    Mucosa associated lymphoid tissue [MALT]
    Nodal marginal zone B-cell lymphoma
    Splenic marginal zone B-cell lymphoma

√5ᵗʰ **200.4 Mantle cell lymphoma**
[0-8]

√5ᵗʰ **200.5 Primary central nervous system lymphoma**
[0-8]

√5ᵗʰ **200.6 Anaplastic large cell lymphoma**
[0-8]

√5ᵗʰ **200.7 Large cell lymphoma**
[0-8]

√5ᵗʰ **200.8 Other named variants**
[0-8]
    Lymphoma (malignant):
        lymphoplasmacytoid type
        mixed lymphocytic-histiocytic (diffuse)
    Lymphosarcoma, mixed cell type (diffuse)
    Reticulolymphosarcoma (diffuse)

√4ᵗʰ **201 Hodgkin's disease**

DEF: Painless, progressive enlargement of lymph nodes, spleen and general lymph tissue; symptoms include anorexia, lassitude, weight loss, fever, pruritis, night sweats, anemia.

√5ᵗʰ **201.0 Hodgkin's paragranuloma**
[0-8]

√5ᵗʰ **201.1 Hodgkin's granuloma**
[0-8]

√5ᵗʰ **201.2 Hodgkin's sarcoma**
[0-8]

√5ᵗʰ **201.4 Lymphocytic-histiocytic predominance**
[0-8]

√5ᵗʰ **201.5 Nodular sclerosis**
[0-8]
    Hodgkin's disease, nodular sclerosis:
        NOS
        cellular phase

√5ᵗʰ **201.6 Mixed cellularity**
[0-8]

√5ᵗʰ **201.7 Lymphocytic depletion**
[0-8]
    Hodgkin's disease, lymphocytic depletion:
        NOS
        diffuse fibrosis
        reticular type

√5ᵗʰ **201.9 Hodgkin's disease, unspecified**
[0-8]
    Hodgkin's: Malignant:
        disease NOS   lymphogranuloma
        lymphoma NOS   lymphogranulomatosis

√4ᵗʰ **202 Other malignant neoplasms of lymphoid and histiocytic tissue**

√5ᵗʰ **202.0 Nodular lymphoma**
[0-8]
    Brill-Symmers disease
    Lymphoma:
        follicular (giant) (large cell)
        lymphocytic, nodular
    Lymphosarcoma:
        follicular (giant)
        nodular

DEF: Lymphomatous cells clustered into nodules within the lymph node; usually occurs in older adults and may involve all nodes and possibly extranodal sites.

√5ᵗʰ **202.1 Mycosis fungoides**
[0-8]
> **EXCLUDES** *peripheral T-cell lymphoma (202.7)*

DEF: Type of cutaneous T-cell lymphoma; may evolve into generalized lymphoma; formerly thought to be of fungoid origin.

√5ᵗʰ **202.2 Sézary's disease**
[0-8]

DEF: Type of cutaneous T-cell lymphoma with erythroderma, intense pruritus, peripheral lymphadenopathy, abnormal hyperchromatic mononuclear cells in skin, lymph nodes and peripheral blood.

√5ᵗʰ **202.3 Malignant histiocytosis**
[0-8]
    Histiocytic medullary reticulosis
    Malignant:
        reticuloendotheliosis
        reticulosis

√5ᵗʰ **202.4 Leukemic reticuloendotheliosis**
[0-8]
    Hairy-cell leukemia

DEF: Chronic leukemia with large, mononuclear cells with "hairy" appearance in marrow, spleen, liver, blood.

√5ᵗʰ **202.5 Letterer-Siwe disease**
[0-8]
    Acute:
        differentiated progressive histiocytosis
        histiocytosis X (progressive)
        infantile reticuloendotheliosis
        reticulosis of infancy

> **EXCLUDES** *adult pulmonary Langerhans cell histiocytosis (516.5)*
>   *Hand-Schüller-Christian disease (277.89)*
>   *histiocytosis (acute) (chronic) (277.89)*
>   *histiocytosis X (chronic) (277.89)*

DEF: A recessive reticuloendotheliosis of early childhood, with a hemorrhagic tendency, eczema-like skin eruption, hepatosplenomegaly, lymph node enlargement, and progressive anemia; often a fatal disease with no established cause.

√5ᵗʰ **202.6 Malignant mast cell tumors**
[0-8]
    Malignant:
        mastocytoma
        mastocytosis
    Mast cell sarcoma
    Systemic tissue mast cell disease
> **EXCLUDES** *mast cell leukemia (207.8)*

√5ᵗʰ **202.7 Peripheral T-cell lymphoma**
[0-8]

√5ᵗʰ **202.8 Other lymphomas**
[0-8]
    Lymphoma (malignant):
        NOS
        diffuse
> **EXCLUDES** *benign lymphoma (229.0)*

√5ᵗʰ **202.9 Other and unspecified malignant neoplasms of lymphoid and histiocytic tissue**
[0-8]
    Follicular dendritic cell sarcoma
    Interdigitating dendritic cell sarcoma
    Langerhans cell sarcoma
    Malignant neoplasm of bone marrow NOS

Neoplasms

203–208.1

✓4ᵗʰ **203 Multiple myeloma and immunoproliferative neoplasms**

The following fifth-digit subclassification is for use with category 203:

    0 without mention of having achieved remission
      Failed remission
    1 in remission
    2 in relapse

✓5ᵗʰ **203.0 Multiple myeloma**
[0-2]   Kahler's disease   Myelomatosis
       EXCLUDES   solitary myeloma (238.6)

✓5ᵗʰ **203.1 Plasma cell leukemia**
[0-2]   Plasmacytic leukemia

✓5ᵗʰ **203.8 Other immunoproliferative neoplasms**
[0-2]

✓4ᵗʰ **204 Lymphoid leukemia**
    INCLUDES   leukemia:
           lymphatic
           lymphoblastic
           lymphocytic
           lymphogenous

The following fifth-digit subclassification is for use with category 204:

    0 without mention of having achieved remission
      Failed remission
    1 in remission
    2 in relapse

✓5ᵗʰ **204.0 Acute**
[0-2]   **EXCLUDES**   acute exacerbation of chronic lymphoid leukemia (204.1)

✓5ᵗʰ **204.1 Chronic**
[0-2]

✓5ᵗʰ **204.2 Subacute**
[0-2]

✓5ᵗʰ **204.8 Other lymphoid leukemia**
[0-2]   Aleukemic leukemia: Aleukemic leukemia:
         lymphatic   lymphoid
         lymphocytic

✓5ᵗʰ **204.9 Unspecified lymphoid leukemia**
[0-2]

✓4ᵗʰ **205 Myeloid leukemia**
    INCLUDES   leukemia:
           granulocytic
           myeloblastic
           myelocytic
           myelogenous
           myelomonocytic
           myelosclerotic
           myelosis

The following fifth-digit subclassification is for use with category 205:

    0 without mention of having achieved remission
      Failed remission
    1 in remission
    2 in relapse

✓5ᵗʰ **205.0 Acute**
[0-2]   Acute promyelocytic leukemia
       EXCLUDES   acute exacerbation of chronic myeloid leukemia (205.1)

✓5ᵗʰ **205.1 Chronic**
[0-2]   Eosinophilic leukemia
       Neutrophilic leukemia

✓5ᵗʰ **205.2 Subacute**
[0-2]

✓5ᵗʰ **205.3 Myeloid sarcoma**
[0-2]   Chloroma
       Granulocytic sarcoma

✓5ᵗʰ **205.8 Other myeloid leukemia**
[0-2]   Aleukemic leukemia: Aleukemic leukemia:
         granulocytic   myeloid
         myelogenous   Aleukemic myelosis

✓5ᵗʰ **205.9 Unspecified myeloid leukemia**
[0-2]

✓4ᵗʰ **206 Monocytic leukemia**
    INCLUDES   leukemia:
           histiocytic
           monoblastic
           monocytoid

The following fifth-digit subclassification is for use with category 206:

    0 without mention of having achieved remission
      Failed remission
    1 in remission
    2 in relapse

✓5ᵗʰ **206.0 Acute**
[0-2]   **EXCLUDES**   acute exacerbation of chronic monocytic leukemia (206.1)

✓5ᵗʰ **206.1 Chronic**
[0-2]

✓5ᵗʰ **206.2 Subacute**
[0-2]

✓5ᵗʰ **206.8 Other monocytic leukemia**
[0-2]   Aleukemic:
         monocytic leukemia
         monocytoid leukemia

✓5ᵗʰ **206.9 Unspecified monocytic leukemia**
[0-2]

✓4ᵗʰ **207 Other specified leukemia**
    EXCLUDES   leukemic reticuloendotheliosis (202.4)
                  plasma cell leukemia (203.1)

The following fifth-digit subclassification is for use with category 207:

    0 without mention of having achieved remission
      Failed remission
    1 in remission
    2 in relapse

✓5ᵗʰ **207.0 Acute erythremia and erythroleukemia**
[0-2]   Acute erythremic myelosis
       Di Guglielmo's disease
       Erythremic myelosis
       DEF: Erythremia: polycythemia vera.
       DEF: Erythroleukemia: a malignant blood dyscrasia (a myeloproliferative disorder).

✓5ᵗʰ **207.1 Chronic erythremia**
[0-2]   Heilmeyer-Schöner disease

✓5ᵗʰ **207.2 Megakaryocytic leukemia**
[0-2]   Megakaryocytic myelosis
       Thrombocytic leukemia

✓5ᵗʰ **207.8 Other specified leukemia**
[0-2]   Lymphosarcoma cell leukemia

✓4ᵗʰ **208 Leukemia of unspecified cell type**

The following fifth-digit subclassification is for use with category 208:

    0 without mention of having achieved remission
      Failed remission
    1 in remission
    2 in relapse

✓5ᵗʰ **208.0 Acute**
[0-2]   Acute leukemia NOS
       Blast cell leukemia
       Stem cell leukemia
       EXCLUDES   acute exacerbation of chronic unspecified leukemia (208.1)

✓5ᵗʰ **208.1 Chronic**
[0-2]   Chronic leukemia NOS

√5ᵗʰ **208.2 Subacute**
[0-2]   Subacute leukemia NOS

√5ᵗʰ **208.8 Other leukemia of unspecified cell type**
[0-2]

√5ᵗʰ **208.9 Unspecified leukemia**
[0-2]   Leukemia NOS

NEUROENDOCRINE TUMORS (209)

√4ᵗʰ **209 Neuroendocrine tumors**
Code first any associated multiple endocrine neoplasia syndrome (258.01-258.03)
Use additional code to identify associated endocrine syndrome, such as:
carcinoid syndrome (259.2)
> **EXCLUDES** *benign pancreatic islet cell tumors (211.7)*
> *malignant pancreatic islet cell tumors (157.4)*

√5ᵗʰ **209.0 Malignant carcinoid tumors of the small intestine**

     209.00 Malignant carcinoid tumor of the small intestine, unspecified portion

     209.01 Malignant carcinoid tumor of the duodenum

     209.02 Malignant carcinoid tumor of the jejunum

     209.03 Malignant carcinoid tumor of the ileum

√5ᵗʰ **209.1 Malignant carcinoid tumors of the appendix, large intestine, and rectum**

     209.10 Malignant carcinoid tumor of the large intestine, unspecified portion
         Malignant carcinoid tumor of the colon NOS

     209.11 Malignant carcinoid tumor of the appendix

     209.12 Malignant carcinoid tumor of the cecum

     209.13 Malignant carcinoid tumor of the ascending colon

     209.14 Malignant carcinoid tumor of the transverse colon

     209.15 Malignant carcinoid tumor of the descending colon

     209.16 Malignant carcinoid tumor of the sigmoid colon

     209.17 Malignant carcinoid tumor of the rectum

√5ᵗʰ **209.2 Malignant carcinoid tumors of other and unspecified sites**

     209.20 Malignant carcinoid tumor of the unknown primary site

     209.21 Malignant carcinoid tumor of the bronchus and lung

     209.22 Malignant carcinoid tumor of the thymus

     209.23 Malignant carcinoid tumor of the stomach

     209.24 Malignant carcinoid tumor of the kidney

     209.25 Malignant carcinoid tumor of the foregut NOS

     209.26 Malignant carcinoid tumor of the midgut NOS

     209.27 Malignant carcinoid tumor of the hindgut NOS

     209.29 Malignant carcinoid tumor of the other sites

√5ᵗʰ **209.3 Malignant poorly differentiated neuroendocrine tumors**

     209.30 Malignant poorly differentiated neuroendocrine carcinoma, any site
         High grade neuroendocrine carcinoma, any site
         Malignant poorly differentiated neuroendocrine tumor NOS
>   **EXCLUDES** *Merkel cell carcinoma (209.31-209.36)*

     209.31 Merkel cell carcinoma of the face
         Merkel cell carcinoma of the ear
         Merkel cell carcinoma of the eyelid, including canthus
         Merkel cell carcinoma of the lip

     209.32 Merkel cell carcinoma of the scalp and neck

     209.33 Merkel cell carcinoma of the upper limb

     209.34 Merkel cell carcinoma of the lower limb

     209.35 Merkel cell carcinoma of the trunk

     209.36 Merkel cell carcinoma of other sites
         Merkel cell carcinoma of the buttock
         Merkel cell carcinoma of the genitals
         Merkel cell carcinoma NOS

√5ᵗʰ **209.4 Benign carcinoid tumors of the small intestine**

     209.40 Benign carcinoid tumor of the small intestine, unspecified portion

     209.41 Benign carcinoid tumor of the duodenum

     209.42 Benign carcinoid tumor of the jejunum

     209.43 Benign carcinoid tumor of the ileum

√5ᵗʰ **209.5 Benign carcinoid tumors of the appendix, large intestine, and rectum**

     209.50 Benign carcinoid tumor of the large intestine, unspecified portion
         Benign carcinoid tumor of the colon NOS

     209.51 Benign carcinoid tumor of the appendix

     209.52 Benign carcinoid tumor of the cecum

     209.53 Benign carcinoid tumor of the ascending colon

     209.54 Benign carcinoid tumor of the transverse colon

     209.55 Benign carcinoid tumor of the descending colon

     209.56 Benign carcinoid tumor of the sigmoid colon

     209.57 Benign carcinoid tumor of the rectum

√5ᵗʰ **209.6 Benign carcinoid tumors of other and unspecified sites**

     209.60 Benign carcinoid tumor of unknown primary site
         Carcinoid tumor NOS
         Neuroendocrine tumor NOS

     209.61 Benign carcinoid tumor of the bronchus and lung

     209.62 Benign carcinoid tumor of the thymus

     209.63 Benign carcinoid tumor of the stomach

     209.64 Benign carcinoid tumor of the kidney

     209.65 Benign carcinoid tumor of the foregut NOS

     209.66 Benign carcinoid tumor of the midgut NOS

     209.67 Benign carcinoid tumor of the hindgut NOS

     209.69 Benign carcinoid tumors of other sites

√5ᵗʰ **209.7 Secondary neuroendocrine tumors**
Secondary carcinoid tumors

     209.70 Secondary neuroendocrine tumor, unspecified site

     209.71 Secondary neuroendocrine tumor of distant lymph nodes

     209.72 Secondary neuroendocrine tumor of liver

     209.73 Secondary neuroendocrine tumor of bone

     209.74 Secondary neuroendocrine tumor of peritoneum
         Mesentery metastasis of neuroendocrine tumor

     209.75 Secondary Merkel cell carcinoma
         Merkel cell carcinoma nodal presentation
         Merkel cell carcinoma visceral metastatic presentation
         Secondary Merkel cell carcinoma, any site

     209.79 Secondary neuroendocrine tumor of other sites

Neoplasms

210–212.2

BENIGN NEOPLASMS (210-229)

✓4ᵗʰ **210   Benign neoplasm of lip, oral cavity, and pharynx**
     EXCLUDES   cyst (of):
            jaw (526.0-526.2, 526.89)
            oral soft tissue (528.4)
            radicular (522.8)

210.0   Lip
     Frenulum labii
     Lip (inner aspect) (mucosa) (vermilion border)
     EXCLUDES   labial commissure (210.4)
            skin of lip (216.0)

210.1   Tongue
     Lingual tonsil

210.2   Major salivary glands
     Gland: Gland:
       parotid   submandibular
       sublingual
     EXCLUDES   benign neoplasms of minor salivary glands:
            NOS (210.4)
            buccal mucosa (210.4)
            lips (210.0)
            palate (hard) (soft) (210.4)
            tongue (210.1)
            tonsil, palatine (210.5)

210.3   Floor of mouth

210.4   Other and unspecified parts of mouth
     Gingiva   Oral mucosa
     Gum (upper) (lower)   Palate (hard) (soft)
     Labial commissure   Uvula
     Oral cavity NOS
     EXCLUDES   benign odontogenic neoplasms of bone
            (213.0-213.1)
            developmental odontogenic cysts (526.0)
            mucosa of lips (210.0)
            nasopharyngeal [posterior] [superior] surface
            of soft palate (210.7)

210.5   Tonsil
     Tonsil (faucial) (palatine)
     EXCLUDES   lingual tonsil (210.1)
            pharyngeal tonsil (210.7)
            tonsillar:
            fossa (210.6)
            pillars (210.6)

210.6   Other parts of oropharynx
     Branchial cleft or vestiges   Tonsillar:
     Epiglottis, anterior aspect   fossa
     Fauces NOS   pillars
     Mesopharynx NOS   Vallecula
     EXCLUDES   epiglottis:
            NOS (212.1)
            suprahyoid portion (212.1)

210.7   Nasopharynx
     Adenoid tissue   Pharyngeal tonsil
     Lymphadenoid tissue   Posterior nasal septum

210.8   Hypopharynx
     Arytenoid fold   Postcricoid region
     Laryngopharynx   Pyriform fossa

210.9   Pharynx, unspecified
     Throat NOS

✓4ᵗʰ **211   Benign neoplasm of other parts of digestive system**
     EXCLUDES   benign stromal tumors of digestive system (215.5)

211.0   Esophagus

211.1   Stomach
     Body
     Cardia   } of stomach
     Fundus
     Cardiac orifice
     Pylorus
     EXCLUDES   benign carcinoid tumors of the stomach
            (209.63)

211.2   Duodenum, jejunum, and ileum
     Small intestine NOS
     EXCLUDES   ampulla of Vater (211.5)
            benign carcinoid tumors of the small intestine
            (209.40-209.43)
            ileocecal valve (211.3)

211.3   Colon
     Appendix   Ileocecal valve
     Cecum   Large intestine NOS
     EXCLUDES   benign carcinoid tumors of the large intestine
            (209.50-209.56)
            rectosigmoid junction (211.4)

211.4   Rectum and anal canal
     Anal canal or sphincter
     Anus NOS
     Rectosigmoid junction
     EXCLUDES   anus:
            margin (216.5)
            skin (216.5)
            benign carcinoid tumors of the rectum
            (209.57)
            perianal skin (216.5)

211.5   Liver and biliary passages
     Ampulla of Vater   Gallbladder
     Common bile duct   Hepatic duct
     Cystic duct   Sphincter of Oddi

211.6   Pancreas, except islets of Langerhans

211.7   Islets of Langerhans
     Islet cell tumor
     Use additional code to identify any functional activity

211.8   Retroperitoneum and peritoneum
     Mesentery   Omentum
     Mesocolon   Retroperitoneal tissue

211.9   Other and unspecified site
     Alimentary tract NOS
     Digestive system NOS
     Gastrointestinal tract NOS
     Intestinal tract NOS
     Intestine NOS
     Spleen, not elsewhere classified

✓4ᵗʰ **212   Benign neoplasm of respiratory and intrathoracic organs**

212.0   Nasal cavities, middle ear, and accessory sinuses
     Cartilage of nose   Sinus:
     Eustachian tube   ethmoidal
     Nares   frontal
     Septum of nose   maxillary
                        sphenoidal
     EXCLUDES   auditory canal (external) (216.2)
            bone of:
            ear (213.0)
            nose [turbinates] (213.0)
            cartilage of ear (215.0)
            ear (external) (skin) (216.2)
            nose NOS (229.8)
            skin (216.3)
            olfactory bulb (225.1)
            polyp of:
            accessory sinus (471.8)
            ear (385.30-385.35)
            nasal cavity (471.0)
            posterior margin of septum and choanae
            (210.7)

212.1   Larynx
     Cartilage: Epiglottis (suprahyoid
       arytenoid   portion) NOS
       cricoid   Glottis
       cuneiform   Vocal cords (false)(true)
       thyroid
     EXCLUDES   epiglottis, anterior aspect (210.6)
            polyp of vocal cord or larynx (478.4)

212.2   Trachea

212.3 **Bronchus and lung**
Carina
Hilus of lung
EXCLUDES *benign carcinoid tumors of bronchus and*
lung (209.61)

212.4 **Pleura**

212.5 **Mediastinum**

212.6 **Thymus**
EXCLUDES *benign carcinoid tumors of thymus (209.62)*

212.7 **Heart**
EXCLUDES *great vessels (215.4)*

212.8 **Other specified sites**

212.9 **Site unspecified**
Respiratory organ NOS
Upper respiratory tract NOS
EXCLUDES *intrathoracic NOS (229.8)*
thoracic NOS (229.8)

√4ᵗʰ 213 **Benign neoplasm of bone and articular cartilage**
INCLUDES cartilage (articular) (joint)
periosteum
EXCLUDES *cartilage of:*
ear (215.0)
eyelid (215.0))
larynx (212.1)
nose (212.0)
exostosis NOS (726.91)
synovia (215.0-215.9)

213.0 **Bones of skull and face**
EXCLUDES *lower jaw bone (213.1)*

213.1 **Lower jaw bone**

213.2 **Vertebral column, excluding sacrum and coccyx**

213.3 **Ribs, sternum, and clavicle**

213.4 **Scapula and long bones of upper limb**

213.5 **Short bones of upper limb**

213.6 **Pelvic bones, sacrum, and coccyx**

213.7 **Long bones of lower limb**

213.8 **Short bones of lower limb**

213.9 **Bone and articular cartilage, site unspecified**

√4ᵗʰ 214 **Lipoma**
INCLUDES angiolipoma
fibrolipoma
hibernoma
lipoma (fetal) (infiltrating) (intramuscular)
myelolipoma
myxolipoma

DEF: Benign tumor frequently composed of mature fat cells; may occasionally be composed of fetal fat cells.

214.0 **Skin and subcutaneous tissue of face**

214.1 **Other skin and subcutaneous tissue**

214.2 **Intrathoracic organs**

214.3 **Intra-abdominal organs**

214.4 **Spermatic cord**

214.8 **Other specified sites**

214.9 **Lipoma, unspecified site**

√4ᵗʰ 215 **Other benign neoplasm of connective and other soft tissue**
INCLUDES blood vessel
bursa
fascia
ligament
muscle
peripheral, sympathetic, and parasympathetic
nerves and ganglia
synovia
tendon (sheath)
EXCLUDES *cartilage:*
articular (213.0-213.9)
larynx (212.1)
nose (212.0)
connective tissue of:
breast (217)
internal organ, except lipoma and hemangioma–
code to benign neoplasm of the site
lipoma (214.0-214.9)

215.0 **Head, face, and neck**

215.2 **Upper limb, including shoulder**

215.3 **Lower limb, including hip**

215.4 **Thorax**
EXCLUDES *heart (212.7)*
mediastinum (212.5)
thymus (212.6)

215.5 **Abdomen**
Abdominal wall
Benign stromal tumors of abdomen
Hypochondrium

215.6 **Pelvis**
Buttock
Groin
Inguinal region
Perineum
EXCLUDES *uterine:*
leiomyoma (218.0-218.9)
ligament, any (221.0)

215.7 **Trunk, unspecified**
Back NOS   Flank NOS

215.8 **Other specified sites**

215.9 **Site unspecified**

√4ᵗʰ 216 **Benign neoplasm of skin**
INCLUDES blue nevus
dermatofibroma
hydrocystoma
pigmented nevus
syringoadenoma
syringoma
EXCLUDES *skin of genital organs (221.0-222.9)*

216.0 **Skin of lip**
EXCLUDES *vermilion border of lip (210.0)*

216.1 **Eyelid, including canthus**
EXCLUDES *cartilage of eyelid (215.0)*

216.2 **Ear and external auditory canal**
Auricle (ear)   External meatus
Auricular canal, external   Pinna
EXCLUDES *cartilage of ear (215.0)*

216.3 **Skin of other and unspecified parts of face**
Cheek, external   Nose, external
Eyebrow   Temple

216.4 **Scalp and skin of neck**

216.5 Skin of trunk, except scrotum
Axillary fold
Perianal skin
Skin of:
  abdominal wall
  anus
  back
  breast
Skin of:
  buttock
  chest wall
  groin
  perineum
  Umbilicus
> EXCLUDES anal canal (211.4)
> anus NOS (211.4)
> skin of scrotum (222.4)

216.6 Skin of upper limb, including shoulder

216.7 Skin of lower limb, including hip

216.8 Other specified sites of skin

216.9 Skin, site unspecified

217 Benign neoplasm of breast
Breast (male) (female):
  connective tissue
  glandular tissue
Breast (male) (female):
  soft parts
> EXCLUDES adenofibrosis (610.2)
> benign cyst of breast (610.0)
> fibrocystic disease (610.1)
> skin of breast (216.5)

✓4ᵗʰ 218 Uterine leiomyoma
> INCLUDES fibroid (bleeding) (uterine)
> uterine:
>   fibromyoma
>   myoma

DEF: Benign tumor primarily derived from uterine smooth muscle tissue; may contain fibrous, fatty, or epithelial tissue; also called uterine fibroid or myoma.

218.0 Submucous leiomyoma of uterus

218.1 Intramural leiomyoma of uterus
Interstitial leiomyoma of uterus

218.2 Subserous leiomyoma of uterus

218.9 Leiomyoma of uterus, unspecified

✓4ᵗʰ 219 Other benign neoplasm of uterus

219.0 Cervix uteri

219.1 Corpus uteri
Endometrium   Myometrium
Fundus

219.8 Other specified parts of uterus

219.9 Uterus, part unspecified

220 Benign neoplasm of ovary
Use additional code to identify any functional activity
(256.0-256.1)
> EXCLUDES cyst:
>   corpus albicans (620.2)
>   corpus luteum (620.1)
>   endometrial (617.1)
>   follicular (atretic) (620.0)
>   graafian follicle (620.0)
>   ovarian NOS (620.2)
>   retention (620.2)

Types of Uterine Fibroids

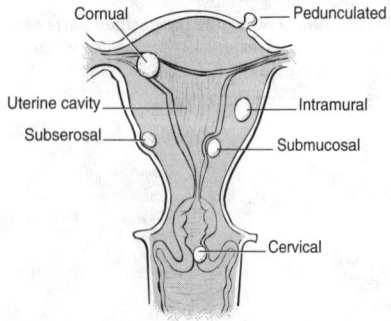

✓4ᵗʰ 221 Benign neoplasm of other female genital organs
> INCLUDES adenomatous polyp
> benign teratoma
> EXCLUDES cyst:
>   epoophoron (752.11)
>   fimbrial (752.11)
>   Gartner's duct (752.11)
>   parovarian (752.11)

221.0 Fallopian tube and uterine ligaments
Oviduct
Parametruim
Uterine ligament (broad) (round) (uterosacral)
Uterine tube

221.1 Vagina

221.2 Vulva
Clitoris
External female genitalia NOS
Greater vestibular [Bartholin's] gland
Labia (majora) (minora)
Pudendum
> EXCLUDES Bartholin's (duct) (gland) cyst (616.2)

221.8 Other specified sites of female genital organs

221.9 Female genital organ, site unspecified
Female genitourinary tract NOS

✓4ᵗʰ 222 Benign neoplasm of male genital organs

222.0 Testis
Use additional code to identify any functional activity

222.1 Penis
Corpus cavernosum   Prepuce
Glans penis

222.2 Prostate
> EXCLUDES adenomatous hyperplasia of prostate
>   (600.20-600.21)
> prostatic:
>   adenoma (600.20-600.21)
>   enlargement (600.00-600.01)
>   hypertrophy (600.00-600.01)

222.3 Epididymis

222.4 Scrotum
Skin of scrotum

222.8 Other specified sites of male genital organs
Seminal vesicle
Spermatic cord

222.9 Male genital organ, site unspecified
Male genitourinary tract NOS

✓4ᵗʰ 223 Benign neoplasm of kidney and other urinary organs

223.0 Kidney, except pelvis
Kidney NOS
> EXCLUDES benign carcinoid tumors of kidney (209.64)
> renal:
>   calyces (223.1)
>   pelvis (223.1)

223.1 Renal pelvis

223.2 Ureter
> EXCLUDES ureteric orifice of bladder (223.3)

223.3 Bladder

✓5ᵗʰ 223.8 Other specified sites of urinary organs

223.81 Urethra
> EXCLUDES urethral orifice of bladder (223.3)

223.89 Other
Paraurethral glands

223.9 Urinary organ, site unspecified
Urinary system NOS

Eyeball

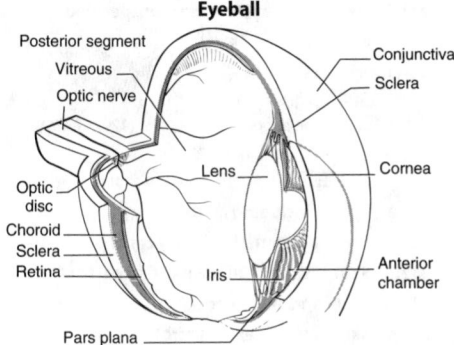

Posterior segment
Vitreous
Optic nerve

Optic disc
Choroid
Sclera
Retina

Conjunctiva
Sclera

Lens
Cornea

Iris
Anterior chamber

Pars plana

✓4ᵗʰ **224 Benign neoplasm of eye**

> *EXCLUDES* *cartilage of eyelid (215.0)*
> *eyelid (skin) (216.1)*
> *optic nerve (225.1)*
> *orbital bone (213.0)*

224.0 Eyeball, except conjunctiva, cornea, retina, and choroid
Ciliary body   Sclera
Iris   Uveal tract

224.1 Orbit
> *EXCLUDES* *bone of orbit (213.0)*

224.2 Lacrimal gland

224.3 Conjunctiva

224.4 Cornea

224.5 Retina
> *EXCLUDES* *hemangioma of retina (228.03)*

224.6 Choroid

224.7 Lacrimal duct
Lacrimal sac
Nasolacrimal duct

224.8 Other specified parts of eye

224.9 Eye, part unspecified

✓4ᵗʰ **225 Benign neoplasm of brain and other parts of nervous system**

> *EXCLUDES* *hemangioma (228.02)*
> *neurofibromatosis (237.70-237.79)*
> *peripheral, sympathetic, and parasympathetic nerves*
> *and ganglia (215.0-215.9)*
> *retrobulbar (224.1)*

225.0 Brain

225.1 Cranial nerves
Acoustic neuroma

225.2 Cerebral meninges
Meninges NOS
Meningioma (cerebral)

225.3 Spinal cord
Cauda equina

225.4 Spinal meninges
Spinal meningioma

225.8 Other specified sites of nervous system

225.9 Nervous system, part unspecified
Nervous system (central) NOS
> *EXCLUDES* *meninges NOS (225.2)*

226 Benign neoplasm of thyroid glands
Use additional code to identify any functional activity

✓4ᵗʰ **227 Benign neoplasm of other endocrine glands and related structures**
Use additional code to identify any functional activity
> *EXCLUDES* *ovary (220)*
> *pancreas (211.6)*
> *testis (222.0)*

227.0 Adrenal gland
Suprarenal gland

227.1 Parathyroid gland

227.3 Pituitary gland and craniopharyngeal duct (pouch)
Craniobuccal pouch   Rathke's pouch
Hypophysis   Sella turcica

227.4 Pineal gland
Pineal body

227.5 Carotid body

227.6 Aortic body and other paraganglia
Coccygeal body   Para-aortic body
Glomus jugulare

227.8 Other

227.9 Endocrine gland, site unspecified

✓4ᵗʰ **228 Hemangioma and lymphangioma, any site**
> *INCLUDES* angioma (benign) (cavernous) (congenital) NOS
> cavernous nevus
> glomus tumor
> hemangioma (benign) (congenital)
> *EXCLUDES* *benign neoplasm of spleen, except hemangioma and*
> *lymphangioma (211.9)*
> *glomus jugulare (227.6)*
> *nevus:*
> *NOS (216.0-216.9)*
> *blue or pigmented (216.0-216.9)*
> *vascular (757.32)*

✓5ᵗʰ **228.0 Hemangioma, any site**
> **DEF:** A common benign tumor usually occurring in infancy; composed of newly formed blood vessels due to malformation of angioblastic tissue.

228.00 Of unspecified site

228.01 Of skin and subcutaneous tissue

228.02 Of intracranial structures

228.03 Of retina

228.04 Of intra-abdominal structures
Peritoneum
Retroperitoneal tissue

228.09 Of other sites
Systemic angiomatosis

228.1 Lymphangioma, any site
Congenital lymphangioma
Lymphatic nevus

✓4ᵗʰ **229 Benign neoplasm of other and unspecified sites**

229.0 Lymph nodes
> *EXCLUDES* *lymphangioma (228.1)*

229.8 Other specified sites
Intrathoracic NOS
Thoracic NOS

229.9 Site unspecified
> **DEF:** A neoplastic type; with tumor cells confined to epithelium of origin; without further invasion.

Neoplasms

CARCINOMA IN SITU (230-234)

INCLUDES   Bowen's disease
erythroplasia
Queyrat's erythroplasia
EXCLUDES   *leukoplakia–see Alphabetic Index*

DEF: A neoplastic type; with tumor cells confined to epithelium of origin; without further invasion.

230   Carcinoma in situ of digestive organs

230.0   Lip, oral cavity, and pharynx
Gingiva   Oropharynx
Hypopharynx   Salivary gland or duct
Mouth [any part]   Tongue
Nasopharynx
EXCLUDES   *aryepiglottic fold or interarytenoid fold,*
laryngeal aspect (231.0)
epiglottis:
NOS (231.0)
suprahyoid portion (231.0)
skin of lip (232.0)

230.1   Esophagus

230.2   Stomach
Body
Cardia } of stomach
Fundus
Cardiac orifice
Pylorus

230.3   Colon
Appendix   Ileocecal valve
Cecum   Large intestine NOS
EXCLUDES   *rectosigmoid junction (230.4)*

230.4   Rectum
Rectosigmoid junction

230.5   Anal canal
Anal sphincter

230.6   Anus, unspecified
EXCLUDES   *anus:*
margin (232.5)
skin (232.5)
perianal skin (232.5)

230.7   Other and unspecified parts of intestine
Duodenum   Jejunum
Ileum   Small intestine NOS
EXCLUDES   *ampulla of Vater (230.8)*

230.8   Liver and biliary system
Ampulla of Vater   Gallbladder
Common bile duct   Hepatic duct
Cystic duct   Sphincter of Oddi

230.9   Other and unspecified digestive organs
Digestive organ NOS   Pancreas
Gastrointestinal tract NOS   Spleen

231   Carcinoma in situ of respiratory system

231.0   Larynx
Cartilage: Epiglottis:
   arytenoid   NOS
   cricoid   posterior surface
   cuneiform   suprahyoid portion
   thyroid   Vocal cords (false)(true)
EXCLUDES   *aryepiglottic fold or interarytenoid fold:*
NOS (230.0)
hypopharyngeal aspect (230.0)
marginal zone (230.0)

231.1   Trachea

231.2   Bronchus and lung
Carina   Hilus of lung

231.8   Other specified parts of respiratory system
Accessory sinuses   Nasal cavities
Middle ear   Pleura
EXCLUDES   *ear (external) (skin) (232.2)*
nose NOS (234.8)
skin (232.3)

231.9   Respiratory system, part unspecified
Respiratory organ NOS

232   Carcinoma in situ of skin
INCLUDES   pigment cells
EXCLUDES   *melanoma in situ of skin (172.0-172.9)*

232.0   Skin of lip
EXCLUDES   *vermilion border of lip (230.0)*

232.1   Eyelid, including canthus

232.2   Ear and external auditory canal

232.3   Skin of other and unspecified parts of face

232.4   Scalp and skin of neck

232.5   Skin of trunk, except scrotum
Anus, margin   Skin of:
Axillary fold   breast
Perianal skin   buttock
Skin of: chest wall
   abdominal wall   groin
   anus   perineum
   back   Umbilicus
EXCLUDES   *anal canal (230.5)*
anus NOS (230.6)
skin of genital organs (233.30-233.39,
233.5-233.6)

232.6   Skin of upper limb, including shoulder

232.7   Skin of lower limb, including hip

232.8   Other specified sites of skin

232.9   Skin, site unspecified

233   Carcinoma in situ of breast and genitourinary system

233.0   Breast
EXCLUDES   *Paget's disease (174.0-174.9)*
skin of breast (232.5)

233.1   Cervix uteri
Adenocarcinoma in situ of cervix
Cervical intraepithelial glandular neoplasia, grade III
Cervical intraepithelial neoplasia III [CIN III]
Severe dysplasia of cervix
EXCLUDES   *cervical intraepithelial neoplasia II [CIN II]*
(622.12)
cytologic evidence of malignancy without
histologic confirmation (795.06)
high grade squamous intraepithelial lesion
(HGSIL) (795.04)
moderate dysplasia of cervix (622.12)

233.2   Other and unspecified parts of uterus

233.3   Other and unspecified female genital organs

  233.30   Unspecified female genital organ

  233.31   Vagina
Severe dysplasia of vagina
Vaginal intraepithelial neoplasia III [VAIN III]

  233.32   Vulva
Severe dysplasia of vulva
Vulvar intraepithelial neoplasia III [VIN III]

  233.39   Other female genital organ

233.4   Prostate

233.5   Penis

233.6   Other and unspecified male genital organs

233.7   Bladder

233.9   Other and unspecified urinary organs

234   Carcinoma in situ of other and unspecified sites

234.0   Eye
EXCLUDES   *cartilage of eyelid (234.8)*
eyelid (skin) (232.1)
optic nerve (234.8)
orbital bone (234.8)

234.8   Other specified sites
Endocrine gland [any]

234.9   **Site unspecified**
Carcinoma in situ NOS

NEOPLASMS OF UNCERTAIN BEHAVIOR (235-238)

Note: Categories 235–238 classify by site certain histomorphologically well-defined neoplasms, the subsequent behavior of which cannot be predicted from the present appearance.

✓4ᵗʰ **235   Neoplasm of uncertain behavior of digestive and respiratory systems**

EXCLUDES   stromal tumors of uncertain behavior of digestive system (238.1)

235.0   **Major salivary glands**
Gland:
parotid
sublingual
submandibular
EXCLUDES   minor salivary glands (235.1)

235.1   **Lip, oral cavity, and pharynx**
Gingiva   Nasopharynx
Hypopharynx   Oropharynx
Minor salivary glands   Tongue
Mouth
EXCLUDES   aryepiglottic fold or interarytenoid fold, laryngeal aspect (235.6)
epiglottis:
NOS (235.6)
suprahyoid portion (235.6)
skin of lip (238.2)

235.2   **Stomach, intestines, and rectum**

235.3   **Liver and biliary passages**
Ampulla of Vater   Gallbladder
Bile ducts [any]   Liver

235.4   **Retroperitoneum and peritoneum**

235.5   **Other and unspecified digestive organs**
Anal: Esophagus
canal   Pancreas
sphincter   Spleen
Anus NOS
EXCLUDES   anus:
margin (238.2)
skin (238.2)
perianal skin (238.2)

235.6   **Larynx**
EXCLUDES   aryepiglottic fold or interarytenoid fold:
NOS (235.1)
hypopharyngeal aspect (235.1)
marginal zone (235.1)

235.7   **Trachea, bronchus, and lung**

235.8   **Pleura, thymus, and mediastinum**

235.9   **Other and unspecified respiratory organs**
Accessory sinuses
Middle ear
Nasal cavities
Respiratory organ NOS
EXCLUDES   ear (external) (skin) (238.2)
nose (238.8)
skin (238.2)

✓4ᵗʰ **236   Neoplasm of uncertain behavior of genitourinary organs**

236.0   **Uterus**

236.1   **Placenta**
Chorioadenoma (destruens)
Invasive mole
Malignant hydatid mole
Malignant hydatidiform mole

236.2   **Ovary**
Use additional code to identify any functional activity

236.3   **Other and unspecified female genital organs**

236.4   **Testis**
Use additional code to identify any functional activity

236.5   **Prostate**

236.6   **Other and unspecified male genital organs**

236.7   **Bladder**

✓5ᵗʰ 236.9   **Other and unspecified urinary organs**
236.90   **Urinary organ, unspecified**
236.91   **Kidney and ureter**
236.99   **Other**

✓4ᵗʰ **237   Neoplasm of uncertain behavior of endocrine glands and nervous system**

237.0   **Pituitary gland and craniopharyngeal duct**
Use additional code to identify any functional activity

237.1   **Pineal gland**

237.2   **Adrenal gland**
Suprarenal gland
Use additional code to identify any functional activity

237.3   **Paraganglia**
Aortic body   Coccygeal body
Carotid body   Glomus jugulare

237.4   **Other and unspecified endocrine glands**
Parathyroid gland   Thyroid gland

237.5   **Brain and spinal cord**

237.6   **Meninges**
Meninges: Meninges:
NOS   spinal
cerebral

✓5ᵗʰ 237.7   **Neurofibromatosis**
DEF: An inherited condition with developmental changes in the nervous system, muscles, bones and skin; multiple soft tumors (neurofibromas) distributed over the entire body.

237.70   **Neurofibromatosis, unspecified**
237.71   **Neurofibromatosis, type 1 [von Recklinghausen's disease]**
237.72   **Neurofibromatosis, type 2 [acoustic neurofibromatosis]**
DEF: Inherited condition with cutaneous lesions, benign tumors of peripheral nerves and bilateral 8th nerve masses.
237.73   **Schwannomatosis**
DEF: A genetic mutation (SMARCB1/INI1) causing multiple benign tumors along nerve pathways, yet characterized by the exception of the 8th cranial nerve involvement.
237.79   **Other neurofibromatosis**

237.9   **Other and unspecified parts of nervous system**
Cranial nerves
EXCLUDES   peripheral, sympathetic, and parasympathetic nerves and ganglia (238.1)

✓4ᵗʰ **238   Neoplasm of uncertain behavior of other and unspecified sites and tissues**

238.0   **Bone and articular cartilage**
EXCLUDES   cartilage:
ear (238.1)
eyelid (238.1)
larynx (235.6)
nose (235.9)
synovia (238.1)

238.1   **Connective and other soft tissue**
Peripheral, sympathetic, and parasympathetic nerves and ganglia
Stromal tumors of digestive system
EXCLUDES   cartilage (of):
articular (238.0)
larynx (235.6)
nose (235.9)
connective tissue of breast (238.3)

238.2   **Skin**
EXCLUDES   anus NOS (235.5)
skin of genital organs (236.3, 236.6)
vermilion border of lip (235.1)

Neoplasms

238.3–239.9

238.3 Breast
> EXCLUDES   skin of breast (238.2)

238.4 Polycythemia vera
> DEF: Abnormal proliferation of all bone marrow elements, increased red cell mass and total blood volume; unknown etiology, frequently associated with splenomegaly, leukocytosis, and thrombocythemia.

238.5 Histiocytic and mast cells
Mast cell tumor NOS   Mastocytoma NOS

238.6 Plasma cells
Plasmacytoma NOS   Solitary myeloma

√5ᵗʰ   **238.7 Other lymphatic and hematopoietic tissues**
> EXCLUDES   acute myelogenous leukemia (205.0)
> chronic myelomonocytic leukemia (205.1)
> myelosclerosis NOS (289.89)
> myelosis:
>   NOS (205.9)
>   megakaryocytic (207.2)

238.71 Essential thrombocythemia
Essential hemorrhagic thrombocythemia
Essential thrombocytosis
Idiopathic (hemorrhagic) thrombocythemia
Primary thrombocytosis

238.72 Low grade myelodysplastic syndrome lesions
Refractory anemia (RA)
Refractory anemia with excess blasts-1 (RAEB-1)
Refractory anemia with ringed sideroblasts (RARS)
Refractory cytopenia with multilineage dysplasia (RCMD)
Refractory cytopenia with multilineage dysplasia and ringed sideroblasts (RCMD-RS)
> DEF: Refractory anemia (RA): Form of bone marrow disorder (myelodysplastic syndrome) that interferes with red blood cell production in the bone marrow; unresponsive to hematinics; characteristic normal or hypercellular marrow with abnormal erythrocyte development and reticulocytopenia.

238.73 High grade myelodysplastic syndrome lesions
Refractory anemia with excess blasts-2 (RAEB-2)

238.74 Myelodysplastic syndrome with 5q deletion
5q minus syndrome NOS
> EXCLUDES   constitutional 5q deletion (758.39)
> high grade myelodysplastic syndrome with 5q deletion (238.73)

238.75 Myelodysplastic syndrome, unspecified

238.76 Myelofibrosis with myeloid metaplasia
Agnogenic myeloid metaplasia
Idiopathic myelofibrosis (chronic)
Myelosclerosis with myeloid metaplasia
Primary myelofibrosis
> EXCLUDES   myelofibrosis NOS (289.83)
> myelophthisic anemia (284.2)
> myelophthisis (284.2)
> secondary myelofibrosis (289.83)

238.77 Post-transplant lymphoproliferative disorder [PTLD]
Code first complications of transplant (996.80-996.89)
> DEF: Excessive proliferation of B-cell lymphocytes following Epstein-Barr virus infection in organ transplant patients; may progress to non-Hodgkins lymphoma.

238.79 Other lymphatic and hematopoietic tissues
Lymphoproliferative disease (chronic) NOS
Megakaryocytic myelosclerosis
Myeloproliferative disease (chronic) NOS
Panmyelosis (acute)

238.8 Other specified sites
Eye
Heart
> EXCLUDES   eyelid (skin) (238.2)
> cartilage (238.1)

238.9 Site unspecified

NEOPLASMS OF UNSPECIFIED NATURE (239)

√4ᵗʰ   **239 Neoplasms of unspecified nature**
Note: Category 239 classifies by site neoplasms of unspecified morphology and behavior. The term "mass,"unless otherwise stated, is not to be regarded as a neoplastic growth.
> INCLUDES   "growth" NOS
> neoplasm NOS
> new growth NOS
> tumor NOS

239.0 Digestive system
> EXCLUDES   anus:
>   margin (239.2)
>   skin (239.2)
>   perianal skin (239.2)

239.1 Respiratory system

239.2 Bone, soft tissue, and skin
> EXCLUDES   anal canal (239.0)
> anus NOS (239.0)
> bone marrow (202.9)
> cartilage:
>   larynx (239.1)
>   nose (239.1)
> connective tissue of breast (239.3)
> skin of genital organs (239.5)
> vermilion border of lip (239.0)

239.3 Breast
> EXCLUDES   skin of breast (239.2)

239.4 Bladder

239.5 Other genitourinary organs

239.6 Brain
> EXCLUDES   cerebral meninges (239.7)
> cranial nerves (239.7)

239.7 Endocrine glands and other parts of nervous system
> EXCLUDES   peripheral, sympathetic, and parasympathetic nerves and ganglia (239.2)

√5ᵗʰ   **239.8 Other specified sites**
> EXCLUDES   eyelid (skin) (239.2)
> cartilage (239.2)
> great vessels (239.2)
> optic nerve (239.7)

239.81 Retina and choroid
Dark area on retina
Retinal freckle

239.89 Other specified sites

239.9 Site unspecified

Chapter 3: Endocrine, Nutritional and Metabolic Diseases, and Immunity Disorders (240–279)

Coding Guidance

Disorders of the endocrine system include a variety of specific glandular disorders that can affect any body system. Diseases of the endocrine system include hormonal disturbances that affect some of the body's most important physiological functions, including reproduction, growth and development, and energy balance. Nutritional deficiencies include dietary and nutritional disorders such as protein-calorie malnutrition, vitamin deficiencies, and mineral deficiencies. Nutritional deficiencies due to problems relating to intestinal malabsorption normally are classified to category 579 in the digestive system chapter.

Metabolic disorders include disturbances in any of the chemical processes that take place in the human body. Metabolism is divided into two phases: anabolism, the constructive phase in which smaller molecules such as amino acids are converted into larger molecules such as proteins, and catabolism, the destructive phase in which the process is reversed. The result is growth and regeneration of tissue, elimination of waste products, energy production, and energy conservation (stored reserves).

Disorders of the Thyroid Gland (240–246)

Disorders of the thyroid gland include goiter, thyrotoxicosis, hypothyroidism, thyroiditis, congenital goiter, cysts of the thyroid, hemorrhage, and infarction of the thyroid.

Congenital Hypothyroidism (243)

Congenital hypothyroidism is classified to chapter 3 rather than to chapter 14, "Congenital Anomalies," because congenital hypothyroid is not a structural anomaly but rather a functional anomaly. Severe congenital hypothyroidism in infants leads to cretinism, which is marked by arrested physical and mental development, dystrophy of the bones and lowered basal metabolism.

When coding congenital hypothyroidism use additional codes to describe any associated mental retardation. For example, a patient with mild retardation due to congenital hypothyroidism is coded 243 Congenital hypothyroidism, and 317 Mild mental retardation.

Acquired Hypothyroidism (244)

Acquired hypothyroidism (244) is a thyroid hormone deficiency also known as myxedema. The most common cause of hypothyroidism is secondary hypothyroidism due to pituitary failure (code 244.8). Acquired hypothyroidism also may be caused by surgical resection, external beam irradiation, radioactive iodine ablation, and antithyroid medications. For example, acquired hypothyroidism due to surgical resection of the thyroid to remove primary cancer is coded 244.0, Postsurgical hypothyroidism, and V10.87 History of malignant neoplasm of the thyroid.

Thyroiditis (245)

This is the inflammation of the thyroid gland. Acute thyroiditis is caused by staphylococcal, streptococcal, or other infection. Other thyroiditis results from an autoimmune response or as a result of treatment (iatrogenic), or of unknown etiology. Use an additional code to identify infectious organism. For example, acute thyroiditis due to staphylococcal infection is coded 245.0 and 041.10.

Diseases of Other Endocrine Glands (249–259)

This section covers diabetes mellitus, disorders of the pancreas, parathyroid gland, pituitary gland, thymus gland, adrenal glands, ovarian dysfunction, testicular dysfunction, polyglandular dysfunction, and other endocrine disorders.

The most complex coding issue concerning this section is coding diabetes mellitus. Each subcategory of diabetes is discussed separately since coding issues need to be addressed specifically.

Secondary Diabetes Mellitus (249)

Secondary diabetes develops due to damage or destruction of insulin-producing cells in the pancreas by the presence of chronic disease, drugs, trauma, hormonal disturbances, genetic disorders, and other conditions. Secondary diabetes mellitus presents with the same symptoms as diabetes mellitus and carries the same risks as primary diabetes, including complications such as heart conditions, stroke, diabetic retinopathy, diabetic nephropathy, diabetic neuropathy, and sexual dysfunction. Treatment of secondary diabetes involves treating the underlying cause. When the underlying cause cannot be resolved or remains unidentified, the diabetes is treated similarly to primary diabetes, with consideration given to pre-existing comorbidities. In general, this treatment focuses on controlling the level of glucose (blood sugar) with a combination of diet and exercise, and may involve insulin therapy and antidiabetic agents. Code category 249 Secondary diabetes mellitus includes 20 codes that parallel category 250. Similarly, all of the manifestation coding that applies to category 250 also applies to 249. In the same manner, instructional notes at subcategories 249.4–249.8 direct the coder to "Use additional code to identify manifestation." Sequencing of category 249 codes depends on the documentation in the medical record and forthcoming official coding guidelines.

For postpancreatectomy diabetes mellitus (lack of insulin due to the surgical removal of all or part of the pancreas), assign code 251.3 Postsurgical hypoinsulinemia, followed by a code from subcategory 249. Use additional codes to identify any and all diabetic manifestations (e.g., diabetic nephrosis 581.81). Also assign code V88.11 Acquired total absence of pancreas, or V88.12 Acquired partial absence of pancreas, as appropriate as additional codes.

After a pancreatic transplant the patient's diabetes may no longer be an issue; however, manifestations of diabetes may still be. Assign the appropriate code from the 249 category. Assign additional codes for any manifestations and code V88.11 Acquired total absence of pancreas, or V88.12 Acquired partial absence of pancreas, as appropriate.

Diabetes Mellitus (250)

Diabetes mellitus results in a chronic and progressive course of serious systemic complications. Type I patients have a complete absence of insulin secretion from the beta cells within the islets of Langerhans and have virtually no endogenous circulating insulin. This type is commonly referred to as juvenile diabetes and can be very difficult to regulate. These patients are dependent on exogenous insulin. Type II patients have some ability to secrete insulin and produce enough endogenous circulating insulin to prevent ketosis. Onset of type II diabetes is generally later in life and is commonly referred to as adult-onset diabetes. These patients may not produce sufficient amounts or may be unable to effectively utilize the insulin produced.

The fact that a patient is receiving insulin is not the determining factor to assign a fifth digit indicating type I, insulin-dependent diabetes. In some cases Type II supplemental insulin is required.

The first axis of coding for category 250 is the identification of complications present due to the diabetes. Patients with diabetes mellitus can have a variety of complications, which may or may not be due to the diabetic condition. When the condition is caused by the diabetes, ICD-9-CM provides codes to designate a causal relationship between the condition and the disease. For example, 250.4X Diabetes with renal manifestations. The source document must support the causal relationship to assign these codes. When a casual relationship is established, the diabetic code from category 250 is sequenced first followed by the code describing the complication or manifestation.

The second axis of coding is the fifth-digit assignment for the category 250, which indicates both type of diabetes and status of control of the disease. The physician MUST document the type of diabetes in order to assign a fifth-digit. The status of uncontrolled must also be stated by the physician in order to assign a fifth-digit indicating uncontrolled status. When the physician specifically states that the patient has uncontrolled diabetes, then and only then is a fifth-digit assignment of 2 or 3 made.

Both type I and type II diabetes may exist without complications.

Diabetes with Ketoacidosis (250.1)

Ketoacidosis is a form of metabolic acidosis characterized by raised levels of circulating ketone (acetone) bodies. Ketone bodies accumulate due to metabolization of fatty acids in place of carbohydrates. The carbohydrates are not being utilized due to a lack of insulin to metabolize them.

Endocrine, Nutritional and Metabolic Diseases, and Immunity

Diabetes with Hyperosmolarity (250.2)
Coma due to very high glucose concentrations in the blood and an increased concentration of osmotically active particles (e.g., sodium and potassium). For example, hyperosmolar coma in type II diabetic patient, stated as out of control, is coded 250.22.

Diabetes with Renal Manifestations (250.4)
Diabetes with renal manifestation presents as severe thickening of the capillary basement membrane of the kidney which eventually impairs renal function. There are two basic types of diabetic nephropathy, diffuse and nodular, which may coexist. In the diffuse type, the entire suspensory structure of the renal glomerulus thickens, causing glomerulosclerosis. With nodular diabetic nephropathy (also known as Kimmelstiel-Wilson syndrome and intercapillary glomerulosclerosis), fibrin caps, capsular drops, and adhesions form in one or several areas of the glomerulus, causing glomerulosclerosis. Clinical manifestations as a result of glomerulosclerosis are known as nephrotic syndrome.

Nephritis is the first stage of kidney disease that may progress to nephrosis leading to chronic kidney disease (CKD). Code only to the most severe stage exhibited by the patient's condition. For example, type I diabetes stated as uncontrolled with diabetic nephritis and nephrosis is coded 250.43 and 583.81.

Diabetes with Ophthalmic Manifestations (250.5)
Ophthalmic disorders such as retinopathy and cataracts can result as complications of diabetes. Diabetic retinopathy is the most common ophthalmic complication and a leading cause of blindness in the United States. There are two basic types of diabetic retinopathy: background (nonproliferative or simple) and proliferative. For example, type I diabetes stated as uncontrolled with proliferative diabetic retinopathy is coded 250.53 and 362.02.

Cataracts or retinopathies are classified to this subcategory only when the physician specifies a cause and effect relationship with diabetes mellitus. Do not code cataracts as diabetic cataracts in the presence of diabetes mellitus unless the record supports a relationship between the disease and the manifestation. Diabetics may develop senile cataracts that have no causal relationship to the diabetes.

Diabetes with Neurological Manifestations (250.6)
Common long-term complications of diabetes encompass several distinct syndromes that differ with respect to anatomical distribution, neurological deficits, and clinical course. Diabetic neuropathy can affect the peripheral nerves alone or in combination with the autonomic nerves. Involvement of just a single nerve trunk is called mononeuropathy. Mononeuropathies usually are acute, self-limiting disorders most often affecting the extraocular muscles, but they can affect any single nerve trunk.

Involvement of the nerves of the peripheral nervous system is called polyneuropathy or peripheral polyneuropathy. Diabetic neuropathy affecting the part of the nervous system that regulates involuntary vital functions, particularly in the gastrointestinal system, urogenital system, and cardiovascular system, are called autonomic neuropathies. Since the autonomic nervous system includes the peripheral nerves involved in regulating cardiovascular, respiratory, endocrine, and other autonomic body functions, the term "peripheral autonomic neuropathy" (polyneuropathy) often is used.

Diabetes with Peripheral Circulatory Disorders (250.7)
Complications of diabetes that affect the blood vessels outside the heart and the lymphatic vessels are coded to this subcategory. Peripheral circulatory disorders usually are attributed to atherosclerosis and can generally be divided into two groups: macroangiopathy and microangiopathy. Macroangiopathy is disease that affects the major arterial systems; microangiopathy is disease that affects the capillary basement membranes and is a characteristic lesion of diabetes. Diabetics are more likely than nondiabetics to develop atherosclerosis and arteriosclerosis, and they tend to develop the diseases earlier.

Diabetes and Insulin Pump Malfunction
An underdose of insulin due to an insulin pump failure should be assigned 996.57 Mechanical complication due to insulin pump, as the principal or first-listed code, followed by the appropriate diabetes mellitus code based on documentation. The principal or first-listed code for an encounter due to an insulin pump malfunction resulting in an overdose of insulin should also be assigned 996.57 Mechanical complication due to insulin pump, followed by code 962.3 Poisoning by insulins and antidiabetic agents, and the appropriate diabetes mellitus code based on documentation.

Diabetic Ulcers
The instructional note under category 707.1 Ulcer of lower limbs, except pressure ulcer, indicates that the causal condition must be reported first. For diabetic ulcers, assign a code for either the 250 or 249 categories as determined by the documentation. Do not assign a code from category 707.2 Pressure ulcer staging with diabetic ulcers. Not all ulcers in diabetic patients are related to the diabetes. Documentation must state the relationship or the physician should be queried.

Nutritional Deficiencies (260–269)
Nutritionally related diseases are reported with code 260–269. Categories 262 and 263 describe protein-caloric malnutrition. Note that categories 264–269 report the lack of specific nutrients and may identify their manifestation or associated disease process.

Gout (274)
Gout is a chronic disorder of uric metabolism manifested by hyperuricemia and recurrent characteristic inflammatory arthritis. Monosodium urate or monohydrate crystals may be deposited in and around joints. Pseudogout (chondrocalcinosis), classified to code 275.49, is a disorder of calcium metabolism. Joint disease due to deposits of dicalcium phosphate or pyrophosphate crystals is a manifestation of pseudogout. Dual coding is required to indicate joint involvement. For example, pseudogout of the ankle and foot due to dicalcium phosphate crystal deposits is coded 275.49 and 712.17.

Hungry Bone Syndrome (275.5)
Hungry bone syndrome (HBS) describes a state of severe or long-standing hypocalcemia, most commonly due to primary or secondary (including post-surgical) hypoparathyroidism. Elevated levels of parathyroid hormone and bone demineralization cause the bone to sequester calcium. This results in increased bone formation (density) and decreased bone resorption, characterized by a rapid fall in plasma calcium, phosphorus, and magnesium levels. The resultant metabolic imbalance may precede osteoporosis and associated pathological fracture, tetany, or seizures. Other causal conditions for HBS include neoplasm or associated therapies, systemic metabolic acidosis, or other chronic disease (e.g., chronic renal disease). Code any causal conditions such as neoplasm, chronic disease, or certain postsurgical states (e.g., parathyroidectomy) documented in the medical record. Code also any other specified manifestations, as appropriate.

Volume Depletion (276.5)
Disorders of fluid, electrolyte, and acid-base balance dehydration (276.51), volume depletion (276.50), or hypovolemia (276.52) are imbalances of homeostasis brought on by depletion of water in the body. The manifestations of dehydration (276.51) include lethargy, weakness, and reduced alertness. Since dehydration is usually a result of another condition (i.e., gastroenteritis, renal failure, burns, urinary tract infection, and so forth), code sequencing can be confusing. Physician documentation is the deciding factor in sequencing the condition, since the physician must make the determination of the condition that necessitates reason for the visit.

Fluid overload due to dialysis noncompliance must be documented as such to distinguish this condition from cardiogenic fluid overload associated with CHF. Sequence the code for fluid overload first if the fluid overload (276.69) is the reason for the visit along with V45.12 Noncompliance with renal dialysis.

Graft-versus-Host Disease (279.5)
Graft-versus-host disease (GVHD) was previously classified exclusively to code 996.85 Complications of transplanted organ, Bone marrow. GVHD does occur most often as a complication of bone marrow transplant. However, GVHD can also occur following blood transfusion or any organ transplant when white blood cells are present in the organ that is transplanted. GVHD may be either acute or chronic in nature. Acute on chronic GVHD describes an acute exacerbation of a chronic GVHD status. Acute GVHD may affect the skin (ranging from maculopapular rash to desquamation), gastrointestinal tract (with diarrhea), and liver (with elevated bilirubin), and cause increased susceptibility to infection (which may be in part a direct effect and in part due to treatment of GVHD). Chronic GVHD with onset more than three months after transplant may exhibit manifestations similar to acute GVHD. The chronic nature of the disease increases the severity of the symptoms. Treatment of GVHD involves corticosteroids and other immune suppressants. Since GVHD is a manifestation of an underlying condition, mandatory dual coding is required. Also, multiple codes may be required to describe associated manifestations.

3. ENDOCRINE, NUTRITIONAL AND METABOLIC DISEASES, AND IMMUNITY DISORDERS (240-279)

> **EXCLUDES** *endocrine and metabolic disturbances specific to the fetus and newborn (775.0-775.9)*

Note: All neoplasms, whether functionally active or not, are classified in Chapter 2. Codes in Chapter 3 (i.e., 242.8, 246.0, 251-253, 255-259) may be used to identify such functional activity associated with any neoplasm, or by ectopic endocrine tissue.

DISORDERS OF THYROID GLAND (240-246)

✓4ᵗʰ 240 Simple and unspecified goiter

> **DEF:** An enlarged thyroid gland often caused by an inadequate dietary intake of iodine.

240.0 Goiter, specified as simple

Any condition classifiable to 240.9, specified as simple

240.9 Goiter, unspecified

Enlargement of thyroid
Goiter or struma:
  NOS
  diffuse colloid
  endemic

Goiter or struma:
  hyperplastic
  nontoxic (diffuse)
  parenchymatous
  sporadic

> **EXCLUDES** *congenital (dyshormonogenic) goiter (246.1)*

✓4ᵗʰ 241 Nontoxic nodular goiter

> **EXCLUDES** *adenoma of thyroid (226)*
> *cystadenoma of thyroid (226)*

241.0 Nontoxic uninodular goiter

Thyroid nodule   Uninodular goiter (nontoxic)

> **DEF:** Enlarged thyroid, commonly due to decreased thyroid production, with single nodule; no clinical hypothyroidism.

241.1 Nontoxic multinodular goiter

Multinodular goiter (nontoxic)

> **DEF:** Enlarged thyroid, commonly due to decreased thyroid production with multiple nodules; no clinical hypothyroidism.

241.9 Unspecified nontoxic nodular goiter

Adenomatous goiter
Nodular goiter (nontoxic) NOS
Struma nodosa (simplex)

✓4ᵗʰ 242 Thyrotoxicosis with or without goiter

> **EXCLUDES** *neonatal thyrotoxicosis (775.3)*

> **DEF:** A condition caused by excess quantities of thyroid hormones being introduced into the tissues

The following fifth-digit subclassification is for use with categories 242:

  0 without mention of thyrotoxic crisis or storm
  1 with mention of thyrotoxic crisis or storm

✓5ᵗʰ 242.0 Toxic diffuse goiter
[0-1]
Basedow's disease
Exophthalmic or toxic goiter NOS
Graves' disease
Primary thyroid hyperplasia

> **DEF:** Diffuse thyroid enlargement accompanied by hyperthyroidism, bulging eyes, and dermopathy.

✓5ᵗʰ 242.1 Toxic uninodular goiter
[0-1]
Thyroid nodule
Uninodular goiter } toxic or with hyperthyroidism

> **DEF:** Symptomatic hyperthyroidism with a single nodule on the enlarged thyroid gland. Abrupt onset of symptoms; including extreme nervousness, insomnia, weight loss, tremors, and psychosis or coma.

✓5ᵗʰ 242.2 Toxic multinodular goiter
[0-1]
Secondary thyroid hyperplasia

> **DEF:** Symptomatic hyperthyroidism with multiple nodules on the enlarged thyroid gland. Abrupt onset of symptoms; including extreme nervousness, insomnia, weight loss, tremors, and psychosis or coma.

The Endocrine System

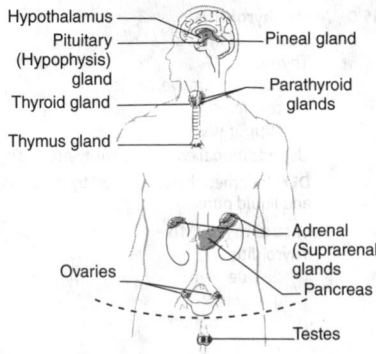

✓5ᵗʰ 242.3 Toxic nodular goiter, unspecified
[0-1]
Adenomatous goiter
Nodular goiter } toxic or with hyperthyroidism
Struma nodosa

Any condition classifiable to 241.9 specified as toxic or with hyperthyroidism

✓5ᵗʰ 242.4 Thyrotoxicosis from ectopic thyroid nodule
[0-1]

✓5ᵗʰ 242.8 Thyrotoxicosis of other specified origin
[0-1]
Overproduction of thyroid-stimulating hormone [TSH]
Thyrotoxicosis:
  factitia from ingestion of excessive thyroid material
Use additional E code to identify cause, if drug-induced

✓5ᵗʰ 242.9 Thyrotoxicosis without mention of goiter
[0-1] **or other cause**
Hyperthyroidism NOS
Thyrotoxicosis NOS

243 Congenital hypothyroidism

Congenital thyroid insufficiency
Cretinism (athyrotic) (endemic)
Use additional code to identify associated intellectual disabilities

> **EXCLUDES** *congenital (dyshormonogenic) goiter (246.1)*

> **DEF:** Underproduction of thyroid hormone present from birth.

✓4ᵗʰ 244 Acquired hypothyroidism

> **INCLUDES** athyroidism (acquired)
> hypothyroidism (acquired)
> myxedema (adult) (juvenile)
> thyroid (gland) insufficiency (acquired)

244.0 Postsurgical hypothyroidism

> **DEF:** Underproduction of thyroid hormone due to surgical removal of all or part of the thyroid gland.

244.1 Other postablative hypothyroidism

Hypothyroidism following therapy, such as irradiation

244.2 Iodine hypothyroidism

Hypothyroidism resulting from administration or ingestion of iodide
Use additional E code to identify drug

> **EXCLUDES** *hypothyroidism resulting from administration of radioactive iodine (244.1)*

244.3 Other iatrogenic hypothyroidism

Hypothyroidism resulting from:
  P-aminosalicylic acid [PAS]
  Phenylbutazone
  Resorcinol
Iatrogenic hypothyroidism NOS
Use additional E code to identify drug

244.8 Other specified acquired hypothyroidism

Secondary hypothyroidism NEC

244.9 Unspecified hypothyroidism

Hypothyroidism
Myxedema } primary or NOS

Endocrine, Nutritional and Metabolic Diseases, and Immunity

245–249.7

☑4ᵗʰ **245 Thyroiditis**

245.0 Acute thyroiditis
Abscess of thyroid
Thyroiditis:
 nonsuppurative, acute
 pyogenic
 suppurative
Use additional code to identify organism
DEF: Inflamed thyroid caused by infection, with abscess and liquid puris.

245.1 Subacute thyroiditis
Thyroiditis:
 de Quervain's
 giant cell
 granulomatous
 viral
DEF: Inflammation of the thyroid, characterized by fever and painful enlargement of the thyroid gland, with granulomas in the gland.

245.2 Chronic lymphocytic thyroiditis
Hashimoto's disease
Struma lymphomatosa
Thyroiditis:
 autoimmune
 lymphocytic (chronic)
DEF: Autoimmune disease of thyroid; lymphocytes infiltrate the gland and thyroid antibodies are produced; women more often affected.

245.3 Chronic fibrous thyroiditis
Struma fibrosa
Thyroiditis:
 invasive (fibrous)
 ligneous
 Riedel's
DEF: Persistent fibrosing inflammation of thyroid with adhesions to nearby structures; rare condition.

245.4 Iatrogenic thyroiditis
Use additional code to identify cause
DEF: Thyroiditis resulting from treatment or intervention by physician or in a patient intervention setting.

245.8 Other and unspecified chronic thyroiditis
Chronic thyroiditis:
 NOS
 nonspecific

245.9 Thyroiditis, unspecified
Thyroiditis NOS

☑4ᵗʰ **246 Other disorders of thyroid**

246.0 Disorders of thyrocalcitonin secretion
Hypersecretion of calcitonin or thyrocalcitonin

246.1 Dyshormonogenic goiter
Congenital (dyshormonogenic) goiter
Goiter due to enzyme defect in synthesis of thyroid hormone
Goitrous cretinism (sporadic)

246.2 Cyst of thyroid
 EXCLUDES *cystadenoma of thyroid (226)*

246.3 Hemorrhage and infarction of thyroid

246.8 Other specified disorders of thyroid
Abnormality of thyroid-binding globulin
Atrophy of thyroid
Hyper-TBG-nemia
Hypo-TBG-nemia

246.9 Unspecified disorder of thyroid

DISEASES OF OTHER ENDOCRINE GLANDS (249-259)

☑4ᵗʰ **249 Secondary diabetes mellitus**
 INCLUDES diabetes mellitus (due to) (in) (secondary) (with):
  drug-induced or chemical induced
  infection
Use additional code to identify any associated insulin use (V58.67)
 EXCLUDES *gestational diabetes (648.8)*
  hyperglycemia NOS (790.29)
  neonatal diabetes mellitus (775.1)
  nonclinical diabetes (790.29)
  Type I diabetes – see category 250
  Type II diabetes – see category 250

The following fifth-digit subclassification is for use with category 249:
  0 not stated as uncontrolled, or unspecified
  1 uncontrolled

☑5ᵗʰ **249.0 Secondary diabetes mellitus without mention**
[0-1] **of complication**
  Secondary diabetes mellitus without mention of complication or manifestation classifiable to 249.1-249.9
  Secondary diabetes mellitus NOS

☑5ᵗʰ **249.1 Secondary diabetes mellitus with ketoacidosis**
[0-1] Secondary diabetes mellitus with diabetic acidosis without mention of coma
  Secondary diabetes mellitus with diabetic ketosis without mention of coma

☑5ᵗʰ **249.2 Secondary diabetes mellitus with hyperosmolarity**
[0-1] Secondary diabetes mellitus with hyperosmolar (nonketotic) coma

☑5ᵗʰ **249.3 Secondary diabetes mellitus with other coma**
[0-1] Secondary diabetes mellitus with diabetic coma (with ketoacidosis)
  Secondary diabetes mellitus with diabetic hypoglycemic coma
  Secondary diabetes mellitus with insulin coma NOS
   EXCLUDES *secondary diabetes mellitus with hyperosmolar coma (249.2)*

☑5ᵗʰ **249.4 Secondary diabetes mellitus with renal manifestations**
[0-1] Use additional code to identify manifestation, as:
   chronic kidney disease (585.1-585.9)
   diabetic nephropathy NOS (583.81)
   diabetic nephrosis (581.81)
   intercapillary glomerulosclerosis (581.81)
   Kimmelstiel-Wilson syndrome (581.81)

☑5ᵗʰ **249.5 Secondary diabetes mellitus with ophthalmic**
[0-1] **manifestations**
  Use additional code to identify manifestation, as:
   diabetic blindness (369.00-369.9)
   diabetic cataract (366.41)
   diabetic glaucoma (365.44)
   diabetic macular edema (362.07)
   diabetic retinal edema (362.07)
   diabetic retinopathy (362.01-362.07)

☑5ᵗʰ **249.6 Secondary diabetes mellitus with neurological**
[0-1] **manifestations**
  Use additional code to identify manifestation, as:
   diabetic amyotrophy (353.5)
   diabetic gastroparalysis (536.3)
   diabetic gastroparesis (536.3)
   diabetic mononeuropathy (354.0-355.9)
   diabetic neurogenic arthropathy (713.5)
   diabetic peripheral autonomic neuropathy (337.1)
   diabetic polyneuropathy (357.2)

☑5ᵗʰ **249.7 Secondary diabetes mellitus with peripheral**
[0-1] **circulatory disorders**
  Use additional code to identify manifestation, as:
   diabetic gangrene (785.4)
   diabetic peripheral angiopathy (443.81)

√5th **249.8** **Secondary diabetes mellitus with other**
[0-1] **specified manifestations**
Secondary diabetic hypoglycemia in diabetes mellitus
Secondary hypoglycemic shock in diabetes mellitus
Use additional code to identify manifestation, as:
any associated ulceration (707.10-707.19, 707.8, 707.9)
diabetic bone changes (731.8)

√5th **249.9** **Secondary diabetes mellitus with unspecified**
[0-1] **complication**

√4th **250** **Diabetes mellitus**
EXCLUDES *gestational diabetes (648.8)*
hyperglycemia NOS (790.29)
neonatal diabetes mellitus (775.1)
nonclinical diabetes (790.29)
secondary diabetes (249.0-249.9)

The following fifth-digit subclassification is for use with category 250:
0 type II or unspecified type, not state as uncontrolled
Fifth-digit 0 is for use for type II patients, even if the patient requires insulin
Use additional code, if applicable, for associated long-term (current) insulin use (V58.67)
1 type I [juvenile type], not stated as uncontrolled
2 type II or unspecified type, uncontrolled
Fifth-digit 2 is for use for type II patients, even if the patient requires insulin
Use additional code, if applicable, for associated long-term (current) insulin use (V58.67)
3 type I [juvenile type], uncontrolled

DEF: Diabetes mellitus: Inability to metabolize carbohydrates, proteins, and fats due to insufficient secretion of insulin. Symptoms may be unremarkable, with long-term complications involving kidneys, nerves, blood vessels, and eyes.
DEF: Uncontrolled diabetes: A nonspecific term indicating that the current treatment regimen does not keep the blood sugar level of a patient within acceptable levels.

√5th **250.0** **Diabetes mellitus without mention of complication**
[0-3] Diabetes mellitus without mention of complication or manifestation classifiable to 250.1-250.9
Diabetes (mellitus) NOS

√5th **250.1** **Diabetes with ketoacidosis**
[0-3] Diabetic:
acidosis } without mention of coma
ketosis
DEF: Diabetic hyperglycemic crisis causing ketone presence in body fluids.

√5th **250.2** **Diabetes with hyperosmolarity**
[0-3] Hyperosmolar (nonketotic) coma

√5th **250.3** **Diabetes with other coma**
[0-3] Diabetic coma (with ketoacidosis)
Diabetic hypoglycemic coma
Insulin coma NOS
EXCLUDES *diabetes with hyperosmolar coma (250.2)*
DEF: Coma (not hyperosmolar) caused by hyperglycemia or hypoglycemia as complication of diabetes.

√5th **250.4** **Diabetes with renal manifestations**
[0-3] Use additional code to identify manifestation, as:
chronic kidney disease (585.1-585.9)
diabetic:
nephropathy NOS (583.81)
nephrosis (581.81)
intercapillary glomerulosclerosis (581.81)
Kimmelstiel-Wilson syndrome (581.81)

√5th **250.5** **Diabetes with ophthalmic manifestations**
[0-3] Use additional code to identify manifestation, as:
diabetic:
blindness (369.00-369.9)
cataract (366.41)
glaucoma (365.44)
macular edema (362.07)
retinal edema (362.07)
retinopathy (362.01-362.07)

√5th **250.6** **Diabetes with neurological manifestations**
[0-3] Use additional code to identify manifestation, as:
diabetic:
amyotrophy (353.5)
gastroparalysis (536.3)
gastroparesis (536.3)
mononeuropathy (354.0-355.9)
neurogenic arthropathy (713.5)
peripheral autonomic neuropathy (337.1)
polyneuropathy (357.2)

√5th **250.7** **Diabetes with peripheral circulatory disorders**
[0-3] Use additional code to identify manifestation, as:
diabetic:
gangrene (785.4)
peripheral angiopathy (443.81)
DEF: Blood vessel damage or disease, usually in the feet, legs, or hands, as a complication of diabetes.

√5th **250.8** **Diabetes with other specified manifestations**
[0-3] Diabetic hypoglycemia NOS
Hypoglycemic shock NOS
Use additional code to identify manifestation, as:
any associated ulceration (707.10-707.19, 707.8, 707.9)
diabetic bone changes (731.8)

√5th **250.9** **Diabetes with unspecified complication**
[0-3]

√4th **251** **Other disorders of pancreatic internal secretion**

251.0 **Hypoglycemic coma**
Iatrogenic hyperinsulinism
Non-diabetic insulin coma
Use additional E code to identify cause, if drug-induced
EXCLUDES *hypoglycemic coma in diabetes mellitus (249.3, 250.3)*
DEF: Coma induced by low blood sugar in non-diabetic patient.

251.1 **Other specified hypoglycemia**
Hyperinsulinism:
NOS
ectopic
functional
Hyperplasia of pancreatic islet beta cells NOS
Use additional E code to identify cause, if drug-induced.
EXCLUDES *hypoglycemia:*
in diabetes mellitus (249.8, 250.8)
in infant of diabetic mother (775.0)
hypoglycemic coma (251.0)
neonatal hypoglycemia (775.6)
DEF: Excessive production of insulin by the pancreas; associated with obesity and insulin-producing tumors.

251.2 **Hypoglycemia, unspecified**
Hypoglycemia: Hypoglycemia:
NOS   spontaneous
reactive
EXCLUDES *hypoglycemia:*
with coma (251.0)
in diabetes mellitus (249.8, 250.8)
leucine-induced (270.3)

251.3 **Postsurgical hypoinsulinemia**
Hypoinsulinemia following complete or partial pancreatectomy
Postpancreatectomy hyperglycemia
Use additional code to identify (any associated):
acquired absence of pancreas (V88.11-V88.12)
insulin use (V58.67)
secondary diabetes mellitus (249.00-249.91)
EXCLUDES *transient hyperglycemia post procedure (790.29)*
transient hypoglycemia post procedure (251.2)

251.4 Abnormality of secretion of glucagon
Hyperplasia of pancreatic islet alpha cells with glucagon excess

DEF: Production malfunction of a pancreatic hormone secreted by cells of the islets of Langerhans.

251.5 Abnormality of secretion of gastrin
Hyperplasia of pancreatic alpha cells with gastrin excess
Zollinger-Ellison syndrome

251.8 Other specified disorders of pancreatic internal secretion

251.9 Unspecified disorder of pancreatic internal secretion
Islet cell hyperplasia NOS

√4ᵗʰ **252 Disorders of parathyroid gland**
EXCLUDES   *hungry bone syndrome (275.5)*

√5ᵗʰ **252.0 Hyperparathyroidism**
EXCLUDES   *ectopic hyperparathyroidism (259.3)*

DEF: Abnormally high secretion of parathyroid hormones causing bone deterioration, reduced renal function, kidney stones.

252.00 Hyperparathyroidism, unspecified

252.01 Primary hyperparathyroidism
Hyperplasia of parathyroid

DEF: Parathyroid dysfunction commonly caused by hyperplasia of two or more glands; characteristic hypercalcemia and increased parathyroid hormone levels.

252.02 Secondary hyperparathyroidism, non-renal
EXCLUDES   *secondary hyperparathyroidism (of renal origin) (588.81)*

DEF: Underlying disease of nonrenal origin decreases blood levels of calcium causing the parathyroid to release increased levels of parathyroid hormone; parathyroid hormone levels return to normal once underlying condition is treated and blood calcium levels are normal.

252.08 Other hyperparathyroidism
Tertiary hyperparathyroidism

DEF: Tertiary hyperparathyroidism: chronic secondary hyperparathyroidism with adenomatous parathyroid causing irreversible abnormal production of parathyroid hormone (PTH); PTH remains high after the serum calcium levels are brought under control.

252.1 Hypoparathyroidism
Parathyroiditis (autoimmune)
Tetany:
    parathyroid
    parathyroprival
EXCLUDES   *pseudohypoparathyroidism (275.4)*
    pseudopseudohypoparathyroidism (275.4)
    tetany NOS (781.7)
    transitory neonatal hypoparathyroidism (775.4)

DEF: Abnormally low secretion of parathyroid hormones which causes decreased calcium and increased phosphorus in the blood, resulting in muscle cramps, tetany, urinary frequency and cataracts.

Dorsal View of Parathyroid Glands

Pharynx

Thyroid gland

Parathyroid glands

Trachea

Esophagus

Parathyroid glands
↓
Parathyroid hormone (PTH)
↓
Calcium in bones ———→ Calcium in blood

252.8 Other specified disorders of parathyroid gland
Cyst
Hemorrhage } of parathyroid

252.9 Unspecified disorder of parathyroid gland

√4ᵗʰ **253 Disorders of the pituitary gland and its hypothalamic control**
INCLUDES   the listed conditions whether the disorder is in the pituitary or the hypothalamus
EXCLUDES   *Cushing's syndrome (255.0)*

253.0 Acromegaly and gigantism
Overproduction of growth hormone

DEF: Acromegaly: chronic, middle age condition; caused by hypersecretion of the pituitary growth hormone; enlarged parts of skeleton, especially the nose, ears, jaws, fingers and toes.

DEF: Gigantism: pituitary gigantism caused by excess growth of short flat bones; men may grow 78 to 80 inches tall.

253.1 Other and unspecified anterior pituitary hyperfunction
Forbes-Albright syndrome
EXCLUDES   *overproduction of:*
    ACTH (255.3)
    thyroid-stimulating hormone [TSH] (242.8)

DEF: Spontaneous galactorrhea-amenorrhea syndrome unrelated to pregnancy; usually related to presence of pituitary tumor.

253.2 Panhypopituitarism
Cachexia, pituitary   Pituitary insufficiency NOS
Necrosis of pituitary   Sheehan's syndrome
   (postpartum)   Simmonds' disease
EXCLUDES   *iatrogenic hypopituitarism (253.7)*

DEF: Damage to or absence of pituitary gland leading to impaired sexual function, weight loss, fatigue, bradycardia, hypotension, pallor, depression, and impaired growth in children; called Simmonds' disease if cachexia is prominent.

253.3 Pituitary dwarfism
Isolated deficiency of (human) growth hormone [HGH]
Lorain-Levi dwarfism

DEF: Dwarfism with infantile physical characteristics due to abnormally low secretion of growth hormone and gonadotropin deficiency.

253.4 Other anterior pituitary disorders
Isolated or partial deficiency of an anterior pituitary hormone, other than growth hormone
Prolactin deficiency

253.5 Diabetes insipidus
Vasopressin deficiency
EXCLUDES   *nephrogenic diabetes insipidus (588.1)*

DEF: Metabolic disorder causing insufficient antidiuretic hormone release; symptoms include frequent urination, thirst, ravenous hunger, loss of weight, fatigue.

253.6 Other disorders of neurohypophysis
Syndrome of inappropriate secretion of antidiuretic hormone [ADH]
EXCLUDES   *ectopic antidiuretic hormone secretion (259.3)*

253.7 Iatrogenic pituitary disorders
Hypopituitarism:
    hormone-induced
    hypophysectomy-induced
    postablative
    radiotherapy-induced
Use additional E code to identify cause

DEF: Pituitary dysfunction that results from drug therapy, radiation therapy, or surgery, causing mild to severe symptoms.

253.8 Other disorders of the pituitary and other syndromes of diencephalohypophyseal origin
Abscess of pituitary
Adiposogenital dystrophy
Cyst of Rathke's pouch
Fröhlich's syndrome
EXCLUDES   *craniopharyngioma (237.0)*

253.9 Unspecified
Dyspituitarism

✓4ᵗʰ 254 Diseases of thymus gland

> *EXCLUDES*   *aplasia or dysplasia with immunodeficiency (279.2)*
> *hypoplasia with immunodeficiency (279.2)*
> *myasthenia gravis (358.00-358.01)*

254.0 Persistent hyperplasia of thymus
Hypertrophy of thymus

> **DEF:** Continued abnormal growth of the twin lymphoid lobes that produce T lymphocytes.

254.1 Abscess of thymus

254.8 Other specified diseases of thymus gland
Astrophy } of thymus
Cyst

> *EXCLUDES*   *thymoma (212.6)*

254.9 Unspecified disease of thymus gland

✓4ᵗʰ 255 Disorders of adrenal glands

> *INCLUDES*   the listed conditions whether the basic disorder is in the adrenals or is pituitary-induced

255.0 Cushing's syndrome
Adrenal hyperplasia due to excess ACTH
Cushing's syndrome:
NOS
iatrogenic
idiopathic
pituitary-dependent
Ectopic ACTH syndrome
Iatrogenic syndrome of excess cortisol
Overproduction of cortisol
Use additional E code to identify cause, if drug-induced

> *EXCLUDES*   *congenital adrenal hyperplasia (255.2)*

> **DEF:** Due to adrenal cortisol oversecretion or glucocorticoid medications; may cause excess fatty tissue of the face, neck and body; osteoporosis and curvature of spine, hypertension, diabetes mellitus, female genitourinary problems, male impotence, degeneration of muscle tissues, weakness.

✓5ᵗʰ 255.1 Hyperaldosteronism

> **DEF:** Oversecretion of aldosterone causing fluid retention, hypertension.

255.10 Hyperaldosteronism, unspecified
Aldosteronism NOS
Primary aldosteronism, unspecified

> *EXCLUDES*   *Conn's syndrome (255.12)*

255.11 Glucocorticoid-remediable aldosteronism
Familial aldosteronism type I

> *EXCLUDES*   *Conn's syndrome (255.12)*

> **DEF:** Rare autosomal dominant familial form of primary aldosteronism in which the secretion of aldosterone is under the influence of adrenocortiotrophic hormone (ACTH) rather than the renin-angiotensin mechanism; moderate hypersecretion of aldosterone and suppressed plasma renin activity rapidly reversed by administration of glucosteroids; symptoms include hypertension and mild hypokalemia.

255.12 Conn's syndrome

> **DEF:** A type of primary aldosteronism caused by an adenoma of the glomerulosa cells in the adrenal cortex; presence of hypertension.

255.13 Bartter's syndrome

> **DEF:** A cluster of symptoms caused by a defect in the ability of the kidney to reabsorb potassium; signs include alkalosis (hypokalemic alkalosis), increased aldosterone, increased plasma renin, and normal blood pressure; symptoms include muscle cramping, weakness, constipation, frequency of urination, and failure to grow; also known as urinary potassium wasting or juxtaglomerular cell hyperplasia.

255.14 Other secondary aldosteronism

255.2 Adrenogenital disorders
Achard-Thiers syndrome
Adrenogenital syndromes, virilizing or feminizing, whether acquired or associated with congenital adrenal hyperplasia consequent on inborn enzyme defects in hormone synthesis
Congenital adrenal hyperplasia
Female adrenal pseudohermaphroditism
Male:
macrogenitosomia praecox
sexual precocity with adrenal hyperplasia
Virilization (female) (suprarenal)

> *EXCLUDES*   *adrenal hyperplasia due to excess ACTH (255.0)*
> *isosexual virilization (256.4)*

255.3 Other corticoadrenal overactivity
Acquired benign adrenal androgenic overactivity
Overproduction of ACTH

✓5ᵗʰ 255.4 Corticoadrenal insufficiency

> *EXCLUDES*   *tuberculous Addison's disease (017.6)*

> **DEF:** Underproduction of adrenal hormones causing low blood pressure.

255.41 Glucocorticoid deficiency
Addisonian crisis
Addison's disease NOS
Adrenal atrophy (autoimmune)
Adrenal calcification
Adrenal crisis
Adrenal hemorrhage
Adrenal infarction
Adrenal insufficiency NOS
Combined glucocorticoid and mineralocorticoid deficiency
Corticoadrenal insufficiency NOS

> **DEF:** Decreased function of the adrenal cortex resulting in insufficient production of glucocorticoid, the hormone regulating carbohydrate, fat, and protein metabolism; manifestations: hyponatremia, hyperpigmentation, orthostatic hypotension, anemia, loss of appetite, and malaise.

255.42 Mineralocorticoid deficiency
Hypoaldosteronism

> *EXCLUDES*   *combined glucocorticoid and mineralocorticoid deficiency (255.41)*

> **DEF:** Decreased function of the adrenal cortex resulting in insufficient production of mineralocorticoid, which regulates electrolyte and water balance; manifestations: hyponatremia, hyperkalemia, and mild acidosis.

255.5 Other adrenal hypofunction
Adrenal medullary insufficiency

> *EXCLUDES*   *Waterhouse-Friderichsen syndrome (meningococcal) (036.3)*

255.6 Medulloadrenal hyperfunction
Catecholamine secretion by pheochromocytoma

255.8 Other specified disorders of adrenal glands
Abnormality of cortisol-binding globulin

255.9 Unspecified disorder of adrenal glands

✓4ᵗʰ 256 Ovarian dysfunction

256.0 Hyperestrogenism

> **DEF:** Excess secretion of estrogen by the ovaries; characterized by ovaries containing multiple follicular cysts filled with serous fluid.

256.1 Other ovarian hyperfunction
Hypersecretion of ovarian androgens

256.2 Postablative ovarian failure
Ovarian failure:
  iatrogenic
  postirradiation
  postsurgical
Use additional code for states associated with artificial menopause (627.4)
  EXCLUDES *acquired absence of ovary (V45.77)*
  asymptomatic age-related (natural) postmenopausal status (V49.81)
DEF: Failed ovarian function after medical or surgical intervention.

√5ᵗʰ **256.3 Other ovarian failure**
Use additional code for states associated with natural menopause (627.2)
  EXCLUDES *asymptomatic age-related (natural) postmenopausal status (V49.81)*

256.31 Premature menopause
  DEF: Permanent cessation of ovarian function before the age of 40 occuring naturally of unknown cause.

256.39 Other ovarian failure
  Delayed menarche
  Ovarian hypofunction
  Primary ovarian failure NOS

256.4 Polycystic ovaries
  Isosexual virilization
  Stein-Leventhal syndrome
  DEF: Multiple serous filled cysts of ovary; symptoms of infertility, hirsutism, oligomenorrhea or amenorrhea.

256.8 Other ovarian dysfunction

256.9 Unspecified ovarian dysfunction

√4ᵗʰ **257 Testicular dysfunction**

257.0 Testicular hyperfunction
  Hypersecretion of testicular hormones

257.1 Postablative testicular hypofunction
Testicular hypofunction:
  iatrogenic
  postirradiation
  postsurgical

257.2 Other testicular hypofunction
  Defective biosynthesis of testicular androgen
  Eunuchoidism:
    NOS
    hypogonadotropic
  Failure:
    Leydig's cell, adult
    seminiferous tubule, adult
  Testicular hypogonadism
  EXCLUDES *azoospermia (606.0)*

257.8 Other testicular dysfunction
  EXCLUDES *androgen insensitivity syndromes (259.50-259.52)*

257.9 Unspecified testicular dysfunction

√4ᵗʰ **258 Polyglandular dysfunction and related disorders**

√5ᵗʰ **258.0 Polyglandular activity in multiple endocrine adenomatosis**
  Multiple endocrine neoplasia [MEN] syndromes
  Use additional codes to identify any malignancies and other conditions associated with the syndromes

258.01 Multiple endocrine neoplasia [MEN] type I
  Wermer's syndrome
  DEF: Wermer's syndrome: A rare hereditary condition characterized by the presence of adenomas or hyperplasia in more than one endocrine gland causing premature aging.

258.02 Multiple endocrine neoplasia [MEN] type IIA
  Sipple's syndrome
  DEF: Sipple's syndrome: A hereditary disorder caused by a defect in the RET gene causing overactivity of the thyroid, adrenal, and parathyroid glands, resulting in adrenal pheochromocytoma and thyroid medullary carcinoma.

258.03 Multiple endocrine neoplasia [MEN] type IIB

258.1 Other combinations of endocrine dysfunction
  Lloyd's syndrome
  Schmidt's syndrome

258.8 Other specified polyglandular dysfunction

258.9 Polyglandular dysfunction, unspecified

√4ᵗʰ **259 Other endocrine disorders**

259.0 Delay in sexual development and puberty, not elsewhere classified
  Delayed puberty

259.1 Precocious sexual development and puberty, not elsewhere classified
  Sexual precocity: Sexual precocity:
    NOS   cryptogenic
    constitutional   idiopathic

259.2 Carcinoid syndrome
  Hormone secretion by carcinoid tumors
  DEF: Presence of carcinoid tumors that spread to liver; characterized by cyanotic flushing of skin, diarrhea, bronchospasm, acquired tricuspid and pulmonary stenosis, sudden drops in blood pressure, edema, ascites.

259.3 Ectopic hormone secretion, not elsewhere classified
  Ectopic:
    antidiuretic hormone secretion [ADH]
    hyperparathyroidism
  EXCLUDES *ectopic ACTH syndrome (255.0)*

259.4 Dwarfism, not elsewhere classified
  Dwarfism:
    NOS
    constitutional
  EXCLUDES *dwarfism:*
    achondroplastic (756.4)
    intrauterine (759.7)
    nutritional (263.2)
    pituitary (253.3)
    renal (588.0)
    progeria (259.8)

√5ᵗʰ **259.5 Androgen insensitivity syndrome**
  DEF: X chromosome abnormality that prohibits the body from recognizing androgen; XY genotype with ambiguous genitalia.

259.50 Androgen insensitivity, unspecified

259.51 Androgen insensitivity syndrome
  Complete androgen insensitivity
  de Quervain's syndrome
  Goldberg-Maxwell Syndrome

259.52 Partial androgen insensitivity
  Partial androgen insensitivity syndrome
  Reifenstein syndrome

259.8 Other specified endocrine disorders
  Pineal gland dysfunction
  Progeria
  Werner's syndrome

259.9 Unspecified endocrine disorder
  Disturbance:
    endocrine NOS
    hormone NOS
  Infantilism NOS

NUTRITIONAL DEFICIENCIES (260-269)

EXCLUDES *deficiency anemias (280.0-281.9)*

260 Kwashiorkor
Nutritional edema with dyspigmentation of skin and hair

DEF: Syndrome, particularly of children; excessive carbohydrate with inadequate protein intake, inhibited growth potential, anomalies in skin and hair pigmentation, edema and liver disease.

261 Nutritional marasmus
Nutritional atrophy
Severe calorie deficiency
Severe malnutrition NOS

DEF: Protein-calorie malabsorption or malnutrition in children; characterized by tissue wasting, dehydration, and subcutaneous fat depletion; may occur with infectious disease; also called infantile atrophy.

262 Other severe, protein-calorie malnutrition
Nutritional edema without mention of dyspigmentation of skin and hair

✓4ᵗʰ 263 Other and unspecified protein-calorie malnutrition

263.0 Malnutrition of moderate degree
DEF: Malnutrition characterized by biochemical changes in electrolytes, lipids, blood plasma.

263.1 Malnutrition of mild degree

263.2 Arrested development following protein-calorie malnutrition
Nutritional dwarfism
Physical retardation due to malnutrition

263.8 Other protein-calorie malnutrition

263.9 Unspecified protein-calorie malnutrition
Dystrophy due to malnutrition
Malnutrition (calorie) NOS
EXCLUDES *nutritional deficiency NOS (269.9)*

✓4ᵗʰ 264 Vitamin A deficiency

264.0 With conjunctival xerosis
DEF: Vitamin A deficiency with conjunctival dryness.

264.1 With conjunctival xerosis and Bitot's spot
Bitot's spot in the young child
DEF: Vitamin A deficiency with conjunctival dryness, superficial spots of keratinized epithelium.

264.2 With corneal xerosis
DEF: Vitamin A deficiency with corneal dryness.

264.3 With corneal ulceration and xerosis
DEF: Vitamin A deficiency with corneal dryness, epithelial ulceration.

264.4 With keratomalacia
DEF: Vitamin A deficiency creating corneal dryness; progresses to corneal insensitivity, softness, necrosis; usually bilateral.

264.5 With night blindness
DEF: Vitamin A deficiency causing vision failure in dim light.

264.6 With xerophthalmic scars of cornea
DEF: Vitamin A deficiency with corneal scars from dryness.

264.7 Other ocular manifestations of vitamin A deficiency
Xerophthalmia due to vitamin A deficiency

264.8 Other manifestations of vitamin A deficiency
Follicular keratosis } due to vitamin A deficiency
Xeroderma

264.9 Unspecified vitamin A deficiency
Hypovitaminosis A NOS

✓4ᵗʰ 265 Thiamine and niacin deficiency states

265.0 Beriberi
DEF: Inadequate vitamin B1 (thiamine) intake, affects heart and peripheral nerves; individual may become edematous and develop cardiac disease due to the excess fluid; affects alcoholics and people with a diet of excessive polished rice.

265.1 Other and unspecified manifestations of thiamine deficiency
Other vitamin B₁ deficiency states

265.2 Pellagra
Deficiency:
niacin (-tryptophan)
nicotinamide
nicotinic acid
vitamin PP
Pellagra (alcoholic)
DEF: Niacin deficiency causing dermatitis, inflammation of mucous membranes, diarrhea, and psychic disturbances.

✓4ᵗʰ 266 Deficiency of B-complex components

266.0 Ariboflavinosis
Riboflavin [vitamin B₂] deficiency
DEF: Vitamin B2 (riboflavin) deficiency marked by swollen lips and tongue fissures, corneal vascularization, scaling lesions, and anemia.

266.1 Vitamin B₆ deficiency
Deficiency:
pyridoxal
pyridoxamine
pyridoxine
Vitamin B₆ deficiency syndrome
EXCLUDES *vitamin B₆-responsive sideroblastic anemia (285.0)*
DEF: Vitamin B6 deficiency causing skin, lip, and tongue disturbances, peripheral neuropathy; and convulsions in infants.

266.2 Other B-complex deficiencies
Deficiency:
cyanocobalamin
folic acid
vitamin B₁₂
EXCLUDES *combined system disease with anemia (281.0-281.1)*
deficiency anemias (281.0-281.9)
subacute degeneration of spinal cord with anemia (281.0-281.1)

266.9 Unspecified vitamin B deficiency

267 Ascorbic acid deficiency
Deficiency of vitamin C
Scurvy
EXCLUDES *scorbutic anemia (281.8)*
DEF: Vitamin C deficiency causing swollen gums, myalgia, weight loss, and weakness.

✓4ᵗʰ 268 Vitamin D deficiency
EXCLUDES *vitamin D-resistant:*
osteomalacia (275.3)
rickets (275.3)

268.0 Rickets, active
EXCLUDES *celiac rickets (579.0)*
renal rickets (588.0)
DEF: Inadequate vitamin D intake, usually in pediatrics, that affects bones most involved with muscular action; may cause nodules on ends and sides of bones; delayed closure of fontanels in infants; symptoms may include muscle soreness, and profuse sweating.

268.1 Rickets, late effect
Any condition specified as due to rickets and stated to be a late effect or sequela of rickets
Code first the nature of late effect
DEF: Distorted or demineralized bones as a result of vitamin D deficiency.

268.2 Osteomalacia, unspecified
DEF: Softening of bones due to decrease in calcium; marked by pain, tenderness, muscular weakness, anorexia, and weight loss.

268.9 Unspecified vitamin D deficiency
Avitaminosis D

269   Other nutritional deficiencies

269.0   Deficiency of vitamin K
> EXCLUDES deficiency of coagulation factor due to
> vitamin K deficiency (286.7)
> vitamin K deficiency of newborn (776.0)

269.1   Deficiency of other vitamins
Deficiency:
vitamin E
vitamin P

269.2   Unspecified vitamin deficiency
Multiple vitamin deficiency NOS

269.3   Mineral deficiency, not elsewhere classified
Deficiency:
calcium, dietary
iodine
> EXCLUDES deficiency:
> calcium NOS (275.4)
> potassium (276.8)
> sodium (276.1)

269.8   Other nutritional deficiency
> EXCLUDES adult failure to thrive (783.7)
> failure to thrive in childhood (783.41)
> feeding problems (783.3)
> newborn (779.31-779.34)

269.9   Unspecified nutritional deficiency

OTHER METABOLIC AND IMMUNITY DISORDERS (270-279)

Use additional code to identify any associated intellectual
disabilities

270   Disorders of amino-acid transport and metabolism
> EXCLUDES abnormal findings without manifest disease
> (790.0-796.9)
> disorders of purine and pyrimidine metabolism
> (277.1-277.2)
> gout (274.00-274.9)

270.0   Disturbances of amino-acid transport
Cystinosis
Cystinuria
Fanconi (-de Toni) (-Debré) syndrome
Glycinuria (renal)
Hartnup disease

270.1   Phenylketonuria [PKU]
Hyperphenylalaninemia
DEF: Inherited metabolic condition causing excess
phenylpyruvic and other acids in urine; results in mental
retardation, neurological manifestations, including
spasticity and tremors, light pigmentation, eczema, and
mousy odor.

270.2   Other disturbances of aromatic amino-acid metabolism
Albinism
Alkaptonuria
Alkaptonuric ochronosis
Disturbances of metabolism of tyrosine and tryptophan
Homogentisic acid defects
Hydroxykynureninuria
Hypertyrosinemia
Indicanuria
Kynureninase defects
Oasthouse urine disease
Ochronosis
Tyrosinosis
Tyrosinuria
Waardenburg syndrome
> EXCLUDES vitamin B_6-deficiency syndrome (266.1)

270.3   Disturbances of branched-chain amino-acid metabolism
Disturbances of metabolism of leucine, isoleucine, and
valine
Hypervalinemia
Intermittent branched-chain ketonuria
Leucine-induced hypoglycemia
Leucinosis
Maple syrup urine disease

270.4   Disturbances of sulphur-bearing amino-acid metabolism
Cystathioninemia
Cystathioninuria
Disturbances of metabolism of methionine,
homocystine, and cystathionine
Homocystinuria
Hypermethioninemia
Methioninemia

270.5   Disturbances of histidine metabolism
Carnosinemia
Histidinemia
Hyperhistidinemia
Imidazole aminoaciduria

270.6   Disorders of urea cycle metabolism
Argininosuccinic aciduria
Citrullinemia
Disorders of metabolism of ornithine, citrulline,
argininosuccinic acid, arginine, and ammonia
Hyperammonemia
Hyperomithinemia

270.7   Other disturbances of straight-chain amino-acid metabolism
Glucoglycinuria
Glycinemia (with methyl-malonic acidemia)
Hyperglycinemia
Hyperlysinemia
Other disturbances of metabolism of glycine, threonine,
serine, glutamine, and lysine
Pipecolic acidemia
Saccharopinuria

270.8   Other specified disorders of amino-acid metabolism

Alaninemia	Iminoacidopathy
Ethanolaminuria	Prolinemia
Glycoprolinuria	Prolinuria
Hydroxyprolinemia	Sarcosinemia
Hyperprolinemia	

270.9   Unspecified disorder of amino-acid metabolism

271   Disorders of carbohydrate transport and metabolism
> EXCLUDES abnormality of secretion of glucagon (251.4)
> diabetes mellitus (249.0-249.9, 250.0-250.9)
> hypoglycemia NOS (251.2)
> mucopolysaccharidosis (277.5)

271.0   Glycogenosis
Amylopectinosis
Glucose-6-phosphatase deficiency
Glycogen storage disease
McArdle's disease
Pompe's disease
von Gierke's disease
DEF: Excess glycogen storage; rare inherited trait affects
liver, kidneys; causes various symptoms depending on
type, though often weakness and muscle cramps.

271.1   Galactosemia
Galactose-1-phosphate uridyl transferase deficiency
Galactosuria
DEF: Any of three genetic disorders due to defective
galactose metabolism; symptoms include failure to thrive
in infancy, jaundice, liver and spleen damage, cataracts,
and mental retardation.

271.2   Hereditary fructose intolerance
Essential benign fructosuria
Fructosemia
DEF: Chromosome recessive disorder of carbohydrate
metabolism; in infants, occurs after dietary sugar
introduced; characterized by enlarged spleen, yellowish
cast to skin, and progressive inability to thrive.

271.3   Intestinal disaccharidase deficiencies and disaccharide malabsorption
Intolerance or malabsorption (congenital) (of):
glucose-galactose
lactose
sucrose-isomaltose

271.4 Renal glycosuria
Renal diabetes

DEF: Persistent abnormal levels of glucose in urine, with normal blood glucose levels; caused by failure of the renal tubules to reabsorb glucose.

271.8 Other specified disorders of carbohydrate transport and metabolism

Essential benign pentosuria   Mannosidosis
Fucosidosis   Oxalosis
Glycolic aciduria   Xylosuria
Hyperoxaluria (primary)   Xylulosuria

271.9 Unspecified disorder of carbohydrate transport and metabolism

✓4ᵗʰ **272 Disorders of lipoid metabolism**

     EXCLUDES *localized cerebral lipidoses (330.1)*

272.0 Pure hypercholesterolemia
Familial hypercholesterolemia
Fredrickson Type IIa hyperlipoproteinemia
Hyperbetalipoproteinemia
Hyperlipidemia, Group A
Low-density-lipoid-type [LDL] hyperlipoproteinemia

272.1 Pure hyperglyceridemia
Endogenous hyperglyceridemia
Fredrickson Type IV hyperlipoproteinemia
Hyperlipidemia, Group B
Hyperprebetalipoproteinemia
Hypertriglyceridemia, essential
Very-low-density-lipoid-type [VLDL]
     hyperlipoproteinemia

272.2 Mixed hyperlipidemia
Broad- or floating-betalipoproteinemia
Combined hyperlipidemia
Elevated cholesterol with elevated triglycerides NEC
Fredrickson Type IIb or III hyperlipoproteinemia
Hypercholesterolemia with endogenous
     hyperglyceridemia
Hyperbetalipoproteinemia with prebetalipoproteinemia
Tubo-eruptive xanthoma
Xanthoma tuberosum

DEF: Elevated levels of lipoprotein, a complex of fats and proteins, in blood due to inherited metabolic disorder.

272.3 Hyperchylomicronemia
Bürger-Grütz syndrome
Fredrickson type I or V hyperlipoproteinemia
Hyperlipidemia, Group D
Mixed hyperglyceridemia

272.4 Other and unspecified hyperlipidemia
Alpha-lipoproteinemia
Hyperlipidemia NOS
Hyperlipoproteinemia NOS

DEF: Hyperlipoproteinemia: elevated levels of transient chylomicrons in the blood which are a form of lipoproteins that transport dietary cholesterol and triglycerides from the small intestine to the blood.

272.5 Lipoprotein deficiencies
Abetalipoproteinemia
Bassen-Kornzweig syndrome
High-density lipoid deficiency
Hypoalphalipoproteinemia
Hypobetalipoproteinemia (familial)

DEF: Abnormally low levels of lipoprotein, a complex of fats and protein, in the blood.

272.6 Lipodystrophy
Barraquer-Simons disease
Progressive lipodystrophy
Use additional E code to identify cause, if iatrogenic
     EXCLUDES *intestinal lipodystrophy (040.2)*

DEF: Disturbance of fat metabolism resulting in loss of fatty tissue in some areas of the body.

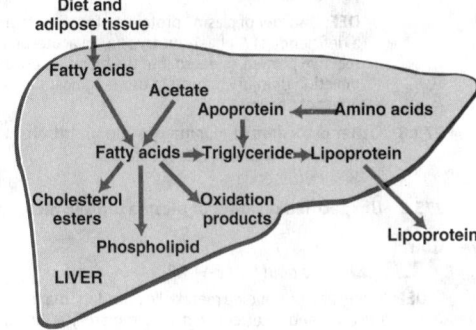

Lipid Metabolism

272.7 Lipidoses
Chemically-induced lipidosis
Disease:
     Anderson's
     Fabry's
     Gaucher's
     I cell [mucolipidosis I]
     lipoid storage NOS
     Niemann-Pick
     pseudo-Hurler's or mucolipidosis III
     triglyceride storage, Type I or II
     Wolman's or triglyceride storage, Type III
Mucolipidosis II
Primary familial xanthomatosis
     EXCLUDES *cerebral lipidoses (330.1)*
                      Tay-Sachs disease (330.1)

DEF: Lysosomal storage diseases marked by an abnormal amount of lipids in reticuloendothelial cells.

272.8 Other disorders of lipoid metabolism
Hoffa's disease or liposynovitis prepatellaris
Launois-Bensaude's lipomatosis
Lipoid dermatoarthritis

272.9 Unspecified disorder of lipoid metabolism

✓4ᵗʰ **273 Disorders of plasma protein metabolism**

     EXCLUDES *agammaglobulinemia and hypogammaglobulinemia*
                   (279.0-279.2)
                 coagulation defects (286.0-286.9)
                 hereditary hemolytic anemias (282.0-282.9)

273.0 Polyclonal hypergammaglobulinemia
Hypergammaglobulinemic purpura:
     benign primary
     Waldenström's

DEF: Elevated blood levels of gamma globulins, frequently found in patients with chronic infectious diseases.

273.1 Monoclonal paraproteinemia
Benign monoclonal hypergammaglobulinemia [BMH]
Monoclonal gammopathy:
     NOS
     associated with lymphoplasmacytic dyscrasias
     benign
Paraproteinemia:
     benign (familial)
     secondary to malignant or inflammatory disease

273.2 Other paraproteinemias
Cryoglobulinemic:
     purpura
     vasculitis
Mixed cryoglobulinemia

273.3 Macroglobulinemia
Macroglobulinemia (idiopathic) (primary)
Waldenström's macroglobulinemia

DEF: Elevated blood levels of macroglobulins (plasma globulins of high weight); characterized by malignant neoplasms of bone marrow, spleen, liver, or lymph nodes; symptoms include weakness, fatigue, bleeding disorders, and vision problems.

273.4 Alpha-1-antitrypsin deficiency
AAT deficiency

DEF: Disorder of plasma protein metabolism that results in a deficiency of Alpha-1-antitrypsin, an acute-phase reactive protein, released into the blood in response to infection or injury to protect tissue against the harmful effect of enzymes.

273.8 Other disorders of plasma protein metabolism
Abnormality of transport protein
Bisalbuminemia

273.9 Unspecified disorder of plasma protein metabolism

✓4th **274 Gout**

EXCLUDES *lead gout (984.0-984.9)*

DEF: Purine and pyrimidine metabolic disorders; manifested by hyperuricemia and recurrent acute inflammatory arthritis; monosodium urate or monohydrate crystals may be deposited in and around the joints, leading to joint destruction, and severe crippling.

✓5th **274.0 Gouty arthropathy**

274.00 Gouty arthropathy, unspecified

274.01 Acute gouty arthropathy
Acute gout
Gout attack
Gout flare
Podagra

274.02 Chronic gouty arthropathy without mention of tophus (tophi)
Chronic gout

274.03 Chronic gouty arthropathy with tophus (tophi)
Chronic tophaceous gout
Gout with tophi NOS

✓5th **274.1 Gouty nephropathy**

274.10 Gouty nephropathy, unspecified

274.11 Uric acid nephrolithiasis

DEF: Sodium urate stones in the kidney.

274.19 Other

✓5th **274.8 Gout with other specified manifestations**

274.81 Gouty tophi of ear

DEF: Chalky sodium urate deposit in the ear due to gout; produces chronic inflammation of external ear.

274.82 Gouty tophi of other sites
Gouty tophi of heart

EXCLUDES *gout with tophi NOS (274.03)*
gouty arthropathy with tophi (274.03)

274.89 Other
Use additional code to identify manifestations, as:
gouty:
iritis (364.11)
neuritis (357.4)

274.9 Gout, unspecified

✓4th **275 Disorders of mineral metabolism**

EXCLUDES *abnormal findings without manifest disease (790.0-796.9)*

✓5th **275.0 Disorders of iron metabolism**

EXCLUDES *anemia:*
iron deficiency (280.0-280.9)
sideroblastic (285.0)

275.01 Hereditary hemochromatosis
Bronzed diabetes
Pigmentary cirrhosis (of liver)
Primary (hereditary) hemochromatosis

275.02 Hemochromatosis due to repeated red blood cell transfusions
Iron overload due to repeated red blood cell transfusions
Transfusion (red blood cell) associated hemochromatosis

275.03 Other hemochromatosis
Hemochromatosis NOS

275.09 Other disorders of iron metabolism

275.1 Disorders of copper metabolism
Hepatolenticular degeneration
Wilson's disease

275.2 Disorders of magnesium metabolism
Hypermagnesemia   Hypomagnesemia

275.3 Disorders of phosphorus metabolism
Familial hypophosphatemia
Hypophosphatasia
Vitamin D-resistant:
osteomalacia
rickets

✓5th **275.4 Disorders of calcium metabolism**

EXCLUDES *hungry bone syndrome (275.5)*
parathyroid disorders (252.00-252.9)
vitamin D deficiency (268.0-268.9)

275.40 Unspecified disorder of calcium metabolism

275.41 Hypocalcemia

DEF: Abnormally decreased blood calcium level; symptoms include hyperactive deep tendon reflexes, muscle, abdominal cramps, and carpopedal spasm.

275.42 Hypercalcemia

DEF: Abnormally increased blood calcium level; symptoms include muscle weakness, fatigue, nausea, depression, and constipation.

275.49 Other disorders of calcium metabolism
Nephrocalcinosis
Pseudohypoparathyroidism
Pseudopseudohypoparathyroidism

DEF: Nephrocalcinosis: calcium phosphate deposits in the tubules of the kidney with resultant renal insufficiency.

DEF: Pseudohypoparathyroidism: inherited hypoparathyroidismdisorder; caused by inadequate response to parathyroid hormone, not hormonal deficiency; includes muscle cramps, tetany, urinary frequency, blurred vision due to cataracts, and dry scaly skin.

DEF: Pseudopseudohypoparathyroidism: clinical manifestations of hypoparathyroidism without affecting blood calcium levels.

275.5 Hungry bone syndrome

DEF: Marked and prolonged hypocalcemia; usually involves an extended history of elevated levels of parathyroid hormone, related bone demineralization causing the bone to sequester calcium.

275.8 Other specified disorders of mineral metabolism

275.9 Unspecified disorder of mineral metabolism

✓4th **276 Disorders of fluid, electrolyte, and acid-base balance**

EXCLUDES *diabetes insipidus (253.5)*
familial periodic paralysis (359.3)

276.0 Hyperosmolality and/or hypernatremia
Sodium [Na] excess
Sodium [Na] overload

276.1 Hyposmolality and/or hyponatremia
Sodium [Na] deficiency

276.2 Acidosis
Acidosis:
NOS
lactic
metabolic
respiratory

EXCLUDES *diabetic acidosis (249.1, 250.1)*

DEF: Disorder involves decrease of pH (hydrogen ion) concentration in blood and cellular tissues; caused by increase in acid and decrease in bicarbonate.

276.3 Alkalosis
Alkalosis:
NOS
metabolic
respiratory

DEF: Increased blood alkalinity (base) without relative loss of base in body fluids; caused by increased arterial plasma bicarbonate concentration or loss of carbon dioxide due to hyperventilation.

276.4 Mixed acid-base balance disorder
Hypercapnia with mixed acid-base disorder

√5ᵗʰ **276.5 Volume depletion**
EXCLUDES *hypovolemic shock:*
postoperative (998.09)
traumatic (958.4)

276.50 Volume depletion, unspecified
DEF: Depletion of total body water (dehydration) and/or contraction of total intravascular plasma (hypovolemia).

276.51 Dehydration
DEF: Depletion of total body water; blood volume may be normal while fluid is pulled from other tissues.

276.52 Hypovolemia
Depletion of volume of plasma
DEF: Depletion of volume plasma; depletion of total blood volume.

√5ᵗʰ **276.6 Fluid overload**
EXCLUDES *ascites (789.51-789.59)*
localized edema (782.3)

276.61 Transfusion associated circulatory overload
Fluid overload due to transfusion (blood)
(blood components)
TACO

276.69 Other fluid overload
Fluid retention

276.7 Hyperpotassemia
Hyperkalemia
Potassium [K]:
excess
intoxication
overload

DEF: Elevated blood levels of potassium; symptoms include abnormal EKG readings, weakness; related to defective renal excretion.

276.8 Hypopotassemia
Hypokalemia
Potassium [K] deficiency
DEF: Decreased blood levels of potassium; symptoms include neuromuscular disorders.

276.9 Electrolyte and fluid disorders not elsewhere classified
Electrolyte imbalance
Hyperchloremia
Hypochloremia
EXCLUDES *electrolyte imbalance:*
associated with hyperemesis gravidarum (643.1)
complicating labor and delivery (669.0)
following abortion and ectopic or molar pregnancy (634-638 with .4, 639.4)

√4ᵗʰ **277 Other and unspecified disorders of metabolism**

√5ᵗʰ **277.0 Cystic fibrosis**
Fibrocystic disease of the pancreas
Mucoviscidosis
DEF: Genetic disorder of infants, children, and young adults marked by exocrine gland dysfunction; characterized by chronic pulmonary disease with excess mucus production, pancreatic deficiency, and high levels of electrolytes in the sweat.

277.00 Without mention of meconium ileus
Cystic fibrosis NOS

277.01 With meconium ileus
Meconium:
ileus (of newborn)
obstruction of intestine in mucoviscidosis

277.02 With pulmonary manifestations
Cystic fibrosis with pulmonary exacerbation
Use additional code to identify any infectious organism present, such as:
pseudomonas (041.7)

277.03 With gastrointestinal manifestations
EXCLUDES *with meconium ileus (277.01)*

277.09 With other manifestations

277.1 Disorders of porphyrin metabolism
Hematoporphyria
Hematoporphyrinuria
Hereditary coproporphyria
Porphyria
Porphyrinuria
Protocoproporphyria
Protoporphyria
Pyrroloporphyria

277.2 Other disorders of purine and pyrimidine metabolism
Hypoxanthine-guanine-phosphoribosyltransferase deficiency [HG-PRT deficiency]
Lesch-Nyhan syndrome
Xanthinuria
EXCLUDES *gout (274.00-274.9)*
orotic aciduric anemia (281.4)

√5ᵗʰ **277.3 Amyloidosis**
DEF: Conditions of diverse etiologies characterized by the accumulation of insoluble fibrillar proteins (amyloid) in various organs and tissues of the body, compromising vital functions.

277.30 Amyloidosis, unspecified
Amyloidosis NOS

277.31 Familial Mediterranean fever
Benign paroxysmal peritonitis
Hereditary amyloid nephropathy
Periodic familial polyserositis
Recurrent polyserositis
DEF: Early-life onset of recurrent attacks characterized by high fevers with pain and inflammation of chest and abdominal cavities, skin and joints, also rash or vasculitis. Etiology unknown, possibly genetic, but may be precipitated by stress, trauma or exertion.

277.39 Other amyloidosis
Hereditary cardiac amyloidosis
Inherited systemic amyloidosis
Neuropathic (Portuguese) (Swiss) amyloidosis
Secondary amyloidosis

277.4 Disorders of bilirubin excretion
Hyperbilirubinemia:
congenital
constitutional
Syndrome:
Crigler-Najjar
Dubin-Johnson
Gilbert's
Rotor's
EXCLUDES *hyperbilirubinemias specific to the perinatal period (774.0-774.7)*

277.5 Mucopolysaccharidosis
Gargoylism
Hunter's syndrome
Hurler's syndrome
Lipochondrodystrophy
Maroteaux-Lamy syndrome
Morquio-Brailsford disease
Osteochondrodystrophy
Sanfilippo's syndrome
Scheie's syndrome

DEF: Metabolic disorders evidenced by excretion of various mucopolysaccharides in urine and infiltration of these substances into connective tissue, with resulting defects of bone, cartilage and connective tissue.

277.6 Other deficiencies of circulating enzymes
Hereditary angioedema

277.7 Dysmetabolic syndrome X
Use additional code for associated manifestation, such as:
cardiovascular disease (414.00-414.07)
obesity (278.00-278.03)

DEF: A specific group of metabolic disorders that are related to the state of insulin resistance (decreased cellular response to insulin) without elevated blood sugars; often related to elevated cholesterol and triglycerides, obesity, cardiovascular disease, and high blood pressure.

√5ᵗʰ **277.8 Other specified disorders of metabolism**

277.81 Primary carnitine deficiency

277.82 Carnitine deficiency due to inborn errors of metabolism

277.83 Iatrogenic carnitine deficiency
Carnitine deficiency due to:
hemodialysis
valproic acid therapy

277.84 Other secondary carnitine deficiency

277.85 Disorders of fatty acid oxidation
Carnitine palmitoyltransferase deficiencies (CPT1, CPT2)
Glutaric aciduria type II (type IIA, IIB, IIC)
Long chain 3-hydroxyacyl CoA dehydrogenase deficiency (LCHAD)
Long chain/very long chain acyl CoA dehydrogenase deficiency (LCAD, VLCAD)
Medium chain acyl CoA dehydrogenase deficiency (MCAD)
Short chain acyl CoA dehydrogenase deficiency (SCAD)
EXCLUDES   primary carnitine deficiency (277.81)

277.86 Peroxisomal disorders
Adrenomyeloneuropathy
Neonatal adrenoleukodystrophy
Rhizomelic chrondrodysplasia punctata
X-linked adrenoleukodystrophy
Zellweger syndrome
EXCLUDES   infantile Refsum disease (356.3)

277.87 Disorders of mitochondrial metabolism
Kearns-Sayre syndrome
Mitochondrial Encephalopathy, Lactic Acidosis and Stroke-like episodes (MELAS syndrome)
Mitochondrial Neurogastrointestinal Encephalopathy syndrome (MNGIE)
Myoclonus with Epilepsy and with Ragged Red Fibers (MERRF syndrome)
Neuropathy, Ataxia and Retinitis Pigmentosa (NARP syndrome)
Use additional code for associated conditions
EXCLUDES   disorders of pyruvate metabolism (271.8)
Leber's optic atrophy (377.16)
Leigh's subacute necrotizing encephalopathy (330.8)
Reye's syndrome (331.81)

277.88 Tumor lysis syndrome
Spontaneous tumor lysis syndrome
Tumor lysis syndrome following antineoplastic drug therapy
Use additional E code to identify cause, if drug-induced

DEF: A potentially fatal metabolic complication of tumor necrosis caused by either spontaneous or treatment-related accumulation of byproducts from dying cancer cells; symptoms include hyperkalemia, hyperphosphatemia, hypocalcemia, hyperuricemia, and hyperuricosuria.

277.89 Other specified disorders of metabolism
Hand-Schüller-Christian disease
Histiocytosis (acute) (chronic)
Histiocytosis X (chronic)
EXCLUDES   histiocytosis:
acute differentiated progressive (202.5)
adult pulmonary Langerhans cell (516.5)
X, acute (progressive) (202.5)

277.9 Unspecified disorder of metabolism
Enzymopathy NOS

√4ᵗʰ **278 Overweight, obesity and other hyperalimentation**
EXCLUDES   hyperalimentation NOS (783.6)
poisoning by vitamins NOS (963.5)
polyphagia (783.6)

√5ᵗʰ **278.0 Overweight and obesity**
Use additional code to identify Body Mass Index (BMI), if known (V85.0-V85.54)
EXCLUDES   adiposogenital dystrophy (253.8)
obesity of endocrine origin NOS (259.9)

278.00 Obesity, unspecified
Obesity NOS

DEF: BMI (body mass index) between 30.0 and 39.9.

278.01 Morbid obesity
Severe obesity

DEF: BMI (body mass index) 40 or greater.

278.02 Overweight

DEF: BMI (body mass index) between 25 and 29.9.

278.03 Obesity hypoventilation syndrome
Pickwickian syndrome

DEF: Hypoventilation, somnolence and erythrocytosis due to excessive weight against the chest wall.

278.1 Localized adiposity
Fat pad

278.2 Hypervitaminosis A

278.3 Hypercarotinemia

DEF: Elevated blood carotene level due to ingesting excess carotenoids or the inability to convert carotenoids to vitamin A.

278.4 Hypervitaminosis D

DEF: Weakness, fatigue, loss of weight, and other symptoms resulting from ingesting excessive amounts of vitamin D.

278.8 Other hyperalimentation

√4ᵗʰ **279 Disorders involving the immune mechanism**
Use additional code for associated manifestations

√5ᵗʰ **279.0 Deficiency of humoral immunity**

DEF: Inadequate immune response to bacterial infections with potential reinfection by viruses due to lack of circulating immunoglobulins (acquired antibodies).

279.00 Hypogammaglobulinemia, unspecified
Agammaglobulinemia NOS

279.01 Selective IgA immunodeficiency

279.02 Selective IgM immunodeficiency

279.03 Other selective immunoglobulin deficiencies
Selective deficiency of IgG

279.04 Congenital hypogammaglobulinemia
Agammaglobulinemia:
  Bruton's type
  X-linked

279.05 Immunodeficiency with increased IgM
Immunodeficiency with hyper-IgM:
  autosomal recessive
  X-linked

279.06 Common variable immunodeficiency
Dysgammaglobulinemia (acquired)
  (congenital) (primary)
Hypogammaglobulinemia:
  acquired primary
  congenital non-sex-linked
  sporadic

279.09 Other
Transient hypogammaglobulinemia of infancy

√5ᵗʰ **279.1 Deficiency of cell-mediated immunity**

279.10 Immunodeficiency with predominant T-cell defect, unspecified

279.11 DiGeorge's syndrome
Pharyngeal pouch syndrome
Thymic hypoplasia
DEF: Congenital hypoplasia or aplasia of the thymus, parathyroid glands; related heart defects, anomalies of the great vessels, esophageal atresia, and abnormalities of facial structures.

279.12 Wiskott-Aldrich syndrome
DEF: A disease characterized by chronic conditions, such as eczema, suppurative otitis media and anemia; results from an X-linked recessive gene and is classified as an immune deficiency syndrome.

279.13 Nezelof's syndrome
Cellular immunodeficiency with abnormal immunoglobulin deficiency
DEF: Immune system disorder characterized by a pathological deficiency in cellular immunity and humoral antibodies resulting in inability to fight infectious diseases.

279.19 Other
EXCLUDES ataxia-telangiectasia (334.8)

279.2 Combined immunity deficiency
Agammaglobulinemia:
  autosomal recessive
  Swiss-type
  x-linked recessive
Severe combined immunodeficiency [SCID]
Thymic:
  alymphoplasia
  aplasia or dysplasia with immunodeficiency
EXCLUDES thymic hypoplasia (279.11)
DEF: Agammaglobulinemia: No immunoglobulins in the blood.
DEF: Thymic alymphoplasia: Severe combined immunodeficiency; result of failed lymphoid tissue development.

279.3 Unspecified immunity deficiency

√5ᵗʰ **279.4 Autoimmune disease, not elsewhere classified**
EXCLUDES transplant failure or rejection (996.80-996.89)

279.41 Autoimmune lymphoproliferative syndrome
ALPS
DEF: Rare genetic alteration of the *Fas* protein; impairs normal cellular apoptosis (normal cell death), causing abnormal accumulation of lymphocytes in the lymph glands, liver, and spleen; symptoms include neutropenia, anemia, and thrombocytopenia.

279.49 Autoimmune disease, not elsewhere classified
Autoimmune disease NOS

√5ᵗʰ **279.5 Graft-versus-host disease**
Code first underlying cause, such as:
  complication of blood transfusion (999.89)
  complication of transplanted organ (996.80-996.89)
Use additional code to identify associated manifestations, such as:
  desquamative dermatitis (695.89)
  diarrhea (787.91)
  elevated bilirubin (782.4)
  hair loss (704.09)
DEF: A complication of transplantation, most commonly bone marrow; may involve skin, GI tract, liver and cause increased susceptibility to infection; results when donor cells responsible for immune response attack the cells of the transplant recipient.

279.50 Graft-versus-host disease, unspecified

279.51 Acute graft-versus-host disease

279.52 Chronic graft-versus-host disease

279.53 Acute on chronic graft-versus-host disease

279.8 Other specified disorders involving the immune mechanism
Single complement [C_1-C_9] deficiency or dysfunction

279.9 Unspecified disorder of immune mechanism

Chapter 4: Diseases of the Blood and Blood-Forming Organs (280–289)

Coding Guidance

This ICD-9-CM chapter classifies diseases and disorders of blood and blood-forming (hemopoietic) organs, including the following:

- Anemias
- Coagulation defects
- Purpura and other hemorrhagic conditions
- Diseases of white blood cells
- Other diseases of blood and blood-forming organs

The term "anemia" refers to a lower than normal erythrocyte count or level of hemoglobin in the circulating blood. A clinical sign rather than a diagnostic entity, anemia can be classified by three morphological variations of the erythrocyte: size (volume), hemoglobin content, and shape.

In laboratory blood tests, erythrocyte size is gauged by estimating the volume of red cells in the circulating blood. Red cell volume, or mean corpuscular volume, is estimated by dividing the patient's hematocrit (percentage of red blood cells in whole blood) by the red blood cell count. Normal values are normocytic; abnormally low values are microcytic; and abnormally high values are macrocytic.

Hemoglobin content refers to the average amount of hemoglobin in each red blood cell. This value, called the mean cell hemoglobin, is calculated by dividing the patient's hemoglobin by the number of red blood cells. Normal values are normochromic, less than normal values are hypochromic, and greater than normal values are hyperchromic.

Shape is determined by microscopy. Normally, red blood cells have a smooth concave shape. Erythrocytes with irregular shapes are called poikilocytes, a general term meaning abnormally shaped. Terms referring to specific abnormal cell shapes include acanthocytes, leptocytes, nucleated erythrocytes, macro-ovalocytes, schistocytes, helmet cells, teardrop cells, sickle cells, and target cells.

Once the cell morphology is determined, the anemia can be classified further based on certain physiological and pathological criteria. For example, constitutional aplastic anemia (subcategory 284.0) is classified physiologically as an anemia of hypoproliferation and pathologically as an inborn error of heredity.

The "coagulation defects" refers to deficiencies or disorders of hemostasis. A complicated process involving substances in the injured tissues, formed elements of blood (platelets, monocytes) and the coagulation proteins, coagulation requires the production of thrombin, a substance that stabilizes the platelet plug and forms the fibrin clot. Together they mechanically block the extravasation of blood from ruptured vessels. The coagulation process can be interrupted by a genetic or disease-caused protein deficiency, interrupted by an increase in the catabolism of coagulation proteins or inhibited by antibodies directed against the coagulation proteins. There are many proteins involved in coagulation, many of which are identified by the term "factor" followed by a roman numeral. The activated form of a coagulation factor is indicated by the appropriate roman numeral followed by the suffix "a." For example, the protein factor II (prothrombin) is activated by the enzyme thrombin; when this occurs, it is designated factor IIa.

Iron Deficiency Anemias (280) and Other Deficiency Anemias (281)

Iron deficiency anemia is a chronic hypochromic, microcytic anemia characterized by small, pale erythrocytes and a depletion of iron stores. In adults, iron deficiency anemia is almost always due to blood loss; loss of as little as 2 to 4 ml of blood per day may deplete iron stores. This condition is also known as hypoferric anemia, hypochromic or microcytic anemia, and chlorosis.

Iron deficiency anemias secondary to inadequate dietary iron intake (280.1) is due to excretion of iron that exceeds normal dietary intake. Iron is recycled metabolically so that less than 1 mg is lost through excretion per day. A normal diet consists of 12–15 mg of iron, of which 0.6–1.5 mg are absorbed. Neonates and young children may develop iron deficiency anemia due to new blood formation and increased iron utilization that exceeds dietary intake.

Other specified iron deficiency anemias (280.8) are iron deficiency anemias of other specified types and causes, such as gastrectomy, excessive blood donation, and upper small-bowel malabsorption syndromes.

Iron deficiency anemia, unspecified (280.9) is a hypochromic anemia or iron deficiency anemia due to an unspecified or unknown cause. Included are microcytic or hypochromic anemias not otherwise specified and iron deficiency anemia due to impaired iron absorption not otherwise specified.

Pernicious anemia (281.0) is a progressive anemia of vitamin B-12 deficiency due to an absorption defect. Also known as Addison's or Biermer's anemia, it rarely occurs before the fourth decade of life. The condition may be due to an inherited genetic defect characterized by a deficiency of intrinsic factor, a substance essential for B-12 absorption.

Folate deficiency anemia (281.2) is macrocytic anemia caused by a deficiency of the anionic form of folic acid. If drug induced, use an additional E code to identify the drug.

Hereditary Hemolytic Anemias (282)

Thalassemia (282.4x) is a microcytic, hypochromic hemolytic anemia that results from a hereditary defect causing deficient hemoglobin synthesis. The severity, treatment, and prognosis of thalassemia depends on the globin gene arrangement and deletion type. Thalassemia major, also known as beta thalessemia, the most severe form, is evident soon after birth.

Sickle-cell trait (282.5) is a heterozygous carrier of both the hemoglobin S and hemoglobin A genes. The condition rarely is associated with a clinical disorder.

Sickle-cell disease (282.6x) is a severe, chronic, and incurable form of anemia occurring in patients who inherit hemoglobin S genes from both parents. Less severe variations of the disease occur when the patient inherits a hemoglobin S gene from one parent and a hemoglobin C, D, or E gene from the other.

Acquired Hemolytic Anemias (283)

Acquired hemolytic anemia is characterized by the premature destruction of erythrocytes, exclusive of an inherited erythrocyte disorder. Hemolytic anemias may be acquired through infection, drugs, blood transfusions (autoimmune), or other intrinsic or extrinsic causes. Hemolytic uremic syndrome (hemolytic anemia and thrombocytopenia occurring with acute renal failure) is a common nonautoimmune hemolytic anemia. For example, hemolytic-uremic syndrome with acute renal failure is coded 283.11 Hemolytic-uremic syndrome, and 584.9 Acute renal failure, unspecified.

Aplastic Anemia and Other Bone Marrow Failure Syndromes (284)

Aplastic anemia is the failure of bone marrow to generate blood cells, resulting in a deficiency of all of the formed elements of the blood (erythrocytes, platelets, and leukocytes).

Aplastic anemia may be a direct result of chemotherapy for a malignant tumor. If treatment is directed toward the anemia, code as 284.89 and E933.1. This should not be confused with anemia due to the neoplastic process (e.g., 285.22).

Pure red cell aplasia (PRCA) describes a condition in which RBC precursors in bone marrow are nearly absent, while megakaryocytes and WBC precursors are usually present at normal levels. This condition is recognized as being a different entity from aplastic anemia. Although separate classifications exist for congenital red cell aplasia, the default code for the disease is the acquired form, code 284.81 Red cell aplasia. Code 284.89 Other specified aplastic anemia classifies other aplastic anemia due to chronic systemic disease or other external factors. Use an additional code to identify cause, such as drugs and radiation.

Other and Unspecified Anemias (285)

Secondary anemia caused by chronic illness (infections and neoplastic disease) or treatment for disease is assigned code 285.2x Anemia in chronic disease, only when no further information concerning the specific anemia is available. When the type of anemia is specified, the more specific anemia code should be assigned. In addition, assign codes to describe the specific chronic condition or specific malignancy (unless it's ESRD, which is contained in the code description) and an appropriate E code, if due to treatment.

Code 285.22 Anemia in neoplastic disease, excludes anemia caused by antineoplastic chemotherapy.

Purpura and Other Hemorrhagic Conditions (287)

Purpura is hemorrhages of the skin. Initially red, the lesions darken to purple, fade to brownish-yellow and typically disappear in two to three weeks. Causes include allergic reactions, blood disorders, vascular abnormalities, and trauma.

Thrombocytopenia is a disorder distinguished by an abnormal decrease in the number of blood platelets and the presence of purpural skin hemorrhages. Secondary thrombocytopenia (287.49) may be caused by underlying conditions such as lupus erythematosus, Gaucher's disease, tuberculosis, or may be a result of massive blood transfusion, extracorporeal circulation of the blood, drugs, and platelet alloimmunization.

Diseases of White Blood Cells (288)

Neutropenia, also known as granulocytopenia or agranulocytosis, is a condition in which the neutrophil or granulocyte count in the blood is diminished, resulting in an increased susceptibility to bacterial and fungal infections. Elevated and decreased white blood cell counts are often clinical findings that lead to further patient assessment. Separate codes classify the various forms of neutropenia. Instructional notes direct the coder to use an additional E code to identify the drug in drug-induced neutropenia, or an additional code to report fever associated (but not inherent to) neutropenia.

Bandemia is a CBC laboratory finding in which there is an increase in early neutrophil cells, or band cells. The nucleus is not segmented but forms a continuous band. Code 288.66 Bandemia, is intended for reporting when a definitive diagnosis such as infection has not yet been established. If documentation states that bandemia is associated with a confirmed cause such as infection, code only the infection.

Other Diseases of Blood and Blood-forming Organs (289)

Polycythemia, secondary (289.0) is the increase in the normal number of red blood cells. Secondary polycythemia is also known as secondary erythrocytosis, spurious polycythemia and reactive polycythemia. Spurious polycythemia, which is characterized by increased hematocrit and normal or increased erythrocyte total mass, results from a decrease in plasma volume and hemoconcentration. Reactive polycythemia is a condition characterized by excessive production of circulating erythrocytes due to an identifiable secondary condition such as hypoxia or an underlying disease such as a neoplasm.

Chronic lymphadenitis (289.1) is an inflammation of the lymph nodes. Any pathogen can cause lymphadenitis. Lymphadenitis may be generalized or restricted to regional lymph nodes and may occur with systemic infections.

Nonspecific mesenteric lymphadenitis (289.2) is a lymphadenitis occurring in the double layer of peritoneum attached to the abdominal wall, which encloses a portion or all of one of the abdominal viscera.

Hypersplenism (289.4) is a clinical syndrome characterized by splenic hyperactivity and splenomegaly. The condition results in a peripheral blood cell deficiency because the spleen traps and destroys the circulating peripheral blood cells.

Code 289.84 distinguishes heparin-induced thrombocytopenia (HIT) from other forms of secondary thrombocytopenia (287.49).Heparin is one of the most frequently prescribed medications, and its usage can lead to a particularly challenging adverse thrombocytopenic reaction (HIT). It is one of the three most common causes of iatrogenic thrombocytopenia, along with sepsis (with or without DIC) and the adverse effects of other drugs. Fifty percent or more of those with HIT will have thrombotic complications. These thromboembolic events may be arterial or venous and can lead to limb amputation, pulmonary emboli, strokes, and myocardial infarction. Although treatment should be initiated immediately if HIT is clinically suspected, the diagnosis can be confirmed by serologic tests for the pathogenic antibody. The serologic tests include commercially available ELISAs that detect the pathogenic antibodies to modified PF4, or functional assays demonstrating the activation of platelets in the presence of patient serum and heparin. Treatment includes the initiation of an alternative anticoagulant with thrombin inhibitors. Prolonged anticoagulation after recovery is essential to prevent thromboembolic events. Assign 287.49 for secondary thrombocytopenia due to drugs other than heparin or due to other treatment such as extracorporeal circulation of blood or massive blood transfusion. While clinically the same, heparin-induced thrombocytopenia has been given its own code due to the prevalence of heparin treatment and increased rate of subsequent adverse reactions.

4. DISEASES OF THE BLOOD AND BLOOD-FORMING ORGANS (280-289)

EXCLUDES *anemia complicating pregnancy or the puerperium (648.2)*

✓4ᵗʰ 280 Iron deficiency anemias

INCLUDES anemia:
   asiderotic
   hypochromic-microcytic
   sideropenic
EXCLUDES *familial microcytic anemia (282.49)*

280.0 Secondary to blood loss (chronic)
Normocytic anemia due to blood loss
EXCLUDES *acute posthemorrhagic anemia (285.1)*

280.1 Secondary to inadequate dietary iron intake

280.8 Other specified iron deficiency anemias
Paterson-Kelly syndrome
Plummer-Vinson syndrome
Sideropenic dysphagia

280.9 Iron deficiency anemia, unspecified
Anemia:
   achlorhydric
   chlorotic
   idiopathic hypochromic
   iron [Fe] deficiency NOS

✓4ᵗʰ 281 Other deficiency anemias

281.0 Pernicious anemia
Anemia:
   Addison's
   Biermer's
   congenital pernicious
Congenital intrinsic factor [Castle's] deficiency
EXCLUDES *combined system disease without mention of anemia (266.2)*
subacute degeneration of spinal cord without mention of anemia (266.2)

DEF: Chronic progressive anemia due to Vitamin B12 malabsorption; caused by lack of a secretion of intrinsic factor, which is produced by the gastric mucosa of the stomach.

281.1 Other vitamin B$_{12}$ deficiency anemia
Anemia:
   vegan's
   vitamin B$_{12}$ deficiency (dietary)
   due to selective vitamin B$_{12}$ malabsorption with proteinuria
Syndrome:
   Imerslund's
   Imerslund-Gräsbeck
EXCLUDES *combined system disease without mention of anemia (266.2)*
subacute degeneration of spinal cord without mention of anemia (266.2)

281.2 Folate-deficiency anemia
Congenital folate malabsorption
Folate or folic acid deficiency anemia:
   NOS
   dietary
   drug-induced
Goat's milk anemia
Nutritional megaloblastic anemia (of infancy)
Use additional E code to identify drug

DEF: Macrocytic anemia resembles pernicious anemia but without absence of hydrochloric acid secretions; responsive to folic acid therapy.

281.3 Other specified megaloblastic anemias not elsewhere classified
Combined B$_{12}$ and folate-deficiency anemia
Refractory megaloblastic anemia

DEF: Megaloblasts predominant in bone marrow with few normoblasts; rare familial type associated with proteinuria and genitourinary tract anomalies.

281.4 Protein-deficiency anemia
Amino-acid-deficiency anemia

281.8 Anemia associated with other specified nutritional deficiency
Scorbutic anemia

281.9 Unspecified deficiency anemia
Anemia:
   dimorphic
   macrocytic
   megaloblastic NOS
   nutritional NOS
   simple chronic

✓4ᵗʰ 282 Hereditary hemolytic anemias

DEF: Escalated rate of erythrocyte destruction; similar to all anemias, occurs when imbalance exists between blood loss and blood production.

282.0 Hereditary spherocytosis
Acholuric (familial) jaundice
Congenital hemolytic anemia (spherocytic)
Congenital spherocytosis
Minkowski-Chauffard syndrome
Spherocytosis (familial)
EXCLUDES *hemolytic anemia of newborn (773.0-773.5)*

DEF: Hereditary, chronic illness marked by abnormal red blood cell membrane; symptoms include enlarged spleen, jaundice; and anemia in severe cases.

282.1 Hereditary elliptocytosis
Elliptocytosis (congenital)
Ovalocytosis (congenital) (hereditary)

DEF: Genetic hemolytic anemia characterized by malformed, elliptical erythrocytes; there is increased destruction of red cells with resulting anemia.

282.2 Anemias due to disorders of glutathione metabolism
Anemia:
   6-phosphogluconic dehydrogenase deficiency
   enzyme deficiency, drug-induced
   erythrocytic glutathione deficiency
   glucose-6-phosphate dehydrogenase [G-6-PD] deficiency
   glutathione-reductase deficiency
   hemolytic nonspherocytic (hereditary), type I
Disorder of pentose phosphate pathway
Favism

282.3 Other hemolytic anemias due to enzyme deficiency
Anemia:
   hemolytic nonspherocytic (hereditary), type II
   hexokinase deficiency
   pyruvate kinase [PK] deficiency
   triosephosphate isomerase deficiency

✓5ᵗʰ 282.4 Thalassemias

EXCLUDES *sickle-cell:*
disease (282.60-282.69)
trait (282.5)

DEF: Inherited hemolytic disorders characterized by decreased production of at least one polypeptide globin chain results in defective hemoglobin synthesis; symptoms include severe anemia, expanded marrow spaces, transfusional and absorptive iron overload, impaired growth rate, thickened cranial bones, and pathologic fractures.

282.40 Thalassemia, unspecified
Thalassemia NOS

282.41 Sickle-cell thalassemia without crisis
Microdrepanocytosis
Sickle-cell thalassemia NOS
Thalassemia Hb-S disease without crisis

282.42 Sickle-cell thalassemia with crisis
Sickle-cell thalassemia with vaso-occlusive pain
Thalassemia Hb-S disease with crisis
Use additional code for type of crisis, such as:
   acute chest syndrome (517.3)
   splenic sequestration (289.52)

Diseases of the Blood and Blood-Forming Organs

282.43–282.69

282.43 Alpha thalassemia
Alpha thalassemia major
Hemoglobin H Constant Spring
Hemoglobin H disease
Hydrops fetalis due to alpha thalassemia
Severe alpha thalassemia
Triple gene defect alpha thalassemia

> **EXCLUDES** *alpha thalassemia trait or minor (282.46)*
> *hydrops fetalis due to isoimmunization (773.3)*
> *hydrops fetalis not due to immune hemolysis (778.0)*

DEF: HBA1 and HBA2 genetic variant of chromosome 16 prevalent among those of West African and South Asian descent; associated with a wide spectrum of anemic presentation, includes hemoglobin H disease subtypes.

282.44 Beta thalassemia
Beta thalassemia major
Cooley's anemia
Homozygous beta thalassemia
Severe beta thalassemia
Thalassemia intermedia
Thalassemia major

> **EXCLUDES** *beta thalassemia minor (282.46)*
> *beta thalassemia trait (282.46)*
> *delta-beta thalassemia (282.45)*
> *hemoglobin E-beta thalassemia (282.47)*
> *sickle-cell beta thalassemia (282.41, 282.42)*

DEF: Diversity of mutations of HBB gene on chromosome 11 prevalent among those of Mediterranean and certain South Asian descent with significant cellular damage can result in toxicity and increased disease severity (e.g., severe beta thalassemia, thalassemia major).

282.45 Delta-beta thalassemia
Homozygous delta-beta thalassemia

> **EXCLUDES** *delta-beta thalassemia trait (282.46)*

282.46 Thalassemia minor
Alpha thalassemia minor
Alpha thalassemia trait
Alpha thalassemia silent carrier
Beta thalassemia minor
Beta thalassemia trait
Delta-beta thalassemia trait
Thalassemia trait NOS

> **EXCLUDES** *alpha thalassemia (282.43)*
> *beta thalassemia (282.44)*
> *delta-beta thalassemia (282.45)*
> *hemoglobin E-beta thalassemia (282.47)*
> *sickle-cell trait (282.5)*

DEF: Solitary abnormal gene that identifies a carrier of the disease, yet with an absence of symptoms or a clinically mild anemic presentation.

282.47 Hemoglobin E-beta thalassemia

> **EXCLUDES** *beta thalassemia (282.44)*
> *beta thalassemia minor (282.46)*
> *beta thalassemia trait (282.46)*
> *delta-beta thalassemia (282.45)*
> *delta-beta thalassemia trait (282.46)*
> *hemoglobin E disease (282.7)*
> *other hemoglobinopathies (282.7)*
> *sickle-cell beta thalassemia (282.41, 282.42)*

DEF: Clinically similar phenotype to B thalassemia major that is prevalent among those of Southeast Asian and certain Indian descent; results in severe transfusion-dependent anemia when present with certain B mutations.

282.49 Other thalassemia
Dominant thalassemia
Hemoglobin C thalassemia
Hereditary leptocytosis
Mediterranean anemia (with other hemoglobinopathy)
Mix thalassemia
Thalassemia with other hemoglobinopathy

> **EXCLUDES** *hemoglobin C disease (282.7)*
> *hemoglobin E disease (282.7)*
> *other hemoglobinopathies (282.7)*
> *sickle-cell anemias (282.60-282.69)*
> *sickle-cell beta thalassemia (282.41-282.42)*

282.5 Sickle-cell trait
Hb-AS genotype
Hemoglobin S [Hb-S] trait
Heterozygous:
  hemoglobin S
  Hb-S

> **EXCLUDES** *that with other hemoglobinopathy (282.60-282.69)*
> *that with thalassemia (282.41-282.42)*

DEF: Heterozygous genetic makeup characterized by one gene for normal hemoglobin and one for sickle-cell hemoglobin; clinical disease rarely present.

√5ᵗʰ **282.6 Sickle-cell disease**
Sickle-cell anemia

> **EXCLUDES** *sickle-cell thalassemia (282.41-282.42)*
> *sickle-cell trait (282.5)*

DEF: Inherited blood disorder; sickle-shaped red blood cells are hard and pointed, clogging blood flow; anemia characterized by periodic episodes of pain, acute abdominal discomfort, skin ulcerations of the legs, increased infections.

282.60 Sickle-cell disease, unspecified
Sickle-cell anemia NOS

282.61 Hb-SS disease without crisis

282.62 Hb-SS disease with crisis
Hb-SS disease with vaso-occlusive pain
Sickle-cell crisis NOS
Use additional code for type of crisis, such as:
  acute chest syndrome (517.3)
  splenic sequestration (289.52)

282.63 Sickle-cell/Hb-C disease without crisis
Hb-S/Hb-C disease without crisis

282.64 Sickle-cell/Hb-C disease with crisis
Hb-S/Hb-C disease with crisis
Sickle-cell/Hb-C disease with vaso-occlusive pain
Use additional code for type of crisis, such as:
  acute chest syndrome (517.3)
  splenic sequestration (289.52)

282.68 Other sickle-cell disease without crisis
Hb-S/Hb-D
Hb-S/Hb-E   } diseases without
Sickle-cell/Hb-D   } crisis
Sickle-cell/Hb-E

282.69 Other sickle-cell disease with crisis
Hb-S/Hb-D
Hb-S/Hb-E   } diseases with crisis
Sickle-cell/Hb-D
Sickle-cell/Hb-E
Other sickle-cell disease with vaso-occlusive pain
Use additional code for type of crisis, such as:
  acute chest syndrome (517.3)
  splenic sequestration (289.52)

282.7 Other hemoglobinopathies
Abnormal hemoglobin NOS
Congenital Heinz-body anemia
Disease:
    hemoglobin C [Hb-C]
    hemoglobin D [Hb-D]
    hemoglobin E [Hb-E]
    hemoglobin Zurich [Hb-Zurich]
Hemoglobinopathy NOS
Hereditary persistence of fetal hemoglobin [HPFH]
Unstable hemoglobin hemolytic disease

> **EXCLUDES** *familial polycythemia (289.6)*
> *hemoglobin E-beta thalassemia (282.47)*
> *hemoglobin M [Hb-M] disease (289.7)*
> *high-oxygen-affinity hemoglobin (289.0)*
> *other hemoglobinopathies with thalassemia (282.49)*

> **DEF:** Any disorder of hemoglobin due to alteration of molecular structure; may include overt anemia.

282.8 Other specified hereditary hemolytic anemias
Stomatocytosis

282.9 Hereditary hemolytic anemia, unspecified
Hereditary hemolytic anemia NOS

√4ᵗʰ **283 Acquired hemolytic anemias**

> **DEF:** Nonhereditary anemia characterized by premature destruction of red blood cells; caused by infectious organisms, poisons, and physical agents.

283.0 Autoimmune hemolytic anemias
Autoimmune hemolytic disease (cold type) (warm type)
Chronic cold hemagglutinin disease
Cold agglutinin disease or hemoglobinuria
Hemolytic anemia:
    cold type (secondary) (symptomatic)
    drug-induced
    warm type (secondary) (symptomatic)
Use additional E code to identify cause, if drug-induced

> **EXCLUDES** *Evans' syndrome (287.32)*
> *hemolytic disease of newborn (773.0-773.5)*

√5ᵗʰ **283.1 Non-autoimmune hemolytic anemias**
Use additional E code to identify cause

> **DEF:** Hemolytic anemia and thrombocytopenia with acute renal failure; relatively rare condition; 50 percent of patients require renal dialysis.

283.10 Non-autoimmune hemolytic anemia, unspecified

283.11 Hemolytic-uremic syndrome
Use additional code to identify associated:
    E. coli infection (041.41-041.49)
    Pneumococcal pnemonia (481)
    Shigella dysenteriae (004.0)

283.19 Other non-autoimmune hemolytic anemias
Hemolytic anemia:
    mechanical
    microangiopathic
    toxic

283.2 Hemoglobinuria due to hemolysis from external causes
Acute intravascular hemolysis
Hemoglobinuria:
    from exertion
    march
    paroxysmal (cold) (nocturnal)
    due to other hemolysis
Marchiafava-Micheli syndrome
Use additional E code to identify cause

283.9 Acquired hemolytic anemia, unspecified
Acquired hemolytic anemia NOS
Chronic idiopathic hemolytic anemia

√4ᵗʰ **284 Aplastic anemia and other bone marrow failure syndromes**

> **DEF:** Bone marrow failure to produce the normal amount of blood components; generally non-responsive to usual therapy.

√5ᵗʰ **284.0 Constitutional aplastic anemia**

284.01 Constitutional red blood cell aplasia
Aplasia, (pure) red cell:
    congenital
    of infants
    primary
Blackfan-Diamond syndrome
Familial hypoplastic anemia

284.09 Other constitutional aplastic anemia
Fanconi's anemia
Pancytopenia with malformations

√5ᵗʰ **284.1 Pancytopenia**

> **EXCLUDES** *pancytopenia (due to) (with):*
> *aplastic anemia NOS (284.9)*
> *bone marrow infiltration (284.2)*
> *constitutional red blood cell aplasia (284.01)*
> *hairy cell leukemia (202.4)*
> *human immunodeficiency virus disease (042)*
> *leukoerythroblastic anemia (284.2)*
> *malformations (284.09)*
> *myelodysplastic syndromes (238.72-238.75)*
> *myeloproliferative disease (238.79)*
> *other constitutional aplastic anemia (284.09)*

284.11 Antineoplastic chemotherapy induced pancytopenia

> **EXCLUDES** *aplastic anemia due to antineoplastic chemotherapy (284.89)*

284.12 Other drug-induced pancytopenia

> **EXCLUDES** *aplastic anemia due to drugs (284.89)*

284.19 Other pancytopenia

284.2 Myelophthisis
Leukoerythroblastic anemia
Myelophthisic anemia
Code first the underlying disorder, such as:
    malignant neoplasm of breast (174.0-174.9, 175.0-175.9)
    tuberculosis (015.0-015.9)

> **EXCLUDES** *idiopathic myelofibrosis (238.76)*
> *myelofibrosis NOS (289.83)*
> *myelofibrosis with myeloid metaplasia (238.76)*
> *primary myelofibrosis (238.76)*
> *secondary myelofibrosis (289.83)*

> **DEF:** A secondary disease process involving replacement of normal hematopoeitic tissue in the bone marrow with abnormal tissue, such as fibrous tissue or tumors. Occurs with advanced-stage neoplasms, granulomatous diseases such as miliary tuberculosis, and other inflammatory diseases.

√5ᵗʰ **284.8 Other specified aplastic anemias**

284.81 Red cell aplasia (acquired) (adult) (with thymoma)
Red cell aplasia NOS

284.89 Other specified aplastic anemias
Aplastic anemia (due to):
    chronic systemic disease
    drugs
    infection
    radiation
    toxic (paralytic)
Use additional E code to identify cause

284.9 Aplastic anemia, unspecified
Anemia:
    aplastic (idiopathic) NOS
    aregenerative
    hypoplastic NOS
    nonregenerative
Medullary hypoplasia

> **EXCLUDES** *refractory anemia (238.72)*

Diseases of the Blood and Blood-Forming Organs

285–286.52

✓4ᵗʰ **285 Other and unspecified anemias**

285.0 Sideroblastic anemia
Anemia:
   hypochromic with iron loading
   sideroachrestic
   sideroblastic:
      acquired
      congenital
      hereditary
      primary
      secondary (drug-induced) (due to disease)
      sex-linked hypochromic
      vitamin B6-responsive
Pyridoxine-responsive (hypochromic) anemia
Use additional E code to identify cause, if drug induced
   EXCLUDES   refractory sideroblastic anemia (238.72)
   DEF: Characterized by a disruption of final heme synthesis; results in iron overload of reticuloendothelial tissues.

285.1 Acute posthemorrhagic anemia
Anemia due to acute blood loss
   EXCLUDES   anemia due to chronic blood loss (280.0)
               blood loss anemia NOS (280.0)

✓5ᵗʰ **285.2 Anemia of chronic disease**
Anemia in (due to) (with) chronic illness

   285.21 Anemia in chronic kidney disease
   Anemia in end stage renal disease
   Erythropoietin-resistant anemia (EPO resistant anemia)

   285.22 Anemia in neoplastic disease
      EXCLUDES   anemia due to antineoplastic chemotherapy (285.3)
                  aplastic anemia due to antineoplastic chemotherapy (284.89)

   285.29 Anemia of other chronic disease
   Anemia in other chronic illness

285.3 Antineoplastic chemotherapy induced anemia
Anemia due to antineoplastic chemotherapy
   EXCLUDES   anemia due to drug NEC–code to type of anemia
               anemia in neoplastic disease (285.22)
               aplastic anemia due to antineoplastic chemotherapy (284.89)
   DEF: Reversible adverse effect of chemotherapy, causing inhibition of bone marrow production; decrease in red blood cell production prevents adequate oxygenation of the tissues and organs, causing fatigue, SOB, and exacerbation of other medical conditions.

285.8 Other specified anemias
Anemia:
   dyserythropoietic (congenital)
   dyshematopoietic (congenital)
   von Jaksch's
Infantile pseudoleukemia

285.9 Anemia, unspecified
Anemia:
   NOS
   essential
   normocytic, not due to blood loss
   profound
   progressive
   secondary
Oligocythemia
   EXCLUDES   anemia (due to):
               blood loss:
                  acute (285.1)
                  chronic or unspecified (280.0)
               iron deficiency (280.0-280.9)

✓4ᵗʰ **286 Coagulation defects**

286.0 Congenital factor VIII disorder
Antihemophilic globulin [AHG] deficiency
Factor VIII (functional)deficiency
Hemophilia:
   NOS
   A
   classical
   familial
   hereditary
Subhemophilia
   EXCLUDES   factor VIII deficiency with vascular defect (286.4)
   DEF: Hereditary, sex-linked, results in missing antihemophilic globulin (AHG) (factor VIII); causes abnormal coagulation characterized by increased bleeding, large bruises of skin, bleeding in mouth, nose, gastrointestinal tract; hemorrhages into joints, resulting in swelling and impaired function.

286.1 Congenital factor IX disorder
Christmas disease
Deficiency:
   factor IX (functional)
   plasma thromboplastin component [PTC]
Hemophilia B
   DEF: Deficiency of plasma thromboplastin component (PTC) (factor IX) and plasma thromboplastin antecedent (PTA); PTC deficiency clinically indistinguishable from classical hemophilia.

286.2 Congenital factor XI deficiency
Hemophilia C
Plasma thromboplastin antecedent [PTA] deficiency
Rosenthal's disease

286.3 Congenital deficiency of other clotting factors
Congenital afibrinogenemia
Deficiency:
   AC globulin factor:
      I [fibrinogen]
      II [prothrombin]
      V [labile]
      VII [stable]
      X [Stuart-Prower]
      XII [Hageman]
      XIII [fibrin stabilizing]
   Laki-Lorand factor
   proaccelerin
Disease:
   Owren's
   Stuart-Prower
Dysfibrinogenemia (congenital)
Dysprothrombinemia (constitutional)
Hypoproconvertinemia
Hypoprothrombinemia (hereditary)
Parahemophilia

286.4 von Willebrand's disease
Angiohemophilia (A) (B)
Constitutional thrombopathy
Factor VIII deficiency with vascular defect
Pseudohemophilia type B
Vascular hemophilia
von Willebrand's (-Jürgens') disease
   EXCLUDES   factor VIII deficiency:
               NOS (286.0)
               with functional defect (286.0)
               hereditary capillary fragility (287.8)
   DEF: Abnormal blood coagulation caused by deficient blood Factor VII; congenital; symptoms include excess or prolonged bleeding.

✓5ᵗʰ **286.5 Hemorrhagic disorder due to intrinsic circulating anticoagulants, antibodies, or inhibitors**

   286.52 Acquired hemophilia
      Autoimmune hemophilia
      Autoimmune inhibitors to clotting factors
      Secondary hemophilia

286.53 Antiphospholipid antibody with hemorrhagic disorder

Lupus anticoagulant [LAC] with hemorrhagic disorder

Systemic lupus erythematosus [SLE] inhibitor with hemorrhagic disorder

EXCLUDES   *anti-phospholipid antibody, finding without diagnosis (795.79)*
anti-phospholipid antibody syndrome (289.81)
anti-phospholipid antibody with hypercoagulable state (289.81)
lupus anticoagulant [LAC] finding without diagnosis (795.79)
lupus anticoagulant [LAC] with hypercoagulable state (289.81)
systemic lupus erythematosus [SLE] inhibitor finding without diagnosis (795.79)
systemic lupus erythematosus [SLE] inhibitor with hypercoagulable state (289.81)

286.59 Other hemorrhagic disorder due to intrinsic circulating anticoagulants, antibodies, or inhibitors

Antithrombinemia
Antithromboplastinemia
Antithromboplastinogenemia
Increase in:
    anti-II (prothrombin)
    anti-VIIIa
    anti-IXa
    anti-XIa

286.6 Defibrination syndrome

Afibrinogenemia, acquired
Consumption coagulopathy
Diffuse or disseminated intravascular coagulation [DIC syndrome]
Fibrinolytic hemorrhage, acquired
Hemorrhagic fibrinogenolysis
Pathologic fibrinolysis
Purpura:
    fibrinolytic
    fulminans

EXCLUDES   *that complicating:*
abortion (634-638 with .1, 639.1)
pregnancy or the puerperium (641.3, 666.3)
disseminated intravascular coagulation in newborn (776.2)

DEF: Characterized by destruction of circulating fibrinogen; often precipitated by other conditions, such as injury, causing release of thromboplastic particles in blood stream.

286.7 Acquired coagulation factor deficiency

Deficiency of coagulation factor due to:
    liver disease
    vitamin K deficiency
Hypoprothrombinemia, acquired
Use additional E code to identify cause, if drug induced

EXCLUDES   *vitamin K deficiency of newborn (776.0)*

286.9 Other and unspecified coagulation defects

Defective coagulation NOS   Disorder:
Deficiency, coagulation   coagulation
    factor NOS   hemostasis
Delay, coagulation

EXCLUDES   *abnormal coagulation profile (790.92)*
hemorrhagic disease of newborn (776.0)
that complicating:
abortion (634-638 with .1, 639.1)
pregnancy or the puerperium (641.3, 666.3)

√4ᵗʰ **287 Purpura and other hemorrhagic conditions**

EXCLUDES   *hemorrhagic thrombocythemia (238.71)*
purpura fulminans (286.6)

287.0 Allergic purpura

Peliosis rheumatica
Purpura:
    anaphylactoid
    autoimmune
    Henoch's
    nonthrombocytopenic:
      hemorrhagic
      idiopathic
    rheumatica
    Schönlein-Henoch
    vascular
Vasculitis, allergic

EXCLUDES   *hemorrhagic purpura (287.39)*
purpura annularis telangiectodes (709.1)

DEF: Any hemorrhagic condition, thrombocytic or nonthrombocytopenic in origin, caused by a presumed allergic reaction.

287.1 Qualitative platelet defects

Thrombasthenia (hemorrhagic) (hereditary)
Thrombocytasthenia
Thrombocytopathy (dystrophic)
Thrombopathy (Bernard-Soulier)

EXCLUDES   *von Willebrand's disease (286.4)*

287.2 Other nonthrombocytopenic purpuras

Purpura:
    NOS
    senile
    simplex

√5ᵗʰ **287.3 Primary thrombocytopenia**

EXCLUDES   *thrombotic thrombocytopenic purpura (446.6)*
transient thrombocytopenia of newborn (776.1)

DEF: Decrease in number of blood platelets in circulating blood and purpural skin hemorrhages.

287.30 Primary thrombocytopenia, unspecified

Megakaryocytic hypoplasia

287.31 Immune thrombocytopenic purpura

Idiopathic thrombocytopenic purpura
Tidal platelet dysgenesis

DEF: Tidal platelet dysgenesis: Platelet counts fluctuate from normal to very low within periods of 20 to 40 days and may involve autoimmune platelet destruction.

287.32 Evans' syndrome

DEF: Combination of immunohemolytic anemia and autoimmune hemolytic anemia, sometimes with neutropenia.

287.33 Congenital and hereditary thrombocytopenic purpura

Congenital and hereditary thrombocytopenia
Thrombocytopenia with absent radii (TAR) syndrome

EXCLUDES   *Wiskott-Aldrich syndrome (279.12)*

DEF: Thrombocytopenia with absent radii (TAR) syndrome: autosomal recessive syndrome characterized by thrombocytopenia and bilateral radial aplasia; manifestations include skeletal, gastrointestinal, hematologic, and cardiac system abnormalities.

287.39 Other primary thrombocytopenia

Diseases of the Blood and Blood-Forming Organs

287.4–288.69

√5ᵗʰ **287.4 Secondary thrombocytopenia**
Use additional E code to identify cause
EXCLUDES   *heparin-induced thrombocytopenia (HIT)*
                (289.84)
                transient thrombocytopenia of newborn
                (776.1)

287.41 Posttransfusion purpura
Posttransfusion purpura from whole blood
    (fresh) or blood products
PTP

DEF: A potentially fatal transfusion complication
characterized by sudden onset of severe
thrombocytopenia, fever, chills, and cutaneous
hemorrhaging.

287.49 Other secondary thrombocytopenia
Thrombocytopenia (due to):
    dilutional
    drugs
    extracorporeal circulation of blood
    massive blood transfusion
    platelet alloimmunization
    secondary NOS

DEF: Reduced number of platelets in circulating
blood as consequence of an underlying disease
or condition.

287.5 Thrombocytopenia, unspecified

287.8 Other specified hemorrhagic conditions
Capillary fragility (hereditary)
Vascular pseudohemophilia

287.9 Unspecified hemorrhagic conditions
Hemorrhagic diathesis (familial)

√4ᵗʰ **288 Diseases of white blood cells**
EXCLUDES   *leukemia (204.0-208.9)*

√5ᵗʰ **288.0 Neutropenia**
Decreased absolute neutrophil count [ANC]
Use additional code for any associated:
    fever (780.61)
    mucositis (478.11, 528.00-528.09, 538, 616.81)
EXCLUDES   *neutropenic splenomegaly (289.53)*
                transitory neonatal neutropenia (776.7)

DEF: Sudden, severe condition characterized by reduced
number of white blood cells; results in sores in the throat,
stomach or skin; symptoms include chills, fever.

288.00 Neutropenia, unspecified

288.01 Congenital neutropenia
Congenital agranulocytosis
Infantile genetic agranulocytosis
Kostmann's syndrome

288.02 Cyclic neutropenia
Cyclic hematopoiesis
Periodic neutropenia

288.03 Drug induced neutropenia
Use additional E code to identify drug

288.04 Neutropenia due to infection

288.09 Other neutropenia
Agranulocytosis
Neutropenia:
    immune
    toxic

**288.1 Functional disorders of polymorphonuclear
neutrophils**
Chronic (childhood) granulomatous disease
Congenital dysphagocytosis
Job's syndrome
Lipochrome histiocytosis (familial)
Progressive septic granulomatosis

288.2 Genetic anomalies of leukocytes
Anomaly (granulation) (granulocyte) or syndrome:
    Alder's (-Reilly)
    Chédiak-Steinbrinck (-Higashi)
    Jordan's
    May-Hegglin
    Pelger-Huet
Hereditary:
    hypersegmentation
    hyposegmentation
    leukomelanopathy

288.3 Eosinophilia
Eosinophilia:
    allergic
    hereditary
    idiopathic
    secondary
Eosinophilic leukocytosis
EXCLUDES   *Löffler's syndrome (518.3)*
                pulmonary eosinophilia (518.3)

DEF: Elevated number of eosinophils in the blood;
characteristic of allergic states and various parasitic
infections.

288.4 Hemophagocytic syndromes
Familial hemophagocytic lymphohistiocytosis
Familial hemophagocytic reticulosis
Hemophagocytic syndrome, infection-associated
Histiocytic syndromes
Macrophage activation syndrome

√5ᵗʰ **288.5 Decreased white blood cell count**
EXCLUDES   *neutropenia (288.01-288.09)*

288.50 Leukocytopenia, unspecified
Decreased leukocytes, unspecified
Decreased white blood cell count, unspecified
Leukopenia NOS

288.51 Lymphocytopenia
Decreased lymphocytes

288.59 Other decreased white blood cell count
Basophilic leukopenia
Eosinophilic leukopenia
Monocytopenia
Plasmacytopenia

√5ᵗʰ **288.6 Elevated white blood cell count**
EXCLUDES   *eosinophilia (288.3)*

288.60 Leukocytosis, unspecified
Elevated leukocytes, unspecified
Elevated white blood cell count, unspecified

288.61 Lymphocytosis (symptomatic)
Elevated lymphocytes

288.62 Leukemoid reaction
Basophilic leukemoid reaction
Lymphocytic leukemoid reaction
Monocytic leukemoid reaction
Myelocytic leukemoid reaction
Neutrophilic leukemoid reaction

288.63 Monocytosis (symptomatic)
EXCLUDES   *infectious mononucleosis (075)*

288.64 Plasmacytosis

288.65 Basophilia

288.66 Bandemia
Bandemia without diagnosis of specific
    infection
EXCLUDES   *confirmed infection–code to*
                infection
                leukemia (204.00-208.9)

DEF: Increase in early neutrophil cells, called
band cells; may indicate infection.

288.69 Other elevated white blood cell count

288.8 Other specified disease of white blood cells

> EXCLUDES *decreased white blood cell counts (288.50-288.59)*
> *elevated white blood cell counts (288.60-288.69)*
> *immunity disorders (279.0-279.9)*

288.9 Unspecified disease of white blood cells

√4th **289 Other diseases of blood and blood-forming organs**

289.0 Polycythemia, secondary

High-oxygen-affinity hemoglobin
Polycythemia:
    acquired
    benign
    due to:
        fall in plasma volume
        high altitude
    emotional
    erythropoietin
    hypoxemic
    nephrogenous
    relative
    spurious
    stress

> EXCLUDES *polycythemia:*
> *neonatal (776.4)*
> *primary (238.4)*
> *vera (238.4)*

DEF: Elevated number of red blood cells in circulating blood as result of reduced oxygen supply to the tissues.

289.1 Chronic lymphadenitis

Chronic:
    adenitis   } any lymph node, except
    lymphadenitis }   mesenteric

> EXCLUDES *acute lymphadenitis (683)*
> *mesenteric (289.2)*
> *enlarged glands NOS (785.6)*

DEF: Persistent inflammation of lymph node tissue; origin of infection is usually elsewhere.

289.2 Nonspecific mesenteric lymphadenitis

Mesenteric lymphadenitis (acute) (chronic)

DEF: Inflammation of the lymph nodes in peritoneal fold that encases abdominal organs; disease resembles acute appendicitis; unknown etiology.

289.3 Lymphadenitis, unspecified, except mesenteric

289.4 Hypersplenism

"Big spleen" syndrome
Dyssplenism
Hypersplenia

> EXCLUDES *primary splenic neutropenia (289.53)*

DEF: An overactive spleen causing a deficiency of the peripheral blood components, an increase in bone marrow cells and sometimes a notable increase in the size of the spleen.

√5th **289.5 Other diseases of spleen**

289.50 Disease of spleen, unspecified

289.51 Chronic congestive splenomegaly

289.52 Splenic sequestration

Code first sickle-cell disease in crisis (282.42, 282.62, 282.64, 282.69)

DEF: Blood is entrapped in the spleen due to vessel occlusion; most often associated with sickle-cell disease; spleen becomes enlarged and there is a sharp drop in hemoglobin.

289.53 Neutropenic splenomegaly

289.59 Other

Lien migrans
Perisplenitis
Splenic:
    abscess
    atrophy
    cyst
    fibrosis
    infarction
    rupture, nontraumatic
Splenitis
Wandering spleen

> EXCLUDES *bilharzial splenic fibrosis (120.0-120.9)*
> *hepatolienal fibrosis (571.5)*
> *splenomegaly NOS (789.2)*

289.6 Familial polycythemia

Familial:
    benign polycythemia
    erythrocytosis

DEF: Elevated number of red blood cells.

289.7 Methemoglobinemia

Congenital NADH [DPNH]-methemoglobin- reductase deficiency
Hemoglobin M [Hb-M] disease
Methemoglobinemia:
    NOS
    acquired (with sulfhemoglobinemia)
    hereditary
    toxic
Stokvis' disease
Sulfhemoglobinemia

Use additional E code to identify cause

DEF: Presence of blood methemoglobin, a chemically altered form of hemoglobin; causes cyanosis, headache, ataxia, dyspnea, tachycardia, nausea, stupor, and coma.

Diseases of the Blood and Blood-Forming Organs

289.8–289.9

√5ᵗʰ **289.8 Other specified diseases of blood and blood-forming organs**

DEF: Hypercoagulable states: a group of inherited or acquired abnormalities of specific proteins and anticoagulant factors; also called thromboembolic states or thrombotic disorders; result in abnormal development of blood clots.

289.81 Primary hypercoagulable state

Activated protein C resistance
Antiphospholipid antibody syndrome
Antithrombin III deficiency
Factor V Leiden mutation
Lupus anticoagulant with hypercoagulable state
Protein C deficiency
Protein S deficiency
Prothrombin gene mutation
Systemic lupus erythematosus [SLE] inhibitor with hypercoagulable state

EXCLUDES anti-phospholipid antibody, finding without diagnosis (795.79)
anti-phospholipid antibody with hemorrhagic disorder (286.53)
lupus anticoagulant (LAC) finding without diagnosis (795.79)
lupus anticoagulant (LAC) with hemorrhagic disorder (286.53)
secondary activated protein C resistance (289.82)
secondary antiphospholipid antibody syndrome (289.82)
secondary lupus anticoagulant with hypercoagulable state (289.82)
secondary systemic lupus erythematosus [SLE] inhibitor with hypercoagulable state (289.82)
systemic lupus erythematosus [SLE] inhibitor finding without diagnosis (795.79)
systemic lupus erythematosus [SLE] inhibitor with hypercoagulable state (286.53)

DEF: Activated protein C resistance: decreased effectiveness of protein C to degrade factor V, necessary to inhibit clotting cascade; also called Factor V Leiden mutation.

DEF: Antithrombin III deficiency: deficiency in plasma antithrombin III one of six naturally occurring antithrombins that limit coagulation.

DEF: Factor V Leiden mutation: also called activated protein C resistance.

DEF: Lupus anticoagulant: autoimmune deficiency in a circulating anticoagulant that inhibits the conversion of prothrombin into thrombin; also called anti-phospholipid syndrome.

DEF: Protein C deficiency: deficiency of activated protein C which functions to bring the blood-clotting process into balance; same outcome as factor V Leiden mutation.

DEF: Protein S deficiency: similar to protein C deficiency; protein S is a vitamin K dependent cofactor in the activation of protein C.

DEF: Prothrombin gene mutation: increased levels of prothrombin, or factor II, a plasma protein that is converted to thrombin, which acts upon fibrinogen to form the fibrin.

289.82 Secondary hypercoagulable state

EXCLUDES heparin-induced thrombocytopenia (HIT) (289.84)

289.83 Myelofibrosis

Myelofibrosis NOS
Secondary myelofibrosis
Code first the underlying disorder, such as:
malignant neoplasm of breast (174.0-174.9, 175.0-175.9)
Use additional code for associated therapy-related myelodysplastic syndrome, if applicable (238.72, 238.73)
Use additional external cause code if due to anti-neoplastic chemotherapy (E933.1)

EXCLUDES idiopathic myelofibrosis (238.76)
leukoerythroblastic anemia (284.2)
myelofibrosis with myeloid metaplasia (238.76)
myelophthisic anemia (284.2)
myelophthisis (284.2)
primary myelofibrosis (238.76)

DEF: A progressive bone marrow disease characterized by the replacement of bone marrow with the overgrowth of neoplastic stem cells and fibrotic tissue, also progressive anemia and enlarged spleen.

289.84 Heparin-induced thrombocytopenia [HIT]

DEF: Immune-mediated reaction to heparin therapy causing an abrupt fall in platelet count and serious complications such as pulmonary embolism, stroke, AMI or DVT.

289.89 Other specified diseases of blood and blood-forming organs

Hypergammaglobulinemia
Pseudocholinesterase deficiency

289.9 Unspecified diseases of blood and blood-forming organs

Blood dyscrasia NOS
Erythroid hyperplasia

Chapter 5: Mental, Behavioral, and Neurodevelopmental Disorders (290–319)

Coding Guidance

The fifth chapter of ICD-9-CM includes the following mental, behavioral, and neurodevelopmental disorders:

- Psychoses
- Neuroses
- Transient stress disorders
- Personality disorders
- Sexual deviation and dysfunction
- Psychophysiological disorders

A suggested hierarchy for coding psychiatric disorders is provided by the World Health Organization as follows: All organically based psychiatric illnesses are given precedence over functional ones, and within the functional group the order then may be psychoses, neuroses, personality disorders, and others.

The American Psychiatric Association has developed a classification system to record diagnostic and statistical data on psychiatric patients. The Diagnostic and Statistical Manual (DSM-V) is based on a multiaxial system which evaluates each patient on five axes. Psychiatric hospitals and treatment centers frequently use both DSM-V and ICD-9-CM to record diagnosis and statistical data on their patients. Physician offices, however, should use the ICD-9-CM coding system to code for reimbursement. The clinical definitions of the diagnostic codes between ICD-9-CM and DSM-V are nearly identical. Differences occur in the other axes, such as axis IV for psychosocial and environmental factors and axis V for global assessment of functioning (GAF).

When coding mental disorders associated with physical conditions, assign as many codes as necessary to fully describe the condition.

The following sections are included in chapter 5, "Mental, Behavioral, and Neurodevelopmental Disorders."

- Psychoses (290–299)
  - organic psychotic conditions (290–294)
  - other psychoses (295–299)
- Neurotic disorders, personality disorders, and other nonpsychotic mental disorders (300–316)
- Intellectual disabilities (317–319)

Organic Psychotic Conditions (290–294)

Organic psychotic conditions are defined as impairments of mental function to a degree that interferes with the activities of daily living and the ability to maintain contact with reality. Note that this section classifies conditions that are referred to as psychotic, a gross impairment of reality. Nonpsychotic organic brain syndromes are classified to categories 310–316. Conditions classified to this section include senile and presenile dementia, arteriosclerotic dementia, alcoholic dementia and withdrawal hallucinosis, drug psychosis and withdrawal syndromes, and organic brain syndromes.

Senile and presenile organic psychotic conditions (290) are characterized by severely impaired mental and social function. Signs and symptoms include memory loss, impaired comprehension, impaired orientation, poor judgment, and changes in personality or mood.

Category 290 lists multiple exclusions. If the nature or underlying cause of dementia is documented as arteriosclerotic (294), due to alcohol or drugs (291, 292), or attributed to transient organic psychoses (293), assign specific codes classifiable to other categories.

Vascular dementia (290.4x) results from multiple infarcts and is attributable to degenerative arterial disease of the brain. Use an additional code to identify cerebral atherosclerosis. For example, vascular dementia with delirium due to cerebral arteriosclerosis is coded 290.41 Arteriosclerotic dementia with delirium, and 437.0, Cerebral arteriosclerosis.

Alcohol-Induced Mental Disorders (291)

Alcohol-induced psychoses result from excessive alcohol consumption, usually in association with nutritional deficits. This category excludes alcoholism without psychosis, which is classified to category 303. However, when alcohol dependence or abuse results in a psychotic condition, code both the psychotic condition and the dependence (303) or abuse (305.0x). For example, alcoholic withdrawal due to chronic alcoholism is coded 291.81 and 303.90.

Alcohol withdrawal delirium (291.0) is delirium resulting from the abrupt cessation of the use of alcohol by an individual who habitually consumes alcohol.

Alcohol-induced persisting amnestic syndrome (291.1) is the prominent and lasting reduction of memory span, including loss of recent memory, disordered time appreciation and confabulation, occurring in alcoholics, usually as a sequel to alcoholic psychosis.

Other alcohol-induced persisting dementia (291.2) is a nonhallucinatory dementia associated with alcoholism but without features of delirium tremens or Korsakov's psychosis.

Alcohol-induced psychotic disorder with hallucinations (291.3) is a psychosis usually lasting less than six months with slight or no clouding of consciousness in which auditory hallucinations predominate.

Idiosyncratic alcohol intoxication (291.4) is a unique behavioral pattern including belligerence, after the intake of relatively small amounts of alcohol. This behavior is not due to excessive consumption and is without conspicuous neurological signs of intoxication.

Drug-Induced Mental Disorders (292)

Drug psychoses include drug-induced mental disorders and organic brain disorders associated with drug abuse, dependence, or use. Additional E codes identify the drug. Assign additional codes to indicate associated drug dependence (304.0x–304.9x). The coding guidelines to assign drug-induced mental disorders is very similar to the guidelines to code alcohol induced psychoses.

The subcategories include drug withdrawal (292.0), paranoid and/or hallucinatory states induced by drugs (292.1x), pathological drug intoxication (292.2), and other (292.8x) and unspecified (292.9x) drug-induced mental disorders.

Other Organic Mental Disorders Due to Conditions Classified Elsewhere (Persistent) (294)

This category includes dementia in conditions classified elsewhere, amnestic syndrome, and other chronic organic brain syndromes not classified elsewhere.

The term behavioral disturbances in subcategory 294.1 Dementia in conditions classified elsewhere with and without behavioral disturbances, is defined as aggressive, combative, violent, or wandering-off behavior as distinguished from more organic psychotic conditions such as hallucinations, delirium, and delusions. The more specific organic psychotic conditions (hallucinations, delirium, and delusions) are included in the code descriptions for the conditions that produce them. For example, arteriosclerotic dementia, presenile and senile dementia, alcohol and drug psychoses have code options specific to the manifestation of an organic psychotic conditions.

Behavioral disturbances are patterns of activity that interfere with normal functioning and increase resource utilization in cases of long term care. The existence of behavioral conditions in dementia in conditions classified elsewhere is a mandatory multiple coding situation. Code first the underlying condition followed by the dementia code.

Schizophrenic Disorders (295)

These are mental disorders characterized by disturbances in thinking, feeling and behavior. Informally, schizophrenia is referred to as "split personality." Signs and symptoms include: hypersensitivity, shyness, unsociability, lack of affect, paranoia, auditory hallucinations, difficulties in personal relationships, thought disorders such as unclear thinking, perplexity, affective emotional changes such as blunting, mood disturbances, and inappropriateness.

To support a diagnosis of schizophrenia, a characteristic disturbance of at least two of these areas is seen: thought, perception, mood, conduct, and personality.

The first axis of coding schizophrenia is to identify the type (i.e., simple, disordered, paranoid, latent, residual, etc.). Identify the course of illness with a fifth digit.

Episodic Mood Disorder (296)

Bipolar I disorder is a recurrent, severe disturbances of mood accompanied by one or more of the following: delusions, perplexity, disturbed attitude to self, disorder of perception and behavior. Patients with bipolar I disorder have a strong characteristic toward suicide. This category includes mild disorders of mood if the symptoms closely match the descriptions.

Subcategories identify the type (i.e., manic or major depressive, bipolar, etc.) and episodic nature (i.e., single, recurrent, etc.). A fifth-digit assignment identifies severity of the episode.

Neurotic Disorders, Personality Disorders and Other Nonpsychotic Mental Disorders (300–316)

Neurotic disorders (300) are mental disorders without any obvious evidence of an organic etiology. In neurotic disorders, fantasies are not confused with reality, nor is personality disorganized. These include panic disorder, neurotic depression, hysteria, conversion disorder, psychogenic fugue, phobic disorders, obsessive-compulsive disorders, hypochondriasis and others.

Personality disorders (301) include paranoid, affective, chronic hypomanic, schizoid, explosive, compulsive, histrionic, dependent, antisocial, narcissistic, avoidant, borderline, and passive-aggressive types.

Sexual deviations and disorders (302) include ego-dystonic homosexuality, zoophilia, pedophilia, transvestism, exhibitionism, transexualism, psychosexual identity disorder, fetishism, voyeurism, sadism, and others.

Alcohol Dependence Syndrome (303)

Alcohol dependence syndrome is a psychotic and often physical state caused by alcohol. It is characterized by behavioral and other responses that always include the need to consume alcohol on a continuous or periodic basis. Fifth-digit assignment indicates pattern of use.

Use additional codes to identify any associated condition such as alcoholic psychoses (291.0–291.9), drug dependence (304.0x–304.9x), or physical complications such as cerebral degeneration (331.7), cirrhosis of the liver (571.2), epilepsy and recurrent seizures (345.0x– 345.9x), hepatitis (571.1), and liver damage (571.3).

Dependence (304)

The first axis of classification in this category is the class of drug to which the patient is addicted (e.g. opioids, hallucinogens). Fifth-digit assignment indicates pattern of use.

Nondependent Drug Abuse (305)

Nondependent abuse is the maladaptive, but nondependent, effect of a drug taken by a patient on his or her own to the detriment of health and/or social functioning. The subcategories reflect the type of drug, and the fifth-digit subclassification identifies the documented pattern of use.

Tobacco dependence (305.1) is included in this category. Tobacco dependence is included here rather than under category 304, because tobacco differs from other drugs of dependence in its psychotoxic effects.

Post-concussion Syndrome (310.2)

Post-concussion syndrome is a nonpsychotic disorder due to brain trauma that causes symptoms unrelated to any disease process. Symptoms include amnesia, serial headaches, rapid heartbeat, fatigue, disrupted sleep patterns, and inability to concentrate. Use an additional code to identify associated post-traumatic headache, if applicable (339.20–339.22). Subcategory 339.2 Post-traumatic headache includes three codes that classify post-traumatic headache by severity as acute, chronic, or unspecified. Headache is a common symptom of post-concussion syndrome. According to the instructional note, it is appropriate to report an additional code for post-traumatic headache when associated with postconcussion syndrome.

Specific Delays in Development (315)

Code category 315 classifies certain specific developmental delay disorders. These disorders are separate from delays of an intellectual, educational, or neurological nature, and instead are often the result of other biological or nonbiological factors.

Children born with hearing loss or deafness, whether permanent or intermittent, are at significantly greater risk for not acquiring normal, age-appropriate language and speech abilities. Code 315.34 Speech and language developmental delay due to hearing loss should be reported for cases specific to congenital hearing loss that results in developmental delays.

Intellectual Disabilities (317–319)

Intellectual disabilities is the condition of arrested or incomplete development of the mind characterized by subnormal intelligence.

Assign a code based on the individual's current level of function without regard to the nature or cause of intellectual disabilities. However, when intellectual disabilities involves psychiatric disturbances or develops as a result of some physical disease or injury, use an additional code or codes to identify the associated condition.

5. MENTAL, BEHAVIORAL AND NEURODEVELOPMENTAL DISORDERS (290-319)

PSYCHOSES (290-299)

EXCLUDES   *intellectual disabilities (317-319)*

ORGANIC PSYCHOTIC CONDITIONS (290-294)

INCLUDES   psychotic organic brain syndrome
EXCLUDES   *nonpsychotic syndromes of organic etiology*
(310.0-310.9)
psychoses classifiable to 295-298 and without
impairment of orientation, comprehension,
calculation, learning capacity, and judgment,
but associated with physical disease, injury, or
condition affecting the brain [eg., following
childbirth] (295.0-298.8)

√4ᵗʰ **290   Dementias**
Code first the associated neurological condition
EXCLUDES   *dementia due to alcohol (291.0-291.2)*
dementia due to drugs (292.82)
dementia not classified as senile, presenile, or
arteriosclerotic (294.10-294.11)
psychoses classifiable to 295-298 occurring in the
senium without dementia or delirium
(295.0-298.8)
senility with mental changes of nonpsychotic severity
(310.1)
transient organic psychotic conditions (293.0-293.9)

290.0   Senile dementia, uncomplicated
Senile dementia: Senile dementia:
NOS   simple type
EXCLUDES   *mild memory disturbances, not amounting to*
dementia, associated with senile brain
disease (310.89)
senile dementia with:
delirium or confusion (290.3)
delusional [paranoid] features (290.20)
depressive features (290.21)

√5ᵗʰ **290.1   Presenile dementia**
Brain syndrome with presenile brain disease
EXCLUDES   *arteriosclerotic dementia (290.40-290.43)*
dementia associated with other cerebral
conditions (294.10-294.11)

290.10   Presenile dementia, uncomplicated
Presenile dementia:
NOS
simple type

290.11   Presenile dementia with delirium
Presenile dementia with acute confusional
state

290.12   Presenile dementia with delusional features
Presenile dementia, paranoid type

290.13   Presenile dementia with depressive features
Presenile dementia, depressed type

√5ᵗʰ **290.2   Senile dementia with delusional or depressive features**
EXCLUDES   *senile dementia:*
NOS (290.0)
with delirium and/or confusion (290.3)

290.20   Senile dementia with delusional features
Senile dementia, paranoid type
Senile psychosis NOS

290.21   Senile dementia with depressive features

290.3   Senile dementia with delirium
Senile dementia with acute confusional state
EXCLUDES   *senile:*
dementia NOS (290.0)
psychosis NOS (290.20)

√5ᵗʰ **290.4   Vascular dementia**
Multi-infarct dementia or psychosis
Use additional code to identify cerebral atherosclerosis
(437.0)
EXCLUDES   *suspected cases with no clear evidence of*
arteriosclerosis (290.9)

290.40   Vascular dementia, uncomplicated
Arteriosclerotic dementia:
NOS
simple type

290.41   Vascular dementia with delirium
Arteriosclerotic dementia with acute
confusional state

290.42   Vascular dementia with delusions
Arteriosclerotic dementia, paranoid type

290.43   Vascular dementia with depressed mood
Arteriosclerotic dementia, depressed type

290.8   Other specified senile psychotic conditions
Presbyophrenic psychosis

290.9   Unspecified senile psychotic condition

√4ᵗʰ **291   Alcohol induced mental disorders**
EXCLUDES   *alcoholism without psychosis (303.0-303.9)*

291.0   Alcohol withdrawal delirium
Alcoholic delirium
Delirium tremens
EXCLUDES   *alcohol withdrawal (291.81)*

291.1   Alcohol induced persisting amnestic disorder
Alcoholic polyneuritic psychosis
Korsakoff's psychosis, alcoholic
Wernicke-Korsakoff syndrome (alcoholic)
DEF: Prominent and lasting reduced memory span,
disordered time appreciation and confabulation, occurring
in alcoholics, as sequel to acute alcoholic psychosis.

291.2   Alcohol induced persisting dementia
Alcoholic dementia NOS
Alcoholism associated with dementia NOS
Chronic alcoholic brain syndrome

291.3   Alcohol induced psychotic disorder with hallucinations
Alcoholic:
hallucinosis (acute)
psychosis with hallucinosis
EXCLUDES   *alcohol withdrawal with delirium (291.0)*
schizophrenia (295.0-295.9) and paranoid
states (297.0-297.9) taking the form of
chronic hallucinosis with clear
consciousness in an alcoholic
DEF: Psychosis lasting less than six months with slight or
no clouding of consciousness in which auditory
hallucinations predominate.

291.4   Idiosyncratic alcohol intoxication
Pathologic: Pathologic:
alcohol intoxication   drunkenness
EXCLUDES   *acute alcohol intoxication (305.0)*
in alcoholism (303.0)
simple drunkenness (305.0)
DEF: Unique behavioral patterns, like belligerence, after
intake of relatively small amounts of alcohol; behavior not
due to excess consumption.

291.5   Alcohol induced psychotic disorder with delusions
Alcoholic: Alcoholic:
paranoia   psychosis, paranoid type
EXCLUDES   *nonalcoholic paranoid states (297.0-297.9)*
schizophrenia, paranoid type (295.3)

√5ᵗʰ **291.8   Other specified alcohol induced mental disorders**

291.81   Alcohol withdrawal
Alcohol:
abstinence syndrome or symptoms
withdrawal syndrome or symptoms
EXCLUDES   *alcohol withdrawal:*
delirium (291.0)
hallucinosis (291.3)
delirium tremens (291.0)

Mental, Behavioral, & Neurodevelopmental Disorders

291.82–294.0

291.82 Alcohol induced sleep disorders
Alcohol induced circadian rhythm sleep
disorders
Alcohol induced hypersomnia
Alcohol induced insomnia
Alcohol induced parasomnia

291.89 Other
Alcohol induced anxiety disorder
Alcohol induced mood disorder
Alcohol induced sexual dysfunction

291.9 Unspecified alcohol induced mental disorders
Alcoholic:
mania NOS
psychosis NOS
Alcoholism (chronic) with psychosis
Alcohol related disorder NOS

√4ᵗʰ **292 Drug induced mental disorders**
INCLUDES organic brain syndrome associated with
consumption of drugs
Use additional code for any associated drug dependence
(304.0-304.9)
Use additional E code to identify drug

292.0 Drug withdrawal
Drug:
abstinence syndrome or symptoms
withdrawal syndrome or symptoms

√5ᵗʰ **292.1 Drug induced psychotic disorders**

**292.11 Drug induced psychotic disorder with
delusions**
Paranoid state induced by drugs

**292.12 Drug induced psychotic disorder with
hallucinations**
Hallucinatory state induced by drugs
EXCLUDES *states following LSD or other
hallucinogens, lasting only a
few days or less ["bad trips"]
(305.3)*

292.2 Pathological drug intoxication
Drug reaction:
NOS ⎫
idiosyncratic ⎬ resulting in brief psychotic
pathologic ⎭ states
EXCLUDES *expected brief psychotic reactions to
hallucinogens ["bad trips"] (305.3)
physiological side-effects of drugs (e.g.,
dystonias)*

√5ᵗʰ **292.8 Other specified drug induced mental disorders**

292.81 Drug induced delirium

292.82 Drug induced persisting dementia

292.83 Drug induced persisting amnestic disorder

292.84 Drug induced mood disorder
Depressive state induced by drugs

292.85 Drug induced sleep disorders
Drug induced circadian rhythm sleep disorder
Drug induced hypersomnia
Drug induced insomnia
Drug induced parasomnia

292.89 Other
Drug induced anxiety disorder
Drug induced organic personality syndrome
Drug induced sexual dysfunction
Drug intoxication

292.9 Unspecified drug induced mental disorder
Drug related disorder NOS
Organic psychosis NOS due to or associated with drugs

√4ᵗʰ **293 Transient mental disorders due to conditions classified
elsewhere**
INCLUDES transient organic mental disorders not associated
with alcohol or drugs
Code first the associated physical or neurological condition
EXCLUDES *confusional state or delirium superimposed on senile
dementia (290.3)
dementia due to:
alcohol (291.0-291.9)
arteriosclerosis (290.40-290.43)
drugs (292.82)
senility (290.0)*

293.0 Delirium due to conditions classified elsewhere
Acute:
confusional state
infective psychosis
organic reaction
posttraumatic organic psychosis
psycho-organic syndrome
Acute psychosis associated with endocrine, metabolic,
or cerebrovascular disorder
Epileptic:
confusional state
twilight state

293.1 Subacute delirium
Subacute:
confusional state
infective psychosis
organic reaction
posttraumatic organic psychosis
psycho-organic syndrome
psychosis associated with endocrine or metabolic
disorder

√5ᵗʰ **293.8 Other specified transient mental disorders due to
conditions classified elsewhere**

**293.81 Psychotic disorder with delusions in
conditions classified elsewhere**
Transient organic psychotic condition, paranoid
type

**293.82 Psychotic disorder with hallucinations in
conditions classified elsewhere**
Transient organic psychotic condition,
hallucinatory type

**293.83 Mood disorder in conditions classified
elsewhere**
Transient organic psychotic condition,
depressive type

**293.84 Anxiety disorder in conditions classified
elsewhere**

293.89 Other
Catatonic disorder in conditions classified
elsewhere

**293.9 Unspecified transient mental disorder in conditions
classified elsewhere**
Organic psychosis:
infective NOS
posttraumatic NOS
transient NOS
Psycho-organic syndrome

√4ᵗʰ **294 Persistent mental disorders due to conditions classified
elsewhere**
INCLUDES organic psychotic brain syndromes (chronic), not
elsewhere classified

294.0 Amnestic disorder in conditions classified elsewhere
Korsakoff's psychosis or syndrome (nonalcoholic)
Code first underlying condition
EXCLUDES *alcoholic:
amnestic syndrome (291.1)
Korsakoff's psychosis (291.1)*

294.1 Dementia in conditions classified elsewhere
Dementia of the Alzheimer's type
Code first any underlying physical condition, as:
    Alzheimer's disease (331.0)
    cerebral lipidoses (330.1)
    dementia with Lewy bodies (331.82)
    dementia with Parkinsonism (331.82)
    epilepsy (345.0-345.9)
    frontal dementia (331.19)
    frontotemporal dementia (331.19)
    general paresis [syphilis] (094.1)
    hepatolenticular degeneration (275.1)
    Huntington's chorea (333.4)
    Jakob-Creutzfeldt disease (046.11-046.19)
    multiple sclerosis (340)
    Parkinson's disease (332.0)
    Pick's disease of the brain (331.11)
    polyarteritis nodosa (446.0)
    syphilis (094.1)
    EXCLUDES *dementia:*
        arteriosclerotic (290.40-290.43)
        presenile (290.10-290.13)
        senile (290.0)
        epileptic psychosis NOS (294.8)

294.10 *Dementia in conditions classified elsewhere without behavioral disturbance*
    Dementia in conditions classified elsewhere NOS

294.11 *Dementia in conditions classified elsewhere with behavioral disturbance*
    Aggressive behavior
    Combative behavior
    Violent behavior
    Use additional code, where applicable, to identify:
        wandering in conditions classified elsewhere (V40.31)

294.2 Dementia, unspecified
    EXCLUDES *mild memory disturbances, not amounting to dementia (310.89)*

294.20 Dementia, unspecified, without behavioral disturbance
    Dementia NOS

294.21 Dementia, unspecified, with behavioral disturbance
    Aggressive behavior
    Combative behavior
    Violent behavior
    Use additional code, where applicable, to identify:
        wandering in conditions classified elsewhere (V40.31)

294.8 Other persistent mental disorders due to conditions classified elsewhere
    Amnestic disorder NOS
    Epileptic psychosis NOS
    Mixed paranoid and affective organic psychotic states
    Use additional code for associated epilepsy (345.0-345.9)
    EXCLUDES *mild memory disturbances, not amounting to dementia (310.89)*

294.9 Unspecified persistent mental disorders due to conditions classified elsewhere
    Cognitive disorder NOS
    Organic psychosis (chronic)

OTHER PSYCHOSES (295-299)

Use additional code to identify any associated physical disease, injury, or condition affecting the brain with psychoses classifiable to 295-298

295 Schizophrenic disorders
    INCLUDES schizophrenia of the types described in 295.0-295.9 occurring in children
    EXCLUDES *childhood type schizophrenia (299.9)*
        infantile autism (299.0)

The following fifth-digit subclassification is for use with category 295:
    0 unspecified
    1 subchronic
    2 chronic
    3 subchronic with acute exacerbation
    4 chronic with acute exacerbation
    5 in remission

DEF: Group of disorders with disturbances in thought (delusions, hallucinations), mood (blunted, flattened, inappropriate affect), sense of self; also bizarre, purposeless behavior, repetitive activity, or inactivity.

295.0 Simple type
[0-5]   Schizophrenia simplex
    EXCLUDES *latent schizophrenia (295.5)*

295.1 Disorganized type
[0-5]   Hebephrenia
    Hebephrenic type schizophrenia

    DEF: Inappropriate behavior; results in extreme incoherence and disorganization of time, place and sense of social appropriateness; withdrawal from routine social interaction may occur.

295.2 Catatonic type
[0-5]   Catatonic (schizophrenia):
        agitation
        excitation
        excited type
        stupor
        withdrawn type
    Schizophrenic:
        catalepsy
        catatonia
        flexibilitas cerea

    DEF: Extreme changes in motor activity; one extreme is decreased response or reaction to the environment and the other is spontaneous activity.

295.3 Paranoid type
[0-5]   Paraphrenic schizophrenia
    EXCLUDES *involutional paranoid state (297.2)*
        paranoia (297.1)
        paraphrenia (297.2)

    DEF: Preoccupied with delusional suspicions and auditory hallucinations related to single theme; usually hostile, grandiose, overly religious, occasionally hypochondriacal.

295.4 Schizophreniform disorder
[0-5]   Oneirophrenia   Schizophreniform:
    Schizophreniform: psychosis, confusional type
        attack
    EXCLUDES *acute forms of schizophrenia of:*
        catatonic type (295.2)
        hebephrenic type (295.1)
        paranoid type (295.3)
        simple type (295.0)
        undifferentiated type (295.8)

295.5 Latent schizophrenia
[0-5]   Latent schizophrenic reaction
    Schizophrenia:
        borderline
        incipient
        prepsychotic
        prodromal
        pseudoneurotic
        pseudopsychopathic
    EXCLUDES *schizoid personality (301.20-301.22)*

√5ᵗʰ **295.6 Residual type**
[0-5] Chronic undifferentiated schizophrenia
Restzustand (schizophrenic)
Schizophrenic residual state

√5ᵗʰ **295.7 Schizoaffective disorder**
[0-5] Cyclic schizophrenia
Mixed schizophrenic and affective psychosis
Schizo-affective psychosis
Schizophreniform psychosis, affective type

√5ᵗʰ **295.8 Other specified types of schizophrenia**
[0-5] Acute (undifferentiated) schizophrenia
Atypical schizophrenia
Cenesthopathic schizophrenia
EXCLUDES *infantile autism (299.0)*

√5ᵗʰ **295.9 Unspecified schizophrenia**
[0-5] Schizophrenia:
NOS
mixed NOS
undifferentiated NOS
undifferentiated type
Schizophrenic reaction NOS
Schizophreniform psychosis NOS

√4ᵗʰ **296 Episodic mood disorders**
INCLUDES episodic affective disorders
EXCLUDES *neurotic depression (300.4)*
reactive depressive psychosis (298.0)
reactive excitation (298.1)

The following fifth-digit subclassification is for use with categories 296.0-296.6:
0 unspecified
1 mild
2 moderate
3 severe, without mention of psychotic behavior
4 severe, specified as with psychotic behavior
5 in partial or unspecified remission
6 in full remission

√5ᵗʰ **296.0 Bipolar I disorder, single manic episode**
[0-6] Hypomania (mild) NOS
Hypomanic psychosis
Mania (monopolar) NOS   single episode or
Manic-depressive psychosis or   unspecified
reaction:
hypomanic
manic
EXCLUDES *circular type, if there was a previous attack of*
depression (296.4)
DEF: Mood disorder identified by hyperactivity; may show extreme agitation or exaggerated excitability; speech and thought processes may be accelerated.

√5ᵗʰ **296.1 Manic disorder, recurrent episode**
[0-6] Any condition classifiable to 296.0, stated to be recurrent
EXCLUDES *circular type, if there was a previous attack of*
depression (296.4)

√5ᵗʰ **296.2 Major depressive disorder, single episode**
[0-6] Depressive psychosis
Endogenous depression
Involutional melancholia
Manic-depressive psychosis or   single episode or
reaction, depressed type   unspecified
Monopolar depression
Psychotic depression
EXCLUDES *circular type, if previous attack was of manic*
type (296.5)
depression NOS (311)
reactive depression (neurotic) (300.4)
psychotic (298.0)
DEF: Mood disorder that produces depression; may exhibit as sadness, low self-esteem, or guilt feelings; other manifestations may be withdrawal from friends and family; interrupted sleep.

√5ᵗʰ **296.3 Major depressive disorder, recurrent episode**
[0-6] Any condition classifiable to 296.2, stated to be recurrent
EXCLUDES *circular type, if previous attack was of manic*
type (296.5)
depression NOS (311)
reactive depression (neurotic) (300.4)
psychotic (298.0)

√5ᵗʰ **296.4 Bipolar I disorder, most recent episode**
[0-6] **(or current) manic**
Bipolar disorder, now manic
Manic-depressive psychosis, circular type but currently manic
EXCLUDES *brief compensatory or rebound mood swings*
(296.99)

√5ᵗʰ **296.5 Bipolar I disorder, most recent episode**
[0-6] **(or current) depressed**
Bipolar disorder, now depressed
Manic-depressive psychosis, circular type but currently depressed
EXCLUDES *brief compensatory or rebound mood swings*
(296.99)

√5ᵗʰ **296.6 Bipolar I disorder, most recent episode (or current)**
[0-6] **mixed**
Manic-depressive psychosis, circular type, mixed

296.7 Bipolar I disorder, most recent episode (or current)
unspecified
Atypical bipolar affective disorder NOS
Manic-depressive psychosis, circular type, current condition not specified as either manic or depressive
DEF: Manic-depressive disorder referred to as bipolar because of the mood range from manic to depressive.

√5ᵗʰ **296.8 Other and unspecified bipolar disorders**
296.80 Bipolar disorder, unspecified
Bipolar disorder NOS
Manic-depressive:
reaction NOS
syndrome NOS

296.81 Atypical manic disorder

296.82 Atypical depressive disorder

296.89 Other
Bipolar II disorder
Manic-depressive psychosis, mixed type

√5ᵗʰ **296.9 Other and unspecified episodic mood disorder**
EXCLUDES *psychogenic affective psychoses*
(298.0-298.8)

296.90 Unspecified episodic mood disorder
Affective psychosis NOS
Melancholia NOS
Mood disorder NOS

296.99 Other specified episodic mood disorder
Mood swings:
brief compensatory
rebound

√4ᵗʰ **297 Delusional disorders**
INCLUDES paranoid disorders
EXCLUDES *acute paranoid reaction (298.3)*
alcoholic jealousy or paranoid state (291.5)
paranoid schizophrenia (295.3)

297.0 Paranoid state, simple

297.1 Delusional disorder
Chronic paranoid psychosis
Sander's disease
Systematized delusions
EXCLUDES *paranoid personality disorder (301.0)*

297.2 Paraphrenia
Involutional paranoid state
Late paraphrenia
Paraphrenia (involutional)
DEF: Paranoid schizophrenic disorder that persists over a prolonged period but does not distort personality despite persistent delusions.

297.3 Shared psychotic disorder
Folie à deux
Induced psychosis or paranoid disorder
DEF: Mental disorder two people share; first person with the delusional disorder convinces second person because of a close relationship and shared experiences to accept the delusions.

297.8 Other specified paranoid states
Paranoia querulans
Sensitiver Beziehungswahn
EXCLUDES *acute paranoid reaction or state (298.3)*
senile paranoid state (290.20)

297.9 Unspecified paranoid state
Paranoid:
   disorder NOS
   psychosis NOS
   reaction NOS
   state NOS

√4th **298 Other nonorganic psychoses**
INCLUDES psychotic conditions due to or provoked by:
   emotional stress
   environmental factors as major part of etiology

298.0 Depressive type psychosis
Psychogenic depressive psychosis
Psychotic reactive depression
Reactive depressive psychosis
EXCLUDES *manic-depressive psychosis, depressed type (296.2-296.3)*
neurotic depression (300.4)
reactive depression NOS (300.4)

298.1 Excitative type psychosis
Acute hysterical psychosis
Psychogenic excitation
Reactive excitation
EXCLUDES *manic-depressive psychosis, manic type (296.0-296.1)*
DEF: Affective disorder similar to manic-depressive psychosis, in the manic phase, seemingly brought on by stress.

298.2 Reactive confusion
Psychogenic confusion
Psychogenic twilight state
EXCLUDES *acute confusional state (293.0)*
DEF: Confusion, disorientation, cloudiness in consciousness; brought on by severe emotional upheaval.

298.3 Acute paranoid reaction
Acute psychogenic paranoid psychosis
Bouffée délirante
EXCLUDES *paranoid states (297.0-297.9)*

298.4 Psychogenic paranoid psychosis
Protracted reactive paranoid psychosis

298.8 Other and unspecified reactive psychosis
Brief psychotic disorder
Brief reactive psychosis NOS
Hysterical psychosis
Psychogenic psychosis NOS
Psychogenic stupor
EXCLUDES *acute hysterical psychosis (298.1)*

298.9 Unspecified psychosis
Atypical psychosis
Psychosis NOS
Psychotic disorder NOS

√4th **299 Pervasive developmental disorders**
EXCLUDES *adult type psychoses occurring in childhood, as:*
affective disorders (296.0-296.9)
manic-depressive disorders (296.0-296.9)
schizophrenia (295.0-295.9)

The following fifth-digit subclassification is for use with category 299:
  0 current or active state
  1 residual state

√5th **299.0 Autistic disorder**
[0-1]
Childhood autism
Infantile psychosis
Kanner's syndrome
EXCLUDES *disintegrative psychosis (299.1)*
Heller's syndrome (299.1)
schizophrenic syndrome of childhood (299.9)
DEF: Severe mental disorder of children, results in impaired social behavior; abnormal development of communicative skills, appears to be unaware of the need for emotional support and little emotional response to family members.

√5th **299.1 Childhood disintegrative disorder**
[0-1]
Heller's syndrome
Use additional code to identify any associated neurological disorder
EXCLUDES *infantile autism (299.0)*
schizophrenic syndrome of childhood (299.9)
DEF: Mental disease of children identified by impaired development of reciprocal social skills, verbal and nonverbal communication skills, imaginative play.

√5th **299.8 Other specified pervasive developmental disorders**
[0-1]
Asperger's disorder
Atypical childhood psychosis
Borderline psychosis of childhood
EXCLUDES *simple stereotypes without psychotic disturbance (307.3)*

√5th **299.9 Unspecified pervasive developmental disorder**
[0-1]
Child psychosis NOS
Pervasive developmental disorder NOS
Schizophrenia, childhood type NOS
Schizophrenic syndrome of childhood NOS
EXCLUDES *schizophrenia of adult type occurring in childhood (295.0-295.9)*

NEUROTIC DISORDERS, PERSONALITY DISORDERS, AND OTHER NONPSYCHOTIC MENTAL DISORDERS (300-316)

√4th **300 Anxiety, dissociative and somatoform disorders**

√5th **300.0 Anxiety states**
EXCLUDES *anxiety in:*
acute stress reaction (308.0)
transient adjustment reaction (309.24)
neurasthenia (300.5)
psychophysiological disorders (306.0-306.9)
separation anxiety (309.21)
DEF: Mental disorder characterized by anxiety and avoidance behavior not particularly related to any specific situation or stimulus; symptoms include emotional instability, apprehension, fatigue.

300.00 Anxiety state, unspecified
Anxiety:
   neurosis
   reaction
   state (neurotic)
Atypical anxiety disorder

Mental, Behavioral, & Neurodevelopmental Disorders

300.01–300.5

300.01 Panic disorder without agoraphobia
Panic:
    attack
    state
    EXCLUDES   *panic disorder with agoraphobia*
                      (300.21)

DEF: Neurotic disorder characterized by recurrent panic or anxiety, apprehension, fear or terror; symptoms include shortness of breath, palpitations, dizziness, shakiness; fear of dying may persist.

300.02 Generalized anxiety disorder

300.09 Other

✓5ᵗʰ **300.1 Dissociative, conversion and factitious disorders**
    EXCLUDES   *adjustment reaction (309.0-309.9)*
                   anorexia nervosa (307.1)
                   gross stress reaction (308.0-308.9)
                   hysterical personality (301.50-301.59)
                   psychophysiologic disorders (306.0-306.9)

300.10 Hysteria, unspecified

300.11 Conversion disorder
Astasia-abasia, hysterical
Conversion hysteria or reaction
Hysterical:
    blindness
    deafness
    paralysis

DEF: Mental disorder that impairs physical functions with no physiological basis; sensory motor symptoms include seizures, paralysis, temporary blindness; increase in stress or avoidance of unpleasant responsibilities may precipitate onset of symptoms.

300.12 Dissociative amnesia
Hysterical amnesia

300.13 Dissociative fugue
Hysterical fugue

DEF: Dissociative hysteria; identified by loss of memory, flight from familiar surroundings; conscious activity is not associated with perception of surroundings, no later memory of episode.

300.14 Dissociative identity disorder

300.15 Dissociative disorder or reaction, unspecified

DEF: Hysterical neurotic episode; sudden but temporary changes in perceived identity, memory, consciousness, segregated memory patterns exist separate from dominant personality.

300.16 Factitious disorder with predominantly psychological signs and symptoms
Compensation neurosis
Ganser's syndrome, hysterical

DEF: A disorder characterized by the purposeful assumption of mental illness symptoms; which are acted out more often when another person is present.

300.19 Other and unspecified factitious illness
Factitious disorder (with combined psychological and physical signs and symptoms) (with predominantly physical signs and symptoms) NOS
    EXCLUDES   *multiple operations or hospital*
                   addiction syndrome (301.51)

✓5ᵗʰ **300.2 Phobic disorders**
    EXCLUDES   *anxiety state not associated with a specific*
                   situation or object (300.00-300.09)
                   obsessional phobias (300.3)

300.20 Phobia, unspecified
Anxiety-hysteria NOS
Phobia NOS

300.21 Agoraphobia with panic disorder
Fear of:
    open spaces
    streets   } with panic attacks
    travel
Panic disorder with agoraphobia
    EXCLUDES   *agoraphobia without panic disorder*
                   (300.22)
                   panic disorder without agoraphobia
                   (300.01)

300.22 Agoraphobia without mention of panic attacks
Any condition classifiable to 300.21 without mention of panic attacks

300.23 Social phobia
Fear of:
    eating in public
    public speaking
    washing in public

300.29 Other isolated or specific phobias
Acrophobia
Animal phobias
Claustrophobia
Fear of crowds

300.3 Obsessive-compulsive disorders
Anancastic neurosis
Compulsive neurosis
Obsessional phobia [any]
    EXCLUDES   *obsessive-compulsive symptoms occurring in:*
                   endogenous depression (296.2-296.3)
                   organic states (eg., encephalitis)
                   schizophrenia (295.0-295.9)

300.4 Dysthymic disorder
Anxiety depression
Depression with anxiety
Depressive reaction
Neurotic depressive state
Reactive depression
    EXCLUDES   *adjustment reaction with depressive*
                   symptoms (309.0-309.1)
                   depression NOS (311)
                   manic-depressive psychosis, depressed type
                   (296.2-296.3)
                   reactive depressive psychosis (298.0)

DEF: Depression without psychosis; less severe depression related to personal change or unexpected circumstances; also referred to as "reactional depression."

300.5 Neurasthenia
Fatigue neurosis
Nervous debility
Psychogenic:
    asthenia
    general fatigue
Use additional code to identify any associated physical disorder
    EXCLUDES   *anxiety state (300.00-300.09)*
                   neurotic depression (300.4)
                   psychophysiological disorders (306.0-306.9)
                   specific nonpsychotic mental disorders
                   following organic brain damage
                   (310.0-310.9)

DEF: Physical and mental symptoms caused primarily by what is known as mental exhaustion; symptoms include chronic weakness, fatigue.

300.6   Depersonalization disorder
Derealization (neurotic)
Neurotic state with depersonalization episode
> EXCLUDES   *depersonalization associated with:*
> *anxiety (300.00-300.09)*
> *depression (300.4)*
> *manic-depressive disorder or psychosis*
> *(296.0-296.9)*
> *schizophrenia (295.0-295.9)*

DEF: Dissociative disorder characterized by feelings of strangeness about self or body image; symptoms include dizziness, anxiety, fear of insanity, loss of reality of surroundings.

300.7   Hypochondriasis
Body dysmorphic disorder
> EXCLUDES   *hypochondriasis in:*
> *hysteria (300.10-300.19)*
> *manic-depressive psychosis, depressed*
> *type (296.2-296.3)*
> *neurasthenia (300.5)*
> *obsessional disorder (300.3)*
> *schizophrenia (295.0-295.9)*

√5ᵗʰ   **300.8   Somatoform disorders**

300.81   Somatization disorder
Briquet's disorder
Severe somatoform disorder

300.82   Undifferentiated somatoform disorder
Atypical somatoform disorder
Somatoform disorder NOS
DEF: Disorders in which patients have symptoms that suggest an organic disease but no evidence of physical disorder after repeated testing.

300.89   Other somatoform disorders
Occupational neurosis, including writers' cramp
Psychasthenia
Psychasthenic neurosis

300.9   Unspecified nonpsychotic mental disorder
Psychoneurosis NOS

√4ᵗʰ   **301   Personality disorders**
> INCLUDES   character neurosis
Use additional code to identify any associated neurosis or psychosis, or physical condition
> EXCLUDES   *nonpsychotic personality disorder associated with*
> *organic brain syndromes (310.0-310.9)*

301.0   Paranoid personality disorder
Fanatic personality
Paranoid personality (disorder)
Paranoid traits
> EXCLUDES   *acute paranoid reaction (298.3)*
> *alcoholic paranoia (291.5)*
> *paranoid schizophrenia (295.3)*
> *paranoid states (297.0-297.9)*

√5ᵗʰ   **301.1   Affective personality disorder**
> EXCLUDES   *affective psychotic disorders (296.0-296.9)*
> *neurasthenia (300.5)*
> *neurotic depression (300.4)*

301.10   Affective personality disorder, unspecified

301.11   Chronic hypomanic personality disorder
Chronic hypomanic disorder
Hypomanic personality

301.12   Chronic depressive personality disorder
Chronic depressive disorder
Depressive character or personality

301.13   Cyclothymic disorder
Cycloid personality
Cyclothymia
Cyclothymic personality

√5ᵗʰ   **301.2   Schizoid personality disorder**
> EXCLUDES   *schizophrenia (295.0-295.9)*

301.20   Schizoid personality disorder, unspecified

301.21   Introverted personality

301.22   Schizotypal personality disorder

301.3   Explosive personality disorder
Aggressive:
personality
reaction
Aggressiveness
Emotional instability (excessive)
Pathological emotionality
Quarrelsomeness
> EXCLUDES   *dyssocial personality (301.7)*
> *hysterical neurosis (300.10-300.19)*

301.4   Obsessive-compulsive personality disorder
Anancastic personality
Obsessional personality
> EXCLUDES   *obsessive-compulsive disorder (300.3)*
> *phobic state (300.20-300.29)*

√5ᵗʰ   **301.5   Histrionic personality disorder**
> EXCLUDES   *hysterical neurosis (300.10-300.19)*

DEF: Extreme emotional behavior, often theatrical; often concerned about own appeal; may demand attention, exhibit seductive behavior.

301.50   Histrionic personality disorder, unspecified
Hysterical personality NOS

301.51   Chronic factitious illness with physical symptoms
Hospital addiction syndrome
Multiple operations syndrome
Munchausen syndrome

301.59   Other histrionic personality disorder
Personality:
emotionally unstable
labile
psychoinfantile

301.6   Dependent personality disorder
Asthenic personality
Inadequate personality
Passive personality
> EXCLUDES   *neurasthenia (300.5)*
> *passive-aggressive personality (301.84)*

DEF: Overwhelming feeling of helplessness; fears of abandonment may persist; difficulty in making personal decisions without confirmation by others; low self-esteem due to irrational sensitivity to criticism.

301.7   Antisocial personality disorder
Amoral personality
Asocial personality
Dyssocial personality
Personality disorder with predominantly sociopathic or asocial manifestation
> EXCLUDES   *disturbance of conduct without specifiable*
> *personality disorder (312.0-312.9)*
> *explosive personality (301.3)*

DEF: Continuous antisocial behavior that violates rights of others; social traits include extreme aggression, total disregard for traditional social rules.

√5ᵗʰ   **301.8   Other personality disorders**

301.81   Narcissistic personality disorder
DEF: Grandiose fantasy or behavior, lack of social empathy, hypersensitive to the lack of others' judgment, exploits others; need for continual admiration.

301.82   Avoidant personality disorder
DEF: Personality disorder marked by feelings of social inferiority; sensitivity to criticism, emotionally restrained due to fear of rejection.

301.83   Borderline personality disorder
DEF: Personality disorder characterized by unstable moods, self-image, and interpersonal relationships; uncontrolled anger, impulsive and self-destructive acts, fears of abandonment, feelings of emptiness and boredom, recurrent suicide threats or self-mutilation.

Mental, Behavioral, & Neurodevelopmental Disorders

301.84–303.9

301.84 Passive-aggressive personality

DEF: Pattern of procrastination and refusal to meet standards; introduce own obstacles to success and exploit failure.

301.89 Other

Personality:
eccentric
"haltlose" type
immature
masochistic
psychoneurotic
EXCLUDES *psychoinfantile personality (301.59)*

301.9 Unspecified personality disorder

Pathological personality NOS
Personality disorder NOS
Psychopathic:
constitutional state
personality (disorder)

√4ᵗʰ **302 Sexual and gender identity disorders**

EXCLUDES *sexual disorder manifest in:*
organic brain syndrome (290.0-294.9, 310.0-310.9)
psychosis (295.0-298.9)

302.0 Ego-dystonic sexual orientation

Ego-dystonic lesbianism
Sexual orientation conflict disorder
EXCLUDES *homosexual pedophilia (302.2)*

302.1 Zoophilia

Bestiality

DEF: A sociodeviant disorder marked by engaging in sexual intercourse with animals.

302.2 Pedophilia

DEF: A sociodeviant condition of adults characterized by sexual activity with children.

302.3 Transvestic fetishism

EXCLUDES *trans-sexualism (302.5)*

DEF: The desire to dress in clothing of opposite sex.

302.4 Exhibitionism

DEF: Sexual deviant behavior; exposure of genitals to strangers; behavior prompted by intense sexual urges and fantasies.

√5ᵗʰ **302.5 Trans-sexualism**

Sex reassignment surgery status
EXCLUDES *transvestism (302.3)*

DEF: Gender identity disturbance; overwhelming desire to change anatomic sex, due to belief that individual is a member of the opposite sex.

302.50 With unspecified sexual history

302.51 With asexual history

302.52 With homosexual history

302.53 With heterosexual history

302.6 Gender identity disorder in children

Feminism in boys
Gender identity disorder NOS
EXCLUDES *gender identity disorder in adult (302.85)*
trans-sexualism (302.50-302.53)
transvestism (302.3)

√5ᵗʰ **302.7 Psychosexual dysfunction**

EXCLUDES *impotence of organic origin (607.84)*
normal transient symptoms from ruptured hymen
transient or occasional failures of erection due to fatigue, anxiety, alcohol, or drugs

302.70 Psychosexual dysfunction, unspecified

Sexual dysfunction NOS

302.71 Hypoactive sexual desire disorder

EXCLUDES *decreased sexual desire NOS (799.81)*

302.72 With inhibited sexual excitement

Female sexual arousal disorder
Frigidity
Impotence
Male erectile disorder

302.73 Female orgasmic disorder

302.74 Male orgasmic disorder

302.75 Premature ejaculation

302.76 Dyspareunia, psychogenic

DEF: Difficult or painful sex due to psychosomatic state.

302.79 With other specified psychosexual dysfunctions

Sexual aversion disorder

√5ᵗʰ **302.8 Other specified psychosexual disorders**

302.81 Fetishism

DEF: Psychosexual disorder noted for intense sexual urges and arousal precipitated by fantasies; use of inanimate objects, such as clothing, to stimulate sexual arousal, orgasm.

302.82 Voyeurism

DEF: Psychosexual disorder characterized by uncontrollable impulse to observe others, without their knowledge, who are nude or engaged in sexual activity.

302.83 Sexual masochism

DEF: Psychosexual disorder noted for need to achieve sexual gratification through humiliating or hurtful acts inflicted on self.

302.84 Sexual sadism

DEF: Psychosexual disorder noted for need to achieve sexual gratification through humiliating or hurtful acts inflicted on someone else.

302.85 Gender identity disorder in adolescents or adults

Use additional code to identify sex reassignment surgery status (302.5)
EXCLUDES *gender identity disorder NOS (302.6)*
gender identity disorder in children (302.6)

302.89 Other

Frotteurism
Nymphomania
Satyriasis

302.9 Unspecified psychosexual disorder

Paraphilia NOS
Pathologic sexuality NOS
Sexual deviation NOS
Sexual disorder NOS

√4ᵗʰ **303 Alcohol dependence syndrome**

Use additional code to identify any associated condition, as:
alcoholic psychoses (291.0-291.9)
drug dependence (304.0-304.9)
physical complications of alcohol, such as:
cerebral degeneration (331.7)
cirrhosis of liver (571.2)
epilepsy (345.0-345.9)
gastritis (535.3)
hepatitis (571.1)
liver damage NOS (571.3)
EXCLUDES *drunkenness NOS (305.0)*

The following fifth-digit subclassification is for use with category 303:
0 unspecified
1 continuous
2 episodic
3 in remission

√5ᵗʰ **303.0 Acute alcoholic intoxication**

[0-3] Acute drunkenness in alcoholism

√5ᵗʰ **303.9 Other and unspecified alcohol dependence**

[0-3] Chronic alcoholism
Dipsomania

✓4ᵗʰ **304 Drug dependence**

    EXCLUDES *nondependent abuse of drugs (305.1-305.9)*

    The following fifth-digit subclassification is for use with category 304:

       0 unspecified
       1 continuous
       2 episodic
       3 in remission

✓5ᵗʰ **304.0 Opioid type dependence**
    [0-3]

       Heroin
       Meperidine
       Methadone
       Morphine
       Opium
       Opium alkaloids and their derivatives
       Synthetics with morphine-like effects

✓5ᵗʰ **304.1 Sedative, hypnotic or anxiolytic dependence**
    [0-3]

       Barbiturates
       Nonbarbiturate sedatives and tranquilizers with a similar effect:
          chlordiazepoxide
          diazepam
          glutethimide
          meprobamate
          methaqualone

✓5ᵗʰ **304.2 Cocaine dependence**
    [0-3]   Coca leaves and derivatives

✓5ᵗʰ **304.3 Cannabis dependence**
    [0-3]   Hashish   Marihuana
            Hemp

✓5ᵗʰ **304.4 Amphetamine and other psychostimulant dependence**
    [0-3]
       Methylphenidate   Phenmetrazine

✓5ᵗʰ **304.5 Hallucinogen dependence**
    [0-3]
       Dimethyltryptamine [DMT]
       Lysergic acid diethylamide [LSD] and derivatives
       Mescaline
       Psilocybin

✓5ᵗʰ **304.6 Other specified drug dependence**
    [0-3]
       Absinthe addiction
       Glue sniffing
       Inhalant dependence
       Phencyclidine dependence
       EXCLUDES *tobacco dependence (305.1)*

✓5ᵗʰ **304.7 Combinations of opioid type drug with any other**
    [0-3]

✓5ᵗʰ **304.8 Combinations of drug dependence excluding opioid type drug**
    [0-3]

✓5ᵗʰ **304.9 Unspecified drug dependence**
    [0-3]
       Drug addiction NOS
       Drug dependence NOS

✓4ᵗʰ **305 Nondependent abuse of drugs**

    Note: Includes cases where a person, for whom no other diagnosis is possible, has come under medical care because of the maladaptive effect of a drug on which he is not dependent and that he has taken on his own initiative to the detriment of his health or social functioning.

    EXCLUDES *alcohol dependence syndrome (303.0-303.9)*
          drug dependence (304.0-304.9)
          drug withdrawal syndrome (292.0)
          poisoning by drugs or medicinal substances (960.0-979.9)

    The following fifth-digit subclassification is for use with codes 305.0, 305.2-305.9:
       0 unspecified
       1 continuous
       2 episodic
       3 in remission

✓5ᵗʰ **305.0 Alcohol abuse**
    [0-3]
       Drunkenness NOS
       Excessive drinking of alcohol NOS
       "Hangover" (alcohol)
       Inebriety NOS
       EXCLUDES *acute alcohol intoxication in alcoholism (303.0)*
          alcoholic psychoses (291.0-291.9)

305.1 Tobacco use disorder
    Tobacco dependence
    EXCLUDES *history of tobacco use (V15.82)*
          smoking complicating pregnancy (649.0)
          tobacco use disorder complicating pregnancy (649.0)

✓5ᵗʰ **305.2 Cannabis abuse**
    [0-3]

✓5ᵗʰ **305.3 Hallucinogen abuse**
    [0-3]
       Acute intoxication from hallucinogens ["bad trips"]
       LSD reaction

✓5ᵗʰ **305.4 Sedative, hypnotic or anxiolytic abuse**
    [0-3]

✓5ᵗʰ **305.5 Opioid abuse**
    [0-3]

✓5ᵗʰ **305.6 Cocaine abuse**
    [0-3]

✓5ᵗʰ **305.7 Amphetamine or related acting sympathomimetic abuse**
    [0-3]

✓5ᵗʰ **305.8 Antidepressant type abuse**
    [0-3]

✓5ᵗʰ **305.9 Other, mixed, or unspecified drug abuse**
    [0-3]
       Caffeine intoxication   Nonprescribed use of drugs or
       Inhalant abuse   patent medicinals
       "Laxative habit"   Phencyclidine abuse
       Misuse of drugs NOS

✓4ᵗʰ **306 Physiological malfunction arising from mental factors**

    INCLUDES psychogenic:
          physical symptoms   } not involving tissue
          physiological   } damage
             manifestations

    EXCLUDES *hysteria (300.11-300.19)*
          physical symptoms secondary to a psychiatric disorder classified elsewhere
          psychic factors associated with physical conditions involving tissue damage classified elsewhere (316)
          specific nonpsychotic mental disorders following organic brain damage (310.0-310.9)

    DEF: Functional disturbances or interruptions due to mental or psychological causes; no tissue damage sustained in these conditions.

306.0 Musculoskeletal
    Psychogenic paralysis
    Psychogenic torticollis
    EXCLUDES *Gilles de la Tourette's syndrome (307.23)*
          paralysis as hysterical or conversion reaction (300.11)
          tics (307.20-307.22)

306.1 Respiratory
    Psychogenic: Psychogenic:
      air hunger   hyperventilation
      cough   yawning
      hiccough
    EXCLUDES *psychogenic asthma (316 and 493.9)*

306.2 Cardiovascular
Cardiac neurosis
Cardiovascular neurosis
Neurocirculatory asthenia
Psychogenic cardiovascular disorder
EXCLUDES *psychogenic paroxysmal tachycardia (316 and 427.2)*

DEF: Neurocirculatory asthenia: functional nervous and circulatory irregularities with palpitations, dyspnea, fatigue, rapid pulse, precordial pain, fear of effort, discomfort during exercise, anxiety; also called DaCosta's syndrome, Effort syndrome, Irritable or Soldier's Heart.

306.3 Skin
Psychogenic pruritus
EXCLUDES *psychogenic:*
alopecia (316 and 704.00)
dermatitis (316 and 692.9)
eczema (316 and 691.8 or 692.9)
urticaria (316 and 708.0-708.9)

306.4 Gastrointestinal
Aerophagy
Cyclical vomiting, psychogenic
Diarrhea, psychogenic
Nervous gastritis
Psychogenic dyspepsia
EXCLUDES *cyclical vomiting NOS (536.2)*
associated with migraine (346.2)
globus hystericus (300.11)
mucous colitis (316 and 564.9)
psychogenic:
cardiospasm (316 and 530.0)
duodenal ulcer (316 and 532.0-532.9)
gastric ulcer (316 and 531.0-531.9)
peptic ulcer NOS (316 and 533.0-533.9)
vomiting NOS (307.54)

DEF: Aerophagy: excess swallowing of air, usually unconscious; related to anxiety; results in distended abdomen or belching, often interpreted by the patient as a physical disorder.

√5ᵗʰ **306.5 Genitourinary**
EXCLUDES *enuresis, psychogenic (307.6)*
frigidity (302.72)
impotence (302.72)
psychogenic dyspareunia (302.76)

306.50 Psychogenic genitourinary malfunction, unspecified

306.51 Psychogenic vaginismus
Functional vaginismus
DEF: Psychogenic response resulting in painful contractions of vaginal canal muscles; can be severe enough to prevent sexual intercourse.

306.52 Psychogenic dysmenorrhea

306.53 Psychogenic dysuria

306.59 Other

306.6 Endocrine

306.7 Organs of special sense
EXCLUDES *hysterical blindness or deafness (300.11)*
psychophysical visual disturbances (368.16)

306.8 Other specified psychophysiological malfunction
Bruxism
Teeth grinding

306.9 Unspecified psychophysiological malfunction
Psychophysiologic disorder NOS
Psychosomatic disorder NOS

√4ᵗʰ **307 Special symptoms or syndromes, not elsewhere classified**
Note: This category is intended for use if the psychopathology is manifested by a single specific symptom or group of symptoms which is not part of an organic illness or other mental disorder classifiable elsewhere.
EXCLUDES *those due to mental disorders classified elsewhere*
those of organic origin

307.0 Adult onset fluency disorder
EXCLUDES *childhood onset fluency disorder (315.35)*
dysphasia (784.59)
fluency disorder due to late effect of cerebrovascular accident (438.14)
fluency disorder in conditions classified elsewhere (784.52)
lisping or lalling (307.9)
retarded development of speech (315.31-315.39)

307.1 Anorexia nervosa
EXCLUDES *eating disturbance NOS (307.50)*
feeding problem (783.3)
of nonorganic origin (307.59)
loss of appetite (783.0)
of nonorganic origin (307.59)

√5ᵗʰ **307.2 Tics**
EXCLUDES *nail-biting or thumb-sucking (307.9)*
stereotypes occurring in isolation (307.3)
tics of organic origin (333.3)

DEF: Involuntary muscle response usually confined to the face, shoulders.

307.20 Tic disorder, unspecified
Tic disorder NOS

307.21 Transient tic disorder

307.22 Chronic motor or vocal tic disorder

307.23 Tourette's disorder
Motor-verbal tic disorder
DEF: Syndrome of facial and vocal tics in childhood; progresses to spontaneous or involuntary jerking, obscene utterances, other uncontrollable actions considered inappropriate.

307.3 Stereotypic movement disorder
Body-rocking
Head banging
Spasmus nutans
Stereotypes NOS
EXCLUDES *tics (307.20-307.23)*
of organic origin (333.3)

√5ᵗʰ **307.4 Specific disorders of sleep of nonorganic origin**
EXCLUDES *narcolepsy (347.00-347.11)*
organic hypersomnia (327.10-327.19)
organic insomnia (327.00-327.09)
those of unspecified cause (780.50-780.59)

307.40 Nonorganic sleep disorder, unspecified

307.41 Transient disorder of initiating or maintaining sleep
Adjustment insomnia
Hyposomnia ⎫ associated with intermittent
Insomnia ⎬ emotional reactions or
Sleeplessness ⎭ conflicts

307.42 Persistent disorder of initiating or maintaining sleep
Hyposomnia, insomnia, or sleeplessness associated with:
anxiety
conditioned arousal
depression (major) (minor)
psychosis
Idiopathic insomnia
Paradoxical insomnia
Primary insomnia
Psychophysiological insomnia

307.43 Transient disorder of initiating or maintaining wakefulness
Hypersomnia associated with acute or intermittent emotional reactions or conflicts

307.44 Persistent disorder of initiating or maintaining wakefulness
Hypersomnia associated with depression (major) (minor)
Insufficient sleep syndrome
Primary hypersomnia
> EXCLUDES   sleep deprivation (V69.4)

307.45 Circadian rhythm sleep disorder of nonorganic origin

307.46 Sleep arousal disorder
Night terror disorder
Night terrors
Sleep terror disorder
Sleepwalking
Somnambulism
> DEF: Sleepwalking marked by extreme terror, panic, screaming, confusion; no recall of event upon arousal; term may refer to simply the act of sleepwalking.

307.47 Other dysfunctions of sleep stages or arousal from sleep
Nightmare disorder
Nightmares:
  NOS
  REM-sleep type
  Sleep drunkenness

307.48 Repetitive intrusions of sleep
Repetitive intrusion of sleep with:
  atypical polysomnographic features
  environmental disturbances
  repeated REM-sleep interruptions

307.49 Other
"Short-sleeper"
Subjective insomnia complaint

307.5 Other and unspecified disorders of eating
> EXCLUDES   anorexia:
>   nervosa (307.1)
>   of unspecified cause (783.0)
>   overeating, of unspecified cause (783.6)
>   vomiting:
>   NOS (787.03)
>   cyclical (536.2)
>   associated with migraine (346.2)
>   psychogenic (306.4)

307.50 Eating disorder, unspecified
Eating disorder NOS

307.51 Bulimia nervosa
Overeating of nonorganic origin
> DEF: Mental disorder commonly characterized by binge eating followed by self-induced vomiting; perceptions of being fat; and fear the inability to stop eating voluntarily.

307.52 Pica
Perverted appetite of nonorganic origin
> DEF: Compulsive eating disorder characterized by craving for substances other than food, such as paint chips or dirt.

307.53 Rumination disorder
Regurgitation, of nonorganic origin, of food with reswallowing
> EXCLUDES   obsessional rumination (300.3)

307.54 Psychogenic vomiting

307.59 Other
Feeding disorder of infancy or early childhood of nonorganic origin
Infantile feeding disturbances } of nonorganic origin
Loss of appetite

307.6 Enuresis
Enuresis (primary) (secondary) of nonorganic origin
> EXCLUDES   enuresis of unspecified cause (788.3)
> DEF: Involuntary urination past age of normal control; also called bedwetting; no trace to biological problem; focus on psychological issues.

307.7 Encopresis
Encopresis (continuous) (discontinuous) of nonorganic origin
> EXCLUDES   encopresis of unspecified cause (787.60-787.63)
> DEF: Inability to control bowel movements; cause traced to psychological, not biological, problems.

307.8 Pain disorders related to psychological factors

307.80 Psychogenic pain, site unspecified

307.81 Tension headache
> EXCLUDES   headache:
>   NOS (784.0)
>   migraine (346.0-346.9)
>   syndromes (339.00-339.89)
>   tension type (339.10-339.12)

307.89 Other
Code first to type or site of pain
> EXCLUDES   pain disorder exclusively attributed to psychological factors (307.80)
>   psychogenic pain (307.80)

307.9 Other and unspecified special symptoms or syndromes, not elsewhere classified
Communication disorder NOS
Hair plucking
Lalling
Lisping
Masturbation
Nail-biting
Thumb-sucking

308 Acute reaction to stress
> INCLUDES   combat and operational stress reaction
> EXCLUDES   adjustment reaction or disorder (309.0-309.9)
>   chronic stress reaction (309.1-309.9)

308.0 Predominant disturbance of emotions
Anxiety
Emotional crisis } as acute reaction to exceptional [gross] stress
Panic state

308.1 Predominant disturbance of consciousness
Fugues as acute reaction to exceptional [gross] stress

308.2 Predominant psychomotor disturbance
Agitation states } as acute reaction to exceptional
Stupor } [gross] stress

308.3 Other acute reactions to stress
Acute situational disturbance
Acute stress disorder
> EXCLUDES   prolonged posttraumatic emotional disturbance (309.81)

308.4 Mixed disorders as reaction to stress

308.9 Unspecified acute reaction to stress

309 Adjustment reaction
> INCLUDES   adjustment disorders
>   reaction (adjustment) to chronic stress
> EXCLUDES   acute reaction to major stress (308.0-308.9)
>   neurotic disorders (300.0-300.9)

309.0 Adjustment disorder with depressed mood
Grief reaction
> EXCLUDES   affective psychoses (296.0-296.9)
>   neurotic depression (300.4)
>   prolonged depressive reaction (309.1)
>   psychogenic depressive psychosis (298.0)

309.1 Prolonged depressive reaction
> EXCLUDES   affective psychoses (296.0-296.9)
>   brief depressive reaction (309.0)
>   neurotic depression (300.4)
>   psychogenic depressive psychosis (298.0)

309.2 With predominant disturbance of other emotions

309.21 Separation anxiety disorder
> DEF: Abnormal apprehension by a child when physically separated from support environment; byproduct of abnormal symbiotic child-parent relationship.

Mental, Behavioral, & Neurodevelopmental Disorders

309.22–311

309.22 Emancipation disorder of adolescence and early adult life

DEF: Adjustment reaction of late adolescence; conflict over independence from parental supervision; symptoms include difficulty in making decisions, increased reliance on parental advice, deliberate adoption of values in opposition of parents.

309.23 Specific academic or work inhibition

309.24 Adjustment disorder with anxiety

309.28 Adjustment disorder with mixed anxiety and depressed mood

Adjustment reaction with anxiety and depression

309.29 Other

Culture shock

309.3 Adjustment disorder with disturbance of conduct

Conduct disturbance ⎱
Destructiveness ⎰ as adjustment reaction

EXCLUDES destructiveness in child (312.9)
disturbance of conduct NOS (312.9)
dyssocial behavior without manifest psychiatric disorder (V71.01-V71.02)
personality disorder with predominantly sociopathic or asocial manifestations (301.7)

309.4 Adjustment disorder with mixed disturbance of emotions and conduct

√5ᵗʰ **309.8 Other specified adjustment reactions**

309.81 Posttraumatic stress disorder

Chronic posttraumatic stress disorder
Concentration camp syndrome
Posttraumatic stress disorder NOS
Post-traumatic stress disorder (PTSD)

EXCLUDES acute stress disorder (308.3)
posttraumatic brain syndrome:
nonpsychotic (310.2)
psychotic (293.0-293.9)

DEF: Preoccupation with traumatic events beyond normal experience; i.e., rape, personal assault, etc.; also recurring flashbacks of trauma; symptoms include difficulty remembering, sleeping, or concentrating, and guilt feelings for surviving.

309.82 Adjustment reaction with physical symptoms

309.83 Adjustment reaction with withdrawal

Elective mutism as adjustment reaction
Hospitalism (in children) NOS

309.89 Other

309.9 Unspecified adjustment reaction

Adaptation reaction NOS
Adjustment reaction NOS

√4ᵗʰ **310 Specific nonpsychotic mental disorders due to brain damage**

EXCLUDES neuroses, personality disorders, or other nonpsychotic conditions occurring in a form similar to that seen with functional disorders but in association with a physical condition (300.0-300.9, 301.0-301.9)

310.0 Frontal lobe syndrome

Lobotomy syndrome
Postleucotomy syndrome [state]

EXCLUDES postcontusion syndrome (310.2)

310.1 Personality change due to conditions classified elsewhere

Cognitive or personality change of other type, of nonpsychotic severity
Organic psychosyndrome of nonpsychotic severity
Presbyophrenia NOS
Senility with mental changes of nonpsychotic severity

EXCLUDES mild cognitive impairment (331.83)
postconcussion syndrome (310.2)
signs and symptoms involving emotional state (799.21-799.29)

DEF: Personality disorder caused by organic factors, such as brain lesions, head trauma, or cerebrovascular accident (CVA).

310.2 Postconcussion syndrome

Postcontusion syndrome or encephalopathy
Posttraumatic brain syndrome, nonpsychotic
Status postcommotio cerebri

Use additional code to identify associated post-traumatic headache, if applicable (339.20-339.22)

EXCLUDES any organic psychotic conditions following head injury (293.0-294.0)
frontal lobe syndrome (310.0)
postencephalitic syndrome (310.89)

DEF: Nonpsychotic disorder due to brain trauma, causes symptoms unrelated to any disease process; symptoms include amnesia, serial headaches, rapid heartbeat, fatigue, disrupted sleep patterns, inability to concentrate.

√5ᵗʰ **310.8 Other specified nonpsychotic mental disorders following organic brain damage**

310.81 Pseudobulbar affect

Involuntary emotional expression disorder
Code first underlying cause, such as:
amyotrophic lateral sclerosis (335.20)
late effect of cerebrovascular accident (438.89)
late effect of traumatic brain injury (907.0)
mutiple sclerosis (340)

310.89 Other specified nonpsychotic mental disorders following organic brain damage

Mild memory disturbance
Other focal (partial) organic psychosyndromes
Postencephalitic syndrome

EXCLUDES memory loss of unknown cause (780.93)

310.9 Unspecified nonpsychotic mental disorder following organic brain damage

311 Depressive disorder, not elsewhere classified

Depressive disorder NOS   Depression NOS
Depressive state NOS

EXCLUDES acute reaction to major stress with depressive symptoms (308.0)
affective personality disorder (301.10-301.13)
affective psychoses (296.0-296.9)
brief depressive reaction (309.0)
depressive states associated with stressful events (309.0-309.1)
disturbance of emotions specific to childhood and adolescence, with misery and unhappiness (313.1)
mixed adjustment reaction with depressive symptoms (309.4)
neurotic depression (300.4)
prolonged depressive adjustment reaction (309.1)
psychogenic depressive psychosis (298.0)

✓4ᵗʰ 312 Disturbance of conduct, not elsewhere classified
     EXCLUDES   *adjustment reaction with disturbance of conduct*
           (309.3)
           drug dependence (304.0-304.9)
           dyssocial behavior without manifest psychiatric
              disorder (V71.01-V71.02)
           personality disorder with predominantly sociopathic or
              asocial manifestations (301.7)
           sexual deviations (302.0-302.9)

> The following fifth-digit subclassification is for use with categories
> 312.0-312.2
>   **0**   **unspecified**
>   **1**   **mild**
>   **2**   **moderate**
>   **3**   **severe**

✓5ᵗʰ 312.0 Undersocialized conduct disorder, aggressive type
   [0-3]   Aggressive outburst
          Anger reaction
          Unsocialized aggressive disorder

          DEF: Mental condition identified by behaviors
          disrespectful of others' rights and of age-appropriate
          social norms or rules; symptoms include bullying,
          vandalism, verbal and physical abusiveness, lying, stealing,
          defiance.

✓5ᵗʰ 312.1 Undersocialized conduct disorder, unaggressive type
   [0-3]   Childhood truancy, unsocialized
          Solitary stealing
          Tantrums

✓5ᵗʰ 312.2 Socialized conduct disorder
   [0-3]   Childhood truancy, socialized
          Group delinquency
          EXCLUDES   *gang activity without manifest psychiatric*
                     disorder (V71.01)

✓5ᵗʰ 312.3 Disorders of impulse control, not elsewhere classified
     312.30 Impulse control disorder, unspecified
     312.31 Pathological gambling
     312.32 Kleptomania
     312.33 Pyromania
     312.34 Intermittent explosive disorder
     312.35 Isolated explosive disorder
     312.39 Other
            Trichotillomania

312.4 Mixed disturbance of conduct and emotions
       Neurotic delinquency
       EXCLUDES   *compulsive conduct disorder (312.3)*

✓5ᵗʰ 312.8 Other specified disturbances of conduct, not elsewhere classified
     312.81 Conduct disorder, childhood onset type
     312.82 Conduct disorder, adolescent onset type
     312.89 Other conduct disorder
            Conduct disorder of unspecified onset

312.9 Unspecified disturbance of conduct
       Delinquency (juvenile)
       Disruptive behavior disorder NOS

✓4ᵗʰ 313 Disturbance of emotions specific to childhood and adolescence
     EXCLUDES   *adjustment reaction (309.0-309.9)*
          emotional disorder of neurotic type (300.0-300.9)
          masturbation, nail-biting, thumbsucking, and other
              isolated symptoms (307.0-307.9)

313.0 Overanxious disorder
       Anxiety and fearfulness } of childhood and
       Overanxious disorder   }   adolescence
       EXCLUDES   *abnormal separation anxiety (309.21)*
          anxiety states (300.00-300.09)
          hospitalism in children (309.83)
          phobic state (300.20-300.29)

313.1 Misery and unhappiness disorder
       EXCLUDES   *depressive neurosis (300.4)*

✓5ᵗʰ 313.2 Sensitivity, shyness, and social withdrawal disorder
     EXCLUDES   *infantile autism (299.0)*
          schizoid personality (301.20-301.22)
          schizophrenia (295.0-295.9)

     313.21 Shyness disorder of childhood
            Sensitivity reaction of childhood or
              adolescence

     313.22 Introverted disorder of childhood
            Social withdrawal } of childhood and
            Withdrawal reaction }   adolescence

     313.23 Selective mutism
            EXCLUDES   *elective mutism as adjustment*
                     reaction (309.83)

313.3 Relationship problems
       Sibling jealousy
       EXCLUDES   *relationship problems associated with*
                     aggression, destruction, or other forms
                     of conduct disturbance (312.0-312.9)

✓5ᵗʰ 313.8 Other or mixed emotional disturbances of childhood or adolescence
     313.81 Oppositional defiant disorder
            DEF: Mental disorder of children noted for
            pervasive opposition, defiance of authority.

     313.82 Identity disorder
            Identity problem
            DEF: Distress of adolescents caused by inability
            to form acceptable self-identity; uncertainty
            about career choice, sexual orientation, moral
            values.

     313.83 Academic underachievement disorder

     313.89 Other
            Reactive attachment disorder of infancy or
            early childhood

313.9 Unspecified emotional disturbance of childhood or adolescence
       Mental disorder of infancy, childhood or adolescence
       NOS

✓4ᵗʰ 314 Hyperkinetic syndrome of childhood
     EXCLUDES   *hyperkinesis as symptom of underlying disorder–code*
               the underlying disorder

✓5ᵗʰ 314.0 Attention deficit disorder
       Adult
       Child
       DEF: A behavioral disorder usually diagnosed at an early
       age; characterized by the inability to focus attention for a
       normal period of time.

     314.00 Without mention of hyperactivity
            Predominantly inattentive type

     314.01 With hyperactivity
            Combined type
            Overactivity NOS
            Predominantly hyperactive/impulsive type
            Simple disturbance of attention with
              overactivity

314.1 Hyperkinesis with developmental delay
       Developmental disorder of hyperkinesis
       Use additional code to identify any associated
       neurological disorder

314.2 Hyperkinetic conduct disorder
       Hyperkinetic conduct disorder without developmental
       delay
       EXCLUDES   *hyperkinesis with significant delays in specific*
                skills (314.1)

314.8 Other specified manifestations of hyperkinetic syndrome

314.9 Unspecified hyperkinetic syndrome
       Hyperkinetic reaction of childhood or adolescence NOS
       Hyperkinetic syndrome NOS

Mental, Behavioral, & Neurodevelopmental Disorders

315–319

√4ᵗʰ **315 Specific delays in development**
     EXCLUDES   that due to a neurological disorder (320.0-389.9)

√5ᵗʰ **315.0 Specific reading disorder**

     315.00 Reading disorder, unspecified

     315.01 Alexia
        DEF: Lack of ability to understand written language; manifestation of aphasia.

     315.02 Developmental dyslexia
        DEF: Serious impairment of reading skills unexplained in relation to general intelligence and teaching processes.

     315.09 Other
        Specific spelling difficulty

315.1 Mathematics disorder
     Dyscalculia

315.2 Other specific learning difficulties
     Disorder of written expression
     EXCLUDES   specific arithmetical disorder (315.1)
             specific reading disorder (315.00-315.09)

√5ᵗʰ **315.3 Developmental speech or language disorder**

     315.31 Expressive language disorder
        Developmental aphasia
        Word deafness
        EXCLUDES   acquired aphasia (784.3)
               elective mutism (309.83, 313.0, 313.23)

     315.32 Mixed receptive-expressive language disorder
        Central auditory processing disorder
        EXCLUDES   acquired auditory processing disorder (388.45)

     315.34 Speech and language developmental delay due to hearing loss

     315.35 Childhood onset fluency disorder
        Cluttering NOS
        Stuttering NOS
        EXCLUDES   adult onset fluency disorder (307.0)
               fluency disorder due to late effect of cerebrovascular accident (438.14)
               fluency disorder in conditions classified elsewhere (784.52)

     315.39 Other
        Developmental articulation disorder
        Dyslalia
        Phonological disorder
        EXCLUDES   lisping and lalling (307.9)

315.4 Developmental coordination disorder
     Clumsiness syndrome
     Dyspraxia syndrome
     Specific motor development disorder

315.5 Mixed development disorder

315.8 Other specified delays in development

315.9 Unspecified delay in development
     Developmental disorder NOS
     Learning disorder NOS

316 Psychic factors associated with diseases classified elsewhere
     Psychologic factors in physical conditions classified elsewhere
     Use additional code to identify the associated physical condition, as:
     psychogenic:
        asthma (493.9)
        dermatitis (692.9)
        duodenal ulcer (532.0-532.9)
        eczema (691.8, 692.9)
        gastric ulcer (531.0-531.9)
        mucous colitis (564.9)
        paroxysmal tachycardia (427.2)
        ulcerative colitis (556)
        urticaria (708.0-708.9)
     psychosocial dwarfism (259.4)
     EXCLUDES   physical symptoms and physiological malfunctions, not involving tissue damage, of mental origin (306.0-306.9)

INTELLECTUAL DISABILITIES (317-319)
     Use additional code(s) to identify any associated psychiatric or physical condition(s)

317 Mild intellectual disabilities
     High-grade defect
     IQ 50-70
     Mild mental subnormality

√4ᵗʰ **318 Other specified intellectual disabilities**

     318.0 Moderate intellectual disabilities
        IQ 35-49
        Moderate mental subnormality

     318.1 Severe intellectual disabilities
        IQ 20-34
        Severe mental subnormality

     318.2 Profound intellectual disabilities
        IQ under 20
        Profound mental subnormality

319 Unspecified intellectual disabilities
     Mental deficiency NOS
     Mental subnormality NOS

Chapter 6: Diseases of the Nervous System and Sense Organs (320–389)

Coding Guidance
This chapter classifies diseases and disorders of the nervous system and the sense organs.

Inflammatory Diseases of the Central Nervous System (320–326)
Inflammatory diseases such as meningitis, encephalitis, cerebral abscesses, late effects of infections of the central nervous system and other types of inflammations such as meningitis due to sarcoidosis, and lead poisoning (toxic) encephalitis are grouped together in this subchapter. However, many infections of the central nervous system considered communicable or transmissable are excluded from this section and are classified to chapter 1, "Infectious and Parasitic Diseases."

Meningitis (320)
Bacterial meningitis is the inflammation of the covering of the meninges due to a bacterial organism. Bacterial meningitis can be caused by a variety of pyogenic bacterial organisms, most commonly Haemophilus influenzae (type B), Streptococcus pneumoniae, Pneumococcus, Neisseria meningitidis, Staphylococcus aureus, Klebsiella, Pseudomonas, and Escherichia coli.

Encephalitis, Myelitis, and Encephalomyelitis (323)
These are inflammations of the central nervous system that alter the function of various portions of the brain (encephalitis), spinal cord (myelitis), or both (encephalomyelitis). These diseases usually result from either a direct invasion of the central nervous system by a virus or postinfection involvement of the central nervous system after a viral disease. They also may be caused by bacteria, medications, toxic substances, and parasites. Encephalitis or myelitis infection resulting from direct invasion is most often caused by arthropod-borne viruses as seen in mosquito or tick bites classified to categories 062, 063, and 064.

Assign fourth and fifth digits to identify the causative organism. Since encephalitis classified to codes 323.0x, 323.1, 323.2, 323.4x, 323.6x, and 323.7x is a manifestation of another disease process, code the underlying disease first. If the organism is unspecified or the encephalitis has a noninfectious or toxic etiology, see codes 323.5, 323.8, and 323.9.

Late Effects of Intracranial Abscess or Pyogenic Infection (326)
This category is used to indicate late effects of meningitis, encephalitis, myelitis, encephalomyelitis, intracranial and intraspinal abscess, phlebitis or thrombophlebitis of the intracranial sinuses except when these conditions are manifestations of another disease process identified by italics in the ICD-9-CM tabular list. These late effects include conditions specified as such and may occur any time after the resolution of the causal condition. Use an additional code to identify the residual condition.

Hereditary and Degenerative Diseases of the Central Nervous System (330–337)
Alzheimer's disease (331.0) is a form of presenile dementia caused by the destruction of the subcortical white matter of the brain and characterized by increasing loss of intellectual functioning beginning with minor memory loss and eventually resulting in total loss of ability to function. Assign an additional code to identify any mental condition, such as presenile dementia (290.10), associated with the current condition.

Other Cerebral Degenerations (331)
Code category 331 classifies Alzheimer's disease (331.0), frontotemporal dementias (331.1x), acquired hydrocephalus, and senile and other degenerative cerebral disorders.

Normal pressure hydrocephalus (NPH) results from a disruption in the CSF circulation, leading to gradual enlargement of the ventricles and emergence of symptoms. This syndrome, when secondary to disease processes such as subarachnoid hemorrhage, traumatic brain injury, cerebral infarction, and meningitis, is referred to as secondary NPH, or communicating hydrocephalus. Secondary NPH is appropriately coded as communicating hydrocephalus, 331.3. Hydrocephalus in patients without known etiologies may be documented as idiopathic normal pressure hydrocephalus (INPH), which is reported with code 331.5. Congenital hydrocephalus associated with spina bifida (741.0) and congenital obstructive hydrocephalus (742.3) are classified to chapter 14, "Congenital Anomalies."

Parkinson's Disease (332)
Paralysis agitans (332.0) is an idiopathic neurological disease causing degeneration and dysfunction of the basal ganglia. This disease, also known as Parkinsonism or Parkinson's disease, is due to a toxic degeneration of the nigral neurons, a group of specialized cells in the midbrain that contain neuromelanin and manufacture the neurotransmitter substance dopamine. When 75 percent to 80 percent of the dopamine innervation is destroyed, signs and symptoms of Parkinsonism appear. When Parkinsonism is accompanied by dementia, assign code 331.82 Dementia with Lewy bodies, instead of code 332.0. Secondary Parkinsonism (332.1) is a neurologic disease with features similar to paralysis agitans affecting the central nervous system. Secondary Parkinsonism caused by a number of diseases or by the adverse affect of certain drugs and chemicals.

Huntington's Chorea (333.4)
This is a fatal hereditary disease affecting the basal ganglia and cerebral cortex. The onset varies but usually begins in the fourth decade of life. Death usually follows within 15 years of onset.

Disorders of the Autonomic Nervous System (337)
This category includes disorders of the peripheral autonomic, sympathetic, and parasympathetic nervous system.

Subcategory 337 includes fifth-digit subclassification codes for unspecified (337.00) and other (337.09) idiopathic peripheral neuropathies, and a specific code to report carotid sinus syndrome (337.01). Carotid sinus syndrome (CSS) (a.k.a., carotid sinus syncope, carotid sinus hypersensitivity) is an idiopathic peripheral autonomic neuropathy that exhibits as exaggerated vagal response stimulation due to pressure on the carotid sinus. CSS is characterized by recurrent dizziness, syncope or near syncope, unexplained falls, and symptoms associated with head turning or constriction of the neck. CSS contributes to increased incidence of falls, fracture, and other injury.

Peripheral autonomic neuropathy is a chronic and progressive disorder of the peripheral autonomic nerves most often associated with diabetes mellitus, usually insulin dependent or of long-standing duration. Other common etiologies include amyloidosis, botulism, porphyria, and multiple endocrine adenomas. Code the etiology of the peripheral autonomic neuropathy first, such as diabetes mellitus (250.6x) or amyloidosis (277.3), then code 337.1.

Pain (338)
Category 338 is assigned for pain that is specified as acute or chronic and cannot be classified elsewhere, except for post-thoracotomy pain, postoperative pain, neoplasm-related pain, or central pain syndrome. Category 338 codes may be used in conjunction with codes from other categories and chapters to provide detailed reporting of the acute or chronic pain. Headache syndromes (339.00–339.89), migraines (346.0–346.9), vulvodynia (625.70–625.79), and localized pain, which should be coded to pain by site. Use an additional code (307.89) to identify pain associated with psychological factors. A code from subcategories 338.1 and 338.2 should not be assigned if the underlying (definitive) diagnosis is known and the encounter is for management of the underlying condition. However, if the reason for the encounter is pain control or management, subcategory 338 codes may be sequenced as a first-listed or principal diagnosis. An encounter for a procedure aimed at treating an underlying condition (e.g., fracture) is reported with the code for the underlying condition assigned as the first-listed diagnosis. In these cases, do not report an additional code from category 338.

Routine or expected postoperative pain immediately after surgery should not be coded. However, postoperative pain not associated with a specific postoperative complication is assigned to the appropriate postoperative pain code in category 338. If the pain is associated with a specific postoperative complication of devices, implants or grafts, then assign the appropriate code from chapter 17. Use additional code(s) from category 338 to identify acute or chronic pain due to presence of the device, implant or graft (338.18–338.19 or 338.28–338.29).

Chronic pain is classified to subcategory 338.2. There is no time frame defining when pain becomes chronic pain. The provider's documentation should be used to guide use of these codes. Chronic pain syndrome is different from the term "chronic pain," and therefore this code should be used only when the provider has specifically documented this condition. Assign code 338.4 for chronic pain syndrome.

Code 338.3 is reported for pain that is documented as being related, associated with, or due to primary or secondary malignancy or tumor and is assigned regardless of whether the pain is acute or chronic. This code may be assigned as the principal or first-listed code when the stated reason for the admission/encounter is documented as pain control/pain management, and the underlying neoplasm should be reported as an additional diagnosis.

Other Disorders of the Central Nervous System (340–349)

Other Headache Syndromes (339)
Diagnostic differentiation between the various types of headache, such as cluster headache and migraine (346), can be difficult. To further complicate matters, patients may experience overlapping types of headache, such as a migraine and cluster headache combination. There are many clinical variations of headache pain with distinct characteristics and treatments. Treatment is reliant upon accurate diagnosis; therefore, differentiation between headache syndromes is essential.

Cluster headaches that have been formerly classified to 346.2 are now more appropriately classifiable to codes 339.00–339.02.When reporting 339.3 Drug induced headache, assign the appropriate E code to report the causal drug or medication. Category 339 specifically excludes migraine headache (346.0–346.9), headache NOS (784.0), and headache due to lumbar puncture (349.0). Also note the classification difference between tension headache (307.81) and tension **type** headache (339.10-339.12). Tension headache triggered by psychological factors is classified to pain disorders due to psychological factors (307.8). This is the default classification for tension headache NOS. Tension type headache is due to physiological factors rather than psychological.

Hemiplegia and Hemiparesis (342)
Hemiplegia and hemiparesis codes are used when hemiplegia (complete) (incomplete) is reported without further specification, or is stated to be old or long standing but of unspecified cause. The category is used also in multiple coding to identify these types of hemiplegia resulting from any cause. Hemiplegia and hemiparesis resulting from cerebrovascular disease is classified to subcategory 438.2x.

Epilepsy and Recurrent Seizures (345)
Epilepsy is a disorder characterized by recurrent transient disturbances of the cerebral function. An abnormal paroxysmal neuronal discharge in the brain usually results in convulsive seizures, but may result in loss of consciousness, abnormal behavior, sensory disturbances, or any combination. Epilepsy may be secondary to prior trauma, hemorrhage, intoxication (toxins), chemical imbalances, anoxia, infections, neoplasms, or congenital defects.

A series of seizures at intervals too brief to allow consciousness between attacks is known as status epilepticus and can result in death. Status epilepticus, not otherwise specified, is classified to code 345.3 Grand mal status. However, status epilepticus can occur in other specified forms of epilepsy.

Migraine (346)
Migraine is a vascular-type headache usually located in the temporal lobe and unilateral in nature. These headaches are commonly associated with irritability, nausea, vomiting, and often photophobia. Preceding the attacks, the cranial arteries constrict resulting in warning sensory symptoms. In addition to classic and common, migraine headache can take several other forms. The terms "classic" and "common" have been replaced by "with aura" and "without aura" in the titles of codes 346.0 and 346.1. Fifth-digit subclassifications describe migraines with or without associated complications. Status migrainosus describes a severe, debilitating migraine lasting more than 72 hours. This is a relatively rare, but life-threatening, migraine complication that could result in a potentially fatal ischemic stroke. Except for its prolonged duration, the headache characteristics are the same as for typical migraine. Intractable migraine describes frequently occurring, continuous, unremitting, or other migraine recalcitrant to conventional medical therapy that often requires acute care to resolve.

Disorders of the Peripheral Nervous System (350–359)
This subchapter classifies disorders of the peripheral nervous system based upon the specific nerve or nerve complex, involvement, or condition.

Categories 356–359 are hereditary and idiopathic peripheral neuropathies, inflammatory neuropathies, myoneural and myotonic disorders, and muscular dystrophies. Many of the conditions included in this subchapter are manifestations of other diseases and are used in addition to the code for the underlying condition. For example, polyneuropathy in diabetes, code 357.2, is used in addition to the code for the underlying condition, diabetes, 250.6x.

Acute infective polyneuritis (357.0) is a polyneuropathy due to an infective organism, most commonly herpes zoster. Guillain-Barre syndrome (357.0), usually preceded by a herpes infection, is the most common diagnosis classified here.

Disorders of the Eye and Adnexa (360–379)
Retinopathy of prematurity (ROP) is a progressive vasoproliferative disorder in premature infants and is a leading cause of blindness in children. ROP (formerly called retrolental fibroplasia) is caused by injury to the retina from O_2 therapy for the treatment of hypoxia associated with delayed lung maturation. Severe forms may progress to vision loss due to the retinal scarring and damage. Stage 5 is the end stage of the disease with a completely detached retina and severe vision loss. The term "retrolental fibroplasia" applies only to scarred retina (cicatrical disease) and has been differentiated from the more appropriate term "retinopathy of prematurity" (362.20–362.27) for this vasoproliferative condition. Retrolental fibroplasia is coded to 362. 21.

Plateau iris (364.82) is a common secondary angle-closure glaucoma characterized by closing of the anterior chamber angle due to a large or anteriorly positioned ciliary body that mechanically alters the position of the peripheral iris in relation to the trabecular meshwork. If the angle remains capable of closure after iridotomy, the condition is then termed plateau iris syndrome, a postoperative condition that increases the risk of glaucoma.

Glaucoma (365)
Glaucoma is a condition often characterized by increased intraocular pressure (IOP) that, when untreated, results in optic nerve damage with subsequent loss of vision. Glaucoma can be clinically differentiated as primary or secondary in nature and further divided into a constellation of subtypes, the most common of which are primary open angle glaucoma (POAG) and primary angle closure glaucoma:

- Primary open angle glaucoma (POAG) is characterized by high IOP, despite free flow of aqueous. This occurs due to a partially obstructed trabecular meshwork and impairs the drainage of the aqueous humor.
- Angle closure glaucoma (in acute presentation) is characterized by an abnormally narrow iris opening or displacement of the iris (bulging) that obstructs the drainage apparatus.

Although a certain degree of variance or overlap occurs among the constellation of glaucoma types, disease stage (when determinable) can be broadly classified from mild to severe with relative degrees of optic nerve impairment or damage. In general, during the *pre-glaucoma* and initial stages of disease, pathological alterations begin to take place in a previously normal aqueous outflow system. In *mild glaucoma*, the changes become more prominent and begin to cause a mild degree of obstruction, resulting in a mild decrease in aqueous outflow, with an elevation in IOP. In *moderate glaucoma* the increased IOP progresses in severity with a moderate loss of vision in one or both eyes yet with preservation of central vision. *Severe, advanced or end-stage glaucoma* refers to significant optic nerve damage with resultant loss of vision in both eyes or loss of sight in one eye. Do not confuse indeterminate stage (365.74) with unspecified stage (365.74). There are specific guidelines for reporting bilateral glaucoma, depending on whether the glaucoma type or stage is the same or different in each eye. Glaucoma that evolves from one stage to the next during an admission is coded to the highest stage documented.

Codes 365.05 and 365.06 provide a mechanism to report POAG and primary angle closure glaucoma at additional stages of severity. When reporting glaucoma, assign an additional code to identify the specific stage of glaucoma (365.7) as appropriate. Subcategory 365.7 includes sequencing instruction to code first the glaucoma, by type. Report code V19.11 Family history of glaucoma, when documented.

6. DISEASES OF THE NERVOUS SYSTEM AND SENSE ORGANS (320-389)

INFLAMMATORY DISEASES OF THE CENTRAL NERVOUS SYSTEM (320-326)

✓4ᵗʰ **320 Bacterial meningitis**

> INCLUDES   arachnoiditis
> leptomeningitis
> meningitis   } bacterial
> meningoencephalitis
> meningomyelitis
> pachymeningitis

> **DEF:** Bacterial infection causing inflammation of the lining of the brain and/or spinal cord.

320.0 Hemophilus meningitis
> Meningitis due to Hemophilus influenzae [H. influenzae]

320.1 Pneumococcal meningitis

320.2 Streptococcal meningitis

320.3 Staphylococcal meningitis

320.7 Meningitis in other bacterial diseases classified elsewhere

> Code first underlying disease, as:
> actinomycosis (039.8)
> listeriosis (027.0)
> typhoid fever (002.0)
> whooping cough (033.0-033.9)
> EXCLUDES   meningitis (in):
> epidemic (036.0)
> gonococcal (098.82)
> meningococcal (036.0)
> salmonellosis (003.21)
> syphilis:
> NOS (094.2)
> congenital (090.42)
> meningovascular (094.2)
> secondary (091.81)
> tuberculous (013.0)

✓5ᵗʰ **320.8 Meningitis due to other specified bacteria**

320.81 Anaerobic meningitis
> Bacteroides (fragilis)
> Gram-negative anaerobes

320.82 Meningitis due to gram-negative bacteria, not elsewhere classified
> Aerobacter aerogenes pneumoniae
> Escherichia coli [E. coli]
> Friedländer bacillus
> Klebsiella
> Proteus morganii
> Pseudomonas
> EXCLUDES   gram-negative anaerobes (320.81)

320.89 Meningitis due to other specified bacteria
> Bacillus pyocyaneus

320.9 Meningitis due to unspecified bacterium
> Meningitis: Meningitis:
> bacterial NOS   pyogenic NOS
> purulent NOS   suppurative NOS

✓4ᵗʰ **321 Meningitis due to other organisms**

> INCLUDES   arachnoiditis
> leptomeningitis   } due to organisms other
> meningitis   than bacterial
> pachymeningitis

> **DEF:** Infection causing inflammation of the lining of the brain and/or spinal cord, due to organisms other than bacteria.

321.0 Cryptococcal meningitis
> Code first underlying disease (117.5)

321.1 Meningitis in other fungal diseases
> Code first underlying disease (110.0-118)
> EXCLUDES   meningitis in:
> candidiasis (112.83)
> coccidioidomycosis (114.2)
> histoplasmosis (115.01, 115.11, 115.91)

321.2 Meningitis due to viruses not elsewhere classified
> Code first underlying disease, as:
> meningitis due to arbovirus (060.0-066.9)
> EXCLUDES   meningitis (due to):
> abacterial (047.0-047.9)
> adenovirus (049.1)
> aseptic NOS (047.9)
> Coxsackie (virus)(047.0)
> ECHO virus (047.1)
> enterovirus (047.0-047.9)
> herpes simplex virus (054.72)
> herpes zoster virus (053.0)
> lymphocytic choriomeningitis virus (049.0)
> mumps (072.1)
> viral NOS (047.9)
> meningo-eruptive syndrome (047.1)

321.3 Meningitis due to trypanosomiasis
> Code first underlying disease (086.0-086.9)

321.4 Meningitis in sarcoidosis
> Code first underlying disease (135)

321.8 Meningitis due to other nonbacterial organisms classified elsewhere
> Code first underlying disease
> EXCLUDES   leptospiral meningitis (100.81)

✓4ᵗʰ **322 Meningitis of unspecified cause**

> INCLUDES   arachnoiditis
> leptomeningitis   } with no organism
> meningitis   specified as cause
> pachymeningitis

> **DEF:** Infection causing inflammation of the lining of the brain and/or spinal cord, due to unspecified cause.

322.0 Nonpyogenic meningitis
> Meningitis with clear cerebrospinal fluid

322.1 Eosinophilic meningitis

322.2 Chronic meningitis

322.9 Meningitis, unspecified

✓4ᵗʰ **323 Encephalitis, myelitis, and encephalomyelitis**

> INCLUDES   acute disseminated encephalomyelitis
> meningoencephalitis, except bacterial
> meningomyelitis, except bacterial
> myelitis:
> ascending
> transverse
> EXCLUDES   acute transverse myelitis NOS (341.20)
> acute transverse myelitis in conditions classified
> elsewhere (341.21)
> bacterial:
> meningoencephalitis (320.0-320.9)
> meningomyelitis (320.0-320.9)
> idiopathic transverse myelitis (341.22)

> **DEF:** Encephalitis: inflammation of brain tissues.
> **DEF:** Myelitis: inflammation of the spinal cord.
> **DEF:** Encephalomyelitis: inflammation of brain and spinal cord.

Diseases of the Nervous System and Sense Organs

323.0–324.9

√5ᵗʰ **323.0 Encephalitis, myelitis, and encephalomyelitis in viral diseases classified elsewhere**

Code first underlying disease, as:
cat-scratch disease (078.3)
human immunodeficiency virus [HIV] disease (042)
infectious mononucleosis (075)
ornithosis (073.7)

323.01 Encephalitis and encephalomyelitis in viral diseases classified elsewhere

EXCLUDES encephalitis (in):
arthropod-borne viral (062.0-064)
herpes simplex (054.3)
mumps (072.2)
other viral diseases of central nervous system (049.8-049.9)
poliomyelitis (045.0-045.9)
rubella (056.01)
slow virus infections of central nervous system (046.0-046.9)
viral NOS (049.9)
West Nile (066.41)

323.02 Myelitis in viral diseases classified elsewhere

EXCLUDES myelitis (in):
herpes simplex (054.74)
herpes zoster (053.14)
poliomyelitis (045.0-045.9)
rubella (056.01)
other viral diseases of central nervous system (049.8-049.9)

323.1 Encephalitis, myelitis, and encephalomyelitis in rickettsial diseases classified elsewhere

Code first underlying disease (080-083.9)

DEF: Inflammation of the brain caused by rickettsial disease carried by louse, tick, or mite.

323.2 Encephalitis, myelitis, and encephalomyelitis in protozoal diseases classified elsewhere

Code first underlying disease, as:
malaria (084.0-084.9)
trypanosomiasis (086.0-086.9)

DEF: Inflammation of the brain caused by protozoal disease carried by mosquitoes and flies.

√5ᵗʰ **323.4 Other encephalitis, myelitis, and encephalomyelitis due to other infections classified elsewhere**

Code first underlying disease

323.41 Other encephalitis and encephalomyelitis due to other infections classified elsewhere

EXCLUDES encephalitis (in):
meningococcal (036.1)
syphilis:
NOS (094.81)
congenital (090.41)
toxoplasmosis (130.0)
tuberculosis (013.6)
meningoencephalitis due to free-living ameba [Naegleria] (136.29)

323.42 Other myelitis due to other infections classified elsewhere

EXCLUDES myelitis (in):
syphilis (094.89)
tuberculosis (013.6)

√5ᵗʰ **323.5 Encephalitis, myelitis, and encephalomyelitis following immunization procedures**

Use additional E code to identify vaccine

323.51 Encephalitis and encephalomyelitis following immunization procedures

Encephalitis postimmunization or postvaccinal
Encephalomyelitis postimmunization or postvaccinal

323.52 Myelitis following immunization procedures

Myelitis postimmunization or postvaccinal

√5ᵗʰ **323.6 Postinfectious encephalitis, myelitis, and encephalomyelitis**

Code first underlying disease

DEF: Infection, inflammation of brain several weeks following the outbreak of a systemic infection.

323.61 Infectious acute disseminated encephalomyelitis [ADEM]

Acute necrotizing hemorrhagic encephalopathy

EXCLUDES noninfectious acute disseminated encephalomyelitis (ADEM) (323.81)

323.62 Other postinfectious encephalitis and encephalomyelitis

EXCLUDES encephalitis:
postchickenpox (052.0)
postmeasles (055.0)

323.63 Postinfectious myelitis

EXCLUDES postchickenpox myelitis (052.2)
herpes simplex myelitis (054.74)
herpes zoster myelitis (053.14)

√5ᵗʰ **323.7 Toxic encephalitis, myelitis, and encephalomyelitis**

Code first underlying cause, as:
carbon tetrachloride (982.1)
hydroxyquinoline derivatives (961.3)
lead (984.0-984.9)
mercury (985.0)
thallium (985.8)

323.71 Toxic encephalitis and encephalomyelitis

323.72 Toxic myelitis

√5ᵗʰ **323.8 Other causes of encephalitis, myelitis, and encephalomyelitis**

323.81 Other causes of encephalitis and encephalomyelitis

Noninfectious acute disseminated encephalomyelitis (ADEM)

323.82 Other causes of myelitis

Transverse myelitis NOS

323.9 Unspecified cause of encephalitis, myelitis, and encephalomyelitis

√4ᵗʰ **324 Intracranial and intraspinal abscess**

324.0 Intracranial abscess

Abscess (embolic):
cerebellar
cerebral
Abscess (embolic) of brain [any part]:
epidural
extradural
otogenic
subdural

EXCLUDES tuberculous (013.3)

324.1 Intraspinal abscess

Abscess (embolic) of spinal cord [any part]:
epidural
extradural
subdural

EXCLUDES tuberculous (013.5)

324.9 Of unspecified site

Extradural or subdural abscess NOS

325 Phlebitis and thrombophlebitis of intracranial venous sinuses

Embolism
Endophlebitis
Phlebitis, septic or suppurative
Thrombophlebitis
Thrombosis
} of cavernous, lateral or other intracranial or unspecified intracranial venous sinus

> *EXCLUDES* *that specified as:*
> *complicating pregnancy, childbirth, or the puerperium (671.5)*
> *of nonpyogenic origin (437.6)*

DEF: Inflammation and formation of blood clot in a vein within the brain or its lining.

326 Late effects of intracranial abscess or pyogenic infection

Note: This category is to be used to indicate conditions whose primary classification is to 320-325 [excluding 320.7, 321.0-321.8, 323.01-323.42, 323.6-323.7] as the cause of late effects, themselves classifiable elsewhere. The "late effects" include conditions specified as such, or as sequelae, which may occur at any time after the resolution of the causal condition.

Use additional code to identify condition, as:
hydrocephalus (331.4)
paralysis (342.0-342.9, 344.0-344.9)

ORGANIC SLEEP DISORDERS (327)

✓4ᵗʰ 327 Organic sleep disorders

✓5ᵗʰ 327.0 Organic disorders of initiating and maintaining sleep [Organic insomnia]
> *EXCLUDES* *insomnia NOS (780.52)*
> *insomnia not due to a substance or known physiological condition (307.41-307.42)*
> *insomnia with sleep apnea NOS (780.51)*

327.00 Organic insomnia, unspecified

327.01 *Insomnia due to medical condition classified elsewhere*
> *Code first underlying condition*
> > *EXCLUDES* *insomnia due to mental disorder (327.02)*

327.02 *Insomnia due to mental disorder*
> *Code first mental disorder*
> > *EXCLUDES* *alcohol induced insomnia (291.82)*
> > *drug induced insomnia (292.85)*

327.09 Other organic insomnia

✓5ᵗʰ 327.1 Organic disorder of excessive somnolence [Organic hypersomnia]
> *EXCLUDES* *hypersomnia NOS (780.54)*
> *hypersomnia not due to a substance or known physiological condition (307.43-307.44)*
> *hypersomnia with sleep apnea NOS (780.53)*

327.10 Organic hypersomnia, unspecified

327.11 Idiopathic hypersomnia with long sleep time

327.12 Idiopathic hypersomnia without long sleep time

327.13 Recurrent hypersomnia
Kleine-Levin syndrome
Menstrual related hypersomnia

327.14 *Hypersomnia due to medical condition classified elsewhere*
> *Code first underlying condition*
> > *EXCLUDES* *hypersomnia due to mental disorder (327.15)*

327.15 *Hypersomnia due to mental disorder*
> *Code first mental disorder*
> > *EXCLUDES* *alcohol induced hypersomnia (291.82)*
> > *drug induced hypersomnia (292.85)*

327.19 Other organic hypersomnia

✓5ᵗʰ 327.2 Organic sleep apnea
> *EXCLUDES* *Cheyne-Stokes breathing (786.04)*
> *hypersomnia with sleep apnea NOS (780.53)*
> *insomnia with sleep apnea NOS (780.51)*
> *sleep apnea in newborn (770.81-770.82)*
> *sleep apnea NOS (780.57)*

327.20 Organic sleep apnea, unspecified

327.21 Primary central sleep apnea

327.22 High altitude periodic breathing

327.23 Obstructive sleep apnea (adult) (pediatric)

327.24 Idiopathic sleep related nonobstructive alveolar hypoventilation
Sleep related hypoxia

327.25 Congenital central alveolar hypoventilation syndrome

327.26 *Sleep related hypoventilation/ hypoxemia in conditions classifiable elsewhere*
> *Code first underlying condition*

327.27 *Central sleep apnea in conditions classified elsewhere*
> *Code first underlying condition*

327.29 Other organic sleep apnea

✓5ᵗʰ 327.3 Circadian rhythm sleep disorder
Organic disorder of sleep wake cycle
Organic disorder of sleep wake schedule
> *EXCLUDES* *alcohol induced circadian rhythm sleep disorder (291.82)*
> *circadian rhythm sleep disorder of nonorganic origin (307.45)*
> *disruption of 24 hour sleep wake cycle NOS (780.55)*
> *drug induced circadian rhythm sleep disorder (292.85)*

327.30 Circadian rhythm sleep disorder, unspecified

327.31 Circadian rhythm sleep disorder, delayed sleep phase type

327.32 Circadian rhythm sleep disorder, advanced sleep phase type

327.33 Circadian rhythm sleep disorder, irregular sleep-wake type

327.34 Circadian rhythm sleep disorder, free-running type

327.35 Circadian rhythm sleep disorder, jet lag type

327.36 Circadian rhythm sleep disorder, shift work type

327.37 *Circadian rhythm sleep disorder in conditions classified elsewhere*
> *Code first underlying condition*

327.39 Other circadian rhythm sleep disorder

✓5ᵗʰ 327.4 Organic parasomnia
> *EXCLUDES* *alcohol induced parasomnia (291.82)*
> *drug induced parasomnia (292.85)*
> *parasomnia not due to a known physiological condition (307.47)*

327.40 Organic parasomnia, unspecified

327.41 Confusional arousals

327.42 REM sleep behavior disorder

327.43 Recurrent isolated sleep paralysis

327.44 *Parasomnia in conditions classified elsewhere*
> *Code first underlying condition*

327.49 Other organic parasomnia

✓5ᵗʰ 327.5 Organic sleep related movement disorders
> *EXCLUDES* *restless legs syndrome (333.94)*
> *sleep related movement disorder NOS (780.58)*

327.51 Periodic limb movement disorder
Periodic limb movement sleep disorder

Diseases of the Nervous System and Sense Organs

327.52–331.81

327.52   Sleep related leg cramps

327.53   Sleep related bruxism

327.59   Other organic sleep related movement disorders

327.8   Other organic sleep disorders

HEREDITARY AND DEGENERATIVE DISEASES OF THE CENTRAL NERVOUS SYSTEM (330-337)

> **EXCLUDES**   *hepatolenticular degeneration (275.1)*
> *multiple sclerosis (340)*
> *other demyelinating diseases of central nervous system (341.0-341.9)*

√4ᵗʰ **330**   **Cerebral degenerations usually manifest in childhood**

Use additional code to identify associated intellectual disabilities

330.0   **Leukodystrophy**

Krabbe's disease

Leukodystrophy:
NOS
globoid cell
metachromatic
sudanophilic

Pelizaeus-Merzbacher disease

Sulfatide lipidosis

DEF: Hereditary disease of arylsulfatase or cerebroside sulfatase; characterized by a diffuse loss of myelin in CNS; infantile form causes blindness, motor disturbances, rigidity, mental deterioration and, occasionally, convulsions.

330.1   **Cerebral lipidoses**

Amaurotic (familial) idiocy

Disease:
Batten
Jansky-Bielschowsky
Kufs'
Spielmeyer-Vogt
Tay-Sachs

Gangliosidosis

DEF: Genetic disorder causing abnormal lipid accumulation in the reticuloendothelial cells of the brain.

330.2   *Cerebral degeneration in generalized lipidoses*

Code first underlying disease, as:
Fabry's disease (272.7)
Gaucher's disease (272.7)
Niemann-Pick disease (272.7)
sphingolipidosis (272.7)

330.3   *Cerebral degeneration of childhood in other diseases classified elsewhere*

Code first underlying disease, as:
Hunter's disease (277.5)
mucopolysaccharidosis (277.5)

330.8   **Other specified cerebral degenerations in childhood**

Alpers' disease or gray-matter degeneration
Infantile necrotizing encephalomyelopathy
Leigh's disease
Subacute necrotizing encephalopathy or encephalomyelopathy

330.9   **Unspecified cerebral degeneration in childhood**

√4ᵗʰ **331**   **Other cerebral degenerations**

Use additional code, where applicable, to identify dementia:
with behavioral disturbance (294.11)
without behavioral disturbance (294.10)

331.0   **Alzheimer's disease**

DEF: Diffuse atrophy of cerebral cortex; causing a progressive decline in intellectual and physical functions, including memory loss, personality changes and profound dementia.

√5ᵗʰ **331.1**   **Frontotemporal dementia**

DEF: Rare, progressive degenerative brain disease, similar to Alzheimer's; cortical atrophy affects the frontal and temporal lobes.

331.11   **Pick's disease**

DEF: A progressive frontotemporal dementia with asymmetrical atrophy of the frontal and temporal regions of the cerebral cortex, abnormal rounded brain cells called Pick cells with the presence of abnormal staining of protein (called tau); symptoms include prominent apathy, behavioral changes such as disinhibition and restlessness, echolalia, impairment of language, memory, and intellect, increased carelessness, poor personal hygiene, and decreased attention span.

331.19   **Other frontotemporal dementia**

Frontal dementia

331.2   **Senile degeneration of brain**

> **EXCLUDES**   *senility NOS (797)*

331.3   **Communicating hydrocephalus**

Secondary normal pressure hydrocephalus

> **EXCLUDES**   *congenital hydrocephalus (742.3)*
> *idiopathic normal pressure hydrocephalus (331.5)*
> *normal pressure hydrocephalus (331.5)*
> *spina bifida with hydrocephalus (741.0)*

DEF: Subarachnoid hemorrhage and meningitis causing excess buildup of cerebrospinal fluid in cavities due to nonabsorption of fluid back through fluid pathways.

331.4   **Obstructive hydrocephalus**

Acquired hydrocephalus NOS

> **EXCLUDES**   *congenital hydrocephalus (742.3)*
> *idiopathic normal pressure hydrocephalus (331.5)*
> *normal pressure hydrocephalus (331.5)*
> *spina bifida with hydrocephalus (741.0)*

DEF: Obstruction of cerebrospinal fluid passage from brain into spinal canal.

331.5   **Idiopathic normal pressure hydrocephalus [INPH]**

Normal pressure hydrocephalus NOS

> **EXCLUDES**   *congenital hydrocephalus (742.3)*
> *secondary normal pressure hydrocephalus (331.3)*
> *spina bifida with hydrocephalus (741.0)*

DEF: Abnormal increase of cerebrospinal fluid in the brain's ventricles; results in dementia, progressive mental impairment, gait disturbance, and impaired bladder control.

331.6   **Corticobasal degeneration**

331.7   *Cerebral degeneration in diseases classified elsewhere*

Code first underlying disease, as:
alcoholism (303.0-303.9)
beriberi (265.0)
cerebrovascular disease (430-438)
congenital hydrocephalus (741.0, 742.3)
myxedema (244.0-244.9)
neoplastic disease (140.0-239.9)
vitamin B12 deficiency (266.2)

> **EXCLUDES**   *cerebral degeneration in:*
> *Jakob-Creutzfeldt disease (046.11-046.19)*
> *progressive multifocal leukoencephalopathy (046.3)*
> *subacute spongiform encephalopathy (046.1)*

√5ᵗʰ **331.8**   **Other cerebral degeneration**

331.81   **Reye's syndrome**

DEF: Rare childhood illness, often developed after a viral upper respiratory infection; characterized by vomiting, elevated serum transaminase, changes in liver and other viscera; brain swelling, disturbances of consciousness and seizures; can be fatal.

331.82　Dementia with Lewy bodies
　　　　Dementia with Parkinsonism
　　　　Lewy body dementia
　　　　Lewy body disease
　　　　DEF: A cerebral dementia with neurophysiologic
　　　　changes, increased hippocampal volume,
　　　　hypoperfusion in the occipital lobes, and beta
　　　　amyloid deposits with neurofibrillary tangles,
　　　　atrophy of cortex and brainstem, hallmark
　　　　neuropsychologic characteristics are fluctuating
　　　　cognition with pronounced variation in attention
　　　　and alertness; recurrent hallucinations; and
　　　　parkinsonism.

331.83　Mild cognitive impairment, so stated
　　　　EXCLUDES　*altered mental status (780.97)*
　　　　　　　　cerebral degeneration (331.0-331.9)
　　　　　　　　change in mental status (780.97)
　　　　　　　　cognitive deficits following (late
　　　　　　　　　effects of) cerebral
　　　　　　　　　hemorrhage or infarction
　　　　　　　　　(438.0)
　　　　　　　　cognitive impairment due to
　　　　　　　　　intracranial or head injury
　　　　　　　　　(850-854, 959.01)
　　　　　　　　cognitive impairment due to late
　　　　　　　　　effect of intracranial injury
　　　　　　　　　(907.0)
　　　　　　　　cognitive impairment due to skull
　　　　　　　　　fracture (800-801, 803-804)
　　　　　　　　dementia (290.0-290.43,
　　　　　　　　　294.20-294.21)
　　　　　　　　mild memory disturbance (310.89)
　　　　　　　　neurologic neglect syndrome
　　　　　　　　　(781.8)
　　　　　　　　personality change, nonpsychotic
　　　　　　　　　(310.1)

331.89　Other
　　　　Cerebral ataxia

331.9　Cerebral degeneration, unspecified

√4ᵗʰ **332　Parkinson's disease**
　　　　EXCLUDES　*dementia with Parkinsonism (331.82)*

332.0　Paralysis agitans
　　　　Parkinsonism or Parkinson's disease:
　　　　　NOS
　　　　　idiopathic
　　　　　primary
　　　　DEF: Form of progressive parkinsonism characterized by
　　　　mask-like facial expressions, inability to stand or walk
　　　　smoothly, muscle weakness, and involuntary trembling
　　　　movement.

332.1　Secondary Parkinsonism
　　　　Neuroleptic-induced Parkinsonism
　　　　Parkinsonism due to drugs
　　　　Use additional E code to identify drug, if drug-induced
　　　　EXCLUDES　*Parkinsonism (in):*
　　　　　　　　Huntington's disease (333.4)
　　　　　　　　progressive supranuclear palsy (333.0)
　　　　　　　　Shy-Drager syndrome (333.0)
　　　　　　　　syphilitic (094.82)

√4ᵗʰ **333　Other extrapyramidal disease and abnormal movement
　　　disorders**
　　　　INCLUDES　other forms of extrapyramidal, basal ganglia, or
　　　　　　　　striatopallidal disease
　　　　EXCLUDES　*abnormal movements of head NOS (781.0)*
　　　　　　　　sleep related movement disorders (327.51-327.59)

333.0　Other degenerative diseases of the basal ganglia
　　　　Atrophy or degeneration:
　　　　　olivopontocerebellar [Déjérine-Thomas syndrome]
　　　　　pigmentary pallidal [Hallervorden-Spatz disease]
　　　　　striatonigral
　　　　Parkinsonian syndrome associated with:
　　　　　idiopathic orthostatic hypotension
　　　　　symptomatic orthostatic hypotension
　　　　Progressive supranuclear ophthalmoplegia
　　　　Shy-Drager syndrome

333.1　Essential and other specified forms of tremor
　　　　Benign essential tremor
　　　　Familial tremor
　　　　Medication-induced postural tremor
　　　　Use additional E code to identify drug, if drug-induced
　　　　EXCLUDES　*tremor NOS (781.0)*

333.2　Myoclonus
　　　　Familial essential myoclonus
　　　　Palatal myoclonus
　　　　EXCLUDES　*progressive myoclonic epilepsy (345.1)*
　　　　　　　　Unverricht-Lundborg disease (345.1)
　　　　Use additional E code to identify drug, if drug-induced
　　　　DEF: Spontaneous movements or contractions of muscles.

333.3　Tics of organic origin
　　　　Use additional E code to identify drug, if drug-induced
　　　　EXCLUDES　*Gilles de la Tourette's syndrome (307.23)*
　　　　　　　　habit spasm (307.22)
　　　　　　　　tic NOS (307.20)

333.4　Huntington's chorea
　　　　DEF: Genetic disease characterized by chronic progressive
　　　　mental deterioration; dementia and death within 15 years
　　　　of onset.

333.5　Other choreas
　　　　Hemiballism(us)
　　　　Paroxysmal choreo-athetosis
　　　　Use additional E code to identify drug, if drug-induced
　　　　EXCLUDES　*Sydenham's or rheumatic chorea*
　　　　　　　　(392.0-392.9)

333.6　Genetic torsion dystonia
　　　　Dystonia:
　　　　　deformans progressiva
　　　　　musculorum deformans
　　　　(Schwalbe-) Ziehen-Oppenheim disease
　　　　DEF: Sustained muscular contractions, causing twisting
　　　　and repetitive movements that result in abnormal
　　　　postures of trunk and limbs; etiology unknown.

√5ᵗʰ **333.7　Acquired torsion dystonia**

333.71　Athetoid cerebral palsy
　　　　Double athetosis (syndrome)
　　　　Vogt's disease
　　　　EXCLUDES　*infantile cerebral palsy*
　　　　　　　　(343.0-343.9)

333.72　Acute dystonia due to drugs
　　　　Acute dystonic reaction due to drugs
　　　　Neuroleptic induced acute dystonia
　　　　Use additional E code to identify drug
　　　　EXCLUDES　*blepharospasm due to drugs*
　　　　　　　　(333.85)
　　　　　　　　orofacial dyskinesia due to drugs
　　　　　　　　(333.85)
　　　　　　　　secondary Parkinsonism (332.1)
　　　　　　　　subacute dyskinesia due to drugs
　　　　　　　　(333.85)
　　　　　　　　tardive dyskinesia (333.85)

333.79　Other acquired torsion dystonia

√5ᵗʰ **333.8　Fragments of torsion dystonia**
　　　　Use additional E code to identify drug, if drug-induced

333.81　Blepharospasm
　　　　EXCLUDES　*blepharospasm due to drugs*
　　　　　　　　(333.85)
　　　　　　　　DEF: Uncontrolled winking or blinking due to
　　　　　　　　orbicularis oculi muscle spasm.

333.82　Orofacial dyskinesia
　　　　EXCLUDES　*orofacial dyskinesia due to drugs*
　　　　　　　　(333.85)
　　　　　　　　DEF: Uncontrolled movement of mouth or facial
　　　　　　　　muscles.

333.83 Spasmodic torticollis
> EXCLUDES torticollis:
> NOS (723.5)
> hysterical (300.11)
> psychogenic (306.0)

DEF: Uncontrolled movement of head due to spasms of neck muscle.

333.84 Organic writers' cramp
> EXCLUDES pychogenic (300.89)

333.85 Subacute dyskinesia due to drugs
Blepharospasm due to drugs
Orofacial dyskinesia due to drugs
Tardive dyskinesia
Use additional E code to identify drug
> EXCLUDES acute dystonia due to drugs
> (333.72)
> acute dystonic reaction due to drugs
> (333.72)
> secondary Parkinsonism (332.1)

333.89 Other

√5ᵗʰ **333.9 Other and unspecified extrapyramidal diseases and abnormal movement disorders**

333.90 Unspecified extrapyramidal disease and abnormal movement disorder
Medication-induced movement disorders NOS
Use additional E code to identify drug, if drug-induced

333.91 Stiff-man syndrome

333.92 Neuroleptic malignant syndrome
Use additional E code to identify drug
> EXCLUDES neuroleptic induced Parkinsonism
> (332.1)

333.93 Benign shuddering attacks

333.94 Restless legs syndrome [RLS]
DEF: Neurological disorder of unknown etiology with an irresistible urge to move the legs, which may temporarily relieve the symptoms, is accompanied by motor restlessness and sensations of pain, burning, prickling, or tingling.

333.99 Other
Neuroleptic-induced acute akathisia
Use additional E code to identify drug, if drug-induced

√4ᵗʰ **334 Spinocerebellar disease**
> EXCLUDES olivopontocerebellar degeneration (333.0)
> peroneal muscular atrophy (356.1)

334.0 Friedreich's ataxia
DEF: Genetic recessive disease of children; sclerosis of dorsal, lateral spinal cord columns; characterized by ataxia, speech impairment, swaying and irregular movements, with muscle paralysis, especially of lower limbs.

334.1 Hereditary spastic paraplegia

334.2 Primary cerebellar degeneration
Cerebellar ataxia:
Marie's
Sanger-Brown
Dyssynergia cerebellaris myoclonica
Primary cerebellar degeneration:
NOS
hereditary
sporadic

334.3 Other cerebellar ataxia
Cerebellar ataxia NOS
Use additional E code to identify drug, if drug-induced

334.4 *Cerebellar ataxia in diseases classified elsewhere*
Code first underlying disease, as:
alcoholism (303.0-303.9)
myxedema (244.0-244.9)
neoplastic disease (140.0-239.9)

334.8 Other spinocerebellar diseases
Ataxia-telangiectasia [Louis-Bar syndrome]
Corticostriatal-spinal degeneration

334.9 Spinocerebellar disease, unspecified

√4ᵗʰ **335 Anterior horn cell disease**

335.0 Werdnig-Hoffmann disease
Infantile spinal muscular atrophy
Progressive muscular atrophy of infancy
DEF: Spinal muscle atrophy manifested in prenatal period or shortly after birth; symptoms include hypotonia, atrophy of skeletal muscle; death occurs in infancy.

√5ᵗʰ **335.1 Spinal muscular atrophy**

335.10 Spinal muscular atrophy, unspecified

335.11 Kugelberg-Welander disease
Spinal muscular atrophy:
familial
juvenile
DEF: Hereditary; juvenile muscle atrophy; appears during first two decades of life; due to lesions of anterior horns of spinal cord; includes wasting, diminution of lower body muscles and twitching.

335.19 Other
Adult spinal muscular atrophy

√5ᵗʰ **335.2 Motor neuron disease**

335.20 Amyotrophic lateral sclerosis
Motor neuron disease (bulbar) (mixed type)

335.21 Progressive muscular atrophy
Duchenne-Aran muscular atrophy
Progressive muscular atrophy (pure)

335.22 Progressive bulbar palsy

335.23 Pseudobulbar palsy

335.24 Primary lateral sclerosis

335.29 Other

335.8 Other anterior horn cell diseases

335.9 Anterior horn cell disease, unspecified

√4ᵗʰ **336 Other diseases of spinal cord**

336.0 Syringomyelia and syringobulbia

336.1 Vascular myelopathies
Acute infarction of spinal cord (embolic) (nonembolic)
Arterial thrombosis of spinal cord
Edema of spinal cord
Hematomyelia
Subacute necrotic myelopathy

336.2 *Subacute combined degeneration of spinal cord in diseases classified elsewhere*
Code first underlying disease, as:
pernicious anemia (281.0)
other vitamin B₁₂ deficiency anemia (281.1)
vitamin B₁₂ deficiency (266.2)

336.3 *Myelopathy in other diseases classified elsewhere*
Code first underlying disease, as:
myelopathy in neoplastic disease (140.0-239.9)
> EXCLUDES myelopathy in:
> intervertebral disc disorder
> (722.70-722.73)
> spondylosis (721.1, 721.41-721.42, 721.91)

336.8 Other myelopathy
Myelopathy:
drug-induced
radiation-induced
Use additonal E code to identify cause

336.9 Unspecified disease of spinal cord
Cord compression NOS   Myelopathy NOS
> EXCLUDES myelitis (323.02, 323.1, 323.2, 323.42, 323.52,
> 323.63, 323.72, 323.82, 323.9)
> spinal (canal) stenosis (723.0, 724.00-724.09)

√4ᵗʰ **337　Disorders of the autonomic nervous system**
　　INCLUDES　disorders of peripheral autonomic, sympathetic, parasympathetic, or vegetative system
　　EXCLUDES　familial dysautonomia [Riley-Day syndrome] (742.8)

√5ᵗʰ **337.0　Idiopathic peripheral autonomic neuropathy**

　　337.00　Idiopathic peripheral autonomic neuropathy, unspecified

　　337.01　Carotid sinus syndrome
　　　　Carotid sinus syncope
　　　　DEF: Vagal activation caused by pressure on the carotid sinus baroreceptors; sympathetic nerve impulses may cause sinus arrest or AV block.

　　337.09　Other idiopathic peripheral autonomic neuropathy
　　　　Cervical sympathetic dystrophy or paralysis

337.1　Peripheral autonomic neuropathy in disorders classified elsewhere
　　　　Code first underlying disease, as:
　　　　　amyloidosis (277.30-277.39)
　　　　　diabetes (249.6, 250.6)

√5ᵗʰ **337.2　Reflex sympathetic dystrophy**
　　　　DEF: Disturbance of the sympathetic nervous system evidenced by sweating, pain, pallor and edema following injury to nerves or blood vessels.

　　337.20　Reflex sympathetic dystrophy, unspecified
　　　　Complex regional pain syndrome type I, unspecified

　　337.21　Reflex sympathetic dystrophy of the upper limb
　　　　Complex regional pain syndrome type I of the upper limb

　　337.22　Reflex sympathetic dystrophy of the lower limb
　　　　Complex regional pain syndrome type I of the lower limb

　　337.29　Reflex sympathetic dystrophy of other specified site
　　　　Complex regional pain syndrome type I of other specified site

337.3　Autonomic dysreflexia
　　　　Use additional code to identify the cause, such as:
　　　　　pressure ulcer (707.00-707.09)
　　　　　fecal impaction (560.32)
　　　　　urinary tract infection (599.0)
　　　　DEF: Noxious stimuli evokes paroxysmal hypertension, bradycardia, excess sweating, headache, pilomotor responses, facial flushing, and nasal congestion due to uncontrolled parasympathetic nerve response; occurs in patients with spinal cord injury above sympathetic outflow tract (T6).

337.9　Unspecified disorder of autonomic nervous system

PAIN (338)

√4ᵗʰ **338　Pain, not elsewhere classified**
　　　　Use additional code to identify:
　　　　　pain associated with psychological factors (307.89)
　　　　EXCLUDES　generalized pain (780.96)
　　　　　headache syndromes (339.00-339.89)
　　　　　localized pain, unspecified type–code to pain by site
　　　　　migraines (346.0-346.9)
　　　　　pain disorder exclusively attributed to psychological factors (307.80)
　　　　　vulvar vestibulitis (625.71)
　　　　　vulvodynia (625.70-625.79)

338.0　Central pain syndrome
　　　　Déjérine-Roussy syndrome
　　　　Myelopathic pain syndrome
　　　　Thalamic pain syndrome (hyperesthetic)

√5ᵗʰ **338.1　Acute pain**

　　338.11　Acute pain due to trauma

　　338.12　Acute post-thoracotomy pain
　　　　Post-thoracotomy pain NOS

　　338.18　Other acute postoperative pain
　　　　Postoperative pain NOS

　　338.19　Other acute pain
　　　　EXCLUDES　neoplasm related acute pain (338.3)

√5ᵗʰ **338.2　Chronic pain**
　　　　EXCLUDES　causalgia (355.9)
　　　　　lower limb (355.71)
　　　　　upper limb (354.4)
　　　　chronic pain syndrome (338.4)
　　　　myofascial pain syndrome (729.1)
　　　　neoplasm related chronic pain (338.3)
　　　　reflex sympathetic dystrophy (337.20-337.29)

　　338.21　Chronic pain due to trauma

　　338.22　Chronic post-thoracotomy pain

　　338.28　Other chronic postoperative pain

　　338.29　Other chronic pain

338.3　Neoplasm related pain (acute) (chronic)
　　　　Cancer associated pain
　　　　Pain due to malignancy (primary) (secondary)
　　　　Tumor associated pain

338.4　Chronic pain syndrome
　　　　Chronic pain associated with significant psychosocial dysfunction

OTHER HEADACHE SYNDROMES (339)

√4ᵗʰ **339　Other headache syndromes**
　　　　EXCLUDES　headache:
　　　　　NOS (784.0)
　　　　　due to lumbar puncture (349.0)
　　　　　migraine (346.0-346.9)

√5ᵗʰ **339.0　Cluster headaches and other trigeminal autonomic cephalgias**
　　　　TACS

　　339.00　Cluster headache syndrome, unspecified
　　　　Ciliary neuralgia　　　　Lower half migraine
　　　　Cluster headache NOS　　Migrainous neuralgia
　　　　Histamine cephalgia

　　339.01　Episodic cluster headache

　　339.02　Chronic cluster headache

　　339.03　Episodic paroxysmal hemicrania
　　　　Paroxysmal hemicrania NOS

　　339.04　Chronic paroxysmal hemicrania

　　339.05　Short lasting unilateral neuralgiform headache with conjunctival injection and tearing
　　　　SUNCT

　　339.09　Other trigeminal autonomic cephalgias

√5ᵗʰ **339.1　Tension type headache**
　　　　EXCLUDES　tension headache NOS (307.81)
　　　　　tension headache related to psychological factors (307.81)

　　339.10　Tension type headache, unspecified

　　339.11　Episodic tension type headache

　　339.12　Chronic tension type headache

√5ᵗʰ **339.2　Post-traumatic headache**

　　339.20　Post-traumatic headache, unspecified

　　339.21　Acute post-traumatic headache

　　339.22　Chronic post-traumatic headache

339.3　Drug induced headache, not elsewhere classified
　　　　Medication overuse headache　Rebound headache

√5ᵗʰ **339.4　Complicated headache syndromes**

　　339.41　Hemicrania continua

　　339.42　New daily persistent headache
　　　　NDPH

　　339.43　Primary thunderclap headache

　　339.44　Other complicated headache syndrome

✓5th **339.8 Other specified headache syndromes**

339.81 Hypnic headache

339.82 Headache associated with sexual activity
Orgasmic headache
Preorgasmic headache

339.83 Primary cough headache

339.84 Primary exertional headache

339.85 Primary stabbing headache

339.89 Other specified headache syndromes

OTHER DISORDERS OF THE CENTRAL NERVOUS SYSTEM
(340-349)

340 Multiple sclerosis
Disseminated or multiple sclerosis:
NOS
brain stem
cord
generalized

✓4th **341 Other demyelinating diseases of central nervous system**

341.0 Neuromyelitis optica

341.1 Schilder's disease
Baló's concentric sclerosis
Encephalitis periaxialis:
concentrica [Baló's]
diffusa [Schilder's]

DEF: Chronic leukoencephalopathy of children and adolescents; symptoms include blindness, deafness, bilateral spasticity and progressive mental deterioration.

✓5th **341.2 Acute (transverse) myelitis**

*EXCLUDES acute (transverse) myelitis (in) (due to):
following immunization procedures (323.52)
infection classified elsewhere (323.42)
postinfectious (323.63)
protozoal diseases classified elsewhere (323.2)
rickettsial diseases classified elsewhere (323.1)
toxic (323.72)
viral diseases classified elsewhere (323.02)
transverse myelitis NOS (323.82)*

341.20 Acute (transverse) myelitis NOS

341.21 Acute (transverse) myelitis in conditions classified elsewhere
Code first underlying condition

341.22 Idiopathic transverse myelitis

341.8 Other demyelinating diseases of central nervous system
Central demyelination of corpus callosum
Central pontine myelinosis
Marchiafava (-Bignami) disease

341.9 Demyelinating disease of central nervous system, unspecified

✓4th **342 Hemiplegia and hemiparesis**
Note: This category is to be used when hemiplegia (complete) (incomplete) is reported without further specification, or is stated to be old or long-standing but of unspecified cause. The category is also for use in multiple coding to identify these types of hemiplegia resulting from any cause.

*EXCLUDES congenital (343.1)
hemiplegia due to late effect of cerebrovascular accident (438.20-438.22)
infantile NOS (343.4)*

The following fifth digits are for use with codes 342.0-342.9:
0 affecting unspecified side
1 affecting dominant side
2 affecting nondominant side

✓5th **342.0 Flaccid hemiplegia**
[0-2]

✓5th **342.1 Spastic hemiplegia**
[0-2]

✓5th **342.8 Other specified hemiplegia**
[0-2]

✓5th **342.9 Hemiplegia, unspecified**
[0-2]

✓4th **343 Infantile cerebral palsy**
INCLUDES cerebral:
palsy NOS
spastic infantile paralysis
congenital spastic paralysis (cerebral)
Little's disease
paralysis (spastic) due to birth injury:
intracranial
spinal

*EXCLUDES athetoid cerebral palsy (333.71)
hereditary cerebral paralysis, such as:
hereditary spastic paraplegia (334.1)
Vogt's disease (333.71)
spastic paralysis specified as noncongenital or noninfantile (344.0-344.9)*

343.0 Diplegic
Congenital diplegia   Congenital paraplegia
DEF: Paralysis affecting both sides of the body simultaneously.

343.1 Hemiplegic
Congenital hemiplegia
EXCLUDES infantile hemiplegia NOS (343.4)

343.2 Quadriplegic
Tetraplegic

343.3 Monoplegic

343.4 Infantile hemiplegia
Infantile hemiplegia (postnatal) NOS

343.8 Other specified infantile cerebral palsy

343.9 Infantile cerebral palsy, unspecified
Cerebral palsy NOS

✓4th **344 Other paralytic syndromes**
Note: This category is to be used when the listed conditions are reported without further specification or are stated to be old or long-standing but of unspecified cause. The category is also for use in multiple coding to identify these conditions resulting from any cause.

INCLUDES paralysis (complete) (incomplete), except as classifiable to 342 and 343
*EXCLUDES congenital or infantile cerebral palsy (343.0-343.9)
hemiplegia (342.0-342.9)
congenital or infantile (343.1, 343.4)*

✓5th **344.0 Quadriplegia and quadriparesis**

344.00 Quadriplegia unspecified

344.01 C_1-C_4 complete

344.02 C_1-C_4 incomplete

344.03 C_5-C_7 complete

344.04 C_5-C_7 incomplete

344.09 Other

344.1 Paraplegia
Paralysis of both lower limbs
Paraplegia (lower)

344.2 Diplegia of upper limbs
Diplegia (upper)
Paralysis of both upper limbs

✓5th **344.3 Monoplegia of lower limb**
Paralysis of lower limb
EXCLUDES monoplegia of lower limb due to late effect of cerebrovascular accident (438.40-438.42)

344.30 Affecting unspecified side

344.31 Affecting dominant side

344.32 Affecting nondominant side

√5ᵗʰ **344.4 Monoplegia of upper limb**
Paralysis of upper limb
EXCLUDES *monoplegia of upper limb due to late effect of cerebrovascular accident (438.30-438.32)*

344.40 Affecting unspecified side

344.41 Affecting dominant side

344.42 Affecting nondominant side

344.5 Unspecified monoplegia

√5ᵗʰ **344.6 Cauda equina syndrome**
DEF: Dull pain and paresthesias in sacrum, perineum and bladder due to compression of spinal nerve roots; pain radiates down buttocks, back of thigh, calf of leg and into foot with prickling, burning sensations.

344.60 Without mention of neurogenic bladder

344.61 With neurogenic bladder
Acontractile bladder
Autonomic hyperreflexia of bladder
Cord bladder
Detrusor hyperreflexia

√5ᵗʰ **344.8 Other specified paralytic syndromes**

344.81 Locked-in state
DEF: State of consciousness where patients are paralyzed and unable to respond to environmental stimuli; patients have eye movements, and stimuli can enter the brain but patients unable to respond.

344.89 Other specified paralytic syndrome

344.9 Paralysis, unspecified

√4ᵗʰ **345 Epilepsy and recurrent seizures**
The following fifth-digit subclassification is for use with categories 345.0, .1, .4-.9:
0 without mention of intractable eilepsy
1 with intractable epilepsy
pharmacoresistant (pharmacologically resistant)
poorly controlled
refractory (medically)
treatment resistant

EXCLUDES *hippocampal sclerosis (348.81)*
mesial temporal sclerosis (348.81)
temporal sclerosis (348.81)

DEF: Brain disorder characterized by electrical-like disturbances; may include occasional impairment or loss of consciousness, abnormal motor phenomena and psychic or sensory disturbances.

√5ᵗʰ **345.0 Generalized nonconvulsive epilepsy**
[0-1] Absences: Pykno-epilepsy
         atonic   Seizures:
         typical   akinetic
       Minor epilepsy   atonic
       Petit mal

√5ᵗʰ **345.1 Generalized convulsive epilepsy**
[0-1] Epileptic seizures:
         clonic
         myoclonic
         tonic
         tonic-clonic
       Grand mal
       Major epilepsy
       Progressive myoclonic epilepsy
       Unverricht-Lundborg disease
       EXCLUDES *convulsions:*
                   NOS (780.39)
                   infantile (780.39)
                   newborn (779.0)
               infantile spasms (345.6)

DEF: Convulsive seizures with tension of limbs (tonic) or rhythmic contractions (clonic).

345.2 Petit mal status
Epileptic absence status
DEF: Minor myoclonic spasms and sudden momentary loss of consciousness in epilepsy.

345.3 Grand mal status
Status epilepticus NOS
EXCLUDES *epilepsia partialis continua (345.7)*
status:
    psychomotor (345.7)
    temporal lobe (345.7)
DEF: Sudden loss of consciousness followed by generalized convulsions in epilepsy.

√5ᵗʰ **345.4 Localization-related (focal) (partial) epilepsy**
[0-1] **and epileptic syndromes with complex partial seizures**
Epilepsy:
  limbic system
  partial:
    secondarily generalized
    with impairment of consciousness
    with memory and ideational disturbances
  psychomotor
  psychosensory
  temporal lobe
Epileptic automatism

√5ᵗʰ **345.5 Localization-related (focal) (partial) epilepsy**
[0-1] **and epileptic syndromes with simple partial seizures**
Epilepsy:
  Bravais-Jacksonian NOS
  focal (motor) NOS
  Jacksonian NOS
  motor partial
  partial NOS:
    without impairment of consciousness
  sensory-induced
  somatomotor
  somatosensory
  visceral
  visual

√5ᵗʰ **345.6 Infantile spasms**
[0-1] Hypsarrhythmia   Salaam attacks
       Lightning spasms
       EXCLUDES *salaam tic (781.0)*

√5ᵗʰ **345.7 Epilepsia partialis continua**
[0-1] Kojevnikov's epilepsy
       DEF: Continuous muscle contractions and relaxation; result of abnormal neural discharge.

√5ᵗʰ **345.8 Other forms of epilepsy and recurrent seizures**
[0-1] Epilepsy: Epilepsy:
       cursive [running]   gelastic

√5ᵗʰ **345.9 Epilepsy, unspecified**
[0-1] Epileptic convulsions, fits, or seizures NOS
       Seizure disorder NOS
       EXCLUDES *convulsion (convulsive) disorder (780.39)*
                   convulsive seizure or fit NOS (780.39)
                   recurrent convulsions (780.39)

Diseases of the Nervous System and Sense Organs

344.4–345.9

Diseases of the Nervous System and Sense Organs

346–348.9

√4ᵗʰ **346 Migraine**

> **EXCLUDES** headache:
> NOS (784.0)
> syndromes (339.00-339.89)

> The following fifth-digit subclassification is for use with category 346:
>> **0 without mention of intractable migraine without mention of status migrainosus**
>>> without mention of refractory migraine without mention of status migrainosus
>> **1 with intractable migraine, so stated, without mention of status migrainosus**
>>> with refractory migraine, so stated, without mention of status migrainosus
>> **2 without mention of intractable migraine with status migrainosus**
>>> without mention of refractory migraine with status migrainosus
>> **3 with intractable migraine, so stated, with status migrainosus**
>>> with refractory migraine, so stated, with status migrainosus

DEF: Benign vascular headache of extreme pain; commonly associated with irritability, nausea, vomiting and often photophobia; premonitory visual hallucination of a crescent in the visual field (scotoma).

√5ᵗʰ **346.0 Migraine with aura**
[0-3]
Basilar migraine
Classic migraine
Migraine preceded or accompanied by transient focal neurological phenomena
Migraine triggered seizures
Migraine with acute-onset aura
Migraine with aura without headache (migraine equivalents)
Migraine with prolonged aura
Migraine with typical aura
Retinal migraine

> **EXCLUDES** persistent migraine aura (346.5, 346.6)

√5ᵗʰ **346.1 Migraine without aura**
[0-3]
Common migraine

√5ᵗʰ **346.2 Variants of migraine, not elsewhere classified**
[0-3]
Abdominal migraine
Cyclical vomiting associated with migraine
Ophthalmoplegic migraine
Periodic headache syndromes in child or adolescent

> **EXCLUDES** cyclical vomiting NOS (536.2)
> psychogenic cyclical vomiting (306.4)

√5ᵗʰ **346.3 Hemiplegic migraine**
[0-3]
Familial migraine   Sporadic migraine

√5ᵗʰ **346.4 Menstrual migraine**
[0-3]
Menstrual headache
Menstrually related migraine
Premenstrual headache
Premenstrual migraine
Pure menstrual migraine

√5ᵗʰ **346.5 Persistent migraine aura without cerebral infarction**
[0-3]
Persistent migraine aura NOS

√5ᵗʰ **346.6 Persistent migraine aura with cerebral infarction**
[0-3]

√5ᵗʰ **346.7 Chronic migraine without aura**
[0-3]
Transformed migraine without aura

√5ᵗʰ **346.8 Other forms of migraine**
[0-3]

√5ᵗʰ **346.9 Migraine, unspecified**
[0-3]

√4ᵗʰ **347 Cataplexy and narcolepsy**

DEF: Cataplexy: Sudden onset of muscle weakness with loss of tone and strength; caused by aggressive or spontaneous emotions.
DEF: Narcolepsy: Brief, recurrent, uncontrollable episodes of sound sleep.

√5ᵗʰ **347.0 Narcolepsy**

347.00 Without cataplexy
Narcolepsy NOS

347.01 With cataplexy

√5ᵗʰ **347.1 Narcolepsy in conditions classified elsewhere**
Code first underlying condition

347.10 Without cataplexy

347.11 With cataplexy

√4ᵗʰ **348 Other conditions of brain**

348.0 Cerebral cysts
Arachnoid cyst   Porencephaly, acquired
Porencephalic cyst   Pseudoporencephaly
> **EXCLUDES** porencephaly (congenital) (742.4)

348.1 Anoxic brain damage
Use additional E code to identify cause
> **EXCLUDES** that occurring in:
> abortion (634-638 with .7, 639.8)
> ectopic or molar pregnancy (639.8)
> labor or delivery (668.2, 669.4)
> that of newborn (767.0, 768.0-768.9, 772.1-772.2)

DEF: Brain injury due to lack of oxygen, other than birth trauma.

348.2 Benign intracranial hypertension
Pseudotumor cerebri
> **EXCLUDES** hypertensive encephalopathy (437.2)

DEF: Elevated pressure in brain due to fluid retention in brain cavities.

√5ᵗʰ **348.3 Encephalopathy, not elsewhere classified**

348.30 Encephalopathy, unspecified

348.31 Metabolic encephalopathy
Septic encephalopathy
> **EXCLUDES** toxic metabolic encephalopathy (349.82)

348.39 Other encephalopathy
> **EXCLUDES** encephalopathy:
> alcoholic (291.2)
> hepatic (572.2)
> hypertensive (437.2)
> toxic (349.82)

348.4 Compression of brain
Compression ⎫
Herniation ⎬ brain (stem)

Posterior fossa compression syndrome
DEF: Elevated pressure in brain due to blood clot, tumor, fracture, abscess, other condition.

348.5 Cerebral edema
DEF: Elevated pressure in the brain due to fluid retention in brain tissues.

√5ᵗʰ **348.8 Other conditions of brain**

348.81 Temporal sclerosis
Hippocampal sclerosis
Mesial temporal sclerosis
DEF: Abnormal hardening or scarring of frontal lobe tissues due to injury, tumor, congenital anomaly, or hypoxia, resulting in loss of functional neurons; commonly associated with temporal lobe epilepsy.

348.82 Brain death

348.89 Other conditions of brain
Cerebral: Cerebral:
calcification   fungus
> **EXCLUDES** brain death (348.82)

348.9 Unspecified condition of brain

✓4ᵗʰ **349 Other and unspecified disorders of the nervous system**

349.0 Reaction to spinal or lumbar puncture
Headache following lumbar puncture

349.1 Nervous system complications from surgically implanted device
EXCLUDES immediate postoperative complications (997.00-997.09)
mechanical complications of nervous system device (996.2)

349.2 Disorders of meninges, not elsewhere classified
Adhesions, meningeal (cerebral) (spinal)
Cyst, spinal meninges
Meningocele, acquired
Pseudomeningocele, acquired

✓5ᵗʰ **349.3 Dural tear**

349.31 Accidental puncture or laceration of dura during a procedure
Incidental (inadvertent) durotomy

349.39 Other dural tear

✓5ᵗʰ **349.8 Other specified disorders of nervous system**

349.81 Cerebrospinal fluid rhinorrhea
EXCLUDES cerebrospinal fluid otorrhea (388.61)
DEF: Cerebrospinal fluid discharging from the nose; caused by fracture of frontal bone with tearing of dura mater and arachnoid.

349.82 Toxic encephalopathy
Toxic metabolic encephalopathy
Use additional E code to identify cause
DEF: Brain tissue degeneration due to toxic substance.

349.89 Other

349.9 Unspecified disorders of nervous system
Disorder of nervous system (central) NOS

DISORDERS OF THE PERIPHERAL NERVOUS SYSTEM (350-359)

EXCLUDES diseases of:
acoustic [8th] nerve (388.5)
oculomotor [3rd, 4th, 6th] nerves (378.0-378.9)
optic [2nd] nerve (377.0-377.9)
peripheral autonomic nerves (337.0-337.9)
neuralgia
neuritis   } NOS or "rheumatic" (729.2)
radiculitis
peripheral neuritis in pregnancy (646.4)

✓4ᵗʰ **350 Trigeminal nerve disorders**
INCLUDES disorders of 5th cranial nerve

350.1 Trigeminal neuralgia
Tic douloureux   Trigeminal neuralgia NOS
Trifacial neuralgia
EXCLUDES postherpetic (053.12)

350.2 Atypical face pain

350.8 Other specified trigeminal nerve disorders

350.9 Trigeminal nerve disorder, unspecified

✓4ᵗʰ **351 Facial nerve disorders**
INCLUDES disorders of 7th cranial nerve
EXCLUDES that in newborn (767.5)

351.0 Bell's palsy
Facial palsy
DEF: Unilateral paralysis of face due to lesion on facial nerve; produces facial distortion.

351.1 Geniculate ganglionitis
Geniculate ganglionitis NOS
EXCLUDES herpetic (053.11)
DEF: Inflammation of tissue at bend in facial nerve.

351.8 Other facial nerve disorders
Facial myokymia   Melkersson's syndrome

351.9 Facial nerve disorder, unspecified

✓4ᵗʰ **352 Disorders of other cranial nerves**

352.0 Disorders of olfactory [lst] nerve

352.1 Glossopharyngeal neuralgia
DEF: Pain between throat and ear along petrosal and jugular ganglia.

352.2 Other disorders of glossopharyngeal [9th] nerve

352.3 Disorders of pneumogastric [10th] nerve
Disorders of vagal nerve
EXCLUDES paralysis of vocal cords or larynx (478.30-478.34)
DEF: Nerve disorder affecting ear, tongue, pharynx, larynx, esophagus, viscera and thorax.

352.4 Disorders of accessory [11th] nerve
DEF: Nerve disorder affecting palate, pharynx, larynx, thoracic viscera, sternocleidomastoid and trapezius muscles.

352.5 Disorders of hypoglossal [12th] nerve
DEF: Nerve disorder affecting tongue muscles.

352.6 Multiple cranial nerve palsies
Collet-Sicard syndrome
Polyneuritis cranialis

352.9 Unspecified disorder of cranial nerves

✓4ᵗʰ **353 Nerve root and plexus disorders**
EXCLUDES conditions due to:
intervertebral disc disorders (722.0-722.9)
spondylosis (720.0-721.9)
vertebrogenic disorders (723.0-724.9)

353.0 Brachial plexus lesions
Cervical rib syndrome
Costoclavicular syndrome
Scalenus anticus syndrome
Thoracic outlet syndrome
EXCLUDES brachial neuritis or radiculitis NOS (723.4)
that in newborn (767.6)
DEF: Acquired disorder in tissue along nerves in shoulder; causes corresponding motor and sensory dysfunction.

Cranial Nerves

Olfactory bulb (I)
Optic nerve (II)
Oculomotor nerve (III)
Trochlear nerve (IV)
Trigeminal nerve (V)
Abducens nerve (VI)
Facial nerve (VII)
Vestibulocochlear nerve (VIII)
Glossopharyngeal nerve (IX)
Vagus nerve (X)
Accessory nerve (XI)
Hypoglossal nerve (XII)
Pons

Trigeminal and Facial Nerve Branches

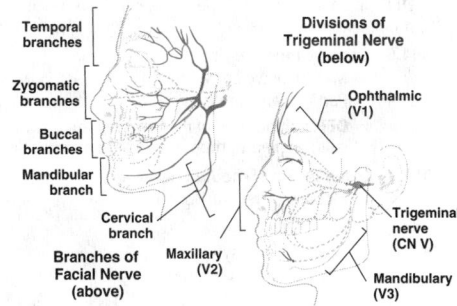

Temporal branches
Zygomatic branches
Buccal branches
Mandibular branch
Cervical branch
Branches of Facial Nerve (above)
Maxillary (V2)
Divisions of Trigeminal Nerve (below)
Ophthalmic (V1)
Trigeminal nerve (CN V)
Mandibulary (V3)

Peripheral Nervous System

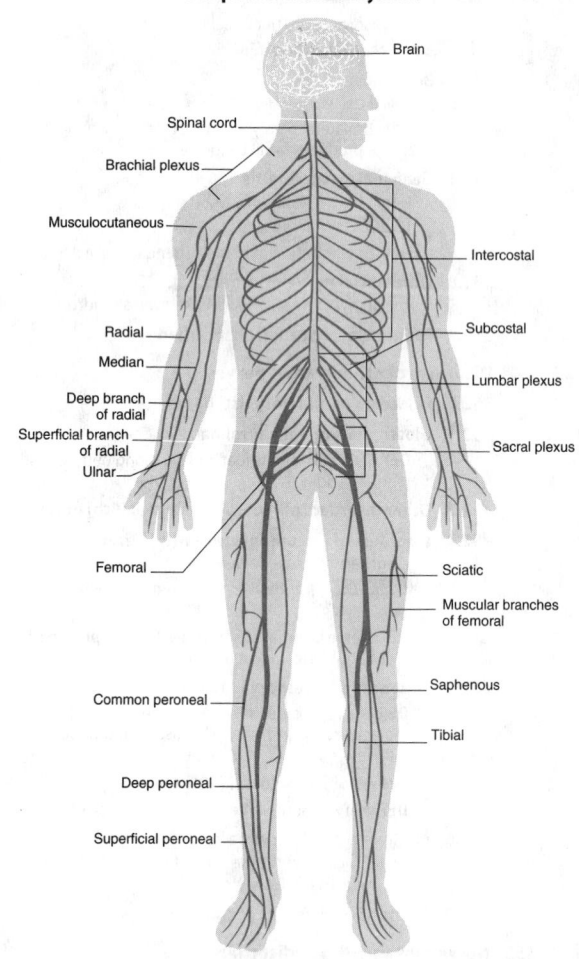

Brain
Spinal cord
Brachial plexus
Musculocutaneous
Intercostal
Radial
Subcostal
Median
Lumbar plexus
Deep branch of radial
Superficial branch of radial
Sacral plexus
Ulnar
Femoral
Sciatic
Muscular branches of femoral
Saphenous
Common peroneal
Tibial
Deep peroneal
Superficial peroneal

353.1 Lumbosacral plexus lesions
DEF: Acquired disorder in tissue along nerves in lower back; causes corresponding motor and sensory dysfunction.

353.2 Cervical root lesions, not elsewhere classified

353.3 Thoracic root lesions, not elsewhere classified

353.4 Lumbosacral root lesions, not elsewhere classified

353.5 Neuralgic amyotrophy
Parsonage-Aldren-Turner syndrome
Code first any associated underlying disease, such as: diabetes mellitus (249.6, 250.6)

353.6 Phantom limb (syndrome)
DEF: Abnormal tingling or a burning sensation, transient aches, and intermittent or continuous pain perceived as originating in the absent limb.

353.8 Other nerve root and plexus disorders

353.9 Unspecified nerve root and plexus disorder

√4ᵗʰ **354 Mononeuritis of upper limb and mononeuritis multiplex**
DEF: Inflammation of a single nerve; known as mononeuritis multiplex when several nerves in unrelated body areas are affected.

354.0 Carpal tunnel syndrome
Median nerve entrapment
Partial thenar atrophy
DEF: Compression of median nerve by tendons; causes pain, tingling, numbness and burning sensation in hand.

354.1 Other lesion of median nerve
Median nerve neuritis

354.2 Lesion of ulnar nerve
Cubital tunnel syndrome
Tardy ulnar nerve palsy

354.3 Lesion of radial nerve
Acute radial nerve palsy

354.4 Causalgia of upper limb
Complex regional pain syndrome type II of the upper limb
EXCLUDES   causalgia:
NOS (355.9)
lower limb (355.71)
complex regional pain syndrome type II of the lower limb (355.71)
DEF: Peripheral nerve damage, upper limb; usually due to injury; causes burning sensation and trophic skin changes.

354.5 Mononeuritis multiplex
Combinations of single conditions classifiable to 354 or 355

354.8 Other mononeuritis of upper limb

354.9 Mononeuritis of upper limb, unspecified

√4ᵗʰ **355 Mononeuritis of lower limb**

355.0 Lesion of sciatic nerve
EXCLUDES   sciatica NOS (724.3)
DEF: Acquired disorder of sciatic nerve; causes motor and sensory dysfunction in back, buttock and leg.

355.1 Meralgia paresthetica
Lateral cutaneous femoral nerve of thigh compression or syndrome
DEF: Inguinal ligament entraps lateral femoral cutaneous nerve; causes tingling, pain and numbness along outer thigh.

355.2 Other lesion of femoral nerve

355.3 Lesion of lateral popliteal nerve
Lesion of common peroneal nerve

355.4 Lesion of medial popliteal nerve

355.5 Tarsal tunnel syndrome
DEF: Compressed, entrapped posterior tibial nerve; causes tingling, pain and numbness in sole of foot.

355.6 Lesion of plantar nerve
Morton's metatarsalgia, neuralgia, or neuroma

√5ᵗʰ **355.7 Other mononeuritis of lower limb**

355.71 Causalgia of lower limb
EXCLUDES   causalgia:
NOS (355.9)
upper limb (354.4)
complex regional pain syndrome type II of upper limb (354.4)
DEF: Dysfunction of lower limb peripheral nerve, usually due to injury; causes burning pain and trophic skin changes.

355.79 Other mononeuritis of lower limb

355.8 Mononeuritis of lower limb, unspecified

355.9 Mononeuritis of unspecified site
Causalgia NOS
Complex regional pain syndrome NOS
EXCLUDES   causalgia:
lower limb (355.71)
upper limb (354.4)
complex regional pain syndrome:
lower limb (355.71)
upper limb (354.4)

√4ᵗʰ **356 Hereditary and idiopathic peripheral neuropathy**

356.0 Hereditary peripheral neuropathy
Déjérine-Sottas disease

356.1 Peroneal muscular atrophy
Charcôt-Marie-Tooth disease
Neuropathic muscular atrophy
DEF: Genetic disorder, in muscles innervated by peroneal nerves; symptoms include muscle wasting in lower limbs and locomotor difficulties.

356.2 Hereditary sensory neuropathy
DEF: Inherited disorder in dorsal root ganglia, optic nerve, and cerebellum, causing sensory losses, shooting pains, and foot ulcers.

356.3 Refsum's disease
Heredopathia atactica polyneuritiformis
DEF: Genetic disorder of lipid metabolism; causes persistent, painful inflammation of nerves and retinitis pigmentosa.

356.4 Idiopathic progressive polyneuropathy

356.8 Other specified idiopathic peripheral neuropathy
Supranuclear paralysis

356.9 Unspecified

357 Inflammatory and toxic neuropathy

357.0 Acute infective polyneuritis
Guillain-Barré syndrome
Postinfectious polyneuritis
DEF: Guillain-Barré syndrome: acute demyelinating polyneuropathy preceded by viral illness (i.e., herpes, cytomegalovirus [CMV], Epstein-Barr virus [EBV]) or a bacterial illness; areflexic motor paralysis with mild sensory disturbance and acellular rise in spinal fluid protein.

357.1 *Polyneuropathy in collagen vascular disease*
Code first underlying disease, as:
disseminated lupus erythematosus (710.0)
polyarteritis nodosa (446.0)
rheumatoid arthritis (714.0)

357.2 *Polyneuropathy in diabetes*
Code first underlying disease (249.6, 250.6)

357.3 *Polyneuropathy in malignant disease*
Code first underlying disease (140.0-208.9)

357.4 *Polyneuropathy in other diseases classified elsewhere*
Code first underlying disease, as:
amyloidosis (277.30-277.39)
beriberi (265.0)
chronic uremia (585.9)
deficiency of B vitamins (266.0-266.9)
diphtheria (032.0-032.9)
hypoglycemia (251.2)
pellagra (265.2)
porphyria (277.1)
sarcoidosis (135)
uremia NOS (586)
    EXCLUDES *polyneuropathy in:*
herpes zoster (053.13)
mumps (072.72)

357.5 Alcoholic polyneuropathy

357.6 Polyneuropathy due to drugs
Use additional E code to identify drug

357.7 Polyneuropathy due to other toxic agents
Use additional E code to identify toxic agent

357.8 Other

357.81 Chronic inflammatory demyelinating polyneuritis
DEF: Inflammation of peripheral nerves resulting in destruction of myelin sheath; associated with diabetes mellitus, dysproteinemias, renal failure and malnutrition; symptoms include tingling, numbness, burning pain, diminished tendon reflexes, weakness of lower extremities.

357.82 Critical illness polyneuropathy
Acute motor neuropathy
DEF: An acute axonal neuropathy, both sensory and motor, that is associated with Systemic Inflammatory Response Syndrome (SIRS).

357.89 Other inflammatory and toxic neuropathy

357.9 Unspecified

358 Myoneural disorders

358.0 Myasthenia gravis
DEF: Autoimmune disorder of acetylcholine at neuromuscular junction; causing fatigue of voluntary muscles.

358.00 Myasthenia gravis without (acute) exacerbation
Myasthenia gravis NOS

358.01 Myasthenia gravis with (acute) exacerbation
Myasthenia gravis in crisis

358.1 *Myasthenic syndromes in diseases classified elsewhere*
Code first underlying disease, as:
botulism (005.1, 040.41-040.42)
hypothyroidism (244.0-244.9)
malignant neoplasm (140.0-208.9)
pernicious anemia (281.0)
thyrotoxicosis (242.0-242.9)

358.2 Toxic myoneural disorders
Use additional E code to identify toxic agent

358.3 Lambert-Eaton syndrome
Eaton-Lambert syndrome

358.30 Lambert-Eaton syndrome, unspecified
Lambert-Eaton syndrome NOS

358.31 Lambert-Eaton syndrome in neoplastic disease
Code first the underlying neoplastic disease

358.39 *Lambert-Eaton syndrome in other diseases classified elsewhere*
Code first the underlying condition

358.8 Other specified myoneural disorders

358.9 Myoneural disorders, unspecified

359 Muscular dystrophies and other myopathies
    EXCLUDES *idiopathic polymyositis (710.4)*

359.0 Congenital hereditary muscular dystrophy
Benign congenital myopathy
Central core disease
Centronuclear myopathy
Myotubular myopathy
Nemaline body disease
    EXCLUDES *arthrogryposis multiplex congenita (754.89)*
DEF: Genetic disorder; causing progressive or nonprogressive muscle weakness.

359.1 Hereditary progressive muscular dystrophy
Muscular dystrophy:
NOS
distal
Duchenne
Erb's
fascioscapulohumeral
Gower's
Landouzy-Déjérine
limb-girdle
ocular
oculopharyngeal
DEF: Genetic degenerative, muscle disease; causes progressive weakness, wasting of muscle with no nerve involvement.

359.2 Myotonic disorders
    EXCLUDES *periodic paralysis (359.3)*
DEF: Impaired movement due to spasmatic, rigid muscles.

359.21 Myotonic muscular dystrophy
Dystrophia myotonica
Myotonia atrophica
Myotonic dystrophy
Proximal myotonic myopathy [PROMM]
Steinert's disease

359.22 Myotonia congenita
Acetazolamide responsive myotonia congenita
Dominant form [Thomsen's disease]
Myotonia levior
Recessive form [Becker's disease]

Diseases of the Nervous System and Sense Organs

359.23–360.29

359.23 Myotonic chondrodystrophy
Congenital myotonic chondrodystrophy
Schwartz-Jampel disease

359.24 Drug induced myotonia
Use additional E code to identify drug

359.29 Other specified myotonic disorder
Myotonia fluctuans
Myotonia permanens
Paramyotonia congenita (of von Eulenburg)

359.3 Periodic paralysis
Familial periodic paralysis
Hypokalemic familial periodic paralysis
Hyperkalemic periodic paralysis
Hypokalemic periodic paralysis
Potassium sensitive periodic paralysis
EXCLUDES *paramyotonia congenita (of von Eulenburg) (359.29)*
DEF: Genetic disorder; characterized by rapidly progressive flaccid paralysis; attacks often occur after exercise or exposure to cold or dietary changes.

359.4 Toxic myopathy
Use additional E code to identify toxic agent
DEF: Muscle disorder caused by toxic agent.

359.5 *Myopathy in endocrine diseases classified elsewhere*
Code first underlying disease, as:
Addison's disease (255.41)
Cushing's syndrome (255.0)
hypopituitarism (253.2)
myxedema (244.0-244.9)
thyrotoxicosis (242.0-242.9)
DEF: Muscle disorder secondary to dysfunction in hormone secretion.

359.6 *Symptomatic inflammatory myopathy in diseases classified elsewhere*
Code first underlying disease, as:
amyloidosis (277.30-277.39)
disseminated lupus erythematosus (710.0)
malignant neoplasm (140.0-208.9)
polyarteritis nodosa (446.0)
rheumatoid arthritis (714.0)
sarcoidosis (135)
scleroderma (710.1)
Sjögren's disease (710.2)

√5ᵗʰ **359.7 Inflammatory and immune myopathies, NEC**

359.71 Inclusion body myositis
IBM
DEF: Progressive, debilitating inflammatory muscle disease characterized by dysphagia, chronic muscle swelling, weakness, and atrophy (wasting); impairs fine motor functions.

359.79 Other inflammatory and immune myopathies, NEC
Inflammatory myopathy NOS

√5ᵗʰ **359.8 Other myopathies**

359.81 Critical illness myopathy
Acute necrotizing myopathy
Acute quadriplegic myopathy
Intensive care (ICU) myopathy
Myopathy of critical illness

359.89 Other myopathies

359.9 Myopathy, unspecified

DISORDERS OF THE EYE AND ADNEXA (360-379)
Use additional external cause code, if applicable, to identify the cause of the eye condition

√4ᵗʰ **360 Disorders of the globe**
INCLUDES disorders affecting multiple structures of eye

√5ᵗʰ **360.0 Purulent endophthalmitis**
EXCLUDES *bleb associated endophthalmitis (379.63)*

360.00 Purulent endophthalmitis, unspecified

360.01 Acute endophthalmitis

360.02 Panophthalmitis

360.03 Chronic endophthalmitis

360.04 Vitreous abscess

√5ᵗʰ **360.1 Other endophthalmitis**
EXCLUDES *bleb associated endophthalmitis (379.63)*

360.11 Sympathetic uveitis
DEF: Inflammation of vascular layer of uninjured eye; follows injury to other eye.

360.12 Panuveitis
DEF: Inflammation of entire vascular layer of eye, including choroid, iris and ciliary body.

360.13 Parasitic endophthalmitis NOS
DEF: Parasitic infection causing inflammation of the entire eye.

360.14 Ophthalmia nodosa
DEF: Conjunctival inflammation caused by embedded hairs.

360.19 Other
Phacoanaphylactic endophthalmitis

√5ᵗʰ **360.2 Degenerative disorders of globe**

360.20 Degenerative disorder of globe, unspecified

360.21 Progressive high (degenerative) myopia
Malignant myopia
DEF: Severe, progressive nearsightedness in adults, complicated by serious disease of the choroid; leads to retinal detachment and blindness.

360.23 Siderosis
DEF: Iron pigment deposits within tissue of eyeball; caused by high iron content of blood.

360.24 Other metallosis
Chalcosis
DEF: Metal deposits, other than iron, within eyeball tissues.

360.29 Other
EXCLUDES *xerophthalmia (264.7)*

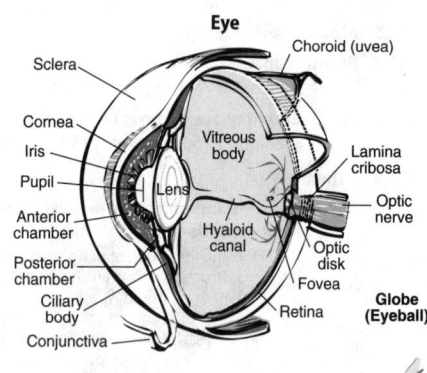

Eye

Sclera — Choroid (uvea) — Cornea — Iris — Pupil — Anterior chamber — Posterior chamber — Ciliary body — Conjunctiva — Vitreous body — Lens — Hyaloid canal — Lamina cribosa — Optic nerve — Optic disk — Fovea — Retina — **Globe (Eyeball)**

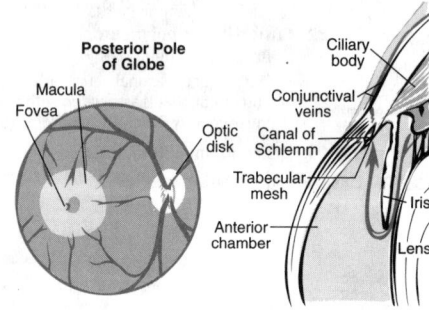

Posterior Pole of Globe

Macula — Fovea — Optic disk — Ciliary body — Conjunctival veins — Canal of Schlemm — Trabecular mesh — Anterior chamber — Iris — Lens

Flow of Aqueous Humor

Adnexa

Upper eyelid
Orbicularis oculi muscle
Orbital septum
Tarsal plate (cartilage)
Conjunctival fornix
Lower eyelid
Tarsal plate
Orbital septum
Orbital floor
Orbital roof
Levator palpebri muscle
Müller's muscle
Globe (eyeball)
Optic nerve
Retrobulbar space
Fascia bulbi (Tenon's capsule)
Extraocular muscle

√5ᵗʰ **360.3 Hypotony of eye**

   360.30 Hypotony, unspecified

      DEF: Low osmotic pressure causing lack of tone, tension and strength.

      360.32

      DEF: Low intraocular pressure due to leak through abnormal passage.

   360.31 Primary hypotony

   360.32 Ocular fistula causing hypotony

      DEF: Low intraocular pressure due to leak through abnormal passage.

   360.33 Hypotony associated with other ocular disorders

   360.34 Flat anterior chamber

      DEF: Low pressure behind cornea, causing compression.

√5ᵗʰ **360.4 Degenerated conditions of globe**

   360.40 Degenerated globe or eye, unspecified

   360.41 Blind hypotensive eye
      Atrophy of globe
      Phthisis bulbi

      DEF: Vision loss due to extremely low intraocular pressure.

   360.42 Blind hypertensive eye
      Absolute glaucoma

      DEF: Vision loss due to painful, high intraocular pressure.

   360.43 Hemophthalmos, except current injury
      EXCLUDES traumatic (871.0-871.9, 921.0-921.9)

      DEF: Pool of blood within eyeball, not from current injury.

   360.44 Leucocoria

      DEF: Whitish mass or reflex in the pupil behind lens; also called cat's eye reflex; often indicative of retinoblastoma.

√5ᵗʰ **360.5 Retained (old) intraocular foreign body, magnetic**
      Use additional code to identify foreign body (V90.11)
      EXCLUDES current penetrating injury with magnetic foreign body (871.5)
                  retained (old) foreign body of orbit (376.6)

   360.50 Foreign body, magnetic, intraocular, unspecified

   360.51 Foreign body, magnetic, in anterior chamber

   360.52 Foreign body, magnetic, in iris or ciliary body

   360.53 Foreign body, magnetic, in lens

   360.54 Foreign body, magnetic, in vitreous

   360.55 Foreign body, magnetic, in posterior wall

   360.59 Foreign body, magnetic, in other or multiple sites

√5ᵗʰ **360.6 Retained (old) intraocular foreign body, nonmagnetic**
      Retained (old) foreign body:
        NOS
        nonmagnetic
      Use additional code to identify foreign body (V90.01-V90.10, V90.12, V90.2-V90.9)
      EXCLUDES current penetrating injury with (nonmagnetic) foreign body (871.6)
                  retained (old) foreign body in orbit (376.6)

   360.60 Foreign body, intraocular, unspecified

   360.61 Foreign body in anterior chamber

   360.62 Foreign body in iris or ciliary body

   360.63 Foreign body in lens

   360.64 Foreign body in vitreous

   360.65 Foreign body in posterior wall

   360.69 Foreign body in other or multiple sites

√5ᵗʰ **360.8 Other disorders of globe**

   360.81 Luxation of globe

      DEF: Displacement of eyeball.

   360.89 Other

   360.9 Unspecified disorder of globe

√4ᵗʰ **361 Retinal detachments and defects**

   DEF: Disorders of light-sensitive layer at back of eye, which separates from blood supply, disrupting vision.

√5ᵗʰ **361.0 Retinal detachment with retinal defect**
      Rhegmatogenous retinal detachment
      EXCLUDES detachment of retinal pigment epithelium (362.42-362.43)
                  retinal detachment (serous) (without defect) (361.2)

   361.00 Retinal detachment with retinal defect, unspecified

   361.01 Recent detachment, partial, with single defect

   361.02 Recent detachment, partial, with multiple defects

   361.03 Recent detachment, partial, with giant tear

   361.04 Recent detachment, partial, with retinal dialysis
      Dialysis (juvenile) of retina (with detachment)

   361.05 Recent detachment, total or subtotal

   361.06 Old detachment, partial
      Delimited old retinal detachment

   361.07 Old detachment, total or subtotal

√5ᵗʰ **361.1 Retinoschisis and retinal cysts**
      EXCLUDES juvenile retinoschisis (362.73)
                  microcystoid degeneration of retina (362.62)
                  parasitic cyst of retina (360.13)

   361.10 Retinoschisis, unspecified

      DEF: Separation of retina due to degenerative process of aging; should not be confused with acute retinal detachment.

   361.11 Flat retinoschisis

      DEF: Slow, progressive split of retinal sensory layers.

   361.12 Bullous retinoschisis

      DEF: Fluid retention between split retinal sensory layers.

   361.13 Primary retinal cysts

   361.14 Secondary retinal cysts

   361.19 Other
      Pseudocyst of retina

   361.2 Serous retinal detachment
      Retinal detachment without retinal defect
      EXCLUDES central serous retinopathy (362.41)
                  retinal pigment epithelium detachment (362.42-362.43)

Diseases of the Nervous System and Sense Organs

361.3–362.42

√5th **361.3 Retinal defects without detachment**
> EXCLUDES *chorioretinal scars after surgery for detachment (363.30-363.35)*
> *peripheral retinal degeneration without defect (362.60-362.66)*

361.30 Retinal defect, unspecified
Retinal break(s) NOS

361.31 Round hole of retina without detachment

361.32 Horseshoe tear of retina without detachment
Operculum of retina without mention of detachment

361.33 Multiple defects of retina without detachment

√5th **361.8 Other forms of retinal detachment**

361.81 Traction detachment of retina
Traction detachment with vitreoretinal organization

361.89 Other

361.9 Unspecified retinal detachment

√4th **362 Other retinal disorders**
> EXCLUDES *chorioretinal scars (363.30-363.35)*
> *chorioretinitis (363.0-363.2)*

√5th **362.0 Diabetic retinopathy**
Code first diabetes (249.5, 250.5)
DEF: Retinal changes in diabetes of long duration; causes hemorrhages, microaneurysms, waxy deposits and proliferative noninflammatory degenerative disease of retina.

362.01 Background diabetic retinopathy
Diabetic retinal microaneurysms
Diabetic retinopathy NOS

362.02 Proliferative diabetic retinopathy
DEF: Occurrence of the ischemic effects of vessel blockages result in neovascularization; new blood vessels begin to form to compensate for restricted blood flow; multiple areas of the retina and inner vitreous may be affected.

362.03 Nonproliferative diabetic retinopathy NOS

362.04 Mild nonproliferative diabetic retinopathy
DEF: Early stages of degenerative condition of the retina due to diabetes; microaneurysm formation; small balloon-like swelling of the retinal vessels.

362.05 Moderate nonproliferative diabetic retinopathy
DEF: Stage of degenerative condition of the retina due to diabetes with pronounced microaneurysms; vessel blockages can occur.

362.06 Severe nonproliferative diabetic retinopathy
DEF: Stage of degenerative condition of the retina due to diabetes in which vascular breakdown in the retina results in multiple vascular blockages, or "beadings," with intraretinal hemorrhages.

362.07 Diabetic macular edema
Note: Code 362.07 must be used with a code for diabetic retinopathy (362.01-362.06)
Diabetic retinal edema
DEF: Leakage from retinal blood vessels causes swelling of the macula and impaired vision; exudates or plaques may develop in the posterior pole of the retina due to the breakdown of retinal vasculature.

√5th **362.1 Other background retinopathy and retinal vascular changes**

362.10 Background retinopathy, unspecified

362.11 Hypertensive retinopathy
DEF: Retinal irregularities caused by systemic hypertension.

362.12 Exudative retinopathy
Coats' syndrome

362.13 Changes in vascular appearance
Vascular sheathing of retina
Use additional code for any associated atherosclerosis (440.8)

362.14 Retinal microaneurysms NOS
DEF: Microscopic dilation of retinal vessels in nondiabetic.

362.15 Retinal telangiectasia
DEF: Dilation of blood vessels of the retina.

362.16 Retinal neovascularization NOS
Neovascularization: Neovascularization:
choroidal subretinal
DEF: New and abnormal vascular growth in the retina.

362.17 Other intraretinal microvascular abnormalities
Retinal sclerosis Retinal varices

362.18 Retinal vasculitis
Eales' disease Retinal:
Retinal: perivasculitis
arteritis phlebitis
endarteritis
DEF: Inflammation of retinal blood vessels.

√5th **362.2 Other proliferative retinopathy**

362.20 Retinopathy of prematurity, unspecified
Retinopathy of prematurity NOS

362.21 Retrolental fibroplasia
Cicatricial retinopathy of prematurity
DEF: Fibrous tissue in vitreous, from retina to lens, causing blindness; associated with premature infants requiring high amounts of oxygen.

362.22 Retinopathy of prematurity, stage 0

362.23 Retinopathy of prematurity, stage 1

362.24 Retinopathy of prematurity, stage 2

362.25 Retinopathy of prematurity, stage 3

362.26 Retinopathy of prematurity, stage 4

362.27 Retinopathy of prematurity, stage 5

362.29 Other nondiabetic proliferative retinopathy

√5th **362.3 Retinal vascular occlusion**
DEF: Obstructed blood flow to and from retina.

362.30 Retinal vascular occlusion, unspecified

362.31 Central retinal artery occlusion

362.32 Arterial branch occlusion

362.33 Partial arterial occlusion
Hollenhorst plaque
Retinal microembolism

362.34 Transient arterial occlusion
Amaurosis fugax

362.35 Central retinal vein occlusion

362.36 Venous tributary (branch) occlusion

362.37 Venous engorgement
Occlusion:
incipient } of retinal vein
partial

√5th **362.4 Separation of retinal layers**
> EXCLUDES *retinal detachment (serous) (361.2)*
> *rhegmatogenous (361.00-361.07)*

362.40 Retinal layer separation, unspecified

362.41 Central serous retinopathy
DEF: Serous-filled blister causing detachment of retina from pigment epithelium.

362.42 Serous detachment of retinal pigment epithelium
Exudative detachment of retinal pigment epithelium
DEF: Blister of fatty fluid causing detachment of retina from pigment epithelium.

362.43 Hemorrhagic detachment of retinal pigment epithelium
  DEF: Blood-filled blister causing detachment of retina from pigment epithelium.

√5ᵗʰ **362.5 Degeneration of macula and posterior pole**
  EXCLUDES degeneration of optic disc (377.21-377.24)
  hereditary retinal degeneration [dystrophy] (362.70-362.77)

362.50 Macular degeneration (senile), unspecified

362.51 Nonexudative senile macular degeneration
  Senile macular degeneration:
    atrophic
    dry

362.52 Exudative senile macular degeneration
  Kuhnt-Junius degeneration
  Senile macular degeneration:
    disciform
    wet
  DEF: Leakage in macular blood vessels with loss of visual acuity.

362.53 Cystoid macular degeneration
  Cystoid macular edema
  DEF: Retinal swelling and cyst formation in macula.

362.54 Macular cyst, hole, or pseudohole

362.55 Toxic maculopathy
  Use additional E code to identify drug, if drug induced

362.56 Macular puckering
  Preretinal fibrosis

362.57 Drusen (degenerative)
  DEF: White, hyaline deposits on Bruch's membrane (lamina basalis choroideae).

√5ᵗʰ **362.6 Peripheral retinal degenerations**
  EXCLUDES hereditary retinal degeneration [dystrophy] (362.70-362.77)
  retinal degeneration with retinal defect (361.00-361.07)

362.60 Peripheral retinal degeneration, unspecified

362.61 Paving stone degeneration
  DEF: Degeneration of peripheral retina; causes thinning through which choroid is visible.

362.62 Microcystoid degeneration
  Blessig's cysts   Iwanoff's cysts

362.63 Lattice degeneration
  Palisade degeneration of retina
  DEF: Degeneration of retina; often bilateral, usually benign; characterized by lines intersecting at irregular intervals in peripheral retina; retinal thinning and retinal holes may occur.

362.64 Senile reticular degeneration
  DEF: Net-like appearance of retina; sign of degeneration.

362.65 Secondary pigmentary degeneration
  Pseudoretinitis pigmentosa

362.66 Secondary vitreoretinal degenerations

√5ᵗʰ **362.7 Hereditary retinal dystrophies**
  DEF: Genetically induced progressive changes in retina.

362.70 Hereditary retinal dystrophy, unspecified

362.71 Retinal dystrophy in systemic or cerebroretinal lipidoses
  Code first underlying disease, as:
    cerebroretinal lipidoses (330.1)
    systemic lipidoses (272.7)

362.72 Retinal dystrophy in other systemic disorders and syndromes
  Code first underlying disease, as:
    Bassen-Kornzweig syndrome (272.5)
    Refsum's disease (356.3)

362.73 Vitreoretinal dystrophies
  Juvenile retinoschisis

362.74 Pigmentary retinal dystrophy
  Retinal dystrophy, albipunctate
  Retinitis pigmentosa

362.75 Other dystrophies primarily involving the sensory retina
  Progressive cone(-rod) dystrophy
  Stargardt's disease

362.76 Dystrophies primarily involving the retinal pigment epithelium
  Fundus flavimaculatus
  Vitelliform dystrophy

362.77 Dystrophies primarily involving Bruch's membrane
  Dystrophy:
    hyaline
    pseudoinflammatory foveal
  Hereditary drusen

√5ᵗʰ **362.8 Other retinal disorders**
  EXCLUDES chorioretinal inflammations (363.0-363.2)
  chorioretinal scars (363.30-363.35)

362.81 Retinal hemorrhage
  Hemorrhage:
    preretinal
    retinal (deep) (superficial)
    subretinal

362.82 Retinal exudates and deposits

362.83 Retinal edema
  Retinal:
    cotton wool spots
    edema (localized) (macular) (peripheral)
  DEF: Retinal swelling due to fluid accumulation.

362.84 Retinal ischemia
  DEF: Reduced retinal blood supply.

362.85 Retinal nerve fiber bundle defects

362.89 Other retinal disorders

362.9 Unspecified retinal disorder

√4ᵗʰ **363 Chorioretinal inflammations, scars, and other disorders of choroid**

√5ᵗʰ **363.0 Focal chorioretinitis and focal retinochoroiditis**
  EXCLUDES focal chorioretinitis or retinochoroiditis in:
    histoplasmosis (115.02, 115.12, 115.92)
    toxoplasmosis (130.2)
      congenital infection (771.2)

363.00 Focal chorioretinitis, unspecified
  Focal:
    choroiditis or chorioretinitis NOS
    retinitis or retinochoroiditis NOS

363.01 Focal choroiditis and chorioretinitis, juxtapapillary

363.03 Focal choroiditis and chorioretinitis of other posterior pole

363.04 Focal choroiditis and chorioretinitis, peripheral

363.05 Focal retinitis and retinochoroiditis, juxtapapillary
  Neuroretinitis

363.06 Focal retinitis and retinochoroiditis, macular or paramacular

363.07 Focal retinitis and retinochoroiditis of other posterior pole

363.08 Focal retinitis and retinochoroiditis, peripheral

Diseases of the Nervous System and Sense Organs

363.1–364.10

√5ᵗʰ **363.1　Disseminated chorioretinitis and disseminated retinochoroiditis**

> **EXCLUDES**　disseminated choroiditis or chorioretinitis in secondary syphilis (091.51)
> neurosyphilitic disseminated retinitis or retinochoroiditis (094.83)
> retinal (peri)vasculitis (362.18)

363.10　Disseminated chorioretinitis, unspecified
Disseminated:
choroiditis or chorioretinitis NOS
retinitis or retinochoroiditis NOS

363.11　Disseminated choroiditis and chorioretinitis, posterior pole

363.12　Disseminated choroiditis and chorioretinitis, peripheral

363.13　Disseminated choroiditis and chorioretinitis, generalized
Code first any underlying disease, as:
tuberculosis (017.3)

363.14　Disseminated retinitis and retinochoroiditis, metastatic

363.15　Disseminated retinitis and retinochoroiditis, pigment epitheliopathy
Acute posterior multifocal placoid pigment epitheliopathy
DEF: Widespread inflammation of retina and choroid; characterized by pigmented epithelium involvement.

√5ᵗʰ **363.2　Other and unspecified forms of chorioretinitis and retinochoroiditis**

> **EXCLUDES**　panophthalmitis (360.02)
> sympathetic uveitis (360.11)
> uveitis NOS (364.3)

363.20　Chorioretinitis, unspecified
Choroiditis NOS
Retinitis NOS
Uveitis, posterior NOS

363.21　Pars planitis
Posterior cyclitis
DEF: Inflammation of peripheral retina and ciliary body; characterized by bands of white cells.

363.22　Harada's disease
DEF: Retinal detachment and bilateral widespread exudative choroiditis; symptoms include headache, vomiting, increased lymphocytes in cerebrospinal fluid; with temporary or permanent deafness.

√5ᵗʰ **363.3　Chorioretinal scars**
Scar (postinflammatory) (postsurgical) (posttraumatic):
choroid
retina

363.30　Chorioretinal scar, unspecified

363.31　Solar retinopathy
DEF: Retinal scarring caused by solar radiation.

363.32　Other macular scars

363.33　Other scars of posterior pole

363.34　Peripheral scars

363.35　Disseminated scars

√5ᵗʰ **363.4　Choroidal degenerations**

363.40　Choroidal degeneration, unspecified
Choroidal sclerosis NOS

363.41　Senile atrophy of choroid
DEF: Wasting away of choroid; due to aging.

363.42　Diffuse secondary atrophy of choroid
DEF: Wasting away of choroid in systemic disease.

363.43　Angioid streaks of choroid
DEF: Degeneration of choroid; characterized by dark brown streaks radiating from optic disc; occurs with pseudoxanthoma, elasticum or Paget's disease.

√5ᵗʰ **363.5　Hereditary choroidal dystrophies**
Hereditary choroidal atrophy:
partial [choriocapillaris]
total [all vessels]

363.50　Hereditary choroidal dystrophy or atrophy, unspecified

363.51　Circumpapillary dystrophy of choroid, partial

363.52　Circumpapillary dystrophy of choroid, total
Helicoid dystrophy of choroid

363.53　Central dystrophy of choroid, partial
Dystrophy, choroidal:
central areolar
circinate

363.54　Central choroidal atrophy, total
Dystrophy, choroidal:　　Dystrophy, choroidal:
central gyrate　　　　　serpiginous

363.55　Choroideremia
DEF: Hereditary choroid degeneration, occurs in first decade; characterized by constricted visual field and ultimately blindness in males; less debilitating in females.

363.56　Other diffuse or generalized dystrophy, partial
Diffuse choroidal sclerosis

363.57　Other diffuse or generalized dystrophy, total
Generalized gyrate atrophy, choroid

√5ᵗʰ **363.6　Choroidal hemorrhage and rupture**

363.61　Choroidal hemorrhage, unspecified

363.62　Expulsive choroidal hemorrhage

363.63　Choroidal rupture

√5ᵗʰ **363.7　Choroidal detachment**

363.70　Choroidal detachment, unspecified

363.71　Serous choroidal detachment
DEF: Detachment of choroid from sclera; due to blister of serous fluid.

363.72　Hemorrhagic choroidal detachment
DEF: Detachment of choroid from sclera; due to blood-filled blister.

363.8　Other disorders of choroid

363.9　Unspecified disorder of choroid

√4ᵗʰ **364　Disorders of iris and ciliary body**

√5ᵗʰ **364.0　Acute and subacute iridocyclitis**
Anterior uveitis
Cylitis　　　　　　　┐
Iridocyclitis　　　　├ acute, subacute
Iritis　　　　　　　 ┘

> **EXCLUDES**　gonococcal (098.41)
> herpes simplex (054.44)
> herpes zoster (053.22)

364.00　Acute and subacute iridocyclitis, unspecified

364.01　Primary iridocyclitis

364.02　Recurrent iridocyclitis

364.03　Secondary iridocyclitis, infectious

364.04　Secondary iridocyclitis, noninfectious
Aqueous:　　　　　Aqueous:
cells　　　　　　　flare
fibrin

364.05　Hypopyon
DEF: Accumulation of white blood cells between cornea and lens.

√5ᵗʰ **364.1　Chronic iridocyclitis**

> **EXCLUDES**　posterior cyclitis (363.21)

364.10　Chronic iridocyclitis, unspecified

364.11 **_Chronic iridocyclitis in diseases classified elsewhere_**

Code first underlying disease, as:
sarcoidosis (135)
tuberculosis (017.3)
EXCLUDES _syphilitic iridocyclitis (091.52)_
DEF: Persistent inflammation of iris and ciliary body; due to underlying disease or condition.

√5ᵗʰ **364.2** **Certain types of iridocyclitis**
EXCLUDES _posterior cyclitis (363.21)_
sympathetic uveitis (360.11)

364.21 **Fuchs' heterochromic cyclitis**
DEF: Chronic cyclitis characterized by differences in the color of the two irises; the lighter iris appears in the inflamed eye.

364.22 **Glaucomatocyclitic crises**
DEF: An uncommon inflammatory unilateral eye condition, characteristic recurrent episodes of high intraocular pressure accompanied by mild inflammation.

364.23 **Lens-induced iridocyclitis**
DEF: Inflammation of iris; due to immune reaction to proteins in lens following trauma or other lens abnormality.

364.24 **Vogt-Koyanagi syndrome**
DEF: Uveomeningitis with exudative iridocyclitis and choroiditis; causes depigmentation of hair and skin, detached retina; tinnitus and loss of hearing.

364.3 **Unspecified iridocyclitis**
Uveitis NOS

√5ᵗʰ **364.4** **Vascular disorders of iris and ciliary body**
364.41 **Hyphema**
Hemorrhage of iris or ciliary body
DEF: Hemorrhage in anterior chamber; also called hyphemia or "blood shot" eyes.

364.42 **Rubeosis iridis**
Neovascularization of iris or ciliary body
DEF: Blood vessel and connective tissue formation on surface of iris; symptomatic of diabetic retinopathy, central retinal vein occlusion and retinal detachment.

√5ᵗʰ **364.5** **Degenerations of iris and ciliary body**
364.51 **Essential or progressive iris atrophy**

364.52 **Iridoschisis**
DEF: Splitting of the iris into two layers.

364.53 **Pigmentary iris degeneration**
Acquired heterochromia
Pigment dispersion syndrome } of iris
Translucency

364.54 **Degeneration of pupillary margin**
Atrophy of sphincter
Ectropion of pigment epithelium } of iris

364.55 **Miotic cysts of pupillary margin**
DEF: Serous-filled sacs in pupillary margin of iris.

364.56 **Degenerative changes of chamber angle**

364.57 **Degenerative changes of ciliary body**

364.59 **Other iris atrophy**
Iris atrophy (generalized) (sector shaped)

√5ᵗʰ **364.6** **Cysts of iris, ciliary body, and anterior chamber**
EXCLUDES _miotic pupillary cyst (364.55)_
parasitic cyst (360.13)

364.60 **Idiopathic cysts**
DEF: Fluid-filled sacs in iris or ciliary body; unknown etiology.

364.61 **Implantation cysts**
Epithelial down-growth, anterior chamber
Implantation cysts (surgical) (traumatic)

364.62 **Exudative cysts of iris or anterior chamber**

364.63 **Primary cyst of pars plana**
DEF: Fluid-filled sacs of outermost ciliary ring.

364.64 **Exudative cyst of pars plana**
DEF: Protein, fatty-filled sacs of outermost ciliary ring; due to fluid leak from blood vessels.

√5ᵗʰ **364.7** **Adhesions and disruptions of iris and ciliary body**
EXCLUDES _flat anterior chamber (360.34)_

364.70 **Adhesions of iris, unspecified**
Synechiae (iris) NOS

364.71 **Posterior synechiae**
DEF: Adhesion binding iris to lens.

364.72 **Anterior synechiae**
DEF: Adhesion binding the iris to cornea.

364.73 **Goniosynechiae**
Peripheral anterior synechiae
DEF: Adhesion binding the iris to cornea at the angle of the anterior chamber.

364.74 **Pupillary membranes**
Iris bombé   Pupillary:
Pupillary: seclusion
   occlusion
DEF: Membrane traversing the pupil and blocking vision.

364.75 **Pupillary abnormalities**
Deformed pupil   Rupture of sphincter,
Ectopic pupil   pupil

364.76 **Iridodialysis**
DEF: Separation of the iris from the ciliary body base; due to trauma or surgical accident.

364.77 **Recession of chamber angle**
DEF: Receding of anterior chamber angle of the eye; restricts vision.

√5ᵗʰ **364.8** **Other disorders of iris and ciliary body**
364.81 **Floppy iris syndrome**
Intraoperative floppy iris syndrome [IFIS]
Use additional E code to identify cause, such as:
sympatholytics [antiadrenergics] causing adverse effect in therapeutic use (E941.3)
DEF: Condition complicating cataract surgery for patients who have received alpha blocker treatment for urinary retention problems; iris dilator muscle fails to dilate, and the iris may billow or flap.

364.82 **Plateau iris syndrome**
DEF: A postoperative chronic angle-closure glaucoma characterized by closing of the anterior chamber angle secondary to a large or anteriorly positioned ciliary body that impairs the normal flow of aqueous fluid.

364.89 **Other disorders of iris and ciliary body**
Prolapse of iris NOS
EXCLUDES _prolapse of iris in recent wound (871.1)_

364.9 **Unspecified disorder of iris and ciliary body**

Plateau Iris Syndrome

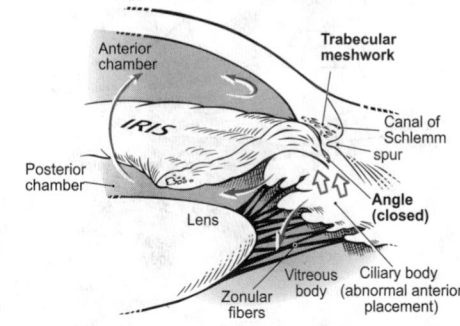

✓4th **365 Glaucoma**

> **EXCLUDES** *blind hypertensive eye [absolute glaucoma] (360.42)*
> *congenital glaucoma (743.20-743.22)*
>
> **DEF:** Rise in intraocular pressure restricting blood flow; multiple causes.

✓5th **365.0 Borderline glaucoma [glaucoma suspect]**

365.00 Preglaucoma, unspecified

365.01 Open angle with borderline findings, low risk
Open angle, low risk
> **DEF:** Minor block of aqueous outflow from eye.

365.02 Anatomical narrow angle
Primary angle closure suspect

365.03 Steroid responders

365.04 Ocular hypertension
> **DEF:** High fluid pressure within eye; no clear cause.

365.05 Open angle with borderline findings, high risk
Open angle, high risk

365.06 Primary angle closure without glaucoma damage

✓5th **365.1 Open-angle glaucoma**

365.10 Open-angle glaucoma, unspecified
Wide-angle glaucoma NOS
Use additional code to identify glaucoma stage (365.70-365.74)

365.11 Primary open angle glaucoma
Chronic simple glaucoma
Use additional code to identify glaucoma stage (365.70-365.74)
> **DEF:** High intraocular pressure, despite free flow of aqueous.

365.12 Low tension glaucoma
Use additional code to identify glaucoma stage (365.70-365.74)

365.13 Pigmentary glaucoma
Use additional code to identify glaucoma stage (365.70-365.74)
> **DEF:** High intraocular pressure; due to iris pigment granules blocking aqueous flow.

365.14 Glaucoma of childhood
Infantile or juvenile glaucoma

365.15 Residual stage of open angle glaucoma

✓5th **365.2 Primary angle-closure glaucoma**
> **DEF:** Glaucoma caused by a shift in the position of the iris of the eye that blocks the surface of the trabecular meshwork causing impairment of the normal flow of aqueous fluid.

365.20 Primary angle-closure glaucoma, unspecified
Use additional code to identify glaucoma stage (365.70-365.74)

Normal Aqueous Flow

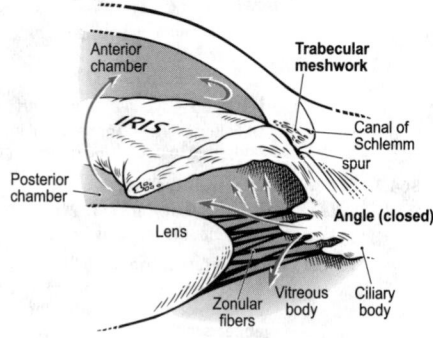

Angle-Closure Glaucoma

365.21 Intermittent angle-closure glaucoma
Angle-closure glaucoma:
interval
subacute
> **DEF:** Recurring attacks of high intraocular pressure; due to blocked aqueous flow.

365.22 Acute angle-closure glaucoma
Acute angle-closure glaucoma attack
Acute angle-closure glaucoma crisis
> **DEF:** Sudden, severe rise in intraocular pressure due to blockage in aqueous drainage.

365.23 Chronic angle-closure glaucoma
Chronic primary angle closure glaucoma
Use additional code to identify glaucoma stage (365.70-365.74)

365.24 Residual stage of angle-closure glaucoma

✓5th **365.3 Corticosteroid-induced glaucoma**
> **DEF:** Elevated intraocular pressure; due to long-term corticosteroid therapy.

365.31 Glaucomatous stage
Use additional code to identify glaucoma stage (365.70-365.74)

365.32 Residual stage

✓5th **365.4 Glaucoma associated with congenital anomalies, dystrophies, and systemic syndromes**

365.41 Glaucoma associated with chamber angle anomalies

365.42 Glaucoma associated with anomalies of iris

365.43 Glaucoma associated with other anterior segment anomalies

365.44 *Glaucoma associated with systemic syndromes*

Code first associated disease, as
neurofibromatosis (237.70-237.79)
Sturge-Weber (-Dimitri) syndrome (759.6)

✓5th **365.5 Glaucoma associated with disorders of the lens**

365.51 Phacolytic glaucoma
> **DEF:** Elevated intraocular pressure; due to lens protein blocking aqueous flow.

Cataract

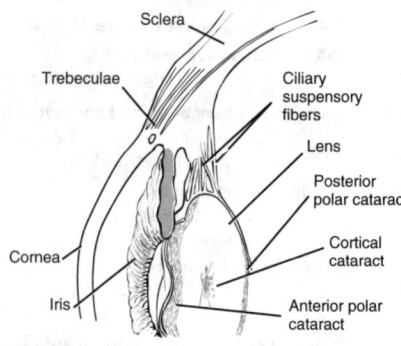

365.52 Pseudoexfoliation glaucoma
Use additional code to identify glaucoma stage (365.70-365.74)

> **DEF:** Glaucoma characterized by small grayish particles deposited on the lens.

365.59 Glaucoma associated with other lens disorders

✓5ᵗʰ **365.6 Glaucoma associated with other ocular disorders**

365.60 Glaucoma associated with unspecified ocular disorder

365.61 Glaucoma associated with pupillary block

> **DEF:** Acute, open-angle glaucoma caused by mature cataract; aqueous flow is blocked by lens material and macrophages.

365.62 Glaucoma associated with ocular inflammations
Use additional code to identify glaucoma stage (365.70-365.74)

365.63 Glaucoma associated with vascular disorders
Use additional code to identify glaucoma stage (365.70-365.74)

365.64 Glaucoma associated with tumors or cysts

365.65 Glaucoma associated with ocular trauma
Use additional code to identify glaucoma stage (365.70-365.74)

✓5ᵗʰ **365.7 Glaucoma stage**
Code first associated type of glaucoma (365.10-365.13, 365.20, 365.23, 365.31, 365.52, 365.62-365.63, 365.65)

365.70 Glaucoma stage, unspecified
Glaucoma stage NOS

365.71 Mild stage glaucoma
Early stage glaucoma

365.72 Moderate stage glaucoma

365.73 Severe stage glaucoma
Advanced stage glaucoma
End-stage glaucoma

365.74 Indeterminate stage glaucoma

✓5ᵗʰ **365.8 Other specified forms of glaucoma**

365.81 Hypersecretion glaucoma

365.82 Glaucoma with increased episcleral venous pressure

365.83 Aqueous misdirection
Malignant glaucoma

> **DEF:** A form of secondary angle-closure glaucoma that occurs when aqueous humor flows into the posterior chamber of the eye (vitreous) rather than through the normal recycling channels.

365.89 Other specified glaucoma

365.9 Unspecified glaucoma

✓4ᵗʰ **366 Cataract**
> *EXCLUDES* congenital cataract (743.30-743.34)

> **DEF:** A variety of conditions that create a cloudy, or calcified lens that obstructs vision.

✓5ᵗʰ **366.0 Infantile, juvenile, and presenile cataract**

366.00 Nonsenile cataract, unspecified

366.01 Anterior subcapsular polar cataract
> **DEF:** Defect within the front, center lens surface.

366.02 Posterior subcapsular polar cataract
> **DEF:** Defect within the rear, center lens surface.

366.03 Cortical, lamellar, or zonular cataract
> **DEF:** Opacities radiating from center to edge of lens; appear as thin, concentric layers of lens.

366.04 Nuclear cataract

366.09 Other and combined forms of nonsenile cataract

✓5ᵗʰ **366.1 Senile cataract**

366.10 Senile cataract, unspecified

366.11 Pseudoexfoliation of lens capsule

366.12 Incipient cataract

Cataract:	Cataract:
coronary	punctate
immature NOS	Water clefts

> **DEF:** Minor disorders of lens not affecting vision; due to aging.

366.13 Anterior subcapsular polar senile cataract

366.14 Posterior subcapsular polar senile cataract

366.15 Cortical senile cataract

366.16 Nuclear sclerosis
Cataracta brunescens
Nuclear cataract

366.17 Total or mature cataract

366.18 Hypermature cataract
Morgagni cataract

366.19 Other and combined forms of senile cataract

✓5ᵗʰ **366.2 Traumatic cataract**

366.20 Traumatic cataract, unspecified

366.21 Localized traumatic opacities
Vossius' ring

366.22 Total traumatic cataract

366.23 Partially resolved traumatic cataract

✓5ᵗʰ **366.3 Cataract secondary to ocular disorders**

366.30 Cataracta complicata, unspecified

366.31 Glaucomatous flecks (subcapsular)
Code first underlying glaucoma (365.0-365.9)

366.32 Cataract in inflammatory disorders
Code first underlying condition, as:
chronic choroiditis (363.0-363.2)

366.33 Cataract with neovascularization
Code first underlying condition, as:
chronic iridocyclitis (364.10)

366.34 Cataract in degenerative disorders
Sunflower cataract
Code first underlying condition, as:
chalcosis (360.24)
degenerative myopia (360.21)
pigmentary retinal dystrophy (362.74)

✓5ᵗʰ **366.4 Cataract associated with other disorders**

366.41 *Diabetic cataract*
Code first diabetes (249.5, 250.5)

366.42 *Tetanic cataract*
Code first underlying disease, as:
calcinosis (275.4)
hypoparathyroidism (252.1)

366.43 *Myotonic cataract*
Code first underlying disorder (359.21, 359.23)

366.44 *Cataract associated with other syndromes*
Code first underlying condition, as:
craniofacial dysostosis (756.0)
galactosemia (271.1)

366.45 Toxic cataract
Drug-induced cataract
Use additional E code to identify drug or other toxic substance

366.46 Cataract associated with radiation and other physical influences
Use additional E code to identify cause

√5ᵗʰ **366.5 After-cataract**

366.50 After-cataract, unspecified
Secondary cataract NOS

366.51 Soemmering's ring
DEF: A donut-shaped lens remnant and a capsule behind the pupil as a result of cataract surgery or trauma.

366.52 Other after-cataract, not obscuring vision

366.53 After-cataract, obscuring vision

366.8 Other cataract
Calcification of lens

366.9 Unspecified cataract

√4ᵗʰ **367 Disorders of refraction and accommodation**

367.0 Hypermetropia
Far-sightedness   Hyperopia
DEF: Refraction error, called also hyperopia, focal point is posterior to retina; abnormally short anteroposterior diameter or subnormal refractive power; causes farsightedness.

367.1 Myopia
Near-sightedness
DEF: Refraction error, focal point is anterior to retina; causes near-sightedness.

√5ᵗʰ **367.2 Astigmatism**

367.20 Astigmatism, unspecified

367.21 Regular astigmatism

367.22 Irregular astigmatism

√5ᵗʰ **367.3 Anisometropia and aniseikonia**

367.31 Anisometropia
DEF: Eyes with refractive powers that differ by at least one diopter.

367.32 Aniseikonia
DEF: Eyes with unequal retinal imaging; usually due to refractive error.

367.4 Presbyopia
DEF: Loss of crystalline lens elasticity; causes errors of accommodation; due to aging.

√5ᵗʰ **367.5 Disorders of accommodation**

367.51 Paresis of accommodation
Cycloplegia
DEF: Partial paralysis of ciliary muscle, causing focus problems.

367.52 Total or complete internal ophthalmoplegia
DEF: Total paralysis of ciliary muscle; large pupil incapable of focus.

367.53 Spasm of accommodation
DEF: Abnormal contraction of ciliary muscle; causes focus problems.

√5ᵗʰ **367.8 Other disorders of refraction and accommodation**

367.81 Transient refractive change

367.89 Other
Drug-induced ⎫ disorders of refraction and
Toxic   ⎬ accommodation

367.9 Unspecified disorder of refraction and accommodation

√4ᵗʰ **368 Visual disturbances**
EXCLUDES *electrophysiological disturbances (794.11-794.14)*

√5ᵗʰ **368.0 Amblyopia ex anopsia**
DEF: Vision impaired due to disuse; esotropia often cause.

368.00 Amblyopia, unspecified

368.01 Strabismic amblyopia
Suppression amblyopia

368.02 Deprivation amblyopia
DEF: Decreased vision associated with suppressed retinal image of one eye.

368.03 Refractive amblyopia

√5ᵗʰ **368.1 Subjective visual disturbances**

368.10 Subjective visual disturbance, unspecified

368.11 Sudden visual loss

368.12 Transient visual loss
Concentric fading   Scintillating scotoma

368.13 Visual discomfort
Asthenopia   Photophobia
Eye strain

368.14 Visual distortions of shape and size
Macropsia   Micropsia
Metamorphopsia

368.15 Other visual distortions and entoptic phenomena
Photopsia   Refractive:
Refractive: polyopia
  diplopia   Visual halos

368.16 Psychophysical visual disturbances
Prosopagnosia
Visual:
  agnosia
  disorientation syndrome
  hallucinations
  object agnosia

368.2 Diplopia
Double vision

√5ᵗʰ **368.3 Other disorders of binocular vision**

368.30 Binocular vision disorder, unspecified

368.31 Suppression of binocular vision

368.32 Simultaneous visual perception without fusion

368.33 Fusion with defective stereopsis
DEF: Faulty depth perception though normal ability to focus.

368.34 Abnormal retinal correspondence

√5ᵗʰ **368.4 Visual field defects**

368.40 Visual field defect, unspecified

368.41 Scotoma involving central area
Scotoma: Scotoma:
  central   paracentral
  centrocecal
DEF: Vision loss (blind spot) in central five degrees of visual field.

368.42 Scotoma of blind spot area
Enlarged: Paracecal scotoma
  angioscotoma
  blind spot

368.43 Sector or arcuate defects
Scotoma: Scotoma:
  arcuate   Seidel
  Bjerrum
DEF: Arc-shaped blind spot caused by retinal nerve damage.

368.44 Other localized visual field defect
Scotoma: Visual field defect:
  NOS   nasal step
  ring   peripheral

368.45 Generalized contraction or constriction

368.46 Homonymous bilateral field defects
Hemianopsia (altitudinal) (homonymous)
Quadrant anopia
DEF: Disorders found in the corresponding vertical halves of the visual fields of both eyes.

368.47 Heteronymous bilateral field defects
Hemianopsia: Hemianopsia:
  binasal   bitemporal
DEF: Disorders in the opposite halves of the visual fields of both eyes.

√5ᵗʰ **368.5 Color vision deficiencies**
Color blindness

368.51 Protan defect
Protanomaly   Protanopia
DEF: Mild difficulty distinguishing green and red hues with shortened spectrum; sex-linked affecting one percent of males.

368.52 Deutan defect
Deuteranomaly   Deuteranopia
DEF: Male-only disorder; difficulty in distinguishing green and red, no shortened spectrum.

368.53 Tritan defect
Tritanomaly   Tritanopia
DEF: Difficulty in distinguishing blue and yellow; occurs often due to drugs, retinal detachment and central nervous system diseases.

368.54 Achromatopsia
Monochromatism (cone) (rod)
DEF: Complete color blindness; caused by disease, injury to retina, optic nerve or pathway.

368.55 Acquired color vision deficiencies

368.59 Other color vision deficiencies

√5ᵗʰ **368.6 Night blindness**
Nyctalopia
DEF: Nyctalopia: disorder of vision in dim light or night blindness.

368.60 Night blindness, unspecified

368.61 Congenital night blindness
Hereditary night blindness
Oguchi's disease

368.62 Acquired night blindness
EXCLUDES that due to vitamin A deficiency (264.5)

368.63 Abnormal dark adaptation curve
Abnormal threshold
Delayed adaptation } of cones or rods

368.69 Other night blindness

368.8 Other specified visual disturbances
Blurred vision NOS

368.9 Unspecified visual disturbance

√4ᵗʰ **369 Blindness and low vision**
Note: Visual impairment refers to a functional limitation of the eye (e.g., limited visual acuity or visual field). It should be distinguished from visual disability, indicating a limitation of the abilities of the individual (e.g., limited reading skills, vocational skills), and from visual handicap, indicating a limitation of personal and socioeconomic indepen- dence (e.g., limited mobility, limited employability).

The levels of impairment defined in the table on the next page are based on the recommendations of the WHO Study Group on Prevention of Blindness (Geneva, November 6-10, 1972; WHO Technical Report Series 518), and of the International Council of Ophthalmology (1976). Note that definitions of blindness vary in different settings. For international reporting WHO defines blindness as profound impairment. This definition can be applied to blindness of one eye (369.1, 369.6) and to blindness of the individual (369.0).

For determination of benefits in the U.S.A., the definition of legal blindness as severe impairment is often used. This definition applies to blindness of the individual only.
EXCLUDES correctable impaired vision due to refractive errors (367.0-367.9)

√5ᵗʰ **369.0 Profound impairment, both eyes**

369.00 Impairment level not further specified
Blindness:
NOS according to WHO definition
both eyes

369.01 Better eye: total impairment; lesser eye: total impairment

369.02 Better eye: near-total impairment; lesser eye: not further specified

369.03 Better eye: near-total impairment; lesser eye: total impairment

369.04 Better eye: near-total impairment; lesser eye: near-total impairment

369.05 Better eye: profound impairment; lesser eye: not further specified

369.06 Better eye: profound impairment; lesser eye: total impairment

369.07 Better eye: profound impairment; lesser eye: near-total impairment

369.08 Better eye: profound impairment; lesser eye: profound impairment

√5ᵗʰ **369.1 Moderate or severe impairment, better eye, profound impairment lesser eye**

369.10 Impairment level not further specified
Blindness, one eye, low vision other eye

369.11 Better eye: severe impairment; lesser eye: blind, not further specified

369.12 Better eye: severe impairment; lesser eye: total impairment

369.13 Better eye: severe impairment; lesser eye: near-total impairment

369.14 Better eye: severe impairment; lesser eye: profound impairment

369.15 Better eye: moderate impairment; lesser eye: blind, not further specified

369.16 Better eye: moderate impairment; lesser eye: total impairment

369.17 Better eye: moderate impairment; lesser eye: near-total impairment

369.18 Better eye: moderate impairment; lesser eye: profound impairment

√5ᵗʰ **369.2 Moderate or severe impairment, both eyes**

369.20 Impairment level not further specified
Low vision, both eyes NOS

369.21 Better eye: severe impairment; lesser eye: not further specified

369.22 Better eye: severe impairment; lesser eye: severe impairment

369.23 Better eye: moderate impairment; lesser eye: not further specified

369.24 Better eye: moderate impairment; lesser eye: severe impairment

369.25 Better eye: moderate impairment; lesser eye: moderate impairment

369.3 Unqualified visual loss, both eyes
EXCLUDES blindness NOS:
legal [U.S.A. definition] (369.4)
WHO definition (369.00)

369.4 Legal blindness, as defined in U.S.A.
Blindness NOS according to U.S.A. definition
EXCLUDES legal blindness with specification of impairment level (369.01-369.08, 369.11-369.14, 369.21-369.22)

√5ᵗʰ **369.6 Profound impairment, one eye**

369.60 Impairment level not further specified
Blindness, one eye

369.61 One eye: total impairment; other eye: not specified

369.62 One eye: total impairment; other eye: near normal vision

369.63 One eye: total impairment; other eye: normal vision

369.64 One eye: near-total impairment; other eye: not specified

Diseases of the Nervous System and Sense Organs

369.65–370.49

369.65 One eye: near-total impairment; other eye: near-normal vision

369.66 One eye: near-total impairment; other eye: normal vision

369.67 One eye: profound impairment; other eye: not specified

369.68 One eye: profound impairment; other eye: near-normal vision

369.69 One eye: profound impairment; other eye: normal vision

√5ᵗʰ **369.7 Moderate or severe impairment, one eye**

369.70 Impairment level not further specified
Low vision, one eye

369.71 One eye: severe impairment; other eye: not specified

369.72 One eye: severe impairment; other eye: near-normal vision

369.73 One eye: severe impairment; other eye: normal vision

369.74 One eye: moderate impairment; other eye: not specified

369.75 One eye: moderate impairment; other eye: near-normal vision

369.76 One eye: moderate impairment; other eye: normal vision

369.8 Unqualified visual loss, one eye

369.9 Unspecified visual loss

√4ᵗʰ **370 Keratitis**

√5ᵗʰ **370.0 Corneal ulcer**
    EXCLUDES *that due to vitamin A deficiency (264.3)*

370.00 Corneal ulcer, unspecified

370.01 Marginal corneal ulcer

370.02 Ring corneal ulcer

370.03 Central corneal ulcer

370.04 Hypopyon ulcer
Serpiginous ulcer
DEF: Corneal ulcer with an accumulation of pus in the eye's anterior chamber.

370.05 Mycotic corneal ulcer
DEF: Fungal infection causing corneal tissue loss.

370.06 Perforated corneal ulcer
DEF: Tissue loss through all layers of cornea.

370.07 Mooren's ulcer
DEF: Tissue loss, with chronic inflammation, at junction of cornea and sclera; seen in elderly.

√5ᵗʰ **370.2 Superficial keratitis without conjunctivitis**
    EXCLUDES *dendritic [herpes simplex] keratitis (054.42)*

370.20 Superficial keratitis, unspecified

370.21 Punctate keratitis
Thygeson's superficial punctate keratitis
DEF: Formation of cellular and fibrinous deposits (keratic precipitates) on posterior surface; deposits develop after injury or iridocyclitis.

370.22 Macular keratitis
Keratitis: Keratitis:
areolar   stellate
nummular   striate

370.23 Filamentary keratitis
DEF: Keratitis characterized by twisted filaments of mucoid material on the cornea's surface.

370.24 Photokeratitis
Snow blindness
Welders' keratitis
DEF: Painful, inflamed cornea; due to extended exposure to ultraviolet light.

Classification		LEVELS OF VISUAL IMPAIRMENT	Additional descriptors which may be encountered
"legal"	WHO	Visual acuity and/or visual field limitation (whichever is worse)	
	(NEAR-) NORMAL VISION	RANGE OF NORMAL VISION 20/10 20/13 20/16 20/20 20/25 2.0 1.6 1.25 1.0 0.8	
		NEAR-NORMAL VISION 20/30 20/40 20/50 20/60 0.7 0.6 0.5 0.4 0.3	
	LOW VISION	MODERATE VISUAL IMPAIRMENT 20/70 20/80 20/100 20/125 20/160 0.25 0.20 0.16 0.12	Moderate low vision
		SEVERE VISUAL IMPAIRMENT 20/200 20/250 20/320 20/400 0.10 0.08 0.06 0.05 Visual field: 20 degrees or less	Severe low vision, "Legal" blindness
LEGAL BLINDNESS (U.S.A.) both eyes	BLINDNESS (WHO) one or both eyes	PROFOUND VISUAL IMPAIRMENT 20/500 20/630 20/800 20/1000 0.04 0.03 0.025 0.02 Count fingers at: less than 3m (10 ft.) Visual field: 10 degrees or less	Profound low vision, Moderate blindness
		NEAR-TOTAL VISUAL IMPAIRMENT Visual acuity: less than 0.02 (20/1000) Count fingers at: 1m (3 ft.) or less Hand movements: 5m (15 ft.) or less Light projection, light perception Visual field: 5 degrees or less	Severe blindness Near-total blindness
		TOTAL VISUAL IMPAIRMENT No light perception (NLP)	Total blindness

Visual acuity refers to best achievable acuity with correction.
Non-listed Snellen fractions may be classified by converting to the nearest decimal equivalent, e.g. 10/200 = 0.05, 6/30 = 0.20.
CF (count fingers) without designation of distance, may be classified to profound impairment.
HM (hand motion) without designation of distance, may be classified to near-total impairment.
Visual field measurements refer to the largest field diameter for a 1/100 white test object.

√5ᵗʰ **370.3 Certain types of keratoconjunctivitis**

370.31 Phlyctenular keratoconjunctivitis
Phlyctenulosis
Use additional code for any associated tuberculosis (017.3)
DEF: Miniature blister on conjunctiva or cornea; associated with tuberculosis and malnutrition disorders.

370.32 Limbar and corneal involvement in vernal conjunctivitis
Use additional code for vernal conjunctivitis (372.13)
DEF: Corneal itching and inflammation in conjunctivitis; often limited to lining of eyelids.

370.33 Keratoconjunctivitis sicca, not specified as Sjögren's
    EXCLUDES *Sjögren's syndrome (710.2)*
DEF: Inflammation of conjunctiva and cornea; characterized by "horny" looking tissue and excess blood in these areas; decreased flow of lacrimal (tear) is a contributing factor.

370.34 Exposure keratoconjunctivitis
DEF: Incomplete closure of eyelid causing dry, inflamed eye.

370.35 Neurotrophic keratoconjunctivitis

√5ᵗʰ **370.4 Other and unspecified keratoconjunctivitis**

370.40 Keratoconjunctivitis, unspecified
Superficial keratitis with conjunctivitis NOS

370.44 *Keratitis or keratoconjunctivitis in exanthema*
Code first underlying condition (050.0-052.9)
    EXCLUDES *herpes simplex (054.43)*
herpes zoster (053.21)
measles (055.71)

370.49 Other
    EXCLUDES *epidemic keratoconjunctivitis (077.1)*

√5ᵗʰ **370.5 Interstitial and deep keratitis**

370.50 Interstitial keratitis, unspecified

370.52 Diffuse interstitial keratitis
Cogan's syndrome
DEF: Inflammation of cornea; with deposits in middle corneal layers; may obscure vision.

370.54 Sclerosing keratitis
DEF: Chronic corneal inflammation leading to opaque scarring.

370.55 Corneal abscess
DEF: Pocket of pus and inflammation on the cornea.

370.59 Other
EXCLUDES   *disciform herpes simplex keratitis (054.43)*
syphilitic keratitis (090.3)

√5ᵗʰ **370.6 Corneal neovascularization**

370.60 Corneal neovascularization, unspecified

370.61 Localized vascularization of cornea
DEF: Limited infiltration of cornea by new blood vessels.

370.62 Pannus (corneal)
DEF: Buildup of superficial vascularization and granulated tissue under epithelium of cornea.

370.63 Deep vascularization of cornea
DEF: Deep infiltration of cornea by new blood vessels.

370.64 Ghost vessels (corneal)

370.8 Other forms of keratitis
Code first underlying condition, such as:
Acanthamoeba (136.21)
Fusarium (118)

370.9 Unspecified keratitis

√4ᵗʰ **371 Corneal opacity and other disorders of cornea**

√5ᵗʰ **371.0 Corneal scars and opacities**
EXCLUDES   *that due to vitamin A deficiency (264.6)*

371.00 Corneal opacity, unspecified
Corneal scar NOS

371.01 Minor opacity of cornea
Corneal nebula

371.02 Peripheral opacity of cornea
Corneal macula not interfering with central vision

371.03 Central opacity of cornea
Corneal:
leucoma ⎫ interfering with central
macula ⎭ vision

371.04 Adherent leucoma
DEF: Dense, opaque corneal growth adhering to the iris; also spelled as leukoma.

371.05 *Phthisical cornea*
Code first underlying tuberculosis (017.3)

√5ᵗʰ **371.1 Corneal pigmentations and deposits**

371.10 Corneal deposit, unspecified

371.11 Anterior pigmentations
Stähli's lines

371.12 Stromal pigmentations
Hematocornea

371.13 Posterior pigmentations
Krukenberg spindle

371.14 Kayser-Fleischer ring
DEF: Copper deposits forming ring at outer edge of cornea; seen in Wilson's disease and other liver disorders.

371.15 Other deposits associated with metabolic disorders

371.16 Argentous deposits
DEF: Silver deposits in cornea.

√5ᵗʰ **371.2 Corneal edema**

371.20 Corneal edema, unspecified

371.21 Idiopathic corneal edema
DEF: Corneal swelling and fluid retention of unknown cause.

371.22 Secondary corneal edema
DEF: Corneal swelling and fluid retention caused by an underlying disease, injury, or condition.

371.23 Bullous keratopathy
DEF: Corneal degeneration; characterized by recurring, rupturing epithelial "blisters;" ruptured blebs expose corneal nerves; occurs in glaucoma, iridocyclitis and Fuchs' epithelial dystrophy.

371.24 Corneal edema due to wearing of contact lenses

√5ᵗʰ **371.3 Changes of corneal membranes**

371.30 Corneal membrane change, unspecified

371.31 Folds and rupture of Bowman's membrane

371.32 Folds in Descemet's membrane

371.33 Rupture in Descemet's membrane

√5ᵗʰ **371.4 Corneal degenerations**

371.40 Corneal degeneration, unspecified

371.41 Senile corneal changes
Arcus senilis   Hassall-Henle bodies

371.42 Recurrent erosion of cornea
EXCLUDES   *Mooren's ulcer (370.07)*

371.43 Band-shaped keratopathy
DEF: Horizontal bands of superficial corneal calcium deposits.

371.44 Other calcerous degenerations of cornea

371.45 Keratomalacia NOS
EXCLUDES   *that due to vitamin A deficiency (264.4)*
DEF: Destruction of the cornea by keratinization of the epithelium with ulceration and perforation of the cornea; seen in cases of vitamin A deficiency.

371.46 Nodular degeneration of cornea
Salzmann's nodular dystrophy

371.48 Peripheral degenerations of cornea
Marginal degeneration of cornea [Terrien's]

371.49 Other
Discrete colliquative keratopathy

√5ᵗʰ **371.5 Hereditary corneal dystrophies**
DEF: Genetic disorder; leads to opacities, edema or lesions of cornea.

371.50 Corneal dystrophy, unspecified

371.51 Juvenile epithelial corneal dystrophy

371.52 Other anterior corneal dystrophies
Corneal dystrophy: Corneal dystrophy:
microscopic cystic   ring-like

371.53 Granular corneal dystrophy

371.54 Lattice corneal dystrophy

371.55 Macular corneal dystrophy

371.56 Other stromal corneal dystrophies
Crystalline corneal dystrophy

371.57 Endothelial corneal dystrophy
Combined corneal dystrophy
Cornea guttata
Fuchs' endothelial dystrophy

371.58 Other posterior corneal dystrophies
Polymorphous corneal dystrophy

Diseases of the Nervous System and Sense Organs

371.6–372.52

√5ᵗʰ **371.6 Keratoconus**

>**DEF:** Bilateral bulging protrusion of anterior cornea; often due to noninflammatory thinning.

371.60 Keratoconus, unspecified

371.61 Keratoconus, stable condition

371.62 Keratoconus, acute hydrops

√5ᵗʰ **371.7 Other corneal deformities**

371.70 Corneal deformity, unspecified

371.71 Corneal ectasia

>**DEF:** Bulging protrusion of thinned, scarred cornea.

371.72 Descemetocele

>**DEF:** Protrusion of Descemet's membrane into cornea.

371.73 Corneal staphyloma

>**DEF:** Protrusion of cornea into adjacent tissue.

√5ᵗʰ **371.8 Other corneal disorders**

371.81 Corneal anesthesia and hypoesthesia

>**DEF:** Decreased or absent sensitivity of cornea.

371.82 Corneal disorder due to contact lens

>**EXCLUDES** corneal edema due to contact lens (371.24)
>
>**DEF:** Contact lens wear causing cornea disorder, excluding swelling.

371.89 Other

371.9 Unspecified corneal disorder

√4ᵗʰ **372 Disorders of conjunctiva**

>**EXCLUDES** keratoconjunctivitis (370.3-370.4)

√5ᵗʰ **372.0 Acute conjunctivitis**

372.00 Acute conjunctivitis, unspecified

372.01 Serous conjunctivitis, except viral

>**EXCLUDES** viral conjunctivitis NOS (077.9)

372.02 Acute follicular conjunctivitis
>Conjunctival folliculosis NOS
>
>**EXCLUDES** conjunctivitis:
>   adenoviral (acute follicular) (077.3)
>   epidemic hemorrhagic (077.4)
>   inclusion (077.0)
>   Newcastle (077.8)
>   epidemic keratoconjunctivitis (077.1)
>   pharyngoconjunctival fever (077.2)
>
>**DEF:** Severe conjunctival inflammation with dense infiltrations of lymphoid tissues of inner eyelids; may be traced to a viral or chlamydial etiology.

372.03 Other mucopurulent conjunctivitis
>Catarrhal conjunctivitis
>
>**EXCLUDES** blennorrhea neonatorum (gonococcal) (098.40)
>   neonatal conjunctivitis (771.6)
>   ophthalmia neonatorum NOS (771.6)

372.04 Pseudomembranous conjunctivitis
>Membranous conjunctivitis
>
>**EXCLUDES** diphtheritic conjunctivitis (032.81)
>
>**DEF:** Severe inflammation of conjunctiva; false membrane develops on inner surface of eyelid; membrane can be removed without harming epithelium, due to bacterial infections, toxic and allergic factors, and viral infections.

372.05 Acute atopic conjunctivitis

>**DEF:** Sudden, severe conjunctivitis due to allergens.

372.06 Acute chemical conjunctivitis
>Acute toxic conjunctivitis
>Use additional E code to identify the chemical or toxic agent
>
>**EXCLUDES** burn of eye and adnexa (940.0-940.9)
>   chemical corrosion injury of eye (940.2-940.3)

√5ᵗʰ **372.1 Chronic conjunctivitis**

372.10 Chronic conjunctivitis, unspecified

372.11 Simple chronic conjunctivitis

372.12 Chronic follicular conjunctivitis

>**DEF:** Persistent conjunctival inflammation with dense, localized infiltrations of lymphoid tissues of inner eyelids.

372.13 Vernal conjunctivitis

372.14 Other chronic allergic conjunctivitis

372.15 Parasitic conjunctivitis

>Code first underlying disease, as:
>   filariasis (125.0-125.9)
>   mucocutaneous leishmaniasis (085.5)

√5ᵗʰ **372.2 Blepharoconjunctivitis**

372.20 Blepharoconjunctivitis, unspecified

372.21 Angular blepharoconjunctivitis

>**DEF:** Inflammation at junction of upper and lower eyelids; may block lacrimal secretions.

372.22 Contact blepharoconjunctivitis

√5ᵗʰ **372.3 Other and unspecified conjunctivitis**

372.30 Conjunctivitis, unspecified

372.31 Rosacea conjunctivitis

>Code first underlying rosacea dermatitis (695.3)

372.33 Conjunctivitis in mucocutaneous disease

>Code first underlying disease, as:
>   erythema multiforme (695.10-695.19)
>   Reiter's disease (099.3)
>
>**EXCLUDES** ocular pemphigoid (694.61)

372.34 Pingueculitis

>**EXCLUDES** pinguecula (372.51)

372.39 Other

√5ᵗʰ **372.4 Pterygium**

>**EXCLUDES** pseudopterygium (372.52)
>
>**DEF:** Wedge-shaped, conjunctival thickening that advances from the inner corner of the eye toward the cornea.

372.40 Pterygium, unspecified

372.41 Peripheral pterygium, stationary

372.42 Peripheral pterygium, progressive

372.43 Central pterygium

372.44 Double pterygium

372.45 Recurrent pterygium

√5ᵗʰ **372.5 Conjunctival degenerations and deposits**

372.50 Conjunctival degeneration, unspecified

372.51 Pinguecula

>**EXCLUDES** pingueculitis (372.34)
>
>**DEF:** Proliferative spot on the bulbar conjunctiva located near the sclerocorneal junction, usually on the nasal side; it is seen in elderly people.

372.52 Pseudopterygium

>**DEF:** Conjunctival scar joined to the cornea; it looks like a pterygium but is not attached to the tissue.

372.53 Conjunctival xerosis

EXCLUDES *conjunctival xerosis due to vitamin A deficiency (264.0, 264.1, 264.7)*

DEF: Dry conjunctiva due to vitamin A deficiency; related to Bitot's spots; may develop into xerophthalmia and keratomalacia.

372.54 Conjunctival concretions

DEF: Calculus or deposit on conjunctiva.

372.55 Conjunctival pigmentations
Conjunctival argyrosis

DEF: Color deposits in conjunctiva.

372.56 Conjunctival deposits

√5th **372.6 Conjunctival scars**

372.61 Granuloma of conjunctiva

372.62 Localized adhesions and strands of conjunctiva

DEF: Abnormal fibrous connections in conjunctiva.

372.63 Symblepharon
Extensive adhesions of conjunctiva

DEF: Adhesion of the eyelids to the eyeball.

372.64 Scarring of conjunctiva
Contraction of eye socket (after enucleation)

√5th **372.7 Conjunctival vascular disorders and cysts**

372.71 Hyperemia of conjunctiva

DEF: Conjunctival blood vessel congestion causing eye redness.

372.72 Conjunctival hemorrhage
Hyposphagma
Subconjunctival hemorrhage

372.73 Conjunctival edema
Chemosis of conjunctiva
Subconjunctival edema

DEF: Fluid retention and swelling in conjunctival tissue.

372.74 Vascular abnormalities of conjunctiva
Aneurysm(ata) of conjunctiva

372.75 Conjunctival cysts

DEF: Abnormal sacs of fluid in conjunctiva.

√5th **372.8 Other disorders of conjunctiva**

372.81 Conjunctivochalasis

DEF: Bilateral condition of redundant conjunctival tissue between globe and lower eyelid margin; may cover lower punctum, interfering with normal tearing.

372.89 Other disorders of conjunctiva

372.9 Unspecified disorder of conjunctiva

√4th **373 Inflammation of eyelids**

√5th **373.0 Blepharitis**

EXCLUDES *blepharoconjunctivitis (372.20-372.22)*

373.00 Blepharitis, unspecified

373.01 Ulcerative blepharitis

373.02 Squamous blepharitis

√5th **373.1 Hordeolum and other deep inflammation of eyelid**

DEF: Purulent, localized, staphylococcal infection in sebaceous glands of eyelids.

373.11 Hordeolum externum
Hordeolum NOSStye

DEF: Infection of the oil glands in the eyelash follicles.

373.12 Hordeolum internum
Infection of meibomian gland

DEF: Infection of the oil gland of the eyelid margin.

373.13 Abscess of eyelid
Furuncle of eyelid

DEF: Inflamed pocket of pus on the eyelid.

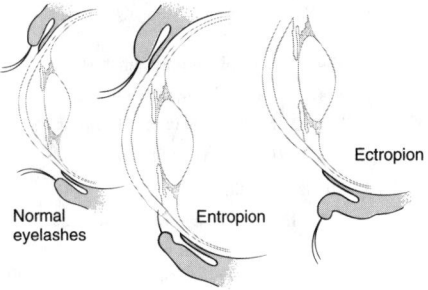

Entropion and Ectropion

Normal eyelashes   Entropion   Ectropion

373.2 Chalazion
Meibomian (gland) cyst

EXCLUDES *infected meibomian gland (373.12)*

DEF: Chronic inflammation of the meibomian gland, causing an eyelid mass.

√5th **373.3 Noninfectious dermatoses of eyelid**

373.31 Eczematous dermatitis of eyelid

373.32 Contact and allergic dermatitis of eyelid

373.33 Xeroderma of eyelid

373.34 Discoid lupus erythematosus of eyelid

373.4 Infective dermatitis of eyelid of types resulting in deformity

Code first underlying disease, as:
leprosy (030.0-030.9)
lupus vulgaris (tuberculous) (017.0)
yaws (102.0-102.9)

373.5 Other infective dermatitis of eyelid

Code first underlying disease, as:
actinomycosis (039.3)
impetigo (684)
mycotic dermatitis (110.0-111.9)
vaccinia (051.0)
postvaccination (999.0)

EXCLUDES *herpes:*
simplex (054.41)
zoster (053.20)

373.6 Parasitic infestation of eyelid

Code first underlying disease, as:
leishmaniasis (085.0-085.9)
loiasis (125.2)
onchocerciasis (125.3)
pediculosis (132.0)

373.8 Other inflammations of eyelids

373.9 Unspecified inflammation of eyelid

√4th **374 Other disorders of eyelids**

√5th **374.0 Entropion and trichiasis of eyelid**

DEF: Entropion: turning inward of eyelid edge toward eyeball.

DEF: Trichiasis: ingrowing eyelashes marked by irritation with possible distortion of sight.

374.00 Entropion, unspecified

374.01 Senile entropion

374.02 Mechanical entropion

374.03 Spastic entropion

374.04 Cicatricial entropion

374.05 Trichiasis without entropion

√5th **374.1 Ectropion**

DEF: Turning outward (eversion) of eyelid edge; exposes palpebral conjunctiva; dryness irritation result.

374.10 Ectropion, unspecified

374.11 Senile ectropion

374.12 Mechanical ectropion

374.13 Spastic ectropion

374.14 Cicatricial ectropion

√5ᵗʰ **374.2 Lagophthalmos**

> **DEF:** Incomplete closure of eyes; causes dry eye and other complications.

374.20 Lagophthalmos, unspecified

374.21 Paralytic lagophthalmos

374.22 Mechanical lagophthalmos

374.23 Cicatricial lagophthalmos

√5ᵗʰ **374.3 Ptosis of eyelid**

374.30 Ptosis of eyelid, unspecified

374.31 Paralytic ptosis

> **DEF:** Drooping of upper eyelid due to nerve disorder.

374.32 Myogenic ptosis

> **DEF:** Drooping of upper eyelid due to muscle disorder.

374.33 Mechanical ptosis

> **DEF:** Outside force causes drooping of upper eyelid.

374.34 Blepharochalasis
Pseudoptosis

> **DEF:** Loss of elasticity, thickened or indurated skin of eyelids associated with recurrent episodes of idiopathic edema causing intracellular tissue atrophy.

√5ᵗʰ **374.4 Other disorders affecting eyelid function**

> EXCLUDES   *blepharoclonus (333.81)*
> *blepharospasm (333.81)*
> *facial nerve palsy (351.0)*
> *third nerve palsy or paralysis (378.51-378.52)*
> *tic (psychogenic) (307.20-307.23)*
> *organic (333.3)*

374.41 Lid retraction or lag

374.43 Abnormal innervation syndrome
Jaw-blinking
Paradoxical facial movements

374.44 Sensory disorders

374.45 Other sensorimotor disorders
Deficient blink reflex

374.46 Blepharophimosis
Ankyloblepharon

> **DEF:** Narrowing of palpebral fissure horizontally; caused by laterally displaced inner canthi; either acquired or congenital.

√5ᵗʰ **374.5 Degenerative disorders of eyelid and periocular area**

374.50 Degenerative disorder of eyelid, unspecified

374.51 *Xanthelasma*
Xanthoma (planum) (tuberosum) of eyelid
Code first underlying condition (272.0-272.9)

> **DEF:** Fatty tumors of the eyelid linked to high fat content of blood.

374.52 Hyperpigmentation of eyelid
Chloasma
Dyspigmentation

> **DEF:** Excess pigment of eyelid.

374.53 Hypopigmentation of eyelid
Vitiligo of eyelid

> **DEF:** Lack of color pigment of the eyelid.

374.54 Hypertrichosis of eyelid

> **DEF:** Excessive eyelash growth.

374.55 Hypotrichosis of eyelid
Madarosis of eyelid

> **DEF:** Less than normal, or absent, eyelashes.

374.56 Other degenerative disorders of skin affecting eyelid

√5ᵗʰ **374.8 Other disorders of eyelid**

374.81 Hemorrhage of eyelid

> EXCLUDES   *black eye (921.0)*

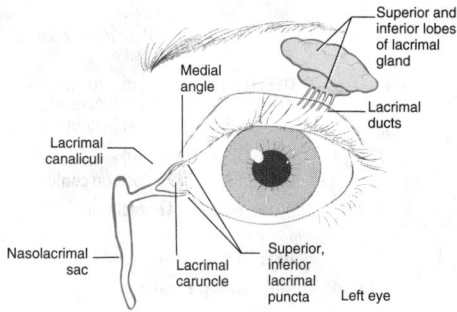

Lacrimal System

374.82 Edema of eyelid
Hyperemia of eyelid

> **DEF:** Swelling and fluid retention in eyelid.

374.83 Elephantiasis of eyelid

> **DEF:** Filarial disease causing dermatitis and enlargement of eyelid.

374.84 Cysts of eyelids
Sebaceous cyst of eyelid

374.85 Vascular anomalies of eyelid

374.86 Retained foreign body of eyelid

> Use additional code to identify foreign body (V90.01-V90.9)

374.87 Dermatochalasis

> **DEF:** Acquired form of connective tissue disorder associated with decreased elastic tissue and abnormal elastin formation resulting in loss of elasticity of the skin of the eyelid, generally associated with aging.

374.89 Other disorders of eyelid

374.9 Unspecified disorder of eyelid

√4ᵗʰ **375 Disorders of lacrimal system**

√5ᵗʰ **375.0 Dacryoadenitis**

375.00 Dacryoadenitis, unspecified

375.01 Acute dacryoadenitis

> **DEF:** Severe, sudden inflammation of the lacrimal gland.

375.02 Chronic dacryoadenitis

> **DEF:** Persistent inflammation of the lacrimal gland.

375.03 Chronic enlargement of lacrimal gland

√5ᵗʰ **375.1 Other disorders of lacrimal gland**

375.11 Dacryops

> **DEF:** Overproduction and constant flow of tears; may cause distended lacrimal duct.

375.12 Other lacrimal cysts and cystic degeneration

375.13 Primary lacrimal atrophy

375.14 Secondary lacrimal atrophy

> **DEF:** Wasting away of the lacrimal gland due to another disease.

375.15 Tear film insufficiency, unspecified
Dry eye syndrome

> **DEF:** Eye dryness and irritation from insufficient tear production.

375.16 Dislocation of lacrimal gland

√5ᵗʰ **375.2 Epiphora**

> **DEF:** Abnormal development of tears due to stricture of lacrimal passages.

375.20 Epiphora, unspecified as to cause

375.21 Epiphora due to excess lacrimation

> **DEF:** Tear overflow due to overproduction.

375.22 Epiphora due to insufficient drainage

> **DEF:** Tear overflow due to blocked drainage.

√5ᵗʰ **375.3** **Acute and unspecified inflammation of lacrimal passages**
   EXCLUDES *neonatal dacryocystitis (771.6)*
   375.30 **Dacryocystitis, unspecified**
   375.31 **Acute canaliculitis, lacrimal**
   375.32 **Acute dacryocystitis**
      Acute peridacryocystitis
   375.33 **Phlegmonous dacryocystitis**
      DEF: Infection of the tear sac with pockets of pus.

√5ᵗʰ **375.4** **Chronic inflammation of lacrimal passages**
   375.41 **Chronic canaliculitis**
   375.42 **Chronic dacryocystitis**
   375.43 **Lacrimal mucocele**

√5ᵗʰ **375.5** **Stenosis and insufficiency of lacrimal passages**
   375.51 **Eversion of lacrimal punctum**
      DEF: Abnormal turning outward of the tear duct.
   375.52 **Stenosis of lacrimal punctum**
      DEF: Abnormal narrowing of the tear duct.
   375.53 **Stenosis of lacrimal canaliculi**
   375.54 **Stenosis of lacrimal sac**
      DEF: Abnormal narrowing of the tear sac.
   375.55 **Obstruction of nasolacrimal duct, neonatal**
      EXCLUDES *congenital anomaly of nasolacrimal duct (743.65)*
      DEF: Acquired abnormal obstruction of tear drainage system from the eye to the nose; in an infant.
   375.56 **Stenosis of nasolacrimal duct, acquired**
   375.57 **Dacryolith**
      DEF: Concretion or stone anywhere in lacrimal system.

√5ᵗʰ **375.6** **Other changes of lacrimal passages**
   375.61 **Lacrimal fistula**
      DEF: Abnormal communication from the lacrimal system.
   375.69 **Other**

√5ᵗʰ **375.8** **Other disorders of lacrimal system**
   375.81 **Granuloma of lacrimal passages**
      DEF: Abnormal nodules within lacrimal system.
   375.89 **Other**

375.9 **Unspecified disorder of lacrimal system**

√4ᵗʰ **376** **Disorders of the orbit**

√5ᵗʰ **376.0** **Acute inflammation of orbit**
   376.00 **Acute inflammation of orbit, unspecified**
   376.01 **Orbital cellulitis**
      Abscess of orbit
      DEF: Infection of tissue between the orbital bone and eyeball.
   376.02 **Orbital periostitis**
      DEF: Inflammation of connective tissue covering the orbital bone.
   376.03 **Orbital osteomyelitis**
      DEF: Inflammation of the orbital bone.
   376.04 **Tenonitis**

√5ᵗʰ **376.1** **Chronic inflammatory disorders of orbit**
   376.10 **Chronic inflammation of orbit, unspecified**
   376.11 **Orbital granuloma**
      Pseudotumor (inflammatory) of orbit
      DEF: Abnormal nodule between orbital bone and eyeball.
   376.12 **Orbital myositis**
      DEF: Painful inflammation of the muscles of the eye.

376.13 *Parasitic infestation of orbit*
   Code first underlying disease, as:
      hydatid infestation of orbit (122.3, 122.6, 122.9)
      myiasis of orbit (134.0)

√5ᵗʰ **376.2** **Endocrine exophthalmos**
   Code first underlying thyroid disorder (242.0-242.9)
   376.21 *Thyrotoxic exophthalmos*
      DEF: Painful inflammation of eye muscles.
   376.22 *Exophthalmic ophthalmoplegia*
      DEF: Inability to rotate eye as a result of bulging eyes.

√5ᵗʰ **376.3** **Other exophthalmic conditions**
   376.30 **Exophthalmos, unspecified**
      DEF: Abnormal protrusion of eyeball.
   376.31 **Constant exophthalmos**
      DEF: Continuous, abnormal protrusion or bulging of eyeball.
   376.32 **Orbital hemorrhage**
      DEF: Bleeding behind the eyeball, causing it to bulge forward.
   376.33 **Orbital edema or congestion**
      DEF: Fluid retention behind eyeball, causing forward bulge.
   376.34 **Intermittent exophthalmos**
   376.35 **Pulsating exophthalmos**
      DEF: Bulge or protrusion; associated with a carotid-cavernous fistula.
   376.36 **Lateral displacement of globe**
      DEF: Abnormal displacement of the eyeball away from nose, toward temple.

√5ᵗʰ **376.4** **Deformity of orbit**
   376.40 **Deformity of orbit, unspecified**
   376.41 **Hypertelorism of orbit**
      DEF: Abnormal increase in interorbital distance; associated with congenital facial deformities; may be accompanied by mental deficiency.
   376.42 **Exostosis of orbit**
      DEF: Abnormal bony growth of orbit.
   376.43 **Local deformities due to bone disease**
      DEF: Acquired abnormalities of orbit; due to bone disease.
   376.44 **Orbital deformities associated with craniofacial deformities**
   376.45 **Atrophy of orbit**
      DEF: Wasting away of bone tissue of orbit.
   376.46 **Enlargement of orbit**
   376.47 **Deformity due to trauma or surgery**

√5ᵗʰ **376.5** **Enophthalmos**
      DEF: Recession of eyeball deep into eye socket.
   376.50 **Enophthalmos, unspecified as to cause**
   376.51 **Enophthalmos due to atrophy of orbital tissue**
   376.52 **Enophthalmos due to trauma or surgery**

376.6 **Retained (old) foreign body following penetrating wound of orbit**
   Retrobulbar foreign body
   Use additional code to identify foreign body (V90.01-V90.9)

√5ᵗʰ **376.8** **Other orbital disorders**
   376.81 **Orbital cysts**
      Encephalocele of orbit
   376.82 **Myopathy of extraocular muscles**
      DEF: Disease in the muscles that control eyeball movement.
   376.89 **Other**

376.9 **Unspecified disorder of orbit**

✓4ᵗʰ **377   Disorders of optic nerve and visual pathways**

✓5ᵗʰ **377.0   Papilledema**

377.00   Papilledema, unspecified

377.01   Papilledema associated with increased intracranial pressure

377.02   Papilledema associated with decreased ocular pressure

377.03   Papilledema associated with retinal disorder

377.04   Foster-Kennedy syndrome

     DEF: Retrobulbar optic neuritis, central scotoma and optic atrophy; caused by tumors in frontal lobe of brain that press downward.

✓5ᵗʰ **377.1   Optic atrophy**

377.10   Optic atrophy, unspecified

377.11   Primary optic atrophy

     EXCLUDES   neurosyphilitic optic atrophy (094.84)

377.12   Postinflammatory optic atrophy

     DEF: Adverse effect of inflammation causing wasting away of eye.

377.13   Optic atrophy associated with retinal dystrophies

     DEF: Progressive changes in retinal tissue due to metabolic disorder causing wasting away of eye.

377.14   Glaucomatous atrophy [cupping] of optic disc

377.15   Partial optic atrophy

     Temporal pallor of optic disc

377.16   Hereditary optic atrophy

     Optic atrophy:
        dominant hereditary
        Leber's

✓5ᵗʰ **377.2   Other disorders of optic disc**

377.21   Drusen of optic disc

377.22   Crater-like holes of optic disc

377.23   Coloboma of optic disc

     DEF: Ocular malformation caused by the failure of fetal fissure of optic stalk to close.

377.24   Pseudopapilledema

✓5ᵗʰ **377.3   Optic neuritis**

     EXCLUDES   meningococcal optic neuritis (036.81)

377.30   Optic neuritis, unspecified

377.31   Optic papillitis

     DEF: Swelling and inflammation of the optic disc.

377.32   Retrobulbar neuritis (acute)

     EXCLUDES   syphilitic retrobulbar neuritis (094.85)

     DEF: Inflammation of optic nerve immediately behind the eyeball.

377.33   Nutritional optic neuropathy

     DEF: Malnutrition causing optic nerve disorder.

377.34   Toxic optic neuropathy

     Toxic amblyopia

     DEF: Toxic substance causing optic nerve disorder.

377.39   Other

     EXCLUDES   ischemic optic neuropathy (377.41)

✓5ᵗʰ **377.4   Other disorders of optic nerve**

377.41   Ischemic optic neuropathy

     DEF: Decreased blood flow affecting optic nerve.

377.42   Hemorrhage in optic nerve sheaths

     DEF: Bleeding in meningeal lining of optic nerve.

377.43   Optic nerve hypoplasia

377.49   Other

     Compression of optic nerve

Eye Musculature

Superior rectus   Superior oblique
Lateral rectus   Medial rectus
Inferior oblique   Inferior rectus

Muscles and actions (right eye)

R.   L.
Monocular (one eye only) esotropia (inward)

Monocular exotropia (outward)

Monocular hypertropia (upward)

✓5ᵗʰ **377.5   Disorders of optic chiasm**

377.51   Associated with pituitary neoplasms and disorders

     DEF: Abnormal pituitary growth causing disruption in nerve chain from retina to brain.

377.52   Associated with other neoplasms

     DEF: Abnormal growth, other than pituitary, causing disruption in nerve chain from retina to brain.

377.53   Associated with vascular disorders

     DEF: Vascular disorder causing disruption in nerve chain from retina to brain.

377.54   Associated with inflammatory disorders

     DEF: Inflammatory disease causing disruption in nerve chain from retina to brain.

✓5ᵗʰ **377.6   Disorders of other visual pathways**

377.61   Associated with neoplasms

377.62   Associated with vascular disorders

377.63   Associated with inflammatory disorders

✓5ᵗʰ **377.7   Disorders of visual cortex**

     EXCLUDES   visual:
        agnosia (368.16)
        hallucinations (368.16)
        halos (368.15)

377.71   Associated with neoplasms

377.72   Associated with vascular disorders

377.73   Associated with inflammatory disorders

377.75   Cortical blindness

     DEF: Blindness due to brain disorder, rather than eye disorder.

377.9   Unspecified disorder of optic nerve and visual pathways

✓4ᵗʰ **378   Strabismus and other disorders of binocular eye movements**

     EXCLUDES   nystagmus and other irregular eye movements (379.50-379.59)

     DEF: Misalignment of the eyes due to imbalance in extraocular muscles.

✓5ᵗʰ **378.0   Esotropia**

     Convergent concomitant strabismus

     EXCLUDES   intermittent esotropia (378.20-378.22)

     DEF: Visual axis deviation created by one eye fixing upon an image and the other eye deviating inward.

378.00   Esotropia, unspecified

378.01   Monocular esotropia

378.02   Monocular esotropia with A pattern

378.03   Monocular esotropia with V pattern

378.04   Monocular esotropia with other noncomitancies

     Monocular esotropia with X or Y pattern

378.05   Alternating esotropia

378.06   Alternating esotropia with A pattern

378.07 **Alternating esotropia with V pattern**

378.08 **Alternating esotropia with other noncomitancies**
　　　　 Alternating esotropia with X or Y pattern

✓5ᵗʰ 378.1 **Exotropia**
　　　　Divergent concomitant strabismus
　　　　EXCLUDES *intermittent exotropia (378.20, 378.23-378.24)*
　　　　DEF: Visual axis deviation created by one eye fixing upon an image and the other eye deviating outward.

378.10 **Exotropia, unspecified**

378.11 **Monocular exotropia**

378.12 **Monocular exotropia with A pattern**

378.13 **Monocular exotropia with V pattern**

378.14 **Monocular exotropia with other noncomitancies**
　　　　 Monocular exotropia with X or Y pattern

378.15 **Alternating exotropia**

378.16 **Alternating exotropia with A pattern**

378.17 **Alternating exotropia with V pattern**

378.18 **Alternating exotropia with other noncomitancies**
　　　　 Alternating exotropia with X or Y pattern

✓5ᵗʰ 378.2 **Intermittent heterotropia**
　　　　EXCLUDES *vertical heterotropia (intermittent) (378.31)*
　　　　DEF: Deviation of eyes seen only at intervals; it is also called strabismus.

378.20 **Intermittent heterotropia, unspecified**
　　　　 Intermittent:
　　　　　 esotropia NOS
　　　　　 exotropia NOS

378.21 **Intermittent esotropia, monocular**

378.22 **Intermittent esotropia, alternating**

378.23 **Intermittent exotropia, monocular**

378.24 **Intermittent exotropia, alternating**

✓5ᵗʰ 378.3 **Other and unspecified heterotropia**

378.30 **Heterotropia, unspecified**

378.31 **Hypertropia**
　　　　 Vertical heterotropia (constant) (intermittent)

378.32 **Hypotropia**

378.33 **Cyclotropia**

378.34 **Monofixation syndrome**
　　　　 Microtropia

378.35 **Accommodative component in esotropia**

✓5ᵗʰ 378.4 **Heterophoria**
　　　　DEF: Deviation occurring only when the other eye is covered.

378.40 **Heterophoria, unspecified**

378.41 **Esophoria**

378.42 **Exophoria**

378.43 **Vertical heterophoria**

378.44 **Cyclophoria**

378.45 **Alternating hyperphoria**

✓5ᵗʰ 378.5 **Paralytic strabismus**
　　　　DEF: Deviation of the eye due to nerve paralysis affecting muscle.

378.50 **Paralytic strabismus, unspecified**

378.51 **Third or oculomotor nerve palsy, partial**

378.52 **Third or oculomotor nerve palsy, total**

378.53 **Fourth or trochlear nerve palsy**

378.54 **Sixth or abducens nerve palsy**

378.55 **External ophthalmoplegia**

378.56 **Total ophthalmoplegia**

✓5ᵗʰ 378.6 **Mechanical strabismus**
　　　　DEF: Deviation of the eye due to an outside force upon the extraocular muscles.

378.60 **Mechanical strabismus, unspecified**

378.61 **Brown's (tendon) sheath syndrome**
　　　　DEF: Congenital or acquired shortening of the anterior sheath of superior oblique muscle; eye is unable to move upward and inward; usually unilateral.

378.62 **Mechanical strabismus from other musculofascial disorders**

378.63 **Limited duction associated with other conditions**

✓5ᵗʰ 378.7 **Other specified strabismus**

378.71 **Duane's syndrome**
　　　　DEF: Congenital, affects one eye; due to abnormal fibrous bands attached to rectus muscle; inability to abduct affected eye with retraction of globe.

378.72 **Progressive external ophthalmoplegia**
　　　　DEF: Paralysis progressing from one eye muscle to another.

378.73 **Strabismus in other neuromuscular disorders**

✓5ᵗʰ 378.8 **Other disorders of binocular eye movements**
　　　　EXCLUDES *nystagmus (379.50-379.56)*

378.81 **Palsy of conjugate gaze**
　　　　DEF: Paralysis progressing from one eye muscle to another.

378.82 **Spasm of conjugate gaze**
　　　　DEF: Muscle contractions impairing parallel movement of eye.

378.83 **Convergence insufficiency or palsy**

378.84 **Convergence excess or spasm**

378.85 **Anomalies of divergence**

378.86 **Internuclear ophthalmoplegia**
　　　　DEF: Eye movement anomaly due to brainstem lesion.

378.87 **Other dissociated deviation of eye movements**
　　　　 Skew deviation

378.9 **Unspecified disorder of eye movements**
　　　　 Ophthalmoplegia NOS　　　　Strabismus NOS

✓4ᵗʰ 379 **Other disorders of eye**

✓5ᵗʰ 379.0 **Scleritis and episcleritis**
　　　　EXCLUDES *syphilitic episcleritis (095.0)*

379.00 **Scleritis, unspecified**
　　　　 Episcleritis NOS

379.01 **Episcleritis periodica fugax**
　　　　DEF: Hyperemia (engorgement) of the sclera and overlying conjunctiva characterized by a sudden onset and short duration.

379.02 **Nodular episcleritis**
　　　　DEF: Inflammation of the outermost layer of the sclera, with formation of nodules.

379.03 **Anterior scleritis**

379.04 **Scleromalacia perforans**
　　　　DEF: Scleral thinning, softening and degeneration; seen with rheumatoid arthritis.

379.05 **Scleritis with corneal involvement**
　　　　 Scleroperikeratitis

379.06 **Brawny scleritis**
　　　　DEF: Severe scleral inflammation with thickening corneal margins.

379.07 **Posterior scleritis**
　　　　 Sclerotenonitis

379.09 **Other**
　　　　 Scleral abscess

Diseases of the Nervous System and Sense Organs

379.1–380.03

√5ᵗʰ **379.1   Other disorders of sclera**
EXCLUDES   blue sclera (743.47)

379.11   Scleral ectasia
Scleral staphyloma NOS
DEF: Protrusion of the contents of the eyeball where the sclera has thinned.

379.12   Staphyloma posticum
DEF: Ring-shaped protrusion or bulging of sclera and uveal tissue at posterior pole of eye.

379.13   Equatorial staphyloma
DEF: Ring-shaped protrusion or bulging of sclera and uveal tissue midway between front and back of eye.

379.14   Anterior staphyloma, localized

379.15   Ring staphyloma

379.16   Other degenerative disorders of sclera

379.19   Other

√5ᵗʰ **379.2   Disorders of vitreous body**
DEF: Disorder of clear gel that fills space between retina and lens.

379.21   Vitreous degeneration
Vitreous: Vitreous:
   cavitation   liquefaction
   detachment

379.22   Crystalline deposits in vitreous
Asteroid hyalitis   Synchysis scintillans

379.23   Vitreous hemorrhage

379.24   Other vitreous opacities
Vitreous floaters

379.25   Vitreous membranes and strands

379.26   Vitreous prolapse
DEF: Slipping of vitreous from normal position.

379.27   Vitreomacular adhesion
Vitreomacular traction
EXCLUDES   traction detachment with vitreoretinal organization (361.81)

379.29   Other disorders of vitreous
EXCLUDES   vitreous abscess (360.04)

√5ᵗʰ **379.3   Aphakia and other disorders of lens**
EXCLUDES   after-cataract (366.50-366.53)

379.31   Aphakia
EXCLUDES   cataract extraction status (V45.61)
DEF: Absence of eye's crystalline lens.

379.32   Subluxation of lens

379.33   Anterior dislocation of lens
DEF: Lens displaced toward iris.

379.34   Posterior dislocation of lens
DEF: Lens displaced backward toward vitreous.

379.39   Other disorders of lens

√5ᵗʰ **379.4   Anomalies of pupillary function**

379.40   Abnormal pupillary function, unspecified

379.41   Anisocoria
DEF: Unequal pupil diameter.

379.42   Miosis (persistent), not due to miotics
DEF: Abnormal contraction of pupil less than 2 mil.

379.43   Mydriasis (persistent), not due to mydriatics
DEF: Morbid dilation of pupil.

379.45   Argyll Robertson pupil, atypical
Argyll Robertson phenomenon or pupil, nonsyphilitic
EXCLUDES   Argyll Robertson pupil (syphilitic) (094.89)
DEF: Failure of pupil to respond to light; affects both eyes; may be caused by diseases such as syphilis of the central nervous system or miosis.

379.46   Tonic pupillary reaction
Adie's pupil or syndrome

379.49   Other
Hippus
Pupillary paralysis

√5ᵗʰ **379.5   Nystagmus and other irregular eye movements**

379.50   Nystagmus, unspecified
DEF: Involuntary, rapid, rhythmic movement of eyeball; vertical, horizontal, rotatory or mixed; cause may be congenital, acquired, physiological, neurological, myopathic, or due to ocular diseases.

379.51   Congenital nystagmus

379.52   Latent nystagmus

379.53   Visual deprivation nystagmus

379.54   Nystagmus associated with disorders of the vestibular system

379.55   Dissociated nystagmus

379.56   Other forms of nystagmus

379.57   Deficiencies of saccadic eye movements
Abnormal optokinetic response
DEF: Saccadic eye movements; small, rapid, involuntary movements by both eyes simultaneously, due to changing point of fixation on visualized object.

379.58   Deficiencies of smooth pursuit movements

379.59   Other irregularities of eye movements
Opsoclonus

√5ᵗʰ **379.6   Inflammation (infection) of postprocedural bleb**
Postprocedural blebitis

379.60   Inflammation (infection) of postprocedural bleb, unspecified

379.61   Inflammation (infection) of postprocedural bleb, stage 1

379.62   Inflammation (infection) of postprocedural bleb, stage 2

379.63   Inflammation (infection) of postprocedural bleb, stage 3
Bleb associated endophthalmitis

379.8   Other specified disorders of eye and adnexa

√5ᵗʰ **379.9   Unspecified disorder of eye and adnexa**

379.90   Disorder of eye, unspecified

379.91   Pain in or around eye

379.92   Swelling or mass of eye

379.93   Redness or discharge of eye

379.99   Other ill-defined disorders of eye
EXCLUDES   blurred vision NOS (368.8)

DISEASES OF THE EAR AND MASTOID PROCESS (380-389)
Use additional external cause code, if applicable, to identify the cause of the ear condition

√4ᵗʰ **380   Disorders of external ear**

√5ᵗʰ **380.0   Perichondritis and chondritis of pinna**
Chondritis of auricle   Perichondritis of auricle

380.00   Perichondritis of pinna, unspecified

380.01   Acute perichondritis of pinna

380.02   Chronic perichondritis of pinna

380.03   Chondritis of pinna
DEF: Infection that has progressed into the cartilage; presents as indurated and edematous skin over the pinna; vascular compromise occurs with tissue necrosis and deformity.

Ear and Mastoid Process

Helix

Antihelix

Concha

Mastoid process

External auditory meatus

Tragus

Antitragus

√5ᵗʰ **380.1 Infective otitis externa**

380.10 Infective otitis externa, unspecified
Otitis externa (acute):
NOS
circumscribed
diffuse
hemorrhagica
infective NOS

380.11 Acute infection of pinna
EXCLUDES   furuncular otitis externa (680.0)

380.12 Acute swimmers' ear
Beach ear   Tank ear
DEF: Otitis externa due to swimming.

380.13 Other acute infection of external ear
Code first underlying disease, as:
erysipelas (035)
impetigo (684)
seborrheic dermatitis (690.10-690.18)
EXCLUDES   herpes simplex (054.73)
herpes zoster (053.71)

380.14 Malignant otitis externa
DEF: Severe necrotic otitis externa; due to bacteria.

380.15 Chronic mycotic otitis externa
Code first underlying disease, as:
aspergillosis (117.3)
otomycosis NOS (111.9)
EXCLUDES   candidal otitis externa (112.82)

380.16 Other chronic infective otitis externa
Chronic infective otitis externa NOS

√5ᵗʰ **380.2 Other otitis externa**

380.21 Cholesteatoma of external ear
Keratosis obturans of external ear (canal)
EXCLUDES   cholesteatoma NOS
(385.30-385.35)
postmastoidectomy (383.32)
DEF: Cystlike mass filled with debris, including cholesterol; rare, congenital condition.

380.22 Other acute otitis externa
Acute otitis externa: Acute otitis externa:
actinic   eczematoid
chemical   reactive
contact

380.23 Other chronic otitis externa
Chronic otitis externa NOS

√5ᵗʰ **380.3 Noninfectious disorders of pinna**

380.30 Disorder of pinna, unspecified

380.31 Hematoma of auricle or pinna

380.32 Acquired deformities of auricle or pinna
EXCLUDES   cauliflower ear (738.7)

380.39 Other
EXCLUDES   gouty tophi of ear (274.81)

380.4 Impacted cerumen
Wax in ear

√5ᵗʰ **380.5 Acquired stenosis of external ear canal**
Collapse of external ear canal

380.50 Acquired stenosis of external ear canal, unspecified as to cause

380.51 Secondary to trauma
DEF: Narrowing of the external ear canal; due to trauma.

380.52 Secondary to surgery
DEF: Postsurgical narrowing of the external ear canal.

380.53 Secondary to inflammation
DEF: Narrowing of the external ear canal; due to chronic inflammation.

√5ᵗʰ **380.8 Other disorders of external ear**

380.81 Exostosis of external ear canal

380.89 Other

380.9 Unspecified disorder of external ear

√4ᵗʰ **381 Nonsuppurative otitis media and Eustachian tube disorders**

√5ᵗʰ **381.0 Acute nonsuppurative otitis media**
Acute tubotympanic catarrh
Otitis media, acute or subacute:
catarrhal
exudative
transudative
with effusion
EXCLUDES   otitic barotrauma (993.0)

381.00 Acute nonsuppurative otitis media, unspecified

381.01 Acute serous otitis media
Acute or subacute secretory otitis media
DEF: Sudden, severe infection of the middle ear.

381.02 Acute mucoid otitis media
Acute or subacute seromucinous otitis media
Blue drum syndrome
DEF: Sudden, severe infection of the middle ear, with mucous.

381.03 Acute sanguinous otitis media
DEF: Sudden, severe infection of the middle ear, with blood.

381.04 Acute allergic serous otitis media

381.05 Acute allergic mucoid otitis media

381.06 Acute allergic sanguinous otitis media

√5ᵗʰ **381.1 Chronic serous otitis media**
Chronic tubotympanic catarrh

381.10 Chronic serous otitis media, simple or unspecified
DEF: Persistent infection of the middle ear, without pus.

381.19 Other
Serosanguinous chronic otitis media

√5ᵗʰ **381.2 Chronic mucoid otitis media**
Glue ear
EXCLUDES   adhesive middle ear disease (385.10-385.19)
DEF: Chronic condition; characterized by viscous fluid in middle ear; due to obstructed Eustachian tube.

381.20 Chronic mucoid otitis media, simple or unspecified

381.29 Other
Mucosanguinous chronic otitis media

381.3 Other and unspecified chronic nonsuppurative otitis media
Otitis media, chronic: Otitis media, chronic:
allergic   seromucinous
exudative   transudative
secretory   with effusion

381.4   Nonsuppurative otitis media, not specified as acute or chronic

Otitis media:	Otitis media:
allergic	secretory
catarrhal	seromucinous
exudative	serous
mucoid	transudative
	with effusion

√5th **381.5   Eustachian salpingitis**

381.50   Eustachian salpingitis, unspecified

381.51   Acute Eustachian salpingitis
> **DEF:** Sudden, severe inflammation of the Eustachian tube.

381.52   Chronic Eustachian salpingitis
> **DEF:** Persistent inflammation of the Eustachian tube.

√5th **381.6   Obstruction of Eustachian tube**

Stenosis } of Eustachian tube
Stricture

381.60   Obstruction of Eustachian tube, unspecified

381.61   Osseous obstruction of Eustachian tube
> Obstruction of Eustachian tube from cholesteatoma, polyp, or other osseous lesion

381.62   Intrinsic cartilaginous obstruction of Eustachian tube
> **DEF:** Blockage of Eustachian tube; due to cartilage overgrowth.

381.63   Extrinsic cartilaginous obstruction of Eustachian tube
> Compression of Eustachian tube

381.7   Patulous Eustachian tube
> **DEF:** Distended, oversized Eustachian tube.

√5th **381.8   Other disorders of Eustachian tube**

381.81   Dysfunction of Eustachian tube

381.89   Other

381.9   Unspecified Eustachian tube disorder

√4th **382   Suppurative and unspecified otitis media**

√5th **382.0   Acute suppurative otitis media**

Otitis media, acute:	Otitis media, acute:
necrotizing NOS	purulent

382.00   Acute suppurative otitis media without spontaneous rupture of ear drum
> **DEF:** Sudden, severe inflammation of middle ear, with pus.

382.01   Acute suppurative otitis media with spontaneous rupture of ear drum
> **DEF:** Sudden, severe inflammation of middle ear, with pressure tearing ear drum tissue.

382.02   *Acute suppurative otitis media in diseases classified elsewhere*
> *Code first underlying disease, as:*
> influenza (487.8, 488.09, 488.19)
> scarlet fever (034.1)
> **EXCLUDES**   *postmeasles otitis (055.2)*

382.1   Chronic tubotympanic suppurative otitis media

Benign chronic suppurative } (with anterior
     ottis media   perforation of
Chronic tubotympanic disease } ear drum)

> **DEF:** Inflammation of tympanic cavity and auditory tube; with pus formation.

382.2   Chronic atticoantral suppurative otitis media

Chronic atticoantral disease } (with posterior or superior
Persistent mucosal disease } maginal perforation
     of ear drum)

> **DEF:** Inflammation of upper tympanic membrane and mastoid antrum with pus formation.

382.3   Unspecified chronic suppurative otitis media
> Chronic purulent otitis media
> **EXCLUDES**   *tuberculous otitis media (017.4)*

382.4   Unspecified suppurative otitis media
> Purulent otitis media NOS

382.9   Unspecified otitis media

Otitis media:	Otitis media:
NOS	chronic NOS
acute NOS	

√4th **383   Mastoiditis and related conditions**

√5th **383.0   Acute mastoiditis**

Abscess of mastoid	Empyema of mastoid

383.00   Acute mastoiditis without complications
> **DEF:** Sudden, severe inflammation of mastoid air cells.

383.01   Subperiosteal abscess of mastoid
> **DEF:** Pocket of pus within the mastoid bone.

383.02   Acute mastoiditis with other complications
> Gradenigo's syndrome

383.1   Chronic mastoiditis

Caries of mastoid	Fistula of mastoid

> **EXCLUDES**   *tuberculous mastoiditis (015.6)*
> **DEF:** Persistent inflammation of the mastoid air cells.

√5th **383.2   Petrositis**

Coalescing osteitis }
Inflammation } of petrous bone
Osteomyelitis }

383.20   Petrositis, unspecified

383.21   Acute petrositis
> **DEF:** Sudden, severe inflammation of dense bone behind the ear.

383.22   Chronic petrositis
> **DEF:** Persistent inflammation of dense bone behind the ear.

√5th **383.3   Complications following mastoidectomy**

383.30   Postmastoidectomy complication, unspecified

383.31   Mucosal cyst of postmastoidectomy cavity
> **DEF:** Mucous-lined cyst cavity following removal of mastoid bone.

383.32   Recurrent cholesteatoma of postmastoidectomy cavity
> **DEF:** Cystlike mass of cell debris in cavity following removal of mastoid bone.

383.33   Granulations of postmastoidectomy cavity
> Chronic inflammation of postmastoidectomy cavity
> **DEF:** Granular tissue in cavity following removal of mastoid bone.

√5th **383.8   Other disorders of mastoid**

383.81   Postauricular fistula
> **DEF:** Abnormal passage behind mastoid cavity.

383.89   Other

383.9   Unspecified mastoiditis

√4th **384   Other disorders of tympanic membrane**

√5th **384.0   Acute myringitis without mention of otitis media**

384.00   Acute myringitis, unspecified
> Acute tympanitis NOS
> **DEF:** Sudden, severe inflammation of ear drum.

384.01   Bullous myringitis
> Myringitis bullosa hemorrhagica
> **DEF:** Type of viral otitis media characterized by the appearance of serous or hemorrhagic blebs on the tympanic membrane.

384.09   Other

384.1 Chronic myringitis without mention of otitis media
Chronic tympanitis
DEF: Persistent inflammation of ear drum; with no evidence of middle ear infection.

√5ᵗʰ **384.2 Perforation of tympanic membrane**
Perforation of ear drum:
  NOS
  persistent posttraumatic
  postinflammatory
  EXCLUDES *otitis media with perforation of tympanic membrane (382.00-382.9)*
    traumatic perforation [current injury] (872.61)

384.20 Perforation of tympanic membrane, unspecified

384.21 Central perforation of tympanic membrane

384.22 Attic perforation of tympanic membrane
Pars flaccida

384.23 Other marginal perforation of tympanic membrane

384.24 Multiple perforations of tympanic membrane

384.25 Total perforation of tympanic membrane

√5ᵗʰ **384.8 Other specified disorders of tympanic membrane**

384.81 Atrophic flaccid tympanic membrane
Healed perforation of ear drum

384.82 Atrophic nonflaccid tympanic membrane

384.9 Unspecified disorder of tympanic membrane

√4ᵗʰ **385 Other disorders of middle ear and mastoid**
  EXCLUDES *mastoiditis (383.0-383.9)*

√5ᵗʰ **385.0 Tympanosclerosis**

385.00 Tympanosclerosis, unspecified as to involvement

385.01 Tympanosclerosis involving tympanic membrane only
DEF: Tough, fibrous tissue impeding functions of ear drum.

385.02 Tympanosclerosis involving tympanic membrane and ear ossicles
DEF: Tough, fibrous tissue impeding functions of middle ear bones (stapes, malleus, incus).

385.03 Tympanosclerosis involving tympanic membrane, ear ossicles, and middle ear
DEF: Tough, fibrous tissue impeding functions of ear drum, middle ear bones and middle ear canal.

385.09 Tympanosclerosis involving other combination of structures

√5ᵗʰ **385.1 Adhesive middle ear disease**
Adhesive otitis   Otitis media:
Otitis media: fibrotic
  chronic adhesive
  EXCLUDES *glue ear (381.20-381.29)*
DEF: Adhesions of middle ear structures.

385.10 Adhesive middle ear disease, unspecified as to involvement

385.11 Adhesions of drum head to incus

385.12 Adhesions of drum head to stapes

385.13 Adhesions of drum head to promontorium

385.19 Other adhesions and combinations

√5ᵗʰ **385.2 Other acquired abnormality of ear ossicles**

385.21 Impaired mobility of malleus
Ankylosis of malleus

385.22 Impaired mobility of other ear ossicles
Ankylosis of ear ossicles, except malleus

385.23 Discontinuity or dislocation of ear ossicles
DEF: Disruption in auditory chain; created by malleus, incus and stapes.

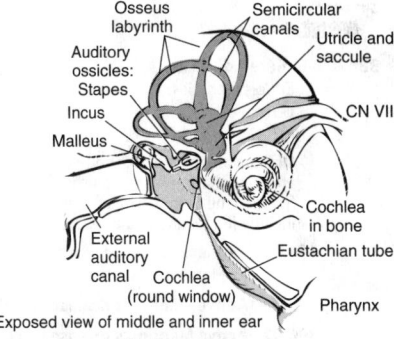

Middle and Inner Ear
Osseous labyrinth
Semicircular canals
Utricle and saccule
Auditory ossicles:
Stapes
Incus
CN VIII
Malleus
Cochlea in bone
Eustachian tube
External auditory canal
Cochlea (round window)
Pharynx
Exposed view of middle and inner ear

Cholesteatoma
Middle ear chamber
Cholesteatoma sac   Ear drum

385.24 Partial loss or necrosis of ear ossicles
DEF: Tissue loss in malleus, incus and stapes.

√5ᵗʰ **385.3 Cholesteatoma of middle ear and mastoid**
Cholesterosis
Epidermosis   } of (middle) ear
Keratosis
Polyp
  EXCLUDES *cholesteatoma:*
    external ear canal (380.21)
    recurrent of postmastoidectomy cavity (383.32)
DEF: Cystlike mass of middle ear and mastoid antrum filled with debris, including cholesterol.

385.30 Cholesteatoma, unspecified

385.31 Cholesteatoma of attic

385.32 Cholesteatoma of middle ear

385.33 Cholesteatoma of middle ear and mastoid
DEF: Cystlike mass of cell debris in middle ear and mastoid air cells behind ear.

385.35 Diffuse cholesteatosis

√5ᵗʰ **385.8 Other disorders of middle ear and mastoid**

385.82 Cholesterin granuloma
DEF: Granuloma formed of fibrotic tissue; contains cholesterol crystals surrounded by foreign-body cells; found in the middle ear and mastoid area.

385.83 Retained foreign body of middle ear
Use additional code to identify foreign body (V90.01-V90.9)

385.89 Other

385.9 Unspecified disorder of middle ear and mastoid

√4ᵗʰ 386 Vertiginous syndromes and other disorders of vestibular system
EXCLUDES vertigo NOS (780.4)

√5ᵗʰ 386.0 Ménière's disease
Endolymphatic hydrops
Lermoyez's syndrome
Ménière's syndrome or vertigo
DEF: Distended membranous labyrinth of middle ear from endolymphatic hydrops; causes ischemia, failure of nerve function; hearing and balance dysfunction; symptoms include fluctuating deafness, ringing in ears and dizziness.

386.00 Ménière's disease, unspecified
Ménière's disease (active)

386.01 Active Ménière's disease, cochleovestibular

386.02 Active Ménière's disease, cochlear

386.03 Active Ménière's disease, vestibular

386.04 Inactive Ménière's disease
Ménière's disease in remission

√5ᵗʰ 386.1 Other and unspecified peripheral vertigo
EXCLUDES epidemic vertigo (078.81)

386.10 Peripheral vertigo, unspecified

386.11 Benign paroxysmal positional vertigo
Benign paroxysmal positional nystagmus

386.12 Vestibular neuronitis
Acute (and recurrent) peripheral vestibulopathy
DEF: Transient benign vertigo, unknown cause; characterized by response to caloric stimulation on one side, nystagmus with rhythmic movement of eyes; normal auditory function present.

386.19 Other
Aural vertigo
Otogenic vertigo

386.2 Vertigo of central origin
Central positional nystagmus
Malignant positional vertigo

√5ᵗʰ 386.3 Labyrinthitis

386.30 Labyrinthitis, unspecified

386.31 Serous labyrinthitis
Diffuse labyrinthitis
DEF: Inflammation of labyrinth; with fluid buildup.

386.32 Circumscribed labyrinthitis
Focal labyrinthitis

386.33 Suppurative labyrinthitis
Purulent labyrinthitis
DEF: Inflammation of labyrinth; with pus.

386.34 Toxic labyrinthitis
DEF: Inflammation of labyrinth; due to toxic reaction.

386.35 Viral labyrinthitis

√5ᵗʰ 386.4 Labyrinthine fistula

386.40 Labyrinthine fistula, unspecified

386.41 Round window fistula

386.42 Oval window fistula

386.43 Semicircular canal fistula

386.48 Labyrinthine fistula of combined sites

√5ᵗʰ 386.5 Labyrinthine dysfunction

386.50 Labyrinthine dysfunction, unspecified

386.51 Hyperactive labyrinth, unilateral
DEF: Abnormal increased sensitivity of labyrinth to stimuli such as sound, pressure or gravitational change, affecting one ear.

386.52 Hyperactive labyrinth, bilateral
DEF: Abnormal increased sensitivity of labyrinth to stimuli such as sound, pressure or gravitational change, affecting one ear.

386.53 Hypoactive labyrinth, unilateral
DEF: Abnormal decreased sensitivity of labyrinth to stimuli such as sound, pressure or gravitational change, affecting one ear.

386.54 Hypoactive labyrinth, bilateral
DEF: Abnormal decreased sensitivity of labyrinth to stimuli such as sound, pressure or gravitational change, affecting both ears.

386.55 Loss of labyrinthine reactivity, unilateral
DEF: Decreased function of the labyrinth sensors, affecting one ear

386.56 Loss of labyrinthine reactivity, bilateral
DEF: Decreased function of the labyrinth sensors, affecting both ears

386.58 Other forms and combinations

386.8 Other disorders of labyrinth

386.9 Unspecified vertiginous syndromes and labyrinthine disorders

√4ᵗʰ 387 Otosclerosis
INCLUDES otospongiosis
DEF: Synonym for otospongiosis, spongy bone formation in the labyrinth bones of the ear; it causes progressive hearing impairment.

387.0 Otosclerosis involving oval window, nonobliterative
DEF: Tough, fibrous tissue impeding functions of oval window.

387.1 Otosclerosis involving oval window, obliterative
DEF: Tough, fibrous tissue blocking oval window.

387.2 Cochlear otosclerosis
Otosclerosis involving:
otic capsule
round window
DEF: Tough, fibrous tissue impeding functions of cochlea.

387.8 Other otosclerosis

387.9 Otosclerosis, unspecified

√4ᵗʰ 388 Other disorders of ear

√5ᵗʰ 388.0 Degenerative and vascular disorders of ear

388.00 Degenerative and vascular disorders, unspecified

388.01 Presbyacusis
DEF: Progressive, bilateral perceptive hearing loss caused by advancing age; it is also known as presbycusis.

388.02 Transient ischemic deafness
DEF: Restricted blood flow to auditory organs causing temporary hearing loss.

√5ᵗʰ 388.1 Noise effects on inner ear

388.10 Noise effects on inner ear, unspecified

388.11 Acoustic trauma (explosive) to ear
Otitic blast injury

388.12 Noise-induced hearing loss

388.2 Sudden hearing loss, unspecified

√5ᵗʰ 388.3 Tinnitus
DEF: Abnormal noises in ear; may be heard by others beside the affected individual; noises include ringing, clicking, roaring and buzzing.

388.30 Tinnitus, unspecified

388.31 Subjective tinnitus

388.32 Objective tinnitus

√5ᵗʰ 388.4 Other abnormal auditory perception

388.40 Abnormal auditory perception, unspecified

388.41 Diplacusis
DEF: Perception of a single auditory sound as two sounds at two different levels of intensity.

388.42 Hyperacusis

DEF: Exceptionally acute sense of hearing caused by such conditions as Bell's palsy; this term may also refer to painful sensitivity to sounds.

388.43 Impairment of auditory discrimination

DEF: Impaired ability to distinguish tone of sound.

388.44 Recruitment

DEF: Perception of abnormally increased loudness caused by a slight increase in sound intensity; it is a term used in audiology.

388.45 Acquired auditory processing disorder

Auditory processing disorder NOS

EXCLUDES central auditory processing disorder (315.32)

DEF: Difficulty in recognizing and interpreting sounds; a failure of the brain to process auditory information; due to neurological problems due to injury, infection, and degenerative conditions.

388.5 Disorders of acoustic nerve

Acoustic neuritis
Degeneration } of acoustic or eighth nerve
Disorder

EXCLUDES acoustic neuroma (225.1)
syphilitic acoustic neuritis (094.86)

√5ᵗʰ **388.6 Otorrhea**

388.60 Otorrhea, unspecified

Discharging ear NOS

388.61 Cerebrospinal fluid otorrhea

EXCLUDES cerebrospinal fluid rhinorrhea (349.81)

DEF: Spinal fluid leakage from ear.

388.69 Other

Otorrhagia

√5ᵗʰ **388.7 Otalgia**

388.70 Otalgia, unspecified

Earache NOS

388.71 Otogenic pain

388.72 Referred pain

388.8 Other disorders of ear

388.9 Unspecified disorder of ear

√4ᵗʰ **389 Hearing loss**

√5ᵗʰ **389.0 Conductive hearing loss**

Conductive deafness

EXCLUDES mixed conductive and sensorineural hearing loss (389.20-389.22)

DEF: Dysfunction in sound-conducting structures of external or middle ear causing hearing loss.

389.00 Conductive hearing loss, unspecified

389.01 Conductive hearing loss, external ear

389.02 Conductive hearing loss, tympanic membrane

389.03 Conductive hearing loss, middle ear

389.04 Conductive hearing loss, inner ear

389.05 Conductive hearing loss, unilateral

389.06 Conductive hearing loss, bilateral

389.08 Conductive hearing loss of combined types

√5ᵗʰ **389.1 Sensorineural hearing loss**

Perceptive hearing loss or deafness

EXCLUDES abnormal auditory perception (388.40-388.44)
mixed conductive and sensorineural hearing loss (389.20-389.22)
psychogenic deafness (306.7)

DEF: Nerve conduction causing hearing loss.

389.10 Sensorineural hearing loss, unspecified

389.11 Sensory hearing loss, bilateral

389.12 Neural hearing loss, bilateral

389.13 Neural hearing loss, unilateral

389.14 Central hearing loss

389.15 Sensorineural hearing loss, unilateral

389.16 Sensorineural hearing loss, asymmetrical

389.17 Sensory hearing loss, unilateral

389.18 Sensorineural hearing loss, bilateral

√5ᵗʰ **389.2 Mixed conductive and sensorineural hearing loss**

Deafness or hearing loss of type classifiable to 389.00-389.08 with type classifiable to 389.10-389.18

389.20 Mixed hearing loss, unspecified

389.21 Mixed hearing loss, unilateral

389.22 Mixed hearing loss, bilateral

389.7 Deaf, non-speaking, not elsewhere classifiable

389.8 Other specified forms of hearing loss

389.9 Unspecified hearing loss

Deafness NOS

Chapter 7: Diseases of the Circulatory System (390–459)

Coding Guidance

Very specific guidelines and instructions affect assignment of codes within this category. Pay careful attention to instruction notes in both the alphabetic index and the tabular list. Many of the conditions within this chapter are complex and interrelated. Physicians may use a variety of terms and phrases to describe a diagnosis.

Acute Rheumatic Fever (390–392)

Rheumatic fever is a febrile disease occurring mainly in children or young adults following throat infection by Group A Streptococci. Symptoms include sudden occurrence of fever and joint pain; followed by lesions of the heart, blood vessels, and joint connective tissue, abdominal pain, skin changes, and chorea.

The instructional notes below each of the subcategories further define and clarify the subcategory. These instructional notes assist the user to assign codes accurately even though a variety of terms and phrases may be used to describe diagnosis. For example, the "Includes" notes below category 390 indicate that the conditions rheumatic arthritis (acute or subacute), rheumatic fever (active or acute), and articular rheumatism (acute or subacute) are included in this category. "Excludes" notes under category 392 indicate that if the medical documentation states the condition to be chorea, NOS, or Huntington's chorea, a code from category 392 is not an appropriate assignment.

Chronic Rheumatic Heart Disease (393–398)

Heart disease as a consequence of acute rheumatic fever commonly involves damage to the heart valves during the acute phase of the streptococcal infection. ICD-9-CM makes the presumption that certain conditions of the mitral valve such as stenosis, stenosis with insufficiency, and failure of unknown etiology are of rheumatic fever origin. None of the disorders of the aortic valve are presumed to be of rheumatic origin, however, and must be specified by documentation as "rheumatic" to be classified to these categories. However, when disorders to both mitral and aortic valves are described with the terms stenosis, stenosis with insufficiency, and failure, then ICD-9-CM presumes rheumatic origin.

Hypertensive Disease (401–405)

Hypertension is the condition of abnormally elevated arterial blood pressure. The blood pressure range considered to be hypertensive varies, but most commonly a 140/ 90 mm. Hg. is considered hypertensive.

Hypertension is classified using three axes: First, by type (i.e., primary or secondary); second is by nature of hypertension (i.e., benign, malignant, or unspecified); and third indicates associated heart disease, renal disease, or both heart and renal disease. Refer to instructional notes in coding hypertension. There are many diagnostic terms used to describe the types of hypertension.

The hypertension table, a complete list of diagnoses associated with or due to hypertension, is located in the alphabetic index under the main term "Hypertension."

Three terms "malignant," "benign," and "unspecified," serve as headings in the table to assist the user to select the most specific code to describe the diagnosis. They are defined as follows:

*   Malignant: This type of hypertension is considered the most severe and difficult to treat. A malignant diagnosis is made when the patient's diastolic blood pressure is consistently greater than 140 and if other clinical features are present, such as cardiac and renal involvement, and neuroretinopathy.
*   Benign: This type of hypertension is considered relatively mild and usually is chronic or occurs over a prolonged period of time.
*   Unspecified: This term is selected when the physician does not specify the type of hypertension as benign or malignant. If the physician has not specified the type, request clarification of the diagnosis.

Essential hypertension (401) is also referred to as primary, idiopathic, or systolic hypertension, and is defined as hypertension without apparent cause. The physician must document in the medical record whether the hypertension is malignant or benign to assign a fourth digit of 0 or 1 respectively. When no entry in the medical record supports either designation, assign a fifth digit of 9, unspecified.

Hypertensive heart disease is assigned to category 402. Chronic elevated blood pressure often produces changes in the heart myocardium as a result of the increased workload against the elevated blood pressure in the vessels. Hypertensive heart disease includes cardiomegaly, cardiopathy, cardiovascular disease, and heart failure. The first axis of coding is the kind of hypertension (i.e., malignant, benign, or unspecified). The second axis indicates hypertension, with or without heart failure.

In order to assign a code from the 402 category, the diagnostic statement must indicate a causal relationship between the hypertension and the heart disease. Phrases such as "due to hypertension" and "hypertensive" indicate a causal relationship. For example, hypertensive heart disease without heart failure, unspecified, is coded 402.90.

A diagnostic statement "with hypertension" does not indicate a casual relationship between the heart disease and the hypertension and the combination code 402 is inappropriate. In this case, code the heart disease and the hypertension separately. For example, congestive heart failure with hypertension, unspecified, is coded 428.0, 401.9.

Heart disease in combination with an associated hypertensive heart condition classifiable to 428, 429.0–429.3, 429.8, 429.9 is presumed by ICD-9-CM to be hypertensive. For example, congestive heart failure with unspecified hypertensive cardiovascular disease is coded 402.91.

A causal relationship between hypertension and kidney disease is assumed when the diagnostic statement indicates both conditions, even though the statement does not specify hypertensive kidney disease. Hypertensive chronic kidney disease is assigned to the category 403. Fourth-digit assignment, as with other hypertension subcategories, indicates malignant (0), benign (1), or unspecified (9). Fifth-digit assignment indicates without mention of chronic kidney disease (0) or with chronic kidney disease (1). To report chronic renal insufficiency (CRI) with hypertension, assign 403.90 Hypertensive chronic kidney disease stage I through stage IV, or unspecified and code 585.9 Chronic kidney disease, unspecified.

Category 404 includes conditions of hypertensive heart and kidney disease. This category is reviewed when the diagnostic statement indicates both hypertensive heart disease (402) and hypertensive kidney disease (403). Fifth-digit assignment in this category indicates the presence of congestive heart failure, chronic kidney disease, both conditions, or neither. Assign codes from combination category 404 Hypertensive heart and kidney disease, when both hypertensive kidney disease and hypertensive heart disease are stated in the diagnosis. Assume a relationship between the hypertension and the kidney disease, whether or not the condition is so designated.

A patient may have an elevated blood pressure reading during an outpatient visit without having a known diagnosis of hypertension. In this situation, code 796.2, which describes an elevated blood pressure reading that may be the result of emotional problems or stress. This diagnosis code can be found in the alphabetic index under the main term "Elevation" and subterms "blood pressure," "reading," and "no diagnosis of hypertension."

For hypertensive cerebrovascular disease, first assign codes from 430–438 Cerebrovascular disease, then the appropriate hypertension code from categories 401–405.

Hypertensive retinopathy requires two codes to identify the condition. First assign the code from subcategory 362.11 Hypertensive retinopathy, then the appropriate code from categories 401–405 to indicate the type of hypertension.

Secondary hypertension defined as high blood pressure due to or with a variety of primary diseases requires two codes: one to identify the underlying etiology and one from category 405 to identify the hypertension.

The terms "controlled" or "uncontrolled" hypertension refer to whether the hypertension is responding to current therapeutic regimen or not. In either case, code to the type of hypertension, and assign an appropriate code from categories 401–405.

Ischemic Heart Disease (410–414)

Myocardial Infarction (410)

An acute myocardial infarction (AMI) results from an interruption of the blood supply to an area of the myocardium. Physicians associate the condition as part

Diseases of the Circulatory System

of acute ischemic heart disease, which is classified to category 410. Category 410 has subcategories that identify the site of the myocardial infarction and fifth digits to indicate the episode of care involved with the myocardial infarction. ICD-9-CM classifies myocardial infarctions according to the site involved as identified by EKG, such as anterolateral wall.

The fifth digits indicate new acute myocardial infarctions and patients who are admitted within eight weeks of an acute myocardial infarction. The fifth digit of "1" (initial episode of care) covers all care during the acute phase of treatment, and is used principally in acute facility care.

The fifth digit of "2" (subsequent episode of care) covers further observation, evaluation, or treatment rendered after the initial treatment (discharge), but within an eight week period since the myocardial infarction. For example, AMI of anterolateral wall, occurring two weeks ago is coded 410.02. Acute myocardial infarctions within eight weeks or that are unspecified require the use of a fifth digit of "2" or "0 (unspecified)." A myocardial infarction of greater than eight weeks duration with persistent symptoms is coded to 414.8.

Ischemic Heart Disease (411)
Intermediate coronary syndrome (411.1) is a condition representing an intermediate stage between angina of effort and acute myocardial infarction. It is often documented by the physician as "unstable angina." Other terms for this condition are impending infarction, preinfarction angina, and preinfarction syndrome.

Old myocardial infarction, code 412, is assigned for diagnosis of an old or healed myocardial infarction diagnosed by EKG but currently presenting no symptoms.

Other Forms of Chronic Ischemic Heart Disease (414)
Fifth-digit subclassifications are required when reporting coronary atherosclerosis. The fifth digit specifies the type of vessel affected by atherosclerotic disease; whether a native vessel, previously grafted vessel, or vessel of a transplanted heart.

A complete blockage of a coronary artery that has been present for an extended duration is known as a chronic total occlusion of the coronary artery (414.2). Collateral flow may avoid myocardial infarction, despite the chronic total occlusion of the coronary artery. However, this flow could not likely increase much during exercise and so would be likely to greatly limit activity.

Chronic total occlusion of a coronary artery may be treated with angioplasty or stent placement, usually with a drug-eluting stent. When reporting chronic total occlusion of coronary artery (414.2), code first the appropriate code for coronary atherosclerosis classifiable to codes 414.00–414.07.

Lipid-rich atherosclerotic plaques (414.3) are particularly unstable and vulnerable to rupture, increasing the risk of acute coronary events such as thrombosis, arrhythmia, and myocardial infarction. Atherosclerotic plaques containing lipid-rich cores have been identified as a cause of arterial filling defects during angiography procedures. In atherogenesis, plaque stability depends on multiple factors, including plaque composition, size and location of the core, arterial wall stress, and relationship of plaque to blood flow. Since lipid-rich plaque is present in some coronary atherosclerotic diseased vessels (but perhaps not all vessels), the presence of this code is an indicator of disease severity. Lipid-rich plaque of coronary vessels cannot be present without coronary atherosclerosis. Therefore, the appropriate coronary atherosclerosis code from subcategory 414.0 should be sequenced first, followed by code 414.3, when documented as such.

Congestive Heart Failure (428)
Congestive heart failure (CHF) is a syndrome of impaired contraction, or power failure (in pumping of the heart), pressure volume overload, and impaired filling of the heart, in which the heart may be functioning normally otherwise.

Congestive heart failure affects either the left or right ventricles of the heart. Left heart failure is the inability of the heart to meet the metabolic demands of the body. It occurs when the left ventricle has an overload of fluid due to the inability of the ventricle to contract, or pump, blood from the lungs.

Right heart failure occurs secondary to left heart failure when the left ventricle has failed completely to contract and move blood into systemic circulation. Once

the left ventricle fails, patients evolving into heart failure have a grave prognosis, since the pumping mechanism of the heart is so severely damaged.

In some instances the heart muscle may "compensate" during heart failure by increasing the force of the contraction, raising the arterial pressure, or increasing ventricular dilation. The heart may perform at near normal functional levels. When these compensating factors no longer are effective, decompensation is said to occur. The heart can no longer work at increased levels. Heart failure may be stated as compensated or decompensated, but ICD-9-CM code selection is still 428.0.

Heart failure not otherwise specified is assigned code 428.9 and should not be confused with congestive heart failure.

Cerebrovascular Disease (430–438)

Occlusion and Stenosis of Precerebral and Cerebral Arteries (433–434)
Determine the artery where the site of the stenosis or occlusion occurs before coding from this section. The code category 433 includes occlusion and stenosis of the precerebral arteries. The second step is to determine the presence of cerebral infarction. A fifth-digit assignment of "0" indicates "without mention of infarction" and the fifth-digit assignment of "1" indicates "with cerebral infarction."

The same general guidelines apply to occlusion and stenosis of the cerebral arteries (434), although the first axis of classification differentiates between thrombosis and embolism instead of identification of the cerebral artery. CVA and stroke NOS are assigned code 434.9x since the vast majority of strokes and CVA are attributed to cerebral artery occlusion. Additional codes should be assigned for any neurologic deficits associated with acute CVA, whether or not the neurologic deficit resolved prior to discharge.

Report V45.88 for the administration of tPA (rtPA) to patients transferred from a different facility within the last 24 hours. Code V45.88 is reported in addition to the code for the acute condition requiring tPA administration, such as acute cerebral infarction classifiable to categories 433 and 434.

Late Effects of Cerebrovascular Disease (438)
The instructional note at the beginning of this category explains the use of these codes.This category is used to indicate conditions in categories 430–437 as the cause of the late effect, which is classifiable elsewhere. The "late effect" includes conditions specified as such, or as sequelae, which may occur any time after the onset of the causal condition. Assignment of a code from the 438 category is inappropriate in cases of past history of cerebrovascular disease which resulted in no neurological deficits. The appropriate code assignment is V12.54 Personal history of other diseases of the circulatory system.

 "Late effects" include neurologic deficits that persist after initial onset of conditions classifiable to 430–437. The neurologic deficits caused by cerebrovascular disease may be present from the onset or may arise at any time after the onset of the condition classifiable to 430–437. A code from category 438 may be assigned on a medical record with codes from 430–437, if the patient has a current CVA and deficits from an old CVA.

Diseases of Arteries, Arterioles, and Capillaries (440-449)
This section includes conditions affecting the arterial vasculature, which include atherosclerosis, thrombus, and embolism (clots) and other forms of peripheral vascular disease.

Atherosclerosis (440)
Atherosclerosis may be loosely defined as "hardening" of the arteries, whereby plaque formations adhere to the arterial walls, impairing their elasticity, patency, and functionality. Arteriosclerosis (occlusive) of the extremities is reported with code 440.2x. However, chronic total occlusion of an artery in the extremities (440.4) generally develops over a long time period, with partial occlusion present initially. This can cause symptoms such as intermittent claudication (leg pain with exercise) when arteries to the lower extremities are involved.

When reporting chronic occlusive disease (440.4), code first the underlying disease, atherosclerosis of arteries of extremities (440.20–440.29, 440.30–440.32). Code 440.4 excludes acute occlusion of artery of extremity documented as embolism or thrombosis (444.2x).

7. DISEASES OF THE CIRCULATORY SYSTEM (390-459)

ACUTE RHEUMATIC FEVER (390-392)

DEF: Febrile disease occurs mainly in children or young adults following throat infection by group A *streptococci*; symptoms include fever, joint pain, lesions of heart, blood vessels and joint connective tissue, abdominal pain, skin changes, and chorea.

390 Rheumatic fever without mention of heart involvement
Arthritis, rheumatic, acute or subacute
Rheumatic fever (active) (acute)
Rheumatism, articular, acute or subacute
  EXCLUDES *that with heart involvement (391.0-391.9)*

✓4ᵗʰ **391 Rheumatic fever with heart involvement**
  EXCLUDES *chronic heart diseases of rheumatic origin (393-398.99)*
      unless rheumatic fever is also present or there is
      evidence of recrudescence or activity of the
      rheumatic process

391.0 Acute rheumatic pericarditis
Rheumatic:
  fever (active) (acute) with pericarditis
  pericarditis (acute)
Any condition classifiable to 390 with pericarditis
  EXCLUDES *that not specified as rheumatic (420.0-420.9)*
DEF: Sudden, severe inflammation of heart lining due to rheumatic fever.

391.1 Acute rheumatic endocarditis
Rheumatic:
  endocarditis, acute
  fever (active) (acute) with endocarditis or valvulitis
  valvulitis acute
Any condition classifiable to 390 with endocarditis or valvulitis
DEF: Sudden, severe inflammation of heart cavities due to rheumatic fever.

391.2 Acute rheumatic myocarditis
Rheumatic fever (active) (acute) with myocarditis
Any condition classifiable to 390 with myocarditis
DEF: Sudden, severe inflammation of heart muscles due to rheumatic fever.

391.8 Other acute rheumatic heart disease
Rheumatic:
  fever (active) (acute) with other or multiple types of
    heart involvement
  pancarditis, acute
Any condition classifiable to 390 with other or multiple types of heart involvement

391.9 Acute rheumatic heart disease, unspecified
Rheumatic:
  carditis, acute
  fever (active) (acute) with unspecified type of heart
    involvement
  heart disease, active or acute
Any condition classifiable to 390 with unspecified type of heart involvement

✓4ᵗʰ **392 Rheumatic chorea**
  INCLUDES Sydenham's chorea
  EXCLUDES *chorea:*
      NOS (333.5)
      Huntington's (333.4)
DEF: Childhood disease linked with rheumatic fever and streptococcal infections; symptoms include spasmodic, involuntary movements of limbs or facial muscles, psychic symptoms, and irritability.

392.0 With heart involvement
Rheumatic chorea with heart involvement of any type classifiable to 391

392.9 Without mention of heart involvement

CHRONIC RHEUMATIC HEART DISEASE (393-398)

393 Chronic rheumatic pericarditis
Adherent pericardium, rheumatic
Chronic rheumatic:
  mediastinopericarditis
  myopericarditis
  EXCLUDES *pericarditis NOS or not specified as rheumatic*
      (423.0-423.9)
DEF: Persistent inflammation of heart lining due to rheumatic heart disease.

✓4ᵗʰ **394 Diseases of mitral valve**
  EXCLUDES *that with aortic valve involvement (396.0-396.9)*

394.0 Mitral stenosis
Mitral (valve):
  obstruction (rheumatic)
  stenosis NOS
DEF: Narrowing, of mitral valve between left atrium and left ventricle; due to rheumatic heart disease.

394.1 Rheumatic mitral insufficiency
Rheumatic mitral:
  incompetence
  regurgitation
  EXCLUDES *that not specified as rheumatic (424.0)*
DEF: Malfunction of mitral valve between left atrium and left ventricle; due to rheumatic heart disease.

394.2 Mitral stenosis with insufficiency
Mitral stenosis with incompetence or regurgitation
DEF: A narrowing or stricture of the mitral valve situated between the left atrium and left ventricle; valve does not completely close ,is insufficient (inadequate)in preventing regurgitation into the atrium; also called incompetence.

394.9 Other and unspecified mitral valve diseases
Mitral (valve):
  disease (chronic)
  failure

✓4ᵗʰ **395 Diseases of aortic valve**
  EXCLUDES *that not specified as rheumatic (424.1)*
      that with mitral valve involvement (396.0-396.9)

395.0 Rheumatic aortic stenosis
Rheumatic aortic (valve) obstruction
DEF: Narrowing of the aortic valve; results in backflow into ventricle; due to rheumatic heart disease.

395.1 Rheumatic aortic insufficiency
Rheumatic aortic:
  incompetence
  regurgitation
DEF: Malfunction of the aortic valve; results in backflow into left ventricle; due to rheumatic heart disease.

395.2 Rheumatic aortic stenosis with insufficiency
Rheumatic aortic stenosis with incompetence or regurgitation
DEF: Malfunction and narrowing, of the aortic valve; results in backflow into left ventricle; due to rheumatic heart disease.

395.9 Other and unspecified rheumatic aortic diseases
Rheumatic aortic (valve) disease

✓4ᵗʰ **396 Diseases of mitral and aortic valves**
  INCLUDES involvement of both mitral and aortic valves,
      whether specified as rheumatic or not

396.0 Mitral valve stenosis and aortic valve stenosis
Atypical aortic (valve) stenosis
Mitral and aortic (valve) obstruction (rheumatic)

396.1 Mitral valve stenosis and aortic valve insufficiency

396.2 Mitral valve insufficiency and aortic valve stenosis

396.3 Mitral valve insufficiency and aortic valve insufficiency
Mitral and aortic (valve):
  incompetence
  regurgitation

Diseases of the Circulatory System

396.8–403.9

396.8 Multiple involvement of mitral and aortic valves
Stenosis and insufficiency of mitral or aortic valve with stenosis or insufficiency, or both, of the other valve

396.9 Mitral and aortic valve diseases, unspecified

√4th **397 Diseases of other endocardial structures**

397.0 Diseases of tricuspid valve
Tricuspid (valve) (rheumatic):
disease
insufficiency
obstruction
regurgitation
stenosis
DEF: Malfunction of the valve between right atrium and right ventricle; due to rheumatic heart disease.

397.1 Rheumatic diseases of pulmonary valve
EXCLUDES *that not specified as rheumatic (424.3)*

397.9 Rheumatic diseases of endocardium, valve unspecified
Rheumatic: Rheumatic:
endocarditis (chronic)   valvulitis (chronic)
EXCLUDES *that not specified as rheumatic (424.90-424.99)*

√4th **398 Other rheumatic heart disease**

398.0 Rheumatic myocarditis
Rheumatic degeneration of myocardium
EXCLUDES *myocarditis not specified as rheumatic (429.0)*
DEF: Chronic inflammation of heart muscle; due to rheumatic heart disease.

√5th **398.9 Other and unspecified rheumatic heart diseases**

398.90 Rheumatic heart disease, unspecified
Rheumatic:
carditis
heart disease NOS
EXCLUDES *carditis not specified as rheumatic (429.89)*
heart disease NOS not specified as rheumatic (429.9)

398.91 Rheumatic heart failure (congestive)
Rheumatic left ventricular failure
DEF: Decreased cardiac output, edema and hypertension; due to rheumatic heart disease.

398.99 Other

HYPERTENSIVE DISEASE (401-405)
EXCLUDES *that complicating pregnancy, childbirth, or the puerperium (642.0-642.9)*
that involving coronary vessels (410.00-414.9)

√4th **401 Essential hypertension**
INCLUDES high blood pressure
hyperpiesia
hyperpiesis
hypertension (arterial) (essential) (primary) (systemic)
hypertensive vascular:
degeneration
disease
EXCLUDES *elevated blood pressure without diagnosis of hypertension (796.2)*
pulmonary hypertension (416.0-416.9)
that involving vessels of:
brain (430-438)
eye (362.11)
DEF: Hypertension that occurs without apparent organic cause; idiopathic.

401.0 Malignant
DEF: Severe high arterial blood pressure; results in necrosis in kidney, retina, etc.; hemorrhages occur and death commonly due to uremia or rupture of cerebral vessel.

401.1 Benign
DEF: Mildly elevated arterial blood pressure.

401.9 Unspecified

√4th **402 Hypertensive heart disease**
INCLUDES hypertensive:
cardiomegaly
cardiopathy
cardiovascular disease
heart (disease) (failure)
any condition classifiable to 429.0-429.3, 429.8, 429.9 due to hypertension
Use additional code to specify type of heart failure (428.0-428.43), if known

√5th **402.0 Malignant**
402.00 Without heart failure
402.01 With heart failure

√5th **402.1 Benign**
402.10 Without heart failure
402.11 With heart failure

√5th **402.9 Unspecified**
402.90 Without heart failure
402.91 With heart failure

√4th **403 Hypertensive chronic kidney disease**
INCLUDES arteriolar nephritis
arteriosclerosis of:
kidney
renal arterioles
arteriosclerotic nephritis (chronic) (interstitial)
hypertensive:
nephropathy
renal failure
uremia (chronic)
nephrosclerosis
renal sclerosis with hypertension
any condition classifiable to 585 and 587 with any condition classifiable to 401
EXCLUDES *acute kidney failure (584.5-584.9)*
renal disease stated as not due to hypertension
renovascular hypertension (405.0-405.9 with fifth-digit 1)

The following fifth-digit subclassification is for use with category 403:
0 **with chronic kidney disease stage I through stage IV, or unspecified**
Use additional code to identify the stage of chronic kidney disease (585.1-585.4, 585.9)
1 **with chronic kidney disease stage V or end stage renal disease**
Use additional code to identify the stage of chronic kidney disease (585.5, 585.6)

√5th **403.0 Malignant**
[0-1]

√5th **403.1 Benign**
[0-1]

√5th **403.9 Unspecified**
[0-1]

√4ᵗʰ **404 Hypertensive heart and chronic kidney disease**

[INCLUDES] disease:
          cardiorenal
          cardiovascular renal
       any condition classifiable to 402 with any condition
          classifiable to 403
Use additional code to specify type of heart failure
    (428.0-428.43), if known

> The following fifth-digit subclassification is for use with category
> 404:
>   **0 without heart failure and with chronic kidney disease
>   stage I through stage IV, or unspecified**
>   Use additional code to identify the stage of chronic
>   kidney disease (585.1-585.4, 585.9)
>   **1 with heart failure and with chronic kidney disease
>   stage I through stage IV, or unspecified**
>   Use additional code to identify the stage of chronic
>   kidney disease (585.1-585.4, 585.9)
>   **2 without heart failure and with chronic kidney disease
>   stage V or end stage renal disease**
>   Use additional code to identify the stage of chronic
>   kidney disease (585.5, 585.6)
>   **3 with heart failure and chronic kidney disease stage V
>   or end stage renal disease**
>   Use additional code to identify the stage of chronic
>   kidney disease (585.5, 585.6)

√5ᵗʰ **404.0 Malignant**
     [0-3]

√5ᵗʰ **404.1 Benign**
     [0-3]

√5ᵗʰ **404.9 Unspecified**
     [0-3]

√4ᵗʰ **405 Secondary hypertension**
     DEF: High arterial blood pressure due to or with a variety of primary
     diseases, such as renal disorders, CNS disorders, endocrine, and
     vascular diseases.

√5ᵗʰ **405.0 Malignant**
       405.01 Renovascular
       405.09 Other

√5ᵗʰ **405.1 Benign**
       405.11 Renovascular
       405.19 Other

√5ᵗʰ **405.9 Unspecified**
       405.91 Renovascular
       405.99 Other

Acute Myocardial Infarction

ISCHEMIC HEART DISEASE (410-414)

[INCLUDES] that with mention of hypertension
Use additional code to identify presence of hypertension
    (401.0-405.9)

√4ᵗʰ **410 Acute myocardial infarction**

[INCLUDES] cardiac infarction
       coronary (artery):
          embolism
          occlusion
          rupture
          thrombosis
       infarction of heart, myocardium, or ventricle
       rupture of heart, myocardium, or ventricle
       ST elevation (STEMI) and non-ST elevation (NSTEMI)
          myocardial infarction
       any condition classifiable to 414.1-414.9 specified as
          acute or with a stated duration of 8 weeks or
          less

> The following fifth-digit subclassification is for use with category
> 410:
>   **0 episode of care unspecified**
>   Use when the source document does not contain
>   sufficient information for the assigment of
>   fifth-digit 1 or 2.
>   **1 initial episode of care**
>   Use fifth-digit 1 to designate the first episode of care
>   (regardless of facility site) for a newly diagnosed
>   myocardial infarction. The fifth-digit 1 is assigned
>   regardless of the number of times a patient may
>   be transferred during the initial episode of care.
>   **2 subsequent episode of care**
>   Use fifth-digit 2 to designate an episode of care
>   following the initial episode when the patient is
>   admitted for further observation, evaluation or
>   treatment for a myocardial infarction that has
>   received initial treatment, but is still less than 8
>   weeks old.

DEF: A sudden insufficiency of blood supply to an area of the heart
muscle; usually due to a coronary artery occlusion.

√5ᵗʰ **410.0 Of anterolateral wall**
     [0-2]   ST elevation myocardial infarction (STEMI) of
               anterolateral wall

√5ᵗʰ **410.1 Of other anterior wall**
     [0-2]   Infarction:
               anterior (wall) NOS ⎫ (with contiguous portion of
               anteroapical   ⎬   intraventricular
               anteroseptal   ⎭   septum)
               ST elevation myocardial infarction (STEMI) of other
                  anterior wall

√5ᵗʰ **410.2 Of inferolateral wall**
     [0-2]   ST elevation myocardial infarction (STEMI) of
               inferolateral wall

√5ᵗʰ **410.3 Of inferoposterior wall**
     [0-2]   ST elevation myocardial infarction (STEMI) of
               inferoposterior wall

√5ᵗʰ **410.4 Of other inferior wall**
     [0-2]   Infarction:
               diaphragmatic wall ⎫ (with contiguous portion of
                  NOS   ⎬   intraventricular
               inferior (wall) NOS ⎭   septum)
               ST elevation myocardial infarction (STEMI) of other
                  inferior wall

√5ᵗʰ **410.5 Of other lateral wall**
     [0-2]   Infarction:
               apical-lateral
               basal-lateral
               high lateral
               posterolateral
               ST elevation myocardial infarction (STEMI) of other
                  lateral wall

Diseases of the Circulatory System

410.6–414.19

√5th **410.6 True posterior wall infarction**
[0-2]   Infarction:
              posterobasal
              strictly posterior
         ST elevation myocardial infarction (STEMI) of true
              posterior wall

√5th **410.7 Subendocardial infarction**
[0-2]   Non-ST elevation myocardial infarction (NSTEMI)
         Nontransmural infarction

√5th **410.8 Of other specified sites**
[0-2]   Infarction of:
              atrium
              papillary muscle
              septum alone
         ST elevation myocardial infarction (STEMI) of other
              specified sites

√5th **410.9 Unspecified site**
[0-2]   Acute myocardial infarction NOS
         Coronary occlusion NOS
         Myocardial infarction NOS

√4th **411 Other acute and subacute forms of ischemic heart disease**

411.0 Postmyocardial infarction syndrome
         Dressler's syndrome

         DEF: Complication developing several days/weeks after
         myocardial infarction; symptoms include fever,
         leukocytosis, chest pain, pericarditis, pleurisy, and
         pneumonitis; tendency to recur.

411.1 Intermediate coronary syndrome
         Impending infarction
         Preinfarction angina
         Preinfarction syndrome
         Unstable angina
         EXCLUDES angina (pectoris) (413.9)
                       decubitus (413.0)

         DEF: A condition representing an intermediate stage
         between angina of effort and acute myocardial infarction.
         It is often documented by the physician as "unstable
         angina."

√5th **411.8 Other**

**411.81 Acute coronary occlusion without myocardial
          infarction**
          Acute coronary (artery):
              embolism   ⎤ without or not
              obstruction   ⎥ resulting in
              occlusion   ⎥ myocardial
              thrombosis   ⎦ infarction
          EXCLUDES obstruction without infarction due
                        to atherosclerosis
                        (414.00-414.07)
                        occlusion without infarction due to
                        atherosclerosis
                        (414.00-414.07)

          DEF: Interrupted blood flow to a portion of the
          heart; without tissue death.

411.89 Other
          Coronary insufficiency (acute)
          Subendocardial ischemia

412 Old myocardial infarction
     Healed myocardial infarction
     Past myocardial infarction diagnosed on ECG [EKG] or other
          special investigation, but currently presenting no
          symptoms

√4th **413 Angina pectoris**
     DEF: Severe constricting pain in the chest, often radiating from the
     precordium to the left shoulder and down the arm, due to ischemia
     of the heart muscle; usually caused by coronary disease; pain is
     often precipitated by effort or excitement.

413.0 Angina decubitus
         Nocturnal angina
         DEF: Angina occurring only in the recumbent position.

413.1 Prinzmetal angina
         Variant angina pectoris
         DEF: Angina occurring when patient is recumbent;
         associated with ST-segment elevations.

413.9 Other and unspecified angina pectoris
         Angina: Anginal syndrome
              NOS   Status anginosus
              cardiac   Stenocardia
              equivalent   Syncope anginosa
              of effort
         Use additional code(s) for symptoms associated with
              angina equivalent
         EXCLUDES preinfarction angina (411.1)

√4th **414 Other forms of chronic ischemic heart disease**
     EXCLUDES arteriosclerotic cardiovascular disease [ASCVD] (429.2)
                   cardiovascular:
                       arteriosclerosis or sclerosis (429.2)
                       degeneration or disease (429.2)

√5th **414.0 Coronary atherosclerosis**
         Arteriosclerotic heart disease [ASHD]
         Atherosclerotic heart disease
         Coronary (artery):
              arteriosclerosis
              arteritis or endarteritis
              atheroma
              sclerosis
              stricture
         Use additional code, if applicable, to identify chronic
              total occlusion of coronary artery (414.2)
         EXCLUDES embolism of graft (996.72)
                       occlusion NOS of graft (996.72)
                       thrombus of graft (996.72)

         DEF: A chronic condition marked by thickening and loss of
         elasticity of the coronary artery; caused by deposits of
         plaque containing cholesterol, lipoid material and
         lipophages.

414.00 Of unspecified type of vessel, native or graft

414.01 Of native coronary artery
          DEF: Plaque deposits in natural heart vessels.

414.02 Of autologous vein bypass graft
          DEF: Plaque deposit in grafted vein originating
          within patient.

414.03 Of nonautologous biological bypass graft
          DEF: Plaque deposits in grafted vessel
          originating outside patient.

414.04 Of artery bypass graft
          Internal mammary artery
          DEF: Plaque deposits in grafted artery
          originating within patient.

414.05 Of unspecified type of bypass graft
          Bypass graft NOS

**414.06 Of native coronary artery of transplanted
          heart**

**414.07 Of bypass graft (artery) (vein) of transplanted
          heart**

√5th **414.1 Aneurysm and dissection of heart**

414.10 Aneurysm of heart (wall)
          Aneurysm (arteriovenous):
              mural
              ventricular

414.11 Aneurysm of coronary vessels
          Aneurysm (arteriovenous) of coronary vessels
          DEF: Dilatation of all three-vessel wall layers
          forming a sac filled with blood.

414.12 Dissection of coronary artery
          DEF: A tear in the intimal arterial wall of a
          coronary artery resulting in the sudden intrusion
          of blood within the layers of the wall.

414.19 Other aneurysm of heart
          Arteriovenous fistula, acquired, of heart

Arteries of the Heart

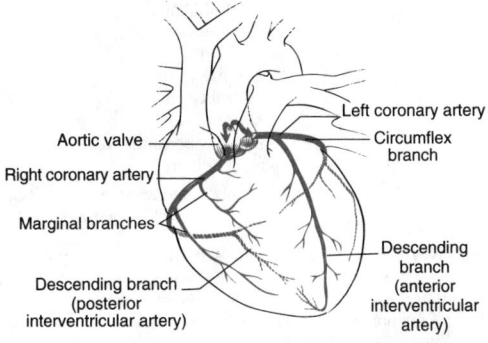

414.2 Chronic total occlusion of coronary artery
Complete occlusion of coronary artery
Total occlusion of coronary artery
Code first coronary atherosclerosis (414.00-414.07)
EXCLUDES   *acute coronary occlusion with myocardial*
infarction (410.00-410.92)
acute coronary occlusion without myocardial
infarction (411.81)

DEF: Complete blockage of coronary artery due to plaque
accumulation over an extended period of time; results in
substantial reduction of blood flow.

414.3 Coronary atherosclerosis due to lipid rich plaque
Code first coronary atherosclerosis (414.00-414.07)

**414.4 Coronary atherosclerosis due to calcified coronary
lesion**
Coronary atherosclerosis due to severely calcified
coronary lesion
Code first coronary atherosclerosis (414.00-414.07)

414.8 Other specified forms of chronic ischemic heart disease
Chronic coronary insufficiency
Ischemia, myocardial (chronic)
Any condition classifiable to 410 specified as chronic, or
presenting with symptoms after 8 weeks from
date of infarction
EXCLUDES   *coronary insufficiency (acute) (411.89)*

414.9 Chronic ischemic heart disease, unspecified
Ischemic heart disease NOS

DISEASES OF PULMONARY CIRCULATION (415-417)

✔4ᵗʰ **415 Acute pulmonary heart disease**

415.0 Acute cor pulmonale
EXCLUDES   *cor pulmonale NOS (416.9)*

DEF: A heart-lung disease marked by dilation and failure
of the right side of heart; due to pulmonary embolism;
ventilatory function is impaired and pulmonary
hypertension results.

✔5ᵗʰ **415.1 Pulmonary embolism and infarction**
Pulmonary (artery) (vein):   Pulmonary (artery) (vein):
apoplexy   infarction (hemorrhagic)
embolism   thrombosis
EXCLUDES   *chronic pulmonary embolism (416.2)*
personal history of pulmonary embolism
(V12.55)
that complicating:
abortion (634-638 with .6, 639.6)
ectopic or molar pregnancy (639.6)
pregnancy, childbirth, or the puerperium
(673.0-673.8)

DEF: Embolism: Closure of the pulmonary artery or
branch; due to thrombosis (blood clot).
DEF: Infarction: Necrosis of lung tissue; due to obstructed
arterial blood supply, most often by pulmonary embolism.

**415.11 Iatrogenic pulmonary embolism and
infarction**
Use additional code for associated septic pulmonary embolism, if applicable, 415.12

415.12 Septic pulmonary embolism
Septic embolism NOS
Code first underlying infection, such as:
septicemia (038.0-038.9)
EXCLUDES   *septic arterial embolism (449)*

415.13 Saddle embolus of pulmonary artery

415.19 Other

✔4ᵗʰ **416 Chronic pulmonary heart disease**

416.0 Primary pulmonary hypertension
Idiopathic pulmonary arteriosclerosis
Pulmonary hypertension (essential) (idiopathic)
(primary)
EXCLUDES   *pulmonary hypertension NOS (416.8)*
secondary pulmonary hypertension (416.8)

DEF: A rare increase in pulmonary circulation, often
resulting in right ventricular failure or fatal syncope.

416.1 Kyphoscoliotic heart disease

DEF: High blood pressure within the lungs as a result of
curvature of the spine.

416.2 Chronic pulmonary embolism
Use additional code, if applicable, for associated
long-term (current) use of anticoagulants (V58.61)
EXCLUDES   *personal history of pulmonary embolism*
(V12.55)

DEF: A long-standing condition commonly associated
with pulmonary hypertension in which small blood clots
travel to the lungs repeatedly over many weeks, months,
or years, requiring continuation of established
anticoagulant or thrombolytic therapy.

416.8 Other chronic pulmonary heart diseases
Pulmonary hypertension NOS
Pulmonary hypertension, secondary

416.9 Chronic pulmonary heart disease, unspecified
Chronic cardiopulmonary disease
Cor pulmonale (chronic) NOS

✔4ᵗʰ **417 Other diseases of pulmonary circulation**

417.0 Arteriovenous fistula of pulmonary vessels
EXCLUDES   *congenital arteriovenous fistula (747.32)*

DEF: Abnormal communication between blood vessels
within lung.

417.1 Aneurysm of pulmonary artery
EXCLUDES   *congenital aneurysm (747.39)*
congenital arteriovenous aneurysm (747.32)

417.8 Other specified diseases of pulmonary circulation
Pulmonary:
arteritis
endarteritis
Rupture   } of pulmonary vessel
Stricture

417.9 Unspecified disease of pulmonary circulation

Diseases of the Circulatory System

420–422.91

OTHER FORMS OF HEART DISEASE (420-429)

✓4ᵗʰ **420 Acute pericarditis**

INCLUDES acute:
- mediastinopericarditis
- myopericarditis
- pericardial effusion
- pleuropericarditis
- pneumopericarditis

EXCLUDES *acute rheumatic pericarditis (391.0)*
postmyocardial infarction syndrome [Dressler's] (411.0)

DEF: Inflammation of the pericardium (heart sac); pericardial friction rub results from this inflammation and is heard as a scratchy or leathery sound.

420.0 *Acute pericarditis in diseases classified elsewhere*

Code first underlying disease, as:
- actinomycosis (039.8)
- amebiasis (006.8)
- chronic uremia (585.9)
- nocardiosis (039.8)
- tuberculosis (017.9)
- uremia NOS (586)

EXCLUDES *pericarditis (acute) (in):*
   Coxsackie (virus) (074.21)
   gonococcal (098.83)
   histoplasmosis (115.0-115.9 with
      fifth-digit 3)
   meningococcal infection (036.41)
   syphilitic (093.81)

✓5ᵗʰ **420.9 Other and unspecified acute pericarditis**

420.90 Acute pericarditis, unspecified
Pericarditis (acute):
- NOS
- infective NOS
- sicca

420.91 Acute idiopathic pericarditis
Pericarditis, acute:
- benign
- nonspecific
- viral

Anatomy

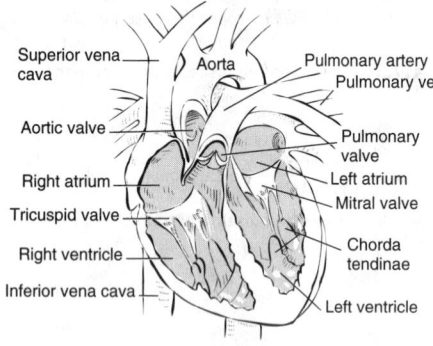

- Superior vena cava
- Aorta
- Pulmonary artery
- Pulmonary vein
- Aortic valve
- Pulmonary valve
- Right atrium
- Left atrium
- Tricuspid valve
- Mitral valve
- Right ventricle
- Chorda tendinae
- Inferior vena cava
- Left ventricle

Blood Flow

420.99 Other
Pericarditis (acute):
- pneumococcal
- purulent
- staphylococcal
- streptococcal
- suppurative
Pneumopyopericardium
Pyopericardium

EXCLUDES *pericarditis in diseases classified*
   elsewhere (420.0)

✓4ᵗʰ **421 Acute and subacute endocarditis**

DEF: Bacterial inflammation of the endocardium (intracardiac area); major symptoms include fever, fatigue, heart murmurs, splenomegaly, embolic episodes and areas of infarction.

421.0 Acute and subacute bacterial endocarditis
Endocarditis (acute)(chronic) (subacute):
- bacterial
- infective NOS
- lenta
- malignant
- purulent
- septic
- ulcerative
- vegetative
Infective aneurysm
Subacute bacterial endocarditis [SBE]

Use additional code to identify infectious organism [e.g., Streptococcus 041.0, Staphylococcus 041.1]

421.1 *Acute and subacute infective endocarditis in diseases classified elsewhere*

Code first underlying disease, as:
- blastomycosis (116.0)
- Q fever (083.0)
- typhoid (fever) (002.0)

EXCLUDES *endocarditis (in):*
   Coxsackie (virus) (074.22)
   gonococcal (098.84)
   histoplasmosis (115.0-115.9 with
      fifth-digit 4)
   meningococcal infection (036.42)
   monilial (112.81)

421.9 Acute endocarditis, unspecified
Endocarditis
Myoendocarditis   } acute or subacute
Periendocarditis

EXCLUDES *acute rheumatic endocarditis (391.1)*

✓4ᵗʰ **422 Acute myocarditis**

EXCLUDES *acute rheumatic myocarditis (391.2)*

DEF: Acute inflammation of the muscular walls of the heart (myocardium).

422.0 *Acute myocarditis in diseases classified elsewhere*

Code first underlying disease, as:
myocarditis (acute):
- influenzal (487.8, 488.09, 488.19)
- tuberculous (017.9)

EXCLUDES *myocarditis (acute) (due to):*
   aseptic, of newborn (074.23)
   Coxsackie (virus) (074.23)
   diphtheritic (032.82)
   meningococcal infection (036.43)
   syphilitic (093.82)
   toxoplasmosis (130.3)

✓5ᵗʰ **422.9 Other and unspecified acute myocarditis**

422.90 Acute myocarditis, unspecified
Acute or subacute (interstitial) myocarditis

422.91 Idiopathic myocarditis
Myocarditis (acute or subacute):
- Fiedler's
- giant cell
- isolated (diffuse) (granulomatous)
- nonspecific granulomatous

Cardiac Tamponade

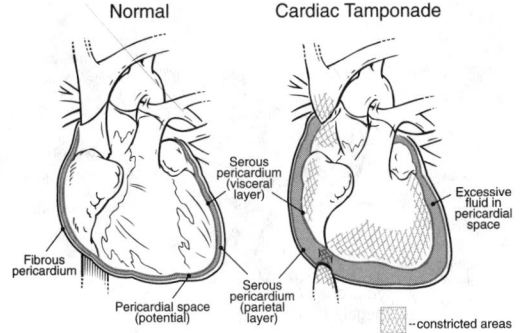

Normal

Cardiac Tamponade

Serous pericardium (visceral layer)

Excessive fluid in pericardial space

Fibrous pericardium

Pericardial space (potential)

Serous pericardium (parietal layer)

▨ --constricted areas

Heart Valve Disorders

Incompetent valve (trouble closing)

causes regurgitation (backflow of blood)

Valve stenosis (trouble opening)

Insufficient valve (unable to close completely)

Shortened, fused chorda tendinae

Ventricular hypertrophy

Normal Heart Valve Function

Atrium contracts

Valve leaflet (cusp)

Chorda tendinae

Papillary muscle

Great artery (aorta or pulmonary artery)

Ventricle fills

Atrium fills

Great vein (vena cava or pulmonary vein)

Ventricle contracts

Great artery (blood to body or lungs)

422.92 Septic myocarditis
Myocarditis, acute or subacute:
pneumococcal
staphylococcal
Use additional code to identify infectious organism [e.g., Staphylococcus 041.1]
EXCLUDES   *myocarditis, acute or subacute:*
in bacterial diseases classified elsewhere (422.0)
streptococcal (391.2)

422.93 Toxic myocarditis
DEF: Inflammation of the heart muscle due to an adverse reaction to certain drugs or chemicals reaching the heart through the bloodstream.

422.99 Other

✓4ᵗʰ **423 Other diseases of pericardium**
EXCLUDES   *that specified as rheumatic (393)*

423.0 Hemopericardium
DEF: Blood in the pericardial sac (pericardium).

423.1 Adhesive pericarditis
Adherent pericardium
Fibrosis of pericardium
Milk spots
Pericarditis:
adhesive
obliterative
Soldiers' patches
DEF: Two layers of serous pericardium adhere to each other by fibrous adhesions.

423.2 Constrictive pericarditis
Concato's disease
Pick's disease of heart (and liver)
DEF: Inflammation identified by a rigid, thickened and sometimes calcified pericardium; ventricles of the heart not adequately filled; congestive heart failure may result.

423.3 Cardiac tamponade
Code first the underlying cause
DEF: Life-threatening condition in which fluid or blood accumulates between the muscle of the heart (myocardium) and the outer sac (pericardium), resulting in compression of the heart, which decreases cardiac output.

423.8 Other specified diseases of pericardium
Calcification
Fistula   } of pericardium

423.9 Unspecified disease of pericardium

✓4ᵗʰ **424 Other diseases of endocardium**
EXCLUDES   *bacterial endocarditis (421.0-421.9)*
rheumatic endocarditis (391.1, 394.0-397.9)
syphilitic endocarditis (093.20-093.24)

424.0 Mitral valve disorders
Mitral (valve):
incompetence
insufficiency   } NOS of specified cause, except rheumatic
regurgitation
EXCLUDES   *mitral (valve):*
disease (394.9)
failure (394.9)
stenosis (394.0)
the listed conditions:
specified as rheumatic (394.1)
unspecified as to cause but with mention of:
diseases of aortic valve (396.0-396.9)
mitral stenosis or obstruction (394.2)

424.1 Aortic valve disorders
Aortic (valve):
incompetence
insufficiency
regurgitation   } NOS of specified cause, except rheumatic
stenosis
EXCLUDES   *hypertrophic subaortic stenosis (425.11)*
that specified as rheumatic (395.0-395.9)
that of unspecified cause but with mention of diseases of mitral valve (396.0-396.9)

424.2 Tricuspid valve disorders, specified as nonrheumatic
Tricuspid valve:
incompetence
insufficiency   } of specified cause, except rheumatic
regurgitation
stenosis
EXCLUDES   *rheumatic or of unspecified cause (397.0)*

424.3 Pulmonary valve disorders
Pulmonic:
incompetence NOS
insufficiency NOS
regurgitation NOS
stenosis NOS
EXCLUDES   *that specified as rheumatic (397.1)*

✓5ᵗʰ **424.9 Endocarditis, valve unspecified**

424.90 Endocarditis, valve unspecified, unspecified cause

Endocarditis (chronic):
NOS
nonbacterial thrombotic
Valvular:
incompetence ⎫
insufficiency ⎬ of unspecified valve,
regurgitation ⎬ unspecified cause
stenosis ⎭
Valvulitis (chronic)

424.91 *Endocarditis in diseases classified elsewhere*

Code first underlying disease as:
atypical verrucous endocarditis
[Libman-Sacks] (710.0)
disseminated lupus erythematosus (710.0)
tuberculosis (017.9)

> EXCLUDES   syphilitic (093.20-093.24)

424.99 Other

Any condition classifiable to 424.90 with
specified cause, except rheumatic

> EXCLUDES   endocardial fibroelastosis (425.3)
> that specified as rheumatic (397.9)

✓4ᵗʰ **425 Cardiomyopathy**

INCLUDES   myocardiopathy

425.0 Endomyocardial fibrosis

✓5ᵗʰ **425.1 Hypertrophic cardiomyopathy**

> EXCLUDES   ventricular hypertrophy (429.3)

DEF: Cardiomyopathy marked by left ventricle
hypertrophy, enlarged septum; results in obstructed blood
flow.

425.11 Hypertrophic obstructive cardiomyopathy
Hypertrophic subaortic stenosis (idiopathic)

425.18 Other hypertrophic cardiomyopathy
Nonobstructive hypertrophic cardiomyopathy

425.2 Obscure cardiomyopathy of Africa
Becker's disease
Idiopathic mural endomyocardial disease

425.3 Endocardial fibroelastosis
Elastomyofibrosis

DEF: A condition marked by left ventricle hypertrophy and
conversion of the endocardium into a thick fibroelastic
coat; capacity of the ventricle may be reduced, but is often
increased.

425.4 Other primary cardiomyopathies
Cardiomyopathy:
NOS
congestive
constrictive
familial
idiopathic
obstructive
restrictive
Cardiovascular collagenosis

425.5 Alcoholic cardiomyopathy

DEF: Heart disease as result of excess alcohol
consumption.

425.7 *Nutritional and metabolic cardiomyopathy*

Code first underlying disease, as:
amyloidosis (277.30-277.39)
beriberi (265.0)
cardiac glycogenosis (271.0)
mucopolysaccharidosis (277.5)
thyrotoxicosis (242.0-242.9)

> EXCLUDES   gouty tophi of heart (274.82)

Nerve Conduction of the Heart

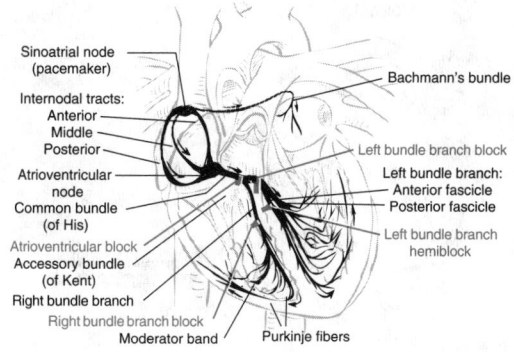

425.8 *Cardiomyopathy in other diseases classified elsewhere*

Code first underlying disease, as:
Friedreich's ataxia (334.0)
myotonia atrophica (359.21)
progressive muscular dystrophy (359.1)
sarcoidosis (135)

> EXCLUDES   cardiomyopathy in Chagas' disease (086.0)

425.9 Secondary cardiomyopathy, unspecified

✓4ᵗʰ **426 Conduction disorders**

DEF: Disruption or disturbance in the electrical impulses that
regulate heartbeats.

426.0 Atrioventricular block, complete
Third degree atrioventricular block

✓5ᵗʰ **426.1 Atrioventricular block, other and unspecified**

426.10 Atrioventricular block, unspecified
Atrioventricular [AV] block (incomplete)
(partial)

426.11 First degree atrioventricular block
Incomplete atrioventricular block, first degree
Prolonged P-R interval NOS

426.12 Mobitz (type) II atrioventricular block
Incomplete atrioventricular block:
Mobitz (type) II
second degree, Mobitz (type) II

DEF: Impaired conduction of excitatory impulse
from cardiac atrium to ventricle through AV
node.

426.13 Other second degree atrioventricular block
Incomplete atrioventricular block:
Mobitz (type) I [Wenckebach's]
second degree:
NOS
Mobitz (type) I
with 2:1 atrioventricular response [block]
Wenckebach's phenomenon

DEF: Wenckebach's phenomenon: impulses
generated at constant rate to sinus node, P-R
interval lengthens; results in cycle of ventricular
inadequacy and shortened P-R interval;
second-degree A-V block commonly called
"Mobitz type 1."

426.2 Left bundle branch hemiblock
Block:
left anterior fascicular
left posterior fascicular

426.3 Other left bundle branch block
Left bundle branch block:
NOS
anterior fascicular with posterior fascicular
complete
main stem

426.4 Right bundle branch block

✓5ᵗʰ **426.5 Bundle branch block, other and unspecified**

426.50 Bundle branch block, unspecified

Diseases of the Circulatory System

426.51–428.0

Normal and Long QT Electrocardiogram

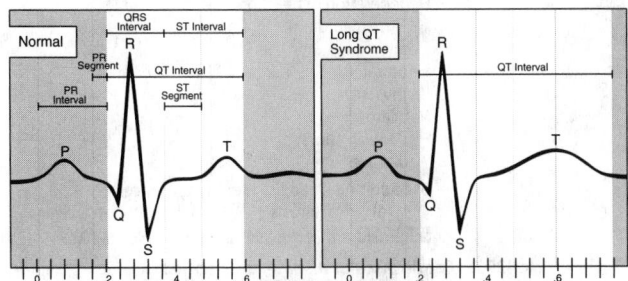

426.51 **Right bundle branch block and left posterior fascicular block**

426.52 **Right bundle branch block and left anterior fascicular block**

426.53 **Other bilateral bundle branch block**
Bifascicular block NOS
Bilateral bundle branch block NOS
Right bundle branch with left bundle branch block (incomplete) (main stem)

426.54 **Trifascicular block**

426.6 **Other heart block**
Intraventricular block: Sinoatrial block
NOS   Sinoauricular block
diffuse
myofibrillar

426.7 **Anomalous atrioventricular excitation**
Atrioventricular conduction:
accelerated
accessory
pre-excitation
Ventricular pre-excitation
Wolff-Parkinson-White syndrome
DEF: Wolff-Parkinson-White: normal conduction pathway is bypassed; results in short P-R interval on EKG; tendency to supraventricular tachycardia.

✓5ᵗʰ **426.8** **Other specified conduction disorders**

426.81 **Lown-Ganong-Levine syndrome**
Syndrome of short P-R interval, normal QRS complexes, and supraventricular tachycardias

426.82 **Long QT syndrome**
DEF: Condition characterized by recurrent syncope, malignant arrhythmias, and sudden death; characteristic prolonged Q-T interval on electrocardiogram.

426.89 **Other**
Dissociation:
atrioventricular [AV]
interference
isorhythmic
Nonparoxysmal AV nodal tachycardia

426.9 **Conduction disorder, unspecified**
Heart block NOS
Stokes-Adams syndrome

✓4ᵗʰ **427** **Cardiac dysrhythmias**
EXCLUDES *that complicating:*
abortion (634-638 with .7, 639.8)
ectopic or molar pregnancy (639.8)
labor or delivery (668.1, 669.4)
DEF: Disruption or disturbance in the rhythm of heartbeats.

427.0 **Paroxysmal supraventricular tachycardia**
Paroxysmal tachycardia: Paroxysmal tachycardia:
atrial [PAT]   junctional
atrioventricular [AV]   nodal
DEF: Rapid atrial rhythm.

427.1 **Paroxysmal ventricular tachycardia**
Ventricular tachycardia (paroxysmal)
DEF: Rapid ventricular rhythm.

427.2 **Paroxysmal tachycardia, unspecified**
Bouveret-Hoffmann syndrome
Paroxysmal tachycardia:
essential
NOS

✓5ᵗʰ **427.3** **Atrial fibrillation and flutter**
427.31 **Atrial fibrillation**
DEF: Irregular, rapid atrial contractions.

427.32 **Atrial flutter**
DEF: Regular, rapid atrial contractions.

✓5ᵗʰ **427.4** **Ventricular fibrillation and flutter**
427.41 **Ventricular fibrillation**
DEF: Irregular, rapid ventricular contractions.

427.42 **Ventricular flutter**
DEF: Regular, rapid, ventricular contractions.

427.5 **Cardiac arrest**
Cardiorespiratory arrest

✓5ᵗʰ **427.6** **Premature beats**
427.60 **Premature beats, unspecified**
Ectopic beats
Extrasystoles
Extrasystolic arrhythmia
Premature contractions or systoles NOS

427.61 **Supraventricular premature beats**
Atrial premature beats, contractions, or systoles

427.69 **Other**
Ventricular premature beats, contractions, or systoles

✓5ᵗʰ **427.8** **Other specified cardiac dysrhythmias**
427.81 **Sinoatrial node dysfunction**
Sinus bradycardia:
persistent
severe
Syndrome:
sick sinus
tachycardia-bradycardia
EXCLUDES *sinus bradycardia NOS (427.89)*
DEF: Complex cardiac arrhythmia; appears as severe sinus bradycardia, sinus bradycardia with tachycardia, or sinus bradycardia with atrioventricular block.

427.89 **Other**
Rhythm disorder:
coronary sinus
ectopic
nodal
Wandering (atrial) pacemaker
EXCLUDES *carotid sinus syncope (337.0)*
neonatal bradycardia (779.81)
neonatal tachycardia (779.82)
reflex bradycardia (337.0)
tachycardia NOS (785.0)

427.9 **Cardiac dysrhythmia, unspecified**
Arrhythmia (cardiac) NOS

✓4ᵗʰ **428** **Heart failure**
Code, if applicable, heart failure due to hypertension first (402.0-402.9, with fifth-digit 1 or 404.0-404.9 with fifth-digit 1 or 3)
EXCLUDES *following cardiac surgery (429.4)*
rheumatic (398.91)
that complicating:
abortion (634-638 with .7, 639.8)
ectopic or molar pregnancy (639.8)
labor or delivery (668.1, 669.4)

428.0 **Congestive heart failure, unspecified**
Congestive heart disease
Right heart failure (secondary to left heart failure)
EXCLUDES *fluid overload NOS (276.69)*
DEF: Mechanical inadequacy; caused by inability of heart to pump and circulate blood; results in fluid collection in lungs, hypertension, congestion and edema of tissue.

Diseases of the Circulatory System

428.1–429.81

Echocardiography of Heart Failure

Four-chamber echocardiograms, two-dimensional views.
LV: Left ventricle
RV: Right ventricle
RA: Right atrium
LA: Left atrium

Systolic dysfunction with dilated LV

Diastolic dysfunction with LV hypertrophy

428.1 Left heart failure
Acute edema of lung
Acute pulmonary edema } with heart disease NOS or heart failure
Cardiac asthma
Left ventricular failure
DEF: Mechanical inadequacy of left ventricle; causing fluid in lungs.

√5ᵗʰ **428.2 Systolic heart failure**
EXCLUDES combined systolic and diastolic heart failure (428.40-428.43)
DEF: Heart failure due to a defect in expulsion of blood caused by an abnormality in systolic function, or ventricular contractile dysfunction.
428.20 Unspecified
428.21 Acute
428.22 Chronic
428.23 Acute on chronic

√5ᵗʰ **428.3 Diastolic heart failure**
EXCLUDES combined systolic and diastolic heart failure (428.40-428.43)
DEF: Heart failure due to resistance to ventricular filling caused by an abnormality in the diastolic function.
428.30 Unspecified
428.31 Acute
428.32 Chronic
428.33 Acute on chronic

√5ᵗʰ **428.4 Combined systolic and diastolic heart failure**
428.40 Unspecified
428.41 Acute
428.42 Chronic
428.43 Acute on chronic

428.9 Heart failure, unspecified
Cardiac failure NOS
Heart failure NOS
Myocardial failure NOS
Weak heart

√4ᵗʰ **429 Ill-defined descriptions and complications of heart disease**
429.0 Myocarditis, unspecified
Myocarditis:
  NOS
  chronic (interstitial } (with mention of
  fibroid   arteriosclerosis)
  senile
Use additional code to identify presence of arteriosclerosis
EXCLUDES acute or subacute (422.0-422.9)
         rheumatic (398.0)
             acute (391.2)
         that due to hypertension (402.0-402.9)

429.1 Myocardial degeneration
Degeneration of heart or myocardium:
  fatty
  mural   } (with mention of
  muscular   arteriosclerosis)
Myocardial:
  degeneration
  disease
Use additional code to identify presence of arteriosclerosis
EXCLUDES that due to hypertension (402.0-402.9)

429.2 Cardiovascular disease, unspecified
Arteriosclerotic cardiovascular disease [ASCVD]
Cardiovascular arteriosclerosis
Cardiovascular:
  degeneration
  disease   } (with mention of
  sclerosis   arteriosclerosis)
Use additional code to identify presence of arteriosclerosis
EXCLUDES that due to hypertension (402.0-402.9)

429.3 Cardiomegaly
Cardiac:
  dilatation
  hypertrophy
Ventricular dilatation
EXCLUDES that due to hypertension (402.0-402.9)

429.4 Functional disturbances following cardiac surgery
Cardiac insufficiency } following cardiac surgery or
Heart failure   } due to prosthesis
Postcardiotomy syndrome
Postvalvulotomy syndrome
EXCLUDES cardiac failure in the immediate postoperative period (997.1)

429.5 Rupture of chordae tendineae
DEF: Torn tissue, between heart valves and papillary muscles.

429.6 Rupture of papillary muscle
DEF: Torn muscle, between chordae tendineae and heart wall.

√5ᵗʰ **429.7 Certain sequelae of myocardial infarction, not elsewhere classified**
Use additional code to identify the associated myocardial infarction:
  with onset of 8 weeks or less (410.00-410.92)
  with onset of more than 8 weeks (414.8)
EXCLUDES congenital defects of heart (745, 746)
         coronary aneurysm (414.11)
         disorders of papillary muscle (429.6, 429.81)
         postmyocardial infarction syndrome (411.0)
         rupture of chordae tendineae (429.5)
429.71 Acquired cardiac septal defect
EXCLUDES acute septal infarction (410.00-410.92)
DEF: Abnormal communication, between opposite heart chambers; due to defect of septum; not present at birth.
429.79 Other
Mural thrombus (atrial) (ventricular), acquired, following myocardial infarction

√5ᵗʰ **429.8 Other ill-defined heart diseases**
429.81 Other disorders of papillary muscle
Papillary muscle:
  atrophy
  degeneration
  dysfunction
  incompetence
  incoordination
  scarring

429.82 Hyperkinetic heart disease
DEF: Condition of unknown origin in young adults; marked by increased cardiac output at rest, increased rate of ventricular ejection; may lead to heart failure.

429.83 Takotsubo syndrome
Broken heart syndrome
Reversible left ventricular dysfunction following sudden emotional stress
Stress induced cardiomyopathy
Transient left ventricular apical ballooning syndrome

429.89 Other
Carditis
> **EXCLUDES** that due to hypertension (402.0-402.9)

429.9 Heart disease, unspecified
Heart disease (organic) NOS
Morbus cordis NOS
> **EXCLUDES** that due to hypertension (402.0-402.9)

CEREBROVASCULAR DISEASE (430-438)
INCLUDES with mention of hypertension (conditions classifiable to 401-405)
Use additional code to identify presence of hypertension
> **EXCLUDES** any condition classifiable to 430-434, 436, 437 occurring during pregnancy, childbirth, or the puerperium, or specified as puerperal (674.0)
> iatrogenic cerebrovascular infarction or hemorrhage (997.02)

430 Subarachnoid hemorrhage
Meningeal hemorrhage
Ruptured:
   berry aneurysm
   (congenital) cerebral aneurysm NOS
> **EXCLUDES** berry aneurysm, nonruptured (437.3)
> syphilitic ruptured cerebral aneurysm (094.87)

DEF: Bleeding in space between brain and lining.

431 Intracerebral hemorrhage
Hemorrhage (of):   Hemorrhage (of):
basilar   internal capsule
bulbar   intrapontine
cerebellar   pontine
cerebral   subcortical
cerebromeningeal   ventricular
cortical   Rupture of blood vessel in brain

DEF: Bleeding within the brain.

432 Other and unspecified intracranial hemorrhage
432.0 Nontraumatic extradural hemorrhage
Nontraumatic epidural hemorrhage
DEF: Bleeding, nontraumatic, between skull and brain lining.

432.1 Subdural hemorrhage
Subdural hematoma, nontraumatic
DEF: Bleeding, between outermost and other layers of brain lining.

432.9 Unspecified intracranial hemorrhage
Intracranial hemorrhage NOS

Berry Aneurysms

Berry aneurysm
Anterior communicating artery — 40 %
34%
Internal carotid — 20 %
4%
Posterior cerebral arteries
Basilar artery
Vertebral arteries
Arrows depict blood flow

433 Occlusion and stenosis of precerebral arteries
INCLUDES
embolism
narrowing   } of basilar, carotid, and vertebral
obstruction   arteries
thrombosis

Use additional code, if applicable, to identify status post administration of tPA (rtPA) in a different facility within the last 24 hours prior to admission to current facility (V45.88)
> **EXCLUDES** insufficiency NOS of precerebral arteries (435.0-435.9)

The following fifth-digit subclassification is for use with category 433:
  0 without mention of cerebral infarction
  1 with cerebral infarction

DEF: Blockage, stricture, arteries branching into brain.

433.0 Basilar artery
[0-1]

433.1 Carotid artery
[0-1]

433.2 Vertebral artery
[0-1]

433.3 Multiple and bilateral
[0-1]

433.8 Other specified precerebral artery
[0-1]

433.9 Unspecified precerebral artery
[0-1] Precerebral artery NOS

434 Occlusion of cerebral arteries
Use additional code, if applicable, to identify status post administration of tPA (rtPA) in a different facility within the last 24 hours prior to admission to current facility (V45.88)

The following fifth-digit subclassification is for use with category 434:
  0 without mention of cerebral infarction
  1 with cerebral infarction

434.0 Cerebral thrombosis
[0-1] Thrombosis of cerebral arteries

434.1 Cerebral embolism
[0-1]

434.9 Cerebral artery occlusion, unspecified
[0-1]

435 Transient cerebral ischemia
INCLUDES cerebrovascular insufficiency (acute) with transient focal neurological signs and symptoms
insufficiency of basilar, carotid, and vertebral arteries
spasm of cerebral arteries
> **EXCLUDES** acute cerebrovascular insufficiency NOS (437.1)
> that due to any condition classifiable to 433 (433.0-433.9)

435.0 Basilar artery syndrome

435.1 Vertebral artery syndrome

Cerebrovascular Arteries

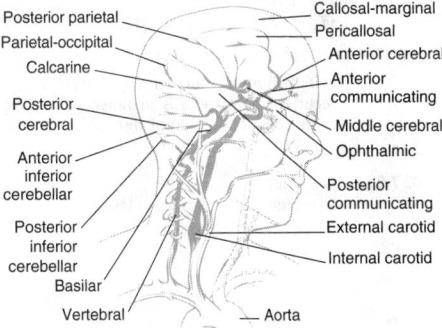

Posterior parietal
Parietal-occipital
Calcarine
Posterior cerebral
Anterior inferior cerebellar
Posterior inferior cerebellar
Basilar
Vertebral
Callosal-marginal
Pericallosal
Anterior cerebral
Anterior communicating
Middle cerebral
Ophthalmic
Posterior communicating
External carotid
Internal carotid
Aorta

435.2 Subclavian steal syndrome

DEF: Cerebrovascular insufficiency, due to occluded subclavian artery; symptoms include pain in mastoid and posterior head regions, flaccid paralysis of arm and diminished or absent radial pulse on affected side.

435.3 Vertebrobasilar artery syndrome

DEF: Transient ischemic attack; due to brainstem dysfunction; symptoms include confusion, vertigo, binocular blindness, diplopia, unilateral or bilateral weakness and paresthesis of extremities.

435.8 Other specified transient cerebral ischemias

435.9 Unspecified transient cerebral ischemia

Impending cerebrovascular accident
Intermittent cerebral ischemia
Transient ischemic attack [TIA]

DEF: Temporary restriction of blood flow to arteries branching into brain.

436 Acute, but ill-defined, cerebrovascular disease

Apoplexy, apoplectic:
  NOS
  attack
  cerebral
  seizure
Cerebral seizure

EXCLUDES   any condition classifiable to categories 430-435
  cerebrovascular accident (434.91)
  CVA (ischemic) (434.91)
    embolic (434.11)
    hemorrhagic (430, 431, 432.0-432.9)
    thrombotic (434.01)
  postoperative cerebrovascular accident (997.02)
  stroke (ischemic) (434.91)
    embolic (434.11)
    hemorrhagic (430, 431, 432.0-432.9)
    thrombotic (434.01)

√4ᵗʰ 437 Other and ill-defined cerebrovascular disease

437.0 Cerebral atherosclerosis

Atheroma of cerebral arteries
Cerebral arteriosclerosis

437.1 Other generalized ischemic cerebrovascular disease

Acute cerebrovascular insufficiency NOS
Cerebral ischemia (chronic)

437.2 Hypertensive encephalopathy

DEF: Cerebral manifestations (such as visual disturbances and headache) due to high blood pressure.

437.3 Cerebral aneurysm, nonruptured

Internal carotid artery, intracranial portion
Internal carotid artery NOS

EXCLUDES   congenital cerebral aneurysm, nonruptured (747.81)
  internal carotid artery, extracranial portion (442.81)

437.4 Cerebral arteritis

DEF: Inflammation of a cerebral artery or arteries.

437.5 Moyamoya disease

DEF: Cerebrovascular ischemia; vessels occlude and rupture causing tiny hemorrhages at base of brain; predominantly affects Japanese.

437.6 Nonpyogenic thrombosis of intracranial venous sinus

EXCLUDES   pyogenic (325)

437.7 Transient global amnesia

DEF: Episode of short-term memory loss, not often recurrent; pathogenesis unknown; with no signs or symptoms of neurological disorder.

437.8 Other

437.9 Unspecified

Cerebrovascular disease or lesion NOS

√4ᵗʰ 438 Late effects of cerebrovascular disease

Note: This category is to be used to indicate conditions in 430-437 as the cause of late effects. The "late effects" include conditions specified as such, as sequelae, which may occur at any time after the onset of the causal condition.

EXCLUDES   personal history of:
  cerebral infarction without residual deficits (V12.54)
  PRIND [Prolonged reversible ischemic neurologic deficit] (V12.54)
  RIND [Reversible ischemic neurological deficit] (V12.54)
  transient ischemic attack [TIA] (V12.54)

438.0 Cognitive deficits

√5ᵗʰ 438.1 Speech and language deficits

438.10 Speech and language deficit, unspecified

438.11 Aphasia

DEF: Impairment or absence of the ability to communicate by speech, writing or signs or to comprehend the spoken or written language due to disease or injury to the brain.

438.12 Dysphasia

DEF: Impaired speech; marked by inability to sequence language.

438.13 Dysarthria

DEF: Speech disorder caused by paralysis, spasticity, or other nerve damage resulting in difficulty expressing words or sounds; characterized by slurring, interrupted rhythm of speech, or distorted vowel sounds.

438.14 Fluency disorder

Stuttering due to late effect of cerebrovascular accident

DEF: Interruption in the flow of speech that significantly interferes with communication; characterized by primary sound and syllable repetitions, articulatory fixations, and abnormal prolongation of speech sounds.

438.19 Other speech and language deficits

√5ᵗʰ 438.2 Hemiplegia/hemiparesis

DEF: Paralysis of one side of the body.

438.20 Hemiplegia affecting unspecified side

438.21 Hemiplegia affecting dominant side

438.22 Hemiplegia affecting nondominant side

√5ᵗʰ 438.3 Monoplegia of upper limb

DEF: Paralysis of one limb or one muscle group.

438.30 Monoplegia of upper limb affecting unspecified side

438.31 Monoplegia of upper limb affecting dominant side

438.32 Monoplegia of upper limb affecting nondominant side

√5ᵗʰ 438.4 Monoplegia of lower limb

438.40 Monoplegia of lower limb affecting unspecified side

438.41 Monoplegia of lower limb affecting dominant side

438.42 Monoplegia of lower limb affecting nondominant side

√5ᵗʰ 438.5 Other paralytic syndrome

Use additional code to identify type of paralytic syndrome, such as:
  locked-in state (344.81)
  quadriplegia (344.00-344.09)

EXCLUDES   late effects of cerebrovascular accident with:
  hemiplegia/hemiparesis (438.20-438.22)
  monoplegia of lower limb (438.40-438.42)
  monoplegia of upper limb (438.30-438.32)

438.50 Other paralytic syndrome affecting unspecified side

Map of Major Arteries

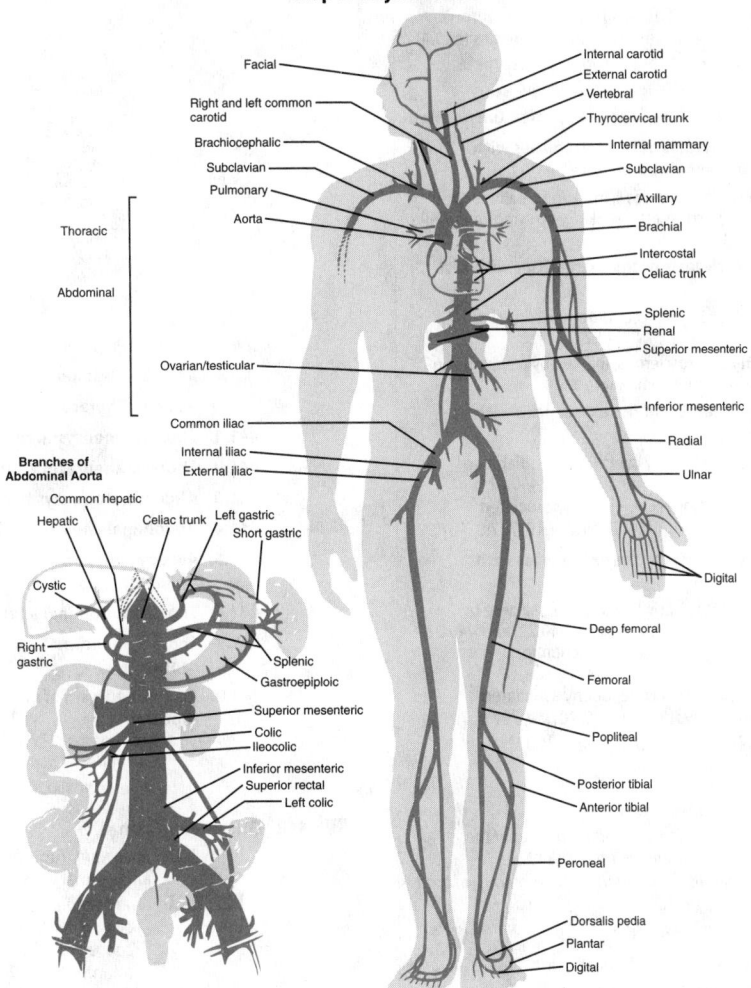

438.51 **Other paralytic syndrome affecting dominant side**

438.52 **Other paralytic syndrome affecting nondominant side**

438.53 **Other paralytic syndrome, bilateral**

438.6 **Alterations of sensations**
Use additional code to identify the altered sensation

438.7 **Disturbances of vision**
Use additional code to identify the visual disturbance

√5th **438.8** **Other late effects of cerebrovascular disease**

438.81 **Apraxia**
DEF: Inability to activate learned movements; no known sensory or motor impairment.

438.82 **Dysphagia**
Use additional code to identify the type of dysphagia, if known (787.20-787.29)
DEF: Inability or difficulty in swallowing.

438.83 **Facial weakness**
Facial droop

438.84 **Ataxia**

438.85 **Vertigo**

438.89 **Other late effects of cerebrovascular disease**
Use additional code to identify the late effect

438.9 **Unspecified late effects of cerebrovascular disease**

DISEASES OF ARTERIES, ARTERIOLES, AND CAPILLARIES (440-449)

√4th **440** **Atherosclerosis**

INCLUDES   arteriolosclerosis
arteriosclerosis (obliterans) (senile)
arteriosclerotic vascular disease
atheroma
degeneration:
  arterial
  arteriovascular
  vascular
endarteritis deformans or obliterans
senile:
  arteritis
  endarteritis

EXCLUDES   *atheroembolism (445.01-445.89)*
atherosclerosis of bypass graft of the extremities (440.30-440.32)

DEF: Stricture and reduced elasticity of artery; due to plaque deposits.

440.0 **Of aorta**

440.1 **Of renal artery**
EXCLUDES   *atherosclerosis of renal arterioles (403.00-403.91)*

Diseases of the Circulatory System

440.2–442.84

√5ᵗʰ **440.2 Of native arteries of the extremities**

Use additional code, if applicable, to identify chronic total occlusion of artery of the extremities (440.4)

EXCLUDES   *atherosclerosis of bypass graft of the extremities (440.30-440.32)*

440.20 Atherosclerosis of the extremities, unspecified

440.21 Atherosclerosis of the extremities with intermittent claudication

DEF: Atherosclerosis; marked by pain, tension and weakness after walking; no symptoms while at rest.

440.22 Atherosclerosis of the extremities with rest pain

INCLUDES   any condition classifiable to 440.21

DEF: Atherosclerosis, marked by pain, tension and weakness while at rest.

440.23 Atherosclerosis of the extremities with ulceration

INCLUDES   any condition classifiable to 440.21 and 440.22

Use additional code for any associated ulceration (707.10-707.19, 707.8, 707.9)

440.24 Atherosclerosis of the extremities with gangrene

INCLUDES   any condition classifiable to 440.21, 440.22, and 440.23 with ischemic gangrene 785.4

Use additional code for any associated ulceration (707.10-707.19, 707.8, 707.9)

EXCLUDES   *gas gangrene (040.0)*

440.29 Other

√5ᵗʰ **440.3 Of bypass graft of extremities**

EXCLUDES   *atherosclerosis of native arteries of the extremities (440.21-440.24)*
embolism [occlusion NOS] [thrombus] of graft (996.74)

440.30 Of unspecified graft

440.31 Of autologous vein bypass graft

440.32 Of nonautologous biological bypass graft

440.4 Chronic total occlusion of artery of the extremities

Complete occlusion of artery of the extremities

Total occlusion of artery of the extremities

Code first atherosclerosis of arteries of the extremities (440.20-440.29, 440.30-440.32)

EXCLUDES   *acute occlusion of artery of extremity (444.21-444.22)*

440.8 Of other specified arteries

EXCLUDES   *basilar (433.0)*
carotid (433.1)
cerebral (437.0)
coronary (414.00-414.07)
mesenteric (557.1)
precerebral (433.0-433.9)
pulmonary (416.0)
vertebral (433.2)

440.9 Generalized and unspecified atherosclerosis

Arteriosclerotic vascular disease NOS

EXCLUDES   *arteriosclerotic cardiovascular disease [ASCVD] (429.2)*

√4ᵗʰ **441 Aortic aneurysm and dissection**

EXCLUDES   *aortic ectasia (447.70-447.73)*
syphilitic aortic aneurysm (093.0)
traumatic aortic aneurysm (901.0, 902.0)

√5ᵗʰ **441.0 Dissection of aorta**

DEF: Dissection or splitting of wall of the aorta; due to blood entering through intimal tear or interstitial hemorrhage.

441.00 Unspecified site

441.01 Thoracic

Thoracic and Abdominal Aortic Aneurysm

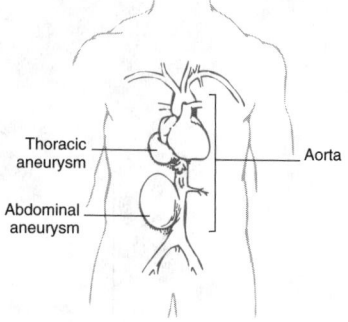

Thoracic aneurysm

Abdominal aneurysm

Aorta

441.02 Abdominal

441.03 Thoracoabdominal

441.1 Thoracic aneurysm, ruptured

441.2 Thoracic aneurysm without mention of rupture

441.3 Abdominal aneurysm, ruptured

441.4 Abdominal aneurysm without mention of rupture

441.5 Aortic aneurysm of unspecified site, ruptured

Rupture of aorta NOS

441.6 Thoracoabdominal aneurysm, ruptured

441.7 Thoracoabdominal aneurysm, without mention of rupture

441.9 Aortic aneurysm of unspecified site without mention of rupture

Aneurysm
Dilatation } of aorta
Hyaline necrosis

√4ᵗʰ **442 Other aneurysm**

INCLUDES   aneurysm (ruptured) (cirsoid) (false) (varicose)
aneurysmal varix

EXCLUDES   *arteriovenous aneurysm or fistula:*
acquired (447.0)
congenital (747.60-747.69)
traumatic (900.0-904.9)

DEF: Dissection or splitting of arterial wall; due to blood entering through intimal tear or interstitial hemorrhage.

442.0 Of artery of upper extremity

442.1 Of renal artery

442.2 Of iliac artery

442.3 Of artery of lower extremity

Aneurysm:
femoral artery
popliteal artery

√5ᵗʰ **442.8 Of other specified artery**

442.81 Artery of neck

Aneurysm of carotid artery (common) (external) (internal, extracranial portion)

EXCLUDES   *internal carotid artery, intra- cranial portion (437.3)*

442.82 Subclavian artery

442.83 Splenic artery

442.84 Other visceral artery

Aneurysm:
celiac
gastroduodenal
gastroepiploic
hepatic } artery
pancreaticoduodenal
superior mesenteric

442.89   Other
Aneurysm:
mediastinal artery
spinal artery

> EXCLUDES *cerebral (nonruptured) (437.3)*
> *congenital (747.81)*
> *ruptured (430)*
> *coronary (414.11)*
> *heart (414.10)*
> *pulmonary (417.1)*

442.9   Of unspecified site

✓4ᵗʰ **443   Other peripheral vascular disease**

443.0   Raynaud's syndrome
Raynaud's:
disease
phenomenon (secondary)
Use additional code to identify gangrene (785.4)

DEF: Constriction of the arteries, due to cold or stress; bilateral ischemic attacks of fingers, toes, nose or ears; symptoms include pallor, paresthesia and pain.

443.1   Thromboangiitis obliterans [Buerger's disease]
Presenile gangrene

DEF: Inflammatory disease of extremity blood vessels, mainly the lower; occurs primarily in young men and leads to tissue ischemia and gangrene.

✓5ᵗʰ **443.2   Other arterial dissection**

> EXCLUDES *dissection of aorta (441.00-441.03)*
> *dissection of coronary arteries (414.12)*

443.21   Dissection of carotid artery

443.22   Dissection of iliac artery

443.23   Dissection of renal artery

443.24   Dissection of vertebral artery

443.29   Dissection of other artery

✓5ᵗʰ **443.8   Other specified peripheral vascular diseases**

443.81   *Peripheral angiopathy in diseases classified elsewhere*
Code first underlying disease, as:
diabetes mellitus (249.7, 250.7)

443.82   Erythromelalgia
DEF: Rare syndrome of paroxysmal vasodilation; maldistribution of blood flow causes redness, pain, increased skin temperature, and burning sensations in various parts of the body.

443.89   Other
Acrocyanosis
Acroparesthesia:
simple [Schultze's type]
vasomotor [Nothnagel's type]
Erythrocyanosis

> EXCLUDES *chilblains (991.5)*
> *frostbite (991.0-991.3)*
> *immersion foot (991.4)*

443.9   Peripheral vascular disease, unspecified
Intermittent claudication NOS
Peripheral:
angiopathy NOS
vascular disease NOS
Spasm of artery

> EXCLUDES *atherosclerosis of the arteries of the extremities (440.20-440.22)*
> *spasm of cerebral artery (435.0-435.9)*

Arterial Diseases and Disorders

Lipids / Calcium deposits — Intimal proliferation — Atherosclerosis narrowing lumen — Thrombus (clot) forming in lumen — Organization of thrombus and recanalization — Embolus (from elsewhere) occluding lumen — Aneurysm bypasses lumen or… …bulges from arterial wall — Arteriovenous fistula

✓4ᵗʰ **444   Arterial embolism and thrombosis**

> INCLUDES infarction:
> embolic
> thrombotic
> occlusion

> EXCLUDES *atheroembolism (445.01-445.89)*
> *that complicating:*
> *abortion (634-638 with .6, 639.6)*
> *ectopic or molar pregnancy (639.6)*
> *pregnancy, childbirth, or the pueperium (673.0-673.8)*
> *septic arterial embolism (449)*

✓5ᵗʰ **444.0   Of abdominal aorta**

444.01   Saddle embolus of abdominal aorta

444.09   Other arterial embolism and thrombosis of abdominal aorta
Aortic bifurcation syndrome
Aortoiliac obstruction
Leriche's syndrome

444.1   Of thoracic aorta
Embolism or thrombosis of aorta (thoracic)

✓5ᵗʰ **444.2   Of arteries of the extremities**

444.21   Upper extremity

444.22   Lower extremity
Arterial embolism or thrombosis:
femoral
peripheral NOS
popliteal

> EXCLUDES *iliofemoral (444.81)*

✓5ᵗʰ **444.8   Of other specified artery**

444.81   Iliac artery

444.89   Other

> EXCLUDES *basilar (433.0)*
> *carotid (433.1)*
> *cerebral (434.0-434.9)*
> *coronary (410.00-410.92)*
> *mesenteric (557.0)*
> *ophthalmic (362.30-362.34)*
> *precerebral (433.0-433.9)*
> *pulmonary (415.11-415.19)*
> *renal (593.81)*
> *retinal (362.30-362.34)*
> *vertebral (433.2)*

444.9   Of unspecified artery

✓4ᵗʰ **445   Atheroembolism**

> INCLUDES atherothrombotic microembolism
> cholesterol embolism

✓5ᵗʰ **445.0   Of extremities**

445.01   Upper extremity

445.02   Lower extremity

Diseases of the Circulatory System

445.8–448.1

☑5ᵗʰ **445.8 Of other sites**

445.81 Kidney

Use additional code for any associated acute kidney failure or chronic kidney disease (584, 585)

445.89 Other site

☑4ᵗʰ **446 Polyarteritis nodosa and allied conditions**

446.0 Polyarteritis nodosa

Disseminated necrotizing periarteritis
Necrotizing angiitis
Panarteritis (nodosa)
Periarteritis (nodosa)

DEF: Inflammation of small and mid-size arteries; symptoms related to involved arteries in kidneys, muscles, gastrointestinal tract and heart; results in tissue death.

446.1 Acute febrile mucocutaneous lymph node syndrome [MCLS]

Kawasaki disease

DEF: Acute febrile disease of children; marked by erythema of conjunctiva and mucous membranes of upper respiratory tract, skin eruptions and edema.

☑5ᵗʰ **446.2 Hypersensitivity angiitis**

EXCLUDES *antiglomerular basement membrane disease without pulmonary hemorrhage (583.89)*

446.20 Hypersensitivity angiitis, unspecified

446.21 Goodpasture's syndrome

Antiglomerular basement membrane antibody-mediated nephritis with pulmonary hemorrhage

Use additional code to identify renal disease (583.81)

DEF: Glomerulonephritis associated with hematuria, progresses rapidly; results in death from renal failure.

446.29 Other specified hypersensitivity angiitis

446.3 Lethal midline granuloma

Malignant granuloma of face

DEF: Granulomatous lesion; in nose or paranasal sinuses; often fatal; occurs chiefly in males.

446.4 Wegener's granulomatosis

Necrotizing respiratory granulomatosis
Wegener's syndrome

DEF: A disease occurring mainly in men; marked by necrotizing granulomas and ulceration of the upper respiratory tract; cause is a vasculitis affecting small vessels due to an immune disorder.

446.5 Giant cell arteritis

Bagratuni's syndrome
Cranial arteritis
Horton's disease
Temporal arteritis

DEF: Inflammation of arteries; due to giant cells affecting carotid artery branches, resulting in occlusion; symptoms include fever, headache and neurological problems.

446.6 Thrombotic microangiopathy

Moschcowitz's syndrome
Thrombotic thrombocytopenic purpura

DEF: Blockage of small blood vessels; due to hyaline deposits; symptoms include purpura, CNS disorders; results in protracted disease or rapid death.

446.7 Takayasu's disease

Aortic arch arteritis
Pulseless disease

DEF: Progressive obliterative arteritis of brachiocephalic trunk, left subclavian, and left common carotid arteries above aortic arch; results in ischemia in brain, heart and arm.

☑4ᵗʰ **447 Other disorders of arteries and arterioles**

447.0 Arteriovenous fistula, acquired

Arteriovenous aneurysm, acquired

EXCLUDES *cerebrovascular (437.3)*
coronary (414.19)
pulmonary (417.0)
surgically created arteriovenous shunt or fistula:
complication (996.1, 996.61-996.62)
status or presence (V45.11)
traumatic (900.0-904.9)

DEF: Communication between an artery and vein caused by error in healing.

447.1 Stricture of artery

447.2 Rupture of artery

Erosion
Fistula, except arteriovenous } of artery
Ulcer

EXCLUDES *traumatic rupture of artery (900.0-904.9)*

447.3 Hyperplasia of renal artery

Fibromuscular hyperplasia of renal artery

DEF: Overgrowth of cells in muscular lining of renal artery.

447.4 Celiac artery compression syndrome

Celiac axis syndrome
Marable's syndrome

447.5 Necrosis of artery

447.6 Arteritis, unspecified

Aortitis NOS
Endarteritis NOS

EXCLUDES *arteritis, endarteritis:*
aortic arch (446.7)
cerebral (437.4)
coronary (414.00-414.07)
deformans (440.0-440.9)
obliterans (440.0-440.9)
pulmonary (417.8)
senile (440.0-440.9)
polyarteritis NOS (446.0)
syphilitic aortitis (093.1)

☑5ᵗʰ **447.7 Aortic ectasia**

Ectasis aorta

EXCLUDES *aortic aneurysm and dissection (441.00-441.9)*

DEF: A diffuse, irregular dilation of the aorta less than 3 cm in diameter; increases the patient's risk of developing an aortic aneurysm.

447.70 Aortic ectasia, unspecified site

447.71 Thoracic aortic ectasia

447.72 Abdominal aortic ectasia

447.73 Thoracoabdominal aortic ectasia

447.8 Other specified disorders of arteries and arterioles

Fibromuscular hyperplasia of arteries, except renal

447.9 Unspecified disorders of arteries and arterioles

☑4ᵗʰ **448 Disease of capillaries**

448.0 Hereditary hemorrhagic telangiectasia

Rendu-Osler-Weber disease

DEF: Genetic disease with onset after puberty; results in multiple telangiectases, dilated venules on skin and mucous membranes; recurrent bleeding may occur.

448.1 Nevus, non-neoplastic

Nevus:	Nevus:
araneus	spider
senile	stellar

EXCLUDES *neoplastic (216.0-216.9)*
port wine (757.32)
strawberry (757.32)

DEF: Enlarged or malformed blood vessels of skin; results in reddish swelling, skin patch, or birthmark.

Map of Major Veins

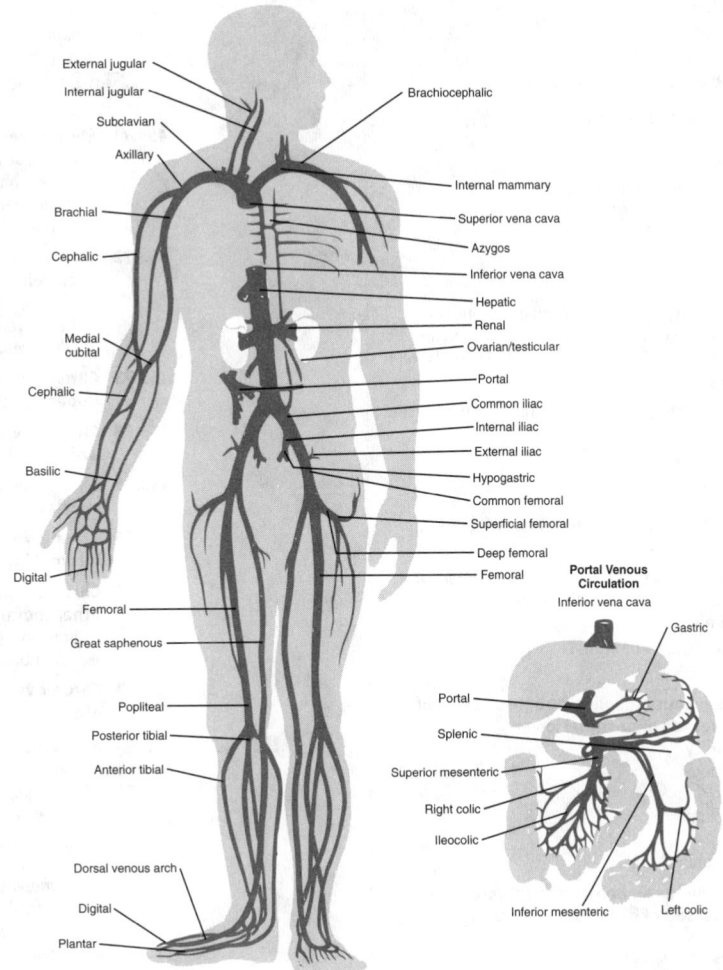

448.9   Other and unspecified capillary diseases
Capillary:
    hemorrhage
    hyperpermeability
    thrombosis
    EXCLUDES *capillary fragility (hereditary) (287.8)*

449   Septic arterial embolism
Code first underlying infection, such as:
    infective endocarditis (421.0)
    lung abscess (513.0)
Use additional code to identify the site of the embolism
    (433.0-433.9, 444.01-444.9)
    EXCLUDES *septic pulmonary embolism (415.12)*

DISEASES OF VEINS AND LYMPHATICS, AND OTHER DISEASES OF CIRCULATORY SYSTEM (451-459)

√4ᵗʰ 451   Phlebitis and thrombophlebitis
    INCLUDES endophlebitis
        inflammation, vein
        periphlebitis
        suppurative phlebitis
Use additional E code to identify drug, if drug-induced
    EXCLUDES *that complicating:*
        abortion (634-638 with .7, 639.8)
        ectopic or molar pregnancy (639.8)
        pregnancy, childbirth, or the puerperium
            (671.0-671.9)
    that due to or following:
        implant or catheter device (996.61-996.62)
        infusion, perfusion, or transfusion (999.2)
DEF: Inflammation of a vein (phlebitis) with formation of a
thrombus (thrombophlebitis).

451.0   Of superficial vessels of lower extremities
Saphenous vein (greater) (lesser)

√5ᵗʰ 451.1   Of deep vessels of lower extremities

451.11   Femoral vein (deep) (superficial)

451.19   Other
    Femoropopliteal vein
    Popliteal vein
    Tibial vein

451.2   Of lower extremities, unspecified

√5ᵗʰ 451.8   Of other sites
    EXCLUDES *intracranial venous sinus (325)*
        nonpyogenic (437.6)
        portal (vein) (572.1)

451.81   Iliac vein

451.82   Of superficial veins of upper extremities
    Antecubital vein
    Basilic vein
    Cephalic vein

451.83   Of deep veins of upper extremities
    Brachial vein
    Radial vein
    Ulnar vein

451.84   Of upper extremities, unspecified

451.89   Other
    Axillary vein
    Jugular vein
    Subclavian vein
    Thrombophlebitis of breast (Mondor's disease)

451.9   Of unspecified site

Diseases of the Circulatory System

452–453.9

452   Portal vein thrombosis
Portal (vein) obstruction
EXCLUDES   *hepatic vein thrombosis (453.0)*
     phlebitis of portal vein (572.1)
DEF: Formation of a blood clot in main vein of liver.

453   Other venous embolism and thrombosis
EXCLUDES   *that complicating:*
     abortion (634-638 with .7, 639.8)
     ectopic or molar pregnancy (639.8)
     pregnancy, childbirth, or the puerperium
       (671.0-671.9)

453.0   Budd-Chiari syndrome
Hepatic vein thrombosis
DEF: Thrombosis or other obstruction of hepatic vein; symptoms include enlarged liver, extensive collateral vessels, intractable ascites and severe portal hypertension.

453.1   Thrombophlebitis migrans
DEF: Slow, advancing thrombophlebitis; appearing first in one vein then another.

453.2   Of inferior vena cava

453.3   Of renal vein

453.4   Acute venous embolism and thrombosis of deep vessels of lower extremity

453.40   Acute venous embolism and thrombosis of unspecified deep vessels of lower extremity
Deep vein thrombosis NOS
DVT NOS

453.41   Acute venous embolism and thrombosis of deep vessels of proximal lower extremity
Femoral
Iliac
Popliteal
Thigh
Upper leg NOS

453.42   Acute venous embolism and thrombosis of deep vessels of distal lower extremity
Calf
Lower leg NOS
Peroneal
Tibial

453.5   Chronic venous embolism and thrombosis of deep vessels of lower extremity
Use additional code, if applicable, for associated long-term (current) use of anticoagulants (V58.61)
EXCLUDES   *personal history of venous thrombosis and embolism (V12.51)*

453.50   Chronic venous embolism and thrombosis of unspecified deep vessels of lower extremity

453.51   Chronic venous embolism and thrombosis of deep vessels of proximal lower extremity
Femoral
Iliac
Popliteal
Thigh
Upper leg NOS

453.52   Chronic venous embolism and thrombosis of deep vessels of distal lower extremity
Calf
Lower leg NOS
Peroneal
Tibial

453.6   Venous embolism and thrombosis of superficial vessels of lower extremity
Saphenous vein (greater) (lesser)
Use additional code, if applicable, for associated long-term (current) use of anticoagulants (V58.61)

453.7   Chronic venous embolism and thrombosis of other specified vessels
Use additional code, if applicable, for associated long-term (current) use of anticoagulants (V58.61)
EXCLUDES   *personal history of venous thrombosis and embolism (V12.51)*

453.71   Chronic venous embolism and thrombosis of superficial veins of upper extremity
Antecubital vein
Basilic vein
Cephalic vein

453.72   Chronic venous embolism and thrombosis of deep veins of upper extremity
Brachial vein
Radial vein
Ulnar vein

453.73   Chronic venous embolism and thrombosis of upper extremity, unspecified

453.74   Chronic venous embolism and thrombosis of axillary veins

453.75   Chronic venous embolism and thrombosis of subclavian veins

453.76   Chronic venous embolism and thrombosis of internal jugular veins

453.77   Chronic venous embolism and thrombosis of other thoracic veins
Brachiocephalic (innominate)
Superior vena cava

453.79   Chronic venous embolism and thrombosis of other specified veins

453.8   Acute venous embolism and thrombosis of other specified veins
EXCLUDES   *cerebral (434.0-434.9)*
     coronary (410.00-410.92)
     intracranial venous sinus (325)
       nonpyogenic (437.6)
     mesenteric (557.0)
     portal (452)
     precerebral (433.0-433.9)
     pulmonary (415.19)

453.81   Acute venous embolism and thrombosis of superficial veins of upper extremity
Antecubital vein
Basilic vein
Cephalic vein

453.82   Acute venous embolism and thrombosis of deep veins of upper extremity
Brachial vein
Radial vein
Ulnar vein

453.83   Acute venous embolism and thrombosis of upper extremity, unspecified

453.84   Acute venous embolism and thrombosis of axillary veins

453.85   Acute venous embolism and thrombosis of subclavian veins

453.86   Acute venous embolism and thrombosis of internal jugular veins

453.87   Acute venous embolism and thrombosis of other thoracic veins
Brachiocephalic (innominate)
Superior vena cava

453.89   Acute venous embolism and thrombosis of other specified veins

453.9   Of unspecified site
Embolism of vein
Thrombosis (vein)

✓4ᵗʰ **454   Varicose veins of lower extremities**

> **EXCLUDES** *that complicating pregnancy, childbirth, or the puerperium (671.0)*

DEF: Dilated leg veins; due to incompetent vein valves that allow reversed blood flow and cause tissue erosion or weakness of wall; may be painful.

454.0   With ulcer
Varicose ulcer (lower extremity, any part)
Varicose veins with ulcer of lower extremity [any part] or of unspecified site
Any condition classifiable to 454.9 with ulcer or specified as ulcerated

454.1   With inflammation
Stasis dermatitis
Varicose veins with inflammation of lower extremity [any part] or of unspecified site
Any condition classifiable to 454.9 with inflammation or specified as inflamed

454.2   With ulcer and inflammation
Varicose veins with ulcer and inflammation of lower extremity [any part] or of unspecified site
Any condition classifiable to 454.9 with ulcer and inflammation

454.8   With other complications
Edema
Pain
Swelling

454.9   Asymptomatic varicose veins
Phlebectasia   ⎫
Varicose veins ⎬ of lower extremity [any part] or of unspecified site
Varix   ⎭
Varicose veins NOS

✓4ᵗʰ **455   Hemorrhoids**

> **INCLUDES** hemorrhoids (anus) (rectum)
> piles
> varicose veins, anus or rectum
> **EXCLUDES** *that complicating pregnancy, childbirth, or the puerperium (671.8)*

DEF: Varicose condition of external hemorrhoidal veins causing painful swellings at the anus.

455.0   Internal hemorrhoids without mention of complication

455.1   Internal thrombosed hemorrhoids

455.2   Internal hemorrhoids with other complication
Internal hemorrhoids:
bleeding
prolapsed
strangulated
ulcerated

455.3   External hemorrhoids without mention of complication

455.4   External thrombosed hemorrhoids

455.5   External hemorrhoids with other complication
External hemorrhoids:
bleeding
prolapsed
strangulated
ulcerated

455.6   Unspecified hemorrhoids without mention of complication
Hemorrhoids NOS

455.7   Unspecified thrombosed hemorrhoids
Thrombosed hemorrhoids, unspecified whether internal or external

455.8   Unspecified hemorrhoids with other complication
Hemorrhoids, unspecified whether internal or external:
bleeding
prolapsed
strangulated
ulcerated

455.9   Residual hemorrhoidal skin tags
Skin tags, anus or rectum

Veins of Head and Neck

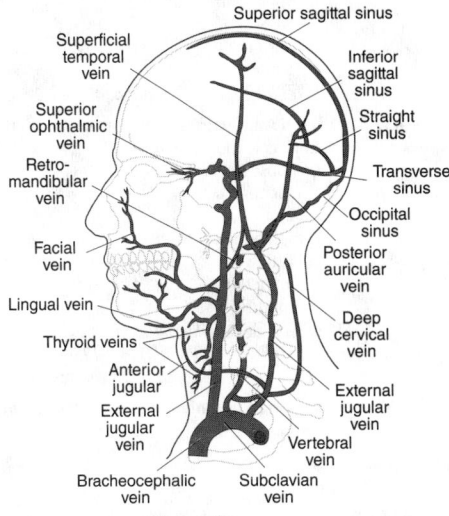

✓4ᵗʰ **456   Varicose veins of other sites**

456.0   Esophageal varices with bleeding
DEF: Distended, tortuous, veins of lower esophagus, usually due to portal hypertension.

456.1   Esophageal varices without mention of bleeding

✓5ᵗʰ **456.2   Esophageal varices in diseases classified elsewhere**
Code first underlying cause, as:
cirrhosis of liver (571.0-571.9)
portal hypertension (572.3)

  456.20   With bleeding

  456.21   Without mention of bleeding

456.3   Sublingual varices
DEF: Distended, tortuous veins beneath tongue.

456.4   Scrotal varices
Varicocele

456.5   Pelvic varices
Varices of broad ligament

456.6   Vulval varices
Varices of perineum
> **EXCLUDES** *that complicating pregnancy, childbirth, or the puerperium (671.1)*

456.8   Varices of other sites
Varicose veins of nasal septum (with ulcer)
> **EXCLUDES** *placental varices (656.7)*
> *retinal varices (362.17)*
> *varicose ulcer of unspecified site (454.0)*
> *varicose veins of unspecified site (454.9)*

✓4ᵗʰ **457   Noninfectious disorders of lymphatic channels**

457.0   Postmastectomy lymphedema syndrome
Elephantiasis   ⎫
Obliteration of lymphatic ⎬ due to mastectomy
vessel   ⎭

DEF: Reduced lymphatic circulation following mastectomy; symptoms include swelling of the arm on the operative side.

457.1   Other lymphedema
Elephantiasis (nonfilarial) NOS
Lymphangiectasis
Lymphedema:
acquired (chronic)
praecox
secondary
Obliteration, lymphatic vessel
> **EXCLUDES** *elephantiasis (nonfilarial):*
> *congenital (757.0)*
> *eyelid (374.83)*
> *vulva (624.8)*

DEF: Fluid retention due to reduced lymphatic circulation; due to other than mastectomy.

Diseases of the Circulatory System

457.2–459.9

457.2   **Lymphangitis**
Lymphangitis:
    NOS
    chronic
    subacute
    EXCLUDES   *acute lymphangitis (682.0-682.9)*

457.8   **Other noninfectious disorders of lymphatic channels**
Chylocele (nonfilarial)
Chylous:
    ascites
    cyst
Lymph node or vessel:
    fistula
    infarction
    rupture
    EXCLUDES   *chylocele:*
       filarial (125.0-125.9)
       tunica vaginalis (nonfilarial) (608.84)

457.9   **Unspecified noninfectious disorder of lymphatic channels**

458   **Hypotension**
    INCLUDES   hypopiesis
    EXCLUDES   *cardiovascular collapse (785.50)*
       maternal hypotension syndrome (669.2)
       shock (785.50-785.59)
       Shy-Drager syndrome (333.0)

458.0   **Orthostatic hypotension**
Hypotension:
    orthostatic (chronic)
    postural
DEF: Low blood pressure; occurs when standing.

458.1   **Chronic hypotension**
Permanent idiopathic hypotension
DEF: Persistent low blood pressure.

458.2   **Iatrogenic hypotension**
DEF: Abnormally low blood pressure; due to medical treatment.

    458.21   **Hypotension of hemodialysis**
       Intra-dialytic hypotension

    458.29   **Other iatrogenic hypotension**
       Postoperative hypotension

458.8   **Other specified hypotension**

458.9   **Hypotension, unspecified**
Hypotension (arterial) NOS

459   **Other disorders of circulatory system**

459.0   **Hemorrhage, unspecified**
Rupture of blood vessel NOS
Spontaneous hemorrhage NEC
    EXCLUDES   *hemorrhage:*
       gastrointestinal NOS (578.9)
       in newborn NOS (772.9)
       secondary or recurrent following trauma (958.2)
       traumatic rupture of blood vessel (900.0-904.9)
       nontraumatic hematoma of soft tissue (729.92)

459.1   **Postphlebitic syndrome**
Chronic venous hypertension due to deep vein thrombosis
    EXCLUDES   *chronic venous hypertension without deep vein thrombosis (459.30-459.39)*
DEF: Various conditions following deep vein thrombosis; including edema, pain, stasis dermatitis, cellulitis, varicose veins and ulceration of the lower leg.

    459.10   **Postphlebitic syndrome without complications**
       Asymptomatic postphlebitic syndrome
       Postphlebitic syndrome NOS

    459.11   **Postphlebitic syndrome with ulcer**

    459.12   **Postphlebitic syndrome with inflammation**

    459.13   **Postphlebitic syndrome with ulcer and inflammation**

    459.19   **Postphlebitic syndrome with other complication**

459.2   **Compression of vein**
Stricture of vein
Vena cava syndrome (inferior) (superior)

459.3   **Chronic venous hypertension (idiopathic)**
Stasis edema
    EXCLUDES   *chronic venous hypertension due to deep vein thrombosis (459.10-459.9)*
       varicose veins (454.0-454.9)

    459.30   **Chronic venous hypertension without complications**
       Asymptomatic chronic venous hypertension
       Chronic venous hypertension NOS

    459.31   **Chronic venous hypertension with ulcer**

    459.32   **Chronic venous hypertension with inflammation**

    459.33   **Chronic venous hypertension with ulcer and inflammation**

    459.39   **Chronic venous hypertension with other complication**

459.8   **Other specified disorders of circulatory system**

    459.81   **Venous (peripheral) insufficiency, unspecified**
       Chronic venous insufficiency NOS
       Use additional code for any associated ulceration (707.10-707.19, 707.8, 707.9)
       DEF: Insufficient drainage, venous blood, any part of body, results in edema or dermatosis.

    459.89   **Other**
       Collateral circulation (venous), any site
       Phlebosclerosis
       Venofibrosis

459.9   **Unspecified circulatory system disorder**

Chapter 8: Diseases of the Respiratory System (460–519)

Coding Guidance

Conditions related to the respiratory system may be difficult to code because some conditions are classified in chapter 1, "Infectious and Parasitic Diseases." All other conditions are classified to this chapter, Diseases of the Respiratory System, with use of an additional code from category 041 or 079 if an infectious organism is known.

This complex of organs includes pulmonary ventilation and the exchange of oxygen and carbon dioxide between the lungs and the ambient air. The organs of the respiratory system also perform nonrespiratory functions such as warming and moisturizing air passing into the lungs, air flow for the larynx and vocal cords for speech and thermoregulation, and homeostasis through release of excess body heat. The lung also performs important metabolic and embolic filtering functions.

Acute Respiratory Infections (460–466)
This subchapter includes infections of the respiratory tract, excluding pneumonia and influenza, and is organized by site.

Common Cold (460)
Acute infective nasopharyngitis, or the common cold, is classified to category 460. This category excludes allergic and chronic rhinitis, acute and chronic pharyngitis and sore throat.

Sore Throat (462)
Acute pharyngitis is a prolonged inflammatory disorder of the throat, which may be caused by a virus or bacteria.

Acute Tonsillitis (463)
Acute tonsillitis is classified to code 463. This includes follicular, gangrenous, infective, pneumococcal, septic, staphylococcal, suppurative, ulcerative, and viral tonsillitis. Chronic tonsillitis is classified to category 474. The alphabetic index directs the coder to code acute adenoiditis to 463 as well.

Acute Upper Respiratory Infection of Multiple or Unspecified Sites (URI) (465)
Category 465 classifies those upper respiratory infections of multiple or unspecified sites such as acute larygopharyngitis, multiple upper respiratory infection (URI) and acute URI, NOS.

Other Diseases of the Upper Respiratory Tract (470–478)
This section includes the noninfective disorders and chronic conditions of the upper respiratory tract.

Chronic Tonsillitis and Adenoiditis (474)
This category classifies chronic tonsillitis, chronic adenoiditis or a combination of the two conditions. Acute conditions are classified to 463.

Pneumonia and Influenza (480–488)
Pneumonia and influenza are inflammations in the alveolar parenchyma of the lung caused by microbial infection, irradiation or physicochemical agents. Microbial agents include viral, bacterial, fungal, protozoa mycobacterial, mycoplasmal or rickettsial pathogens. Physicochemical agents may be inhaled or reach the lung via the bloodstream. Inhaled agents include toxic gases, irritant particles, or irritant fluids such as gastric juice.

Pneumonia (480–486)
Pneumonia is classified by infective organism such as:

- Viral (480)
- Streptococcal (481)
- Other bacterial (482)
- Other specified organisms (483)

or classified as:

- Pneumonia in infectious disease classified elsewhere (484)
- Bronchopneumonia (485)
- Pneumonia unspecified (486)

Many forms of pneumonia are classified to other chapters of ICD-9-CM because of their etiology. Always refer to the Index under the main terms "Pneumonia" and "Pneumonitis" as a first step in coding pneumonia.

Methicillin-resistant *Staphylococcus aureus* (MRSA) is a variant form of the bacterium *Staphylococcus aureus (S. aureus)* that is resistant to traditional beta-lactam antibiotic therapies for *S. aureus* infections, which include penicillin, methicillin, and cephalosporins. The term methicillin-susceptible *Staphylococcus aureus* (MSSA) identifies certain strains of *Staphylococcus aureus* that are penicillin-resistant, yet susceptible or treatable with methicillin. Due to the clinical challenges MRSA poses, it is sometimes referred to as a "superbug." Previously limited to nosocomial infections, community-acquired pneumonia (CAP) caused by the *Staphylococcus aureus (S. aureus)* bacterium is occurring with increasing frequency, including that caused by antibiotic-resistant and antibiotic-susceptible (MRSA and MSSA) strains. Although rare, MRSA pneumonia can be particularly severe and rapidly fatal, affecting otherwise healthy young people. Some MRSA strains contain toxins (e.g., Panton-Valentine leukocidin) that have been identified as responsible for the severity of illness.

Certain genetic elements for methicillin resistance have been identified in specific, highly virulent MSSA strains, posing significant public health concern. The presence of a toxin may contribute to the changing epidemiology and clinical presentation of staphylococcal pneumonia whether it is due to MSSA or MRSA. Community-acquired MRSA strains have an increased genetic predisposition for such concomitant toxins, although not all currently known MRSA strains are toxin-producing. Increased risk is associated with certain strains of influenza, or patients with a history of MRSA skin infections, or those who have had exposure to persons with MRSA infection. Diagnosis relies upon early recognition, empiric treatment, and microbiological confirmation to ensure appropriate infection control precautions. Treatment includes vancomycin or linezolid therapies when MRSA community-acquired pneumonia is suspected. Assign code 482.42 for methicillin resistant pneumonia due to *Staphylococcus aureus* (MRSA). Code 482.41 reports pneumonia due to methicillin susceptible *Staphylococcus aureus* (MSSA). Pneumonia due to *Staphylococcus aureus* NOS is classified as methicillin susceptible, not methicillin resistant. V codes have been created to report MRSA (V02.53) and MSSA (V02.54) colonization status and personal history of MRSA infection (V12.04).

Influenza (487–488)
Influenza is an acute viral respiratory infection characterized by the abrupt onset of tracheobronchitis. The severity of the disease varies from a mild upper respiratory infection to an extensive pneumonia. Influenza virus type A is the most common and can cause epidemics of varying severity. Influenza virus type B is associated with more limited epidemics and has been linked to Reye's syndrome. Influenza virus type C is an uncommon strain that causes very mild upper respiratory symptoms.

Four-digit subclassification identifies associated manifestations such as influenzal laryngitis, pharyngitis, or URI (487.1).

Influenza type A affects a number of different animal species, with the largest variety found among birds. Waterfowl are considered a natural reservoir for influenza type A viruses. Only three subtypes of influenza type A are currently known to be circulating in humans: H1N1, H1N2, and H3N2. Human influenza due to H5N1 has generally been associated with close contact with birds. The diagnosis of avian influenza should be definitive before assigning code 488 Influenza due to identified avian influenza virus. Code 488.1x is used to report confirmed cases of H1N1 (Swine) flu.

The 2009 pandemic influenza is now regularly referred to as 2009 H1N1 influenza, rather than novel H1N1 influenza, and is reported using a code from subcategory 488.1x.

Novel influenza A viruses that are different from currently circulating human influenza viruses, that are of a subtyped as nonhuman in origin, and are unsubtypable with standard laboratory methods are reported using a code from subcategory 488.8x.

"Confirmation" does not require documentation of positive laboratory testing specific for avian or novel H1N1 influenza. The provider's diagnostic statement that the patient has avian or novel H1N1 (H1N1 or swine flu) influenza is sufficient. If the provider records "suspected or possible or probable avian or novel H1N1 influenza (H1N1 or swine flu)," the appropriate influenza code from category 487 should be assigned.

Both subcategories 488.0 and 488.1 include fifth-digit code options identifying the influenza with pneumonia, other respiratory manifestations, or other manifestations.

Chronic obstructive pulmonary disease (COPD) is a term that causes confusion for many coders. COPD describes many disorders that cause persistent obstruction of the bronchial air flow. This general term, COPD, may refer to the following conditions:

Code	Conditions
491.20	Emphysematous chronic bronchitis, obstructive chronic bronchitis, bronchitis with airway obstruction, bronchitis with emphysema
491.21	COPD with acute exacerbation.
491.22	Chronic obstructive bronchitis with acute bronchitis, acute bronchitis with COPD
491.8	Chronic tracheitis, chronic tracheobronchitis
493.2x	Chronic obstructive asthma, asthma with chronic obstructive pulmonary disease (COPD), chronic asthmatic bronchitis
495.9	Chronic obstructive lung disease with allergic alveolitis
496	Chronic airway obstruction NOS, nonspecific chronic lung disease, obstructive lung disease, COPD NOS, diffuse chronic obstructive lung disease with fibrosis

Obstructive Chronic Bronchitis (491.2x)
Chronic bronchitis combined with obstructive lung disease is defined as a persistent cough with sputum production occurring on most days for at least three months of the year and for at least two years. Obstructive lung disease is defined as a chronic or recurrent reduction in expiratory airflow within the lung. Obstructive chronic bronchitis is characterized by an increased mass of mucous glands in the lung, resulting in an increase in the thickness of the bronchial mucosa. Its most common etiology is cigarette smoking, but it also may be caused by environmental pollution or inhalation of irritant chemicals.

Emphysema (492)
The term "emphysema" refers to any condition in which air is present in a small area of an organ or tissue, for example, subcutaneous emphysema, characterized by air in the subcutaneous tissue. Emphysema classified to category 492 refers to pulmonary emphysema only.

Asthma (493)
Asthma is a narrowing of the airways due to increased responsiveness of the trachea and bronchi to various stimuli. Asthma is reversible, changing in severity either spontaneously or as a result of treatment. Asthma is associated with bronchospasm and pathologic features such as increased mucous secretion, mucosal edema and hyperemia, hypertrophy of bronchial smooth muscle, and acute inflammation. The most serious condition is "status asthmaticus," in which attacks are severe and prolonged.

Asthma has traditionally been classified as extrinsic, intrinsic, or unspecified. This differentiation is considered archaic by many clinicians because manifestations of both extrinsic and intrinsic disease commonly occur in the same patient.

The following fifth-digit assignment is used with category 493:

- 0 without mention of status asthmaticus or acute exacerbation or unspecified
- 1 with status asthmaticus
- 2 with acute exacerbation

Status asthmaticus is severe and does not respond to normal therapeutic measures.

Pneumoconioses (500–505)
Pneumoconioses are diseases marked by permanent deposits of particulate matter within the lungs. The sources of the matter are usually environmental or occupational.

Other Diseases of Respiratory System (510–519)

Empyema (510)
Empyema is the accumulation of pus within the pleural space. Use an additional code to identify the infectious organism from category 041.

Pleurisy (511)
Pleurisy is the inflammation of the serous membrane of the lungs and lining of the thoracic cavity. Exudation develops in the cavity or on the surface of the membrane. This category excludes pleurisy mentioned with tuberculosis (012.0). Use an additional code to identify any causal organism. Malignant pleural effusion is an abnormal accumulation of fluid in the pleura. The pleural space lies between the outside of the lung and the wall of the chest cavity. Malignant pleural effusion commonly occurs as a result of a cancerous neoplastic process in the lung, breast, lymph glands, and vessels or within the chest cavity. Malignant pleural effusions may be attributed to the presence of a metastatic secondary neoplasm of the pleura from primary tumors elsewhere in the body, or they may arise as a primary neoplasm of the pleura, as a thoracic lymphoma, or as an integral part of progressive primary lung cancer. As the malignant fluid accumulates in the pleural space, the lung collapses, resulting in chest pain, cough, hypoxia, and shortness of breath.

Prior to October 1, 2008, malignant pleural effusion defaulted to code 197.2 as a secondary malignant neoplasm of the pleura. Clinically, this was not a valid default code. Therefore, a unique classification has been created to report malignant pleural effusion (511.81). Additionally, malignant pleural effusion is a sign used in the staging of lung cancer. An instructional note has been listed at code 511.81 to "code first malignant neoplasm, if known."

Pneumothorax (512)
Pneumothorax is an accumulation of gas or air in the pleural space. The degree of lung collapse is determined by the amount of air or gas trapped in the intrapleural space. Postoperative pneumothorax is coded as 512.1, whereas postoperative air leak is coded to 512.2. Traumatic pneumothorax is classified to 860.0–860.1 and 860.4–860.5.

Acute Respiratory Failure (518.81)
Acute respiratory failure is the failure of oxygenation and/or ventilation severe enough to impair or threaten the function of vital organs.

Associated conditions include:

- Chronic obstructive lung disease such as chronic obstructive bronchitis, emphysema, cystic fibrosis
- Acute obstructive lung disease such as asthma, pneumonia, acute bronchitis
- Disorder of respiratory control such as drug overdose, cerebrovascular accident
- Neuromuscular abnormalities such as poliomyelitis, myasthenia gravis, Guillain-Barre syndrome
- Chest wall trauma such as flail chest

If both acute respiratory failure and pneumonia are present on admission and both conditions are treated equally, either condition may be sequenced as the principal diagnosis. According to *The Official Guidelines for Coding and Reporting* (section II.C. Selection of Principal Diagnosis), "In the unusual instance when two or more diagnoses equally meet the criteria for principal diagnosis as determined by the circumstances of admission, diagnostic workup, and/or therapy provided, and the Alphabetic Index, Tabular List, or another coding guideline does not provide sequencing direction, any one of the diagnoses may be sequenced first."

Acute Bronchospasm (519.11)
By definition, bronchospasm is an abnormal contraction of the smooth muscle of the bronchi, resulting in an acute narrowing and obstruction of the respiratory airway. This is chiefly characterized by a cough with generalized wheezing and a sensation of tightness in the chest. Bronchospasm is a component of asthma and bronchitis, and thought to be a precursor to diagnosis. However, many other conditions exhibit manifestation of bronchospasm, including abscess of bronchus, atrophy of trachea, bronchostenosis and calcification of bronchus. Code 519.11 Acute bronchospasm, is used to report and monitor incidences and recurrences of bronchospasm in patients that have not yet been diagnosed with asthma, and/or do not meet bronchitis criteria.

8. DISEASES OF THE RESPIRATORY SYSTEM (460-519)

Use additional code to identify infectious organism

ACUTE RESPIRATORY INFECTIONS (460-466)

EXCLUDES *pneumonia and influenza (480.0-488.19)*

460 Acute nasopharyngitis [common cold]

Coryza (acute)
Nasal catarrh, acute
Nasopharyngitis:
  NOS
  acute
  infective NOS
Rhinitis:
  acute
  infective

EXCLUDES *nasopharyngitis, chronic (472.2)*
pharyngitis:
  acute or unspecified (462)
  chronic (472.1)
rhinitis:
  allergic (477.0-477.9)
  chronic or unspecified (472.0)
sore throat:
  acute or unspecified (462)
  chronic (472.1)

DEF: Acute inflammation of mucous membranes; extends from nares to pharynx.

✓4ᵗʰ 461 Acute sinusitis

INCLUDES abscess
empyema
infection   acute, of sinus
inflammation   (accessory) (nasal)
suppuration

EXCLUDES *chronic or unspecified sinusitis (473.0-473.9)*

461.0 Maxillary
Acute antritis

461.1 Frontal

461.2 Ethmoidal

461.3 Sphenoidal

461.8 Other acute sinusitis
Acute pansinusitis

461.9 Acute sinusitis, unspecified
Acute sinusitis NOS

462 Acute pharyngitis

Acute sore throat NOS   Pharyngitis (acute):
Pharyngitis (acute):   staphylococca
  NOS   suppurative
  gangrenous   ulcerative
  infective   Sore throat (viral) NOS
  phlegmonous   Viral pharyngitis
  pneumococcal

EXCLUDES *abscess:*
  peritonsillar [quinsy] (475)
  pharyngeal NOS (478.29)
  retropharyngeal (478.24)
chronic pharyngitis (472.1)
infectious mononucleosis (075)
that specified as (due to):
  Coxsackie (virus) (074.0)
  gonococcus (098.6)
  herpes simplex (054.79)
  influenza (487.1, 488.02, 488.12)
  septic (034.0)
  streptococcal (034.0)

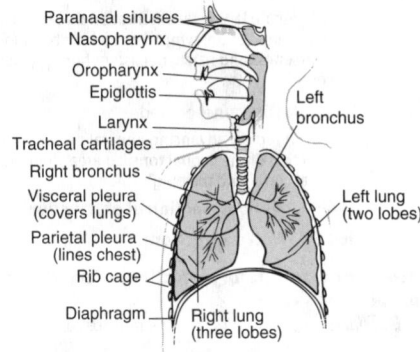

Respiratory System

Paranasal sinuses
Nasopharynx
Oropharynx
Epiglottis
Larynx   Left bronchus
Tracheal cartilages
Right bronchus
Visceral pleura (covers lungs)   Left lung (two lobes)
Parietal pleura (lines chest)
Rib cage
Diaphragm   Right lung (three lobes)

463 Acute tonsillitis

Tonsillitis (acute):
  NOS
  follicular
  gangrenous
  infective
  pneumococcal
  septic
  staphylococcal
  suppurative
  ulcerative
  viral

EXCLUDES *chronic tonsillitis (474.0)*
hypertrophy of tonsils (474.1)
peritonsillar abscess [quinsy] (475)
sore throat:
  acute or NOS (462)
  septic (034.0)
streptococcal tonsillitis (034.0)

✓4ᵗʰ 464 Acute laryngitis and tracheitis

EXCLUDES *that associated with influenza (487.1, 488.02, 488.12)*
that due to Streptococcus (034.0)

✓5ᵗʰ 464.0 Acute laryngitis

Laryngitis (acute):
  NOS
  edematous
  Hemophilus influenzae [H. influenzae]
  pneumococcal
  septic
  suppurative
  ulcerative

EXCLUDES *chronic laryngitis (476.0-476.1)*
influenzal laryngitis (487.1, 488.02, 488.12)

464.00 Without mention of obstruction

464.01 With obstruction

✓5ᵗʰ 464.1 Acute tracheitis

Tracheitis (acute):
  NOS
  catarrhal
  viral

EXCLUDES *chronic tracheitis (491.8)*

464.10 Without mention of obstruction

464.11 With obstruction

✓5ᵗʰ 464.2 Acute laryngotracheitis

Laryngotracheitis (acute)
Tracheitis (acute) with laryngitis (acute)

EXCLUDES *chronic laryngotracheitis (476.1)*

464.20 Without mention of obstruction

464.21 With obstruction

✓5ᵗʰ 464.3 Acute epiglottitis

Viral epiglottitis

EXCLUDES *epiglottitis, chronic (476.1)*

464.30 Without mention of obstruction

464.31 With obstruction

Diseases of the Respiratory System

464.4–472.2

464.4 Croup
Croup syndrome
DEF: Acute laryngeal obstruction due to allergy, foreign body or infection; symptoms include barking cough, hoarseness and harsh, persistent high-pitched respiratory sound.

√5ᵗʰ **464.5 Supraglottitis, unspecified**
DEF: A rapidly advancing generalized upper respiratory infection of the lingual tonsillar area, epiglottic folds, false vocal cords, and the epiglottis.

464.50 Without mention of obstruction
464.51 With obstruction

√4ᵗʰ **465 Acute upper respiratory infections of multiple or unspecified sites**
EXCLUDES upper respiratory infection due to:
influenza (487.1, 488.02, 488.12)
Streptococcus (034.0)

465.0 Acute laryngopharyngitis
DEF: Acute infection of the vocal cords and pharynx.

465.8 Other multiple sites
Multiple URI

465.9 Unspecified site
Acute URI NOS
Upper respiratory infection (acute)

√4ᵗʰ **466 Acute bronchitis and bronchiolitis**
INCLUDES that with:
bronchospasm
obstruction

466.0 Acute bronchitis
Bronchitis, acute or subacute:
fibrinous
membranous
pneumococcal
purulent
septic
viral
with tracheitis
Croupous bronchitis
Tracheobronchitis, acute
EXCLUDES acute bronchitis with chronic obstructive pulmonary disease (491.22)
DEF: Acute inflammation of main branches of bronchial tree due to infectious or irritant agents; symptoms include cough with a varied production of sputum, fever, substernal soreness, and lung rales.

√5ᵗʰ **466.1 Acute bronchiolitis**
Bronchiolitis (acute)
Capillary pneumonia
EXCLUDES respiratory bronchiolitis interstitial lung disease (516.34)
DEF: Acute inflammation of the smallest branches of bronchial tree due to infectious or irritant agents; symptoms include cough, tachycardia, labored breathing, and lung crackles.

466.11 Acute bronchiolitis due to respiratory syncytial virus (RSV)

466.19 Acute bronchiolitis due to other infectious organisms
Use additional code to identify organism

OTHER DISEASES OF THE UPPER RESPIRATORY TRACT (470-478)

470 Deviated nasal septum
Deflected septum (nasal) (acquired)
EXCLUDES congenital (754.0)

√4ᵗʰ **471 Nasal polyps**
EXCLUDES adenomatous polyps (212.0)

471.0 Polyp of nasal cavity
Polyp:
choanal
nasopharyngeal

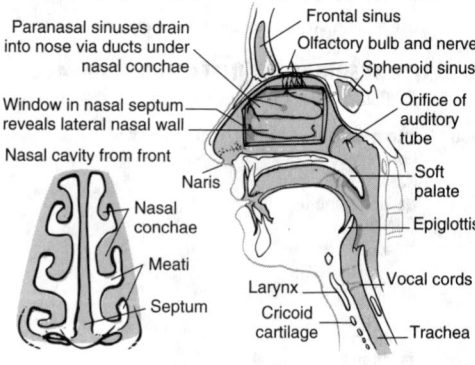

Upper Respiratory System

471.1 Polypoid sinus degeneration
Woakes' syndrome or ethmoiditis

471.8 Other polyp of sinus
Polyp of sinus::
accessory
ethmoidal
maxillary
sphenoidal

471.9 Unspecified nasal polyp
Nasal polyp NOS

√4ᵗʰ **472 Chronic pharyngitis and nasopharyngitis**
472.0 Chronic rhinitis
Ozena
Rhinitis:
NOS
atrophic
granulomatous
hypertrophic
obstructive
purulent
ulcerative
EXCLUDES allergic rhinitis (477.0-477.9)
DEF: Persistent inflammation of mucous membranes of nose.

472.1 Chronic pharyngitis
Chronic sore throat
Pharyngitis:
atrophic
granular (chronic)
hypertrophic

472.2 Chronic nasopharyngitis
EXCLUDES acute or unspecified nasopharyngitis (460)
DEF: Persistent inflammation of mucous membranes extending from nares to pharynx.

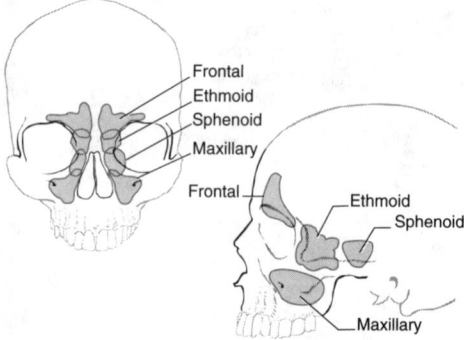

Paranasal Sinuses

√4ᵗʰ **473 Chronic sinusitis**

> **INCLUDES**   abscess   ⎱ (chronic) of sinus
> empyema   (accessory)
> infection   (nasal)
> suppuration   ⎰
>
> **EXCLUDES**   acute sinusitis (461.0-461.9)

473.0 Maxillary
Antritis (chronic)

473.1 Frontal

473.2 Ethmoidal
> **EXCLUDES**   Woakes' ethmoiditis (471.1)

473.3 Sphenoidal

473.8 Other chronic sinusitis
Pansinusitis (chronic)

473.9 Unspecified sinusitis (chronic)
Sinusitis (chronic) NOS

√4ᵗʰ **474 Chronic disease of tonsils and adenoids**

√5ᵗʰ **474.0 Chronic tonsillitis and adenoiditis**
> **EXCLUDES**   acute or unspecified tonsillitis (463)

474.00 Chronic tonsillitis

474.01 Chronic adenoiditis

474.02 Chronic tonsillitis and adenoiditis

√5ᵗʰ **474.1 Hypertrophy of tonsils and adenoids**
Enlargement   ⎱
Hyperplasia   of tonsils or adenoids
Hypertrophy   ⎰
> **EXCLUDES**   that with:
> adenoiditis (474.01)
> adenoiditis and tonsillitis (474.02)
> tonsillitis (474.00)

474.10 Tonsils with adenoids

474.11 Tonsils alone

474.12 Adenoids alone

474.2 Adenoid vegetations
> **DEF:** Fungus-like growth of lymph tissue between the nares and pharynx.

474.8 Other chronic disease of tonsils and adenoids
Amygdalolith
Calculus, tonsil
Cicatrix of tonsil (and adenoid)
Tonsillar tag
Ulcer, tonsil

474.9 Unspecified chronic disease of tonsils and adenoids
Disease (chronic) of tonsils (and adenoids)

475 Peritonsillar abscess
Abscess of tonsil
Peritonsillar cellulitis
Quinsy
> **EXCLUDES**   tonsillitis:
> acute or NOS (463)
> chronic (474.0)

√4ᵗʰ **476 Chronic laryngitis and laryngotracheitis**

476.0 Chronic laryngitis
Laryngitis:
catarrhal
hypertrophic
sicca

476.1 Chronic laryngotracheitis
Laryngitis, chronic, with tracheitis (chronic)
Tracheitis, chronic, with laryngitis
> **EXCLUDES**   chronic tracheitis (491.8)
> laryngitis and tracheitis, acute or unspecified
> (464.00-464.51)

√4ᵗʰ **477 Allergic rhinitis**

> **INCLUDES**   allergic rhinitis (nonseasonal) (seasonal)
> hay fever
> spasmodic rhinorrhea
>
> **EXCLUDES**   allergic rhinitis with asthma (bronchial) (493.0)
>
> **DEF:** True immunoglobulin E (IgE)-mediated allergic reaction of nasal mucosa; seasonal (typical hay fever) or perennial (year-round allergens: dust, food, dander).

477.0 Due to pollen
Pollinosis

477.1 Due to food

477.2 Due to animal (cat) (dog) hair and dander

477.8 Due to other allergen

477.9 Cause unspecified

√4ᵗʰ **478 Other diseases of upper respiratory tract**

478.0 Hypertrophy of nasal turbinates
> **DEF:** Overgrowth, enlargement of shell-shaped bones in nasal cavity.

√5ᵗʰ **478.1 Other diseases of nasal cavity and sinuses**
> **EXCLUDES**   varicose ulcer of nasal septum (456.8)

478.11 Nasal mucositis (ulcerative)
Use additional E code to identify adverse effects of therapy, such as:
antineoplastic and immunosuppressive drugs (E930.7, E933.1)
radiation therapy (E879.2)

478.19 Other diseases of nasal cavity and sinuses
Abscess   ⎱
Necrosis   of nose (septum)
Ulcer   ⎰
Cyst or mucocele of sinus (nasal)
Rhinolith

√5ᵗʰ **478.2 Other diseases of pharynx, not elsewhere classified**

478.20 Unspecified disease of pharynx

478.21 Cellulitis of pharynx or nasopharynx

478.22 Parapharyngeal abscess

478.24 Retropharyngeal abscess
> **DEF:** Purulent infection, behind pharynx and front of precerebral fascia.

478.25 Edema of pharynx or nasopharynx

478.26 Cyst of pharynx or nasopharynx

478.29 Other
Abscess of pharynx or nasopharynx
> **EXCLUDES**   ulcerative pharyngitis (462)

√5ᵗʰ **478.3 Paralysis of vocal cords or larynx**
> **DEF:** Loss of motor ability of vocal cords or larynx; due to nerve or muscle damage.

478.30 Paralysis, unspecified
Laryngoplegia   Paralysis of glottis

478.31 Unilateral, partial

478.32 Unilateral, complete

478.33 Bilateral, partial

478.34 Bilateral, complete

478.4 Polyp of vocal cord or larynx
> **EXCLUDES**   adenomatous polyps (212.1)

478.5 Other diseases of vocal cords
Abscess   ⎱
Cellulitis   of vocal cords
Granuloma
Leukoplakia   ⎰
Chorditis (fibrinous) (nodosa) (tuberosa)
Singers' nodes

478.6 Edema of larynx
Edema (of):   Edema (of):
glottis   supraglottic
subglottic

Diseases of the Respiratory System

478.7–484.6

√5ᵗʰ **478.7 Other diseases of larynx, not elsewhere classified**

478.70 Unspecified disease of larynx

478.71 Cellulitis and perichondritis of larynx
> DEF: Inflammation of deep soft tissues or lining of bone of the larynx.

478.74 Stenosis of larynx

478.75 Laryngeal spasm
Laryngismus (stridulus)
> DEF: Involuntary muscle contraction of the larynx.

478.79 Other
Abscess
Necrosis
Obstruction } of larynx
Pachyderma
Ulcer
> EXCLUDES   ulcerative laryngitis (464.00-464.01)

478.8 Upper respiratory tract hypersensitivity reaction, site unspecified
> EXCLUDES   hypersensitivity reaction of lower respiratory tract, as:
> extrinsic allergic alveolitis (495.0-495.9)
> pneumoconiosis (500-505)

478.9 Other and unspecified diseases of upper respiratory tract
Abscess } of trachea
Cicatrix

PNEUMONIA AND INFLUENZA (480-488)
> EXCLUDES   pneumonia:
> allergic or eosinophilic (518.3)
> aspiration:
>   NOS (507.0)
>   newborn (770.18)
>   solids and liquids (507.0-507.8)
> congenital (770.0)
> lipoid (507.1)
> passive (514)
> rheumatic (390)
> ventilator-associated (997.31)

√4ᵗʰ **480 Viral pneumonia**

480.0 Pneumonia due to adenovirus

480.1 Pneumonia due to respiratory syncytial virus

480.2 Pneumonia due to parainfluenza virus

480.3 Pneumonia due to SARS-associated coronavirus
> DEF: A severe adult respiratory syndrome caused by the coronavirus, specified as inflammation of the lungs with consolidation.

480.8 Pneumonia due to other virus not elsewhere classified
> EXCLUDES   congenital rubella pneumonitis (771.0)
> pneumonia complicating viral diseases classified elsewhere (484.1-484.8)

480.9 Viral pneumonia, unspecified

481 Pneumococcal pneumonia [Streptococcus pneumoniae pneumonia]
Lobar pneumonia, organism unspecified

√4ᵗʰ **482 Other bacterial pneumonia**

482.0 Pneumonia due to Klebsiella pneumoniae

482.1 Pneumonia due to Pseudomonas

482.2 Pneumonia due to Hemophilus influenzae [H. influenzae]

√5ᵗʰ **482.3 Pneumonia due to Streptococcus**
> EXCLUDES   Streptococcus pneumoniae (481)

482.30 Streptococcus, unspecified

482.31 Group A

482.32 Group B

482.39 Other Streptococcus

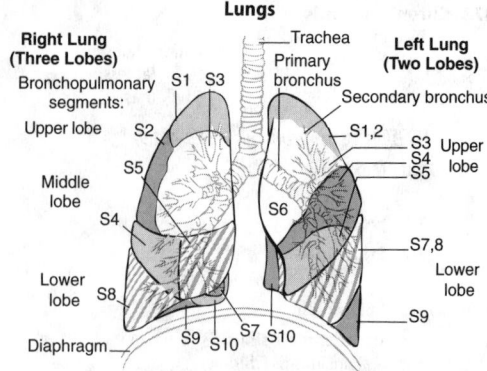

Lungs

Right Lung (Three Lobes) — Trachea — Left Lung (Two Lobes)
Bronchopulmonary segments: — Primary bronchus — Secondary bronchus
Upper lobe S1 S3 S1,2 S3 S4 S5 Upper lobe
S2 S5 S6 Middle lobe S4 S7,8 Lower lobe
Lower lobe S8 S7 S10 S9
Diaphragm S9 S10

√5ᵗʰ **482.4 Pneumonia due to Staphylococcus**

482.40 Pneumonia due to Staphylococcus, unspecified

482.41 Methicillin susceptible pneumonia due to Staphylococcus aureus
Staphylococcus aureus
MSSA pneumonia
Pneumonia due to Staphylococcus aureus NOS

482.42 Methicillin resistant pneumonia due to Staphylococcus aureus

482.49 Other Staphylococcus pneumonia

√5ᵗʰ **482.8 Pneumonia due to other specified bacteria**
> EXCLUDES   pneumonia, complicating infectious disease classified elsewhere (484.1-484.8)

482.81 Anaerobes
Bacteroides (melaninogenicus)
Gram-negative anaerobes

482.82 Escherichia coli [E. coli]

482.83 Other gram-negative bacteria
Gram-negative pneumonia NOS
Proteus
Serratia marcescens
> EXCLUDES   gram-negative anaerobes (482.81)
> Legionnaires' disease (482.84)

482.84 Legionnaires' disease
> DEF: Severe and often fatal infection by Legionella pneumophilia; symptoms include high fever, gastrointestinal pain, headache, myalgia, dry cough, and pneumonia; usually transmitted airborne via air conditioning systems.

482.89 Other specified bacteria

482.9 Bacterial pneumonia unspecified

√4ᵗʰ **483 Pneumonia due to other specified organism**

483.0 Mycoplasma pneumoniae
Eaton's agent
Pleuropneumonia-like organism [PPLO]

483.1 Chlamydia

483.8 Other specified organism

√4ᵗʰ **484 Pneumonia in infectious diseases classified elsewhere**

484.1 *Pneumonia in cytomegalic inclusion disease*
Code first underlying disease (078.5)

484.3 *Pneumonia in whooping cough*
Code first underlying disease (033.0-033.9)

484.5 *Pneumonia in anthrax*
Code first underlying disease (022.1)

484.6 *Pneumonia in aspergillosis*
Code first underlying disease (117.3)

484.7 **Pneumonia in other systemic mycoses**
Code first underlying disease
EXCLUDES pneumonia in:
candidiasis (112.4)
coccidioidomycosis (114.0)
histoplasmosis (115.0-115.9 with
fifth-digit 5)

484.8 **Pneumonia in other infectious diseases classified elsewhere**
Code first underlying disease, as:
Q fever (083.0)
typhoid fever (002.0)
EXCLUDES pneumonia in:
actinomycosis (039.1)
measles (055.1)
nocardiosis (039.1)
ornithosis (073.0)
Pneumocystis carinii (136.3)
salmonellosis (003.22)
toxoplasmosis (130.4)
tuberculosis (011.6)
tularemia (021.2)
varicella (052.1)

485 **Bronchopneumonia, organism unspecified**
Bronchopneumonia: Pneumonia:
hemorrhagic   lobular
terminal   segmental
Pleurobronchopneumonia
EXCLUDES bronchiolitis (acute) (466.11-466.19)
chronic (491.8)
lipoid pneumonia (507.1)

486 **Pneumonia, organism unspecified**
EXCLUDES hypostatic or passive pneumonia (514)
inhalation or aspiration pneumonia due to foreign
materials (507.0-507.8)
pneumonitis due to fumes and vapors (506.0)

√4ᵗʰ **487** **Influenza**
Influenza caused by unspecified influenza virus
EXCLUDES Hemophilus influenzae [H. influenzae]:
infection NOS (041.5)
influenza due to identified avian influenza virus
(488.01-488.09)
influenza due to 2009 H1N1 [swine] influenza virus
(488.11-488.19)
influenza due to identified (novel) 2009 H1N1
influenza virus (488.11-488.19)
laryngitis (464.00-464.01)
meningitis (320.0)

487.0 **With pneumonia**
Influenza with pneumonia, any form
Influenzal:
bronchopneumonia
pneumonia
Use additional code to identify the type of pneumonia
(480.0-480.9, 481, 482.0-482.9, 483.0-483.8, 485)

487.1 **With other respiratory manifestations**
Influenza NEC
Influenza NOS
Influenzal:
laryngitis
pharyngitis
respiratory infection (upper) (acute)

487.8 **With other manifestations**
Encephalopathy due to influenza
Influenza with involvement of gastrointestinal tract
EXCLUDES "intestinal flu" [viral gastroenteritis] (008.8)

Bronchioli and Alveoli

To trachea
Pulmonary arteriole
Terminal bronchiolus
Elastic fibers
Capillary
network
over all
alveoli
Alveoli
Alveolus

√4ᵗʰ **488** **Influenza due to certain identified influenza viruses**
EXCLUDES influenza caused by unspecified or seasonal influenza
viruses (487.0-487.8)

√5ᵗʰ **488.0** **Influenza due to identified avian influenza virus**
Avian influenza
Bird flu
Influenza A/H5N1
DEF: Infection caused by contact with bird influenza
viruses; results in flu-like symptoms that may progress to
other severe and life-threatening complications.

488.01 **Influenza due to identified avian influenza
virus with pneumonia**
Avian influenzal:
bronchopneumonia
pneumonia
Influenza due to identified avian influenza virus
with pneumonia, any form
Use additional code to identify the type of
pneumonia (480.0- 480.9, 481,
482.0-482.9, 483.0-483.8, 485)

488.02 **Influenza due to identified avian influenza
virus with other respiratory manifestations**
Avian influenzal:
laryngitis
pharyngitis
respiratory infection (acute) (upper)
Identified avian influenza NOS

488.09 **Influenza due to identified avian influenza
virus with other manifestations**
Avian influenza with involvement of
gastrointestinal tract
Encephalopathy due to identified avian
influenza
EXCLUDES "intestinal flu" [viral gastroenteritis]
(008.8)

√5ᵗʰ **488.1** **Influenza due to identified 2009 H1N1 influenza virus**
2009 H1N1 swine influenza virus
(Novel) 2009 influenza H1N1
Novel H1N1 influenza
Novel influenza A/H1N1
EXCLUDES bird influenza virus infection (488.01-488.09)
influenza A/H5N1 (488.01-488.09)
other human infection with influenza virus of
animal origin (488.81-488.89)
swine influenza virus infection
(488.81-488.89)

488.11 **Influenza due to identified 2009 H1N1
influenza virus with pneumonia**
Influenza due to identified (novel) 2009 H1N1
with pneumonia, any form
(Novel) 2009 H1N1 influenzal:
bronchopneumonia
pneumonia
Use additional code to identify the type of
pneumonia (480.0- 480.9, 481,
482.0-482.9, 483.0-483.8, 485)

Diseases of the Respiratory System

488.12–492.0

488.12 Influenza due to identified 2009 H1N1 influenza virus with other respiratory manifestations

(Novel) 2009 H1N1 influenza NOS
(Novel) 2009 H1N1 influenzal:
  laryngitis
  pharyngitis
  respiratory infection (acute) (upper)

488.19 Influenza due to identified 2009 H1N1 influenza virus with other manifestations

Encephalopathy due to identified (novel) 2009 H1N1 influenza
(Novel) 2009 H1N1 influenza with involvement of gastrointestinal tract

> *EXCLUDES*   *"intestinal flu" [viral gastroenteritis] (008.8)*

✓5ᵗʰ **488.8 Influenza due to novel influenza A**

Influenza due to animal origin influenza virus
Infection with influenza viruses occurring in pigs or other animals
Other novel influenza A viruses not previously found in humans

> *EXCLUDES*   *bird influenza virus infection (488.01-488.09)*
> *influenza A/H5N1 (488.01-488.09)*
> *influenza due to identified 2009 H1N1 influenza virus (488.11- 488.19)*

488.81 Influenza due to identified novel influenza A virus with pneumonia

Influenza due to animal origin influenza virus with pneumonia, any form
Novel influenza A:
  bronchopneumonia
  pneumonia
Use additional code to identify the type of pneumonia (480.0-480.9, 481, 482.0-482.9, 483.0-483.8, 485)

488.82 Influenza due to identified novel influenza A virus with other respiratory manifestations

Influenza due to animal origin influenza A virus with other respiratory manifestations
Novel influenza A:
  laryngitis
  pharyngitis
  respiratory infection (acute) (upper)

488.89 Influenza due to identified novel influenza A virus with other manifestations

Encephalopathy due to novel influenza A
Influenza due to animal origin influenza virus with encephalopathy
Influenza due to animal origin influenza virus with involvement of gastrointestinal tract
Novel influenza A with involvement of gastrointestinal tract

> *EXCLUDES*   *"intestinal flu" [viral gastroenteritis] (008.8)*

CHRONIC OBSTRUCTIVE PULMONARY DISEASE AND ALLIED CONDITIONS (490-496)

490 Bronchitis, not specified as acute or chronic

Bronchitis NOS:
  catarrhal
  with tracheitis NOS
Tracheobronchitis NOS

> *EXCLUDES*   *bronchitis:*
> *allergic NOS (493.9)*
> *asthmatic NOS (493.9)*
> *due to fumes and vapors (506.0)*

✓4ᵗʰ **491 Chronic bronchitis**

> *EXCLUDES*   *chronic obstructive asthma (493.2)*

491.0 Simple chronic bronchitis

Catarrhal bronchitis, chronic
Smokers' cough

Interrelationship Between Chronic Airway Obstruction, Chronic Bronchitis, and Emphysema

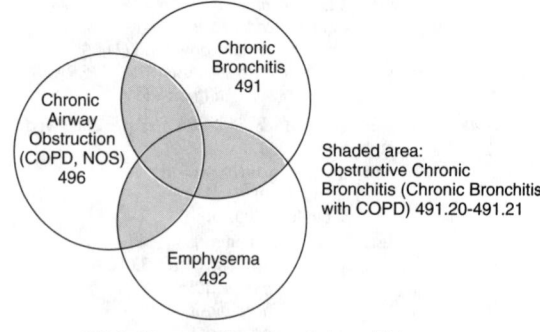

Shaded area:
Obstructive Chronic Bronchitis (Chronic Bronchitis with COPD) 491.20-491.21

491.1 Mucopurulent chronic bronchitis

Bronchitis (chronic) (recurrent):
  fetid
  mucopurulent
  purulent

DEF: Chronic bronchial infection characterized by both mucus and pus secretions in the bronchial tree; recurs after asymptomatic periods; signs are coughing, expectoration and secondary changes in the lung.

✓5ᵗʰ **491.2 Obstructive chronic bronchitis**

Bronchitis:
  emphysematous
  obstructive (chronic) (diffuse)
Bronchitis with:
  chronic airway obstruction
  emphysema

> *EXCLUDES*   *asthmatic bronchitis (acute) NOS (493.9)*
> *chronic obstructive asthma (493.2)*

491.20 Without exacerbation

Emphysema with chronic bronchitis

491.21 With (acute) exacerbation

Acute exacerbation of chronic obstructive pulmonary disease [COPD]
Decompensated chronic obstructive pulmonary disease [COPD]
Decompensated chronic obstructive pulmonary disease [COPD] with exacerbation

> *EXCLUDES*   *chronic obstructive asthma with acute exacerbation (493.22)*

491.22 With acute bronchitis

491.8 Other chronic bronchitis

Chronic:
  tracheitis
  tracheobronchitis

491.9 Unspecified chronic bronchitis

✓4ᵗʰ **492 Emphysema**

492.0 Emphysematous bleb

Giant bullous emphysema
Ruptured emphysematous bleb
Tension pneumatocele
Vanishing lung

DEF: Formation of vesicle or bulla in emphysematous lung, more than one millimeter; contains serum or blood.

492.8 Other emphysema
Emphysema
(lung or pulmonary):
NOS
centriacinar
centrilobular
obstructive
panacinar
panlobular
unilateral
vesicular
MacLeod's syndrome
Swyer-James syndrome
Unilateral hyperlucent lung
EXCLUDES   *emphysema:*
with chronic bronchitis (491.20-491.22)
compensatory (518.2)
due to fumes and vapors (506.4)
interstitial (518.1)
newborn (770.2)
mediastinal (518.1)
surgical (subcutaneous) (998.81)
traumatic (958.7)

√4ᵗʰ 493 Asthma
EXCLUDES   *wheezing NOS (786.07)*

The following fifth-digit subclassification is for use with codes 493.0-493.2, 493.9:
   0 unspecified
   1 with status asthmaticus
   2 with (acute) exacerbation

DEF: Status asthmaticus: severe, intractable episode of asthma unresponsive to normal therapeutic measures.

√5ᵗʰ 493.0 Extrinsic asthma
[0-2]   Asthma:
allergic with stated cause
atopic
childhood
hay
platinum
Hay fever with asthma
EXCLUDES   *asthma:*
allergic NOS (493.9)
detergent (507.8)
miners' (500)
wood (495.8)

DEF: Transient stricture of airway diameters of bronchi; due to environmental factor; also called allergic (bronchial) asthma.

√5ᵗʰ 493.1 Intrinsic asthma
[0-2]   Late-onset asthma

DEF: Transient stricture of airway diameters of bronchi; due to pathophysiological disturbances.

√5ᵗʰ 493.2 Chronic obstructive asthma
[0-2]   Asthma with chronic obstructive pulmonary disease [COPD]
Chronic asthmatic bronchitis
EXCLUDES   *acute bronchitis (466.0)*
chronic obstructive bronchitis (491.20-491.22)

DEF: Persistent narrowing of airway diameters in the bronchial tree, restricting airflow and causing constant labored breathing.

√5ᵗʰ 493.8 Other forms of asthma
   493.81 Exercise induced bronchospasm
   493.82 Cough variant asthma

√5ᵗʰ 493.9 Asthma, unspecified
[0-2]   Asthma (bronchial) (allergic NOS)
Bronchitis:
allergic
asthmatic

√4ᵗʰ 494 Bronchiectasis
Bronchiectasis (fusiform) (postinfectious) (recurrent)
Bronchiolectasis
EXCLUDES   *congenital (748.61)*
tuberculous bronchiectasis (current disease) (011.5)

DEF: Dilation of bronchi; due to infection or chronic conditions; causes decreased lung capacity and recurrent infections of lungs.

   494.0 Bronchiectasis without acute exacerbation
   494.1 Bronchiectasis with acute exacerbation

√4ᵗʰ 495 Extrinsic allergic alveolitis
INCLUDES   allergic alveolitis and pneumonitis due to inhaled organic dust particles of fungal, thermophilic actinomycete, or other origin

DEF: Pneumonitis due to particles inhaled into lung, often at workplace; symptoms include cough, chills, fever, increased heart and respiratory rates; develops within hours of exposure.

   495.0 Farmers' lung
   495.1 Bagassosis
   495.2 Bird-fanciers' lung
      Budgerigar-fanciers' disease or lung
      Pigeon-fanciers' disease or lung
   495.3 Suberosis
      Cork-handlers' disease or lung
   495.4 Malt workers' lung
      Alveolitis due to Aspergillus clavatus
   495.5 Mushroom workers' lung
   495.6 Maple bark-strippers' lung
      Alveolitis due to Cryptostroma corticale
   495.7 "Ventilation" pneumonitis
      Allergic alveolitis due to fungal, thermophilic actinomycete, and other organisms growing in ventilation [air conditioning] systems
   495.8 Other specified allergic alveolitis and pneumonitis
      Cheese-washers' lung
      Coffee workers' lung
      Fish-meal workers' lung
      Furriers' lung
      Grain-handlers' disease or lung
      Pituitary snuff-takers' disease
      Sequoiosis or red-cedar asthma
      Wood asthma
   495.9 Unspecified allergic alveolitis and pneumonitis
      Alveolitis, allergic (extrinsic)
      Hypersensitivity pneumonitis

496 Chronic airway obstruction, not elsewhere classified
Note: This code is not to be used with any code from categories 491-493
Chronic:
nonspecific lung disease
obstructive lung disease
obstructive pulmonary disease [COPD] NOS
EXCLUDES   *chronic obstructive lung disease [COPD] specified (as) (with):*
allergic alveolitis (495.0-495.9)
asthma (493.20-493.22)
bronchiectasis (494.0-494.1)
bronchitis (491.20-491.22)
with emphysema (491.20-491.22)
decompensated (491.21)
emphysema (492.0-492.8)

PNEUMOCONIOSES AND OTHER LUNG DISEASES DUE TO EXTERNAL AGENTS (500-508)

DEF: Permanent deposits of particulate matter, within lungs; due to occupational or environmental exposure; results in chronic induration and fibrosis. (See specific listings in 500-508 code range.

500 Coal workers' pneumoconiosis
Anthracosilicosis
Anthracosis
Black lung disease
Coal workers' lung
Miner's asthma

Diseases of the Respiratory System

501–511.1

501   Asbestosis

502   Pneumoconiosis due to other silica or silicates
Pneumoconiosis due to talc
Silicotic fibrosis (massive) of lung
Silicosis (simple) (complicated)

503   Pneumoconiosis due to other inorganic dust
Aluminosis (of lung)
Baritosis
Bauxite fibrosis (of lung)
Berylliosis
Graphite fibrosis (of lung)
Siderosis
Stannosis

504   Pneumonopathy due to inhalation of other dust
Byssinosis
Cannabinosis
Flax-dressers' disease
EXCLUDES   *allergic alveolitis (495.0-495.9)*
asbestosis (501)
bagassosis (495.1)
farmers' lung (495.0)

505   Pneumoconiosis, unspecified

√4ᵗʰ **506   Respiratory conditions due to chemical fumes and vapors**
Use additonal E code to identify cause
Use additional code to identify associated respiratory conditions,
such as:
acute respiratory failure (518.81)

506.0   Bronchitis and pneumonitis due to fumes and vapors
Chemical bronchitis (acute)

506.1   Acute pulmonary edema due to fumes and vapors
Chemical pulmonary edema (acute)
EXCLUDES   *acute pulmonary edema NOS (518.4)*
chronic or unspecified pulmonary edema
(514)

506.2   Upper respiratory inflammation due to fumes and vapors

506.3   Other acute and subacute respiratory conditions due to fumes and vapors

506.4   Chronic respiratory conditions due to fumes and vapors
Emphysema (diffuse)
(chronic)   } due to inhalation
Obliterative bronchiolitis   of chemical
(chronic) (subacute)   fumes and
Pulmonary fibrosis (chronic)   vapors

506.9   Unspecified respiratory conditions due to fumes and vapors
Silo-fillers' disease

√4ᵗʰ **507   Pneumonitis due to solids and liquids**
EXCLUDES   *fetal aspiration pneumonitis (770.18)*
postprocedural pneumonitis (997.32)

507.0   Due to inhalation of food or vomitus
Aspiration pneumonia (due to):
NOS
food (regurgitated)
gastric secretions
milk
saliva
vomitus

507.1   Due to inhalation of oils and essences
Lipoid pneumonia (exogenous)
EXCLUDES   *endogenous lipoid pneumonia (516.8)*

507.8   Due to other solids and liquids
Detergent asthma

√4ᵗʰ **508   Respiratory conditions due to other and unspecified external agents**
Use additonal E code to identify cause
Use additional code to identify associated respiratory conditions,
such as:
acute respiratory failure (518.81)

508.0   Acute pulmonary manifestations due to radiation
Radiation pneumonitis

508.1   Chronic and other pulmonary manifestations due to radiation
Fibrosis of lung following radiation

508.2   Respiratory conditions due to smoke inhalation
Smoke inhalation NOS
EXCLUDES   *smoke inhalation due to chemical fumes and*
vapors (506.9)

508.8   Respiratory conditions due to other specified external agents

508.9   Respiratory conditions due to unspecified external agent

OTHER DISEASES OF RESPIRATORY SYSTEM (510-519)

√4ᵗʰ **510   Empyema**
Use additional code to identify infectious organism (041.0-041.9)
EXCLUDES   *abscess of lung (513.0)*
DEF: Purulent infection within pleural space.

510.0   With fistula
Fistula:
bronchocutaneous
bronchopleural
hepatopleural
mediastinal
pleural
thoracic
Any condition classifiable to 510.9 with fistula
DEF: Purulent infection of respiratory cavity, with
communication from cavity to another structure.

510.9   Without mention of fistula
Abscess:
pleura
thorax
Empyema (chest) (lung) (pleura)
Fibrinopurulent pleurisy
Pleurisy:
purulent
septic
seropurulent
suppurative
Pyopneumothorax
Pyothorax

√4ᵗʰ **511   Pleurisy**
EXCLUDES   *pleurisy with mention of tuberculosis, current disease*
(012.0)
DEF: Inflammation of serous membrane of lungs and lining of
thoracic cavity; causes exudation in cavity or membrane surface.

511.0   Without mention of effusion or current tuberculosis
Adhesion, lung or pleura
Calcification of pleura
Pleurisy (acute) (sterile):
diaphragmatic
fibrinous
interlobar
NOS
pneumococcal
staphylococcal
streptococcal
Thickening of pleura

511.1   With effusion, with mention of a bacterial cause other than tuberculosis
Pleurisy with effusion (exudative) (serous):
other specified nontuberculous bacterial cause
pneumococcal
staphylococcal
streptococcal

Lower Respiratory System

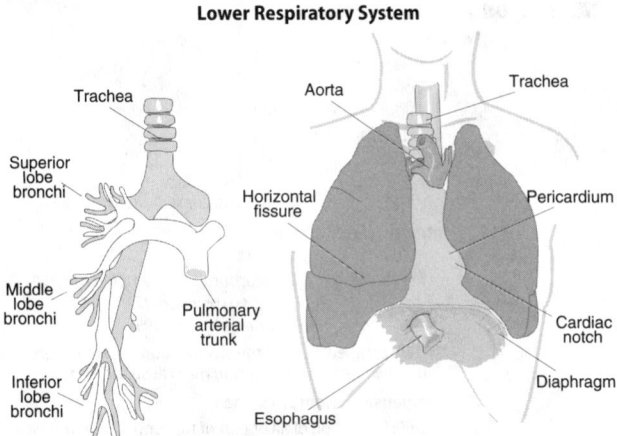

√5ᵗʰ 511.8 Other specified forms of effusion, except tuberculous
EXCLUDES *traumatic (860.2-860.5, 862.29, 862.39)*

511.81 Malignant pleural effusion
Code first malignant neoplasm, if known

511.89 Other specified forms of effusion, except tuberculous
Encysted pleurisy
Hemopneumothorax
Hemothorax
Hydropneumothorax
Hydrothorax

511.9 Unspecified pleural effusion
Pleural effusion NOS   Pleurisy:
Pleurisy: serous
  exudative   with effusion NOS
  serofibrinous

√4ᵗʰ 512 Pneumothorax and air leak
DEF: Collapsed lung; due to gas or air in pleural space.

512.0 Spontaneous tension pneumothorax
DEF: Leaking air from lung into lining causing collapse.

512.1 Iatrogenic pneumothorax
Postoperative pneumothorax
DEF: Air trapped in the lining of the lung following surgery.

512.2 Postoperative air leak

√5ᵗʰ 512.8 Other pneumothorax and air leak
EXCLUDES *pneumothorax:*
congenital (770.2)
traumatic (860.0-860.1, 860.4-860.5)
tuberculous, current disease (011.7)

512.81 Primary spontaneous pneumothorax

512.82 Secondary spontaneous pneumothorax
Code first underlying condition, such as:
cancer metastatic to lung (197.0)
catamenial pneumothorax due to endometriosis (617.8)
cystic fibrosis (277.02)
eosinophilic pneumonia (518.3)
lymphangioleiomyomatosis (516.4)
Marfan syndrome (759.82)
pneumocystis carinii pneumonia (136.3)
primary lung cancer (162.3-162.9)
spontaneous rupture of the esophagus (530.4)

512.83 Chronic pneumothorax

512.84 Other air leak
Persistent air leak

512.89 Other pneumothorax
Acute pneumothorax
Pneumothorax NOS
Spontaneous pneumothorax NOS

√4ᵗʰ 513 Abscess of lung and mediastinum

513.0 Abscess of lung
Abscess (multiple) of lung
Gangrenous or necrotic pneumonia
Pulmonary gangrene or necrosis

513.1 Abscess of mediastinum

514 Pulmonary congestion and hypostasis
Hypostatic:
bronchopneumonia
pneumonia
Passive pneumonia
Pulmonary congestion (chronic) (passive)
Pulmonary edema:
NOS
chronic
EXCLUDES *acute pulmonary edema:*
NOS (518.4)
with mention of heart disease or failure (428.1)
hypostatic pneumonia due to or specified as a specific type of pneumonia — code to the type of pneumonia (480.0-480.9, 481, 482.0-482.9, 483.0-483.8, 487.0, 488.01, 488.11)
DEF: Excessive retention of interstitial fluid in the lungs and pulmonary vessels; due to poor circulation.

515 Postinflammatory pulmonary fibrosis
Cirrhosis of lung
Fibrosis of lung (atrophic) (confluent) (massive) (perialveolar) (peribronchial) } chronic or unspecified
Induration of lung
DEF: Fibrosis and scarring of the lungs due to inflammatory reaction.

√4ᵗʰ 516 Other alveolar and parietoalveolar pneumonopathy

516.0 Pulmonary alveolar proteinosis
DEF: Reduced ventilation; due to proteinaceous deposits on alveoli; symptoms include dyspnea, cough, chest pain, weakness, weight loss, and hemoptysis.

516.1 *Idiopathic pulmonary hemosiderosis*
Code first underlying disease (275.01-275.09)
Essential brown induration of lung
EXCLUDES *acute idiopathic pulmonary hemorrhage in infants [AIPHI] (786.31)*
DEF: Fibrosis of alveolar walls; marked by abnormal amounts hemosiderin in lungs; primarily affects children; symptoms include anemia, fluid in lungs, and blood in sputum; etiology unknown.

516.2 Pulmonary alveolar microlithiasis
DEF: Small calculi in pulmonary alveoli resembling sand-like particles on x-ray.

√5ᵗʰ 516.3 Idiopathic interstitial pneumonia

516.30 Idiopathic interstitial pneumonia, not otherwise specified
Idiopathic fibrosing alveolitis

516.31 Idiopathic pulmonary fibrosis
Cryptogenic fibrosing alveolitis
DEF: Chronic disease of unknown causation characterized by scarring and thickening of the lungs that affects males over age 50; symptoms include progressive dyspnea, pleuritic chest pain, dry paroxysmal cough, and shortness of breath.

516.32 Idiopathic non-specific interstitial pneumonitis
EXCLUDES *non-specific interstitial pneumonia NOS, or due to known underlying cause (516.8)*

516.33 Acute interstitial pneumonitis
Hamman-Rich syndrome
EXCLUDES *pneumocystis pneumonia (136.3)*

516.34 Respiratory bronchiolitis interstitial lung disease

Diseases of the Respiratory System

516.35–518.53

516.35   Idiopathic lymphoid interstitial pneumonia
Idiopathic lymphocytic interstitial pneumonitis
EXCLUDES   *lymphoid interstitial pneumonia*
NOS, or due to known
underlying cause (516.8)
pneumocystis pneumonia (136.3)

516.36   Cryptogenic organizing pneumonia
EXCLUDES   *organizing pneumonia NOS, or due*
to known underlying cause
(516.8)

516.37   Desquamative interstitial pneumonia

516.4   Lymphangioleiomyomatosis
Lymphangiomyomatosis

516.5   Adult pulmonary Langerhans cell histiocytosis
Adult PLCH

√5ᵗʰ   516.6   Interstitial lung diseases of childhood

516.61   Neuroendocrine cell hyperplasia of infancy

516.62   Pulmonary interstitial glycogenosis

516.63   Surfactant mutations of the lung
DEF: Group of genetic disorders resulting in
potentially fatal pediatric lung disease with
onset typically within the perinatal period,
although it can be diagnosed later in childhood,
depending on the specific surfactant mutation;
leading indication for pediatric lung
transplantation.

**516.64   Alveolar capillary dysplasia with vein
misalignment**

516.69   Other interstitial lung diseases of childhood

**516.8   Other specified alveolar and parietoalveolar
pneumonopathies**
Endogenous lipoid pneumonia
Interstitial pneumonia
Lymphoid interstitial pneumonia due to known
underlying cause
Lymphoid interstitial pneumonia NOS
Non-specific interstitial pneumonia due to known
underlying cause
Non-specific interstitial pneumonia NOS
Organizing pneumonia due to known underlying cause
Organizing pneumonia NOS
Code first, if applicable, underlying cause of
pneumonopathy, if known
Use additional E code, if applicable, for drug-induced or
toxic pneumonopathy
EXCLUDES   *cryptogenic organizing pneumonia (516.36)*
idiopathic lymphoid interstitial pneumonia
(516.35)
idiopathic non-specific interstitial
pneumonitis (516.32)
lipoid pneumonia, exogenous or unspecified
(507.1)

**516.9   Unspecified alveolar and parietoalveolar
pneumonopathy**

√4ᵗʰ   517   Lung involvement in conditions classified elsewhere
EXCLUDES   *rheumatoid lung (714.81)*

517.1   Rheumatic pneumonia
Code first underlying disease (390)

517.2   Lung involvement in systemic sclerosis
Code first underlying disease (710.1)

517.3   Acute chest syndrome
*Code first sickle-cell disease in crisis (282.42, 282.62,
282.64, 282.69)*

**517.8   Lung involvement in other diseases
classified elsewhere**
Code first underlying disease, as:
amyloidosis (277.30-277.39)
polymyositis (710.4)
sarcoidosis (135)
Sjögren's disease (710.2)
systemic lupus erythematosus (710.0)
EXCLUDES   *syphilis (095.1)*

√4ᵗʰ   518   Other diseases of lung

518.0   Pulmonary collapse
Atelectasis
Collapse of lung
Middle lobe syndrome
EXCLUDES   *atelectasis:*
congenital (partial) (770.5)
primary (770.4)
tuberculous, current disease (011.8)

518.1   Interstitial emphysema
Mediastinal emphysema
EXCLUDES   *surgical (subcutaneous) emphysema (998.81)*
that in fetus or newborn (770.2)
traumatic emphysema (958.7)
DEF: Escaped air from the alveoli trapped in the interstices
of the lung; trauma or cough may cause the disease.

518.2   Compensatory emphysema
DEF: Distention of all or part of the lung caused by disease
processes or surgical intervention that decreased volume
in another part of the lung; overcompensation reaction to
the loss of capacity in another part of the lung.

518.3   Pulmonary eosinophilia
Eosinophilic asthma
Löffler's syndrome
Pneumonia:
allergic
eosinophilic
Tropical eosinophilia
EXCLUDES   *pulmonary infiltrate NOS (793.19)*
DEF: Infiltration, into pulmonary parenchyma of
eosinophils; results in cough, fever, and dyspnea.

518.4   Acute edema of lung, unspecified
Acute pulmonary edema NOS
Pulmonary edema, postoperative
EXCLUDES   *pulmonary edema:*
acute, with mention of heart disease or
failure (428.1)
chronic or unspecified (514)
due to external agents (506.0-508.9)
DEF: Severe, sudden fluid retention within lung tissues.

√5ᵗʰ   518.5   Pulmonary insufficiency following trauma and surgery
EXCLUDES   *adult respiratory distress syndrome*
associated with other conditions
(518.82)
pneumonia:
aspiration (507.0)
hypostatic (514)
*respiratory failure in other conditions (518.81,
518.83-518.84)*

**518.51   Acute respiratory failure following trauma and
surgery**
Respiratory failure, not otherwise specified,
following trauma and surgery
EXCLUDES   *acute respiratory failure in other
conditions (518.81)*

**518.52   Other pulmonary insufficiency, not elsewhere
classified, following trauma and surgery**
Adult respiratory distress syndrome
Pulmonary insufficiency following surgery
Pulmonary insufficiency following trauma
Shock lung related to trauma and surgery
EXCLUDES   *adult respiratory distress syndrome
associated with other
conditions (518.82)*
aspiration pneumonia (507.0)
hypostatic pneumonia (514)
*shock lung, not related to trauma or
surgery (518.82)*

**518.53   Acute and chronic respiratory failure following
trauma and surgery**
EXCLUDES   *acute and chronic respiratory
failure in other conditions
(518.84)*

518.6 Allergic bronchopulmonary aspergillosis

> **DEF:** Noninvasive hypersensitive reaction; due to allergic reaction to *Aspergillus fumigatus* (mold).

518.7 Transfusion related acute lung injury [TRALI]

> **DEF:** A relatively rare, but serious pulmonary complication of blood transfusion, with acute respiratory distress, noncardiogenic pulmonary edema, cyanosis, hypoxemia, hypotension, fever and chills.

√5ᵗʰ **518.8 Other diseases of lung**

  518.81 Acute respiratory failure

> Respiratory failure NOS
>
> **EXCLUDES** acute and chronic respiratory failure (518.84)
> acute respiratory distress (518.82)
> acute respiratory failure following trauma and surgery (518.51)
> chronic respiratory failure (518.83)
> respiratory arrest (799.1)
> respiratory failure, newborn (770.84)

  518.82 Other pulmonary insufficiency, not elsewhere classified

> Acute respiratory distress
> Acute respiratory insufficiency
> Adult respiratory distress syndrome NEC
>
> **EXCLUDES** acute interstitial pneumonitis (516.33)
> adult respiratory distress syndrome associated with trauma or surgery (518.52)
> pulmonary insufficiency following trauma or surgery (518.52)
> respiratory distress:
> NOS (786.09)
> newborn (770.89)
> syndrome, newborn (769)

  518.83 Chronic respiratory failure

  518.84 Acute and chronic respiratory failure

> Acute on chronic respiratory failure
>
> **EXCLUDES** acute and chronic respiratory failure following trauma or surgery (518.53)

  518.89 Other diseases of lung, not elsewhere classified

> Broncholithiasis
> Calcification of lung
> Lung disease NOS
> Pulmolithiasis
>
> **DEF:** Broncholithiasis: calculi in lumen of transbronchial tree.
> **DEF:** Pulmolithiasis: calculi in lung.

√4ᵗʰ **519 Other diseases of respiratory system**

√5ᵗʰ **519.0 Tracheostomy complications**

  519.00 Tracheostomy complication, unspecified

  519.01 Infection of tracheostomy

> Use additional code to identify type of infection, such as:
> abscess or cellulitis of neck (682.1)
> septicemia (038.0-038.9)
> Use additional code to identify organism (041.00-041.9)

  519.02 Mechanical complication of tracheostomy

> Tracheal stenosis due to tracheostomy

  519.09 Other tracheostomy complications

> Hemorrhage due to tracheostomy
> Tracheoesophageal fistula due to tracheostomy

√5ᵗʰ **519.1 Other diseases of trachea and bronchus, not elsewhere classified**

  519.11 Acute bronchospasm

> Bronchospasm NOS
>
> **EXCLUDES** acute bronchitis with bronchospasm (466.0)
> asthma (493.00-493.92)
> exercise induced bronchospasm (493.81)

  519.19 Other diseases of trachea and bronchus

> Calcification
> Stenosis } of bronchus or trachea
> Ulcer

519.2 Mediastinitis

> **DEF:** Inflammation of tissue between organs behind sternum.

519.3 Other diseases of mediastinum, not elsewhere classified

> Fibrosis
> Hernia } of mediastinum
> Retraction

519.4 Disorders of diaphragm

> Diaphragmitis
> Paralysis of diaphragm
> Relaxation of diaphragm
>
> **EXCLUDES** congenital defect of diaphragm (756.6)
> diaphragmatic hernia (551-553 with .3)
> congenital (756.6)

519.8 Other diseases of respiratory system, not elsewhere classified

519.9 Unspecified disease of respiratory system

> Respiratory disease (chronic) NOS

Chapter 9: Diseases of the Digestive System (520–579)

Coding Guidance

This chapter classifies diseases and disorders of all of the organs along the alimentary (digestive) tract - the long, muscular tube beginning at the oral cavity and ending at the anus. The major digestive organs include the pharynx, esophagus, stomach, and intestines. Accessory, or secondary, organs include the salivary and parotid glands, jaw, teeth and the supporting structures of teeth, liver, gallbladder and biliary tract, pancreas, and peritoneum.

The primary function of the digestive system is to mechanically break down and chemically dissolve food in order to provide the body with essential vitamins, proteins, minerals, and water. Diseases and disorders that interfere with this function are classified here, along with diseases and disorders that affect the organs of the digestive tract, even though they may have no direct affect on digestion. For example, dental caries have a direct effect on digestion because they interfere with mastication, the mechanical breakdown of food by chewing. Portal hypertension does not directly affect digestion, but is included here because it represents a disease of a digestive system organ.

The main subchapters of chapter 9, "Diseases of the Digestive System," are as follows:

*   Diseases of oral cavity, salivary glands, and jaws (520–529)
*   Diseases of esophagus, stomach, and duodenum (530–538)
*   Appendicitis (540–543)
*   Hernia of abdominal cavity (550–553)
*   Noninfectious enteritis and colitis (555–558)
*   Other diseases of intestines and peritoneum (560–569)
*   Other diseases of digestive system (570–579)

Diseases of Oral Cavity, Salivary Glands, and Jaws (520–529)

This category includes diseases and disorders of the jaw, salivary and parotid glands, teeth, gingiva and periodontium, lips, oral mucosa, and tongue.

Disorders of Tooth Development and Eruption (520)

Disorders of tooth development and eruption in all patients regardless of age are included in this category. This is one of the few categories in ICD-9-CM that classifies congenital anomalies and hereditary disturbances outside of chapter 14, "Congenital Anomalies."

Dentofacial Anomalies, Including Malocclusion (524)

Anomalies in the alignment of the jaw to the cranium can cause problems with the ability to chew food, may obstruct swallowing, and obstruct opening or closure of the mouth and cause physical distortion to the appearance of the face. Also included in this category are disorders of the temporomandibular joint.

Diseases of the Salivary Glands (527)

Diseases of the salivary glands include atrophy, hypertrophy, sialoadenitis, abscess, fistula, sialolithiasis, and disturbances of salivary secretion.

Diseases of the Oral Soft Tissues (528)

Excluded from this category are lesions specific to the gingiva and tongue, which are included in category 529. Included are cellulitis of the mouth, cysts, diseases of the lips, leukoplakia, and others.

Diseases of Esophagus, Stomach, and Duodenum (530–538)

This category includes diseases and disorders of the esophagus, the muscular, tubular structure that serves as a conduit for the passage of food and water from the pharynx to the stomach. The esophagus functions by transporting food and fluids from the mouth to the stomach (and sometimes in the reverse direction). The esophagus is equipped with two sphincters. The first is the pharyngoesophageal sphincter located at the level of the cricoid cartilage; the second is the gastroesophageal sphincter (also known as the lower esophageal sphincter) located at the level of the esophageal hiatus of the diaphragm.

Esophagitis (530.1)

Esophagitis is the inflammation of the esophagus due to reflux, chemicals and infection. Reflux esophagitis, is the most common form and is caused by acid and pepsin from the stomach rising past the gastroesophageal sphincter into the esophagus. Underlying causes include: hiatal hernia, pregnancy, certain drugs

(e.g., calcium channel blockers, beta-adrenergic agonists), scleroderma, obesity, and surgeries.

Barrett's esophagus is a common metaplastic condition that develops as a result of chronic gastroesophageal reflux disease (GERD) or inflammation of the esophagus (esophagitis). Barrett's esophagus carries a greater potential risk of the development of cancer. Assign code 530.89 for Barrett's esophagus.

Gastric Ulcer (531)

Gastric ulcer is a condition formed by tissue destruction within the lumen of the stomach. The destruction is due to the action of hydrochloric (gastric) acid and pepsin on areas of gastric mucosa having a decreased resistance to ulceration. Also known as pyloric ulcer, stomach ulcer or prepyloric ulcer. Note peptic ulcer NOS is classified to category 533 when the site is unspecified. Fifth-digit assignment for category 531 indicates whether there is mention of obstruction.

Gastric ulcers are classified according to four axes: site; acute vs. chronic; with and without hemorrhage; and with or without obstruction.

Gastric outlet obstruction (GOO) is an obstruction at the level of the pylorus. Gastric outlet obstruction is characterized by recurrent vomiting of food that accumulates in the stomach because the obstruction prevents the food from moving into the small intestine. Assign fifth digit 1 to indicate obstruction for category 531.

Peptic Ulcer, Site Unspecified (533)

A peptic ulcer is an acute or chronic benign ulcer occurring in a portion of the digestive tract accessible to gastric secretions. Peptic ulcers result from the corrosive action of acid gastric juice on vulnerable epithelium. This category (533) includes only peptic ulcers for which no site has been specified. Peptic ulcers may occur in the esophagus (530.2), stomach (531), duodenum (532), jejunum and gastrojejunum (534), and ileum (569.82). Fifth-digit assignment for category 533 indicates whether there is mention of obstruction. When ulcers are drug induced, an additional E code is assigned.

A common cause of peptic ulcer is the presence of *H. pylori*, which is treated with bismuth salicylate and oral amoxicillin. The *H. pylori* should be reported as an additional code 041.86 Helicobacter pylori [H. pylori].

Gastritis and Duodenitis (535)

Gastritis and duodenitis are self-limiting illnesses characterized by nausea, vomiting, anorexia, epigastric pain, and some systemic symptoms. Report the type of gastritis as documented. Diagnosis of underlying etiology will determine the treatment plan.

Eosinophilic gastrointestinal disorders (EGIDs) selectively affect the lining of the gastrointestinal tract through the accumulation of eosinophil cells in the intestinal tissue, causing inflammation. In this disease, eosinophil accumulation occurs in the absence of known causes for eosinophilia (e.g., drug reactions, parasitic infection, connective tissue disease, or malignancy). EGIDs are characterized by inflammation of the esophagus, stomach, or intestine. Symptoms and features of EGIDs mimic those of food allergy and immune dysregulation but do not clearly fit those disease categories. While these conditions may be difficult to diagnose, they are being identified with increasing frequency. Inflammation may not always be present visually during an endoscopic exam, but it may be seen under the microscope. Abnormally high numbers of eosinophils within the digestive tract may not provide a conclusive diagnosis of an EGID. Fifth-digit assignment for subcategory 535.7 identifies the complication of hemorrhage.

Gastroparesis (536.3)

Gastroparesis, a slight degree of paralysis within the muscular lining of the stomach, is most often a complication of type I diabetes. Symptoms include nausea, vomiting, early satiation, weight loss, abdominal bloating, and abdominal discomfort. Coding gastroparesis requires the assignment of an appropriate diabetes code (249.6x, 250.6x) and 536.3 Gastroparesis.

Appendicitis (540–543)

Appendicitis is an inflammation of the vermiform appendix and is usually initiated by obstruction. The obstruction is then followed by infection, edema, and frequently infarction of the appendiceal wall.

Subcategory levels of 540 indicate whether there is peritonitis or peritoneal abscess.

Hernia of Abdominal Cavity (550–553)

Hernias included in this section are acquired and congenital except diaphragmatic or hiatal.

Steps for coding hernias are as follows:

1. Determine the site.
2. Determine if gangrene is a complication.
3. Determine if there is obstruction.
4. For some categories, fifth-digit assignment identifies the nature (recurrent or not) and laterality (unilateral or bilateral).

Noninfectious Enteritis and Colitis (555–558)

Regional enteritis is a form of inflammatory bowel disease and is also known as Crohn's disease. Regional enteritis most often affects the large intestines but may occur anywhere along the gastrointestinal tract. Often, enteritis, gastroenteritis and diarrhea, when specified as due to an underlying condition, should be classified to a category other than 555. Infectious disease is the most frequent cause of gastritis and gastroenteritis and is classified to chapter 1, "Infectious and Parasitic Diseases."

Commonly caused by infection, diarrhea may also be caused by numerous disorders such as chronic bowel disease, malabsorption, food poisoning, adverse reactions to medications, dietary factors such as malnutrition and food allergy, pancreatic disease, metabolic disease, neurological disease, psychogenic disorders, heavy metal poisoning, laxative abuse, and immunodeficiency disease.

Enteritis and colitis due to infectious cause is more appropriately classified to chapter 1, "Infectious and Parasitic Diseases." Follow the guidance in the Alphabetic Index to code gastroenteritis and colitis to the specific underlying cause or type.

Other Diseases of Intestines and Peritoneum (560–579)

Intussusception and Volvulus (560)

Intussusception is the prolapse of one part of the intestine into another part below. It occurs primarily in children and its chief symptoms are paroxysmal pain, vomiting, and passage of blood and mucus via the rectum.

Volvulus is a looped or entangled bowel causing intestinal obstruction, particularly in the sigmoid flexure. Circulation of the bowel may be severely compromised in severe cases.

Diverticula of Colon (562.1)

Diverticula is the formation of a pouch or sac in the colon. Acquired diverticula are herniations of the mucosa through the muscle. Congenital diverticula are herniations of the entire thickness of the intestinal wall. This tends to occur in higher pressure areas such as the sigmoid colon. Diverticulosis is the presence of diverticula in the absence of inflammation. Diverticulitis is the inflammation of the diverticula.

Functional Digestive Disorders (564)

Conditions classified to category 564 include constipation, irritable bowel syndrome, functional diarrhea, postgastric surgery syndromes, and vomiting following gastrointestinal surgery.

Constipation (564.0) is further subdivided by type of constipation, slow transit (564.01), outlet dysfunction (564.02), and unspecified (564.00). Excluded from this is fecal impaction (560.32), fecal incontinence (787.60), fecal urgency (767.62), and incomplete defecation (787.61).

Peritonitis and Retroperitoneal Infections (567)

Peritonitis is the acute or chronic inflammation of the peritoneum. Inflammation and infection may be in response to agents such as bacteria, viruses, bile, hydrochloric acid, chemicals, parasites, fungi, and foreign bodies such as barium sulfate used in diagnostic imaging studies. Ruptured viscus and surgical procedures are two common underlying factors in secondary peritonitis and retroperitoneal abscess. Chronic peritonitis can lead to dense, widespread abdominal adhesions.

Other Disorders of Intestine (569)

This section includes other intestinal disorders not classifiable elsewhere, including anorectal disorders, intestinal abscesses, fistula and angiodysplasias, and colostomy complications.

Colostomy and enterostomy complications in subcategory 569.6 include mechanical, infection, and other. Note that ICD-9-CM does not classify these complications in chapter 17 under complications of surgical and medical care

(996–999). However, the same rules apply as when coding complications in the 996–999 series. If the complication is an infection, codes are assigned to identify the infectious organism and the type of infection. Mechanical complications include obstruction, leakage, malfunction, breakdown, etc. Do not assign code 997.4 in addition to the 569.6 series.

Anal Sphincter Tear (Healed) (Old) (Nontraumatic) (569.43)

Anal sphincter tears often result in fecal incontinence. Fecal incontinence may be the first symptom that leads to a diagnosis of an old, nonhealed anal sphincter tear. Anal sphincter tears can occur during delivery independent of third-degree lacerations, and such tears may not be identified until they complicate a subsequent delivery. Report code 569.43 Anal sphincter tear (healed) (old), for nongravid patients presenting for treatment of complications of an old tear. Report code 664.6x Anal sphincter tear complicating delivery, when not associated with third-degree perineal laceration. When reporting code 569.43, use an additional code for any associated fecal incontinence (787.60–787.63).

Chronic Liver Disease and Cirrhosis (571)

Cirrhosis of the liver is a chronic, progressive disease characterized by damage to the hepatic parenchymal cells and nodular regeneration, fibrosis formation, and disturbance of the normal architecture. Two different types of cirrhosis have been described based on the amount of regenerative activity in the liver: chronic sclerosing cirrhosis, in which the liver is small and hard, and nodular cirrhosis in which the liver may be quite enlarged initially.

Chronic hepatitis is defined as an inflammation and necrosis of the liver. Chronic hepatitis due to viral infection (070) is classified with the infectious and parasitic diseases of chapter 1. There are several forms of nonviral chronic hepatitis, based upon localization and extent of liver injury: active, aggressive, recurrent, and persistent. Code assignment is based upon the form of chronic hepatitis or upon the etiology of the liver disease.

Example:

> Chronic liver disease due to chronic persistent hepatitis is coded as 571.41.
>
> Acute alcoholic hepatitis is coded as 571.1.
>
> Acute viral hepatitis C without hepatic coma is coded as 070.51.
>
> Nonalcoholic cirrhosis of the liver is coded as 571.5.
>
> Autoimmune hepatitis is coded to 571.42.

Acute Cholecystitis (575.0)

Acute cholecystitis without mention of cholelithiasis (calculi or "gallstones" of the gallbladder or bile ducts) is classified to 575.0. This condition may be caused by obstruction of the cystic duct by another process (such as a malignant tumor), bile stasis ("sludge" formation), or infection due to organisms such as Escherichia coli, Clostridia, or Salmonella typhi.

Most cases (95 percent) of acute cholecystitis are due to obstruction of the cystic duct by an impacted gallstone and are classified to category 574.

Gastrointestinal Hemorrhage (578)

Gastrointestinal hemorrhage is bleeding of the stomach, ileum, jejunum, duodenum, and/or colon. The condition may be described as acute or chronic and involve a grossly bloody (visible) appearance or be detected by laboratory examination only (occult bleeding). GI bleeding is classified as either hematemesis (vomiting of blood) or blood in stool, which includes melena (partially digested blood showing as dark tarry stools) and hematochezia (passage of red blood in stools not specified as hematemesis or blood in stool).

This category excludes bleeding of the anus and rectum for classification purposes.

The terms "upper" and "lower" have no value as modifiers for classification of GI bleeding; the codes are distinguished by the presentation of the GI bleeding, not the site. Unspecified GI bleeding must be assigned to code 578.9 Hemorrhage of gastrointestinal tract, unspecified, when not stated as hematemesis or blood in stool (melena).

Hematemesis (578.0)

Hematemesis is the vomiting of frank red or partially digested blood and is usually indicative of bleeding of the upper gastrointestinal tract. Occult bleeding can be detected by analysis of vomitus or nasogastric tube aspiration.

Blood in Stool (578.1)

Blood in stool is the passage of frank red or partially digested blood in the stools, which may be due to a lower GI bleed. Blood in the stool without further documentation of GI bleeding is classified to code 792.1 Nonspecific abnormal findings in stool contents.

9. DISEASES OF THE DIGESTIVE SYSTEM (520-579)

DISEASES OF ORAL CAVITY, SALIVARY GLANDS, AND JAWS (520-529)

✓4ᵗʰ **520 Disorders of tooth development and eruption**

520.0 Anodontia
Absence of teeth (complete) (congenital) (partial)
Hypodontia
Oligodontia
EXCLUDES acquired absence of teeth (525.10-525.19)

520.1 Supernumerary teeth
Distomolar
Fourth molar
Mesiodens
Paramolar
Supplemental teeth
EXCLUDES supernumerary roots (520.2)

520.2 Abnormalities of size and form
Concrescence
Fusion } of teeth
Gemination

Dens evaginatus
Dens in dente
Dens invaginatus
Enamel pearls
Macrodontia
Microdontia
Peg-shaped [conical] teeth
Supernumerary roots
Taurodontism
Tuberculum paramolare
EXCLUDES that due to congenital syphilis (090.5)
tuberculum Carabelli, which is regarded as a
normal variation

520.3 Mottled teeth
Mottling of enamel
Dental fluorosis
Nonfluoride enamel opacities

Digestive System

The Oral Cavity

Teeth

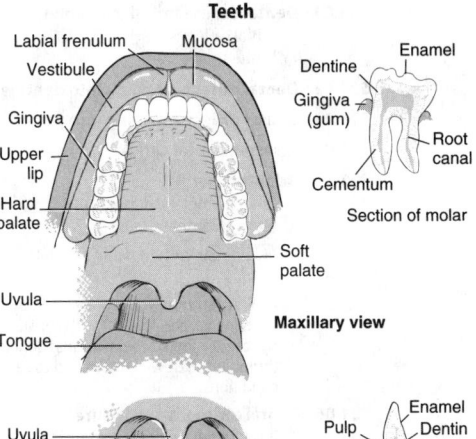

Section of molar

Maxillary view

Section of incisor

Mandibulary view

520.4 Disturbances of tooth formation
Aplasia and hypoplasia of cementum
Dilaceration of tooth
Enamel hypoplasia (neonatal) (postnatal) (prenatal)
Horner's teeth
Hypocalcification of teeth
Regional odontodysplasia
Turner's tooth
EXCLUDES Hutchinson's teeth and mulberry molars in
congenital syphilis (090.5)
mottled teeth (520.3)

**520.5 Hereditary disturbances in tooth structure, not
elsewhere classified**
Amelogensis
Dentinogenesis } imperfecta
Odontogenesis

Dentinal dysplasia
Shell teeth

520.6 Disturbances in tooth eruption

Teeth:	Tooth eruption:
embedded	late
impacted	obstructed
natal	premature
neonatal	
prenatal	
primary [deciduous]:	
persistent	
shedding, premature	

EXCLUDES exfoliation of teeth (attributable to disease of
surrounding tissues) (525.0-525.19)

520.7 Teething syndrome

**520.8 Other specified disorders of tooth development and
eruption**
Color changes during tooth formation
Pre-eruptive color changes
EXCLUDES posteruptive color changes (521.7)

**520.9 Unspecified disorder of tooth development
and eruption**

✓4ᵗʰ **521 Diseases of hard tissues of teeth**

✓5ᵗʰ **521.0 Dental caries**

521.00 Dental caries, unspecified

521.01 Dental caries limited to enamel
Initial caries
White spot lesion

521.02 Dental caries extending into dentine

521.03 Dental caries extending into pulp

521.04 Arrested dental caries

521.05 Odontoclasia
Infantile melanodontia
Melanodontoclasia
EXCLUDES *internal and external resorption of teeth (521.40-521.49)*
DEF: A pathological dental condition described as stained areas, loss of tooth substance, and hypoplasia linked to nutritional deficiencies during tooth development and to cariogenic oral conditions.

521.06 Dental caries pit and fissure
Primary dental caries, pit and fissure origin

521.07 Dental caries of smooth surface
Primary dental caries, smooth surface origin

521.08 Dental caries of root surface
Primary dental caries, root surface

521.09 Other dental caries

√5ᵗʰ **521.1 Excessive attrition (approximal wear) (occlusal wear)**

521.10 Excessive attrition, unspecified

521.11 Excessive attrition, limited to enamel

521.12 Excessive attrition, extending into dentine

521.13 Excessive attrition, extending into pulp

521.14 Excessive attrition, localized

521.15 Excessive attrition, generalized

√5ᵗʰ **521.2 Abrasion**
Abrasion:
dentifrice
habitual
occupational } of teeth
ritual
traditional
Wedge defect NOS

521.20 Abrasion, unspecified

521.21 Abrasion, limited to enamel

521.22 Abrasion, extending into dentine

521.23 Abrasion, extending into pulp

521.24 Abrasion, localized

521.25 Abrasion, generalized

√5ᵗʰ **521.3 Erosion**
Erosion of teeth:
NOS
due to:
medicine
persistent vomiting
idiopathic
occupational

521.30 Erosion, unspecified

521.31 Erosion, limited to enamel

521.32 Erosion, extending into dentine

521.33 Erosion, extending into pulp

521.34 Erosion, localized

521.35 Erosion, generalized

√5ᵗʰ **521.4 Pathological resorption**
DEF: Loss of dentin and cementum due to disease process.

521.40 Pathological resorption, unspecified

521.41 Pathological resorption, internal

521.42 Pathological resorption, external

521.49 Other pathological resorption
Internal granuloma of pulp

521.5 Hypercementosis
Cementation hyperplasia
DEF: Excess deposits of cementum, on tooth root.

521.6 Ankylosis of teeth
DEF: Adhesion of tooth to surrounding bone.

521.7 Intrinsic posteruptive color changes
Staining [discoloration] of teeth:
NOS
due to:
drugs
metals
pulpal bleeding
EXCLUDES *accretions [deposits] on teeth (523.6)*
extrinsic color changes (523.6)
pre-eruptive color changes (520.8)

√5ᵗʰ **521.8 Other specified diseases of hard tissues of teeth**

521.81 Cracked tooth
EXCLUDES *asymptomatic craze lines in enamel — omit code*
broken tooth due to trauma (873.63, 873.73)
fractured tooth due to trauma (873.63, 873.73)

521.89 Other specified diseases of hard tissues of teeth
Irradiated enamel
Sensitive dentin

521.9 Unspecified disease of hard tissues of teeth

√4ᵗʰ **522 Diseases of pulp and periapical tissues**

522.0 Pulpitis
Pulpal:
abscess
polyp
Pulpitis:
acute
chronic (hyperplastic) (ulcerative)
suppurative

522.1 Necrosis of the pulp
Pulp gangrene
DEF: Death of pulp tissue.

522.2 Pulp degeneration
Denticles
Pulp calcifications
Pulp stones

522.3 Abnormal hard tissue formation in pulp
Secondary or irregular dentin

522.4 Acute apical periodontitis of pulpal origin
DEF: Severe inflammation of periodontal ligament due to pulpal inflammation or necrosis.

522.5 Periapical abscess without sinus
Abscess:
dental
dentoalveolar
EXCLUDES *periapical abscess with sinus (522.7)*

522.6 Chronic apical periodontitis
Apical or periapical granuloma
Apical periodontitis NOS

522.7 Periapical abscess with sinus
Fistula:
alveolar process
dental

522.8 Radicular cyst
Cyst:
apical (periodontal)
periapical
radiculodental
residual radicular
EXCLUDES *lateral developmental or lateral periodontal cyst (526.0)*
DEF: Cyst in tissue around tooth apex due to chronic infection of granuloma around root.

© 2014 OptumInsight, Inc.

522.9   **Other and unspecified diseases of pulp and periapical tissues**

√4ᵗʰ **523**   **Gingival and periodontal diseases**

√5ᵗʰ **523.0**   **Acute gingivitis**
     EXCLUDES   *acute necrotizing ulcerative gingivitis (101)*
                    herpetic gingivostomatitis (054.2)

     523.00   **Acute gingivitis, plaque induced**
           Acute gingivitis NOS

     523.01   **Acute gingivitis, non-plaque induced**

√5ᵗʰ **523.1**   **Chronic gingivitis**
     Gingivitis (chronic):
       desquamative
       hyperplastic
       simple marginal
       ulcerative
     EXCLUDES   *herpetic gingivostomatitis (054.2)*

     523.10   **Chronic gingivitis, plaque induced**
           Chronic gingivitis NOS
           Gingivitis NOS

     523.11   **Chronic gingivitis, non-plaque induced**

√5ᵗʰ **523.2**   **Gingival recession**
     Gingival recession (postinfective) (postoperative)

     523.20   **Gingival recession, unspecified**

     523.21   **Gingival recession, minimal**

     523.22   **Gingival recession, moderate**

     523.23   **Gingival recession, severe**

     523.24   **Gingival recession, localized**

     523.25   **Gingival recession, generalized**

√5ᵗʰ **523.3**   **Aggressive and acute periodontitis**
     Acute:
       pericementitis
       pericoronitis
     EXCLUDES   *acute apical periodontitis (522.4)*
                    periapical abscess (522.5, 522.7)
     DEF: Severe inflammation of tissues supporting teeth.

     523.30   **Aggressive periodontitis, unspecified**

     523.31   **Aggressive periodontitis, localized**
           Periodontal abscess

     523.32   **Aggressive periodontitis, generalized**

     523.33   **Acute periodontitis**

√5ᵗʰ **523.4**   **Chronic periodontitis**
     Chronic pericoronitis
     Pericementitis (chronic)
     Periodontitis:
       complex
       simplex
       NOS
     EXCLUDES   *chronic apical periodontitis (522.6)*

     523.40   **Chronic periodontitis, unspecified**

     523.41   **Chronic periodontitis, localized**

     523.42   **Chronic periodontitis, generalized**

523.5   **Periodontosis**

523.6   **Accretions on teeth**
     Dental calculus:
       subgingival
       supragingival
     Deposits on teeth:
       betel
       materia alba
       soft
       tartar
       tobacco
     Extrinsic discoloration of teeth
     EXCLUDES   *intrinsic discoloration of teeth (521.7)*
     DEF: Foreign material on tooth surface, usually plaque or calculus.

523.8   **Other specified periodontal diseases**
     Giant cell:
       epulis
       peripheral granuloma
     Gingival:
       cysts
       enlargement NOS
       fibromatosis
     Gingival polyp
     Periodontal lesions due to traumatic occlusion
     Peripheral giant cell granuloma
     EXCLUDES   *leukoplakia of gingiva (528.6)*

523.9   **Unspecified gingival and periodontal disease**

√4ᵗʰ **524**   **Dentofacial anomalies, including malocclusion**

√5ᵗʰ **524.0**   **Major anomalies of jaw size**
     EXCLUDES   *hemifacial atrophy or hypertrophy (754.0)*
                    unilateral condylar hyperplasia or hypoplasia
                    of mandible (526.89)

     524.00   **Unspecified anomaly**
           DEF: Unspecified deformity of jaw size.

     524.01   **Maxillary hyperplasia**
           DEF: Overgrowth or over development of upper jaw bone.

     524.02   **Mandibular hyperplasia**
           DEF: Overgrowth or over development of lower jaw bone.

     524.03   **Maxillary hypoplasia**
           DEF: Incomplete or underdeveloped upper jaw bone.

     524.04   **Mandibular hypoplasia**
           DEF: Incomplete or underdeveloped lower jaw bone.

     524.05   **Macrogenia**
           DEF: Enlarged jaw, especially chin; affects bone, soft tissue, or both.

     524.06   **Microgenia**
           DEF: Underdeveloped mandible characterized by an extremely small chin.

     524.07   **Excessive tuberosity of jaw**
           Entire maxillary tuberosity

     524.09   **Other specified anomaly**

√5ᵗʰ **524.1**   **Anomalies of relationship of jaw to cranial base**

     524.10   **Unspecified anomaly**
           Prognathism
           Retrognathism
           DEF: Prognathism: protrusion of lower jaw.
           DEF: Retrognathism: jaw is located posteriorly to a normally positioned jaw; backward position of mandible.

     524.11   **Maxillary asymmetry**
           DEF: Absence of symmetry of maxilla.

     524.12   **Other jaw asymmetry**

     524.19   **Other specified anomaly**

Angle's Classification of Malocclusion

Normal occlusion

Class I Malocclusion

Class II Malocclusion

Class III Malocclusion

√5th **524.2 Anomalies of dental arch relationship**
Anomaly of dental arch
EXCLUDES hemifacial atrophy or hypertrophy (754.0)
soft tissue impingement (524.81-524.82)
unilateral condylar hyperplasia or hypoplasia
of mandible (526.89)

524.20 Unspecified anomaly of dental arch relationship

524.21 Malocclusion, Angle's class I
Neutro-occlusion

524.22 Malocclusion, Angle's class II
Disto-occlusion Division I
Disto-occlusion Division II

524.23 Malocclusion, Angle's class III
Mesio-occlusion

524.24 Open anterior occlusal relationship
Anterior open bite

524.25 Open posterior occlusal relationship
Posterior open bite

524.26 Excessive horizontal overlap
Excessive horizontal overjet

524.27 Reverse articulation
Anterior articulation
Crossbite
Posterior articulation

524.28 Anomalies of interarch distance
Excessive interarch distance
Inadequate interarch distance

524.29 Other anomalies of dental arch relationship
Other anomalies of dental arch

√5th **524.3 Anomalies of tooth position of fully erupted teeth**
EXCLUDES impacted or embedded teeth with abnormal
position of such teeth or adjacent teeth
(520.6)

524.30 Unspecified anomaly of tooth position
Diastema of teeth NOS
Displacement of teeth NOS
Transposition of teeth NOS

524.31 Crowding of teeth

524.32 Excessive spacing of teeth

524.33 Horizontal displacement of teeth
Tipped teeth
Tipping of teeth

524.34 Vertical displacement of teeth
Extruded tooth
Infraeruption of teeth
Intruded tooth
Supraeruption of teeth

524.35 Rotation of tooth/teeth

524.36 Insufficient interocclusal distance of teeth (ridge)
Lack of adequate intermaxillary vertical dimension

524.37 Excessive interocclusal distance of teeth
Excessive intermaxillary vertical dimension
Loss of occlusal vertical dimension

524.39 Other anomalies of tooth position

524.4 Malocclusion, unspecified
DEF: Malposition of top and bottom teeth; interferes with chewing.

√5th **524.5 Dentofacial functional abnormalities**

524.50 Dentofacial functional abnormality, unspecified

524.51 Abnormal jaw closure

524.52 Limited mandibular range of motion

524.53 Deviation in opening and closing of the mandible

524.54 Insufficient anterior guidance
Insufficient anterior occlusal guidance

524.55 Centric occlusion maximum intercuspation discrepancy
Centric occlusion of teeth discrepancy

524.56 Non-working side interference
Balancing side interference

524.57 Lack of posterior occlusal support

524.59 Other dentofacial functional abnormalities
Abnormal swallowing
Mouth breathing
Sleep postures
Tongue, lip, or finger habits

√5th **524.6 Temporomandibular joint disorders**
EXCLUDES current temporomandibular joint:
dislocation (830.0-830.1)
strain (848.1)

524.60 Temporomandibular joint disorders, unspecified
Temporomandibular joint-pain-dysfunction syndrome [TMJ]

524.61 Adhesions and ankylosis (bony or fibrous)
DEF: Stiffening or union of temporomandibular joint due to bony or fibrous union across joint.

524.62 Arthralgia of temporomandibular joint
DEF: Pain in temporomandibular joint; not inflammatory in nature.

524.63 Articular disc disorder (reducing or non-reducing)

524.64 Temporomandibular joint sounds on opening and/or closing the jaw

524.69 Other specified temporomandibular joint disorders

√5th **524.7 Dental alveolar anomalies**

524.70 Unspecified alveolar anomaly

524.71 Alveolar maxillary hyperplasia
DEF: Excessive tissue formation in the dental alveoli of upper jaw.

524.72 Alveolar mandibular hyperplasia
DEF: Excessive tissue formation in the dental alveoli of lower jaw.

524.73 Alveolar maxillary hypoplasia
DEF: Incomplete or underdeveloped alveolar tissue of upper jaw.

524.74 Alveolar mandibular hypoplasia
DEF: Incomplete or underdeveloped alveolar tissue of lower jaw.

524.75 Vertical displacement of alveolus and teeth
Extrusion of alveolus and teeth

524.76 Occlusal plane deviation

524.79 Other specified alveolar anomaly

√5th **524.8 Other specified dentofacial anomalies**

524.81 Anterior soft tissue impingement

524.82 Posterior soft tissue impingement

524.89 Other specified dentofacial anomalies

524.9 Unspecified dentofacial anomalies

√4th **525 Other diseases and conditions of the teeth and supporting structures**

525.0 Exfoliation of teeth due to systemic causes
DEF: Deterioration of teeth and surrounding structures due to systemic disease.

√5th **525.1 Loss of teeth due to trauma, extraction, or periodontal disease**
Code first class of edentulism (525.40-525.44, 525.50-525.54)

525.10 Acquired absence of teeth, unspecified
Tooth extraction status, NOS

525.11 Loss of teeth due to trauma

525.12 Loss of teeth due to periodontal disease

525.13   *Loss of teeth due to caries*

525.19   *Other loss of teeth*

√5ᵗʰ   **525.2   Atrophy of edentulous alveolar ridge**

525.20   Unspecified atrophy of edentulous alveolar ridge
Atrophy of the mandible NOS
Atrophy of the maxilla NOS

525.21   Minimal atrophy of the mandible

525.22   Moderate atrophy of the mandible

525.23   Severe atrophy of the mandible

525.24   Minimal atrophy of the maxilla

525.25   Moderate atrophy of the maxilla

525.26   Severe atrophy of the maxilla

525.3   Retained dental root

√5ᵗʰ   **525.4   Complete edentulism**
Use additional code to identify cause of edentulism (525.10-525.19)

525.40   Complete edentulism, unspecified
Edentulism NOS

525.41   Complete edentulism, class I

525.42   Complete edentulism, class II

525.43   Complete edentulism, class III

525.44   Complete edentulism, class IV

√5ᵗʰ   **525.5   Partial edentulism**
Use additional code to identify cause of edentulism (525.10-525.19)

525.50   Partial edentulism, unspecified

525.51   Partial edentulism, class I

525.52   Partial edentulism, class II

525.53   Partial edentulism, class III

525.54   Partial edentulism, class IV

√5ᵗʰ   **525.6   Unsatisfactory restoration of tooth**
Defective bridge, crown, fillings
Defective dental restoration
EXCLUDES   *dental restoration status (V45.84)*
unsatisfactory endodontic treatment (526.61-526.69)

525.60   Unspecified unsatisfactory restoration of tooth
Unspecified defective dental restoration

525.61   Open restoration margins
Dental restoration failure of marginal integrity
Open margin on tooth restoration

525.62   Unrepairable overhanging of dental restorative materials
Overhanging of tooth restoration

525.63   Fractured dental restorative material without loss of material
EXCLUDES   *cracked tooth (521.81)*
fractured tooth (873.63, 873.73)

525.64   Fractured dental restorative material with loss of material
EXCLUDES   *cracked tooth (521.81)*
fractured tooth (873.63, 873.73)

525.65   Contour of existing restoration of tooth biologically incompatible with oral health
Dental restoration failure of periodontal anatomical integrity
Unacceptable contours of existing restoration
Unacceptable morphology of existing restoration

525.66   Allergy to existing dental restorative material
Use additional code to identify the specific type of allergy

525.67   Poor aesthetics of existing restoration
Dental restoration aesthetically inadequate or displeasing

525.69   Other unsatisfactory restoration of existing tooth

√5ᵗʰ   **525.7   Endosseous dental implant failure**

525.71   Osseointegration failure of dental implant
Failure of dental implant due to infection
Failure of dental implant due to unintentional loading
Failure of dental implant osseointegration due to premature loading
Failure of dental implant to osseointegrate prior to intentional prosthetic loading
Hemorrhagic complications of dental implant placement
Iatrogenic osseointegration failure of dental implant
Osseointegration failure of dental implant due to complications of systemic disease
Osseointegration failure of dental implant due to poor bone quality
Pre-integration failure of dental implant NOS
Pre-osseointegration failure of dental implant

525.72   Post-osseointegration biological failure of dental implant
Failure of dental implant due to lack of attached gingiva
Failure of dental implant due to occlusal trauma (caused by poor prosthetic design)
Failure of dental implant due to parafunctional habits
Failure of dental implant due to periodontal infection (peri-implantitis)
Failure of dental implant due to poor oral hygiene
Failure of dental implant to osseointegrate following intentional prosthetic loading
Iatrogenic post-osseointegration failure of dental implant
Post-osseointegration failure of dental implant due to complications of systemic disease

525.73   Post-osseointegration mechanic failure of dental implant
Failure of dental prosthesis causing loss of dental implant
Fracture of dental implant
Mechanical failure of dental implant NOS
EXCLUDES   *cracked tooth (521.81)*
fractured dental restorative material with loss of material (525.64)
fractured dental restorative material without loss of material (525.63)
fractured tooth (873.63, 873.73)

525.79   Other endosseous dental implant failure
Dental implant failure NOS

525.8   Other specified disorders of the teeth and supporting structures
Enlargement of alveolar ridge NOS
Irregular alveolar process

525.9   Unspecified disorder of the teeth and supporting structures

√4ᵗʰ   **526   Diseases of the jaws**

526.0   Developmental odontogenic cysts
Cyst:
     dentigerous
     eruption
     follicular
     lateral developmental
     lateral periodontal
     primordial
Keratocyst
EXCLUDES   *radicular cyst (522.8)*

Diseases of the Digestive System

526.1–528.2

526.1 Fissural cysts of jaw
Cyst:
globulomaxillary
incisor canal
median anterior maxillary
median palatal
nasopalatine
palatine of papilla
EXCLUDES   *cysts of oral soft tissues (528.4)*

526.2 Other cysts of jaws
Cyst of jaw:
NOS
aneurysmal
hemorrhagic
traumatic

526.3 Central giant cell (reparative) granuloma
EXCLUDES   *peripheral giant cell granuloma (523.8)*

526.4 Inflammatory conditions
Abscess
Osteitis   } of jaw (acute) (chronic)
Osteomyelitis (neonatal)   (suppurative)
Periostitis

Sequestrum of jaw bone
EXCLUDES   *alveolar osteitis (526.5)*
osteonecrosis of jaw (733.45)

526.5 Alveolitis of jaw
Alveolar osteitis
Dry socket
DEF: Inflammation of alveoli or tooth socket.

√5ᵗʰ **526.6 Periradicular pathology associated with previous endodontic treatment**
526.61 Perforation of root canal space
526.62 Endodontic overfill
526.63 Endodontic underfill
526.69 Other periradicular pathology associated with previous endodontic treatment

√5ᵗʰ **526.8 Other specified diseases of the jaws**
526.81 Exostosis of jaw
Torus mandibularis
Torus palatinus
DEF: Spur or bony outgrowth on the jaw.

526.89 Other
Cherubism
Fibrous dysplasia   } of jaw(s)
Latent bone cyst
Osteoradionecrosis

Unilateral condylar hyperplasia or hypoplasia of mandible

526.9 Unspecified disease of the jaws

√4ᵗʰ **527 Diseases of the salivary glands**
527.0 Atrophy
DEF: Wasting away, necrosis of salivary gland tissue.

527.1 Hypertrophy
DEF: Overgrowth or overdeveloped salivary gland tissue.

527.2 Sialoadenitis
Parotitis:
NOS
allergic
toxic
Sialoangitis
Sialodochitis
EXCLUDES   *epidemic or infectious parotitis (072.0-072.9)*
uveoparotid fever (135)
DEF: Inflammation of salivary gland.

527.3 Abscess

527.4 Fistula
EXCLUDES   *congenital fistula of salivary gland (750.24)*

527.5 Sialolithiasis
Calculus } of salivary gland or duct
Stone
Sialodocholithiasis

527.6 Mucocele
Mucous:
extravasation cyst of salivary gland
retention cyst of salivary gland
Ranula
DEF: Dilated salivary gland cavity filled with mucous.

527.7 Disturbance of salivary secretion
Hyposecretion
Ptyalism
Sialorrhea
Xerostomia

527.8 Other specified diseases of the salivary glands
Benign lymphoepithelial lesion of salivary gland
Sialectasia
Sialosis
Stenosis } of salivary duct
Stricture

527.9 Unspecified disease of the salivary glands

√4ᵗʰ **528 Diseases of the oral soft tissues, excluding lesions specific for gingiva and tongue**

√5ᵗʰ **528.0 Stomatitis and mucositis (ulcerative)**
EXCLUDES   *cellulitis and abscess of mouth (528.3)*
diphtheritic stomatitis (032.0)
epizootic stomatitis (078.4)
gingivitis (523.0-523.1)
oral thrush (112.0)
Stevens-Johnson syndrome (695.13)
stomatitis:
acute necrotizing ulcerative (101)
aphthous (528.2)
gangrenous (528.1)
herpetic (054.2)
Vincent's (101)

DEF: Stomatitis: Inflammation of oral mucosa; labial and buccal mucosa, tongue, palate, floor of the mouth, and gingivae.

528.00 Stomatitis and mucositis, unspecified
Mucositis NOS
Ulcerative mucositis NOS
Ulcerative stomatitis NOS
Vesicular stomatitis NOS

528.01 Mucositis (ulcerative) due to antineoplastic therapy
Use additional E code to identify adverse effects of therapy, such as:
antineoplastic and immunosuppressive drugs (E930.7, E933.1)
radiation therapy (E879.2)

528.02 Mucositis (ulcerative) due to other drugs
Use additional E code to identify drug

528.09 Other stomatitis and mucositis (ulcerative)

528.1 Cancrum oris
Gangrenous stomatitis
Noma
DEF: A severely gangrenous lesion of mouth due to fusospirochetal infection; destroys buccal, labial and facial tissues; can be fatal; found primarily in debilitated and malnourished children.

528.2 Oral aphthae
Aphthous stomatitis
Canker sore
Periadenitis mucosa necrotica recurrens
Recurrent aphthous ulcer
Stomatitis herpetiformis
EXCLUDES   *herpetic stomatitis (054.2)*
DEF: Small oval or round ulcers of the mouth marked by a grayish exudate and a red halo effect.

528.3 Cellulitis and abscess
Cellulitis of mouth (floor)
Ludwig's angina
Oral fistula
> **EXCLUDES** abscess of tongue (529.0)
> cellulitis or abscess of lip (528.5)
> fistula (of):
>   dental (522.7)
>   lip (528.5)
> gingivitis (523.00-523.11)

528.4 Cysts
Dermoid cyst
Epidermoid cyst
Epstein's pearl   } of mouth
Lymphoepithelial cyst
Nasoalveolar cyst
Nasolabial cyst
> **EXCLUDES** cyst:
>   gingiva (523.8)
>   tongue (529.8)

528.5 Diseases of lips
Abscess
Cellulitis   } of lips
Fistula
Hypertrophy
Cheilitis:
   NOS
   angular
Cheilodynia
Cheilosis
> **EXCLUDES** actinic cheilitis (692.79)
> congenital fistula of lip (750.25)
> leukoplakia of lips (528.6)

528.6 Leukoplakia of oral mucosa, including tongue
Leukokeratosis of oral mucosa
Leukoplakia of:
   gingiva
   lips
   tongue
> **EXCLUDES** carcinoma in situ (230.0, 232.0)
> leukokeratosis nicotina palati (528.79)

DEF: Thickened white patches of epithelium on mucous membranes of mouth.

√5ᵗʰ **528.7 Other disturbances of oral epithelium, including tongue**
> **EXCLUDES** carcinoma in situ (230.0, 232.0)
> leukokeratosis NOS (702.8)

528.71 Minimal keratinized residual ridge mucosa
Minimal keratinization of alveolar ridge mucosa

528.72 Excessive keratinized residual ridge mucosa
Excessive keratinization of alveolar ridge mucosa

528.79 Other disturbances of oral epithelium, including tongue
Erythroplasia of mouth or tongue
Focal epithelial hyperplasia of mouth or tongue
Leukoedema of mouth or tongue
Leukokeratosis nicotina palate
Other oral epithelium disturbances

528.8 Oral submucosal fibrosis, including of tongue

528.9 Other and unspecified diseases of the oral soft tissues
Cheek and lip biting
Denture sore mouth
Denture stomatitis
Melanoplakia
Papillary hyperplasia of palate
Eosinophilic granuloma
Irritative hyperplasisa   } of oral mucosa
Pyogenic granuloma
Ulcer (traumatic)

√4ᵗʰ **529 Diseases and other conditions of the tongue**

529.0 Glossitis
Abscess
Ulceration (traumatic)   } of tongue
> **EXCLUDES** glossitis:
>   benign migratory (529.1)
>   Hunter's (529.4)
>   median rhomboid (529.2)
>   Moeller's (529.4)

529.1 Geographic tongue
Benign migratory glossitis
Glossitis areata exfoliativa
DEF: Chronic glossitis; marked by filiform papillae atrophy and inflammation; no known etiology.

529.2 Median rhomboid glossitis
DEF: A noninflammatory, congenital disease characterized by rhomboid-like lesions at the middle third of the tongue's dorsal surface.

529.3 Hypertrophy of tongue papillae
Black hairy tongue
Coated tongue
Hypertrophy of foliate papillae
Lingua villosa nigra

529.4 Atrophy of tongue papillae
Bald tongue
Glazed tongue
Glossitis:
   Hunter's
   Moeller's
Glossodynia exfoliativa
Smooth atrophic tongue

529.5 Plicated tongue
Fissured
Furrowed   } tongue
Scrotal
> **EXCLUDES** fissure of tongue, congenital (750.13)

DEF: Cracks, fissures or furrows, on dorsal surface of tongue.

529.6 Glossodynia
Glossopyrosis
Painful tongue
> **EXCLUDES** glossodynia exfoliativa (529.4)

529.8 Other specified conditions of the tongue
Atrophy
Crenated   } (of) tongue
Enlargement
Hypertrophy
Glossocele
Glossoptosis
> **EXCLUDES** erythroplasia of tongue (528.79)
> leukoplakia of tongue (528.6)
> macroglossia (congenital) (750.15)
> microglossia (congenital) (750.16)
> oral submucosal fibrosis (528.8)

529.9 Unspecified condition of the tongue

DISEASES OF ESOPHAGUS, STOMACH, AND DUODENUM (530-539)

√4ᵗʰ **530 Diseases of esophagus**
> **EXCLUDES** esophageal varices (456.0-456.2)

530.0 Achalasia and cardiospasm
Achalasia (of cardia)
Aperistalsis of esophagus
Megaesophagus
> **EXCLUDES** congenital cardiospasm (750.7)

DEF: Failure of smooth muscle fibers to relax at gastrointestinal junctures, such as esophagogastric sphincter when swallowing.

Diseases of the Digestive System

530.1–531.6

Esophagus

Pharyngeal constrictors

Front view

Epiglottis

Cricoid cartilage

C6

Trachea

Gastroesophageal sphincter

Pharyngoesophageal sphincter

Diaphragm

Side view

Stomach

✓5ᵗʰ **530.1 Esophagitis**

Esophagitis: Esophagitis:
   chemical   postoperative
   peptic   regurgitant

Use additional E code to identify cause, if induced by chemical

EXCLUDES   tuberculous esophagitis (017.8)

530.10 Esophagitis, unspecified
Esophagitis NOS

530.11 Reflux esophagitis
DEF: Inflammation of lower esophagus; due to regurgitated gastric acid.

530.12 Acute esophagitis
DEF: An acute invflammation of the mucous lining or submucosal coat of the esophagus.

530.13 Eosinophilic esophagitis

530.19 Other esophagitis
Abscess of esophagus

✓5ᵗʰ **530.2 Ulcer of esophagus**

Ulcer of esophagus:
   fungal
   peptic
Ulcer of esophagus due to ingestion of:
   aspirin
   chemicals
   medicines
Use additional E code to identify cause, if induced by chemical or drug

530.20 Ulcer of esophagus without bleeding
Ulcer of esophagus NOS

530.21 Ulcer of esophagus with bleeding
EXCLUDES   bleeding esophageal varices (456.0, 456.20)

530.3 Stricture and stenosis of esophagus
Compression of esophagus
Obstruction of esophagus
EXCLUDES   congenital stricture of esophagus (750.3)

530.4 Perforation of esophagus
Rupture of esophagus
EXCLUDES   traumatic perforation of esophagus (862.22, 862.32, 874.4-874.5)

530.5 Dyskinesia of esophagus
Corkscrew esophagus   Esophagospasm
Curling esophagus   Spasm of esophagus
EXCLUDES   cardiospasm (530.0)
DEF: Difficulty performing voluntary esophageal movements.

530.6 Diverticulum of esophagus, acquired
Diverticulum, acquired:
   epiphrenic
   pharyngoesophageal
   pulsion
   subdiaphragmatic
   traction
   Zenker's (hypopharyngeal)
Esophageal pouch, acquired
Esophagocele, acquired
EXCLUDES   congenital diverticulum of esophagus (750.4)

530.7 Gastroesophageal laceration-hemorrhage syndrome
Mallory-Weiss syndrome
DEF: Laceration of distal esophagus and proximal stomach due to vomiting, hiccups or other sustained activity.

✓5ᵗʰ **530.8 Other specified disorders of esophagus**

530.81 Esophageal reflux
Gastroesophageal reflux
EXCLUDES   reflux esophagitis (530.11)
DEF: Regurgitation of the gastric contents into esophagus and possibly pharynx.

530.82 Esophageal hemorrhage
EXCLUDES   hemorrhage due to esophageal varices (456.0-456.2)

530.83 Esophageal leukoplakia

530.84 Tracheoesophageal fistula
EXCLUDES   congenital tracheoesophageal fistula (750.3)

530.85 Barrett's esophagus
DEF: A metaplastic disorder in which specialized columnar epithelial cells replace the normal squamous epithelial cells; secondary to chronic gastroesophageal reflux damage to the mucosa; increases risk of developing adenocarcinoma.

530.86 Infection of esophagostomy
Use additional code to specify infection

530.87 Mechanical complication of esophagostomy
Malfunction of esophagostomy

530.89 Other
EXCLUDES   Paterson-Kelly syndrome (280.8)

530.9 Unspecified disorder of esophagus

✓4ᵗʰ **531 Gastric ulcer**
INCLUDES   ulcer (peptic):
   prepyloric
   pylorus
   stomach
Use additional E code to identify drug, if drug-induced
EXCLUDES   peptic ulcer NOS (533.0-533.9)

> The following fifth-digit subclassification is for use with category 531:
>   **0 without mention of obstruction**
>   **1 with obstruction**

DEF: Destruction of tissue in lumen of stomach due to action of gastric acid and pepsin on gastric mucosa decreasing resistance to ulcers.

✓5ᵗʰ **531.0 Acute with hemorrhage**
[0-1]

✓5ᵗʰ **531.1 Acute with perforation**
[0-1]

✓5ᵗʰ **531.2 Acute with hemorrhage and perforation**
[0-1]

✓5ᵗʰ **531.3 Acute without mention of hemorrhage or perforation**
[0-1]

✓5ᵗʰ **531.4 Chronic or unspecified with hemorrhage**
[0-1]

✓5ᵗʰ **531.5 Chronic or unspecified with perforation**
[0-1]

✓5ᵗʰ **531.6 Chronic or unspecified with hemorrhage and perforation**
[0-1]

Stomach

Esophagus

Diaphragm

Cardiac portion

Stomach

Fundus

Pylorus

Greater curvature

Pancreas

Sphincter of Oddi

Pancreatic duct

Common bile duct

Proximal duodenum

√5ᵗʰ **531.7** **Chronic without mention of hemorrhage or perforation**
[0-1]

√5ᵗʰ **531.9** **Unspecified as acute or chronic, without mention of hemorrhage or perforation**
[0-1]

√4ᵗʰ **532** **Duodenal ulcer**

INCLUDES   erosion (acute) of duodenum
ulcer (peptic):
    duodenum
    postpyloric

Use additional E code to identify drug, if drug-induced

EXCLUDES   *peptic ulcer NOS (533.0-533.9)*

The following fifth-digit subclassification is for use with category 532:
    0 **without mention of obstruction**
    1 **with obstruction**

DEF: Ulcers in duodenum due to action of gastric acid and pepsin on mucosa decreasing resistance to ulcers.

√5ᵗʰ **532.0** **Acute with hemorrhage**
[0-1]

√5ᵗʰ **532.1** **Acute with perforation**
[0-1]

√5ᵗʰ **532.2** **Acute with hemorrhage and perforation**
[0-1]

√5ᵗʰ **532.3** **Acute without mention of hemorrhage or perforation**
[0-1]

√5ᵗʰ **532.4** **Chronic or unspecified with hemorrhage**
[0-1]

√5ᵗʰ **532.5** **Chronic or unspecified with perforation**
[0-1]

√5ᵗʰ **532.6** **Chronic or unspecified with hemorrhage and perforation**
[0-1]

√5ᵗʰ **532.7** **Chronic without mention of hemorrhage or perforation**
[0-1]

√5ᵗʰ **532.9** **Unspecified as acute or chronic, without mention of hemorrhage or perforation**
[0-1]

√4ᵗʰ **533** **Peptic ulcer, site unspecified**

INCLUDES   gastroduodenal ulcer NOS
peptic ulcer NOS
stress ulcer NOS

Use additional E code to identify drug, if drug-induced

EXCLUDES   *peptic ulcer:*
    duodenal (532.0-532.9)
    gastric (531.0-531.9)

The following fifth-digit subclassification is for use with category 533:
    0 **without mention of obstruction**
    1 **with obstruction**

DEF: Ulcer of mucous membrane of esophagus, stomach or duodenum due to gastric acid secretion.

√5ᵗʰ **533.0** **Acute with hemorrhage**
[0-1]

√5ᵗʰ **533.1** **Acute with perforation**
[0-1]

√5ᵗʰ **533.2** **Acute with hemorrhage and perforation**
[0-1]

√5ᵗʰ **533.3** **Acute without mention of hemorrhage and perforation**
[0-1]

√5ᵗʰ **533.4** **Chronic or unspecified with hemorrhage**
[0-1]

√5ᵗʰ **533.5** **Chronic or unspecified with perforation**
[0-1]

√5ᵗʰ **533.6** **Chronic or unspecified with hemorrhage and perforation**
[0-1]

√5ᵗʰ **533.7** **Chronic without mention of hemorrhage or perforation**
[0-1]

√5ᵗʰ **533.9** **Unspecified as acute or chronic, without mention of hemorrhage or perforation**
[0-1]

√4ᵗʰ **534** **Gastrojejunal ulcer**

INCLUDES   ulcer (peptic) or erosion:
    anastomotic
    gastrocolic
    gastrointestinal
    gastrojejunal
    jejunal
    marginal
    stomal

EXCLUDES   *primary ulcer of small intestine (569.82)*

The following fifth-digit subclassification is for use with category 534:
    0 **without mention of obstruction**
    1 **with obstruction**

√5ᵗʰ **534.0** **Acute with hemorrhage**
[0-1]

√5ᵗʰ **534.1** **Acute with perforation**
[0-1]

√5ᵗʰ **534.2** **Acute with hemorrhage and perforation**
[0-1]

√5ᵗʰ **534.3** **Acute without mention of hemorrhage or perforation**
[0-1]

√5ᵗʰ **534.4** **Chronic or unspecified with hemorrhage**
[0-1]

√5ᵗʰ **534.5** **Chronic or unspecified with perforation**
[0-1]

√5ᵗʰ **534.6** **Chronic or unspecified with hemorrhage and perforation**
[0-1]

√5ᵗʰ **534.7** **Chronic without mention of hemorrhage or perforation**
[0-1]

√5ᵗʰ **534.9** **Unspecified as acute or chronic, without mention of hemorrhage or perforation**
[0-1]

√4ᵗʰ **535** **Gastritis and duodenitis**

The following fifth-digit subclassification is for use with category 535:
    0 **without mention of hemorrhage**
    1 **with hemorrhage**

√5ᵗʰ **535.0** **Acute gastritis**
[0-1]   **DEF:** Inflammation of stomach, with mucous membrane atrophy and peptic gland destruction.

√5ᵗʰ **535.1** **Atrophic gastritis**
[0-1]   Gastritis:
    atrophic-hyperplastic
    chronic (atrophic)

    DEF: Inflammation of stomach, with mucous membrane atrophy and peptic gland destruction.

√5ᵗʰ **535.2** **Gastric mucosal hypertrophy**
[0-1]   Hypertrophic gastritis

√5ᵗʰ **535.3** **Alcoholic gastritis**
[0-1]

Diseases of the Digestive System

535.4–538

√5ᵗʰ **535.4 Other specified gastritis**
[0-1] Gastritis: Gastritis:
    allergic   superficial
    bile induced   toxic
    irritant
    EXCLUDES *eosinophilic gastritis (535.7)*

√5ᵗʰ **535.5 Unspecified gastritis and gastroduodenitis**
[0-1]

√5ᵗʰ **535.6 Duodenitis**
[0-1] **DEF:** Inflammation of intestine, between pylorus and
jejunum.

√5ᵗʰ **535.7 Eosinophilic gastritis**
[0-1]

√4ᵗʰ **536 Disorders of function of stomach**
EXCLUDES *functional disorders of stomach specified as*
psychogenic (306.4)

536.0 Achlorhydria
DEF: Absence of gastric acid due to gastric mucosa
atrophy; unresponsive to histamines; also known as gastric
anacidity.

536.1 Acute dilatation of stomach
Acute distention of stomach

536.2 Persistent vomiting
Cyclical vomiting
Habit vomiting
Persistent vomiting [not of pregnancy]
Uncontrollable vomiting
EXCLUDES *bilious emesis (vomiting) (787.04)*
excessive vomiting in pregnancy
(643.0-643.9)
vomiting NOS (787.03)
cyclical, associated with migraine (346.2)
vomiting of fecal matter (569.87)

536.3 Gastroparesis
Gastroparalysis
Code first underlying disease, if known, such as:
diabetes mellitus (249.6, 250.6)
DEF: Slight degree of paralysis within muscular coat of
stomach.

√5ᵗʰ **536.4 Gastrostomy complications**

536.40 Gastrostomy complication, unspecified

536.41 Infection of gastrostomy
Use additional code to identify organism
(041.00-041.9)
Use additional code to specify type of infection,
such as:
abscess or cellulitis of abdomen (682.2)
septicemia (038.0-038.9)

536.42 Mechanical complication of gastrostomy

536.49 Other gastrostomy complications

**536.8 Dyspepsia and other specified disorders of function of
stomach**
Achylia gastrica   Hyperchlorhydria
Hourglass contraction   Hypochlorhydria
  of stomach   Indigestion
Hyperacidity   Tachygastria
EXCLUDES *achlorhydria (536.0)*
heartburn (787.1)

536.9 Unspecified functional disorder of stomach
Functional gastrointestinal:
  disorder
  disturbance
  irritation

√4ᵗʰ **537 Other disorders of stomach and duodenum**

537.0 Acquired hypertrophic pyloric stenosis
Constriction   ⎫
Obstruction   ⎬ of pylorus, acquired or adult
Stricture   ⎭
EXCLUDES *congenital or infantile pyloric stenosis (750.5)*

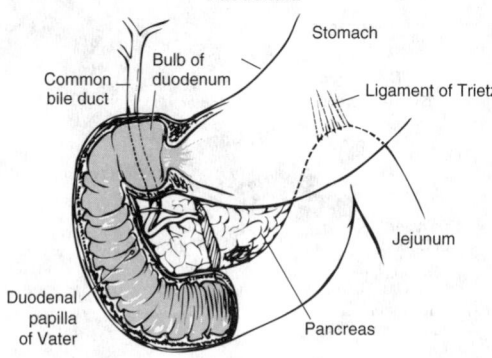
Duodenum

Stomach

Bulb of
duodenum

Common
bile duct

Ligament of Trietz

Jejunum

Duodenal
papilla
of Vater

Pancreas

537 .1 Gastric diverticulum
EXCLUDES *congenital diverticulum of stomach (750.7)*
DEF: Herniated sac or pouch within stomach or
duodenum.

537.2 Chronic duodenal ileus
DEF: Persistent obstruction between pylorus and jejunum.

537.3 Other obstruction of duodenum
Cicatrix   ⎫
Stenosis   ⎬ of duodenum
Stricture   ⎪
Volvulus   ⎭
EXCLUDES *congenital obstruction of duodenum (751.1)*

537.4 Fistula of stomach or duodenum
Gastrocolic fistula
Gastrojejunocolic fistula

537.5 Gastroptosis
DEF: Downward displacement of stomach.

537.6 Hourglass stricture or stenosis of stomach
Cascade stomach
EXCLUDES *congenital hourglass stomach (750.7)*
hourglass contraction of stomach (536.8)

√5ᵗʰ **537.8 Other specified disorders of stomach and duodenum**

537.81 Pylorospasm
EXCLUDES *congenital pylorospasm (750.5)*
DEF: Spasm of the pyloric sphincter.

**537.82 Angiodysplasia of stomach and duodenum
(without mention of hemorrhage)**

**537.83 Angiodysplasia of stomach and duodenum
with hemorrhage**
DEF: Bleeding of stomach and duodenum due to
vascular abnormalities.

**537.84 Dieulafoy lesion (hemorrhagic) of stomach
and duodenum**
DEF: An abnormally large and convoluted
submucosal artery protruding through a defect
in the mucosa in the stomach or intestines that
can erode the epithelium causing hemorrhaging.

537.89 Other
Gastric or duodenal:
  prolapse
  rupture
Intestinal metaplasia of gastric mucosa
Passive congestion of stomach
EXCLUDES *diverticula of duodenum*
(562.00-562.01)
gastrointestinal hemorrhage
(578.0-578.9)

537.9 Unspecified disorder of stomach and duodenum

538 Gastrointestinal mucositis (ulcerative)
Use additional E code to identify adverse effects of therapy, such
as:
antineoplastic and immunosuppressive drugs (E930.7, E933.1)
radiation therapy (E879.2)
EXCLUDES *mucositis (ulcerative) of mouth and oral soft tissue*
(528.00- 528.09)

√4ᵗʰ **539 Complications of bariatric procedures**

√5ᵗʰ **539.0 Complications of gastric band procedure**

539.01 Infection due to gastric band procedure
Use additional code to specify type of infection, such as:
abscess or cellulitis of abdomen (682.2)
septicemia (038.0-038.9)
Use additional code to identify organism (041.00-041.9)

539.09 Other complications of gastric band procedure
Use additional code(s) to further specify the complication

√5ᵗʰ **539.8 Complications of other bariatric procedure**
EXCLUDES *complications of gastric band procedure (539.01-539.09)*

539.81 Infection due to other bariatric procedure
Use additional code to specify type of infection, such as:
abscess or cellulitis of abdomen (682.2)
septicemia (038.0-038.9)
Use additional code to identify organism (041.00-041.9)

539.89 Other complications of other bariatric procedure
Use additional code(s) to further specify the complication

APPENDICITIS (540-543)

√4ᵗʰ **540 Acute appendicitis**
DEF: Inflammation of vermiform appendix due to fecal obstruction, neoplasm or foreign body of appendiceal lumen; causes infection, edema and infarction of appendiceal wall; may result in mural necrosis, and perforation.

540.0 With generalized peritonitis
Appendicitis (acute) with: perforation, peritonitis (generalized), rupture, fulminating, gangrenous, obstructive
Cecitis (acute) with perforation, peritonitis (generalized), rupture
Rupture of appendix
EXCLUDES *acute appendicitis with peritoneal abscess (540.1)*

540.1 With peritoneal abscess
Abscess of appendix
With generalized peritonitis

540.9 Without mention of peritonitis
Acute appendicitis without mention of perforation, peritonitis, or rupture:
fulminating
gangrenous
inflamed
obstructive
Acute cecitis without mention of perforation, peritonitis, or rupture

541 Appendicitis, unqualified

542 Other appendicitis
Appendicitis: Appendicitis:
chronic   relapsing
recurrent   subacute
EXCLUDES *hyperplasia (lymphoid) of appendix (543.0)*

√4ᵗʰ **543 Other diseases of appendix**

543.0 Hyperplasia of appendix (lymphoid)
DEF: Proliferation of cells in appendix tissue.

Appendix
- Appendicular artery
- Mesoappendix
- Cecum
- Vermiform appendix

Hernias of Abdominal Cavity
- Hiatal hernia
- Diaphragm
- Epigastric hernia
- Incisional hernia
- Umbilical hernia
- Inguinal hernia

543.9 Other and unspecified diseases of appendix
Appendicular or appendiceal:
colic
concretion
fistula
Diverticulum
Fecalith
Intussusception   of appendix
Mucocele
Stercolith

HERNIA OF ABDOMINAL CAVITY (550-553)

INCLUDES hernia:
acquired
congenital, except diaphragmatic or hiatal

√4ᵗʰ **550 Inguinal hernia**
INCLUDES bubonocele
inguinal hernia (direct) (double) (indirect) (oblique) (sliding)
scrotal hernia

The following fifth-digit subclassification is for use with category 550:
0 unilateral or unspecified (not specified as recurrent)
Unilateral NOS
1 unilateral or unspecified, recurrent
2 bilateral (not specified as recurrent)
Bilateral NOS
3 bilateral, recurrent

DEF: Hernia protrusion of an abdominal organ or tissue through inguinal canal.
DEF: Indirect inguinal hernia: (external or oblique) leaves abdomen through deep inguinal ring, passes through inguinal canal lateral to the inferior epigastric artery.
DEF: Direct inguinal hernia: (internal) emerges between inferior epigastric artery and rectus muscle edge.

√5ᵗʰ **550.0 Inguinal hernia, with gangrene**
[0-3]   Inguinal hernia with gangrene (and obstruction)

√5ᵗʰ **550.1 Inguinal hernia, with obstruction, without**
[0-3]   **mention of gangrene**
Inguinal hernia with mention of incarceration, irreducibility, or strangulation

√5ᵗʰ **550.9 Inguinal hernia, without mention of**
[0-3]   **obstruction or gangrene**
Inguinal hernia NOS

Diseases of the Digestive System

551–552.9

Inguinal Hernias

- Abdominal wall
- Spermatic cord
- Inguinal ligament
- Internal inguinal ring
- Deep inferior epigastric artery and vein
- Indirect hernia (internal inguinal ring)
- Direct inguinal hernia (between deep inferior epigastric vessels and rectus fascia)
- Incarcerated hernia

Femoral Hernia

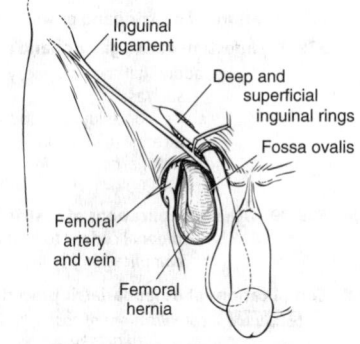

- Inguinal ligament
- Deep and superficial inguinal rings
- Fossa ovalis
- Femoral artery and vein
- Femoral hernia

Diaphragmatic Hernias

- Esophagus
- Gastroesophageal junction (remains in place)
- Stomach
- Diaphragm
- Gastroesophageal junction (slides up and down)
- Paraesophageal Hiatal Hernia
- Sliding Hiatal Hernia

☑4ᵗʰ   **551**   **Other hernia of abdominal cavity, with gangrene**
     INCLUDES   *that with gangrene (and obstruction)*

   ☑5ᵗʰ   **551.0**   **Femoral hernia with gangrene**

       551.00   **Unilateral or unspecified (not specified as recurrent)**
           Femoral hernia NOS with gangrene

       551.01   **Unilateral or unspecified, recurrent**

       551.02   **Bilateral (not specified as recurrent)**

       551.03   **Bilateral, recurrent**

   551.1   **Umbilical hernia with gangrene**
      Parumbilical hernia specified as gangrenous

   ☑5ᵗʰ   **551.2**   **Ventral hernia with gangrene**

       551.20   **Ventral, unspecified, with gangrene**

       551.21   **Incisional, with gangrene**
         Hernia:
           postoperative ⎫
           recurrent, ventral ⎬ specified as gangrenous
           ⎭

       551.29   **Other**
         Epigastric hernia specified as gangrenous

   551.3   **Diaphragmatic hernia with gangrene**
      Hernia:
       hiatal (esophageal) ⎫
       (sliding)   ⎬ specified as
       paraesophageal   ⎭ gangrenous
       Thoracic stomach
       EXCLUDES   *congenital diaphragmatic hernia (756.6)*

   551.8   **Hernia of other specified sites, with gangrene**
      Any condition classifiable to 553.8 if specified as gangrenous

   551.9   **Hernia of unspecified site, with gangrene**
      Any condition classifiable to 553.9 if specified as gangrenous

☑4ᵗʰ   **552**   **Other hernia of abdominal cavity, with obstruction, but without mention of gangrene**
     EXCLUDES   *that with mention of gangrene (551.0-551.9)*

   ☑5ᵗʰ   **552.0**   **Femoral hernia with obstruction**
      Femoral hernia specified as incarcerated, irreducible, strangulated, or causing obstruction

       552.00   **Unilateral or unspecified (not specified as recurrent)**

       552.01   **Unilateral or unspecified, recurrent**

       552.02   **Bilateral (not specified as recurrent)**

       552.03   **Bilateral, recurrent**

   552.1   **Umbilical hernia with obstruction**
      Parumbilical hernia specified as incarcerated, irreducible, strangulated, or causing obstruction

   ☑5ᵗʰ   **552.2**   **Ventral hernia with obstruction**
      Ventral hernia specified as incarcerated, irreducible, strangulated, or causing obstruction

       552.20   **Ventral, unspecified, with obstruction**

       552.21   **Incisional, with obstruction**
         Hernia:
           postoperative ⎫ specified as incarcerated,
           recurrent,   ⎬ irreducible,
           ventral   ⎭ strangulated, or
                    causing obstruction

       552.29   **Other**
         Epigastric hernia specified as incarcerated, irreducible, strangulated, or causing obstruction

   552.3   **Diaphragmatic hernia with obstruction**
      Hernia:
       hiatal (esophageal) ⎫ specified as caracerated,
       (sliding)   ⎬ irreducible,
       paraesophageal   ⎪ strangulated, or causing
       Thoracic stomach ⎭ obstruction
       EXCLUDES   *congenital diaphragmatic hernia (756.6)*

   552.8   **Hernia of other specified sites, with obstruction**
      Any condition classifiable to 553.8 if specified as incarcerated, irreducible, strangulated, or causing obstruction

   552.9   **Hernia of unspecified site, with obstruction**
      Any condition classifiable to 553.9 if specified as incarcerated, irreducible, strangulated, or causing obstruction

√4ᵗʰ **553 Other hernia of abdominal cavity without mention of obstruction or gangrene**

> **EXCLUDES** *the listed conditions with mention of:*
> *gangrene (and obstruction) (551.0-551.9)*
> *obstruction (552.0-552.9)*

√5ᵗʰ **553.0 Femoral hernia**

553.00 Unilateral or unspecified (not specified as recurrent)
Femoral hernia NOS

553.01 Unilateral or unspecified, recurrent

553.02 Bilateral (not specified as recurrent)

553.03 Bilateral, recurrent

553.1 Umbilical hernia
Parumbilical hernia

√5ᵗʰ **553.2 Ventral hernia**

553.20 Ventral, unspecified

553.21 Incisional
Hernia:
postoperative
recurrent, ventral

553.29 Other
Hernia:
epigastric
spigelian

553.3 Diaphragmatic hernia
Hernia: Thoracic stomach
hiatal (esophageal)
(sliding)
paraesophageal
> **EXCLUDES** *congenital:*
> *diaphragmatic hernia (756.6)*
> *hiatal hernia (750.6)*
> *esophagocele (530.6)*

553.8 Hernia of other specified sites
Hernia: Hernia:
ischiatic   pudendal
ischiorectal   retroperitoneal
lumbar   sciatic
obturator
Other abdominal hernia of specified site
> **EXCLUDES** *vaginal enterocele (618.6)*

553.9 Hernia of unspecified site
Enterocele   Hernia:
Epiplocele   intestinal
Hernia: intra-abdominal
NOS   Rupture (nontraumatic)
interstitial   Sarcoepiplocele

NONINFECTIOUS ENTERITIS AND COLITIS (555-558)

√4ᵗʰ **555 Regional enteritis**

> **INCLUDES** Crohn's disease
> granulomatous enteritis
> **EXCLUDES** *ulcerative colitis (556)*

DEF: Inflammation of intestine; classified to site.

555.0 Small intestine
Ileitis:
regional
segmental
terminal
Regional enteritis or Crohn's disease of:
duodenum
ileum
jejunum

555.1 Large intestine
Colitis:
granulmatous
regional
transmural
Regional enteritis or Crohn's disease of:
colon
large bowel
rectum

Large Intestine

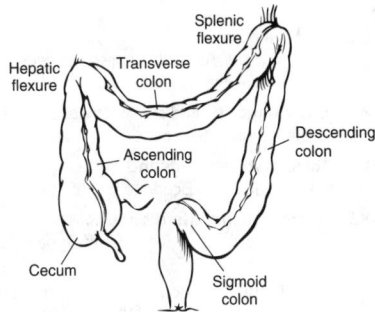

555.2 Small intestine with large intestine
Regional ileocolitis

555.9 Unspecified site
Crohn's disease NOS
Regional enteritis NOS

√4ᵗʰ **556 Ulcerative colitis**

DEF: Chronic inflammation of mucosal lining of intestinal tract; may be single area or entire colon.

556.0 Ulcerative (chronic) enterocolitis

556.1 Ulcerative (chronic) ileocolitis

556.2 Ulcerative (chronic) proctitis

556.3 Ulcerative (chronic) proctosigmoiditis

556.4 Pseudopolyposis of colon

556.5 Left-sided ulcerative (chronic) colitis

556.6 Universal ulcerative (chronic) colitis
Pancolitis

556.8 Other ulcerative colitis

556.9 Ulcerative colitis, unspecified
Ulcerative enteritis NOS

√4ᵗʰ **557 Vascular insufficiency of intestine**

> **EXCLUDES** *necrotizing enterocolitis of the newborn (777.50-777.53)*

DEF: Inadequacy of intestinal vessels.

557.0 Acute vascular insufficiency of intestine
Acute:
hemorrhagic enterocolitis
ischemic colitis, enteritis, or enterocolitis
massive necrosis of intestine
Bowel infarction
Embolism of mesenteric artery
Fulminant enterocolitis
Hemorrhagic necrosis of intestine
Infarction of appendices epiploicae
Intestinal gangrene
Intestinal infarction (acute) (agnogenic) (hemorrhagic) (nonocclusive)
Mesenteric infarction (embolic) (thrombotic)
Necrosis of intestine
Terminal hemorrhagic enteropathy
Thrombosis of mesenteric artery

557.1 Chronic vascular insufficiency of intestine
Angina, abdominal
Chronic ischemic colitis, enteritis, or enterocolitis
Ischemic stricture of intestine
Mesenteric:
angina
artery syndrome (superior)
vascular insufficiency

557.9 Unspecified vascular insufficiency of intestine
Alimentary pain due to vascular insufficiency
Ischemic colitis, enteritis, or enterocolitis NOS

✓4ᵗʰ **558   Other and unspecified noninfectious gastroenteritis and colitis**

> EXCLUDES   infectious:
>> colitis, enteritis, or gastroenteritis (009.0-009.1)
>> diarrhea (009.2-009.3)

558.1   Gastroenteritis and colitis due to radiation
Radiation enterocolitis

558.2   Toxic gastroenteritis and colitis
Use additional E code to identify cause

558.3   Allergic gastroenteritis and colitis
Use additional code to identify type of food allergy (V15.01-V15.05)

> **DEF:** True immunoglobulin E (IgE)-mediated allergic reaction of the lining of the stomach, intestines, or colon to food proteins; causes nausea, vomiting, diarrhea, and abdominal cramping.

✓5ᵗʰ **558.4   Eosinophilic gastroenteritis and colitis**

558.41   Eosinophilic gastroenteritis
Eosinophilic enteritis

558.42   Eosinophilic colitis

558.9   Other and unspecified noninfectious gastroenteritis and colitis

Colitis
Enteritis
Gastroenteritis } NOS, dietetic, or noninfectious
Ileitis
Jejunitis
Sigmoiditis

OTHER DISEASES OF INTESTINES AND PERITONEUM (560-569)

✓4ᵗʰ **560   Intestinal obstruction without mention of hernia**

> EXCLUDES   duodenum (537.2-537.3)
>> inguinal hernia with obstruction (550.1)
>> intestinal obstruction complicating hernia (552.0-552.9)
>> mesenteric:
>>> embolism (557.0)
>>> infarction (557.0)
>>> thrombosis (557.0)
>> neonatal intestinal obstruction (277.01, 777.1-777.2, 777.4)

560.0   Intussusception
Intussusception (colon) (intestine) (rectum)
Invagination of intestine or colon

> EXCLUDES   intussusception of appendix (543.9)

> **DEF:** Prolapse of a bowel section into adjacent section; occurs primarily in children; symptoms include paroxysmal pain, vomiting, presence of blood, and mucous passage from rectum.

560.1   Paralytic ileus
Adynamic ileus
Ileus (of intestine) (of bowel) (of colon)
Paralysis of intestine or colon

> EXCLUDES   gallstone ileus (560.31)

> **DEF:** Obstruction of ileus due to inhibited bowel motility.

560.2   Volvulus
Knotting
Strangulation } of intestine, bowel, or colon
Torsion
Twist

> **DEF:** Entanglement of bowel; causes obstruction; may compromise bowel circulation.

✓5ᵗʰ **560.3   Impaction of intestine**

560.30   Impaction of intestine, unspecified
Impaction of colon

560.31   Gallstone ileus
Obstruction of intestine by gallstone

560.32   Fecal impaction

> EXCLUDES   constipation (564.00-564.09)
>> incomplete defecation (787.61)

Volvulus and Diverticulitis

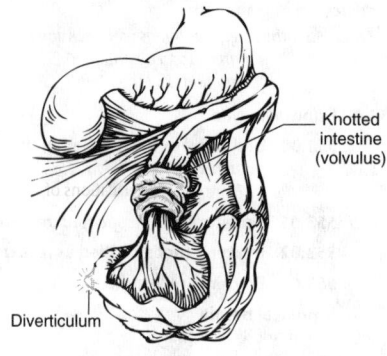

Knotted intestine (volvulus)

Diverticulum

560.39   Other
Concretion of intestine
Enterolith

✓5ᵗʰ **560.8   Other specified intestinal obstruction**

560.81   Intestinal or peritoneal adhesions with obstruction (postoperative) (postinfection)

> EXCLUDES   adhesions without obstruction (568.0)

> **DEF:** Obstruction of peritoneum or intestine due to abnormal union of tissues.

560.89   Other
Acute pseudo-obstruction of intestine
Mural thickening causing obstruction

> EXCLUDES   ischemic stricture of intestine (557.1)

560.9   Unspecified intestinal obstruction
Enterostenosis
Obstruction
Occlusion } of intestine or colon
Stenosis
Stricture

> EXCLUDES   congenital stricture or stenosis of intestine (751.1-751.2)

✓4ᵗʰ **562   Diverticula of intestine**
Use additional code to identify any associated:
peritonitis (567.0-567.9)

> EXCLUDES   congenital diverticulum of colon (751.5)
>> diverticulum of appendix (543.9)
>> Meckel's diverticulum (751.0)

✓5ᵗʰ **562.0   Small intestine**

562.00   Diverticulosis of small intestine (without mention of hemorrhage)
Diverticulosis:
duodenum
ileum } without mention of diverticulitis
jejunum

> **DEF:** Saclike herniations of mucous lining of small intestine.

562.01   Diverticulitis of small intestine (without mention of hemorrhage)
Diverticulitis (with diverticulosis):
duodenum
ileum
jejunum
small intestine

> **DEF:** Inflamed saclike herniations of mucous lining of small intestine

562.02   Diverticulosis of small intestine with hemorrhage

562.03   Diverticulitis of small intestine with hemorrhage

✓5ᵗʰ **562.1 Colon**

562.10 Diverticulosis of colon (without mention of hemorrhage)
Diverticulosis:
NOS   } without mention of
intestine (large)   diverticulitis
Diverticular disease (colon) without mention of diverticulitis
DEF: Saclike herniations of mucous lining of large intestine.

562.11 Diverticulitis of colon (without mention of hemorrhage)
Diverticulitis (with diverticulosis):
NOS
colon
intestine (large)
DEF: Inflamed saclike herniations of mucosal lining of large intestine.

562.12 Diverticulosis of colon with hemorrhage

562.13 Diverticulitis of colon with hemorrhage

✓4ᵗʰ **564 Functional digestive disorders, not elsewhere classified**
EXCLUDES *functional disorders of stomach (536.0-536.9)*
those specified as psychogenic (306.4)

✓5ᵗʰ **564.0 Constipation**
EXCLUDES *fecal impaction (560.32)*
incomplete defecation (787.61)

564.00 Constipation, unspecified

564.01 Slow transit constipation
DEF: Delay in the transit of fecal material through the colon secondary to smooth muscle dysfunction or decreased peristaltic contractions along the colon: also called colonic inertia or delayed transit.

564.02 Outlet dysfunction constipation
DEF: Failure to relax the paradoxical contractions of the striated pelvic floor muscles during the attempted defecation.

564.09 Other constipation

564.1 Irritable bowel syndrome
Irritable colon
Spastic colon
DEF: Functional gastrointestinal disorder (FGID); symptoms include diarrhea, constipation, abdominal pain, gas, distended abdomen, nausea, vomiting, emotional distress, and depression.

564.2 Postgastric surgery syndromes
Dumping syndrome
Jejunal syndrome
Postgastrectomy syndrome
Postvagotomy syndrome
EXCLUDES *malnutrition following gastrointestinal surgery (579.3)*
postgastrojejunostomy ulcer (534.0-534.9)

564.3 Vomiting following gastrointestinal surgery
Vomiting (bilious) following gastrointestinal surgery

564.4 Other postoperative functional disorders
Diarrhea following gastrointestinal surgery
EXCLUDES *colostomy and enterostomy complications (569.60-569.69)*

564.5 Functional diarrhea
EXCLUDES *diarrhea:*
NOS (787.91)
psychogenic (306.4)
DEF: Diarrhea with no detectable organic cause.

564.6 Anal spasm
Proctalgia fugax

Anal Fistula and Abscess

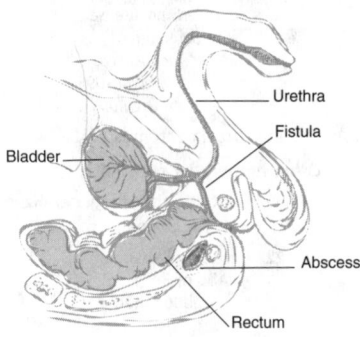

Urethra
Fistula
Bladder
Abscess
Rectum

564.7 Megacolon, other than Hirschsprung's
Dilatation of colon
EXCLUDES *megacolon:*
congenital [Hirschsprung's] (751.3)
toxic (556)
DEF: Enlarged colon; congenital or acquired; can occur acutely or become chronic.

✓5ᵗʰ **564.8 Other specified functional disorders of intestine**
EXCLUDES *malabsorption (579.0-579.9)*

564.81 Neurogenic bowel
DEF: Disorder of bowel due to spinal cord lesion above conus medullaris; symptoms include precipitous micturition, nocturia, headache, sweating, nasal obstruction and spastic contractions.

564.89 Other functional disorders of intestine
Atony of colon
DEF: Absence of normal bowel tone or strength.

564.9 Unspecified functional disorder of intestine

✓4ᵗʰ **565 Anal fissure and fistula**

565.0 Anal fissure
EXCLUDES *anal sphincter tear (healed) (non-traumatic) (old) (569.43)*
traumatic (863.89, 863.99)
DEF: Ulceration of cleft at anal mucosa; causes pain, itching, bleeding, infection, and sphincter spasm; may occur with hemorrhoids.

565.1 Anal fistula
Fistula:
anorectal
rectal
rectum to skin
EXCLUDES *fistula of rectum to internal organs–see Alphabetic Index*
ischiorectal fistula (566)
rectovaginal fistula (619.1)
DEF: Abnormal opening on cutaneous surface near anus; may lack connection with rectum.

566 Abscess of anal and rectal regions
Abscess: Cellulitis:
ischiorectal   anal
perianal   perirectal
perirectal   rectal
                                   Ischiorectal fistula

✓4ᵗʰ **567 Peritonitis and retroperitoneal infections**
EXCLUDES *peritonitis:*
benign paroxysmal (277.31)
pelvic, female (614.5, 614.7)
periodic familial (277.31)
puerperal (670.8)
with or following:
abortion (634-638 with .0, 639.0)
appendicitis (540.0-540.1)
ectopic or molar pregnancy (639.0)
DEF: Inflammation of the peritoneal cavity.

Diseases of the Digestive System

567.0   *Peritonitis in infectious diseases classified elsewhere*
  Code first underlying disease
  EXCLUDES peritonitis:
    gonococcal (098.86)
    syphilitic (095.2)
    tuberculous (014.0)

567.1 Pneumococcal peritonitis

√5ᵗʰ **567.2 Other suppurative peritonitis**

567.21 Peritonitis (acute) generalized
  Pelvic peritonitis, male

567.22 Peritoneal abscess
  Abscess (of):
    abdominopelvic
    mesenteric
    omentum
    peritoneum
    retrocecal
    subdiaphragmatic
    subhepatic
    subphrenic

567.23 Spontaneous bacterial peritonitis
  EXCLUDES bacterial peritonitis NOS (567.29)

567.29 Other suppurative peritonitis
  Subphrenic peritonitis

√5ᵗʰ **567.3 Retroperitoneal infections**

567.31 Psoas muscle abscess
  DEF: Infection that extends into or around the psoas muscle that connects the lumbar vertebrae to the femur.

567.38 Other retroperitoneal abscess

567.39 Other retroperitoneal infections

√5ᵗʰ **567.8 Other specified peritonitis**

567.81 Choleperitonitis
  Peritonitis due to bile
  DEF: Inflammation or infection due to presence of bile in the peritoneum resulting from rupture of the bile passages or gallbladder.

567.82 Sclerosing mesenteritis
  Fat necrosis of peritoneum
  (Idiopathic) sclerosing mesenteric fibrosis
  Mesenteric lipodystrophy
  Mesenteric panniculitis
  Retractile mesenteritis
  DEF: Inflammatory processes involving the mesenteric fat; progresses to fibrosis and necrosis of tissue.

567.89 Other specified peritonitis
  Chronic proliferative peritonitis
  Mesenteric saponification
  Peritonitis due to urine

567.9 Unspecified peritonitis
  Peritonitis NOS
  Peritonitis of unspecified cause

√4ᵗʰ **568 Other disorders of peritoneum**

568.0 Peritoneal adhesions (postoperative) (postinfection)
  Adhesions (of):   Adhesions (of):
    abdominal (wall)   mesenteric
    diaphragm   omentum
    intestine   stomach
    male pelvis   Adhesive bands
  EXCLUDES adhesions:
    pelvic, female (614.6)
    with obstruction:
      duodenum (537.3)
      intestine (560.81)
  DEF: Abnormal union of tissues in peritoneum.

√5ᵗʰ **568.8 Other specified disorders of peritoneum**

568.81 Hemoperitoneum (nontraumatic)

568.82 Peritoneal effusion (chronic)
  EXCLUDES ascites NOS (789.51-789.59)
  DEF: Persistent leakage of fluid within peritoneal cavity.

568.89 Other
  Peritoneal: Peritoneal:
    cyst   granuloma

568.9 Unspecified disorder of peritoneum

√4ᵗʰ **569 Other disorders of intestine**

569.0 Anal and rectal polyp
  Anal and rectal polyp NOS
  EXCLUDES adenomatous anal and rectal polyp (211.4)

569.1 Rectal prolapse
  Procidentia: Prolapse:
    anus (sphincter)   anal canal
    rectum (sphincter)   rectal mucosa
  Proctoptosis
  EXCLUDES prolapsed hemorrhoids (455.2, 455.5)

569.2 Stenosis of rectum and anus
  Stricture of anus (sphincter)

569.3 Hemorrhage of rectum and anus
  EXCLUDES gastrointestinal bleeding NOS (578.9)
    melena (578.1)

√5ᵗʰ **569.4 Other specified disorders of rectum and anus**

569.41 Ulcer of anus and rectum
  Solitary ulcer   ⎫ of anus (sphincter) or
  Stercoral ulcer ⎬   rectum (sphincter)

569.42 Anal or rectal pain

569.43 Anal sphincter tear (healed) (old)
  Tear of anus, nontraumatic
  Use additional code for any associated fecal incontinence (787.60-787.63)
  EXCLUDES anal fissure (565.0)
    anal sphincter tear (healed) (old)
      complicating delivery (654.8)

Psoas Muscle Abscess

Rectum and Anus

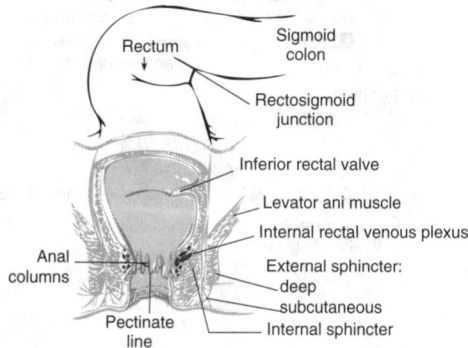

569.44 Dysplasia of anus
Anal intraepithelial neoplasia I and II
(AIN I and II) (histologically confirmed)
Dysplasia of anus NOS
Mild and moderate dysplasia of anus
(histologically confirmed)

> **EXCLUDES** *abnormal results from anal cytologic examination without histologic confirmation (796.70-796.79)*
> *anal intraepithelial neoplasia III (230.5, 230.6)*
> *carcinoma in situ of anus (230.5, 230.6)*
> *HGSIL of anus (796.74)*
> *severe dysplasia of anus (230.5, 230.6)*

569.49 Other
Granuloma } of rectum (sphincter)
Rupture

Hypertrophy of anal papillae
Proctitis NOS
Use additional code for any associated fecal
incontinence (787.60-787.63)

> **EXCLUDES** *fistula of rectum to:*
> *internal organs — see Alphabetic Index*
> *skin (565.1)*
> *hemorrhoids (455.0-455.9)*

569.5 Abscess of intestine
> **EXCLUDES** *appendiceal abscess (540.1)*

√5ᵗʰ **569.6 Colostomy and enterostomy complications**
> **DEF:** Complication in a surgically created opening, from intestine to surface skin.

569.60 Colostomy and enterostomy complication, unspecified

569.61 Infection of colostomy or enterostomy
Use additional code to identify organism
(041.00-041.9)
Use additional code to specify type of infection,
such as:
abscess or cellulitis of abdomen (682.2)
septicemia (038.0-038.9)

569.62 Mechanical complication of colostomy and enterostomy
Malfunction of colostomy and enterostomy

569.69 Other complication
Fistula   Prolapse
Hernia

√5ᵗʰ **569.7 Complications of intestinal pouch**

569.71 Pouchitis
Inflammation of internal ileoanal pouch
> **DEF:** Inflammatory complication of an existing surgically created ileoanal pouch, resulting in multiple GI complaints, including diarrhea, abdominal pain, rectal bleeding, fecal urgency, or incontinence.

569.79 Other complications of intestinal pouch

√5ᵗʰ **569.8 Other specified disorders of intestine**

569.81 Fistula of intestine, excluding rectum and anus
Fistula: Fistula:
abdominal wall   enteroenteric
enterocolic   ileorectal

> **EXCLUDES** *fistula of intestine to internal organs–see Alphabetic Index*
> *persistent postoperative fistula (998.6)*

569.82 Ulceration of intestine
Primary ulcer of intestine
Ulceration of colon
> **EXCLUDES** *that with perforation (569.83)*

569.83 Perforation of intestine

569.84 Angiodysplasia of intestine (without mention of hemorrhage)
> **DEF:** Small vascular abnormalities of the intestinal tract without bleeding problems.

569.85 Angiodysplasia of intestine with hemorrhage
> **DEF:** Small vascular abnormalities of the intestinal tract with bleeding problems.

569.86 Dieulafoy lesion (hemorrhagic) of intestine

569.87 Vomiting of fecal matter
> **DEF:** Spasmodic expulsion of partially digested substance with similar odor to fecal matter; often suggestive of bowel obstruction or other underlying causal pathology.

569.89 Other
Enteroptosis
Granuloma }
Prolapse   } of intestine

Pericolitis
Perisigmoiditis
Visceroptosis

> **EXCLUDES** *gangrene of intestine, mesentery, or omentum (557.0)*
> *hemorrhage of intestine NOS (578.9)*
> *obstruction of intestine (560.0-560.9)*

569.9 Unspecified disorder of intestine

OTHER DISEASES OF DIGESTIVE SYSTEM (570-579)

570 Acute and subacute necrosis of liver
Acute hepatic failure
Acute or subacute hepatitis, not specified as infective
Necrosis of liver (acute) (diffuse) (massive) (subacute)
Parenchymatous degeneration of liver
Yellow atrophy (liver) (acute) (subacute)
> **EXCLUDES** *icterus gravis of newborn (773.0-773.2)*
> *serum hepatitis (070.2-070.3)*
> *that with:*
> *abortion (634-638 with .7, 639.8)*
> *ectopic or molar pregnancy (639.8)*
> *pregnancy, childbirth, or the puerperium (646.7)*
> *viral hepatitis (070.0-070.9)*

√4ᵗʰ **571 Chronic liver disease and cirrhosis**

571.0 Alcoholic fatty liver

571.1 Acute alcoholic hepatitis
Acute alcoholic liver disease

571.2 Alcoholic cirrhosis of liver
Florid cirrhosis
Laennec's cirrhosis (alcoholic)
> **DEF:** Fibrosis and dysfunction of liver; due to alcoholic liver disease.

571.3 Alcoholic liver damage, unspecified

√5ᵗʰ **571.4 Chronic hepatitis**
> **EXCLUDES** *viral hepatitis (acute) (chronic) (070.0-070.9)*

571.40 Chronic hepatitis, unspecified

571.41 Chronic persistent hepatitis

571.42 Autoimmune hepatitis

571.49 Other
Chronic hepatitis:
active
aggressive
Recurrent hepatitis

Liver

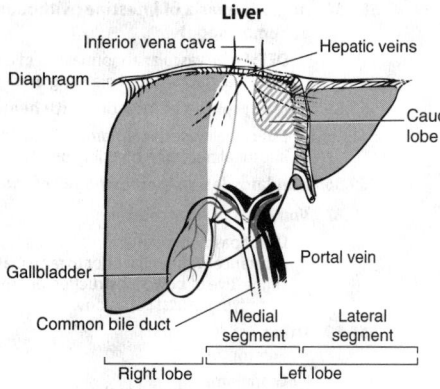

571.5 Cirrhosis of liver without mention of alcohol

Cirrhosis of liver:
NOS
cryptogenic
macronodular
micronodular
posthepatitic
postnecrotic

Healed yellow atrophy
(liver)
Portal cirrhosis

Code first, if applicable, viral hepatitis (acute) (chronic) (070.0–070.9)

DEF: Fibrosis and dysfunction of liver; not alcohol related.

571.6 Biliary cirrhosis

Chronic nonsuppurative destructive cholangitis
Cirrhosis:
cholangitic
cholestatic

571.8 Other chronic nonalcoholic liver disease

Chronic yellow atrophy (liver)
Fatty liver, without mention of alcohol

571.9 Unspecified chronic liver disease without mention of alcohol

√4ᵗʰ 572 Liver abscess and sequelae of chronic liver disease

572.0 Abscess of liver
EXCLUDES   *amebic liver abscess (006.3)*

572.1 Portal pyemia
Phlebitis of portal vein   Pylephlebitis
Portal thrombophlebitis   Pylethrombophlebitis

DEF: Inflammation of portal vein or branches; may be due to intestinal disease; symptoms include fever, chills, jaundice, sweating, and abscess in various body parts.

572.2 Hepatic encephalopathy
Hepatic coma
Hepatocerebral intoxication
Portal-systemic encephalopathy
EXCLUDES   *hepatic coma associated with viral hepatitis—see category 070*

Hepatic Portal Veins

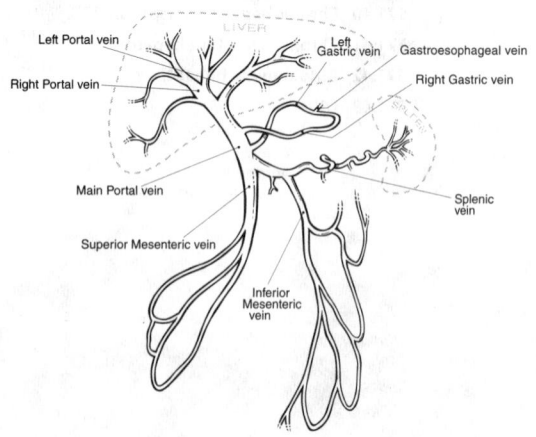

572.3 Portal hypertension

Use additional code for any associated complications, such as:
portal hypertensive gastropathy (537.89)

DEF: Abnormally high blood pressure in the portal vein.

572.4 Hepatorenal syndrome
EXCLUDES   *that following delivery (674.8)*

DEF: Hepatic and renal failure characterized by cirrhosis with ascites or obstructive jaundice, oliguria, and low sodium concentration.

572.8 Other sequelae of chronic liver disease
EXCLUDES   *hepatopulmonary syndrome (573.5)*

√4ᵗʰ 573 Other disorders of liver
EXCLUDES   *amyloid or lardaceous degeneration of liver (277.39)*
congenital cystic disease of liver (751.62)
glycogen infiltration of liver (271.0)
hepatomegaly NOS (789.1)
portal vein obstruction (452)

573.0 Chronic passive congestion of liver
DEF: Blood accumulation in liver tissue.

573.1 *Hepatitis in viral diseases classified elsewhere*
Code first underlying disease as:
Coxsackie virus disease (074.8)
cytomegalic inclusion virus disease (078.5)
infectious mononucleosis (075)
EXCLUDES   *hepatitis (in):*
mumps (072.71)
viral (070.0–070.9)
yellow fever (060.0–060.9)

573.2 *Hepatitis in other infectious diseases classified elsewhere*
Code first underlying disease, as:
malaria (084.9)
EXCLUDES   *hepatitis in:*
late syphilis (095.3)
secondary syphilis (091.62)
toxoplasmosis (130.5)

573.3 Hepatitis, unspecified
Toxic (noninfectious) hepatitis
Use additional E code to identify cause

573.4 Hepatic infarction

573.5 Hepatopulmonary syndrome
Code first underlying liver disease, such as:
alcoholic cirrhosis of liver (571.2)
cirrhosis of liver without mention of alcohol (571.5)

573.8 Other specified disorders of liver
Hepatoptosis

573.9 Unspecified disorder of liver

√4ᵗʰ 574 Cholelithiasis

The following fifth-digit subclassification is for use with category 574:
  0 without mention of obstruction
  1 with obstruction

EXCLUDES   *retained cholelithiasis following cholecystectomy (997.41)*

√5ᵗʰ 574.0 Calculus of gallbladder with acute cholecystitis
[0-1]
Billary calculus
Calculus of cystic duct   } with acute cholecystitis
Cholelithiasis

Any condition classifiable to 574.2 with acute cholecystitis

√5ᵗʰ 574.1 Calculus of gallbladder with other cholecystitis
[0-1]
Billary calculus
Calculus of cystic duct   } with cholecystitis
Choleithiasis

Cholecystitis with cholelithiasis NOS

Any condition classifiable to 574.2 with cholecystitis (chronic)

Gallbladder and Bile Ducts

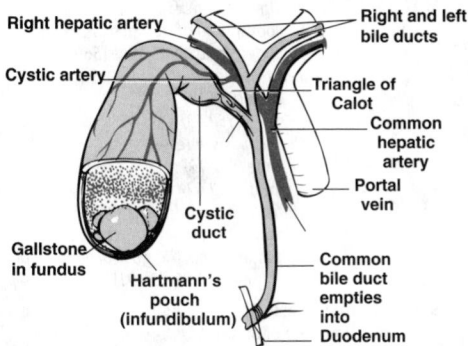

√5ᵗʰ **574.2** **Calculus of gallbladder without mention of**
[0-1] **cholecystitis**
Biliary:
calculus NOS
colic NOS
Calculus of cystic duct
Cholelithiasis NOS
Colic (recurrent) of gallbladder
Gallstone (impacted)

√5ᵗʰ **574.3** **Calculus of bile duct with acute cholecystitis**
[0-1] Calculus of bile duct (any) ⎫ with acute cholecystitis
Choledocholithiasis ⎭

Any condition classifiable to 574.5 with acute
cholecystitis

√5ᵗʰ **574.4** **Calculus of bile duct with other cholecystitis**
[0-1] Calculus of bile duct (any) ⎫ with cholecystitis (chronic)
Choledocholithiasis ⎭

Any condition classifiable to 574.5 with cholecystitis
(chronic)

√5ᵗʰ **574.5** **Calculus of bile duct without mention of**
[0-1] **cholecystitis**
Calculus of:
bile duct [any]   common duct   hepatic duct
Choledocholithiasis
Hepatic:
colic (recurrent)   lithiasis

√5ᵗʰ **574.6** **Calculus of gallbladder and bile duct with**
[0-1] **acute cholecystitis**
Any condition classifiable to 574.0 and 574.3

√5ᵗʰ **574.7** **Calculus of gallbladder and bile duct with**
[0-1] **other cholecystitis**
Any condition classifiable to 574.1 and 574.4

√5ᵗʰ **574.8** **Calculus of gallbladder and bile duct**
[0-1] **with acute and chronic cholecystitis**
Any condition classifiable to 574.6 and 574.7

√5ᵗʰ **574.9** **Calculus of gallbladder and bile duct**
[0-1] **without cholecystitis**
Any condition classifiable to 574.2 and 574.5

√4ᵗʰ **575** **Other disorders of gallbladder**

575.0 **Acute cholecystitis**
Abscess of gallbladder
Angiocholecystitis
Cholecystitis:
emphysematous (acute) ⎫ without mention of
gangrenous   ⎬ calculus
suppurative   ⎭
Empyema of gallbladder
Gangrene of gallbladder

EXCLUDES *that with:*
acute and chronic cholecystitis (575.12)
choledocholithiasis (574.3)
choledocholithiasis and cholelithiasis
(574.6)
cholelithiasis (574.0)

√5ᵗʰ **575.1** **Other cholecystitis**
Cholecystitis:
NOS   ⎫ without mention of calculus
chronic ⎭

EXCLUDES *that with:*
choledocholithiasis (574.4)
choledocholithiasis and cholelithiasis
(574.8)
cholelithiasis (574.1)

575.10 **Cholecystitis, unspecified**
Cholecystitis NOS

575.11 **Chronic cholecystitis**

575.12 **Acute and chronic cholecystitis**

575.2 **Obstruction of gallbladder**
Occlusion ⎫ of cystic duct or gallbladder without
Stenosis   ⎬ mention of calculus
Stricture ⎭

EXCLUDES *that with calculus (574.0-574.2 with*
fifth-digit 1)

575.3 **Hydrops of gallbladder**
Mucocele of gallbladder

DEF: Serous fluid accumulation in bladder.

575.4 **Perforation of gallbladder**
Rupture of cystic duct or gallbladder

575.5 **Fistula of gallbladder**
Fistula:
cholecystoduodenal
cholecystoenteric

575.6 **Cholesterolosis of gallbladder**
Strawberry gallbladder

DEF: Cholesterol deposits in gallbladder tissue.

575.8 **Other specified disorders of gallbladder**
Adhesions ⎫
Atrophy   ⎪
Cyst   ⎬ of cystic duct or gallbladder
Hypertrophy⎪
Nonfunctioning
Ulcer   ⎭

Biliary dyskinesia

EXCLUDES *Hartmann's pouch of intestine (V44.3)*
nonvisualization of gallbladder (793.3)

575.9 **Unspecified disorder of gallbladder**

√4ᵗʰ **576** **Other disorders of biliary tract**

EXCLUDES *that involving the:*
cystic duct (575.0-575.9)
gallbladder (575.0-575.9)

576.0 **Postcholecystectomy syndrome**

DEF: Jaundice or abdominal pain following
cholecystectomy.

576.1 **Cholangitis**
Cholangitis:
NOS
acute
ascending
chronic
primary
recurrent
sclerosing
secondary
stenosing
suppurative

576.2 **Obstruction of bile duct**
Occlusion ⎫ of bile duct, except cystic duct, without
Stenosis   ⎬ mention of calculus
Stricture ⎭

EXCLUDES *congenital (751.61)*
that with calculus (574.3-574.5 with
fifth-digit 1)

576.3 **Perforation of bile duct**
Rupture of bile duct, except cystic duct

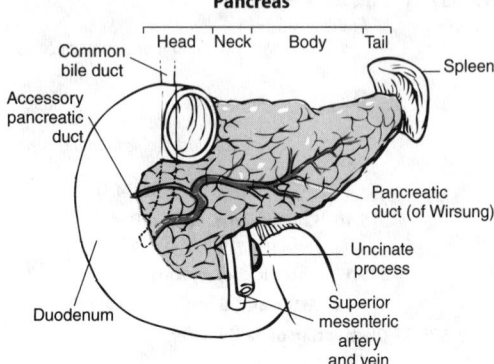

Pancreas

Head   Neck   Body   Tail

Common bile duct

Accessory pancreatic duct

Spleen

Pancreatic duct (of Wirsung)

Uncinate process

Superior mesenteric artery and vein

Duodenum

576.4 Fistula of bile duct
Choledochoduodenal fistula

576.5 Spasm of sphincter of Oddi

576.8 Other specified disorders of biliary tract
Adhesions
Atrophy
Cyst
Hypertrophy   } of bile duct (any)
Nonfunctioning
Ulcer

EXCLUDES *congenital choledochal cyst (751.69)*

576.9 Unspecified disorder of biliary tract

✓4th **577 Diseases of pancreas**

577.0 Acute pancreatitis
Abscess of pancreas
Necrosis of pancreas:
   acute
   infective
Pancreatitis:
   NOS
   acute (recurrent)
   apoplectic
   hemorrhagic
   subacute
   suppurative
EXCLUDES *mumps pancreatitis (072.3)*

577.1 Chronic pancreatitis

Chronic pancreatitis: Pancreatitis:
   NOS   painless
   infectious   recurrent
   interstitial   relapsing

577.2 Cyst and pseudocyst of pancreas

577.8 Other specified diseases of pancreas
Atrophy
Calculus
Cirrhosis   } of pancreas
Fibrosis

Pancreatic:
   infantilism
   necrosis:
      NOS
      aseptic
      fat
Pancreatolithiasis
EXCLUDES *fibrocystic disease of pancreas (277.00-277.09)*
islet cell tumor of pancreas (211.7)
pancreatic steatorrhea (579.4)

577.9 Unspecified disease of pancreas

✓4th **578 Gastrointestinal hemorrhage**
EXCLUDES *that with mention of:*
angiodysplasia of stomach and duodenum (537.83)
angiodysplasia of intestine (569.85)
diverticulitis, intestine:
large (562.13)
small (562.03)
diverticulosis, intestine:
large (562.12)
small (562.02)
gastritis and duodenitis (535.0-535.6)
ulcer:
duodenal, gastric, gastrojejunal or peptic (531.00-534.91)

578.0 Hematemesis
Vomiting of blood

578.1 Blood in stool
Melena
EXCLUDES *melena of the newborn (772.4, 777.3)*
occult blood (792.1)

578.9 Hemorrhage of gastrointestinal tract, unspecified
Gastric hemorrhage
Intestinal hemorrhage

✓4th **579 Intestinal malabsorption**

579.0 Celiac disease
Celiac:
   crisis
   infantilism
   rickets
Gee (-Herter) disease
Gluten enteropathy
Idiopathic steatorrhea
Nontropical sprue

DEF: Malabsorption syndrome due to gluten consumption; symptoms include fetid, bulky, frothy, oily stools, distended abdomen, gas, asthenia, electrolyte depletion and vitamin B, D and K deficiency.

579.1 Tropical sprue
Sprue:
   NOS
   tropical
Tropical steatorrhea

DEF: Diarrhea, occurs in tropics; may be due to enteric infection and malnutrition.

579.2 Blind loop syndrome
Postoperative blind loop syndrome

DEF: Obstruction or impaired passage in small intestine due to alterations, from strictures or surgery; causes stasis, abnormal bacterial flora, diarrhea, weight loss, multiple vitamin deficiency, and megaloblastic anemia.

579.3 Other and unspecified postsurgical nonabsorption
Hypoglycemia
Malnutrition   } following gastrointestinal surgery

579.4 Pancreatic steatorrhea
DEF: Excess fat in feces due to absence of pancreatic secretions in intestine.

579.8 Other specified intestinal malabsorption
Enteropathy:
   exudative
   protein-losing
Steatorrhea (chronic)

579.9 Unspecified intestinal malabsorption
Malabsorption syndrome NOS

Coding Guidance

Diseases of the genitourinary system are classified to chapter 10 of ICD-9-CM and include the following subchapters:

- Nephritis, nephrotic syndrome and nephrosis (580–589)
- Other diseases of urinary system (590–599)
- Diseases of male genital organs (600–608)
- Disorders of breast (610–612)
- Inflammatory disease of female pelvic organs (614–616)
- Other disorders of female genital tract (617–629)

Conditions relating to the female genitourinary system complicating pregnancy, childbirth, and the puerperium are classified to chapter 11, "Complications of Pregnancy, Childbirth and the Puerperium." Some infectious diseases affecting the genitourinary system are also classified to chapter 1, "Infectious and Parasitic Diseases." The nephritis, nephrotic syndrome and nephrosis (580–589) section classifies those conditions affecting the kidney, excluding those conditions associated with hypertensive renal disease (403.00–403.91).

Acute Glomerulonephritis (580)

Acute glomerulonephritis is a prolonged inflammation in the glomeruli of the kidney and may also be known as acute hemorrhagic glomerulonephritis or acute nephritis. Acute glomerulonephritis with lesion or rapidly progressive glomerulonephritis (580.4) is characterized by rapid deterioration of kidney function.

Acute exacerbation of chronic glomerulonephritis is classified to chronic glomerulonephritis (582). Do not assign a code from 580 Acute glomerulonephritis, with 582 unless documentation specifically identifies acute and chronic conditions.

Nephrotic Syndrome (581)

Usually due to some form of glomerulonephritis, nephrotic syndrome may result in chronic renal failure. The nephrotic syndrome is the end point of the glomerulonephritis and should not be coded in addition to the syndrome.

Example:

> Nephrotic syndrome with lesions of proliferative glomerulonephritis is coded as 581.0.
>
> Do not assign an additional code for the proliferative glomerulnephritis (580.0, acute or 582.0, chronic).

Nephrotic syndrome may or may not be present with chronic renal failure, code only when nephrotic syndrome is stated by the physician.

Chronic Glomerulonephritis (582)

Chronic glomerulonephritis is a slowly progressing disease characterized by inflammation of the glomeruli, which results in sclerosis, scarring, and eventual chronic renal failure. Etiologies for chronic glomerulonephritis include primary renal disorders (classified to categories 580 and 581) and systemic diseases, such as lupus erythematosus, amyloidosis, and hemolytic-uremic syndrome.

If the cause of the acute exacerbation of the chronic glomerulonephritis is known, such as infection (e.g., streptococcal septicemia, 038.0), report the infection with the code from category 582.

Acute Renal Failure (584)

Acute renal failure is the sudden interruption of renal function following any one of a variety or conditions affecting the normal kidney. Although usually reversible with treatment, acute renal failure may progress to chronic renal insufficiency, chronic renal failure or death.

The causes of acute renal failure are classified as prerenal, intrinsic (renal), or postrenal. Prerenal failure is due to diminished blood flow to the kidneys and may be caused by conditions such as dehydration, shock, or other emergent conditions. Intrinsic failure results from diseases and disorders of the kidneys themselves, such as acute tubular necrosis. Postrenal failure is caused by bilateral obstruction of urinary outflow, as caused by stones, clots, neoplasms, strictures, or benign prostatic hypertrophy. This category excludes renal failure due to trauma, which is classified to 958.5.

Chronic Kidney Disease (585)

Chronic kidney disease (CKD) can be defined as structural or functional abnormalities of the kidneys over a period of three months or greater and is indicated by pathologic or laboratory abnormalities. The condition is divided into five stages of increasing severity based on the GFR. At the final stage, there is total or near-total loss of kidney function, necessitating dialysis or transplantation.

The GFR is a standard measure of how well the kidneys filter waste products from the blood, and is an overall expression of kidney function. The GFR falls from its normal values of approximately 100–140 mL/min in men, and 85–115 mL/min in women as CKD progresses. These values are estimated using calculations that include factoring in the serum creatinine, blood urea nitrogen, serum albumin, and a patient's age, race, and sex. ESRD is a term defined by the federal government that indicates a patient is undergoing chronic treatment by dialysis or transplantation for stage 5 chronic kidney disease. The GFR may be an indicator of the stage of CKD, but confirmation and documentation from the physician must be obtained before assigning a code for a specific stage of disease.

If documentation identifies CKD with hypertension, assign codes from category 403 Hypertensive chronic kidney disease, when conditions classified to category 585 are present. Unlike hypertension with heart disease, ICD-9-CM presumes a cause-and-effect relationship and classifies chronic kidney disease (CKD) with hypertension as hypertensive chronic kidney disease. If CKD and hypertension are documented as unrelated, the CKD (585) and hypertension (401, 402) are reported separately.

When documentation identifies CKD with hypertensive heart disease, code first the hypertensive CKD with heart disease (404.0x–404.9x); then assign the appropriate fifth digit to identify the presence of heart failure (if present) and stage of CKD. Assign in addition the appropriate 585 code along with a code to identify the type of heart failure (428.0–428.9), if applicable.

When a causal relationship between diabetes and the CKD has been established, the diabetes code 249.4x or 250.4x is sequenced first, followed by the appropriate renal failure code.

Urinary Tract Infection (599.0)

Urinary tract infection, site not specified, covers a wide variety of clinical conditions characterized by a significant number of micro-organisms in an unspecified part of the urinary tract. Predisposing factors include calculi or other urinary tract obstructions or foreign bodies, pregnancy, and diabetes mellitus among many others. Many urinary tract infections recur due to bacterial persistence or reinfection from new organisms outside the urinary tract.

When the bacterial organism is identified, an additional code should be used (E.coli, 041.4).

Urinalysis and urine culture are the most important indicators for urinary tract infection.

Hematuria (599.7)

Hematuria is a common presenting symptom of multiple genitourinary diseases, including bladder cancer. Hematuria may be visible to the naked eye (gross) or visible only under a microscope (microscopic). It is usually painless, but patients presenting with hematuria are at high risk for bladder cancer and may have other distinct risk factors for bladder cancer. A number of these risk factors include smoking, voiding dysfunction, exposure to toxic metals and chemicals, and personal history of urinary disorder or disease. Several conditions can cause hematuria, many of which are not serious. Hematuria may also occur in the absence of any other related health problems. Treatment for hematuria depends on establishing the underlying cause by further diagnostic examination. Code 599.7 Hematuria has fifth-digit subclassifications to provide unique codes for gross (599.71), microscopic (599.72), and unspecified (599.70) hematuria. Review of personal history may indicate factors associated with an increased risk of bladder cancer. A V code should be assigned to indicate factors influencing health.

Diseases of Male Genital Organs (600–608)

Conditions classified to this section include prostate disease, disorders of the penis, disorders of the testes, and other structural and functional disorders of the male genital system.

Hyperplasia of Prostate (600)

Hyperplasia of prostate describes several conditions believed to arise as fibrostromal proliferation in the periurethral glands. The etiology is unknown, but a relationship between aging and prostate enlargement is well documented.

Other terms used to describe hyperplasia of the prostate include: hypertrophy (benign) of the prostate (BPH) (600.0); nodular prostate (600.1); adenoma (benign) of the prostate (600.2); cyst of prostate (600.3); and prostatic obstruction (600.9).

Fifth-digit subclassifications indicate the presence of LUTS (lower urinary tract symptoms) or obstruction with certain conditions classified to category 600 Hyperplasia of prostate. An instructional note directs the coder to assign a code for each symptom in addition to the code for the underlying condition (BPH).

Disorders of Breast (610-612)

Other Specified Disorders of Breast (611.8)

Historically, ICD-9-CM codes have not clearly identified the various stages for which a breast reconstruction encounter may occur, or distinguished between the disorders of reconstructed breasts and native breasts. This subcategory includes codes which provide unique classifications for the following conditions:

Breast ptosis (611.81): Drooping breasts. In general, it is a naturally occurring process of aging coinciding with loosening of the skin and suspensory ligaments. Early ptosis can occur from reduction in the volume of breast tissue, such as after pregnancy or significant weight loss.

Breast hypoplasia (611.82): May refer to postpubertal underdevelopment of breast tissue, although many surgeons use this diagnosis in reference to small breasts for patients who wish to undergo elective augmentation procedures. Clinically, there is no objective definition of hypoplasia, as normal breast development is relatively unrelated to breast size. True hypoplasia refers to the congenital underdevelopment of the pectoral muscle.

Capsular contracture of breast implant (611.83): An abnormal response of the immune system to an artificial breast implant. Collagen fibers form around the implant as a normal immune response to a foreign body. Contracture occurs when the collagen fibers form too tightly around the implant, causing a painful compression of the implant capsule, with possible associated distortion and asymmetry. Risk factors include rupture, leakage, and hematoma formation. Surgery is normally required to correct capsular contractures.

Deformity and Disproportion of Reconstructed Breast (612)

Breast reconstruction procedures are often performed to correct defects as a result of prior surgery or trauma to the breast. Depending on the nature of the defect and type of procedure indicated, breast reconstructive procedures may be performed in a single operative episode or separately, in staged procedures over the course of months or years. When a patient undergoes mastectomy, breast tissue is removed according to the size, location, and nature of the tumor. The patient may also have a biopsy scar to consider in the reconstructive surgery plan. When significant breast tissue is excised, tissue expanders are routinely inserted over time into the chest wall to create a soft pocket for a permanent implant. Attaining symmetry and aesthetic balance with the natural breast can pose a challenge for the surgeon. Post-mastectomy, circulation and healing of breast tissue may be compromised, delaying the insertion of a permanent implant or resulting in an unfavorable anatomic appearance. Examples of breast reconstructive procedures include insertion of tissue expanders or implants, revisions involving matching or balancing procedures to mimic the appearance of the native breast and areolar and nipple grafting, or tattooing. When these procedures result in a deformity or disproportion when compared with the native breast, surgical revision is usually required to restore desired anatomic appearance.

Category 612 contains two fourth-digit subclassification codes for deformities (612.0) and disproportions (612.1) of a reconstructed breast. Coding options for acquired breast deformity not related to reconstruction are found under category 611.

Inflammatory Disease of Female Pelvic Organs (614–616)

Use additional codes to identify the infectious organism such as Staphylococcus (041.1x) or Streptococcus (041.0x). This section excludes conditions complicating pregnancy, childbirth and the puerperium. Also excluded from this section are endometriosis (617) and gonococcal (098) and tuberculous (016) infections.

Other Disorders of Female Genital Tract (617-629)

Endometriosis (617)

Endometriosis is the presence of tissues that ordinarily line only the uterine cavity occurring outside of the uterine vault. The etiology is unknown, but previous uterine surgery or heredity may be predisposing factors. Endometriosis is classified by site, such as the rectovaginal septum (617.4) and intestine (617.5).

Genital Prolapse (618)

Genital prolapse includes vaginal wall, uterine, uterovaginal, and vaginal enterocele. Prolapse may cause urinary incontinence, which should be identified by using an additional code from 625.6, 788.31, or 788.33–788.39.

Use an additional code for associated fecal incontinence (787.60–787.63).

Dystrophy of Vulva (624.0x)

Vulvar intraepithelial neoplasia (VIN), a precancerous condition of the vulva, is a pathological process within the vulva's epithelial cells that results in the formation and growth of a tumor. VIN is relatively rare but appears to have a high risk of becoming cancerous if left untreated. HPV-16, a prevalent causative agent of cervical cancer, can cause vulvar intraepithelial neoplasia. Subcategory 624.0 classifies vulvar intraepithelial neoplasia type I, II and other dystrophies of vulva not classifiable elsewhere. This subcategory excludes vulvar carcinoma in situ, severe dysplasia, and VIN III, all of which are appropriately reported with code 233.32.

Vulvodynia (625.7)

Vulvodynia may be defined as persistent vulvar pain without an identifiable cause. The most commonly reported symptoms include severe and persistent burning, stinging and/or rawness, itching, and dyspareunia. Symptoms include constant or intermittent pain lasting for months or even years, which can vanish as mysteriously as it started. As a result, the patient's quality of life is affected by sexual, physical, and psychological limitations. Although the underlying cause is unknown, contributing factors have been identified such as previous injury to pelvic nerves, history of infection, allergies or localized hypersensitivity, muscle spasm, or hormonal changes associated with menopause. Vulvar vestibulitis (625.71) is a specific type of vulvodynia often associated with premenopausal hormone changes that is characterized by localized tenderness within the vulvar vestibulum, and focal or diffuse vestibular erythema. History of certain procedures such as carbon dioxide laser therapy, cryotherapy, or allergic drug reactions, including recent use of chemical irritants, have also been identified as possible precipitating factors. Other vulvodynia is indexed to code 625.79.

10. DISEASES OF THE GENITOURINARY SYSTEM (580-629)

NEPHRITIS, NEPHROTIC SYNDROME, AND NEPHROSIS (580-589)

EXCLUDES *hypertensive chronic kidney disease (403.00-403.91, 404.00-404.93)*

✓4ᵗʰ **580 Acute glomerulonephritis**

INCLUDES acute nephritis

DEF: Acute, severe inflammation in tuft of capillaries that filter the kidneys.

580.0 With lesion of proliferative glomerulonephritis
Acute (diffuse) proliferative glomerulonephritis
Acute poststreptococcal glomerulonephritis

580.4 With lesion of rapidly progressive glomerulonephritis
Acute nephritis with lesion of necrotizing glomerulitis

DEF: Acute glomerulonephritis; progresses to ESRD with diffuse epithelial proliferation.

✓5ᵗʰ **580.8 With other specified pathological lesion in kidney**

580.81 Acute glomerulonephritis in diseases classified elsewhere

Code first underlying disease, as:
infectious hepatitis (070.0-070.9)
mumps (072.79)
subacute bacterial endocarditis (421.0)
typhoid fever (002.0)

580.89 Other
Glomerulonephritis, acute, with lesion of:
exudative nephritis
interstitial (diffuse) (focal) nephritis

580.9 Acute glomerulonephritis with unspecified pathological lesion in kidney
Glomerulonephritis
NOS
hemorrhagic } specified as acute
Nephritis
Nephropathy

✓4ᵗʰ **581 Nephrotic syndrome**

DEF: Disease process marked by symptoms such as extensive edema, notable proteinuria, hypoalbuminemia, and susceptibility to intercurrent infections.

581.0 With lesion of proliferative glomerulonephritis

581.1 With lesion of membranous glomerulonephritis
Epimembranous nephritis
Idiopathic membranous glomerular disease
Nephrotic syndrome with lesion of:
focal glomerulosclerosis
sclerosing membranous glomerulonephritis
segmental hyalinosis

581.2 With lesion of membranoproliferative glomerulonephritis
Nephrotic syndrome with lesion (of):
endothelial
hypocomplementemic
persistent
lobular } glomerulonephritis
mesangiocapillary
mixed membranous and
proliferative

DEF: Glomerulonephritis combined with clinical features of nephrotic syndrome; characterized by uneven thickening of glomerular capillary walls and mesangial cell increase; slowly progresses to ESRD.

581.3 With lesion of minimal change glomerulonephritis
Foot process disease
Lipoid nephrosis
Minimal change:
glomerular disease
glomerulitis
nephrotic syndrome

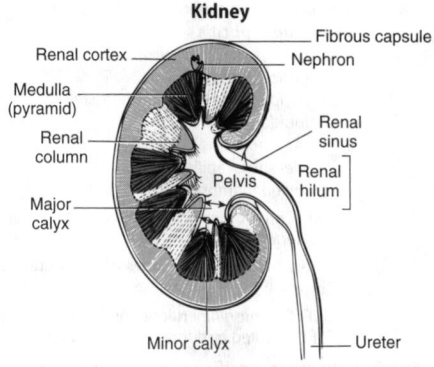

Kidney

Fibrous capsule
Renal cortex
Nephron
Medulla (pyramid)
Renal column
Renal sinus
Renal hilum
Major calyx
Pelvis
Minor calyx
Ureter

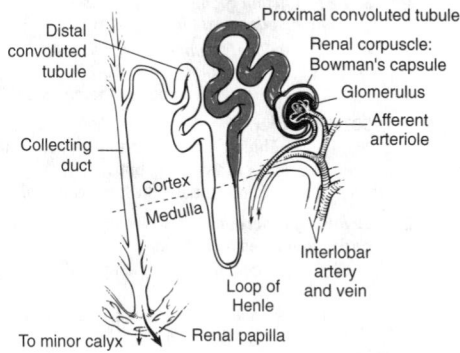

Nephron

Distal convoluted tubule
Proximal convoluted tubule
Renal corpuscle: Bowman's capsule
Glomerulus
Afferent arteriole
Collecting duct
Cortex
Medulla
Interlobar artery and vein
Loop of Henle
To minor calyx
Renal papilla

✓5ᵗʰ **581.8 With other specified pathological lesion in kidney**

581.81 Nephrotic syndrome in diseases classified elsewhere

Code first underlying disease, as:
amyloidosis (277.30-277.39)
diabetes mellitus (249.4, 250.4)
malaria (084.9)
polyarteritis (446.0)
systemic lupus erythematosus (710.0)

EXCLUDES *nephrosis in epidemic hemorrhagic fever (078.6)*

581.89 Other
Glomerulonephritis with edema and lesion of:
exudative nephritis
interstitial (diffuse) (focal) nephritis

581.9 Nephrotic syndrome with unspecified pathological lesion in kidney
Glomerulonephritis with edema NOS
Nephritis:
nephrotic NOS
with edema NOS
Nephrosis NOS
Renal disease with edema NOS

✓4ᵗʰ **582 Chronic glomerulonephritis**

INCLUDES chronic nephritis

DEF: Slow progressive type of nephritis characterized by inflammation of the capillary loops in the glomeruli of the kidney, which leads to renal failure.

582.0 With lesion of proliferative glomerulonephritis
Chronic (diffuse) proliferative glomerulonephritis

582.1 With lesion of membranous glomerulonephritis
Chronic glomerulonephritis:
membranous
sclerosing
Focal glomerulosclerosis
Segmental hyalinosis

582.2 With lesion of membranoproliferative glomerulonephritis
Chronic glomerulonephritis:
    endothelial
    hypocomplementemic persistent
    lobular
    membranoproliferative
    mesangiocapillary
    mixed membranous and proliferative
> **DEF:** Chronic glomerulonephritis with mesangial cell proliferation.

582.4 With lesion of rapidly progressive glomerulonephritis
Chronic nephritis with lesion of necrotizing glomerulitis
> **DEF:** Chronic glomerulonephritis rapidly progresses to ESRD; marked by diffuse epithelial proliferation.

√5ᵗʰ **582.8 With other specified pathological lesion in kidney**

    582.81 *Chronic glomerulonephritis in diseases classified elsewhere*
        Code first underlying disease, as:
          amyloidosis (277.30-277.39)
          systemic lupus erythematosus (710.0)

    582.89 Other
        Chronic glomerulonephritis with lesion of:
          exudative nephritis
          interstitial (diffuse) (focal) nephritis

582.9 Chronic glomerulonephritis with unspecified pathological lesion in kidney
Glomerulonephritis:
    NOS
    hemorrhagic
Nephritis   } specified as chronic
Nephropathy

√4ᵗʰ **583 Nephritis and nephropathy, not specified as acute or chronic**
> **INCLUDES** "renal disease" so stated, not specified as acute or chronic but with stated pathology or cause

583.0 With lesion of proliferative glomerulonephritis
Proliferative:
    glomerulonephritis (diffuse) NOS
    nephritis NOS
    nephropathy NOS

583.1 With lesion of membranous glomerulonephritis
Membranous:
    glomerulonephritis NOS
    nephritis NOS
Membranous nephropathy NOS
> **DEF:** Kidney inflammation or dysfunction with deposits on glomerular capillary basement membranes.

583.2 With lesion of membranoproliferative glomerulonephritis
Membranoproliferative:
    glomerulonephritis NOS
    nephritis NOS
    nephropathy NOS
Nephritis NOS, with lesion of:
    hypocomplementemic
        persistant
    lobular
    mesangiocapillary   } glomerulonephritis
    mixed membranous and
        proliferative
> **DEF:** Kidney inflammation or dysfunction with mesangial cell proliferation.

583.4 With lesion of rapidly progressive glomerulonephritis
Necrotizing or rapidly progressive:
    glomerulitis NOS
    glomerulonephritis NOS
    nephritis NOS
    nephropathy NOS
Nephritis, unspecified, with lesion of necrotizing glomerulitis
> **DEF:** Kidney inflammation or dysfunction; rapidly progresses to ESRD marked by diffuse epithelial proliferation.

583.6 With lesion of renal cortical necrosis
Nephritis, NOS   } with (renal) cortical necrosis
Nephropathy NS
Renal cortical necrosis NOS

583.7 With lesion of renal medullary necrosis
Nephritis, NOS   } with (renal) medullary
Nephropathy NOS   [papillary] necrosis

√5ᵗʰ **583.8 With other specified pathological lesion in kidney**

    583.81 *Nephritis and nephropathy, not specified as acute or chronic, in diseases classified elsewhere*
        Code first underlying disease, as:
          amyloidosis (277.30-277.39)
          diabetes mellitus (249.4, 250.4)
          gonococcal infection (098.19)
          Goodpasture's syndrome (446.21)
          systemic lupus erythematosus (710.0)
          tuberculosis (016.0)
        EXCLUDES *gouty nephropathy (274.10)*
                  syphilitic nephritis (095.4)

    583.89 Other
        Glomerulitis   } with lesions of:
        Glomerulonephritis   exudative
        Nephritis   nephritis
        Nephropathy   interstitial
        Renal disease   nephritis

583.9 With unspecified pathological lesion in kidney
Glomerulitis
Glomerulonephritis   } NOS
Nephritis
Nephropathy
> **EXCLUDES** *nephropathy complicating pregnancy, labor, or the puerperium (642.0-642.9, 646.2) renal disease NOS with no stated cause (593.9)*

√4ᵗʰ **584 Acute kidney failure**
> **INCLUDES** acute renal failure
> **EXCLUDES** *following labor and delivery (669.3)*
> *posttraumatic (958.5)*
> *that complicating:*
>   *abortion (634-638 with .3, 639.3)*
>   *ectopic or molar pregnancy (639.3)*

> **DEF:** State resulting from increasing urea and related substances from the blood (azotemia), often with urine output of less than 500 ml per day.

584.5 Acute kidney failure with lesion of tubular necrosis
Lower nephron nephrosis
Renal failure with (acute) tubular necrosis
Tubular necrosis:
    NOS
    acute
> **DEF:** Acute decline in kidney efficiency with destruction of tubules.

584.6 Acute kidney failure with lesion of renal cortical necrosis
> **DEF:** Acute decline in kidney efficiency with destruction of renal tissues that filter blood.

584.7 Acute kidney failure with lesion of renal medullary [papillary] necrosis
Necrotizing renal papillitis
> **DEF:** Acute decline in kidney efficiency with destruction of renal tissues that collect urine.

584.8 Acute kidney failure with other specified pathological lesion in kidney

584.9 Acute kidney failure, unspecified
Acute kidney injury (nontraumatic)
> **EXCLUDES** *traumatic kidney injury (866.00-866.13)*

☑4ᵗʰ **585　Chronic kidney disease [CKD]**
Chronic uremia
Code first hypertensive chronic kidney disease, if applicable,
　(403.00-403.91, 404.00-404.93)
Use additional code to identify kidney transplant status, if
　applicable (V42.0)
Use additional code to identify manifestation as:
　uremic:
　　neuropathy (357.4)
　　pericarditis (420.0)

585.1　Chronic kidney disease, Stage I
DEF: Some kidney damage; normal or slightly increased
GFR (> 90).

585.2　Chronic kidney disease, Stage II (mild)
DEF: Kidney damage with mild decrease in GFR (60–89).

585.3　Chronic kidney disease, Stage III (moderate)
DEF: Kidney damage with moderate decrease in GFR
(30–59).

585.4　Chronic kidney disease, Stage IV (severe)
DEF: Kidney damage with severe decrease in GFR (15–29).

585.5　Chronic kidney disease, Stage V
EXCLUDES　*chronic kidney disease, stage V requiring
chronic dialysis (585.6)*
DEF: Kidney failure with GFR value of less than 15.

585.6　End stage renal disease
Chronic kidney disease requiring chronic dialysis
DEF: Federal government indicator of a stage V CKD
patient undergoing treatment by dialysis or
transplantation.

585.9　Chronic kidney disease, unspecified
Chronic renal disease
Chronic renal failure NOS
Chronic renal insufficiency

586　Renal failure, unspecified
Uremia NOS
EXCLUDES　*following labor and delivery (669.3)*
posttraumatic renal failure (958.5)
that complicating:
　abortion (634-638 with .3, 639.3)
　ectopic or molar pregnancy (639.3)
uremia:
　extrarenal (788.9)
　prerenal (788.9)
DEF: Renal failure: kidney functions cease; malfunction may be due
to inability to excrete metabolized substances or retain level of
electrolytes.
DEF: Uremia: excess urea, creatinine and other nitrogenous
products of protein and amino acid metabolism in blood due to
reduced excretory function in bilateral kidney disease; also called
azotemia.

587　Renal sclerosis, unspecified
Atrophy of kidney
Contracted kidney
Renal:
　cirrhosis
　fibrosis

☑4ᵗʰ **588　Disorders resulting from impaired renal function**

588.0　Renal osteodystrophy
Azotemic osteodystrophy
Phosphate-losing tubular disorders
Renal:
　dwarfism
　infantilism
　rickets
DEF: Condition resulting from chronic renal failure results
in osteomalacia, osteoporosis or osteosclerosis; an
abnormal level of phosphorus in the blood and impaired
stimulation of the parathyroid.

588.1　Nephrogenic diabetes insipidus
EXCLUDES　*diabetes insipidus NOS (253.5)*
DEF: Type of diabetes due to renal tubules inability to
reabsorb water; not responsive to vasopressin; may
develop into chronic renal insufficiency.

☑5ᵗʰ **588.8　Other specified disorders resulting from impaired renal
function**
EXCLUDES　*secondary hypertension (405.0-405.9)*

**588.81　Secondary hyperparathyroidism (of renal
origin)**
Secondary hyperparathyroidism NOS
DEF: Parathyroid dysfunction caused by chronic
renal failure; phosphate clearance is impaired,
phosphate is released from bone, vitamin D is
not produced, intestinal calcium absorption is
low, and blood levels of calcium are lowered
causing excessive production of parathyroid
hormone.

**588.89　Other specified disorders resulting from
impaired renal function**
Hypokalemic nephropathy

**588.9　Unspecified disorder resulting from impaired renal
function**

☑4ᵗʰ **589　Small kidney of unknown cause**
589.0　Unilateral small kidney
589.1　Bilateral small kidneys
589.9　Small kidney, unspecified

OTHER DISEASES OF URINARY SYSTEM (590-599)

☑4ᵗʰ **590　Infections of kidney**
Use additional code to identify organism, such as Escherichia coli
[E. coli] (041.41-041.49)

☑5ᵗʰ **590.0　Chronic pyelonephritis**
Chronic pyelitis
Chronic pyonephrosis
Code, if applicable, any casual condition first

590.00　Without lesion of renal medullary necrosis
590.01　With lesion of renal medullary necrosis

☑5ᵗʰ **590.1　Acute pyelonephritis**
Acute pyelitis
Acute pyonephrosis

590.10　Without lesion of renal medullary necrosis
590.11　With lesion of renal medullary necrosis

590.2　Renal and perinephric abscess
Abscess:
　kidney
　nephritic
　perirenal
Carbuncle of kidney

590.3　Pyeloureteritis cystica
Infection of renal pelvis and ureter
Ureteritis cystica
DEF: Inflammation and formation of submucosal cysts in
the kidney, pelvis, and ureter.

☑5ᵗʰ **590.8　Other pyelonephritis or pyonephrosis, not specified as
acute or chronic**

590.80　Pyelonephritis, unspecified
Pyelitis NOS
Pyelonephritis NOS

Genitourinary System

Inferior vena cava — — Aorta
Right kidney — — Left kidney
— Ureter
Anterior
division
of internal
iliac artery
— Ovarian or
testicular
artery
and vein
Superior
and
Inferior
vesicular
arteries
— Urinary
bladder
Ureteral orifice — — Urogenital
diaphragm
Urethra

Diseases of the Genitourinary System

590.81–595.3

> **590.81 Pyelitis or pyelonephritis in diseases classified elsewhere**
> Code first underlying disease, as:
> tuberculosis (016.0)

590.9 Infection of kidney, unspecified
EXCLUDES   urinary tract infection NOS (599.0)

591 Hydronephrosis
Hydrocalycosis   Hydroureteronephrosis
Hydronephrosis
EXCLUDES   congenital hydronephrosis (753.29)
            hydroureter (593.5)

DEF: Distention of kidney and pelvis, with urine build-up due to ureteral obstruction; pyonephrosis may result.

✓4ᵗʰ 592 Calculus of kidney and ureter
EXCLUDES   nephrocalcinosis (275.4)

592.0 Calculus of kidney
Nephrolithiasis NOS   Staghorn calculus
Renal calculus or stone   Stone in kidney
EXCLUDES   uric acid nephrolithiasis (274.11)

592.1 Calculus of ureter
Ureteric stone   Ureterolithiasis

592.9 Urinary calculus, unspecified

✓4ᵗʰ 593 Other disorders of kidney and ureter

593.0 Nephroptosis
Floating kidney
Mobile kidney

593.1 Hypertrophy of kidney

593.2 Cyst of kidney, acquired
Cyst (multiple) (solitary) of kidney, not congenital
Peripelvic (lymphatic) cyst
EXCLUDES   calyceal or pyelogenic cyst of kidney (591)
            congenital cyst of kidney (753.1)
            polycystic (disease of) kidney (753.1)

DEF: Abnormal, fluid-filled sac in the kidney, not present at birth.

593.3 Stricture or kinking of ureter
Angulation   } of ureter (post-operative)
Constriction
Stricture of pelviureteric junction

DEF: Stricture or knot in tube connecting kidney to bladder.

593.4 Other ureteric obstruction
Idiopathic retroperitoneal fibrosis
Occlusion NOS of ureter
EXCLUDES   that due to calculus (592.1)

593.5 Hydroureter
EXCLUDES   congenital hydroureter (753.22)
            hydroureteronephrosis (591)

593.6 Postural proteinuria
Benign postural proteinuria   Orthostatic proteinuria
EXCLUDES   proteinuria NOS (791.0)

DEF: Excessive amounts of serum protein in the urine caused by the body position, e.g., orthostatic and lordotic.

✓5ᵗʰ 593.7 Vesicoureteral reflux
DEF: Backflow of urine, from bladder into ureter due to obstructed bladder neck.

593.70 Unspecified or without reflux nephropathy

593.71 With reflux nephropathy, unilateral

593.72 With reflux nephropathy, bilateral

593.73 With reflux nephropathy NOS

✓5ᵗʰ 593.8 Other specified disorders of kidney and ureter

593.81 Vascular disorders of kidney
Renal (artery):   Renal (artery):
  embolism   thrombosis
  hemorrhage   Renal infarction

593.82 Ureteral fistula
Intestinoureteral fistula
EXCLUDES   fistula between ureter and female genital tract (619.0)

DEF: Abnormal communication, between tube connecting kidney to bladder and another structure.

593.89 Other
Adhesions, kidney or ureter
Periureteritis
Polyp of ureter
Pyelectasia
Ureterocele
EXCLUDES   tuberculosis of ureter (016.2)
            ureteritis cystica (590.3)

593.9 Unspecified disorder of kidney and ureter
Acute renal disease
Acute renal insufficiency
Renal disease NOS
Salt-losing nephritis or syndrome
EXCLUDES   chronic renal insufficiency (585.9)
            cystic kidney disease (753.1)
            nephropathy, so stated (583.0-583.9)
            renal disease:
              arising in pregnancy or the puerperium
                (642.1-642.2, 642.4-642.7, 646.2)
              not specified as acute or chronic, but with
                stated pathology or cause
                (583.0-583.9)

✓4ᵗʰ 594 Calculus of lower urinary tract

594.0 Calculus in diverticulum of bladder
DEF: Stone or mineral deposit in abnormal sac on the bladder wall.

594.1 Other calculus in bladder
Urinary bladder stone
EXCLUDES   staghorn calculus (592.0)

DEF: Stone or mineral deposit in bladder.

594.2 Calculus in urethra
DEF: Stone or mineral deposit in tube that empties urine from bladder.

594.8 Other lower urinary tract calculus

594.9 Calculus of lower urinary tract, unspecified
EXCLUDES   calculus of urinary tract NOS (592.9)

✓4ᵗʰ 595 Cystitis
Use additional code to identify organism, such as Escherichia coli [E. coli] (041.41-041.49)
EXCLUDES   prostatocystitis (601.3)

595.0 Acute cystitis
EXCLUDES   trigonitis (595.3)
DEF: Acute inflammation of bladder.

595.1 Chronic interstitial cystitis
Hunner's ulcer
Panmural fibrosis of bladder
Submucous cystitis
DEF: Inflamed lesion affecting bladder wall; symptoms include urinary frequency, pain on bladder filling, nocturia, and distended bladder.

595.2 Other chronic cystitis
Chronic cystitis NOS   Subacute cystitis
EXCLUDES   trigonitis (595.3)
DEF: Persistent inflammation of bladder.

595.3 Trigonitis
Follicular cystitis
Trigonitis (acute) (chronic)
Urethrotrigonitis
DEF: Inflammation of the triangular area of the bladder called the trigonum vesicae.

595.4   **Cystitis in diseases classified elsewhere**

Code first underlying disease, as:
    actinomycosis (039.8)
    amebiasis (006.8)
    bilharziasis (120.0-120.9)
    Echinococcus infestation (122.3, 122.6)

EXCLUDES   *cystitis:*
    diphtheritic (032.84)
    gonococcal (098.11, 098.31)
    monilial (112.2)
    trichomonal (131.09)
    tuberculous (016.1)

√5ᵗʰ   **595.8**   **Other specified types of cystitis**

    595.81   **Cystitis cystica**

        DEF: Inflammation of the bladder characterized by formation of multiple cysts.

    595.82   **Irradiation cystitis**

        Use additional E code to identify cause

        DEF: Inflammation of the bladder due to effects of radiation.

    595.89   **Other**

        Abscess of bladder
        Cystitis:
            bullous
            emphysematous
            glandularis

    595.9   **Cystitis, unspecified**

√4ᵗʰ   **596**   **Other disorders of bladder**

    Use additional code to identify urinary incontinence (625.6, 788.30-788.39)

    596.0   **Bladder neck obstruction**

        Contracture (acquired) ⎫
        Obstruction (acquired) ⎬ of bladder neck or vesicourethral orifice
        Stenosis (acquired)   ⎭

        EXCLUDES   *congenital (753.6)*

        DEF: Bladder outlet and vesicourethral obstruction; occurs as a consequence of benign prostatic hypertrophy or prostatic cancer; may also occur in either sex due to strictures, following radiation, cystoscopy, catheterization, injury, infection, blood clots, bladder cancer, impaction or disease compressing bladder neck.

    596.1   **Intestinovesical fistula**

        Fistula: Fistula:
           enterovesical   vesicoenteric
           vesicocolic   vesicorectal

        DEF: Abnormal communication, between intestine and bladder.

    596.2   **Vesical fistula, not elsewhere classified**

        Fistula: Fistula:
           bladder NOS   vesicocutaneous
           urethrovesical   vesicoperineal

        EXCLUDES   *fistula between bladder and female genital tract (619.0)*

        DEF: Abnormal communication between bladder and another structure.

    596.3   **Diverticulum of bladder**

        Diverticulitis   ⎫
        Diverticulum (acquired) (false) ⎬ of bladder

        EXCLUDES   *that with calculus in diverticulum of bladder (594.0)*

        DEF: Abnormal pouch in bladder wall.

    596.4   **Atony of bladder**

        High compliance bladder
        Hypotonicity ⎫
        Inertia   ⎬ of bladder

        EXCLUDES   *neurogenic bladder (596.54)*

        DEF: Distended, bladder with loss of expulsive force; linked to CNS disease.

Bladder

Anterior View

Fundus — Right ureter — Left ureter — Lateral wall — Ureteral orifice — Trigone — Uvula of bladder — Urethra

Lateral View

Urachus — Left ureter — Peritoneum — Pubic bone — Urogenital diaphragm

√5ᵗʰ   **596.5**   **Other functional disorders of bladder**

    EXCLUDES   *cauda equina syndrome with neurogenic bladder (344.61)*

    596.51   **Hypertonicity of bladder**

        Hyperactivity   Overactive bladder

        DEF: Abnormal tension of muscular wall of bladder; may appear after surgery of voluntary nerve.

    596.52   **Low bladder compliance**

        DEF: Low bladder capacity; causes increased pressure and frequent urination.

    596.53   **Paralysis of bladder**

        DEF: Impaired bladder motor function due to nerve or muscle damage.

    596.54   **Neurogenic bladder NOS**

        DEF: Unspecified dysfunctional bladder due to lesion of central, peripheral nervous system; may result in incontinence, residual urine retention, urinary infection, stones and renal failure.

    596.55   **Detrusor sphincter dyssynergia**

        DEF: Instability of the urinary bladder sphincter muscle associated with urinary incontinence.

    596.59   **Other functional disorder of bladder**

        Detrusor instability

        DEF: Detrusor instability: instability of bladder; marked by uninhibited contractions often leading to incontinence.

    596.6   **Rupture of bladder, nontraumatic**

    596.7   **Hemorrhage into bladder wall**

        Hyperemia of bladder

        EXCLUDES   *acute hemorrhagic cystitis (595.0)*

√5ᵗʰ   **596.8**   **Other specified disorders of bladder**

    EXCLUDES   *cystocele, female (618.01-618.02, 618.09, 618.2-618.4)*
            hernia or prolapse of bladder, female (618.01-618.02, 618.09, 618.2-618.4)

    596.81   **Infection of cystostomy**

        Use additional code to specify type of infection, such as:
            abscess or cellulitis of abdomen (682.2)
            septicemia (038.0-038.9)
        Use additional code to identify organism (041.00-041.9)

    596.82   **Mechanical complication of cystostomy**

        Malfunction of cystostomy

596.83 Other complication of cystostomy
Fistula
Hernia
Prolapse

596.89 Other specified disorders of bladder
Bladder hemorrhage
Bladder hypertrophy
Calcified bladder
Contracted bladder

596.9 Unspecified disorder of bladder

√4ᵗʰ **597 Urethritis, not sexually transmitted, and urethral syndrome**
EXCLUDES   *nonspecific urethritis, so stated (099.4)*

597.0 Urethral abscess
Abscess:
periurethral
urethral (gland)
Abscess of:
bulbourethral gland
Cowper's gland
Littré's gland
Periurethral cellulitis
EXCLUDES   *urethral caruncle (599.3)*
DEF: Pocket of pus in tube that empties urine from the bladder.

√5ᵗʰ **597.8 Other urethritis**

597.80 Urethritis, unspecified

597.81 Urethral syndrome NOS

597.89 Other
Adenitis, Skene's glands
Cowperitis
Meatitis, urethral
Ulcer, urethra (meatus)
Verumontanitis
EXCLUDES   *trichomonal (131.02)*

√4ᵗʰ **598 Urethral stricture**
Use additional code to identify urinary incontinence (625.6, 788.30-788.39)
INCLUDES   pinhole meatus
stricture of urinary meatus
EXCLUDES   *congenital stricture of urethra and urinary meatus (753.6)*
DEF: Narrowing of tube that empties urine from bladder.

√5ᵗʰ **598.0 Urethral stricture due to infection**

598.00 Due to unspecified infection

598.01 *Due to infective diseases classified elsewhere*
Code first underlying disease, as:
gonococcal infection (098.2)
schistosomiasis (120.0-120.9)
syphilis (095.8)

598.1 Traumatic urethral stricture
Stricture of urethra:
late effect of injury
postobstetric
EXCLUDES   *postoperative following surgery on genitourinary tract (598.2)*

598.2 Postoperative urethral stricture
Postcatheterization stricture of urethra

598.8 Other specified causes of urethral stricture

598.9 Urethral stricture, unspecified

√4ᵗʰ **599 Other disorders of urethra and urinary tract**

599.0 Urinary tract infection, site not specified
Use additional code to identify organism, such as Escherichia coli [E. coli] (041.41-041.49)
EXCLUDES   *candidiasis of urinary tract (112.2)*
urinary tract infection of newborn (771.82)

599.1 Urethral fistula
Fistula:
urethroperineal
urethrorectal
Urinary fistula NOS
EXCLUDES   *fistula:*
urethroscrotal (608.89)
urethrovaginal (619.0)
urethrovesicovaginal (619.0)

599.2 Urethral diverticulum
DEF: Abnormal pouch in urethral wall.

599.3 Urethral caruncle
Polyp of urethra

599.4 Urethral false passage
DEF: Abnormal opening in urethra due to surgery; trauma or disease.

599.5 Prolapsed urethral mucosa
Prolapse of urethra
Urethrocele
EXCLUDES   *urethrocele, female (618.03, 618.09, 618.2-618.4)*

√5ᵗʰ **599.6 Urinary obstruction**
Use additional code to identify urinary incontinence (625.6, 788.30-788.39)
EXCLUDES   *obstructive nephropathy NOS (593.89)*

599.60 Urinary obstruction, unspecified
Obstructive uropathy NOS
Urinary (tract) obstruction NOS

599.69 Urinary obstruction, not elsewhere classified
Code, if applicable, any causal condition first, such as:
hyperplasia of prostate (600.0-600.9 with fifth-digit 1)

√5ᵗʰ **599.7 Hematuria**
Hematuria (benign) (essential)
EXCLUDES   *hemoglobinuria (791.2)*

599.70 Hematuria, unspecified

599.71 Gross hematuria

599.72 Microscopic hematuria

√5ᵗʰ **599.8 Other specified disorders of urethra and urinary tract**
Use additional code to identify urinary incontinence (625.6, 788.30-788.39), if present
EXCLUDES   *symptoms and other conditions classifiable to 788.0-788.2, 788.4-788.9, 791.0-791.9*

599.81 Urethral hypermobility
DEF: Hyperactive urethra.

599.82 Intrinsic (urethral) sphincter deficiency [ISD]
DEF: Malfunctioning urethral sphincter.

599.83 Urethral instability
DEF: Inconsistent functioning of urethra.

599.84 Other specified disorders of urethra
Rupture of urethra (nontraumatic)
Urethral:
cyst
granuloma
DEF: Rupture of urethra due to herniation or breaking down of tissue; not due to trauma.
DEF: Urethral cyst: abnormal sac in urethra; usually fluid filled.
DEF: Granuloma: inflammatory cells forming small nodules in urethra.

599.89 Other specified disorders of urinary tract

599.9 Unspecified disorder of urethra and urinary tract

Male Pelvic Organs

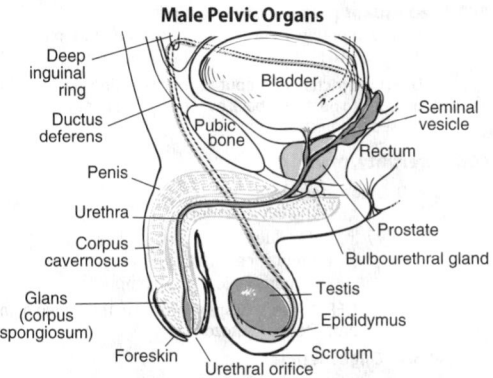

Deep inguinal ring
Ductus deferens
Penis
Urethra
Corpus cavernosus
Glans (corpus spongiosum)
Foreskin
Bladder
Pubic bone
Seminal vesicle
Rectum
Prostate
Bulbourethral gland
Testis
Epididymus
Scrotum
Urethral orifice

DISEASES OF MALE GENITAL ORGANS (600-608)

✓4ᵗʰ 600 Hyperplasia of prostate

INCLUDES enlarged prostate

DEF: Fibrostromal proliferation in periurethral glands, causes blood in urine; etiology unknown.

✓5ᵗʰ 600.0 Hypertrophy (benign) of prostate
Benign prostatic hypertrophy
Enlargement of prostate
Smooth enlarged prostate
Soft enlarged prostate

600.00 Hypertrophy (benign) of prostate without urinary obstruction and other lower urinary tract symptoms [LUTS]
Hypertrophy (benign) of prostate NOS

600.01 Hypertrophy (benign) of prostate with urinary obstruction and other lower urinary tract symptoms [LUTS]
Hypertrophy (benign) of prostate with urinary retention
Use additional code to identify symptoms:
incomplete bladder emptying (788.21)
nocturia (788.43)
straining on urination (788.65)
urinary frequency (788.41)
urinary hesitancy (788.64)
urinary incontinence (788.30-788.39)
urinary obstruction (599.69)
urinary retention (788.20)
urinary urgency (788.63)
weak urinary stream (788.62)

✓5ᵗʰ 600.1 Nodular prostate
Hard, firm prostate
Multinodular prostate
EXCLUDES malignant neoplasm of prostate (185)
DEF: Hard, firm nodule in prostate.

600.10 Nodular prostate without urinary obstruction
Nodular prostate NOS

600.11 Nodular prostate with urinary obstruction
Nodular prostate with urinary retention

✓5ᵗʰ 600.2 Benign localized hyperplasia of prostate
Adenofibromatous hypertrophy of prostate
Adenoma of prostate
Fibroadenoma of prostate
Fibroma of prostate
Myoma of prostate
Polyp of prostate
EXCLUDES benign neoplasms of prostate (222.2)
hypertrophy of prostate (600.00-600.01)
malignant neoplasm of prostate (185)
DEF: Benign localized hyperplasia clearly defined epithelial tumor.

600.20 Benign localized hyperplasia of prostate without urinary obstruction and other lower urinary tract symptoms [LUTS]
Benign localized hyperplasia of prostate NOS

600.21 Benign localized hyperplasia of prostate with urinary obstruction and other lower urinary tract symptoms [LUTS]
Benign localized hyperplasia of prostate with urinary retention
Use additional code to identify symptoms:
incomplete bladder emptying (788.21)
nocturia (788.43)
straining on urination (788.65)
urinary frequency (788.41)
urinary hesitancy (788.64)
urinary incontinence (788.30-788.39)
urinary obstruction (599.69)
urinary retention (788.20)
urinary urgency (788.63)
weak urinary stream (788.62)

600.3 Cyst of prostate
DEF: Sacs of fluid, which differentiate this from either nodular or adenomatous tumors.

✓5ᵗʰ 600.9 Hyperplasia of prostate, unspecified
Median bar
Prostatic obstruction NOS

600.90 Hyperplasia of prostate, unspecified, without urinary obstruction and other lower urinary tract symptoms [LUTS]
Hyperplasia of prostate NOS

600.91 Hyperplasia of prostate, unspecified with urinary obstruction and other lower urinary tract symptoms [LUTS]
Hyperplasia of prostate, unspecified, with urinary retention
Use additional code to identify symptoms:
incomplete bladder emptying (788.21)
nocturia (788.43)
straining on urination (788.65)
urinary frequency (788.41)
urinary hesitancy (788.64)
urinary incontinence (788.30-788.39)
urinary obstruction (599.69)
urinary retention (788.20)
urinary urgency (788.63)
weak urinary stream (788.62)

✓4ᵗʰ 601 Inflammatory diseases of prostate
Use additional code to identify organism, such as Staphylococcus (041.1), or Streptococcus (041.0)

601.0 Acute prostatitis

601.1 Chronic prostatitis

601.2 Abscess of prostate

601.3 Prostatocystitis

601.4 *Prostatitis in diseases classified elsewhere*
Code first underlying disease, as:
actinomycosis (039.8)
blastomycosis (116.0)
syphilis (095.8)
tuberculosis (016.5)
EXCLUDES *prostatitis:*
gonococcal (098.12, 098.32)
monilial (112.2)
trichomonal (131.03)

601.8 Other specified inflammatory diseases of prostate
Prostatitis:
cavitary
diverticular
granulomatous

601.9 Prostatitis, unspecified
Prostatitis NOS

✓4ᵗʰ 602 Other disorders of prostate

602.0 Calculus of prostate
Prostatic stone
DEF: Stone or mineral deposit in prostate.

602.1 Congestion or hemorrhage of prostate
DEF: Bleeding or fluid collection in prostate.

Diseases of the Genitourinary System

602.2–607.85

Common Inguinal Canal Anomalies

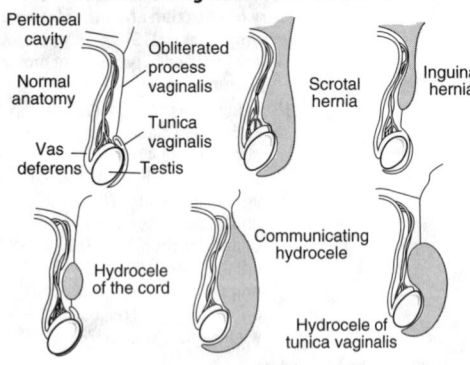

602.2 Atrophy of prostate

602.3 Dysplasia of prostate
Prostatic intraepithelial neoplasia I (PIN I)
Prostatic intraepithelial neoplasia II (PIN II)
EXCLUDES *prostatic intraepithelial neoplasia III (PIN III) (233.4)*

DEF: Abnormality of shape and size of the intraepithelial tissues of the prostate; premalignant condition characterized by stalks and absence of a basilar cell layer; synonyms are intraductal dysplasia, large acinar atypical hyperplasia, atypical primary hyperplasia, hyperplasia with malignant changes, marked atypia, or duct-acinar dysplasia.

602.8 Other specified disorders of prostate
Fistula
Infarction   } of prostate
Stricture
Periprostatic adhesions

602.9 Unspecified disorder of prostate

✓4ᵗʰ 603 Hydrocele
INCLUDES hydrocele of spermatic cord, testis or tunica vaginalis
EXCLUDES *congenital (778.6)*

DEF: Circumscribed collection of fluid in tunica vaginalis, spermatic cord or testis.

603.0 Encysted hydrocele

603.1 Infected hydrocele
Use additional code to identify organism

603.8 Other specified types of hydrocele

603.9 Hydrocele, unspecified

✓4ᵗʰ 604 Orchitis and epididymitis
Use additional code to identify organism, such as:
Escherichia coli [E. coli] (041.41-041.49)
Staphylococcus (041.10-041.19)
Streptococcus (041.00-041.09)

604.0 Orchitis, epididymitis, and epididymoorchitis, with abscess
Abscess of epididymis or testis

✓5ᵗʰ 604.9 Other orchitis, epididymitis, and epididymo-orchitis, without mention of abscess

604.90 Orchitis and epididymitis, unspecified

604.91 Orchitis and epididymitis in diseases classified elsewhere
Code first underlying disease, as:
diphtheria (032.89)
filariasis (125.0-125.9)
syphilis (095.8)
EXCLUDES *orchitis:*
gonococcal (098.13, 098.33)
mumps (072.0)
tuberculous (016.5)
tuberculous epididymitis (016.4)

604.99 Other

605 Redundant prepuce and phimosis
Adherent prepuce   Phimosis (congenital)
Paraphimosis   Tight foreskin

DEF: Constriction of preputial orifice causing inability of the prepuce to be drawn back over the glans; it may be congenital or caused by infection.

✓4ᵗʰ 606 Infertility, male

606.0 Azoospermia
Absolute infertility
Infertility due to:
germinal (cell) aplasia
spermatogenic arrest (complete)
DEF: Absence of spermatozoa in the semen or inability to produce spermatozoa.

606.1 Oligospermia
Infertility due to:
germinal cell desquamation
hypospermatogenesis
incomplete spermatogenic arrest
DEF: Insufficient number of sperm in semen.

606.8 Infertility due to extratesticular causes
Infertility due to:
drug therapy
infection
obstruction of efferent ducts
radiation
systemic disease

606.9 Male infertility, unspecified

✓4ᵗʰ 607 Disorders of penis
EXCLUDES *phimosis (605)*

607.0 Leukoplakia of penis
Kraurosis of penis
EXCLUDES *carcinoma in situ of penis (233.5)*
erythroplasia of Queyrat (233.5)

DEF: White, thickened patches on glans penis.

607.1 Balanoposthitis
Balanitis
Use additional code to identify organism
DEF: Inflammation of glans penis and prepuce.

607.2 Other inflammatory disorders of penis
Abscess
Boil
Carbuncle   } of corpus cavernosum or penis
Cellulitis
Cavernitis (penis)
Use additional code to identify organism
EXCLUDES *herpetic infection (054.13)*

607.3 Priapism
Painful erection
DEF: Prolonged penile erection without sexual stimulation.

✓5ᵗʰ 607.8 Other specified disorders of penis

607.81 Balanitis xerotica obliterans
Induratio penis plastica
DEF: Inflammation of the glans penis, caused by stricture of the opening of the prepuce.

607.82 Vascular disorders of penis
Embolisim
Hematoma
(nontraumatic) } of corpus cavernosum
Hemorrhage   or penis
Thrombosis

607.83 Edema of penis
DEF: Fluid retention within penile tissues.

607.84 Impotence of organic origin
EXCLUDES *nonorganic (302.72)*
DEF: Physiological cause interfering with erection.

607.85 Peyronie's disease
DEF: A severe curvature of the erect penis due to fibrosis of the cavernous sheaths.

Torsion of the Testis

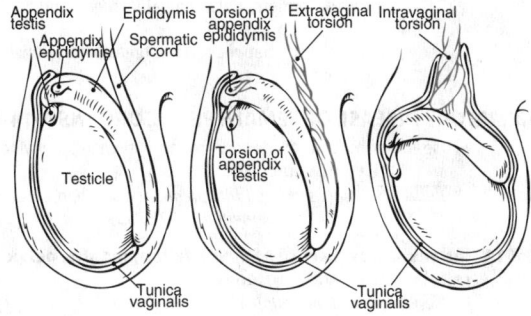

607.89 Other

Atrophy
Fibrosis
Hypertrophy
Ulcer (chronic)
} of corpus cavernosum or penis

607.9 Unspecified disorder of penis

✓4ᵗʰ **608 Other disorders of male genital organs**

608.0 Seminal vesiculitis

Abscess
Cellulitis
} of seminal vesicle

Vesiculitis (seminal)
Use additional code to identify organism
EXCLUDES *gonococcal infection (098.14, 098.34)*
DEF: Inflammation of seminal vesicle.

608.1 Spermatocele

DEF: Cystic enlargement of the epididymis or the testis; the cysts contain spermatozoa.

✓5ᵗʰ **608.2 Torsion of testis**

DEF: Twisted or rotated testis; may compromise blood flow.

608.20 Torsion of testis, unspecified

608.21 Extravaginal torsion of spermatic cord

DEF: Torsion of the spermatic cord just below the tunica vaginalis attachments.

608.22 Intravaginal torsion of spermatic cord
Torsion of spermatic cord NOS

DEF: Torsion within the tunica vaginalis also called the "bell-clapper" anomaly. It usually occurs in older children.

608.23 Torsion of appendix testis

DEF: Torsion of small solid projection of tissue on the upper outer surface of the testis (hydatid of Morgagni); a remnant of the embryologic Müllerian duct.

608.24 Torsion of appendix epididymis

DEF: Torsion of small stalked appendage of the head of the epididymis (pedunculated hydatid); a detached embryologic efferent duct.

608.3 Atrophy of testis

608.4 Other inflammatory disorders of male genital organs

Abscess
Boil
Carbuncle
Cellulitis
} of scrotum, spermatic cord, testis [except abscess], tunica vaginalis, or vas deferens

Vasitis
Use additional code to identify organism
EXCLUDES *abscess of testis (604.0)*

✓5ᵗʰ **608.8 Other specified disorders of male genital organs**

608.81 Disorders of male genital organs in diseases classified elsewhere

Code first underlying disease, as:
filariasis (125.0-125.9)
tuberculosis (016.5)

608.82 Hematospermia

DEF: Presence of blood in the ejaculate; relatively common, affecting men of any age after puberty; cause is often the result of a viral or bacterial infection and inflammation.

608.83 Vascular disorders

Hematoma (non-traumatic)
Hemorrhage
Thrombosis
} of seminal vessel, spermatic cord, testis, scrotum, tunica vaginalis, or vas deferens

Hematocele NOS, male

608.84 Chylocele of tunica vaginalis

DEF: Chylous effusion into tunica vaginalis; due to infusion of lymphatic fluids.

608.85 Stricture

Stricture of:
spermatic cord
tunica vaginalis

Stricture of:
vas deferens

608.86 Edema

608.87 Retrograde ejaculation

DEF: Condition where the semen travels to the bladder rather than out through the urethra due to damaged nerves causing the bladder neck to remain open during ejaculation.

608.89 Other

Atrophy
Fibrosis
Hypertrophy
Ulcer
} of seminal vessel, spermatic cord, testis, scrotum, tunica vaginalis, or vas deferens

EXCLUDES *atrophy of testis (608.3)*

608.9 Unspecified disorder of male genital organs

DISORDERS OF BREAST (610-612)

✓4ᵗʰ **610 Benign mammary dysplasias**

610.0 Solitary cyst of breast
Cyst (solitary) of breast

610.1 Diffuse cystic mastopathy
Chronic cystic mastitis
Cystic breast
Fibrocystic disease of breast

DEF: Extensive formation of nodular cysts in breast tissue; symptoms include tenderness, change in size and hyperplasia of ductal epithelium.

610.2 Fibroadenosis of breast
Fibroadenosis of breast:
NOS
chronic
cystic
diffuse
periodic
segmental

DEF: Non-neoplastic nodular condition of breast.

610.3 Fibrosclerosis of breast

DEF: Fibrous tissue in breast.

610.4 Mammary duct ectasia
Comedomastitis
Duct ectasia

Mastitis:
periductal
plasma cell

DEF: Atrophy of duct epithelium; causes distended collecting ducts of mammary gland, drying up of breast secretion, intraductal inflammation and periductal and interstitial chronic inflammatory reaction.

610.8 Other specified benign mammary dysplasias
Mazoplasia   Sebaceous cyst of breast

610.9 Benign mammary dysplasia, unspecified

Diseases of the Genitourinary System

611–614.9

☑4ᵗʰ **611 Other disorders of breast**
> EXCLUDES   *that associated with lactation or the puerperium (675.0-676.9)*

611.0 Inflammatory disease of breast
Abscess (acute) (chronic) (nonpuerperal) of:
    areola
    breast
Mammillary fistula
Mastitis (acute) (subacute) (nonpuerperal):
    NOS
    infective
    retromammary
    submammary
> EXCLUDES   *carbuncle of breast (680.2)*
> *chronic cystic mastitis (610.1)*
> *neonatal infective mastitis (771.5)*
> *thrombophlebitis of breast [Mondor's disease] (451.89)*

611.1 Hypertrophy of breast
Gynecomastia
Hypertrophy of breast:
    NOS
    massive pubertal
> EXCLUDES   *breast engorgement in newborn (778.7)*
> *disproportion of reconstructed breast (612.1)*

611.2 Fissure of nipple

611.3 Fat necrosis of breast
Fat necrosis (segmental) of breast
Code first breast necrosis due to breast graft (996.79)
DEF: Splitting of neutral fats in adipose tissue cells as a result of trauma; a firm circumscribed mass is then formed in the breast.

611.4 Atrophy of breast

611.5 Galactocele
DEF: Milk-filled cyst in breast due to blocked duct.

611.6 Galactorrhea not associated with childbirth
DEF: Flow of milk not associated with childbirth or pregnancy.

☑5ᵗʰ **611.7 Signs and symptoms in breast**

  611.71 Mastodynia
    Pain in breast

  611.72 Lump or mass in breast

  611.79 Other
    Induration of breast
    Inversion of nipple
    Nipple discharge
    Retraction of nipple

☑5ᵗʰ **611.8 Other specified disorders of breast**

  611.81 Ptosis of breast
> EXCLUDES   *ptosis of native breast in relation to reconstructed breast (612.1)*

  611.82 Hypoplasia of breast
    Micromastia
> EXCLUDES   *congenital absence of breast (757.6)*
> *hypoplasia of native breast in relation to reconstructed breast (612.1)*

  611.83 Capsular contracture of breast implant

  611.89 Other specified disorders of breast
    Hematoma (nontraumatic) of breast
    Infarction of breast
    Occlusion of breast duct
    Subinvolution of breast (postlactational) (postpartum)

611.9 Unspecified breast disorder

☑4ᵗʰ **612 Deformity and disproportion of reconstructed breast**

612.0 Deformity of reconstructed breast
Contour irregularity in reconstructed breast
Excess tissue in reconstructed breast
Misshapen reconstructed breast

612.1 Disproportion of reconstructed breast
Breast asymmetry between native breast and reconstructed breast
Disproportion between native breast and reconstructed breast

INFLAMMATORY DISEASE OF FEMALE PELVIC ORGANS (614-616)

Use additional code to identify organism, such as Staphylococcus (041.1), or Streptococcus (041.0)
> EXCLUDES   *that associated with pregnancy, abortion, childbirth, or the puerperium (630-676.9)*

☑4ᵗʰ **614 Inflammatory disease of ovary, fallopian tube, pelvic cellular tissue, and peritoneum**
> EXCLUDES   *endometritis (615.0-615.9)*
> *major infection following delivery (670.0-670.8)*
> *that complicating:*
>   *abortion (634-638 with .0, 639.0)*
>   *ectopic or molar pregnancy (639.0)*
>   *pregnancy or labor (646.6)*

614.0 Acute salpingitis and oophoritis
Any condition classifiable to 614.2, specified as acute or subacute
DEF: Acute inflammation of ovary and fallopian tube.

614.1 Chronic salpingitis and oophoritis
Hydrosalpinx
Salpingitis:
    follicularis
    isthmica nodosa
Any condition classifiable to 614.2, specified as chronic
DEF: Persistent inflammation of ovary and fallopian tube.

614.2 Salpingitis and oophoritis not specified as acute, subacute, or chronic

Abscess (of):	Perisalpingitis
fallopian tube	Pyosalpinx
ovary	Salpingitis
tubo-ovarian	Salpingo-oophoritis
Oophoritis	Tubo-ovarian inflammatory
Perioophoritis	disease

> EXCLUDES   *gonococcal infection (chronic) (098.37)*
> *acute (098.17)*
> *tuberculous (016.6)*

614.3 Acute parametritis and pelvic cellulitis
Acute inflammatory pelvic disease
Any condition classifiable to 614.4, specified as acute
DEF: Parametritis: inflammation of the parametrium; pelvic cellulitis is a synonym for parametritis.

614.4 Chronic or unspecified parametritis and pelvic cellulitis
Abscess (of):
    broad ligament
    parametrium   } chronic or NOS
    pelvis, femal
    pouch of Douglas
Chronic inflammatory pelvic disease
Pelvic cellulitis, female
> EXCLUDES   *tuberculous (016.7)*

614.5 Acute or unspecified pelvic peritonitis, female

614.6 Pelvic peritoneal adhesions, female (postoperative) (postinfection)
Adhesions:
    peritubal
    tubo-ovarian
Use additional code to identify any associated infertility (628.2)
DEF: Fibrous scarring abnormally joining structures within abdomen.

614.7 Other chronic pelvic peritonitis, female
> EXCLUDES   *tuberculous (016.7)*

614.8 Other specified inflammatory disease of female pelvic organs and tissues

614.9 Unspecified inflammatory disease of female pelvic organs and tissues
Pelvic infection or inflammation, female NOS
Pelvic inflammatory disease [PID]

☑4ᵗʰ 615 Inflammatory diseases of uterus, except cervix

> **EXCLUDES** *following delivery (670.0-670.8)*
> *hyperplastic endometritis (621.30-621.35)*
> *that complicating:*
> *abortion (634-638 with .0, 639.0)*
> *ectopic or molar pregnancy (639.0)*
> *pregnancy or labor (646.6)*

615.0 Acute

> Any condition classifiable to 615.9, specified as acute or subacute

615.1 Chronic

> Any condition classifiable to 615.9, specified as chronic

615.9 Unspecified inflammatory disease of uterus

> Endometritis
> Endomyometritis
> Intrauterine infection
> Metritis
> Myometritis
> Perimetritis
> Pyometra
> Uterine abscess

☑4ᵗʰ 616 Inflammatory disease of cervix, vagina, and vulva

> **EXCLUDES** *that complicating:*
> *abortion (634-638 with .0, 639.0)*
> *ectopic or molar pregnancy (639.0)*
> *pregnancy, childbirth, or the puerperium (646.6)*

616.0 Cervicitis and endocervicitis

> Cervicitis ⎫ with or without mention of
> Endocervicitis ⎬ erosion or ectropion
>
> Nabothian (gland) cyst or follicle
> **EXCLUDES** *erosion or ectropion without mention of cervicitis (622.0)*

☑5ᵗʰ 616.1 Vaginitis and vulvovaginitis

> **EXCLUDES** *vulvar vestibulitis (625.71)*
> **DEF:** Inflammation or infection of vagina or external female genitalia.

616.10 Vaginitis and vulvovaginitis, unspecified

> Vaginitis:
> NOS
> postirradiation
> Vulvitis NOS
> Vulvovaginitis NOS
> Use additional code to identify organism, such as:
> Escherichia coli [E. coli] (041.41-041.49)
> Staphylococcus (041.10-041.19)
> Streptococcus (041.00-041.09)
> **EXCLUDES** *noninfective leukorrhea (623.5)*
> *postmenopausal or senile vaginitis (627.3)*

616.11 Vaginitis and vulvovaginitis in diseases classified elsewhere

> Code first underlying disease, as:
> pinworm vaginitis (127.4)
> **EXCLUDES** *herpetic vulvovaginitis (054.11)*
> *monilial vulvovaginitis (112.1)*
> *trichomonal vaginitis or vulvovaginitis (131.01)*

616.2 Cyst of Bartholin's gland

> Bartholin's duct cyst
> **DEF:** Fluid-filled sac within gland of vaginal orifice.

616.3 Abscess of Bartholin's gland

> Vulvovaginal gland abscess

616.4 Other abscess of vulva

> Abscess ⎫
> Carbuncle ⎬ of vulva
> Furuncle ⎭

☑5ᵗʰ 616.5 Ulceration of vulva

616.50 Ulceration of vulva, unspecified

> Ulcer NOS of vulva

616.51 Ulceration of vulva in diseases classified elsewhere

> Code first underlying disease, as:
> Behçet's syndrome (136.1)
> tuberculosis (016.7)
> **EXCLUDES** *vulvar ulcer (in):*
> *gonococcal (098.0)*
> *herpes simplex (054.12)*
> *syphilitic (091.0)*

☑5ᵗʰ 616.8 Other specified inflammatory diseases of cervix, vagina, and vulva

> **EXCLUDES** *noninflammatory disorders of:*
> *cervix (622.0-622.9)*
> *vagina (623.0-623.9)*
> *vulva (624.0-624.9)*

616.81 Mucositis (ulcerative) of cervix, vagina, and vulva

> Use additional E code to identify adverse effects of therapy, such as:
> antineoplastic and immunosuppressive drugs (E930.7, E933.1)
> radiation therapy (E879.2)

616.89 Other inflammatory disease of cervix, vagina and vulva

> Caruncle, vagina or labium
> Ulcer, vagina

616.9 Unspecified inflammatory disease of cervix, vagina, and vulva

OTHER DISORDERS OF FEMALE GENITAL TRACT (617-629)

☑4ᵗʰ 617 Endometriosis

617.0 Endometriosis of uterus

> Adenomyosis
> Endometriosis:
> cervix
> Endometriosis:
> internal
> myometrium
> **EXCLUDES** *stromal endometriosis (236.0)*
> **DEF:** Aberrant uterine mucosal tissue; creating products of menses and inflamed uterine tissues.

Female Genitourinary System

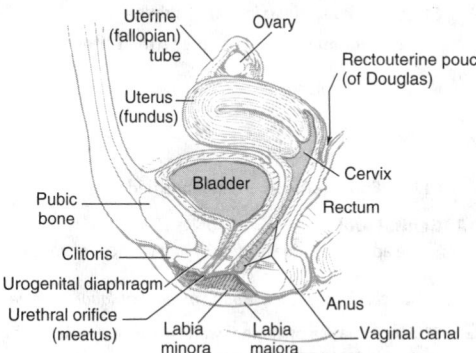

Uterine (fallopian) tube — Ovary — Rectouterine pouch (of Douglas) — Uterus (fundus) — Cervix — Bladder — Rectum — Pubic bone — Clitoris — Urogenital diaphragm — Anus — Urethral orifice (meatus) — Labia minora — Labia majora — Vaginal canal

Common Sites of Endometriosis

Common sites of endometriosis, in descending order of frequency:
(1) ovary
(2) cul de sac
(3) uterosacral ligaments
(4) broad ligaments
(5) fallopian tube
(6) uterovesical fold
(7) round ligament
(8) vermiform appendix
(9) vagina
(10) rectovaginal septum

Vaginal Midline Cystocele

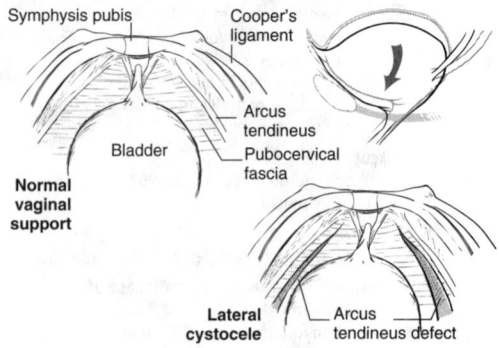

Vaginal Lateral Cystocele

Types of Vaginal Hernias

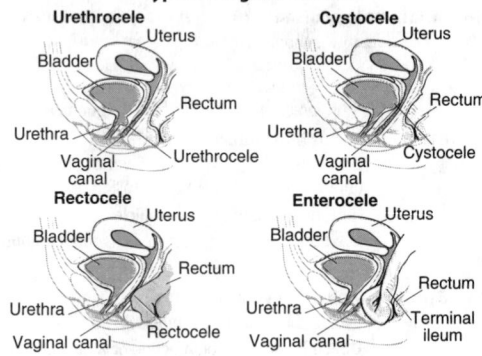

617.1 Endometriosis of ovary
Chocolate cyst of ovary
Endometrial cystoma of ovary
DEF: Aberrant uterine tissue; creating products of menses and inflamed ovarian tissues.

617.2 Endometriosis of fallopian tube
DEF: Aberrant uterine tissue; creating products of menses and inflamed tissues of fallopian tubes.

617.3 Endometriosis of pelvic peritoneum
Endometriosis:
broad ligament
cul-de-sac (Douglas')
parametrium
round ligament
DEF: Aberrant uterine tissue; creating products of menses and inflamed peritoneum tissues.

617.4 Endometriosis of rectovaginal septum and vagina
DEF: Aberrant uterine tissue; creating products of menses and inflamed tissues in and behind vagina.

617.5 Endometriosis of intestine
Endometriosis: Endometriosis:
appendix   rectum
colon
DEF: Aberrant uterine tissue; creating products of menses and inflamed intestinal tissues.

617.6 Endometriosis in scar of skin

617.8 Endometriosis of other specified sites
Endometriosis:
bladder
lung
umbilicus
vulva

617.9 Endometriosis, site unspecified

✓4ᵗʰ **618 Genital prolapse**
Use additional code to identify urinary incontinence (625.6, 788.31, 788.33-788.39)
EXCLUDES *that complicating pregnancy, labor, or delivery (654.4)*

✓5ᵗʰ **618.0 Prolapse of vaginal walls without mention of uterine prolapse**
EXCLUDES *that with uterine prolapse (618.2-618.4)*
enterocele (618.6)
vaginal vault prolapse following hysterectomy (618.5)

618.00 Unspecified prolapse of vaginal walls
Vaginal prolapse NOS

618.01 Cystocele, midline
Cystocele NOS
DEF: Defect in the pubocervical fascia, the supportive layer of the bladder, causing bladder drop and herniated into the vagina along the midline.

618.02 Cystocele, lateral
Paravaginal
DEF: Loss of support of the lateral attachment of the vagina at the arcus tendinous results in bladder drop; bladder herniates into the vagina laterally.

618.03 Urethrocele

618.04 Rectocele
Proctocele
Use additional code for any associated fecal incontinence (787.60-787.63)

618.05 Perineocele

618.09 Other prolapse of vaginal walls without mention of uterine prolapse
Cystourethrocele

618.1 Uterine prolapse without mention of vaginal wall prolapse
Descensus uteri
Uterine prolapse:
NOS
complete
first degree
second degree
third degree
EXCLUDES *that with mention of cystocele, urethrocele, or rectocele (618.2-618.4)*

618.2 Uterovaginal prolapse, incomplete
DEF: Downward displacement of uterus downward into vagina.

618.3 Uterovaginal prolapse, complete
DEF: Downward displacement of uterus exposed within external genitalia.

618.4 Uterovaginal prolapse, unspecified

618.5 Prolapse of vaginal vault after hysterectomy

618.6 Vaginal enterocele, congenital or acquired
Pelvic enterocele, congenital or acquired
DEF: Vaginal vault hernia formed by the loop of the small intestine protruding into the rectal vaginal pouch; can also accompany uterine prolapse or follow hysterectomy.

618.7 Old laceration of muscles of pelvic floor

✓5ᵗʰ **618.8 Other specified genital prolapse**

618.81 Incompetence or weakening of pubocervical tissue

618.82   **Incompetence or weakening of rectovaginal tissue**

618.83   **Pelvic muscle wasting**
Disuse atrophy of pelvic muscles and anal sphincter

618.84   **Cervical stump prolapse**

618.89   **Other specified genital prolapse**

618.9   **Unspecified genital prolapse**

√4ᵗʰ **619   Fistula involving female genital tract**
EXCLUDES   *vesicorectal and intestinovesical fistula (596.1)*

619.0   **Urinary-genital tract fistula, femal**
Fistula:
cervicovesical
ureterovaginal
urethrovaginal
urethrovesicovaginal
uteroureteric
uterovesical
vesicocervicovaginal
vesicovaginal

619.1   **Digestive-genital tract fistula, female**
Fistula: Fistula:
intestinouterine   rectovulval
intestinovaginal   sigmoidovaginal
rectovaginal   uterorectal

619.2   **Genital tract-skin fistula, female**
Fistula:
uterus to abdominal wall
vaginoperineal

619.8   **Other specified fistulas involving female genital tract**
Fistula:
cervix
cul-de-sac (Douglas')
uterus
vagina
DEF: Abnormal communication between female reproductive tract and skin.

619.9   **Unspecified fistula involving female genital tract**

√4ᵗʰ **620   Noninflammatory disorders of ovary, fallopian tube, and broad ligament**
EXCLUDES   *hydrosalpinx (614.1)*

620.0   **Follicular cyst of ovary**
Cyst of graafian follicle
DEF: Fluid-filled, encapsulated cyst due to occluded follicle duct that secretes hormones into ovaries.

620.1   **Corpus luteum cyst or hematoma**
Corpus luteum hemorrhage or rupture
Lutein cyst
DEF: Fluid-filled cyst due to serous developing from corpus luteum or clotted blood.

620.2   **Other and unspecified ovarian cyst**
Cyst:
NOS
corpus albicans
retention NOS   } of ovary
serous
theca-lutein
Simple cystoma of ovary
EXCLUDES   *cystadenoma (benign) (serous) (220)*
developmental cysts (752.0)
neoplastic cysts (220)
polycystic ovaries (256.4)
Stein-Leventhal syndrome (256.4)

620.3   **Acquired atrophy of ovary and fallopian tube**
Senile involution of ovary

620.4   **Prolapse or hernia of ovary and fallopian tube**
Displacement of ovary and fallopian tube
Salpingocele

620.5   **Torsion of ovary, ovarian pedicle, or fallopian tube**
Torsion:
accessory tube
hydatid of Morgagni

Uterus and Ovaries

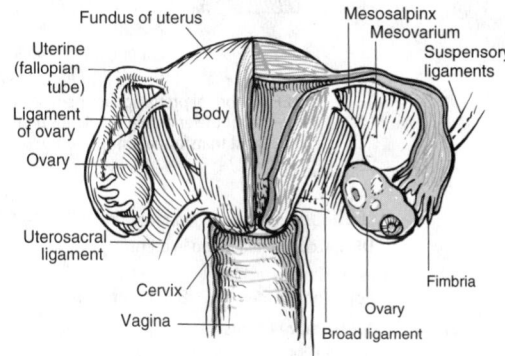

620.6   **Broad ligament laceration syndrome**
Masters-Allen syndrome

620.7   **Hematoma of broad ligament**
Hematocele, broad ligament
DEF: Blood within peritoneal fold that supports uterus.

620.8   **Other noninflammatory disorders of ovary, fallopian tube, and broad ligament**
Cyst
Polyp   } of broad ligament or fallopian tube

Infarction
Rupture   } of ovary or fallopian tube
Hematosalpinx
EXCLUDES   *hematosalpinx in ectopic pregnancy (639.2)*
peritubal adhesions (614.6)
torsion of ovary, ovarian pedicle, or fallopian tube (620.5)

620.9   **Unspecified noninflammatory disorder of ovary, fallopian tube, and broad ligament**

√4ᵗʰ **621   Disorders of uterus, not elsewhere classified**

621.0   **Polyp of corpus uteri**
Polyp:
endometrium
uterus NOS
EXCLUDES   *cervical polyp NOS (622.7)*

621.1   **Chronic subinvolution of uterus**
EXCLUDES   *puerperal (674.8)*
DEF: Abnormal size of uterus after delivery; the uterus does not return to its normal size after the birth of a child.

621.2   **Hypertrophy of uterus**
Bulky or enlarged uterus
EXCLUDES   *puerperal (674.8)*

√5ᵗʰ 621.3   **Endometrial hyperplasia**
DEF: Abnormal cystic overgrowth of endometrial tissue.

621.30   **Endometrial hyperplasia, unspecified**
Endometrial hyperplasia NOS
Hyperplasia (adenomatous) (cystic) (glandular) of endometrium
Hyperplastic endometritis

621.31   **Simple endometrial hyperplasia without atypia**
EXCLUDES   *benign endometrial hyperplasia (621.34)*

621.32   **Complex endometrial hyperplasia without atypia**
EXCLUDES   *benign endometrial hyperplasia (621.34)*

621.33   **Endometrial hyperplasia with atypia**
EXCLUDES   *endometrial intraepithelial neoplasia [EIN] (621.35)*

621.34   **Benign endometrial hyperplasia**
DEF: Excessive cell growth of the endometrium due to primary hormonal changes (menopause) that result in secondary effects to the endometrial stroma and associated structures.

Diseases of the Genitourinary System

621.35–623.4

621.35 Endometrial intraepithelial neoplasia [EIN]
EXCLUDES malignant neoplasm of endometrium with endometrial intraepithelial neoplasia [EIN] (182.0)

DEF: Abnormal premalignant neoplastic changes of the endometrial glands prone to malignant transformation.

621.4 Hematometra
Hemometra
EXCLUDES that in congenital anomaly (752.2-752.39)
DEF: Accumulated blood in uterus.

621.5 Intrauterine synechiae
Adhesions of uterus   Band(s) of uterus

621.6 Malposition of uterus
Anteversion
Retroflexion   } of uterus
Retroversion
EXCLUDES malposition complicating pregnancy, labor, or delivery (654.3-654.4)

621.7 Chronic inversion of uterus
EXCLUDES current obstetrical trauma (665.2)
prolapse of uterus (618.1-618.4)

621.8 Other specified disorders of uterus, not elsewhere classified
Atrophy, acquired
Cyst
Fibrosis NOS   } of uterus
Old laceration (postpartum)
Ulcer
EXCLUDES bilharzial fibrosis (120.0-120.9)
endometriosis (617.0)
fistulas (619.0-619.8)
inflammatory diseases (615.0-615.9)

621.9 Unspecified disorder of uterus

✓4ᵗʰ **622 Noninflammatory disorders of cervix**
EXCLUDES abnormality of cervix complicating pregnancy, labor, or delivery (654.5-654.6)
fistula (619.0-619.8)

622.0 Erosion and ectropion of cervix
Eversion
Ulcer   } of cervix
EXCLUDES that in chronic cervicitis (616.0)
DEF: Ulceration or turning outward of uterine cervix.

✓5ᵗʰ **622.1 Dysplasia of cervix (uteri)**
EXCLUDES abnormal results from cervical cytologic examination without histologic confirmation (795.00-795.09)
carcinoma in situ of cervix (233.1)
cervical intraepithelial neoplasia III [CIN III] (233.1)
HGSIL of cervix (795.04)
DEF: Abnormal cell structures in portal between uterus and vagina.

622.10 Dysplasia of cervix, unspecified
Anaplasia of cervix
Cervical atypism
Cervical dysplasia NOS

622.11 Mild dysplasia of cervix
Cervical intraepithelial neoplasia I [CIN I]

622.12 Moderate dysplasia of cervix
Cervical intraepithelial neoplasia II [CIN II]
EXCLUDES carcinoma in situ of cervix (233.1)
cervical intraepithelial neo-plasia III [CIN III] (233.1)
severe dysplasia (233.1)

622.2 Leukoplakia of cervix (uteri)
EXCLUDES carcinoma in situ of cervix (233.1)
DEF: Thickened, white patches on portal between uterus and vagina.

622.3 Old laceration of cervix
Adhesions
Band(s)   } of cervix
Cicatrix (postpartum)
EXCLUDES current obstetrical trauma (665.3)
DEF: Scarring or other evidence of old wound on cervix.

622.4 Stricture and stenosis of cervix
Atresia (acquired)
Contracture   } of cervix
Occlusion
Pinpoint os uteri
EXCLUDES congenital (752.49)
that complicating labor (654.6)

622.5 Incompetence of cervix
EXCLUDES complicating pregnancy (654.5)
that affecting fetus or newborn (761.0)
DEF: Inadequate functioning of cervix; marked by abnormal widening during pregnancy; causing miscarriage.

622.6 Hypertrophic elongation of cervix
DEF: Overgrowth of cervix tissues extending down into vagina.

622.7 Mucous polyp of cervix
Polyp NOS of cervix
EXCLUDES adenomatous polyp of cervix (219.0)

622.8 Other specified noninflammatory disorders of cervix
Atrophy (senile)
Cyst
Fibrosis   } of cervix
Hemorrhage
EXCLUDES endometriosis (617.0)
fistula (619.0-619.8)
inflammatory diseases (616.0)

622.9 Unspecified noninflammatory disorder of cervix

✓4ᵗʰ **623 Noninflammatory disorders of vagina**
EXCLUDES abnormality of vagina complicating pregnancy, labor, or delivery (654.7)
congenital absence of vagina (752.49)
congenital diaphragm or bands (752.49)
fistulas involving vagina (619.0-619.8)

623.0 Dysplasia of vagina
Mild and moderate dysplasia of vagina
Vaginal intraepithelial neoplasia I and II [VAIN I and II]
EXCLUDES abnormal results from vaginal cytological examination without histologic confirmation (795.10-795.19)
carcinoma in situ of vagina (233.31)
HGSIL of vagina (795.14)
severe dysplasia of vagina (233.31)
vaginal intraepithelial neoplasia III [VAIN III] (233.31)

623.1 Leukoplakia of vagina
DEF: Thickened white patches on vaginal canal.

623.2 Stricture or atresia of vagina
Adhesions (postoperative) (postradiation) of vagina
Occlusion of vagina
Stenosis, vagina
Use additional E code to identify any external cause
EXCLUDES congenital atresia or stricture (752.49)

623.3 Tight hymenal ring
Rigid hymen
Tight hymenal ring   } acquired or congenital
Tight introitus
EXCLUDES imperforate hymen (752.42)

623.4 Old vaginal laceration
EXCLUDES old laceration involving muscles of pelvic floor (618.7)
DEF: Scarring or other evidence of old wound on vagina.

623.5   **Leukorrhea, not specified as infective**
Leukorrhea NOS of vagina
Vaginal discharge NOS
EXCLUDES   trichomonal (131.00)
DEF: Viscid whitish discharge from vagina.

623.6   **Vaginal hematom**
EXCLUDES   current obstetrical trauma (665.7)

623.7   **Polyp of vagina**

623.8   **Other specified noninflammatory disorders of vagina**
Cyst
Hemorrhage } of vagina

623.9   **Unspecified noninflammatory disorder of vagina**

√4ᵗʰ   **624**   **Noninflammatory disorders of vulva and perineum**
EXCLUDES   abnormality of vulva and perineum complicating
pregnancy, labor, or delivery (654.8)
condyloma acuminatum (078.11)
fistulas involving:
perineum–see Alphabetic Index
vulva (619.0-619.8)
vulval varices (456.6)
vulvar involvement in skin conditions (690-709.9)

√5ᵗʰ   **624.0**   **Dystrophy of vulva**
EXCLUDES   carcinoma in situ of vulva (233.32)
severe dysplasia of vulva (233.32)
vulvar intraepithelial neoplasia III
[VIN III] (233.32)

     624.01   **Vulvar intraepithelial neoplasia I [VIN I]**
Mild dysplasia of vulva

     624.02   **Vulvar intraepithelial neoplasia II [VIN II]**
Moderate dysplasia of vulva

     624.09   **Other dystrophy of vulva**
Kraurosis of vulva
Leukoplakia of vulva

624.1   **Atrophy of vulva**

624.2   **Hypertrophy of clitoris**
EXCLUDES   that in endocrine disorders (255.2, 256.1)

624.3   **Hypertrophy of labia**
Hypertrophy of vulva NOS
DEF: Overgrowth of fleshy folds on either side of vagina.

624.4   **Old laceration or scarring of vulva**
DEF: Scarring or other evidence of old wound on external
female genitalia.

624.5   **Hematoma of vulva**
EXCLUDES   that complicating delivery (664.5)
DEF: Blood in tissue of external genitalia.

624.6   **Polyp of labia and vulva**

624.8   **Other specified noninflammatory disorders of vulva
and perineum**
Cyst
Edema } of vulva
Stricture

624.9   **Unspecified noninflammatory disorder of vulva and
perineum**

√4ᵗʰ   **625**   **Pain and other symptoms associated with female genital
organs**

625.0   **Dyspareunia**
EXCLUDES   psychogenic dyspareunia (302.76)
DEF: Difficult or painful sexual intercourse.

625.1   **Vaginismus**
Colpospasm
Vulvismus
EXCLUDES   psychogenic vaginismus (306.51)
DEF: Vaginal spasms; due to involuntary contraction of
musculature; prevents intercourse.

625.2   **Mittelschmerz**
Intermenstrual pain
Ovulation pain
DEF: Pain occurring between menstrual periods.

625.3   **Dysmenorrhea**
Painful menstruation
EXCLUDES   psychogenic dysmenorrhea (306.52)

625.4   **Premenstrual tension syndromes**
Menstrual molimen
Premenstrual dysphoric disorder
Premenstrual syndrome
Premenstrual tension NOS
EXCLUDES   menstrual migraine (346.4)

625.5   **Pelvic congestion syndrome**
Congestion-fibrosis syndrome
Taylor's syndrome
DEF: Excessive accumulation of blood in vessels of pelvis;
may occur after orgasm; causes abnormal menstruation,
lower back pain and vaginal discharge.

625.6   **Stress incontinence, female**
EXCLUDES   mixed incontinence (788.33)
stress incontinence, male (788.32)
DEF: Involuntary leakage of urine due to insufficient
sphincter control; occurs upon sneezing, laughing,
coughing, sudden movement or lifting.

√5ᵗʰ   **625.7**   **Vulvodynia**
DEF: Vulvar pain without an identifiable cause that
persists for three months or longer.

     625.70   **Vulvodynia, unspecified**
Vulvodynia NOS

     625.71   **Vulvar vestibulitis**

     625.79   **Other vulvodynia**

625.8   **Other specified symptoms associated with female
genital organs**

625.9   **Unspecified symptom associated with female genital
organs**

√4ᵗʰ   **626**   **Disorders of menstruation and other abnormal bleeding
from female genital tract**
EXCLUDES   menopausal and premenopausal bleeding (627.0)
pain and other symptoms associated with menstrual
cycle (625.2-625.4)
postmenopausal bleeding (627.1)
precocious puberty (259.1)

626.0   **Absence of menstruation**
Amenorrhea (primary) (secondary)

626.1   **Scanty or infrequent menstruation**
Hypomenorrhea   Oligomenorrhea

626.2   **Excessive or frequent menstruation**
Heavy periods
Menometrorrhagia
Menorrhagia
Plymenorrhea
EXCLUDES   premenopausal (627.0)
that in puberty (626.3)

626.3   **Puberty bleeding**
Excessive bleeding associated with onset of menstrual
periods
Pubertal menorrhagia

626.4   **Irregular menstrual cycle**
Irregular:
bleeding NOS
menstruation
periods

626.5   **Ovulation bleeding**
Regular intermenstrual bleeding

626.6   **Metrorrhagia**
Bleeding unrelated to menstrual cycle
Irregular intermenstrual bleeding

626.7   **Postcoital bleeding**
DEF: Bleeding from vagina after sexual intercourse.

626.8   **Other**
Dysfunctional or functional uterine hemorrhage NOS
Menstruation:
retained
suppression of

626.9　**Unspecified**

√4ᵗʰ　**627　Menopausal and postmenopausal disorders**
　　EXCLUDES　*asymptomatic age-related (natural)*
　　　　　　postmenopausal status (V49.81)

627.0　**Premenopausal menorrhagia**
　　Excessive bleeding associated with onset of menopause
　　Menorrhagia:
　　　climacteric
　　　menopausal
　　　preclimacteric

627.1　**Postmenopausal bleeding**

627.2　**Symptomatic menopausal or female climacteric states**
　　Symptoms, such as flushing, sleeplessness, headache,
　　　lack of concentration, associated with the
　　　menopause

627.3　**Postmenopausal atrophic vaginitis**
　　Senile (atrophic) vaginitis

627.4　**Symptomatic states associated with artificial menopause**
　　Postartificial menopause syndromes
　　Any condition classifiable to 627.1, 627.2, or 627.3 which
　　　follows induced menopause
　　DEF: Conditions arising after hysterectomy.

627.8　**Other specified menopausal and postmenopausal disorders**
　　　EXCLUDES　*premature menopause NOS (256.31)*

627.9　**Unspecified menopausal and postmenopausal disorder**

√4ᵗʰ　**628　Infertility, female**
　　INCLUDES　primary and secondary sterility
　　DEF: Infertility: inability to conceive for at least one year with
　　regular intercourse.
　　DEF: Primary infertility: occurring in patients who have never
　　conceived.
　　DEF: Secondary infertility: occurring in patients who have
　　previously conceived.

628.0　**Associated with anovulation**
　　Anovulatory cycle
　　Use additional code for any associated Stein-Leventhal
　　　syndrome (256.4)

628.1　*Of pituitary-hypothalamic origin*
　　Code first underlying cause, as:
　　　adiposogenital dystrophy (253.8)
　　　anterior pituitary disorder (253.0-253.4)

628.2　**Of tubal origin**
　　Infertility associated with congenital anomaly of tube
　　Tubal:
　　　block
　　　occlusion
　　　stenosis
　　Use additional code for any associated peritubal
　　　adhesions (614.6)

628.3　**Of uterine origin**
　　Infertility associated with congenital anomaly of uterus
　　Nonimplantation
　　Use additional code for any associated tuberculous
　　　endometritis (016.7)

628.4　**Of cervical or vaginal origin**
　　Infertility associated with:
　　　anomaly of cervical mucus
　　　congenital structural anomaly
　　　dysmucorrhea

628.8　**Of other specified origin**

628.9　**Of unspecified origin**

√4ᵗʰ　**629　Other disorders of female genital organs**

629.0　**Hematocele, female, not elsewhere classified**
　　　EXCLUDES　*hematocele or hematoma:*
　　　　　broad ligament (620.7)
　　　　　fallopian tube (620.8)
　　　　　that associated with ectopic pregnancy
　　　　　　(633.00-633.91)
　　　　　uterus (621.4)
　　　　　vagina (623.6)
　　　　　vulva (624.5)

629.1　**Hydrocele, canal of Nuck**
　　Cyst of canal of Nuck (acquired)
　　　EXCLUDES　*congenital (752.41)*

√5ᵗʰ　629.2　**Female genital mutilation status**
　　Female circumcision status
　　Female genital cutting

629.20　**Female genital mutilation status, unspecified**
　　Female genital cutting status, unspecified
　　Female genital mutilation status NOS

629.21　**Female genital mutilation Type I status**
　　Clitorectomy status
　　Female genital cutting Type I status
　　DEF: Female genital mutilation involving
　　clitorectomy, with part or all of the clitoris
　　removed.

629.22　**Female genital mutilation Type II status**
　　Clitorectomy with excision of labia
　　　minora status
　　Female genital cutting Type II status
　　DEF: Female genital mutilation involving clitoris
　　and the labia minora amputation.

629.23　**Female genital mutilation Type III status**
　　Female genital cutting Type III status
　　Infibulation status
　　DEF: Female genital mutilation involving
　　removal, most or all of the labia minora excised,
　　labia majora incised which is then made into a
　　hood of skin over the urethral and vaginal
　　opening.

629.29　**Other female genital mutilation status**
　　Female genital cutting Type IV status
　　Female genital mutilation Type IV status
　　Other female genital cutting status

√5ᵗʰ　629.3　**Complication of implanted vaginal mesh and other prosthetic materials**

629.31　**Erosion of implanted vaginal mesh and other prosthetic materials to surrounding organ or tissue**
　　Erosion of implanted vaginal mesh and other
　　　prosthetic materials into pelvic floor
　　　muscles

629.32　**Exposure of implanted vaginal mesh and other prosthetic materials into vagina**
　　Exposure of vaginal mesh and other prosthetic
　　　materials through vaginal wall

√5ᵗʰ　629.8　**Other specified disorders of female genital organs**

629.81　**Recurrent pregnancy loss without current pregnancy**
　　　EXCLUDES　*recurrent pregnancy loss with*
　　　　　current pregnancy (646.3)

629.89　**Other specified disorders of female genital organs**

629.9　**Unspecified disorder of female genital organs**

Chapter 11: Complications of Pregnancy, Childbirth, and the Puerperium (630–679)

Coding Guidance

Chapter 11 of the tabular list provides codes for normal delivery as well as for obstetrical complications. Obstetrical terms can be found in the alphabetic index under the main terms "Pregnancy," Delivery," "Labor," and "Puerperal." The coder must decide whether the condition specified in the diagnostic statement is a complication of the pregnancy, labor or delivery, or whether it occurred after delivery.

The categories in chapter 11 are:

- Ectopic and molar pregnancy (630–633)
- Other pregnancy with abortive outcome (634–639)
- Complications mainly related to pregnancy (640–649)
- Normal delivery, and other indications for care in pregnancy, labor and delivery (650–659)
- Complications occurring mainly in the course of labor and delivery (660–669)
- Complications of the puerperium (670–677)
- Other maternal and fetal complications contains two categories: 678 Other fetal conditions and 679 Complications of in utero procedures.

Ectopic and Molar Pregnancy (630–633)

An hydatidiform mole (630) is an abnormal product of conception that results in a mass of cells that resembles a bunch of grapes. This condition is also called cystic or vesicular mole.

Missed abortion (632) is the retention of a fetus before completion of 22 weeks of gestation for at least four weeks after fetal demise. (This period of time varies according to state law. It may be as few as 19 weeks.) This excludes retained products of conception following spontaneous (634) or induced abortion (637), delivery, or missed delivery (656.4x).

Ectopic pregnancy (633) is the implantation of fertilized ovum in an anatomic location other than the uterus. The most common site of ectopic pregnancy is the fallopian tube, but it may occur in other locations of the body such as the abdomen, ovary, or cervix.

Legally Induced Abortion (635)

Legally induced abortion is the termination of a pregnancy with removal of some but not all of the products of conception, with or without an identifiable fetus weighing less than 500 grams or before completion of 22 weeks of gestation for therapeutic or elective reasons.

Terms that apply to this category are:

- Termination of pregnancy
- Elective abortion
- Legal abortion
- Therapeutic abortion

Fourth-digit subcategories specify complications that arise during the current episode of care.

Fifth-digit assignment indicates the stage of the abortion as, unspecified, incomplete, or complete. Generally, induced abortions are complete at the time of initial episode of care and a fifth digit of "2" is assigned.

Use an additional code from categories 640–648 and 651–657 to identify the complication or reason for the induced abortion. When assigning these additional codes use the fifth digit of "3," antepartum condition or complication. For example the reason for the termination of pregnancy is maternal primary genital syphilis. Code as follows:

Example:

635.42   Legally induced abortion complicated by metabolic disorder, complete

647.03   Maternal syphilis complicating pregnancy, childbirth or puerperium, antepartum condition, or complication

091.0   Genital syphilis, primary

Complications Following Abortion and Ectopic and Molar Pregnancy (639)

Complications under the 639 category include:

- Genital tract and pelvic infection (639.0)
- Delayed or excessive hemorrhage (639.1)
- Damage to the pelvic organs or tissues (639.2)
- Renal failure (639.3)
- Metabolic disorders (electrolyte imbalance) (639.4)
- Shock (639.5)
- Embolism (639.6)
- Other specified complication (cardiac arrest, UTI, cerebral anoxia, etc.) (639.8)
- Unspecified complication (639.9)

Complications Mainly Related to Pregnancy (640–649)

These codes describe conditions that affect the management of labor, pregnancy or delivery, and the puerperium, even if the condition was present before pregnancy. Multiple coding may be necessary to fully describe complications relating to the pregnancy. Sequencing of the codes depends upon the main focus of and the reason for the episode of care.

Categories include:

- Hemorrhage in early pregnancy (640)
- Antepartum hemorrhage, abruptio placentae and placenta previa (641)
- Hypertension complicating pregnancy, childbirth, and the puerperium (642)
- Excessive vomiting in pregnancy (643)
- Early or threatened labor (644)
- Late pregnancy (645)
- Other complications, not elsewhere classified (646)
- Infectious and parasitic conditions in the mother classifiable elsewhere but complicating pregnancy, childbirth, or the puerperium (647)
- Other current conditions in the mother classifiable elsewhere but complicating pregnancy, childbirth or the puerperium (648)
- Other conditions or status of the mother complicating pregnancy, childbirth or puerperium (649) are general guidelines to follow when coding complications of pregnancy, childbirth or the puerperium classifiable to categories 640–649.

The following are general guidelines to follow when coding complications of pregnancy, childbirth, or the puerperium classifiable to categories 640–649:

First, the fourth-digit subcategories generally add specificity to the described complication.

The fifth-digit subclassification denotes the current episode of care or the stage of pregnancy, childbirth or puerperium at which the complication occurred.

0   Unspecified as to episode of care or not applicable

1   Delivered, with or without mention of antepartum condition

2   Delivered, with mention of postpartum complication

3   Antepartum condition or complication (delivery does not occur during this episode of care)

4   Postpartum condition or complication (following previous episode of care resulting in delivery)

Multiple coding is used to fully describe the complications affecting the pregnancy, childbirth, and the puerperium. Appropriate fifth-digit assignment is needed to specify the episode of care and the stage during which the complication arose.

A postpartum complication is any complication occurring within the six-week period following delivery. Codes from this section may also be used to describe pregnancy-related complications after the six-week period should the physician document that a condition is pregnancy related. Postpartum complications that occur during the same admission as the delivery are identified with a fifth digit of "2." Subsequent admissions for postpartum complications should be identified with a fifth digit of "4."

Complications Occurring Mainly in the Course of Labor and Delivery (660-669)

Anal Sphincter Tear Complicating Delivery, Not Associated with Third-Degree Perineal Laceration (664.6x)

Anal sphincter tears can occur during delivery independent of third-degree lacerations, and such tears may not be identified until they complicate a subsequent delivery. Conversely, a third-degree tear may occur independently of an anal sphincter tear. Report code 664.6x Anal sphincter tear complicating delivery, when the anal sphincter tear complicates delivery but is not associated with a third-degree perineal laceration. When reporting code 664.6, assign the appropriate fifth digit to indicate episode of care.

Other Maternal and Fetal Complications (678–679)

Other Fetal Conditions (678)

Section "Other Maternal and Fetal Complications" includes categories 678 and 679. Valid fifth-digit subclassifications 0–4 are listed at the beginning of the section and are required to denote the episode of care. Category 679 contains two subcategories: one representing maternal complications and one representing fetal complications from in utero procedures.

Category 678 includes two subcategories that classify both fetal hematological conditions (678.0) and fetal conjoined twins (678.1). Fetal hemorrhagic conditions classified under this subcategory include only conditions affecting the fetus during pregnancy or affecting the management of the mother during delivery. These codes are reported on the mother's medical record. This subcategory excludes isoimmunization incompatability and fetal-maternal hemorrhage. Fetal hematological disorders include fetal anemia, whereby red blood cells are inadequately produced or are destroyed faster than they can be produced. Causal conditions include maternal-fetal incompatibility, viral infection, or other infectious process. If anemia is diagnosed or suspected, the pregnancy will require close observation, as it can be fatal for the fetus. Treatment of severe fetal anemia may include intrauterine blood transfusion.

Fetal thrombocytopenia is a potentially fatal condition whereby the fetus's platelet (blood clotting) cell count is abnormally low or deficient, possibly due to maternal-fetal immune incompatibility. Risks include fetal hemorrhage which, if it occurs in the central nervous system, can result in a fetal stroke. Early detection and treatment of fetal hematological disorders (678.0X) is essential to optimal outcomes. However, the procedures used to manage these diagnoses carry some risk to the pregnancy and fetus. Anemic infants may have short-term

complications from their anemia or low platelet counts after birth, requiring transfusions or other specialized treatments.

A pregnancy complicated by twin-to-twin transfusion syndrome (TTTS) carries significant risk of severe disabilities or death of one or both twins. TTTS occurs when monozygotic (identical) twins share the same placenta and blood vessels and results from an intrauterine blood transfusion from one twin to the other. If TTTS develops after 26 weeks, the babies can usually be delivered and have a greater chance of survival without disability. There are a number of different therapies used to treat TTTS, with varying rates of success, including serial amniocentesis from recipient twin, or fetoscopic laser ablation of communicating blood vessels.

Conjoined twins (678.1X) are identical twins that fail to completely separate into two individuals. They are most often joined at the head, chest, or pelvis and may share one or more internal organs. The success of separation surgery often depends on the anatomic site or sites of connection and which or how many organs are shared. Conjoined twins pose significant risks during pregnancy. Identification can be made by ultrasound imaging as early as the 12th week of pregnancy, with specific anatomic details apparent by the 20th week. Approximately half of conjoined twins develop excessive amniotic fluid (polyhydramnios), which increases the risk of premature rupture of the membranes, problems with the umbilical cord, and stillbirth. About 40 percent of conjoined twins are stillborn. Vaginal delivery is rarely possible. If the parents choose to continue the pregnancy, cesarean section delivery is usually required.

Complications from In Utero Procedures (679)

Fetal surgery is a relatively new surgical specialty that enables treatment of certain fetal conditions and anomalies previously considered untreatable. Diagnostic imaging technologies help in early detection of fetal anomalies and associated gestational risks. Conditions treatable by in utero surgery include:

- Twin-to-twin transfusion syndrome (TTTS) by laser photocoagulation
- Vasa previa by YAG laser photocoagulation of placental blood vessels
- Bladder outlet obstruction by cystoscopy-guided laser incision or vesicoamniotic shunting
- Myelomeningocele by open neurosurgical repair by hysterotomy
- Congenital cystic pulmonary adenoma by resection or thoracoamniotic shunt
- Sacrococcygeal teratoma by open surgical repair via hysterotomy
- Congenital diaphragmatic hernia repair by fetal tracheal occlusion

In utero interventional procedures provide opportunities to improve outcomes for pregnancies complicated by fetal conditions previously not amenable to treatment. However, these procedures are not without risk for both the fetus and the mother, depending on the nature of the diagnosis and type of intervention. The greatest risk is loss of fetal life by preterm labor, hemorrhage, or other surgical complication. For the mother, damage can occur to the uterus, precluding or complicating future pregnancies.

11. COMPLICATIONS OF PREGNANCY, CHILDBIRTH, AND THE PUERPERIUM (630-679)

ECTOPIC AND MOLAR PREGNANCY (630-633)

Use additional code from category 639 to identify any complications

630 Hydatidiform mole

Trophoblastic disease NOS
Vesicular mole

> **EXCLUDES** chorioadenoma (destruens) (236.1)
> chorionepithelioma (181)
> malignant hydatidiform mole (236.1)

DEF: Abnormal product of pregnancy; marked by mass of cysts resembling bunch of grapes due to chorionic villi proliferation, and dissolution; must be surgically removed.

✓4ᵗʰ 631 Other abnormal product of conception

631.0 Inappropriate change in quantitative human chorionic gonadotropin (hCG) in early pregnancy

Biochemical pregnancy
Chemical pregnancy
Inappropriate level of quantitative human chorionic gonadotropin (hCG) for gestational age in early pregnancy

> **EXCLUDES** blighted ovum (631.8)
> molar pregnancy (631.8)

631.8 Other abnormal products of conception

Blighted ovum

632 Missed abortion

Early fetal death before completion of 22 weeks' gestation with retention of dead fetus
Retained products of conception, not following spontaneous or induced abortion or delivery

> **EXCLUDES** failed induced abortion (638.0-638.9)
> fetal death (intrauterine) (late) (656.4)
> missed delivery (656.4)
> that with hydatidiform mole (630)
> that with other abnormal products of conception (631.8)

✓4ᵗʰ 633 Ectopic pregnancy

> **INCLUDES** ruptured ectopic pregnancy

DEF: Fertilized egg develops outside uterus.

✓5ᵗʰ 633.0 Abdominal pregnancy

Intraperitoneal pregnancy

633.00 Abdominal pregnancy without intrauterine pregnancy

633.01 Abdominal pregnancy with intrauterine pregnancy

✓5ᵗʰ 633.1 Tubal pregnancy

Fallopian pregnancy
Rupture of (fallopian) tube due to pregnancy
Tubal abortion

633.10 Tubal pregnancy without intrauterine pregnancy

633.11 Tubal pregnancy with intrauterine pregnancy

✓5ᵗʰ 633.2 Ovarian pregnancy

633.20 Ovarian pregnancy without intrauterine pregnancy

633.21 Ovarian pregnancy with intrauterine pregnancy

✓5ᵗʰ 633.8 Other ectopic pregnancy

Pregnancy:
  cervical
  combined
  cornual

Pregnancy:
  intraligamentous
  mesometric
  mural

Ectopic Pregnancy Sites

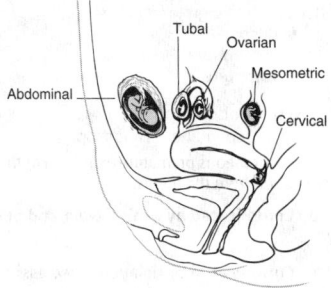

633.80 Other ectopic pregnancy without intrauterine pregnancy

633.81 Other ectopic pregnancy with intrauterine pregnancy

✓5ᵗʰ 633.9 Unspecified ectopic pregnancy

633.90 Unspecified ectopic pregnancy without intrauterine pregnancy

633.91 Unspecified ectopic pregnancy with intrauterine pregnancy

OTHER PREGNANCY WITH ABORTIVE OUTCOME (634-639)

The following fourth-digit subdivisions are for use with categories 634-638:

.0 Complicated by genital tract and pelvic infection

Endometritis
Salpingo-oophoritis
Sepsis NOS
Septicemia NOS
Any condition classifiable to 639.0 with condition classifiable to 634-638

> **EXCLUDES** urinary tract infection (634-638 with .7)

.1 Complicated by delayed or excessive hemorrhage

Afibrinogenemia
Defibrination syndrome
Intravascular hemolysis
Any condition classifiable to 639.1 with condition classifiable to 634-638

.2 Complicated by damage to pelvic organs and tissues

Laceration, perforation, or tear of:
  bladder
  uterus
Any condition classifiable to 639.2 with condition classifiable to 634-638

.3 Complicated by renal failure

Oliguria
Uremia
Any condition classifiable to 639.3, with condition classifiable to 634-638

.4 Complicated by metabolic disorder

Electrolyte imbalance with conditions classfiable to 634-638

.5 Complicated by shock

Circulatory collapse
Shock (postoperative) (septic)
Any condition classifiable to 639.5 with condition classifiable to 634-638

.6 Complicated by embolism

Embolism:
  NOS
  amniotic fluid
  pulmonary
Any condition classifiable to 639.6, with condition classifiable to 634-638

.7 With other specified complications

Cardiac arrest or failure
Urinary tract infection
Any condition classiable to 639.8 with condition classifiable to 634-638

.8 With unspecified complication

.9 Without mention of complication

Complications of Pregnancy, Childbirth, and the Puerperium   634–638.1

√4ᵗʰ **634 Spontaneous abortion**

Requires fifth digit to identify stage:
- **0 unspecified**
- **1 incomplete**
- **2 complete**

INCLUDES miscarriage
spontaneous abortion

DEF: Spontaneous premature expulsion of the products of conception from the uterus.

√5ᵗʰ **634.0 Complicated by genital tract and pelvic infection**
[0-2]

√5ᵗʰ **634.1 Complicated by delayed or excessive hemorrhage**
[0-2]

√5ᵗʰ **634.2 Complicated by damage to pelvic organs or tissues**
[0-2]

√5ᵗʰ **634.3 Complicated by renal failure**
[0-2]

√5ᵗʰ **634.4 Complicated by metabolic disorder**
[0-2]

√5ᵗʰ **634.5 Complicated by shock**
[0-2]

√5ᵗʰ **634.6 Complicated by embolism**
[0-2]

√5ᵗʰ **634.7 With other specified complications**
[0-2]

√5ᵗʰ **634.8 With unspecified complication**
[0-2]

√5ᵗʰ **634.9 Without mention of complication**
[0-2]

√4ᵗʰ **635 Legally induced abortion**

Requires fifth digit to identify stage:
- **0 unspecified**
- **1 incomplete**
- **2 complete**

INCLUDES abortion or termination of pregnancy:
elective
legal
therapeutic

EXCLUDES *menstrual extraction or regulation (V25.3)*

DEF: Intentional expulsion of products of conception from uterus performed by medical professionals inside boundaries of law.

√5ᵗʰ **635.0 Complicated by genital tract and pelvic infection**
[0-2]

√5ᵗʰ **635.1 Complicated by delayed or excessive hemorrhage**
[0-2]

√5ᵗʰ **635.2 Complicated by damage to pelvic organs or tissues**
[0-2]

√5ᵗʰ **635.3 Complicated by renal failure**
[0-2]

√5ᵗʰ **635.4 Complicated by metabolic disorder**
[0-2]

√5ᵗʰ **635.5 Complicated by shock**
[0-2]

√5ᵗʰ **635.6 Complicated by embolism**
[0-2]

√5ᵗʰ **635.7 With other specified complications**
[0-2]

√5ᵗʰ **635.8 With unspecified complication**
[0-2]

√5ᵗʰ **635.9 Without mention of complication**
[0-2]

√4ᵗʰ **636 Illegally induced abortion**

Requires fifth digit to identify stage:
- **0 unspecified**
- **1 incomplete**
- **2 complete**

INCLUDES abortion:
criminal
illegal
self-induced

DEF: Intentional expulsion of products of conception from uterus; outside boundaries of law.

√5ᵗʰ **636.0 Complicated by genital tract and pelvic infection**
[0-2]

√5ᵗʰ **636.1 Complicated by delayed or excessive hemorrhage**
[0-2]

√5ᵗʰ **636.2 Complicated by damage to pelvic organs or tissues**
[0-2]

√5ᵗʰ **636.3 Complicated by renal failure**
[0-2]

√5ᵗʰ **636.4 Complicated by metabolic disorder**
[0-2]

√5ᵗʰ **636.5 Complicated by shock**
[0-2]

√5ᵗʰ **636.6 Complicated by embolism**
[0-2]

√5ᵗʰ **636.7 With other specified complications**
[0-2]

√5ᵗʰ **636.8 With unspecified complication**
[0-2]

√5ᵗʰ **636.9 Without mention of complication**
[0-2]

√4ᵗʰ **637 Unspecified abortion**

Requires fifth digit to identify stage:
- **0 unspecified**
- **1 incomplete**
- **2 complete**

INCLUDES abortion NOS
retained products of conception following abortion, not classifiable elsewhere

√5ᵗʰ **637.0 Complicated by genital tract and pelvic infection**
[0-2]

√5ᵗʰ **637.1 Complicated by delayed or excessive hemorrhage**
[0-2]

√5ᵗʰ **637.2 Complicated by damage to pelvic organs or tissues**
[0-2]

√5ᵗʰ **637.3 Complicated by renal failure**
[0-2]

√5ᵗʰ **637.4 Complicated by metabolic disorder**
[0-2]

√5ᵗʰ **637.5 Complicated by shocc**
[0-2]

√5ᵗʰ **637.6 Complicated by embolism**
[0-2]

√5ᵗʰ **637.7 With other specified complications**
[0-2]

√5ᵗʰ **637.8 With unspecified complication**
[0-2]

√5ᵗʰ **637.9 Without mention of complication**
[0-2]

√4ᵗʰ **638 Failed attempted abortion**

INCLUDES failure of attempted induction of (legal) abortion
EXCLUDES *incomplete abortion (634.0-637.9)*

DEF: Continued pregnancy despite an attempted legal abortion.

638.0 Complicated by genital tract and pelvic infection

638.1 Complicated by delayed or excessive hemorrhage

638.2   **Complicated by damage to pelvic organs or tissues**

638.3   **Complicated by renal failure**

638.4   **Complicated by metabolic disorder**

638.5   **Complicated by shock**

638.6   **Complicated by embolism**

638.7   **With other specified complications**

638.8   **With unspecified complication**

638.9   **Without mention of complication**

√4th 639   **Complications following abortion and ectopic and molar pregnancies**

Note: This category is provided for use when it is required to classify separately the complications classifiable to the fourth-digit level in categories 634-638; for example:

a)   when the complication itself was responsible for an episode of medical care, the abortion, ectopic or molar pregnancy itself having been dealt with at a previous episode

b)   when these conditions are immediate complications of ectopic or molar pregnancies classifiable to 630-633 where they cannot be identified at fourth-digit level.

639.0   **Genital tract and pelvic infection**

Endometritis
Parametritis
Pelvic peritonitis
Salpingitis
Salpingo-oophoritis
Sepsis NOS
Septicemia NOS
} following conditions classifiable to 630-638

EXCLUDES *urinary tract infection (639.8)*

639.1   **Delayed or excessive hemorrhage**

Afibrinogenemia
Defibrination syndrome
Intravascular
} following conditions classifiable to 630-638

639.2   **Damage to pelvic organs and tissues**

Laceration, perforation, or tear of:
bladder
bowel
broad ligament
cervix
periurethral tissue
uterus
vagina
} following conditions classifiable to 630-638

639.3   **Kidney failure**

Oliguria
Renal (kidney):
failure (acute)
shutdown
tubular necrosis
Uremia
} following conditions classifiable to 630-638

639.4   **Metabolic disorders**

Electrolyte imbalance following conditions classifiable to 630-638

639.5   **Shock**

Circulatory collapse
Shock (postoperative)
(septic)
} following conditions classifiable to 630-638

639.6   **Embolism**

Embolism:
NOS
air
amniotic fluid
blood-clot
fat
pulmonary
pyemic
septic
soap
} following conditions classifiable to 630-638

Placenta Previa

Low (marginal) implantation   Partial placenta previa   Total placenta previa

Abruptio Placentae

Partial separation (concealed bleeding)   Partial separation (apparent hemorrhage)   Complete separation (concealed hemorrhage)

639.8   **Other specified complications following abortion or ectopic and molar pregnancy**

Acute yellow atrophy or necrosis of liver
Cardiac arrest or failure
Cerebral anoxia
Urinary tract infection
} following conditons classifiable to 630-638

639.9   **Unspecified complication following abortion or ectopic and molar pregnancy**

Complication(s) not further specified following conditions classifiable to 630-638

COMPLICATIONS MAINLY RELATED TO PREGNANCY (640-649)

INCLUDES   the listed conditions even if they arose or were present during labor, delivery, or the puerperium

The following fifth-digit subclassification is for use with categories 640-649 to denote the current episode of care. Valid fifth-digits are in [brackets] under each code.

0   **unspecified as to episode of care or not applicable**

1   **delivered, with or without mention of antepartum condition**

Antepartum condition with delivery
Delivery NOS (with mention of antepartum complication during current episode of care)
Intrapartum obstetric condition (with mention of antepartum complication during current episode of care)
Pregnancy, delivered (with mention of antepartum complication during current episode of care)

2   **delivered, with mention of postpartum complication**

Delivery with mention of puerperal complication during current episode of care

3   **antepartum condition or complication**

Antepartum obstetric condtion, not delivered during the current episode of care

4   **postpartum condition or complication**

Postpartum or puerperal obstetric condition or complication following delivery that occurred:
during previous episode of care
outside hospital, with subsequent admission for observation or care

√4th 640   **Hemorrhage in early pregnancy**

INCLUDES   hemorrhage before completion of 22 weeks' gestation

√5th 640.0   **Threatened abortion**

[0,1,3]   **DEF:** Bloody discharge during pregnancy; cervix may be dilated and pregnancy is threatened, but the pregnancy is not terminated.

Complications of Pregnancy, Childbirth, and the Puerperium

640.8–643.8

√5ᵗʰ **640.8 Other specified hemorrhage in early pregnancy**
[0,1,3]

√5ᵗʰ **640.9 Unspecified hemorrhage in early pregnancy**
[0,1,3]

√4ᵗʰ **641 Antepartum hemorrhage, abruptio placentae, and placenta previa**

√5ᵗʰ **641.0 Placenta previa without hemorrhage**
[0,1,3]
Low implantation of placenta
Placenta previa noted: } without
   during pregnancy   hemorrhage
   before labor (and delivered
     by caesarean delivery

DEF: Placenta implanted in lower segment of uterus; commonly causes hemorrhage in the last trimester of pregnancy.

√5ᵗʰ **641.1 Hemorrhage from placenta previa**
[0,1,3]
Low-lying placenta
Placenta previa
  incomplete } NOS or with hemorrhage
  marginal   (intrapartum)
  partial
  total
EXCLUDES *hemorrhage from vasa previa (663.5)*

√5ᵗʰ **641.2 Premature separation of placenta**
[0,1,3]
Ablatio placentae
Abruptio placentae
Accidental antepartum hemorrhage
Couvelaire uterus
Detachment of placenta (premature)
Premature separation of normally implanted placenta
DEF: Abruptio placentae: premature detachment of the placenta, characterized by shock, oliguria and decreased fibrinogen.

√5ᵗʰ **641.3 Antepartum hemorrhage associated with**
[0,1,3] **coagulation defects**
Antepartum or intrapartum hemorrhage associated with:
  afibrinogenemia
  hyperfibrinolysis
  hypofibrinogenemia
EXCLUDES *coagulation defects not associated with antepartum hemorrhage (649.3)*
DEF: Uterine hemorrhage prior to delivery.

√5ᵗʰ **641.8 Other antepartum hemorrhage**
[0,1,3]
Antepartum or intrapartum hemorrhage associated with:
  trauma
  uterine leiomyoma

√5ᵗʰ **641.9 Unspecified antepartum hemorrhage**
[0,1,3]
Hemorrhage: Hemorrhage:
  antepartum NOS   of pregnancy NOS
  intrapartum NOS

√4ᵗʰ **642 Hypertension complicating pregnancy, childbirth, and the puerperium**

√5ᵗʰ **642.0 Benign essential hypertension complicating**
[0-4] **pregnancy, childbirth, and the puerperium**
Hypertension   specified as complicating, or as
  benign essential   reason for obstetric care
  chronic NOS } during pregnancy,
  essential   childbirth, or the
  pre-existing NOS   puerperium

√5ᵗʰ **642.1 Hypertension secondary to renal disease, complicating**
[0-4] **pregnancy, childbirth, and the puerperium**
Hypertension secondary to renal disease, specified as complicating, or as a reason for obstetric care during pregnancy, childbirth, or the puerperium

√5ᵗʰ **642.2 Other pre-existing hypertension complicating**
[0-4] **pregnancy, childbirth, and the puerperium**
Hypertensive   specified as complicating,
  chronic kidney disease   or as a reason for
  heart and chronic } obstetric care during
   kidney disease   pregnancy,
  heart disease   childbirth, or the
Malignant hypertension   puerperium

√5ᵗʰ **642.3 Transient hypertension of pregnancy**
[0-4]
Gestational hypertension
Transient hypertension, so described, in pregnancy, childbirth, or the puerperium

√5ᵗʰ **642.4 Mild or unspecified pre-eclampsia**
[0-4]
Hypertension in pregnancy, childbirth, or the puerperium, not specified as pre-existing, with either albuminuria or edema, or both; mild or unspecified
Pre-eclampsia:
  NOS
  mild
Toxemia (pre-eclamptic):
  NOS
  mild
EXCLUDES *albuminuria in pregnancy, without mention of hypertension (646.2)*
edema in pregnancy, without mention of hypertension (646.1)

√5ᵗʰ **642.5 Severe pre-eclampsia**
[0-4]
Hypertension in pregnancy, childbirth, or the puerperium, not specified as pre-existing, with either albuminuria or edema, or both; specified as severe
Pre-eclampsia, severe
Toxemia (pre-eclamptic), severe

√5ᵗʰ **642.6 Eclampsia**
[0-4]
Toxemia:
  eclamptic
  with convulsions

√5ᵗʰ **642.7 Pre-eclampsia or eclampsia superimposed**
[0-4] **on pre-existing hypertension**
Conditions classifiable to 642.4-642.6, with conditions classifiable to 642.0-642.2

√5ᵗʰ **642.9 Unspecified hypertension complicating pregnancy,**
[0-4] **childbirth, or the puerperium**
Hypertension NOS, without mention of albuminuria or edema, complicating pregnancy, childbirth, or the puerperium

√4ᵗʰ **643 Excessive vomiting in pregnancy**
INCLUDES hyperemesis
  vomiting: } arising during pregnancy
   persistent
   vicious
  hyperemesis gravidarum

√5ᵗʰ **643.0 Mild hyperemesis gravidarum**
[0,1,3]
Hyperemesis gravidarum, mild or unspecified, starting before the end of the 22nd week of gestation
DEF: Detrimental vomiting and nausea.

√5ᵗʰ **643.1 Hyperemesis gravidarum with metabolic disturbance**
[0,1,3]
Hyperemesis gravidarum, starting before the end of the 22nd week of gestation, with metabolic disturbance, such as:
  carbohydrate depletion
  dehydration
  electrolyte imbalance

√5ᵗʰ **643.2 Late vomiting of pregnancy**
[0,1,3]
Excessive vomiting starting after 22 completed weeks of gestation

√5ᵗʰ **643.8 Other vomiting complicating pregnancy**
[0,1,3]
Vomiting due to organic disease or other cause, specified as complicating pregnancy, or as a reason for obstetric care during pregnancy
Use additional code to specify cause

✓5ᵗʰ 643.9 Unspecified vomiting of pregnancy
[0,1,3]   Vomiting as a reason for care during pregnancy, length of gestation unspecified

✓4ᵗʰ 644 Early or threatened labor

✓5ᵗʰ 644.0 Threatened premature labor
[0,3]   Premature labor after 22 weeks, but before 37 completed weeks of gestation without delivery
    EXCLUDES *that occurring before 22 completed weeks of gestation (640.0)*

✓5ᵗʰ 644.1 Other threatened labor
[0,3]   False labor:
      NOS
      after 37 completed weeks of gestation ⎫ without delivery
      Threatened labor NOS ⎭

✓5ᵗʰ 644.2 Early onset of delivery
[0,1]   Onset (spontaneous) of delivery ⎫ before 37 completed weeks
      Premature labor with onset of delivery ⎭ of gestation

✓4ᵗʰ 645 Late pregnancy

✓5ᵗʰ 645.1 Post term pregnancy
[0,1,3]   Pregnancy over 40 completed weeks to 42 completed weeks gestation

✓5ᵗʰ 645.2 Prolonged pregnancy
[0,1,3]   Pregnancy which has advanced beyond 42 completed weeks gestation

✓4ᵗʰ 646 Other complications of pregnancy, not elsewhere classified
Use additional code(s) to further specify complication

✓5ᵗʰ 646.0 Papyraceous fetus
[0,1,3]   **DEF:** Fetus that dies in the second trimester of pregnancy and is retained in the uterus, with subsequent atrophy and mummification; commonly occurs in twin pregnancy, nonviable fetus becomes compressed by growth of living twin.

✓5ᵗʰ 646.1 Edema or excessive weight gain in pregnancy, without mention of hypertension
[0-4]
    Gestational edema
    Maternal obesity syndrome
    EXCLUDES *that with mention of hypertension (642.0-642.9)*

✓5ᵗʰ 646.2 Unspecified renal disease in pregnancy, without mention of hypertension
[0-4]
    Albuminuria ⎫ in pregnancy or the
    Nephropathy NOS ⎪ puerperium, without
    Renal disease NOS ⎬ mention of
    Uremia ⎭ hypertension
    Gestational proteinuria
    EXCLUDES *that with mention of hypertension (642.0-642.9)*

✓5ᵗʰ 646.3 Recurrent pregnancy loss
[0,1,3]   **EXCLUDES** *with current abortion (634.0-634.9)*
         without current pregnancy (629.81)
    DEF: Three or more consecutive spontaneous abortions.

✓5ᵗʰ 646.4 Peripheral neuritis in pregnancy
[0-4]

✓5ᵗʰ 646.5 Asymptomatic bacteriuria in pregnancy
[0-4]

✓5ᵗʰ 646.6 Infections of genitourinary tract in pregnancy
[0-4]   Conditions classifiable to 590, 595, 597, 599.0, 616 complicating pregnancy, childbirth, or the puerperium
    Conditions classifiable to 614.0-614.5, 614.7-614.9, 615 complicating pregnancy or labor
    EXCLUDES *major puerperal infection (670.0-670.8)*

✓5ᵗʰ 646.7 Liver and biliary tract disorders in pregnancy
[0,1,3]
    Acute yellow atrophy of liver (obstetric) (true) ⎫
    Icterus gravis ⎬ of pregnancy
    Necrosis of liver ⎭
    EXCLUDES *hepatorenal syndrome following delivery (674.8)*
         viral hepatitis (647.6)

✓5ᵗʰ 646.8 Other specified complications of pregnancy
    Fatigue during pregnancy
    Herpes gestationis
    Insufficient weight gain of pregnancy

✓5ᵗʰ 646.9 Unspecified complication of pregnancy
[0,1,3]

✓4ᵗʰ 647 Infectious and parasitic conditions in the mother classifiable elsewhere, but complicating pregnancy, childbirth, or the puerperium
    INCLUDES the listed conditions when complicating the pregnant state, aggravated by the pregnancy, or when a main reason for obstetric care
    EXCLUDES *those conditions in the mother known or suspected to have affected the fetus (655.0-655.9)*
    Use additional code(s) to further specify complication

✓5ᵗʰ 647.0 Syphilis
[0-4]   Conditions classifiable to 090-097

✓5ᵗʰ 647.1 Gonorrhea
[0-4]   Conditions classifiable to 098

✓5ᵗʰ 647.2 Other venereal diseases
[0-4]   Conditions classifiable to 099

✓5ᵗʰ 647.3 Tuberculosis
[0-4]   Conditions classifiable to 010-018

✓5ᵗʰ 647.4 Malaria
[0-4]   Conditions classifiable to 084

✓5ᵗʰ 647.5 Rubella
[0-4]   Conditions classifiable to 056

✓5ᵗʰ 647.6 Other viral diseases
[0-4]   Conditions classifiable to 042, 050-055, 057-079, 795.05, 795.15, 796.75

✓5ᵗʰ 647.8 Other specified infectious and parasitic diseases
[0-4]

✓5ᵗʰ 647.9 Unspecified infection or infestation
[0-4]

✓4ᵗʰ 648 Other current conditions in the mother classifiable elsewhere, but complicating pregnancy, childbirth, or the puerperium
    INCLUDES the listed conditions when complicating the pregnant state, aggravated by the pregnancy, or when a main reason for obstetric care
    Use additional code(s) to identify the condition
    EXCLUDES *those conditions in the mother known or suspected to have affected the fetus (655.0-655.9)*

✓5ᵗʰ 648.0 Diabetes mellitus
[0-4]   Conditions classifiable to 249, 250
    EXCLUDES *gestational diabetes (648.8)*

✓5ᵗʰ 648.1 Thyroid dysfunction
[0-4]   Conditions classifiable to 240-246

✓5ᵗʰ 648.2 Anemia
[0-4]   Conditions classifiable to 280-285

✓5ᵗʰ 648.3 Drug dependence
[0-4]   Conditions classifiable to 304

✓5ᵗʰ 648.4 Mental disorders
[0-4]   Conditions classifiable to 290-303, 305.0, 305.2-305.9, 306-316, 317-319

✓5ᵗʰ 648.5 Congenital cardiovascular disorders
[0-4]   Conditions classifiable to 745-747

√5ᵗʰ **648.6 Other cardiovascular diseases**
[0-4]   Conditions classifiable to 390-398, 410-429
           EXCLUDES *cerebrovascular disorders in the puerperium (674.0)*
                         peripartum cardiomyopathy (674.5)
                         venous complications (671.0-671.9)

√5ᵗʰ **648.7 Bone and joint disorders of back,**
[0-4]   **pelvis, and lower limbs**
           Conditions classifiable to 720-724, and those classifiable to 711-719 or 725-738, specified as affecting the lower limbs

√5ᵗʰ **648.8 Abnormal glucose tolerance**
[0-4]   Conditions classifiable to 790.21-790.29
           Gestational diabetes
           Use additional code, if applicable, for associated long-term (current) insulin use (V58.67)
           DEF: Glucose intolerance arising in pregnancy, resolving at end of pregnancy.

√5ᵗʰ **648.9 Other current conditions classifiable elsewhere**
[0-4]   Conditions classifiable to 440-459, 795.01-795.04, 795.06, 795.10-795.14, 795.16, 796.70-796.74, 796.76
           Nutritional deficiencies [conditions classifiable to 260-269]

√4ᵗʰ **649 Other conditions or status of the mother complicating pregnancy, childbirth, or the puerperium**

√5ᵗʰ **649.0 Tobacco use disorder complicating**
[0-4]   **pregnancy, childbirth, or the puerperium**
           Smoking complicating pregnancy, childbirth, or the puerperium

√5ᵗʰ **649.1 Obesity complicating pregnancy, childbirth,**
[0-4]   **or the puerperium**
           Use additional code to identify the obesity (278.00-278.03)

√5ᵗʰ **649.2 Bariatric surgery status complicating**
[0-4]   **pregnancy, childbirth, or the puerperium**
           Gastric banding status complicating pregnancy, childbirth, or the puerperium
           Gastric bypass status for obesity complicating pregnancy, childbirth, or the puerperium
           Obesity surgery status complicating pregnancy, childbirth, or the puerperium

√5ᵗʰ **649.3 Coagulation defects complicating**
[0-4]   **pregnancy, childbirth, or the puerperium**
           Conditions classifiable to 286, 287, 289
           Use additional code to identify the specific coagulation defect (286.0-286.9, 287.0-287.9, 289.0-289.9)
           EXCLUDES *coagulation defects causing antepartum hemorrhage (641.3)*
                         postpartum coagulation defects (666.3)

√5ᵗʰ **649.4 Epilepsy complicating pregnancy,**
[0-4]   **childbirth, or the puerperium**
           Conditions classifiable to 286, 287, 289
           Use additional code to identify specific type of epilepsy (345.00-345.91)
           EXCLUDES *eclampsia (642.6)*

√5ᵗʰ **649.5 Spotting complicating pregnancy**
[0,1,3]   **EXCLUDES** *antepartum hemorrhage (641.0-641.9)*
                         hemorrhage in early pregnancy (640.0-640.9)

√5ᵗʰ **649.6 Uterine size date discrepancy**
[0-4]   **EXCLUDES** *suspected problem with fetal growth not found (V89.04)*

√5ᵗʰ **649.7 Cervical shortening**
[0,1,3]   **EXCLUDES** *suspected cervical shortening not found (V89.05)*
           DEF: A cervix that has shortened to < 25 mm in length by the 16th week of pregnancy; warning sign for impending premature delivery; treated by cervical cerclage placement or progesterone.

√5ᵗʰ **649.8 Onset (spontaneous) of labor after 37 completed**
[1,2]   **weeks of gestation but before 39 completed weeks gestation, with delivery by (planned) cesarean section**
           Delivery by (planned) cesarean section occurring after 37 completed weeks of gestation but before 39 completed weeks gestation due to (spontaneous) onset of labor
           Use additional code to specify reason for planned cesarean section such as:
           cephalopelvic disproportion (normally formed fetus) (653.4)
           previous cesarean delivery (654.2)

NORMAL DELIVERY, AND OTHER INDICATIONS FOR CARE IN PREGNANCY, LABOR, AND DELIVERY (650-659)

The following fifth-digit subclassification is for use with categories 651-659 to denote the current episode of care. Valid fifth-digits are in [brackets] under each code.

0 **unspecified as to episode of care or not applicable**
1 **delivered, with or without mention of antepartum condition**
2 **delivered, with mention of postpartum complication**
3 **antepartum condition or complication**
4 **postpartum condition or complication**

650 Normal delivery
           Delivery requiring minimal or no assistance, with or without episiotomy, without fetal manipulation [e.g., rotation version] or instrumentation [forceps] of spontaneous, cephalic, vaginal, full-term, single, live-born infant. This code is for use as a single diagnosis code and is not to be used with any other code in the range 630-676.
           Use additional code to indicate outcome of delivery (V27.0)
           EXCLUDES *breech delivery (assisted) (spontaneous) NOS (652.2)*
                         delivery by vacuum extractor, forceps, cesarean section, or breech extraction, without specified complication (669.5-669.7)

√4ᵗʰ **651 Multiple gestation**
           Use additional code to specify placenta status (V91.00-V91.99)

√5ᵗʰ **651.0 Twin pregnancy**
[0,1,3]   **EXCLUDES** *fetal conjoined twins (678.1)*

√5ᵗʰ **651.1 Triplet pregnancy**
[0,1,3]

√5ᵗʰ **651.2 Quadruplet pregnancy**
[0,1,3]

√5ᵗʰ **651.3 Twin pregnancy with fetal loss and retention of one**
[0,1,3] **fetus**
           Vanishing twin syndrome (651.33)

√5ᵗʰ **651.4 Triplet pregnancy with fetal loss and retention of one**
[0,1,3] **or more fetus(es)**

√5ᵗʰ **651.5 Quadruplet pregnancy with fetal loss and retention of**
[0,1,3] **one or more fetus(es)**

√5ᵗʰ **651.6 Other multiple pregnancy with fetal loss and retention**
[0,1,3] **of one or more fetus(es)**

√5ᵗʰ **651.7 Multiple gestation following (elective) fetal**
[0,1,3] **reduction**
           Fetal reduction of multiple fetuses reduced to single fetus

√5ᵗʰ **651.8 Other specified multiple gestation**
[0,1,3]

√5ᵗʰ **651.9 Unspecified multiple gestation**
[0,1,3]

√4ᵗʰ **652 Malposition and malpresentation of fetus**
           Code first any associated obstructed labor (660.0)

√5ᵗʰ **652.0 Unstable lie**
[0,1,3] **DEF:** Changing fetal position.

√5ᵗʰ **652.1 Breech or other malpresentation successfully**
[0,1,3] **converted to cephalic presentation**
           Cephalic version NOS

Malposition and Malpresentation

Breech

Mother's pelvis

Face (mentum)

Shoulder (arm prolapse)

Compound (extremity together with head)

Oblique

Cephalopelvic Disproportion

Pubic symphysis

Ischial tuberosity

Contraction of pelvic outlet (from below)

Cephalopelvic disproportion due to: Contraction of pelvic inlet, or large fetus, or hydrocephalus

Pubic symphysis

Pelvic inlet from above

√5ᵗʰ **652.2 Breech presentation without mention of version**
[0,1,3]   Breech delivery (assisted) (spontaneous) NOS
            Buttocks presentation
            Complete breech
            Frank breech
            EXCLUDES *footling presentation (652.8)*
                        incomplete breech (652.8)
            DEF: Fetal presentation of buttocks or feet at birth canal.

√5ᵗʰ **652.3 Transverse or oblique presentation**
[0,1,3]   Oblique lie   Transverse lie
            EXCLUDES *transverse arrest of fetal head (660.3)*
            DEF: Delivery of fetus, shoulder first.

√5ᵗʰ **652.4 Face or brow presentation**
[0,1,3]   Mentum presentation

√5ᵗʰ **652.5 High head at term**
[0,1,3]   Failure of head to enter pelvic brim

√5ᵗʰ **652.6 Multiple gestation with malpresentation**
[0,1,3] **of one fetus or more**

√5ᵗʰ **652.7 Prolapsed arm**
[0,1,3]

√5ᵗʰ **652.8 Other specified malposition or malpresentation**
[0,1,3]   Compound presentation

√5ᵗʰ **652.9 Unspecified malposition or malpresentation**
[0,1,3]

√4ᵗʰ **653 Disproportion**
        Code first any associated obstructed labor (660.1)

√5ᵗʰ **653.0 Major abnormality of bony pelvis, not further specified**
[0,1,3]   Pelvic deformity NOS

√5ᵗʰ **653.1 Generally contracted pelvis**
[0,1,3]   Contracted pelvis NOS

√5ᵗʰ **653.2 Inlet contraction of pelvis**
[0,1,3]   Inlet contraction (pelvis)

√5ᵗʰ **653.3 Outlet contraction of pelvis**
[0,1,3]   Outlet contraction (pelvis)

√5ᵗʰ **653.4 Fetopelvic disproportion**
[0,1,3]   Cephalopelvic disproportion NOS
            Disproportion of mixed maternal and fetal origin, with
                normally formed fetus

√5ᵗʰ **653.5 Unusually large fetus causing disproportion**
[0,1,3]   Disproportion of fetal origin with normally formed fetus
            Fetal disproportion NOS
            EXCLUDES *that when the reason for medical care was*
                        concern for the fetus (656.6)

√5ᵗʰ **653.6 Hydrocephalic fetus causing disproportion**
[0,1,3]   **EXCLUDES** *that when the reason for medical care was*
                        concern for the fetus (655.0)

√5ᵗʰ **653.7 Other fetal abnormality causing disproportion**
[0,1,3]   Fetal:
                ascites
                hydrops
                myelomeningocele
                sacral teratoma
                tumor
            EXCLUDES *conjoined twins causing disproportion (678.1)*

√5ᵗʰ **653.8 Disproportion of other origin**
[0,1,3]   **EXCLUDES** *shoulder (girdle) dystocia (660.4)*

√5ᵗʰ **653.9 Unspecified disproportion**
[0,1,3]

√4ᵗʰ **654 Abnormality of organs and soft tissues of pelvis**
        INCLUDES the listed conditions during pregnancy, childbirth, or
                    the puerperium
        Code first any associated obstructed labor (660.2)
        EXCLUDES *trauma to perineum and vulva complicating current*
                    delivery (664.0-664.9)

√5ᵗʰ **654.0 Congenital abnormalities of uterus**
[0-4]   Double uterus
            Uterus bicornis

√5ᵗʰ **654.1 Tumors of body of uterus**
[0-4]   Uterine fibroids

√5ᵗʰ **654.2 Previous cesarean delivery**
[0,1,3]   Uterine scar from previous cesarean delivery

√5ᵗʰ **654.3 Retroverted and incarcerated gravid uterus**
[0-4]   **DEF:** Retroverted: tilted back uterus; no change in angle of
            longitudinal axis.
            DEF: Incarcerated: immobile, fixed uterus.

√5ᵗʰ **654.4 Other abnormalities in shape or position**
[0-4] **of gravid uterus and of neighboring structures**
            Cystocele
            Pelvic floor repair
            Pendulous abdomen
            Prolapse of gravid uterus
            Rectocele
            Rigid pelvic floor

√5ᵗʰ **654.5 Cervical incompetence**
[0-4]   Presence of Shirodkar suture with or without mention of
                cervical incompetence
            DEF: Abnormal cervix; tendency to dilate in second
            trimester; causes premature fetal expulsion.
            DEF: Shirodkar suture: purse-string suture used to
            artificially close incompetent cervix.

√5ᵗʰ **654.6 Other congenital or acquired abnormality of cervix**
[0-4]   Cicatricial cervix
            Polyp of cervix
            Previous surgery to cervix
            Rigid cervix (uteri)
            Stenosis or stricture of cervix
            Tumor of cervix

√5ᵗʰ **654.7 Congenital or acquired abnormality of vagina**
[0-4]   Previous surgery to vagina
            Septate vagina
            Stenosis of vagina (acquired) (congenital)
            Stricture of vagina
            Tumor of vagina

Complications of Pregnancy, Childbirth, and the Puerperium

654.8–658.4

√5ᵗʰ **654.8 Congenital or acquired abnormality of vulva**
[0-4]   Anal sphincter tear (healed) (old) complicating delivery
          Fibrosis of perineum
          Persistent hymen
          Previous surgery to perineum or vulva
          Rigid perineum
          Tumor of vulva
          EXCLUDES *anal sphincter tear (healed) (old) not*
                          associated with delivery (569.43)
                        varicose veins of vulva (671.1)

√5ᵗʰ **654.9 Other and unspecified**
[0-4]   Uterine scar NEC

√4ᵗʰ **655 Known or suspected fetal abnormality affecting**
        management of mother
        INCLUDES the listed conditions in the fetus as a reason for
                      observation or obstetrical care of the mother,
                      or for termination of pregnancy

√5ᵗʰ **655.0 Central nervous system malformation in fetus**
[0,1,3]   Fetal or suspected fetal:
          anencephaly
          hydrocephalus
          spina bifida (with myelomeningocele)

√5ᵗʰ **655.1 Chromosomal abnormality in fetus**
[0,1,3]

√5ᵗʰ **655.2 Hereditary disease in family possibly affecting fetus**
[0,1,3]

√5ᵗʰ **655.3 Suspected damage to fetus from viral disease in**
[0,1,3]   **the mother**
          Suspected damage to fetus from maternal rubella

√5ᵗʰ **655.4 Suspected damage to fetus from other disease in**
[0,1,3]   **the mother**
          Suspected damage to fetus from maternal:
          alcohol addiction
          listeriosis
          toxoplasmosis

√5ᵗʰ **655.5 Suspected damage to fetus from drugs**
[0,1,3]

√5ᵗʰ **655.6 Suspected damage to fetus from radiation**
[0,1,3]

√5ᵗʰ **655.7 Decreased fetal movements**

√5ᵗʰ **655.8 Other known or suspected fetal abnormality, not**
[0,1,3]   **elsewhere classified**
          Suspected damage to fetus from:
          environmental toxins
          intrauterine contraceptive device

√5ᵗʰ **655.9 Unspecified**
[0,1,3]

√4ᵗʰ **656 Other known or suspected fetal and placental problems**
        affecting management of mother
        EXCLUDES *fetal hematologic conditions (678.0)*
                      suspected placental problems not found (V89.02)

√5ᵗʰ **656.0 Fetal-maternal hemorrhage**
[0,1,3]   Leakage (microscopic) of fetal blood into maternal
          circulation

√5ᵗʰ **656.1 Rhesus isoimmunization**
[0,1,3]   Anti-D [Rh] antibodies
          Rh incompatibility
          DEF: Antibodies developing against Rh factor; mother
          with Rh negative develops antibodies against Rh positive
          fetus.

√5ᵗʰ **656.2 Isoimmunization from other and**
[0,1,3]   **unspecified blood-group incompatibility**
          ABO isoimmunization

√5ᵗʰ **656.3 Fetal distress**
[0,1,3]   Fetal metabolic acidemia
          EXCLUDES *abnormal fetal acid-base balance (656.8)*
                        abnormality in fetal heart rate or rhythm
                          (659.7)
                        fetal bradycardia (659.7)
                        fetal tachycardia (659.7)
                        meconium in liquor (656.8)
          DEF: Life-threatening disorder; fetal anoxia, hemolytic
          disease and other miscellaneous diseases cause fetal
          distress.

√5ᵗʰ **656.4 Intrauterine death**
[0,1,3]   Fetal death:
          NOS
          after completion of 22 weeks' gestation
          late
          Missed delivery
          EXCLUDES *missed abortion (632)*

√5ᵗʰ **656.5 Poor fetal growth**
[0,1,3]   "Light-for-dates"
          "Placental insufficiency"
          "Small-for-dates"

√5ᵗʰ **656.6 Excessive fetal growth**
[0,1,3]   "Large-for-dates"

√5ᵗʰ **656.7 Other placental conditions**
[0,1,3]   Abnormal placenta
          Placental infarct
          EXCLUDES *placental polyp (674.4)*
                        placentitis (658.4)

√5ᵗʰ **656.8 Other specified fetal and placental problems**
[0,1,3]   Abnormal acid-base balance
          Intrauterine acidosis
          Lithopedian
          Meconium in liquor
          Subchorionic hematoma
          DEF: Lithopedion: Calcified fetus; not expelled by mother.

√5ᵗʰ **656.9 Unspecified fetal and placental problem**
[0,1,3]

√4ᵗʰ **657 Polyhydramnios**
[0,1,3]

√5ᵗʰ   Use 0 as fourth-digit for this category
          Hydramnios
          EXCLUDES *suspected polyhydramnios not found (V89.01)*
          DEF: Excess amniotic fluid.

√4ᵗʰ **658 Other problems associated with amniotic cavity and**
        membranes
        EXCLUDES *amniotic fluid embolism (673.1)*
                      suspected problems with amniotic cavity and
                        membranes not found (V89.01)

√5ᵗʰ **658.0 Oligohydramnios**
[0,1,3]   Oligohydramnios without mention of
          rupture of membranes
          DEF: Deficient amount of amniotic fluid.

√5ᵗʰ **658.1 Premature rupture of membranes**
[0,1,3]   Rupture of amniotic sac less than 24
          hours prior to the onset of labor

√5ᵗʰ **658.2 Delayed delivery after spontaneous or**
[0,1,3]   **unspecified rupture of membranes**
          Prolonged rupture of membranes NOS
          Rupture of amniotic sac 24 hours or more prior to the
          onset of labor

√5ᵗʰ **658.3 Delayed delivery after artificial rupture**
[0,1,3]   **of membranes**

√5ᵗʰ **658.4 Infection of amniotic cavity**
[0,1,3]   Amnionitis
          Chorioamnionitis
          Membranitis
          Placentitis

√5ᵗʰ **658.8 Other**
[0,1,3]   Amnion nodosum
     Amniotic cyst

√5ᵗʰ **658.9 Unspecified**
[0,1,3]

√4ᵗʰ **659 Other indications for care or intervention related to labor and delivery, not elsewhere classified**

√5ᵗʰ **659.0 Failed mechanical induction**
[0,1,3]   Failure of induction of labor by surgical or other instrumental methods

√5ᵗʰ **659.1 Failed medical or unspecified induction**
[0,1,3]   Failed induction NOS
     Failure of induction of labor by medical methods, such as oxytocic drugs

√5ᵗʰ **659.2 Maternal pyrexia during labor, unspecified**
[0,1,3]   **DEF:** Fever during labor.

√5ᵗʰ **659.3 Generalized infection during labor**
[0,1,3]   Septicemia during labor

√5ᵗʰ **659.4 Grand multiparity**
[0,1,3]   EXCLUDES *supervision only, in pregnancy (V23.3)*
     without current pregnancy (V61.5)
     DEF: Having borne six or more children previously.

√5ᵗʰ **659.5 Elderly primigravida**
[0,1,3]   First pregnancy in a woman who will be 35 years of age or older at expected date of delivery
     EXCLUDES *supervision only, in pregnancy (V23.81)*

√5ᵗʰ **659.6 Elderly multigravida**
[0,1,3]   Second or more pregnancy in a woman who will be 35 years of age or older at expected date of delivery
     EXCLUDES *elderly primigravida 659.5*
     supervision only, in pregnancy (V23.82)

√5ᵗʰ **659.7 Abnormality in fetal heart rate or rhythm**
[0,1,3]   Depressed fetal heart tones
     Fetal:
       bradycardia
       tachycardia
     Fetal heart rate decelerations
     Non-reassuring fetal heart rate or rhythm

√5ᵗʰ **659.8 Other specified indications for care or**
[0,1,3] **intervention related to labor and delivery**
     Pregnancy in a female less than 16 years old at expected date of delivery
     Very young maternal age

√5ᵗʰ **659.9 Unspecified indication for care or**
[0,1,3] **intervention related to labor and delivery**

COMPLICATIONS OCCURRING MAINLY IN THE COURSE OF LABOR AND DELIVERY (660-669)

The following fifth-digit subclassification is for use with categories 660-669 to denote the current episode of care. Valid fifth-digits are in [brackets] under each code.

   0 unspecified as to episode of care or not applicable
   1 delivered, with or without mention of antepartum condition
   2 delivered, with mention of postpartum complication
   3 antepartum condition or complication
   4 postpartum condition or complication

√4ᵗʰ **660 Obstructed labor**

√5ᵗʰ **660.0 Obstruction caused by malposition of**
[0,1,3] **fetus at onset of labor**
     Any condition classifiable to 652, causing obstruction during labor
     Use additional code from 652.0-652.9 to identify condition

√5ᵗʰ **660.1 Obstruction by bony pelvis**
[0,1,3]   Any condition classifiable to 653, causing obstruction during labor
     Use additional code from 653.0-653.9 to identify condition

√5ᵗʰ **660.2 Obstruction by abnormal pelvic soft**
[0,1,3] **tissues**
     Prolapse of anterior lip of cervix
     Any condition classifiable to 654, causing obstruction during labor
     Use additional code from 654.0-654.9 to identify condition

√5ᵗʰ **660.3 Deep transverse arrest and persistent**
[0,1,3] **occipitoposterior position**

√5ᵗʰ **660.4 Shoulder (girdle) dystocia**
[0,1,3]   Impacted shoulders
     DEF: Obstructed labor due to impacted fetal shoulders.

√5ᵗʰ **660.5 Locced twins**
[0,1,3]

√5ᵗʰ **660.6 Failed trial of labor, unspecified**
[0,1,3]   Failed trial of labor, without mention of condition or suspected condition

√5ᵗʰ **660.7 Failed forceps or vacuum extractor, unspecified**
[0,1,3]   Application of ventouse or forceps, without mention of condition

√5ᵗʰ **660.8 Other causes of obstructed labor**
[0,1,3]   Use additional code to identify condition

√5ᵗʰ **660.9 Unspecified obstructed labor**
[0,1,3]   Dystocia:
     NOS
     fetal NOS
     maternal NOS

√4ᵗʰ **661 Abnormality of forces of labor**

√5ᵗʰ **661.0 Primary uterine inertia**
[0,1,3]   Failure of cervical dilation
     Hypotonic uterine dysfunction, primary
     Prolonged latent phase of labor
     DEF: Lack of efficient contractions during labor causing prolonged labor.

√5ᵗʰ **661.1 Secondary uterine inertia**
[0,1,3]   Arrested active phase of labor
     Hypotonic uterine dysfunction, secondary

√5ᵗʰ **661.2 Other and unspecified uterine inertia**
[0,1,3]   Atony of uterus without hemorrhage
     Desultory labor
     Irregular labor
     Poor contractions
     Slow slope active phase of labor
     EXCLUDES *atony of uterus with hemorrhage (666.1)*
     postpartum atony of uterus without hemorrhage (669.8)

√5ᵗʰ **661.3 Precipitate labor**
[0,1,3]   **DEF:** Rapid labor and delivery.

√5ᵗʰ **661.4 Hypertonic, incoordinate, or prolonged**
[0,1,3] **uterine contractions**
     Cervical spasm
     Contraction ring (dystocia)
     Dyscoordinate labor
     Hourglass contraction of uterus
     Hypertonic uterine dysfunction
     Incoordinate uterine action
     Retraction ring (Bandl's) (pathological)
     Tetanic contractions
     Uterine dystocia NOS
     Uterine spasm

√5ᵗʰ **661.9 Unspecified abnormality of labor**
[0,1,3]

√4ᵗʰ **662 Long labor**

√5ᵗʰ **662.0 Prolonged first stage**
[0,1,3]

√5ᵗʰ **662.1 Prolonged labor, unspecified**
[0,1,3]

√5ᵗʰ **662.2 Prolonged second stage**
[0,1,3]

Complications of Pregnancy, Childbirth, and the Puerperium

662.3–666.2

✓5ᵗʰ **662.3 Delayed delivery of second twin, triplet, etc.**
[0,1,3]

✓4ᵗʰ **663 Umbilical cord complications**

✓5ᵗʰ **663.0 Prolapse of cord**
[0,1,3]   Presentation of cord
     DEF: Abnormal presentation of fetus; marked by protruding umbilical cord during labor; can cause fetal death.

✓5ᵗʰ **663.1 Cord around neck, with compression**
[0,1,3]   Cord tightly around neck

✓5ᵗʰ **663.2 Other and unspecified cord entanglement,**
[0,1,3] **with compression**
     Entanglement of cords of twins in mono-amniotic sac
     Knot in cord (with compression)

✓5ᵗʰ **663.3 Other and unspecified cord entanglement,**
[0,1,3] **without mention of compression**

✓5ᵗʰ **663.4 Short cord**
[0,1,3]

✓5ᵗʰ **663.5 Vasa previa**
[0,1,3]   **DEF:** Abnormal presentation of fetus marked by blood vessels of umbilical cord in front of fetal head.

✓5ᵗʰ **663.6 Vascular lesions of cord**
[0,1,3]   Bruising of cord   Thrombosis of vessels
     Hematoma of cord   of cord

✓5ᵗʰ **663.8 Other umbilical cord complications**
[0,1,3]   Velamentous insertion of umbilical cord

✓5ᵗʰ **663.9 Unspecified umbilical cord complication**
[0,1,3]

✓4ᵗʰ **664 Trauma to perineum and vulva during delivery**
    INCLUDES   damage from instruments
          that from extension of episiotomy

✓5ᵗʰ **664.0 First-degree perineal laceration**
[0,1,4]   Perineal laceration, rupture, or tear involving:
     fourchette   skin
     hymen   vagina
     labia   vulva

✓5ᵗʰ **664.1 Second-degree perineal laceration**
[0,1,4]   Perineal laceration, rupture, or tear (following episiotomy) involving:
     pelvic floor
     perineal muscles
     vaginal muscles
     EXCLUDES   *that involving anal sphincter (664.2)*

✓5ᵗʰ **664.2 Third-degree perineal laceration**
[0,1,4]   Perineal laceration, rupture, or tear (following episiotomy) involving:
     anal sphincter
     rectovaginal septum
     sphincter NOS
     EXCLUDES   *anal sphincter tear during delivery not associated with third-degree perineal laceration (664.6)*
                  that with anal or rectal mucosal laceration (664.3)

Perineal Lacerations

First degree
Second degree
Anus
Third degree
Fourth degree

✓5ᵗʰ **664.3 Fourth-degree perineal laceration**
[0,1,4]   Perineal laceration, rupture, or tear as classifiable to 664.2 and involving also:
     anal mucosa
     rectal mucosa

✓5ᵗʰ **664.4 Unspecified perineal laceration**
[0,1,4]   Central laceration

✓5ᵗʰ **664.5 Vulval and perineal hematoma**
[0,1,4]

✓5ᵗʰ **664.6 Anal sphincter tear complicating delivery,**
[0,1,4] **not associated with third-degree perineal laceration**
     EXCLUDES   *third-degree perineal laceration (664.2)*

✓5ᵗʰ **664.8 Other specified trauma to perineum and vulva**
[0,1,4]   Periurethral trauma

✓5ᵗʰ **664.9 Unspecified trauma to perineum and vulva**
[0,1,4]

✓4ᵗʰ **665 Other obstetrical trauma**
    INCLUDES   damage from instruments

✓5ᵗʰ **665.0 Rupture of uterus before onset of labor**
[0,1,3]

✓5ᵗʰ **665.1 Rupture of uterus during labor**
[0,1]   Rupture of uterus NOS

✓5ᵗʰ **665.2 Inversion of uterus**
[0,2,4]

✓5ᵗʰ **665.3 Laceration of cervix**
[0,1,4]

✓5ᵗʰ **665.4 High vaginal laceration**
[0,1,4]   Laceration of vaginal wall or sulcus without mention of perineal laceration

✓5ᵗʰ **665.5 Other injury to pelvic organs**
[0,1,4]   Injury to:
     bladder
     urethra
     EXCLUDES   *periurethral trauma (664.8)*

✓5ᵗʰ **665.6 Damage to pelvic joints and ligaments**
[0,1,4]   Avulsion of inner symphyseal cartilage
     Damage to coccyx
     Separation of symphysis (pubis)

✓5ᵗʰ **665.7 Pelvic hematoma**
[0,1,2,4]   Hematoma of vagina

✓5ᵗʰ **665.8 Other specified obstetrical trauma**
[0–4]

✓5ᵗʰ **665.9 Unspecified obstetrical trauma**
[0–4]

✓4ᵗʰ **666 Postpartum hemorrhage**

✓5ᵗʰ **666.0 Third-stage hemorrhage**
[0,2,4]   Hemorrhage associated with retained, trapped, or adherent placenta
     Retained placenta NOS

✓5ᵗʰ **666.1 Other immediate postpartum hemorrhage**
[0,2,4]   Atony of uterus with hemorrhage
     Hemorrhage within the first 24 hours following delivery of placenta
     Postpartum atony of uterus with hemorrhage
     Postpartum hemorrhage (atonic) NOS
     EXCLUDES   *atony of uterus without hemorrhage (661.2)*
                  postpartum atony of uterus without hemorrhage (669.8)

✓5ᵗʰ **666.2 Delayed and secondary postpartum hemorrhage**
[0,2,4]   Hemorrhage:
     after the first 24 hours following delivery
     associated with retained portions of placenta or membranes
     Postpartum hemorrhage specified as delayed or secondary
     Retained products of conception NOS, following delivery

✓5ᵗʰ **666.3 Postpartum coagulation defects**
[0,2,4]   Postpartum:
                afibrinogenemia
                fibrinolysis

✓4ᵗʰ **667 Retained placenta or membranes, without hemorrhage**
     DEF: Postpartum condition resulting from failure to expel placental membrane tissues due to failed contractions of uterine wall.

✓5ᵗʰ **667.0 Retained placenta without hemorrhage**
[0,2,4]   Placenta accreta
                Retained placenta: ⎫
                   NOS   ⎬ without hemorrhage
                   total   ⎭

✓5ᵗʰ **667.1 Retained portions of placenta or membranes,**
[0,2,4] **without hemorrhage**
                Retained products of conception following delivery, without hemorrhage

✓4ᵗʰ **668 Complications of the administration of anesthetic or other sedation in labor and delivery**
     INCLUDES   complications arising from the administration of a general or local anesthetic, analgesic, or other sedation in labor and delivery
     Use additional code(s) to further specify complication
     EXCLUDES   reaction to spinal or lumbar puncture (349.0)
                spinal headache (349.0)

✓5ᵗʰ **668.0 Pulmonary complications**
[0-4]   Inhalation (aspiration) of   ⎫
                stomach contents or   ⎬ following anesthesia
                secretions   ⎬ or other
             Mendelson's syndrome   ⎬ sedation in
             Pressure collapse of lung   ⎭ labor or delivery

✓5ᵗʰ **668.1 Cardiac complications**
[0-4]   Cardiac arrest or failure following anesthesia or other sedation in labor and delivery

✓5ᵗʰ **668.2 Central nervous system complications**
[0-4]   Cerebral anoxia following anesthesia or other sedation in labor and delivery

✓5ᵗʰ **668.8 Other complications of anesthesia or other sedation in labor and delivery**
[0-4]

✓5ᵗʰ **668.9 Unspecified complication of anesthesia and other sedation**
[0-4]

✓4ᵗʰ **669 Other complications of labor and delivery, not elsewhere classified**

✓5ᵗʰ **669.0 Maternal distress**
[0-4]   Metabolic disturbance in labor and delivery

✓5ᵗʰ **669.1 Shock during or following labor and delivery**
[0-4]   Obstetric shock

✓5ᵗʰ **669.2 Maternal hypotension syndrome**
[0-4]   **DEF:** Low arterial blood pressure in mother during labor and delivery.

✓5ᵗʰ **669.3 Acute kidney failure following labor and delivery**
[0,2,4]

✓5ᵗʰ **669.4 Other complications of obstetrical surgery and procedures**
[0-4]   Cardiac:
                arrest   ⎫ following cesarean or other
                failure   ⎬ obstetrical surgery or
             Cerebral   ⎬ procedure, including delivery
                anoxia   ⎭ NOS
             EXCLUDES   complications of obstetrical surgical wounds (674.1-674.3)

✓5ᵗʰ **669.5 Forceps or vacuum extractor delivery without mention of indication**
[0,1]   Delivery by ventouse, without mention of indication

✓5ᵗʰ **669.6 Breech extraction, without mention of indication**
[0,1]   EXCLUDES   breech delivery NOS (652.2)

✓5ᵗʰ **669.7 Cesarean delivery, without mention of indication**
[0,1]

✓5ᵗʰ **669.8 Other complications of labor and delivery**
[0-4]

✓5ᵗʰ **669.9 Unspecified complication of labor and delivery**
[0-4]

COMPLICATIONS OF THE PUERPERIUM (670-677)

Note: Categories 671 and 673-676 include the listed conditions even if they occur during pregnancy or childbirth.

The following fifth-digit subclassification is for use with categories 670-676 to denote the current episode of care. Valid fifth-digits are in [brackets] under each code.
   0 unspecified as to episode of care or not applicable
   1 delivered, with or without mention of antepartum condition
   2 delivered, with mention of postpartum complication
   3 antepartum condition or complication
   4 postpartum condition or complication

✓4ᵗʰ **670 Major puerperal infection**
     EXCLUDES   infection following abortion (639.0)
                minor genital tract infection following delivery (646.6)
                puerperal pyrexia NOS (672)
                puerperal fever NOS (672)
                puerperal pyrexia of unknown origin (672)
                urinary tract infection following delivery (646.6)
     DEF: Infection and inflammation following childbirth.

✓5ᵗʰ **670.0 Major puerperal infection, unspecified**
[0,2,4]

✓5ᵗʰ **670.1 Puerperal endometritis**
[0,2,4]

✓5ᵗʰ **670.2 Puerperal sepsis**
[0,2,4]   Puerperal pyemia
                Use additional code to identify severe sepsis (995.92) and any associated acute organ dysfunction, if applicable

✓5ᵗʰ **670.3 Puerperal septic thrombophlebitis**
[0,2,4]

✓5ᵗʰ **670.8 Other major puerperal infection**
[0,2,4]   Puerperal:
                pelvic cellulitis
                peritonitis
                salpingitis

✓4ᵗʰ **671 Venous complications in pregnancy and the puerperium**
     EXCLUDES   personal history of venous complications prior to pregnancy, such as:
                thrombophlebitis (V12.52)
                thrombosis and embolism (V12.51)

✓5ᵗʰ **671.0 Varicose veins of legs**
[0-4]   Varicose veins NOS
             DEF: Distended, tortuous veins on legs associated with pregnancy.

✓5ᵗʰ **671.1 Varicose veins of vulva and perineum**
[0-4]   **DEF:** Distended, tortuous veins on external female genitalia associated with pregnancy.

✓5ᵗʰ **671.2 Superficial thrombophlebitis**
[0-4]   Phlebitis NOS
             Thrombophlebitis (superficial)
             Thrombosis NOS
             Use additional code to identify the superficial thrombophlebitis (453.6, 453.71, 453.81)

✓5ᵗʰ **671.3 Deep phlebothrombosis, antepartum**
[0,1,3]   Deep vein thrombosis antepartum
             Use additional code to identify the deep vein thrombosis (453.40-453.42, 453.50-453.52, 453.72-453.79, 453.82-453.89)
             Use additional code for long term (current) use of anticoagulants, if applicable (V58.61)

Complications of Pregnancy, Childbirth, and the Puerperium

671.4–676.5

✓5ᵗʰ **671.4 Deep phlebothrombosis, postpartum**
[0,2,4]   Deep-vein thrombosis, postpartum
Pelvic thrombophlebitis, postpartum
Phlegmasia alba dolens (puerperal)
Use additional code to identify the deep vein thrombosis (453.40-453.42, 453.50-453.52, 453.72-453.79, 453.82-453.89)
Use additional code for long term (current) use of anticoagulants, if applicable (V58.61)

✓5ᵗʰ **671.5 Other phlebitis and thrombosis**
[0-4]   Cerebral venous thrombosis
Thrombosis of intracranial venous sinus

✓5ᵗʰ **671.8 Other venous complications**
[0-4]   Hemorrhoids

✓5ᵗʰ **671.9 Unspecified venous complication**
[0-4]

✓4ᵗʰ **672 Pyrexia of unknown origin during the puerperium**
[0,2,4]

✓5ᵗʰ   Use 0 as fourth-digit for this category
Postpartum fever NOS
Puerperal fever NOS
Puerperal pyrexia NOS
DEF: Fever of unknown origin experienced by the mother after childbirth.

✓4ᵗʰ **673 Obstetrical pulmonary embolism**
INCLUDES   pulmonary emboli in pregnancy, childbirth, or the puerperium, or specified as puerperal
EXCLUDES   *embolism following abortion (639.6)*

✓5ᵗʰ **673.0 Obstetrical air embolism**
[0-4]   **DEF:** Sudden blocking of pulmonary artery with air or nitrogen bubbles during puerperium.

✓5ᵗʰ **673.1 Amniotic fluid embolism**
[0-4]   **DEF:** Sudden onset of pulmonary artery blockage from amniotic fluid entering the mother's circulation near the end of pregnancy due to strong uterine contractions.

✓5ᵗʰ **673.2 Obstetrical blood-clot embolism**
[0-4]   Puerperal pulmonary embolism NOS
DEF: Blood clot blocking artery in the lung; associated with pregnancy.

✓5ᵗʰ **673.3 Obstetrical pyemic and septic embolism**
[0-4]

✓5ᵗʰ **673.8 Other pulmonary embolism**
[0-4]   Fat embolism

✓4ᵗʰ **674 Other and unspecified complications of the puerperium, not elsewhere classified**

✓5ᵗʰ **674.0 Cerebrovascular disorders in the puerperium**
[0-4]   Any condition classifiable to 430-434, 436-437 occurring during pregnancy, childbirth, or the puerperium, or specified as puerperal
EXCLUDES   *intracranial venous sinus thrombosis (671.5)*

✓5ᵗʰ **674.1 Disruption of cesarean wound**
[0,2,4]   Dehiscence or disruption of uterine wound
EXCLUDES   *uterine rupture before onset of labor (665.0)*
uterine rupture during labor (665.1)

✓5ᵗʰ **674.2 Disruption of perineal wound**
[0,2,4]   Breakdown of perineum
Disruption of wound of:
episiotomy
perineal laceration
Secondary perineal tear

✓5ᵗʰ **674.3 Other complications of obstetrical**
[0,2,4] **surgical wounds**
Hematoma
Hemorrhage } of cesarean section or perineal
Infection } wound
EXCLUDES   *damage from instruments in delivery (664.0-665.9)*

✓5ᵗʰ **674.4 Placental polyp**
[0,2,4]

✓5ᵗʰ **674.5 Peripartum cardiomyopathy**
[0-4]   Postpartum cardiomyopathy
DEF: Any structural or functional abnormality of the ventricular myocardium, non-inflammatory disease of obscure or unknown etiology with onset during the postpartum period.

✓5ᵗʰ **674.8 Other**
[0,2,4]   Hepatorenal syndrome, following delivery
Postpartum:
subinvolution of uterus
uterine hypertrophy

✓5ᵗʰ **674.9 Unspecified**
[0,2,4]   Sudden death of unknown cause during the puerperium

✓4ᵗʰ **675 Infections of the breast and nipple associated with childbirth**
INCLUDES   the listed conditions during pregnancy, childbirth, or the puerperium

✓5ᵗʰ **675.0 Infections of nipple**
[0-4]   Abscess of nipple

✓5ᵗʰ **675.1 Abscess of breast**
[0-4]   Abscess:
mammary
subareolar
submammary
purulent
retromammary
submammary

✓5ᵗʰ **675.2 Nonpurulent mastitis**
[0-4]   Lymphangitis of breast
Mastitis:
NOS
interstitial
parenchymatous

✓5ᵗʰ **675.8 Other specified infections of the breast and nipple**
[0-4]

✓5ᵗʰ **675.9 Unspecified infection of the breast and nipple**
[0-4]

✓4ᵗʰ **676 Other disorders of the breast associated with childbirth and disorders of lactation**
INCLUDES   the listed conditions during pregnancy, the puerperium, or lactation

✓5ᵗʰ **676.0 Retracted nipple**
[0-4]

✓5ᵗʰ **676.1 Cracked nipple**
[0-4]   Fissure of nipple

✓5ᵗʰ **676.2 Engorgement of breasts**
[0-4]   **DEF:** Abnormal accumulation of milk in ducts of breast.

✓5ᵗʰ **676.3 Other and unspecified disorder of breast**
[0-4]

✓5ᵗʰ **676.4 Failure of lactation**
[0-4]   Agalactia
DEF: Abrupt ceasing of milk secretion by breast.

✓5ᵗʰ **676.5 Suppressed lactation**
[0-4]

Lactation Process: Ejection Reflex Arc

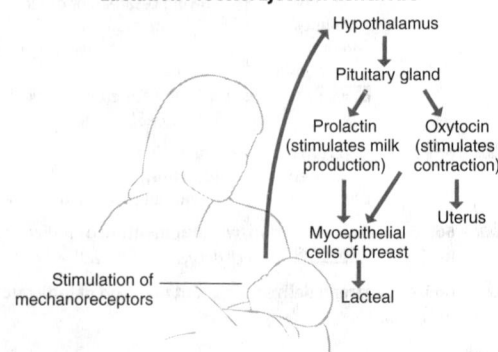

√5ᵗʰ **676.6 Galactorrhea**
[0-4]   **EXCLUDES**   *galactorrhea not associated with childbirth (611.6)*

      DEF: Excessive or persistent milk secretion by breast; may be in absence of nursing.

√5ᵗʰ **676.8 Other disorders of lactation**
[0-4]   Galactocele

      DEF: Galactocele: Obstructed mammary gland, creating retention cyst, results in milk-filled cysts enlarging mammary gland.

√5ᵗʰ **676.9 Unspecified disorder of lactation**
[0-4]

677 Late effect of complication of pregnancy, childbirth, and the puerperium

      Note: This category is to be used to indicate conditions in 632-648.9 and 651-676.9 as the cause of the late effect, themselves classifiable elsewhere. The "late effects" include conditions specified as such, or as sequelae, which may occur at any time after puerperium.

      Code first any sequelae

OTHER MATERNAL AND FETAL COMPLICATIONS (678-679)

The following fifth-digit subclassification is for use with categories 678-679 to denote the current episode of care. Valid fifth-digits are in [brackets] under each code.

   0 unspecified as to episode of care or not applicable
   1 delivered, with or without mention of antepartum condition
   2 delivered, with mention of postpartum complication
   3 antepartum condition or complication
   4 postpartum condition or complication

√4ᵗʰ **678 Other fetal conditions**

√5ᵗʰ **678.0 Fetal hematologic conditions**
[0,1,3]   Fetal anemia
      Fetal thrombocytopenia
      Fetal twin to twin transfusion
      EXCLUDES   *fetal and neonatal hemorrhage (772.0-772.9)*
           fetal hematologic disorders affecting newborn (776.0-776.9)
           fetal-maternal hemorrhage (656.00-656.03)
           isoimmunization incompatibility (656.10-656.13, 656.20-656.23)

√5ᵗʰ **678.1 Fetal conjoined twins**
[0,1,3]

√4ᵗʰ **679 Complications of in utero procedures**

√5ᵗʰ **679.0 Maternal complications from in utero procedure**
[0-4]
      EXCLUDES   *maternal history of in utero procedure during previous pregnancy (V23.86)*

√5ᵗʰ **679.1 Fetal complications from in utero procedure**
[0-4]
      Fetal complications from amniocentesis
      EXCLUDES   *newborn affected by in utero procedure (760.61-760.64)*

Chapter 12: Diseases of the Skin and Subcutaneous Tissue (680–709)

Coding Guidance

This chapter classifies diseases and disorders of the epidermis, dermis, subcutaneous tissue, nails, scar tissue, sebaceous glands, sweat glands, hair, and hair follicles. The sections of this chapter are as follows:

- Infections of skin and subcutaneous tissue (680–686)
- Other inflammatory conditions of skin and subcutaneous tissue (690–698)
- Other diseases of skin and subcutaneous tissue (700–709)

Infections of the Skin and Subcutaneous Tissue (680–686)

Certain infections and parasitic diseases of the skin and subcutaneous tissue such as herpes simplex and herpes zoster, viral warts, and molluscum contagiosum are classified to chapter 1. Refer to the alphabetic index for instruction concerning the correct classification of infectious conditions of the skin and subcutaneous tissue.

This subchapter classifies diseases and disorders such as boils, carbuncles, furuncles, cellulitis, abscess, lymphadenitis, local infections, and pilonidal cysts.

When assigning a code from categories 680–686, also assign a code (as a secondary code) to identify the infective organism, such as Staphylococcus (subcategory 041.1).

Carbuncle and Furuncle (680)

Carbuncle and furuncle are infections caused by either aerobic or anaerobic bacterial organisms. A carbuncle is a collection of pus contained in a cavity or sac. A furuncle is a painful nodule formed by circumscribed inflammation of the skin and subcutaneous tissue, which encloses a central core.

Use an additional code to identify the infective organism, typically Streptococcus or Staphylococcus. Use the appropriate fourth digit to indicate the anatomic location of the furuncle or carbuncle.

Cellulitis and Abscess (681–682)

Cellulitis is a diffuse infection of the dermis and subcutaneous tissues often caused by group A Strep or Staphylococcus aureus, but sometimes caused by other organisms. Cellulitis may be associated with an abscess, which is a collection of pus resulting from an acute or chronic localized infection with tissue destruction. Category 681 includes lymphangitis and abscess and is often associated with cellulitis of the skin affecting fingers and toes.

Use an additional code to identify the infective organism, typically Streptococcus or Staphylococcus.

Abscess and lymphangitis are included in category 681. Do not code in addition to the cellulitis.

When cellulitis occurs with chronic skin ulcer (category 707), code both conditions.

Example:

Chronic pressure ulcer of the heel with cellulitis, unspecified organism, is coded 707.07 Pressure ulcer, heel and 682. 7. Sequencing is dependent upon circumstances of the episode of care. Code also the stage of pressure ulcer (707.20–707.25).

When cellulitis occurs secondary to a superficial injury (e.g., frostbite or burn) two codes are required sequenced according to the circumstances of the episode of care.

Example:

Patient seen for care of staphylococcal cellulitis of a second-degree burn on the hand is coded:

682.4	Cellulitis of the hand, except fingers and thumb
944.20	Burn, second degree of hand, unspecified site
041.10	Staphylococcus, unspecified

There are sites other than skin and subcutaneous tissue where cellulitis may occur. These sites include the cervix, larynx, nose, penis and tonsils. Coders should follow the instructions in the alphabetic index to code these sites.

Other Inflammatory Conditions of Skin and Subcutaneous Tissue (690–698)

Other inflammatory conditions that affect the skin such as dermatitis, eczema, sunburn, rosacea, lupus erythematosus, psoriasis, and lichen are classified to this section.

Contact Dermatitis and Other Eczema (692)

Contact dermatitis is classified by agent. The fourth digit specifies the agent such as detergents, solvents, medicines and drugs, food in contact with skin, solar radiation, and metals.

Palmar Plantar Erythrodysesthesia (693.0)

Palmar plantar erythrodysesthesia (PPE), also called hand and foot syndrome, may be described as an adverse effect of certain cancer therapies that occurs as a result of small amounts of antineoplastic or biologic drugs leaking from the capillaries into the tissues. Tissue damage occurs in the palms of the hands and soles of the feet due to the friction and heat generated during the course of normal daily activities. Symptoms include tenderness, redness, and peeling skin resembling a sunburn. Palmar plantar erythrodysesthesia is reported as drug dermatitis, with code 693.0 Dermatitis due to substances taken internally. Assign the appropriate E code for the adverse effect of drug. In addition, report the malignancy.

Erythematous Conditions (695.1)

Clinical classifications for erythema multiforme are based on the pattern and distribution of cutaneous lesions. Different causes, characteristics, and risk factors exist between erythema multiforme, Stevens-Johnson syndrome, and toxic epidermal necrolysis. The term "erythema multiforme" (EM) refers to the "multiple forms" in which these conditions, characterized by redness of the skin, are manifest. The characteristic redness (erythema) is produced by congestion of the capillaries. The "multiforme" portion of the diagnosis refers to the wide range of clinical presentation in which it appears, from the nature of symptoms and associated conditions to the variance in degrees of severity.

Erythema multiforme (695.10–695.12) is a hypersensitivity (allergic) reaction that can occur at any age but primarily affects children or young adults. It may occur in response to medications, infections, or illness. The causal agent induces damage to dermal blood vessels and tissues. Clinical presentation may range from a mild, self-limited rash (minor) to a more severe, life-threatening form involving mucous membranes. These erythematous conditions are characterized by the sudden onset of multiple, symmetrical pruritic (itching) skin lesions of the limbs and face that may spread and form blisters. Other associated symptoms include fever, malaise, and joint pain. Facial lesions are often associated with painful conjunctivitis, vision abnormalities, and buccal lesions. Erythema multiforme minor accounts for approximately 80 percent of EM cases.

In Stevens-Johnson syndrome (695.13–695.14), the lesions are more extensive than those characteristic of erythema multiforme major, and the systemic symptoms are more severe. Multiple body areas are usually involved, especially the mucous membranes. An overlap condition with an intermediate percent of body surface area affected (10 to 30 percent) is identified as SJS-TEN overlap syndrome (695.14). TEN (toxic epidermal necrolysis) (695.15) (also called Lyell's syndrome) involves multiple large blisters with exfoliation of all or most of the skin and mucous membranes, generally involving over 30 percent of the body surface area—similar to the skin loss with a severe burn, necessitating treatment in a burn unit.

SJS is part of the same spectrum of disease as TEN, although it generally involves body surface area of less than 10 percent. Erythema multiforme major has been strongly associated with herpes virus infection, while Stevens-Johnson syndrome and TEN have been associated with severe adverse drug reactions to certain medications that cause an extreme immunologically mediated abnormal metabolic reaction in sensitive people.

Three instructional notes at subcategory 695.1 Erythema multiforme provide important coding and sequencing information. Multiple codes may be necessary to report any associated manifestations, causal drug E codes, and the percentage of skin exfoliation.

Lupus Erythematosus (695.4)

Lupus erythematosus is a chronic disease that causes inflammation of the connective tissue of the skin only. This disease affects nine times as many women as men, usually those of childbearing age.

Note that this subcategory includes discoid lupus erythematosus, but excludes systemic lupus erythematosus.

Exfoliation Due to Erythematous Conditions According to Extent of Body Surface Involved (695.5)

Erythematous conditions are skin disorders characterized by diffuse redness (erythema). Exfoliation describes scaling and flaking off of the epidermal layers of the skin. Many of the conditions classified to code subcategory 695.1 result in scaling and flaking of the skin. The percentage of body surface involved correlates to the severity of presentation and represents the level of clinical care required. Specific codes indicate the severity of erythematous conditions. To help indicate severity, the percentage of skin exfoliation due to these conditions is reported with an additional code from subcategory 695.5. An instructional note is included with this subcategory to "Code first the erythematous condition causing exfoliation." These additional codes report the percentage of body surface involved, ranging from less than 10 percent to 90 percent or more of body surface.

Psoriasis (696)

Psoriasis is a common skin disease characterized by patches of inflamed, red skin, covered by silvery scales and sometimes accompanied by painful swelling and stiffness of joints (arthritis). The skin stratum becomes thickened, particularly over the elbows, knees, scalp, and trunk.

Other Diseases of Skin and Subcutaneous Tissue (700–709)

These codes describe conditions of the skin and subcutaneous tissues. The conditions in this section are benign but may require treatment.

Categories include:

- Corns and callosities (700)
- Other hypertrophic and atrophic conditions of skin (701)

Chronic Ulcer of Skin (707) and Pressure [Decubitus] Ulcer Staging (707.2)

Subclassification 707.0 reports conditions also known as bedsores or pressure sores. These lesions initially affect superficial tissues and, depending on the state of patient's health and other circumstances, may progress to affect muscle and bone. Patients at risk for developing pressure ulcers include the bedridden, those who are unconscious or immobile such as stroke patients, or those with paralysis and limited motion. Intrinsic loss of pain and pressure sensations, disuse atrophy, malnutrition, anemia, and infection contribute to the formation and progression of pressure ulcers. In the early stages, the condition is reversible, but left untended, the pressure ulcer can become extensively infected, necrotic and, ultimately, irreversible.

Code assignment reflects the National Pressure Ulcer Advisory Panel (NPUAP) definition and staging of pressure ulcers. A pressure ulcer is defined as a "localized injury to the skin and/or underlying tissue, usually over a bony prominence, as a result of pressure, or pressure in combination with shear and/or friction." Clinicians ordinarily characterize pressure ulcers by location, shape, depth, and healing status. The depth of the lesion or stage of ulcer is the most important element in clinical measurement:

- Unstageable (707.25): Lesion inaccessible for evaluation due to nonremovable dressings, eschar, sterile blister, or suspected deep injury in evolution are unstageable. Deep tissue injury may be difficult to detect in individuals with dark skin tones, and as such evolution of the wound may progress rapidly. Suspected deep tissue injury may be characterized by purple or maroon discoloration of the skin with or without blistering. Affected tissue may be painful and variant in temperature and texture from surrounding normal tissue.
- Stage I (707.21): Nonblanching erythema (a reddened area on the skin)
- Stage II (707.22): Abrasion, blister, shallow open crater, or other partial-thickness skin loss
- Stage III (707.23): Full-thickness skin loss involving damage or necrosis into subcutaneous soft tissues
- Stage IV (707.24): Full-thickness skin loss with necrosis of soft tissues through to the muscle, tendons, or tissues around underlying bone

Previous ICD-9-CM coding did not differentiate stages, with unique codes only for pressure ulcers for the more common anatomic sites (707.05 for buttock, for example). This method of classification precluded the use of coded records to accurately reflect severity data for quality improvement initiatives. Assign the appropriate code for the site of ulcer from subcategory 707.0 with an additional code from subcategory 707.2 to specify the stage of the ulcer.

Subcategory 707.1 Ulcer of lower limb, except pressure ulcer, includes skin ulcers of the lower limb due to other conditions such as diabetes, postphlebitic syndrome, and chronic venous hypertension. Code first the underlying condition. Do not assign a pressure ulcer stage code (707.20–707.25) with a code from 707.10–707.19.

12. DISEASES OF THE SKIN AND SUBCUTANEOUS TISSUE (680-709)

INFECTIONS OF SKIN AND SUBCUTANEOUS TISSUE (680-686)

EXCLUDES *certain infections of skin classified under "Infectious and Parasitic Diseases," such as:*
erysipelas (035)
erysipeloid of Rosenbach (027.1)
herpes:
  simplex (054.0-054.9)
  zoster (053.0-053.9)
molluscum contagiosum (078.0)
viral warts (078.10-078.19)

√4ᵗʰ 680 Carbuncle and furuncle

INCLUDES boil
furunculosis

DEF: Carbuncle: necrotic boils in skin and subcutaneous tissue of neck or back mainly due to staphylococcal infection.
DEF: Furuncle: circumscribed inflammation of corium and subcutaneous tissue due to staphylococcal infection.

680.0 Face
Ear [any part]
Face [any part, except eye]
Nose (septum)
Temple (region)
EXCLUDES *eyelid (373.13)*
lacrimal apparatus (375.31)
orbit (376.01)

680.1 Neck

680.2 Trunk
Abdominal wall
Back [any part, except buttocks]
Breast
Chest wall
Flank
Groin
Pectoral region
Perineum
Umbilicus
EXCLUDES *buttocks (680.5)*
external genital organs:
female (616.4)
male (607.2, 608.4)

680.3 Upper arm and forearm
Arm [any part, except hand]
Axilla
Shoulder

680.4 Hand
Finger [any]
Thumb
Wrist

680.5 Buttock
Anus
Gluteal region

680.6 Leg, except foot
Ankle
Hip
Knee
Thigh

680.7 Foot
Heel
Toe

680.8 Other specified sites
Head [any part, except face]
Scalp
EXCLUDES *external genital organs:*
female (616.4)
male (607.2, 608.4)

680.9 Unspecified site
Boil NOS
Carbuncle NOS
Furuncle NOS

Skin and Subcutaneous Layer

√4ᵗʰ 681 Cellulitis and abscess of finger and toe

INCLUDES that with lymphangitis
Use additional code to identify organism, such as Staphylococcus (041.1)
DEF: Acute suppurative inflammation and edema in subcutaneous tissue or muscle of finger or toe.

√5ᵗʰ 681.0 Finger
  681.00 Cellulitis and abscess, unspecified
  681.01 Felon
    Pulp abscess
    Whitlow
    EXCLUDES *herpetic whitlow (054.6)*
    DEF: Painful abscess of fingertips caused by infection in the closed space of terminal phalanx.
  681.02 Onychia and paronychia of finger
    Panaritium } of finger
    Perionychia
    DEF: Onychia: inflammation of nail matrix; causes nail loss.
    DEF: Paronychia: inflammation of tissue folds around nail.

√5ᵗʰ 681.1 Toe
  681.10 Cellulitis and abscess, unspecified
  681.11 Onychia and paronychia of toe
    Panaritium } of toe
    Perionychia

681.9 Cellulitis and abscess of unspecified digit
Infection of nail NOS

√4ᵗʰ 682 Other cellulitis and abscess

INCLUDES abscess (acute
cellulitis (diffuse) } (with lymphangitis) except
lymphangitis, acute   of finger or toe
Use additional code to identify organism, such as Staphylococcus (041.1)
EXCLUDES *lymphangitis (chronic) (subacute) (457.2)*
DEF: Cellulitis: Acute suppurative inflammation of deep subcutaneous tissue and sometimes muscle due to infection of wound, burn or other lesion.

682.0 Face
Cheek, external   Nose, external
Chin   Submandibular
Forehead   Temple (region)
EXCLUDES *ear [any part] (380.10-380.16)*
eyelid (373.13)
lacrimal apparatus (375.31)
lip (528.5)
mouth (528.3)
nose (internal) (478.1)
orbit (376.01)

682.1 Neck

Lymphatic System of Head and Neck

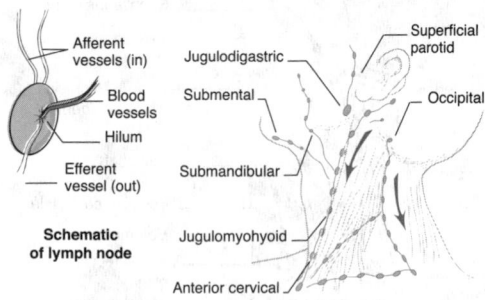

Schematic
of lymph node

Lymphatic drainage of the
head, neck, and face

682.2   **Trunk**
    Abdominal wall
    Back [any part, except buttock]
    Chest wall
    Flank
    Groin
    Pectoral region
    Perineum
    Umbilicus, except newborn
    EXCLUDES   *anal and rectal regions (566)*
             breast:
                NOS (611.0)
                puerperal (675.1)
             external genital organs:
                female (616.3-616.4)
                male (604.0, 607.2, 608.4)
             umbilicus, newborn (771.4)

682.3   **Upper arm and forearm**
    Arm [any part, except hand]
    Axilla
    Shoulder
    EXCLUDES   *hand (682.4)*

682.4   **Hand, except fingers and thumb**
    Wrist
    EXCLUDES   *finger and thumb (681.00-681.02)*

682.5   **Buttock**
    Gluteal region
    EXCLUDES   *anal and rectal regions (566)*

682.6   **Leg, except foot**
    Ankle
    Hip
    Knee
    Thigh

682.7   **Foot, except toes**
    Heel
    EXCLUDES   *toe (681.10-681.11)*

682.8   **Other specified sites**
    Head [except face]
    Scalp
    EXCLUDES   *face (682.0)*

682.9   **Unspecified site**
    Abscess NOS
    Cellulitis NOS
    Lymphangitis, acute NOS
    EXCLUDES   *lymphangitis NOS (457.2)*

683   **Acute lymphadenitis**
    Abscess (acute)   ⎫
    Adenitis, acute   ⎬ lymph gland or node,
    Lymphadenitis, acute ⎭   except mesenteric
    Use additional code to identify organism, such as Staphylococcus
    (041.1)
    EXCLUDES   *enlarged glands NOS (785.6)*
             lymphadenitis:
                chronic or subacute, except mesenteric (289.1)
                mesenteric (acute) (chronic) (subacute) (289.2)
                unspecified (289.3)
    DEF: Acute inflammation of lymph nodes due to primary infection located elsewhere in the body.

Stages of Pilonidal Disease

684   **Impetigo**
    Impetiginization of other dermatoses
    Impetigo (contagiosa) [any site] [any organism]:
       bullous
       circinate
       neonatorum
       simplex
    Pemphigus neonatorum
    EXCLUDES   *impetigo herpetiformis (694.3)*
    DEF: Infectious skin disease commonly occurring in children; caused by group A streptococci or Staphylococcus aureus; skin lesions usually appear on the face and consist of subcorneal vesicles and bullae that burst and form yellow crusts.

√4ᵗʰ **685**   **Pilonidal cyst**
    INCLUDES   fistula ⎫
                  sinus   ⎬ coccygeal or pilonidal
    DEF: Hair-containing cyst or sinus in the tissues of the sacrococcygeal area; often drains through opening at the postanal dimple.

    685.0   **With abscess**

    685.1   **Without mention of abscess**

√4ᵗʰ **686**   **Other local infections of skin and subcutaneous tissue**
    Use additional code to identify any infectious organism (041.0-041.8)

√5ᵗʰ   **686.0**   **Pyoderma**
       Dermatitis:
          purulent
          septic
          suppurative
       DEF: Nonspecific purulent skin disease related most to furuncles, pustules, or possibly carbuncles.

       686.00   **Pyoderma, unspecified**

       686.01   **Pyoderma gangrenosum**
          DEF: Persistent debilitating skin disease characterized by irregular, boggy, blue-red ulcerations, with central healing and undermined edges.

       686.09   **Other pyoderma**

    686.1   **Pyogenic granuloma**
       Granuloma:
          septic
          suppurative
          telangiectaticum
       EXCLUDES   *pyogenic granuloma of oral mucosa (528.9)*
       DEF: Solitary polypoid capillary hemangioma often associated with local irritation, trauma, and superimposed inflammation; located on the skin and gingival or oral mucosa.

    686.8   **Other specified local infections of skin and subcutaneous tissue**
       Bacterid (pustular)
       Dermatitis vegetans
       Ecthyma
       Perlèche
       EXCLUDES   *dermatitis infectiosa eczematoides (690.8)*
                    panniculitis (729.30-729.39)

686.9 Unspecified local infection of skin and subcutaneous tissue
Fistula of skin NOS
Skin infection NOS
EXCLUDES   *fistula to skin from internal organs – see Alphabetic Index*

OTHER INFLAMMATORY CONDITIONS OF SKIN AND SUBCUTANEOUS TISSUE (690-698)
EXCLUDES   *panniculitis (729.30-729.39)*

√4ᵗʰ **690 Erythematosquamous dermatosis**
EXCLUDES   *eczematous dermatitis of eyelid (373.31)*
parakeratosis variegata (696.2)
psoriasis (696.0-696.1)
seborrheic keratosis (702.11-702.19)

√5ᵗʰ **690.1 Seborrheic dermatitis**

    690.10 Seborrheic dermatitis, unspecified
Seborrheic dermatitis NOS

    690.11 Seborrhea capitis
Cradle cap

    690.12 Seborrheic infantile dermatitis

    690.18 Other seborrheic dermatitis

   690.8 Other erythematosquamous dermatosis

√4ᵗʰ **691 Atopic dermatitis and related conditions**
DEF: Atopic dermatitis: chronic, pruritic, inflammatory skin disorder found on the face and antecubital and popliteal fossae; often accompanied by allergic rhinitis, hay fever, asthma, and extreme itching; also called allergic dermatitis, or disseminated neurodermatitis.

   691.0 Diaper or napkin rash
Ammonia dermatitis
Diaper or napkin:
    dermatitis
    erythema
    rash
Psoriasiform napkin eruption

   691.8 Other atopic dermatitis and related conditions
Atopic dermatitis
Besnier's prurigo
Eczema:
    atopic
    flexural
    intrinsic (allergic)
Neurodermatitis:
    atopic
    diffuse (of Brocq)

√4ᵗʰ **692 Contact dermatitis and other eczema**
INCLUDES   dermatitis:
    NOS
    contact
    occupational
    venenata
eczema (acute) (chronic):
    NOS
    allergic
    erythematous
    occupational
EXCLUDES   *allergy NOS (995.3)*
contact dermatitis of eyelids (373.32)
dermatitis due to substances taken internally (693.0-693.9)
eczema of external ear (380.22)
perioral dermatitis (695.3)
urticarial reactions (708.0-708.9, 995.1)
DEF: Contact dermatitis: acute or chronic dermatitis caused by initial irritant effect of a substance, or by prior sensitization to a substance coming once again in contact with skin.

   692.0 Due to detergents

   692.1 Due to oils and greases

   692.2 Due to solvents
Dermatitis due to solvents of:
    chlorocompound
    cyclohexane
    ester
    glycol   } group
    hydrocarbon
    ketone

   692.3 Due to drugs and medicines in contact with skin
Dermatitis (allergic) (contact) due to:
    arnica
    fungicides
    iodine
    keratolytics
    mercurials
    neomycin
    pediculocides
    phenols
    scabicides
    any drug applied to skin
Dermatitis medicamentosa due to drug applied to skin
Use additional E code to identify drug
EXCLUDES   *allergy NOS due to drugs (995.27)*
dermatitis due to ingested drugs (693.0)
dermatitis medicamentosa NOS (693.0)

   692.4 Due to other chemical products
Dermatitis due to:
    acids
    adhesive plaster
    alkalis
    caustics
    dichromate
    insecticide
    nylon
    plastic
    rubber

   692.5 Due to food in contact with skin
Dermatitis, contact, due to:
    cereals
    fish
    flour
    fruit
    meat
    milk
EXCLUDES   *dermatitis due to:*
    dyes (692.89)
    ingested foods (693.1)
    preservatives (692.89)

   692.6 Due to plants [except food]
Dermatitis due to:
    lacquer tree [Rhus verniciflua]
    other plants in contact with the skin
    poison:
      ivy [Rhus toxicodendron]
      oak [Rhus diversiloba]
      sumac [Rhus venenata]
      vine [Rhus radicans]
    primrose [Primula]
    ragweed [Senecio jacobae]
EXCLUDES   *allergy NOS due to pollen (477.0)*
nettle rash (708.8)

√5ᵗʰ **692.7 Due to solar radiation**
EXCLUDES   *sunburn due to other ultraviolet radiation exposure (692.82)*

    692.70 Unspecified dermatitis due to sun

    692.71 Sunburn
First degree sunburn
Sunburn NOS

Diseases of the Skin and Subcutaneous Tissue

692.72–694.60

692.72 Acute dermatitis due to solar radiation
Acute solar skin damage NOS
Berlogue dermatitis
Photoallergic response
Phototoxic response
Polymorphus light eruption
Use additional E code to identify drug, if drug induced

EXCLUDES   sunburn (692.71, 692.76-692.77)

DEF: Berloque dermatitis: Phytophotodermatitis due to sun exposure after use of a product containing bergamot oil; causes red patches, that turn brown.
DEF: Photoallergic response: Dermatitis due to hypersensitivity to the sun; causes papulovesicular, eczematous or exudative eruptions.
DEF: Phototoxic response: Chemically induced sensitivity to sun causes burn-like reaction, occasionally vesiculation and subsequent hyperpigmentation.
DEF: Polymorphous light eruption: Inflammatory skin eruptions due to sunlight exposure; eruptions differ in size and shape.
DEF: Acute solar skin damage (NOS): Rapid, unspecified injury to skin from sun.

692.73 Actinic reticuloid and actinic granuloma

DEF: Actinic reticuloid: Dermatosis aggravated by light, causes chronic eczema-like eruption on exposed skin which extends to other unexposed surfaces; occurs in the elderly.
DEF: Actinic granuloma: Inflammatory response of skin to sun causing small nodule of microphages.

692.74 Other chronic dermatitis due to solar radiation
Chronic solar skin damage NOS
Solar elastosis

EXCLUDES   actinic [solar] keratosis (702.0)

DEF: Solar elastosis: Premature aging of skin of light-skinned people; causes inelasticity, thinning or thickening, wrinkling, dryness, scaling and hyperpigmentation.
DEF: Chronic solar skin damage (NOS): Chronic skin impairment due to exposure to the sun, not otherwise specified.

692.75 Disseminated superficial actinic porokeratosis [DSAP]

DEF: Autosomal dominant skin condition occurring in skin that has been overexposed to the sun; characterized by superficial annular, keratotic, brownish-red spots or thickenings with depressed centers and sharp, ridged borders, may evolve into squamous cell carcinoma.

692.76 Sunburn of second degree

692.77 Sunburn of third degree

692.79 Other dermatitis due to solar radiation
Hydroa aestivale
Photodermatitis
Photosensitiveness   } (due to sun)
Solar skin damage NOS

✓5ᵗʰ 692.8 Due to other specified agents

692.81 Dermatitis due to cosmetics

692.82 Dermatitis due to other radiation
Infrared rays
Light, except from sun
Radiation NOS
Tanning bed
Ultraviolet rays, except from sun
X-rays

EXCLUDES   solar radiation (692.70-692.79)

692.83 Dermatitis due to metals
Jewelry

692.84 Due to animal (cat) (dog) dander
Due to animal (cat) (dog) hair

692.89 Other
Dermatitis due to: Dermatitis due to:
   cold weather   hot weather
   dyes   preservatives

EXCLUDES   allergy (NOS) (rhinitis) due to animal hair or dander (477.2)
allergy to dust (477.8)
sunburn (692.71, 692.76-692.77)

692.9 Unspecified cause
Dermatitis:
   NOS
   contact NOS
   venenata NOS
Eczema NOS

✓4ᵗʰ 693 Dermatitis due to substances taken internally

EXCLUDES   adverse effect NOS of drugs and medicines (995.20)
allergy NOS (995.3)
contact dermatitis (692.0-692.9)
urticarial reactions (708.0-708.9, 995.1)

DEF: Inflammation of skin due to ingested substance.

693.0 Due to drugs and medicines
Dermatitis medicamentosa NOS
Use additional E code to identify drug

EXCLUDES   that due to drugs in contact with skin (692.3)

693.1 Due to food

693.8 Due to other specified substances taken internally

693.9 Due to unspecified substance taken internally

EXCLUDES   dermatitis NOS (692.9)

✓4ᵗʰ 694 Bullous dermatoses

694.0 Dermatitis herpetiformis
Dermatosis herpetiformis   Hydroa herpetiformis
Duhring's disease

EXCLUDES   herpes gestationis (646.8)
dermatitis herpetiformis:
   juvenile (694.2)
   senile (694.5)

DEF: Chronic, multisystem disease manifested most in the cutaneous system; seen as an extremely pruritic eruption of various lesions that frequently heal leaving hyperpigmentation or hypopigmentation and occasionally scarring; usually associated with an asymptomatic gluten-sensitive enteropathy, and immunogenic factors.

694.1 Subcorneal pustular dermatosis
Sneddon-Wilkinson disease or syndrome

DEF: Chronic relapses of sterile pustular blebs beneath the horny skin layer of the trunk and skin folds; resembles dermatitis herpetiformis.

694.2 Juvenile dermatitis herpetiformis
Juvenile pemphigoid

694.3 Impetigo herpetiformis

DEF: Rare dermatosis associated with pregnancy; marked by itching pustules in third trimester, hypocalcemia, tetany, fever and lethargy; may result in maternal or fetal death.

694.4 Pemphigus
Pemphigus: Pemphigus:
   NOS   malignant
   erythematosus   vegetans
   foliaceus   vulgaris

EXCLUDES   pemphigus neonatorum (684)

DEF: Chronic, relapsing, sometimes fatal skin diseases; causes vesicles, bullae; autoantibodies against intracellular connections cause acantholysis.

694.5 Pemphigoid
Benign pemphigus NOS
Bullous pemphigoid
Herpes circinatus bullosus
Senile dermatitis herpetiformis

✓5ᵗʰ 694.6 Benign mucous membrane pemphigoid
Cicatricial pemphigoid
Mucosynechial atrophic bullous dermatitis

694.60 Without mention of ocular involvement

Diseases of the Skin and Subcutaneous Tissue

694.61–696.1

694.61 With ocular involvement
Ocular pemphigus
DEF: Mild self-limiting, subepidermal blistering of mucosa including the conjunctiva, seen predominantly in the elderly, produces adhesions and scarring.

694.8 Other specified bullous dermatoses
EXCLUDES herpes gestationis (646.8)

694.9 Unspecified bullous dermatoses

✓4ᵗʰ **695 Erythematous conditions**

695.0 Toxic erythema
Erythema venenatum

✓5ᵗʰ **695.1 Erythema multiforme**
Use additional code to identify associated manifestations, such as:
arthropathy associated with dermatological disorders (713.3)
conjunctival edema (372.73)
conjunctivitis (372.04, 372.33)
corneal scars and opacities (371.00-371.05)
corneal ulcer (370.00-370.07)
edema of eyelid (374.82)
inflammation of eyelid (373.8)
keratoconjunctivitis sicca (370.33)
mechanical lagophthalmos (374.22)
mucositis (478.11, 528.00, 538, 616.81)
stomatitis (528.00)
symblepharon (372.63)
Use additional E code to identify drug, if drug-induced
Use additional code to identify percentage of skin exfoliation (695.50-695.59)
EXCLUDES (Staphylococcal) scalded skin syndrome (695.81)
DEF: Symptom complex with varied skin eruption pattern of macular, bullous, papular, nodose, or vesicular lesions on the neck, face, and legs; gastritis and rheumatic pains; secondary to number of factors, including infections, ingestants, physical agents, malignancy and pregnancy.

695.10 Erythema multiforme, unspecified
Erythema iris
Herpes iris

695.11 Erythema multiforme minor

695.12 Erythema multiforme major

695.13 Stevens-Johnson syndrome

695.14 Stevens-Johnson syndrome-toxic epidermal necrolysis overlap syndrome
SJS-TEN overlap syndrome

695.15 Toxic epidermal necrolysis
Lyell's syndrome

695.19 Other erythema multiforme

695.2 Erythema nodosum
EXCLUDES tuberculous erythema nodosum (017.1)
DEF: Panniculitis (an inflammatory reaction of the subcutaneous fat) of women, usually seen as a hypersensitivity reaction to infections, drugs, sarcoidosis, and specific enteropathies; the acute stage associated with fever, malaise, and arthralgia; the lesions are pink to blue in color as tender nodules and are found on the front of the legs below the knees.

695.3 Rosacea
Acne: Perioral dermatitis
 erythematosa Rhinophyma
 rosacea
DEF: Chronic skin disease, usually of the face, characterized by persistent erythema and telangiectasis with acute episodes of edema, engorgement papules, and pustules.

695.4 Lupus erythematosus
Lupus:
 erythematodes (discoid)
 erythematosus (discoid), not disseminated
EXCLUDES lupus (vulgaris) NOS (017.0)
systemic [disseminated] lupus erythematosus (710.0)
DEF: Group of connective tissue disorders occurring as various cutaneous diseases of unknown origin; it primarily affects women between the ages of 20 and 40.

✓5ᵗʰ **695.5 Exfoliation due to erythematous conditions according to extent of body surface involved**
Code first erythematous condition causing exfoliation, such as:
Ritter's disease (695.81)
(Staphylococcal) scalded skin syndrome (695.81)
Stevens-Johnson syndrome (695.13)
Stevens-Johnson syndrome-toxic epidermal necrolysis overlap syndrome (695.14)
toxic epidermal necrolysis (695.15)

695.50 Exfoliation due to erythematous condition involving less than 10 percent of body surface
Exfoliation due to erythematous condition NOS

695.51 Exfoliation due to erythematous condition involving 10-19 percent of body surface

695.52 Exfoliation due to erythematous condition involving 20-29 percent of body surface

695.53 Exfoliation due to erythematous condition involving 30-39 percent of body surface

695.54 Exfoliation due to erythematous condition involving 40-49 percent of body surface

695.55 Exfoliation due to erythematous condition involving 50-59 percent of body surface

695.56 Exfoliation due to erythematous condition involving 60-69 percent of body surface

695.57 Exfoliation due to erythematous condition involving 70-79 percent of body surface

695.58 Exfoliation due to erythematous condition involving 80-89 percent of body surface

695.59 Exfoliation due to erythematous condition involving 90 percent or more of body surface

✓5ᵗʰ **695.8 Other specified erythematous conditions**

695.81 Ritter's disease
Dermatitis exfoliativa neonatorum
(Staphylococcal) Scalded skin syndrome
Use additional code to identify percentage of skin exfoliation (695.50-695.59)
DEF: Infectious skin disease of young children marked by eruptions ranging from a localized bullous to widespread of easily ruptured fine vesicles and bullae; results in exfoliation of large planes of skin and leaves raw areas.

695.89 Other
Erythema intertrigo   Pityriasis rubra
Intertrigo   (Hebra)
EXCLUDES mycotic intertrigo (111.0-111.9)

695.9 Unspecified erythematous condition
Erythema NOS   Erythroderma (secondary)

✓4ᵗʰ **696 Psoriasis and similar disorders**

696.0 Psoriatic arthropathy
DEF: Psoriasis associated with inflammatory arthritis; often involves interphalangeal joints.

696.1 Other psoriasis
Acrodermatitis continua   Psoriasis:
Dermatitis repens   NOS
                           any type, except
                           arthropathic
EXCLUDES psoriatic arthropathy (696.0)

696.2   Parapsoriasis
Parakeratosis variegata
Parapsoriasis lichenoides chronica
Pityriasis lichenoides et varioliformis

DEF: Erythrodermas similar to lichen, planus and psoriasis; symptoms include redness and itching; resistant to treatment.

696.3   Pityriasis rosea
Pityriasis circinata (et maculata)

DEF: Common, self-limited rash of unknown etiology marked by a solitary erythematous, salmon or fawn-colored herald plaque on the trunk, arms or thighs; followed by development of papular or macular lesions that tend to peel and form a scaly collarette.

696.4   Pityriasis rubra pilaris
Devergie's disease
Lichen ruber acuminatus

EXCLUDES   pityriasis rubra (Hebra) (695.89)

DEF: Inflammatory disease of hair follicles; marked by firm, red lesions topped by horny plugs; may form patches; occurs on fingers elbows, knees.

696.5   Other and unspecified pityriasis
Pityriasis:
NOS
alba
streptogenes

EXCLUDES   pityriasis:
simplex (690.18)
versicolor (111.0)

696.8   Other

☑4ᵗʰ 697   Lichen

EXCLUDES   lichen:
obtusus corneus (698.3)
pilaris (congenital) (757.39)
ruber acuminatus (696.4)
sclerosus et atrophicus (701.0)
scrofulosus (017.0)
simplex chronicus (698.3)
spinulosus (congenital) (757.39)
urticatus (698.2)

697.0   Lichen planus
Lichen:
planopilaris
ruber planus

DEF: Inflammatory, pruritic skin disease; marked by angular, flat-top, violet-colored papules; may be acute and widespread or chronic and localized.

697.1   Lichen nitidus
Pinkus' disease

DEF: Chronic, inflammatory, asymptomatic skin disorder, characterized by numerous glistening, flat-topped, discrete, skin-colored micropapules most often on penis, lower abdomen, inner thighs, wrists, forearms, breasts and buttocks.

697.8   Other lichen, not elsewhere classified
Lichen:
ruber moniliforme
striata

697.9   Lichen, unspecified

☑4ᵗʰ 698   Pruritus and related conditions

EXCLUDES   pruritus specified as psychogenic (306.3)

DEF: Pruritus: Intense, persistent itching due to irritation of sensory nerve endings from organic or psychogenic causes.

698.0   Pruritus ani
Perianal itch

698.1   Pruritus of genital organs

698.2   Prurigo
Lichen urticatus   Prurigo:
Prurigo: mitis
NOS   simplex
Hebra's   Urticaria papulosa (Hebra)

EXCLUDES   prurigo nodularis (698.3)

698.3   Lichenification and lichen simplex chronicus
Hyde's disease
Neurodermatitis (circumscripta) (local)
Prurigo nodularis

EXCLUDES   neurodermatitis, diffuse (of Brocq) (691.8)

DEF: Lichenification: thickening of skin due to prolonged rubbing or scratching.

DEF: Lichen simplex chronicus: eczematous dermatitis, of face, neck, extremities, scrotum, vulva, and perianal region due to repeated itching, rubbing and scratching; spontaneous or evolves with other dermatoses.

698.4   Dermatitis factitia [artefacta]
Dermatitis ficta
Neurotic excoriation

Use additional code to identify any associated mental disorder

DEF: Various types of self-inflicted skin lesions characterized in appearance as an erythema to a gangrene.

698.8   Other specified pruritic conditions
Pruritus: Winter itch
hiemalis
senilis

698.9   Unspecified pruritic disorder
Itch NOS
Pruritus NOS

OTHER DISEASES OF SKIN AND SUBCUTANEOUS TISSUE (700-709)

EXCLUDES   conditions confined to eyelids (373.0-374.9)
congenital conditions of skin, hair, and nails (757.0-757.9)

700   Corns and callosities
Callus   Clavus

DEF: Corns: Conical or horny thickening of skin on toes, due to friction, pressure from shoes and hosiery; pain and inflammation may develop.

DEF: Callosities: Localized overgrowth (hyperplasia) of the horny epidermal layer due to pressure or friction.

☑4ᵗʰ 701   Other hypertrophic and atrophic conditions of skin

EXCLUDES   dermatomyositis (710.3)
hereditary edema of legs (757.0)
scleroderma (generalized) (710.1)

701.0   Circumscribed scleroderma
Addison's keloid
Dermatosclerosis, localized
Lichen sclerosus et atrophicus
Morphea
Scleroderma, circumscribed or localized

DEF: Thickened, hardened, skin and subcutaneous tissue; may involve musculoskeletal system.

701.1   Keratoderma, acquired
Acquired:
ichthyosis
keratoderma palmaris et plantaris
Elastosis perforans serpiginosa
Hyperkeratosis:
NOS
follicularis in cutem penetrans
palmoplantaris climacterica
Keratoderma:
climactericum
tylodes, progressive
Keratosis (blennorrhagica)

EXCLUDES   Darier's disease [keratosis follicularis] (congenital) (757.39)
keratosis:
arsenical (692.4)
gonococcal (098.81)

701.2 **Acquired acanthosis nigricans**
Keratosis nigricans

DEF: Diffuse velvety hyperplasia of the spinous skin layer of the axilla and other body folds marked by gray, brown, or black pigmentation; in adult form often associated with malignant acanthosis nigricans in a benign, nevoid form relatively generalized.

701.3 **Striae atrophicae**
Atrophic spots of skin
Atrophoderma maculatum
Atrophy blanche (of Milian)
Degenerative colloid atrophy
Senile degenerative atrophy
Striae distensae

DEF: Bands of atrophic, depressed, wrinkled skin associated with stretching of skin from pregnancy, obesity, or rapid growth during puberty.

701.4 **Keloid scar**
Cheloid
Hypertrophic scar
Keloid

DEF: Overgrowth of scar tissue due to excess amounts of collagen during connective tissue repair; occurs mainly on upper trunk, face.

701.5 **Other abnormal granulation tissue**
Excessive granulation

701.8 **Other specified hypertrophic and atrophic conditions of skin**
Acrodermatitis atrophicans chronica
Atrophia cutis senilis
Atrophoderma neuriticum
Confluent and reticulate papillomatosis
Cutis laxa senilis
Elastosis senilis
Folliculitis ulerythematosa reticulata
Gougerot-Carteaud syndrome or disease

701.9 **Unspecified hypertrophic and atrophic conditions of skin**
Atrophoderma
Skin tag

√4ᵗʰ **702** **Other dermatoses**
EXCLUDES *carcinoma in situ (232.0-232.9)*

702.0 **Actinic keratosis**
DEF: Wart-like growth, red or skin-colored; may form a cutaneous horn.

√5ᵗʰ **702.1** **Seborrheic keratosis**
DEF: Common, benign, lightly pigmented, warty growth composed of basaloid cells.

702.11 **Inflamed seborrheic keratosis**

702.19 **Other seborrheic keratosis**
Seborrheic keratosis NOS

702.8 **Other specified dermatoses**

√4ᵗʰ **703** **Diseases of nail**
EXCLUDES *congenital anomalies (757.5)*
onychia and paronychia (681.02, 681.11)

703.0 **Ingrowing nail**
Ingrowing nail with infection
Unguis incarnatus
EXCLUDES *infection, nail NOS (681.9)*

703.8 **Other specified diseases of nail**
Dystrophia unguium
Hypertrophy of nail
Koilonychia
Leukonychia (punctata) (striata)
Onychauxis
Onychogryposis
Onycholysis

703.9 **Unspecified disease of nail**

√4ᵗʰ **704** **Diseases of hair and hair follicles**
EXCLUDES *congenital anomalies (757.4)*

√5ᵗʰ **704.0** **Alopecia**
EXCLUDES *madarosis (374.55)*
syphilitic alopecia (091.82)

DEF: Lack of hair, especially on scalp; often called baldness; may be partial or total; occurs at any age.

704.00 **Alopecia, unspecified**
Baldness
Loss of hair

704.01 **Alopecia areata**
Ophiasis

DEF: Alopecia areata: usually reversible, inflammatory, patchy hair loss found in beard or scalp.

DEF: Ophiasis: alopecia areata of children; marked by band around temporal and occipital scalp margins.

704.02 **Telogen effluvium**
DEF: Shedding of hair from premature telogen development in follicles due to stress, including shock, childbirth, surgery, drugs or weight loss.

704.09 **Other**
Folliculitis decalvans
Hypotrichosis:
  NOS
  postinfectional NOS
Pseudopelade

704.1 **Hirsutism**
Hypertrichosis:
  NOS
  lanuginosa, acquired
Polytrichia
EXCLUDES *hypertrichosis of eyelid (374.54)*
DEF: Excess hair growth; often in unexpected places and amounts.

704.2 **Abnormalities of the hair**
Atrophic hair
Clastothrix
Fragilitas crinium
Trichiasis:
  NOS
  cicatrical
Trichorrhexis (nodosa)
EXCLUDES *trichiasis of eyelid (374.05)*

704.3 **Variations in hair color**
Canities (premature)
Grayness, hair (premature)
Heterochromia of hair
Poliosis:
  NOS
  circumscripta, acquired

√5ᵗʰ **704.4** **Pilar and trichilemmal cysts**

704.41 **Pilar cyst**

704.42 **Trichilemmal cyst**
Trichilemmal proliferating cyst

704.8 **Other specified diseases of hair and hair follicles**
Folliculitis:
  NOS
  abscedens et suffodiens
  pustular
Perifolliculitis:
  NOS
  capitis abscedens et suffodiens
  scalp
Sycosis:
  NOS
  barbae [not parasitic]
  lupoid
  vulgaris

704.9 **Unspecified disease of hair and hair follicles**

√4ᵗʰ **705 Disorders of sweat glands**

705.0 Anhidrosis
Hypohidrosis
Oligohidrosis
DEF: Lack or deficiency of ability to sweat.

705.1 Prickly heat
Heat rash
Miliaria rubra (tropicalis)
Sudamina

√5ᵗʰ **705.2 Focal hyperhidrosis**
EXCLUDES *generalized (secondary) hyperhidrosis (780.8)*

705.21 Primary focal hyperhidrosis
Focal hyperhidrosis NOS
Hyperhidrosis NOS
Hyperhidrosis of:
axilla
face
palms
soles
DEF: A rare disorder of the sweat glands resulting in excessive production of sweat; occurs in the absence of any underlying condition, almost always focal, confined to one or more specific areas of the body.

705.22 Secondary focal hyperhidrosis
Frey's syndrome
DEF: Secondary focal hyperhidrosis: a symptom of an underlying disease process resulting in excessive sweating beyond what the body requires to maintain thermal control, confined to one or more specific areas of the body.
DEF: Frey's syndrome: an auriculotemporal syndrome due to lesion on the parotid gland; characteristic redness and excessive sweating on the cheek in connection with eating.

√5ᵗʰ **705.8 Other specified disorders of sweat glands**

705.81 Dyshidrosis
Cheiropompholyx
Pompholyx
DEF: Vesicular eruption, on hands, feet causing itching and burning.

705.82 Fox-Fordyce disease
DEF: Chronic, usually pruritic disease evidenced by small follicular papular eruptions, especially in the axillary and pubic areas; develops from the closure and rupture of the affected apocrine glands' intraepidermal portion of the ducts.

705.83 Hidradenitis
Hidradenitis suppurativa
DEF: Inflamed sweat glands.

705.89 Other
Bromhidrosis
Chromhidrosis
Granulosis rubra nasi
Urhidrosis
EXCLUDES *generalized hyperhidrosis (780.8)*
hidrocystoma (216.0-216.9)
DEF: Bromhidrosis: foul-smelling axillary sweat due to decomposed bacteria.
DEF: Chromhidrosis: secretion of colored sweat.
DEF: Granulosis rubra nasi: idiopathic condition of children; causes redness, sweating around nose, face and chin; tends to end by puberty.
DEF: Urhidrosis: urinous substance, such as uric acid, in sweat; occurs in uremia.

705.9 Unspecified disorder of sweat glands
Disorder of sweat glands NOS

√4ᵗʰ **706 Diseases of sebaceous glands**

706.0 Acne varioliformis
Acne:
frontalis
necrotica
DEF: Rare form of acne characterized by persistent brown papulo-pustules usually on the brow and temporoparietal part of the scalp.

706.1 Other acne
Acne: Blackhead
NOS   Comedo
conglobata
cystic
pustular
vulgaris
EXCLUDES *acne rosacea (695.3)*

706.2 Sebaceous cyst
Atheroma, skin
Keratin cyst
Wen
EXCLUDES *pilar cyst (704.41)*
trichilemmal (proliferating) cyst (704.42)
DEF: Benign epidermal cyst, contains sebum and keratin; presents as firm, circumscribed nodule.

706.3 Seborrhea
EXCLUDES *seborrhea:*
capitis (690.11)
sicca (690.18)
seborrheic
dermatitis (690.10)
keratosis (702.11-702.19)
DEF: Seborrheic dermatitis marked by excessive secretion of sebum; the sebum forms an oily coating, crusts, or scales on the skin; it is also called hypersteatosis.

706.8 Other specified diseases of sebaceous glands
Asteatosis (cutis)
Xerosis cutis

706.9 Unspecified disease of sebaceous glands

√4ᵗʰ **707 Chronic ulcer of skin**
INCLUDES non-infected sinus of skin
non-healing ulcer
EXCLUDES *varicose ulcer (454.0, 454.2)*

√5ᵗʰ **707.0 Pressure ulcer**
Bed sore
Decubitus ulcer
Plaster ulcer
Use additional code to identify pressure ulcer stage (707.20-707.25)

707.00 Unspecified site

707.01 Elbow

707.02 Upper back
Shoulder blades

707.03 Lower back
Coccyx
Sacrum

707.04 Hip

707.05 Buttock

707.06 Ankle

707.07 Heel

707.09 Other site
Head

Four Stages of Pressure Ulcers

First Stage
Persistent focal erythema

Second Stage
Partial thickness skin loss involving epidermis, dermis, or both

Third Stage
Full thickness skin loss extending through subcutaneous tissue

Fourth Stage
Necrosis of soft tissue extending to muscle and bone

Cutaneous Lesions

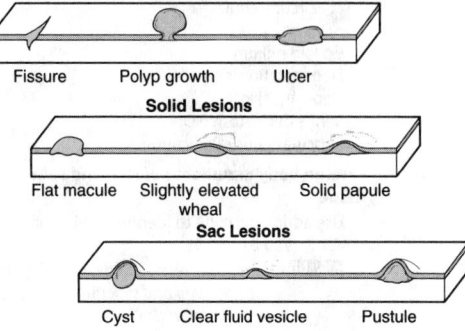

Surface Lesions

Fissure   Polyp growth   Ulcer

Solid Lesions

Flat macule   Slightly elevated wheal   Solid papule

Sac Lesions

Cyst   Clear fluid vesicle   Pustule

√5ᵗʰ 707.1 Ulcer of lower limbs, except pressure ulcer
Ulcer, chronic:
neurogenic
trophic } of lower limb

Code, if applicable, any causal condition first:
atherosclerosis of the extremities with ulceration (440.23)
chronic venous hypertension with ulcer (459.31)
chronic venous hypertension with ulcer and inflammation (459.33)
diabetes mellitus (249.80-249.81, 250.80-250.83)
postphlebitic syndrome with ulcer (459.11)
postphlebitic syndrome with ulcer and inflammation (459.13)

707.10 Ulcer of lower limb, unspecified

707.11 Ulcer of thigh

707.12 Ulcer of calf

707.13 Ulcer of ankle

707.14 Ulcer of heel and midfoot
Plantar surface of midfoot

707.15 Ulcer of other part of foot
Toes

707.19 Ulcer of other part of lower limb

√5ᵗʰ 707.2 Pressure ulcer stages
Code first site of pressure ulcer (707.00-707.09)

707.20 Pressure ulcer, unspecified stage
Healing pressure ulcer NOS
Healing pressure ulcer, unspecified stage

707.21 Pressure ulcer stage I
Healing pressure ulcer, stage I
Pressure pre-ulcer skin changes limited to persistent focal erythema

707.22 Pressure ulcer stage II
Healing pressure ulcer, stage II
Pressure ulcer with abrasion, blister, partial thickness skin loss involving epidermis and/or dermis

707.23 Pressure ulcer stage III
Healing pressure ulcer, stage III
Pressure ulcer with full thickness skin loss involving damage or necrosis of subcutaneous tissue

707.24 Pressure ulcer stage IV
Healing pressure ulcer, stage IV
Pressure ulcer with necrosis of soft tissues through to underlying muscle, tendon, or bone

707.25 Pressure ulcer, unstageable

707.8 Chronic ulcer of other specified sites
Ulcer, chronic:
neurogenic
trophic } of other specified sites

707.9 Chronic ulcer of unspecified site
Chronic ulcer NOS
Trophic ulcer NOS
Tropical ulcer NOS
Ulcer of skin NOS

√4ᵗʰ 708 Urticaria
EXCLUDES edema:
angioneurotic (995.1)
Quincke's (995.1)
hereditary angioedema (277.6)
urticaria:
giant (995.1)
papulosa (Hebra) (698.2)
pigmentosa (juvenile) (congenital) (757.33)

DEF: Skin disorder marked by raised edematous patches of skin or mucous membrane with intense itching; also called hives.

708.0 Allergic urticaria

708.1 Idiopathic urticaria

708.2 Urticaria due to cold and heat
Thermal urticaria

708.3 Dermatographic urticaria
Dermatographia
Factitial urticaria

708.4 Vibratory urticaria

708.5 Cholinergic urticaria

708.8 Other specified urticaria
Nettle rash
Urticaria:
chronic
recurrent periodic

708.9 Urticaria, unspecified
Hives NOS

√4ᵗʰ 709 Other disorders of skin and subcutaneous tissue

√5ᵗʰ 709.0 Dyschromia
EXCLUDES albinism (270.2)
pigmented nevus (216.0-216.9)
that of eyelid (374.52-374.53)

DEF: Pigment disorder of skin or hair.

709.00 Dyschromia, unspecified

709.01 Vitiligo
DEF: Persistent, progressive development of nonpigmented white patches on otherwise normal skin.

709.09 Other

709.1 Vascular disorders of skin
Angioma serpiginosum
Purpura (primary)annularis telangiectodes

709.2 Scar conditions and fibrosis of skin
Adherent scar (skin)
Cicatrix
Disfigurement (due to scar)
Fibrosis, skin NOS
Scar NOS
EXCLUDES keloid scar (701.4)

Diseases of the Skin and Subcutaneous Tissue

709.3–709.9

709.3   **Degenerative skin disorders**
Calcinosis:
     circumscripta
     cutis
Colloid milium
Degeneration, skin
Deposits, skin
Senile dermatosis NOS
Subcutaneous calcification

709.4   **Foreign body granuloma of skin and subcutaneous tissue**
Use additional code to identify foreign body
     (V90.01-V90.9)
     EXCLUDES   *residual foreign body without granuloma of*
                 skin and subcutaneous tissue (729.6)
                 that of muscle (728.82)

709.8   **Other specified disorders of skin**
Epithelial hyperplasia
Menstrual dermatosis
Vesicular eruption
DEF: Epithelial hyperplasia: increased number of epithelial cells.
DEF: Vesicular eruption: liquid-filled structures appearing through skin.

709.9   **Unspecified disorder of skin and subcutaneous tissue**
Dermatosis NOS

Chapter 13: Diseases of the Musculoskeletal System and Connective Tissue (710–739)

Coding Guidance

Diseases and disorders of the bones, muscles, cartilage, fascia, ligaments, synovia, tendons, and bursa are classified to this chapter. The major sections of this chapter are as follows:

- Arthropathies and related disorder (710–719)
- Dorsopathies (720–724)
- Rheumatism, excluding the back (725–729)
- Osteopathies, chondropathies, and acquired musculoskeletal deformities (730–739)

Connective tissue disorders classified to chapter 13 are those primarily affecting the musculoskeletal system. Injuries and certain congenital disorders of the musculoskeletal system are classified elsewhere.

Many codes for the manifestation of musculoskeletal diseases due to specified infections and other diseases and disorders classified elsewhere are included in this chapter. Also included are many codes describing the residuals of previous diseases, disorders, and injuries classified as late effects. These codes often can be identified by the term "acquired" in the description.

Arthropathies and Related Disorders (710–719)

Arthropathy is defined as any joint disease, including arthritis (inflammatory) and arthrosis (noninflammatory). This section excludes myelopathy, disorders of the spinal cord, and dorsopathy, disorders of the spine.

Diffuse Diseases of Connective Tissue (710)

This is a group of diseases in which the primary lesion appears to be damage to collagen, a protein that is the major component of connective tissue. Collagen diseases, attributed largely to disorders of the immune complex mechanisms include dermatomyositis, systemic sclerosis, Sicca syndrome, polymyositis, collagen disease NOS, multifocal fibrosclerosis, and systemic lupus erythematosus. Many of these conditions, such as polyarteritis nodosa (a connective tissue disease that is a form of vasculitis) are classified to other chapters.

Rheumatoid Arthritis (714.0)

Rheumatoid arthritis is a chronic, systemic inflammatory disease of unknown etiology, characterized by a variable but prolonged course with exacerbations and remissions of joint pains and swelling. In early stages, the disease attacks the joints of the hands and feet. As the disease progresses, more joints become involved. Also known as primary progressive arthritis and proliferative arthritis, the disease often leads to progressive deformities, which may develop rapidly, and produce permanent disability.

Osteoarthrosis and Allied Disorders (715)

Osteoarthrosis is a degenerative, rather than inflammatory, disease of one joint or more than one joint. Also known as osteoarthritis and degenerative joint disease, osteoarthrosis is most conspicuous in the large joints and is initiated by local deterioration of the articular cartilage. It progressively destroys the cartilage, remodels the subchondral bone and causes a secondary inflammation of the synovial membrane.

Assignment of the fourth-digit to codes in this category is based on whether the disease is generalized or localized and whether it is primary or secondary. In these subcategories localized includes bilateral involvement of the same site.

Example:

Primary localized osteoarthritis of the hand is coded 715.14, whether unilateral or bilateral and is not considered generalized osteoarthritis because of the bilateral nature of the condition.

Generalized disease is defined as osteoarthrosis involving many joints without any known pre-existing abnormality. There are three code choices for generalized arthritis or osteoarthrosis for unspecified site (715.00), the hand (715.04) or for multiple sites (715.09).

Localized osteoarthrosis is a disease confined to a limited number of sites. The distinction between generalized and localized can be difficult for the clinician because the disease may be generalized, but detectable in only one or two of the larger weight- bearing joints such as the hip or knee. The physician must document localized or generalized, or the coder should assign the unspecified code.

Difficulty in Walking (719.7)

Difficulty in walking (791.7) is a valid four-digit code. No additional digits are required for this subcategory code. Category 719 includes other and unspecified disorders of joints. Do not use this category to report problems with ambulation (abnormality of gait) after hip surgery. Instead, assign 781.2.

Dorsopathies (720–724)

Dorsopathies classified to this section exclude curvature of the spine (737) and osteochondrosis of the spine (732.0 Juvenile, and 732.8 Adult).

Included in this section are:

- Ankylosing spondylitis (720)
- Spondylosis (721)
- Intervertebral disc disorders (722)
- Other disorders of the cervical region (723)
- Other and unspecified disorders of the back (724)

Other Disorders of the Synovium, Tendon and Bursa (727)

Synovitis is the inflammation of a synovial membrane, especially the synovium that lines articular joints. In a normal joint, the smooth and reciprocally shaped cartilaginous opposing surfaces permit a fluid, frictionless and painless articulation. Irregularities, disease, and damage to the articular surfaces lead to progressive degenerative changes resulting in pain and limitation of movement. The joint capsule is particularly sensitive to stretching and increased fluid pressure.

Tenosynovitis is the inflammation of a tendon and its synovial sheath. It is also known as tendosynovitis, tendovaginitis, tenontothecitis, and vaginal or tendinous synovitis. At sites of friction, the tendon is enveloped by a sheath consisting of a visceral and parietal layer of synovial membrane and is lubricated by a synovial-like fluid. The synovial sheath is in turn covered by a dense, fibrous tissue sheath. Irregularities, disease, and damage to the tendon's attachment to the articular joints may lead to progressive degenerative changes with resultant limitation of movement and pain. The synovial membranes of tendon sheaths and bursae are capable of the same inflammatory reactions to abnormal conditions as the synovial membranes of joints.

Ganglions and cysts of synovium, tendon, and bursa (727.4x) are thin-walled cystic lesions of unknown etiology containing thick, clear, mucinous fluid, possibly due to mucoid degeneration. Ganglions are limited to the hands and feet and are most common in the dorsum of the wrist.

Synovial cyst of popliteal space (727.51), such as a Baker's cysts, is sometimes called popliteal cysts. In children, Baker's cysts are common but usually are asymptomatic and regress spontaneously. In adults, Baker's cysts, in conjunction with synovial effusion due to rheumatoid arthritis or degenerative joint disease, may produce significant impairment. Baker's cysts are classified to subcategory 727.5.

Post-traumatic Seroma, Nontraumatic Hematoma of Soft Tissue (729.9)

A nontraumatic hematoma is a localized collection of blood in a tissue or space due to the breakage in the wall of a blood vessel that does not occur as a result of any obvious injury to the affected area. When nontraumatic hematoma occurs in the muscle, it is often characterized by a localized lump or swollen area that may be painful or associated with a decreased range of motion of the affected area. Depending on the depth of hematoma into the muscle and soft tissues, associated skin discoloration may vary. A seroma is a localized accumulation of serum (fluid) within a tissue or space resulting in swelling. As fluid accumulates, a hematoma may subsequently develop with a seroma in the soft tissue of the affected area. Nontraumatic hematoma may be caused by circulatory disorders, vascular anomalies, or the effects of other disease processes. Post-traumatic seroma occurs as a result of injury in which the lymph vessels or lymph nodes sustain damage. In either case, the accumulation of blood (hematoma) and clear fluid (seroma) in the soft tissue may require incision and drainage.

Osteopathies, Chondropathies and Acquired Musculoskeletal Deformities (730–739)

This category includes a broad spectrum of bone infections. Osteomyelitis is an inflammation of bone and/or bone marrow. The condition is virtually always due to a pathogen such as bacteria, virus, protozoa, or fungus. Periostitis is an inflammation of the periosteum, the thick fibrous membrane covering all the surfaces of bones except at the articular cartilage.

Other Disorders of Bone and Cartilage (733)

Osteoporosis (733.0) is a generalized bone disease characterized by decreased formation of matrix combined with increased resorption of bone, resulting in a marked decrease in bone mass. Osteoporosis often presents with osteopenia, which is a decrease in bone mineralization. Clinically, osteoporosis is classified into two major groups: primary and secondary. Primary osteoporosis implies that the condition is a fundamental disease entity itself. Secondary osteoporosis attributes the condition to an underlying clinical disease, medical condition, or medication.

When the osteoporosis is due to drug use, assign the appropriate drug code and E code in addition to the code for osteoporosis.

Pathologic Fractures (733.1)

Pathological fractures occur at a site weakened by pre-existing disease. They are often differentiated from traumatic fractures by clinically assessing the magnitude of the trauma or stress causing the fracture. A relatively minor trauma or stress can cause a pathological fracture in bones diseased by osteoporosis and other metabolic bone disease, disseminated bone disorders, inflammatory bone diseases, or any other condition that can compromise bone strength and integrity. Other terms used to describe pathologic fractures are spontaneous and secondary fractures.

Code the underlying disease in addition to the appropriate code from subcategory 733.1. Sequencing of the codes depends on whether only the fracture or the fracture and the underlying disease were treated. Code the fracture first if the treatment is toward the fracture only. If treatment of the underlying disease is addressed then code the underlying disease first.

Pathologic fractures are reported using subcategory 733.1 when the fracture is newly diagnosed and while the patient is receiving active treatment (surgical treatment, emergency department encounter, evaluation, and treatment by a new physician) for the fracture. Use the aftercare codes (subcategory V54.0, V54.2, V54.8, or V54.9) for encounters after the patient has completed active treatment of the fracture and is receiving routine care for the fracture during the healing or recovery phase, such as cast change or removal, removal of external or internal fixation device, medication adjustment, and follow-up visits following fracture treatment. Care for complications of surgical treatment for fracture repairs during the healing or recovery phase should be coded with the appropriate complication codes. Malunion and nonunion of fractures are reported with the appropriate codes from subcategory 733.8.

Necrosis of Bone; Jaw (733.45)

A possible relationship between osteonecrosis of the jaw (ONJ) and the use of bisphosphonates and other medications is being studied in the oral and maxillofacial surgery (OMS) patient population. Without a specific reporting mechanism, the incidence of this occurrence is not being captured. The American Association of Oral and Maxillofacial Surgeons' (AAOMS) case definition of osteonecrosis is "any patient who has not received radiation therapy to the oral cavity or neck and who has exposed bone in the maxillofacial area that occurred spontaneously or following dental surgery and has no evidence of healing for more than 3–6 weeks after appropriate care." As noted in the definition, osteonecrosis differs from osteoradionecrosis, which is caused by radiation therapy.

Use an additional E code to identify the drug, if drug-induced. Codes E933.6 Oral bisphosphonates and E933.7 Intravenous bisphosphonates, report the adverse effects of these prescribed bisphosphonates. Bisphosphonate drugs include Boniva, Fosamax, and Zometa. Do not assign 733.45 Aseptic necrosis of bone, jaw for osteoradionecrosis of jaw (526.89).

Stress Fracture (733.9)

Stress fractures are classified separately from pathological fractures (733.1X). Stress fractures may occur as a result of overexertion, strenuous, repetitive motion, static positioning, and load-bearing injuries, and sudden traumatic and cumulative trauma injuries. Subcategory 733.9 includes an instructional note to "Use additional external cause code(s) to identify the cause of the stress fracture" with codes 733.93–733.98.

Curvature of the Spine (737)

Kyphosis (737.0–737.1x) is the abnormal increase in the thoracic convexity of the spine as viewed from the side.

Lordosis (737.2x) is the anterior convexity of the cervical and lumbar spine as viewed from the side.

Scoliosis (737.3x) is the lateral curvature of the spine described as structural or nonstructural depending on whether the condition is reversible.

Kyphoscoliosis (737.3x) the lateral curvature of the spine with extensive flexion.

Acquired deformities of the spine associated with disease classified elsewhere are coded to subcategory 737.4. Code first the underlying condition. The fifth digit identifies the type of deformity.

13. DISEASES OF THE MUSCULOSKELETAL SYSTEM AND CONNECTIVE TISSUE (710-739)

Use additional external cause code, if applicable, to identify the cause of the musculoskeletal condition

The following fifth-digit subclassification is for use with categories 711-712, 715-716, 718-719, and 730:

0 site unspecified
1 shoulder region
   Acromioclavicular joint(s)
   Clavicle
   Glenohumeral joint(s)
   Scapula
   Sternoclavicular joint(s)
2 upper arm
   Elbow joint
   Humerus
3 forearm
   Radius
   Ulna
   Wrist joint
4 hand
   Carpus
   Metacarpus
   Phalanges [fingers]
5 pelvic region and thigh
   Buttock
   Femur
   Hip (joint)

6 lower leg
   Fibula
   Knee joint
   Patella
   Tibia
7 ankle and foot
   Ankle joint
   Digits [toes]
   Metatarsus
   Phalanges, foot
   Tarsus
   Other joints in foot
8 other specified sites
   Head
   Neck
   Ribs
   Skull
   Trunk
   Vertebral column
9 multiple sites

ARTHROPATHIES AND RELATED DISORDERS (710-719)

EXCLUDES   disorders of spine (720.0-724.9)

✓4ᵗʰ 710 Diffuse diseases of connective tissue

INCLUDES   all collagen diseases whose effects are not mainly confined to a single system

EXCLUDES   those affecting mainly the cardiovascular system, i.e., polyarteritis nodosa and allied conditions (446.0-446.7)

710.0 Systemic lupus erythematosus
Disseminated lupus erythematosus
Libman-Sacks disease
Use additional code to identify manifestation, as:
   endocarditis (424.91)
   nephritis (583.81)
      chronic (582.81)
   nephrotic syndrome (581.81)
EXCLUDES   lupus erythematosus (discoid) NOS (695.4)

DEF: A chronic multisystemic inflammatory disease affecting connective tissue; marked by anemia, leukopenia, muscle and joint pains, fever, rash of a butterfly pattern around cheeks and forehead area; of unknown etiology.

710.1 Systemic sclerosis
Acrosclerosis   Progressive systemic sclerosis
CRST syndrome   Scleroderma
Use additional code to identify manifestation, as:
   lung involvement (517.2)
   myopathy (359.6)
EXCLUDES   circumscribed scleroderma (701.0)

DEF: Systemic disease, involving excess fibrotic collagen build-up; symptoms include thickened skin, fibrotic degenerative changes in various organs, and vascular abnormalities; condition occurs more often in females.

710.2 Sicca syndrome
Keratoconjunctivitis sicca
Sjögren's disease

DEF: Autoimmune disease; associated with keratoconjunctivitis, laryngopharyngitis, rhinitis, dry mouth, enlarged parotid gland, and chronic polyarthritis.

710.3 Dermatomyositis
Poikilodermatomyositis
Polymyositis with skin involvement

DEF: Polymyositis characterized by flat-top purple papules on knuckles; upper eyelid rash, edema of eyelids and orbit area, red rash on forehead, neck, shoulders, trunk and arms; symptoms include fever, weight loss, aching muscles; visceral cancer.

Joint Structures

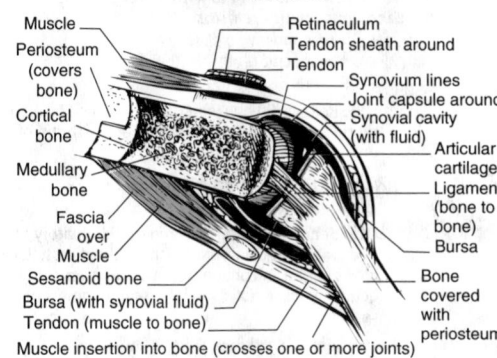

710.4 Polymyositis

DEF: Chronic, progressive, inflammatory skeletal muscle disease; causes weakness of limb girdles, neck, pharynx; may precede or follow scleroderma, Sjogren's disease, systemic lupus erythematosus, arthritis, or malignancy.

710.5 Eosinophilia myalgia syndrome
Toxic oil syndrome
Use additional E code to identify drug, if drug induced

DEF: Eosinophilia myalgia syndrome (EMS): inflammatory, multisystem fibrosis; associated with ingesting elementary L-tryptophan; symptoms include myalgia, weak limbs and bulbar muscles, distal sensory loss, areflexia, arthralgia, cough, fever, fatigue, skin rashes, myopathy, and eosinophil counts greater than 1000/microliter.

DEF: Toxic oil syndrome: syndrome similar to EMS due to ingesting contaminated cooking oil.

710.8 Other specified diffuse diseases of connective tissue
Multifocal fibrosclerosis (idiopathic) NEC
Systemic fibrosclerosing syndrome

710.9 Unspecified diffuse connective tissue disease
Collagen disease NOS

✓4ᵗʰ 711 Arthropathy associated with infections

INCLUDES   arthritis   associated with
              arthropathy   conditions
              polyarthritis   classifiable
              polyarthropathy   below

EXCLUDES   rheumatic fever (390)

The following fifth-digit subclassification is for use with category 711; valid digits are in [brackets] under each code. See list at beginning of chapter for definitions.

0 site unspecified
1 shoulder region
2 upper arm
3 forearm
4 hand
5 pelvic region and thigh
6 lower leg
7 ankle and foot
8 other specified sites
9 multiple sites

✓5ᵗʰ 711.0 Pyogenic arthritis
[0-9]   Arthritis or polyarthritis (due to):
     coliform [Escherichia coli]
     Hemophilus influenzae [H. influenzae]
     pneumococcal
     Pseudomonas
     staphylococcal
     streptococcal
  Pyarthrosis
Use additional code to identify infectious organism (041.0-041.8)

DEF: Infectious arthritis caused by various bacteria; marked by inflamed synovial membranes, and purulent effusion in joints.

√5ᵗʰ **711.1**   **Arthropathy associated with Reiter's disease**
[0-9]   **and nonspecific urethritis**
     Code first underlying disease as:
       nonspecific urethritis (099.4)
       Reiter's disease (099.3)
     DEF: Reiter's disease: joint disease marked by diarrhea, urethritis, conjunctivitis, keratosis and arthritis; of unknown etiology; affects young males.

√5ᵗʰ **711.2**   **Arthropathy in Behçet's syndrome**
[0-9]   Code first underlying disease (136.1)
     DEF: Behçet's syndrome: Chronic inflammatory disorder, of unknown etiology; affects small blood vessels; causes ulcers of oral and pharyngeal mucous membranes and genitalia, skin lesions, retinal vasculitis, optic atrophy and severe uveitis.

√5ᵗʰ **711.3**   **Postdysenteric arthropathy**
[0-9]   Code first underlying disease as:
       dysentery (009.0)
       enteritis, infectious (008.0-009.3)
       paratyphoid fever (002.1-002.9)
       typhoid fever (002.0)
     EXCLUDES   salmonella arthritis (003.23)

√5ᵗʰ **711.4**   **Arthropathy associated with other bacterial diseases**
[0-9]   Code first underlying disease as:
       diseases classifiable to 010-040, 090-099, except as in 711.1, 711.3, and 713.5
       leprosy (030.0-030.9)
       tuberculosis (015.0-015.9)
     EXCLUDES   gonococcal arthritis (098.50)
           meningococcal arthritis (036.82)

√5ᵗʰ **711.5**   **Arthropathy associated with other viral diseases**
[0-9]   Code first underlying disease as:
       diseases classifiable to 045-049, 050-079, 480, 487
       O'nyong nyong (066.3)
     EXCLUDES   that due to rubella (056.71)

√5ᵗʰ **711.6**   **Arthropathy associated with mycoses**
[0-9]   Code first underlying disease (110.0-118)

√5ᵗʰ **711.7**   **Arthropathy associated with helminthiasis**
[0-9]   Code first underlying disease as:
       filariasis (125.0-125.9)

√5ᵗʰ **711.8**   **Arthropathy associated with other**
[0-9]   **infectious and parasitic diseases**
     Code first underlying disease as:
       diseases classifiable to 080-088, 100-104, 130-136
     EXCLUDES   arthropathy associated with sarcoidosis (713.7)

√5ᵗʰ **711.9**   **Unspecified infective arthritis**
[0-9]   Infective arthritis or polyarthritis (acute) (chronic) (subacute) NOS

√4ᵗʰ **712**   **Crystal arthropathies**
     INCLUDES   crystal-induced arthritis and synovitis
     EXCLUDES   gouty arthropathy (274.00-274.03)
     DEF: Joint disease due to urate crystal deposit in joints or synovial membranes.

     The following fifth-digit subclassification is for use with category 712; valid digits are in [brackets] under each code. See list at beginning of chapter for definitions.
       0   site unspecified
       1   shoulder region
       2   upper arm
       3   forearm
       4   hand
       5   pelvic region and thigh
       6   lower leg
       7   ankle and foot
       8   other specified sites
       9   multiple sites

√5ᵗʰ **712.1**   **Chondrocalcinosis due to dicalcium phosphate crystals**
[0-9]   Chondrocalcinosis due to dicalcium phosphate crystals (with other crystals)
     Code first underlying disease (275.4)

√5ᵗʰ **712.2**   **Chondrocalcinosis due to pyrophosphate crystals**
[0-9]   Code first underlying disease (275.4)

√5ᵗʰ **712.3**   **Chondrocalcinosis, unspecified**
[0-9]   Code first underlying disease (275.4)

√5ᵗʰ **712.8**   **Other specified crystal arthropathies**
[0-9]

√5ᵗʰ **712.9**   **Unspecified crystal arthropathy**
[0-9]

√4ᵗʰ **713**   **Arthropathy associated with other disorders classified elsewhere**
     INCLUDES   arthritis
       arthropathy   }   associated with conditions
       polyarthritis   classifiable below
       polyarthropathy

713.0   **Arthropathy associated with other endocrine and metabolic disorders**
     Code first underlying disease as:
       acromegaly (253.0)
       hemochromatosis (275.01-275.09)
       hyperparathyroidism (252.00-252.08)
       hypogammaglobulinemia (279.00-279.09)
       hypothyroidism (243-244.9)
       lipoid metabolism disorder (272.0-272.9)
       ochronosis (270.2)
     EXCLUDES   arthropathy associated with:
           amyloidosis (713.7)
           crystal deposition disorders, except gout (712.1-712.9)
           diabetic neuropathy (713.5)
           gout (274.00-274.03)

713.1   **Arthropathy associated with gastrointestinal conditions other than infections**
     Code first underlying disease as:
       regional enteritis (555.0-555.9)
       ulcerative colitis (556)

713.2   **Arthropathy associated with hematological disorders**
     Code first underlying disease as:
       hemoglobinopathy (282.4-282.7)
       hemophilia (286.0-286.2)
       leukemia (204.0-208.9)
       malignant reticulosis (202.3)
       multiple myelomatosis (203.0)
     EXCLUDES   arthropathy associated with Henoch-Schönlein purpura (713.6)

713.3   **Arthropathy associated with dermatological disorders**
     Code first underlying disease as:
       erythema multiforme (695.10-695.19)
       erythema nodosum (695.2)
     EXCLUDES   psoriatic arthropathy (696.0)

713.4   **Arthropathy associated with respiratory disorders**
     Code first underlying disease as:
       diseases classifiable to 490-519
     EXCLUDES   arthropathy associated with respiratory infections (711.0, 711.4-711.8)

713.5   **Arthropathy associated with neurological disorders**
     Charcôt's arthropathy   }   associated with diseases
     Neuropathic arthritis   classifiable elsewhere
     Code first underlying disease as:
       neuropathic joint disease [Charcôt's joints]:
         NOS (094.0)
         diabetic (249.6, 250.6)
         syringomyelic (336.0)
         tabetic [syphilitic] (094.0)

713.6   **Arthropathy associated with hypersensitivity reaction**
     Code first underlying disease as:
       Henoch (-Schönlein) purpura (287.0)
       serum sickness (999.51-999.59)
     EXCLUDES   allergic arthritis NOS (716.2)

713.7   *Other general diseases with articular involvement*
> *Code first underlying disease as:*
> amyloidosis (277.30-277.39)
> familial Mediterranean fever (277.31)
> sarcoidosis (135)

713.8   *Arthropathy associated with other condition classifiable elsewhere*
> *Code first underlying disease as:*
> conditions classifiable elsewhere except as in 711.1-711.8, 712, and 713.0-713.7

√4ᵗʰ 714   Rheumatoid arthritis and other inflammatory polyarthropathies
> EXCLUDES   *rheumatic fever (390)*
> *rheumatoid arthritis of spine NOS (720.0)*

714.0   Rheumatoid arthritis
> Arthritis or polyarthritis:
> atrophic
> rheumatic (chronic)
> Use additional code to identify manifestation, as:
> myopathy (359.6)
> polyneuropathy (357.1)
> EXCLUDES   *juvenile rheumatoid arthritis NOS (714.30)*
> **DEF:** Chronic systemic disease principally of joints, manifested by inflammatory changes in articular structures and synovial membranes, atrophy, and loss in bone density.

714.1   Felty's syndrome
> Rheumatoid arthritis with splenoadenomegaly and leukopenia
> **DEF:** Syndrome marked by rheumatoid arthritis, splenomegaly, leukopenia, pigmented spots on lower extremity skin, anemia, and thrombocytopenia.

714.2   Other rheumatoid arthritis with visceral or systemic involvement
> Rheumatoid carditis

√5ᵗʰ 714.3   Juvenile chronic polyarthritis
> **DEF:** Rheumatoid arthritis of more than one joint; lasts longer than six weeks in age 17 or younger; symptoms include fever, erythematous rash, weight loss, lymphadenopathy, hepatosplenomegaly and pericarditis.

714.30   Polyarticular juvenile rheumatoid arthritis, chronic or unspecified
> Juvenile rheumatoid arthritis NOS
> Still's disease

714.31   Polyarticular juvenile rheumatoid arthritis, acute

714.32   Pauciarticular juvenile rheumatoid arthritis

714.33   Monoarticular juvenile rheumatoid arthritis

714.4   Chronic postrheumatic arthropathy
> Chronic rheumatoid nodular fibrositis
> Jaccoud's syndrome
> **DEF:** Persistent joint disorder; follows previous rheumatic infection.

√5ᵗʰ 714.8   Other specified inflammatory polyarthropathies

714.81   Rheumatoid lung
> Caplan's syndrome
> Diffuse interstitial rheumatoid disease of lung
> Fibrosing alveolitis, rheumatoid
> **DEF:** Lung disorders associated with rheumatoid arthritis.

714.89   Other

714.9   Unspecified inflammatory polyarthropathy
> Inflammatory polyarthropathy or polyarthritis NOS
> EXCLUDES   *polyarthropathy NOS (716.5)*

√4ᵗʰ 715   Osteoarthrosis and allied disorders
> Note: Localized, in the subcategories below, includes bilateral involvement of the same site.
> INCLUDES   arthritis or polyarthritis:
> degenerative
> hypertrophic
> degenerative joint disease
> osteoarthritis
> EXCLUDES   *Marie-Strümpell spondylitis (720.0)*
> *osteoarthrosis [osteoarthritis] of spine (721.0-721.9)*

> The following fifth-digit subclassification is for use with category 715; valid digits are in [brackets] under each code. See list at beginning of chapter for definitions.
>   0   site unspecified
>   1   shoulder region
>   2   upper arm
>   3   forearm
>   4   hand
>   5   pelvic region and thigh
>   6   lower leg
>   7   ankle and foot
>   8   other specified sites
>   9   multiple sites

√5ᵗʰ 715.0   Osteoarthrosis, generalized
[0,4,9]
> Degenerative joint disease, involving multiple joints
> Primary generalized hypertrophic osteoarthrosis
> **DEF:** Chronic noninflammatory arthritis; marked by degenerated articular cartilage and enlarged bone; symptoms include pain and stiffness with activity.

√5ᵗʰ 715.1   Osteoarthrosis, localized, primary
[0-8]
> Localized osteoarthropathy, idiopathic

√5ᵗʰ 715.2   Osteoarthrosis, localized, secondary
[0-8]
> Coxae malum senilis

√5ᵗʰ 715.3   Osteoarthrosis, localized, not specified whether
[0-8]   **primary or secondary**
> Otto's pelvis

√5ᵗʰ 715.8   Osteoarthrosis involving, or with mention of
[0,9]   **more than one site, but not specified as generalized**

√5ᵗʰ 715.9   Osteoarthrosis, unspecified whether
[0-8]   **generalized or localized**

√4ᵗʰ 716   Other and unspecified arthropathies
> EXCLUDES   *cricoarytenoid arthropathy (478.79)*

> The following fifth-digit subclassification is for use with category 716; valid digits are in [brackets] under each code. See list at beginning of chapter for definitions.
>   0   site unspecified
>   1   shoulder region
>   2   upper arm
>   3   forearm
>   4   hand
>   5   pelvic region and thigh
>   6   lower leg
>   7   ankle and foot
>   8   other specified sites
>   9   multiple sites

√5ᵗʰ 716.0   Kaschin-Beck disease
[0-9]
> Endemic polyarthritis
> **DEF:** Chronic degenerative disease of spine and peripheral joints; occurs in eastern Siberian, northern Chinese, and Korean youth; may be a mycotoxicosis caused by eating cereals infected with fungus.

√5ᵗʰ 716.1   Traumatic arthropathy
[0-9]

√5ᵗʰ 716.2   Allergic arthritis
[0-9]   EXCLUDES   *arthritis associated with Henoch-Schönlein purpura or serum sickness (713.6)*

√5ᵗʰ 716.3   Climacteric arthritis
[0-9]
> Menopausal arthritis
> **DEF:** Ovarian hormone deficiency; causes pain in small joints, shoulders, elbows or knees; affects females at menopause; also called arthropathia ovaripriva.

√5ᵗʰ 716.4 Transient arthropathy
[0-9]   *EXCLUDES*   *palindromic rheumatism (719.3)*

√5ᵗʰ 716.5 Unspecified polyarthropathy or polyarthritis
[0-9]

√5ᵗʰ 716.6 Unspecified monoarthritis
[0-8]   Coxitis

√5ᵗʰ 716.8 Other specified arthropathy
[0-9]

√5ᵗʰ 716.9 Arthropathy, unspecified
[0-9]   Arthritis } (acute) (chronic) (subacute)
             Arthropathy
             Articular rheumatism (chronic)
             Inflammation of joint NOS

√4ᵗʰ 717 Internal derangement of knee
       INCLUDES   degeneration } of articular cartilage or
                    rupture, old   meniscus of knee
                    tear, old

       EXCLUDES   *acute derangement of knee (836.0-836.6)*
                    ankylosis (718.5)
                    contracture (718.4)
                    current injury (836.0-836.6)
                    deformity (736.4-736.6)
                    recurrent dislocation (718.3)

717.0 Old bucket handle tear of medial meniscus
        Old bucket handle tear of unspecified cartilage

717.1 Derangement of anterior horn of medial meniscus

717.2 Derangement of posterior horn of medial meniscus

717.3 Other and unspecified derangement of medial meniscus
        Degeneration of internal semilunar cartilage

√5ᵗʰ 717.4 Derangement of lateral meniscus

717.40 Derangement of lateral meniscus, unspecified

717.41 Bucket handle tear of lateral meniscus

717.42 Derangement of anterior horn of lateral meniscus

717.43 Derangement of posterior horn of lateral meniscus

717.49 Other

Disruption and Tears of Meniscus

Bucket-handle   Flap-type   Peripheral   Radial

Horizontal cleavage   Vertical   Congenital discoid meniscus

Internal Derangements of Knee

Anterior   Posterior

Disruptions of Cruciate Ligament

Chondromalacia of Patella

"Kissing" lesion of femur

717.5 Derangement of meniscus, not elsewhere classified
        Congenital discoid meniscus
        Cyst of semilunar cartilage
        Derangement of semilunar cartilage NOS

717.6 Loose body in knee
        Joint mice, knee
        Rice bodies, knee (joint)
        DEF: The presence in the joint synovial area of a small, frequently calcified, loose body created from synovial membrane, organized fibrin fragments of articular cartilage or arthritis osteophytes.

717.7 Chondromalacia of patella
        Chondromalacia patellae
        Degeneration [softening] of articular cartilage of patella
        DEF: Softened patella cartilage.

√5ᵗʰ 717.8 Other internal derangement of knee

717.81 Old disruption of lateral collateral ligament

717.82 Old disruption of medial collateral ligament

717.83 Old disruption of anterior cruciate ligament

717.84 Old disruption of posterior cruciate ligament

717.85 Old disruption of other ligaments of knee
         Capsular ligament of knee

717.89 Other
         Old disruption of ligaments NOS

717.9 Unspecified internal derangement of knee
        Derangement NOS of knee

√4ᵗʰ 718 Other derangement of joint
       EXCLUDES   *current injury (830.0-848.9)*
                    jaw (524.60-524.69)

The following fifth-digit subclassification is for use with category 718; valid digits are in [brackets] under each code. See list at beginning of chapter for definitions.
    0 site unspecified
    1 shoulder region
    2 upper arm
    3 forearm
    4 hand
    5 pelvic region and thigh
    6 lower leg
    7 ankle and foot
    8 other specified sites
    9 multiple sites

√5ᵗʰ 718.0 Articular cartilage disorder
[0-5,7-9] Meniscus:
             disorder
             rupture, old
             tear, old
           Old rupture of ligament(s) of joint NOS
           EXCLUDES   *articular cartilage disorder:*
                        in ochronosis (270.2)
                        knee (717.0-717.9)
                        chondrocalcinosis (275.4)
                        metastatic calcification (275.4)

Joint Derangements and Disorders

Loose body in joint   Dislocation of joint

Joint contracture   Ankylosis of joint   Synovial effusion (fluid)   Hemarthrosis (blood)

√5ᵗʰ **718.1** **Loose body in joint**
[0-5,7-9]   Joint mice
   EXCLUDES *knee (717.6)*
   DEF: Calcified loose bodies in synovial fluid; due to arthritic osteophytes.

√5ᵗʰ **718.2** **Pathological dislocation**
[0-9]   Dislocation or displacement of joint, not recurrent and not current injury
   Spontaneous dislocation (joint)

√5ᵗʰ **718.3** **Recurrent dislocation of joint**
[0-9]

√5ᵗʰ **718.4** **Contracture of joint**
[0-9]

√5ᵗʰ **718.5** **Ankylosis of joint**
[0-9]   Ankylosis of joint (fibrous) (osseous)
   EXCLUDES *spine (724.9)*
      stiffness of joint without mention of ankylosis (719.5)
   DEF: Immobility and solidification of joint; due to disease, injury or surgical procedure.

√5ᵗʰ **718.6** **Unspecified intrapelvic protrusion of acetabulum**
[5]   Protrusio acetabuli, unspecified
   DEF: Sinking of the floor of acetabulum, causing femoral head to protrude, limits hip movement; of unknown etiology.

√5ᵗʰ **718.7** **Developmental dislocation of joint**
[0-9]   **EXCLUDES** *congenital dislocation of joint (754.0-755.8)*
      traumatic dislocation of joint (830-839)

√5ᵗʰ **718.8** **Other joint derangement, not elsewhere classified**
[0-9]   Flail joint (paralytic)   Instability of joint
   EXCLUDES *deformities classifiable to 736 (736.0-736.9)*

√5ᵗʰ **718.9** **Unspecified derangement of joint**
[0-5,7-9]   **EXCLUDES** *knee (717.9)*

√4ᵗʰ **719** **Other and unspecified disorders of joint**
   EXCLUDES *jaw (524.60-524.69)*

The following fifth-digit subclassification is for use with codes 719.0-719.6, 719.8-719.9; valid digits are in [brackets] under each code. See list at beginning of chapter for definitions.
   0 site unspecified
   1 shoulder region
   2 upper arm
   3 forearm
   4 hand
   5 pelvic region and thigh
   6 lower leg
   7 ankle and foot
   8 other specified sites
   9 multiple sites

√5ᵗʰ **719.0** **Effusion of joint**
[0-9]   Hydrarthrosis
   Swelling of joint, with or without pain
   EXCLUDES *intermittent hydrarthrosis (719.3)*

√5ᵗʰ **719.1** **Hemarthrosis**
[0-9]   **EXCLUDES** *current injury (840.0-848.9)*

√5ᵗʰ **719.2** **Villonodular synovitis**
[0-9]   **DEF:** Overgrowth of synovial tissue, especially at knee joint; due to macrophage infiltration of giant cells in synovial villi and fibrous nodules.

√5ᵗʰ **719.3** **Palindromic rheumatism**
[0-9]   Hench-Rosenberg syndrome
   Intermittent hydrarthrosis
   DEF: Recurrent episodes of afebrile arthritis and periarthritis marked by their complete disappearance after a few days or hours; causes swelling, redness, and disability usually affecting only one joint; no known cause.

√5ᵗʰ **719.4** **Pain in joint**
[0-9]   Arthralgia

√5ᵗʰ **719.5** **Stiffness of joint, not elsewhere classified**
[0-9]

√5ᵗʰ **719.6** **Other symptoms referable to joint**
[0-9]   Joint crepitus
   Snapping hip

719.7 **Difficulty in walking**
   EXCLUDES *abnormality of gait (781.2)*

√5ᵗʰ **719.8** **Other specified disorders of joint**
[0-9]   Calcification of joint
   Fistula of joint
   EXCLUDES *temporomandibular joint-pain-dysfunction syndrome [Costen's syndrome] (524.60)*

√5ᵗʰ **719.9** **Unspecified disorder of joint**
[0-9]

DORSOPATHIES (720-724)
   EXCLUDES *curvature of spine (737.0-737.9)*
      osteochondrosis of spine (juvenile) (732.0)
      adult (732.8)

√4ᵗʰ **720** **Ankylosing spondylitis and other inflammatory spondylopathies**
   720.0 **Ankylosing spondylitis**
      Rheumatoid arthritis of spine NOS
      Spondylitis:
         Marie-Strümpell
         rheumatoid
      DEF: Rheumatoid arthritis of spine and sacroiliac joints; fusion and deformity in spine follows; affects mainly males; cause unknown.

   720.1 **Spinal enthesopathy**
      Disorder of peripheral ligamentous or muscular attachments of spine
      Romanus lesion
      DEF: Tendinous or muscular vertebral bone attachment abnormality.

   720.2 **Sacroiliitis, not elsewhere classified**
      Inflammation of sacroiliac joint NOS
      DEF: Pain due to inflammation in joint, at juncture of sacrum and hip.

√5ᵗʰ **720.8** **Other inflammatory spondylopathies**
      720.81 ***Inflammatory spondylopathies in diseases classified elsewhere***
         Code first underlying disease as:
            tuberculosis (015.0)
      720.89 **Other**

   720.9 **Unspecified inflammatory spondylopathy**
      Spondylitis NOS

√4ᵗʰ **721** **Spondylosis and allied disorders**
   DEF: Degenerative changes in spinal joint.
   721.0 **Cervical spondylosis without myelopathy**
      Cervical or cervicodorsal:
         arthritis
         osteoarthritis
         spondylarthritis

   721.1 **Cervical spondylosis with myelopathy**
      Anterior spinal artery compression syndrome
      Spondylogenic compression of cervical spinal cord
      Vertebral artery compression syndrome

   721.2 **Thoracic spondylosis without myelopathy**
      Thoracic:
         arthritis
         osteoarthritis
         spondylarthritis

   721.3 **Lumbosacral spondylosis without myelopathy**
      Lumbar or lumbosacral:
         arthritis
         osteoarthritis
         spondylarthritis

√5ᵗʰ **721.4** **Thoracic or lumbar spondylosis with myelopathy**
      721.41 **Thoracic region**
         Spondylogenic compression of thoracic spinal cord
      721.42 **Lumbar region**

721.5 Kissing spine
Baastrup's syndrome
DEF: Compression of spinous processes of adjacent vertebrae; due to mutual contact.

721.6 Ankylosing vertebral hyperostosis

721.7 Traumatic spondylopathy
Kümmell's disease or spondylitis

721.8 Other allied disorders of spine

✓5ᵗʰ **721.9 Spondylosis of unspecified site**

721.90 Without mention of myelopathy
Spinal:
    arthritis (deformans) (degenerative)
        (hypertrophic)
    osteoarthritis NOS
Spondylarthrosis NOS

721.91 With myelopathy
Spondylogenic compression of spinal cord NOS

✓4ᵗʰ **722 Intervertebral disc disorders**

722.0 Displacement of cervical intervertebral disc without myelopathy
Neuritis (brachial) or radiculitis due to displacement or rupture of cervical intervertebral disc
Any condition classifiable to 722.2 of the cervical or cervicothoracic intervertebral disc

✓5ᵗʰ **722.1 Displacement of thoracic or lumbar intervertebral disc without myelopathy**

722.10 Lumbar intervertebral disc without myelopathy
Lumbago or sciatica due to displacement of intervertebral disc
Neuritis or radiculitis due to displacement or rupture of lumbar intervertebral disc
Any condition classifiable to 722.2 of the lumbar or lumbosacral intervertebral disc

722.11 Thoracic intervertebral disc without myelopathy
Any condition classifiable to 722.2 of thoracic intervertebral disc

Anatomy of Vertebral Disc

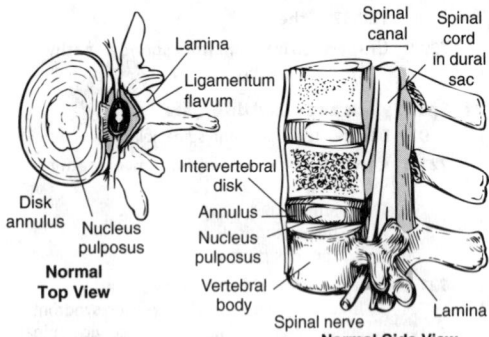

Normal Top View

Normal Side View

Derangement of Vertebral Disc

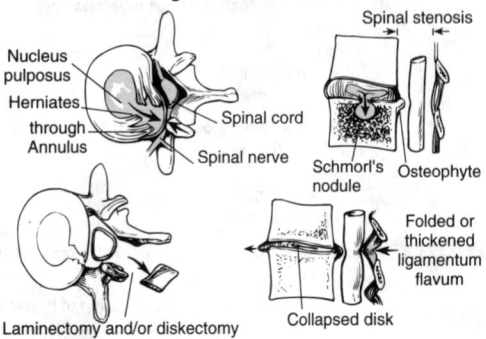

Laminectomy and/or diskectomy decompresses spinal canal

722.2 Displacement of intervertebral disc, site unspecified, without myelopathy
Discogenic syndrome NOS
Herniation of nucleus pulposus NOS
Intervertebral disc NOS:
    extrusion
    prolapse
    protrusion
    rupture
Neuritis or radiculitis due to displacement or rupture of intervertebral disc

✓5ᵗʰ **722.3 Schmorl's nodes**
DEF: Irregular bone defect in the margin of the vertebral body; causes herniation into end plate of vertebral body.

722.30 Unspecified region

722.31 Thoracic region

722.32 Lumbar region

722.39 Other

722.4 Degeneration of cervical intervertebral disc
Degeneration of cervicothoracic intervertebral disc

✓5ᵗʰ **722.5 Degeneration of thoracic or lumbar intervertebral disc**

722.51 Thoracic or thoracolumbar intervertebral disc

722.52 Lumbar or lumbosacral intervertebral disc

722.6 Degeneration of intervertebral disc, site unspecified
Degenerative disc disease NOS
Narrowing of intervertebral disc or space NOS

✓5ᵗʰ **722.7 Intervertebral disc disorder with myelopathy**

722.70 Unspecified region

722.71 Cervical region

722.72 Thoracic region

722.73 Lumbar region

✓5ᵗʰ **722.8 Postlaminectomy syndrome**
DEF: Spinal disorder due to spinal laminectomy surgery.

722.80 Unspecified region

722.81 Cervical region

722.82 Thoracic region

722.83 Lumbar region

✓5ᵗʰ **722.9 Other and unspecified disc disorder**
Calcification of intervertebral cartilage or disc
Discitis

722.90 Unspecified region

722.91 Cervical region

722.92 Thoracic region

722.93 Lumbar region

✓4ᵗʰ **723 Other disorders of cervical region**
EXCLUDES   conditions due to:
    intervertebral disc disorders (722.0-722.9)
    spondylosis (721.0-721.9)

723.0 Spinal stenosis in cervical region

723.1 Cervicalgia
Pain in neck
DEF: Pain in cervical spine or neck region.

723.2 Cervicocranial syndrome
Barré-Liéou syndrome
Posterior cervical sympathetic syndrome
DEF: Neurologic disorder of upper cervical spine and nerve roots.

723.3 Cervicobrachial syndrome (diffuse)
DEF: Complex of symptoms due to scalenus anterior muscle compressing the brachial plexus; pain radiates from shoulder to arm or back of neck.

Stenosis in Cervical Region

723.4 Brachial neuritis or radiculitis NOS
Cervical radiculitis
Radicular syndrome of upper limbs

723.5 Torticollis, unspecified
Contracture of neck
EXCLUDES congenital (754.1)
due to birth injury (767.8)
hysterical (300.11)
ocular torticollis (781.93)
psychogenic (306.0)
spasmodic (333.83)
traumatic, current (847.0)

DEF: Abnormally positioned neck relative to head due to cervical muscle or fascia contractions; also called wryneck.

723.6 Panniculitis specified as affecting neck

DEF: Inflammation of the panniculus adiposus (subcutaneous fat) in the neck.

723.7 Ossification of posterior longitudinal ligament in cervical region

723.8 Other syndromes affecting cervical region
Cervical syndrome NEC
Klippel's disease
Occipital neuralgia

723.9 Unspecified musculoskeletal disorders and symptoms referable to neck
Cervical (region) disorder NOS

√4th **724 Other and unspecified disorders of back**
EXCLUDES collapsed vertebra (code to cause, e.g., osteoporosis, 733.00-733.09)
conditions due to:
intervertebral disc disorders (722.0-722.9)
spondylosis (721.0-721.9)

√5th **724.0 Spinal stenosis, other than cervical**

724.00 Spinal stenosis, unspecified region

724.01 Thoracic region

724.02 Lumbar region, without neurogenic claudication
Lumbar region NOS

724.03 Lumbar region, with neurogenic claudication
DEF: Spinal canal narrowing with nerve root compression causing muscle pain, fatigue, and weakness during extension of the lumbar spine; pain is relieved by sitting or bending.

724.09 Other

724.1 Pain in thoracic spine

724.2 Lumbago
Low back pain
Low back syndrome
Lumbalgia

724.3 Sciatica
Neuralgia or neuritis of sciatic nerve
EXCLUDES specified lesion of sciatic nerve (355.0)

724.4 Thoracic or lumbosacral neuritis or radiculitis, unspecified
Radicular syndrome of lower limbs

724.5 Backache, unspecified
Vertebrogenic (pain) syndrome NOS

724.6 Disorders of sacrum
Ankylosis ⎫
Instability ⎬ lumbosacral or sacroiliac (joint)

√5th **724.7 Disorders of coccyx**

724.70 Unspecified disorder of coccyx

724.71 Hypermobility of coccyx

724.79 Other
Coccygodynia

724.8 Other symptoms referable to back
Ossification of posterior longitudinal ligament NOS
Panniculitis specified as sacral or affecting back

724.9 Other unspecified back disorders
Ankylosis of spine NOS
Compression of spinal nerve root NEC
Spinal disorder NOS
EXCLUDES sacroiliitis (720.2)

RHEUMATISM, EXCLUDING THE BACK (725-729)
INCLUDES disorders of muscles and tendons and their attachments, and of other soft tissues

725 Polymyalgia rheumatica
DEF: Joint and muscle pain, pelvis, and shoulder girdle stiffness, high sedimentation rate and temporal arteritis; occurs in elderly.

√4th **726 Peripheral enthesopathies and allied syndromes**
Note: Enthesopathies are disorders of peripheral ligamentous or muscular attachments.
EXCLUDES spinal enthesopathy (720.1)

726.0 Adhesive capsulitis of shoulder

√5th **726.1 Rotator cuff syndrome of shoulder and allied disorders**

726.10 Disorders of bursae and tendons in shoulder region, unspecified
Rotator cuff syndrome NOS
Supraspinatus syndrome NOS

726.11 Calcifying tendinitis of shoulder

726.12 Bicipital tenosynovitis

726.13 Partial tear of rotator cuff
EXCLUDES complete rupture of rotator cuff, nontraumatic (727.61)

726.19 Other specified disorders
EXCLUDES complete rupture of rotator cuff, nontraumatic (727.61)

726.2 Other affections of shoulder region, not elsewhere classified
Periarthritis of shoulder
Scapulohumeral fibrositis

√5th **726.3 Enthesopathy of elbow region**

726.30 Enthesopathy of elbow, unspecified

726.31 Medial epicondylitis

726.32 Lateral epicondylitis
Epicondylitis NOS
Golfers' elbow
Tennis elbow

726.33 Olecranon bursitis
Bursitis of elbow

726.39 Other

726.4 Enthesopathy of wrist and carpus
Bursitis of hand or wrist
Periarthritis of wrist

726.5 Enthesopathy of hip region
Bursitis of hip
Gluteal tendinitis
Iliac crest spur
Psoas tendinitis
Trochanteric tendinitis

Diseases of the Musculoskeletal System and Connective Tissue

726.6–727.64

√5ᵗʰ **726.6 Enthesopathy of knee**

726.60 Enthesopathy of knee, unspecified
Bursitis of knee NOS

726.61 Pes anserinus tendinitis or bursitis
DEF: Inflamed tendons of sartorius, gracilis and semitendinosus muscles of medial aspect of knee.

726.62 Tibial collateral ligament bursitis
Pellegrini-Stieda syndrome

726.63 Fibular collateral ligament bursitis

726.64 Patellar tendinitis

726.65 Prepatellar bursitis

726.69 Other
Bursitis:
infrapatellar
subpatellar

√5ᵗʰ **726.7 Enthesopathy of ankle and tarsus**

726.70 Enthesopathy of ankle and tarsus, unspecified
Metatarsalgia NOS
EXCLUDES   *Morton's metatarsalgia (355.6)*

726.71 Achilles bursitis or tendinitis

726.72 Tibialis tendinitis
Tibialis (anterior) (posterior) tendinitis

726.73 Calcaneal spur
DEF: Overgrowth of calcaneus bone; causes pain on walking; due to chronic avulsion injury of plantar fascia from calcaneus.

726.79 Other
Peroneal tendinitis

726.8 Other peripheral enthesopathies

√5ᵗʰ **726.9 Unspecified enthesopathy**

726.90 Enthesopathy of unspecified site
Capsulitis NOS
Periarthritis NOS
Tendinitis NOS

726.91 Exostosis of unspecified site
Bone spur NOS

√4ᵗʰ **727 Other disorders of synovium, tendon, and bursa**

√5ᵗʰ **727.0 Synovitis and tenosynovitis**

727.00 Synovitis and tenosynovitis, unspecified
Synovitis NOS
Tenosynovitis NOS

727.01 *Synovitis and tenosynovitis in diseases classified elsewhere*
Code first underlying disease as:
tuberculosis (015.0-015.9)
EXCLUDES   *crystal-induced (275.4)*
gonococcal (098.51)
gout (274.00-274.03)
syphilitic (095.7)

727.02 Giant cell tumor of tendon sheath

727.03 Trigger finger (acquired)
DEF: Stenosing tenosynovitis or nodule in flexor tendon; cessation of flexion or extension movement in finger, followed by snapping into place.

727.04 Radial styloid tenosynovitis
de Quervain's disease

727.05 Other tenosynovitis of hand and wrist

727.06 Tenosynovitis of foot and ankle

727.09 Other

727.1 Bunion
DEF: Enlarged first metatarsal head due to inflamed bursa; results in laterally displaced great toe.

Bunion

Normal metatarsophalangeal joint

Exostosis

Ganglia

Extensor tendon sheaths

Ganglion of wrist (fluid-filled sac)

Baker's cyst connected to knee joint synovial cavity

727.2 Specific bursitides often of occupational origin
Beat:
elbow
hand
knee
Chronic crepitant synovitis of wrist
Miners':
elbow
knee

727.3 Other bursitis
Bursitis NOS
EXCLUDES   *bursitis:*
gonococcal (098.52)
subacromial (726.19)
subcoracoid (726.19)
subdeltoid (726.19)
syphilitic (095.7)
"frozen shoulder" (726.0)

√5ᵗʰ **727.4 Ganglion and cyst of synovium, tendon, and bursa**

727.40 Synovial cyst, unspecified
EXCLUDES   *that of popliteal space (727.51)*

727.41 Ganglion of joint

727.42 Ganglion of tendon sheath

727.43 Ganglion, unspecified

727.49 Other
Cyst of bursa

√5ᵗʰ **727.5 Rupture of synovium**

727.50 Rupture of synovium, unspecified

727.51 Synovial cyst of popliteal space
Baker's cyst (knee)

727.59 Other

√5ᵗʰ **727.6 Rupture of tendon, nontraumatic**

727.60 Nontraumatic rupture of unspecified tendon

727.61 Complete rupture of rotator cuff
EXCLUDES   *partial tear of rotator cuff (726.13)*

727.62 Tendons of biceps (long head)

727.63 Extensor tendons of hand and wrist

727.64 Flexor tendons of hand and wrist

727.65　**Quadriceps tendon**

727.66　**Patellar tendon**

727.67　**Achilles tendon**

727.68　**Other tendons of foot and ankle**

727.69　**Other**

√5ᵗʰ　**727.8**　**Other disorders of synovium, tendon, and bursa**

727.81　**Contracture of tendon (sheath)**
Short Achilles tendon (acquired)

727.82　**Calcium deposits in tendon and bursa**
Calcification of tendon NOS
Calcific tendinitis NOS
　　EXCLUDES　*peripheral ligamentous or muscular attachments (726.0-726.9)*

727.83　**Plica syndrome**
Plica knee
DEF: A fold in the synovial tissue formed before birth, creating a septum between two pockets of synovial tissue; most common are the medial patellar plica and the suprapatellar plica. Plica syndrome, or plica knee, refers to symptomatic plica.

727.89　**Other**
Abscess of bursa or tendon
　　EXCLUDES　*xanthomatosis localized to tendons (272.7)*

727.9　**Unspecified disorder of synovium, tendon, and bursa**

√4ᵗʰ　**728**　**Disorders of muscle, ligament, and fascia**
　　EXCLUDES　*enthesopathies (726.0-726.9)*
　　muscular dystrophies (359.0-359.1)
　　myoneural disorders (358.00-358.9)
　　myopathies (359.2-359.9)
　　nontraumatic hematoma of muscle (729.92)
　　old disruption of ligaments of knee (717.81-717.89)

728.0　**Infective myositis**
Myositis:
　purulent
　suppurative
　　EXCLUDES　*myositis:*
　　　epidemic (074.1)
　　　interstitial (728.81)
　　　syphilitic (095.6)
　　　tropical (040.81)
DEF: Inflamed connective septal tissue of muscle.

√5ᵗʰ　**728.1**　**Muscular calcification and ossification**

728.10　**Calcification and ossification, unspecified**
Massive calcification (paraplegic)

728.11　**Progressive myositis ossificans**
DEF: Progressive myositic disease; marked by bony tissue formed by voluntary muscle; occurs among very young.

728.12　**Traumatic myositis ossificans**
Myositis ossificans (circumscripta)

728.13　**Postoperative heterotopic calcification**
DEF: Abnormal formation of calcium deposits in muscular tissue after surgery, marked by a corresponding loss of muscle tone and tension.

728.19　**Other**
Polymyositis ossificans

728.2　**Muscular wasting and disuse atrophy, not elsewhere classified**
Amyotrophia NOS
Myofibrosis
　　EXCLUDES　*neuralgic amyotrophy (353.5)*
　　pelvic muscle wasting and disuse atrophy (618.83)
　　progressive muscular atrophy (335.0-335.9)

728.3　**Other specific muscle disorders**
Arthrogryposis
Immobility syndrome (paraplegic)
　　EXCLUDES　*arthrogryposis multiplex congenita (754.89)*
　　stiff-man syndrome (333.91)

728.4　**Laxity of ligament**

728.5　**Hypermobility syndrome**

728.6　**Contracture of palmar fascia**
Dupuytren's contracture
DEF: Dupuytren's contracture: flexion deformity of finger, due to shortened, thickened fibrosing of palmar fascia; cause unknown; associated with long-standing epilepsy.

√5ᵗʰ　**728.7**　**Other fibromatoses**

728.71　**Plantar fascial fibromatosis**
Contracture of plantar fascia
Plantar fasciitis (traumatic)
DEF: Plantar fascia fibromatosis; causes nodular swelling and pain; not associated with contractures.

728.79　**Other**
Garrod's or knuckle pads
Nodular fasciitis
Pseudosarcomatous fibromatosis (proliferative) (subcutaneous)
DEF: Knuckle pads: Pea-size nodules on dorsal surface of interphalangeal joints; new growth of fibrous tissue with thickened dermis and epidermis.

√5ᵗʰ　**728.8**　**Other disorders of muscle, ligament, and fascia**

728.81　**Interstitial myositis**
DEF: Inflammation of septal connective parts of muscle tissue.

728.82　**Foreign body granuloma of muscle**
Talc granuloma of muscle
Use additional code to identify foreign body (V90.01-V90.9)

728.83　**Rupture of muscle, nontraumatic**

728.84　**Diastasis of muscle**
Diastasis recti (abdomen)
　　EXCLUDES　*diastasis recti complicating pregnancy, labor, and delivery (665.8)*
DEF: Muscle separation, such as recti abdominis after repeated pregnancies.

728.85　**Spasm of muscle**

728.86　**Necrotizing fasciitis**
Use additional code to identify:
　gangrene (785.4), if applicable
　infectious organism (041.00-041.89)
DEF: Fulminating infection begins with extensive cellulitis, spreads to superficial and deep fascia; causes thrombosis of subcutaneous vessels, and gangrene of underlying tissue.

728.87　**Muscle weakness (generalized)**
　　EXCLUDES　*generalized weakness (780.79)*

728.88　**Rhabdomyolysis**
DEF: A disintegration or destruction of muscle; an acute disease characterized by the excretion of myoglobin into the urine.

728.89　**Other**
Eosinophilic fasciitis
Use additional E code to identify drug, if drug induced
DEF: Eosinophilic fasciitis: inflammation of fascia of extremities associated with eosinophilia, edema, and swelling; occurs alone or as part of myalgia syndrome.

728.9　**Unspecified disorder of muscle, ligament, and fascia**

√4ᵗʰ **729 Other disorders of soft tissues**

EXCLUDES acroparesthesia (443.89)
carpal tunnel syndrome (354.0)
disorders of the back (720.0-724.9)
entrapment syndromes (354.0-355.9)
palindromic rheumatism (719.3)
periarthritis (726.0-726.9)
psychogenic rheumatism (306.0)

729.0 Rheumatism, unspecified and fibrositis

DEF: General term describes diseases of muscle, tendon, nerve, joint, or bone; symptoms include pain and stiffness.

729.1 Myalgia and myositis, unspecified

Fibromyositis NOS

DEF: Myalgia: muscle pain.

DEF: Myositis: inflamed voluntary muscle.

DEF: Fibromyositis: inflamed fibromuscular tissue.

729.2 Neuralgia, neuritis, and radiculitis, unspecified

EXCLUDES brachial radiculitis (723.4)
cervical radiculitis (723.4)
lumbosacral radiculitis (724.4)
mononeuritis (354.0-355.9)
radiculitis due to intervertebral disc
  involvement (722.0-722.2, 722.7)
sciatica (724.3)

DEF: Neuralgia: paroxysmal pain along nerve; symptoms include brief pain and tenderness at point nerve exits.

DEF: Neuritis: inflamed nerve, symptoms include paresthesia, paralysis and loss of reflexes at nerve site.

DEF: Radiculitis: inflamed nerve root.

√5ᵗʰ **729.3 Panniculitis, unspecified**

DEF: Inflammatory reaction of subcutaneous fat; causes nodules; often develops in abdominal region.

729.30 Panniculitis, unspecified site

Weber-Christian disease

DEF: Febrile, nodular, nonsuppurative, relapsing inflammation of subcutaneous fat.

729.31 Hypertrophy of fat pad, knee

Hypertrophy of infrapatellar fat pad

729.39 Other site

EXCLUDES panniculitis specified as (affecting):
back (724.8)
neck (723.6)
sacral (724.8)

729.4 Fasciitis, unspecified

EXCLUDES necrotizing fasciitis (728.86)
nodular fasciitis (728.79)

729.5 Pain in limb

729.6 Residual foreign body in soft tissue

Use additional code to identify foreign body (V90.01-V90.9)

EXCLUDES foreign body granuloma:
muscle (728.82)
skin and subcutaneous tissue (709.4)

√5ᵗʰ **729.7 Nontraumatic compartment syndrome**

Code first, if applicable, postprocedural complication (998.89)

EXCLUDES compartment syndrome NOS (958.90)
traumatic compartment syndrome
  (958.90-958.99)

DEF: Compression of nerves and blood vessels within an enclosed space, leading to impaired blood flow and muscle and nerve damage.

729.71 Nontraumatic compartment syndrome of upper extremity

Nontraumatic compartment syndrome of shoulder, arm, forearm, wrist, hand, and fingers

729.72 Nontraumatic compartment syndrome of lower extremity

Nontraumatic compartment syndrome of hip, buttock, thigh, leg, foot, and toes

729.73 Nontraumatic compartment syndrome of abdomen

729.79 Nontraumatic compartment syndrome of other sites

√5ᵗʰ **729.8 Other musculoskeletal symptoms referable to limbs**

729.81 Swelling of limb

729.82 Cramp

729.89 Other

EXCLUDES abnormality of gait (781.2)
tetany (781.7)
transient paralysis of limb (781.4)

√5ᵗʰ **729.9 Other and unspecified disorders of soft tissue**

729.90 Disorders of soft tissue, unspecified

729.91 Post-traumatic seroma

EXCLUDES seroma complicating a procedure
  (998.13)

729.92 Nontraumatic hematoma of soft tissue

Nontraumatic hematoma of muscle

729.99 Other disorders of soft tissue

Polyalgia

OSTEOPATHIES, CHONDROPATHIES, AND ACQUIRED MUSCULOSKELETAL DEFORMITIES (730-739)

√4ᵗʰ **730 Osteomyelitis, periostitis, and other infections involving bone**

EXCLUDES jaw (526.4-526.5)
petrous bone (383.2)

Use additional code to identify organism, such as Staphylococcus (041.1)

The following fifth-digit subclassification is for use with category 730; valid digits are in [brackets] under each code. See list at beginning of chapter for definitions.

0 site unspecified
1 shoulder region
2 upper arm
3 forearm
4 hand
5 pelvic region and thigh
6 lower leg
7 ankle and foot
8 other specified sites
9 multiple sites

DEF: Osteomyelitis: bacterial inflammation of bone tissue and marrow.

DEF: Periostitis: inflammation of specialized connective tissue; causes swelling of bone and aching pain.

√5ᵗʰ **730.0 Acute osteomyelitis**
[0-9]

Abscess of any bone except accessory sinus, jaw, or mastoid

Acute or subacute osteomyelitis, with or without mention of periostitis

Use additional code to identify major osseous defect, if applicable (731.3)

√5ᵗʰ **730.1 Chronic osteomyelitis**
[0-9]

Brodie's abscess

Chronic or old osteomyelitis, with or without mention of periostitis

Sclerosing osteomyelitis of Garré

Sequestrum of bone

Use additional code to identify major osseous defect, if applicable (731.3)

EXCLUDES aseptic necrosis of bone (733.40-733.49)

√5ᵗʰ **730.2 Unspecified osteomyelitis**
[0-9]

Osteitis or osteomyelitis NOS, with or without mention of periostitis

Use additional code to identify major osseous defect, if applicable (731.3)

√5ᵗʰ **730.3 Periostitis without mention of osteomyelitis**
[0-9]

Abscess of periosteum ⎫ without mention of
Periostosis   ⎬ osteomyelitis

EXCLUDES that in secondary syphilis (091.61)

✓5ᵗʰ **730.7 Osteopathy resulting from poliomyelitis**
[0-9]   *Code first underlying disease (045.0-045.9)*

✓5ᵗʰ **730.8 Other infections involving bone in diseases**
[0-9]   **classified elsewhere**
           Code first underlying disease as:
               tuberculosis (015.0-015.9)
               typhoid fever (002.0)
           EXCLUDES *syphilis of bone NOS (095.5)*

✓5ᵗʰ **730.9 Unspecified infection of bone**
[0-9]

✓4ᵗʰ **731 Osteitis deformans and osteopathies associated with other disorders classified elsewhere**
    DEF: Osteitis deformans: Bone disease marked by episodes of increased bone loss, excessive repair attempts; causes weakened, deformed bones with increased mass, bowed long bones, deformed flat bones, pain and pathological fractures; may be fatal if associated with congestive heart failure, giant cell tumors or bone sarcoma; also called Paget's disease.

731.0 Osteitis deformans without mention of bone tumor
    · Paget's disease of bone

731.1 Osteitis deformans in diseases classified elsewhere
    Code first underlying disease as:
        malignant neoplasm of bone (170.0-170.9)

731.2 Hypertrophic pulmonary osteoarthropathy
    Bamberger-Marie disease
    DEF: Clubbing of fingers and toes; related to enlarged ends of long bones, due to chronic lung and heart disease.

731.3 Major osseous defects
    Code first underlying disease, if known, such as:
        aseptic necrosis (733.40-733.49)
        malignant neoplasm of bone (170.0-170.9)
        osteomyelitis (730.00-730.29)
        osteoporosis (733.00-733.09)
        peri-prosthetic osteolysis (996.45)

731.8 Other bone involvement in diseases classified elsewhere
    Code first underlying disease as:
        diabetes mellitus (249.8, 250.8)
    Use additional code to specify bone condition, such as:
        acute osteomyelitis (730.00-730.09)

✓4ᵗʰ **732 Osteochondropathies**
    DEF: Conditions related to both bone and cartilage, or conditions in which cartilage is converted to bone (enchondral ossification).

732.0 Juvenile osteochondrosis of spine
    Juvenile osteochondrosis (of):
        marginal or vertebral epiphysis (of Scheuermann)
        spine NOS
    Vertebral epiphysitis
    EXCLUDES *adolescent postural kyphosis (737.0)*

732.1 Juvenile osteochondrosis of hip and pelvis
    Coxa plana
    Ischiopubic synchondrosis (of van Neck)
    Osteochondrosis (juvenile) of:
        acetabulum
        head of femur (of Legg-Calvé-Perthes)
        iliac crest (of Buchanan)
        symphysis pubis (of Pierson)
    Pseudocoxalgia

732.2 Nontraumatic slipped upper femoral epiphysis
    Slipped upper femoral epiphysis NOS

732.3 Juvenile osteochondrosis of upper extremity
    Osteochondrosis (juvenile) of:
        capitulum of humerus (of Panner)
        carpal lunate (of Kienbock)
        hand NOS
        head of humerus (of Haas)
        heads of metacarpals (of Mauclaire)
        lower ulna (of Burns)
        radial head (of Brailsford)
        upper extremity NOS

Slipped Femoral Epiphysis

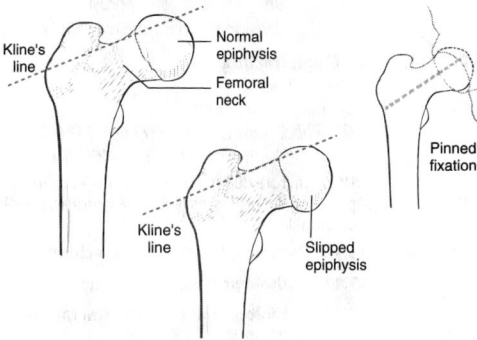

Kline's line — Normal epiphysis — Femoral neck — Pinned fixation — Kline's line — Slipped epiphysis

732.4 Juvenile osteochondrosis of lower extremity, excluding foot
    Osteochondrosis (juvenile) of:
        lower extremity NOS
        primary patellar center (of Köhler)
        proximal tibia (of Blount)
        secondary patellar center (of Sinding-Larsen)
        tibial tubercle (of Osgood-Schlatter)
    Tibia vara

732.5 Juvenile osteochondrosis of foot
    Calcaneal apophysitis
    Epiphysitis, os calcis
    Osteochondrosis (juvenile) of:
        astragalus (of Diaz)
        calcaneum (of Sever)
        foot NOS
        metatarsal
            second (of Freiberg)
            fifth (of Iselin)
        os tibiale externum (of Haglund)
        tarsal navicular (of Köhler)

732.6 Other juvenile osteochondrosis
    Apophysitis ⎫
    Epiphysitis ⎬ specified as juvenile, of other
    Osteochondritis ⎪   site, or site NOS
    Osteochondrosis ⎭

732.7 Osteochondritis dissecans

732.8 Other specified forms of osteochondropathy
    Adult osteochondrosis of spine

732.9 Unspecified osteochondropathy
    Apophysitis ⎫ NOS
    Epiphysitis ⎬ not specified as adult or
    Osteochondritis ⎪   juvenile, of unspecified
    Osteochondrosis ⎭   site

✓4ᵗʰ **733 Other disorders of bone and cartilage**
    EXCLUDES *bone spur (726.91)*
                  cartilage of, or loose body in, joint (717.0-717.9, 718.0-718.9)
                  giant cell granuloma of jaw (526.3)
                  osteitis fibrosa cystica generalisata (252.01)
                  osteomalacia (268.2)
                  polyostotic fibrous dysplasia of bone (756.54)
                  prognathism, retrognathism (524.1)
                  xanthomatosis localized to bone (272.7)

✓5ᵗʰ **733.0 Osteoporosis**
    Use additional code to identify major osseous defect, if applicable (731.3)
    Use additional code to identify personal history of pathologic (healed) fracture (V13.51)
    DEF: Bone mass reduction that ultimately results in fractures after minimal trauma; dorsal kyphosis or loss of height often occur.

733.00 Osteoporosis, unspecified
    Wedging of vertebra NOS

733.01 Senile osteoporosis
    Postmenopausal osteoporosis

733.02 Idiopathic osteoporosis

733.03 Disuse osteoporosis

Diseases of the Musculoskeletal System and Connective Tissue

733.09–734

733.09 Other
Drug-induced osteoporosis
Use additional E code to identify drug

√5ᵗʰ **733.1 Pathologic fracture**
Chronic fracture
Spontaneous fracture
EXCLUDES stress fracture (733.93-733.95)
traumatic fracture (800-829)
DEF: Fracture due to bone structure weakening by pathological processes (e.g., osteoporosis, neoplasms and osteomalacia).

733.10 Pathologic fracture, unspecified site

733.11 Pathologic fracture of humerus

733.12 Pathologic fracture of distal radius and ulna
Wrist NOS

733.13 Pathologic fracture of vertebrae
Collapse of vertebra NOS

733.14 Pathologic fracture of neck of femur
Femur NOS
Hip NOS

733.15 Pathologic fracture of other specified part of femur

733.16 Pathologic fracture of tibia or fibula
Ankle NOS

733.19 Pathologic fracture of other specified site

√5ᵗʰ **733.2 Cyst of bone**

733.20 Cyst of bone (localized), unspecified

733.21 Solitary bone cyst
Unicameral bone cyst

733.22 Aneurysmal bone cyst
DEF: Solitary bone lesion, bulges into periosteum; marked by calcified rim.

733.29 Other
Fibrous dysplasia (monostotic)
EXCLUDES cyst of jaw (526.0-526.2, 526.89)
osteitis fibrosa cystica (252.01)
polyostotic fibrousdyplasia of bone (756.54)

733.3 Hyperostosis of skull
Hyperostosis interna frontalis
Leontiasis ossium
DEF: Abnormal bone growth on inner aspect of cranial bones.

√5ᵗʰ **733.4 Aseptic necrosis of bone**
Use additional code to identify major osseous defect, if applicable (731.3)
EXCLUDES osteochondropathies (732.0-732.9)
DEF: Infarction of bone tissue due to a noninfectious etiology, such as a fracture, ischemic disorder or administration of immunosuppressive drugs; leads to degenerative joint disease or nonunion of fractures.

733.40 Aseptic necrosis of bone, site unspecified

733.41 Head of humerus

733.42 Head and neck of femur
Femur NOS
EXCLUDES Legg-Calvé-Perthes disease (732.1)

733.43 Medial femoral condyle

733.44 Talus

733.45 Jaw
Use additional E code to identify drug, if drug-induced
EXCLUDES osteoradionecrosis of jaw (526.89)

733.49 Other

733.5 Osteitis condensans
Piriform sclerosis of ilium
DEF: Idiopathic condition marked by low back pain; associated with oval or triangular sclerotic, opaque bone next to sacroiliac joints in the ileum.

733.6 Tietze's disease
Costochondral junction syndrome
Costochondritis
DEF: Painful, idiopathic, nonsuppurative, swollen costal cartilage sometimes confused with cardiac symptoms because the anterior chest pain resembles that of coronary artery disease.

733.7 Algoneurodystrophy
Disuse atrophy of bone
Sudeck's atrophy
DEF: Painful, idiopathic complex reflex sympathetic dystrophy, a chronic progressive disease characterized by severe pain, swelling, and changes in the skin.

√5ᵗʰ **733.8 Malunion and nonunion of fracture**

733.81 Malunion of fracture

733.82 Nonunion of fracture
Pseudoarthrosis (bone)

√5ᵗʰ **733.9 Other unspecified disorders of bone and cartilage**

733.90 Disorder of bone and cartilage

733.91 Arrest of bone development or growth
Epiphyseal arrest

733.92 Chondromalacia
Chondromalacia:
NOS
localized, except patella
systemic
tibial plateau
EXCLUDES chondromalacia of patella (717.7)
DEF: Articular cartilage softening.

733.93 Stress fracture of tibia or fibula
Stress reaction of tibia or fibula
Use additional external cause code(s) to identify the cause of the stress fracture

733.94 Stress fracture of the metatarsals
Stress reaction of metatarsals
Use additional external cause code(s) to identify the cause of the stress fracture

733.95 Stress fracture of other bone
Stress reaction of other bone
Use additional external cause code(s) to identify the cause of the stress fracture
EXCLUDES stress fracture of:
femoral neck (733.96)
fibula (733.93)
metatarsals (733.94)
pelvis (733.98)
shaft of femur (733.97)
tibia (733.93)

733.96 Stress fracture of femoral neck
Stress reaction of femoral neck
Use additional external cause code(s) to identify the cause of the stress fracture

733.97 Stress fracture of shaft of femur
Stress reaction of shaft of femur
Use additional external cause code(s) to identify the cause of the stress fracture

733.98 Stress fracture of pelvis
Stress reaction of pelvis
Use additional external cause code(s) to identify the cause of the stress fracture

733.99 Other
Diaphysitis
Hypertrophy of bone
Relapsing polychondritis

734 Flat foot
Pes planus (acquired)
Talipes planus (acquired)
EXCLUDES congenital (754.61)
rigid flat foot (754.61)
spastic (everted) flat foot (754.61)

Acquired Deformities of Toe

Acquired Deformities of Forearm

√4ᵗʰ **735 Acquired deformities of toe**
　　　EXCLUDES　congenital (754.60-754.69, 755.65-755.66)

735.0 Hallux valgus (acquired)
DEF: Angled displacement of the great toe, causing it to ride over or under other toes.

735.1 Hallux varus (acquired)
DEF: Angled displacement of the great toe toward the body midline, away from the other toes.

735.2 Hallux rigidus
DEF: Limited flexion movement at metatarsophalangeal joint of great toe; due to degenerative joint disease.

735.3 Hallux malleus
DEF: Extended proximal phalanx, flexed distal phalanges of great toe; foot resembles claw or hammer.

735.4 Other hammer toe (acquired)

735.5 Claw toe (acquired)
DEF: Hyperextended proximal phalanges, flexed middle and distal phalanges.

735.8 Other acquired deformities of toe

735.9 Unspecified acquired deformity of toe

√4ᵗʰ **736 Other acquired deformities of limbs**
　　　EXCLUDES　congenital (754.3-755.9)

√5ᵗʰ **736.0 Acquired deformities of forearm, excluding fingers**

736.00 Unspecified deformity
Deformity of elbow, forearm, hand, or wrist (acquired) NOS

736.01 Cubitus valgus (acquired)
DEF: Deviation of the elbow away from the body midline upon extension; it occurs when the palm is turning outward.

736.02 Cubitus varus (acquired)
DEF: Elbow joint displacement angled laterally; when the forearm is extended, it is deviated toward the midline of the body; also called "gun stock" deformity.

736.03 Valgus deformity of wrist (acquired)
DEF: Abnormal angulation away from the body midline.

736.04 Varus deformity of wrist (acquired)
DEF: Abnormal angulation toward the body midline.

736.05 Wrist drop (acquired)
DEF: Inability to extend the hand at the wrist due to extensor muscle paralysis.

736.06 Claw hand (acquired)
DEF: Flexion and atrophy of the hand and fingers; found in ulnar nerve lesions, syringomyelia, and leprosy.

736.07 Club hand, acquired
DEF: Twisting of the hand out of shape or position; caused by the congenital absence of the ulna or radius.

736.09 Other

736.1 Mallet finger
DEF: Permanently flexed distal phalanx.

√5ᵗʰ **736.2 Other acquired deformities of finger**

736.20 Unspecified deformity
Deformity of finger (acquired) NOS

736.21 Boutonniere deformity
DEF: A deformity of the finger caused by flexion of the proximal interphalangeal joint and hyperextension of the distal joint; also called buttonhole deformity.

736.22 Swan-neck deformity
DEF: Flexed distal and hyperextended proximal interphalangeal joint.

736.29 Other
　　EXCLUDES　trigger finger (727.03)

√5ᵗʰ **736.3 Acquired deformities of hip**

736.30 Unspecified deformity
Deformity of hip (acquired) NOS

736.31 Coxa valga (acquired)
DEF: Increase of at least 140 degrees in the angle formed by the axis of the head and the neck of the femur, and the axis of its shaft.

736.32 Coxa vara (acquired)
DEF: The bending downward of the neck of the femur, causing difficulty in movement; a right angle or less may be formed by the axis of the head and neck of the femur and the axis of its shaft.

736.39 Other

√5ᵗʰ **736.4 Genu valgum or varum (acquired)**

736.41 Genu valgum (acquired)
DEF: Abnormally close together and an abnormally large space between the ankles; also called "knock-knees."

736.42 Genu varum (acquired)
DEF: Abnormally separated knees and the inward bowing of the legs; it is also called "bowlegs."

736.5 Genu recurvatum (acquired)
DEF: Hyperextended knees; also called "backknee."

736.6 Other acquired deformities of knee
Deformity of knee (acquired) NOS

√5ᵗʰ **736.7 Other acquired deformities of ankle and foot**
　　　EXCLUDES　deformities of toe (acquired) (735.0-735.9)
　　　　　　　　　pes planus (acquired) (734)

736.70 Unspecified deformity of ankle and foot, acquired

736.71 Acquired equinovarus deformity
Clubfoot, acquired
　　EXCLUDES　clubfoot not specified as acquired (754.5-754.7)

736.72 Equinus deformity of foot, acquired
DEF: A plantar flexion deformity that forces people to walk on their toes.

Acquired Deformities of Hip

Deformities of Lower Limb

Kyphosis and Lordosis

Scoliosis and Kyphoscoliosis

Scoliosis   Kyphoscoliosis

736.73 Cavus deformity of foot

> *EXCLUDES* that with claw foot (736.74)

> **DEF:** Abnormally high longitudinal arch of the foot.

736.74 Claw foot, acquired

> **DEF:** High foot arch with hyperextended toes at metatarsophalangeal joint and flexed toes at distal joints; also called "main en griffe."

736.75 Cavovarus deformity of foot, acquired

> **DEF:** Inward turning of the heel from the midline of the leg and an abnormally high longitudinal arch.

736.76 Other calcaneus deformity

736.79 Other

> Acquired:
> pes
> talipes } not elsewhere classified

√5ᵗʰ **736.8 Acquired deformities of other parts of limbs**

736.81 Unequal leg length (acquired)

736.89 Other

> Deformity (acquired):
> arm or leg, not elsewhere classified
> shoulder

736.9 Acquired deformity of limb, site unspecified

√4ᵗʰ **737 Curvature of spine**

> *EXCLUDES* congenital (754.2)

737.0 Adolescent postural kyphosis

> *EXCLUDES* osteochondrosis of spine (juvenile) (732.0)
> adult (732.8)

√5ᵗʰ **737.1 Kyphosis (acquired)**

737.10 Kyphosis (acquired) (postural)

737.11 Kyphosis due to radiation

737.12 Kyphosis, postlaminectomy

737.19 Other

> *EXCLUDES* that associated with conditions classifiable elsewhere (737.41)

√5ᵗʰ **737.2 Lordosis (acquired)**

> **DEF:** Swayback appearance created by an abnormally increased spinal curvature; it is also referred to as "hollow back" or "saddle back."

737.20 Lordosis (acquired) (postural)

737.21 Lordosis, postlaminectomy

737.22 Other postsurgical lordosis

737.29 Other

> *EXCLUDES* that associated with conditions classifiable elsewhere (737.42)

√5ᵗʰ **737.3 Kyphoscoliosis and scoliosis**

> **DEF:** Kyphoscoliosis: backward and lateral curvature of the spinal column; it is found in vertebral osteochondrosis.
> **DEF:** Scoliosis: an abnormal deviation of the spine to the left or right of the midline.

737.30 Scoliosis [and kyphoscoliosis], idiopathic

737.31 Resolving infantile idiopathic scoliosis

737.32 Progressive infantile idiopathic scoliosis

737.33 Scoliosis due to radiation

737.34 Thoracogenic scoliosis

737.39 Other

> *EXCLUDES* that associated with conditions classifiable elsewhere (737.43)
> that in kyphoscoliotic heart disease (416.1)

√5ᵗʰ **737.4 Curvature of spine associated with other conditions**

> *Code first associated condition as:*
> Charcôt-Marie-Tooth disease (356.1)
> mucopolysaccharidosis (277.5)
> neurofibromatosis (237.70-237.79)
> osteitis deformans (731.0)
> osteitis fibrosa cystica (252.01)
> osteoporosis (733.00-733.09)
> poliomyelitis (138)
> tuberculosis [Pott's curvature] (015.0)

737.40 *Curvature of spine, unspecified*

737.41　*Kyphosis*

737.42　*Lordosis*

737.43　*Scoliosis*

737.8　Other curvatures of spine

737.9　Unspecified curvature of spine
Curvature of spine (acquired) (idiopathic) NOS
Hunchback, acquired
EXCLUDES　*deformity of spine NOS (738.5)*

✓4ᵗʰ **738　Other acquired deformity** ·
EXCLUDES　*congenital (754.0-756.9, 758.0-759.9)*
dentofacial anomalies (524.0-524.9)

738.0　Acquired deformity of nose
Deformity of nose (acquired)
Overdevelopment of nasal bones
EXCLUDES　*deflected or deviated nasal septum (470)*

✓5ᵗʰ **738.1　Other acquired deformity of head**

738.10　Unspecified deformity

738.11　Zygomatic hyperplasia
DEF: Abnormal enlargement of the zygoma (processus zygomaticus temporalis).

738.12　Zygomatic hypoplasia
DEF: Underdevelopment of the zygoma (processus zygomaticus temporalis).

738.19　Other specified deformity

738.2　Acquired deformity of neck

738.3　Acquired deformity of chest and rib
Deformity:
chest (acquired)
rib (acquired)
Pectus:
carinatum, acquired
excavatum, acquired

738.4　Acquired spondylolisthesis
Degenerative spondylolisthesis
Spondylolysis, acquired
EXCLUDES　*congenital (756.12)*
DEF: Vertebra displaced forward over another; due to bilateral defect in vertebral arch, eroded articular surface of posterior facets and elongated pedicle between fifth lumbar vertebra and sacrum.

738.5　Other acquired deformity of back or spine
Deformity of spine NOS
EXCLUDES　*curvature of spine (737.0-737.9)*

738.6　Acquired deformity of pelvis
Pelvic obliquity
EXCLUDES　*intrapelvic protrusion of acetabulum (718.6)*
that in relation to labor and delivery
(653.0-653.4, 653.8-653.9)
DEF: Pelvic obliquity: slanting or inclination of the pelvis at an angle between 55 and 60 degrees between the plane of the pelvis and the horizontal plane.

738.7　Cauliflower ear
DEF: Abnormal external ear; due to injury, subsequent perichondritis.

738.8　Acquired deformity of other specified site
Deformity of clavicle

738.9　Acquired deformity of unspecified site

✓4ᵗʰ **739　Nonallopathic lesions, not elsewhere classified**
INCLUDES　segmental dysfunction
somatic dysfunction
DEF: Disability, loss of function or abnormality of a body part that is neither classifiable to a particular system nor brought about therapeutically to counteract another disease.

739.0　Head region
Occipitocervical region

739.1　Cervical region
Cervicothoracic region

739.2　Thoracic region
Thoracolumbar region

739.3　Lumbar region
Lumbosacral region

739.4　Sacral region
Sacrococcygeal region
Sacroiliac region

739.5　Pelvic region
Hip region
Pubic region

739.6　Lower extremities

739.7　Upper extremities
Acromioclavicular region
Sternoclavicular region

739.8　Rib cage
Costochondral region
Costovertebral region
Sternochondral region

739.9　Abdomen and other

Chapter 14: Congenital Anomalies (740–759)

Coding Guidance

Congenital anomalies may be the result of genetic factors (chromosomes), teratogens (agents causing physical defects in the embryo), or both. The anomalies may be apparent at birth or hidden and identified sometime after birth. Whatever the cause, congenital anomalies can be attributed to nearly 50 percent of deaths to full-term newborn infants.

Codes in Chapter 14 are classified according to a principal or defining defect rather than to the cause (chromosome abnormalities are the exception). Regardless of the origin, dysmorphology (clinical structural abnormality) is generally the primary indication of a congenital anomaly, and in many cases, a syndrome may be classified according to a single anatomic anomaly rather than a complex of symptoms.

ICD-9-CM does not differentiate between abnormalities that are intrinsic — related to the fetus — or extrinsic — as a result of intrauterine problems, although a note in ICD-9-CM prior to rubric 754 Certain congenital musculoskeletal deformities identifies codes as specific to extrinsic factors.

However ICD-9-CM does make a distinction in the classification of an anomaly as compared to a deformity. An anomaly is a malformation caused by abnormal fetal development, as in transposition of great vessels or spina bifida. A deformity is an alteration in structure caused by an extrinsic force, as in uterine compression.

Many congenital anomalies are patterns of multiple malformations that are considered pathogenetically related, meaning the cellular events and mechanical reactions occurring during the development of the disease are linked. These symptom complexes are called syndromes. When syndromes are not specifically indexed in ICD-9-CM, a code is assigned to each presenting manifestation of the syndrome that occurs as a set of symptoms or as multiple malformations.

This chapter classifies conditions present at birth including neurological problems, anomalies of the senses, heart anomalies, respiratory anomalies and digestive system anomalies. The chapter is organized by organ system or anatomical site affected by the congenital anomaly.

The coding guidelines for congenital anomalies follow the general guidelines for ICD-9-CM. Coders should pay close attention to the instructional notes and be aware of the various structural anomalies associated with certain syndromes, so as to not assign unnecessary additional codes. Alternately, instructional notes may also prompt the coder to report additional or separate codes, where necessary, to fully describe the condition.

Codes from chapter 14 may be used throughout the life of the patient. If a congenital anomaly has been corrected, a personal history code should be used to identify the history of the anomaly. Whenever the condition is diagnosed by the physician, it is appropriate to assign a code from codes 740–759 even when a congenital anomaly is identified later in life.

When a congenital anomaly does not have a unique code assignment, assign additional codes for any manifestations that may be present. When the code assignment specifically identifies the congenital anomaly, manifestations that are inherent components of the anomaly should not be coded separately. Additional codes should be assigned for manifestations that are not inherent components.

Anomalies that arise due to the birth process are considered injuries due to the birth process, not congenital anomalies, and are classified to category 767, "Conditions in the Perinatal Period."

Hydrocephalus (742.3)

Congenital hydrocephalus is characterized by ventricular enlargement with an abnormal accumulation of cerebral spinal fluid resulting in increased intracerebral pressure. Other forms of hydrocephalus are coded elsewhere such as secondary normal pressure hydrocephalus (331.3–331.4), hydrocephalus with spina bifida (741.0x), and due to congenital toxoplasmosis (771.2).

Obstructive Anomalies of Heart, NEC (746.84)

Multiple codes may be required to report certain obstructive cardiac anomalies. For example, an instructional note at code 746.84 directs the coder to "Use additional code for associated anomalies, such as:"

- Coarctation of aorta (747.10)

- Congenital mitral stenosis (746.5)
- Subaortic stenosis (746.81)

This instructional note alerts the coder that an additional code is necessary to describe specific anomalies associated with cardiac obstruction classifiable to code 746.84. Code first the obstruction (746.84) followed by an additional code for the specific anomaly. For example, Shone's syndrome with subaortic stenosis is reported with code 746.84, followed by code 746.81.

Patent Ductus Arteriosus (747.0)

Patent ductus arteriosus is the failure of the ductus arteriosus to close. A vessel that allows blood to bypass the nonfunctioning lungs of the fetus, the ductus arteriosus normally constricts rapidly within minutes of birth and closes completely within one to two months after birth. When the ductus arteriosus fails to close, blood from the aorta is allowed to flow into the pulmonary artery where it is recirculated to the lungs and reoxygenated, resulting in an increased workload on the left side of the heart and increased pulmonary vascular congestion.

Cleft Palate (749)

Cleft palate is the fissure or abnormal elongated opening of the palate. Cleft palate can occur either unilaterally or bilaterally and can be partial or involve the entire palate. The most common types of cleft palate are the complete left unilateral and partial midline cleft of the secondary palate. Fifth-digit assignment indicates laterality.

Meckel's Diverticulum (751.0)

Meckel's diverticulum is a diverticulum protruding from the wall of the ileum, arising from any point as close as 3 cm and as far as 100 cm from the cecum. Usually asymptomatic, Meckel's diverticulum is an incidental finding in most people.

Down's Syndrome (758.0)

Down's syndrome is a syndrome of congenital anomalies due to chromosomal abnormality, specifically an extra chromosome, usually at 21 or 22. The condition also is known as trisomy 21 or 22.

Marfan Syndrome (759.82)

Marfan syndrome is a hereditary autosomal trait disorder of connective tissue with many manifestations. It is characterized by elongation of the bones, often with associated abnormalities of the eyes and the cardiovascular system.

Finnish-type Congenital Nephrosis (759.89)

This congenital kidney disease is caused by a rare genetic recessive mutation of chromosome 19, which affects one out of 8,000 births in Finland, usually in premature and low-birth-weight babies. It occurs during the first week of life and develops to end-stage renal disease between 3 and 8 years of age. Treatment may include immune therapy, metabolic support, tube feedings, dialysis, and renal transplant.

Two codes are required to report Finnish-type congenital nephrosis: 759.89 Other specified anomalies and 581.3 Nephrotic syndrome with lesion of minimal change glomerulonephritis.

Borjeson-Forssman-Lehmann Syndrome (759.89)

Borjeson-Forssman-Lehmann syndrome is a rare X-linked recessive disorder described as a mental deficiency, epilepsy-endocrine disorder. Characteristics of this syndrome include severe mental retardation, epilepsy, obesity, hypogonadism, hypometabolism, swelling of facial subcutaneous tissue, visual problems, and large ears. Developmental delays and learning disabilities are common. Borjeson-Forssman-Lehmann syndrome is not classifiable to a single, unique code. Report code 759.89 Other specified anomalies, along with separate codes for each separate manifestation of the syndrome (e.g., mental retardation, obesity, hypogonadism, anatomical deformities).

Congenital Anomalies

740–742.51

14. CONGENITAL ANOMALIES (740-759)

☑️4th **740 Anencephalus and similar anomalies**

740.0 Anencephalus
Acrania
Amyelencephalus
Hemicephaly
Hemianencephaly
DEF: Fetus without cerebrum, cerebellum and flat bones of skull.

740.1 Craniorachischisis
DEF: Congenital slit in cranium and vertebral column.

740.2 Iniencephaly
DEF: Spinal cord passes through enlarged occipital bone (foramen magnum); absent vertebral bone layer and spinal processes; resulting in both reduction in number and proper fusion of the vertebrae.

☑️4th **741 Spina bifida**
<u>EXCLUDES</u>   spina bifida occulta (756.17)

The following fifth-digit subclassification is for use with category 741:

   0 unspecified region
   1 cervical region
   2 dorsal [thoracic] region
   3 lumbar region

DEF: Lack of closure of spinal cord's bony encasement; marked by cord protrusion into lumbosacral area; evident by elevated alpha-fetoprotein of amniotic fluid.

☑️5th **741.0 With hydrocephalus**
[0-3]   Arnold-Chiari syndrome, type II
Chiari malformation, type II
Any condition classifiable to 741.9 with any condition classifiable to 742.3

☑️5th **741.9 Without mention of hydrocephalus**
[0-3]   Hydromeningocele (spinal)
Hydromyelocele
Meningocele (spinal)
Meningomyelocele
Myelocele
Myelocystocele
Rachischisis
Spina bifida (aperta)
Syringomyelocele

☑️4th **742 Other congenital anomalies of nervous system**
<u>EXCLUDES</u>   congenital central alveolar hypoventilation syndrome (327.25)

742.0 Encephalocele
Encephalocystocele
Encephalomyelocele
Hydroencephalocele
Hydromeningocele, cranial
Meningocele, cerebral
Meningoencephalocele
DEF: Brain tissue protrudes through skull defect.

742.1 Microcephalus
Hydromicrocephaly
Micrencephaly
DEF: Extremely small head or brain.

742.2 Reduction deformities of brain
Absence
Agenesis } of part of brain
Aplasia
Hypoplasia

Agyria
Arhinencephaly
Holoprosencephaly
Microgyria

Spina Bifida

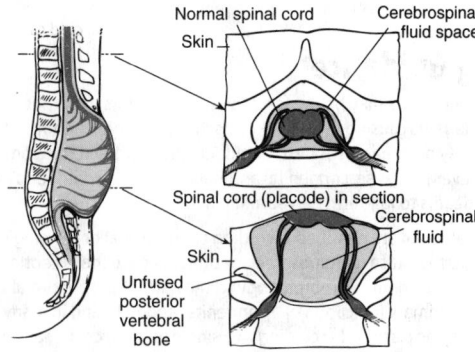

742.3 Congenital hydrocephalus
Aqueduct of Sylvius:
  anomaly
  obstruction, congenital
  stenosis
Atresia of foramina of Magendie and Luschka
Hydrocephalus in newborn
<u>EXCLUDES</u>   hydrocephalus:
   acquired (331.3-331.4)
   due to congenital toxoplasmosis (771.2)
   with any condition classifiable to 741.9 (741.0)
DEF: Fluid accumulation within the skull; involves subarachnoid (external) or ventricular (internal) brain spaces.

742.4 Other specified anomalies of brain
Congenital cerebral cyst
Macroencephaly
Macrogyria
Megalencephaly
Multiple anomalies of brain NOS
Porencephaly
Ulegyria

☑️5th **742.5 Other specified anomalies of spinal cord**
742.51 Diastematomyelia
DEF: Congenital anomaly often associated with spina bifida; the spinal cord is separated into halves by a bony tissue resembling a "spike" (a spicule), each half surrounded by a dural sac.

Normal Ventricles and Hydrocephalus

742.53 Hydromyelia
Hydrorhachis
DEF: Dilated central spinal cord canal; characterized by increased fluid accumulation.

742.59 Other
Amyelia
Atelomyelia
Congenital anomaly of spinal meninges
Defective development of cauda equina
Hypoplasia of spinal cord
Myelatelia
Myelodysplasia

742.8 Other specified anomalies of nervous system
Agenesis of nerve
Displacement of brachial plexus
Familial dysautonomia
Jaw-winking syndrome
Marcus-Gunn syndrome
Riley-Day syndrome
EXCLUDES *neurofibromatosis (237.70-237.79)*

742.9 Unspecified anomaly of brain, spinal cord, and nervous system
Anomaly
Congenital:
  disease   of: { brain
  lesion   nervous system
Deformity   spinal cord

✓4ᵗʰ **743 Congenital anomalies of eye**

✓5ᵗʰ **743.0 Anophthalmos**
DEF: Complete absence of the eyes or the presence of vestigial eyes.

743.00 Clinical anophthalmos, unspecified
Agenesis
Congenital absence } of eye
Anophthalmos NOS

743.03 Cystic eyeball, congenital

743.06 Cryptophthalmos
DEF: Skin is continuous over eyeball, results in apparent absence of eyelids.

✓5ᵗʰ **743.1 Microphthalmos**
Dysplasia
Hypoplasia } of eye
Rudimentary eye
DEF: Abnormally small eyeballs, may be opacities of cornea and lens, scarring of choroid and retina.

743.10 Microphthalmos, unspecified

743.11 Simple microphthalmos

743.12 Microphthalmos associated with other anomalies of eye and adnexa

✓5ᵗʰ **743.2 Buphthalmos**
Glaucoma:
  congenital
  newborn
Hydrophthalmos
EXCLUDES *glaucoma of childhood (365.14)*
traumatic glaucoma due to birth injury (767.8)
DEF: Distended, enlarged fibrous coats of eye; due to intraocular pressure of congenital glaucoma.

743.20 Buphthalmos, unspecified

743.21 Simple buphthalmos

743.22 Buphthalmos associated with other ocular anomalies
Keratoglobus,
  congenital } associated with
Megalocornea   buphthalmos

✓5ᵗʰ **743.3 Congenital cataract and lens anomalies**
EXCLUDES *infantile cataract (366.00-366.09)*
DEF: Opaque eye lens.

743.30 Congenital cataract, unspecified

743.31 Capsular and subcapsular cataract

743.32 Cortical and zonular cataract

743.33 Nuclear cataract

743.34 Total and subtotal cataract, congenital

743.35 Congenital aphakia
Congenital absence of lens

743.36 Anomalies of lens shape
Microphakia
Spherophakia

743.37 Congenital ectopic lens

743.39 Other

✓5ᵗʰ **743.4 Coloboma and other anomalies of anterior segment**
DEF: Coloboma: ocular tissue defect associated with defect of ocular fetal intraocular fissure; may cause small pit on optic disk, major defects of iris, ciliary body, choroid, and retina.

743.41 Anomalies of corneal size and shape
Microcornea
EXCLUDES *that associated with buphthalmos (743.22)*

743.42 Corneal opacities, interfering with vision, congenital

743.43 Other corneal opacities, congenital

743.44 Specified anomalies of anterior chamber, chamber angle, and related structures
Anomaly:
  Axenfeld's
  Peters'
  Rieger's

743.45 Aniridia
DEF: Incompletely formed or absent iris; affects both eyes; dominant trait; also called congenital absence of iris.

743.46 Other specified anomalies of iris and ciliary body
Anisocoria, congenital   Coloboma of iris
Atresia of pupil   Corectopia

743.47 Specified anomalies of sclera

743.48 Multiple and combined anomalies of anterior segment

743.49 Other

✓5ᵗʰ **743.5 Congenital anomalies of posterior segment**

743.51 Vitreous anomalies
Congenital vitreous opacity

743.52 Fundus coloboma
DEF: Absent retinal and choroidal tissue; occurs in lower fundus; a bright white ectatic zone of exposed sclera extends into and changes the optic disk.

743.53 Chorioretinal degeneration, congenital

743.54 Congenital folds and cysts of posterior segment

743.55 Congenital macular changes

743.56 Other retinal changes, congenital

743.57 Specified anomalies of optic disc
Coloboma of optic disc (congenital)

743.58 Vascular anomalies
Congenital retinal aneurysm

743.59 Other

✓5ᵗʰ **743.6 Congenital anomalies of eyelids, lacrimal system, and orbit**

743.61 Congenital ptosis
DEF: Drooping of eyelid.

743.62 Congenital deformities of eyelids
Ablepharon   Congenital:
Absence of eyelid   ectropion
Accessory eyelid   entropion

743.63 Other specified congenital anomalies of eyelid
Absence, agenesis, of cilia

743.64 Specified congenital anomalies of lacrimal gland

743.65 Specified congenital anomalies of lacrimal passages
Absence, agenesis of:
lacrimal apparatus
punctum lacrimale
Accessory lacrimal canal

743.66 Specified congenital anomalies of orbit

743.69 Other
Accessory eye muscles

743.8 Other specified anomalies of eye
EXCLUDES   *congenital nystagmus (379.51)*
ocular albinism (270.2)
optic nerve hypoplasia (377.43)
retinitis pigmentosa (362.74)

743.9 Unspecified anomaly of eye
Congenital:
anomaly NOS } of eye (any part)
deformity NOS

√4ᵗʰ **744 Congenital anomalies of ear, face, and neck**
EXCLUDES   *anomaly of:*
cervical spine (754.2, 756.10-756.19)
larynx (748.2-748.3)
nose (748.0-748.1)
parathyroid gland (759.2)
thyroid gland (759.2)
cleft lip (749.10-749.25)

√5ᵗʰ **744.0 Anomalies of ear causing impairment of hearing**
EXCLUDES   *congenital deafness without mention of cause (389.0-389.9)*

744.00 Unspecified anomaly of ear with impairment of hearing

744.01 Absence of external ear
Absence of:
auditory canal (external)
auricle (ear) (with stenosis or atresia of auditory canal)

744.02 Other anomalies of external ear with impairment of hearing
Atresia or stricture of auditory canal (external)

744.03 Anomaly of middle ear, except ossicles
Atresia or stricture of osseous meatus (ear)

744.04 Anomalies of ear ossicles
Fusion of ear ossicles

744.05 Anomalies of inner ear
Congenital anomaly of:
membranous labyrinth
organ of Corti

744.09 Other
Absence of ear, congenital

744.1 Accessory auricle
Accessory tragus
Polyotia
Preauricular appendage
Supernumerary:
ear
lobule
DEF: Redundant tissue or structures of ear.

√5ᵗʰ **744.2 Other specified anomalies of ear**
EXCLUDES   *that with impairment of hearing (744.00-744.09)*

744.21 Absence of ear lobe, congenital

744.22 Macrotia
DEF: Abnormally large pinna of ear.

744.23 Microtia
DEF: Hypoplasia of pinna; associated with absent or closed auditory canal.

744.24 Specified anomalies of Eustachian tube
Absence of Eustachian tube

744.29 Other
Bat ear
Darwin's tubercle
Pointed ear
Prominence of auricle
Ridge ear
EXCLUDES   *preauricular sinus (744.46)*

744.3 Unspecified anomaly of ear
Congenital:
anomaly NOS } of ear, not elsewhere classified
deformity NOS

√5ᵗʰ **744.4 Branchial cleft cyst or fistula; preauricular sinus**

744.41 Branchial cleft sinus or fistula
Branchial:
sinus (external) (internal)
vestige
DEF: Cyst due to failed closure of embryonic branchial cleft.

744.42 Branchial cleft cyst

744.43 Cervical auricle

744.46 Preauricular sinus or fistula

744.47 Preauricular cyst

744.49 Other
Fistula (of):
auricle, congenital
cervicoaural

744.5 Webbing of neck
Pterygium colli
DEF: Thick, triangular skinfold, stretches from lateral side of neck across shoulder; associated with Turner's and Noonan's syndromes.

√5ᵗʰ **744.8 Other specified anomalies of face and neck**

744.81 Macrocheilia
Hypertrophy of lip, congenital
DEF: Abnormally large lips.

744.82 Microcheilia
DEF: Abnormally small lips.

744.83 Macrostomia
DEF: Bilateral or unilateral anomaly of mouth due to malformed maxillary and mandibular processes; results in mouth extending toward ear.

744.84 Microstomia
DEF: Abnormally small mouth.

744.89 Other
EXCLUDES   *congenital fistula of lip (750.25)*
musculoskeletal anomalies (754.0-754.1, 756.0)

744.9 Unspecified anomalies of face and neck
Congenital:
anomaly NOS } of face [any part] or neck [any
deformity NOS } part]

√4ᵗʰ **745 Bulbus cordis anomalies and anomalies of cardiac septal closure**

745.0 Common truncus
Absent septum } between aorta and
Communication (abnormal) } pulmonary artery
Aortic septal defect
Common aortopulmonary trunk
Persistent truncus arteriosus

√5ᵗʰ **745.1 Transposition of great vessels**

745.10 Complete transposition of great vessels
Transposition of great vessels:
NOS
classical

Heart Defects

Atrial septal defect

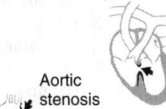
Ventricular septal defect

Aortic stenosis

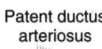
Patent ductus arteriosus

Pulmonary stenosis

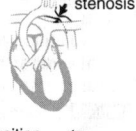
Transposition of the great vessels

Tetralogy of Fallot

745.11 Double outlet right ventricle
Dextratransposition of aorta
Incomplete transposition of great vessels
Origin of both great vessels from right ventricle
Taussig-Bing syndrome or defect

745.12 Corrected transposition of great vessels

745.19 Other

745.2 Tetralogy of Fallot
Fallot's pentalogy
Ventricular septal defect with pulmonary stenosis or atresia, dextraposition of aorta, and hypertrophy of right ventricle
> **EXCLUDES** *Fallot's triad (746.09)*

DEF: Obstructed cardiac outflow causes pulmonary stenosis, interventricular septal defect and right ventricular hypertrophy.

745.3 Common ventricle
Cor triloculare biatriatum
Single ventricle

745.4 Ventricular septal defect
Eisenmenger's defect or complex
Gerbo dedefect
Interventricular septal defect
Left ventricular-right atrial communication
Roger's disease
> **EXCLUDES** *common atrioventricular canal type (745.69)*
> *single ventricle (745.3)*

745.5 Ostium secundum type atrial septal defect
Defect:
  atrium secundum
  fossa ovalis
Lutembacher's syndrome
Patent or persistent:
  foramen ovale
  ostium secundum

DEF: Opening in atrial septum due to failure of the septum secundum and the endocardial cushions to fuse; there is a rim of septum surrounding the defect.

✓5ᵗʰ 745.6 Endocardial cushion defects
DEF: Atrial and/or ventricular septal defects causing abnormal fusion of cushions in atrioventricular canal.

745.60 Endocardial cushion defect, unspecified type
DEF: Septal defect due to imperfect fusion of endocardial cushions.

745.61 Ostium primum defect
Persistent ostium primum
DEF: Opening in low, posterior septum primum; causes cleft in basal portion of atrial septum; associated with cleft mitral valve.

745.69 Other
Absence of atrial septum
Atrioventricular canal type ventricular septal defect
Common atrioventricular canal
Common atrium

745.7 Cor biloculare
Absence of atrial and ventricular septa
DEF: Atrial and ventricular septal defect; marked by heart with two cardiac chambers (one atrium, one ventricle), and one atrioventricular valve.

745.8 Other

745.9 Unspecified defect of septal closure
Septal defect NOS

✓4ᵗʰ 746 Other congenital anomalies of heart
> **EXCLUDES** *endocardial fibroelastosis (425.3)*

✓5ᵗʰ 746.0 Anomalies of pulmonary valve
> **EXCLUDES** *infundibular or subvalvular pulmonic stenosis (746.83)*
> *tetralogy of Fallot (745.2)*

746.00 Pulmonary valve anomaly, unspecified

746.01 Atresia, congenital
Congenital absence of pulmonary valve

746.02 Stenosis, congenital
DEF: Stenosis of opening between pulmonary artery and right ventricle; causes obstructed blood outflow from right ventricle.

746.09 Other
Congenital insufficiency of pulmonary valve
Fallot's triad or trilogy

746.1 Tricuspid atresia and stenosis, congenital
Absence of tricuspid valve

746.2 Ebstein's anomaly
DEF: Malformation of the tricuspid valve characterized by septal and posterior leaflets attaching to the wall of the right ventricle; causing the right ventricle to fuse with the atrium into a large right atrium and a small ventricle; causes heart failure and abnormal cardiac rhythm.

746.3 Congenital stenosis of aortic valve
Congenital aortic stenosis
> **EXCLUDES** *congenital:*
> *subaortic stenosis (746.81)*
> *supravalvular aortic stenosis (747.22)*

DEF: Stenosis of orifice of aortic valve; obstructs blood outflow from left ventricle.

746.4 Congenital insufficiency of aortic valve
Bicuspid aortic valve
Congenital aortic insufficiency
DEF: Impaired functioning of aortic valve due to incomplete closure; causes backflow (regurgitation) of blood from aorta to left ventricle.

746.5 Congenital mitral stenosis
Fused commissure
Parachute deformity ⎫ of mitral valve
Supernumerary cusps ⎭
DEF: Stenosis of left atrioventricular orifice.

746.6 Congenital mitral insufficiency
DEF: Impaired functioning of mitral valve due to incomplete closure; causes backflow of blood from left ventricle to left atrium.

746.7 Hypoplastic left heart syndrome
Atresia, or marked hypoplasia, of aortic orifice or valve, with hypoplasia of ascending aorta and defective development of left ventricle (with mitral valve atresia)

✓5ᵗʰ 746.8 Other specified anomalies of heart

746.81 Subaortic stenosis
DEF: Stenosis, of left ventricular outflow tract due to fibrous tissue ring or septal hypertrophy below aortic valve.

746.82 Cor triatriatum
DEF: Transverse septum divides left atrium due to failed resorption of embryonic common pulmonary vein; results in three atrial chambers.

Congenital Anomalies

746.83–747.5

746.83 Infundibular pulmonic stenosis
Subvalvular pulmonic stenosis
DEF: Stenosis of right ventricle outflow tract within infundibulum due to fibrous diaphragm below valve or long, narrow fibromuscular channel.

746.84 Obstructive anomalies of heart, not elsewhere classified
Shone's syndrome
Uhl's disease
Use additional code for associated anomalies, such as:
coarctation of aorta (747.10)
congenital mitral stenosis (746.5)
subaortic stenosis (746.81)

746.85 Coronary artery anomaly
Anomalous origin or communication of coronary artery
Arteriovenous malformation of coronary artery
Coronary artery:
absence
arising from aorta or pulmonary trunk
single

746.86 Congenital heart block
Complete or incomplete atrioventricular [AV] block
DEF: Impaired conduction of electrical impulses; due to maldeveloped junctional tissue.

746.87 Malposition of heart and cardiac apex
Abdominal heart
Dextrocardia
Ectopia cordis
Levocardia (isolated)
Mesocardia
EXCLUDES *dextrocardia with complete transposition of viscera (759.3)*

746.89 Other
Atresia ⎱ of cardiac vein
Hypoplasia ⎰
Congenital:
cardiomegaly
diverticulum, left ventricle
pericardial defect

746.9 Unspecified anomaly of heart
Congenital:
anomaly of heart NOS
heart disease NOS

✓4ᵗʰ **747 Other congenital anomalies of circulatory system**

747.0 Patent ductus arteriosus
Patent ductus Botalli
Persistent ductus arteriosus
DEF: Open lumen in ductus arteriosus causes arterial blood recirculation in lungs; inhibits blood supply to aorta; symptoms such as shortness of breath more noticeable upon activity.

✓5ᵗʰ **747.1 Coarctation of aorta**
DEF: Localized deformity of aortic media seen as a severe constriction of the vessel lumen; major symptom is high blood pressure in the arms and low pressure in the legs; may result in a CVA, rupture of the aorta, bacterial endocarditis or congestive heart failure.

747.10 Coarctation of aorta (preductal) (postductal)
Hypoplasia of aortic arch

747.11 Interruption of aortic arch

✓5ᵗʰ **747.2 Other anomalies of aorta**

747.20 Anomaly of aorta, unspecified

747.21 Anomalies of aortic arch
Anomalous origin, right subclavian artery
Dextraposition of aorta
Double aortic arch
Kommerell's diverticulum
Overriding aorta
Persistent:
convolutions, aortic arch
right aortic arch
Vascular ring
EXCLUDES *hypoplasia of aortic arch (747.10)*

747.22 Atresia and stenosis of aorta
Absence ⎱
Aplasia ⎰ of aorta
Hypoplasia ⎰
Stricture ⎰
Supra (valvular)-aortic stenosis
EXCLUDES *congenital aortic (valvular) stenosis or stricture, so stated (746.3)*
hypoplasia of aorta in hypoplastic left heart syndrome (746.7)

747.29 Other
Aneurysm of sinus of Valsalva
Congenital:
aneurysm ⎱ of aorta
dilation ⎰

✓5ᵗʰ **747.3 Anomalies of pulmonary artery**

747.31 Pulmonary artery coarctation and atresia
Agenesis of pulmonary artery
Atresia of pulmonary artery
Coarctation of pulmonary artery
Hypoplasia of pulmonary artery
Stenosis of pulmonary artery

747.32 Pulmonary arteriovenous malformation
Pulmonary arteriovenous aneurysm
EXCLUDES *acquired pulmonary arteriovenous fistula (417.0)*

747.39 Other anomalies of pulmonary artery and pulmonary circulation
Anomaly of pulmonary artery

✓5ᵗʰ **747.4 Anomalies of great veins**

747.40 Anomaly of great veins, unspecified
Anomaly NOS of:
pulmonary veins
vena cava

747.41 Total anomalous pulmonary venous connection
Total anomalous pulmonary venous return [TAPVR]:
subdiaphragmatic
supradiaphragmatic

747.42 Partial anomalous pulmonary venous connection
Partial anomalous pulmonary venous return

747.49 Other anomalies of great veins
Absence ⎱
Congenital ⎰ of vena cava (inferior)
stenosis ⎰ (superior)
Persistent:
left posterior cardinal vein
left superior vena cava
Scimitar syndrome
Transposition of pulmonary veins NOS

747.5 Absence or hypoplasia of umbilical artery
Single umbilical artery

√5ᵗʰ 747.6   Other anomalies of peripheral vascular system

Absence ⎫
Anomaly ⎬ of artery or vein, NEC
Atresia ⎭

Arteriovenous aneurysm (peripheral)
Arteriovenous malformation of the peripheral vascular
   system
Congenital:
   aneurysm (peripheral)
   phlebectasia
   stricture, artery
   varix
Multiple renal arteries

   EXCLUDES *anomalies of:*
      cerebral vessels (747.81)
      pulmonary artery (747.39)
      congenital retinal aneurysm (743.58)
      hemangioma (228.00-228.09)
      lymphangioma (228.1)

**747.60   Anomaly of the peripheral vascular system,
         unspecified site**

747.61   Gastrointestinal vessel anomaly

747.62   Renal vessel anomaly

747.63   Upper limb vessel anomaly

747.64   Lower limb vessel anomaly

**747.69   Anomalies of other specified sites of
         peripheral vascular system**

√5ᵗʰ 747.8   Other specified anomalies of circulatory system

747.81   Anomalies of cerebrovascular system
      Arteriovenous malformation of brain
      Cerebral arteriovenous aneurysm, congenital
      Congenital anomalies of cerebral vessels
         EXCLUDES *ruptured cerebral (arteriovenous)*
                  aneurysm (430)

747.82   Spinal vessel anomaly
      Arteriovenous malformation of spinal vessel

747.83   Persistent fetal circulation
      Persistent pulmonary hypertension
      Primary pulmonary hypertension of newborn

      DEF: A return to fetal circulation due to
      constriction of pulmonary arterioles and
      opening of the ductus arteriosus and foramen
      ovale, right-to-left shunting, oxygenation of the
      blood does not occur, and the lungs remain
      constricted after birth; is seen in term or
      post-term infants; causes include asphyxiation,
      meconium aspiration syndrome, acidosis, sepsis,
      and developmental immaturity.

747.89   Other
      Aneurysm, congenital, specified site not
         elsewhere classified
         EXCLUDES *congenital aneurysm:*
                  coronary (746.85)
                  peripheral (747.6)
                  pulmonary (747.39)
                     arteriovenous (747.32)
                  retinal (743.58)

Persistent Fetal Circulation

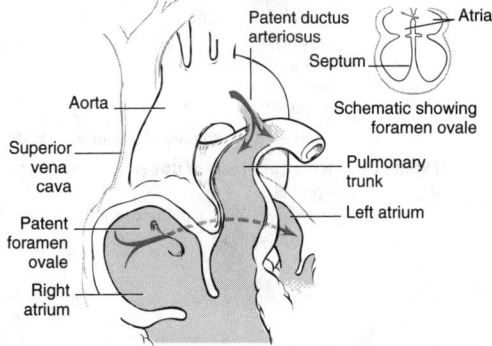

747.9   Unspecified anomaly of circulatory system

√4ᵗʰ 748   Congenital anomalies of respiratory system
   EXCLUDES *congenital central alveolar hypoventilation syndrome*
            (327.25)
            congenital defect of diaphragm (756.6)

748.0   Choanal atresia
      Atresia ⎫
      Congenital stenosis ⎬ of nares (anterior) (posterior)

      DEF: Occluded posterior nares (choana), bony or
      membranous due to failure of embryonic bucconasal
      membrane to rupture.

748.1   Other anomalies of nose
      Absent nose
      Accessory nose
      Cleft nose
      Congenital:
         deformity of nose
         notching of tip of nose
         perforation of wall of nasal sinus
      Deformity of wall of nasal sinus
         EXCLUDES *congenital deviation of nasal septum (754.0)*

748.2   Web of larynx
      Web of larynx: Web of larynx:
         NOS   subglottic
         glottic

      DEF: Malformed larynx; marked by thin, translucent, or
      thick, fibrotic spread between vocal folds; affects speech.

748.3   Other anomalies of larynx, trachea, and bronchus
      Absence or agenesis of: Congenital:
         bronchus   dilation, trachea
         larynx   stenosis:
         trachea   larynx
      Anomaly (of):   trachea
         cricoid cartilage   tracheocele
         epiglottis   Diverticulum:
         thyroid cartilage   bronchus
         tracheal cartilage   trachea
      Atresia (of):   Fissure of epiglottis
         epiglottis   Laryngocele
         glottis   Posterior cleft of cricoid
         larynx   cartilage (congenital)
         trachea   Rudimentary tracheal bronchus
      Cleft thyroid, cartilage, Stridor, laryngeal, congenital
         congenital

748.4   Congenital cystic lung
      Disease, lung:
         cystic, congenital
         polycystic, congenital
      Honeycomb lung, congenital
         EXCLUDES *acquired or unspecified cystic lung (518.89)*
      DEF: Enlarged air spaces of lung parenchyma.

748.5   Agenesis, hypoplasia, and dysplasia of lung
      Absence of lung (fissures) (lobe) (lobe)
      Aplasia of lung
      Hypoplasia of lung
      Sequestration of lung

√5ᵗʰ 748.6   Other anomalies of lung

748.60   Anomaly of lung, unspecified

748.61   Congenital bronchiectasis

748.69   Other
         Accessory lung (lobe)
         Azygos lobe (fissure), lung

748.8   Other specified anomalies of respiratory system
      Abnormal communication between pericardial and
         pleural sacs
      Anomaly, pleural folds
      Atresia of nasopharynx
      Congenital cyst of mediastinum

748.9   Unspecified anomaly of respiratory system
      Anomaly of respiratory system NOS

Cleft Lip and Palate

Unilateral cleft lip

Cleft lip with cleft alveolar ridge

No cleft palate

No cleft palate

Unilateral cleft lip and cleft palate

Alveolar ridge

Cleft palate

Prolabium

Bilateral cleft lip and cleft palate

Isolated cleft palate

✓4ᵗʰ 749   Cleft palate and cleft lip

✓5ᵗʰ 749.0   Cleft palate

     749.00   Cleft palate, unspecified

     749.01   Unilateral, complete

     749.02   Unilateral, incomplete
         Cleft uvula

     749.03   Bilateral, complete

     749.04   Bilateral, incomplete

✓5ᵗʰ 749.1   Cleft lip
     Cheiloschisis
     Congenital fissure of lip
     Harelip
     Labium leporinum

     749.10   Cleft lip, unspecified

     749.11   Unilateral, complete

     749.12   Unilateral, incomplete

     749.13   Bilateral, complete

     749.14   Bilateral, incomplete

✓5ᵗʰ 749.2   Cleft palate with cleft lip
     Cheilopalatoschisis

     749.20   Cleft palate with cleft lip, unspecified

     749.21   Unilateral, complete

     749.22   Unilateral, incomplete

     749.23   Bilateral, complete

     749.24   Bilateral, incomplete

     749.25   Other combinations

✓4ᵗʰ 750   Other congenital anomalies of upper alimentary tract
EXCLUDES   *dentofacial anomalies (524.0-524.9)*

750.0   Tongue tie
     Ankyloglossia
     DEF: Restricted tongue movement due to lingual frenum extending toward tip of tongue. Tongue may be fused to mouth floor affecting speech.

✓5ᵗʰ 750.1   Other anomalies of tongue

     750.10   Anomaly of tongue, unspecified

     750.11   Aglossia
         DEF: Absence of tongue.

     750.12   Congenital adhesions of tongue

     750.13   Fissure of tongue
         Bifid tongue   Double tongue

     750.15   Macroglossia
         Congenital hypertrophy of tongue

     750.16   Microglossia
         Hypoplasia of tongue

     750.19   Other

✓5ᵗʰ 750.2   Other specified anomalies of mouth and pharynx

     750.21   Absence of salivary gland

     750.22   Accessory salivary gland

     750.23   Atresia, salivary duct
         Imperforate salivary duct

     750.24   Congenital fistula of salivary gland

     750.25   Congenital fistula of lip
         Congenital (mucus) lip pits

     750.26   Other specified anomalies of mouth
         Absence of uvula

     750.27   Diverticulum of pharynx
         Pharyngeal pouch

     750.29   Other specified anomalies of pharynx
         Imperforate pharynx

750.3   Tracheoesophageal fistula, esophageal atresia and stenosis
     Absent esophagus
     Atresia of esophagus
     Congenital:
         esophageal ring
         stenosis of esophagus
         stricture of esophagus
     Congenital fistula:
         esophagobronchial
         esophagotracheal
     Imperforate esophagus
     Webbed esophagus

750.4   Other specified anomalies of esophagus
     Dilatation, congenital
     Displacement, congenital
     Diverticulum   } (of) esophagus
     Duplication
     Giant

     Esophageal pouch
     EXCLUDES   *congenital hiatus hernia (750.6)*

750.5   Congenital hypertrophic pyloric stenosis
     Congenital or infantile:
         constriction
         hypertrophy
         spasm   } of pylorus
         stenosis
         stricture

     DEF: Obstructed pylorus due to overgrowth of pyloric muscle.

750.6   Congenital hiatus hernia
     Displacement of cardia through esophageal hiatus
     EXCLUDES   *congenital diaphragmatic hernia (756.6)*

750.7   Other specified anomalies of stomach
     Congenital:
         cardiospasm
         hourglass stomach
     Displacement of stomach
     Diverticulum of stomach, congenital
     Duplication of stomach
     Megalogastria
     Microgastria
     Transposition of stomach

750.8   Other specified anomalies of upper alimentary tract

750.9   Unspecified anomaly of upper alimentary tract
     Congenital:
         anomaly NOS } of upper alimentary tract [any
         deformity NOS }   part, except tongue]

Congenital Anomalies

751–752.11

☑4ᵗʰ **751 Other congenital anomalies of digestive system**

751.0 Meckel's diverticulum
Meckel's diverticulum (displaced) (hypertrophic)
Persistent:
  omphalomesenteric duct
  vitelline duct

DEF: Malformed sacs or appendages of ileum of small intestine; can cause strangulation, volvulus and intussusception.

751.1 Atresia and stenosis of small intestine
Atresia of:
  duodenum
  ileum
  intestine NOS
Congenital:
  absence
  obstruction } of small intestine or intestine
  stenosis   NOS
  stricture
Imperforate jejunum

751.2 Atresia and stenosis of large intestine rectum, and anal canal
Absence:
  anus (congenital)
  appendix, congenital
  large intestine, congenital
  rectum
Atresia of:
  anus
  colon
  rectum
Congenital or infantile:
  obstruction of large intestine
  occlusion of anus
  stricture of anus
Imperforate:
  anus
  rectum
Stricture of rectum, congenital

751.3 Hirschsprung's disease and other congenital functional disorders of colon
Aganglionosis
Congenital dilation of colon
Congenital megacolon
Macrocolon

DEF: Hirschsprung's disease: enlarged or dilated colon (megacolon), with absence of ganglion cells in the narrowed wall distally; causes inability to defecate.

751.4 Anomalies of intestinal fixation
Congenital adhesions:
  omental, anomalous
  peritoneal
Jackson's membrane
Malrotation of colon
Rotation of cecum or colon:
  failure of
  incomplete
  insufficient
Universal mesentery

751.5 Other anomalies of intestine
Congenital diverticulum, colon
Dolichocolon
Duplication of:
  anus
  appendix
  cecum
  intestine
Ectopic anus
Megaloappendix
Megaloduodenum
Microcolon
Persistent cloaca
Transposition of:
  appendix
  colon
  intestine

☑5ᵗʰ **751.6 Anomalies of gallbladder, bile ducts, and liver**

751.60 Unspecified anomaly of gallbladder, bile ducts, and liver

751.61 Biliary atresia
Congenital:
  absence
  hypoplasia } of bile duct (common)
  obstruction   of passage
  stricture

751.62 Congenital cystic disease of liver
Congenital polycystic disease of liver
Fibrocystic disease of liver

751.69 Other anomalies of gallbladder, bile ducts, and liver
Absence of:
  gallbladder, congenital
  liver (lobe)
Accessory:
  hepatic ducts
  liver
Congenital:
  choledochal cyst
  hepatomegaly
Duplication of:
  biliary duct
  cystic duct
  gallbladder
  liver
Floating:
  gallbladder
  liver
Intrahepatic gallbladder

751.7 Anomalies of pancreas
Absence
Accessory
Agenesis } (of) pancreas
Annular
Hypoplasia
Ectopic pancreatic tissue
Pancreatic heterotopia
EXCLUDES diabetes mellitus (249.0-249.9, 250.0-250.9)
  fibrocystic disease of pancreas
    (277.00-277.09)
  neonatal diabetes mellitus (775.1)

751.8 Other specified anomalies of digestive system
Absence (complete) (partial) of alimentary tract NOS
Duplication
Malposition, congenital } of digestive organs NOS
EXCLUDES congenital diaphragmatic hernia (756.6)
  congenital hiatus hernia (750.6)

751.9 Unspecified anomaly of digestive system
Congenital:
  anomaly NOS
  deformity NOS } of digestive system NOS

☑4ᵗʰ **752 Congenital anomalies of genital organs**
EXCLUDES syndromes associated with anomalies in the number and form of chromosomes (758.0-758.9)

752.0 Anomalies of ovaries
Absence, congenital
Accessory
Ectopic } (of) ovary
Streak

☑5ᵗʰ **752.1 Anomalies of fallopian tubes and broad ligaments**

752.10 Unspecified anomaly of fallopian tubes and broad ligaments

752.11 Embryonic cyst of fallopian tubes and broad ligaments
Cyst:
  epoophoron
  fimbrial
  parovarian

Congenital Anomalies

752.19–752.81

752.19 Other

Absence
Accessory   } (of) fallopian tube or broad ligament
Atresia

752.2 Doubling of uterus

Didelphic uterus
Doubling of uterus [any degree] (associated with doubling of cervix and vagina)

√5ᵗʰ **752.3 Other anomalies of uterus**

752.31 Agenesis of uterus

Congenital absence of uterus

752.32 Hypoplasia of uterus

752.33 Unicornuate uterus

Unicornuate uterus with or without a separate uterine horn
Uterus with only one functioning horn

752.34 Bicornuate uterus

Bicornuate uterus, complete or partial

752.35 Septate uterus

Septate uterus, complete or partial

752.36 Arcuate uterus

752.39 Other anomalies of uterus

Aplasia of uterus NOS
Müllerian anomaly of the uterus, NEC

> **EXCLUDES** anomaly of uterus due to exposure to diethylstilbestrol [DES] in utero (760.76)
> didelphic uterus (752.2)
> doubling of uterus (752.2)

DEF: Müllerian anomalies: The failure or disruption of female embryonic Müllerian ducts to transform into the upper vagina, cervix, uterus, and oviducts, resulting in anomalous organ development.

√5ᵗʰ **752.4 Anomalies of cervix, vagina, and external female genitalia**

752.40 Unspecified anomaly of cervix, vagina, and external female genitalia

752.41 Embryonic cyst of cervix, vagina, and external female genitalia

Cyst of:
    canal of Nuck, congenital
    Gartner's duct
    vagina, embryonal
    vulva, congenital

DEF: Embryonic fluid-filled cysts of cervix, vagina or external female genitalia.

752.42 Imperforate hymen

DEF: Complete closure of membranous fold around external opening of vagina.

752.43 Cervical agenesis

Cervical hypoplasia

752.44 Cervical duplication

752.45 Vaginal agenesis

Agenesis of vagina, total or partial

752.46 Transverse vaginal septum

752.47 Longitudinal vaginal septum

Longitudinal vaginal septum with or without obstruction

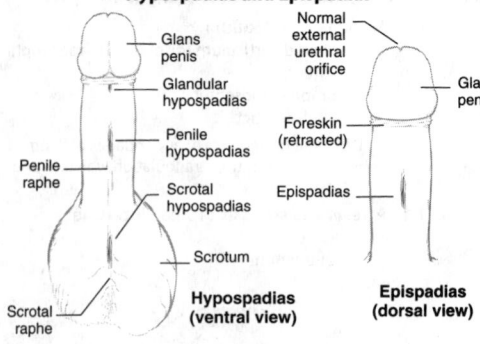

Hypospadias and Epispadias

Hypospadias (ventral view)
Epispadias (dorsal view)

Glans penis · Glandular hypospadias · Penile hypospadias · Scrotal hypospadias · Scrotum · Penile raphe · Scrotal raphe · Normal external urethral orifice · Foreskin (retracted) · Glans penis · Epispadias

752.49 Other anomalies of cervix, vagina, and external female genitalia

Absence of clitoris or vulva
Agenesis of clitoris or vulva
Anomalies of cervix, NEC
Anomalies of hymen, NEC
Congenital stenosis or stricture of:
    cervical canal
    vagina
Müllerian anomalies of the cervix and vagina, NEC

> **EXCLUDES** double vagina associated with total duplication (752.2)

√5ᵗʰ **752.5 Undescended and retractile testicle**

752.51 Undescended testis

Cryptorchism   Ectopic testis

752.52 Retractile testis

√5ᵗʰ **752.6 Hypospadias and epispadias and other penile anomalies**

752.61 Hypospadias

DEF: Abnormal opening of urethra on the ventral surface of the penis or perineum.

752.62 Epispadias

Anaspadias

DEF: Urethra opening on dorsal surface of penis.

752.63 Congenital chordee

DEF: Ventral bowing of penis due to fibrous band along corpus spongiosum; occurs with hypospadias.

752.64 Micropenis

752.65 Hidden penis

752.69 Other penile anomalies

752.7 Indeterminate sex and pseudohermaphroditism

Gynandrism
Hermaphroditism
Ovotestis
Pseudohermaphroditism (male) (female)
Pure gonadal dysgenesis

> **EXCLUDES** androgen insensitivity (259.50-259.52)
> pseudohermaphroditism:
>   female, with adrenocortical disorder (255.2)
>   male, with gonadal disorder (257.8)
>   with specified chromosomal anomaly (758.0-758.9)
>   testicular feminization syndrome (259.50-259.52)

DEF: Pseudohermaphroditism: presence of gonads of one sex and external genitalia of other sex.

√5ᵗʰ **752.8 Other specified anomalies of genital organs**

> **EXCLUDES** congenital hydrocele (778.6)
> penile anomalies (752.61-752.69)
> phimosis or paraphimosis (605)

752.81 Scrotal transposition

752.89 Other specified anomalies of genital organs
Absence of:
prostate
spermatic cord
vas deferens
Anorchism
Aplasia (congenital) of:
prostate
round ligament
testicle
Atresia of:
ejaculatory duct
vas deferens
Fusion of testes
Hypoplasia of testis
Monorchism
Polyorchism

752.9 Unspecified anomaly of genital organs
Congenital:
anomaly NOS ⎫ of genital organ, not
deformity NOS ⎭   elsewhere classified

✓4ᵗʰ **753 Congenital anomalies of urinary system**

753.0 Renal agenesis and dysgenesis
Atrophy of kidney:
congenital
infantile
Congenital absence of kidney(s)
Hypoplasia of kidney(s)

✓5ᵗʰ **753.1 Cystic kidney disease**
EXCLUDES   *acquired cyst of kidney (593.2)*

753.10 Cystic kidney disease, unspecified

753.11 Congenital single renal cyst

753.12 Polycystic kidney, unspecified type

753.13 Polycystic kidney, autosomal dominant
DEF: Slow progressive disease characterized by
bilateral cysts causing increased kidney size and
impaired function.

753.14 Polycystic kidney, autosomal recessive
DEF: Rare disease characterized by multiple cysts
involving kidneys and liver, producing renal and
hepatic failure in childhood or adolescence.

753.15 Renal dysplasia

753.16 Medullary cystic kidney
Nephronopthisis
DEF: Diffuse kidney disease results in uremia
onset prior to age 20.

753.17 Medullary sponge kidney
DEF: Dilated collecting tubules; usually
asymptomatic but calcinosis in tubules may
cause renal insufficiency.

753.19 Other specified cystic kidney disease
Multicystic kidney

✓5ᵗʰ **753.2 Obstructive defects of renal pelvis and ureter**

**753.20 Unspecified obstructive defect of renal pelvis
and ureter**

**753.21 Congenital obstruction of ureteropelvic
junction**
DEF: Stricture at junction of ureter and renal
pelvis.

**753.22 Congenital obstruction of ureterovesical
junction**
Adynamic ureter
Congenital hydroureter
DEF: Stricture at junction of ureter and bladder.

753.23 Congenital ureterocele

753.29 Other

753.3 Other specified anomalies of kidney
Accessory kidney
Congenital:
calculus of kidney
displaced kidney
Discoid kidney
Double kidney with double pelvis
Ectopic kidney
Fusion of kidneys
Giant kidney
Horseshoe kidney
Hyperplasia of kidney
Lobulation of kidney
Malrotation of kidney
Trifid kidney (pelvis)

753.4 Other specified anomalies of ureter
Absent ureter
Accessory ureter
Deviation of ureter
Displaced ureteric orifice
Double ureter
Ectopic ureter
Implantation, anomalous of ureter

753.5 Exstrophy of urinary bladder
Ectopia vesicae
Extroversion of bladder
DEF: Absence of lower abdominal and anterior bladder
walls with posterior bladder wall protrusion.

753.6 Atresia and stenosis of urethra and bladder neck
Congenital obstruction:
bladder neck
urethra
Congenital stricture of:
urethra (valvular)
urinary meatus
vesicourethral orifice
Imperforate urinary meatus
Impervious urethra
Urethral valve formation

753.7 Anomalies of urachus
Cyst ⎫
Fistula ⎬ (of) urachussinus
Patent ⎭

Persistent umbilical sinus

753.8 Other specified anomalies of bladder and urethra
Absence, congenital of:
bladder
urethra
Accessory:
bladder
urethra
Congenital:
diverticulum of bladder
hernia of bladder
urethrorectal fistula
prolapse of:
bladder (mucosa)
urethra
Double:
urethra
urinary meatus

753.9 Unspecified anomaly of urinary system
Congenital:
anomaly NOS ⎫ of urinary system [any part,
deformity NOS ⎭   except urachus]

Congenital Anomalies

754–755.22

√4ᵗʰ **754 Certain congenital musculoskeletal deformities**
         INCLUDES   nonteratogenic deformities which are considered to be due to intrauterine malposition and pressure

     754.0 Of skull, face, and jaw
         Asymmetry of face
         Compression facies
         Depressions in skull
         Deviation of nasal septum, congenital
         Dolichocephaly
         Plagiocephaly
         Potter's facies
         Squashed or bent nose, congenital
         EXCLUDES   dentofacial anomalies (524.0-524.9)
                           syphilitic saddle nose (090.5)

     754.1 Of sternocleidomastoid muscle
         Congenital sternomastoid torticollis
         Congenital wryneck
         Contracture of sternocleidomastoid (muscle)
         Sternomastoid tumor

     754.2 Of spine
         Congenital postural:
            lordosis
            scoliosis

    √5ᵗʰ **754.3 Congenital dislocation of hip**

        754.30 Congenital dislocation of hip, unilateral
            Congenital dislocation of hip NOS

        754.31 Congenital dislocation of hip, bilateral

        754.32 Congenital subluxation of hip, unilateral
            Congenital flexion deformity, hip or thigh
            Predislocation status of hip at birth
            Preluxation of hip, congenital

        754.33 Congenital subluxation of hip, bilateral

        754.35 Congenital dislocation of one hip with subluxation of other hip

    √5ᵗʰ **754.4 Congenital genu recurvatum and bowing of long bones of leg**

        754.40 Genu recurvatum
            DEF: Backward curving of knee joint.

        754.41 Congenital dislocation of knee (with genu recurvatum)

        754.42 Congenital bowing of femur

        754.43 Congenital bowing of tibia and fibula

        754.44 Congenital bowing of unspecified long bones of leg

    √5ᵗʰ **754.5 Varus deformities of feet**
         EXCLUDES   acquired (736.71, 736.75, 736.79)

        754.50 Talipes varus
            Congenital varus deformity of foot, unspecified
            Pes varus
            DEF: Inverted foot marked by outer sole resting on ground.

        754.51 Talipes equinovarus
            Equinovarus (congenital)
            DEF: Elevated, outward rotation of heel; also called clubfoot.

        754.52 Metatarsus primus varus
            DEF: Malformed first metatarsal bone, with bone angled toward body.

        754.53 Metatarsus varus

        754.59 Other
            Talipes calcaneovarus

    √5ᵗʰ **754.6 Valgus deformities of feet**
         EXCLUDES   valgus deformity of foot (acquired) (736.79)

        754.60 Talipes valgus
            Congenital valgus deformity of foot, unspecified

        754.61 Congenital pes planus
            Congenital rocker bottom flat foot
            Flat foot, congenital
            EXCLUDES   pes planus (acquired) (734)

        754.62 Talipes calcaneovalgus

        754.69 Other
            Talipes:
               equinovalgus
               planovalgus

    √5ᵗʰ **754.7 Other deformities of feet**
         EXCLUDES   acquired (736.70-736.79)

        754.70 Talipes, unspecified
            Congenital deformity of foot NOS

        754.71 Talipes cavus
            Cavus foot (congenital)

        754.79 Other
            Asymmetric talipes
            Talipes:
               calcaneus
               equinus

    √5ᵗʰ **754.8 Other specified nonteratogenic anomalies**

        754.81 Pectus excavatum
            Congenital funnel chest

        754.82 Pectus carinatum
            Congenital pigeon chest [breast]

        754.89 Other
            Club hand (congenital)
            Congenital:
               deformity of chest wall
               dislocation of elbow
            Generalized flexion contractures of lower limb joints, congenital
            Spade-like hand (congenital)

√4ᵗʰ **755 Other congenital anomalies of limbs**
         EXCLUDES   those deformities classifiable to 754.0-754.8

    √5ᵗʰ **755.0 Polydactyly**

        755.00 Polydactyly, unspecified digits
            Supernumerary digits

        755.01 Of fingers
            Accessory fingers

        755.02 Of toes
            Accessory toes

    √5ᵗʰ **755.1 Syndactyly**
         Symphalangy
         Webbing of digits

        755.10 Of multiple and unspecified sites

        755.11 Of fingers without fusion of bone

        755.12 Of fingers with fusion of bone

        755.13 Of toes without fusion of bone

        755.14 Of toes with fusion of bone

    √5ᵗʰ **755.2 Reduction deformities of upper limb**

        755.20 Unspecified reduction deformity of upper limb
            Ectromelia NOS } of upper limb
            Hemimelia NOS
            Shortening of arm, congenital

        755.21 Transverse deficiency of upper limb
            Amelia of upper limb
            Congenital absence of:
               fingers, all (complete or partial)
               forearm, including hand and fingers
               upper limb, complete
            Congenital amputation of upper limb
            Transverse hemimelia of upper limb

        755.22 Longitudinal deficiency of upper limb, not elsewhere classified
            Phocomelia NOS of upper limb
            Rudimentary arm

755.23 Longitudinal deficiency, combined, involving humerus, radius, and ulna (complete or incomplete)
>Congenital absence of arm and forearm (complete or incomplete) with or without metacarpal deficiency and/or phalangeal deficiency, incomplete
>Phocomelia, complete, of upper limb

755.24 Longitudinal deficiency, humeral, complete or partial (with or without distal deficiencies, incomplete)
>Congenital absence of humerus (with or without absence of some [but not all] distal elements)
>Proximal phocomelia of upper limb

755.25 Longitudinal deficiency, radioulnar, complete or partial (with or without distal deficiencies, incomplete)
>Congenital absence of radius and ulna (with or without absence of some [but not all] distal elements)
>Distal phocomelia of upper limb

755.26 Longitudinal deficiency, radial, complete or partial (with or without distal deficiencies, incomplete)
>Agenesis of radius
>Congenital absence of radius (with or without absence of some [but not all] distal elements)

755.27 Longitudinal deficiency, ulnar, complete or partial (with or without distal deficiencies, incomplete)
>Agenesis of ulna
>Congenital absence of ulna (with or without absence of some [but not all] distal elements)

755.28 Longitudinal deficiency, carpals or metacarpals, complete or partial (with or without incomplete phalangeal deficiency)

755.29 Longitudinal deficiency, phalanges, complete or partial
>Absence of finger, congenital
>Aphalangia of upper limb, terminal, complete or partial
>>**EXCLUDES**   *terminal deficiency of all five digits (755.21)*
>>*transverse deficiency of phalanges (755.21)*

☑5ᵗʰ **755.3 Reduction deformities of lower limb**

755.30 Unspecified reduction deformity of lower limb
>Ectromelia NOS ⎫
>Hemimelia NOS ⎬ of lower limb
>Shortening of leg, congenital

755.31 Transverse deficiency of lower limb
>Amelia of lower limb
>Congenital absence of:
>>foot
>>leg, including foot and toes
>>lower limb, complete
>>toes, all, complete
>Transverse hemimelia of lower limb

755.32 Longitudinal deficiency of lower limb, not elsewhere classified
>Phocomelia NOS of lower limb

755.33 Longitudinal deficiency, combined, involving femur, tibia, and fibula (complete or incomplete)
>Congenital absence of thigh and (lower) leg (complete or incomplete) with or without metacarpal deficiency and/or phalangeal deficiency, incomplete
>Phocomelia, complete, of lower limb

755.34 Longitudinal deficiency, femoral, complete or partial (with or without distal deficiencies, incomplete)
>Congenital absence of femur (with or without absence of some [but not all] distal elements)
>Proximal phocomelia of lower limb

755.35 Longitudinal deficiency, tibiofibular, complete or partial (with or without distal deficiencies, incomplete)
>Congenital absence of tibia and fibula (with or without absence of some [but not all] distal elements)
>Distal phocomelia of lower limb

755.36 Longitudinal deficiency, tibia, complete or partial (with or without distal deficiencies, incomplete)
>Agenesis of tibia
>Congenital absence of tibia (with or without absence of some [but not all] distal elements)

755.37 Longitudinal deficiency, fibular, complete or partial (with or without distal deficiencies, incomplete)
>Agenesis of fibula
>Congenital absence of fibula (with or without absence of some [but not all] distal elements)

755.38 Longitudinal deficiency, tarsals or metatarsals, complete or partial (with or without incomplete phalangeal deficiency)

755.39 Longitudinal deficiency, phalanges, complete or partial
>Absence of toe, congenital
>Aphalangia of lower limb, terminal, complete or partial
>>**EXCLUDES**   *terminal deficiency of all five digits (755.31)*
>>*transverse deficiency of phalanges (755.31)*

755.4 Reduction deformities, unspecified limb
>Absence, congenital (complete or partial) of limb NOS
>Amelia ⎫
>Ectromelia ⎬ of unspecified limb
>Hemimelia ⎪
>Phocomelia ⎭

☑5ᵗʰ **755.5 Other anomalies of upper limb, including shoulder girdle**

755.50 Unspecified anomaly of upper limb

755.51 Congenital deformity of clavicle

755.52 Congenital elevation of scapula
>Sprengel's deformity

755.53 Radioulnar synostosis
>**DEF:** Osseous adhesion of radius and ulna.

755.54 Madelung's deformity
>**DEF:** Distal ulnar overgrowth or radial shortening; also called carpus curvus.

755.55 Acrocephalosyndactyly
>Apert's syndrome
>**DEF:** Premature cranial suture fusion (craniostenosis); marked by cone-shaped or pointed (acrocephaly) head and webbing of the fingers (syndactyly); similar to craniofacial dysostosis.

755.56 Accessory carpal bones

755.57 Macrodactylia (fingers)
>**DEF:** Abnormally large fingers, toes.

755.58 Cleft hand, congenital
>Lobster-claw hand
>**DEF:** Extended separation between fingers into metacarpus; also may refer to large fingers and absent middle fingers of hand.

Congenital Anomalies

755.59–756.3

755.59 Other
Cleidocranial dysostosis
Cubitus:
  valgus, congenital
  varus, congenital
  EXCLUDES club hand (congenital) (754.89)
    congenital dislocation of elbow
    (754.89)

√5ᵗʰ **755.6 Other anomalies of lower limb, including pelvic girdle**

755.60 Unspecified anomaly of lower limb

755.61 Coxa valga, congenital
DEF: Abnormally wide angle between the neck and shaft of the femur.

755.62 Coxa vara, congenital
DEF: Diminished angle between neck and shaft of femur.

755.63 Other congenital deformity of hip (joint)
Congenital anteversion of femur (neck)
EXCLUDES congenital dislocation of hip
    (754.30-754.35)

755.64 Congenital deformity of knee (joint)
Congenital:
  absence of patella
  genu valgum [knock-knee]
  genu varum [bowleg]
  Rudimentary patella

755.65 Macrodactylia of toes
DEF: Abnormally large toes.

755.66 Other anomalies of toes
Congenital:
  hallux valgus
  hallux varus
  hammer toe

755.67 Anomalies of foot, not elsewhere classified
Astragaloscaphoid synostosis
Calcaneonavicular bar
Coalition of calcaneus
Talonavicular synostosis
Tarsal coalitions

755.69 Other
Congenital:
  angulation of tibia
  deformity (of):
    ankle (joint)
    sacroiliac (joint)
  fusion of sacroiliac joint

755.8 Other specified anomalies of unspecified limb

755.9 Unspecified anomaly of unspecified limb
Congenital:
  anomaly NOS }
  deformity NOS } of unspecified limb
  EXCLUDES reduction deformity of unspecified limb
    (755.4)

√4ᵗʰ **756 Other congenital musculoskeletal anomalies**
EXCLUDES congenital myotonic chondrodystrophy (359.23)
  those deformities classifiable to 754.0-754.8

756.0 Anomalies of skull and face bones
Absence of skull bones
Acrocephaly
Congenital deformity of forehead
Craniosynostosis
Crouzon's disease
Hypertelorism
Imperfect fusion of skull
Oxycephaly
Platybasia
Premature closure of cranial sutures
Tower skull
Trigonocephaly
EXCLUDES acrocephalosyndactyly [Apert's syndrome]
    (755.55)
  dentofacial anomalies (524.0-524.9)
  skull defects associated with brain anomalies,
    such as:
    anencephalus (740.0)
    encephalocele (742.0)
    hydrocephalus (742.3)
    microcephalus (742.1)

√5ᵗʰ **756.1 Anomalies of spine**

756.10 Anomaly of spine, unspecified

756.11 Spondylolysis, lumbosacral region
Prespondylolisthesis (lumbosacral)
DEF: Bilateral or unilateral defect through the pars interarticularis of a vertebra causes spondylolisthesis.

756.12 Spondylolisthesis
DEF: Downward slipping of lumbar vertebra over next vertebra; usually related to pelvic deformity.

756.13 Absence of vertebra, congenital

756.14 Hemivertebra
DEF: Incomplete development of one side of a vertebra.

756.15 Fusion of spine [vertebra], congenital

756.16 Klippel-Feil syndrome
DEF: Short, wide neck; limits range of motion due to abnormal number of cervical vertebra or fused hemivertebrae.

756.17 Spina bifida occulta
EXCLUDES spina bifida (aperta) (741.0-741.9)
DEF: Spina bifida marked by a bony spinal canal defect without a protrusion of the cord or meninges; it is diagnosed by radiography and has no symptoms.

756.19 Other
Platyspondylia
Supernumerary vertebra

756.2 Cervical rib
Supernumerary rib in the cervical region
DEF: Costa cervicalis: extra rib attached to cervical vertebra.

756.3 Other anomalies of ribs and sternum
Congenital absence of:
  rib
  sternum
Congenital:
  fissure of sternum
  fusion of ribs
Sternum bifidum
EXCLUDES nonteratogenic deformity of chest wall
    (754.81-754.89)

756.4 Chondrodystrophy
Achondroplasia
Chondrodystrophia (fetalis)
Dyschondroplasia
Enchondromatosis
Ollier's disease
> EXCLUDES   congenital myotonic chondrodystrophy (359.23)
> lipochondrodystrophy [Hurler's syndrome] (277.5)
> Morquio's disease (277.5)

DEF: Abnormal development of cartilage.

√5ᵗʰ **756.5 Osteodystrophies**

756.50 Osteodystrophy, unspecified

756.51 Osteogenesis imperfecta
Fragilitas ossium
Osteopsathyrosis
DEF: A collagen disorder commonly characterized by brittle, osteoporotic, easily fractured bones, hypermobility of joints, blue sclerae, and a tendency to hemorrhage.

756.52 Osteopetrosis
DEF: Abnormally dense bone, optic atrophy, hepatosplenomegaly, deafness; sclerosing depletes bone marrow and nerve foramina of skull; often fatal.

756.53 Osteopoikilosis
DEF: Multiple sclerotic foci on ends of long bones, stippling in round, flat bones; identified by x-ray.

756.54 Polyostotic fibrous dysplasia of bone
DEF: Fibrous tissue displaces bone results in segmented ragged-edge café-au-lait spots; occurs in girls of early puberty.

756.55 Chondroectodermal dysplasia
Ellis-van Creveld syndrome
DEF: Inadequate enchondral bone formation; impaired development of hair and teeth, polydactyly, and cardiac septum defects.

756.56 Multiple epiphyseal dysplasia

756.59 Other
Albright (-McCune)-Sternberg syndrome

756.6 Anomalies of diaphragm
Absence of diaphragm
Congenital hernia:
  diaphragmatic
  foramen of Morgagni
Eventration of diaphragm
> EXCLUDES   congenital hiatus hernia (750.6)

√5ᵗʰ **756.7 Anomalies of abdominal wall**

756.70 Anomaly of abdominal wall, unspecified

Omphalocele

Gastroschisis

756.71 Prune belly syndrome
Eagle-Barrett syndrome
Prolapse of bladder mucosa
DEF: Prune belly syndrome: absence of lower rectus abdominis muscle and lower and medial oblique muscles; results in dilated bladder and ureters, dysplastic kidneys and hydronephrosis; common in male infants with undescended testicles.

756.72 Omphalocele
Exomphalos
DEF: Exomphalos: umbilical hernia prominent navel.
DEF: Omphalocele: hernia of umbilicus due to impaired abdominal wall; results in membrane-covered intestine protruding through peritoneum and amnion.

756.73 Gastroschisis
DEF: Fissure of abdominal wall, results in protruding small or large intestine.

756.79 Other congenital anomalies of abdominal wall
> EXCLUDES   umbilical hernia (551-553 with .1)

√5ᵗʰ **756.8 Other specified anomalies of muscle, tendon, fascia, and connective tissue**

756.81 Absence of muscle and tendon
Absence of muscle (pectoral)

756.82 Accessory muscle

756.83 Ehlers-Danlos syndrome
DEF: Danlos syndrome: connective tissue disorder causes hyperextended skin and joints; results in fragile blood vessels with bleeding, poor wound healing and subcutaneous pseudotumors.

756.89 Other
Amyotrophia congenita
Congenital shortening of tendon

756.9 Other and unspecified anomalies of musculoskeletal system
Congenital:
  anomaly NOS } of musculoskeletal system, not
  deformity NOS } elsewhere classified

√4ᵗʰ **757 Congenital anomalies of the integument**
> INCLUDES   anomalies of skin, subcutaneous tissue, hair, nails, and breast
> EXCLUDES   hemangioma (228.00-228.09)
> pigmented nevus (216.0-216.9)

757.0 Hereditary edema of legs
Congenital lymphedema
Hereditary trophedema
Milroy's disease

757.1 Ichthyosis congenita
Congenital ichthyosis
Harlequin fetus
Ichthyosiform erythroderma
DEF: Overproduction of skin cells causes scaling of skin; may result in stillborn fetus or death soon after birth.

Congenital Anomalies

757.2–759.1

757.2 Dermatoglyphic anomalies
Abnormal palmar creases

DEF: Abnormal skin-line patterns of fingers, palms, toes and soles; initial finding of possible chromosomal abnormalities.

✓5ᵗʰ 757.3 Other specified anomalies of skin

757.31 Congenital ectodermal dysplasia
DEF: Tissues and structures originate in embryonic ectoderm; includes anhidrotic and hidrotic ectodermal dysplasia and EEC syndrome.

757.32 Vascular hamartomas
Birthmarks
Port-wine stain
Strawberry nevus

DEF: Benign tumor of blood vessels; due to malformed angioblastic tissues.

757.33 Congenital pigmentary anomalies of skin
Congenital poikiloderma
Urticaria pigmentosa
Xeroderma pigmentosum
EXCLUDES   albinism (270.2)

757.39 Other
Accessory skin tags, congenital
Congenital scar
Epidermolysis bullosa
Keratoderma (congenital)
EXCLUDES   pilonidal cyst (685.0-685.1)

757.4 Specified anomalies of hair
Congenital:
  alopecia
  atrichosis
  beaded hair
  hypertrichosis
  monilethrix
Persistent lanugo

757.5 Specified anomalies of nails
Anonychia
Congenital:
  clubnail
  koilonychia
  leukonychia
  onychauxis
  pachyonychia

757.6 Specified congenital anomalies of breast
Accessory
Congenital absent } breast or nipple
Supernumerary

EXCLUDES   absence of pectoral muscle (756.81)
          hypoplasia of breast (611.82)
          micromastia (611.82)

757.8 Other specified anomalies of the integument

757.9 Unspecified anomaly of the integument
Congenital:
  anomaly NOS
  deformity NOS } of integument

✓4ᵗʰ 758 Chromosomal anomalies
INCLUDES   syndromes associated with anomalies in the number and form of chromosomes

Use additional codes for conditions associated with the chromosomal anomalies

758.0 Down's syndrome
Mongolism
Translocation Down's syndrome
Trisomy:
  21 or 22
  G

758.1 Patau's syndrome
Trisomy:
  13
  D₁

DEF: Trisomy of 13th chromosome; characteristic failure to thrive, severe mental impairment, seizures, abnormal eyes, low-set ears and sloped forehead.

758.2 Edwards' syndrome
Trisomy:
  18
  E₃

DEF: Trisomy of 18th chromosome; characteristic mental and physical impairments; mainly affects females.

✓5ᵗʰ 758.3 Autosomal deletion syndromes

758.31 Cri-du-chat syndrome
Deletion 5p

DEF: Hereditary congenital syndrome caused by a microdeletion of short arm of chromosome 5; characterized by catlike cry in newborn, microencephaly, severe mental deficiency, and hypertelorism.

758.32 Velo-cardio-facial syndrome
Deletion 22q11.2

DEF: Microdeletion syndrome affecting multiple organs; characteristic cleft palate, heart defects, elongated face with almond-shaped eyes, wide nose, small ears, weak immune systems, weak musculature, hypothyroidism, short stature, and scoliosis; deletion at q11.2 on the long arm of the chromosome 22.

758.33 Other microdeletions
Miller-Dieker syndrome
Smith-Magenis syndrome

DEF: Miller-Dieker syndrome: deletion from the short arm of chromosome 17; characteristic mental retardation, speech and motor development delays, neurological complications, and multiple abnormalities affecting the kidneys, heart, gastrointestinal tract; death in infancy or early childhood.

DEF: Smith-Magenis syndrome: deletion in a certain area of chromosome 17 that results in craniofacial changes, speech delay, hoarse voice, hearing loss and behavioral problems, such as self-destructive head banging, wrist biting, and tearing at nails.

758.39 Other autosomal deletions

758.4 Balanced autosomal translocation in normal individual

758.5 Other conditions due to autosomal anomalies
Accessory autosomes NEC

758.6 Gonadal dysgenesis
Ovarian dysgenesis   XO syndrome
Turner's syndrome
EXCLUDES   pure gonadal dysgenesis (752.7)

758.7 Klinefelter's syndrome
XXY syndrome

DEF: Impaired embryonic development of seminiferous tubes; results in small testes, azoospermia, infertility and enlarged mammary glands.

✓5ᵗʰ 758.8 Other conditions due to chromosome anomalies

758.81 Other conditions due to sex chromosome anomalies

758.89 Other

758.9 Conditions due to anomaly of unspecified chromosome

✓4ᵗʰ 759 Other and unspecified congenital anomalies

759.0 Anomalies of spleen
Aberrant
Absent } spleen
Accessory

Congenital splenomegaly
Ectopic spleen
Lobulation of spleen

759.1 Anomalies of adrenal gland
Aberrant
Absent } adrenal gland
Accessory

EXCLUDES   adrenogenital disorders (255.2)
          congenital disorders of steroid metabolism
            (255.2)

759.2   Anomalies of other endocrine glands
   Absent parathyroid gland
   Accessory thyroid gland
   Persistent thyroglossal or thyrolingual duct
   Thyroglossal (duct) cyst
   EXCLUDES   *congenital:*
                 goiter (246.1)
                 hypothyroidism (243)

759.3   Situs inversus
   Situs inversus or transversus:
      abdominalis
      thoracis
   Transposition of viscera:
      abdominal
      thoracic
   EXCLUDES   *dextrocardia without mention of complete*
                 transposition (746.87)
   DEF: Laterally transposed thoracic and abdominal viscera.

759.4   Conjoined twins
   Craniopagus
   Dicephalus
   Pygopagus
   Thoracopagus
   Xiphopagus

759.5   Tuberous sclerosis
   Bourneville's disease
   Epiloia
   DEF: Hamartomas of brain, retina and viscera, impaired mental ability, seizures and adenoma sebaceum.

759.6   Other hamartoses, not elsewhere classified
   Syndrome:
      Peutz-Jeghers
      Sturge-Weber (-Dimitri)
      von Hippel-Lindau
   EXCLUDES   *neurofibromatosis (237.70-237.79)*
   DEF: Peutz-Jeghers: hereditary syndrome characterized by hamartomas of small intestine.
   DEF: Sturge-Weber: congenital syndrome characterized by unilateral port-wine stain over trigeminal nerve, underlying meninges and cerebral cortex.
   DEF: von Hipple-Lindau: hereditary syndrome of congenital angiomatosis of the retina and cerebellum.

759.7   Multiple congenital anomalies, so described
   Congenital:
      anomaly, multiple NOS
      deformity, multiple NOS

√5ᵗʰ **759.8   Other specified anomalies**

   759.81   Prader-Willi syndrome

   759.82   Marfan syndrome

   759.83   Fragile X syndrome

   759.89   Other
      Congenital malformation syndromes affecting multiple systems, not elsewhere classified
      Laurence-Moon-Biedl syndrome

759.9   Congenital anomaly, unspecified

Chapter 15: Certain Conditions Originating in the Perinatal Period (760–779)

Coding Guidance

This chapter classifies conditions that begin during the perinatal period even if death or morbidity occurs later. The perinatal period is defined as the period of time occurring before, during, through the first 28 days following birth. These codes are used to classify causes or morbidity, and mortality in the fetus or newborn and should not be used on the mother's coded profile.

ICD-9-CM divides this chapter into the following sections:

- Maternal causes of perinatal morbidity and mortality (760–763)
- Other conditions originating in the perinatal period (764–779)

All clinically significant conditions noted on routine newborn examination should be coded. A condition is clinically significant if it requires one of the following:

- Clinical evaluation
- Therapeutic treatment
- Diagnostic procedures
- Extended length of hospital stay
- Increased nursing care and/or monitoring
- Has implications for future health care needs (Codes should be assigned for conditions that the provider has specified as having implications for future health care needs.)

Maternal Causes of Perinatal Morbidity and Mortality (760–763)

Fetal or newborn conditions caused by systemic, metabolic, or infectious diseases of the mother are classified to this section. Maternal diseases that can affect the health or life of the fetus or newborn include hypertension, renal disease, urinary or respiratory tract infections, and chronic respiratory or circulatory diseases (e.g., pulmonary embolism, thrombophlebitis). Categories 760–763 also include fetal or newborn conditions caused by maternal nutritional disorders; maternal injury, surgery or death, maternal ingestion of drugs, chemicals, or alcohol; and maternal complications of labor, delivery, or both.

Assign an additional code to identify the condition that was a result of the maternal condition described by codes in this section, unless the resultant condition code already specifies the maternal condition.

Example:

Syndrome of "infant of diabetic mother" need only be assigned code 775.0 rather than a code from the 760–763 range.

These codes may be used regardless of the patient's age. For example, it is not uncommon for the daughters of women who ingested DES during pregnancy to develop ovarian cancer from exposure through the placenta while in utero. Code 760.76 is assigned to women affected by DES exposure. E-code assignment is made only for first generation users of DES.

Surgical Operation on Mother and Fetus (760.6)

Subcategory 760.6 describes conditions in which a liveborn infant has been affected in some manner by interventional procedures or surgeries performed during the pregnancy, to diagnose or treat either a fetal condition or a maternal complication of the pregnancy. Fetal surgery is a relatively new surgical specialty that enables treatment of certain conditions that were previously considered untreatable. Diagnostic imaging technologies help in early detection of fetal anomalies and associated gestational risks. In utero interventional procedures provide alternatives to improve outcomes for pregnancies complicated by fetal conditions not previously amenable to treatment. However, these procedures are not without risk for both the fetus and the mother, depending on the nature of the diagnosis and type of intervention. The primary risk for the newborn is premature birth or injury as a result of a procedural intervention during the pregnancy. Premature infants face an increased risk of potentially serious complications and typically require neonatal intensive care unit (NICU) care. Some studies have suggested that amniocentesis and other interventional procedures increase the risk for clubfoot, hip dislocation, and respiratory problems in the infant. Infection of the amniotic fluid is possible, although extremely rare, less than one occurring in 1,000 procedures. Chronic infections such as HIV, cytomegalovirus, hepatitis C, and toxoplasmosis are suspected to be transmittable during in utero interventions.

Slow Fetal Growth and Fetal Malnutrition (764)

Slow fetal growth and fetal malnutrition is a condition in which a fetus is considerably below the normal weight expected for a fetus of the same gestational age. Malnutrition in a fetus may be due to defective assimilation or utilization of nutrients or to a maternal diet that is unbalanced or insufficient, as well as other factors.

This condition may be described with such terms as "small for gestational age," "intrauterine growth retardation" or "IUGR."

Conditions Originating in the Perinatal Period (764-779)

Monochorionic Gestation Complicated by Inter-twin Vascular Communication

Twin-twin transfusion syndrome (TTTS) is a complication of fetal cardiovascular development that results in a hostile intrauterine fluid volume environment. Due to the abnormal development of anastomotic blood vessels, one twin is polyhydramniotic and the other is oligohydramniotic, creating a donor-recipient situation with associated complicating conditions for each fetus. Amnioreduction can be performed to treat the polyhydramniotic twin, reducing the fluid volume and pressure. However, the definitive surgery is fetoscopic laser photocoagulation, which is performed to ablate and correct the underlying chorionic vascular anomalies that cause TTTS, and prevent further fluid loss for the oligohydramniotic twin.

Separate diagnoses are required to report a pregnancy complicated by inter-twin vascular communication and the resultant manifestations of oligohydramnios and polyhydramnios.

Code assignment for mother's record:

651.03 Twin pregnancy, antepartum complication

655.83 Other known or suspected fetal abnormality NEC, antepartum complication

657.03 Polyhydramnios, antepartum condition

658.03 Oligohydramnios, antepartum condition.

If one fetus is terminated as a result of TTTS, report code 651.73 Multiple gestation following elective reduction, antepartum condition, for the reduction diagnosis, with a secondary diagnosis of 655.83 Other known or suspected fetal abnormality.

Code assignment for newborn record:

762.3   Placental transfusion syndromes

Use an additional code to indicate any resultant condition in the fetus or newborn, such as fetal blood loss (772.0) or polycythemia neonatorum (776.4)

Post-term and Prolonged Gestation Infant (766.2x)

Post-term infant is defined as an infant with a gestation period of more than 40 to 42 completed weeks. Prolonged gestation is defined as an infant with a gestation period of more than 42 completed weeks. The definitions relate to length of gestation and not to associated conditions that may arise due to the length of gestation.

Codes 766.21 Post-term infant and 766.22 Prolonged gestation of infant may be assigned based only on the gestational age of the newborn. A specific condition or disorder does not have to be associated with the longer gestational period to assign these codes.

Necrotizing Enterocolitis (777.5)

Necrotizing enterocolitis (NEC) is a serious and life-threatening condition in premature infants. It is a gastrointestinal illness associated with some very low birth-weight (VLBW) infants. In NEC, the lining of the intestinal wall dies and the tissue sloughs off. The cause for this disorder is unknown, but it is thought that a decrease in blood flow to the bowel keeps the bowel from producing mucus that protects the gastrointestinal tract. Bacteria in the intestine may also be a contributing factor. NEC without pneumatosis (defined as gas in the bowel wall) or perforation is a vague disorder and may resolve with medical treatment. NEC with pneumatosis places the patient at higher risk for mortality and progression to serious complications, such as portal vein gas or perforation.

Stages of NEC may be classified as follows:

- Stage 1 (suspected) (777.51): Nonspecific systemic signs, including lethargy, abdominal distention, blood in stool. Radiology studies may be normal or positive for bowel dilation.

- Stage 2 (proven) (777.52): Absent bowel sounds. Radiology studies positive for intestinal dilation, ileus, pneumatosis, and possibly ascites.

- Stage 3 (advanced) (777.53): Critical illness with hypotension or shock, bradycardia, apnea, peritonitis, or bowel perforation. Appropriate use of treatments such as antenatal steroids, standardized enteric feeding regimens with human milk, and probiotics, along with careful monitoring, could substantially reduce the incidence of this serious disease. When perforation or necrotic bowel occurs, emergent surgery is necessary.

Due to the fragility of premature infants, those who suffer intestinal perforation often have high mortality rates. Assign the appropriate code for the clinical stage of disease only as documented in the medical record.

15. CERTAIN CONDITIONS ORIGINATING IN THE PERINATAL PERIOD (760-779)

INCLUDES   conditions which have their origin in the perinatal period, before birth through the first 28 days after birth, even though death or morbidity occurs later

Use additional code(s) to further specify condition

MATERNAL CAUSES OF PERINATAL MORBIDITY AND MORTALITY (760-763)

√4ᵗʰ **760   Fetus or newborn affected by maternal conditions which may be unrelated to present pregnancy**

INCLUDES   the listed maternal conditions only when specified as a cause of mortality or morbidity of the fetus or newborn

EXCLUDES   *maternal endocrine and metabolic disorders affecting fetus or newborn (775.0-775.9)*

760.0   Maternal hypertensive disorders
Fetus or newborn affected by maternal conditions classifiable to 642

760.1   Maternal renal and urinary tract diseases
Fetus or newborn affected by maternal conditions classifiable to 580-599

760.2   Maternal infections
Fetus or newborn affected by maternal infectious disease classifiable to 001-136 and 487, but fetus or newborn not manifesting that disease

EXCLUDES   *congenital infectious diseases (771.0-771.8)*
maternal genital tract and other localized infections (760.8)

760.3   Other chronic maternal circulatory and respiratory diseases
Fetus or newborn affected by chronic maternal conditions classifiable to 390-459, 490-519, 745-748

760.4   Maternal nutritional disorders
Fetus or newborn affected by:
maternal disorders classifiable to 260-269
maternal malnutrition NOS

EXCLUDES   *fetal malnutrition (764.10-764.29)*

760.5   Maternal injury
Fetus or newborn affected by maternal conditions classifiable to 800-995

√5ᵗʰ **760.6   Surgical operation on mother and fetus**

EXCLUDES   *cesarean section for present delivery (763.4)*
damage to placenta from amniocentesis, cesarean section, or surgical induction (762.1)

760.61   Newborn affected by amniocentesis

EXCLUDES   *fetal complications from amniocentesis (679.1)*

760.62   Newborn affected by other in utero procedure

EXCLUDES   *fetal complications of in utero procedure (679.1)*

760.63   Newborn affected by other surgical operations on mother during pregnancy

EXCLUDES   *newborn affected by previous surgical procedure on mother not associated with pregnancy (760.64)*

760.64   Newborn affected by previous surgical procedure on mother not associated with pregnancy

√5ᵗʰ **760.7   Noxious influences affecting fetus or newborn via placenta or breast milk**
Fetus or newborn affected by noxious substance transmitted via placenta or breast milk

EXCLUDES   *anesthetic and analgesic drugs administered during labor and delivery (763.5)*
drug withdrawal syndrome in newborn (779.5)

760.70   Unspecified noxious substance
Fetus or newborn affected by:
Drug NEC

760.71   Alcohol
Fetal alcohol syndrome

760.72   Narcotics

760.73   Hallucinogenic agents

760.74   Anti-infectives
Antibiotics
Antifungals

760.75   Cocaine

760.76   Diethylstilbestrol [DES]

760.77   Anticonvulsants
Carbamazepine
Phenobarbital
Phenytoin
Valproic acid

760.78   Antimetabolic agents
Methotrexate
Retinoic acid
Statins

760.79   Other
Fetus or newborn affected by:
immune sera   ⎤ transmitted via
medicinal agents NEC   ⎬ placenta
toxic substance NEC   ⎦ or breast

760.8   Other specified maternal conditions affecting fetus or newborn
Maternal genital tract and other localized infection affecting fetus or newborn, but fetus or newborn not manifesting that disease

EXCLUDES   *maternal urinary tract infection affecting fetus or newborn (760.1)*

760.9   Unspecified maternal condition affecting fetus or newborn

√4ᵗʰ **761   Fetus or newborn affected by maternal complications of pregnancy**

INCLUDES   the listed maternal conditions only when specified as a cause of mortality or morbidity of the fetus or newborn

761.0   Incompetent cervix
DEF: Inadequate functioning of uterine cervix.

761.1   Premature rupture of membranes

761.2   Oligohydramnios

EXCLUDES   *that due to premature rupture of membranes (761.1)*

DEF: Deficient amniotic fluid.

761.3   Polyhydramnios
Hydramnios (acute) (chronic)
DEF: Excess amniotic fluid.

761.4   Ectopic pregnancy
Pregnancy:
abdominal
intraperitoneal
tubal

761.5   Multiple pregnancy
Triplet (pregnancy)
Twin (pregnancy)

761.6   Maternal death

Certain Conditions Originating in the Perinatal Period

761.7–763.9

761.7 Malpresentation before labor
Breech presentation
External version
Oblique lie
Transverse lie
Unstable lie
} before labor

761.8 Other specified maternal complications of pregnancy affecting fetus or newborn
Spontaneous abortion, fetus

761.9 Unspecified maternal complication of pregnancy affecting fetus or newborn

762 Fetus or newborn affected by complications of placenta, cord, and membranes
INCLUDES the listed maternal conditions only when specified as a cause of mortality or morbidity in the fetus or newborn

762.0 Placenta previa
DEF: Placenta developed in lower segment of uterus; causes hemorrhaging in last trimester.

762.1 Other forms of placental separation and hemorrhage
Abruptio placentae
Antepartum hemorrhage
Damage to placenta from amniocentesis, cesarean section, or surgical induction
Maternal blood loss
Premature separation of placenta
Rupture of marginal sinus

762.2 Other and unspecified morphological and functional abnormalities of placenta
Placental: dysfunction, infarction
Placental: insufficiency

762.3 Placental transfusion syndromes
Placental and cord abnormality resulting in twin-to-twin or other transplacental transfusion
Use additional code to indicate resultant condition in newborn:
fetal blood loss (772.0)
polycythemia neonatorum (776.4)

762.4 Prolapsed cord
Cord presentation

762.5 Other compression of umbilical cord
Cord around neck   Knot in cord
Entanglement of cord   Torsion of cord

762.6 Other and unspecified conditions of umbilical cord
Short cord
Thrombosis
Varices
Velamentous insertion
Vasa previa
} of umbilical cord
EXCLUDES infection of umbilical cord (771.4)
single umbilical artery (747.5)

762.7 Chorioamnionitis
Amnionitis   Placentitis
Membranitis
DEF: Inflamed fetal membrane.

762.8 Other specified abnormalities of chorion and amnion

762.9 Unspecified abnormality of chorion and amnion

763 Fetus or newborn affected by other complications of labor and delivery
INCLUDES the listed conditions only when specified as a cause of mortality or morbidity in the fetus or newborn
EXCLUDES newborn affected by surgical procedures on mother (760.61-760.64)

763.0 Breech delivery and extraction

763.1 Other malpresentation, malposition, and disproportion during labor and delivery
Fetus or newborn affected by:
abnormality of bony pelvis
contracted pelvis
persistent occipitoposterior position
shoulder presentation
transverse lie
Fetus or newborn affected by conditions classifiable to 652, 653, and 660

763.2 Forceps delivery
Fetus or newborn affected by forceps extraction

763.3 Delivery by vacuum extractor

763.4 Cesarean delivery
EXCLUDES placental separation or hemorrhage from cesarean section (762.1)

763.5 Maternal anesthesia and analgesia
Reactions and intoxications from maternal opiates and tranquilizers during labor and delivery
EXCLUDES drug withdrawal syndrome in newborn (779.5)

763.6 Precipitate delivery
Rapid second stage

763.7 Abnormal uterine contractions
Fetus or newborn affected by:
contraction ring
hypertonic labor
hypotonic uterine dysfunction
uterine inertia or dysfunction
Fetus or newborn affected by conditions classifiable to 661, except 661.3

763.8 Other specified complications of labor and delivery affecting fetus or newborn

763.81 Abnormality in fetal heart rate or rhythm before the onset of labor

763.82 Abnormality in fetal heart rate or rhythm during labor

763.83 Abnormality in fetal heart rate or rhythm, unspecified as to time of onset

763.84 Meconium passage during delivery
EXCLUDES meconium aspiration (770.11, 770.12)
meconium staining (779.84)
DEF: Fetal intestinal activity that increases in response to a distressed state during delivery; anal sphincter relaxes, and meconium is passed into the amniotic fluid.

763.89 Other specified complications of labor and delivery affecting fetus or newborn
Fetus or newborn affected by:
abnormality of maternal soft tissues
destructive operation on live fetus to facilitate delivery
induction of labor (medical)
other procedures used in labor and delivery
Fetus or newborn affected by other conditions classifiable to 650-699

763.9 Unspecified complication of labor and delivery affecting fetus or newborn

OTHER CONDITIONS ORIGINATING IN THE PERINATAL PERIOD (764-779)

The following fifth-digit subclassification is for use with category 764 and codes 765.0-765.1 to denote birthweight:
0 unspecified [weight]
1 less than 500 grams
2 500-749 grams
3 750-999 grams
4 1,000-1,249 grams
5 1,250-1,499 grams
6 1,500-1,749 grams
7 1,750-1,999 grams
8 2,000-2,499 grams
9 2,500 grams and over

✓4ᵗʰ **764 Slow fetal growth and fetal malnutrition**

✓5ᵗʰ **764.0 "Light-for-dates" without mention of fetal**
[0-9] **malnutrition**
Infants underweight for gestational age
"Small-for-dates"

✓5ᵗʰ **764.1 "Light-for-dates" with signs of fetal malnutrition**
[0-9] Infants "light-for-dates" classifiable to 764.0, who in
addition show signs of fetal malnutrition, such as
dry peeling skin and loss of subcutaneous tissue

✓5ᵗʰ **764.2 Fetal malnutrition without mention of**
[0-9] **"light-for-dates"**
Infants, not underweight for gestational age, showing
signs of fetal malnutrition, such as dry peeling skin
and loss of subcutaneous tissue
Intrauterine malnutrition

✓5ᵗʰ **764.9 Fetal growth retardation, unspecified**
[0-9] Intrauterine growth retardation

✓4ᵗʰ **765 Disorders relating to short gestation and low birthweight**
INCLUDES the listed conditions, without further specification, as
causes of mortality, morbidity, or additional
care, in fetus or newborn

✓5ᵗʰ **765.0 Extreme immaturity**
[0-9] Note: Usually implies a birthweight of less than
1000 grams.
Use additional code for weeks of gestation
(765.20-765.29)

✓5ᵗʰ **765.1 Other preterm infants**
[0-9] Note: Usually implies a birthweight of 1000-2499 grams.
Prematurity NOS
Prematurity or small size, not classifiable to 765.0 or as
"light-for-dates" in 764
Use additional code for weeks of gestation
(765.20-765.29)

✓5ᵗʰ **765.2 Weeks of gestation**

765.20 Unspecified weeks of gestation

765.21 Less than 24 completed weeks of gestation

765.22 24 completed weeks of gestation

765.23 25-26 completed weeks of gestation

765.24 27-28 completed weeks of gestation

765.25 29-30 completed weeks of gestation

765.26 31-32 completed weeks of gestation

765.27 33-34 completed weeks of gestation

765.28 35-36 completed weeks of gestation

765.29 37 or more completed weeks of gestation

✓4ᵗʰ **766 Disorders relating to long gestation and high birthweight**
INCLUDES the listed conditions, without further specification, as
causes of mortality, morbidity, or additional
care, in fetus or newborn

766.0 Exceptionally large baby
Note: Usually implies a birthweight of 4500 grams or
more.

766.1 Other "heavy-for-dates" infants
Other fetus or infant "heavy-" or "large-for-dates"
regardless of period of gestation

✓5ᵗʰ **766.2 Late infant, not "heavy-for-dates"**

766.21 Post-term infant
Infant with gestation period over 40 completed
weeks to 42 completed weeks

766.22 Prolonged gestation of infant
Infant with gestation period over 42 completed
weeks
Postmaturity NOS

✓4ᵗʰ **767 Birth trauma**

767.0 Subdural and cerebral hemorrhage
Subdural and cerebral hemorrhage, whether described
as due to birth trauma or to intrapartum anoxia or
hypoxia
Subdural hematoma (localized)
Tentorial tear
Use additional code to identify cause
EXCLUDES *intraventricular hemorrhage (772.10-772.14)*
subarachnoid hemorrhage (772.2)

✓5ᵗʰ **767.1 Injuries to scalp**

767.11 Epicranial subaponeurotic hemorrhage
(massive)
Subgaleal hemorrhage
DEF: A hemorrhage that occurs within the space
between the galea aponeurotica, or epicranial
aponeurosis, a thin tendinous structure that is
attached to the skull laterally, and the
periosteum of the skull.

767.19 Other injuries to scalp
Caput succedaneum
Cephalhematoma
Chignon (from vacuum extraction)

767.2 Fracture of clavicle

767.3 Other injuries to skeleton
Fracture of:
long bones
skull
EXCLUDES *congenital dislocation of hip (754.30-754.35)*
fracture of spine, congenital (767.4)

767.4 Injury to spine and spinal cord
Dislocation
Fracture } of spine or spinal cord due to
Laceration   birth trauma
Rupture

767.5 Facial nerve injury
Facial palsy

767.6 Injury to brachial plexus
Palsy or paralysis:
brachial
Erb (-Duchenne)
Klumpke (-Déjérine)

767.7 Other cranial and peripheral nerve injuries
Phrenic nerve paralysis

767.8 Other specified birth trauma
Eye damage
Hematoma of:
liver (subcapsular)
testes
vulva
Rupture of:
liver
spleen
Scalpel wound
Traumatic glaucoma
EXCLUDES *hemorrhage classifiable to 772.0-772.9*

767.9 Birth trauma, unspecified
Birth injury NOS

Epicranial Aponeurosis

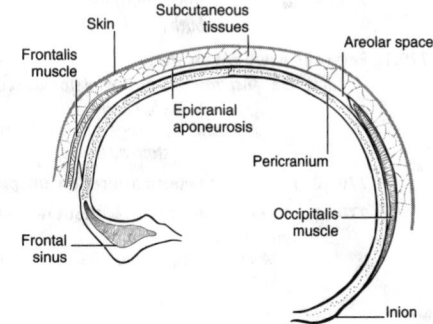

Certain Conditions Originating in the Perinatal Period

768–770.7

√4ᵗʰ **768   Intrauterine hypoxia and birth asphyxia**
Use only when associated with newborn morbidity classifiable elsewhere

     EXCLUDES   *acidemia NOS of newborn (775.81)*
acidosis NOS of newborn (775.81)
cerebral ischemia NOS (779.2)
hypoxia NOS of newborn (770.88)
mixed metabolic and respiratory acidosis of newborn (775.81)
respiratory arrest of newborn (770.87)

     DEF: Oxygen intake insufficiency due to interrupted placental circulation or premature separation of placenta.

768.0   Fetal death from asphyxia or anoxia before onset of labor or at unspecified time

768.1   Fetal death from asphyxia or anoxia during labor

768.2   Fetal distress before onset of labor, in liveborn infant
Fetal metabolic acidemia before onset of labor, in liveborn infant

768.3   Fetal distress first noted during labor and delivery, in liveborn infant
Fetal metabolic acidemia first noted during labor and delivery, in liveborn infant

768.4   Fetal distress, unspecified as to time of onset, in liveborn infant
Fetal metabolic acidemia unspecified as to time of onset, in liveborn infant

768.5   Severe birth asphyxia
Birth asphyxia with neurologic involvement

     EXCLUDES   *hypoxic-ischemic encephalopathy [HIE] (768.70-768.73)*

768.6   Mild or moderate birth asphyxia
Birth asphyxia (without mention of neurologic involvement)

     EXCLUDES   *hypoxic-ischemic encephalopathy [HIE] (768.70-768.73)*

√5ᵗʰ **768.7   Hypoxic-ischemic encephalopathy [HIE]**

     768.70   Hypoxic-ischemic encephalopathy, unspecified

     768.71   Mild hypoxic-ischemic encephalopathy

     768.72   Moderate hypoxic-ischemic encephalopathy

     768.73   Severe hypoxic-ischemic encephalopathy

768.9   Unspecified birth asphyxia in liveborn infant
Anoxia
Asphyxia   } NOS, in liveborn infant

769   Respiratory distress syndrome
Cardiorespiratory distress syndrome of newborn
Hyaline membrane disease (pulmonary)
Idiopathic respiratory distress syndrome [IRDS or RDS] of newborn
Pulmonary hypoperfusion syndrome

     EXCLUDES   *transient tachypnea of newborn (770.6)*

     DEF: Severe chest contractions upon air intake and expiratory grunting; infant appears blue due to oxygen deficiency and has rapid respiratory rate; formerly called hyaline membrane disease.

√4ᵗʰ **770   Other respiratory conditions of fetus and newborn**

770.0   Congenital pneumonia
Infective pneumonia acquired prenatally

     EXCLUDES   *pneumonia from infection acquired after birth (480.0-486)*

√5ᵗʰ **770.1   Fetal and newborn aspiration**

     EXCLUDES   *aspiration of postnatal stomach contents (770.85, 770.86)*
meconium passage during delivery (763.84)
meconium staining (779.84)

     770.10   Fetal and newborn aspiration, unspecified

     770.11   Meconium aspiration without respiratory symptoms
Meconium aspiration NOS

     770.12   Meconium aspiration with respiratory symptoms
Meconium aspiration pneumonia
Meconium aspiration pneumonitis
Meconium aspiration syndrome NOS
Use additional code to identify any secondary pulmonary hypertension (416.8), if applicable

         DEF: Meconium aspiration syndrome: aspiration of fetal intestinal material during or prior to delivery, usually a complication of placental insufficiency, causing pneumonitis and bronchial obstruction (inflammatory reaction of lungs).

     770.13   Aspiration of clear amniotic fluid without respiratory symptoms
Aspiration of clear amniotic fluid NOS

     770.14   Aspiration of clear amniotic fluid with respiratory symptoms
Aspiration of clear amniotic fluid with pneumonia
Aspiration of clear amniotic fluid with pneumonitis
Use additional code to identify any secondary pulmonary hypertension (416.8), if applicable

     770.15   Aspiration of blood without respiratory symptoms
Aspiration of blood NOS

     770.16   Aspiration of blood with respiratory symptoms
Aspiration of blood with pneumonia
Aspiration of blood with pneumonitis
Use additional code to identify any secondary pulmonary hypertension (416.8), if applicable

     770.17   Other fetal and newborn aspiration without respiratory symptoms

     770.18   Other fetal and newborn aspiration with respiratory symptoms
Other aspiration pneumonia
Other aspiration pneumonitis
Use additional code to identify any secondary pulmonary hypertension (416.8), if applicable

770.2   Interstitial emphysema and related conditions
Pneumomediastinum
Pneumopericardium   } originating in the perinatal period
Pneumothorax

770.3   Pulmonary hemorrhage
Hemorrhage:
   alveolar (lung)
   intra-alveolar (lung)   } originating in the perinatal period
   massive pulmonary

770.4   Primary atelectasis
Pulmonary immaturity NOS

     DEF: Alveoli fail to expand causing insufficient air intake by newborn.

770.5   Other and unspecified atelectasis
Atelectasis:
   NOS
   partial   } originating in the perinatal period
   secondary
Pulmonary collapse

770.6   Transitory tachypnea of newborn
Idiopathic tachypnea of newborn
Wet lung syndrome

     EXCLUDES   *respiratory distress syndrome (769)*

     DEF: Quick, shallow breathing of newborn; short-term problem.

770.7   Chronic respiratory disease arising in the perinatal period
Bronchopulmonary dysplasia
Interstitial pulmonary fibrosis of prematurity
Wilson-Mikity syndrome

☑5ᵗʰ **770.8 Other respiratory problems after birth**
   EXCLUDES *mixed metabolic and respiratory acidosis of newborn (775.81)*

  770.81 Primary apnea of newborn
    Apneic spells of newborn NOS
    Essential apnea of newborn
    Sleep apnea of newborn
    DEF: Cessation of breathing when a neonate makes no respiratory effort for 15 seconds, resulting in cyanosis and bradycardia.

  770.82 Other apnea of newborn
    Obstructive apnea of newborn

  770.83 Cyanotic attacks of newborn

  770.84 Respiratory failure of newborn
    EXCLUDES *respiratory distress syndrome (769)*

  770.85 Aspiration of postnatal stomach contents without respiratory symptoms
    Aspiration of postnatal stomach contents NOS

  770.86 Aspiration of postnatal stomach contents with respiratory symptoms
    Aspiration of postnatal stomach contents with pneumonia
    Aspiration of postnatal stomach contents with pneumonitis
    Use additional code to identify any secondary pulmonary hypertension (416.8), if applicable

  770.87 Respiratory arrest of newborn

  770.88 Hypoxemia of newborn
    Hypoxia NOS of newborn

  770.89 Other respiratory problems after birth

770.9 Unspecified respiratory condition of fetus and newborn

☑4ᵗʰ **771 Infections specific to the perinatal period**
  INCLUDES infections acquired before or during birth or via the umbilicus or during the first 28 days after birth
  EXCLUDES *congenital pneumonia (770.0)*
   congenital syphilis (090.0-090.9)
   infant botulism (040.41)
   maternal infectious disease as a cause of mortality or morbidity in fetus or newborn, but fetus or newborn not manifesting the disease (760.2)
   ophthalmia neonatorum due to gonococcus (098.40)
   other infections not specifically classified to this category

771.0 Congenital rubella
  Congenital rubella pneumonitis

771.1 Congenital cytomegalovirus infection
  Congenital cytomegalic inclusion disease

771.2 Other congenital infections
  Congenital: herpes simplex, listeriosis, malaria
  Congenital: toxoplasmosis, tuberculosis

771.3 Tetanus neonatorum
  Tetanus omphalitis
  EXCLUDES *hypocalcemic tetany (775.4)*
  DEF: Severe infection of central nervous system; due to exotoxin of tetanus bacillus from navel infection prompted by nonsterile technique during umbilical ligation.

771.4 Omphalitis of the newborn
  Infection: navel cord, umbilical stump
  EXCLUDES *tetanus omphalitis (771.3)*
  DEF: Inflamed umbilicus.

771.5 Neonatal infective mastitis
  EXCLUDES *noninfective neonatal mastitis (778.7)*

771.6 Neonatal conjunctivitis and dacryocystitis
  Ophthalmia neonatorum NOS
  EXCLUDES *ophthalmia neonatorum due to gonococcus (098.40)*

771.7 Neonatal Candida infection
  Neonatal moniliasis
  Thrush in newborn

☑5ᵗʰ **771.8 Other infection specific to the perinatal period**
  Use additional code to identify organism or specific infection

  771.81 Septicemia [sepsis] of newborn
    Use additional codes to identify severe sepsis (995.92) and any associated acute organ dysfunction, if applicable

  771.82 Urinary tract infection of newborn

  771.83 Bacteremia of newborn

  771.89 Other infections specific to the perinatal period
    Intra-amniotic infection of fetus NOS
    Infection of newborn NOS

☑4ᵗʰ **772 Fetal and neonatal hemorrhage**
  EXCLUDES *fetal hematologic conditions complicating pregnancy (678.0)*
   hematological disorders of fetus and newborn (776.0-776.9)

772.0 Fetal blood loss affecting newborn
  Fetal blood loss from: cut end of co-twin's cord, placenta, ruptured cord, vasa previa
  Fetal exsanguination
  Fetal hemorrhage into: co-twin, mother's circulation

☑5ᵗʰ **772.1 Intraventricular hemorrhage**
  Intraventricular hemorrhage from any perinatal cause

  772.10 Unspecified grade

  772.11 Grade I
    Bleeding into germinal matrix

  772.12 Grade II
    Bleeding into ventricle

  772.13 Grade III
    Bleeding with enlargement of ventricle

  772.14 Grade IV
    Bleeding into cerebral cortex

772.2 Subarachnoid hemorrhage
  Subarachnoid hemorrhage from any perinatal cause
  EXCLUDES *subdural and cerebral hemorrhage (767.0)*

772.3 Umbilical hemorrhage after birth
  Slipped umbilical ligature

772.4 Gastrointestinal hemorrhage
  EXCLUDES *swallowed maternal blood (777.3)*

772.5 Adrenal hemorrhage

772.6 Cutaneous hemorrhage
  Bruising, Ecchymoses, Petechiae, Superficial hematoma } in fetus or newborn

772.8 Other specified hemorrhage of fetus or newborn
  EXCLUDES *hemorrhagic disease of newborn (776.0)*
   pulmonary hemorrhage (770.3)

772.9 Unspecified hemorrhage of newborn

Certain Conditions Originating in the Perinatal Period

773–776.0

√4ᵗʰ **773 Hemolytic disease of fetus or newborn, due to isoimmunization**

DEF: Hemolytic anemia of fetus or newborn due to maternal antibody formation against fetal erythrocytes; infant blood contains nonmaternal antigen.

773.0 Hemolytic disease due to Rh isoimmunization

Anemia — due to RH:
Erythroblastosis (fetalis) — antibodies
Hemolytic disease (fetus) — isoimmunization
(newborn) — maternal/fetal
Jaundice — incompatibility
Rh hemolytic disease
Rh isoimmunization

773.1 Hemolytic disease due to ABO isoimmunization

ABO hemolytic disease
ABO isoimmunization
Anemia — due to ABO:
Erythroblastosis (fetalis) — antibodies
Hemolytic disease (fetus) — isoimmunization
(newborn) — maternal/fetal
Jaundice — incompatibility

DEF: Incompatible Rh fetal-maternal blood grouping; prematurely destroys red blood cells; detected by Coombs test.

773.2 Hemolytic disease due to other and unspecified isoimmunization

Eythroblastosis (fetalis) (neonatorum) NOS
Hemolytic disease (fetus) (newborn) NOS
Jaundice or anemia due to other and unspecified blood-group incompatibility

773.3 Hydrops fetalis due to isoimmunization

Use additional code to identify type of isoimmunization (773.0-773.2)

DEF: Massive edema of entire body and severe anemia; may result in fetal death or stillbirth.

773.4 Kernicterus due to isoimmunization

Use additional code to identify type of isoimmunization (773.0-773.2)

DEF: Complication of erythroblastosis fetalis associated with severe neural symptoms, high blood bilirubin levels and nerve cell destruction; results in bilirubin-pigmented gray matter of central nervous system.

773.5 Late anemia due to isoimmunization

√4ᵗʰ **774 Other perinatal jaundice**

774.0 Perinatal jaundice from hereditary hemolytic anemias
Code first underlying disease (282.0-282.9)

774.1 Perinatal jaundice from other excessive hemolysis
Fetal or neonatal jaundice from:
bruising
drugs or toxins transmitted from mother
infection
polycythemia
swallowed maternal blood
Use additional code to identify cause
EXCLUDES *jaundice due to isoimmunization (773.0-773.2)*

774.2 Neonatal jaundice associated with preterm delivery
Hyperbilirubinemia of prematurity
Jaundice due to delayed conjugation associated with preterm delivery

√5ᵗʰ **774.3 Neonatal jaundice due to delayed conjugation from other causes**

774.30 Neonatal jaundice due to delayed conjugation, cause unspecified
DEF: Jaundice of newborn with abnormal bilirubin metabolism; causes excess accumulated unconjugated bilirubin in blood.

774.31 Neonatal jaundice due to delayed conjugation in diseases classified elsewhere
Code first underlying diseases as:
congenital hypothyroidism (243)
Crigler-Najjar syndrome (277.4)
Gilbert's syndrome (277.4)

774.39 Other
Jaundice due to delayed conjugation from causes, such as:
breast milk inhibitors
delayed development of conjugating system

774.4 Perinatal jaundice due to hepatocellular damage
Fetal or neonatal hepatitis   Inspissated bile syndrome
Giant cell hepatitis

774.5 Perinatal jaundice from other causes
Code first underlying cause as:
congenital obstruction of bile duct (751.61)
galactosemia (271.1)
mucoviscidosis (277.00-277.09)

774.6 Unspecified fetal and neonatal jaundice
Icterus neonatorum
Neonatal hyperbilirubinemia (transient)
Physiologic jaundice NOS in newborn
EXCLUDES *that in preterm infants (774.2)*

774.7 Kernicterus not due to isoimmunization
Bilirubin encephalopathy
Kernicterus of newborn NOS
EXCLUDES *kernicterus due to isoimmunization (773.4)*

√4ᵗʰ **775 Endocrine and metabolic disturbances specific to the fetus and newborn**
INCLUDES transitory endocrine and metabolic disturbances caused by the infant's response to maternal endocrine and metabolic factors, its removal from them, or its adjustment to extrauterine existence

775.0 Syndrome of "infant of a diabetic mother"
Maternal diabetes mellitus affecting fetus or newborn (with hypoglycemia)

775.1 Neonatal diabetes mellitus
Diabetes mellitus syndrome in newborn infant

775.2 Neonatal myasthenia gravis

775.3 Neonatal thyrotoxicosis
Neonatal hyperthydroidism (transient)

775.4 Hypocalcemia and hypomagnesemia of newborn
Cow's milk hypocalcemia
Hypocalcemic tetany, neonatal
Neonatal hypoparathyroidism
Phosphate-loading hypocalcemia

775.5 Other transitory neonatal electrolyte disturbances
Dehydration, neonatal

775.6 Neonatal hypoglycemia
EXCLUDES *infant of mother with diabetes mellitus (775.0)*

775.7 Late metabolic acidosis of newborn

√5ᵗʰ **775.8 Other neonatal endocrine and metabolic disturbances**

775.81 Other acidosis of newborn
Acidemia NOS of newborn
Acidosis of newborn NOS
Mixed metabolic and respiratory acidosis of newborn

775.89 Other neonatal endocrine and metabolic disturbances
Amino-acid metabolic disorders described as transitory

775.9 Unspecified endocrine and metabolic disturbances specific to the fetus and newborn

√4ᵗʰ **776 Hematological disorders of newborn**
INCLUDES disorders specific to the newborn though possibly originating in utero
EXCLUDES *fetal hematologic conditions (678.0)*

776.0 Hemorrhagic disease of newborn
Hemorrhagic diathesis of newborn
Vitamin K deficiency of newborn
EXCLUDES *fetal or neonatal hemorrhage (772.0-772.9)*

776.1 Transient neonatal thrombocytopenia
Neonatal thrombocytopenia due to:
    exchange transfusion
    idiopathic maternal thrombocytopenia
    isoimmunization
DEF: Temporary decrease in blood platelets of newborn.

776.2 Disseminated intravascular coagulation in newborn
DEF: Disseminated intravascular coagulation of newborn: clotting disorder due to excess thromboplastic agents in blood as a result of disease or trauma; causes blood clotting within vessels and reduces available elements necessary for blood coagulation.

776.3 Other transient neonatal disorders of coagulation
Transient coagulation defect, newborn

776.4 Polycythemia neonatorum
Plethora of newborn
Polycythemia due to:
    donor twin transfusion
    maternal-fetal transfusion
DEF: Abnormal increase of total red blood cells of newborn.

776.5 Congenital anemia
Anemia following fetal blood loss
EXCLUDES *anemia due to isoimmunization (773.0-773.2, 773.5)*
hereditary hemolytic anemias (282.0-282.9)

776.6 Anemia of prematurity

776.7 Transient neonatal neutropenia
Isoimmune neutropenia
Maternal transfer neutropenia
EXCLUDES *congenital neutropenia (nontransient) (288.01)*
DEF: Decreased neutrophilic leukocytes in blood of newborn.

776.8 Other specified transient hematological disorders

776.9 Unspecified hematological disorder specific to newborn

√4ᵗʰ **777 Perinatal disorders of digestive system**
INCLUDES disorders specific to the fetus and newborn
EXCLUDES *intestinal obstruction classifiable to 560.0-560.9*

777.1 Meconium obstruction
Congenital fecaliths
Delayed passage of meconium
Meconium ileus NOS
Meconium plug syndrome
EXCLUDES *meconium ileus in cystic fibrosis (277.01)*
DEF: Meconium blocked digestive tract of newborn.

777.2 Intestinal obstruction due to inspissated milk

777.3 Hematemesis and melena due to swallowed maternal blood
Swallowed blood syndrome in newborn
EXCLUDES *that not due to swallowed maternal blood (772.4)*

777.4 Transitory ileus of newborn
EXCLUDES *Hirschsprung's disease (751.3)*

√5ᵗʰ **777.5 Necrotizing enterocolitis in newborn**
DEF: Serious intestinal infection and inflammation in preterm infants; severity is measured by stages and may progress to life-threatening perforation or peritonitis; resection surgical treatment may be necessary.

777.50 Necrotizing enterocolitis in newborn, unspecified
Necrotizing enterocolitis in newborn, NOS

777.51 Stage I necrotizing enterocolitis in newborn
Necrotizing enterocolitis without pneumatosis, without perforation
DEF: Broad-spectrum symptoms with non-specific signs including feeding intolerance, sepsis, gastroenteritis, ileus, metabolic abnormalities.

777.52 Stage II necrotizing enterocolitis in newborn
Necrotizing enterocolitis with pneumatosis, without perforation
DEF: Radiographic confirmation of necrotizing enterocolitis showing intestinal dilatation, fixed loops of bowels, pneumatosis intestinalis, metabolic acidosis, and thrombocytopenia.

777.53 Stage III necrotizing enterocolitis in newborn
Necrotizing enterocolitis with perforation
Necrotizing enterocolitis with pneumatosis and perforation
DEF: Advanced stage in which infant demonstrates signs of bowel perforation, septic shock, metabolic acidosis, ascites, disseminated intravascular coagulopathy, neutropenia.

777.6 Perinatal intestinal perforation
Meconium peritonitis

777.8 Other specified perinatal disorders of digestive system

777.9 Unspecified perinatal disorder of digestive system

√4ᵗʰ **778 Conditions involving the integument and temperature regulation of fetus and newborn**

778.0 Hydrops fetalis not due to isoimmunization
Idiopathic hydrops
EXCLUDES *hydrops fetalis due to isoimmunization (773.3)*
DEF: Edema of entire body, unrelated to immune response.

778.1 Sclerema neonatorum
Subcutaneous fat necrosis
DEF: Diffuse, rapidly progressing white, waxy, nonpitting hardening of tissue, usually of legs and feet, life-threatening; found in preterm or debilitated infants; unknown etiology.

778.2 Cold injury syndrome of newborn

778.3 Other hypothermia of newborn

778.4 Other disturbances of temperature regulation of newborn
Dehydration fever in newborn
Environmentally-induced pyrexia
Hyperthermia in newborn
Transitory fever of newborn

778.5 Other and unspecified edema of newborn
Edema neonatorum

778.6 Congenital hydrocele
Congenital hydrocele of tunica vaginalis

778.7 Breast engorgement in newborn
Noninfective mastitis of newborn
EXCLUDES *infective mastitis of newborn (771.5)*

778.8 Other specified conditions involving the integument of fetus and newborn
Urticaria neonatorum
EXCLUDES *impetigo neonatorum (684)*
pemphigus neonatorum (684)

778.9 Unspecified condition involving the integument and temperature regulation of fetus and newborn

√4ᵗʰ **779 Other and ill-defined conditions originating in the perinatal period**

779.0 Convulsions in newborn
Fits ⎫
Seizures ⎬ in newborn

779.1 Other and unspecified cerebral irritability in newborn

779.2 Cerebral depression, coma, and other abnormal cerebral signs
Cerebral ischemia NOS of newborn
CNS dysfunction in newborn NOS
EXCLUDES *cerebral ischemia due to birth trauma (767.0)*
intrauterine cerebral ischemia (768.2-768.9)
intraventricular hemorrhage (772.10-772.14)

Certain Conditions Originating in the Perinatal Period

779.3–779.9

√5ᵗʰ **779.3 Disorder of stomach function and feeding problems in newborn**

779.31 Feeding problems in newborn
Slow feeding in newborn
EXCLUDES   feeding problem in child over 28 days old (783.3)

779.32 Bilious vomiting in newborn
EXCLUDES   bilious vomiting in child over 28 days old (787.04)

779.33 Other vomiting in newborn
Regurgitation of food in newborn
EXCLUDES   vomiting in child over 28 days old (536.2, 787.01-787.04)

779.34 Failure to thrive in newborn
EXCLUDES   failure to thrive in child over 28 days old (783.41)

779.4 Drug reactions and intoxications specific to newborn
Gray syndrome from chloramphenicol administration in newborn
EXCLUDES   fetal alcohol syndrome (760.71)
reactions and intoxications from maternal opiates and tranquilizers (763.5)

779.5 Drug withdrawal syndrome in newborn
Drug withdrawal syndrome in infant of dependent mother
EXCLUDES   fetal alcohol syndrome (760.71)

779.6 Termination of pregnancy (fetus)
Fetal death due to:
induced abortion
termination of pregnancy
EXCLUDES   spontaneous abortion (fetus) (761.8)

779.7 Periventricular leukomalacia
DEF: Necrosis of white matter adjacent to lateral ventricles with the formation of cysts; cause of PVL has not been firmly established, but thought to be related to inadequate blood flow in certain areas of the brain.

√5ᵗʰ **779.8 Other specified conditions originating in the perinatal period**

779.81 Neonatal bradycardia
EXCLUDES   abnormality in fetal heart rate or rhythm complicating labor and delivery (763.81-763.83)
bradycardia due to birth asphyxia (768.5-768.9)

779.82 Neonatal tachycardia
EXCLUDES   abnormality in fetal heart rate or rhythm complicating labor and delivery (763.81-763.83)

779.83 Delayed separation of umbilical cord

779.84 Meconium staining
EXCLUDES   meconium aspiration (770.11, 770.12)
meconium passage during delivery (763.84)

779.85 Cardiac arrest of newborn

779.89 Other specified conditions originating in the perinatal period
Use additional code to specify condition

779.9 Unspecified condition originating in the perinatal period
Congenital debility NOS
Stillbirth NEC

Chapter 16: Symptoms, Signs, and Ill-defined Conditions (780–799)

Coding Guidance

This chapter includes symptoms, signs, and abnormal results of laboratory or other investigative procedures, as well as ill-defined conditions for which there are no other, more specific diagnoses classifiable elsewhere.

Symptoms are subjective observations reported to the physician by the patient. These observations depart from the structure, function or sensation that the patient normally experiences.

In general, codes from this chapter are used to report symptoms, signs, and ill-defined conditions that point with equal suspicion to two or more diagnoses or represent important problems in medical care that may affect management of the patient.

In addition, this chapter provides codes to classify abnormal findings that are reported without a corresponding definitive diagnosis. Codes for such findings can be located in the alphabetic index under such terms as "Abnormal, abnormality, abnormalities," "Decrease, decreased," "Elevation" and "Findings, abnormal, without diagnosis."

Codes from this chapter also are used to report:

- Symptoms and signs that existed on initial encounter but proved to be transient and whose causes could not be determined
- Provisional diagnoses for patients who fail to return for further investigation
- Cases referred elsewhere for further investigation before being diagnosed
- Cases in which a more definitive diagnosis was not available for other reasons

Do not assign a code from categories 780–799 when the symptoms, signs, and abnormal findings pertain to and are integral to a definitive diagnosis.

Example:

A patient with acute appendicitis would not need additional codes for abdominal pain (789.00) and abdominal rigidity (789.40). These signs and symptoms are integral to acute appendicitis and add no value to the patient's coding profile when assigned as secondary codes.

However, you may use a code from this chapter to report symptoms, signs, and abnormal findings that pertain to a particular clinical diagnosis if they represent important problems in medical care. Such problems may be useful to record because they may affect treatment plans.

A symptom, sign, or abnormal finding that is not integral to the principal diagnosis but coexist at the time of current episode of care and affects treatment, clinical evaluation, or increased monitoring or care may be listed as a secondary diagnosis.

Example:

A patient with benign prostatic hypertrophy NOS (600.00) seen for urinary retention may have acute urinary retention listed as a secondary diagnosis (788.20). Acute urinary retention is not integral to the disease process for benign prostatic hypertrophy, but it is an indication for an aggressive treatment plan. Acute urinary retention can be viewed as an "important medical problem" when the medical record documentation indicates the need for diagnostic procedures, therapeutic treatment, or monitoring to determine the cause.

List as the principal diagnosis any symptoms, signs, and abnormal findings that, after study, cannot be attributed to a definitive diagnosis classifiable to another chapter. The official coding guideline for coding symptoms, signs, and ill-defined conditions for outpatient services states that codes describing symptoms and signs, as opposed to diagnoses, are acceptable for reporting purposes when an established diagnosis has not been confirmed by the physician.

Symptoms that are integral to the disease process should not be assigned additional codes. However, those symptoms that are not routinely exhibited by patients with the disease may be coded in addition.

Example:

Patients with Crohn's disease do not routinely exhibit intestinal obstruction. In some cases the intestinal obstruction occurs with Crohn's disease and both conditions should be coded.

The alphabetic index should be consulted to determine which symptoms and signs are to be classified here and which should be classified to more specific sections of ICD-9-CM. The residual subcategories designated as .9 subcategories are provided for other relevant symptoms that are not elsewhere classified.

Symptoms (780-789)

Convulsions and Seizures

Subcategory 780.6 includes convulsive disorders and seizures that are ill-defined, sudden, acute symptomatic manifestations of other conditions. Excluded from this subcategory are seizures related to epilepsy that are irreversible, recurrent, chronic, or requiring maintenance with phenobarbitol or Dilantin for control.

Seizures documented as recurrent, not otherwise specified, convulsive, epileptiform, or repetitive are assigned code 780.39. Posttraumatic seizures are assigned code 780.33. If the documentation is not clear as to whether the seizures are epileptic in nature and should be coded to the 345 category, the physician should be queried.

Fever and Other Physiologic Disturbances of Temperature Regulation (780.6)

While inherent in a number of conditions, fever is considered a significant complication when associated with many chronic conditions, such as leukemia and sickle cell disease. In these chronic conditions, the presence of a fever may be a warning sign that the disease is being exacerbated or that a complicating infectious or inflammatory process is occurring in the body. Fever in chronic disease may also indicate an adverse drug or transfusion reaction, or the cause may not be known. However, the presence of a fever often affects the resources and intensity of required treatment. Code first the underlying condition when reporting code 780.61.

Postprocedural fevers are assigned code 780.62. Posttransfusion fever is assigned code 780.66 Febrile nonhemolytic transfusion reaction.

Functional Quadriplegia (780.72)

Functional quadriplegia is the inability to move due to another condition (e.g., dementia, severe contractures, arthritis, etc.) excluding neurological conditions. Functionally, the patient is the same as a paralyzed person. The inability to move and perform routine daily tasks for themselves renders patients immobile. This state poses certain associated health risks such as pressure ulcer, contractures, and pneumonia. The amount and type of care required to attend to these patients is greater than that of a patient with similar state of health but who is more mobile or has a greater degree of physical function.

Dysphagia (787.2x)

Dysphagia is a dynamic disorder, whereby the symptoms vary significantly depending on the affected phase of swallow. Oral-phase disorders typically result from impaired tongue control. Patients may experience trouble chewing solid food and initiating swallows. When drinking, there may be difficulty in containing the liquid in the oral cavity before swallowing, resulting in aspiration. In pharyngeal-phase dysphagia, the patient may be unable to ingest sufficiently life-sustaining amounts of food when pharyngeal clearance is severely limited. Impairment of esophageal function may cause food and liquid to be retained in the esophagus after swallowing. This can result from mechanical obstruction, motility disorder, or impaired opening of the lower esophageal sphincter.

Unique subclassification codes are available to facilitate reporting of dysphagia by the affected phase(s) of swallow as well as options for unspecified (787.20) and other (787.29) dysphagia. Dysphagia due to late effect of cerebrovascular accident (438.82) is sequenced first, if applicable.

Fecal Incontinence (786.6x)

Fecal incontinence can be the result of several conditions such as rectoceles or anal sphincter and rectal problems manifesting as fecal smears, fecal urgency, and incomplete defecation. Subcategory 786.6 includes these conditions: fecal incontinence (787.60), fecal urgency (767.62), and incomplete defecation (787.61). This subcategory excludes constipation (564.0x) and fecal impaction (560.32).

Functional Urinary Incontinence (788.9)

Functional urinary incontinence (FUI) is defined as leakage of urine related to impairment in cognitive function or other physical disability that makes the patient unable to control bladder function. FUI may be a temporary or permanent condition, depending on the underlying cause and contributing factors. This type of urinary incontinence is common among the elderly population, particularly those who suffer from dementia or mobility issues. Precipitating causes include stroke, neurological deficits (Parkinson's, Alzheimer's), severe depression, effects of medication, or musculoskeletal deconditioning due to aging.

Ascites (789.5x)

Subcategory 789.5 includes classifications for malignant (789.51) and nonmalignant ascites (789.59).

Malignant ascites (789.51) is most often seen in patients with ovarian, endometrial, breast, colon, gastric, and pancreatic cancer. Management of malignant ascites can include systemic chemotherapy, instillation of radioisotopes or chemotherapeutic drugs into the peritoneal fluid, and peritoneal venous shunting procedures. Code first the associated causal malignancy (e.g., 183.0, 197.6) when reporting malignant ascites.

Nonspecific Abnormal Findings (790–796)

Included in this section are nonspecific findings on examination of:

- Blood (790)
- Urine (791)
- Other body substances (792)
- Radiological and other examinations of body structure (793)
- Function studies (794)
- Immunological studies (795)
- Other (796)

Abnormal findings (laboratory, x-ray, pathologic, and other diagnostic results) are not assigned and reported unless the physician indicates a clinical significance or if a definitive diagnosis cannot be made. If the findings are outside the normal range and the physician has ordered other tests to evaluate the condition or prescribed treatment, it is appropriate to ask the physician whether the diagnosis should be added.

Abnormal Cytologies (795, 796)

Cytology samples may be obtained from the vagina, cervix, vulva, or anorectal canal to screen for human papillomavirus (HPV), abnormal growth such as dysplasia, anal intraepithelial neoplasia (AIN), and perianal intraepithelial neoplasia (PAIN). The correlation between abnormal cytologic smears and the risk of dysplasia and carcinoma is the same for the anus as it is for the cervix. Many pathophysiological parallels exist between cervical-vaginal and anal-rectal screening. For example, there is a transformation zone in the anus (similar to that of the cervix), which is the area between the keratinized and nonkeratinized epithelia. It is important to obtain a cytological sample from these tissues. Transformational zone tissue samples contain either squamous metaplastic and/or rectal columnar cells. Cellular analysis of transformation zone cells help diagnose and classify dysplastic changes. The histological and immunological cell changes reported with the Bethesda system are determined by cytology studies of the cell samples of the anus, cervix, vagina, and vulva as obtained by smear tests. The Bethesda system classifies cell changes by type and severity, from normal tissue to the identification of malignant cells. A pathologist interprets the findings and places the samples into the following categories:

- No pathologic change (normal) or inflammation (e.g., infection): Cells indicate the presence of inflammation that may be due to infection
- Atypical squamous cells of undetermined significance (ASCUS): Minor changes of the thin, flat surface cells due to unknown causes; may be followed up with DNA testing to identify the presence of a human papillomavirus (HPV)
- Atypical glandular cells (AGC): Abnormal mucus-producing cells due to unknown cause; favorable conditions for neoplastic growth
- Low-grade squamous intraepithelial lesion (LGSIL): Minor cellular changes unlikely to progress to cancer. Includes HPV infection, mild dysplasia, and intraepithelial neoplasia (CIN 1); may be followed up with DNA testing to identify the presence of a high-risk HPV infection
- High-grade squamous intraepithelial lesion (HSGIL): Cellular changes with a likelihood of progressing to cancer. Includes moderate to severe dysplasia, carcinoma in situ (CIS), CIN 2 and CIN 3, or changes suspicious for invasive cancer
- Malignant cells identified

Definitive diagnoses of carcinoma, intraepithelial neoplasia, and dysplasia are excluded from subcategory 795.0. Assign the appropriate chapter 2 neoplasm code or chapter 10 genitourinary disease code. When reporting abnormal vaginal smears, use an additional code from new category V88 to identify the acquired absence of the uterus or cervix, if applicable. Use an additional code to report associated HPV when reporting 795.19 or 796.79, when appropriate.

16. SYMPTOMS, SIGNS, AND ILL-DEFINED CONDITIONS (780-799)

This section includes symptoms, signs, abnormal results of laboratory or other investigative procedures, and ill-defined conditions regarding which no diagnosis classifiable elsewhere is recorded.

Signs and symptoms that point rather definitely to a given diagnosis are assigned to some category in the preceding part of the classification. In general, categories 780-796 include the more ill-defined conditions and symptoms that point with perhaps equal suspicion to two or more diseases or to two or more systems of the body, and without the necessary study of the case to make a final diagnosis. Practically all categories in this group could be designated as "not otherwise specified," or as "unknown etiology," or as "transient." The Alphabetic Index should be consulted to determine which symptoms and signs are to be allocated here and which to more specific sections of the classification; the residual subcategories numbered .9 are provided for other relevant symptoms which cannot be allocated elsewhere in the classification.

The conditions and signs or symptoms included in categories 780-796 consist of: (a) cases for which no more specific diagnosis can be made even after all facts bearing on the case have been investigated; (b) signs or symptoms existing at the time of initial encounter that proved to be transient and whose causes could not be determined; (c) provisional diagnoses in a patient who failed to return for further investigation or care; (d) cases referred elsewhere for investigation or treatment before the diagnosis was made; (e) cases in which a more precise diagnosis was not available for any other reason; (f) certain symptoms which represent important problems in medical care and which it might be desired to classify in addition to a known cause.

SYMPTOMS (780-789)

✓4ᵗʰ 780 General symptoms

✓5ᵗʰ 780.0 Alteration of consciousness

EXCLUDES   alteration of consciousness due to:
intracranial injuries (850.0-854.19)
skull fractures (800.00-801.99, 803.00-804.99)
coma:
diabetic (249.2-249.3, 250.2-250.3)
hepatic (572.2)
originating in the perinatal period (779.2)

780.01 Coma
DEF: State of unconsciousness from which the patient cannot be awakened.

780.02 Transient alteration of awareness
DEF: Temporary, recurring spells of reduced consciousness.

780.03 Persistent vegetative state
DEF: Persistent wakefulness without consciousness due to nonfunctioning cerebral cortex.

780.09 Other
Drowsiness   Stupor
Semicoma   Unconsciousness
Somnolence

780.1 Hallucinations
Hallucinations:
NOS
auditory
gustatory
olfactory
tactile
EXCLUDES   those associated with mental disorders, as
functional psychoses (295.0-298.9)
organic brain syndromes (290.0-294.9, 310.0-310.9)
visual hallucinations (368.16)
DEF: Perception of external stimulus in absence of stimulus; inability to distinguish between real and imagined.

780.2 Syncope and collapse
Blackout
Fainting
(Near) (Pre) syncope
Vasovagal attack
EXCLUDES   carotid sinus syncope (337.0)
heat syncope (992.1)
neurocirculatory asthenia (306.2)
orthostatic hypotension (458.0)
shock NOS (785.50)
DEF: Sudden unconsciousness due to reduced blood flow to brain.

✓5ᵗʰ 780.3 Convulsions
EXCLUDES   convulsions:
epileptic (345.10-345.91)
in newborn (779.0)
DEF: Sudden, involuntary contractions of the muscles.

780.31 Febrile convulsions (simple), unspecified
Febrile seizure NOS

780.32 Complex febrile convulsions
Febrile seizure:
atypical
complex
complicated
EXCLUDES   status epilepticus (345.3)

780.33 Post traumatic seizures
EXCLUDES   post traumatic epilepsy (345.00-345.91)

780.39 Other convulsions
Convulsive disorder NOS
Fit NOS
Recurrent convulsions NOS
Seizure NOS

780.4 Dizziness and giddiness
Light-headedness
Vertigo NOS
EXCLUDES   Ménière's disease and other specified
vertiginous syndromes (386.0-386.9)
DEF: Whirling sensations in head with feeling of falling.

✓5ᵗʰ 780.5 Sleep disturbances
EXCLUDES   circadian rhythm sleep disorders
(327.30-327.39)
organic hypersomnia (327.10-327.19)
organic insomnia (327.00-327.09)
organic sleep apnea (327.20-327.29)
organic sleep related movement disorders
(327.51-327.59)
parasomnias (327.40-327.49)
that of nonorganic origin (307.40-307.49)

780.50 Sleep disturbance, unspecified

780.51 Insomnia with sleep apnea, unspecified
DEF: Transient cessation of breathing disturbing sleep.

780.52 Insomnia, unspecified
DEF: Inability to maintain adequate sleep cycle.

780.53 Hypersomnia with sleep apnea, unspecified
DEF: Autonomic response inhibited during sleep; causes insufficient oxygen intake, acidosis and pulmonary hypertension.

780.54 Hypersomnia, unspecified
DEF: Prolonged sleep cycle.

780.55 Disruptions of 24 hour sleep wake cycle, unspecified

780.56 Dysfunctions associated with sleep stages or arousal from sleep

780.57 Unspecified sleep apnea

780.58 Sleep related movement disorder, unspecified
EXCLUDES   restless legs syndrome (333.94)

780.59 Other

√5ᵗʰ **780.6 Fever and other physiologic disturbances of temperature regulation**

> EXCLUDES   *effects of reduced environmental temperature (991.0-991.9)*
> *effects of heat and light (992.0-992.9)*
> *fever, chills or hypothermia associated with confirmed infection – code to infection*

780.60 Fever, unspecified
Chills with fever
Fever NOS
Fever of unknown origin (FUO)
Hyperpyrexia NOS
Pyrexia NOS
Pyrexia of unknown origin

> EXCLUDES   *chills without fever (780.64)*
> *neonatal fever (778.4)*
> *pyrexia of unknown origin (during):*
> *in newborn (778.4)*
> *labor (659.2)*
> *the puerperium (672)*

780.61 Fever presenting with conditions classified elsewhere
Code first underlying condition when associated fever is present, such as with:
leukemia (conditions classifiable to 204-208)
neutropenia (288.00-288.09)
sickle-cell disease (282.60-282.69)

780.62 Postprocedural fever

> EXCLUDES   *posttransfusion fever (780.66)*
> *postvaccination fever (780.63)*

780.63 Postvaccination fever
Postimmunization fever

780.64 Chills (without fever)
Chills NOS

> EXCLUDES   *chills with fever (780.60)*

780.65 Hypothermia not associated with low environmental temperature

> EXCLUDES   *hypothermia:*
> *associated with low environmental temperature (991.6)*
> *due to anesthesia (995.89)*
> *of newborn (778.2, 778.3)*

780.66 Febrile nonhemolytic transfusion reaction
FNHTR
Posttransfusion fever

√5ᵗʰ **780.7 Malaise and fatigue**

> EXCLUDES   *debility, unspecified (799.3)*
> *fatigue (during):*
> *combat (308.0-308.9)*
> *heat (992.6)*
> *pregnancy (646.8)*
> *neurasthenia (300.5)*
> *senile asthenia (797)*

780.71 Chronic fatigue syndrome
> DEF: Persistent fatigue, symptoms include weak muscles, sore throat, lymphadenitis, headache, depression and mild fever; no known cause; also called chronic mononucleosis, benign myalgic encephalomyelitis, Iceland disease and neurosthenia.

780.72 Functional quadriplegia
Complete immobility due to severe physical disability or frailty

> EXCLUDES   *hysterical paralysis (300.11)*
> *immobility syndrome (728.3)*
> *neurologic quadriplegia (344.00-344.09)*
> *quadriplegia NOS (344.00)*

> DEF: Inability to move due to another condition such as dementia, severe contractures, or arthritis, not a physiologic one; no mental ability to move independently; typically found in severely demented patients.

780.79 Other malaise and fatigue
Asthenia NOS
Lethargy
Postviral (asthenic) syndrome
Tiredness

> DEF: Asthenia: Any weakness, lack of strength or loss of energy, especially neuromuscular.
> DEF: Lethargy: Listlessness, drowsiness, stupor and apathy.
> DEF: Malaise: Vague feeling of debility or lack of good health.
> DEF: Postviral (asthenic) syndrome: Listlessness, drowsiness, stupor and apathy; follows acute viral infection.
> DEF: Tiredness: General exhaustion or fatigue.

780.8 Generalized hyperhidrosis
Diaphoresis
Excessive sweating
Secondary hyperhidrosis

> EXCLUDES   *focal (localized) (primary) (secondary) hyperhidrosis (705.21-705.22)*
> *Frey's syndrome (705.22)*

> DEF: Excessive sweating, appears as droplets on skin; general or localized.

√5ᵗʰ **780.9 Other general symptoms**

> EXCLUDES   *hypothermia:*
> *NOS (accidental) (991.6)*
> *due to anesthesia (995.89)*
> *of newborn (778.2-778.3)*
> *memory disturbance as part of a pattern of mental disorder*

780.91 Fussy infant (baby)

780.92 Excessive crying of infant (baby)

> EXCLUDES   *excessive crying of child, adolescent or adult (780.95)*

780.93 Memory loss
Amnesia (retrograde)
Memory loss NOS

> EXCLUDES   *memory loss due to:*
> *intracranial injuries (850.0-854.19)*
> *skull fractures (800.00-801.99, 803.00-804.99)*
> *mild memory disturbance due to organic brain damage (310.89)*
> *transient global amnesia (437.7)*

780.94 Early satiety
> DEF: The premature feeling of being full; mechanism of satiety is multifactorial.

780.95 Excessive crying of child, adolescent, or adult

> EXCLUDES   *excessive crying of infant (baby) (780.92)*

780.96 Generalized pain
Pain NOS

780.97 Altered mental status
Change in mental status

> EXCLUDES   *altered level of consciousness (780.01-780.09)*
> *altered mental status due to known condition–code to condition*
> *delirium NOS (780.09)*

780.99 Other general symptoms

✓4ᵗʰ **781 Symptoms involving nervous and musculoskeletal systems**

> EXCLUDES   *depression NOS (311)*
> *disorders specifically relating to:*
> > *back (724.0-724.9)*
> > *hearing (388.0-389.9)*
> > *joint (718.0-719.9)*
> > *limb (729.0-729.9)*
> > *neck (723.0-723.9)*
> > *vision (368.0-369.9)*
> > *pain in limb (729.5)*

781.0 Abnormal involuntary movements
Abnormal head movements
Fasciculation
Spasms NOS
Tremor NOS

> EXCLUDES   *abnormal reflex (796.1)*
> *chorea NOS (333.5)*
> *infantile spasms (345.60-345.61)*
> *spastic paralysis (342.1, 343.0-344.9)*
> *specified movement disorders classifiable to 333 (333.0-333.9)*
> *that of nonorganic origin (307.2-307.3)*

781.1 Disturbances of sensation of smell and taste
Anosmia
Parageusia
Parosmia

DEF: Anosmia: loss of sense of smell due to organic factors, including loss of olfactory nerve conductivity, cerebral disease, nasal fossae formation and peripheral olfactory nerve diseases; can also be psychological disorder.

DEF: Parageusia: distorted sense of taste, or bad taste in mouth.

DEF: Parosmia: distorted sense of smell.

781.2 Abnormality of gait
Gait:
> ataxic
> paralytic
> spastic
> staggering

> EXCLUDES   *ataxia:*
> > *NOS (781.3)*
> > *locomotor (progressive) (094.0)*
> *difficulty in walking (719.7)*

DEF: Abnormal, asymmetric gait.

781.3 Lack of coordination
Ataxia NOS
Muscular incoordination

> EXCLUDES   *ataxic gait (781.2)*
> *cerebellar ataxia (334.0-334.9)*
> *difficulty in walking (719.7)*
> *vertigo NOS (780.4)*

781.4 Transient paralysis of limb
Monoplegia, transient NOS

> EXCLUDES   *paralysis (342.0-344.9)*

781.5 Clubbing of fingers

DEF: Enlarged soft tissue of distal fingers.

781.6 Meningismus
Dupré's syndrome
Meningism

DEF: Condition with signs and symptoms that resemble meningeal irritation; it is associated with febrile illness and dehydration with no evidence of infection.

781.7 Tetany
Carpopedal spasm

> EXCLUDES   *tetanus neonatorum (771.3)*
> *tetany:*
> > *hysterical (300.11)*
> > *newborn (hypocalcemic) (775.4)*
> > *parathyroid (252.1)*
> > *psychogenic (306.0)*

DEF: Nerve and muscle hyperexcitability; symptoms include muscle spasms, twitching, cramps, laryngospasm with inspiratory stridor, hyperreflexia and choreiform movements.

781.8 Neurologic neglect syndrome
Asomatognosia	Left-sided neglect
Hemi-akinesia	Sensory extinction
Hemi-inattention	Sensory neglect
Hemispatial neglect	Visuospatial neglect

> EXCLUDES   *visuospatial deficit (799.53)*

✓5ᵗʰ **781.9 Other symptoms involving nervous and musculoskeletal systems**

781.91 Loss of height

> EXCLUDES   *osteoporosis (733.00-733.09)*

781.92 Abnormal posture

781.93 Ocular torticollis

DEF: Abnormal head posture as a result of a contracted state of cervical muscles to correct a visual disturbance; either double vision or a visual field defect.

781.94 Facial weakness
Facial droop

> EXCLUDES   *facial weakness due to late effect of cerebrovascular accident (438.83)*

781.99 Other symptoms involving nervous and musculoskeletal systems

✓4ᵗʰ **782 Symptoms involving skin and other integumentary tissue**

> EXCLUDES   *symptoms relating to breast (611.71-611.79)*

782.0 Disturbance of skin sensation
Anesthesia of skin
Burning or prickling sensation
Hyperesthesia
Hypoesthesia
Numbness
Paresthesia
Tingling

782.1 Rash and other nonspecific skin eruption
Exanthem

> EXCLUDES   *vesicular eruption (709.8)*

782.2 Localized superficial swelling, mass, or lump
Subcutaneous nodules

> EXCLUDES   *localized adiposity (278.1)*

782.3 Edema
Anasarca	Localized edema NOS
Dropsy	

> EXCLUDES   *ascites (789.51-789.59)*
> *edema of:*
> > *newborn NOS (778.5)*
> > *pregnancy (642.0-642.9, 646.1)*
> *fluid retention (276.69)*
> *hydrops fetalis (773.3, 778.0)*
> *hydrothorax (511.81-511.89)*
> *nutritional edema (260, 262)*

DEF: Edema: excess fluid in intercellular body tissue.

DEF: Anasarca: massive edema in all body tissues.

DEF: Dropsy: serous fluid accumulated in body cavity or cellular tissue.

DEF: Localized edema: edema in specific body areas.

782.4 Jaundice, unspecified, not of newborn
Cholemia NOS
Icterus NOS

> EXCLUDES   *jaundice in newborn (774.0-774.7)*
> > *due to isoimmunization (773.0-773.2, 773.4)*

DEF: Bilirubin deposits of skin, causing yellow cast.

782.5 Cyanosis

> EXCLUDES   *newborn (770.83)*

DEF: Deficient oxygen of blood; causes blue cast to skin.

✓5ᵗʰ **782.6 Pallor and flushing**

782.61 Pallor

782.62 Flushing
Excessive blushing

782.7　Spontaneous ecchymoses
Petechiae
EXCLUDES　ecchymosis in fetus or newborn (772.6)
　　　purpura (287.0-287.9)
DEF: Hemorrhagic spots of skin; resemble freckles.

782.8　Changes in skin texture
Induration　⎫
Thickening　⎬ of skin
　　　　　⎭

782.9　Other symptoms involving skin and integumentary tissues

✓4ᵗʰ **783　Symptoms concerning nutrition, metabolism, and development**

783.0　Anorexia
Loss of appetite
EXCLUDES　anorexia nervosa (307.1)
　　　loss of appetite of nonorganic origin (307.59)

783.1　Abnormal weight gain
EXCLUDES　excessive weight gain in pregnancy (646.1)
　　　obesity (278.00)
　　　　　morbid (278.01)

✓5ᵗʰ **783.2　Abnormal loss of weight and underweight**
Use additional code to identify Body Mass Index (BMI), if known (V85.0-V85.54)

　783.21　Loss of weight

　783.22　Underweight

783.3　Feeding difficulties and mismanagement
Feeding problem (elderly) (infant)
EXCLUDES　feeding disturbance or problems:
　　　in newborn (779.31-779.34)
　　　of nonorganic origin (307.50-307.59)

✓5ᵗʰ **783.4　Lack of expected normal physiological development in childhood**
EXCLUDES　delay in sexual development and puberty (259.0)
　　　gonadal dysgenesis (758.6)
　　　pituitary dwarfism (253.3)
　　　slow fetal growth and fetal malnutrition (764.00-764.99)
　　　specific delays in mental development (315.0-315.9)

　783.40　Lack of normal physiological development, unspecified
　　Inadequate development
　　Lack of development

　783.41　Failure to thrive
　　Failure to gain weight
　　EXCLUDES　failure to thrive in newborn (779.34)
　　DEF: Organic failure to thrive: acute or chronic illness that interferes with nutritional intake, absorption, metabolism excretion and energy requirements. Nonorganic FTT is symptom of neglect or abuse.

　783.42　Delayed milestones
　　Late talker
　　Late walker

　783.43　Short stature
　　Growth failure　　　Lack of growth
　　Growth retardation　Physical retardation
　　DEF: Constitutional short stature: stature inconsistent with chronological age. Genetic short stature is when skeletal maturation matches chronological age.

783.5　Polydipsia
Excessive thirst

783.6　Polyphagia
Excessive eating
Hyperalimentation NOS
EXCLUDES　disorders of eating of nonorganic origin (307.50-307.59)

783.7　Adult failure to thrive

783.9　Other symptoms concerning nutrition, metabolism, and development
Hypometabolism
EXCLUDES　abnormal basal metabolic rate (794.7)
　　　dehydration (276.51)
　　　other disorders of fluid, electrolyte, and acid-base balance (276.0-276.9)

✓4ᵗʰ **784　Symptoms involving head and neck**
EXCLUDES　encephalopathy NOS (348.30)
　　　specific symptoms involving neck classifiable to 723 (723.0-723.9)

784.0　Headache
Facial pain
Pain in head NOS
EXCLUDES　atypical face pain (350.2)
　　　migraine (346.0-346.9)
　　　tension headache (307.81)

784.1　Throat pain
EXCLUDES　dysphagia (787.20-787.29)
　　　neck pain (723.1)
　　　sore throat (462)
　　　　chronic (472.1)

784.2　Swelling, mass, or lump in head and neck
Space-occupying lesion, intracranial NOS

784.3　Aphasia
EXCLUDES　aphasia due to late effects of cerebrovascular disease (438.11)
　　　developmental aphasia (315.31)
DEF: Inability to communicate through speech, written word, or sign language.

✓5ᵗʰ **784.4　Voice and resonance disorders**

　784.40　Voice and resonance disorder, unspecified

　784.41　Aphonia
　　Loss of voice

　784.42　Dysphonia
　　Hoarseness

　784.43　Hypernasality

　784.44　Hyponasality

　784.49　Other voice and resonance disorders
　　Change in voice

✓5ᵗʰ **784.5　Other speech disturbance**
EXCLUDES　speech disorder due to late effect of cerebrovascular accident (438.10-438.19)
　　　stuttering (315.35)

　784.51　Dysarthria
　　EXCLUDES　dysarthria due to late effect of cerebrovascular accident (438.13)

　784.52　Fluency disorder in conditions classified elsewhere
　　Stuttering in conditions classified elsewhere
　　Code first underlying disease or condition, such as:
　　Parkinson's disease (332.0)
　　EXCLUDES　adult onset fluency disorder (307.0)
　　　childhood onset fluency disorder (315.35)
　　　fluency disorder due to late effect of cerebrovascular accident (438.14)

　784.59　Other speech disturbance
　　Dysphasia
　　Slurred speech
　　Speech disturbance NOS

✓5ᵗʰ **784.6　Other symbolic dysfunction**
EXCLUDES　developmental learning delays (315.0-315.9)

　784.60　Symbolic dysfunction, unspecified

784.61 Alexia and dyslexia
Alexia (with agraphia)
DEF: Alexia: Inability to understand written word due to central brain lesion.
DEF: Dyslexia: Ability to recognize letters but inability to read, spell, and write words; genetic.

784.69 Other
Acalculia   Agraphia NOS
Agnosia   Apraxia

784.7 Epistaxis
Hemorrhage from nose   Nosebleed

784.8 Hemorrhage from throat
    EXCLUDES hemoptysis (786.30-786.39)

√5ᵗʰ **784.9 Other symptoms involving head and neck**

784.91 Postnasal drip

784.92 Jaw pain
Mandibular pain
Maxilla pain
    EXCLUDES temporomandibular joint arthralgia (524.62)

784.99 Other symptoms involving head and neck
Choking sensation
Feeling of foreign body in throat
Halitosis
Mouth breathing
Sneezing
    EXCLUDES foreign body in throat (933.0)

√4ᵗʰ **785 Symptoms involving cardiovascular system**
    EXCLUDES heart failure NOS (428.9)

785.0 Tachycardia, unspecified
Rapid heart beat
    EXCLUDES neonatal tachycardia (779.82)
             paroxysmal tachycardia (427.0-427.2)
DEF: Excessively rapid heart rate.

785.1 Palpitations
Awareness of heart beat
    EXCLUDES specified dysrhythmias (427.0-427.9)

785.2 Undiagnosed cardiac murmurs
Heart murmurs NOS

785.3 Other abnormal heart sounds
Cardiac dullness, increased or decreased
Friction fremitus, cardiac
Precordial friction

785.4 Gangrene
Gangrene:
    NOS
    spreading cutaneous
Gangrenous cellulitis
Phagedena
Code first any associated underlying condition
    EXCLUDES gangrene of certain sites – see Alphabetic Index
             gangrene with atherosclerosis of the extremities (440.24)
             gas gangrene (040.0
DEF: Gangrene: necrosis of skin tissue due to bacterial infection, diabetes, embolus and vascular supply loss.
DEF: Gangrenous cellulitis: group A streptococcal infection; begins with severe cellulitis, spreads to superficial and deep fascia; produces gangrene of underlying tissues.

√5ᵗʰ **785.5 Shock without mention of trauma**

785.50 Shock, unspecified
Failure of peripheral circulation
DEF: Peripheral circulatory failure due to heart insufficiencies.

785.51 Cardiogenic shock
DEF: Shock syndrome: associated with myocardial infarction, cardiac tamponade and massive pulmonary embolism; symptoms include mental confusion, reduced blood pressure, tachycardia, pallor and cold, clammy skin.

785.52 Septic shock
Shock:
    endotoxic
    gram-negative
Code first underlying infection
Use additional code, if applicable, to identify systemic inflammatory response syndrome due to infectious process with organ dysfunction (995.92)

785.59 Other
Shock:
    hypovolemic
    EXCLUDES shock (due to):
             anesthetic (995.4)
             anaphylactic (995.0)
                due to serum (999.41-999.49)
             electric (994.8)
             following abortion (639.5)
             lightning (994.0)
             obstetrical (669.1)
             postoperative (998.00-998.09)
             traumatic (958.4)

785.6 Enlargement of lymph nodes
Lymphadenopathy
"Swollen glands"
    EXCLUDES lymphadenitis (chronic) (289.1-289.3)
             acute (683)

785.9 Other symptoms involving cardiovascular system
Bruit (arterial)
Weak pulse

√4ᵗʰ **786 Symptoms involving respiratory system and other chest symptoms**

√5ᵗʰ **786.0 Dyspnea and respiratory abnormalities**

786.00 Respiratory abnormality, unspecified

786.01 Hyperventilation
    EXCLUDES hyperventilation, psychogenic (306.1)
DEF: Rapid breathing causes carbon dioxide loss from blood.

786.02 Orthopnea
DEF: Difficulty breathing except in upright position.

786.03 Apnea
    EXCLUDES apnea of newborn (770.81, 770.82)
             sleep apnea (780.51, 780.53, 780.57)
DEF: Cessation of breathing.

786.04 Cheyne-Stokes respiration
DEF: Rhythmic increase of depth and frequency of breathing with apnea; occurs in frontal lobe and diencephalic dysfunction.

786.05 Shortness of breath
DEF: Inability to take in sufficient oxygen.

786.06 Tachypnea
    EXCLUDES transitory tachypnea of newborn (770.6)
DEF: Abnormal rapid respiratory rate; called hyperventilation.

786.07 Wheezing
    EXCLUDES asthma (493.00-493.92)
DEF: Stenosis of respiratory passageway; causes whistling sound; due to asthma, coryza, croup, emphysema, hay fever, edema, and pleural effusion.

Symptoms, Signs, and Ill-Defined Conditions

786.09–787.61

786.09 **Other**
Respiratory:
  distress
  insufficiency
    EXCLUDES   *respiratory distress:*
        following trauma and surgery
          (518.52)
        newborn (770.89)
        syndrome (newborn) (769)
          adult (518.52)
        respiratory failure (518.81,
          518.83-518.84)
        newborn (770.84)

786.1 **Stridor**
    EXCLUDES   *congenital laryngeal stridor (748.3)*
  DEF: Obstructed airway causes harsh sound.

786.2 **Cough**
    EXCLUDES   *cough:*
        psychogenic (306.1)
        smokers' (491.0)
        with hemorrhage (786.39)

√5ᵗʰ 786.3 **Hemoptysis**
  DEF: Coughing up blood or blood-stained sputum.

786.30 **Hemoptysis, unspecified**
Pulmonary hemorrhage NOS

786.31 **Acute idiopathic pulmonary hemorrhage in infants [AIPHI]**
Acute idiopathic pulmonary hemorrhage in infant over 28 days old
    EXCLUDES   *pulmonary hemorrhage of newborn*
        under 28 days old (770.3)
        von Willebrand's disease (286.4)
  DEF: An abrupt onset of bleeding or blood in the airway with acute respiratory distress or failure in a patient with no prior history of an identifiable causal condition.

786.39 **Other hemoptysis**
Cough with hemorrhage

786.4 **Abnormal sputum**
Abnormal:
  amount
  color   } sputum
  odor
Excessive septum

√5ᵗʰ 786.5 **Chest pain**

786.50 **Chest pain, unspecified**

786.51 **Precordial pain**
  DEF: Chest pain over heart and lower thorax.

786.52 **Painful respiration**
Pain:
  anterior chest wall
  pleuritic
Pleurodynia
    EXCLUDES   *epidemic pleurodynia (074.1)*

786.59 **Other**
Discomfort
Pressure   } in chest
Tightness
    EXCLUDES   *pain in breast (611.71)*

786.6 **Swelling, mass, or lump in chest**
    EXCLUDES   *lump in breast (611.72)*

786.7 **Abnormal chest sounds**
Abnormal percussion, chest
Friction sounds, chest
Rales
Tympany, chest
    EXCLUDES   *wheezing (786.07)*

786.8 **Hiccough**
    EXCLUDES   *psychogenic hiccough (306.1)*

786.9 **Other symptoms involving respiratory system and chest**
Breath-holding spell

√4ᵗʰ 787 **Symptoms involving digestive system**
    EXCLUDES   *constipation (564.00-564.09)*
        pylorospasm (537.81)
          congenital (750.5)

√5ᵗʰ 787.0 **Nausea and vomiting**
Emesis
    EXCLUDES   *hematemesis NOS (578.0)*
        vomiting:
          bilious, following gastrointestinal surgery
            (564.3)
          cyclical (536.2)
            associated with migraine (346.2)
            psychogenic (306.4)
          excessive, in pregnancy (643.0-643.9)
          fecal matter (569.87)
          habit (536.2)
          of newborn (779.32, 779.33)
          persistent (536.2)
          psychogenic NOS (307.54)

787.01 **Nausea with vomiting**

787.02 **Nausea alone**

787.03 **Vomiting alone**

787.04 **Bilious emesis**
Bilious vomiting
    EXCLUDES   *bilious emesis (vomiting) in*
        newborn (779.32)

787.1 **Heartburn**
Pyrosis
Waterbrash
    EXCLUDES   *dyspepsia or indigestion (536.8)*

√5ᵗʰ 787.2 **Dysphagia**
Code first, if applicable, dysphagia due to late effect of cerebrovascular accident (438.82)

787.20 **Dysphagia, unspecified**
Difficulty in swallowing NOS

787.21 **Dysphagia, oral phase**

787.22 **Dysphagia, oropharyngeal phase**

787.23 **Dysphagia, pharyngeal phase**

787.24 **Dysphagia, pharyngoesophageal phase**

787.29 **Other dysphagia**
Cervical dysphagia
Neurogenic dysphagia

787.3 **Flatulence, eructation, and gas pain**
Abdominal distention (gaseous)
Bloating
Tympanites (abdominal) (intestinal)
    EXCLUDES   *aerophagy (306.4)*
  DEF: Flatulence: excess air or gas in intestine or stomach.
  DEF: Eructation: belching, expelling gas through mouth.
  DEF: Gas pain: gaseous pressure affecting gastrointestinal system.

787.4 **Visible peristalsis**
Hyperperistalsis
  DEF: Increase in involuntary movements of intestines.

787.5 **Abnormal bowel sounds**
Absent bowel sounds
Hyperactive bowel sounds

√5ᵗʰ 787.6 **Incontinence of feces**
Encopresis NOS
Incontinence of sphincter ani
    EXCLUDES   *that of nonorganic origin (307.7)*

787.60 **Full incontinence of feces**
Fecal incontinence NOS

787.61 **Incomplete defecation**
    EXCLUDES   *constipation (564.00-564.09)*
        fecal impaction (560.32)

Phases of Swallowing

Oral phase

Oropharyngeal phase

Pharyngeal phase

Pharyngeoesophageal phase

787.62 Fecal smearing
Fecal soiling

787.63 Fecal urgency

787.7 Abnormal feces
Bulky stools
EXCLUDES *abnormal stool content (792.1)*
melena:
NOS (578.1)
newborn (772.4, 777.3)

√5ᵗʰ **787.9 Other symptoms involving digestive system**
EXCLUDES *gastrointestinal hemorrhage (578.0-578.9)*
intestinal obstruction (560.0-560.9)
specific functional digestive disorders:
esophagus (530.0-530.9)
stomach and duodenum (536.0-536.9)
those not elsewhere classified
(564.00-564.9)

787.91 Diarrhea
Diarrhea NOS

787.99 Other
Change in bowel habits
Tenesmus (rectal)
DEF: Tenesmus: Painful, ineffective straining at the rectum with limited passage of fecal matter.

√4ᵗʰ **788 Symptoms involving urinary system**
EXCLUDES *hematuria (599.70-599.72)*
nonspecific findings on examination of the urine (791.0-791.9)
small kidney of unknown cause (589.0-589.9)
uremia NOS (586)
urinary obstruction (599.60, 599.69)

788.0 Renal colic
Colic (recurrent) of:
kidney
ureter
DEF: Kidney pain.

788.1 Dysuria
Painful urination
Strangury

√5ᵗʰ **788.2 Retention of urine**
Code, if applicable, any causal condition first, such as:
hyperplasia of prostate (600.0-600.9 with fifth-digit 1)
DEF: Accumulation of urine in the bladder due to inability to void.

788.20 Retention of urine, unspecified

788.21 Incomplete bladder emptying

788.29 Other specified retention of urine

√5ᵗʰ **788.3 Urinary incontinence**
Code, if applicable, any causal condition first, such as:
congenital ureterocele (753.23)
genital prolapse (618.00-618.9)
hyperplasia of prostate (600.0-600.9 with fifth-digit 1)
EXCLUDES *functional urinary incontinence (788.91)*
that of nonorganic origin (307.6)
urinary incontinence associated with cognitive impairment (788.91)

788.30 Urinary incontinence, unspecified
Enuresis NOS

788.31 Urge incontinence
DEF: Inability to control urination, upon urge to urinate.

788.32 Stress incontinence, male
EXCLUDES *stress incontinence, female (625.6)*
DEF: Inability to control urination associated with weak sphincter in males.

788.33 Mixed incontinence, (male) (female)
Urge and stress
DEF: Urge, stress incontinence: involuntary discharge of urine due to anatomic displacement.

788.34 Incontinence without sensory awareness
DEF: Involuntary discharge of urine without sensory warning.

788.35 Post-void dribbling
DEF: Involuntary discharge of residual urine after voiding.

788.36 Nocturnal enuresis
DEF: Involuntary discharge of urine during the night.

788.37 Continuous leakage
DEF: Continuous, involuntary urine seepage.

788.38 Overflow incontinence
DEF: Leakage caused by pressure of retained urine in the bladder after the bladder has fully contracted due to weakened bladder muscles or an obstruction of the urethra.

788.39 Other urinary incontinence

√5ᵗʰ **788.4 Frequency of urination and polyuria**
Code, if applicable, any causal condition first, such as:
hyperplasia of prostate (600.0-600.9 with fifth-digit 1)

788.41 Urinary frequency
Frequency of micturition

788.42 Polyuria
DEF: Excessive urination.

788.43 Nocturia
DEF: Urination affecting sleep patterns.

788.5 Oliguria and anuria
Deficient secretion of urine
Suppression of urinary secretion
EXCLUDES *that complicating:*
abortion (634-638 with .3, 639.3)
ectopic or molar pregnancy (639.3)
pregnancy, childbirth, or the puerperium (642.0-642.9, 646.2)
DEF: Oliguria: diminished urinary secretion related to fluid intake.
DEF: Anuria: lack of urinary secretion due to renal failure or obstructed urinary tract.

√5ᵗʰ **788.6 Other abnormality of urination**
Code, if applicable, any causal condition first, such as:
hyperplasia of prostate (600.0-600.9 with fifth-digit 1)

788.61 Splitting of urinary stream
Intermittent urinary stream

788.62 Slowing of urinary stream
Weak stream

Symptoms, Signs, and Ill-Defined Conditions

788.63–790.5

788.63 Urgency of urination
> *EXCLUDES* urge incontinence (788.31, 788.33)
>
> **DEF:** Feeling of intense need to urinate; abrupt sensation of imminent urination.

788.64 Urinary hesitancy

788.65 Straining on urination

788.69 Other

788.7 Urethral discharge
> Penile discharge
> Urethrorrhea

788.8 Extravasation of urine
> **DEF:** Leaking or infiltration of urine into tissues.

√5ᵗʰ **788.9 Other symptoms involving urinary system**

788.91 Functional urinary incontinence
> Urinary incontinence due to cognitive impairment, or severe physical disability or immobility
> *EXCLUDES* urinary incontinence due to physiologic condition (788.30-788.39)

788.99 Other symptoms involving urinary system
> Extrarenal uremia   Vesical:
> Vesical: tenesmus
>   pain

√4ᵗʰ **789 Other symptoms involving abdomen and pelvis**
> *EXCLUDES* symptoms referable to genital organs:
> female (625.0-625.9)
> male (607.0-608.9)
> psychogenic (302.70-302.79))

> The following fifth-digit subclassification is to be used for codes 789.0. 789.3, 789.4, 789.6:
> **0 unspecified site**
> **1 right upper quadrant**
> **2 left upper quadrant**
> **3 right lower quadrant**
> **4 left lower quadrant**
> **5 periumbilic**
> **6 epigastric**
> **7 generalized**
> **9 other specified site**
>   Multiple sites

√5ᵗʰ **789.0 Abdominal pain**
[0-7, 9]   Cramps, abdominal

789.1 Hepatomegaly
> Enlargement of liver

789.2 Splenomegaly
> Enlargement of spleen

√5ᵗʰ **789.3 Abdominal or pelvic swelling, mass, or lump**
[0-7, 9]   Diffuse or generalized swelling or mass:
> abdominal NOS
> umbilical
> *EXCLUDES* abdominal distention (gaseous) (787.3)
> ascites (789.51-789.59)

√5ᵗʰ **789.4 Abdominal rigidity**
[0-7, 9]

√5ᵗʰ **789.5 Ascites**
> Fluid in peritoneal cavity
> **DEF:** Serous fluid effusion and accumulation in abdominal cavity.

789.51 Malignant ascites
> Code first malignancy, such as:
> malignant neoplasm of ovary (183.0)
> secondary malignant neoplasm of retroperitoneum and peritoneum (197.6)

789.59 Other ascites

√5ᵗʰ **789.6 Abdominal tenderness**
[0-7, 9]   Rebound tenderness

789.7 Colic
> Colic NOS
> Infantile colic
> *EXCLUDES* colic in adult and child over 12 months old (789.0)
> renal colic (788.0)

789.9 Other symptoms involving abdomen and pelvis
> Umbilical: Umbilical:
> bleeding   discharge

NONSPECIFIC ABNORMAL FINDINGS (790-796)

√4ᵗʰ **790 Nonspecific findings on examination of blood**
> *EXCLUDES* abnormality of:
> platelets (287.0-287.9)
> thrombocytes (287.0-287.9)
> white blood cells (288.00-288.9)

√5ᵗʰ **790.0 Abnormality of red blood cells**
> *EXCLUDES* anemia:
> congenital (776.5)
> newborn, due to isoimmunization (773.0-773.2, 773.5)
> of premature infant (776.6)
> other specified types (280.0-285.9)
> hemoglobin disorders (282.5-282.7)
> polycythemia:
> familial (289.6)
> neonatorum (776.4)
> secondary (289.0)
> vera (238.4)

790.01 Precipitous drop in hematocrit
> Drop in hematocrit
> Drop in hemoglobin

790.09 Other abnormality of red blood cells
> Abnormal red cell morphology NOS
> Abnormal red cell volume NOS
> Anisocytosis
> Poikilocytosis

790.1 Elevated sedimentation rate

√5ᵗʰ **790.2 Abnormal glucose**
> *EXCLUDES* diabetes mellitus (249.00-249.91, 250.00-250.93)
> dysmetabolic syndrome X (277.7)
> gestational diabetes (648.8)
> glycosuria (791.5)
> hypoglycemia (251.2)
> that complicating pregnancy, childbirth, or puerperium (648.8)

790.21 Impaired fasting glucose
> Elevated fasting glucose

790.22 Impaired glucose tolerance test (oral)
> Elevated glucose tolerance test

790.29 Other abnormal glucose
> Abnormal glucose NOS
> Abnormal non-fasting glucose
> Hyperglycemia NOS
> Pre-diabetes NOS

790.3 Excessive blood level of alcohol
> Elevated blood-alcohol

790.4 Nonspecific elevation of levels of transaminase or lactic acid dehydrogenase [LDH]

790.5 Other nonspecific abnormal serum enzyme levels
> Abnormal serum level of:
> acid phosphatase
> alkaline phosphatase
> amylase
> lipase
> *EXCLUDES* deficiency of circulating enzymes (277.6)

790.6   Other abnormal blood chemistry

Abnormal blood level of: Abnormal blood level of:
cobalt   lithium
copper   magnesium
iron   mineral
lead   zinc

> EXCLUDES   abnormality of electrolyte or acid-base
> balance (276.0-276.9)
> hypoglycemia NOS (251.2)
> lead poisoning (984.0-984.9)
> specific finding indicating abnormality of:
> amino-acid transport and metabolism
> (270.0-270.9)
> carbohydrate transport and metabolism
> (271.0-271.9)
> lipid metabolism (272.0-272.9)
> uremia NOS (586)

790.7   Bacteremia

> EXCLUDES   bacteremia of newborn (771.83)
> septicemia (038)

Use additional code to identify organism (041)

DEF: Laboratory finding of bacteria in the blood in the absence of two or more signs of sepsis; transient in nature, progresses to septicemia with severe infectious process.

790.8   Viremia, unspecified

DEF: Presence of a virus in the blood stream.

√5th **790.9   Other nonspecific findings on examination of blood**

790.91   Abnormal arterial blood gases

790.92   Abnormal coagulation profile

Abnormal or prolonged:
bleeding time
coagulation time
partial thromboplastin time [PTT]
prothrombin time [PT]

> EXCLUDES   coagulation (hemorrhagic)
> disorders (286.0-286.9)

790.93   Elevated prostate specific antigen, [PSA]

790.94   Euthyroid sick syndrome

DEF: Transient alteration of thyroid hormone metabolism due to nonthyroid illness or stress.

790.95   Elevated C-reactive protein [CRP]

DEF: Inflammation in an arterial wall results in elevated C-reactive protein (CRP) in the blood; CRP is a recognized risk factor in cardiovascular disease.

790.99   Other

√4th **791   Nonspecific findings on examination of urine**

> EXCLUDES   hematuria NOS (599.70-599.72)
> specific findings indicating abnormality of:
> amino-acid transport and metabolism (270.0-270.9)
> carbohydrate transport and metabolism
> (271.0-271.9)

791.0   Proteinuria

Albuminuria   Bence-Jones proteinuria

> EXCLUDES   postural proteinuria (593.6)
> that arising during pregnancy or the
> puerperium (642.0-642.9, 646.2)

DEF: Excess protein in urine.

791.1   Chyluria

> EXCLUDES   filarial (125.0-125.9)

DEF: Excess chyle in urine.

791.2   Hemoglobinuria

DEF: Free hemoglobin in blood due to rapid hemolysis of red blood cells.

791.3   Myoglobinuria

DEF: Myoglobin (oxygen-transporting pigment) in urine.

791.4   Biliuria

DEF: Bile pigments in urine.

791.5   Glycosuria

> EXCLUDES   renal glycosuria (271.4)

DEF: Sugar in urine.

791.6   Acetonuria

Ketonuria

DEF: Excess acetone in urine.

791.7   Other cells and casts in urine

791.9   Other nonspecific findings on examination of urine

Crystalluria
Elevated urine levels of:
17-ketosteroids
catecholamines
indolacetic acid
vanillylmandelic acid [VMA]
Melanuria

√4th **792   Nonspecific abnormal findings in other body substances**

> EXCLUDES   that in chromosomal analysis (795.2)

792.0   Cerebrospinal fluid

792.1   Stool contents

Abnormal stool color   Occult stool
Fat in stool   Pus in stool
Mucus in stool

> EXCLUDES   blood in stool [melena] (578.1)
> newborn (772.4, 777.3)

792.2   Semen

Abnormal spermatozoa

> EXCLUDES   azoospermia (606.0)
> oligospermia (606.1)

792.3   Amniotic fluid

DEF: Nonspecific abnormal findings in amniotic fluid.

792.4   Saliva

> EXCLUDES   that in chromosomal analysis (795.2)

792.5   Cloudy (hemodialysis) (peritoneal) dialysis effluent

792.9   Other nonspecific abnormal findings in body substances

Peritoneal fluid   Synovial fluid
Pleural fluid   Vaginal fluids

√4th **793   Nonspecific (abnormal) findings on radiological and other examination of body structure**

> INCLUDES   nonspecific abnormal findings of:
> thermography
> ultrasound examination [echogram]
> x-ray examination

> EXCLUDES   abnormal results of function studies and radioisotope
> scans (794.0-794.9)

793.0   Skull and head

> EXCLUDES   nonspecific abnormal echoencephalogram
> (794.01)

√5th **793.1   Lung field**

793.11   Solitary pulmonary nodule

Coin lesion lung
Solitary pulmonary nodule, subsegmental
branch of the bronchial tree

793.19   Other nonspecific abnormal finding of lung field

Pulmonary infiltrate NOS
Shadow, lung

793.2   Other intrathoracic organ

Abnormal:
echocardiogram
heart shadow
ultrasound cardiogram
Mediastinal shift

793.3   Biliary tract

Nonvisualization of gallbladder

793.4   Gastrointestinal tract

793.5   Genitourinary organs

Filling defect:
bladder
kidney
ureter

793.6   Abdominal area, including retroperitoneum

793.7   Musculoskeletal system

Symptoms, Signs, and Ill-Defined Conditions

793.8–795.07

√5ᵗʰ **793.8 Breast**

793.80 Abnormal mammogram, unspecified

793.81 Mammographic microcalcification

EXCLUDES   *mammographic calcification (793.89)*
mammographic calculus (793.89)

DEF: Calcium and cellular debris deposits in the breast that cannot be felt but can be detected on a mammogram; can be a sign of cancer, benign conditions, or changes in the breast tissue as a result of inflammation, injury, or obstructed duct.

793.82 Inconclusive mammogram
Dense breasts NOS
Inconclusive mammogram NEC
Inconclusive mammography due to dense breasts
Inconclusive mammography NEC

793.89 Other (abnormal) findings on radiological examination of breast
Mammographic calcification
Mammographic calculus

√5ᵗʰ **793.9 Other**

EXCLUDES   *abnormal finding by radioisotope localization of placenta (794.9)*

793.91 Image test inconclusive due to excess body fat
Use additional code to identify Body Mass Index (BMI), if known (V85.0-V85.54)

793.99 Other nonspecific (abnormal) findings on radiological and other examinations of body structure
Abnormal:
placental finding by x-ray or ultrasound method
radiological findings in skin and subcutaneous tissue

√4ᵗʰ **794 Nonspecific abnormal results of function studies**

INCLUDES   radioisotope:
scans
uptake studies
scintiphotography

√5ᵗʰ **794.0 Brain and central nervous system**

794.00 Abnormal function study, unspecified

794.01 Abnormal echoencephalogram

794.02 Abnormal electroencephalogram [EEG]

794.09 Other
Abnormal brain scan

√5ᵗʰ **794.1 Peripheral nervous system and special senses**

794.10 Abnormal response to nerve stimulation, unspecified

794.11 Abnormal retinal function studies
Abnormal electroretinogram [ERG]

794.12 Abnormal electro-oculogram [EOG]

794.13 Abnormal visually evoked potential

794.14 Abnormal oculomotor studies

794.15 Abnormal auditory function studies

794.16 Abnormal vestibular function studies

794.17 Abnormal electromyogram [EMG]

EXCLUDES   *that of eye (794.14)*

794.19 Other

794.2 Pulmonary
Abnormal lung scan
Reduced:
ventilatory capacity
vital capacity

√5ᵗʰ **794.3 Cardiovascular**

794.30 Abnormal function study, unspecified

794.31 Abnormal electrocardiogram [ECG] [EKG]

EXCLUDES   *long QT syndrome (426.82)*

794.39 Other
Abnormal:
ballistocardiogram
phonocardiogram
vectorcardiogram

794.4 Kidney
Abnormal renal function test

794.5 Thyroid
Abnormal thyroid:
scan
uptake

794.6 Other endocrine function study

794.7 Basal metabolism
Abnormal basal metabolic rate [BMR]

794.8 Liver
Abnormal liver scan

794.9 Other
Bladder
Pancreas
Placenta
Spleen

√4ᵗʰ **795 Other and nonspecific abnormal cytological, histological, immunological and DNA test findings**

EXCLUDES   *abnormal cytologic smear of anus and anal HPV (796.70-796.79)*
nonspecific abnormalities of red blood cells (790.01-790.09)

√5ᵗʰ **795.0 Abnormal Papanicolaou smear of cervix and cervical HPV**
Abnormal thin preparation smear of cervix
Abnormal cervical cytology

EXCLUDES   *abnormal cytologic smear of vagina and vaginal HPV (795.10-795.19)*
carcinoma in situ of cervix (233.1)
cervical intraepithelial neoplasia I (CIN I) (622.11)
cervical intraepithelial neoplasia II (CIN II) (622.12)
cervical intraepithelial neoplasia III (CIN III) (233.1)
dysplasia (histologically confirmed) of cervix (uteri) NOS (622.10)
mild cervical dysplasia (histologically confirmed) (622.11)
moderate cervical dysplasia (histologically confirmed) (622.12)
severe cervical dysplasia (histologically confirmed) (233.1)

795.00 Abnormal glandular Papanicolaou smear of cervix
Atypical endocervical cells NOS
Atypical endometrial cells NOS
Atypical cervical glandular cells NOS

795.01 Papanicolaou smear of cervix with atypical squamous cells of undetermined significance [ASC-US]

795.02 Papanicolaou smear of cervix with atypical squamous cells cannot exclude high grade squamous intraepithelial lesion [ASC-H]

795.03 Papanicolaou smear of cervix with low grade squamous intraepithelial lesion [LGSIL]

795.04 Papanicolaou smear of cervix with high grade squamous intraepithelial lesion [HGSIL]

795.05 Cervical high risk human papillomavirus [HPV] DNA test positive

795.06 Papanicolaou smear of cervix with cytologic evidence of malignancy

795.07 Satisfactory cervical smear but lacking transformation zone

795.08 Unsatisfactory cervical cytology smear
Inadequate cervical cytology sample

795.09 Other abnormal Papanicolaou smear of cervix and cervical HPV
Cervical low risk human papillomavirus (HPV) DNA test positive
Use additional code for associated human papillomavirus (079.4)

> **EXCLUDES** encounter for Papanicolaou cervical smear to confirm findings of recent normal smear following initial abnormal smear (V72.32)

√5ᵗʰ **795.1 Abnormal Papanicolaou smear of vagina and vaginal HPV**
Abnormal thin preparation smear of vagina NOS
Abnormal vaginal cytology NOS
Use additional code to identify acquired absence of uterus and cervix, if applicable (V88.01-V88.03)

> **EXCLUDES** abnormal cytologic smear of cervix and cervical HPV (795.00-795.09)
> carcinoma in situ of vagina (233.31)
> carcinoma in situ of vulva (233.32)
> dysplasia (histologically confirmed) of vagina NOS (623.0, 233.31)
> dysplasia (histologically confirmed) of vulva NOS (624.01, 624.02, 233.32)
> mild vaginal dysplasia (histologically confirmed) (623.0)
> mild vulvar dysplasia (histologically confirmed) (624.01)
> moderate vaginal dysplasia (histologically confirmed) (623.0)
> moderate vulvar dysplasia (histologically confirmed) (624.02)
> severe vaginal dysplasia (histologically confirmed) (233.31)
> severe vulvar dysplasia (histologically confirmed) (233.32)
> vaginal intraepithelial neoplasia I (VAIN I) (623.0)
> vaginal intraepithelial neoplasia II (VAIN II) (623.0)
> vaginal intraepithelial neoplasia III (VAIN III) (233.31)
> vulvar intraepithelial neoplasia I (VIN I) (624.01)
> vulvar intraepithelial neoplasia II (VIN II) (624.02)
> vulvar intraepithelial neoplasia III (VIN III) (233.32)

795.10 Abnormal glandular Papanicolaou smear of vagina
Atypical vaginal glandular cells NOS

795.11 Papanicolaou smear of vagina with atypical squamous cells of undetermined significance [ASC-US]

795.12 Papanicolaou smear of vagina with atypical squamous cells cannot exclude high grade squamous intraepithelial lesion [ASC-H]

795.13 Papanicolaou smear of vagina with low grade squamous intraepithelial lesion [LGSIL]

795.14 Papanicolaou smear of vagina with high grade squamous intraepithelial lesion [HGSIL]

795.15 Vaginal high risk human papillomavirus [HPV] DNA test positive

> **EXCLUDES** condyloma acuminatum (078.11)
> genital warts (078.11)

795.16 Papanicolaou smear of vagina with cytologic evidence of malignancy

795.18 Unsatisfactory vaginal cytology smear
Inadequate vaginal cytology sample

795.19 Other abnormal Papanicolaou smear of vagina and vaginal HPV
Vaginal low risk human papillomavirus (HPV) DNA test positive
Use additional code for associated human papillomavirus (079.4)

795.2 Nonspecific abnormal findings on chromosomal analysis
Abnormal karyotype

√5ᵗʰ **795.3 Nonspecific positive culture findings**
Positive culture findings in:
nose
throat
sputum
wound

> **EXCLUDES** that of:
> blood (790.7-790.8)
> urine (791.9)

795.31 Nonspecific positive findings for anthrax
Positive findings by nasal swab

795.39 Other nonspecific positive culture findings

> **EXCLUDES** colonization status (V02.0-V02.9)

795.4 Other nonspecific abnormal histological findings

√5ᵗʰ **795.5 Nonspecific reaction to test for tuberculosis**

795.51 Nonspecific reaction to tuberculin skin test without active tuberculosis
Abnormal result of Mantoux test
PPD positive
Tuberculin (skin test) positive
Tuberculin (skin test) reactor

> **EXCLUDES** nonspecific reaction to cell mediated immunity measurement of gamma interferon antigen response without active tuberculosis (795.52)

795.52 Nonspecific reaction to cell mediated immunity measurement of gamma interferon antigen response without active tuberculosis
Nonspecific reaction to QuantiFERON-TB test (QFT) without active tuberculosis

> **EXCLUDES** nonspecific reaction to tuberculin skin test without active tuberculosis (795.51)
> positive tuberculin skin test (795.51)

795.6 False positive serological test for syphilis
False positive Wassermann reaction

√5ᵗʰ **795.7 Other nonspecific immunological findings**

> **EXCLUDES** abnormal tumor markers (795.81-795.89)
> elevated prostate specific antigen [PSA] (790.93)
> elevated tumor associated antigens (795.81-795.89)
> isoimmunization, in pregnancy (656.1-656.2)
> affecting fetus or newborn (773.0-773.2)

795.71   Nonspecific serologic evidence of human immunodeficiency virus [HIV]

Inclusive human immunodeficiency [HIV] test (adult) (infant)

Note: This code is **only** to be used when a test finding is reported as nonspecific. Asymptomatic positive findings are coded to V08. If any HIV infection symptom or condition is present, see code 042. Negative findings are not coded.

> **EXCLUDES**   *acquired immunodeficiency syndrome [AIDS] (042)*
> *asymptomatic human immunodeficiency virus, [HIV] infection status (V08)*
> *HIV infection, symptomatic (042)*
> *human immunodeficiency virus [HIV] disease (042)*
> *positive (status) NOS (V08)*

795.79   Other and unspecified nonspecific immunological findings

Raised antibody titer
Raised level of immunoglobulins

√5ᵗʰ **795.8   Abnormal tumor markers**

Elevated tumor associated antigens [TAA]
Elevated tumor specific antigens [TSA]

> **EXCLUDES**   *elevated prostate specific antigen [PSA] (790.93)*

795.81   Elevated carcinoembryonic antigen [CEA]

795.82   Elevated cancer antigen 125 [CA 125]

795.89   Other abnormal tumor markers

√4ᵗʰ **796   Other nonspecific abnormal findings**

796.0   Nonspecific abnormal toxicological findings

Abnormal levels of heavy metals or drugs in blood, urine, or other tissue

Use additional code for retained foreign body, if applicable, (V90.01-V90.9)

> **EXCLUDES**   *excessive blood level of alcohol (790.3)*

796.1   Abnormal reflex

796.2   Elevated blood pressure reading without diagnosis of hypertension

Note: This category is to be used to record an episode of elevated blood pressure in a patient in whom no formal diagnosis of hypertension has been made, or as an incidental finding.

796.3   Nonspecific low blood pressure reading

796.4   Other abnormal clinical findings

796.5   Abnormal finding on antenatal screening

796.6   Abnormal findings on neonatal screening

> **EXCLUDES**   *nonspecific serologic evidence of human immunodeficiency virus [HIV] (795.71)*

√5ᵗʰ **796.7   Abnormal cytologic smear of anus and anal HPV**

> **EXCLUDES**   *abnormal cytologic smear of cervix and cervical HPV (795.00-795.09)*
> *abnormal cytologic smear of vagina and vaginal HPV (795.10-795.19)*
> *anal intraepithelial neoplasia I (AIN I) (569.44)*
> *anal intraepithelial neoplasia II (AIN II) (569.44)*
> *anal intraepithelial neoplasia III (AIN III) (230.5, 230.6)*
> *carcinoma in situ of anus (230.5, 230.6)*
> *dysplasia (histologically confirmed) of anus NOS (569.44)*
> *mild anal dysplasia (histologically confirmed) (569.44)*
> *moderate anal dysplasia (histologically confirmed) (569.44)*
> *severe anal dysplasia (histologically confirmed) (230.5, 230.6)*

796.70   Abnormal glandular Papanicolaou smear of anus

Atypical anal glandular cells NOS

796.71   Papanicolaou smear of anus with atypical squamous cells of undetermined significance [ASC-US]

796.72   Papanicolaou smear of anus with atypical squamous cells cannot exclude high grade squamous intraepithelial lesion [ASC-H]

796.73   Papanicolaou smear of anus with low grade squamous intraepithelial lesion [LGSIL]

796.74   Papanicolaou smear of anus with high grade squamous intraepithelial lesion [HGSIL]

796.75   Anal high risk human papillomavirus [HPV] DNA test positive

796.76   Papanicolaou smear of anus with cytologic evidence of malignancy

796.77   Satisfactory anal smear but lacking transformation zone

796.78   Unsatisfactory anal cytology smear

Inadequate anal cytology sample

796.79   Other abnormal Papanicolaou smear of anus and anal HPV

Anal low risk human papillomavirus (HPV) DNA test positive

Use additional code for associated human papillomavirus (079.4)

796.9   Other

ILL-DEFINED AND UNKNOWN CAUSES OF MORBIDITY AND MORTALITY (797-799)

797   Senility without mention of psychosis

Frailty
Old age
Senescence
Senile asthenia
Senile:
     debility
     exhaustion

> **EXCLUDES**   *senile psychoses (290.0-290.9)*

√4ᵗʰ **798   Sudden death, cause unknown**

798.0   Sudden infant death syndrome

Cot death
Crib death
Sudden death of nonspecific cause in infancy

DEF: Death of infant under age one due to nonspecific cause.

798.1   Instantaneous death

798.2   Death occurring in less than 24 hours from onset of symptoms, not otherwise explained

Death known not to be violent or instantaneous, for which no cause could be discovered
Died without sign of disease

798.9   Unattended death

Death in circumstances where the body of the deceased was found and no cause could be discovered
Found dead

√4ᵗʰ **799   Other ill-defined and unknown causes of morbidity and mortality**

√5ᵗʰ **799.0   Asphyxia and hypoxemia**

> **EXCLUDES**   *asphyxia and hypoxemia (due to):*
> *carbon monoxide (986)*
> *hypercapnia (786.09)*
> *inhalation of food or foreign body (932-934.9)*
> *newborn (768.0-768.9)*
> *traumatic (994.7)*

799.01   Asphyxia

DEF: Lack of oxygen in inspired air, causing a deficiency of oxygen in tissues (hypoxia) and elevated levels of arterial carbon dioxide (hypercapnia).

799.02   Hypoxemia

DEF: Deficient oxygenation of the blood.

799.1   Respiratory arrest
Cardiorespiratory failure
EXCLUDES   *cardiac arrest (427.5)*
failure of peripheral circulation (785.50)
respiratory distress:
NOS (786.09)
acute (518.82)
following trauma and surgery (518.52)
newborn (770.89)
syndrome (newborn) (769)
adult (following trauma and surgery)
(518.52)
other (518.82)
respiratory failure (518.81, 518.83-518.84)
newborn (770.84)
respiratory insufficiency (786.09)
acute (518.82)

√5ᵗʰ   **799.2   Signs and symptoms involving emotional state**
EXCLUDES   *anxiety (293.84, 300.00-300.09)*
depression (311)

799.21   Nervousness
Nervous

799.22   Irritability
Irritable

799.23   Impulsiveness
Impulsive
EXCLUDES   *impulsive neurosis (300.3)*

799.24   Emotional lability

799.25   Demoralization and apathy
Apathetic

799.29   Other signs and symptoms involving emotional state

799.3   Debility, unspecified
EXCLUDES   *asthenia (780.79)*
nervous debility (300.5)
neurasthenia (300.5)
senile asthenia (797)

799.4   Cachexia
Wasting disease
Code first underlying condition, if known
DEF: General ill health and poor nutrition.

√5ᵗʰ   **799.5   Signs and symptoms involving cognition**
EXCLUDES   *amnesia (780.93)*
amnestic syndrome (294.0)
attention deficit disorder (314.00-314.01)
late effects of cerebrovascular disease (438.0)
memory loss (780.93)
mild cognitive impairment, so stated (331.83)
specific problems in developmental delay
(315.00-315.9)
transient global amnesia (437.7)
visuospatial neglect (781.8)

799.51   Attention or concentration deficit

799.52   Cognitive communication deficit

799.53   Visuospatial deficit

799.54   Psychomotor deficit

799.55   Frontal lobe and executive function deficit

799.59   Other signs and symptoms involving cognition

√5ᵗʰ   **799.8   Other ill-defined conditions**

799.81   Decreased libido
Decreased sexual desire
EXCLUDES   *psychosexual dysfunction with*
inhibited sexual desire
(302.71)

799.82   Apparent life threatening event in infant
ALTE
Apparent life threatening event in newborn and infant
Code first confirmed diagnosis, if known
Use additional code(s) for associated signs and symptoms if no confirmed diagnosis established, or if signs and symptoms are not associated routinely with confirmed diagnosis, or provide additional information for cause of ALTE

799.89   Other ill-defined conditions

799.9   Other unknown and unspecified cause
Undiagnosed disease, not specified as to site or system involved
Unknown cause of morbidity or mortality

Symptoms, Signs, and Ill-Defined Conditions

799.1–799.9

Chapter 17: Injury and Poisoning (800–999)

Coding Guidance

This chapter classifies:

- Fractures, dislocations, sprains, and strains
- Intracranial, internal, superficial, blood vessel, nerve and spinal cord, crush, and foreign body injuries
- Contusions, open wounds, and burns
- Late effects of injuries, poisonings, toxic effects, and other external causes
- Certain traumatic complications and unspecified injuries
- Poisonings and toxic effects of nonmedicinal substances
- Other and unspecified effects of external causes
- Complications of surgical and medical care, not elsewhere classified

Injuries, burns, poisoning and adverse effects, and complications of surgery and medical care are all covered in this one chapter of ICD-9-CM. Each of these areas is governed by specific coding guidelines and are discussed separately.

Injuries (800–959)

Multiple coding is encouraged in ICD-9-CM to provide specific detail regarding the nature and extent of injuries. Combination categories for multiple injuries are provided for use when there is insufficient detail available to record a code for each component. When the component sites of injury are specified, the term "with" indicates involvement of both sites, and the term "and" indicates involvement of either or both sites. For example, in category 823, fracture of tibia and fibula, the term "and" between tibia and fibula indicates fractures of the tibia alone, fibula alone, or fibula with tibia. The fifth-digit assignment for this category emphasizes this point. A fifth-digit assignment of "0" indicates tibia involvement alone, "1" indicates fibula involvement alone, and "2" indicates that both fibula and tibia are involved.

Code fractures and other injuries as current conditions during the healing phase as long as they continue to require monitoring and treatment.

The sequencing of codes for fractures and other injuries depends on the circumstances of the admission.

Example:

A patient is seen for treatment of a pressure ulcer of the elbow (code 707.01) but also has a plaster cast on his left arm for a fracture of the humerus suffered six weeks prior to the visit. Only if the patient requires additional care because of the cast would code V54.11, Aftercare for healing traumatic fracture of upper arm, be listed as a secondary diagnosis since the condition had a bearing on the episode of care.

Example:

A patient is seen for treatment of a new displacement of humeral fracture initially suffered six weeks prior. At the time of the visit, the patient also is noted to have pressure ulcers requiring application of a dressing. In this case, the humeral fracture would be listed as the principal diagnosis, followed by a secondary code for pressure ulcer.

Fracture (800–829)

A fracture is a structural break in the continuity of a bone that occurs as the result of physical forces exerted on the rigid bone tissue beyond its ability to accommodate by resistance, elasticity, or bending. ICD-9-CM classifies fractures by anatomic site: skull (800–804), neck and trunk (805–809), upper limb (810–819), and lower limb (820–829).

Fractures may occur as a result of direct injury, such as a forceful blow to the bone by a heavy object, or indirect injury, such as indirect transmission of force through one or more joints (e.g., a stress fracture of the distal tibia caused by jogging).

Fractures may be defined as closed or open. A closed fracture is one in which the skin is intact at the site of the fracture. An open fracture is one in which there is a wound communicating from the skin surface to the fracture site. Open fractures may occur when an external object penetrates the skin to fracture the bone or when a bone or bone fragment penetrates the skin from within.

Clinically, the term "fracture" may be used more broadly to include injuries classified elsewhere in the chapter. "Fracture of cartilage of knee" (836.2) is a tear of the cartilage or "fractured liver" (864) is an injury to the liver. Fractures with dislocation of the joint are classified to the fracture category only.

Fractures designated as pathological fractures are classified to subcategory 733.1 and are defined as fractures due to bone structure weakening by pathological processes (e.g., osteoporosis).

Terms normally used to describe open and closed fractures are listed in the notes to this subchapter. However, these terms are not restricted. Coders should read the documentation to determine whether the fracture should be classified as open or closed.

Example:

A "depressed skull fracture with exposed skull fragments" is coded as an open fracture of the skull, even though the term "depressed" is grouped with the terms describing closed fractures.

Note that an open wound associated with a fracture does not necessarily indicate an open fracture.

Example:

A patient with a fractured femur secondary to a motorcycle accident may also have an open wound or skin avulsion over or near the fracture site. If the wound or avulsion is superficial and does not reach and expose the fracture site, the fracture is coded as closed.

Skull Fracture (800–804)

Skull fracture (800–804) is a fracture of any of the bones of the cranial vault and facial bones. Closed skull fractures most often result from blunt trauma to the head; open skull fractures usually result from extreme trauma or missile injuries such as gunshot wounds.

A concussion is a clinical syndrome caused by a blow or whiplash injury to the head, causing the brain to strike against the skull, but not hard enough to cause a cerebral contusion. Most concussion patients recover uneventfully within 48 hours. Code category 850 is used for concussion uncomplicated by cerebral hemorrhage, laceration, or contusion.

Sprains and Strains of Joint and Adjacent Muscles (840–848)

A sprain is a complete or an incomplete tear in any one or more of the ligaments that surround and support a joint. A strain is an ill-defined injury caused by overuse or overextension of the muscles or tendons of a joint. A "charleyhorse" is an idiom for a strain of a muscle, usually one of the major muscles such as the quadriceps femoris or gastrocnemius. A "slap" lesion refers to the detachment of the superior glenoid labrum (shoulder region), and is considered an injury. These categories also include muscle, tendon, ligament, or joint capsule ruptures.

Strains and sprains are classified according to site (e.g., wrist, foot, knee, leg, etc.) at the category level. Subcategory and subclassification further specify site or structure (e.g., joint or ligament).

Open Wounds (870–897)

Open wounds are bites, avulsions, lacerations, puncture wounds, and traumatic amputations. Excluded injuries are burns, crushing injuries, puncture of internal organs, superficial injuries, and those incidental to dislocation, fracture, and intracranial injury.

Complicated, when described in the fourth digit subcategory, is used to distinguish wounds documented as having delayed healing, delayed treatment, foreign body, or infection. Any wound complicated by infection requires an additional code to identify the infection.

Many types and sites of open wounds are excluded from this code range. Review the ICD-9-CM index under "Wound, open" for "see" and "see category" instructions, as well as the excludes note at the beginning of the code range in the tabular list for proper code assignment.

Injury to Blood Vessels (900–904)

Injuries to any artery or vein due to or associated with traumatic injury are classified to this section. Penetrating trauma with injury of the blood vessel usually involves disruption of the blood vessel with extravasation of blood. Contusions and crush injuries may produce blood vessel injuries such as intimal damage or intramural hematomas with no extravasation of blood.

Late Effects of Injury, Poisoning, Toxic Effects and Other External Causes (905–909)

This category is to be used to indicate conditions classifiable to 800–999 (chapter 17, "Injury and Poisoning") as the cause of the late effects, which themselves are classified elsewhere. The "late effects" include those specified as such, or as sequelae, which may occur at any time after the acute injury.

Each section of chapter 17 has correlating "late effects" categories. For example, injuries classifiable to skull fracture (800–804) have "late effect" codes in the subcategory 905.0 Late effect of fracture of the skull and face bones. Instructional notes within each subcategory alert the coder as to the nature of the acute injury that resulted in the residual condition classifiable to that subcategory.

Burns (940–949)

Burns are injury or destruction of tissue due to the effects of thermal energy, chemicals, electricity or radiation. This section includes current unhealed burns from electricity, flame, hot object, lightening, radiation, chemicals, and scalds. Excluded are friction burns and sunburns, which are classified elsewhere.

First-degree burn, or erythema, is injury limited to tissue damage to the outer layer of the epidermis. Second-degree burn is injury extending beyond the epidermis to partial thickness of the dermis. Third-degree burn is a full thickness skin loss. Third-degree burn with presence of necrotic tissue is termed deep necrosis and is further specified as with or without loss of body parts.

Categories 940–947 classify burns by degree and site. This section is subdivided by general anatomical site at the category level. Subcategory subdivision is according to either more specific site designation (scalp, shoulder, foot), causal agent (chemical) or degree of burn (first, second, third). "Excludes" notes direct coders to the appropriate site category for such areas as mouth (947, internal organs), and scapula (943, upper arm).

Category 948 classifies burns according to the extent of body surface involved. This category is to be used when the site of the burn is unspecified or with categories 940– 947 when the site is specified.

The percentage of body surface is calculated using the "Rule of Nines." The Rule of Nines is a method of estimating the percent of body surface as illustrated. Fourth-digit subdivision indicates the total percent of body surface involved in the burn injury regardless of degree.

Poisoning by Drugs, Medicinal and Biological Substances (960–979)

These categories include situations in which a patient suffers an adverse reaction, or poisoning, from a drug, medicine, or biological substance taken in error or a correct substance improperly administered.

These codes are used primarily in inpatient and emergency settings. However, office coders should be aware of the general guidelines for these categories. E codes from the table of drugs and chemicals are used to identify the circumstances under which the poisoning occurred: accidental, suicide (attempt), assault, or undetermined. Codes identifying suicide or assault should never be assigned without specific physician documentation. Note that an E code from the therapeutic use column is never paired with a poisoning code.

Chronic conditions occurring as a result of substance abuse or dependence are not classified as poisonings. Use codes from 303–305 to classify chronic abuse or dependence.

Late effects of poisoning due to drugs, medicinal, or biological substances are coded to subcategory 909.0. Code the residual first, then the late effect code, followed by the E code for poisoning.

Adverse Effects of Drugs, Medicinal, and Biological Substances

Adverse effects of incorrectly administered drugs are not classified to this section. Note: The interaction of a prescribed drug and an over the counter drug is coded as an adverse effect if both were used correctly and both prescribed by a physician. Adverse effects are described by the following terms:

- Allergic reaction
- Toxicity (cumulative effect of a drug)
- Hypersensitivity
- Idiosyncratic reaction
- Paradoxical reaction
- Synergistic reaction

To code adverse effects, code the condition and assign an E code from the therapeutic use column in the drug table. Do not assign a code from the 960–979 categories. If the adverse effect is unspecified, use code from subcategory 995.2x Unspecified effect of drug, medicinal, and biological substance to identify that an adverse effect occurred.

If the drug is specified but not elsewhere classified, refer to the drug table under the main term "Drug" and choose the appropriate E code from the therapeutic use column. To locate drugs not listed as a main entry in the table refer to the AHFS listing in appendix C of the disease tabular section. Locate the appropriate AHFS number under the main entry "Drug."

Late Effects of Poisoning or Adverse Reactions

Late effects of either poisoning or adverse reactions to drugs, medicinal, and biological substances are classified elsewhere under the appropriate late effect categories. Refer to the alphabetic index for code assignment under main term "Late, effect(s) (of)" and subterm "adverse effect of drug, medicinal or biological substance; or poisoning due to drug, medicinal or biological substance." Code the residual condition first, then the late effect code, followed by the E code to identify the drug.

Examples:

Urticaria due to allergic reaction to penicillin taken as prescribed is coded 708.0 Urticaria, and E930.0 External cause due to therapeutic use of penicillin.

Scarring due to extreme urticaria as a late effect result of an adverse reaction to penicillin is coded 709.2, 909.5, and E930.0.

Complications of Surgical and Medical Care, Not Elsewhere Classified (996–999)

This section classifies complications of medical and surgical care not classified elsewhere. Code assignment should be based on the provider's documentation of the relationship between the condition and the procedure. Not all conditions that occur following a procedure or treatment are considered complications. Complications include those conditions that exceed routine postoperative or post-interventional expectations and those conditions in which a cause-and-effect relationship is documented by the provider. The term "complication" does not imply that the condition is a result of a mishap or other occurrence on the part of the provider. There is no time limit associated with the development of a complication. Depending on the nature of the complication, it may occur immediately, following the procedure or other care provided, or years later. Sequencing is determined by the circumstances of the admission/encounter. Complications occurring during the current episode of care, following treatment, should be reported as an additional code. When the complication is the reason for the admission/encounter, the complication may be designated as the first-listed diagnosis. Instructional notes are provided throughout this section to help the coder appropriately report complication codes.

17. INJURY AND POISONING (800-999)

Use E code(s) to identify the cause and intent of the injury or poisoning (E800-E999)

Use additional code for retained foreign body, if applicable, V90.01-V90.9)

Note:

1. The principle of multiple coding of injuries should be followed wherever possible. Combination categories for multiple injuries are provided for use when there is insufficient detail as to the nature of the individual conditions, or for primary tabulation purposes when it is more convenient to record a single code; otherwise, the component injuries should be coded separately.

   Where multiple sites of injury are specified in the titles, the word "with" indicates involvement of both sites, and the word "and" indicates involvement of either or both sites. The word "finger" includes thumb.

2. Categories for "late effect" of injuries are to be found at 905-909.

FRACTURES (800-829)

> **EXCLUDES** malunion (733.81)
> nonunion (733.82)
> pathological or spontaneous fracture (733.10-733.19)
> stress fractures (733.93-733.95)

The terms "condyle," "coronoid process," "ramus," and "symphysis" indicate the portion of the bone fractured, not the name of the bone involved.

The descriptions "closed" and "open" used in the fourth-digit subdivisions include the following terms:

closed (with or without delayed healing):

comminuted	impacted
depressed	linear
elevated	simple
fissured	slipped epiphysis
fracture NOS	spiral
greenstick	

open (with or without delayed healing):

compound	puncture
infected	with foreign body
missile	

Note: A fracture not indicated as closed or open should be classified as closed.

FRACTURE OF SKULL (800-804)

> **INCLUDES** traumatic brain injury due to fracture of skull

The following fifth-digit subclassification is for use with the appropriate codes in category 800, 801, 803, and 804:
- **0 unspecified state of consciousness**
- **1 with no loss of consciousness**
- **2 with brief [less than one hour] loss of consciousness**
- **3 with moderate [1-24 hours] loss of consciousness**
- **4 with prolonged [more than 24 hours] loss of consciousness and return to pre-existing conscious level**
- **5 with prolonged [more than 24 hours] loss of consciousness, without return to pre-existing conscious level**
  Use fifth-digit 5 to designate when a patient is unconscious and dies before regaining consciousness, regardless of the duration of the loss of consciousness
- **6 with loss of consciousness of unspecified duration**
- **9 with concussion, unspecified**

√4ᵗʰ **800　Fracture of vault of skull**
> **INCLUDES** frontal bone
> parietal bone
> **DEF:** Fracture of bone that forms skull dome and protects brain.

√5ᵗʰ **800.0　Closed without mention of intracranial injury**
[0-6, 9]

√5ᵗʰ **800.1　Closed with cerebral laceration and contusion**
[0-6, 9]

√5ᵗʰ **800.2　Closed with subarachnoid, subdural, and extradural**
[0-6, 9] **hemorrhage**

√5ᵗʰ **800.3　Closed with other and unspecified intracranial**
[0-6, 9] **hemorrhage**

√5ᵗʰ **800.4　Closed with intracranial injury of other and unspecified**
[0-6, 9] **nature**

Fractures

√5ᵗʰ **800.5　Open without mention of intracranial injury**
[0-6, 9]

√5ᵗʰ **800.6　Open with cerebral laceration and contusion**
[0-6, 9]

√5ᵗʰ **800.7　Open with subarachnoid, subdural, and extradural**
[0-6, 9] **hemorrhage**

√5ᵗʰ **800.8　Open with other and unspecified intracranial**
[0-6, 9] **hemorrhage**

√5ᵗʰ **800.9　Open with intracranial injury of other and unspecified**
[0-6, 9] **nature**

√4ᵗʰ **801　Fracture of base of skull**
> **INCLUDES** fossa:
> anterior
> middle
> posterior
> occiput bone
> orbital roof
> sinus:
> ethmoid
> frontal
> sphenoid bone
> temporal bone
> **DEF:** Fracture of bone that forms skull floor.

√5ᵗʰ **801.0　Closed without mention of intracranial injury**
[0-6, 9]

√5ᵗʰ **801.1　Closed with cerebral laceration and contusion**
[0-6, 9]

√5ᵗʰ **801.2　Closed with subarachnoid, subdural, and extradural**
[0-6, 9] **hemorrhage**

√5ᵗʰ **801.3　Closed with other and unspecified intracranial**
[0-6, 9] **hemorrhage**

√5ᵗʰ **801.4　Closed with intracranial injury of other and unspecified**
[0-6, 9] **nature**

√5ᵗʰ **801.5　Open without mention of intracranial injury**
[0-6, 9]

√5ᵗʰ **801.6　Open with cerebral laceration and contusion**
[0-6, 9]

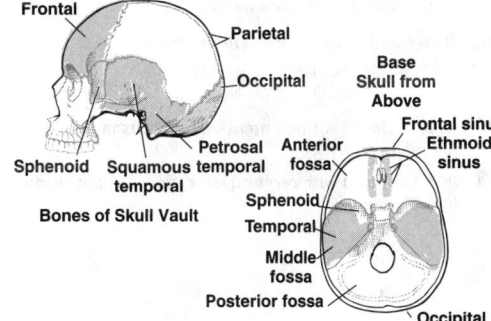

Skull

Injury and Poisoning

801.7–804.9

☑5ᵗʰ **801.7 Open with subarachnoid, subdural, and extradural**
[0-6, 9] **hemorrhage**

☑5ᵗʰ **801.8 Open with other and unspecified intracranial**
[0-6, 9] **hemorrhage**

☑5ᵗʰ **801.9 Open with intracranial injury of other and unspecified**
[0-6, 9] **nature**

☑4ᵗʰ **802 Fracture of face bones**

802.0 Nasal bones, closed

802.1 Nasal bones, open

☑5ᵗʰ **802.2 Mandible, closed**
Inferior maxilla
Lower jaw (bone)

    802.20 Unspecified site

    802.21 Condylar process

    802.22 Subcondylar

    802.23 Coronoid process

    802.24 Ramus, unspecified

    802.25 Angle of jaw

    802.26 Symphysis of body

    802.27 Alveolar border of body

    802.28 Body, other and unspecified

    802.29 Multiple sites

☑5ᵗʰ **802.3 Mandible, open**

    802.30 Unspecified site

    802.31 Condylar process

    802.32 Subcondylar

    802.33 Coronoid process

    802.34 Ramus, unspecified

    802.35 Angle of jaw

    802.36 Symphysis of body

    802.37 Alveolar border of body

    802.38 Body, other and unspecified

    802.39 Multiple sites

802.4 Malar and maxillary bones, closed
Superior maxilla
Upper jaw (bone)
Zygoma
Zygomatic arch

802.5 Malar and maxillary bones, open

802.6 Orbital floor (blow-out), closed

802.7 Orbital floor (blow-out), open

802.8 Other facial bones, closed
Alveolus
Orbit:
  NOS
  part other than roof or floor
Palate
EXCLUDES orbital:
  floor (802.6)
  roof (801.0-801.9)

802.9 Other facial bones, open

☑4ᵗʰ **803 Other and unqualified skull fractures**
INCLUDES skull NOS
skull multiple NOS

☑5ᵗʰ **803.0 Closed without mention of intracranial injury**
[0-6, 9]

☑5ᵗʰ **803.1 Closed with cerebral laceration and contusion**
[0-6, 9]

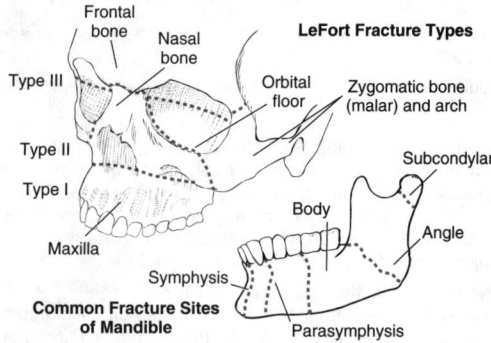

Facial Fracture

Common Fracture Sites of Mandible

☑5ᵗʰ **803.2 Closed with subarachnoid, subdural, and extradural**
[0-6, 9] **hemorrhage**

☑5ᵗʰ **803.3 Closed with other and unspecified intracranial**
[0-6, 9] **hemorrhage**

☑5ᵗʰ **803.4 Closed with intracranial injury of other and unspecified**
[0-6, 9] **nature**

☑5ᵗʰ **803.5 Open without mention of intracranial injury**
[0-6, 9]

☑5ᵗʰ **803.6 Open with cerebral laceration and contusion**
[0-6, 9]

☑5ᵗʰ **803.7 Open with subarachnoid, subdural, and extradural**
[0-6, 9] **hemorrhage**

☑5ᵗʰ **803.8 Open with other and unspecified intracranial**
[0-6, 9] **hemorrhage**

☑5ᵗʰ **803.9 Open with intracranial injury of other and unspecified**
[0-6, 9] **nature**

☑4ᵗʰ **804 Multiple fractures involving skull or face with other bones**

☑5ᵗʰ **804.0 Closed without mention of intracranial injury**
[0-6, 9]

☑5ᵗʰ **804.1 Closed with cerebral laceration and contusion**
[0-6, 9]

☑5ᵗʰ **804.2 Closed with subarachnoid, subdural, and extradural**
[0-6, 9] **hemorrhage**

☑5ᵗʰ **804.3 Closed with other and unspecified intracranial**
[0-6, 9] **hemorrhage**

☑5ᵗʰ **804.4 Closed with intracranial injury of other and**
[0-6, 9] **unspecified nature**

☑5ᵗʰ **804.5 Open without mention of intracranial injury**
[0-6, 9]

☑5ᵗʰ **804.6 Open with cerebral laceration and contusion**
[0-6, 9]

☑5ᵗʰ **804.7 Open with subarachnoid, subdural, and extradural**
[0-6, 9] **hemorrage**

☑5ᵗʰ **804.8 Open with other and unspecified intracranial**
[0-6, 9] **hemorrhage**

☑5ᵗʰ **804.9 Open with intracranial injury of other and unspecified**
[0-6, 9] **nature**

Vertebral Column

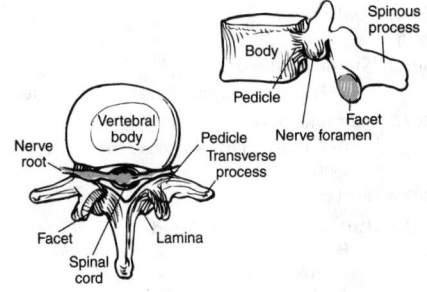

FRACTURE OF NECK AND TRUNK (805-809)

√4th **805 Fracture of vertebral column without mention of spinal cord injury**

INCLUDES   neural arch
              spine
              spinous process
              transverse process
              vertebra

The following fifth-digit subclassification is for use with codes 805.0-805.1:

  0 cervical vertebra, unspecified level
  1 first cervical vertebra
  2 second cervical vertebra
  3 third cervical vertebra
  4 fourth cervical vertebra
  5 fifth cervical vertebra
  6 sixth cervical vertebra
  7 seventh cervical vertebra
  8 multiple cervical vertebrae

√5th **805.0 Cervical, closed**
[0-8]   Atlas
         Axis

√5th **805.1 Cervical, open**
[0-8]

805.2 Dorsal [thoracic], closed

805.3 Dorsal [thoracic], open

805.4 Lumbar, closed

805.5 Lumbar, open

805.6 Sacrum and coccyx, closed

805.7 Sacrum and coccyx, open

805.8 Unspecified, closed

805.9 Unspecified, open

√4th **806 Fracture of vertebral column with spinal cord injury**

INCLUDES   any condition classifiable to 805 with:
            complete or incomplete transverse lesion (of cord)
            hematomyelia
            injury to:
               cauda equina
               nerve
            paralysis
            paraplegia
            quadriplegia
            spinal concussion

√5th **806.0 Cervical, closed**

806.00 C_1-C_4 level with unspecified spinal cord injury
Cervical region NOS with spinal cord injury NOS

806.01 C_1-C_4 level with complete lesion of cord

806.02 C_1-C_4 level with anterior cord syndrome

806.03 C_1-C_4 level with central cord syndrome

806.04 C_1-C_4 level with other specified spinal cord injury
C_1-C_4 level with:
    incomplete spinal cord lesion NOS
    posterior cord syndrome

806.05 C_5-C_7 level with unspecified spinal cord injury

806.06 C_5-C_7 level with complete lesion of cord

806.07 C_5-C_7 level with anterior cord syndrome

806.08 C_5-C_7 level with central cord syndrome

806.09 C_5-C_7 level with other specified spinal cord injury
C_5-C_7 level with:
    incomplete spinal cord lesion NOS
    posterior cord syndrome

√5th **806.1 Cervical, open**

806.10 C_1-C_4 level with unspecified spinal cord injury

806.11 C_1-C_4 level with complete lesion of cord

806.12 C_1-C_4 level with anterior cord syndrome

806.13 C_1-C_4 level with central cord syndrome

806.14 C_1-C_4 level with other specified spinal cord injury
C_1-C_4 level with:
    incomplete spinal cord lesion NOS
    posterior cord syndrome

806.15 C_5-C_7 level with unspecified spinal cord injury

806.16 C_5-C_7 level with complete lesion of cord

806.17 C_5-C_7 level with anterior cord syndrome

806.18 C_5-C_7 level with central cord syndrome

806.19 C_5-C_7 level with other specified spinal cord injury
C_5-C_7 level with:
    incomplete spinal cord lesion NOS
    posterior cord syndrome

√5th **806.2 Dorsal [thoracic], closed**

806.20 T_1-T_6 level with unspecified spinal cord injury
Thoracic region NOS with spinal cord injury NOS

806.21 T_1-T_6 level with complete lesion of cord

806.22 T_1-T_6 level with anterior cord syndrome

806.23 T_1-T_6 level with central cord syndrome

806.24 T_1-T_6 level with other specified spinal cord injury
T_1-T_6 level with:
    incomplete spinal cord lesion NOS
    posterior cord syndrome

806.25 T_7-T_{12} level with unspecified spinal cord injury

806.26 T_7-T_{12} level with complete lesion of cord

806.27 T_7-T_{12} level with anterior cord syndrome

806.28 T_7-T_{12} level with central cord syndrome

806.29 T_7-T_{12} level with other specified spinal cord injury

> T_7-T_{12} level with:
> incomplete spinal cord lesion NOS
> posterior cord syndrome

✓5th   806.3   Dorsal [thoracic], open

806.30 T_1-T_6 level with unspecified spinal cord injury

806.31 T_1-T_6 level with complete lesion of cord

806.32 T_1-T_6 level with anterior cord syndrome

806.33 T_1-T_6 level with central cord syndrome

806.34 T_1-T_6 level with other specified spinal cord injury

> T_1-T_6 level with:
> incomplete spinal cord lesion NOS
> posterior cord syndrome

806.35 T_7-T_{12} level with unspecified spinal cord injury

806.36 T_7-T_{12} level with complete lesion of cord

806.37 T_7-T_{12} level with anterior cord syndrome

806.38 T_7-T_{12} level with central cord syndrome

806.39 T_7-T_{12} level with other specified spinal cord injury

> T_7-T_{12} level with:
> incomplete spinal cord lesion NOS
> posterior cord syndrome

806.4   Lumbar, closed

806.5   Lumbar, open

✓5th   806.6   Sacrum and coccyx, closed

806.60   With unspecified spinal cord injury

806.61   With complete cauda equina lesion

806.62   With other cauda equina injury

806.69   With other spinal cord injury

✓5th   806.7   Sacrum and coccyx, open

806.70   With unspecified spinal cord injury

806.71   With complete cauda equina lesion

806.72   With other cauda equina injury

806.79   With other spinal cord injury

806.8   Unspecified, closed

806.9   Unspecified, open

✓4th   807   Fracture of rib(s), sternum, larynx, and trachea

> The following fifth-digit subclassification is for use with codes 807.0-807.1:
> 0   rib(s) unspecifed
> 1   one rib
> 2   two ribs
> 3   three ribs
> 4   four ribs
> 5   five ribs
> 6   six ribs
> 7   seven ribs
> 8   eight or more ribs
> 9   multiple ribs, unspecified

✓5th   807.0   Rib(s), closed
[0-9]

Ribs, Sternum, Larynx, and Trachea

Pelvis and Pelvic Fractures

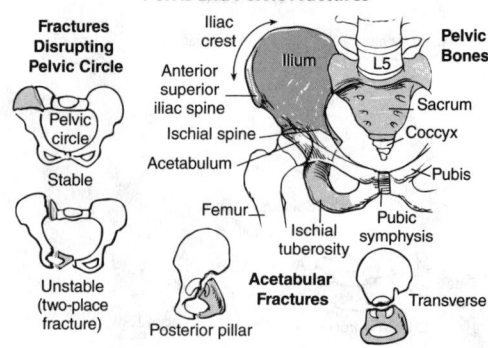

✓5th   807.1   Rib(s), open
[0-9]

807.2   Sternum, closed
> DEF: Break in flat bone (breast bone) in anterior thorax.

807.3   Sternum, open
> DEF: Break, with open wound, in flat bone in mid anterior thorax.

807.4   Flail chest

807.5   Larynx and trachea, closed
> Hyoid bone
> Thyroid cartilage
> Trachea

807.6   Larynx and trachea, open

✓4th   808   Fracture of pelvis

808.0   Acetabulum, closed

808.1   Acetabulum, open

808.2   Pubis, closed

808.3   Pubis, open

✓5th   808.4   Other specified part, closed

808.41   Ilium

808.42   Ischium

808.43   Multiple closed pelvic fractures with disruption of pelvic circle
> Multiple closed pelvic fractures with disruption of pelvic ring

808.44   Multiple closed pelvic fractures without disruption of pelvic circle
> Multiple closed pelvic fractures without disruption of pelvic ring

808.49   Other
> Innominate bone
> Pelvic rim

✓5th   808.5   Other specified part, open

808.51   Ilium

808.52   Ischium

808.53   Multiple open pelvic fractures with disruption of pelvic circle
> Multiple open pelvic fractures with disruption of pelvic ring

808.54   Multiple open pelvic fractures without disruption of pelvic circle
> Multiple open pelvic fractures without disruption of pelvic ring

808.59   Other

808.8   Unspecified, closed

808.9   Unspecified, open

Right Clavicle and Scapula, Anterior View

Right Humerus, Anterior View

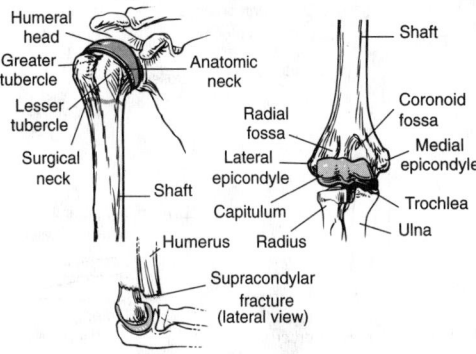

√4ᵗʰ **809 Ill-defined fractures of bones of trunk**

INCLUDES   bones of trunk with other bones except those of skull and face
multiple bones of trunk

EXCLUDES   *multiple fractures of:*
pelvic bones alone (808.0-808.9)
ribs alone (807.0-807.1, 807.4)
ribs or sternum with limb bones (819.0-819.1, 828.0-828.1)
skull or face with other bones (804.0-804.9)

809.0 Fracture of bones of trunk, closed

809.1 Fracture of bones of trunk, open

FRACTURE OF UPPER LIMB (810-819)

√4ᵗʰ **810 Fracture of clavicle**

INCLUDES   collar bone
interligamentous part of clavicle

The following fifth-digit subclassification is for use with category 810:

   0 unspecified part
     Clavicle NOS
   1 sternal end of clavicle
   2 shaft of clavicle
   3 acromial end of clavicle

√5ᵗʰ **810.0 Closed**
[0-3]

√5ᵗʰ **810.1 Open**
[0-3]

√4ᵗʰ **811 Fracture of scapula**

INCLUDES   shoulder blade

The following fifth-digit subclassification is for use with category 811:

   0 unspecified part
   1 acromial process
     Acromion (process)
   2 coracoid process
   3 glenoid cavity and neck of scapula
   9 other

√5ᵗʰ **811.0 Closed**
[0-3, 9]

√5ᵗʰ **811.1 Open**
[0-3, 9]

√4ᵗʰ **812 Fracture of humerus**

√5ᵗʰ **812.0 Upper end, closed**

   812.00 Upper end, unspecified part
     Proximal end
     Shoulder

   812.01 Surgical neck
     Neck of humerus NOS

   812.02 Anatomical neck

   812.03 Greater tuberosity

   812.09 Other
     Head   Upper epiphysis
     Lesser tuberosity

√5ᵗʰ **812.1 Upper end, open**

   812.10 Upper end, unspecified part

   812.11 Surgical neck

   812.12 Anatomical neck

   812.13 Greater tuberosity

   812.19 Other

√5ᵗʰ **812.2 Shaft or unspecified part, closed**

   812.20 Unspecified part of humerus
     Humerus NOS
     Lesser tuberosity
     Upper arm NOS

   812.21 Shaft of humerus

√5ᵗʰ **812.3 Shaft or unspecified part, open**

   812.30 Unspecified part of humerus

   812.31 Shaft of humerus

√5ᵗʰ **812.4 Lower end, closed**
     Distal end of humerus
     Elbow

   812.40 Lower end, unspecified part

   812.41 Supracondylar fracture of humerus

   812.42 Lateral condyle
     External condyle

   812.43 Medial condyle
     Internal epicondyle

   812.44 Condyle(s), unspecified
     Articular process NOS
     Lower epiphysis NOS

   812.49 Other
     Multiple fractures of lower end
     Trochlea

√5ᵗʰ **812.5 Lower end, open**

   812.50 Lower end, unspecified part

   812.51 Supracondylar fracture of humerus

   812.52 Lateral condyle

   812.53 Medial condyle

   812.54 Condyle(s), unspecified

   812.59 Other

√4ᵗʰ **813 Fracture of radius and ulna**

√5ᵗʰ **813.0 Upper end, closed**
     Proximal end

   813.00 Upper end of forearm, unspecified

   813.01 Olecranon process of ulna

   813.02 Coronoid process of ulna

   813.03 Monteggia's fracture
     DEF: Fracture near the head of the ulnar shaft, causing dislocation of the radial head.

   813.04 Other and unspecified fractures of proximal end of ulna (alone)
     Multiple fractures of ulna, upper end

Injury and Poisoning

813.05–815.0

Right Radius and Ulna, Anterior View

Hand Fractures

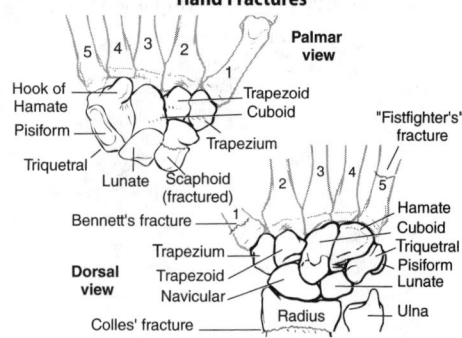

813.05   **Head of radius**

813.06   **Neck of radius**

813.07   **Other and unspecified fractures of proximal end of radius (alone)**
Multiple fractures of radius, upper end

813.08   **Radius with ulna, upper end [any part]**

√5th   **813.1**   **Upper end, open**

813.10   **Upper end of forearm, unspecified**

813.11   **Olecranon process of ulna**

813.12   **Coronoid process of ulna**

813.13   **Monteggia's fracture**

813.14   **Other and unspecified fractures of proximal end of ulna**

813.15   **Head of radius**

813.16   **Neck of radius**

813.17   **Other and unspecified fractures of proximal end of radius (alone)**

813.18   **Radius with ulna, upper end [any part]**

√5th   **813.2**   **Shaft, closed**

813.20   **Shaft, unspecified**

813.21   **Radius (alone)**

813.22   **Ulna (alone)**

813.23   **Radius with ulna**

√5th   **813.3**   **Shaft, open**

813.30   **Shaft, unspecified**

813.31   **Radius (alone)**

813.32   **Ulna (alone)**

813.33   **Radius with ulna**

√5th   **813.4**   **Lower end, closed**
Distal end

813.40   **Lower end of forearm, unspecified**

813.41   **Colles' fracture**
Smith's fracture

DEF: Break of lower end of radius; associated with backward movement of the radius lower section.

813.42   **Other fractures of distal end of radius (alone)**
Dupuytren's fracture, radius
Radius, lower end

DEF: Dupuytren's fracture: fracture and dislocation of the forearm; the fracture is of the radius above the wrist, and the dislocation is of the ulna at the lower end.

813.43   **Distal end of ulna (alone)**
Ulna: Ulna:
head   lower epiphysis
lower end   styloid process

813.44   **Radius with ulna, lower end**

813.45   **Torus fracture of radius (alone)**
EXCLUDES   *torus fracture of radius and ulna (813.47)*

813.46   **Torus fracture of ulna (alone)**
EXCLUDES   *torus fracture of radius and ulna (813.47)*

813.47   **Torus fracture of radius and ulna**

√5th   **813.5**   **Lower end, open**

813.50   **Lower end of forearm, unspecified**

813.51   **Colles' fracture**

813.52   **Other fractures of distal end of radius (alone)**

813.53   **Distal end of ulna (alone)**

813.54   **Radius with ulna, lower end**

√5th   **813.8**   **Unspecified part, closed**

813.80   **Forearm, unspecified**

813.81   **Radius (alone)**

813.82   **Ulna (alone)**

813.83   **Radius with ulna**

√5th   **813.9**   **Unspecified part, open**

813.90   **Forearm, unspecified**

813.91   **Radius (alone)**

813.92   **Ulna (alone)**

813.93   **Radius with ulna**

√4th   **814**   **Fracture of carpal bone(s)**

The following fifth-digit subclassification is for use with category 814:

0   **carpal bone, unspecified**
    Wrist NOS
1   **navicular [scaphoid] of wrist**
2   **lunate [semilunar] bone of wrist**
3   **triquetral [cuneiform] bone of wrist**
4   **pisiform**
5   **trapezium bone [larger multangular]**
6   **trapezoid bone [smaller multangular]**
7   **capitate bone [os magnum]**
8   **hamate [unciform] bone**
9   **other**

√5th   **814.0**   **Closed**
[0-9]

√5th   **814.1**   **Open**
[0-9]

√4th   **815**   **Fracture of metacarpal bone(s)**
INCLUDES   hand [except finger]
             metacarpus

The following fifth-digit subclassification is for use with category 815:

0   **metacarpal bone(s), site unspecified**
1   **base of thumb [first] metacarpal**
    Bennett's fracture
2   **base of other metacarpal bone(s)**
3   **shaft of metacarpal bone(s)**
4   **neck of metacarpal bone(s)**
9   **multiple sites of metacarpus**

√5th   **815.0**   **Closed**
[0-4, 9]

✓5th **815.1 Open**
[0-4, 9]

✓4th **816 Fracture of one or more phalanges of hand**
INCLUDES finger(s)
thumb

> The following fifth-digit subclassification is for use with category 816:
> **0 phalanx or phalanges, unspecified**
> **1 middle or proximal phalanx or phalanges**
> **2 distal phalanx or phalanges**
> **3 multiple sites**

✓5th **816.0 Closed**
[0-3]

✓5th **816.1 Open**
[0-3]

✓4th **817 Multiple fractures of hand bones**
INCLUDES metacarpal bone(s) with phalanx or phalanges of same hand

817.0 Closed

817.1 Open

✓4th **818 Ill-defined fractures of upper limb**
INCLUDES arm NOS
multiple bones of same upper limb
EXCLUDES *multiple fractures of:*
metacarpal bone(s) with phalanx or phalanges (817.0-817.1)
phalanges of hand alone (816.0-816.1)
radius with ulna (813.0-813.9)

818.0 Closed

818.1 Open

✓4th **819 Multiple fractures involving both upper limbs, and upper limb with rib(s) and sternum**
INCLUDES arm(s) with rib(s) or sternum
both arms [any bones]

819.0 Closed

819.1 Open

FRACTURE OF LOWER LIMB (820-829)

✓4th **820 Fracture of neck of femur**

✓5th **820.0 Transcervical fracture, closed**

820.00 Intracapsular section, unspecified

820.01 Epiphysis (separation) (upper)
Transepiphyseal

820.02 Midcervical section
Transcervical NOS

820.03 Base of neck
Cervicotrochanteric section

820.09 Other
Head of femur
Subcapital

✓5th **820.1 Transcervical fracture, open**

820.10 Intracapsular section, unspecified

820.11 Epiphysis (separation) (upper)

820.12 Midcervical section

820.13 Base of neck

820.19 Other

✓5th **820.2 Pertrochanteric fracture, closed**

820.20 Trochanteric section, unspecified
Trochanter: Trochanter:
  NOS   lesser
  greater

820.21 Intertrochanteric section

820.22 Subtrochanteric section

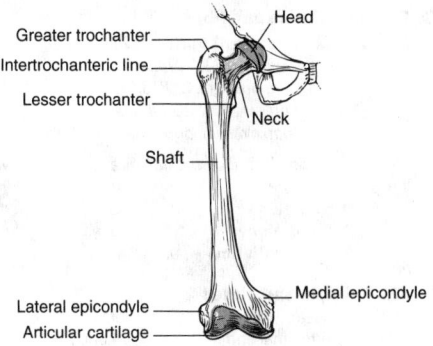

Right Femur, Anterior View

Greater trochanter
Head
Intertrochanteric line
Lesser trochanter
Neck
Shaft
Medial epicondyle
Lateral epicondyle
Articular cartilage

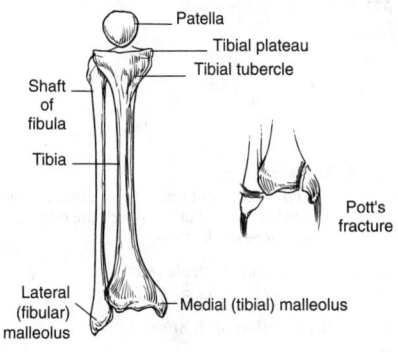

Right Tibia and Fibula, Anterior View

Patella
Tibial plateau
Tibial tubercle
Shaft of fibula
Tibia
Pott's fracture
Lateral (fibular) malleolus
Medial (tibial) malleolus

✓5th **820.3 Pertrochanteric fracture, open**

820.30 Trochanteric section, unspecified

820.31 Intertrochanteric section

820.32 Subtrochanteric section

820.8 Unspecified part of neck of femur, closed
Hip NOS   Neck of femur NOS

820.9 Unspecified part of neck of femur, open

✓4th **821 Fracture of other and unspecified parts of femur**

✓5th **821.0 Shaft or unspecified part, closed**

821.00 Unspecified part of femur
Thigh
Upper leg
EXCLUDES *hip NOS (820.8)*

821.01 Shaft

✓5th **821.1 Shaft or unspecified part, open**

821.10 Unspecified part of femur

821.11 Shaft

✓5th **821.2 Lower end, closed**
Distal end

821.20 Lower end, unspecified part

821.21 Condyle, femoral

821.22 Epiphysis, lower (separation)

821.23 Supracondylar fracture of femur

821.29 Other
Multiple fractures of lower end

✓5th **821.3 Lower end, open**

821.30 Lower end, unspecified part

821.31 Condyle, femoral

821.32 Epiphysis, lower (separation)

821.33 Supracondylar fracture of femur

821.39 Other

✓4th **822 Fracture of patella**

822.0 Closed

822.1 **Open**

✓4th **823 Fracture of tibia and fibula**
 EXCLUDES *Dupuytren's fracture (824.4-824.5)*
  ankle (824.4-824.5)
  radius (813.42, 813.52)
  Pott's fracture (824.4-824.5)
  that involving ankle (824.0-824.9)

The following fifth-digit subclassification is for use with category 823:
 0 tibia alone
 1 fibula alone
 2 fibula with tibia

✓5th **823.0 Upper end, closed**
 [0-2] Head Tibia:
  Proximal end condyles
    tuberosity

✓5th **823.1 Upper end, open**
 [0-2]

✓5th **823.2 Shaft, closed**
 [0-2]

✓5th **823.3 Shaft, open**
 [0-2]

✓5th **823.4 Torus fracture**
 [0-2] **DEF:** A bone deformity in children, occurring commonly in the tibia and fibula, in which the bone bends and buckles but does not fracture.

✓5th **823.8 Unspecified part, closed**
 [0-2] Lower leg NOS

✓5th **823.9 Unspecified part, open**
 [0-2]

✓4th **824 Fracture of ankle**
 824.0 Medial malleolus, closed
  Tibia involving:
   ankle
   malleolus

 824.1 Medial malleolus, open

 824.2 Lateral malleolus, closed
  Fibula involving:
   ankle
   malleolus

 824.3 Lateral malleolus, open

 824.4 Bimalleolar, closed
  Dupuytren's fracture, fibula
  Pott's fracture
  DEF: Bimalleolar, closed: Breaking of both nodules (malleoli) on either side of ankle joint, without an open wound.
  DEF: Dupuytren's fracture (Pott's fracture): The breaking of the farthest end of the lower leg bone (fibula), with injury to the farthest end joint of the other lower leg bone (tibia).

 824.5 Bimalleolar, open

 824.6 Trimalleolar, closed
  Lateral and medial malleolus with anterior or posterior lip of tibia

 824.7 Trimalleolar, open

Torus Fracture

Fibula — — Tibia
  — Diaphysis
  — Direction of force
  — Torus, bulging, fracture

Anterior views of torus compression fracture

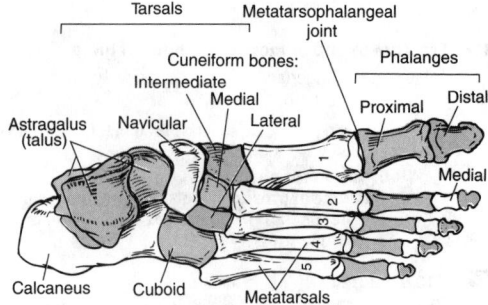

Right Foot, Dorsal

Tarsals Metatarsophalangeal joint
  Cuneiform bones: Phalanges
  Intermediate Medial
Astragalus (talus) Navicular Medial Lateral Proximal Distal
  Medial
Calcaneus Cuboid Metatarsals

 824.8 Unspecified, closed
  Ankle NOS

 824.9 Unspecified, open

✓4th **825 Fracture of one or more tarsal and metatarsal bones**
 825.0 Fracture of calcaneus, closed
  Heel bone
  Os calcis

 825.1 Fracture of calcaneus, open

✓5th **825.2 Fracture of other tarsal and metatarsal bones, closed**
  825.20 Unspecified bone(s) of foot [except toes]
   Instep

  825.21 Astragalus
   Talus

  825.22 Navicular [scaphoid], foot

  825.23 Cuboid

  825.24 Cuneiform, foot

  825.25 Metatarsal bone(s)

  825.29 Other
   Tarsal with metatarsal bone(s) only
   EXCLUDES *calcaneus (825.0)*

✓5th **825.3 Fracture of other tarsal and metatarsal bones, open**
  825.30 Unspecified bone(s) of foot [except toes]

  825.31 Astragalus

  825.32 Navicular [scaphoid], foot

  825.33 Cuboid

  825.34 Cuneiform, foot

  825.35 Metatarsal bone(s)

  825.39 Other

✓4th **826 Fracture of one or more phalanges of foot**
 INCLUDES toe(s)

 826.0 Closed

 826.1 Open

✓4th **827 Other, multiple, and ill-defined fractures of lower limb**
 INCLUDES leg NOS
  multiple bones of same lower limb
 EXCLUDES *multiple fractures of:*
  ankle bones alone (824.4-824.9)
  phalanges of foot alone (826.0-826.1)
  tarsal with metatarsal bones (825.29, 825.39)
  tibia with fibula (823.0-823.9 with fifth-digit 2)

 827.0 Closed

 827.1 Open

✓4th **828 Multiple fractures involving both lower limbs, lower with upper limb, and lower limb(s) with rib(s) and sternum**
 INCLUDES arm(s) with leg(s) [any bones]
  both legs [any bones]
  leg(s) with rib(s) or sternum

 828.0 Closed

 828.1 Open

✓4ᵗ **829 Fracture of unspecified bones**

829.0 **Unspecified bone, closed**

829.1 **Unspecified bone, open**

DISLOCATION (830-839)

INCLUDES   displacement
          subluxation

EXCLUDES   *congenital dislocation (754.0-755.8)*
          pathological dislocation (718.2)
          recurrent dislocation (718.3)

Note: The descriptions "closed" and "open," used in the fourth-digit subdivisions, include the following terms:

closed:	open:
complete	compound
dislocation NOS	infected
partial	with foreign body
simple	
uncomplicated	

A dislocation not indicated as closed or open should be classified as closed.

✓4ᵗ **830 Dislocation of jaw**

INCLUDES   jaw (cartilage) (meniscus)
          mandible
          maxilla (inferior)
          temporomandibular (joint)

830.0 **Closed dislocation**

830.1 **Open dislocation**

✓4ᵗ **831 Dislocation of shoulder**

EXCLUDES   *sternoclavicular joint (839.61, 839.71)*
          sternum (839.61, 839.71)

The following fifth-digit subclassification is for use with category 831:

   0 **shoulder, unspecified**
        Humerus NOS
   1 **anterior dislocation of humerus**
   2 **posterior dislocation of humerus**
   3 **inferior dislocation of humerus**
   4 **acromioclavicular (joint)**
        Clavicle
   9 **other**
        Scapula

✓5ᵗ 831.0 **Closed dislocation**
[0-4, 9]

✓5ᵗ 831.1 **Open dislocation**
[0-4, 9]

✓4ᵗ **832 Dislocation of elbow**

The following fifth-digit subclassification is for use with subcategories 832.0 and 832.1
   0 **elbow, unspecified**
   1 **anterior dislocation of elbow**
   2 **posterior dislocation of elbow**
   3 **medial dislocation of elbow**
   4 **lateral dislocation of elbow**
   9 **other**

✓5ᵗ 832.0 **Closed dislocation**
[0-4, 9]

✓5ᵗ 832.1 **Open dislocation**
[0-4, 9]

832.2 **Nursemaid's elbow**
        Subluxation of radial head

✓4ᵗ **833 Dislocation of wrist**

The following fifth-digit subclassification is for use with category 833:
   0 **wrist unspecified part**
        Carpal (bone)
        Radius, distal end
   1 **radioulnar (joint), distal**
   2 **radiocarpal (joint)**
   3 **midcarpal (joint)**
   4 **carpometacarpal (joint)**
   5 **metacarpal (bone), proximal end**
   9 **other**
        Ulna, distal end

✓5ᵗ 833.0 **Closed dislocation**
[0-5, 9]

✓5ᵗ 833.1 **Open dislocation**
[0-5, 9]

✓4ᵗ **834 Dislocation of finger**

INCLUDES   finger(s)
          phalanx of hand
          thumb

The following fifth-digit subclassification is for use with category 834:
   0 **finger unspecified part**
   1 **metacarpophalangeal (joint)**
        Metacarpal (bone), distal end
   2 **interphalangeal (joint), hand**

✓5ᵗ 834.0 **Closed dislocation**
[0-2]

✓5ᵗ 834.1 **Open dislocation**
[0-2]

✓4ᵗ **835 Dislocation of hip**

The following fifth-digit subclassification is for use with category 835:
   0 **dislocation of hip, unspecified**
   1 **posterior dislocation**
   2 **obturator dislocation**
   3 **other anterior dislocation**

✓5ᵗ 835.0 **Closed dislocation**
[0-3]

✓5ᵗ 835.1 **Open dislocation**
[0-3]

✓4ᵗ **836 Dislocation of knee**

EXCLUDES   *dislocation of knee:*
          old or pathological (718.2)
          recurrent (718.3)
          internal derangement of knee joint (717.0-717.5,
          717.8-717.9)
          old tear of cartilage or meniscus of knee (717.0-717.5,
          717.8-717.9)

836.0 **Tear of medial cartilage or meniscus of knee, current**
        Bucket handle tear:
          NOS   ⎫ current injury
          medial meniscus ⎭

836.1 **Tear of lateral cartilage or meniscus of knee, current**

836.2 **Other tear of cartilage or meniscus of knee, current**
        Tear of:
          cartilage (semilunar) ⎫ current injury, not specified
          meniscus   ⎭ as medial or lateral

836.3 **Dislocation of patella, closed**

836.4 **Dislocation of patella, open**

✓5ᵗ 836.5 **Other dislocation of knee, closed**

836.50 **Dislocation of knee, unspecified**

836.51 **Anterior dislocation of tibia, proximal end**
        Posterior dislocation of femur, distal end, closed

836.52 **Posterior dislocation of tibia, proximal end**
        Anterior dislocation of femur, distal end, closed

836.53 **Medial dislocation of tibia, proximal end**

Injury and Poisoning

836.54–841.1

836.54   Lateral dislocation of tibia, proximal end

836.59   Other

√5th   836.6   **Other dislocation of knee, open**

836.60   **Dislocation of knee, unspecified**

836.61   **Anterior dislocation of tibia, proximal end**
Posterior dislocation of femur, distal end, open

836.62   **Posterior dislocation of tibia, proximal end**
Anterior dislocation of femur, distal end, open

836.63   **Medial dislocation of tibia, proximal end**

836.64   **Lateral dislocation of tibia, proximal end**

836.69   **Other**

√4th   **837**   **Dislocation of ankle**

INCLUDES   astragalus
fibula, distal end
navicular, foot
scaphoid, foot
tibia, distal end

837.0   **Closed dislocation**

837.1   **Open dislocation**

√4th   **838**   **Dislocation of foot**

The following fifth-digit subclassification is for use with category 838:

   0   **foot unspecified**
   1   **tarsal (bone), joint unspecified**
   2   **midtarsal (joint)**
   3   **tarsometatarsal (joint)**
   4   **metatarsal (bone), joint unspecified**
   5   **metatarsophalangeal (joint)**
   6   **interphalangeal (joint), foot**
   9   **other**
     Phalanx of foot
     Toe(s)

√5th   838.0   **Closed dislocation**
[0-6, 9]

√5th   838.1   **Open dislocation**
[0-6, 9]

√4th   **839**   **Other, multiple, and ill-defined dislocations**

√5th   839.0   **Cervical vertebra, closed**
Cervical spine
Neck

839.00   **Cervical vertebra, unspecified**

839.01   **First cervical vertebra**

839.02   **Second cervical vertebra**

839.03   **Third cervical vertebra**

839.04   **Fourth cervical vertebra**

839.05   **Fifth cervical vertebra**

839.06   **Sixth cervical vertebra**

839.07   **Seventh cervical vertebra**

839.08   **Multiple cervical vertebrae**

√5th   839.1   **Cervical vertebra, open**

839.10   **Cervical vertebra, unspecified**

839.11   **First cervical vertebra**

839.12   **Second cervical vertebra**

839.13   **Third cervical vertebra**

839.14   **Fourth cervical vertebra**

839.15   **Fifth cervical vertebra**

839.16   **Sixth cervical vertebra**

839.17   **Seventh cervical vertebra**

839.18   **Multiple cervical vertebrae**

√5th   839.2   **Thoracic and lumbar vertebra, closed**

839.20   **Lumbar vertebra**

839.21   **Thoracic vertebra**
Dorsal [thoracic] vertebra

√5th   839.3   **Thoracic and lumbar vertebra, open**

839.30   **Lumbar vertebra**

839.31   **Thoracic vertebra**

√5th   839.4   **Other vertebra, closed**

839.40   **Vertebra, unspecified site**
Spine NOS

839.41   **Coccyx**

839.42   **Sacrum**
Sacroiliac (joint)

839.49   **Other**

√5th   839.5   **Other vertebra, open**

839.50   **Vertebra, unspecified site**

839.51   **Coccyx**

839.52   **Sacrum**

839.59   **Other**

√5th   839.6   **Other location, closed**

839.61   **Sternum**
Sternoclavicular joint

839.69   **Other**
Pelvis

√5th   839.7   **Other location, open**

839.71   **Sternum**

839.79   **Other**

839.8   **Multiple and ill-defined, closed**
Arm
Back
Hand
Multiple locations, except fingers or toes alone
Other ill-defined locations
Unspecified location

839.9   **Multiple and ill-defined, open**

SPRAINS AND STRAINS OF JOINTS AND ADJACENT MUSCLES (840-848)

INCLUDES   avulsion
hemarthrosis   of:
laceration   joint capsule
rupture   ligament
sprain   muscle
strain   tendon
tear

EXCLUDES   *laceration of tendon in open wounds (880-884 and 890-894 with .2)*

√4th   **840**   **Sprains and strains of shoulder and upper arm**

840.0   **Acromioclavicular (joint) (ligament)**

840.1   **Coracoclavicular (ligament)**

840.2   **Coracohumeral (ligament)**

840.3   **Infraspinatus (muscle) (tendon)**

840.4   **Rotator cuff (capsule)**
EXCLUDES   *complete rupture of rotator cuff, nontraumatic (727.61)*

840.5   **Subscapularis (muscle)**

840.6   **Supraspinatus (muscle) (tendon)**

840.7   **Superior glenoid labrum lesion**
SLAP lesion
DEF: Detachment injury of the superior aspect of the glenoid labrum which is the ring of fibrocartilage attached to the rim of the glenoid cavity of the scapula.

840.8   **Other specified sites of shoulder and upper arm**

840.9   **Unspecified site of shoulder and upper arm**
Arm NOS   Shoulder NOS

√4th   **841**   **Sprains and strains of elbow and forearm**

841.0   **Radial collateral ligament**

841.1   **Ulnar collateral ligament**

841.2   Radiohumeral (joint)

841.3   Ulnohumeral (joint)

841.8   Other specified sites of elbow and forearm

841.9   Unspecified site of elbow and forearm
        Elbow NOS

√4th **842   Sprains and strains of wrist and hand**

√5th   842.0   Wrist

        842.00   Unspecified site

        842.01   Carpal (joint)

        842.02   Radiocarpal (joint) (ligament)

        842.09   Other
                 Radioulnar joint, distal

√5th   842.1   Hand

        842.10   Unspecified site

        842.11   Carpometacarpal (joint)

        842.12   Metacarpophalangeal (joint)

        842.13   Interphalangeal (joint)

        842.19   Other
                 Midcarpal (joint)

√4th **843   Sprains and strains of hip and thigh**

        843.0   Iliofemoral (ligament)

        843.1   Ischiocapsular (ligament)

        843.8   Other specified sites of hip and thigh

        843.9   Unspecified site of hip and thigh
                Hip NOS
                Thigh NOS

√4th **844   Sprains and strains of knee and leg**

        844.0   Lateral collateral ligament of knee

        844.1   Medial collateral ligament of knee

        844.2   Cruciate ligament of knee

        844.3   Tibiofibular (joint) (ligament), superior

        844.8   Other specified sites of knee and leg

        844.9   Unspecified site of knee and leg
                Knee NOS
                Leg NOS

√4th **845   Sprains and strains of ankle and foot**

√5th   845.0   Ankle

        845.00   Unspecified site

        845.01   Deltoid (ligament), ankle
                 Internal collateral (ligament), ankle

        845.02   Calcaneofibular (ligament)

        845.03   Tibiofibular (ligament), distal

        845.09   Other
                 Achilles tendon

√5th   845.1   Foot

        845.10   Unspecified site

        845.11   Tarsometatarsal (joint) (ligament)

        845.12   Metatarsophalangeal (joint)

        845.13   Interphalangeal (joint), toe

        845.19   Other

√4th **846   Sprains and strains of sacroiliac region**

        846.0   Lumbosacral (joint) (ligament)

        846.1   Sacroiliac ligament

        846.2   Sacrospinatus (ligament)

        846.3   Sacrotuberous (ligament)

        846.8   Other specified sites of sacroiliac region

        846.9   Unspecified site of sacroiliac region

√4th **847   Sprains and strains of other and unspecified parts of back**
        EXCLUDES   lumbosacral (846.0)

        847.0   Neck
                Anterior longitudinal (ligament), cervical
                Atlanto-axial (joints)
                Atlanto-occipital (joints)
                Whiplash injury
                EXCLUDES   neck injury NOS (959.0)
                           thyroid region (848.2)

        847.1   Thoracic

        847.2   Lumbar

        847.3   Sacrum
                Sacrococcygeal (ligament)

        847.4   Coccyx

        847.9   Unspecified site of back
                Back NOS

√4th **848   Other and ill-defined sprains and strains**

        848.0   Septal cartilage of nose

        848.1   Jaw
                Temporomandibular (joint) (ligament)

        848.2   Thyroid region
                Cricoarytenoid (joint) (ligament)
                Cricothyroid (joint) (ligament)
                Thyroid cartilage

        848.3   Ribs
                Chondrocostal (joint) ⎤ without mention of injury
                Costal cartilage   ⎦ to sternum

√5th   848.4   Sternum

        848.40   Unspecified site

        848.41   Sternoclavicular (joint) (ligament)

        848.42   Chondrosternal (joint)

        848.49   Other
                 Xiphoid cartilage

        848.5   Pelvis
                Symphysis pubis
                EXCLUDES   that in childbirth (665.6)

        848.8   Other specified sites of sprains and strains

        848.9   Unspecified site of sprain and strain

INTRACRANIAL INJURY, EXCLUDING THOSE WITH SKULL FRACTURE (850-854)

        INCLUDES   traumatic brain injury without skull fracture
        EXCLUDES   intracranial injury with skull fracture (800-801 and
                   803-804, except .0 and .5)
                   open wound of head without intracranial injury
                   (870.0-873.9)
                   skull fracture alone (800-801 and 803-804 with .0, .5)
        Note: The description "with open intracranial wound," used in the
              fourth-digit subdivisions, includes those specified as open
              or with mention of infection or foreign body.

The following fifth-digit subclassification is for use with categories 851-854:
   0 unspecified state of consciousness
   1 with no loss of consciousness
   2 with brief [less than one hour] loss of consciousness
   3 with moderate [1-24 hours] loss of consciousness
   4 with prolonged [more than 24 hours] loss of consciousness and
      return to pre-existing conscious level
   5 with prolonged [more than 24 hours] loss of consciousness
      without return to pre-existing conscious level
        Use fifth-digit 5 to designate when a patient is unconscious and dies
        before regaining consciousness, regardless of the duration of
        the loss of consciousness
   6 with loss of consciousness of unspecified duration
   9 with concussion, unspecified

√4th **850   Concussion**

        INCLUDES   commotio cerebri
        EXCLUDES   concussion with:
                   cerebral laceration or contusion (851.0-851.9)
                   cerebral hemorrhage (852-853)
                   head injury NOS (959.01)

Brain

850.0 **With no loss of consciousness**
Concussion with mental confusion or disorientation, without loss of consciousness

√5ᵗʰ 850.1 **With brief loss of consciousness**
Loss of consciousness for less than one hour

850.11 **With loss of consciousness of 30 minutes or less**

850.12 **With loss of consciousness from 31 to 59 minutes**

850.2 **With moderate loss of consciousness**
Loss of consciousness for 1-24 hours

850.3 **With prolonged loss of consciousness and return to pre-existing conscious level**
Loss of consciousness for more than 24 hours with complete recovery

850.4 **With prolonged loss of consciousness, without return to pre-existing conscious level**

850.5 **With loss of consciousness of unspecified duration**

850.9 **Concussion, unspecified**

√4ᵗʰ 851 **Cerebral laceration and contusion**

√5ᵗʰ 851.0 **Cortex (cerebral) contusion without mention of open**
[0-6, 9] **intracranial wound**

√5ᵗʰ 851.1 **Cortex (cerebral) contusion with open intracranial**
[0-6, 9] **wound**

√5ᵗʰ 851.2 **Cortex (cerebral) laceration without mention of open**
[0-6, 9] **intracranial wound**

√5ᵗʰ 851.3 **Cortex (cerebral) laceration with open intracranial**
[0-6, 9] **wound**

√5ᵗʰ 851.4 **Cerebellar or brain stem contusion without mention of**
[0-6, 9] **open intracranial wound**

√5ᵗʰ 851.5 **Cerebellar or brain stem contusion with open**
[0-6, 9] **intracranial wound**

√5ᵗʰ 851.6 **Cerebellar or brain stem laceration without mention of**
[0-6, 9] **open intracranial wound**

√5ᵗʰ 851.7 **Cerebellar or brain stem laceration with open**
[0-6, 9] **intracranial wound**

√5ᵗʰ 851.8 **Other and unspecified cerebral laceration and**
[0-6, 9] **contusion, without mention of open intracranial**
wound
Brain (membrane) NOS

√5ᵗʰ 851.9 **Other and unspecified cerebral laceration and**
[0-6, 9] **contusion, with open intracranial wound**

√4ᵗʰ 852 **Subarachnoid, subdural, and extradural hemorrhage,**
following injury
EXCLUDES *Cerebral contusion or laceration (with hemorrhage)*
(851.0-851.9)
DEF: Bleeding from lining of brain; due to injury.

√5ᵗʰ 852.0 **Subarachnoid hemorrhage following injury without**
[0-6, 9] **mention of open intracranial wound**
Middle meningeal hemorrhage following injury

√5ᵗʰ 852.1 **Subarachnoid hemorrhage following injury with open**
[0-6, 9] **intracranial wound**

√5ᵗʰ 852.2 **Subdural hemorrhage following injury without**
[0-6, 9] **mention of open intracranial wound**

√5ᵗʰ 852.3 **Subdural hemorrhage following injury with open**
[0-6, 9] **intracranial wound**

√5ᵗʰ 852.4 **Extradural hemorrhage following injury without**
[0-6, 9] **mention of open intracranial wound**
Epidural hematoma following injury

√5ᵗʰ 852.5 **Extradural hemorrhage following injury with open**
[0-6, 9] **intracranial wound**

√4ᵗʰ 853 **Other and unspecified intracranial hemorrhage following**
injury

√5ᵗʰ 853.0 **Without mention of open intracranial wound**
[0-6, 9] Cerebral compression due to injury
Intracranial hematoma following injury
Traumatic cerebral hemorrhage

√5ᵗʰ 853.1 **With open intracranial wound**
[0-6, 9]

√4ᵗʰ 854 **Intracranial injury of other and unspecified nature**
INCLUDES injury:
brain NOS
cavernous sinus
intracranial
traumatic brain NOS
EXCLUDES *any condition classifiable to 850-853*
head injury NOS (959.01)

√5ᵗʰ 854.0 **Without mention of open intracranial wound**
[0-6, 9]

√5ᵗʰ 854.1 **With open intracranial wound**
[0-6, 9]

INTERNAL INJURY OF THORAX, ABDOMEN, AND PELVIS (860-869)

INCLUDES	blast injuries	
	blunt trauma	
	bruise	
	concussion injuries (except cerebral)	
	crushing	of internal
	hematoma	organs
	laceration	
	puncture	
	tear	
	traumatic rupture	

EXCLUDES *concussion NOS (850.0-850.9)*
flail chest (807.4)
foreign body entering through orifice (930.0-939.9)
injury to blood vessels (901.0-902.9)

Note: The description "with open wound," used in the fourth-digit subdivisions, includes those with mention of infection or foreign body.

☑4ᵗ **860 Traumatic pneumothorax and hemothorax**
> **DEF:** Traumatic pneumothorax: air or gas leaking into pleural space of lung due to trauma.
> **DEF:** Traumatic hemothorax: blood buildup in pleural space of lung due to trauma.

860.0 Pneumothorax without mention of open wound into thorax

860.1 Pneumothorax with open wound into thorax

860.2 Hemothorax without mention of open wound into thorax

860.3 Hemothorax with open wound into thorax

860.4 Pneumohemothorax without mention of open wound into thorax

860.5 Pneumohemothorax with open wound into thorax

☑4ᵗ **861 Injury to heart and lung**
> EXCLUDES   *injury to blood vessels of thorax (901.0-901.9)*

☑5ᵗ **861.0 Heart, without mention of open wound into thorax**

861.00 Unspecified injury

861.01 Contusion
> Cardiac contusion
> Myocardial contusion
> **DEF:** Bruising within the pericardium with no mention of open wound.

861.02 Laceration without penetration of heart chambers
> **DEF:** Tearing injury of heart tissue, without penetration of chambers; no open wound.

861.03 Laceration with penetration of heart chambers

☑5ᵗ **861.1 Heart, with open wound into thorax**

861.10 Unspecified injury

861.11 Contusion

861.12 Laceration without penetration of heart chambers

861.13 Laceration with penetration of heart chambers

☑5ᵗ **861.2 Lung, without mention of open wound into thorax**

861.20 Unspecified injury

861.21 Contusion
> **DEF:** Bruising of lung without mention of open wound.

861.22 Laceration

☑5ᵗ **861.3 Lung, with open wound into thorax**

861.30 Unspecified injury

861.31 Contusion

861.32 Laceration

☑4ᵗ **862 Injury to other and unspecified intrathoracic organs**
> EXCLUDES   *injury to blood vessels of thorax (901.0-901.9)*

862.0 Diaphragm, without mention of open wound into cavity

862.1 Diaphragm, with open wound into cavity

☑5ᵗ **862.2 Other specified intrathoracic organs, without mention of open wound into cavity**

862.21 Bronchus

862.22 Esophagus

862.29 Other
> Pleura
> Thymus gland

☑5ᵗ **862.3 Other specified intrathoracic organs, with open wound into cavity**

862.31 Bronchus

862.32 Esophagus

862.39 Other

862.8 Multiple and unspecified intrathoracic organs, without mention of open wound into cavity
> Crushed chest
> Multiple intrathoracic organs

862.9 Multiple and unspecified intrathoracic organs, with open wound into cavity

☑4ᵗ **863 Injury to gastrointestinal tract**
> EXCLUDES   *anal sphincter laceration during delivery (664.2)*
> *bile duct (868.0-868.1 with fifth-digit 2)*
> *gallbladder (868.0-868.1 with fifth-digit 2)*

863.0 Stomach, without mention of open wound into cavity

863.1 Stomach, with open wound into cavity

☑5ᵗ **863.2 Small intestine, without mention of open wound into cavity**

863.20 Small intestine, unspecified site

863.21 Duodenum

863.29 Other

☑5ᵗ **863.3 Small intestine, with open wound into cavity**

863.30 Small intestine, unspecified site

863.31 Duodenum

863.39 Other

☑5ᵗ **863.4 Colon or rectum, without mention of open wound into cavity**

863.40 Colon, unspecified site

863.41 Ascending [right] colon

863.42 Transverse colon

863.43 Descending [left] colon

863.44 Sigmoid colon

863.45 Rectum

863.46 Multiple sites in colon and rectum

863.49 Other

☑5ᵗ **863.5 Colon or rectum, with open wound into cavity**

863.50 Colon, unspecified site

863.51 Ascending [right] colon

863.52 Transverse colon

863.53 Descending [left] colon

863.54 Sigmoid colon

863.55 Rectum

863.56 Multiple sites in colon and rectum

863.59 Other

☑5ᵗ **863.8 Other and unspecified gastrointestinal sites, without mention of open wound into cavity**

863.80 Gastrointestinal tract, unspecified site

863.81 Pancreas, head

863.82 Pancreas, body

863.83 Pancreas, tail

863.84 Pancreas, multiple and unspecified sites

863.85 Appendix

863.89 Other
> Intestine NOS

☑5ᵗ **863.9 Other and unspecified gastrointestinal sites, with open wound into cavity**

863.90 Gastrointestinal tract, unspecified site

863.91 Pancreas, head

863.92 Pancreas, body

863.93 Pancreas, tail

863.94 Pancreas, multiple and unspecified sites

863.95 Appendix

863.99 Other

Injury and Poisoning

864–871.5

√4th **864 Injury to liver**

> The following fifth-digit subclassification is for use with category 864:
>
> 0 **unspecified injury**
> 1 **hematoma and contusion**
> 2 **laceration, minor**
> > Laceration involving capsule only, or without significant involvement of hepatic parenchyma [i.e., less than 1 cm deep]
> 3 **laceration, moderate**
> > Laceration involving parenchyma but without major disruption of parenchyma [i.e., less than 10 cm long and less than 3 cm deep]
> 4 **laceration, major**
> > Laceration with significant disruption of hepatic parenchyma [i.e., 10 cm long and 3 cm deep]
> > Multiple moderate lacerations, with or without hematoma
> > Stellate lacerations of liver
> 5 **laceration, unspecified**
> 9 **other**

√5th **864.0 Without mention of open wound into cavity**
[0-5, 9]

√5th **864.1 With open wound into cavity**
[0-5, 9]

√4th **865 Injury to spleen**

> The following fifth-digit subclassification is for use with category 865:
>
> 0 **unspecified injury**
> 1 **hematoma without rupture of capsule**
> 2 **capsular tears, without major disruption of parenchyma**
> 3 **laceration extending into parenchyma**
> 4 **massive parenchymal disruption**
> 9 **other**

√5th **865.0 Without mention of wound into cavity**
[0-4, 9]

√5th **865.1 With open wound into cavity**
[0-4, 9]

√4th **866 Injury to kidney**
> EXCLUDES *acute kidney injury (nontraumatic) (584.9)*

> The following fifth-digit subclassification is for use with category 866:
>
> 0 **unspecified injury**
> 1 **hematoma without rupture of capsule**
> 2 **laceration**
> 3 **complete disruption of kidney parenchyma**

√5th **866.0 Without mention of open wound into cavity**
[0-3]

√5th **866.1 With open wound into cavity**
[0-3]

√4th **867 Injury to pelvic organs**
> EXCLUDES *injury during delivery (664.0-665.9)*

867.0 Bladder and urethra, without mention of open wound into cavity

867.1 Bladder and urethra, with open wound into cavity

867.2 Ureter, without mention of open wound into cavity

867.3 Ureter, with open wound into cavity

867.4 Uterus, without mention of open wound into cavity

867.5 Uterus, with open wound into cavity

867.6 Other specified pelvic organs, without mention of open wound into cavity
> Fallopian tube   Seminal vesicle
> Ovary   Vas deferens
> Prostate

867.7 Other specified pelvic organs, with open wound into cavity

867.8 Unspecified pelvic organ, without mention of open wound into cavity

867.9 Unspecified pelvic organ, with open wound into cavity

√4th **868 Injury to other intra-abdominal organs**

> The following fifth-digit subclassification is for use with category 868:
>
> 0 **unspecified intra-abdominal organ**
> 1 **adrenal gland**
> 2 **bile duct and gallbladder**
> 3 **peritoneum**
> 4 **retroperitoneum**
> 9 **other and multiple intra-abdominal organs**

√5th **868.0 Without mention of open wound into cavity**
[0-4, 9]

√5th **868.1 With open wound into cavity**
[0-4, 9]

√4th **869 Internal injury to unspecified or ill-defined organs**
> INCLUDES   internal injury NOS
>   multiple internal injury NOS

869.0 Without mention of open wound into cavity

869.1 With open wound into cavity

OPEN WOUND (870-897)

> INCLUDES   animal bite
>   avulsion
>   cut
>   laceration
>   puncture wound
>   traumatic amputation
> EXCLUDES   *burn (940.0-949.5)*
>   *crushing (925-929.9)*
>   *puncture of internal organs (860.0-869.1)*
>   *superficial injury (910.0-919.9)*
>   *that incidental to:*
>   *dislocation (830.0-839.9)*
>   *fracture (800.0-829.1)*
>   *internal injury (860.0-869.1)*
>   *intracranial injury (851.0-854.1)*

Note: The description "complicated" used in the fourth-digit subdivisions includes those with mention of delayed healing, delayed treatment, foreign body, or infection.

OPEN WOUND OF HEAD, NECK, AND TRUNK (870-879)

√4th **870 Open wound of ocular adnexa**

870.0 Laceration of skin of eyelid and periocular area

870.1 Laceration of eyelid, full-thickness, not involving lacrimal passages

870.2 Laceration of eyelid involving lacrimal passages

870.3 Penetrating wound of orbit, without mention of foreign body

870.4 Penetrating wound of orbit with foreign body
> EXCLUDES   *retained (old) foreign body in orbit (376.6)*

870.8 Other specified open wounds of ocular adnexa

870.9 Unspecified open wound of ocular adnexa

√4th **871 Open wound of eyeball**
> EXCLUDES   *2nd cranial nerve [optic] injury (950.0-950.9)*
>   *3rd cranial nerve [oculomotor] injury (951.0)*

871.0 Ocular laceration without prolapse of intraocular tissue
> DEF: Tear in ocular tissue without displacing structures.

871.1 Ocular laceration with prolapse or exposure of intraocular tissue

871.2 Rupture of eye with partial loss of intraocular tissue
> DEF: Forcible tearing of eyeball, with tissue loss.

871.3 Avulsion of eye
> Traumatic enucleation
> DEF: Traumatic extraction of eyeball from socket.

871.4 Unspecified laceration of eye

871.5 Penetration of eyeball with magnetic foreign body
> EXCLUDES   *retained (old) magnetic foreign body in globe (360.50-360.59)*

871.6   **Penetration of eyeball with (nonmagnetic) foreign body**
   EXCLUDES   *retained (old) (nonmagnetic) foreign body in globe (360.60-360.69)*

871.7   **Unspecified ocular penetration**

871.9   **Unspecified open wound of eyeball**

√4th **872   Open wound of ear**

√5th **872.0   External ear, without mention of complication**

   872.00   **External ear, unspecified site**

   872.01   **Auricle, ear**
      Pinna
      DEF: Open wound of fleshy, outer ear.

   872.02   **Auditory canal**
      DEF: Open wound of passage from external ear to eardrum.

√5th **872.1   External ear, complicated**

   872.10   **External ear, unspecified site**

   872.11   **Auricle, ear**

   872.12   **Auditory canal**

√5th **872.6   Other specified parts of ear, without mention of complication**

   872.61   **Ear drum**
      Drumhead
      Tympanic membrane

   872.62   **Ossicles**

   872.63   **Eustachian tube**
      DEF: Open wound of channel between nasopharynx and tympanic cavity.

   872.64   **Cochlea**
      DEF: Open wound of snail shell shaped tube of inner ear.

   872.69   **Other and multiple sites**

√5th **872.7   Other specified parts of ear, complicated**

   872.71   **Ear drum**

   872.72   **Ossicles**

   872.73   **Eustachian tube**

   872.74   **Cochlea**

   872.79   **Other and multiple sites**

872.8   **Ear, part unspecified, without mention of complication**
   Ear NOS

872.9   **Ear, part unspecified, complicated**

√4th **873   Other open wound of head**

873.0   **Scalp, without mention of complication**

873.1   **Scalp, complicated**

√5th **873.2   Nose, without mention of complication**

   873.20   **Nose, unspecified site**

   873.21   **Nasal septum**
      DEF: Open wound between nasal passages.

   873.22   **Nasal cavity**
      DEF: Open wound of nostrils.

   873.23   **Nasal sinus**
      DEF: Open wound of mucous-lined respiratory cavities.

   873.29   **Multiple sites**

√5th **873.3   Nose, complicated**

   873.30   **Nose, unspecified site**

   873.31   **Nasal septum**

   873.32   **Nasal cavity**

   873.33   **Nasal sinus**

   873.39   **Multiple sites**

√5th **873.4   Face, without mention of complication**

   873.40   **Face, unspecified site**

   873.41   **Cheek**

   873.42   **Forehead**
      Eyebrow

   873.43   **Lip**

   873.44   **Jaw**

   873.49   **Other and multiple sites**

√5th **873.5   Face, complicated**

   873.50   **Face, unspecified site**

   873.51   **Cheek**

   873.52   **Forehead**

   873.53   **Lip**

   873.54   **Jaw**

   873.59   **Other and multiple sites**

√5th **873.6   Internal structures of mouth, without mention of complication**

   873.60   **Mouth, unspecified site**

   873.61   **Buccal mucosa**
      DEF: Open wound of inside of cheek.

   873.62   **Gum (alveolar process)**

   873.63   **Tooth (broken) (fractured) (due to trauma)**
      EXCLUDES   *cracked tooth (521.81)*

   873.64   **Tongue and floor of mouth**

   873.65   **Palate**
      DEF: Open wound of roof of mouth.

   873.69   **Other and multiple sites**

√5th **873.7   Internal structures of mouth, complicated**

   873.70   **Mouth, unspecified site**

   873.71   **Buccal mucosa**

   873.72   **Gum (alveolar process)**

   873.73   **Tooth (broken) (fractured) (due to trauma)**
      EXCLUDES   *cracked tooth (521.81)*

   873.74   **Tongue and floor of mouth**

   873.75   **Palate**

   873.79   **Other and multiple sites**

873.8   **Other and unspecified open wound of head without mention of complication**
   Head NOS

873.9   **Other and unspecified open wound of head, complicated**

√4th **874   Open wound of neck**

√5th **874.0   Larynx and trachea, without mention of complication**

   874.00   **Larynx with trachea**

   874.01   **Larynx**

   874.02   **Trachea**

√5th **874.1   Larynx and trachea, complicated**

   874.10   **Larynx with trachea**

   874.11   **Larynx**

   874.12   **Trachea**

874.2   **Thyroid gland, without mention of complication**

874.3   **Thyroid gland, complicated**

874.4   **Pharynx, without mention of complication**
   Cervical esophagus

874.5   **Pharynx, complicated**

874.8   **Other and unspecified parts, without mention of complication**
   Nape of neck
   Supraclavicular region
   Throat NOS

874.9   **Other and unspecified parts, complicated**

Injury and Poisoning

875–887.3

✓4th **875 Open wound of chest (wall)**
    EXCLUDES   *open wound into thoracic cavity (860.0-862.9)*
                   traumatic pneumothorax and hemothorax (860.1,
                     860.3, 860.5)

    875.0 Without mention of complication

    875.1 Complicated

✓4th **876 Open wound of back**
    INCLUDES   loin
                lumbar region
    EXCLUDES   *open wound into thoracic cavity (860.0-862.9)*
                    traumatic pneumothorax and hemothorax (860.1,
                     860.3, 860.5)

    876.0 Without mention of complication

    876.1 Complicated

✓4th **877 Open wound of buttock**
    INCLUDES   sacroiliac region

    877.0 Without mention of complication

    877.1 Complicated

✓4th **878 Open wound of genital organs (external), including traumatic amputation**
    EXCLUDES   *injury during delivery (664.0-665.9)*
                    internal genital organs (867.0-867.9)

    878.0 Penis, without mention of complication

    878.1 Penis, complicated

    878.2 Scrotum and testes, without mention of complication

    878.3 Scrotum and testes, complicated

    878.4 Vulva, without mention of complication
        Labium (majus) (minus)

    878.5 Vulva, complicated

    878.6 Vagina, without mention of complication

    878.7 Vagina, complicated

    878.8 Other and unspecified parts, without mention of complication

    878.9 Other and unspecified parts, complicated

✓4th **879 Open wound of other and unspecified sites, except limbs**

    879.0 Breast, without mention of complication

    879.1 Breast, complicated

    879.2 Abdominal wall, anterior, without mention of complication
        Abdominal wall NOS
        Epigastric region
        Hypogastric region
        Pubic region
        Umbilical region

    879.3 Abdominal wall, anterior, complicated

    879.4 Abdominal wall, lateral, without mention of complication
        Flank
        Groin
        Hypochondrium
        Iliac (region)
        Inguinal region

    879.5 Abdominal wall, lateral, complicated

    879.6 Other and unspecified parts of trunk, without mention of complication
        Pelvic region
        Perineum
        Trunk NOS

    879.7 Other and unspecified parts of trunk, complicated

    879.8 Open wound(s) (multiple) of unspecified site(s) without mention of complication
        Multiple open wounds NOS
        Open wound NOS

    879.9 Open wound(s) (multiple) of unspecified site(s), complicated

OPEN WOUND OF UPPER LIMB (880-887)

✓4th **880 Open wound of shoulder and upper arm**
    The following fifth-digit subclassification is for use with category 880:
        0   shoulder region
        1   scapular region
        2   axillary region
        3   upper arm
        9   multiple sites

    ✓5th **880.0 Without mention of complication**
        [0-3,9]

    ✓5th **880.1 Complicated**
        [0-3,9]

    ✓5th **880.2 With tendon involvement**
        [0-3,9]

✓4th **881 Open wound of elbow, forearm, and wrist**
    The following fifth-digit subclassification is for use with category 881:
        0   forearm
        1   elbow
        2   wrist

    ✓5th **881.0 Without mention of complication**
        [0-2]

    ✓5th **881.1 Complicated**
        [0-2]

    ✓5th **881.2 With tendon involvement**
        [0-2]

✓4th **882 Open wound of hand except finger(s) alone**

    882.0 Without mention of complication

    882.1 Complicated

    882.2 With tendon involvement

✓4th **883 Open wound of finger(s)**
    INCLUDES   fingernail
                thumb (nail)

    883.0 Without mention of complication

    883.1 Complicated

    883.2 With tendon involvement

✓4th **884 Multiple and unspecified open wound of upper limb**
    INCLUDES   arm NOS
                multiple sites of one upper limb
                upper limb NOS

    884.0 Without mention of complication

    884.1 Complicated

    884.2 With tendon involvement

✓4th **885 Traumatic amputation of thumb (complete) (partial)**
    INCLUDES   thumb(s) (with finger(s) of either hand)

    885.0 Without mention of complication

    885.1 Complicated

✓4th **886 Traumatic amputation of other finger(s) (complete) (partial)**
    INCLUDES   finger(s) of one or both hands, without mention of thumb(s)

    886.0 Without mention of complication

    886.1 Complicated

✓4th **887 Traumatic amputation of arm and hand (complete) (partial)**

    887.0 Unilateral, below elbow, without mention of complication

    887.1 Unilateral, below elbow, complicated

    887.2 Unilateral, at or above elbow, without mention of complication

    887.3 Unilateral, at or above elbow, complicated

887.4 Unilateral, level not specified, without mention of complication

887.5 Unilateral, level not specified, complicated

887.6 Bilateral [any level], without mention of complication
   One hand and other arm

887.7 Bilateral [any level], complicated

OPEN WOUND OF LOWER LIMB (890-897)

√4ᵗʰ **890 Open wound of hip and thigh**

890.0 Without mention of complication

890.1 Complicated

890.2 With tendon involvement

√4ᵗʰ **891 Open wound of knee, leg [except thigh], and ankle**
   INCLUDES leg NOS
      multiple sites of leg, except thigh
   EXCLUDES that of thigh (890.0-890.2)
      with multiple sites of lower limb (894.0-894.2)

891.0 Without mention of complication

891.1 Complicated

891.2 With tendon involvement

√4ᵗʰ **892 Open wound of foot except toe(s) alone**
   INCLUDES heel

892.0 Without mention of complication

892.1 Complicated

892.2 With tendon involvement

√4ᵗʰ **893 Open wound of toe(s)**
   INCLUDES toenail

893.0 Without mention of complication

893.1 Complicated

893.2 With tendon involvement

√4ᵗʰ **894 Multiple and unspecified open wound of lower limb**
   INCLUDES lower limb NOS
      multiple sites of one lower limb, with thigh

894.0 Without mention of complication

894.1 Complicated

894.2 With tendon involvement

√4ᵗʰ **895 Traumatic amputation of toe(s) (complete) (partial)**
   INCLUDES toe(s) of one or both feet

895.0 Without mention of complication

895.1 Complicated

√4ᵗʰ **896 Traumatic amputation of foot (complete) (partial)**

896.0 Unilateral, without mention of complication

896.1 Unilateral, complicated

896.2 Bilateral, without mention of complication
   EXCLUDES one foot and other leg (897.6-897.7)

896.3 Bilateral, complicated

√4ᵗʰ **897 Traumatic amputation of leg(s) (complete) (partial)**

897.0 Unilateral, below knee, without mention complication

897.1 Unilateral, below knee, complicated

897.2 Unilateral, at or above knee, without mention of complication

897.3 Unilateral, at or above knee, complicated

897.4 Unilateral, level not specified, without mention of complication

897.5 Unilateral, level not specified, complicated

897.6 Bilateral [any level], without mention of complication
   One foot and other leg

897.7 Bilateral [any level], complicated

INJURY TO BLOOD VESSELS (900-904)

INCLUDES arterial hematoma
   avulsion
   cut   of blood vessel
   laceration   secondary to
   rupture   other injuries,
   traumatic aneurysm or fistula   e.g.; fracture
      (arteriovenous)   or open
                                    wound

EXCLUDES accidental puncture or laceration during medical
      procedure (998.2)
   intracranial hemorrhage following injury (851.0-854.1)

√4ᵗʰ **900 Injury to blood vessels of head and neck**

√5ᵗʰ 900.0 Carotid artery

900.00 Carotid artery, unspecified

900.01 Common carotid artery

900.02 External carotid artery

900.03 Internal carotid artery

900.1 Internal jugular vein

√5ᵗʰ 900.8 Other specified blood vessels of head and neck

900.81 External jugular vein
   Jugular vein NOS

900.82 Multiple blood vessels of head and neck

900.89 Other

900.9 Unspecified blood vessel of head and neck

√4ᵗʰ **901 Injury to blood vessels of thorax**
   EXCLUDES traumatic hemothorax (860.2-860.5)

901.0 Thoracic aorta

901.1 Innominate and subclavian arteries

901.2 Superior vena cava

901.3 Innominate and subclavian veins

√5ᵗʰ 901.4 Pulmonary blood vessels

901.40 Pulmonary vessel(s), unspecified

901.41 Pulmonary artery

901.42 Pulmonary vein

√5ᵗʰ 901.8 Other specified blood vessels of thorax

901.81 Intercostal artery or vein

901.82 Internal mammary artery or vein

901.83 Multiple blood vessels of thorax

901.89 Other
   Azygos vein
   Hemiazygos vein

901.9 Unspecified blood vessel of thorax

√4ᵗʰ **902 Injury to blood vessels of abdomen and pelvis**

902.0 Abdominal aorta

√5ᵗʰ 902.1 Inferior vena cava

902.10 Inferior vena cava, unspecified

902.11 Hepatic veins

902.19 Other

√5ᵗʰ 902.2 Celiac and mesenteric arteries

902.20 Celiac and mesenteric arteries, unspecified

902.21 Gastric artery

902.22 Hepatic artery

902.23 Splenic artery

902.24 Other specified branches of celiac axis

902.25 Superior mesenteric artery (trunk)

902.26 Primary branches of superior mesenteric artery
   Ileocolic artery

902.27 Inferior mesenteric artery

902.29 Other

Injury and Poisoning

902.3–906.8

☑5ᵗʰ **902.3 Portal and splenic veins**

    902.31 Superior mesenteric vein and primary subdivisions
        Ileocolic vein

    902.32 Inferior mesenteric vein

    902.33 Portal vein

    902.34 Splenic vein

    902.39 Other
        Cystic vein
        Gastric vein

☑5ᵗʰ **902.4 Renal blood vessels**

    902.40 Renal vessel(s), unspecified

    902.41 Renal artery

    902.42 Renal vein

    902.49 Other
        Suprarenal arteries

☑5ᵗʰ **902.5 Iliac blood vessels**

    902.50 Iliac vessel(s), unspecified

    902.51 Hypogastric artery

    902.52 Hypogastric vein

    902.53 Iliac artery

    902.54 Iliac vein

    902.55 Uterine artery

    902.56 Uterine vein

    902.59 Other

☑5ᵗʰ **902.8 Other specified blood vessels of abdomen and pelvis**

    902.81 Ovarian artery

    902.82 Ovarian vein

    902.87 Multiple blood vessels of abdomen and pelvis

    902.89 Other

    902.9 Unspecified blood vessel of abdomen and pelvis

☑4ᵗʰ **903 Injury to blood vessels of upper extremity**

☑5ᵗʰ **903.0 Axillary blood vessels**

    903.00 Axillary vessel(s), unspecified

    903.01 Axillary artery

    903.02 Axillary vein

    903.1 Brachial blood vessels

    903.2 Radial blood vessels

    903.3 Ulnar blood vessels

    903.4 Palmar artery

    903.5 Digital blood vessels

    903.8 Other specified blood vessels of upper extremity
        Multiple blood vessels of upper extremity

    903.9 Unspecified blood vessel of upper extremity

☑4ᵗʰ **904 Injury to blood vessels of lower extremity and unspecified sites**

    904.0 Common femoral artery
        Femoral artery above profunda origin

    904.1 Superficial femoral artery

    904.2 Femoral veins

    904.3 Saphenous veins
        Saphenous vein (greater) (lesser)

☑5ᵗʰ **904.4 Popliteal blood vessels**

    904.40 Popliteal vessel(s), unspecified

    904.41 Popliteal artery

    904.42 Popliteal vein

☑5ᵗʰ **904.5 Tibial blood vessels**

    904.50 Tibial vessel(s), unspecified

    904.51 Anterior tibial artery

    904.52 Anterior tibial vein

    904.53 Posterior tibial artery

    904.54 Posterior tibial vein

    904.6 Deep plantar blood vessels

    904.7 Other specified blood vessels of lower extremity
        Multiple blood vessels of lower extremity

    904.8 Unspecified blood vessel of lower extremity

    904.9 Unspecified site
        Injury to blood vessel NOS

LATE EFFECTS OF INJURIES, POISONINGS, TOXIC EFFECTS, AND OTHER EXTERNAL CAUSES (905-909)

Note: These categories are to be used to indicate conditions classifiable to 800-999 as the cause of late effects, which are themselves classified elsewhere. The "late effects" include those specified as such, or as sequelae, which may occur at any time after the acute injury.

☑4ᵗʰ **905 Late effects of musculoskeletal and connective tissue injuries**

    905.0 Late effect of fracture of skull and face bones
        Late effect of injury classifiable to 800-804

    905.1 Late effect of fracture of spine and trunk without mention of spinal cord lesion
        Late effect of injury classifiable to 805, 807-809

    905.2 Late effect of fracture of upper extremities
        Late effect of injury classifiable to 810-819

    905.3 Late effect of fracture of neck of femur
        Late effect of injury classifiable to 820

    905.4 Late effect of fracture of lower extremities
        Late effect of injury classifiable to 821-827

    905.5 Late effect of fracture of multiple and unspecified bones
        Late effect of injury classifiable to 828-829

    905.6 Late effect of dislocation
        Late effect of injury classifiable to 830-839

    905.7 Late effect of sprain and strain without mention of tendon injury
        Late effect of injury classifiable to 840-848, except tendon injury

    905.8 Late effect of tendon injury
        Late effect of tendon injury due to:
            open wound [injury classifiable to 880-884 with .2, 890-894 with .2]
            sprain and strain [injury classifiable to 840-848]

    905.9 Late effect of traumatic amputation
        Late effect of injury classifiable to 885-887, 895-897
        EXCLUDES *late amputation stump complication (997.60-997.69)*

☑4ᵗʰ **906 Late effects of injuries to skin and subcutaneous tissues**

    906.0 Late effect of open wound of head, neck, and trunk
        Late effect of injury classifiable to 870-879

    906.1 Late effect of open wound of extremities without mention of tendon injury
        Late effect of injury classifiable to 880-884, 890-894 except .2

    906.2 Late effect of superficial injury
        Late effect of injury classifiable to 910-919

    906.3 Late effect of contusion
        Late effect of injury classifiable to 920-924

    906.4 Late effect of crushing
        Late effect of injury classifiable to 925-929

    906.5 Late effect of burn of eye, face, head, and neck
        Late effect of injury classifiable to 940-941

    906.6 Late effect of burn of wrist and hand
        Late effect of injury classifiable to 944

    906.7 Late effect of burn of other extremities
        Late effect of injury classifiable to 943 or 945

    906.8 Late effect of burns of other specified sites
        Late effect of injury classifiable to 942, 946-947

906.9   **Late effect of burn of unspecified site**
Late effect of injury classifiable to 948-949

✓4ᵗʰ **907 Late effects of injuries to the nervous system**

907.0   **Late effect of intracranial injury without mention of skull fracture**
Late effect of injury classifiable to 850-854

907.1   **Late effect of injury to cranial nerve**
Late effect of injury classifiable to 950-951

907.2   **Late effect of spinal cord injury**
Late effect of injury classifiable to 806, 952

907.3   **Late effect of injury to nerve root(s), spinal plexus(es), and other nerves of trunk**
Late effect of injury classifiable to 953-954

907.4   **Late effect of injury to peripheral nerve of shoulder girdle and upper limb**
Late effect of injury classifiable to 955

907.5   **Late effect of injury to peripheral nerve of pelvic girdle and lower limb**
Late effect of injury classifiable to 956

907.9   **Late effect of injury to other and unspecified nerve**
Late effect of injury classifiable to 957

✓4ᵗʰ **908 Late effects of other and unspecified injuries**

908.0   **Late effect of internal injury to chest**
Late effect of injury classifiable to 860-862

908.1   **Late effect of internal injury to intra-abdominal organs**
Late effect of injury classifiable to 863-866, 868

908.2   **Late effect of internal injury to other internal organs**
Late effect of injury classifiable to 867 or 869

908.3   **Late effect of injury to blood vessel of head, neck, and extremities**
Late effect of injury classifiable to 900, 903-904

908.4   **Late effect of injury to blood vessel of thorax, abdomen, and pelvis**
Late effect of injury classifiable to 901-902

908.5   **Late effect of foreign body in orifice**
Late effect of injury classifiable to 930-939

908.6   **Late effect of certain complications of trauma**
Late effect of complications classifiable to 958

908.9   **Late effect of unspecified injury**
Late effect of injury classifiable to 959

✓4ᵗʰ **909 Late effects of other and unspecified external causes**

909.0   **Late effect of poisoning due to drug, medicinal or biological substance**
Late effect of conditions classifiable to 960-979
EXCLUDES   *late effect of adverse effect of drug, medicinal or biological substance (909.5)*

909.1   **Late effect of toxic effects of nonmedical substances**
Late effect of conditions classifiable to 980-989

909.2   **Late effect of radiation**
Late effect of conditions classifiable to 990

909.3   **Late effect of complications of surgical and medical care**
Late effect of conditions classifiable to 996-999

909.4   **Late effect of certain other external causes**
Late effect of conditions classifiable to 991-994

909.5   **Late effect of adverse effect of drug, medical or biological substance**
EXCLUDES   *late effect of poisoning due to drug, medicinal or biological substance (909.0)*

909.9   **Late effect of other and unspecified external causes**

SUPERFICIAL INJURY (910-919)

EXCLUDES   *burn (blisters) (940.0-949.5)*
contusion (920-924.9)
foreign body:
   granuloma (728.82)
   inadvertently left in operative wound (998.4)
   residual in soft tissue (729.6)
insect bite, venomous (989.5)
open wound with incidental foreign body (870.0-897.7)

✓4ᵗʰ **910 Superficial injury of face, neck, and scalp except eye**

INCLUDES   cheek
ear
gum
lip
nose
throat

EXCLUDES   *eye and adnexa (918.0-918.9)*

910.0   **Abrasion or friction burn without mention of infection**

910.1   **Abrasion or friction burn, infected**

910.2   **Blister without mention of infection**

910.3   **Blister, infected**

910.4   **Insect bite, nonvenomous, without mention of infection**

910.5   **Insect bite, nonvenomous, infected**

910.6   **Superficial foreign body (splinter) without major open wound and without mention of infection**

910.7   **Superficial foreign body (splinter) without major open wound, infected**

910.8   **Other and unspecified superficial injury of face, neck, and scalp without mention of infection**

910.9   **Other and unspecified superficial injury of face, neck, and scalp, infected**

✓4ᵗʰ **911 Superficial injury of trunk**

INCLUDES   abdominal wall   interscapular region
anus   labium (majus) (minus)
back   penis
breast   perineum
buttock   scrotum
chest wall   testis
flank   vagina
groin   vulva

EXCLUDES   *hip (916.0-916.9)*
scapular region (912.0-912.9)

911.0   **Abrasion or friction burn without mention of infection**

911.1   **Abrasion or friction burn, infected**

911.2   **Blister without mention of infection**

911.3   **Blister, infected**

911.4   **Insect bite, nonvenomous, without mention of infection**

911.5   **Insect bite, nonvenomous, infected**

911.6   **Superficial foreign body (splinter) without major open wound and without mention of infection**

911.7   **Superficial foreign body (splinter) without major open wound, infected**

911.8   **Other and unspecified superficial injury of trunk without mention of infection**

911.9   **Other and unspecified superficial injury of trunk, infected**

✓4ᵗʰ **912 Superficial injury of shoulder and upper arm**

INCLUDES   axilla
scapular region

912.0   **Abrasion or friction burn without mention of infection**

912.1   **Abrasion or friction burn, infected**

912.2   **Blister without mention of infection**

912.3   **Blister, infected**

912.4   **Insect bite, nonvenomous, without mention of infection**

912.5   Insect bite, nonvenomous, infected

912.6   Superficial foreign body (splinter) without major open wound and without mention of infection

912.7   Superficial foreign body (splinter) without major open wound, infected

912.8   Other and unspecified superficial injury of shoulder and upper arm without mention of infection

912.9   Other and unspecified superficial injury of shoulder and upper arm, infected

√4ᵗʰ **913   Superficial injury of elbow, forearm, and wrist**

913.0   Abrasion or friction burn without mention of infection

913.1   Abrasion or friction burn, infected

913.2   Blister without mention of infection

913.3   Blister, infected

913.4   Insect bite, nonvenomous, without mention of infection

913.5   Insect bite, nonvenomous, infected

913.6   Superficial foreign body (splinter) without major open wound and without mention of infection

913.7   Superficial foreign body (splinter) without major open wound, infected

913.8   Other and unspecified superficial injury of elbow, forearm, and wrist without mention of infection

913.9   Other and unspecified superficial injury of elbow, forearm, and wrist, infected

√4ᵗʰ **914   Superficial injury of hand(s) except finger(s) alone**

914.0   Abrasion or friction burn without mention of infection

914.1   Abrasion or friction burn, infected

914.2   Blister without mention of infection

914.3   Blister, infected

914.4   Insect bite, nonvenomous, without mention of infection

914.5   Insect bite, nonvenomous, infected

914.6   Superficial foreign body (splinter) without major open wound and without mention of infection

914.7   Superficial foreign body (splinter) without major open wound, infected

914.8   Other and unspecified superficial injury of hand without mention of infection

914.9   Other and unspecified superficial injury of hand, infected

√4ᵗʰ **915   Superficial injury of finger(s)**

INCLUDES   fingernail
           thumb (nail)

915.0   Abrasion or friction burn without mention of infection

915.1   Abrasion or friction burn, infected

915.2   Blister without mention of infection

915.3   Blister, infected

915.4   Insect bite, nonvenomous, without mention of infection

915.5   Insect bite, nonvenomous, infected

915.6   Superficial foreign body (splinter) without major open wound and without mention of infection

915.7   Superficial foreign body (splinter) without major open wound, infected

915.8   Other and unspecified superficial injury of fingers without mention of infection

915.9   Other and unspecified superficial injury of fingers, infected

√4ᵗʰ **916   Superficial injury of hip, thigh, leg, and ankle**

916.0   Abrasion or friction burn without mention of infection

916.1   Abrasion or friction burn, infected

916.2   Blister without mention of infection

916.3   Blister, infected

916.4   Insect bite, nonvenomous, without mention of infection

916.5   Insect bite, nonvenomous, infected

916.6   Superficial foreign body (splinter) without major open wound and without mention of infection

916.7   Superficial foreign body (splinter) without major open wound, infected

916.8   Other and unspecified superficial injury of hip, thigh, leg, and ankle without mention of infection

916.9   Other and unspecified superficial injury of hip, thigh, leg, and ankle, infected

√4ᵗʰ **917   Superficial injury of foot and toe(s)**

INCLUDES   heel
           toenail

917.0   Abrasion or friction burn without mention of infection

917.1   Abrasion or friction burn, infected

917.2   Blister without mention of infection

917.3   Blister, infected

917.4   Insect bite, nonvenomous, without mention of infection

917.5   Insect bite, nonvenomous, infected

917.6   Superficial foreign body (splinter) without major open wound and without mention of infection

917.7   Superficial foreign body (splinter) without major open wound, infected

917.8   Other and unspecified superficial injury of foot and toes without mention of infection

917.9   Other and unspecified superficial injury of foot and toes, infected

√4ᵗʰ **918   Superficial injury of eye and adnexa**

EXCLUDES   burn (940.0-940.9)
           foreign body on external eye (930.0-930.9)

918.0   Eyelids and periocular area
        Abrasion
        Insect bite
        Superficial foreign body (splinter)

918.1   Cornea
        Corneal abrasion
        Superficial laceration
        EXCLUDES   corneal injury due to contact lens (371.82)

918.2   Conjunctiva

918.9   Other and unspecified superficial injuries of eye
        Eye (ball) NOS

√4ᵗʰ **919   Superficial injury of other, multiple, and unspecified sites**

EXCLUDES   multiple sites classifiable to the same three-digit category (910.0-918.9)

919.0   Abrasion or friction burn without mention of infection

919.1   Abrasion or friction burn, infected

919.2   Blister without mention of infection

919.3   Blister, infected

919.4   Insect bite, nonvenomous, without mention of infection

919.5   Insect bite, nonvenomous, infected

919.6   Superficial foreign body (splinter) without major open wound and without mention of infection

919.7   Superficial foreign body (splinter) without major open wound, infected

919.8   Other and unspecified superficial injury without mention of infection

919.9   Other and unspecified superficial injury, infected

CONTUSION WITH INTACT SKIN SURFACE (920-924)

INCLUDES	bruise } without fracture or open
	hematoma } wound

EXCLUDES	concussion (850.0-850.9)
	hemarthrosis (840.0-848.9)
	internal organs (860.0-869.1)
	that incidental to:
	crushing injury (925-929.9)
	dislocation (830.0-839.9)
	fracture (800.0-829.1)
	internal injury (860.0-869.1)
	intracranial injury (850.0-854.1)
	nerve injury (950.0-957.9)
	open wound (870.0-897.7)

920 Contusion of face, scalp, and neck except eye(s)

Cheek	Mandibular joint area
Ear (auricle)	Nose
Gum	Throat
Lip	

√4th **921 Contusion of eye and adnexa**

   921.0 Black eye, not otherwise specified

   921.1 Contusion of eyelids and periocular area

   921.2 Contusion of orbital tissues

   921.3 Contusion of eyeball

   921.9 Unspecified contusion of eye
      Injury of eye NOS

√4th **922 Contusion of trunk**

   922.0 Breast

   922.1 Chest wall

   922.2 Abdominal wall
      Flank   Groin

√5th   **922.3 Back**

      922.31 Back

	EXCLUDES	interscapular region (922.33)

      922.32 Buttock

      922.33 Interscapular region

   922.4 Genital organs

Labium (majus) (minus)	Testis
Penis	Vagina
Perineum	Vulva
Scrotum	

   922.8 Multiple sites of trunk

   922.9 Unspecified part
      Trunk NOS

√4th **923 Contusion of upper limb**

√5th   **923.0 Shoulder and upper arm**

      923.00 Shoulder region

      923.01 Scapular region

      923.02 Axillary region

      923.03 Upper arm

      923.09 Multiple sites

√5th   **923.1 Elbow and forearm**

      923.10 Forearm

      923.11 Elbow

√5th   **923.2 Wrist and hand(s), except finger(s) alone**

      923.20 Hand(s)

      923.21 Wrist

   923.3 Finger
      Fingernail
      Thumb (nail)

   923.8 Multiple sites of upper limb

   923.9 Unspecified part of upper limb
      Arm NOS

√4th **924 Contusion of lower limb and of other and unspecified sites**

√5th   **924.0 Hip and thigh**

      924.00 Thigh

      924.01 Hip

√5th   **924.1 Knee and lower leg**

      924.10 Lower leg

      924.11 Knee

√5th   **924.2 Ankle and foot, excluding toe(s)**

      924.20 Foot
         Heel

      924.21 Ankle

   924.3 Toe
      Toenail

   924.4 Multiple sites of lower limb

   924.5 Unspecified part of lower limb
      Leg NOS

   924.8 Multiple sites, not elsewhere classified

   924.9 Unspecified site

CRUSHING INJURY (925-929)

Use additional code to identify any associated injuries, such as:
   fractures (800-829)
   internal injuries (860.0-869.1)
   intracranial injuries (850.0-854.1)

√4th **925 Crushing injury of face, scalp, and neck**

Cheek	Pharynx
Ear	Throat
Larynx	

   925.1 Crushing injury of face and scalp
      Cheek   Ear

   925.2 Crushing injury of neck

Larynx	Throat
Pharynx	

√4th **926 Crushing injury of trunk**

   926.0 External genitalia

Labium (majus) (minus)	Testis
Penis	Vulva
Scrotum	

√5th   **926.1 Other specified sites**

      926.11 Back

      926.12 Buttock

      926.19 Other
         Breast

   926.8 Multiple sites of trunk

   926.9 Unspecified site
      Trunk NOS

√4th **927 Crushing injury of upper limb**

√5th   **927.0 Shoulder and upper arm**

      927.00 Shoulder region

      927.01 Scapular region

      927.02 Axillary region

      927.03 Upper arm

      927.09 Multiple sites

√5th   **927.1 Elbow and forearm**

      927.10 Forearm

      927.11 Elbow

√5th   **927.2 Wrist and hand(s), except finger(s) alone**

      927.20 Hand(s)

      927.21 Wrist

   927.3 Finger(s)

   927.8 Multiple sites of upper limb

927.9 Unspecified site
Arm NOS

√4ᵗʰ **928 Crushing injury of lower limb**

√5ᵗʰ **928.0 Hip and thigh**

928.00 Thigh

928.01 Hip

√5ᵗʰ **928.1 Knee and lower leg**

928.10 Lower leg

928.11 Knee

√5ᵗʰ **928.2 Ankle and foot, excluding toe(s) alone**

928.20 Foot
Heel

928.21 Ankle

928.3 Toe(s)

928.8 Multiple sites of lower limb

928.9 Unspecified site
Leg NOS

√4ᵗʰ **929 Crushing injury of multiple and unspecified sites**

929.0 Multiple sites, not elsewhere classified

929.9 Unspecified site

EFFECTS OF FOREIGN BODY ENTERING THROUGH ORIFICE (930-939)

EXCLUDES *foreign body:*
granuloma (728.82)
inadvertently left in operative wound (998.4, 998.7)
in open wound (800-839, 851-897)
residual in soft tissues (729.6)
superficial without major open wound (910-919 with .6 or .7)

√4ᵗʰ **930 Foreign body on external eye**
EXCLUDES *foreign body in penetrating wound of:*
eyeball (871.5-871.6)
retained (old) (360.5-360.6)
ocular adnexa (870.4)
retained (old) (376.6)

930.0 Corneal foreign body

930.1 Foreign body in conjunctival sac

930.2 Foreign body in lacrimal punctum

930.8 Other and combined sites

930.9 Unspecified site
External eye NOS

931 Foreign body in ear
Auditory canal
Auricle

932 Foreign body in nose
Nasal sinus
Nostril

√4ᵗʰ **933 Foreign body in pharynx and larynx**

933.0 Pharynx
Nasopharynx
Throat NOS

933.1 Larynx
Asphyxia due to foreign body
Choking due to:
food (regurgitated)
phlegm

√4ᵗʰ **934 Foreign body in trachea, bronchus, and lung**

934.0 Trachea

934.1 Main bronchus

934.8 Other specified parts
Bronchioles
Lung

934.9 Respiratory tree, unspecified
Inhalation of liquid or vomitus, lower respiratory tract NOS

√4ᵗʰ **935 Foreign body in mouth, esophagus, and stomach**

935.0 Mouth

935.1 Esophagus

935.2 Stomach

936 Foreign body in intestine and colon

937 Foreign body in anus and rectum
Rectosigmoid (junction)

938 Foreign body in digestive system, unspecified
Alimentary tract NOS
Swallowed foreign body

√4ᵗʰ **939 Foreign body in genitourinary tract**

939.0 Bladder and urethra

939.1 Uterus, any part
EXCLUDES *intrauterine contraceptive device:*
complications from (996.32, 996.65)
presence of (V45.51)

939.2 Vulva and vagina

939.3 Penis

939.9 Unspecified site

BURNS (940-949)

INCLUDES burns from:
electrical heating appliance
electricity
flame
hot object
lightning
radiation
chemical burns (external) (internal)
scalds

EXCLUDES *friction burns (910-919 with .0, .1)*
sunburn (692.71, 692.76-692.77)

√4ᵗʰ **940 Burn confined to eye and adnexa**

940.0 Chemical burn of eyelids and periocular area

940.1 Other burns of eyelids and periocular area

940.2 Alkaline chemical burn of cornea and conjunctival sac

940.3 Acid chemical burn of cornea and conjunctival sac

940.4 Other burn of cornea and conjunctival sac

940.5 Burn with resulting rupture and destruction of eyeball

940.9 Unspecified burn of eye and adnexa

√4ᵗʰ **941 Burn of face, head, and neck**
EXCLUDES *mouth (947.0)*

The following fifth-digit subclassification is for use with category 941:

0 face and head, unspecified site
1 ear [any part]
2 eye (with other parts of face, head, and neck)
3 lip(s)
4 chin
5 nose (septum)
6 scalp [any part]
Temple (region)
7 forehead and cheek
8 neck
9 multiple sites [except with eye] of face, head, and neck

√5ᵗʰ **941.0 Unspecified degree**
[0-9]

√5ᵗʰ **941.1 Erythema [first degree]**
[0-9]

√5ᵗʰ **941.2 Blisters, epidermal loss [second degree]**
[0-9]

√5ᵗʰ **941.3 Full-thickness skin loss [third degree NOS]**
[0-9]

√5ᵗʰ **941.4** Deep necrosis of underlying tissues [deep third degree]
[0-9] without mention of loss of a body part

√5ᵗʰ **941.5** Deep necrosis of underlying tissues [deep third degree]
[0-9] with loss of a body part

√4ᵗʰ **942** **Burn of trunk**
EXCLUDES *scapular region (943.0-943.5 with fifth-digit 6)*

The following fifth-digit subclassificaiton is for use with category 942:
- 0 trunk, unspecified
- 1 breast
- 2 chest wall, excluding breast and nipple
- 3 abdominal wall
  - Flank
  - Groin
- 4 back [any part]
  - Buttock
  - Interscapular region
- 5 genitalia
  - Labium (majus) (minus
  - Penis
  - Perineum
  - Scrotum
  - Testis
  - Vulva
- 9 other and multiple sites of trunk

√5ᵗʰ **942.0** Unspecified degree
[0-5, 9]

√5ᵗʰ **942.1** Erythema [first degree]
[0-5, 9]

√5ᵗʰ **942.2** Blisters, epidermal loss [second degree]
[0-5, 9]

√5ᵗʰ **942.3** Full-thickness skin loss [third degree NOS]
[0-5, 9]

√5ᵗʰ **942.4** Deep necrosis of underlying tissues [deep third degree]
[0-5, 9] without mention of loss of a body part

√5ᵗʰ **942.5** Deep necrosis of underlying tissues [deep third degree]
[0-5, 9] with loss of a body part

√4ᵗʰ **943** **Burn of upper limb, except wrist and hand**

The following fifth-digit subclassificaiton is for use with category 943:
- 0 upper limb, unspecified site
- 1 forearm
- 2 elbow
- 3 upper arm
- 4 axilla
- 5 shoulder
- 6 scapular region
- 9 multiple sites of upper limb, except wrist and hand

√5ᵗʰ **943.0** Unspecified degree
[0-6, 9]

√5ᵗʰ **943.1** Erythema [first degree]
[0-6, 9]

√5ᵗʰ **943.2** Blisters, epidermal loss [second degree]
[0-6, 9]

√5ᵗʰ **943.3** Full-thickness skin loss [third degree NOS]
[0-6, 9]

√5ᵗʰ **943.4** Deep necrosis of underlying tissues [deep third degree]
[0-6, 9] without mention of loss of a body part

√5ᵗʰ **943.5** Deep necrosis of underlying tissues [deep third degree]
[0-6, 9] with loss of a body part

√4ᵗʰ **944** **Burn of wrist(s) and hand(s)**

The following fifth-digit subclassification is for use with category 944:
- 0 hand, unspecified site
- 1 single digit [finger (nail)] other than thumb
- 2 thumb (nail)
- 3 two or more digits, not including thumb
- 4 two or more digits including thumb
- 5 palm
- 6 back of hand
- 7 wrist
- 8 multiple sites of wrist(s) and hand(s)

√5ᵗʰ **944.0** Unspecified degree
[0-8]

√5ᵗʰ **944.1** Erythema [first degree]
[0-8]

√5ᵗʰ **944.2** Blisters, epidermal loss [second degree]
[0-8]

√5ᵗʰ **944.3** Full-thickness skin loss [third degree NOS]
[0-8]

√5ᵗʰ **944.4** Deep necrosis of underlying tissues [deep third degree]
[0-8] without mention of loss of a body part

√5ᵗʰ **944.5** Deep necrosis of underlying tissues [deep third degree]
[0-8] with loss of a body part

√4ᵗʰ **945** **Burn of lower limb(s)**

The following fifth-digit subclassification is for use with category 945:
- 0 lower limb [leg], unspecified site
- 1 toe(s) (nail)
- 2 foot
- 3 ankle
- 4 lower leg
- 5 knee
- 6 thigh [any part]
- 9 multiple sites of lower limb(s)

√5ᵗʰ **945.0** Unspecified degree
[0-6, 9]

√5ᵗʰ **945.1** Erythema [first degree]
[0-6, 9]

√5ᵗʰ **945.2** Blisters, epidermal loss [second degree]
[0-6, 9]

√5ᵗʰ **945.3** Full-thickness skin loss [third degree NOS]
[0-6, 9]

√5ᵗʰ **945.4** Deep necrosis of underlying tissues [deep third degree]
[0-6, 9] without mention of loss of a body part

√5ᵗʰ **945.5** Deep necrosis of underlying tissues [deep third degree]
[0-6, 9] with loss of a body part

√4ᵗʰ **946** **Burns of multiple specified sites**
INCLUDES burns of sites classifiable to more than one three-digit category in 940-945
EXCLUDES *multiple burns NOS (949.0-949.5)*

946.0 Unspecified degree

946.1 Erythema [first degree]

946.2 Blisters, epidermal loss [second degree]

946.3 Full-thickness skin loss [third degree NOS]

946.4 Deep necrosis of underlying tissues [deep third degree] without mention of loss of a body part

946.5 Deep necrosis of underlying tissues [deep third degree] with loss of a body part

√4ᵗʰ **947** **Burn of internal organs**
INCLUDES burns from chemical agents (ingested)

947.0 Mouth and pharynx
Gum
Tongue

947.1 Larynx, trachea, and lung

947.2 Esophagus

947.3 Gastrointestinal tract
    Colon   Small intestine
    Rectum   Stomach

947.4 Vagina and uterus

947.8 Other specified sites

947.9 Unspecified site

√4ᵗʰ **948 Burns classified according to extent of body surface involved**

> Note: This category is to be used when the site of the burn is unspecified, or with categories 940-947 when the site is specified.

> **EXCLUDES** *sunburn (692.71, 692.76-692.77)*

> The following fifth-digit subclassification is for use with category 948 to indicate the percent of body surface with third degree burn; valid digits are in [brackets] under each code:
> **0 less than 10 percent or unspecified**
> **1 10-19%**
> **2 20-29%**
> **3 30-39%**
> **4 40-49%**
> **5 50-59%**
> **6 60-69%**
> **7 70-79%**
> **8 80-89%**
> **9 90% or more of body surface**

√5ᵗʰ **948.0** **Burn [any degree] involving less than 10**
[0]   **percent of body surface**

√5ᵗʰ **948.1** **10-19 percent of body surface**
[0-1]

√5ᵗʰ **948.2** **20-29 percent of body surface**
[0-2]

√5ᵗʰ **948.3** **30-39 percent of body surface**
[0-3]

√5ᵗʰ **948.4** **40-49 percent of body surface**
[0-4]

√5ᵗʰ **948.5** **50-59 percent of body surface**
[0-5]

√5ᵗʰ **948.6** **60-69 percent of body surface**
[0-6]

√5ᵗʰ **948.7** **70-79 percent of body surface**
[0-7]

√5ᵗʰ **948.8** **80-89 percent of body surface**
[0-8]

√5ᵗʰ **948.9** **90 percent or more of body surface**
[0-9]

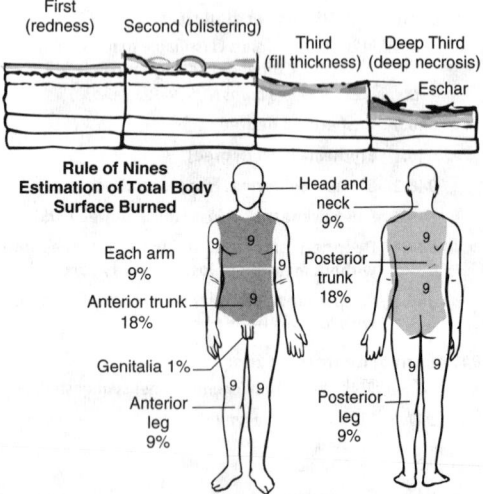

Burns

Degrees of Burns

First (redness)   Second (blistering)   Third (fill thickness)   Deep Third (deep necrosis)

Eschar

Rule of Nines
Estimation of Total Body Surface Burned

Head and neck 9%

Each arm 9%

Anterior trunk 18%

Genitalia 1%

Anterior leg 9%

Posterior trunk 18%

Posterior leg 9%

√4ᵗʰ **949 Burn, unspecified**

> **INCLUDES**   burn NOS
>   multiple burns NOS

> **EXCLUDES**   *burn of unspecified site but with statement of the extent of body surface involved (948.0-948.9)*

949.0 Unspecified degree

949.1 Erythema [first degree]

949.2 Blisters, epidermal loss [second degree]

949.3 Full-thickness skin loss [third degree NOS]

949.4 Deep necrosis of underlying tissues [deep third degree] without mention of loss of a body part

949.5 Deep necrosis of underlying tissues [deep third degree] with loss of a body part

INJURY TO NERVES AND SPINAL CORD (950-957)

> **INCLUDES**   division of nerve
>   lesion in continuity   } (with open
>   traumatic neuroma   wound)
>   traumatic transient paralysis

> **EXCLUDES**   *accidental puncture or laceration during medical procedure (998.2)*

√4ᵗʰ **950 Injury to optic nerve and pathways**

950.0 Optic nerve injury
    Second cranial nerve

950.1 Injury to optic chiasm

950.2 Injury to optic pathways

950.3 Injury to visual cortex

950.9 Unspecified
    Traumatic blindness NOS

√4ᵗʰ **951 Injury to other cranial nerve(s)**

951.0 Injury to oculomotor nerve
    Third cranial nerve

951.1 Injury to trochlear nerve
    Fourth cranial nerve

951.2 Injury to trigeminal nerve
    Fifth cranial nerve

951.3 Injury to abducens nerve
    Sixth cranial nerve

951.4 Injury to facial nerve
    Seventh cranial nerve

951.5 Injury to acoustic nerve
    Auditory nerve
    Eighth cranial nerve
    Traumatic deafness NOS

951.6 Injury to accessory nerve
    Eleventh cranial nerve

951.7 Injury to hypoglossal nerve
    Twelfth cranial nerve

951.8 Injury to other specified cranial nerves
    Glossopharyngeal [9th cranial] nerve
    Olfactory [1st cranial] nerve
    Pneumogastric [10th cranial] nerve
    Traumatic anosmia NOS
    Vagus [10th cranial] nerve

951.9 Injury to unspecified cranial nerve

√4ᵗʰ **952 Spinal cord injury without evidence of spinal bone injury**

√5ᵗʰ **952.0 Cervical**

    952.00 C_1-C_4 level with unspecified spinal cord injury
       Spinal cord injury, cervical region NOS

    952.01 C_1-C_4 level with complete lesion of spinal cord

    952.02 C_1-C_4 level with anterior cord syndrome

    952.03 C_1-C_4 level with central cord syndrome

Spinal Nerve Roots

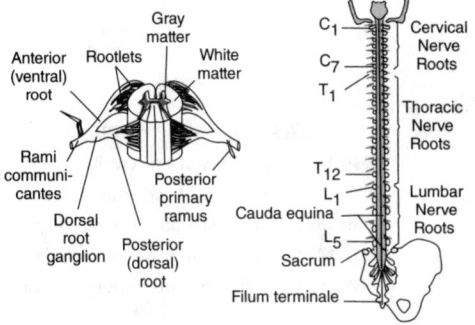

952.04 C_1-C_4 level with other specified spinal cord injury
　Incomplete spinal cord lesion at C_1-C_4 level:
　　NOS
　　with posterior cord syndrome

952.05 C_5-C_7 level with unspecified spinal cord injury

952.06 C_5-C_7 level with complete lesion of spinal cord

952.07 C_5-C_7 level with anterior cord syndrome

952.08 C_5-C_7 level with central cord syndrome

952.09 C_5-C_7 level with other specified spinal cord injury
　Incomplete spinal cord lesion at C_5-C_7 level:
　　NOS
　　with posterior cord syndrome

√5ᵗʰ **952.1** Dorsal [thoracic]

952.10 T_1-T_6 level with unspecified spinal cord injury
　Spinal cord injury, thoracic region NOS

952.11 T_1-T_6 level with complete lesion of spinal cord

952.12 T_1-T_6 level with anterior cord syndrome

952.13 T_1-T_6 level with central cord syndrome

952.14 T_1-T_6 level with other specified spinal cord injury
　Incomplete spinal cord lesion at T_1-T_6 level:
　　NOS
　　with posterior cord syndrome

952.15 T_7-T_{12} level with unspecified spinal cord injury

952.16 T_7-T_{12} level with complete lesion of spinal cord

952.17 T_7-T_{12} level with anterior cord syndrome

952.18 T_7-T_{12} level with central cord syndrome

952.19 T_7-T_{12} level with other specified spinal cord injury
　Incomplete spinal cord lesion at T_7-T_{12} level:
　　NOS
　　with posterior cord syndrome

952.2 Lumbar

952.3 Sacral

952.4 Cauda equina

952.8 Multiple sites of spinal cord

952.9 Unspecified site of spinal cord

√4ᵗʰ **953** Injury to nerve roots and spinal plexus

953.0 Cervical root

953.1 Dorsal root

953.2 Lumbar root

953.3 Sacral root

953.4 Brachial plexus

953.5 Lumbosacral plexus

953.8 Multiple sites

953.9 Unspecified site

√4ᵗʰ **954** Injury to other nerve(s) of trunk, excluding shoulder and pelvic girdles

954.0 Cervical sympathetic

954.1 Other sympathetic
　Celiac ganglion or plexus
　Inferior mesenteric plexus
　Splanchnic nerve(s)
　Stellate ganglion

954.8 Other specified nerve(s) of trunk

954.9 Unspecified nerve of trunk

√4ᵗʰ **955** Injury to peripheral nerve(s) of shoulder girdle and upper limb

955.0 Axillary nerve

955.1 Median nerve

955.2 Ulnar nerve

955.3 Radial nerve

955.4 Musculocutaneous nerve

955.5 Cutaneous sensory nerve, upper limb

955.6 Digital nerve

955.7 Other specified nerve(s) of shoulder girdle and upper limb

955.8 Multiple nerves of shoulder girdle and upper limb

955.9 Unspecified nerve of shoulder girdle and upper limb

√4ᵗʰ **956** Injury to peripheral nerve(s) of pelvic girdle and lower limb

956.0 Sciatic nerve

956.1 Femoral nerve

956.2 Posterior tibial nerve

956.3 Peroneal nerve

956.4 Cutaneous sensory nerve, lower limb

956.5 Other specified nerve(s) of pelvic girdle and lower limb

956.8 Multiple nerves of pelvic girdle and lower limb

956.9 Unspecified nerve of pelvic girdle and lower limb

√4ᵗʰ **957** Injury to other and unspecified nerves

957.0 Superficial nerves of head and neck

957.1 Other specified nerve(s)

957.8 Multiple nerves in several parts
　Multiple nerve injury NOS

957.9 Unspecified site
　Nerve injury NOS

CERTAIN TRAUMATIC COMPLICATIONS AND UNSPECIFIED INJURIES (958-959)

√4ᵗʰ **958** Certain early complications of trauma
　EXCLUDES *adult respiratory distress syndrome (518.52)*
　　flail chest (807.4)
　　post-traumatic seroma (729.91)
　　shock lung related to trauma and surgery (518.52)
　　that occurring during or following medical procedures (996.0-999.9)

958.0 Air embolism
　Pneumathemia
　EXCLUDES *that complicating:*
　　abortion (634-638 with .6, 639.6)
　　ectopic or molar pregnancy (639.6)
　　pregnancy, childbirth, or the puerperium (673.0)

　DEF: Arterial obstruction due to introduction of air bubbles into the veins following surgery or trauma.

958.1 Fat embolism
　EXCLUDES *that complicating:*
　　abortion (634-638 with .6, 639.6)
　　pregnancy, childbirth, or the puerperium (673.8)

　DEF: Arterial blockage due to the entrance of fat in circulatory system, after fracture of large bones or administration of corticosteroids.

958.2 Secondary and recurrent hemorrhage

958.3 Posttraumatic wound infection, not elsewhere classified
EXCLUDES infected open wounds-code to complicated open wound of site

958.4 Traumatic shock
Shock (immediate) (delayed) following injury
EXCLUDES shock:
anaphylactic (995.0)
due to serum (999.41-999.49)
anesthetic (995.4)
electric (994.8)
following abortion (639.5)
lightning (994.0)
nontraumatic NOS (785.50)
obstetric (669.1)
postoperative (998.00-998.09)
DEF: Shock, immediate or delayed following injury.

958.5 Traumatic anuria
Crush syndrome
Renal failure following crushing
EXCLUDES that due to a medical procedure (997.5)
DEF: Complete suppression of urinary secretion by kidneys due to trauma.

958.6 Volkmann's ischemic contracture
Posttraumatic muscle contracture
DEF: Muscle deterioration due to loss of blood supply from injury or tourniquet; causes muscle contraction and results in inability to extend the muscles fully.

958.7 Traumatic subcutaneous emphysema
EXCLUDES subcutaneous emphysema resulting from a procedure (998.81)

958.8 Other early complications of trauma

958.9 Traumatic compartment syndrome
EXCLUDES nontraumatic compartment syndrome (729.71-729.79)
DEF: Compression of nerves and blood vessels within an enclosed space due to previous trauma, which leads to impaired blood flow and muscle and nerve damage.

958.90 Compartment syndrome, unspecified

958.91 Traumatic compartment syndrome of upper extremity
Traumatic compartment syndrome of shoulder, arm, forearm, wrist, hand, and fingers

958.92 Traumatic compartment syndrome of lower extremity
Traumatic compartment syndrome of hip, buttock, thigh, leg, foot, and toes

958.93 Traumatic compartment syndrome of abdomen

958.99 Traumatic compartment syndrome of other sites

959 Injury, other and unspecified
INCLUDES injury NOS
EXCLUDES injury NOS of:
blood vessels (900.0-904.9)
eye (921.0-921.9)
internal organs (860.0-869.1)
intracranial sites (854.0-854.1)
nerves (950.0-951.9, 953.0-957.9)
spinal cord (952.0-952.9)

959.0 Head, face and neck

959.01 Head injury, unspecified
EXCLUDES concussion (850.1-850.9)
with head injury NOS (850.1-850.9)
head injury NOS with loss of consciousness (850.1-850.5)
specified intracranial injuries (850.0-854.1)

959.09 Injury of face and neck
Cheek   Mouth
Ear   Nose
Eyebrow   Throat
Lip

959.1 Trunk
EXCLUDES scapular region (959.2)

959.11 Other injury of chest wall

959.12 Other injury of abdomen

959.13 Fracture of corpus cavernosum penis

959.14 Other injury of external genitals

959.19 Other injury of other sites of trunk
Injury of trunk NOS

959.2 Shoulder and upper arm
Axilla
Scapular region

959.3 Elbow, forearm, and wrist

959.4 Hand, except finger

959.5 Finger
Fingernail
Thumb (nail)

959.6 Hip and thigh
Upper leg

959.7 Knee, leg, ankle, and foot

959.8 Other specified sites, including multiple
EXCLUDES multiple sites classifiable to the same four-digit category (959.0-959.7)

959.9 Unspecified site

POISONING BY DRUGS, MEDICINAL AND BIOLOGICAL SUBSTANCES (960-979)

INCLUDES overdose of these substances
wrong substance given or taken in error
Use additional code to specify the effects of the poisoning
EXCLUDES adverse effects ["hypersensitivity," "reaction," etc.] of correct substance properly administered. Such cases are to be classified according to the nature of the adverse effect, such as:
adverse effect NOS (995.20)
allergic lymphadenitis (289.3)
aspirin gastritis (535.4)
blood disorders (280.0-289.9)
dermatitis:
contact (692.0-692.9)
due to ingestion (693.0-693.9)
nephropathy (583.9)
[The drug giving rise to the adverse effect may be identified by use of categories E930-E949.]
drug dependence (304.0-304.9)
drug reaction and poisoning affecting the newborn (760.0-779.9)
nondependent abuse of drugs (305.0-305.9)
pathological drug intoxication (292.2)

960 Poisoning by antibiotics
EXCLUDES antibiotics:
ear, nose, and throat (976.6)
eye (976.5)
local (976.0)

960.0 Penicillins
Ampicillin   Cloxacillin
Carbenicillin   Penicillin G

960.1 Antifungal antibiotics
Amphotericin B   Nystatin
Griseofulvin   Trichomycin
EXCLUDES preparations intended for topical use (976.0-976.9)

960.2 Chloramphenicol group
Chloramphenicol
Thiamphenicol

960.3 Erythromycin and other macrolides
Oleandomycin
Spiramycin

960.4 Tetracycline group
Doxycycline   Oxytetracycline
Minocycline

960.5 Cephalosporin group
Cephalexin   Cephaloridine
Cephaloglycin   Cephalothin

960.6 Antimycobacterial antibiotics
Cycloserine   Rifampin
Kanamycin   Streptomycin

960.7 Antineoplastic antibiotics
Actinomycin such as: Actinomycin such as:
     Bleomycin   Daunorubicin
     Cactinomycin   Mitomycin
     Dactinomycin

960.8 Other specified antibiotics

960.9 Unspecified antibiotic

√4th **961 Poisoning by other anti-infectives**
EXCLUDES *anti-infectives:*
     ear, nose, and throat (976.6)
     eye (976.5)
     local (976.0)

961.0 Sulfonamides
Sulfadiazine   Sulfamethoxazole
Sulfafurazole

961.1 Arsenical anti-infectives

961.2 Heavy metal anti-infectives
Compounds of: Compounds of:
     antimony   lead
     bismuth   mercury
     EXCLUDES *mercurial diuretics (974.0)*

961.3 Quinoline and hydroxyquinoline derivatives
Chiniofon
Diiodohydroxyquin
EXCLUDES *antimalarial drugs (961.4)*

961.4 Antimalarials and drugs acting on other blood protozoa
Chloroquine   Proguanil [chloroguanide]
Cycloguanil   Pyrimethamine
Primaquine   Quinine

961.5 Other antiprotozoal drugs
Emetine

961.6 Anthelmintics
Hexylresorcinol   Thiabendazole
Piperazine

961.7 Antiviral drugs
Methisazone
EXCLUDES *amantadine (966.4)*
         cytarabine (963.1)
         idoxuridine (976.5)

961.8 Other antimycobacterial drugs
Ethambutol
Ethionamide
Isoniazid
Para-aminosalicylic acid derivatives
Sulfones

961.9 Other and unspecified anti-infectives
Flucytosine
Nitrofuran derivatives

√4th **962 Poisoning by hormones and synthetic substitutes**
EXCLUDES *oxytocic hormones (975.0)*

962.0 Adrenal cortical steroids
Cortisone derivatives
Desoxycorticosterone derivatives
Fluorinated corticosteroids

962.1 Androgens and anabolic congeners
Methandriol   Oxymetholone
Nandrolone   Testosterone

962.2 Ovarian hormones and synthetic substitutes
Contraceptives, oral
Estrogens
Estrogens and progestogens, combined
Progestogens

962.3 Insulins and antidiabetic agents
Acetohexamide
Biguanide derivatives, oral
Chlorpropamide
Glucagon
Insulin
Phenformin
Sulfonylurea derivatives, oral
Tolbutamide

962.4 Anterior pituitary hormones
Corticotropin
Gonadotropin
Somatotropin [growth hormone]

962.5 Posterior pituitary hormones
Vasopressin
EXCLUDES *oxytocic hormones (975.0)*

962.6 Parathyroid and parathyroid derivatives

962.7 Thyroid and thyroid derivatives
Dextrothyroxin   Liothyronine
Levothyroxine sodium   Thyroglobulin

962.8 Antithyroid agents
Iodides
Thiouracil
Thiourea

962.9 Other and unspecified hormones and synthetic substitutes

√4th **963 Poisoning by primarily systemic agents**

963.0 Antiallergic and antiemetic drugs
Antihistamines   Diphenylpyraline
Chlorpheniramine   Thonzylamine
Diphenhydramine   Tripelennamine
EXCLUDES *phenothiazine-based tranquilizers (969.1)*

963.1 Antineoplastic and immunosuppressive drugs
Azathioprine   Cytarabine
Busulfan   Fluorouracil
Chlorambucil   Mercaptopurine
Cyclophosphamide   thio-TEPA
EXCLUDES *antineoplastic antibiotics (960.7)*

963.2 Acidifying agents

963.3 Alkalizing agents

963.4 Enzymes, not elsewhere classified
Penicillinase

963.5 Vitamins, not elsewhere classified
Vitamin A
Vitamin D
EXCLUDES *nicotinic acid (972.2)*
         vitamin K (964.3)

963.8 Other specified systemic agents
Heavy metal antagonists

963.9 Unspecified systemic agent

√4th **964 Poisoning by agents primarily affecting blood constituents**

964.0 Iron and its compounds
Ferric salts
Ferrous sulfate and other ferrous salts

964.1 Liver preparations and other antianemic agents
Folic acid

964.2 Anticoagulants
Coumarin   Phenindione
Heparin   Warfarin sodium

964.3 Vitamin K [phytonadione]

964.4 Fibrinolysis-affecting drugs
Aminocaproic acid   Streptokinase
Streptodornase   Urokinase

964.5 **Anticoagulant antagonists and other coagulants**
Hexadimethrine
Protamine sulfate

964.6 **Gamma globulin**

964.7 **Natural blood and blood products**
Blood plasma   Packed red cells
Human fibrinogen   Whole blood
EXCLUDES *transfusion reactions (999.41-999.8)*

964.8 **Other specified agents affecting blood constituents**
Macromolecular blood substitutes
Plasma expanders

964.9 **Unspecified agent affecting blood constituents**

√4ᵗʰ **965** **Poisoning by analgesics, antipyretics, and antirheumatics**
EXCLUDES *drug dependence (304.0-304.9)*
nondependent abuse (305.0-305.9)

√5ᵗʰ **965.0** **Opiates and related narcotics**

965.00 **Opium (alkaloids), unspecified**

965.01 **Heroin**
Diacetylmorphine

965.02 **Methadone**

965.09 **Other**
Codeine [methylmorphine]
Meperidine [pethidine]
Morphine

965.1 **Salicylates**
Acetylsalicylic acid [aspirin]
Salicylic acid salts

965.4 **Aromatic analgesics, not elsewhere classified**
Acetanilid
Paracetamol [acetaminophen]
Phenacetin [acetophenetidin]

965.5 **Pyrazole derivatives**
Aminophenazone [aminopyrine]
Phenylbutazone

√5ᵗʰ **965.6** **Antirheumatics [antiphlogistics]**
EXCLUDES *salicylates (965.1)*
steroids (962.0-962.9)

965.61 **Propionic acid derivatives**
Fenoprofen   Ketoprofen
Flurbiprofen   Naproxen
Ibuprofen   Oxaprozin

965.69 **Other antirheumatics**
Gold salts
Indomethacin

965.7 **Other non-narcotic analgesics**
Pyrabital

965.8 **Other specified analgesics and antipyretics**
Pentazocine

965.9 **Unspecified analgesic and antipyretic**

√4ᵗʰ **966** **Poisoning by anticonvulsants and anti-Parkinsonism drugs**

966.0 **Oxazolidine derivatives**
Paramethadione
Trimethadione

966.1 **Hydantoin derivatives**
Phenytoin

966.2 **Succinimides**
Ethosuximide
Phensuximide

966.3 **Other and unspecified anticonvulsants**
Primidone
EXCLUDES *barbiturates (967.0)*
sulfonamides (961.0)

966.4 **Anti-Parkinsonism drugs**
Amantadine
Ethopropazine [profenamine]
Levodopa [L-dopa]

√4ᵗʰ **967** **Poisoning by sedatives and hypnotics**
EXCLUDES *drug dependence (304.0-304.9)*
nondependent abuse (305.0-305.9)

967.0 **Barbiturates**
Amobarbital [amylobarbitone]
Barbital [barbitone]
Butabarbital [butabarbitone]
Pentobarbital [pentobarbitone]
Phenobarbital [phenobarbitone]
Secobarbital [quinalbarbitone]
EXCLUDES *thiobarbiturate anesthetics (968.3)*

967.1 **Chloral hydrate group**

967.2 **Paraldehyde**

967.3 **Bromine compounds**
Bromide
Carbromal (derivatives)

967.4 **Methaqualone compounds**

967.5 **Glutethimide group**

967.6 **Mixed sedatives, not elsewhere classified**

967.8 **Other sedatives and hypnotics**

967.9 **Unspecified sedative or hypnotic**
Sleeping:
drug ⎫
pill ⎬ NOS
tablet ⎭

√4ᵗʰ **968** **Poisoning by other central nervous system depressants and anesthetics**
EXCLUDES *drug dependence (304.0-304.9)*
nondependent abuse (305.0-305.9)

968.0 **Central nervous system muscle-tone depressants**
Chlorphenesin (carbamate)
Mephenesin
Methocarbamol

968.1 **Halothane**

968.2 **Other gaseous anesthetics**
Ether
Halogenated hydrocarbon derivatives, except halothane
Nitrous oxide

968.3 **Intravenous anesthetics**
Ketamine
Methohexital [methohexitone]
Thiobarbiturates, such as thiopental sodium

968.4 **Other and unspecified general anesthetics**

968.5 **Surface (topical) and infiltration anesthetics**
Cocaine (topical)
Lidocaine (lignocaine)
Procaine
Tetracaine
EXCLUDES *poisoning by cocaine used as a central nervous system stimulant (970.81)*

968.6 **Peripheral nerve- and plexus-blocking anesthetics**

968.7 **Spinal anesthetics**

968.9 **Other and unspecified local anesthetics**

√4ᵗʰ **969** **Poisoning by psychotropic agents**
EXCLUDES *drug dependence (304.0-304.9)*
nondependent abuse (305.0-305.9)

√5ᵗʰ **969.0** **Antidepressants**

969.00 **Antidepressant, unspecified**

969.01 **Monoamine oxidase inhibitors**
MAOI

969.02 **Selective serotonin and norepinephrine reuptake inhibitors**
SSNRI antidepressants

969.03 **Selective serotonin reuptake inhibitors**
SSRI antidepressants

969.04 **Tetracyclic antidepressants**

969.05 **Tricyclic antidepressants**

    969.09   **Other antidepressants**

969.1   **Phenothiazine-based tranquilizers**
    Chlorpromazine   Prochlorperazine
    Fluphenazine   Promazine

969.2   **Butyrophenone-based tranquilizers**
    Haloperidol
    Spiperone
    Trifluperidol

969.3   **Other antipsychotics, neuroleptics, and major tranquilizers**

969.4   **Benzodiazepine-based tranquilizers**
    Chlordiazepoxide
    Diazepam
    Flurazepam
    Lorazepam
    Medazepam
    Nitrazepam

969.5   **Other tranquilizers**
    Hydroxyzine
    Meprobamate

969.6   **Psychodysleptics [hallucinogens]**
    Cannabis (derivatives)
    Lysergide [LSD]
    Marihuana (derivatives)
    Mescaline
    Psilocin
    Psilocybin

√5ᵗʰ 969.7   **Psychostimulants**
    EXCLUDES   *central appetite depressants (977.0)*

    969.70   **Psychostimulant, unspecified**

    969.71   **Caffeine**

    969.72   **Amphetamines**
        Methamphetamines

    969.73   **Methylphenidate**

    969.79   **Other psychostimulants**

969.8   **Other specified psychotropic agents**

969.9   **Unspecified psychotropic agent**

√4ᵗʰ **970   Poisoning by central nervous system stimulants**

970.0   **Analeptics**
    Lobeline
    Nikethamide

970.1   **Opiate antagonists**
    Levallorphan
    Nalorphine
    Naloxone

√5ᵗʰ 970.8   **Other specified central nervous system stimulants**

    970.81   **Cocaine**
        Crack

    970.89   **Other central nervous system stimulants**

970.9   **Unspecified central nervous system stimulant**

√4ᵗʰ **971   Poisoning by drugs primarily affecting the autonomic nervous system**

971.0   **Parasympathomimetics [cholinergics]**
    Acetylcholine
    Anticholinesterase:
        organophosphorus
        reversible
    Pilocarpine

971.1   **Parasympatholytics [anticholinergics and antimuscarinics] and spasmolytics**
    Atropine
    Homatropine
    Hyoscine [scopolamine]
    Quaternary ammonium derivatives
    EXCLUDES   *papaverine (972.5)*

971.2   **Sympathomimetics [adrenergics]**
    Epinephrine [adrenalin]
    Levarterenol [noradrenalin]

971.3   **Sympatholytics [antiadrenergics]**
    Phenoxybenzamine
    Tolazolinehydrochloride

971.9   **Unspecified drug primarily affecting autonomic nervous system**

√4ᵗʰ **972   Poisoning by agents primarily affecting the cardiovascular system**

972.0   **Cardiac rhythm regulators**
    Practolol
    Procainamide
    Propranolol
    Quinidine
    EXCLUDES   *lidocaine (968.5)*

972.1   **Cardiotonic glycosides and drugs of similar action**
    Digitalis glycosides
    Digoxin
    Strophanthins

972.2   **Antilipemic and antiarteriosclerotic drugs**
    Clofibrate
    Nicotinic acid derivatives

972.3   **Ganglion-blocking agents**
    Pentamethonium bromide

972.4   **Coronary vasodilators**
    Dipyridamole
    Nitrates [nitroglycerin]
    Nitrites

972.5   **Other vasodilators**
    Cyclandelate
    Diazoxide
    Papaverine
    EXCLUDES   *nicotinic acid (972.2)*

972.6   **Other antihypertensive agents**
    Clonidine
    Guanethidine
    Rauwolfia alkaloids
    Reserpine

972.7   **Antivaricose drugs, including sclerosing agents**
    Sodium morrhuate
    Zinc salts

972.8   **Capillary-active drugs**
    Adrenochrome derivatives
    Metaraminol

972.9   **Other and unspecified agents primarily affecting the cardiovascular system**

√4ᵗʰ **973   Poisoning by agents primarily affecting the gastrointestinal system**

973.0   **Antacids and antigastric secretion drugs**
    Aluminum hydroxide
    Magnesium trisilicate

973.1   **Irritant cathartics**
    Bisacodyl
    Castor oil
    Phenolphthalein

973.2   **Emollient cathartics**
    Dioctyl sulfosuccinates

973.3   **Other cathartics, including intestinal atonia drugs**
    Magnesium sulfate

973.4   **Digestants**
    Pancreatin
    Papain
    Pepsin

973.5   **Antidiarrheal drugs**
    Kaolin
    Pectin
    EXCLUDES   *anti-infectives (960.0-961.9)*

973.6   **Emetics**

973.8   **Other specified agents primarily affecting the gastrointestinal system**

973.9   **Unspecified agent primarily affecting the gastrointestinal system**

Injury and Poisoning

974–980.0

☑4ᵗʰ **974 Poisoning by water, mineral, and uric acid metabolism drugs**

974.0 Mercurial diuretics
Chlormerodrin   Mersalyl
Mercaptomerin

974.1 Purine derivative diuretics
Theobromine
Theophylline
EXCLUDES   aminophylline [theophylline ethylenediamine] (975.7)
caffeine (969.71)

974.2 Carbonic acid anhydrase inhibitors
Acetazolamide

974.3 Saluretics
Benzothiadiazides
Chlorothiazide group

974.4 Other diuretics
Ethacrynic acid
Furosemide

974.5 Electrolytic, caloric, and water-balance agents

974.6 Other mineral salts, not elsewhere classified

974.7 Uric acid metabolism drugs
Allopurinol   Probenecid
Colchicine

☑4ᵗʰ **975 Poisoning by agents primarily acting on the smooth and skeletal muscles and respiratory system**

975.0 Oxytocic agents
Ergot alkaloids
Oxytocin
Prostaglandins

975.1 Smooth muscle relaxants
Adiphenine
Metaproterenol [orciprenaline]
EXCLUDES   papaverine (972.5)

975.2 Skeletal muscle relaxants

975.3 Other and unspecified drugs acting on muscles

975.4 Antitussives
Dextromethorphan
Pipazethate

975.5 Expectorants
Acetylcysteine
Guaifenesin
Terpin hydrate

975.6 Anti-common cold drugs

975.7 Antiasthmatics
Aminophylline [theophylline ethylenediamine]

975.8 Other and unspecified respiratory drugs

☑4ᵗʰ **976 Poisoning by agents primarily affecting skin and mucous membrane, ophthalmological, otorhinolaryngological, and dental drugs**

976.0 Local anti-infectives and anti-inflammatory drugs

976.1 Antipruritics

976.2 Local astringents and local detergents

976.3 Emollients, demulcents, and protectants

976.4 Keratolytics, keratoplastics, other hair treatment drugs and preparations

976.5 Eye anti-infectives and other eye drugs
Idoxuridine

976.6 Anti-infectives and other drugs and preparations for ear, nose, and throat

976.7 Dental drugs topically applied
EXCLUDES   anti-infectives (976.0)
local anesthetics (968.5)

976.8 Other agents primarily affecting skin and mucous membrane
Spermicides [vaginal contraceptives]

976.9 Unspecified agent primarily affecting skin and mucous membrane

☑4ᵗʰ **977 Poisoning by other and unspecified drugs and medicinal substances**

977.0 Dietetics
Central appetite depressants

977.1 Lipotropic drugs

977.2 Antidotes and chelating agents, not elsewhere classified

977.3 Alcohol deterrents

977.4 Pharmaceutical excipients
Pharmaceutical adjuncts

977.8 Other specified drugs and medicinal substances
Contrast media used for diagnostic x-ray procedures
Diagnostic agents and kits

977.9 Unspecified drug or medicinal substance

☑4ᵗʰ **978 Poisoning by bacterial vaccines**

978.0 BCG

978.1 Typhoid and paratyphoid

978.2 Cholera

978.3 Plague

978.4 Tetanus

978.5 Diphtheria

978.6 Pertussis vaccine, including combinations with a pertussis component

978.8 Other and unspecified bacterial vaccines

978.9 Mixed bacterial vaccines, except combinations with a pertussis component

☑4ᵗʰ **979 Poisoning by other vaccines and biological substances**
EXCLUDES   gamma globulin (964.6)

979.0 Smallpox vaccine

979.1 Rabies vaccine

979.2 Typhus vaccine

979.3 Yellow fever vaccine

979.4 Measles vaccine

979.5 Poliomyelitis vaccine

979.6 Other and unspecified viral and rickettsial vaccines
Mumps vaccine

979.7 Mixed viral-rickettsial and bacterial vaccines, except combinations with a pertussis component
EXCLUDES   combinations with a pertussis component (978.6)

979.9 Other and unspecified vaccines and biological substances

TOXIC EFFECTS OF SUBSTANCES CHIEFLY NONMEDICINAL AS TO SOURCE (980-989)

Use additional code to identify:
personal history of retained foreign body fully removed (V15.53)
retained foreign body status, if applicable, (V90.01-V90.9)
Use additional code to specify the nature of the toxic effect
EXCLUDES   burns from chemical agents (ingested) (947.0-947.9)
localized toxic effects indexed elsewhere (001.0-799.9)
respiratory conditions due to external agents (506.0-508.9)
respiratory conditions due to smoke inhalation NOS (508.2)

☑4ᵗʰ **980 Toxic effect of alcohol**

980.0 Ethyl alcohol
Denatured alcohol   Grain alcohol
Ethanol
Use additional code to identify any associated:
acute alcohol intoxication (305.0)
in alcoholism (303.0)
drunkenness (simple) (305.0)
pathological (291.4)

980.1 **Methyl alcohol**
Methanol
Wood alcohol

980.2 **Isopropyl alcohol**
Dimethyl carbinol
Isopropanol
Rubbing alcohol

980.3 **Fusel oil**
Alcohol:
amyl
butyl
propyl

980.8 **Other specified alcohols**

980.9 **Unspecified alcohol**

981 **Toxic effect of petroleum products**
Benzine
Gasoline
Kerosene
Paraffin wax
Petroleum:
ether
naphtha
spirit

982 **Toxic effect of solvents other than petroleum-based**

982.0 **Benzene and homologues**

982.1 **Carbon tetrachloride**

982.2 **Carbon disulfide**
Carbon bisulfide

982.3 **Other chlorinated hydrocarbon solvents**
Tetrachloroethylene
Trichloroethylene
EXCLUDES *chlorinated hydrocarbon preparations other than solvents (989.2)*

982.4 **Nitroglycol**

982.8 **Other nonpetroleum-based solvents**
Acetone

983 **Toxic effect of corrosive aromatics, acids, and caustic alkalis**

983.0 **Corrosive aromatics**
Carbolic acid or phenol
Cresol

983.1 **Acids**
Acid:
hydrochloric
nitric
sulfuric

983.2 **Caustic alkalis**
Lye
Potassium hydroxide
Sodium hydroxide

983.9 **Caustic, unspecified**

984 **Toxic effect of lead and its compounds (including fumes)**
INCLUDES that from all sources except medicinal substances

984.0 **Inorganic lead compounds**
Lead dioxide
Lead salts

984.1 **Organic lead compounds**
Lead acetate
Tetraethyl lead

984.8 **Other lead compounds**

984.9 **Unspecified lead compound**

985 **Toxic effect of other metals**
INCLUDES that from all sources except medicinal substances

985.0 **Mercury and its compounds**
Minamata disease

985.1 **Arsenic and its compounds**

985.2 **Manganese and its compounds**

985.3 **Beryllium and its compounds**

985.4 **Antimony and its compounds**

985.5 **Cadmium and its compounds**

985.6 **Chromium**

985.8 **Other specified metals**
Brass fumes   Iron compounds
Copper salts   Nickel compounds

985.9 **Unspecified metal**

986 **Toxic effect of carbon monoxide**
Carbon monoxide from any source

987 **Toxic effect of other gases, fumes, or vapors**

987.0 **Liquefied petroleum gases**
Butane
Propane

987.1 **Other hydrocarbon gas**

987.2 **Nitrogen oxides**
Nitrogen dioxide
Nitrous fumes

987.3 **Sulfur dioxide**

987.4 **Freon**
Dichloromonofluoromethane

987.5 **Lacrimogenic gas**
Bromobenzyl cyanide
Chloroacetophenone
Ethyliodoacetate

987.6 **Chlorine gas**

987.7 **Hydrocyanic acid gas**

987.8 **Other specified gases, fumes, or vapors**
Phosgene
Polyester fumes

987.9 **Unspecified gas, fume, or vapor**

988 **Toxic effect of noxious substances eaten as food**
EXCLUDES *allergic reaction to food, such as:*
gastroenteritis (558.3)
rash (692.5, 693.1)
food poisoning (bacterial) (005.0-005.9)
toxic effects of food contaminants, such as:
aflatoxin and other mycotoxin (989.7)
mercury (985.0)

988.0 **Fish and shellfish**

988.1 **Mushrooms**

988.2 **Berries and other plants**

988.8 **Other specified noxious substances eaten as food**

988.9 **Unspecified noxious substance eaten as food**

989 **Toxic effect of other substances, chiefly nonmedicinal as to source**

989.0 **Hydrocyanic acid and cyanides**
Potassium cyanide
Sodium cyanide
EXCLUDES *gas and fumes (987.7)*

989.1 **Strychnine and salts**

989.2 **Chlorinated hydrocarbons**
Aldrin
Chlordane
DDT
Dieldrin
EXCLUDES *chlorinated hydrocarbon solvents (982.0-982.3)*

989.3 **Organophosphate and carbamate**
Carbaryl
Dichlorvos
Malathion
Parathion
Phorate
Phosdrin

989.4 **Other pesticides, not elsewhere classified**
Mixtures of insecticides

989.5 Venom
Bites of venomous snakes, lizards, and spiders
Tick paralysis

989.6 Soaps and detergents

989.7 Aflatoxin and other mycotoxin [food contaminants]

√5th **989.8 Other substances, chiefly nonmedicinal as to source**

989.81 Asbestos
EXCLUDES *asbestosis (501)*
exposure to asbestos (V15.84)

989.82 Latex

989.83 Silicone
EXCLUDES *silicone used in medical devices, implants and grafts (996.00-996.79)*

989.84 Tobacco

989.89 Other

989.9 Unspecified substance, chiefly nonmedicinal as to source

OTHER AND UNSPECIFIED EFFECTS OF EXTERNAL CAUSES (990-995)

990 Effects of radiation, unspecified
Complication of:
phototherapy
radiation therapy
Radiation sickness
[The type of radiation giving rise to the adverse effect may be identified by use of the E codes.]
EXCLUDES *specified adverse effects of radiation. Such conditions are to be classified according to the nature of the adverse effect, as:*
burns (940.0-949.5)
dermatitis (692.7-692.8)
leukemia (204.0-208.9)
pneumonia (508.0)
sunburn (692.71, 692.76-692.77)

√4th **991 Effects of reduced temperature**

991.0 Frostbite of face

991.1 Frostbite of hand

991.2 Frostbite of foot

991.3 Frostbite of other and unspecified sites

991.4 Immersion foot
Trench foot
DEF: Paresthesia, edema, blotchy cyanosis of foot, the skin is soft (macerated), pale and wrinkled, and the sole is swollen with surface ridging and following sustained immersion in water.

991.5 Chilblains
Erythema pernio
Perniosis
DEF: Red, swollen, itchy skin; follows damp cold exposure; also associated with pruritus and a burning feeling in hands, feet, ears, and face in children, legs and toes in women, and hands and fingers in men.

991.6 Hypothermia
Hypothermia (accidental)
EXCLUDES *hypothermia following anesthesia (995.89)*
hypothermia not associated with low environmental temperature (780.65)
DEF: Reduced body temperature due to low environmental temperatures.

991.8 Other specified effects of reduced temperature

991.9 Unspecified effect of reduced temperature
Effects of freezing or excessive cold NOS

√4th **992 Effects of heat and light**
EXCLUDES *burns (940.0-949.5)*
diseases of sweat glands due to heat (705.0-705.9)
malignant hyperpyrexia following anesthesia (995.86)
sunburn (692.71, 692.76-692.77)

992.0 Heat stroke and sunstroke
Heat apoplexy
Heat pyrexia
Ictus solaris
Siriasis
Thermoplegia
Use additional code(s) to identify any associated complication of heat stroke, such as:
alterations of consciousness (780.01-780.09)
systemic inflammatory response syndrome (995.93-995.94)
DEF: Headache, vertigo, cramps and elevated body temperature due to high environmental temperatures.

992.1 Heat syncope
Heat collapse

992.2 Heat cramps

992.3 Heat exhaustion, anhydrotic
Heat prostration due to water depletion
EXCLUDES *that associated with salt depletion (992.4)*

992.4 Heat exhaustion due to salt depletion
Heat prostration due to salt (and water) depletion

992.5 Heat exhaustion, unspecified
Heat prostration NOS

992.6 Heat fatigue, transient

992.7 Heat edema
DEF: Fluid retention due to high environmental temperatures.

992.8 Other specified heat effects

992.9 Unspecified

√4th **993 Effects of air pressure**

993.0 Barotrauma, otitic
Aero-otitis media
Effects of high altitude on ears
DEF: Ringing ears, deafness, pain and vertigo due to air pressure changes.

993.1 Barotrauma, sinus
Aerosinusitis
Effects of high altitude on sinuses

993.2 Other and unspecified effects of high altitude
Alpine sickness
Andes disease
Anoxia due to high altitude
Hypobaropathy
Mountain sickness

993.3 Caisson disease
Bends
Compressed-air disease
Decompression sickness
Divers' palsy or paralysis
DEF: Rapid reduction in air pressure while breathing compressed air; symptoms include skin lesions, joint pains, respiratory and neurological problems.

993.4 Effects of air pressure caused by explosion

993.8 Other specified effects of air pressure

993.9 Unspecified effect of air pressure

√4th **994 Effects of other external causes**
EXCLUDES *certain adverse effects not elsewhere classified (995.0-995.8)*

994.0 Effects of lightning
Shock from lightning
Struck by lightning NOS
EXCLUDES *burns (940.0-949.5)*

994.1 Drowning and nonfatal submersion
Bathing cramp
Immersion

994.2 Effects of hunger
Deprivation of food
Starvation

994.3 Effects of thirst
Deprivation of water

994.4 Exhaustion due to exposure

994.5 Exhaustion due to excessive exertion
Exhaustion due to overexertion

994.6 Motion sickness
Air sickness
Seasickness
Travel sickness

994.7 Asphyxiation and strangulation
Suffocation (by):   Suffocation (by):
bedclothes   plastic bag
cave-in   pressure
constriction   strangulation
mechanical
EXCLUDES *asphyxia from:*
carbon monoxide (986)
inhalation of food or foreign body
(932-934.9)
other gases, fumes, and vapors
(987.0-987.9)

994.8 Electrocution and nonfatal effects of electric current
Shock from electric current
Shock from electroshock gun (taser)
EXCLUDES *electric burns (940.0-949.5)*

994.9 Other effects of external causes
Effects of:
abnormal gravitational [G] forces or states
weightlessness

√4ᵗʰ **995 Certain adverse effects not elsewhere classified**
EXCLUDES *complications of surgical and medical care*
(996.0-999.9)

995.0 Other anaphylactic reaction
Allergic shock
Anaphylactic reaction
Anaphylactic shock NOS or due to adverse effect of
correct medicinal substance properly
administered
Anaphylactoid reaction, NOS
Anaphylaxis
Use additional E code to identify external cause, such as:
adverse effects of correct medicinal substance
properly administered [E930-E949]
EXCLUDES *anaphylactic reaction to serum*
(999.41-999.49)
anaphylactic shock or reaction due to adverse
food reaction (995.60-995.69)

DEF: Immediate sensitivity response after exposure to
specific antigen; results in life-threatening respiratory
distress; usually followed by vascular collapse, shock,
urticaria, angioedema and pruritus.

995.1 Angioneurotic edema
Allergic angioedema
Giant urticaria
EXCLUDES *urticaria:*
due to serum (999.51-999.59)
other specified (698.2, 708.0-708.9,
757.33)

DEF: Circulatory response of deep dermis, subcutaneous
or submucosal tissues; causes localized edema and
wheals.

√5ᵗʰ **995.2 Other and unspecified adverse effect of drug,
medicinal and biological substance**
EXCLUDES *pathological drug intoxication (292.2)*

**995.20 Unspecified adverse effect of unspecified
drug, medicinal and biological substance**
Unspecified adverse effect of unspecified
medicinal substance properly
administered

995.21 Arthus phenomenon
Arthus reaction

995.22 Unspecified adverse effect of anesthesia

995.23 Unspecified adverse effect of insulin

995.24 Failed moderate sedation during procedure
Failed conscious sedation during procedure

995.27 Other drug allergy
Allergic reaction NEC (due) to correct medical
substance properly administered
Drug allergy NOS
Drug hypersensitivity NOS
Hypersensitivity (due) to correct medical
substance properly administered

**995.29 Unspecified adverse effect of other
drug, medicinal and biological substance**
Unspecified adverse effect of medicinal
substance NEC properly administered

995.3 Allergy, unspecified
Allergic reaction NOS
Hypersensitivity NOS
Idiosyncrasy NOS
EXCLUDES *allergic reaction NOS to correct medicinal*
substance properly administered
(995.27)
allergy to existing dental restorative materials
(525.66)
specific types of allergic reaction, such as:
allergic diarrhea (558.3)
dermatitis (691.0-693.9)
hayfever (477.0-477.9)

995.4 Shock due to anesthesia
Shock due to anesthesia in which the correct substance
was properly administered
EXCLUDES *complications of anesthesia in labor or*
delivery (668.0-668.9)
overdose or wrong substance given
(968.0-969.9)
postoperative shock NOS (998.00)
specified adverse effects of anesthesia
classified elsewhere, such as:
anoxic brain damage (348.1)
hepatitis (070.0-070.9), etc.
unspecified adverse effect of anesthesia
(995.22)

√5ᵗʰ **995.5 Child maltreatment syndrome**
Use additional code(s), if applicable, to identify any
associated injuries
Use additional E code to identify:
nature of abuse (E960-E968)
perpetrator (E967.0-E967.9)

995.50 Child abuse, unspecified

995.51 Child emotional/psychological abuse

995.52 Child neglect (nutritional)

995.53 Child sexual abuse

995.54 Child physical abuse
Battered baby or child syndrome
EXCLUDES *shaken infant syndrome (995.55)*

995.55 Shaken infant syndrome
Use additional code(s) to identify any
associated injuries

995.59 Other child abuse and neglect
Multiple forms of abuse

√5ᵗʰ **995.6 Anaphylactic reaction due to food**
Anaphylactic reaction due to adverse food reaction
Anaphylactic shock or reaction due to nonpoisonous
foods
Anaphylactoid reaction due to food

995.60 Anaphylactic reaction due to unspecified food

995.61 Anaphylactic reaction due to peanuts

995.62 Anaphylactic reaction due to crustaceans

**995.63 Anaphylactic reaction due to fruits and
vegetables**

Injury and Poisoning

995.64–995.94

995.64 Anaphylactic reaction due to tree nuts and seeds

995.65 Anaphylactic reaction due to fish

995.66 Anaphylactic reaction due to food additives

995.67 Anaphylactic reaction due to milk products

995.68 Anaphylactic reaction due to eggs

995.69 Anaphylactic reaction due to other specified food

995.7 Other adverse food reactions, not elsewhere classified

Use additional code to identify the type of reaction, such as:
hives (708.0)
wheezing (786.07)

EXCLUDES   *anaphylactic reaction or shock due to adverse food reaction (995.60-995.69)*
asthma (493.0, 493.9)
dermatitis due to food (693.1)
in contact with skin (692.5)
gastroenteritis and colitis due to food (558.3)
rhinitis due to food (477.1)

√5ᵗʰ **995.8 Other specified adverse effects, not elsewhere classified**

995.80 Adult maltreatment, unspecified

Abused person NOS
Use additional code to identify:
any associated injury
perpetrator (E967.0-E967.9)

995.81 Adult physical abuse

Battered:
person syndrome NEC
man
spouse
woman
Use additional code to identify:
any association injury
nature of abuse (E960-E968)
perpetrator (E967.0-E967.9)

995.82 Adult emotional/psychological abuse

Use additional E code to identify perpetrator (E967.0-E967.9)

995.83 Adult sexual abuse

Use additional code(s) to identify:
any associated injury
perpetrator (E967.0-E967.9)

995.84 Adult neglect (nutritional)

Use additional code(s) to identify:
intent of neglect (E904.0, E968.4)
perpetrator (E967.0-E967.9)

995.85 Other adult abuse and neglect

Multiple forms of abuse and neglect
Use additional code(s) to identify
any associated injury
intent of neglect (E904.0, E968.4)
nature of abuse (E960-E968)
perpetrator (E967.0-E967.9)

995.86 Malignant hyperthermia

Malignant hyperpyrexia due to anesthesia

995.89 Other

Hypothermia due to anesthesia

√5ᵗʰ **995.9 Systemic inflammatory response syndrome (SIRS)**

DEF: Clinical response to infection or trauma that can trigger an acute inflammatory reaction and progresses to coagulation, impaired fibrinolysis, and organ failure; manifested by two or more of the following symptoms: fever, tachycardia, tachypnea, leukocytosis or leukopenia.

995.90 Systemic inflammatory response syndrome, unspecified

SIRS NOS

Continuum of Illness Due to Infection

Bacteremia ➡ Septicemia ➡ Sepsis
Severe Sepsis with Septic Shock ⬅ Severe Sepsis
MODS (Multiple Organ Dysfunction Syndrome) ➡ Death

995.91 Sepsis

Systemic inflammatory response syndrome due to infectious process without acute organ dysfunction
Code first underlying infection

EXCLUDES   *sepsis with acute organ dysfunction (995.92)*
sepsis with multiple organ dysfunction (995.92)
severe sepsis (995.92)

995.92 Severe sepsis

Sepsis with acute organ dysfunction
Sepsis with multiple organ dysfunction (MOD)
Systemic inflammatory response syndrome due to infectious process with acute organ dysfunction
Code first underlying infection
Use additional code to specify acute organ dysfunction, such as:
acute kidney failure (584.5-584.9)
acute respiratory failure (518.81)
critical illness myopathy (359.81)
critical illness polyneuropathy (357.82)
disseminated intravascular coagulopathy [DIC] (286.6)
encephalopathy (348.31)
hepatic failure (570)
septic shock (785.52)

995.93 Systemic inflammatory response syndrome due to noninfectious process without acute organ dysfunction

Code first underlying conditions, such as:
acute pancreatitis (577.0)
trauma

EXCLUDES   *systemic inflammatory response syndrome due to noninfectious process with acute organ dysfunction (995.94)*

995.94 Systemic inflammatory response syndrome due to noninfectious process with acute organ dysfunction

Code first underlying conditions, such as:
acute pancreatitis (577.0)
heat stroke (992.0)
trauma
Use additional code to specify acute organ dysfunction, such as:
acute kidney failure (584.5-584.9)
acute respiratory failure (518.81)
critical illness myopathy (359.81)
critical illness polyneuropathy (357.82)
disseminated intravascular coagulopathy [DIC] syndrome (286.6)
encephalopathy (348.31)
hepatic failure (570)

EXCLUDES   *severe sepsis (995.92)*

COMPLICATIONS OF SURGICAL AND MEDICAL CARE, NOT ELSEWHERE CLASSIFIED (996-999)

> **EXCLUDES** adverse effects of medicinal agents (001.0-799.9, 995.0-995.8)
> burns from local applications and irradiation (940.0-949.5)
> complications of:
>   conditions for which the procedure was performed
>   surgical procedures during abortion, labor, and delivery (630-676.9)
> poisoning and toxic effects of drugs and chemicals (960.0-989.9)
> postoperative conditions in which no complications are present, such as:
>   artificial opening status (V44.0-V44.9)
>   closure of external stoma (V55.0-V55.9)
>   fitting of prosthetic device (V52.0-V52.9)
> specified complications classified elsewhere
>   anesthetic shock (995.4)
>   electrolyte imbalance (276.0-276.9)
>   postlaminectomy syndrome (722.80-722.83)
>   postmastectomy lymphedema syndrome (457.0)
>   postoperative psychosis (293.0-293.9)
>   any other condition classified elsewhere in the Alphabetic Index when described as due to a procedure

✓4ᵗʰ 996 Complications peculiar to certain specified procedures

> **INCLUDES** complications, not elsewhere classified, in the use of artificial substitutes [e.g., Dacron, metal, Silastic, Teflon] or natural sources [e.g., bone] involving:
>   anastomosis (internal)
>   graft (bypass) (patch)
>   implant
>   internal device:
>   catheter
>   electronic
>   fixation
>   prosthetic
>   reimplant
>   transplant

> **EXCLUDES** accidental puncture or laceration during procedure (998.2)
> capsular contracture of breast implant (611.83)
> complications of internal anastomosis of:
>   gastrointestinal tract (997.49)
>   urinary tract (997.5)
> endosseous dental implant failures (525.71-525.79)
> intraoperative floppy iris syndrome [IFIS] (364.81)
> mechanical complication of respirator (V46.14)
> other specified complications classified elsewhere, such as:
>   hemolytic anemia (283.1)
>   functional cardiac disturbances (429.4)
>   serum hepatitis (070.2-070.3)

✓5ᵗʰ 996.0 Mechanical complication of cardiac device, implant, and graft

Breakdown (mechanical)
Displacement
Leakage
Obstruction, mechanical
Perforation
Protrusion

996.00 Unspecified device, implant, and graft

996.01 Due to cardiac pacemaker (electrode)

996.02 Due to heart valve prosthesis

996.03 Due to coronary bypass graft

> **EXCLUDES** atherosclerosis of graft (414.02, 414.03)
> embolism [occlusion NOS] [thrombus] of graft (996.72)

996.04 Due to automatic implantable cardiac defibrillator

996.09 Other

996.1 Mechanical complication of other vascular device, implant, and graft

Mechanical complications involving:
    aortic (bifurcation) graft (replacement)
    arteriovenous:
        dialysis catheter ⎫
        fistula   ⎬ surgically created
        shunt   ⎭
    balloon (counterpulsation) device, intra-aortic
    carotid artery bypass graft
    femoral-popliteal bypass graft
    umbrella device, vena cava

> **EXCLUDES** atherosclerosis of biological graft (440.30-440.32)
> embolism [occlusion NOS] [thrombus] of (biological) (synthetic) graft (996.74)
> peritoneal dialysis catheter (996.56)

996.2 Mechanical complication of nervous system device, implant, and graft

Mechanical complications involving:
    dorsal column stimulator
    electrodes implanted in brain [brain "pacemaker"]
    peripheral nerve graft
    ventricular (communicating) shunt

✓5ᵗʰ 996.3 Mechanical complication of genitourinary device, implant, and graft

996.30 Unspecified device, implant, and graft

996.31 Due to urethral [indwelling] catheter

996.32 Due to intrauterine contraceptive device

996.39 Other

Prosthetic reconstruction of vas deferens
Repair (graft) of ureter without mention of resection

> **EXCLUDES** complications due to:
>   external stoma of urinary tract (596.81-596.83)
>   internal anastomosis of urinary tract (997.5)

✓5ᵗʰ 996.4 Mechanical complication of internal orthopedic device, implant, and graft

Mechanical complications involving:
    external (fixation) device utilizing internal screw(s), pin(s) or other methods of fixation
    grafts of bone, cartilage, muscle, or tendon
    internal (fixation) device such as nail, plate, rod, etc.
Use additional code to identify prosthetic joint with mechanical complication (V43.60-V43.69)

> **EXCLUDES** complications of external orthopedic device, such as:
>   pressure ulcer due to cast (707.00-707.09)

996.40 Unspecified mechanical complication of internal orthopedic device, implant, and graft

996.41 Mechanical loosening of prosthetic joint
Aseptic loosening

996.42 Dislocation of prosthetic joint
Instability of prosthetic joint
Subluxation of prosthetic joint

996.43 Broken prosthetic joint implant
Breakage (fracture) of prosthetic joint

996.44 Peri-prosthetic fracture around prosthetic joint

996.45 Peri-prosthetic osteolysis
Use additional code to identify major osseous defect, if applicable (731.3)

996.46 Articular bearing surface wear of prosthetic joint

996.47 Other mechanical complication of prosthetic joint implant
Mechanical complication of prosthetic joint NOS
Prosthetic joint implant failure NOS

996.49 Other mechanical complication of other internal orthopedic device, implant, and graft
Breakage of internal fixation device in bone
Dislocation of internal fixation device in bone
EXCLUDES *mechanical complication of prosthetic joint implant (996.41-996.47)*

√5ᵗʰ **996.5 Mechanical complication of other specified prosthetic device, implant, and graft**
Mechanical complications involving:
prosthetic implant in:
bile duct
breast
chin
orbit of eye
nonabsorbable surgical material NOS
other graft, implant, and internal device, not elsewhere classified

996.51 Due to corneal graft

996.52 Due to graft of other tissue, not elsewhere classified
Skin graft failure or rejection
EXCLUDES *failure of artificial skin graft (996.55)*
failure of decellularized allodermis (996.55)
sloughing of temporary skin allografts or xenografts (pigskin) — omit code

996.53 Due to ocular lens prosthesis
EXCLUDES *contact lenses–code to condition*

996.54 Due to breast prosthesis
Breast capsule (prosthesis)
Mammary implant

996.55 Due to artificial skin graft and decellularized allodermis
Dislodgement
Displacement
Failure
Non-adherence
Poor incorporation
Shearing

996.56 Due to peritoneal dialysis catheter
EXCLUDES *mechanical complication of arteriovenous dialysis catheter (996.1)*

996.57 Due to insulin pump

996.59 Due to other implant and internal device, not elsewhere classified
Nonabsorbable surgical material NOS
Prosthetic implant in:
bile duct
chin
orbit of eye

√5ᵗʰ **996.6 Infection and inflammatory reaction due to internal prosthetic device, implant, and graft**
Infection (causing obstruction)
Inflammation } due to (presence of) any device, implant, and graft classifiable to 996.0-996.5
Use additional code to identify specified infections

996.60 Due to unspecified device, implant, and graft

996.61 Due to cardiac device, implant, and graft
Cardiac pacemaker or defibrillator:
electrode(s), lead(s)
pulse generator
subcutaneous pocket
Coronary artery bypass graft
Heart valve prosthesis

996.62 Due to other vascular device, implant, and graft
Arterial graft
Arteriovenous fistula or shunt
Infusion pump
Vascular catheter (arterial) (dialysis) (peripheral venous)
EXCLUDES *infection due to:*
central venous catheter (999.31-999.32)
Hickman catheter (999.31-999.32)
peripherally inserted central catheter [PICC] (999.31-999.32)
portacath (port-a-cath) (999.31-999.32)
triple lumen catheter (999.31-999.32)
umbilical venous catheter (999.31-999.32)

996.63 Due to nervous system device, implant, and graft
Electrodes implanted in brain
Peripheral nerve graft
Spinal canal catheter
Ventricular (communicating) shunt (catheter)

996.64 Due to indwelling urinary catheter
Use additional code to identify specified infections, such as:
cystitis (595.0-595.9)
sepsis (038.0-038.9)
EXCLUDES *complications due to:*
external stoma of urinary tract (596.81-596.83)

996.65 Due to other genitourinary device, implant, and graft
Intrauterine contraceptive device

996.66 Due to internal joint prosthesis
Use additional code to identify infected prosthetic joint (V43.60-V43.69)

996.67 Due to other internal orthopedic device, implant, and graft
Bone growth stimulator (electrode)
Internal fixation device (pin) (rod) (screw)

996.68 Due to peritoneal dialysis catheter
Exit-site infection or inflammation

996.69 Due to other internal prosthetic device, implant, and graft
Breast prosthesis
Ocular lens prosthesis
Prosthetic orbital implant

√5ᵗʰ **996.7 Other complications of internal (biological) (synthetic) prosthetic device, implant, and graft**
Complication NOS
Occlusion NOS
Embolism
Fibrosis } due to (presence of) any device, implant, and graft classifiable to 996.0-996.5
Hemorrhage
Pain
Stenosis
Thrombus
Use additional code to identify complication, such as:
pain due to presence of device, implant or graft (338.18-338.19, 338.28-338.29)
venous embolism and thrombosis (453.2-453.9)
EXCLUDES *disruption (dehiscence) of internal suture material (998.31)*
transplant rejection (996.80-996.89)

996.70 Due to unspecified device, implant, and graft

996.71 Due to heart valve prosthesis

996.72 Due to other cardiac device, implant, and graft
Cardiac pacemaker or defibrillator:
electrode(s), lead(s)
subcutaneous pocket
Coronary artery bypass (graft)
EXCLUDES occlusion due to atherosclerosis
(414.02-414.06)

996.73 Due to renal dialysis device, implant, and graft

996.74 Due to other vascular device, implant, and graft
EXCLUDES occlusion of biological graft due to
atherosclerosis
(440.30-440.32)

996.75 Due to nervous system device, implant, and graft

996.76 Due to genitourinary device, implant, and graft
EXCLUDES complications of implanted vaginal
mesh (629.31-629.32)

996.77 Due to internal joint prosthesis
Use additional code to identify prosthetic joint
(V43.60-V43.69)

996.78 Due to other internal orthopedic device, implant, and graft

996.79 Due to other internal prosthetic device, implant, and graft

√5ᵗʰ **996.8 Complications of transplanted organ**
Transplant failure or rejection
Use additional code to identify nature of complication, such as:
cytomegalovirus (CMV) infection (078.5)
graft-versus-host disease (279.50-279.53)
malignancy associated with organ transplant (199.2)
post-transplant lymphoproliferative disorder (PTLD) (238.77)

996.80 Transplanted organ, unspecified

996.81 Kidney

996.82 Liver

996.83 Heart

996.84 Lung

996.85 Bone marrow

996.86 Pancreas

996.87 Intestine

996.88 Stem cell
Complications from stem cells from:
peripheral blood
umbilical cord

996.89 Other specified transplanted organ

√5ᵗʰ **996.9 Complications of reattached extremity or body part**

996.90 Unspecified extremity

996.91 Forearm

996.92 Hand

996.93 Finger(s)

996.94 Upper extremity, other and unspecified

996.95 Foot and toe(s)

996.96 Lower extremity, other and unspecified

996.99 Other specified body part

√4ᵗʰ **997 Complications affecting specified body systems, not elsewhere classified**
Use additional code to identify complications
EXCLUDES the listed conditions when specified as:
causing shock (998.00-998.09)
complications of:
anesthesia:
adverse effect (001.0-799.9, 995.0-995.8)
in labor or delivery (668.0-668.9)
poisoning (968.0-969.9)
implanted device or graft (996.0-996.9)
obstetrical procedures (669.0-669.4)
reattached extremity (996.90-996.96)
transplanted organ (996.80-996.89)

√5ᵗʰ **997.0 Nervous system complications**

997.00 Nervous system complication, unspecified

997.01 Central nervous system complication
Anoxic brain damage
Cerebral hypoxia
EXCLUDES cerebrovascular hemorrhage or
infarction (997.02)

997.02 Iatrogenic cerebrovascular infarction or hemorrhage
Postoperative stroke

997.09 Other nervous system complications

997.1 Cardiac complications
Cardiac:
arrest
insufficiency
Cardiorespiratory failure
Heart failure
} during or resulting from a procedure
EXCLUDES the listed conditions as long-term effects of
cardiac surgery or due to the presence
of cardiac prosthetic device (429.4)

997.2 Peripheral vascular complications
Phlebitis or thrombophlebitis during or resulting from a procedure
EXCLUDES the listed conditions due to:
implant or catheter device (996.62)
infusion, perfusion, or transfusion (999.2)
complications affecting blood vessels
(997.71-997.79)

√5ᵗʰ **997.3 Respiratory complications**
EXCLUDES iatrogenic [postoperative] pneumothorax
(512.1)
iatrogenic pulmonary embolism (415.11)
specified complications classified elsewhere,
such as:
adult respiratory distress syndrome
(518.52)
pulmonary edema, postoperative (518.4)
respiratory insufficiency, acute,
postoperative (518.52)
shock lung related to trauma and surgery
(518.52)
tracheostomy complications (519.00-519.09)
transfusion related acute lung injury [TRALI]
(518.7)

DEF: Mendelson's syndrome: acid pneumonitis due to aspiration of gastric acids, may occur after anesthesia or sedation.

997.31 Ventilator associated pneumonia
Ventilator associated pneumonitis
Use additional code to identify organism

997.32 Postprocedural aspiration pneumonia
Chemical pneumonitis resulting from a procedure
Mendelson's syndrome resulting from a procedure
EXCLUDES aspiration pneumonia during labor
and delivery (668.0)

997.39 Other respiratory complications

> **DEF:** Mendelson's syndrome: acid pneumonitis due to aspiration of gastric acids, may occur after anesthesia or sedation.

√5ᵗʰ **997.4 Digestive system complications**

> Complications of:
> intestinal (internal) anastomosis and bypass, not elsewhere classified, except that involving urinary tract
> Hepatic failure ⎫
> Hepatorenal syndrome ⎬ specified as due to a procedure
> Intestinal obstruction NOS ⎭

> **EXCLUDES** complications of gastric band procedure (539.01-539.09)
> complications of other bariatric procedure (539.81-539.89)
> gastrostomy complications (536.40-536.49)
> specified gastrointestinal complications classified elsewhere, such as:
> blind loop syndrome (579.2)
> colostomy and enterostomy complications (569.60-569.69)
> complications of intestinal pouch (569.71-569.79)
> gastrojejunal ulcer (534.0-534.9)
> infection of esophagostomy (530.86)
> infection of external stoma (569.61)
> mechanical complication of esophagostomy (530.87)
> pelvic peritoneal adhesions, female (614.6)
> peritoneal adhesions (568.0)
> peritoneal adhesions with obstruction (560.81)
> postcholecystectomy syndrome (576.0)
> postgastric surgery syndromes (564.2)
> pouchitis (569.71)
> vomiting following gastrointestinal surgery (564.3)

997.41 Retained cholelithiasis following cholecystectomy

997.49 Other digestive system complications

997.5 Urinary complications

> Complications of:
> internal anastomosis and bypass of urinary tract, including that involving intestinal tract
> Oliguria or anuria ⎫
> Renal (kidney): ⎪
> failure (acute) ⎬ specified as due to procedure
> insufficiency (acute) ⎪
> Tubular necrosis (acute) ⎭

> **EXCLUDES** complications of cystostomy (596.81-596.83)
> complications of external stoma of urinary tract (596.81-596.83)
> specified complications classified elsewhere, such as:
> postoperative stricture of:
> ureter (593.3)
> urethra (598.2)

√5ᵗʰ **997.6 Amputation stump complication**

> **EXCLUDES** admission for treatment for a current traumatic amputation – code to complicated traumatic amputation
> phantom limb (syndrome) (353.6)

997.60 Unspecified complication

997.61 Neuroma of amputation stump

> **DEF:** Hyperplasia generated nerve cell mass following amputation.

997.62 Infection (chronic)

> Use additional code to identify the organism

997.69 Other

√5ᵗʰ **997.7 Vascular complications of other vessels**

> **EXCLUDES** peripheral vascular complications (997.2)

997.71 Vascular complications of mesenteric artery

997.72 Vascular complications of renal artery

997.79 Vascular complications of other vessels

√5ᵗʰ **997.9 Complications affecting other specified body systems, not elsewhere classified**

> **EXCLUDES** specified complications classified elsewhere, such as:
> broad ligament laceration syndrome (620.6)
> postartificial menopause syndrome (627.4)
> postoperative stricture of vagina (623.2)

997.91 Hypertension

> **EXCLUDES** essential hypertension (401.0-401.9)

997.99 Other

> Vitreous touch syndrome
> **DEF:** Vitreous touch syndrome: vitreous protruding through pupil and attaches to corneal epithelium; causes aqueous fluid in vitreous body; marked by corneal edema, loss of lucidity; complication of cataract surgery.

√4ᵗʰ **998 Other complications of procedures, not elsewhere classified**

> **EXCLUDES** fluid overload due to transfusion (blood) (276.61)
> TACO (276.61)
> transfusion associated circulatory overload (276.61)

√5ᵗʰ **998.0 Postoperative shock**

> Shock during or resulting from a surgical procedure
> **EXCLUDES** shock:
> anaphylactic due to serum (999.41-999.49)
> anesthetic (995.4)
> electric (994.8)
> following abortion (639.5)
> obstetric (669.1)
> traumatic (958.4)

998.00 Postoperative shock, unspecified

> Collapse, not otherwise specified, during or resulting from a surgical procedure
> Failure of peripheral circulation, postoperative

998.01 Postoperative shock, cardiogenic

998.02 Postoperative shock, septic

> Postoperative endotoxic shock
> Postoperative gram-negative shock
> Code first underlying infection
> Use additional code, to identify severe sepsis (995.92) and any associated acute organ dysfunction, if applicable

998.09 Postoperative shock, other

> Postoperative hypovolemic shock

√5ᵗʰ **998.1 Hemorrhage or hematoma or seroma complicating a procedure**

> **EXCLUDES** hemorrhage, hematoma, or seroma:
> complicating cesarean section or puerperal perineal wound (674.3)
> due to implanted device or graft (996.70-996.79)

998.11 Hemorrhage complicating a procedure

998.12 Hematoma complicating a procedure

998.13 Seroma complicating a procedure

998.2   Accidental puncture or laceration during a procedure
Accidental perforation by catheter or other instrument
during a procedure on:
blood vessel
nerve
organ

> EXCLUDES   iatrogenic [postoperative] pneumothorax
> (512.1)
> puncture or laceration caused by implanted
> device intentionally left in operation
> wound (996.0-996.5)
> specified complications classified elsewhere,
> such as:
> broad ligament laceration syndrome
> (620.6)
> dural tear (349.31)
> incidental durotomy (349.31)
> trauma from instruments during delivery
> (664.0-665.9)

√5ᵗʰ 998.3   Disruption of wound
Dehiscence   }
Rupture   } of operation wound
Disruption of any suture materials or other closure
method

> EXCLUDES   disruption of:
> cesarean wound (674.1)
> perineal wound, puerperal (674.2)

998.30   Disruption of wound, unspecified
Disruption of wound NOS

**998.31   Disruption of internal operation (surgical)
wound**
Disruption or dehiscence of closure of:
fascia, superficial or muscular
internal organ
muscle or muscle flap
ribs or rib cage
skull or craniotomy
sternum or sternotomy
tendon or ligament
Deep disruption or dehiscence of operation
wound NOS

> EXCLUDES   complications of internal
> anastomosis of:
> gastrointestinal tract (997.49)
> urinary tract (997.5)

**998.32   Disruption of external operation (surgical)
wound**
Disruption of operation wound NOS
Disruption or dehiscence of closure of:
cornea
mucosa
skin
subcutaneous tissue
Full-thickness skin disruption or dehiscence
Superficial disruption or dehiscence of
operation wound

998.33   Disruption of traumatic injury wound repair
Disruption or dehiscence of closure of
traumatic laceration (external) (internal)

998.4   Foreign body accidentally left during a procedure
Adhesions   } due to foreign body accidentally left in
Obstruction   } operative wound or body cavity
Perforation   } during a procedure

> EXCLUDES   obstruction or perforation caused by
> implanted device intentionally left in
> body (996.0-996.5)

√5ᵗʰ 998.5   Postoperative infection

> EXCLUDES   bleb associated endophthalmitis (379.63)
> infection due to:
> implanted device (996.60-996.69)
> infusion, perfusion, or transfusion
> (999.31-999.39)
> postoperative obstetrical wound infection
> (674.3)

998.51   Infected postoperative seroma
Use additional code to identify organism

998.59   Other postoperative infection
Abscess:
intra-abdominal   }
stitch   }
subphrenic   } postoperative
wound   }
Septicemia   }
Use additional code to identify infection

998.6   Persistent postoperative fistula

**998.7   Acute reaction to foreign substance accidentally left
during a procedure**
Peritonitis:
aseptic
chemical

**√5ᵗʰ 998.8   Other specified complications of procedures, not
elsewhere classified**

**998.81   Emphysema (subcutaneous) (surgical)
resulting from a procedure**

**998.82   Cataract fragments in eye following cataract
surgery**

998.83   Non-healing surgical wound

998.89   Other specified complications

**998.9   Unspecified complication of procedure, not elsewhere
classified**
Postoperative complication NOS

> EXCLUDES   complication NOS of obstetrical, surgery or
> procedure (669.4)

√4ᵗʰ 999   Complications of medical care, not elsewhere classified

> INCLUDES   complications, not elsewhere classified, of:
> dialysis (hemodialysis) (peritoneal) (renal)
> extracorporeal circulation
> hyperalimentation therapy
> immunization
> infusion
> inhalation therapy
> injection
> inoculation
> perfusion
> transfusion
> vaccination
> ventilation therapy

Use additional code, where applicable, to identify specific
complication

> EXCLUDES   specified complications classified elsewhere such as:
> complications of implanted device (996.0-996.9)
> contact dermatitis due to drugs (692.3)
> dementia dialysis (294.8)
> transient (293.9)
> dialysis disequilibrium syndrome (276.0-276.9)
> poisoning and toxic effects of drugs and chemicals
> (960.0-989.9)
> postvaccinal encephalitis (323.51)
> water and electrolyte imbalance (276.0-276.9)

999.0   Generalized vaccinia

> EXCLUDES   vaccinia not from vaccine (051.02)

DEF: Skin eruption, self-limiting; follows vaccination; due
to transient viremia with virus localized in skin.

999.1   Air embolism
Air embolism to any site following infusion, perfusion, or
transfusion

> EXCLUDES   embolism specified as:
> complicating:
> abortion (634-638 with .6, 639.6)
> ectopic or molar pregnancy (639.6)
> pregnancy, childbirth, or the
> puerperium (673.0)
> due to implanted device (996.7)
> traumatic (958.0)

Injury and Poisoning

999.2–999.69

999.2   Other vascular complications

Phlebitis   ⎫
Thromboembolism   ⎬   following infusion, perfusion, or transfusion
Thrombophlebitis   ⎭

> **EXCLUDES**   *extravasation of vesicant drugs (999.81, 999.82)*
> *the listed conditions when specified as:*
> *due to implanted device (996.61-996.62. 996.72-996.74)*
> *postoperative NOS (997.2, 997.71-997.79)*

✓5ᵗʰ 999.3   Other infection

Infection   ⎫
Sepsis   ⎬ following infusion, injection, transfusion, or vaccination
Septicemia   ⎭

Use additional code to identify the specified infection, such as:
septicemia (038.0-038.9)

> **EXCLUDES**   *the listed conditions when specified as:*
> *due to implanted device (996.60-996.69)*
> *postoperative NOS (998.51-998.59)*

999.31   Other and unspecified infection due to central venous catheter

Central line-associated infection
Infection due to:
    central venous catheter NOS
    Hickman catheter
    peripherally inserted central catheter (PICC)
    triple lumen catheter
    umbilical venous catheter

> **EXCLUDES**   *infection due to:*
> *arterial catheter (996.62)*
> *catheter NOS (996.69)*
> *peripheral venous catheter (996.62)*
> *urinary catheter (996.64)*

999.32   Bloodstream infection due to central venous catheter

Bloodstream infection due to:
    Hickman catheter
    peripherally inserted central catheter (PICC)
    portacath (port-a-cath)
    triple lumen catheter
    umbilical venous catheter
Catheter-related bloodstream infection (CRBSI) NOS
Central line-associated bloodstream infection (CLABSI)

999.33   Local infection due to central venous catheter

Exit or insertion site infection
Local infection due to:
    Hickman catheter
    peripherally inserted central catheter (PICC)
    portacath (port-a-cath)
    triple lumen catheter
    umbilical venous catheter
Port or reservoir infection
Tunnel infection

999.34   Acute infection following transfusion, infusion, or injection of blood and blood products

999.39   Infection following other infusion, injection, transfusion, or vaccination

✓5ᵗʰ 999.4   Anaphylactic reaction due to serum

Allergic shock
Anaphylactic shock due to serum
Anaphylactoid reaction due to serum
Anaphylaxis

> **EXCLUDES**   *ABO incompatibility reaction due to transfusion of blood or blood products (999.60-999.69)*
> *reaction:*
> *allergic NOS (995.0)*
> *anaphylactic:*
> *NOS (995.0)*
> *due to drugs and chemicals (995.0)*
> *other serum (999.51-999.59)*
> *shock:*
> *allergic NOS (995.0)*
> *anaphylactic:*
> *NOS (995.0)*
> *due to drugs and chemicals (995.0)*

DEF: Life-threatening hypersensitivity to foreign serum; causes respiratory distress, vascular collapse, and shock.

999.41   Anaphylactic reaction due to administration of blood and blood products

999.42   Anaphylactic reaction due to vaccination

999.49   Anaphylactic reaction due to other serum

✓5ᵗʰ 999.5   Other serum reaction

Intoxication by serum
Protein sickness
Serum rash
Serum sickness
Urticaria due to serum

> **EXCLUDES**   *serum hepatitis (070.2-070.3)*

DEF: Serum sickness: Hypersensitivity to foreign serum; causes fever, hives, swelling, and lymphadenopathy.

999.51   Other serum reaction due to administration of blood and blood products

999.52   Other serum reaction due to vaccination

999.59   Other serum reaction

✓5ᵗʰ 999.6   ABO incompatibility reaction due to transfusion of blood or blood products

> **EXCLUDES**   *minor blood group antigens reactions (Duffy) (E) (K(ell)) (Kidd) (Lewis) (M) (N) (P) (S) (999.75-999.79)*

999.60   ABO incompatibility reaction, unspecified

ABO incompatible blood transfusion NOS
Reaction to ABO incompatibility from transfusion NOS

999.61   ABO incompatibility with hemolytic transfusion reaction not specified as acute or delayed

ABO incompatibility with hemolytic transfusion reaction at unspecified time after transfusion
Hemolytic transfusion reaction (HTR) due to ABO incompatibility

999.62   ABO incompatibility with acute hemolytic transfusion reaction

ABO incompatibility with hemolytic transfusion reaction less than 24 hours after transfusion
Acute hemolytic transfusion reaction (AHTR) due to ABO incompatibility

999.63   ABO incompatibility with delayed hemolytic transfusion reaction

ABO incompatibility with hemolytic transfusion reaction 24 hours or more after transfusion
Delayed hemolytic transfusion reaction (DHTR) due to ABO incompatibility

999.69   Other ABO incompatibility reaction

Delayed serologic transfusion reaction (DSTR) from ABO incompatibility
Other ABO incompatible blood transfusion
Other reaction to ABO incompatibility from transfusion

√5ᵗʰ **999.7 Rh and other non-ABO incompatibility reaction due to transfusion of blood or blood products**
Elevation of Rh titer

999.70 Rh incompatibility reaction, unspecified
Reaction due to Rh factor in transfusion NOS
Rh incompatible blood transfusion NOS
Unspecified reaction due to incompatibility related to Rh antigens (C) (c) (D) (E) (e)
Unspecified reaction to Rh incompatibility

999.71 Rh incompatibility with hemolytic transfusion reaction not specified as acute or delayed
Hemolytic transfusion reaction (HTR) due to Rh incompatibility
HTR due to incompatibility related to Rh antigens (C) (c) (D) (E) (e), not specified as acute or delayed
Rh incompatibility with hemolytic transfusion reaction at unspecified time after transfusion

999.72 Rh incompatibility with acute hemolytic transfusion reaction
Acute hemolytic transfusion reaction (AHTR) due to Rh incompatibility
AHTR due to incompatibility related to Rh antigens (C) (c) (D) (E) (e)
Rh incompatibility with hemolytic transfusion reaction less than 24 hours after transfusion

999.73 Rh incompatibility with delayed hemolytic transfusion reaction
Delayed hemolytic transfusion reaction (DHTR) due to Rh incompatibility
DHTR due to incompatibility related to Rh antigens (C) (c) (D) (E) (e)
Rh incompatibility with hemolytic transfusion reaction 24 hours or more after transfusion

999.74 Other Rh incompatibility reaction
Delayed serologic transfusion reaction (DSTR) from Rh incompatibility
Other reaction due to incompatibility related to Rh antigens (C) (c) (D) (E) (e)
Other reaction to Rh incompatible blood transfusion

999.75 Non-ABO incompatibility reaction, unspecified
Non-ABO incompatible blood transfusion NOS
Reaction to non-ABO antigen incompatibility from transfusion NOS
Unspecified reaction due to incompatibility related to minor antigens (Duffy) (Kell) (Kidd) (Lewis) (M) (N) (P) (S)

999.76 Non-ABO incompatibility with hemolytic transfusion reaction not specified as acute or delayed
Hemolytic transfusion reaction (HTR) due to non-ABO incompatibility
HTR from incompatibility related to minor antigens (Duffy) (Kell) (Kidd) (Lewis) (M) (N) (P) (S)
Non-ABO incompatibility with hemolytic transfusion reaction at unspecified time after transfusion

999.77 Non-ABO incompatibility with acute hemolytic transfusion reaction
Acute hemolytic transfusion reaction (AHTR) due to non-ABO incompatibility
AHTR from incompatibility related to minor antigens (Duffy) (Kell) (Kidd) (Lewis) (M) (N) (P) (S)
Non-ABO incompatibility with hemolytic transfusion reaction less than 24 hours after transfusion

999.78 Non-ABO incompatibility with delayed hemolytic transfusion reaction
Delayed hemolytic transfusion reaction(DHTR) due to non-ABO incompatibility
DHTR from incompatibility related to minor antigens (Duffy) (Kell) (Kidd) (Lewis) (M) (N) (P) (S)
Non-ABO incompatibility with hemolytic transfusion reaction 24 hours or more after transfusion

999.79 Other non-ABO incompatibility reaction
Delayed serologic transfusion reaction (DSTR) from non-ABO incompatibility
Other non-ABO incompatible blood transfusion
Other reaction due to incompatibility related to minor antigens (Duffy) (Kell) (Kidd) (Lewis) (M) (N) (P) (S)
Other reaction to non-ABO incompatibility from transfusion

√5ᵗʰ **999.8 Other and unspecified infusion and transfusion reaction**

> **EXCLUDES** *ABO incompatibility reactions (999.60-999.69)*
> *febrile nonhemolytic transfusion reaction (FNHTR) (780.66)*
> *hemochromatosis due to repeated red blood cell transfusions (275.02)*
> *non-ABO incompatibility reactions (999.70-999.79)*
> *postoperative shock (998.00-998.09)*
> *posttransfusion purpura (287.41)*
> *Rh incompatibility reactions (999.70-999.74)*
> *transfusion associated circulatory overload (TACO) (276.61)*
> *transfusion related acute lung injury [TRALI] (518.7)*

999.80 Transfusion reaction, unspecified
Incompatible blood transfusion NOS
Reaction to blood group incompatibility in infusion or transfusion NOS

999.81 Extravasation of vesicant chemotherapy
Infiltration of vesicant chemotherapy

999.82 Extravasation of other vesicant agent
Infiltration of other vesicant agent

999.83 Hemolytic transfusion reaction, incompatibility unspecified
Hemolytic transfusion reaction (HTR) with antigen incompatibility unspecified, not specified as acute or delayed
HTR with incompatibility unspecified at unspecified time after transfusion

999.84 Acute hemolytic transfusion reaction, incompatibility unspecified
Acute hemolytic transfusion reaction (AHTR) with antigen incompatibility unspecified
AHTR, incompatibility unspecified

999.85 Delayed hemolytic transfusion reaction, incompatibility unspecified
Delayed hemolytic transfusion reaction (DHTR) with antigen incompatibility unspecified
DHTR, incompatibility unspecified

999.88 Other infusion reaction

999.89 Other transfusion reaction
Delayed serologic transfusion reaction (DSTR), incompatibility unspecified
Use additional code to identify graft-versus-host reaction (279.5)

Injury and Poisoning

999.9   **Other and unspecified complications of medical care, not elsewhere classified**

Complications, not elsewhere classified, of:

electroshock

inhalation

ultrasound   } therapy

ventilation

Unspecified misadventure of medical care

EXCLUDES   *unspecified complication of:*

phototherapy (990)

radiation therapy (999)

ventilator associated pneumonia (997.31)

V Codes: Supplementary Classification of Factors Influencing Health Status and Contact with Health Service (V01–V91)

Coding Guidance

This chapter classifies the following situations that are not classifiable to categories 001–999, specifically:

- Encounters for health services
- Problems influencing a person's health status
- Facts needed for statistical tabulations

The encounter V codes are used to record a visit or classify a patient who is not acutely ill but needs a health service for a specific purpose, such as prophylactic immunization, routine examination, or counseling. These V codes are not procedure codes. If a procedure is performed as a result of the encounter, then an appropriate procedure code must be assigned.

Example:

> Patient encounter for the purpose of receiving prophylactic tetanus immunization is coded as V03.7 Need for prophylactic vaccination and inoculation, tetanus toxoid alone.

The problem V codes describe circumstances that influence the person's health status but are not a current illness or injury, such as a colostomy status or a past history of mental illness. Except in rare cases, the problem V codes are not reported as a principal diagnosis, nor do they stand alone. They do not describe the reason for the encounter, but rather provide an item of information about the state of the patient. These V codes are used only when the circumstance influences the patient's current condition or treatment.

Example:

> Patient has a history of stomach cancer and the purpose of the encounter is screening; findings are negative. Assign codes V76.49 Special screening for malignant neoplasm and V10.04 Personal history of malignant neoplasm of the stomach.

Other V codes may provide supplementary information that is important to record but is not representative of a problem or service.

V codes are used in both inpatient and outpatient settings. V codes for encounters are more appropriate for outpatient and physician office visits.

The instructions for V code use contained in the official coding guidelines identify only those V codes that can be used only as a PDx. All other V codes may be either SDx or PDx depending upon circumstances of the encounter, by meeting the definition of first-listed or principal diagnosis, and by following any specific V code guidelines in section I.C.18 a-e. With the elimination of the V Code Table, those assigning a V code as a PDx must make sure the circumstances of the encounter meet the definition of first-listed or principal diagnosis, follow all coding instructions, and follow the V-code-specific guidelines.

Persons with Potential Health Hazards Related to Communicable Diseases (V01–V06)

This subchapter contains service and problem V codes and is especially applicable for ambulatory care settings, including the emergency department. Encounters for vaccination, isolation, and prophylactic surgery are classified here.

Encounters for contact or exposure to communicable diseases (V01) are to be used for patients who do not exhibit any signs or symptoms of the disease.

Carriers or suspected carriers of infectious disease are classified to V02. This V code provides supplementary information about the patient that may affect the course of or outcome of treatment.

Categories V03–V06 classify encounters for the reason of inoculation or vaccination as a prophylactic measure.

Persons with Need for Isolation, Other Potential Health Hazards and Prophylactic Measures (V07-V09)

Encounters for the reasons of isolation other prophylactic measures or treatment are classified to V07. This category includes isolation, desentitization to allergens, postmenopausal hormone replacement therapy, prophylactic fluoride treatments, and use of specific drugs for treatment, not just for prophylactic measures.

Code V08 Asymptomatic human immunodeficiency virus (HIV) infection status, is used for patients who have the HIV virus (i.e., have tested positive) but have not ever manifested signs or symptoms of the disease.

Infection with drug-resistant micro-organism, V09, is used to indicate that a patient has a form of infection resistant to drugs.

Persons with Potential Health Hazards Related to Personal and Family History (V10–V19)

Categories V10–V19 contain personal and family history codes. Personal history codes include a history of neoplasms, mental disorders, diseases, and allergies. Family history codes include a history of neoplasms and diseases. Personal history codes are often reported to indicate the need for adjunctive surgery and treatment; family history codes are often used to indicate the need for prophylactic surgery and treatment. Family history codes are frequently used with screening codes to justify a test or procedure. This range of codes should be used as secondary codes if the historical condition or family history has an impact on current care or influences treatment.

Persons Encountering Health Services in Circumstances Related to Reproduction and Development (V20–V29)

This subchapter contains codes to indicate supervision of uncomplicated pregnancy and perceived problems which, after evaluation, are determined to be normal states in development (e.g., onset of menses, teething). Codes to report outcome of delivery on the mother's record (used in addition to codes from the obstetric section of ICD-9-CM) also are included here.

Category V23 Supervision of high-risk pregnancy, is used for pregnancy with a history of conditions classifiable to 634–638 or other conditions with a potential adverse effect on outcome. Recurrent pregnancy loss is coded as 646.3x.

Code V28 Antenatal screening, should be used only if no specific condition is found to exist during the screening process. Code the condition, not the screening, if one is discovered.

Code V29 Observation and evaluation of newborns for suspected condition not found, should be sequenced second after V30 Live born infant. Category V29 codes may be reported as principal diagnoses for newborns or infants admitted or readmitted to the hospital for suspected conditions not found after study, provided no associated signs or symptoms are present. In such cases, code and report the sign or symptom instead of V29.

Liveborn Infants According to Type of Birth (V30–V39)

This section contains codes for the principal diagnosis for an infant and describes the type of birth, single or multiple. These codes are used in the inpatient setting for most patients (fourth digit 0) but may be used for those born before admission (fourth digit 1) or not admitted to the hospital (fourth digit 2). The fifth digit identifies whether the delivery was vaginal (0) or cesarean (1).

Persons with a Condition Influencing Their Health Status (V40–V49)

Category V40–V49 codes are used to describe circumstances other than a disease or an injury that influences a patient's health status. These codes describe the residual of a past disease or a condition that in some way affects the way the patient's treatment is carried out. The status codes are different from the history codes in that a history code indicates that the patient no longer has the disease. These codes should be used when the condition is documented as a diagnosis or problem.

Category V46 Other dependence on machines and devices is assigned to indicate the status of dependence upon machines or devices such as an aspirator, ventilator (respirator), wheelchair, or supplemental oxygen.

Persons Encountering Health Services for Specific Procedures and Aftercare (V50–V59)

This subchapter contains codes to indicate reasons for care in patients who have already been treated for some disease or injury, but may need aftercare or adjunctive treatment to consolidate the treatment, deal with residual states, or prevent recurrence.

Encounters for plastic surgery are classified in two ways: procedures used for cosmetic surgery for conditions that are normal variations rather than the result of pathological states and procedures for the residual conditions of a healed injury or operation.

Also classified here are encounters for services such as chemotherapy, radiotherapy, rehabilitation and physical therapy, fittings and adjustments of devices, orthopedic aftercare, and dialysis.

The subdivision of this section includes the following categories:

Persons Encountering Health Services in Other Circumstances (V60–V69)

Category V60–V68 codes contain additional information that must be included in the medical record regarding family, household, administrative, follow-up, and psychosocial circumstances. Included in this section is category V64 *Persons encountering health services for specific procedures, not carried out*. Code sequencing depends on the reason the procedure was not performed.

Examination and Investigation of Individuals and Populations (V70–V82)

This subchapter contains codes to represent encounters with health services for general physical and mental examinations, routine tests on specific body systems and screenings. The special screening codes are used only when screening procedures are done on defined population groups.

These V codes are especially applicable for ambulatory care settings as well as emergency departments and are largely beyond the scope of office settings.

Genetics (V83–V84)

Category V83 codes are used to report genetic carrier status. The codes are mainly used for women who are pregnant or are considering pregnancy and are known carriers of a disease. The codes listed are for asymptomatic carriers except for V83.02, which is for carriers of hemophilia A, who have trouble with blood coagulation. Category V84 reports genetic susceptibility to disease. Having a genetic susceptibility to a disease, in particular a malignancy, is not the same as being a carrier of a disease that may be passed on to offspring. Those people who are genetically susceptibility is a red flag a person is at higher risk and has a greater chance of getting a disease or malignant growth because of their inborn predisposition. These patients sometimes request to have the particular organ at risk removed prophylactically in the hope that taking such a step will prevent the disease from occurring. Most of these requests are for prophylactic breast or ovary removal. A V code for genetic susceptibility to a disease (V84) is assigned only after positive confirmation through genetic testing.

Body Mass Index (V85)

BMI is measured in kilograms per meters squared. The calculation is based on height and weight determined by dividing a person's weight in kilograms by height in meters squared. The index score can also be calculated by multiplying a patient's weight in kilograms by 704.5, and dividing the result by the patient's height in inches twice. BMI measurements are a guideline for categorizing weight in a more specific manner than relying solely on "overweight" or "obese" terminology. By definition, an adult is generally considered overweight if he or she has a BMI between 25 and 29.9 kg/m2. Obesity is defined as a BMI of 30 or higher. Individual variances such as the presence or absence of muscle mass and the distribution of body fat also need to be taken into consideration. BMI pediatric codes are to be used for persons aged 2 to 20 years only. The percentiles specified above are based on growth charts published by the Centers for Disease Control and Prevention (CDC).

Estrogen Receptor Status (V86)

In breast cancer, the hormone receptor status of the cells is a useful tool for determining treatment and prognosis. Cancers in which the cells express estrogen receptor (ER) in their nuclei generally have a better prognosis, since these cells are better differentiated and can respond to hormonal manipulation. According to the National Cancer Institute, seven out of 10 breast cancer patients have ER-positive tumors.

Other Specified Personal Exposures and History Presenting Hazards to Health (V87)

Patients may be initially asymptomatic following exposures to drugs, chemicals, and other substances, but develop subsequent health concerns as a result. For example, individuals such as firefighters, hair stylists, truck drivers, and textile workers may have more exposure to certain chemicals and dyes, such as

benzenes or aromatic amines, and are therefore at higher risk of developing adverse effects of these exposures for which they may seek medical care. These adverse effects may include medical problems that persist for months or years after treatment ends. Some therapeutic drug therapies for the treatment of cancer may result in infertility, growth problems in children, or cancer treatment-related fatigue.

Acquired Absence of Other Organs and Tissue (V88)

Category V88 codes classify the acquired absence of cervix or uterus. Women who have had a full hysterectomy no longer need cervical Pap smears, but they do require vaginal smears to test for vaginal malignancies. Women with a cervical stump following a hysterectomy still require cervical Pap smears. These codes assist in supporting medical necessity of Pap smears for this population of patients.

Other Suspected Conditions Not Found (V89)

Pregnant patients may be referred to maternal-fetal specialists for further detailed diagnostic tests when an initial prenatal screening test indicates a possible abnormality. However, in many cases the detailed exam shows no abnormality and the suspected condition is ruled out. Category V89 codes help support the medical necessity of tests and encounters for the purpose of ruling out suspected conditions that would require a higher level of care.

Retained Foreign Body (V90)

Retained foreign bodies pose a potential risk of infection, interference with MRI (if the foreign body is magnetic), and even toxic poisoning if the foreign body contains lead or radioactive material. Category V90 covers the status of retained foreign body of a variety of materials.

Sequencing of V Codes

The official coding guidelines includes the following list of V codes that are to be reported as the first-listed diagnosis (Section I.C.18.e.), except when the V code does not meet the definition of a first-listed diagnosis for a health care encounter or more than one V code associated with the encounter meets the definition of first-listed. All V codes not included in the list are sequenced according to the circumstances of the health care encounter.

V codes in the following categories/subcategories/subclassifications are accepted only as first-listed codes:

V20.x	Health supervision of infant or child
V22.0	Supervision of normal first pregnancy
V22.1	Supervision of other normal pregnancy
V24.x	Postpartum care and examination
V26.81	Encounter for assisted reproductive fertility procedure cycle
V26.82	Encounter for fertility preservation procedure
V30–V39	Liveborn infants according to type of birth
V46.12	Encounter for respirator dependence during power failure
V46.13	Encounter for weaning from respirator [ventilator]
V51.0	Encounter for breast reconstruction following mastectomy
V56.0	Extracorporeal dialysis
V57.x	Care involving use of rehabilitation procedures
V58.0	Radiotherapy
V58.11	Encounter for antineoplastic chemotherapy
	V58.0 and V58.11 may be used together on a record with either one being sequenced first, when the patient receives both chemotherapy and radiation therapy during the same session.
V58.12	Encounter for antineoplastic immunotherapy
V59	Donors
V66.x	Convalescence and palliative care
	EXCEPT V66.7 Palliative care
V68.x	Encounters for administrative purposes
V70	General medical examination
	EXCEPT V70.7 Examination of participant in clinical trial
V71	Observation and evaluation for suspected conditions not found

SUPPLEMENTARY CLASSIFICATION OF FACTORS INFLUENCING HEALTH STATUS AND CONTACT WITH HEALTH SERVICES (V01-V91)

This classification is provided to deal with occasions when circumstances other than a disease or injury classifiable to categories 001-999 (the main part of ICD) are recorded as "diagnoses" or "problems." This can arise mainly in three ways:

a) When a person who is not currently sick encounters the health services for some specific purpose, such as to act as a donor of an organ or tissue, to receive prophylactic vaccination, or to discuss a problem which is in itself not a disease or injury. This will be a fairly rare occurrence among hospital inpatients, but will be relatively more common among hospital outpatients and patients of family practitioners, health clinics, etc.

b) When a person with a known disease or injury, whether it is current or resolving, encounters the health care system for a specific treatment of that disease or injury (e.g., dialysis for renal disease; chemotherapy for malignancy; cast change).

c) When some circumstance or problem is present which influences the person's health status but is not in itself a current illness or injury. Such factors may be elicited during population surveys, when the person may or may not be currently sick, or be recorded as an additional factor to be borne in mind when the person is receiving care for some current illness or injury classifiable to categories 001-999.

In the latter circumstances the V code should be used only as a supplementary code and should not be the one selected for use in primary, single cause tabulations. Examples of these circumstances are a personal history of certain diseases, or a person with an artificial heart valve in situ.

PERSONS WITH POTENTIAL HEALTH HAZARDS RELATED TO COMMUNICABLE DISEASES (V01-V06)

> **EXCLUDES** family history of infectious and parasitic diseases (V18.8)
> personal history of infectious and parasitic diseases (V12.0)

√4ᵗʰ **V01 Contact with or exposure to communicable diseases**

V01.0 Cholera
Conditions classifiable to 001

V01.1 Tuberculosis
Conditions classifiable to 010-018

V01.2 Poliomyelitis
Conditions classifiable to 045

V01.3 Smallpox
Conditions classifiable to 050

V01.4 Rubella
Conditions classifiable to 056

V01.5 Rabies
Conditions classifiable to 071

V01.6 Venereal diseases
Conditions classifiable to 090-099

√5ᵗʰ **V01.7 Other viral diseases**
Conditions classifiable to 042-078 and V08, except as above

V01.71 Varicella

V01.79 Other viral diseases

√5ᵗʰ **V01.8 Other communicable diseases**
Conditions classifiable to 001-136, except as above

V01.81 Anthrax

V01.82 Exposure to SARS-associated coronavirus

V01.83 Escherichia coli (E. coli)

V01.84 Meningococcus

V01.89 Other communicable diseases

V01.9 Unspecified communicable diseases

√4ᵗʰ **V02 Carrier or suspected carrier of infectious diseases**
> **INCLUDES** colonization status

V02.0 Cholera

V02.1 Typhoid

V02.2 Amebiasis

V02.3 Other gastrointestinal pathogens

V02.4 Diphtheria

√5ᵗʰ **V02.5 Other specified bacterial diseases**

V02.51 Group B streptococcus

V02.52 Other streptococcus

V02.53 Methicillin susceptible Staphylococcus aureus
MSSA colonization

V02.54 Methicillin resistant Staphylococcus aureus
MRSA colonization

V02.59 Other specified bacterial diseases
Meningococcal
Staphylococcal

√5ᵗʰ **V02.6 Viral hepatitis**
Hepatitis Australian-antigen [HAA] [SH] carrier
Serum hepatitis carrier

V02.60 Viral hepatitis carrier, unspecified

V02.61 Hepatitis B carrier

V02.62 Hepatitis C carrier

V02.69 Other viral hepatitis carrier

V02.7 Gonorrhea

V02.8 Other veneral diseases

V02.9 Other specified infectious organism

√4ᵗʰ **V03 Need for prophylactic vaccination and inoculation against bacterial diseases**
> **EXCLUDES** vaccination not carried out (V64.00-V64.09)
> vaccines against combinations of diseases (V06.0-V06.9)

V03.0 Cholera alone

V03.1 Typhoid-paratyphoid alone [TAB]

V03.2 Tuberculosis [BCG]

V03.3 Plague

V03.4 Tularemia

V03.5 Diphtheria alone

V03.6 Pertussis alone

V03.7 Tetanus toxoid alone

√5ᵗʰ **V03.8 Other specified vaccinations against single bacterial diseases**

V03.81 Hemophilus influenza, type B [Hib]

V03.82 Streptococcus pneumoniae [pneumococcus]

V03.89 Other specified vaccination

V03.9 Unspecified single bacterial disease

√4ᵗʰ **V04 Need for prophylactic vaccination and inoculation against certain viral diseases**
> **EXCLUDES** vaccines against combinations of diseases (V06.0-V06.9)

V04.0 Poliomyelitis

V04.1 Smallpox

V04.2 Measles alone

V04.3 Rubella alone

V04.4 Yellow fever

V04.5 Rabies

V04.6 Mumps alone

V04.7 Common cold

√5ᵗʰ **V04.8 Other viral diseases**

V04.81 Influenza

V04.82 Respiratory syncytial virus (RSV)

V04.89 Other viral diseases

☑4ᵗʰ **V05** **Need for other prophylactic vaccination and inoculation against single diseases**

> EXCLUDES *vaccines against combinations of diseases (V06.0-V06.9)*

V05.0 **Athropod-borne viral encephalitis**

V05.1 **Other arthropod-borne viral diseases**

V05.2 **Leshmaniasis**

V05.3 **Viral hepatitis**

V05.4 **Varicella**
> Chickenpox

V05.8 **Other specified disease**

V05.9 **Unspecified single disease**

☑4ᵗʰ **V06** **Need for prophylactic vaccination and inoculation against combinations of diseases**

> Note: Use additional single vaccination codes from categories V03-V05 to identify any vaccinations not included in a combination code.

V06.0 **Cholera with typhoid-paratyphoid [cholera+TAB]**

V06.1 **Diphtheria-tetanus-pertussis, combined [DTP] [DTaP]**

V06.2 **Diphtheria-tetanus-pertussis with typhoid-paratyphoid [DTP+TAB]**

V06.3 **Diphtheria-tetanus-pertussis with poliomyelitis [DTP+polio]**

V06.4 **Measles-mumps-rubella [MMR]**

V06.5 **Tetanus-diphtheria [Td] [DT]**

V06.6 **Streptococcus pneumoniae [pneumococcus] and influenza**

V06.8 **Other combinations**
> EXCLUDES *multiple single vaccination codes (V03.0-V05.9)*

V06.9 **Unspecified combined vaccine**

PERSONS WITH NEED FOR ISOLATION, OTHER POTENTIAL HEALTH HAZARDS AND PROPHYLACTIC MEASURES (V07-V09)

☑4ᵗʰ **V07** **Need for isolation and other prophylactic or treatment measures**

> EXCLUDES *long-term (current) (prophylactic) use of certain specific drugs (V58.61-V58.69)*
> *prophylactic organ removal (V50.41-V50.49)*

V07.0 **Isolation**
> Admission to protect the individual from his surroundings or for isolation of individual after contact with infectious diseases

V07.1 **Desensitization to allergens**

V07.2 **Prophylactic immunotherapy**
> Administration of:
> antivenin
> immune sera [gamma globulin]
> RhoGAM
> tetanus antitoxin

☑5ᵗʰ **V07.3** **Other prophylactic chemotherapy**

V07.31 **Prophylactic fluoride administration**

V07.39 **Other prophylactic chemotherapy**
> EXCLUDES *maintenance chemotherapy following disease (V58.11)*

V07.4 **Hormone replacement therapy (postmenopausal)**

☑5ᵗʰ **V07.5** **Use of agents affecting estrogen receptors and estrogen levels**
> Code first, if applicable:
> malignant neoplasm of breast (174.0-174.9, 175.0-175.9)
> malignant neoplasm of prostate (185)
> Use additional code, if applicable, to identify:
> estrogen receptor positive status (V86.0)
> family history of breast cancer (V16.3)
> genetic susceptibility to cancer (V84.01-V84.09)
> personal history of breast cancer (V10.3)
> personal history of prostate cancer (V10.46)
> postmenopausal status (V49.81)

> EXCLUDES *hormone replacement therapy (postmenopausal) (V07.4)*

V07.51 **Use of selective estrogen receptor modulators [SERMs]**
> Use of:
> raloxifene (Evista)
> tamoxifen (Nolvadex)
> toremifene (Fareston)

V07.52 **Use of aromatase inhibitors**
> Use of:
> anastrozole (Arimidex)
> exemestane (Aromasin)
> letrozole (Femara)

V07.59 **Use of other agents affecting estrogen receptors and estrogen levels**
> Use of:
> estrogen receptor downregulators
> fulvestrant (Faslodex)
> gonadotropin-releasing hormone (GnRH) agonist
> goserelin acetate (Zoladex)
> leuprolide acetate (leuprorelin) (Lupron)
> megestrol acetate (Megace)

V07.8 **Other specified prophylactic or treatment measure**

V07.9 **Unspecified prophylactic or treatment measure**

V08 **Asymptomatic human immunodeficiency virus [HIV] infection status**
> HIV positive NOS
> Note: This code is only to be used when no HIV infection symptoms or conditions are present. If any HIV infection symptoms or conditions are present, see code 042.

> EXCLUDES *AIDS (042)*
> *human immunodeficiency virus [HIV] disease (042)*
> *exposure to HIV (V01.79)*
> *nonspecific serologic evidence of HIV (795.71)*
> *symptomatic human immunodeficiency virus [HIV] infection (042)*

☑4ᵗʰ **V09** **Infection with drug-resistant microorganisms**
> Note: This category is intended for use as an additional code for infectious conditions classified elsewhere to indicate the presence of drug-resistance of the infectious organism.

V09.0 **Infection with microorganisms resistant to penicillins**

V09.1 **Infection with microorganisms resistant to cephalosporins and other B-lactam antibiotics**

V09.2 **Infection with microorganisms resistant to macrolides**

V09.3 **Infection with microorganisms resistant to tetracyclines**

V09.4 **Infection with microorganisms resistant to aminoglycosides**

☑5ᵗʰ **V09.5** **Infection with microorganisms resistant to quinolones and fluoroquinolones**

V09.50 **Without mention of resistance to multiple quinolones and fluoroquinoles**

V09.51 **With resistance to multiple quinolones and fluoroquinoles**

V09.6 **Infection with microorganisms resistant to sulfonamides**

✓5ᵗʰ **V09.7 Infection with microorganisms resistant to other specified antimycobacterial agents**
EXCLUDES Amikacin (V09.4)
Kanamycin (V09.4)
Streptomycin [SM] (V09.4)

V09.70 Without mention of resistance to multiple antimycobacterial agents

V09.71 With resistance to multiple antimycobacterial agents

✓5ᵗʰ **V09.8 Infection with microorganisms resistant to other specified drugs**
Vancomycin (glycopeptide) intermediate staphylococcus aureus (VISA/GISA)
Vancomycin (glycopeptide) resistant enterococcus (VRE)
Vancomycin (glycopeptide) resistant staphylococcus aureus (VRSA/GRSA)

V09.80 Without mention of resistance to multiple drugs

V09.81 With resistance to multiple drugs

✓5ᵗʰ **V09.9 Infection with drug-resistant microorganisms, unspecified**
Drug resistance, NOS

V09.90 Without mention of multiple drug resistance

V09.91 With multiple drug resistance
Multiple drug resistance NOS

PERSONS WITH POTENTIAL HEALTH HAZARDS RELATED TO PERSONAL AND FAMILY HISTORY (V10-V19)
EXCLUDES obstetric patients where the possibility that the fetus might be affected is the reason for observation or management during pregnancy (655.0-655.9)

✓4ᵗʰ **V10 Personal history of malignant neoplasm**

✓5ᵗʰ **V10.0 Gastrointestinal tract**
History of conditions classifiable to 140-159
EXCLUDES personal history of malignant carcinoid tumor (V10.91)
personal history of malignant neuroendocrine tumor (V10.91)

V10.00 Gastrointestinal tract, unspecified
V10.01 Tongue
V10.02 Other and unspecified oral cavity and pharynx
V10.03 Esophagus
V10.04 Stomach
V10.05 Large intestine
V10.06 Rectum, rectosigmoid junction, and anus
V10.07 Liver
V10.09 Other

✓5ᵗʰ **V10.1 Trachea, bronchus, and lung**
History of conditions classifiable to 162
EXCLUDES personal history of malignant carcinoid tumor (V10.91)
personal history of malignant neurondocrine tumor (V10.91)

V10.11 Bronchus and lung
V10.12 Trachea

✓5ᵗʰ **V10.2 Other respiratory and intrathoracic organs**
History of conditions classifiable to 160, 161, 163-165

V10.20 Respiratory organ, unspecified
V10.21 Larynx
V10.22 Nasal cavities, middle ear, and accessory sinuses
V10.29 Other

V10.3 Breast
History of conditions classifiable to 174 and 175

✓5ᵗʰ **V10.4 Genital organs**
History of conditions classifiable to 179-187

V10.40 Female genital organ, unspecfied
V10.41 Cervix uteri
V10.42 Other parts of uterus
V10.43 Ovary
V10.44 Other female genital organs
V10.45 Male genital organ, unspecfied
V10.46 Prostate
V10.47 Testis
V10.48 Epididymis
V10.49 Other male genital organs

✓5ᵗʰ **V10.5 Urinary organs**
History of conditions classifiable to 188 and 189
EXCLUDES personal history of malignant carcinoid tumor (V10.91)
personal history of malignant neuroendocrine tumor (V10.91)

V10.50 Urinary organ, unspecified
V10.51 Bladder
V10.52 Kidney
EXCLUDES renal pelvis (V10.53)
V10.53 Renal pelvis
V10.59 Other

✓5ᵗʰ **V10.6 Leukemia**
Conditions classifiable to 204-208
EXCLUDES leukemia in remission (204-208)

V10.60 Leukemia, unspecified
V10.61 Lymphoid leukemia
V10.62 Myeloid leukemia
V10.63 Monocytic leukemia
V10.69 Other

✓5ᵗʰ **V10.7 Other lymphatic and hematopoietic neoplasms**
Conditions classifiable to 200-203
EXCLUDES listed conditions in 200-203 in remission

V10.71 Lymphosarcoma and reticulosarcoma
V10.72 Hodgkin's disease
V10.79 Other

✓5ᵗʰ **V10.8 Personal history of malignant neoplasm of other sites**
History of conditions classifiable to 170-173, 190-195
EXCLUDES personal history of malignant carcinoid tumor (V10.91)
personal history of malignant neuroendocrine tumor (V10.91)

V10.81 Bone
V10.82 Malignant melanoma of skin
V10.83 Other malignant neoplasm of skin
V10.84 Eye
V10.85 Brain
V10.86 Other parts of the nervous system
EXCLUDES peripheral sympathetic, and parasympathetic nerves (V10.89)
V10.87 Thyroid
V10.88 Other endocrine glands and related structures
V10.89 Other

☑5ᵗʰ **V10.9** **Other and unspecified personal history of malignant neoplasm**

    V10.90 **Personal history of unspecified malignant neoplasm**
        Personal history of malignant neoplasm NOS
        EXCLUDES *personal history of malignant carcinoid tumor (V10.91)*
           personal history of malignant neuroendocrine tumor (V10.91)
           personal history of Merkel cell carcinoma (V10.91)

    V10.91 **Personal history of malignant neuroendocrine tumor**
        Personal history of malignant carcinoid tumor NOS
        Personal history of malignant neuroendocrine tumor NOS
        Personal history of Merkel cell carcinoma NOS
        Code first any continuing functional activity, such as:
           carcinoid syndrome (259.2)

☑4ᵗʰ **V11** **Personal history of mental disorder**

    V11.0 **Schizophrenia**
        EXCLUDES *that in remission (295.0-295.9 with fifth-digit 5)*

    V11.1 **Affective disorders**
        Personal history of manic-depressive psychosis
        EXCLUDES *that in remission (296.0-296.6 with fifth-digit 5, 6)*

    V11.2 **Neurosis**

    V11.3 **Alcoholism**

    V11.4 **Combat and operational stress reaction**

    V11.8 **Other mental disorders**

    V11.9 **Unspecified mental disorder**

☑4ᵗʰ **V12** **Personal history of certain other diseases**

  ☑5ᵗʰ **V12.0** **Infectious and parasitic diseases**
        EXCLUDES *personal history of infectious diseases specific to a body system*

    V12.00 **Unspecified infectious and parasitic disease**
    V12.01 **Tuberculosis**
    V12.02 **Poliomyelitis**
    V12.03 **Malaria**
    V12.04 **Methicillin resistant Staphylococcus aureus**
        MRSA
    V12.09 **Other**

    V12.1 **Nutritional deficiency**

  ☑5ᵗʰ **V12.2** **Endocrine, metabolic, and immunity disorders**
    V12.21 **Gestational diabetes**
    V12.29 **Other endocrine, metabolic, and immunity disorders**

    V12.3 **Diseases of blood and blood-forming organs**

  ☑5ᵗʰ **V12.4** **Disorders of nervous system and sense organs**
    V12.40 **Unspecified disorder of nervous system and sense organs**
    V12.41 **Benign neoplasm of the brain**
    V12.42 **Infections of the central nervous system**
        Encephalitis Meningitis
    V12.49 **Other disorders of nervous system and sense organs**

  ☑5ᵗʰ **V12.5** **Diseases of circulatory system**
        EXCLUDES *history of anaphylactic shock (V13.81)*
           old myocardial infarction (412)
           postmyocardial infarction syndrome (411.0)
    V12.50 **Unspecified circulatory disease**

    V12.51 **Venous thrombosis and embolism**
        EXCLUDES *pulmonary embolism (V12.55)*
    V12.52 **Thrombophlebitis**
    V12.53 **Sudden cardiac arrest**
        Sudden cardiac death successfully resuscitated
    V12.54 **Transient ischemic attack [TIA], and cerebral infarction without residual deficits**
        Prolonged reversible ischemic neurological deficit [PRIND]
        Reversible ischemic neurologic deficit [RIND]
        Stroke NOS without residual deficits
        EXCLUDES *history of traumatic brain injury (V15.52)*
           late effects of cerebrovascular disease (438.0-438.9)
    V12.55 **Pulmonary embolism**
    V12.59 **Other**

  ☑5ᵗʰ **V12.6** **Diseases of respiratory system**
        EXCLUDES *tuberculosis (V12.01)*
    V12.60 **Unspecified disease of respiratory system**
    V12.61 **Pneumonia (recurrent)**
    V12.69 **Other diseases of respiratory system**

  ☑5ᵗʰ **V12.7** **Diseases of digestive system**
    V12.70 **Unspecified digestive disease**
    V12.71 **Peptic ulcer disease**
    V12.72 **Colonic polyps**
    V12.79 **Other**

☑4ᵗʰ **V13** **Personal history of other diseases**

  ☑5ᵗʰ **V13.0** **Disorders of urinary system**
    V13.00 **Unspecified urinary disorder**
    V13.01 **Urinary calculi**
    V13.02 **Urinary (tract) infection**
    V13.03 **Nephrotic syndrome**
    V13.09 **Other**

    V13.1 **Trophoblastic disease**
        EXCLUDES *supervision during a current pregnancy (V23.1)*

  ☑5ᵗʰ **V13.2** **Other genital system and obstetric disorders**
        EXCLUDES *recurrent pregnancy loss (646.3)*
           without current pregnancy (629.81)
           supervision during a current pregnancy of a woman with poor obstetric history (V23.0-V23.9)
    V13.21 **Personal history of pre-term labor**
        EXCLUDES *current pregnancy with history of pre-term labor (V23.41)*
    V13.22 **Personal history of cervical dysplasia**
        Personal history of conditions classifiable to 622.10-622.12
        EXCLUDES *personal history of malignant neoplasm of cervix uteri (V10.41)*
    V13.23 **Personal history of vaginal dysplasia**
        Personal history of conditions classifiable to 623.0
        EXCLUDES *personal history of malignant neoplasm of vagina (V10.44)*
    V13.24 **Personal history of vulvar dysplasia**
        Personal history of conditions classifiable to 624.01-624.02
        EXCLUDES *personal history of malignant neoplasm of vulva (V10.44)*
    V13.29 **Other genital system and obstetric disorders**

    V13.3 **Diseases of skin and subcutaneous tissue**

    V13.4 **Arthritis**

√5ᵗʰ **V13.5 Other musculoskeletal disorders**

    V13.51 Pathologic fracture
        Healed pathologic fracture
        EXCLUDES *personal history of traumatic fracture (V15.51)*

    V13.52 Stress fracture
        Healed stress fracture
        EXCLUDES *personal history of traumatic fracture (V15.51)*

    V13.59 Other musculoskeletal disorders

√5ᵗʰ **V13.6 Congenital (corrected) malformations**

    V13.61 Personal history of (corrected) hypospadias

    V13.62 Personal history of other (corrected) congenital malformations of genitourinary system

    V13.63 Personal history of (corrected) congenital malformations of nervous system

    V13.64 Personal history of (corrected) congenital malformations of eye, ear, face and neck
        Corrected cleft lip and palate

    V13.65 Personal history of (corrected) congenital malformations of heart and circulatory system

    V13.66 Personal history of (corrected) congenital malformations of respiratory system

    V13.67 Personal history of (corrected) congenital malformations of digestive system

    V13.68 Personal history of (corrected) congenital malformations of integument, limbs, and musculoskeletal systems

    V13.69 Personal history of other (corrected) congenital malformations

V13.7 Perinatal problems
    EXCLUDES *low birth weight status (V21.30-V21.35)*

√5ᵗʰ **V13.8 Other specified diseases**

    V13.81 Anaphylaxis

    V13.89 Other specified diseases

V13.9 Unspecified disease

√4ᵗʰ **V14 Personal history of allergy to medicinal agents**

    V14.0 Penicillin

    V14.1 Other antibiotic agent

    V14.2 Sulfonamides

    V14.3 Other anti-infective agent

    V14.4 Anesthetic agent

    V14.5 Narcotic agent

    V14.6 Analgesic agent

    V14.7 Serum or vaccine

    V14.8 Other specified medicinal agents

    V14.9 Unspecified medicinal agent

√4ᵗʰ **V15 Other personal history presenting hazards to health**
    EXCLUDES *personal history of drug therapy (V87.41-V87.49)*

√5ᵗʰ **V15.0 Allergy, other than to medicinal agents**
    EXCLUDES *allergy to food substance used as base for medicinal agent (V14.0-V14.9)*

    V15.01 Allergy to peanuts

    V15.02 Allergy to milk products
        EXCLUDES *lactose intolerance (271.3)*

    V15.03 Allergy to eggs

    V15.04 Allergy to seafood
        Seafood (octopus) (squid) ink
        Shellfish

    V15.05 Allergy to other foods
        Food additives   Nuts other than peanuts

    V15.06 Allergy to insects and arachnids
        Bugs   Spiders
        Insect bites and stings

    V15.07 Allergy to latex
        Latex sensitivity

    V15.08 Allergy to radiographic dye
        Contrast media used for diagnostic x-ray procedures

    V15.09 Other allergy, other than to medicinal agents

V15.1 Surgery to heart and great vessels
    EXCLUDES *replacement by transplant or other means (V42.1-V42.2, V43.2-V43.4)*

√5ᵗʰ **V15.2 Surgery to other organs**
    EXCLUDES *replacement by transplant or other means (V42.0-V43.8)l*

    V15.21 Personal history of undergoing in utero procedure during pregnancy

    V15.22 Personal history of undergoing in utero procedure while a fetus

    V15.29 Surgery to other organs

V15.3 Irradiation
    Previous exposure to therapeutic or other ionizing radiation

√5ᵗʰ **V15.4 Psychological trauma**
    EXCLUDES *history of condition classifiable to 290-316 (V11.0-V11.9)*

    V15.41 History of physical abuse
        Rape

    V15.42 History of emotional abuse
        Neglect

    V15.49 Other

√5ᵗʰ **V15.5 Injury**

    V15.51 Traumatic fracture
        Healed traumatic fracture
        EXCLUDES *personal history of pathologic and stress fracture (V13.51, V13.52)*

    V15.52 History of traumatic brain injury
        EXCLUDES *personal history of cerebrovascular accident (cerebral infarction) without residual deficits (V12.54)*

    V15.53 Personal history of retained foreign body fully removed

    V15.59 Other injury

V15.6 Poisoning

V15.7 Contraception
    EXCLUDES *current contraceptive management (V25.0-V25.4)*
        presence of intrauterine contraceptive device as incidental finding (V45.5)

√5ᵗʰ **V15.8 Other specified personal history presenting hazards to health**
    EXCLUDES *contact with and (suspected) exposure to:*
        aromatic compounds and dyes (V87.11-V87.19)
        arsenic and other metals (V87.01-V87.09)
        molds (V87.31)

    V15.80 History of failed moderate sedation
        History of failed conscious sedation

    V15.81 Noncompliance with medical treatment
        EXCLUDES *noncompliance with renal dialysis (V45.12)*

    V15.82 History of tobacco use
        EXCLUDES *tobacco dependence (305.1)*

    V15.83 Underimmunization status
        Delinquent immunization status
        Lapsed immunization schedule status

V13.5–V15.83

V15.84 Contact with and (suspected) exposure to asbestos

V15.85 Contact with and (suspected) exposure to potentially hazardous body fluids

V15.86 Contact with and (suspected) exposure to lead

V15.87 History of extracorporeal membrane oxygenation [ECMO]

V15.88 History of fall
At risk for falling

V15.89 Other
EXCLUDES   *contact with and (suspected) exposure to other potentially hazardous:*
chemicals (V87.2)
substances (V87.39)

V15.9 Unspecified personal history presenting hazards to health

✓4ᵗʰ **V16** **Family history of malignant neoplasm**

V16.0 Gastrointestinal tract
Family history of condition classifiable to 140-159

V16.1 Trachea, bronchus, and lung
Family history of condition classifiable to 162

V16.2 Other respiratory and intrathoracic organs
Family history of condition classifiable to 160-161, 163-165

V16.3 Breast
Family history of condition classifiable to 174

✓5ᵗʰ **V16.4** Genital organs
Family history of condition classifiable to 179-187

V16.40 Genital organ, unspecified

V16.41 Ovary

V16.42 Prostate

V16.43 Testis

V16.49 Other

✓5ᵗʰ **V16.5** Urinary organs
Family history of condition classifiable to 188-189

V16.51 Kidney

V16.52 Bladder

V16.59 Other

V16.6 Leukemia
Family history of condition classifiable to 204-208

V16.7 Other lymphatic and hematopoietic neoplasms
Family history of condition classifiable to 200-203

V16.8 Other specified malignant neoplasm
Family history of other condition classifiable to 140-199

V16.9 Unspecified malignant neoplasm

✓4ᵗʰ **V17** **Family history of certain chronic disabling diseases**

V17.0 Psychiatric condition
EXCLUDES   *family history of intellectual disabilities (V18.4)*

V17.1 Stroke (cerebrovascular)

V17.2 Other neurological diseases
Epilepsy   Huntington's chorea

V17.3 Ischemic heart disease

✓5ᵗʰ **V17.4** Other cardiovascular diseases

V17.41 Family history of sudden cardiac death [SCD]
EXCLUDES   *family history of ischemic heart disease (V17.3)*
family history of myocardial infarction (V17.3)

V17.49 Family history of other cardiovascular diseases
Family history of cardiovascular disease NOS

V17.5 Asthma

V17.6 Other chronic respiratory conditions

V17.7 Arthritis

✓5ᵗʰ **V17.8** Other musculoskeletal diseases

V17.81 Osteoporosis

V17.89 Other musculoskeletal diseases

✓4ᵗʰ **V18** **Family history of certain other specific conditions**

V18.0 Diabetes mellitus

✓5ᵗʰ **V18.1** Other endocrine and metabolic diseases

V18.11 Multiple endocrine neoplasia [MEN] syndrome

V18.19 Other endocrine and metabolic diseases

V18.2 Anemia

V18.3 Other blood disorders

V18.4 Intellectual disabilities

✓5ᵗʰ **V18.5** Digestive disorders

V18.51 Colonic polyps
EXCLUDES   *family history of malignant neoplasm of gastrointestinal tract (V16.0)*

V18.59 Other digestive disorders

✓5ᵗʰ **V18.6** Kidney diseases

V18.61 Polycystic kidney

V18.69 Other kidney diseases

V18.7 Other genitourinary diseases

V18.8 Infectious and parasitic diseases

V18.9 Genetic disease carrier

✓4ᵗʰ **V19** **Family history of other conditions**

V19.0 Blindness or visual loss

✓5ᵗʰ **V19.1** Other eye disorders

V19.11 Glaucoma

V19.19 Other specified eye disorder

V19.2 Deafness or hearing loss

V19.3 Other ear disorders

V19.4 Skin conditions

V19.5 Congenital anomalies

V19.6 Allergic disorders

V19.7 Consanguinity

V19.8 Other condition

PERSONS ENCOUNTERING HEALTH SERVICES IN CIRCUMSTANCES RELATED TO REPRODUCTION AND DEVELOPMENT (V20-V29)

✓4ᵗʰ **V20** **Health supervision of infant or child**

V20.0 Foundling

V20.1 Other healthy infant or child receiving care
Medical or nursing care supervision of healthy infant in cases of:
maternal illness, physical or psychiatric
socioeconomic adverse condition at home
too many children at home preventing or interfering with normal care

V20.2 Routine infant or child health check
Developmental testing of infant or child
Health check for child over 28 days old
Immunizations appropriate for age
Routine vision and hearing testing
Use additional code(s) to identify:
special screening examination(s) performed (V73.0-V82.9)
EXCLUDES   *health check for child under 29 days old (V20.31-V20.32)*
newborn health supervision (V20.31-V20.32)
special screening for developmental handicaps (V79.3)

✓5th **V20.3 Newborn health supervision**
Health check for child under 29 days old
EXCLUDES *health check for child over 28 days old (V20.2)*

V20.31 Health supervision for newborn under 8 days old
Health check for newborn under 8 days old

V20.32 Health supervision for newborn 8 to 28 days old
Health check for newborn 8 to 28 days old
Newborn weight check

✓4th **V21 Constitutional states in development**

V21.0 Period of rapid growth in childhood

V21.1 Puberty

V21.2 Other adolecsence

✓5th **V21.3 Low birth weight status**
EXCLUDES *history of perinatal problems*

V21.30 Low birth weight status, unspecified

V21.31 Low birth weight status, less than 500 grams

V21.32 Low birth weight status, 500-999 grams

V21.33 Low birth weight status, 1000-1499 grams

V21.34 Low birth weight status, 1500-1999 grams

V21.35 Low birth weight status, 2000-2500 grams

V21.8 Other specified constitutional states in development

V21.9 Unspecified constitutional state in development

✓4th **V22 Normal pregnancy**
EXCLUDES *pregnancy examination or test, pregnancy unconfirmed (V72.40)*

V22.0 Supervision of normal first pregnancy

V22.1 Supervision of other normal pregnancy

V22.2 Pregnant state, incidental
Pregnant state NOS

✓4th **V23 Supervision of high-risk pregnancy**

V23.0 Pregnancy with history of infertility

V23.1 Pregnancy with history of trophoblastic disease
Pregnancy with history of:
hydatidiform mole
vesicular mole
EXCLUDES *that without current pregnancy (V13.1)*

V23.2 Pregnancy with history of abortion
Pregnancy with history of conditions classifiable to 634-638
EXCLUDES *recurrent pregnancy loss:*
care during pregnancy (646.3)
that without current pregnancy (629.81)

V23.3 Grand multiparity
EXCLUDES *care in relation to labor and delivery (659.4)*
that without current pregnancy (V61.5)

✓5th **V23.4 Pregnancy with other poor obstetric history**
Pregnancy with history of other conditions classifiable to 630-676

V23.41 Pregnancy with history of pre-term labor

V23.42 Pregnancy with history of ectopic pregnancy

V23.49 Pregnancy with other poor obstetric history

V23.5 Pregnancy with other poor reproductive history
Pregnancy with history of stillbirth or neonatal death

V23.7 Insufficient prenatal care
History of little or no prenatal care

✓5th **V23.8 Other high-risk pregnancy**

V23.81 Elderly primigravida
First pregnancy in a woman who will be 35 years of age or older at expected date of delivery
EXCLUDES *elderly primigravida complicating pregnancy (659.5)*

V23.82 Elderly multigravida
Second or more pregnancy in a woman who will be 35 years of age or older at expected date of delivery
EXCLUDES *elderly multigravida complicating pregnancy (659.6)*

V23.83 Young primigravida
First pregnancy in a female less than 16 years old at expected date of delivery
EXCLUDES *young primigravida complicating pregnancy (659.8)*

V23.84 Young multigravida
Second or more pregnancy in a female less than 16 years old at expected date of delivery
EXCLUDES *young multigravida complicating pregnancy (659.8)*

V23.85 Pregnancy resulting from assisted reproductive technology
Pregnancy resulting from in vitro fertilization

V23.86 Pregnancy with history of in utero procedure during previous pregnancy
EXCLUDES *management of pregnancy affected by in utero procedure during current pregnancy (679.0-679.1)*

V23.87 Pregnancy with inconclusive fetal viability
Encounter to determine fetal viability of pregnancy

V23.89 Other high-risk pregnancy

V23.9 Unspecified high-risk pregnancy

✓4th **V24 Postpartum care and examination**

V24.0 Immediately after delivery
Care and observation in uncomplicated cases

V24.1 Lactating mother
Supervision of lactation

V24.2 Routine postpartum follow-up

✓4th **V25 Encounter for contraceptive management**

✓5th **V25.0 General counseling and advice**

V25.01 Prescription of oral contraceptives

V25.02 Initiation of other contraceptive measures
Fitting of diaphragm
Prescription of foams, creams, or other agents

V25.03 Encounter for emergency contraceptive counseling and prescription
Encounter for postcoital contraceptive counseling and prescription

V25.04 Counseling and instruction in natural family planning to avoid pregnancy

V25.09 Other
Family planning advice

✓5th **V25.1 Encounter for insertion or removal of intrauterine contraceptive device**
EXCLUDES *encounter for routine checking of intrauterine contraceptive device (V25.42)*

V25.11 Encounter for insertion of intrauterine contraceptive device

V25.12 Encounter for removal of intrauterine contraceptive device

V25.13 Encounter for removal and reinsertion of intrauterine contraceptive device
Encounter for replacement of intrauterine contraceptive device

V25.2 Sterilization
Admission for interruption of fallopian tubes or vas deferens

V25.3 Menstrual extraction
Menstrual regulation

√5ᵗʰ **V25.4 Surveillance of previously prescribed contraceptive methods**
Checking, reinsertion, or removal of contraceptive device
Repeat prescription for contraceptive method
Routine examination in connection with contraceptive maintenance

V25.40 Contraceptive surveillance, unspecified

V25.41 Contraceptive pill

V25.42 Intrauterine contraceptive device
Checking of intrauterine device
EXCLUDES *insertion or removal of intrauterine contraceptive device (V25.11-V25.13)*
presence of intrauterine contraceptive device as incidental finding (V45.51)

V25.43 Implantable subdermal contraceptive

V25.49 Other contraceptive method

V25.5 Insertion of implantable subdermal contraceptive

V25.8 Other specified contraceptive management
Postvasectomy sperm count
EXCLUDES *sperm count following sterilization reversal (V26.22)*
sperm count for fertility testing (V26.21)

V25.9 Unspecified contraceptive management

√4ᵗʰ **V26 Procreative management**

V26.0 Tuboplasty or vasoplasty after previous sterilization

V26.1 Artificial insemination

√5ᵗʰ **V26.2 Investigation and testing**
EXCLUDES *postvasectomy sperm count (V25.8)*

V26.21 Fertility testing
Fallopian insufflation
Sperm count for fertility testing
EXCLUDES *genetic counseling and testing (V26.31-V26.39)*

V26.22 Aftercare following sterilization reversal
Fallopian insufflation following sterilization reversal
Sperm count following sterilization reversal

V26.29 Other investigation and testing

√5ᵗʰ **V26.3 Genetic counseling and testing**
EXCLUDES *fertility testing (V26.21)*
nonprocreative genetic screening (V82.71, V82.79)

V26.31 Testing of female for genetic disease carrier status

V26.32 Other genetic testing of female
Use additional code to identify recurrent pregnancy loss (629.81, 646.3)

V26.33 Genetic counseling

V26.34 Testing of male for genetic disease carrier status

V26.35 Encounter for testing of male partner of female with recurrent pregnancy loss

V26.39 Other genetic testing of male

√5ᵗʰ **V26.4 General counseling and advice**

V26.41 Procreative counseling and advice using natural family planning

V26.42 Encounter for fertility preservation counseling
Encounter for fertility preservation counseling prior to cancer therapy
Encounter for fertility preservation counseling prior to surgical removal of gonads

V26.49 Other procreative management, counseling and advice

√5ᵗʰ **V26.5 Sterilization status**

V26.51 Tubal ligation status
EXCLUDES *infertility not due to previous tubal ligation (628.0-628.9)*

V26.52 Vasectomy status

√5ᵗʰ **V26.8 Other specified procreative management**

V26.81 Encounter for assisted reproductive fertility procedure cycle
Patient undergoing in vitro fertilization cycle
Use additional code to identify the type of infertility
EXCLUDES *pre-cycle diagnosis and testing— code to reason for encounter*

V26.82 Encounter for fertility preservation procedure
Encounter for fertility preservation procedure prior to cancer therapy
Encounter for fertility preservation procedure prior to surgical removal of gonads

V26.89 Other specified procreative management

V26.9 Unspecified procreative management

√4ᵗʰ **V27 Outcome of delivery**
Note: This category is intended for the coding of the outcome of delivery on the mother's record.

V27.0 Single liveborn

V27.1 Single stillborn

V27.2 Twins, both liveborn

V27.3 Twins, one liveborn and one stillborn

V27.4 Twins, both stillborn

V27.5 Other multiple birth, all liveborn

V27.6 Other multiple birth, some liveborn

V27.7 Other multiple birth, all stillborn

V27.9 Unspecified outcome of delivery
Single birth ⎫
Multiple birth ⎭ outcome to infant unspecified

√4ᵗʰ **V28 Encounter for antenatal screening of mother**
EXCLUDES *abnormal findings on screening — code to findings*
routine prenatal care (V22.0-V23.9)
suspected fetal conditions affecting management of pregnancy (655.00-655.93, 656.00-656.93, 657.00-657.03, 658.00, 658.93)
suspected fetal conditions not found (V89.01-V89.09)

V28.0 Screening for chromosomal anomalies by amniocentesis

V28.1 Screening for raised alpha-fetoprotein levels in amniotic fluid

V28.2 Other screening based on amniocentesis

V28.3 Encounter for routine screening for malformation using ultrasonics
Encounter for routine fetal ultrasound NOS
EXCLUDES *encounter for fetal anatomic survey (V28.81)*
genetic counseling and testing (V26.31-V26.39)

V28.4 Screening for fetal growth retardation using ultrasonics

V28.5 Screening for isoimmunization

V28.6 Screening for Streptococcus B

√5ᵗʰ **V28.8 Other specified antenatal screening**

V28.81 Encounter for fetal anatomic survey

V28.82 Encounter for screening for risk of pre-term labor

V28.89 Other specified antenatal screening
Chorionic villus sampling
Genomic screening
Nuchal translucency testing
Proteomic screening

V28.9 Unspecified antenatal screening

© 2014 OptumInsight, Inc.

✓4ᵗʰ **V29** **Observation and evaluation of newborns and infants for suspected condition not found**

Note: This category is to be used for newborns, within the neonatal period, (the first 28 days of life) who are suspected of having an abnormal condition resulting from exposure from the mother or the birth process, but without signs or symptoms, and, which after examination and observation, is found not to exist.

EXCLUDES *suspected fetal conditions not found (V89.01-V89.09)*

V29.0 **Observation for suspected infectious condition**

V29.1 **Observation for suspected neurological condition**

V29.2 **Observation for suspected respiratory condition**

V29.3 **Observation for suspected genetic or metabolic condition**

V29.8 **Observation for other specified suspected condition**

V29.9 **Observation for unspecified suspected condition**

LIVEBORN INFANTS ACCORDING TO TYPE OF BIRTH (V30-V39)

Note: These categories are intended for the coding of liveborn infants who are consuming health care [e.g., crib or bassinet occupancy].

The following fouth-digit subdivisions are for use with categories V30-V39:

✓5ᵗʰ   0 Born in hospital
    1 Born before admission to hospital
    2 Born outside hospital and not hospitalized

The following two fifth digits are for use with the fourth-digit .0, Born in hospital:

    0 delivered without mention of cesarean delivery
    1 delivered by cesarean delivery

✓4ᵗʰ **V30** **Single liveborn**

✓4ᵗʰ **V31** **Twin, mate liveborn**

✓4ᵗʰ **V32** **Twin, mate stillborn**

✓4ᵗʰ **V33** **Twin, unspecified**

✓4ᵗʰ **V34** **Other multiple, mates all liveborn**

✓4ᵗʰ **V35** **Other multiple, mates all stillborn**

✓4ᵗʰ **V36** **Other multiple, mates live and stillborn**

✓4ᵗʰ **V37** **Other multiple, unspecified**

✓4ᵗʰ **V39** **Unspecified**

PERSONS WITH A CONDITION INFLUENCING THEIR HEALTH STATUS (V40-V49)

Note: These categories are intended for use when these conditions are recorded as "diagnoses" or "problems."

✓4ᵗʰ **V40** **Mental and behavioral problems**

V40.0 **Problems with learning**

V40.1 **Problems with communication [including speech]**

V40.2 **Other mental problems**

✓5ᵗʰ **V40.3** **Other behavioral problems**

V40.31 ***Wandering in diseases classified elsewhere***
Code first underlying disorder such as:
Alzheimer's disease (331.0)
autism or pervasive developmental disorder (299.0-299.9)
dementia, unspecified, with behavioral disturbance (294.21)
intellectual disabilities (317-319)

V40.39 **Other specified behavioral problem**

V40.9 **Unspecified mental or behavioral problem**

✓4ᵗʰ **V41** **Problems with special senses and other special functions**

V41.0 **Problems with sight**

V41.1 **Other eye problems**

V41.2 **Problems with hearing**

V41.3 **Other ear problems**

V41.4 **Problems with voice production**

V41.5 **Problems with smell and taste**

V41.6 **Problems with swallowing and mastication**

V41.7 **Problems with sexual function**
EXCLUDES *marital problems (V61.10)*
psychosexual disorders (302.0-302.9)

V41.8 **Other problems with special functions**

V41.9 **Unspecified problem with special functions**

✓4ᵗʰ **V42** **Organ or tissue replaced by transplant**
INCLUDES *homologous or heterologous (animal) (human) transplant organ status*

V42.0 **Kidney**

V42.1 **Heart**

V42.2 **Heart valve**

V42.3 **Skin**

V42.4 **Bone**

V42.5 **Cornea**

V42.6 **Lung**

V42.7 **Liver**

✓5ᵗʰ **V42.8** **Other specified organ or tissue**

V42.81 **Bone marrow**

V42.82 **Peripheral stem cells**

V42.83 **Pancreas**

V42.84 **Intestines**

V42.89 **Other**

V42.9 **Unspecified organ or tissue**

✓4ᵗʰ **V43** **Organ or tissue replaced by other means**
INCLUDES *organ or tissue assisted by other means*
replacement of organ by:
artificial device
mechanical device
prosthesis
EXCLUDES *cardiac pacemaker in situ (V45.01)*
fitting and adjustment of prosthetic device (V52.0-V52.9)
renal dialysis status (V45.11)

V43.0 **Eye globe**

V43.1 **Lens**
Pseudophakos

✓5ᵗʰ **V43.2** **Heart**

V43.21 **Heart assist device**

V43.22 **Fully implantable artificial heart**

V43.3 **Heart valve**

V43.4 **Blood vessel**

V43.5 **Bladder**

✓5ᵗʰ **V43.6** **Joint**

V43.60 **Unspecified joint**

V43.61 **Shoulder**

V43.62 **Elbow**

V43.63 **Wrist**

V43.64 **Hip**

V43.65 **Knee**

V43.66 **Ankle**

V43.69 **Other**

V43.7 **Limb**

✓5ᵗʰ **V43.8** **Other organ or tissue**

V43.81 **Larynx**

V43.82 **Breast**

V43.83 **Artificial skin**

V43.89 **Other**

✓4ᵗʰ V44 Artificial opening status

> **EXCLUDES** artificial openings requiring attention or management (V55.0-V55.9)

V44.0 Tracheostomy

V44.1 Gastrostomy

V44.2 Ileostomy

V44.3 Colostomy

V44.4 Other artificial opening of gastrointestinal tract

✓5ᵗʰ V44.5 Cystostomy

    V44.50 Cystostomy, unspecified

    V44.51 Cutaneous-vesicostomy

    V44.52 Appendico-vesicostomy

    V44.59 Other cystostomy

V44.6 Other artificial opening of urinary tract
> Nephrostomy
> Ureterostomy
> Urethrostomy

V44.7 Artificial vagina

V44.8 Other artificial opening status

V44.9 Unspecified artificial opening status

✓4ᵗʰ V45 Other postprocedural states

> **EXCLUDES** aftercare management (V51-V58.9)
> malfunction or other complication — code to condition

✓5ᵗʰ V45.0 Cardiac device in situ

> **EXCLUDES** artificial heart (V43.22)
> heart assist device (V43.21)

    V45.00 Unspecified cardiac device

    V45.01 Cardiac pacemaker
> **EXCLUDES** cardiac defibrillator with synchronous cardiac pacemaker (V45.02)

    V45.02 Automatic implantable cardiac defibrillator
> With synchronous cardiac pacemaker

    V45.09 Other specified cardiac device
> Carotid sinus pacemaker in situ

✓5ᵗʰ V45.1 Renal dialysis status

> **EXCLUDES** admission for dialysis treatment or session (V56.0)

    V45.11 Renal dialysis status
> Hemodialysis status
> Patient requiring intermittent renal dialysis
> Peritoneal dialysis status
> Presence of arterial-venous shunt (for dialysis)

    V45.12 Noncompliance with renal dialysis

V45.2 Presence of cerebrospinal fluid drainage device
> Cerebral ventricle (communicating) shunt, valve, or device in situ
> **EXCLUDES** malfunction (996.2)

V45.3 Intestinal bypass or anastomosis status
> **EXCLUDES** bariatric surgery status (V45.86)
> gastric bypass status (V45.86)
> obesity surgery status (V45.86)

V45.4 Arthrodesis status

✓5ᵗʰ V45.5 Presence of contraceptive device

    V45.51 Intrauterine contraceptive device
> **EXCLUDES** checking of device (V25.42)
> complication from device (996.32)
> insertion and removal of device (V25.11-V25.13)

    V45.52 Subdermal contraceptive implant

    V45.59 Other

✓5ᵗʰ V45.6 States following surgery of eye and adnexa

> Cataract extraction
> Filtering bleb   } state following eye surgery
> Surgical eyelid adhesion

> **EXCLUDES** aphakia (379.31)
> artificial eye globe (V43.0)

    V45.61 Cataract extraction status
> Use additional code for associated artificial lens status (V43.1)

    V45.69 Other states following surgery of eye and adnexa

✓5ᵗʰ V45.7 Acquired absence of organ

    V45.71 Acquired absence of breast and nipple
> **EXCLUDES** congenital absence of breast and nipple (757.6)

    V45.72 Acquired absence of intestine (large) (small)

    V45.73 Acquired absence of kidney

    V45.74 Other parts of urinary tract
> Bladder

    V45.75 Stomach

    V45.76 Lung

    V45.77 Genital organs
> **EXCLUDES** acquired absence of cervix and uterus (V88.01-V88.03)
> female genital mutilation status (629.20-629.29)

    V45.78 Eye

    V45.79 Other acquired absence of organ
> **EXCLUDES** acquired absence of pancreas (V88.11-V88.12)

✓5ᵗʰ V45.8 Other postprocedural status

    V45.81 Aortocoronary bypass status

    V45.82 Percutaneous transluminal coronary angioplasty status

    V45.83 Breast implant removal status

    V45.84 Dental restoration status
> Dental crowns status   Dental fillings status

    V45.85 Insulin pump status

    V45.86 Bariatric surgery status
> Gastric banding status
> Gastric bypass status for obesity
> Obesity surgery status
> **EXCLUDES** bariatric surgery status complicating pregnancy, childbirth or the puerperium (649.2)
> intestinal bypass or anastomosis status (V45.3)

    V45.87 Transplanted organ removal status
> Transplanted organ previously removed due to complication, failure, rejection or infection
> **EXCLUDES** encounter for removal of transplanted organ — code to complication of transplanted organ (996.80-996.89)

    V45.88 Status post administration of tPA (rtPA) in a different facility within the last 24 hours prior to admission to current facility
> Code first condition requiring tPA administration, such as:
> acute cerebral infarction (433.0-433.9 with fifth-digit 1, 434.0-434.9 with fifth digit 1)
> acute myocardial infarction (410.00-410.92)

    V45.89 Other
> Presence of neuropacemaker or other electronic device
> **EXCLUDES** artificial heart valve in situ (V43.3)
> vascular prosthesis in situ (V43.4)

✓4ᵗʰ **V46 Other dependence on machines and devices**

V46.0 Aspirator

✓5ᵗʰ **V46.1 Respirator [Ventilator]**
Iron lung

V46.11 Dependence on respirator, status

V46.12 Encounter for respirator dependence during power failure

V46.13 Encounter for weaning from respirator [ventilator]

V46.14 Mechanical complication of respirator [ventilator]
Mechanical failure of respirator [ventilator]

V46.2 Supplemental oxygen
Long-term oxygen therapy

V46.3 Wheelchair dependence
Wheelchair confinement status
Code first cause of dependence, such as:
muscular dystrophy (359.1)
obesity (278.00-278.03)

V46.8 Other enabling machines
Hyperbaric chamber
Possum [Patient-Operated-Selector-Mechanism]
EXCLUDES   *cardiac pacemaker (V45.0)*
kidney dialysis machine (V45.11)

V46.9 Unspecified machine dependence

✓4ᵗʰ **V47 Other problems with internal organs**

V47.0 Deficiencies of internal organs

V47.1 Mechanical and motor problems with internal organs

V47.2 Other cardiorespiratory problems
Cardiovascular exercise intolerance with pain (with):
at rest
less than ordinary activity
ordinary activity

V47.3 Other digestive problems

V47.4 Other urinary problems

V47.5 Other genital problems

V47.9 Unspecified

✓4ᵗʰ **V48 Problems with head, neck, and trunk**

V48.0 Deficiencies of head
EXCLUDES   *deficiencies of ears, eyelids, and nose (V48.8)*

V48.1 Deficiencies of neck and trunk

V48.2 Mechanical and motor problems with head

V48.3 Mechanical and motor problems with neck and trunk

V48.4 Sensory problem with head

V48.5 Sensory problem with neck and trunk

V48.6 Disfigurements of head

V48.7 Disfigurements of neck and trunk

V48.8 Other problems with head, neck, and trunk

V48.9 Unspecified problem with head, neck, or trunk

✓4ᵗʰ **V49 Other conditions influencing health status**

V49.0 Deficiencies of limbs

V49.1 Mechanical problems with limbs

V49.2 Motor problems with limbs

V49.3 Sensory problems with limbs

V49.4 Disfigurements of limbs

V49.5 Other problems of limbs

✓5ᵗʰ **V49.6 Upper limb amputation status**

V49.60 Unspecified level

V49.61 Thumb

V49.62 Other finger(s)

V49.63 Hand

V49.64 Wrist
Disarticulation of wrist

V49.65 Below elbow

V49.66 Above elbow
Disarticulation of elbow

V49.67 Shoulder
Disarticulation of shoulder

✓5ᵗʰ **V49.7 Lower limb amputation status**

V49.70 Unspecified level

V49.71 Great toe

V49.72 Other toe(s)

V49.73 Foot

V49.74 Ankle
Disarticulation of ankle

V49.75 Below knee

V49.76 Above knee
Disarticulation of knee

V49.77 Hip
Disarticulation of hip

✓5ᵗʰ **V49.8 Other specified conditions influencing health status**

V49.81 Asymptomatic postmenopausal status (age-related) (natural)
EXCLUDES   *menopausal and premenopausal*
disorder (627.0-627.9)
postsurgical menopause (256.2)
premature menopause (256.31)
symptomatic menopause
(627.0-627.9)

V49.82 Dental sealant status

V49.83 Awaiting organ transplant status

V49.84 Bed confinement status

V49.85 Dual sensory impairment
Blindness with deafness
Combined visual hearing impairment
Code first:
hearing impairment (389.00-389.9)
visual impairment (369.00-369.9)

V49.86 Do not resuscitate status

V49.87 Physical restraints status
EXCLUDES   *restraint due to a procedure – omit*
code

V49.89 Other specified conditions influencing health status

V49.9 Unspecified

PERSONS ENCOUNTERING HEALTH SERVICES FOR SPECIFIC PROCEDURES AND AFTERCARE (V50-V59)

Note: Categories V51-V59 are intended for use to indicate a reason for care in patients who may have already been treated for some disease or injury not now present, or who are receiving care to consolidate the treatment, to deal with residual states, or to prevent recurrence.
EXCLUDES   *follow-up examination for medical surveillance*
following treatment (V67.0-V67.9)

✓4ᵗʰ **V50 Elective surgery for purposes other than remedying health states**

V50.0 Hair transplant

V50.1 Other plastic surgery for unacceptable cosmetic appearance
Breast augmentation or reduction
Face-lift
EXCLUDES   *encounter for breast reduction (611.1)*
plastic surgery following healed injury or
operation (V51.0-V51.8)

V50.2 Routine or ritual circumcision
Circumcision in the absence of significant medical indication

V50.3 Ear piercing

√5ᵗʰ V50.4 Prophylactic organ removal
> EXCLUDES   organ donations (V59.0-V59.9)
> therapeutic organ removal — code to condition

    V50.41 Breast

    V50.42 Ovary

    V50.49 Other

V50.8 Other

V50.9 Unspecified

√4ᵗʰ V51 Aftercare involving the use of plastic surgery
Plastic surgery following healed injury or operation
> EXCLUDES   cosmetic plastic surgery (V50.1)
> plastic surgery as treatment for current condtion or injury — code to condition or injury
> repair of scarred tissue — code to scar

V51.0 Encounter for breast reconstruction following mastectomy
> EXCLUDES   deformity and disproportion of reconstructed breast (612.0-612.1)

V51.8 Other aftercare involving the use of plastic surgery

√4ᵗʰ V52 Fitting and adjustment of prosthetic device and implant
> INCLUDES   removal of device
> EXCLUDES   malfunction or complication of prosthetic device (996.0-996.7)
> status only, without need for care (V43.0-V43.8)

V52.0 Artificial arm (complete) (partial)

V52.1 Artificial leg (complete) (partial)

V52.2 Artificial eye

V52.3 Dental prosthetic device

V52.4 Breast prosthesis and implant
Elective implant exchange (different material) (different size)
Removal of tissue expander without synchronous insertion of permanent implant
> EXCLUDES   admission for initial breast implant insertion for breast augmentation (V50.1)
> complications of breast implant (996.54, 996.69, 996.79)
> encounter for breast reconstruction following mastectomy (V51.0)

V52.8 Other specified prosthetic device

V52.9 Unspecified prosthetic device

√4ᵗʰ V53 Fitting and adjustment of other device
> INCLUDES   removal of device
> replacement of device
> EXCLUDES   status only, without need for care (V45.0-V45.8)

√5ᵗʰ V53.0 Devices related to nervous system and special senses

    V53.01 Fitting and adjustment of cerebral ventricular (communicating) shunt

    V53.02 Neuropacemaker (brain) (peripheral nerve) (spinal cord)

    V53.09 Fitting and adjustment of other devices related to nervous system and special senses
        Auditory substitution device
        Visual substitution device

V53.1 Spectacles and contact lenses

V53.2 Hearing aid

√5ᵗʰ V53.3 Cardiac device
Reprogramming

    V53.31 Cardiac pacemaker
> EXCLUDES   automatic implantable cardiac defibrillator with synchronous cardiac pacemaker (V53.32)
> mechanical complication of cardiac pacemaker (996.01)

    V53.32 Automatic implantable cardiac defibrillator
        With synchronous cardiac pacemaker

    V53.39 Other cardiac device

V53.4 Orthodontic devices

√5ᵗʰ V53.5 Other gastrointestinal appliance and device
> EXCLUDES   colostomy (V55.3)
> ileostomy (V55.2)
> other artificial opening of digestive tract (V55.4)

    V53.50 Fitting and adjustment of intestinal appliance and device

    V53.51 Fitting and adjustment of gastric lap band

    V53.59 Fitting and adjustment of other gastrointestinal appliance and device

V53.6 Urinary devices
Urinary catheter
> EXCLUDES   cystostomy (V55.5)
> nephrostomy (V55.6)
> ureterostomy (V55.6)
> urethrostomy (V55.6)

V53.7 Orthopedic devices
Orthopedic: Orthopedic:
  brace   corset
  cast   shoes
> EXCLUDES   other orthopedic aftercare (V54)

V53.8 Wheelchair

√5ᵗʰ V53.9 Other and unspecified device

    V53.90 Unspecified device

    V53.91 Fitting and adjustment of insulin pump
        Insulin pump titration

    V53.99 Other device

√4ᵗʰ V54 Other orthopedic aftercare
> EXCLUDES   fitting and adjustment of orthopedic devices (V53.7)
> malfunction of internal orthopedic device (996.40-996.49)
> other complication of nonmechanical nature (996.60-996.79)

√5ᵗʰ V54.0 Aftercare involving internal fixation device
> EXCLUDES   malfunction of internal orthopedic device (996.40-996.49)
> other complication of nonmechanical nature (996.60-996.79)
> removal of external fixation device (V54.89)

    V54.01 Encounter for removal of internal fixation device

    V54.02 Encounter for lengthening/adjustment of growth rod

    V54.09 Other aftercare involving internal fixation device

√5ᵗʰ V54.1 Aftercare for healing traumatic fracture
> EXCLUDES   aftercare following joint replacement (V54.81)
> aftercare for amputation stump (V54.89)

    V54.10 Aftercare for healing traumatic fracture of arm, unspecified

    V54.11 Aftercare for healing traumatic fracture of upper arm

    V54.12 Aftercare for healing traumatic fracture of lower arm

    V54.13 Aftercare for healing traumatic fracture of hip

    V54.14 Aftercare for healing traumatic fracture of leg, unspecified

    V54.15 Aftercare for healing traumatic fracture of upper leg
> EXCLUDES   aftercare for healing traumatic fracture of hip (V54.13)

    V54.16 Aftercare for healing traumatic fracture of lower leg

V54.17 Aftercare for healing traumatic fracture of vertebrae

V54.19 Aftercare for healing traumatic fracture of other bone

√5ᵗʰ **V54.2 Aftercare for healing pathologic fracture**
> EXCLUDES   aftercare following joint replacement (V54.81)

V54.20 Aftercare for healing pathologic fracture of arm, unspecified

V54.21 Aftercare for healing pathologic fracture of upper arm

V54.22 Aftercare for healing pathologic fracture of lower arm

V54.23 Aftercare for healing pathologic fracture of hip

V54.24 Aftercare for healing pathologic fracture of leg, unspecified

V54.25 Aftercare for healing pathologic fracture of upper leg
> EXCLUDES   aftercare for healing pathologic fracture of hip (V54.23)

V54.26 Aftercare for healing pathologic fracture of lower leg

V54.27 Aftercare for healing pathologic fracture of vertebrae

V54.29 Aftercare for healing pathologic fracture of other bone

√5ᵗʰ **V54.8 Other orthopedic aftercare**

V54.81 Aftercare following joint replacement
Use additional code to identify joint replacement site (V43.60-V43.69)

V54.82 Aftercare following explantation of joint prosthesis
Aftercare following explantation of joint prosthesis, staged procedure
Encounter for joint prosthesis insertion following prior explantation of joint prosthesis

V54.89 Other orthopedic aftercare
Aftercare for healing fracture NOS

V54.9 Unspecified orthopedic aftercare

√4ᵗʰ **V55 Attention to artificial openings**
> INCLUDES   adjustment or repositioning of catheter
> closure
> passage of sounds or bougies
> reforming
> removal or replacement of catheter
> toilet or cleansing
> EXCLUDES   complications of external stoma (519.00-519.09, 569.60-569.69, 596.81-596.83, 997.49)
> status only, without need for care (V44.0-V44.9)

V55.0 Tracheostomy

V55.1 Gastrostomy

V55.2 Ileostomy

V55.3 Colostomy

V55.4 Other artificial opening of digestive tract

V55.5 Cystostomy

V55.6 Other artificial opening of urinary tract
Nephrostomy   Urethrostomy
Ureterostomy

V55.7 Artificial vagina

V55.8 Other specified artificial opening

V55.9 Unspecified artificial opening

√4ᵗʰ **V56 Encounter for dialysis and dialysis catheter care**
Use additional code to identify the associated condition
> EXCLUDES   dialysis preparation — code to condition

V56.0 Extracorporeal dialysis
Dialysis (renal) NOS
> EXCLUDES   dialysis status (V45.11)

V56.1 Fitting and adjustment of extracorporeal dialysis catheter
Removal or replacement of catheter
Toilet or cleansing
Use additional code for any concurrent extracorporeal dialysis (V56.0)

V56.2 Fitting and adjustment of peritoneal dialysis catheter
Use additional code for any concurrent peritoneal dialysis (V56.8)   c

V56.3 Encounter for adequacy testing for dialysis

V56.31 Encounter for adequacy testing for hemodialysis

V56.32 Encounter for adequacy testing for peritoneal dialysis
Peritoneal equilibration test

(handwritten: 996.1)

V56.8 Other dialysis
Peritoneal dialysis

√4ᵗʰ **V57 Care involving use of rehabilitation procedures**
Use additional code to identify underlying condition

V57.0 Breathing exercises

V57.1 Other physical therapy
Therapeutic and remedial exercises, except breathing

√5ᵗʰ **V57.2 Occupational therapy and vocational rehabilitation**

V57.21 Encounter for occupational therapy

V57.22 Encounter for vocational therapy

V57.3 Speech-language therapy

V57.4 Orthoptic training

√5ᵗʰ **V57.8 Other specified rehabilitation procedure**

V57.81 Orthotic training
Gait training in the use of artificial limbs

V57.89 Other
Multiple training or therapy

V57.9 Unspecified rehabilitation procedure

√4ᵗʰ **V58 Encounter for other and unspecified procedures and aftercare**
> EXCLUDES   convalescence and palliative care (V66)

V58.0 Radiotherapy
Encounter or admission for radiotherapy
> EXCLUDES   encounter for radioactive implant — code to condition
> radioactive iodine therapy — code to condition

√5ᵗʰ **V58.1 Encounter for antineoplastic chemotherapy and immunotherapy**
Encounter or admission for chemotherapy
> EXCLUDES   chemotherapy and immunotherapy for nonneoplastic conditions — code to condition

V58.11 Encounter for antineoplastic chemotherapy

V58.12 Encounter for antineoplastic immunotherapy

V58.2 Blood transfusion, without reported diagnosis

√5ᵗʰ **V58.3 Attention to dressings and sutures**
Change or removal of wound packing
> EXCLUDES   attention to drains (V58.49)
> planned postoperative wound closure (V58.41)

V58.30 Encounter for change or removal of nonsurgical wound dressing
Encounter for change or removal of wound dressing NOS

V58.31 Encounter for change or removal of surgical wound dressing

V58.32 Encounter for removal of sutures
Encounter for removal of staples

✓5ᵗʰ **V58.4 Other aftercare following surgery**
Note: Codes from this subcategory should be used in conjunction with other aftercare codes to fully identify the reason for the aftercare encounter
EXCLUDES aftercare following sterilization reversal surgery (V26.22)
attention to artificial openings (V55.0-V55.9)
orthopedic aftercare (V54.0-V54.9)

V58.41 Encounter for planned postoperative wound closure
EXCLUDES disruption of operative wound (998.31-998.32)
encounter for dressings and suture aftercare (V58.30-V58.32)

V58.42 Aftercare following surgery for neoplasm
Conditions classifiable to 140-239

V58.43 Aftercare following surgery for injury and trauma
Conditions classifiable to 800-999
EXCLUDES aftercare for healing traumatic fracture (V54.10-V54.19)

V58.44 Aftercare following organ transplant
Use additional code to identify the organ transplanted (V42.0-V42.9)

V58.49 Other specified aftercare following surgery
Change or removal of drains

V58.5 Orthodontics
EXCLUDES fitting and adjustment of orthodontic device (V53.4)

✓5ᵗʰ **V58.6 Long-term (current) drug use**
Long-term (current) prophylactic drug use
EXCLUDES drug abuse and dependence complicating pregnancy (648.3-648.4)
drug abuse (305.00-305.93)
drug dependence (304.00-304.93)
hormone replacement therapy (postmenopausal) (V07.4)
use of agents affecting estrogen receptors and estrogen levels (V07.51-V07.59)

V58.61 Long-term (current) use of anticoagulants
EXCLUDES long-term (current) use of aspirin (V58.66)

V58.62 Long-term (current) use of antibiotics

V58.63 Long-term (current) use of antiplatelets/antithrombotics
EXCLUDES long-term (current) use of aspirin (V58.66)

V58.64 Long-term (current) use of non-steroidal anti-inflammatories (NSAID)
EXCLUDES long-term (current) use of aspirin (V58.66)

V58.65 Long-term (current) use of steroids

V58.66 Long-term (current) use of aspirin

V58.67 Long-term (current) use of insulin

V58.68 Long term (current) use of bisphosphonates

V58.69 Long-term (current) use of other medications
Other high-risk medications
Long term current use of methadone for pain control
Long term current use of opiate analgesic
EXCLUDES methadone maintenance NOS (304.00)
methadone use NOS (304.00)

✓5ᵗʰ **V58.7 Aftercare following surgery to specified body systems, not elsewhere classified**
Note: Codes from this subcategory should be used in conjunction with other aftercare codes to fully identify the reason for the aftercare encounter
EXCLUDES aftercare following organ transplant (V58.44)
aftercare following surgery for neoplasm (V58.42)

V58.71 Aftercare following surgery of the sense organs, NEC
Conditions classifiable to 360-379, 380-389

V58.72 Aftercare following surgery of the nervous system, NEC
Conditions classifiable to 320-359
EXCLUDES aftercare following surgery of the sense organs, NEC (V58.71)

V58.73 Aftercare following surgery of the circulatory system, NEC
Conditions classifiable to 390-459

V58.74 Aftercare following surgery of the respiratory system, NEC
Conditions classifiable to 460-519

V58.75 Aftercare following surgery of the teeth, oral cavity and digestive system, NEC
Conditions classifiable to 520-579

V58.76 Aftercare following surgery of the genitourinary system, NEC
Conditions classifiable to 580-629
EXCLUDES aftercare following sterilization reversal (V26.22)

V58.77 Aftercare following surgery of the skin and subcutaneous tissue, NEC
Conditions classifiable to 680-709

V58.78 Aftercare following surgery of the musculoskeletal system, NEC
Conditions classifiable to 710-739
EXCLUDES orthopedic aftercare (V54.01-V54.9)

✓5ᵗʰ **V58.8 Other specified procedures and aftercare**

V58.81 Fitting and adjustment of vascular catheter
Removal or replacement of catheter
Toilet or cleansing
EXCLUDES complication of renal dialysis (996.73)
complication of vascular catheter (996.74)
dialysis preparation — code to condition
encounter for dialysis (V56.0-V56.8)
fitting and adjustment of dialysis catheter (V56.1)

V58.82 Fitting and adjustment of nonvascular catheter, NEC
Removal or replacement of catheter
Toilet or cleansing
EXCLUDES fitting and adjustment of peritoneal dialysis catheter (V56.2)
fitting and adjustment of urinary catheter (V53.6)

V58.83 Encounter for therapeutic drug monitoring
Use additional code for any associated long-term (current) drug use (V58.61-V58.69)
EXCLUDES blood-drug testing for medicolegal reasons (V70.4)
DEF: Drug monitoring: Measurement of the level of a specific drug in the body or measurement of a specific function to assess effectiveness of a drug.

V58.89 Other specified aftercare

V58.9 Unspecified aftercare

✓4ᵗʰ **V59 Donors**
> **EXCLUDES** *examination of potential donor (V70.8)*
> *self-donation of organ or tissue — code to condition*

✓5ᵗʰ **V59.0 Blood**

   V59.01 Whole blood

   V59.02 Stem cells

   V59.09 Other

V59.1 Skin

V59.2 Bone

V59.3 Bone marrow

V59.4 Kidney

V59.5 Cornea

V59.6 Liver

✓5ᵗʰ **V59.7 Egg (oocyte) (ovum)**

   V59.70 Egg (oocyte) (ovum) donor, unspecified

   V59.71 Egg (oocyte) (ovum) donor, under age 35, anonymous recipient
   > Egg donor, under age 35 NOS

   V59.72 Egg (oocyte) (ovum) donor, under age 35, designated recipient

   V59.73 Egg (oocyte) (ovum) donor, age 35 and over, anonymous recipient
   > Egg donor, age 35 and over NOS

   V59.74 Egg (oocyte) (ovum) donor, age 35 and over, designated recipient

V59.8 Other specified organ or tissue

V59.9 Unspecified organ or tissue

PERSONS ENCOUNTERING HEALTH SERVICES IN OTHER CIRCUMSTANCES (V60-V69)

✓4ᵗʰ **V60 Housing, household, and economic circumstances**

V60.0 Lack of housing
> Hobos
> Social migrants
> Tramps
> Transients
> Vagabonds

V60.1 Inadequate housing
> Lack of heating
> Restriction of space
> Technical defects in home preventing adequate care

V60.2 Inadequate material resources
> Economic problem
> Poverty NOS

V60.3 Person living alone

V60.4 No other household member able to render care
> Person requiring care (has) (is):
>   family member too handicapped, ill, or otherwise unsuited to render care
>   partner temporarily away from home
>   temporarily away from usual place of abode
> **EXCLUDES** *holiday relief care (V60.5)*

V60.5 Holiday relief care
> Provision of health care facilities to a person normally cared for at home, to enable relatives to take a vacation

V60.6 Person living in residential institution
> Boarding school resident

✓5ᵗʰ **V60.8 Other specified housing or economic circumstances**

   V60.81 Foster care (status)

   V60.89 Other specified housing or economic circumstances

V60.9 Unspecified housing or economic circumstance

✓4ᵗʰ **V61 Other family circumstances**
> **INCLUDES** when these circumstances or fear of them, affecting the person directly involved or others, are mentioned as the reason, justified or not, for seeking or receiving medical advice or care

✓5ᵗʰ **V61.0 Family disruption**

   V61.01 Family disruption due to family member on military deployment
   > Individual or family affected by other family member being on deployment
   > **EXCLUDES** *family disruption due to family member on non-military extended absence from home (V61.08)*

   V61.02 Family disruption due to return of family member from military deployment
   > Individual or family affected by other family member having returned from deployment (current or past conflict)

   V61.03 Family disruption due to divorce or legal separation

   V61.04 Family disruption due to parent-child estrangement
   > **EXCLUDES** *other family estrangement (V61.09)*

   V61.05 Family disruption due to child in welfare custody

   V61.06 Family disruption due to child in foster care or in care of non-parental family member

   V61.07 Family disruption due to death of family member
   > **EXCLUDES** *bereavement (V62.82)*

   V61.08 Family disruption due to other extended absence of family member
   > **EXCLUDES** *family disruption due to family member on military deployment (V61.01)*

   V61.09 Other family disruption
   > Family estrangement NOS

✓5ᵗʰ **V61.1 Counseling for marital and partner problems**
> **EXCLUDES** *problems related to:*
>   *psychosexual disorders (302.0-302.9)*
>   *sexual function (V41.7)*

   V61.10 Counseling for marital and partner problems, unspecified
   > Marital conflict
   > Marital relationship problem
   > Partner conflict
   > Partner relationship problem

   V61.11 Counseling for victim of spousal and partner abuse
   > **EXCLUDES** *encounter for treatment of current injuries due to abuse (995.80-995.85)*

   V61.12 Counseling for perpetrator of spousal and partner abuse

✓5ᵗʰ **V61.2 Parent-child problems**

   V61.20 Counseling for parent-child problem, unspecified
   > Concern about behavior of child
   > Parent-child conflict
   > Parent-child relationship problem

   V61.21 Counseling for victim of child abuse
   > Child battering
   > Child neglect
   > **EXCLUDES** *current injuries due to abuse (995.50-995.59)*

   V61.22 Counseling for perpetrator of parental child abuse
   > **EXCLUDES** *counseling for non-parental abuser (V62.83)*

V61.23 Counseling for parent-biological child problem
Concern about behavior of biological child
Parent-biological child conflict
Parent-biological child relationship problem

V61.24 Counseling for parent-adopted child problem
Concern about behavior of adopted child
Parent-adopted child conflict
Parent-adopted child relationship problem

V61.25 Counseling for parent (guardian)-foster child problem
Concern about behavior of foster child
Parent (guardian)-foster child conflict
Parent (guardian)-foster child relationship problem

V61.29 Other parent-child problems

V61.3 Problems with aged parents or in-laws

✓5ᵗʰ **V61.4 Health problems within family**

V61.41 Alcoholism in family

V61.42 Substance abuse in family

V61.49 Other
Care of ⎫ sick or handicapped person
Presence of ⎭ in family or household

V61.5 Multiparity

V61.6 Illegitimacy or illegitimate pregnancy

V61.7 Other unwanted pregnancy

V61.8 Other specified family circumstances
Problems with family members NEC
Sibling relationship problem

V61.9 Unspecified family circumstance

✓4ᵗʰ **V62 Other psychosocial circumstances**
INCLUDES those circumstances or fear of them, affecting the person directly involved or others, mentioned as the reason, justified or not, for seeking or receiving medical advice or care
EXCLUDES previous psychological trauma (V15.41-V15.49)

V62.0 Unemployment
EXCLUDES circumstances when main problem is economic inadequacy or poverty (V60.2)

V62.1 Adverse effects of work environment

✓5ᵗʰ **V62.2 Other occupational circumstances or maladjustment**

V62.21 Personal current military deployment status
Individual (civilian or military) currently deployed in theater or in support of military war, peacekeeping and humanitarian operations

V62.22 Personal history of return from military deployment
Individual (civilian or military) with past history of military war, peacekeeping and humanitarian deployment (current or past conflict)

V62.29 Other occupational circumstances or maladjustment
Career choice problem
Dissatisfaction with employment
Occupational problem

V62.3 Educational circumstances
Academic problem
Dissatisfaction with school environment
Educational handicap

V62.4 Social maladjustment
Acculturation problem
Cultural deprivation
Political, religious, or sex discrimination
Social:
isolation
persecution

V62.5 Legal circumstances
Imprisonment   Litigation
Legal investigation   Prosecution

V62.6 Refusal of treatment for reasons of religion or conscience

✓5ᵗʰ **V62.8 Other psychological or physical stress, not elsewhere classified**

V62.81 Interpersonal problems, not elsewhere classified
Relational problem NOS

V62.82 Bereavement, uncomplicated
EXCLUDES family disruption due to death of family member (V61.07)

V62.83 Counseling for perpetrator of physical/sexual abuse
EXCLUDES counseling for perpetrator of parental child abuse (V61.22)
counseling for perpetrator of spousal and partner abuse (V61.12)

V62.84 Suicidal ideation
EXCLUDES suicidal tendencies (300.9)
DEF: Thoughts of committing suicide; no actual attempt of suicide has been made.

V62.85 Homicidal ideation

V62.89 Other
Borderline intellectual functioning
Life circumstance problems
Phase of life problems
Religious or spiritual problem

V62.9 Unspecified psychosocial circumstance

✓4ᵗʰ **V63 Unavailability of other medical facilities for care**

V63.0 Residence remote from hospital or other health care facility

V63.1 Medical services in home not available
EXCLUDES no other household member able to render care (V60.4)

V63.2 Person awaiting admission to adequate facility elsewhere

V63.8 Other specified reasons for unavailability of medical facilities
Person on waiting list undergoing social agency investigation

V63.9 Unspecified reason for unavailability of medical facilities

✓4ᵗʰ **V64 Persons encountering health services for specific procedures, not carried out**

✓5ᵗʰ **V64.0 Vaccination not carried out**

V64.00 Vaccination not carried out, unspecified reason

V64.01 Vaccination not carried out because of acute illness

V64.02 Vaccination not carried out because of chronic illness or condition

V64.03 Vaccination not carried out because of immune compromised state

V64.04 Vaccination not carried out because of allergy to vaccine or component

V64.05 Vaccination not carried out because of caregiver refusal
Guardian refusal   Parent refusal
EXCLUDES vaccination not carried out because of caregiver refusal for religious reasons (V64.07)

V64.06 Vaccination not carried out because of patient refusal

V64.07 Vaccination not carried out for religious reasons

V64.08   Vaccination not carried out because patient had disease being vaccinated against

V64.09   Vaccination not carried out for other reason

V64.1   Surgical or other procedure not carried out because of contraindication

V64.2   Surgical or other procedure not carried out because of patient's decision

V64.3   Procedure not carried out for other reasons

√5ᵗʰ **V64.4**   Closed surgical procedure converted to open procedure

V64.41   Laparoscopic surgical procedure converted to open procedure

V64.42   Thoracoscopic surgical procedure converted to open procedure

V64.43   Arthroscopic surgical procedure converted to open procedure

√4ᵗʰ **V65**   **Other persons seeking consultation**

V65.0   Healthy person accompanying sick person
Boarder

√5ᵗʰ **V65.1**   Person consulting on behalf of another person
Advice or treatment for nottending third party
> EXCLUDES   *concern (normal) about sick person in family (V61.41-V61.49)*

V65.11   Pediatric pre-birth visit for expectant parent(s)
Pre-adoption visit for adoptive parent(s)

V65.19   Other person consulting on behalf of another person

V65.2   Person feigning illness
Malingerer
Peregrinating patient

V65.3   Dietary surveillance and counseling
Dietary surveillance and counseling (in):
NOS
colitis
diabetes mellitus
food allergies or intolerance
gastritis
hypercholesterolemia
hypoglycemia
obesity
Use additional code to identify Body Mass Index (BMI), if known (V85.0-V85.54)

√5ᵗʰ **V65.4**   Other counseling, not elsewhere classified
Health: Health:
advice   instruction
education
> EXCLUDES   *counseling (for):*
> *contraception (V25.40-V25.49)*
> *genetic (V26.31-V26.39)*
> *on behalf of third party (V65.11-V65.19)*
> *procreative management (V26.41-V26.49)*

V65.40   Counseling NOS

V65.41   Exercise counseling

V65.42   Counseling on substance use and abuse

V65.43   Counseling on injury prevention

V65.44   Human immunodeficiency virus [HIV] counseling

V65.45   Counseling on other sexually transmitted diseases

V65.46   Encounter for insulin pump training

V65.49   Other specified counseling

V65.5   Person with feared complaint in whom no diagnosis was made
Feared condition not demonstrated
Problem was normal state
"Worried well"

V65.8   Other reasons for seeking consultation
> EXCLUDES   *specified symptoms*

V65.9   Unspecified reason for consultation

√4ᵗʰ **V66**   **Convalescence and palliative care**

V66.0   Following surgery

V66.1   Following radiotherapy

V66.2   Following chemotherapy

V66.3   Following psychotherapy and other treatment for mental disorder

V66.4   Following treatment of fracture

V66.5   Following other treatment

V66.6   Following combined treatment

V66.7   Encounter for palliative care
End of life care   Terminal care
Hospice care
Code first underlying disease

V66.9   Unspecified convalescence

√4ᵗʰ **V67**   **Follow-up examination**
> INCLUDES   surveillance only following completed treatment
> EXCLUDES   *surveillance of contraception (V25.40-V25.49)*

√5ᵗʰ **V67.0**   Following surgery

V67.00   Following surgery, unspecified

V67.01   Follow-up vaginal pap smear
Vaginal pap-smear, status-post hysterectomy for malignant condition
Use additional code to identify:
acquired absence of uterus (V88.01-V88.03)
personal history of malignant neoplasm (V10.40-V10.44)
> EXCLUDES   *vaginal pap smear status-post hysterectomy for non-malignant condition (V76.47)*

V67.09   Following other surgery
> EXCLUDES   *sperm count following sterilization reversal (V26.22)*
> *sperm count for fertility testing (V26.21)*

V67.1   Following radiotherapy

V67.2   Following chemotherapy
Cancer chemotherapy follow-up

V67.3   Following psychotherapy and other treatment for mental disorder

V67.4   Following treatment of healed fracture
> EXCLUDES   *current (healing) fracture aftercare (V54.0-V54.9)*

√5ᵗʰ **V67.5**   Following other treatment

V67.51   Following completed treatment with high-risk medications, not elsewhere classified
> EXCLUDES   *long-term (current) drug use (V58.61-V58.69)*

V67.59   Other

V67.6   Following combined treatment

V67.9   Unspecified follow-up examination

√4ᵗʰ **V68**   **Encounters for administrative purposes**

√5ᵗʰ **V68.0**   Issue of medical certificates
> EXCLUDES   *encounter for general medical examination (V70.0-V70.9)*

V68.01   Disability examination
Use additional code(s) to identify specific examination(s), screening and testing performed (V72.0-V82.9)

V68.09   Other issue of medical certificates

V68.1 Issue of repeat prescriptions
Issue of repeat prescription for:
appliance
glasses
medications
EXCLUDES *repeat prescription for contraceptives (V25.41-V25.49)*

V68.2 Request for expert evidence

√5ᵗʰ **V68.8 Other specified administrative purpose**

V68.81 Referral of patient without examination or treatment

V68.89 Other

V68.9 Unspecified administrative purpose

√4ᵗʰ **V69 Problems related to lifestyle**

V69.0 Lack of physical exercise

V69.1 Inappropriate diet and eating habits
EXCLUDES *anorexia nervosa (307.1)*
bulimia (783.6)
malnutrition and other nutritional deficiencies (260-269.9)
other and unspecified eating disorders (307.50-307.59)

V69.2 High-risk sexual behavior

V69.3 Gambling and betting
EXCLUDES *pathological gambling (312.31)*

V69.4 Lack of adequate sleep
Sleep deprivation
EXCLUDES *insomnia (780.52)*

V69.5 Behavioral insomnia of childhood
DEF: Behaviors on the part of the child or caregivers that cause negative compliance with a child's sleep schedule; results in lack of adequate sleep.

V69.8 Other problems related to lifestyle
Self-damaging behavior

V69.9 Problem related to lifestyle, unspecified

PERSONS WITHOUT REPORTED DIAGNOSIS ENCOUNTERED DURING EXAMINATION AND INVESTIGATION OF INDIVIDUALS AND POPULATIONS (V70-V82)

Note: Nonspecific abnormal findings disclosed at the time of these examinations are classifiable to categories 790-796.

√4ᵗʰ **V70 General medical examination**
Use additional code(s) to identify any special screening examination(s) performed (V73.0-V82.9)

V70.0 Routine general medical examination at a health care facility
Health checkup
EXCLUDES *health checkup of infant or child over 28 days old (V20.2)*
health supervision of newborn 8 to 28 days old (V20.32)
health supervision of newborn under 8 days old (V20.31)
pre-procedural general physical examination (V72.83)

V70.1 General psychiatric examination, requested by the authority

V70.2 General psychiatric examination, other and unspecified

V70.3 Other medical examination for administrative purposes
General medical examination for:
admission to old age home
adoption
camp
driving license
immigration and naturalization
insurance certification
marriage
prison
school admission
sports competition
EXCLUDES *attendance for issue of medical certificates (V68.0)*
pre-employment screening (V70.5)

V70.4 Examination for medicolegal reasons
Blood-alcohol tests   Paternity testing
Blood-drug tests
EXCLUDES *examination and observation following:*
accidents (V71.3, V71.4)
assault (V71.6)
rape (V71.5)

V70.5 Health examination of defined subpopulations
Armed forces personnel
Inhabitants of institutions
Occupational healthexaminations
Pre-employment screening
Preschool children
Prisoners
Prostitutes
Refugees
School children
Students

V70.6 Health examination in population surveys
EXCLUDES *special screening (V73.0-V82.9)*

V70.7 Examination of participant in clinical trial
Examination of participant or control in clinical research

V70.8 Other specified general medical examinations
Examination of potential donor of organ or tissue

V70.9 Unspecified general medical examination

√4ᵗʰ **V71 Observation and evaluation for suspected conditions not found**
INCLUDES This category is to be used when persons without a diagnosis are suspected of having an abnormal condition, without signs or symptoms, which requires study, but after examination and observation, is found not to exist. This category is also for use for administrative and legal observation status.
EXCLUDES *suspected maternal and fetal conditions not found (V89.01-V89.09)*

√5ᵗʰ **V71.0 Observation for suspected mental condition**

V71.01 Adult antisocial behavior
Dyssocial behavior or gang activity in adult without manifest psychiatric disorder

V71.02 Childhood or adolescent antisocial behavior
Dyssocial behavior or gang activity in child or adolescent without manifest psychiatric disorder

V71.09 Other suspected mental condition

V71.1 Observation for suspected malignant neoplasm

V71.2 Observation for suspected tuberculosis

V71.3 Observation following accident at work

V71.4 Observation following other accident
Examination of individual involved in motor vehicle traffic accident

V71.5 Observation following alleged rape or seduction
Examination of victim or culprit

V71.6 Observation following other inflicted injury
Examination of victim or culprit

V71.7 Observation for suspected cardiovascular disease

☑5ᵗʰ **V71.8 Observation and evaluation for other specified suspected conditions**
EXCLUDES contact with and (suspected) exposure to (potentially) hazardous substances (V15.84-V15.86, V87.0-V87.31)

V71.81 Abuse and neglect
EXCLUDES adult abuse and neglect (995.80-995.85)
child abuse and neglect (995.50-995.59)

V71.82 Observation and evaluation for suspected exposure to anthrax

V71.83 Observation and evaluation for suspected exposure to other biological agent

V71.89 Other specified suspected conditions

V71.9 Observation for unspecified suspected condition

☑4ᵗʰ **V72 Special investigations and examinations**
INCLUDES routine examination of specific system
Use additional code(s) to identify any special screening examination(s) performed (V73.0-V82.9)
EXCLUDES general medical examination (V70.0-V70.4)
general screening examination of defined population groups (V70.5, V70.6, V70.7)
health supervision of newborn 8 to 28 days old (V20.32)
health supervision of newborn under 8 days old (V20.31)
routine examination of infant or child over 28 days old (V20.2)

V72.0 Examination of eyes and vision

☑5ᵗʰ **V72.1 Examination of ears and hearing**
V72.11 Encounter for hearing examination following failed hearing screening
V72.12 Encounter for hearing conservation and treatment
V72.19 Other examination of ears and hearing

V72.2 Dental examination

☑5ᵗʰ **V72.3 Gynecological examination**
EXCLUDES cervical Papanicolaou smear without general gynecological examination (V76.2)
routine examination in contraceptive management (V25.40-V25.49)
V72.31 Routine gynecological examination
General gynecological examination with or without Papanicolaou cervical smear
Pelvic examination (annual) (periodic)
Use additional code to identify:
human papillomavirus (HPV) screening (V73.81)
routine vaginal Papanicolaou smear (V76.47)
V72.32 Encounter for Papanicolaou cervical smear to confirm findings of recent normal smear following initial abnormal smear

☑5ᵗʰ **V72.4 Pregnancy examination or test**
V72.40 Pregnancy examination or test, pregnancy unconfirmed
Possible pregnancy, not (yet) confirmed
V72.41 Pregnancy examination or test, negative result
V72.42 Pregnancy examination or test, positive result

V72.5 Radiological examination, not elsewhere classified
Routine chest x-ray
EXCLUDES radiologic examinations as part of pre-procedural testing (V72.81-V72.84)

☑5ᵗʰ **V72.6 Laboratory examination**
Encounters for blood and urine testing
V72.60 Laboratory examination, unspecified

V72.61 Antibody response examination
Immunity status testing
EXCLUDES encounter for allergy testing (V72.7)

V72.62 Laboratory examination ordered as part of a routine general medical examination
Blood tests for routine general physical examination

V72.63 Pre-procedural laboratory examination
Blood tests prior to treatment or procedure
Pre-operative laboratory examination

V72.69 Other laboratory examination

V72.7 Diagnostic skin and sensitization tests
Allergy tests
Skin tests for hypersensitivity
EXCLUDES diagnostic skin tests for bacterial diseases (V74.0-V74.9)

☑5ᵗʰ **V72.8 Other specified examinations**
EXCLUDES pre-procedural laboratory examinations (V72.63)
V72.81 Pre-operative cardiovascular examination
Pre-procedural cardiovascular examination
V72.82 Pre-operative respiratory examination
Pre-procedural respiratory examination
V72.83 Other specified pre-operative examination
Examination prior to chemotherapy
Other pre-procedural examination
Pre-procedural general physical examination
EXCLUDES routine general medical examination (V70.0)
V72.84 Pre-operative examination, unspecified
Pre-procedural examination, unspecified
V72.85 Other specified examination
V72.86 Encounter for blood typing

V72.9 Unspecified examination

☑4ᵗʰ **V73 Special screening examination for viral and chlamydial diseases**
V73.0 Poliomyelitis
V73.1 Smallpox
V73.2 Measles
V73.3 Rubella
V73.4 Yellow fever
V73.5 Other arthropod-borne viral diseases
Dengue fever
Hemorrhagic fever
Viral encephalitis: mosquito-borne
Viral encephalitis: tick-borne
V73.6 Trachoma
☑5ᵗʰ **V73.8 Other specified viral and chlamydial diseases**
V73.81 Human papillomavirus [HPV]
V73.88 Other specified chlamydial diseases
V73.89 Other specified viral diseases
☑5ᵗʰ **V73.9 Unspecified viral and chlamydial disease**
V73.98 Unspecified chlamydial disease
V73.99 Unspecified viral disease

☑4ᵗʰ **V74 Special screening examination for bacterial and spirochetal diseases**
INCLUDES diagnostic skin tests for these diseases
V74.0 Cholera
V74.1 Pulmonary tuberculosis
V74.2 Leprosy [Hansen's disease]
V74.3 Diphtheria
V74.4 Bacterial conjunctivitis

V74.5 Venereal disease
Screening for bacterial and spirochetal sexually transmitted diseases
Screening for sexually transmitted diseases NOS
> EXCLUDES *special screening for nonbacterial sexually transmitted diseases (V73.81-V73.89, V75.4, V75.8)*

V74.6 Yaws

V74.8 Other specified bacterial and spirochetal diseases
Brucellosis	Tetanus
Leptospirosis	Whooping cough
Plague	

V74.9 Unspecified bacterial and spirochetal disease

✓4ᵗʰ **V75 Special screening examination for other infectious diseases**

V75.0 Rickettsial diseases

V75.1 Malaria

V75.2 Leishmaniasis

V75.3 Trypanosomiasis
Chagas' disease
Sleeping sickness

V75.4 Mycotic infections

V75.5 Schistosomiasis

V75.6 Filariasis

V75.7 Intestinal helminthiasis

V75.8 Other specified parasitic infections

V75.9 Unspecified infectious disease

✓4ᵗʰ **V76 Special screening for malignant neoplasms**

V76.0 Respiratory organs

✓5ᵗʰ **V76.1 Breast**

V76.10 Breast screening, unspecified

V76.11 Screening mammogram for high-risk patient

V76.12 Other screening mammogram

V76.19 Other screening breast examination

V76.2 Cervix
Routine cervical Papanicolaou smear
> EXCLUDES *special screening for human papillomavirus (V73.81)*
> *that as part of a general gynecological examination (V72.31)*

V76.3 Bladder

✓5ᵗʰ **V76.4 Other sites**

V76.41 Rectum

V76.42 Oral cavity

V76.43 Skin

V76.44 Prostate

V76.45 Testis

V76.46 Ovary

V76.47 Vagina
Vaginal pap smear status-post hysterectomy for non-malignant condition
Use additional code to identify acquired absence of uterus (V88.01-V88.03)
> EXCLUDES *vaginal pap smear status-post hysterectomy for malignant condition (V67.01)*

V76.49 Other sites

✓5ᵗʰ **V76.5 Intestine**

V76.50 Intestine, unspecified

V76.51 Colon
Screening colonoscopy NOS
> EXCLUDES *rectum (V76.41)*

V76.52 Small intestine

✓5ᵗʰ **V76.8 Other neoplasm**

V76.81 Nervous system

V76.89 Other neoplasm

V76.9 Unspecified

✓4ᵗʰ **V77 Special screening for endocrine, nutritional, metabolic, and immunity disorders**

V77.0 Thyroid disorders

V77.1 Diabetes mellitus

V77.2 Malnutrition

V77.3 Phenylketonuria [PKU]

V77.4 Galactosemia

V77.5 Gout

V77.6 Cystic fibrosis
Screening for mucoviscidosis

V77.7 Other inborn errors of metabolism

V77.8 Obesity

✓5ᵗʰ **V77.9 Other and unspecified endocrine, nutritional, metabolic, and immunity disorders**

V77.91 Screening for lipoid disorders
Screening for cholesterol level
Screening for hypercholesterolemia
Screening for hyperlipidemia

V77.99 Other and unspecified endocrine, nutritional, metabolic, and immunity disorders

✓4ᵗʰ **V78 Special screening for disorders of blood and blood-forming organs**

V78.0 Iron deficiency anemia

V78.1 Other and unspecified deficiency anemia

V78.2 Sickle cell disease or trait

V78.3 Other hemoglobinopathies

V78.8 Other disorders of blood and blood-forming organs

V78.9 Unspecified disorder of blood and blood-forming organs

✓4ᵗʰ **V79 Special screening for mental disorders and developmental handicaps**

V79.0 Depression

V79.1 Alcoholism

V79.2 Intellectual disabilities

V79.3 Developmental handicaps in early childhood

V79.8 Other specified mental disorders and developmental handicaps

V79.9 Unspecified mental disorder and developmental handicap

✓4ᵗʰ **V80 Special screening for neurological, eye, and ear diseases**

✓5ᵗʰ **V80.0 Neurological conditions**

V80.01 Traumatic brain injury

V80.09 Other neurological conditions

V80.1 Glaucoma

V80.2 Other eye conditions
Screening for:	Screening for:
cataract	senile macular
congenital anomaly of eye	lesions
> EXCLUDES *general vision examination (V72.0)*

V80.3 Ear diseases
> EXCLUDES *general hearing examination (V72.11-V72.19)*

✓4ᵗʰ **V81 Special screening for cardiovascular, respiratory, and genitourinary diseases**

V81.0 Ischemic heart disease

V81.1 Hypertension

V81.2 Other and unspecified cardiovascular conditions

V81.3 Chronic bronchitis and emphysema

V81.4 **Other and unspecified respiratory conditions**
> EXCLUDES *screening for:*
> *lung neoplasm (V76.0)*
> *pulmonary tuberculosis (V74.1)*

V81.5 **Nephropathy**
Screening for asymptomatic bacteriuria

V81.6 **Other and unspecified genitourinary conditions**

√4th **V82 Special screening for other conditions**

V82.0 **Skin conditions**

V82.1 **Rheumatoid arthritis**

V82.2 **Other rheumatic disorders**

V82.3 **Congenital dislocation of hip**

V82.4 **Maternal postnatal screening for chromosomal anomalies**
> EXCLUDES *antenatal screening by amniocentesis (V28.0)*

V82.5 **Chemical poisoning and other contamination**
Screening for:
heavy metal poisoning
ingestion of radioactive substance
poisoning from contaminated water supply
radiation exposure

V82.6 **Multiphasic screening**

√5th V82.7 **Genetic screening**
> EXCLUDES *genetic testing for procreative management (V26.31-V26.39)*

V82.71 **Screening for genetic disease carrier status**

V82.79 **Other genetic screening**

√5th V82.8 **Other specified conditions**

V82.81 **Osteoporosis**
Use additional code to identify:
hormone replacement therapy (postmenopausal) status (V07.4)
postmenopausal (age-related) (natural) status (V49.81)

V82.89 **Other specified conditions**

V82.9 **Unspecified condition**

GENETICS (V83-V84)

√4th **V83 Genetic carrier status**

√5th V83.0 **Hemophilia A carrier**

V83.01 **Asymptomatic hemophilia A carrier**

V83.02 **Symptomatic hemophilia A carrier**

√5th V83.8 **Other genetic carrier status**

V83.81 **Cystic fibrosis gene carrier**

V83.89 **Other genetic carrier status**

√4th **V84 Genetic susceptibility to disease**
> INCLUDES confirmed abnormal gene
Use additional code, if applicable, for any associated family history of the disease (V16-V19)
> EXCLUDES *chromosomal anomalies (758.0-758.9)*

√5th V84.0 **Genetic susceptibility to malignant neoplasm**
Code first, if applicable, any current malignant neoplasms (140.0-195.8, 200.0-208.9, 230.0-234.9)
Use additional code, if applicable, for any personal history of malignant neoplasm (V10.0-V10.9)

V84.01 **Genetic susceptibility to malignant neoplasm of breast**

V84.02 **Genetic susceptibility to malignant neoplasm of ovary**

V84.03 **Genetic susceptibility to malignant neoplasm of prostate**

V84.04 **Genetic susceptibility to malignant neoplasm of endometrium**

V84.09 **Genetic susceptibility to other malignant neoplasm**

√5th V84.8 **Genetic susceptibility to other disease**

V84.81 **Genetic susceptibility to multiple endocrine neoplasia [MEN]**
> EXCLUDES *multiple endocrine neoplasia [MEN] syndromes (258.01-258.03)*

V84.89 **Genetic susceptibility to other disease**

BODY MASS INDEX (V85)

√4th **V85 Body Mass Index [BMI]**
Kilograms per meters squared
Note: BMI adult codes are for use for persons over 20 years old

V85.0 **Body Mass Index less than 19, adult**

V85.1 **Body Mass Index between 19-24, adult**

√5th V85.2 **Body Mass Index between 25-29, adult**

V85.21 **Body Mass Index 25.0-25.9, adult**

V85.22 **Body Mass Index 26.0-26.9, adult**

V85.23 **Body Mass Index 27.0-27.9, adult**

V85.24 **Body Mass Index 28.0-28.9, adult**

V85.25 **Body Mass Index 29.0-29.9, adult**

√5th V85.3 **Body Mass Index between 30-39, adult**

V85.30 **Body Mass Index 30.0-30.9, adult**

V85.31 **Body Mass Index 31.0-31.9, adult**

V85.32 **Body Mass Index 32.0-32.9, adult**

V85.33 **Body Mass Index 33.0-33.9, adult**

V85.34 **Body Mass Index 34.0-34.9, adult**

V85.35 **Body Mass Index 35.0-35.9, adult**

V85.36 **Body Mass Index 36.0-36.9, adult**

V85.37 **Body Mass Index 37.0-37.9, adult**

V85.38 **Body Mass Index 38.0-38.9, adult**

V85.39 **Body Mass Index 39.0-39.9, adult**

√5th V85.4 **Body Mass Index 40 and over, adult**

V85.41 **Body Mass Index 40.0-44.9, adult**

V85.42 **Body Mass Index 45.0-49.9, adult**

V85.43 **Body Mass Index 50.0-59.9, adult**

V85.44 **Body Mass Index 60.0-69.9, adult**

V85.45 **Body Mass Index 70 and over, adult**

√5th V85.5 **Body Mass Index, pediatric**
Note: BMI pediatric codes are for use for persons age 2-20 years old. These percentiles are based on the growth charts published by the Centers for Disease Control and Prevention (CDC)

V85.51 **Body Mass Index, pediatric, less than 5th percentile for age**

V85.52 **Body Mass Index, pediatric, 5th percentile to less than 85th percentile for age**

V85.53 **Body Mass Index, pediatric, 85th percentile to less than 95th percentile for age**

V85.54 **Body Mass Index, pediatric, greater than or equal to 95th percentile for age**

ESTROGEN RECEPTOR STATUS (V86)

√4th **V86 Estrogen receptor status**
Code first malignant neoplasm of breast (174.0-174.9, 175.0-175.9)

V86.0 **Estrogen receptor positive status [ER+]**

V86.1 **Estrogen receptor negative status [ER-]**

OTHER SPECIFIED PERSONAL EXPOSURES AND HISTORY PRESENTING HAZARDS TO HEALTH (V87)

√4ᵗʰ **V87 Other specified personal exposures and history presenting hazards to health**

√5ᵗʰ **V87.0 Contact with and (suspected) exposure to hazardous metals**
  EXCLUDES   *exposure to lead (V15.86)*
              toxic effect of metals (984.0-985.9)

V87.01 Arsenic

V87.02 Contact with and (suspected) exposure to uranium
  EXCLUDES   *retained depleted uranium fragments (V90.01)*

V87.09 Other hazardous metals
  Chromium compounds
  Nickel dust

√5ᵗʰ **V87.1 Contact with and (suspected) exposure to hazardous aromatic compounds**
  EXCLUDES   *toxic effects of aromatic compounds (982.0, 983.0)*

V87.11 Aromatic amines

V87.12 Benzene

V87.19 Other hazardous aromatic compounds
  Aromatic dyes NOS
  Polycyclic aromatic hydrocarbons

V87.2 Contact with and (suspected) exposure to other potentially hazardous chemicals
  Dyes NOS
  EXCLUDES   *exposure to asbestos (V15.84)*
              toxic effect of chemicals (980-989)

√5ᵗʰ **V87.3 Contact with and (suspected) exposure to other potentially hazardous substances**
  EXCLUDES   *contact with and (suspected) exposure to potentially hazardous body fluids (V15.85)*
              personal history of retained foreign body fully removed (V15.53)
              toxic effect of substances (980-989)

V87.31 Exposure to mold

V87.32 Contact with and (suspected) exposure to algae bloom

V87.39 Contact with and (suspected) exposure to other potentially hazardous substances

√5ᵗʰ **V87.4 Personal history of drug therapy**
  EXCLUDES   *long-term (current) drug use (V58.61-V58.69)*

V87.41 Personal history of antineoplastic chemotherapy

V87.42 Personal history of monoclonal drug therapy

V87.43 Personal history of estrogen therapy

V87.44 Personal history of inhaled steroid therapy

V87.45 Personal history of systemic steroid therapy
  Personal history of steroid therapy NOS

V87.46 Personal history of immunosuppression therapy
  EXCLUDES   *personal history of steroid therapy (V87.44, V87.45)*

V87.49 Personal history of other drug therapy

ACQUIRED ABSENCE OF OTHER ORGANS AND TISSUE (V88)

√4ᵗʰ **V88 Acquired absence of other organs and tissue**

√5ᵗʰ **V88.0 Acquired absence of cervix and uterus**

V88.01 Acquired absence of both cervix and uterus
  Acquired absence of uterus NOS
  Status post total hysterectomy

V88.02 Acquired absence of uterus with remaining cervical stump
  Status post partial hysterectomy with remaining cervical stump

V88.03 Acquired absence of cervix with remaining uterus

√5ᵗʰ **V88.1 Acquired absence of pancreas**
  Use additional code to identify any associated:
    insulin use (V58.67)
    secondary diabetes mellitus (249.00-249.91)

V88.11 Acquired total absence of pancreas
  Acquired absence of pancreas NOS

V88.12 Acquired partial absence of pancreas

√5ᵗʰ **V88.2 Acquired absence of joint**
  Acquired absence of joint following prior explantation of joint prosthesis
  Joint prosthesis explantation status

V88.21 Acquired absence of hip joint
  Acquired absence of hip joint following explantation of joint prosthesis, with or without presence of antibiotic-impregnated cement spacer

V88.22 Acquired absence of knee joint
  Acquired absence of knee joint following explantation of joint prosthesis, with or without presence of antibiotic-impregnated cement spacer

V88.29 Acquired absence of other joint
  Acquired absence of other joint following explantation of joint prosthesis, with or without presence of antibiotic-impregnated cement spacer

OTHER SUSPECTED CONDITIONS NOT FOUND (V89)

√4ᵗʰ **V89 Other suspected conditions not found**

√5ᵗʰ **V89.0 Suspected maternal and fetal conditions not found**
  EXCLUDES   *known or suspected fetal anomalies affecting management of mother, not ruled out (655.00, 655.93, 656.00-656.93, 657.00-657.03, 658.00-658.93)*
              newborn and perinatal conditions — code to condition

V89.01 Suspected problem with amniotic cavity and membrane not found
  Suspected oligohydramnios not found
  Suspected polyhydramnios not found

V89.02 Suspected placental problem not found

V89.03 Suspected fetal anomaly not found

V89.04 Suspected problem with fetal growth not found

V89.05 Suspected cervical shortening not found

V89.09 Other suspected maternal and fetal condition not found

RETAINED FOREIGN BODY (V90)

✓4ᵗʰ **V90 Retained foreign body**
   Embedded fragment (status)
   Embedded splinter (status)
   Retained foreign body status
   EXCLUDES *artificial joint prosthesis status (V43.60-V43.69)*
      foreign body accidentally left during a procedure (998.4)
      foreign body entering through orifice (930.0-939.9)
      in situ cardiac devices (V45.00-V45.09)
      organ or tissue replaced by other means (V43.0-V43.89)
      organ or tissue replaced by transplant (V42.0-V42.9)
      personal history of retained foreign body removed (V15.53)
      superficial foreign body (splinter) (categories 910-917 and 919 with 4ᵗʰ character 6 or 7, 918.0)

✓5ᵗʰ **V90.0 Retained radioactive fragment**
   V90.01 Retained depleted uranium fragments
   V90.09 Other retained radioactive fragments
      Other retained depleted isotope fragments
      Retained nontherapeutic radioactive fragments

✓5ᵗʰ **V90.1 Retained metal fragments**
   EXCLUDES *retained radioactive metal fragments (V90.01-V90.09)*
   V90.10 Retained metal fragments, unspecified
      Retained metal fragment NOS
   V90.11 Retained magnetic metal fragments
   V90.12 Retained nonmagnetic metal fragments

V90.2 Retained plastic fragments
   Acrylics fragments
   Diethylhexylphthalates fragments
   Isocyanate fragments

✓5ᵗʰ **V90.3 Retained organic fragments**
   V90.31 Retained animal quills or spines
   V90.32 Retained tooth
   V90.33 Retained wood fragments
   V90.39 Other retained organic fragments

✓5ᵗʰ **V90.8 Other specified retained foreign body**
   V90.81 Retained glass fragments
   V90.83 Retained stone or crystalline fragments
      Retained concrete or cement fragments
   V90.89 Other specified retained foreign body
V90.9 Retained foreign body, unspecified material

MULTIPLE GESTATION PLACENTA STATUS (V91)

✓4ᵗʰ **V91 Multiple gestation placenta status**
   Code first multiple gestation (651.0-651.9)

✓5ᵗʰ **V91.0 Twin gestation placenta status**
   V91.00 Twin gestation, unspecified number of placenta, unspecified number of amniotic sacs
   V91.01 Twin gestation, monochorionic/monoamniotic (one placenta, one amniotic sac)
   V91.02 Twin gestation, monochorionic/diamniotic (one placenta, two amniotic sacs)
   V91.03 Twin gestation, dichorionic/diamniotic (two placentae, two amniotic sacs)
   V91.09 Twin gestation, unable to determine number of placenta and number of amniotic sacs

✓5ᵗʰ **V91.1 Triplet gestation placenta status**
   V91.10 Triplet gestation, unspecified number of placenta and unspecified number of amniotic sacs
   V91.11 Triplet gestation, with two or more monochorionic fetuses
   V91.12 Triplet gestation, with two or more monoamniotic fetuses
   V91.19 Triplet gestation, unable to determine number of placenta and number of amniotic sacs

✓5ᵗʰ **V91.2 Quadruplet gestation placenta status**
   V91.20 Quadruplet gestation, unspecified number of placenta and unspecified number of amniotic sacs
   V91.21 Quadruplet gestation, with two or more monochorionic fetuses
   V91.22 Quadruplet gestation, with two or more monoamniotic fetuses
   V91.29 Quadruplet gestation, unable to determine number of placenta and number of amniotic sacs

✓5ᵗʰ **V91.9 Other specified multiple gestation placenta status**
   Placenta status for multiple gestations greater than quadruplets
   V91.90 Other specified multiple gestation, unspecified number of placenta and unspecified number of amniotic sacs
   V91.91 Other specified multiple gestation, with two or more monochorionic fetuses
   V91.92 Other specified multiple gestation, with two or more monoamniotic fetuses
   V91.99 Other specified multiple gestation, unable to determine number of placenta and number of amniotic sacs

E Codes: Supplementary Classification of External Causes of Injury and Poisoning (E000-E999.1)

Coding Guidance

The section titled "Supplementary Classification of External Causes of Injury and Poisoning" is commonly referred to as "E codes." E codes provide a classification of external causes that relate to the condition or injury being coded. E codes may indicate how an accident occurred; what caused an injury; whether a drug overdose was accidental; an adverse drug reaction; or, the location of occurrence of the injury.

Some major categories of E codes include the following:

- Transport accidents
- Poisoning and adverse effects of drugs, medicinal substances, and biologicals
- Accidental falls
- Accidents caused by fire and flames
- Accidents due to natural and environmental factors
- Late effects of accidents, assaults, or self-injury
- Assaults or purposely inflicted injury
- Suicide or self-inflicted injury

Coding Principles for E Codes

Coders should be aware of the principles of E code assignment. The following principles are used to assign E codes: Look for the causes (fire, accident, fall, shooting) in section 3 of the alphabetic index. For adverse reactions to medical or surgical care, look under the main term "Reaction" in the alphabetic index. When listing an E code on a claim, be sure to use the letter "E" with the code number.

E codes are never used alone.

An E code is never used as a primary, principal or first-listed diagnosis.

An E code may be used with any code in the range of 001.0–V91, which indicates an injury, poisoning or adverse effect due to an external cause.

Use the full range of E codes to completely describe the cause, the intent and the place of occurrence, if applicable, for all injuries, poisonings, and adverse effects of drugs. Assign as many E codes as necessary to fully explain each cause. If only one E code can be recorded, assign the E code most related to the principal diagnosis.

Use an additional code from category E849 to identify the place of occurrence, if stated.

Late effect E codes exist for injuries and poisonings but not for adverse effects of drugs, misadventures, and surgical complications. A late effect E code (E929, E959, E969, E977, E989 or E999) should be assigned to report a late effect or sequela resulting from a previous injury or poisoning (905–909) and never to be used with an injury code.

There are several guidelines to follow when assigning multiple E codes. The hierarchy of reporting E codes is as follows:

- E codes for child and adult abuse take priority over all other E codes.
- E codes for terrorism events take priority over all other E codes except child and adult abuse.
- E codes for cataclysmic events take priority over all other E codes except child and adult abuse and terrorism.
- E codes for transport accidents take priority over all other E codes except cataclysmic events and child and adult abuse and terrorism.
- E codes for cause/intent, including medical misadventures, take priority over codes for place, activity, or external status.
- Activity and external cause status codes are assigned following all causal (intent) E codes.

E codes provide information concerning intent (unintentional, or accidental or intentional, such as suicide or assault). If the intent (accident, self-harm, assault) of the cause of an injury or poisoning is unknown, questionable, probable or suspected or unspecified, code the intent as undetermined E980–E989. When reporting assaults, accidents, or self-harm, sequence first the E code which reports the cause of the most serious diagnosis.

External Cause Status (E000)

Only one external cause status code may be reported per encounter. An external cause status should be assigned to report a patient's work status (e.g., civilian activity, military activity, other; including student and volunteer activities, unspecified) at the time the injury or event occurred. These codes are intended to report whether a patient was involved in a military or civilian work or nonwork activity at the time of injury or event. These codes may be reported in addition to transport or fall E codes. However, external cause status codes may not be reported with poisonings, adverse effects, late effects, or other misadventures related to medical or surgical treatment. External cause status E000.9 Unspecified external cause status, should not be reported by default; do not report this code if the status is not documented or stated.

Activity Codes (E001–E030)

Activity codes describe the activity that caused or contributed to the injury or other health condition being reported. These codes are not limited to injury reporting; however, they may not be used to report circumstances of poisonings, adverse effects, misadventures, or late effects. If the causal or contributing activity is not documented, do not report code E030 Unspecified activity.

Transport Accidents (E800–E848)

Transport accidents (E800–E848) involve a vehicle that is used primarily to transport people or products. Agriculture and construction vehicle accidents are considered transport accidents if the machinery is under its own power on a highway. Report the code for the injury sustained in the accident before the E code.

According to ICD-9-CM guidelines, a motor vehicle accident (E810–E819) is a transport accident involving a vehicle that is motorized. A motor vehicle accident is an accident that occurs on the highway and is assumed to have occurred on the highway unless otherwise specified. An accident that involves an off-road vehicle, such as an ATV or a snowmobile, is considered a nontraffic accident (E820–E825) unless otherwise specified. All codes require fourth digits.

Accidental Poisoning by Drugs, Medicinal Substances and Biologicals (E850–E858)

Poisoning by drugs, medicinal, and biological substances is the major cause of childhood accidents in the home and can occur by many routes, including oral ingestion, inhalation, dermal absorption, and ocular instillation.

Accidental poisoning codes identify accidental overdose of a drug, a wrong substance given or taken, a drug taken inadvertently, and accidents in the use of drugs and biologicals in medical and surgical procedures. The alphabetical index of ICD-9-CM can give a more complete list of specific drugs classified under a fourth-digit category; however, codes should not be assigned directly from the table of drugs and chemicals. Always consult the tabular section of ICD-9-CM before assigning the accidental poisoning codes. Many of the common medications can be found in the pharmacological listings found in the back of ICD-9-CM. When coding accidental poisoning use as many codes as necessary to completely describe the drug, medicinal, or biological poisoning. Sequence poisoning first, manifestation second, and the E code third. Assign an additional code for drug dependency, if applicable.

Misadventures to Patients During Surgical and Medical Care (E870–E876)

Many people are incapacitated as a result of medical errors. These errors increase health care costs significantly. The following kinds of errors unfortunately are often made: prescribing the wrong medication, administering an anesthetic improperly, operating a mechanical device incorrectly, causing an infection by improper wound treatment, contaminating blood or other pathological tests, completing a surgical procedure incorrectly. The physician should document clearly that a misadventure occurred and the nature of the complication.

Accidental Falls (E880–E888)

Codes for accidental fall codes are one of the most frequently assigned series of E codes. A fall is the most common cause of fatal injury in the elderly and a common cause of injury in children. Accidental falls are broken down into specific types depending on whether the fall was from a bed, a chair, a ladder, the toilet, or the sidewalk curb. Also included in this category is a fall that results in the person striking against an object. Excluded from this section is a fall in or from a burning building; into a fire; into water with submerging and drowning; in or from operating machinery; on an edged, painted, or sharp object; and in or from a transport or other vehicle.

Environmental Exposure to Harmful Algae and Toxins (E928.6)

Red tide is the reddish-brown color of sea water caused by an overconcentration of microscopic algae. Red tides are not always red but can vary in color or even look normal during a "bloom." Blooms are caused by a multitude of factors, including temperature shifts, rainfall accumulations, and changes in wind currents. A red tide begins offshore and moves shoreward, which accounts for beaches littered with dead marine mammals and fish. Red tides are natural phenomena, apparently unrelated to, though possibly exacerbated by, man-made pollution.

Irritation of the eyes, nose, throat, and tingling lips and tongue are common symptoms that occur in humans from airborne toxins during a red tide. Waves, wind, and boat propellers disperse toxin particles into the air, creating irritants for people along the shore. People suffering from severe or chronic respiratory conditions should avoid red tide areas, as the airborne irritants can exacerbate these conditions. Swimming in a red tide is unadvisable and may cause skin and mucous membrane irritation. Red tide can also be responsible for illnesses caused by consuming contaminated shellfish.

Code E928.6 Environmental exposure to harmful algae and toxins is assigned as a secondary diagnosis to describe the external cause of environmental exposure to harmful algae and toxins. Code first the manifestation (e.g., 462 Acute pharyngitis) and E928.6 Environmental exposure to harmful algae and toxins.

Overexertion and Strenuous Movements (E927)

Overexertion and strenuous movements may cause small tears in the muscle, which are referred to as muscle strain. This occurs when the muscle is suddenly stretched beyond its limit. Muscle strains are graded according to their severity. Muscle strains can heal rapidly in the cases of mild strain or take months to heal for more severe strains. Standard treatment for muscle strains is rest, ice, compression, and elevation. Properly warming up, using correct body mechanics, strengthening muscles, and regular exercise can prevent muscle strains.

Drugs, Medicinal and Biological Substances Causing Adverse Effects in Therapeutic Use (E930–E949)

Codes E930–E949 report adverse medication reactions related to therapeutic use. Use the appropriate "other specified" or "unspecified" code within a category or subcategory to report drugs, medicinal, or biological substances if the reporting format limits the number of codes. However, if the codes are in different three-digit categories, assign the appropriate E code for other multiple drugs and medicinal substances.

This section is not used to report overdoses but rather allergic reaction or hypersensitivity and other adverse effects. Symptoms can range from hives or skin rash to anaphylactic shock. Anaphylaxis is a severe allergic reaction and, in some cases, can produce life-threatening bronchospasm and laryngeal edema.

Adverse Effects of Oral (E933.6) and Intravenous (E933.7) Bisphosphonates

Codes E933.6 and E933.7 enable tracking of adverse effects of bisphosphonates drugs (e.g., Boniva, Fosamax, and Zometa) in therapeutic use. A causal relationship between osteonecrosis of the jaw and bisphosphonate medications is currently under investigation. The route of administration of these external causes is distinguished as either oral (E933.6) or intravenous (E933.7).

Suicide and Self-inflicted Injury (E950–E959)

Codes E950–E959 report suicide and self-inflicted injury, which includes injury and suicide by self-inflicted poisoning, hanging, strangulating, suffocating, shooting, submerging, and drowning, and cutting or piercing. Near drowning is now more commonly referred to as a submersion accident. If the intent is not specified, is unknown, or documented as questionable, probable, or suspected, assign the E code for cause undetermined.

Homicide and Injury Purposely Inflicted by Other Persons (E960–E969)

This section includes fights, rape, assault by corrosive substance, assault by poisoning, and assault by firearm. Also included in this section are codes to describe the perpetrator of child and adult abuse. E codes for child and adult abuse take priority over all other E codes. An E code for the type of abuse should be listed first, followed by the code for perpetrator. Report an accidental neglect code first if the intent is an accidental abandonment of an adult or a child. If the intent is not specified, unknown, or documented as questionable, probable, or suspected, assign the E code for cause undetermined.

Injury Resulting from Operations of War (E990–E999)

Section E990–E999 reports injury resulting from operations of war. Operations of war are injuries to military personnel and civilians caused by war and civil revolt and occurring during the time of war. Excluded from this section are accidents during training of military personnel, manufacture of war material, and transport, unless attributable to enemy action.

SUPPLEMENTARY CLASSIFICATION OF EXTERNAL CAUSES OF INJURY AND POISONING (E000-E999)

This section is provided to permit the classification of environmental events, circumstances, and conditions as the cause of injury, poisoning, and other adverse effects. Where a code from this section is applicable, it is intended that it shall be used in addition to a code from one of the main chapters of ICD-9-CM, indicating the nature of the condition. Certain other conditions which may be stated to be due to external causes are classified in Chapters 1 to 16 of ICD-9-CM. For these, the "E" code classification should be used as an additional code for more detailed analysis.

Machinery accidents [other than those connected with transport] are classifiable to category E919, in which the fourth digit allows a broad classification of the type of machinery involved.

Categories for "late effects" of accidents and other external causes are to be found at E929, E959, E969, E977, E989, and E999.

EXTERNAL CAUSE STATUS (E000)

Note: A code from category E000 may be used in conjunction with the external cause code(s) assigned to a record to indicate the status of the person at the time the event occurred. A single code from category E000 should be assigned for an encounter.

√4ᵗʰ **E000　External cause status**

　　E000.0　Civilian activity done for income or pay
　　　　Civilian activity done for financial or other compensation
　　　　EXCLUDES　　military activity (E000.1)

　　E000.1　Military activity
　　　　EXCLUDES　　activity of off-duty military personnel (E000.8)

　　E000.2　Volunteer activity
　　　　EXCLUDES　　activity of child or other family member assisting in compensated work of other family member

　　E000.8　Other external cause status
　　　　Activity NEC
　　　　Hobby not done for income
　　　　Leisure activity
　　　　Off-duty activity of military personnel
　　　　Recreation or sport not for income or while a student
　　　　Student activity
　　　　EXCLUDES　　Activity of child or other family member assisting in compensated work of other family member
　　　　　　civilian activity done for income or compensation (E000.0)
　　　　　　military activity (E000.1)

　　E000.9　Unspecified external cause status

ACTIVITY (E001-E030)

Note: Categories E001 to E030 are provided for use to indicate the activity of the person seeking healthcare for an injury or health condition, such as a heart attack while shoveling snow, which resulted from, or was contributed to, by the activity. These codes are appropriate for use for both acute injuries, such as those from chapter 17, and conditions that are due to the long-term, cumulative affects of an activity, such as those from chapter 13. They are also appropriate for use with external cause codes for cause and intent if identifying the activity provides additional information on the event.

These codes should be used in conjunction with other external cause codes for external cause status (E000) and place of occurrence (E849).

This section contains the following broad activity categories:

E001　Activities involving walking and running
E002　Activities involving water and water craft
E003　Activities involving ice and snow
E004　Activities involving climbing, rappelling, and jumping off
E005　Activities involving dancing and other rhythmic movement
E006　Activities involving other sports and athletics played individually
E007　Activities involving other sports and athletics played as a team or group
E008　Activities involving other specified sports and athletics
E009　Activity involving other cardiorespiratory exercise
E010　Activity involving other muscle strengthening exercises
E011　Activities involving computer technology and electronic devices
E012　Activities involving arts and handcrafts
E013　Activities involving personal hygiene and household maintenance
E014　Activities involving person providing caregiving
E015　Activities involving food preparation, cooking and grilling
E016　Activities involving property and land maintenance, building and construction
E017　Activities involving roller coasters and other types of external motion
E018　Activities involving playing musical instrument
E019　Activities involving animal care
E029　Other activity
E030　Unspecified activity

√4ᵗʰ **E001　Activities involving walking and running**
　　EXCLUDES　　walking an animal (E019.0)
　　　　walking or running on a treadmill (E009.0)

　　E001.0　Walking, marching and hiking
　　　　Walking, marching and hiking on level or elevated terrain
　　　　EXCLUDES　　mountain climbing (E004.0)

　　E001.1　Running

√4ᵗʰ **E002　Activities involving water and water craft**
　　EXCLUDES　　activities involving ice (E003.0-E003.9)
　　　　boating and other watercraft transport accidents (E830-E838)

　　E002.0　Swimming

　　E002.1　Springboard and platform diving

　　E002.2　Water polo

　　E002.3　Water aerobics and water exercise

　　E002.4　Underwater diving and snorkeling
　　　　SCUBA diving

　　E002.5　Rowing, canoeing, kayaking, rafting and tubing
　　　　Canoeing, kayaking, rafting and tubing in calm and turbulent water

　　E002.6　Water skiing and wake boarding

　　E002.7　Surfing, windsurfing and boogie boarding

　　E002.8　Water sliding

　　E002.9　Other activity involving water and watercraft
　　　　Activity involving water NOS
　　　　Parasailing
　　　　Water survival training and testing

√4ᵗʰ **E003　Activities involving ice and snow**
　　EXCLUDES　　shoveling ice and snow (E016.0)

　　E003.0　Ice skating
　　　　Figure skating (singles) (pairs)
　　　　Ice dancing
　　　　EXCLUDES　　ice hockey (E003.1)

　　E003.1　Ice hockey

　　E003.2　Snow (alpine) (downhill) skiing, snow boarding, sledding, tobogganing and snow tubing
　　　　EXCLUDES　　cross country skiing (E003.3)

　　E003.3　Cross country skiing
　　　　Nordic skiing

　　E003.9　Other activity involving ice and snow
　　　　Activity involving ice and snow NOS

√4ᵗʰ **E004　Activities involving climbing, rappelling, and jumping off**
　　EXCLUDES　　hiking on level or elevated terrain (E001.0)
　　　　jumping rope (E006.5)
　　　　sky diving (E840-E844)
　　　　trampoline jumping (E005.3)

　　E004.0　Mountain climbing, rock climbing and wall climbing

　　E004.1　Rappelling

　　E004.2　BASE jumping
　　　　Building, Antenna, Span, Earth jumping

E004.3 Bungee jumping

E004.4 Hang gliding

E004.9 Other activity involving climbing, rappelling and jumping off

☑4ᵗʰ **E005 Activities involving dancing and other rhythmic movement**
> EXCLUDES   martial arts (E008.4)

E005.0 Dancing

E005.1 Yoga

E005.2 Gymnastics
Rhythmic gymnastics
> EXCLUDES   trampoline (E005.3)

E005.3 Trampoline

E005.4 Cheerleading

E005.9 Other activity involving dancing and other rhythmic movements

☑4ᵗʰ **E006 Activities involving other sports and athletics played individually**
> EXCLUDES   dancing (E005.0)
> gymnastic (E005.2)
> trampoline (E005.3)
> yoga (E005.1)

E006.0 Roller skating (inline) and skateboarding

E006.1 Horseback riding

E006.2 Golf

E006.3 Bowling

E006.4 Bike riding
> EXCLUDES   transport accident involving bike riding (E800-E829)

E006.5 Jumping rope

E006.6 Non-running track and field events
> EXCLUDES   running (any form) (E001.1)

E006.9 Other activity involving other sports and athletics played individually
> EXCLUDES   activities involving climbing, rappelling, and jumping (E004.0-E004.9)
> activities involving ice and snow (E003.0-E003.9)
> activities involving walking and running (E001.0-E001.1)
> activities involving water and watercraft (E002.0-E002.9)

☑4ᵗʰ **E007 Activities involving other sports and athletics played as a team or group**
> EXCLUDES   ice hockey (E003.1)
> water polo (E002.2)

E007.0 American tackle football
Football NOS

E007.1 American flag or touch football

E007.2 Rugby

E007.3 Baseball
Softball

E007.4 Lacrosse and field hockey

E007.5 Soccer

E007.6 Basketball

E007.7 Volleyball (beach) (court)

E007.8 Physical games generally associated with school recess, summer camp and children
Capture the flag
Dodge ball
Four square
Kickball

E007.9 Other activity involving other sports and athletics played as a team or group
Cricket

☑4ᵗʰ **E008 Activities involving other specified sports and athletics**

E008.0 Boxing

E008.1 Wrestling

E008.2 Racquet and hand sports
Handball
Racquetball
Squash
Tennis

E008.3 Frisbee
Ultimate frisbee

E008.4 Martial arts
Combatives

E008.9 Other specified sports and athletics activity
> EXCLUDES   sports and athletics activities specified in categories E001-E007'

☑4ᵗʰ **E009 Activity involving other cardiorespiratory exercise**
Activity involving physical training

E009.0 Exercise machines primarily for cardiorespiratory conditioning
Elliptical and stepper machines
Stationary bike
Treadmill

E009.1 Calisthenics
Jumping jacks
Warm up and cool down

E009.2 Aerobic and step exercise

E009.3 Circuit training

E009.4 Obstacle course
Challenge course
Confidence course

E009.5 Grass drills
Guerilla drills

E009.9 Other activity involving cardiorespiratory exercise
> EXCLUDES   activities involving cardiorespiratory exercise specified in categories E001-E008

☑4ᵗʰ **E010 Activity involving other muscle strengthening exercises**

E010.0 Exercise machines primarily for muscle strengthening

E010.1 Push-ups, pull-ups, sit-ups

E010.2 Free weights
Barbells
Dumbbells

E010.3 Pilates

E010.9 Other activity involving other muscle strengthening exercises
> EXCLUDES   activities involving muscle strengthening specified in categories E001-E009

☑4ᵗʰ **E011 Activities involving computer technology and electronic devices**
> EXCLUDES   electronic musical keyboard or instruments (E018.0)

E011.0 Computer keyboarding
Electronic game playing using keyboard or other stationary device

E011.1 Hand held interactive electronic device
Cellular telephone and communication device
Electronic game playing using interactive device
> EXCLUDES   electronic game playing using keyboard or other stationary device (E011.0)

E011.9 Other activity involving computer technology and electronic devices

☑4ᵗʰ **E012 Activities involving arts and handcrafts**
> EXCLUDES   activities involving playing musical instrument (E018.0-E018.3)

E012.0 Knitting and crocheting

E012.1 Sewing

E012.2 Furniture building and finishing
Furniture repair

E012.9 Activity involving other arts and handcrafts

✓4ᵗʰ **E013 Activities involving personal hygiene and household maintenance**

> EXCLUDES   *activities involving cooking and grilling (E015.0-E015.9)*
> *activities involving property and land maintenance, building and construction (E016.0-E016.9)*
> *activity involving persons providing caregiving (E014.0-E014.9)*
> *dishwashing (E015.0)*
> *food preparation (E015.0)*
> *gardening (E016.1)*

E013.0 Personal bathing and showering

E013.1 Laundry

E013.2 Vacuuming

E013.3 Ironing

E013.4 Floor mopping and cleaning

E013.5 Residential relocation
> Packing up and unpacking involved in moving to a new residence

E013.8 Other personal hygiene activity

E013.9 Other household maintenance

✓4ᵗʰ **E014 Activities involving person providing caregiving**

E014.0 Caregiving involving bathing

E014.1 Caregiving involving lifting

E014.9 Other activity involving person providing caregiving

✓4ᵗʰ **E015 Activities involving food preparation, cooking and grilling**

E015.0 Food preparation and clean up
> Dishwasing

E015.1 Grilling and smoking food

E015.2 Cooking and baking
> Use of stove, oven and microwave oven

E015.9 Other activity involving cooking and grilling

✓4ᵗʰ **E016 Activities involving property and land maintenance, building and construction**

E016.0 Digging, shoveling and raking
> Dirt digging
> Raking leaves
> Snow shoveling

E016.1 Gardening and landscaping
> Pruning, trimming shrubs, weeding

E016.2 Building and construction

E016.9 Other activity involving property and land maintenance, building and construction

✓4ᵗʰ **E017 Activities involving roller coasters and other types of external motion**

E017.0 Roller coaster riding

E017.9 Other activity involving external motion

✓4ᵗʰ **E018 Activities involving playing musical instrument**
> Activity involving playing electric musical instrument

E018.0 Piano playing
> Musical keyboard (electronic) playing

E018.1 Drum and other percussion instrument playing

E018.2 String instrument playing

E018.3 Wind and brass instrument playing

✓4ᵗʰ **E019 Activities involving animal care**

> EXCLUDES   *horseback riding (E006.1)*

E019.0 Walking an animal

E019.1 Milking an animal

E019.2 Grooming and shearing an animal

E019.9 Other activity involving animal care

✓4ᵗʰ **E029 Other activity**

E029.0 Refereeing a sports activity

E029.1 Spectator at an event

E029.2 Rough housing and horseplay

E029.9 Other activity

E030 Unspecified activity

TRANSPORT ACCIDENTS (E800-E848)

DEFINITIONS AND EXAMPLES RELATED TO TRANSPORT ACCIDENTS

(a) A **transport accident** (E800-E848) is any accident involving a device designed primarily for, or being used at the time primarily for, conveying persons or goods from one place to another.

> INCLUDES   accidents involving:
> aircraft and spacecraft (E840-E845)
> watercraft (E830-E838)
> motor vehicle (E810-E825)
> railway (E800-E807)
> other road vehicles (E826-E829)

In classifying accidents which involve more than one kind of transport, the above order of precedence of transport accidents should be used.

Accidents involving agricultural and construction machines, such as tractors, cranes, and bulldozers, are regarded as transport accidents only when these vehicles are under their own power on a highway [otherwise the vehicles are regarded as machinery]. Vehicles which can travel on land or water, such as hovercraft and other amphibious vehicles, are regarded as watercraft when on the water, as motor vehicles when on the highway, and as off-road motor vehicles when on land, but off the highway.

> EXCLUDES   *accidents:*
> *in sports which involve the use of transport but where the transport vehicle itself was not involved in the accident*
> *involving vehicles which are part of industrial equipment used entirely on industrial premises*
> *occurring during transportation but unrelated to the hazards associated with the means of transportation [e.g., injuries received in a fight on board ship; transport vehicle involved in a cataclysm such as an earthquake]*
> *to persons engaged in the maintenance or repair of transport equipment or vehicle not in motion, unlesss injured by another vehicle in motion*

(b) A **railway accident** is a transport accident involving a railway train or other railway vehicle operated on rails, whether in motion or not.

> EXCLUDES   *accidents:*
> *in repair shops*
> *in roundhouse or on turntable*
> *on railway premises but not involving a train or other railway vehicle*

(c) A **railway train** or **railway vehicle** is any device with or without cars coupled to it, desiged for traffic on a railway.

> INCLUDES   interurban:
> electric car ⎫ (operated chiefly on its own
> street car   ⎬   right-of-way, not open to
>   ⎭   other traffic)
> railway train, any power [diesel] [electric] [steam]
> funicular
> monorail or two-rail
> subterranean or elevated
> other vehicle designed to run on a railway track
> EXCLUDES   *interurban electric cars [streetcars] specified to be operating on a right-of-way that forms part of the public street or highway [definition (h)]*

(d) A **railway** or **railroad** is a right-of-way designed for traffic on rails, which is used by carriages or wagons transporting passengers or freight, and by other rolling stock, and which is not open to other public vehicular traffic.

(e) A **motor vehicle accident** is a transport accident involving a motor vehicle. It is defined as a motor vehicle traffic accident or as a motor vehicle nontraffic accident according to whether the accident occurs on a public highway or elsewhere.

> EXCLUDES   *injury or damage due to cataclysm*
> *injury or damage while a motor vehicle, not under its own power, is being loaded on, or unloaded from, another conveyance*

(f) A **motor vehicle traffic accident** is any motor vehicle accident occurring on a public highway [i.e., originating, terminating, or involving a vehicle partially on the highway]. A motor vehicle accident is assumed to have occurred on the highway unless another place is specified, except in the case of accidents involving only off-road motor vehicles which are classified as nontraffic accidents unless the contrary is stated.

(g) A **motor vehicle nontraffic accident** is any motor vehicle accident which occurs entirely in any place other than a public highway.

(h) A **public highway [trafficway]** or **street** is the entire width between property lines [or other boundary lines] of every way or place, of which any part is open to the use of the public for purposes of vehicular traffic as a matter of right or custom. A **roadway** is that part of the public highway designed, improved, and ordinarily used, for vehicular travel.

> INCLUDES   approaches (public) to:
>   docks
>   public building
>   station
> EXCLUDES   driveway (private)
>   parking lot
>   ramp
>   roads in:
>   airfield
>   farm
>   industrial premises
>   mine
>   private grounds
>   quarry

(i) A **motor vehicle** is any mechanically or electrically powered device, not operated on rails, upon which any person or property may be transported or drawn upon a highway. Any object such as a trailer, coaster, sled, or wagon being towed by a motor vehicle is considered a part of the motor vehicle.

> INCLUDES   automobile [any type]
>   bus
>   construction machinery, farm and industrial machinery, steam roller, tractor, army tank, highway grader, or similar vehicle on wheels or treads, while in transport under own power
>   fire engine (motorized)
>   motorcycle
>   motorized bicycle [moped] or scooter
>   trolley bus not operating on rails
>   truck
>   van
> EXCLUDES   devices used solely to move persons or materials within the confines of a building and its premises, such as:
>   building elevator
>   coal car in mine
>   electric baggage or mail truck used solely within a railroad station
>   electric truck used solely within an industrial plant
>   moving overhead crane

(j) A **motorcycle** is a two-wheeled motor vehicle having one or two riding saddles and sometimes having a third wheel for the support of a sidecar. The sidecar is considered part of the motorcycle.

> INCLUDES   motorized:
>   bicycle [moped]
>   scooter
>   tricycle

(k) An **off-road motor vehicle** is a motor vehicle of special design, to enable it to negotiate rough or soft terrain or snow. Examples of special design are high construction, special wheels and tires, driven by treads, or support on a cushion of air.

> INCLUDES   all terrain vehicle [ATV]
>   army tank
>   hovercraft, on land or swamp
>   snowmobile

(l) A **driver** of a motor vehicle is the occupant of the motor vehicle operating it or intending to operate it. A **motorcyclist** is the driver of a motorcycle. Other authorized occupants of a motor vehicle are **passengers**.

(m) An **other road vehicle** is any device, except a motor vehicle, in, on, or by which any person or property may be transported on a highway.

> INCLUDES   animal carrying a person or goods
>   animal-drawn vehicles
>   animal harnessed to conveyance
>   bicycle [pedal cycle]
>   streetcar
>   tricycle (pedal)
> EXCLUDES   pedestrian conveyance [definition (q)]

(n) A **streetcar** is a device designed and used primarily for transporting persons within a municipality, running on rails, usually subject to normal traffic control signals, and operated principally on a right-of-way that forms part of the traffic way. A trailer being towed by a streetcar is considered a part of the streetcar.

> INCLUDES   interurban or intraurban electric or streetcar, when specified to be operating on a street or public highway
>   tram (car)
>   trolley (car)

(o) A **pedal cycle** is any road transport vehicle operated solely by pedals.

> INCLUDES   bicycle
>   pedal cycle
>   tricycle
> EXCLUDES   motorized bicycle [definition (j)]

(p) A **pedal cyclist** is any person riding on a pedal cycle or in a sidecar attached to such a vehicle.

(q) A **pedestrian conveyance** is any human powered device by which a pedestrian may move other than by walking or by which a walking person may move another pedestrian.

> INCLUDES   baby carriage
>   coaster wagon
>   heelies, wheelies
>   ice skates
>   motorized mobility scooter
>   perambulator
>   pushcart
>   pushchair
>   roller skates
>   scooter
>   skateboard
>   skis
>   sled
>   wheelchair (electric)

(r) A **pedestrian** is any person involved in an accident who was not at the time of the accident riding in or on a motor vehicle, railroad train, streetcar, animal-drawn or other vehicle, or on a bicycle or animal.

> INCLUDES   person:
>   changing tire of vehicle
>   in or operating a pedestrian conveyance
>   making adjustment to motor of vehicle
>   on foot

(s) A **watercraft** is any device for transporting passengers or goods on the water.

(t) A **small boat** is any watercraft propelled by paddle, oars, or small motor, with a passenger capacity of less than ten.

> INCLUDES   boat NOS
>   canoe
>   coble
>   dinghy
>   punt
>   raft
>   rowboat
>   rowing shell
>   scull
>   skiff
>   small motorboat
> EXCLUDES   barge
>   lifeboat (used after abandoning ship)
>   raft (anchored) being used as a diving platform
>   yacht

(u) An **aircraft** is any device for transporting passengers or goods in the air.

> **INCLUDES**   airplane [any type]
> balloon
> bomber
> dirigible
> glider (hang)
> military aircraft
> parachute

(v) A **commercial transport aircraft** is any device for collective passenger or freight transportation by air, whether run on commercial lines for profit or by government authorities, with the exception of military craft.

RAILWAY ACCIDENTS (E800-E807)

Note: For definitions of railway accident and related terms see definitions (a) to (d).

> **EXCLUDES**   accidents involving railway train and:
> aircraft (E840.0-E845.9)
> motor vehicle (E810.0-E825.9)
> watercraft (E830.0-E838.9)

The following fourth-digit subdivisions are for use with categories E800-E807 to identify the injured person:

.0   **Railway employee**
     Any person who by virtue of his employment in connection with a railway, whether by the railway company or not, is at increased risk of involvement in a railway accident, such as:
     catering staff of train
     driver
     guard
     porter
     postal staff on train
     railway fireman
     shunter
     sleeping car attendant

.1   **Passenger on railway**
     Any authorized person traveling on a train, except a railway employee.
     EXCLUDES   intending passenger waiting at station (.8)
               unauthorized rider on railway vehicle (.8)

.2   **Pedestrian**
     See definition (r)

.3   **Pedal cyclist**
     See definition (p)

.8   **Other specified person**
     Intending passenger or bystander waiting at station
     Unauthorized rider on railway vehicle

.9   **Unspecified person**

✓4ᵗʰ E800   Railway accident involving collision with rolling stock

> **INCLUDES**   collision between railway trains or railway vehicles, any kind
> collision NOS on railway
> derailment with antecedent collision with rolling stock or NOS

✓4ᵗʰ E801   Railway accident involving collision with other object

> **INCLUDES**   collision of railway train with:
> buffers
> fallen tree on railway
> gates
> platform
> rock on railway
> streetcar
> other nonmotor vehicle
> other object
>
> **EXCLUDES**   collision with:
> aircraft (E840.0-E842.9)
> motor vehicle (E810.0-E810.9, E820.0-E822.9)

✓4ᵗʰ E802   Railway accident involving derailment without antecedent collision

✓4ᵗʰ E803   Railway accident involving explosion, fire, or burning

> **EXCLUDES**   explosion or fire, with antecedent derailment (E802.0-E802.9)
> explosion or fire, with mention of antecedent collision (E800.0-E801.9)

✓4ᵗʰ E804   Fall in, on, or from railway train

> **INCLUDES**   fall while alighting from or boarding railway train
> **EXCLUDES**   fall related to collision, derailment, or explosion of railway train (E800.0-E803.9)

✓4ᵗʰ E805   Hit by rolling stock

> **INCLUDES**   crushed
> injured
> killed   } by railway train or part
> knocked down
> run over
>
> **EXCLUDES**   pedestrian hit by object set in motion by railway train (E806.0-E806.9)

✓4ᵗʰ E806   Other specified railway accident

> **INCLUDES**   hit by object falling in railway train
> injured by door or window on railway train
> nonmotor road vehicle or pedestrian hit by object set in motion by railway train
> railway train hit by falling:
>   earth NOS
>   rock
>   tree
>   other object
>
> **EXCLUDES**   railway accident due to cataclysm (E908-E909)

✓4ᵗʰ E807   Railway accident of unspecified nature

> **INCLUDES**   found dead
> injured   } on railway right-of-way NOS
> railway accident NOS

MOTOR VEHICLE TRAFFIC ACCIDENTS (E810-E819)

Note: For definitions of motor vehicle traffic accident, and related terms, see definitions (e) to (k).

> **EXCLUDES**   accidents involving motor vehicle and aircraft (E840.0-E845.9)

The following fourth-digit subdivisions are for use with categories E810-E819 to identify the injured person:

.0   **Driver of motor vehicle other than motorcycle**
     See definition (l)

.1   **Passenger in motor vehicle other than motorcycle**
     See definition (l)

.2   **Motorcyclist**
     See definition (l)

.3   **Passenger on motorcycle**
     See definition (l)

.4   **Occupant of streetcar**

.5   **Rider of animal; occupant of animal-drawn vehicle**

.6   **Pedal cyclist**
     See definition (p)

.7   **Pedestrian**
     See definition (r)

.8   **Other specified person**
     Occupant of vehicle other than above
     Person in railway train involved in accident
     Unauthorized rider of motor vehicle

.9   **Unspecified person**

✓4ᵗʰ E810   Motor vehicle traffic accident involving collision with train

> **EXCLUDES**   motor vehicle collision with object set in motion by railway train (E815.0-E815.9)
> railway train hit by object set in motion by motor vehicle (E818.0-E818.9)

✓4ᵗʰ E811   Motor vehicle traffic accident involving re-entrant collision with another motor vehicle

> **INCLUDES**   collision between motor vehicle which accidentally leaves the roadway then re-enters the same roadway, or the opposite roadway on a divided highway, and another motor vehicle
>
> **EXCLUDES**   collision on the same roadway when none of the motor vehicles involved have left and re-entered the highway (E812.0-E812.9)

E Codes

E812–E819

✓4ᵗʰ **E812 Other motor vehicle traffic accident involving collision with motor vehicle**

  INCLUDES   collision with another motor vehicle parked, stopped, stalled, disabled, or abandoned on the highway
           motor vehicle collision NOS

  EXCLUDES   *collision with object set in motion by another motor vehicle (E815.0-E815.9)*
           re-entrant collision with another motor vehicle (E811.0-E811.9)

✓4ᵗʰ **E813 Motor vehicle traffic accident involving collision with other vehicle**

  INCLUDES   collision between motor vehicle, any kind, and:
           other road (nonmotor transport) vehicle, such as:
              animal carrying a person
              animal-drawn vehicle
              pedal cycle
              streetcar

  EXCLUDES   *collision with:*
           object set in motion by nonmotor road vehicle (E815.0-E815.9)
           pedestrian (E814.0-E814.9)
           nonmotor road vehicle hit by object set in motion by motor vehicle (E818.0-E818.9)

✓4ᵗʰ **E814 Motor vehicle traffic accident involving collision with pedestrian**

  INCLUDES   collision between motor vehicle, any kind, and pedestrian
           pedestrian dragged, hit, or run over by motor vehicle, any kind

  EXCLUDES   *pedestrian hit by object set in motion by motor vehicle (E818.0-E818.9)*

✓4ᵗʰ **E815 Other motor vehicle traffic accident involving collision on the highway**

  INCLUDES   collision (due to loss of control) (on highway) between motor vehicle, any kind, and:
           abutment (bridge) (overpass)
           animal (herded) (unattended)
           fallen stone, traffic sign, tree, utility pole
           guard rail or boundary fence
           interhighway divider
           landslide (not moving)
           object set in motion by railway train or road vehicle (motor) (nonmotor)
           object thrown in front of motor vehicle
           other object, fixed, movable, or moving
           safety island
           temporary traffic sign or marker
           wall of cut made for road

  EXCLUDES   *collision with:*
           any object off the highway (resulting from loss of control) (E816.0-E816.9)
           any object which normally would have been off the highway and is not stated to have been on it (E816.0-E816.9)
           motor vehicle parked, stopped, stalled, disabled, or abandoned on highway (E812.0-E812.9)
           moving landslide (E909)
           motor vehicle hit by object:
           set in motion by railway train or road vehicle (motor) (nonmotor) (E818.0-E818.9)
           thrown into or on vehicle (E818.0-E818.9)

✓4ᵗʰ **E816 Motor vehicle traffic accident due to loss of control, without collision on the highway**

  INCLUDES   motor vehicle:
           failing to make curve
           going out of control (due to):
              blowout
              burst tire
              driver falling asleep
              drive inattention
              excessive speed
              failure of mechanical part
        and:
           coliding with object off the highway
           overturning
           stopping abruptly off the highway

  EXCLUDES   *collision on highway following loss of control (E810.0-E815.9)*
           loss of control of motor vehicle following collision on the highway (E810.0-E815.9)

✓4ᵗʰ **E817 Noncollision motor vehicle traffic accident while boarding or alighting**

  INCLUDES   fall down stairs of motor bus
           fall from car in street
           injured by moving part of the vehicle
           trapped by door of motor bus
        while boarding or alighting

✓4ᵗʰ **E818 Other noncollision motor vehicle traffic accident**

  INCLUDES   accidental poisoning from exhaust gas generated by
           breakage of any part of
           explosion of any part of
           fall, jump, or being accidentally pushed from
           fire starting in
           hit by object thrown into or on
           injured by being thrown against some part of, or object in
           injury from moving part of
           object falling in or on
           object thrown on
        motor vehicle while in motion

           collision of railway train or road vehicle except motor vehicle, with object set in motion by motor vehicle
           motor vehicle hit by object set in motion by railway train or road vehicle (motor) (nonmotor)
           pedestrian, railway train, or road vehicle (motor) (nonmotor) hit by object set in motion by motor vehicle

  EXCLUDES   *collision between motor vehicle and:*
           object set in motion by railway train or road vehicle (motor) (nonmotor) (E815.0-E815.9)
           object thrown towards the motor vehicle (E815.0-E815.9)
           person overcome by carbon monoxide generated by stationary motor vehicle off the roadway with motor running (E868.2)

✓4ᵗʰ **E819 Motor vehicle traffic accident of unspecified nature**

  INCLUDES   motor vehicle traffic accident NOS
           traffic accident NOS

MOTOR VEHICLE NONTRAFFIC ACCIDENTS (E820-E825)

Note: For definitions of motor vehicle nontraffic accident and related terms see definition (a) to (k).

INCLUDES accidents involving motor vehicles being used in recreational or sporting activities off the highway

collision and noncollision motor vehicle acci- dents occurring entirely off the highway

EXCLUDES *accidents involving motor vehicle and:*
aircraft (E840.0-E845.9)
watercraft (E830.0-E838.9)
accidents, not on the public highway, involving agricultural and construction machinery but not involving another motor vehicle (E919.0, E919.2, E919.7)

The following fourth-digit subdivisions are for use with categories E820-E825 to identify the injured person:

.0 Driver of motor vehicle other than motorcycle
See definition (l)
.1 Passenger in motor vehicle other than motorcycle
See definition (l)
.2 Motorcyclist
See definition (l)
.3 Passenger on motorcycle
See definition (l)
.4 Occupant of streetcar
.5 Rider of animal; occupant of animal-drawn vehicle
.6 Pedal cyclist
See definition (p)
.7 Pedestrian
See definition (r)
.8 Other specified person
Occupant of vehicle other than above
Person in railway train involved in accident
Unauthorized rider of motor vehicle
.9 Unspecified person

✓4ᵗʰ E820 Nontraffic accident involving motor-driven snow vehicle

INCLUDES breakage of part of
fall from
hit by } motor-driven snow vehicle (not on public highway)
overturning of
run over or dragged by

collision of motor-driven snow vehicle with:
animal (being ridden) (-drawn vehicle)
another off-road motor vehicle
other motor vehicle, not on public highway
railway train
other object, fixed or movable
injury caused by rough landing of motor-driven snow vehicle (after leaving ground on rough terrain)

EXCLUDES *accident on the public highway involving motor driven snow vehicle (E810.0-E819.9)*

✓4ᵗʰ E821 Nontraffic accident involving other off-road motor vehicle

INCLUDES breakage of part of
fall from
hit by
overturning of } off-road motorvehicle except snow vehicle (not on public highway)
run over or dragged by
thrown against some part of or object in

collision with:
animal (being ridden) (-drawn vehicle)
another off-road motor vehicle, except snow vehicle
other motor vehicle, not on public highway
other object, fixed or movable

EXCLUDES *accident on public highway involving off-road motor vehicle (E810.0-E819.9)*
collision between motor driven snow vehicle and other off-road motor vehicle (E820.0-E820.9)
hovercraft accident on water (E830.0-E838.9)

✓4ᵗʰ E822 Other motor vehicle nontraffic accident involving collision with moving object

INCLUDES collision, not on public highway, between motor vehicle, except off-road motor vehicle and:
animal
nonmotor vehicle
other motor vehicle, except off-road motor vehicle
pedestrian
railway train
other moving object

EXCLUDES *collision with:*
motor-driven snow vehicle (E820.0-E820.9)
other off-road motor vehicle (E821.0-E821.9)

✓4ᵗʰ E823 Other motor vehicle nontraffic accident involving collision with stationary object

INCLUDES collision, not on public highway, between motor vehicle, except off-road motor vehicle, and any object, fixed or movable, but not in motion

✓4ᵗʰ E824 Other motor vehicle nontraffic accident while boarding and alighting

INCLUDES
fall
injury from oving part of motor vehicle } while boarding or alighting from motor vehicle, except off-road motor vehicle, not on public highway
trapped by door of motor vehhicle

✓4ᵗʰ E825 Other motor vehicle nontraffic accident of other and unspecified nature

INCLUDES accidental poisoning from carbon monoxide generated by
breakage of any part of
explosion of any part of
fall, jump, or being accidentally pushed from
fire starting in } motor vehicle while in motion, not on public highway
hit by object thrown into, towards, or on
injured by being thrown against some part of, or object in
injury from moving part of
object falling in or on

motor vehicle nontraffic accident NOS

EXCLUDES *fall from or in stationary motor vehicle (E884.9, E885.9)*
overcome by carbon monoxide or exhaust gas generated by stationary motor vehicle off the roadway with motor running (E868.2)
struck by falling object from or in stationary motor vehicle (E916)

OTHER ROAD VEHICLE ACCIDENTS (E826-E829)

Note: Other road vehicle accidents are transport accidents involving road vehicles other than motor vehicles. For definitions of other road vehicle and related terms see definitions (m) to (o).

INCLUDES accidents involving other road vehicles being used in recreational or sporting activities

EXCLUDES *collision of other road vehicle [any] with:*
aircraft (E840.0-E845.9)
motor vehicle (E813.0-E813.9, E820.0-E822.9)
railway train (E801.0-E801.9))

The following fourth-digit subdivisions are for use with categories E826-E829 to identify the injured person:
.0 Pedestrian
    See definition (r)
.1 Pedal cyclist
    See definition (p)
.2 Rider of animal
.3 Occupant of animal-drawn vehicle
.4 Occupant of streetcar
.8 Other specified person
.9 Unspecified person

✓4ᵗʰ E826 Pedal cycle accident

[0-9]   **INCLUDES**   breakage of any part of pedal cycle
collision between pedal cycle and:
    animal (being ridden) (herded) (unattended)
    another pedal cycle
    any pedestrian
    nonmotor road vehicle
    other object, fixed, movable, or moving, not set in
        motion by motor vehicle, railway train,
        or aircraft
entanglement in wheel of pedal cycle
fall from pedal cycle
hit by object falling or thrown on the pedal cycle
pedal cycle accident NOS
pedal cycle overturned

✓4ᵗʰ E827 Animal-drawn vehicle accident

[0,2,4,8,9] **INCLUDES** breakage of any part of vehicle
collision between animal-drawn vehicle and:
    animal (being ridden) (herded) (unattended)
    nonmotor road vehicle, except pedal cycle
    pedestrian, pedestrian conveyance, or pedestrian
        vehicle
    other object, fixed, movable, or moving, not set in
        motion by motor vehicle, railway train,
        or aircraft

fall from   ⎫
knocked down by   ⎬ animal drawn vehicle
overturning of   ⎪
running over by   ⎪
thrown from   ⎭

EXCLUDES *collision of animal-drawn vehicle with pedal cycle*
(E826.0-E826.9)

✓4ᵗʰ E828 Accident involving animal being ridden

[0,2,4,8,9] **INCLUDES** collision between animal being ridden and:
    another animal
    nonmotor road vehicle, except pedal cycle, and
        animal-drawn vehicle
    pedestrian, pedestrian conveyance, or pedestrian
        vehicle
    other object, fixed, movable, or moving, not set in
        motion by motor vehicle, railway train,
        or aircraft

fall from   ⎫
knocked down by   ⎬ animal being ridden
thrown from   ⎪
trampled by   ⎭

ridden animal stumbled and fell

EXCLUDES *collision of animal being ridden with:*
animal-drawn vehicle (E827.0-E827.9)
pedal cycle (E826.0-E826.9)

✓4ᵗʰ E829 Other road vehicle accidents

[0,4,8,9]   **INCLUDES**   accident while boarding or   ⎫
    alighting from   ⎪ streetcar
blow from object in   ⎬ nonmotor road
breakage of any part of   ⎪ vehicle not
caught in door of   ⎪ classifiable to
derailment of   ⎪ E826-E828
fall in, on, or from   ⎪
fire in   ⎭
collision between streetcar or nonmotor road vehi-
    cle, except as in E826-E828, and:
    animal (not being ridden)
    another nonmotor road vehicle not classifiable to
        E826-E828
    pedestrian
    other object, fixed, movable, or moving, not set in
        motion by motor vehicle, railway train,
        or aircraft
nonmotor road vehicle accident NOS
streetcar accident NOS

EXCLUDES *collision with:*
animal being ridden (E828.0-E828.9)
animal-drawn vehicle (E827.0-E827.9)
pedal cycle (E826.0-E826.9)

WATER TRANSPORT ACCIDENTS (E830-E838)

Note: For definitions of water transport accident and related terms see definitions (a), (s), and (t).

INCLUDES watercraft accidents in the course of recreational activities

EXCLUDES *accidents involving both aircraft, including objects set in motion by aircraft, and watercraft (E840.0-E845.9)*

The following fourth-digit subdivisions are for use with categories E830-E838 to identify the injured person:
.0 **Occupant of small boat, unpowered**
.1 **Occupant of small boat, powered**
    See definition (t)
    EXCLUDES *water skier (.4)*
.2 **Occupant of other watercraft – crew**
    Persons:
        engaged in operation of watercraft
        providing passenger services [cabin attendants,
            ship's physician, catering personnel]
        working on ship during voyage in other capacity
            [musician in band, operators of shops and
            beauty parlors
.3 **Occupant of other watercraft – other than crew**
    Passenger
    Occupant of lifeboat, other than crew, after
        abandoning ship
.4 **Water skier**
.5 **Swimmer**
.6 **Dockers, stevedores**
    Longshoreman employed on the dock in loading and
        unloading ships
.7 **Occupant of military watercraft, any type**
.8 **Other specified person**
    Immigration and custom officials on board ship
    Person:
        accompanying passenger or member of crew
        visiting boat
    Pilot (guiding ship into port)
.9 **Unspecified person**

✓4ᵗʰ E830 Accident to watercraft causing submersion

INCLUDES submersion and drowning due to:
    boat overturning
    boat submerging
    falling or jumping from burning ship
    falling or jumping from crushed watercraft
    ship sinking
    other accident to watercraft

☑4ᵗʰ **E831 Accident to watercraft causing other injury**

INCLUDES any injury, except submersion and drowning, as a result of an accident to watercraft
burned while ship on fire
crushed between ships in collision
crushed by lifeboat after abandoning ship
fall due to collision or other accident to watercraft
hit by falling object due to accident to watercraft
injured in watercraft accident involving collision
struck by boat or part thereof after fall or jump from damaged boat

EXCLUDES *burns from localized fire or explosion on board ship (E837.0-E837.9)*

☑4ᵗʰ **E832 Other accidental submersion or drowning in water transport accident**

INCLUDES submersion or drowning as a result of an accident other than accident to the watercraft, such as:
fall:
from gangplank
from ship
overboard
thrown overboard by motion of ship
washed overboard

EXCLUDES *submersion or drowning of swimmer or diver who voluntarily jumps from boat not involved in an accident (E910.0-E910.9)*

☑4ᵗʰ **E833 Fall on stairs or ladders in water transport**

EXCLUDES *fall due to accident to watercraft (E831.0-E831.9)*

☑4ᵗʰ **E834 Other fall from one level to another in water transport**

EXCLUDES *fall due to accident to watercraft (E831.0-E831.9)*

☑4ᵗʰ **E835 Other and unspecified fall in water transport**

EXCLUDES *fall due to accident to watercraft (E831.0-E831.9)*

☑4ᵗʰ **E836 Machinery accident in water transport**

INCLUDES injuries in water transport caused by:
deck
engine room
galley } machinery
laundry
loading

☑4ᵗʰ **E837 Explosion, fire, or burning in watercraft**

INCLUDES explosion of boiler on steamship
localized fire on ship

EXCLUDES *burning ship (due to collision or explosion) resulting in:*
submersion or drowning (E830.0-E830.9)
other injury (E831.0-E831.9)

☑4ᵗʰ **E838 Other and unspecified water transport accident**

INCLUDES accidental poisoning by gases or fumes on ship
atomic power plant malfunction in watercraft
crushed between ship and stationary object [wharf]
crushed between ships without accident to watercraft
crushed by falling object on ship or while loading or unloading
hit by boat while water skiing
struck by boat or part thereof (after fall from boat)
watercraft accident NOS

AIR AND SPACE TRANSPORT ACCIDENTS (E840-E845)

Note: For definition of aircraft and related terms see definitions (u) and (v).

The following fourth-digit subdivisions are for use with categories E840-E845 to identify the injured person. Valid fourth digits are in [brackets] under codes E842-E845:

.0 Occupant of spacecraft

.1 Occupant of military aircraft, any
Crew in military aircraft [air force] [army] [national guard] [navy]
Passenger (civilian) (military) in military aircraft [air force] [army] [national guard] [navy]
Troops in military aircraft [air force] [army] [national guard] [navy]
EXCLUDES *occupants of aircraft operated under jurisdiction of police departments (.5)*
parachutist (.7)

.2 Crew of commercial aircraft (powered) in surface to surface transport

.3 Other occupant of commercial aircraft (powered) in surface to surface transport
Flight personnel:
not part of crew
on familiarization flight
Passenger on aircraft (powered) NOS

.4 Occupant of commercial aircraft (powered) in surface to air transport
Occupant [crew] [passenger] of aircraft (powered) engaged in activities, such as:
aerial spraying (crops) (fire retardants)
air drops of emergency supplies
air drops of parachutists, except from military craft
crop dusting
lowering of construction material [bridge or telephone pole]
sky writing

.5 Occupant of other powered aircraft
Occupant [crew] [passenger] of aircraft (powered) engaged in activities, such as:
aerobatic flying
aircraft racing
rescue operation
storm surveillance
traffic surveillance
Occupant of private plane NOS

.6 Occupant of unpowered aircraft, except parachutist
Occupant of aircraft classifiable to E842

.7 Parachutist (military) (other)
Person making voluntary descent
EXCLUDES *person making descent after accident to aircraft (.1-.6)*

.8 Ground crew, airline employee
Persons employed at airfields (civil) (military) or launching pads, not occupants of aircraft

.9 Other person

☑4ᵗʰ **E840 Accident to powered aircraft at takeoff or landing**

INCLUDES collision of aircraft with any object, fixed, movable, or moving
crash
explosion on aircraft } while taking off or landing
fire on aircraft
forced landing

☑4ᵗʰ **E841 Accident to powered aircraft, other and unspecified**

INCLUDES aircraft accident NOS
aircraft crash or wreck NOS
any accident to powered aircraft while in transit or when not specified whether in transit, taking off, or landing
collision of aircraft with another aircraft, bird, or any object, while in transit
explosion on aircraft while in transit
fire on aircraft while in transit

E Codes

E842–E849.5

☑4ᵗʰ **E842 Accident to unpowered aircraft**
[6-9] INCLUDES any accident, except collision with powered aircraft, to:
balloon
glider
hang glider
kite carrying a person
hit by object falling from unpowered aircraft

☑4ᵗʰ **E843 Fall in, on, or from aircraft**
[0-9] INCLUDES accident in boarding or alighting from aircraft, any kind
fall in, on, or from aircraft [any kind], while in transit, taking off, or landing, except when as a result of an accident to aircraft

☑4ᵗʰ **E844 Other specified air transport accidents**
[0-9] INCLUDES hit by:
aircraft
object falling from aircraft
injury by or from:
machinery of aircraft   }
rotating propellar   } without accident
voluntary parachute descent } to aircraft
poisoning by carbon monoxide
from aircraft while in transit
sucked into jet

any accident involving other transport vehicle (motor) (nonmotor) due to being hit by object set in motion by aircraft (powered)
EXCLUDES air sickness (E903)
effects of:
high altitude (E902.0-E902.1)
pressure change (E902.0-E902.1)
injury in parachute descent due to accident to aircraft (E840.0-E842-9)

☑4ᵗʰ **E845 Accident involving spacecraft**
[0,8,9] INCLUDES launching pad accident
EXCLUDES effects of weightlessness in spacecraft (E928.0)

VEHICLE ACCIDENTS NOT ELSEWHERE CLASSIFIABLE (E846-E848)

E846 Accidents involving powered vehicles used solely within the buildings and premises of industrial or commercial establishment
Accident to, on, or involving:
battery powered airport passenger vehicle
battery powered trucks (baggage) (mail)
coal car in mine
logging car
self propelled truck, industrial
station baggage truck (powered)
tram, truck, or tub (powered) in mine or quarry
Collision with:
pedestrian
other vehicle or object within premises
Explosion of
Fall from   } powered vehicle, industrial or
Overturning of } commercial
Struck by
EXCLUDES accidental poisoning by exhaust gas from vehicle not elsewhere classifiable (E868.2)
injury by crane, lift (fork), or elevator (E919.2)

E847 Accidents involving cable cars not running on rails
Accident to, on, or involving:
cable car, not on rails
ski chair-lift
ski-lift with gondola
téléférique
Breakage of cable
Caught or dragged by   }
Fall or jump from   } cable car, not on rails
Object thrown from or in }

E848 Accidents involving other vehicles, not elsewhere classifiable
Accident to, on, or involving:
ice yacht
land yacht
nonmotor, nonroad vehicle NOS

PLACE OF OCCURRENCE (E849)

☑4ᵗʰ **E849 Place of occurrence**
Note: The following category is for use to denote the place where the injury or poisoning occurred.

E849.0 Home
Apartment
Boarding house
Farm house
Home premises
House (residential)
Noninstitutional place of residence
Private:
driveway
garage
garden
home
walk
Swimming pool in private house or garden
Yard of home
EXCLUDES home under construction but not yet occupied (E849.3)
institutional place of residence (E849.7)

E849.1 Farm
Farm:
buildings
land under cultivation
EXCLUDES farm house and home premises of farm (E849.0)

E849.2 Mine and quarry
Gravel pit
Sand pit
Tunnel under construction

E849.3 Industrial place and premises
Building under construction
Dockyard
Dry dock
Factory
building
premises
Garage (place of work)
Industrial yard
Loading platform (factory) (store)
Plant, industrial
Railway yard
Shop (place of work)
Warehouse
Workhouse

E849.4 Place for recreation and sport
Amusement park   Playground, including school
Baseball field   playground
Basketball court   Public park
Beach resort   Racecourse
Cricket ground   Resort NOS
Fives court   Riding school
Football field   Rifle range
Golf course   Seashore resort
Gymnasium   Skating rink
Hockey field   Sports palace
Holiday camp   Stadium
Ice palace   Swimming pool, public
Lake resort   Tennis court
Mountain resort   Vacation resort
EXCLUDES that in private house or garden (E849.0)

E849.5 Street and highway

E849.6 Public building

> *Building (including adjacent grounds) used by the general*
> > *public or by a particular group of the public, such as:*
> > *airport*
> > *bank*
> > *café*
> > *casino*
> > *church*
> > *cinema*
> > *clubhouse*
> > *courthouse*
> > *dance hall*
> > *garage building (for car storage)*
> > *hotel*
> > *market (grocery or other commodity)*
> > *movie house*
> > *music hall*
> > *nightclub*
> > *office*
> > *office building*
> > *opera house*
> > *post office*
> > *public hall*
> > *radio broadcasting station*
> > *restaurant*
> > *school (state) (public) (private)*
> > *shop, commercial*
> > *station (bus) (railway)*
> > *store*
> > *theater*

> EXCLUDES   *home garage (E849.0)*
> > *industrial building or workplace (E849.3)*

E849.7 Residential institution

> *Children's home*
> *Dormitory*
> *Hospital*
> *Jail*
> *Old people's home*
> *Orphanage*
> *Prison*
> *Reform school*

E849.8 Other specified places

Beach NOS	*Pond or pool (natural)*
Canal	*Prairie*
Caravan site NOS	*Public place NOS*
Derelict house	*Railway line*
Desert	*Reservoir*
Dock	*River*
Forest	*Sea*
Harbor	*Seashore NOS*
Hill	*Stream*
Lake NOS	*Swamp*
Mountain	*Trailer court*
Parking lot	*Woods*
Parking place	

E849.9 Unspecified place

ACCIDENTAL POISONING BY DRUGS, MEDICINAL SUBSTANCES, AND BIOLOGICALS (E850-E858)

INCLUDES   accidental overdose of drug, wrong drug given or
> taken in error, and drug taken inadvertently
> accidents in the use of drugs and biologicals in medi-
> cal and surgical procedures

EXCLUDES   *administration with suicidal or homicidal intent or*
> *intent to harm, or in circumstances classifiable to*
> *E980-E989 (E950.0-E950.5, E962.0,*
> *E980.0-E980.5)*
> *correct drug properly administered in therapeutic or*
> *prophylactic dosage, as the cause of adverse*
> *effect (E930.0-E949.9)*

Note: See Alphabetic Index for more complete list of specific
drugs to be classified under the fourth-digit subdivisions.
The American Hospital Formulary numbers can be used to
classify new drugs listed by the American Hospital
Formulary Service (AHFS). See Appendix C.

✓4ᵗʰ **E850 Accidental poisoning by analgesics, antipyretics, and antirheumatics**

E850.0 Heroin
> Diacetylmorphine

E850.1 Methadone

E850.2 Other opiates and related narcotics
> Codeine [methylmorphine]
> Meperidine [pethidine]
> Morphine
> Opium (alkaloids)

E850.3 Salicylates
> Acetylsalicylic acid [aspirin]
> Amino derivatives of salicylic acid
> Salicylic acid salts

E850.4 Aromatic analgesics, not elsewhere classified
> Acetanilid
> Paracetamol [acetaminophen]
> Phenacetin [acetophenetidin]

E850.5 Pyrazole derivatives
> Aminophenazone [amidopyrine]
> Phenylbutazone

E850.6 Antirheumatics [antiphlogistics]
> Gold salts
> Indomethacin
> > EXCLUDES   *salicylates (E850.3)*
> > *steroids (E858.0)*

E850.7 Other non-narcotic analgesics
> Pyrabital

E850.8 Other specified analgesics and antipyretics
> Pentazocine

E850.9 Unspecified analgesic or antipyretic

E851 Accidental poisoning by barbiturates
> Amobarbital [amylobarbitone]
> Barbital [barbitone]
> Butabarbital [butabarbitone]
> Pentobarbital [pentobarbitone]
> Phenobarbital [phenobarbitone]
> Secobarbital [quinalbarbitone]
> > EXCLUDES   *thiobarbiturates (E855.1)*

✓4ᵗʰ **E852 Accidental poisoning by other sedatives and hypnotics**

E852.0 Chloral hydrate group

E852.1 Paraldehyde

E852.2 Bromine compounds
> Bromides
> Carbromal (derivatives)

E852.3 Methaqualone compounds

E852.4 Glutethimide group

E852.5 Mixed sedatives, not elsewhere classified

E852.8 Other specified sedatives and hypnotics

E852.9 Unspecified sedative or hypnotic
> Sleeping:
> > drug
> > pill } NOS
> > tablet

✓4ᵗʰ **E853 Accidental poisoning by tranquilizers**

E853.0 Phenothiazine-based tranquilizers

Chlorpromazine	Prochlorperazine
Fluphenazine	Promazine

E853.1 Butyrophenone-based tranquilizers

Haloperidol	Trifluperidol
Spiperone	

E853.2 Benzodiazepine-based tranquilizers

Chlordiazepoxide	Lorazepam
Diazepam	Medazepam
Flurazepam	Nitrazepam

E853.8 Other specified tranquilizers

Hydroxyzine	Meprobamate

E853.9 Unspecified tranquilizer

☑4ᵗʰ **E854 Accidental poisoning by other psychotropic agents**

E854.0 Antidepressants
    Amitriptyline
    Imipramine
    Monoamine oxidase [MAO] inhibitors

E854.1 Psychodysleptics [hallucinogens]
Cannabis derivatives	Mescaline
Lysergide [LSD]	Psilocin
Marihuana (derivatives)	Psilocybin

E854.2 Psychostimulants
    Amphetamine
    Caffeine

> **EXCLUDES** *central appetite depressants (E858.8)*

E854.3 Central nervous system stimulants
    Analeptics
    Opiate antagonists

E854.8 Other psychotropic agents

☑4ᵗʰ **E855 Accidental poisoning by other drugs acting on central and autonomic nervous system**

E855.0 Anticonvulsant and anti-Parkinsonism drugs
    Amantadine
    Hydantoin derivatives
    Levodopa [L-dopa]
    Oxazolidine derivatives [paramethadione]
        [trimethadione]
    Succinimides

E855.1 Other central nervous system depressants
    Ether
    Gaseous anesthetics
    Halogenated hydrocarbon derivatives
    Intravenous anesthetics
    Thiobarbiturates, such as thiopental sodium

E855.2 Local anesthetics
Cocaine	Procaine
Lidocaine [lignocaine]	Tetracaine

E855.3 Parasympathomimetics [cholinergics]
Acetylcholine	Anticholinesterase:
Anticholinesterase:	reversible
organophosphorus	Pilocarpine

E855.4 Parasympatholytics [anticholinergics and antimuscarinics] and spasmolytics
Atropine	Hyoscine [scopolamine]
Homatropine	Quaternary ammonium
	derivatives

E855.5 Sympathomimetics [adrenergics]
    Epinephrine [adrenalin]
    Levarterenol [noradrenalin]

E855.6 Sympatholytics [antiadrenergics]
    Phenoxybenzamine
    Tolazoline hydrochloride

E855.8 Other specified drugs acting on central and autonomic nervous systems

E855.9 Unspecified drug acting on central and autonomic nervous systems

E856 Accidental poisoning by antibiotics

E857 Accidental poisoning by other anti-infectives

☑4ᵗʰ **E858 Accidental poisoning by other drugs**

E858.0 Hormones and synthetic substitutes

E858.1 Primarily systemic agents

E858.2 Agents primarily affecting blood constituents

E858.3 Agents primarily affecting cardiovascular system

E858.4 Agents primarily affecting gastrointestinal system

E858.5 Water, mineral, and uric acid metabolism drugs

E858.6 Agents primarily acting on the smooth and skeletal muscles and respiratory system

E858.7 Agents primarily affecting skin and mucous membrane, ophthalmological, otorhinolaryngological, and dental drugs

E858.8 Other specified drugs
    Central appetite depressants

E858.9 Unspecified drug

ACCIDENTAL POISONING BY OTHER SOLID AND LIQUID SUBSTANCES, GASES, AND VAPORS (E860-E869)

Note: Categories in this section are intended primarily to indicate the external cause of poisoning states classifiable to 980-989. They may also be used to indicate external causes of localized effects classifiable to 001-799.

☑4ᵗʰ **E860 Accidental poisoning by alcohol, not elsewhere classified**

E860.0 Alcoholic beverages
    Alcohol in preparations intended for consumption

E860.1 Other and unspecified ethyl alcohol and its products
Denatured alcohol	Grain alcohol NOS
Ethanol NOS	Methylated spirit

E860.2 Methyl alcohol
Methanol	Wood alcohol

E860.3 Isopropyl alcohol
Dimethyl carbinol	Rubbing alcohol subsitute
Isopropanol	Secondary propyl alcohol

E860.4 Fusel oil
Alcohol:	Alcohol:
amyl	propyl
butyl	

E860.8 Other specified alcohols

E860.9 Unspecified alcohol

☑4ᵗʰ **E861 Accidental poisoning by cleansing and polishing agents, disinfectants, paints, and varnishes**

E861.0 Synthetic detergents and shampoos

E861.1 Soap products

E861.2 Polishes

E861.3 Other cleansing and polishing agents
    Scouring powders

E861.4 Disinfectants
    Household and other disinfectants not ordinarily used on the person

> **EXCLUDES** *carbolic acid or phenol (E864.0)*

E861.5 Lead paints

E861.6 Other paints and varnishes
Lacquers	Paints, other than lead
Oil colors	White washes

E861.9 Unspecified

☑4ᵗʰ **E862 Accidental poisoning by petroleum products, other solvents and their vapors, not elsewhere classified**

E862.0 Petroleum solvents
Petroleum:	Petroleum:
ether	naphtha
benzine	

E862.1 Petroleum fuels and cleaners
Antiknock additives	Gasoline or petrol
to petroleum fuels	Kerosene
Gas oils	

> **EXCLUDES** *kerosene insecticides (E863.4)*

E862.2 Lubricating oils

E862.3 Petroleum solids
    Paraffin wax

E862.4 Other specified solvents
    Benzene

E862.9 Unspecified solvent

☑4ᵗʰ **E863 Accidental poisoning by agricultural and horticultural chemical and pharmaceutical preparations other than plant foods and fertilizers**

> **EXCLUDES** *plant foods and fertilizers (E866.5)*

E863.0 Insecticides of organochlorine compounds

Benzene hexachloride	Dieldrin
Chlordane	Endrine
DDT	Toxaphene

E863.1 Insecticides of organophosphorus compounds

Demeton	Parathion
Diazinon	Phenylsulphthion
Dichlorvos	Phorate
Malathion	Phosdrin
Methyl parathion	

E863.2 Carbamates

Aldicarb	Propoxur
Carbaryl	

E863.3 Mixtures of insecticides

E863.4 Other and unspecified insecticides
Kerosene insecticides

E863.5 Herbicides
2, 4-Dichlorophenoxyacetic acid [2, 4-D]
2, 4, 5-Trichlorophenoxyacetic acid [2, 4, 5-T]
Chlorates
Diquat
Mixtures of plant foods and fertilizers with herbicides
Paraquat

E863.6 Fungicides
Organic mercurials (used in seed dressing)
Pentachlorophenols

E863.7 Rodenticides

Fluoroacetates	Warfarin
Squill and derivatives	Zinc phosphide
Thallium	

E863.8 Fumigants

Cyanides	Phosphine
Methyl bromide	

E863.9 Other and unspecified

✓4ᵗʰ **E864 Accidental poisoning by corrosives and caustics, not elsewhere classified**
     EXCLUDES *those as components of disinfectants (E861.4)*

E864.0 Corrosive aromatics
Carbolic acid or phenol

E864.1 Acids

Acid:	Acid:
hydrochloric	sulfuric
nitric	

E864.2 Caustic alkalis
Lye

E864.3 Other specified corrosives and caustics

E864.4 Unspecified corrosives and caustics

✓4ᵗʰ **E865 Accidental poisoning from poisonous foodstuffs and poisonous plants**
     INCLUDES *any meat, fish, or shellfish*
               plants, berries, and fungi eaten as, or in mistake for, food, or by a child
     EXCLUDES *anaphylactic shock due to adverse food reaction (995.60-995.69)*
               food poisoning (bacterial) (005.0-005.9)
               poisoning and toxic reactions to venomous plants (E905.6-E905.7)

E865.0 Meat

E865.1 Shellfish

E865.2 Other fish

E865.3 Berries and seeds

E865.4 Other specified plants

E865.5 Mushrooms and other fungi

E865.8 Other specified foods

E865.9 Unspecified foodstuff or poisonous plant

✓4ᵗʰ **E866 Accidental poisoning by other and unspecified solid and liquid substances**
     EXCLUDES *these substances as a component of:*
               medicines (E850.0-E858.9)
               paints (E861.5-E861.6)
               pesticides (E863.0-E863.9)
               petroleum fuels (E862.1)

E866.0 Lead and its compounds and fumes

E866.1 Mercury and its compounds and fumes

E866.2 Antimony and its compounds and fumes

E866.3 Arsenic and its compounds and fumes

E866.4 Other metals and their compounds and fumes
Beryllium (compounds)
Brass fumes
Cadmium (compounds)
Copper salts
Iron (compounds)
Manganese (compounds)
Nickel (compounds)
Thallium (compounds)

E866.5 Plant foods and fertilizers
     EXCLUDES *mixtures with herbicides (E863.5)*

E866.6 Glues and adhesives

E866.7 Cosmetics

E866.8 Other specified solid or liquid substances

E866.9 Unspecified solid or liquid substance

✓4ᵗʰ **E867 Accidental poisoning by gas distributed by pipeline**
Carbon monoxide from incomplete combustion of piped gas
Coal gas NOS
Liquefied petroleum gas distributed through pipes (pure or mixed with air)
Piped gas (natural) (manufactured)

✓4ᵗʰ **E868 Accidental poisoning by other utility gas and other carbon monoxide**

E868.0 Liquefied petroleum gas distributed in mobile containers

Butane	⎫ or carbon monoxide
Liquefied hydrocarbon gas NOS	from incomplete
	conbustion of
Propane	⎭ these gases

E868.1 Other and unspecified utility gas

Acetylene	⎫ or carbon monoxide
Gas NOS used for lighting, heating, or cooking	from incomplete conbustion of
Water gas	⎭ these gases

E868.2 Motor vehicle exhaust gas
Exhaust gas from:
     any type of combustion engine not in watercraft
     farm tractor, not in transit
     gas engine
     motor pump
     motor vehicle, not in transit
     EXCLUDES *poisoning by carbon monoxide from:*
               aircraft while in transit (E844.0-E844.9)
               motor vehicle while in transit (E818.0-E818.9)
               watercraft whether or not in transit (E838.0-E838.9)

E868.3 Carbon monoxide from incomplete combustion of other domestic fuels
Carbon monoxide from incomplete combustion of:

coal	⎫
coke	⎬ in domestic stove or fireplace
kerosene	
wood	⎭

     EXCLUDES *carbon monoxide from smoke and fumes due to conflagration (E890.0-E893.9)*

E868.8 Carbon monoxide from other sources
Carbon monoxide from:
blast furnace gas
incomplete combustion of fuels in industrial use
kiln vapor

E868.9 Unspecified carbon monoxide

☑4ᵗʰ **E869 Accidental poisoning by other gases and vapors**
EXCLUDES *effects of gases used as anesthetics (E855.1, E938.2)*
fumes from heavy metals (E866.0-E866.4)
smoke and fumes due to conflagration or explosion (E890.0-E899)

E869.0 Nitrogen oxides

E869.1 Sulfur dioxide

E869.2 Freon

E869.3 Lacrimogenic gas [tear gas]
Bromobenzyl cyanide
Chloroacetophenone
Ethyliodoacetate

E869.4 Second-hand tobacco smoke

E869.8 Other specified gases and vapors
Chlorine
Hydrocyanic acid gas

E869.9 Unspecified gases and vapors

MISADVENTURES TO PATIENTS DURING SURGICAL AND MEDICAL CARE (E870-E876)
EXCLUDES *accidental overdose of drug and wrong drug given in error (E850.0-E858.9)*
surgical and medical procedures as the cause of abnormal reaction by the patient, without mention of misadventure at the time of procedure (E878.0-E879.9)

☑4ᵗʰ **E870 Accidental cut, puncture, perforation, or hemorrhage during medical care**

E870.0 Surgical operation

E870.1 Infusion or transfusion

E870.2 Kidney dialysis or other perfusion

E870.3 Injection or vaccination

E870.4 Endoscopic examination

E870.5 Aspiration of fluid or tissue, puncture, and catheterization
Abdominal paracentesis
Aspirating needle biopsy
Blood sampling
Lumbar puncture
Thoracentesis
EXCLUDES *heart catheterization (E870.6)*

E870.6 Heart catheterization

E870.7 Administration of enema

E870.8 Other specified medical care

E870.9 Unspecified medical care

☑4ᵗʰ **E871 Foreign object left in body during procedure**

E871.0 Surgical operation

E871.1 Infusion or transfusion

E871.2 Kidney dialysis or other perfusion

E871.3 Injection or vaccination

E871.4 Endoscopic examination

E871.5 Aspiration of fluid or tissue, puncture, and catheterization
Abdominal paracentesis
Aspiration needle biopsy
Blood sampling
Lumbar puncture
Thoracentesis
EXCLUDES *heart catheterization (E871.6)*

E871.6 Heart catheterization

E871.7 Removal of catheter or packing

E871.8 Other specified procedures

E871.9 Unspecified procedure

☑4ᵗʰ **E872 Failure of sterile precautions during procedure**

E872.0 Surgical operation

E872.1 Infusion or transfusion

E872.2 Kidney dialysis and other perfusion

E872.3 Injection or vaccination

E872.4 Endoscopic examination

E872.5 Aspiration of fluid or tissue, puncture, and catheterization
Abdominal paracentesis
Aspiration needle biopsy
Blood sampling
Lumbar puncture
Thoracentesis
EXCLUDES *heart catheterization (E872.6)*

E872.6 Heart catheterization

E872.8 Other specified procedures

E872.9 Unspecified procedure

☑4ᵗʰ **E873 Failure in dosage**
EXCLUDES *accidental overdose of drug, medicinal or biological substance (E850.0-E858.9)*

E873.0 Excessive amount of blood or other fluid during transfusion or infusion

E873.1 Incorrect dilution of fluid during infusion

E873.2 Overdose of radiation in therapy

E873.3 Inadvertent exposure of patient to radiation during medical care

E873.4 Failure in dosage in electroshock or insulin-shock therapy

E873.5 Inappropriate [too hot or too cold] temperature in local application and packing

E873.6 Nonadministration of necessary drug or medicinal substance

E873.8 Other specified failure in dosage

E873.9 Unspecified failure in dosage

☑4ᵗʰ **E874 Mechanical failure of instrument or apparatus during procedure**

E874.0 Surgical operation

E874.1 Infusion and transfusion
Air in system

E874.2 Kidney dialysis and other perfusion

E874.3 Endoscopic examination

E874.4 Aspiration of fluid or tissue, puncture, and catheterization
Abdominal paracentesis   Lumbar puncture
Aspiration needle biopsy   Thoracentesis
Blood sampling
EXCLUDES *heart catheterization (E874.5)*

E874.5 Heart catheterization

E874.8 Other specified procedures

E874.9 Unspecified procedure

☑4ᵗʰ **E875 Contaminated or infected blood, other fluid, drug, or biological substance**
INCLUDES presence of:
bacterial pyrogens
endotoxin-producing bacteria
serum hepatitis-producing agent

E875.0 Contaminated substance transfused or infused

E875.1 Contaminated substance injected or used for vaccination

E875.2 Contaminated drug or biological substance administered by other means

E875.8 Other

E875.9 Unspecified

☑4ᵗʰ **E876 Other and unspecified misadventures during medical care**

E876.0 Mismatched blood in transfusion

E876.1 Wrong fluid in infusion

E876.2 Failure in suture and ligature during surgical operation

E876.3 Endotracheal tube wrongly placed during anesthetic procedure

E876.4 Failure to introduce or to remove other tube or instrument
> EXCLUDES foreign object left in body during procedure (E871.0-E871.9)

E876.5 Performance of wrong operation (procedure) on correct patient
Wrong device implanted into correct surgical site
> EXCLUDES correct operation (procedure) performed on wrong body part (E876.7)

E876.6 Performance of operation (procedure) on patient not scheduled for surgery
Performance of operation (procedure) intended for another patient
Performance of operation (procedure) on wrong patient

E876.7 Performance of correct operation (procedure) on wrong side/body part
Performance of correct operation (procedure) on wrong side
Performance of correct operation (procedure) on wrong site

E876.8 Other specified misadventures during medical care
Performance of inappropriate treatment NEC

E876.9 Unspecified misadventure during medical care

SURGICAL AND MEDICAL PROCEDURES AS THE CAUSE OF ABNORMAL REACTION OF PATIENT OR LATER COMPLICATION, WITHOUT MENTION OF MISADVENTURE AT THE TIME OF PROCEDURE (E878-E879)

> INCLUDES procedures as the cause of abnormal reaction, such as:
> displacement or malfunction of prosthetic device
> hepatorenal failure, postoperative
> malfunction of external stoma
> postoperative intestinal obstruction
> rejection of transplanted organ
>
> EXCLUDES anesthetic management properly carried out as the cause of adverse effect (E937.0-E938.9)
> infusion and transfusion, without mention of misadventure in the technique of procedure (E930.0-E949.9)

☑4ᵗʰ **E878 Surgical operation and other surgical procedures as the cause of abnormal reaction of patient, or of later complication, without mention of misadventure at the time of operation**

E878.0 Surgical operation with transplant of whole organ
Transplantation of: Transplantation of:
    heart   liver
    kidney

E878.1 Surgical operation with implant of artificial internal device
Cardiac pacemaker
Electrodes implanted in brain
Heart valve prosthesis
Internal orthopedic device

E878.2 Surgical operation with anastomosis, bypass, or graft, with natural or artificial tissues used as implant
Anastomosis:
    arteriovenous
    gastrojejunal
Graft of blood vessel, tendon, or skin
> EXCLUDES external stoma (E878.3)

E878.3 Surgical operation with formation of external stoma
Colostomy   Gastrostomy
Cystostomy   Ureterostomy
Duodenostomy

E878.4 Other restorative surgery

E878.5 Amputation of limb(s)

E878.6 Removal of other organ (partial) (total)

E878.8 Other specified surgical operations and procedures

E878.9 Unspecified surgical operations and procedures

☑4ᵗʰ **E879 Other procedures, without mention of misadventure at the time of procedure, as the cause of abnormal reaction of patient, or of later complication**

E879.0 Cardiac catheterization

E879.1 Kidney dialysis

E879.2 Radiological procedure and radiotherapy
> EXCLUDES radio-opaque dyes for diagnostic x-ray procedures (E947.8)

E879.3 Shock therapy
Electroshock therapy   Insulin-shock therapy

E879.4 Aspiration of fluid
Lumbar puncture   Thoracentesis

E879.5 Insertion of gastric or duodenal sound

E879.6 Urinary catheterization

E879.7 Blood sampling

E879.8 Other specified procedures
Blood transfusion

E879.9 Unspecified procedure

ACCIDENTAL FALLS (E880-E888)

> EXCLUDES falls (in or from):
> burning building (E890.8, E891.8)
> into fire (E890.0-E899)
> into water (with submersion or drowning) (E910.0-E910.9)
> machinery (in operation) (E919.0-E919.9)
> on edged, pointed, or sharp object (E920.0-E920.9)
> transport vehicle (E800.0-E845.9)
> vehicle not elsewhere classifiable (E846-E848)

☑4ᵗʰ **E880 Fall on or from stairs or steps**

E880.0 Escalator

E880.1 Fall on or from sidewalk curb
> EXCLUDES fall from moving sidewalk (E885.9)

E880.9 Other stairs or steps

☑4ᵗʰ **E881 Fall on or from ladders or scaffolding**

E881.0 Fall from ladder

E881.1 Fall from scaffolding

E882 Fall from or out of building or other structure
Fall from: Fall from:
    balcony   turret
    bridge   viaduct
    building   wall
    flagpole   window
    tower   Fall through roof
> EXCLUDES collapse of a building or structure (E916)
> fall or jump from burning building (E890.8, E891.8)

☑4ᵗʰ **E883 Fall into hole or other opening in surface**
> INCLUDES fall into: fall into:
> cavity   shaft
> dock   swimming pool
> hole   tank
> pit   well
> quarry
>
> EXCLUDES fall into water NOS (E910.9)
> that resulting in drowning or submersion without mention of injury (E910.0-E910.9)

E883.0 Accident from diving or jumping into water [swimming pool]
Strike or hit:
against bottom when jumping or diving into water
wall or board of swimming pool
water surface
EXCLUDES *diving with insufficient air supply (E913.2)*
effects of air pressure from diving (E902.2)

E883.1 Accidental fall into well

E883.2 Accidental fall into storm drain or manhole

E883.9 Fall into other hole or other opening in surface

√4ᵗʰ **E884 Other fall from one level to another**

E884.0 Fall from playground equipment
EXCLUDES *recreational machinery (E919.8)*

E884.1 Fall from cliff

E884.2 Fall from chair

E884.3 Fall from wheelchair
Fall from motorized mobility scooter
Fall from motorized wheelchair

E884.4 Fall from bed

E884.5 Fall from other furniture

E884.6 Fall from commode
Toilet

E884.9 Other fall from one level to another
Fall from: Fall from:
embankment   stationary vehicle
haystack   tree

√4ᵗʰ **E885 Fall on same level from slipping, tripping, or stumbling**

E885.0 Fall from (nonmotorized) scooter
EXCLUDES *fall from motorized mobility scooter (E884.3)*

E885.1 Fall from roller skates
Heelies
In-line skates
Wheelies

E885.2 Fall from skateboard

E885.3 Fall from skis

E885.4 Fall from snowboard

E885.9 Fall from other slipping, tripping, or stumbling
Fall on moving sidewalk

√4ᵗʰ **E886 Fall on same level from collision, pushing, or shoving, by or with other person**
EXCLUDES *crushed or pushed by a crowd or human stampede (E917.1, E917.6)*

E886.0 In sports
Tackles in sports
EXCLUDES *kicked, stepped on, struck by object, in sports (E917.0, E917.5)*

E886.9 Other and unspecified
Fall from collision of pedestrian (conveyance) with another pedestrian (conveyance)

E887 Fracture, cause unspecified

√4ᵗʰ **E888 Other and unspecified fall**
Accidental fall NOS
Fall on same level NOS

E888.0 Fall resulting in striking against sharp object
Use additional external cause code to identify object (E920)

E888.1 Fall resulting in striking against other object

E888.8 Other fall

E888.9 Unspecified fall
Fall NOS

ACCIDENTS CAUSED BY FIRE AND FLAMES (E890-E899)

INCLUDES asphyxia or poisoning due to conflagration or ignition
burning by fire
secondary fires resulting from explosion
EXCLUDES *arson (E968.0)*
fire in or on:
machinery (in operation) (E919.0-E919.9)
transport vehicle other than stationary vehicle (E800.0-E845.9)
vehicle not elsewhere classifiable (E846-E848)

√4ᵗʰ **E890 Conflagration in private dwelling**
INCLUDES conflagration in:
apartment
boarding house
camping place
caravan
farmhouse
house
lodging house
mobile home
private garage
rooming house
tenement
conflagration originating from sources classifiable to E893-E898 in the above buildings

E890.0 Explosion caused by conflagration

E890.1 Fumes from combustion of polyvinylchloride [PVC] and similar material in conflagration

E890.2 Other smoke and fumes from conflagration
Carbon monoxide
Fumes NOS } from conflagration in private building
Smoke NOS

E890.3 Burning caused by conflagration

E890.8 Other accident resulting from conflagration
Collapse of
Fall from } burning private building
Hit by object falling from
Jump from

E890.9 Unspecified accident resulting from conflagration in private dwelling

√4ᵗʰ **E891 Conflagration in other and unspecified building or structure**
Conflagration in:
barn
church
convalescent and other residential home
dormitory of educational institution
factory
farm outbuildings
hospital
hotel
school
store
theater
Conflagration originating from sources classifiable to E893-E898, in the above buildings

E891.0 Explosion caused by conflagration

E891.1 Fumes from combustion of polyvinylchloride [PVC] and similar material in conflagration

E891.2 Other smoke and fumes from conflagration
Carbon monoxide
Fumes NOS } from conflagration in private building or structure
Smoke NOS

E891.3 Burning caused by conflagration

E891.8 Other accident resulting from conflagration
Collapse of
Fall from } burning private building or structure
Hit by object falling from
Jump from

E891.9 Unspecified accident resulting from conflagration of other and unspecified building or structure

E892 Conflagration not in building or structure
    Fire (uncontrolled) (in) (of):
        forest
        grass
        hay
        lumber
        mine
        prairie
        transport vehicle [any], except while in transit
        tunnel

✓4ᵗʰ **E893 Accident caused by ignition of clothing**
    EXCLUDES *ignition of clothing:*
        from highly inflammable material (E894)
        with conflagration (E890.0-E892)

E893.0 From controlled fire in private dwelling
    Ignition of clothing from:
      normal fire (charcoal) (coal)
        (electric) (gas) (wood)
        in:
      brazier   in private dwelling
      fireplace   (as listed in
      furnace   E890)
      stove

E893.1 From controlled fire in other building or structure
    Ignition of clothing from:
      normal fire (charcoal) (coal)
        (electric) (gas) (wood)
        in:
      brazier   in other building or
      fireplace   structure (as
      furnace   listed in E891)
      stove

E893.2 From controlled fire not in building or structure
    Ignition of clothing from:
        bonfire (controlled)
        brazier fire (controlled), not in building or structure
        trash fire (controlled)
    EXCLUDES *conflagration not in building (E892)*
        trash fire out of control (E892)

E893.8 From other specified sources
    Ignition of clothing from: Ignition of clothing from:
      blowlamp   cigarette
      blowtorch   lighter
      burning bedspread   matches
      candle   pipe
      cigar   welding torch

E893.9 Unspecified source
    Ignition of clothing (from controlled fire NOS) (in
      building NOS) NOS

E894 Ignition of highly inflammable material
    Ignition of:
      benzine
      gasoline
      fat   (with ignition of clothing)
      kerosene
      paraffin
      petrol
    EXCLUDES *ignition of highly inflammable material with:*
        conflagration (E890.0-E892)
        explosion (E923.0-E923.9)

E895 Accident caused by controlled fire in private dwelling
    Burning by (flame of) normal fire (charcoal) (coal) (electric) (gas)
      (wood) in:
      brazier
      fireplace   in private dwelling (as
      furnace   listed in E890)
      stove
    EXCLUDES *burning by hot objects not producing fire or flames*
        (E924.0-E924.9)
        ignition of clothing from these sources (E893.0)
        poisoning by carbon monoxide from incomplete
          combustion of fuel (E867-E868.9)
        that with conflagration (E890.0-E890.9)

E896 Accident caused by controlled fire in other and unspecified building or structure
    Burning by (flame of) normal fire (charcoal)
      (coal)(electric)(gas)(wood) in:
      brazier
      fireplace   in other building or structure (as
      furnace   listed in E891)
      stove
    EXCLUDES *burning by hot objects not producing fire or flames*
        (E924.0-E924.9)
        ignition of clothing from these sources (E893.1)
        poisoning by carbon monoxide from incomplete
          combustion of fuel (E867-E868.9)
        that with conflagration (E891.0-E891.9)

E897 Accident caused by controlled fire not in building or structure
    Burns from flame of:
      bonfire
      brazier fire, not in building or structure   controlled
      trash fire
    EXCLUDES *ignition of clothing from these sources (E893.2)*
        trash fire out of control (E892)
        that with conflagration (E892)

✓4ᵗʰ **E898 Accident caused by other specified fire and flames**
    EXCLUDES *conflagration (E890.0-E892)*
        that with ignition of:
          clothing (E893.0-E893.9)
          highly inflammable material (E894)

E898.0 Burning bedclothes
    Bed set on fire NOS

E898.1 Other
    Burning by: Burning by:
      blowlamp   lamp
      blowtorch   lighter
      candle   matches
      cigar   pipe
      cigarette   welding torch
      fire in room NOS

E899 Accident caused by unspecified fire
    Burning NOS

ACCIDENTS DUE TO NATURAL AND ENVIRONMENTAL FACTORS (E900-E909)

✓4ᵗʰ **E900 Excessive heat**

E900.0 Due to weather conditions
    Excessive heat as the external cause of:
      ictus solaris
      siriasis
      sunstroke

E900.1 Of man-made origin
    Heat (in):
      boiler room
      drying room
      factory
      furnace room
      generated in transport vehicle
      kitchen

E900.9 Of unspecified origin

✓4ᵗʰ **E901 Excessive cold**

E901.0 Due to weather conditions
    Excessive cold as the cause of:
      chilblains NOS
      immersion foot

E901.1 Of man-made origin
    Contact with or   Prolonged exposure in:
      inhalation of: deep freeze unit
      dry ice   refrigerator
      liquid air
      liquid hydrogen
      liquid nitrogen

E901.8 Other specified origin

E901.9 Of unspecified origin

✓4ᵗʰ E902 High and low air pressure and changes in air pressure

E902.0 Residence or prolonged visit at high altitude

Residence or prolonged visit at high altitude as the cause of:

Acosta syndrome
Alpine sickness
altitude sickness
Andes disease
anoxia, hypoxia
barotitis, barodontalgia, barosinusitis, otitic barotrauma
hypobarism, hypobaropathy
mountain sickness
range disease

E902.1 In aircraft

Sudden change in air pressure in aircraft during ascent or descent as the cause of:
aeroneurosis
aviators' disease

E902.2 Due to diving

High air pressure from rapid descent in water

Reduction in atmospheric pressure while surfacing from deep water diving

⎱ as the cause of:
caisson disease
divers' disease
divers' palsy or paralysis

E902.8 Due to other specified causes

Reduction in atmospheric pressure while surfacing from underground

E902.9 Unspecified cause

E903 Travel and motion

✓4ᵗʰ E904 Hunger, thirst, exposure, and neglect

> **EXCLUDES** any condition resulting from homicidal intent (E968.0-E968.9)
> hunger, thirst, and exposure resulting from accidents connected with transport (E800.0-E848)

E904.0 Abandonment or neglect of infants and helpless persons

Exposure to weather conditions

Hunger or thirst

⎱ resulting from abandonment or neglect

Desertion of newborn
Inattention at or after birth
Lack of care (helpless person) (infant)

> **EXCLUDES** criminal [purposeful] neglect (E968.4)

E904.1 Lack of food

Lack of food as the cause of:
inanition
insufficient nourishment
starvation

> **EXCLUDES** hunger resulting from abandonment or neglect (E904.0)

E904.2 Lack of water

Lack of water as the cause of:
dehydration
inanition

> **EXCLUDES** dehydration due to acute fluid loss (276.51)

E904.3 Exposure (to weather conditions), not elsewhere classifiable

Exposure NOS
Humidity
Struck by hailstones

> **EXCLUDES** struck by lightning (E907)

E904.9 Privation, unqualified

Destitution

✓4ᵗʰ E905 Venomous animals and plants as the cause of poisoning and toxic reactions

> **INCLUDES** chemical released by animal
> insects
> release of venom through fangs, hairs, spines, tentacles, and other venom apparatus

> **EXCLUDES** eating of poisonous animals or plants (E865.0-E865.9)

E905.0 Venomous snakes and lizards

Cobra	Mamba
Copperhead snake	Rattlesnake
Coral snake	Sea snake
Fer de lance	Snake (venomous)
Gila monster	Viper
Krait	Water moccasin

> **EXCLUDES** bites of snakes and lizards known to be nonvenomous (E906.2)

E905.1 Venomous spiders

Black widow spider
Brown spider
Tarantula (venomous)

E905.2 Scorpion

E905.3 Hornets, wasps, and bees

Yellow jacket

E905.4 Centipede and venomous millipede (tropical)

E905.5 Other venomous arthropods

Sting of:
ant
caterpillar

E905.6 Venomous marine animals and plants

Puncture by sea urchin spine
Sting of:
coral
jelly fish
nematocysts
sea anemone
sea cucumber
other marine animal or plant

> **EXCLUDES** bites and other injuries caused by nonvenomous marine animal (E906.2-E906.8)
> bite of sea snake (venomous) (E905.0)

E905.7 Poisoning and toxic reactions caused by other plants

Injection of poisons or toxins into or through skin by plant thorns, spines, or other mechanisms

> **EXCLUDES** puncture wound NOS by plant thorns or spines (E920.8)

E905.8 Other specified

E905.9 Unspecified

Sting NOS
Venomous bite NOS

✓4ᵗʰ E906 Other injury caused by animals

> **EXCLUDES** poisoning and toxic reactions caused by venomous animals and insects (E905.0-E905.9)
> road vehicle accident involving animals (E827.0-E828.9)
> tripping or falling over an animal (E885.9)

E906.0 Dog bite

E906.1 Rat bite

E906.2 Bite of nonvenomous snakes and lizards

E906.3 Bite of other animal except arthropod

Cats	Rodents, except rats
Moray eel	Shark

E906.4 Bite of nonvenomous arthropod

Insect bite NOS

E906.5 Bite by unspecified animal

Animal bite NOS

E906.8 Other specified injury caused by animal

Butted by animal
Fallen on by horse or other animal, not being ridden
Gored by animal
Implantation of quills of porcupine
Pecked by bird
Run over by animal, not being ridden
Stepped on by animal, not being ridden

> **EXCLUDES** injury by animal being ridden (E828.0-E828.9)

E906.9 Unspecified injury caused by animal

E907 Lightning
> EXCLUDES   injury from:
> fall of tree or other object caused by lightning (E916)
> fire caused by lightning (E890.0-E892)

✓4ᵗʰ **E908 Cataclysmic storms, and floods resulting from storms**
> EXCLUDES   collapse of dam or man-made structure causing flood
> (E909.3)

E908.0 Hurricane
Storm surge
"Tidal wave" caused by storm action
Typhoon

E908.1 Tornado
Cyclone
Twisters

E908.2 Floods
Torrential rainfall
Flash flood
> EXCLUDES   collapse of dam or man-made structure
> causing flood (E909.3)

E908.3 Blizzard (snow)(ice)

E908.4 Dust storm

E908.8 Other cataclysmic storms
Cloudburst

E908.9 Unspecified cataclysmic storms, and floods resulting from storms
Storm NOS

✓4ᵗʰ **E909 Cataclysmic earth surface movements and eruptions**

E909.0 Earthquakes

E909.1 Volcanic eruptions
Burns from lava
Ash inhalation

E909.2 Avalanche, landslide, or mudslide

E909.3 Collapse of dam or man-made structure

E909.4 Tidalwave caused by earthquake
Tidalwave NOS
Tsunami
> EXCLUDES   tidalwave caused by tropical storm (E908.0)

E909.8 Other cataclysmic earth surface movements and eruptions

E909.9 Unspecified cataclysmic earth surface movements and eruptions

ACCIDENTS CAUSED BY SUBMERSION, SUFFOCATION, AND FOREIGN BODIES (E910-E915)

✓4ᵗʰ **E910 Accidental drowning and submersion**
> INCLUDES   immersion
> swimmers' cramp
> EXCLUDES   diving accident (NOS) (resulting in injury except
> drowning) (E883.0)
> diving with insufficient air supply (E913.2)
> drowning and submersion due to:
> cataclysm (E908-E909)
> machinery accident (E919.0-E919.9)
> transport accident (E800.0-E845.9)
> effect of high and low air pressure (E902.2)
> injury from striking against objects while in running
> water (E917.2)

E910.0 While water-skiing
Fall from water skis with submersion or drowning
> EXCLUDES   accident to water-skier involving a watercraft
> and resulting in submersion or other
> injury (E830.4, E831.4)

E910.1 While engaged in other sport or recreational activity with diving equipment
Scuba diving NOS
Skin diving NOS
Underwater spear fishing NOS

E910.2 While engaged in other sport or recreational activity without diving equipment
Fishing or hunting, except from boat or with diving equipment
Ice skating
Playing in water
Surfboarding
Swimming NOS
Voluntarily jumping from boat, not involved in accident, for swim NOS
Wading in water
> EXCLUDES   jumping into water to rescue another person
> (E910.3)

E910.3 While swimming or diving for purposes other than recreation or sport
Marine salvage
Pearl diving
Placement of fishing nets   } (with diving equipment)
Rescue (attempt) of another person
Underwater construction or repairs

E910.4 In bathtub

E910.8 Other accidental drowning or submersion
Drowning in:
quenching tank
swimming pool

E910.9 Unspecified accidental drowning or submersion
Accidental fall into water NOS
Drowning NOS

E911 Inhalation and ingestion of food causing obstruction of respiratory tract or suffocation
Aspiration and inhalation of food [any] (into respiratory tract) NOS
Asphyxia by
Choked on   } food [including bone, seed in food, regurgitated food]
Suffocation by
Compression of trachea
Interruption of respiration   } by food lodged in esophagus
Obstruction of respiration
Obstruction of pharynx by food (bolus)
> EXCLUDES   injury, except asphyxia and obstruction of respiratory
> passage, caused by food (E915)
> obstruction of esophagus by food without mention of
> asphyxia or obstruction of respiratory passage
> (E915)

E912 Inhalation and ingestion of other object causing obstruction of respiratory tract or suffocation
Aspiration and inhalation of foreign body except food (into respiratory tract) NOS
Foreign object [bean] [marble] in nose
Obstruction of pharynx by foreign body
Compression
Interruption of respiration   } by foreign body in esophagus
Obstruction of respiration
> EXCLUDES   injury, except asphyxia and obstruction of respiratory
> passage, caused by foreign body (E915)
> obstruction of esophagus by foreign body without
> mention of asphyxia or obstruction in respiratory
> passage (E915)

✓4ᵗʰ **E913 Accidental mechanical suffocation**
> EXCLUDES   mechanical suffocation from or by:
> accidental inhalation or ingestion of:
> food (E911)
> foreign object (E912)
> cataclysm (E908-E909)
> explosion (E921.0-E921.9, E923.0-E923.9)
> machinery accident (E919.0-E919.9)

E913.0 In bed or cradle
> EXCLUDES   suffocation by plastic bag (E913.1)

E913.1 By plastic bag

E913.2 Due to lack of air (in closed place)
Accidentally closed up in refrigerator or other airtight enclosed space
Diving with insufficient air supply
EXCLUDES *suffocation by plastic bag (E913.1)*

E913.3 By falling earth or other substance
Cave-in NOS
EXCLUDES *cave-in caused by cataclysmic earth surface movements and eruptions (E909)*
struck by cave-in without asphyxiation or suffocation (E916)

E913.8 Other specified means
Accidental hanging, except in bed or cradle

E913.9 Unspecified means
Asphyxia, mechanical NOS
Strangulation NOS
Suffocation NOS

E914 Foreign body accidentally entering eye and adnexa
EXCLUDES *corrosive liquid (E924.1)*

E915 Foreign body accidentally entering other orifice
EXCLUDES *aspiration and inhalation of foreign body, any, (into respiratory tract) NOS (E911-E912)*

OTHER ACCIDENTS (E916-E928)

E916 Struck accidentally by falling object
Collapse of building, except on fire
Falling:
rock
snowslide NOS
stone
tree
Object falling from:
machine, not in operation
stationary vehicle
Code first:
collapse of building on fire (E890.0-E891.9)
falling object in:
cataclysm (E908-E909)
machinery accidents (E919.0-E919.9)
transport accidents (E800.0-E845.9)
vehicle accidents not elsewhere classifiable (E846-E848)
object set in motion by:
explosion (E921.0-E921.9, E923.0-E923.9)
firearm (E922.0-E922.9)
projected object (E917.0-E917.9)

☑4ᵗʰ E917 Striking against or struck accidentally by objects or persons
INCLUDES bumping into or
against   object (moving) (projected)
colliding with   (stationary)
kicking against   pedestrian conveyance
stepping on   person
struck by
EXCLUDES *fall from:*
collision with another person, except when caused by a crowd (E886.0-E886.9)
stumbling over object (E885.9)
fall resulting in striking against object (E888.0, E888.1)
injury caused by:
assault (E960.0-E960.1, E967.0-E967.9)
cutting or piercing instrument (E920.0-E920.9)
explosion (E921.0-E921.9, E923.0-E923.9)
firearm (E922.0-E922.9)
machinery (E919.0-E919.9)
transport vehicle (E800.0-E845.9)
vehicle not elsewhere classifiable (E846-E848)

E917.0 In sports without subsequent fall
Kicked or stepped on during game (football) (rugby)
Struck by hit or thrown ball
Struck by hockey stick or puck

E917.1 Caused by a crowd, by collective fear or panic without subsequent fall
Crushed
Pushed   } by crowd or human stampede
Stepped on

E917.2 In running water without subsequent fall
EXCLUDES *drowning or submersion (E910.0-E910.9)*
that in sports (E917.0, E917.5)

E917.3 Furniture without subsequent fall
EXCLUDES *fall from furniture (E884.2, E884.4-E884.5)*

E917.4 Other stationary object without subsequent fall
Bath tub
Fence
Lamp-post

E917.5 Object in sports with subsequent fall
Knocked down while boxing

E917.6 Caused by a crowd, by collective fear or panic with subsequent fall

E917.7 Furniture with subsequent fall
EXCLUDES *fall from furniture (E884.2, E884.4-E884.5)*

E917.8 Other stationary object with subsequent fall
Bath tub
Fence
Lamp-post

E917.9 Other striking against with or without subsequent fall

E918 Caught accidentally in or between objects
Caught, crushed, jammed, or pinched in or between moving or stationary objects, such as:
escalator
folding object
hand tools, appliances, or implements
sliding door and door frame
under packing crate
washing machine wringer
EXCLUDES *injury caused by:*
cutting or piercing instrument (E920.0-E920.9)
machinery (E919.0-E919.9)
mechanism or component of firearm and air gun (E928.7)
transport vehicle (E800.0-E845.9)
vehicle not elsewhere classifiable (E846-E848)
struck accidentally by:
falling object (E916)
object (moving) (projected) (E917.0-E917.9)

☑4th **E919 Accidents caused by machinery**

INCLUDES	
burned by	
caught in (moving parts of)	
collapse of	
crushed by	
cut or pierced by	
drowning or submersion caused by	
expolosion of, on, in	
fall from or into moving part of	machinery (accident)
fire starting in or on	
mechanical suffocation caused by	
object falling from, on, in motion by	
overturning of	
pinned under	
run over by	
struck by	
thrown from	

caught between machinery and other object

machinery accident NOS

EXCLUDES	accidents involving machinery, not in operation (E884.9, E916-E918)
	injury caused by:
	electric current in connection with machinery (E925.0-E925.9)
	escalator (E880.0, E918)
	explosion of pressure vessel in connection with machinery (E921.0-E921.9)
	mechanism or component of firearm and air gun (E928.7)
	moving sidewalk (E885.9)
	powered hand tools, appliances, and implements (E916-E918, E920.0-E921.9, E923.0-E926.9)
	transport vehicle accidents involving machinery (E800.0-E848)
	poisoning by carbon monoxide generated by machine (E868.8)

E919.0 Agricultural machines

Animal-powered agricultural machine	Farm tractor
Combine	Harvester
Derrick, hay	Hay mower or rake
Farm machinery NOS	Reaper
	Thresher

EXCLUDES	that in transport under own power on the highway (E810.0-E819.9)
	that being towed by another vehicle on the highway (E810.0-E819.9, E827.0-E827.9, E829.0-E829.9)
	that involved in accident classifiable to E820-E829 (E820.0-E829.9)

E919.1 Mining and earth-drilling machinery

Bore or drill (land) (seabed)

Shaft hoist

Shaft lift

Under-cutter

EXCLUDES	coal car, tram, truck, and tub in mine (E846)

E919.2 Lifting machines and appliances

Chain hoist	
Crane	
Derrick	
Elevator (building) (grain)	except in agricultural or mining operations
Forklift truck	
Lift	
Pulley block	
Winch	

EXCLUDES	that being towed by another vehicle on the highway (E810.0-E819.9, E827.0-E827.9, E829.0-829.9)
	that in transport under own power on the highway (E810.0-E819.9)
	that involved in accident classifiable to E820-E829 (E820.0-E829.9)

E919.3 Metalworking machines

Abrasive wheel	Metal:
Forging machine	milling machine
Lathe	power press
Mechanical shears	rolling-mill
Metal:	sawing machine
drilling machine	

E919.4 Woodworking and forming machines

Band saw	Overhead plane
Bench saw	Powered saw
Circular saw	Radial saw
Molding machine	Sander

EXCLUDES	hand saw (E920.1)

E919.5 Prime movers, except electrical motors

Gas turbine

Internal combustion engine

Steam engine

Water driven turbine

EXCLUDES	that being towed by other vehicle on the highway (E810.0-E819.9, E827.0-E827.9, E829.0-E829.9)
	that in transport under own power on the highway (E810.0-E819.9)

E919.6 Transmission machinery

Transmission:	Transmission:
belt	pinion
cable	pulley
chain	shaft
gear	

E919.7 Earth moving, scraping, and other excavating machines

Bulldozer	Steam shovel
Road scraper	

EXCLUDES	that being towed by other vehicle on the highway (E810.0-E819.9, E827.0-E827.9, E829.0-E829.9)
	that in transport under own power on the highway (E810.0-E819.9)

E919.8 Other specified machinery

Machines for manufacture of:

  clothing

  foodstuffs and beverages

  paper

Printing machine

Recreational machinery

Spinning, weaving, and textile machines

E919.9 Unspecified machinery

☑4th **E920 Accidents caused by cutting and piercing instruments or objects**

INCLUDES		
	accidental injury (by) object	edged
		pointed
		sharp

EXCLUDES	injury caused by mechanism or component of firearm and air gun (E928.7)

E920.0 Powered lawn mower

E920.1 Other powered hand tools

Any powered hand tool [compressed air] [electric] [explosive cartridge] [hydraulic power], such as:

  drill

  hand saw

  hedge clipper

  rivet gun

  snow blower

  staple gun

EXCLUDES	band saw (E919.4)
	bench saw (E919.4)

E920.2 Powered household appliances and implements

Blender	Electric:
Electric:	knife
beater or mixer	sewing machine
can opener	Garbage disposal appliance
fan	

E920.3 Knives, swords, and daggers

E920.4 Other hand tools and implements

Axe	Paper cutter
Can opener NOS	Pitchfork
Chisel	Rake
Fork	Scissors
Hand saw	Screwdriver
Hoe	Sewing machine, not powered
Ice pick	Shovel
Needle (sewing)	

E920.5 Hypodermic needle
Contaminated needle
Needle stick

E920.8 Other specified cutting and piercing instruments or objects

Arrow	Nail
Broken glass	Plant thorn
Dart	Splinter
Edge of stiff paper	Tin can lid
Lathe turnings	

> **EXCLUDES** animal spines or quills (E906.8)
> flying glass due to explosion (E921.0-E923.9)

E920.9 Unspecified cutting and piercing instrument or object

✓4ᵗʰ E921 Accident caused by explosion of pressure vessel

> **INCLUDES** accidental explosion of pressure vessels, whether or not part of machinery
> **EXCLUDES** explosion of pressure vessel on transport vehicle (E800.0-E845.9)

E921.0 Boilers

E921.1 Gas cylinders
Air tank   Pressure gas tank

E921.8 Other specified pressure vessels
Aerosol can   Tin can lid
Automobile tire

E921.9 Unspecified pressure vessel

✓4ᵗʰ E922 Accident caused by firearm, and air gun missile

> **EXCLUDES** injury caused by mechanism or component of firearm and air gun (E928.7)

E922.0 Handgun
Pistol   Revolver
> **EXCLUDES** Verey pistol (E922.8)

E922.1 Shotgun (automatic)

E922.2 Hunting rifle

E922.3 Military firearms
Army rifle   Machine gun

E922.4 Air gun
BB gun   Pellet gun

E922.5 Paintball gun

E922.8 Other specified firearm missile
Verey pistol [flare]

E922.9 Unspecified firearm missile
Gunshot wound NOS
Shot NOS

✓4ᵗʰ E923 Accident caused by explosive material

> **INCLUDES** flash burns and other injuries resulting from explosion of explosive material
> ignition of highly explosive material with explosion
> **EXCLUDES** explosion:
> in or on machinery (E919.0-E919.9)
> on any transport vehicle, except stationary motor vehicle (E800.0-E848)
> with conflagration (E890.0, E891.0,E892)
> injury caused by mechanism or component of firearm and air gun (E928.7)
> secondary fires resulting from explosion (E890.0-E899)

E923.0 Fireworks

E923.1 Blasting materials
Blasting cap   Dynamite
Detonator   Explosive [any] used in blasting operations

E923.2 Explosive gases

Acetylene	Fire damp
Butane	Gasoline fumes
Coal gas	Methane
Explosion in mine NOS	Propane

E923.8 Other explosive materials

Bomb	Torpedo
Explosive missile	Explosion in munitions:
Grenade	dump
Mine	factory
Shell	

E923.9 Unspecified explosive material
Explosion NOS

✓4ᵗʰ E924 Accident caused by hot substance or object, caustic or corrosive material, and steam

> **EXCLUDES** burning NOS (E899)
> chemical burn resulting from swallowing a corrosive substance (E860.0-E864.4)
> fire caused by these substances and objects (E890.0-E894)
> radiation burns (E926.0-E926.9)
> therapeutic misadventures (E870.0-E876.9)

E924.0 Hot liquids and vapors, including steam
Burning or scalding by:
boiling water
hot or boiling liquids not primarily caustic or corrosive
liquid metal
steam
other hot vapor
> **EXCLUDES** hot (boiling) tap water (E924.2)

E924.1 Caustic and corrosive substances
Burning by:
acid [any kind]
ammonia
caustic oven cleaner or other substance
corrosive substance
lye
vitriol

E924.2 Hot (boiling) tap water

E924.8 Other
Burning by:
heat from electric heating appliance
hot object NOS
light bulb
steam pipe

E924.9 Unspecified

✓4ᵗʰ E925 Accident caused by electric current

> **INCLUDES** electric current from exposed wire, faulty appliance, high voltage cable, live rail, or open electric socket as the cause of:
> burn
> cardiac fibrillation
> convulsion
> electric shock
> electrocution
> puncture wound
> respiratory paralysis
> **EXCLUDES** burn by heat from electrical appliance (E924.8)
> lightning (E907)

E925.0 Domestic wiring and appliances

E925.1 Electric power generating plants, distribution stations, transmission lines
Broken power line

E925.2 Industrial wiring, appliances, and electrical machinery
Conductors
Control apparatus
Electrical equipment and machinery
Transformers

E925.8 Other electric current
Wiring and appliances in or on:
farm [not farmhouse]
outdoors
public building
residential institutions
schools

E925.9 Unspecified electric current
Burns or other injury from electric current NOS
Electric shock NOS
Electrocution NOS

✓4ᵗʰ **E926 Exposure to radiation**
EXCLUDES *abnormal reaction to or complication of treatment
without mention of misadventure (E879.2)
atomic power plant malfunction in water transport
(E838.0-E838.9)
misadventure to patient in surgical and medical
procedures (E873.2-E873.3)
use of radiation in war operations (E996-E997.9)*

E926.0 Radiofrequency radiation
Overexposure to: from:
microwave   high-powered radio and
radiation   television
radar radiation   transmitters
radiofrequency   industrial radiofrequency
radiofrequency   induction heaters
radiation   radar installations
[any]

E926.1 Infrared heaters and lamps
Exposure to infrared radiation from heaters and lamps as
the cause of:
blistering
burning
charring
inflammatory change
EXCLUDES *physical contact with heater or lamp (E924.8)*

E926.2 Visible and ultraviolet light sources
Arc lamps
Black light sources
Electrical welding arc
Oxygas welding torch
Sun rays
Tanning bed
EXCLUDES *excessive heat from these sources
(E900.1-E900.9)*

E926.3 X-rays and other electromagnetic ionizing radiation
Gamma rays
X-rays (hard) (soft)

E926.4 Lasers

E926.5 Radioactive isotopes
Radiobiologicals
Radiopharmaceuticals

E926.8 Other specified radiation
Artificially accelerated beams of ionized particles
generated by:
betatrons
synchrotrons

E926.9 Unspecified radiation
Radiation NOS

✓4ᵗʰ **E927 Overexertion and strenuous and repetitive movements or
loads**
Use additional code to identify activity (E001-E030)

E927.0 Overexertion from sudden strenuous movement
Sudden trauma from strenuous movement

E927.1 Overexertion from prolonged static position
Overexertion from maintaining prolonged positions,
such as:
holding
sitting
standing

E927.2 Excessive physical exertion from prolonged activity

E927.3 Cumulative trauma from repetitive motion
Cumulative trauma from repetitive movements

E927.4 Cumulative trauma from repetitive impact

**E927.8 Other overexertion and strenuous and repetitive
movements or loads**

**E927.9 Unspecified overexertion and strenuous and repetitive
movements or loads**

✓4ᵗʰ **E928 Other and unspecified environmental and accidental
causes**

E928.0 Prolonged stay in weightless environment
Weightlessness in spacecraft (simulator)

E928.1 Exposure to noise
Noise (pollution)
Sound waves
Supersonic waves

E928.2 Vibration

E928.3 Human bite

E928.4 External constriction caused by hair

E928.5 External constriction caused by other object

E928.6 Environmental exposure to harmful algae and toxins
Algae bloom NOS   Florida red tide
Blue-green algae bloom   Harmful algae bloom
Brown tide   Pfiesteria piscicida
Cyanobacteria bloom   Red tide

E928.7 Mechanism or component of firearm and air gun
Injury due to:
explosion of gun parts
recoil
Pierced, cut, crushed, or pinched by slide, trigger
mechanism, scope, or other gun part
Powder burn from firearm or air gun
EXCLUDES *accident caused by firearm and air gun
missile (E922.0-E922.9)*

E928.8 Other

E928.9 Unspecified accident
Accident NOS
Blow NOS   stated as accidentally
Casualty (not due to war)   inflicted
Decapitation

Knocked down
Killed   stated as accidentally
Injury [any part of body, or   inflicted, but not
unspecified]   otherwise
Mangled   specified
Wound
EXCLUDES *fracture, cause unspecified (E887)
injuries undetermined whether accidentally
or purposely inflicted (E980.0-E989)*

LATE EFFECTS OF ACCIDENTAL INJURY (E929)

Note: This category is to be used to indicate accidental injury as
the cause of death or disability from late effects, which are
themselves classifiable elsewhere. The "late effects"
include conditions reported as such, or as sequelae which
may occur at any time after the attempted suicide or
self-inflicted injury.

✓4ᵗʰ **E929 Late effects of accidental injury**
EXCLUDES *late effects of:
surgical and medical procedures (E870.0-E879.9)
therapeutic use of drugs and medicines
(E930.0-E949.9)*

E929.0 Late effects of motor vehicle accident
Late effects of accidents classifiable to E810-E825

E929.1 Late effects of other transport accident
Late effects of accidents classifiable to E800-E807,
E826-E838, E840-E848

E929.2 Late effects of accidental poisoning
Late effects of accidents classifiable to E850-E858,
E860-E869

E929.3 Late effects of accidental fall
Late effects of accidents classifiable to E880-E888

E929.4 Late effects of accident caused by fire
Late effects of accidents classifiable to E890-E899

E929.5 Late effects of accident due to natural and environmental factors
Late effects of accidents classifiable to E900-E909

E929.8 Late effects of other accidents
Late effects of accidents classifiable to E910-E928.8

E929.9 Late effects of unspecified accident
Late effects of accidents classifiable to E928.9

DRUGS, MEDICINAL AND BIOLOGICAL SUBSTANCES CAUSING ADVERSE EFFECTS IN THERAPEUTIC USE (E930-E949)

INCLUDES　correct drug properly administered in therapeutic or prophylactic dosage, as the cause of any adverse effect including allergic or hypersensitivity reactions

EXCLUDES　accidental overdose of drug and wrong drug given or taken in error (E850.0-E858.9)
accidents in the technique of administration of drug or biological substance, such as accidental puncture during injection, or contamination of drug (E870.0-E876.9)
administration with suicidal or homicidal intent or intent to harm, or in circumstances classifiable to E950.0-E950.5, E962.0, E980.0-E980.5

Note: See Alphabetic Index for more complete list of specific drugs to be classified under the fourth-digit subdivisions. The American Hospital Formulary numbers can be used to classify new drugs listed by the American Hospital Formulary Service (AHFS). See Appendix C.

✓4ᵗʰ **E930 Antibiotics**
EXCLUDES　that used as eye, ear, nose, and throat [ENT], and local anti-infectives (E946.0-E946.9)

E930.0 Penicillins

Natural	Semisynthetic, such as:
Synthetic	cloxacillin
Semisynthetic, such as:	nafcillin
ampicillin	oxacillin

E930.1 Antifungal antibiotics

Amphotericin B	Hachimycin [trichomycin]
Griseofulvin	Nystatin

E930.2 Chloramphenicol group

Chloramphenicol	Thiamphenicol

E930.3 Erythromycin and other macrolides

Oleandomycin	Spiramycin

E930.4 Tetracycline group

Doxycycline	Oxytetracycline
Minocycline	

E930.5 Cephalosporin group

Cephalexin	Cephaloridine
Cephaloglycin	Cephalothin

E930.6 Antimycobacterial antibiotics

Cycloserine	Rifampin
Kanamycin	Streptomycin

E930.7 Antineoplastic antibiotics
Actinomycins, such as:
Bleomycin
Cactinomycin
Dactinomycin
Daunorubicin
Mitomycin
EXCLUDES　other antineoplastic drugs (E933.1)

E930.8 Other specified antibiotics

E930.9 Unspecified antibiotic

✓4ᵗʰ **E931 Other anti-infectives**
EXCLUDES　ENT, and local anti-infectives (E946.0-E946.9)

E931.0 Sulfonamides

Sulfadiazine	Sulfamethoxazole
Sulfafurazole	

E931.1 Arsenical anti-infectives

E931.2 Heavy metal anti-infectives
Compounds of:
antimony
bismuth
lead
mercury
EXCLUDES　mercurial diuretics (E944.0)

E931.3 Quinoline and hydroxyquinoline derivatives
Chiniofon
Diiodohydroxyquin
EXCLUDES　antimalarial drugs (E931.4)

E931.4 Antimalarials and drugs acting on other blood protozoa

Chloroquine phosphate	Proguanil [chloroguanide]
Cycloguanil	Pyrimethamine
Primaquine	Quinine (sulphate)

E931.5 Other antiprotozoal drugs
Emetine

E931.6 Anthelmintics

Hexylresorcinol	Piperazine
Male fern oleoresin	Thiabendazole

E931.7 Antiviral drugs
Methisazone
EXCLUDES　amantadine (E936.4)
cytarabine (E933.1)
idoxuridine (E946.5)

E931.8 Other antimycobacterial drugs
Ethambutol
Ethionamide
Isoniazid
Para-aminosalicylic acid derivatives
Sulfones

E931.9 Other and unspecified anti-infectives
Flucytosine
Nitrofuranderivatives

✓4ᵗʰ **E932 Hormones and synthetic substitutes**

E932.0 Adrenal cortical steroids
Cortisone derivatives
Desoxycorticosterone derivatives
Fluorinated corticosteroid

E932.1 Androgens and anabolic congeners
Nandrolone phenpropionate
Oxymetholone
Testosterone and preparations

E932.2 Ovarian hormones and synthetic substitutes
Contraceptives, oral
Estrogens
Estrogens and progestogens combined
Progestogens

E932.3 Insulins and antidiabetic agents
Acetohexamide
Biguanide derivatives, oral
Chlorpropamide
Glucagon
Insulin
Phenformin
Sulfonylurea derivatives, oral
Tolbutamide
EXCLUDES　adverse effect of insulin administered for shock therapy (E879.3)

E932.4 Anterior pituitary hormones
Corticotropin
Gonadotropin
Somatotropin [growth hormone]

E932.5 Posterior pituitary hormones
Vasopressin
EXCLUDES　oxytocic agents (E945.0)

E932.6 Parathyroid and parathyroid derivatives

E932.7 Thyroid and thyroid derivatives
Dextrothyroxine
Levothyroxine sodium
Liothyronine
Thyroglobulin

E932.8 Antithyroid agents
Iodides
Thiouracil
Thiourea

E932.9 Other and unspecified hormones and synthetic substitutes

✓4ᵗʰ **E933 Primarily systemic agents**

E933.0 Antiallergic and antiemetic drugs
Antihistamines	Diphenylpyraline
Chlorpheniramine	Thonzylamine
Diphenhydramine	Tripelennamine

EXCLUDES *phenothiazine-based tranquilizers (E939.1)*

E933.1 Antineoplastic and immunosuppressive drugs
Azathioprine
Busulfan
Chlorambucil
Cyclophosphamide
Cytarabine
Fluorouracil
Mechlorethamine hydrochloride
Mercaptopurine
Triethylenethiophosphoramide [thio-TEPA]

EXCLUDES *antineoplastic antibiotics (E930.7)*

E933.2 Acidifying agents

E933.3 Alkalizing agents

E933.4 Enzymes, not elsewhere classified
Penicillinase

E933.5 Vitamins, not elsewhere classified
Vitamin A
Vitamin D

EXCLUDES *nicotinic acid (E942.2)*
vitamin K (E934.3)

E933.6 Oral bisphosphonates

E933.7 Intravenous bisphosphonates

E933.8 Other systemic agents, not elsewhere classified
Heavy metal antagonists

E933.9 Unspecified systemic agent

✓4ᵗʰ **E934 Agents primarily affecting blood constituents**

E934.0 Iron and its compounds
Ferric salts
Ferrous sulphate and other ferrous salts

E934.1 Liver preparations and other antianemic agents
Folic acid

E934.2 Anticoagulants
Coumarin
Heparin
Phenindione
Prothrombin synthesis inhibitor
Warfarin sodium

E934.3 Vitamin K [phytonadione]

E934.4 Fibrinolysis-affecting drugs
| Aminocaproic acid | Streptokinase |
| Streptodornase | Urokinase |

E934.5 Anticoagulant antagonists and other coagulants
Hexadimethrine bromide
Protamine sulfate

E934.6 Gamma globulin

E934.7 Natural blood and blood products
Blood plasma
Human fibrinogen
Packed red cells
Whole blood

E934.8 Other agents affecting blood constituents
Macromolecular blood substitutes

E934.9 Unspecified agent affecting blood constituents

✓4ᵗʰ **E935 Analgesics, antipyretics, and antirheumatics**

E935.0 Heroin
Diacetylmorphine

E935.1 Methadone

E935.2 Other opiates and related narcotics
Codeine [methylmorphine]
Meperidine [pethidine]
Morphine
Opium (alkaloids)

E935.3 Salicylates
Acetylsalicylic acid [aspirin]
Amino derivatives of salicylic acid
Salicylic acid salts

E935.4 Aromatic analgesics, not elsewhere classified
Acetanilid
Paracetamol [acetaminophen]
Phenacetin [acetophenetidin]

E935.5 Pyrazole derivatives
Aminophenazone [aminopyrine]
Phenylbutazone

E935.6 Antirheumatics [antiphlogistics]
Gold salts
Indomethacin

EXCLUDES *salicylates (E935.3)*
steroids (E932.0)

E935.7 Other non-narcotic analgesics
Pyrabital

E935.8 Other specified analgesics and antipyretics
Pentazocine

E935.9 Unspecified analgesic and antipyretic

✓4ᵗʰ **E936 Anticonvulsants and anti-Parkinsonism drugs**

E936.0 Oxazolidine derivatives
Paramethadione
Trimethadione

E936.1 Hydantoin derivatives
Phenytoin

E936.2 Succinimides
Ethosuximide
Phensuximide

E936.3 Other and unspecified anticonvulsants
Beclamide
Primidone

E936.4 Anti-Parkinsonism drugs
Amantadine
Ethopropazine [profenamine]
Levodopa [L-dopa]

✓4ᵗʰ **E937 Sedatives and hypnotics**

E937.0 Barbiturates
Amobarbital [amylobarbitone]
Barbital [barbitone]
Butabarbital [butabarbitone]
Pentobarbital [pentobarbitone]
Phenobarbital [phenobarbitone]
Secobarbital [quinalbarbitone]

EXCLUDES *thiobarbiturates (E938.3)*

E937.1 Chloral hydrate group

E937.2 Paraldehyde

E937.3 Bromine compounds
Bromide
Carbromal (derivatives)

E937.4 Methaqualone compounds

E937.5 Glutethimide group

E937.6 Mixed sedatives, not elsewhere classified

E937.8 Other sedatives and hypnotics

E937.9 Unspecified
Sleeping:
  drug
  pill   } NOS
  tablet

☑4ᵗʰ **E938 Other central nervous system depressants and anesthetics**

E938.0 Central nervous system muscle-tone depressants
Chlorphenesin (carbamate)
Mephenesin
Methocarbamol

E938.1 Halothane

E938.2 Other gaseous anesthetics
Ether
Halogenated hydrocarbon derivatives, except halothane
Nitrous oxide

E938.3 Intravenous anesthetics
Ketamine
Methohexital [methohexitone]
Thiobarbiturates, such as thiopental sodium

E938.4 Other and unspecified general anesthetics

E938.5 Surface and infiltration anesthetics
Cocaine
Lidocaine [lignocaine]
Procaine
Tetracaine

E938.6 Peripheral nerve- and plexus-blocking anesthetics

E938.7 Spinal anesthetics

E938.9 Other and unspecified local anesthetics

☑4ᵗʰ **E939 Psychotropic agents**

E939.0 Antidepressants
Amitriptyline
Imipramine
Monoamine oxidase [MAO] inhibitors

E939.1 Phenothiazine-based tranquilizers
Chlorpromazine   Prochlorperazine
Fluphenazine   Promazine
Phenothiazine

E939.2 Butyrophenone-based tranquilizers
Haloperidol
Spiperone
Trifluperidol

E939.3 Other antipsychotics, neuroleptics, and major tranquilizers

E939.4 Benzodiazepine-based tranquilizers
Chlordiazepoxide   Lorazepam
Diazepam   Medazepam
Flurazepam   Nitrazepam

E939.5 Other tranquilizers
Hydroxyzine
Meprobamate

E939.6 Psychodysleptics [hallucinogens]
Cannabis (derivatives)   Mescaline
Lysergide [LSD]   Psilocin
Marihuana (derivatives)   Psilocybin

E939.7 Psychostimulants
Amphetamine
Caffeine
EXCLUDES *central appetite depressants (E947.0)*

E939.8 Other psychotropic agents

E939.9 Unspecified psychotropic agent

☑4ᵗʰ **E940 Central nervous system stimulants**

E940.0 Analeptics
Lobeline
Nikethamide

E940.1 Opiate antagonists
Levallorphan
Nalorphine
Naloxone

E940.8 Other specified central nervous system stimulants

E940.9 Unspecified central nervous system stimulant

☑4ᵗʰ **E941 Drugs primarily affecting the autonomic nervous system**

E941.0 Parasympathomimetics [cholinergics]
Acetylcholine
Anticholinesterase:
   organophosphorus
   reversible
Pilocarpine

E941.1 Parasympatholytics [anticholinergics and antimuscarinics] and spasmolytics
Atropine
Homatropine
Hyoscine [scopolamine]
Quaternary ammonium derivatives
EXCLUDES *papaverine (E942.5)*

E941.2 Sympathomimetics [adrenergics]
Epinephrine [adrenalin]
Levarterenol [noradrenalin]

E941.3 Sympatholytics [antiadrenergics]
Phenoxybenzamine
Tolazolinehydrochloride

E941.9 Unspecified drug primarily affecting the autonomic nervous system

☑4ᵗʰ **E942 Agents primarily affecting the cardiovascular system**

E942.0 Cardiac rhythm regulators
Practolol   Propranolol
Procainamide   Quinidine

E942.1 Cardiotonic glycosides and drugs of similar action
Digitalis glycosides   Strophanthins
Digoxin

E942.2 Antilipemic and antiarteriosclerotic drugs
Cholestyramine   Nicotinic acid derivatives
Clofibrate   Sitosterols
EXCLUDES *dextrothyroxine (E932.7)*

E942.3 Ganglion-blocking agents
Pentamethonium bromide

E942.4 Coronary vasodilators
Dipyridamole   Nitrites
Nitrates [nitroglycerin]   Prenylamine

E942.5 Other vasodilators
Cyclandelate   Hydralazine
Diazoxide   Papaverine

E942.6 Other antihypertensive agents
Clonidine   Rauwolfia alkaloids
Guanethidine   Reserpine

E942.7 Antivaricose drugs, including sclerosing agents
Monoethanolamine
Zinc salts

E942.8 Capillary-active drugs
Adrenochrome derivatives
Bioflavonoids
Metaraminol

E942.9 Other and unspecified agents primarily affecting the cardiovascular system

☑4ᵗʰ **E943 Agents primarily affecting gastrointestinal system**

E943.0 Antacids and antigastric secretion drugs
Aluminum hydroxide
Magnesium trisilicate

E943.1 Irritant cathartics
Bisacodyl
Castor oil
Phenolphthalein

E943.2 Emollient cathartics
Sodium dioctyl sulfosuccinate

E943.3 Other cathartics, including intestinal atonia drugs
Magnesium sulfate

E943.4 Digestants
Pancreatin
Papain
Pepsin

E943.5 Antidiarrheal drugs
Bismuth subcarbonate Pectin or Kaolin
EXCLUDES *anti-infectives (E930.0-E931.9)*

E943.6 Emetics

E943.8 Other specified agents primarily affecting the gastrointestinal system

E943.9 Unspecified agent primarily affecting the gastrointestinal system

☑4ᵗʰ **E944 Water, mineral, and uric acid metabolism drugs**

E944.0 Mercurial diuretics
Chlormerodrin   Mercurophylline
Mercaptomerin   Mersalyl

E944.1 Purine derivative diuretics
Theobromine
Theophylline
EXCLUDES *aminophylline [theophylline ethylenediamine] (E945.7)*

E944.2 Carbonic acid anhydrase inhibitors
Acetazolamide

E944.3 Saluretics
Benzothiadiazides   Chlorothiazide group

E944.4 Other diuretics
Ethacrynic acid   Furosemide

E944.5 Electrolytic, caloric, and water-balance agents

E944.6 Other mineral salts, not elsewhere classified

E944.7 Uric acid metabolism drugs
Cinchophen and congeners
Colchicine
Phenoquin
Probenecid

☑4ᵗʰ **E945 Agents primarily acting on the smooth and skeletal muscles and respiratory system**

E945.0 Oxytocic agents
Ergot alkaloids
Prostaglandins

E945.1 Smooth muscle relaxants
Adiphenine
Metaproterenol [orciprenaline]
EXCLUDES *papaverine (E942.5)*

E945.2 Skeletal muscle relaxants
Alcuronium chloride
Suxamethonium chloride

E945.3 Other and unspecified drugs acting on muscles

E945.4 Antitussives
Dextromethorphan
Pipazethate hydrochloride

E945.5 Expectorants
Acetylcysteine
Cocillana
Guaifenesin [glyceryl guaiacolate]
Ipecacuanha
Terpin hydrate

E945.6 Anti-common cold drugs

E945.7 Antiasthmatics
Aminophylline [theophylline ethylenediamine]

E945.8 Other and unspecified respiratory drugs

☑4ᵗʰ **E946 Agents primarily affecting skin and mucous membrane, ophthalmological, otorhinolaryngological, and dental drugs**

E946.0 Local anti-infectives and anti-inflammatory drugs

E946.1 Antipruritics

E946.2 Local astringents and local detergents

E946.3 Emollients, demulcents, and protectants

E946.4 Keratolytics, kerstoplastics, other hair treatment drugs and preparations

E946.5 Eye anti-infectives and other eye drugs
Idoxuridine

E946.6 Anti-infectives and other drugs and preparations for ear, nose, and throat

E946.7 Dental drugs topically applied

E946.8 Other agents primarily affecting skin and mucous membrane
Spermicides

E946.9 Unspecified agent primarily affecting skin and mucous membrane

☑4ᵗʰ **E947 Other and unspecified drugs and medicinal substances**

E947.0 Dietetics

E947.1 Lipotropic drugs

E947.2 Antidotes and chelating agents, not elsewhere classified

E947.3 Alcohol deterrents

E947.4 Pharmaceutical excipients

E947.8 Other drugs and medicinal substances
Contrast media used for diagnostic x-ray procedures
Diagnostic agents and kits

E947.9 Unspecified drug or medicinal substance

☑4ᵗʰ **E948 Bacterial vaccines**

E948.0 BCG vaccine

E948.1 Typhoid and paratyphoid

E948.2 Cholera

E948.3 Plague

E948.4 Tetanus

E948.5 Diphtheria

E948.6 Pertussis vaccine, including combinations with a pertussis component

E948.8 Other and unspecified bacterial vaccines

E948.9 Mixed bacterial vaccines, except combinations with a pertussis component

☑4ᵗʰ **E949 Other vaccines and biological substances**
EXCLUDES *gamma globulin (E934.6)*

E949.0 Smallpox vaccine

E949.1 Rabies vaccine

E949.2 Typhus vaccine

E949.3 Yellow fever vaccine

E949.4 Measles vaccine

E949.5 Poliomyelitis vaccine

E949.6 Other and unspecified viral and rickettsial vaccines
Mumps vaccine

E949.7 Mixed viral-rickettsial and bacterial vaccines, except combinations with a pertussis component
EXCLUDES *combinations with a pertussis component (E948.6)*

E949.9 Other and unspecified vaccines and biological substances

SUICIDE AND SELF-INFLICTED INJURY (E950-E959)
INCLUDES injuries in suicide and attempted suicide
self-inflicted injuries specified as intentional

☑4ᵗʰ **E950 Suicide and self-inflicted poisoning by solid or liquid substances**

E950.0 Analgesics, antipyretics, and antirheumatics

E950.1 Barbiturates

E950.2 Other sedatives and hypnotics

E950.3 Tranquilizers and other psychotropic agents

E950.4 Other specified drugs and medicinal substances

E950.5 Unspecified drug or medicinal substance

E950.6 Agricultural and horticultural chemical and pharmaceutical preparations other than plant foods and fertilizers

E950.7 Corrosive and caustic substances
   Suicide and self-inflicted poisoning by substances classifiable to E864

E950.8 Arsenic and its compounds

E950.9 Other and unspecified solid and liquid substances

√4ᵗʰ **E951 Suicide and self-inflicted poisoning by gases in domestic use**

E951.0 Gas distributed by pipeline

E951.1 Liquefied petroleum gas distributed in mobile containers

E951.8 Other utility gas

√4ᵗʰ **E952 Suicide and self-inflicted poisoning by other gases and vapors**

E952.0 Motor vehicle exhaust gas

E952.1 Other carbon monoxide

E952.8 Other specified gases and vapors

E952.9 Unspecified gases and vapors

√4ᵗʰ **E953 Suicide and self-inflicted injury by hanging, strangulation, and suffocation**

E953.0 Hanging

E953.1 Suffocation by plastic bag

E953.8 Other specified means

E953.9 Unspecified means

E954 Suicide and self-inflicted injury by submersion [drowning]

√4ᵗʰ **E955 Suicide and self-inflicted injury by firearms, air guns and explosives**

E955.0 Handgun

E955.1 Shotgun

E955.2 Hunting rifle

E955.3 Military firearms

E955.4 Other and unspecified firearm
   Gunshot NOS
   Shot NOS

E955.5 Explosives

E955.6 Air gun
   BB gun
   Pellet gun

E955.7 Paintball gun

E955.9 Unspecified

E956 Suicide and self-inflicted injury by cutting and piercing instrument

√4ᵗʰ **E957 Suicide and self-inflicted injuries by jumping from high place**

E957.0 Residential premises

E957.1 Other man-made structures

E957.2 Natural sites

E957.9 Unspecified

√4ᵗʰ **E958 Suicide and self-inflicted injury by other and unspecified means**

E958.0 Jumping or lying before moving object

E958.1 Burns, fire

E958.2 Scald

E958.3 Extremes of cold

E958.4 Electrocution

E958.5 Crashing of motor vehicle

E958.6 Crashing of aircraft

E958.7 Caustic substances, except poisoning
   EXCLUDES   *poisoning by caustic substance (E950.7)*

E958.8 Other specified means

E958.9 Unspecified means

E959 Late effects of self-inflicted injury
   Note: This category is to be used to indicate circumstances classifiable to E950-E958 as the cause of death or disability from late effects, which are themselves classifiable elsewhere. The "late effects" include conditions reported as such, or as sequelae which may occur at any time after the attempted suicide or self-inflicted injury.

HOMICIDE AND INJURY PURPOSELY INFLICTED BY OTHER PERSONS (E960-E969)

INCLUDES   injuries inflicted by another person with intent to injure or kill, by any means

EXCLUDES   *injuries due to:*
   legal intervention (E970-E978)
   operations of war (E990-E999)
   terrorism (E979)

√4ᵗʰ **E960 Fight, brawl, rape**

E960.0 Unarmed fight or brawl
   Beatings NOS
   Brawl or fight with hands, fists, feet
   Injured or killed in fight NOS
   EXCLUDES   *homicidal:*
      injury by weapons (E965.0-E966, E969)
      strangulation (E963)
      submersion (E964)

E960.1 Rape

E961 Assault by corrosive or caustic substance, except poisoning
   Injury or death purposely caused by corrosive or caustic substance, such as:
   acid [any]
   corrosive substance
   vitriol
   EXCLUDES   *burns from hot liquid (E968.3)*
      chemical burns from swallowing a corrosive substance (E962.0-E962.9)

√4ᵗʰ **E962 Assault by poisoning**

E962.0 Drugs and medicinal substances
   Homicidal poisoning by any drug or medicinal substance

E962.1 Other solid and liquid substances

E962.2 Other gases and vapors

E962.9 Unspecified poisoning

E963 Assault by hanging and strangulation
   Homicidal (attempt):
   garrotting or ligature
   hanging
   strangulation
   suffocation

E964 Assault by submersion [drowning]

√4ᵗʰ **E965 Assault by firearms and explosives**

E965.0 Handgun
   Pistol
   Revolver

E965.1 Shotgun

E965.2 Hunting rifle

E965.3 Military firearms

E965.4 Other and unspecified firearm

E965.5 Antipersonnel bomb

E965.6 Gasoline bomb

E965.7 Letter bomb

E965.8 Other specified explosive
   Bomb NOS (placed in):
      car
      house
   Dynamite

E965.9 Unspecified explosive

E966 Assault by cutting and piercing instrument
    Assassination (attempt), homicide (attempt) by any instrument
        classifiable under E920
    Homicidal:
        cut
        puncture } any part of the body
        stab
    Stabbed any part of the body

☑4ᵗʰ **E967 Perpetrator of child and adult abuse**
    Note: Selection of the correct perpetrator code is based on the
        relationship between the perpetrator and the victim

    E967.0 By father, stepfather, or boyfriend
        Male partner of child's parent or guardian

    E967.1 By other specified person

    E967.2 By mother, stepmother, or girlfriend
        Female partner of child's parent or guardian

    E967.3 By spouse or partner
        Abuse of spouse or partner by ex-spouse or ex-partner

    E967.4 By child

    E967.5 By sibling

    E967.6 By grandparent

    E967.7 By other relative

    E967.8 By non-related caregiver

    E967.9 By unspecified person

☑4ᵗʰ **E968 Assault by other and unspecified means**
    E968.0 Fire
        Arson
        Homicidal burns NOS
        EXCLUDES   *burns from hot liquid (E968.3)*

    E968.1 Pushing from a high place

    E968.2 Striking by blunt or thrown object

    E968.3 Hot liquid
        Homicidal burns by scalding

    E968.4 Criminal neglect
        Abandonment of child, infant, or other helpless person
            with intent to injure or kill

    E968.5 Transport vehicle
        Being struck by other vehicle or run down with intent to
            injure
        Pushed in front of, thrown from, or dragged by moving
            vehicle with intent to injure

    E968.6 Air gun
        BB gun
        Pellet gun

    E968.7 Human bite

    E968.8 Other specified means

    E968.9 Unspecified means
        Assassination (attempt) NOS
        Homicidal (attempt):
            injury NOS
            wound NOS
        Manslaughter (nonaccidental)
        Murder (attempt) NOS
        Violence, non-accidental

E969 Late effects of injury purposely inflicted by other person
    Note: This category is to be used to indicate circumstances
        classifiable to E960-E968 as the cause of death or disability
        from late effects, which are themselves classifiable
        elsewhere. The "late effects" include conditions reported as
        such, or as sequelae which may occur at any time after
        injury purposely inflicted by another person.

LEGAL INTERVENTION (E970-E978)

    INCLUDES   injuries inflicted by the police or other law-enforcing
                agents, including military on duty, in the
                course of arresting or attempting to arrest
                lawbreakers, suppressing disturbances,
                maintaining order, and other legal action
                legal execution
    EXCLUDES   *injuries caused by civil insurrections (E990.0-E999)*

E970 Injury due to legal intervention by firearms
    Gunshot wound
    Injury by:
        machine gun
        revolver
        rifle pellet or rubber bullet
        shot NOS

E971 Injury due to legal intervention by explosives
    Injury by:
        dynamite
        explosive shell
        grenade
        mortar bomb

E972 Injury due to legal intervention by gas
    Asphyxiation by gas
    Injury by tear gas
    Poisoning by gas

E973 Injury due to legal intervention by blunt object
    Hit, struck by:
        baton (nightstick)
        blunt object
        stave

E974 Injury due to legal intervention by cutting and piercing instrument
    Cut
    Incised wound
    Injured by bayonet
    Stab wound

E975 Injury due to legal intervention by other specified means
    Blow
    Manhandling

E976 Injury due to legal intervention by unspecified means

E977 Late effects of injuries due to legal intervention
    Note: This category is to be used to indicate circumstances
        classifiable to E970-E976 as the cause of death or disability
        from late effects, which are themselves classifiable
        elsewhere. The "late effects" include conditions reported as
        such, or as sequelae, which may occur at any time after the
        injury due to legal intervention.

E978 Legal execution
    All executions performed at the behest of the judiciary or ruling
        authority [whether permanent or temporary] as:
    asphyxiation by gas
    beheading, decapitation (by guillotine)
    capital punishment
    electrocution
    hanging
    poisoning
    shooting
    other specified means

TERRORISM (E979)

☑4ᵗʰ **E979 Terrorism**
    Injuries resulting from the unlawful use of force or violence
        against persons or property to intimidate or coerce a
        Government, the civilian population, or any segment
        thereof, in furtherance of political or social objective

    E979.0 Terrorism involving explosion of marine weapons
        Depth-charge
        Marine mine
        Mine NOS, at sea or in harbour
        Sea-based artillery shell
        Torpedo
        Underwater blast

E979.1 Terrorism involving destruction of aircraft
    Aircraft used as a weapon
    Aircraft:
        burned
        exploded
        shot down
    Crushed by falling aircraft

E979.2 Terrorism involving other explosions and fragments
    Antipersonnel bomb (fragments)
    Blast NOS
    Explosion (of):
        artillery shell
        breech-block
        cannon block
        mortar bomb
        munitions being used in terrorism
        NOS
    Fragments from:
        artillery shell
        bomb
        grenade
        guided missile
        land-mine
        rocket
        shell
        shrapnel
    Mine NOS

E979.3 Terrorism involving fires, conflagration and hot substances
    Burning building or structure:
        collapse of
        fall from
        hit by falling object in
        jump from
    Conflagration NOS
    Fire (causing):
        Asphyxia
        Burns
        NOS
        Other injury
    Melting of fittings and furniture in burning
    Petrol bomb
    Smouldering building or structure

E979.4 Terrorism involving firearms
    Bullet:
        carbine
        machine gun
        pistol
        rifle
        rubber (rifle)
    Pellets (shotgun)

E979.5 Terrorism involving nuclear weapons
    Blast effects
    Exposure to ionizing radiation from nuclear weapon
    Fireball effects
    Heat from nuclear weapon
    Other direct and secondary effects of nuclear weapons

E979.6 Terrorism involving biological weapons
    Anthrax
    Cholera
    Smallpox

E979.7 Terrorism involving chemical weapons
    Gases, fumes, chemicals
    Hydrogen cyanide
    Phosgene
    Sarin

E979.8 Terrorism involving other means
    Drowning and submersion
    Lasers
    Piercing or stabbing instruments
    Terrorism NOS

E979.9 Terrorism, secondary effects
    Note: This code is for use to identify conditions occurring subsequent to a terrorist attack not those that are due to the initial terrorist act
    EXCLUDES *late effect of terrorist attack (E999.1)*

INJURY UNDETERMINED WHETHER ACCIDENTALLY OR PURPOSELY INFLICTED (E980-E989)

Note: Categories E980-E989 are for use when it is unspecified or it cannot be determined whether the injuries are accidental (unintentional), suicide (attempted), or assault.

√4th **E980 Poisoning by solid or liquid substances, undetermined whether accidentally or purposely inflicted**

    E980.0 Analgesics, antipyretics, and antirheumatics

    E980.1 Barbiturates

    E980.2 Other sedatives and hypnotics

    E980.3 Tranquilizers and other psychotropic agents

    E980.4 Other specified drugs and medicinal substances

    E980.5 Unspecified drug or medicinal substance

    E980.6 Corrosive and caustic substances
        Poisoning, undetermined whether accidental or purposeful, by substances classifiable to E864

    E980.7 Agricultural and horticultural chemical and pharmaceutical preparations other than plant foods and fertilizers

    E980.8 Arsenic and its compounds

    E980.9 Other and unspecified solid and liquid substances

√4th **E981 Poisoning by gases in domestic use, undetermined whether accidentally or purposely inflicted**

    E981.0 Gas distributed by pipeline

    E981.1 Liquefied petroleum gas distributed in mobile containers

    E981.8 Other utility gas

√4th **E982 Poisoning by other gases, undetermined whether accidentally or purposely inflicted**

    E982.0 Motor vehicle exhaust gas

    E982.1 Other carbon monoxide

    E982.8 Other specified gases and vapors

    E982.9 Unspecified gases and vapors

√4th **E983 Hanging, strangulation, or suffocation, undetermined whether accidentally or purposely inflicted**

    E983.0 Hanging

    E983.1 Suffocation by plastic bag

    E983.8 Other specified means

    E983.9 Unspecified means

E984 Submersion [drowning], undetermined whether accidentally or purposely inflicted

√4th **E985 Injury by firearms, air guns and explosives, undetermined whether accidentally or purposely inflicted**

    E985.0 Handgun

    E985.1 Shotgun

    E985.2 Hunting rifle

    E985.3 Military firearms

    E985.4 Other and unspecified firearm

    E985.5 Explosives

    E985.6 Air gun
        BB gun   Pellet gun

    E985.7 Paintball gun

E986 Injury by cutting and piercing instruments, undetermined whether accidentally or purposely inflicted

√4th **E987 Falling from high place, undetermined whether accidentally or purposely inflicted**

    E987.0 Residential premises

    E987.1 Other man-made structures

    E987.2 Natural sites

    E987.9 Unspecified site

√4ᵗ **E988 Injury by other and unspecified means, undetermined whether accidentally or purposely inflicted**

E988.0 Jumping or lying before moving object

E988.1 Burns, fire

E988.2 Scald

E988.3 Extremes of cold

E988.4 Electrocution

E988.5 Crashing of motor vehicle

E988.6 Crashing of aircraft

E988.7 Caustic substances, except poisoning

E988.8 Other specified means

E988.9 Unspecified means

E989 Late effects of injury, undetermined whether accidentally or purposely inflicted

Note: This category is to be used to indicate circumstances classifiable to E980-E988 as the cause of death or disability from late effects, which are themselves classifiable elsewhere. The "late effects" include conditions reported as such, or as sequelae, which may occur at any time after injury, undetermined whether accidentally or purposely inflicted.

INJURY RESULTING FROM OPERATIONS OF WAR (E990-E999)

INCLUDES   injuries to military personnel and civilians caused by war and civil insurrections and occurring during the time of war and insurrection, and peacekeeping missions

EXCLUDES   accidents during training of military personnel manufacture of war material and transport, unless attributable to enemy action

√4ᵗ **E990 Injury due to war operations by fires and conflagrations**

INCLUDES   asphyxia, burns, or other injury originating from fire caused by a fire-producing device or indirectly by any conventional weapon

E990.0 From gasoline bomb
Incendiary bomb

E990.1 From flamethrower

E990.2 From incendiary bullet

E990.3 From fire caused indirectly from conventional weapon
EXCLUDES   fire aboard military aircraft (E994.3)

E990.9 From other and unspecified source

√4ᵗ **E991 Injury due to war operations by bullets and fragments**

EXCLUDES   injury due to bullets and fragments due to war operations, but occurring after cessation of hostilities (E998.0)
injury due to explosion of artillery shells and mortars (E993.2)
injury due to explosion of improvised explosive device [IED] (E993.3-E993.5)
injury due to sea-based artillery shell (E992.3)

E991.0 Rubber bullets (rifle)

E991.1 Pellets (rifle)

E991.2 Other bullets
Bullet [any, except rubber bullets and pellets]
carbine
machine gun
pistol
rifle
shotgun

E991.3 Antipersonnel bomb (fragments)

E991.4 Fragments from munitions
Fragments from:
artillery shell
bombs, except antipersonnel
detonation of unexploded ordnance [UXO]
grenade
guided missile
land mine
rockets
shell

E991.5 Fragments from person-borne improvised explosive device [IED]

E991.6 Fragments from vehicle-borne improvised explosive device [IED]
IED borne by land, air, or water transport vehicle

E991.7 Fragments from other improvised explosive device [IED]
Roadside IED

E991.8 Fragments from weapons
Fragments from:
artillery
autocannons
automatic grenade launchers
missile launchers
mortars
small arms

E991.9 Other and unspecified fragments
Shrapnel NOS

√4ᵗ **E992 Injury due to war operations by explosion of marine weapons**

E992.0 Torpedo

E992.1 Depth charge

E992.2 Marine mines
Marine mines at sea or in harbor

E992.3 Sea-based artillery shell

E992.8 Other marine weapons

E992.9 Unspecified marine weapon
Underwater blast NOS

√4ᵗ **E993 Injury due to war operations by other explosion**
Injuries due to direct or indirect pressure or air blast of an explosion occurring during war operations
EXCLUDES   injury due to fragments resulting from an explosion (E991.0-E991.9)
injury due to detonation of unexploded ordnance but occurring after cessation of hostilities (E998.0-E998.9)
injury due to nuclear weapons (E996.0-E996.9)

E993.0 Aerial bomb

E993.1 Guided missile

E993.2 Mortar
Artillery shell

E993.3 Person-borne improvised explosive device [IED]

E993.4 Vehicle-borne improvised explosive device [IED]
IED borne by land, air, or water transport vehicle

E993.5 Other improvised explosive device [IED]
Roadside IED

E993.6 Unintentional detonation of own munitions
Unintentional detonation of own ammunition (artillery) (mortars)

E993.7 Unintentional discharge of own munitions launch device
Unintentional explosion of own:
autocannons
automatic grenade launchers
missile launchers
small arms

E993.8 Other specified explosion
Bomb
Grenade
Land mine

E993.9 Unspecified explosion
Air blast NOS
Blast NOS
Blast wave NOS
Blast wind NOS
Explosion NOS

√4ᵗʰ **E994 Injury due to war operations by destruction of aircraft**

E994.0 Destruction of aircraft due to enemy fire or explosives
Air to air missile
Explosive device placed on aircraft
Rocket propelled grenade [RPG]
Small arms fire
Surface to air missile

E994.1 Unintentional destruction of aircraft due to own onboard explosives

E994.2 Destruction of aircraft due to collision with other aircraft

E994.3 Destruction of aircraft due to onboard fire

E994.8 Other destruction of aircraft

E994.9 Unspecified destruction of aircraft

√4ᵗʰ **E995 Injury due to war operations by other and unspecified forms of conventional warfare**

E995.0 Unarmed hand-to-hand combat
EXCLUDES   *intentional restriction of airway (E995.3)*

E995.1 Struck by blunt object
Baton (nightstick)
Stave

E995.2 Piercing object
Bayonet
Knife
Sword

E995.3 Intentional restriction of air and airway
Intentional submersion
Strangulation
Suffocation

E995.4 Unintentional drowning due to inability to surface or obtain air
Submersion

E995.8 Other forms of conventional warfare

E995.9 Unspecified form of conventional warfare

√4ᵗʰ **E996 Injury due to war operations by nuclear weapons**
Dirty bomb NOS
EXCLUDES   *late effects of injury due to nuclear weapons (E999.0, E999.1)*

E996.0 Direct blast effect of nuclear weapon
Injury to bodily organs due to blast pressure

E996.1 Indirect blast effect of nuclear weapon
Injury due to being thrown by blast
Injury due to being struck or crushed by blast debris

E996.2 Thermal radiation effect of nuclear weapon
Burns due to thermal radiation
Fireball effects
Flash burns
Heat effects

E996.3 Nuclear radiation effects
Acute radiation exposure
Beta burns
Fallout exposure
Radiation sickness
Secondary effects of nuclear weapons

E996.8 Other effects of nuclear weapons

E996.9 Unspecified effect of nuclear weapon

√4ᵗʰ **E997 Injury due to war operations by other forms of unconventional warfare**

E997.0 Lasers

E997.1 Biological warfare

E997.2 Gases, fumes, and chemicals

E997.3 Weapon of mass destruction [WMD], unspecified

E997.8 Other specified forms of unconventional warfare

E997.9 Unspecified form of unconventional warfare

√4ᵗʰ **E998 Injury due to war operations but occurring after cessation of hostilities**
Injuries due to operations of war but occurring after cessation of hostilities by any means classifiable under E990-E997
Injuries by explosion of bombs or mines placed in the course of operations of war, if the explosion occurred after cessation of hostilities

E998.0 Explosion of mines

E998.1 Explosion of bombs

E998.8 Injury due to other war operations but occurring after cessation of hostilities

E998.9 Injury due to unspecified war operations but occurring after cessation of hostilities

√4ᵗʰ **E999 Late effect of injury due to war operations and terrorism**
Note: This category is to be used to indicate circumstances classifiable to E979, E990-E998 as the cause of death or disability from late effects, which are themselves classifiable elsewhere. The "late effects" include conditions reported as such, or as sequelae, which may occur at any time after the injury, resulting from operations of war or terrorism

E999.0 Late effect of injury due to war operations

E999.1 Late effect of injury due to terrorism

Appendix A: Morphology of Neoplasms

The World Health Organization has published an adaptation of the International Classification of Diseases for oncology (ICD-O). It contains a coded nomenclature for the morphology of neoplasms, which is reproduced here for those who wish to use it in conjunction with Chapter 2 of the International Classification of Diseases, 9th Revision, Clinical Modification.

The morphology code numbers consist of five digits; the first four identify the histological type of the neoplasm and the fifth indicates its behavior. The one-digit behavior code is as follows:

/0 Benign
/1 Uncertain whether benign or malignant
   Borderline malignancy
/2 Carcinoma in situ
   Intraepithelial
   Noninfiltrating
   Noninvasive
/3 Malignant, primary site
/6 Malignant, metastatic site
   Secondary site
/9 Malignant, uncertain whether primary or metastatic site

In the nomenclature below, the morphology code numbers include the behavior code appropriate to the histological type of neoplasm, but this behavior code should be changed if other reported information makes this necessary. For example, "chordoma (M9370/3)" is assumed to be malignant; the term "benign chordoma" should be coded M9370/0. Similarly, "superficial spreading adenocarcinoma (M8143/3)" described as "noninvasive" should be coded M8143/2 and "melanoma (M8720/3)" described as "secondary" should be coded M8720/6.

The following table shows the correspondence between the morphology code and the different sections of Chapter 2:

Morphology Code Histology/Behavior		ICD-9-CM Chapter 2	
Any	0	210-229	Benign neoplasms
M8000-M8004	1	239	Neoplasms of unspecified nature
M8010+	1	235-238	Neoplasms of uncertain behavior
Any	2	230-234	Carcinoma in situ
Any	3	140-195 200-208	Malignant neoplasms, stated or presumed to be primary
Any	6	196-198	Malignant neoplasms, stated or presumed to be secondary

The ICD-O behavior digit /9 is inapplicable in an ICD context, since all malignant neoplasms are presumed to be primary (/3) or secondary (/6) according to other information on the medical record. Only the first-listed term of the full ICD-O morphology nomenclature appears against each code number in the list below. The ICD-9-CM Alphabetical Index (Volume 2), however, includes all the ICD-O synonyms as well as a number of other morphological names still likely to be encountered on medical records but omitted from ICD-O as outdated or otherwise undesirable.

A coding difficulty sometimes arises where a morphological diagnosis contains two qualifying adjectives that have different code numbers. An example is "transitional cell epidermoid carcinoma." "Transitional cell carcinoma NOS" is M8120/3 and "epidermoid carcinoma NOS" is M8070/3. In such circumstances, the higher number (M8120/3 in this example) should be used, as it is usually more specific.

Coded Nomenclature for Morphology of Neoplasms

M800   **Neoplasms NOS**
M8000/0   Neoplasm, benign
M8000/1   Neoplasm, uncertain whether benign or malignant
M8000/3   Neoplasm, malignant
M8000/6   Neoplasm, metastatic
M8000/9   Neoplasm, malignant, uncertain whether primary or metastatic
M8001/0   Tumor cells, benign
M8001/1   Tumor cells, uncertain whether benign or malignant
M8001/3   Tumor cells, malignant
M8002/3   Malignant tumor, small cell type
M8003/3   Malignant tumor, giant cell type
M8004/3   Malignant tumor, fusiform cell type

M801-M804   **Epithelial neoplasms NOS**
M8010/0   Epithelial tumor, benign
M8010/2   Carcinoma in situ NOS
M8010/3   Carcinoma NOS
M8010/6   Carcinoma, metastatic NOS
M8010/9   Carcinomatosis
M8011/0   Epithelioma, benign
M8011/3   Epithelioma, malignant
M8012/3   Large cell carcinoma NOS
M8020/3   Carcinoma, undifferentiated type NOS
M8021/3   Carcinoma, anaplastic type NOS
M8022/3   Pleomorphic carcinoma
M8030/3   Giant cell and spindle cell carcinoma
M8031/3   Giant cell carcinoma
M8032/3   Spindle cell carcinoma
M8033/3   Pseudosarcomatous carcinoma
M8034/3   Polygonal cell carcinoma
M8035/3   Spheroidal cell carcinoma
M8040/1   Tumorlet
M8041/3   Small cell carcinoma NOS
M8042/3   Oat cell carcinoma
M8043/3   Small cell carcinoma, fusiform cell type

M805-M808   **Papillary and squamous cell neoplasms**
M8050/0   Papilloma NOS (except Papilloma of urinary bladder M8120/1)
M8050/2   Papillary carcinoma in situ
M8050/3   Papillary carcinoma NOS
M8051/0   Verrucous papilloma
M8051/3   Verrucous carcinoma NOS
M8052/0   Squamous cell papilloma
M8052/3   Papillary squamous cell carcinoma
M8053/0   Inverted papilloma
M8060/0   Papillomatosis NOS
M8070/2   Squamous cell carcinoma in situ NOS
M8070/3   Squamous cell carcinoma NOS
M8070/6   Squamous cell carcinoma, metastatic NOS
M8071/3   Squamous cell carcinoma, keratinizing type NOS
M8072/3   Squamous cell carcinoma, large cell, nonkeratinizing type
M8073/3   Squamous cell carcinoma, small cell, nonkeratinizing type
M8074/3   Squamous cell carcinoma, spindle cell type
M8075/3   Adenoid squamous cell carcinoma
M8076/2   Squamous cell carcinoma in situ with questionable stromal invasion
M8076/3   Squamous cell carcinoma, microinvasive
M8080/2   Queyrat's erythroplasia
M8081/2   Bowen's disease
M8082/3   Lymphoepithelial carcinoma

M809-M811   **Basal cell neoplasms**
M8090/1   Basal cell tumor
M8090/3   Basal cell carcinoma NOS
M8091/3   Multicentric basal cell carcinoma
M8092/3   Basal cell carcinoma, morphea type
M8093/3   Basal cell carcinoma, fibroepithelial type
M8094/3   Basosquamous carcinoma
M8095/3   Metatypical carcinoma
M8096/0   Intraepidermal epithelioma of Jadassohn
M8100/0   Trichoepithelioma
M8101/0   Trichofolliculoma
M8102/0   Tricholemmoma
M8110/0   Pilomatrixoma

M812-M813   **Transitional cell papillomas and carcinomas**
M8120/0   Transitional cell papilloma NOS
M8120/1   Urothelial papilloma
M8120/2   Transitional cell carcinoma in situ
M8120/3   Transitional cell carcinoma NOS
M8121/0   Schneiderian papilloma
M8121/1   Transitional cell papilloma, inverted type
M8121/3   Schneiderian carcinoma
M8122/3   Transitional cell carcinoma, spindle cell type
M8123/3   Basaloid carcinoma
M8124/3   Cloacogenic carcinoma
M8130/3   Papillary transitional cell carcinoma

M814-M838   **Adenomas and adenocarcinomas**
M8140/0   Adenoma NOS
M8140/1   Bronchial adenoma NOS
M8140/2   Adenocarcinoma in situ
M8140/3   Adenocarcinoma NOS
M8140/6   Adenocarcinoma, metastatic NOS
M8141/3   Scirrhous adenocarcinoma
M8142/3   Linitis plastica
M8143/3   Superficial spreading adenocarcinoma
M8144/3   Adenocarcinoma, intestinal type
M8145/3   Carcinoma, diffuse type
M8146/0   Monomorphic adenoma
M8147/0   Basal cell adenoma
M8150/0   Islet cell adenoma
M8150/3   Islet cell carcinoma
M8151/0   Insulinoma NOS

M8151/3	Insulinoma, malignant	M8321/0	Chief cell adenoma	M8441/1	Serous cystadenoma, borderline malignancy
M8152/0	Glucagonoma NOS	M8322/0	Water-clear cell adenoma	M8441/3	Serous cystadenocarcinoma NOS
M8152/3	Glucagonoma, malignant	M8322/3	Water-clear cell adenocarcinoma	M8450/0	Papillary cystadenoma NOS
M8153/1	Gastrinoma NOS	M8323/0	Mixed cell adenoma	M8450/1	Papillary cystadenoma, borderline malignancy
M8153/3	Gastrinoma, malignant	M8323/3	Mixed cell adenocarcinoma	M8450/3	Papillary cystadenocarcinoma NOS
M8154/3	Mixed islet cell and exocrine adenocarcinoma	M8324/0	Lipoadenoma	M8460/0	Papillary serous cystadenoma NOS
M8160/0	Bile duct adenoma	M8330/0	Follicular adenoma	M8460/1	Papillary serous cystadenoma, borderline malignancy
M8160/3	Cholangiocarcinoma	M8330/3	Follicular adenocarcinoma NOS	M8460/3	Papillary serous cystadenocarcinoma
M8161/0	Bile duct cystadenoma	M8331/3	Follicular adenocarcinoma, well differentiated type	M8461/0	Serous surface papilloma NOS
M8161/3	Bile duct cystadenocarcinoma	M8332/3	Follicular adenocarcinoma, trabecular type	M8461/1	Serous surface papilloma, borderline malignancy
M8170/0	Liver cell adenoma	M8333/0	Microfollicular adenoma	M8461/3	Serous surface papillary carcinoma
M8170/3	Hepatocellular carcinoma NOS	M8334/0	Macrofollicular adenoma	M8470/0	Mucinous cystadenoma NOS
M8180/0	Hepatocholangioma, benign	M8340/3	Papillary and follicular adenocarcinoma	M8470/1	Mucinous cystadenoma, borderline malignancy
M8180/3	Combined hepatocellular carcinoma and cholangiocarcinoma	M8350/3	Nonencapsulated sclerosing carcinoma	M8470/3	Mucinous cystadenocarcinoma NOS
M8190/0	Trabecular adenoma	M8360/1	Multiple endocrine adenomas	M8471/0	Papillary mucinous cystadenoma NOS
M8190/3	Trabecular adenocarcinoma	M8361/1	Juxtaglomerular tumor	M8471/1	Papillary mucinous cystadenoma, borderline malignancy
M8191/0	Embryonal adenoma	M8370/0	Adrenal cortical adenoma NOS	M8471/3	Papillary mucinous cystadenocarcinoma
M8200/0	Eccrine dermal cylindroma	M8370/3	Adrenal cortical carcinoma		
M8200/3	Adenoid cystic carcinoma	M8371/0	Adrenal cortical adenoma, compact cell type	M8480/0	Mucinous adenoma
M8201/3	Cribriform carcinoma	M8372/0	Adrenal cortical adenoma, heavily pigmented variant	M8480/3	Mucinous adenocarcinoma
M8210/0	Adenomatous polyp NOS			M8480/6	Pseudomyxoma peritonei
M8210/3	Adenocarcinoma in adenomatous polyp	M8373/0	Adrenal cortical adenoma, clear cell type	M8481/3	Mucin-producing adenocarcinoma
M8211/0	Tubular adenoma NOS	M8374/0	Adrenal cortical adenoma, glomerulosa cell type	M8490/3	Signet ring cell carcinoma
M8211/3	Tubular adenocarcinoma	M8375/0	Adrenal cortical adenoma, mixed cell type	M8490/6	Metastatic signet ring cell carcinoma
M8220/0	Adenomatous polyposis coli			**M850-M854**	**Ductal, lobular, and medullary neoplasms**
M8220/3	Adenocarcinoma in adenomatous polyposis coli	M8380/0	Endometrioid adenoma NOS		
M8221/0	Multiple adenomatous polyps	M8380/1	Endometrioid adenoma, borderline malignancy	M8500/2	Intraductal carcinoma, noninfiltrating NOS
M8230/3	Solid carcinoma NOS	M8380/3	Endometrioid carcinoma	M8500/3	Infiltrating duct carcinoma
M8231/3	Carcinoma simplex	M8381/0	Endometrioid adenofibroma NOS	M8501/2	Comedocarcinoma, noninfiltrating
M8240/1	Carcinoid tumor NOS	M8381/1	Endometrioid adenofibroma, borderline malignancy	M8501/3	Comedocarcinoma NOS
M8240/3	Carcinoid tumor, malignant	M8381/3	Endometrioid adenofibroma, malignant	M8502/3	Juvenile carcinoma of the breast
M8241/1	Carcinoid tumor, argentaffin NOS			M8503/0	Intraductal papilloma
M8241/3	Carcinoid tumor, argentaffin, malignant	**M839-M842**	**Adnexal and skin appendage neoplasms**	M8503/2	Noninfiltrating intraductal papillary adenocarcinoma
M8242/1	Carcinoid tumor, nonargentaffin NOS	M8390/0	Skin appendage adenoma	M8504/0	Intracystic papillary adenoma
M8242/3	Carcinoid tumor, nonargentaffin, malignant	M8390/3	Skin appendage carcinoma	M8504/2	Noninfiltrating intracystic carcinoma
M8243/3	Mucocarcinoid tumor, malignant	M8400/0	Sweat gland adenoma	M8505/0	Intraductal papillomatosis NOS
M8244/3	Composite carcinoid	M8400/1	Sweat gland tumor NOS	M8506/0	Subareolar duct papillomatosis
M8250/1	Pulmonary adenomatosis	M8400/3	Sweat gland adenocarcinoma	M8510/3	Medullary carcinoma NOS
M8250/3	Bronchiolo-alveolar adenocarcinoma	M8401/0	Apocrine adenoma	M8511/3	Medullary carcinoma with amyloid stroma
M8251/0	Alveolar adenoma	M8401/3	Apocrine adenocarcinoma	M8512/3	Medullary carcinoma with lymphoid stroma
M8251/3	Alveolar adenocarcinoma	M8402/0	Eccrine acrospiroma		
M8260/0	Papillary adenoma NOS	M8403/0	Eccrine spiradenoma	M8520/2	Lobular carcinoma in situ
M8260/3	Papillary adenocarcinoma NOS	M8404/0	Hidrocystoma	M8520/3	Lobular carcinoma NOS
M8261/1	Villous adenoma NOS	M8405/0	Papillary hydradenoma	M8521/3	Infiltrating ductular carcinoma
M8261/3	Adenocarcinoma in villous adenoma	M8406/0	Papillary syringadenoma	M8530/3	Inflammatory carcinoma
M8262/3	Villous adenocarcinoma	M8407/0	Syringoma NOS	M8540/3	Paget's disease, mammary
M8263/0	Tubulovillous adenoma	M8410/0	Sebaceous adenoma	M8541/3	Paget's disease and infiltrating duct carcinoma of breast
M8270/0	Chromophobe adenoma	M8410/3	Sebaceous adenocarcinoma		
M8270/3	Chromophobe carcinoma	M8420/0	Ceruminous adenoma	M8542/3	Paget's disease, extramammary (except Paget's disease of bone)
M8280/0	Acidophil adenoma	M8420/3	Ceruminous adenocarcinoma		
M8280/3	Acidophil carcinoma			**M855**	**Acinar cell neoplasms**
M8281/0	Mixed acidophil-basophil adenoma	**M843**	**Mucoepidermoid neoplasms**	M8550/0	Acinar cell adenoma
M8281/3	Mixed acidophil-basophil carcinoma	M8430/1	Mucoepidermoid tumor	M8550/1	Acinar cell tumor
M8290/0	Oxyphilic adenoma	M8430/3	Mucoepidermoid carcinoma	M8550/3	Acinar cell carcinoma
M8290/3	Oxyphilic adenocarcinoma			**M856-M858**	**Complex epithelial neoplasms**
M8300/0	Basophil adenoma	**M844-M849**	**Cystic, mucinous, and serous neoplasms**	M8560/3	Adenosquamous carcinoma
M8300/3	Basophil carcinoma			M8561/0	Adenolymphoma
M8310/0	Clear cell adenoma	M8440/0	Cystadenoma NOS	M8570/3	Adenocarcinoma with squamous metaplasia
M8310/3	Clear cell adenocarcinoma NOS	M8440/3	Cystadenocarcinoma NOS		
M8311/1	Hypernephroid tumor	M8441/0	Serous cystadenoma NOS		
M8312/3	Renal cell carcinoma				
M8313/0	Clear cell adenofibroma				
M8320/3	Granular cell carcinoma				

M8571/3	Adenocarcinoma with cartilaginous and osseous metaplasia	M8742/3	Malignant melanoma in Hutchinson's melanotic freckle	M8860/3	Angiomyoliposarcoma
M8572/3	Adenocarcinoma with spindle cell metaplasia	M8743/3	Superficial spreading melanoma	M8861/0	Angiolipoma NOS
		M8750/0	Intradermal nevus	M8861/1	Angiolipoma, infiltrating
M8573/3	Adenocarcinoma with apocrine metaplasia	M8760/0	Compound nevus	M8870/0	Myelolipoma
		M8761/1	Giant pigmented nevus	M8880/0	Hibernoma
M8580/0	Thymoma, benign	M8761/3	Malignant melanoma in giant pigmented nevus	M8881/0	Lipoblastomatosis
M8580/3	Thymoma, malignant				

M859-M867   Specialized gonadal neoplasms

M8590/1	Sex cord-stromal tumor
M8600/0	Thecoma NOS
M8600/3	Theca cell carcinoma
M8610/0	Luteoma NOS
M8620/1	Granulosa cell tumor NOS
M8620/3	Granulosa cell tumor, malignant
M8621/1	Granulosa cell-theca cell tumor
M8630/0	Androblastoma, benign
M8630/1	Androblastoma NOS
M8630/3	Androblastoma, malignant
M8631/0	Sertoli-Leydig cell tumor
M8632/1	Gynandroblastoma
M8640/0	Tubular androblastoma NOS
M8640/3	Sertoli cell carcinoma
M8641/0	Tubular androblastoma with lipid storage
M8650/0	Leydig cell tumor, benign
M8650/1	Leydig cell tumor NOS
M8650/3	Leydig cell tumor, malignant
M8660/0	Hilar cell tumor
M8670/0	Lipid cell tumor of ovary
M8671/0	Adrenal rest tumor

M868-M871   Paragangliomas and glomus tumors

M8680/1	Paraganglioma NOS
M8680/3	Paraganglioma, malignant
M8681/1	Sympathetic paraganglioma
M8682/1	Parasympathetic paraganglioma
M8690/1	Glomus jugulare tumor
M8691/1	Aortic body tumor
M8692/1	Carotid body tumor
M8693/1	Extra-adrenal paraganglioma NOS
M8693/3	Extra-adrenal paraganglioma, malignant
M8700/0	Pheochromocytoma NOS
M8700/3	Pheochromocytoma, malignant
M8710/3	Glomangiosarcoma
M8711/0	Glomus tumor
M8712/0	Glomangioma

M872-M879   Nevi and melanomas

M8720/0	Pigmented nevus NOS
M8720/3	Malignant melanoma NOS
M8721/3	Nodular melanoma
M8722/0	Balloon cell nevus
M8722/3	Balloon cell melanoma
M8723/0	Halo nevus
M8724/0	Fibrous papule of the nose
M8725/0	Neuronevus
M8726/0	Magnocellular nevus
M8730/0	Nonpigmented nevus
M8730/3	Amelanotic melanoma
M8740/0	Junctional nevus
M8740/3	Malignant melanoma in junctional nevus
M8741/2	Precancerous melanosis NOS
M8741/3	Malignant melanoma in precancerous melanosis
M8742/2	Hutchinson's melanotic freckle

M8770/0	Epithelioid and spindle cell nevus
M8771/3	Epithelioid cell melanoma
M8772/3	Spindle cell melanoma NOS
M8773/3	Spindle cell melanoma, type A
M8774/3	Spindle cell melanoma, type B
M8775/3	Mixed epithelioid and spindle cell melanoma
M8780/0	Blue nevus NOS
M8780/3	Blue nevus, malignant
M8790/0	Cellular blue nevus

M880   Soft tissue tumors and sarcomas NOS

M8800/0	Soft tissue tumor, benign
M8800/3	Sarcoma NOS
M8800/9	Sarcomatosis NOS
M8801/3	Spindle cell sarcoma
M8802/3	Giant cell sarcoma (except of bone M9250/3)
M8803/3	Small cell sarcoma
M8804/3	Epithelioid cell sarcoma

M881-M883   Fibromatous neoplasms

M8810/0	Fibroma NOS
M8810/3	Fibrosarcoma NOS
M8811/0	Fibromyxoma
M8811/3	Fibromyxosarcoma
M8812/0	Periosteal fibroma
M8812/3	Periosteal fibrosarcoma
M8813/0	Fascial fibroma
M8813/3	Fascial fibrosarcoma
M8814/3	Infantile fibrosarcoma
M8820/0	Elastofibroma
M8821/1	Aggressive fibromatosis
M8822/1	Abdominal fibromatosis
M8823/1	Desmoplastic fibroma
M8830/0	Fibrous histiocytoma NOS
M8830/1	Atypical fibrous histiocytoma
M8830/3	Fibrous histiocytoma, malignant
M8831/0	Fibroxanthoma NOS
M8831/1	Atypical fibroxanthoma
M8831/3	Fibroxanthoma, malignant
M8832/0	Dermatofibroma NOS
M8832/1	Dermatofibroma protuberans
M8832/3	Dermatofibrosarcoma NOS

M884   Myxomatous neoplasms

M8840/0	Myxoma NOS
M8840/3	Myxosarcoma

M885-M888   Lipomatous neoplasms

M8850/0	Lipoma NOS
M8850/3	Liposarcoma NOS
M8851/0	Fibrolipoma
M8851/3	Liposarcoma, well differentiated type
M8852/0	Fibromyxolipoma
M8852/3	Myxoid liposarcoma
M8853/3	Round cell liposarcoma
M8854/3	Pleomorphic liposarcoma
M8855/3	Mixed type liposarcoma
M8856/0	Intramuscular lipoma
M8857/0	Spindle cell lipoma
M8860/0	Angiomyolipoma

M889-M892   Myomatous neoplasms

M8890/0	Leiomyoma NOS
M8890/1	Intravascular leiomyomatosis
M8890/3	Leiomyosarcoma NOS
M8891/1	Epithelioid leiomyoma
M8891/3	Epithelioid leiomyosarcoma
M8892/1	Cellular leiomyoma
M8893/0	Bizarre leiomyoma
M8894/0	Angiomyoma
M8894/3	Angiomyosarcoma
M8895/0	Myoma
M8895/3	Myosarcoma
M8900/0	Rhabdomyoma NOS
M8900/3	Rhabdomyosarcoma NOS
M8901/3	Pleomorphic rhabdomyosarcoma
M8902/3	Mixed type rhabdomyosarcoma
M8903/0	Fetal rhabdomyoma
M8904/0	Adult rhabdomyoma
M8910/3	Embryonal rhabdomyosarcoma
M8920/3	Alveolar rhabdomyosarcoma

M893-M899   Complex mixed and stromal neoplasms

M8930/3	Endometrial stromal sarcoma
M8931/1	Endolymphatic stromal myosis
M8932/0	Adenomyoma
M8940/0	Pleomorphic adenoma
M8940/3	Mixed tumor, malignant NOS
M8950/3	Mullerian mixed tumor
M8951/3	Mesodermal mixed tumor
M8960/1	Mesoblastic nephroma
M8960/3	Nephroblastoma NOS
M8961/3	Epithelial nephroblastoma
M8962/3	Mesenchymal nephroblastoma
M8970/3	Hepatoblastoma
M8980/3	Carcinosarcoma NOS
M8981/3	Carcinosarcoma, embryonal type
M8982/3	Myoepithelioma
M8990/0	Mesenchymoma, benign
M8990/1	Mesenchymoma NOS
M8990/3	Mesenchymoma, malignant
M8991/3	Embryonal sarcoma

M900-M903   Fibroepithelial neoplasms

M9000/0	Brenner tumor NOS
M9000/1	Brenner tumor, borderline malignancy
M9000/3	Brenner tumor, malignant
M9010/0	Fibroadenoma NOS
M9011/0	Intracanalicular fibroadenoma NOS
M9012/0	Pericanalicular fibroadenoma
M9013/0	Adenofibroma NOS
M9014/0	Serous adenofibroma
M9015/0	Mucinous adenofibroma
M9020/0	Cellular intracanalicular fibroadenoma
M9020/1	Cystosarcoma phyllodes NOS
M9020/3	Cystosarcoma phyllodes, malignant
M9030/0	Juvenile fibroadenoma

M904   Synovial neoplasms

M9040/0	Synovioma, benign
M9040/3	Synovial sarcoma NOS
M9041/3	Synovial sarcoma, spindle cell type
M9042/3	Synovial sarcoma, epithelioid cell type

M9043/3	Synovial sarcoma, biphasic type
M9044/3	Clear cell sarcoma of tendons and aponeuroses

M905 — **Mesothelial neoplasms**

M9050/0	Mesothelioma, benign
M9050/3	Mesothelioma, malignant
M9051/0	Fibrous mesothelioma, benign
M9051/3	Fibrous mesothelioma, malignant
M9052/0	Epithelioid mesothelioma, benign
M9052/3	Epithelioid mesothelioma, malignant
M9053/0	Mesothelioma, biphasic type, benign
M9053/3	Mesothelioma, biphasic type, malignant
M9054/0	Adenomatoid tumor NOS

M906-M909 — **Germ cell neoplasms**

M9060/3	Dysgerminoma
M9061/3	Seminoma NOS
M9062/3	Seminoma, anaplastic type
M9063/3	Spermatocytic seminoma
M9064/3	Germinoma
M9070/3	Embryonal carcinoma NOS
M9071/3	Endodermal sinus tumor
M9072/3	Polyembryoma
M9073/1	Gonadoblastoma
M9080/0	Teratoma, benign
M9080/1	Teratoma NOS
M9080/3	Teratoma, malignant NOS
M9081/3	Teratocarcinoma
M9082/3	Malignant teratoma, undifferentiated type
M9083/3	Malignant teratoma, intermediate type
M9084/0	Dermoid cyst
M9084/3	Dermoid cyst with malignant transformation
M9090/0	Struma ovarii NOS
M9090/3	Struma ovarii, malignant
M9091/1	Strumal carcinoid

M910 — **Trophoblastic neoplasms**

M9100/0	Hydatidiform mole NOS
M9100/1	Invasive hydatidiform mole
M9100/3	Choriocarcinoma
M9101/3	Choriocarcinoma combined with teratoma
M9102/3	Malignant teratoma, trophoblastic

M911 — **Mesonephromas**

M9110/0	Mesonephroma, benign
M9110/1	Mesonephric tumor
M9110/3	Mesonephroma, malignant
M9111/1	Endosalpingioma

M912-M916 — **Blood vessel tumors**

M9120/0	Hemangioma NOS
M9120/3	Hemangiosarcoma
M9121/0	Cavernous hemangioma
M9122/0	Venous hemangioma
M9123/0	Racemose hemangioma
M9124/0	Kupffer cell sarcoma
M9130/0	Hemangioendothelioma, benign
M9130/1	Hemangioendothelioma NOS
M9130/3	Hemangioendothelioma, malignant
M9131/0	Capillary hemangioma
M9132/0	Intramuscular hemangioma
M9140/3	Kaposi's sarcoma
M9141/0	Angiokeratoma
M9142/0	Verrucous keratotic hemangioma
M9150/0	Hemangiopericytoma, benign
M9150/1	Hemangiopericytoma NOS

M9150/3	Hemangiopericytoma, malignant
M9160/0	Angiofibroma NOS
M9161/1	Hemangioblastoma

M917 — **Lymphatic vessel tumors**

M9170/0	Lymphangioma NOS
M9170/3	Lymphangiosarcoma
M9171/0	Capillary lymphangioma
M9172/0	Cavernous lymphangioma
M9173/0	Cystic lymphangioma
M9174/0	Lymphangiomyoma
M9174/1	Lymphangiomyomatosis
M9175/0	Hemolymphangioma

M918-M920 — **Osteomas and osteosarcomas**

M9180/0	Osteoma NOS
M9180/3	Osteosarcoma NOS
M9181/3	Chondroblastic osteosarcoma
M9182/3	Fibroblastic osteosarcoma
M9183/3	Telangiectatic osteosarcoma
M9184/3	Osteosarcoma in Paget's disease of bone
M9190/3	Juxtacortical osteosarcoma
M9191/0	Osteoid osteoma NOS
M9200/0	Osteoblastoma

M921-M924 — **Chondromatous neoplasms**

M9210/0	Osteochondroma
M9210/1	Osteochondromatosis NOS
M9220/0	Chondroma NOS
M9220/1	Chondromatosis NOS
M9220/3	Chondrosarcoma NOS
M9221/0	Juxtacortical chondroma
M9221/3	Juxtacortical chondrosarcoma
M9230/0	Chondroblastoma NOS
M9230/3	Chondroblastoma, malignant
M9240/3	Mesenchymal chondrosarcoma
M9241/0	Chondromyxoid fibroma

M925 — **Giant cell tumors**

M9250/1	Giant cell tumor of bone NOS
M9250/3	Giant cell tumor of bone, malignant
M9251/1	Giant cell tumor of soft parts NOS
M9251/3	Malignant giant cell tumor of soft parts

M926 — **Miscellaneous bone tumors**

M9260/3	Ewing's sarcoma
M9261/3	Adamantinoma of long bones
M9262/0	Ossifying fibroma

M927-M934 — **Odontogenic tumors**

M9270/0	Odontogenic tumor, benign
M9270/1	Odontogenic tumor NOS
M9270/3	Odontogenic tumor, malignant
M9271/0	Dentinoma
M9272/0	Cementoma NOS
M9273/0	Cementoblastoma, benign
M9274/0	Cementifying fibroma
M9275/0	Gigantiform cementoma
M9280/0	Odontoma NOS
M9281/0	Compound odontoma
M9282/0	Complex odontoma
M9290/0	Ameloblastic fibro-odontoma
M9290/3	Ameloblastic odontosarcoma
M9300/0	Adenomatoid odontogenic tumor
M9301/0	Calcifying odontogenic cyst
M9310/0	Ameloblastoma NOS
M9310/3	Ameloblastoma, malignant
M9311/0	Odontoameloblastoma
M9312/0	Squamous odontogenic tumor
M9320/0	Odontogenic myxoma

M9321/0	Odontogenic fibroma NOS
M9330/0	Ameloblastic fibroma
M9330/3	Ameloblastic fibrosarcoma
M9340/3	Calcifying epithelial odontogenic tumor

M935-M937 — **Miscellaneous tumors**

M9350/1	Craniopharyngioma
M9360/1	Pinealoma
M9361/1	Pineocytoma
M9362/3	Pineoblastoma
M9363/0	Melanotic neuroectodermal tumor
M9370/3	Chordoma

M938-M948 — **Gliomas**

M9380/3	Glioma, malignant
M9381/3	Gliomatosis cerebri
M9382/3	Mixed glioma
M9383/1	Subependymal glioma
M9384/1	Subependymal giant cell astrocytoma
M9390/0	Choroid plexus papilloma NOS
M9390/3	Choroid plexus papilloma, malignant
M9391/3	Ependymoma NOS
M9392/3	Ependymoma, anaplastic type
M9393/1	Papillary ependymoma
M9394/1	Myxopapillary ependymoma
M9400/3	Astrocytoma NOS
M9401/3	Astrocytoma, anaplastic type
M9410/3	Protoplasmic astrocytoma
M9411/3	Gemistocytic astrocytoma
M9420/3	Fibrillary astrocytoma
M9421/3	Pilocytic astrocytoma
M9422/3	Spongioblastoma NOS
M9423/3	Spongioblastoma polare
M9430/3	Astroblastoma
M9440/3	Glioblastoma NOS
M9441/3	Giant cell glioblastoma
M9442/3	Glioblastoma with sarcomatous component
M9443/3	Primitive polar spongioblastoma
M9450/3	Oligodendroglioma NOS
M9451/3	Oligodendroglioma, anaplastic type
M9460/3	Oligodendroblastoma
M9470/3	Medulloblastoma NOS
M9471/3	Desmoplastic medulloblastoma
M9472/3	Medullomyoblastoma
M9480/3	Cerebellar sarcoma NOS
M9481/3	Monstrocellular sarcoma

M949-M952 — **Neuroepitheliomatous neoplasms**

M9490/0	Ganglioneuroma
M9490/3	Ganglioneuroblastoma
M9491/0	Ganglioneuromatosis
M9500/3	Neuroblastoma NOS
M9501/3	Medulloepithelioma NOS
M9502/3	Teratoid medulloepithelioma
M9503/3	Neuroepithelioma NOS
M9504/3	Spongioneuroblastoma
M9505/1	Ganglioglioma
M9506/0	Neurocytoma
M9507/0	Pacinian tumor
M9510/3	Retinoblastoma NOS
M9511/3	Retinoblastoma, differentiated type
M9512/3	Retinoblastoma, undifferentiated type
M9520/3	Olfactory neurogenic tumor
M9521/3	Esthesioneurocytoma
M9522/3	Esthesioneuroblastoma
M9523/3	Esthesioneuroepithelioma

M953	**Meningiomas**
M9530/0	*Meningioma NOS*
M9530/1	*Meningiomatosis NOS*
M9530/3	*Meningioma, malignant*
M9531/0	*Meningotheliomatous meningioma*
M9532/0	*Fibrous meningioma*
M9533/0	*Psammomatous meningioma*
M9534/0	*Angiomatous meningioma*
M9535/0	*Hemangioblastic meningioma*
M9536/0	*Hemangiopericytic meningioma*
M9537/0	*Transitional meningioma*
M9538/1	*Papillary meningioma*
M9539/3	*Meningeal sarcomatosis*

M954-M957	**Nerve sheath tumor**
M9540/0	*Neurofibroma NOS*
M9540/1	*Neurofibromatosis NOS*
M9540/3	*Neurofibrosarcoma*
M9541/0	*Melanotic neurofibroma*
M9550/0	*Plexiform neurofibroma*
M9560/0	*Neurilemmoma NOS*
M9560/1	*Neurinomatosis*
M9560/3	*Neurilemmoma, malignant*
M9570/0	*Neuroma NOS*

M958	**Granular cell tumors and alveolar soft part sarcoma**
M9580/0	*Granular cell tumor NOS*
M9580/3	*Granular cell tumor, malignant*
M9581/3	*Alveolar soft part sarcoma*

M959-M963	**Lymphomas, NOS or diffuse**
M9590/0	*Lymphomatous tumor, benign*
M9590/3	*Malignant lymphoma NOS*
M9591/3	*Malignant lymphoma, non Hodgkin's type*
M9600/3	*Malignant lymphoma, undifferentiated cell type NOS*
M9601/3	*Malignant lymphoma, stem cell type*
M9602/3	*Malignant lymphoma, convoluted cell type NOS*
M9610/3	*Lymphosarcoma NOS*
M9611/3	*Malignant lymphoma, lymphoplasmacytoid type*
M9612/3	*Malignant lymphoma, immunoblastic type*
M9613/3	*Malignant lymphoma, mixed lymphocytic-histiocytic NOS*
M9614/3	*Malignant lymphoma, centroblastic-centrocytic, diffuse*
M9615/3	*Malignant lymphoma, follicular center cell NOS*
M9620/3	*Malignant lymphoma, lymphocytic, well differentiated NOS*
M9621/3	*Malignant lymphoma, lymphocytic, intermediate differentiation NOS*
M9622/3	*Malignant lymphoma, centrocytic*
M9623/3	*Malignant lymphoma, follicular center cell, cleaved NOS*
M9630/3	*Malignant lymphoma, lymphocytic, poorly differentiated NOS*
M9631/3	*Prolymphocytic lymphosarcoma*
M9632/3	*Malignant lymphoma, centroblastic type NOS*
M9633/3	*Malignant lymphoma, follicular center cell, noncleaved NOS*

M964	**Reticulosarcomas**
M9640/3	*Reticulosarcoma NOS*
M9641/3	*Reticulosarcoma, pleomorphic cell type*
M9642/3	*Reticulosarcoma, nodular*

M965-M966	**Hodgkin's disease**
M9650/3	*Hodgkin's disease NOS*
M9651/3	*Hodgkin's disease, lymphocytic predominance*
M9652/3	*Hodgkin's disease, mixed cellularity*
M9653/3	*Hodgkin's disease, lymphocytic depletion NOS*
M9654/3	*Hodgkin's disease, lymphocytic depletion, diffuse fibrosis*
M9655/3	*Hodgkin's disease, lymphocytic depletion, reticular type*
M9656/3	*Hodgkin's disease, nodular sclerosis NOS*
M9657/3	*Hodgkin's disease, nodular sclerosis, cellular phase*
M9660/3	*Hodgkin's paragranuloma*
M9661/3	*Hodgkin's granuloma*
M9662/3	*Hodgkin's sarcoma*

M969	**Lymphomas, nodular or follicular**
M9690/3	*Malignant lymphoma, nodular NOS*
M9691/3	*Malignant lymphoma, mixed lymphocytic-histiocytic, nodular*
M9692/3	*Malignant lymphoma, centroblastic-centrocytic, follicular*
M9693/3	*Malignant lymphoma, lymphocytic, well differentiated, nodular*
M9694/3	*Malignant lymphoma, lymphocytic, intermediate differentiation, nodular*
M9695/3	*Malignant lymphoma, follicular center cell, cleaved, follicular*
M9696/3	*Malignant lymphoma, lymphocytic, poorly differentiated, nodular*
M9697/3	*Malignant lymphoma, centroblastic type, follicular*
M9698/3	*Malignant lymphoma, follicular center cell, noncleaved, follicular*

M970	**Mycosis fungoides**
M9700/3	*Mycosis fungoides*
M9701/3	*Sezary's disease*

M971-M972	**Miscellaneous reticuloendothelial neoplasms**
M9710/3	*Microglioma*
M9720/3	*Malignant histiocytosis*
M9721/3	*Histiocytic medullary reticulosis*
M9722/3	*Letterer-Siwe's disease*

M973	**Plasma cell tumors**
M9730/3	*Plasma cell myeloma*
M9731/0	*Plasma cell tumor, benign*
M9731/1	*Plasmacytoma NOS*
M9731/3	*Plasma cell tumor, malignant*

M974	**Mast cell tumors**
M9740/1	*Mastocytoma NOS*
M9740/3	*Mast cell sarcoma*
M9741/3	*Malignant mastocytosis*

M975	**Burkitt's tumor**
M9750/3	*Burkitt's tumor*

M980-M994	**Leukemias NOS**
M9800/3	Leukemias NOS
M9800/3	*Leukemia NOS*
M9801/3	*Acute leukemia NOS*
M9802/3	*Subacute leukemia NOS*
M9803/3	*Chronic leukemia NOS*
M9804/3	*Aleukemic leukemia NOS*

M981	**Compound leukemias**
M9810/3	*Compound leukemia*

M982	**Lymphoid leukemias**
M9820/3	*Lymphoid leukemia NOS*
M9821/3	*Acute lymphoid leukemia*
M9822/3	*Subacute lymphoid leukemia*
M9823/3	*Chronic lymphoid leukemia*
M9824/3	*Aleukemic lymphoid leukemia*
M9825/3	*Prolymphocytic leukemia*

M983	**Plasma cell leukemias**
M9830/3	*Plasma cell leukemia*

M984	**Erythroleukemias**
M9840/3	*Erythroleukemia*
M9841/3	*Acute erythremia*
M9842/3	*Chronic erythremia*

M985	**Lymphosarcoma cell leukemias**
M9850/3	*Lymphosarcoma cell leukemia*

M986	**Myeloid leukemias**
M9860/3	*Myeloid leukemia NOS*
M9861/3	*Acute myeloid leukemia*
M9862/3	*Subacute myeloid leukemia*
M9863/3	*Chronic myeloid leukemia*
M9864/3	*Aleukemic myeloid leukemia*
M9865/3	*Neutrophilic leukemia*
M9866/3	*Acute promyelocytic leukemia*

M987	**Basophilic leukemias**
M9870/3	*Basophilic leukemia*

M988	**Eosinophilic leukemias**
M9880/3	*Eosinophilic leukemia*

M989	**Monocytic leukemias**
M9890/3	*Monocytic leukemia NOS*
M9891/3	*Acute monocytic leukemia*
M9892/3	*Subacute monocytic leukemia*
M9893/3	*Chronic monocytic leukemia*
M9894/3	*Aleukemic monocytic leukemia*

M990-M994	**Miscellaneous leukemias**
M9900/3	*Mast cell leukemia*
M9910/3	*Megakaryocytic leukemia*
M9920/3	*Megakaryocytic myelosis*
M9930/3	*Myeloid sarcoma*
M9940/3	*Hairy cell leukemia*

M995-M997	**Miscellaneous myeloproliferative and lymphoproliferative disorders**
M9950/1	*Polycythemia vera*
M9951/1	*Acute panmyelosis*
M9960/1	*Chronic myeloproliferative disease*
M9961/1	*Myelosclerosis with myeloid metaplasia*
M9962/1	*Idiopathic thrombocythemia*
M9970/1	*Chronic lymphoproliferative disease*

Appendix B: Glossary of Mental Disorders

was officially deleted October 1, 2004

Appendix C: Classification of Drugs by American Hospital Formulary Service List Number and Their ICD-9-CM Equivalents

The coding of adverse effects of drugs is keyed to the continually revised Hospital Formulary of the American Hospital Formulary Service (AHFS) published under the direction of the American Society of Hospital Pharmacists.

The following section gives the ICD-9-CM diagnosis code for each AHFS list.

AHFS* List		ICD-9-CM Dx Code
4:00	ANTIHISTAMINE DRUGS	963.0
8:00	ANTI-INFECTIVE AGENTS	
8:04	Amebacides	961.5
	hydroxyquinoline derivatives	961.3
	arsenical anti-infectives	961.1
	quinoline derivatives	961.3
8:12.04	Antifungal Antibiotics	960.1
	nonantibiotics	961.9
8:12.06	Cephalosporins	960.5
8:12.08	Chloramphenicol	960.2
8:12.12	The Erythromycins	960.3
8:12.16	The Penicillins	960.0
8:12.20	The Streptomycins	960.6
8:12.24	The Tetracyclines	960.4
8:12.28	Other Antibiotics	960.8
	antimycobacterial antibiotics	960.6
	macrolides	960.3
8:16	Antituberculars	961.8
	antibiotics	960.6
8:18	Antivirals	961.7
8:20	Plasmodicides (antimalarials)	961.4
8:24	Sulfonamides	961.0
8:26	The Sulfones	961.8
8:28	Treponemicides	961.2
8:32	Trichomonacides	961.5
	hydroxyquinoline derivatives	961.3
	nitrofuran derivatives	961.9
8:36	Urinary Germicides	961.9
	quinoline derivatives	961.3
8:40	Other Anti-Infectives	961.9
10:00	ANTINEOPLASTIC AGENTS	963.1
	antibiotics	960.7
	progestogens	962.2
12:00	AUTONOMIC DRUGS	
12:04	Parasympathomimetic (Cholinergic) Agents	971.0
12:08	Parasympatholytic (Cholinergic Blocking Agents	971.1
12:12	Sympathomimetic (Adrenergic) Agents	971.2
12:16	Sympatholytic (Adrenergic Blocking) Agents	971.3
12:20	Skeletal Muscle Relaxants	975.2
	central nervous system muscle-tone depressants	968.0
16:00	BLOOD DERIVATIVES	964.7
20:00	BLOOD FORMATION AND COAGULATION	
20:04	Antianemia Drugs	964.1
20:04.04	Iron Preparations	964.0
20:04.08	Liver and Stomach Preparations	964.1
20:12.04	Anticoagulants	964.2
20:12.08	Antiheparin Agents	964.5
20:12.12	Coagulants	964.5
20.12.16	Hemostatics	964.5
	capillary-active drugs	972.8
	fibrinolysis-affecting agents	964.4
	natural products	964.7
24:00	CARDIOVASCULAR DRUGS	
24:04	Cardiac Drugs	972.9
	cardiotonic agents	972.1
	rhythm regulators	972.0

AHFS* List		ICD-9-CM Dx Code
24:06	Antilipemic Agents	972.2
	thyroid derivatives	962.7
24:08	Hypotensive Agents	972.6
	adrenergic blocking agents	971.3
	ganglion-blocking agents	972.3
	vasodilators	972.5
24:12	Vasodilating Agents	972.5
	coronary	972.4
	nicotinic acid derivatives	972.2
24:16	Sclerosing Agents	972.7
28:00	CENTRAL NERVOUS SYSTEM DRUGS	
28:04	General Anesthetics	968.4
	gaseous anesthetics	968.2
	halothane	968.1
	intravenous anesthetics	968.3
28:08	Analgesics and Antipyretics	965.9
	antirheumatics	965.61-965.69
	aromatic analgesics	965.4
	non-narcotics NEC	965.7
	opium alkaloids	965.00
	heroin	965.01
	methadone	965.02
	specified type NEC	965.09
	pyrazole derivatives	965.5
	salicylates	965.1
	specified type NEC	965.8
28:10	Narcotic Antagonists	970.1
28:12	Anticonvulsants	966.3
	barbiturates	967.0
	benzodiazepine-based tranquilizers	969.4
	bromides	967.3
	hydantoin derivatives	966.1
	oxazolidine derivative	966.0
	succinimides	966.2
28:16.04	Antidepressants	969.00-969.09
28:16.08	Tranquilizers	969.5
	benzodiazepine-based	969.4
	butyrophenone-based	969.2
	major NEC	969.3
	phenothiazine-based	969.1
28:16.12	Other Psychotherapeutic Agents	969.8
28:20	Respiratory and Cerebral Stimulants	970.9
	analeptics	970.0
	anorexigenic agents	977.0
	psychostimulants	969.70-969.79
	specified type NEC	970.81-970.89
28:24	Sedatives and Hypnotics	967.9
	barbiturates	967.0
	benzodiazepine-based tranquilizers	969.4
	chloral hydrate group	967.1
	glutethamide group	967.5
	intravenous anesthetics	968.3
	methaqualone	967.4
	paraldehyde	967.2
	phenothiazine-based tranquilizers	969.1
	specified type NEC	967.8
	thiobarbiturates	968.3
	tranquilizer NEC	969.5
36:00	DIAGNOSTIC AGENTS	977.8
40:00	ELECTROLYTE, CALORIC, AND WATER BALANCE AGENTS NEC	974.5
40:04	Acidifying Agents	963.2
40:08	Alkalinizing Agents	963.3
40:10	Ammonia Detoxicants	974.5
40:12	Replacement Solutions NEC	974.5
	plasma volume expanders	964.8
40:16	Sodium-Removing Resins	974.5

40:18	Potassium-Removing Resins	974.5

AHFS* List		**ICD-9-CM Dx Code**
40:20	Caloric Agents	974.5
40:24	Salt and Sugar Substitutes	974.5
40:28	Diuretics NEC	974.4
	carbonic acid anhydrase inhibitors	974.2
	mercurials	974.0
	purine derivatives	974.1
	saluretics	974.3
40:36	Irrigating Solutions	974.5
40:40	Uricosuric Agents	974.7
44:00	ENZYMES NEC	963.4
	fibrinolysis-affecting agents	964.4
	gastric agents	973.4
48:00	EXPECTORANTS AND COUGH PREPARATIONS	
	antihistamine agents	963.0
	antitussives	975.4
	codeine derivatives	965.09
	expectorants	975.5
	narcotic agents NEC	965.09
52:00	EYE, EAR, NOSE, AND THROAT PREPARATIONS	
52:04	Anti-Infectives	
	ENT	976.6
	ophthalmic	976.5
52:04.04	Antibiotics	
	ENT	976.6
	ophthalmic	976.5
52:04.06	Antivirals	
	ENT	976.6
	ophthalmic	976.5
52:04.08	Sulfonamides	
	ENT	976.6
	ophthalmic	976.5
52:04.12	Miscellaneous Anti-Infectives	
	ENT	976.6
	ophthalmic	976.5
52:08	Anti-Inflammatory Agents	
	ENT	976.6
	ophthalmic	976.5
52:10	Carbonic Anhydrase Inhibitors	974.2
52:12	Contact Lens Solutions	976.5
52:16	Local Anesthetics	968.5
52:20	Miotics	971.0
52:24	Mydriatics	
	adrenergics	971.2
	anticholinergics	971.1
	antimuscarinics	971.1
	parasympatholytics	971.1
	spasmolytics	971.1
	sympathomimetics	971.2
52:28	Mouth Washes and Gargles	976.6
52:32	Vasoconstrictors	971.2
52:36	Unclassified Agents	
	ENT	976.6
	ophthalmic	976.5
56:00	GASTROINTESTINAL DRUGS	
56:04	Antacids and Absorbents	973.0
56:08	Anti-Diarrhea Agents	973.5
56:10	Antiflatulents	973.8
56:12	Cathartics NEC	973.3
	emollients	973.2
	irritants	973.1
56:16	Digestants	973.4
56:20	Emetics and Antiemetics	
	antiemetics	963.0
	emetics	973.6
56:24	Lipotropic Agents	977.1
60:00	GOLD COMPOUNDS	965.69
64:00	HEAVY METAL ANTAGONISTS	963.8
68:00	HORMONES AND SYNTHETIC SUBSTITUTES	
68:04	Adrenals	962.0

68:08	Androgens	962.1

AHFS* List		**ICD-9-CM Dx Code**
68:12	Contraceptives	962.2
68:16	Estrogens	962.2
68:18	Gonadotropins	962.4
68:20	Insulins and Antidiabetic Agents	962.3
68:20.08	Insulins	962.3
68:24	Parathyroid	962.6
68:28	Pituitary	
	anterior	962.4
	posterior	962.5
68:32	Progestogens	962.2
68:34	Other Corpus Luteum Hormones	962.2
68:36	Thyroid and Antithyroid	
	antithyroid	962.8
	thyroid	962.7
72:00	LOCAL ANESTHETICS NEC	968.9
	topical (surface) agents	968.5
	infiltrating agents (intradermal) (subcutaneous) (submucosal)	968.5
	nerve blocking agents (peripheral) (plexus) (regional)	968.6
	spinal	968.7
76:00	OXYTOCICS	975.0
78:00	RADIOACTIVE AGENTS	990
80:00	SERUMS, TOXOIDS, AND VACCINES	
80:04	Serums	979.9
	immune globulin (gamma) (human)	964.6
80:08	Toxoids NEC	978.8
	diphtheria	978.5
	and tetanus	978.9
	with pertussis component	978.6
	tetanus	978.4
	and diphtheria	978.9
	with pertussis component	978.6
80:12	Vaccines NEC	979.9
	bacterial NEC	978.8
	with other bacterial component	978.9
	pertussis component	978.6
	viral and rickettsial component	979.7
	rickettsial NEC	979.6
	with bacterial component	979.7
	pertussis component	978.6
	viral component	979.7
	viral NEC	979.6
	with bacterial component	979.7
	pertussis component	978.6
	rickettsial component	979.7
84:00	SKIN AND MUCOUS MEMBRANE PREPARATIONS	
84:04	Anti-Infectives	976.0
84:04.04	Antibiotics	976.0
84:04.08	Fungicides	976.0
84:04.12	Scabicides and Pediculicides	976.0
84:04.16	Miscellaneous Local Anti-Infectives	976.0
84:06	Anti-Inflammatory Agents	976.0
84:08	Antipruritics and Local Anesthetics	
	antipruritics	976.1
	local anesthetics	968.5
84:12	Astringents	976.2
84:16	Cell Stimulants and Proliferants	976.8
84:20	Detergents	976.2
84:24	Emollients, Demulcents, and Protectants	976.3
84:28	Keratolytic Agents	976.4
84:32	Keratoplastic Agents	976.4
84:36	Miscellaneous Agents	976.8
86:00	SPASMOLYTIC AGENTS	975.1
	antiasthmatics	975.7
	papaverine	972.5
	theophyllin	974.1
88:00	VITAMINS	
88:04	Vitamin A	963.5

AHFS* List		ICD-9-CM Dx Code
88:08	Vitamin B Complex	963.5
	hematopoietic vitamin	964.1
	nicotinic acid derivatives	972.2
88:12	Vitamin C	963.5
88:16	Vitamin D	963.5

AHFS* List		ICD-9-CM Dx Code
88:20	Vitamin E	963.5
88:24	Vitamin K Activity	964.3
88:28	Multivitamin Preparations	963.5
92:00	UNCLASSIFIED THERAPEUTIC AGENTS	977.8

* American Hospital Formulary Service

Appendix D: Classification of Industrial Accidents According to Agency

Annex B to the Resolution concerning Statistics of Employment Injuries adopted by the Tenth International Conference of Labor Statisticians on 12 October 1962

1 Machines

11	*Prime-Movers, except Electrical Motors*
111	*Steam engines*
112	*Internal combustion engines*
119	*Others*
12	*Transmission Machinery*
121	*Transmission shafts*
122	*Transmission belts, cables, pulleys, pinions, chains, gears*
129	*Others*
13	*Metalworking Machines*
131	*Power presses*
132	*Lathes*
133	*Milling machines*
134	*Abrasive wheels*
135	*Mechanical shears*
136	*Forging machines*
137	*Rolling-mills*
139	*Others*
14	*Wood and Assimilated Machines*
141	*Circular saws*
142	*Other saws*
143	*Molding machines*
144	*Overhand planes*
149	*Others*
15	*Agricultural Machines*
151	*Reapers (including combine reapers)*
152	*Threshers*
159	*Others*
16	*Mining Machinery*
161	*Under-cutters*
169	*Others*
19	*Other Machines Not Elsewhere Classified*
191	*Earth-moving machines, excavating and scraping machines, except means of transport*
192	*Spinning, weaving and other textile machines*
193	*Machines for the manufacture of food- stuffs and beverages*
194	*Machines for the manufacture of paper*
195	*Printing machines*
199	*Others*

2 Means of Transport and Lifting Equipment

21	*Lifting Machines and Appliances*
211	*Cranes*
212	*Lifts and elevators*
213	*Winches*
214	*Pulley blocks*
219	*Others*
22	*Means of Rail Transport*
221	*Inter-urban railways*
222	*Rail transport in mines, tunnels, quarries, industrial establishments, docks, etc.*
229	*Others*
23	*Other Wheeled Means of Transport, Excluding Rail Transport*
231	*Tractors*
232	*Lorries*
233	*Trucks*
234	*Motor vehicles, not elsewhere classified*
235	*Animal-drawn vehicles*
236	*Hand-drawn vehicles*
239	*Others*
24	*Means of Air Transport*
25	*Means of Water Transport*
251	*Motorized means of water transport*
252	*Non-motorized means of water transport*
26	*Other Means of Transport*
261	*Cable-cars*
262	*Mechanical conveyors, except cable-cars*
269	*Others*

3 Other Equipment

31	*Pressure Vessels*
311	*Boilers*
312	*Pressurized containers*
313	*Pressurized piping and accessories*
314	*Gas cylinders*
315	*Caissons, diving equipment*
319	*Others*
32	*Furnaces, Ovens, Kilns*
321	*Blast furnaces*
322	*Refining furnaces*
323	*Other furnaces*
324	*Kilns*
325	*Ovens*
33	*Refrigerating Plants*
34	*Electrical Installations, Including Electric Motors, but Excluding Electric Hand Tools*
341	*Rotating machines*
342	*Conductors*
343	*Transformers*
344	*Control apparatus*
349	*Others*
35	*Electric Hand Tools*
36	*Tools, Implements, and Appliances, Except Electric Hand Tools*
361	*Power-driven hand tools, except electrichand tools*
362	*Hand tools, not power-driven*
369	*Others*
37	*Ladders, Mobile Ramps*
38	*Scaffolding*
39	*Other Equipment, Not Elsewhere Classified*

4 Materials, Substances and Radiations

41	*Explosives*
42	*Dusts, Gases, Liquids and Chemicals, Excluding Explosives*
421	*Dusts*
422	*Gases, vapors, fumes*
423	*Liquids, not elsewhere classified*
424	*Chemicals, not elsewhere classified*
43	*Flying Fragments*
44	*Radiations*
441	*Ionizing radiations*
449	*Others*
49	*Other Materials and Substances Not Elsewhere Classified*

5 Working Environment

51	*Outdoor*
511	*Weather*
512	*Traffic and working surfaces*
513	*Water*
519	*Others*
52	*Indoor*
521	*Floors*
522	*Confined quarters*
523	*Stairs*
524	*Other traffic and working surfaces*
525	*Floor openings and wall openings*
526	*Environmental factors (lighting, ventilation, temperature, noise, etc.)*
529	*Others*
53	*Underground*
531	*Roofs and faces of mine roads and tunnels, etc.*
532	*Floors of mine roads and tunnels, etc.*
533	*Working-faces of mines, tunnels, etc.*
534	*Mine shafts*
535	*Fire*
536	*Water*
539	*Others*

6 Other Agencies, Not Elsewhere Classified

61	*Animals*
611	*Live animals*
612	*Animal products*
69	*Other Agencies, Not Elsewhere Classified*

7 Agencies Not Classified for Lack of Sufficient Data

Appendix E: List of Three-digit Categories

1. Infectious and Parasitic Diseases

Intestinal infectious diseases (001-009)
001   Cholera
002   Typhoid and paratyphoid fevers
003   Other salmonella infections
004   Shigellosis
005   Other food poisoning (bacterial)
006   Amebiasis
007   Other protozoal intestinal diseases
008   Intestinal infections due to other organisms
009   Ill-defined intestinal infections

Tuberculosis (010-018)
010   Primary tuberculous infection
011   Pulmonary tuberculosis
012   Other respiratory tuberculosis
013   Tuberculosis of meninges and central nervous system
014   Tuberculosis of intestines, peritoneum, and mesenteric glands
015   Tuberculosis of bones and joints
016   Tuberculosis of genitourinary system
017   Tuberculosis of other organs
018   Miliary tuberculosis

Zoonotic bacterial diseases (020-027)
020   Plague
021   Tularemia
022   Anthrax
023   Brucellosis
024   Glanders
025   Melioidosis
026   Rat-bite fever
027   Other zoonotic bacterial diseases

Other bacterial diseases (030-041)
030   Leprosy
031   Diseases due to other mycobacteria
032   Diphtheria
033   Whooping cough
034   Streptococcal sore throat and scarlet fever
035   Erysipelas
036   Meningococcal infection
037   Tetanus
038   Septicemia
039   Actinomycotic infections
040   Other bacterial diseases
041   Bacterial infection in conditions classified elsewhere and of unspecified site

Human immunodeficiency virus (042)
042   Human immunodeficiency virus [HIV] disease

Poliomyelitis and other non-arthropod-borne viral diseases and prion diseases of central nervous system (045-049)
045   Acute poliomyelitis
046   Slow virus infections and prion diseases of central nervous system
047   Meningitis due to enterovirus
048   Other enterovirus diseases of central nervous system
049   Other non-arthropod-borne viral diseases of central nervous system

Viral diseases generally accompanied by exanthem (050-059)
050   Smallpox
051   Cowpox and paravaccinia
052   Chickenpox
053   Herpes zoster
054   Herpes simplex
055   Measles
056   Rubella
057   Other viral exanthemata
058   Other human herpesvirus
059   Other poxvirus infections

Arthropod-borne viral diseases (060-066)
060   Yellow fever
061   Dengue
062   Mosquito-borne viral encephalitis
063   Tick-borne viral encephalitis
064   Viral encephalitis transmitted by other and unspecified arthropods
065   Arthropod-borne hemorrhagic fever
066   Other arthropod-borne viral diseases

Other diseases due to viruses and Chlamydiae (070-079)
070   Viral hepatitis
071   Rabies
072   Mumps
073   Ornithosis
074   Specific diseases due to Coxsackie virus
075   Infectious mononucleosis
076   Trachoma
077   Other diseases of conjunctiva due to viruses and Chlamydiae
078   Other diseases due to viruses and Chlamydiae
079   Viral and chlamydial infection in conditions classified elsewhere and of unspecified site

Rickettsioses and other arthropod-borne diseases (080-088)
080   Louse-borne [epidemic] typhus
081   Other typhus
082   Tick-borne rickettsioses
083   Other rickettsioses
084   Malaria
085   Leishmaniasis
086   Trypanosomiasis
087   Relapsing fever
088   Other arthropod-borne diseases

Syphilis and other venereal diseases (090-099)
090   Congenital syphilis
091   Early syphilis, symptomatic
092   Early syphilis, latent
093   Cardiovascular syphilis
094   Neurosyphilis
095   Other forms of late syphilis, with symptoms
096   Late syphilis, latent
097   Other and unspecified syphilis
098   Gonococcal infections
099   Other venereal diseases

Other spirochetal diseases (100-104)
100   Leptospirosis
101   Vincent's angina
102   Yaws
103   Pinta
104   Other spirochetal infection

Mycoses (110-118)
110   Dermatophytosis
111   Dermatomycosis, other and unspecified
112   Candidiasis
114   Coccidioidomycosis
115   Histoplasmosis
116   Blastomycotic infection
117   Other mycoses
118   Opportunistic mycoses

Helminthiases (120-129)
120   Schistosomiasis [bilharziasis]
121   Other trematode infections
122   Echinococcosis
123   Other cestode infection
124   Trichinosis
125   Filarial infection and dracontiasis
126   Ancylostomiasis and necatoriasis
127   Other intestinal helminthiases
128   Other and unspecified helminthiases
129   Intestinal parasitism, unspecified

Other infectious and parasitic diseases (130-136)
130   Toxoplasmosis
131   Trichomoniasis
132   Pediculosis and phthirus infestation
133   Acariasis
134   Other infestation
135   Sarcoidosis
136   Other and unspecified infectious and parasitic diseases

Late effects of infectious and parasitic diseases (137-139)
137   Late effects of tuberculosis
138   Late effects of acute poliomyelitis
139   Late effects of other infectious and parasitic diseases

2. Neoplasms

Malignant neoplasm of lip, oral cavity, and pharynx (140-149)
140   Malignant neoplasm of lip
141   Malignant neoplasm of tongue
142   Malignant neoplasm of major salivary glands
143   Malignant neoplasm of gum
144   Malignant neoplasm of floor of mouth
145   Malignant neoplasm of other and unspecified parts of mouth
146   Malignant neoplasm of oropharynx
147   Malignant neoplasm of nasopharynx
148   Malignant neoplasm of hypopharynx
149   Malignant neoplasm of other and ill-defined sites within the lip, oral cavity, and pharynx

Malignant neoplasm of digestive organs and peritoneum (150-159)
150   Malignant neoplasm of esophagus
151   Malignant neoplasm of stomach
152   Malignant neoplasm of small intestine, including duodenum
153   Malignant neoplasm of colon
154   Malignant neoplasm of rectum, rectosigmoid junction, and anus
155   Malignant neoplasm of liver and intrahepatic bile ducts
156   Malignant neoplasm of gallbladder and extrahepatic bile ducts
157   Malignant neoplasm of pancreas
158   Malignant neoplasm of retroperitoneum and peritoneum
159   Malignant neoplasm of other and ill-defined sites within the digestive organs and peritoneum

Malignant neoplasm of respiratory and intrathoracic organs (160-165)
160   Malignant neoplasm of nasal cavities, middle ear, and accessory sinuses
161   Malignant neoplasm of larynx
162   Malignant neoplasm of trachea, bronchus, and lung
163   Malignant neoplasm of pleura
164   Malignant neoplasm of thymus, heart, and mediastinum
165   Malignant neoplasm of other and ill-defined sites within the respiratory system and intrathoracic organs

Malignant neoplasm of bone, connective tissue, skin, and breast (170-176)
170   Malignant neoplasm of bone and articular cartilage

171 Malignant neoplasm of connective and other soft tissue
172 Malignant melanoma of skin
173 Other and unspecified malignant neoplasm of skin
174 Malignant neoplasm of female breast
175 Malignant neoplasm of male breast
176 Kaposi's sarcoma

Malignant neoplasm of genitourinary organs (179-189)
179 Malignant neoplasm of uterus, part unspecified
180 Malignant neoplasm of cervix uteri
181 Malignant neoplasm of placenta
182 Malignant neoplasm of body of uterus
183 Malignant neoplasm of ovary and other uterine adnexa
184 Malignant neoplasm of other and unspecified female genital organs
185 Malignant neoplasm of prostate
186 Malignant neoplasm of testis
187 Malignant neoplasm of penis and other male genital organs
188 Malignant neoplasm of bladder
189 Malignant neoplasm of kidney and other unspecified urinary organs

Malignant neoplasm of other and unspecified sites (190-199)
190 Malignant neoplasm of eye
191 Malignant neoplasm of brain
192 Malignant neoplasm of other and unspecified parts of nervous system
193 Malignant neoplasm of thyroid gland
194 Malignant neoplasm of other endocrine glands and related structures
195 Malignant neoplasm of other and ill-defined sites
196 Secondary and unspecified malignant neoplasm of lymph nodes
197 Secondary malignant neoplasm of respiratory and digestive systems
198 Secondary malignant neoplasm of other specified sites
199 Malignant neoplasm without specification of site

Malignant neoplasm of lymphatic and hematopoietic tissue (200-208)
200 Lymphosarcoma and reticulosarcoma and other specified malignant tumors of lymphatic tissue
201 Hodgkin's disease
202 Other malignant neoplasm of lymphoid and histiocytic tissue
203 Multiple myeloma and immunoproliferative neoplasms
204 Lymphoid leukemia
205 Myeloid leukemia
206 Monocytic leukemia
207 Other specified leukemia
208 Leukemia of unspecified cell type

Neuroendocrine tumors (209)
209 Neuroendocrine tumors

Benign neoplasms (210-229)
210 Benign neoplasm of lip, oral cavity, and pharynx
211 Benign neoplasm of other parts of digestive system
212 Benign neoplasm of respiratory and intrathoracic organs
213 Benign neoplasm of bone and articular cartilage
214 Lipoma

215 Other benign neoplasm of connective and other soft tissue
216 Benign neoplasm of skin
217 Benign neoplasm of breast
218 Uterine leiomyoma
219 Other benign neoplasm of uterus
220 Benign neoplasm of ovary
221 Benign neoplasm of other female genital organs
222 Benign neoplasm of male genital organs
223 Benign neoplasm of kidney and other urinary organs
224 Benign neoplasm of eye
225 Benign neoplasm of brain and other parts of nervous system
226 Benign neoplasm of thyroid gland
227 Benign neoplasm of other endocrine glands and related structures
228 Hemangioma and lymphangioma, any site
229 Benign neoplasm of other and unspecified sites

Carcinoma in situ (230-234)
230 Carcinoma in situ of digestive organs
231 Carcinoma in situ of respiratory system
232 Carcinoma in situ of skin
233 Carcinoma in situ of breast and genitourinary system
234 Carcinoma in situ of other and unspecified sites

Neoplasms of uncertain behavior (235-238)
235 Neoplasm of uncertain behavior of digestive and respiratory systems
236 Neoplasm of uncertain behavior of genitourinary organs
237 Neoplasm of uncertain behavior of endocrine glands and nervous system
238 Neoplasm of uncertain behavior of other and unspecified sites and tissues

Neoplasms of unspecified nature (239)
239 Neoplasm of unspecified nature

3. Endocrine, Nutritional and Metabolic Diseases, and Immunity Disorders

Disorders of thyroid gland (240-246)
240 Simple and unspecified goiter
241 Nontoxic nodular goiter
242 Thyrotoxicosis with or without goiter
243 Congenital hypothyroidism
244 Acquired hypothyroidism
245 Thyroiditis
246 Other disorders of thyroid

Diseases of other endocrine glands (249-259)
249 Secondary diabetes mellitus
250 Diabetes mellitus
251 Other disorders of pancreatic internal secretion
252 Disorders of parathyroid gland
253 Disorders of the pituitary gland and its hypothalamic control
254 Diseases of thymus gland
255 Disorders of adrenal glands
256 Ovarian dysfunction
257 Testicular dysfunction
258 Polyglandular dysfunction and related disorders
259 Other endocrine disorders

Nutritional deficiencies (260-269)
260 Kwashiorkor
261 Nutritional marasmus
262 Other severe protein-calorie malnutrition

263 Other and unspecified protein-calorie malnutrition
264 Vitamin A deficiency
265 Thiamine and niacin deficiency states
266 Deficiency of B-complex components
267 Ascorbic acid deficiency
268 Vitamin D deficiency
269 Other nutritional deficiencies

Other metabolic disorders and immnity disorders (270-279)
270 Disorders of amino-acid transport and metabolism
271 Disorders of carbohydrate transport and metabolism
272 Disorders of lipoid metabolism
273 Disorders of plasma protein metabolism
274 Gout
275 Disorders of mineral metabolism
276 Disorders of fluid, electrolyte, and acid-base balance
277 Other and unspecified disorders of metabolism
278 Overweight, obesity and other hyperalimentation
279 Disorders involving the immune mechanism

4. Diseases of Blood and Blood-forming Organs (280-289)
280 Iron deficiency anemias
281 Other deficiency anemias
282 Hereditary hemolytic anemias
283 Acquired hemolytic anemias
284 Aplastic anemia and other bone marrow failure syndromes
285 Other and unspecified anemias
286 Coagulation defects
287 Purpura and other hemorrhagic conditions
288 Diseases of white blood cells
289 Other diseases of blood and blood-forming organs

5. Mental, Behavioral and Neurodevelopmental Disorders

Organic psychotic conditions (290-294)
290 Dementias
291 Alcoholic induced mental disorders
292 Drug induced mental disorders
293 Transient mental disorders due to conditions classified elsewhere
294 Persistent mental disorders due to conditions classified elsewhere

Other psychoses (295-299)
295 Schizophrenic disorders
296 Episodic mood disorders
297 Delusional disorders
298 Other nonorganic psychoses
299 Pervasive developmental disorders

Neurotic disorders, personality disorders, and other nonpsychotic mental disorders (300-316)
300 Anxiety, dissociative and somatoform disorders
301 Personality disorders
302 Sexual and gender identity disorders
303 Alcohol dependence syndrome
304 Drug dependence
305 Nondependent abuse of drugs
306 Physiological malfunction arising from mental factors
307 Special symptoms or syndromes, not elsewhere classified
308 Acute reaction to stress
309 Adjustment reaction

310 Specific nonpsychotic mental disorders due to brain damage
311 Depressive disorder, not elsewhere classified
312 Disturbance of conduct, not elsewhere classified
313 Disturbance of emotions specific to childhood and adolescence
314 Hyperkinetic syndrome of childhood
315 Specific delays in development
316 Psychic factors associated with diseases classified elsewhere

Intellectual Disabilities (317-319)
317 Mild intellectual disabilities
318 Other specified intellectual disabilities
319 Unspecified intellectual disabilities

6. Diseases of the Nervous System and Sense Organs

Inflammatory diseases of the central nervous system (320-326)
320 Bacterial meningitis
321 Meningitis due to other organisms
322 Meningitis of unspecified cause
323 Encephalitis, myelitis, and encephalomyelitis
324 Intracranial and intraspinal abscess
325 Phlebitis and thrombophlebitis of intracranial venous sinuses
326 Late effects of intracranial abscess or pyogenic infection

Organic Sleep Disorders (327)
327 Organic sleep disorders

Hereditary and degenerative diseases of the central nervous system (330-337)
330 Cerebral degenerations usually manifest in childhood
331 Other cerebral degenerations
332 Parkinson's disease
333 Other extrapyramidal diseases and abnormal movement disorders
334 Spinocerebellar disease
335 Anterior horn cell disease
336 Other diseases of spinal cord
337 Disorders of the autonomic nervous system

Pain (338)
338 Pain, not elsewhere classified

Other headache syndromes (339)
339 Other headache syndromes

Other disorders of the central nervous system (340-349)
340 Multiple sclerosis
341 Other demyelinating diseases of central nervous system
342 Hemiplegia and hemiparesis
343 Infantile cerebral palsy
344 Other paralytic syndromes
345 Epilepsy and recurrent seizures
346 Migraine
347 Cataplexy and narcolepsy
348 Other conditions of brain
349 Other and unspecified disorders of the nervous system

Disorders of the peripheral nervous system (350-359)
350 Trigeminal nerve disorders
351 Facial nerve disorders
352 Disorders of other cranial nerves
353 Nerve root and plexus disorders
354 Mononeuritis of upper limb and mononeuritis multiplex
355 Mononeuritis of lower limb

356 Hereditary and idiopathic peripheral neuropathy
357 Inflammatory and toxic neuropathy
358 Myoneural disorders
359 Muscular dystrophies and other myopathies

Disorders of the eye and adnexa (360-379)
360 Disorders of the globe
361 Retinal detachments and defects
362 Other retinal disorders
363 Chorioretinal inflammations and scars and other disorders of choroid
364 Disorders of iris and ciliary body
365 Glaucoma
366 Cataract
367 Disorders of refraction and accommodation
368 Visual disturbances
369 Blindness and low vision
370 Keratitis
371 Corneal opacity and other disorders of cornea
372 Disorders of conjunctiva
373 Inflammation of eyelids
374 Other disorders of eyelids
375 Disorders of lacrimal system
376 Disorders of the orbit
377 Disorders of optic nerve and visual pathways
378 Strabismus and other disorders of binocular eye movements
379 Other disorders of eye

Diseases of the ear and mastoid process (380-389)
380 Disorders of external ear
381 Nonsuppurative otitis media and Eustachian tube disorders
382 Suppurative and unspecified otitis media
383 Mastoiditis and related conditions
384 Other disorders of tympanic membrane
385 Other disorders of middle ear and mastoid
386 Vertiginous syndromes and other disorders of vestibular system
387 Otosclerosis
388 Other disorders of ear
389 Hearing loss

7. Diseases of the Circulatory System

Acute rheumatic fever (390-392)
390 Rheumatic fever without mention of heart involvement
391 Rheumatic fever with heart involvement
392 Rheumatic chorea

Chronic rheumatic heart disease (393-398)
393 Chronic rheumatic pericarditis
394 Diseases of mitral valve
395 Diseases of aortic valve
396 Diseases of mitral and aortic valves
397 Diseases of other endocardial structures
398 Other rheumatic heart disease

Hypertensive disease (401-405)
401 Essential hypertension
402 Hypertensive heart disease
403 Hypertensive chronic kidney disease
404 Hypertensive heart and chronic kidney disease
405 Secondary hypertension

Ischemic heart disease (410-414)
410 Acute myocardial infarction
411 Other acute and subacute forms of ischemic heart disease
412 Old myocardial infarction
413 Angina pectoris
414 Other forms of chronic ischemic heart disease

Diseases of pulmonary circulation (415-417)
415 Acute pulmonary heart disease
416 Chronic pulmonary heart disease
417 Other diseases of pulmonary circulation

Other forms of heart disease (420-429)
420 Acute pericarditis
421 Acute and subacute endocarditis
422 Acute myocarditis
423 Other diseases of pericardium
424 Other diseases of endocardium
425 Cardiomyopathy
426 Conduction disorders
427 Cardiac dysrhythmias
428 Heart failure
429 Ill-defined descriptions and complications of heart disease

Cerebrovascular disease (430-438)
430 Subarachnoid hemorrhage
431 Intracerebral hemorrhage
432 Other and unspecified intracranial hemorrhage
433 Occlusion and stenosis of precerebral arteries
434 Occlusion of cerebral arteries
435 Transient cerebral ischemia
436 Acute, but ill-defined, cerebrovascular disease
437 Other and ill-defined cerebrovascular disease
438 Late effects of cerebrovascular disease

Diseases of arteries, arterioles, and capillaries (440-449)
440 Atherosclerosis
441 Aortic aneurysm and dissection
442 Other aneurysm
443 Other peripheral vascular disease
444 Arterial embolism and thrombosis
445 Atheroembolism
446 Polyarteritis nodosa and allied conditions
447 Other disorders of arteries and arterioles
448 Diseases of capillaries
449 Septic arterial embolism

Diseases of veins and lymphatics, and other diseases of circulatory system (451-459)
451 Phlebitis and thrombophlebitis
452 Portal vein thrombosis
453 Other venous embolism and thrombosis
454 Varicose veins of lower extremities
455 Hemorrhoids
456 Varicose veins of other sites
457 Noninfectious disorders of lymphatic channels
458 Hypotension
459 Other disorders of circulatory system

8. Diseases of the Respiratory System

Acute respiratory infections (460-466)
460 Acute nasopharyngitis [common cold]
461 Acute sinusitis
462 Acute pharyngitis
463 Acute tonsillitis
464 Acute laryngitis and tracheitis
465 Acute upper respiratory infections of multiple or unspecified sites
466 Acute bronchitis and bronchiolitis

Other diseases of upper respiratory tract (470-478)
470 Deviated nasal septum
471 Nasal polyps
472 Chronic pharyngitis and nasopharyngitis
473 Chronic sinusitis
474 Chronic disease of tonsils and adenoids
475 Peritonsillar abscess

476 Chronic laryngitis and laryngotracheitis
477 Allergic rhinitis
478 Other diseases of upper respiratory tract

Pneumonia and influenza (480-488)
480 Viral pneumonia
481 Pneumococcal pneumonia [Streptococcus pneumoniae pneumonia]
482 Other bacterial pneumonia
483 Pneumonia due to other specified organism
484 Pneumonia in infectious diseases classified elsewhere
485 Bronchopneumonia, organism unspecified
486 Pneumonia, organism unspecified
487 Influenza
488 Influenza due to certain identified influenza viruses

Chronic obstructive pulmonary disease and allied conditions (490-496)
490 Bronchitis, not specified as acute or chronic
491 Chronic bronchitis
492 Emphysema
493 Asthma
494 Bronchiectasis
495 Extrinsic allergic alveolitis
496 Chronic airways obstruction, not elsewhere classified

Pneumoconioses and other lung diseases due to external agents (500-508)
500 Coal workers' pneumoconiosis
501 Asbestosis
502 Pneumoconiosis due to other silica or silicates
503 Pneumoconiosis due to other inorganic dust
504 Pneumopathy due to inhalation of other dust
505 Pneumoconiosis, unspecified
506 Respiratory conditions due to chemical fumes and vapors
507 Pneumonitis due to solids and liquids
508 Respiratory conditions due to other and unspecified external agents

Other diseases of respiratory system (510-519)
510 Empyema
511 Pleurisy
512 Pneumothorax and air leak
513 Abscess of lung and mediastinum
514 Pulmonary congestion and hypostasis
515 Postinflammatory pulmonary fibrosis
516 Other alveolar and parietoalveolar pneumopathy
517 Lung involvement in conditions classified elsewhere
518 Other diseases of lung
519 Other diseases of respiratory system

9. Diseases of the Digestive System

Diseases of oral cavity, salivary glands, and jaws (520-529)
520 Disorders of tooth development and eruption
521 Diseases of hard tissues of teeth
522 Diseases of pulp and periapical tissues
523 Gingival and periodontal diseases
524 Dentofacial anomalies, including malocclusion
525 Other diseases and conditions of the teeth and supporting structures
526 Diseases of the jaws
527 Diseases of the salivary glands
528 Diseases of the oral soft tissues, excluding lesions specific for gingiva and tongue
529 Diseases and other conditions of the tongue

Diseases of esophagus, stomach, and duodenum (530-539)
530 Diseases of esophagus
531 Gastric ulcer
532 Duodenal ulcer
533 Peptic ulcer, site unspecified
534 Gastrojejunal ulcer
535 Gastritis and duodenitis
536 Disorders of function of stomach
537 Other disorders of stomach and duodenum
538 Gastrointestinal mucositis (ulcerative)
539 Complications of bariatric procedures

Appendicitis (540-543)
540 Acute appendicitis
541 Appendicitis, unqualified
542 Other appendicitis
543 Other diseases of appendix

Hernia of abdominal cavity (550-553)
550 Inguinal hernia
551 Other hernia of abdominal cavity, with gangrene
552 Other hernia of abdominal cavity, with obstruction, but without mention of gangrene
553 Other hernia of abdominal cavity without mention of obstruction or gangrene

Noninfective enteritis and colitis (555-558)
555 Regional enteritis
556 Ulcerative colitis
557 Vascular insufficiency of intestine
558 Other noninfective gastroenteritis and colitis

Other diseases of intestines and peritoneum (560-569)
560 Intestinal obstruction without mention of hernia
562 Diverticula of intestine
564 Functional digestive disorders, not elsewhere classified
565 Anal fissure and fistula
566 Abscess of anal and rectal regions
567 Peritonitis and retroperitoneal infections
568 Other disorders of peritoneum
569 Other disorders of intestine

Other diseases of digestive system (570-579)
570 Acute and subacute necrosis of liver
571 Chronic liver disease and cirrhosis
572 Liver abscess and sequelae of chronic liver disease
573 Other disorders of liver
574 Cholelithiasis
575 Other disorders of gallbladder
576 Other disorders of biliary tract
577 Diseases of pancreas
578 Gastrointestinal hemorrhage
579 Intestinal Malabsorption

10. Diseases of the Genitourinary System

Nephritis, nephrotic syndrome, and nephrosis (580-589)
580 Acute gloerulonephritis
581 Nephrotic syndrome
582 Chronic glomerulonephritis
583 Nephritis and nephropathy, not specified as acute or chronic
584 Acute kidney failure
585 Chronic kidney disease (CKD)
586 Renal failure, unspecified
587 Renal sclerosis, unspecified
588 Disorders resulting from impaired renal function
589 Small kidney of unknown cause

Other diseases of urinary system (590-599)
590 Infections of kidney
591 Hydronephrosis
592 Calculus of kidney and ureter
593 Other disorders of kidney and ureter
594 Calculus of lower urinary tract
595 Cystitis
596 Other disorders of bladder
597 Urethritis, not sexually transmitted, and urethral syndrome
598 Urethral stricture
599 Other disorders of urethra and urinary tract

Diseases of male genital organs (600-608)
600 Hyperplasia of prostate
601 Inflammatory diseases of prostate
602 Other disorders of prostate
603 Hydrocele
604 Orchitis and epididymitis
605 Redundant prepuce and phimosis
606 Infertility, male
607 Disorders of penis
608 Other disorders of male genital organs

Disorders of breast (610-612)
610 Benign mammary dysplasias
611 Other disorders of breast
612 Deformity and disproportion of reconstructed breast

Inflammatory disease of female pelvic organs (614-616)
614 Inflammatory disease of ovary, fallopian tube, pelvic cellular tissue, and peritoneum
615 Inflammatory diseases of uterus, except cervix
616 Inflammatory disease of cervix, vagina, and vulva

Other disorders of female genital tract (617-629)
617 Endometriosis
618 Genital prolapse
619 Fistula involving female genital tract
620 Noninflammatory disorders of ovary, fallopian tube, and broad ligament
621 Disorders of uterus, not elsewhere classified
622 Noninflammatory disorders of cervix
623 Noninflammatory disorders of vagina
624 Noninflammatory disorders of vulva and perineum
625 Pain and other symptoms associated with female genital organs
626 Disorders of menstruation and other abnormal bleeding from female genital tract
627 Menopausal and postmenopausal disorders
628 Infertility, female
629 Other disorders of female genital organs

11. Complications of Pregnancy, Childbirth and the Puerperium

Ectopic and molar pregnancy (630-633)
630 Hydatidiform mole
631 Other abnormal product of conception
632 Missed abortion
633 Ectopic pregnancy

Other pregnancy with abortive outcome (634-639)
634 Spontaneous abortion
635 Legally induced abortion
636 Illegally induced abortion
637 Unspecified abortion
638 Failed attempted abortion
639 Complications following abortion and ectopic and molar pregnancies

Complications mainly related to pregnancy (640-649)
640 Hemorrhage in early pregnancy
641 Antepartum hemorrhage, abruptio placentae, and placenta previa
642 Hypertension complicating pregnancy, childbirth, and the puerperium
643 Excessive vomiting in pregnancy
644 Early or threatened labor
645 Late pregnancy
646 Other complications of pregnancy, not elsewhere classified
647 Infectious and parasitic conditions in the mother classifiable elsewhere, but complicating pregnancy, childbirth, and the puerperium
648 Other current conditions in the mother classifiable elsewhere, but complicating pregnancy, childbirth, and the puerperium
649 Other conditions or status of the mother complicating pregnancy, childbirth, or the puerperium

Normal delivery, and other indications for care in pregnancy, labor, and delivery (650-659)
650 Normal delivery
651 Multiple gestation
652 Malposition and malpresentation of fetus
653 Disproportion
654 Abnormality of organs and soft tissues of pelvis
655 Known or suspected fetal abnormality affecting management of mother
656 Other known or suspected fetal and placental problems affecting management of mother
657 Polyhydramnios
658 Other problems associated with amniotic cavity and membranes
659 Other indications for care or intervention related to labor and delivery, not elsewhere classified

Complications occurring mainly in the course of labor and delivery (660-669)
660 Obstructed labor
661 Abnormality of forces of labor
662 Long labor
663 Umbilical cord complications
664 Trauma to perineum and vulva during delivery
665 Other obstetrical trauma
666 Postpartum hemorrhage
667 Retained placenta or membranes, without hemorrhage
668 Complications of the administration of anesthetic or other sedation in labor and delivery
669 Other complications of labor and delivery, not elsewhere classified

Complications of the puerperium (670-677)
670 Major puerperal infection
671 Venous complications in pregnancy and the puerperium
672 Pyrexia of unknown origin during the puerperium
673 Obstetrical pulmonary embolism
674 Other and unspecified complications of the puerperium, not elsewhere classified
675 Infections of the breast and nipple associated with childbirth
676 Other disorders of the breast associated with childbirth, and disorders of lactation
677 Late effect of complication of pregnancy, childbirth, and the puerperium

Other maternal and fetal complications (678-679)
678 Other fetal conditions
679 Complications of in utero procedures

12. Diseases of the Skin and Subcutaneous Tissue

Infections of skin and subcutaneous tissue (680-686)
680 Carbuncle and furuncle
681 Cellulitis and abscess of finger and toe
682 Other cellulitis and abscess
683 Acute lymphadenitis
684 Impetigo
685 Pilonidal cyst
686 Other local infections of skin and subcutaneous tissue

Other inflammatory conditions of skin and subcutaneous tissue (690-698)
690 Erythematosquamous dermatosis
691 Atopic dermatitis and related conditions
692 Contact dermatitis and other eczema
693 Dermatitis due to substances taken internally
694 Bullous dermatoses
695 Erythematous conditions
696 Psoriasis and similar disorders
697 Lichen
698 Pruritus and related conditions

Other diseases of skin and subcutaneous tissue (700-709)
700 Corns and callosities
701 Other hypertrophic and atrophic conditions of skin
702 Other dermatoses
703 Diseases of nail
704 Diseases of hair and hair follicles
705 Disorders of sweat glands
706 Diseases of sebaceous glands
707 Chronic ulcer of skin
708 Urticaria
709 Other disorders of skin and subcutaneous tissue

13. Diseases of the Musculoskeletal System and Connective Tissue

Arthropathies and related disorders (710-719)
710 Diffuse diseases of connective tissue
711 Arthropathy associated with infections
712 Crystal arthropathies
713 Arthropathy associated with other disorders classified elsewhere
714 Rheumatoid arthritis and other inflammatory polyarthropathies
715 Osteoarthrosis and allied disorders
716 Other and unspecified arthropathies
717 Internal derangement of knee
718 Other derangement of joint
719 Other and unspecified disorder of joint

Dorsopathies (720-724)
720 Ankylosing spondylitis and other inflammatory spondylopathies
721 Spondylosis and allied disorders
722 Intervertebral disc disorders
723 Other disorders of cervical region
724 Other and unspecified disorders of back

Rheumatism, excluding the back (725-729)
725 Polymyalgia rheumatica
726 Peripheral enthesopathies and allied syndromes
727 Other disorders of synovium, tendon, and bursa
728 Disorders of muscle, ligament, and fascia
729 Other disorders of soft tissues

Osteopathies, chondropathies, and acquired musculoskeletal deformities (730-739)
730 Osteomyelitis, periostitis, and other infections involving bone
731 Osteitis deformans and osteopathies associated with other disorders classified elsewhere
732 Osteochondropathies
733 Other disorders of bone and cartilage
734 Flat foot
735 Acquired deformities of toe
736 Other acquired deformities of limbs
737 Curvature of spine
738 Other acquired deformity
739 Nonallopathic lesions, not elsewhere classified

14. Congenital Anomalies
740 Anencephalus and similar anomalies
741 Spina bifida
742 Other congenital anomalies of nervous system
743 Congenital anomalies of eye
744 Congenital anomalies of ear, face, and neck
745 Bulbus cordis anomalies and anomalies of cardiac septal closure
746 Other congenital anomalies of heart
747 Other congenital anomalies of circulatory system
748 Congenital anomalies of respiratory system
749 Cleft palate and cleft lip
750 Other congenital anomalies of upper alimentary tract
751 Other congenital anomalies of digestive system
752 Congenital anomalies of genital organs
753 Congenital anomalies of urinary system
754 Certain congenital musculoskeletal deformities
755 Other congenital anomalies of limbs
756 Other congenital musculoskeletal anomalies
757 Congenital anomalies of the integument
758 Chromosomal anomalies
759 Other and unspecified congenital anomalies

15. Certain Conditions Originating in the Perinatal Period

Maternal causes of perinatal morbidity and mortality (760-763)
760 Fetus or newborn affected by maternal conditions which may be unrelated to present pregnancy
761 Fetus or newborn affected by maternal complications of pregnancy
762 Fetus or newborn affected by complications of placenta, cord, and membranes
763 Fetus or newborn affected by other complications of labor and delivery

Other conditions originating in the perinatal period (764-779)
764 Slow fetal growth and fetal malnutrition
765 Disorders relating to short gestation and unspecified low birthweight
766 Disorders relating to long gestation and high birthweight
767 Birth trauma
768 Intrauterine hypoxia and birth asphyxia
769 Respiratory distress syndrome

770 Other respiratory conditions of fetus and newborn
771 Infections specific to the perinatal period
772 Fetal and neonatal hemorrhage
773 Hemolytic disease of fetus or newborn, due to isoimmunization
774 Other perinatal jaundice
775 Endocrine and metabolic disturbances specific to the fetus and newborn
776 Hematological disorders of newborn
777 Perinatal disorders of digestive system
778 Conditions involving the integument and temperature regulation of fetus and newborn
779 Other and ill-defined conditions originating in the perinatal period

16. Symptoms, Signs, and Ill-defined Conditions

Symptoms (780-789)
780 General symptoms
781 Symptoms involving nervous and musculoskeletal systems
782 Symptoms involving skin and other integumentary tissue
783 Symptoms concerning nutrition, metabolism, and development
784 Symptoms involving head and neck
785 Symptoms involving cardiovascular system
786 Symptoms involving respiratory system and other chest symptoms
787 Symptoms involving digestive system
788 Symptoms involving urinary system
789 Other symptoms involving abdomen and pelvis

Nonspecific abnormal findings (790-796)
790 Nonspecific findings on examination of blood
791 Nonspecific findings on examination of urine
792 Nonspecific abnormal findings in other body substances
793 Nonspecific (abnormal) findings on radiological and other examination of body structure
794 Nonspecific abnormal results of function studies
795 Other and nonspecific abnormal cystological, histological, immunological and DNA test findings
796 Other nonspecific abnormal findings

Ill-defined and unknown causes of morbidity and mortality (797-799)
797 Senility without mention of psychosis
798 Sudden death, cause unknown
799 Other ill-defined and unknown causes of morbidity and mortality

17. Injury and Poisoning

Fracture of skull (800-804)
800 Fracture of vault of skull
801 Fracture of base of skull
802 Fracture of face bones
803 Other and unqualified skull fractures
804 Multiple fractures involving skull or face with other bones

Fracture of spine and trunk (805-809)
805 Fracture of vertebral column without mention of spinal cord injury
806 Fracture of vertebral column with spinal cord injury
807 Fracture of rib(s), sternum, larynx, and trachea
808 Fracture of pelvis
809 Ill-defined fractures of bones of trunk

Fracture of upper limb (810-819)
810 Fracture of clavicle
811 Fracture of scapula
812 Fracture of humerus
813 Fracture of radius and ulna
814 Fracture of carpal bone(s)
815 Fracture of metacarpal bone(s)
816 Fracture of one or more phalanges of hand
817 Multiple fractures of hand bones
818 Ill-defined fractures of upper limb
819 Multiple fractures involving both upper limbs, and upper limb with rib(s) and sternum

Fracture of lower limb (820-829)
820 Fracture of neck of femur
821 Fracture of other and unspecified parts of femur
822 Fracture of patella
823 Fracture of tibia and fibula
824 Fracture of ankle
825 Fracture of one or more tarsal and metatarsal bones
826 Fracture of one or more phalanges of foot
827 Other, multiple, and ill-defined fractures of lower limb
828 Multiple fractures involving both lower limbs, lower with upper limb, and lower limb(s) with rib(s) and sternum
829 Fracture of unspecified bones

Dislocation (830-839)
830 Dislocation of jaw
831 Dislocation of shoulder
832 Dislocation of elbow
833 Dislocation of wrist
834 Dislocation of finger
835 Dislocation of hip
836 Dislocation of knee
837 Dislocation of ankle
838 Dislocation of foot
839 Other, multiple, and ill-defined dislocations

Sprains and strains of joints and adjacent muscles (840-848)
840 Sprains and strains of shoulder and upper arm
841 Sprains and strains of elbow and forearm
842 Sprains and strains of wrist and hand
843 Sprains and strains of hip and thigh
844 Sprains and strains of knee and leg
845 Sprains and strains of ankle and foot
846 Sprains and strains of sacroiliac region
847 Sprains and strains of other and unspecified parts of back
848 Other and ill-defined sprains and strains

Intracranial injury, excluding those with skull fracture (850-854)
850 Concussion
851 Cerebral laceration and contusion
852 Subarachnoid, subdural, and extradural hemorrhage, following injury
853 Other and unspecified intracranial hemorrhage following injury
854 Intracranial injury of other and unspecified nature

Internal injury of thorax, abdomen, and pelvis (860-869)
860 Traumatic pneumothorax and hemothorax
861 Injury to heart and lung
862 Injury to other and unspecified intrathoracic organs
863 Injury to gastrointestinal tract
864 Injury to liver
865 Injury to spleen
866 Injury to kidney
867 Injury to pelvic organs
868 Injury to other intra-abdominal organs
869 Internal injury to unspecified or ill-defined organs

Open wound of head, neck, and trunk (870-879)
870 Open wound of ocular adnexa
871 Open wound of eyeball
872 Open wound of ear
873 Other open wound of head
874 Open wound of neck
875 Open wound of chest (wall)
876 Open wound of back
877 Open wound of buttock
878 Open wound of genital organs (external), including traumatic amputation
879 Open wound of other and unspecified sites, except limbs

Open wound of upper limb (880-887)
880 Open wound of shoulder and upper arm
881 Open wound of elbow, forearm, and wrist
882 Open wound of hand except finger(s) alone
883 Open wound of finger(s)
884 Multiple and unspecified open wound of upper limb
885 Traumatic amputation of thumb (complete) (partial)
886 Traumatic amputation of other finger(s) (complete) (partial)
887 Traumatic amputation of arm and hand (complete) (partial)

Open wound of lower limb (890-897)
890 Open wound of hip and thigh
891 Open wound of knee, leg [except thigh], and ankle
892 Open wound of foot except toe(s) alone
893 Open wound of toe(s)
894 Multiple and unspecified open wound of lower limb
895 Traumatic amputation of toe(s) (complete) (partial)
896 Traumatic amputation of foot (complete) (partial)
897 Traumatic amputation of leg(s) (complete) (partial)

Injury to blood vessels (900-904)
900 Injury to blood vessels of head and neck
901 Injury to blood vessels of thorax
902 Injury to blood vessels of abdomen and pelvis
903 Injury to blood vessels of upper extremity
904 Injury to blood vessels of lower extremity and unspecified sites

Late effects of injuries, poisonings, toxic effects, and other external causes (905-909)
905 Late effects of musculoskeletal and connective tissue injuries
906 Late effects of injuries to skin and subcutaneous tissues
907 Late effects of injuries to the nervous system
908 Late effects of other and unspecified injuries
909 Late effects of other and unspecified external causes

Superficial injury (910-919)
910 Superficial injury of face, neck, and scalp except eye
911 Superficial injury of trunk
912 Superficial injury of shoulder and upper arm
913 Superficial injury of elbow, forearm, and wrist
914 Superficial injury of hand(s) except finger(s) alone
915 Superficial injury of finger(s)
916 Superficial injury of hip, thigh, leg, and ankle
917 Superficial injury of foot and toe(s)
918 Superficial injury of eye and adnexa

919 Superficial injury of other, multiple, and unspecified sites

Contusion with intact skin surface (920-924)
920 Contusion of face, scalp, and neck except eye(s)
921 Contusion of eye and adnexa
922 Contusion of trunk
923 Contusion of upper limb
924 Contusion of lower limb and of other and unspecified sites

Crushing injury (925-929)
925 Crushing injury of face, scalp, and neck
926 Crushing injury of trunk
927 Crushing injury of upper limb
928 Crushing injury of lower limb
929 Crushing injury of multiple and unspecified sites

Effects of foreign body entering through orifice (930-939)
930 Foreign body on external eye
931 Foreign body in ear
932 Foreign body in nose
933 Foreign body in pharynx and larynx
934 Foreign body in trachea, bronchus, and lung
935 Foreign body in mouth, esophagus, and stomach
936 Foreign body in intestine and colon
937 Foreign body in anus and rectum
938 Foreign body in digestive system, unspecified
939 Foreign body in genitourinary tract

Burns (940-949)
940 Burn confined to eye and adnexa
941 Burn of face, head, and neck
942 Burn of trunk
943 Burn of upper limb, except wrist and hand
944 Burn of wrist(s) and hand(s)
945 Burn of lower limb(s)
946 Burns of multiple specified sites
947 Burn of internal organs
948 Burns classified according to extent of body surface involved
949 Burn, unspecified

Injury to nerves and spinal cord (950-957)
950 Injury to optic nerve and pathways
951 Injury to other cranial nerve(s)
952 Spinal cord injury without evidence of spinal bone injury
953 Injury to nerve roots and spinal plexus
954 Injury to other nerve(s) of trunk excluding shoulder and pelvic girdles
955 Injury to peripheral nerve(s) of shoulder girdle and upper limb
956 Injury to peripheral nerve(s) of pelvic girdle and lower limb
957 Injury to other and unspecified nerves

Certain traumatic complications and unspecified injuries (958-959)
958 Certain early complications of trauma
959 Injury, other and unspecified

Poisoning by drugs, medicinals and biological substances (960-979)
960 Poisoning by antibiotics
961 Poisoning by other anti-infectives
962 Poisoning by hormones and synthetic substitutes
963 Poisoning by primarily systemic agents
964 Poisoning by agents primarily affecting blood constituents
965 Poisoning by analgesics, antipyretics, and antirheumatics
966 Poisoning by anticonvulsants and anti-Parkinsonism drugs

967 Poisoning by sedatives and hypnotics
968 Poisoning by other central nervous system depressants and anesthetics
969 Poisoning by psychotropic agents
970 Poisoning by central nervous system stimulants
971 Poisoning by drugs primarily affecting the autonomic nervous system
972 Poisoning by agents primarily affecting the cardiovascular system
973 Poisoning by agents primarily affecting the gastrointestinal system
974 Poisoning by water, mineral, and uric acid metabolism drugs
975 Poisoning by agents primarily acting on the smooth and skeletal muscles and respiratory system
976 Poisoning by agents primarily affecting skin and mucous membrane, ophthalmological, otorhinolaryngological, and dental drugs
977 Poisoning by other and unspecified drugs and medicinals
978 Poisoning by bacterial vaccines
979 Poisoning by other vaccines and biological substances

Toxic effects of substances chiefly nonmedicinal as to source (980-989)
980 Toxic effect of alcohol
981 Toxic effect of petroleum products
982 Toxic effect of solvents other than petroleum-based
983 Toxic effect of corrosive aromatics, acids, and caustic alkalis
984 Toxic effect of lead and its compounds (including fumes)
985 Toxic effect of other metals
986 Toxic effect of carbon monoxide
987 Toxic effect of other gases, fumes, or vapors
988 Effect of noxious substances eaten as food
989 Toxic effect of other substances, chiefly nonmedicinal as to source

Other and unspecified effects of external causes (990-995)
990 Effects of radiation, unspecified
991 Effects of reduced temperature
992 Effects of heat and light
993 Effects of air pressure
994 Effects of other external causes
995 Certain adverse effects, not elsewhere classified

Complications of surgical and medical care, not elsewhere classified (996-999)
996 Complications peculiar to certain specified procedures
997 Complications affecting specified body systems, not elsewhere classified
998 Other complications of procedures, not elsewhere classified
999 Complications of medical care, not elsewhere classified

Supplementary Classification of Factors Influencing Health Status and Contact With Health Services

Persons with potential health hazards related to communicable diseases (V01-V06)
V01 Contact with or exposure to communicable diseases
V02 Carrier or suspected carrier of infectious diseases
V03 Need for prophylactic vaccination and inoculation against bacterial diseases

V04 Need for prophylactic vaccination and inoculation against certain viral diseases
V05 Need for other prophylactic vaccination and inoculation against single diseases
V06 Need for prophylactic vaccination and inoculation against combinations of diseases

Persons with need for isolation, other potential health hazards, and prophylactic measures (V07-V09)
V07 Need for isolation and other prophylactic or treatment measures
V08 Asymptomatic human immunodeficiency virus [HIV] infection status
V09 Infection with drug-resistant microorganisms

Persons with potential health hazards related to personal and family history (V10-V19)
V10 Personal history of malignant neoplasm
V11 Personal history of mental disorder
V12 Personal history of certain other diseases
V13 Personal history of other diseases
V14 Personal history of allergy to medicinal agents
V15 Other personal history presenting hazards to health
V16 Family history of malignant neoplasm
V17 Family history of certain chronic disabling diseases
V18 Family history of certain other specific conditions
V19 Family history of other conditions

Persons encountering health services in circumstances related to reproduction and development (V20-V29)
V20 Health supervision of infant or child
V21 Constitutional states in development
V22 Normal pregnancy
V23 Supervision of high-risk pregnancy
V24 Postpartum care and examination
V25 Encounter for contraceptive management
V26 Procreative management
V27 Outcome of delivery
V28 Encounter for antenatal screening of mother
V29 Observation and evaluation of newborns and infants for suspected condition not found

Liveborn infants according to type of birth (V30-V39)
V30 Single liveborn
V31 Twin, mate liveborn
V32 Twin, mate stillborn
V33 Twin, unspecified
V34 Other multiple, mates all liveborn
V35 Other multiple, mates all stillborn
V36 Other multiple, mates live and stillborn
V37 Other multiple, unspecified
V39 Unspecified

Persons with a condition influencing their health status (V40-V49)
V40 Mental and behavioral problems
V41 Problems with special senses and other special functions
V42 Organ or tissue replaced by transplant
V43 Organ or tissue replaced by other means
V44 Artificial opening status
V45 Other postprocedural states
V46 Other dependence on machines and devices
V47 Other problems with internal organs
V48 Problems with head, neck, and trunk
V49 Other conditions influencing health status

Persons encountering health services for specific procedures and aftercare (V50-V59)
V50 Elective surgery for purposes other than remedying health states
V51 Aftercare involving the use of plastic surgery

Appendix E: List of Three-digit Categories

V52 Fitting and adjustment of prosthetic device and implant
V53 Fitting and adjustment of other device
V54 Other orthopedic aftercare
V55 Attention to artificial openings
V56 Encounter for dialysis and dialysis catheter care
V57 Care involving use of rehabilitation procedures
V58 Encounter for other and unspecified procedures and aftercare
V59 Donors

Persons encountering health services in other circumstances (V60-V69)
V60 Housing, household, and economic circumstances
V61 Other family circumstances
V62 Other psychosocial circumstances
V63 Unavailability of other medical facilities for care
V64 Persons encountering health services for specific procedures, not carried out
V65 Other persons seeking consultation
V66 Convalescence and palliative care
V67 Follow-up examination
V68 Encounters for administrative purposes
V69 Problems related to lifestyle

Persons without reported diagnosis encountered during examination and investigation of individuals and populations (V70-V82)
V70 General medical examination
V71 Observation and evaluation for suspected conditions not found
V72 Special investigations and examinations
V73 Special screening examination for viral and chlamydial diseases
V74 Special screening examination for bacterial and spirochetal diseases
V75 Special screening examination for other infectious diseases
V76 Special screening for malignant neoplasms
V77 Special screening for endocrine, nutritional, metabolic, and immunity disorders
V78 Special screening for disorders of blood and blood-forming organs
V79 Special screening for mental disorders and developmental handicaps
V80 Special screening for neurological, eye, and ear diseases
V81 Special screening for cardiovascular, respiratory, and genitourinary diseases
V82 Special screening for other conditions

Genetics (V83-V84)
V83 Genetic carrier status
V84 Genetic susceptibility to disease

Body mass index (V85)
V85 Body Mass Index [BMI]

Estrogen receptor status (V86)
V86 Estrogen receptor status

Other specified personal exposures and history presenting hazards to health (V87)
V87 Other specified personal exposures and history presenting hazards to health

Acquired absence of other organs and tissue (V88)
V88 Acquired absence of other organs and tissue

Other suspected conditions not found (V89)
V89 Other suspected conditions not found

Retained Foreign Body (V90)
V90 Retained foreign body

Multiple Gestation Placenta Status (V91)
V91 Multiple gestation placenta status

Supplementary Classification of External Causes of Injury and Poisoning

External Cause Status (E000)
E000 External cause status

Activity (E001-E030)
E001 Activities involving walking and running
E002 Activities involving water and water craft
E003 Activities involving ice and snow
E004 Activities involving climbing, rappelling, and jumping off
E005 Activities involving dancing and other rhythmic movement
E006 Activities involving other sports and athletics played individually
E007 Activities involving other sports and athletics played as a team or group
E008 Activities involving other specified sports and athletics
E009 Activity involving other cardiorespiratory exercise
E010 Activity involving other muscle strengthening exercises
E011 Activities involving computer technology and electronic devices
E012 Activities involving arts and handcrafts
E013 Activities involving personal hygiene and household maintenance
E014 Activities involving person providing caregiving
E015 Activities involving food preparation, cooking and grilling
E016 Activities involving property and land maintenance, building and construction
E017 Activities involving roller coasters and other types of external motion
E018 Activities involving playing musical instrument
E019 Activities involving animal care
E029 Other activity
E030 Unspecified activity

Transport Accidents (E800-E848)

Railway accidents (E800-E807)
E800 Railway accident involving collision with roling stock
E801 Railway accident involving collision with other object
E802 Railway accident involving derailment without antecedent collision
E803 Railway accident involving explosion, fire, or burning
E804 Fall in, on, or from railway train
E805 Hit by rolling stock
E806 Other specified railway accident
E807 Railway accident of unspecified nature

Motor vehicle traffic accidents (E810-E819)
E810 Motor vehicle traffic accident involving collision with train
E811 Motor vehicle traffic accident involving re-entrant collision with another motor vehicle
E812 Other motor vehicle traffic accident involving collision with another motor vehicle
E813 Motor vehicle traffic accident involving collision with other vehicle
E814 Motor vehicle traffic accident involving collision with pedestrian
E815 Other motor vehicle traffic accident involving collision on the highway
E816 Motor vehicle traffic accident due to loss of control, without collision on the highway
E817 Noncollision motor vehicle traffic accident while boarding or alighting
E818 Other noncollision motor vehicle traffic accident
E819 Motor vehicle traffic accident of unspecified nature

Motor vehicle nontraffic accidents (E820-E825)
E820 Nontraffic accident involving motor-driven snow vehicle
E821 Nontraffic accident involving other off-road motor vehicle
E822 Other motor vehicle nontraffic accident involving collision with moving object
E823 Other motor vehicle nontraffic accident involving collision with stationary object
E824 Other motor vehicle nontraffic accident while boarding and alighting
E825 Other motor vehicle nontraffic accident of other and unspecified nature

Other road vehicle accidents (E826-E829)
E826 Pedal cycle accident
E827 Animal-drawn vehicle accident
E828 Accident involving animal being ridden
E829 Other road vehicle accidents

Water transport accidents (E830-E838)
E830 Accident to watercraft causing submersion
E831 Accident to watercraft causing other injury
E832 Other accidental submersion or drowning in water transport accident
E833 Fall on stairs or ladders in water transport
E834 Other fall from one level to another in water transport
E835 Other and unspecified fall in water transport
E836 Machinery accident in water transport
E837 Explosion, fire, or burning in watercraft
E838 Other and unspecified water transport accident

Air and space transport accidents (E840-E845)
E840 Accident to powered aircraft at takeoff or landing
E841 Accident to powered aircraft, other and unspecified
E842 Accident to unpowered aircraft
E843 Fall in, on, or from aircraft
E844 Other specified air transport accidents
E845 Accident involving spacecraft

Vehicle accidents, not elsewhere classfiable (E846-E849)
E846 Accidents involving powered vehicles used solely within the buildings and premises of an industrial or commercial establishment
E847 Accidents involving cable cars not running on rails
E848 Accidents involving other vehicles, not elsewhere classifiable
E849 Place of occurrence

Accidental poisoning by drugs, medicinal substances, and biologicals (E850-E858)
E850 Accidental poisoning by analgesics, antipyretics, and antirheumatics
E851 Accidental poisoning by barbiturates
E852 Accidental poisoning by other sedatives and hypnotics
E853 Accidental poisoning by tranquilizers
E854 Accidental poisoning by other psychotropic agents
E855 Accidental poisoning by other drugs acting on central and autonomic nervous systems
E856 Accidental poisoning by antibiotics

E857   Accidental poisoning by anti-infectives
E858   Accidental poisoning by other drugs

Accidental poisoning by other solid and liquid substances, gases, and vapors (E860-E869)

E860   Accidental poisoning by alcohol, not elsewhere classified
E861   Accidental poisoning by cleansing and polishing agents, disinfectants, paints, and varnishes
E862   Accidental poisoning by petroleum products, other solvents and their vapors, not elsewhere classified
E863   Accidental poisoning by agricultural and horticultural chemical and pharmaceutical preparations other than plant foods and fertilizers
E864   Accidental poisoning by corrosives and caustics, not elsewhere classified
E865   Accidental poisoning from poisonous foodstuffs and poisonous plants
E866   Accidental poisoning by other and unspecified solid and liquid substances
E867   Accidental poisoning by gas distributed by pipeline
E868   Accidental poisoning by other utility gas and other carbon monoxide
E869   Accidental poisoning by other gases and vapors

Misadventures to patients during surgical and medical care (E870-E876)

E870   Accidental cut, puncture, perforation, or hemorrhage during medical care
E871   Foreign object left in body during procedure
E872   Failure of sterile precautions during procedure
E873   Failure in dosage
E874   Mechanical failure of instrument or apparatus during procedure
E875   Contaminated or infected blood, other fluid, drug, or biological substance
E876   Other and unspecified misadventures during medical care

Surgical and medical procedures as the cause of abnormal reaction of patient or later complication, without mention of misadventure at the time of procedure (E878-E879)

E878   Surgical operation and other surgical procedures as the cause of abnormal reaction of patient, or of later complication, without mention of misadventure at the time of operation
E879   Other procedures, without mention of misadventure at the time of procedure, as the cause of abnormal reaction of patient, or of later complication

Accidental falls (E880-E888)

E880   Fall on or from stairs or steps
E881   Fall on or from ladders or scaffolding
E882   Fall from or out of building or other structure
E883   Fall into hole or other opening in surface
E884   Other fall from one level to another
E885   Fall on same level from slipping, tripping, or stumbling
E886   Fall on same level from collision, pushing or shoving, by or with other person
E887   Fracture, cause unspecified
E888   Other and unspecified fall

Accidents caused by fire and flames (E890-E899)

E890   Conflagration in private dwelling
E891   Conflagration in other and unspecified building or structure
E892   Conflagration not in building or structure
E893   Accident caused by ignition of clothing

E894   Ignition of highly inflammable material
E895   Accident caused by controlled fire in private dwelling
E896   Accident caused by controlled fire in other and unspecified building or structure
E897   Accident caused by controlled fire not in building or structure
E898   Accident caused by other specified fire and flames
E899   Accident caused by unspecified fire

Accidents due to natural and environmental factors (E900-E909)

E900   Excessive heat
E901   Excessive cold
E902   High and low air pressure and changes in air pressure
E903   Travel and motion
E904   Hunger, thirst, exposure, and neglect
E905   Venomous animals and plants as the cause of poisoning and toxic reactions
E906   Other injury caused by animals
E907   Lightning
E908   Cataclysmic storms, and floods resulting from storms
E909   Cataclysmic earth surface movements and eruptions

Accidents caused by submersion, suffocation, and foreign bodies (E910-E915)

E910   Accidental drowning and submersion
E911   Inhalation and ingestion of food causing obstruction of respiratory tract or suffocation
E912   Inhalation and ingestion of other object causing obstruction of respiratory tract or suffocation
E913   Accidental mechanical suffocation
E914   Foreign body accidentally entering eye and adnexa
E915   Foreign body accidentally entering other orifice

Other accidents (E916-E928)

E916   Struck accidentally by falling object
E917   Striking against or struck accidentally by objects or persons
E918   Caught accidentally in or between objects
E919   Accidents caused by machinery
E920   Accidents caused by cutting and piercing instruments or objects
E921   Accident caused by explosion of pressure vessel
E922   Accident caused by firearm and air gun missile
E923   Accident caused by explosive material
E924   Accident caused by hot substance or object, caustic or corrosive material, and steam
E925   Accident caused by electric current
E926   Exposure to radiation
E927   Overexertion and strenuous and repetitive movements or loads
E928   Other and unspecified environmental and accidental causes

Late effects of accidental injury (E929)

E929   Late effects of accidental injury

Drugs, medicinal and biological substances causing adverse effects in therapeutic use (E930-E949)

E930   Antibiotics
E931   Other anti-infectives
E932   Hormones and synthetic substitutes
E933   Primarily systemic agents
E934   Agents primarily affecting blood constituents
E935   Analgesics, antipyretics, and antirheumatics
E936   Anticonvulsants and anti-Parkinsonism drugs
E937   Sedatives and hypnotics

E938   Other central nervous system depressants and anesthetics
E939   Psychotropic agents
E940   Central nervous system stimulants
E941   Drugs primarily affecting the autonomic nervous system
E942   Agents primarily affecting the cardiovascular system
E943   Agents primarily affecting gastrointestinal system
E944   Water, mineral, and uric acid metabolism drugs
E945   Agents primarily acting on the smooth and skeletal muscles and respiratory system
E946   Agents primarily affecting skin and mucous membrane, ophthalmological, otorhinolaryngological, and dental drugs
E947   Other and unspecified drugs and medicinal substances
E948   Bacterial vaccines
E949   Other vaccines and biological substances

Suicide and self-inflicted injury (E950-E959)

E950   Suicide and self-inflicted poisoning by solid or liquid substances
E951   Suicide and self-inflicted poisoning by gases in domestic use
E952   Suicide and self-inflicted poisoning by other gases and vapors
E953   Suicide and self-inflicted injury by hanging, strangulation, and suffocation
E954   Suicide and self-inflicted injury by submersion [drowning]
E955   Suicide and self-inflicted injury by firearms, air guns and explosives
E956   Suicide and self-inflicted injury by cutting and piercing instruments
E957   Suicide and self-inflicted injuries by jumping from high place
E958   Suicide and self-inflicted injury by other and unspecified means
E959   Late effects of self-inflicted injury

Homicide and injury purposely inflicted by other persons (E960-E969)

E960   Fight, brawl, and rape
E961   Assault by corrosive or caustic substance, except poisoning
E962   Assault by poisoning
E963   Assault by hanging and strangulation
E964   Assault by submersion [drowning]
E965   Assault by firearms and explosives
E966   Assault by cutting and piercing instrument
E967   Perpetrator of child and adult abuse
E968   Assault by other and unspecified means
E969   Late effects of injury purposely inflicted by other person

Legal intervention (E970-E978)

E970   Injury due to legal intervention by firearms
E971   Injury due to legal intervention by explosives
E972   Injury due to legal intervention by gas
E973   Injury due to legal intervention by blunt object
E974   Injury due to legal intervention by cutting and piercing instruments
E975   Injury due to legal intervention by other specified means
E976   Injury due to legal intervention by unspecified means
E977   Late effects of injuries due to legal intervention
E978   Legal execution

Terrorism (E979)

E979   Terrorism

Injury undetermined whether accidentally or purposely inflicted (E980-E989)

E980 Poisoning by solid or liquid substances, undetermined whether accidentally or purposely inflicted

E981 Poisoning by gases in domestic use, undetermined whether accidentally or purposely inflicted

E982 Poisoning by other gases, undetermined whether accidentally or purposely inflicted

E983 Hanging, strangulation, or suffocation, undetermined whether accidentally or purposely inflicted

E984 Submersion [drowning], undetermined whether accidentally or purposely inflicted

E985 Injury by firearms and explosives, undetermined whether accidentally or purposely inflicted

E986 Injury by cutting and piercing instruments, undetermined whether accidentally or purposely inflicted

E987 Falling from high place, undetermined whether accidentally or purposely inflicted

E988 Injury by other and unspecified means, undetermined whether accidentally or purposely inflicted

E989 Late effects of injury, undetermined whether accidentally or purposely inflicted

Injury resulting from operations of war (E990-E999)

E990 Injury due to war operations by fires and conflagrations

E991 Injury due to war operations by bullets and fragments

E992 Injury due to war operations by explosion of marine weapons

E993 Injury due to war operations by other explosion

E994 Injury due to war operations by destruction of aircraft

E995 Injury due to war operations by other and unspecified forms of conventional warfare

E996 Injury due to war operations by nuclear weapons

E997 Injury due to war operations by other forms of unconventional warfare

E998 Injury due to war operations but occurring after cessation of hostilities

E999 Late effects of injury due to war operations and terrorism

A

Abbe operation
  construction of vagina 70.61
    with graft or prosthesis 70.63
  intestinal anastomosis — see Anastomosis, intestine
Abciximab, infusion 99.20
Abdominocentesis 54.91
Abdominohysterectomy 68.49
  laparoscopic 68.41
Abdominoplasty 86.83
Abdominoscopy 54.21
Abdominouterotomy 68.0
  obstetrical 74.99
Abduction, arytenoid 31.69
AbioCor® total replacement heart 37.52
Ablation
  biliary tract (lesion) by ERCP 51.64
  endometrial (hysteroscopic) 68.23
  inner ear (cryosurgery) (ultrasound) 20.79
    by injection 20.72
  lesion
    esophagus 42.39
      endoscopic 42.33
    heart
      by peripherally inserted catheter 37.34
      endovascular approach 37.34
      maze procedure (Cox-maze)
        endovascular approach 37.34
        open approach 37.33
        thoracoscopic approach 37.37
      thoracoscopic approach 37.37
    intestine
      large 45.49
        endoscopic 45.43
    large intestine 45.49
      endoscopic 45.43
    liver 50.26
      laparoscopic 50.25
      open 50.23
      percutaneous 50.24
    lung 32.26
      bronchoscopic thermoplasty 32.27
      open 32.23
      percutaneous 32.24
      thoracoscopic 32.25
    renal 55.35
      laparoscopic 55.34
      open 55.32
      percutaneous 55.33
  pituitary 07.69
    by
      Cobalt 60 92.32
      implantation (strontium-yttrium) (Y) NEC 07.68
        transfrontal approach 07.64
        transphenoidal approach 07.65
      proton beam (Bragg peak) 92.33
  prostate
    by
      cryoablation 60.62
      laser, transurethral 60.21
      radical cryosurgical ablation (RCSA) 60.62
      radiofrequency thermotherapy 60.97
      transurethral needle ablation (TUNA) 60.97
  tissue
    heart — see Ablation, lesion, heart
    liver — see Ablation, lesion, liver
    lung — see Ablation, lesion, lung
    renal — see Ablation, lesion, renal
Abortion, therapeutic 69.51
  by
    aspiration curettage 69.51
    dilation and curettage 69.01
    hysterectomy — see Hysterectomy
    hysterotomy 74.91
    insertion
      laminaria 69.93
      prostaglandin suppository 96.49
    intra-amniotic injection (saline) 75.0
Abrasion
  corneal epithelium 11.41
    for smear or culture 11.21

Abrasion — continued
  epicardial surface 36.39
  pleural 34.6
  skin 86.25
Abscission, cornea 11.49
Absorptiometry
  photon (dual) (single) 88.98
Aburel operation (intra-amniotic injection for abortion) 75.0
Accouchement forcé 73.99
Acetabulectomy 77.85
Acetabuloplasty NEC 81.40
  with prosthetic implant 81.52
Achillorrhaphy 83.64
  delayed 83.62
Achillotenotomy 83.11
  plastic 83.85
Achillotomy 83.11
  plastic 83.85
Acid peel, skin 86.24
Acromionectomy 77.81
Acromioplasty 81.83
  for recurrent dislocation of shoulder 81.82
  partial replacement 81.81
  total replacement, NEC 81.80
    other 81.80
    reverse 81.88
Actinotherapy 99.82
Activities of daily living (ADL)
  therapy 93.83
  training for the blind 93.78
Acupuncture 99.92
  with smouldering moxa 93.35
  for anesthesia 99.91
Adams operation
  advancement of round ligament 69.22
  crushing of nasal septum 21.88
  excision of palmar fascia 82.35
Adenectomy — see also Excision, by site
  prostate NEC 60.69
    retropubic 60.4
Adenoidectomy (without tonsillectomy) 28.6
  with tonsillectomy 28.3
Adhesiolysis — see also Lysis, adhesions
  for collapse of lung 33.39
  middle ear 20.23
Adipectomy 86.83
Adjustment
  cardiac pacemaker program (reprogramming) — omit code
  cochlear prosthetic device (external components) 95.49
  dental 99.97
  gastric restrictive device (laparoscopic) 44.98
  occlusal 24.8
  orthopedic device (noninvasive)
    external fixator — omit code
  spectacles 95.31
Administration (of) — see also Injection
  Activase® 99.10
  adhesion barrier substance 99.77
  Alteplase (tPA, generic) 99.10
  Anistreplase (tPA, generic) 99.10
  antitoxins NEC 99.58
    botulism 99.57
    diphtheria 99.58
    gas gangrene 99.58
    scarlet fever 99.58
    tetanus 99.56
  Bender Visual-Motor Gestalt test 94.02
  Benton Visual Retention test 94.02
  DrotAA 00.11
  Eminase® 99.10
  inhaled nitric oxide 00.12
  intelligence test or scale (Stanford-Binet) (Wechsler) (adult) (children) 94.01
  Minnesota Multiphasic Personality Inventory (MMPI) 94.02
  MMPI (Minnesota Multiphasic Personality Inventory) 94.02
  neuroprotective agent 99.75
  Proleukin® (low-dose) 99.28
    high-dose 00.15
  psychologic test 94.02
  Retavase® 99.10

Administration — see also Injection — continued
  Reteplase (tPA, generic) 99.10
  Stanford-Binet test 94.01
  Streptase® 99.10
  Streptokinase (tPA, generic) 99.10
  Tenecteplase (tPA, generic) 99.10
  TNKase™ 99.10
  toxoid
    diphtheria 99.36
      with tetanus and pertussis, combined (DTP) 99.39
    tetanus 99.38
      with diphtheria and pertussis, combined (DTP) 99.39
  vaccine (see also Vaccination)
    BCG 99.33
    measles-mumps-rubella (MMR) 99.48
    poliomyelitis 99.41
    TAB 99.32
  Wechsler
    Intelligence Scale (adult) (children) 94.01
    Memory Scale 94.02
  Xigris® 00.11
Adrenalectomy (unilateral) 07.22
  with partial removal of remaining gland 07.29
  bilateral 07.3
    partial 07.29
    subtotal 07.29
  complete 07.3
  partial NEC 07.29
  remaining gland 07.3
  subtotal NEC 07.29
  total 07.3
Adrenalorrhaphy 07.44
Adrenalotomy (with drainage) 07.41
Advancement
  extraocular muscle 15.12
    multiple (with resection or recession) 15.3
  eyelid muscle 08.59
  eye muscle 15.12
    multiple (with resection or recession) 15.3
  graft — see Graft
  leaflet (heart) 35.10
  pedicle (flap) 86.72
  profundus tendon (Wagner) 82.51
  round ligament 69.22
  tendon 83.71
    hand 82.51
    profundus (Wagner) 82.51
  Wagner (profundus tendon) 82.51
AESOP® (Automated Endoscopic System for Optimal Positioning) — see category 17.4 ☑
Albee operation
  bone peg, femoral neck 78.05
  graft for slipping patella 78.06
  sliding inlay graft, tibia 78.07
Albert operation (arthrodesis of knee) 81.22
Aldridge (-Studdiford) operation (urethral sling) 59.5
Alexander-Adams operation (shortening of round ligaments) 69.22
Alexander operation
  prostatectomy
    perineal 60.62
    suprapubic 60.3
  shortening of round ligaments 69.22
Alimentation, parenteral 99.29
Allograft — see Graft
Almoor operation (extrapetrosal drainage) 20.22
Altemeier operation (perineal rectal pull-through) 48.49
Alveolectomy (interradicular) (intraseptal) (radical) (simple) (with graft) (with implant) 24.5
Alveoloplasty (with graft or implant) 24.5
Alveolotomy (apical) 24.0
Ambulatory cardiac monitoring (ACM) 89.50
Ammon operation (dacryocystotomy) 09.53
Amniocentesis (transuterine) (diagnostic) 75.1
  with intra-amniotic injection of saline 75.0

Amniography 87.81
Amnioinfusion 75.37
Amnioscopy, internal 75.31
Amniotomy 73.09
  to induce labor 73.01
Amputation (cineplastic) (closed flap) (guillotine) (kineplastic) (open) 84.91
  abdominopelvic 84.19
  above-elbow 84.07
  above-knee (AK) 84.17
  ankle (disarticulation) 84.13
    through malleoli of tibia and fibula 84.14
  arm NEC 84.00
    through
      carpals 84.03
      elbow (disarticulation) 84.06
      forearm 84.05
      humerus 84.07
      shoulder (disarticulation) 84.08
      wrist (disarticulation) 84.04
    upper 84.07
  Batch-Spittler-McFaddin (knee disarticulation) 84.16
  below-knee (BK) NEC 84.15
    conversion into above-knee amputation 84.17
  Boyd (hip disarticulation) 84.18
  Burgess operation (amputation of ankle) 84.14
  Callander's (knee disarticulation) 84.16
  carpals 84.03
  cervix 67.4
  Chopart's (midtarsal) 84.12
  clitoris 71.4
  Dieffenbach (hip disarticulation) 84.18
  Dupuytren's (shoulder disarticulation) 84.08
  ear, external 18.39
  elbow (disarticulation) 84.06
  finger, except thumb 84.01
    thumb 84.02
  foot (middle) 84.12
  forearm 84.05
  forefoot 84.12
  forequarter 84.09
  Gordon-Taylor (hindquarter) 84.19
  Gritti-Stokes (knee disarticulation) 84.16
  Guyon (ankle) 84.13
  hallux 84.11
  hand 84.03
  Hey's (foot) 84.12
  hindquarter 84.19
  hip (disarticulation) 84.18
  humerus 84.07
  interscapulothoracic 84.09
  interthoracoscapular 84.09
  King-Steelquist (hindquarter) 84.19
  Kirk (thigh) 84.17
  knee (disarticulation) 84.16
  Kutler (revision of current traumatic amputation of finger) 84.01
  Larry (shoulder disarticulation) 84.08
  leg NEC 84.10
    above knee (AK) 84.17
    below knee (BK) 84.15
    through
      ankle (disarticulation) 84.13
      femur (AK) 84.17
      foot 84.12
      hip (disarticulation) 84.18
      tibia and fibula (BK) 84.15
  Lisfranc
    foot 84.12
    shoulder (disarticulation) 84.08
  Littlewood (forequarter) 84.09
  lower limb NEC (see also Amputation, leg) 84.10
  Mazet (knee disarticulation) 84.16
  metacarpal 84.03
  metatarsal 84.11
    head (bunionectomy) 77.59
  metatarsophalangeal (joint) 84.11
  midtarsal 84.12
  nose 21.4
  penis (circle) (complete) (flap) (partial) (radical) 64.3

☑ Additional Digit Required — Refer to the Tabular List for Digit Selection   ▽ Subterms under main terms may continue to next column or page

2014 ICD-9-CM   825

Aneurysmorrhaphy — *continued*
by or with — *continued*
excision or resection (*see also* Aneurysmectomy, by site) — *continued*
with — *continued*
graft replacement — *see* Aneurysmectomy, with graft replacement, by site
filipuncture 39.52
graft replacement — *see* Aneurysmectomy, with graft replacement, by site
methyl methacrylate 39.52
suture 39.52
wiring 39.52
wrapping 39.52
Matas' 39.52
Aneurysmotomy — *see* Aneurysmectomy
Angiectomy
with
anastomosis 38.30
abdominal
artery 38.36
vein 38.37
aorta (arch) (ascending) (descending) 38.34
head and neck NEC 38.32
intracranial NEC 38.31
lower limb
artery 38.38
vein 38.39
thoracic vessel NEC 38.35
upper limb (artery) (vein) 38.33
graft replacement (interposition) 38.40
abdominal
aorta 38.44
artery 38.46
vein 38.47
aorta (arch) (ascending) (descending) (thoracic)
abdominal 38.44
thoracic 38.45
thoracoabdominal 38.45 [38.44]
head and neck NEC 38.42
intracranial NEC 38.41
lower limb
artery 38.48
vein 38.49
thoracic vessel NEC 38.45
upper limb (artery) (vein) 38.43
Angiocardiography (selective) 88.50
carbon dioxide (negative contrast) 88.58
combined right and left heart 88.54
intra-operative coronary fluorescence vascular 88.59
left heart (aortic valve) (atrium) (ventricle) (ventricular outflow tract) 88.53
combined with right heart 88.54
right heart (atrium) (pulmonary valve) (ventricle) (ventricular outflow tract) 88.52
combined with left heart 88.54
SPY, coronary 88.59
vena cava (inferior) (superior) 88.51
Angiography (arterial) — *see also* Arteriography 88.40
by C.A.T. — *see* Scan, C.A.T., by site
by computed tomography — *see* Scan, C.A.T., by site
by magnetic resonance — *see* Imaging, magnetic resonance, by site
by radioisotope — *see* Scan, radioisotope, by site
by ultrasound — *see* Ultrasonography, by site
basilar 88.41
brachial 88.49
carotid (internal) 88.41
celiac 88.47
cerebral (posterior circulation) 88.41
coronary NEC 88.57
intra-operative fluorescence vascular 88.59
eye (fluorescein) 95.12
femoral 88.48

Angiography — *see also* Arteriography — *continued*
heart 88.50
intra-abdominal NEC 88.47
intracranial 88.41
intrathoracic vessels NEC 88.44
lower extremity NEC 88.48
neck 88.41
non-coronary, intra-operative fluorescence 17.71
placenta 88.46
pulmonary 88.43
renal 88.45
specified artery NEC 88.49
transfemoral 88.48
upper extremity NEC 88.49
veins — *see* Phlebography
vertebral 88.41
Angioplasty (laser) — *see also* Repair, blood vessel

Note — Also use 00.40, 00.41, 00.42, or 00.43 to show the total number of vessels treated. Use code 00.44 once to show procedure on a bifurcated vessel. In addition, use 00.45, 00.46, 00.47, or 00.48 to show the number of vascular stents inserted.

balloon (percutaneous transluminal) NEC 39.50
coronary artery 00.66
multiple vessels
coronary 36.09
open chest approach 36.03
percutaneous transluminal (balloon) 00.66
percutaneous transluminal (balloon)
basilar 00.62
carotid 00.61
cerebrovascular
extracranial 00.61
intracranial 00.62
carotid 00.61
coronary (balloon) 00.66
extracranial 00.61
femoropopliteal 39.50
iliac 39.50
intracranial 00.62
lower extremity NOS 39.50
mesenteric 39.50
peripheral NEC 39.50
renal 39.50
subclavian 39.50
upper extremity NOS 39.50
vertebral 00.61
intracranial portion 00.62
specified site 39.50
cerebrovascular
extracranial 00.61
intracranial 00.62
peripheral 39.50
Angiorrhaphy 39.30
artery 39.31
vein 39.32
Angioscopy, percutaneous 38.22
eye (fluorescein) 95.12
Angiotomy 38.00
abdominal
artery 38.06
vein 38.07
aorta (arch) (ascending) (descending) 38.04
head and neck NEC 38.02
intracranial NEC 38.01
lower limb
artery 38.08
vein 38.09
thoracic NEC 38.05
upper limb (artery) (vein) 38.03
Angiotripsy 39.98
Ankylosis, production of — *see* Arthrodesis
Annuloplasty (heart) (posteromedial) 35.33
Anoplasty 49.79
with hemorrhoidectomy 49.46
Anoscopy 49.21
Antibiogram — *see* Examination, microscopic
Antiembolic filter, vena cava 38.7
Antiphobic treatment 94.39

Antrectomy
mastoid 20.49
maxillary 22.39
radical 22.31
pyloric 43.6
Antrostomy — *see* Antrotomy
Antrotomy (exploratory) (nasal sinus) 22.2
Caldwell-Luc (maxillary sinus) 22.39
with removal of membrane lining 22.31
intranasal 22.2
with external approach (Caldwell-Luc) 22.39
radical 22.31
maxillary (simple) 22.2
with Caldwell-Luc approach 22.39
with removal of membrane lining 22.31
external (Caldwell-Luc approach) 22.39
with removal of membrane lining 22.31
radical (with removal of membrane lining) 22.31
Antrum window operation — *see* Antrotomy, maxillary
Aorticopulmonary window operation 39.59
Aortogram, aortography (abdominal) (retrograde) (selective) (translumbar) 88.42
Aortoplasty (aortic valve) (gusset type) 35.11
Aortotomy 38.04
Apexcardiogram (with ECG lead) 89.57
Apheresis, therapeutic — *see* category 99.7 ☑
Apicectomy
lung 32.39
thoracoscopic 32.30
petrous pyramid 20.59
tooth (root) 23.73
with root canal therapy 23.72
Apicoectomy 23.73
with root canal therapy 23.72
Apicolysis (lung) 33.39
Apicostomy, alveolar 24.0
Aponeurectomy 83.42
hand 82.33
Aponeurorrhaphy — *see also* Suture, tendon 83.64
hand (*see also* Suture, tendon, hand) 82.45
Aponeurotomy 83.13
hand 82.11
Appendectomy (with drainage) 47.09
incidental 47.19
laparoscopic 47.11
laparoscopic 47.01
Appendicectomy (with drainage) 47.09
incidental 47.19
laparoscopic 47.11
laparoscopic 47.01
Appendicocecostomy 47.91
Appendicoenterostomy 47.91
Appendicolysis 54.59
with appendectomy 47.09
laparoscopic 47.01
other 47.09
laparoscopic 54.51
Appendicostomy 47.91
closure 47.92
Appendicotomy 47.2
Application
adhesion barrier substance 99.77
anti-shock trousers 93.58
arch bars (orthodontic) 24.7
for immobilization (fracture) 93.55
barrier substance, adhesion 99.77
Barton's tongs (skull) (with synchronous skeletal traction) 02.94
bone growth stimulator (surface) (transcutaneous) 99.86
bone morphogenetic protein (Infuse™) (OP-1™) (recombinant) (rhBMP) 84.52
Bryant's traction 93.44
with reduction of fracture or dislocation — *see* Reduction, fracture *and* Reduction, dislocation
Buck's traction 93.46
caliper tongs (skull) (with synchronous skeletal traction) 02.94

Application — *continued*
cast (fiberglass) (plaster) (plastic) NEC 93.53
with reduction of fracture or dislocation — *see* Reduction, fracture *and* Reduction, dislocation
spica 93.51
cervical collar 93.52
with reduction of fracture or dislocation — *see* Reduction, fracture *and* Reduction, dislocation
clamp, cerebral aneurysm (Crutchfield) (Silverstone) 39.51
croupette, croup tent 93.94
crown (artificial) 23.41
Crutchfield tongs (skull) (with synchronous skeletal traction) 02.94
Dunlop's traction 93.44
with reduction of fracture or dislocation — *see* Reduction, fracture *and* Reduction, dislocation
elastic stockings 93.59
electronic gaiter 93.59
external fixator device (bone) 78.10
carpal, metacarpal 78.14
clavicle 78.11
computer assisted (dependent) 84.73
femur 78.15
fibula 78.17
humerus 78.12
hybrid device or system 84.73
Ilizarov type 84.72
monoplanar system or device 84.71
patella 78.16
pelvic 78.19
phalanges (foot) (hand) 78.19
radius 78.13
ring device or system 84.72
scapula 78.11
Sheffield type 84.72
specified site NEC 78.19
tarsal, metatarsal 78.18
thorax (ribs) (sternum) 78.11
tibia 78.17
ulna 78.13
vertebrae 78.19
forceps, with delivery — *see* Delivery, forceps
graft — *see* Graft
gravity (G-) suit 93.59
intermittent pressure device 93.59
Jewett extension brace 93.59
Jobst pumping unit (reduction of edema) 93.59
Lyman Smith traction 93.44
with reduction of fracture or dislocation — *see* Reduction, fracture *and* Reduction, dislocation
MAST (military anti-shock trousers) 93.58
Minerva jacket 93.52
minifixator device (bone) — *see* category 78.1 ☑
neck support (molded) 93.52
obturator (orthodontic) 24.7
orthodontic appliance (obturator) (wiring) 24.7
pelvic sling 93.44
with reduction of fracture or dislocation — *see* Reduction, fracture *and* Reduction, dislocation
peridontal splint (orthodontic) 24.7
plaster jacket 93.51
Minerva 93.52
pressure
dressing (bandage) (Gibney) (Robert Jones') (Shanz) 93.56
trousers (anti-shock) (MAST) 93.58
prosthesis for missing ear 18.71
Russell's traction 93.44
with reduction of fracture or dislocation — *see* Reduction, fracture *and* Reduction, dislocation
splint, for immobilization (plaster) (pneumatic) (tray) 93.54
with fracture reduction — *see* Reduction, fracture
stereotactic head frame 93.59

Biopsy — *continued*

duodenum — *continued*
  closed (endoscopic) 45.14
  open 45.15
ear (external) 18.12
  middle or inner 20.32
endocervix 67.11
endometrium NEC 68.16
  by
    aspiration curettage 69.59
    dilation and curettage 69.09
  closed (endoscopic) 68.16
  open 68.13
epididymis 63.01
esophagus 42.24
  closed (endoscopic) 42.24
  open 42.25
extraocular muscle or tendon 15.01
eye 16.23
  muscle (oblique) (rectus) 15.01
eyelid 08.11
fallopian tube 66.11
fascia 83.21
fetus 75.33
gallbladder 51.12
  closed (endoscopic) 51.14
  open 51.13
  percutaneous (needle) 51.12
ganglion (cranial) (peripheral) NEC 04.11
  closed 04.11
  open 04.12
  percutaneous (needle) 04.11
  sympathetic nerve 05.11
gum 24.11
heart 37.25
hypophysis (*see also* Biopsy, pituitary gland) 07.15
ileum 45.14
  brush 45.14
  closed (endoscopic) 45.14
  open 45.15
intestine NEC 45.27
  large 45.25
    brush 45.25
    closed (endoscopic) 45.25
    open 45.26
  small 45.14
    brush 45.14
    closed (endoscopic) 45.14
    open 45.15
intra-abdominal mass 54.24
  closed 54.24
  percutaneous (needle) 54.24
iris 12.22
jejunum 45.14
  brush 45.14
  closed (endoscopic) 45.14
  open 45.15
joint structure (aspiration) 80.30
  ankle 80.37
  elbow 80.32
  foot and toe 80.38
  hand and finger 80.34
  hip 80.35
  knee 80.36
  shoulder 80.31
  specified site NEC 80.39
  spine 80.39
  wrist 80.33
kidney 55.23
  closed 55.23
  open 55.24
  percutaneous (aspiration) (needle) 55.23
labia 71.11
lacrimal
  gland 09.11
  sac 09.12
larynx 31.43
  brush 31.43
  closed (endoscopic) 31.43
  open 31.45
lip 27.23
liver 50.11
  closed 50.11
  laparoscopic 50.14
  open 50.12

Biopsy — *continued*

liver — *continued*
  percutaneous (aspiration) (needle) 50.11
  transjugular 50.13
  transvenous 50.13
lung NEC 33.27
  brush 33.24
  closed (percutaneous) (needle) 33.26
    brush 33.24
    endoscopic 33.27
      brush 33.24
  endoscopic 33.27
    brush 33.24
  open 33.28
  thoracoscopic 33.20
  transbronchial 33.27
  transthoracic 33.26
lymphatic structure (channel) (node) (vessel) 40.11
mediastinum NEC 34.25
  closed 34.25
  open 34.26
  percutaneous (needle) 34.25
meninges (cerebral) NEC 01.11
  closed 01.11
  open 01.12
  percutaneous (needle) 01.11
  spinal 03.32
mesentery 54.23
mouth NEC 27.24
muscle 83.21
  extraocular 15.01
  ocular 15.01
nasopharynx 29.12
nerve (cranial) (peripheral) NEC 04.11
  closed 04.11
  open 04.12
  percutaneous (needle) 04.11
  sympathetic 05.11
nose, nasal 21.22
  sinus 22.11
    closed (endoscopic) (needle) 22.11
    open 22.12
ocular muscle or tendon 15.01
omentum
  closed 54.24
  open 54.23
  percutaneous (needle) 54.24
orbit 16.23
  by aspiration 16.22
ovary 65.12
  by aspiration 65.11
  laparoscopic 65.13
palate (bony) 27.21
  soft 27.22
pancreas 52.11
  closed (endoscopic) 52.11
  open 52.12
  percutaneous (aspiration) (needle) 52.11
pancreatic duct 52.14
  closed (endoscopic) 52.14
parathyroid gland 06.13
penis 64.11
perianal tissue 49.22
pericardium 37.24
periprostatic 60.15
perirectal tissue 48.26
perirenal tissue 59.21
peritoneal implant
  closed 54.24
  open 54.23
  percutaneous (needle) 54.24
peritoneum
  closed 54.24
  open 54.23
  percutaneous (needle) 54.24
periurethral tissue 58.24
perivesical tissue 59.21
pharynx, pharyngeal 29.12
pineal gland 07.17
pituitary gland 07.15
  transfrontal approach 07.13
  transsphenoidal approach 07.14
pleura, pleural 34.24
  thoracoscopic 34.20
prostate NEC 60.11

Biopsy — *continued*

prostate — *continued*
  closed (transurethral) 60.11
  open 60.12
  percutaneous (needle) 60.11
  transrectal 60.11
rectum 48.24
  brush 48.24
  closed (endoscopic) 48.24
  open 48.25
retroperitoneal tissue 54.24
salivary gland or duct 26.11
  closed (needle) 26.11
  open 26.12
scrotum 61.11
seminal vesicle NEC 60.13
  closed 60.13
  open 60.14
  percutaneous (needle) 60.13
sigmoid colon 45.25
  brush 45.25
  closed (endoscopic) 45.25
  open 45.26
sinus, nasal 22.11
  closed (endoscopic) (needle) 22.11
  open 22.12
skin (punch) 86.11
skull 01.15
soft palate 27.22
soft tissue NEC 86.11
  closed (needle) (punch) 86.11
  open 83.21
spermatic cord 63.01
sphincter of Oddi 51.14
  closed (endoscopic) 51.14
  open 51.13
spinal cord (meninges) 03.32
spleen 41.32
  closed 41.32
  open 41.33
  percutaneous (aspiration) (needle) 41.32
stomach 44.14
  brush 44.14
  closed (endoscopic) 44.14
  open 44.15
subcutaneous tissue (punch) 86.11
supraglottic mass 29.12
sympathetic nerve 05.11
tendon 83.21
  extraocular 15.01
  ocular 15.01
testis NEC 62.11
  closed 62.11
  open 62.12
  percutaneous (needle) 62.11
thymus 07.16
thyroid gland NEC 06.11
  closed 06.11
  open 06.12
  percutaneous (aspiration) (needle) 06.11
tongue 25.01
  closed (needle) 25.01
  open 25.02
tonsil 28.11
trachea 31.44
  brush 31.44
  closed (endoscopic) 31.44
  open 31.45
tunica vaginalis 61.11
umbilicus 54.22
ureter 56.33
  closed (percutaneous) 56.32
    endoscopic 56.33
    open 56.34
  transurethral 56.33
urethra 58.23
uterus, uterine (endometrial) 68.16
  by
    aspiration curettage 69.59
    dilation and curettage 69.09
  closed (endoscopic) 68.16
  ligaments 68.15
    closed (endoscopic) 68.15
    open 68.14
  open 68.13
uvula 27.22

Biopsy — *continued*

vagina 70.24
vas deferens 63.01
vein (any site) 38.21
vulva 71.11
BiPAP 93.90
  delivered by
    endotracheal tube — *see category* 96.7 ☑
    tracheostomy — *see category* 96.7 ☑
Bischoff operation (spinal myelotomy) 03.29
Bischoff operation (ureteroneocystostomy) 56.74
Bisection — *see also* Excision
  hysterectomy 68.39
    laparoscopic 68.31
  ovary 65.29
    laparoscopic 65.25
  stapes foot plate 19.19
    with incus replacement 19.11
BIS (bispectral index) **monitoring** 00.94 *[89.14]*
Blalock-Hanlon operation (creation of atrial septal defect) 35.42
Blalock operation (systemic-pulmonary anastomosis) 39.0
Blalock-Taussig operation (subclavian-pulmonary anastomosis) 39.0
Blascovic operation (resection and advancement of levator palpebrae superioris) 08.33
Blepharectomy 08.20
Blepharoplasty — *see also* Reconstruction, eyelid 08.70
  extensive 08.44
Blepharorrhaphy 08.52
  division or severing 08.02
Blepharotomy 08.09
Blind rehabilitation therapy NEC 93.78
Block
  caudal — *see* Injection, spinal
  celiac ganglion or plexus 05.31
  dissection
    breast
      bilateral 85.46
      unilateral 85.45
    bronchus 32.6
    larynx 30.3
    lymph nodes 40.50
    neck 40.40
    vulva 71.5
  epidural, spinal — *see* Injection, spinal
  gasserian ganglion 04.81
  intercostal nerves 04.81
  intrathecal — *see* Injection, spinal
  nerve (cranial) (peripheral) NEC 04.81
  paravertebral stellate ganglion 05.31
  peripheral nerve 04.81
  spinal nerve root (intrathecal) — *see* Injection, spinal
  stellate (ganglion) 05.31
  subarachnoid, spinal — *see* Injection, spinal
  sympathetic nerve 05.31
  trigeminal nerve 04.81
Blood
  flow study, Doppler-type (ultrasound) — *see* Ultrasonography
  patch, spine (epidural) 03.95
  transfusion
    antihemophilic factor 99.06
    autologous
      collected prior to surgery 99.02
      intraoperative 99.00
      perioperative 99.00
      postoperative 99.00
      previously collected 99.02
      salvage 99.00
    blood expander 99.08
    blood surrogate 99.09
    coagulation factors 99.06
    exchange 99.01
    granulocytes 99.09
    hemodilution 99.03
    other substance 99.09
    packed cells 99.04
    plasma 99.07
    platelets 99.05

☑ **Additional Digit Required — Refer to the Tabular List for Digit Selection**   ▽ **Subterms under main terms may continue to next column or page**

830   **2014 ICD-9-CM**

☑ Additional Digit Required — Refer to the Tabular List for Digit Selection   ▽ Subterms under main terms may continue to next column or page

2014 ICD-9-CM   **831**

☑ **Additional Digit Required — Refer to the Tabular List for Digit Selection**

▽ **Subterms under main terms may continue to next column or page**

☑ **Additional Digit Required** — Refer to the Tabular List for Digit Selection   ▽ **Subterms under main terms may continue to next column or page**

2014 ICD-9-CM   833

Closure — see also Repair — continued
  stoma
    bile duct 51.79
    bladder 57.82
    bronchus 33.42
    common duct 51.72
    esophagus 42.83
    gallbladder 51.92
    hepatic duct 51.79
    intestine 46.50
      large 46.52
      small 46.51
    kidney 55.82
    larynx 31.62
    rectum 48.72
    stomach 44.62
    thorax 34.72
    trachea 31.72
    ureter 56.83
    urethra 58.42
  thoracostomy 34.72
  tracheostomy 31.72
  ulcer (bleeding) (peptic) (perforated) 44.40
    duodenum 44.42
    gastric 44.41
    intestine (perforated) 46.79
    skin 86.59
    stomach 44.41
  ureterostomy 56.83
  urethrostomy 58.42
  vagina 70.8
  vascular
    percutaneous puncture — omit code
  vesicostomy 57.22
  wound (see also Suture, by site)
    with graft — see Graft
    with tissue adhesive 86.59
Coagulation, electrocoagulation — see also
    Destruction, lesion, by site
  aneurysm (cerebral) (peripheral vessel)
    39.52
  arteriovenous fistula 39.53
  brain tissue (incremental) (radio-frequency)
    01.59
  broad ligament 69.19
  cervix 67.32
  ear
    external 18.29
    inner 20.79
    middle 20.51
  fallopian tube 66.61
  gasserian ganglion 04.05
  nose for epistaxis (with packing) 21.03
  ovary 65.29
    laparoscopic 65.25
  pharynx (by diathermy) 29.39
  prostatic bed 60.94
  rectum (polyp) 48.32
    radical 48.31
  retina (for)
    destruction of lesion 14.21
    reattachment 14.51
    repair of tear 14.31
  round ligament 69.19
  semicircular canals 20.79
  spinal cord (lesion) 03.4
  urethrovesical junction, transurethral 57.49
  uterosacral ligament 69.19
  uterus 68.29
  vagina 70.33
  vulva 71.3
Coating, aneurysm of brain 39.52
Cobalt-60 therapy (treatment) 92.23
Coccygectomy (partial) 77.89
  total 77.99
Coccygotomy 77.39
"Cocked hat" procedure (metacarpal lengthening and transfer of local flap) 82.69
Cockett operation (varicose vein)
  lower limb 38.59
  upper limb 38.53
Cody tack (perforation of footplate) 19.0
Coffey operation (uterine suspension) (Meig's
  modification) 69.22

Colectomy (partial) (segmental) (subtotal)
  cecum (with terminal ileum)
    laparoscopic 17.32
    open and other 45.72
  laparoscopic 17.39
  left (Hartmann) (lower) (radical)
    laparoscopic 17.35
    open and other 45.75
  multiple segmental
    laparoscopic 17.31
    open and other 45.71
  open and other 45.79
  right (radical)
    laparoscopic 17.33
    open and other 45.73
  sigmoid
    laparoscopic 17.36
    open and other 45.76
  terminal ileum with cecum
    laparoscopic 17.32
    open and other 45.72
  total
    laparoscopic 45.81
    open 45.82
    other 45.83
    unspecified 45.83
  transverse
    laparoscopic 17.34
    open and other 45.74
Cole operation (anterior tarsal wedge osteotomy) 77.28
Collapse, lung, surgical 33.39
  by
    destruction of phrenic nerve 33.31
    pneumoperitoneum 33.33
    pneumothorax, artificially-induced 33.32
    thoracoplasty 33.34
Collection, sperm for artificial insemination
  99.96
Collis-Nissen operation (hiatal hernia repair
  with esophagogastroplasty) 53.80
Colocentesis 45.03
Colocolostomy 45.94
  proximal to distal segment 45.79
Colocystoplasty 57.87 [45.52]
Colofixation 46.64
Coloileotomy 45.00
Colonna operation
  adductor tenotomy (first stage) 83.12
  hip arthroplasty (second stage) 81.40
  reconstruction of hip (second stage) 81.40
Colonoscopy 45.23
  with
    biopsy 45.25
      rectum 48.24
    stent — see Insertion, stent, colon
  fiberoptic (flexible) 45.23
  intraoperative 45.21
  through stoma (artificial) 45.22
  transabdominal 45.21
Colopexy 46.63
Coloplication 46.64
Coloproctostomy 45.94
Colorectosigmoidostomy 45.94
Colorectostomy 45.94
Colorrhaphy 46.75
Coloscopy — see Colonoscopy
Colosigmoidostomy 45.94
Colostomy (ileo-ascending) (ileo-transverse)
    (perineal) (transverse) 46.10
  with anterior rectal resection 48.62
  delayed opening 46.14
  loop 46.03
  permanent (magnetic) 46.13
  temporary 46.11
Colotomy 45.03
Colpectomy 70.4
Colpoceliocentesis 70.0
Colpocentesis 70.0
Colpocleisis (complete) (partial) 70.8
Colpohysterectomy 68.59
  laparoscopically assisted (LAVH) 68.51
Colpoperineoplasty 70.79
  with repair of urethrocele 70.51
    with graft or prosthesis 70.53
Colpoperineorrhaphy 70.71

Colpoperineorrhaphy — continued
  following delivery 75.69
Colpopexy 70.77
  with graft or prosthesis 70.78
Colpoplasty 70.79
Colpopoiesis 70.61
  vaginal construction 70.61
    with graft or prosthesis 70.63
Colporrhaphy 70.71
  anterior (cystocele repair) 70.51
    with graft or prosthesis 70.54
  for repair of
    cystocele 70.51
      with rectocele 70.50
        with graft or prosthesis 70.53
      enterocele 70.92
        with graft or prosthesis 70.93
      rectocele 70.52
        with cystocele 70.50
          with graft or prosthesis 70.53
      urethrocele 70.51
        with graft or prosthesis 70.54
  posterior (rectocele repair) 70.52
    with graft or prosthesis 70.55
Colposcopy 70.21
Colpotomy 70.14
  for pelvic peritoneal drainage 70.12
Commando operation (radical glossectomy)
  25.4
Commissurotomy
  closed heart technique — see Valvulotomy,
    heart
  open heart technique — see Valvuloplasty,
    heart
Compression, trigeminal nerve 04.02
Conchectomy 21.69
Conchotomy 21.1
Conduction study, nerve 89.15
Conduitogram, ileum 87.78
Condylectomy — see category 77.8 ☑
  mandible 76.5
Condylotomy NEC — see also Division, joint
    capsule 80.40
  mandible (open) 76.62
    closed 76.61
Conization
  cervix (knife) (sharp) (biopsy) 67.2
    by
      cryosurgery 67.33
      electroconization 67.32
Conjunctivocystorhinostomy 09.82
  with insertion of tube or stent 09.83
Conjunctivodacryocystorhinostomy (CDCR)
  09.82
  with insertion of tube or stent 09.83
Conjunctivodacryocystostomy 09.82
  with insertion of tube or stent 09.83
Conjunctivoplasty 10.49
Conjunctivorhinostomy 09.82
  with insertion of tube or stent 09.83
Constriction of globe, for scleral buckling
  — see also Buckling, scleral 14.49
Construction
  auricle, ear (with graft) (with implant) 18.71
  ear
    auricle (with graft) (with implant) 18.71
    meatus (osseous) (skin-lined) 18.6
  endorectal ileal pouch (J-pouch) (H-pouch)
    (S-pouch) (with anastomosis to anus)
    45.95
  esophagus, artificial — see Anastomosis,
    esophagus
  ileal bladder (open) 56.51
    closed 57.87 [45.51]
  ileal conduit 56.51
  larynx, artificial 31.75
  patent meatus (ear) 18.6
  penis (rib graft) (skin graft) (myocutaneous
    flap) 64.43
  pharyngeal valve, artificial 31.75
  urethra 58.46
  vagina, artificial 70.61
    with graft or prosthesis 70.63
  venous valves (peripheral) 39.59
Consultation 89.09
  comprehensive 89.07

Consultation — continued
  limited (single organ system) 89.06
  specified type NEC 89.08
Continuous positive airway pressure [CPAP]
  (non-invasive) 93.90
  delivered by
    endotracheal tube — see category
      96.7 ☑
    tracheostomy — see category 96.7 ☑
Control
  atmospheric pressure and composition NEC
    93.98
    antigen-free air conditioning 93.98
    decompression chamber 93.97
    mountain sanatorium 93.98
  epistaxis 21.00
    by
      cauterization (and packing) 21.03
      coagulation (with packing) 21.03
      electrocoagulation (with packing)
        21.03
      excision of nasal mucosa with graft-
        ing 21.07
      ligation of artery 21.09
        ethmoidal 21.04
        external carotid 21.06
        maxillary (transantral) 21.05
      packing (nasal) (anterior) 21.01
        posterior (and anterior) 21.02
      specified means NEC 21.09
  hemorrhage 39.98
    abdominal cavity 54.19
    adenoids (postoperative) 28.7
    anus (postoperative) 49.95
    bladder (postoperative) 57.93
    chest 34.09
    colon 45.49
      endoscopic 45.43
    duodenum (ulcer) 44.49
      by
        embolization (transcatheter)
          44.44
        suture (ligation) 44.42
      endoscopic 44.43
    esophagus 42.39
      endoscopic 42.33
    gastric (ulcer) 44.49
      by
        embolization (transcatheter)
          44.44
        suture (ligation) 44.41
      endoscopic 44.43
    intrapleural 34.09
      postoperative (recurrent) 34.03
    laparotomy site 54.12
    nose (see also Control, epistaxis) 21.00
    peptic (ulcer) 44.49
      by
        embolization (transcatheter)
          44.44
        suture (ligation) 44.40
      endoscopic 44.43
    pleura, pleural cavity 34.09
      postoperative (recurrent) 34.03
    postoperative NEC 39.98
    postvascular surgery 39.41
    prostate 60.94
    specified site NEC 39.98
    stomach — see Control, hemorrhage,
      gastric
    thorax NEC 34.09
      postoperative (recurrent) 34.03
    thyroid (postoperative) 06.02
    tonsils (postoperative) 28.7
Conversion
  anastomosis — see Revision, anastomosis
  atrial rhythm (to sinus rhythm) 99.61
  cardiac rhythm NEC 99.69
    to sinus rhythm 99.62
  gastrostomy to jejunostomy (endoscopic)
    for feeding tube placement 46.32
  obstetrical position — see Version
Cooling, gastric 96.31
CorCap™ 37.41
Cordectomy, vocal 30.22
Cordopexy, vocal 31.69

☑ Additional Digit Required — Refer to the Tabular List for Digit Selection
▽ Subterms under main terms may continue to next column or page

834
2014 ICD-9-CM

Cordotomy
spinal (bilateral) NEC 03.29
  percutaneous 03.21
  vocal 31.3
Corectomy 12.12
Corelysis 12.35
Coreoplasty 12.35
Corneoconjunctivoplasty 11.53
Corpectomy, (vertebral) 80.99
  with diskectomy 80.99
Correction — *see also* Repair
atresia
  esophageal 42.85
    by magnetic forces 42.99
  external meatus (ear) 18.6
  nasopharynx, nasopharyngeal 29.4
  rectum 48.0
  tricuspid 35.94
atrial septal defect (*see also* Repair, atrial
  septal defect) 35.71
  combined with repair of valvular and
    ventricular septal defects — *see*
    Repair, endocardial cushion de-
    fect
blepharoptosis (*see also* Repair, blepharoptosis) 08.36
bunionette (with osteotomy) 77.54
chordee 64.42
claw toe 77.57
cleft
  lip 27.54
  palate 27.62
clubfoot NEC 83.84
coarctation of aorta
  with
    anastomosis 38.34
    graft replacement 38.44
cornea NEC 11.59
  refractive NEC 11.79
    epikeratophakia 11.76
    keratomileusis 11.71
    keratophakia 11.72
    radial keratotomy 11.75
esophageal atresia 42.85
  by magnetic forces 42.99
everted lacrimal punctum 09.71
eyelid
  ptosis (*see also* Repair, blepharoptosis)
    08.36
  retraction 08.38
fetal defect 75.36
forcible, of musculoskeletal deformity NEC
  93.29
hammer toe 77.56
hydraulic pressure, open surgery for penile
  inflatable prosthesis 64.99
  urinary artificial sphincter 58.99
intestinal malrotation 46.80
  large 46.82
  small 46.81
inverted uterus — *see* Repair, inverted
  uterus
lymphedema (of limb) 40.9
  excision with graft 40.9
  obliteration of lymphatics 40.9
  transplantation of autogenous lymphat-
    ics 40.9
nasopharyngeal atresia 29.4
overlapping toes 77.58
palate (cleft) 27.62
prognathism NEC 76.64
prominent ear 18.5
punctum (everted) 09.71
spinal pseudarthrosis — *see* Refusion, spinal
syndactyly 86.85
tetralogy of Fallot
  one-stage 35.81
  partial — *see* specific procedure
  total 35.81
total anomalous pulmonary venous connection
  one-stage 35.82
  partial — *see* specific procedure
  total 35.82
transposition, great arteries, total 35.84
tricuspid atresia 35.94

Correction — *see also* Repair — *continued*
truncus arteriosus
  one-stage 35.83
  partial — *see* specific procedure
  total 35.83
ureteropelvic junction 55.87
ventricular septal defect (*see also* Repair,
  ventricular septal defect) 35.72
  combined with repair of valvular and
    atrial septal defects — *see* Repair,
    endocardial cushion defect
Costectomy 77.91
with lung excision — *see* Excision, lung
associated with thoracic operation — *omit
  code*
Costochondrectomy 77.91
associated with thoracic operation — *omit
  code*
Costosternoplasty (pectus excavatum repair)
  34.74
Costotomy 77.31
Costotransversectomy 77.91
associated with thoracic operation — *omit
  code*
Counseling (for) NEC 94.49
alcoholism 94.46
drug addiction 94.45
employers 94.49
family (medical) (social) 94.49
marriage 94.49
ophthalmologic (with instruction) 95.36
pastoral 94.49
Countershock, cardiac NEC 99.62
Coventry operation (tibial wedge osteotomy)
  77.27
CPAP (continuous positive airway pressure)
  93.90
delivered by
  endotracheal tube — *see* category
    96.7 ☑
  tracheostomy — *see* category 96.7 ☑
Craniectomy 01.25
linear (opening of cranial suture) 02.01
reopening of site 01.23
strip (opening of cranial suture) 02.01
Cranioclasis, fetal 73.8
Cranioplasty 02.06
with synchronous repair of encephalocele
  02.12
Craniotomy 01.24
as operative approach — omit code
fetal 73.8
for decompression of fracture 02.02
reopening of site 01.23
Craterization, bone — *see also* Excision, lesion,
  bone 77.60
Crawford operation (tarso-frontalis sling of
  eyelid) 08.32
Creation — *see also* Formation
cardiac device (defibrillator) (pacemaker)
  pocket
  with initial insertion of cardiac device —
    omit code
  new site (skin) (subcutaneous) 37.79
conduit
  apical-aortic (AAC) 35.93
  ileal (urinary) NEC 56.51
  left ventricle and aorta 35.93
  right atrium and pulmonary artery 35.94
  right ventricle and pulmonary (distal)
    artery 35.92
  in repair of
    pulmonary artery atresia 35.92
    transposition of great vessels
      35.92
    truncus arteriosus 35.83
endorectal ileal pouch (J-pouch) (H-pouch)
  (S-pouch) (with anastomosis to anus)
  45.95
esophagogastric sphincteric competence
  NEC 44.66
  laparoscopic 44.67
Hartmann pouch — *see* Colectomy, by site
interatrial fistula 35.42
pericardial window 37.12
pleural window, for drainage 34.09

Creation — *see also* Formation —
  continued
pocket
  cardiac device (defibrillator) (pacemaker)
    with initial insertion of cardiac device
      — *omit code*
    new site (skin) (subcutaneous) 37.79
  loop recorder 37.79
  thalamic stimulator pulse generator
    with initial insertion of battery pack-
      age — *omit code*
    new site (skin) (subcutaneous) 86.09
shunt (*see also* Shunt)
  arteriovenous fistula, for dialysis 39.93
  left-to-right (systemic to pulmonary cir-
    culation) 39.0
subcutaneous tunnel for esophageal anastomosis 42.86
  with anastomosis — *see* Anastomosis,
    esophagus, antesternal
syndactyly (finger) (toe) 86.89
thalamic stimulator pulse generator pocket
  with initial insrtion of battery package
    — omit code
  new site (skin) (subcutaneous) 86.09
tracheoesophageal fistula 31.95
window
  pericardial 37.12
  pleura, for drainage 34.09
Credé maneuver 73.59
Cricoidectomy 30.29
Cricothyreotomy (for assistance in breathing)
  31.1
Cricothyroidectomy 30.29
Cricothyrostomy 31.1
Cricothyrotomy (for assistance in breathing)
  31.1
Cricotomy (for assistance in breathing) 31.1
Cricotracheotomy (for assistance in breathing)
  31.1
Crisis intervention 94.35
Croupette, croup tent 93.94
Crown, dental (ceramic) (gold) 23.41
Crushing
bone — *see* category 78.4 ☑
calculus
  bile (hepatic) passage 51.49
    endoscopic 51.88
  bladder (urinary) 57.0
  pancreatic duct 52.09
    endoscopic 52.94
fallopian tube (*see also* Ligation, fallopian
  tube) 66.39
ganglion — *see* Crushing, nerve
hemorrhoids 49.45
nasal septum 21.88
nerve (cranial) (peripheral) NEC 04.03
  acoustic 04.01
  auditory 04.01
  phrenic 04.03
    for collapse of lung 33.31
  sympathetic 05.0
  trigeminal 04.02
  vestibular 04.01
vas deferens 63.71
Cryoablation — *see* Ablation
Cryoanalgesia
nerve (cranial) (peripheral) 04.2
Cryoconization, cervix 67.33
Cryodestruction — *see* Destruction, lesion, by
  site
Cryoextraction, lens — *see also* Extraction,
  cataract, intracapsular 13.19
Cryohypophysectomy (complete) (total) —
  see also Hypophysectomy 07.69
Cryoleucotomy 01.32
Cryopexy, retinal — *see* Cryotherapy, retina
Cryoprostatectomy 60.62
Cryoretinopexy (for)
reattachment 14.52
repair of tear or defect 14.32
Cryosurgery — *see* Cryotherapy
Cryothalamectomy 01.41
Cryotherapy — *see also* Destruction, lesion,
  by site
bladder 57.59

Cryotherapy — *see also* Destruction, lesion, by
  site — *continued*
brain 01.59
cataract 13.19
cervix 67.33
choroid — *see* Cryotherapy, retina
ciliary body 12.72
corneal lesion (ulcer) 11.43
  to reshape cornea 11.79
ear
  external 18.29
  inner 20.79
esophagus 42.39
  endoscopic 42.33
eyelid 08.25
hemorrhoids 49.44
iris 12.41
nasal turbinates 21.61
palate (bony) 27.31
prostate 60.62
retina (for)
  destruction of lesion 14.22
  reattachment 14.52
  repair of tear 14.32
skin 86.3
stomach 43.49
  endoscopic 43.41
subcutaneous tissue 86.3
turbinates (nasal) 21.61
warts 86.3
  genital 71.3
Cryptectomy (anus) 49.39
endoscopic 49.31
Cryptorchidectomy (unilateral) 62.3
bilateral 62.41
Cryptotomy (anus) 49.39
endoscopic 49.31
Cuirass 93.99
Culdocentesis 70.0
Culdoplasty 70.92
with graft or prosthesis 70.93
Culdoscopy (exploration) (removal of foreign
  body or lesion) 70.22
Culdotomy 70.12
Culp-Deweerd operation (spiral flap pyeloplasty) 55.87
Culp-Scardino operation (ureteral flap
  pyeloplasty) 55.87
Culture (and sensitivity) — *see* Examination,
  microscopic
Curettage (with packing) (with secondary closure) — *see also* Dilation and curettage
adenoids 28.6
anus 49.39
  endoscopic 49.31
bladder 57.59
  transurethral 57.49
bone (*see also* Excision, lesion, bone) 77.60
brain 01.59
bursa 83.39
  hand 82.29
cartilage (*see also* Excision, lesion, joint)
  80.80
cerebral meninges 01.51
chalazion 08.25
conjunctiva (trachoma follicles) 10.33
corneal epithelium 11.41
  for smear or culture 11.21
ear, external 18.29
eyelid 08.25
joint (*see also* Excision, lesion, joint) 80.80
meninges (cerebral) 01.51
  spinal 03.4
muscle 83.32
  hand 82.22
nerve (peripheral) 04.07
  sympathetic 05.29
sclera 12.84
skin 86.3
spinal cord (meninges) 03.4
subgingival 24.31
tendon 83.39
  sheath 83.31
    hand 82.21
uterus (with dilation) 69.09
  aspiration (diagnostic) NEC 69.59

☑ **Additional Digit Required** — Refer to the Tabular List for Digit Selection   ▽ **Subterms under main terms may continue to next column or page**

2014 ICD-9-CM   **835**

Curettage — *see also* Dilation and curettage
— *continued*
  uterus — *continued*
    aspiration — *continued*
      after abortion or delivery 69.52
      to terminate pregnancy 69.51
      following delivery or abortion 69.02
Curette evacuation, lens 13.2
Curtis operation (interphalangeal joint arthroplasty) 81.72
Cutaneolipectomy 86.83
Cutdown, venous 38.94
Cutting
  nerve (cranial) (peripheral) NEC 04.03
    acoustic 04.01
    auditory 04.01
    root, spinal 03.1
    sympathetic 05.0
    trigeminal 04.02
    vestibular 04.01
  pedicle (flap) graft 86.71
  pylorus (with wedge resection) 43.3
  spinal nerve root 03.1
  ureterovesical orifice 56.1
  urethral sphincter 58.5
CVP (central venous pressure monitoring) 89.62
Cyclectomy (ciliary body) 12.44
  eyelid margin 08.20
Cyclicotomy 12.55
Cycloanemization 12.74
Cyclocryotherapy 12.72
Cyclodialysis (initial) (subsequent) 12.55
Cyclodiathermy (penetrating) (surface) 12.71
Cycloelectrolysis 12.71
Cyclophotocoagulation 12.73
Cyclotomy 12.55
Cystectomy — *see also* Excision, lesion, by site
  gallbladder — *see* Cholecystectomy
  urinary (partial) (subtotal) 57.6
    complete (with urethrectomy) 57.79
    radical 57.71
      with pelvic exenteration (female) 68.8
    total (with urethrectomy) 57.79
Cystocolostomy 57.88
Cystogram, cystography NEC 87.77
Cystolitholapaxy 57.0
Cystolithotomy 57.19
Cystometrogram 89.22
Cystopexy NEC 57.89
Cystoplasty NEC 57.89
Cystoproctostomy 57.88
Cystoprostatectomy, radical 57.71
Cystopyelography 87.74
Cystorrhaphy 57.81
Cystoscopy (transurethral) 57.32
  for
    control of hemorrhage
      bladder 57.93
      prostate 60.94
    retrograde pyelography 87.74
  with biopsy 57.33
  ileal conduit 56.35
  through stoma (artificial) 57.31
Cystostomy
  closed (suprapubic) (percutaneous) 57.17
  open (suprapubic) 57.18
  percutaneous (closed) (suprapubic) 57.17
  suprapubic
    closed 57.17
    open 57.18
Cystotomy (open) (for removal of calculi) 57.19
Cystourethrogram (retrograde) (voiding) 87.76
Cystourethropexy (by) 59.79
  levator muscle sling 59.71
  retropubic suspension 59.5
  suprapubic suspension 59.4
Cystourethroplasty 57.85
Cystourethroscopy 57.32
  with biopsy
    bladder 57.33
    ureter 56.33
Cytology — *see* Examination, microscopic

D

Dacryoadenectomy 09.20
  partial 09.22
  total 09.23
Dacryoadenotomy 09.0
Dacryocystectomy (complete) (partial) 09.6
Dacryocystogram 87.05
Dacryocystorhinostomy (DCR) (by intubation) (external) (intranasal) 09.81
Dacryocystostomy 09.53
Dacryocystosyringotomy 09.53
Dacryocystotomy 09.53
Dahlman operation (excision of esophageal diverticulum) 42.31
Dana operation (posterior rhizotomy) 03.1
Danforth operation (fetal) 73.8
Darrach operation (ulnar resection) 77.83
da Vinci® (S HD) Surgical System — *see* category 17.4 ☑
Davis operation (intubated ureterotomy) 56.2
Deaf training 95.49
Debridement, NOS 86.28
  excisional, NOS 86.22
    abdominal wall 54.3
    bone (*see also* Excision, lesion, bone) 77.60
      fracture — *see* Debridement, open fracture
    brain 01.59
    burn (skin) 86.22
    bursa 83.5
    cerebral meninges 01.51
    fascia 83.44
    flap graft 86.75
    graft (flap) (pedicle) 86.75
    heart valve (calcified) — *see* Valvuloplasty, heart
    infection (skin) 86.22
      nail bed or fold 86.27
    joint — *see* Excision, lesion, joint
    meninges (cerebral) 01.51
      spinal 03.4
    muscle 83.45
      hand 82.36
    nail 86.27
    nerve (peripheral) 04.07
    open fracture (compound) 79.60
      arm NEC 79.62
      carpal, metacarpal 79.63
      facial bone 76.2
      femur 79.65
      fibula 79.66
      foot NEC 79.67
      hand NEC 79.63
      humerus 79.61
      leg NEC 79.66
      phalanges
        foot 79.68
        hand 79.64
      radius 79.62
      specified site NEC 79.69
      tarsal, metatarsal 79.67
      tibia 79.66
      ulna 79.62
    patella 77.66
    pedicle graft 86.75
    skin or subcutaneous tissue (burn) (infection) (wound) 86.22
      cardioverter/defibrillator (automatic) pocket 37.79
      graft 86.75
      nail, nail bed, nail fold 86.27
      pacemaker pocket 37.79
      pocket
        cardiac device NEC 37.79
        cardiac pacemaker 37.79
        cardioverter/defibrillator (automatic) 37.79
    skull 01.25
      compound fracture 02.02
    spinal cord (meninges) 03.4
    tendon 83.39
    wound (skin) 86.22
  nonexcisional, NOS 86.28
    burn (skin) 86.28
    dental 96.54

Debridement, — *continued*
  nonexcisional, — *continued*
    infection (skin) 86.28
    skin or subcutaneous tissue (burn) (infection) (wound) 86.28
    ultrasonic, ultrasound 86.28
    VersaJet™ 86.28
    wound (skin) 86.28
Decapitation, fetal 73.8
Decapsulation, kidney 55.91
Declotting — *see also* Removal, thrombus
  arteriovenous cannula or shunt 39.49
Decompression
  anus (imperforate) 48.0
  biliary tract 51.49
    by intubation 51.43
      endoscopic 51.87
      percutaneous 51.98
  brain 01.24
  carpal tunnel 04.43
  cauda equina 03.09
  chamber 93.97
  colon 96.08
    by incision 45.03
    endoscopic (balloon) 46.85
  common bile duct 51.42
    by intubation 51.43
      endoscopic 51.87
      percutaneous 51.98
  cranial 01.24
    for skull fracture 02.02
  endolymphatic sac 20.79
  ganglion (peripheral) NEC 04.49
    cranial NEC 04.42
  gastric 96.07
  heart 37.0
  intestine 96.08
    by incision 45.00
    endoscopic (balloon) 46.85
  intracranial 01.24
  labyrinth 20.79
  laminectomy 03.09
  laminotomy 03.09
  median nerve 04.43
  muscle 83.02
    hand 82.02
  nerve (peripheral) NEC 04.49
    auditory 04.42
    cranial NEC 04.42
    median 04.43
    trigeminal (root) 04.41
  orbit (*see also* Orbitotomy) 16.09
  pancreatic duct 52.92
    endoscopic 52.93
  pericardium 37.0
  rectum 48.0
  skull fracture 02.02
  spinal cord (canal) 03.09
  tarsal tunnel 04.44
  tendon (sheath) 83.01
    hand 82.01
  thoracic outlet
    by
      myotomy (division of scalenus anticus muscle) 83.19
      tenotomy 83.13
  trigeminal (nerve root) 04.41
Decortication
  arterial 05.25
  brain 01.51
  cerebral meninges 01.51
  heart 37.31
  kidney 55.91
  lung (partial) (total) 34.51
    thoracoscopic 34.52
  nasal turbinates — *see* Turbinectomy
  nose 21.89
  ovary 65.29
    laparoscopic 65.25
  periarterial 05.25
  pericardium 37.31
  ventricle, heart (complete) 37.31
Decoy, E2F 00.16
Deepening
  alveolar ridge 24.5
  buccolabial sulcus 24.91

Deepening — *continued*
  lingual sulcus 24.91
Defatting, flap or pedicle graft 86.75
Defibrillation, electric (external) (internal) 99.62
  automatic cardioverter/defibrillator — *see* category 37.9 ☑
de Grandmont operation (tarsectomy) 08.35
Delaying of pedicle graft 86.71
Delivery (with)
  assisted spontaneous 73.59
  breech extraction (assisted) 72.52
    partial 72.52
      with forceps to aftercoming head 72.51
    total 72.54
      with forceps to aftercoming head 72.53
  unassisted (spontaneous delivery) — *omit code*
  cesarean section — *see* Cesarean section
  Credé maneuver 73.59
  De Lee maneuver 72.4
  forceps 72.9
    application to aftercoming head (Piper) 72.6
    with breech extraction
      partial 72.51
      total 72.53
    Barton's 72.4
    failed 73.3
    high 72.39
      with episiotomy 72.31
    low (outlet) 72.0
      with episiotomy 72.1
    mid 72.29
      with episiotomy 72.21
    outlet (low) 72.0
      with episiotomy 72.1
    rotation of fetal head 72.4
    trial 73.3
  instrumental NEC 72.9
    specified NEC 72.8
  key-in-lock rotation 72.4
  Kielland rotation 72.4
  Malström's extraction 72.79
    with episiotomy 72.71
  manually assisted (spontaneous) 73.59
  spontaneous (unassisted) 73.59
    assisted 73.59
  vacuum extraction 72.79
    with episiotomy 72.71
Delorme operation
  pericardiectomy 37.31
  proctopexy 48.76
  repair of prolapsed rectum 48.76
  thoracoplasty 33.34
Denervation
  aortic body 39.89
  carotid body 39.89
  facet, percutaneous (radiofrequency) 03.96
  ovarian 65.94
  paracervical uterine 69.3
  uterosacral 69.3
Denker operation (radical maxillary antrotomy) 22.31
Dennis-Barco operation — *see* Repair, hernia, femoral
Denonvillier operation (limited rhinoplasty) 21.86
Densitometry, bone (serial) (radiographic) 88.98
Depilation, skin 86.92
Derlacki operation (tympanoplasty) 19.4
Dermabond 86.59
Dermabrasion (laser) 86.25
  for wound debridement 86.28
Derotation — *see* Reduction, torsion
Desensitization
  allergy 99.12
  psychologic 94.33
Desmotomy — *see also* Division, ligament 80.40
Destruction
  breast 85.20

Destruction — *continued*
　chorioretinopathy (*see also* Destruction, lesion, choroid) 14.29
　ciliary body 12.74
　epithelial downgrowth, anterior chamber 12.93
　fallopian tube 66.39
　　with
　　　crushing (and ligation) 66.31
　　　　by endoscopy (laparoscopy) 66.21
　　　division (and ligation) 66.32
　　　　by endoscopy (culdoscopy) (hysteroscopy) (laparoscopy) (peritoneoscopy) 66.22
　　　ligation 66.39
　　　　with
　　　　　crushing 66.31
　　　　　　by endoscopy (laparoscopy) 66.21
　　　　　division 66.32
　　　　　　by endoscopy (culdoscopy) (hysteroscopy) (laparoscopy) (peritoneoscopy) 66.22
　fetus 73.8
　hemorrhoids 49.49
　　by
　　　cryotherapy 49.44
　　　sclerotherapy 49.42
　inner ear NEC 20.79
　　by injection 20.72
　intervertebral disc (NOS) 80.50
　　by injection 80.52
　　by other specified method 80.59
　　herniated (nucleus pulposus) 80.51
　LAA 37.36
　lacrimal sac 09.6
　left atrial appendage 37.36
　lesion (local)
　　anus 49.39
　　　endoscopic 49.31
　　Bartholin's gland 71.24
　　　by
　　　　aspiration 71.21
　　　　excision 71.24
　　　　incision 71.22
　　　　marsupialization 71.23
　　biliary ducts 51.69
　　　endoscopic 51.64
　　bladder 57.59
　　　transurethral 57.49
　　bone — *see* Excision, lesion, bone
　　bowel — *see* Destruction, lesion, intestine
　　brain (transtemporal approach) NEC 01.59
　　　by stereotactic radiosurgery 92.30
　　　　cobalt 60 92.32
　　　　linear accelerator (LINAC) 92.31
　　　　multi-source 92.32
　　　　particle beam 92.33
　　　　particulate 92.33
　　　　radiosurgery NEC 92.39
　　　　single source photon 92.31
　　breast NEC 85.20
　　bronchus NEC 32.09
　　　endoscopic 32.01
　　cerebral NEC 01.59
　　　meninges 01.51
　　cervix 67.39
　　　by
　　　　cauterization 67.32
　　　　cryosurgery, cryoconization 67.33
　　　　electroconization 67.32
　　choroid 14.29
　　　by
　　　　cryotherapy 14.22
　　　　diathermy 14.21
　　　　implantation of radiation source 14.27
　　　　photocoagulation 14.25
　　　　　laser 14.24
　　　　　xenon arc 14.23
　　　　radiation therapy 14.26

Destruction — *continued*
　lesion — *continued*
　　ciliary body (nonexcisional) 12.43
　　　by excision 12.44
　　conjunctiva 10.32
　　　by excision 10.31
　　cornea NEC 11.49
　　　by
　　　　cryotherapy 11.43
　　　　electrocauterization 11.42
　　　　thermocauterization 11.42
　　cul-de-sac 70.32
　　duodenum NEC 45.32
　　　by excision 45.31
　　　endoscopic 45.30
　　　endoscopic 45.30
　　esophagus (chemosurgery) (cryosurgery) (electroresection) (fulguration) NEC 42.39
　　　by excision 42.32
　　　endoscopic 42.33
　　　endoscopic 42.33
　　eyebrow 08.25
　　eyelid 08.25
　　　excisional — *see* Excision, lesion, eyelid
　　eye NEC 16.93
　　heart
　　　by catheter ablation 37.34
　　　by endovascular approach 37.34
　　　by open approach 37.33
　　　by thoracoscopic approach 37.37
　　　left atrial appendage 37.36
　　intestine (large) 45.49
　　　by excision 45.41
　　　　endoscopic 45.43
　　　　　polypectomy 45.42
　　　endoscopic 45.43
　　　　polypectomy 45.42
　　　small 45.34
　　　　by excision 45.33
　　intranasal 21.31
　　iris (nonexcisional) NEC 12.41
　　　by excision 12.42
　　kidney 55.39
　　　by marsupialization 55.31
　　lacrimal sac 09.6
　　larynx 30.09
　　liver 50.29
　　lung 32.29
　　　endoscopic 32.28
　　meninges (cerebral) 01.51
　　　spinal 03.4
　　nerve (peripheral) 04.07
　　　sympathetic 05.29
　　nose 21.30
　　　intranasal 21.31
　　　specified NEC 21.32
　　ovary
　　　by
　　　　aspiration 65.91
　　　　excision 65.29
　　　　　laparoscopic 65.25
　　　cyst by rupture (manual) 65.93
　　palate (bony) (local) 27.31
　　　wide 27.32
　　pancreas 52.22
　　　by marsupialization 52.3
　　　endoscopic 52.21
　　pancreatic duct 52.22
　　　endoscopic 52.21
　　penis 64.2
　　pharynx (excisional) NEC 29.39
　　pituitary gland
　　　by stereotactic radiosurgery 92.30
　　　　cobalt 60 92.32
　　　　linear accelerator (LINAC) 92.31
　　　　multi-source 92.32
　　　　particle beam 92.33
　　　　particulate 92.33
　　　　radiosurgery NEC 92.39
　　　　single source photon 92.31
　　rectum (local) 48.32
　　　by
　　　　cryosurgery 48.34
　　　　electrocoagulation 48.32

Destruction — *continued*
　lesion — *continued*
　　rectum — *continued*
　　　by — *continued*
　　　　excision 48.35
　　　　fulguration 48.32
　　　　laser (Argon) 48.33
　　　　polyp 48.36
　　　　radical 48.31
　　retina 14.29
　　　by
　　　　cryotherapy 14.22
　　　　diathermy 14.21
　　　　implantation of radiation source 14.27
　　　　photocoagulation 14.25
　　　　　laser 14.24
　　　　　xenon arc 14.23
　　　　radiation therapy 14.26
　　salivary gland NEC 26.29
　　　by marsupialization 26.21
　　sclera 12.84
　　scrotum 61.3
　　skin NEC 86.3
　　sphincter of Oddi 51.69
　　　endoscopic 51.64
　　spinal cord (meninges) 03.4
　　spleen 41.42
　　　by marsupialization 41.41
　　stomach NEC 43.49
　　　by excision 43.42
　　　　endoscopic 43.41
　　　endoscopic 43.41
　　subcutaneous tissue NEC 86.3
　　testis 62.2
　　tongue 25.1
　　urethra (excisional) 58.39
　　　endoscopic 58.31
　　uterus 68.29
　　nerve (cranial) (peripheral) (by cryoanalgesia) by radiofrequency 04.2
　　sympathetic, by injection of neurolytic agent 05.32
　　neuroma
　　　acoustic 04.01
　　　　by craniotomy 04.01
　　　　by stereotactic radiosurgery 92.30
　　　　　cobalt 60 92.32
　　　　　linear accelerator (LINAC) 92.31
　　　　　multi-source 92.32
　　　　　particle beam 92.33
　　　　　particulate 92.33
　　　　　radiosurgery NEC 92.39
　　　　　single source photon 92.31
　　　cranial 04.07
　　　Morton's 04.07
　　　peripheral
　　　　Morton's 04.07
　　prostate (prostatic tissue)
　　　by
　　　　cryotherapy 60.62
　　　　microwave 60.96
　　　　radiofrequency 60.97
　　　　transurethral microwave thermotherapy (TUMT) 60.96
　　　　transurethral needle ablation (TUNA) 60.97
　　　　TULIP (transurethral (ultrasound) guided laser induced prostatectomy) 60.21
　　　　TUMT (transurethral microwave thermotherapy) 60.96
　　　　TUNA (transurethral needle ablation) 60.97
　　semicircular canals, by injection 20.72
　　tissue of heart — *see* Excision, lesion, heart
　　vestibule, by injection 20.72
Detachment, uterosacral ligaments 69.3
Determination
　mental status (clinical) (medicolegal) (psychiatric) NEC 94.11
　psychologic NEC 94.09
　vital capacity (pulmonary) 89.37
Detorsion
　intestine (twisted) (volvulus) 46.80
　　large 46.82

Detorsion — *continued*
　intestine — *continued*
　　large — *continued*
　　　endoscopic (balloon) 46.85
　　small 46.81
　kidney 55.84
　ovary 65.95
　spermatic cord 63.52
　　with orchiopexy 62.5
　testis 63.52
　　with orchiopexy 62.5
　volvulus 46.80
　　endoscopic (balloon) 46.85
Detoxification therapy 94.25
　alcohol 94.62
　　with rehabilitation 94.63
　　combined alcohol and drug 94.68
　　　with rehabilitation 94.69
　drug 94.65
　　with rehabilitation 94.66
　　combined alcohol and drug 94.68
　　　with rehabilitation 94.69
Devascularization, stomach 44.99
Device
　CorCap™ 37.41
　external fixator — *see* Fixator, external
Dewebbing
　esophagus 42.01
　syndactyly (fingers) (toes) 86.85
Dextrorotation — *see* Reduction, torsion
Dialysis
　hemodiafiltration, hemofiltration (extracorporeal) 39.95
　kidney (extracorporeal) 39.95
　liver 50.92
　peritoneal 54.98
　renal (extracorporeal) 39.95
Diaphanoscopy
　nasal sinuses 89.35
　skull (newborn) 89.16
Diaphysectomy — *see* category 77.8 ☑
Diathermy 93.34
　choroid — *see* Diathermy, retina
　nasal turbinates 21.61
　retina
　　for
　　　destruction of lesion 14.21
　　　reattachment 14.51
　　　repair of tear 14.31
　　surgical — *see* Destruction, lesion, by site
　turbinates (nasal) 21.61
Dickson-Diveley operation (tendon transfer and arthrodesis to correct claw toe) 77.57
Dickson operation (fascial transplant) 83.82
Dieffenbach operation (hip disarticulation) 84.18
Dilation
　achalasia 42.92
　ampulla of Vater 51.81
　　endoscopic 51.84
　anus, anal (sphincter) 96.23
　biliary duct
　　endoscopic 51.84
　　pancreatic duct 52.99
　　　endoscopic 52.98
　　percutaneous (endoscopy) 51.98
　　sphincter
　　　of Oddi 51.81
　　　　endoscopic 51.84
　　　pancreatic 51.82
　　　　endoscopic 51.85
　bladder 96.25
　　neck 57.92
　bronchus 33.91
　cervix (canal) 67.0
　　obstetrical 73.1
　　to assist delivery 73.1
　choanae (nasopharynx) 29.91
　colon (endoscopic) (balloon) 46.85
　　with insertion of colonic stent
　　　endoscopic 46.86
　　　other 46.87
　colostomy stoma 96.24
　duodenum (endoscopic) (balloon) 46.85

☑ **Additional Digit Required** — Refer to the Tabular List for Digit Selection　　　　　　　　🔻 **Subterms under main terms may continue to next column or page**

2014 ICD-9-CM　　　　　　　　　　　　　　　　　　　　　　　　　　　　　　　837

☑ **Additional Digit Required — Refer to the Tabular List for Digit Selection**

▽ **Subterms under main terms may continue to next column or page**

Division — *continued*
 vein — *continued*
  head and neck NEC 38.82
  intracranial NEC 38.81
  lower limb 38.89
   varicose 38.59
  thoracic NEC 38.85
  upper limb 38.83
  varicose 38.50
   abdominal 38.57
   head and neck NEC 38.52
   intracranial NEC 38.51
   lower limb 38.59
   thoracic NEC 38.55
   upper limb 38.53
  vitreous, cicatricial bands (posterior approach) 14.74
   anterior approach 14.73
Doleris operation (shortening of round ligaments) 69.22
D'Ombrain operation (excision of pterygium with corneal graft) 11.32
Domestic tasks therapy 93.83
Dopplergram, Doppler flow mapping — *see also* Ultrasonography
 aortic arch 88.73
 head and neck 88.71
 heart 88.72
 intraoperative transcranial 00.94
 thorax NEC 88.73
Dorrance operation (push-back operation for cleft palate) 27.62
Dotter operation (transluminal angioplasty) 39.59
Douche, vaginal 96.44
Douglas' operation (suture of tongue to lip for micrognathia) 25.59
Downstream® System (AO therapy) (aqueous oxygen) 00.49
Doyle operation (paracervical uterine denervation) 69.3
Drainage
 by
  anastomosis — *see* Anastomosis
  aspiration — *see* Aspiration
  incision — *see* Incision
 abdomen 54.19
  percutaneous 54.91
 abscess (*see also* Drainage, by site *and* Incision, by site)
  appendix 47.2
   with appendectomy 47.09
    laparoscopic 47.01
  parapharyngeal (oral) (transcervical) 28.0
  peritonsillar (oral) (transcervical) 28.0
  retropharyngeal (oral) (transcervical) 28.0
  thyroid (field) (gland) 06.09
   percutaneous (needle) 06.01
   postoperative 06.02
  tonsil, tonsillar (oral) (transcervical) 28.0
 antecubital fossa 86.04
 appendix 47.91
  with appendectomy 47.09
   laparoscopic 47.01
  abscess 47.2
   with appendectomy 47.09
    laparoscopic 47.01
 axilla 86.04
 bladder (without incision) 57.0
  by indwelling catheter 57.94
   percutaneous suprapubic (closed) 57.17
   suprapubic NEC 57.18
 buccal space 27.0
 bursa 83.03
  by aspiration 83.94
   hand 82.92
  hand 82.03
   by aspiration 82.92
  radial 82.03
  ulnar 82.03
 cerebrum, cerebral (meninges) (ventricle) (incision) (trephination) 01.39
  by
   anastomosis — *see* Shunt, ventricular

Drainage — *continued*
 cerebrum, cerebral — *continued*
  by — *continued*
   aspiration 01.09
    through previously implanted catheter 01.02
 chest (closed) 34.04
  open (by incision) 34.09
  thoracoscopic 34.06
 cranial sinus (incision) (trephination) 01.21
  by aspiration 01.09
 cul-de-sac 70.12
  by aspiration 70.0
 cyst (*see also* Drainage, by site and Incision, by site)
  pancreas (by catheter) 52.01
   by marsupialization 52.3
   internal (anastomosis) 52.4
  pilonidal 86.03
  spleen, splenic (by marsupialization) 41.41
 duodenum (tube) 46.39
  by incision 45.01
 ear
  external 18.09
  inner 20.79
  middle (by myringotomy) 20.09
   with intubation 20.01
 epidural space, cerebral (incision) (trephination) 01.24
  by aspiration 01.09
 extradural space, cerebral (incision) (trephination) 01.24
  by aspiration 01.09
 extraperitoneal 54.0
 facial region 27.0
 fascial compartments, head and neck 27.0
 fetal hydrocephalic head (needling) (trocar) 73.8
 fluid (blood) (cerebrospinal) (CSF)
  by
   external ventricular drain (EVD) placement 02.21
 gallbladder 51.04
  by
   anastomosis 51.35
   aspiration 51.01
   incision 51.04
 groin region (abdominal wall) (inguinal) 54.0
  skin 86.04
  subcutaneous tissue 86.04
 hematoma — *see* Drainage, by site *and* Incision, by site
 hydrocephalic head (needling) (trocar) 73.8
 hypochondrium 54.0
  intra-abdominal 54.19
 iliac fossa 54.0
 infratemporal fossa 27.0
 intracranial space (epidural) (extradural) (incision) (trephination) 01.24
  by aspiration 01.09
  subarachnoid or subdural (incision) (trephination) 01.31
   by aspiration 01.09
 intraperitoneal 54.19
  percutaneous 54.91
 kidney (by incision) 55.01
  by
   anastomosis 55.86
   catheter 59.8
  pelvis (by incision) 55.11
 liver 50.0
  by aspiration 50.91
 Ludwig's angina 27.0
 lung (by incision) 33.1
  by punch (needle) (trocar) 33.93
 midpalmar space 82.04
 mouth floor 27.0
 mucocele, nasal sinus 22.00
  by puncture 22.01
  through natural ostium 22.02
 omentum 54.19
  percutaneous 54.91
 ovary (aspiration) 65.91
  by incision 65.09

Drainage — *continued*
 ovary — *continued*
  laparoscopic 65.01
 palmar space (middle) 82.04
 pancreas (by catheter) 52.01
  by anastomosis 52.96
 parapharyngeal 28.0
 paronychia 86.04
 parotid space 27.0
 pelvic peritoneum (female) 70.12
  male 54.19
 pericardium 37.0
 perigastric 54.19
  percutaneous 54.91
 perineum
  female 71.09
  male 86.04
 perisplenic tissue 54.19
  percutaneous 54.91
 peritoneum 54.19
  pelvic (female) 70.12
  percutaneous 54.91
 peritonsillar 28.0
 pharyngeal space, lateral 27.0
 pilonidal cyst or sinus 86.03
 pleura (closed) 34.04
  open (by incision) 34.09
  thoracoscopic 34.06
 popliteal space 86.04
 postural 93.99
 postzygomatic space 27.0
 pseudocyst, pancreas 52.3
  by anastomosis 52.4
 pterygopalatine fossa 27.0
 retropharyngeal 28.0
 scrotum 61.0
 skin 86.04
 spinal (canal) (cord) 03.09
  by anastomosis — *see* Shunt, spinal
  diagnostic 03.31
 spleen 41.2
  cyst (by marsupialization) 41.41
 subarachnoid space, cerebral (incision) (trephination) 01.31
  by aspiration 01.09
 subcutaneous tissue 86.04
 subdiaphragmatic 54.19
  percutaneous 54.91
 subdural space, cerebral (incision) (trephination) 01.31
  by aspiration 01.09
 subhepatic space 54.19
  percutaneous 54.91
 sublingual space 27.0
 submental space 27.0
 subphrenic space 54.19
  percutaneous 54.91
 supraclavicular fossa 86.04
 temporal pouches 27.0
 tendon (sheath) 83.01
  hand 82.01
 thenar space 82.04
 thorax (closed) 34.04
  open (by incision) 34.09
  thoracoscopic 34.06
 thyroglossal tract (by incision) 06.09
  by aspiration 06.01
 thyroid (field) (gland) (by incision) 06.09
  by aspiration 06.01
  postoperative 06.02
 tonsil 28.0
 tunica vaginalis 61.0
 ureter (by catheter) 59.8
  by
   anastomosis NEC (*see also* Anastomosis, ureter) 56.79
   incision 56.2
 ventricle (cerebral) (incision)
  by
   anastomosis — *see* Shunt, ventricular
   aspiration 01.09
    through previously implanted catheter 01.02
   extracranial ventricular shunt — *see* category 02.3
 vertebral column 03.09

Drawing test 94.08
Dressing
 burn 93.57
 ulcer 93.56
 wound 93.57
Drilling
 bone (*see also* Incision, bone) 77.10
 ovary 65.99
Drotrecogin alfa (activated), infusion 00.11
Ductogram, mammary 87.35
Duhamel operation (abdominoperineal pullthrough) 48.65
Dührssen's
 incisions (cervix, to assist delivery) 73.93
 operation (vaginofixation of uterus) 69.22
Dunn operation (triple arthrodesis) 81.12
Duodenectomy 45.62
 with
  gastrectomy — *see* Gastrectomy
  pancreatectomy — *see* Pancreatectomy
Duodenocholedochotomy 51.51
Duodenoduodenostomy 45.91
 proximal to distal segment 45.62
Duodenoileostomy 45.91
Duodenojejunostomy 45.91
Duodenoplasty 46.79
Duodenorrhaphy 46.71
Duodenoscopy 45.13
 through stoma (artificial) 45.12
 transabdominal (operative) 45.11
Duodenostomy 46.39
Duodenotomy 45.01
Dupuytren operation
 fasciectomy 82.35
 fasciotomy 82.12
  with excision 82.35
 shoulder disarticulation 84.08
Durabond 86.59
Duraplasty 02.12
Durham (-Caldwell) operation (transfer of biceps femoris tendon) 83.75
DuToit and Roux operation (staple capsulorrhaphy of shoulder) 81.82
DuVries operation (tenoplasty) 83.88
Dwyer operation
 fasciotomy 83.14
 soft tissue release NEC 83.84
 wedge osteotomy, calcaneus 77.28

E

E2F decoy 00.16
Eagleton operation (extrapetrosal drainage) 20.22
ECG — *see* Electrocardiogram
Echocardiography 88.72
 intracardiac (heart chambers) (ICE) 37.28
 intravascular (coronary vessels) 00.24
 transesophageal 88.72
  monitoring (Doppler) (ultrasound) 89.68
Echoencephalography 88.71
Echography — *see* Ultrasonography
Echogynography 88.79
Echoplacentogram 88.78
EC-IC vascular bypass 39.28
ECMO (extracorporeal membrane oxygenation) 39.65
Eden-Hybinette operation (glenoid bone block) 78.01
Educational therapy (bed-bound children) (handicapped) 93.82
EEG (electroencephalogram) 89.14
 monitoring (radiographic) (video) 89.19
Effler operation (heart) 36.2
Effleurage 93.39
EGD (esophagogastroduodenoscopy) 45.13
 with closed biopsy 45.16
Eggers operation
 tendon release (patellar retinacula) 83.13
 tendon transfer (biceps femoris tendon) (hamstring tendon) 83.75
EKG — *see also* Electrocardiogram 89.52
Elastic hosiery 93.59
Electrocardiogram (with 12 or more leads) 89.52
 with vectorcardiogram 89.53
 fetal (scalp), intrauterine 75.32

☑ **Additional Digit Required** — Refer to the Tabular List for Digit Selection   ▽ **Subterms under main terms may continue to next column or page**

2014 ICD-9-CM   **839**

☑ Additional Digit Required — Refer to the Tabular List for Digit Selection   ▽ Subterms under main terms may continue to next column or page

2014 ICD-9-CM   841

☑ **Additional Digit Required — Refer to the Tabular List for Digit Selection**   ▽ **Subterms under main terms may continue to next column or page**

842   **2014 ICD-9-CM**

F

Fistulectomy — *see also* Closure, fistula, by site
  — *continued*
  subcutaneous tissue 86.3
  thoracoabdominal 34.83
  thoracogastric 34.83
  thoracointestinal 34.83
  thorax NEC 34.73
  trachea NEC 31.73
  tracheoesophageal 31.73
  ureter 56.84
  urethra 58.43
  uteroenteric 69.42
  uterointestinal 69.42
  uterorectal 69.42
  uterovaginal 69.42
  vagina 70.75
  vesicosigmoidovaginal 57.83
  vocal cords 31.62
  vulvorectal 71.72

Fistulization
  appendix 47.91
  arteriovenous 39.27
  cisterna chyli 40.62
  endolymphatic sac (for decompression) 20.79
  esophagus, external 42.10
    cervical 42.11
    specified technique NEC 42.19
  interatrial 35.41
  labyrinth (for decompression) 20.79
  lacrimal sac into nasal cavity 09.81
  larynx 31.29
  lymphatic duct, left (thoracic) 40.62
  orbit 16.09
  peritoneal 54.93
  salivary gland 26.49
  sclera 12.69
    by trephination 12.61
    with iridectomy 12.65
  sinus, nasal NEC 22.9
  subarachnoid space 02.22
  thoracic duct 40.62
  trachea 31.29
  tracheoesophageal 31.95
  urethrovaginal 58.0
  ventricle, cerebral (*see also* Shunt, ventricular) 02.22

Fistulogram
  abdominal wall 88.03
  chest wall 87.38
  retroperitoneum 88.14
  specified site NEC 88.49

Fistulotomy, anal 49.11

Fitting
  arch bars (orthodontic) 24.7
    for immobilization (fracture) 93.55
  artificial limb 84.40
  contact lens 95.32
  denture (total) 99.97
    bridge (fixed) 23.42
      removable 23.43
    partial (fixed) 23.42
      removable 23.43
  hearing aid 95.48
  obturator (orthodontic) 24.7
  ocular prosthetics 95.34
  orthodontic
    appliance 24.7
    obturator 24.7
    wiring 24.7
  orthotic device 93.23
  periodontal splint (orthodontic) 24.7
  prosthesis, prosthetic device
    above knee 84.45
    arm 84.43
      lower (and hand) 84.42
      upper (and shoulder) 84.41
    below knee 84.46
    hand (and lower arm) 84.42
    leg 84.47
      above knee 84.45
      below knee 84.46
    limb NEC 84.40
    ocular 95.34
    penis (external) 64.94
    shoulder (and upper arm) 84.41

Fitting — *continued*
  spectacles 95.31

Five-in-one repair, knee 81.42

Fixation
  bone
    external, without reduction 93.59
      with fracture reduction — *see* Reduction, fracture
      cast immobilization NEC 93.53
      external fixator — *see* Fixator, external
      splint 93.54
      traction (skeletal) NEC 93.44
        intermittent 93.43
    internal (without fracture reduction) 78.50
      with fracture reduction — *see* Reduction, fracture
      carpal, metacarpal 78.54
      clavicle 78.51
      femur 78.55
      fibula 78.57
      humerus 78.52
      patella 78.56
      pelvic 78.59
      phalanges (foot) (hand) 78.59
      radius 78.53
      scapula 78.51
      specified site NEC 78.59
      tarsal, metatarsal 78.58
      thorax (ribs) (sternum) 78.51
        sternal fixation device with rigid plates 84.94
      tibia 78.57
      ulna 78.53
      vertebrae 78.59
  breast (pendulous) 85.6
  cardinal ligaments 69.22
  cervical collar 93.52
  duodenum 46.62
    to abdominal wall 46.61
  external (without manipulation for reduction) 93.59
    with fracture reduction — *see* Reduction, fracture
    cast immobilization NEC 93.53
    pressure dressing 93.56
    splint 93.54
    strapping (non-traction) 93.59
    traction (skeletal) NEC 93.44
      intermittent 93.43
  hip 81.40
  ileum 46.62
    to abdominal wall 46.61
  internal
    with fracture reduction — *see* Reduction, fracture
    without fracture reduction — *see* Fixation, bone, internal
  intestine 46.60
    large 46.64
      to abdominal wall 46.63
    small 46.62
      to abdominal wall 46.60
  iris (bombé) 12.11
  jejunum 46.62
    to abdominal wall 46.61
  joint — *see* Arthroplasty
  kidney 55.7
  ligament
    cardinal 69.22
    palpebrae 08.36
  omentum 54.74
  parametrial 69.22
  plaster jacket 93.51
    other cast 93.53
  rectum (sling) 48.76
  spine, with fusion (*see also* Fusion, spinal) 81.00
  spleen 41.95
  splint 93.54
  tendon 83.88
    hand 82.85
  testis in scrotum 62.5
  tongue 25.59

Fixation — *continued*
  urethrovaginal (to Cooper's ligament) 70.77
    with graft or prosthesis 70.78
  uterus (abdominal) (vaginal) (ventrofixation) 69.22
  vagina 70.77
    with graft or prosthesis 70.78

Fixator, external
  computer assisted (dependent) 84.73
  hybrid device or system 84.73
  Ilizarov type 84.72
  monoplanar system 84.71
  ring device or system 84.72
  Sheffield type 84.72

Flooding (psychologic desensitization) 94.33

Flowmetry, Doppler (ultrasonic) — *see also* Ultrasonography
  aortic arch 88.73
  head and neck 88.71
  heart 88.72
  thorax NEC 88.73

Fluoroscopy — *see* Radiography

Fog therapy (respiratory) 93.94

Folding, eye muscle 15.22
  multiple (two or more muscles) 15.4

Foley operation (pyeloplasty) 55.87

Fontan operation (creation of conduit between right atrium and pulmonary artery) 35.94

Foraminotomy 03.09

Forced extension, limb 93.25

Forceps delivery — *see* Delivery, forceps

Formation
  adhesions
    pericardium 36.39
    pleura 34.6
  anus, artificial — *see* Colostomy
    duodenostomy 46.39
    ileostomy — *see* Ileostomy
    jejunostomy 46.39
      percutaneous (endoscopic) (PEJ) 46.32
  arteriovenous fistula (for kidney dialysis) (peripheral) (shunt) 39.27
    external cannula 39.93
  bone flap, cranial 02.03
  cardiac device (defibrillator) (pacemaker) pocket
    with initial insertion of cardiac device — *omit code*
    new site (skin) (subcutaneous) 37.79
  colostomy — *see* Colostomy
  conduit
    apical-aortic (AAC) 35.93
    ileal (urinary) 56.51
    left ventricle and aorta 35.93
    right atrium and pulmonary artery 35.94
    right ventricle and pulmonary (distal) artery 35.92
    in repair of
      pulmonary artery atresia 35.92
      transposition of great vessels 35.92
      truncus arteriosus 35.83
  endorectal ileal pouch (J-pouch) (H-pouch) (S-pouch) (with anastomosis to anus) 45.95
  fistula
    arteriovenous (for kidney dialysis) (peripheral shunt) 39.27
      external cannula 39.93
    bladder to skin NEC 57.18
      with bladder flap 57.21
      percutaneous 57.17
    cutaneoperitoneal 54.93
    gastric 43.19
      percutaneous (endoscopic) (transabdominal) 43.11
    mucous — *see* Colostomy
    rectovaginal 48.99
    tracheoesophageal 31.95
    tubulovalvular (Beck-Jianu) (Frank's) (Janeway) (Spivack's) (Ssabanejew-Frank) 43.19
    urethrovaginal 58.0

Formation — *continued*
  ileal
    bladder
      closed 57.87 [45.51]
      open 56.51
    conduit 56.51
  interatrial fistula 35.42
  mucous fistula — *see* Colostomy
  pericardial
    baffle, interatrial 35.91
    window 37.12
  pleural window (for drainage) 34.09
  pocket
    cardiac device (defibrillator) (pacemaker)
      with initial insertion of cardiac device — *omit code*
      new site (skin) (subcutaneous) 37.79
    loop recorder 37.79
    thalamic stimulator pulse generator
      with initial insertion of battery package — *omit code*
      new site (skin) (subcutaneous) 86.09
  pupil 12.39
    by iridectomy 12.14
  rectovaginal fistula 48.99
  reversed gastric tube (intrathoracic) (retrosternal) 42.58
    antesternal or antethoracic 42.68
  septal defect, interatrial 35.42
  shunt
    abdominovenous 54.94
    arteriovenous 39.93
    peritoneojugular 54.94
    peritoneo-vascular 54.94
    pleuroperitoneal 34.05
    transjugular intrahepatic portosystemic [TIPS] 39.1
  subcutaneous tunnel
    esophageal 42.86
      with anastomosis — *see* Anastomosis, esophagus, antesternal
    pulse generator lead wire 86.99
      with initial procedure — *omit code*
    thalamic stimulator pulse generator pocket
      with initial insertion of battery package — *omit code*
      new site (skin) (subcutaneous) 86.09
  syndactyly (finger) (toe) 86.89
  tracheoesophageal 31.95
  tubulovalvular fistula (Beck-Jianu) (Frank's) (Janeway) (Spivack's) (Ssabanejew-Frank) 43.19
  uretero-ileostomy, cutaneous 56.51
  ureterostomy, cutaneous 56.61
    ileal 56.51
  urethrovaginal fistula 58.0
  window
    pericardial 37.12
    pleural (for drainage) 34.09
    thoracoscopic 34.06

Fothergill (-Donald) operation (uterine suspension) 69.22

Fowler operation
  arthroplasty of metacarpophalangeal joint 81.72
  release (mallet finger repair) 82.84
  tenodesis (hand) 82.85
  thoracoplasty 33.34

Fox operation (entropion repair with wedge resection) 08.43

Fracture, surgical — *see also* Osteoclasis 78.70
  turbinates (nasal) 21.62

Fragmentation
  lithotriptor — *see* Lithotripsy
  mechanical
    cataract (with aspiration) 13.43
      posterior route 13.42
      secondary membrane 13.66
    secondary membrane (after cataract) 13.66
  ultrasonic
    cataract (with aspiration) 13.41
    stones, urinary (Kock pouch) 59.95
    urinary stones 59.95
      percutaneous nephrostomy 55.04

☑ **Additional Digit Required** — Refer to the Tabular List for Digit Selection   ▽ **Subterms under main terms may continue to next column or page**

2014 ICD-9-CM   847

Girdlestone operation — *continued*
  resection of femoral head and neck — *continued*
    with replacement prosthesis — *see* Implant, joint, hip
  resection of hip prosthesis 80.05
    with replacement prosthesis — *see* Implant, joint, hip
Girdlestone-Taylor operation (muscle transfer for claw toe repair) 77.57
Glenn operation (anastomosis of superior vena cava to right pulmonary artery) 39.21
Glenoplasty, shoulder 81.83
  with
    partial replacement 81.81
    total replacement, NEC 81.80
      other 81.80
      reverse 81.88
  for recurrent dislocation 81.82
Glomectomy
  carotid 39.89
  jugulare 20.51
Glossectomy (complete) (total) 25.3
  partial or subtotal 25.2
  radical 25.4
Glossopexy 25.59
Glossoplasty NEC 25.59
Glossorrhaphy 25.51
Glossotomy NEC 25.94
  for tongue tie 25.91
Glycoprotein IIb/IIIa inhibitor 99.20
Goebel-Frangenheim-Stoeckel operation (urethrovesical suspension) 59.4
Goldner operation (clubfoot release) 80.48
Goldthwaite operation
  ankle stabilization 81.11
  patellar stabilization 81.44
  tendon transfer for stabilization of patella 81.44
Gonadectomy
  ovary
    bilateral 65.51
      laparoscopic 65.53
    unilateral 65.39
      laparoscopic 65.31
  testis 62.3
    bilateral 62.41
    unilateral 62.3
Goniopuncture 12.51
  with goniotomy 12.53
Gonioscopy 12.29
Goniospasis 12.59
Goniotomy (Barkan's) 12.52
  with goniopuncture 12.53
Goodal-Power operation (vagina) 70.8
Gordon-Taylor operation (hindquarter amputation) 84.19
GP IIb/IIIa inhibitor, infusion 99.20
Graber-Duvernay operation (drilling of femoral head) 77.15
Graft, grafting
  aneurysm 39.52
    endovascular
      abdominal aorta 39.71
        fenestrated (branching) graft 39.78
      lower extremity artery(s) 39.79
      thoracic aorta 39.73
      upper extremity artery(s) 39.79
  artery, arterial (patch) 39.58
    with
      excision or resection of vessel — *see* Arteriectomy, with graft replacement
      synthetic patch (Dacron) (Teflon) 39.57
      tissue patch (vein) (autogenous) (homograft) 39.56
  blood vessel (patch) 39.58
    with
      excision or resection of vessel — *see* Angiectomy, with graft replacement
      synthetic patch (Dacron) (Teflon) 39.57

Graft, grafting — *continued*
  blood vessel — *continued*
    with — *continued*
      tissue patch (vein) (autogenous) (homograft) 39.56
  bone (autogenous) (bone bank) (dual onlay) (heterogenous) (inlay) (massive onlay) (multiple) (osteoperiosteal) (peg) (subperiosteal) (with metallic fixation) 78.00
    with
      arthrodesis — *see* Arthrodesis
      arthroplasty — *see* Arthroplasty
      gingivoplasty 24.2
      lengthening — *see* Lengthening, bone
    carpals, metacarpals 78.04
    clavicle 78.01
    facial NEC 76.91
      with total ostectomy 76.44
    femur 78.05
    fibula 78.07
    humerus 78.02
    joint — *see* Arthroplasty
    mandible 76.91
      with total mandibulectomy 76.41
    marrow — *see* Transplant, bone, marrow
    nose — *see* Graft, nose
    patella 78.06
    pelvic 78.09
    pericranial 02.04
    phalanges (foot) (hand) 78.09
    radius 78.03
    scapula 78.01
    skull 02.04
    specified site NEC 78.09
    spine 78.09
      with fusion — *see* Fusion, spinal
    tarsal, metatarsal 78.08
    thorax (ribs) (sternum) 78.01
    thumb (with transfer of skin flap) 82.69
    tibia 78.07
    ulna 78.03
    vertebrae 78.09
      with fusion — *see* Fusion, spinal
  breast (*see also* Mammoplasty) 85.89
    fat graft 85.55
  buccal sulcus 27.99
  cartilage (joint) (*see also* Arthroplasty)
    nose — *see* Graft, nose
  chest wall (mesh) (silastic) 34.79
  conjunctiva (free) (mucosa) 10.44
    for symblepharon repair 10.41
  cornea (*see also* Keratoplasty) 11.60
  dermal-fat 86.69
  dermal regenerative 86.67
  dura 02.12
  ear
    auricle 18.79
  esophagus NEC 42.87
    with interposition (intrathoracic) NEC 42.58
      antesternal or antethoracic NEC 42.68
      colon (intrathoracic) 42.55
        antesternal or antethoracic 42.65
      small bowel (intrathoracic) 42.53
        antesternal or antethoracic 42.63
  external auditory meatus 18.6
    inner 20.61
    pedicle preparation 86.71
  eyebrow (*see also* Reconstruction, eyelid, with graft) 08.69
  eyelid (*see also* Reconstruction, eyelid, with graft) 08.69
    free mucous membrane 08.62
  eye socket (skin) (cartilage) (bone) 16.63
  fallopian tube 66.79
  fascia 83.82
    with hernia repair — *see* Repair, hernia
    eyelid 08.32
    hand 82.72
    tarsal cartilage 08.69
  fat pad NEC 86.89
    with skin graft — *see* Graft, skin, full-thickness

Graft, grafting — *continued*
  flap (advanced) (rotating) (sliding) (*see also* Graft, skin, pedicle)
    tarsoconjunctival 08.64
  hair-bearing skin 86.64
  hand
    fascia 82.72
    free skin 86.62
    muscle 82.72
    pedicle (flap) 86.73
    tendon 82.79
  heart, for revascularization — *see* category 36.3 ☑
  joint — *see* Arthroplasty
  larynx 31.69
  lip 27.56
    full-thickness 27.55
  lymphatic structure(s) (channel) (node) (vessel) 40.9
  mediastinal fat to myocardium 36.39
  meninges (cerebral) 02.12
  mouth, except palate 27.56
    full-thickness 27.55
  muscle 83.82
    hand 82.72
  myocardium, for revascularization 36.39
  nasolabial flaps 21.86
  nerve (cranial) (peripheral) 04.5
  nipple 85.86
  nose 21.89
    with
      augmentation 21.85
      rhinoplasty — *see* Rhinoplasty
      total reconstruction 21.83
    septum 21.88
    tip 21.86
  omentum 54.74
    to myocardium 36.39
  orbit (bone) (cartilage) (skin) 16.63
  outflow tract (patch) (pulmonary valve) 35.26
    in total repair of tetralogy of Fallot 35.81
  ovary 65.92
  palate 27.69
    for cleft palate repair 27.62
  pedicle — *see* Graft, skin, pedicle
  penis (rib) (skin) 64.49
  pigskin 86.65
  pinch — *see* Graft, skin, free
  pocket — *see* Graft, skin, pedicle
  porcine 86.65
  postauricular (Wolff) 18.79
  razor — *see* Graft, skin, free
  rope — *see* Graft, skin, pedicle
  saphenous vein in aortocoronary bypass — *see* Bypass, aortocoronary
  scrotum 61.49
  skin (partial-thickness) (split-thickness) 86.69
    amnionic membrane 86.66
    auditory meatus (ear) 18.6
    dermal-fat 86.69
      for breast augmentation 85.50
    dermal regenerative 86.67
    ear
      auditory meatus 18.6
      postauricular 18.79
    eyelid 08.61
    fat 86.87
    flap — *see* Graft, skin, pedicle
    free (autogenous) NEC 86.60
      breast
        deep inferior epigastric artery perforator (DIEP) flap, free 85.74
        gluteal artery perforator (GAP) flap, free 85.76
        superficial inferior epigastric artery (SIEA) flap, free 85.75
        transverse rectus abdominis musculocutaneous (TRAM) flap, free 85.73
      lip 27.56
      thumb 86.62

Graft, grafting — *continued*
  skin — *continued*
    free — *continued*
      thumb — *continued*
        for
          pollicization 82.61
          reconstruction 82.69
    full-thickness 86.63
      breast 85.83
      hand 86.61
    hair-bearing 86.64
      eyelid or eyebrow 08.63
    hand 86.62
      full-thickness 86.61
    heterograft 86.65
    homograft 86.66
    island flap 86.70
    mucous membrane 86.69
      eyelid 08.62
    nose — *see* Graft, nose
    pedicle (flap) (tube) 86.70
      advancement 86.72
      attachment to site (advanced) (double) (rotating) (sliding) 86.74
        hand (cross finger) (pocket) 86.73
        lip 27.57
        mouth 27.57
        thumb 86.73
          for
            pollicization 82.61
            reconstruction NEC 82.69
      breast 85.84
        deep inferior epigastric artery perforator (DIEP) flap, free 85.74
        gluteal artery perforator (GAP) flap, free 85.76
        latissimus dorsi myocutaneous flap 85.71
        superficial inferior epigastric artery (SIEA) flap, free 85.75
        transverse rectus abdominis musculocutaneous (TRAM) flap, free 85.73
        transverse rectus abdominis myocutaneous (TRAM) flap, pedicled 85.72
      defatting 86.75
      delayed 86.71
      design and raising 86.71
      elevation 86.71
      preparation of (cutting) 86.71
      revision 86.75
      sculpturing 86.71
      transection 86.71
      transfer 86.74
      trimming 86.71
    postauricular 18.79
    rotation flap 86.70
    specified site NEC 86.69
      full-thickness 86.63
  tarsal cartilage 08.69
  temporalis muscle to orbit 16.63
    with exenteration of orbit 16.59
  tendon 83.81
    for joint repair — *see* Arthroplasty
    hand 82.79
  testicle 62.69
  thumb (for reconstruction) NEC 82.69
  tongue (mucosal) (skin) 25.59
  trachea 31.79
  tubular (tube) — *see* Graft, skin, pedicle
  tunnel — *see* Graft, skin, pedicle
  tympanum (*see also* Tympanoplasty) 19.4
  ureter 56.89
  vagina
    biological 70.94
    synthetic 70.95
  vein (patch) 39.58
    with
      excision or resection of vessel — *see* Phlebectomy, with graft replacement
      synthetic patch (Dacron) (Teflon) 39.57

☑ Additional Digit Required — Refer to the Tabular List for Digit Selection   ▽ Subterms under main terms may continue to next column or page

2014 ICD-9-CM

849

Girdlestone operation — Graft, grafting

Graft, grafting — *continued*
  vein — *continued*
    with — *continued*
      tissue patch (vein) (autogenous)
        (homograft) 39.56
      vermilion border (lip) 27.56
Grattage, conjunctiva 10.31
Green operation (scapulopexy) 78.41
Grice operation (subtalar arthrodesis) 81.13
Grip, strength 93.04
Gritti-Stokes operation (knee disarticulation)
  84.16
Gross operation (herniorrhaphy)
  laparoscopic 53.43
    with graft or prosthesis 53.42
  other and open with graft or prosthesis
    53.41
  other open 53.49
Group therapy 94.44
Guttering, bone — *see also* Excision, lesion,
  bone 77.60
Guyon operation (amputation of ankle) 84.13

H

Hagner operation (epididymotomy) 63.92
Halsted operation — *see* Repair, hernia, inguinal
Hampton operation (anastomosis small intestine to rectal stump) 45.92
Hanging hip operation (muscle release) 83.19
Harelip operation 27.54
Harrison-Richardson operation (vaginal suspension) 70.77
  with graft or prosthesis 70.78
Hartmann resection (of intestine) (with pouch)
  — *see* Colectomy, by site
Harvesting
  bone marrow 41.91
  fat for grafting or banking 86.90
  stem cells 99.79
Hauser operation
  achillotenotomy 83.11
  bunionectomy with adductor tendon
    transfer 77.53
  stabilization of patella 81.44
Heaney operation (vaginal hysterectomy)
  68.59
  laparoscopically assisted (LAVH) 68.51
Hearing aid (with battery replacement) 95.49
Hearing test 95.47
HeartMate® II left ventricular assist system
  [LVAS] 37.66
HeartMate® implantable heart assist system
  37.66
Hegar operation (perineorrhaphy) 71.79
Heineke-Mikulicz operation (pyloroplasty)
  44.29
Heine operation (cyclodialysis) 12.55
Heller operation (esophagomyotomy) 42.7
Hellström operation (transplantation of
  aberrant renal vessel) 39.55
Hemicolectomy
  left
    laparoscopic 17.35
    open and other 45.75
  right (extended)
    laparoscopic 17.33
    open and other 45.73
Hemicystectomy 57.6
Hemigastrectomy — *see* Gastrectomy
Hemiglossectomy 25.2
Hemilaminectomy (decompression) (explo-
  ration) 03.09
Hemilaryngectomy (anterior) (lateral) (vertical)
  30.1
Hemimandibulectomy 76.31
Hemimastectomy (radical) 85.23
Hemimaxillectomy (with bone graft) (with
  prosthesis) 76.39
Heminephrectomy 55.4
Hemipelvectomy 84.19
Hemispherectomy (cerebral) 01.52
Hemithyroidectomy (with removal of isthmus)
  (with removal of portion of remaining
  lobe) 06.2
Hemodiafiltration (extracorporeal) 39.95

Hemodialysis (extracorporeal) 39.95
Hemodilution 99.03
Hemofiltration (extracorporeal) 39.95
Hemorrhage control — *see* Control, hemor-
  rhage
Hemorrhoidectomy 49.46
  by
    cautery, cauterization 49.43
    crushing 49.45
    cryotherapy, cryosurgery 49.44
    excision 49.46
    injection 49.42
    ligation 49.45
Hemostasis — *see* Control, hemorrhage
Henley operation (jejunal transposition) 43.81
Hepatectomy (complete) (total) 50.4
  partial or subtotal 50.22
Hepatic assistance, extracorporeal 50.92
Hepaticocholangiojejunostomy 51.37
Hepaticocystoduodenostomy 51.37
Hepaticodochotomy 51.59
Hepaticoduodenostomy 51.37
Hepaticojejunostomy 51.37
Hepaticolithectomy 51.49
  endoscopic 51.88
Hepaticolithotomy 51.49
  endoscopic 51.88
Hepaticostomy 51.59
Hepaticotomy 51.59
Hepatocholangiocystoduodenostomy 51.37
Hepatocholedochostomy 51.43
  endoscopic 51.87
Hepatoduodenostomy 50.69
Hepatogastrostomy 50.69
Hepatojejunostomy 50.69
Hepatolithotomy
  hepatic duct 51.49
  liver 50.0
Hepatopexy 50.69
Hepatorrhaphy 50.61
Hepatostomy (external) (internal) 50.69
Hepatotomy (with packing) 50.0
Hernioplasty — *see* Repair, hernia
Herniorrhaphy — *see* Repair, hernia
Herniotomy — *see* Repair, hernia
Heterograft — *see* Graft
Heterotransplant, heterotransplantation
  — *see* Transplant
Hey-Groves operation (reconstruction of an-
  terior cruciate ligament) 81.45
Heyman-Herndon (-Strong) operation (correc-
  tion of metatarsus varus) 80.48
Heymen operation (soft tissue release for
  clubfoot) 83.84
Hey operation (amputation of foot) 84.12
Hibbs operation (lumbar spinal fusion) — *see*
  Fusion, lumbar
Higgins operation — *see* Repair, hernia,
  femoral
High forceps delivery 72.39
  with episiotomy 72.31
Hill-Allison operation (hiatal hernia repair,
  transpleural approach) 53.80
Hinging, mitral valve 35.12
His bundle recording 37.29
Hitchcock operation (anchoring tendon of
  biceps) 83.88
Hofmeister operation (gastrectomy) 43.7
Hoke operation
  midtarsal fusion 81.14
  triple arthrodesis 81.12
Holth operation
  iridencleisis 12.63
  sclerectomy 12.65
Homan operation (correction of lymphedema)
  40.9
Homograft — *see* Graft
Homotransplant, homotransplantation —
  see Transplant
Hosiery, elastic 93.59
Hutch operation (ureteroneocystostomy)
  56.74
Hybinette-Eden operation (glenoid bone
  block) 78.01
Hydrocelectomy
  canal of Nuck (female) 69.19

Hydrocelectomy — *continued*
  canal of Nuck — *continued*
    male 63.1
    round ligament 69.19
    spermatic cord 63.1
    tunica vaginalis 61.2
Hydrotherapy 93.33
  assisted exercise in pool 93.31
  whirlpool 93.32
Hymenectomy 70.31
Hymenoplasty 70.76
Hymenorrhaphy 70.76
Hymenotomy 70.11
Hyperalimentation (parenteral) 99.15
Hyperbaric oxygenation 93.95
  wound 93.59
Hyperextension, joint 93.25
Hyperthermia NEC 93.35
  for cancer treatment (interstitial) (local) (ra-
    diofrequency) (regional) (ultrasound)
    (whole-body) 99.85
Hypnodrama, psychiatric 94.32
Hypnosis (psychotherapeutic) 94.32
  for anesthesia — *omit code*
Hypnotherapy 94.32
Hypophysectomy (complete) (total) 07.69
  partial or subtotal 07.63
    transfrontal approach 07.61
    transsphenoidal approach 07.62
  specified approach NEC 07.68
  transfrontal approach (complete) (total)
    07.64
    partial 07.61
  transsphenoidal approach (complete) (total)
    07.65
    partial 07.62
Hypothermia (central) (local) 99.81
  gastric (cooling) 96.31
    freezing 96.32
  systemic (in open heart surgery) 39.62
Hypotympanotomy 20.23
Hysterectomy, NOS 68.9
  abdominal
    laparoscopic (total) (TLH) 68.41
    other (total) 68.49
    partial or subtotal (supracervical)
      (supravaginal) 68.39
    radical (modified) (Wertheim's) 68.69
      laparoscopic (total) (TLRH) 68.61
    supracervical 68.39
      classic infrafascial SEMM hysterecto-
        my (CISH) 68.31
      laparoscopically assisted (LASH)
        68.31
  laparoscopic
    abdominal
      radical (total) (TLRH) 68.61
      total (TLH) 68.41
    supracervical (LASH) (LSH) 68.31
    total (TLH) 68.41
    vaginal, assisted (LAVH) 68.51
      radical (LRVH) 68.71
  radical
    abdominal
      laparoscopic 68.61
      other (modified) (Wertheim's) 68.69
    vaginal
      laparoscopic (LRVH) 68.71
      other 68.79
  vaginal (complete) (partial) (subtotal) (total)
    68.59
    laparoscopically assisted (LAVH) 68.51
    radical (Schauta) 68.79
    laparoscopic (LRVH) 68.71
Hysterocolpectomy (radical) (vaginal) 68.79
  abdominal 68.69
    laparoscopic 68.61
  laparoscopic 68.71
Hysterogram NEC 87.85
  percutaneous 87.84
Hysterolysis 54.59
  laparoscopic 54.51
Hysteromyomectomy 68.29
Hysteropexy 69.22
Hysteroplasty 69.49
Hysterorrhaphy 69.41

Hysterosalpingography gas (contrast) 87.82
  opaque dye (contrast) 87.83
Hysterosalpingostomy 66.74
Hysteroscopy 68.12
  with
    ablation
      endometrial 68.23
    biopsy 68.16
Hysterotomy (with removal of foreign body)
  (with removal of hydatidiform mole) 68.0
  for intrauterine transfusion 75.2
  obstetrical 74.99
    for termination of pregnancy 74.91
Hysterotrachelectomy 67.4
Hysterotracheloplasty 69.49
Hysterotrachelorrhaphy 69.41
Hysterotrachelotomy 69.95

I

IAEMT (intraoperative anesthetic effect moni-
  toring and titration) 00.94 *[89.14]*
ICCE (intracapsular cataract extraction) 13.19
Ileal
  bladder
    closed 57.87 *[45.51]*
      open (ileoureterostomy) 56.51
  conduit (ileoureterostomy) 56.51
Ileocecostomy 45.93
Ileocolectomy
  laparoscopic 17.33
  open and other 45.73
Ileocolostomy 45.93
Ileocolotomy 45.00
Ileocystoplasty (isolated segment anastomo-
  sis) (open loop) 57.87 *[45.51]*
Ileoduodenotomy 45.01
Ileoectomy (partial) 45.62
  with cecectomy
    laparoscopic 17.32
    open and other 45.72
Ileoentectropy 46.99
Ileoesophagostomy 42.54
Ileoileostomy 45.91
  proximal to distal segment 45.62
Ileoloopogram 87.78
Ileopancreatostomy 52.96
Ileopexy 46.61
Ileoproctostomy 45.93
Ileorectostomy 45.93
Ileorrhaphy 46.73
Ileoscopy 45.13
  through stoma (artificial) 45.12
  transabdominal (operative) 45.11
Ileosigmoidostomy 45.93
Ileostomy 46.20
  continent (permanent) 46.22
    for urinary diversion 56.51
  delayed opening 46.24
  Hendon (temporary) 46.21
  loop 46.01
  Paul (temporary) 46.21
  permanent 46.23
    continent 46.22
  repair 46.41
  revision 46.41
  tangential (temporary) 46.21
  temporary 46.21
  transplantation to new site 46.23
  tube (temporary) 46.21
  ureteral
    external 56.51
    internal 56.71
Ileotomy 45.02
Ileotransversostomy 45.93
Ileoureterostomy (Bricker's) (ileal bladder)
  56.51
Imaging (diagnostic)
  by
    optical coherence tomography (OCT) —
      see OCT and Tomography, optical
      coherence
  diagnostic, not elsewhere classified 88.90
  endovascular ultrasound — *see* Imaging,
    intravascular ultrasound

Imaging — *continued*
  intraoperative
    iMRI — *see* Imaging, magnetic resonance
    intravascular — *see* Imaging, intravascular ultrasound
  intravascular ultrasound (IVUS) 00.29
    aorta 00.22
    aortic arch 00.22
    carotid vessel 00.21
    cerebral vessel, extracranial 00.21
    coronary vessel 00.24
    intrathoracic vessel 00.22
    other specified vessel 00.28
    peripheral vessel 00.23
    renal vessel 00.25
    vena cava (inferior) (superior) 00.22
  magnetic resonance (nuclear) (proton) NEC 88.97
    abdomen 88.97
    bladder (urinary) 88.95
    bone marrow blood supply 88.94
    brain (brain stem) 88.91
      intraoperative (iMRI) 88.96
      real-time 88.96
    chest (hilar) (mediastinal) 88.92
    computer assisted surgery (CAS) with MR/MRA 00.32
    extremity (upper) (lower) 88.94
    eye orbit 88.97
    face 88.97
    head NEC 88.97
    musculoskeletal 88.94
    myocardium 88.92
    neck 88.97
    orbit of eye 88.97
    prostate 88.95
    specified site NEC 88.97
    spinal canal (cord) (spine) 88.93
  VH™-IVUS — *see* Imaging (diagnostic), intravascular ultrasound (IVUS), by site
  virtual histology intravascular ultrasound — *see* Imaging (diagnostic), intravascular ultrasound (IVUS), by site

Immobilization (by)
  with fracture-reduction — *see* Reduction, fracture
  bandage 93.59
  bone 93.53
  cast NEC 93.53
    with reduction of fracture or dislocation — *see* Reduction, fracture, *and* Reduction, dislocation
  device NEC 93.59
  pressure dressing 93.56
  splint (plaster) (tray) 93.54
    with reduction of fracture or dislocation — *see* Reduction, fracture, *and* Reduction, dislocation
  stereotactic head frame 93.59
  strapping (non-traction) 93.59

Immunization — *see also* Vaccination
  allergy 99.12
  autoimmune disease 99.13
  BCG 99.33
  brucellosis 99.55
  cholera 99.31
  diphtheria 99.36
  DPT 99.39
  epidemic parotitis 99.46
  German measles 99.47
  Hemophilus influenzae 99.52
  influenza 99.52
  measles 99.45
  meningococcus 99.55
  mumps 99.46
  pertussis 99.37
  plague 99.34
  poliomyelitis 99.41
  rabies 99.44
  rubella 99.47
  salmonella 99.55
  smallpox 99.42
  staphylococcus 99.55
  TAB 99.32
  tetanus 99.38

Immunization — *see also* Vaccination — *continued*
  triple vaccine 99.48
  tuberculosis 99.33
  tularemia 99.35
  typhoid-paratyphoid 99.32
  typhus 99.55
  viral NEC 99.55
  whooping cough 99.37
  yellow fever 99.43

Immunoadsorption
  extracorporeal (ECI) 99.76

Immunotherapy, antineoplastic 99.28
  C-Parvum 99.28
  Interferon 99.28
  interleukin-2 (low-dose) 99.28
    high-dose 00.15
  Levamisole 99.28
  Proleukin (low-dose) 99.28
    high-dose 00.15
  Thymosin 99.28

Impella® percutaneous external heart assist device 37.68

Implant, implantation
  abdominal artery to coronary artery 36.17
  artery
    aortic branches to heart muscle 36.2
    mammary to ventricular wall (Vineberg) 36.2
  baffle, atrial or interatrial 35.91
  biliary fistulous tract into stomach or intestine 51.39
  bipolar endoprosthesis (femoral head) 81.52
  bladder sphincter, artificial (inflatable) 58.93
  blood vessels to myocardium 36.2
  bone growth stimulator (invasive) (percutaneous) (semi-invasive) — *see* category 78.9 ☑
  bone morphogenetic protein (Infuse™) (OP-1™) (recombinant) (rhBMP) 84.52
  bone void filler 84.55
    that with percutaneous vertebral augmentation 81.66
    that with percutaneous vertebroplasty 81.65
  breast (for augmentation) (bilateral) 85.54
    unilateral 85.53
  cardiac contractility modulation (CCM)
    rechargeable pulse generator only 17.52
    total system 17.51
  cardiac resynchronization device
    defibrillator (biventricular) (BiV ICD) (BiV pacemaker with defibrillator) (BiV pacing with defibrillator) (CRT-D) (device and one or more leads) (total system) 00.51
      left ventricular coronary venous lead only 00.52
      pulse generator only 00.54
    pacemaker (BiV) (biventricular) (CRT-P) (device and one or more leads) (total system) 00.50
      left ventricular coronary venous lead only 00.52
      pulse generator only 00.53
  cardiac support device (CSD) 37.41
  cardiomyostimulation system 37.67
  cardioverter/defibrillator (automatic) 37.94
    leads only (patch electrodes) (sensing) (pacing) 37.95
    pulse generator only 37.96
    total system 37.94
  CCM (cardiac contractility modulation)
    rechargeable pulse generator only 17.52
    total system 17.51
  chemotherapeutic agent 00.10
  chest wall (mesh) (silastic) 34.79
  chin (polyethylene) (silastic) 76.68
  cochlear (electrode) 20.96
    prosthetic device (electrode and receiver) 20.96
    channel (single) 20.97
      multiple 20.98
    electrode only 20.99
    internal coil only 20.99
  coil(s), endovascular 39.79

Implant, implantation — *continued*
  coil(s), endovascular — *continued*
    head or neck vessels
      bare metal 39.75
      bioactive 39.76
  CorCap™ 37.41
  cornea 11.73
  CRT-D (biventricular defibrillator) (BiV ICD) (BiV pacepaker with defibrillator) (BiV pacing with defibrillator) (cardiac resynchronization defibrillator) (device and one or more leads) 00.51
    left ventricular coronary venous lead only 00.52
    pulse generator only 00.54
  CRT-P (biventricular pacemaker) (BiV pacemaker) (cardiac resynchronization pacemaker) (device and one or more leads) 00.50
    left ventricular coronary venous lead only 00.52
    pulse generator only 00.53
  custodis eye 14.41
  dental (endosseous) (prosthetic) 23.6
  device
    adjustable gastric band and port 44.95
    bronchial device NOS 33.79
    bronchial substance NOS 33.79
    bronchial valve(s)
      multiple lobes 33.73
      single lobe 33.71
    cardiac support device (CSD) 37.41
    CorCap™ 37.41
    epicardial support device 37.41
    Lap-Band® 44.95
    left atrial appendage 37.90
    left atrial filter 37.90
    left atrial occluder 37.90
    MitraClip® percutaneous mitral valve leaflet clip 35.97
    prosthetic cardiac support device 37.41
    sternal fixation device with rigid plates 84.94
    subcutaneous for intracardiac or great vessel hemodynamic monitoring 00.57
    vascular access 86.07
    ventricular support device 37.41
  diaphragmatic pacemaker 34.85
  Dynesys® 84.82
  electrode(s)
    brain 02.93
      depth 02.93
      foramen ovale 02.93
      sphenoidal 02.93
    cardiac (initial) (transvenous) 37.70
      atrium (initial) 37.73
        replacement 37.76
      atrium and ventricle (initial) 37.72
        replacement 37.76
      epicardium (sternotomy or thoracotomy approach) 37.74
      left ventricular coronary venous system 00.52
      temporary transvenous pacemaker system 37.78
        during and immediately following cardiac surgery 39.64
      ventricle (initial) 37.71
        replacement 37.76
    carotid sinus 39.82
      with synchronous pulse generator implantation (total system) 39.81
    depth 02.93
    foramen ovale 02.96
    gastric 04.92
    heart (*see also* Implant, electrode(s), cardiac) 37.70
    intracranial 02.93
    osteogenic (invasive) for bone growth stimulation — *see* category 78.9 ☑
    peripheral nerve 04.92
    sacral nerve 04.92
    sphenoidal 02.96

Implant, implantation — *continued*
  electrode(s) — *continued*
    spine 03.93
  electroencephalographic receiver
    brain 02.93
    intracranial 02.93
  electronic stimulator
    anus (subcutaneous) 49.92
    bladder 57.96
    bone growth (invasive) (percutaneous) (semi-invasive) 78.9 ☑
    brain — *see* Implant, neurostimulator, brain
    carotid sinus 39.83
      with synchronous lead(s) implantation (total system) 39.81
    cochlear 20.96
      channel (single) 20.97
        multiple 20.98
    gastric 04.92
    intracranial — *see* Implant, neurostimulator, intracranial
    peripheral nerve — *see* Implant, neurostimulator, peripheral nerve
    phrenic nerve 34.85
    skeletal muscle 83.92
    spine — *see* Implant, neurostimulator, spine
    ureter 56.92
  electrostimulator — *see* Implant, electronic stimulator, by site
  endoprosthesis
    bile duct 51.87
    femoral head (bipolar) 81.52
    pancreatic duct 52.93
  endosseous (dental) 23.6
  epidural pegs 02.93
  epikeratoprosthesis 11.73
  epiretinal visual prosthesis 14.81
  estradiol (pellet) 99.23
  eye (Iowa type) 16.61
    integrated 16.41
  facial bone, synthetic (alloplastic) 76.92
  fallopian tube (Mulligan hood) (silastic tube) (stent) 66.93
    into uterus 66.74
  gastroepiploic artery to coronary artery 36.17
  hearing device, electromagnetic 20.95
  heart
    artificial 37.52
      total internal biventricular replacement system 37.52
        AbioCor® 37.52
        CardioWest™ (TAH-t) 37.52
    assist system
      CentriMag® — *see* Insertion, circulatory support device
      external heart assist device, percutaneous — *see* Insertion, circulatory support device
      external heart assist system, open approach 37.65
      extrinsic 37.68
      HeartMate® II left ventricular assist system [LVAS] 37.66
      HeartMate® implantable heart assist system 37.66
      Impella® percutaneous external circulatory assist device — *see* Insertion, circulatory support device
      implantable 37.66
      non-implantable — *see* Insertion, circulatory support device
      percutaneous external circulatory assist device — *see* Insertion, circulatory support device
      pulsation balloon 37.61
      pVAD (percutaneous VAD) — *see* Insertion, circulatory support device
      TandemHeart® — *see* Insertion, circulatory support device

Implant, implantation — continued
heart — continued
  assist system — continued
    temporary non-implantable circulatory assist device — see Insertion, circulatory support device
    that for destination therapy (DT) 37.66
    auxiliary ventricle 37.62
    cardiac support device (CSD) 37.41
    circulatory assist system — see Implant, heart, assist system
    CorCap™ 37.41
    epicardial support device 37.41
    pacemaker (see also Implant, pacemaker, cardiac) 37.80
    prosthetic cardiac support device 37.41
    total internal biventricular replacement system 37.52
  valve(s)
    prosthesis or synthetic device (partial) (synthetic) (total) 35.20
      aortic 35.22
      mitral 35.24
      pulmonary 35.26
      tricuspid 35.28
    tissue graft 35.20
      aortic 35.21
      mitral 35.23
      pulmonary 35.25
      tricuspid 35.27
  ventricular support device 37.41
inert material
  breast (for augmentation) (bilateral) 85.54
    unilateral 85.53
  larynx 31.0
  nose 21.85
  orbit (eye socket) 16.69
    reinsertion 16.62
  scleral shell (cup) (with evisceration of eyeball) 16.31
    reinsertion 16.62
  Tenon's capsule (with enucleation of eyeball) 16.42
    with attachment of muscles 16.41
    reinsertion 16.62
  urethra 59.79
  vocal cord(s) 31.0
infusion pump 86.06
interbody spinal fusion device 84.51
intracardiac or great vessel hemodynamic monitor, subcutaneous 00.57
joint (prosthesis) (silastic) (Swanson type) NEC 81.96
  ankle (total) 81.56
    revision 81.59
  carpocarpal, carpometacarpal 81.74
  elbow (total) 81.84
    revision 81.97
  extremity (bioelectric) (cineplastic) (kineplastic) 84.40
    lower 84.48
      revision 81.59
    upper 84.44
      revision 81.97
  femoral (bipolar endoprosthesis) 81.52
    revision NOS 81.53
      acetabular and femoral components (total) 00.70
      acetabular component only 00.71
      acetabular liner and/or femoral head only 00.73
      femoral component only 00.72
      femoral head only and/or acetabular liner 00.73
      total (acetabular and femoral components) 00.70
  finger 81.71
  hand (metacarpophalangeal) (interphalangeal) 81.71
    revision 81.97
  hip (partial) 81.52
    revision NOS 81.53

Implant, implantation — continued
joint — continued
  hip — continued
    revision — continued
      acetabular and femoral components (total) 00.70
      acetabular component only 00.71
      acetabular liner and/or femoral head only 00.73
      femoral component only 00.72
      femoral head only and/or acetabular liner 00.73
      partial
        acetabular component only 00.71
        acetabular liner and/or femoral head only 00.73
        femoral component only 00.72
        femoral head only and/or acetabular liner 00.73
      total (acetabular and femoral components) 00.70
    total 81.51
      revision (acetabular and femoral components) 00.70
  interphalangeal 81.71
    revision 81.97
  knee (partial) (total) 81.54
    revision NOS 81.55
      femoral component 00.82
      partial
        femoral component 00.82
        patellar component 00.83
        tibial component 00.81
        tibial insert 00.84
      patellar component 00.83
      tibial component 00.81
      tibial insert 00.84
      total (all components) 00.80
  metacarpophalangeal 81.71
    revision 81.97
  shoulder (partial) 81.81
    revision 81.97
    total replacement, NEC 81.80
      other 81.80
      reverse 81.88
  toe 81.57
    for hallux valgus repair 77.59
    revision 81.59
  wrist (partial) 81.74
    revision 81.97
    total replacement 81.73
kidney, mechanical 55.97
Lap-Band™ 44.95
larynx 31.0
leads (cardiac) — see Implant, electrode(s), cardiac
limb lengthening device, internal (NOS) 84.54
  with kinetic distraction 84.53
mammary artery
  in ventricle (Vineberg) 36.2
  to coronary artery (single vessel) 36.15
    double vessel 36.16
M-Brace™ 84.82
Mulligan hood, fallopian tube 66.93
nerve (peripheral) 04.79
neuropacemaker — see Implant, neurostimulator, by site
neurostimulator
  brain 02.93
  electrodes
    brain 02.93
    gastric 04.92
    intracranial 02.93
    peripheral nerve 04.92
    sacral nerve 04.92
    spine 03.93
  intracranial 02.93
  peripheral nerve 04.92
  pulse generator (subcutaneous) 86.96
    cranial 01.20
    multiple array 86.95
      rechargeable 86.98

Implant, implantation — continued
neurostimulator — continued
  pulse generator — continued
    single array 86.94
      rechargeable 86.97
    spine 03.93
  nose 21.85
Ommaya reservoir 02.22
orbit 16.69
  reinsertion 16.62
outflow tract prosthesis (heart) (gusset type) in
  pulmonary valvuloplasty 35.26
  total repair of tetralogy of Fallot 35.81
ovary into uterine cavity 65.72
  laparoscopic 65.75
pacemaker
  brain — see Implant, neurostimulator, brain
  cardiac (device) (initial) (permanent) (replacement) 37.80
    dual-chamber device (initial) 37.83
      replacement 37.87
    resynchronization device (biventricular pacemaker) (BiV pacemaker) (CRT-P)
      device only (initial) (replacement) 00.53
      total system (device and one or more leads) 00.50
      transvenous lead into left ventricular coronary venous system 00.52
    single-chamber device (initial) 37.81
      rate responsive 37.82
      replacement 37.85
        rate responsive 37.86
    temporary transvenous pacemaker system 37.78
      during and immediately following cardiac surgery 39.64
  carotid sinus 39.89
  diaphragm 34.85
  gastric 04.92
  intracranial — see Implant, neurostimulator, intracranial
  neural — see Implant, neurostimulator, by site
  peripheral nerve — see Implant, neurostimulator, peripheral nerve
  spine — see Implant, neurostimulator, spine
pancreas (duct) 52.96
penis, prosthesis (internal)
  inflatable 64.97
  non-inflatable 64.95
port, vascular access device 86.07
premaxilla 76.68
progesterone (subdermal) 99.23
prosthesis, prosthetic device
  acetabulum (Aufranc-Turner) 81.52
  ankle (total) 81.56
  arm (bioelectric) (cineplastic) (kineplastic) 84.44
  breast (Cronin) (Dow-Corning) (Perras-Pappillon) (bilateral) 85.54
    unilateral 85.53
  cardiac support device (CSD) (CorCap™) 37.41
  cochlear 20.96
    channel (single) 20.97
      multiple 20.98
  epiretinal visual 14.81
  extremity (bioelectric) (cineplastic) (kineplastic) 84.40
    lower 84.48
    upper 84.44
  fallopian tube (Mulligan hood) (stent) 66.93
  femoral head (Austin-Moore) (bipolar) (Eicher) (Thompson) 81.52
    revision NOS 81.53
      acetabular and femoral components (total) 00.70
      acetabular component only 00.71

Implant, implantation — continued
prosthesis, prosthetic device — continued
  femoral head — continued
    revision — continued
      acetabular liner and/or femoral head only 00.73
      femoral component only 00.72
      femoral head only and/or acetabular liner 00.73
      partial
        acetabular component only 00.71
        acetabular liner and/or femoral head only 00.73
        femoral component only 00.72
        femoral head only and/or acetabular liner 00.73
      total (acetabular and femoral components) 00.70
  joint (Swanson type) NEC 81.96
    ankle (total) 81.56
    carpocarpal, carpometacarpal 81.74
    elbow (total) 81.84
    finger 81.71
    hand (metacarpophalangeal) (interphalangeal) 81.71
    hip (partial) 81.52
      revision NOS 81.53
        acetabular and femoral components (total) 00.70
        acetabular component only 00.71
        acetabular liner and/or femoral head only 00.73
        femoral component only 00.72
        femoral head only and/or acetabular liner 00.73
        partial
          acetabular component only 00.71
          acetabular liner and/or femoral head only 00.73
          femoral component only 00.72
          femoral head only and/or acetabular liner 00.73
        total (acetabular and femoral components) 00.70
    total 81.51
      revision (acetabular and femoral components) 00.70
    interphalangeal 81.71
    knee (partial) (total) 81.54
      revision NOS 81.55
        femoral component 00.82
        partial
          femoral component 00.82
          patellar component 00.83
          tibial component 00.81
          tibial insert 00.84
        patellar component 00.83
        tibial component 00.81
        tibial insert 00.84
        total (all components) 00.80
    metacarpophalangeal 81.71
    shoulder (partial) 81.81
      total, NEC 81.80
        other 81.80
        reverse 81.88
    spine NEC 84.59
      interspinous process decompression device
    toe 81.57
      for hallux valgus repair 77.59
    wrist (partial) 81.74
      total 81.73
  leg (bioelectric) (cineplastic) (kineplastic) 84.48

☑ **Additional Digit Required — Refer to the Tabular List for Digit Selection**
    ▽ **Subterms under main terms may continue to next column or page**
854
    2014 ICD-9-CM

Insertion — *continued*
  catheter — *continued*
    spinal canal space (epidural) (subarachnoid) (subdural) for infusion of therapeutic or palliative substances 03.90
    Swan-Ganz (pulmonary) 89.64
    temporary occlusion, abdominal aorta 39.77
    transtracheal for oxygenation 31.99
    vein NEC 38.93
      for renal dialysis 38.95
  chest tube 34.04
    thoracoscopic 34.06
  choledochohepatic tube (for decompression) 51.43
    endoscopic 51.87
  circulatory support device
    CentriMag® 37.62
    external heart assist device
      biventricular 37.60
      Impella® 37.68
      percutaneous 37.68
      temporary 37.62
    non-implantable 37.62
    pVAD (percutaneous VAD) 37.68
    TandemHeart® 37.68
    temporary non-implantable circulatory assist device 37.62
  cochlear prosthetic device — *see* Implant, cochlear prosthetic device
  contraceptive device (intrauterine) 69.7
  CorCap™ 37.41
  cordis cannula 54.98
  coronary (artery)

> *Note: Also use 00.40, 00.41, 00.42, or 00.43 to show the total number of vessels treated. Use code 00.44 once to show procedure on a bifurcated vessel. In addition, use 00.45, 00.46, 00.47, or 00.48 to show the number of vascular stents inserted.*

    stent, drug-eluting 36.07
    stent, non-drug-eluting 36.06
  Crosby-Cooney button 54.98
  CRT-D (biventricular defibrillator) (BiV ICD) (BiV pacemaker with defibrillator) (BiV pacing with defibrillator) (cardiac resynchronization defibrillator) (device and one or more leads) 00.51
    left ventricular coronary venous lead only 00.52
    pulse generator only 00.54
  CRT-P (biventricular pacemaker) (BiV pacemaker) (cardiac resynchronization pacemaker) (device and one or more leads) 00.50
    left ventricular coronary venous lead only 00.52
    pulse generator only 00.53
  Crutchfield tongs (skull) (with synchronous skeletal traction) 02.94
  Davidson button 54.98
  denture (total) 99.97
  device
    adjustable gastric band and port 44.95
    bronchial device NOS 33.79
    bronchial substance NOS 33.79
    bronchial valve(s)
      multiple lobes 33.73
      single lobe 33.71
    cardiac resynchronization — *see* Insertion, cardiac resynchronization device
    cardiac support device (CSD) 37.41
    CorCap™ 37.41
    epicardial support device 37.41
    Lap-Band™ 44.95
    left atrial appendage 37.90
    left atrial filter 37.90
    left atrial occluder 37.90
    MitraClip® mitral leaflet clip 35.97
    prosthetic cardiac support device 37.41
    sternal fixation device with rigid plates 84.94
    vascular access 86.07

Insertion — *continued*
  device — *continued*
    ventricular support device 37.41
  diaphragm, vagina 96.17
  drainage tube
    kidney 55.02
      pelvis 55.12
    renal pelvis 55.12
  Dynesys® 84.82
  elbow prosthesis (total) 81.84
    revision 81.97
  electrode(s)
    bone growth stimulator (invasive) (percutaneous) (semi-invasive) — *see* category 78.9 ☑
    brain 02.93
      depth 02.93
      foramen ovale 02.93
      sphenoidal 02.96
    depth 02.93
    foramen ovale 02.93
    gastric 04.92
    heart (initial) (transvenous) 37.70
      atrium (initial) 37.73
        replacement 37.76
      atrium and ventricle (initial) 37.72
        replacement 37.76
      epicardium (sternotomy or thoracotomy approach) 37.74
      left ventricular coronary venous system 00.52
      temporary transvenous pacemaker system 37.78
        during and immediately following cardiac surgery 39.64
      ventricle (initial) 37.71
        replacement 37.76
    intracranial 02.93
    osteogenic (for bone growth stimulation) — *see* category 78.9 ☑
    peripheral nerve 04.92
    sacral nerve 04.92
    sphenoidal 02.96
    spine 03.93
  electroencephalographic receiver — *see* Implant, electroencephalographic receiver, by site
  electronic stimulator — *see* Implant, electronic stimulator, by site
  electrostimulator — *see* Implant, electronic stimulator, by site
  endograft(s), endovascular graft(s)
    endovascular, abdominal aorta 39.71
      fenestrated (branching) 39.78
    endovascular, head and neck vessels 39.72
    endovascular, other vessels (for aneurysm) 39.79
    endovascular, thoracic aorta 39.73
  endoprosthesis
    bile duct 51.87
    femoral head (bipolar) 81.52
    pancreatic duct 52.93
  envelope, antimicrobial 17.81
  epidural pegs 02.93
  external fixation device (bone) — *see* category 78.1 ☑
  eye valve implant 12.67
  facial bone implant (alloplastic) (synthetic) 76.92
  filling material, skin (filling of defect) 86.02
  filter
    vena cava (inferior) (superior) (transvenous) 38.7
  fixator, mini device (bone) — *see* category 78.1 ☑
  frame (stereotactic)
    for radiosurgery 93.59
  Gardner Wells tongs (skull) (with synchronous skeletal traction) 02.94
  gastric bubble (balloon) 44.93
  globe, into eye socket 16.69
  Greenfield filter 38.7
  halo device (skull) (with synchronous skeletal traction) 02.94

Insertion — *continued*
  Harrington rod (*see also* Fusion, spinal, by level)
    with dorsal, dorsolumbar fusion 81.05
  Harris pin 79.15
  heart
    assist system — *see* Implant, heart assist system
    cardiac support device (CSD) 37.41
    circulatory assist system — *see* Implant, heart assist system
    CorCap™ 37.41
    epicardial support device 37.41
    Impella® 37.68
    pacemaker — *see* Insertion, pacemaker, cardiac
    prosthetic cardiac support device 37.41
    pump (Kantrowitz) 37.62
    valve — *see* Replacement, heart valve
    ventricular support device 37.41
  hip prosthesis (partial) 81.52
    revision NOS 81.53
      acetabular and femoral components (total) 00.70
      acetabular component only 00.71
      acetabular liner and/or femoral head only 00.73
      femoral component only 00.72
      femoral head only and/or acetabular liner 00.73
      partial
        acetabular component only 00.71
        acetabular liner and/or femoral head only 00.73
        femoral component only 00.72
        femoral head only and/or acetabular liner 00.73
      total (acetabular and femoral components) 00.70
    total 81.51
      revision
        acetabular and femoral components (total) 00.70
        total (acetabular and femoral components) 00.70
  Holter valve 02.22
  Hufnagel valve — *see* Replacement, heart valve
  implant — *see* Insertion, prosthesis
  infusion pump 86.06
  interbody spinal fusion device 84.51
  intercostal catheter (with water seal), for drainage 34.04
    revision (with lysis of adhesions) 34.04
    thoracoscopic 34.06
  intra-arterial blood gas monitoring system 89.60
  intrauterine
    contraceptive device 69.7
    radium (intracavitary) 69.91
    tamponade (nonobstetric) 69.91
  Kantrowitz
    heart pump 37.62
    pulsation balloon (phase-shift) 37.61
  keratoprosthesis 11.73
  King-Mills umbrella device (heart) 35.52
  Kirschner wire 93.44
    with reduction of fracture or dislocation — *see* Reduction, fracture *and* Reduction, dislocation
  knee prosthesis (partial) (total) 81.54
    revision NOS 81.55
      femoral component 00.82
      partial
        femoral component 00.82
        patellar component 00.83
        tibial component 00.81
        tibial insert 00.84
      patellar component 00.83
      tibial component 00.81
      tibial insert 00.84
      total (all components) 00.80
  laminaria, cervix 69.93
  Lap-Band™ 44.95
  larynx, valved tube 31.75
  leads — *see* Insertion, electrode(s)

Insertion — *continued*
  lens, prosthetic (intraocular) 13.70
    with cataract extraction, one-stage 13.71
    secondary (subsequent to cataract extraction) 13.72
  limb lengthening device, internal, NOS 84.54
    with kinetic distraction 84.53
  loop recorder 37.79
  M-Brace™ 84.82
  metal staples into epiphyseal plate (*see also* Stapling, epiphyseal plate) 78.20
  minifixator device (bone) — *see* category 78.1 ☑
  Mobitz-Uddin umbrella, vena cava 38.7
  mold, vagina 96.15
  Moore (cup) 81.52
  Myringotomy device (button) (tube) 20.01
    with intubation 20.01
  nasobiliary drainage tube (endoscopic) 51.86
  nasogastric tube
    for
      decompression, intestinal 96.07
      feeding 96.6
  naso-intestinal tube 96.08
  nasolacrimal tube or stent 09.44
  nasopancreatic drainage tube (endoscopic) 52.97
  neuropacemaker — *see* Implant, neurostimulator, by site
  neurostimulator — *see* Implant, neurostimulator, by site
  non-coronary vessel
    stent(s) (stent graft)

> *Note: Also use 00.40, 00.41, 00.42, or 00.43 to show the total number of vessels treated. Use code 00.44 once to show procedure on a bifurcated vessel. In addition, use 00.45, 00.46, 00.47, or 00.48 to show the number of vascular stents inserted.*

    with
      angioplasty 39.50
      atherectomy 17.56
    basilar 00.64
    bypass — *omit code*
    carotid 00.63
    extracranial 00.64
    intracranial 00.65
    peripheral 39.90
      bare, drug-coated 39.90
      drug-eluting 00.55
    vertebral 00.64
  non-invasive (transcutaneous) (surface) stimulator 99.86
  obturator (orthodontic) 24.7
  ocular implant
    with synchronous
      enucleation 16.42
        with muscle attachment to implant 16.41
      evisceration 16.31
    following or secondary to enucleation 16.61
      evisceration 16.61
  Ommaya reservoir 02.22
  orbital implant (stent) (outside muscle cone) 16.69
    with orbitotomy 16.02
  orthodontic appliance (obturator) (wiring) 24.7
  outflow tract prosthesis (gusset type) (heart)
    in
      pulmonary valvuloplasty 35.26
      total repair of tetralogy of Fallot 35.81
  pacemaker
    brain — *see* Implant, neurostimulator, brain
    cardiac (device) (initial) (permanent) (replacement) 37.80
      dual-chamber device (initial) 37.83
        replacement 37.87
      during and immediately following cardiac surgery 39.64

Insertion — Insertion

Insertion — *continued*
  pacemaker — *continued*
    cardiac — *continued*
      resynchronization (biventricular
        pacemaker) (BiV pacemaker)
        (CRT-P) (device)
        device only (initial) (replacement)
          00.53
        total system (device and one or
          more leads) 00.50
        transvenous lead into left ventric-
          ular coronary venous sys-
          tem 00.52
      single-chamber device (initial) 37.81
        rate responsive 37.82
        replacement 37.85
          rate responsive 37.86
      temporary transvenous pacemaker
        system 37.78
        during and immediately follow-
          ing cardiac surgery 39.64
    carotid 39.89
    gastric 04.92
    heart — *see* Insertion, pacemaker, car-
      diac
    intracranial — *see* Implant, neurostimu-
      lator, intracranial
    neural — *see* Implant, neurostimulator,
      by site
    peripheral nerve — *see* Implant, neu-
      rostimulator, peripheral nerve
    spine — *see* Implant, neurostimulator,
      spine
    pacing catheter — *see* Insertion, pacemaker,
      cardiac
  pack
    auditory canal, external 96.11
    cervix (nonobstetrical) 67.0
      after delivery or abortion 75.8
      to assist delivery or induce labor 73.1
    rectum 96.19
    sella turcica 07.79
    vagina (nonobstetrical) 96.14
      after delivery or abortion 75.8
  palatal implant 27.64
  penile prosthesis (non-inflatable) (internal)
    64.95
    inflatable (internal) 64.97
  peridontal splint (orthodontic) 24.7
  peripheral blood vessel — *see* non-coronary vessel
  pessary
    cervix 96.18
      to assist delivery or induce labor 73.1
    vagina 96.18
  pharyngeal valve, artificial 31.75
  port, vascular access 86.07
  prostaglandin suppository (for abortion)
    96.49
  prosthesis, prosthetic device
    acetabulum (partial) 81.52
      hip 81.52
        revision NOS 81.53
          acetabular and femoral com-
            ponents (total) 00.70
          acetabular component only
            00.71
          acetabular liner and/or
            femoral head only
            00.73
          femoral component only
            00.72
          femoral head only and/or ac-
            etabular liner 00.73
          partial
            acetabular component
              only 00.71
            acetabular liner and/or
              femoral head only
              00.73
            femoral component only
              00.72
            femoral head only and/or
              acetabular liner
              00.73
          total (acetabular and femoral
            components) 00.70

Insertion — *continued*
  prosthesis, prosthetic device — *contin-
    ued*
    acetabulum — *continued*
      revision 81.53
    ankle (total) 81.56
    arm (bioelectric) (cineplastic) (kineplas-
      tic) 84.44
    biliary tract 51.99
    breast (bilateral) 85.54
      unilateral 85.53
    cardiac support device (CSD) (CorCap™)
      37.41
    chin (polyethylene) (silastic) 76.68
    elbow (total) 81.84
      revision 81.97
    extremity (bioelectric) (cineplastic)
      (kineplastic) 84.40
      lower 84.48
      upper 84.44
    fallopian tube 66.93
    femoral head (Austin-Moore) (bipolar)
      (Eicher) (Thompson) 81.52
    hip (partial) 81.52
      revision NOS 81.53
        acetabular and femoral compo-
          nents (total) 00.70
        acetabular component only 00.71
        acetabular liner and/or femoral
          head only 00.73
        femoral component only 00.72
        femoral head only and/or acetab-
          ular liner 00.73
        partial
          acetabular component only
            00.71
          acetabular liner and/or
            femoral head only
            00.73
          femoral component only
            00.72
          femoral head only and/or ac-
            etabular liner 00.73
        total (acetabular and femoral
          components) 00.70
      total 81.51
        revision
          acetabular and femoral com-
            ponents (total) 00.70
          total (acetabular and femoral
            components) 00.70
    joint — *see* Arthroplasty
    knee (partial) (total) 81.54
      revision NOS 81.55
        femoral component 00.82
        partial
          femoral component 00.82
          patellar component 00.83
          tibial component 00.81
          tibial insert 00.84
        patellar component 00.83
        tibial component 00.81
        tibial insert 00.84
        total (all components) 00.80
    leg (bioelectric) (cineplastic) (kineplastic)
      84.48
    lens 13.91
    ocular (secondary) 16.61
      with orbital exenteration 16.42
    outflow tract (gusset type) (heart)
      in
        pulmonary valvuloplasty 35.26
        total repair of tetralogy of Fallot
          35.81
    penis (internal) (noninflatable) 64.95
      with
        construction 64.43
        reconstruction 64.44
      inflatable (internal) 64.97
    Rosen (for urinary incontinence) 59.79
    shoulder
      partial 81.81
      revision 81.97
      total, NEC 81.80
        other 81.80
        reverse 81.88

Insertion — *continued*
  prosthesis, prosthetic device — *contin-
    ued*
    spine
      artificial disc, NOS 84.60
        cervical 84.62
          nucleus 84.61
          partial 84.61
          total 84.62
        lumbar, lumbosacral 84.65
          nucleus 84.64
          partial 84.64
          total 84.65
        thoracic (partial) (total) 84.63
      other device 84.59
    testicular (bilateral) (unilateral) 62.7
    toe 81.57
      hallux valgus repair 77.59
    vagina
      synthetic 70.95
  pseudophakos (*see also* Insertion, lens) 13.70
  pump, infusion 86.06
  radioactive isotope 92.27
  radium 92.27
  radon seeds 92.27
  Reuter bobbin (with intubation) 20.01
  Rickham reservoir 02.22
  Rosen prosthesis (for urinary incontinence)
    59.79
  Scribner shunt 39.93
  Sengstaken-Blakemore tube 96.06
  sensor (lead)
    intra-aneurysm sac pressure monitoring
      device 00.58
    intra-arterial, for continuous blood gas
      monitoring 89.60
    intracardiac or great vessel hemodynam-
      ic monitoring
      with lead 00.56
      without lead 38.26
  shunt — *see* Shunt
  sieve, vena cava 38.7
  skeletal muscle stimulator 83.92
  skull
    plate 02.05
    stereotactic frame 93.59
    tongs (Barton) (caliper) (Garder Wells)
      (Vinke) (with synchronous skele-
      tal traction) 02.94
  spacer (cement) (joint) (methylmethacry-
    late) 84.56
    spine 84.51
  sphenoidal electrodes 02.96
  spine
    bone void filler
      that with percutaneous vertebral
        augmentation 81.66
      that with percutaneous vertebroplas-
        ty 81.65
    cage (BAK) 84.51
    facet replacement device(s) 84.84
    interbody spinal fusion device 84.51
    interspinous process decompression
      device 84.80
    non-fusion stabilization device — *see*
      category 84.8
    pedicle-based dynamic stabilization de-
      vice(s) 84.82
    posterior motion preservation device(s)
      — *see* category 84.8
    spacer 84.51
  Spitz-Holter valve 02.2 ☑
  Steinmann pin 93.44
    with reduction of fracture or dislocation
      — *see* Reduction, fracture *and*
      Reduction, dislocation
  stent(s) (stent graft)
    aqueous drainage 12.67

Insertion — *continued*
  stent(s) — *continued*
    artery (bare) (bonded) (drug-coated)
      (non-drug-eluting)

> *Note — Also use 00.40, 00.41, 00.42,
> or 00.43 to show the total number of
> vessels treated. Use code 00.44 once to
> show procedure on a bifurcated vessel.
> In addition, use 00.45, 00.46, 00.47, or
> 00.48 to show the number of vascular
> stents inserted.*

      basilar 00.64
      carotid 00.63
      cerebrovascular
        cerebral (intracranial) 00.65
        precerebral (extracranial) 00.64
          carotid 00.63
      coronary (bare) (bonded) (drug-
        coated) (non-drug-eluting)
        36.06
        drug-eluting 36.07
      extracranial 00.64
        carotid 00.63
      femoral artery, superficial 39.90
        drug-eluting 00.60
        non-drug-eluting 39.90
      intracranial 00.65
      non-coronary vessel
        basilar 00.64
        carotid 00.63
        extracranial 00.64
        intracranial 00.65
        peripheral 39.90
          bare, drug-coated 39.90
          drug-eluting 00.55
        vertebral 00.64
    bile duct 51.43
      endoscopic 51.87
      percutaneous transhepatic 51.98
    colon
      endoscopic (fluoroscopic guidance)
        46.86
      other 46.87
    coronary (artery) (bare) (bonded) (drug-
      coated) (non-drug-eluting) 36.06

> *Note — Also use 00.40, 00.41, 00.42,
> or 00.43 to show the total number of
> vessels treated. Use code 00.44 once to
> show procedure on a bifurcated vessel.
> In addition, use 00.45, 00.46, 00.47, or
> 00.48 to show the number of vascular
> stents inserted.*

      drug-eluting 36.07
    esophagus (endoscopic) (fluoroscopic)
      42.81
    mesenteric 39.90
      bare, drug-coated 39.90
      drug-eluting 00.55
    non-coronary vessel

> *Note — Also use 00.40, 00.41, 00.42,
> or 00.43 to show the total number of
> vessels treated. Use code 00.44 once to
> show procedure on a bifurcated vessel.
> In addition, use 00.45, 00.46, 00.47, or
> 00.48 to show the number of vascular
> stents inserted.*

      with angioplasty or atherectomy
        39.50
      with bypass — *omit code*
      basilar 00.64
      carotid 00.63
      extracranial 00.64
      femoral artery, superficial 39.90
        drug-eluting 00.60
        non-drug-eluting 39.90
      intracranial 00.65
      mesenteric 39.90
        bare, drug-coated 39.90
        drug-eluting 00.55
      peripheral 39.90
        bare, drug-coated 39.90
        drug-eluting 00.55
      renal 39.90
        bare, drug-coated 39.90

☑ **Additional Digit Required — Refer to the Tabular List for Digit Selection**   ▽ **Subterms under main terms may continue to next column or page**

Insertion — *continued*
  stent(s) — *continued*
    non-coronary vessel — *continued*
      renal — *continued*
        drug-eluting 00.55
      vertebral 00.64
    pancreatic duct 52.92
      endoscopic 52.93
    peripheral vessel 39.90

> Note — Also use 00.40, 00.41, 00.42, or 00.43 to show the total number of vessels treated. Use code 00.44 once to show procedure on a bifurcated vessel. In addition, use 00.45, 00.46, 00.47, or 00.48 to show the number of vascular stents inserted.

      bare, drug-coated 39.90
      drug-eluting 00.55
      femoral artery, superficial, drug-eluting 00.60
      precerebral 00.64

> Note — Also use 00.40, 00.41, 00.42, or 00.43 to show the total number of vessels treated. Use code 00.44 once to show procedure on a bifurcated vessel. In addition, use 00.45, 00.46, 00.47, or 00.48 to show the number of vascular stents inserted.

      renal 39.90
      bare, drug-coated 39.90
      drug-eluting 00.55
      subclavian 39.90

> Note — Also use 00.40, 00.41, 00.42, or 00.43 to show the total number of vessels treated. Use code 00.44 once to show procedure on a bifurcated vessel In addition, use 00.45, 00.46, 00.47, or 00.48 to show the number of vascular stents inserted.

      bare, drug-coated 39.90
      drug-eluting 00.55
      tracheobronchial 96.05
      vertebral 00.64

> Note — Also use 00.40, 00.41, 00.42, or 00.43 to show the total number of vessels treated. Use code 00.44 once to show procedure on a bifurcated vessel. In addition, use 00.45, 00.46, 00.47, or 00.48 to show the number of vascular stents inserted.

  sternal fixation device with rigid plates 84.94
  stimoceiver — *see* Implant, neurostimulator, by site
  stimulator for bone growth — *see* category 78.9 ☑
  subdural
    grids 02.93
    strips 02.93
  suppository
    prostaglandin (for abortion) 96.49
    vagina 96.49
  Swan-Ganz catheter (pulmonary) 89.64
  tampon
    esophagus 96.06
    uterus 69.91
    vagina 96.14
      after delivery or abortion 75.8
  Tandem™ heart 37.68
  telescope (IMT) (miniature) 13.91
  testicular prosthesis (bilateral) (unilateral) 62.7
  tissue expander (skin) NEC 86.93
    breast 85.95
  tissue mandril (peripheral vessel) (Dacron) (Spark's type) 39.99
    with
      blood vessel repair 39.56
      vascular bypass or shunt — *see* Bypass, vascular
  tongs, skull (with synchronous skeletal traction) 02.94

Insertion — *continued*
  totally implanted device for bone growth (invasive) — *see* category 78.9 ☑
  tube (*see also* Catheterization and Intubation)
    bile duct 51.43
      endoscopic 51.87
    chest 34.04
      revision (with lysis of adhesions) 34.04
        thoracoscopic 34.06
      thoracoscopic 34.06
    endotracheal 96.04
    esophagus (nonoperative) (Sengstaken) 96.06
      permanent (silicone) (Souttar) 42.81
    feeding
      esophageal 42.81
      gastric 96.6
      nasogastric 96.6
    gastric
      by gastrostomy — *see* category 43.1 ☑
      for
        decompression, intestinal 96.07
        feeding 96.6
    intercostal catheter (with water seal), for drainage 34.04
      revision (with lysis of adhe-sions) 34.04
        thoracoscopic 34.06
      thoracoscopic 34.06
    Miller-Abbott (for intestinal decompression) 96.08
    nasobiliary (drainage) 51.86
    nasogastric (for intestinal decompression) NEC 96.07
    naso-intestinal 96.08
    nasopancreatic drainage (endoscopic) 52.97
    pancreatic duct 52.92
      endoscopic 52.93
    rectum 96.09
    stomach (nasogastric) (for intestinal decompression) NEC 96.07
      for feeding 96.6
    tracheobronchial 96.05
  umbrella device
    atrial septum (King-Mills) 35.52
    vena cava (Mobitz-Uddin) 38.7
  ureteral stent (transurethral) 59.8
    with ureterotomy 59.8 *[56.2]*
  urinary sphincter, artificial (AUS) (inflatable) 58.93
  vaginal mold 96.15
  valve(s)
    bronchus
      multiple lobes 33.73
      single lobe 33.71
    Holter 02.22
    Hufnagel — *see* Replacement, heart valve
    pharyngeal (artificial) 31.75
    Spitz-Holter 02.22
    vas deferens 63.95
  vascular access device, totally implantable 86.07
  vena cava sieve or umbrella 38.7
  Vinke tongs (skull) (with synchronous skeletal traction) 02.94
  X Stop™ 84.80

Instillation
  bladder 96.49
  digestive tract, except gastric gavage 96.43
  genitourinary NEC 96.49
  radioisotope (intracavitary) (intravenous) 92.28
  thoracic cavity 34.92

Insufflation
  Eustachian tube 20.8
  fallopian tube (air) (dye) (gas) (saline) 66.8
    for radiography — *see* Hysterosalpingography
    therapeutic substance 66.95
  lumbar retroperitoneal, bilateral 88.15

Intubation — *see also* Catheterization and Insertion

Intercricothyroidotomy (for assistance in breathing) 31.1
Interleukin-2, infusion
  high-dose 00.15
  low-dose 99.28
Intermittent positive pressure breathing (IPPB) 93.91
Interposition operation
  antesternal or antethoracic NEC (*see also* Anastomosis, esophagus, antesternal, with, interposition) 42.68
  esophageal reconstruction (intrathoracic) (retrosternal) NEC (*see also* Anastomosis, esophagus, with, interposition) 42.58
  uterine suspension 69.21
Interrogation
  cardioverter-defibrillator, automatic (AICD)
    with catheter based invasive electrophysiologic testing 37.26
    with NIPS (arrhythmia induction) 37.20
    interrogation only (bedside device check) 89.49
  CRT-D (cardiac resynchronization defibrillator)
    with catheter based invasive electrophysiologic testing 37.26
    with NIPS (arrhythmia induction) 37.20
    interrogation only (bedside device check) 89.49
  CRT-P (cardiac resynchronization pacemaker)
    with catheter based invasive electrophysiologic testing 37.26
    with NIPS (arrhythmia induction) 37.20
    interrogation only (bedside device check) 89.45
  pacemaker
    with catheter based invasive electrophysiologic testing 37.26
    with NIPS (arrhythmia induction) 37.20
    interrogation only (bedside device check) 89.45
Interruption
  vena cava (inferior) (superior) 38.7
Interview (evaluation) (diagnostic)
  medical, except psychiatric 89.05
    brief (abbreviated history) 89.01
    comprehensive (history and evaluation of new problem) 89.03
    limited (interval history) 89.02
    specified type NEC 89.04
  psychiatric NEC 94.19
    follow-up 94.19
    initial 94.19
    pre-commitment 94.13
Intimectomy 38.10
  abdominal 38.16
  aorta (arch) (ascending) (descending) 38.14
  head and neck NEC 38.12
  intracranial NEC 38.11
  lower limb 38.18
  thoracic NEC 38.15
  upper limb 38.13
Intraoperative anesthetic effect monitoring and titration (IAEMT) 00.94 *[89.14]*
Introduction
  orthodontic appliance 24.7
  therapeutic substance (acting locally or systemically) NEC 99.29
    bursa 83.96
      hand 82.94
    fascia 83.98
      hand 82.96
    heart 37.92
    joint 81.92
      temporomandibular 76.96
    ligament (joint) 81.92
    pericardium 37.93
    soft tissue NEC 83.98
      hand 82.96
    tendon 83.97
      hand 82.95
    vein 39.92
Intubation — *see also* Catheterization and Insertion

Intubation — *see also* Catheterization and Insertion — *continued*
  bile duct(s) 51.59
    common 51.51
      endoscopic 51.87
    endoscopic 51.87
  esophagus (nonoperative) (Sengstaken) 96.06
    permanent tube (silicone) (Souttar) 42.81
  Eustachian tube 20.8
  intestine (for decompression) 96.08
  lacrimal for
    dilation 09.42
    tear drainage, intranasal 09.81
  larynx 96.05
  nasobiliary (drainage) 51.86
  nasogastric
    for
      decompression, intestinal 96.07
      feeding 96.6
  naso-intestinal 96.08
  nasolacrimal (duct) (with irrigation) 09.44
  nasopancreatic drainage (endoscopic) 52.97
  respiratory tract NEC 96.05
  small intestine (Miller-Abbott) 96.08
  stomach (nasogastric) (for intestinal decompression) NEC 96.07
    for feeding 96.6
  trachea 96.04
  ventriculocisternal 02.22
Invagination, diverticulum
  gastric 44.69
    laparoscopic 44.68
  pharynx 29.59
  stomach 44.69
    laparoscopic 44.68
Inversion
  appendix 47.99
  diverticulum
    gastric 44.69
      laparoscopic 44.68
    intestine
      large 45.49
        endoscopic 45.43
      small 45.34
    stomach 44.69
      laparoscopic 44.68
  tunica vaginalis 61.49
IOERT (intra-operative electron radiation therapy) 92.41
IOM (intra-operative neurophysiologic monitoring) 00.94
Ionization, medical 99.27
Iontherapy 99.27
Iontophoresis 99.27
Iridectomy (basal) (buttonhole) (optical) (peripheral) (total) 12.14
  with
    capsulectomy 13.65
    cataract extraction — *see* Extraction, cataract
    filtering operation (for glaucoma) NEC 12.65
    scleral
      fistulization 12.65
      thermocauterization 12.62
      trephination 12.61
Iridencleisis 12.63
Iridesis 12.63
Irido-capsulectomy 13.65
Iridocyclectomy 12.44
Iridocystectomy 12.42
Iridodesis 12.63
Iridoplasty NEC 12.39
Iridosclerectomy 12.65
Iridosclerotomy 12.69
Iridotasis 12.63
Iridotomy 12.12
  by photocoagulation 12.12
  with transfixion 12.11
  for iris bombé 12.11
  specified type NEC 12.12
Iron lung 93.99
Irradiation
  gamma, stereotactic 92.32

Irrigation

anterior chamber (eye) 12.91
bronchus NEC 96.56
canaliculus 09.42
catheter
  ureter 96.46
  urinary, indwelling NEC 96.48
  vascular 96.57
  ventricular 02.41
  wound 96.58
cholecystostomy 96.41
cornea 96.51
  with removal of foreign body 98.21
corpus cavernosum 64.98
cystostomy 96.47
ear (removal of cerumen) 96.52
enterostomy 96.36
eye 96.51
  with removal of foreign body 98.21
gastrostomy 96.36
lacrimal
  canaliculi 09.42
  punctum 09.41
muscle 83.02
  hand 82.02
nasal
  passages 96.53
  sinus 22.00
nasolacrimal duct 09.43
  with insertion of tube or stent 09.44
nephrostomy 96.45
peritoneal 54.25
pyelostomy 96.45
rectal 96.39
stomach 96.33
tendon (sheath) 83.01
  hand 82.01
trachea NEC 96.56
traumatic cataract 13.3
tube
  biliary NEC 96.41
  nasogastric NEC 96.34
  pancreatic 96.42
ureterostomy 96.46
ventricular shunt 02.41
wound (cleaning) NEC 96.59
Irving operation (tubal ligation) 66.32
Irwin operation — *see also* Osteotomy 77.30
Ischiectomy (partial) 77.89
  total 77.99
Ischiopubiotomy 77.39
Isolation
  after contact with infectious disease 99.84
  ileal loop 45.51
  intestinal segment or pedicle flap
    large 45.52
    small 45.51
Isthmectomy, thyroid — *see also* Thyroidectomy, partial 06.39
IVUS — *see* Ultrasound, intravascular, by site

J

Jaboulay operation (gastroduodenostomy) 44.39
  laparoscopic 44.38
Janeway operation (permanent gastrostomy) 43.19
Jatene operation (arterial switch) 35.84
Jejunectomy 45.62
Jejunocecostomy 45.93
Jejunocholecystostomy 51.32
Jejunocolostomy 45.93
Jejunoileostomy 45.91
Jejunojejunostomy 45.91
Jejunopexy 46.61
Jejunorrhaphy 46.73
Jejunostomy (feeding) 46.39
  delayed opening 46.31
  loop 46.01
  percutaneous (endoscopic) (PEJ) 46.32
  revision 46.41
Jejunotomy 45.02
Johanson operation (urethral reconstruction) 58.46

Jones operation

claw toe (transfer of extensor hallucis longus tendon) 77.57
  modified (with arthrodesis) 77.57
  unilateral 77.61
dacryocystorhinostomy 09.81
hammer toe (interphalangeal fusion) 77.56
modified (tendon transfer with arthrodesis) 77.57
repair of peroneal tendon 83.88
Joplin operation (exostectomy with tendon transfer) 77.53

K

Kader operation (temporary gastrostomy) 43.19
Kasai portoenterostomy 51.37
Kaufman operation (for urinary stress incontinence) 59.79
Kazanjiian operation (buccal vestibular sulcus extension) 24.91
Kehr operation (hepatopexy) 50.69
Keller operation (bunionectomy) 77.59
Kelly (-Kennedy) operation (urethrovesical plication) 59.3
Kelly-Stoeckel operation (urethrovesical plication) 59.3
Kelotomy 53.9
Keratectomy (complete) (partial) (superficial) 11.49
  for pterygium 11.39
    with corneal graft 11.32
Keratocentesis (for hyphema) 12.91
Keratomileusis 11.71
Keratophakia 11.72
Keratoplasty (tectonic) (with autograft) (with homograft) 11.60
  lamellar (nonpenetrating) (with homograft) 11.62
    with autograft 11.61
  penetrating (full-thickness) (with homograft) 11.64
    with autograft 11.63
  perforating — *see* Keratoplasty, penetrating
  refractive 11.71
  specified type NEC 11.69
Keratoprosthesis 11.73
Keratotomy (delimiting) (posterior) 11.1
  radial (refractive) 11.75
Kerr operation (low cervical cesarean section) 74.1
Kessler operation (arthroplasty, carpometacarpal joint) 81.74
Kidner operation (excision of accessory navicular bone) (with tendon transfer) 77.98
Killian operation (frontal sinusotomy) 22.41
Kineplasty — *see* Cineplasty
King-Steelquist operation (hind-quarter amputation) 84.19
Kirk operation (amputation through thigh) 84.17
Kockogram (ileal conduitogram) 87.78
Kockoscopy 45.12
Kock pouch
  bowel anastomosis — *omit code*
  continent ileostomy 46.22
  cutaneous uretero-ileostomy 56.51
  ESWL (extracorporeal shockwave lithotripsy) 98.51
  removal, calculus 57.19
  revision, cutaneous uretero-ileostomy 56.52
  urinary diversion procedure 56.51
Kondoleon operation (correction of lymphedema) 40.9
Krause operation (sympathetic denervation) 05.29
Kroener operation (partial salpingectomy) 66.69
Kroenlein operation (lateral orbitotomy) 16.01
Krönig operation (low cervical cesarean section) 74.1
Krukenberg operation (reconstruction of below-elbow amputation) 82.89
Kuhnt-Szymanowski operation (ectropion repair with lid reconstruction) 08.44
Kyphoplasty 81.66

L

Labbe operation (gastrotomy) 43.0
Labiectomy (bilateral) 71.62
  unilateral 71.61
Labyrinthectomy (transtympanic) 20.79
Labyrinthotomy (transtympanic) 20.79
Ladd operation (mobilization of intestine) 54.95
Lagrange operation (iridosclerectomy) 12.65
Lambrinudi operation (triple arthrodesis) 81.12
Laminectomy (decompression) (for exploration) 03.09
  as operative approach — *omit code*
  with
    excision of herniated intervertebral disc (nucleus pulposus) 80.51
    excision of other intraspinal lesion (tumor) 03.4
  reopening of site 03.02
Laminography — *see* Radiography
Laminoplasty, expansile 03.09
Laminotomy (decompression) (for exploration) 03.09
  as operative approach — *omit code*
  reopening of site 03.02
Langenbeck operation (cleft palate repair) 27.62
Laparoamnioscopy 75.31
Laparorrhaphy 54.63
Laparoscopy 54.21
  with
    biopsy (intra-abdominal) 54.24
      uterine ligaments 68.15
      uterus 68.16
    destruction of fallopian tubes — *see* Destruction, fallopian tube
Laparotomy NEC 54.19
  as operative approach — *omit code*
  exploratory (pelvic) 54.11
  reopening of recent operative site (for control of hemorrhage) (for exploration) (for incision of hematoma) 54.12
Laparotrachelotomy 74.1
Lapidus operation (bunionectomy with metatarsal osteotomy) 77.51
Larry operation (shoulder disarticulation) 84.08
Laryngectomy
  with radical neck dissection (with synchronous thyroidectomy) (with synchronous tracheostomy) 30.4
  complete (with partial laryngectomy) (with synchronous tracheostomy) 30.3
    with radical neck dissection (with synchronous thyroidectomy) (with synchronous tracheostomy) 30.4
  frontolateral partial (extended) 30.29
  glottosupraglottic partial 30.29
  lateral partial 30.29
  partial (frontolateral) (glottosupraglottic) (lateral) (submucous) (supraglottic) (vertical) 30.29
  radical (with synchronous thyroidectomy) (with synchronous tracheostomy) 30.4
  submucous (partial) 30.29
  supraglottic partial 30.29
  total (with partial pharyngectomy) (with synchronous tracheostomy) 30.3
    with radical neck dissection (with synchronous thyroidectomy) (with synchronous tracheostomy) 30.4
  vertical partial 30.29
  wide field 30.3
Laryngocentesis 31.3
Laryngoesophagectomy 30.4
Laryngofissure 30.29
Laryngogram 87.09
  contrast 87.07
Laryngopharyngectomy (with synchronous tracheostomy) 30.3
  radical (with synchronous thyroidectomy) 30.4
Laryngopharyngoesophagectomy (with synchronous tracheostomy) 30.3

Laryngopharyngoesophagectomy — *continued*
  with radical neck dissection (with synchronous thyroidectomy) 30.4
Laryngoplasty 31.69
Laryngorrhaphy 31.61
Laryngoscopy (suspension) (through artificial stoma) 31.42
Laryngostomy (permanent) 31.29
  revision 31.63
  temporary (emergency) 31.1
Laryngotomy 31.3
Laryngotracheobronchoscopy 33.23
  with biopsy 33.24
Laryngotracheoscopy 31.42
Laryngotracheostomy (permanent) 31.29
  temporary (emergency) 31.1
Laryngotracheotomy (temporary) 31.1
  permanent 31.29
Laser — *see also* Coagulation, Destruction, and Photocoagulation by site
  angioplasty, percutaneous transluminal 39.59
  coronary — *see* Angioplasty, coronary
Laser interstitial thermal therapy (LITT) **under guidance**
  lesion
    brain 17.61
    breast 17.69
    head and neck 17.62
    liver 17.63
    lung 17.69
    prostate 17.69
    thyroid 17.62
Lash operation
  internal cervical os repair 67.59
  laparoscopic supracervical hysterectomy 68.31
LASIK (laser-assisted in situ keratomileusis) 11.71
Latzko operation
  cesarean section 74.2
  colpocleisis 70.8
Lavage
  antral 22.00
  bronchus NEC 96.56
    diagnostic (endoscopic) bronchoalveolar lavage (BAL) (Mini-BAL) 33.24
  endotracheal 96.56
  gastric 96.33
  lung (total) (whole) 33.99
    diagnostic (endoscopic) bronchoalveolar lavage (BAL) 33.24
  nasal sinus(es) 22.00
    by puncture 22.01
    through natural ostium 22.02
  peritoneal (diagnostic) 54.25
  trachea NEC 96.56
Leadbetter operation (urethral reconstruction) 58.46
Leadbetter-Politano operation (ureteroneocystostomy) 56.74
LEEP (loop electrosurgical excision procedure) of cervix 67.32
Le Fort operation (colpocleisis) 70.8
LeMesurier operation (cleft lip repair) 27.54
Lengthening
  bone (with bone graft) 78.30
    femur 78.35
    for reconstruction of thumb 82.69
    specified site NEC (*see also* category 78.3 ☑)
    tibia 78.37
    ulna 78.33
  extraocular muscle NEC 15.21
    multiple (two or more muscles) 15.4
  fascia 83.89
    hand 82.89
  hamstring NEC 83.85
  heel cord 83.85
  leg
    femur 78.35
    tibia 78.37
  levator palpebrae muscle 08.38
  muscle 83.85
    extraocular 15.21

Lengthening — *continued*
- muscle — *continued*
  - extraocular — *continued*
    - multiple (two or more muscles) 15.4
    - hand 82.55
  - palate 27.62
    - secondary or subsequent 27.63
  - tendon 83.85
    - for claw toe repair 77.57
    - hand 82.55

Leriche operation (periarterial sympathectomy) 05.25

Leucotomy, leukotomy 01.32

Leukopheresis, therapeutic 99.72

Lid suture operation (blepharoptosis) 08.31

Ligation
- adrenal vessel (artery) (vein) 07.43
- aneurysm 39.52
- appendages, dermal 86.26
- arteriovenous fistula 39.53
  - coronary artery 36.99
- artery 38.80
  - abdominal 38.86
  - adrenal 07.43
  - aorta (arch) (ascending) (descending) 38.84
  - coronary (anomalous) 36.99
  - ethmoidal 21.04
  - external carotid 21.06
  - for control of epistaxis — *see* Control, epistaxis
  - head and neck NEC 38.82
  - intracranial NEC 38.81
  - lower limb 38.88
  - maxillary (transantral) 21.05
  - middle meningeal 02.13
  - thoracic NEC 38.85
  - thyroid 06.92
  - upper limb 38.83
- atrium, heart 37.99
- auricle, heart 37.99
- bleeding vessel — *see* Control, hemorrhage
- blood vessel 38.80
  - abdominal
    - artery 38.86
    - vein 38.87
  - adrenal 07.43
  - aorta (arch) (ascending) (descending) 38.84
  - esophagus 42.91
    - endoscopic 42.33
  - head and neck NEC 38.82
  - intracranial NEC 38.81
  - lower limb
    - artery 38.88
    - vein 38.89
  - meningeal (artery) (longitudinal sinus) 02.13
  - thoracic NEC 38.85
  - thyroid 06.92
  - upper limb (artery) (vein) 38.83
- bronchus 33.92
- cisterna chyli 40.64
- coronary
  - artery (anomalous) 36.99
  - sinus 36.39
- dermal appendage 86.26
- ductus arteriosus, patent 38.85
- esophageal vessel 42.91
  - endoscopic 42.33
- ethmoidal artery 21.04
- external carotid artery 21.06
- fallopian tube (bilateral) (remaining) (solitary) 66.39
  - by endoscopy (culdoscopy) (hysteroscopy) (laparoscopy) (peritoneoscopy) 66.29
  - with
    - crushing 66.31
      - by endoscopy (laparoscopy) 66.21
    - division 66.32
      - by endoscopy (culdoscopy) (laparoscopy) (peritoneoscopy) 66.22
    - Falope ring 66.39

Ligation — *continued*
- fallopian tube — *continued*
  - with — *continued*
    - Falope ring — *continued*
      - by endoscopy (laparoscopy) 66.29
    - unilateral 66.92
- fistula, arteriovenous 39.53
  - coronary artery 36.99
- gastric
  - artery 38.86
  - varices 44.91
    - endoscopic 43.41
- hemorrhoids 49.45
- longitudinal sinus (superior) 02.13
- lymphatic (channel) (peripheral) 40.9
  - thoracic duct 40.64
- maxillary artery 21.05
- meningeal vessel 02.13
- spermatic
  - cord 63.72
    - varicocele 63.1
  - vein (high) 63.1
- splenic vessels 38.86
- subclavian artery 38.85
- superior longitudinal sinus 02.13
- supernumerary digit 86.26
- thoracic duct 40.64
- thyroid vessel (artery) (vein) 06.92
- toes (supernumerary) 86.26
- tooth 93.55
  - impacted 24.6
- ulcer (peptic) (base) (bed) (bleeding vessel) 44.40
  - duodenal 44.42
  - gastric 44.41
- ureter 56.95
- varices
  - esophageal 42.91
    - endoscopic 42.33
  - gastric 44.91
    - endoscopic 43.41
  - peripheral vein (lower limb) 38.59
  - upper limb 38.53
- varicocele 63.1
- vas deferens 63.71
- vein 38.80
  - abdominal 38.87
  - adrenal 07.43
  - head and neck NEC 38.82
  - intracranial NEC 38.81
  - lower limb 38.89
  - spermatic, high 63.1
  - thoracic NEC 38.85
  - thyroid 06.92
  - upper limb 38.83
  - varicose 38.50
    - abdominal 38.57
    - esophagus 42.91
      - endoscopic 42.33
    - gastric 44.91
      - endoscopic 43.41
    - head and neck NEC 38.52
    - intracranial NEC 38.51
    - lower limb 38.59
    - stomach 44.91
    - thoracic NEC 38.55
    - upper limb 38.53
- vena cava, inferior 38.7
- venous connection between anomalous vein to
  - left innominate vein 35.82
  - superior vena cava 35.82
- wart 86.26

Light coagulation — *see* Photocoagulation

Lindholm operation (repair of ruptured tendon) 83.88

Lingulectomy, lung 32.39

Linton operation (varicose vein) 38.59

Lipectomy (subcutaneous tissue) (abdominal) (submental) 86.83

Liposuction 86.83

Lip reading training 95.49

Lip shave 27.43

Lisfranc operation
- foot amputation 84.12

Lisfranc operation — *continued*
- shoulder disarticulation 84.08

Litholapaxy, bladder 57.0
- by incision 57.19

Lithotomy
- bile passage 51.49
- bladder (urinary) 57.19
- common duct 51.41
  - percutaneous 51.96
- gallbladder 51.04
- hepatic duct 51.49
- kidney 55.01
  - percutaneous 55.03
- ureter 56.2

Lithotripsy
- bile duct NEC 51.49
  - extracorporeal shockwave (ESWL) 98.52
- bladder 57.0
  - with ultrasonic fragmentation 57.0 [59.95]
  - extracorporeal shockwave (ESWL) 98.51
- extracorporeal shockwave (ESWL) NEC 98.59
  - bile duct 98.52
  - bladder (urinary) 98.51
  - gallbladder 98.52
  - kidney 98.51
  - Kock pouch 98.51
  - renal pelvis 98.51
  - specified site NEC 98.59
  - ureter 98.51
- gallbladder NEC 51.04
  - endoscopic 51.88
  - extracorporeal shockwave (ESWL) 98.52
- kidney 56.0
  - extracorporeal shockwave (ESWL) 98.51
  - percutaneous nephrostomy with fragmentation (laser) (ultrasound) 55.04
- renal pelvis 56.0
  - extracorporeal shockwave (ESWL) 98.51
  - percutaneous nephrostomy with fragmentation (laser) (ultrasound) 55.04
- ureter 56.0
  - extracorporeal shockwave (ESWL) 98.51

Littlewood operation (forequarter amputation) 84.09

LITT (laser interstitial thermal therapy) **under guidance**
- lesion
  - brain 17.61
  - breast 17.69
  - head and neck 17.62
  - liver 17.63
  - lung 17.69
  - prostate 17.69
  - thyroid 17.62

LLETZ (large loop excision of the transformation zone) of cervix 67.32

Lloyd-Davies operation (abdominoperineal resection), NOS 48.50
- laparoscopic 48.51
- open 48.52
- other 48.59

Lobectomy
- brain 01.53
  - partial 01.59
- liver (with partial excision of adjacent lobes) 50.3
- lung (complete) 32.49
  - partial 32.39
    - thoracoscopic 32.30
  - segmental (with resection of adjacent lobes) 32.49
    - thoracoscopic 32.41
  - thoracoscopic 32.41
- thyroid (total) (unilateral) (with removal of isthmus) (with removal of portion of remaining lobe) 06.2
  - partial (*see also* Thyroidectomy, partial) 06.39
  - substernal 06.51
  - subtotal (*see also* Thyroidectomy, partial) 06.39

Lobotomy, brain 01.32

Localization, placenta 88.78
- by RISA injection 92.17

Longmire operation (bile duct anastomosis) 51.39

Loop ileal stoma — *see also* Ileostomy 46.01

Loopogram 87.78

Looposcopy (ileal conduit) 56.35

Lord operation
- dilation of anal canal for hemorrhoids 49.49
- hemorrhoidectomy 49.49
- orchidopexy 62.5

Lower GI series (x-ray) 87.64

Lucas and Murray operation (knee arthrodesis with plate) 81.22

Lumpectomy
- breast 85.21
- specified site — *see* Excision, lesion, by site

Lymphadenectomy (simple) — *see also* Excision, lymph, node 40.29

Lymphadenotomy 40.0

Lymphangiectomy (radical) — *see also* Excision, lymph, node, by site, radical 40.50

Lymphangiogram
- abdominal 88.04
- cervical 87.08
- intrathoracic 87.34
- lower limb 88.36
- pelvic 88.04
- upper limb 88.34

Lymphangioplasty 40.9

Lymphangiorrhaphy 40.9

Lymphangiotomy 40.0

Lymphaticostomy 40.9
- thoracic duct 40.62

Lysis
- adhesions

> *Note:*
> *blunt — omit code*
> *digital — omit code*
> *manual — omit code*
> *mechanical — omit code*
> *without instrumentation — omit code*

- abdominal 54.59
  - laparoscopic 54.51
- appendiceal 54.59
  - laparoscopic 54.51
- artery-vein-nerve bundle 39.91
- biliary tract 54.59
  - laparoscopic 54.51
- bladder (neck) (intraluminal) 57.12
  - external 59.11
    - laparoscopic 59.12
  - transurethral 57.41
- blood vessels 39.91
- bone — *see* category 78.4 ☑
- bursa 83.91
  - by stretching or manipulation 93.28
  - hand 82.91
- cartilage of joint 93.26
- chest wall 33.99
- choanae (nasopharynx) 29.54
- conjunctiva 10.5
- corneovitreal 12.34
- cortical (brain) 02.91
- ear, middle 20.23
- Eustachean tube 20.8
- extraocular muscle 15.7
- extrauterine 54.59
  - laparoscopic 54.51
- eyelid 08.09
  - and conjunctiva 10.5
- eye muscle 15.7
- fallopian tube 65.89
  - laparoscopic 65.81
- fascia 83.91
  - hand 82.91
  - by stretching or manipulation 93.26
- gallbladder 54.59
  - laparoscopic 54.51
- ganglion (peripheral) NEC 04.49
  - cranial NEC 04.42
- hand 82.91
  - by stretching or manipulation 93.26
- heart 37.10
- intestines 54.59

☑ Additional Digit Required — Refer to the Tabular List for Digit Selection
▽ Subterms under main terms may continue to next column or page
2014 ICD-9-CM
861

Index

Lysis — Measurement

Nephrostomy — *continued*
  percutaneous — *continued*
    with fragmentation (ultrasound) 55.04
Nephrotomogram, nephrotomography NEC 87.72
Nephrotomy 55.01
Nephroureterectomy (with bladder cuff) 55.51
Nephroureterocystectomy 55.51 *[57.79]*
Nerve block (cranial) (peripheral) NEC — *see also* Block, by site 04.81
Neurectasis (cranial) (peripheral) 04.91
Neurectomy (cranial) (infraorbital) (occipital) (peripheral) (spinal) NEC 04.07
  gastric (vagus) (*see also* Vagotomy) 44.00
  opticociliary 12.79
  paracervical 05.22
  presacral 05.24
  retrogasserian 04.07
  sympathetic — *see* Sympathectomy
  trigeminal 04.07
  tympanic 20.91
Neurexeresis NEC 04.07
Neuroablation
  radiofrequency 04.2
Neuroanastomosis (cranial) (peripheral) NEC 04.74
  accessory-facial 04.72
  accessory-hypoglossal 04.73
  hypoglossal-facial 04.71
NeuroFlo™ catheter for partial (temporary) **abdominal aorta occlusion** 39.77
Neurolysis (peripheral nerve) NEC 04.49
  carpal tunnel 04.43
  cranial nerve NEC 04.42
  spinal (cord) (nerve roots) 03.6
  tarsal tunnel 04.44
  trigeminal nerve 04.41
Neuromonitoring
  intra-operative 00.94
Neuroplasty (cranial) (peripheral) NEC 04.79
  of old injury (delayed repair) 04.76
  revision 04.75
Neurorrhaphy (cranial) (peripheral) 04.3
Neurotomy (cranial) (peripheral) (spinal) NEC 04.04
  acoustic 04.01
  glossopharyngeal 29.92
  lacrimal branch 05.0
  retrogasserian 04.02
  sympathetic 05.0
  vestibular 04.01
Neurotripsy (peripheral) NEC 04.03
  trigeminal 04.02
Nicola operation (tenodesis for recurrent dislocation of shoulder) 81.82
Nimodipine, infusion 99.75
NIPS (non-invasive programmed electrical stimulation) 37.20
Nissen operation (fundoplication of stomach) 44.66
  laparoscopic 44.67
Noble operation (plication of small intestine) 46.62
Norman Miller operation (vaginopexy) 70.77
  with graft or prosthesis 70.78
Norton operation (extraperitoneal cesarean section) 74.2
Nuclear magnetic resonance imaging — *see* Imaging, magnetic resonance
Nutrition, concentrated substances
  enteral infusion (of) 96.6
  parenteral, total 99.15
  peripheral parenteral 99.15

O

Ober (-Yount) operation (gluteal-iliotibial fasciotomy) 83.14
Obliteration
  bone cavity (*see also* Osteoplasty) 78.40
  calyceal diverticulum 55.39
  canaliculi 09.6
  cerebrospinal fistula 02.12
  cul-de-sac 70.92
    with graft or prosthesis 70.93
  frontal sinus (with fat) 22.42
  lacrimal punctum 09.91

Obliteration — *continued*
  lumbar pseudomeningocele 03.51
  lymphatic structure(s) (peripheral) 40.9
  maxillary sinus 22.31
  meningocele (sacral) 03.51
  pelvic 68.8
  pleural cavity 34.6
  sacral meningocele 03.51
  Skene's gland 71.3
  tympanomastoid cavity 19.9
  vagina, vaginal (partial) (total) 70.4
    vault 70.8
Occlusal molds (dental) 89.31
Occlusion
  artery
    by embolization — *see* Embolization, artery
    by endovascular approach — *see* Embolization, artery
    by ligation — *see* Ligation, artery
  fallopian tube — *see* Ligation, fallopian tube
  patent ductus arteriosus (PDA) 38.85
  vein
    by embolization — *see* Embolization, vein
    by endovascular approach — *see* Embolization, vein
    by ligation — *see* Ligation, vein
  vena cava (surgical) 38.7
Occupational therapy 93.83
OCT (optical coherence tomography) (intravascular imaging)
  coronary vessel(s) 38.24
  non-coronary vessel(s) 38.25
O'Donoghue operation (triad knee repair) 81.43
Odontectomy NEC — *see also* Removal, tooth, surgical 23.19
Oleothorax 33.39
Olshausen operation (uterine suspension) 69.22
Omentectomy 54.4
Omentofixation 54.74
Omentopexy 54.74
Omentoplasty 54.74
Omentorrhaphy 54.74
Omentotomy 54.19
Omphalectomy 54.3
Onychectomy 86.23
Onychoplasty 86.86
Onychotomy 86.09
  with drainage 86.04
Oophorectomy (unilateral) 65.39
  with salpingectomy 65.49
    laparoscopic 65.41
  bilateral (same operative episode) 65.51
    with salpingectomy 65.61
      laparoscopic 65.63
    laparoscopic 65.53
  laparoscopic 65.31
  partial 65.29
    laparoscopic 65.25
    wedge 65.22
      that by laparoscope 65.24
  remaining ovary 65.52
    with tube 65.62
      laparoscopic 65.64
    laparoscopic 65.54
Oophorocystectomy 65.29
  laparoscopic 65.25
Oophoropexy 65.79
Oophoroplasty 65.79
Oophororrhaphy 65.71
  laparoscopic 65.74
Oophorostomy 65.09
  laparoscopic 65.01
Oophorotomy 65.09
  laparoscopic 65.01
Opening
  bony labyrinth (ear) 20.79
  cranial suture 02.01
  heart valve
    closed heart technique — *see* Valvulotomy, by site
    open heart technique — *see* Valvuloplasty, by site

Opening — *continued*
  spinal dura 03.09
Operation
  Abbe
    construction of vagina 70.61
      with graft or prosthesis 70.63
    intestinal anastomosis — *see* Anastomosis, intestine
  abdominal (region) NEC 54.99
  abdominoperineal, NOS 48.50
    laparoscopic 48.51
    open 48.52
    other 48.49
  Aburel (intra-amniotic injection for abortion) 75.0
  Adams
    advancement of round ligament 69.22
    crushing of nasal septum 21.88
    excision of palmar fascia 82.35
  adenoids NEC 28.99
  adrenal (gland) (nerve) (vessel) NEC 07.49
  Albee
    bone peg, femoral neck 78.05
    graft for slipping patella 78.06
    sliding inlay graft, tibia 78.07
  Albert (arthrodesis, knee) 81.22
  Aldridge (-Studdiford) (urethral sling) 59.5
  Alexander
    prostatectomy
      perineal 60.62
      suprapubic 60.3
    shortening of round ligaments of uterus 69.22
  Alexander-Adams (shortening of round ligaments of uterus) 69.22
  Almoor (extrapetrosal drainage) 20.22
  Altemeier (perineal rectal pull-through) 48.49
  Ammon (dacryocystotomy) 09.53
  Anderson (tibial lengthening) 78.37
  Anel (dilation of lacrimal duct) 09.42
  anterior chamber (eye) NEC 12.99
  anti-incontinence NEC 59.79
  antrum window (nasal sinus) 22.2
    with Caldwell-Luc approach 22.39
  anus NEC 49.99
  aortic body NEC 39.89
  aorticopulmonary window 39.59
  appendix NEC 47.99
  Arslan (fenestration of inner ear) 20.61
  artery NEC 39.99
  Asai (larynx) 31.75
  Baffes (interatrial transposition of venous return) 35.91
  Baldy-Webster (uterine suspension) 69.22
  Ball
    herniorrhaphy — *see* Repair, hernia, inguinal
    undercutting 49.02
  Bankhart (capsular repair into glenoid, for shoulder dislocation) 81.82
  Bardenheurer (ligation of innominate artery) 38.85
  Barkan (goniotomy) 12.52
    with goniopuncture 12.53
  Barr (transfer of tibialis posterior tendon) 83.75
  Barsky (closure of cleft hand) 82.82
  Bassett (vulvectomy with inguinal lymph node dissection) 71.5 *[40.3]*
  Bassini (herniorrhaphy) — *see* Repair, hernia, inguinal
  Batch-Spittler-McFaddin (knee disarticulation) 84.16
  Batista (partial ventriculectomy) (ventricular reduction) (ventricular remodeling) 37.35
  Beck I (epicardial poudrage) 36.39
  Beck II (aorta-coronary sinus shunt) 36.39
  Beck-Jianu (permanent gastrostomy) 43.19
  Bell-Beuttner (subtotal abdominal hysterectomy) 68.39
  Belsey (esophagogastric sphincter) 44.65
  Benenenti (rotation of bulbous urethra) 58.49
  Berke (levator resection eyelid) 08.33

Operation — *continued*
  Biesenberger (size reduction of breast, bilateral) 85.32
    unilateral 85.31
  Bigelow (litholapaxy) 57.0
  biliary (duct) (tract) NEC 51.99
  Billroth I (partial gastrectomy with gastroduodenostomy) 43.6
  Billroth II (partial gastrectomy with gastrojejunostomy) 43.7
  Binnie (hepatopexy) 50.69
  Bischoff (ureteroneocystostomy) 56.74
  bisection hysterectomy 68.39
    laparoscopic 68.31
  Bishoff (spinal myelotomy) 03.29
  bladder NEC 57.99
    flap 56.74
  Blalock (systemic-pulmonary anastomosis) 39.0
  Blalock-Hanlon (creation of atrial septal defect) 35.42
  Blalock-Taussig (subclavian-pulmonary anastomosis) 39.0
  Blascovic (resection and advancement of levator palpebrae superioris) 08.33
  blood vessel NEC 39.99
  Blount
    by epiphyseal stapling 78.25
    femoral shortening (with blade plate) 78.25
  Boari (bladder flap) 56.74
  Bobb (cholelithotomy) 51.04
  bone NEC — *see category* 78.4 ☑
    facial 76.99
    injury NEC — *see category* 79.9 ☑
    marrow NEC 41.98
    skull NEC 02.99
  Bonney (abdominal hysterectomy) 68.49
    laparoscopic 68.41
  Borthen (iridotasis) 12.63
  Bost
    plantar dissection 80.48
    radiocarpal fusion 81.26
  Bosworth
    arthroplasty for acromioclavicular separation 81.83
    fusion of posterior lumbar spine 81.08
      for pseudarthrosis 81.38
    resection of radial head ligaments (for tennis elbow) 80.92
    shelf procedure, hip 81.40
  Bottle (repair of hydrocele of tunica vaginalis) 61.2
  Boyd (hip disarticulation) 84.18
  brain NEC 02.99
  Brauer (cardiolysis) 37.10
  breast NEC 85.99
  Bricker (ileoureterostomy) 56.51
  Bristow (repair of shoulder dislocation) 81.82
  Brock (pulmonary valvulotomy) 35.03
  Brockman (soft tissue release for clubfoot) 83.84
  bronchus NEC 33.98
  Browne (-Denis) (hypospadias repair) 58.45
  Brunschwig (temporary gastrostomy) 43.19
  buccal cavity NEC 27.99
  Bunnell (tendon transfer) 82.56
  Burch procedure (retropubic urethral suspension for urinary stress incontinence) 59.5
  Burgess (amputation of ankle) 84.14
  bursa NEC 83.99
    hand 82.99
  bypass — *see* Bypass
  Caldwell (sulcus extension) 24.91
  Caldwell-Luc (maxillary sinusotomy) 22.39
    with removal of membrane lining 22.31
  Callander (knee disarticulation) 84.16
  Campbell
    bone block, ankle 81.11
    fasciotomy (iliac crest) 83.14
    reconstruction of anterior cruciate ligaments 81.45
  canthus NEC 08.99
  cardiac NEC 37.99

Operation — *continued*

cardiac — *continued*
  septum NEC 35.98
  valve NEC 35.99
carotid body or gland NEC 39.89
Carroll and Taber (arthroplasty proximal interphalangeal joint) 81.72
Cattell (herniorrhaphy) 53.51
Cecil (urethral reconstruction) 58.46
cecum NEC 46.99
cerebral (meninges) NEC 02.99
cervix NEC 69.99
Chandler (hip fusion) 81.21
Charles (correction of lymphedema) 40.9
Charnley (compression arthrodesis)
  ankle 81.11
  hip 81.21
  knee 81.22
Cheatle-Henry — *see* Repair, hernia, femoral
chest cavity NEC 34.99
Chevalier-Jackson (partial laryngectomy) 30.29
Child (radical subtotal pancreatectomy) 52.53
Chopart (midtarsal amputation) 84.12
chordae tendineae NEC 35.32
choroid NEC 14.9
ciliary body NEC 12.98
cisterna chyli NEC 40.69
Clagett (closure of chest wall following open flap drainage) 34.72
Clayton (resection of metatarsal heads and bases of phalanges) 77.88
clitoris NEC 71.4
cocked hat (metacarpal lengthening and transfer of local flap) 82.69
Cockett (varicose vein)
  lower limb 38.59
  upper limb 38.53
Cody tack (perforation of footplate) 19.0
Coffey (uterine suspension) (Meigs' modification) 69.22
Cole (anterior tarsal wedge osteotomy) 77.28
Collis-Nissen (hiatal hernia repair) 53.80
Colonna
  adductor tenotomy (first stage) 83.12
  hip arthroplasty (second stage) 81.40
  reconstruction of hip (second stage) 81.40
colon NEC 46.99
commando (radical glossectomy) 25.4
conjunctiva NEC 10.99
  destructive NEC 10.33
cornea NEC 11.99
Coventry (tibial wedge osteotomy) 77.27
Cox-maze procedure (ablation or destruction of heart tissue) — *see* Operation, maze procedure
Crawford (tarso-frontalis sling of eyelid) 08.32
cul-de-sac NEC 70.92
Culp-Deweerd (spiral flap pyeloplasty) 55.87
Culp-Scardino (ureteral flap pyeloplasty) 55.87
Curtis (interphalangeal joint arthroplasty) 81.72
cystocele NEC 70.51
Dahlman (excision of esophageal diverticulum) 42.31
Dana (posterior rhizotomy) 03.1
Danforth (fetal) 73.8
Darrach (ulnar resection) 77.83
Davis (intubated ureterotomy) 56.2
de Grandmont (tarsectomy) 08.35
Delorme
  pericardiectomy 37.31
  proctopexy 48.76
  repair of prolapsed rectum 48.76
  thoracoplasty 33.34
Denker (radical maxillary antrotomy) 22.31
Dennis-Varco (herniorrhaphy) — *see* Repair, hernia, femoral
dental NEC 24.99
  orthodontic NEC 24.8

Operation — *continued*

Derlacki (tympanoplasty) 19.4
diaphragm NEC 34.89
Dickson (fascial transplant) 83.82
Dickson-Diveley (tendon transfer and arthrodesis to correct claw toe) 77.57
Dieffenbach (hip disarticulation) 84.18
digestive tract NEC 46.99
Doléris (shortening of round ligaments) 69.22
D'Ombrain (excision of pterygium with corneal graft) 11.32
Dorrance (push-back operation for cleft palate) 27.62
Dotter (transluminal angioplasty) 39.59
Douglas (suture of tongue to lip for micrognathia) 25.59
Doyle (paracervical uterine denervation) 69.3
Duhamel (abdominoperineal pull-through) 48.65
Dührssen (vaginofixation of uterus) 69.22
Dunn (triple arthrodesis) 81.12
duodenum NEC 46.99
Dupuytren
  fasciectomy 82.35
  fasciotomy 82.12
    with excision 82.35
  shoulder disarticulation 84.08
Durham (-Caldwell) (transfer of biceps femoris tendon) 83.75
DuToit and Roux (staple capsulorrhaphy of shoulder) 81.82
DuVries (tenoplasty) 83.88
Dwyer
  fasciotomy 83.14
  soft tissue release NEC 83.84
  wedge osteotomy, calcaneus 77.28
Eagleton (extrapetrosal drainage) 20.22
ear (external) NEC 18.9
  middle or inner NEC 20.99
Eden-Hybinette (glenoid bone block) 78.01
Effler (heart) 36.2
Eggers
  tendon release (patellar retinacula) 83.13
  tendon transfer (biceps femoris tendon) (hamstring tendon) 83.75
Elliot (scleral trephination with iridectomy) 12.61
Ellis Jones (repair of peroneal tendon) 83.88
Ellison (reinforcement of collateral ligament) 81.44
Elmslie-Cholmeley (tarsal wedge osteotomy) 77.28
Eloesser
  thoracoplasty 33.34
  thoracostomy 34.09
Emmet (cervix) 67.61
endorectal pull-through 48.41
epididymis NEC 63.99
esophagus NEC 42.99
Estes (ovary) 65.72
  laparoscopic 65.75
Estlander (thoracoplasty) 33.34
Evans (release of clubfoot) 83.84
extraocular muscle NEC 15.9
  multiple (two or more muscles) 15.4
    with temporary detachment from globe 15.3
  revision 15.6
  single 15.29
    with temporary detachment from globe 15.19
eyeball NEC 16.99
eyelid(s) NEC 08.99
face NEC 27.99
facial bone or joint NEC 76.99
fallopian tube NEC 66.99
Farabeuf (ischiopubiotomy) 77.39
Fasanella-Servatt (blepharoptosis repair) 08.35
fascia NEC 83.99
  hand 82.99
female (genital organs) NEC 71.9
  hysterectomy NEC 68.9
fenestration (aorta) 39.54

Operation — *continued*

Ferguson (hernia repair) 53.00
Fick (perforation of footplate) 19.0
filtering (for glaucoma) 12.79
  with iridectomy 12.65
Finney (pyloroplasty) 44.29
fistulizing, sclera NEC 12.69
Foley (pyeloplasty) 55.87
Fontan (creation of conduit between right atrium and pulmonary artery) 35.94
Fothergill (-Donald) (uterine suspension) 69.22
Fowler
  arthroplasty of metacarpophalangeal joint 81.72
  release (mallet finger repair) 82.84
  tenodesis (hand) 82.85
  thoracoplasty 33.34
Fox (entropion repair with wedge resection) 08.43
Franco (suprapubic cystotomy) 57.18
Frank (permanent gastrostomy) 43.19
Frazier (-Spiller) (subtemporal trigeminal rhizotomy) 04.02
Fredet-Ramstedt (pyloromyotomy) (with wedge resection) 43.3
Frenckner (intrapetrosal drainage) 20.22
Frickman (abdominal proctopexy) 48.75
Frommel (shortening of uterosacral ligaments) 69.22
Gabriel (abdominoperineal resection of rectum), NOS 48.50
  laparoscopic 48.51
  open 48.52
  other 48.59
gallbladder NEC 51.99
ganglia NEC 04.99
  sympathetic 05.89
Gant (wedge osteotomy of trochanter) 77.25
Garceau (tibial tendon transfer) 83.75
Gardner (spinal meningocele repair) 03.51
gastric NEC 44.99
Gelman (release of clubfoot) 83.84
genital organ NEC
  female 71.9
  male 64.99
Ghormley (hip fusion) 81.21
Gifford
  destruction of lacrimal sac 09.6
  keratotomy (delimiting) 11.1
Gill
  arthrodesis of shoulder 81.23
  laminectomy 03.09
Gilliam (uterine suspension) 69.22
Gill-Stein (carporadial arthrodesis) 81.25
Girdlestone
  laminectomy with spinal fusion 81.00
  muscle transfer for claw toe 77.57
  resection of femoral head and neck (without insertion of joint prosthesis) 77.85
    with replacement prosthesis — *see* Implant, joint, hip
  resection of hip prosthesis 80.05
    with replacement prosthesis — *see* Implant, joint, hip
Girdlestone-Taylor (muscle transfer for claw toe repair) 77.57
glaucoma NEC 12.79
Glenn (anastomosis of superior vena cava to right pulmonary artery) 39.21
globus pallidus NEC 01.42
Goebel-Frangenheim-Stoeckel (urethrovesical suspension) 59.4
Goldner (clubfoot release) 80.48
Goldthwait
  ankle stabilization 81.11
  patella stabilization 81.44
  tendon transfer for patella dislocation 81.44
Goodall-Power (vagina) 70.4
Gordon-Taylor (hindquarter amputation) 84.19
Graber-Duvernay (drilling femoral head) 77.15
Green (scapulopexy) 78.41

Operation — *continued*

Grice (subtalar arthrodesis) 81.13
Gritti-Stokes (knee disarticulation) 84.16
Gross (herniorrhaphy)
  laparoscopic 53.43
    with graft or prosthesis 53.42
    other and open with graft or prosthesis 53.41
  other open 53.49
gum NEC 24.39
Guyon (amputation of ankle) 84.13
Hagner (epididymotomy) 63.92
Halsted — *see* Repair, hernia, inguinal
Halsted mastectomy 85.45
Hampton (anastomosis small intestine to rectal stump) 45.92
hanging hip (muscle release) 83.19
harelip 27.54
Harrison-Richardson (vaginal suspension) 70.77
  with graft or prosthesis 70.78
Hartmann — *see* Colectomy, by site
Hauser
  achillotenotomy 83.11
  bunionectomy with adductor tendon transfer 77.53
  stabilization of patella 81.44
Heaney (vaginal hysterectomy) 68.59
  laparoscopically assisted (LAVH) 68.51
heart NEC 37.99
  valve NEC 35.99
    adjacent structure NEC 35.39
Hegar (perineorrhaphy) 71.79
Heine (cyclodialysis) 12.55
Heineke-Mikulicz (pyloroplasty) — *see* category 44.2 ☑
Heller (esophagomyotomy) 42.7
Hellström (transplantation of aberrant renal vessel) 39.55
hemorrhoids NEC 49.49
Henley (jejunal transposition) 43.81
hepatic NEC 50.99
hernia — *see* Repair, hernia
Hey (amputation of foot) 84.12
Hey-Groves (reconstruction of anterior cruciate ligament) 81.45
Heyman (soft tissue release for clubfoot) 83.84
Heyman-Herndon (-Strong) (correction of metatarsus varus) 80.48
Hibbs (lumbar spinal fusion) — *see* Fusion, lumbar
Higgins — *see* Repair, hernia, femoral
Hill-Allison (hiatal hernia repair, transpleural approach) 53.80
Hitchcock (anchoring tendon of biceps) 83.88
Hofmeister (gastrectomy) 43.7
Hoke
  midtarsal fusion 81.14
  triple arthrodesis 81.12
Holth
  iridencleisis 12.63
  sclerectomy 12.65
Homan (correction of lymphedema) 40.9
Hutch (ureteroneocystostomy) 56.74
Hybinette-eden (glenoid bone block) 78.01
hymen NEC 70.91
hypopharynx NEC 29.99
hypophysis NEC 07.79
ileal loop 56.51
ileum NEC 46.99
intestine NEC 46.99
iris NEC 12.97
  inclusion 12.63
Irving (tubal ligation) 66.32
Irwin (*see also* Osteotomy) 77.30
Jaboulay (gastroduodenostomy) 44.39
  laparoscopic 44.38
Janeway (permanent gastrostomy) 43.19
Jatene (arterial switch) 35.84
jejunum NEC 46.99
Johanson (urethral reconstruction) 58.46
joint (capsule) (ligament) (structure) NEC 81.99
  facial NEC 76.99

☑ Additional Digit Required — Refer to the Tabular List for Digit Selection   ▽ Subterms under main terms may continue to next column or page

2014 ICD-9-CM 865

Operation — Operation

Patch — continued
subdural, brain 02.12
Patellapexy 78.46
Patellaplasty NEC 78.46
Patellectomy 77.96
partial 77.86
Pattee operation (auditory canal) 18.6
PDT (percutaneous dilatational tracheostomy) — see Tracheostomy
Pectenotomy — see also Sphincterotomy, anal 49.59
Pedicle flap — see Graft, skin, pedicle
Peet operation (splanchnic resection) 05.29
PEG (percutaneous endoscopic gastrostomy) 43.11
PEGJJ (percutaneous [endoscopic] gastrojejunostomy) 44.32
PEJ (percutaneous endoscopic jejunostomy) 46.32
Pelvectomy, kidney (partial) 55.4
Pelvimetry 88.25
gynecological 89.26
Pelviolithotomy 55.11
Pelvioplasty, kidney 55.87
Pelviostomy 55.12
closure 55.82
Pelviotomy 77.39
to assist delivery 73.94
Pelvi-ureteroplasty 55.87
Pemberton operation
osteotomy of ilium 77.39
rectum (mobilization and fixation for prolapse repair) 48.76
Penectomy 64.3
Pereyra operation (paraurethral suspension) 59.6
Perforation
stapes footplate 19.0
Perfusion NEC 39.97
for
chemotherapy NEC 99.25
hormone therapy NEC 99.24
carotid artery 39.97
coronary artery 39.97
head 39.97
hyperthermic (lymphatic), localized region or site 93.35
intestine (large) (local) 46.96
small 46.95
kidney, local 55.95
limb (lower) (upper) 39.97
liver, localized 50.93
neck 39.97
subarachnoid (spinal cord) (refrigerated saline) 03.92
total body 39.96
Pericardiectomy 37.31
Pericardiocentesis 37.0
Pericardiolysis 37.12
Pericardioplasty 37.49
Pericardiorrhaphy 37.49
Pericardiostomy (tube) 37.12
Pericardiotomy 37.12
Peridectomy 10.31
Perilimbal suction 89.11
Perimetry 95.05
Perineoplasty 71.79
Perineorrhaphy 71.71
obstetrical laceration (current) 75.69
Perineotomy (nonobstetrical) 71.09
to assist delivery — see Episiotomy
Periosteotomy — see also Incision, bone 77.10
facial bone 76.09
Perirectofistulectomy 48.93
Peritectomy 10.31
Peritomy 10.1
Peritoneocentesis 54.91
Peritoneoscopy 54.21
Peritoneotomy 54.19
Peritoneumectomy 54.4
Phacoemulsification (ultrasonic) (with aspiration) 13.41
Phacofragmentation (mechanical) (with aspiration) 13.43
posterior route 13.42
ultrasonic 13.41

Phalangectomy (partial) 77.89
claw toe 77.57
cockup toe 77.58
hammer toe 77.56
overlapping toe 77.58
total 77.99
Phalangization (fifth metacarpal) 82.81
Pharyngeal flap operation (cleft palate repair) 27.62
secondary or subsequent 27.63
Pharyngectomy (partial) 29.33
with laryngectomy 30.3
Pharyngogram 87.09
contrast 87.06
Pharyngolaryngectomy 30.3
Pharyngoplasty (with silastic implant) 29.4
for cleft palate 27.62
secondary or subsequent 27.63
Pharyngorrhaphy 29.51
for cleft palate 27.62
Pharyngoscopy 29.11
Pharyngotomy 29.0
Phenopeel (skin) 86.24
Phlebectomy 38.60
with
anastomosis 38.30
abdominal 38.37
head and neck NEC 38.32
intracranial NEC 38.31
lower limb 38.39
thoracic NEC 38.35
upper limb 38.33
graft replacement 38.4 ☑
abdominal 38.47
head and neck NEC 38.42
intracranial NEC 38.41
lower limb 38.49
thoracic NEC 38.45
upper limb 38.43
abdominal 38.67
head and neck NEC 38.62
intracranial NEC 38.61
lower limb 38.69
thoracic NEC 38.65
upper limb 38.63
varicose 38.50
abdominal 38.57
head and neck NEC 38.52
intracranial NEC 38.51
lower limb 38.59
thoracic NEC 38.55
upper limb 38.53
Phlebogoniostomy 12.52
Phlebography (contrast) (retrograde) 88.60
by radioisotope — see Scan, radioisotope, by site
adrenal 88.65
femoral 88.66
head 88.61
hepatic 88.64
impedance 88.68
intra-abdominal NEC 88.65
intrathoracic NEC 88.63
lower extremity NEC 88.66
neck 88.61
portal system 88.64
pulmonary 88.62
specified site NEC 88.67
vena cava (inferior) (superior) 88.51
Phleborrhaphy 39.32
Phlebotomy 38.99
Phonocardiogram, with ECG lead 89.55
Photochemotherapy NEC 99.83
extracorporeal 99.88
Photocoagulation
ciliary body 12.73
eye, eyeball 16.99
iris 12.41
macular hole — see Photocoagulation, retina
orbital lesion 16.92
retina
for
destruction of lesion 14.25
reattachment 14.55
repair of tear or defect 14.35

Photocoagulation — continued
retina — continued
laser (beam)
for
destruction of lesion 14.24
reattachment 14.54
repair of tear or defect 14.34
xenon arc
for
destruction of lesion 14.23
reattachment 14.53
repair of tear or defect 14.33
Photography 89.39
fundus 95.11
Photopheresis, therapeutic 99.88
Phototherapy NEC 99.83
newborn 99.83
ultraviolet 99.82
Phrenemphraxis 04.03
for collapse of lung 33.31
Phrenicectomy 04.03
for collapse of lung 33.31
Phrenicoexeresis 04.03
for collapse of lung 33.31
Phrenicotomy 04.03
for collapse of lung 33.31
Phrenicotripsy 04.03
for collapse of lung 33.31
Phrenoplasty 34.84
Physical medicine — see Therapy, physical
Physical therapy — see Therapy, physical
Physiotherapy, chest 93.99
PICC (peripherally inserted central catheter) 38.93
Piercing ear, external (pinna) 18.01
Pigmenting, skin 86.02
Pilojection (aneurysm) (Gallagher) 39.52
Pinealectomy (complete) (total) 07.54
partial 07.53
Pinealotomy (with drainage) 07.52
Pinning
bone — see Fixation, bone, internal
ear 18.5
Pinsker operation (obliteration of nasoseptal telangiectasia) 21.07
Piper operation (forceps) 72.6
Pirogoff operation (ankle amputation through malleoli of tibia and fibula) 84.14
Pituitectomy (complete) (total) — see also Hypophysectomy 07.69
Placentogram, placentography 88.46
with radioisotope (RISA) 92.17
Planing, skin 86.25
Plantation, tooth (bud) (germ) 23.5
prosthetic 23.6
Plasma exchange 99.07
Plasmapheresis, therapeutic 99.71
Plastic repair — see Repair, by site
Plasty — see also Repair, by site
bladder neck (V-Y) 57.85
skin (without graft) 86.89
subcutaneous tissue 86.89
Platelet inhibitor (GP IIb/IIIa inhibitor only), infusion 99.20
Plateletpheresis, therapeutic 99.74
Play
psychotherapy 94.36
therapy 93.81
Pleating
eye muscle 15.22
multiple (two or more muscles) 15.4
sclera, for buckling (see also Buckling, scleral) 14.49
Plethysmogram (carotid) 89.58
air-filled (pneumatic) 89.58
capacitance 89.58
cerebral 89.58
differential 89.58
oculoplethysmogram 89.58
penile 89.58
photoelectric 89.58
regional 89.58
respiratory function measurement (body) 89.38
segmental 89.58
strain-gauge 89.58

Plethysmogram — continued
thoracic impedance 89.38
venous occlusion 89.58
water-filled 89.58
Plethysmography
CaverMap™ 89.58
penile 89.58
Pleurectomy NEC 34.59
Pleurocentesis 34.91
Pleurodesis 34.6
chemical 34.92
with cancer chemotherapy substance 34.92 [99.25]
tetracycline 34.92 [99.21]
Pleurolysis (for collapse of lung) 33.39
Pleuropexy 34.99
Pleurosclerosis 34.6
chemical 34.92
with cancer chemotherapy substance 34.92 [99.25]
tetracycline 34.92 [99.21]
Pleurotomy 34.09
Plexectomy
choroid 02.14
hypogastric 05.24
Plication
aneurysm
heart 37.32
annulus, heart valve 35.33
bleb (emphysematous), lung 32.21
broad ligament 69.22
diaphragm (for hernia repair) (thoracic approach) (thoracoabdominal approach) 53.81
eye muscle (oblique) (rectus) 15.22
multiple (two or more muscles) 15.4
fascia 83.89
hand 82.89
inferior vena cava 38.7
intestine (jejunum) (Noble) 46.62
Kelly (-Stoeckel) (urethrovesical junction) 59.3
levator, for blepharoptosis 08.34
ligament (see also Arthroplasty) 81.96
broad 69.22
round 69.22
uterosacral 69.22
mesentery 54.75
round ligament 69.22
sphincter, urinary bladder 57.85
stomach 44.69
laparoscopic 44.68
superior vena cava 38.7
tendon 83.85
hand 82.55
tricuspid valve (with repositioning) 35.14
ureter 56.89
urethra 58.49
urethrovesical junction 59.3
vein (peripheral) 39.59
vena cava (inferior) (superior) 38.7
ventricle (heart)
aneurysm 37.32
Plicotomy, tympanum 20.23
Plombage, lung 33.39
Pneumocentesis 33.93
Pneumocisternogram 87.02
Pneumoencephalogram 87.01
Pneumogram, pneumography
extraperitoneal 88.15
mediastinal 87.33
orbit 87.14
pelvic 88.13
peritoneum NEC 88.13
presacral 88.15
retroperitoneum 88.15
Pneumogynecography 87.82
Pneumomediastinography 87.33
Pneumonectomy (extended) (radical) (standard) (total) (with mediastinal dissection) 32.59
partial
complete excision, one lobe 32.49
resection (wedge), one lobe 32.39
thoracoscopic 32.50
Pneumonolysis (for collapse of lung) 33.39

Pubococcygeoplasty — Reattachment

☑ **Additional Digit Required — Refer to the Tabular List for Digit Selection**   ▽ **Subterms under main terms may continue to next column or page**

870   **2014 ICD-9-CM**

Reattachment — *continued*
  extremity — *continued*
    forearm 84.23
    hand 84.23
    leg (lower) NEC 84.27
    thigh 84.28
    thumb 84.21
    toe 84.25
    wrist 84.23
  finger 84.22
    thumb 84.21
  foot 84.26
  forearm 84.23
  hand 84.23
  joint capsule (*see also* Arthroplasty) 81.96
  leg (lower) NEC 84.27
  ligament (*see also* Arthroplasty)
    uterosacral 69.22
  muscle 83.74
    hand 82.54
    papillary (heart) 35.31
  nerve (peripheral) 04.79
  nose (amputated) 21.89
  papillary muscle (heart) 35.31
  penis (amputated) 64.45
  retina (and choroid) NEC 14.59
    by
      cryotherapy 14.52
      diathermy 14.51
      electrocoagulation 14.51
      photocoagulation 14.55
        laser 14.54
        xenon arc 14.53
  tendon (to tendon) 83.73
    hand 82.53
    to skeletal attachment 83.88
      hand 82.85
  thigh 84.28
  thumb 84.21
  toe 84.25
  tooth 23.5
  uterosacral ligament(s) 69.22
  vessels (peripheral) 39.59
    renal, aberrant 39.55
  wrist 84.23
Recession
  extraocular muscle 15.11
    multiple (two or more muscles) (with advancement or resection) 15.3
  gastrocnemius tendon (Strayer operation) 83.72
  levator palpebrae (superioris) muscle 08.38
  prognathic jaw 76.64
  tendon 83.72
    hand 82.52
Reclosure — *see also* Closure
  disrupted abdominal wall (postoperative) 54.61
Reconstruction (plastic) — *see also* Construction and Repair, by site
  alveolus, alveolar (process) (ridge) (with graft or implant) 24.5
  artery (graft) — *see* Graft, artery
  artificial stoma, intestine 46.40
  auditory canal (external) 18.6
  auricle (ear) 18.71
  bladder 57.87
    with
      ileum 57.87 *[45.51]*
      sigmoid 57.87 *[45.52]*
  bone, except facial (*see also* Osteoplasty) 78.40
  facial NEC 76.46
    with total ostectomy 76.44
    mandible 76.43
      with total mandibulectomy 76.41
  breast, total NOS 85.70
    deep inferior epigastric artery perforator (DIEP) flap, free 85.74
    gluteal artery perforator (GAP) flap, free 85.76
    latissimus dorsi myocutaneous flap 85.71
    other 85.79
    superficial inferior epigastric artery (SIEA) flap, free 85.75

Reconstruction — *see also* Construction and Repair, by site — *continued*
  breast, total — *continued*
    transverse rectus abdominis musculocutaneous (TRAM) flap, free 85.73
    transverse rectus abdominis myocutaneous (TRAM) flap, pedicled 85.72
  bronchus 33.48
  canthus (lateral) 08.59
  cardiac annulus 35.33
  chest wall (mesh) (silastic) 34.79
  cleft lip 27.54
  conjunctival cul-de-sac 10.43
    with graft (buccal mucous membrane) (free) 10.42
  cornea NEC 11.79
  diaphragm 34.84
  ear (external) (auricle) 18.71
    external auditory canal 18.6
    meatus (new) (osseous skin-lined) 18.6
    ossicles 19.3
    prominent or protruding 18.5
  eyebrow 08.70
  eyelid 08.70
    with graft or flap 08.69
      hair follicle 08.63
      mucous membrane 08.62
      skin 08.61
      tarsoconjunctival (one-stage) (two-stage) 08.64
    full-thickness 08.74
      involving lid margin 08.73
    partial-thickness 08.72
      involving lid margin 08.71
  eye socket 16.64
    with graft 16.63
  fallopian tube 66.79
  foot and toes (with fixation device) 81.57
    with prosthetic implant 81.57
  frontonasal duct 22.79
  hip (total) (with prosthesis) 81.51
  intraoral 27.59
  joint — *see* Arthroplasty
  lymphatic (by transplantation) 40.9
  mandible 76.43
    with total mandibulectomy 76.41
  mastoid cavity 19.9
  mouth 27.59
  nipple NEC 85.87
  nose (total) (with arm flap) (with forehead flap) 21.83
  ossicles (graft) (prosthesis) NEC 19.3
    with
      stapedectomy 19.19
      tympanoplasty 19.53
  pelvic floor 71.79
  penis (rib graft) (skin graft) (myocutaneous flap) 64.44
  pharynx 29.4
  scrotum (with pedicle flap) (with rotational flap) 61.49
  skin (plastic) (without graft) NEC 86.89
    with graft — *see* Graft, skin
  subcutaneous tissue (plastic) (without skin graft) NEC 86.89
    with graft — *see* Graft, skin
  tendon pulley — (with graft) (with local tissue) 83.83
    for opponensplasty 82.71
    hand 82.71
  thumb (osteoplastic) (with bone graft) (with skin graft) 82.69
  trachea (with graft) 31.75
  umbilicus
    laparoscopic 53.43
      with graft or prosthesis 53.42
    other and open with graft or prosthesis 53.41
    other open 53.49
  ureteropelvic junction 55.87
  urethra 58.46
  vagina 70.62
    with graft or prosthesis 70.64
  vas deferens, surgically divided 63.82
Recontour, gingiva 24.2
Recreational therapy 93.81

Rectectomy — *see also* Resection, rectum 48.69
Rectopexy (Delorme) 48.76
  abdominal (Ripstein) 48.75
Rectoplasty 48.79
Rectorectostomy 48.74
Rectorrhaphy 48.71
Rectosigmoidectomy — *see also* Resection, rectum 48.69
  transsacral 48.61
Rectosigmoidostomy 45.94
Rectostomy 48.1
  closure 48.72
Red cell survival studies 92.05
Reduction
  adipose tissue 86.83
  batwing arms 86.83
  breast (bilateral) 85.32
    unilateral 85.31
  bulbous tuberosities (mandible) (maxilla) (fibrous) (osseous) 24.31
  buttocks 86.83
  diastasis, ankle mortise (closed) 79.77
    open 79.87
  dislocation (of joint) (manipulation) (with cast) (with splint) (with traction device) (closed) 79.70
    with fracture — *see* Reduction, fracture, by site
    ankle (closed) 79.77
      open 79.87
    elbow (closed) 79.72
      open 79.82
    finger (closed) 79.74
      open 79.84
    foot (closed) 79.78
      open 79.88
    hand (closed) 79.74
      open 79.84
    hip (closed) 79.75
      open 79.85
    knee (closed) 79.76
      open 79.86
    open (with external fixation) (with internal fixation) 79.80
      specified site NEC 79.89
    shoulder (closed) 79.71
      open 79.81
    specified site (closed) NEC 79.79
      open 79.89
    temporomandibular (closed) 76.93
      open 76.94
    toe (closed) 79.78
      open 79.88
    wrist (closed) 79.73
      open 79.83
  elephantiasis, scrotum 61.3
  epistaxis (*see also* Control, epistaxis) 21.00
  fracture (bone) (with cast) (with splint) (with traction device) (closed) 79.00
    with internal fixation 79.10
    alveolar process (with stabilization of teeth)
      mandible (closed) 76.75
        open 76.77
      maxilla (closed) 76.73
        open 76.77
    ankle — *see* Reduction, fracture, leg
    arm (closed) NEC 79.02
      with internal fixation 79.12
      open 79.22
        with internal fixation 79.32
    blow-out — *see* Reduction, fracture, orbit
    carpal, metacarpal (closed) 79.03
      with internal fixation 79.13
      open 79.23
        with internal fixation 79.33
    epiphysis — *see* Reduction, separation
    facial (bone) NEC 76.70
      closed 76.78
      open 76.79
    femur (closed) 79.05
      with internal fixation 79.15
      open 79.25

Reduction — *continued*
  fracture — *continued*
    femur — *continued*
      open — *continued*
        with internal fixation 79.35
    fibula (closed) 79.06
      with internal fixation 79.16
      open 79.26
        with internal fixation 79.36
    foot (closed) NEC 79.07
      with internal fixation 79.17
      open 79.27
        with internal fixation 79.37
    hand (closed) NEC 79.03
      with internal fixation 79.13
      open 79.23
        with internal fixation 79.33
    humerus (closed) 79.01
      with internal fixation 79.11
      open 79.21
        with internal fixation 79.31
    jaw (lower) (*see also* Reduction, fracture, mandible)
      upper — *see* Reduction, fracture, maxilla
    larynx 31.64
    leg (closed) NEC 79.06
      with internal fixation 79.16
      open 79.26
        with internal fixation 79.36
    malar (closed) 76.71
      open 76.72
    mandible (with dental wiring) (closed) 76.75
      open 76.76
    maxilla (with dental wiring) (closed) 76.73
      open 76.74
    nasal (closed) 21.71
      open 21.72
    open 79.20
      with internal fixation 79.30
      specified site NEC 79.29
        with internal fixation 79.39
    orbit (rim) (wall) (closed) 76.78
      open 76.79
    patella (open) (with internal fixation) 79.36
    phalanges
      foot (closed) 79.08
        with internal fixation 79.18
        open 79.28
          with internal fixation 79.38
      hand (closed) 79.04
        with internal fixation 79.14
        open 79.24
          with internal fixation 79.34
    radius (closed) 79.02
      with internal fixation 79.12
      open 79.22
        with internal fixation 79.32
    skull 02.02
    specified site (closed) NEC 79.09
      with internal fixation 79.19
      open 79.29
        with internal fixation 79.39
    spine 03.53
    tarsal, metatarsal (closed) 79.07
      with internal fixation 79.17
      open 79.27
        with internal fixation 79.37
    tibia (closed) 79.06
      with internal fixation 79.16
      open 79.26
        with internal fixation 79.36
    ulna (closed) 79.02
      with internal fixation 79.12
      open 79.22
        with internal fixation 79.32
    vertebra 03.53
    zygoma, zygomatic arch (closed) 76.71
      open 76.72
  fracture-dislocation — *see* Reduction, fracture
  heart volume 37.35
  hemorrhoids (manual) 49.41

☑ **Additional Digit Required — Refer to the Tabular List for Digit Selection**

▽ Subterms under main terms may continue to next column or page

Reduction — *continued*
　hernia (*see also* Repair, hernia)
　　manual 96.27
　intussusception (open) 46.80
　　with
　　　fluoroscopy 96.29
　　　ionizing radiation enema 96.29
　　　ultrasonography guidance 96.29
　　hydrostatic 96.29
　　large intestine 46.82
　　　endoscopic (balloon) 46.85
　　pneumatic 96.29
　　small intestine 46.81
　lung volume 32.22
　　biologic lung volume reduction (BLVR)
　　　— *see* category 33.7 ☑
　malrotation, intestine (manual) (surgical)
　　46.80
　　large 46.82
　　　endoscopic (balloon) 46.85
　　small 46.81
　mammoplasty (bilateral) 85.32
　　unilateral 85.31
　prolapse
　　anus (operative) 49.94
　　colostomy (manual) 96.28
　　enterostomy (manual) 96.28
　　ileostomy (manual) 96.28
　　rectum (manual) 96.26
　　uterus
　　　by pessary 96.18
　　　surgical 69.22
　ptosis overcorrection 08.37
　retroversion, uterus by pessary 96.18
　separation, epiphysis (with internal fixation)
　　(closed) 79.40
　　femur (closed) 79.45
　　　open 79.55
　　fibula (closed) 79.46
　　　open 79.56
　　humerus (closed) 79.41
　　　open 79.51
　　open 79.50
　　specified site (closed) NEC (*see also* category) 79.4 ☑
　　　open — *see* category 79.5 ☑
　　tibia (closed) 79.46
　　　open 79.56
　size
　　abdominal wall (adipose) (pendulous)
　　　86.83
　　arms (adipose) (batwing) 86.83
　　breast (bilateral) 85.32
　　　unilateral 85.31
　　buttocks (adipose) 86.83
　　finger (macrodactyly repair) 82.83
　　skin 86.83
　　subcutaneous tissue 86.83
　　thighs (adipose) 86.83
　torsion
　　intestine (manual) (surgical) 46.80
　　　large 46.82
　　　　endoscopic (balloon) 46.85
　　　small 46.81
　　kidney pedicle 55.84
　　omentum 54.74
　　spermatic cord 63.52
　　　with orchiopexy 62.5
　　testis 63.52
　　　with orchiopexy 62.5
　　uterus NEC 69.98
　　　gravid 75.99
　ventricular 37.35
　volvulus
　　intestine 46.80
　　　large 46.82
　　　　endoscopic (balloon) 46.85
　　　small 46.81
　　stomach 44.92
Reefing, joint capsule — *see also* Arthroplasty
　81.96
Re-entry operation (aorta) 39.54
Re-establishment, continuity — *see also*
　Anastomosis
　bowel 46.50
　fallopian tube 66.79

Re-establishment, continuity — *see also*
　Anastomosis — *continued*
　vas deferens 63.82
Referral (for)
　psychiatric aftercare (halfway house) (outpatient clinic) 94.52
　psychotherapy 94.51
　rehabilitation
　　alcoholism 94.53
　　drug addiction 94.54
　　psychologic NEC 94.59
　　vocational 94.55
Reformation
　cardiac pacemaker pocket, new site (skin)
　　(subcutaneous) 37.79
　cardioverter/defibrillator (automatic) pocket, new site (skin) (subcutaneous)
　　37.79
　chamber of eye 12.99
Refracture
　bone (for faulty union) (*see also* Osteoclasis)
　　78.70
　nasal bones 21.88
Refusion
　spinal, NOS 81.30

> *Note: Also use either 81.62, 81.63, or 81.64 as an additional code to show the total number of vertebrae fused*

　atlas-axis (anterior) (transoral) (posterior)
　　81.31
　axial lumbar interbody fusion (AxiaLIF®)
　　81.38
　cervical (C$_2$ level or below) NEC 81.32
　　anterior column (interbody), anterolateral (anterior) technique
　　　81.32
　　C$_1$-C$_2$ level (anterior) (posterior)
　　　81.31
　　posterior column, posterolateral
　　　(posterior) technique 81.33
　craniocervical (anterior) (transoral)
　　(posterior) 81.31
　direct lateral interbody fusion (DLIF)
　　81.36
　dorsal, dorsolumbar NEC 81.35
　　anterior column (interbody), anterolateral (anterior) (extracavitary) technique 81.34
　　posterior column, posterolateral
　　　(posterior) technique 81.35
　extreme lateral interbody fusion (XLIF®)
　　81.36
　facet 81.37
　lumbar, lumbosacral NEC 81.38
　　anterior column (interbody)
　　　anterolateral (anterior) technique
　　　81.36
　　　posterior technique 81.38
　　anterior lumbar interbody fusion
　　　(ALIF) 81.36
　　lateral transverse process technique
　　　81.37
　　posterior column, posterior (posterolateral) (transverse process)
　　　technique 81.37
　　posterior lumbar interbody fusion
　　　(PLIF) 81.38
　　posterior (interbody), posterolateral
　　　technique 81.38
　　transforaminal lumbar interbody fusion (TLIF) 81.38
　number of vertebrae — *see* codes 81.62-
　　81.64
　occiput — C$_2$ (anterior) (transoral) (posterior) 81.31
　refusion NEC 81.39
Regional blood flow study 92.05
Regulation, menstrual 69.6
Rehabilitation programs NEC 93.89
　alcohol 94.61
　　with detoxification 94.63
　　combined alcohol and drug 94.67
　　　with detoxification 94.69
　drug 94.64
　　with detoxification 94.66

Rehabilitation programs — *continued*
　drug — *continued*
　　combined drug and alcohol 94.67
　　　with detoxification 94.69
　　sheltered employment 93.85
　　vocational 93.85
Reimplantation
　adrenal tissue (heterotopic) (orthotopic)
　　07.45
　artery 39.59
　　renal, aberrant 39.55
　bile ducts following excision of ampulla of
　　Vater 51.62
　extremity — *see* Reattachment, extremity
　fallopian tube into uterus 66.74
　kidney 55.61
　lung 33.5 ☑
　ovary 65.72
　　laparoscopic 65.75
　pancreatic tissue 52.81
　parathyroid tissue (heterotopic) (orthotopic)
　　06.95
　pulmonary artery for hemitruncus repair
　　35.83
　renal vessel, aberrant 39.55
　testis in scrotum 62.5
　thyroid tissue (heterotopic) (orthotopic)
　　06.94
　tooth 23.5
　ureter into bladder 56.74
Reinforcement — *see also* Repair, by site
　sclera NEC 12.88
　　with graft 12.87
Reinsertion — *see also* Insertion or Revision
　cystostomy tube 59.94
　fixation device (internal) (*see also* Fixation,
　　bone, internal) 78.50
　heart valve (prosthetic) 35.95
　Holter (-Spitz) valve 02.42
　implant (expelled) (extruded)
　　eyeball (with conjunctival graft) 16.62
　　orbital 16.62
　nephrostomy tube 55.93
　pyelostomy tube 55.94
　ureteral stent (transurethral) 59.8
　　with ureterotomy 59.8 *[56.2]*
　ureterostomy tube 59.93
　valve
　　heart (prosthetic) 35.95
　　ventricular (cerebral) 02.42
Relaxation — *see also* Release training 94.33
Release
　carpal tunnel (for nerve decompression)
　　04.43
　celiac artery axis 39.91
　central slip, extensor tendon hand (mallet
　　finger repair) 82.84
　chordee 64.42
　clubfoot NEC 83.84
　de Quervain's tenosynovitis 82.01
　Dupuytren's contracture (by palmar fasciectomy) 82.35
　　by fasciotomy (subcutaneous) 82.12
　　　with excision 82.35
　Fowler (mallet finger repair) 82.84
　joint (capsule) (adherent) (constrictive) (*see
　　also* Division, joint capsule) 80.40
　laryngeal 31.92
　ligament (*see also* Division, ligament) 80.40
　　median arcuate 39.91
　median arcuate ligament 39.91
　muscle (division) 83.19
　　hand 82.19
　nerve (peripheral) NEC 04.49
　　cranial NEC 04.42
　　trigeminal 04.41
　pressure, intraocular 12.79
　scar tissue
　　skin 86.84
　　stoma — *see* Revision, stoma
　tarsal tunnel 04.44
　tendon 83.13
　　hand 82.11
　　　extensor, central slip (repair mallet
　　　　finger) 82.84
　　sheath 83.01

Release — *continued*
　tendon — *continued*
　　sheath — *continued*
　　　hand 82.01
　　tenosynovitis 83.01
　　　abductor pollicis longus 82.01
　　　de Quervain's 82.01
　　　external pollicis brevis 82.01
　　　hand 82.01
　　torsion
　　　intestine 46.80
　　　　large 46.82
　　　　　endoscopic (balloon) 46.85
　　　　small 46.81
　　　kidney pedicle 55.84
　　　ovary 65.95
　　　testes 63.52
　　transverse carpal ligament (for nerve decompression) 04.43
　　trigger finger or thumb 82.01
　　urethral stricture 58.5
　　Volkmann's contracture
　　　excision of scar, muscle 83.32
　　　fasciotomy 83.14
　　　muscle transplantation 83.77
　　web contracture (skin) 86.84
Relief — *see* Release
Relocation — *see also* Revision
　cardiac device (CRT-D) (CRT-P) (defibrillator)
　　(pacemaker) pocket, new site (skin)
　　(subcutaneous) 37.79
　CRT-D pocket 37.79
　CRT-P pocket 37.79
　subcutaneous device pocket NEC 86.09
Remobilization
　joint 93.16
　stapes 19.0
Remodel
　ventricle 37.35
Removal — *see also* Excision
　Abrams bar (chest wall) 34.01
　abscess — *see* Incision, by site
　adenoid tag(s) 28.6
　anal sphincter
　　with revision 49.75
　　without revision 49.76
　arch bars (orthodontic) 24.8
　　immobilization device 97.33
　arterial graft or prosthesis 39.49
　arteriovenous shunt (device) 39.43
　　with creation of new shunt 39.42
　artificial heart
　　internal biventricular replacement system 37.55
　Barton's tongs (skull) 02.95
　　with synchronous replacement 02.94
　bladder sphincter, artificial 58.99
　　with replacement 58.93
　blood clot (*see also* Incision, by site)
　　bladder (by incision) 57.19
　　　without incision 57.0
　　kidney (without incision) 56.0
　　　by incision 55.01
　　ureter
　　　by incision 56.2
　bone fragment (chip) (*see also* Incision,
　　bone) 77.10
　　joint (*see also* Arthrotomy) 80.10
　　necrotic (*see also* Sequestrectomy, bone)
　　　77.00
　　　joint (*see also* Arthrotomy) 80.10
　　skull 01.25
　　　with debridement compound fracture 02.02
　bone growth stimulator — *see* category
　　78.6 ☑
　bony spicules, spinal canal 03.53
　brace 97.88
　breast implant 85.94
　　tissue expander 85.96
　bronchial device or substance
　　endoscopic 33.78
　calcareous deposit
　　bursa 83.03
　　　hand 82.03
　　tendon, intratendinous 83.39

☑ **Additional Digit Required** — Refer to the Tabular List for Digit Selection　　　　　　　▽ **Subterms under main terms may continue to next column or page**

872　　　　　　　　　　　　　　　　　　　　　　　　　　　　　　　　　　　　　　**2014 ICD-9-CM**

Removal — *see also* Excision — *continued*
calcareous deposit — *continued*
tendon, intratendinous — *continued*
hand 82.29
calcification, heart valve leaflets — *see* Valvuloplasty, heart
calculus
bile duct (by incision) 51.49
endoscopic 51.88
laparoscopic 51.88
percutaneous 51.98
bladder (by incision) 57.19
without incision 57.0
common duct (by incision) 51.41
endoscopic 51.88
laparoscopic 51.88
percutaneous 51.96
gallbladder 51.04
endoscopic 51.88
laparoscopic 51.88
kidney (by incision) 55.01
without incision (transurethral) 56.0
percutaneous 55.03
with fragmentation (ultrasound) 55.04
renal pelvis (by incision) 55.11
percutaneous nephrostomy 55.03
with fragmentation 55.04
transurethral 56.0
lacrimal
canaliculi 09.42
by incision 09.52
gland 09.3
by incision 09.0
passage(s) 09.49
by incision 09.59
punctum 09.41
by incision 09.51
sac 09.49
by incision 09.53
pancreatic duct (by incision) 52.09
endoscopic 52.94
perirenal tissue 59.09
pharynx 29.39
prostate 60.0
salivary gland (by incision) 26.0
by probe 26.91
ureter (by incision) 56.2
without incision 56.0
urethra (by incision) 58.0
without incision 58.6
caliper tongs (skull) 02.95
cannula
for extracorporeal membrane oxygenation (ECMO) — *omit code*
cardiac pacemaker (device) (initial) (permanent) (cardiac resynchronization device, CRT-P) 37.89
with replacement
cardiac resynchronization pacemaker (CRT-P)
device only 00.53
total system 00.50
dual-chamber 37.87
single-chamber device 37.85
rate responsive 37.86
cardioverter/defibrillator pulse generator
without replacement (cardiac resynchronization defibrillator device (CRT-D) 37.79
cast 97.88
with reapplication 97.13
lower limb 97.12
upper limb 97.11
catheter (indwelling) (*see also* Removal, tube)
bladder 97.64
cranial cavity 01.27
middle ear (tympanum) 20.1
ureter 97.62
urinary 97.64
CCM (cardiac contractility modulation)
without replacement (rechargeable pulse generator) (total system) 37.79
cerclage material, cervix 69.96
cerumen, ear 96.52

Removal — *see also* Excision — *continued*
corneal epithelium 11.41
for smear or culture 11.21
coronary artery obstruction (thrombus) 36.09
direct intracoronary artery infusion 36.04
open chest approach 36.03
percutaneous transluminal (balloon) 00.66

Note — Also use 00.40, 00.41, 00.42, or 00.43 to show the total number of vessels treated. Use code 00.44 once to show procedure on a bifurcated vessel. In addition, use 00.45, 00.46, 00.47, or 00.48 to show the number of vascular stents inserted.

Crutchfield tongs (skull) 02.95
with synchronous replacement 02.94
cyst (*see also* Excision, lesion, by site)
dental 24.4
lung 32.29
endoscopic 32.28
thoracoscopic 32.20
cystic duct remnant 51.61
decidua (by)
aspiration curettage 69.52
curettage (D and C) 69.02
manual 75.4
dental wiring (immobilization device) 97.33
orthodontic 24.8
device (therapeutic) NEC 97.89
abdomen NEC 97.86
bronchus 33.78
valve 33.78
digestive system NEC 97.59
drainage — *see* Removal, tube
external fixation device 97.88
mandibular NEC 97.36
minifixator (bone) — *see* category 78.6 ☑
for musculoskeletal immobilization NEC 97.88
genital tract NEC 97.79
head and neck NEC 97.39
intrauterine contraceptive 97.71
spine 80.09
thorax NEC 97.49
trunk NEC 97.87
urinary system NEC 97.69
diaphragm, vagina 97.73
drainage device — *see* Removal, tube
dye, spinal canal 03.31
ectopic fetus (from) 66.02
abdominal cavity 74.3
extraperitoneal (intraligamentous) 74.3
fallopian tube (by salpingostomy) 66.02
by salpingotomy 66.01
with salpingectomy 66.62
intraligamentous 74.3
ovarian 74.3
peritoneal (following uterine or tubal rupture) 74.3
site NEC 74.3
tubal (by salpingostomy) 66.02
by salpingotomy 66.01
with salpingectomy 66.62
electrodes
bone growth stimulator — *see* category 78.6 ☑
brain 01.22
depth 01.22
with synchronous replacement 02.93
foramen ovale 01.22
with synchronous replacement 02.93
sphenoidal — *omit code*
with synchronous replacement 02.96
cardiac pacemaker (atrial) (transvenous) (ventricular) 37.77
with replacement 37.76
carotid sinus 39.87
with synchronous pulse generator removal (total system) 39.86
with synchronous replacement 39.82

Removal — *see also* Excision — *continued*
electrodes — *continued*
depth 01.22
with synchronous replacement 02.93
epicardial (myocardial) 37.77
with replacement (by)
atrial and/or ventricular lead(s) (electrode) 37.76
epicardial lead 37.74
epidural pegs 01.22
with synchronous replacement 02.93
foramen ovale 01.22
with synchronous replacement 02.93
gastric 04.93
with synchronous replacement 04.92
intracranial 01.22
with synchronous replacement 02.93
peripheral nerve 04.93
with synchronous replacement 04.92
sacral nerve 04.93
sphenoidal — *omit code*
with synchronous replacement 02.96
spinal 03.94
with synchronous replacement 03.93
temporary transvenous pacemaker system — *omit code*
electroencephalographic receiver (brain) (intracranial) 01.22
with synchronous replacement 02.93
electronic
stimulator — *see* Removal, neurostimulator, by site
bladder 57.98
bone 78.6 ☑
skeletal muscle 83.93
with synchronous replacement 83.92
ureter 56.94
electrostimulator — *see* Removal, electronic, stimulator, by site
embolus 38.00
with endarterectomy — *see* Endarterectomy
abdominal
artery 38.06
vein 38.07
aorta (arch) (ascending) (descending) 38.04
arteriovenous shunt or cannula 39.49
bovine graft 39.49
head and neck vessel
endovascular approach 39.74
open approach, intracranial vessels 38.01
open approach, other vessels of head and neck 38.02
intracranial vessel
endovascular approach 39.74
open approach, intracranial vessels 38.01
open approach, other vessels of head and neck 38.02
lower limb
artery 38.08
vein 38.09
pulmonary (artery) (vein) 38.05
thoracic vessel NEC 38.05
upper limb (artery) (vein) 38.03
embryo — *see* Removal, ectopic fetus
encircling tube, eye (episcleral) 14.6
epithelial downgrowth, anterior chamber 12.93
external fixation device 97.88
mandibular NEC 97.36
minifixator (bone) — *see* category 78.6 ☑
extrauterine embryo — *see* Removal, ectopic fetus
eyeball 16.49
with implant 16.42
with attachment of muscles 16.41
fallopian tube — *see* Salpingectomy
feces (impacted) (by flushing) (manual) 96.38
fetus, ectopic — *see* Removal, ectopic fetus
fingers, supernumerary 86.26

Removal — *see also* Excision — *continued*
fixation device
external 97.88
mandibular NEC 97.36
minifixator (bone) — *see* category 78.6 ☑
internal 78.60
carpal, metacarpal 78.64
clavicle 78.61
facial (bone) 76.97
femur 78.65
fibula 78.67
humerus 78.62
patella 78.66
pelvic 78.69
phalanges (foot) (hand) 78.69
radius 78.63
scapula 78.61
specified site NEC 78.69
tarsal, metatarsal 78.68
thorax (ribs) (sternum) 78.61
tibia 78.67
ulna 78.63
vertebrae 78.69
foreign body NEC (*see also* Incision, by site) 98.20
abdominal (cavity) 54.92
wall 54.0
adenoid 98.13
by incision 28.91
alveolus, alveolar bone 98.22
by incision 24.0
antecubital fossa 98.27
by incision 86.05
anterior chamber 12.00
by incision 12.02
with use of magnet 12.01
anus (intraluminal) 98.05
by incision 49.93
artifical stoma (intraluminal) 98.18
auditory canal, external 18.02
axilla 98.27
by incision 86.05
bladder (without incision) 57.0
by incision 57.19
bone, except fixation device (*see also* Incision, bone) 77.10
alveolus, alveolar 98.22
by incision 24.0
brain 01.39
without incision into brain 01.24
breast 85.0
bronchus (intraluminal) 98.15
by incision 33.0
bursa 83.03
hand 82.03
canthus 98.22
by incision 08.51
cerebral meninges 01.31
cervix (intraluminal) NEC 98.16
penetrating 69.97
choroid (by incision) 14.00
with use of magnet 14.01
without use of magnet 14.02
ciliary body (by incision) 12.00
with use of magnet 12.01
without use of magnet 12.02
conjunctiva (by magnet) 98.22
by incision 10.0
cornea 98.21
by
incision 11.1
magnet 11.0
duodenum 98.03
by incision 45.01
ear (intraluminal) 98.11
with incision 18.09
epididymis 63.92
esophagus (intraluminal) 98.02
by incision 42.09
extrapleural (by incision) 34.01
eye, eyeball (by magnet) 98.21
anterior segment (by incision) 12.00
with use of magnet 12.01
without use of magnet 12.02
posterior segment (by incision) 14.00

☑ **Additional Digit Required** — Refer to the Tabular List for Digit Selection

▼ **Subterms under main terms may continue to next column or page**

Index

Removal — Removal

Removal — *see also* Excision — *continued*
  foreign body (*see also* Incision, by site) — *continued*
    eye, eyeball — *continued*
      posterior segment — *continued*
        with use of magnet 14.01
        without use of magnet 14.02
      superficial 98.21
    eyelid 98.22
      by incision 08.09
    fallopian tube
      by salpingostomy 66.02
      by salpingotomy 66.01
    fascia 83.09
      hand 82.09
    foot 98.28
    gall bladder 51.04
    groin region (abdominal wall) (inguinal) 54.0
    gum 98.22
      by incision 24.0
    hand 98.26
    head and neck NEC 98.22
    heart 37.11
    internal fixation device — *see* Removal, fixation device, internal
    intestine
      by incision 45.00
      large (intraluminal) 98.04
        by incision 45.03
      small (intraluminal) 98.03
        by incision 45.02
    intraocular (by incision) 12.00
      with use of magnet 12.01
      without use of magnet 12.02
    iris (by incision) 12.00
      with use of magnet 12.01
      without use of magnet 12.02
    joint structures (*see also* Arthrotomy) 80.10
    kidney (transurethral) (by endoscopy) 56.0
      by incision 55.01
      pelvis (transurethral) 56.0
        by incision 55.11
    labia 98.23
      by incision 71.09
    lacrimal
      canaliculi 09.42
        by incision 09.52
      gland 09.3
        by incision 09.0
      passage(s) 09.49
        by incision 09.59
      punctum 09.41
        by incision 09.51
      sac 09.49
        by incision 09.53
    large intestine (intraluminal) 98.04
      by incision 45.03
    larynx (intraluminal) 98.14
      by incision 31.3
    lens 13.00
      by incision 13.02
        with use of magnet 13.01
    liver 50.0
    lower limb, except foot 98.29
      foot 98.28
    lung 33.1
    mediastinum 34.1
    meninges (cerebral) 01.31
      spinal 03.01
    mouth (intraluminal) 98.01
      by incision 27.92
    muscle 83.02
      hand 82.02
    nasal sinus 22.50
      antrum 22.2
        with Caldwell-Luc approach 22.39
      ethmoid 22.51
      frontal 22.41
      maxillary 22.2
        with Caldwell-Luc approach 22.39
      sphenoid 22.52
    nerve (cranial) (peripheral) NEC 04.04
      root 03.01

Removal — *see also* Excision — *continued*
  foreign body (*see also* Incision, by site) — *continued*
    nose (intraluminal) 98.12
      by incision 21.1
    oral cavity (intraluminal) 98.01
      by incision 27.92
    orbit (by magnet) 98.21
      by incision 16.1
    palate (penetrating) 98.22
      by incision 27.1
    pancreas 52.09
    penis 98.24
      by incision 64.92
    pericardium 37.12
    perineum (female) 98.23
      by incision 71.09
      male 98.25
        by incision 86.05
    perirenal tissue 59.09
    peritoneal cavity 54.92
    perivesical tissue 59.19
    pharynx (intraluminal) 98.13
      by pharyngotomy 29.0
    pleura (by incision) 34.09
    popliteal space 98.29
      by incision 86.05
    rectum (intraluminal) 98.05
      by incision 48.0
    renal pelvis (transurethral) 56.0
      by incision 56.1
    retina (by incision) 14.00
      with use of magnet 14.01
      without use of magnet 14.02
    retroperitoneum 54.92
    sclera (by incision) 12.00
      with use of magnet 12.01
      without use of magnet 12.02
    scrotum 98.24
      by incision 61.0
    sinus (nasal) 22.50
      antrum 22.2
        with Caldwell-Luc approach 22.39
      ethmoid 22.51
      frontal 22.41
      maxillary 22.2
        with Caldwell-Luc approach 22.39
      sphenoid 22.52
    skin NEC 98.20
      by incision 86.05
    skull 01.24
      with incision into brain 01.39
    small intestine (intraluminal) 98.03
      by incision 45.02
    soft tissue NEC 83.09
      hand 82.09
    spermatic cord 63.93
    spinal (canal) (cord) (meninges) 03.01
    stomach (intraluminal) 98.03
      by incision 43.0
      bubble (balloon) 44.94
    subconjunctival (by magnet) 98.22
      by incision 10.0
    subcutaneous tissue NEC 98.20
      by incision 86.05
    supraclavicular fossa 98.27
      by incision 86.05
    tendon (sheath) 83.01
      hand 82.01
    testis 62.0
    thorax (by incision) 34.09
    thyroid (field) (gland) (by incision) 06.09
    tonsil 98.13
      by incision 28.91
    trachea (intraluminal) 98.15
      by incision 31.3
    trunk NEC 98.25
    tunica vaginalis 98.24
    upper limb, except hand 98.27
      hand 98.26
    ureter (transurethral) 56.0
      by incision 56.2
    urethra (intraluminal) 98.19
      by incision 58.0
    uterus (intraluminal) 98.16
    vagina (intraluminal) 98.17

Removal — *see also* Excision — *continued*
  foreign body (*see also* Incision, by site) — *continued*
    vagina — *continued*
      by incision 70.14
    vas deferens 63.6
    vitreous (by incision) 14.00
      with use of magnet 14.01
      without use of magnet 14.02
    vulva 98.23
      by incision 71.09
  gallstones
    bile duct (by incision) NEC 51.49
      endoscopic 51.88
    common duct (by incision) 51.41
      endoscopic 51.88
      percutaneous 51.96
    duodenum 45.01
    gallbladder 51.04
      endoscopic 51.88
      laparoscopic 51.88
    hepatic ducts 51.49
      endoscopic 51.88
    intestine 45.00
      large 45.03
      small NEC 45.02
    liver 50.0
  Gardner Wells tongs (skull) 02.95
    with synchronous replacement 02.94
  gastric band (adjustable), laparoscopic 44.97
  gastric bubble (balloon) 44.94
  granulation tissue (*see also* Excision, lesion, by site)
    with repair — *see* Repair, by site
    cranial 01.6
    skull 01.6
  halo traction device (skull) 02.95
    with synchronous replacement 02.94
  heart assist system
    with replacement 37.63
    intra-aortic balloon pump (IABP) 97.44
    nonoperative 97.44
    open removal 37.64
    percutaneous external device 97.44
  heart replacement system
    internal biventricular 37.55
  hematoma — *see* Drainage, by site
  Hoffman minifixator device (bone) — *see* category 78.6 ☑
  hydatidiform mole 68.0
  impacted
    feces (rectum) (by flushing) (manual) 96.38
    tooth 23.19
      from nasal sinus (maxillary) 22.61
  implant
    breast 85.94
    cochlear prosthetic device 20.99
    cornea 11.92
    lens (prosthetic) 13.8
    middle ear NEC 20.99
    ocular 16.71
      posterior segment 14.6
    orbit 16.72
    retina 14.6
    tympanum 20.1
  implantable hemodynamic sensor (lead) and monitor device 37.79
  internal biventricular heart replacement system 37.55
  internal fixation device — *see* Removal, fixation device, internal
  intra-aortic balloon pump (IABP) 97.44
  intrauterine contraceptive device (IUD) 97.71
  joint (structure) NOS 80.90
    ankle 80.97
    elbow 80.92
    foot and toe 80.98
    hand and finger 80.94
    hip 80.95
    knee 80.96
    other specified sites 80.99
    shoulder 80.91
    spine 80.99
    toe 80.98

Removal — *see also* Excision — *continued*
  joint — *continued*
    wrist 80.93
  Kantrowitz heart pump 37.64
    nonoperative 97.44
  keel (tantalum plate), larynx 31.98
  kidney (*see also* Nephrectomy)
    mechanical 55.98
    transplanted or rejected 55.53
  laminaria (tent), uterus 97.79
  leads (cardiac) — *see* Removal, electrodes, cardiac pacemaker
  lesion — *see* Excision, lesion, by site
  ligamentum flavum (spine) — *omit code*
  ligature
    fallopian tube 66.79
    ureter 56.86
    vas deferens 63.84
  limb lengthening device, internal — *see* category 78.6 ☑
  loop recorder 86.05
  loose body
    bone — *see* Sequestrectomy, bone
    joint 80.10
    mesh (surgical) — *see* Removal, foreign body, by site
  lymph node — *see* Excision, lymph, node
  minifixator device (bone) — *see* category 78.6 ☑
    external fixation device 97.88
  Mulligan hood, fallopian tube 66.94
    with synchronous replacement 66.93
  muscle stimulator (skeletal) 83.93
    with replacement 83.92
  myringotomy device or tube 20.1
  nail (bed) (fold) 86.23
    internal fixation device — *see* Removal, fixation device, internal
  necrosis
    skin 86.28
      excisional 86.22
  neuropacemaker — *see* Removal, neurostimulator, by site
  neurostimulator
    brain 01.22
      with synchronous replacement 02.93
    electrodes
      brain 01.22
        with synchronous replacement 02.93
      gastric 04.93
        with synchronous replacement 04.92
      intracranial 01.22
        with synchronous replacement 02.93
      peripheral nerve 04.93
        with synchronous replacement 04.92
      sacral nerve 04.93
        with synchronous replacement 04.92
      spinal 03.94
        with synchronous replacement 03.93
    intracranial 01.22
      with synchronous replacement 02.93
    peripheral nerve 04.93
      with synchronous replacement 04.92
    pulse generator (subcutaneous single array, multiple array) 86.05
      with synchronous replacement 86.96
      multiple array 86.95
        rechargeable 86.98
      single array 86.94
        rechargeable 86.97
    cranial 01.29
      with synchronous replacement 01.20
    spinal 03.94
      with synchronous replacement 03.93
  nonabsorbable surgical material NEC — *see* Removal, foreign body, by site
  odontoma (tooth) 24.4
  orbital implant 16.72

☑ Additional Digit Required — Refer to the Tabular List for Digit Selection
▽ Subterms under main terms may continue to next column or page
2014 ICD-9-CM
875

Repair — *continued*
  aneurysm — *continued*
    by or with — *continued*
      endovascular graft — *continued*
        abdominal aorta — *continued*
          fenestrated (branching) 39.78
        head and neck 39.72
        lower extremity artery(s) 39.79
        thoracic aorta 39.73
        upper extremity artery(s) 39.79
      filipuncture 39.52
      graft replacement — *see* Aneurysmectomy, with graft replacement, by site
      ligation 39.52
      liquid tissue adhesive (glue) 39.79
        endovascular approach 39.79
          head and neck 39.72
      methyl methacrylate 39.52
        endovascular approach 39.79
          head and neck 39.72
      occlusion 39.52
        endovascular approach 39.79
          head and neck 39.72
      suture 39.52
      trapping 39.52
      wiring 39.52
      wrapping (gauze) (methyl methacrylate) (plastic) 39.52
    coronary artery 36.91
    heart 37.32
    sinus of Valsalva 35.39
    thoracic aorta (dissecting), by fenestration 39.54
  anomalous pulmonary venous connection (total)
    one-stage 35.82
    partial — *see* specific procedure
    total 35.82
  anular disc 80.54
    with graft or prosthesis 80.53
  anulus fibrosus 80.54
    with graft or prosthesis 80.53
  anus 49.79
    laceration (by suture) 49.71
      obstetric (current) 75.62
      old 49.79
  aorta 39.31
  aorticopulmonary window 39.59
  arteriovenous fistula 39.53
    by or with
      clipping 39.53
      coagulation 39.53
      coil, NEC (endovascular approach) 39.79
        head and neck vessels
          bare coils 39.75
          bioactive coils 39.76
      division 39.53
      excision or resection (*see also* Aneurysmectomy, by site)
        with
          anastomosis — *see* Aneurysmectomy, with anastomosis, by site
          graft replacement — *see* Aneurysmectomy, with graft replacement, by site
      ligation 39.53
        coronary artery 36.99
      occlusion 39.53
        endovascular approach 39.79
          head and neck 39.72
      suture 39.53
  artery NEC 39.59
    by
      endovascular approach
        abdominal aorta 39.71
          fenestrated (branching) graft 39.78
        head and neck (total embolization or occlusion) 39.72
        other repair (of aneurysm) 39.79

Repair — *continued*
  artery — *continued*
    by — *continued*
      endovascular approach — *continued*
        percutaneous repair of extracranial vessel(s) (for stent insertion) 00.61

Note — Also use 00.40, 00.41, 00.42, or 00.43 to show the total number of vessels treated. Use code 00.44 once to show procedure on a bifurcated vessel. In addition, use 00.45, 00.46, 00.47, or 00.48 to show the number of vascular stents inserted.

        percutaneous repair of intracranial vessel(s) (for stent insertion) 00.62

Note — Also use 00.40, 00.41, 00.42, or 00.43 to show the total number of vessels treated. Use code 00.44 once to show procedure on a bifurcated vessel. In addition, use 00.45, 00.46, 00.47, or 00.48 to show the number of vascular stents inserted.

        thoracic aorta 39.73
      non-coronary percutaneous transluminal approach

Note — Also use 00.40, 00.41, 00.42, or 00.43 to show the total number of vessels treated. Use code 00.44 once to show procedure on a bifurcated vessel. In addition, use 00.45, 00.46, 00.47, or 00.48 to show the number of vascular stents inserted.

        angioplasty
          basilar 00.62
          carotid 00.61
          femoropopliteal 39.50
          iliac 39.50
          lower extremity NOS 39.50
          mesenteric 39.50
          renal 39.50
          upper extremity 39.50
          vertebral 00.61
            intracranial portion 00.62
        atherectomy 17.56
      with
        patch graft 39.58
          with excision or resection of vessel — *see* Arteriectomy, with graft replacement, by site
          synthetic (Dacron) (Teflon) 39.57
          tissue (vein) (autogenous) (homograft) 39.56
        suture 39.31
      coronary NEC 36.99
        by angioplasty — *see* Angioplasty, coronary
        by atherectomy
          percutaneous transluminal 17.55
  artificial opening — *see* Repair, stoma
  atrial septal defect 35.71
    with
      prosthesis (open heart technique) 35.51
        closed heart technique 35.52
      tissue graft 35.61
    combined with repair of valvular and ventricular septal defects — *see* Repair, endocardial cushion defect
    in total repair of total anomalous pulmonary venous connection 35.82
  atrioventricular canal defect (any type) 35.73
    with
      prosthesis 35.54
      tissue graft 35.63
  bifid digit (finger) 82.89
  bile duct NEC 51.79
    laceration (by suture) NEC 51.79
      common bile duct 51.71
  bladder NEC 57.89

Repair — *continued*
  bladder — *continued*
    exstrophy 57.86
    for stress incontinence — *see* Repair, stress incontinence
    laceration (by suture) 57.81
      obstetric (current) 75.61
      old 57.89
    neck 57.85
  blepharophimosis 08.59
  blepharoptosis 08.36
    by
      frontalis muscle technique (with)
        fascial sling 08.32
        suture 08.31
      levator muscle technique 08.34
        with resection or advancement 08.33
      orbicularis oculi muscle sling 08.36
      tarsal technique 08.35
  blood vessel NEC 39.59
    with
      patch graft 39.58
        with excision or resection — *see* Angiectomy, with graft replacement
        synthetic (Dacron) (Teflon) 39.57
        tissue (vein) (autogenous) (homograft) 39.56
      resection — *see* Angiectomy
      suture 39.30
    coronary artery NEC 36.99
      by angioplasty — *see* Angioplasty, coronary
      by atherectomy
        percutaneous transluminal 17.55
    peripheral vessel NEC 39.59
      by angioplasty 39.50

Note — Also use 00.40, 00.41, 00.42, or 00.43 to show the total number of vessels treated. Use code 00.44 once to show procedure on a bifurcated vessel. In addition, use 00.45, 00.46, 00.47, or 00.48 to show the number of vascular stents inserted.

      by atherectomy 17.56

Note — Also use 00.40, 00.41, 00.42, or 00.43 to show the total number of vessels treated. Use code 00.44 once to show procedure on a bifurcated vessel. In addition, use 00.45, 00.46, 00.47, or 00.48 to show the number of vascular stents inserted.

      by endovascular approach 39.79
  bone NEC (*see also* Osteoplasty) — *see* category 78.4 ☑
    by synostosis technique — *see* Arthrodesis
    accessory sinus 22.79
    cranium NEC 02.06
      with
        flap (bone) 02.03
        graft (bone) 02.04
    for malunion, nonunion, or delayed union of fracture — *see* Repair, fracture, malunion or nonunion
    nasal 21.89
    skull NEC 02.06
      with
        flap (bone) 02.03
        graft (bone) 02.04
  bottle, hydrocele of tunica vaginalis 61.2
  brain (trauma) NEC 02.92
  breast (plastic) (*see also* Mammoplasty) 85.89
  broad ligament 69.29
  bronchus NEC 33.48
    laceration (by suture) 33.41
  bunionette (with osteotomy) 77.54
  canaliculus, lacrimal 09.73
  canthus (lateral) 08.59
  cardiac pacemaker NEC 37.89
    electrode(s) (lead) NEC 37.75
  cardioverter/defibrillator (automatic) pocket (skin) (subcutaneous) 37.99
  cerebral meninges 02.12

Repair — *continued*
  cervix 67.69
    internal os 67.59
      transabdominal 67.51
      transvaginal 67.59
    laceration (by suture) 67.61
      obstetric (current) 75.51
      old 67.69
  chest wall (mesh) (silastic) NEC 34.79
  chordae tendineae 35.32
  choroid NEC 14.9
    with retinal repair — *see* Repair, retina
  cisterna chyli 40.69
  claw toe 77.57
  cleft
    hand 82.82
    laryngotracheal 31.69
    lip 27.54
    palate 27.62
      secondary or subsequent 27.63
  coarctation of aorta — *see* Excision, coarctation of aorta
  cochlear prosthetic device 20.99
    external components only 95.49
  cockup toe 77.58
  colostomy 46.43
  conjunctiva NEC 10.49
    with scleral repair 12.81
    laceration 10.6
      with repair of sclera 12.81
    late effect of trachoma 10.49
  cornea NEC 11.59
    with
      conjunctival flap 11.53
      transplant — *see* Keratoplasty
    postoperative dehiscence 11.52
  coronary artery NEC 36.99
    by angioplasty — *see* Angioplasty, coronary
    by atherectomy
      percutaneous transluminal 17.55
  cranium NEC 02.06
    with
      flap (bone) 02.03
      graft (bone) 02.04
  cusp, valve — *see* Repair, heart, valve
  cystocele 70.51
    with graft or prosthesis 70.54
    and rectocele 70.50
      with graft or prosthesis 70.53
  dental arch 24.8
  diaphragm NEC 34.84
  diastasis recti 83.65
  diastematomyelia 03.59
  ear (external) 18.79
    auditory canal or meatus 18.6
    auricle NEC 18.79
    cartilage NEC 18.79
    laceration (by suture) 18.4
    lop ear 18.79
    middle NEC 19.9
    prominent or protruding 18.5
  ectropion 08.49
    by or with
      lid reconstruction 08.44
      suture (technique) 08.42
      thermocauterization 08.41
      wedge resection 08.43
  encephalocele (cerebral) 02.12
  endocardial cushion defect 35.73
    with
      prosthesis (grafted to septa) 35.54
      tissue graft 35.63
  enterocele (female) 70.92
    with graft or prosthesis 70.93
    male 53.9
  enterostomy 46.40
  entropion 08.49
    by or with
      lid reconstruction 08.44
      suture (technique) 08.42
      thermocauterization 08.41
      wedge resection 08.43
  epicanthus (fold) 08.59
  epididymis (and spermatic cord) NEC 63.59
    with vas deferens 63.89

☑ Additional Digit Required — Refer to the Tabular List for Digit Selection   ▽ Subterms under main terms may continue to next column or page

878   2014 ICD-9-CM

☑ Additional Digit Required — Refer to the Tabular List for Digit Selection   ▽ Subterms under main terms may continue to next column or page

2014 ICD-9-CM   **879**

Replacement — continued
electrode(s) — see Implant, electrode or lead
by site or name of device — continued
foramen ovale 02.93
gastric 04.92
intracranial 02.93
pacemaker — see Replacement, pacemaker, electrode(s)
peripheral nerve 04.92
sacral nerve 04.92
sphenoidal 02.96
spine 03.93
electroencephalographic receiver (brain) (intracranial) 02.93
electronic
cardioverter/defibrillator — see Replacement, cardioverter/defibrillator
leads (electrode) (s) — see Replacement, electrode(s)
stimulator (see also Implant, electronic stimulator, by site)
bladder 57.97
muscle (skeletal) 83.92
ureter 56.93
electrostimulator — see Implant, electronic stimulator by site
enterostomy device (tube)
large intestine 97.04
small intestine 97.03
epidural pegs 02.93
femoral head, by prosthesis 81.52
revision 81.53
Gardner Wells tongs (skull) 02.94
gastric band, laparoscopic 44.96
gastric port device (subcutaneous) 44.96
graft — see Graft
halo traction device (skull) 02.94
Harrington rod (with refusion of spine) — see Refusion, spinal
heart
artificial
total internal biventricular replacement system 37.52
implantable battery 37.54
implantable controller 37.54
thoracic unit 37.53
transcutaneous energy transfer (TET) device 37.54
total internal biventricular replacement system 37.52
implantable battery 37.54
implantable controller 37.54
thoracic unit 37.53
transcutaneous energy transfer (TET) device 37.54
valve, NOS (with prosthesis) (with tissue graft) 35.20
aortic, NOS 35.22
with
prosthesis 35.22
tissue graft 35.21
endovascular 35.05
endovascular (TAVI) (TAVR) (transarterial) (transcatheter) (transfemoral) (with tissue graft) 35.05
transapical (intercostal) (transcatheter) (transthoracic) (transventricular) (with tissue graft) 35.06
endovascular, NOS 35.09
mitral, NOS 35.24
with
prosthesis 35.24
tissue graft 35.23
poppet (prosthetic) 35.95
pulmonary, NOS 35.26
with
prosthesis 35.26
tissue graft 35.25
endovascular (percutaneous) (PPVI) (TPVR) (transcatheter) (transfemoral) (transvenous) 35.07

Replacement — continued
heart — continued
valve, — continued
pulmonary, — continued
in total repair of tetralogy of Fallot 35.81
transapical (intercostal) (transcatheter) (transthoracic) (transventricular) 35.08
tricuspid, NOS 35.28
with
prosthesis 35.28
tissue graft 35.27
hip (partial) (with fixation device) (with prosthesis) (with traction) 81.52
acetabulum 81.52
revision 81.53
femoral head 81.52
revision 81.53
total 81.51
revision 81.53
intervertebral disc
artificial, NOS 84.60
cervical 84.62
nucleus 84.61
partial 84.61
total 84.62
lumbar, lumbosacral 84.65
nucleus 84.64
partial 84.64
total 84.65
thoracic (partial) (total) 84.63
inverted uterus — see Repair, inverted uterus
iris NEC 12.39
kidney, mechanical 55.97
knee (bicompartmental) (hemijoint) (partial) (total) (tricompartmental) (unicompartmental) 81.54
revision 81.55
laryngeal stent 31.93
leads (electrode) (s) — see Replacement, electrode(s)
mechanical kidney 55.97
mitral valve, NOS 35.24
with
prosthesis 35.24
tissue graft 35.23
Mulligan hood, fallopian tube 66.93
muscle stimulator (skeletal) 83.92
nephrostomy tube 55.93
neuropacemaker — see Implant, neurostimulator, by site
neurostimulator — see Implant, neurostimulator, by site
skeletal muscle 83.92
pacemaker
brain — see Implant, neurostimulator, brain
cardiac device (initial) (permanent)
dual-chamber device 37.87
resynchronization — see Replacement, CRT-P
single-chamber device 37.85
rate responsive 37.86
electrode(s), cardiac (atrial) (transvenous) (ventricular) 37.76
epicardium (myocardium) 37.74
left ventricular coronary venous system 00.52
gastric — see Implant, neurostimulator, gastric
intracranial — see Implant, neurostimulator, intracranial
neural — see Implant, neurostimulator, by site
peripheral nerve — see Implant, neurostimulator, peripheral nerve
sacral nerve — see Implant, neurostimulator, sacral nerve
spine — see Implant, neurostimulator, spine
temporary transvenous pacemaker system 37.78
pack or bag
nose 97.21

Replacement — continued
pack or bag — continued
teeth, tooth 97.22
vagina 97.26
vulva 97.26
wound 97.16
pessary, vagina NEC 97.25
prosthesis
acetabulum 81.53
arm (bioelectric) (cineplastic) (kineplastic) 84.44
biliary tract 51.99
channel (single) 20.97
multiple 20.98
cochlear 20.96
elbow 81.97
epiretinal visual 14.83
extremity (bioelectric) (cineplastic) (kineplastic) 84.40
lower 84.48
upper 84.44
fallopian tube (Mulligan hood) (stent) 66.93
femur 81.53
knee 81.55
leg (bioelectric) (cineplastic) (kineplastic) 84.48
penis (internal) (non-inflatable) 64.95
inflatable (internal) 64.97
pulmonary valve, NOS 35.26
with
prosthesis 35.26
tissue graft 35.25
endovascular (percutaneous) (PPVI) (TPVR) (transcatheter) (transfemoral) (transvenous) 35.07
in total repair of tetralogy of Fallot 35.81
transapical (intercostal) (transcatheter) (transthoracic) (transventricular) 35.08
pyelostomy tube 55.94
rectal tube 96.09
Rheos™ carotid sinus baroreflex activation device 39.81
sensor (lead)
intracardiac or great vessel hemodynamic monitoring 00.56
shoulder NEC 81.83
partial 81.81
total, NEC 81.80
other 81.80
reverse 81.88
skull
plate 02.05
tongs 02.94
spacer (cement) (joint) (methylmethacrylate) 84.56
specified appliance or device NEC 97.29
spinal motion preservation device
facet replacement device(s) 84.84
interspinous process device(s) 84.80
pedicle-based dynamic stabilization device(s) 84.82
splint 97.14
stent
bile duct 97.05
fallopian tube 66.93
larynx 31.93
pancreatic duct 97.05
trachea 31.93
stimoceiver — see Implant, stimoceiver, by site
stimulator
electrode(s)
carotid sinus 39.82
with synchronous pulse generator replacement (total system) 39.81
pulse generator
carotid sinus 39.83
with synchronous electrode(s) replacement (total system) 39.81
subdural
grids 02.93
strips 02.93

Replacement — continued
testis in scrotum 62.5
tongs, skull 02.94
tracheal stent 31.93
tricuspid valve (with prosthesis) 35.28
with tissue graft 35.27
tube
bile duct 97.05
bladder 57.95
cystostomy 59.94
esophagostomy 97.01
gastrostomy 97.02
large intestine 97.04
nasogastric 97.01
nephrostomy 55.93
pancreatic duct 97.05
pyelostomy 55.94
rectal 96.09
small intestine 97.03
tracheostomy 97.23
ureterostomy 59.93
ventricular (cerebral) 02.42
umbilical cord, prolapsed 73.92
ureter (with)
bladder flap 56.74
ileal segment implanted into bladder 56.89 [45.51]
ureterostomy tube 59.93
urethral sphincter, artificial 58.93
urinary sphincter, artificial 58.93
valve
heart (see also Replacement, heart valve)
poppet (prosthetic) 35.95
ventricular (cerebral) 02.42
ventricular shunt (valve) 02.42
Vinke tongs (skull) 02.94
vitreous (silicone) 14.75
for retinal reattachment 14.59
Replant, replantation — see also Reattachment
extremity — see Reattachment, extremity
penis 64.45
scalp 86.51
tooth 23.5
Reposition
cardiac pacemaker
electrode(s) (atrial) (transvenous) (ventricular) 37.75
pocket 37.79
cardiac resynchronization defibrillator (CRT-D) — see Revision, cardiac resynchronization defibrillator
cardiac resynchronization pacemaker (CRT-P) — see Revision, cardiac resynchronization pacemaker
cardioverter/defibrillator (automatic)
lead(s) (sensing) (pacing) (epicardial patch) 37.75
pocket 37.79
pulse generator 37.79
cilia base 08.71
implantable hemodynamic sensor (lead) and monitor device 37.79
iris 12.39
neurostimulator
leads
subcutaneous, without device replacement 86.09
within brain 02.93
within or over gastric nerve 04.92
within or over peripheral nerve 04.92
within or over sacral nerve 04.92
within spine 03.93
pulse generator
subcutaneous, without device replacement 86.09
renal vessel, aberrant 39.55
subcutaneous device pocket NEC 86.09
thyroid tissue 06.94
tricuspid valve (with plication) 35.14
Resection — see also Excision, by site
abdominoendorectal (combined), NOS 48.50
laparoscopic 48.51
open 48.52
other 48.59

Resection — *see also* Excision, by site — *continued*
abdominoperineal (rectum), NOS 48.50
  pull-through (Altemeier) (Swenson) NEC 48.49
    Duhamel type 48.65
    laparoscopic 48.42
    not otherwise specified 48.40
    open 48.43
alveolar process and palate (en bloc) 27.32
aneurysm — *see* Aneurysmectomy
aortic valve (for subvalvular stenosis) 35.11
artery — *see* Arteriectomy
bile duct NEC 51.69
  common duct NEC 51.63
bladder (partial) (segmental) (transvesical) (wedge) 57.6
  complete or total 57.79
  lesion NEC 57.59
    transurethral approach 57.49
  neck 57.59
    transurethral approach 57.49
blood vessel — *see* Angiectomy
brain 01.59
  by
    stereotactic radiosurgery 92.30
      cobalt 60 92.32
      linear accelerator (LINAC) 92.31
      multi-source 92.32
      particle beam 92.33
      particulate 92.33
      radiosurgery NEC 92.39
      single source photon 92.31
  hemisphere 01.52
  lobe 01.53
breast (*see also* Mastectomy)
  quadrant 85.22
  segmental 85.23
broad ligament 69.19
bronchus (sleeve) (wide sleeve) 32.1
  block (en bloc) (with radical dissection of brachial plexus, bronchus, lobe of lung, ribs, and sympathetic nerves) 32.6
bursa 83.5
  hand 82.31
cecum (and terminal ileum)
  laparoscopic 17.32
  open and other 45.72
cerebral meninges 01.51
chest wall 34.4
clavicle 77.81
clitoris 71.4
colon (partial) (segmental)
  ascending (cecum and terminal ileum)
    laparoscopic 17.32
    open and other 45.72
  cecum (and terminal ileum)
    laparoscopic 17.32
    open and other 45.72
  complete
    laparoscopic 45.81
    open 45.82
    other 45.83
    unspecified 45.83
  descending (sigmoid)
    laparoscopic 17.36
    open and other 45.76
  for interposition 45.52
  Hartmann
    laparoscopic 17.35
    open and other 45.75
  hepatic flexure
    laparoscopic 17.33
    open and other 45.73
  laparoscopic 17.39
  left radical (hemicolon)
    laparoscopic 17.35
    open and other 45.75
  multiple segmental
    laparoscopic 17.31
    open and other 45.71
  open and other 45.79
  right radical (hemicolon) (ileocolectomy)
    laparoscopic 17.33
    open and other 45.73

Resection — *see also* Excision, by site — *continued*
colon — *continued*
  segmental NEC
    laparoscopic 17.39
    multiple
      laparoscopic 17.31
      open and other 45.71
    open and other 45.79
  sigmoid
    laparascopic 17.36
    open and other 45.76
  splenic flexure
    laparoscopic 17.35
    open and other 45.75
  total
    laparoscopic 45.81
    open 45.82
    other 45.83
    unspecified 45.83
  transverse
    laparoscopic 17.34
    open and other 45.74
conjunctiva, for pterygium 11.39
  corneal graft 11.32
cornual (fallopian tube) (unilateral) 66.69
  bilateral 66.63
diaphragm 34.81
endaural 20.79
endorectal (pull-through) (Soave) 48.41
  combined abdominal, NOS 48.50
    laparoscopic 48.51
    open 48.52
    other 48.59
esophagus (partial) (subtotal) (*see also* Esophagectomy) 42.41
  total 42.42
exteriorized intestine — *see* Resection, intestine, exteriorized
fascia 83.44
  for graft 83.43
    hand 82.34
  hand 82.35
    for graft 82.34
gallbladder (total) 51.22
gastric (partial) (sleeve) (subtotal) NEC (*see also* Gastrectomy) 43.89
  with anastomosis NEC 43.89
    esophagogastric 43.5
    gastroduodenal 43.6
    gastrogastric 43.89
    gastrojejunal 43.7
  complete or total NEC 43.99
    with intestinal interposition 43.91
  laparoscopic 43.82
  radical NEC 43.99
    with intestinal interposition 43.91
  wedge 43.42
  endoscopic 43.41
hallux valgus (joint) (*see also* Bunionectomy)
  with prosthetic implant 77.59
hepatic
  duct 51.69
  flexure (colon)
    laparoscopic 17.33
    open and other 45.73
infundibula, heart (right) 35.34
intestine (partial) NEC
  cecum (with terminal ileum)
    laparoscopic 17.32
    open and other 45.72
  exteriorized (large intestine) 46.04
    small intestine 46.02
  for interposition 45.50
    large intestine 45.52
    small intestine 45.51
  hepatic flexure
    laparoscopic 17.33
    open and other 45.73
  ileum 45.62
    with cecum
      laparoscopic 17.32
      open and other 45.72
    laparoscopic 17.39
  large (partial) (segmental) NEC
    for interposition 45.52

Resection — *see also* Excision, by site — *continued*
intestine — *continued*
  large — *continued*
    laparoscopic 17.39
    multiple segmental
      laparoscopic 17.31
      open and other 45.71
    other 45.79
    total
      laparoscopic 45.81
      open 45.82
      other 45.83
      unspecified 45.83
    unspecified 45.79
  left hemicolon
    laparoscopic 17.35
    open and other 45.75
  multiple segmental (large intestine)
    laparoscopic 17.31
    open and other 45.71
    small intestine 45.61
  open and other 45.79
  right hemicolon
    laparoscopic 17.33
    open and other 45.73
  segmental (large intestine)
    laparoscopic 17.39
    multiple
      laparoscopic 17.31
      open and other 45.71
    open and other 45.79
    small intestine 45.62
      multiple 45.61
  sigmoid
    laparoscopic 17.36
    open and other 45.76
  small (partial) (segmental) NEC 45.62
    for interposition 45.51
    multiple segmental 45.61
    total 45.63
  total
    large intestine
      laparoscopic 45.81
      open 45.82
      other 45.83
      unspecified 45.83
    small intestine 45.63
joint structure NEC (*see also* Arthrectomy) 80.90
kidney (segmental) (wedge) 55.4
larynx (*see also* Laryngectomy)
  submucous 30.29
lesion — *see* Excision, lesion, by site
levator palpebrae muscle 08.33
ligament (*see also* Arthrectomy) 80.90
  broad 69.19
  round 69.19
  uterine 69.19
lip (wedge) 27.43
liver (partial) (wedge) 50.22
  lobe (total) 50.3
  total 50.4
lung (wedge) NEC 32.29
  endoscopic 32.28
  segmental (any part) 32.39
    thoracoscopic 32.30
  thoracoscopic 32.20
  volume reduction 32.22
    biologic lung volume reduction (BLVR) — *see* category 33.7 ☑
meninges (cerebral) 01.51
  spinal 03.4
mesentery 54.4
muscle 83.45
  extraocular 15.13
    with
      advancement or recession of other eye muscle 15.3
      suture of original insertion 15.13
    levator palpebrae 08.33
    Müller's, for blepharoptosis 08.35
    orbicularis oculi 08.20
    tarsal, for blepharoptosis 08.35
  for graft 83.43

Resection — *see also* Excision, by site — *continued*
muscle — *continued*
  for graft — *continued*
    hand 82.34
    hand 82.36
      for graft 82.34
  ocular — *see* Resection, muscle, extraocular
  myocardium 37.33
nasal septum (submucous) 21.5
nerve (cranial) (peripheral) NEC 04.07
  phrenic 04.03
    for collapse of lung 33.31
  sympathetic 05.29
  vagus — *see* Vagotomy
nose (complete) (extended) (partial) (radical) 21.4
omentum 54.4
orbitomaxillary, radical 16.51
ovary (*see also* Oophorectomy, wedge) 65.22
  laparoscopic 65.24
palate (bony) (local) 27.31
  by wide excision 27.32
  soft 27.49
pancreas (total) (with synchronous duodenectomy) 52.6
  partial NEC 52.59
    distal (tail) (with part of body) 52.52
    proximal (head) (with part of body) (with synchronous duodenectomy) 52.51
  radical subtotal 52.53
  radical (one-stage) (two-stage) 52.7
  subtotal 52.53
pancreaticoduodenal (*see also* Pancreatectomy) 52.6
pelvic viscera (en masse) (female) 68.8
  male 57.71
penis 64.3
pericardium (partial) (for)
  chronic constrictive pericarditis 37.31
  drainage 37.12
  removal of adhesions 37.31
peritoneum 54.4
pharynx (partial) 29.33
phrenic nerve 04.03
  for collapse of lung 33.31
prostate (*see also* Prostatectomy)
  transurethral (punch) 60.29
pterygium 11.39
radial head 77.83
rectosigmoid (*see also* Resection, rectum) 48.69
rectum (partial) NEC 48.69
  with
    pelvic exenteration 68.8
    transsacral sigmoidectomy 48.61
  abdominoendorectal (combined), NOS 48.50
    laparoscopic 48.51
    open 48.52
    other 48.59
  abdominoperineal, NOS 48.50
    laparoscopic 48.51
    open 48.52
    other 48.59
    pull-through NEC 48.49
      Duhamel type 48.65
      laparoscopic 48.42
      not otherwise specified 48.40
      open 48.43
  anterior 48.63
    with colostomy (synchronous) 48.62
  Duhamel 48.65
  endorectal 48.41
    combined abdominal, NOS 48.50
      laparoscopic 48.51
      open 48.52
      other 48.59
  posterior 48.64
  pull-through NEC 48.49
    endorectal 48.41
    laparoscopic 48.42
    not otherwise specified 48.40
    open 48.43

☑ **Additional Digit Required** — Refer to the Tabular List for Digit Selection   ▽ **Subterms under main terms may continue to next column or page**

2014 ICD-9-CM   **881**

Resection — *see also* Excision, by site — *continued*
- rectum — *continued*
  - STARR procedure 48.74
  - submucosal (Soave) 48.41
    - combined abdominal, NOS 48.50
      - laparoscopic 48.51
      - open 48.52
      - other 48.59
- rib (transaxillary) 77.91
  - as operative approach — *omit code*
  - incidental to thoracic operation — *omit code*
- right ventricle (heart), for infundibular stenosis 35.34
- root (tooth) (apex) 23.73
  - with root canal therapy 23.72
  - residual or retained 23.11
- round ligament 69.19
- sclera 12.65
  - with scleral buckling (*see also* Buckling, scleral) 14.49
  - lamellar (for retinal reattachment) 14.49
  - with implant 14.41
- scrotum 61.3
- soft tissue NEC 83.49
  - hand 82.39
- sphincter of Oddi 51.89
- spinal cord (meninges) 03.4
- splanchnic 05.29
- splenic flexure (colon) 45.75
- sternum 77.81
- stomach (partial) (sleeve) (subtotal) NEC (*see also* Gastrectomy) 43.89
  - with anastomosis NEC 43.89
    - esophagogastric 43.5
    - gastroduodenal 43.6
    - gastrogastric 43.89
    - gastrojejunal 43.7
  - complete or total NEC 43.99
    - with intestinal interposition 43.91
  - fundus 43.89
  - laparoscopic 43.82
  - radical NEC 43.99
    - with intestinal interposition 43.91
  - wedge 43.42
    - endoscopic 43.41
- submucous
  - larynx 30.29
  - nasal septum 21.5
  - vocal cords 30.22
- synovial membrane (complete) (partial) (*see also* Synovectomy) 80.70
- tarsolevator 08.33
- tendon 83.42
  - hand 82.33
- thoracic structures (block) (en bloc) (radical) (brachial plexus, bronchus, lobes of lung, ribs, and sympathetic nerves) 32.6
- thorax 34.4
- tongue 25.2
  - wedge 25.1
- tooth root 23.73
  - with root canal therapy 23.72
  - apex (abscess) 23.73
    - with root canal therapy 23.72
  - residual or retained 23.11
- trachea 31.5
- transurethral
  - bladder NEC 57.49
  - prostate 60.29
- transverse colon
  - laparoscopic 17.34
  - open and other 45.74
- turbinates — *see* Turbinectomy
- ureter (partial) 56.41
  - total 56.42
- uterus — *see* Hysterectomy
- vein — *see* Phlebectomy
- ventricle (heart) 37.35
  - infundibula 35.34
- vesical neck 57.59
  - transurethral 57.49
- vocal cords (punch) 30.22

Respirator, volume-controlled (Bennett) (Byrd) — *see* Ventilation

Restoration
- cardioesophageal angle 44.66
  - laparoscopic 44.67
- dental NEC 23.49
  - by
    - application of crown (artificial) 23.41
    - insertion of bridge (fixed) 23.42
      - removable 23.43
- extremity — *see* Reattachment, extremity
- eyebrow 08.70
  - with graft 08.63
- eye socket 16.64
  - with graft 16.63
- tooth NEC 23.2
  - by
    - crown (artificial) 23.41
    - filling (amalgam) (plastic) (silicate) 23.2
    - inlay 23.3

Restrictive
- gastric band, laparoscopic 44.95

Resurfacing, hip 00.86
- acetabulum 00.87
  - with femoral head 00.85
- femoral head 00.86
  - with acetabulum 00.85
- partial NOS 00.85
  - acetabulum 00.87
  - femoral head 00.86
- total (acetabulum and femoral head) 00.85

Resuscitation
- artificial respiration 93.93
- cardiac 99.60
  - cardioversion 99.62
    - atrial 99.61
  - defibrillation 99.62
  - external massage 99.63
    - open chest 37.91
  - intracardiac injection 37.92
- cardiopulmonary 99.60
- endotracheal intubation 96.04
- manual 93.93
- mouth-to-mouth 93.93
- pulmonary 93.93

Resuture
- abdominal wall 54.61
- cardiac septum prosthesis 35.95
- chest wall 34.71
- heart valve prosthesis (poppet) 35.95
- wound (skin and subcutaneous tissue) (without graft) NEC 86.59

Retavase, infusion 99.10
Reteplase, infusion 99.10
Retightening (noninvasive)
- external fixator device — *omit code*

Retinaculotomy NEC — *see also* Division, ligament 80.40
- carpal tunnel (flexor) 04.43

Retraining
- cardiac 93.36
- vocational 93.85

Retrogasserian neurotomy 04.02

Revascularization
- cardiac (heart muscle) (myocardium) (direct) 36.10
  - with
    - bypass anastomosis
      - abdominal artery to coronary artery 36.17
      - aortocoronary (catheter stent) (homograft) (prosthesis) (saphenous vein graft) 36.10
        - one coronary vessel 36.11
        - two coronary vessels 36.12
        - three coronary vessels 36.13
        - four coronary vessels 36.14
      - gastroepiploic artery to coronary artery 36.17
      - internal mammary-coronary artery (single vessel) 36.15
        - double vessel 36.16
      - specified type NEC 36.19

Revascularization — *continued*
- cardiac — *continued*
  - with — *continued*
    - bypass anastomosis — *continued*
      - thoracic artery-coronary artery (single vessel) 36.15
        - double vessel 36.16
      - implantation of artery into heart (muscle) (myocardium) (ventricle) 36.2
    - indirect 36.2
    - specified type NEC 36.39
    - transmyocardial
      - endoscopic 36.33
      - endovascular 36.34
      - open chest 36.31
      - percutaneous 36.34
      - specified type NEC 36.32
      - thoracoscopic 36.33

Reversal, intestinal segment 45.50
- large 45.52
- small 45.51

Revision
- amputation stump 84.3
  - current traumatic — *see* Amputation
- anastomosis
  - biliary tract 51.94
  - blood vessel 39.49
  - gastric, gastrointestinal (with jejunal interposition) 44.5
  - intestine (large) 46.94
    - small 46.93
  - pleurothecal 03.97
  - pyelointestinal 56.72
  - salpingothecal 03.97
  - subarachnoid-peritoneal 03.97
  - subarachnoid-ureteral 03.97
  - ureterointestinal 56.72
- ankle replacement (prosthesis) 81.59
- anterior segment (eye) wound (operative) NEC 12.83
- arteriovenous shunt (cannula) (for dialysis) 39.42
- arthroplasty — *see* Arthroplasty
- bone flap, skull 02.06
- breast implant 85.93
- bronchostomy 33.42
- bypass graft (vascular) 39.49
  - abdominal-coronary artery 36.17
  - aortocoronary (catheter stent) (with prosthesis) (with saphenous vein graft) (with vein graft) 36.10
    - one coronary vessel 36.11
    - three coronary vessels 36.13
    - four coronary vessels 36.14
    - two coronary vessels 36.12
  - CABG — *see* Revision, aortocoronary bypass graft
  - chest tube — *see* intercostal catheter
  - coronary artery bypass graft (CABG) — *see* Revision, aortocoronary bypass graft, abdominal-coronary artery bypass, and internal mammary-coronary artery bypass
  - intercostal catheter (with lysis of adhesions) 34.04
    - thoracoscopic 34.06
  - internal mammary-coronary artery (single) 36.15
    - double vessel 36.16
- cannula, vessel-to-vessel (arteriovenous) 39.94
- canthus, lateral 08.59
- cardiac pacemaker
  - device (permanent) 37.89
  - electrode(s) (atrial) (transvenous) (ventricular) 37.75
  - pocket 37.79
- cardiac resynchronization defibrillator (CRT-D)
  - device 37.79
  - electrode(s) 37.75
  - pocket 37.79
- cardiac resynchronization pacemaker (CRT-P)
  - device (permanent) 37.89

Revision — *continued*
- cardiac resynchronization pacemaker — *continued*
  - electrode(s) (atria) (transvenous) (ventricular) 37.75
  - pocket 37.79
- cardioverter/defibrillator (automatic) pocket 37.79
- cholecystostomy 51.99
- cleft palate repair 27.63
- colostomy 46.43
- conduit, urinary 56.52
- cystostomy (stoma) 57.22
- disc — *see* Revision, intervertebral disc
- elbow replacement (prosthesis) 81.97
- enterostomy (stoma) 46.40
  - large intestine 46.43
  - small intestine 46.41
- enucleation socket 16.64
  - with graft 16.63
- esophagostomy 42.83
- exenteration cavity 16.66
  - with secondary graft 16.65
- extraocular muscle surgery 15.6
- fenestration, inner ear 20.62
- filtering bleb 12.66
- fixation device (broken) (displaced) (*see also* Fixation, bone, internal) 78.50
- flap or pedicle graft (skin) 86.75
- foot replacement (prosthesis) 81.59
- gastric anastomosis (with jejunal interposition) 44.5
- gastric band, laparoscopic 44.96
- gastric port device
  - laparoscopic 44.96
- gastroduodenostomy (with jejunal interposition) 44.5
- gastrointestinal anastomosis (with jejunal interposition) 44.5
- gastrojejunostomy 44.5
- gastrostomy 44.69
  - laparoscopic 44.68
- hand replacement (prosthesis) 81.97
- heart procedure NEC 35.95
- hip replacement NOS 81.53
  - acetabular and femoral components (total) 00.70
  - acetabular component only 00.71
  - acetabular liner and/or femoral head only 00.73
  - femoral component only 00.72
  - femoral head only and/or acetabular liner 00.73
  - partial
    - acetabular component only 00.71
    - acetabular liner and/or femoral head only 00.73 *continued*
    - femoral component only 00.72
    - femoral head only and/or acetabular liner 00.73
  - total (acetabular and femoral components) 00.70
- Holter (-Spitz) valve 02.42
- ileal conduit 56.52
- ileostomy 46.41
- intervertebral disc, artificial (partial) (total) NOS 84.69
  - cervical 84.66
  - lumbar, lumbosacral 84.68
  - thoracic 84.67
- jejunoileal bypass 46.93
- jejunostomy 46.41
- joint replacement
  - acetabular and femoral components (total) 00.70
  - acetabular component only 00.71
  - acetabular liner and/or femoral head only 00.73
  - ankle 81.59
  - elbow 81.97
  - femoral component only 00.72
  - femoral head only and/or acetabular liner 00.73
  - foot 81.59
  - hand 81.97
  - hip 81.53

☑ **Additional Digit Required — Refer to the Tabular List for Digit Selection**
▽ **Subterms under main terms may continue to next column or page**
Resection — Revision
Index
882
2014 ICD-9-CM

☑ **Additional Digit Required** — Refer to the Tabular List for Digit Selection   ▽ **Subterms under main terms may continue to next column or page**

2014 ICD-9-CM   **883**

Revision — Scalenectomy

Study — continued
- bundle of His 37.29
- color vision 95.06
- conduction, nerve (median) 89.15
- dark adaptation, eye 95.07
- electrophysiologic stimulation and recording, cardiac
  - as part of intraoperative testing — omit code
  - catheter based invasive electrophysiologic testing 37.26
  - device interrogation only without arrhythmia induction (bedside check) 89.45-89.49
  - noninvasive programmed electrical stimulation (NIPS) 37.20
- function (see also Function, study)
  - radioisotope — see Scan, radioisotope
- lacrimal flow (radiographic) 87.05
- ocular motility 95.15
- pulmonary
  - airway flow measurement, endoscopic 33.72
  - function — see categories 89.37-89.38
- radiographic — see Radiography
- radio-iodinated triolein 92.04
- renal clearance 92.03
- spirometer 89.37
- tracer (see also Scan, radioisotope eye (P^{32})) 95.16
- ultrasonic — see Ultrasonography
- visual field 95.05
- xenon flow NEC 92.19
  - cardiovascular 92.05
  - pulmonary 92.15

Sturmdorf operation (conization of cervix) 67.2

Submucous resection
- larynx 30.29
- nasal septum 21.5

Summerskill operation (dacryocystorhinostomy by intubation) 09.81

Surgery
- computer assisted (CAS) 00.39
  - with robotics — see category 17.4 ☑
  - CAS with CT/CTA 00.31
  - CAS with fluoroscopy 00.33
  - CAS with MR/MRA 00.32
  - CAS with multiple datasets 00.35
    - imageless 00.34
  - other CAS 00.39
- IGS — see Surgery, computer assisted
- image guided — see Surgery, computer assisted
- navigation (CT-free, IGN image guided, imageless) — see Surgery, computer assisted
- robotic assisted — see category 17.4 ☑

Surmay operation (jejunostomy) 46.39

Suspension
- balanced, for traction 93.45
- bladder NEC 57.89
- diverticulum, pharynx 29.59
- kidney 55.7
- Olshausen (uterus) 69.22
- ovary 65.79
- paraurethral (Pereyra) 59.6
- periurethral 59.6
- urethra (retropubic) (sling) 59.5
- urethrovesical
  - Goebel-Frangenheim-Stoeckel 59.4
  - gracilis muscle transplant 59.71
  - levator muscle sling 59.71
  - Marshall-Marchetti (-Krantz) 59.5
  - Millin-Read 59.4
  - suprapubic 59.4
- uterus (abdominal or vaginal approach) 69.22
- vagina 70.77
  - with graft or prosthesis 70.78

Suture (laceration)
- abdominal wall 54.63
  - secondary 54.61
- adenoid fossa 28.7
- adrenal (gland) 07.44
- aneurysm (cerebral) (peripheral) 39.52

Suture — continued
- anus 49.71
  - obstetric laceration (current) 75.62
  - old 49.79
- aorta 39.31
- aponeurosis (see also Suture, tendon) 83.64
- arteriovenous fistula 39.53
- artery 39.31
  - percutaneous puncture closure — omit code
- bile duct 51.79
- bladder 57.81
  - obstetric laceration (current) 75.61
- blood vessel NEC 39.30
  - artery 39.31
  - percutaneous puncture closure — omit code
  - vein 39.32
- breast (skin) 85.81
- bronchus 33.41
- bursa 83.99
  - hand 82.99
- canaliculus 09.73
- cecum 46.75
- cerebral meninges 02.11
- cervix (traumatic laceration) 67.61
  - internal os, encirclement 67.59
  - obstetric laceration (current) 75.51
  - old 67.69
- chest wall 34.71
- cleft palate 27.62
- clitoris 71.4
- colon 46.75
- common duct 51.71
- conjunctiva 10.6
- cornea 11.51
  - with conjunctival flap 11.53
- corneoscleral 11.51
  - with conjunctival flap 11.53
- diaphragm 34.82
- duodenum 46.71
  - ulcer (bleeding) (perforated) 44.42
    - endoscopic 44.43
- dura mater (cerebral) 02.11
  - spinal 03.59
- ear, external 18.4
- enterocele 70.92
  - with graft or prosthesis 70.93
- entropion 08.42
- epididymis (and)
  - spermatic cord 63.51
  - vas deferens 63.81
- episiotomy — see Episiotomy
- esophagus 42.82
- eyeball 16.89
- eyebrow 08.81
- eyelid 08.81
  - with entropion or ectropion repair 08.42
- fallopian tube 66.71
- fascia 83.65
  - hand 82.46
  - to skeletal attachment 83.89
    - hand 82.89
- gallbladder 51.91
- ganglion, sympathetic 05.81
- gingiva 24.32
- great vessel 39.30
  - artery 39.31
  - vein 39.32
- gum 24.32
- heart 37.49
- hepatic duct 51.79
- hymen 70.76
- ileum 46.73
- intestine 46.79
  - large 46.75
  - small 46.73
- jejunum 46.73
- joint capsule 81.96
  - with arthroplasty — see Arthroplasty
  - ankle 81.94
  - foot 81.94
  - lower extremity NEC 81.95
  - upper extremity 81.93
- kidney 55.81
- labia 71.71

Suture — continued
- laceration — see Suture, by site
- larynx 31.61
- ligament 81.96
  - with arthroplasty — see Arthroplasty
  - ankle 81.94
  - broad 69.29
  - Cooper's 54.64
  - foot and toes 81.94
  - gastrocolic 54.73
  - knee 81.95
  - lower extremity NEC 81.95
  - sacrouterine 69.29
  - upper extremity 81.93
  - uterine 69.29
- ligation — see Ligation
- lip 27.51
- liver 50.61
- lung 33.43
- meninges (cerebral) 02.11
  - spinal 03.59
- mesentery 54.75
- mouth 27.52
- muscle 83.65
  - hand 82.46
  - ocular (oblique) (rectus) 15.7
- nerve (cranial) (peripheral) 04.3
  - sympathetic 05.81
- nose (external) (internal) 21.81
  - for epistaxis 21.09
- obstetric laceration NEC 75.69
  - bladder 75.61
  - cervix 75.51
  - corpus uteri 75.52
  - pelvic floor 75.69
  - perineum 75.69
  - periurethral 75.69
  - rectum 75.62
  - sphincter ani 75.62
  - urethra 75.61
  - uterus 75.50
  - vagina 75.69
  - vulva 75.69
- omentum 54.64
- ovary 65.71
  - laparoscopic 65.74
- palate 27.61
  - cleft 27.62
- palpebral fissure 08.59
- pancreas 52.95
- pelvic floor 71.71
  - obstetric laceration (current) 75.69
- penis 64.41
- peptic ulcer (bleeding) (perforated) 44.40
- pericardium 37.49
- perineum (female) 71.71
  - after delivery 75.69
    - episiotomy repair — see Episiotomy
  - male 86.59
- periosteum 78.20
  - carpal, metacarpal 78.24
  - femur 78.25
  - fibula 78.27
  - humerus 78.22
  - pelvic 78.29
  - phalanges (foot) (hand) 78.29
  - radius 78.23
  - specified site NEC 78.29
  - tarsal, metatarsal 78.28
  - tibia 78.27
  - ulna 78.23
  - vertebrae 78.29
- peritoneum 54.64
- periurethral tissue to symphysis pubis 59.5
- pharynx 29.51
- pleura 34.93
- rectum 48.71
  - obstetric laceration (current) 75.62
- retina (for reattachment) 14.59
- sacrouterine ligament 69.29
- salivary gland 26.41
- scalp 86.59
  - replantation 86.51
- sclera (with repair of conjunctiva) 12.81
- scrotum (skin) 61.41

Suture — continued
- secondary
  - abdominal wall 54.61
  - episiotomy 75.69
  - peritoneum 54.64
- sigmoid 46.75
- skin (mucous membrane) (without graft) 86.59
  - with graft — see Graft, skin
  - breast 85.81
  - ear 18.4
  - eyebrow 08.81
  - eyelid 08.81
  - nose 21.81
  - penis 64.41
  - scalp 86.59
    - replantation 86.51
  - scrotum 61.41
  - vulva 71.71
- specified site NEC — see Repair, by site
- spermatic cord 63.51
- sphincter ani 49.71
  - obstetric laceration (current) 75.62
  - old 49.79
- spinal meninges 03.59
- spleen 41.95
- stomach 44.61
  - ulcer (bleeding) (perforated) 44.41
    - endoscopic 44.43
- subcutaneous tissue (without skin graft) 86.59
  - with graft — see Graft, skin
- tendon (direct) (immediate) (primary) 83.64
  - delayed (secondary) 83.62
    - hand NEC 82.43
      - flexors 82.42
  - hand NEC 82.45
    - delayed (secondary) 82.43
    - flexors 82.44
      - delayed (secondary) 82.42
  - ocular 15.7
  - rotator cuff 83.63
  - sheath 83.61
    - hand 82.41
  - supraspinatus (rotator cuff repair) 83.63
  - to skeletal attachment 83.88
    - hand 82.85
- Tenon's capsule 15.7
- testis 62.61
- thymus 07.93
- thyroid gland 06.93
- tongue 25.51
- tonsillar fossa 28.7
- trachea 31.71
- tunica vaginalis 61.41
- ulcer (bleeding) (perforated) (peptic) 44.40
  - duodenum 44.42
    - endoscopic 44.43
  - gastric 44.41
    - endoscopic 44.43
  - intestine 46.79
  - skin 86.59
  - stomach 44.41
    - endoscopic 44.43
- ureter 56.82
- urethra 58.41
  - obstetric laceration (current) 75.61
- uterosacral ligament 69.29
- uterus 69.41
  - obstetric laceration (current) 75.50
  - old 69.49
- uvula 27.73
- vagina 70.71
  - obstetric laceration (current) 75.69
  - old 70.79
- vas deferens 63.81
- vein 39.32
- vulva 71.71
  - obstetric laceration (current) 75.69
  - old 71.79

Suture-ligation — see also Ligation
- blood vessel — see Ligation, blood vessel

Sweep, anterior iris 12.97

Swenson operation
- bladder reconstruction 57.87
- proctectomy 48.49

Therapy — *continued*
  domestic tasks — *continued*
    for the blind 93.78
  Downstream® system 00.49
  educational (bed-bound children) (handi-capped) 93.82
  electroconvulsive (ECT) 94.27
  electroshock (EST) 94.27
    subconvulsive 94.26
  electrotonic (ETT) 94.27
  encounter group 94.44
  extinction 94.33
  family 94.42
  fog (inhalation) 93.94
  gamma ray 92.23
  group 94.44
    for psychosexual dysfunctions 94.41
  hearing NEC 95.49
  heat NEC 93.35
    for cancer treatment 99.85
  helium 93.98
  hot pack(s) 93.35
  hyperbaric oxygen 93.95
    wound 93.59
  hyperthermia NEC 93.35
    for cancer treatment 99.85
  individual, psychiatric NEC 94.39
    for psychosexual dysfunction 94.34
  industrial 93.89
  infrared irradiation 93.35
  inhalation NEC 93.96
    nitric oxide 00.12
  insulin shock 94.24
  intermittent positive pressure breathing (IPPB) 93.91
  IPPB (intermittent positive pressure breathing) 93.91
  leech 99.99
  lithium 94.22
  LITT (laser interstitial thermal therapy) under guidance
    lesion
      brain 17.61
      breast 17.69
      head and neck 17.62
      liver 17.63
      lung 17.69
      prostate 17.69
      thyroid 17.62
  maggot 86.28
  manipulative, osteopathic (*see also* Manipulation, osteopathic) 93.67
  manual arts 93.81
  methadone 94.25
  mist (inhalation) 93.94
  music 93.84
  nebulizer 93.94
  neuroleptic 94.23
  nitric oxide 00.12
  occupational 93.83
  oxygen 93.96
    aqueous 00.49
    catalytic 93.96
    hyperbaric 93.95
      wound 93.59
    SuperSaturated 00.49
    wound (hyperbaric) 93.59
  paraffin bath 93.35
  physical NEC 93.39
    combined (without mention of components) 93.38
    diagnostic NEC 93.09
  play 93.81
    psychotherapeutic 94.36
  positive end expiratory pressure — *see* category 96.7 ☑
  psychiatric NEC 94.39
    drug NEC 94.25
    lithium 94.22
  radiation 92.29
    contact (150 KVP or less) 92.21
    deep (200-300 KVP) 92.22
    electron, intra-operative 92.41
    high voltage (200-300 KVP) 92.22
    low voltage (150 KVP or less) 92.21
    megavoltage 92.24

Therapy — *continued*
  radiation — *continued*
    orthovoltage 92.22
    particle source NEC 92.26
    photon 92.24
    radioisotope (teleradiotherapy) 92.23
    retinal lesion 14.26
    superficial (150 KVP or less) 92.21
    supervoltage 92.24
  radioisotope, radioisotopic NEC 92.29
    implantation or insertion 92.27
    injection or instillation 92.28
    teleradiotherapy 92.23
  radium (radon) 92.23
  recreational 93.81
  rehabilitation NEC 93.89
  respiratory NEC 93.99
    bi-level positive airway pressure [BiPAP] 93.90
      delivered by
        endotracheal tube — *see* category 96.7 ☑
        tracheostomy — *see* category 96.7 ☑
    continuous positive airway pressure [CPAP] 93.90
      delivered by
        endotracheal tube — *see* category 96.7 ☑
        tracheostomy — *see* category 96.7 ☑
    endotracheal respiratory assistance — *see* category 96.7 ☑
    intermittent positive pressure breathing [IPPB] 93.91
    negative pressure (continuous) [CNP] 93.99
    nitric oxide 00.12
    non-invasive positive pressure (NIPPV) 93.90
    other continuous invasive (unspecified duration) 96.70
      for 96 consecutive hours or more 96.72
      for less than 96 consecutive hours 96.71
    positive end expiratory pressure [PEEP]
      invasive — *see* category 96.7 ☑
      non-invasive [NIPPV] 93.90
  root canal 23.70
    with
      apicoectomy 23.72
      irrigation 23.71
  shock
    chemical 94.24
    electric 94.27
      subconvulsive 94.26
    insulin 94.24
  speech 93.75
    for correction of defect 93.74
  SuperOxygenation (SSO₂) 00.49
  SuperSaturated oxygen 00.49
  ultrasound
    heat therapy 93.35
    hyperthermia for cancer treatment 99.85
    physical therapy 93.35
    therapeutic — *see* Ultrasound
  ultraviolet light 99.82
Thermocautery — *see* Cauterization
Thermography 88.89
  blood vessel 88.86
  bone 88.83
  breast 88.85
  cerebral 88.81
  eye 88.82
  lymph gland 88.89
  muscle 88.84
  ocular 88.82
  osteoarticular 88.83
  specified site NEC 88.89
  vein, deep 88.86
Thermokeratoplasty 11.74
Thermoplasty
  bronchoscopic, bronchial (lung) 32.27
Thermosclerectomy 12.62

Thermotherapy (hot packs) (paraffin bath) NEC 93.35
  prostate
    by
      microwave 60.96
      radiofrequency 60.97
    transurethral microwave thermotherapy (TUMT) 60.96
    transurethral needle ablation (TUNA) 60.97
    TUMT (transurethral microwave thermotherapy) 60.96
    TUNA (transurethral needle ablation) 60.97
Thiersch operation
  anus 49.79
  skin graft 86.69
    hand 86.62
Thompson operation
  cleft lip repair 27.54
  correction of lymphedema 40.9
  quadricepsplasty 83.86
  thumb apposition with bone graft 82.69
Thoracectomy 34.09
  for lung collapse 33.34
Thoracentesis 34.91
Thoracocentesis 34.91
Thoracolysis (for collapse of lung) 33.39
Thoracoplasty (anterior) (extrapleural) (paravertebral) (posterolateral) (complete) (partial) 33.34
Thoracoscopy, transpleural (for exploration) 34.21
Thoracostomy 34.09
  for lung collapse 33.32
Thoracotomy (with drainage) 34.09
  as operative approach — *omit code*
  exploratory 34.02
Thoratec® implantable ventricular assist device (IVAD™) 37.66
Thoratec® ventricular assist device (VAD) system 37.66
Three-snip operation, punctum 09.51
Thrombectomy 38.00
  with endarterectomy — *see* Endarterectomy
  abdominal
    artery 38.06
    vein 38.07
  aorta (arch) (ascending) (descending) 38.04
  arteriovenous shunt or cannula 39.49
  bovine graft 39.49
  coronary artery 36.09
  head and neck vessel NEC 38.02
  intracranial vessel NEC 38.01
  lower limb
    artery 38.08
    vein 38.09
  mechanical
    endovascular
      head and neck 39.74
  pulmonary vessel 38.05
  thoracic vessel NEC 38.05
  upper limb (artery) (vein) 38.03
Thromboendarterectomy 38.10
  abdominal 38.16
  aorta (arch) (ascending) (descending) 38.14
  coronary artery 36.09
    open chest approach 36.03
  head and neck NEC 38.12
  intracranial NEC 38.11
  lower limb 38.18
  thoracic NEC 38.15
  upper limb 38.13
Thymectomy 07.80
  partial (open) (other) 07.81
    thoracoscopic 07.83
  total (open) (other) 07.82
    thoracoscopic 07.84
  transcervical 07.99
Thyrochondrotomy 31.3
Thyrocricoidectomy 30.29
Thyrocricotomy (for assistance in breathing) 31.1
Thyroidectomy NEC 06.39
  by mediastinotomy (*see also* Thyroidectomy, substernal) 06.50

Thyroidectomy — *continued*
  with laryngectomy — *see* Laryngectomy
  complete or total 06.4
    substernal (by mediastinotomy) (transsternal route) 06.52
    transoral route (lingual) 06.6
  lingual (complete) (partial) (subtotal) (total) 06.6
  partial or subtotal NEC 06.39
    with complete removal of remaining lobe 06.2
    submental route (lingual) 06.6
    substernal (by mediastinotomy) (transsternal route) 06.51
  remaining tissue 06.4
  submental route (lingual) 06.6
  substernal (by mediastinotomy) (transsternal route) 06.50
    complete or total 06.52
    partial or subtotal 06.51
  transoral route (lingual) 06.6
  transsternal route (*see also* Thyroidectomy, substernal) 06.50
  unilateral (with removal of isthmus) (with removal of portion of other lobe) 06.2
Thyroidorrhaphy 06.93
Thyroidotomy (field) (gland) NEC 06.09
  postoperative 06.02
Thyrotomy 31.3
  with tantalum plate 31.69
Tirofiban (HCl), infusion 99.20
Toilette
  skin — *see* Debridement, skin or subcutaneous tissue
  tracheostomy 96.55
Token economy (behavior therapy) 94.33
Tomkins operation (metroplasty) 69.49
Tomography — *see also* Radiography
  abdomen NEC 88.02
  cardiac 87.42
  computerized axial NEC 88.38
    abdomen 88.01
    bone 88.38
      quantitative 88.98
    brain 87.03
    cardiac 87.41
    coronary 87.41
    head 87.03
    kidney 87.71
    skeletal 88.38
      quantitative 88.98
    thorax 87.41
  head NEC 87.04
  kidney NEC 87.72
  lung 87.42
  optical coherence (intravascular imaging)
    coronary vessel(s) 38.24
    non-coronary vessel(s) 38.25
  thorax NEC 87.42
Tongue tie operation 25.91
Tonography 95.26
Tonometry 89.11
Tonsillectomy 28.2
  with adenoidectomy 28.3
Tonsillotomy 28.0
Topectomy 01.32
Torek (-Bevan) operation (orchidopexy) (first stage) (second stage) 62.5
Torkildsen operation (ventriculocisternal shunt) 02.2 ☑
Torpin operation (cul-de-sac resection) 70.92
Toti operation (dacryocystorhinostomy) 09.81
Touchas operation 86.83
Touroff operation (ligation of subclavian artery) 38.85
Toxicology — *see* Examination, microscopic
TPN (total parenteral nutrition) 99.15
Trabeculectomy ab externo 12.64
Trabeculodialysis 12.59
Trabeculotomy ab externo 12.54
Trachelectomy 67.4
Trachelopexy 69.22
Tracheloplasty 67.69
Trachelorrhaphy (Emmet) (suture) 67.61
  obstetrical 75.51

☑ **Additional Digit Required — Refer to the Tabular List for Digit Selection**   ▽ **Subterms under main terms may continue to next column or page**

☑ **Additional Digit Required — Refer to the Tabular List for Digit Selection**   ▽ **Subterms under main terms may continue to next column or page**

890   **2014 ICD-9-CM**

Vaginoscopy 70.21
Vaginotomy 70.14
  for
    culdocentesis 70.0
    pelvic abscess 70.12
Vagotomy (gastric) 44.00
  parietal cell 44.02
  selective NEC 44.03
    highly 44.02
    Holle's 44.02
    proximal 44.02
  truncal 44.01
Valvotomy — *see* Valvulotomy
Valvulectomy, heart — *see* Valvuloplasty, heart
Valvuloplasty
  heart, unspecified (without valve replacement) 35.10
    with prosthesis or tissue graft — *see* Replacement, heart, valve, by site
  aortic valve 35.11
    percutaneous (balloon) 35.96
  balloon, percutaneous 35.96
  combined with repair of atrial and ventricular septal defects — *see* Repair, endocardial cushion defect
  mitral valve
    balloon, percutaneous repair 35.96
    endovascular repair with implant 35.97
    open, without replacement 35.12
    percutaneous repair
      with implant (leaflet clip) 35.97
    transcatheter repair with implant 35.97
  open heart technique 35.10
  percutaneous (balloon) 35.96
  pulmonary valve 35.13
    in total repair of tetralogy of Fallot 35.81
    percutaneous (balloon) 35.96
  tricuspid valve 35.14
Valvulotomy
  heart (closed heart technique) (transatrial) (transventricular) 35.00
  aortic valve 35.01
  mitral valve 35.02
  open heart technique — *see* Valvuloplasty, heart
  pulmonary valve 35.03
    in total repair of tetralogy of Fallot 35.81
  tricuspid valve 35.04
Varicocelectomy, spermatic cord 63.1
Varicotomy, peripheral vessels (lower limb) 38.59
  upper limb 38.53
Vascular access device, totally implantable 86.07
Vascular closure, percutaneous puncture — *omit code*
Vascularization — *see* Revascularization
Vasectomy (complete) (partial) 63.73
Vasogram 87.94
Vasoligation 63.71
  gastric 38.86
Vasorrhaphy 63.81
Vasostomy 63.6
Vasotomy 63.6
Vasotripsy 63.71
Vasovasostomy 63.82
Vectorcardiogram (VCG) (with ECG) 89.53
Vectra® vascular access graft 86.07
Venectomy — *see* Phlebectomy
Venipuncture NEC 38.99
  for injection of contrast material — *see* Phlebography
Venography — *see* Phlebography
Venorrhaphy 39.32
Venotomy 38.00
  abdominal 38.07
  head and neck NEC 38.02
  intracranial NEC 38.01
  lower limb 38.09
  thoracic NEC 38.05
  upper limb 38.03

Venotripsy 39.98
Venovenostomy 39.29
Ventilation
  bi-level positive airway pressure [BiPAP] 93.90
  delivered by
    endotracheal tube — *see* category 96.7 ☑
    tracheostomy — *see* category 96.7 ☑
  continuous positive airway pressure [CPAP] 93.90
  delivered by
    endotracheal tube — *see* category 96.7 ☑
    tracheostomy — *see* category 96.7 ☑
  endotracheal respiratory assistance — *see* category 96.7 ☑
  intermittent positive pressure breathing [IPPB] 93.91
  mechanical, NOS 93.90
    by endotracheal tube — *see* category 96.7 ☑
    by tracheostomy — *see* category 96.7 ☑
    endotracheal respiratory assistance — *see* category 96.7 ☑
    invasive — *see* category 96.7 ☑
    non-invasive [NIPPV] 93.90
    other continuous invasive (unspecified duration) 96.70
      for 96 consecutive hours or more 96.72
      for less than 96 consecutive hours 96.71
    positive end expiratory pressure [PEEP]
      invasive — *see* category 96.7 ☑
      non-invasive [NIPPV] 93.90
  negative pressure (continuous) [CNP] 93.99
  non-invasive positive pressure (NIPPV) 93.90
Ventriculectomy, heart
  partial 37.35
Ventriculocholecystostomy 02.34
Ventriculocisternostomy 02.22
Ventriculocordectomy 30.29
Ventriculogram, ventriculography (cerebral) 87.02
  cardiac
    left ventricle (outflow tract) 88.53
      combined with right heart 88.54
    right ventricle (outflow tract) 88.52
      combined with left heart 88.54
  radionuclide cardiac 92.05
Ventriculomyocardiotomy 37.11
Ventriculoperitoneostomy 02.34
Ventriculopuncture 01.09
  through previously implanted catheter or reservoir (Ommaya) (Rickham) 01.02
Ventriculoseptopexy — *see also* Repair, ventricular septal defect 35.72
Ventriculoseptoplasty — *see also* Repair, ventricular septal defect 35.72
Ventriculostomy
  for
    external ventricular drainage (EVD) 02.21
    placement of ventricular catheter 02.21
  third (endoscopic) 02.22
Ventriculotomy
  cerebral 02.22
  heart 37.11
Ventriculoureterostomy 02.35
Ventriculovenostomy 02.32
Ventrofixation, uterus 69.22
Ventrohysteropexy 69.22
Ventrosuspension, uterus 69.22
VEP (visual evoked potential) 95.23
Version, obstetrical (bimanual) (cephalic) (combined) (internal) (podalic) 73.21
  with extraction 73.22
  Braxton Hicks 73.21
    with extraction 73.22
  external (bipolar) 73.91
  Potter's (podalic) 73.21
    with extraction 73.22
  Wigand's (external) 73.91

Version, obstetrical — *continued*
  Wright's (cephalic) 73.21
    with extraction 73.22
Vertebroplasty, percutaneous 81.65
Vesicolithotomy (suprapubic) 57.19
Vesicostomy 57.21
Vesicourethroplasty 57.85
Vesiculectomy 60.73
  with radical prostatectomy 60.5
Vesiculogram, seminal 87.92
  contrast 87.91
Vesiculotomy 60.72
Vestibuloplasty (buccolabial) (lingual) 24.91
Vestibulotomy 20.79
VH™-IVUS — *see* Ultrasound, intravascular, by site
Vicq D'azyr operation (larynx) 31.1
Vidal operation (varicocele ligation) 63.1
Vidianectomy 05.21
Villusectomy — *see also* Synovectomy 80.70
Vision check 95.09
Visual evoked potential (VEP) 95.23
Vitrectomy (mechanical) (posterior approach) 14.74
  with scleral buckling 14.49
  anterior approach 14.73
Vocational
  assessment 93.85
  retraining 93.85
  schooling 93.82
Voice training (postlaryngectomy) 93.73
von Kraske operation (proctectomy) 48.64
Voss operation (hanging hip operation) 83.19
Vulpius (-Compere) operation (lengthening of gastrocnemius muscle) 83.85
Vulvectomy (bilateral) (simple) 71.62
  partial (unilateral) 71.61
  radical (complete) 71.5
  unilateral 71.61
V-Y operation (repair)
  bladder 57.89
  neck 57.85
  ectropion 08.44
  lip 27.59
  skin (without graft) 86.89
  subcutaneous tissue (without skin graft) 86.89
  tongue 25.59

W

Wada test (hemispheric function) 89.10
Wang needle aspiration biopsy
  bronchus 33.24
  lung 33.27
Wardill operation 27.62
Ward-Mayo operation (vaginal hysterectomy) 68.59
  laparoscopically assisted (LAVH) 68.51
Washing — *see* Lavage and Irrigation
Waterston operation (aorta-right pulmonary artery anastomosis) 39.0
Watkins (-Wertheim) operation (uterus interposition) 69.21
Watson-Jones operation
  hip arthrodesis 81.21
  reconstruction of lateral ligaments, ankle 81.49
  shoulder arthrodesis (extra-articular) 81.23
  tenoplasty 83.88
Webbing (syndactylization) 86.89
Weir operation
  appendicostomy 47.91
  correction of nostrils 21.86
Wertheim operation (radical hysterectomy) 68.69
  laparoscopic 68.61
West operation (dacryocystorhinostomy) 09.81
Wheeler operation
  entropion repair 08.44
  halving procedure (eyelid) 08.24
Whipple operation (radical pancreaticoduodenectomy) 52.7
  Child modification (radical subtotal pancreatectomy) 52.53

Whipple operation — *continued*
  Rodney Smith modification (radical subtotal pancreatectomy) 52.53
Whitehead operation
  glossectomy, radical 25.4
  hemorrhoidectomy 49.46
White operation (lengthening of tendo calcaneus by incomplete tenotomy) 83.11
Whitman operation
  foot stabilization (talectomy) 77.98
  hip reconstruction 81.40
  repair of serratus anterior muscle 83.87
  talectomy 77.98
  trochanter wedge osteotomy 77.25
Wier operation (entropion repair) 08.44
Williams-Richardson operation (vaginal construction) 70.61
  with graft or prosthesis 70.63
Wilms operation (thoracoplasty) 33.34
Wilson operation (angulation osteotomy for hallux valgus) 77.51
Window operation
  antrum (nasal sinus) — *see* Antrotomy, maxillary
  aorticopulmonary 39.59
  bone cortex (*see also* Incision, bone) 77.10
    facial 76.09
  nasoantral — *see* Antrotomy, maxillary
  pericardium 37.12
  pleura 34.09
Winiwarter operation (cholecystoenterostomy) 51.32
Wiring
  aneurysm 39.52
  dental (for immobilization) 93.55
    with fracture-reduction — *see* Reduction, fracture
  orthodontic 24.7
Wirsungojejunostomy 52.96
Witzel operation (temporary gastrostomy) 43.19
Woodward operation (release of high riding scapula) 81.83
Wrapping, aneurysm (gauze) (methyl methacrylate) (plastic) 39.52

X

Xenograft 86.65
Xerography, breast 87.36
Xeromammography 87.36
Xiphoidectomy 77.81
X-ray
  chest (routine) 87.44
    wall NEC 87.39
  contrast — *see* Radiography, contrast
  diagnostic — *see* Radiography
  injection of radio-opaque substance — *see* Radiography, contrast
  skeletal series, whole or complete 88.31
  therapeutic — *see* Therapy, radiation

Y

Young operation
  epispadias repair 58.45
  tendon transfer (anterior tibialis) (repair of flat foot) 83.75
Yount operation (division of iliotibial band) 83.14

Z

Zancolli operation
  capsuloplasty 81.72
  tendon transfer (biceps) 82.56
Zeus® Robotic Surgical System — *see* category 17.4 ☑
Ziegler operation (iridectomy) 12.14
Zonulolysis (with lens extraction) — *see also* Extraction, cataract, intracapsular 13.19
Z-plasty
  epicanthus 08.59
  eyelid (*see also* Reconstruction, eyelid) 08.70
  hypopharynx 29.4
  skin (scar) (web contracture) 86.84
    with excision of lesion 86.3

☑ **Additional Digit Required** — Refer to the Tabular List for Digit Selection   ▽ **Subterms under main terms may continue to next column or page**

2014 ICD-9-CM   **891**

0. PROCEDURES AND INTERVENTIONS, NOT ELSEWHERE CLASSIFIED (00)

✓3ᵗʰ **00 Procedures and interventions, not elsewhere classified**

✓4ᵗʰ **00.0 Therapeutic ultrasound**

> *EXCLUDES*   *diagnostic ultrasound (non-invasive) (88.71-88.79)*
> *intracardiac echocardiography [ICE] (heart chamber(s)) (37.28)*
> *intravascular imaging (adjunctive) (00.21-00.29)*

> **DEF:** Interventional treatment modality using lower frequency and higher intensity levels of ultrasound energy than used in diagnostic ultrasound modality for the purpose of limiting intimal hyperplasia, or restenosis, associated with atherosclerotic vascular disease.

00.01 Therapeutic ultrasound of vessels of head and neck

> Anti-restenotic ultrasound
> Intravascular non-ablative ultrasound
> *EXCLUDES*   *diagnostic ultrasound of:*
> *eye (95.13)*
> *head and neck (88.71)*
> *that of inner ear (20.79)*
> *ultrasonic:*
> *angioplasty of non-coronary vessel (39.50)*
> *embolectomy (38.01, 38.02)*
> *endarterectomy (38.11, 38.12)*
> *thrombectomy (38.01, 38.02)*

00.02 Therapeutic ultrasound of heart

> Anti-restenotic ultrasound
> Intravascular non-ablative ultrasound
> *EXCLUDES*   *diagnostic ultrasound of heart (88.72)*
> *ultrasonic ablation of heart lesion (37.34)*
> *ultrasonic angioplasty of coronary vessels (00.66, 36.09)*

00.03 Therapeutic ultrasound of peripheral vascular vessels

> Anti-restenotic ultrasound
> Intravascular non-ablative ultrasound
> *EXCLUDES*   *diagnostic ultrasound of peripheral vascular system (88.77)*
> *ultrasonic angioplasty of:*
> *non-coronary vessel (39.50)*

00.09 Other therapeutic ultrasound

> *EXCLUDES*   *ultrasonic:*
> *fragmentation of urinary stones (59.95)*
> *percutaneous nephrostomy with fragmentation (55.04)*
> *physical therapy (93.35)*
> *transurethral guided laser induced prostatectomy (TULIP) (60.21)*

✓4ᵗʰ **00.1 Pharmaceuticals**

00.10 Implantation of chemotherapeutic agent

> Brain wafer chemotherapy
> Interstitial/intracavitary
> *EXCLUDES*   *injection or infusion of cancer chemotherapeutic substance (99.25)*

> **DEF:** Brain wafer chemotherapy: Placement of wafers containing antineoplastic agent against the wall of the resection cavity subsequent to the surgeon completing a tumor excision to deliver chemotherapy directly to the tumor site; used to treat glioblastoma multiforme (GBM).

00.11 Infusion of drotrecogin alfa (activated)

> Infusion of recombinant protein

00.12 Administration of inhaled nitric oxide

> Nitric oxide therapy

00.13 Injection or infusion of nesiritide

> Human B-type natriuretic peptide (hBNP)

00.14 Injection or infusion of oxazolidinone class of antibiotics

> Linezolid injection

00.15 High-dose infusion interleukin-2 [IL-2]

> Infusion (IV bolus, CIV) interleukin
> Injection of aldesleukin
> *EXCLUDES*   *low-dose infusion interleukin-2 (99.28)*

> **DEF:** A high-dose anti-neoplastic therapy using a biological response modifier (BRM); the body naturally produces substances called interleukins, which are multi-function cytokines in the generation of an immune response.

00.16 Pressurized treatment of venous bypass graft [conduit] with pharmaceutical substance

> Ex-vivo treatment of vessel
> Hyperbaric pressurized graft [conduit]
> **DEF:** Ex-vivo process of delivering small nucleic acid molecules that block protein transcription factors essential for the expression of genes controlling cell proliferation into graft tissue under nondistending pressure; reduces intimal hyperplasia and vein graft failure.

00.17 Infusion of vasopressor agent

00.18 Infusion of immunosuppressive antibody therapy

> Monoclonal antibody therapy
> Polyclonal antibody therapy
> *INCLUDES*   *during induction phase of solid organ transplantation*

00.19 Disruption of blood brain barrier via infusion [BBBD]

> Infusion of substance to disrupt blood brain barrier
> Code also chemotherapy (99.25)
> *EXCLUDES*   *other perfusion (39.97)*

> **DEF:** Infusion of chemotherapy drug that temporarily allows the transport of materials into the brain through the blood brain barrier (BBB), which is the protective mechanism that limits transport of toxins while allowing necessary nutrients to pass from the blood vessels into the brain tissue; used in the treatment of brain cancers.

✓4ᵗʰ **00.2 Intravascular imaging of blood vessels**

> Note: Real-time imaging of lumen of blood vessel(s) using sound waves
> Endovascular ultrasonography
> Intravascular [ultrasound] imaging of blood vessels
> Intravascular ultrasound (IVUS)
> Virtual histology intravascular ultrasound [VH-IVUS]
> Code also any synchronous diagnostic or therapeutic procedures
> *EXCLUDES*   *adjunct vascular system procedures, number of vessels treated (00.40-00.43)*
> *diagnostic procedures on blood vessels (38.21-38.29)*
> *diagnostic ultrasound of peripheral vascular system (88.77)*
> *intravascular imaging of vessel(s) by OCT (38.24-38.25)*
> *magnetic resonance imaging (MRI) (88.91-88.97)*
> *therapeutic ultrasound (00.01-00.09)*

00.21 Intravascular imaging of extracranial cerebral vessels

> Common carotid vessels and branches
> Intravascular ultrasound (IVUS), extracranial cerebral vessels
> *EXCLUDES*   *diagnostic ultrasound (non-invasive) of head and neck (88.71)*

00.22 Intravascular imaging of intrathoracic vessels

> Aorta and aortic arch
> Intravascular ultrasound (IVUS), intrathoracic vessels
> Vena cava (superior) (inferior)
> *EXCLUDES*   *diagnostic ultrasound (non-invasive) of other sites of thorax (88.73)*

00.23 Intravascular imaging of peripheral vessels
Imaging of:
  vessels of arm(s)
  vessels of leg(s)
Intravascular ultrasound (IVUS), peripheral vessels
> **EXCLUDES**   *diagnostic ultrasound (non-invasive) of peripheral vascular system (88.77)*

00.24 Intravascular imaging of coronary vessels
Intravascular ultrasound (IVUS), coronary vessels
> **EXCLUDES**   *diagnostic ultrasound (non-invasive) of heart (88.72)*
>   *intracardiac echocardiography [ICE] (ultrasound of heart chamber(s)) (37.28)*

00.25 Intravascular imaging of renal vessels
Intravascular ultrasound (IVUS), renal vessels
Renal artery
> **EXCLUDES**   *diagnostic ultrasound (non-invasive) of urinary system (88.75)*

00.28 Intravascular imaging, other specified vessel(s)

00.29 Intravascular imaging, unspecified vessel(s)

√4ᵗʰ **00.3 Computer assisted surgery [CAS]**
CT-free navigation
Image guided navigation (IGN)
Image guided surgery (IGS)
Imageless navigation
That without the use of robotic(s) technology
Code also diagnostic or therapeutic procedure
> **EXCLUDES**   *robotic assisted procedures (17.41-17.49)*
>   *stereotactic frame application only (93.59)*

00.31 Computer assisted surgery with CT/CTA

00.32 Computer assisted surgery with MR/MRA

00.33 Computer assisted surgery with fluoroscopy

00.34 Imageless computer assisted surgery

00.35 Computer assisted surgery with multiple datasets

00.39 Other computer assisted surgery
Computer assisted surgery NOS

√4ᵗʰ **00.4 Adjunct vascular system procedures**
Note: These codes can apply to both coronary and peripheral vessels. These codes are to be used in conjunction with other therapeutic procedure codes to provide additional information on the number of vessels upon which a procedure was performed and/or the number of stents inserted. As appropriate, code both the number of vessels operated on (00.40-00.43), and the number of stents inserted (00.45-00.48).
Code also any:
  angioplasty (00.61-00.62, 00.66, 39.50)
  atherectomy (17.53-17.56)
  endarterectomy (38.10-38.18)
  insertion of vascular stent(s) (00.55, 00.63-00.65, 36.06-36.07, 39.90)
  other removal of coronary artery obstruction (36.09)

00.40 Procedure on single vessel
Number of vessels, unspecified
> **EXCLUDES**   *(aorto)coronary bypass (36.10-36.19)*
>   *intravascular imaging of blood vessels (00.21-00.29)*

Stenting Techniques on Vessel Bifurcation

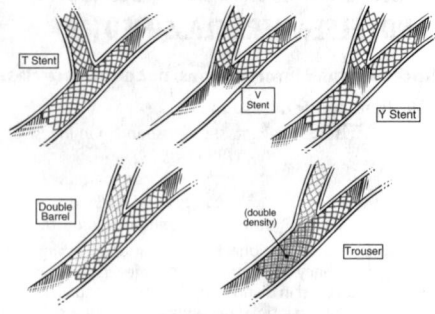

00.41 Procedure on two vessels
> **EXCLUDES**   *(aorto)coronary bypass (36.10-36.19)*
>   *intravascular imaging of blood vessels (00.21-00.29)*

00.42 Procedure on three vessels
> **EXCLUDES**   *(aorto)coronary bypass (36.10-36.19)*
>   *intravascular imaging of blood vessels (00.21-00.29)*

00.43 Procedure on four or more vessels
> **EXCLUDES**   *(aorto)coronary bypass (36.10-36.19)*
>   *intravascular imaging of blood vessels (00.21-00.29)*

00.44 Procedure on vessel bifurcation
Note: This code is to be used to identify the presence of a vessel bifurcation; it does not describe a specific bifurcation stent. Use this code only once per operative episode, irrespective of the number of bifurcations in vessels.

00.45 Insertion of one vascular stent
Number of stents, unspecified

00.46 Insertion of two vascular stents

00.47 Insertion of three vascular stents

00.48 Insertion of four or more vascular stents

00.49 SuperSaturated oxygen therapy
Aqueous oxygen (AO) therapy
SSO_2
SuperOxygenation infusion therapy
Code also any:
  injection or infusion of thrombolytic agent (99.10)
  insertion of coronary artery stent(s) (36.06-36.07)
  intracoronary artery thrombolytic infusion (36.04)
  number of vascular stents inserted (00.45-00.48)
  number of vessels treated (00.40-00.43)
  open chest coronary artery angioplasty (36.03)
  other removal of coronary obstruction (36.09)
  percutaneous transluminal coronary angioplasty [PTCA] (00.66)
  procedure on vessel bifurcation (00.44)
  transluminal coronary atherectomy (17.55)
> **EXCLUDES**   *other oxygen enrichment (93.96)*
>   *other perfusion (39.97)*

DEF: Method of reducing myocardial tissue damage via infusion of super-oxygenated blood directly to oxygen-deprived myocardial tissue in MI patients; typically performed as an adjunct procedure during PTCA or stent insertion.

✓4ᵗʰ **00.5 Other cardiovascular procedures**

00.50 Implantation of cardiac resynchronization pacemaker without mention of defibrillation, total system [CRT-P]

Note: Device testing during procedure — *omit code*
Biventricular pacemaker
Biventricular pacing without internal cardiac defibrillator
BiV pacemaker
Implantation of cardiac resynchronization (biventricular) pulse generator pacing device, formation of pocket, transvenous leads including placement of lead into left ventricular coronary venous system, and intraoperative procedures for evaluation of lead signals
That with CRT-P generator and one or more leads

EXCLUDES *implantation of cardiac resynchronization defibrillator, total system [CRT-D] (00.51)*
insertion or replacement of any type pacemaker device (37.80-37.87)
replacement of cardiac resynchronization:
defibrillator, pulse generator only [CRT-D] (00.54)
pacemaker, pulse generator only [CRT-P] (00.53)

DEF: Cardiac resynchronization pacemaker: CRT-P, or bi-ventricular pacing, adds a third lead to traditional pacemaker designs that connects to the left ventricle. The device provides electrical stimulation and coordinates ventricular contractions to improve cardiac output.

00.51 Implantation of cardiac resynchronization defibrillator, total system [CRT-D]

Note: Device testing during procedure — *omit code*
BiV defibrillator
Biventricular defibrillator
Biventricular pacing with internal cardiac defibrillator
BiV ICD
BiV pacemaker with defibrillator
BiV pacing with defibrillator
Implantation of cardiac resynchronization (biventricular) pulse generator with defibrillator [AICD], formation of pocket, transvenous leads, including placement of lead into left ventricular coronary venous system, intraoperative procedures for evaluation of lead signals, and obtaining defibrillator threshold measurements
That with CRT-D generator and one or more leads

EXCLUDES *implantation of cardiac resynchronization pacemaker, total system [CRT-P] (00.50)*
implantation or replacement of automatic cardioverter/ defibrillator, total system [AICD] (37.94)
replacement of cardiac resynchronization defibrillator, pulse generator only [CRT-D] (00.54)

00.52 Implantation or replacement of transvenous lead [electrode] into left ventricular coronary venous system

EXCLUDES *implantation of cardiac resynchronization:*
defibrillator, total system [CRT-D] (00.51)
pacemaker, total system [CRT-P] (00.50)
initial insertion of transvenous lead [electrode] (37.70-37.72)
replacement of transvenous atrial and/or ventricular lead(s) [electrodes] (37.76)

00.53 Implantation or replacement of cardiac resynchronization pacemaker, pulse generator only [CRT-P]

Note: Device testing during procedure — *omit code*
Implantation of CRT-P device with removal of any existing CRT-P or other pacemaker device

EXCLUDES *implantation of cardiac resynchronization pacemaker, total system [CRT-P] (00.50)*
implantation or replacement of cardiac resynchronization defibrillator, pulse generator only [CRT-D] (00.54)
insertion or replacement of any type pacemaker device (37.80-37.87)

00.54 Implantation or replacement of cardiac resynchronization defibrillator, pulse generator device only [CRT-D]

Note: Device testing during procedure — *omit code*
Implantation of CRT-D device with removal of any existing CRT-D, CRT-P, pacemaker, or defibrillator device

EXCLUDES *implantation of automatic cardioverter/defibrillator pulse generator only (37.96)*
implantation of cardiac resynchronization defibrillator, total system [CRT-D] (00.51)
implantation or replacement of cardiac resynchronization pacemaker, pulse generator only [CRT-P] (00.53)

00.55 Insertion of drug-eluting stent(s) of other peripheral vessel(s)

Endograft(s)
Endovascular graft(s)
Stent graft(s)
Code also any:
angioplasty of other non-coronary vessel(s) (39.50)
atherectomy of other non-coronary vessel(s) (17.56)
number of vascular stents inserted (00.45-00.48)
number of vessels treated (00.40-00.43)
procedure on vessel bifurcation (00.44)

EXCLUDES *drug-coated peripheral stents, e.g., heparin coated (39.90)*
insertion of cerebrovascular stent(s) (00.63-00.65)
insertion of drug-eluting coronary artery stent (36.07)
insertion of drug-eluting stent(s) of superficial femoral artery (00.60)
insertion of non-drug-eluting stent(s):
coronary artery (36.06)
peripheral vessel (39.90)
that for other endovascular procedure (39.71-39.79)

00.56 **Insertion or replacement of implantable pressure sensor with lead for intracardiac or great vessel hemodynamic monitoring**

Note: The sensor is physically connected by a lead to a separately implanted monitor

Code also any associated implantation or replacement of subcutaneous monitor (00.57)

> **EXCLUDES** *circulatory monitoring (blood gas, arterial or venous pressure, cardiac output and coronary blood flow) (89.60-89.69)*
>
> *insertion of implantable pressure sensor without lead for intracardiac or great vessel hemodynamic monitoring (38.26)*

DEF: Insertion of an implantable device consisting of a data storage system, a single lead with a pressure sensor tip and a wireless antenna that continuously collects data on heart rate, pressures, physical activity and temperature.

00.57 **Implantation or replacement of subcutaneous device for intracardiac or great vessel hemodynamic monitoring**

Implantation of monitoring device with formation of subcutaneous pocket and connection to intracardiac pressure sensor via lead

Code also any associated insertion or replacement of implanted pressure sensor with lead (00.56)

00.58 **Insertion of intra-aneurysm sac pressure monitoring device (intraoperative)**

Insertion of pressure sensor during endovascular repair of abdominal or thoracic aortic aneurysm(s)

DEF: Placement of a device in an aortic aneurysm sac during aneurysm repair to evaluate sac pressure before and after stent graft placement; helps detect endoleaks and prevents serious aneurysm complications.

00.59 **Intravascular pressure measurement of coronary arteries**

> **INCLUDES** fractional flow reserve (FFR)

Code also any synchronous diagnostic or therapeutic procedures

> **EXCLUDES** *intravascular pressure meas- urement of intrathoracic arteries (00.67)*

√4ᵗʰ **00.6** **Procedures on blood vessels**

00.60 **Insertion of drug-eluting stent(s) of superficial femoral artery**

Code also any:
> angioplasty of other non-coronary vessel(s) (39.50)
>
> atherectomy of other non-coronary vessel(s) (17.56)
>
> non-drug-eluting peripheral stents (39.90)
>
> number of vascular stents inserted (00.45-00.48)
>
> number of vessels treated (00.40-00.43)
>
> procedure on vessel bifurcation (00.44)

> **EXCLUDES** *insertion of drug-eluting stent(s) of other peripheral vessel (00.55)*
>
> *that for other endovascular procedure (39.71-39.79)*

DEF: A self-expanding device made of nitinol, a thin, specialized durable metal that targets delivery of a drug directly to the arterial lesion to restore blood flow.

00.61 **Percutaneous angioplasty of extracranial vessel(s)**

Carotid   Vertebral

Code also any:
> injection or infusion of thrombolytic agent (99.10)
>
> number of vascular stents inserted (00.45-00.48)
>
> number of vessels treated (00.40-00.43)
>
> percutaneous atherectomy of extracranial vessel(s) (17.53)
>
> percutaneous insertion of carotid artery stent(s) (00.63)
>
> percutaneous insertion of other extracranial artery stent(s) (00.64)
>
> procedure on vessel bifurcation (00.44)

> **EXCLUDES** *angioplasty of other non-coronary vessel(s) (39.50)*
>
> *atherectomy of other non-coronary vessel(s) (17.56)*
>
> *removal of cerebrovascular obstruction of vessel(s) by open approach (38.01-38.02, 38.11-38.12, 38.31-38.32, 38.41-38.42)*

00.62 **Percutaneous angioplasty of intracranial vessel(s)**

Basilar artery

Intracranial portion of vertebral artery

Code also any:
> injection or infusion of thrombolytic agent (99.10)
>
> number of vascular stents inserted (00.45-00.48)
>
> number of vessels treated (00.40-00.43)
>
> percutaneous atherectomy of intracranial vessel(s) (17.54)
>
> percutaneous insertion of intracranial stent(s) (00.65)
>
> procedure on vessel bifurcation (00.44)

> **EXCLUDES** *angioplasty of other non-coronary vessel(s) (39.50)*
>
> *atherectomy of other non-coronary vessel(s) (17.56)*
>
> *removal of cerebrovascular obstruction of vessel(s) by open approach (38.01-38.02, 38.11-38.12, 38.31-38.32, 38.41-38.42)*

00.63 **Percutaneous insertion of carotid artery stent(s)**

Includes the use of any embolic protection device, distal protection device, filter device, or stent delivery system

Non-drug-eluting stent

Code also any:
> number of vascular stents inserted (00.45-00.48)
>
> number of vessels treated (00.40-00.43)
>
> percutaneous angioplasty of extracranial vessel(s) (00.61)
>
> percutaneous atherectomy of extracranial vessel(s) (17.53)
>
> procedure on vessel bifurcation (00.44)

> **EXCLUDES** *angioplasty of other non-coronary vessel(s) (39.50)*
>
> *atherectomy of other non-coronary vessel(s) (17.56)*
>
> *insertion of coil-retention or embolization stent (39.72)*
>
> *insertion of drug-eluting peripheral vessel stent(s) (00.55)*

00.64   Percutaneous insertion of other extracranial artery stent(s)

Includes the use of any embolic protection device, distal protection device, filter device, or stent delivery system

Vertebral stent

Code also any:

number of vascular stents inserted (00.45-00.48)

number of vessels treated (00.40-00.43)

percutaneous angioplasty of extracranial vessel(s) (00.61)

percutaneous atherectomy of extracranial vessel(s) (17.53)

procedure on vessel bifurcation (00.44)

> **EXCLUDES**   *angioplasty of other non-coronary vessel(s) (39.50)*
> *atherectomy of other non-coronary vessel(s) (17.56)*
> *insertion of coil-retention or embolization stent (39.72)*
> *insertion of drug-eluting peripheral vessel stent(s) (00.55)*

00.65   Percutaneous insertion of intracranial vascular stent(s)

Includes the use of any embolic protection device, distal protection device, filter device, or stent delivery system

Basilar stent

Code also any:

number of vascular stents inserted (00.45-00.48)

number of vessels treated (00.40-00.43)

percutaneous angioplasty of intracranial vessel(s) (00.62)

percutaneous atherectomy of intracranial vessel(s) (17.54)

procedure on vessel bifurcation (00.44)

> **EXCLUDES**   *angioplasty of other non-coronary vessel(s) (39.50)*
> *atherectomy of other non-coronary vessel(s) (17.56)*
> *insertion of coil-retention or embolization stent (39.72)*
> *insertion of drug-eluting peripheral vessel stent(s) (00.55)*

00.66   Percutaneous transluminal coronary angioplasty [PTCA]

Balloon angioplasty of coronary artery

Percutaneous coronary angioplasty NOS

PTCA NOS

Code also any:

injection or infusion of thrombolytic agent (99.10)

insertion of coronary artery stent(s) (36.06-36.07)

intracoronary artery thrombolytic infusion (36.04)

number of vascular stents inserted (00.45-00.48)

number of vessels treated (00.40-00.43)

procedure on vessel bifurcation (00.44)

SuperSaturated oxygen therapy (00.49)

transluminal coronary atherectomy (17.55)

DEF: Balloon angioplasty: Insertion of catheter with inflation of balloon to flatten plaque and widen vessels.

00.67   Intravascular pressure measurement of intrathoracic arteries

Assessment of:

aorta and aortic arch

carotid

Code also any synchronous diagnostic or therapeutic procedures

PTCA (Balloon Angioplasty)

Aorta

Left coronary artery

Right coronary artery

Plaque

Inflated balloon

00.68   Intravascular pressure measurement of peripheral arteries

Assessment of:

other peripheral vessels

vessels of arm(s)

vessels of leg(s)

Code also any synchronous diagnostic or therapeutic procedures

00.69   Intravascular pressure measurement, other specified and unspecified vessels

Assessment of: Assessment of:

iliac vessels   mesenteric vessels

intra-abdominal vessels   renal vessels

Code also any synchronous diagnostic or therapeutic procedures

> **EXCLUDES**   *intravascular pressure measurement of:*
> *coronary arteries (00.59)*
> *intrathoracic arteries (00.67)*
> *peripheral arteries (00.68)*

✓4ᵗʰ 00.7   Other hip procedures

00.70   Revision of hip replacement, both acetabular and femoral components

Total hip revision

Code also any:

removal of (cement) (joint) spacer (84.57)

type of bearing surface, if known (00.74-00.77)

> **EXCLUDES**   *revision of hip replacement, acetabular component only (00.71)*
> *revision of hip replacement, fem- oral component only (00.72)*
> *revision of hip replacement, not otherwise specified (81.53)*
> *revision with replacement of acetabular liner and/or femoral head only (00.73)*

00.71   Revision of hip replacement, acetabular component

Partial, acetabular component only

That with:

exchange of acetabular cup and liner

exchange of femoral head

Code also any type of bearing surface, if known (00.74-00.77)

> **EXCLUDES**   *revision of hip replacement, both acetabular and femoral components (00.70)*
> *revision of hip replacement, femoral component (00.72)*
> *revision of hip replacement, not otherwise specified (81.53)*
> *revision with replacement of acetabular liner and/or femoral head only (00.73)*

00.72 Revision of hip replacement, femoral component
Partial, femoral component only
That with:
exchange of acetabular liner
exchange of femoral stem and head
Code also any type of bearing surface, if known
(00.74-00.77)
EXCLUDES revision of hip replacement, acetabular
component (00.71)
revision of hip replacement, both
acetabular and femoral
components (00.70)
revision of hip replacement, not
otherwise specified (81.53)
revision with replacement of acetabular
liner and/or femoral head only
(00.73)

00.73 Revision of hip replacement, acetabular liner and/or femoral head only
Code also any type of bearing surface, if known
(00.74-00.77)

00.74 Hip bearing surface, metal-on- polyethylene

00.75 Hip bearing surface, metal-on-metal

00.76 Hip bearing surface, ceramic-on-ceramic

00.77 Hip bearing surface, ceramic-on- polyethylene
Hip bearing surface, oxidized
zirconium-on-polyethylene

√4ᵗʰ **00.8 Other knee and hip procedures**
Note: Report up to two components using 00.81-00.83 to
describe revision of knee replacements. If all three
components are revised, report 00.80.

00.80 Revision of knee replacement, total (all components)
Replacement of femoral, tibial, and patellar
components (all components)
Code also any removal of (cement) (joint) spacer
(84.57)
EXCLUDES revision of only one or two components
(tibial, femoral or patellar
component) (00.81-00.84)

00.81 Revision of knee replacement, tibial component
Replacement of tibial baseplate and tibial insert
(liner)
EXCLUDES revision of knee replacement, total (all
components) (00.80)

00.82 Revision of knee replacement, femoral component
That with replacement of tibial insert (liner)
EXCLUDES revision of knee replacement, total (all
components) (00.80)

00.83 Revision of knee replacement, patellar component
EXCLUDES revision of knee replacement, total (all
components) (00.80)

00.84 Revision of total knee replacement, tibial insert (liner)
Replacement of tibial insert (liner)
EXCLUDES that with replacement of tibial
component (tibial base plate and
liner) (00.81)

00.85 Resurfacing hip, total, acetabulum and femoral head
Hip resurfacing arthroplasty, total

00.86 Resurfacing hip, partial, femoral head
Hip resurfacing arthroplasty, NOS
Hip resurfacing arthroplasty, partial, femoral head
EXCLUDES that with resurfacing of acetabulum
(00.85)

00.87 Resurfacing hip, partial, acetabulum
Hip resurfacing arthroplasty, partial, acetabulum
EXCLUDES that with resurfacing of femoral head
(00.85)

√4ᵗʰ **00.9 Other procedures and interventions**

00.91 Transplant from live related donor
Code also organ transplant procedure

00.92 Transplant from live non-related donor
Code also organ transplant procedure

00.93 Transplant from cadaver
Code also organ transplant procedure

00.94 Intra-operative neurophysiologic monitoring
INCLUDES Cranial nerve, peripheral nerve and
spinal cord testing performed
intra-operatively
Intra-operative neurophysiologic testing
IOM
Nerve monitoring
Neuromonitoring
That by:
brainstem auditory evoked potentials [BAEP]
electroencephalogram [EEG]
electromyogram [EMG]
motor evoked potentials [MEP]
nerve conduction study
somatosensory evoked potentials [SSEP]
transcranial Doppler
EXCLUDES brain temperature monitoring (01.17)
intracranial oxygen monitoring (01.16)
intracranial pressure monitoring (01.10)
plethysmogram (89.58)

DEF: Real-time testing techniques used in brain,
spinal cord, and nerve procedures to assist in lesion
excision and provide ongoing neurological
functioning information and/or warning of
impending neural structure injury.

00.95 Injection or infusion of glucarpidase

00.96 Infusion of 4-Factor Prothrombin Complex Concentrate
Infusion of 4F-PCC
EXCLUDES transfusion of coagulation factors (99.06)
transfusion of Factor IX complex (99.06)

1. OPERATIONS ON THE NERVOUS SYSTEM (01-05)

√3ʳᵈ **01 Incision and excision of skull, brain, and cerebral meninges**

√4ᵗʰ **01.0 Cranial puncture**

01.01 Cisternal puncture

Cisternal aspiration   Cisternal tap

EXCLUDES *pneumocisternogram (87.02)*

DEF: Needle insertion through subarachnoid space to withdraw cerebrospinal fluid.

01.02 Ventriculopuncture through previously implanted catheter

Puncture of ventricular shunt tubing

DEF: Piercing of artificial, fluid-diverting tubing in the brain for withdrawal of cerebrospinal fluid.

01.09 Other cranial puncture

Aspiration of:
subarachnoid space
subdural space
Cranial aspiration NOS
Puncture of anterior fontanel
Subdural tap (through fontanel)

√4ᵗʰ **01.1 Diagnostic procedures on skull, brain, and cerebral meninges**

01.10 Intracranial pressure monitoring

INCLUDES insertion of catheter or probe for monitoring

01.11 Closed [percutaneous] [needle] biopsy of cerebral meninges

Burr hole approach

DEF: Needle excision of tissue sample through skin into cerebral membranes; no other procedure performed.

01.12 Open biopsy of cerebral meninges

DEF: Open surgical excision of tissue sample from cerebral membrane.

01.13 Closed [percutaneous] [needle] biopsy of brain

Burr hole approach   Stereotactic method

DEF: Removal by needle of brain tissue sample through skin.

01.14 Open biopsy of brain

DEF: Open surgical excision of brain tissue sample.

01.15 Biopsy of skull

01.16 Intracranial oxygen monitoring

Partial pressure of brain oxygen ($PbtO_2$)

INCLUDES insertion of catheter or probe for monitoring

01.17 Brain temperature monitoring

INCLUDES insertion of catheter or probe for monitoring

01.18 Other diagnostic procedures on brain and cerebral meninges

EXCLUDES *brain temperature monitoring (01.17)*
cerebral:
arteriography (88.41)
thermography (88.81)
contrast radiogram of brain (87.01-87.02)
echoencephalogram (88.71)
electroencephalogram (89.14)
intracranial oxygen monitoring (01.16)
intracranial pressure monitoring (01.10)
microscopic examination of specimen from nervous system and of spinal fluid (90.01-90.09)
neurologic examination (89.13)
phlebography of head and neck (88.61)
pneumoencephalogram (87.01)
radioisotope scan:
cerebral (92.11)
head NEC (92.12)
tomography of head:
C.A.T. scan (87.03)
other (87.04)

01.19 Other diagnostic procedures on skull

EXCLUDES *transillumination of skull (89.16)*
x-ray of skull (87.17)

√4ᵗʰ **01.2 Craniotomy and craniectomy**

EXCLUDES *decompression of skull fracture (02.02)*
exploration of orbit (16.01-16.09)
that as operative approach — omit code

DEF: Craniotomy: Incision into skull.

DEF: Craniectomy: Excision of part of skull.

01.20 Cranial implantation or replacement of neurostimulator pulse generator

Code also any associated lead implantation (02.93)

EXCLUDES *implantation or replacement of subcutaneous neurostimulator pulse generator (86.94-86.98)*

DEF: A small, curved device designed to be implanted within the skull near the patient's specific foci (point of origin) of seizure.

01.21 Incision and drainage of cranial sinus

DEF: Incision for drainage, including drainage of air cavities in skull bones.

01.22 Removal of intracranial neurostimulator lead(s)

Code also any removal of neurostimulator pulse generator (86.05)

EXCLUDES *removal with synchronous replacement (02.93)*

01.23 Reopening of craniotomy site

DEF: Reopening of skull incision.

01.24 Other craniotomy

Cranial: Craniotomy with removal of:
decompression   epidural abscess
exploration   extradural hematoma
trephination   foreign body of skull
Craniotomy NOS

EXCLUDES *removal of foreign body with incision into brain (01.39)*

01.25 Other craniectomy

Debridement of skull NOS
Sequestrectomy of skull

EXCLUDES *debridement of compound fracture of skull (02.02)*
strip craniectomy (02.01)

01.26 Insertion of catheter(s) into cranial cavity or tissue

Code also any concomitant procedure (e.g. resection (01.59))

EXCLUDES *placement of intracerebral catheter(s) via burr hole(s) (01.28)*

01.27 Removal of catheter(s) from cranial cavity or tissue

01.28 Placement of intracerebral catheter(s) via burr hole(s)

Convection enhanced delivery
Stereotactic placement of intracerebral catheter(s)
Code also infusion of medication

EXCLUDES *insertion of catheter(s) into cranial cavity or tissue(s) (01.26)*

DEF: The strategic neurosurgical placement of catheters via burr holes into targeted brain tissue, through which therapeutic agents such as antineoplastics are microinfused.

01.29 Removal of cranial neurostimulator pulse generator

√4ᵗʰ **01.3 Incision of brain and cerebral meninges**

01.31 Incision of cerebral meninges

Drainage of:
intracranial hygroma
subarachnoid abscess (cerebral)
subdural empyema

Operations on the Nervous System

01.32–02.22

01.32 Lobotomy and tractotomy
Division of:
brain tissue
cerebral tracts
Percutaneous (radiofrequency) cingulotomy
DEF: Lobotomy: Incision of nerve fibers of brain lobe, usually frontal.
DEF: Tractotomy: Severing of a nerve fiber group to relieve pain.

01.39 Other incision of brain
Amygdalohippocampotomy
Drainage of intracerebral hematoma
Incision of brain NOS
EXCLUDES *division of cortical adhesions (02.91)*

√4th **01.4 Operations on thalamus and globus pallidus**

01.41 Operations on thalamus
Chemothalamectomy
Thalamotomy
EXCLUDES *that by stereotactic radiosurgery (92.30-92.39)*

01.42 Operations on globus pallidus
Pallidoansectomy
Pallidotomy
EXCLUDES *that by stereotactic radiosurgery (92.30-92.39)*

√4th **01.5 Other excision or destruction of brain and meninges**

01.51 Excision of lesion or tissue of cerebral meninges
Decortication
Resection } of (cerebral) meninges
Stripping of subdural
membrane
EXCLUDES *biopsy of cerebral meninges (01.11-01.12)*

01.52 Hemispherectomy
DEF: Removal of one half of the brain. Most often performed for malignant brain tumors or intractable epilepsy.

01.53 Lobectomy of brain
DEF: Excision of a brain lobe.

01.59 Other excision or destruction of lesion or tissue of brain
Amygdalohippocampectomy
Curettage of brain
Debridement of brain
Marsupialization of brain cyst
Transtemporal (mastoid) excision of brain tumor
EXCLUDES *biopsy of brain (01.13-01.14)*
laser interstitial thermal therapy [LITT] of lesion or tissue of brain under guidance (17.61)
that by stereotactic radiosurgery (92.30-92.39)

01.6 Excision of lesion of skull
Removal of granulation tissue of cranium
EXCLUDES *biopsy of skull (01.15)*
sequestrectomy (01.25)

√3rd **02 Other operations on skull, brain, and cerebral meninges**

√4th **02.0 Cranioplasty**
EXCLUDES *that with synchronous repair of encephalocele (02.12)*

02.01 Opening of cranial suture
Linear craniectomy
Strip craniectomy
DEF: Opening of the lines of junction between the bones of the skull for removal of strips of skull bone.

02.02 Elevation of skull fracture fragments
Debridement of compound fracture of skull
Decompression of skull fracture
Reduction of skull fracture
Code also any synchronous debridement of brain (01.59)
EXCLUDES *debridement of skull NOS (01.25)*
removal of granulation tissue of cranium (01.6)

02.03 Formation of cranial bone flap
Repair of skull with flap

02.04 Bone graft to skull
Pericranial graft (autogenous) (heterogenous)

02.05 Insertion of skull plate
Replacement of skull plate

02.06 Other cranial osteoplasty
Repair of skull NOS
Revision of bone flap of skull
DEF: Plastic surgery repair of skull bones.

02.07 Removal of skull plate
EXCLUDES *removal with synchronous replacement (02.05)*

√4th **02.1 Repair of cerebral meninges**
EXCLUDES *marsupialization of cerebral lesion (01.59)*

02.11 Simple suture of dura mater of brain

02.12 Other repair of cerebral meninges
Closure of fistula of cerebrospinal fluid
Dural graft
Repair of encephalocele including synchronous cranioplasty
Repair of meninges NOS
Subdural patch

02.13 Ligation of meningeal vessel
Ligation of:
longitudinal sinus
middle meningeal artery

02.14 Choroid plexectomy
Cauterization of choroid plexus
DEF: Excision or destruction of the ependymal cells that form the membrane lining in the third, fourth, and lateral ventricles of the brain and secrete cerebrospinal fluid.

√4th **02.2 Ventriculostomy**

02.21 Insertion or replacement of external ventricular drain [EVD]
External ventricular drainage [EVD] setup
Replacement of external ventricular drain
Ventricular catheter placement for:
drainage of cerebrospinal fluid [CSF]
injection of medication or other substance
sampling of cerebrospinal fluid [CSF]
EXCLUDES *extracranial ventricular shunt (02.31-02.35, 02.39)*
intracranial ventricular shunt (02.22)
other cranial puncture (01.09)
ventricular shunt replacement (02.41-02.43)
DEF: Placement of a catheter into the ventricles for external drainage of cerebrospinal fluid into a container outside the body.

02.22 Intracranial ventricular shunt or anastomosis
Anastomosis of ventricle to:
cervical subarachnoid space
cistern magna
Insertion of Holter valve into intracranial system
Shunt between two intracranial ventricles
That by endoscopy
Third ventriculostomy
Ventriculocisternostomy
DEF: Surgical creation of an opening of ventricle; often performed to drain cerebrospinal fluid in treating hydrocephalus.

✓4ᵗʰ **02.3 Extracranial ventricular shunt**

    INCLUDES   that with insertion of valve

    DEF: Placement of shunt or creation of artificial passage leading from skull cavities to site outside skull to relieve excess cerebrospinal fluid created in the chorioid plexuses of the third and fourth ventricles of the brain.

02.31 Ventricular shunt to structure in head and neck
    Ventricle to nasopharynx shunt
    Ventriculomastoid anastomosis

02.32 Ventricular shunt to circulatory system
    Ventriculoatrial anastomosis
    Ventriculocaval shunt

02.33 Ventricular shunt to thoracic cavity
    Ventriculopleural anastomosis

02.34 Ventricular shunt to abdominal cavity and organs
    Ventriculocholecystostomy
    Ventriculoperitoneostomy

02.35 Ventricular shunt to urinary system
    Ventricle to ureter shunt

02.39 Ventricular shunt to extracranial site NEC
    Ventricle to bone marrow shunt

✓4ᵗʰ **02.4 Revision, removal, and irrigation of ventricular shunt**

    EXCLUDES   revision of distal catheter of ventricular shunt (54.95)

02.41 Irrigation and exploration of ventricular shunt
    Exploration of ventriculoperitoneal shunt at ventricular site
    Re-programming of ventriculoperitoneal shunt

02.42 Replacement of ventricular shunt
    Reinsertion of Holter valve
    Revision of ventriculoperitoneal shunt at ventricular site

02.43 Removal of ventricular shunt

✓4ᵗʰ **02.9 Other operations on skull, brain, and cerebral meninges**

    EXCLUDES   operations on:
        pineal gland (07.17, 07.51-07.59)
        pituitary gland [hypophysis] (07.13-07.15, 07.61-07.79)

02.91 Lysis of cortical adhesions
    DEF: Breaking up of fibrous structures in brain outer layer.

02.92 Repair of brain

02.93 Implantation or replacement of intracranial neurostimulator lead(s)
    Implantation, insertion, placement, or replacement of intracranial:
        brain pacemaker [neuropacemaker]
        depth electrodes
        epidural pegs
        electroencephalographic receiver
        foramen ovale electrodes
        intracranial electrostimulator
        subdural grids
        subdural strips
    Code also any:
        insertion of cranial implantation or replacement of neurostimulator pulse generator (01.20)
        insertion of subcutaneous neurostimulator pulse generator (86.94-86.98)

02.94 Insertion or replacement of skull tongs or halo traction device
    DEF: Halo traction device: Metal or plastic band encircles the head or neck secured to the skull with four pins and attached to a metal chest plate by rods; provides support and stability for the head and neck.
    DEF: Skull tongs: Device inserted into each side of the skull used to apply parallel traction to the long axis of the cervical spine.

02.95 Removal of skull tongs or halo traction device

02.96 Insertion of sphenoidal electrodes

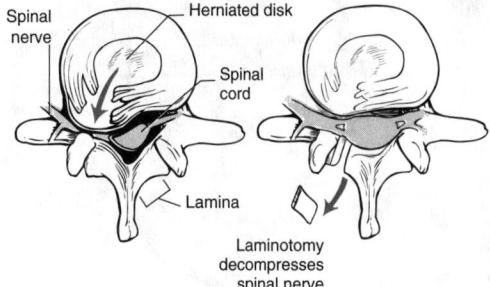
Laminotomy with Decompression

Spinal nerve · Herniated disk · Spinal cord · Lamina · Laminotomy decompresses spinal nerve

02.99 Other
    EXCLUDES   chemical shock therapy (94.24)
        electroshock therapy:
            subconvulsive (94.26)
            other (94.27)

✓3ʳᵈ **03 Operations on spinal cord and spinal canal structures**
    Code also any application or administration of an adhesion barrier substance (99.77).

✓4ᵗʰ **03.0 Exploration and decompression of spinal canal structures**

03.01 Removal of foreign body from spinal canal

03.02 Reopening of laminectomy site

03.09 Other exploration and decompression of spinal canal
    Decompression:
        laminectomy
        laminotomy
    Expansile laminoplasty
    Exploration of spinal nerve root
    Foraminotomy
    Code also any synchronous insertion, replacement and revision of posterior spinal motion preservation device(s), if performed (84.80-84.85)
    EXCLUDES   drainage of spinal fluid by anastomosis (03.71-03.79)
        laminectomy with excision of intervertebral disc (80.51)
        spinal tap (03.31)
        that as operative approach — omit code
    DEF: Decompression of spinal canal: Excision of bone pieces, hematoma or other lesion to relieve spinal cord pressure.
    DEF: Expansile laminoplasty: Lamina is incised at the level of the pedicle to relieve pressure; no tissue is excised.
    DEF: Foraminotomy: Removal of root opening between vertebrae to relieve nerve root pressure.

03.1 Division of intraspinal nerve root
    Rhizotomy
    DEF: Rhizotomy: Surgical severing of spinal nerve roots within spinal canal for pain relief.

✓4ᵗʰ **03.2 Chordotomy**
    DEF: Chordotomy: Surgical cutting of lateral spinothalamic tract of spinal cord to relieve pain.

03.21 Percutaneous chordotomy
    Stereotactic chordotomy
    DEF: Percutaneous chordotomy: Insertion of hollow needle through skin to interrupt spinal nerve root.
    DEF: Stereotactic chordotomy: Use of three-dimensional imaging to locate spinal nerve root for surgical interruption.

03.29 Other chordotomy
    Chordotomy NOS
    Tractotomy (one-stage) (two-stage) of spinal cord
    Transection of spinal cord tracts
    DEF: Tractotomy (one stage) (two stages) of the spinal cord: Surgical incision or severing of a nerve tract of spinal cord.
    DEF: Transection of spinal cord tracts: Use of transverse incision to divide spinal nerve root.

Lumbar Spinal Puncture

Cut edge of dura mater
"Cauda equina" (shown cut)

Injection site

Sacrum

L-4

L-5

Filum terminale

✓4th **03.3 Diagnostic procedures on spinal cord and spinal canal structures**

03.31 Spinal tap
Lumbar puncture for removal of dye
EXCLUDES lumbar puncture for injection of dye [myelogram] (87.21)

DEF: Puncture into lumbar subarachnoid space to tap cerebrospinal fluid.

03.32 Biopsy of spinal cord or spinal meninges

03.39 Other diagnostic procedures on spinal cord and spinal canal structures
EXCLUDES microscopic examination of specimen from nervous system or of spinal fluid (90.01-90.09)
x-ray of spine (87.21-87.29)

03.4 Excision or destruction of lesion of spinal cord or spinal meninges
Curettage
Debridement   } of spinal cord or spinal
Marsupialization of cyst   meninges
Resection
EXCLUDES biopsy of spinal cord or meninges (03.32)

✓4th **03.5 Plastic operations on spinal cord structures**

03.51 Repair of spinal meningocele
Repair of meningocele NOS
DEF: Restoration of hernial protrusion of spinal meninges through defect in vertebral column.

03.52 Repair of spinal myelomeningocele
DEF: Restoration of hernial protrusion of spinal cord and meninges through defect in vertebral column.

03.53 Repair of vertebral fracture
Elevation of spinal bone fragments
Reduction of fracture of vertebrae
Removal of bony spicules from spinal canal
EXCLUDES percutaneous vertebral augmentation (81.66)
percutaneous vertebroplasty (81.65)

03.59 Other repair and plastic operations on spinal cord structures
Repair of: Repair of:
diastematomyelia   spinal meninges NOS
spina bifida NOS   vertebral arch defect
spinal cord NOS

03.6 Lysis of adhesions of spinal cord and nerve roots

✓4th **03.7 Shunt of spinal theca**
INCLUDES that with valve
DEF: Surgical passage created from spinal cord dura mater to another channel.

03.71 Spinal subarachnoid-peritoneal shunt

03.72 Spinal subarachnoid-ureteral shunt

03.79 Other shunt of spinal theca
Lumbar-subarachnoid shunt NOS
Pleurothecal anastomosis
Salpingothecal anastomosis

03.8 Injection of destructive agent into spinal canal

✓4th **03.9 Other operations on spinal cord and spinal canal structures**

03.90 Insertion of catheter into spinal canal for infusion of therapeutic or palliative substances
Insertion of catheter into epidural, subarachnoid, or subdural space of spine with intermittent or continuous infusion of drug (with creation of any reservoir)
Code also any implantation of infusion pump (86.06)

03.91 Injection of anesthetic into spinal canal for analgesia
EXCLUDES that for operative anesthesia — omit code

03.92 Injection of other agent into spinal canal
Intrathecal injection of steroid
Subarachnoid perfusion of refrigerated saline
EXCLUDES injection of:
contrast material for myelogram (87.21)
destructive agent into spinal canal (03.8)

03.93 Implantation or replacement of spinal neurostimulator lead(s)
Code also any insertion of neurostimulator pulse generator (86.94-86.98)

03.94 Removal of spinal neurostimulator lead(s)
Code also any removal of neurostimulator pulse generator (86.05)

03.95 Spinal blood patch
DEF: Injection of blood into epidural space to patch hole in outer spinal membrane made by previous spinal puncture; blood clots and fills hole.

03.96 Percutaneous denervation of facet

03.97 Revision of spinal thecal shunt

03.98 Removal of spinal thecal shunt

03.99 Other

✓3rd **04 Operations on cranial and peripheral nerves**

✓4th **04.0 Incision, division, and excision of cranial and peripheral nerves**
EXCLUDES opticociliary neurectomy (12.79)
sympathetic ganglionectomy (05.21-05.29)

04.01 Excision of acoustic neuroma
That by craniotomy
EXCLUDES that by stereotactic radiosurgery (92.3)

04.02 Division of trigeminal nerve
Retrogasserian neurotomy
DEF: Transection of sensory root fibers of trigeminal nerve for relief of trigeminal neuralgia.

04.03 Division or crushing of other cranial and peripheral nerves
EXCLUDES that of:
glossopharyngeal nerve (29.92)
laryngeal nerve (31.91)
nerves to adrenal glands (07.42)
phrenic nerve for collapse of lung (33.31)
vagus nerve (44.00-44.03)

04.04 Other incision of cranial and peripheral nerves

04.05 Gasserian ganglionectomy

04.06 Other cranial or peripheral ganglionectomy
EXCLUDES sympathetic ganglionectomy (05.21-05.29)

04.07   Other excision or avulsion of cranial and peripheral nerves
    Curettage ⎫
    Debridement ⎬ of peripheral nerve
    Resection ⎭
    Excision of peripheral neuroma [Morton's]
    EXCLUDES *biopsy of cranial or peripheral nerve (04.11-04.12)*

✓4ᵗʰ **04.1   Diagnostic procedures on peripheral nervous system**

    04.11   Closed [percutaneous] [needle] biopsy of cranial or peripheral nerve or ganglion

    04.12   Open biopsy of cranial or peripheral nerve or ganglion

    04.19   Other diagnostic procedures on cranial and peripheral nerves and ganglia
        EXCLUDES *microscopic examination of specimen from nervous system (90.01-90.09)*
        neurologic examination (89.13)

04.2   Destruction of cranial and peripheral nerves
    Destruction of cranial or peripheral nerves by:
        cryoanalgesia
        injection of neurolytic agent
        radiofrequency
        Radiofrequency ablation
    DEF: Radiofrequency ablation: High frequency radio waves are applied to injure the nerve resulting in interruption of the pain signal.

04.3   Suture of cranial and peripheral nerves

✓4ᵗʰ **04.4   Lysis of adhesions and decompression of cranial and peripheral nerves**

    04.41   Decompression of trigeminal nerve root

    04.42   Other cranial nerve decompression

    04.43   Release of carpal tunnel

    04.44   Release of tarsal tunnel

    04.49   Other peripheral nerve or ganglion decompression or lysis of adhesions
        Peripheral nerve neurolysis NOS

04.5   Cranial or peripheral nerve graft

04.6   Transposition of cranial and peripheral nerves
    Nerve transplantation
    DEF: Relocation of cranial or peripheral nerves without detaching or severing them.

✓4ᵗʰ **04.7   Other cranial or peripheral neuroplasty**

    04.71   Hypoglossal-facial anastomosis
        DEF: Surgical connection of hypoglossal nerve to facial nerve.

    04.72   Accessory-facial anastomosis
        DEF: Surgical connection of accessory nerve to facial nerve.

    04.73   Accessory-hypoglossal anastomosis
        DEF: Surgical connection of accessory nerve to hypoglossal nerve.

    04.74   Other anastomosis of cranial or peripheral nerve

    04.75   Revision of previous repair of cranial and peripheral nerves

    04.76   Repair of old traumatic injury of cranial and peripheral nerves

    04.79   Other neuroplasty

04.8   Injection into peripheral nerve
    EXCLUDES *destruction of nerve (by injection of neurolytic agent) (04.2)*

    04.80   Peripheral nerve injection, not otherwise specified

    04.81   Injection of anesthetic into peripheral nerve for analgesia
        EXCLUDES *that for operative anesthesia — omit code*

    04.89   Injection of other agent, except neurolytic
        EXCLUDES *injection of neurolytic agent (04.2)*

Release of Carpal Tunnel

Median nerve

(Deep) transverse carpal ligament being cut

✓4ᵗʰ **04.9   Other operations on cranial and peripheral nerves**

    04.91   Neurectasis
        DEF: Surgical stretching of peripheral or cranial nerve.

    04.92   Implantation or replacement of peripheral neurostimulator lead(s)
        Code also any insertion of neurostimulator pulse generator (86.94-86.98)
        EXCLUDES *implantation or replacement of carotid sinus stimulation lead(s) (39.82)*
        DEF: Placement of or removal and replacement of neurostimulator lead(s) during the same episode.

    04.93   Removal of peripheral neurostimulator lead(s)
        Code also any removal of neurostimulator pulse generator (86.05)

    04.99   Other

✓3ʳᵈ **05   Operations on sympathetic nerves or ganglia**
    EXCLUDES *paracervical uterine denervation (69.3)*

    05.0   Division of sympathetic nerve or ganglion
        EXCLUDES *that of nerves to adrenal glands (07.42)*

✓4ᵗʰ **05.1   Diagnostic procedures on sympathetic nerves or ganglia**

    05.11   Biopsy of sympathetic nerve or ganglion

    05.19   Other diagnostic procedures on sympathetic nerves or ganglia

✓4ᵗʰ **05.2   Sympathectomy**
    DEF: Sympathectomy: Division of nerve pathway at a specific site of a sympathetic nerve.

    05.21   Sphenopalatine ganglionectomy

    05.22   Cervical sympathectomy

    05.23   Lumbar sympathectomy
        DEF: Excision, resection of lumber chain nerve group to relieve causalgia, Raynaud's disease, or lower extremity thromboangiitis.

    05.24   Presacral sympathectomy
        DEF: Excision or resection of hypogastric nerve network.

    05.25   Periarterial sympathectomy
        DEF: Removal of arterial sheath containing sympathetic nerve fibers.

    05.29   Other sympathectomy and ganglionectomy
        Excision or avulsion of sympathetic nerve NOS
        Sympathetic ganglionectomy NOS
        EXCLUDES *biopsy of sympathetic nerve or ganglion (05.11)*
        opticociliary neurectomy (12.79)
        periarterial sympathectomy (05.25)
        tympanosympathectomy (20.91)

✓4ᵗʰ **05.3   Injection into sympathetic nerve or ganglion**
    EXCLUDES *injection of ciliary sympathetic ganglion (12.79)*

    05.31   Injection of anesthetic into sympathetic nerve for analgesia

    05.32   Injection of neurolytic agent into sympathetic nerve

05.39   Other injection into sympathetic nerve or ganglion

✓4ᵗʰ 05.8   Other operations on sympathetic nerves or ganglia

05.81   Repair of sympathetic nerve or ganglion

05.89   Other

05.9   Other operations on nervous system

2. OPERATIONS ON THE ENDOCRINE SYSTEM (06-07)

√3ʳᵈ **06   Operations on thyroid and parathyroid glands**
    INCLUDES   incidental resection of hyoid bone

√4ᵗʰ **06.0   Incision of thyroid field**
    EXCLUDES   *division of isthmus (06.91)*

    06.01   Aspiration of thyroid field
        Percutaneous or needle drainage of thyroid field
        EXCLUDES   *aspiration biopsy of thyroid (06.11)*
                   drainage by incision (06.09)
                   postoperative aspiration of field (06.02)

    06.02   Reopening of wound of thyroid field
        Reopening of wound of thyroid field for:
           control of (postoperative) hemorrhage
           examination
           exploration
           removal of hematoma

    06.09   Other incision of thyroid field
        Drainage of hematoma
        Drainage of thyroglossal tract
        Exploration
           neck   } by incision
           thyroid (field)
        Removal of foreign body
        Thyroidotomy NOS
        EXCLUDES   *postoperative exploration (06.02)*
                   removal of hematoma by aspiration
                       (06.01)

√4ᵗʰ **06.1   Diagnostic procedures on thyroid and parathyroid glands**

    06.11   Closed [percutaneous] [needle] biopsy of thyroid gland
        Aspiration biopsy of thyroid
        DEF: Insertion of needle-type device for removal of thyroid tissue sample.

    06.12   Open biopsy of thyroid gland

    06.13   Biopsy of parathyroid gland

    06.19   Other diagnostic procedures on thyroid and parathyroid glands
        EXCLUDES   *radioisotope scan of:*
                   parathyroid (92.13)
                   thyroid (92.01)
             soft tissue x-ray of thyroid field (87.09)

06.2   Unilateral thyroid lobectomy
    Complete removal of one lobe of thyroid (with removal of isthmus or portion of other lobe)
    Hemithyroidectomy
    EXCLUDES   *partial substernal thyroidectomy (06.51)*
    DEF: Excision of thyroid lobe.

√4ᵗʰ **06.3   Other partial thyroidectomy**

    06.31   Excision of lesion of thyroid
        EXCLUDES   *biopsy of thyroid (06.11-06.12)*
                   laser interstitial thermal therapy [LITT] of
                     lesion or tissue of neck under
                     guidance (17.62)
        DEF: Removal of growth on thyroid.

Thyroidectomy

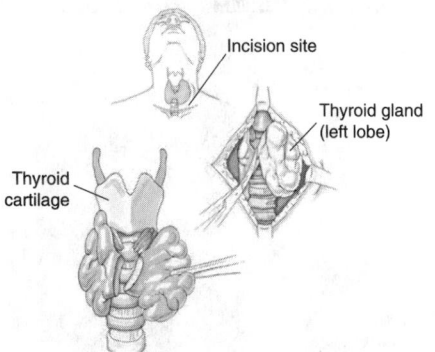

Incision site

Thyroid gland (left lobe)

Thyroid cartilage

    06.39   Other
        Isthmectomy
        Partial thyroidectomy NOS
        EXCLUDES   *partial substernal thyroidectomy (06.51)*

06.4   Complete thyroidectomy
    EXCLUDES   *complete substernal thyroidectomy (06.52)*
              that with laryngectomy (30.3-30.4)

√4ᵗʰ **06.5   Substernal thyroidectomy**
    DEF: Removal of thyroid tissue below breastbone.

    06.50   Substernal thyroidectomy, not otherwise specified

    06.51   Partial substernal thyroidectomy

    06.52   Complete substernal thyroidectomy

06.6   Excision of lingual thyroid
    Excision of thyroid by: Excision of thyroid by:
      submental route   transoral route
    DEF: Excision of thyroid tissue at base of tongue.

06.7   Excision of thyroglossal duct or tract

√4ᵗʰ **06.8   Parathyroidectomy**
    DEF: Removal of parathyroid glands.

    06.81   Complete parathyroidectomy

    06.89   Other parathyroidectomy
        Parathyroidectomy NOS
        Partial parathyroidectomy
        EXCLUDES   *biopsy of parathyroid (06.13)*

√4ᵗʰ **06.9   Other operations on thyroid (region) and parathyroid**

    06.91   Division of thyroid isthmus
        Transection of thyroid isthmus
        DEF: Cutting or division of tissue at narrowest point of thyroid.

    06.92   Ligation of thyroid vessels

    06.93   Suture of thyroid gland

    06.94   Thyroid tissue reimplantation
        Autotransplantation of thyroid tissue
        DEF: Placement of thyroid tissue graft into functional site.
        DEF: Autotransplantation of thyroid tissue: Tissue graft from patient's own thyroid tissue to another site on thyroid.

    06.95   Parathyroid tissue reimplantation
        Autotransplantation of parathyroid tissue

    06.98   Other operations on thyroid glands

    06.99   Other operations on parathyroid glands

√3ʳᵈ **07   Operations on other endocrine glands**
    INCLUDES   operations on:
                adrenal glands
                pineal gland
                pituitary gland
                thymus
    EXCLUDES   *operations on:*
                aortic and carotid bodies (39.81-39.89)
                ovaries (65.0-65.99)
                pancreas (52.01-52.99)
                testes (62.0-62.99)

√4ᵗʰ **07.0   Exploration of adrenal field**
    EXCLUDES   *incision of adrenal (gland) (07.41)*

    07.00   Exploration of adrenal field, not otherwise specified

    07.01   Unilateral exploration of adrenal field
        DEF: Investigation of one adrenal gland for diagnostic reasons.

    07.02   Bilateral exploration of adrenal field
        DEF: Investigation of both adrenal glands for diagnostic reasons.

√4ᵗʰ **07.1   Diagnostic procedures on adrenal glands, pituitary gland, pineal gland, and thymus**

    07.11   Closed [percutaneous] [needle] biopsy of adrenal gland

    07.12   Open biopsy of adrenal gland

Operations on the Endocrine System

07.13–07.84

07.13　Biopsy of pituitary gland, transfrontal approach
　DEF: Excision of pituitary gland tissue for exam through frontal bone.

07.14　Biopsy of pituitary gland, transsphenoidal approach
　DEF: Excision of pituitary gland tissue for exam through sphenoid bone.

07.15　Biopsy of pituitary gland, unspecified approach

07.16　Biopsy of thymus

07.17　Biopsy of pineal gland

07.19　Other diagnostic procedures on adrenal glands, pituitary gland, pineal gland, and thymus
　EXCLUDES　*microscopic examination of specimen from endocrine gland (90.11-90.19)*
　　　　　　radioisotope scan of pituitary gland (92.11)

✓4ᵗʰ **07.2　Partial adrenalectomy**

07.21　Excision of lesion of adrenal gland
　EXCLUDES　*biopsy of adrenal gland (07.11-07.12)*

07.22　Unilateral adrenalectomy
　Adrenalectomy NOS
　EXCLUDES　*excision of remaining adrenal gland (07.3)*
　DEF: Excision of one adrenal gland.

07.29　Other partial adrenalectomy
　Partial adrenalectomy NOS

07.3　Bilateral adrenalectomy
　Excision of remaining adrenal gland
　EXCLUDES　*bilateral partial adrenalectomy (07.29)*

✓4ᵗʰ **07.4　Other operations on adrenal glands, nerves, and vessels**

07.41　Incision of adrenal gland
　Adrenalotomy (with drainage)

07.42　Division of nerves to adrenal glands

07.43　Ligation of adrenal vessels

07.44　Repair of adrenal gland

07.45　Reimplantation of adrenal tissue
　Autotransplantation of adrenal tissue
　DEF: Autotransplantation of adrenal tissue: Use of tissue graft from the patient's own body.

07.49　Other

✓4ᵗʰ **07.5　Operations on pineal gland**

07.51　Exploration of pineal field
　EXCLUDES　*that with incision of pineal gland (07.52)*

07.52　Incision of pineal gland

07.53　Partial excision of pineal gland
　EXCLUDES　*biopsy of pineal gland (07.17)*

07.54　Total excision of pineal gland
　Pinealectomy (complete) (total)

07.59　Other operations on pineal gland

✓4ᵗʰ **07.6　Hypophysectomy**
　DEF: Excision, destruction of pituitary gland.

07.61　Partial excision of pituitary gland, transfrontal approach
　Cryohypophysectomy, partial
　Division of hypophyseal stalk
　Excision of lesion of pituitary [hypophysis]　} transfrontal approach
　Hypophysectomy subtotal
　Infundibulectomy, hypophyseal
　EXCLUDES　*biopsy of pituitary gland, transfrontal approach (07.13)*
　DEF: Removal of partial pituitary gland through frontal bone.

07.62　Partial excision of pituitary gland, transsphenoidal approach
　EXCLUDES　*biopsy of pituitary gland, transsphenoidal approach (07.14)*
　DEF: Removal of partial pituitary gland through sphenoid bone.

07.63　Partial excision of pituitary gland, unspecified approach
　EXCLUDES　*biopsy of pituitary gland NOS (07.15)*

07.64　Total excision of pituitary gland, transfrontal approach
　Ablation of pituitary by implantation (strontium-yttrium)(Y)　} transfrontal approach
　Cryohypophysectomy, complete
　DEF: Removal of total pituitary gland through frontal bone.

07.65　Total excision of pituitary gland, transsphenoidal approach
　DEF: Removal of total pituitary gland through sphenoid bone.

07.68　Total excision of pituitary gland, other specified approach
　DEF: Destroy or remove pituitary gland by a specified approach, other than those listed.

07.69　Total excision of pituitary gland, unspecified approach
　Hypophysectomy NOS
　Pituitectomy NOS

✓4ᵗʰ **07.7　Other operations on hypophysis**

07.71　Exploration of pituitary fossa
　EXCLUDES　*exploration with incision of pituitary gland (07.72)*
　DEF: Exploration of region of pituitary gland.

07.72　Incision of pituitary gland
　Aspiration of:　　　　Aspiration of:
　craniobuccal pouch　　pituitary gland
　craniopharyngioma　　Rathke's pouch
　hypophysis

07.79　Other
　Insertion of pack into sella turcica

✓4ᵗʰ **07.8　Thymectomy**

07.80　Thymectomy, not otherwise specified

07.81　Other partial excision of thymus
　Open partial excision of thymus
　EXCLUDES　*biopsy of thymus (07.16)*
　　　　　　thoracoscopic partial excision of thymus (07.83)

07.82　Other total excision of thymus
　Open total excision of thymus
　EXCLUDES　*thoracoscopic total excision of thymus (07.84)*

07.83　Thoracoscopic partial excision of thymus
　EXCLUDES　*other partial excision of thymus (07.81)*

07.84　Thoracoscopic total excision of thymus
　EXCLUDES　*other total excision of thymus (07.82)*

√4ᵗʰ **07.9 Other operations on thymus**

07.91 Exploration of thymus field
> *EXCLUDES*   *exploration with incision of thymus (07.92)*

07.92 Other incision of thymus
> Open incision of thymus
> *EXCLUDES*   *thoracoscopic incision of thymus (07.95)*

07.93 Repair of thymus

07.94 Transplantation of thymus
> **DEF:** Placement of thymus tissue grafts into functional area of gland.

07.95 Thoracoscopic incision of thymus
> *EXCLUDES*   *other incision of thymus (07.92)*

07.98 Other and unspecified thoracoscopic operations on thymus

07.99 Other and unspecified operations on thymus
> Transcervical thymectomy
> *EXCLUDES*   *other thoracoscopic operations on thymus (07.98)*

3. OPERATIONS ON THE EYE (08-16)

✓3ʳᵈ **08   Operations on eyelids**
INCLUDES   operations on the eyebrow

✓4ᵗʰ **08.0   Incision of eyelid**

08.01   Incision of lid margin
DEF: Cutting into eyelid edge.

08.02   Severing of blepharorrhaphy
DEF: Freeing of eyelids previously sutured shut.

08.09   Other incision of eyelid

✓4ᵗʰ **08.1   Diagnostic procedures on eyelid**

08.11   Biopsy of eyelid

08.19   Other diagnostic procedures on eyelid

✓4ᵗʰ **08.2   Excision or destruction of lesion or tissue of eyelid**
Code also any synchronous reconstruction (08.61-08.74)
EXCLUDES   biopsy of eyelid (08.11)

08.20   Removal of lesion of eyelid, not otherwise specified
Removal of meibomian gland NOS

08.21   Excision of chalazion

08.22   Excision of other minor lesion of eyelid
Excision of:
verruca
wart

08.23   Excision of major lesion of eyelid, partial-thickness
Excision involving one-fourth or more of lid margin, partial-thickness
DEF: Excision of lesion not in all eyelid layers.

08.24   Excision of major lesion of eyelid, full-thickness
Excision involving one-fourth or more of lid margin, full-thickness
Wedge resection of eyelid
DEF: Excision of growth in all eyelid layers, full thickness.

08.25   Destruction of lesion of eyelid

✓4ᵗʰ **08.3   Repair of blepharoptosis and lid retraction**

08.31   Repair of blepharoptosis by frontalis muscle technique with suture
DEF: Correction of drooping upper eyelid with suture of frontalis muscle.

08.32   Repair of blepharoptosis by frontalis muscle technique with fascial sling
DEF: Correction of drooping upper eyelid with fascial tissue sling of frontalis muscle.

08.33   Repair of blepharoptosis by resection or advancement of levator muscle or aponeurosis
DEF: Correction of drooping upper eyelid with levator muscle, extended, cut, or by expanded tendon.

08.34   Repair of blepharoptosis by other levator muscle techniques

08.35   Repair of blepharoptosis by tarsal technique
DEF: Correction of drooping upper eyelid with tarsal muscle.

08.36   Repair of blepharoptosis by other techniques
Correction of eyelid ptosis NOS
Orbicularis oculi muscle sling for correction of blepharoptosis

08.37   Reduction of overcorrection of ptosis
DEF: Correction, release of previous plastic repair of drooping eyelid.

08.38   Correction of lid retraction
DEF: Fixing of withdrawn eyelid into normal position.

✓4ᵗʰ **08.4   Repair of entropion or ectropion**

08.41   Repair of entropion or ectropion by thermocauterization
DEF: Restoration of eyelid margin to normal position with heat cautery.

08.42   Repair of entropion or ectropion by suture technique
DEF: Restoration of eyelid margin to normal position by suture.

08.43   Repair of entropion or ectropion with wedge resection
DEF: Restoration of eyelid margin to normal position by removing tissue.

08.44   Repair of entropion or ectropion with lid reconstruction
DEF: Reconstruction of eyelid margin.

08.49   Other repair of entropion or ectropion

✓4ᵗʰ **08.5   Other adjustment of lid position**

08.51   Canthotomy
DEF: Incision into outer canthus of eye.

08.52   Blepharorrhaphy
Canthorrhaphy
Tarsorrhaphy
DEF: Eyelids are partially sutured together; done to shorten palpebral fissure or protect cornea.

08.59   Other
Canthoplasty NOS
Repair of epicanthal fold

✓4ᵗʰ **08.6   Reconstruction of eyelid with flaps or grafts**
EXCLUDES   that associated with repair of entropion and ectropion (08.44)

08.61   Reconstruction of eyelid with skin flap or graft
DEF: Rebuild of eyelid by graft or flap method.

08.62   Reconstruction of eyelid with mucous membrane flap or graft
DEF: Rebuild of eyelid with mucous membrane graft or flap method.

08.63   Reconstruction of eyelid with hair follicle graft
DEF: Rebuild of eyelid with hair follicle graft.

08.64   Reconstruction of eyelid with tarsoconjunctival flap
Transfer of tarsoconjunctival flap from opposing lid
DEF: Recreation of eyelid with tarsoconjunctival tissue.

08.69   Other reconstruction of eyelid with flaps or grafts

✓4ᵗʰ **08.7   Other reconstruction of eyelid**
EXCLUDES   that associated with repair of entropion and ectropion (08.44)

08.70   Reconstruction of eyelid, not otherwise specified

08.71   Reconstruction of eyelid involving lid margin, partial-thickness
DEF: Repair of eyelid margin not using all lid layers.

08.72   Other reconstruction of eyelid, partial-thickness
DEF: Reshape of eyelid not using all lid layers.

08.73   Reconstruction of eyelid involving lid margin, full-thickness
DEF: Repair of eyelid and margin using all tissue layers.

08.74   Other reconstruction of eyelid, full-thickness
DEF: Other repair of eyelid using all tissue layers.

✓4ᵗʰ **08.8   Other repair of eyelid**

08.81   Linear repair of laceration of eyelid or eyebrow

08.82   Repair of laceration involving lid margin, partial-thickness
DEF: Repair of laceration not involving all layers of eyelid margin.

08.83   Other repair of laceration of eyelid, partial thickness
DEF: Repair of eyelid tear not involving all eyelid layers.

08.84   Repair of laceration involving lid margin, full-thickness
DEF: Repair of eyelid margin tear involving all margin layers.

08.85 Other repair of laceration of eyelid, full-thickness
DEF: Repair of eyelid tear involving all layers.

08.86 Lower eyelid rhytidectomy
DEF: Removal of wrinkles from lower eyelid.

08.87 Upper eyelid rhytidectomy
DEF: Removal of wrinkles from upper eyelid.

08.89 Other eyelid repair

✓4ᵗʰ **08.9 Other operations on eyelids**

08.91 Electrosurgical epilation of eyelid
DEF: Electrical removal of eyelid hair roots.

08.92 Cryosurgical epilation of eyelid
DEF: Removal of eyelid hair roots by freezing.

08.93 Other epilation of eyelid

08.99 Other

✓3ʳᵈ **09 Operations on lacrimal system**

09.0 Incision of lacrimal gland
Incision of lacrimal cyst (with drainage)

✓4ᵗʰ **09.1 Diagnostic procedures on lacrimal system**

09.11 Biopsy of lacrimal gland

09.12 Biopsy of lacrimal sac

09.19 Other diagnostic procedures on lacrimal system
EXCLUDES *contrast dacryocystogram (87.05)*
soft tissue x-ray of nasolacrimal duct (87.09)

✓4ᵗʰ **09.2 Excision of lesion or tissue of lacrimal gland**

09.20 Excision of lacrimal gland, not otherwise specified

09.21 Excision of lesion of lacrimal gland
EXCLUDES *biopsy of lacrimal gland (09.11)*

09.22 Other partial dacryoadenectomy
EXCLUDES *biopsy of lacrimal gland (09.11)*
DEF: Partial excision of tear gland.

09.23 Total dacryoadenectomy
DEF: Total excision of tear gland.

09.3 Other operations on lacrimal gland

✓4ᵗʰ **09.4 Manipulation of lacrimal passage**
INCLUDES removal of calculus
that with dilation
EXCLUDES *contrast dacryocystogram (87.05)*

09.41 Probing of lacrimal punctum
DEF: Exploration of tear duct entrance with flexible rod.

09.42 Probing of lacrimal canaliculi
DEF: Exploration of tear duct with flexible rod.

09.43 Probing of nasolacrimal duct
EXCLUDES *that with insertion of tube or stent (09.44)*
DEF: Exploration of passage between tear sac and nose with flexible rod.

09.44 Intubation of nasolacrimal duct
Insertion of stent into nasolacrimal duct

09.49 Other manipulation of lacrimal passage

✓4ᵗʰ **09.5 Incision of lacrimal sac and passages**

09.51 Incision of lacrimal punctum

09.52 Incision of lacrimal canaliculi

09.53 Incision of lacrimal sac
DEF: Cutting into lacrimal pouch of tear gland.

09.59 Other incision of lacrimal passages
Incision (and drainage) of nasolacrimal duct NOS

09.6 Excision of lacrimal sac and passage
EXCLUDES *biopsy of lacrimal sac (09.12)*
DEF: Removal of pouch and passage of tear gland.

✓4ᵗʰ **09.7 Repair of canaliculus and punctum**
EXCLUDES *repair of eyelid (08.81-08.89)*

09.71 Correction of everted punctum
DEF: Repair of an outwardly turned tear duct entrance.

09.72 Other repair of punctum

09.73 Repair of canaliculus

✓4ᵗʰ **09.8 Fistulization of lacrimal tract to nasal cavity**

09.81 Dacryocystorhinostomy [DCR]
DEF: Creation of entrance between tear gland and nasal passage for tear flow.

09.82 Conjunctivocystorhinostomy
Conjunctivodacryocystorhinostomy [CDCR]
EXCLUDES *that with insertion of tube or stent (09.83)*
DEF: Creation of tear drainage path from lacrimal sac to nasal cavity through conjunctiva.

09.83 Conjunctivorhinostomy with insertion of tube or stent
DEF: Creation of passage between eye sac membrane and nasal cavity with tube or stent.

✓4ᵗʰ **09.9 Other operations on lacrimal system**

09.91 Obliteration of lacrimal punctum
DEF: Total destruction of tear gland opening in eyelid.

09.99 Other

✓3ʳᵈ **10 Operations on conjunctiva**

10.0 Removal of embedded foreign body from conjunctiva by incision
EXCLUDES *removal of:*
embedded foreign body without incision (98.22)
superficial foreign body (98.21)

10.1 Other incision of conjunctiva

✓4ᵗʰ **10.2 Diagnostic procedures on conjunctiva**

10.21 Biopsy of conjunctiva

10.29 Other diagnostic procedures on conjunctiva

✓4ᵗʰ **10.3 Excision or destruction of lesion or tissue of conjunctiva**

10.31 Excision of lesion or tissue of conjunctiva
Excision of ring of conjunctiva around cornea
EXCLUDES *biopsy of conjunctiva (10.21)*
DEF: Removal of growth or tissue from eye membrane.

10.32 Destruction of lesion of conjunctiva
EXCLUDES *excision of lesion (10.31)*
thermocauterization for entropion (08.41)
DEF: Destruction of eye membrane growth; not done by excision.

10.33 Other destructive procedures on conjunctiva
Removal of trachoma follicles

✓4ᵗʰ **10.4 Conjunctivoplasty**
DEF: Correction of conjunctiva by plastic surgery.

10.41 Repair of symblepharon with free graft

10.42 Reconstruction of conjunctival cul-de-sac with free graft
EXCLUDES *revision of enucleation socket with graft (16.63)*
DEF: Rebuilding of eye membrane fold with graft of unattached tissue.

10.43 Other reconstruction of conjunctival cul-de-sac
EXCLUDES *revision of enucleation socket (16.64)*

10.44 Other free graft to conjunctiva

10.49 Other conjunctivoplasty
EXCLUDES *repair of cornea with conjunctival flap (11.53)*

10.5 Lysis of adhesions of conjunctiva and eyelid
Division of symblepharon (with insertion of conformer)

10.6 Repair of laceration of conjunctiva
EXCLUDES   *that with repair of sclera (12.81)*

√4th **10.9 Other operations on conjunctiva**

10.91 Subconjunctival injection

10.99 Other

√3rd **11 Operations on cornea**

11.0 Magnetic removal of embedded foreign body from cornea
EXCLUDES   *that with incision (11.1)*

11.1 Incision of cornea
Incision of cornea for removal of foreign body

√4th **11.2 Diagnostic procedures on cornea**

11.21 Scraping of cornea for smear or culture

11.22 Biopsy of cornea

11.29 Other diagnostic procedures on cornea

√4th **11.3 Excision of pterygium**

11.31 Transposition of pterygium
DEF: Cutting into membranous structure extending from eye membrane to cornea and suturing it in a downward position.

11.32 Excision of pterygium with corneal graft
DEF: Surgical removal and repair of membranous structure extending from eye membrane to cornea using corneal tissue graft.

11.39 Other excision of pterygium

√4th **11.4 Excision or destruction of tissue or other lesion of cornea**

11.41 Mechanical removal of corneal epithelium
That by chemocauterization
EXCLUDES   *that for smear or culture (11.21)*
DEF: Removal of outer layer of cornea by mechanical means.

11.42 Thermocauterization of corneal lesion
DEF: Destruction of corneal lesion by electrical cautery.

11.43 Cryotherapy of corneal lesion
DEF: Destruction of corneal lesion by freezing.

11.49 Other removal or destruction of corneal lesion
Excision of cornea NOS
EXCLUDES   *biopsy of cornea (11.22)*

√4th **11.5 Repair of cornea**

11.51 Suture of corneal laceration

11.52 Repair of postoperative wound dehiscence of cornea
DEF: Repair of ruptured postoperative corneal wound.

11.53 Repair of corneal laceration or wound with conjunctival flap
DEF: Correction corneal wound or tear with conjunctival tissue.

11.59 Other repair of cornea

√4th **11.6 Corneal transplant**
EXCLUDES   *excision of pterygium with corneal graft (11.32)*

11.60 Corneal transplant, not otherwise specified
Note: To report donor sources – see codes 00.91-00.93
Keratoplasty NOS

11.61 Lamellar keratoplasty with autograft
DEF: Restoration of sight using patient's own corneal tissue, partial thickness.

11.62 Other lamellar keratoplasty
DEF: Restoration of sight using donor corneal tissue, partial thickness.

11.63 Penetrating keratoplasty with autograft
Perforating keratoplasty with autograft

11.64 Other penetrating keratoplasty
Perforating keratoplasty (with homograft)

11.69 Other corneal transplant

√4th **11.7 Other reconstructive and refractive surgery on cornea**

11.71 Keratomileusis
DEF: Restoration of corneal shape by removing portion of cornea, freezing, reshaping curve and reattaching it.

11.72 Keratophakia
DEF: Correction of eye lens loss by dissecting the central zone of the cornea and replacing it with a thickened graft of the cornea.

11.73 Keratoprosthesis
DEF: Placement of corneal artificial implant.

11.74 Thermokeratoplasty
DEF: Reshaping and reforming cornea by heat application.

11.75 Radial keratotomy
DEF: Incisions around cornea radius to correct nearsightedness.

11.76 Epikeratophakia
DEF: Repair lens loss by cornea graft sutured to central corneal zone.

11.79 Other

√4th **11.9 Other operations on cornea**

11.91 Tattooing of cornea

11.92 Removal of artificial implant from cornea

11.99 Other

√3rd **12 Operations on iris, ciliary body, sclera, and anterior chamber**
EXCLUDES   *operations on cornea (11.0-11.99)*

√4th **12.0 Removal of intraocular foreign body from anterior segment of eye**

12.00 Removal of intraocular foreign body from anterior segment of eye, not otherwise specified

12.01 Removal of intraocular foreign body from anterior segment of eye with use of magnet

12.02 Removal of intraocular foreign body from anterior segment of eye without use of magnet

√4th **12.1 Iridotomy and simple iridectomy**
EXCLUDES   *iridectomy associated with:*
cataract extraction (13.11-13.69)
removal of lesion (12.41-12.42)
scleral fistulization (12.61-12.69)

12.11 Iridotomy with transfixion

12.12 Other iridotomy
Corectomy   Iridotomy NOS
Discission of iris
DEF: Corectomy: Incision into iris (also called iridectomy).

12.13 Excision of prolapsed iris
DEF: Removal of downwardly placed portion of iris.

12.14 Other iridectomy
Iridectomy (basal) (peripheral) (total)
DEF: Partial or total removal of iris.

√4th **12.2 Diagnostic procedures on iris, ciliary body, sclera, and anterior chamber**

12.21 Diagnostic aspiration of anterior chamber of eye
DEF: Suction withdrawal of fluid from anterior eye chamber for diagnostic reasons.

12.22 Biopsy of iris

12.29 Other diagnostic procedures on iris, ciliary body, sclera, and anterior chamber

√4th **12.3 Iridoplasty and coreoplasty**
DEF: Correction of abnormal iris or pupil by plastic surgery.

12.31 Lysis of goniosynechiae
Lysis of goniosynechiae by injection of air or liquid
DEF: Freeing of fibrous structures between cornea and iris by injecting air or liquid.

12.32 Lysis of other anterior synechiae
Lysis of anterior synechiae:
NOS
by injection of air or liquid

12.33 Lysis of posterior synechiae
Lysis of iris adhesions NOS

12.34 Lysis of corneovitreal adhesions
DEF: Release of adhesions of cornea and vitreous body.

12.35 Coreoplasty
Needling of pupillary membrane
DEF: Correction of an iris defect.

12.39 Other iridoplasty

12.4 Excision or destruction of lesion of iris and ciliary body

12.40 Removal of lesion of anterior segment of eye, not otherwise specified

12.41 Destruction of lesion of iris, nonexcisional
Destruction of lesion of iris by:
cauterization
cryotherapy
photocoagulation

12.42 Excision of lesion of iris
EXCLUDES biopsy of iris (12.22)

12.43 Destruction of lesion of ciliary body, nonexcisional

12.44 Excision of lesion of ciliary body

12.5 Facilitation of intraocular circulation

12.51 Goniopuncture without goniotomy
DEF: Stab incision into anterior chamber of eye to relieve optic pressure.

12.52 Goniotomy without goniopuncture
DEF: Incision into Schlemm's canal to drain aqueous and relieve pressure.

12.53 Goniotomy with goniopuncture

12.54 Trabeculotomy ab externo
DEF: Incision into supporting connective tissue strands of eye capsule, via exterior approach.

12.55 Cyclodialysis
DEF: Creation of passage between anterior chamber and suprachoroidal space.

12.59 Other facilitation of intraocular circulation

12.6 Scleral fistulization
EXCLUDES exploratory sclerotomy (12.89)

12.61 Trephination of sclera with iridectomy
DEF: Cut around sclerocornea to remove part of the iris.

12.62 Thermocauterization of sclera with iridectomy
DEF: Destruction of outer eyeball layer with partial excision of iris using heat.

12.63 Iridencleisis and iridotasis
DEF: Creation of permanent drain in iris by transposing or stretching iris tissue.

12.64 Trabeculectomy ab externo
DEF: Excision of supporting connective tissue strands of eye capsule, via exterior approach.

Trabeculectomy Ab Externo

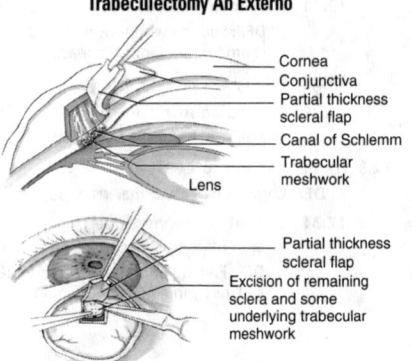

Cornea
Conjunctiva
Partial thickness scleral flap
Canal of Schlemm
Trabecular meshwork
Lens

Partial thickness scleral flap
Excision of remaining sclera and some underlying trabecular meshwork

12.65 Other scleral fistulization with iridectomy
Holth's sclerectomy
DEF: Creation of outer eyeball layer passage with partial excision of iris.

12.66 Postoperative revision of scleral fistulization procedure
Revision of filtering bleb
EXCLUDES repair of fistula (12.82)

12.67 Insertion of aqueous drainage device
Anterior chamber drainage device
Aqueous drainage shunt or stent
Eye valve implant
Filtration canal shunt or device
DEF: Placement of glaucoma drainage devices, shunts, or valves that shunt aqueous fluid from the anterior chamber of the eye for absorption into the lymph and blood vessels around the eye.

12.69 Other fistulizing procedure

12.7 Other procedures for relief of elevated intraocular pressure

12.71 Cyclodiathermy
DEF: Destruction of ciliary body tissue with heat.

12.72 Cyclocryotherapy
DEF: Destruction of ciliary body tissue by freezing.

12.73 Cyclophotocoagulation
DEF: Destruction of ciliary body tissue by high energy light source.

12.74 Diminution of ciliary body, not otherwise specified

12.79 Other glaucoma procedures

12.8 Operations on sclera
EXCLUDES those associated with:
retinal reattachment (14.41-14.59)
scleral fistulization (12.61-12.69)

12.81 Suture of laceration of sclera
Suture of sclera with synchronous repair of conjunctiva

12.82 Repair of scleral fistula
EXCLUDES postoperative revision of scleral fistulization procedure (12.66)

12.83 Revision of operative wound of anterior segment, not elsewhere classified
EXCLUDES postoperative revision of scleral fistulization procedure (12.66)

12.84 Excision or destruction of lesion of sclera

12.85 Repair of scleral staphyloma with graft
DEF: Repair of protruding outer eyeball layer with a graft.

12.86 Other repair of scleral staphyloma

12.87 Scleral reinforcement with graft
DEF: Restoration of outer eyeball shape with tissue graft.

12.88 Other scleral reinforcement

12.89 Other operations on sclera
Exploratory sclerotomy

12.9 Other operations on iris, ciliary body, and anterior chamber

12.91 Therapeutic evacuation of anterior chamber
Paracentesis of anterior chamber
EXCLUDES diagnostic aspiration (12.21)

12.92 Injection into anterior chamber
Injection of:
air
liquid } into anterior chamber
medication

12.93 Removal or destruction of epithelial downgrowth from anterior chamber
EXCLUDES that with iridectomy (12.41-12.42)
DEF: Excision or destruction of epithelial overgrowth in anterior eye chamber.

Extraction of Lens (with insertion of intraocular lens prosthesis)

Iris

Lens cataract removed

Iris

Lens

Intraocular lens insertion

12.97　**Other operations on iris**

12.98　**Other operations on ciliary body**

12.99　**Other operations on anterior chamber**

√3ʳᵈ **13　Operations on lens**

√4ᵗʰ **13.0　Removal of foreign body from lens**
　EXCLUDES *removal of pseudophakos (13.8)*

　13.00　Removal of foreign body from lens, not otherwise specified

　13.01　Removal of foreign body from lens with use of magnet

　13.02　Removal of foreign body from lens without use of magnet

√4ᵗʰ **13.1　Intracapsular extraction of lens**
　Code also any synchronous insertion of pseudophakos (13.71)

　13.11　Intracapsular extraction of lens by temporal inferior route
　　DEF: Extraction of lens and capsule via anterior approach through outer side of eyeball.

　13.19　Other intracapsular extraction of lens
　　Cataract extraction NOS
　　Cryoextraction of lens
　　Erysiphake extraction of cataract
　　Extraction of lens NOS

13.2　Extracapsular extraction of lens by linear extraction technique
　Code also any synchronous insertion of pseudophakos (13.71)
　DEF: Excision of lens without the posterior capsule at junction between the cornea and outer eyeball layer by means of a linear incision.

13.3　Extracapsular extraction of lens by simple aspiration (and irrigation) technique
　Irrigation of traumatic cataract
　Code also any synchronous insertion of pseudophakos (13.71)
　DEF: Removal of lens without the posterior capsule by suctioning and flushing out the area.

√4ᵗʰ **13.4　Extracapsular extraction of lens by fragmentation and aspiration technique**
　Code also any synchronous insertion of pseudophakos (13.71)
　DEF: Removal of lens after division into smaller pieces with posterior capsule left intact.

　13.41　Phacoemulsification and aspiration of cataract

　13.42　Mechanical phacofragmentation and aspiration of cataract by posterior route
　　Code also any synchronous vitrectomy (14.74)

　13.43　Mechanical phacofragmentation and other aspiration of cataract

√4ᵗʰ **13.5　Other extracapsular extraction of lens**
　Code also any synchronous insertion of pseudophakos (13.71)

　13.51　Extracapsular extraction of lens by temporal inferior route
　　DEF: Removal of lens through outer eyeball with posterior capsule left intact.

　13.59　Other extracapsular extraction of lens

√4ᵗʰ **13.6　Other cataract extraction**
　Code also any synchronous insertion of pseudophakos (13.71)

　13.64　Discission of secondary membrane [after cataract]
　　DEF: Breaking up of fibrotic lens capsule developed after previous lens extraction.

　13.65　Excision of secondary membrane [after cataract]
　　Capsulectomy
　　DEF: Capsulectomy: Excision of lens capsule membrane after previous lens extraction.

　13.66　Mechanical fragmentation of secondary membrane [after cataract]
　　DEF: Breaking up and removal of fibrotic lens capsule developed after previous lens extraction.

　13.69　Other cataract extraction

√4ᵗʰ **13.7　Insertion of prosthetic lens [pseudophakos]**
　EXCLUDES *implantation of intraocular telescope prosthesis (13.91)*
　DEF: Insertion of ocular implant, following lens extraction.

　13.70　Insertion of pseudophakos, not otherwise specified

　13.71　Insertion of intraocular lens prosthesis at time of cataract extraction, one-stage
　　Code also synchronous extraction of cataract (13.11-13.69)

　13.72　Secondary insertion of intraocular lens prosthesis

13.8　Removal of implanted lens
　Removal of pseudophakos

√4ᵗʰ **13.9　Other operations on lens**

　13.90　Operation on lens, not elsewhere classified

　13.91　Implantation of intraocular telescope prosthesis
　　Implantable miniature telescope
　　INCLUDES removal of lens, any method
　　EXCLUDES *secondary insertion of ocular implant (16.61)*

√3ʳᵈ **14　Operations on retina, choroid, vitreous, and posterior chamber**

√4ᵗʰ **14.0　Removal of foreign body from posterior segment of eye**
　EXCLUDES *removal of surgically implanted material (14.6)*

　14.00　Removal of foreign body from posterior segment of eye, not otherwise specified

　14.01　Removal of foreign body from posterior segment of eye with use of magnet

　14.02　Removal of foreign body from posterior segment of eye without use of magnet

√4ᵗʰ **14.1　Diagnostic procedures on retina, choroid, vitreous, and posterior chamber**

　14.11　Diagnostic aspiration of vitreous

　14.19　Other diagnostic procedures on retina, choroid, vitreous, and posterior chamber

√4ᵗʰ **14.2　Destruction of lesion of retina and choroid**
　INCLUDES destruction of chorioretinopathy or isolated chorioretinal lesion
　EXCLUDES *that for repair of retina (14.31-14.59)*
　DEF: Destruction of damaged retina and choroid tissue.

　14.21　Destruction of chorioretinal lesion by diathermy

　14.22　Destruction of chorioretinal lesion by cryotherapy

　14.23　Destruction of chorioretinal lesion by xenon arc photocoagulation

Laser Surgery (YAG)

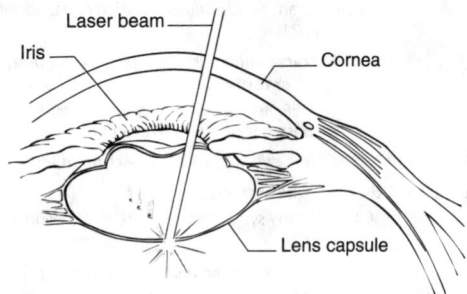

Scleral Buckling with Implant

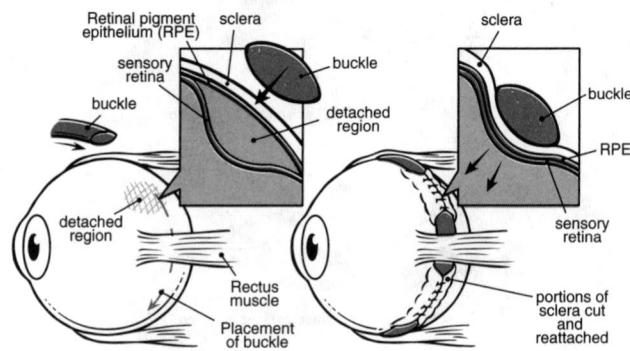

14.24   **Destruction of chorioretinal lesion by laser photocoagulation**

14.25   **Destruction of chorioretinal lesion by photocoagulation of unspecified type**

14.26   **Destruction of chorioretinal lesion by radiation therapy**

14.27   **Destruction of chorioretinal lesion by implantation of radiation source**

14.29   **Other destruction of chorioretinal lesion**
Destruction of lesion of retina and choroid NOS

✓4th **14.3**   **Repair of retinal tear**
INCLUDES   repair of retinal defect
EXCLUDES   *repair of retinal detachment (14.41-14.59)*

14.31   **Repair of retinal tear by diathermy**

14.32   **Repair of retinal tear by cryotherapy**

14.33   **Repair of retinal tear by xenon arc photocoagulation**

14.34   **Repair of retinal tear by laser photocoagulation**

14.35   **Repair of retinal tear by photocoagulation of unspecified type**

14.39   **Other repair of retinal tear**

✓4th **14.4**   **Repair of retinal detachment with scleral buckling and implant**
DEF: Placement of material around eye to indent sclera and close a hole or tear or to reduce vitreous traction.

14.41   **Scleral buckling with implant**

14.49   **Other scleral buckling**
Scleral buckling with: Scleral buckling with:
   air tamponade   vitrectomy
   resection of sclera

✓4th **14.5**   **Other repair of retinal detachment**
INCLUDES   that with drainage

14.51   **Repair of retinal detachment with diathermy**

14.52   **Repair of retinal detachment with cryotherapy**

14.53   **Repair of retinal detachment with xenon arc photocoagulation**

14.54   **Repair of retinal detachment with laser photocoagulation**

14.55   **Repair of retinal detachment with photocoagulation of unspecified type**

14.59   **Other**

14.6   **Removal of surgically implanted material from posterior segment of eye**

✓4th **14.7**   **Operations on vitreous**

14.71   **Removal of vitreous, anterior approach**
Open sky technique
Removal of vitreous, anterior approach (with replacement)
DEF: Removal of all or part of the eyeball fluid via the anterior segment of the eyeball.

14.72   **Other removal of vitreous**
Aspiration of vitreous by posterior sclerotomy

14.73   **Mechanical vitrectomy by anterior approach**
DEF: Removal of abnormal tissue in eyeball fluid to control fibrotic overgrowth in severe intraocular injury.

14.74   **Other mechanical vitrectomy**
Posterior approach

14.75   **Injection of vitreous substitute**
EXCLUDES   *that associated with removal (14.71-14.72)*

14.79   **Other operations on vitreous**

✓4th **14.8**   **Implantation of epiretinal visual prosthesis**

14.81   **Implantation of epiretinal visual prosthesis**
Note: Includes lens removal if present, scleral buckling, vitrectomy, epiretinal membrane peeling and pericardial grafting
EXCLUDES   *implantation of intraocular telescope prosthesis (13.91)*
other operations on retina, choroid, and posterior chamber (14.9)
replacement of epiretinal visual prosthesis (14.83)

14.82   **Removal of epiretinal visual prosthesis**
Note: Includes 360-degree limbal peritomy and vitrectomy if performed, and device extraction
EXCLUDES   *removal of eye prosthesis (97.31)*

14.83   **Revision or replacement of epiretinal visual prosthesis**
Note: Includes tack replacement, device relocation, and replacement of pericardial grafting, if needed
EXCLUDES   *implantation of epiretinal visual prosthesis (14.81)*

14.9   **Other operations on retina, choroid, and posterior chamber**

✓3rd **15**   **Operations on extraocular muscles**

✓4th **15.0**   **Diagnostic procedures on extraocular muscles or tendons**

15.01   **Biopsy of extraocular muscle or tendon**

15.09   **Other diagnostic procedures on extraocular muscles and tendons**

✓4th **15.1**   **Operations on one extraocular muscle involving temporary detachment from globe**

15.11   **Recession of one extraocular muscle**
DEF: Detachment of exterior eye muscle with posterior reattachment to correct strabismus.

15.12   **Advancement of one extraocular muscle**
DEF: Detachment of exterior eye muscle with forward reattachment to correct strabismus.

15.13   **Resection of one extraocular muscle**

15.19   **Other operations on one extraocular muscle involving temporary detachment from globe**
EXCLUDES   *transposition of muscle (15.5)*

Lengthening Procedure on One Extraocular Muscle

Shortening Procedure on One Extraocular Muscle

✓4ᵗʰ 15.2 Other operations on one extraocular muscle

    15.21 Lengthening procedure on one extraocular muscle
        DEF: Extension of exterior eye muscle length.

    15.22 Shortening procedure on one extraocular muscle
        DEF: Shortening of exterior eye muscle.

    15.29 Other

15.3 Operations on two or more extraocular muscles involving temporary detachment from globe, one or both eyes

15.4 Other operations on two or more extraocular muscles, one or both eyes

15.5 Transposition of extraocular muscles
    EXCLUDES *that for correction of ptosis (08.31-08.36)*
    DEF: Relocation of exterior eye muscle to a more functional site.

15.6 Revision of extraocular muscle surgery
    DEF: Repair of previous exterior eye muscle surgery.

15.7 Repair of injury of extraocular muscle
    Freeing of entrapped extraocular muscle
    Lysis of adhesions of extraocular muscle
    Repair of laceration of extraocular muscle, tendon, or Tenon's capsule

15.9 Other operations on extraocular muscles and tendons

✓3ʳᵈ 16 Operations on orbit and eyeball
    EXCLUDES *reduction of fracture of orbit (76.78-76.79)*

✓4ᵗʰ 16.0 Orbitotomy

    16.01 Orbitotomy with bone flap
        Orbitotomy with lateral approach
        DEF: Incision into orbital bone with insertion of small bone piece.

    16.02 Orbitotomy with insertion of orbital implant
        EXCLUDES *that with bone flap (16.01)*

    16.09 Other orbitotomy

16.1 Removal of penetrating foreign body from eye, not otherwise specified
    EXCLUDES *removal of nonpenetrating foreign body (98.21)*
    DEF: Removal of foreign body from an unspecified site in eye.

✓4ᵗʰ 16.2 Diagnostic procedures on orbit and eyeball

    16.21 Ophthalmoscopy

    16.22 Diagnostic aspiration of orbit

    16.23 Biopsy of eyeball and orbit

    16.29 Other diagnostic procedures on orbit and eyeball
        EXCLUDES *examination of form and structure of eye (95.11-95.16)*
        general and subjective eye examination (95.01-95.09)
        microscopic examination of specimen from eye (90.21-90.29)
        objective functional tests of eye (95.21-95.26)
        ocular thermography (88.82)
        tonometry (89.11)
        x-ray of orbit (87.14, 87.16)

✓4ᵗʰ 16.3 Evisceration of eyeball
    DEF: Removal of eyeball, leaving sclera and occasionally cornea.

    16.31 Removal of ocular contents with synchronous implant into scleral shell
        DEF: Removal of eyeball leaving outer eyeball layer with ocular implant into shell.

    16.39 Other evisceration of eyeball

✓4ᵗʰ 16.4 Enucleation of eyeball
    DEF: Removal of entire eyeball after severing eye muscles and optic nerves.

    16.41 Enucleation of eyeball with synchronous implant into Tenon's capsule with attachment of muscles
        Integrated implant of eyeball
        DEF: Removal of eyeball with insertion of ocular implant and muscle attachment.

    16.42 Enucleation of eyeball with other synchronous implant

    16.49 Other enucleation of eyeball
        Removal of eyeball NOS

✓4ᵗʰ 16.5 Exenteration of orbital contents

    16.51 Exenteration of orbit with removal of adjacent structures
        Radical orbitomaxillectomy
        DEF: Removal of contents of bony cavity of eye as well as related tissues and structures.
        DEF: Radical orbitomaxillectomy: Removal of contents of bony cavity of eye, related tissues and structures, and a portion of maxillary bone.

    16.52 Exenteration of orbit with therapeutic removal of orbital bone

    16.59 Other exenteration of orbit
        Evisceration of orbit NOS
        Exenteration of orbit with temporalis muscle transplant

✓4ᵗʰ 16.6 Secondary procedures after removal of eyeball
    EXCLUDES *that with synchronous:*
        enucleation of eyeball (16.41-16.42)
        evisceration of eyeball (16.31)

    16.61 Secondary insertion of ocular implant
        DEF: Insertion of ocular implant after previous eye removal.

    16.62 Revision and reinsertion of ocular implant
        DEF: Reimplant or correction of ocular implant.

    16.63 Revision of enucleation socket with graft
        DEF: Implant of tissue to correct socket after eye removal.

    16.64 Other revision of enucleation socket

    16.65 Secondary graft to exenteration cavity
        DEF: Implant of tissue in place of eye after removal.

    16.66 Other revision of exenteration cavity

    16.69 Other secondary procedures after removal of eyeball

√4ᵗʰ **16.7 Removal of ocular or orbital implant**

16.71 Removal of ocular implant

16.72 Removal of orbital implant

√4ᵗʰ **16.8 Repair of injury of eyeball and orbit**

16.81 Repair of wound of orbit

EXCLUDES *reduction of orbital fracture*
(76.78-76.79)
repair of extraocular muscles (15.7)

16.82 Repair of rupture of eyeball
Repair of multiple structures of eye

EXCLUDES *repair of laceration of:*
cornea (11.51-11.59)
sclera (12.81)

16.89 Other repair of injury of eyeball or orbit

√4ᵗʰ **16.9 Other operations on orbit and eyeball**

EXCLUDES *irrigation of eye (96.51)*
prescription and fitting of low vision aids
(95.31-95.33)
removal of:
eye prosthesis NEC (97.31)
nonpenetrating foreign body from eye without
incision (98.21)

16.91 Retrobulbar injection of therapeutic agent

EXCLUDES *injection of radiographic contrast*
material (87.14)
opticociliary injection (12.79)

16.92 Excision of lesion of orbit

EXCLUDES *biopsy of orbit (16.23)*

16.93 Excision of lesion of eye, unspecified structure

EXCLUDES *biopsy of eye NOS (16.23)*

16.98 Other operations on orbit

16.99 Other operations on eyeball

3A. OTHER MISCELLANEOUS DIAGNOSTIC AND THERAPEUTIC PROCEDURES (17)

✓3ʰ **17　Other miscellaneous procedures**

✓4ʰ **17.1　Laparoscopic unilateral repair of inguinal hernia**
EXCLUDES *other and open unilateral repair of hernia (53.00-53.05)*

17.11　Laparoscopic repair of direct inguinal hernia with graft or prosthesis
Laparoscopic repair of direct and indirect inguinal hernia with graft or prosthesis

17.12　Laparoscopic repair of indirect inguinal hernia with graft or prosthesis

17.13　Laparoscopic repair of inguinal hernia with graft or prosthesis, not otherwise specified

✓4ʰ **17.2　Laparoscopic bilateral repair of inguinal hernia**
EXCLUDES *other and open bilateral repair of hernia (53.10-53.17)*

17.21　Laparoscopic bilateral repair of direct inguinal hernia with graft or prosthesis

17.22　Laparoscopic bilateral repair of indirect inguinal hernia with graft or prosthesis

17.23　Laparoscopic bilateral repair of inguinal hernia, one direct and one indirect, with graft or prosthesis

17.24　Laparoscopic bilateral repair of inguinal hernia with graft or prosthesis, not otherwise specified

✓4ʰ **17.3　Laparoscopic partial excision of large intestine**
EXCLUDES *other and open partial excision of large intestine (45.71-45.79)*

17.31　Laparoscopic multiple segmental resection of large intestine

17.32　Laparoscopic cecectomy

17.33　Laparoscopic right hemicolectomy

17.34　Laparoscopic resection of transverse colon

17.35　Laparoscopic left hemicolectomy

17.36　Laparoscopic sigmoidectomy

17.39　Other laparoscopic partial excision of large intestine

✓4ʰ **17.4　Robotic assisted procedures**
Note: This category includes use of a computer console with (3-D) imaging, software, camera(s), visualization and instrumentation *combined* with the use of robotic arms, device(s), or system(s) at the time of the procedure.
Computer assisted robotic surgery
Computer-enhanced robotic surgery
Robotic procedure with computer assistance
Surgeon-controlled robotic surgery
Code first primary procedure
EXCLUDES *computer assisted surgery (00.31-00.35, 00.39)*

17.41　Open robotic assisted procedure
Robotic assistance in open procedure

17.42　Laparoscopic robotic assisted procedure
Robotic assistance in laparoscopic procedure

17.43　Percutaneous robotic assisted procedure
Robotic assistance in percutaneous procedure

17.44　Endoscopic robotic assisted procedure
Robotic assistance in endoscopic procedure

17.45　Thoracoscopic robotic assisted procedure
Robotic assistance in thoracoscopic procedure

17.49　Other and unspecified robotic assisted procedure
Robotic assistance in other and unspecified procedure
EXCLUDES *endoscopic robotic assisted procedure (17.44)*
laparoscopic robotic assisted procedure (17.42)
open robotic assisted procedure (17.41)
percutaneous robotic assisted procedure (17.43)
thoracoscopic robotic assisted procedure (17.45)

✓4ʰ **17.5　Additional cardiovascular procedures**

17.51　Implantation of rechargeable cardiac contractility modulation [CCM], total system
Note: Device testing during procedure — *omit code*
Implantation of CCM system includes formation of pocket, transvenous leads, including placement of leads, placement of catheter into left ventricle, intraoperative procedures for evaluation of lead signals, obtaining sensing threshold measurements, obtaining defibrillator threshold measurements.
Includes implantation of device with removal of existing device
Code also any concomitant:
coronary bypass (36.10-36.19)
extracorporeal circulation (39.61)
insertion or replacement of automatic cardioverter/defibrillator, total system [AICD] 37.94
EXCLUDES *implantation of CCM pulse generator only (17.52)*
DEF: Device that delivers nonexcitatory impulses to the right ventricular septum during the absolute refractory period and signals that enhance myocardial strength and performance.

17.52　Implantation or replacement of cardiac contractility modulation [CCM] rechargeable pulse generator only
Note: Device testing during procedure — *omit code*
Implantation of CCM device with removal of any existing CCM device
Code also any concomitant:
revision of device pocket (37.79)
revision of lead [electrode] (37.75)

17.53　Percutaneous atherectomy of extracranial vessel(s)
Directional atherectomy
Excimer laser atherectomy
Rotational atherectomy
That by laser
That by transluminal extraction
Code also any:
injection or infusion of thrombolytic agent (99.10)
number of vascular stents inserted (00.45-00.48)
number of vessels treated (00.40-00.43)
percutaneous insertion of carotid artery stent(s) (00.63)
percutaneous insertion of other extracranial artery stent(s) (00.64)
procedure on vessel bifurcation (00.44)
EXCLUDES *angioplasty of other non-coronary vessel(s) (39.50)*
atherectomy of intracranial vessel(s) (17.54)
atherectomy of other non-coronary vessel(s) (17.56)
removal of cerebrovascular obstruction of vessel(s) by open approach (38.01-38.02, 38.11-38.12, 38.31-38.32, 38.41-38.42)

17.54 Percutaneous atherectomy of intracranial vessel(s)
Directional atherectomy
Excimer laser atherectomy
Rotational atherectomy
That by laser
That by transluminal extraction
Code also any:
   injection or infusion of thrombolytic agent
      (99.10)
   number of vascular stents inserted (00.45-00.48)
   number of vessels treated (00.40-00.43)
   percutaneous insertion of intracranial vascular
      stent(s) (00.65)
   procedure on vessel bifurcation (00.44)
   EXCLUDES   *angioplasty of other non-coronary*
      vessel(s) (39.50)
      atherectomy of extracranial vessel(s)
         (17.53)
      atherectomy of other non-coronary
         vessel(s) (17.56)
      removal of cerebrovascular obstruction
         of vessel(s) by open approach
         (38.01-38.02, 38.11-38.12,
         38.31-38.32, 38.41-38.42)

17.55 Transluminal coronary atherectomy
Directional atherectomy
Excimer laser atherectomy
Rotational atherectomy
That by laser
That by percutaneous approach
That by transluminal extraction
Code also any:
   injection or infusion of thrombolytic agent
      (99.10)
   insertion of coronary artery stent (36.06-36.07)
   intracoronary artery thrombolytic infusion
      (36.04)
   number of vascular stents inserted (00.45-00.48)
   number of vessels treated (00.40-00.43)
   procedure on vessel bifurcation (00.44)
   SuperSaturated oxygen therapy (00.49)
   transluminal coronary angioplasty (00.66)

17.56 Atherectomy of other non-coronary vessel(s)
Percutaneous transluminal angioplasty of:
   lower extremity vessels
   mesenteric artery
   renal artery
   upper extremity vessels
   INCLUDES   directional atherectomy
      excimer laser atherectomy
      rotational atherectomy
      that by laser
      that by transluminal extraction
Code also any:
   injection or infusion of thrombolytic agent
      (99.10)
   insertion of drug-eluting peripheral vessel stent
      (00.55)
   insertion of non-drug-eluting peripheral vessel
      stent(s) or stent graft(s) (39.90)
   number of vascular stents inserted (00.45-00.48)
   number of vessels treated (00.40-00.43)
   procedure on vessel bifurcation (00.44)
   EXCLUDES   *percutaneous angioplasty of extracranial*
      or intracranial vessel(s)
         (00.61-00.62)
      percutaneous atherectomy of
         extracranial vessel(s) (17.53)
      percutaneous atherectomy of
         intracranial vessel(s) (17.54)

Laser Interstitial Thermal Therapy

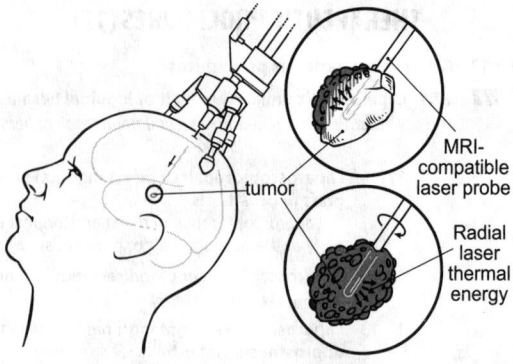

MRI-compatible laser probe

tumor

Radial laser thermal energy

☑4ᵗʰ **17.6 Laser interstitial thermal therapy [LITT] under guidance**
Focused laser interstitial thermal therapy [f-LITT] under MRI
   guidance
MRI-guided LITT
DEF: Selective, real-time thermal ablation of tumors using a
laser probe placed directly into the tumor, avoiding damage
to surrounding tissue.

**17.61 Laser interstitial thermal therapy [LITT] of lesion
or tissue of brain under guidance**
Focused laser interstitial thermal therapy [f-LITT]
   under MRI guidance
MRI-guided LITT of lesion or tissue of brain
   EXCLUDES   *laser interstitial thermal therapy [LITT] of*
      lesion or tissue of head under
      guidance (17.62)

**17.62 Laser interstitial thermal therapy [LITT] of lesion
or tissue of head and neck under guidance**
Focused laser interstitial thermal therapy [f-LITT]
   under MRI guidance
MRI-guided LITT of lesion or tissue of head and neck
   EXCLUDES   *laser interstitial thermal therapy [LITT] of*
      lesion or tissue of brain under
      guidance (17.61)

**17.63 Laser interstitial thermal therapy [LITT] of lesion
or tissue of liver under guidance**
Focused laser interstitial thermal therapy [f-LITT]
   under MRI guidance
MRI-guided LITT of lesion or tissue of liver

**17.69 Laser interstitial thermal therapy [LITT] of lesion
or tissue of other and unspecified site under
guidance**
Focused laser interstitial thermal therapy [f-LITT]
   under MRI guidance
MRI-guided LITT of lesion or tissue of breast
MRI-guided LITT of lesion or tissue of lung
MRI-guided LITT of lesion or tissue of prostate
   EXCLUDES   *laser interstitial thermal therapy [LITT] of*
      lesion or tissue of brain under
      guidance (17.61)
      laser interstitial thermal therapy [LITT] of
         lesion or tissue of head and neck
         under guidance (17.62)
      laser interstitial thermal therapy [LITT] of
         lesion or tissue of liver under
         guidance (17.63)

☑4ᵗʰ **17.7 Other diagnostic and therapeutic procedures**

17.70 Intravenous infusion of clofarabine
   EXCLUDES   *injection or infusion of cancer*
      chemotherapeutic substance
      (99.25)

**17.71 Non-coronary intra-operative fluorescence
vascular angiography [IFVA]**
Intraoperative laser arteriogram
SPY arteriogram
SPY arteriography
   EXCLUDES   *intra-operative coronary fluorescence*
      vascular angiography (88.59)

☑4ᵗʰ **17.8 Other adjunct procedures**

Note: These codes are to be used in conjunction with other therapeutic procedure codes to provide additional information on devices used as part of a procedure.

17.81 Insertion of antimicrobial envelope

Use of anti-microbial (mesh) (prophylactic antibiotics embedded) envelope with the insertion of cardiovascular implantable electronic devices [CIED]

Code first primary procedure:

Insertion of cardiovascular implantable electronic device(s) [CIED] (00.51, 00.53, 00.54, 37.94, 37.96, 37.98)

DEF: Biocompatible mesh pouches coated with antibiotics that elute within a seven- to 10-day period post-implantation that serve a dual purpose, stabilization of the device by reducing migration and reduction of postoperative infections by providing localized antibiotic prophylaxis in the surgically created subcutaneous "pocket."

4. OPERATIONS ON THE EAR (18-20)

√3ʳᵈ **18 Operations on external ear**
  INCLUDES   operations on:
              external auditory canal
              skin and cartilage of:
                auricle
                meatus

√4ᵗʰ **18.0 Incision of external ear**
  EXCLUDES   *removal of intraluminal foreign body (98.11)*

  18.01 Piercing of ear lobe
          Piercing of pinna

  18.02 Incision of external auditory canal

  18.09 Other incision of external ear

√4ᵗʰ **18.1 Diagnostic procedures on external ear**

  18.11 Otoscopy
          DEF: Exam of the ear with instrument designed for
          visualization.

  18.12 Biopsy of external ear

  18.19 Other diagnostic procedures on external ear
          EXCLUDES   *microscopic examination of specimen*
                     from ear (90.31-90.39)

√4ᵗʰ **18.2 Excision or destruction of lesion of external ear**

  18.21 Excision of preauricular sinus
          Radical excision of preauricular sinus or cyst
          EXCLUDES   *excision of preauricular remnant*
                     [appendage] (18.29)

          DEF: Excision of preauricular sinus or cyst with
          adjacent tissues.

  **18.29 Excision or destruction of other lesion of external
          ear**
          Cauterization
          Coagulation
          Cryosurgery   } of external ear
          Curettage
          Electrocoagulation
          Enucleation

          Excision of:
            exostosis of external auditory canal
            preauricular remnant [appendage]
          Partial excision of ear
          EXCLUDES   *biopsy of external ear (18.12)*
                     radical excision of lesion (18.31)
                     removal of cerumen (96.52)

√4ᵗʰ **18.3 Other excision of external ear**
  EXCLUDES   *biopsy of external ear (18.12)*

  18.31 Radical excision of lesion of external ear
          EXCLUDES   *radical excision of preauricular sinus*
                     (18.21)

          DEF: Removal of damaged, diseased ear and adjacent
          tissue.

  18.39 Other
          Amputation of external ear
          EXCLUDES   *excision of lesion (18.21-18.29, 18.31)*

  18.4 Suture of laceration of external ear

  18.5 Surgical correction of prominent ear
          Ear: Ear:
            pinning   setback
          DEF: Reformation of protruding outer ear.

  18.6 Reconstruction of external auditory canal
          Canaloplasty of external auditory meatus
          Construction [reconstruction] of external meatus of ear:
            osseous portion
            skin-lined portion (with skin graft)
          DEF: Repair of outer ear canal.

Stapedectomy with Incus Replacement

■ Area excised

√4ᵗʰ **18.7 Other plastic repair of external ear**

  18.71 Construction of auricle of ear
          Prosthetic appliance for absent ear
          Reconstruction:
            auricle
            ear
          DEF: Reformation or repair of external ear flap.

  18.72 Reattachment of amputated ear

  18.79 Other plastic repair of external ear
          Otoplasty NOS
          Postauricular skin graft
          Repair of lop ear
          DEF: Postauricular skin graft: Graft repair behind ear.
          DEF: Repair of lop ear: Reconstruction of ear that is at
          right angle to head.

  18.9 Other operations on external ear
          EXCLUDES   *irrigation of ear (96.52)*
                     packing of external auditory canal (96.11)
                     removal of:
                       cerumen (96.52)
                       foreign body (without incision) (98.11)

√3ʳᵈ **19 Reconstructive operations on middle ear**

  19.0 Stapes mobilization
          Division, otosclerotic: Remobilization of stapes
            material   Stapediolysis
            process   Transcrural stapes mobilization
          EXCLUDES   *that with synchronous stapedectomy*
                     (19.11-19.19)

          DEF: Repair of innermost bone of middle ear to enable
          movement and response to sound.

√4ᵗʰ **19.1 Stapedectomy**
          EXCLUDES   *revision of previous stapedectomy (19.21-19.29)*
                     stapes mobilization only (19.0)

          DEF: Removal of innermost bone of middle ear.

  19.11 Stapedectomy with incus replacement
          Stapedectomy with incus:
            homograft
            prosthesis
          DEF: Removal of innermost bone of middle ear with
          autograft or prosthesis replacement.

  19.19 Other stapedectomy

√4ᵗʰ **19.2 Revision of stapedectomy**

  19.21 Revision of stapedectomy with incus replacement

  19.29 Other revision of stapedectomy

  19.3 Other operations on ossicular chain
          Incudectomy NOS
          Ossiculectomy NOS
          Reconstruction of ossicles, second stage
          DEF: Incudectomy: Excision of middle bone of middle ear, not
          otherwise specified.
          DEF: Ossiculectomy: Excision of middle ear bones, not
          otherwise specified.
          DEF: Reconstruction of ossicles, second stage: Repair of
          middle ear bones following previous surgery.

Operations on the Ear

19.4–20.79

19.4 Myringoplasty
Epitympanic, type I
Myringoplasty by:
  cauterization
  graft
Tympanoplasty (type I)
DEF: Epitympanic, type I: Repair over or upon eardrum.
DEF: Myringoplasty by cauterization: Plastic repair of tympanic membrane of eardrum by heat.
DEF: Graft: Plastic repair using implanted tissue.
DEF: Tympanoplasty (type I): Reconstruction of eardrum to restore hearing.

√4ᵗʰ **19.5 Other tympanoplasty**

19.52 Type II tympanoplasty
Closure of perforation with graft against incus or malleus

19.53 Type III tympanoplasty
Graft placed in contact with mobile and intact stapes

19.54 Type IV tympanoplasty
Mobile footplate left exposed with air pocket between round window and graft

19.55 Type V tympanoplasty
Fenestra in horizontal semicircular canal covered by graft

19.6 Revision of tympanoplasty
DEF: Repair or correction of previous plastic surgery on eardrum.

19.9 Other repair of middle ear
Closure of mastoid fistula
Mastoid myoplasty
Obliteration of tympanomastoid cavity
DEF: Closure of mastoid fistula: Closing of abnormal channel in mastoid.
DEF: Mastoid myoplasty: Restoration or repair of mastoid muscle.
DEF: Obliteration of tympanomastoid cavity: Removal, total, of functional elements of middle ear.

√3ʳᵈ **20 Other operations on middle and inner ear**

√4ᵗʰ **20.0 Myringotomy**
DEF: Myringotomy: Puncture of tympanic membrane or eardrum, also called tympanocentesis

20.01 Myringotomy with insertion of tube
Myringostomy

20.09 Other myringotomy
Aspiration of middle ear NOS

20.1 Removal of tympanostomy tube

√4ᵗʰ **20.2 Incision of mastoid and middle ear**

20.21 Incision of mastoid

20.22 Incision of petrous pyramid air cells

20.23 Incision of middle ear
Atticotomy
Division of tympanum
Lysis of adhesions of middle ear
EXCLUDES *division of otosclerotic process (19.0)*
stapediolysis (19.0)
that with stapedectomy (19.11-19.19)

√4ᵗʰ **20.3 Diagnostic procedures on middle and inner ear**

20.31 Electrocochleography
DEF: Measure of electric potential of eighth cranial nerve by electrode applied sound.

20.32 Biopsy of middle and inner ear

20.39 Other diagnostic procedures on middle and inner ear
EXCLUDES *auditory and vestibular function tests (89.13, 95.41-95.49)*
microscopic examination of specimen from ear (90.31-90.39)

√4ᵗʰ **20.4 Mastoidectomy**
Code also any:
  skin graft (18.79)
  tympanoplasty (19.4-19.55)
EXCLUDES *that with implantation of cochlear prosthetic device (20.96-20.98)*
DEF: Mastoidectomy: Excision of bony protrusion behind ear.

20.41 Simple mastoidectomy

20.42 Radical mastoidectomy

20.49 Other mastoidectomy
Atticoantrostomy
Mastoidectomy:
  NOS
  modified radical
DEF: Atticoantrotomy: Opening of cavity of mastoid bone and middle ear.

√4ᵗʰ **20.5 Other excision of middle ear**
EXCLUDES *that with synchronous mastoidectomy (20.41-20.49)*

20.51 Excision of lesion of middle ear
EXCLUDES *biopsy of middle ear (20.32)*

20.59 Other
Apicectomy of petrous pyramid
Tympanectomy

√4ᵗʰ **20.6 Fenestration of inner ear**

20.61 Fenestration of inner ear (initial)
Fenestration of:
  labyrinth   with graft (skin)
  semicircular canals   (vein)
  vestibule
EXCLUDES *that with tympanoplasty, type V (19.55)*
DEF: Creation of inner ear opening.

20.62 Revision of fenestration of inner ear

√4ᵗʰ **20.7 Incision, excision, and destruction of inner ear**

20.71 Endolymphatic shunt
DEF: Insertion of tube to drain fluid in inner ear cavities.

20.72 Injection into inner ear
Destruction by injection (alcohol):
  inner ear
  semicircular canals
  vestibule

20.79 Other incision, excision, and destruction of inner ear
Decompression of labyrinth
Drainage of inner ear
Fistulization:
  endolymphatic sac
  labyrinth
Incision of endolymphatic sac
Labyrinthectomy (transtympanic)
Opening of bony labyrinth
Perilymphatic tap
EXCLUDES *biopsy of inner ear (20.32)*
DEF: Decompression of labyrinth: Controlled relief of pressure in cavities of inner ear.
DEF: Drainage of inner ear: Removal of fluid from inner ear.
DEF: Fistulization of endolymphatic sac: Creation of passage to fluid sac in inner ear cavities.
DEF: Fistulization of labyrinth: Creation of passage to inner ear cavities.
DEF: Incision of endolymphatic sac: Cutting into fluid sac in inner ear cavities.
DEF: Labyrinthectomy (transtympanic): Excision of cavities across eardrum.
DEF: Opening of bony labyrinth: Cutting into inner ear bony cavities.
DEF: Perilymphatic tap: Puncture or incision into fluid sac of inner ear cavities.

20.8 Operations on Eustachian tube

Catheterization
Inflation
Injection (Teflon paste)
Insufflation (boric   } of Eustachian tube
    acid-salicylic acid)
Intubation
Politzerization

DEF: Catheterization: Passing catheter into passage between pharynx and middle ear.

DEF: Inflation: Blowing air, gas or liquid into passage between pharynx and middle ear to inflate.

DEF: Injection (Teflon paste): Forcing fluid (Teflon paste) into passage between pharynx and middle ear.

DEF: Insufflation (boric acid-salicylic acid): Blowing gas or liquid into passage between pharynx and middle ear.

DEF: Intubation: Placing tube into passage between pharynx and middle ear.

DEF: Politzerization: Inflating passage between pharynx and middle ear with Politzer bag.

√4ᵗʰ **20.9 Other operations on inner and middle ear**

20.91 Tympanosympathectomy

DEF: Excision or chemical suppression of impulses of middle ear nerves.

20.92 Revision of mastoidectomy

DEF: Correction of previous removal of mastoid cells from temporal or mastoid bone.

20.93 Repair of oval and round windows

Closure of fistula:
    oval window
    perilymph
    round window

DEF: Restoration of middle ear openings.

20.94 Injection of tympanum

20.95 Implantation of electromagnetic hearing device

Bone conduction hearing device

EXCLUDES *cochlear prosthetic device (20.96-20.98)*

20.96 Implantation or replacement of cochlear prosthetic device, not otherwise specified

INCLUDES mastoidectomy

Implantation of receiver (within skull) and insertion of electrode(s) in the cochlea

EXCLUDES *electromagnetic hearing device (20.95)*

20.97 Implantation or replacement of cochlear prosthetic device, single channel

INCLUDES mastoidectomy

Implantation of receiver (within skull) and insertion of electrode in the cochlea

EXCLUDES *electromagnetic hearing device (20.95)*

20.98 Implantation or replacement of cochlear prosthetic device, multiple channel

INCLUDES mastoidectomy

Implantation of receiver (within skull) and insertion of electrodes in the cochlea

EXCLUDES *electromagnetic hearing device (20.95)*

20.99 Other operations on middle and inner ear

Attachment of percutaneous abutment (screw) for prosthetic device

Repair or removal of cochlear prosthetic device (receiver) (electrode)

EXCLUDES *adjustment (external components) of cochlear prosthetic device (95.49)*
    fitting of hearing aid (95.48)

5. OPERATIONS ON THE NOSE, MOUTH, AND PHARYNX (21-29)

✓3ʳᵈ **21 Operations on nose**

> **INCLUDES** operations on:
> bone
> skin } of nose

✓4ᵗʰ **21.0 Control of epistaxis**

21.00 Control of epistaxis, not otherwise specified

21.01 Control of epistaxis by anterior nasal packing

21.02 Control of epistaxis by posterior (and anterior) packing

21.03 Control of epistaxis by cauterization (and packing)

21.04 Control of epistaxis by ligation of ethmoidal arteries

21.05 Control of epistaxis by (transantral) ligation of the maxillary artery

21.06 Control of epistaxis by ligation of the external carotid artery

21.07 Control of epistaxis by excision of nasal mucosa and skin grafting of septum and lateral nasal wall

21.09 Control of epistaxis by other means

21.1 Incision of nose
> Chondrotomy
> Incision of skin of nose
> Nasal septotomy
> **DEF:** Chondrotomy: Incision or division of nasal cartilage.
> **DEF:** Nasal septotomy: Incision into bone dividing nose into two chambers.

✓4ᵗʰ **21.2 Diagnostic procedures on nose**

21.21 Rhinoscopy
> **DEF:** Visualization of nasal passage with nasal speculum.

21.22 Biopsy of nose

21.29 Other diagnostic procedures on nose
> **EXCLUDES** *microscopic examination of specimen from nose (90.31-90.39)*
> *nasal:*
> *function study (89.12)*
> *x-ray (87.16)*
> *rhinomanometry (89.12)*

✓4ᵗʰ **21.3 Local excision or destruction of lesion of nose**
> **EXCLUDES** *biopsy of nose (21.22)*
> *nasal fistulectomy (21.82)*

21.30 Excision or destruction of lesion of nose, not otherwise specified

21.31 Local excision or destruction of intranasal lesion
> Nasal polypectomy

21.32 Local excision or destruction of other lesion of nose

21.4 Resection of nose
> Amputation of nose

21.5 Submucous resection of nasal septum
> **DEF:** Partial resection of nasal septum with mucosa reimplanted after excision.

✓4ᵗʰ **21.6 Turbinectomy**
> **DEF:** Partial or total removal of turbinate bones; inferior turbinate is most often excised.

21.61 Turbinectomy by diathermy or cryosurgery
> **DEF:** Destruction of turbinate bone by heat or freezing.

21.62 Fracture of the turbinates
> **DEF:** Surgical breaking of turbinate bones.

21.69 Other turbinectomy
> **EXCLUDES** *turbinectomy associated with sinusectomy (22.31-22.39, 22.42, 22.60-22.64)*

Excision of Turbinate

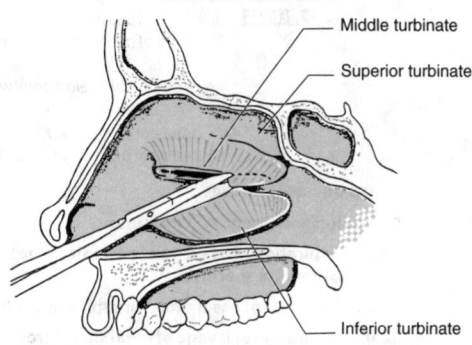

Middle turbinate
Superior turbinate
Inferior turbinate

✓4ᵗʰ **21.7 Reduction of nasal fracture**

21.71 Closed reduction of nasal fracture

21.72 Open reduction of nasal fracture

✓4ᵗʰ **21.8 Repair and plastic operations on the nose**

21.81 Suture of laceration of nose

21.82 Closure of nasal fistula
> Nasolabial
> Nasopharyngeal } fistulectomy
> Oronasal
> **DEF:** Sealing off crack or hole between nose and lip, nose and pharynx, or nose and mouth.

21.83 Total nasal reconstruction
> Reconstruction of nose with:
> arm flap
> forehead flap
> **DEF:** Plastic reformation of nasal structure with tissue flap from arm or forehead.

21.84 Revision rhinoplasty
> Rhinoseptoplasty
> Twisted nose rhinoplasty
> **DEF:** Rhinoseptoplasty: Repair of nose and the bone dividing the nose into two chambers.
> **DEF:** Twisted nose rhinoplasty: Repair of nose alignment following reconstructive surgery.

21.85 Augmentation rhinoplasty
> Augmentation rhinoplasty with:
> graft
> synthetic implant
> **DEF:** Implant of tissue or synthetic graft to enlarge nose.

21.86 Limited rhinoplasty
> Plastic repair of nasolabial flaps
> Tip rhinoplasty
> **DEF:** Plastic repair of nasolabial flaps: Reconstruction of nasal area above lips.
> **DEF:** Tip rhinoplasty: Reconstruction or restoration of nasal tip.

21.87 Other rhinoplasty
> Rhinoplasty NOS

21.88 Other septoplasty
> Crushing of nasal septum
> Repair of septal perforation
> **EXCLUDES** *septoplasty associated with submucous resection of septum (21.5)*
> **DEF:** Crushing of nasal septum: Division and reconstruction of defects in bone dividing nasal chambers.
> **DEF:** Repair of septal perforation: Repair of hole in bone dividing nasal chambers with adjacent tissue.

21.89 Other repair and plastic operations on nose
> Reattachment of amputated nose

✓4ᵗʰ **21.9 Other operations on nose**

21.91 Lysis of adhesions of nose
> Posterior nasal scrub
> **DEF:** Posterior nasal scrub: Clearing out of abnormal adhesions in posterior nasal area.

Operations on the Nose, Mouth, and Pharynx

21.99–24.2

21.99 Other
> EXCLUDES   dilation of frontonasal duct (96.21)
> irrigation of nasal passages (96.53)
> removal of:
> > intraluminal foreign body without
> > incision (98.12)
> > nasal packing (97.32)
> > replacement of nasal packing (97.21)

√3ʳᵈ **22 Operations on nasal sinuses**

√4ᵗʰ **22.0 Aspiration and lavage of nasal sinus**

22.00 Aspiration and lavage of nasal sinus, not otherwise specified

22.01 Puncture of nasal sinus for aspiration or lavage

22.02 Aspiration or lavage of nasal sinus through natural ostium
> **DEF:** Withdrawal of fluid and washing of nasal cavity through natural opening.

√4ᵗʰ **22.1 Diagnostic procedures on nasal sinus**

22.11 Closed [endoscopic] [needle] biopsy of nasal sinus

22.12 Open biopsy of nasal sinus

22.19 Other diagnostic procedures on nasal sinuses
> Endoscopy without biopsy
> EXCLUDES   transillumination of sinus (89.35)
> x-ray of sinus (87.15-87.16)

22.2 Intranasal antrotomy
> EXCLUDES   antrotomy with external approach (22.31-22.39)
> **DEF:** Incision of intranasal sinus.

√4ᵗʰ **22.3 External maxillary antrotomy**

22.31 Radical maxillary antrotomy
> Removal of lining membrane of maxillary sinus using Caldwell-Luc approach
> **DEF:** Caldwell-Luc approach: Removal of membrane lining the maxillary cavity through incision above canine teeth.

22.39 Other external maxillary antrotomy
> Exploration of maxillary antrum with Caldwell-Luc approach

√4ᵗʰ **22.4 Frontal sinusotomy and sinusectomy**

22.41 Frontal sinusotomy

22.42 Frontal sinusectomy
> Excision of lesion of frontal sinus
> Obliteration of frontal sinus (with fat)
> EXCLUDES   biopsy of nasal sinus (22.11-22.12)

√4ᵗʰ **22.5 Other nasal sinusotomy**

22.50 Sinusotomy, not otherwise specified

22.51 Ethmoidotomy

22.52 Sphenoidotomy

22.53 Incision of multiple nasal sinuses

√4ᵗʰ **22.6 Other nasal sinusectomy**
> INCLUDES   that with incidental turbinectomy
> EXCLUDES   biopsy of nasal sinus (22.11-22.12)

22.60 Sinusectomy, not otherwise specified

22.61 Excision of lesion of maxillary sinus with Caldwell-Luc approach

22.62 Excision of lesion of maxillary sinus with other approach

22.63 Ethmoidectomy
> **DEF:** Partial or total removal of ethmoid cells and bone; includes excising partial or total mucosal lining.

22.64 Sphenoidectomy
> **DEF:** Removal of wedge shaped sphenoid bone at base of brain.

√4ᵗʰ **22.7 Repair of nasal sinus**

22.71 Closure of nasal sinus fistula
> Repair of oro-antral fistula

22.79 Other repair of nasal sinus
> Reconstruction of frontonasal duct
> Repair of bone of accessory sinus

22.9 Other operations on nasal sinuses
> Exteriorization of maxillary sinus
> Fistulization of sinus
> EXCLUDES   dilation of frontonasal duct (96.21)
> **DEF:** Exteriorization of maxillary sinus: Creation of external maxillary cavity opening.
> **DEF:** Fistulization of sinus: Creation of fistula canal in nasal cavity.

√3ʳᵈ **23 Removal and restoration of teeth**

√4ᵗʰ **23.0 Forceps extraction of tooth**

23.01 Extraction of deciduous tooth

23.09 Extraction of other tooth
> Extraction of tooth NOS

√4ᵗʰ **23.1 Surgical removal of tooth**

23.11 Removal of residual root

23.19 Other surgical extraction of tooth
> Odontectomy NOS
> Removal of impacted tooth
> Tooth extraction with elevation of mucoperiosteal flap

23.2 Restoration of tooth by filling

23.3 Restoration of tooth by inlay
> **DEF:** Restoration of tooth by cementing in a molded filling.

√4ᵗʰ **23.4 Other dental restoration**

23.41 Application of crown

23.42 Insertion of fixed bridge

23.43 Insertion of removable bridge

23.49 Other

23.5 Implantation of tooth
> **DEF:** Insertion of a sound tooth to replace extracted tooth.

23.6 Prosthetic dental implant
> Endosseous dental implant
> **DEF:** Implant of artificial denture within bone covering tooth socket.

√4ᵗʰ **23.7 Apicoectomy and root canal therapy**

23.70 Root canal, not otherwise specified

23.71 Root canal therapy with irrigation

23.72 Root canal therapy with apicoectomy
> **DEF:** Removal of tooth root to treat damaged root canal tissue.

23.73 Apicoectomy

√3ʳᵈ **24 Other operations on teeth, gums, and alveoli**

24.0 Incision of gum or alveolar bone
> Apical alveolotomy

√4ᵗʰ **24.1 Diagnostic procedures on teeth, gums, and alveoli**

24.11 Biopsy of gum

24.12 Biopsy of alveolus

24.19 Other diagnostic procedures on teeth, gums, and alveoli
> EXCLUDES   dental:
> > examination (89.31)
> > x-ray:
> > > full-mouth (87.11)
> > > other (87.12)
> > microscopic examination of dental specimen (90.81-90.89)

24.2 Gingivoplasty
> Gingivoplasty with bone or soft tissue graft
> **DEF:** Repair of gum tissue.

24.3 Other operations on gum

    24.31 Excision of lesion or tissue of gum
        EXCLUDES biopsy of gum (24.11)
                    excision of odontogenic lesion (24.4)

    24.32 Suture of laceration of gum

    24.39 Other

24.4 Excision of dental lesion of jaw
    Excision of odontogenic lesion

24.5 Alveoloplasty
    Alveolectomy (interradicular) (intraseptal) (radical) (simple)
        (with graft or implant)
    EXCLUDES biopsy of alveolus (24.12)
               en bloc resection of alveolar process and palate
                 (27.32)
    DEF: Repair or correction of bony tooth socket.

24.6 Exposure of tooth

24.7 Application of orthodontic appliance
    Application, insertion, or fitting of:
        arch bars
        orthodontic obturator
        orthodontic wiring
        periodontal splint
    EXCLUDES nonorthodontic dental wiring (93.55)

24.8 Other orthodontic operation
    Closure of diastema (alveolar) (dental)
    Occlusal adjustment
    Removal of arch bars
    Repair of dental arch
    EXCLUDES removal of nonorthodontic wiring (97.33)

24.9 Other dental operations

    24.91 Extension or deepening of buccolabial or lingual sulcus

    24.99 Other
        EXCLUDES dental:
                debridement (96.54)
                examination (89.31)
                prophylaxis (96.54)
                scaling and polishing (96.54)
                wiring (93.55)
            fitting of dental appliance [denture]
                (99.97)
            microscopic examination of dental
                specimen (90.81-90.89)
            removal of dental:
                packing (97.34)
                prosthesis (97.35)
                wiring (97.33)
            replacement of dental packing (97.22)

25 Operations on tongue

25.0 Diagnostic procedures on tongue

    25.01 Closed [needle] biopsy of tongue

    25.02 Open biopsy of tongue
        Wedge biopsy

    25.09 Other diagnostic procedures on tongue

25.1 Excision or destruction of lesion or tissue of tongue
    EXCLUDES biopsy of tongue (25.01-25.02)
               frenumectomy:
                labial (27.41)
                lingual (25.92)

25.2 Partial glossectomy

25.3 Complete glossectomy
    Glossectomy NOS
    Code also any neck dissection (40.40-40.42)

25.4 Radical glossectomy
    Code also any:
        neck dissection (40.40-40.42)
        tracheostomy (31.1-31.29)

25.5 Repair of tongue and glossoplasty

    25.51 Suture of laceration of tongue

    25.59 Other repair and plastic operations on tongue
        Fascial sling of tongue
        Fusion of tongue (to lip)
        Graft of mucosa or skin to tongue
        EXCLUDES lysis of adhesions of tongue (25.93)

25.9 Other operations on tongue

    25.91 Lingual frenotomy
        EXCLUDES labial frenotomy (27.91)
        DEF: Extension of groove between cheek and lips or
        cheek and tongue.

    25.92 Lingual frenectomy
        EXCLUDES labial frenectomy (27.41)
        DEF: Frenectomy: Removal of vertical membrane
        attaching tongue to floor of mouth.

    25.93 Lysis of adhesions of tongue

    25.94 Other glossotomy

    25.99 Other

26 Operations on salivary glands and ducts
    INCLUDES operations on:
            lesser salivary
            parotid
            sublingual } gland and duct
            submaxillry
    Code also any neck dissection (40.40-40.42)

26.0 Incision of salivary gland or duct

26.1 Diagnostic procedures on salivary glands and ducts

    26.11 Closed [needle] biopsy of salivary gland or duct

    26.12 Open biopsy of salivary gland or duct

    26.19 Other diagnostic procedures on salivary glands and ducts
        EXCLUDES x-ray of salivary gland (87.09)

26.2 Excision of lesion of salivary gland

    26.21 Marsupialization of salivary gland cyst
        DEF: Creation of pouch of salivary gland cyst to drain
        and promote healing.

    26.29 Other excision of salivary gland lesion
        EXCLUDES biopsy of salivary gland (26.11-26.12)
               salivary fistulectomy (26.42)

26.3 Sialoadenectomy
    DEF: Removal of salivary gland.

    26.30 Sialoadenectomy, not otherwise specified

    26.31 Partial sialoadenectomy

    26.32 Complete sialoadenectomy
        En bloc excision of salivary gland lesion
        Radical sialoadenectomy

26.4 Repair of salivary gland or duct

    26.41 Suture of laceration of salivary gland

    26.42 Closure of salivary fistula
        DEF: Closing of abnormal opening in salivary gland.

    26.49 Other repair and plastic operations on salivary gland or duct
        Fistulization of salivary gland
        Plastic repair of salivary gland or duct NOS
        Transplantation of salivary duct opening

26.9 Other operations on salivary gland or duct

    26.91 Probing of salivary duct

    26.99 Other

√3ʳᵈ **27**   **Other operations on mouth and face**
>INCLUDES   operations on:
>>lips
>>palate
>>soft tissue of face and mouth, except tongue and
>>gingiva
>
>EXCLUDES   operations on:
>>gingiva (24.0-24.99)
>>tongue (25.01-25.99)

27.0   **Drainage of face and floor of mouth**
>Drainage of:
>facial region (abscess)
>fascial compartment of face
>Ludwig's angina
>>EXCLUDES   drainage of thyroglossal tract (06.09)

27.1   **Incision of palate**

√4ᵗʰ **27.2**   **Diagnostic procedures on oral cavity**

     27.21   **Biopsy of bony palate**

     27.22   **Biopsy of uvula and soft palate**

     27.23   **Biopsy of lip**

     27.24   **Biopsy of mouth, unspecified structure**

     27.29   **Other diagnostic procedures on oral cavity**
>>EXCLUDES   soft tissue x-ray (87.09)

√4ᵗʰ **27.3**   **Excision of lesion or tissue of bony palate**

     27.31   **Local excision or destruction of lesion or tissue of bony palate**
>>Local excision or destruction of palate by:
>>cautery
>>chemotherapy
>>cryotherapy
>>>EXCLUDES   biopsy of bony palate (27.21)

     27.32   **Wide excision or destruction of lesion or tissue of bony palate**
>>En bloc resection of alveolar process and palate

√4ᵗʰ **27.4**   **Excision of other parts of mouth**

     27.41   **Labial frenectomy**
>>EXCLUDES   division of labial frenum (27.91)
>>
>>DEF: Removal of mucous membrane fold of lip.

     27.42   **Wide excision of lesion of lip**

     27.43   **Other excision of lesion or tissue of lip**

     27.49   **Other excision of mouth**
>>EXCLUDES   biopsy of mouth NOS (27.24)
>>>excision of lesion of:
>>>palate (27.31-27.32)
>>>tongue (25.1)
>>>uvula (27.72)
>>>fistulectomy of mouth (27.53)
>>>frenectomy of:
>>>lip (27.41)
>>>tongue (25.92)

√4ᵗʰ **27.5**   **Plastic repair of lip and mouth**
>EXCLUDES   palatoplasty (27.61-27.69)

     27.51   **Suture of laceration of lip**

     27.52   **Suture of laceration of other part of mouth**

     27.53   **Closure of fistula of mouth**
>>EXCLUDES   fistulectomy:
>>>nasolabial (21.82)
>>>oro-antral (22.71)
>>>oronasal (21.82)

     27.54   **Repair of cleft lip**

     27.55   **Full-thickness skin graft to lip and mouth**

     27.56   **Other skin graft to lip and mouth**

     27.57   **Attachment of pedicle or flap graft to lip and mouth**
>>DEF: Repair of lip or mouth with tissue pedicle or flap still connected to original vascular base.

     27.59   **Other plastic repair of mouth**

√4ᵗʰ **27.6**   **Palatoplasty**

     27.61   **Suture of laceration of palate**

     27.62   **Correction of cleft palate**
>>Correction of cleft palate by push-back operation
>>>EXCLUDES   revision of cleft palate repair (27.63)

     27.63   **Revision of cleft palate repair**
>>Secondary:
>>>attachment of pharyngeal flap
>>>lengthening of palate

     27.64   **Insertion of palatal implant**
>>DEF: Nonabsorbable polyester implants placed into the soft palate at the back of the roof of the mouth; one implant placed at the soft palate midline and two are positioned on either side; used to support and stiffen the palate, reducing vibration (snoring).

     27.69   **Other plastic repair of palate**
>>Code also any insertion of palatal implant (27.64)
>>>EXCLUDES   fistulectomy of mouth (27.53)

√4ᵗʰ **27.7**   **Operations on uvula**

     27.71   **Incision of uvula**

     27.72   **Excision of uvula**
>>EXCLUDES   biopsy of uvula (27.22)

     27.73   **Repair of uvula**
>>EXCLUDES   that with synchronous cleft palate repair (27.62)
>>>uranostaphylorrhaphy (27.62)

     27.79   **Other operations on uvula**

√4ᵗʰ **27.9**   **Other operations on mouth and face**

     27.91   **Labial frenotomy**
>>Division of labial frenum
>>>EXCLUDES   lingual frenotomy (25.91)
>>
>>DEF: Division of labial frenum: Cutting and separating mucous membrane fold of lip.

     27.92   **Incision of mouth, unspecified structure**
>>EXCLUDES   incision of:
>>>gum (24.0)
>>>palate (27.1)
>>>salivary gland or duct (26.0)
>>>tongue (25.94)
>>>uvula (27.71)

     27.99   **Other operations on oral cavity**
>>Graft of buccal sulcus
>>>EXCLUDES   removal of:
>>>intraluminal foreign body (98.01)
>>>penetrating foreign body from mouth without incision (98.22)
>>
>>DEF: Graft of buccal sulcus: Implant of tissue into groove of interior cheek lining.

√3ʳᵈ **28**   **Operations on tonsils and adenoids**

28.0   **Incision and drainage of tonsil and peritonsillar structures**
>Drainage (oral) (transcervical) of:
>parapharyngeal ⎤
>peritonsillar |
>retropharyngeal | abscess
>tonsillar   ⎦

√4ᵗʰ **28.1**   **Diagnostic procedures on tonsils and adenoids**

     28.11   **Biopsy of tonsils and adenoids**

     28.19   **Other diagnostic procedures on tonsils and adenoids**
>>EXCLUDES   soft tissue x-ray (87.09)

28.2   **Tonsillectomy without adenoidectomy**

28.3   **Tonsillectomy with adenoidectomy**

28.4   **Excision of tonsil tag**

28.5   **Excision of lingual tonsil**

28.6   **Adenoidectomy without tonsillectomy**
>Excision of adenoid tag

28.7   **Control of hemorrhage after tonsillectomy and adenoidectomy**

√4ᵗʰ **28.9　Other operations on tonsils and adenoids**

28.91　Removal of foreign body from tonsil and adenoid by incision
> **EXCLUDES**　*that without incision (98.13)*

28.92　Excision of lesion of tonsil and adenoid
> **EXCLUDES**　*biopsy of tonsil and adenoid (28.11)*

28.99　Other

√3ʳᵈ **29　Operations on pharynx**
> **INCLUDES**　operations on:
> hypopharynx
> nasopharynx
> oropharynx
> pharyngeal pouch
> pyriform sinus

29.0　Pharyngotomy
Drainage of pharyngeal bursa
> **EXCLUDES**　*incision and drainage of retropharyngeal abscess (28.0)*
> *removal of foreign body (without incision) (98.13)*

√4ᵗʰ **29.1　Diagnostic procedures on pharynx**

29.11　Pharyngoscopy

29.12　Pharyngeal biopsy
Biopsy of supraglottic mass

29.19　Other diagnostic procedures on pharynx
> **EXCLUDES**　*x-ray of nasopharynx:*
> *contrast (87.06)*
> *other (87.09)*

29.2　Excision of branchial cleft cyst or vestige
> **EXCLUDES**　*branchial cleft fistulectomy (29.52)*

√4ᵗʰ **29.3　Excision or destruction of lesion or tissue of pharynx**

29.31　Cricopharyngeal myotomy
> **EXCLUDES**　*that with pharyngeal diverticulectomy (29.32)*
> **DEF:** Removal of outward pouching of throat.

29.32　Pharyngeal diverticulectomy

29.33　Pharyngectomy (partial)
> **EXCLUDES**　*laryngopharyngectomy (30.3)*

29.39　Other excision or destruction of lesion or tissue of pharynx

29.4　Plastic operation on pharynx
Correction of nasopharyngeal atresia
> **EXCLUDES**　*pharyngoplasty associated with cleft palate repair (27.62-27.63)*
> **DEF:** Correction of nasopharyngeal atresia: Construction of normal opening for throat stricture behind nose.

√4ᵗʰ **29.5　Other repair of pharynx**

29.51　Suture of laceration of pharynx

29.52　Closure of branchial cleft fistula
> **DEF:** Sealing off an abnormal opening of the branchial fissure in throat.

29.53　Closure of other fistula of pharynx
Pharyngoesophageal fistulectomy

29.54　Lysis of pharyngeal adhesions

29.59　Other

√4ᵗʰ **29.9　Other operations on pharynx**

29.91　Dilation of pharynx
Dilation of nasopharynx

29.92　Division of glossopharyngeal nerve

29.99　Other
> **EXCLUDES**　*insertion of radium into pharynx and nasopharynx (92.27)*
> *removal of intraluminal foreign body (98.13)*

6. OPERATIONS ON THE RESPIRATORY SYSTEM (30-34)

√3ʳᵈ **30 Excision of larynx**

√4ᵗʰ **30.0 Excision or destruction of lesion or tissue of larynx**

30.01 Marsupialization of laryngeal cyst
DEF: Incision of cyst of larynx with the edges sutured open to create pouch.

30.09 Other excision or destruction of lesion or lesion or tissue of larynx
Stripping of vocal cords
EXCLUDES   *biopsy of larynx (31.43)*
laryngeal fistulectomy (31.62)
laryngotracheal fistulectomy (31.62)

30.1 Hemilaryngectomy
DEF: Excision of one side (half) of larynx.

√4ᵗʰ **30.2 Other partial laryngectomy**

30.21 Epiglottidectomy

30.22 Vocal cordectomy
Excision of vocal cords

30.29 Other partial laryngectomy
Excision of laryngeal cartilage

30.3 Complete laryngectomy
Block dissection of larynx (with thyroidectomy) (with synchronous tracheostomy)
Laryngopharyngectomy
EXCLUDES   *that with radical neck dissection (30.4)*

30.4 Radical laryngectomy
Complete [total] laryngectomy with radical neck dissection (with thyroidectomy) (with synchronous tracheostomy)

√3ʳᵈ **31 Other operations on larynx and trachea**

31.0 Injection of larynx
Injection of inert material into larynx or vocal cords

31.1 Temporary tracheostomy
Temporary percutaneous dilatational tracheostomy [PDT]
Tracheotomy for assistance in breathing
Code also any synchronous bronchoscopy, if performed (33.21-33.24, 33.27)

√4ᵗʰ **31.2 Permanent tracheostomy**

31.21 Mediastinal tracheostomy
DEF: Placement of artificial breathing tube in windpipe through mediastinum, for long-term use.

31.29 Other permanent tracheostomy
Permanent percutaneous dilatational tracheostomy [PDT]
Code also any synchronous bronchoscopy, if performed (33.21-33.24, 33.27)
EXCLUDES   *that with laryngectomy (30.3-30.4)*

31.3 Other incision of larynx or trachea
EXCLUDES   *that for assistance in breathing (31.1-31.29)*

√4ᵗʰ **31.4 Diagnostic procedures on larynx and trachea**

31.41 Tracheoscopy through artificial stoma
EXCLUDES   *that with biopsy (31.43-31.44)*
DEF: Exam of trachea by scope through an artificial opening.

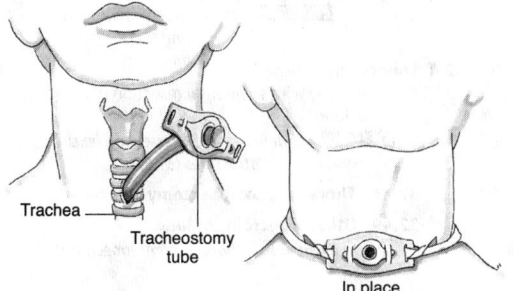

Temporary Tracheostomy

Trachea
Tracheostomy tube
In place

Closed Endoscopic Biopsy of Larynx

Laryngoscope
Trachea
Palate

Growth on vocal cord

31.42 Laryngoscopy and other tracheoscopy
EXCLUDES   *that with biopsy (31.43-31.44)*

31.43 Closed [endoscopic] biopsy of larynx

31.44 Closed [endoscopic] biopsy of trachea

31.45 Open biopsy of larynx or trachea

31.48 Other diagnostic procedures on larynx
EXCLUDES   *contrast laryngogram (87.07)*
microscopic examination of specimen from larynx (90.31-90.39)
soft tissue x-ray of larynx NEC (87.09)

31.49 Other diagnostic procedures on trachea
EXCLUDES   *microscopic examination of specimen from trachea (90.41-90.49)*
x-ray of trachea (87.49)

31.5 Local excision or destruction of lesion or tissue of trachea
EXCLUDES   *biopsy of trachea (31.44-31.45)*
laryngotracheal fistulectomy (31.62)
tracheoesophageal fistulectomy (31.73)

√4ᵗʰ **31.6 Repair of larynx**

31.61 Suture of laceration of larynx

31.62 Closure of fistula of larynx
Laryngotracheal fistulectomy
Take-down of laryngostomy
DEF: Laryngotracheal fistulectomy: Excision and closing of passage between voice box and trachea.
DEF: Take-down of laryngostomy: Removal of laryngostomy tube and restoration of voice box.

31.63 Revision of laryngostomy

31.64 Repair of laryngeal fracture
DEF: Alignment and positioning of harder structures of larynx such as hyoid bone, following fracture.

31.69 Other repair of larynx
Arytenoidopexy   Graft of larynx
Cordopexy   Transposition of vocal cords
EXCLUDES   *construction of artificial larynx (31.75)*
DEF: Arytenoidopexy: Fixation of pitcher-shaped cartilage in voice box.
DEF: Graft of larynx: Implant of graft tissue into voice box.
DEF: Transposition of the vocal cords: Placement of vocal cords into more functional positions.

√4ᵗʰ **31.7 Repair and plastic operations on trachea**

31.71 Suture of laceration of trachea

31.72 Closure of external fistula of trachea
Closure of tracheotomy

31.73 Closure of other fistula of trachea
Tracheoesophageal fistulectomy
EXCLUDES   *laryngotracheal fistulectomy (31.62)*
DEF: Tracheoesophageal fistulectomy: Excision and closure of abnormal opening between windpipe and esophagus.

31.74 Revision of tracheostomy

Operations on the Respiratory System

31.75–32.49

31.75   **Reconstruction of trachea and construction of artificial larynx**
Tracheoplasty with artificial larynx

31.79   **Other repair and plastic operations on trachea**

√4th **31.9**   **Other operations on larynx and trachea**

31.91   **Division of laryngeal nerve**

31.92   **Lysis of adhesions of trachea or larynx**

31.93   **Replacement of laryngeal or tracheal stent**
DEF: Removal and substitution of tubed molding into larynx or trachea.

31.94   **Injection of locally-acting therapeutic substance into trachea**

31.95   **Tracheoesophageal fistulization**
DEF: Creation of passage between trachea and esophagus.

31.98   **Other operations on larynx**
Dilation
Division of congenital web } of larynx
Removal of keel or stent
EXCLUDES   *removal of intraluminal foreign body from larynx without incision (98.14)*
DEF: Dilation: Increasing larynx size by stretching.
DEF: Division of congenital web: Cutting and separating congenital membranes around larynx.
DEF: Removal of keel or stent: Removal of prosthetic device from larynx.

31.99   **Other operations on trachea**
EXCLUDES   *removal of:*
intraluminal foreign body from trachea without incision (98.15)
tracheostomy tube (97.37)
replacement of tracheostomy tube (97.23)
tracheostomy toilette (96.55)

√3rd **32**   **Excision of lung and bronchus**
INCLUDES   rib section
sternotomy
sternum-splitting incision } as operative approach
thoracotomy
Code also any synchronous bronchoplasty (33.48)
DEF: Rib resection: Cutting of ribs to access operative field.
DEF: Sternotomy: Cut through breastbone as an operative approach.
DEF: Sternum-splitting incision: Breaking through breastbone to access operative field.

√4th **32.0**   **Local excision or destruction of lesion or tissue of bronchus**
EXCLUDES   *biopsy of bronchus (33.24-33.25)*
bronchial fistulectomy (33.42)

32.01   **Endoscopic excision or destruction of lesion or tissue of bronchus**

32.09   **Other local excision or destruction of lesion or tissue of bronchus**
EXCLUDES   *that by endoscopic approach (32.01)*

32.1   **Other excision of bronchus**
Resection (wide sleeve) of bronchus
EXCLUDES   *radical dissection [excision] of bronchus (32.6)*
DEF: Resection (wide sleeve) of bronchus: Excision and partial, lengthwise removal of a lung branch.

√4th **32.2**   **Local excision or destruction of lesion or tissue of lung**

32.20   **Thoracoscopic excision of lesion or tissue of lung**
Thoracoscopic wedge resection

32.21   **Plication of emphysematous bleb**
DEF: Stitching of a swollen vesicle into folds or tuck.

32.22   **Lung volume reduction surgery**
DEF: Excision of portion of lung(s) to reduce respiratory effort in moderate to severe emphysema.

32.23   **Open ablation of lung lesion or tissue**

Lung Volume Reduction

Chest wall
Diaphragm (dome-shaped)
Normal lungs
Flattened diaphragm
Lungs with emphysema
Original lung area
Staples
Diaphragm resumes a more domed shape
Lungs after surgery

32.24   **Percutaneous ablation of lung lesion or tissue**

32.25   **Thoracoscopic ablation of lung lesion or tissue**
EXCLUDES   *thoracoscopic excision of lesion or tissue of lung (32.20)*

32.26   **Other and unspecified ablation of lung lesion or tissue**
EXCLUDES   *bronchoscopic bronchial thermoplasty, ablation of smooth airway muscle (32.27)*

32.27   **Bronchoscopic bronchial thermoplasty, ablation of airway smooth muscle**
DEF: A transcatheter radiofrequency (RF)-based technology for severe asthma in which therapeutic heat is applied to the smooth muscle of the tracheobronchial tree and lungs.

32.28   **Endoscopic excision or destruction of lesion or tissue of lung**
EXCLUDES   *ablation of lung lesion or tissue:*
open (32.23)
other (32.26)
percutaneous (32.24)
thoracoscopic (32.25)
biopsy of lung (33.26-33.27)

32.29   **Other local excision or destruction of lesion or tissue of lung**
Resection of lung:
NOS
wedge
EXCLUDES   *ablation of lung lesion or tissue:*
open (32.23)
other (32.26)
percutaneous (32.24)
thoracoscopic (32.25)
biopsy of lung (33.26-33.27)
laser interstitial thermal therapy [LITT] of lesion or tissue of lung under guidance (17.69)
that by endoscopic approach (32.28)
thoracoscopic excision of lesion or tissue of lung (32.20)
wide excision of lesion of lung (32.3)

√4th **32.3**   **Segmental resection of lung**
Partial lobectomy

32.30   **Thoracoscopic segmental resection of lung**

32.39   **Other and unspecified segmental resection of lung**
EXCLUDES   *thoracoscopic segmental resection of lung (32.30)*

√4th **32.4**   **Lobectomy of lung**
Lobectomy with segmental resection of adjacent lobes of lung
EXCLUDES   *that with radical dissection [excision] of thoracic structures (32.6)*

32.41   **Thoracoscopic lobectomy of lung**

32.49   **Other lobectomy of lung**
EXCLUDES   *thoracoscopic lobectomy of lung (32.41)*

✓4ᵗʰ 32.5 Pneumonectomy
    Excision of lung NOS
    Pneumonectomy (with mediastinal dissection)

32.50 Thoracoscopic pneumonectomy

32.59 Other and unspecified pneumonectomy
    EXCLUDES   *thoracoscopic pneumonectomy (32.50)*

32.6 Radical dissection of thoracic structures
    Block [en bloc] dissection of bronchus, lobe of lung, brachial
    plexus, intercostal structure, ribs (transverse process),
    and sympathetic nerves

32.9 Other excision of lung
    EXCLUDES   *biopsy of lung and bronchus (33.24-33.27)*
        pulmonary decortication (34.51)

✓3ʳᵈ 33 Other operations on lung and bronchus
    INCLUDES   rib section
        sternotomy   as operative
        sternum-splitting incision   approach
        thoracotomy

33.0 Incision of bronchus

33.1 Incision of lung
    EXCLUDES   *puncture of lung (33.93)*

✓4ᵗʰ 33.2 Diagnostic procedures on lung and bronchus

33.20 Thoracoscopic lung biopsy
    EXCLUDES   *closed endoscopic biopsy of lung (33.27)*
        closed [percutaneous] [needle] biopsy of
            lung (33.26)
        open biopsy of lung (33.28)

33.21 Bronchoscopy through artificial stoma
    EXCLUDES   *that with biopsy (33.24, 33.27)*
    DEF: Visual exam of lung and its branches via tube
    through artificial opening.

33.22 Fiber-optic bronchoscopy
    EXCLUDES   *that with biopsy (33.24, 33.27)*
    DEF: Exam of lung and bronchus via flexible optical
    instrument for visualization.

33.23 Other bronchoscopy
    EXCLUDES   *that for:*
        aspiration (96.05)
        biopsy (33.24, 33.27)

33.24 Closed [endoscopic] biopsy of bronchus
    Bronchoscopy (fiberoptic) (rigid) with:
        brush biopsy of "lung"
        brushing or washing for specimen collection
        excision (bite) biopsy
    Diagnostic bronchoalveolar lavage [BAL]
    Mini-bronchoalveolar lavage [mini-BAL]
    Transbronchoscopic needle aspiration [TBNA] of
        bronchus
    EXCLUDES   *closed biopsy of lung, other than brush*
            biopsy of "lung" (33.26, 33.27)
        whole lung lavage (33.99)
    DEF: Bronchoalveolar lavage (BAL): Saline is
    introduced into the subsegment of a lobe and
    retrieved using gentle suction; also called 'liquid
    biopsy'.
    DEF: Brush biopsy: Obtaining cell or tissue samples
    via bristled instrument without incision.

33.25 Open biopsy of bronchus
    EXCLUDES   *open biopsy of lung (33.28)*

33.26 Closed [percutaneous] [needle] biopsy of lung
    Fine needle aspiration [FNA] of lung
    Transthoracic needle biopsy of lung [TTNB]
    EXCLUDES   *endoscopic biopsy of lung (33.27)*
        thoracoscopic lung biopsy (33.20)

Bronchoscopy with Bite Biopsy

33.27 Closed endoscopic biopsy of lung
    Fiber-optic (flexible) bronchoscopy with
        fluoroscopic guidance with biopsy
    Transbronchial lung biopsy
    Transbronchoscopic needle aspiration [TBNA] of
        lung
    EXCLUDES   *brush biopsy of "lung" (33.24)*
        percutaneous biopsy of lung (33.26)
        thoracoscopic lung biopsy (33.20)

33.28 Open biopsy of lung

**33.29 Other diagnostic procedures on lung and
    bronchus**
    EXCLUDES   *bronchoalveolar lavage [BAL] (33.24)*
        contrast bronchogram:
            endotracheal (87.31)
            other (87.32)
        endoscopic pulmonary airway flow
            measurement (33.72)
        lung scan (92.15)
        magnetic resonance imaging (88.92)
        microscopic examination of specimen
            from bronchus or lung
            (90.41-90.49)
        routine chest x-ray (87.44)
        ultrasonography of lung (88.73)
        vital capacity determination (89.37)
        x-ray of bronchus or lung NOS (87.49)

✓4ᵗʰ 33.3 Surgical collapse of lung

33.31 Destruction of phrenic nerve for collapse of lung
    DEF: Therapeutic deadening or destruction of
    diaphragmatic nerve to collapse the lung.

33.32 Artificial pneumothorax for collapse of lung
    Thoracotomy for collapse of lung
    DEF: Forcing air or gas into diaphragmatic space to
    achieve therapeutic collapse of lung.
    DEF: Thoracotomy for collapse of lung: Incision into
    chest for therapeutic collapse of lung.

33.33 Pneumoperitoneum for collapse of lung
    DEF: Forcing air or gas into abdominal serous
    membrane to achieve therapeutic collapse of lung.

33.34 Thoracoplasty
    DEF: Removal of ribs for therapeutic collapse of
    lungs.

33.39 Other surgical collapse of lung
    Collapse of lung NOS

✓4ᵗʰ **33.4** **Repair and plastic operation on lung and bronchus**

33.41 **Suture of laceration of bronchus**

33.42 **Closure of bronchial fistula**
Closure of bronchostomy
Fistulectomy:
bronchocutaneous
bronchoesophageal
bronchovisceral
EXCLUDES *closure of fistula:*
bronchomediastinal (34.73)
bronchopleural (34.73)
bronchopleuromediastinal (34.73)
DEF: Closure of bronchostomy: Removal of bronchostomy tube and repair of surgical wound.
DEF: Fistulectomy: Closure of abnormal passage.
Bronchocutaneous: Between skin and lung branch.
Bronchoesophagus: Between esophagus and lung branch.
Bronchovisceral: Between an internal organ and lung branch.

33.43 **Closure of laceration of lung**

33.48 **Other repair and plastic operations on bronchus**

33.49 **Other repair and plastic operations on lung**
EXCLUDES *closure of pleural fistula (34.73)*

✓4ᵗʰ **33.5** **Lung transplant**
Note: To report donor source – *see* codes 00.91-00.93
Code also cardiopulmonary bypass [extracorporeal circulation] [heart-lung machine] [39.61]
EXCLUDES *combined heart-lung transplantation (33.6)*

33.50 **Lung transplantation, not otherwise specified**

33.51 **Unilateral lung transplantation**

33.52 **Bilateral lung transplantation**
Double-lung transplantation
En bloc transplantation
DEF: Sequential excision and implant of both lungs.

33.6 **Combined heart-lung transplantation**
Note: To report donor source – *see* codes 00.91-00.93
Code also cardiopulmonary bypass [extracorporeal circulation] [heart-lung machine] (39.61)

✓4ᵗʰ **33.7** **Other endoscopic procedures in bronchus or lung**
EXCLUDES *insertion of tracheobronchial stent (96.05)*

33.71 **Endoscopic insertion or replacement of bronchial valve(s), single lobe**
Endobronchial airflow redirection valve
Intrabronchial airflow redirection valve
EXCLUDES *endoscopic insertion or replacement of bronchial valve(s), multiple lobes (33.73)*

33.72 **Endoscopic pulmonary airway flow measurement**
Assessment of pulmonary airway flow
Code also any diagnostic or therapeutic procedure, if performed

33.73 **Endoscopic insertion or replacement of bronchial valve(s), multiple lobes**
Endobronchial airflow redirection valve
Intrabronchial airflow redirection valve
EXCLUDES *endoscopic insertion or replacement of bronchial valve(s), single lobe (33.71)*
DEF: Minimally invasive treatment of air leaks resulting from disease, injury, or surgical intervention by the endoscopic placement of more than one bronchial valve.

33.78 **Endoscopic removal of bronchial device(s) or substances**

33.79 **Endoscopic insertion of other bronchial device or substances**
Biologic lung volume reduction NOS (BLVR)

✓4ᵗʰ **33.9** **Other operations on lung and bronchus**

33.91 **Bronchial dilation**

33.92 **Ligation of bronchus**
DEF: Tying off of a lung branch.

33.93 **Puncture of lung**
EXCLUDES *needle biopsy (33.26)*
DEF: Piercing of lung with surgical instrument.

33.98 **Other operations on bronchus**
EXCLUDES *bronchial lavage (96.56)*
removal of intraluminal foreign body from bronchus without incision (98.15)

33.99 **Other operations on lung**
Whole lung lavage
EXCLUDES *other continuous mechanical ventilation (96.70-96.72)*
respiratory therapy (93.90-93.99)

✓3ʳᵈ **34** **Operations on chest wall, pleura, mediastinum, and diaphragm**
EXCLUDES *operations on breast (85.0-85.99)*

✓4ᵗʰ **34.0** **Incision of chest wall and pleura**
EXCLUDES *that as operative approach — omit code*

34.01 **Incision of chest wall**
Extrapleural drainage
EXCLUDES *incision of pleura (34.09)*
DEF: Extrapleural drainage: Incision to drain fluid from external pleura.

34.02 **Exploratory thoracotomy**

34.03 **Reopening of recent thoracotomy site**

34.04 **Insertion of intercostal catheter for drainage**
Chest tube
Closed chest drainage
Revision of intercostal catheter (chest tube) (with lysis of adhesions)
EXCLUDES *thoracoscopic drainage of pleural cavity (34.06)*
DEF: Insertion of catheter between ribs for drainage.

34.05 **Creation of pleuroperitoneal shunt**

34.06 **Thoracoscopic drainage of pleural cavity**
Evacuation of empyema

34.09 **Other incision of pleura**
Creation of pleural window for drainage
Intercostal stab
Open chest drainage
EXCLUDES *thoracoscopy (34.21)*
thoracotomy for collapse of lung (33.32)
DEF: Creation of pleural window: Creation of circumscribed drainage hole in serous membrane of chest.
DEF: Intercostal stab: Creation of penetrating stab wound between ribs.
DEF: Open chest drainage: Insertion of tube through ribs and serous membrane of chest for drainage.

34.1 **Incision of mediastinum**
Code also any biopsy, if performed
EXCLUDES *mediastinoscopy (34.22)*
mediastinotomy associated with pneumonectomy (32.5)

✓4ᵗʰ **34.2** **Diagnostic procedures on chest wall, pleura, mediastinum, and diaphragm**

34.20 **Thoracoscopic pleural biopsy**

34.21 **Transpleural thoracoscopy**
DEF: Exam of chest through serous membrane using scope.

34.22 **Mediastinoscopy**
Code also any biopsy, if performed
DEF: Exam of lung cavity and heart using scope.

34.23 **Biopsy of chest wall**

34.24　Other pleural biopsy
　　EXCLUDES　*thoracoscopic pleural biopsy (34.20)*

34.25　Closed [percutaneous] [needle] biopsy of mediastinum

34.26　Open biopsy of mediastinum

34.27　Biopsy of diaphragm

34.28　Other diagnostic procedures on chest wall, pleura, and diaphragm
　　EXCLUDES　*angiocardiography (88.50-88.58)*
　　　　　　　aortography (88.42)
　　　　　　　arteriography of:
　　　　　　　　intrathoracic vessels NEC (88.44)
　　　　　　　　pulmonary arteries (88.43)
　　　　　　　microscopic examination of specimen from chest wall, pleura, and diaphragm (90.41-90.49)
　　　　　　　phlebography of:
　　　　　　　　intrathoracic vessels NEC (88.63)
　　　　　　　　pulmonary veins (88.62)
　　　　　　　radiological examinations of thorax:
　　　　　　　　C.A.T. scan (87.41)
　　　　　　　　diaphragmatic x-ray (87.49)
　　　　　　　　intrathoracic lymphangiogram (87.34)
　　　　　　　　routine chest x-ray (87.44)
　　　　　　　　sinogram of chest wall (87.38)
　　　　　　　　soft tissue x-ray of chest wall NEC (87.39)
　　　　　　　　tomogram of thorax NEC (87.42)
　　　　　　　　ultrasonography of thorax (88.73)

34.29　Other diagnostic procedures on mediastinum
　　EXCLUDES　*mediastinal:*
　　　　　　　　pneumogram (87.33)
　　　　　　　　x-ray NEC (87.49)

34.3　Excision or destruction of lesion or tissue of mediastinum
　　EXCLUDES　*biopsy of mediastinum (34.25-34.26)*
　　　　　　　mediastinal fistulectomy (34.73)

34.4　Excision or destruction of lesion of chest wall
　　Excision of lesion of chest wall NOS (with excision of ribs)
　　EXCLUDES　*biopsy of chest wall (34.23)*
　　　　　　　costectomy not incidental to thoracic procedure (77.91)
　　　　　　　excision of lesion of:
　　　　　　　　breast (85.20-85.25)
　　　　　　　　cartilage (80.89)
　　　　　　　　skin (86.2-86.3)
　　　　　　　fistulectomy (34.73)

✓4th **34.5　Pleurectomy**

34.51　Decortication of lung
　　EXCLUDES　*thoracoscopic decortication of lung (34.52)*
　　DEF: Removal of thickened serous membrane for lung expansion.

34.52　Thoracoscopic decortication of lung

34.59　Other excision of pleura
　　Excision of pleural lesion
　　EXCLUDES　*biopsy of pleura (34.24)*
　　　　　　　pleural fistulectomy (34.73)

34.6　Scarification of pleura
　　Pleurosclerosis
　　EXCLUDES　*injection of sclerosing agent (34.92)*
　　DEF: Destruction of fluid-secreting serous membrane cells of chest.

✓4th **34.7　Repair of chest wall**

34.71　Suture of laceration of chest wall
　　EXCLUDES　*suture of skin and subcutaneous tissue alone (86.59)*

34.72　Closure of thoracostomy

34.73　Closure of other fistula of thorax
　　Closure of:
　　　bronchopleural ⎫
　　　bronchopleurocutaneous ⎬ fistula
　　　bronchopleuromediastinal ⎭

34.74　Repair of pectus deformity
　　Repair of:
　　　pectus carinatum ⎫ (with implant)
　　　pectus excavatum ⎭
　　DEF: Pectus carinatum repair: Restoration of prominent chest bone defect with implant.
　　DEF: Pectus excavatum: Restoration of depressed chest bone defect with implant.

34.79　Other repair of chest wall
　　Repair of chest wall NOS

✓4th **34.8　Operations on diaphragm**

34.81　Excision of lesion or tissue of diaphragm
　　EXCLUDES　*biopsy of diaphragm (34.27)*

34.82　Suture of laceration of diaphragm

34.83　Closure of fistula of diaphragm
　　Thoracicoabdominal ⎫
　　Thoracicogastric ⎬ fistulectomy
　　Thoracicointestinal ⎭
　　DEF: Fistulectomy: Closure of abnormal passage.

34.84　Other repair of diaphragm
　　EXCLUDES　*repair of diaphragmatic hernia (53.7-53.82)*

34.85　Implantation of diaphragmatic pacemaker

34.89　Other operations on diaphragm

✓4th **34.9　Other operations on thorax**

34.91　Thoracentesis
　　DEF: Puncture of pleural cavity for fluid aspiration, also called pleurocentesis.

34.92　Injection into thoracic cavity
　　Chemical pleurodesis
　　Injection of cytotoxic agent or tetracycline
　　Instillation into thoracic cavity
　　Requires additional code for any cancer chemotherapeutic substance (99.25)
　　EXCLUDES　*that for collapse of lung (33.32)*
　　DEF: Chemical pleurodesis: Tetracycline hydrochloride injections to create adhesions between parietal and visceral pleura for treatment of pleural effusion.

34.93　Repair of pleura

34.99　Other
　　EXCLUDES　*removal of:*
　　　　　　　　mediastinal drain (97.42)
　　　　　　　　sutures (97.43)
　　　　　　　　thoracotomy tube (97.41)
　　DEF: Pleural tent: Extrapleural mobilization of parietal pleura that allows draping of membrane over visceral pleura to eliminate intrapleural dead space and seal visceral pleura.

7. OPERATIONS ON THE CARDIOVASCULAR SYSTEM (35-39)

√3ᵈ **35　Operations on valves and septa of heart**

INCLUDES　　sternotomy (median)
　　　　　　　　　　　(tranverse)　　} as operative approach
　　　　　　　　thoracotomy

Code also any cardiopulmonary bypass [extracorporeal circulation] [heart-lung machine] (39.61)

√4ᵗʰ **35.0　Closed heart valvotomy or transcatheter replacement of heart valve**

　　EXCLUDES　　*percutaneous (balloon) valvuloplasty (35.96)*
　　DEF: Incision into valve to restore function.

35.00　Closed heart valvotomy, unspecified valve

35.01　Closed heart valvotomy, aortic valve

35.02　Closed heart valvotomy, mitral valve

35.03　Closed heart valvotomy, pulmonary valve

35.04　Closed heart valvotomy, tricuspid valve

35.05　Endovascular replacement of aortic valve
　　　　NOTE: Includes that with any balloon valvuloplasty; do not code separately
　　　　Implantation of transcatheter aortic valve
　　　　Replacement of aortic valve with tissue graft (autograft) (bioprosthetic) (heterograft) (homograft):
　　　　　　transarterial approach
　　　　　　transfemoral approach
　　　　TAVI (transcatheter aortic valve implantation)
　　　　TAVR (transcatheter aortic valve replacement)
　　　　EXCLUDES　　*open and other replacement of heart valve (35.20-35.28)*

35.06　Transapical replacement of aortic valve
　　　　NOTE: Includes that with any balloon valvuloplasty; do not code separately
　　　　Implantation of transcatheter aortic valve
　　　　Replacement of aortic valve with tissue graft (autograft) (bioprosthetic) (heterograft) (homograft):
　　　　　　intercostal approach
　　　　　　transventricular approach
　　　　That via transthoracic exposure, i.e. thoracotomy, sternotomy, or subxiphoid approach
　　　　EXCLUDES　　*open and other replacement of heart valve (35.20-35.28)*

35.07　Endovascular replacement of pulmonary valve
　　　　NOTE: Includes that with any balloon valvuloplasty; do not code separately
　　　　Implantation of transcatheter pulmonary valve
　　　　PPVI (percutaneous pulmonary valve implantation)
　　　　Replacement of pulmonary valve:
　　　　　　transfemoral approach
　　　　　　transvenous approach
　　　　That within previously created right ventricle-to-pulmonary artery conduit
　　　　TPVI (transcatheter pulmonary valve implantation)
　　　　EXCLUDES　　*open and other replacement of heart valve (35.20-35.28)*

35.08　Transapical replacement of pulmonary valve
　　　　NOTE: Includes that with any balloon valvuloplasty; do not code separately
　　　　Implantation of transcatheter pulmonary valve
　　　　Replacement of pulmonary valve:
　　　　　　intercostal approach
　　　　　　transventricular approach
　　　　That via transthoracic exposure, i.e. thoracotomy, sternotomy, or subxiphoid approach
　　　　EXCLUDES　　*open and other replacement of heart valve (35.20-35.28)*

35.09　Endovascular replacement of unspecified heart valve
　　　　NOTE: Includes that with any balloon valvuloplasty; do not code separately
　　　　Replacement of valve via:
　　　　　　intercostal approach
　　　　　　transventricular approach
　　　　EXCLUDES　　*open and other replacement of heart valve (35.20-35.28)*

√4ᵗʰ **35.1　Open heart valvuloplasty without replacement**

　　INCLUDES　　open heart valvotomy
Code also cardiopulmonary bypass, if performed [extracorporeal circulation] [heart-lung machine] (39.61)
　　EXCLUDES　　*that associated with repair of:*
　　　　　　endocardial cushion defect (35.54,35.63,35.73)
　　　　　　percutaneous (balloon) valvuloplasty (35.96)
　　　　　　valvular defect associated with atrial and ventricular septal defects (35.54, 35.63, 35.73)
　　DEF: Incision into heart for plastic valve repair without replacing valve.

35.10　Open heart valvuloplasty without replacement, unspecified valve

35.11　Open heart valvuloplasty of aortic valve

35.12　Open heart valvuloplasty of mitral valve without replacement

35.13　Open heart valvuloplasty of pulmonary valve without replacement

35.14　Open heart valvuloplasty of tricuspid valve without replacemen

√4ᵗʰ **35.2　Open and other replacement of heart valve**

　　INCLUDES　　excision of heart valve with replacement
Code also cardiopulmonary bypass [extracorporeal circulation] [heart-lung machine] (39.61)
　　EXCLUDES　　*that associated with repair of:*
　　　　　　endocardial cushion defect (35.54,35.63, 35.73)
　　　　　　valvular defect associated with atrial and ventricular septal defects (35.54, 35.63, 35.73)
　　　　　　transapical replacement of heart valve (35.06, 35.08)
　　　　　　transcatheter replacement of heart valve (35.05, 35.07)
　　DEF: Removal and replacement of valve with tissue from patient, animal, other human, or prosthetic (synthetic) valve.

35.20　Open and other replacement of unspecified heart valve
　　　　That with tissue graft or prosthetic implant
　　　　EXCLUDES　　*endovascular replacement of unspecified heart valve (35.09)*

35.21　Open and other replacement of aortic valve with tissue graft
　　　　Includes that by:
　　　　　　autograft
　　　　　　heterograft
　　　　　　homograft
　　　　EXCLUDES　　*endovascular replacement of aortic valve (35.05)*
　　　　　　transapical replacement of aortic valve (35.06)

35.22　Open and other replacement of aortic valve
　　　　Replacement of aortic valve, NOS
　　　　That with prosthetic (partial) (synthetic) (total)
　　　　EXCLUDES　　*endovascular replacement of aortic valve (35.05)*
　　　　　　transapical replacement of aortic valve (35.06)

Operations on the Cardiovascular System

35.23–35.55

35.23　Open and other replacement of mitral valve with tissue graft
Includes that by:
autograft
heterograft
homograft

35.24　Open and other replacement of mitral valve
Replacement of mitral valve, NOS
That with prosthetic (partial) (synthetic) (total)
EXCLUDES　percutaneous repair with implant or leaflet clip (35.97)

35.25　Open and other replacement of pulmonary valve with tissue graft
Includes that by:
autograft
heterograft
homograft
EXCLUDES　endovascular replacement of pulmonary valve (35.07)
transapical replacement of pulmonary valve (35.08)

35.26　Open and other replacement of pulmonary valve
Replacement of pulmonary valve, NOS
That with prosthetic (partial) (synthetic) (total)
EXCLUDES　endovascular replacement of pulmonary valve (35.07)
transapical replacement of pulmonary valve (35.08)

35.27　Open and other replacement of tricuspid valve with tissue graft
Includes that by:
autograft
heterograft
homograft

35.28　Open and other replacement of tricuspid valve
Replacement of tricuspid valve, NOS
That with prosthetic (partial) (synthetic) (total)

√4ᵗʰ　35.3　Operations on structures adjacent to heart valves
Code also cardiopulmonary bypass [extracorporeal circulation] [heart-lung machine] (39.61)

35.31　Operations on papillary muscle
Division
Reattachment } of papillary muscle
Repair

35.32　Operations on chordae tendineae
Division
Repair } chordae tendineae

35.33　Annuloplasty
Plication of annulus
DEF: Plication of annulus: Tuck stitched in valvular ring for tightening.

35.34　Infundibulectomy
Right ventricular infundibulectomy
DEF: Infundibulectomy: Excision of funnel-shaped heart passage.
DEF: Right ventricular infundibulectomy: Excision of funnel-shaped passage in right upper heart chamber.

35.35　Operations on trabeculae carneae cordis
Division
Excision } of trabeculae carneae cordis
Excision of aortic subvalvular ring

35.39　Operations on other structures adjacent to valves of heart
Repair of sinus of Valsalva (aneurysm)

√4ᵗʰ　35.4　Production of septal defect in heart

35.41　Enlargement of existing atrial septal defect
Rashkind procedure
Septostomy (atrial) (balloon)
DEF: Enlargement of partition wall defect in lower heart chamber to improve function.
DEF: Rashkind procedure: Enlargement of partition wall defect between the two lower heart chambers by balloon catheter.

35.42　Creation of septal defect in heart
Blalock-Hanlon operation
DEF: Blalock-Hanlon operation: Removal of partition wall defect in lower heart chamber.

√4ᵗʰ　35.5　Repair of atrial and ventricular septa with prosthesis
INCLUDES　repair of septa with synthetic implant or patch
Code also cardiopulmonary bypass [extracorporeal circulation] [heart-lung machine] (39.61)

35.50　Repair of unspecified septal defect of heart with prosthesis
EXCLUDES　that associated with repair of:
endocardial cushion defect (35.54)
septal defect associated with valvular defect (35.54)

35.51　Repair of atrial septal defect with prosthesis, open technique
Atrioseptoplasty
Correction of atrial septal defect
Repair: } with prosthesis
foramen ovale (patent)
ostium secundum defect
EXCLUDES　that associated with repair of:
atrial septal defect associated with valvular and ventricular septal defects (35.54)
endocardial cushion defect (35.54)
DEF: Repair of opening or weakening in septum separating the atria; prosthesis implanted through heart incision.

35.52　Repair of atrial septal defect with prosthesis, closed technique
Insertion of atrial septal umbrella [King-Mills]
DEF: Correction of partition wall defect in lower heart chamber with artificial material, without incision into heart.
DEF: Insertion of atrial septal umbrella (King-Mills): Correction of partition wall defect in lower heart chamber with atrial septal umbrella.

35.53　Repair of ventricular septal defect with prosthesis, open technique
Correction of ventricular septal defect } with prosthesis
Repair of supracristal defect
EXCLUDES　that associated with repair of:
endocardial cushion defect (35.54)
ventricular defect associated with valvular and atrial septal defects (35.54)

35.54　Repair of endocardial cushion defect with prosthesis
Repair:
atrioventricular canal
ostium primum defect
valvular defect } with prosthesis
associated with } (grafted to
atrial and } septa)
ventricular septal
defects
EXCLUDES　repair of isolated:
atrial septal defect (35.51-35.52)
valvular defect (35.20, 35.22, 35.24, 35.26, 35.28)
ventricular septal defect (35.53)

35.55　Repair of ventricular septal defect with prosthesis, closed technique

☑4ᵗʰ 35.6 Repair of atrial and ventricular septa with tissue graft
Code also cardiopulmonary bypass [extracorporeal circulation] [heart-lung machine] (39.61)

35.60 Repair of unspecified septal defect of heart with tissue graft
EXCLUDES *that associated with repair of:*
endocardial cushion defect (35.63)
septal defect associated with valvular defect (35.63)

35.61 Repair of atrial septal defect with tissue graft
Atrioseptoplasty
Correction of atrial septal defect } with tissue graft
Repair:
foramen ovale (patent)
ostium secundum defect
EXCLUDES *that associated with repair of:*
atrial septal defect associated with valvular and ventricular septal defects (35.63)
endocardial cushion defect (35.63)

35.62 Repair of ventricular septal defect with tissue graft
Correction of ventricular
septal defect } with tissue graft
Repair of supracristal defect
EXCLUDES *that associated with repair of:*
endocardial cushion defect (35.63)
ventricular defect associated with valvular and atrial septal defects (35.63)

35.63 Repair of endocardial cushion defect with tissue graft
Repair of:
artrioventricular canal
ostium primum defect } with tissue graft
valvular defect associated with atrial and ventricular septal defects
EXCLUDES *repair of isolated:*
atrial septal defect (35.61)
valvular defect (35.20-35.21, 35.23, 35.25, 35.27)
ventricular septal defect (35.62)

☑4ᵗʰ 35.7 Other and unspecified repair of atrial and ventricular septa
Code also cardiopulmonary bypass [extracorporeal circulation] [heart-lung machine] (39.61)

35.70 Other and unspecified repair of unspecified septal defect of heart
Repair of septal defect NOS
EXCLUDES *that associated with repair of:*
endocardial cushion defect (35.73)
septal defect associated with valvular defect (35.73)

35.71 Other and unspecified repair of atrial septal defect
Repair NOS: Repair NOS:
atrial septum   ostium secundum defect
foramen ovale (patent)
EXCLUDES *that associated with repair of:*
atrial septal defect associated with valvular and ventricular septal defects (35.73)
endocardial cushion defect (35.73)

35.72 Other and unspecified repair of ventricular septal defect
Repair NOS:
supracristal defect
ventricular septum
EXCLUDES *that associated with repair of:*
endocardial cushion defect (35.73)
ventricular septal defect associated with valvular and atrial septal defects (35.73)

35.73 Other and unspecified repair of endocardial cushion defect
Repair NOS:
atrioventricular canal
ostium primum defect
valvular defect associated with atrial and ventricular septal defects
EXCLUDES *repair of isolated:*
atrial septal defect (35.71)
valvular defect (35.20, 35.22, 35.24, 35.26, 35.28)
ventricular septal defect (35.72)

☑4ᵗʰ 35.8 Total repair of certain congenital cardiac anomalies
Note: For partial repair of defect [e.g. repair of atrial septal defect in tetralogy of Fallot] – code to specific procedure

35.81 Total repair of tetralogy of Fallot
One-stage total correction of tetralogy of Fallot with or without:
commissurotomy of pulmonary valve
infundibulectomy
outflow tract prosthesis
patch graft of outflow tract
prosthetic tube for pulmonary artery
repair of ventricular septal defect (with prosthesis)
take-down of previous systemic-pulmonary artery anastomosis

35.82 Total repair of total anomalous pulmonary venous connection
One-stage total correction of total anomalous pulmonary venous connection with or without:
anastomosis between (horizontal) common pulmonary trunk and posterior wall of left atrium (side-to-side)
enlargement of foramen ovale
incision [excision] of common wall between posterior left atrium and coronary sinus and roofing of resultant defect with patch graft (synthetic)
ligation of venous connection (descending anomalous vein) (to left innominate vein) (to superior vena cava)
repair of atrial septal defect (with prosthesis)

35.83 Total repair of truncus arteriosus
One-stage total correction of truncus arteriosus with or without:
construction (with aortic homograft) (with prosthesis) of a pulmonary artery placed from right ventricle to arteries supplying the lung
ligation of connections between aorta and pulmonary artery
repair of ventricular septal defect (with prosthesis)

35.84 Total correction of transposition of great vessels, not elsewhere classified
Arterial switch operation [Jatene]
Total correction of transposition of great arteries at the arterial level by switching the great arteries, including the left or both coronary arteries, implanted in the wall of the pulmonary artery
EXCLUDES *baffle operation [Mustard] [Senning] (35.91)*
creation of shunt between right ventricle and pulmonary artery [Rastelli] (35.92)

Operations on the Cardiovascular System

35.9–36.06

☑4ᵗʰ **35.9　Other operations on valves and septa of heart**
Code also cardiopulmonary bypass, if performed [extracorporeal circulation] [heart-lung machine] (39.61)

35.91　Interatrial transposition of venous return
Baffle:
  atrial
  interatrial
Mustard's operation
Resection of atrial septum and insertion of patch to direct systemic venous return to tricuspid valve and pulmonary venous return to mitral valve

DEF: Atrial baffle: Correction of venous flow of abnormal or deviated lower heart chamber.

DEF: Interatrial baffle: Correction of venous flow between abnormal lower heart chambers.

DEF: Mustard's operation: Creates intra-atrial baffle using pericardial tissue to correct transposition of the great vessels.

35.92　Creation of conduit between right ventricle and pulmonary artery
Creation of shunt between right ventricle and (distal) pulmonary artery
EXCLUDES　that associated with total repair of truncus arteriosus (35.83)

35.93　Creation of conduit between left ventricle and aorta
Creation of apicoaortic shunt
Shunt between apex of left ventricle and aorta

35.94　Creation of conduit between atrium and pulmonary artery
Fontan procedure

35.95　Revision of corrective procedure on heart
Replacement of prosthetic heart valve poppet
Resuture of prosthesis of:
  septum
  valve
EXCLUDES　complete revision – code to specific procedure
replacement of prosthesis or graft of:
  septum (35.50-35.63)
  valve (35.20-35.28)

DEF: Replacement of prosthetic heart valve poppet: Removal and replacement of valve-supporting prosthesis.

DEF: Resuture of prosthesis of septum: Restitching of prosthesis in partition wall.

DEF: Resuture of prosthesis of valve: Restitching of prosthetic valve.

35.96　Percutaneous balloon valvuloplasty
Balloon dilation of valve
EXCLUDES　endovascular replacement of heart valve (35.05, 35.07)
mitral valve repair with implant (35.97)
transapical replacement of heart valve (35.06, 35.08)

DEF: Percutaneous balloon valvuloplasty: Repair of valve with inflatable catheter.

35.97　Percutaneous mitral valve repair with implant
Endovascular mitral valve repair
Implantation of mitral valve leaflet clip
Transcatheter mitral valve repair
Code also any transesophageal echocardiography [TEE] (88.72)
EXCLUDES　percutaneous balloon valvuloplasty (35.96)

35.98　Other operations on septa of heart

35.99　Other operations on valves of heart

☑3ᵗʰ **36　Operations on vessels of heart**
INCLUDES　sternotomy (median)
  (transverse)
  thoracotomy
  } as operative approach
Code also any:
  injection or infusion of platelet inhibitor (99.20)
  injection or infusion of thrombolytic agent (99.10)
Code also cardiopulmonary bypass, if performed [extra- corporeal circulation] [heart-lung machine] (39.61)

☑4ᵗʰ **36.0　Removal of coronary artery obstruction and insertion of stent(s)**

36.03　Open chest coronary artery angioplasty
Coronary (artery):
  endarterectomy (with patch graft)
  thromboendarterectomy (with patch graft)
Open surgery for direct relief of coronary artery obstruction
Code also any:
  insertion of drug-eluting coronary stent(s) (36.07)
  insertion of non-drug-eluting coronary stent(s) (36.06)
  number of vascular stents inserted (00.45-00.48)
  number of vessels treated (00.40-00.43)
  procedure on vessel bifurcation (00.44)
EXCLUDES　that with coronary artery bypass graft (36.10-36.19)

DEF: Endarterectomy (with patch graft): Excision of thickened material within coronary artery; repair with patch graft.

DEF: Thromboendarterectomy (with patch graft): Excision of blood clot and thickened material within coronary artery; repair with patch graft.

DEF: Open surgery for direct relief of coronary artery obstruction: Removal of coronary artery obstruction through opening in chest.

36.04　Intracoronary artery thrombolytic infusion
Enzyme infusion
Platelet inhibitor
That by direct coronary artery injection, infusion, or catheterization
EXCLUDES　infusion of platelet inhibitor (99.20)
infusion of thrombolytic agent (99.10)
that associated with any procedure in 36.03

DEF: Infusion of clot breaking solution into intracoronary artery.

36.06　Insertion of non-drug-eluting coronary atery stent(s)
Bare stent(s)　　　　　　Endograft(s)
Bonded stent(s)　　　　　Endovascular graft(s)
Drug-coated stent(s),e.g.,　Stent graft(s)
  heparin coated
Code also any:
  number of vascular stents inserted (00.45-00.48)
  number of vessels treated (00.40-00.43)
  open chest coronary artery angioplasty (36.03)
  percutaneous transluminal coronary angioplasty [PTCA] (00.66)
  procedure on vessel bifurcation (00.44)
  transluminal coronary atherectomy (17.55)
EXCLUDES　insertion of drug-eluting coronary artery stent(s) (36.07)

DEF: Percutaneous implant of metal stent via catheter, to enlarge, maintain lumen size of coronary artery.

36.07   **Insertion of drug-eluting coronary artery stent(s)**
     Endograft(s)   Stent graft(s)
     Endovascular graft(s)
     Code also any:
       number of vascular stents inserted (00.45-00.48)
       number of vessels treated (00.40-00.43)
       open chest coronary artery angioplasty (36.03)
       percutaneous transluminal coronary angioplasty
         [PTCA] (00.66)
       procedure on vessel bifurcation (00.44)
       transluminal coronary atherectomy (17.55)
       EXCLUDES   *drug-coated stents, e.g., heparin coated*
           (36.06)
           insertion of non-drug-eluting coronary
           artery stent(s) (36.06)

     DEF: Drug-eluting stent technology developed to prevent the accumulation of scar tissue that can narrow reopened coronary arteries. A special polymer is used to coat the drug onto the stent, which slowly releases into the coronary artery wall tissue.

36.09   **Other removal of coronary artery obstruction**
     Coronary angioplasty NOS
     Code also any:
       number of vascular stents inserted (00.45-00.48)
       number of vessels treated (00.40-00.43)
       procedure on vessel bifurcation (00.44)
       EXCLUDES   *that by open angioplasty (36.03)*
           that by percutaneous transluminal
           coronary angioplasty [PTCA]
           (00.66)
           transluminal coronary atherectomy
           (17.55)

✓4ᵗʰ   **36.1**   **Bypass anastomosis for heart revascularization**
     Note: Do not assign codes from series 00.40-00.43 with codes from series 36.10-36.19
     Code also:
       cardiopulmonary bypass [extracorporeal circulation] [heart-lung machine] (39.61)
       pressurized treatment of venous bypass graft [conduit] with pharmaceutical substance, if performed (00.16)

     DEF: Insertion of alternate vessel to bypass blocked coronary artery, correct coronary blood flow.

36.10   **Aortocoronary bypass for heart revascularization, not otherwise specified**
     Direct revascularization:
       cardiac
       coronary   } with catheter stent,
       hear muscle   prosthesis, or vein
       myocardial   graft
     Heart revascularization NOS

36.11   **Aorto)coronary bypass of one coronary artery**

36.12   **(Aorto)coronary bypass of two coronary arteries**

36.13   **(Aorto)coronary bypass of three coronary arteries**

36.14   **(Aorto)coronary bypass of four or more coronary arteries**

36.15   **Single internal mammary-coronary artery bypass**
     Anastomosis (single):
       mammary artery to coronary artery
       thoracic artery to coronary artery

36.16   **Double internal mammary-coronary artery bypass**
     Anastomosis, double:
       mammary artery to coronary artery
       thoracic artery to coronary artery

36.17   **Abdominal-coronary artery bypass**
     Anastomosis:
       gastroepiploic artery to coronary artery

36.19   **Other bypass anastomosis for heart revascularization**

Coronary Bypass

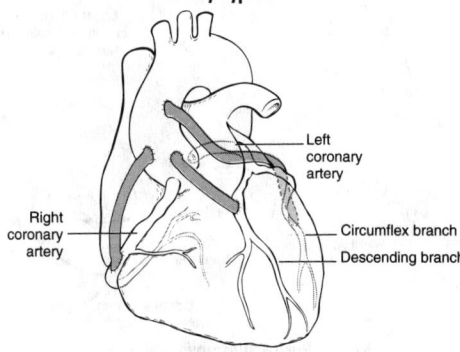

Left coronary artery
Right coronary artery
Circumflex branch
Descending branch

36.2   **Heart revascularization by arterial implant**
     Implantation of:
       aortic branches [ascending aortic branches] into heart muscle
       blood vessels into myocardium
       internal mammary artery [internal thoracic artery] into:
         heart muscle
         myocardium
         ventricle
         ventricular wall
     Indirect heart revascularization NOS

✓4ᵗʰ   **36.3**   **Other heart revascularization**

36.31   **Open chest transmyocardial revascularization**
     DEF: Transmyocardial revascularization (TMR): Laser creation of channels through myocardium allows oxygenated blood flow from sinusoids to myocardial tissue.

36.32   **Other transmyocardial revascularization**

36.33   **Endoscopic transmyocardial revascularization**
     Thoracoscopic transmyocardial revascularization

36.34   **Percutaneous transmyocardial revascularization**
     Endovascular transmyocardial revascularization

36.39   **Other heart revascularization**
     Abrasion of epicardium   Myocardial graft:
     Cardio-omentopexy   mediastinal fat
     Intrapericardial poudrage   omentum
                       pectoral muscles

     DEF: Cardio-omentopexy: Suture of omentum segment to heart after drawing segment through incision in diaphragm to improve blood supply.
     DEF: Intrapericardial poudrage: Application of powder to heart lining to promote fusion.

✓4ᵗʰ   **36.9**   **Other operations on vessels of heart**
     Code also cardiopulmonary bypass [extracorporeal circulation] [heart-lung machine] (39.61)

36.91   **Repair of aneurysm of coronary vessel**

36.99   **Other operations on vessels of heart**
     Exploration
     Incision   } of coronary artery
     Ligation
     Repair of arteriovenous fistula

✓3ʳᵈ   **37**   **Other operations on heart and pericardium**
     Code also any injection or infusion of platelet inhibitor (99.20)

37.0   **Pericardiocentesis**
     DEF: Puncture of the heart lining to withdraw fluid.

✓4ᵗʰ   **37.1**   **Cardiotomy and pericardiotomy**
     Code also cardiopulmonary bypass [extracorporeal circulation] [heart-lung machine] (39.61)

37.10   **Incision of heart, not otherwise specified**
     Cardiolysis NOS

37.11   **Cardiotomy**
     Incision of: Incision of:
       atrium   myocardium
       endocardium   ventricle

Operations on the Cardiovascular System

37.12–37.33

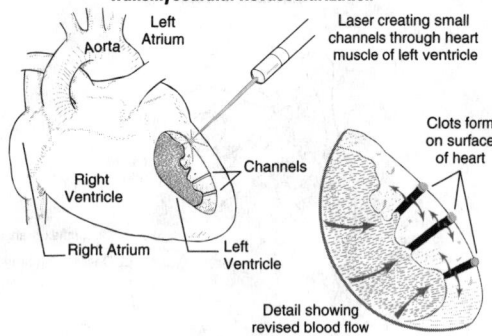

Transmyocardial Revascularization

Left Atrium

Aorta

Laser creating small channels through heart muscle of left ventricle

Right Ventricle

Channels

Clots form on surface of heart

Right Atrium

Left Ventricle

Detail showing revised blood flow

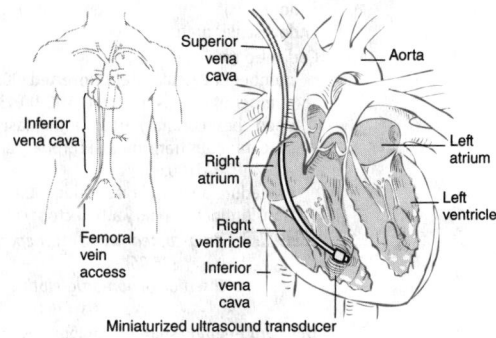

Intracardiac Echocardiography

Superior vena cava

Aorta

Inferior vena cava

Right atrium

Left atrium

Femoral vein access

Right ventricle

Left ventricle

Inferior vena cava

Miniaturized ultrasound transducer

37.12 Pericardiotomy
Pericardial window operation
Pericardiolysis
Pericardiotomy

DEF: Pericardial window operation: Incision into heart lining for drainage.

DEF: Pericardiolysis: Destruction of heart tissue lining.

✓4ᵗʰ **37.2 Diagnostic procedures on heart and pericardium**

37.20 Non-invasive programmed electrical stimulation [NIPS]

EXCLUDES catheter based invasive electro-physiologic testing (37.26)
device interrogation only without arrhythmia induction (bedside check) (89.45-89.49)
that as part of intraoperative testing — omit code

DEF: Non-invasive testing of a previously implanted cardioverter-defibrillator to ensure proper lead placement and system function.

37.21 Right heart cardiac catheterization
Cardiac catheterization NOS

EXCLUDES that with catheterization of left heart (37.23)

37.22 Left heart cardiac catheterization

EXCLUDES that with catheterization of right heart (37.23)

37.23 Combined right and left heart cardiac catheterization

37.24 Biopsy of pericardium

37.25 Biopsy of heart

37.26 Catheter based invasive electrophysiologic testing
Electrophysiologic studies [EPS]
Code also any concomitant procedure

EXCLUDES device interrogation only without arrhythmia induction (bedside check) (89.45-89.49)
His bundle recording (37.29)
non-invasive programmed electrical stimulation (NIPS) (37.20)
that as part of intraoperative testing — omit code

DEF: Diagnostic mapping and measurement of intracardiac electrical activity; requires inserting three to six catheters into heart blood vessels and positioning catheters under fluoroscopic guidance to determine site of the tachycardia or abnormal impulse pathway; may also be used to terminate arrhythmias.

37.27 Cardiac mapping
Code also any concomitant procedure

EXCLUDES electrocardiogram (89.52)
His bundle recording (37.29)

37.28 Intracardiac echocardiography
Echocardiography of heart chambers
ICE
Code also any synchronous Doppler flow mapping (88.72)

EXCLUDES intravascular imaging of coronary vessels (intravascular ultra-sound) (IVUS) (00.24)

DEF: Creation of a two-dimensional graphic of heart using endoscopic echocardiographic equipment.

37.29 Other diagnostic procedures on heart and pericardium

EXCLUDES angiocardiography (88.50-88.58)
cardiac function tests (89.41-89.69)
cardiovascular radioisotopic scan and function study (92.05)
coronary arteriography (88.55-88.57)
diagnostic pericardiocentesis (37.0)
diagnostic ultrasound of heart (88.72)
x-ray of heart (87.49)

✓4ᵗʰ **37.3 Pericardiectomy and excision of lesion of heart**
Code also cardiopulmonary bypass [extracorporeal circulation] [heart-lung machine], if performed (39.61)

37.31 Pericardiectomy
Excision of:
adhesions of pericardium
constricting scar of:
epicardium
pericardium

DEF: Excision of a portion of heart lining.

37.32 Excision of aneurysm of heart
Repair of aneurysm of heart

37.33 Excision or destruction of other lesion or tissue of heart, open approach
Ablation or incision of heart tissue (cryoablation) (electrocurrent) (laser) (microwave) (radiofrequency) (resection) (ultrasound), open chest approach
Cox-maze procedure
Maze procedure
That by median sternotomy
That by thoracotomy without use of thoracoscope

EXCLUDES ablation, excision or destruction of lesion or tissue of heart:
endovascular approach (37.34)
thoracoscopic approach (37.37)
excision or destruction of left atrial appendage (LAA) (37.36)

Ventricular Reduction Surgery

Enlarged Heart

Total Internal Biventricular Heart Replacement System

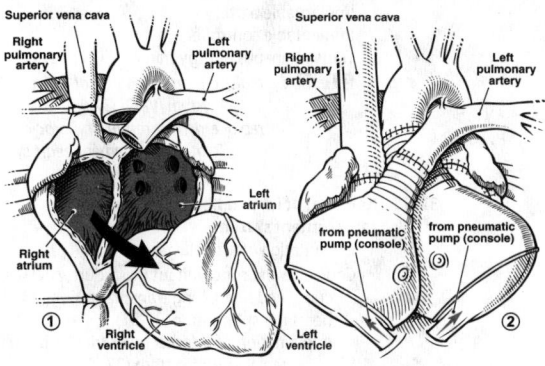

37.34 Excision or destruction of other lesion or tissue of heart, endovascular approach

Ablation of heart tissue (cryoablation) (electrocurrent) (laser) (microwave) (radiofrequency) (ultrasound), via peripherally inserted catheter

Modified maze procedure, percutaneous approach

EXCLUDES *ablation, excision or destruction of lesion of tissue of heart:*
open approach (37.33)
thoracoscopic approach (37.37)

DEF: Destruction of heart tissue or lesion by freezing, electric current or resection.

37.35 Partial ventriculectomy

Ventricular reduction surgery
Ventricular remodeling

Code also any synchronous:
mitral valve repair (35.02, 35.12)
mitral valve replacement (35.23-35.24)

DEF: Removal of elliptical slice of ventricle between anterior and posterior papillary muscle; also called Batiste operation.

37.36 Excision, destruction, or exclusion of left atrial appendage [LAA]

INCLUDES thoracoscopic approach, minithoracotomy approach, percutaneous approach, endovascular approach, or subxiphoid approach

Clipping of left atrial appendage
Oversewing of left atrial appendage
Stapling of left atrial appendage
That by fastener or suture

Code also any:
concomitant (open) procedure performed
fluoroscopy (87.49)
transesophageal echocardiography (TEE) (88.72)

EXCLUDES *ablation, excision or destruction of lesion or tissue of heart, endovascular approach (37.34)*
excision or destruction of other lesion or tissue of heart, thoracoscopic approach (37.37)
insertion of left atrial appendage device (37.90)

DEF: Closure of LAA tissue via use of stapler, clip, or suture; performed for patients with atrial fibrillation for whom traditional anticoagulant therapies are contraindicated; prevents strokes and other embolic events.

37.37 Excision or destruction of other lesion or tissue of heart, thoracoscopic approach

Ablation or incision of heart tissue (cryoablation) (electrocautery) (laser) (microwave) (radiofrequency) (resection) (ultrasound), via thoracoscope

Modified maze procedure, thoracoscopic approach

That via thoracoscopically-assisted approach (without thoracotomy) (with port access) (with sub-xiphoid incision)

EXCLUDES *ablation, excision or destruction of lesion or tissue of heart:*
open approach (37.33)
endovascular approach (37.34)
thoracoscopic excision or destruction of left atrial appendage [LAA] (37.36)

✓4ᵗʰ **37.4 Repair of heart and pericardium**

37.41 Implantation of prosthetic cardiac support device around the heart

Cardiac support device [CSD]
Epicardial support device
Fabric (textile) (mesh) device
Ventricular support device on surface of heart

Code also any:
cardiopulmonary bypass [extracorporeal circulation] [heart-lung machine] if performed (39.61)
mitral valve repair (35.02, 35.12)
mitral valve replacement (35.23-35.24)
transesophageal echocardiography (88.72)

EXCLUDES *circulatory assist systems (37.61-37.68)*

DEF: Cardiac support device: any device implanted around the ventricles of the heart for cardiac support

DEF: Fabric (textile) (mesh) device: textile mesh net sutured around the heart for support.

37.49 Other repair of heart and pericardium

✓4ᵗʰ **37.5 Heart replacement procedures**

37.51 Heart transplantation

EXCLUDES *combined heart-lung transplantation (33.6)*

37.52 Implantation of total internal biventricular heart replacement system

Note: This procedure includes substantial removal of part or all of the biological heart. Both ventricles are resected, and the native heart is no longer intact. Ventriculectomy is included in this procedure; do not code separately.

Artificial heart

EXCLUDES *implantation of heart assist system [VAD] (37.62, 37.65, 37.66, 37.68)*

37.53 Replacement or repair of thoracic unit of (total) replacement heart system

EXCLUDES *replacement and repair of heart assist system [VAD] (37.63)*

Operations on the Cardiovascular System

37.54–37.65

37.54 Replacement or repair of other implantable component of (total) replacement heart system
Implantable battery
Implantable controller
Transcutaneous energy transfer [TET] device
EXCLUDES *replacement and repair of heart assist system [VAD] (37.63)*
replacement or repair of thoracic unit of (total) replacement heart system (37.53)

37.55 Removal of internal biventricular heart replacement system
Explantation of artificial heart
Code also any concomitant procedure, such as:
combined heart-lung transplantation (33.6)
heart transplantation (37.51)
implantation of internal biventricular heart replacement system (37.52)
EXCLUDES *explantation [removal] of external heart assist system (37.64)*
explantation [removal] of percutaneous external heart assist device (97.44)
nonoperative removal of heart assist system (97.44)
that with replacement or repair of heart replacement system (37.53, 37.54)

√4ᵗʰ **37.6 Implantation of heart and circulatory assist system(s)**
EXCLUDES *implantation of prosthetic cardiac support system (37.41)*

DEF: Implant of device for assisting heart in circulating blood.

37.60 Implantation or insertion of biventricular external heart assist system
Note: Device (outside the body but connected to heart) with external circulation pump. Ventriculotomy is included; do not code separately.
INCLUDES open chest (sternotomy) procedure for cannulae attachments
Temporary cardiac support for both left and right ventricles, inserted in the same operative episode
EXCLUDES *implantation of internal biventricular heart replacement system (artificial heart) (37.52)*
implant of pulsation balloon (37.61)
insertion of percutaneous external heart assist device (37.68)
insertion of temporary non-implantable extracorporeal circulatory assist device (37.62)

37.61 Implant of pulsation balloon

37.62 Insertion of temporary non-implantable extracorporeal circulatory assist device
Note: Includes explantation of this device; do not code separately.
Insertion of heart assist system, NOS
Insertion of heart pump
EXCLUDES *implantation of total internal biventricular heart replacement system [artificial heart] (37.52)*
implant of external heart assist system (37.65)
insertion of implantable extracorporeal heart assist system (37.66)
insertion of percutaneous external heart assist device (37.68)
removal of heart assist system (37.64)

Ventricular Assist Devices

Continuous flow pump
Lead to power source
VAD
Balloon inserted into descending aorta
pVAD **IABP**

37.63 Repair of heart assist system
Replacement of parts of an existing ventricular assist device (VAD)
EXCLUDES *replacement or repair of other implantable component of (total) replacement heart system [artificial heart] (37.54)*
replacement or repair of thoracic unit of (total) replacement heart system [artificial heart] (37.53)

37.64 Removal of external heart assist system(s) or device(s)
Explantation of external device(s) providing left and right ventricular support
Explantation of single external device and cannulae
EXCLUDES *explantation [removal] of percutaneous external heart assist device (97.44)*
nonoperative removal of heart assist system (97.44)
temporary non-implantable extracorporeal circulatory assist device (37.62)
that with replacement of implant (37.63)

37.65 Implant of single ventricular (extracorporeal) external heart assist system
Note: Device (outside the body but connected to heart) with external circulation and pump
Note: Insertion or implantation of one external VAD for left or right heart support
INCLUDES open chest (sternotomy) procedure for cannulae attachments
Insertion of one device into one ventricle
EXCLUDES *implantation of total internal biventricular heart replace- ment system (37.52)*
implant of pulsation balloon (37.61)
insertion of implantable heart assist system (37.66)
insertion or implantation of two external VADs for simultaneous right and left heart support (37.60)
insertion of percutaneous external heart assist device (37.68)
that without sternotomy (37.62)

DEF: Insertion of short-term circulatory support device with pump outside body.

37.66   Insertion of implantable heart assist system

Note: Device directly connected to the heart and implanted in the upper left quadrant of peritoneal cavity.This device can be used for either destination therapy (DT) or bridge-to-transplant (BTT).

Axial flow heart assist system

Diagonal pump heart assist system

Left ventricular assist device (LVAD)

Pulsatile heart assist system

Right ventricular assist device (RVAD)

Rotary pump heart assist system

Transportable, implantable heart assist system

Ventricular assist device (VAD) not otherwise specified

EXCLUDES   *implantation of total internal biventricular heart replacement system [artificial heart] (37.52)*
implant of pulsation balloon (37.61)
insertion of percutaneous external heart assist device (37.68)

DEF: Insertion of long-term circulatory support device with pump in body.

37.67   Implantation of cardiomyostimulation system

Note: Two-step open procedure consisting of tranfer of one end of the latissimus dorsi muscle; wrapping it around the heart; rib resection; implantation of epicardial cardiac pacing leads into the right ventricle; tunneling and pocket creation for the cardiomyostimulator.

37.68   Insertion of percutaneous external heart assist device

INCLUDES   percutaneous [femoral] insertion of cannulae attachments

Circulatory assist device

Extrinsic heart assist device

Percutaneous heart assist device

pVAD

√4th **37.7   Insertion, revision, replacement, and removal of leads; insertion of temporary pacemaker system; or revision of cardiac device pocket**

Code also any insertion and replacement of pacemaker device (37.80-37.87)

EXCLUDES   *implantation or replacement of transvenous lead [electrode] into left ventricular cardiac venous system (00.52)*

37.70   Initial insertion of lead [electrode], not otherwise specified

EXCLUDES   *insertion of temporary transvenous pacemaker system (37.78)*
replacement of atrial and/or ventricular lead(s) (37.76)

37.71   Initial insertion of transvenous lead [electrode] into ventricle

EXCLUDES   *insertion of temporary transvenous pacemaker system (37.78)*
replacement of atrial and/or ventricular lead(s) (37.76)

37.72   Initial insertion of transvenous leads [electrodes] into atrium and ventricle

EXCLUDES   *insertion of temporary transvenous pacemaker system (37.78)*
replacement of atrial and/or ventricular lead(s) (37.76)

37.73   Initial insertion of transvenous lead [electrode] into atrium

EXCLUDES   *insertion of temporary transvenous pacemaker system (37.78)*
replacement of atrial and/or ventricular lead(s) (37.76)

37.74   Insertion or replacement of epicardial lead [electrode] into epicardium

Insertion or replacement of epicardial lead by:
sternotomy
thoracotomy

EXCLUDES   *replacement of atrial and/or ventricular lead(s) (37.76)*

37.75   Revision of lead [electrode]

Repair of electrode [removal with re-insertion]

Repositioning of lead(s) (AICD) (cardiac device) (CRT-D) (CRT-P) (defibrillator) (pacemaker) (pacing) (sensing) [electrode]

Revision of lead NOS

EXCLUDES   *repositioning of temporary transvenous pacemaker system — omit code*

37.76   Replacement of transvenous atrial and/or ventricular lead(s) [electrode]

Removal or abandonment of existing transvenous or epicardial lead(s) with transvenous lead(s) replacement

EXCLUDES   *replacement of epicardial lead [electrode] (37.74)*

37.77   Removal of lead(s) [electrode] without replacement

Removal:
epicardial lead (transthoracic approach)
transvenous lead(s)

EXCLUDES   *removal of temporary transvenous pacemaker system — omit code*
that with replacement of:
atrial and/or ventricular lead(s) [electrode] (37.76)
epicardial lead [electrode] (37.74)

37.78   Insertion of temporary transvenous pacemaker system

EXCLUDES   *intraoperative cardiac pacemaker (39.64)*

37.79   Revision or relocation of cardiac device pocket

Debridement and reforming pocket (skin and subcutaneous tissue)

Insertion of loop recorder

Relocation of pocket [creation of new pocket] pacemaker or CRT-P

Removal of cardiac device/pulse generator without replacement

Removal of implantable hemodynamic pressure sensor [lead] and monitor device

Removal without replacement of cardiac resynchronization defibrillator device

Repositioning of implantable hemodynamic pressure sensor [lead] and monitor device

Repositioning of pulse generator

Revision of cardioverter/defibrillator (automatic) pocket

Revision of pocket for intracardiac hemodynamic monitoring

Revision or relocation of CRT-D pocket

Revision or relocation of pacemaker, defibrillator, or other implanted cardiac device pocket

EXCLUDES   *removal of loop recorder (86.05)*

√4th **37.8   Insertion, replacement, removal, and revision of pacemaker device**

Note: Device testing during procedure — omit code

Code also any lead insertion, lead replacement, lead removal and/or lead revision (37.70-37.77)

EXCLUDES   *implantation of cardiac resynchronization pacemaker, total system [CRT-P] (00.50)*
implantation or replacement of cardiac resynchronization pacemaker pulse generator only [CRT-P] (00.53)

37.80   Insertion of permanent pacemaker, initial or replacement, type of device not specified

37.81   Initial insertion of single-chamber device, not specified as rate responsive

EXCLUDES   *replacement of existing pacemaker device (37.85-37.87)*

Operations on the Cardiovascular System

37.82–37.97

Insertion of Pacemaker

Left Atrial Appendage Device Insertion

Automatic Implantable Cardioverter/Defibrillator

37.82 Initial insertion of single-chamber device, rate responsive
Rate responsive to physiologic stimuli other than atrial rate
EXCLUDES *replacement of existing pacemaker device (37.85-37.87)*

37.83 Initial insertion of dual-chamber device
Atrial ventricular sequential device
EXCLUDES *replacement of existing pacemaker device (37.85-37.87)*

37.85 Replacement of any type pacemaker device with single-chamber device, not specified as rate responsive

37.86 Replacement of any type pacemaker device with single-chamber device, rate responsive
Rate responsive to physiologic stimuli other than atrial rate

37.87 Replacement of any type pacemaker device with dual-chamber device
Atrial ventricular sequential device

37.89 Revision or removal of pacemaker device
Removal without replacement of cardiac re-synchronization pacemaker device [CRT-P]
Repair of pacemaker device
EXCLUDES *removal of temporary transvenous pacemaker system — omit code*
replacement of existing pacemaker device (37.85-37.87)
replacement of existing pacemaker device with CRT-P pacemaker device (00.53)

✓4ᵗʰ 37.9 Other operations on heart and pericardium

37.90 Insertion of left atrial appendage device
Left atrial filter
Left atrial occluder
Transseptal catheter technique
DEF: Implantation of a filtering device within the left atrial appendage (LAA) to block emboli from exiting the LAA causing stroke or systemic thromboembolism.

37.91 Open chest cardiac massage
EXCLUDES *closed chest cardiac massage (99.63)*
DEF: Massage of heart through opening in chest wall to reinstate or maintain circulation.

37.92 Injection of therapeutic substance into heart

37.93 Injection of therapeutic substance into pericardium

37.94 Implantation or replacement of automatic cardioverter/defibrillator, total system [AICD]
Note: Device testing during procedure — omit code
Implantation of defibrillator with leads (epicardial patches), formation of pocket (abdominal fascia) (subcutaneous), any transvenous leads, intra-operative procedures for evaluation of lead signals, and obtaining defibrillator threshold measurements
Techniques:
lateral thoracotomy
medial sternotomy
subxiphoid procedure
Code also extracorporeal circulation, if performed (39.61)
Code also any concomitant procedure [e.g., coronary bypass (36.10-36.19) or CCM, total system (17.51)]
EXCLUDES *implantation of cardiac resynchronization defibrillator, total system [CRT-D] (00.51)*
DEF: Direct insertion of defibrillator/cardioverter system to deliver shock and restore heart rhythm.

37.95 Implantation of automatic cardioverter/defibrillator lead(s) only

37.96 Implantation of automatic cardioverter/defibrillator pulse generator only
Note: Device testing during procedure — omit code
EXCLUDES *implantation or replacement of cardiac resynchronization defibrillator, pulse generator device only [CRT-D] (00.54)*

37.97 Replacement of automatic cardioverter/defibrillator lead(s) only
EXCLUDES *replacement of epicardial lead [electrode] into epicardium (37.74)*
replacement of transvenous lead [electrode] into left ventricular coronary venous system (00.52)

37.98 Replacement of automatic cardioverter defibrillator pulse generator only

Note: Device testing during procedure — *omit code*

EXCLUDES   *replacement of cardiac resynchronization defibrillator, pulse generator device only [CRT-D] (00.54)*

37.99 Other

EXCLUDES   *cardiac retraining (93.36)*
conversion of cardiac rhythm (99.60-99.69)
implantation of prosthetic cardiac support device (37.41)
insertion of left atrial appendage device (37.90)
maze procedure (Cox-maze), open (37.33)
maze procedure, endovascular approach (37.34)
repositioning of pulse generator (37.79)
revision of lead(s) (37.75)
revision or relocation of pacemaker, defibrillator or other implanted cardiac device pocket (37.79)

√3ʳᵈ **38 Incision, excision, and occlusion of vessels**

Code also any application or administration of an adhesion barrier substance (99.77)

Code also cardiopulmonary bypass [extracorporeal circulation] [heart-lung machine] (39.61)

EXCLUDES   *that of coronary vessels (00.66, 36.03, 36.04, 36.09, 36.10-36.99)*

The following fourth-digit subclassification is for use with appropriate categories in section 38.0, 38.1, 38.3, 38.5, 38.6, and 38.8 according to site. Valid fourth-digits are in [brackets] under each code.

0 unspecified
1 intracranial vessels
    Cerebral (anterior) (middle)
    Circle of Willis
    Posterior communicating artery
2 other vessels of head and neck
    Carotid artery (common) (external) (internal)
    Jugular vein (external) (internal)
3 upper limb vessels
    Axilllary   Radial
    Brachial   Ulnar
4 aorta
5 other thoracic vessels
    Innominate   Subclavian
    Pulmonary (artery) (vein)   Vena cava, superior
6 abdominal arteries
    Celiac   Mesenteric
    Gastric   Renal
    Hepatic   Splenic
    Iliac   Umbilical
    EXCLUDES *abdominal aorta (4)*
7 abdominal veins
    Iliac   Splenic
    Portal   Vena cava (inferior)
    Renal
8 lower limb arteries
    Femoral (common)   Popliteal
        (superficial) Tibial
9 lower limb veins
    Femoral   Saphenous
    Popliteal   Tibial

√4ᵗʰ **38.0 Incision of vessel**
[0-9]   Embolectomy
         Thrombectomy
    EXCLUDES   *endovascular removal of obstruction from head and neck vessel(s) (39.74)*
    puncture or catheterization of any:
    artery (38.91, 38.98)
    vein (38.92-38.95, 38.99)

Endarterectomy of Aortic Bifurcation

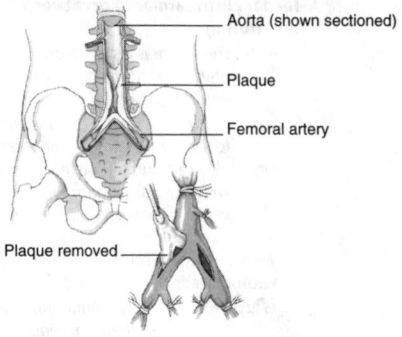

Aorta (shown sectioned)
Plaque
Femoral artery
Plaque removed

√4ᵗʰ **38.1 Endarterectomy**
[0-6,8]   Endarterectomy with:
    embolectomy
    patch graft
    temporary bypass during procedure
    thrombectomy
Code also any:
    number of vascular stents inserted (00.45-00.48)
    number of vessels treated (00.40-00.43)
    procedure on vessel bifurcation (00.44)
    DEF: Excision of tunica intima of artery to relieve arterial walls thickened by plaque or chronic inflammation.

√4ᵗʰ **38.2 Diagnostic procedures on blood vessels**
    EXCLUDES   *adjunct vascular system procedures (00.40-00.43)*

38.21 Biopsy of blood vessel

38.22 Percutaneous angioscopy
    EXCLUDES   *angioscopy of eye (95.12)*
    DEF: Exam with fiberoptic catheter inserted through peripheral artery to visualize inner lining of blood vessels.

38.23 Intravascular spectroscopy
    INCLUDES   spectroscopy of both coronary and peripheral vessels
    Intravascular chemography
    Near infrared (NIR) spectroscopy
    EXCLUDES   *intravascular imaging of:*
    coronary vessels (00.24, 38.24)
    peripheral vessels (00.23, 38.25)
    DEF: Method of identifying the chemical composition of coronary plaques by shining a near infrared (NIR) light at the plaque and measuring the amount of light reflected at different wavelengths.

38.24 Intravascular imaging of coronary vessel(s) by optical coherence tomography [OCT]
    DEF: Use of fiberoptic catheter probes that employ near-infrared electromagnetic radiation light to produce cross-sectional and enhanced resolution images of vessel plaque and intraluminal thrombus.

38.25 Intravascular imaging of non-coronary vessel(s) by optical coherence tomography [OCT]
    EXCLUDES   *intravascular imaging of coronary vessel(s) by OCT (38.24)*
    DEF: Use of fiberoptic catheter probes that employ near-infrared electromagnetic radiation light to produce cross-sectional and enhanced resolution images of vessel plaque and intraluminal thrombus.

Operations on the Cardiovascular System

38.26–38.7

38.26 Insertion of implantable pressure sensor without lead for intracardiac or great vessel hemodynamic monitoring

Note: The sensor is a standalone device and is not physically connected to a separately implanted monitor.

Leadless pressure sensor not physically connected to a separately implanted monitor

Single device combination leadless pressure sensor with integral monitor for intracardiac or great vessel (or branch thereof) hemodynamic monitoring

With or without internal batteries

Without leads

EXCLUDES *circulatory monitoring (blood gas, arterial or venous pressure, cardiac output and coronary blood flow (89.60-89.69)*
hemodynamic monitoring system with sensor and separately implanted monitor (00.56-00.57)
insertion or replacement of implantable pressure sensor with lead for intracardiac or great vessel hemodynamic monitoring (00.56)

38.29 Other diagnostic procedures on blood vessels

EXCLUDES *blood vessel thermography (88.86)*
circulatory monitoring (89.61-89.69)
contrast:
angiocardiography (88.50-88.58)
arteriography (88.40-88.49)
phlebography (88.60-88.67)
impedance phlebography (88.68)
peripheral vascular ultrasonography (88.77)
plethysmogram (89.58)

☑4ᵗʰ **38.3 Resection of vessel with anastomosis**
[0-9]

Angiectomy

Excision of:
aneurysm (arteriovenous)
blood vessel (lesion)
} with anastomosis

DEF: Reconstruction and reconnection of vessel after partial excision.

Methods of Vessel Anastomoses

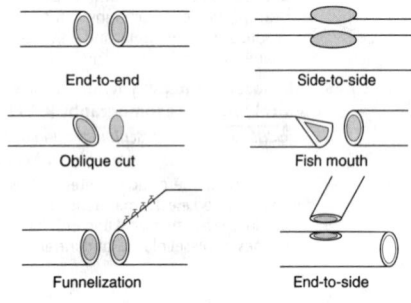

End-to-end   Side-to-side

Oblique cut   Fish mouth

Funnelization   End-to-side

☑4ᵗʰ **38.4 Resection of vessel with replacement**
[0-9]

Angiectomy

Excision of:
aneurysm (arteriovenous) or
blood vessel (lesion)
} with replacement

Partial resection with replacement

EXCLUDES *endovascular repair of aneurysm (39.71-39.79)*

Subcategory 38.4 requires the use of one of the following fourth-digit subclassifications to identify site:

0 unspecified

1 intracranial vessels
Cerebral (anterior) (middle)
Circle of Willis
Posterior communicating artery

2 other vessels of head and neck
Carotid artery (common) (external) (internal)
Jugular vein (external) (internal)

3 upper limb vessels
Axilllary   Radial
Brachial   Ulnar

4 aorta, abdominal
Code also any thoracic vessel involvement (thoracoabdominal procedure) (38.45)

5 other thoracic vessels
Aorta (thoracic)   Subclavian
Innominate   Vena cava, superior
Pulmonary (artery) (vein)
Code also any abdominal aorta involvement (thoracoabdominal procedure) (38.44)

6 abdominal arteries
Celiac   Mesenteric
Gastric   Renal
Hepatic   Splenic
Iliac   Umbilical
EXCLUDES *abdominal aorta (4)*

7 abdominal veins
Iliac   Splenic
Portal   Vena cava (inferior)
Renal

8 lower limb arteries
Femoral (common)(superficial)
Tibial

9 lower limb veins
Femoral   Saphenous
Popliteal   Tibial

DEF: Excision of aneurysm (arteriovenous): Excision and replacement of segment of stretched or bulging blood vessel.
DEF: Excision of blood vessel (lesion): Excision and replacement of segment of vessel containing lesion.

☑4ᵗʰ **38.5 Ligation and stripping of varicose veins**
[0-3,5,7,9]*EXCLUDES* *ligation of varices:*
esophageal (42.91)
gastric (44.91)

DEF: Ligation of varicose veins: Typing off vein with thread or wire to eliminate blood flow; stripping involves excising length of vein.

☑4ᵗʰ **38.6 Other excision of vessels**
[0-9]

Excision of blood vessel (lesion) NOS
EXCLUDES *excision of vessel for aortocoronary bypass (36.10-36.14)*
excision with:
anastomosis (38.30-38.39)
graft replacement (38.40-38.49)
implant (38.40-38.49)

38.7 Interruption of the vena cava

Insertion of implant or sieve in vena cava
Ligation of vena cava (inferior) (superior)
Plication of vena cava

DEF: Interruption of the blood flow through the venous heart vessels to prevent clots from reaching the chambers of the heart by means of implanting a sieve or implant, separating off a portion or by narrowing the venous blood vessels.

✓4ᵗʰ **38.8 Other surgical occlusion of vessels**
[0-9]

Clamping
Division
Ligation
Occlusion
} of blood vessel

EXCLUDES   *adrenal vessels (07.43)*
esophageal varices (42.91)
gastric or duodenal vessel for ulcer (44.40-44.49)
gastric varices (44.91)
meningeal vessel (02.13)
percutaneous transcatheter infusion
    embolization (99.29)
spermatic vein for varicocele (63.1)
surgical occlusion of vena cava (38.7)
that for chemoembolization (99.25)
that for control of (postoperative) hemorrhage:
    anus (49.95)
    bladder (57.93)
    following vascular procedure (39.41)
    nose (21.00-21.09)
    prostate (60.94)
    tonsil (28.7)
    thyroid vessel (06.92)
transcatheter (infusion) 99.29

✓4ᵗʰ **38.9 Puncture of vessel**
EXCLUDES   *that for circulatory monitoring (89.60-89.69)*

38.91 Arterial catheterization

38.92 Umbilical vein catheterization

38.93 Venous catheterization, not elsewhere classified
EXCLUDES   *that for cardiac catheterization*
    (37.21-37.23)
that for renal dialysis (38.95)
that with guidance (electrocardiogram)
    (fluoroscopy) (ultrasound) (38.97)

38.94 Venous cutdown
DEF: Incision of vein to place needle or catheter.

38.95 Venous catheterization for renal dialysis
EXCLUDES   *insertion of totally implantable vascular*
    access device [VAD] (86.07)

38.97 Central venous catheter placement with guidance
INCLUDES   guidance by:
    electrocardiogram
    fluoroscopy
    ultrasound

38.98 Other puncture of artery
EXCLUDES   *that for:*
    arteriography (88.40-88.49)
    coronary arteriography (88.55-88.57)

38.99 Other puncture of vein
Phlebotomy
EXCLUDES   *that for:*
    angiography of veins (88.60-88.68)
    extracorporeal circulation (39.61,
      50.92)
    injection or infusion of:
    sclerosing solution (39.92)
    therapeutic or prophylactic substance
      (99.11-99.29)
    perfusion (39.96, 39.97)
    phlebography 88.60-88.68
    transfusion (99.01-99.09)

Typical Venous Cutdown

Vein mobilized, opened by oblique cut, catheter inserted

Distal vein tied

Saphenous vein (typical site) accessed by transverse incision

✓3ʳᵈ **39 Other operations on vessels**
EXCLUDES   *those on coronary vessels (36.03-36.99)*

39.0 Systemic to pulmonary artery shunt
Descending aorta-pulmonary artery }
Left to right } anastomosis (graft)
Subclavian-pulmonary }

Code also cardiopulmonary bypass [extracorporeal circulation] [heart-lung machine] (39.61)

DEF: Descending aorta-pulmonary artery anastomosis (graft): Connection of descending main heart artery to pulmonary artery.

DEF: Left to right anastomosis (graft): Connection of systemic arterial blood vessel to venous pulmonary system.

DEF: Subclavian-pulmonary anastomosis (graft): Connection of subclavian artery to pulmonary artery

39.1 Intra-abdominal venous shunt
Anastomosis:
   mesocaval
   portacaval
   portal vein to inferior vena cava
   splenic and renal veins
   transjugular intrahepatic portosystemic shunt [TIPS]
EXCLUDES   *peritoneovenous shunt (54.94)*
DEF: Connection of two venous blood vessels within abdominal cavity.

✓4ᵗʰ **39.2 Other shunt or vascular bypass**
Code also pressurized treatment of venous bypass graft [conduit] with pharmaceutical substance, if performed (00.16)
DEF: Creation of supplemental blood flow to area with inadequate blood supply due to disease or injury of vessels.

39.21 Caval-pulmonary artery anastomosis
Code also cardiopulmonary bypass (39.61)

39.22 Aorta-subclavian-carotid bypass
Bypass (arterial):
   aorta to carotid and brachial
   aorta to subclavian and carotid
   carotid to subclavian

39.23 Other intrathoracic vascular shunt or bypass
Intrathoracic (arterial) bypass graft NOS
EXCLUDES   *coronary artery bypass (36.10-36.19)*

39.24 Aorta-renal bypass

39.25 Aorta-iliac-femoral bypass
Bypass: Bypass:
aortofemoral   aortopopliteal
aortoiliac   iliofemoral [iliac-femoral]
aortoiliac to popliteal

39.26 Other intra-abdominal vascular shunt or bypass
Bypass:
   aortoceliac
   aortic-superior mesenteric
   common hepatic-common iliac-renal
Intra-abdominal arterial bypass graft NOS
EXCLUDES   *peritoneovenous shunt (54.94)*

Operations on the Cardiovascular System

39.27–39.53

39.27 Arteriovenostomy for renal dialysis
Anastomosis for renal dialysis
Formation of (peripheral) arteriovenous fistula for renal [kidney] dialysis
Code also any renal dialysis (39.95)

39.28 Extracranial-intracranial (EC-IC) vascular bypass

39.29 Other (peripheral) vascular shunt or bypass
Bypass (graft):
axillary-brachial
axillary-femoral [axillofemora] (superficial)
brachial
femoral-femoral
femoroperoneal
femoropopliteal (arteries)
femorotibial (anterior) (posterior)
popliteal
vascular NOS
EXCLUDES *peritoneovenous shunt (54.94)*

✓4ᵗʰ **39.3 Suture of vessel**
Repair of laceration of blood vessel
EXCLUDES *any other vascular puncture closure device — omit code*
suture of aneurysm (39.52)
that for control of hemorrhage (postoperative):
anus (49.95)
bladder (57.93)
following vascular procedure (39.41)
nose (21.00-21.09)
prostate (60.94)
tonsil (28.7)

39.30 Suture of unspecified blood vessel

39.31 Suture of artery

39.32 Suture of vein

✓4ᵗʰ **39.4 Revision of vascular procedure**

39.41 Control of hemorrhage following vascular surgery
EXCLUDES *that for control of hemorrhage (postoperative):*
anus (49.95)
bladder (57.93)
nose (21.00-21.09)
prostate (60.94)
tonsil (28.7)

39.42 Revision of arteriovenous shunt for renal dialysis
Conversion of renal dialysis:
end-to-end anastomosis to end-to-side
end-to-side anastomosis to end-to-end
vessel-to-vessel cannula to arteriovenous shunt
Removal of old arteriovenous shunt and creation of new shunt
EXCLUDES *replacement of vessel-to-vessel cannula (39.94)*

39.43 Removal of arteriovenous shunt for renal dialysis
EXCLUDES *that with replacement [revision] of shunt (39.42)*

39.49 Other revision of vascular procedure
Declotting (graft)
Revision of:
anastomosis of blood vessel
vascular procedure (previous)
DEF: Declotting (graft): Removal of clot from graft.

✓4ᵗʰ **39.5 Other repair of vessels**

39.50 Angioplasty of other non-coronary vessel(s)
Percutaneous transluminal angioplasty (PTA) of non-coronary vessels:
lower extremity vessels
mesenteric artery
renal artery
upper extremity vessels
Code also any:
atherectomy of other non-coronary vessels(s) (17.56)
injection or infusion of thrombolytic agent (99.10)
insertion of drug-eluting peripheral vessel stent (00.55)
insertion of non-drug-eluting peripheral vessel stent(s) or stent grafts(s) (39.90)
number of vascular stents inserted (00.45-00.48)
number of vessels treated (00.40-00.43)
procedure on vessel bifurcation (00.44)
EXCLUDES *percutaneous angioplasty of extracranial or intracranial vessel(s) (00.61-00.62)*
percutaneous atherectomy of extracranial or intracranial vessel(s) (17.53-17.54)

39.51 Clipping of aneurysm
EXCLUDES *clipping of arteriovenous fistula (39.53)*

39.52 Other repair of aneurysm
Repair of aneurysm by:
coagulation
electrocoagulation
filipuncture
methyl methacrylate
suture
wiring
wrapping
EXCLUDES *endovascular repair of aneurysm (39.71-39.79)*
re-entry operation (aorta) (39.54)
that with:
graft replacement (38.40-38.49)
resection (38.30-38.49, 38.60-38.69)
DEF: Application of device to repair abnormally stretched blood vessel and prevent hemorrhage from vessel.
DEF: Repair of aneurysm by: Coagulation: Clotting or solidifying. Electrocoagulation: Electrically produced clotting. Filipuncture: Insertion of wire or thread. Methyl methacrylate: Injection or insertion of plastic material. Suture: Stitching. Wiring: Insertion of wire. Wrapping: Compression.

39.53 Repair of arteriovenous fistula
Embolization of carotid cavernous fistula
Repair of arteriovenous fistula by:
clipping
coagulation
ligation and division
EXCLUDES *repair of:*
arteriovenous shunt for renal dialysis (39.42)
head and neck vessels, endovascular approach (39.72)
that with:
graft replacement (38.40-38.49)
resection (38.30-38.49, 38.60-38.69)
DEF: Correction of arteriovenous fistula by application of clamps, causing coagulation or by tying off and dividing the connection.

39.54   **Re-entry operation (aorta)**

Fenestration of dissecting aneurysm of thoracic aorta

Code also cardiopulmonary bypass [extracorporeal circulation] [heart-lung machine] (39.61)

DEF: Re-entry operation: Creation of passage between stretched wall of the vessel and major arterial channel to heart.

DEF: Fenestration of dissecting aneurysm of thoracic aorta: Creation of passage between stretched arterial heart vessel and functional part of vessel.

39.55   **Reimplantation of aberrant renal vessel**

DEF: Reimplant of renal vessel into normal position.

39.56   **Repair of blood vessel with tissue patch graft**

EXCLUDES   *that with resection (38.40-38.49)*

39.57   **Repair of blood vessel with synthetic patch graft**

EXCLUDES   *that with resection (38.40-38.49)*

39.58   **Repair of blood vessel with unspecified type of patch graft**

EXCLUDES   *that with resection (38.40-38.49)*

39.59   **Other repair of vessel**

Aorticopulmonary window operation
Arterioplasty NOS
Construction of venous valves (peripheral)
Plication of vein (peripheral)
Reimplantation of artery

Code also cardiopulmonary bypass [extracorporeal circulation] [heart-lung machine] (39.61)

EXCLUDES   *interruption of the vena cava (38.7)*
reimplantation of renal artery (39.55)
that with:
    graft (39.56-39.58)
    resection (38.30-38.49, 38.60-38.69)

DEF: Aorticopulmonary window operation: Repair of abnormal opening between major heart arterial vessel above valves and pulmonary artery.

DEF: Construction of venous valves (peripheral): Reconstruction of valves within peripheral veins.

DEF: Plication of vein (peripheral): Shortening of peripheral vein.

DEF: Reimplantation of artery: Reinsertion of artery into its normal position.

√4ᵗʰ **39.6**   **Extracorporeal circulation and procedures auxiliary to heart surgery**

39.61   **Extracorporeal circulation auxiliary to open heart surgery**

Artificial heart and lung   Pump oxygenator
Cardiopulmonary bypass

EXCLUDES   *extracorporeal hepatic assistance (50.92)*
extracorporeal membrane oxygenation [ECMO] (39.65)
hemodialysis (39.95)
percutaneous cardiopulmonary bypass (39.66)

39.62   **Hypothermia (systemic) incidental to open heart surgery**

39.63   **Cardioplegia**

Arrest: Arrest:
   anoxic   circulatory

DEF: Purposely inducing electromechanical cardiac arrest.

39.64   **Intraoperative cardiac pacemaker**

Temporary pacemaker used during and immediately following cardiac surgery

39.65   **Extracorporeal membrane oxygenation [ECMO]**

EXCLUDES   *extracorporeal circulation auxiliary to open heart surgery (39.61)*
percutaneous cardiopulmonary bypass (39.66)

DEF: Creation of closed-chest, heart-lung bypass or Bard cardiopulmonary assist system with tube insertion.

39.66   **Percutaneous cardiopulmonary bypass**

Closed chest

EXCLUDES   *extracorporeal circulation auxiliary to open heart surgery (39.61)*
extracorporeal hepatic assistance (50.92)
extracorporeal membrane oxygenation [ECMO] (39.65)
hemodialysis (39.95)

DEF: Use of mechanical pump system to oxygenate and pump blood throughout the body via catheter in the femoral artery and vein.

√4ᵗʰ **39.7**   **Endovascular procedures on vessel(s)**

Embolization   Occlusion
Endoluminal repair   Removal
Implantation   Repair

EXCLUDES   *angioplasty of other non-coronary vessel(s) (39.50)*
atherectomy of other non-coronary vessel(s) (17.56)
insertion of non-drug-eluting peripheral vessel stent(s) (39.90)
other repair of aneurysm (39.52)
percutaneous insertion of carotid artery stent(s) (00.63)
percutaneous insertion of intracranial stent(s) (00.65)
percutaneous insertion of other precerebral artery stent(s) (00.64)
resection of abdominal aorta with replacement (38.44)
resection of lower limb arteries with replacement (38.48)
resection of thoracic aorta with replacement (38.45)
resection of upper limb vessels with replacement (38.43)
temporary therapeutic partial occlusion of vessel (39.77)

39.71   **Endovascular implantation of other graft in abdominal aorta**

Endovascular repair of abdominal aortic aneurysm with graft
Stent graft(s)

Code also intra-aneurysm sac pressure monitoring (intraoperative) (00.58)

EXCLUDES   *endovascular implantation of branching or fenestrated graft in aorta (39.78)*

DEF: Replacement of a section of abdominal aorta with mesh graft via catheters inserted through femoral arteries.

39.72   **Endovascular (total) embolization or occlusion of head and neck vessels**

Coil-retention stent
Embolization stent
Endograft(s)
Endovascular graft(s)
Liquid tissue adhesive (glue) embolization or occlusion
Other implant or substance for repair, embolization or occlusion
That for repair of aneurysm, arteriovenous malformation [AVM] or fistula

EXCLUDES   *embolization of head or neck vessels using bare coils (39.75)*
embolization of head or neck vessels using bioactive coils (39.76)
mechanical thrombectomy of precerebral and cerebral vessels (39.74)

DEF: Coil embolization or occlusion: Utilizing x-ray guidance a neuro-microcatheter is guided from entry in the femoral artery in the groin to the site of the aneurysm of the head and neck vessels for delivery of micro-coils that stop blood flow to the arteriovenous malfomation (AVM).

Operations on the Cardiovascular System

39.54–39.72

Operations on the Cardiovascular System

39.73–39.81

Endovascular Repair of Abdominal Aortic Aneurysm

Renal arteries

Stent

Abdominal aortic aneurysm

Common iliac arteries

39.73 Endovascular implantation of graft in thoracic aorta
Endograft(s)
Endovascular graft(s)
Endovascular repair of defect of thoracic aorta with graft(s) or device(s)
Stent graft(s) or device(s)
That for repair of aneurysm, dissection, or injury
Code also intra-aneurysm sac pressure monitoring (intraoperative) (00.58)
EXCLUDES *fenestration of dissecting aneurysm of thoracic aorta (39.54)*
DEF: Intravascular transcatheter deployment of an expanding stent-graft for repair of thoracic aortic aneurysm, performed without opening the chest.

39.74 Endovascular removal of obstruction from head and neck vessel(s)
Endovascular embolectomy
Endovascular thrombectomy of pre-cerebral and cerebral vessels
Mechanical embolectomy or thrombectomy
Code also:
any injection or infusion of thrombolytic agent (99.10)
number of vessels treated (00.40-00.43)
procedure on vessel bifurcation (00.44)
EXCLUDES *endarterectomy of intracranial vessels and other vessels of head and neck (38.11-38.12)*
occlusive endovascular embolization of head or neck vessel(s) using bare coils (39.75)
occlusive endovascular embolization of head or neck vessel(s) using bioactive coils (39.76)
open embolectomy or thrombectomy (38.01-38.02)

39.75 Endovascular embolization or occlusion of vessel(s) of head or neck using bare coils
Bare metal coils
Bare platinum coils [BPC]
That for treatment of aneurysm, arteriovenous malformation [AVM] or fistula

39.76 Endovascular embolization or occlusion of vessel(s) of head or neck using bioactive coils
Biodegradable inner luminal polymer coils
Coil embolization or occlusion utilizing bioactive coils
Coils containing polyglycolic acid [PGA]
That for treatment of aneurysm, arteriovenous malformation [AVM] or fistula
DEF: Enhanced aneurysm treatment by deployment of coils packed with novel polyglycol acid (PGA) or other bioactive substance to improve healing response.

39.77 Temporary (partial) therapeutic endovascular occlusion of vessel
Includes that of aorta
That by balloon catheter
Code also any: diagnostic arteriogram (88.40-88.49)
EXCLUDES *any endovascular head or neck vessel procedure (39.72, 39.74-39.76)*
diagnostic procedures on blood vessels (38.21-38.29)
permanent endovascular procedure (39.79)

39.78 Endovascular implantation of branching or fenestrated graft(s) in aorta
DEF: A tubular, fabric graft with specialized reinforced openings allowing physicians to custom fit and position the stent into vessel branches or bifurcations at complex anatomic sites.

39.79 Other endovascular procedures on other vessels
Endograft(s)
Endovascular graft(s)
Liquid tissue adhesive (glue) embolization or occlusion
Other coil embolization or occlusion
Other implant or substance for repair, embolization or occlusion
Repair of aneurysm
EXCLUDES *abdominal aortic aneurysm resection [AAA] (38.44)*
endovascular implantation of graft in abdominal aorta (39.71)
endovascular implantation of graft in thoracic aorta (39.73)
endovascular embolization or occlusion of head and neck vessels, bare metal coils (39.75)
endovascular embolization or occlusion of head and neck vessels, bioactive coils (39.76)
insertion of drug-eluting peripheral vessel stent(s) (00.55)
insertion of non-drug-eluting peripheral vessel stent(s) (for other than aneurysm repair) (39.90)
non-endovascular repair of arteriovenous fistula (39.53)
other surgical occlusion of vessels – see category 38.8
percutaneous transcatheter infusion (99.29)
thoracic aortic aneurysm resection (38.45)
transcatheter embolization for gastric or duodenal bleeding (44.44)
uterine artery embolization with coils (68.24)

✓4ᵗʰ 39.8 Operations on carotid body, carotid sinus and other vascular bodies

39.81 Implantation or replacement of carotid sinus stimulation device, total system
INCLUDES carotid explorations
Carotid sinus baroreflex activation device
Implantation of carotid sinus stimulator and lead(s)
EXCLUDES *implantation or replacement of carotid sinus stimulation lead(s) only (39.82)*
implantation or replacement of carotid sinus stimulation pulse generator only (39.83)
DEF: A surgically implantable medical device that electrically activates the baroreflex; the system that helps regulate cardiovascular function to treat primary hypertension and hypertensive heart failure recalcitrant to medical therapy.

39.82 **Implantation or replacement of carotid sinus stimulation lead(s) only**
EXCLUDES   *implantation or replacement of carotid sinus stimulation device, total system (39.81)*

39.83 **Implantation or replacement of carotid sinus stimulation pulse generator only**
EXCLUDES   *implantation or replacement of carotid sinus stimulation device, total system (39.81)*

39.84 **Revision of carotid sinus stimulation lead(s) only**
Repair of electrode [removal with re-insertion]
Repositioning of lead(s) [electrode]

39.85 **Revision of carotid sinus stimulation pulse generator**
Debridement and reforming pocket (skin and subcutaneous tissue)
Relocation of pocket [creation of new pocket]
Repositioning of pulse generator
Revision of carotid sinus stimulation pulse generator pocket

39.86 **Removal of carotid sinus stimulation device, total system**

39.87 **Removal of carotid sinus stimulation lead(s) only**

39.88 **Removal of carotid sinus stimulation pulse generator only**

39.89 **Other operations on carotid body, carotid sinus and other vascular bodies**
Chemodectomy   Glomectomy, carotid
Denervation of:
   aortic body
   carotid body
Glomectomy, carotid
EXCLUDES   *excision of glomus jugulare (20.51)*
DEF: Chemodectomy: Removal of a chemoreceptor vascular body.
DEF: Denervation of aortic body: Destruction of nerves attending the major heart blood vessels.
DEF: Denervation of carotid body: Destruction of nerves of carotid artery.
DEF: Glomectomy, carotid: Removal of the carotid artery framework.

√4ᵗʰ **39.9** **Other operations on vessels**

39.90 **Insertion of non-drug-eluting peripheral (non-coronary) vessel stent(s)**
Bare stent(s)
Bonded stent(s)
Drug-coated stent(s), i.e., heparin coated
Endograft(s)
Endovascular graft(s)
Endovascular recanalization techniques
Stent graft(s)
Code also any:
   non-coronary angioplasty or atherectomy (39.50)
   number of vascular stents inserted (00.45-00.48)
   number of vessels treated (00.40-00.43)
   procedure on vessel bifurcation (00.44)
EXCLUDES   *insertion of drug-eluting, peripheral vessel stent(s) (00.55)*
     percutaneous insertion of carotid artery stent(s) (00.63)
     percutaneous insertion of intracranial stent(s) (00.65)
     percutaneous insertion of other precerebral artery stent(s) (00.64)
     that for aneurysm repair (39.71-39.79)

External Arteriovenous Shunt
Cephalic vein
Radial artery

39.91 **Freeing of vessel**
Dissection and freeing of adherent tissue:
   artery-vein-nerve bundle
   vascular bundle

39.92 **Injection of sclerosing agent into vein**
EXCLUDES   *injection:*
     esophageal varices (42.33)
     hemorrhoids (49.42)

39.92 **Injection of sclerosing agent into vein**
EXCLUDES   *injection:*
     esophageal varices (42.33)
     hemorrhoids (49.42)

39.93 **Insertion of vessel-to-vessel cannula**
Formation of:
   arteriovenous:
     fistula } by external cannula
     shunt
Code also any renal dialysis (39.95)

39.94 **Replacement of vessel-to-vessel cannula**
Revision of vessel-to-vessel cannula

39.95 **Hemodialysis**
Artificial kidney   Hemofiltration
Hemodiafiltration   Renal dialysis
EXCLUDES   *peritoneal dialysis (54.98)*
DEF: Filtration process to treat acute and chronic renal failure by eliminating toxic end products of nitrogen metabolism from blood.

39.96 **Total body perfusion**
Code also substance perfused (99.21-99.29)

39.97 **Other perfusion**
Perfusion NOS
Perfusion, local [regional] of:
   carotid artery
   coronary artery
   head
   lower limb
   neck
   upper limb
Code also substance perfused (99.21-99.29)
EXCLUDES   *perfusion of:*
     kidney (55.95)
     large intestine (46.96)
     liver (50.93)
     small intestine (46.95)
     SuperSaturated oxygen therapy (00.49)

39.98 **Control of hemorrhage, not otherwise specified**
Angiotripsy
Control of postoperative hemorrhage NOS
Venotripsy

   EXCLUDES   *control of hemorrhage (postoperative):*
      anus (49.95)
      bladder (57.93)
      following vascular procedure (39.41)
      nose (21.00-21.09)
      prostate (60.94)
      tonsil (28.7)
    that by:
      ligation (38.80-38.89)
      suture (39.30-39.32)

DEF: Angiotripsy: Clamping of tissue to stop arterial blood flow.

DEF: Venotripsy: Clamping of tissue to stop venous blood flow.

39.99 **Other operations on vessels**

   EXCLUDES   *injection or infusion of therapeutic or prophylactic substance (99.11-99.29)*
    transfusion of blood and blood components (99.01-99.09)

8. OPERATIONS ON THE HEMIC AND LYMPHATIC SYSTEMS (40-41)

√3ʳᵈ **40 Operations on lymphatic system**

40.0 Incision of lymphatic structures

√4ᵗʰ **40.1 Diagnostic procedures on lymphatic structures**

40.11 Biopsy of lymphatic structure
Transbronchoscopic needle aspiration [TBNA] of lymph node

40.19 Other diagnostic procedures on lymphatic structures
EXCLUDES   *lymphangiogram:*
abdominal (88.04)
cervical (87.08)
intrathoracic (87.34)
lower limb (88.36)
upper limb (88.34)
microscopic examination of specimen (90.71-90.79)
radioisotope scan (92.16)
thermography (88.89)

√4ᵗʰ **40.2 Simple excision of lymphatic structure**
EXCLUDES   *biopsy of lymphatic structure (40.11)*
DEF: Removal of lymphatic structure only.

40.21 Excision of deep cervical lymph node

40.22 Excision of internal mammary lymph node

40.23 Excision of axillary lymph node

40.24 Excision of inguinal lymph node

40.29 Simple excision of other lymphatic structure
Excision of:
cystic hygroma
lymphangioma
Simple lymphadenectomy
DEF: Lymphangioma: Removal of benign congenital lymphatic malformation.
DEF: Simple lymphadenectomy: Removal of lymph node.

40.3 Regional lymph node excision
Extended regional lymph node excision
Regional lymph node excision with excision of lymphatic drainage area including skin, subcutaneous tissue, and fat
DEF: Extended regional lymph node excision: Removal of lymph node group, including area around nodes.

√4ᵗʰ **40.4 Radical excision of cervical lymph nodes**
Resection of cervical lymph nodes down to muscle and deep fascia
EXCLUDES   *that associated with radical laryngectomy (30.4)*

40.40 Radical neck dissection, not otherwise specified

40.41 Radical neck dissection, unilateral
DEF: Total dissection of cervical lymph nodes on one side of neck.

40.42 Radical neck dissection, bilateral
DEF: Total dissection of cervical lymph nodes on both sides of neck.

√4ᵗʰ **40.5 Radical excision of other lymph nodes**
EXCLUDES   *that associated with radical mastectomy (85.45-85.48)*

40.50 Radical excision of lymph nodes, not otherwise specified
Radical (lymph) node dissection NOS

40.51 Radical excision of axillary lymph nodes

40.52 Radical excision of periaortic lymph nodes

40.53 Radical excision of iliac lymph nodes

40.54 Radical groin dissection

40.59 Radical excision of other lymph nodes
EXCLUDES   *radical neck dissection (40.40-40.42)*

√4ᵗʰ **40.6 Operations on thoracic duct**

40.61 Cannulation of thoracic duct
DEF: Placement of cannula in main lymphatic duct of chest.

40.62 Fistulization of thoracic duct
DEF: Creation of passage in main lymphatic duct of chest.

40.63 Closure of fistula of thoracic duct
DEF: Closure of fistula in main lymphatic duct of chest.

40.64 Ligation of thoracic duct
DEF: Tying off main lymphatic duct of chest.

40.69 Other operations on thoracic duct

40.9 Other operations on lymphatic structures
Anastomosis
Dilation
Ligation
Obliteration   } of peripheral lymphatics
Reconstruction
Repair
Transplantation
Correction of lymphedema of limb, NOS
EXCLUDES   *reduction of elephantiasis of scrotum (61.3)*

√3ʳᵈ **41 Operations on bone marrow and spleen**

√4ᵗʰ **41.0 Bone marrow or hematopoietic stem cell transplant**
Note: To report donor source – see codes 00.91-00.93
EXCLUDES   *aspiration of bone marrow from donor (41.91)*

41.00 Bone marrow transplant, not otherwise specified

41.01 Autologous bone marrow transplant without purging
EXCLUDES   *that with purging (41.09)*
DEF: Transplant of patient's own bone marrow.

41.02 Allogeneic bone marrow transplant with purging
Allograft of bone marrow with in vitro removal (purging) of T-cells
DEF: Transplant of bone marrow from donor to patient after donor marrow purged of undesirable cells.

41.03 Allogeneic bone marrow transplant without purging
Allograft of bone marrow NOS

41.04 Autologous hematopoietic stem cell transplant without purging
EXCLUDES   *that with purging (41.07)*

41.05 Allogeneic hematopoietic stem cell transplant without purging
EXCLUDES   *that with purging (41.08)*

41.06 Cord blood stem cell transplant

41.07 Autologous hematopoietic stem cell transplant with purging
Cell depletion

41.08 Allogeneic hematopoietic stem cell transplant with purging
Cell depletion

41.09 Autologous bone marrow transplant with purging
With extracorporeal purging of malignant cells from marrow
Cell depletion

41.1 Puncture of spleen
EXCLUDES   *aspiration biopsy of spleen (41.32)*

41.2 Splenotomy

√4ᵗʰ **41.3 Diagnostic procedures on bone marrow and spleen**

41.31 Biopsy of bone marrow

41.32 Closed [aspiration] [percutaneous] biopsy of spleen
Needle biopsy of spleen

41.33 Open biopsy of spleen

Operations on the Hemic and Lymphatic Systems

41.38–41.99

Partial Splenectomy

Total Splenectomy

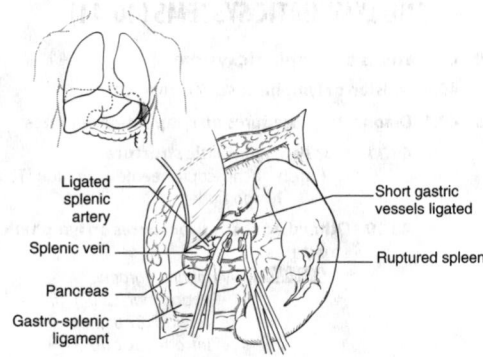

41.38 Other diagnostic procedures on bone marrow
> *EXCLUDES*   *microscopic examination of specimen from bone marrow (90.61-90.69)*
> *radioisotope scan (92.05)*

41.39 Other diagnostic procedures on spleen
> *EXCLUDES*   *microscopic examination of specimen from spleen (90.61-90.69)*
> *radioisotope scan (92.05)*

✓4ᵗʰ **41.4 Excision or destruction of lesion or tissue of spleen**
> Code also any application or administration of an adhesion barrier substance (99.77)
> *EXCLUDES*   *excision of accessory spleen (41.93)*

41.41 Marsupialization of splenic cyst
> **DEF:** Incision of cyst of spleen with edges sutured open to create pouch.

41.42 Excision of lesion or tissue of spleen
> *EXCLUDES*   *biopsy of spleen (41.32-41.33)*

41.43 Partial splenectomy
> **DEF:** Partial removal of spleen.

41.5 Total splenectomy
> Splenectomy NOS
> Code also any application or administration of an adhesion barrier substance (99.77)

✓4ᵗʰ **41.9 Other operations on spleen and bone marrow**
> Code also any application or administration of an adhesion barrier substance (99.77)

41.91 Aspiration of bone marrow from donor for transplant
> *EXCLUDES*   *biopsy of bone marrow (41.31)*

41.92 Injection into bone marrow
> *EXCLUDES*   *bone marrow transplant (41.00-41.03)*

41.93 Excision of accessory spleen

41.94 Transplantation of spleen

41.95 Repair and plastic operations on spleen

41.98 Other operations on bone marrow

41.99 Other operations on spleen

9. OPERATIONS ON THE DIGESTIVE SYSTEM (42-54)

√3rd **42 Operations on esophagus**

√4th **42.0 Esophagotomy**

42.01 Incision of esophageal web
DEF: Cutting into congenital esophageal membrane.

42.09 Other incision of esophagus
Esophagotomy NOS
EXCLUDES   *esophagomyotomy (42.7)*
esophagostomy (42.10-42.19)

√4th **42.1 Esophagostomy**

42.10 Esophagostomy, not otherwise specified

42.11 Cervical esophagostomy
DEF: Creation of opening into upper region of esophagus.

42.12 Exteriorization of esophageal pouch
DEF: Transfer of section of esophageal pouch to exterior of the body.

42.19 Other external fistulization of esophagus
Thoracic esophagostomy
Code also any resection (42.40-42.42)

√4th **42.2 Diagnostic procedures on esophagus**

42.21 Operative esophagoscopy by incision
DEF: Esophageal examination with an endoscope through incision.

42.22 Esophagoscopy through artificial stoma
EXCLUDES   *that with biopsy (42.24)*

42.23 Other esophagoscopy
EXCLUDES   *that with biopsy (42.24)*

42.24 Closed [endoscopic] biopsy of esophagus
Brushing or washing for specimen collection
Esophagoscopy with biopsy
Suction biopsy of the esophagus
EXCLUDES   *esophagogastroduodenoscopy [EGD] with closed biopsy (45.16)*
DEF: Scope passed through mouth and throat to obtain biopsy specimen, usually by brushing and swabbing.

42.25 Open biopsy of esophagus

42.29 Other diagnostic procedures on esophagus
EXCLUDES   *barium swallow (87.61)*
esophageal manometry (89.32)
microscopic examination of specimen from esophagus (90.81-90.89)

√4th **42.3 Local excision or destruction of lesion or tissue of esophagus**

42.31 Local excision of esophageal diverticulum

42.32 Local excision of other lesion or tissue of esophagus
EXCLUDES   *biopsy of esophagus (42.24-42.25)*
esophageal fistulectomy (42.84)

42.33 Endoscopic excision or destruction of lesion or tissue of esophagus
Ablation of esophageal neoplasm
Control of esophageal bleeding
Esophageal polypectomy
Espohageal varices
Injection of esophageal varies
} by endoscopic approach
EXCLUDES   *biopsy of esophagus (42.24-42.25)*
fistulectomy (42.84)
open ligation of esophageal varices (42.91)

42.39 Other destruction of lesion or tissue of esophagus
EXCLUDES   *that by endoscopic approach (42.33)*

√4th **42.4 Excision of esophagus**
EXCLUDES   *esophagogastrectomy NOS 43.99)*

42.40 Esophagectomy, not otherwise specified

42.41 Partial esophagectomy
Code also any synchronous:
anastomosis other than end-to-end (42.51-42.69)
esophagostomy (42.10-42.19)
gastrostomy (43.11-43.19)
DEF: Surgical removal of any part of esophagus.

42.42 Total esophagectomy
Code also any synchronous:
gastrostomy (43.11-43.19)
interposition or anastomosis other than end-to-end (42.51-42.69)
EXCLUDES   *esophagogastrectomy (43.99)*
DEF: Surgical removal of entire esophagus.

√4th **42.5 Intrathoracic anastomosis of esophagus**
Code also any synchronous:
esophagectomy (42.40-42.42)
gastrostomy (43.1)
DEF: Connection of esophagus to conduit within chest.

42.51 Intrathoracic esophagoesophagostomy
DEF: Connection of both ends of esophagus within chest cavity.

42.52 Intrathoracic esophagogastrostomy
DEF: Connection of esophagus to stomach within chest; follows esophagogastrectomy.

42.53 Intrathoracic esophageal anastomosis with interposition of small bowel

42.54 Other intrathoracic esophagoenterostomy
Anastomosis of esophagus to intestinal segment NOS

42.55 Intrathoracic esophageal anastomosis with interposition of colon

42.56 Other intrathoracic esophagocolostomy
Esophagocolostomy NOS

42.58 Intrathoracic esophageal anastomosis with other interposition
Construction of artificial esophagus
Retrosternal formation of reversed gastric tube
DEF: Retrosternal anastomosis of reversed gastric tube: Formation of gastric tube behind breastbone.

42.59 Other intrathoracic anastomosis of esophagus

√4th **42.6 Antesternal anastomosis of esophagus**
Code also any synchronous:
esophagectomy (42.40-42.42)
gastrostomy (43.1)

42.61 Antesternal esophagoesophagostomy

42.62 Antesternal esophagogastrostomy

42.63 Antesternal esophageal anastomosis with interposition of small bowel

42.64 Other antesternal esophagoenterostomy
Antethoracic:
esophagoenterostomy
esophagoileostomy
esophagojejunostomy

42.65 Antesternal esophageal anastomosis with interposition of colon
DEF: Connection of esophagus with colon segment.

42.66 Other antesternal esophagocolostomy
Antethoracic esophagocolostomy

42.68 Other antesternal esophageal anastomosis with interposition

42.69 Other antesternal anastomosis of esophagus

42.7 Esophagomyotomy
DEF: Division of esophageal muscle, usually distal.

√4th **42.8 Other repair of esophagus**

42.81 Insertion of permanent tube into esophagus

42.82 Suture of laceration of esophagus

42.83 Closure of esophagostomy

Operations on the Digestive System

42.84–43.99

42.84　Repair of esophageal fistula, not elsewhere classified
　　EXCLUDES　repair of fistula:
　　　　　　bronchoesophageal (33.42)
　　　　　　esophagopleurocutaneous (34.73)
　　　　　　pharyngoesophageal (29.53)
　　　　　　tracheoesophageal (31.73)

42.85　Repair of esophageal stricture

42.86　Production of subcutaneous tunnel without esophageal anastomosis
　　DEF: Surgical formation of esophageal passage, without cutting, and reconnection.

42.87　Other graft of esophagus
　　EXCLUDES　antesternal esophageal anastomosis with interposition of:
　　　　　　colon (42.65)
　　　　　　small bowel (42.63)
　　　　antesternal esophageal anastomosis with other interposition (42.68)
　　　　intrathoracic esophageal anastomosis with interposition of:
　　　　　　colon (42.55)
　　　　　　small bowel (42.53)
　　　　intrathoracic esophageal anastomosis with other interposition (42.58)

42.89　Other repair of esophagus

✓4ᵗʰ **42.9　Other operations on esophagus**

42.91　Ligation of esophageal varices
　　EXCLUDES　that by endoscopic approach (42.33)
　　DEF: Destruction of dilated veins by suture strangulation.

42.92　Dilation of esophagus
　　Dilation of cardiac sphincter
　　EXCLUDES　intubation of esophagus (96.03, 96.06-96.08)
　　DEF: Passing of balloon or hydrostatic dilators through esophagus to enlarge esophagus and relieve obstruction.

42.99　Other
　　EXCLUDES　insertion of Sengstaken tube (96.06)
　　　　　　intubation of esophagus (96.03, 96.06-96.08)
　　　　　　removal of intraluminal foreign body from esophagus without incision (98.02)
　　　　　　tamponade of esophagus (96.06)

✓3ʳᵈ **43　Incision and excision of stomach**
　　Code also any application or administration of an adhesion barrier substance (99.77)

43.0　Gastrotomy
　　EXCLUDES　gastrostomy (43.11-43.19)
　　　　　　that for control of hemorrhage (44.49)

✓4ᵗʰ **43.1　Gastrostomy**

43.11　Percutaneous [endoscopic] gastrostomy [PEG]
　　Percutaneous transabdominal gastrostomy
　　DEF: Endoscopic positioning of tube through abdominal wall into stomach.

43.19　Other gastrostomy
　　EXCLUDES　percutaneous [endoscopic] gastrostomy [PEG] (43.11)

43.3　Pyloromyotomy
　　DEF: Cutting into longitudinal and circular muscular membrane between stomach and small intestine.

✓4ᵗʰ **43.4　Local excision or destruction of lesion or tissue of stomach**

43.41　Endoscopic excision or destruction of lesion or tissue of stomach
　　Gastric polypectomy by endoscopic approach
　　Gastric varices by endoscopic approach
　　EXCLUDES　biopsy of stomach (44.14-44.15)
　　　　　　control of hemorrhage (44.43)
　　　　　　open ligation of gastric varices (44.91)

Partial Gastrectomy with Anastomosis to Duodenum

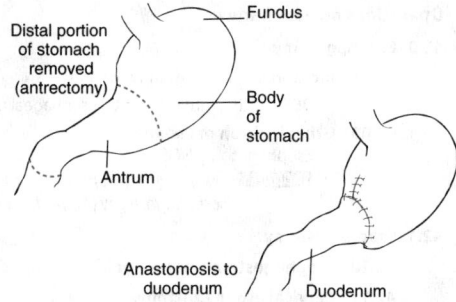

43.42　Local excision of other lesion or tissue of stomach
　　EXCLUDES　biopsy of stomach (44.14-44.15)
　　　　　　gastric fistulectomy (44.62-44.63)
　　　　　　partial gastrectomy (43.5-43.89)

43.49　Other destruction of lesion or tissue of stomach
　　EXCLUDES　that by endoscopic approach (43.41)

43.5　Partial gastrectomy with anastomosis to esophagus
　　Proximal gastrectomy

43.6　Partial gastrectomy with anastomosis to duodenum
　　Billroth I operation
　　Distal gastrectomy
　　Gastropylorectomy

43.7　Partial gastrectomy with anastomosis to jejunum
　　Billroth II operation

✓4ᵗʰ **43.8　Other partial gastrectomy**

43.81　Partial gastrectomy with jejunal transposition
　　Henley jejunal transposition operation
　　Code also any synchronous intestinal resection (45.51)

43.82　Laparoscopic vertical (sleeve) gastrectomy
　　EXCLUDES　laparoscopic banding (44.95)
　　　　　　laparoscopic gastric restrictive procedure (44.95)
　　DEF: Removal of the majority of the stomach, the greater curvature, resulting in a long vertical shape with preservation of the pyloric valve and nerves of the stomach.

43.89　Open and other partial gastrectomy
　　Partial gastrectomy with bypass gastrogastrostomy
　　Sleeve resection of stomach
　　EXCLUDES　laparoscopic sleeve gastrectomy (43.82)

✓4ᵗʰ **43.9　Total gastrectomy**

43.91　Total gastrectomy with intestinal interposition

43.99　Other total gastrectomy
　　Complete gastroduodenectomy
　　Esophagoduodenostomy with complete gastrectomy
　　Esophagogastrectomy NOS
　　Esophagojejunostomy with complete gastrectomy
　　Radical gastrectomy

Biliopancreatic Diversion Without Duodenal Switch

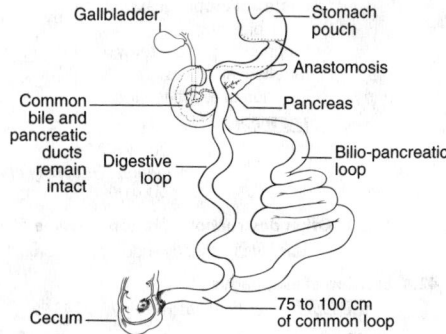

Biliopancreatic Diversion with Duodenal Switch

Types of Vagotomy Procedures

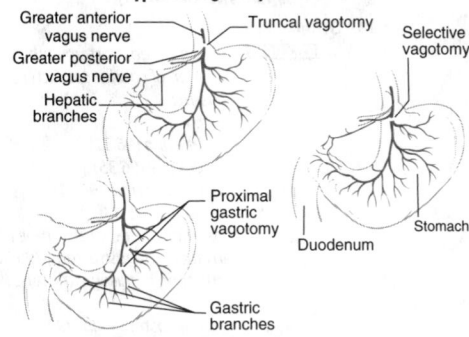

Roux-en-Y Operation (Gastrojejunostomy without gastrectomy)

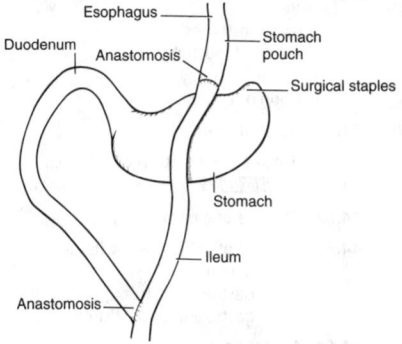

✓3ʳᵈ **44   Other operations on stomach**

Code also any application or administration of an adhesion barrier substance (99.77)

✓4ᵗʰ **44.0   Vagotomy**

44.00   Vagotomy, not otherwise specified

Division of vagus nerve NOS

DEF: Cutting of vagus nerve to reduce acid production.

44.01   Truncal vagotomy

DEF: Surgical removal of vagus nerve segment near stomach branches.

44.02   Highly selective vagotomy

Parietal cell vagotomy
Selective proximal vagotomy

DEF: Cutting select gastric branches of vagus nerve to reduce acid production and preserve other nerve functions.

44.03   Other selective vagotomy

✓4ᵗʰ **44.1   Diagnostic procedures on stomach**

44.11   Transabdominal gastroscopy

Intraoperative gastroscopy

EXCLUDES   *that with biopsy (44.14)*

44.12   Gastroscopy through artificial stoma

EXCLUDES   *that with biopsy (44.14)*

44.13   Other gastroscopy

EXCLUDES   *that with biopsy (44.14)*

44.14   Closed [endoscopic] biopsy of stomach

Brushing or washing for specimen collection

EXCLUDES   *esophagogastroduodenoscopy [EGD] with closed biopsy (45.16)*

44.15   Open biopsy of stomach

44.19   Other diagnostic procedures on stomach

EXCLUDES   *gastric lavage (96.33)*
microscopic examination of specimen from stomach (90.81-90.89)
upper GI series (87.62)

✓4ᵗʰ **44.2   Pyloroplasty**

44.21   Dilation of pylorus by incision

DEF: Cutting and suturing pylorus to relieve obstruction.

44.22   Endoscopic dilation of pylorus

Dilation with balloon endoscope
Endoscopic dilation of gastrojejunostomy site

44.29   Other pyloroplasty

Pyloroplasty NOS
Revision of pylorus

✓4ᵗʰ **44.3   Gastroenterostomy without gastrectomy**

44.31   High gastric bypass

Printen and Mason gastric bypass

DEF: Connection of middle part of small intestine to upper stomach to divert food passage from upper intestine.

44.32   Percutaneous [endoscopic] gastrojejunostomy

Bypass:
    gastroduodenostomy
PEGJJ

EXCLUDES   *percutaneous (endoscopic) feeding jejunostomy (46.32)*

DEF: Percutaneous insertion of an endoscopically guided gastrostomy tube that provides an artificial opening into the gastric lumen and portion of the jejunum via the exterior abdominal wall.

44.38   Laparoscopic gastroenterostomy

Bypass:
    gastroduodenostomy
    gastroenterostomy
    gastrogastrostomy
Laparoscopic gastrojejunostomy without gastrectomy NEC

EXCLUDES   *gastroenterostomy, open approach (44.39)*

44.39   Other gastroenterostomy

Bypass:
    gastroduodenostomy
    gastroenterostomy
    gastrogastrostomy
Gastrojejunostomy without gastrectomy NOS

✓4ᵗʰ **44.4   Control of hemorrhage and suture of ulcer of stomach or duodenum**

44.40   Suture of peptic ulcer, not otherwise specified

44.41   Suture of gastric ulcer site

EXCLUDES   *ligation of gastric varices (44.91)*

44.42   Suture of duodenal ulcer site

44.43   Endoscopic control of gastric or duodenal bleeding

44.44   Transcatheter embolization for gastric or duodenal bleeding

EXCLUDES   *surgical occlusion of abdominal vessels (38.86-38.87)*

DEF: Therapeutic blocking of stomach or upper small intestine blood vessel to stop hemorrhaging; accomplished by introducing various substances using a catheter.

44.49   Other control of hemorrhage of stomach or duodenum

That with gastrotomy

44.5   Revision of gastric anastomosis
Closure of:
gastric anastomosis
gastroduodenostomy
gastrojejunostomy
Pantaloon operation

√4ᵗʰ **44.6   Other repair of stomach**

44.61   Suture of laceration of stomach
EXCLUDES   *that of ulcer site (44.41)*

44.62   Closure of gastrostomy

44.63   Closure of other gastric fistula
Closure of:
gastrocolic fistula
gastrojejunocolic fistula

44.64   Gastropexy
DEF: Suturing of stomach into position.

44.65   Esophagogastroplasty
Belsey operation
Esophagus and stomach cardioplasty

44.66   Other procedures for creation of esophagogastric sphincteric competence
Fundoplication
Gastric cardioplasty
Nissen's fundoplication
Restoration of cardio-esophageal angle
EXCLUDES   *that by laparoscopy (44.67)*

44.67   Laparoscopic procedures for creation of esophagogastric sphincteric competence
Fundoplication
Gastric cardioplasty
Nissen's fundoplication
Restoration of cardio-esophageal angle

44.68   Laparoscopic gastroplasty
Banding
Silastic vertical banding
Vertical banded gastroplasty (VBG)
Code also any synchronous laparoscopic gastroenterostomy (44.38)
EXCLUDES   *insertion, laparoscopic adjustable gastric band (restrictive procedure) (44.95)*
other repair of stomach, open approach (44.61-44.65, 44.69)

44.69   Other
Inversion of gastric diverticulum
Repair of stomach NOS
DEF: Inversion of gastric diverticulum: Turning stomach inward to repair outpouch of wall.

√4ᵗʰ **44.9   Other operations on stomach**

44.91   Ligation of gastric varices
EXCLUDES   *that by endoscopic approach (43.41)*
DEF: Destruction of dilated veins by suture or strangulation.

44.92   Intraoperative manipulation of stomach
Reduction of gastric volvulus

44.93   Insertion of gastric bubble (balloon)

44.94   Removal of gastric bubble (balloon)

44.95   Laparoscopic gastric restrictive procedure
Adjustable gastric band and port insertion
EXCLUDES   *laparoscopic gastroplasty (44.68)*
other repair of stomach (44.69)

44.96   Laparoscopic revision of gastric restrictive procedure
Revision or replacement of:
adjustable gastric band
subcutaneous gastric port device

44.97   Laparoscopic removal of gastric restrictive device(s)
Removal of either or both:
adjustable gastric band
subcutaneous port device
EXCLUDES   *nonoperative removal of gastric restrictive device(s) (97.86)*
open removal of gastric restrictive device(s) (44.99)

44.98   (Laparoscopic) adjustment of size of adjustable gastric restrictive device
Infusion of saline for device tightening
Withdrawal of saline for device loosening
Code also any:
abdominal ultrasound (88.76)
abdominal wall fluoroscopy (88.09)
barium swallow (87.61)

44.99   Other
EXCLUDES   *change of gastrostomy tube (97.02)*
dilation of cardiac sphincter (42.92)
gastric:
cooling (96.31)
freezing (96.32)
gavage (96.35)
hypothermia (96.31)
lavage (96.33)
insertion of nasogastric tube (96.07)
irrigation of gastrostomy (96.36)
irrigation of nasogastric tube (96.34)
removal of:
gastrostomy tube (97.51)
intraluminal foreign body from stomach without incision (98.03)
replacement of:
gastrostomy tube (97.02)
(naso-)gastric tube (97.01)

√3ʳᵈ **45   Incision, excision, and anastomosis of intestine**
Code also any application or administration of an adhesion barrier substance (99.77)

√4ᵗʰ **45.0   Enterotomy**
EXCLUDES   *duodenocholedochotomy (51.41-51.42, 51.51)*
that for destruction of lesion (45.30-45.34)
that of exteriorized intestine (46.14, 46.24, 46.31)

45.00   Incision of intestine, not otherwise specified

45.01   Incision of duodenum

45.02   Other incision of small intestine

45.03   Incision of large intestine
EXCLUDES   *proctotomy (48.0)*

√4ᵗʰ **45.1   Diagnostic procedures on small intestine**
Code also any laparotomy (54.11-54.19)

45.11   Transabdominal endoscopy of small intestine
Intraoperative endoscopy of small intestine
EXCLUDES   *that with biopsy (45.14)*
DEF: Endoscopic exam of small intestine through abdominal wall.
DEF: Intraoperative endoscope of small intestine: Endoscopic exam of small intestine during surgery.

45.12   Endoscopy of small intestine through artificial stoma
EXCLUDES   *that with biopsy (45.14)*

45.13   Other endoscopy of small intestine
Esophagogastroduodenoscopy [EGD]
EXCLUDES   *that with biopsy (45.14, 45.16)*

© 2014 OptumInsight, Inc.

Esophagogastroduodenoscopy

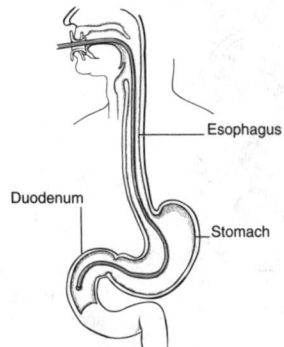

Esophagus

Duodenum

Stomach

45.14 Closed [endoscopic] biopsy of small intestine
Brushing or washing for specimen collection
EXCLUDES   *esophagogastroduodenoscopy [EGD] with closed biopsy (45.16)*

45.15 Open biopsy of small intestine

45.16 Esophagogastroduodenoscopy [EGD] with closed biopsy
Biopsy of one or more sites involving esophagus, stomach, and/or duodenum

45.19 Other diagnostic procedures on small intestine
EXCLUDES   *microscopic examination of specimen from small intestine (90.91-90.99)*
radioisotope scan (92.04)
ultrasonography (88.74)
x-ray (87.61-87.69)

✓4ᵗʰ **45.2 Diagnostic procedures on large intestine**
Code also any laparotomy (54.11-54.19)

45.21 Transabdominal endoscopy of large intestine
Intraoperative endoscopy of large intestine
EXCLUDES   *that with biopsy (45.25)*
DEF: Endoscopic exam of large intestine through abdominal wall.
DEF: Intraoperative endoscopy of large intestine: Endoscopic exam of large intestine during surgery.

45.22 Endoscopy of large intestine through artificial stoma
EXCLUDES   *that with biopsy (45.25)*
DEF: Endoscopic exam of large intestine lining from rectum to cecum via colostomy stoma.

45.23 Colonoscopy
Flexible fiberoptic colonoscopy
EXCLUDES   *endoscopy of large intestine through artificial stoma (45.22)*
flexible sigmoidoscopy (45.24)
rigid proctosigmoidoscopy (48.23)
transabdominal endoscopy of large intestine (45.21)
DEF: Endoscopic exam of descending colon, splenic flexure, transverse colon, hepatic flexure and cecum.

45.24 Flexible sigmoidoscopy
Endoscopy of descending colon
EXCLUDES   *rigid proctosigmoidoscopy (48.23)*
DEF: Endoscopic exam of anus, rectum and sigmoid colon.

45.25 Closed [endoscopic] biopsy of large intestine
Biopsy, closed, of unspecified intestinal site
Brushing or washing for specimen collection
Colonoscopy with biopsy
EXCLUDES   *proctosigmoidoscopy with biopsy (48.24)*

45.26 Open biopsy of large intestine

45.27 Intestinal biopsy, site unspecified

45.28 Other diagnostic procedures on large intestine

45.29 Other diagnostic procedures on intestine, site unspecified
EXCLUDES   *microscopic examination of specimen (90.91-90.99)*
scan and radioisotope function study (92.04)
ultrasonography (88.74)
x-ray (87.61-87.69)

✓4ᵗʰ **45.3 Local excision or destruction of lesion or tissue of small intestine**

45.30 Endoscopic excision or destruction of lesion of duodenum
EXCLUDES   *biopsy of duodenum (45.14-45.15)*
control of hemorrhage (44.43)
fistulectomy (46.72)

45.31 Other local excision of lesion of duodenum
EXCLUDES   *biopsy of duodenum (45.14-45.15)*
fistulectomy (46.72)
multiple segmental resection (45.61)
that by endoscopic approach (45.30)

45.32 Other destruction of lesion of duodenum
EXCLUDES   *that by endoscopic approach (45.30)*

45.33 Local excision of lesion or tissue of small intestine, except duodenum
Excision of redundant mucosa of ileostomy
EXCLUDES   *biopsy of small intestine (45.14-45.15)*
fistulectomy (46.74)
multiple segmental resection (45.61)

45.34 Other destruction of lesion of small intestine, except duodenum

✓4ᵗʰ **45.4 Local excision or destruction of lesion or tissue of large intestine**

45.41 Excision of lesion or tissue of large intestine
Excision of redundant mucosa of colostomy
EXCLUDES   *biopsy of large intestine (45.25-45.27)*
endoscopic polypectomy of large intestine (45.42)
fistulectomy (46.76)
multiple segmental resection (17.31, 45.71)
that by endoscopic approach (45.42-45.43)

45.42 Endoscopic polypectomy of large intestine
EXCLUDES   *that by open approach (45.41)*
DEF: Endoscopic removal of polyp from large intestine.

45.43 Endoscopic destruction of other lesion or tissue of large intestine
Endoscopic ablation of tumor of large intestine
Endoscopic control of colonic bleeding
EXCLUDES   *endoscopic polypectomy of large intestine (45.42)*

45.49 Other destruction of lesion of large intestine
EXCLUDES   *that by endoscopic approach (45.43)*

✓4ᵗʰ **45.5 Isolation of intestinal segment**
Code also any synchronous:
anastomosis other than end-to-end (45.90-45.94)
enterostomy (46.10-46.39)

45.50 Isolation of intestinal segment, not otherwise specified
Isolation of intestinal pedicle flap
Reversal of intestinal segment
DEF: Isolation of small intestinal pedicle flap: Separation of intestinal pedicle flap.
DEF: Reversal of intestinal segment: Separation of intestinal segment.

45.51 Isolation of segment of small intestine
Isolation of ileal loop
Resection of small intestine for interposition

45.52 Isolation of segment of large intestine
Resection of colon for interposition

Operations on the Digestive System

45.6–46.20

Colectomy

Intestinal Anastomosis

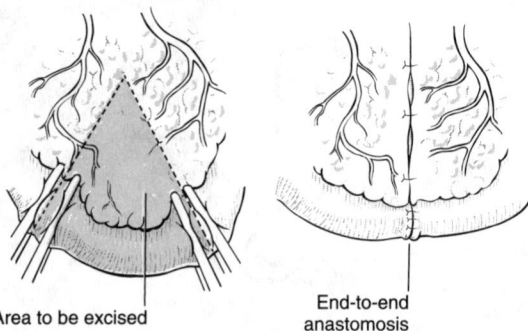

Area to be excised

End-to-end anastomosis

√4th **45.6 Other excision of small intestine**
Code also any synchronous:
anastomosis other than end-to-end (45.90-45.93, 45.95)
colostomy (46.10-46.13)
enterostomy (46.10-46.39)
> EXCLUDES   cecectomy (17.32, 45.72)
> enterocolectomy (17.39, 45.79)
> gastroduodenectomy (43.6-43.99)
> ileocolectomy (17.33, 45.73)
> pancreatoduodenectomy (52.51-52.7)

45.61 Multiple segmental resection of small intestine
Segmental resection for multiple traumatic lesions of small intestine

45.62 Other partial resection of small intestine
Duodenectomy   Jejunectomy
Ileectomy
> EXCLUDES   duodenectomy with synchronous pancreatectomy (52.51-52.7)
> resection of cecum and terminal ileum (17.32, 45.72)

45.63 Total removal of small intestine

√4th **45.7 Open and other partial excision of large intestine**
Code also any synchronous:
anastomosis other than end-to-end (45.92-45.94)
enterostomy (46.10-46.39)
> EXCLUDES   laparoscopic partial excision of large intestine (17.31-17.39)

45.71 Open and other multiple segmental resection of large intestine
Segmental resection for multiple traumatic lesions of large intestine

45.72 Open and other cecectomy
Resection of cecum and terminal ileum

45.73 Open and other right hemicolectomy
Ileocolectomy
Right radical colectomy

45.74 Open and other resection of transverse colon

45.75 Open and other left hemicolectomy
> EXCLUDES   proctosigmoidectomy (48.41-48.69)
> second stage Mikulicz operation (46.04)
> DEF: Excision of left descending large intestine.

45.76 Open and other sigmoidectomy

45.79 Other and unspecified partial excision of large intestine
Enterocolectomy NEC

√4th **45.8 Total intra-abdominal colectomy**
Excision of cecum, colon, and sigmoid
> EXCLUDES   coloproctectomy (48.41-48.69)

45.81 Laparoscopic total intra-abdominal colectomy

45.82 Open total intra-abdominal colectomy

45.83 Other and unspecified total intra- abdominal colectomy

√4th **45.9 Intestinal anastomosis**
Code also any synchronous resection (45.31-45.8, 48.41-48.69)
> EXCLUDES   end-to-end anastomosis — omit code

45.90 Intestinal anastomosis, not otherwise specified

45.91 Small-to-small intestinal anastomosis

45.92 Anastomosis of small intestine to rectal stump
Hampton procedure

45.93 Other small-to-large intestinal anastomosis

45.94 Large-to-large intestinal anastomosis
> EXCLUDES   rectorectostomy (48.74)

45.95 Anastomosis to anus
Formation of endorectal ileal pouch (J-pouch) (H-pouch) (S-pouch) with anastomosis of small intestine to anus

√3rd **46 Other operations on intestine**
Code also any application or administration of an adhesion barrier substance (99.77)

√4th **46.0 Exteriorization of intestine**
> INCLUDES   loop enterostomy
> multiple stage resection of intestine
> DEF: Bringing intestinal segment to body surface.

46.01 Exteriorization of small intestine
Loop ileostomy

46.02 Resection of exteriorized segment of small intestine

46.03 Exteriorization of large intestine
Exteriorization of intestine NOS
First stage Mikulicz exteriorization of intestine
Loop colostomy

46.04 Resection of exteriorized segment of large intestine
Resection of exteriorized segment of intestine NOS
Second stage Mikulicz operation

√4th **46.1 Colostomy**
Code also any synchronous resection (45.49, 45.71-45.79, 45.8)
> EXCLUDES   loop colostomy (46.03)
> that with abdominoperineal resection of rectum (48.5)
> that with synchronous anterior rectal resection (48.62)
> DEF: Creation of opening from large intestine through abdominal wall to body surface.

46.10 Colostomy, not otherwise specified

46.11 Temporary colostomy

46.13 Permanent colostomy

46.14 Delayed opening of colostomy

√4th **46.2 Ileostomy**
Code also any synchronous resection (45.34, 45.61-45.63)
> EXCLUDES   loop ileostomy (46.01)
> DEF: Creation of artificial anus by bringing ileum through abdominal wall to body surface.

46.20 Ileostomy, not otherwise specified

46.21   **Temporary ileostomy**

46.22   **Continent ileostomy**

> **DEF:** Creation of opening from third part of small intestine through abdominal wall, with pouch outside abdomen.

46.23   **Other permanent ileostomy**

46.24   **Delayed opening of ileostomy**

✓4ᵗʰ **46.3**   **Other enterostomy**

> Code also any synchronous resection (45.61-45.8)

46.31   **Delayed opening of other enterostomy**

46.32   **Percutaneous (endoscopic) jejunostomy [PEJ]**

> Endoscopic conversion of gastrostomy to jejunostomy
> Percutaneous (endoscopic) feeding enterostomy
>
> EXCLUDES   *percutaneous [endoscopic] gastrojejunostomy (bypass) (44.32)*
>
> **DEF:** Percutaneous feeding enterostomy: Surgical placement of a (feeding) tube through the midsection of the small intestine through the abdominal wall.
>
> **DEF:** Conversion of gastrostomy to jejunostomy: Endoscopic advancement of a jejunostomy tube through an existing gastrostomy tube into the proximal jejunum.

46.39   **Other**

> Duodenostomy
> Feeding enterostomy

✓4ᵗʰ **46.4**   **Revision of intestinal stoma**

> **DEF:** Revision of opening surgically created from intestine through abdominal wall, to skin surface.

46.40   **Revision of intestinal stoma, not otherwise specified**

> Plastic enlargement of intestinal stoma
> Reconstruction of stoma of intestine
> Release of scar tissue of intestinal stoma
>
> EXCLUDES   *excision of redundant mucosa (45.41)*

46.41   **Revision of stoma of small intestine**

> EXCLUDES   *excision of redundant mucosa (45.33)*

46.42   **Repair of pericolostomy hernia**

46.43   **Other revision of stoma of large intestine**

> EXCLUDES   *excision of redundant mucosa (45.41)*

✓4ᵗʰ **46.5**   **Closure of intestinal stoma**

> Code also any synchronous resection (45.34, 45.49, 45.61-45.8)

46.50   **Closure of intestinal stoma, not otherwise specified**

46.51   **Closure of stoma of small intestine**

46.52   **Closure of stoma of large intestine**

> Closure or take-down of cecostomy
> Closure or take-down of colostomy
> Closure or take-down of sigmoidostomy

✓4ᵗʰ **46.6**   **Fixation of intestine**

46.60   **Fixation of intestine, not otherwise specified**

> Fixation of intestine to abdominal wall

46.61   **Fixation of small intestine to abdominal wall**

> Ileopexy

46.62   **Other fixation of small intestine**

> Noble plication of small intestine
> Plication of jejunum
>
> **DEF:** Noble plication of small intestine: Fixing small intestine into place with tuck in small intestine.
>
> **DEF:** Plication of jejunum: Fixing small intestine into place with tuck in midsection.

46.63   **Fixation of large intestine to abdominal wall**

> Cecocoloplicopexy
> Sigmoidopexy (Moschowitz)

46.64   **Other fixation of large intestine**

> Cecofixation
> Colofixation

✓4ᵗʰ **46.7**   **Other repair of intestine**

> EXCLUDES   closure of:
>   *ulcer of duodenum (44.42)*
>   *vesicoenteric fistula (57.83)*

46.71   **Suture of laceration of duodenum**

46.72   **Closure of fistula of duodenum**

46.73   **Suture of laceration of small intestine, except duodenum**

46.74   **Closure of fistula of small intestine, except duodenum**

> EXCLUDES   closure of:
>   *artificial stoma (46.51)*
>   *vaginal fistula (70.74)*
>   *repair of gastrojejunocolic fistula (44.63)*

46.75   **Suture of laceration of large intestine**

46.76   **Closure of fistula of large intestine**

> EXCLUDES   closure of:
>   *gastrocolic fistula (44.63)*
>   *rectal fistula (48.73)*
>   *sigmoidovesical fistula (57.83)*
>   *stoma (46.52)*
>   *vaginal fistula (70.72-70.73)*
>   *vesicocolic fistula (57.83)*
>   *vesicosigmoidovaginal fistula (57.83)*

46.79   **Other repair of intestine**

> Duodenoplasty

✓4ᵗʰ **46.8**   **Dilation and manipulation of intestine**

46.80   **Intra-abdominal manipulation of intestine, not otherwise specified**

> Correction of intestinal malrotation   Reduction of:
> Reduction of: intestinal volvulus
>   intestinal torsion   intussusception
>
> EXCLUDES   *reduction of intussusception with:*
>   *fluoroscopy (96.29)*
>   *ionizing radiation enema (96.29)*
>   *ultrasonography guidance (96.29)*
>
> **DEF:** Correction of intestinal malrotation: Repair of abnormal rotation.
>
> **DEF:** Reduction of: Intestinal torsion: Repair of twisted segment. Intestinal volvulus: Repair of a knotted segment. Intussusception: Repair of prolapsed segment.

46.81   **Intra-abdominal manipulation of small intestine**

46.82   **Intra-abdominal manipulation of large intestine**

46.85   **Dilation of intestine**

> Dilation (balloon) of duodenum
> Dilation (balloon) of jejunum
> Endoscopic dilation (balloon) of large intestine
> That through rectum or colostomy
>
> EXCLUDES   *with insertion of colonic stent (46.86-46.87)*

46.86   **Endoscopic insertion of colonic stent(s)**

> Colonoscopy (flexible) (through stoma) with transendoscopic stent placement
> Combined with fluoroscopic-guided insertion
> Stent endoprosthesis of colon
> Through the scope [TTS] technique
>
> EXCLUDES   *other non-endoscopic insertion of colonic stent (46.87)*

46.87   **Other insertion of colonic stent(s)**

> INCLUDES   that by:
>   fluoroscopic guidance only
>   rectal guiding tube
> Non-endoscopic insertion
> Code also any synchronous diagnostic procedure(s)
>
> EXCLUDES   *endoscopic insertion of colonic stent (46.86)*

✓4ᵗʰ **46.9**   **Other operations on intestines**

46.91   **Myotomy of sigmoid colon**

46.92   **Myotomy of other parts of colon**

46.93   **Revision of anastomosis of small intestine**

Operations on the Digestive System

46.94–48.43

46.94   Revision of anastomosis of large intestine

46.95   Local perfusion of small intestine
Code also substance perfused (99.21-99.29)

46.96   Local perfusion of large intestine
Code also substance perfused (99.21-99.29)

46.97   Transplant of intestine
Note: To report donor source – see codes 00.91-00.93

46.99   Other
Ileoentectropy
EXCLUDES   *diagnostic procedures on intestine (45.11-45.29)*
dilation of enterostomy stoma (96.24)
intestinal intubation (96.08)
removal of:
intraluminal foreign body from large intestine without incision (98.04)
intraluminal foreign body from small intestine without incision (98.03)
tube from large intestine (97.53)
tube from small intestine (97.52)
replacement of:
large intestine tube or enterostomy device (97.04)
small intestine tube or enterostomy device (97.03)

√3ʳᵈ **47   Operations on appendix**
INCLUDES   appendiceal stump
Code also any application or administration of an adhesion barrier substance (99.77)

√4ᵗʰ **47.0   Appendectomy**
EXCLUDES   *incidental appendectomy, so described*
laparoscopic (47.11)
other (47.19)

47.01   Laparoscopic appendectomy

47.09   Other appendectomy

√4ᵗʰ **47.1   Incidental appendectomy**
DEF: Removal of appendix during abdominal surgery as prophylactic measure, without significant appendiceal pathology.

47.11   Laparoscopic incidental appendectomy

47.19   Other incidental appendectomy

47.2   Drainage of appendiceal abscess
EXCLUDES   *that with appendectomy (47.0)*

√4ᵗʰ **47.9   Other operations on appendix**

47.91   Appendicostomy

47.92   Closure of appendiceal fistula

47.99   Other
Anastomosis of appendix
EXCLUDES   *diagnostic procedures on appendix (45.21-45.29)*

√3ʳᵈ **48   Operations on rectum, rectosigmoid, and perirectal tissue**
Code also any application or administration of an adhesion barrier substance (99.77)

48.0   Proctotomy
Decompression of imperforate anus
Panas' operation [linear proctotomy]
EXCLUDES   *incision of perirectal tissue (48.81)*
DEF: Incision into rectal portion of large intestine.
DEF: Decompression of imperforate anus: opening a closed anus by means of an incision.
DEF: Panas' operation (linear proctotomy): Linear incision into rectal portion of large intestine.

48.1   Proctostomy

√4ᵗʰ **48.2   Diagnostic procedures on rectum, rectosigmoid, and perirectal tissue**

48.21   Transabdominal proctosigmoidoscopy
Intraoperative proctosigmoidoscopy
EXCLUDES   *that with biopsy (48.24)*

48.22   Proctosigmoidoscopy through artificial stoma
EXCLUDES   *that with biopsy (48.24)*

48.23   Rigid proctosigmoidoscopy
EXCLUDES   *flexible sigmoidoscopy (45.24)*
DEF: Endoscopic exam of anus, rectum and lower sigmoid colon.

48.24   Closed [endoscopic] biopsy of rectum
Brushing or washing for specimen collection
Proctosigmoidoscopy with biopsy

48.25   Open biopsy of rectum

48.26   Biopsy of perirectal tissue

48.29   Other diagnostic procedures on rectum, rectosigmoid, and perirectal tissue
EXCLUDES   *digital examination of rectum (89.34)*
lower GI series (87.64)
microscopic examination of specimen from rectum (90.91-90.99)

√4ᵗʰ **48.3   Local excision or destruction of lesion or tissue of rectum**

48.31   Radical electrocoagulation of rectal lesion or tissue
DEF: Destruction of lesion or tissue of rectal part of large intestine.

48.32   Other electrocoagulation of rectal lesion or tissue

48.33   Destruction of rectal lesion or tissue by laser

48.34   Destruction of rectal lesion or tissue by cryosurgery

48.35   Local excision of rectal lesion or tissue
EXCLUDES   *biopsy of rectum (48.24-48.25)*
[endoscopic] polypectomy of rectum (48.36)
excision of perirectal tissue (48.82)
hemorrhoidectomy (49.46)
rectal fistulectomy (48.73)

48.36   [Endoscopic] polypectomy of rectum

√4ᵗʰ **48.4   Pull-through resection of rectum**
Code also any synchronous anastomosis other than end-to-end (45.90, 45.92-45.95)

48.40   Pull-through resection of rectum, not otherwise specified
Pull-through resection NOS
EXCLUDES   *abdominoperineal pull-through NOS (48.50)*

48.41   Soave submucosal resection of rectum
Endorectal pull-through operation
DEF: Soave submucosal resection: Resection of submucosal rectal part of large intestine by pull-through technique.
DEF: Endorectal pull-through operation: Resection of interior large intestine by pull-through technique.

48.42   Laparoscopic pull-through resection of rectum

48.43   Open pull-through resection of rectum

48.49 Other pull-through resection of rectum
Abdominoperineal pull-through
Altemeier operation
Swenson proctectomy
> *EXCLUDES*   *Duhamel abdominoperineal*
> *pull-through (48.65)*
> *laparoscopic pull-through resection of*
> *rectum (48.42)*
> *open pull-through resection of rectum*
> *(48.43)*
> *pull-through resection of rectum, not*
> *otherwise specified (48.40)*

> **DEF:** Abdominoperineal pull-through: Resection of
> large intestine, latter part, by pull-through of
> abdomen, scrotum or vulva and anus.
> **DEF:** Swenson proctectomy: Excision of large
> intestine, rectal by pull-through and preserving
> muscles that close the anus.

√4ᵗʰ 48.5 Abdominoperineal resection of rectum
> *INCLUDES*   with synchronous colostomy
Combined abdominoendorectal resection
Complete proctectomy
Code also any synchronous anastomosis other than
end-to-end (45.90, 45.92-45.95)
> *EXCLUDES*   *Duhamel abdominoperineal pull-through (48.65)*
> *that as part of pelvic exenteration (68.8)*

> **DEF:** Rectal excision through cavities formed by abdomen,
> anus, vulva or scrotum.

48.50 Abdominoperineal resection of the rectum, not otherwise specified

48.51 Laparoscopic abdominoperineal resection of the rectum

48.52 Open abdominoperineal resection of the rectum

48.59 Other abdominoperineal resection of the rectum
> *EXCLUDES*   *abdominoperineal resection of the*
> *rectum, NOS (48.50)*
> *laparoscopic abdominoperineal*
> *resection of the rectum (48.51)*
> *open abdominoperineal resection of the*
> *rectum (48.52)*

√4ᵗʰ 48.6 Other resection of rectum
Code also any synchronous anastomosis other than
end-to-end (45.90, 45.92-45.95)

48.61 Transsacral rectosigmoidectomy
> **DEF:** Excision through sacral bone area of sigmoid
> and last parts of large intestine.

48.62 Anterior resection of rectum with synchronous colostomy
> **DEF:** Resection of front terminal end of large intestine
> and creation of colostomy.

48.63 Other anterior resection of rectum
> *EXCLUDES*   *that with synchronous colostomy (48.62)*

48.64 Posterior resection of rectum

48.65 Duhamel resection of rectum
Duhamel abdominoperineal pull-through

48.69 Other
Partial proctectomy
Rectal resection NOS

√4ᵗʰ 48.7 Repair of rectum
> *EXCLUDES*   *repair of:*
> *current obstetric laceration (75.62)*
> *vaginal rectocele (70.50, 70.52, 70.53, 70.55)*

48.71 Suture of laceration of rectum

48.72 Closure of proctostomy

48.73 Closure of other rectal fistula
> *EXCLUDES*   *fistulectomy:*
> *perirectal (48.93)*
> *rectourethral (58.43)*
> *rectovaginal (70.73)*
> *rectovesical (57.83)*
> *rectovesicovaginal (57.83)*

48.74 Rectorectostomy
Rectal anastomosis NOS
Stapled transanal rectal resection (STARR)
> **DEF:** Rectal anastomosis: Connection of two cut
> portions of large intestine, rectal end.

48.75 Abdominal proctopexy
Frickman procedure
Ripstein repair of rectal prolapse
> **DEF:** Fixation of rectum to adjacent abdominal
> structures.

48.76 Other proctopexy
Delorme repair of prolapsed rectum
Proctosigmoidopexy
Puborectalis sling operation
> *EXCLUDES*   *manual reduction of rectal prolapse*
> *(96.26)*

> **DEF:** Delorme repair of prolapsed rectum: Fixation of
> rectal part of collapsed large intestine.
> **DEF:** Proctosigmoidopexy: Suturing of rectal part of
> twisted large intestine.
> **DEF:** Puborectalis sling operation: Fixation of rectal
> part of large intestine by forming puborectalis muscle
> into sling.

48.79 Other repair of rectum
Repair of old obstetric laceration of rectum
> *EXCLUDES*   *anastomosis to:*
> *large intestine (45.94)*
> *small intestine (45.92-45.93)*
> *repair of:*
> *current obstetrical laceration (75.62)*
> *vaginal rectocele (70.50, 70.52)*

√4ᵗʰ 48.8 Incision or excision of perirectal tissue or lesion
> *INCLUDES*   pelvirectal tissue
> rectovaginal septum

48.81 Incision of perirectal tissue
Incision of rectovaginal septum

48.82 Excision of perirectal tissue
> *EXCLUDES*   *perirectal biopsy (48.26)*
> *perirectofistulectomy (48.93)*
> *rectal fistulectomy (48.73)*

√4ᵗʰ 48.9 Other operations on rectum and perirectal tissue

48.91 Incision of rectal stricture

48.92 Anorectal myectomy
> **DEF:** Excision of anorectal muscle.

48.93 Repair of perirectal fistula
> *EXCLUDES*   *that opening into rectum (48.73)*

> **DEF:** Closure of abdominal passage in tissue around
> rectal part of large intestine.

48.99 Other
> *EXCLUDES*   *digital examination of rectum (89.34)*
> *dilation of rectum (96.22)*
> *insertion of rectal tube (96.09)*
> *irrigation of rectum (96.38-96.39)*
> *manual reduction of rectal prolapse*
> *(96.26)*
> *proctoclysis (96.37)*
> *rectal massage (99.93)*
> *rectal packing (96.19)*
> *removal of:*
> *impacted feces (96.38)*
> *intraluminal foreign body from rec-*
> *tum without incision (98.05)*
> *rectal packing (97.59)*
> *transanal enema (96.39)*

√3ʳᵈ 49 Operations on anus
Code also any application or administration of an adhesion barrier
substance (99.77)

√4ᵗʰ 49.0 Incision or excision of perianal tissue

49.01 Incision of perianal abscess

49.02 Other incision of perianal tissue
Undercutting of perianal tissue
> *EXCLUDES*   *anal fistulotomy (49.11)*

Operations on the Digestive System

49.03–50.13

49.03   **Excision of perianal skin tags**

49.04   **Other excision of perianal tissue**
> *EXCLUDES*   *anal fistulectomy (49.12)*
> *biopsy of perianal tissue (49.22)*

√4ᵗʰ **49.1**   **Incision or excision of anal fistula**
> *EXCLUDES*   *closure of anal fistula (49.73)*

49.11   **Anal fistulotomy**

49.12   **Anal fistulectomy**

√4ᵗʰ **49.2**   **Diagnostic procedures on anus and perianal tissue**

49.21   **Anoscopy**

49.22   **Biopsy of perianal tissue**

49.23   **Biopsy of anus**

49.29   **Other diagnostic procedures on anus and perianal tissue**
> *EXCLUDES*   *microscopic examination of specimen from anus (90.91-90.99)*

√4ᵗʰ **49.3**   **Local excision or destruction of other lesion or tissue of anus**
> Anal cryptotomy
> Cauterization of lesion of anus
> *EXCLUDES*   *biopsy of anus (49.23)*
> *control of (postoperative) hemorrhage of anus (49.95)*
> *hemorrhoidectomy (49.46)*

49.31   **Endoscopic excision or destruction of lesion or tissue of anus**

49.39   **Other local excision or destruction of lesion or tissue of anus**
> *EXCLUDES*   *that by endoscopic approach (49.31)*

√4ᵗʰ **49.4**   **Procedures on hemorrhoids**

49.41   **Reduction of hemorrhoids**
> **DEF:** Manual manipulation to reduce hemorrhoids.

49.42   **Injection of hemorrhoids**

49.43   **Cauterization of hemorrhoids**
> Clamp and cautery of hemorrhoids

49.44   **Destruction of hemorrhoids by cryotherapy**

49.45   **Ligation of hemorrhoids**

49.46   **Excision of hemorrhoids**
> Hemorrhoidectomy NOS

49.47   **Evacuation of thrombosed hemorrhoids**
> **DEF:** Removal of clotted material from hemorrhoid.

49.49   **Other procedures on hemorrhoids**
> Lord procedure

√4ᵗʰ **49.5**   **Division of anal sphincter**

49.51   **Left lateral anal sphincterotomy**

49.52   **Posterior anal sphincterotomy**

49.59   **Other anal sphincterotomy**
> Division of sphincter NOS

49.6   **Excision of anus**

√4ᵗʰ **49.7**   **Repair of anus**
> *EXCLUDES*   *repair of current obstetric laceration (75.62)*

49.71   **Suture of laceration of anus**

49.72   **Anal cerclage**
> **DEF:** Removal of clotted material from hemorrhoid.

49.73   **Closure of anal fistula**
> *EXCLUDES*   *excision of anal fistula (49.12)*

49.74   **Gracilis muscle transplant for anal incontinence**
> **DEF:** Moving pubic attachment of gracilis muscle to restore anal control.

49.75   **Implantation or revision of artificial anal sphincter**
> Removal with subsequent replacement
> Replacement during same or subsequent operative episode

Dynamic Graciloplasty

Rectum — Generator — Electrodes — Gracilis muscle (transpositional) — Neosphincter — Anal opening

49.76   **Removal of artificial anal sphincter**
> Explantation or removal without replacement
> *EXCLUDES*   *revision with implantation during same operative episode (49.75)*

49.79   **Other repair of anal sphincter**
> Repair of old obstetric laceration of anus
> *EXCLUDES*   *anoplasty with synchronous hemorrhoidectomy (49.46)*
> *repair of current obstetric laceration (75.62)*

√4ᵗʰ **49.9**   **Other operations on anus**
> *EXCLUDES*   *dilation of anus (sphincter) (96.23)*

49.91   **Incision of anal septum**

49.92   **Insertion of subcutaneous electrical anal stimulator**

49.93   **Other incision of anus**
> Removal of:
>   foreign body from anus with incision
>   seton from anus
> *EXCLUDES*   *anal fistulotomy (49.11)*
> *removal of intraluminal foreign body without incision (98.05)*

49.94   **Reduction of anal prolapse**
> *EXCLUDES*   *manual reduction of rectal prolapse (96.26)*
> **DEF:** Manipulation of displaced anal tissue to normal position.

49.95   **Control of (postoperative) hemorrhage of anus**

49.99   **Other**

√3ʳᵈ **50**   **Operations on liver**
> Code also any application or administration of an adhesion barrier substance (99.77)

50.0   **Hepatotomy**
> Incision of abscess of liver
> Removal of gallstones from liver
> Stromeyer-Little operation

√4ᵗʰ **50.1**   **Diagnostic procedures on liver**

50.11   **Closed (percutaneous) (needle) biopsy of liver**
> Diagnostic aspiration of liver

50.12   **Open biopsy of liver**
> Wedge biopsy

50.13   **Transjugular liver biopsy**
> Transvenous liver biopsy
> *EXCLUDES*   *closed (percutaneous) [needle] biopsy of liver (50.11)*
> *laparoscopic liver biopsy (50.14)*

Closed Liver Biopsy

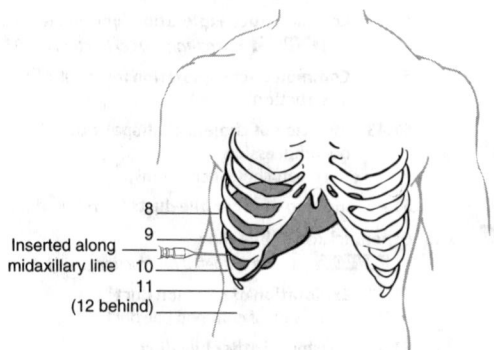

Inserted along midaxillary line

8
9
10
11
(12 behind)

Liver Biopsy (Open, Wedge)

Right lobe — Left lobe

Liver — Caudate lobe

Gallbladder

Typical wedge biopsy sites

50.14 Laparoscopic liver biopsy
> *EXCLUDES* *closed (percutaneous) [needle] biopsy of liver (50.11)*
> *open biopsy of liver (50.12)*
> *transjugular liver biopsy (50.13)*

50.19 Other diagnostic procedures on liver
> *EXCLUDES* *laparoscopic liver biopsy (50.14)*
> *liver scan and radioisotope function study (92.02)*
> *microscopic examination of specimen from liver (91.01-91.09)*
> *transjugular liver biopsy (50.13)*

√4ᵗʰ **50.2 Local excision or destruction of liver tissue or lesion**

50.21 Marsupialization of lesion of liver
> **DEF:** Exteriorizing lesion by incision and suturing cut edges to skin to create opening.

50.22 Partial hepatectomy
> Wedge resection of liver
> *EXCLUDES* *biopsy of liver (50.11-50.12)*
> *hepatic lobectomy (50.3)*

50.23 Open ablation of liver lesion or tissue

50.24 Percutaneous ablation of liver lesion or tissue

50.25 Laparoscopic ablation of liver lesion or tissue

50.26 Other and unspecified ablation of liver lesion or tissue

50.29 Other destruction of lesion of liver
> Cauterization
> Enucleation } of hepatic lesion
> Evacuation
> *EXCLUDES* *ablation of liver lesion or tissue:*
> *laparoscopic (50.25)*
> *open (50.23)*
> *other (50.26)*
> *percutaneous (50.24)*
> *laser interstitial thermal therapy [LITT] of lesion or tissue of liver under guidance (17.63)*
> *percutaneous aspiration of lesion (50.91)*

50.3 Lobectomy of liver
> Total hepatic lobectomy with partial excision of other lobe

50.4 Total hepatectomy

√4ᵗʰ **50.5 Liver transplant**
> Note: To report donor source – see codes 00.91-00.93

50.51 Auxiliary liver transplant
> Auxiliary hepatic transplantation leaving patient's own liver in situ

50.59 Other transplant of liver

√4ᵗʰ **50.6 Repair of liver**

50.61 Closure of laceration of liver

50.69 Other repair of liver
> Hepatopexy

√4ᵗʰ **50.9 Other operations on liver**
> *EXCLUDES* *lysis of adhesions (54.5)*

50.91 Percutaneous aspiration of liver
> *EXCLUDES* *percutaneous biopsy (50.11)*
> **DEF:** Incision into liver through body wall to withdraw fluid.

50.92 Extracorporeal hepatic assistance
> Liver dialysis
> **DEF:** Devices used outside body to assist liver function.

50.93 Localized perfusion of liver

50.94 Other injection of therapeutic substance into liver

50.99 Other

√3ʳᵈ **51 Operations on gallbladder and biliary tract**
> *INCLUDES* operations on:
> ampulla of Vater
> common bile duct
> cystic duct
> hepatic duct
> intrahepatic bile duct
> sphincter of Oddi
> Code also any application or administration of an adhesion barrier substance (99.77)

√4ᵗʰ **51.0 Cholecystotomy and cholecystostomy**

51.01 Percutaneous aspiration of gallbladder
> Percutaneous cholecystostomy for drainage
> That by: needle or catheter
> *EXCLUDES* *needle biopsy (51.12)*

51.02 Trocar cholecystostomy
> **DEF:** Creating opening in gallbladder with catheter.

51.03 Other cholecystostomy

51.04 Other cholecystotomy
> Cholelithotomy NOS

√4ᵗʰ **51.1 Diagnostic procedures on biliary tract**
> *EXCLUDES* *that for endoscopic procedures classifiable to 51.64, 51.84-51.88, 52.14, 52.21, 52.93 -52.94, 52.97-52.98*

51.10 Endoscopic retrograde cholangiopancreatography [ERCP]
> *EXCLUDES* *endoscopic retrograde:*
> *cholangiography [ERC] (51.11)*
> *pancreatography [ERP] (52.13)*
> **DEF:** Endoscopic and radioscopic exam of pancreatic and common bile ducts with contrast material injected through catheter in opposite direction of normal flow.

51.11 Endoscopic retrograde cholangiography [ERC]
> Laparoscopic exploration of common bile duct
> *EXCLUDES* *endoscopic retrograde:*
> *cholangiopancreatography [ERCP] (51.10)*
> *pancreatography [ERP] (52.13)*
> **DEF:** Endoscopic and radioscopic exam of common bile ducts with contrast material injected through catheter in opposite direction of normal flow.

51.12 Percutaneous biopsy of gallbladder or bile ducts
> Needle biopsy of gallbladder

Laparoscopic Cholecystectomy by Laser

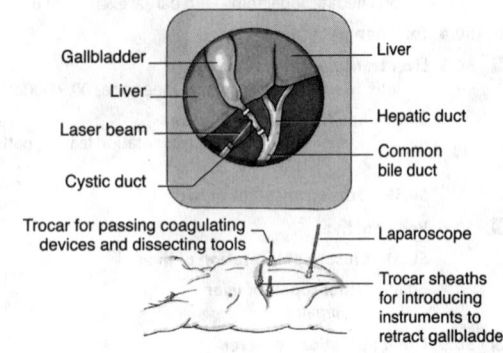

Gallbladder — Liver
Liver — Hepatic duct
Laser beam — Common bile duct
Cystic duct

Trocar for passing coagulating devices and dissecting tools — Laparoscope

Trocar sheaths for introducing instruments to retract gallbladder

51.13 Open biopsy of gallbladder or bile ducts

51.14 Other closed [endoscopic] biopsy of biliary duct or sphincter of Oddi
Brushing or washing for specimen collection
Closed biopsy of biliary duct or sphincter of Oddi by procedures classifiable to 51.10-51.11, 52.13
DEF: Endoscopic biopsy of muscle tissue around pancreatic and common bile ducts.

51.15 Pressure measurement of sphincter of Oddi
Pressure measurement of sphincter by procedures classifiable to 51.10-51.11, 52.13
DEF: Pressure measurement tests of muscle tissue surrounding pancreatic and common bile ducts.

51.19 Other diagnostic procedures on biliary tract
EXCLUDES biliary tract x-ray (87.51-87.59)
microscopic examination of specimen from biliary tract (91.01-91.09)

✓4ᵗʰ 51.2 Cholecystectomy

51.21 Other partial cholecystectomy
Revision of prior cholecystectomy
EXCLUDES that by laparoscope (51.24)

51.22 Cholecystectomy
EXCLUDES laparoscopic cholecystectomy (51.23)

51.23 Laparoscopic cholecystectomy
That by laser
DEF: Endoscopic removal of gallbladder.

51.24 Laparoscopic partial cholecystectomy

✓4ᵗʰ 51.3 Anastomosis of gallbladder or bile duct
EXCLUDES resection with end-to-end anastomosis (51.61-51.69)

51.31 Anastomosis of gallbladder to hepatic ducts

51.32 Anastomosis of gallbladder to intestine

51.33 Anastomosis of gallbladder to pancreas

51.34 Anastomosis of gallbladder to stomach

51.35 Other gallbladder anastomosis
Gallbladder anastomosis NOS

51.36 Choledochoenterostomy
DEF: Connection of common bile duct to intestine.

51.37 Anastomosis of hepatic duct to gastrointestinal tract
Kasai portoenterostomy
DEF: Kaisi portoenterostomy: A duct to drain bile from the liver is formed by anastomosing the porta hepatis to a loop of bowel.

51.39 Other bile duct anastomosis
Anastomosis of bile duct NOS
Anastomosis of unspecified bile duct to:
intestine
liver
pancreas
stomach

✓4ᵗʰ 51.4 Incision of bile duct for relief of obstruction

51.41 Common duct exploration for removal of calculus
EXCLUDES percutaneous extraction (51.96)

51.42 Common duct exploration for relief of other obstruction

51.43 Insertion of choledochohepatic tube for decompression
Hepatocholedochostomy

51.49 Incision of other bile ducts for relief of obstruction

✓4ᵗʰ 51.5 Other incision of bile duct
EXCLUDES that for relief of obstruction (51.41-51.49)

51.51 Exploration of common duct
Incision of common bile duct

51.59 Incision of other bile duct

✓4ᵗʰ 51.6 Local excision or destruction of lesion or tissue of biliary ducts and sphincter of Oddi
Code also anastomosis other than end-to-end (51.31, 51.36-51.39)
EXCLUDES biopsy of bile duct (51.12-51.13)

51.61 Excision of cystic duct remnant

51.62 Excision of ampulla of Vater (with reimplantation of common duct)

51.63 Other excision of common duct
Choledochectomy
EXCLUDES fistulectomy (51.72)

51.64 Endoscopic excision or destruction of lesion of biliary ducts or sphincter of Oddi
Excision or destruction of lesion of biliary duct by procedures classifiable to 51.10-51.11, 52.13

51.69 Excision of other bile duct
Excision of lesion of bile duct NOS
EXCLUDES fistulectomy (51.79)

✓4ᵗʰ 51.7 Repair of bile ducts

51.71 Simple suture of common bile duct

51.72 Choledochoplasty
Repair of fistula of common bile duct

51.79 Repair of other bile ducts
Closure of artificial opening of bile duct NOS
Suture of bile duct NOS
EXCLUDES operative removal of prosthetic device (51.95)

✓4ᵗʰ 51.8 Other operations on biliary ducts and sphincter of Oddi

51.81 Dilation of sphincter of Oddi
Dilation of ampulla of Vater
EXCLUDES that by endoscopic approach (51.84)
DEF: Dilation of muscle around common bile and pancreatic ducts; to mitigate constriction obstructing bile flow.

51.82 Pancreatic sphincterotomy
Incision of pancreatic sphincter
Transduodenal ampullary sphincterotomy
EXCLUDES that by endoscopic approach (51.85)
DEF: Pancreatic sphincterotomy: Division of muscle around common bile and pancreatic ducts.
DEF: Transduodenal ampullary sphincterotomy: Incision into muscle around common bile and pancreatic ducts, closing approach through first section of small intestine.

51.83 Pancreatic sphincteroplasty

51.84 Endoscopic dilation of ampulla and biliary duct
Dilation of ampulla and biliary duct by procedures classifiable to 51.10-51.11, 52.13

51.85 Endoscopic sphincterotomy and papillotomy
Sphincterotomy and papillotomy by procedures classifiable to 51.10-51.11, 52.13
DEF: Incision of muscle around common bile and pancreatic ducts and closing the duodenal papilla.

51.86 Endoscopic insertion of nasobiliary drainage tube
Insertion of nasobiliary tube by procedures classifiable to 51.10-51.11, 52.13

51.87 Endoscopic insertion of stent (tube) into bile duct
Endoprosthesis of bile duct
Insertion of stent into bile duct by procedures classifiable to 51.10-51.11, 52.13
EXCLUDES nasobiliary drainage tube (51.86)
replacement of stent (tube) (97.05)

51.88 Endoscopic removal of stone(s) from biliary tract
Laparoscopic removal of stone(s) from biliary tract
Removal of biliary tract stone(s) by procedures classifiable to 51.10-51.11, 52.13
EXCLUDES percutaneous extraction of common duct stones (51.96)

51.89 Other operations on sphincter of Oddi

51.9 Other operations on biliary tract

51.91 Repair of laceration of gallbladder

51.92 Closure of cholecystostomy

51.93 Closure of other biliary fistula
Cholecystogastroenteric fistulectomy

51.94 Revision of anastomosis of biliary tract

51.95 Removal of prosthetic device from bile duct
EXCLUDES nonoperative removal (97.55)

51.96 Percutaneous extraction of common duct stones

51.98 Other percutaneous procedures on biliary tract
Percutaneous biliary endoscopy via existing T-tube or other tract for:
dilation of biliary duct stricture
removal of stone(s) except common duct stone
exploration (postoperative)
Percutaneous transhepatic biliary drainage
EXCLUDES percutaneous aspiration of gallbladder (51.01)
percutaneous biopsy and/or collection of specimen by brushing or washing (51.12)
percutaneous removal of common duct stone(s) (51.96)

51.99 Other
Insertion or replacement of biliary tract prosthesis
EXCLUDES biopsy of gallbladder (51.12-51.13)
irrigation of cholecystostomy and other biliary tube (96.41)
lysis of peritoneal adhesions (54.5)
nonoperative removal of:
cholecystostomy tube (97.54)
tube from biliary tract or liver (97.55)

52 Operations on pancreas
INCLUDES operations on pancreatic duct
Code also any application or administration of an adhesion barrier substance (99.77)

52.0 Pancreatotomy

52.01 Drainage of pancreatic cyst by catheter

52.09 Other pancreatotomy
Pancreatolithotomy
EXCLUDES drainage by anastomosis (52.4, 52.96)
incision of pancreatic sphincter (51.82)
marsupialization of cyst (52.3)
DEF: Pancreatolithotomy: Incision into pancreas to remove stones.

52.1 Diagnostic procedures on pancreas

52.11 Closed [aspiration] [needle] [percutaneous] biopsy of pancreas

52.12 Open biopsy of pancreas

52.13 Endoscopic retrograde pancreatography [ERP]
EXCLUDES endoscopic retrograde:
cholangiography [ERC] (51.11)
cholangiopancreatography [ERCP] (51.10)
that for procedures classifiable to 51.14-51.15, 51.64, 51.84-51.88, 52.14, 52.21, 52.92-52.94, 52.97-52.98

52.14 Closed [endoscopic] biopsy of pancreatic duct
Closed biopsy of pancreatic duct by procedures classifiable to 51.10-51.11, 52.13

52.19 Other diagnostic procedures on pancreas
EXCLUDES contrast pancreatogram (87.66)
endoscopic retrograde pancreatography [ERP] (52.13)
microscopic examination of specimen from pancreas (91.01-91.09)

52.2 Local excision or destruction of pancreas and pancreatic duct
EXCLUDES biopsy of pancreas (52.11-52.12, 52.14)
pancreatic fistulectomy (52.95)

52.21 Endoscopic excision or destruction of lesion or tissue of pancreatic duct
Excision or destruction of lesion or tissue of pancreatic duct by procedures classifiable to 51.10-51.11, 52.13

52.22 Other excision or destruction of lesion or tissue of pancreas or pancreatic duct

52.3 Marsupialization of pancreatic cyst
EXCLUDES drainage of cyst by catheter (52.01)
DEF: Incision into pancreas and suturing edges to form pocket; promotes drainage and healing.

52.4 Internal drainage of pancreatic cyst
Pancreaticocystoduodenostomy
Pancreaticocystogastrostomy
Pancreaticocystojejunostomy
DEF: Withdrawing fluid from pancreatic cyst by draining it through a created passage to another organ.
DEF: Pancreaticocystoduodenostomy: Creation of passage from pancreatic cyst to first portion of small intestine.
DEF: Pancreaticocystogastrostomy: Creation of passage from pancreatic cyst to stomach.
DEF: Pancreaticocystojejunostomy: Creation of passage from pancreatic cyst to midsection of small intestine.

52.5 Partial pancreatectomy
EXCLUDES pancreatic fistulectomy (52.95)

52.51 Proximal pancreatectomy
Excision of head of pancreas (with part of body)
Proximal pancreatectomy with synchronous duodenectomy

52.52 Distal pancreatectomy
Excision of tail of pancreas (with part of body)

52.53 Radical subtotal pancreatectomy

52.59 Other partial pancreatectomy

52.6 Total pancreatectomy
Pancreatectomy with synchronous duodenectomy

52.7 Radical pancreaticoduodenectomy
One-stage pancreaticoduodenal resection with choledochojejunal anastomosis, pancreaticojejunal anastomosis, and gastrojejunostomy
Two-stage pancreaticoduodenal resection (first stage) (second stage)
Radical resection of the pancreas
Whipple procedure
EXCLUDES radical subtotal pancreatectomy (52.53)
DEF: Whipple procedure: pancreaticoduodenectomy involving the removal of the head of the pancreas and part of the small intestines; pancreaticojejunostomy, choledochojejunal anastomosis, and gastrojejunostomy included in the procedure.

Operations on the Digestive System

52.8–53.29

✓4ᵗʰ **52.8 Transplant of pancreas**
Note: To report donor source–see codes 00.91-00.93

52.80 Pancreatic transplant, not otherwise specified

52.81 Reimplantation of pancreatic tissue

52.82 Homotransplant of pancreas

52.83 Heterotransplant of pancreas

52.84 Autotransplantation of cells of islets of Langerhans
Homotransplantation of islet cells of pancreas
DEF: Transplantation of Islet cells from pancreas to another location of same patient.

52.85 Allotransplantation of cells of islets of Langerhans
Heterotransplantation of islet cells of pancreas
DEF: Transplantation of Islet cells from one individual to another.

52.86 Transplantation of cells of islets of Langerhans, not otherwise specified

✓4ᵗʰ **52.9 Other operations on pancreas**
DEF: Placement of tube into pancreatic duct, without an endoscope.

52.92 Cannulation of pancreatic duct
EXCLUDES *that by endoscopic approach (52.93)*
DEF: Placement of tube into pancreatic duct, without an endoscope.

52.93 Endoscopic insertion of stent (tube) into pancreatic duct
Insertion of cannula or stent into pancreatic duct by procedures classifiable to 51.10-51.11, 52.13
EXCLUDES *endoscopic insertion of nasopancreatic drainage tube (52.97)*
replacement of stent (tube) (97.05)

52.94 Endoscopic removal of stone(s) from pancreatic duct
Removal of stone(s) from pancreatic duct by procedures classifiable to 51.10-51.11, 52.13

52.95 Other repair of pancreas
Fistulectomy } of pancreas
Simple suture }

52.96 Anastomosis of pancreas
Anastomosis of pancreas (duct) to:
    intestine
    jejunum
    stomach
EXCLUDES *anastomosis to:*
bile duct (51.39)
gallbladder (51.33)

52.97 Endoscopic insertion of nasopancreatic drainage tube
Insertion of nasopancreatic drainage tube by procedures classifiable to 51.10-51.11, 52.13
EXCLUDES *drainage of pancreatic cyst by catheter (52.01)*
replacement of stent (tube) (97.05)

52.98 Endoscopic dilation of pancreatic duct
Dilation of Wirsung's duct by procedures classifiable to 51.10-51.11, 52.13

52.99 Other
Dilation of pancreatic }
  [Wirsung's] duct } by open approach
Repair of pancreatic }
  [Wirsung's] duct }
EXCLUDES *irrigation of pancreatic tube (96.42)*
removal of pancreatic tube (97.56)

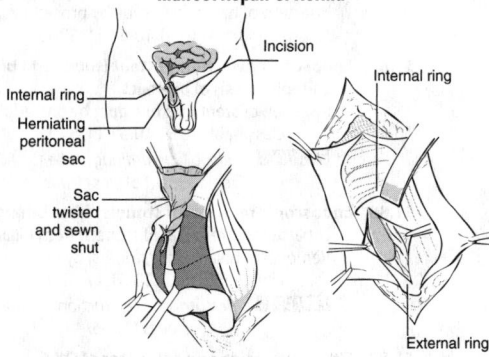

Indirect Repair of Hernia

✓3ʳᵈ **53 Repair of hernia**
INCLUDES herisplasty
           herniorrhaphy
Code also any application or administration of an adhesion barrier substance (99.77)
EXCLUDES *manual reduction of hernia (96.27)*
DEF: Repair of hernia: Restoration of abnormally protruding organ or tissue.
DEF: Herniorrhaphy: Repair of hernia.
DEF: Herniotomy: Division of constricted, strangulated, irreducible hernia.

✓4ᵗʰ **53.0 Other unilateral repair of inguinal hernia**
EXCLUDES *laparoscopic unilateral repair of inguinal hernia (17.11-17.13)*

53.00 Unilateral repair of inguinal hernia, not otherwise specified
Inguinal herniorrhaphy NOS

53.01 Other and open repair of direct inguinal hernia
Direct and indirect inguinal hernia

53.02 Other and open repair of indirect inguinal hernia

53.03 Other and open repair of direct inguinal hernia with graft or prosthesis

53.04 Other and open repair of indirect inguinal hernia with graft or prosthesis

53.05 Repair of inguinal hernia with graft or prosthesis, not otherwise specified

✓4ᵗʰ **53.1 Other bilateral repair of inguinal hernia**
EXCLUDES *laparoscopic bilateral repair of inguinal hernia (17.21-17.24)*

53.10 Bilateral repair of inguinal hernia, not otherwise specified

53.11 Other and open bilateral repair of direct inguinal hernia

53.12 Other and open bilateral repair of indirect inguinal hernia

53.13 Other and open bilateral repair of inguinal hernia, one direct and one indirect

53.14 Other and open bilateral repair of direct inguinal hernia with graft or prosthesis

53.15 Other and open bilateral repair of indirect inguinal hernia with graft or prosthesis

53.16 Other and open bilateral repair of inguinal hernia, one direct and one indirect, with graft or prosthesis

53.17 Bilateral inguinal hernia repair with graft or prosthesis, not otherwise specified

✓4ᵗʰ **53.2 Unilateral repair of femoral hernia**

53.21 Unilateral repair of femoral hernia with graft or prosthesis

53.29 Other unilateral femoral herniorrhaphy

Indirect Inguinal Hernia

Direct Inguinal Hernia

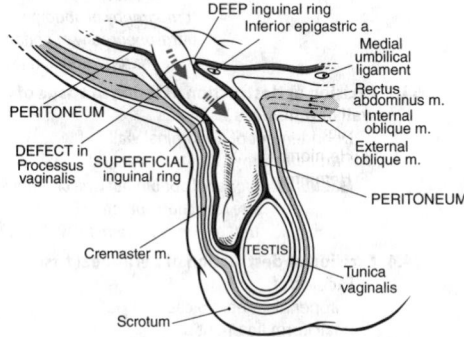

✓4ᵗʰ **53.3 Bilateral repair of femoral hernia**

  53.31 Bilateral repair of femoral hernia with graft or prosthesis

  53.39 Other bilateral femoral herniorrhaphy

✓4ᵗʰ **53.4 Repair of umbilical hernia**

  EXCLUDES *repair of gastroschisis (54.71)*

  53.41 Other and open repair of umbilical hernia with graft or prosthesis

  53.42 Laparoscopic repair of umbilical hernia with graft or prosthesis

  53.43 Other laparoscopic umbilical herniorrhaphy

  53.49 Other open umbilical herniorrhaphy

   EXCLUDES *other laparoscopic umbilical herniorrhaphy (53.43)*
   repair of umbilical hernia with graft or prosthesis (53.41, 53.42)

✓4ᵗʰ **53.5 Repair of other hernia of anterior abdominal wall (without graft or prosthesis)**

  53.51 Incisional hernia repair

  53.59 Repair of other hernia of anterior abdominal wall
   Repair of hernia:
    epigastric
    hypogastric
    spigelian
    ventral
   That by laparoscopic approach

✓4ᵗʰ **53.6 Repair of other hernia of anterior abdominal wall with graft or prosthesis**

  53.61 Other open incisional hernia repair with graft or prosthesis
   EXCLUDES *laparoscopic incisional hernia repair with graft or prosthesis (53.62)*

  53.62 Laparoscopic incisional hernia repair with graft or prosthesis

  53.63 Other laparoscopic repair of other hernia of anterior abdominal wall with graft or prosthesis

  53.69 Other and open repair of other hernia of anterior abdominal wall with graft or prosthesis
   EXCLUDES *other laparoscopic repair of other hernia of anterior abdominal wall with graft or prosthesis (53.63)*

✓4ᵗʰ **53.7 Repair of diaphragmatic hernia, abdominal approach**

  53.71 Laparoscopic repair of diaphragmatic hernia, abdominal approach

  53.72 Other and open repair of diaphragmatic hernia, abdominal approach

  53.75 Repair of diaphragmatic hernia, abdominal approach, not otherwise specified
   EXCLUDES *laparoscopic repair of diaphragmatic hernia (53.71)*
   other and open repair of diaphragmatic hernia (53.72)

✓4ᵗʰ **53.8 Repair of diaphragmatic hernia, thoracic approach**
  DEF: Repair of diaphragmatic hernia though abdomen and thorax.

  53.80 Repair of diaphragmatic hernia with thoracic approach, not otherwise specified
   Thoracoabdominal repair of diaphragmatic hernia

  53.81 Plication of the diaphragm
   DEF: Tuck repair of diaphragmatic hernia.

  53.82 Repair of parasternal hernia
   DEF: Repair of hernia protruding into breastbone area.

  53.83 Laparoscopic repair of diaphragmatic hernia, with thoracic approach

  53.84 Other and open repair of diaphragmatic hernia, with thoracic approach
   EXCLUDES *repair of diaphragmatic hernia with thoracic approach, NOS, (53.80)*

 53.9 Other hernia repair
  Repair of hernia: Repair of hernia:
   ischiatic   omental
   ischiorectal   retroperitoneal
   lumbar   sciatic
   obturator
  EXCLUDES *relief of strangulated hernia with exteriorization of intestine (46.01, 46.03)*
   repair of pericolostomy hernia (46.42)
   repair of vaginal enterocele (70.92)

✓3ʳᵈ **54 Other operations on abdominal region**
  INCLUDES operations on:
    epigastric region
    flank
    groin region
    hypochondrium
    inguinal region
    loin region
    mesentery
    omentum
    pelvic cavity
    peritoneum
    retroperitoneal tissue space
  Code also any application or administration of an adhesion barrier substance (99.77)
  EXCLUDES *hernia repair (53.00-53.9)*
   obliteration of cul-de-sac (70.92)
   retroperitoneal tissue dissection (59.00-59.09)
   skin and subcutaneous tissue of abdominal wall (86.01-86.99)

 54.0 Incision of abdominal wall
  Drainage of: Drainage of:
   abdominal wall   retroperitoneal abscess
   extraperitoneal abscess
  EXCLUDES *incision of peritoneum (54.95)*
   laparotomy (54.11-54.19)

✓4ᵗʰ **54.1 Laparotomy**
> **DEF:** Incision into abdomen.

54.11 Exploratory laparotomy
> *EXCLUDES*   exploration incidental to
> intra-abdominal surgery — omit
> code
>
> **DEF:** Exam of peritoneal cavity through incision into
> abdomen.

54.12 Reopening of recent laparotomy site
> Reopening of recent laparotomy site for:
>   control of hemorrhage
>   exploration
>   incision of hematoma

54.19 Other laparotomy
> Drainage of intraperitoneal abscess or hematoma
> *EXCLUDES*   culdocentesis (70.0)
> drainage of appendiceal abscess (47.2)
> exploration incidental to
> intra-abdominal surgery — omit
> code
> Ladd operation (54.95)
> percutaneous drainage of abdomen
> (54.91)
> removal of foreign body (54.92)

✓4ᵗʰ **54.2 Diagnostic procedures of abdominal region**

54.21 Laparoscopy
> Peritoneoscopy
> *EXCLUDES*   laparoscopic cholecystectomy (51.23)
> that incidental to destruction of fallopian
> tubes (66.21-66.29)
>
> **DEF:** Endoscopic exam of peritoneal cavity through
> abdominal portal.

54.22 Biopsy of abdominal wall or umbilicus

54.23 Biopsy of peritoneum
> Biopsy of:
>   mesentery
>   omentum
>   peritoneal implant
> *EXCLUDES*   closed biopsy of:
>   omentum (54.24)
>   peritoneum (54.24)

**54.24 Closed [percutaneous] [needle] biopsy of
intra-abdominal mass**
> Closed biopsy of:
>   omentum
>   peritoneal implant
>   peritoneum
> *EXCLUDES*   that of:
>   fallopian tube (66.11)
>   ovary (65.11)
>   uterine ligaments (68.15)
>   uterus (68.16)

54.25 Peritoneal lavage
> Diagnostic peritoneal lavage
> *EXCLUDES*   peritoneal dialysis (54.98)
>
> **DEF:** Irrigation of peritoneal cavity with siphoning of
> liquid contents for analysis.

54.29 Other diagnostic procedures on abdominal region
> *EXCLUDES*   abdominal lymphangiogram (88.04)
> abdominal x-ray NEC (88.19)
> angiocardiography of venae cavae
>   (88.51)
> C.A.T. scan of abdomen (88.01)
> contrast x-ray of abdominal cavity
>   (88.11-88.15)
> intra-abdominal arteriography NEC
>   (88.47)
> microscopic examination of peritoneal
>   and retroperitoneal specimen
>   (91.11-91.19)
> phlebography of:
>   intra-abdominal vessels NEC (88.65)
>   portal venous system (88.64)
> sinogram of abdominal wall (88.03)
> soft tissue x-ray of abdominal wall NEC
>   (88.09)
> tomography of abdomen NEC (88.02)
> ultrasonography of abdomen and
>   retroperitoneum (88.76)

**54.3 Excision or destruction of lesion or tissue of abdominal
wall or umbilicus**
> Debridement of abdominal wall
> Omphalectomy
> *EXCLUDES*   biopsy of abdominal wall or umbilicus (54.22)
> size reduction operation (86.83)
> that of skin of abdominal wall (86.22, 86.26, 86.3)

54.4 Excision or destruction of peritoneal tissue
> Excision of:
>   appendices epiploicae
>   falciform ligament
>   gastrocolic ligament
>   lesion of:
>   mesentery
>   omentum
>   peritoneum
>   presacral lesion NOS
>   retroperitoneal lesion NOS
> *EXCLUDES*   biopsy of peritoneum (54.23)
> endometrectomy of cul-de-sac (70.32)

✓4ᵗʰ **54.5 Lysis of peritoneal adhesions**
> Freeing of adhesions of:
>   biliary tract
>   intestines
>   liver
>   pelvic peritoneum
>   peritoneum
>   spleen
>   uterus
> *EXCLUDES*   lysis of adhesions of:
>   bladder (59.11)
>   fallopian tube and ovary (65.81, 65.89)
>   kidney (59.02)
>   ureter (59.02-59.03)

54.51 Laparoscopic lysis of peritoneal adhesions

54.59 Other lysis of peritoneal adhesions

✓4ᵗʰ **54.6 Suture of abdominal wall and peritoneum**

**54.61 Reclosure of postoperative disruption of
abdominal wall**

54.62 Delayed closure of granulating abdominal wound
> Tertiary subcutaneous wound closure
> **DEF:** Closure of outer layers of abdominal wound;
> follows procedure to close initial layers of wound.

54.63 Other suture of abdominal wall
> Suture of laceration of abdominal wall
> *EXCLUDES*   closure of operative wound — omit code

54.64 Suture of peritoneum
> Secondary suture of peritoneum
> *EXCLUDES*   closure of operative wound — omit code

✓4ᵗʰ **54.7 Other repair of abdominal wall and peritoneum**

54.71 Repair of gastroschisis
> **DEF:** Repair of congenital fistula of abdominal wall.

54.72 Other repair of abdominal wall

54.73 Other repair of peritoneum
> Suture of gastrocolic ligament

54.74 Other repair of omentum
> Epiplorrhaphy
> Graft of omentum
> Omentopexy
> Reduction of torsion of omentum
> **EXCLUDES** cardio-omentopexy (36.39)
>
> **DEF:** Epiplorrhaphy: Suture of abdominal serous membrane.
> **DEF:** Graft of omentum: Implantation of tissue into abdominal serous membrane.
> **DEF:** Omentopexy: Anchoring of abdominal serous membrane.
> **DEF:** Reduction of torsion of omentum: Reduction of twisted abdominal serous membrane.

54.75 Other repair of mesentery
> Mesenteric plication
> Mesenteropexy
>
> **DEF:** Creation of folds in mesentery for shortening.
> **DEF:** Mesenteriopexy: Fixation of torn, incised mesentery.

✓4ᵗʰ **54.9 Other operations of abdominal region**
> **EXCLUDES** removal of ectopic pregnancy (74.3)

54.91 Percutaneous abdominal drainage
> Paracentesis
> **EXCLUDES** creation of cutaneoperitoneal fistula (54.93)
>
> **DEF:** Puncture for removal of fluid.

54.92 Removal of foreign body from peritoneal cavity

54.93 Creation of cutaneoperitoneal fistula
> **DEF:** Creation of opening between skin and peritoneal cavity.

54.94 Creation of peritoneovascular shunt
> Peritoneovenous shunt
>
> **DEF:** Peritoneal vascular shunt: Construction of shunt to connect peritoneal cavity with vascular system.
> **DEF:** Peritoneovenous shunt: Construction of shunt to connect peritoneal cavity with vein.

54.95 Incision of peritoneum
> Exploration of ventriculoperitoneal shunt at peritoneal site
> Ladd operation
> Revision of distal catheter of ventricular shunt
> Revision of ventriculoperitoneal shunt at peritoneal site
> **EXCLUDES** that incidental to laparotomy (54.11-54.19)
>
> **DEF:** Ladd operation: Peritoneal attachment of incompletely rotated cecum, obstructing duodenum.

54.96 Injection of air into peritoneal cavity
> Pneumoperitoneum
> **EXCLUDES** that for:
>> collapse of lung (33.33)
>> radiography (88.12-88.13, 88.15)

54.97 Injection of locally-acting therapeutic substance into peritoneal cavity
> **EXCLUDES** peritoneal dialysis (54.98)

54.98 Peritoneal dialysis
> **EXCLUDES** peritoneal lavage (diagnostic) (54.25)
>
> **DEF:** Separation of blood elements by diffusion through membrane.

54.99 Other
> **EXCLUDES** removal of:
>> abdominal wall sutures (97.83)
>> peritoneal drainage device (97.82)
>> retroperitoneal drainage device (97.81)

10. OPERATIONS ON THE URINARY SYSTEM (55-59)

√3rd 55 Operations on kidney

     INCLUDES operations on renal pelvis

     Code also any application or administration of an adhesion barrier substance (99.77)

     EXCLUDES *perirenal tissue (59.00-59.09, 59.21-59.29, 59.91-59.92)*

√4th 55.0 Nephrotomy and nephrostomy

     EXCLUDES *drainage by:*
         anastomosis (55.86)
         aspiration (55.92)

     55.01 Nephrotomy
         Evacuation of renal cyst
         Exploration of kidney
         Nephrolithotomy
         DEF: Nephrotomy: Incision into kidney.
         DEF: Evacuation of renal cyst: Draining contents of cyst.
         DEF: Exploration of kidney: Exploration through incision.
         DEF: Nephrolithotomy: Removal of kidney stone through incision.

     55.02 Nephrostomy

     55.03 Percutaneous nephrostomy without fragmentation
         Nephrostolithotomy, percutaneous (nephroscopic)
         Percutaneous removal of kidney stone(s) by:
             forceps extraction (nephroscopic)
             basket extraction
         Pyelostolithotomy, percutaneous (nephroscopic)
         With placement of catheter down ureter
         EXCLUDES *percutaneous removal by fragmentation (55.04)*
             repeat nephroscopic removal during current episode (55.92)
         DEF: Insertion of tube through abdominal wall without breaking up stones.
         DEF: Nephrostolithotomy: Insertion of tube through the abdominal wall to remove stones.
         DEF: Basket extraction: Percutaneous removal of stone with grasping forceps.
         DEF: Pyelostolithotomy: Percutaneous removal of stones from funnel-shaped portion of kidney.

     55.04 Percutaneous nephrostomy with fragmentation
         Percutaneous nephrostomy with disruption of kidney stone by ultrasonic energy and extraction (suction) through endoscope
         With placement of catheter down ureter
         With fluoroscopic guidance
         EXCLUDES *repeat fragmentation during current episode (59.95)*
         DEF: Insertion of tube through abdominal wall into kidney to break up stones.

√4th 55.1 Pyelotomy and pyelostomy

     EXCLUDES *drainage by anastomosis (55.86)*
         percutaneous pyelostolithotomy (55.03)
         removal of calculus without incision (56.0)

     55.11 Pyelotomy
         Exploration of renal pelvis
         Pyelolithotomy

     55.12 Pyelostomy
         Insertion of drainage tube into renal pelvis

√4th 55.2 Diagnostic procedures on kidney

     55.21 Nephroscopy
         DEF: Endoscopic exam of renal pelvis; retrograde through ureter, percutaneous or open exposure.

     55.22 Pyeloscopy
         DEF: Fluoroscopic exam of kidney pelvis, calyces and ureters; follows IV or retrograde injection of contrast.

     55.23 Closed [percutaneous] [needle] biopsy of kidney
         Endoscopic biopsy via existing nephrostomy, nephrotomy, pyelostomy, or pyelotomy

     55.24 Open biopsy of kidney

     55.29 Other diagnostic procedures on kidney
         EXCLUDES *microscopic examination of specimen from kidney (91.21-91.29)*
             pyelogram:
                 intravenous (87.73)
                 percutaneous (87.75)
                 retrograde (87.74)
             radioisotope scan (92.03)
             renal arteriography (88.45)
             tomography:
                 C.A.T scan (87.71)
                 other (87.72)

√4th 55.3 Local excision or destruction of lesion or tissue of kidney

     55.31 Marsupialization of kidney lesion
         DEF: Exteriorization of lesion by incising anterior wall and suturing cut edges to create open pouch.

     55.32 Open ablation of renal lesion or tissue

     55.33 Percutaneous ablation of renal lesion or tissue

     55.34 Laparoscopic ablation of renal lesion or tissue

     55.35 Other and unspecified ablation of renal lesion or tissue

     55.39 Other local destruction or excision of renal lesion or tissue
         Obliteration of calyceal diverticulum
         EXCLUDES *ablation of renal lesion or tissue:*
             laparoscopic (55.34)
             open (55.32)
             other (55.35)
             percutaneous (55.33)
         biopsy of kidney (55.23-55.24)
         partial nephrectomy (55.4)
         percutaneous aspiration of kidney (55.92)
         wedge resection of kidney (55.4)

55.4 Partial nephrectomy
     Calycectomy
     Wedge resection of kidney
     Code also any synchronous resection of ureter (56.40-56.42)
     DEF: Surgical removal of a part of the kidney.
     DEF: Calycectomy: Removal of indentations in kidney.

√4th 55.5 Complete nephrectomy
     Code also any synchronous excision of:
         adrenal gland (07.21-07.3)
         bladder segment (57.6)
         lymph nodes (40.3, 40.52-40.59)

     55.51 Nephroureterectomy
         Nephroureterectomy with bladder cuff
         Total nephrectomy (unilateral)
         EXCLUDES *removal of transplanted kidney (55.53)*
         DEF: Complete removal of the kidney and all or portion of the ureter.
         DEF: Nephroureterectomy with bladder cuff: Removal of kidney, ureter, and portion of bladder attached to ureter.
         DEF: Total nephrectomy (unilateral): Complete excision of one kidney.

     55.52 Nephrectomy of remaining kidney
         Removal of solitary kidney
         EXCLUDES *removal of transplanted kidney (55.53)*

     55.53 Removal of transplanted or rejected kidney

     55.54 Bilateral nephrectomy
         EXCLUDES *complete nephrectomy NOS (55.51)*
         DEF: Removal of both kidneys same operative session.

√4th 55.6 Transplant of kidney
     Note: To report donor source – see codes 00.91-00.93

     55.61 Renal autotransplantation

     55.69 Other kidney transplantation

55.7 Nephropexy
     Fixation or suspension of movable [floating] kidney

Operations on the Urinary System

55.8–56.42

Symphysiostomy for Horseshoe Kidney

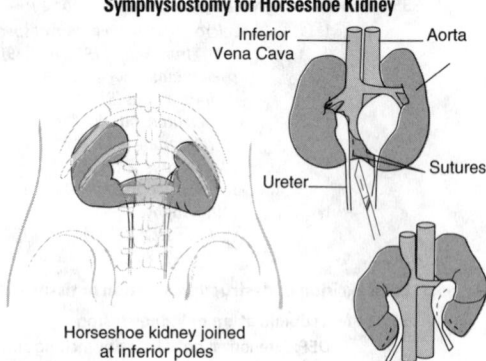

Inferior Vena Cava — Aorta — Sutures — Ureter

Horseshoe kidney joined
at inferior poles

✓4ᵗʰ 55.8 Other repair of kidney

55.81 Suture of laceration of kidney

55.82 Closure of nephrostomy and pyelostomy
DEF: Removal of tube from kidney and closure of site of tube insertion.

55.83 Closure of other fistula of kidney

55.84 Reduction of torsion of renal pedicle
DEF: Restoration of twisted renal pedicle into normal position.

55.85 Symphysiotomy for horseshoe kidney
DEF: Division of congenitally malformed kidney into two parts.

55.86 Anastomosis of kidney
Nephropyeloureterostomy
Pyeloureterovesical anastomosis
Ureterocalyceal anastomosis
> *EXCLUDES*   *nephrocystanastomosis NOS (56.73)*

DEF: Nephropyeloureterostomy: Creation of passage between kidney and ureter.
DEF: Pyeloureterovesical anastomosis: Creation of passage between kidney and bladder.
DEF: Ureterocalyceal anastomosis: Creation of passage between ureter and kidney indentations.

55.87 Correction of ureteropelvic junction

55.89 Other

✓4ᵗʰ 55.9 Other operations on kidney
> *EXCLUDES*   *lysis of perirenal adhesions (59.02)*

55.91 Decapsulation of kidney
Capsulectomy ⎫
Decortication ⎭ of kidney

55.92 Percutaneous aspiration of kidney (pelvis)
Aspiration of renal cyst
Renipuncture
> *EXCLUDES*   *percutaneous biopsy of kidney (55.23)*

DEF: Insertion of needle into kidney to withdraw fluid.

55.93 Replacement of nephrostomy tube

55.94 Replacement of pyelostomy tube

55.95 Local perfusion of kidney
DEF: Fluid passage through kidney.

55.96 Other injection of therapeutic substance into kidney
Injection into renal cyst

55.97 Implantation or replacement of mechanical kidney

55.98 Removal of mechanical kidney

55.99 Other
> *EXCLUDES*   *removal of pyelostomy or nephrostomy tube (97.61)*

✓3ʳ 56 Operations on ureter
Code also any application or administration of an adhesion barrier substance (99.77)

56.0 Transurethral removal of obstruction from ureter and renal pelvis
Removal of:
blood clot ⎫
calculus ⎬ from ureter or renal pelvis
foreign body ⎭ without incision
> *EXCLUDES*   *manipulation without removal of obstruction (59.8)*
> *that by incision (55.11,56.2)*
> *transurethral insertion of ureteral stent for passage of calculus (59.8)*

DEF: Removal of obstruction by tube inserted through urethra to ureter.

56.1 Ureteral meatotomy
DEF: Incision into ureteral meatus to enlarge passage.

56.2 Ureterotomy
Incision of ureter for:
drainage
exploration
removal of calculus
> *EXCLUDES*   *cutting of ureterovesical orifice (56.1)*
> *removal of calculus without incision (56.0)*
> *transurethral insertion of ureteral stent for passage of calculus (59.8)*
> *urinary diversion (56.51-56.79)*

✓4ᵗʰ 56.3 Diagnostic procedures on ureter

56.31 Ureteroscopy

56.32 Closed percutaneous biopsy of ureter
> *EXCLUDES*   *endoscopic biopsy of ureter (56.33)*

56.33 Closed endoscopic biopsy of ureter
Cystourethroscopy with ureteral biopsy
Transurethral biopsy of ureter
Ureteral endoscopy with biopsy through ureterotomy
Ureteroscopy with biopsy
> *EXCLUDES*   *percutaneous biopsy of ureter (56.32)*

56.34 Open biopsy of ureter

56.35 Endoscopy (cystoscopy) (looposcopy) of ileal conduit
DEF: Endoscopic exam of created opening between ureters and one end of small intestine; other end used to form artificial opening.

56.39 Other diagnostic procedures on ureter
> *EXCLUDES*   *microscopic examination of specimen from ureter (91.21-91.29)*

✓4ᵗʰ 56.4 Ureterectomy
Code also anastomosis other than end-to-end (56.51-56.79)
> *EXCLUDES*   *fistulectomy (56.84)*
> *nephroureterectomy (55.51-55.54)*

56.40 Ureterectomy, not otherwise specified

56.41 Partial ureterotomy
Excision of lesion of ureter
Shortening of ureter with reimplantation
> *EXCLUDES*   *biopsy of ureter (56.32-56.34)*

56.42 Total ureterectomy

√4ᵗʰ **56.5 Cutaneous uretero-ileostomy**

    56.51 Formation of cutaneous uretero-ileostomy
        Construction of ileal conduit
        External ureteral ileostomy
        Formation of open ileal bladder
        Ileal loop operation
        Ileoureterostomy (Bricker's) (ileal bladder)
        Transplantation of ureter into ileum with external
           diversion
          EXCLUDES *closed ileal bladder (57.87)*
                replacement of ureteral defect by ileal
                    segment (56.89)
        DEF: Creation of urinary passage by connecting the
        terminal end of small intestine to ureter, then
        connecting to opening through abdominal wall.
        DEF: Construction of ileal conduit: Formation of
        conduit from terminal end of small intestine.

    56.52 Revision of cutaneous uretero-ileostomy

√4ᵗʰ **56.6 Other external urinary diversion**

    56.61 Formation of other cutaneous ureterostomy
        Anastomosis of ureter to skin
        Ureterostomy NOS

    56.62 Revision of other cutaneous ureterostomy
        Revision of ureterostomy stoma
        EXCLUDES *nonoperative removal of ureterostomy*
              tube (97.62)

√4ᵗʰ **56.7 Other anastomosis or bypass of ureter**
        EXCLUDES *ureteropyelostomy (55.86)*

    56.71 Urinary diversion to intestine
        Anastomosis of ureter to intestine
        Internal urinary diversion NOS
        Code also any synchronous colostomy (46.10-46.13)
        EXCLUDES *external ureteral ileostomy (56.51)*

    56.72 Revision of ureterointestinal anastomosis
        EXCLUDES *revision of external ureteral ileostomy*
              (56.52)

    56.73 Nephrocystanastomosis, not otherwise specified
        DEF: Connection of kidney to bladder.

    56.74 Ureteroneocystostomy
        Replacement of ureter with bladder flap
        Ureterovesical anastomosis
        DEF: Transfer of ureter to another site in bladder.
        DEF: Ureterovesical anastomosis: Implantation of
        ureter into bladder.

    56.75 Transureteroureterostomy
        EXCLUDES *ureteroureterostomy associated with*
              partial resection (56.41)
        DEF: Separating one ureter and joining the ends to
        the opposite ureter.

    56.79 Other

√4ᵗʰ **56.8 Repair of ureter**

    56.81 Lysis of intraluminal adhesions of ureter
        EXCLUDES *lysis of periureteral adhesions*
              (59.02-59.03)
              ureterolysis (59.02-59.03)
        DEF: Destruction of adhesions within ureteral cavity.

    56.82 Suture of laceration of ureter

    56.83 Closure of ureterostomy

    56.84 Closure of other fistula of ureter

    56.85 Ureteropexy

    56.86 Removal of ligature from ureter

    56.89 Other repair of ureter
        Graft of ureter
        Replacement of ureter with ileal segment
           implanted into bladder
        Ureteroplication
        DEF: Graft of ureter: Tissue from another site for graft
        replacement or repair of ureter.
        DEF: Replacement of ureter with ileal segment
        implanted into bladder and ureter replacement with
        terminal end of small intestine.
        DEF: Ureteroplication: Creation of tucks in ureter.

√4ᵗʰ **56.9 Other operations on ureter**

    56.91 Dilation of ureteral meatus

    56.92 Implantation of electronic ureteral stimulator

    56.93 Replacement of electronic ureteral stimulator

    56.94 Removal of electronic ureteral stimulator
        EXCLUDES *that with synchronous replacement*
              (56.93)

    56.95 Ligation of ureter

    56.99 Other
        EXCLUDES *removal of ureterostomy tube and*
              ureteral catheter (97.62)
              ureteral catheterization (59.8)

√3ʳᵈ **57 Operations on urinary bladder**
    Code also any application or administration of an adhesion barrier
    substance (99.77)
    EXCLUDES *perivesical tissue (59.11-59.29, 59.91-59.92)*
             ureterovesical orifice (56.0-56.99)

    57.0 Transurethral clearance of bladder
        Drainage of bladder without incision
        Removal of:
           blood clot
           calculus ⎫ from bladder without incision
           foreign body ⎭
        EXCLUDES *that by incision (57.19)*
        DEF: Insertion of device through urethra to cleanse bladder.

√4ᵗʰ **57.1 Cystotomy and cystostomy**
        EXCLUDES *cystotomy and cystostomy as operative approach*
              — omit code
        DEF: Cystotomy: Incision of bladder.
        DEF: Cystostomy: Creation of opening into bladder.

    57.11 Percutaneous aspiration of bladder

    57.12 Lysis of intraluminal adhesions with incision into
        bladder
        EXCLUDES *transurethral lysis of intraluminal*
              adhesions (57.41)
        DEF: Incision into bladder to destroy lesions.

    57.17 Percutaneous cystostomy
        Closed cystostomy
        Percutaneous suprapubic cystostomy
        EXCLUDES *removal of cystostomy tube (97.63)*
              replacement of cystostomy tube (59.94)
        DEF: Incision through body wall into bladder to insert
        tube.
        DEF: Percutaneous (closed) suprapubic cystostomy:
        Incision above pubic arch, through body wall, into the
        bladder to insert tube.

    57.18 Other suprapubic cystostomy
        EXCLUDES *percutaneous cystostomy (57.17)*
              removal of cystostomy tube (97.63)
              replacement of cystostomy tube (59.94)

    57.19 Other cystotomy
        Cystolithotomy
        EXCLUDES *percutaneous cystostomy (57.17)*
              suprapubic cystostomy (57.18)

Operations on the Urinary System

57.2–57.89

Transurethral Cystourethroscopy

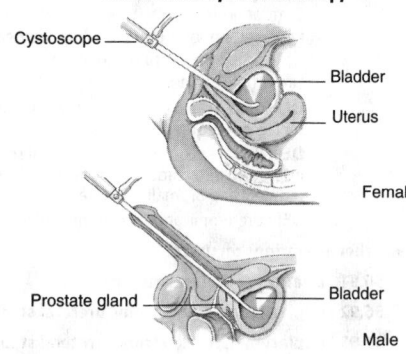

Cystoscope

Bladder

Uterus

Female

Prostate gland

Bladder

Male

✓4ᵗʰ **57.2 Vesicostomy**
> EXCLUDES   *percutaneous cystostomy (57.17)*
> *suprapubic cystostomy (57.18)*

57.21 Vesicostomy
Creation of permanent opening from bladder to skin using a bladder flap
> DEF: Creation of permanent opening from the bladder to the skin.

57.22 Revision or closure of vesicostomy
> EXCLUDES   *closure of cystostomy (57.82)*

✓4ᵗʰ **57.3 Diagnostic procedures on bladder**

57.31 Cystoscopy through artificial stoma

57.32 Other cystoscopy
Transurethral cystoscopy
> EXCLUDES   *cystourethroscopy with ureteral biopsy (56.33)*
> *retrograde pyelogram (87.74)*
> *that for control of hemorrhage (postoperative):*
> *bladder (57.93)*
> *prostate (60.94)*

57.33 Closed [transurethral] biopsy of bladder

57.34 Open biopsy of bladder

57.39 Other diagnostic procedures on bladder
> EXCLUDES   *cystogram NEC (87.77)*
> *microscopic examination of specimen from bladder (91.31-91.39)*
> *retrograde cystourethrogram (87.76)*
> *therapeutic distention of bladder (96.25)*

✓4ᵗʰ **57.4 Transurethral excision or destruction of bladder tissue**
> DEF: Destruction of bladder tissue with instrument inserted into urethra.

57.41 Transurethral lysis of intraluminal adhesions

57.49 Other transurethral excision or destruction of lesion or tissue of bladder
Endoscopic resection of bladder lesion
> EXCLUDES   *transurethral biopsy of bladder (57.33)*
> *transurethral fistulectomy (57.83-57.84)*

✓4ᵗʰ **57.5 Other excision or destruction of bladder tissue**
> EXCLUDES   *that with transurethral approach (57.41-57.49)*

57.51 Excision of urachus
Excision of urachal sinus of bladder
> EXCLUDES   *excision of urachal cyst of abdominal wall (54.3)*

57.59 Open excision or destruction of other lesion or tissue of bladder
Endometrectomy of bladder
Suprapubic excision of bladder lesion
> EXCLUDES   *biopsy of bladder (57.33-57.34)*
> *fistulectomy of bladder (57.83-57.84)*
> DEF: Endometrectomy of bladder: Removal of inner lining.
> DEF: Suprapubic excision of bladder lesion: Removal of lesion by excision above suprapubic bone arch.

57.6 Partial cystectomy
Excision of bladder dome   Wedge resection of bladder
Trigonectomy

✓4ᵗʰ **57.7 Total cystectomy**
> INCLUDES   total cystectomy with urethrectomy

57.71 Radical cystectomy
Pelvic exenteration in male
Removal of bladder, prostate, seminal vesicles and fat
Removal of bladder, urethra, and fat in a female
Code also any:
lymph node dissection (40.3, 40.5)
urinary diversion (56.51-56.79)
> EXCLUDES   *that as part of pelvic exenteration in female (68.8)*
> DEF: Radical cystectomy: Removal of bladder and surrounding tissue.
> DEF: Pelvic exenteration in male: Excision of bladder, prostate, seminal vessels and fat.

57.79 Other total cystectomy

✓4ᵗʰ **57.8 Other repair of urinary bladder**
> EXCLUDES   *repair of:*
> *current obstetric laceration (75.61)*
> *cystocele (70.50-70.51)*
> *that for stress incontinence (59.3-59.79)*

57.81 Suture of laceration of bladder

57.82 Closure of cystostomy

57.83 Repair of fistula involving bladder and intestine
Rectovesicovaginal   ⎫
Vesicosigmoidovaginal ⎬ fistulectomy

57.84 Repair of other fistula of bladder
Cervicovesical   ⎫
Urethroperineovesical ⎬ fistulectomy
Uterovesical ⎪
Vaginovesical ⎭
> EXCLUDES   *vesicoureterovaginal fistulectomy (56.84)*

57.85 Cystourethroplasty and plastic repair of bladder neck
Plication of sphincter of urinary bladder
V-Y plasty of bladder neck
> DEF: Cystourethroplasty: Reconstruction of narrowed portion of bladder.
> DEF: Plication of sphincter or urinary bladder: Creation of tuck in bladder sphincter.
> DEF: V-Y plasty of bladder neck: Surgical reconstruction of the narrowed portion of bladder by V-Y technique.

57.86 Repair of bladder exstrophy
> DEF: Surgical correction of a congenital bladder wall defect.

57.87 Reconstruction of urinary bladder
Anastomosis of bladder with isolated segment of ileum
Augmentation of bladder
Replacement of bladder with ileum or sigmoid [closed ileal bladder]
Code also resection of intestine (45.50-45.52)
> DEF: Anastomosis of bladder with isolated segment of ileum: Creation of connection between bladder and separated terminal end of small intestine.

57.88 Other anastomosis of bladder
Anastomosis of bladder to intestine NOS
Cystocolic anastomosis
> EXCLUDES   *formation of closed ileal bladder (57.87)*

57.89 Other repair of bladder
Bladder suspension, not elsewhere classified
Cystopexy NOS
Repair of old obstetric laceration of bladder
> EXCLUDES   *repair of current obstetric laceration (75.61)*

✓4ᵗʰ **57.9　Other operations on bladder**

57.91　Sphincterotomy of bladder
　　　　Division of bladder neck

57.92　Dilation of bladder neck

57.93　Control of (postoperative) hemorrhage of bladder

57.94　Insertion of indwelling urinary catheter

57.95　Replacement of indwelling urinary catheter

57.96　Implantation of electronic bladder stimulator

57.97　Replacement of electronic bladder stimulator

57.98　Removal of electronic bladder stimulator
　　　　EXCLUDES　*that with synchronous replacement (57.97)*

57.99　Other
　　　　EXCLUDES　*irrigation of:*
　　　　　　　cystostomy (96.47)
　　　　　　　other indwelling urinary catheter (96.48)
　　　　　　lysis of external adhesions (59.11)
　　　　　　removal of:
　　　　　　　cystostomy tube (97.63)
　　　　　　　other urinary drainage device (97.64)
　　　　　　therapeutic distention of bladder (96.25)

✓3ʳᵈ **58　Operations on urethra**
　　　INCLUDES　operations on:
　　　　　　bulbourethral gland [Cowper's gland]
　　　　　　periurethral tissue
　　　Code also any application or administration of an adhesion barrier substance (99.77)

58.0　Urethrotomy
　　　Excision of urethral septum
　　　Formation of urethrovaginal fistula
　　　Perineal urethrostomy
　　　Removal of calculus from urethra by incision
　　　EXCLUDES　*drainage of bulbourethral gland or periurethral tissue (58.91)*
　　　　　　internal urethral meatotomy (58.5)
　　　　　　removal of urethral calculus without incision (58.6)

58.1　Urethral meatotomy
　　　EXCLUDES　*internal urethral meatotomy (58.5)*
　　　DEF: Incision of urethra to enlarge passage.

✓4ᵗʰ **58.2　Diagnostic procedures on urethra**

58.21　Perineal urethroscopy

58.22　Other urethroscopy

58.23　Biopsy of urethra

58.24　Biopsy of periurethral tissue
　　　　DEF: Removal of tissue around urethra for biopsy.

58.29　Other diagnostic procedures on urethra and periurethral tissue
　　　　EXCLUDES　*microscopic examination of specimen from urethra (91.31-91.39)*
　　　　　　retrograde cystourethrogram (87.76)
　　　　　　urethral pressure profile (89.25)
　　　　　　urethral sphincter electromyogram (89.23)

✓4ᵗʰ **58.3　Excision or destruction of lesion or tissue of urethra**
　　　EXCLUDES　*biopsy of urethra (58.23)*
　　　　　excision of bulbourethral gland (58.92)
　　　　　fistulectomy (58.43)
　　　　　urethrectomy as part of:
　　　　　　complete cystectomy (57.79)
　　　　　　pelvic evisceration (68.8)
　　　　　　radical cystectomy (57.71)

58.31　Endoscopic excision or destruction of lesion or tissue of urethra
　　　　Fulguration of urethral lesion

58.39　Other local excision or destruction of lesion or tissue of urethra
　　　Excision of:
　　　　congenital valve
　　　　lesion　　　} of urethra
　　　　stricture
　　　Urethrectomy
　　　　EXCLUDES　*that by endoscopic approach (58.31)*

✓4ᵗʰ **58.4　Repair of urethra**
　　　EXCLUDES　*repair of current obstetric laceration (75.61)*

58.41　Suture of laceration of urethra

58.42　Closure of urethrostomy

58.43　Closure of other fistula of urethra
　　　　EXCLUDES　*repair of urethroperineovesical fistula (57.84)*

58.44　Reanastomosis of urethra
　　　　Anastomosis of urethra
　　　　DEF: Repair of severed urethra.

58.45　Repair of hypospadias or epispadias
　　　　DEF: Repair of abnormal urethral opening.

58.46　Other reconstruction of urethra
　　　　Urethral construction

58.47　Urethral meatoplasty
　　　　DEF: Reconstruction of urethral opening.

58.49　Other repair of urethra
　　　　Benenenti rotation of bulbous urethra
　　　　Repair of old obstetric laceration of urethra
　　　　Urethral plication
　　　　EXCLUDES　*repair of:*
　　　　　　current obstetric laceration (75.61)
　　　　　　urethrocele (70.50-70.51)

58.5　Release of urethral stricture
　　　Cutting of urethral sphincter
　　　Internal urethral meatotomy
　　　Urethrolysis

58.6　Dilation of urethra
　　　Dilation of urethrovesical junction
　　　Passage of sounds through urethra
　　　Removal of calculus from urethra without incision
　　　EXCLUDES　*urethral calibration (89.29)*

✓4ᵗʰ **58.9　Other operations on urethra and periurethral tissue**

58.91　Incision of periurethral tissue
　　　　Drainage of bulbourethral gland
　　　　DEF: Incision of tissue around urethra.

58.92　Excision of periurethral tissue
　　　　EXCLUDES　*biopsy of periurethral tissue (58.24)*
　　　　　　lysis of periurethral adhesions (59.11-59.12)

58.93　Implantation of artificial urinary sphincter [AUS]
　　　　Placement of inflatable:
　　　　　urethral sphincter
　　　　　bladder sphincter
　　　　Removal with replacement of sphincter device [AUS]
　　　　With pump and/or reservoir

58.99　Other
　　　　Repair of inflatable sphincter pump and/or reservoir
　　　　Surgical correction of hydraulic pressure of inflatable sphincter device
　　　　Removal of inflatable urinary sphincter without replacement
　　　　EXCLUDES　*removal of:*
　　　　　　intraluminal foreign body from urethra without incision (98.19)
　　　　　　urethral stent (97.65)

√3ʳᵈ **59 Other operations on urinary tract**

Code also any application or administration of an adhesion barrier substance (99.77)

√4ᵗʰ **59.0 Dissection of retroperitoneal tissue**

59.00 Retroperitoneal dissection, not otherwise specified

59.02 Other lysis of perirenal or periureteral adhesions

> *EXCLUDES*   *that by laparoscope (59.03)*

59.03 Laparoscopic lysis of perirenal or periureteral adhesions

59.09 Other incision of perirenal or periureteral tissue

Exploration of perinephric area
Incision of perirenal abscess

DEF: Exploration of the perinephric area: Exam of tissue around the kidney by incision.

DEF: Incision of perirenal abscess: Incising abscess in tissue around kidney.

√4ᵗʰ **59.1 Incision of perivesical tissue**

DEF: Incising tissue around bladder.

59.11 Other lysis of perivesical adhesions

59.12 Laparoscopic lysis of perivesical adhesions

59.19 Other incision of perivesical tissue

Exploration of perivesical tissue
Incision of hematoma of space of Retzius
Retropubic exploration

√4ᵗʰ **59.2 Diagnostic procedures on perirenal and perivesical tissue**

59.21 Biopsy of perirenal or perivesical tissue

59.29 Other diagnostic procedures on perirenal tissue, perivesical tissue, and retroperitoneum

> *EXCLUDES*   *microscopic examination of specimen from:*
>> *perirenal tissue (91.21-91.29)*
>> *perivesical tissue (91.31-91.39)*
>> *retroperitoneum NEC (91.11-91.19)*
>> *retroperitoneal x-ray (88.14-88.16)*

59.3 Plication of urethrovesical junction

Kelly-Kennedy operation on urethra
Kelly-Stoeckel urethral plication

DEF: Suturing a tuck in tissues around urethra at junction with bladder; changes angle of junction and provides support.

59.4 Suprapubic sling operation

Goebel-Frangenheim-Stoeckel urethrovesical suspension
Millin-Read urethrovesical suspension
Oxford operation for urinary incontinence
Urethrocystopexy by suprapubic suspension

DEF: Suspension of urethra from suprapubic periosteum to restore support to bladder and urethra.

59.5 Retropubic urethral suspension

Burch procedure
Marshall-Marchetti-Krantz operation
Suture of periurethral tissue to symphysis pubis
Urethral suspension NOS

DEF: Suspension of urethra from pubic bone with suture placed from symphysis pubis to paraurethral tissues; elevates urethrovesical angle, restores urinary continence.

59.6 Paraurethral suspension

Pereyra paraurethral suspension
Periurethral suspension

DEF: Suspension of bladder neck from fibrous membranes of anterior abdominal wall; upward traction applied; changes angle of urethra, improves urinary control.

√4ᵗʰ **59.7 Other repair of urinary stress incontinence**

59.71 Levator muscle operation for urethrovesical suspension

Cystourethropexy with levator muscle sling
Gracilis muscle transplant for urethrovesical suspension
Pubococcygeal sling

59.72 Injection of implant into urethra and/or bladder neck

Collagen implant   Fat implant
Endoscopic injection   Polytef implant
    of implant

DEF: Injection of collagen into submucosal tissues to increase tissue bulk and improve urinary control.

59.79 Other

Anterior urethropexy
Repair of stress incontinence NOS
Tudor "rabbit ear" urethropexy

DEF: Pubovaginal sling for treatment of stress incontinence: A strip of fascia is harvested and the vaginal epithelium is mobilized and then sutured to the midline at the urethral level to the rectus muscle to create a sling supporting the bladder.

DEF: Vaginal wall sling with bone anchors for treatment of stress incontinence: A sling for the bladder is formed by a suture attachment of vaginal wall to the abdominal wall. In addition, a suture is run from the vagina to a bone anchor placed in the pubic bone.

DEF: Transvaginal endoscopic bladder neck suspension for treatment of stress incontinence: Endoscopic surgical suturing of the vaginal epithelium and the pubocervical fascia at the bladder neck level on both sides of the urethra. Two supporting sutures are run from the vagina to an anchor placed in the pubic bone on each side.

59.8 Ureteral catheterization

Drainage of kidney by catheter
Insertion of ureteral stent
Ureterovesical orifice dilation
Code also any ureterotomy (56.2)

> *EXCLUDES*   *that for:*
>> *retrograde pyelogram (87.74)*
>> *transurethral removal of calculus or clot from ureter and renal pelvis (56.0)*

√4ᵗʰ **59.9 Other operations on urinary system**

> *EXCLUDES*   *nonoperative removal of therapeutic device (97.61-97.69)*

59.91 Excision of perienal or perivesical tissue

> *EXCLUDES*   *biopsy of perirenal or perivesical tissue (59.21)*

59.92 Other operations on perirenal or perivesical tissue

59.93 Replacement of ureterostomy tube

Change of ureterostomy tube
Reinsertion of ureterostomy tube

> *EXCLUDES*   *nonoperative removal of ureterostomy tube (97.62)*

59.94 Replacement of cystostomy tube

> *EXCLUDES*   *nonoperative removal of cystostomy tube (97.63)*

59.95 Ultrasonic fragmentation of urinary stones

Shattered urinary stones

> *EXCLUDES*   *percutaneous nephrostomy with fragmentation (55.04)*
>> *shockwave disintegration (98.51)*

59.99 Other

> *EXCLUDES*   *instillation of medication into urinary tract (96.49)*
>> *irrigation of urinary tract (96.45-96.48)*

11. OPERATIONS ON THE MALE GENITAL ORGANS (60-64)

√3rd **60 Operations on prostate and seminal vesicles**

> **INCLUDES**   operations on periprostatic tissue
>
> Code also any application or administration of an adhesion barrier substance (99.77)
>
> **EXCLUDES**   *that associated with radical cystectomy (57.71)*

60.0 Incision of prostate

> Drainage of prostatic abscess
> Prostatolithotomy
> **EXCLUDES**   *drainage of periprostatic tissue only (60.81)*

√4th **60.1 Diagnostic procedures on prostate and seminal vesicles**

60.11 Closed [percutaneous] [needle] biopsy of prostate

> Approach:
>> transrectal
>> transurethral
> Punch biopsy
> **DEF:** Excision of prostate tissue by closed technique for biopsy.

60.12 Open biopsy of prostate

60.13 Closed [percutaneous] biopsy of seminal vesicles

> Needle biopsy of seminal vesicles

60.14 Open biopsy of seminal vesicles

60.15 Biopsy of periprostatic tissue

60.18 Other diagnostic procedures on prostate and periprostatic tissue

> **EXCLUDES**   *microscopic examination of specimen from prostate (91.31-91.39)*
>> *x-ray of prostate (87.92)*

60.19 Other diagnostic procedures on seminal vesicles

> **EXCLUDES**   *microscopic examination of specimen from seminal vesicles (91.31-91.39)*
>> *x-ray:*
>>> *contrast seminal vesiculogram (87.91)*
>>> *other (87.92)*

√4th **60.2 Transurethral prostatectomy**

> **EXCLUDES**   *local excision of lesion of prostate (60.61)*

60.21 Transurethral (ultrasound) guided laser induced prostatectomy [TULIP]

> Ablation (contact) (noncontact) by laser

60.29 Other transurethral prostatectomy

> Excision of median bar by transurethral approach
> Transurethral electrovaporization of prostate (TEVAP)
> Transurethral enucleative procedure
> Transurethral prostatectomy NOS
> Transurethral resection of prostate (TURP)
> **DEF:** Excision of median bar by transurethral approach: Removal of fibrous structure of prostate.
> **DEF:** Transurethral enucleative procedure: Transurethral prostatectomy.

60.3 Suprapubic prostatectomy

> Transvesical prostatectomy
> **EXCLUDES**   *local excision of lesion of prostate (60.61)*
>> *radical prostatectomy (60.5)*
> **DEF:** Resection of prostate through incision in abdomen above pubic arch.

60.4 Retropubic prostatectomy

> **EXCLUDES**   *local excision of lesion of prostate (60.61)*
>> *radical prostatectomy (60.5)*
> **DEF:** Removal of the prostate using an abdominal approach with direct cutting into prostatic capsule.

60.5 Radical prostatectomy

> Prostatovesiculectomy
> Radical prostatectomy by any approach
> **EXCLUDES**   *cystoprostatectomy (57.71)*
> **DEF:** Removal of prostate, epididymis and vas ampullae.
> **DEF:** Prostatovesiculectomy: Removal of prostate and epididymis.

Transurethral Prostatectomy

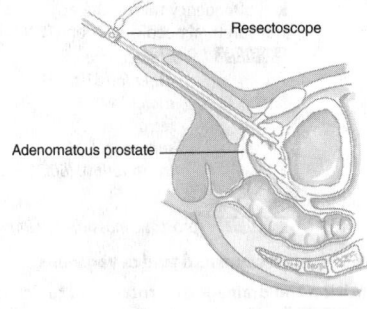

Resectoscope

Adenomatous prostate

√4th **60.6 Other prostatectomy**

60.61 Local excision of lesion of prostate

> **EXCLUDES**   *biopsy of prostate (60.11-60.12)*
>> *laser interstitial thermal therapy [LITT] of lesion or tissue of prostate under guidance (17.69)*

60.62 Perineal prostatectomy

> Cryoablation of prostate
> Cryoprostatectomy
> Cryosurgery of prostate
> Radical cryosurcial ablation of prostate (RCSA)
> **EXCLUDES**   *local excision of lesion of prostate (60.61)*
> **DEF:** Excision of prostate tissue through incision between scrotum and anus.

60.69 Other

√4th **60.7 Operations on seminal vesicles**

60.71 Percutaneous aspiration of seminal vesicle

> **EXCLUDES**   *needle biopsy of seminal vesicle (60.13)*

60.72 Incision of seminal vesicle

60.73 Excision of seminal vesicle

> Excision of Müllerian duct cyst
> Spermatocystectomy
> **EXCLUDES**   *biopsy of seminal vesicle (60.13-60.14)*
>> *prostatovesiculectomy (60.5)*

60.79 Other operations on seminal vesicles

√4th **60.8 Incision or excision of periprostatic tissue**

60.81 Incision of periprostatic tissue

> Drainage of periprostatic abscess

60.82 Excision of periprostatic tissue

> Excision of lesion of periprostatic tissue
> **EXCLUDES**   *biopsy of periprostatic tissue (60.15)*

√4th **60.9 Other operations on prostate**

60.91 Percutaneous aspiration of prostate

> **EXCLUDES**   *needle biopsy of prostate (60.11)*

60.92 Injection into prostate

60.93 Repair of prostate

60.94 Control of (postoperative) hemorrhage of prostate

> Coagulation of prostatic bed
> Cystoscopy for control of prostatic hemorrhage

60.95 Transurethral balloon dilation of the prostatic urethra

> **DEF:** Insertion and inflation of balloon to stretch the portion of the urethra that passes through the prostate.

60.96 Transurethral destruction of prostate tissue by microwave thermotherapy

> Transurethral microwave thermotherapy [TUMT] of prostate
> **EXCLUDES**   *Prostatectomy:*
>> *other (60.61-60.69)*
>> *radical (60.5)*
>> *retropubic (60.4)*
>> *suprapubic (60.3)*
>> *transurethral (60.21-60.29)*

Operations on the Male Genital Organs

60.97   Other transurethral destruction of prostate tissue by other thermotherapy
Radiofrequency thermotherapy
Transurethral needle ablation [TUNA] of prostate
EXCLUDES   *Prostatectomy:*
     other (60.61-60.69)
     radical (60.5)
     retropubic (60.4)
     suprapubic (60.3)
     transurethral (60.21-60.29)

60.99   Other
EXCLUDES   *prostatic massage (99.94)*

√3ʳᵈ **61   Operations on scrotum and tunica vaginalis**

61.0   Incision and drainage of scrotum and tunica vaginalis
EXCLUDES   *percutaneous aspiration of hydrocele (61.91)*

√4ᵗʰ **61.1   Diagnostic procedures on scrotum and tunica vaginalis**

61.11   Biopsy of scrotum or tunica vaginalis

61.19   Other diagnostic procedures on scrotum and tunica vaginalis

61.2   Excision of hydrocele (of tunica vaginalis)
Bottle repair of hydrocele of tunica vaginalis
EXCLUDES   *percutaneous aspiration of hydrocele (61.91)*
DEF: Removal of fluid collected in serous membrane of testes.

61.3   Excision or destruction of lesion or tissue of scrotum
Fulguration of lesion ⎫
Reduction of elephantiasis ⎬ of scrotum
Partial scrotectomy ⎭
EXCLUDES   *biopsy of scrotum (61.11)*
     scrotal fistulectomy (61.42)

√4ᵗʰ **61.4   Repair of scrotum and tunica vaginalis**

61.41   Suture of laceration of scrotum and tunica vaginalis

61.42   Repair of scrotal fistula

61.49   Other repair of scrotum and tunica vaginalis
Reconstruction with rotational or pedicle flaps

√4ᵗʰ **61.9   Other operations on scrotum and tunica vaginalis**

61.91   Percutaneous aspiration of tunica vaginalis
Aspiration of hydrocele of tunica vaginalis

61.92   Excision of lesion of tunica vaginalis other than hydrocele
Excision of hematocele of tunica vaginalis
DEF: Removal of blood (hematocele) collected in tunica vaginalis.

61.99   Other
EXCLUDES   *removal of foreign body from scrotum without incision (98.24)*

√3ʳᵈ **62   Operations on testes**

62.0   Incision of testis

√4ᵗʰ **62.1   Diagnostic procedures on testes**

62.11   Closed [percutaneous] [needle] biopsy of testis

62.12   Open biopsy of testis

62.19   Other diagnostic procedures on testes

Hydrocelectomy

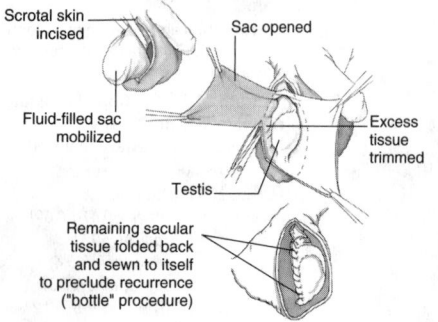

Scrotal skin incised
Sac opened
Fluid-filled sac mobilized
Excess tissue trimmed
Testis
Remaining sacular tissue folded back and sewn to itself to preclude recurrence ("bottle" procedure)

Orchiopexy with Detorsion of Testes

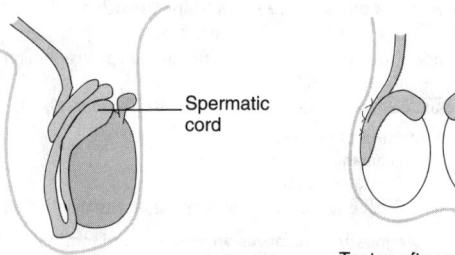

Spermatic cord

Torsion of testis

Testes after correction showing bilateral fixation

62.2   Excision or destruction of testicular lesion
Excision of appendix testis
Excision of cyst of Morgagni in the male
Excision of hydatid of Morgagni in the male
EXCLUDES   *biopsy of testis (62.11-62.12)*

62.3   Unilateral orchiectomy
Orchidectomy (with epididymectomy) NOS

√4ᵗʰ **62.4   Bilateral orchiectomy**
Male castration
Radical bilateral orchiectomy (with epididymectomy)
Code also any synchronous lymph node dissection (40.3, 40.5)
DEF: Removal of both testes.
DEF: Radical bilateral orchiectomy (with epididymectomy): Excision of both testes and structures that store sperm.

62.41   Removal of both testes at same operative episode
Bilateral orchidectomy NOS

62.42   Removal of remaining testis
Removal of solitary testis

62.5   Orchiopexy
Mobilization and replacement of testis in scrotum
Orchiopexy with detorsion of testis
Torek (-Bevan) operation (orchidopexy) (first stage) (second stage)
Transplantation to and fixation of testis in scrotum
DEF: Fixation of testis in scrotum.
DEF: Orchiopexy with detorsion of testis: Fixation and placement of testis in scrotum after correcting angle.
DEF: Torek operation (first stage) (second stage): Transfer of congenitally undescended testis from inguinal canal to scrotum.
DEF: Transplantation to and fixation of testis in scrotum: Transfer of displaced testis to scrotum.

√4ᵗʰ **62.6   Repair of testes**
EXCLUDES   *reduction of torsion (63.52)*

62.61   Suture of laceration of testis

62.69   Other repair of testis
Testicular graft

62.7   Insertion of testicular prosthesis

√4ᵗʰ **62.9   Other operations on testes**

62.91   Aspiration of testis
EXCLUDES   *percutaneous biopsy of testis (62.11)*

62.92   Injection of therapeutic substanc into testis

62.99   Other

√3ʳᵈ **63   Operations on spermatic cord, epididymis, and vas deferens**

√4ᵗʰ **63.0   Diagnostic procedures on spermatic cord, epididymis, and vas deferens**

63.01   Biopsy of spermatic cord, epididymis, or vas deferens

63.09   Other diagnostic procedures on spermatic cord, epididymis, and vas deferens
EXCLUDES   *contrast epididymogram (87.93)*
     contrast vasogram (87.94)
     other x-ray of epididymis and vas deferens (87.95)

Varicocelectomy

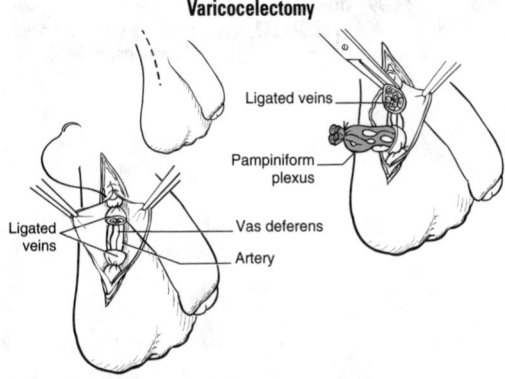

- Ligated veins
- Pampiniform plexus
- Ligated veins
- Vas deferens
- Artery

63.1 Excision of varicocele and hydrocele of spermatic cord
High ligation of spermatic vein
Hydrocelectomy of canal of Nuck
DEF: Removal of a swollen vein and collected fluid from spermatic cord.
DEF: High ligation of spermatic vein: Tying off of spermatic vein.
DEF: Hydrocelectomy of canal of Nuck: Removal of fluid collected from serous membrane of inguinal canal.

63.2 Excision of cyst of epididymis
Spermatocelectomy

63.3 Excision of other lesion or tissue of spermatic cord and epididymis
Excision of appendix epididymis
EXCLUDES *biopsy of spermatic cord or epididymis (63.01)*

63.4 Epididymectomy
EXCLUDES *that synchronous with orchiectomy (62.3-62.42)*

√4ᵗʰ 63.5 Repair of spermatic cord and epididymis
    63.51 Suture of laceration of spermatic cord and epididymis
    63.52 Reduction of torsion of testis or spermatic cord
        EXCLUDES *that associated with orchiopexy (62.5)*
        DEF: Correction of twisted testicle or spermatic cord.
    63.53 Transplantation of spermatic cord
    63.59 Other repair of spermatic cord and epididymis

63.6 Vasotomy
Vasostomy
DEF: Vasotomy: Incision of ducts carrying sperm from testicles.
DEF: Vasostomy: Creation of an opening into duct.

√4ᵗʰ 63.7 Vasectomy and ligation of vas deferens
    63.70 Male sterilization procedure, not otherwise specified
    63.71 Ligation of vas deferens
        Crushing of vas deferens
        Division of vas deferens
    63.72 Ligation of spermatic cord
    63.73 Vasectomy

√4ᵗʰ 63.8 Repair of vas deferens and epididymis
    63.81 Suture of laceration of vas deferens and epididymis
    63.82 Reconstruction of surgically divided vas deferens
    63.83 Epididymovasostomy
        DEF: Creation of new connection between vas deferens and epididymis.
    63.84 Removal of ligature from vas deferens
    63.85 Removal of valve from vas deferens
    63.89 Other repair of vas deferens and epididymis

√4ᵗʰ 63.9 Other operations on spermatic cord, epididymis, and vas deferens
    63.91 Aspiration of spermatocele
        DEF: Puncture of cystic distention of epididymis.
    63.92 Epididymotomy
        DEF: Incision of epididymis.
    63.93 Incision of spermatic cord
        DEF: Incision into sperm storage structure.
    63.94 Lysis of adhesions of spermatic cord
    63.95 Insertion of valve in vas deferens
    63.99 Other

√3ʳᵈ 64 Operations on penis
    INCLUDES operations on:
        corpora cavernosa
        glans penis
        prepuce

64.0 Circumcision
DEF: Removal of penis foreskin.

√4ᵗʰ 64.1 Diagnostic procedures on the penis
    64.11 Biopsy of penis
    64.19 Other diagnostic procedures on penis

64.2 Local excision or destruction of lesion of penis
EXCLUDES *biopsy of penis (64.11)*

64.3 Amputation of penis

√4ᵗʰ 64.4 Repair and plastic operation on penis
    64.41 Suture of laceration of penis
    64.42 Release of chordee
        DEF: Correction of downward displacement of penis.
    64.43 Construction of penis
    64.44 Reconstruction of penis
    64.45 Replantation of penis
        Reattachment of amputated penis
    64.49 Other repair of penis
        EXCLUDES *repair of epispadias and hypospadias (58.45)*

64.5 Operations for sex transformation, not elsewhere classified

√4ᵗʰ 64.9 Other operations on male genital organs
    64.91 Dorsal or lateral slit of prepuce
    64.92 Incision of penis
    64.93 Division of penile adhesions
    64.94 Fitting of external prosthesis of penis
        Penile prosthesis NOS
    64.95 Insertion or replacement of non-inflatable penile prosthesis
        Insertion of semi-rigid rod prosthesis into shaft of penis
        EXCLUDES *external penile prosthesis (64.94)*
                 inflatable penile prosthesis (64.97)
                 plastic repair, penis (64.43-64.49)
                 that associated with:
                    construction (64.43)
                    reconstruction (64.44)
    64.96 Removal of internal prosthesis of penis
        Removal without replacement of non-inflatable or inflatable penile prosthesis
    64.97 Insertion or replacement of inflatable penile prosthesis
        Insertion of cylinders into shaft of penis and placement of pump and reservoir
        EXCLUDES *external penile prosthesis (64.94)*
                 non-inflatable penile prosthesis (64.95)
                 plastic repair, penis (64.43-64.49)

64.98   Other operations on penis

Corpora cavernosa-corpus spongiosum shunt

Corpora-saphenous shunt

Irrigation of corpus cavernosum

EXCLUDES   *removal of foreign body:*
intraluminal (98.19)
without incision (98.24)
stretching of foreskin (99.95)

DEF: Corpora cavernosa-corpus spongiosum shunt: Insertion of shunt between erectile tissues of penis.

DEF: Corpora-saphenous shunt: Insertion of shunt between erectile tissue and vein of penis.

DEF: Irrigation of corpus cavernosum: Washing of erectile tissue forming dorsum and side of penis.

64.99   Other

EXCLUDES   *collection of sperm for artificial*
insemination (99.96)

12. OPERATIONS ON THE FEMALE GENITAL ORGANS (65-71)

√3ʳᵈ **65 Operations on ovary**
Code also any application or administration of an adhesion barrier substance (99.77)

√4ᵗʰ **65.0 Oophorotomy**
Salpingo-oophorotomy
DEF: Incision into ovary.
DEF: Salpingo-oophorotomy: Incision into ovary and the fallopian tube.

     65.01 Laparoscopic oophorotomy

     65.09 Other oophorotomy

√4ᵗʰ **65.1 Diagnostic procedures on ovaries**

     65.11 Aspiration biopsy of ovary

     65.12 Other biopsy of ovary

     65.13 Laparoscopic biopsy of ovary

     65.14 Other laparoscopic diagnostic procedures on ovaries

     65.19 Other diagnostic procedures on ovaries
         EXCLUDES *microscopic examination of specimen from ovary (91.41-91.49)*

√4ᵗʰ **65.2 Local excision or destruction of ovarian lesion or tissue**

     65.21 Marsupialization of ovarian cyst
         EXCLUDES *that by laparoscope (65.23)*
         DEF: Exteriorized cyst to outside by incising anterior wall and suturing cut edges to create open pouch.

     65.22 Wedge resection of ovary
         EXCLUDES *that by laparoscope (65.24)*

     65.23 Laparoscopic marsupialization of ovarian cyst

     65.24 Laparoscopic wedge resection of ovary

     65.25 Other laparoscopic local excision or destruction of ovary

     65.29 Other local excision or destruction of ovary
         Bisection
         Cauterization } of ovary
         Parial excision
         EXCLUDES *biopsy of ovary (65.11-65.13)*
         that by laparoscope (65.25)

√4ᵗʰ **65.3 Unilateral oophorectomy**

     65.31 Laparoscopic unilateral oophorectomy

     65.39 Other unilateral oophorectomy
         EXCLUDES *that by laparoscope (65.31)*

√4ᵗʰ **65.4 Unilateral salpingo-oophorectomy**

     65.41 Laparoscopic unilateral salpingo-oophorectomy

     65.49 Other unilateral salpingo-oophorectomy

√4ᵗʰ **65.5 Bilateral oophorectomy**

     65.51 Other removal of both ovaries at same operative episode
         Female castration
         EXCLUDES *that by laparoscope (65.53)*

     65.52 Other removal of remaining ovary
         Removal of solitary ovary
         EXCLUDES *that by laparoscope (65.54)*

     65.53 Laparoscopic removal of both ovaries at same operative episode

     65.54 Laparoscopic removal of remaining ovary

Oophorectomy

√4ᵗʰ **65.6 Bilateral salpingo-oophorectomy**

     65.61 Other removal of both ovaries and tubes at same operative episode
         EXCLUDES *that by laparoscope (65.53)*

     65.62 Other removal of remaining ovary and tube
         Removal of solitary ovary and tube
         EXCLUDES *that by laparoscope (65.54)*

     65.63 Laparoscopic removal of both ovaries and tubes at the same operative episode

     65.64 Laparoscopic removal of remaining ovary and tube

√4ᵗʰ **65.7 Repair of ovary**
     EXCLUDES *salpingo-oophorostomy (66.72)*

     65.71 Other simple suture of ovary
         EXCLUDES *that by laparoscope (65.74)*

     65.72 Other reimplantation of ovary
         EXCLUDES *that by laparoscope (65.75)*
         DEF: Grafting and repositioning of ovary at same site.

     65.73 Other salpingo-oophoroplasty
         EXCLUDES *that by laparoscope (65.76)*

     65.74 Laparoscopic simple suture of ovary

     65.75 Laparoscopic reimplantation of ovary

     65.76 Laparoscopic salpingo-oophoroplasty

     65.79 Other repair of ovary
         Oophoropexy

√4ᵗʰ **65.8 Lysis of adhesions of ovary and fallopian tube**

     65.81 Laparoscopic lysis of adhesions of ovary and fallopian tube

     65.89 Other lysis of adhesions of ovary and fallopian tube
         EXCLUDES *that by laparoscope (65.81)*

√4ᵗʰ **65.9 Other operations on ovary**

     65.91 Aspiration of ovary
         EXCLUDES *aspiration biopsy of ovary (65.11)*

     65.92 Transplantation of ovary
         EXCLUDES *reimplantation of ovary (65.72, 65.75)*

     65.93 Manual rupture of ovarian cyst
         DEF: Breaking up an ovarian cyst using manual technique or blunt instruments.

     65.94 Ovarian denervation
         DEF: Destruction of nerve tracts to ovary.

     65.95 Release of torsion of ovary

     65.99 Other
         Ovarian drilling

√3ʳᵈ **66 Operations on fallopian tubes**
Code also any application or administration of an adhesion barrier substance (99.77)

√4ᵗʰ **66.0 Salpingotomy and salpingostomy**

     66.01 Salpingotomy

     66.02 Salpingostomy

√4ᵗʰ **66.1 Diagnostic procedures on fallopian tubes**

     66.11 Biopsy of fallopian tube

     66.19 Other diagnostic procedures on fallopian tubes
         EXCLUDES *microscopic examination of specimen from fallopian tubes (91.41-91.49)*
         radiography of fallopian tubes (87.82-87.83, 87.85)
         Rubin's test (66.8)

Endoscopic Ligation of Fallopian Tubes

Uterus

Ovary

Ligated fallopian tube

Monitor view

Laparoscopic procedure

√4ᵗʰ **66.2 Bilateral endoscopic destruction or occlusion of fallopian tubes**

INCLUDES bilateral endoscopic destruction or occlusion of fallopian tubes by:
culdoscopy
endoscopy
hysteroscopy
laparoscopy
peritoneoscopy
endoscopic destruction of solitary fallopian tube

DEF: Endoscopic blockage or destruction of both fallopian tubes.

DEF: Bilateral endoscopic destruction or occlusion of fallopian tubes by:

Culdoscopy: Endoscopic insertion through posterior structure of vagina.

Endoscopic destruction of solitary fallopian tube: Endoscopic destruction of one fallopian tube.

Hysteroscopy: Endoscopic insertion through uterus.

Laparoscopy: Endoscopic insertion through abdomen.

Peritoneoscopy: Endoscopic insertion through abdominal serous membrane cavity.

66.21 Bilateral endoscopic ligation and crushing of fallopian tubes

66.22 Bilateral endoscopic ligation and division of fallopian tubes

66.29 Other bilateral endoscopic destruction or occlusion of fallopian tubes

√4ᵗʰ **66.3 Other bilateral destruction or occlusion of fallopian tubes**

INCLUDES destruction of solitary fallopian tube
EXCLUDES *endoscopic destruction or occlusion of fallopian tubes (66.21-66.29)*

66.31 Other bilateral ligation and crushing of fallopian tubes

66.32 Other bilateral ligation and division of fallopian tubes
Pomeroy operation

66.39 Other bilateral destruction or occlusion of fallopian tubes
Female sterilization operation NOS

66.4 Total unilateral salpingectomy

√4ᵗʰ **66.5 Total bilateral salpingectomy**

EXCLUDES *bilateral partial salpingectomy for sterilization (66.39)*
that with oophorectomy (65.61-65.64)

66.51 Removal of both fallopian tubes at same operative episode

66.52 Removal of remaining fallopian tube
Removal of solitary fallopian tube

√4ᵗʰ **66.6 Other salpingectomy**

INCLUDES salpingectomy by:
cauterization
coagulation
electrocoagulation
excision
EXCLUDES *fistulectomy (66.73)*

66.61 Excision or destruction of lesion of fallopian tube
EXCLUDES *biopsy of fallopian tube (66.11)*

66.62 Salpingectomy with removal of tubal pregnancy
Code also any synchronous oophorectomy (65.31, 65.39)

66.63 Bilateral partial salpingectomy, not otherwise specified

66.69 Other partial salpingectomy

√4ᵗʰ **66.7 Repair of fallopian tube**

66.71 Simple suture of fallopian tube

66.72 Salpingo-oophorostomy

66.73 Salpingo-salpingostomy

66.74 Salpingo-uterostomy

66.79 Other repair of fallopian tube
Graft of fallopian tube
Reopening of divided fallopian tube
Salpingoplasty

DEF: Graft of fallopian: Repair of fallopian tube with implanted graft.

DEF: Reopening of divided fallopian tube: Reconnection of severed fallopian tube to restore patency.

DEF: Salpingoplasty: Plastic reconstruction of fallopian tube defect.

66.8 Insufflation of fallopian tube
Insufflation of fallopian tube with:
air
dye
gas
saline
Rubin's test
EXCLUDES *insufflation of therapeutic agent (66.95)*
that for hysterosalpingography (87.82-87.83)

DEF: Forceful blowing of gas or liquid into fallopian tubes to test patency.

DEF: Rubin's test: Introduction of carbon dioxide gas into fallopian tubes to test patency.

√4ᵗʰ **66.9 Other operations on fallopian tubes**

66.91 Aspiration of fallopian tube

66.92 Unilateral destruction or occlusion of fallopian tube
EXCLUDES *that of solitary tube (66.21-66.39)*

66.93 Implantation or replacement of prosthesis of fallopian tube

66.94 Removal of prosthesis of fallopian tube

66.95 Insufflation of therapeutic agent into fallopian tubes

66.96 Dilation of fallopian tube

66.97 Burying of fimbriae in uterine wall
DEF: Implantation of fringed edges of fallopian tube into uterine wall.

66.99 Other
EXCLUDES *lysis of adhesions of ovary and tube (65.81, 65.89)*

√3ʳᵈ **67 Operations on cervix**
Code also any application or administration of an adhesion barrier substance (99.77)

67.0 Dilation of cervical canal
EXCLUDES *dilation and curettage (69.01-69.09)*
that for induction of labor (73.1)

√4ᵗʰ **67.1** **Diagnostic procedures on cervix**

67.11 **Endocervical biopsy**
EXCLUDES   *conization of cervix (67.2)*

67.12 **Other cervical biopsy**
Punch biopsy of cervix NOS
EXCLUDES   *conization of cervix (67.2)*

67.19 **Other diagnostic procedures on cervix**
EXCLUDES   *microscopic examination of specimen from cervix (91.41-91.49)*

67.2 **Conization of cervix**
EXCLUDES   *that by:*
     cryosurgery (67.33)
     electrosurgery (67.32)
DEF: Removal of cone-shaped section from distal cervix; cervical function preserved.

√4ᵗʰ **67.3** **Other excision or destruction of lesion or tissue of cervix**

67.31 **Marsupialization of cervical cyst**
DEF: Incision and then suturing open of a cyst in the neck of the uterus.

67.32 **Destruction of lesion of cervix by cauterization**
Electroconization of cervix
LEEP (loop electrosurgical excision procedure)
LLETZ (large loop excision of the transformation zone)
DEF: Destruction of lesion of uterine neck by applying intense heat. **DEF:** Electroconization of cervix: Electrocautery excision of multilayer cone-shaped section from uterine neck.

67.33 **Destruction of lesion of cervix by cryosurgery**
Cryoconization of cervix
DEF: Destruction of lesion of uterine neck by freezing.
DEF: Cryoconization of cervix: Excision by freezing of multilayer cone-shaped section of abnormal tissue in uterine neck.

67.39 **Other excision or destruction of lesion or tissue of cervix**
EXCLUDES   *biopsy of cervix (67.11-67.12)*
     cervical fistulectomy (67.62)
     conization of cervix (67.2)

67.4 **Amputation of cervix**
Cervicectomy with synchronous colporrhaphy
DEF: Excision of lower uterine neck.
DEF: Cervicectomy with synchronous colporrhaphy: Excision of lower uterine neck with suture of vaginal stump.

√4ᵗʰ **67.5** **Repair of internal cervical os**
DEF: Repair of cervical opening defect.

67.51 **Transabdominal cerclage of cervix**

67.59 **Other repair of internal cervical os**
Cerclage of isthmus uteri   Shirodkar operation
McDonald operation   Transvaginal cerclage
EXCLUDES   *laparoscopically assisted supracervical hysterectomy [LASH] (68.31)*
     transabdominal cerclage of cervix (67.51)
DEF: Cerclage of isthmus uteri: Placement of encircling suture between neck and body of uterus.
DEF: Shirodkar operation: Placement of purse-string suture in internal cervical opening.

Cerclage of Cervix

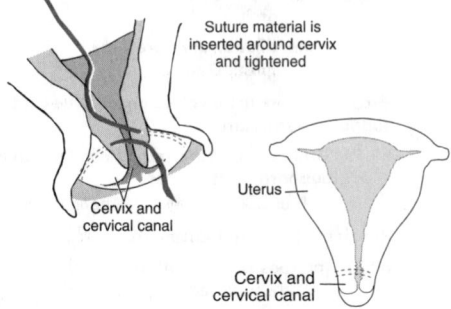

Suture material is inserted around cervix and tightened

Cervix and cervical canal

Uterus

Cervix and cervical canal

√4ᵗʰ **67.6** **Other repair of cervix**
EXCLUDES   *repair of current obstetric laceration (75.51)*

67.61 **Suture of laceration of cervix**

67.62 **Repair of fistula of cervix**
Cervicosigmoidal fistulectomy
EXCLUDES   *fistulectomy:*
     cervicovesical (57.84)
     ureterocervical (56.84)
     vesicocervicovaginal (57.84)
DEF: Closure of fistula in lower uterus.
DEF: Cervicosigmoidal fistulectomy: Excision of abnormal passage between uterine neck and torsion of large intestine.

67.69 **Other repair of cervix**
Repair of old obstetric laceration of cervix

√3ʳᵈ **68** **Other incision and excision of uterus**
Code also any application or administration of an adhesion barrier substance (99.77)

68.0 **Hysterotomy**
Hysterotomy with removal of hydatidiform mole
EXCLUDES   *hysterotomy for termination of pregnancy (74.91)*
DEF: Incision into the uterus.

√4ᵗʰ **68.1** **Diagnostic procedures on uterus and supporting structures**

68.11 **Digital examination of uterus**
EXCLUDES   *pelvic examination, so described (89.26)*
     postpartal manual exploration of uterine cavity (75.7)

68.12 **Hysteroscopy**
EXCLUDES   *that with biopsy (68.16)*

68.13 **Open biopsy of uterus**
EXCLUDES   *closed biopsy of uterus (68.16)*

68.14 **Open biopsy of uterine ligaments**
EXCLUDES   *closed biopsy of uterine ligaments (68.15)*

68.15 **Closed biopsy of uterine ligaments**
Endoscopic (laparoscopy) biopsy of uterine adnexa, except ovary and fallopian tube

68.16 **Closed biopsy of uterus**
Endoscopic (laparoscopy) (hysteroscopy) biopsy of uterus
EXCLUDES   *open biopsy of uterus (68.13)*

68.19 **Other diagnostic procedures on uterus and supporting structures**
EXCLUDES   *diagnostic:*
     aspiration curettage (69.59)
     dilation and curettage (69.09)
     microscopic examination of specimen from uterus (91.41-91.49)
     pelvic examination (89.26)
     radioisotope scan of:
       placenta (92.17)
       uterus (92.19)
     ultrasonography of uterus (88.78-88.79)
     x-ray of uterus (87.81-87.89)

√4ᵗʰ **68.2** **Excision or destruction of lesion or tissue of uterus**

68.21 **Division of endometrial synechiae**
Lysis of intraluminal uterine adhesions
DEF: Separation of uterine adhesions.
DEF: Lysis of intraluminal uterine adhesion: Surgical destruction of adhesive, fibrous structures inside uterine cavity.

68.22 **Incision or excision of congenital septum of uterus**

68.23 **Endometrial ablation**
Dilation and curettage
Hysteroscopic endometrial ablation
DEF: Removal or destruction of uterine lining; usually by electrocautery or loop electrosurgical excision procedure (LEEP).

68.24 **Uterine artery embolization [UAE] with coils**
EXCLUDES   *that without coils (68.25)*

Operations on the Female Genital Organs

68.25–69.21

68.25 Uterine artery embolization [UAE] without coils
> INCLUDES that by:
>> gelatin sponge
>> gelfoam
>> microspheres
>> particulate agent NOS
>> polyvinyl alcohol [PVA]
>> spherical embolics
> EXCLUDES *that with coils (68.24)*

68.29 Other excision or destruction of lesion of uterus
> Uterine myomectomy
> EXCLUDES *biopsy of uterus (68.13)*
>> *uterine fistulectomy (69.42)*

✓4ᵗʰ **68.3 Subtotal abdominal hysterectomy**

68.31 Laparoscopic supracervical hysterectomy [LSH]
> Classic infrafascial SEMM hysterectomy [CISH]
> Laparoscopically assisted supracervical hysterectomy [LASH]
>
> **DEF:** A hysterectomy that spares the cervix and maintains the integrity of the pelvic floor; SEMM version of the supracervical hysterectomy, also called the classic infrafascial SEMM hysterectomy [CISH]; the cardinal ligaments, or lateral cervical ligaments that merge with the pelvic diaphragm remain intact.

68.39 Other and unspecified subtotal abdominal hysterectomy
> Supracervical hysterectomy
> EXCLUDES *classic infrafascial SEMM hysterectomy [CISH] (68.31)*
>> *laparoscopic supracervical hysterectomy [LSH] (68.31)*

✓4ᵗʰ **68.4 Total abdominal hysterectomy**
> Code also any synchronous removal of tubes and ovaries (65.31-65.64)
> EXCLUDES *radical abdominal hysterectomy, any approach (68.61-68.69)*
>
> **DEF:** Complete excision of uterus and uterine neck through abdominal approach.

68.41 Laparoscopic total abdominal hysterectomy
> Total laparoscopic hysterectomy [TLH]

68.49 Other and unspecified total abdominal hysterectomy
> Hysterectomy:
>> extended
> EXCLUDES *laparoscopic total abdominal hysterectomy (68.41)*

✓4ᵗʰ **68.5 Vaginal hysterectomy**
> Code also any synchronous:
>> removal of tubes and ovaries (65.31-65.64)
>> repair of cystocele or rectocele (70.50-70.52)
>> repair of pelvic floor (70.79)
>
> **DEF:** Complete excision of the uterus by a vaginal approach.

68.51 Laparoscopically assisted vaginal hysterectomy [LAVH]

68.59 Other and unspecified vaginal hysterectomy
> EXCLUDES *laparoscopically assisted vaginal hysterectomy (68.51)*
>> *radical vaginal hysterectomy (68.71-68.79)*

✓4ᵗʰ **68.6 Radical abdominal hysterectomy**
> Code also any synchronous:
>> lymph gland dissection (40.3, 40.5)
>> removal of tubes and ovaries (65.31-65.64)
> EXCLUDES *pelvic evisceration (68.8)*
>
> **DEF:** Excision of uterus, loose connective tissue and smooth muscle around uterus and vagina via abdominal approach.

68.61 Laparoscopic radical abdominal hysterectomy
> Laparoscopic modified radical hysterectomy
> Total laparoscopic radical hysterectomy [TLRH]

Vaginal Hysterectomy

Total hysterectomy (uterus only removed)

Total hysterectomy with bilateral salpingectomy (uterus and tubes removed)

Total hysterectomy with bilateral salpingo-oophorectomy (uterus, tubes, and ovaries removed)

68.69 Other and unspecified radical abdominal hysterectomy
> Modified radical hysterectomy
> Wertheim's operation
> EXCLUDES *laparoscopic radical abdominal hysterectomy (68.61)*
>> *laparoscopic total abdominal hysterectomy (68.41)*

✓4ᵗʰ **68.7 Radical vaginal hysterectomy**
> Code also any synchronous:
>> lymph gland dissection (40.3, 40.5)
>> removal of tubes and ovaries (65.31-65.64)
> EXCLUDES *abdominal hysterectomy, any approach (68.31-68.39, 68.41-68.49, 68.61-68.69, 68.9)*
>
> **DEF:** Excision of uterus, loose connective tissue and smooth muscle around uterus and vagina via vaginal approach.

68.71 Laparoscopic radical vaginal hysterectomy [LRVH]

68.79 Other and unspecified radical vaginal hysterectomy
> Hysterocolpectomy
> Schauta operation

68.8 Pelvic evisceration
> Removal of ovaries, tubes, uterus, vagina, bladder, and urethra (with removal of sigmoid colon and rectum)
> Code also any synchronous:
>> colostomy (46.10-46.13)
>> lymph gland dissection (40.3, 40.5)
>> urinary diversion (56.51-56.79)

68.9 Other and unspecified hysterectomy
> Hysterectomy NOS
> EXCLUDES *abdominal hysterectomy, any approach (68.31-68.39, 68.41-68.49, 68.61-68.69)*
>> *vaginal hysterectomy, any approach (68.51-68.59, 68.71-68.79)*

✓3ʳᵈ **69 Other operations on uterus and supporting structures**
> Code also any application or administration of an adhesion barrier substance (99.77)

✓4ᵗʰ **69.0 Dilation and curettage of uterus**
> EXCLUDES *aspiration curettage of uterus (69.51-69.59)*
> **DEF:** Stretching of uterine neck to scrape tissue from walls.

69.01 Dilation and curettage for termination of pregnancy

69.02 Dilation and curettage following delivery or abortion

69.09 Other dilation and curettage
> Diagnostic D and C

✓4ᵗʰ **69.1 Excision or destruction of lesion or tissue of uterus and supporting structures**

69.19 Other excision or destruction of uterus and supporting structures
> EXCLUDES *biopsy of uterine ligament (68.14)*

✓4ᵗʰ **69.2 Repair of uterine supporting structures**

69.21 Interposition operation
> Watkins procedure

Dilation and Curettage

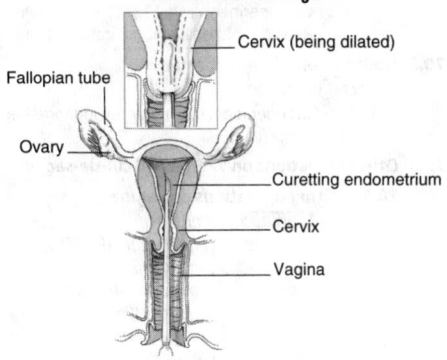

Cervix (being dilated)

Fallopian tube

Ovary

Curetting endometrium

Cervix

Vagina

69.22   **Other uterine suspension**
Hysteropexy
Manchester operation
Plication of uterine ligament
DEF: Hysteropexy: Fixation or anchoring of uterus.
DEF: Manchester operation: Fixation or anchoring of uterus with supportive banding tissue of uterine neck and vagina.
DEF: Plication of uterine ligament: Creation of tucks in suppurative uterine banding tissue.
DEF: Repositioning or realignment of bladder and uterus.

69.23   **Vaginal repair of chronic inversion of uterus**
DEF: Repositioning of inverted uterus via vaginal approach.

69.29   **Other repair of uterus and supporting structures**

69.3   **Paracervical uterine denervation**

√4ᵗʰ   **69.4**   **Uterine repair**
EXCLUDES   *repair of current obstetric laceration (75.50-75.52)*

69.41   **Suture of laceration of uterus**

69.42   **Closure of fistula of uterus**
EXCLUDES   *uterovesical fistulectomy (57.84)*

69.49   **Other repair of uterus**
Repair of old obstetric laceration of uterus

√4ᵗʰ   **69.5**   **Aspiration curettage of uterus**
EXCLUDES   *menstrual extraction (69.6)*

69.51   **Aspiration curettage of uterus for termination of pregnancy**
Therapeutic abortion NOS

69.52   **Aspiration curettage following delivery or abortion**

69.59   **Other aspiration curettage of uterus**

69.6   **Menstrual extraction or regulation**
DEF: Induction of menstruation by low pressure suction.

69.7   **Insertion of intrauterine contraceptive device**

√4ᵗʰ   **69.9**   **Other operations on uterus, cervix, and supporting structures**
EXCLUDES   *obstetric dilation or incision of cervix (73.1, 73.93)*

69.91   **Insertion of therapeutic device into uterus**
EXCLUDES   *insertion of:*
intrauterine contraceptive device (69.7)
laminaria (69.93)
obstetric insertion of bag, bougie, or pack (73.1)

69.92   **Artificial insemination**

69.93   **Insertion of laminaria**
DEF: Placement of laminaria, a sea kelp, in cervical os to induce labor; applied for six to 12 hours.

69.94   **Manual replacement of inverted uterus**
EXCLUDES   *that in immediate postpartal period (75.94)*

69.95   **Incision of cervix**
EXCLUDES   *that to assist delivery (73.93)*

69.96   **Removal of cerclage material from cervix**
DEF: Removal of ring inserted to restore uterine neck competency.

69.97   **Removal of other penetrating foreign body from cervix**
EXCLUDES   *removal of intraluminal foreign body from cervix (98.16)*

69.98   **Other operations on supporting structures of uterus**
EXCLUDES   *biopsy of uterine ligament (68.14)*

69.99   **Other operations on cervix and uterus**
EXCLUDES   *removal of:*
foreign body (98.16)
intrauterine contraceptive device (97.71)
obstetric bag, bougie, or pack (97.72)
packing (97.72)

√3ʳᵈ   **70**   **Operations on vagina and cul-de-sac**
Code also any application or administration of an adhesion barrier substance (99.77)

70.0   **Culdocentesis**
DEF: Insertion of needle into upper vaginal vault encircling cervix to withdraw fluid.

√4ᵗʰ   **70.1**   **Incision of vagina and cul-de-sac**

70.11   **Hymenotomy**

70.12   **Culdotomy**
DEF: Incision into pocket between terminal end of large intestine and posterior uterus.

70.13   **Lysis of intraluminal adhesions of vagina**

70.14   **Other vaginotomy**
Division of vaginal septum
Drainage of hematoma of vaginal cuff
DEF: Division of vaginal septum: Incision into partition of vaginal walls.
DEF: Drainage of hematoma of vaginal cuff: Incision into vaginal tissue to drain collected blood.

√4ᵗʰ   **70.2**   **Diagnostic procedures on vagina and cul-de-sac**

70.21   **Vaginoscopy**

70.22   **Culdoscopy**
DEF: Endoscopic exam of pelvic viscera through incision in posterior vaginal wall.

70.23   **Biopsy of cul-de-sac**

70.24   **Vaginal biopsy**

70.29   **Other diagnostic procedures on vagina and cul-de-sac**

√4ᵗʰ   **70.3**   **Local excision or destruction of vagina and cul-de-sac**

70.31   **Hymenectomy**

70.32   **Excision or destruction of lesion of cul-de-sac**
Endometrectomy of cul-de-sac
EXCLUDES   *biopsy of cul-de-sac (70.23)*

70.33   **Excision or destruction of lesion of vagina**
EXCLUDES   *biopsy of vagina (70.24)*
vaginal fistulectomy (70.72-70.75)

70.4   **Obliteration and total excision of vagina**
Vaginectomy
EXCLUDES   *obliteration of vaginal vault (70.8)*
DEF: Vaginectomy: Removal of vagina.

√4ᵗʰ   **70.5**   **Repair of cystocele and rectocele**

70.50   **Repair of cystocele and rectocele**
EXCLUDES   *repair of cystocele and rectocele with graft or prosthesis (70.53)*
DEF: Repair of anterior and posterior vaginal wall bulges.

Operations on the Female Genital Organs

70.51–71.09

70.51   **Repair of cystocele**
Anterior colporrhaphy (with urethrocele repair)
EXCLUDES   *repair of cystocele and rectocele with*
graft or prosthesis (70.53)
repair of cystocele with graft or prosthesis
(70.54)

70.52   **Repair of rectocele**
Posterior colporrhaphy
EXCLUDES   *repair of cystocele and rectocele with*
graft or prosthesis (70.53)
repair of rectocele with graft or prosthesis
(70.55)
STARR procedure (48.74)

70.53   **Repair of cystocele and rectocele with graft or**
prosthesis
Use additional code for biological substance (70.94)
or synthetic substance (70.95), if known

70.54   **Repair of cystocele with graft or prosthesis**
Anterior colporrhaphy (with urethrocele repair)
Use additional code for biological substance (70.94)
or synthetic substance (70.95), if known

70.55   **Repair of rectocele with graft or prosthesis**
Posterior colporrhaphy
Use additional code for biological substance (70.94)
or synthetic substance (70.95), if known

✓4ᵗʰ **70.6**   **Vaginal construction and reconstruction**

70.61   **Vaginal construction**

70.62   **Vaginal reconstruction**

70.63   **Vaginal construction with graft or prosthesis**
Use additional code for biological substance (70.94)
or synthetic substance (70.95), if known
EXCLUDES   *vaginal construction (70.61)*

70.64   **Vaginal reconstruction with graft or prosthesis**
Use additional code for biological substance (70.94)
or synthetic substance (70.95), if known
EXCLUDES   *vaginal reconstruction (70.62)*

✓4ᵗʰ **70.7**   **Other repair of vagina**
EXCLUDES   *lysis of intraluminal adhesions (70.13)*
repair of current obstetric laceration (75.69)
that associated with cervical amputation (67.4)

70.71   **Suture of laceration of vagina**

70.72   **Repair of colovaginal fistula**
DEF: Correction of abnormal opening between
midsection of large intestine and vagina.

70.73   **Repair of rectovaginal fistula**
DEF: Correction of abnormal opening between last
section of large intestine and vagina.

70.74   **Repair of other vaginoenteric fistula**
DEF: Correction of abnormal opening between
vagina and intestine other than mid or last sections.

70.75   **Repair of other fistula of vagina**
EXCLUDES   *repair of fistula:*
rectovesicovaginal (57.83)
ureterovaginal (56.84)
urethrovaginal (58.43)
uterovaginal (69.42)
vesicocervicovaginal (57.84)
vesicosigmoidovaginal (57.83)
vesicoureterovaginal (56.84)
vesicovaginal (57.84)

70.76   **Hymenorrhaphy**
DEF: Closure of vagina with suture of hymenal ring or
hymenal remnant flaps.

70.77   **Vaginal suspension and fixation**
DEF: Repair of vaginal protrusion, sinking or laxity by
suturing vagina into position.

70.78   **Vaginal suspension and fixation with graft or**
prosthesis
Use additional code for biological substance (70.94)
or synthetic substance (70.95), if known

70.79   **Other repair of vagina**
Colpoperineoplasty
Repair of old obstetric laceration of vagina

70.8   **Obliteration of vaginal vault**
LeFort operation
DEF: LeFort operation: Uniting or sewing together vaginal
walls.

✓4ᵗʰ **70.9**   **Other operations on vagina and cul-de-sac**

70.91   **Other operations on vagina**
EXCLUDES   *insertion of:*
diaphragm (96.17)
mold (96.15)
pack (96.14)
pessary (96.18)
suppository (96.49)
removal of:
diaphragm (97.73)
foreign body (98.17)
pack (97.75)
pessary (97.74)
replacement of:
diaphragm (97.24)
pack (97.26)
pessary (97.25)
vaginal dilation (96.16)
vaginal douche (96.44)

70.92   **Other operations on cul-de-sac**
Obliteration of cul-de-sac
Repair of vaginal enterocele
DEF: Repair of vaginal enterocele: Elimination of
herniated cavity within pouch between last part of
large intestine and posterior uterus.

70.93   **Other operations on cul-de-sac with graft or**
prosthesis
Repair of vaginal enterocele with graft or prosthesis
Use additional code for biological substance (70.94)
or synthetic substance (70.95), if known

70.94   **Insertion of biological graft**
Allogenic material or substance
Allograft
Autograft
Autologous material or substance
Heterograft
Xenogenic material or substance
Code first these procedures when done with graft or
prosthesis:
Other operations on cul-de-sac (70.93)
Repair of cystocele (70.54)
Repair of cystocele and rectocele (70.53)
Repair of rectocele (70.55)
Vaginal construction (70.63)
Vaginal reconstruction (70.64)
Vaginal suspension and fixation (70.78)

70.95   **Insertion of synthetic graft or prosthesis**
Artificial tissue
Code first these procedures when done with graft or
prosthesis:
Other operations on cul-de-sac (70.93)
Repair of cystocele (70.54)
Repair of cystocele and rectocele (70.53)
Repair of rectocele (70.55)
Vaginal construction (70.63)
Vaginal reconstruction (70.64)
Vaginal suspension and fixation (70.78)

✓3ʳᵈ **71**   **Operations on vulva and perineum**
Code also any application or administration of an adhesion barrier
substance (99.77)

✓4ᵗʰ **71.0**   **Incision of vulva and perineum**

71.01   **Lysis of vulvar adhesions**

71.09   **Other incision of vulva and perineum**
Enlargement of introitus NOS
EXCLUDES   *removal of foreign body without incision*
(98.23)

Marsupialization

Portion of cyst and overlying skin to be excised

Cyst "unroofed"

Cyst walls sutured to skin

✓4ᵗʰ 71.1 Diagnostic procedures on vulva

  71.11 Biopsy of vulva

  71.19 Other diagnostic procedures on vulva

✓4ᵗʰ 71.2 Operations on Bartholin's gland

  71.21 Percutaneous aspiration of Bartholin's gland (cyst)

  71.22 Incision of Bartholin's gland (cyst)

  71.23 Marsupialization of Bartholin's gland (cyst)

   DEF: Incision and suturing open a Bartholin's gland cyst.

  71.24 Excision or other destruction of Bartholin's gland (cyst)

  71.29 Other operations on Bartholin's gland

71.3 Other local excision or destruction of vulva and perineum

   Division of Skene's gland

   EXCLUDES biopsy of vulva (71.11)
             vulvar fistulectomy (71.72)

71.4 Operations on clitoris

   Amputation of clitoris   Female circumcision
   Clitoridotomy

   DEF: Amputation of clitoris: Removal of clitoris.
   DEF: Clitoridotomy: Incision into clitoris.
   DEF: Female circumcision: Incision of skin fold over clitoris.

71.5 Radical vulvectomy

   Code also any synchronous lymph gland dissection (40.3, 40.5)

   DEF: Removal of over 80 percent of deep tissue from vulva, including tissue of abdomen, groin, labia minora, labia majora, clitoris, mons veneris, and terminal portions of urethra, vagina and other vulvar organs.

✓4ᵗʰ 71.6 Other vulvectomy

  71.61 Unilateral vulvectomy

  71.62 Bilateral vulvectomy

   Vulvectomy NOS

✓4ᵗʰ 71.7 Repair of vulva and perineum

   EXCLUDES repair of current obstetric laceration (75.69)

  71.71 Suture of laceration of vulva or perineum

  71.72 Repair of fistula of vulva or perineum

   EXCLUDES repair of fistula:
             urethroperineal (58.43)
             urethroperineovesical (57.84)
             vaginoperineal (70.75)

  71.79 Other repair of vulva and perineum

   Repair of old obstetric laceration of vulva or perineum

71.8 Other operations on vulva

   EXCLUDES removal of:
             foreign body without incision (98.23)
             packing (97.75)
             replacement of packing (97.26)

71.9 Other operations on female genital organs

Obstetrical Procedures

13. OBSTETRICAL PROCEDURES (72-75)

☑3ʳᵈ **72 Forceps, vacuum, and breech delivery**

72.0 Low forceps operation
Outlet forceps operation

72.1 Low forceps operation with episiotomy
Outlet forceps operation with episiotomy

☑4ᵗʰ **72.2 Mid forceps operation**

72.21 Mid forceps operation with episiotomy

72.29 Other mid forceps operation

☑4ᵗʰ **72.3 High forceps operation**

72.31 High forceps operation with episiotomy

72.39 Other high forceps operation

72.4 Forceps rotation of fetal head
DeLee maneuver
Key-in-lock rotation
Kielland rotation
Scanzoni's maneuver
Code also any associated forceps extraction (72.0-72.39)

☑4ᵗʰ **72.5 Breech extraction**

72.51 Partial breech extraction with forceps to aftercoming head

72.52 Other partial breech extraction

72.53 Total breech extraction with forceps to aftercoming head

72.54 Other total breech extraction

72.6 Forceps application to aftercoming head
Piper forceps operation
EXCLUDES partial breech extraction with forceps to
aftercoming head (72.51)
total breech extraction with forceps to
aftercoming head (72.53)

☑4ᵗʰ **72.7 Vacuum extraction**
INCLUDES Malström's extraction

72.71 Vacuum extraction with episiotomy

72.79 Other vacuum extraction

72.8 Other specified instrumental delivery

72.9 Unspecified instrumental delivery

☑3ʳᵈ **73 Other procedures inducing or assisting delivery**

☑4ᵗʰ **73.0 Artificial rupture of membranes**

73.01 Induction of labor by artificial rupture of membranes
Surgical induction NOS
EXCLUDES artificial rupture of membranes after
onset of labor (73.09)

73.09 Other artificial rupture of membranes
Artificial rupture of membranes at time of delivery

73.1 Other surgical induction of labor
Induction by cervical dilation
EXCLUDES injection for abortion (75.0)
insertion of suppository for abortion (96.49)

Breech Extraction

Breech presentation

Delivery of legs

Baby rotated for delivery of arms

Umbilicus

☑4ᵗʰ **73.2 Internal and combined version and extraction**

73.21 Internal and combined version without extraction
Version NOS

73.22 Internal and combined version with extraction

73.3 Failed forceps
Application of forceps without delivery
Trial forceps

73.4 Medical induction of labor
EXCLUDES medication to augment active labor — omit code

☑4ᵗʰ **73.5 Manually assisted delivery**

73.51 Manual rotation of fetal head

73.59 Other manually assisted delivery
Assisted spontaneous delivery
Credé maneuver

73.6 Episiotomy
Episioproctotomy
Episiotomy with subsequent episiorrhaphy
EXCLUDES that with:
high forceps (72.31)
low forceps (72.1)
mid forceps (72.21)
outlet forceps (72.1)
vacuum extraction (72.71)

73.8 Operations on fetus to facilitate delivery
Clavicotomy on fetus
Destruction of fetus
Needling of hydrocephalic head

☑4ᵗʰ **73.9 Other operations assisting delivery**

73.91 External version

73.92 Replacement of prolapsed umbilical cord

73.93 Incision of cervix to assist delivery
Dührssen's incisions

73.94 Pubiotomy to assist delivery
Obstetrical symphysiotomy

73.99 Other
EXCLUDES dilation of cervix, obstetrical, to induce
labor (73.1)
insertion of bag or bougie to induce labor
(73.1)
removal of cerclage material (69.96)

☑3ʳᵈ **74 Cesarean section and removal of fetus**
Code also any synchronous:
hysterectomy (68.3-68.4, 68.6, 68.8)
myomectomy (68.29)
sterilization (66.31-66.39, 66.63)

74.0 Classical cesarean section
Transperitoneal classical cesarean section

74.1 Low cervical cesarean section
Lower uterine segment cesarean section

74.2 Extraperitoneal cesarean section
Supravesical cesarean section

74.3 Removal of extratubal ectopic pregnancy
Removal of:
ectopic abdominal pregnancy
fetus from peritoneal or extraperitoneal cavity following
uterine or tubal rupture
EXCLUDES that by salpingostomy (66.02)
that by salpingotomy (66.01)
that with synchronous salpingectomy (66.62)

74.4 Cesarean section of other specified type
Peritoneal exclusion cesareansection
Transperitoneal cesarean section NOS
Vaginal cesarean section

☑4ᵗʰ **74.9 Cesarean section of unspecified type**

74.91 Hysterotomy to terminate pregnancy
Therapeutic abortion by hysterotomy

74.99 Other cesarean section of unspecified type
Cesarean section NOS
Obstetrical abdominouterotomy
Obstetrical hysterotomy

Obstetrical Procedures

75–75.99

Amniocentesis

Amniotic
sac

Aspiration of amniotic fluid

√3ʳᵈ 75 Other obstetric operations

75.0 Intra-amniotic injection for abortion

Injection of:

prostaglandin
saline } for induction of abortion

Termination of pregnancy by intrauterine injection

EXCLUDES *insertion of prostaglandin suppository for
abortion (96.49)*

75.1 Diagnostic amniocentesis

75.2 Intrauterine transfusion

Exchange transfusion in utero
Insertion of catheter into abdomen of fetus for transfusion
Code also any hysterotomy approach (68.0)

√4ᵗʰ 75.3 Other intrauterine operations on fetus and amnion

Code also any hysterotomy approach (68.0)

75.31 Amnioscopy

Fetoscopy
Laparoamnioscopy

75.32 Fetal EKG (scalp)

75.33 Fetal blood sampling and biopsy

75.34 Other fetal monitoring

Antepartum fetal nonstress test
Fetal monitoring, not otherwise specified

EXCLUDES *fetal pulse oximetry (75.38)*

75.35 Other diagnostic procedures on fetus and amnion

Intrauterine pressure determination

EXCLUDES *amniocentesis (75.1)*
*diagnostic procedures on gravid uterus
and placenta (87.81, 88.46, 88.78,
92.17)*

75.36 Correction of fetal defect

75.37 Amnioinfusion

Code also injection of antibiotic (99.21)

75.38 Fetal pulse oximetry

Transcervical fetal oxygen saturation monitoring
Transcervical fetal SpO₂ monitoring

DEF: Single-use sensor inserted through the birth
canal and positioned to rest against the fetal cheek,
forehead, or temple; infrared beam of light aimed at
the fetal skin is reflected back through the sensor for
analysis.

75.4 Manual removal of retained placenta

EXCLUDES *aspiration curettage (69.52)*
dilation and curettage (69.02)

√4ᵗʰ 75.5 Repair of current obstetric laceration of uterus

**75.50 Repair of current obstetric laceration of uterus,
not otherwise specified**

75.51 Repair of current obstetric laceration of cervix

**75.52 Repair of current obstetric laceration of corpus
uteri**

√4ᵗʰ 75.6 Repair of other current obstetric laceration

Code also episiotomy, if performed (73.6)

**75.61 Repair of current obstetric laceration of bladder
and urethra**

**75.62 Repair of current obstetric laceration of rectum
and sphincter ani**

75.69 Repair of other current obstetric laceration

Episioperineorrhaphy
Repair of:
pelvic floor
perineum

Repair of:
vagina
vulva
Secondary repair of
episiotomy

75.7 Manual exploration of uterine cavity, postpartum

75.8 Obstetric tamponade of uterus or vagina

EXCLUDES *antepartum tamponade (73.1)*

√4ᵗʰ 75.9 Other obstetric operations

**75.91 Evacuation of obstetrical incisional hematoma of
perineum**

Evacuation of hematoma of:
episiotomy
perineorrhaphy

75.92 Evacuation of other hematoma of vulva or vagina

75.93 Surgical correction of inverted uterus

Spintelli operation

EXCLUDES *vaginal repair of chronic inversion of
uterus (69.23)*

75.94 Manual replacement of inverted uterus

75.99 Other

14. OPERATIONS ON THE MUSCULOSKELETAL SYSTEM (76-84)

√3ʳᵈ **76 Operations on facial bones and joints**
> **EXCLUDES** *accessory sinuses (22.00-22.9)*
> *nasal bones (21.00-21.99)*
> *skull (01.01-02.99)*

√4ᵗʰ **76.0 Incision of facial bone without division**

> **76.01 Sequestrectomy of facial bone**
> Removal of necrotic bone chip from facial bone

> **76.09 Other incision of facial bone**
> Reopening of osteotomy site of facial bone
> > **EXCLUDES** *osteotomy associated with orthognathic surgery (76.61-76.69)*
> > *removal of internal fixation device (76.97)*

√4ᵗʰ **76.1 Diagnostic procedures on facial bones and joints**

> **76.11 Biopsy of facial bone**

> **76.19 Other diagnostic procedures on facial bones and joints**
> > **EXCLUDES** *contrast arthrogram of temporomandibular joint (87.13)*
> > *other x-ray (87.11-87.12, 87.14-87.16)*

76.2 Local excision or destruction of lesion of facial bone
> **EXCLUDES** *biopsy of facial bone (76.11)*
> *excision of odontogenic lesion (24.4)*

√4ᵗʰ **76.3 Partial ostectomy of facial bone**

> **76.31 Partial mandibulectomy**
> Hemimandibulectomy
> > **EXCLUDES** *that associated with temporomandibular arthroplasty (76.5)*
> > **DEF:** Partial excision of lower jawbone.
> > **DEF:** Hemimandibulectomy: Excision of one-half of lower jawbone.

> **76.39 Partial ostectomy of other facial bone**
> Hemimaxillectomy (with bonegraft or prosthesis)
> > **DEF:** Partial excision of facial bone other than lower jawbone.
> > **DEF:** Hemimaxillectomy (with bone graft or prosthesis): Excision of one side of upper jawbone and restoration with bone graft or prosthesis.

√4ᵗʰ **76.4 Excision and reconstruction of facial bones**

> **76.41 Total mandibulectomy with synchronous reconstruction**

> **76.42 Other total mandibulectomy**

> **76.43 Other reconstruction of mandible**
> > **EXCLUDES** *genioplasty (76.67-76.68)*
> > *that with synchronous total mandibulectomy (76.41)*

> **76.44 Total ostectomy of other facial bone with synchronous reconstruction**
> > **DEF:** Total facial bone excision with reconstruction during same operative session.

> **76.45 Other total ostectomy of other facial bone**

> **76.46 Other reconstruction of other facial bone**
> > **EXCLUDES** *that with synchronous total ostectomy (76.44)*

76.5 Temporomandibular arthroplasty

√4ᵗʰ **76.6 Other facial bone repair and orthognathic surgery**
> Code also any synchronous:
> bone graft (76.91)
> synthetic implant (76.92)
> > **EXCLUDES** *reconstruction of facial bones (76.41-76.46)*

> **76.61 Closed osteoplasty [osteotomy] of mandibular ramus**
> Gigli saw osteotomy
> > **DEF:** Reshaping and restoration of lower jawbone projection; closed surgical field, which is a limited keyhole incision.
> > **DEF:** Gigli saw osteotomy: Plastic repair using a flexible wire with saw teeth.

> **76.62 Open osteoplasty [osteotomy] of mandibular ramus**

> **76.63 Osteoplasty [osteotomy] of body of mandible**

> **76.64 Other orthognathic surgery on mandible**
> Mandibular osteoplasty NOS
> Segmental or subapical osteotomy

> **76.65 Segmental osteoplasty [osteotomy] of maxilla**
> Maxillary osteoplasty NOS

> **76.66 Total osteoplasty [osteotomy] of maxilla**

> **76.67 Reduction genioplasty**
> Reduction mentoplasty
> > **DEF:** Reduction of protruding chin or lower jawbone.

> **76.68 Augmentation genioplasty**
> Mentoplasty:
> NOS
> with graft or implant
> > **DEF:** Extension of the lower jawbone to a functional position by means of plastic surgery.

> **76.69 Other facial bone repair**
> Osteoplasty of facial bone NOS

√4ᵗʰ **76.7 Reduction of facial fracture**
> **INCLUDES** internal fixation
> Code also any synchronous:
> bone graft (76.91)
> synthetic implant (76.92)
> > **EXCLUDES** *that of nasal bones (21.71-21.72)*

> **76.70 Reduction of facial fracture, not otherwise specified**

> **76.71 Closed reduction of malar and zygomatic fracture**

> **76.72 Open reduction of malar and zygomatic fracture**

> **76.73 Closed reduction of maxillary fracture**

> **76.74 Open reduction of maxillary fracture**

> **76.75 Closed reduction of mandibular fracture**

> **76.76 Open reduction of mandibular fracture**

> **76.77 Open reduction of alveolar fracture**
> Reduction of alveolar fracture with stabilization of teeth

> **76.78 Other closed reduction of facial fracture**
> Closed reduction of orbital fracture
> > **EXCLUDES** *nasal bone (21.71)*

> **76.79 Other open reduction of facial fracture**
> Open reduction of orbit rim or wall
> > **EXCLUDES** *nasal bone (21.72)*

√4ᵗʰ **76.9 Other operations on facial bones and joints**

> **76.91 Bone graft to facial bone**
> Autogenous
> Bone bank } graft to facial bone
> Heterogenous

> **76.92 Insertion of synthetic implant in facial bone**
> Alloplastic implant to facial bone

> **76.93 Closed reduction of temporomandibular dislocation**

> **76.94 Open reduction of temporomandibular dislocation**

> **76.95 Other manipulation of temporomandibular joint**

> **76.96 Injection of therapeutic substance into temporomandibular joint**

76.97   **Removal of internal fixation device from facial bone**

> EXCLUDES   removal of:
> dental wiring (97.33)
> external mandibular fixation device NEC (97.36)

76.99   **Other**

✓3ʳᵈ **77**   **Incision, excision, and division of other bones**

> EXCLUDES   laminectomy for decompression (03.09)
> operations on:
> accessory sinuses (22.00-22.9)
> ear ossicles (19.0-19.55)
> facial bones (76.01-76.99)
> joint structures (80.00-81.99)
> mastoid (19.9-20.99)
> nasal bones (21.00-21.99)
> skull (01.01-02.99)

The following fourth-digit subclassification is for use with appropriate categories in section 77 to identify the site. Valid fourth-digit categories are in [brackets] under each code.

0 unspecified site	6 patella
1 scapula, clavicle, and thorax [ribs and sternum]	7 tibia and fibula
	8 tarsals and metatarsals
2 humerus	9 other
3 radius and ulna	Pelvic bones
4 carpals and metacarpals	Phalanges (of foot) (of hand)
5 femur	Vertebrae

✓4ᵗʰ **77.0**   **Sequestrectomy**

[0-9]   **DEF:** Excision and removal of dead bone.

✓4ᵗʰ **77.1**   **Other incision of bone without division**

[0-9]   Reopening of osteotomy site

> EXCLUDES   aspiration of bone marrow, (41.31, 41.91)
> removal of internal fixation device (78.60-78.69)

DEF: Incision into bone without division of site.

✓4ᵗʰ **77.2**   **Wedge osteotomy**

[0-9]   EXCLUDES   that for hallux valgus (77.51)

DEF: Removal of wedge-shaped piece of bone.

✓4ᵗʰ **77.3**   **Other division of bone**

[0-9]   Osteoarthrotomy

> EXCLUDES   clavicotomy of fetus (73.8)
> laminotomy or incision of vertebra (03.01-03.09)
> pubiotomy to assist delivery (73.94)
> sternotomy incidental to thoracic operation — omit code

✓4ᵗʰ **77.4**   **Biopsy of bone**

[0-9]

✓4ᵗʰ **77.5**   **Excision and repair of bunion and other toe deformities**

77.51   **Bunionectomy with soft tissue correction and osteotomy of the first metatarsal**

DEF: Incision and removal of big toe bony prominence and reconstruction with soft tissue.

77.52   **Bunionectomy with soft tissue correction and arthrodesis**

DEF: Removal of big toe bony prominence and reconstruction with soft tissue and joint fixation.

77.53   **Other bunionectomy with soft tissue correction**

77.54   **Excision or correction of bunionette**

That with osteotomy

DEF: Resection of fifth metatarsal head via exposure of joint; includes imbrication of capsule.

77.56   **Repair of hammer toe**

Filleting ⎫
Fusion ⎬ of hammer toe
Phalangectomy (partial) ⎭

DEF: Repair of clawlike toe defect by joint fusion, or partial removal of toe via traction technique.

Repair of Hammer Toe

Corn

Hammertoe

Callus

Hemiphalengectomy

After

77.57   **Repair of claw toe**

Capsulotomy ⎫
Fusion ⎬ of claw toe
Phalangectomy (partial) ⎪
Tendon lenghening ⎭

DEF: Repair of clawlike toe defect by joint fusion, partial removal of toe, joint capsule incision or lengthening of fibrous muscle attachment.

77.58   **Other excision, fusion, and repair of toes**

Cockup toe repair
Overlapping toe repair
That with use of prosthetic materials

77.59   **Other bunionectomy**

Resection of hallux valgus joint with insertion of prosthesis

DEF: Resection of hallux valgus joint with insertion of prosthesis: Cutting away part of big toe with prosthesis insertion to correct bony prominence.

✓4ᵗʰ **77.6**   **Local excision of lesion or tissue of bone**

[0-9]   EXCLUDES   biopsy of bone (77.40-77.49)
debridement of compound fracture (79.60-79.69)

✓4ᵗʰ **77.7**   **Excision of bone for graft**

[0-9]

✓4ᵗʰ **77.8**   **Other partial ostectomy**

[0-9]   Condylectomy

> EXCLUDES   amputation (84.00-84.19, 84.91)
> arthrectomy (80.90-80.99)
> excision of bone ends associated with:
> arthrodesis (81.00-81.39, 81.62-81.66)
> arthroplasty (81.40-81.59, 81.71-81.85)
> excision of cartilage (80.5-80.6, 80.80-80.99)
> excision of head of femur with synchronous replacement (00.70-00.73, 81.51-81.53)
> hemilaminectomy (03.01-03.09)
> laminectomy (03.01-03.09)
> ostectomy for hallux valgus (77.51-77.59)
> partial amputation:
> finger (84.01)
> thumb (84.02)
> toe (84.11)
> resection of ribs incidental to thoracic operation — omit code
> that incidental to other operation — omit code

✓4ᵗʰ **77.9**   **Total ostectomy**

[0-9]   EXCLUDES   amputation of limb (84.00-84.19, 84.91)
that incidental to other operation — omit code

☑3ʳᵈ **78 Other operations on bones, except facial bones**

> EXCLUDES *operations on:*
> *accessory sinuses (22.00-22.9)*
> *facial bones (76.01-76.99)*
> *joint structures (80.00-81.99)*
> *nasal bones (21.00-21.99)*
> *skull (01.01-02.99)*

> The following fourth-digit subclassification is for use with appropriate categories in section 78 to identify the site. Valid fourth-digit categories are in [brackets] under each code.
>
> | | |
> |---|---|
> | 0 unspecified site | 6 patella |
> | 1 scapula, clavicle, and thorax [ribs and sternum] | 7 tibia and fibula |
> | | 8 tarsals and metatarsals |
> | 2 humerus | 9 other |
> | 3 radius and ulna | Pelvic bones |
> | 4 carpals and metacarpals | Phalanges (of foot) (of hand) |
> | 5 femur | Vertebrae |

☑4ᵗʰ **78.0 Bone graft**

[0-9] Bone:
    bank graft
    graft (autogenous) (heterogenous)
That with debridement of bone graft site (removal of sclerosed, fibrous, or necrotic bone or tissue)
Transplantation of bone
Code also any excision of bone for graft (77.70-77.79)
> EXCLUDES *that for bone lengthening (78.30-78.39)*

☑4ᵗʰ **78.1 Application of external fixator device**

[0-9] Fixator with insertion of pins/wires/screws into bone
Code also any type of fixator device, if known (84.71-84.73)
> EXCLUDES *other immobilization, pressure, and attention to wound (93.51-93.59)*

☑4ᵗʰ **78.2 Limb shortening procedures**

[0,2-5, 7-9] Epiphyseal stapling
Open epiphysiodesis
Percutaneous epiphysiodesis
Resection/osteotomy

☑4ᵗʰ **78.3 Limb lengthening procedures**

[0,2-5, 7-9] Bone graft with or without internal fixation devices or osteotomy
Distraction technique with or without corticotomy/osteotomy
Code also any application of an external fixation device (78.10-78.19)

☑4ᵗʰ **78.4 Other repair or plastic operations on bone**

[0-9] Other operation on bone NEC
Repair of malunion or nonunion fracture NEC
> EXCLUDES *application of external fixation device (78.10-78.19)*
> *limb lengthening procedures (78.30-78.39)*
> *limb shortening procedures (78.20-78.29)*
> *osteotomy (77.3)*
> *reconstruction of thumb (82.61-82.69)*
> *repair of pectus deformity (34.74)*
> *repair with bone graft (78.00-78.09)*

☑4ᵗʰ **78.5 Internal fixation of bone without fracture reduction**

[0-9] Internal fixation of bone (prophylactic)
Reinsertion of internal fixation device
Revision of displaced or broken fixation device
> EXCLUDES *arthroplasty and arthrodesis (81.00-81.85)*
> *bone graft (78.00-78.09)*
> *insertion of sternal fixation device with rigid plates (84.94)*
> *limb shortening procedures (78.20-78.29)*
> *that for fracture reduction (79.10-79.19, 79.30-79.59)*

☑4ᵗʰ **78.6 Removal of implanted devices from bone**

[0-9] External fixator device (invasive)
Internal fixation device
Removal of bone growth stimulator (invasive)
Removal of internal limb lengthening device
Removal of pedicle screw(s) used in spinal fusion
> EXCLUDES *removal of cast, splint, and traction device (Kirschner wire) (Steinmann pin) (97.88)*
> *removal of posterior spinal motion preservation (facet replacement, pedicle-based dynamic stabilization, interspinous process) device(s) (80.09)*
> *removal of skull tongs or halo traction device (02.95)*

☑4ᵗʰ **78.7 Osteoclasis**

[0-9] DEF: Surgical breaking or rebreaking of bone.

☑4ᵗʰ **78.8 Diagnostic procedures on bone, not elsewhere classified**

[0-9] EXCLUDES *biopsy of bone (77.40-77.49)*
> *magnetic resonance imaging (88.94)*
> *microscopic examination of specimen from bone (91.51-91.59)*
> *radioisotope scan (92.14)*
> *skeletal x-ray (87.21-87.29, 87.43, 88.21-88.33)*
> *thermography (88.83)*

☑4ᵗʰ **78.9 Insertion of bone growth stimulator**

[0-9] Insertion of:
bone stimulator (electrical) to aid bone healing
osteogenic electrodes for bone growth stimulation
totally implanted device (invasive)
> EXCLUDES *non-invasive (transcutaneous) (surface) stimulator (99.86)*

☑3ʳᵈ **79 Reduction of fracture and dislocation**

> INCLUDES application of cast or splint
> reduction with insertion of traction device (Kirschner wire) (Steinmann pin)

Code also any:
application of external fixator device (78.10-78.19)
type of fixator device, if known (84.71-84.73)
> EXCLUDES *external fixation alone for immobilization of fracture (93.51-93.56, 93.59)*
> *internal fixation without reduction of fracture (78.50-78.59)*
> *operations on:*
> *facial bones(76.70-76.79)*
> *nasal bones (21.71-21.72)*
> *orbit (76.78-76.79)*
> *skull (02.02)*
> *vertebrae (03.53)*
> *removal of cast or splint (97.88)*
> *replacement of cast or splint (97.11-97.14)*
> *traction alone for reduction of fracture (93.41-93.46)*

> The following fourth-digit subclassification is for use with appropriate categories in section 79 to identify the site. Valid fourth-digit categories are in [brackets] under each code.
>
> | | |
> |---|---|
> | 0 unspecified site | 5 femur |
> | 1 humerus | 6 tibia and fibula |
> | 2 radius and ulna | Leg NOS |
> | Arm NOS | 7 tarsals and metatarsals |
> | 3 carpals and metacarpals | Foot NOS |
> | Hand NOS | 8 phalanges of foot |
> | 4 phalanges of hand | 9 other specified bone |

☑4ᵗʰ **79.0 Closed reduction of fracture without internal fixation**

[0-9] EXCLUDES *that for separation of epiphysis (79.40-79.49)*
DEF: Manipulative realignment of fracture; without incision or internal fixation.

☑4ᵗʰ **79.1 Closed reduction of fracture with internal fixation**

[0-9] EXCLUDES *that for separation of epiphysis (79.40-79.49)*
DEF: Manipulative realignment of fracture; with internal fixation but without incision.

☑4ᵗʰ **79.2 Open reduction of fracture without internal fixation**

[0-9] EXCLUDES *that for separation of epiphysis (79.50-79.59)*

Operations on the Musculoskeletal System

79.3–80.50

√4ᵗʰ **79.3 Open reduction of fracture with internal fixation**
[0-9]   **EXCLUDES**   *that for separation of epiphysis (79.50-79.59)*
     DEF: Realignment of fracture with incision and internal fixation.

√4ᵗʰ **79.4 Closed reduction of separated epiphysis**
[0-2,   Reduction with or without internal fixation
5,6,9]   **DEF:** Manipulative reduction of expanded joint end of long bone to normal position without incision.

√4ᵗʰ **79.5 Open reduction of separated epiphysis**
[0-2,   Reduction with or without internal fixation
5,6,9]   **DEF:** Reduction of expanded joint end of long bone with incision.

√4ᵗʰ **79.6 Debridement of open fracture site**
[0-9]   Debridement of compound fracture
     DEF: Removal of damaged tissue at fracture site.

√4ᵗʰ **79.7 Closed reduction of dislocation**
     INCLUDES   closed reduction (with external traction device)
     EXCLUDES   *closed reduction of dislocation of temporomandibular joint (76.93)*
     DEF: Manipulative reduction of displaced joint without incision; with or without external traction.

   79.70 Closed reduction of dislocation of unspecified site
   79.71 Closed reduction of dislocation of shoulder
   79.72 Closed reduction of dislocation of elbow
   79.73 Closed reduction of dislocation of wrist
   79.74 Closed reduction of dislocation of hand and finger
   79.75 Closed reduction of dislocation of hip
   79.76 Closed reduction of dislocation of knee
   79.77 Closed reduction of dislocation of ankle
   79.78 Closed reduction of dislocation of foot and toe
   79.79 Closed reduction of dislocation of other specified sites

√4ᵗʰ **79.8 Open reduction of dislocation**
     INCLUDES   open reduction (with internal and external fixation devices)
     EXCLUDES   *open reduction of dislocation of temporomandibular joint (76.94)*
     DEF: Reduction of displaced joint via incision; with or without internal and external fixation.

   79.80 Open reduction of dislocation of unspecified site
   79.81 Open reduction of dislocation of shoulder
   79.82 Open reduction of dislocation of elbow
   79.83 Open reduction of dislocation of wrist
   79.84 Open reduction of dislocation of hand and finger
   79.85 Open reduction of dislocation of hip
   79.86 Open reduction of dislocation of knee
   79.87 Open reduction of dislocation of ankle
   79.88 Open reduction of dislocation of foot and toe
   79.89 Open reduction of dislocation of other specified sites

√4ᵗʰ **79.9 Unspecified operation on bone injury**
[0-9]

√3ʳᵈ **80 Incision and excision of joint structures**
     INCLUDES   operations on:
           capsule of joint
           cartilage
           condyle
           ligament
           meniscus
           synovial membrane
     EXCLUDES   *cartilage of:*
           ear (18.01-18.9)
           nose (21.00-21.99)
           temporomandibular joint (76.01-76.99)

The following fourth-digit subclassification is for use with appropriate categories in section 80 to identify the site:

0	unspecified site	6	knee
1	shoulder	7	ankle
2	elbow	8	foot and toe
3	wrist	9	other specified sites
4	hand and finger		Spine
5	hip		

√4ᵗʰ **80.0 Arthrotomy for removal of prosthesis, without**
[0-9] **replacement**
     INCLUDES   removal of posterior spinal motion preservation (dynamic stabilization, facet replacement, interspinous process) device(s)
     Code also any:
       insertion of (cement) (joint) (methylmethacrylate) spacer (84.56)
       removal of (cement) (joint) (methylmethacrylate) spacer (84.57)
     EXCLUDES   *removal of pedicle screws used in spinal fusion (78.69)*
     DEF: Incision into joint to remove prosthesis.

√4ᵗʰ **80.1 Other arthrotomy**
[0-9]   Arthrostomy
     EXCLUDES   *that for:*
         arthrography (88.32)
         arthroscopy (80.20-80.29)
         injection of drug (81.92)
         operative approach — omit code
     DEF: Incision into joint; other than to remove prosthesis.
     DEF: Arthrostomy: Creation of opening into joint.

√4ᵗʰ **80.2 Arthroscopy**
[0-9]

√4ᵗʰ **80.3 Biopsy of joint structure**
[0-9]   Aspiration biopsy

√4ᵗʰ **80.4 Division of joint capsule, ligament, or cartilage**
[0-9]   Goldner clubfoot release
     Heyman-Herndon(-Strong) correction of metatarsus varus
     Release of:
       adherent or constrictive joint capsule
       joint
       ligament
     EXCLUDES   *symphysiotomy to assist delivery (73.94)*
         that for:
           carpal tunnel syndrome (04.43)
           tarsal tunnel syndrome (04.44)
     DEF: Incision and separation of joint tissues, including capsule, fibrous bone attachment or cartilage.

√4ᵗʰ **80.5 Excision, destruction and other repair of intervertebral disc**

   80.50 Excision, destruction and other repair of intervertebral disc, unspecified
       Unspecified as to excision or destruction

80.51 Excision of intervertebral disc

Note: Requires additional code for any concomitant decompression of spinal nerve root at different level from excision site

Diskectomy
Level:
    cervical
    thoracic
    lumbar (lumbosacral)
Removal of herniated nucleus pulposus
That by laminotomy or hemilaminectomy
That with decompression of spinal nerve root at same level

Code also any:
    concurrent spinal fusion (81.00-81.08)
    repair of the anulus fibrosus (80.53-80.54)

    EXCLUDES   *intervertebral chemonucleolysis (80.52)*
       laminectomy for exploration of intraspinal canal (03.09)
       laminotomy for decompression of spinal nerve root only (03.09)
       that for insertion of (non-fusion) spinal disc replacement device (84.60-84.69)
       that with corpectomy, (vertebral) (80.99)

DEF: Discectomy: Removal of intervertebral disc.

DEF: Removal of a herniated nucleus pulposus: Removal of displaced intervertebral disc, central part.

80.52 Intervertebral chemonucleolysis

With aspiration of disc fragments
With diskography
Injection of proteolytic enzyme into intervertebral space (chymopapain)

    EXCLUDES   *injection of anesthestic substance (03.91)*
       injection of other substances (03.92)

DEF: Destruction of intervertebral disc via injection of enzyme.

80.53 Repair of the anulus fibrosus with graft or prosthesis

    INCLUDES   microsurgical suture repair with fascial autograft
       soft tissue re-approximation repair with tension bands
       surgical mesh repair

Anular disc repair
Closure (sealing) of the anulus fibrosus defect
Code also any:
    application or administration of adhesion barrier substance, if performed (99.77)
    intervertebral discectomy, if performed (80.51)
    locally harvested fascia for graft (83.43)

DEF: Adjunct procedure involving closure of defect in annulus fibrosis (ring of cartilage and fibrous tissue surrounding nucleus pulposus of IV disc) following discectomy surgery; prevents later disc herniation.

Types of Grafts for Anterior Arthrodesis

Anteroposterior   Anteroposterior   Anteroposterior

Lateral   Lateral   Lateral

80.54 Other and unspecified repair of the anulus fibrosus

Anular disc repair
Closure (sealing) of the anulus fibrosus defect
Microsurgical suture repair without fascial autograft
Percutaneous repair of the anulus fibrosus
Code also any:
    application or administration of adhesion barrier substance, if performed (99.77)
    intervertebral discectomy, if performed (80.51)

DEF: Adjunct procedure involving closure of defect in annulus fibrosis (ring of cartilage and fibrous tissue surrounding nucleus pulposus of IV disc) following discectomy surgery; prevents later disc herniation.

80.59 Other destruction of intervertebral disc

Destruction NEC   That by laser

80.6 Excision of semilunar cartilage of knee

Excision of meniscus of knee

✓4ᵗʰ 80.7 Synovectomy
[0-9]
Complete or partial resection of synovial membrane
    EXCLUDES   *excision of Baker's cyst (83.39)*

DEF: Excision of inner membrane of joint capsule.

✓4ᵗʰ 80.8 Other local excision or destruction of lesion of joint
[0-9]

✓4ᵗʰ 80.9 Other excision of joint
[0-9]
    EXCLUDES   *cheilectomy of joint (77.80-77.89)*
       excision of bone ends (77.80-77.89)

✓3ʳᵈ 81 Repair and plastic operations on joint structures

✓4ᵗʰ 81.0 Spinal fusion

Note: Spinal fusion is classified by the anatomic portion (column) fused and the technique (approach) used to perform the fusion.

For the anterior column, the body (corpus) of adjacent vertebrae are fused (interbody fusion). The anterior column can be fused using an anterior, lateral, or posterior technique.

For the posterior column, posterior structures of adjacent vertebrae are fused (pedicle, lamina, facet, transverse process, or "gutter" fusion). A posterior column fusion can be performed using a posterior, posterolateral, or lateral transverse technique.

    INCLUDES   arthrodesis of spine with:
       bone graft
       internal fixation

Code also any:
    insertion of interbody spinal fusion device (84.51)
    insertion of recombinant bone morphogenetic protein (84.52)
    synchronous excision of (locally) harvested bone for graft (77.70-77.79)
    the total number of vertebrae fused (81.62-81.64)

    EXCLUDES   *corrections of pseudarthrosis of spine (81.30-81.39)*
       refusion of spine (81.30-81.39)

DEF: Spinal fusion: Immobilization of spinal column.

DEF: Anterior interbody fusion: Arthrodesis by excising disc and cartilage end plates with bone graft insertion between two vertebrae.

DEF: Lateral fusion: Arthrodesis by decorticating and bone grafting lateral surface of zygapophysial joint, pars interarticularis and transverse process.

DEF: Posterior fusion: Arthrodesis by decorticating and bone grafting of neural arches between right and left zygapophysial joints.

DEF: Posterolateral fusion: Arthrodesis by decorticating and bone grafting zygapophysial joint, pars interarticularis and transverse processes

81.00 Spinal fusion, not otherwise specified

81.01 Atlas-axis spinal fusion

Craniocervical fusion   ⎫ by anterior transoral
C1–C2 fusion   ⎬ or posterior
Occiput C2 fusion   ⎭ technique

Subtalar Joint Arthroereisis

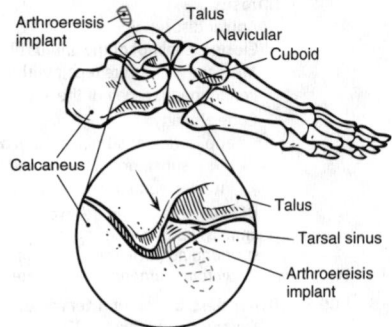

81.02   Other cervical fusion of the anterior column, anterior technique
Arthrodesis of C2 level or below:
     anterior interbody fusion
     anterolateral technique

81.03   Other cervical fusion of the posterior column, posterior technique
Arthrodesis of C2 level or below, posterolateral technique

81.04   Dorsal and dorsolumbar fusion of the anterior column, anterior technique
Arthrodesis of thoracic or thoracolumbar region:
     anterior interbody fusion
     anterolateral technique
Extracavitary technique

81.05   Dorsal and dorsolumbar fusion of the posterior column, posterior technique
Arthrodesis of thoracic or thoracolumbar region, posterolateral technique

81.06   Lumbar and lumbosacral fusion of the anterior column, anterior technique
Anterior lumbar interbody fusion [ALIF]
Arthrodesis of lumbar or lumbosacral region:
     anterior interbody fusion
     anterolateral technique
     retroperitoneal
     transperitoneal
Direct lateral interbody fusion [DLIF]
Extreme lateral interbody fusion [XLIF]

81.07   Lumbar and lumbosacral fusion of the posterior column, posterior technique
Facet fusion
Posterolateral technique
Transverse process technique

81.08   Lumbar and lumbosacral fusion of the anterior column, posterior technique
Arthrodesis of lumbar or lumbosacral region, posterior interbody fusion
Axial lumbar interbody fusion [AxiaLIF]
Posterior lumbar interbody fusion [PLIF]
Transforaminal lumbar interbody fusion [TLIF]

√4ᵗʰ 81.1   Arthrodesis and arthroereisis of foot and ankle
INCLUDES   arthrodesis of foot and ankle with:
     bone graft
     external fixation device
DEF: Fixation of foot or ankle joints.

81.11   Ankle fusion
Tibiotalar fusion

81.12   Triple arthrodesis
Talus to calcaneus and calcaneus to cuboid and navicular

81.13   Subtalar fusion
EXCLUDES   arthroereisis (81.18)

81.14   Midtarsal fusion

81.15   Tarsometatarsal fusion

81.16   Metatarsophalangeal fusion

81.17   Other fusion of foot

81.18   Subtalar joint arthroereisis
DEF: Insertion of an endoprosthesis to limit excessive valgus motion of the subtalar joint; nonfusion procedure to prevent pronation.

√4ᵗʰ 81.2   Arthrodesis of other joint
INCLUDES   arthrodesis with:
     bone graft
     external fixation device
     excision of bone ends and compression

81.20   Arthrodesis of unspecified joint

81.21   Arthrodesis of hip

81.22   Arthrodesis of knee

81.23   Arthrodesis of shoulder

81.24   Arthrodesis of elbow

81.25   Carporadial fusion

81.26   Metacarpocarpal fusion

81.27   Metacarpophalangeal fusion

81.28   Interphalangeal fusion

81.29   Arthrodesis of other specified joints

√4ᵗʰ 81.3   Refusion of spine
Note: Spine fusion is classified by the anatomic portion (column) fused and the technique (approach) used to perform the fusion.
For the anterior column, the body (corpus) of adjacent vertebrae are fused (interbody fusion). The anterior column can be fused using an anterior, lateral, or posterior technique.
For the posterior column, posterior structures of adjacent vertebrae are fused (pedicle, lamina, facet, transverse process, or "gutter" fusion). A posterior column fusion can be performed using a posterior, posterolateral, or lateral transverse technique.
INCLUDES   arthrodesis of spine with:
     bone graft
     internal fixation
     correction of pseudarthrosis of spine
Code also any:
     insertion of interbody spinal fusion device (84.51)
     insertion of recombinant bone morphogenetic protein (84.52)
     synchronous excision of (locally) harvested bone for graft (77.70-77.79)
     the total number of vertebrae fused (81.62-81.64)

81.30   Refusion of spine, not otherwise specified

81.31   Refusion of atlas-axis spine
Craniocervical fusion   }   by anterior transoral or
C1-C2 fusion   posterior
Occiput C2 fusion   }   technique

81.32   Refusion of other cervical spine, anterior column, anterior technique
Arthrodesis of C2 level or below:
     anterior interbody fusion
     anterolateral technique

81.33   Refusion of other cervical spine, posterior column, posterior technique
Arthrodesis of C2 level or below, posterolateral technique

81.34   Refusion of dorsal and dorsolumbar spine, anterior column, anterior technique
Arthrodesis of thoracic or thoracolumbar region:
     anterior interbody fusion
     anterolateral technique
Extracavitary technique

81.35   Refusion of dorsal and dorsolumbar spine, posterior column, posterior technique
Arthrodesis of thoracic or thoracolumbar region, posterolateral technique

81.36 Refusion of lumbar and lumbosacral spine, anterior column, anterior technique
Anterior lumbar interbody fusion [ALIF]
Arthrodesis of lumbar or lumbosacral region:
  anterior interbody fusion
  anterolateral technique
  retroperitoneal
  transperitoneal
Direct lateral interbody fusion [DLIF]
Extreme lateral interbody fusion [XLIF]

81.37 Refusion of lumbar and lumbosacral spine, posterior column, posterior technique
Facet fusion
Posterolateral technique
Transverse process technique

81.38 Refusion of lumbar and lumbosacral spine, anterior column, posterior technique
Arthrodesis of lumbar or lumbosacral region, posterior interbody fusion
Axial lumbar interbody fusion [AxiaLIF]
Posterior lumbar interbody fusion [PLIF]
Transforaminal lumbar interbody fusion [TLIF]

81.39 Refusion of spine, not elsewhere classified

√4ᵗʰ **81.4 Other repair of joint of lower extremity**
INCLUDES arthroplasty of lower extremity with:
  external traction or fixation
  graft of bone (chips) or cartilage
  internal fixation device

81.40 Repair of hip, not elsewhere classified

81.42 Five-in-one repair of knee
Medial meniscectomy, medial collateral ligament repair, vastus medialis advancement, semitendinosus advancement, and pes anserinus transfer

81.43 Triad knee repair
Medial meniscectomy with repair of the anterior cruciate ligament and the medial collateral ligament
O'Donoghue procedure

81.44 Patellar stabilization
Roux-Goldthwait operation for recurrent dislocation of patella
DEF: Roux-Goldthwait operation: Stabilization of patella via lateral ligament transposed at insertion beneath undisturbed medial insertion; excision of capsule ellipse and medial patella retinaculum; capsule reefed for lateral patella hold.

81.45 Other repair of the cruciate ligaments

81.46 Other repair of the collateral ligaments

81.47 Other repair of knee

81.49 Other repair of ankle

√4ᵗʰ **81.5 Joint replacement of lower extremity**
Note: Removal of prior prothesis — omit code
INCLUDES arthroplasty of lower extremity with:
  external traction or fixation
  graft of bone (chips) or cartilage
  internal fixation device or prosthesis

81.51 Total hip replacement
Replacement of both femoral head and acetabulum by prosthesis
Total reconstruction of hip
Code also any type of bearing surface, if known (00.74-00.77)
DEF: Repair of both surfaces of hip joint with prosthesis.

81.52 Partial hip replacement
Bipolar endoprosthesis
Code also any type of bearing surface, if known (00.74-00.77)
DEF: Repair of single surface of hip joint with prosthesis.

Total Hip Replacement

Damaged femur head ("ball") in degenerated socket (acetabulum)

Cuplike acetabular component of prosthesis fixed into hip bone

Prosthesis anchored into shaft of long bone

Damaged femur head replaced with prosthesis

Partial Hip Replacement

Acetabulum remains intact

Prosthesis

81.53 Revision of hip replacement, not otherwise specified
Revision of hip replacement, not specified as to component(s) replaced, (acetabular, femoral or both)
Code also any:
  removal of (cement) (joint) spacer (84.57)
  type of bearing surface, if known (00.74-00.77)
EXCLUDES revision of hip replacement, components specified (00.70-00.73)

81.54 Total knee replacement
Bicompartmental
Partial knee replacement
Tricompartmental
Unicompartmental (hemijoint)
DEF: Repair of a knee joint with prosthetic implant in one, two, or three compartments.

81.55 Revision of knee replacement, not otherwise specified
Code also any removal of (cement) (joint) spacer (84.57)
EXCLUDES arthrodesis of knee (81.22)
  revision of knee replacement, components specified (00.80-00.84)

81.56 Total ankle replacement

81.57 Replacement of joint of foot and toe

81.59 Revision of joint replacement of lower extremity, not elsewhere classified

Total Knee Replacement

Condyle component
Femur
Prosthesis
Patella
Tibia
Plateau component

Operations on the Musculoskeletal System

81.6–81.94

Vertebroplasty

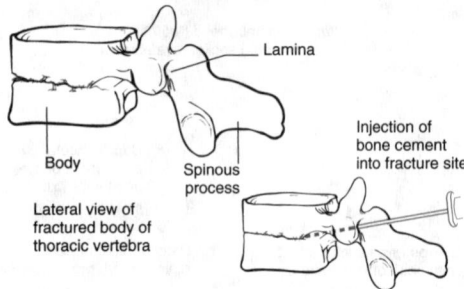

Lateral view of fractured body of thoracic vertebra

Body · Lamina · Spinous process · Injection of bone cement into fracture site

Percutaneous Vertebral Augmentation

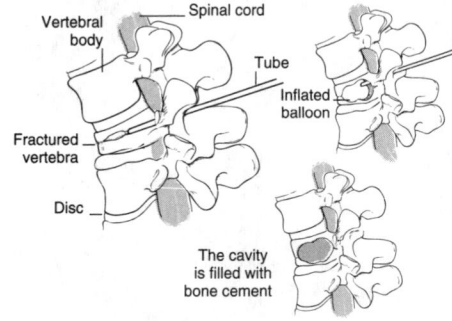

Vertebral body · Spinal cord · Tube · Inflated balloon · Fractured vertebra · Disc · The cavity is filled with bone cement

81.6 Other procedures on spine

Note: Number of vertebrae
The vertebral spine consists of 25 vertebrae in the following order and number:
cervical: C1 (atlas), C2 (axis), C3, C4, C5, C6, C7
thoracic or dorsal: T1, T2, T3, T4, T5, T6, T7, T8, T9, T10, T11, T12
lumbar and sacral: L1, L2, L3, L4, L5, S1
Coders should report only one code from the series 81.62-81.64 to show the total number of vertebrae fused on the patient.
Code also the level and approach of the fusion or refusion (81.00-81.08, 81.30-81.39)

DEF: A combined posterior and anterior fusion performed by a surgeon through one incision: lateral transverse, posterior, or anterior.

81.62 Fusion or refusion of 2-3 vertebrae

81.63 Fusion or refusion of 4-8 vertebrae

81.64 Fusion or refusion of 9 or more vertebrae

81.65 Percutaneous vertebroplasty
Injection of bone void filler (cement) (polymethylmethacrylate) (PMMA) into the diseased or fractured vertebral body
EXCLUDES   *kyphoplasty (81.66)*
percutaneous vertebral augmentation (81.66)

81.66 Percutaneous vertebral augmentation
Arcuplasty
Insertion of inflatable balloon, bone tamp, or other device displacing (removing) (compacting) bone to create a space (cavity) (void) prior to the injection of bone void filler (cement) (polymethyl- methacrylate) (PMMA) or other substance
Kyphoplasty
Skyphoplasty
Spineoplasty
EXCLUDES   *percutaneous vertebroplasty (81.65)*

81.7 Arthroplasty and repair of hand, fingers, and wrist
INCLUDES   arthroplasty of hand and finger with:
external traction or fixation
graft of bone (chips) or cartilage
internal fixation device or prosthesis
EXCLUDES   *operations on muscle, tendon, and fascia of hand (82.01-82.99)*
DEF: Plastic surgery of hand, fingers and wrist joints.

81.71 Arthroplasty of metacarpophalangeal and interphalangeal joint with implant

81.72 Arthroplasty of metacarpophalangeal and interphalangeal joint without implant

81.73 Total wrist replacement

81.74 Arthroplasty of carpocarpal or carpometacarpal joint with implant

81.75 Arthroplasty of carpocarpal or carpometacarpal joint without implant

81.79 Other repair of hand, fingers, and wrist

81.8 Arthroplasty and repair of shoulder and elbow
INCLUDES   arthroplasty of upper limb NEC with:
external traction or fixation
graft of bone (chips) or cartilage
internal fixation device or prosthesis

81.80 Other total shoulder replacement
EXCLUDES   *reverse total shoulder replacement (81.88)*

81.81 Partial shoulder replacement

81.82 Repair of recurrent dislocation of shoulder

81.83 Other repair of shoulder

81.84 Total elbow replacement
Partial elbow replacement

81.85 Other repair of elbow

81.88 Reverse total shoulder replacement
Reverse ball-and-socket of the shoulder
EXCLUDES   *conversion of prior (failed) total shoulder replacement (arthroplasty) to reverse total shoulder replacement (81.97)*

81.9 Other operations on joint structures

81.91 Arthrocentesis
Joint aspiration
EXCLUDES   *that for:*
arthrography (88.32)
biopsy of joint structure (80.30-80.39)
injection of drug (81.92)
DEF: Insertion of needle to withdraw fluid from joint.

81.92 Injection of therapeutic substance into joint or ligament

81.93 Suture of capsule or ligament of upper extremity
EXCLUDES   *that associated with arthroplasty (81.71-81.75, 81.80-81.81, 81.84)*

81.94 Suture of capsule or ligament of ankle and foot
EXCLUDES   *that associated with arthroplasty (81.56-81.59)*

Arthrocentesis

Femur · Needle access into fluid filled knee joint · Patella (kneecap) · Fluid-filled joint capsule · Tibia

81.95 Suture of capsule or ligament of other lower extremity
> EXCLUDES *that associated with arthroplasty (81.51-81.55, 81.59)*

81.96 Other repair of joint

81.97 Revision of joint replacement of upper extremity
Partial
Removal of cement spacer
Revision of arthroplasty of shoulder
Total

81.98 Other diagnostic procedures on joint structures
> EXCLUDES *arthroscopy (80.20-80.29)*
> *biopsy of joint structure (80.30-80.39)*
> *microscopic examination of specimen from joint (91.51-91.59)*
> *thermography (88.83)*
> *x-ray (87.21-87.29, 88.21-88.33)*

81.99 Other

√3rd **82 Operations on muscle, tendon, and fascia of hand**
> INCLUDES operations on:
> aponeurosis
> synovial membrane (tendon sheath)
> tendon sheath

√4th **82.0 Incision of muscle, tendon, fascia, and bursa of hand**

82.01 Exploration of tendon sheath of hand
Incision of   } tendon sheath of
Removal of rice bodies in   } hand
> EXCLUDES *division of tendon (82.11)*
> DEF: Incision into and exploration of the hand's muscle and its accompanying supportive, connective tissue, bands, and sacs.

82.02 Myotomy of hand
> EXCLUDES *myotomy for division (82.19)*
> DEF: Incision into hand muscle.

82.03 Bursotomy of hand

82.04 Incision and drainage of palmar or thenar space

82.09 Other incision of soft tissue of hand
> EXCLUDES *incision of skin and subcutaneous tissue alone (86.01-86.09)*

√4th **82.1 Division of muscle, tendon, and fascia of hand**

82.11 Tenotomy of hand
Division of tendon of hand

82.12 Fasciotomy of hand
Division of fascia of hand

82.19 Other division of soft tissue of hand
Division of muscle of hand

√4th **82.2 Excision of lesion of muscle, tendon, and fascia of hand**

82.21 Excision or lesion of tendon sheath of hand
Ganglionectomy of tendon sheath (wrist)

82.22 Excision of lesion of muscle of hand

82.29 Excision of other lesion of soft tissue of hand
> EXCLUDES *excision of lesion of skin and subcutaneous tissue (86.21-86.3)*

√4th **82.3 Other excision of soft tissue of hand**
Code also any skin graft (86.61-86.62, 86.73)
> EXCLUDES *excision of skin and subcutaneous tissue (86.21-86.3)*

82.31 Bursectomy of hand

82.32 Excision of tendon of hand for graft
> DEF: Resection and excision of fibrous tissue connecting bone to hand muscle for grafting.

82.33 Other tenonectomy of hand
Tenosynovectomy of hand
> EXCLUDES *excision of lesion of:*
> *tendon (82.29)*
> *sheath (82.21)*
> DEF: Removal of fibrous bands connecting muscle to bone of hand.
> DEF: Tenosynovectomy of hand: Excision of fibrous band connecting muscle and bone of hand and removal of coverings.

82.34 Excision of muscle or fascia of hand for graft

82.35 Other fasciectomy of hand
Release of Dupuytren's contracture
> EXCLUDES *excision of lesion of fascia (82.29)*
> DEF: Excision of fibrous connective tissue; other than for grafting or removing lesion.
> DEF: Release of Dupuytren's contracture: Excision of fibrous connective tissue to correct flexion of fingers.

82.36 Other myectomy of hand
> EXCLUDES *excision of lesion of muscle (82.22)*

82.39 Other excision of soft tissue of hand
> EXCLUDES *excision of skin (86.21-86.3)*
> *excision of soft tissue lesion (82.29)*

√4th **82.4 Suture of muscle, tendon, and fascia of hand**

82.41 Suture of tendon sheath of hand

82.42 Delayed suture of flexor tendon of hand
> DEF: Suture of fibrous band between flexor muscle and bone; following initial repair.

82.43 Delayed suture of other tendon of hand

82.44 Other suture of flexor tendon of hand
> EXCLUDES *delayed suture of flexor tendon of hand (82.42)*

82.45 Other suture of other tendon of hand
> EXCLUDES *delayed suture of other tendon of hand (82.43)*

82.46 Suture of muscle or fascia of hand

√4th **82.5 Transplantation of muscle and tendon of hand**

82.51 Advancement of tendon of hand
> DEF: Detachment of fibrous connective muscle band and bone with reattachment at advanced point of hand.

82.52 Recession of tendon of hand
> DEF: Detachment of fibrous band of muscle and bone with reattachment at drawn-back point of hand.

82.53 Reattachment of tendon of hand

82.54 Reattachment of muscle of hand

82.55 Other change in hand muscle or tendon length

82.56 Other hand tendon transfer or transplantation
> EXCLUDES *pollicization of thumb (82.61)*
> *transfer of finger, except thumb (82.81)*

82.57 Other hand tendon transposition

82.58 Other hand muscle transfer or transplantation

82.59 Other hand muscle transposition

√4th **82.6 Reconstruction of thumb**
> INCLUDES digital transfer to act as thumb
Code also any amputation for digital transfer (84.01, 84.11)

82.61 Pollicization operation carrying over nerves and blood supply
> DEF: Creation or reconstruction of a thumb with another digit, commonly the index finger.

82.69 Other reconstruction of thumb
"Cocked-hat" procedure [skin flap and bone]
Grafts:
bone   } to thumb
skin (pedicle) }

Operations on the Musculoskeletal System

82.7–83.21

☑4ᵗʰ **82.7 Plastic operation on hand with graft or implant**

     82.71 Tendon pulley reconstruction
         Reconstruction for opponensplasty
         DEF: Reconstruction of fibrous band between muscle and bone of hand.

     82.72 Plastic operation on hand with graft of muscle or fascia

     82.79 Plastic operation on hand with other graft or implant
         Tendon graft to hand

☑4ᵗʰ **82.8 Other plastic operations on hand**

     82.81 Transfer of finger, except thumb
         EXCLUDES   *pollicization of thumb (82.61)*

     82.82 Repair of cleft hand
         DEF: Correction of fissure defect of hand.

     82.83 Repair of macrodactyly
         DEF: Reduction in size of abnormally large fingers.

     82.84 Repair of mallet finger
         DEF: Repair of flexed little finger.

     82.85 Other tenodesis of hand
         Tendon fixation of hand NOS
         DEF: Fixation of fibrous connective band between muscle and bone of hand.

     82.86 Other tenoplasty of hand
         Myotenoplasty of hand
         DEF: Myotenoplasty of hand: Plastic repair of muscle and fibrous band connecting muscle to bone.

     82.89 Other plastic operations on hand
         Plication of fascia
         Repair of fascial hernia
         EXCLUDES   *that with graft or implant (82.71-82.79)*

☑4ᵗʰ **82.9 Other operations on muscle, tendon, and fascia of hand**
     EXCLUDES   *diagnostic procedures on soft tissue of hand (83.21-83.29)*

     82.91 Lysis of adhesions of hand
         Freeing of adhesions of fascia, muscle, and tendon of hand
         EXCLUDES   *decompression of carpal tunnel (04.43)*
                           that by stretching or manipulation only (93.26)

     82.92 Aspiration of bursa of hand

     82.93 Aspiration of other soft tissue of hand
         EXCLUDES   *skin and subcutaneous tissue (86.01)*

     82.94 Injection of therapeutic substance into bursa of hand

     82.95 Injection of therapeutic substance into tendon of hand

     82.96 Other injection of locally-acting therapeutic substance into soft tissue of hand
         EXCLUDES   *subcutaneous or intramuscular injection (99.11-99.29)*

     82.99 Other operations on muscle, tendon, and fascia of hand

☑3ʳᵈ **83 Operations on muscle, tendon, fascia, and bursa, except hand**
     INCLUDES   operations on:
                 aponeurosis
                 synovial membrane of bursa and tendon sheaths
                 tendon sheaths
     EXCLUDES   *diaphragm (34.81-34.89)*
                     hand (82.01-82.99)
                     muscles of eye (15.01-15.9)

☑4ᵗʰ **83.0 Incision of muscle, tendon, fascia, and bursa**

     83.01 Exploration of tendon sheath
         Incision of tendon sheath
         Removal of rice bodies from tendon sheath
         DEF: Incision of external covering of fibrous cord for exam.
         DEF: Removal of rice bodies from tendon sheath: Incision and removal of small bodies resembling grains of rice.

     83.02 Myotomy
         EXCLUDES   *cricopharyngeal myotomy (29.31)*

     83.03 Bursotomy
         Removal of calcareous deposit of bursa
         EXCLUDES   *aspiration of bursa (percutaneous) (83.94)*

     83.09 Other incision of soft tissue
         Incision of fascia
         EXCLUDES   *incision of skin and subcutaneous tissue alone (86.01-86.09)*

☑4ᵗʰ **83.1 Division of muscle, tendon, and fascia**

     83.11 Achillotenotomy

     83.12 Adductor tenotomy of hip
         DEF: Incision into fibrous attachment between adductor muscle and hip bone.

     83.13 Other tenotomy
         Aponeurotomy   Tendon transection
         Division of tendon   Tenotomy for thoracic
         Tendon release   outlet decompression
         DEF: Aponeurotomy: Incision and separation of fibrous cords attaching a muscle to bone to aid movement.
         DEF: Division of tendon: Separation of fibrous band connecting muscle to bone.
         DEF: Tendon release: Surgical detachment of fibrous band from muscle and/or bone.
         DEF: Tendon transection: Incision across width of fibrous bands between muscle and bone.
         DEF: Tenotomy for thoracic outlet decompression: Incision of fibrous muscle with separation from bone to relieve compressed thoracic outlet.

     83.14 Fasciotomy
         Division of fascia
         Division of iliotibial band
         Fascia stripping
         Release of Volkmann's contracture by fasciotomy
         DEF: Division of fascia: Incision to separate fibrous connective tissue.
         DEF: Division of iliotibial band: Incision to separate fibrous band connecting tibial bone to muscle in flank.
         DEF: Fascia stripping: Incision and lengthwise separation of fibrous connective tissue.
         DEF: Release of Volkmann's contracture by fasciotomy: Divisional incision of connective tissue to correct defect in flexion of finger(s).

     83.19 Other division of soft tissue
         Division of muscle
         Muscle release
         Myotomy for thoracic outlet decompression
         Myotomy with division
         Scalenotomy
         Transection of muscle

☑4ᵗʰ **83.2 Diagnostic procedures on muscle, tendon, fascia, and bursa, including that of hand**

     83.21 Open biopsy of soft tissue
         EXCLUDES   *biopsy of chest wall (34.23)*
                           closed biopsy of skin and subcutaneous tissue (86.11)

83.29   Other diagnostic procedures on muscle, tendon, fascia, and bursa, including that of hand
> *EXCLUDES*   *microscopic examination of specimen (91.51-91.-59)*
> *soft tissue x-ray (87.09, 87.38-87.39, 88.09, 88.35, 88.37)*
> *thermography of muscle (88.84)*

✓4ᵗʰ **83.3   Excision of lesion of muscle, tendon, fascia, and bursa**
> *EXCLUDES*   *biopsy of soft tissue (83.21)*

83.31   Excision of lesion of tendon sheath
> Excision of ganglion of tendon sheath, except of hand

83.32   Excision of lesion of muscle
> Excision of:
>> heterotopic bone
>> muscle scar for release of Volkmann's contracture
>> myositis ossificans
>
> **DEF:** Heterotopic bone: Bone lesion in muscle.
> **DEF:** Muscle scar for release of Volkmann's contracture: Scarred muscle tissue interfering with finger flexion.
> **DEF:** Myositis ossificans: Bony deposits in muscle.

83.39   Excision of lesion of other soft tissue
> Excision of Baker's cyst
> *EXCLUDES*   *bursectomy (83.5)*
> *excision of lesion of skin and subcutaneous tissue (86.3)*
> *synovectomy (80.70-80.79)*

✓4ᵗʰ **83.4   Other excision of muscle, tendon, and fascia**

83.41   Excision of tendon for graft

83.42   Other tenonectomy
> Excision of: Tenosynovectomy
>> aponeurosis
>> tendon sheath

83.43   Excision of muscle or fascia for graft

83.44   Other fasciectomy
> **DEF:** Excision of fascia; other than for graft.

83.45   Other myectomy
> Debridement of muscle NOS
> Scalenectomy
> **DEF:** Scalenectomy: Removal of thoracic scaleni muscle tissue.

83.49   Other excision of soft tissue

83.5   Bursectomy

✓4ᵗʰ **83.6   Suture of muscle, tendon, and fascia**

83.61   Suture of tendon sheath

83.62   Delayed suture of tendon

83.63   Rotator cuff repair
> **DEF:** Repair of musculomembranous structure around shoulder joint capsule.

83.64   Other suture of tendon
> Achillorrhaphy   Aponeurorrhaphy
> *EXCLUDES*   *delayed suture of tendon (83.62)*
> **DEF:** Achillorrhaphy: Suture of fibrous band connecting Achilles tendon to heel bone.
> **DEF:** Aponeurorrhaphy: Suture of fibrous cords connecting muscle to bone.

83.65   Other suture of muscle or fascia
> Repair of diastasis recti

✓4ᵗʰ **83.7   Reconstruction of muscle and tendon**
> *EXCLUDES*   *reconstruction of muscle and tendon associated with arthroplasty*

83.71   Advancement of tendon
> **DEF:** Detaching fibrous cord between muscle and bone with reattachment at advanced point.

83.72   Recession of tendon
> **DEF:** Detaching fibrous cord between muscle and bone with reattachment at drawn-back point.

83.73   Reattachment of tendon

83.74   Reattachment of muscle

83.75   Tendon transfer or transplantation

83.76   Other tendon transposition

83.77   Muscle transfer or transplantation
> Release of Volkmann's contracture by muscle transplantation

83.79   Other muscle transposition

✓4ᵗʰ **83.8   Other plastic operations on muscle, tendon, and fascia**
> *EXCLUDES*   *plastic operations on muscle, tendon, and fascia associated with arthroplasty*

83.81   Tendon graft

83.82   Graft of muscle or fascia

83.83   Tendon pulley reconstruction
> **DEF:** Reconstruction of fibrous cord between muscle and bone at any site other than hand.

83.84   Release of clubfoot, not elsewhere classified
> Evans operation on clubfoot

83.85   Other change in muscle or tendon length
> Hamstring lengthening   Plastic achillotenotomy
> Heel cord shortening   Tendon plication
> **DEF:** Plastic achillotenotomy: Increase in heel cord length.
> **DEF:** Tendon plication: Surgical tuck of tendon.

83.86   Quadricepsplasty
> **DEF:** Correction of quadriceps femoris muscle.

83.87   Other plastic operations on muscle
> Musculoplasty
> Myoplasty

83.88   Other plastic operations on tendon
> Myotenoplasty   Tenodesis
> Tendon fixation   Tenoplasty

83.89   Other plastic operations on fascia
> Fascia lengthening   Plication of fascia
> Fascioplasty

✓4ᵗʰ **83.9   Other operations on muscle, tendon, fascia, and bursa**
> *EXCLUDES*   *nonoperative:*
> *manipulation (93.25-93.29)*
> *stretching (93.27-93.29)*

83.91   Lysis of adhesions of muscle, tendon, fascia, and bursa
> *EXCLUDES*   *that for tarsal tunnel syndrome (04.44)*
> **DEF:** Separation of created fibrous structures from muscle, connective tissues, bands and sacs.

83.92   Insertion or replacement of skeletal muscle stimulator
> Implantation, insertion, placement, or replacement of skeletal muscle:
>> electrodes
>> stimulator

83.93   Removal of skeletal muscle stimulator

83.94   Aspiration of bursa

83.95   Aspiration of other soft tissue
> *EXCLUDES*   *that of skin and subcutaneous tissue (86.01)*

83.96   Injection of therapeutic substance into bursa

83.97   Injection of therapeutic substance into tendon

83.98   Injection of locally-acting therapeutic substance into other soft tissue
> *EXCLUDES*   *subcutaneous or intramuscular injection (99.11-99.29)*

83.99   Other operations on muscle, tendon, fascia, and bursa
> Suture of bursa

✓3ʳᵈ **84   Other procedures on musculoskeletal system**

✓4ᵗʰ **84.0   Amputation of upper limb**

> EXCLUDES   *revision of amputation stump (84.3)*

84.00   Upper limb amputation, not otherwise specified

Closed flap amputation
Kineplastic amputation
Open or guillotine amputation
Revision of current traumatic
    amputation
} of upper limb NOS

DEF: Closed flap amputation: Sewing a created skin flap over stump end of upper limb.

DEF: Kineplastic amputation: Amputation and preparation of stump of upper limb to permit movement.

DEF: Open or guillotine amputation: Straight incision across upper limb; used when primary closure is contraindicated.

DEF: Revision of current traumatic amputation: Reconstruction of traumatic amputation of upper limb to enable closure.

84.01   Amputation and disarticulation of finger

> EXCLUDES   *ligation of supernumerary finger (86.26)*

84.02   Amputation and disarticulation of thumb

84.03   Amputation through hand

Amputation through carpals

84.04   Disarticulation of wrist

84.05   Amputation through forearm

Forearm amputation

84.06   Disarticulation of elbow

DEF: Amputation of forearm through elbow joint.

84.07   Amputation through humerus

Upper arm amputation

84.08   Disarticulation of shoulder

DEF: Amputation of arm through shoulder joint.

84.09   Interthoracoscapular amputation

Forequarter amputation

DEF: Removal of upper arm, shoulder bone and collarbone.

✓4ᵗʰ **84.1   Amputation of lower limb**

> EXCLUDES   *revision of amputation stump (84.3)*

84.10   Lower limb amputation, not otherwise specified

Closed flap amputation
Kineplastic amputation
Open or guillotine amputation
Revision of current traumatic
    amputation
} of lower limb NOS

DEF: Closed flap amputation: Sewing a created skin flap over stump of lower limb.

DEF: Kineplastic amputation: Amputation and preparation of stump of lower limb to permit movement.

DEF: Open or guillotine amputation: Straight incision across lower limb; used when primary closure is contraindicated.

DEF: Revision of current traumatic amputation: Reconstruction of traumatic amputation of lower limb to enable closure.

84.11   Amputation of toe

Amputation through metatarsophalangeal joint
Disarticulation of toe
Metatarsal head amputation
Ray amputation of foot (disarticulation of the
    metatarsal head of the toe extending across
    the forefoot, just proximal to the
    metatarsophalangeal crease)

> EXCLUDES   *ligation of supernumerary toe (86.26)*

84.12   Amputation through foot

Amputation of forefoot
Amputation through middle of foot
Chopart's amputation
Midtarsal amputation
Transmetatarsal amputation (amputation of the
    forefoot, including the toes)

> EXCLUDES   *Ray amputation of foot (84.11)*

DEF: Amputation of forefoot: Removal of foot in front of joint between toes and body of foot.

DEF: Chopart's amputation: Removal of foot with retention of heel, ankle and other associated ankle bones.

DEF: Midtarsal amputation: Amputation of foot through tarsals.

DEF: Transmetatarsal amputation: Amputation of foot through metatarsals.

84.13   Disarticulation of ankle

DEF: Removal of foot through ankle bone.

84.14   Amputation of ankle through malleoli of tibia and fibula

84.15   Other amputation below knee

Amputation of leg through tibia and fibula NOS

84.16   Disarticulation of knee

Batch, Spitler, and McFaddin amputation
Mazet amputation
S.P. Roger's amputation

DEF: Removal of lower leg through knee joint.

84.17   Amputation above knee

Amputation of leg through femur
Amputation of thigh
Conversion of below-knee amputation into
    above-knee amputation
Supracondylar above-knee amputation

84.18   Disarticulation of hip

DEF: Removal of leg through hip joint.

84.19   Abdominopelvic amputation

Hemipelvectomy
Hindquarter amputation

DEF: Removal of leg and portion of pelvic bone.

DEF: Hemipelvectomy: Removal of leg and lateral pelvis.

✓4ᵗʰ **84.2   Reattachment of extremity**

84.21   Thumb reattachment

84.22   Finger reattachment

84.23   Forearm, wrist, or hand reattachment

84.24   Upper arm reattachment

Reattachment of arm NOS

84.25   Toe reattachment

84.26   Foot reattachment

84.27   Lower leg or ankle reattachment

Reattachment of leg NOS

84.28   Thigh reattachment

84.29   Other reattachment

84.3   Revision of amputation stump

Reamputation
Secondary closure
Trimming
} of stump

> EXCLUDES   *revision of current traumatic amputation [revision by further amputation of current injury] (84.00-84.19, 84.91)*

✓4ᵗʰ **84.4   Implantation or fitting of prosthetic limb device**

84.40   Implantation or fitting of prosthetic limb device, not otherwise specified

84.41   Fitting of prosthesis of upper arm and shoulder

84.42   Fitting of prosthesis of lower arm and hand

84.43   Fitting of prosthesis of arm, not otherwise specified

84.44   Implantation of prosthetic device of arm

84.45   **Fitting of prosthesis above knee**

84.46   **Fitting of prosthesis below knee**

84.47   **Fitting of prosthesis of leg, not otherwise specified**

84.48   **Implantation of prosthetic device of leg**

✓4ᵗʰ **84.5**   **Implantation of other musculoskeletal devices and substances**

> **EXCLUDES**   *insertion of (non-fusion) spinal disc replacement device (84.60-84.69)*

84.51   **Insertion of interbody spinal fusion device**

Insertion of:
     cages (carbn, ceramic, metal, plastic or titanium)
     interbody fusion cage
     synthetic cages or spacers
     threaded bone dowels
Code also refusion of spine (81.30-81.39)
Code also spinal fusion (81.00-81.08)

84.52   **Insertion of recombinant bone morphogenetic protein**

rhBMP
That via collagen sponge, coral, ceramic and other carriers
Code also primary procedure performed:
     fracture repair (79.00-79.99)
     spinal fusion (81.00-81.08)
     spinal refusion (81.30-81.39)

DEF: Surgical implantation of bone morphogenetic proteins (BMP) and recombinant BMP (rhBMP) to induce new bone growth formation; clinical applications include delayed unions and nonunions, fractures, and spinal fusions.

84.53   **Implantation of internal limb lengthening device with kinetic distraction**

Code also limb lengthening procedure (78.30-78.39)

84.54   **Implantation of other internal limb lengthening device**

Implantation of internal limb lengthening device, not otherwise specified (NOS)
Code also limb lengthening procedure (78.30-78.39)

84.55   **Insertion of bone void filler**

Insertion of:
     acrylic cement (PMMA)
     bone void cement
     calcium based bone void filler
     polymethylmethacrylate (PMMA)

> **EXCLUDES**   *that with percutaneous vertebral augmentation (81.66)*
> *that with percutaneous vertebroplasty (81.65)*

84.56   **Insertion or replacement of (cement) spacer**

Insertion or replacement of joint (methylmethacrylate) spacer

84.57   **Removal of (cement) spacer**

Removal of joint (methylmethacrylate) spacer

84.59   **Insertion of other spinal devices**

> **EXCLUDES**   *initial insertion of pedicle screws with spinal fusion — omit code*
> *insertion of facet replacement device(s) (84.84)*
> *insertion of interspinous process device(s) (84.80)*
> *insertion of pedicle-based dynamic stabilization device(s) (84.82)*

Spinal Fusion with Metal Cage

Metal cages support spine until fusion occurs

Anterior view

Lateral view

Spinal fusion with metal cages

Detail

✓4ᵗʰ **84.6**   **Replacement of spinal disc**

> **INCLUDES**   non-fusion arthroplasty of the spine with insertion of artificial disc prosthesis

84.60   **Insertion of spinal disc prosthesis, not otherwise specified**

> **INCLUDES**   diskectomy (discectomy)
> Replacement of spinal disc, NOS

84.61   **Insertion of partial spinal disc prosthesis, cervical**

> **INCLUDES**   diskectomy (discectomy)
> Nuclear replacement device, cervical
> Partial artificial disc prosthesis (flexible), cervical
> Replacement of nuclear disc (nucleus pulposus), cervical

84.62   **Insertion of total spinal disc prosthesis, cervical**

> **INCLUDES**   diskectomy (discectomy)
> Replacement of cervical spinal disc, NOS
> Replacement of total spinal disc, cervical
> Total artificial disc prosthesis (flexible), cervical

84.63   **Insertion of spinal disc prosthesis, thoracic**

> **INCLUDES**   diskectomy (discectomy)
> Artificial disc prosthesis (flexible), thoracic
> Replacement of thoracic spinal disc, partial or total

84.64   **Insertion of partial spinal disc prosthesis, lumbosacral**

> **INCLUDES**   diskectomy (discectomy)
> Nuclear replacement device, lumbar
> Partial artificial disc prosthesis (flexible), lumbar
> Replacement of nuclear disc (nucleus pulposus), lumbar

84.65   **Insertion of total spinal disc prosthesis, lumbosacral**

> **INCLUDES**   diskectomy (discectomy)
> Replacement of lumbar spinal disc, NOS
> Replacement of total spinal disc, lumbar
> Total artificial disc prosthesis (flexible), lumbar

84.66   **Revision or replacement of artificial spinal disc prosthesis, cervical**

Removal of (partial) (total) spinal disc prosthesis with synchronous insertion of new (partial) (total) spinal disc prosthesis, cervical
Repair of previously inserted spinal disc prosthesis, cervical

84.67   **Revision or replacement of artificial spinal disc prosthesis, thoracic**

Removal of (partial) (total) spinal disc prosthesis with synchronous insertion of new (partial) (total) spinal disc prosthesis, thoracic
Repair of previously inserted spinal disc prosthesis, thoracic

84.68   **Revision or replacement of artificial spinal disc prosthesis, lumbosacral**

Removal of (partial) (total) spinal disc prosthesis with synchronous insertion of new (partial) (total) spinal disc prosthesis, lumbosacral
Repair of previously inserted spinal disc prosthesis, lumbosacral

External Fixator Devices

Monoplanar   Ring system   Hybrid

Posterior Spinal Motion Preservation Devices

Interspinous devices   Dynamic stabilization   Facet replacement

84.69 **Revision or replacement of artificial spinal disc prosthesis, not otherwise specified**
Removal of (partial) (total) spinal disc prosthesis with synchronous insertion of new (partial) (total) spinal disc prosthesis
Repair of previously inserted spinal disc prosthesis

√4ᵗʰ **84.7** **Adjunct codes for external fixator devices**
Code also any primary procedure performed:
application of external fixator device (78.10, 78.12-78.13, 78.15, 78.17-78.19)
reduction of fracture and dislocation (79.00-79.89)

84.71 **Application of external fixator device, monoplanar system**
EXCLUDES   other hybrid device or system (84.73)
ring device or system (84.72)

DEF: Instrumentation that provides percutaneous neutralization, compression, and /or distraction of bone in a single plane by applying force within that plane.

84.72 **Application of external fixator device, ring system**
Ilizarov type   Sheffield type
EXCLUDES   monoplanar device or system (84.71)
other hybrid device or system (84.73)

DEF: Instrumentation that provides percutaneous neutralization, compression, and/or distraction of bone through 360 degrees of force application.

84.73 **Application of hybrid external fixator device**
Computer (assisted) (dependent) external fixator device
Hybrid system using both ring and monoplanar devices
EXCLUDES   monoplanar device or system, when used alone (84.71)
ring device or system, when used alone (84.72)

DEF: Instrumentation that provides percutaneous neutralization, compression, and /or distraction of bone by applying multiple external forces using monoplanar and ring device combinations.

√4ᵗʰ **84.8** **Insertion, replacement and revision of posterior spinal motion preservation device(s)**
INCLUDES   any synchronous facetectomy (partial, total) performed at the same level
Dynamic spinal stabilization device(s)
Code also any synchronous surgical decompression (foraminotomy, laminectomy, laminotomy), if performed (03.09)
EXCLUDES   fusion of spine (81.00-81.08, 81.30-81.39)
insertion of artificial disc prosthesis (84.60-84.69)
insertion of interbody spinal fusion device (84.51)

84.80 **Insertion or replacement of interspinous process device(s)**
Interspinous process decompression device(s)
Interspinous process distraction device(s)
EXCLUDES   insertion or replacement of facet replacement device (84.84)
insertion or replacement of pedicle-based dynamic stabilization device (84.82)

84.81 **Revision of interspinous process device(s)**
Repair of previously inserted interspinous process device(s)
EXCLUDES   revision of facet replacement device(s) (84.85)
revision of pedicle-based dynamic stabilization device (84.83)

84.82 **Insertion or replacement of pedicle-based dynamic stabilization device(s)**
EXCLUDES   initial insertion of pedicle screws with spinal fusion — omit code
insertion or replacement of facet replacement device(s) (84.84)
insertion or replacement of interspinous process device(s) (84.80)
replacement of pedicle screws used in spinal fusion (78.59)

84.83 **Revision of pedicle-based dynamic stabilization device(s)**
Repair of previously inserted pedicle-based dynamic stabilization device(s)
EXCLUDES   removal of pedicle screws used in spinal fusion (78.69)
replacement of pedicle screws used in spinal fusion (78.59)
revision of facet replacement device(s) (84.85)
revision of interspinous process device(s) (84.81)

84.84 **Insertion or replacement of facet replacement device(s)**
Facet arthroplasty
EXCLUDES   initial insertion of pedicle screws with spinal fusion — omit code
insertion or replacement of interspinous process device(s) (84.80)
insertion or replacement of pedicle-based dynamic stabilization device(s) (84.82)
replacement of pedicle screws used in spinal fusion (78.59)

84.85 **Revision of facet replacement device(s)**
Repair of previously inserted facet replacement device(s)
EXCLUDES   removal of pedicle screws used in spinal fusion (78.69)
replacement of pedicle screws used in spinal fusion (78.59)
revision of interspinous process device(s) (84.81)
revision of pedicle-based dynamic stabilization device(s) (84.83)

Operations on the Musculoskeletal System

84.69–84.85

√4ᵗʰ **84.9 Other operations on musculoskeletal system**
    EXCLUDES nonoperative manipulation (93.25-93.29)

84.91 Amputation, not otherwise specified

84.92 Separation of equal conjoined twins

84.93 Separation of unequal conjoined twins
    Separation of conjoined twins NOS

84.94 Insertion of sternal fixation device with rigid plates
    EXCLUDES insertion of sternal fixation device for internal fixation of fracture (79.39)
    internal fixation of bone without fracture reduction (78.59)

84.99 Other

15. OPERATIONS ON THE INTEGUMENTARY SYSTEM (85-86)

√3ʳᵈ **85 Operations on the breast**

INCLUDES operations on the skin and subcutaneous tissue of:
breast
previous mastectomy site } female or male
revision of previous mastectomy site

85.0 Mastotomy
Incision of breast (skin)
Mammotomy
EXCLUDES aspiration of breast (85.91)
removal of implant (85.94)

√4ᵗʰ **85.1 Diagnostic procedures on breast**

85.11 Closed [percutaneous] [needle] biopsy of breast
DEF: Mammatome biopsy: Excision of breast tissue using a needle inserted through a small incision, followed by a full cut circle of tissue surrounding the core biopsy to obtain multiple contiguous directional sampling for definitive diagnosis and staging of cancer.

85.12 Open biopsy of breast
DEF: Excision of breast tissue for examination.

85.19 Other diagnostic procedures on breast
EXCLUDES mammary ductogram (87.35)
mammography NEC (87.37)
manual examination (89.36)
microscopic examination of specimen (91.61-91.69)
thermography (88.85)
ultrasonography (88.73)
xerography (87.36)

√4ᵗʰ **85.2 Excision or destruction of breast tissue**
EXCLUDES mastectomy (85.41-85.48)
reduction mammoplasty (85.31-85.32)

85.20 Excision or destruction of breast tissue, not otherwise specified
EXCLUDES laser interstitial thermal therapy [LITT] of lesion or tissue of breast under guidance (17.69)

85.21 Local excision of lesion of breast
Lumpectomy
Removal of area of fibrosis from breast
EXCLUDES biopsy of breast (85.11-85.12)

85.22 Resection of quadrant of breast

85.23 Subtotal mastectomy
EXCLUDES quadrant resection (85.22)
DEF: Excision of a large portion of breast tissue.

85.24 Excision of ectopic breast tissue
Excision of accessory nipple
DEF: Excision of breast tissue outside normal breast region.

85.25 Excision of nipple
EXCLUDES excision of accessory nipple (85.24)

√4ᵗʰ **85.3 Reduction mammoplasty and subcutaneous mammectomy**

85.31 Unilateral reduction mammoplasty
Unilateral:
amputative mammoplasty
size reduction mammoplasty

85.32 Bilateral reduction mammoplasty
Amputative mammoplasty
Biesenberger operation
Reduction mammoplasty (for gynecomastia)

85.33 Unilateral subcutaneous mammectomy with synchronous implant
EXCLUDES that without synchronous implant (85.34)
DEF: Removal of mammary tissue, leaving skin and nipple intact with implant of prosthesis.

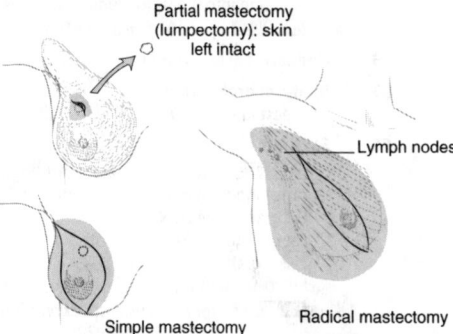

Mastectomy

Partial mastectomy (lumpectomy): skin left intact

Lymph nodes

Simple mastectomy

Radical mastectomy

85.34 Other unilateral subcutaneous mammectomy
Removal of breast tissue with preservation of skin and nipple
Subcutaneous mammectomy NOS
DEF: Excision of mammary tissue, leaving skin and nipple intact.

85.35 Bilateral subcutaneous mammectomy with synchronous implant
EXCLUDES that without synchronous implant (85.36)
DEF: Excision of mammary tissue, both breasts, leaving skin and nipples intact; with prostheses.

85.36 Other bilateral subcutaneous mammectomy

√4ᵗʰ **85.4 Mastectomy**

85.41 Unilateral simple mastectomy
Mastectomy:
NOS
complete
DEF: Removal of one breast.

85.42 Bilateral simple mastectomy
Bilateral complete mastectomy
DEF: Removal of both breasts.

85.43 Unilateral extended simple mastectomy
Extended simple mastectomy NOS
Modified radical mastectomy
Simple mastectomy with excision of regional lymph nodes
DEF: Removal of one breast and lymph nodes under arm.

85.44 Bilateral extended simple mastectomy

85.45 Unilateral radical mastectomy
Excision of breast, pectoral muscles, and regional lymph nodes [axillary, clavicular, supraclavicular]
Radical mastectomy NOS
DEF: Removal of one breast and regional lymph nodes, pectoral muscle and adjacent tissue.

85.46 Bilateral radical mastectomy

85.47 Unilateral extended radical mastectomy
Excision of breast, muscles, and lymph nodes [axillary, clavicular, supraclavicular, internal mammary, and mediastinal]
Extended radical mastectomy NOS
DEF: Removal of one breast, regional and middle chest lymph nodes, chest muscle and adjacent tissue.

85.48 Bilateral extended radical mastectomy
DEF: Removal of both breasts, regional and middle chest lymph nodes, chest muscle and adjacent tissue.

√4ᵗʰ **85.5 Augmentation mammoplasty**
EXCLUDES that associated with subcutaneous mammectomy (85.33, 85.35)
DEF: Plastic surgery to increase breast size.

85.50 Augmentation mammoplasty, not otherwise specified

85.51 Unilateral injection into breast for augmentation
EXCLUDES injection of fat graft of breast (85.55)

85.52   **Bilateral injection into breast for augmentation**
Injection into breast for augmentation NOS
EXCLUDES   *injection of fat graft of breast (85.55)*

85.53   **Unilateral breast implant**

85.54   **Bilateral breast implant**
Breast implant NOS

85.55   **Fat graft to breast**
INCLUDES   extraction of fat for autologous graft
Autologous fat transplantation or transfer
Fat graft to breast NOS
Fat graft to breast with or without use of enriched graft
Micro-fat grafting
EXCLUDES   *that with reconstruction of breast (85.70-85.79)*

85.6   **Mastopexy**
DEF: Anchoring of pendulous breast.

√4ᵗʰ **85.7**   **Total reconstruction of breast**

85.70   **Total reconstruction of breast, not otherwise specified**
Perforator flap, free

85.71   **Latissimus dorsi myocutaneous flap**

85.72   **Transverse rectus abdominis myocutaneous [TRAM] flap, pedicled**
EXCLUDES   *transverse rectus abdominis myocutaneous (TRAM) flap, free (85.73)*

85.73   **Transverse rectus abdominis myocutaneous [TRAM] flap, free**
EXCLUDES   *transverse rectus abdominis myocutaneous (TRAM) flap, pedicled (85.72)*

85.74   **Deep inferior epigastric artery perforator [DIEP] flap, free**

85.75   **Superficial inferior epigastric artery [SIEA] flap, free**

85.76   **Gluteal artery perforator [GAP] flap, free**

85.79   **Other total reconstruction of breast**
EXCLUDES   *deep inferior epigastric artery perforator [DIEP] flap, free (85.74)*
gluteal artery perforator [GAP] flap, free (85.76)
latissimus dorsi myocutaneous flap (85.71)
perforator flap, free (85.70)
superficial inferior epigastric artery [SIEA] flap, free (85.75)
total reconstruction of breast, not otherwise specified (85.70)
transverse rectus abdominis myocutaneous [TRAM] flap, free (85.73)
transverse rectus abdominis myocutaneous [TRAM] flap, pedicled (85.72)

√4ᵗʰ **85.8**   **Other repair and plastic operations on breast**
EXCLUDES   *that for:*
augmentation (85.50-85.54)
reconstruction (85.70-85.76, 85.79)
reduction (85.31-85.32)

85.81   **Suture of laceration of breast**

85.82   **Split-thickness graft to breast**

85.83   **Full-thickness graft to breast**

85.84   **Pedicle graft to breast**
DEF: Implantation of transferred muscle tissue still connected to vascular source.

85.85   **Muscle flap graft to breast**
DEF: Relocation of nipple.

85.86   **Transposition of nipple**
DEF: Relocation of nipple.

85.87   **Other repair or reconstruction of nipple**

85.89   **Other mammoplasty**

√4ᵗʰ **85.9**   **Other operations on the breast**

85.91   **Aspiration of breast**
EXCLUDES   *percutaneous biopsy of breast (85.11)*

85.92   **Injection of therapeutic agent into breast**
EXCLUDES   *that for augmentation of breast (85.51-85.52, 85.55)*

85.93   **Revision of implant of breast**

85.94   **Removal of implant of breast**

85.95   **Insertion of breast tissue expander**
Insertion (soft tissue) of tissue expander (one or more) under muscle or platysma to develop skin flaps for donor use

85.96   **Removal of breast tissue expander(s)**

85.99   **Other**

√3ʳᵈ **86**   **Operations on skin and subcutaneous tissue**
INCLUDES   operations on:
hair follicles
male perineum
nails
sebaceous glands
subcutaneous fat pads
sudoriferous glands
superficial fossae
EXCLUDES   *those on skin of:*
anus (49.01-49.99)
breast (mastectomy site) (85.0-85.99)
ear (18.01-18.9)
eyebrow (08.01-08.99)
eyelid (08.01-08.99)
female perineum (71.01-71.9)
lips (27.0-27.99)
nose (21.00-21.99)
penis (64.0-64.99)
scrotum (61.0-61.99)
vulva (71.01-71.9)

√4ᵗʰ **86.0**   **Incision of skin and subcutaneous tissue**

86.01   **Aspiration of skin and subcutaneous tissue**
Aspiration of:
abscess
hematoma } of nail, skin, or subcutaneous tissue
seroma

86.02   **Injection or tattooing of skin lesion or defect**
Insertion
Injection } of filling material
Pigmenting of skin
DEF: Pigmenting of skin: Adding color to skin.

86.03   **Incision of pilonidal sinus or cyst**
EXCLUDES   *marsupialization (86.21)*

86.04   **Other incision with drainage of skin and subcutaneous tissue**
EXCLUDES   *drainage of:*
fascial compartments of face and mouth (27.0)
palmar or thenar space (82.04)
pilonidal sinus or cyst (86.03)

86.05   **Incision with removal of foreign body or device from skin and subcutaneous tissue**
Removal of carotid sinus baroreflex activation device
Removal of loop recorder
Removal of neurostimulator pulse generator (single array, dual array)
Removal of tissue expander(s) from skin or soft tissue other than breast tissue
EXCLUDES   *removal of foreign body without incision (98.20-98.29)*

86.06 Insertion of totally implantable infusion pump
Code also any associated catheterization
> *EXCLUDES* *insertion of totally implantable vascular access device (86.07)*

86.07 Insertion of totally implantable vascular access device [VAD]
Totally implanted port
> *EXCLUDES* *insertion of totally implantable infusion pump (86.06)*

DEF: Placement of vascular access infusion catheter system under skin to allow for frequent manual infusions into blood vessel.

86.09 Other incision of skin and subcutaneous tissue
Creation of thalamic stimulator pulse generator pocket, new site
Escharotomy
Exploration:
  sinus tract, skin
  superficial fossa
Relocation of subcutaneous device pocket NEC
Reopening subcutaneous pocket for device revision without replacement
Undercutting of hair follicle
> *EXCLUDES* *creation of loop recorder pocket, new site and insertion/relocation of device (37.79)*
> *creation of pocket for implantable, patient-activated cardiac event recorder and insertion/relocation of device (37.79)*
> *removal of catheter from cranial cavity (01.27)*
> *that for drainage (86.04)*
> *that of:*
>   *cardiac pacemaker pocket, new site (37.79)*
>   *fascial compartments of face and mouth (27.0)*

☑4ᵗʰ **86.1 Diagnostic procedures on skin and subcutaneous tissue**

86.11 Closed biopsy of skin and subcutaneous tissue

86.19 Other diagnostic procedures on skin and subcutaneous tissue
> *EXCLUDES* *microscopic examination of specimen from skin and subcutaneous tissue (91.61-91.79)*

☑4ᵗʰ **86.2 Excision or destruction of lesion or tissue of skin and subcutaneous tissue**

86.21 Excision of pilonidal cyst or sinus
Marsupialization of cyst
> *EXCLUDES* *incision of pilonidal cyst or sinus (86.03)*
DEF: Marsupialization of cyst: Incision of cyst and suturing edges to skin to open site.

86.22 Excisional debridement of wound, infection, or burn
Removal by excision of:
  devitalized tissue
  necrosis
  slough
> *EXCLUDES* *debridement of:*
>   *abdominal wall (wound) (54.3)*
>   *bone (77.60-77.69)*
>   *muscle (83.45)*
>   *of hand (82.36)*
>   *nail (bed) (fold) (86.27)*
>   *nonexcisional debridement of wound, infection, or burn (86.28)*
>   *open fracture site (79.60-79.69)*
>   *pedicle or flap graft (86.75)*

86.23 Removal of nail, nail bed, or nail fold

86.24 Chemosurgery of skin
Chemical peel of skin
DEF: Chemicals applied to destroy skin tissue.
DEF: Chemical peel of skin: Chemicals used to peel skin layers.

86.25 Dermabrasion
That with laser
> *EXCLUDES* *dermabrasion of wound to remove embedded debris (86.28)*
DEF: Removal of wrinkled or scarred skin with fine sandpaper, wire, brushes or laser.

86.26 Ligation of dermal appendage
> *EXCLUDES* *excision of preauricular appendage (18.29)*
DEF: Tying off extra skin.

86.27 Debridement of nail, nail bed, or nail fold
Removal of:
  necrosis
  slough
> *EXCLUDES* *removal of nail, nail bed, or nail fold (86.23)*

86.28 Nonexcisional debridement of wound, infection, or burn
Debridement NOS
Maggot therapy
Removal of devitalized tissue, necrosis, and slough by such methods as:
  brushing
  irrigation (under pressure)
  scrubbing
  washing
Ultrasonic debridement
Water scalpel (jet)
DEF: Removal of damaged skin by methods other than excision.

86.3 Other local excision or destruction of lesion or tissue of skin and subcutaneous tissue
Destruction of skin by:
  cauterization
  cryosurgery
  fulguration
  laser beam
That with Z-plasty
> *EXCLUDES* *adipectomy (86.83)*
> *biopsy of skin (86.11)*
> *wide or radical excision of skin (86.4)*
> *Z-plasty without excision (86.84)*

86.4 Radical excision of skin lesion
Wide excision of skin lesion involving underlying or adjacent structure
Code also any lymph node dissection (40.3-40.5)

☑4ᵗʰ **86.5 Suture or other closure of skin and subcutaneous tissue**

86.51 Replantation of scalp

86.59 Closure of skin and subcutaneous tissue of other sites
Adhesives (surgical)(tissue)
Staples
Sutures
> *EXCLUDES* *application of adhesive strips (butterfly) — omit code*

☑4ᵗʰ **86.6 Free skin graft**
> *INCLUDES* *excision of skin for autogenous graft*
> *EXCLUDES* *construction or reconstruction of:*
>   *penis (64.43-64.44)*
>   *trachea (31.75)*
>   *vagina (70.61-70.64)*
DEF: Transplantation of skin to another site.

86.60 Free skin graft, not otherwise specified

86.61 Full-thickness skin graft to hand
> *EXCLUDES* *heterograft (86.65)*
> *homograft (86.66)*

86.62 Other skin graft to hand
> *EXCLUDES* *heterograft (86.65)*
> *homograft (86.66)*

86.63 Full-thickness skin graft to other sites
> *EXCLUDES* *heterograft (86.65)*
> *homograft (86.66)*

86.64 Hair transplant
> *EXCLUDES* hair follicle transplant to eyebrow or
> eyelash (08.63)

86.65 Heterograft to skin
Pigskin graft
Porcine graft
> *EXCLUDES* application of dressing only (93.57)

DEF: Implantation of nonhuman tissue.

86.66 Homograft to skin
Graft to skin of:
amnionic membrane } from donor
skin }

DEF: Implantation of tissue from human donor.

86.67 Dermal regenerative graft
Artificial skin, NOS
Creation of "neodermis"
Decellularized allodermis
Integumentary matrix implants
Prosthetic implant of dermal layer of skin
Regenerate dermal layer of skin
> *EXCLUDES* heterograft to skin (86.65)
> homograft to skin (86.66)

DEF: Replacement of dermis and epidermal layer of
skin by cultured or regenerated autologous tissue;
used to treat full-thickness or deep partial-thickness
burns; also called cultured epidermal autograft (CEA).

86.69 Other skin graft to other sites
> *EXCLUDES* heterograft (86.65)
> homograft (86.66)

√4ᵗʰ 86.7 Pedicle grafts or flaps
> *EXCLUDES* construction or reconstruction of:
> penis (64.43-64.44)
> trachea (31.75)
> vagina (70.61-70.64)

DEF: Full thickness skin and subcutaneous tissue partially
attached to the body by a narrow strip of tissue so that it
retains its blood supply. The unattached portion is sutured to
the defect.

86.70 Pedicle or flap graft, not otherwise specified

86.71 Cutting and preparation of pedicle grafts or flaps
Elevation of pedicle from its bed
Flap design and raising
Partial cutting of pedicle or tube
Pedicle delay
> *EXCLUDES* pollicization or digital transfer
> (82.61,82.81)
> revision of pedicle (86.75)

DEF: Elevation of pedicle from its bed: Separation of
tissue implanted from its bed.
DEF: Flap design and raising: Planing and elevation of
tissue to be implanted.
DEF: Pedicle delay: Elevation and preparation of
tissue still attached to vascular bed; delayed implant.

86.72 Advancement of pedicle graft

86.73 Attachment of pedicle or flap graft to hand
> *EXCLUDES* pollicization or digital transfer (82.61,
> 82.81)

86.74 Attachment of pedicle or flap graft to other sites
Attachment by:
advanced flap
double pedicled flap
pedicle graft
rotating flap
sliding flap
tube graft

DEF: Advanced flap: Sliding tissue implant into new
position.
DEF: Double pedicle flap: Implant connected to two
vascular beds.
DEF: Pedicle graft: Implant connected to vascular
bed.
DEF: Rotating flap: Implant rotated along curved
incision.
DEF: Sliding flap: Sliding implant to site.
DEF: Tube graft: Double tissue implant to form tube
with base connected to original site.

86.75 Revision of pedicle or flap graft
Debridement } of pedicle or flap graft
Defatting }

DEF: Connection of implant still attached to its
vascular tissue.

**√4ᵗʰ 86.8 Other repair and reconstruction of skin and subcutaneous
tissue**

86.81 Repair for facial weakness

86.82 Facial rhytidectomy
Face lift
> *EXCLUDES* rhytidectomy of eyelid (08.86-08.87)

DEF: Revision and tightening of excess, wrinkled
facial skin.

86.83 Size reduction plastic operation
Liposuction
Reduction of adipose tissue of:
abdominal wall (pendulous)
arms (batwing)
buttock
thighs (trochanteric lipomatosis)
> *EXCLUDES* breast (85.31-85.32)
> liposuction to harvest fat graft (86.90)

DEF: Excision and plastic repair of excess skin and
underlying tissue.

86.84 Relaxation of scar or web contracture of skin
Z-plasty of skin
> *EXCLUDES* Z-plasty with excision of lesion (86.3)

86.85 Correction of syndactyly
DEF: Plastic repair of webbed fingers or toes.

86.86 Onychoplasty
DEF: Plastic repair of nail or nail bed.

86.87 Fat graft of skin and subcutaneous tissue
> **INCLUDES** extraction of fat for autologous graft
Autologous fat transplantation or transfer
Fat graft NOS
Fat graft of skin and subcutaneous tissue with or
without use of enriched graft
Micro-fat grafting
> *EXCLUDES* fat graft to breast (85.55)

**86.89 Other repair and reconstruction of skin and
subcutaneous tissue**
> *EXCLUDES* mentoplasty (76.67-76.68)

√4ᵗʰ 86.9 Other operations on skin and subcutaneous tissue

86.90 Extraction of fat for graft or banking
Harvest of fat for extraction of cells for future use
Liposuction to harvest fat graft
> *EXCLUDES* that with graft at same operative episode
> (85.55, 86.87)

86.91 Excision of skin for graft
Excision of skin with closure of donor site
> *EXCLUDES* that with graft at same operative episode
> (86.60-86.69)

86.92   **Electrolysis and other epilation of skin**
>> **EXCLUDES**   *epilation of eyelid (08.91-08.93)*

86.93   **Insertion of tissue expander**
>> Insertion (subcutaneous) (soft tissue) of expander (one or more) in scalp (subgaleal space), face, neck, trunk except breast, and upper and lower extremities for development of skin flaps for donor use
>>
>> **EXCLUDES**   *flap graft preparation (86.71)*
>>   *tissue expander, breast (85.95)*

86.94   **Insertion or replacement of single array neurostimulator pulse generator, not specified as rechargeable**
>> Pulse generator (single array, single channel, single port) for intracranial, spinal, and peripheral neurostimulator
>>
>> Code also any associated lead implantation (02.93, 03.93, 04.92)
>>
>> **EXCLUDES**   *cranial implantation or replacement of neurostimulator pulse generator (01.20)*
>>   *insertion or replacement of single array rechargeable neurostimulator pulse generator (86.97)*

86.95   **Insertion or replacement of multiple array neurostimulator pulse generator, not specified as rechargeable**
>> Pulse generator (multiple array, multiple channel, multiple port) for intracranial, spinal, and peripheral neurostimulator
>>
>> Code also any associated lead implantation (02.93, 03.93, 04.92)
>>
>> **EXCLUDES**   *cranial implantation or replacement of neurostimulator pulse generator (01.20)*
>>   *insertion or replacement of (multiple array) rechargeable neurostimulator pulse generator (86.98)*

86.96   **Insertion or replacement of other neurostimulator pulse generator**
>> Code also any associated lead implantation (02.93, 03.93, 04.92)
>>
>> **EXCLUDES**   *cranial implantation or replacement of neurostimulator pulse generator (01.20)*
>>   *insertion of multiple array neurostimulator pulse generator (86.95, 86.98)*
>>   *insertion of single array neurostimulator pulse generator (86.94, 86.97)*

86.97   **Insertion or replacement of single array rechargeable neurostimulator pulse generator**
>> Rechargeable pulse generator (single array, single channel, single port) for intracranial, spinal, and peripheral neurostimulator
>>
>> Code also any associated lead implantation (02.93, 03.93, 04.92)
>>
>> **EXCLUDES**   *cranial implantation or replacement of neurostimulator pulse generator (01.20)*

86.98   **Insertion or replacement of multiple array (two or more) rechargeable neurostimulator pulse generator**
>> Rechargeable pulse generator (multiple array, multiple channel, multiple port) for intracranial, spinal, and peripheral neurostimulator
>>
>> Code also any associated lead implantation (02.93, 03.93, 04.92)
>>
>> **EXCLUDES**   *cranial implantation or replacement of neurostimulator pulse generator (01.20)*

86.99   **Other**
>> **EXCLUDES**   *removal of sutures from:*
>>   *abdomen (97.83)*
>>   *head and neck (97.38)*
>>   *thorax (97.43)*
>>   *trunk NEC (97.84)*
>>   *wound catheter:*
>>   *irrigation (96.58)*
>>   *replacement (97.15)*

16. MISCELLANEOUS DIAGNOSTIC AND THERAPEUTIC PROCEDURES (87-99)

√3ʳᵈ **87 Diagnostic radiology**

√4ᵗʰ **87.0 Soft tissue x-ray of face, head, and neck**
>   EXCLUDES   *angiography (88.40-88.68)*

87.01 Pneumoencephalogram
>   DEF: Radiographic exam of cerebral ventricles and subarachnoid spaces with injection of air or gas for contrast.

87.02 Other contrast radiogram of brain and skull
> Pneumocisternogram
> Pneumoventriculogram
> Posterior fossa myelogram
>   DEF: Pneumocisternogram: radiographic exam of subarachnoid spaces after injection of gas or contrast.
>   DEF: Pneumoventriculography: radiographic exam of cerebral ventricles after injection of gas or contrast.
>   DEF: Posterior fossa myelogram: radiographic exam of posterior channel of spinal cord after injection of gas or contrast.

87.03 Computerized axial tomography of head
> C.A.T. scan of head

87.04 Other tomography of head

87.05 Contrast dacryocystogram
>   DEF: Radiographic exam of tear sac after injection of contrast.

87.06 Contrast radiogram of nasopharynx

87.07 Contrast laryngogram

87.08 Cervical lymphangiogram
>   DEF: Radiographic exam of lymph vessels of neck, with or without contrast.

87.09 Other soft tissue x-ray of face, head, and neck
> Noncontrast x-ray of:
>   adenoid
>   larynx
>   nasolacrimal duct
>   nasopharynx
>   salivary gland
>   thyroid region
>   uvula
>   EXCLUDES   *x-ray study of eye (95.14)*

√4ᵗʰ **87.1 Other x-ray of face, head, and neck**
>   EXCLUDES   *angiography (88.40-88.68)*

87.11 Full-mouth x-ray of teeth

87.12 Other dental x-ray
> Orthodontic cephalogram or cephalometrics
> Panorex examination of mandible
> Root canal x-ray

87.13 Temporomandibular contrast arthrogram

87.14 Contrast radiogram of orbit

87.15 Contrast radiogram of sinus

87.16 Other x-ray of facial bones
> X-ray of:
>   frontal area
>   mandible
>   maxilla
>   nasal sinuses
>   nose
>   orbit
>   supraorbital area
>   symphysis menti
>   zygomaticomaxillary complex

87.17 Other x-ray of skull
> Lateral projection ⎫
> Sagittal projection ⎬ of skull
> Tangential projection ⎭
>   DEF: Lateral projection: Side to side view of head.
>   DEF: Sagittal projection: View of body in plane running midline from front to back.
>   DEF: Tangential projection: Views from adjacent skull surfaces.

√4ᵗʰ **87.2 X-ray of spine**

87.21 Contrast myelogram
>   DEF: Radiographic exam of space between middle and outer spinal cord coverings after injection of contrast.

87.22 Other x-ray of cervical spine

87.23 Other x-ray of thoracic spine

87.24 Other x-ray of lumbosacral spine
> Sacrococcygeal x-ray

87.29 Other x-ray of spine
> Spinal x-ray NOS

√4ᵗʰ **87.3 Soft tissue x-ray of thorax**
>   EXCLUDES   *angiocardiography (88.50-88.58)*
>   *angiography (88.40-88.68)*

87.31 Endotracheal bronchogram
>   DEF: Radiographic exam of main branch of lung, with contrast introduced through windpipe.

87.32 Other contrast bronchogram
> Transcricoid bronchogram
>   DEF: Transcricoid bronchogram: Radiographic exam of main branch of lung, with contrast introduced through cartilage of neck.

87.33 Mediastinal pneumogram
>   DEF: Radiographic exam of cavity containing heart, esophagus and adjacent structures.

87.34 Intrathoracic lymphangiogram
>   DEF: Radiographic exam of lymphatic vessels within chest; with or without contrast.

87.35 Contrast radiogram of mammary ducts
>   DEF: Radiographic exam of mammary ducts; with contrast.

87.36 Xerography of breast
>   DEF: Radiographic exam of breast via selenium-coated plates.

87.37 Other mammography

87.38 Sinogram of chest wall
> Fistulogram of chest wall
>   DEF: Fistulogram of chest wall: Radiographic exam of abnormal opening in chest.

87.39 Other soft tissue x-ray of chest wall

√4ᵗʰ **87.4 Other x-ray of thorax**
>   EXCLUDES   *angiocardiography (88.50-88.58)*
>   *angiography (88.40-88.68)*

87.41 Computerized axial tomography of thorax
> C.A.T. scan of heart
> C.A.T. scan ⎫
> Crystal linea scan of x-ray beam ⎪
> Electronic subtraction ⎬ of thorax
> Photoelectric response ⎪
> Tomography with use of computer, ⎭
>   x-rays, and camera

87.42 Other tomography of thorax
> Cardiac tomogram
>   EXCLUDES   *C.A.T. scan of heart (87.41)*
>   DEF: Radiographic exam of chest plane.

87.43 X-ray of ribs, sternum, and clavicle
> Examination for:
>   cervical rib
>   fracture

87.44 Routine chest x-ray, so described
> X-ray of chest NOS

87.49   **Other chest x-ray**

X-ray of: X-ray of:
   bronchus NOS   lung NOS
   diaphragm NOS   mediastinum NOS
   heart NOS   trachea NOS

✓4ᵗʰ **87.5**   **Biliary tract x-ray**

87.51   **Percutaneous hepatic cholangiogram**
DEF: Radiographic exam of bile tract of gallbladder; with needle injection of contrast into bile duct of liver.

87.52   **Intravenous cholangiogram**
DEF: Radiographic exam of bile ducts; with intravenous contrast injection.

87.53   **Intraoperative cholangiogram**
DEF: Radiographic exam of bile ducts with contrast, following gallbladder removal.

87.54   **Other cholangiogram**

87.59   **Other biliary tract x-ray**
Cholecystogram

✓4ᵗʰ **87.6**   **Other x-ray of digestive system**

87.61   **Barium swallow**

87.62   **Upper GI series**

87.63   **Small bowel series**

87.64   **Lower GI series**

87.65   **Other x-ray of intestine**

87.66   **Contrast pancreatogram**

87.69   **Other digestive tract x-ray**

✓4ᵗʰ **87.7**   **X-ray of urinary system**
EXCLUDES   *angiography of renal vessels (88.45, 88.65)*

87.71   **Computerized axial tomography of kidney**
C.A.T. scan of kidney

87.72   **Other nephrotomogram**
DEF: Radiographic exam of kidney plane.

87.73   **Intravenous pyelogram**
Diuretic infusion pyelogram
DEF: Radiographic exam of lower kidney, with intravenous contrast injection.
DEF: Diuretic infusion pyelogram: Radiographic exam of lower kidney with diuretic contrast.

87.74   **Retrograde pyelogram**

87.75   **Percutaneous pyelogram**

87.76   **Retrograde cystourethrogram**
DEF: Radiographic exam of bladder and urethra with contrast injected through catheter into bladder.

87.77   **Other cystogram**

87.78   **Ileal conduitogram**
DEF: Radiographic exam of passage created between ureter and artificial opening into abdomen.

87.79   **Other x-ray of the urinary system**
KUB x-ray

✓4ᵗʰ **87.8**   **X-ray of female genital organs**

87.81   **X-ray of gravid uterus**
Intrauterine cephalometry by x-ray

87.82   **Gas contrast hysterosalpingogram**
DEF: Radiographic exam of uterus and fallopian tubes with gas contrast.

87.83   **Opaque dye contrast hysterosalpingogram**

87.84   **Percutaneous hysterogram**
DEF: Radiographic exam of uterus with contrast injected through body wall.

87.85   **Other x-ray of fallopian tubes and uterus**

87.89   **Other x-ray of female genital organs**

✓4ᵗʰ **87.9**   **X-ray of male genital organs**

87.91   **Contrast seminal vesiculogram**

87.92   **Other x-ray of prostate and seminal vesicles**

87.93   **Contrast epididymogram**

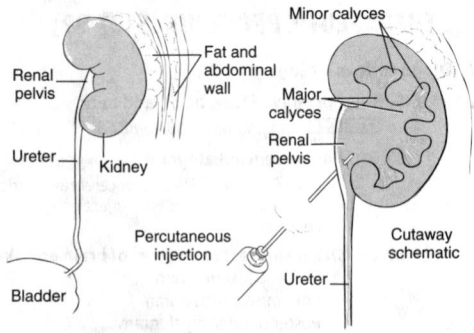

Ureteropyelography

87.94   **Contrast vasogram**

87.95   **Other x-ray of epididymis and vas deferens**

87.99   **Other x-ray of male genital organs**

✓3ʳᵈ **88**   **Other diagnostic radiology and related techniques**

✓4ᵗʰ **88.0**   **Soft tissue x-ray of abdomen**
EXCLUDES   *angiography (88.40-88.68)*

88.01   **Computerized axial tomography of abdomen**
C.A.T. scan of abdomen
EXCLUDES   *C.A.T. scan of kidney (87.71)*

88.02   **Other abdomen tomography**
EXCLUDES   *nephrotomogram (87.72)*

88.03   **Sinogram of abdominal wall**
Fistulogram of abdominal wall
DEF: Radiographic exam of abnormal abdominal passage.

88.04   **Abdominal lymphangiogram**
DEF: Radiographic exam of abdominal lymphatic vessels with contrast.

88.09   **Other soft tissue x-ray of abdominal wall**

✓4ᵗʰ **88.1**   **Other x-ray of abdomen**

88.11   **Pelvic opaque dye contrast radiography**

88.12   **Pelvic gas contrast radiography**
Pelvic pneumoperitoneum

88.13   **Other peritoneal pneumogram**

88.14   **Retroperitoneal fistulogram**

88.15   **Retroperitoneal pneumogram**

88.16   **Other retroperitoneal x-ray**

88.19   **Other x-ray of abdomen**
Flat plate of abdomen

✓4ᵗʰ **88.2**   **Skeletal x-ray of extremities and pelvis**
EXCLUDES   *contrast radiogram of joint (88.32)*

88.21   **Skeletal x-ray of shoulder and upper arm**

88.22   **Skeletal x-ray of elbow and forearm**

88.23   **Skeletal x-ray of wrist and hand**

88.24   **Skeletal x-ray of upper limb, not otherwise specified**

88.25   **Pelvimetry**
DEF: Imaging of pelvic bones to measure pelvic capacity.

88.26   **Other skeletal x-ray of pelvis and hip**

88.27   **Skeletal x-ray of thigh, knee, and lower leg**

88.28   **Skeletal x-ray of ankle and foot**

88.29   **Skeletal x-ray of lower limb, not otherwise specified**

✓4ᵗʰ **88.3**   **Other x-ray**

88.31   **Skeletal series**
X-ray of whole skeleton

88.32   **Contrast arthrogram**
EXCLUDES   *that of temporomandibular joint (87.13)*

88.33　Other skeletal x-ray
　　EXCLUDES　*skeletal x-ray of:*
　　　　　extremities and pelvis (88.21-88.29)
　　　　　face, head, and neck (87.11-87.17)
　　　　　spine (87.21-87.29)
　　　　　thorax (87.43)

88.34　Lymphangiogram of upper limb

88.35　Other soft tissue x-ray of upper limb

88.36　Lymphangiogram of lower limb

88.37　Other soft tissue x-ray of lower limb
　　EXCLUDES　*femoral angiography (88.48, 88.66)*

88.38　Other computerized axial tomography
　　C.A.T. scan NOS
　　EXCLUDES　*C.A.T. scan of:*
　　　　　abdomen (88.01)
　　　　　head (87.03)
　　　　　heart (87.41)
　　　　　kidney (87.71)
　　　　　thorax (87.41)

88.39　X-ray, other and unspecified

√4ᵗʰ **88.4　Arteriography using contrast material**
　　Note: The fourth-digit subclassification identifies the site to
　　　　be viewed, not the site of injection.
　　INCLUDES　angiography of arteries
　　　　　arterial puncture for injection of contrast
　　　　　　material
　　　　　radiography of arteries (by fluoroscopy)
　　　　　retrograde arteriography
　　EXCLUDES　*arteriography using:*
　　　　　radioisotopes or radionuclides (92.01-92.19)
　　　　　ultrasound (88.71-88.79)
　　　　　fluorescein angiography of eye (95.12)

　　DEF: Electromagnetic wave photography of arteries with
　　contrast.

**88.40　Arteriography using contrast material, unspecified
　　site**

88.41　Arteriography of cerebral arteries
　　Angiography of:
　　　basilar artery
　　　carotid (internal)
　　　posterior cerebral circulation
　　　vertebral artery

88.42　Aortography
　　Arteriography of aorta and aortic arch

88.43　Arteriography of pulmonary arteries

88.44　Arteriography of other intrathoracic vessels
　　EXCLUDES　*angiocardiography (88.50-88.58)*
　　　　　arteriography of coronary arteries
　　　　　　(88.55-88.57)

88.45　Arteriography of renal arteries

88.46　Arteriography of placenta
　　Placentogram using contrast material

88.47　Arteriography of other intra-abdominal arteries

**88.48　Arteriography of femoral and other lower
　　extremity arteries**

88.49　Arteriography of other specified sites

√4ᵗʰ **88.5　Angiocardiography using contrast material**
　　INCLUDES　arterial puncture and insertion of arterial
　　　　　　catheter for injection of contrast material
　　　　　cineangiocardiography
　　　　　selective angiocardiography
　　Code also synchronous cardiac catheterization
　　　　(37.21-37.23)
　　EXCLUDES　*angiography of pulmonary vessels (88.43, 88.62)*
　　DEF: Electromagnetic wave photography of heart and great
　　vessels with contrast.

88.50　Angiocardiography, not otherwise specified

88.51　Angiocardiography of venae cavae
　　Inferior vena cavography
　　Phlebography of vena cava (inferior) (superior)

88.52　Angiocardiography of right heart structures
　　Angiocardiography of:
　　　pulmonary valve
　　　right atrium
　　　right ventricle (outflow tract)
　　EXCLUDES　*intra-operative fluorescence vascular*
　　　　　angiography (88.59)
　　　　　that combined with left heart
　　　　　angiocardiography (88.54)

88.53　Angiocardiography of left heart structures
　　Angiocardiography of:
　　　aortic valve
　　　left atrium
　　　left ventricle (outflow tract)
　　EXCLUDES　*intra-operative fluorescence vascular*
　　　　　angiography (88.59)
　　　　　that combined with right heart
　　　　　angiocardiography (88.54)

88.54　Combined right and left heart angiocardiography
　　EXCLUDES　*intra-operative fluorescence vascular*
　　　　　angiography (88.59)

88.55　Coronary arteriography using a single catheter
　　Coronary arteriography by Sones technique
　　Direct selective coronary arteriography using a
　　　single catheter
　　EXCLUDES　*intra-operative fluorescence vascular*
　　　　　angiography (88.59)

88.56　Coronary arteriography using two catheters
　　Coronary arteriography by:
　　　Judkins technique
　　　Ricketts and Abrams technique
　　Direct selective coronary arteriography using two
　　　catheters
　　EXCLUDES　*intra-operative fluorescence vascular*
　　　　　angiography (88.59)

88.57　Other and unspecified coronary arteriography
　　Coronary arteriography NOS
　　EXCLUDES　*intra-operative fluorescence vascular*
　　　　　angiography (88.59)

88.58　Negative-contrast cardiac roentgenography
　　Cardiac roentgenography with injection of carbon
　　　dioxide

**88.59　Intra-operative coronary fluorescence vascular
　　angiography**
　　Intraoperative laser arteriogram (SPY)
　　SPY arteriogram
　　SPY arteriography

　　DEF: Coronary artery bypass grafting (CABG)
　　procedure imaging technology; utilizes dye with
　　high-speed digital infrared photography. Sequence is
　　performed for each graft; provides information on
　　graft patency, vessel size, blood flow velocities.

√4ᵗʰ **88.6　Phlebography**
　　Note: The fourth-digit subclassification (88.60-88.67)
　　　　identifies the site to be viewed, not the site of
　　　　injection.
　　INCLUDES　angiography of veins
　　　　　radiography of veins (by fluoroscopy)
　　　　　retrograde phlebography
　　　　　venipuncture for injection of contrast material
　　　　　venography using contrast material
　　EXCLUDES　*angiography using:*
　　　　　radioisotopes or radionuclides (92.01-92.19)
　　　　　ultrasound (88.71-88.79)
　　　　　fluorescein angiography of eye (95.12)

　　DEF: Electromagnetic wave photography of veins with
　　contrast.

**88.60　Phlebography using contrast material, unspecified
　　site**

**88.61　Phlebography of veins of head and neck using
　　contrast material**

**88.62　Phlebography of pulmonary veins using contrast
　　material**

88.63   **Phlebography of other intrathoracic veins using contrast material**

88.64   **Phlebography of the portal venous system using contrast material**
Splenoportogram (by splenic arteriography)

88.65   **Phlebography of other intra-abdominal veins using contrast material**

88.66   **Phlebography of femoral and other lower extremity veins using contrast material**

88.67   **Phlebography of other specified sites using contrast material**

88.68   **Impedance phlebography**

√4ᵗʰ **88.7**   **Diagnostic ultrasound**

INCLUDES   echography
for intraoperative monitoring 00.94
non-invasive ultrasound
ultrasonic angiography
ultrasonography

EXCLUDES   *intravascular imaging (adjunctive) (IVUS) (00.21-00.29)*
that for intraoperative monitoring (00.94)
therapeutic ultrasound (00.01-00.09)

DEF: Graphic recording of anatomical structures via high frequency, sound-wave imaging and computer graphics.

88.71   **Diagnostic ultrasound of head and neck**
Determination of midline shift of brain
Echoencephalography
EXCLUDES   *eye (95.13)*

88.72   **Diagnostic ultrasound of heart**
Echocardiography
Transesophageal echocardiography
EXCLUDES   *echocardiography of heart chambers (37.28)*
intracardiac echocardiography (ICE) (37.28)
intravascular (IVUS) imaging of coronary vessels (00.24)

88.73   **Diagnostic ultrasound of other sites of thorax**
Aortic arch
Breast   } ultrasonography
Lung

88.74   **Diagnostic ultrasound of digestive system**

88.75   **Diagnostic ultrasound of urinary system**

88.76   **Diagnostic ultrasound of abdomen and retroperitoneum**

88.77   **Diagnostic ultrasound of peripheral vascular system**
Deep vein thrombosis ultrasonic scanning
EXCLUDES   *adjunct vascular system procedures (00.40-00.43)*

88.78   **Diagnostic ultrasound of gravid uterus**
Intrauterine cephalometry:
echo
ultrasonic
Placental localization by ultrasound

88.79   **Other diagnostic ultrasound**
Ultrasonography of: Ultrasonography of:
multiple sites   total body
nongravid uterus

√4ᵗʰ **88.8**   **Thermography**
DEF: Infrared photography to determine various body temperatures.

88.81   **Cerebral thermography**

88.82   **Ocular thermography**

88.83   **Bone thermography**
Osteoarticular thermography

88.84   **Muscle thermography**

88.85   **Breast thermography**

88.86   **Blood vessel thermography**
Deep vein thermography

88.89   **Thermographay of other sites**
Lymph gland thermography
Thermography NOS

√4ᵗʰ **88.9**   **Other diagnostic imaging**

88.90   **Diagnostic imaging, not elsewhere classified**

88.91   **Magnetic resonance imaging of brain and brain stem**
EXCLUDES   *intraoperative magnetic resonance imaging (88.96)*
laser interstitial thermal therapy [LITT] of lesion or tissue of brain under guidance (17.61)
real-time magnetic resonance imaging (88.96)

88.92   **Magnetic resonance imaging of chest and myocardium**
For evaluation of hilar and mediastinal lymphadenopathy
EXCLUDES   *laser interstitial thermal therapy [LITT] of lesion or tissue of breast under guidance (17.69)*
laser interstitial thermal therapy [LITT] of lesion or tissue of lung under guidance (17.69)

88.93   **Magnetic resonance imaging of spinal canal**
Spinal cord levels: Spinal cord
cervical   Spine
thoracic
lumbar (lumbosacral)

88.94   **Magnetic resonance imaging of musculoskeletal**
Bone marrow blood supply
Extremities (upper) (lower)

88.95   **Magnetic resonance imaging of pelvis, prostate, and bladder**
EXCLUDES   *laser interstitial thermal therapy (LITT) of lesion or tissue of prostate under guidance (17.69)*

88.96   **Other intraoperative magnetic resonance imaging**
iMRI
Real-time magnetic resonance imaging

88.97   **Magnetic resonance imaging of other and unspecified sites**
Abdomen
Eye orbit
Face
Neck
EXCLUDES   *laser interstitial thermal therapy (LITT) of lesion or tissue of other and unspecified site under guidance (17.69)*

88.98   **Bone mineral density studies**
Dual photon absorptiometry
Quantitative computed tomography (CT) studies
Radiographic densitometry
Single photon absorptiometry
DEF: Dual photon absorptiometry: Measurement of bone mineral density by comparing dissipation of emission from two separate photoelectric energy peaks.
DEF: Quantitative computed tomography (CT) studies: Computer assisted analysis of x-ray absorption through bone to determine density.
DEF: Radiographic densiometry: Measurement of bone mineral density by degree of bone radiopacity.
DEF: Single photon absorptiometry: Measurement of bone mineral density by degree of dissipation of emission from one photoelectric energy peak emitted by gadolinium 153.

√3ʳᵈ **89**   **Interview, evaluation, consultation, and examination**

√4ᵗʰ **89.0**   **Diagnostic interview, consultation, and evaluation**
EXCLUDES   *psychiatric diagnostic interview (94.11-94.19)*

89.01   **Interview and evaluation, described as brief**
Abbreviated history and evaluation

89.02 Interview and evaluation, described as limited
Interval history and evaluation

89.03 Interview and evaluation, described as comprehensive
History and evaluation of new problem

89.04 Other interview and evaluation

89.05 Diagnostic interview and evaluation, not otherwise specified

89.06 Consultation, described as limited
Consultation on a single organ system

89.07 Consultation, described as comprehensive

89.08 Other consultation

89.09 Consulation, not otherwise specified

√4th 89.1 Anatomic and physiologic measurements and manual examinations — nervous system and sense organs
EXCLUDES *ear examination (95.41-95.49)*
eye examination (95.01-95.26)
the listed procedures when done as part of a general physical examination (89.7)

89.10 Intracarotid amobarbital test
Wada test
DEF: Amobarbital injections into internal carotid artery to induce hemiparalysis to determine the hemisphere that controls speech and language.

89.11 Tonometry
DEF: Pressure measurements inside eye.

89.12 Nasal function study
Rhinomanometry
DEF: Rhinomanometry: Measure of degree of nasal cavity obstruction.

89.13 Neurologic examination

89.14 Electroencephalogram
EXCLUDES *that with polysomnogram (89.17)*
DEF: Recording of electrical currents in brain via electrodes to detect epilepsy, lesions and other encephalopathies.

89.15 Other nonoperative neurologic function tests

89.16 Transillumination of newborn skull
DEF: Light passed through newborn skull for diagnostic purposes.

89.17 Polysomnogram
Sleep recording
DEF: Graphic studies of sleep patterns.

89.18 Other sleep disorder function tests
Multiple sleep latency test [MSLT]

89.19 Video and radio-telemetered electroencephalographic monitoring
Radiographic
Video } EEG Monitoring
EXCLUDES *intraoperative monitoring (00.94)*

√4th 89.2 Anatomic and physiologic measurements and manual examinations — genitourinary system
EXCLUDES *the listed procedures when done as part of a general physical examination (89.7)*

89.21 Urinary manometry
Manometry through:
indwelling ureteral catheter
nephrostomy
pyelostomy
ureterostomy
DEF: Measurement of urinary pressure by:
Indwelling urinary catheter: Semipermanent urinary catheter.
Nephrostomy: Opening into pelvis of kidney.
Pyelostomy: Opening in lower kidney.
Ureterostomy: Opening into ureter.

89.22 Cystometrogram
DEF: Pressure recordings at various stages of bladder filling.

89.23 Urethral sphincter electromyogram

89.24 Uroflowmetry [UFR]
DEF: Continuous recording of urine flow.

89.25 Urethral pressure profile [UPP]

89.26 Gynecological examination
Pelvic examination

89.29 Other nonoperative genitourinary system measurements
Bioassay of urine   Urine chemistry
Renal clearance

√4th 89.3 Other anatomic and physiologic measurements and manual examinations
EXCLUDES *the listed procedures when done as part of a general physical examination (89.7)*

89.31 Dental examination
Oral mucosal survey
Periodontal survey

89.32 Esophageal manometry
DEF: Measurement of esophageal fluid and gas pressures.

89.33 Digital examination of enterostomy stoma
Digital examination of colostomy stoma

89.34 Digital examination of rectum

89.35 Transillumination of nasal sinuses

89.36 Manual examination of breast

89.37 Vital capacity determination
EXCLUDES *endoscopic pulmonary airway flow measurement (33.72)*
DEF: Measurement of expelled gas volume after full inhalation.

89.38 Other nonoperative respiratory measurements
Plethysmography for measurement of respiratory function
Thoracic impedance plethysmography
EXCLUDES *endoscopic pulmonary airway flow measurement (33.72)*
DEF: Plethysmography for measurement of respiratory function: Registering changes in respiratory function as noted in blood circulation.

89.39 Other nonoperative measurements and examinations
^{14}C-Urea breath test
Basal metabolic rate [BMR]
Gastric:
analysis
function NEC
EXCLUDES *body measurement (93.07)*
cardiac tests (89.41-89.69)
fundus photography (95.11)
limb length measurement (93.06)

√4th 89.4 Cardiac stress tests, pacemaker and defibrillator checks

89.41 Cardiovascular stress test using treadmill

89.42 Masters' two-step stress test

89.43 Cardiovascular stress test using bicycle ergometer
DEF: Electrocardiogram during exercise on bicycle with device capable of measuring muscular, metabolic and respiratory effects of exercise.

89.44 Other cardiovascular stress test
Thallium stress test with or without transesophageal pacing

89.45 Artificial pacemaker rate check
Artificial pacemaker function check NOS
Bedside device check of pacemaker or cardiac resynchronization pacemaker [CRT-P]
Interrogation only without arrhythmia induction
EXCLUDES *catheter based invasive electrophysiologic testing (37.26)*
non-invasive programmed electrical stimulation [NIPS] (arrhythmia induction) (37.20)

89.46 Artificial pacemaker artifact wave form check

89.47 Artificial pacemaker electrode impedance check

Miscellaneous Diagnostic and Therapeutic Procedures

89.48–90.1

89.48 Artificial pacemaker voltage or amperage threshold check

89.49 Automatic implantable cardioverter/ defibrillator (AICD) check
Bedside check of an AICD or cardiac resynchronization defibrillator [CRT-D]
Checking pacing thresholds of device
Interrogation only without arrhythmia induction
EXCLUDES   *catheter based invasive electrophysiologic testing (37.26)*
    non-invasive programmed electrical stimulation [NIPS] (arrhythmia induction) (37.20)

✓4ᵗʰ **89.5 Other nonoperative cardiac and vascular diagnostic procedures**
EXCLUDES   *fetal EKG (75.32)*

89.50 Ambulatory cardiac monitoring
Analog devices [Holter-type]

89.51 Rhythm electrocardiogram
Rhythm EKG (with one to three leads)

89.52 Electrocardiogram
ECG NOS
EKG (with 12 or more leads)

89.53 Vectorcardiogram (with ECG)

89.54 Electrographic monitoring
Telemetry
EXCLUDES   *ambulatory cardiac monitoring (89.50)*
    electrographic monitoring during surgery — omit code
DEF: Evaluation of heart electrical activity by continuous screen monitoring.
DEF: Telemetry: Evaluation of heart electrical activity; with radio signals at distance from patient.

89.55 Phonocardiogram with ECG lead

89.56 Carotid pulse tracing with ECG lead
EXCLUDES   *oculoplethysmography (89.58)*

89.57 Apexcardiogram (with ECG lead)

89.58 Plethysmogram
Penile plethysmography with nerve stimulation
EXCLUDES   *plethysmography (for):*
    measurement of respiratory function (89.38)
    thoracic impedance (89.38)
DEF: Determination and recording of blood pressure variations present or passing through an organ.

89.59 Other nonoperative cardiac and vascular measurements

✓4ᵗʰ **89.6 Circulatory monitoring**
EXCLUDES   *electrocardiographic monitoring during surgery — omit code*
    implantation or replacement of subcutaneous device for intracardiac hemodynamic monitoring (00.57)
    insertion or replacement of implantable pressure sensor (lead) for intracardiac hemodynamic monitoring (00.56)

89.60 Continuous intra-arterial blood gas monitoring
Insertion of blood gas monitoring system and continuous monitoring of blood gases through an intra-arterial sensor

89.61 Systemic arterial pressure monitoring
EXCLUDES   *intra-aneurysm sac pressure monitoring (intraoperative) (00.58)*
    intravascular pressure measurement of intrathoracic arteries (00.67)
    intravascular pressure measurement of peripheral arteries (00.68)

Central Venous Pressure Monitoring

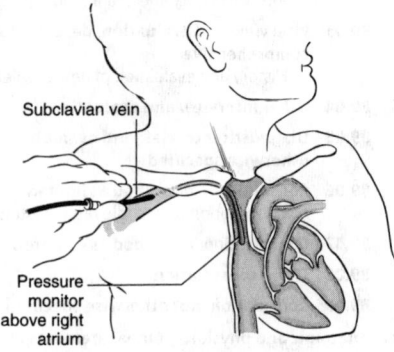

Subclavian vein

Pressure monitor above right atrium

89.62 Central venous pressure monitoring
EXCLUDES   *intravascular pressure measurement, other specified and unspecified vessels (00.69)*

89.63 Pulmonary artery pressure monitoring
EXCLUDES   *pulmonary artery wedge monitoring (89.64)*

89.64 Pulmonary artery wedge monitoring
Pulmonary capillary wedge [PCW] monitoring
Swan-Ganz catheterization
DEF: Monitoring pulmonary artery pressure via catheter inserted through right lower and upper heart chambers into pulmonary artery and advancing the balloon-tip to wedge it in the distal pulmonary artery branch.

89.65 Measurement of systemic arterial blood gases
EXCLUDES   *continuous intra-arterial blood gas monitoring (89.60)*

89.66 Measurement of mixed venous blood gases

89.67 Monitoring of cardiac output by oxygen consumption technique
Fick method
DEF: Fick method: Indirect measure of cardiac output through blood volume flow over pulmonary capillaries; determines oxygen absorption by measurement of arterial oxygen content versus venous oxygen content.

89.68 Monitoring of cardiac output by other technique
Cardiac output monitor by thermodilution indicator
DEF: Cardiac output monitor by thermodilution indicator: Injection of ice cold dextrose solution into right lower heart chamber; temperature sensitive catheter monitors disappearance from beat to beat to measure expelled blood volume.

89.69 Monitoring of coronary blood flow
Coronary blood flow monitoring by coincidence counting technique
EXCLUDES   *intravascular pressure measurement of coronary arteries (00.59)*

89.7 General physical examination

89.8 Autopsy

✓3ʳᵈ **90 Microscopic examination - I**

The following fourth-digit subclassification is for use with categories in section 90 to identify type of examination:
1 **bacterial smear**
2 **culture**
3 **culture and sensitivity**
4 **parasitology**
5 **toxicology**
6 **cell block and Papanicolaou smear**
9 **other microscopic examination**

✓4ᵗʰ **90.0 Microscopic examination of specimen from nervous**
[1-6,9] **system and of spinal fluid**

✓4ᵗʰ **90.1 Microscopic examination of specimen from endocrine**
[1-6,9] **gland, not elsewhere classified**

√4ᵗʰ **90.2 Microscopic examination of specimen from eye**
[1-6,9]

√4ᵗʰ **90.3 Microscopic examination of specimen from ear, nose,**
[1-6,9] **throat, and larynx**

√4ᵗʰ **90.4 Microscopic examination of specimen from trachea,**
[1-6,9] **bronchus, pleura, lung, and other thoracic specimen, and of sputum**

√4ᵗʰ **90.5 Microscopic examination of blood**
[1-6,9]

√4ᵗʰ **90.6 Microscopic examination of specimen from spleen and of**
[1-6,9] **bone marrow**

√4ᵗʰ **90.7 Microscopic examination of specimen from lymph node**
[1-6,9] **and of lymph**

√4ᵗʰ **90.8 Microscopic examination of specimen from upper**
[1-6,9] **gastrointestinal tract and of vomitus**

√4ᵗʰ **90.9 Microscopic examination of specimen from lower**
[1-6,9] **gastrointestinal tract and of stool**

√3ʳᵈ **91 Microscopic examination - II**

The following fourth-digit subclassification is for use with categories in section 91 to identify type of examination:
1 **bacterial smear**
2 **culture**
3 **culture and sensitivity**
4 **parasitology**
5 **toxicology**
6 **cell block and Papanicolaou smear**
9 **other microscopic examination**

√4ᵗʰ **91.0 Microscopic examination of specimen from liver, biliary**
[1-6,9] **tract, and pancreas**

√4ᵗʰ **91.1 Microscopic examination of peritoneal and**
[1-6,9] **retroperitoneal specimen**

√4ᵗʰ **91.2 Microscopic examination of specimen from kidney,**
[1-6,9] **ureter, perirenal and periureteral tissue**

√4ᵗʰ **91.3 Microscopic examination of specimen from bladder,**
[1-6,9] **urethra, prostate, seminal vesicle, perivesical tissue, and of urine and semen**

√4ᵗʰ **91.4 Microscopic examination of specimen from**
[1-6,9] **female genital tract**
    Amnionic sac
    Fetus

√4ᵗʰ **91.5 Microscopic examination of specimen from**
[1-6,9] **musculoskeletal system and of joint fluid**
    Microscopic examination of:
      bone
      bursa
      cartilage
      fascia
      ligament
      muscle
      synovial membrane
      tendon

√4ᵗʰ **91.6 Microscopic examination of specimen from skin and**
[1-6,9] **Other integument**
    Microscopic examination of:
      hair
      nails
      skin
    EXCLUDES *mucous membrane — code to organ site that of operative wound (91.71-91.79)*

√4ᵗʰ **91.7 Microscopic examination of specimen from operative**
[1-6,9] **wound**

√4ᵗʰ **91.8 Microscopic examination of specimen from other site**
[1-6,9]

√4ᵗʰ **91.9 Microscopic examination of specimen from unspecified**
[1-6,9] **site**

√3ʳᵈ **92 Nuclear medicine**

√4ᵗʰ **92.0 Radioisotope scan and function study**

  92.01 Thyroid scan and radioisotope function studies
    Iodine-131 uptake
    Protein-bound iodine
    Radio-iodine uptake

  92.02 Liver scan and radioisotope function study

  92.03 Renal scan and radioisotope function study
    Renal clearance study

  92.04 Gastrointestinal scan and radioisotope function study
    Radio-cobalt B_{12} Schilling test
    Radio-iodinated triolein study

  92.05 Cardiovascular and hematopoietic scan and radioisotope function study
    Bone marrow
    Cardiac output
    Circulation time   ⎫ scan or function
    Radionuclide cardiac   ⎬ study
      ventriculogram
    Spleen   ⎭

  92.09 Other radioisotope function studies

√4ᵗʰ **92.1 Other radioisotope scan**

  92.11 Cerebral scan
    Pituitary

  92.12 Scan of other sites of head
    EXCLUDES *eye (95.16)*

  92.13 Parathyroid scan

  92.14 Bone scan

  92.15 Pulmonary scan

  92.16 Scan of lymphatic system

  92.17 Placental scan

  92.18 Total body scan

  92.19 Scan of other sites

√4ᵗʰ **92.2 Therapeutic radiology and nuclear medicine**
    EXCLUDES *that for:*
        ablation of pituitary gland (07.64-07.69)
        destruction of chorioretinal lesion (14.26-14.27)
    DEF: Radiation and nuclear isotope treatment of diseased tissue.

  92.20 Infusion of liquid brachytherapy radioisotope
    I-125 radioisotope
    Intracavitary brachytherapy
    EXCLUDES *removal of radioisotope*

  92.21 Superficial radiation
    Contact radiation [up to 150 KVP]

  92.22 Orthovoltage radiation
    Deep radiation [200-300 KVP]

  92.23 Radioisotopic teleradiotherapy
    Teleradiotherapy using:
      cobalt-60
      iodine-125
      radioactive cesium

  92.24 Teleradiotherapy using photons
    Megavoltage NOS
    Supervoltage NOS
    Use of:
      Betatron
      linear accelerator

  92.25 Teleradiotherapy using electrons
    Beta particles
    EXCLUDES *intra-operative electron radiation therapy (92.41)*

  92.26 Teleradiotherapy of other particulate radiation
    Neutrons
    Protons NOS

92.27 Implantation or insertion of radioactive elements
Intravascular brachytherapy
Code also incision of site
EXCLUDES *infusion of liquid brachytherapy radioisotope (92.20)*

92.28 Injection or instillation of radioisotopes
Injection or infusion of radioimmunoconjugate
Intracavitary injection or instillation
Intravenous injection or instillation
Iodine-131 [I-131] tositumomab
Radioimmunotherapy
Ytrium-90 [Y-90] ibritumomab tiuxetan
EXCLUDES *infusion of liquid brachytherapy radioisotope (92.20)*

92.29 Other radiotherapeutic procedure

√4ᵗʰ **92.3 Stereotactic radiosurgery**
Code also stereotactic head frame application (93.59)
EXCLUDES *stereotactic biopsy*
DEF: Ablation of deep intracranial lesions; single procedure; placement of head frame for 3-D analysis of lesion, followed by radiation treatment from helmet attached to frame.

92.30 Stereotactic radiosurgery, not otherwise specified

92.31 Single source photon radiosurgery
High energy x-rays
Linear accelerator (LINAC)

92.32 Multi-source photon radiosurgery
Cobalt 60 radiation
Gamma irradiation

92.33 Particulate radiosurgery
Particle beam radiation (cyclotron)
Proton accelerator

92.39 Stereotactic radiosurgery, not elsewhere classified

√4ᵗʰ **92.4 Intra-operative radiation procedures**

92.41 Intra-operative electron radiation therapy
IOERT
That using a mobile linear accelerator
DEF: Use of a mobile linear accelerator unit that delivers precision electron radiation beam radiation to highly focused anatomic sites, protecting the normal surrounding tissues from exposure.

√3ʳᵈ **93 Physical therapy, respiratory therapy, rehabilitation, and related procedures**

√4ᵗʰ **93.0 Diagnostic physical therapy**

93.01 Functional evaluation

93.02 Orthotic evaluation

93.03 Prosthetic evaluation

93.04 Manual testing of muscle function

93.05 Range of motion testing

93.06 Measurement of limb length

93.07 Body measurement
Girth measurement
Measurement of skull circumference

93.08 Electromyography
EXCLUDES *eye EMG (95.25)*
that for intraoperative monitoring (00.94)
that with polysomnogram (89.17)
urethral sphincter EMG (89.23)
DEF: Graphic recording of electrical activity of muscle.

93.09 Other diagnostic physical therapy procedure

√4ᵗʰ **93.1 Physical therapy exercises**

93.11 Assisting exercise
EXCLUDES *assisted exercise in pool (93.31)*

93.12 Other active musculoskeletal exercise

93.13 Resistive exercise

93.14 Training in joint movements

93.15 Mobilization of spine

93.16 Mobilization of other joints
EXCLUDES *manipulation of temporomandibular joint (76.95)*

93.17 Other passive musculoskeletal exercise

93.18 Breathing exercise

93.19 Exercise, not elsewhere classified

√4ᵗʰ **93.2 Other physical therapy musculoskeletal manipulation**

93.21 Manual and mechanical traction
EXCLUDES *skeletal traction (93.43-93.44)*
skin traction (93.45-93.46)
spinal traction (93.41-93.42)

93.22 Ambulation and gait training

93.23 Fitting of orthotic device

93.24 Training in use of prosthetic or orthotic device
Training in crutch walking

93.25 Forced extension of limb

93.26 Manual rupture of joint adhesions
DEF: Therapeutic application of force to rupture adhesions restricting movement.

93.27 Stretching of muscle or tendon

93.28 Stretching of fascia

93.29 Other forcible correction of deformity

√4ᵗʰ **93.3 Other physical therapy therapeutic procedures**

93.31 Assisted exercise in pool

93.32 Whirlpool treatment

93.33 Other hydrotherapy

93.34 Diathermy

93.35 Other heat therapy
Acupuncture with smouldering moxa
Hot packs
Hyperthermia NEC
Infrared irradiation
Moxibustion
Paraffin bath
EXCLUDES *hyperthermia for treatment of cancer (99.85)*
DEF: Moxibustion: Igniting moxa, a Chinese plant, for counterirritation of skin.
DEF: Paraffin bath: Hot wax treatment.

93.36 Cardiac retraining
DEF: Cardiac rehabilitation regimen following myocardial infarction or coronary bypass graft procedure.

93.37 Prenatal training
Training for natural childbirth

93.38 Combined physical therapy without mention of the components

93.39 Other physical therapy

√4ᵗʰ **93.4 Skeletal traction and other traction**

93.41 Spinal traction using skull device
Traction using:
caliper tongs
Crutchfield tongs
halo device
Vinke tongs
EXCLUDES *insertion of tongs or halo traction device (02.94)*
DEF: Applying device to head to exert pulling force on spine.

93.42 Other spinal traction
Cotrel's traction
EXCLUDES *cervical collar (93.52)*
DEF: Pulling force exerted on spine without skull device.

93.43 Intermittent skeletal traction

93.44 Other skeletal traction
Bryant's
Dunlop's } traction
Lyman Smith
Russell's

93.45 Thomas' splint traction
DEF: Thomas splint: Placement of ring around thigh, attached to rods running length of leg for therapeutic purposes.

93.46 Other skin traction of limbs
Adhesive tape traction
Boot traction
Buck's traction
Gallows traction

✓4ᵗʰ **93.5 Other immobilization, pressure, and attention to wound**
EXCLUDES external fixator device (84.71-84.73)
wound cleansing (96.58-96.59)

93.51 Application of plaster jacket
EXCLUDES Minerva jacket (93.52)

93.52 Application of neck support
Application of:
cervical collar
Minerva jacket
molded neck support

93.53 Application of other cast

93.54 Application of splint
Plaster splint
Tray splint
EXCLUDES periodontal splint (24.7)

93.55 Dental wiring
EXCLUDES that for orthodontia (24.7)

93.56 Application of pressure dressing
Application of:
Gibney bandage
Robert Jones' bandage
Shanz dressing

93.57 Application of other wound dressing
Porcine wound dressing

93.58 Application of pressure trousers
Application of:
anti-shock trousers
MAST trousers
vasopneumatic device

93.59 Other immobilization, pressure, and attention to wound
Elastic stockings
Electronic gaiter
Intermittent pressure device
Oxygenation of wound (hyperbaric)
Stereotactic head frame application
Strapping (non-traction)
Velpeau dressing

✓4ᵗʰ **93.6 Osteopathic manipulative treatment**

93.61 Osteopathic manipulative treatment for general mobilization
General articulatory treatment

93.62 Osteopathic manipulative treatment using high-velocity, low-amplitude forces
Thrusting forces

93.63 Osteopathic manipulative treatment using low-velocity, high-amplitude forces
Springing forces

93.64 Osteopathic manipulative treatment using isotonic, isometric forces

93.65 Osteopathic manipulative treatment using indirect forces

93.66 Osteopathic manipulative treatment to move tissue fluids
Lymphatic pump

93.67 Other specified osteopathic manipulative treatment

✓4ᵗʰ **93.7 Speech and reading rehabilitation and rehabilitation of the blind**

93.71 Dyslexia training

93.72 Dysphasia training
DEF: Speech training to coordinate and arrange words in proper sequence.

93.73 Esophageal speech training
DEF: Speech training after voice box removal; sound is produced by vibration of air column in esophagus against the cricopharangeal sphincter.

93.74 Speech defect training

93.75 Other speech training and therapy

93.76 Training in use of lead dog for the blind

93.77 Training in braille or Moon

93.78 Other rehabilitation for the blind

✓4ᵗʰ **93.8 Other rehabilitation therapy**

93.81 Recreational therapy
Diversional therapy
Play therapy
EXCLUDES play psychotherapy (94.36)

93.82 Educational therapy
Education of bed-bound children
Special schooling for the handicapped

93.83 Occupational therapy
Daily living activities therapy
EXCLUDES training in activities of daily living for the blind (93.78)

93.84 Music therapy

93.85 Vocational rehabilitation
Sheltered employment
Vocational:
assessment
retraining
training

93.89 Rehabilitation, not elsewhere classified

✓4ᵗʰ **93.9 Respiratory therapy**
EXCLUDES insertion of airway (96.01-96.05)
other continuous invasive (through endotracheal tube or tracheostomy) mechanical ventilation (96.70-96.72)

93.90 Non-invasive mechanical ventilation
Note: Patients admitted on *non-invasive* mechanical ventilation that subsequently require *invasive* mechanical ventilation; code both types of mechanical ventilation
Bi-level airway pressure
BiPAP without (delivery through) endotracheal tube or tracheostomy
CPAP without (delivery through) endotracheal tube or tracheostomy
Mechanical ventilation NOS
Non-invasive positive pressure (NIPPV)
Non-invasive PPV
NPPV
That delivered by non-invasive interface:
face mask
nasal mask
nasal pillow
oral mouthpiece
oronasal mask
EXCLUDES invasive (through endotracheal tube or tracheostomy) continuous mechanical ventilation (96.70-96.72)
DEF: Noninvasive ventilation support system that augments the ability to breathe spontaneously without the insertion of an endotracheal tube or tracheostomy.

93.91 Intermittent positive pressure breathing [IPPB]

Miscellaneous Diagnostic and Therapeutic Procedures

93.93–95.02

93.93 Nonmechanical methods of resuscitation
Artificial respiration
Manual resuscitation
Mouth-to-mouth resuscitition

93.94 Respiratory medication administered by nebulizer
Mist therapy

93.95 Hyperbaric oxygenation
EXCLUDES   oxygenation of wound (93.59)

93.96 Other oxygen enrichment
Catalytic oxygen therapy
Cytoreductive effect
Oxygenators
Oxygen therapy
EXCLUDES   oxygenation of wound (93.59)
        SuperSaturated oxygen therapy (00.49)

93.97 Decompression chamber

93.98 Other control of atmospheric pressure and composition
Antigen-free air conditioning
Helium therapy
EXCLUDES   inhaled nitric oxide therapy (INO) (00.12)

93.99 Other respiratory procedures
Continuous negative pressure ventilation [CNP]
Postural drainage

√3ʳᵈ **94 Procedures related to the psyche**

√4ᵗʰ **94.0 Psychologic evaluation and testing**

94.01 Administration of intelligence test
Administration of:
Stanford-Binet
Wechsler Adult Intelligence Scale
Wechsler Intelligence Scale for Children

94.02 Administration of psychologic test
Administration of:
Bender Visual-Motor Gestalt Test
Benton Visual Retention Test
Minnesota Multiphasic Personality Inventory
Wechsler Memory Scale

94.03 Character analysis

94.08 Other psychologic evaluation and testing

94.09 Psychologic mental status determination, not otherwise specified

√4ᵗʰ **94.1 Psychiatric interviews, consultations, and evaluations**

94.11 Psychiatric mental status determination
Clinical psychiatric mental status determination
Evaluation for criminal responsibility
Evaluation for testimentary capacity
Medicolegal mental status determination
Mental status determination NOS

94.12 Routine psychiatric visit, not otherwise specified

94.13 Psychiatric commitment evaluation
Pre-commitment interview

94.19 Other psychiatric interview and evaluation
Follow-up psychiatric interview NOS

√4ᵗʰ **94.2 Psychiatric somatotherapy**
DEF: Biological treatment of mental disorders.

94.21 Narcoanalysis
Narcosynthesis

94.22 Lithium therapy

94.23 Neuroleptic therapy

94.24 Chemical shock therapy

94.25 Other psychiatric drug therapy

94.26 Subconvulsive electroshock therapy

94.27 Other electroshock therapy
Electroconvulsive therapy (ECT)
EST

94.29 Other psychiatric somatotherapy

√4ᵗʰ **94.3 Individual psychotherapy**

94.31 Psychoanalysis

94.32 Hypnotherapy
Hypnodrome
Hypnosis

94.33 Behavior therapy
Aversion therapy
Behavior modification
Desensitization therapy
Relaxation training
Token economy
Extinction therapy

94.34 Individual therapy for psychosexual dysfunction
EXCLUDES   that performed in group setting (94.41)

94.35 Crisis intervention

94.36 Play psychotherapy

94.37 Exploratory verbal psychotherapy

94.38 Supportive verbal psychotherapy

94.39 Other individual psychotherapy
Biofeedback

√4ᵗʰ **94.4 Other psychotherapy and counseling**

94.41 Group therapy for psychosexual dysfunction

94.42 Family therapy

94.43 Psychodrama

94.44 Other group therapy

94.45 Drug addiction counseling

94.46 Alcoholism counseling

94.49 Other counseling

√4ᵗʰ **94.5 Referral for psychologic rehabilitation**

94.51 Referral for psychotherapy

94.52 Referral for psychiatric aftercare
That in:
halfway house
outpatient (clinic) facility

94.53 Referral for alcoholism rehabilitation

94.54 Referral for drug addiction rehabilitation

94.55 Referral for vocational rehabilitation

94.59 Referral for other psychologic rehabilitation

√4ᵗʰ **94.6 Alcohol and drug rehabilitation and detoxification**

94.61 Alcohol rehabilitation
DEF: Program designed to restore social and physical functioning, free of the dependence of alcohol.

94.62 Alcohol detoxification
DEF: Treatment of physical symptoms during withdrawal from alcohol dependence.

94.63 Alcohol rehabilitation and detoxification

94.64 Drug rehabilitation
DEF: Program designed to restore social and physical functioning, free of the dependence of drugs.

94.65 Drug detoxification
DEF: Treatment of physical symptoms during withdrawal from drug dependence.

94.66 Drug rehabilitation and detoxification

94.67 Combined alcohol and drug rehabilitation

94.68 Combined alcohol and drug detoxification

94.69 Combined alcohol and drug rehabilitation and detoxification

√3ʳᵈ **95 Ophthalmologic and otologic diagnosis and treatment**

√4ᵗʰ **95.0 General and subjective eye examination**

95.01 Limited eye examination
Eye examination with prescription of spectacles

95.02 Comprehensive eye examination
Eye examination covering all aspects of the visual system

95.03 Extended ophthalmologic work-up
Examination (for):
glaucoma
neuro-ophthalmology
retinal disease

95.04 Eye examination under anesthesia
Code also type of examination

95.05 Visual field study

95.06 Color vision study

95.07 Dark adaptation study
DEF: Exam of eye's adaption to dark.

95.09 Eye examination, not otherwise specified
Vision check NOS

✓4th **95.1 Examinations of form and structure of eye**

95.11 Fundus photography

95.12 Fluorescein angiography or angioscopy of eye

95.13 Ultrasound study of eye

95.14 X-ray study of eye

95.15 Ocular motility study

95.16 P$_{32}$ and other tracer studies of eye

✓4th **95.2 Objective functional tests of eye**
EXCLUDES that with polysomnogram (89.17)

95.21 Electroretinogram [ERG]

95.22 Electro-oculogram [EOG]

95.23 Visual evoked potential [VEP]
DEF: Measuring and recording evoked visual responses of body and senses.

95.24 Electronystagmogram [ENG]
DEF: Monitoring of brain waves to record induced and spontaneous eye movements.

95.25 Electromyogram of eye [EMG]

95.26 Tonography, provocative tests, and other glaucoma testing

✓4th **95.3 Special vision services**

95.31 Fitting and dispensing of spectacles

95.32 Prescription, fitting, and dispensing of contact lens

95.33 Dispensing of other low vision aids

95.34 Ocular prosthetics

95.35 Orthoptic training

95.36 Ophthalmologic counselling and instruction
Counselling in:
adaptation to visual loss
use of low vision aids

✓4th **95.4 Nonoperative procedures related to hearing**

95.41 Audiometry
Békésy 5-tone audiometry
Impedance audiometry
Stapedial reflex response
Subjective audiometry
Tympanogram

95.42 Clinical test of hearing
Tuning fork test
Whispered speech test

95.43 Audiological evaluation
Audiological evaluation by:
Bárány noise machine
blindfold test
delayed feedback
masking
Weber lateralization

95.44 Clinical vestibular function tests
Thermal test of vestibular function

95.45 Rotation tests
Bárány chair
DEF: Irrigation of ear canal with warm or cold water to evaluate vestibular function.

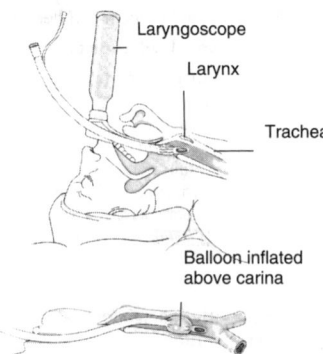

Endotracheal Intubation

Laryngoscope

Larynx

Trachea

Balloon inflated above carina

95.46 Other auditory and vestibular function tests

95.47 Hearing examination, not otherwise specified

95.48 Fitting of hearing aid
EXCLUDES implantation of electromagnetic hearing device (20.95)

95.49 Other nonoperative procedures related to hearing
Adjustment (external components) of cochlear prosthetic device

✓3rd **96 Nonoperative intubation and irrigation**

✓4th **96.0 Nonoperative intubation of gastrointestinal and respiratory tracts**

96.01 Insertion of nasopharyngeal airway

96.02 Insertion of oropharyngeal airway

96.03 Insertion of esophageal obturator airway

96.04 Insertion of endotracheal tube

96.05 Other intubation of respiratory tract
EXCLUDES endoscopic insertion or replacement of bronchial device or substance (33.71, 33.79)

96.06 Insertion of Sengstaken tube
Esophageal tamponade
DEF: Insertion of Sengstaken tube: Nonsurgical emergency measure to stop esophageal bleeding using compression exerted by inflated balloons; additional tube ports to aspirate blood and clots.

96.07 Insertion of other (naso-) gastric tube
Intubation for decompression
EXCLUDES that for enteral infusion of nutritional substance (96.6)

96.08 Insertion of (naso-) intestinal tube
Miller-Abbott tube (for decompression)

96.09 Insertion of rectal tube
Replacement of rectal tube

✓4th **96.1 Other nonoperative insertion**
EXCLUDES nasolacrimal intubation (09.44)

96.11 Packing of external auditory canal

96.14 Vaginal packing

96.15 Insertion of vaginal mold

96.16 Other vaginal dilation

96.17 Insertion of vaginal diaphragm

96.18 Insertion of other vaginal pessary

96.19 Rectal packing

✓4th **96.2 Nonoperative dilation and manipulation**

96.21 Dilation of frontonasal duct

96.22 Dilation of rectum

96.23 Dilation of anal sphincter

96.24 Dilation and manipulation of enterostomy stoma

96.25 Therapeutic distention of bladder
Intermittent distention of bladder

Miscellaneous Diagnostic and Therapeutic Procedures

96.26–97.03

96.26 Manual reduction of rectal prolapse

96.27 Manual reduction of hernia

96.28 Manual reduction of enterostomy prolapse

96.29 Reduction of intussusception of alimentary tract
With:
    fluoroscopy
    ionizing radiation enema
    ultrasonography guidance
Hydrostatic reduction
Pneumatic reduction
> **EXCLUDES** *intra-abdominal manipulation of intestine, not otherwise specified (46.80)*

✓4ᵗʰ **96.3 Nonoperative alimentary tract irrigation, cleaning, and local instillation**

96.31 Gastric cooling
Gastric hypothermia
DEF: Reduction of internal stomach temperature.

96.32 Gastric freezing

96.33 Gastric lavage

96.34 Other irrigation of (naso-)gastric tube

96.35 Gastric gavage
DEF: Food forced into stomach.

96.36 Irrigation of gastrostomy or enterostomy

96.37 Proctoclysis
DEF: Slow introduction of large amounts of fluids into lower large intestine.

96.38 Removal of impacted feces
Removal of impaction:
    by flushing manually

96.39 Other transanal enema
Rectal irrigation
> **EXCLUDES** *reduction of intussusception of alimentary tract by ionizing radiation enema (96.29)*

✓4ᵗʰ **96.4 Nonoperative irrigation, cleaning, and local instillation of other digestive and genitourinary organs**

96.41 Irrigation of cholecystostomy and other biliary tube

96.42 Irrigation of pancreatic tube

96.43 Digestive tract instillation, except gastric gavage

96.44 Vaginal douche

96.45 Irrigation of nephrostomy and pyelostomy

96.46 Irrigation of ureterostomy and ureteral catheter

96.47 Irrigation of cystostomy

96.48 Irrigation of other indwelling urinary catheter

96.49 Other genitourinary instillation
Insertion of prostaglandin suppository

✓4ᵗʰ **96.5 Other nonoperative irrigation and cleaning**

96.51 Irrigation of eye
Irrigation of cornea
> **EXCLUDES** *irrigation with removal of foreign body (98.21)*

96.52 Irrigation of ear
Irrigation with removal of cerumen

96.53 Irrigation of nasal passages

96.54 Dental scaling, polishing, and debridement
Dental prophylaxis   Plaque removal

96.55 Tracheostomy toilette

96.56 Other lavage of bronchus and trachea
> **EXCLUDES** *diagnostic bronchoalveolar lavage (BAL) (33.24)*
> *whole lung lavage (33.99)*

96.57 Irrigation of vascular catheter

96.58 Irrigation of wound catheter

96.59 Other irrigation of wound
Wound cleaning NOS
> **EXCLUDES** *debridement (86.22, 86.27-86.28)*

96.6 Enteral infusion of concentrated-nutritional substances

✓4ᵗʰ **96.7 Other continuous invasive mechanical ventilation**
BiPAP delivered through endotracheal tube or tracheostomy (invasive interface)
CPAP delivered through endotracheal tube or tracheostomy (invasive interface)
Endotracheal respiratory assistance
Invasive positive pressure ventilation [IPPV]
Mechanical ventilation through invasive interface
That by tracheostomy
Weaning of an intubated (endotracheal tube) patient
Code also any associated:
    endotracheal tube insertion (96.04)
    tracheostomy (31.1-31.29)
> **EXCLUDES** *continuous negative pressure ventilation [CNP] (iron lung) (cuirass) (93.99)*
> *intermittent positive pressure breathing [IPPB] (93.91)*
> *non-invasive bi-level positive airway pressure [BiPAP] (93.90)*
> *non-invasive continuous positive airway pressure [CPAP] (93.90)*
> *non-invasive positive pressure (NIPPV) (93.90)*
> *that by face mask (93.90-93.99)*
> *that by nasal cannula (93.90-93.99)*
> *that by nasal catheter (93.90-93.99)*

Note: Endotracheal intubation

To calculate the number of hours (duration) of continuous mechanical ventilation during a hospitalization, begin the count from the start of the (endotracheal) intubation. The duration ends with (endotracheal) extubation.

If a patient is intubated prior to admission, begin counting the duration from the time of the admission. If a patient is transferred (discharged) while intubated, the duration would end at the time of transfer (discharge).

For patients who begin on (endotracheal) intubation and subsequently have a tracheostomy performed for mechanical ventilation, the duration begins with the (endotracheal) intubation and ends when the mechanical ventilation is turned off (after the weaning period).

Note: Tracheostomy

To calculate the number of hours of continuous mechanical ventilation during a hospitalization, begin counting the duration when mechanical ventilation is started. The duration ends when the mechanical ventilator is turned off (after the weaning period).

If a patient has received a tracheostomy prior to admission and is on mechanical ventilation at the time of admission, begin counting the duration from the time of admission. If a patient is transferred (discharged) while still on mechanical ventilation via tracheostomy, the duration would end at the time of the transfer (discharge).

96.70 Continuous invasive mechanical ventilation of unspecified duration
Invasive mechanical ventilation NOS

96.71 Continuous invasive mechanical ventilation for less than 96 consecutive hours

96.72 Continuous invasive mechanical ventilation for 96 consecutive hours or more

✓3ʳᵈ **97 Replacement and removal of therapeutic appliances**

✓4ᵗʰ **97.0 Nonoperative replacement of gastrointestinal appliance**

97.01 Replacement of (naso-)gastric or esophagostomy tube

97.02 Replacement of gastrostomy tube

97.03 Replacement of tube or enterostomy device of small intestine

97.04   **Replacement of tube or enterostomy device of large intestine**

97.05   **Replacement of stent (tube) in biliary or pancreatic duct**

√4ᵗʰ **97.1 Nonoperative replacement of musculoskeletal and integumentary system appliance**

97.11   **Replacement of cast on upper limb**

97.12   **Replacement of cast on lower limb**

97.13   **Replacement of other cast**

97.14   **Replacement of other device for musculoskeletal immobilization**
     Splinting   Strapping

97.15   **Replacement of wound catheter**

97.16   **Replacement of wound packing or drain**
     EXCLUDES   *repacking of:*
         dental wound (97.22)
         vulvar wound (97.26)

√4ᵗʰ **97.2 Other nonoperative replacement**

97.21   **Replacement of nasal packing**

97.22   **Replacement of dental packing**

97.23   **Replacement of tracheostomy tube**

97.24   **Replacement and refitting of vagina diaphragm**

97.25   **Replacement of other vaginal pessary**

97.26   **Replacement of vaginal or vulvar packing or drain**

97.29   **Other nonoperative replacements**

√4ᵗʰ **97.3 Nonoperative removal of therapeutic device from head and neck**

97.31   **Removal of eye prosthesis**
     EXCLUDES   *removal of ocular implant (16.71)*
         removal of orbital implant (16.72)

97.32   **Removal of nasal packing**

97.33   **Removal of dental wiring**

97.34   **Removal of dental packing**

97.35   **Removal of dental prosthesis**

97.36   **Removal of other external mandibular fixation device**

97.37   **Removal of tracheostomy tube**

97.38   **Removal of sutures from head and neck**

97.39   **Removal of other therapeutic device from head and neck**
     EXCLUDES   *removal of skull tongs (02.94)*

√4ᵗʰ **97.4 Nonoperative removal of therapeutic device from thorax**

97.41   **Removal of thoracotomy tube or pleural cavity drain**

97.42   **Removal of mediastinal drain**

97.43   **Removal of sutures from thorax**

97.44   **Nonoperative removal of heart assist system**
     Explantation [removal] of circulatory assist device
     Explantation [removal] of percutaneous external heart assist device
     Removal of extrinsic heart assist device
     Removal of pVAD
     Removal of percutaneous heart assist device
     DEF: Non-invasive removal of ventricular assist systems, or intraaortic balloon pump, which is a balloon catheter placed into the descending thoracic aorta and timed to inflate and deflate with the patient's own heart rhythm to aid in blood circulation.

Intraaortic Balloon Pump

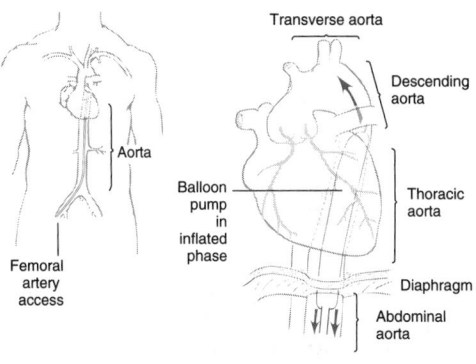

97.49   **Removal of other device from thorax**
     EXCLUDES   *endoscopic removal of bronchial device(s) or substances (33.78)*

√4ᵗʰ **97.5 Nonoperative removal of therapeutic device from digestive system**

97.51   **Removal of gastrostomy tube**

97.52   **Removal of tube from small intestine**

97.53   **Removal of tube from large intestine or appendix**

97.54   **Removal of cholecystostomy tube**

97.55   **Removal of T-tube, other bile duct tube, or liver tube**
     Removal of bile duct stent

97.56   **Removal of pancreatic tube or drain**

97.59   **Removal of other device from digestive system**
     Removal of rectal packing

√4ᵗʰ **97.6 Nonoperative removal of therapeutic device from urinary system**

97.61   **Removal of pyelostomy and nephrostomy tube**
     DEF: Nonsurgical removal of tubes from lower part of kidney.

97.62   **Removal of ureterostomy tube and ureteral catheter**

97.63   **Removal of cystostomy tube**

97.64   **Removal of other urinary drainage device**
     Removal of indwelling urinary catheter

97.65   **Removal of urethral stent**

97.69   **Removal of other device from urinary system**

√4ᵗʰ **97.7 Nonoperative removal of therapeutic device from genital system**

97.71   **Removal of intrauterine contraceptive device**

97.72   **Removal of intrauterine pack**

97.73   **Removal of vaginal diaphragm**

97.74   **Removal of other vaginal pessary**

97.75   **Removal of vaginal or vulvar packing**

97.79   **Removal of other device from genital tract**
     Removal of sutures

√4ᵗʰ **97.8 Other nonoperative removal of therapeutic device**

97.81   **Removal of retroperitoneal drainage device**

97.82   **Removal of peritoneal drainage device**

97.83   **Removal of abdominal wall sutures**

97.84   **Removal of sutures from trunk, not elsewhere classified**

97.85   **Removal of packing from trunk, not elsewhere classified**

97.86   **Removal of other device from abdomen**

97.87   **Removal of other device from trunk**

Miscellaneous Diagnostic and Therapeutic Procedures

97.88–99.06

97.88   **Removal of external immobilization device**
Removal of:
     brace
     cast
     splint

97.89   **Removal of other therapeutic device**

✓3rd   **98**   **Nonoperative removal of foreign body or calculus**

✓4th   **98.0**   **Removal of intraluminal foreign body from digestive system without incision**
     EXCLUDES   *removal of therapeutic device (97.51-97.59)*
     DEF: Retrieval of foreign body from digestive system lining without incision.

   98.01   **Removal of intraluminal foreign body from mouth without incision**

   98.02   **Removal of intraluminal foreign body from esophagus without incision**

   98.03   **Removal of intraluminal foreign body from stomach and small intestine without incision**

   98.04   **Removal of intraluminal foreign body from large intestine without incision**

   98.05   **Removal of intraluminal foreign body from rectum and anus without incision**

✓4th   **98.1**   **Removal of intraluminal foreign body from other sites without incision**
     EXCLUDES   *removal of therapeutic device (97.31-97.49, 97.61-97.89)*

   98.11   **Removal of intraluminal foreign body from ear without incision**

   98.12   **Removal of intraluminal foreign body from nose without incision**

   98.13   **Removal of intraluminal foreign body from pharynx without incision**

   98.14   **Removal of intraluminal foreign body from larynx without incision**

   98.15   **Removal of intraluminal foreign body from trachea and bronchus without incision**
     EXCLUDES   *endoscopic removal of bronchial device(s) or substances (33.78)*

   98.16   **Removal of intraluminal foreign body from uterus without incision**
     EXCLUDES   *removal of intrauterine contraceptive device (97.71)*

   98.17   **Removal of intraluminal foreign body from vagina without incision**

   98.18   **Removal of intraluminal foreign body from artificial stoma without incision**

   98.19   **Removal of intraluminal foreign body from urethra without incision**

✓4th   **98.2**   **Removal of other foreign body without incision**
     EXCLUDES   *removal of intraluminal foreign body (98.01-98.19)*

   98.20   **Removal of foreign body, not otherwise specified**

   98.21   **Removal of superficial foreign body from eye without incision**

   98.22   **Removal of other foreign body without incision from head and neck**
     Removal of embedded foreign body from eyelid or conjunctiva without incision

   98.23   **Removal of foreign body from vulva without incision**

   98.24   **Removal of foreign body from scrotum or penis without incision**

   98.25   **Removal of other foreign body without incision from trunk except scrotum, penis, or vulva**

Extracorporeal Shock Wave Lithotripsy

   98.26   **Removal of foreign body from hand without incision**

   98.27   **Removal of foreign body without incision from upper limb, except hand**

   98.28   **Removal of foreign body from foot without incision**

   98.29   **Removal of foreign body without incision from lower limb, except foot**

✓4th   **98.5**   **Extracorporeal shockwave lithotripsy [ESWL]**
     Lithotriptor tank procedure
     Disintegration of stones by extracorporeal induced shockwaves
     That with insertion of stent
     DEF: Breaking of stones with high voltage condenser device synchronized with patient R waves.

   98.51   **Extracorporeal shockwave lithotripsy [ESWL] of the kidney, ureter and/or bladder**

   98.52   **Extracorporeal shockwave lithotripsy [ESWL] of the gallbladder and/or bile duct**

   98.59   **Extracorporeal shockwave lithotripsy of other sites**

✓3rd   **99**   **Other nonoperative procedures**

✓4th   **99.0**   **Transfusion of blood and blood components**
     Use additional code for that done via catheter or cutdown (38.92-38.94)

   99.00   **Perioperative autologous transfusion of whole blood or blood components**
     Intraoperative blood collection
     Postoperative blood collection
     Salvage
     DEF: Salvaging patient blood with reinfusion during perioperative period.

   99.01   **Exchange transfusion**
     Transfusion:
       exsanguination
       replacement
     DEF: Repetitive withdrawal of blood, replaced by donor blood.

   99.02   **Transfusion of previously collected autologous blood**
     Blood component
     DEF: Transfusion with patient's own previously withdrawn and stored blood.

   99.03   **Other transfusion of whole blood**
     Transfusion:
       blood NOS
       hemodilution
       NOS

   99.04   **Transfusion of packed cells**

   99.05   **Transfusion of platelets**
     Transfusion of thrombocytes

   99.06   **Transfusion of coagulation factors**
     Transfusion of antihemophilic factor
     EXCLUDES   *infusion of 4-Factor Prothrombin Complex Concentrate (00.96)*

99.07   **Transfusion of other serum**
Transfusion of plasma
EXCLUDES   *injection [transfusion] of:*
    antivenin (99.16)
    gamma globulin (99.14)

99.08   **Transfusion of blood expander**
Transfusion of Dextran

99.09   **Transfusion of other substance**
Transfusion of:
    blood surrogate
    granulocytes
EXCLUDES   *transplantation [transfusion] of bone marrow (41.00-41.09)*

√4th **99.1**   **Injection or infusion of therapeutic or prophylactic substance**
INCLUDES   injection or infusion given:
    hypodermically
    intramuscularly   } acting locally or systemically
    intravenously

99.10   **Injection or infusion of thrombolytic agent**
Alteplase
Anistreplase
Reteplase
Streptokinase
Tenecteplase
Tissue plasminogen activator (TPA)
Urokinase
EXCLUDES   *aspirin — omit code*
    GP IIb/IIIa platelet inhibitors (99.20)
    heparin (99.19)
    SuperSaturated oxygen therapy (00.49)
    warfarin — omit code

99.11   **Injection of Rh immune globulin**
Injection of:
    Anti-D (Rhesus) globulin
    RhoGAM

99.12   **Immunization for allergy**
Desensitization

99.13   **Immunization for autoimmune disease**

99.14   **Injection or infusion of immunoglobulin**
Injection of immune sera
Injection or infusion of gamma globulin

99.15   **Parenteral infusion of concentrated nutritional substances**
Hyperalimentation
Total parenteral nutrition [TPN]
Peripheral parenteral nutrition [PPN]
DEF: Administration of greater than necessary amount of nutrients via other than the alimentary canal (e.g., infusion).

99.16   **Injection of antidote**
Injection of:
    antivenin
    heavy metal antagonist

99.17   **Injection of insulin**

99.18   **Injection or infusion of electrolytes**

99.19   **Injection of anticoagulant**
EXCLUDES   *infusion of drotrecogin alfa (activated) (00.11)*

√4th **99.2**   **Injection or infusion of other therapeutic or prophylactic substance**
INCLUDES   injection or infusion given:
    hypodermically
    intramuscularly   } acting locally or systemically
    intravenously
Use additional code for:
  injection (into):
    breast (85.92)
    bursa (82.94, 83.96)
    intraperitoneal (cavity) (54.97)
    intrathecal (03.92)
    joint (76.96, 81.92)
    kidney (55.96)
    liver (50.94)
    orbit (16.91)
    other sites — see Alphabetic Index
  perfusion:
    NOS (39.97)
    intestine (46.95, 46.96)
    kidney (55.95)
    liver (50.93)
    total body (39.96)
EXCLUDES   *SuperSaturated oxygen therapy (00.49)*

99.20   **Injection or infusion of platelet inhibitor**
Glycoprotein IIb/IIIa inhibitor
GP IIb-IIIa inhibitor
GP IIb/IIIa inhibitor
EXCLUDES   *infusion of heparin (99.19)*
    injection or infusion of thrombolytic agent (99.10)

99.21   **Injection of antibiotic**
EXCLUDES   *injection or infusion of oxazolidinone class of antibiotics (00.14)*

99.22   **Injection of other anti-infective**
EXCLUDES   *injection or infusion of oxazolidinone class of antibiotics (00.14)*

99.23   **Injection of steroid**
Injection of cortisone
Subdermal implantation of progesterone

99.24   **Injection of other hormone**

99.25   **Injection or infusion of cancer chemotherapeutic substance**
Chemoembolization
Injection or infusion of antineoplastic agent
Use additional code for disruption of blood brain barrier, if performed [BBBD] (00.19)
EXCLUDES   *immunotherapy, antineoplastic (00.15, 99.28)*
    implantation of chemotherapeutic agent (00.10)
    injection of radioisotope (92.28)
    injection or infusion of biological response modifier [BRM] as an antineoplastic agent (99.28)
    intravenous infusion of clofarabine (17.70)

99.26   **Injection of tranquilizer**

99.27   **Iontophoresis**
DEF: Iontophoresis: Introduction of soluble salts into tissues via electric current.

99.28   **Injection or infusion of biological response modifier [BRM] as an antineoplastic agent**
Immunotherapy, antineoplastic
Infusion of cintredekin besudotox
Interleukin therapy
Low-dose interleukin-2 [IL-2] therapy
Tumor vaccine
EXCLUDES   *high-dose infusion interleukin-2 [IL-2] (00.15)*

99.29　**Injection or infusion of other therapeutic or prophylactic substance**
　　EXCLUDES　administration of neuroprotective agent (99.75)
　　　　immunization (99.31-99.59)
　　　　infusion of blood brain barrier disruption substance (00.19)
　　　　injection of sclerosing agent into:
　　　　　esophageal varices (42.33)
　　　　　hemorrhoids (49.42)
　　　　　veins (39.92)
　　　　injection or infusion of:
　　　　　human B-type natriuretic peptide (hBNP) (00.13)
　　　　　nesiritide (00.13)
　　　　　platelet inhibitor (99.20)
　　　　　thrombolytic agent (99.10)
　　　　uterine artery embolization without coils (68.25)

✓4ᵗʰ　99.3　**Prophylactic vaccination and inoculation against certain bacterial diseases**
　　DEF: Administration of a killed bacteria suspension to produce immunity.

99.31　**Vaccination against cholera**

99.32　**Vaccination against typhoid and paratyphoid fever**
　　Administration of TAB vaccine

99.33　**Vaccination against tuberculosis**
　　Administration of BCG vaccine

99.34　**Vaccination against plague**

99.35　**Vaccination against tularemia**

99.36　**Administration of diphtheria toxoid**
　　EXCLUDES　administration of:
　　　　diphtheria antitoxin (99.58)
　　　　diphtheria-tetanus-pertussis, combined (99.39)

99.37　**Vaccination against pertussis**
　　EXCLUDES　administration of diphtheria-tetanus-pertussis, combined (99.39)

99.38　**Administration of tetanus toxoid**
　　EXCLUDES　administration of:
　　　　diphtheria-tetanus-pertussis, combined (99.39)
　　　　tetanus antitoxin (99.56)

99.39　**Administration of diphtheria-tetanus- pertussis, combined**

✓4ᵗʰ　99.4　**Prophylactic vaccination and inoculation against certain viral diseases**
　　DEF: Administration of a killed virus suspension to produce immunity.

99.41　**Administration of poliomyelitis vaccine**

99.42　**Vaccination against smallpox**

99.43　**Vaccination against yellow fever**

99.44　**Vaccination against rabies**

99.45　**Vaccination against measles**
　　EXCLUDES　administration of measles-mumps-rubella vaccine (99.48)

99.46　**Vaccination against mumps**
　　EXCLUDES　administration of measles-mumps-rubella vaccine (99.48)

99.47　**Vaccination against rubella**
　　EXCLUDES　administration of measles-mumps-rubella vaccine (99.48)

99.48　**Administration of measles-mumps-rubella vaccine**

✓4ᵗʰ　99.5　**Other vaccination and inoculation**

99.51　**Prophylactic vaccination against the common cold**

99.52　**Prophylactic vaccination against influenza**

99.53　**Prophylactic vaccination against arthropod-borne viral encephalitis**

99.54　**Prophylactic vaccination against other arthropod-borne viral diseases**

99.55　**Prophylactic administration of vaccine against other diseases**
　　Vaccination against:
　　　anthrax
　　　brucellosis
　　　Rocky Mountain spotted fever
　　　Staphylococcus
　　　Streptococcus
　　　typhus

99.56　**Administration of tetanus antitoxin**

99.57　**Administration of botulism antitoxin**

99.58　**Administration of other antitoxins**
　　Administration of:
　　　diphtheria antitoxin
　　　gas gangrene antitoxin
　　　scarlet fever antitoxin

99.59　**Other vaccination and inoculation**
　　Vaccination NOS
　　EXCLUDES　injection of:
　　　　gamma globulin (99.14)
　　　　Rh immune globulin (99.11)
　　　immunization for:
　　　　allergy (99.12)
　　　　autoimmune disease (99.13)

✓4ᵗʰ　99.6　**Conversion of cardiac rhythm**
　　EXCLUDES　open chest cardiac:
　　　　electric stimulation (37.91)
　　　　massage (37.91)
　　DEF: Correction of cardiac rhythm.

99.60　**Cardiopulmonary resuscitation, not otherwise specified**

99.61　**Atrial cardioversion**
　　DEF: Application of electric shock to upper heart chamber to restore normal heart rhythm.

99.62　**Other electric countershock of heart**
　　Cardioversion:
　　　NOS
　　　external
　　Conversion to sinus rhythm
　　Defibrillation
　　　External electrode stimulation

99.63　**Closed chest cardiac massage**
　　Cardiac massage NOS
　　Manual external cardiac massage
　　DEF: Application of alternating manual pressure over breastbone to restore normal heart rhythm.

99.64　**Carotid sinus stimulation**

99.69　**Other conversion of cardiac rhythm**

✓4ᵗʰ　99.7　**Therapeutic apheresis or other injection, administration, or infusion of other therpeutic or prophylactic substance**

99.71　**Therapeutic plasmapheresis**
　　EXCLUDES　extracorporeal immunoadsorption [ECI] (99.76)

99.72　**Therapeutic leukopheresis**
　　Therapeutic leukocytapheresis

99.73　**Therapeutic erythrocytapheresis**
　　Therapeutic erythropheresis

99.74　**Therapeutic plateletpheresis**

99.75　**Administration of neuroprotective agent**
　　DEF: Direct application of neuroprotective agent (e.g., nimodipine) to minimize ischemic injury by inhibiting toxic neurotransmitters, blocking free ions, removing free radicals, and causing vasodilation.

99.76 Extracorporeal immunoadsorption
Removal of antibodies from plasma with protein A columns

99.77 Application or administration of adhesion barrier substance

99.78 Aquapheresis
Plasma water removal
Ultrafiltration [for water removal]
> **EXCLUDES** *hemodiafiltration (39.95)*
> *hemodialysis (39.95)*
> *therapeutic plasmapheresis (99.71)*

99.79 Other
Apheresis (harvest) of stem cells

✓4ᵗʰ **99.8 Miscellaneous physical procedures**

99.81 Hypothermia (central) (local)
> **EXCLUDES** *gastric cooling (96.31)*
> *gastric freezing (96.32)*
> *that incidental to open heart surgery (39.62)*

99.82 Ultraviolet light therapy
Actinotherapy

99.83 Other phototherapy
Phototherapy of the newborn
> **EXCLUDES** *extracorporeal photochemotherapy (99.88)*
> *photocoagulation of retinal lesion (14.23-14.25, 14.33-14.35, 14.53-14.55)*

DEF: Treating disease with light rays of various concentrations.

99.84 Isolation
Isolation after contact with infectious disease
Protection of individual from his surroundings
Protection of surroundings from individual

99.85 Hyperthermia for treatment of cancer
Hyperthermia (adjunct therapy) induced by microwave, ultrasound, low energy radio frequency, probes (interstitial), or other means in the treatment of cancer
Code also any concurrent chemotherapy or radiation therapy

99.86 Non-invasive placement of bone growth stimulator
Transcutaneous (surface) placement of pads or patches for stimulation to aid bone healing
> **EXCLUDES** *insertion of invasive or semi-invasive bone growth stimulators (device) (percutaneous electrodes) (78.90-78.99)*

99.88 Therapeutic photopheresis
Extracorporeal photochemotherapy
Extracorporeal photopheresis
> **EXCLUDES** *other phototherapy (99.83)*
> *ultraviolet light therapy (99.82)*

DEF: Extracorporeal photochemotherapy: Treating disease with drugs that react to ultraviolet radiation or sunlight.

✓4ᵗʰ **99.9 Other miscellaneous procedures**

99.91 Acupuncture for anesthesia

99.92 Other acupuncture
> **EXCLUDES** *that with smouldering moxa (93.35)*

99.93 Rectal massage (for levator spasm)

99.94 Prostatic massage

99.95 Stretching of foreskin

99.96 Collection of sperm for artificial insemination

99.97 Fitting of denture

99.98 Extraction of milk from lactating breast

99.99 Other
Leech therapy

HCPCS Introduction

All experienced medical coders know and use the tools to report medical procedures and services and the diagnoses that justify the treatment. Sometimes overlooked in training, though, is another area of medical coding: nonphysician services, specific supplies, and the administration of select drugs. HCPCS Level II codes are the tools to report these types of services and supplies.

The term HCPCS (pronounced "hick-picks") is most accurately used as the acronym for the entire two-level Healthcare Common Procedure Coding System. The federal government refers to all procedure codes as the HCPCS system. But HCPCS is also commonly used to specifically identify HCPCS Level II national codes, the topic of this chapter. (CPT codes are Level I of the system.) The HCPCS Level II codes are maintained by the Centers for Medicare and Medicaid Services (CMS) and are updated throughout the year, with the major update effective the first of each year. Because the Level I CPT coding system does not include codes for nonphysician services many of these services are identified with a Level II code as well as specific supplies, procedures which do not have a specific CPT code and drugs.

HCPCS LEVEL II/NATIONAL CODES

More than 5,900 codes comprise the HCPCS Level II national codes. If an appropriate HCPCS Level II code exists, it usually takes precedence over a CPT code in Medicare billing. These codes are updated annually but new codes may be introduced through out the year as necessary. Codes may also be changed or deleted throughout the year.

The alphanumeric codes represent groups of services or supplies. HCPCS codes are now required to report most medical services and supplies provided in outpatient settings to Medicare and Medicaid patients. An increasing number of private insurance carriers also encourage or require the use of HCPCS codes. Most of the larger national payers, including workers' compensation, recognize HCPCS codes. HCPCS codes are available from the CMS website, Medicare contractor, or from commercial publishers such as Ingenix. For Medicare, Level II codes usually supercede Level 1 codes. Many private payers prefer Level 1 codes to Level II codes when similar codes exist.

THE HCPCS NATIONAL CODES IN DETAIL

HCPCS Level II-national codes may be used throughout the United States in all Medicare regions. National codes consist of one alpha character (A through V) followed by four digits (A0000–V9999). HCPCS Level II provides specific codes for supplies, services, injections and certain drugs, durable medical equipment (DME), orthotics, prosthetics, etc. HCPCS Level II codes are designed to provide more specificity than CPT codes. The HCPCS Level II coding system also contains an Index. In addition, all prescription drugs are listed in the table of drugs. In the index, under "Drugs(s)," the user is directed to this table.

HCPCS Codes

Each section of codes is designated by a letter code except for the last section, the table of drugs.

A codes include ambulance and transportation services, medical and surgical supplies, administrative, and miscellaneous and investigational services and supplies.

B codes include enteral and parenteral therapy.

C codes are used for facility (technical) services.

Note: D codes for diagnostic, preventative, restorative, endodontic, periodontic, prosthodontic, prosthetic, orthodontic, and surgical dental procedures are not included in the official 2014 HCPCS Level II code set. The American Dental Association (ADA) holds the copyright on those codes and instructed CMS to remove them. As a result, Optum has removed them from this product.

E codes include durable medical equipment such as canes, crutches, walkers, commodes, decubitus care, bath and toilet aids, hospital beds, oxygen and related respiratory equipment, monitoring equipment, pacemakers, patient lifts, safety equipment, restraints, traction equipment, fracture frames, wheelchairs, and artificial kidney machines.

G codes include temporary procedures and professional services that are under review prior to inclusion in the CPT coding system.

H codes describe alcohol and drug abuse treatment services. These are temporary codes for state or federal agencies other than Medicare and Medicaid.

J codes include drugs that cannot ordinarily be self-administered, chemotherapy drugs, immunosuppressive drugs, inhalation solutions, and other miscellaneous drugs and solutions.

K codes are temporary codes for durable medical equipment and drugs. Once these codes are approved for permanent inclusion in HCPCS, they typically become A, E, or J codes.

L codes include orthotic and prosthetic procedures and devices, as well as scoliosis equipment, orthopedic shoes, and prosthetic implants.

M codes include office services and cardiovascular and other medical services.

P codes include certain pathology and laboratory services.

Q codes are miscellaneous temporary codes.

R codes are diagnostic radiology services codes.

S codes are not accepted by Medicare and have been developed by Blue cross/Blue Shield and other commercial payers to report drugs, services and supplies. Often these codes are replaced by a CPT code within several years of development.

T codes are for use by state Medicaid agencies and are not valid for Medicare.

V codes include vision, hearing, and speech-language pathology services.

The table of drugs lists all drugs found in HCPCS by their generic name, with amount, route of administration, and code number. Brand name drugs are also listed in the table with a reference to the appropriate generic drug.

The HCPCS Level II coding system also contains modifiers. These modifiers are two-digit suffixes that can be appended to all procedure codes (i.e., HCPCS level I or HCPCS Level II codes). HCPCS modifiers may be alpha or alphanumeric.

There are also two-character modifiers used on claims that are created by combining two single-character modifiers. These are used for ambulance services, the first digit indicating the origin and the second the destination.

USE OF HCPCS

The following points summarize why practices use HCPCS:

- HCPCS codes are mandated by CMS for use on Medicare claims and are also required by most state Medicaid offices.
- HCPCS codes improve a provider's ability to communicate services or supplies correctly without resorting to narrative descriptions.
- The codes reduce resubmission of claims for correction or review.
- Up-to-date and accurate HCPCS codes on office routing slips allow office staff to assign fees quickly and efficiently to services and supplies, saving both time and money.
- Consistent submission of "clean claims" (claims having all correct information necessary for processing) helps avoid an audit by a carrier due to lack of specificity of claims.
- Use of HCPCS is essential for accurate and complete reimbursement from Medicare.
- Supplies billed to Medicare as "other than incidental to an office visit" (CPT code 99070) are not reimbursed unless identified with Level II/HCPCS or Level III/local codes.

The Index

The index is of tremendous help to both new and experienced HCPCS coders. All main terms are in boldface type in the Index. Main term entries include tests, services, supplies, orthotics, prostheses, medical equipment, drugs, therapies, and some medical and surgical procedures. Subterms are listed under the main term to which they apply. Where possible, entries are listed under a common main term. In some instances, the common term is a noun, while in others, the main term is a descriptor.

The steps to follow for searching the index are:

1. Analyze the provided statement or description that designates the term to be coded.

2. Identify the main term.

3. Locate the main term in the index.

4. Check for relevant subterms under the main term. Verify the meaning of any unfamiliar abbreviations.

5. Note the codes found after the selected main term or subterm.

6. Locate the code in the alphanumeric list to ensure the specificity of the code. If a code range is provided, locate the code range and review all code narratives in that code range for specificity.

7. In some cases, an entry may be listed under more than one main term. When this occurs, review all code choices suggested.

8. Never code directly from the index. Always verify the main choice in the alphanumeric list.

Tabular—Color Coding

Red   Codes that are "Not Covered" or invalid for Medicare are designated by a red color bar. Any pertinent Medicare manual references are provided. Please see the resources to review the corresponding manual citations.

Grey   Codes that have "Special Coverage Instructions" are designated by a gray color bar. Any pertinent Medicare manual references are provided. Please see the resources to review the corresponding citations.

No Color   Codes not designated by a color bar are covered at "Carrier Discretion." Contact the carrier for specific instructions.

MED: This notation precedes an instruction pertaining to this code in the Centers for Medicare and Medicaid Services [CMS] Publication 100 (Pub 100) electronic manual. These CMS sources present the rules for submitting these services to the federal goverment or its contractors. See Appendix-4 of this manual for the Pub-100 references.

AHA: The Central Office on HCPCS issues a quarterly publication, *AHA's Coding Clinic for HCPCS* to provide consistent and accurate advice for proper application of HCPCS. References to specfic HCPCS coding issues are identified by the symbol AHA: followed by the issue, year, and page number. For example code A9600 includes AHA: 2Q, '02, 9. This means that in the second quarted publication in 2002 on page 9 there is information regarding assignment of A9600 Strontium Sr-89 chloride, therapeutic, per millicurie.

HCPCS in the Physician's Office

While many of the HCPCS codes relate to supplies, such as durable medical equipment, there are a lot of codes that are used to report the provision of services and pharmaceuticals.

Providers should carefully review the codes in the G section each year. For example, many of the screening codes and services are reported from this section. As previously noted, where there is a HCPCS Level II code, it supersedes a HCPCS Level I (CPT) code for Medicare. Some of those services are listed below:

G0101	Cervical or vaginal cancer screening: pelvic and clinical breast examination
G0102	Prostate cancer screening; digital rectal examination
G0104	Colorectal cancer screening; flexible sigmoidoscopy
G0108	Diabetes outpatient self-management training services, individual per 30 minutes
G0117	Glaucoma screening for high-risk patients furnished by an optometrist or ophthalmologist
G0168	Wound closure utilizing tissue adhesive(s) only

For example, physician who performs a pelvic exam with cervical cancer screening (Pap smear) and clinical breast examination would report G0101 and not an E/M service office visit or preventive medicine examination.

Health intervention and behavioral health services for Medicare patients are reported with the codes starting with "H." Specific prenatal care codes are also included in this section as well as foster care for children and supported housing for adults. State Medicaid programs also require many of these codes. Providers should review these codes and the guidelines from their state program to correctly report services.

Perhaps the best-known set of HCPCS codes by the physician practice is the J code set for pharmaceuticals. Most of these drugs are in the injectable or intravenous format. Oral forms of the medications listed are not in this section of codes and are not covered by Medicare. The drugs are also listed in generic terms and it may be necessary to convert the drug brand name to its generic name. It is also important to verify the dosage. Some drugs are listed with multiple options for dosage. If the entire dose is not used on a single dose vial the modifier JW should be reported to indicate that the remainder was discarded and not given to another patient.

Chemotherapy drugs are also listed as J codes. Again the generic name is used and many have multiple dosing options to choose from.

Many of the current HCPCS codes are considered temporary and changes are made in these sections on a yearly basis. It is important for the provider to verify these codes on a yearly basis to verify that only current codes are used. Many of these codes are assigned while the CPT process determines if a permanent CPT code will be assigned. Some of these codes replace state level codes for Medicaid that were deleted as a result of HIPAA legislation.

Modifiers

Modifiers should, or in some cases must, be used to identify circumstances that alter or enhance the description of a service or supply. As mentioned earlier, the HCPCS level II coding system also contains modifiers. These modifiers can and should be used when appropriate with either CPT or HCPCS Level II codes. In certain circumstances, modifiers must be used to report the alteration of a procedure or service.

In HCPCS Level II, modifiers are composed of two alpha- or alphanumeric characters that range from "A1" to "VP."

> E0260-NU Hospital bed, semi-electric (head and foot adjustment), with any type side rails, with mattress
>
> NU: Identifies the hospital bed as new equipment

When reporting ambulance services, separate one-character codes are used together to form a two-character modifier. The first letter indicates the origination of the patient, and the second identifies the destination.

Although both alpha and numeric modifiers are common throughout the country, some regional carriers do not recognize their use due to software limitations. It may be necessary to provide a cover letter, an invoice, or other specific documentation with the claim for clarification.

Unlisted HCPCS Codes

Unlisted HCPCS codes are unique to a section or a subsection of codes. Third-party payers designate as unlisted all HCPCS codes that include the term unlisted in the definition. In addition, payers often apply the unlisted codes to services and supplies that are described in indefinite terms, do not have a precise meaning, and/or have language open to differing interpretations. Terms and phrases commonly found in the descriptions of these unlisted HCPCS codes include the following:

- Miscellaneous
- NES (not elsewhere specified)
- NOC (not otherwise classified)
- Unclassified
- Unspecified

The DMEPOS Industry

Wheelchairs, artificial limbs, braces, surgical dressings, and medications are all examples of durable medical equipment, prosthetics, orthotics, and supplies, known by the acronyms DME and POS, or simply DMEPOS.

The DMEPOS industry includes manufacturers, pharmaceutical companies, medical equipment and supply companies (suppliers and vendors), and providers. Entities peripheral to the DMEPOS industry–but having direct impact on its operations–include the Food and Drug Administration (FDA), which approves the use of medical devices and pharmaceuticals in the United States, and federal and state health care programs, such as Medicare and Medicaid, which provide DMEPOS coverage and/or reimbursement for millions of beneficiaries. Other third-party payers, such as Blue Cross/Blue Shield, various preferred provider organizations (PPOs), workers' compensation carriers, and managed care organizations (MCOs), also influence the DMEPOS industry.

Special Federal and Third-party Payer Definitions

For federally funded health care programs, such as Medicare and the Children's Health Insurance Program (CHIP), and for programs that are partially funded by the federal government, such as some state Medicaid programs, strict definitions of what constitutes DMEPOS are delineated. A number of commercial insurance plans and MCOs also follow this same framework–or a similar one–constructed around the prescription, dispensation, reporting, and reimbursement of DMEPOS.

DEFINING DME

According to CMS, the federal agency that operates the Medicare program, DME must meet specific criteria to be eligible for coverage. These criteria are shown here in the form of questions. The provider or supplier must answer yes to all of these questions for the equipment or device to be recognized as eligible for reimbursement under the Medicare program:

- Can the medical equipment withstand repeated use?
- Is the medical equipment primarily and customarily used for medical purposes?
- Is the medical equipment not of use to a person without illness or injury or in need of improvement of a malformed body part?
- Is the medical equipment appropriate for home use?

An answer of no to any of the preceding questions could render the DME ineligible for Medicare coverage.

(Special exceptions can be made by the Medicare program, some state Medicaid programs, and other third-party payers even when the DME equipment or device does not meet the accepted definition: (1) the equipment or devices are not primarily and customarily used for medical purposes, and/or (2) the equipment or devices can be used in the absence of illness, injury, or deformity. A DMEPOS item, described by one or both of these contradicting criteria, may be eligible for Medicare coverage if the therapeutic purpose is clearly distinguished, such as use of a heat lamp where the medical need for heat therapy has been established. The fact that the patient's course of treatment is under the supervision of the physician must also be in evidence.)

DEFINING PROSTHESES

Prosthetic devices, as recognized by CMS and many third-party payers, are those devices that replace all or part of an internal body organ, or replace all or part of the function of a permanently inoperative or malfunctioning internal body organ. This category of devices includes:

- Artificial limbs
- Breast and eye prostheses
- Maxillofacial devices
- Joint implants
- Devices that replace all or part of the ear or nose
- Ostomy and colostomy bags
- Irrigation and flushing equipment directly related to ostomy/colostomy care

An example of a prosthesis is a urinary collection and retention system that replaces the function of the bladder in cases of permanent urinary incontinence. Replacement of a prosthetic device may be covered, but only when the replacement is required because of a change in the beneficiary's physical condition. Adjustments to an artificial limb or other prosthetic device required by wear or by a change in the beneficiary's physical condition may likewise be covered when ordered by a physician.

DEFINING ORTHOSES

An orthosis or orthotic device is used for the correction or prevention of skeletal deformities. This includes braces for the neck, shoulder and arm, forearm, wrist

and hand, hip, leg, ankle, and foot, as well as spinal or back devices. If there is a change in the beneficiary's physical condition that requires replacements and adjustments, those may also be covered. However, according to CMS, to be classified as an orthotic the brace must be a rigid or semi-rigid device used to support a weak or deformed body member, or to restrict or eliminate motion in a diseased or injured part of the body.

DEFINING SUPPLIES

Within the DMEPOS industry, a supply is an item or accessory needed for the effective use of a DME, prosthetic or orthotic device, or appliance. Such supplies include those drugs and biologicals that must be placed directly into equipment to achieve the therapeutic benefit of the DME or to ensure the proper function of the equipment. An example of this is the use of heparin within a home dialysis system. To be eligible for coverage by Medicare, Medicaid, and third-party payers, supplies must be medically necessary and must be prescribed by the treating provider. Supplies eligible for reimbursement by these programs and payers are typically not those bought off-the-shelf or over-the-counter at local drug stores and grocery stores. Exceptions include recent additions to covered supplies for a patient's home use, such as supplies needed with a glucometer to monitor diabetes mellitus.

DEFINING CUSTOMIZED DME

CMS's clarification of the definition of customized durable medical equipment was implemented July 19, 2013, but retroactive to January 1, 1992. The agency believes that customized items are rarely necessary and are rarely furnished.

In accordance with a longstanding definition in 42 CFR, section 414.224, the criteria listed in 42 CFR, section 414.224(a) state that "[t]o be considered a customized item for payment purposes under paragraph (b) of this section, a covered item (including a wheelchair) must be uniquely constructed or substantially modified for a specific beneficiary according to the description and orders of a physician and be so different from another item used for the same purpose that the two items cannot be grouped together for pricing purposes. (b) Payment is made on a lump sum basis for the purchase of a customized item based on the carrier's individual consideration and judgment of a reasonable payment amount for each customized item. The carrier's individual consideration takes into account written documentation on the costs of the item including at least the cost of labor and materials used in customizing an item."

The Omnibus Budget Reconciliation Act (OBRA) of November 1990 amended the criteria for treating wheelchairs as customized items. This alternative definition of customized wheelchairs was never adopted for Medicare payment purposes and should not be confused with the definition of customized items referenced above. (*Medicare Claims Processing Manual*, Pub. 100-04, chap. 20, sec. 30.3 [Trans. 2687, April 19, 2013]; *Medicare Program Integrity Manual*, Pub. 100-08, chap. 5, sec. 5.15 [Trans. 460, April 19,2013]; *Medicare One-time Notification*, Pub. 100-20 [Trans.1239, May 21, 2013]).

DMEPOS FOR HOSPITAL INPATIENTS

Medicare does not allow separate payment for durable medical equipment, prosthetics, orthotics, and supplies (DMEPOS) when a patient is in a covered inpatient stay. These claims were related to DME dates of service greater than two days prior to the Part A discharge date or the Part A discharge status was not to home. Effective July 1, 2013, the DME claim will either be rejected or, if paid, the contractor will recover payment when all of the following conditions are met:

- There is a covered Medicare Part A inpatient claim with a TOB of 111.
- The DME and the inpatient claims are for the same beneficiary HICN.
- The DME claim has a line item within the HCPCS Level II category 03 for orthotics and/or prosthesis.
- The from date of service (DOS) of the durable medical equipment item is within the Part A admit and discharge dates.
- The from DOS of the durable medical equipment line items is greater than two days prior to the beneficiary's Part A inpatient discharge date.
- The from DOS of the DME line items is within the beneficiary's Part A inpatient admission and discharge date and the patient discharge status (FL 17) is *not* equal to 01 Discharged to home or self-care (routine discharge).

(*Medicare One-time Notification*, Pub. 100-20 [trans. 1183, February 8, 2013])

The CMS Recovery Audit Contractor (RAC) Program, which is responsible for identifying and correcting improper payments in the Medicare fee-for-service payment process, identified this issue. The contractor identified DMEPOS claims for patients who received DMEPOS items while in an inpatient stay in a hospital.

Since Medicare does not allow separate payments for DMEPOS for the patient during a covered inpatient hospital stay, these payments associated with these claims are considered overpayments.

HCPCS Self Test

1. A patient is transported by helicopter 50 miles from the site of his automobile accident to a hospital. How are the transport and mileage reported?

   a. A0430 and A0435   c. A0431 and A0435
   b. A0431 and A0436   d. A0430 and A0436

2. A patient receives a 1000 ml parenteral solution of 3.5% amino acids for use at home.

   a. B4168, 2 units   c. B4172, 2 units
   b. B4185, 2 units   d. B4180, 2 units

3. A physician administers an emergency injection of 30 mg of FIRAZYR to a patient with hereditary angioedema.

   a. G9158-CI   c. G9168-CN
   b. G8996-CJ   d. G9168-CJ

4. A 45-50 minute group psychotherapy service provided in a partial hospitalization setting should be billed by a hospital using one of the HCPCS codes below:

   a. H0036   c. G0410
   b. Q5008   d. G0164

5. The definition of HCPCS is:

   a.   Health Code Practice Country System
   b.   Hickpicks Common Practice Coding System
   c.   Healthcare Current Procedural Coding System
   d.   Healthcare Common Procedure Coding System

6. Level I HCPCS refers to:

   a.   HCPCS alpha numeric codes
   b.   CPT® codes
   c.   ICD-9 codes
   d.   a and c

7. Level II HCPCS refers to:

   a.   HCPCS alphanumeric codes
   b.   CPT® codes
   c.   ICD-9 codes
   d.   a and c

8. Which of the following is not a step in coding HCPCS:

   a.   Locate main term from index
   b.   Code from index
   c.   Identify the main term
   d.   Locate any subterms under the main term

9. J codes describe:

   a. Ambulance codes   c. Temporary codes
   b. DME   d. Drugs

10. Assign the HCPCS codes for a disposable surgical tray:

    a. A4550   c. A4354
    b. A4310   d. A6206

11. A patient receives an injection of 600,000 units of Bicillin C-R. Assign the correct HCPCS code for the medication.

    a. J0561, units 2   c. J0558, units 6
    b. J0561, units 6   d. J0558

12. A patient presents to his physician's office for the administration of a pneumococcal vaccine. Assign the HCPCS code for the administration:

    a. G0008   c. G0009
    b. G0101   d. G0010

13. A postoperative patient receives 30 mg of Toradol IV for pain relief. Assign the HCPCS code used for the medication:

    a. J1885   c. J3301, 3 units
    b. J3280, 3 units   d. J1885, 2 units

14. A 68-year-old female presents to the outpatient department of the hospital to receive a 60 mg injection of Prolia for her treatment of her osteoporosis. Assign the HCPCS code used for the service:

    a. J0897 X 60   c. J0897 X 30
    b. J1740 X 60   d. J1740 X 30

15. HCPCS modifiers can be used with:

    a. CPT codes   c. ICD-9 codes
    b. HCPCS codes   d. a and b

16. A 65-year-old male patient presents to his physician for a 200 mg injection of Cimzia for treatment of severe Rheumatoid Arthritis.

    a. J0717 X 200   c. J9328 X 200
    b. J9171 X 200   d. J3489 X 200

17. A patient presents for fitting of a below-knee 40–50 mm Hg gradient compression stocking for the right leg. Assign the HCPCS code for this supply:

    a. A6532-RT   c. A6532
    b. A6535-RT   d. A6537-RT

18. A patient is directly admitted to a hospital's observation unit with a diagnosis of head injury. Assign the HCPCS code for this service:

    a. H0033   c. G0407
    b. G0378   d. G0379

19. A head injury patient presents for a protective helmet. The patient is given a hard prefabricated helmet with chin strap. Assign the HCPCS code for this service:

    a. A7036 and A8001   c. A7036 and A8003
    b. A8003   d. A8001

20. A patient receives hospice care in his home. Assign the HCPCS code for this place of service:

    a. Q5004   c. Q5009
    b. Q5002   d. Q5001

21. A patient injured from a biking accident is referred by his physician to the hospital radiology clinic for an MRA of the spinal canal and contents. The physician requests this MRA to include contrast. One of the below HCPCS codes should be used:

    a. C8914   c. C8920
    b. C8931   d. C8934

22. A patient with an MRSA infection in an open skin wound of his leg was placed on an infusion of 600 mg of Teflaro every 12 hours in the outpatient hospital infusion department. What is the correct HCPCS code and units for a 24-hour dose?

    a. J0712 X 2   c. C9254 X 1200
    b. J0290 X 10   d. J0712 X 120

23. A patient presents to the hospital outpatient department to receive 400 mg of NULOJIX by IV infusion. What is the correct HCPCS code and units for the medication.

    a. J0490 X 400   c. J0490 X 40
    b. J0475 X 10   d. Q0139 X 400

24. What is the code and modifier used by a therapist to report a patient's current memory functional limitation status of 30 percent impairment at the time of initial therapy?

    a. G9158-CI   c. G9168-CN
    b. G8996-CJ   d. G9168-CJ

Answer Key can be found in the back of the book.

Childbirth — *continued*
early induction, G9355-G9356
elective delivery, G9355-G9356
Lamaze, S9436
post-partum education, G9357-G9358
post-partum evaluation, G9357-G9358
post-partum screening, G9357-G9358
preparation, S9436
refresher, S9437
VBAC (vaginal birth after cesarean), S9439
Childcare, T2026-T2027
parents in treatment, T1009
Chin
cup, cervical, L0150
strap (for CPAP device), A7036
Chlorhexidine, A4248
Chondrocyte cell harvest, arthroscopic, S2112
Chopart prosthetic
ankle, L5050, L5060
below knee, L5100
Chore services, S5130-S5131
Christian Science provider services, S9900
Chromic phosphate, A9564
Chux, A4554
Clamp
external urethral, A4356
Classes, S9441-S9446
asthma, S9441
birthing, S9442
exercise, S9451
infant safety, S9447
lactation, S9443
nutrition, S9452
parenting, S9444
smoking cessation, S9453
stress management, S9454
weight management, S9449
Clavicle
splint, L3650
Cleaning solvent, Nu-Hope
4 oz bottle, A4455
16 oz bottle, A4455
Cleanser, wound, A6260
Cleft palate, feeder, S8265
Clevis, hip orthotic, L2570, L2600, L2610
Clinical trials
lodging costs, S9994
meals, S9996
phase II, S9990
phase III, S9991
service, S9988
transportation costs, S9992
Clinic visit/encounter, T1015
hospital outpatient, G0463
multidisciplinary, child services, T1025
Closure device, vascular, C1760
Clotting time tube, A4771
Clubfoot wedge, L3380
Cochlear implant, L8614
battery
alkaline, L8622
lithium, L8623-L8624
zinc, L8621
headset, L8615
microphone, L8616
replacement, L8619
transmitter cable, L8618
transmitting coil, L8617
zinc, L8621
Coil, imaging, C1770
Collagen
implant, urinary tract, L8603
microporous nonhuman origin, C9352-C9353
skintest, Q3031
wound dressing, A6021-A6024
Collar
cervical
contour (low, standard), L0120
multiple post, L0180-L0200
nonadjustable foam, L0120
Philadelphia tracheotomy, L0172
Philly one-piece extraction, L0150
tracheotomy, L0172
traction, E0856
turtle neck safety, E0942

Colonoscopy, cancer screening
adenoma or neoplasm detected, G9252-G9253
patient at high risk, G0105
patient not at high risk, G0121
Coloplast
closed pouch, A5051
drainable pouch, A5061
closed, A5054
small, A5063
skin barrier
4 x 4, A4362
6 x 6, A5121
8 x 8, A5122
stoma cap, A5055
Coma stimulation, S9056
Combo-Seat universal raised toilet seat, E0244
Commode, E0160-E0171
chair, E0163-E0165, E0170-E0171
lift, E0172, E0625
pail, E0167
seat, wheelchair, E0968
Communication board, E1902
Companion care, S5135-S5136
Composite
dressing, A6203-A6205
Compressed gas system, E0424-E0480
Compression
bandage
high, A6452
light, A6448
medium, A6451
burn garment, A6501-A6512
burn mask, A6513
stockings, A6530-A6549
wrap, A6545
Compressogrip prosthetic shrinker, L8440-L8465
Compressor, E0565, E0570, E0650-E0652, E0670, K0738
Concentrator
oxygen, E1390-E1392
rental, E1392
Condom
female, A4268
male, A4267
Conductive
garment (for TENS), E0731
paste or gel, A4558
Conductivity meter (for dialysis), E1550
Conference
interdisciplinary team, G0175
Conforming bandage, A6442-A6447
Congenital torticollis orthotic, L0112
Congo red, blood, P2029
Consultation
telehealth, G0406-G0408, G0425-G0427
Contact layer, A6206-A6208
Contact lens, S0500, S0512-S0514, V2500-V2599
Continent device, A5081, A5082
Continuous intraoperative neurophysiology monitoring, G0453
Continuous passive motion exercise device, E0936
Continuous positive airway pressure (CPAP) device, E0601
chin strap, A7036
face mask, A7030-A7031
filter, A7038-A7039
headgear, A7035
nasal application accessories, A7032-A7034
oral interface, A7044
tubing, A7037
Contraceptive
cervical cap, A4261
condom
female, A4268
male, A4267
diaphragm, A4266
foam, A4269
gel, A4269
hormone patch, J7304
implant, A4264, J7306
intratubal occlusion device, A4264
intrauterine, copper, J7300
Levonorgestrel, implants and supplies, J7301-J7302, J7306
pills, S4993

Contraceptive — *continued*
spermicide, A4269
vaginal ring, J7303
Contracts, maintenance, ESRD, A4890
Contrast material
high osmolar, Q9958-Q9964
injection during MRI, A9575-A9579, Q9953
low osmolar, Q9951, Q9965-Q9967
nonradioactive NOC, A9698
oral MRI, Q9954
Controlyte, enteral nutrition, B4155
Coordinated care fee
home monitoring, G9006
initial rate, G9001
maintenance rate, G9002
physician oversight, G9008
risk adjusted, G9003-G9005
scheduled team conference, G9007
Copying fee, medical records, S9981-S9982
Corneal tissue processing, V2785
Corn, trim or remove, S0390
Coronary artery bypass surgery, direct
with coronary arterial and venous grafts
single, each, S2208
two arterial and single venous, S2209
with coronary arterial grafts, only
single, S2205
two grafts, S2206
with coronary venous grafts, only
single, S2207
Corset, spinal orthotic, L0970-L0976
Cough stimulation device, E0482
Counseling
alcohol, G0443
cardiovascular disease risk, G0446
end of life, S0257
genetic, S0265
obesity, G0447
prevention
sexually transmitted infection, G0445
Coupling gel/paste, A4559
Cover, shower
ventricular assist device, Q0501
Cover, wound
alginate dressing, A6196-A6198
foam dressing, A6209-A6214
hydrocolloid dressing, A6234-A6239
hydrogel dressing, A6242-A6248
specialty absorptive dressing, A6251-A6256
CPAP (continuous positive airway pressure) device, E0601
chin strap, A7036
exhalation port, A7045
face mask, A7030-A7031
headgear, A7035
humidifier, E0561-E0562
nasal application accessories, A7032-A7034
oral interface, A7044
supplies, E0470-E0472, E0561-E0562
tubing, A7037
Cradle, bed, E0280
Crisis intervention, H2011, S9484-S9485, T2034
Criticare HN, enteral nutrition, B4153
Crutch
substitute
lower leg platform, E0118
Crutches, E0110-E0116
accessories, A4635-A4637, E2207
aluminum, E0114
articulating, spring assisted, E0117
forearm, E0111
Ortho-Ease, E0111
underarm, other than wood, pair, E0114
Quikfit Custom Pack, E0114
Red Dot, E0114
underarm, wood, single, E0113
Ready-for-use, E0113
wooden, E0112
Cryoprecipitate, each unit, P9012
CTLSO, L0700, L0710, L1000-L1120
Cuirass, E0457
Culture sensitivity study, P7001
Curasorb, alginate dressing, A6196-A6199
Cushion
decubitus care, E0190
Oral/Nasal, A7029

Cushion — *continued*
positioning, E0190
wheelchair
AK addition, L5648
BK addition, L5646
Custom
DME, K0900
wheelchair/base, K0008, K0013
Customized item (in addition to code for basic item), S1002
Custom Masterhinge Hip Hinge 3, L2999
Cyanocobalamin cobalt, A9546, A9559
Cycler
disposable set, A4671
Cycler dialysis machine, E1594
Cylinder tank carrier, E2208
Cystourethroscopy
for uteral calculi, S2070
Cytopathology, screening, G0123, G0124, G0141, G0143-G0148

D

Day care services, S5100-S5102, S5105
Decompression
disc, S2348
hip core, S2325
vertebral axial, S9090
Decubitus care equipment, E0181
cushion or pillow, E0190
mattress
AquaPedic Sectional Gel Flotation, E0196
Iris Pressure Reduction/Relief, dry, E0184
PressureGuard II, air, E0186
TenderFlo II, E0187
TenderGel II, E0196
pressure pads, overlays, E0197-E0199
Body Wrap, E0199
Geo-Matt, E0199
Iris, E0199
PressureKair, E0197
Richfoam Convoluted and Flat, E0199
pressure pads, with pumps, E0181
Bio Flote, E0181
KoalaKair, E0181
protectors
heel or elbow, E0191
Body Wrap Foam Positioners, E0191
Pre-Vent, E0191
pump, E0182
Bio Flote, E0182
Pillo, E0182
TenderCloud, E0182
Deionizer, water purification system, E1615
Delivery/set-up/dispensing, A9901
Delivery system
kidney, E1510
oxygen, topical, E0446
Delivery to high risk area requiring escort, S9381
Delta-Cast Elite Casting Material, A4590
Delta-Lite Conformable Casting Tape, A4590
Delta-Lite C-Splint Fiberglass Immobilizer, A4590
Delta-Lite "S" Fiberglass Casting Tape, A4590
Deluxe item, S1001
Demonstration project
clinic, G9140
Oseltamivir phosphate oral, G9019, G9035
Rimantadine HCl oral, G9036
Zanamivir inhalation powder, G9018, G9034
Dennis Browne, foot orthotic, L3140, L3150
Depression, G9193-G9195, G9212-G9213, G9232
Derata injection device, A4210
Destruction
lesion, G0186
tumor, S2095
Detector, blood leak, dialysis, E1560
Device
auditory osseointegrated, L8691, L8695
continuous passive motion, E0936
electrical stimulation device for cancer treatment, E0766
endoscope colonoscope implantable, C1749
intermittent limb compression, E0676
joint, C1776
medication management, T1505
occlusive device placement, G0269
ocular, C1784

Device — *continued*
  reaching/grabbing, A9281
  retrieval, C1773
  speech generating, E2500
  tissue localization and excision, C1819
  urinary incontinence repair, C1771, C2631
  ventricular assist device
    supply, Q0507-Q0509
Dextrostick, A4772
Diabetes
  alcohol swabs, per box, A4245
  battery for blood glucose monitor, A4233-
    A4236
  bent needle set for insulin pump infusion,
    A4231
  blood glucose monitor, E0607
    with integrated lancer, E2101
    with voice synthesizer, E2100
  blood glucose test strips, box of 50, A4253
  drugs
    Humalin, J1815, J1817
    Humalog, J1817, S5551
    insulin, J1815, J1817, S5551
    Novolin, J1815, J1817
  evaluation and management LOPS, G0245
  injection device, needle-free, A4210
  insulin pump, external, E0784
    infusion set, A4231
    syringe with needle, A4232
  lancet device, A4258
  lancets, box of 100, A4259
  non-needle cannula for insulin infusion, A4232
  retinal exam, S3000
  self management training
    group, G0109
    individual, G0108
  shoe
    fitting, A5500
    inlay, A5508
    insert, A5512-A5513
    modification, A5503-A5507
  syringe, disposable
    box of 100, S8490
    each, A4206
  urine glucose/ketone test strips, box of 100,
    A4250
Diabetic management program
  dietitian visit, S9465
  E/M of sensory neuropathy, G0246-G0247
  follow-up visit to MD provider, S9141
  follow-up visit to non-MD provider, S9140
  foot care, G0247
  group session, S9455
  insulin pump initiation, S9145
  nurse visit, S9460
Dialet lancet device, A4258
Dialysate
  concentrate additives, A4765
  peritoneal dialysis solution, A4720-A4726,
    A4766
  solution, A4728
  testing solution, A4760
Dialysis
  access system, C1881
  air bubble detector, E1530
  anesthetic, A4736-A4737
  bath conductivity, meter, E1550
  blood leak detector, E1560
  centrifuge, E1500
  cleaning solution, A4674
  concentrate
    acetate, A4708
    acid, A4709
    bicarbonate, A4706-A4707
  documentation, G9231
  drain bag/bottle, A4911
  emergency treatment, G0257
  equipment, E1510-E1699
  extension line, A4672-A4673
  filter, A4680
  fluid barrier, E1575
  heating pad, E0210
  hemostats, E1637
  home equipment repair, A4890
  infusion pump, E1520
  mask, surgical, A4928

Dialysis — *continued*
  peritoneal
    clamps, E1634
    pressure alarm, E1540
    scale, E1639
    shunt accessory, A4740
    supplies, A4671-A4918
    surgical mask, A4928
    syringe, A4657
    tourniquet, A4929
    unipuncture control system, E1580
Dialyzer, artificial kidney, A4690
Diaper service, T4538
Diaphragm, contraceptive, A4266
Dietary education, S9449, S9452
Disarticulation
  lower extremities, prosthesis, L5000-L5999
  upper extremities, prosthesis, L6000-L6692
Discharge, patient, G9254-G9255
Disease management program, S0315, S0317,
    S0320
Disetronic
  glass cartridge syringe for insulin pump, each,
    A4232
  H-Tron insulin pump, E0784
  insulin infusion set with bent needle, with or
    without wings, each, A4231
Diskard head halter, E0940
Disk decompression, lumbar, S2348
Diskectomy, lumbar, S2350, S2351
  single interspace, S2350
Dispensing fee
  BICROS, V5240
  binaural, V5160
  CROS, V5200
  monaural hearing aid, V5241
  new spectacle lenses, S0595
  pharmacy
    inhalation drugs, G0333, Q0513-Q0514
Disposable
  diapers, A4335
  glucose monitor, A9275
  supplies, ambulance, A0382-A0398
  underpads, A4554
DNA analysis, S3840
  fecal, S3890
Documentation
  antibiotic regimen, G9286-G9287
  aspirin use or non use, G9277-G9278
  maintenance hemodialysis with catheter,
    G9239
  non-reporting of histological type, G9282,
    G9288
  non-tobacco user, G9275
  patient death, G9256, G9260, G9262
  patient discharged home, G9254-G9255
  patient pain, G9250-G9251
  patient survival, G9259, G9261, G9263
  patient with complications, G9267-G9268
  patient without complications, G9269-G9270
  tobacco user, G9276
  viral load, G9242-G9243
Dome
  and mouthpiece (for nebulizer), A7016
Don-Joy
  cervical support collar, L0150
  deluxe knee immobilizer, L1830
  wrist forearm splint, L3984
Donor cadaver
  harvesting multivisceral organs, with allografts,
    S2055
Doppler, transesophageal, G9157
Dornix Plus, E0601
Dorsiwedge Night Splint, A4570, T2999, L4398
Dose optimization, for infusion, S3722
Dosimeter, implantable radiation, ea, A4650
Double bar
  AK, knee-ankle-foot orthotic, L2020, L2030
  BK, ankle-foot orthotic, L1990
Drainage
  bag, A4357, A4358, A4911
  board, postural, E0606
  bottle, A4911, A5102
Dressing — *see also* Bandage, A6021-A6404
  absorptive, for use with suction pump, K0744-
    K0746

Dressing — *see also* Bandage — *continued*
  alginate, A6196-A6199
  composite, A6203-A6205
  contact layer, A6206-A6208
  film, A6257-A6259
  foam, A6209-A6215
  gauze, A6216-A6230, A6402-A6404
  holder/binder, A4461, A4463
  hydrocolloid, A6234-A6241
  hydrogel, A6242-A6248
  specialty absorptive, A6251-A6256
  tape, A4450, A4452
  transparent film, A6257-A6259
  tubular, A6457
Dropper, A4649
Drug delivery system
  controlled dose delivery system, K0730
  disposable, A4306
Drug screen, G0431, G0434
Drugs - see Table of Drugs
  administered through a metered dose inhaler,
    J3535
  disposable delivery system, 50 ml or greater
    per hour, A4305
  disposable delivery system, 5 ml or less per
    hour, A4306
  infusion supplies, A4221, A4222, A4230-A4232
  not otherwise classified, J3490, J7599, J7699,
    J7799, J8499, J8999, J9999
  Part B drug CAP NOC, Q4082
Dry pressure pad/mattress, E0184, E0199
DSM IV criteria major depressive disorder,
    G9212-G9213
Dunlap
  heating pad, E0210
Duolock curved tail closures, A4421
Durable medical equipment (DME), E0100-E8002
Duratest
  -100, J1070
  -200, J1080
Durr-Fillauer
  cervical collar, L0140
  Pavlik harness, L1620

Ear wax removal, G0268
Easy Care
  folding walker, E0143
  quad cane, E0105
ECG
  initial Medicare ECG, G0403-G0405
Echocardiogram
  transesophageal, C8925-C8928
  transthoracic, C8921-C8924, C8929-C8930
Echosclerotherapy, S2202
Economy knee splint, L1830
Edetate
  calcium disodium, J0600
  edetate disodium, J3520
Education
  asthma, S9441
  birthing, S9436-S9439, S9442
  chronic kidney disease, G0420-G0421
  diabetes, S9145
  exercise, S9451
  family planning
    individualized programs, school based,
      T1018
    nonmedical, H1010
  infant safety, S9447
  lactation, S9443
  Lamaze, S9436
  mental health problems, G0177
  parenting, S9444
  smoking cessation, S9453
  stress management, S9454
  weight management, S9449
EEG
  automated monitoring, S9015
Eggcrate dry pressure pad/mattress, E0184,
    E0199
Elastic garment/covering, A4466
Elastic support, A6530-A6549
Elbow
  brace, universal rehabilitation, L3720
  disarticulation, endoskeletal, L6450

Elbow — *continued*
  Masterhinge Elbow Brace 3, L3999
  orthotic
    EO, E1800, L3702-L3740, L3760-L3762
    EWHO, L3764-L3766
  protector, E0191
Electrical stimulation, S8930
Electrical stimulation device for cancer treat-
    ment, E0766
Electrical work, dialysis equipment, A4870
Electric hand
  adult, L7007
  independently articulating digits, L6880
  pediatric, L7008
Electric heat pad for peritoneal dialysis, E0210
Electric hook, L7009
Electric stimulator supplies, A4595
Electrode
  Electrodes, per pair, A4556
  Electrode/transducer, A4555
Electrodes, per pair, A4556
Electromagnetic therapy, G0295, G0329
Electron beam computed tomography, S8092
Elevating leg rest, K0195
Elevator, air pressure, heel, E0370
Embolization, protection system, C1884
  for tumor destruction, S2095
Embryo
  cryopreserved transferred, S4037
  monitor/store cryopreserved, S4040
  storage, S4027
Emergency response system, S5160-S5162
EMG
  biofeedback device, E0746
  surface, S3900
Encounter, clinic, T1015
Endarterectomy, chemical, M0300
End of life care planning, S0257
Endoscope
  colonoscope device (implantable), C1749
  sheath, A4270
Endoscopy
  full thickness plication stomach, C9724
  nasal, S2342
Endoskeletal system, addition, L5925, L5984
Enema
  bag, reusable, A4458
  barium, G0106
  cancer screening, G0120
Enrich, enteral nutrition, B4150
Ensure, enteral nutrition, B4150
  HN, B4150
  Plus, B4152
  Plus HN, B4152
  powder, B4150
Enteral
  administration services, feeding, S9340-S9343
  feeding supply kit (syringe) (pump) (gravity),
    B4034-B4036
  fiber or additive, B4104
  formulae, B4150-B4162
    electrolytes, B4102, B4103
    for metabolic disease, B4157
    intact nutrients, B4149, B4150, B4152
    pediatric, B4158-B4162
  gastronomy tube, B4087-B4088
  nutrition infusion pump (with alarm) (without),
    B9000, B9002
  supplies, not otherwise classified, B9998
Enterostomal therapy, S9474
Eosinophil count, S3630
Equestrian/hippotherapy, S8940
ESRD End Stage Renal Disease — *see also* Dialysis
  bundle demo/basic, G9013
    expanded, G9014
  documentation, G9231
  machines and accessories, E1510-E1699
  plumbing, A4870
  supplies, A4651-A4913
Evaluation
  comprehensive, multi-discipline, H2000
  for power mobility device, G0372
  ocularist, S9150
  risk factors, G9298-G9299
  self assessment, depression, S3005
  team for handicapped, T1024

Integra — *continued*
  meshed bilayer wound matrix, C9363
  osteoconductive scaffold putty, C9359
  osteoconductive scaffold strip, C9362
Interface
  cough stimulating device, A7020
  oral with suction pump, A7047
Intermittent
  limb compression device, E0676
  peritoneal dialysis system, E1592
  positive pressure breathing (IPPB) machine, E0500
Interphalangeal joint, prosthetic implant, L8658
Interscapular thoracic prosthesis
  endoskeletal, L6570
  upper limb, L6350-L6370
Interspinous process distraction device, C1821
Intervention
  alcohol and/or drug, H0050
  leak of endoluminal contents, G9305-G9306
Intrafallopian transfer
  complete cycle, gamete, S4013
  complete cycle, zygote, S4014
  donor egg cycle, S4023
  incomplete cycle, S4017
Intraocular lenses, C1780, C1840, Q1004-Q1005, S0596, V2630-V2632
  new technology
    category 4, Q1004
    category 5, Q1005
  presbyopia correcting function, V2788
  refractive correcting, S0596
  telescopic, C1840
Intratubal occlusion device, A4264
Intrauterine device
  copper contraceptive, J7300
  other, S4989
  Progestacert, S4989
Introducer sheath
  guiding, C1766, C1892, C1893
  other than guiding, C1894, C2629
In vitro fertilization, S4011
Iodine 125, A9527, A9532, C2638-C2639
Iodine I-131
  albumin, A9524
  iobenguane sulfate, A9508
  sodium iodide, A9517
Iodine swabs/wipes, A4247
IPD
  system, E1592
IPPB machine, E0500
  delivery device, A9274, E0784, S5560-S5561, S5565-S5571
  home infusion administration, S9353
  intermediate acting, S5552
  long acting, S5553
  NPH, J1815, S5552
  outpatient IV treatment, G9147
  rapid onset, S5550-S5551
Ipratropium bromide
  administered through DME, J7644-J7645
Iris Preventix pressure relief/reduction mattress, E0184
Iris therapeutic overlays, E0199
IRM ankle-foot orthotic, L1950
Iron
  sucrose, J1756
Irrigation/evacuation system, bowel
  control unit, E0350
  disposable supplies for, E0352
Irrigation supplies, A4320, A4322, A4355, A4397-A4400
  Surfit
    irrigation sleeve, A4397
    night drainage container set, A5102
  Visi-flow irrigator, A4398, A4399
Islet cell transplant
  laparoscopy, G0342
  laparotomy, G0343
  percutaneous, G0341
Isocal, enteral nutrition, B4150
  HCN, B4152
Isoetharine
  inhalation solution
    concentrated, J7647
    unit dose, J7649-J7650

Isolates, B4150, B4152
Isoproterenol HCl
  administered through DME, J7657-J7660
Isosulfan blue, Q9968
Isotein, enteral nutrition, B4153
IV, G0459
  administration set, non-PVC, S1016
  infusion, OPPS, C8957
  pole, E0776, K0105
  solution
    5% dextrose/normal saline, J7042
    10% LMD, J7100
    D-5-W, J7070
    dextran, J7100, J7110
    Gentran, J7100, J7110
    normal saline, A4217, J7030-J7040, J7050
    Rheomacrodex, J7100
    Ringer's lactate, J7120
  tubing extension set, S1015

J

Jace tribrace, L1832
Jacket
  scoliosis, L1300, L1310
J-cell battery, replacement for blood glucose monitor, A4234
Jejunostomy tube, B4087-B4088
Joint device, C1776
  transcutaneous electrical stimulation, E0762

K

Kaltostat, alginate dressing, A6196-A6199
Kartop Patient Lift, toilet or bathroom (*see also* Lift), E0625
Keratectomy photorefractive, S0810
Keratoprosthesis, C1818
Keto-Diastix, box of 100 glucose/ketone urine test strips, A4250
Key-Pred
  -25,-50, J2650
Kidney
  ESRD supply, A4651-A4913
  system, E1510
  wearable artificial, E1632
Kingsley gloves, above hands, L6890
Kits
  asthma, S8097
  enteral feeding supply (syringe) (pump) (gravity), B4034-B4036
  fistula cannulation (set), A4730
  parenteral nutrition, B4220-B4224
  surgical dressing (tray), A4550
  tracheostomy, A4625
Knee
  Adjustabrace 3, L2999
  disarticulation, prosthesis, L5150-L5160, L5312
  extension/flexion device, E1812
  functional status residual score, G8647
  immobilizer, L1830
  joint, miniature, L5826
  Knee-O-Prene Hinged Wraparound Knee Support, L1810
  locks, L2405-L2425
  Masterbrace 3, L2999
  Masterhinge Adjustabrace 3, L2999
  orthotic (KO), E1810, L1810, L1820, L1830-L1860
Knee-O-Prene Hinged Knee Sleeve, L1810
Knee-O-Prene Hinged Wraparound Knee Support, L1810
Knee Support, L2000-L2038, L2126-L2136
KnitRite
  prosthetic
    sheath, L8400-L8415
    sock, L8420-L8435
    stump sock, L8470-L8485
K-Y Lubricating Jelly, A4332, A4402
Kyphosis pad, L1020, L1025

L

Laboratory tests
  chemistry, P2028-P2038
  microbiology, P7001
  miscellaneous, P9010-P9615, Q0111-Q0115
  toxicology, P3000-P3001, Q0091

Labor care (not resulting in delivery), S4005
Lacrimal duct implant
  permanent, A4263
  temporary, A4262
Lancet, A4258, A4259
Laparoscopy, surgical
  esophageal sphincter augmentation, C9737
  esophagomyotomy, S2079
Laryngectomy
  tube, A7520-A7522
Larynx, artifcial, L8500
Laser
  application, S8948
  assisted uvulopalatoplasty (LAUP), S2080
  in situ keratomileusis, S0800
  myringotomy, S2225
Laser skin piercing device, for blood collection, E0620
  replacement lens, A4257
LAUP, S2080
Lead
  adaptor
    neurostimulator, C1883
    pacing, C1883
  cardioverter, defibrillator, C1777, C1895, C1896
  environmental, home evaluation, T1029
  neurostimulator, C1778
  neurostimulator/test kit, C1897
  pacemaker, C1779, C1898, C1899
  ventricular, C1900
Leg
  bag, A4358, A5112
  extensions for walker, E0158
  Nextep Contour Lower Leg Walker, L2999
  Nextep Low Silhouette Lower Leg Walkers, L2999
  rest, elevating, K0195
  rest, wheelchair, E0990
  strap, A5113, A5114, K0038, K0039
Legg Perthes orthotic, A4565, L1700-L1755
Lens
  aniseikonic, V2118, V2318
  contact, V2500-V2599
  deluxe feature, V2702
  eye, S0504-S0508, S0580-S0590, S0596, V2100-V2615, V2700-V2799
  intraocular, C1780, C1840, V2630-V2632
  low vision, V2600-V2615
  mirror coating, V2761
  occupational multifocal, V2786
  polarization, V2762
  polycarbonate, V2784
  progressive, V2781
  skin piercing device, replacement, A4257
  telescopic, C1840
  tint, V2744
    addition, V2745
Lenticular lens
  bifocal, V2221
  single vision, V2121
  trifocal, V2321
Lerman Minerva spinal orthotic, L0174
Lesion
  destruction, G0186
Leukocyte
  poor blood, each unit, P9016
Levine, stomach tube, B4087-B4088
Levonorgestrel, contraceptive implants and supplies, J7302, J7306
Lice infestation treatment, A9180
Lifescan lancets, box of 100, A4259
Lifestand manual wheelchair, K0009
Lifestyle modification program, coronary heart disease, S0340-S0342
Lift
  combination, E0637
  patient, and seat, E0621-E0635
  Hoyer
    Home Care, E0621
    Partner All-Purpose, hydraulic, E0630
    Partner Power Multifunction, E0625
  shoe, L3300-L3334
  standing frame system, E0638
Lift-Aid patient lifts, E0621
Light box, E0203
Lispro insulin, S5551

Lithium battery for blood glucose monitor, A4233-A4236
Lithrotripsy, gallstones, S9034
Little Ones
  drainable pouch, A5063
  mini-pouch, A5054
  one-piece custom drainable pouch, A5061
  one-piece custom urostomy pouch, A5071
  pediatric belt, A4367
  pediatric urine collector, A4335
  urostomy pouch, transparent, A5073
Lively, knee-ankle-foot orthotic, L2038
Lobectomy, lung, donor, S2061
Lodging
  recipient, escort nonemergency transport, A0180, A0200
  transplant-related, S9975
  NOS, S9976
Lomustine, S0178
Lonalac powder, enteral nutrition, B4150
Lower limb, prosthesis, addition, L5968
Low osmolar contrast
  100-199 mgs iodine, Q9965
  200-299 mgs iodine, Q9966
  300-399 mgs iodine, Q9967
  400 or greater mgs iodine, Q9951
LPN services, T1003
Lubricant, A4332, A4402
Lumbar
  orthotic, L0625-L0627
  pad, L1030, L1040
  sacral orthotic (LSO), L0628-L0640
Lung volume reduction surgery services, G0302-G0305
LVRS services, G0302-G0305
Lymphedema therapy, S8950

M

Madamist II medication compressor/nebulizer, E0570
Magnacal, enteral nutrition, B4152
Magnetic
  resonance angiography, C8900, C8901-C8914, C8918-C8920, C8931-C8936
  resonance cholangiopancreatography, S8037
  resonance imaging, low field, S8042
  source imaging, S8035
Maintenance contract, ESRD, A4890
Male erection system, L7900
Malibu cervical turtleneck safety collar, L0150
Mammography, G0202-G0206
Management
  disease, S0316-S0317
Mapping
  topographic brain, S8040
  vessels, G0365
Marker
  tissue, A4648
Mask
  burn compression, A6513
  CPAP, A7027
  oxygen, A4620
  surgical, for dialysis, A4928
Mastectomy
  bra, L8002
  camisole, S8460
  form, L8020
  prosthesis, L8000-L8039, L8600
  sleeve, L8010
Masterbrace 3, L2999
Masterfoot Walking Cast Sole, L3649
Masterhinge Adjustabrace 3, L2999
Masterhinge Elbow Brace 3, L3999
Masterhinge Hip Hinge 3, L2999
Masterhinge Shoulder Brace 3, L3999
Masters 2 step, S3904
Mattress
  air pressure, E0186, E0197
  alternating pressure, E0277
    pad, Bio Flote, E0181
    pad, KoalaKair, E0181
  AquaPedic Sectional, E0196
  decubitus care, E0196
  dry pressure, E0184
  flotation, E0184
  gel pressure, E0196

Orthomedics
ankle-foot orthotic, L1900
pediatric hip abduction splint, L1640
plastic foot drop brace, L1960
single axis shoe insert, L2180
ultralight airplane arm abduction splint, L3960
upper extremity fracture orthotic
combination, L3763
humeral, L3980
radius/ulnar, L3982
Orthomerica
below knee test socket, L5620
pediatric hip abduction splint, L1640
plastic foot drop brace, L1960
single axis shoe insert, L2180
upper extremity fracture orthotic
humeral, L3980
radius/ulnar, L3982
Orthopedic devices, E0910-E0948
cervical
Diskard head halters, E0942
Turtle Neck safety collars, E0942
Orthopedic shoes
arch support, L3040-L3100
footwear, L3201-L3265
insert, L3000-L3030
lift, L3300-L3334
miscellaneous additions, L3500-L3595
positioning device, L3140-L3170
transfer, L3600-L3649
wedge, L3340-L3420
Orthoplast Splints (and Orthoplast II Splints),
A4590
Orthotic additions
ankle/foot, L5969
carbon graphite lamination, L2755
cervical congenital torticollis, L0112
electric lock, L6638
electronic elbow with microprocessor, L7181
endoskeletal knee-shin system, L5848
with microprocessor, L5856, L5857
fracture, L2180-L2192, L3995
halo, L0859
lock mechanism for elbow, L6698
lower extremity, K0672, L2200-L2999, L5646-
L5648, L5781-L5782, L5984
ratchet lock, L2430
removable soft interface, K0672
replacement strap, L4002
rocker bottom for ankle, L2232
scoliosis, L1010-L1120, L1210-L1290
shoe, L3300-L3595, L3649
shoulder lock, L6646-L6648
socket insert for elbow, L6694-L6697
spinal, L0970-L0999
suspension sleeve for knee, L5685
upper extremity joint, L3956
upper limb, E2631-E2633, L3956, L3995
vacuum pump, L5781-L5782
Orthotic devices
additions, L1005-L1120, L1210-L1290, L5961,
L5988-L5990, L6611, L6624
ankle-foot (see also Orthopedic shoes), E1815,
E1830, L1900-L1990, L2108-L2116,
L3160, L4396-L4397, L4631
anterior-posterior-lateral, L0700, L0710
cervical, L0112, L0180-L0200
cervical-thoracic-lumbar-sacral, L0700, L0710,
L1000-L1001
congenital torticollis, L0112
cranial-cervical, L0113
cranial remolding, S1040
elbow, E1800, L3702-L3740
finger, L3925, L3927
fracture, L3980-L3984
halo, L0810-L0830
hand, E1805, E1825, L3900-L3930
hip, L1600-L1686
hip-knee-ankle-foot, L2040-L2090
interface material, E1820
knee, E1810, L1810-L1820, L1830-L1860
knee-ankle-foot, L2000-L2038, L2126-L2136
Legg Perthes, A4565, L1700-L1755
lumbar, L0625-L0627
lumbar-sacral, L0628-L0651
lumbar-sacral, hip, femur, L1690

Orthotic devices — continued
multiple post collar, L0180-L0200
not otherwise specified, L0999, L1499, L2999,
L3999, L5999, L7499, L8039
pneumatic splint, L4350-L4370
preparatory below knee, L5535
repair or replacement, L4000-L4210
replace soft interface material, L4392-L4394
sacroiliac, L0621-L0624
scoliosis, L1000, L1200, L1300-L1499
shoulder, L3650-L3671, L3674-L3678
shoulder-elbow-wrist-hand, L3960-L3962
spinal, cervical, L0112, L0180-L0200
thoracic belt, L0220
thoracic-lumbar-sacral, L0450-L0492, L1200
toe, E1830
transfer (shoe orthotic), L3600-L3640
walking splint, nonpneumatic, L4386
wrist hand, L3150, L3905-L3908, L3916
wrist hand finger, L3806-L3809, L3900-L3904,
L3931
Oseltamivir phosphate, G9019, G9035
Osmolite, enteral nutrition, B4150
HN, B4150
Ossicula prosthetic implant, L8613
Osteogenic stimulator, E0747-E0749, E0760
Osteotomy, periacetabular, S2115
Ostomy
absorbent material, A4422
accessories, A5093
adhesive remover wipes, A4456
appliance belt, A4367
clamp, A4363
cone/catheter, A4399
filter, A4368
irrigation supply, A4398, A4399
pediatric one-piece system, A5061, A5062
pediatric two-piece drainable pouch, A5063
pouch, A4416-A4420, A4423-A4434
drainable, A4412-A4413, A5056-A5057
pediatric, A5061-A5062
skin barrier, A4411, A4414-A4415
extended wear, A4407-A4410
paste, A4405-A4406
wipes or swabs, A5120
vent, A4366
Otto Bock prosthesis
battery charger, six volt, L7362
battery, six volt, L7360
hook adapter, L6628
lamination collar, L6629
pincher tool, L6810
wrist, L6629, L7260
Outpatient hospital clinic visit, G0463
Overlay, mattress, E0371-E0373
Ovulation induction, S4042
Owens & Minor
cervical collar, L0140
cervical helmet, L0120
Oximeter, E0445
probe, A4606
Oxi-Uni-Pak, E0430
Oxygen
accessory, E1352
ambulance, A0422
battery
charger, E1357
pack, E1356
chamber, hyperbaric, topical, A4575
concentrator, E1390, E1391
portable, rental, E1392
gaseous, K0738, S8120
liquid, S8121
mask, A4620
medication supplies, A4611-A4627
portable, E0433, E0443-E0444, K0738
power adapter, E1358
rack/stand, E1355
regulator, E1353
respiratory equipment/supplies, A4611-A4627,
E0424-E0480
Argyle Sentinel seal chest drainage unit,
E0460
Oxi-Uni-Pak, E0430
supplies and equipment, E0425-E0444, E0433,
E0455, E1353-E1406

Oxygen — continued
tent, E0455
tubing, A4616
water vapor enriching system, E1405, E1406
wheeled cart, E1354

P

Pacemaker
dual chamber
non-rate responsive, C2619
rate responsive, C1785
lead, C1779, C1898, C1899
monitor, E0610, E0615
other than single or dual chamber, C2621
single chamber
non-rate responsive, C2620
rate responsive, C1786
Pacer manual wheelchair, K0003
Packing strips, A6407
Pad
abdominal, L1270
adhesive, A6203-A6205, A6212-A6214, A6219-
A6221, A6237-A6239, A6245-A6247,
A6254-A6256
alginate, A6196-A6199
alternating pressure, E0181
arm, K0019
Asis, L1250
condylar, L2810
crutch, A4635
gel pressure, E0185, E0196
gluteal, L2650
gradient pressure pads, S8421-S8429
heating, E0210, E0215, E0217, E0249
heel, L3480, L3485
kyphosis, L1020, L1025
lumbar, L1030, L1040, L1240
nonadhesive (dressing), A6209-A6211, A6216-
A6218, A6222-A6224, A6228-A6230,
A6234-A6236, A6242-A6244
orthotic device interface, E1820
pressure, E0181-E0182
replacement, infrared heat system, A4639
rib gusset, L1280
sheepskin, E0188, E0189
shoe, L3430-L3485
stabilizer, L3170
sternal, L1050
thoracic, L1060, L1260
triceps, L6100
trocanteric, L1290
truss, L8320, L8330
water circulating, cold, with pump, E0218
water circulating, heat, unit, E0249
water circulating, heat, with pump, E0217
water pressure, E0198
Pail, for use with commode chair, E0167
Pain, G9250-G9251
Palladium, C2640-C2641
Panel
gene
for management of breast cancer, S3854
Pan, for use with commode chair, E0167
Pantoprazole sodium, C9113, S0164
Papanicolaou (Pap) screening smear, P3000,
P3001, Q0091
Paraffin, A4265
bath unit, E0235
Paramedic intercept, S0207-S0208
Paranasal sinus ultrasound, S9024
Parenteral nutrition
administration kit, B4224
home infusion therapy, S9364-S9368
pump, B9004, B9006
solution, B4164-B5200
supplies, not otherwise classified, B9999
supply kit, B4220, B4222
Parenting class, S9444
infant safety, S9447
Parking fee, nonemergency transport, A0170
Partial hospitalization, S0201
PASRR, T2010-T2011
Passive motion
continuous exercise device, E0936
Paste, conductive, A4558
conductive, A4558

Paste, conductive — continued
coupling for ultrasound, A4559
Pathology and laboratory tests
molecular pathology, G0452
surgical
prostate, G0416-G0419
Patient
complications, G9267-G9270
daily aspirin regimen, G9277-G9278
death, G9256, G9260, G9262
decision making, G9296-G9297
discharged to home, G9254-G9255
stroke, G9257-G9259
survival, G9259, G9261, G9263
tobacco non-user, G9276
tobacco user, G9275
Patient lift, E0625, E0637, E0639, E0640
Patten Bottom, Legg Perthes orthotic, L1755
Pavlik harness, hip orthotic, L1650
**Payment, home health bundled care improve-
ment initiative**, G9187
PCA3 testing, S3721
PCP prophylaxis, G9216-G9218
Peak flow meter, S8110
portable, S8096
Pediatric hip abduction splint
Orthomedics, L1640
Orthomerica, L1640
Pediculosis treatment, A9180
PEFR, peak expiratory flow rate meter, A4614
Pelvic and breast exam, G0101
Pelvic belt/harness/boot, E0944
Penicillin G
potassium, J2540
procaine, aqueous, J2510
Penlet II lancet device, A4258
Penlet lancet device, A4258
Percussor, E0480
Percutaneous
access system, A4301
transluminal coronary atherectomy, C9602-
C9603
transluminal revascularizaton, C9604-C9608
vertebroplasty, S2360-S2361
Perflexane lipid microspheres, Q9955
Perflutren lipid microsphere, Q9957
Peripheral
catheter infusion, C1751
Perlstein, ankle-foot orthotic, L1920
Permacol, C9364
Peroneal strap, L0980
Peroxide, A4244
Personal care item, S5199
Personal care services, T1019-T1020
Pessary, A4561-A4562
PET imaging
any site, NOS, G0235
breast, G0252
whole body, G0219
Pharmacy
compounding and dispensing, S9430
dispensing fee
inhalation drugs
per 30 days, Q0513
per 90 days, Q0514
supply fee
initial immunosuppressive drugs, Q0510
oral anticancer antiemetic or immunosuppressive drug, Q0511-Q0512
**Pharmaplast disposable insulin syringes, per
syringe**, A4206
Phelps, ankle-foot orthotic, L1920
Philadelphia tracheotomy cervical collar, L0172
Philly One-piece Extrication collar, L0150
pHisoHex solution, A4246
Photocoagulation, G0186
Phototherapy
home visit service (Bili-Lite), S9098
keratectomy (PKT), S0812
light (bilirubin), E0202
Physical exam
for college, S0622
related to surgical procedure, S0260
Physical therapy, S8990
shoulder stretch device, E1841

Physical therapy/therapist
home health setting, G0151, S9131
Physician management
home care
episodic, S0272
hospice monthly, S0271
standard monthly, S0270
Physician quality reporting system (PQRS)
ACE or ARB therapy, G8473-G8475, G8506, G8935-G8937
amoxicillin with/without clavulanate as first line antibiotic, G9313-G9315
antibiotic, G8629-G8632, G8702-G8703, G8708-G8712, G8916-G8918, G9286-G9287, G9301-G9302
anticoagulation, G8967-G8969, G8971
antidepressant medication, G8126-G8128
antilipid treatment, G8585-G8586
antimicrobial prophylaxis, G9196-G9198
antiplatelet therapy, G8579-G8581
antiretroviral, G9244-G9245
antithrombotic therapy, G8598-G8599, G8696-G8698, G8895-G8897
anti-TNF therapy, G8868-G8871
antivirals, G8458
aspirin/antithrombotic therapy, G8598-G8599, G8895-G8897, G9277-G9278
assessment, patient, G0921
bone loss, G8863
depression severity, G8930-G8931
functional outcomes, G8942
pain, G8732, G8939
suicide risk, G8932-G8933
asthma, G8645-G8646
AV fistula, G8530-G8532
back pain, G8493, G8502
beta-blocker, G8450-G8452, G8582-G8584, G9188-G9192
biopsy, G8872-G8874, G8878, G8880, G8882-G8885, G8946, G9282-G9285, G9288-G9291
blood pressure, G8476-G8478, G8752-G8756, G8783-G8785, G8886-G8889, G8950-G8952, G9273-G9274
BMI, G8417-G8422, G8938
bone loss, G8863
breast cancer, G8875-G8877, G8879, G8881, G8946
cardiac stress test imaging, G8961-G8966
cardiovascular disease, G8764, G8905
care improvement initiative home visit, G9187
case management service NEC, G9012
cataract, G0916-G0918, G8765, G8906
cataract surgery, G0915-G0916, G0918, G8627-G8628
CEA, G8838
chemotherapy, G8927-G8929
colonoscopy, G9252-G9253
complications, G9267-G9270
coordinated care fee
home monitoring, G9006
initial rate, G9001
maintenance rate, G9002
physician oversight, G9008
risk adjusted, G9003-G9005, G9009-G9011
scheduled team conference, G9007
COPD, G8757, G8898
coronary artery bypass graft (CABG), G8497, G8544
coronary artery disease (CAD), G8489, G8498
corticosteroids, G8859-G8860, G8862
counseling, G8780-G8782, G8949
CT and myocardial perfusion studies in 12 months prior to current test, G9321-G9323
CT studies reported to a radiation dose index registry, G9324-G9327
current medications, G8427-G8428
dementia, G8761, G8902
depression, G8431-G8433, G8510-G8511, G8940, G8959-G8960, G9193-G9195, G9212-G9213, G9232
DEXA, G8399-G8400, G8861
diabetes, G8485, G8494, G8777-G8779
dialysis documentation, G9231
Dicom format image data, G9328-G9329, G9340

Physician quality reporting system (PQRS) — *continued*
discharge, patient, G8818, G8825-G8826, G8833-G8834, G8838, G9254-G9255
documentation, G0920-G0922, G8427-G8464, G8474, G8478, G8629-G8631, G8702-G8703, G8722, G8724, G8768-G8772, G8778, G8781, G8840, G8907-G8915, G9224, G9231, G9239, G9250-G9251, G9254-G9264, G9275-G9278, G9282, G9286, G9288, G9292, G9316-G9317, G9320, G9323, G9359
durable medical equipment (DME), G0454
ear drainage, G8560, G8562
early induction, G9355-G9356
elder maltreatment, G8535-G8536, G8733-G8735, G8941
elective delivery, G9355-G9356
electrocardiogram (ECG), G8704-G8707
ESRD documentation, G9231
exposure to ionizing radiation, G9236, G9238
foot exam, G9224-G9226
footwear evaluation, G8410, G8415-G8416
functional outcome, G8539-G8543, G9227
functional status, risk adjusted
elbow, wrist or hand, G8670
hip, G8654
knee, G8650
lower leg, foot, or ankle, G8658
lumbar spine, G8662
neck, cranium or mandible, G8674
other general orthopedic impairment, G8674
shoulder, G8666
thoracic spine or ribs, G8674
general surgery, G9235, G9237
hearing loss, G8565, G8567
heart failure patient, G8548, G8551
hemodialysis, G8714, G8956-G8957, G9239-G9241, G9264-G9266
hemoglobin, G0908-G0910, G8973-G8976
hepatitis C, G8545, G8549, G9202-G9211
hospital readmission, G9309-G9310
hypertension, G8763, G8904, G8950-G8952
inflammatory bowel disease, G8758, G8899
influenza vaccination, G0919, G8482-G8484
intervention, leak of endoluminal contents, G9305-G9306
ischemic vascular disease, G8547, G8552
kidney disease, G8487, G8495, G8771
Kt/V, G8720
LDL, G9271-G9272
LDL-C, G8943
left ventricular ejection fraction (LVEF), G8395-G8396, G8450-G8452, G8694, G8738-G8740, G8923, G8934
left ventricular testing, G8682-G8683, G8685
level of activity, G0920
lipid assessment, G8593-G8597, G8725-G8726, G8728, G8736-G8737, G8767-G8769, G8890-G8894
lymph node, G8878, G8880, G8882
medical visit, G0463, G9246-G9249
medication list/review, G8427-G8430
melanoma, G8749, G8944
mitotic rate, G9292-G9294
neurological exam, G8404-G8406
neuropsychiatric, G8947-G8948
oncology, G8953, G8977
osteoporosis, G8401, G8635, G8861, G8863
otology referrals, G8559, G8561, G8563-G8564, G8566, G8568, G8856-G8858
pain, G8442, G8509, G8730-G8732, G9250-G9251
paranasal sinus CT
at time of or within 28 days of diagnosis, G9348-G9350
more than once within 90 days of diagnosis, G9351-G9354
Parkinson's, G8762, G8903
patient care survey, G0914, G0917
patient death, G9256, G9260, G9262
patient decision making, G9296-G9297
patient-specific risk assessment, G9316-G9317
patient stroke, G9257-G9258
patient survival, G9259, G9261, G9263

Physician quality reporting system (PQRS) — *continued*
perioperative care, G8492, G8501
pharmacological therapy, G8633-G8635
pneumococcal vaccine, G8864-G8867, G9279-G9280
positive airway pressure, G8845, G8849-G8855
post partum education, G9357-G9358
post partum evaluation, G9357-G9358
post partum screening, G9357-G9358
pregnancy documentation, G9231
pregnancy test, G8806
preoperative order, IV antibiotic, G8916-G8918
preventive care, G8486, G8496
prolonged intubation, G8569-G8570
prophylactic antibiotics, G8629-G8632, G8702-G8703
prostate cancer, G8464-G8465
prosthetic implant, G9303-G9305
recommended guidelines for incidental pulmonary nodule, G9345-G9347
reexploration, G8577-G8578
rehabilitation services, G8699-G8701
renal failure, G8575-G8576
renal transplant documentation, G9231
respiratory, G8842-G8846, G8849-G8855
retinopathy, G8397-G8398
return to the operating room, G9307-G9308
rheumatoid arthritis, G8490, G8499
Rh immune globulin (RhoGam), G8809-G8811
risk adjusted functional status, G8648-G8674
risk factor evaluation, G9298-G9299
search for patient prior imaging studies, G9341-G9344
serum creatinine, G8774-G8776
sexually transmitted disease, G9228-G9230
single-pool clearance (SpKt/V), G8713, G8717
sleep apnea, G8759, G8839-G8855, G8900
specimen site, G8797-G8798, G9295
spirometry, G8924-G8926
standard nomenclature for imaging study, G9318-G9320
statin therapy, G8815-G8817
stroke/CVA/TIA, G8573-G8574, G9257-G9259, G9261
surgical site infection, G9311-G9312
thromboembolism prophylaxis, G9199-G9201
thromboembolism risk factor, G8970, G8972
tobacco use, G8751, G9275-G9276
total clearance of urea, G8718, G8720
total knee replacement, G9233-G9234
TPA, G8600-G8602
tuberculosis screening, G9359-G9360
tumor, G8721-G8724
ultrasound, G8807-G8808
urine protein, G8770, G8772-G8773
vaccination, G9279-G9281
viral load, G9242-G9243
visual function, G0913, G0915
volume management, G8955, G8958
wheelchair evaluation, G9156
wound infection, G8571-G8572
Physician review
home INR testing, G0250
Physician supervision, G0181-G0182
Pillow
abduction, E1399
decubitus care, E0190
nasal, A7029
positioning, E0190
Pinworm examination, Q0113
Placement
applicator, breast, C9726
interstitial device radiotherapy, other than prostate, C9728
occlusive, G0269
Planning
cancer treatment, S0353-S0354
Plan of care, T2024
Plasma
autologous platelet rich plasma, G0460
frozen, P9058-P9060
multiple donor, pooled, frozen, P9023
protein fraction, P9048
single donor, fresh frozen, P9017

Plastazote, L3002, L3252, L3253, L3265, L5654-L5658
Plaster
bandages
Orthoflex Elastic Plaster Bandages, A4580
Specialist Plaster Bandages, A4580
Genmould Creamy Plaster, A4580
Specialist J-Splint Plaster Roll Immobilizer, A4580
Specialist Plaster Roll Immobilizer, A4580
Specialist Plaster Splints, A4580
Platelet
concentrate, each unit, P9019
rich plasma, each unit, P9020
Platelets, P9032-P9040, P9052-P9053
Platform attachment
forearm crutch, E0153
walker, E0154
Platform, for home blood glucose monitor, A4255
Pleural catheter, A7042
drainage bottle, A7043
Plumbing, for home ESRD equipment, A4870
Pneumatic nebulizer
administration set
small volume
disposable, A7004
filtered, A7006
non-disposable, A7005
non-filtered, A7003
Pneumococcal conjugate vaccine, S0195
Pneumocystis Jiroveci pneumonia, G9219-G9223
Polaris, E0601
Polaris Lt, E0601
Polycose, enteral nutrition
liquid, B4155
powder, B4155
Poor blood, each unit, P9016
Port
indwelling, C1788
Portable
equipment transfer, R0070-R0076
hemodialyzer system, E1635
home suction pump, K0743
liquid oxygen system, E0433
nebulizer, E0570
x-ray equipment, Q0092
Portagen Powder, enteral nutrition, B4150
Posey restraints, E0700
Positive airway pressure device supply, A7046
Post-coital examination, Q0115
Postdischarge services
LVRS surgery, G0305
Postural drainage board, E0606
Potassium
hydroxide (KOH) preparation, Q0112
Pouch
Active Life convex one-piece urostomy, A4421
closed, A4387, A5052
drainable, A4388-A4389, A5056-A5057, A5061
fecal collection, A4330
Little Ones Sur-fit mini, A5054
ostomy, A4375-A4378, A4387-A4391, A4416-A4420, A4423-A4434, A4435, A5051-A5054, A5061-A5063
pediatric, drainable, A5061
Pouchkins pediatric ostomy system, A5061, A5062, A5073
Sur-Fit, drainable, A5063
urinary, A4379-A4383, A4391, A5071-A5073
urostomy, A5073
Power
mist nebulizer, E0580
mobility device, K0800-K0812, K0899
wheelchair, K0813-K0898
pediatric, E1239
Power mobility device
does not meet criteria, K0899
group 1, K0800-K0802, K0813-K0816
group 2, K0806-K0808, K0820-K0843
group 3, K0849-K0864
group 4, K0868-K0886
group 5, K0890-K0891
not coded by DME PDAC, K0899
not otherwise classified (NOC), K0812, K0898

Stent
  coated
    with delivery system, C1874
    without delivery system, C1875
      with delivery system, C1876
      without delivery system, C1877
  noncoronary
    temporary, C2617, C2625
Stent placement
  intracoronary, C9600-C9601
    with percutaneous transluminal coronary
      atherectomy, C9602-C9603
Stereotactic radiosurgery, G0251
  therapy, G0173, G0339, G0340
Sterile water, A4216-A4218
Stimulated intrauterine insemination, S4035
Stimulation
  electrical, G0281-G0283
    acupuncture, S8930
  electromagnetic, G0295
Stimulators
  cough, device, E0482
  electric, supplies, A4595
  interferential current, S8130-S8131
  joint, E0762
  neuromuscular, E0744, E0745, E0764
  osteogenesis, electrical, E0747-E0749
  salivary reflex, E0755
  transcutaneous, E0770
  ultrasound, E0760
Stocking
  gradient compression, A6530-A6549
Stoma
  cap, A5055
  catheter, A5082
  cone, A4399
  plug, A5081
Stomach tube, B4083
Stomahesive
  skin barrier, A4362, A5122
  sterile wafer, A4362
  strips, A4362
Storm Arrow power wheelchair, K0014
Storm Torque power wheelchair, K0011
Stress management class, S9454
Stretch device, E1801, E1811, E1816, E1818, E1831,
  E1841
Strip(s)
  blood, A4253
  glucose test, A4253, A4772
  Nu-Hope
    adhesive, 1 oz bottle with applicator, A4364
    adhesive, 3 oz bottle with applicator, A4364
  urine reagent, A4250
Stroke, G9257-G9258
Study
  gastrointestinal fat absorption, S3708
  sleep, G0398-G0400
Stump sock, L8470-L8485
Stylet, A4212
Substance abuse treatment, T1006-T1012
  ambulatory setting, S9475
  childcare during, T1009
  couples counseling, T1006
  family counseling, T1006
  meals during, T1010
  other than tobacco, G0396, G0397
  skills development, T1012
  treatment plan, T1007
Suction
  wound, A9272, K0743
Sulfamethoxazole and trimethoprim, S0039
Sullivan
  CPAP, E0601
Sumacal, enteral nutrition, B4155
Sunbeam moist/dry heat pad, E0215
Sunglass frames, S0518
Supplies
  infection control NOS, S8301
  Medicare IVIG demonstration, Q2052
  miscellaneous DME, A9999
  ventricular assist device, Q0507-Q0509
Supply/accessory/service, A9900

Supply fee
  pharmacy
    anticancer oral antiemetic or immunosup-
      pressive drug, Q0511-Q0512
    immunosuppressive drugs, Q0510
Support
  arch, L3040-L3090
  cervical, L0120
  elastic, A6530-A6549
  ongoing to maintain employment, H2025-
    H2026
  spinal, L0970-L0999
  vaginal, A4561-A4562
Supported housing, H0043-H0044
Supportive device
  foot pressure off loading, A9283
Supreme bG Meter, E0607
Sure-Gait folding walker, E0141, E0143
Sure-Safe raised toilet seat, E0244
SureStep blood glucose monitor, E0607
Sur-Fit
  closed-end pouch, A5054
  disposable convex inserts, A5093
  drainable pouch, A5063
  flange cap, A5055
  irrigation sleeve, A4397
  urostomy pouch, A5073
Sur-Fit/Active Life tail closures, A4421
Surgery
  stereotactic, G0251
Surgical
  arthroscopy
    knee, G0289, S2112
    shoulder, S2300
  boot, L3208-L3211
  mask, for dialysis, A4928
  procedure, return/no return to OR, G9307-
    G9308
  site infection, G9311-G9312
  stocking, A4490-A4510
  supplies, miscellaneous, A4649
  tray, A4550
SurgiMend Collagen Matrix
  fetal, C9358
  neonatal, C9360
Survival, G9259, G9261, G9263
Sustacal, enteral nutrition, B4150
  HC, B4152
Sustagen Powder, enteral nutrition, B4150
Swabs, betadine or iodine, A4247
Swede, ACT, Cross, or Elite manual wheelchair,
  K0005
Swede Basic F# manual wheelchair, K0004
Swedish knee orthotic, L1850
Swivel adaptor, S8186
Syringe, A4213
  with needle, A4206-A4209
  dialysis, A4657
  insulin, box of 100, S8490
System2 zippered body holder, E0700

T

Table
  bed, E0274, E0315
  sit-to-stand, E0637
  standing, E0637-E0638, E0641-E0642
Tachdijan, Legg Perthes orthotic, L1720
Tamoxifen citrate, S0187
Tamponade
  retinal, C1814
Tantalum rings scleral application, S8030
Tape
  nonwaterproof, A4450
  waterproof, A4452
Taxi, nonemergency transportation, A0100
Tc-99 from non-highly enriched uranium, Q9969
Team conference, G0175, G9007, S0220-S0221
TechneScan, A9512
Technetium Tc 99
  arcitumomab, A9568
  biscate, A9557
  depreotide, A9536
  disofenin, A9510
  exametazime, A9521, A9569
  fanolesomab, A9566
  glucepatate, A9550

Technetium Tc 99 — *continued*
  labeled red blood cells, A9560
  macroaggregated albumin, A9540
  mebrofenin, A9537
  medronate, A9503
  mertiatide, A9562
  oxidronate, A9561
  pentetate, A9539, A9567
  pertechretate, A9512
  pyrophosphate, A9538
  sestamibi, A9500
  succimer, A9551
  sulfur colloid, A9541
  teboroxime, A9501
  tetrofosmin, A9502
  tilmanocept, A9520
Technol
  Colles splint, L3763
  wrist and forearm splint, L3906
Telehealth
  consultation
    emergency department, G0425-G0427
    inpatient, G0406-G0408, G0425-G0427
  facility fee, Q3014
  inpatient pharmacologic management, G0459
  transmission, T1014
Telemonitoring
  patient in home, includes equipment, S9110
Television
  amplifier, V5270
  caption decoder, V5271
TenderCloud electric air pump, E0182
TenderFlo II, E0187
TenderGel II, E0196
Tenderlet lancet device, A4258
TenoGlide Tendon Protector Sheet, C9356
TENS, A4595, E0720-E0749
  Neuro-Pulse, E0720
Tent, oxygen, E0455
Terminal devices, L6703-L6715, L6721-L6722
**Terumo disposable insulin syringes, up to 1 cc,
  per syringe**, A4206
Testing
  comparative genomic hybridization, S3870
  developmental, G0451
  genetic, S3800, S3840-S3842, S3844-S3846,
    S3849-S3850, S3852-S3855, S3861
  PCA3, S3721
  prostate cancer antigen 3 (PCA3), S3721
  Warfarin responsiveness, genetic technique,
    G9143
Test materials, home monitoring, G0249
Testoject
  -50, J3140
  -LA, J1070, J1080
Testone
  LA 100, J3120
  LA 200, J3130
Testosterone
  aqueous, J3140
  cypionate, J1070, J1080
  cypionate and estradiol cypionate, J1060
  enanthate and estradiol valerate, J0900, J3120,
    J3130
  pellet, S0189
  propionate, J3150
  suspension, J3140
Thalassemia, genetic test
  alpha, S3845
  hemoglobin E beta, S3846
Thallous chloride Tl 201, A9505
Therapeutic
  agent, A4321
  procedures, respiratory, G0239
Therapeutic radiopharmaceutical
  I-131 tositumomab, A9545
  sodium iodide I-131, A9530
Therapy
  activity, G0176, H2032
  antiretroviral, G9244-G9245
  beta-blocker, G9188-G9192
  infusion, Q0081
  lymphedema, S8950
  nutrition, reassessment, G0270-G0271
  respiratory, G0237-G0239
Thermalator T-12-M, E0239

Thermometer
  oral, A4931
  rectal, A4932
Thickener, food, B4100
Thinning solvent, NuHope, 2 oz bottle, A4455
Thomas
  heel wedge, foot orthotic, L3465, L3470
Thoracic-lumbar-sacral orthotic (TLSO)
  flexible with trunk support, L0450-L0457
  sagittal control, L0466-L0467
  sagittal-coronal control, L0468-L0469, L0490-
    L0492
  scoliosis, L1200-L1290
  triplanar control, L0458-L0464, L0470-L0488
Threshold
  current perception, G0255
Thumb-O-Prene Splint, L3999
Thymol turbidity, blood, P2033
Thyrotropin
  alpha, J3240
Tibia
  Specialist Tibial Pre-formed Fracture Brace,
    L2116
  Toad finger splint, A4570
Ticarcillin disodium and clavulanate potassium,
  S0040
Tip (cane, crutch, walker) replacement, A4637
Tire, wheelchair, E2214, E2220
Tissue
  connective
    human, C1762
    non-human, C1763
  localization and excision device, C1819
  marker, A4648
Tissue marker, A4648
TLSO, L0450-L0492, L1200-L1290
Tobramycin
  inhalation solution, J7682, J7685
  sulfate, J3260
  unit dose, J7682
Toe
  holder, E0952
  Specialist Toe Insert for Specialist Closed-Back
    Cast Boot and Specialist Health/Post
    Operative Shoe, A9270
Toilet accessories, E0167-E0175, E0243, E0244,
  E0625
  raised toilet seat, E0244
    Combo-Seat Universal, E0244
    Moore, E0244
    Sure-Safe, E0244
  seat lift, E0172
  transfer bench, E0247, E0248
Toll, non-emergency transport, A0170
Topical hyperbaric oxygen chamber, A4575
Topographic brain mapping, S8040
Toronto, Legg Perthes orthotic, L1700
Total hip resurfacing, S2118
Total Universal Buck's Boot, E0870
Tourniquet, for dialysis, A4929
TPN, home infusion therapy, S9364-S9368
Tracer blood glucose
  meter, E0607
  strips, box of 50, A4253
Tracer II Diabetes Care System, E0607
Tracer Wheelchairs, E1240, E1250, E1260, E1270,
  E1280, E1285, E1290, E1295
Tracheal suction catheter, A4624
Tracheoesophageal prosthesis supplies, L8511-
  L8514
Tracheostoma
  adhesive disc, A7506
  filter, A7504
  filter holder, A7503, A7507, A7509
  housing, A7505, A7508
  replacement diaphragm, faceplate, A7502
  valve, A7501
Tracheostomy
  care kit, A4629
  filter, A4481
  mask, A7525
  speaking valve, L8501
  supplies, A4623-A4626, A4628, A4629, A7523-
    A7526, S8189
  tube, A7520-A7522
Traction equipment, E0840-E0948

Wheelchair — *continued*
  cushion
    back, E2291, E2293, E2605, E2606, E2608-E2617, E2620, E2621
    custom, E2609
    seat, E2610, E2622-E2625
      general, E2601, E2602
      positioning, E2605, E2606, E2607
      replacement cover, E2619
      skin protection, E2603, E2604, E2607, E2622-E2625
  cylinder tank carrier, E2208
  elevating proximal arm, E2631
  hand rim, E0967, E2205
  heavy-duty
    shock absorber, E1015-E1016
    Tracer, E1280, E1285, E1290, E1295
  lightweight, E1240-E1270
    EZ Lite, E1250
    Tracer, E1240, E1250, E1260, E1270
  manual, adult, E1161
    accessories, E2201-E2204, E2300-E2392, E2394-E2397
  motorized, E1239, K0010-K0898
  narrowing device, E0969
  pediatric, E1229, E1231-E1238
    back
      contoured, E2293
      planar, E2291
    modification, E1011
    power, E1239
    power, NOS, E1239
    seat
      contoured, E2294

Wheelchair — *continued*
  pediatric — *continued*
    seat — *continued*
      planar, E2292
  power, accessories, E2300-E2392, E2378, E2394-E2397
    battery, E2358-E2359
    gear box, E2369
    motor, E2368
    motor and gear box, E2370
  reclining back, E1014
  residual limb support, E1020
  rocker arm, E2632
  seat or back cushion, K0669
  specially sized, E1220-E1230
  supinator, E2633
  support, E1020, E2626-E2633
  tire, E2211, E2214, E2220-E2222, E2381-E2392
  transfer board or device, E0705
  transport chair, E1037-E1038
  van, nonemergency, A0130, S0209
  wheel, E2227, E2394-E2395
  wheel drive, E0988
WHFO, with inflatable air chamber, L3807
Whirlpool equipment, E1300-E1310
Wig, A9282
Wipes, A4245, A4247
  Adhesive remover, A4456
  Allkare protective barrier, A5120
Wire, guide, C1769
WIZZ-ard manual wheelchair, K0006
Wooden canes, E0100
Wound
  cleanser, A6260

Wound — *continued*
  cover
    alginate dressing, A6196-A6198
    collagen dressing, A6021-A6024
    foam dressing, A6209-A6214
    hydrocolloid dressing, A6234-A6239
    hydrogel dressing, A6242-A6248
    packing strips, A6407
    specialty absorptive dressing, A6251-A6256
      warming card, E0232
    warming device, E0231
      non-contact warming cover, A6000
  electrical stimulation, E0769
  filler
    alginate, A6199
    foam, A6215
    gel/paste, A6011
    hydrocolloid, A6240-A6241
    hydrogel, A6242-A6248
    not elsewhere classified, A6261-A6262
  healing
    other growth factor preparation, S9055
  matrix, Q4102, Q4114, Q4118-Q4120
    dressing, Q4104
    Ultra Trilayer, Q4104
  negative pressure therapy, G0456-G0457
  packing strips, A6407
  pouch, A6154
    warming device, E0231
      cover, A6000
      warming card, E0232
  suction, A9272
  suction pump, K0743

Wound — *continued*
  therapy
    negative pressure
      supplies, A6550
Wrap
  abdominal aneurysm, M0301
  compression, A6545
Wrist
  brace, cock-up, L3908
  disarticulation prosthesis, L6050, L6055
  hand/finger orthotic (WHFO), E1805, E1825, L3806-L3808
  Specialist Pre-Formed Ulnar Fracture Brace, L3982

X

Xcaliber power wheelchair, K0014
Xenon Xe-133, A9558
X-ray
  equipment
    portable, Q0092, R0070, R0075

Y

Y set tubing for peritoneal dialysis, A4719
Yttrium 90
  ibritumomab tiuxeton, A9543
  microsphere
    brachytherapy, C2616
    procedure, S2095

Z

ZIFT, S4014

TRANSPORTATION SERVICES INCLUDING AMBULANCE
A0021-A0999

This code range includes ground and air ambulance, nonemergency transportation (taxi, bus, automobile, wheelchair van), and ancillary transportation-related fees.

HCPCS Level II codes for ambulance services must be reported with modifiers that indicate pick-up origins and destinations. The modifier describing the arrangement (QM, QN) is listed first. The modifiers describing the origin and destination are listed second. Origin and destination modifiers are created by combining two alpha characters from the following list. Each alpha character, with the exception of X, represents either an origin or a destination. Each pair of alpha characters creates one modifier. The first position represents the origin and the second the destination. The modifiers most commonly used are:

D   Diagnostic or therapeutic site other than "P" or "H" when these are used as origin codes

E   Residential, domiciliary, custodial facility (other than 1819 facility)

G   Hospital-based ESRD facility

H   Hospital

I   Site of transfer (e.g., airport or helicopter pad) between modes of ambulance transport

J   Free standing ESRD facility

N   Skilled nursing facility (SNF)

P   Physician's office

R   Residence

S   Scene of accident or acute event

X   Intermediate stop at physician's office on way to hospital (destination code only)

Note: Modifier X can only be used as a destination code in the second position of a modifier.

See S0215. For Medicaid, see T codes and T modifiers.

AMBULANCE TRANSPORT AND SUPPLIES

A0021 Ambulance service, outside state per mile, transport (Medicaid only)

A0080 Nonemergency transportation, per mile - vehicle provided by volunteer (individual or organization), with no vested interest

A0090 Nonemergency transportation, per mile - vehicle provided by individual (family member, self, neighbor) with vested interest

A0100 Nonemergency transportation; taxi

A0110 Nonemergency transportation and bus, intra- or interstate carrier

A0120 Nonemergency transportation: mini-bus, mountain area transports, or other transportation systems

A0130 Nonemergency transportation: wheelchair van

A0140 Nonemergency transportation and air travel (private or commercial) intra- or interstate

A0160 Nonemergency transportation: per mile - caseworker or social worker

A0170 Transportation ancillary: parking fees, tolls, other

A0180 Nonemergency transportation: ancillary: lodging-recipient

A0190 Nonemergency transportation: ancillary: meals, recipient

A0200 Nonemergency transportation: ancillary: lodging, escort

A0210 Nonemergency transportation: ancillary: meals, escort

A0225 Ambulance service, neonatal transport, base rate, emergency transport, one way
MED: 100-4,1,10.1.4.1

A0380 BLS mileage (per mile)
See code(s): A0425
MED: 100-2,10,10.3.3; 100-4,1,10.1.4.1; 100-4,15,20.2; 100-4,15,30.2

A0382 BLS routine disposable supplies
MED: 100-2,10,30.1.1

A0384 BLS specialized service disposable supplies; defibrillation (used by ALS ambulances and BLS ambulances in jurisdictions where defibrillation is permitted in BLS ambulances)

A0390 ALS mileage (per mile)
See code(s): A0425
MED: 100-2,10,10.3.3; 100-4,1,10.1.4.1; 100-4,15,20.2; 100-4,15,30.2

A0392 ALS specialized service disposable supplies; defibrillation (to be used only in jurisdictions where defibrillation cannot be performed in BLS ambulances)
MED: 100-2,10,30.1.1

A0394 ALS specialized service disposable supplies; IV drug therapy

A0396 ALS specialized service disposable supplies; esophageal intubation

A0398 ALS routine disposable supplies

WAITING TIME

Units	Time
1	1/2 to 1 hr.
2	1 to 1-1/2 hrs.
3	1-1/2 to 2 hrs.
4	2 to 2-1/2 hrs.
5	2-1/2 to 3 hrs.
6	3 to 3-1/2 hrs.
7	3-1/2 to 4 hrs.
8	4 to 4-1/2 hrs.
9	4-1/2 to 5 hrs.
10	5 to 5-1/2 hrs.

A0420 Ambulance waiting time (ALS or BLS), one-half (1/2) hour increments

OTHER AMBULANCE SERVICES

A0422 Ambulance (ALS or BLS) oxygen and oxygen supplies, life sustaining situation

A0424 Extra ambulance attendant, ground (ALS or BLS) or air (fixed or rotary winged); (requires medical review)
Pertinent documentation to evaluate medical appropriateness should be included when this code is reported.
MED: 100-4,15,30.2.1

A0425 Ground mileage, per statute mile

A0426 Ambulance service, advanced life support, nonemergency transport, level 1 (ALS 1)
MED: 100-2,10,20; 100-4,1,10.1.4.1; 100-4,15,20.1.4; 100-4,15,30.2; 100-4,15,30.2.1

A0427 Ambulance service, advanced life support, emergency transport, level 1 (ALS 1 - emergency)
MED: 100-2,10,20; 100-4,1,10.1.4.1; 100-4,15,30.2.1

A0428 Ambulance service, basic life support, nonemergency transport, (BLS)
MED: 100-2,10,20; 100-4,1,10.1.4.1; 100-4,15,20.6; 100-4,15,30.2.1

A0429 Ambulance service, basic life support, emergency transport (BLS, emergency)
MED: 100-2,10,20; 100-4,1,10.1.4.1; 100-4,15,30.2.1

Medical and Surgical Supplies

A0430 — A4256

A0430 Ambulance service, conventional air services, transport, one way (fixed wing)
MED: 100-2,10,20; 100-4,1,10.1.4.1; 100-4,15,20.3; 100-4,15,30.2.1

A0431 Ambulance service, conventional air services, transport, one way (rotary wing)
MED: 100-2,10,20; 100-4,1,10.1.4.1; 100-4,15,30.2.1

A0432 Paramedic intercept (PI), rural area, transport furnished by a volunteer ambulance company which is prohibited by state law from billing third-party payers
MED: 100-2,10,20; 100-2,10,30.1.1; 100-4,15,30.2.1

A0433 Advanced life support, level 2 (ALS 2)
MED: 100-2,10,20; 100-4,15,30.2.1

A0434 Specialty care transport (SCT)
MED: 100-2,10,20; 100-4,15,30.2.1

A0435 Fixed wing air mileage, per statute mile
MED: 100-2,10,20; 100-4,15,20.2; 100-4,15,20.3; 100-4,15,30.2; 100-4,15,30.2.1

A0436 Rotary wing air mileage, per statute mile
MED: 100-2,10,20; 100-4,15,20.2; 100-4,15,30.2.1

A0888 Noncovered ambulance mileage, per mile (e.g., for miles traveled beyond closest appropriate facility)
MED: 100-2,10,20; 100-4,15,20.2; 100-4,15,30.1.2; 100-4,15,30.2.4

A0998 Ambulance response and treatment, no transport

A0999 Unlisted ambulance service
MED: 100-2,10,20

MEDICAL AND SURGICAL SUPPLIES A4206-A9999

This section covers a wide variety of medical, surgical, and some durable medical equipment (DME) related supplies and accessories. DME-related supplies, accessories, maintenance, and repair required to ensure the proper functioning of this equipment is generally covered by Medicare under the prosthetic devices provision.

INJECTION SUPPLIES

A4206 Syringe with needle, sterile, 1 cc or less, each

A4207 Syringe with needle, sterile 2 cc, each

A4208 Syringe with needle, sterile 3 cc, each

A4209 Syringe with needle, sterile 5 cc or greater, each

A4210 Needle-free injection device, each
Sometimes covered by commercial payers with preauthorization and physician letter stating need (e.g., for insulin injection in young children).

A4211 Supplies for self-administered injections
When a drug that is usually injected by the patient (e.g., insulin or calcitonin) is injected by the physician, it is excluded from Medicare coverage unless administered in an emergency situation (e.g., diabetic coma).

A4212 Noncoring needle or stylet with or without catheter

A4213 Syringe, sterile, 20 cc or greater, each

A4215 Needle, sterile, any size, each

A4216 Sterile water, saline and/or dextrose, diluent/flush, 10 ml

A4217 Sterile water/saline, 500 ml

A4218 Sterile saline or water, metered dose dispenser, 10 ml

A4220 Refill kit for implantable infusion pump

A4221 Supplies for maintenance of drug infusion catheter, per week (list drug separately)

A4222 Infusion supplies for external drug infusion pump, per cassette or bag (list drugs separately)

A4223 Infusion supplies not used with external infusion pump, per cassette or bag (list drugs separately)

A4230 Infusion set for external insulin pump, nonneedle cannula type
Covered by some commercial payers as ongoing supply to preauthorized pump.

A4231 Infusion set for external insulin pump, needle type
Covered by some commercial payers as ongoing supply to preauthorized pump.

A4232 Syringe with needle for external insulin pump, sterile, 3 cc
Covered by some commercial payers as ongoing supply to preauthorized pump.

BATTERIES

A4233 Replacement battery, alkaline (other than J cell), for use with medically necessary home blood glucose monitor owned by patient, each
MED: 100-4,23,60.3

A4234 Replacement battery, alkaline, J cell, for use with medically necessary home blood glucose monitor owned by patient, each

A4235 Replacement battery, lithium, for use with medically necessary home blood glucose monitor owned by patient, each

A4236 Replacement battery, silver oxide, for use with medically necessary home blood glucose monitor owned by patient, each

OTHER SUPPLIES

A4244 Alcohol or peroxide, per pint

A4245 Alcohol wipes, per box

A4246 Betadine or pHisoHex solution, per pint

A4247 Betadine or iodine swabs/wipes, per box

A4248 Chlorhexidine containing antiseptic, 1 ml

Dipstick urinalysis: The strip is dipped and color-coded squares are read at timed intervals (e.g., pH immediately; ketones at 15 sec., etc.). Results are compared against a reference chart

Tablet reagents turn specific colors when urine droplets are placed on them

A4250 Urine test or reagent strips or tablets (100 tablets or strips)
MED: 100-2,15,110

A4252 Blood ketone test or reagent strip, each

A4253 Blood glucose test or reagent strips for home blood glucose monitor, per 50 strips
Medicare covers glucose strips for diabetic patients using home glucose monitoring devices prescribed by their physicians.
MED: 100-4,23,60.3

A4255 Platforms for home blood glucose monitor, 50 per box
Some Medicare contractors cover monitor platforms for diabetic patients using home glucose monitoring devices prescribed by their physicians. Some commercial payers also provide this coverage to noninsulin dependent diabetics.

A4256 Normal, low, and high calibrator solution/chips
Some Medicare contractors cover calibration solutions or chips for diabetic patients using home glucose monitoring devices prescribed by their physicians. Some commercial payers also provide this coverage to noninsulin dependent diabetics.
MED: 100-4,23,60.3

A4257 Replacement lens shield cartridge for use with laser skin piercing device, each

A4258 Spring-powered device for lancet, each

Some Medicare contractors cover lancing devices for diabetic patients using home glucose monitoring devices prescribed by their physicians. Medicare jurisdiction: DME regional contractor. Some commercial payers also provide this coverage to noninsulin dependent diabetics.

MED: 100-4,23,60.3

A4259 Lancets, per box of 100

Medicare covers lancets for diabetic patients using home glucose monitoring devices prescribed by their physicians. Medicare jurisdiction: DME regional contractor. Some commercial payers also provide this coverage to noninsulin dependent diabetics.

A4261 Cervical cap for contraceptive use

A4262 Temporary, absorbable lacrimal duct implant, each

Always report concurrent to the implant procedure.

A4263 Permanent, long-term, nondissolvable lacrimal duct implant, each

Always report concurrent to the implant procedure.

A4264 Permanent implantable contraceptive intratubal occlusion device(s) and delivery system

A4265 Paraffin, per pound

A4266 Diaphragm for contraceptive use

A4267 Contraceptive supply, condom, male, each

A4268 Contraceptive supply, condom, female, each

A4269 Contraceptive supply, spermicide (e.g., foam, gel), each

A4270 Disposable endoscope sheath, each

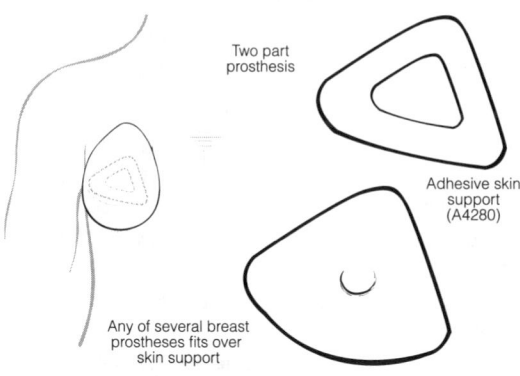

Two part prosthesis

Adhesive skin support (A4280)

Any of several breast prostheses fits over skin support

A4280 Adhesive skin support attachment for use with external breast prosthesis, each

A4281 Tubing for breast pump, replacement

A4282 Adapter for breast pump, replacement

A4283 Cap for breast pump bottle, replacement

A4284 Breast shield and splash protector for use with breast pump, replacement

A4285 Polycarbonate bottle for use with breast pump, replacement

A4286 Locking ring for breast pump, replacement

A4290 Sacral nerve stimulation test lead, each

MED: 100-4,32,40.1
AHA: 1Q,'02,9

VASCULAR CATHETERS AND DRUG DELIVERY SYSTEMS

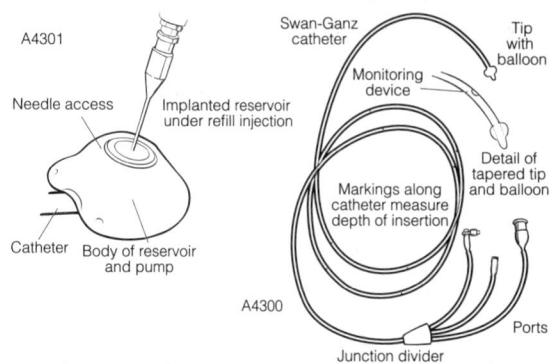

A4301   Needle access   Implanted reservoir under refill injection

Swan-Ganz catheter   Monitoring device   Tip with balloon

Detail of tapered tip and balloon

Markings along catheter measure depth of insertion

Catheter   Body of reservoir and pump

A4300   Junction divider   Ports

A4300 Implantable access catheter, (e.g., venous, arterial, epidural subarachnoid, or peritoneal, etc.) external access

A4301 Implantable access total catheter, port/reservoir (e.g., venous, arterial, epidural, subarachnoid, peritoneal, etc.)

A4305 Disposable drug delivery system, flow rate of 50 ml or greater per hour

A4306 Disposable drug delivery system, flow rate of less than 50 ml per hour

INCONTINENNCE APPLIANCES AND CARE SUPPLIES

Covered by Medicare when the medical record indicates incontinence is permanent, or of long and indefinite duration.

A4310 Insertion tray without drainage bag and without catheter (accessories only)

A4311 Insertion tray without drainage bag with indwelling catheter, Foley type, 2-way latex with coating (Teflon, silicone, silicone elastomer or hydrophilic, etc.)

A4312 Insertion tray without drainage bag with indwelling catheter, Foley type, 2-way, all silicone

A4313 Insertion tray without drainage bag with indwelling catheter, Foley type, 3-way, for continuous irrigation

A4314 Insertion tray with drainage bag with indwelling catheter, Foley type, 2-way latex with coating (Teflon, silicone, silicone elastomer or hydrophilic, etc.)

A4315 Insertion tray with drainage bag with indwelling catheter, Foley type, 2-way, all silicone

A4316 Insertion tray with drainage bag with indwelling catheter, Foley type, 3-way, for continuous irrigation

A4320 Irrigation tray with bulb or piston syringe, any purpose

A4321 Therapeutic agent for urinary catheter irrigation

A4322 Irrigation syringe, bulb or piston, each

A4326 Male external catheter with integral collection chamber, any type, each

A4327 Female external urinary collection device; meatal cup, each

A4328 Female external urinary collection device; pouch, each

A4330 Perianal fecal collection pouch with adhesive, each

A4331 Extension drainage tubing, any type, any length, with connector/adaptor, for use with urinary leg bag or urostomy pouch, each

A4332 Lubricant, individual sterile packet, each

A4333 Urinary catheter anchoring device, adhesive skin attachment, each

A4334 Urinary catheter anchoring device, leg strap, each

A4335 Incontinence supply; miscellaneous

Medical and Surgical Supplies

A4336 — A4402

A4336   Incontinence supply, urethral insert, any type, each

A4338   Indwelling catheter; Foley type, 2-way latex with coating (Teflon, silicone, silicone elastomer, or hydrophilic, etc.), each

A4340   Indwelling catheter; specialty type, (e.g., Coude, mushroom, wing, etc.), each

A4344   Indwelling catheter, Foley type, 2-way, all silicone, each

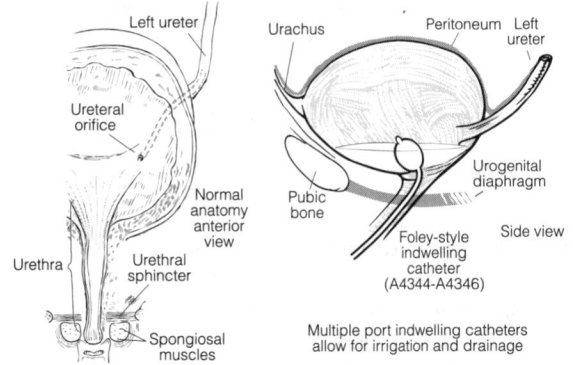

A4346   Indwelling catheter; Foley type, 3-way for continuous irrigation, each

A4349   Male external catheter, with or without adhesive, disposable, each

A4351   Intermittent urinary catheter; straight tip, with or without coating (Teflon, silicone, silicone elastomer, or hydrophilic, etc.), each

A4352   Intermittent urinary catheter; Coude (curved) tip, with or without coating (Teflon, silicone, silicone elastomeric, or hydrophilic, etc.), each

A4353   Intermittent urinary catheter, with insertion supplies

A4354   Insertion tray with drainage bag but without catheter

A4355   Irrigation tubing set for continuous bladder irrigation through a 3-way indwelling Foley catheter, each

A4356   External urethral clamp or compression device (not to be used for catheter clamp), each

A4357   Bedside drainage bag, day or night, with or without antireflux device, with or without tube, each

A4358   Urinary drainage bag, leg or abdomen, vinyl, with or without tube, with straps, each

A4360   Disposable external urethral clamp or compression device, with pad and/or pouch, each

OSTOMY SUPPLIES

A4361   Ostomy faceplate, each

A4362   Skin barrier; solid, 4 x 4 or equivalent; each

A4363   Ostomy clamp, any type, replacement only, each

A4364   Adhesive, liquid or equal, any type, per oz

A4366   Ostomy vent, any type, each

A4367   Ostomy belt, each

A4368   Ostomy filter, any type, each

A4369   Ostomy skin barrier, liquid (spray, brush, etc.), per oz

A4371   Ostomy skin barrier, powder, per oz

A4372   Ostomy skin barrier, solid 4 x 4 or equivalent, standard wear, with built-in convexity, each

A4373   Ostomy skin barrier, with flange (solid, flexible or accordian), with built-in convexity, any size, each

A4375   Ostomy pouch, drainable, with faceplate attached, plastic, each

A4376   Ostomy pouch, drainable, with faceplate attached, rubber, each

A4377   Ostomy pouch, drainable, for use on faceplate, plastic, each

A4378   Ostomy pouch, drainable, for use on faceplate, rubber, each

A4379   Ostomy pouch, urinary, with faceplate attached, plastic, each

A4380   Ostomy pouch, urinary, with faceplate attached, rubber, each

A4381   Ostomy pouch, urinary, for use on faceplate, plastic, each

A4382   Ostomy pouch, urinary, for use on faceplate, heavy plastic, each

A4383   Ostomy pouch, urinary, for use on faceplate, rubber, each

A4384   Ostomy faceplate equivalent, silicone ring, each

A4385   Ostomy skin barrier, solid 4 x 4 or equivalent, extended wear, without built-in convexity, each

A4387   Ostomy pouch, closed, with barrier attached, with built-in convexity (1 piece), each

A4388   Ostomy pouch, drainable, with extended wear barrier attached, (1 piece), each

A4389   Ostomy pouch, drainable, with barrier attached, with built-in convexity (1 piece), each

A4390   Ostomy pouch, drainable, with extended wear barrier attached, with built-in convexity (1 piece), each

A4391   Ostomy pouch, urinary, with extended wear barrier attached (1 piece), each

A4392   Ostomy pouch, urinary, with standard wear barrier attached, with built-in convexity (1 piece), each

A4393   Ostomy pouch, urinary, with extended wear barrier attached, with built-in convexity (1 piece), each

A4394   Ostomy deodorant, with or without lubricant, for use in ostomy pouch, per fl oz

A4395   Ostomy deodorant for use in ostomy pouch, solid, per tablet

A4396   Ostomy belt with peristomal hernia support

A4397   Irrigation supply; sleeve, each

A4398   Ostomy irrigation supply; bag, each

A4399   Ostomy irrigation supply; cone/catheter, with or without brush

A4400   Ostomy irrigation set

A4402   Lubricant, per oz

A4404   Ostomy ring, each

A4405   Ostomy skin barrier, nonpectin-based, paste, per oz

A4406   Ostomy skin barrier, pectin-based, paste, per oz

A4407   Ostomy skin barrier, with flange (solid, flexible, or accordion), extended wear, with built-in convexity, 4 x 4 in or smaller, each

A4408   Ostomy skin barrier, with flange (solid, flexible or accordion), extended wear, with built-in convexity, larger than 4 x 4 in, each

A4409   Ostomy skin barrier, with flange (solid, flexible or accordion), extended wear, without built-in convexity, 4 x 4 in or smaller, each

A4410   Ostomy skin barrier, with flange (solid, flexible or accordion), extended wear, without built-in convexity, larger than 4 x 4 in, each

A4411   Ostomy skin barrier, solid 4 x 4 or equivalent, extended wear, with built-in convexity, each

A4412   Ostomy pouch, drainable, high output, for use on a barrier with flange (2 piece system), without filter, each

A4413   Ostomy pouch, drainable, high output, for use on a barrier with flange (2-piece system), with filter, each

A4414   Ostomy skin barrier, with flange (solid, flexible or accordion), without built-in convexity, 4 x 4 in or smaller, each

A4415   Ostomy skin barrier, with flange (solid, flexible or accordion), without built-in convexity, larger than 4 x 4 in, each

A4416   Ostomy pouch, closed, with barrier attached, with filter (1 piece), each

A4417   Ostomy pouch, closed, with barrier attached, with built-in convexity, with filter (1 piece), each

A4418   Ostomy pouch, closed; without barrier attached, with filter (1 piece), each

A4419   Ostomy pouch, closed; for use on barrier with nonlocking flange, with filter (2 piece), each

A4420   Ostomy pouch, closed; for use on barrier with locking flange (2 piece), each

A4421   Ostomy supply; miscellaneous
Determine if an alternative HCPCS Level II or a CPT code better describes the service being reported. This code should be used only if a more specific code is unavailable.

A4422   Ostomy absorbent material (sheet/pad/crystal packet) for use in ostomy pouch to thicken liquid stomal output, each

A4423   Ostomy pouch, closed; for use on barrier with locking flange, with filter (2 piece), each

A4424   Ostomy pouch, drainable, with barrier attached, with filter (1 piece), each

A4425   Ostomy pouch, drainable; for use on barrier with nonlocking flange, with filter (2-piece system), each

A4426   Ostomy pouch, drainable; for use on barrier with locking flange (2-piece system), each

A4427   Ostomy pouch, drainable; for use on barrier with locking flange, with filter (2-piece system), each

A4428   Ostomy pouch, urinary, with extended wear barrier attached, with faucet-type tap with valve (1 piece), each

A4429   Ostomy pouch, urinary, with barrier attached, with built-in convexity, with faucet-type tap with valve (1 piece), each

A4430   Ostomy pouch, urinary, with extended wear barrier attached, with built-in convexity, with faucet-type tap with valve (1 piece), each

A4431   Ostomy pouch, urinary; with barrier attached, with faucet-type tap with valve (1 piece), each

A4432   Ostomy pouch, urinary; for use on barrier with nonlocking flange, with faucet-type tap with valve (2 piece), each

A4433   Ostomy pouch, urinary; for use on barrier with locking flange (2 piece), each

A4434   Ostomy pouch, urinary; for use on barrier with locking flange, with faucet-type tap with valve (2 piece), each

A4435   Ostomy pouch, drainable, high output, with extended wear barrier (one-piece system), with or without filter, each

MISCELLANEOUS SUPPLIES

A4450   Tape, nonwaterproof, per 18 sq in
See also code A4452.

A4452   Tape, waterproof, per 18 sq in
See also code A4450.

A4455   Adhesive remover or solvent (for tape, cement or other adhesive), per oz

A4456   Adhesive remover, wipes, any type, each

A4458   Enema bag with tubing, reusable

A4461   Surgical dressing holder, nonreusable, each

A4463   Surgical dressing holder, reusable, each

A4465   Nonelastic binder for extremity

A4466   Garment, belt, sleeve or other covering, elastic or similar stretchable material, any type, each

A4470   Gravlee jet washer

A4480   VABRA aspirator

A4481   Tracheostoma filter, any type, any size, each

A4483   Moisture exchanger, disposable, for use with invasive mechanical ventilation

A4490   Surgical stockings above knee length, each
MED: 100-2,15,110

A4495   Surgical stockings thigh length, each
MED: 100-2,15,110

A4500   Surgical stockings below knee length, each
MED: 100-2,15,110

A4510   Surgical stockings full-length, each
MED: 100-2,15,110

A4520   Incontinence garment, any type, (e.g., brief, diaper), each

A4550   Surgical trays

A4554   Disposable underpads, all sizes

A4555   Electrode/transducer for use with electrical stimulation device used for cancer treatment, replacement only

A4556   Electrodes (e.g., apnea monitor), per pair

A4557   Lead wires (e.g., apnea monitor), per pair

A4558   Conductive gel or paste, for use with electrical device (e.g., TENS, NMES), per oz

A4559   Coupling gel or paste, for use with ultrasound device, per oz

A4561   Pessary, rubber, any type

A4562   Pessary, nonrubber, any type
Medicare jurisdiction: DME regional contractor.

A4565   Slings

A4566   Shoulder sling or vest design, abduction restrainer, with or without swathe control, prefabricated, includes fitting and adjustment

A4570   Splint
Dressings applied by a physician are included as part of the professional service.

A4575   Topical hyperbaric oxygen chamber, disposable

A4580   Cast supplies (e.g., plaster)
See Q4001-Q4048.

A4590   Special casting material (e.g., fiberglass)
        See Q4001-Q4048.

A4595   Electrical stimulator supplies, 2 lead, per month, (e.g., TENS, NMES)
        MED: 100-3,10.2

A4600   Sleeve for intermittent limb compression device, replacement only, each

A4601   Lithium ion battery for nonprosthetic use, replacement

A4604   Tubing with integrated heating element for use with positive airway pressure device
        MED: 100-4,23,60.3; 100-4,36,50.14

A4605   Tracheal suction catheter, closed system, each

A4606   Oxygen probe for use with oximeter device, replacement

A4608   Transtracheal oxygen catheter, each
        MED: 100-4,23,60.3

SUPPLIES FOR OXYGEN AND RELATED RESPIRATORY EQUIPMENT

A4611   Battery, heavy-duty; replacement for patient-owned ventilator

A4612   Battery cables; replacement for patient-owned ventilator

A4613   Battery charger; replacement for patient-owned ventilator

A4614   Peak expiratory flow rate meter, hand held

A4615   Cannula, nasal
        MED: 100-4,20,100.2; 100-4,23,60.3

A4616   Tubing (oxygen), per foot
        MED: 100-4,20,100.2

A4617   Mouthpiece
        MED: 100-4,20,100.2

A4618   Breathing circuits
        MED: 100-4,20,100.2

A4619   Face tent
        MED: 100-4,20,100.2

A4620   Variable concentration mask
        MED: 100-4,20,100.2; 100-4,23,60.3

A4623   Tracheostomy, inner cannula

A4624   Tracheal suction catheter, any type other than closed system, each

A4625   Tracheostomy care kit for new tracheostomy

A4626   Tracheostomy cleaning brush, each

A4627   Spacer, bag or reservoir, with or without mask, for use with metered dose inhaler
        MED: 100-2,15,110

A4628   Oropharyngeal suction catheter, each

A4629   Tracheostomy care kit for established tracheostomy

REPLACEMENT SUPPLIES FOR DME

A4630   Replacement batteries, medically necessary, transcutaneous electrical stimulator, owned by patient

A4633   Replacement bulb/lamp for ultraviolet light therapy system, each

A4634   Replacement bulb for therapeutic light box, tabletop model

A4635   Underarm pad, crutch, replacement, each

A4636   Replacement, handgrip, cane, crutch, or walker, each
        MED: 100-4,23,60.3; 100-4,36,50,15

A4637   Replacement, tip, cane, crutch, walker, each

A4638   Replacement battery for patient-owned ear pulse generator, each

A4639   Replacement pad for infrared heating pad system, each

A4640   Replacement pad for use with medically necessary alternating pressure pad owned by patient

RADIOPHARMACEUTICALS

A4641   Radiopharmaceutical, diagnostic, not otherwise classified
        MED: 100-4,13,60.3; 100-4,13,60.3.1; 100-4,13,60.3.2

A4642   Indium In-111 satumomab pendetide, diagnostic, per study dose, up to 6 millicuries
        Use this code for Oncoscint.

MISCELLANEOUS SUPPLIES

A4648   Tissue marker, implantable, any type, each

A4649   Surgical supply; miscellaneous
        Determine if an alternative HCPCS Level II or a CPT code better describes the service being reported. This code should be used only if a more specific code is unavailable.

A4650   Implantable radiation dosimeter, each

A4651   Calibrated microcapillary tube, each

A4652   Microcapillary tube sealant

DIALYSIS SUPPLIES

A4653   Peritoneal dialysis catheter anchoring device, belt, each

A4657   Syringe, with or without needle, each
        MED: 100-4,8,60.4.4; 100-4,8,60.4.6.3; 100-4,8,60.7; 100-4,8,60.7.3; 100-4,13,60.7.1

A4660   Sphygmomanometer/blood pressure apparatus with cuff and stethoscope

A4663   Blood pressure cuff only

A4670   Automatic blood pressure monitor

A4671   Disposable cycler set used with cycler dialysis machine, each

A4672   Drainage extension line, sterile, for dialysis, each

A4673   Extension line with easy lock connectors, used with dialysis

A4674   Chemicals/antiseptics solution used to clean/sterilize dialysis equipment, per 8 oz

A4680   Activated carbon filter for hemodialysis, each

A4690   Dialyzer (artificial kidneys), all types, all sizes, for hemodialysis, each

A4706   Bicarbonate concentrate, solution, for hemodialysis, per gallon

A4707   Bicarbonate concentrate, powder, for hemodialysis, per packet

A4708   Acetate concentrate solution, for hemodialysis, per gallon

A4709   Acid concentrate, solution, for hemodialysis, per gallon

A4714   Treated water (deionized, distilled, or reverse osmosis) for peritoneal dialysis, per gallon

A4719   "Y set" tubing for peritoneal dialysis

A4720   Dialysate solution, any concentration of dextrose, fluid volume greater than 249 cc, but less than or equal to 999 cc, for peritoneal dialysis

A4721   Dialysate solution, any concentration of dextrose, fluid volume greater than 999 cc but less than or equal to 1999 cc, for peritoneal dialysis

A4722   Dialysate solution, any concentration of dextrose, fluid volume greater than 1999 cc but less than or equal to 2999 cc, for peritoneal dialysis

A4723   Dialysate solution, any concentration of dextrose, fluid volume greater than 2999 cc but less than or equal to 3999 cc, for peritoneal dialysis

A4724   Dialysate solution, any concentration of dextrose, fluid volume greater than 3999 cc but less than or equal to 4999 cc, for peritoneal dialysis

A4725   Dialysate solution, any concentration of dextrose, fluid volume greater than 4999 cc but less than or equal to 5999 cc, for peritoneal dialysis

A4726   Dialysate solution, any concentration of dextrose, fluid volume greater than 5999 cc, for peritoneal dialysis

A4728   Dialysate solution, nondextrose containing, 500 ml

A4730   Fistula cannulation set for hemodialysis, each

A4736   Topical anesthetic, for dialysis, per g

A4737   Injectable anesthetic, for dialysis, per 10 ml

A4740   Shunt accessory, for hemodialysis, any type, each

A4750   Blood tubing, arterial or venous, for hemodialysis, each

A4755   Blood tubing, arterial and venous combined, for hemodialysis, each

A4760   Dialysate solution test kit, for peritoneal dialysis, any type, each

A4765   Dialysate concentrate, powder, additive for peritoneal dialysis, per packet

A4766   Dialysate concentrate, solution, additive for peritoneal dialysis, per 10 ml

A4770   Blood collection tube, vacuum, for dialysis, per 50

A4771   Serum clotting time tube, for dialysis, per 50

A4772   Blood glucose test strips, for dialysis, per 50

A4773   Occult blood test strips, for dialysis, per 50

A4774   Ammonia test strips, for dialysis, per 50

A4802   Protamine sulfate, for hemodialysis, per 50 mg

A4860   Disposable catheter tips for peritoneal dialysis, per 10

A4870   Plumbing and/or electrical work for home hemodialysis equipment

A4890   Contracts, repair and maintenance, for hemodialysis equipment

A4911   Drain bag/bottle, for dialysis, each

A4913   Miscellaneous dialysis supplies, not otherwise specified

     Pertinent documentation to evaluate medical appropriateness should be included when this code is reported. Determine if an alternative HCPCS Level II or a CPT code better describes the service being reported. This code should be used only if a more specific code is unavailable.

A4918   Venous pressure clamp, for hemodialysis, each

A4927   Gloves, nonsterile, per 100

A4928   Surgical mask, per 20

A4929   Tourniquet for dialysis, each

A4930   Gloves, sterile, per pair

A4931   Oral thermometer, reusable, any type, each

A4932   Rectal thermometer, reusable, any type, each

OSTOMY POUCHES AND SUPPLIES

A5051   Ostomy pouch, closed; with barrier attached (1 piece), each

A5052   Ostomy pouch, closed; without barrier attached (1 piece), each

A5053   Ostomy pouch, closed; for use on faceplate, each

A5054   Ostomy pouch, closed; for use on barrier with flange (2 piece), each

A5055   Stoma cap

A5056   Ostomy pouch, drainable, with extended wear barrier attached, with filter, (1 piece), each

A5057   Ostomy pouch, drainable, with extended wear barrier attached, with built in convexity, with filter, (1 piece), each

A5061   Ostomy pouch, drainable; with barrier attached, (1 piece), each

A5062   Ostomy pouch, drainable; without barrier attached (1 piece), each

A5063   Ostomy pouch, drainable; for use on barrier with flange (2-piece system), each

A5071   Ostomy pouch, urinary; with barrier attached (1 piece), each

A5072   Ostomy pouch, urinary; without barrier attached (1 piece), each

A5073   Ostomy pouch, urinary; for use on barrier with flange (2 piece), each

A5081   Stoma plug or seal, any type

A5082   Continent device; catheter for continent stoma

A5083   Continent device, stoma absorptive cover for continent stoma

A5093   Ostomy accessory; convex insert

INCONTINENCE SUPPLIES

A5102   Bedside drainage bottle with or without tubing, rigid or expandable, each

A5105   Urinary suspensory with leg bag, with or without tube, each

A5112   Urinary drainage bag, leg or abdomen, latex, with or without tube, with straps, each

A5113   Leg strap; latex, replacement only, per set

A5114   Leg strap; foam or fabric, replacement only, per set

A5120   Skin barrier, wipes or swabs, each

A5121   Skin barrier; solid, 6 x 6 or equivalent, each

A5122   Skin barrier; solid, 8 x 8 or equivalent, each

A5126   Adhesive or nonadhesive; disk or foam pad

A5131   Appliance cleaner, incontinence and ostomy appliances, per 16 oz

A5200   Percutaneous catheter/tube anchoring device, adhesive skin attachment

DIABETIC SHOES, FITTING, AND MODIFICATIONS

According to Medicare, documentation from the prescribing physician must certify the diabetic patient has one of the following conditions: peripheral neuropathy with evidence of callus formation; history of preulcerative calluses; history of ulceration; foot deformity; previous amputation; or poor circulation. The footwear must be fitted and furnished by a podiatrist, pedorthist, orthotist, or prosthetist.

A5500   For diabetics only, fitting (including follow-up), custom preparation and supply of off-the-shelf depth-inlay shoe manufactured to accommodate multidensity insert(s), per shoe

     MED: 100-2,15,140

A5501   For diabetics only, fitting (including follow-up), custom preparation and supply of shoe molded from cast(s) of patient's foot (custom molded shoe), per shoe

     MED: 100-2,15,140

A5503   For diabetics only, modification (including fitting) of off-the-shelf depth-inlay shoe or custom molded shoe with roller or rigid rocker bottom, per shoe

     MED: 100-2,15,140

A5504   For diabetics only, modification (including fitting) of off-the-shelf depth-inlay shoe or custom molded shoe with wedge(s), per shoe

     MED: 100-2,15,140

A5505   For diabetics only, modification (including fitting) of off-the-shelf depth-inlay shoe or custom molded shoe with metatarsal bar, per shoe

     MED: 100-2,15,140

A5506   For diabetics only, modification (including fitting) of off-the-shelf depth-inlay shoe or custom molded shoe with off-set heel(s), per shoe

     MED: 100-2,15,140

A5507 For diabetics only, not otherwise specified modification (including fitting) of off-the-shelf depth-inlay shoe or custom molded shoe, per shoe
MED: 100-2,15,140

A5508 For diabetics only, deluxe feature of off-the-shelf depth-inlay shoe or custom molded shoe, per shoe
MED: 100-2,15,140

A5510 For diabetics only, direct formed, compression molded to patient's foot without external heat source, multiple-density insert(s) prefabricated, per shoe
MED: 100-2,15,140

A5512 For diabetics only, multiple density insert, direct formed, molded to foot after external heat source of 230 degrees Fahrenheit or higher, total contact with patient's foot, including arch, base layer minimum of 1/4 inch material of shore a 35 durometer or 3/16 inch material of shore a 40 durometer (or higher), prefabricated, each

A5513 For diabetics only, multiple density insert, custom molded from model of patient's foot, total contact with patient's foot, including arch, base layer minimum of 3/16 inch material of shore a 35 durometer or higher), includes arch filler and other shaping material, custom fabricated, each

DRESSINGS

A6000 Noncontact wound-warming wound cover for use with the noncontact wound-warming device and warming card

A6010 Collagen based wound filler, dry form, sterile, per g of collagen

A6011 Collagen based wound filler, gel/paste, per g of collagen

A6021 Collagen dressing, sterile, size 16 sq in or less, each

A6022 Collagen dressing, sterile, size more than 16 sq in but less than or equal to 48 sq in, each

A6023 Collagen dressing, sterile, size more than 48 sq in, each

A6024 Collagen dressing wound filler, sterile, per 6 in

A6025 Gel sheet for dermal or epidermal application, (e.g., silicone, hydrogel, other), each

A6154 Wound pouch, each

A6196 Alginate or other fiber gelling dressing, wound cover, sterile, pad size 16 sq in or less, each dressing

A6197 Alginate or other fiber gelling dressing, wound cover, sterile, pad size more than 16 sq in but less than or equal to 48 sq in, each dressing

A6198 Alginate or other fiber gelling dressing, wound cover, sterile, pad size more than 48 sq in, each dressing

A6199 Alginate or other fiber gelling dressing, wound filler, sterile, per 6 in

A6203 Composite dressing, sterile, pad size 16 sq in or less, with any size adhesive border, each dressing

A6204 Composite dressing, sterile, pad size more than 16 sq in, but less than or equal to 48 sq in, with any size adhesive border, each dressing

A6205 Composite dressing, sterile, pad size more than 48 sq in, with any size adhesive border, each dressing

A6206 Contact layer, sterile, 16 sq in or less, each dressing

A6207 Contact layer, sterile, more than 16 sq in but less than or equal to 48 sq in, each dressing

A6208 Contact layer, sterile, more than 48 sq in, each dressing

A6209 Foam dressing, wound cover, sterile, pad size 16 sq in or less, without adhesive border, each dressing

A6210 Foam dressing, wound cover, sterile, pad size more than 16 sq in but less than or equal to 48 sq in, without adhesive border, each dressing

A6211 Foam dressing, wound cover, sterile, pad size more than 48 sq in, without adhesive border, each dressing

A6212 Foam dressing, wound cover, sterile, pad size 16 sq in or less, with any size adhesive border, each dressing

A6213 Foam dressing, wound cover, sterile, pad size more than 16 sq in but less than or equal to 48 sq in, with any size adhesive border, each dressing

A6214 Foam dressing, wound cover, sterile, pad size more than 48 sq in, with any size adhesive border, each dressing

A6215 Foam dressing, wound filler, sterile, per g

A6216 Gauze, nonimpregnated, nonsterile, pad size 16 sq in or less, without adhesive border, each dressing

A6217 Gauze, nonimpregnated, nonsterile, pad size more than 16 sq in but less than or equal to 48 sq in, without adhesive border, each dressing

A6218 Gauze, nonimpregnated, nonsterile, pad size more than 48 sq in, without adhesive border, each dressing

A6219 Gauze, nonimpregnated, sterile, pad size 16 sq in or less, with any size adhesive border, each dressing

A6220 Gauze, nonimpregnated, sterile, pad size more than 16 sq in but less than or equal to 48 sq in, with any size adhesive border, each dressing

A6221 Gauze, nonimpregnated, sterile, pad size more than 48 sq in, with any size adhesive border, each dressing

A6222 Gauze, impregnated with other than water, normal saline, or hydrogel, sterile, pad size 16 sq in or less, without adhesive border, each dressing

A6223 Gauze, impregnated with other than water, normal saline, or hydrogel, sterile, pad size more than 16 sq in, but less than or equal to 48 sq in, without adhesive border, each dressing

A6224 Gauze, impregnated with other than water, normal saline, or hydrogel, sterile, pad size more than 48 sq in, without adhesive border, each dressing

A6228 Gauze, impregnated, water or normal saline, sterile, pad size 16 sq in or less, without adhesive border, each dressing

A6229 Gauze, impregnated, water or normal saline, sterile, pad size more than 16 sq in but less than or equal to 48 sq in, without adhesive border, each dressing

A6230 Gauze, impregnated, water or normal saline, sterile, pad size more than 48 sq in, without adhesive border, each dressing

A6231 Gauze, impregnated, hydrogel, for direct wound contact, sterile, pad size 16 sq in or less, each dressing

A6232 Gauze, impregnated, hydrogel, for direct wound contact, sterile, pad size greater than 16 sq in, but less than or equal to 48 sq in, each dressing

A6233 Gauze, impregnated, hydrogel, for direct wound contact, sterile, pad size more than 48 sq in, each dressing

A6234 Hydrocolloid dressing, wound cover, sterile, pad size 16 sq in or less, without adhesive border, each dressing

A6235 Hydrocolloid dressing, wound cover, sterile, pad size more than 16 sq in but less than or equal to 48 sq in, without adhesive border, each dressing

A6236 Hydrocolloid dressing, wound cover, sterile, pad size more than 48 sq in, without adhesive border, each dressing

A6237 Hydrocolloid dressing, wound cover, sterile, pad size 16 sq in or less, with any size adhesive border, each dressing

A6238 Hydrocolloid dressing, wound cover, sterile, pad size more than 16 sq in but less than or equal to 48 sq in, with any size adhesive border, each dressing

A6239 Hydrocolloid dressing, wound cover, sterile, pad size more than 48 sq in, with any size adhesive border, each dressing

A6240   Hydrocolloid dressing, wound filler, paste, sterile, per oz

A6241   Hydrocolloid dressing, wound filler, dry form, sterile, per g

A6242   Hydrogel dressing, wound cover, sterile, pad size 16 sq in or less, without adhesive border, each dressing

A6243   Hydrogel dressing, wound cover, sterile, pad size more than 16 sq in but less than or equal to 48 sq in, without adhesive border, each dressing

A6244   Hydrogel dressing, wound cover, sterile, pad size more than 48 sq in, without adhesive border, each dressing

A6245   Hydrogel dressing, wound cover, sterile, pad size 16 sq in or less, with any size adhesive border, each dressing

A6246   Hydrogel dressing, wound cover, sterile, pad size more than 16 sq in but less than or equal to 48 sq in, with any size adhesive border, each dressing

A6247   Hydrogel dressing, wound cover, sterile, pad size more than 48 sq in, with any size adhesive border, each dressing

A6248   Hydrogel dressing, wound filler, gel, per fl oz

A6250   **Skin sealants, protectants, moisturizers, ointments, any type, any size**
Surgical dressings applied by a physician are included as part of the professional service. Surgical dressings obtained by the patient to perform homecare as prescribed by the physician are covered.

A6251   Specialty absorptive dressing, wound cover, sterile, pad size 16 sq in or less, without adhesive border, each dressing

A6252   Specialty absorptive dressing, wound cover, sterile, pad size more than 16 sq in but less than or equal to 48 sq in, without adhesive border, each dressing

A6253   Specialty absorptive dressing, wound cover, sterile, pad size more than 48 sq in, without adhesive border, each dressing

A6254   Specialty absorptive dressing, wound cover, sterile, pad size 16 sq in or less, with any size adhesive border, each dressing

A6255   Specialty absorptive dressing, wound cover, sterile, pad size more than 16 sq in but less than or equal to 48 sq in, with any size adhesive border, each dressing

A6256   Specialty absorptive dressing, wound cover, sterile, pad size more than 48 sq in, with any size adhesive border, each dressing

A6257   **Transparent film, sterile, 16 sq in or less, each dressing**
Surgical dressings applied by a physician are included as part of the professional service. Surgical dressings obtained by the patient to perform homecare as prescribed by the physician are covered. Use this code for Polyskin, Tegaderm, and Tegaderm HP.

A6258   **Transparent film, sterile, more than 16 sq in but less than or equal to 48 sq in, each dressing**
Surgical dressings applied by a physician are included as part of the professional service. Surgical dressings obtained by the patient to perform homecare as prescribed by the physician are covered.

A6259   **Transparent film, sterile, more than 48 sq in, each dressing**
Surgical dressings applied by a physician are included as part of the professional service. Surgical dressings obtained by the patient to perform homecare as prescribed by the physician are covered.

A6260   **Wound cleansers, any type, any size**
Surgical dressings applied by a physician are included as part of the professional service. Surgical dressings obtained by the patient to perform homecare as prescribed by the physician are covered.

A6261   **Wound filler, gel/paste, per fl oz, not otherwise specified**
Surgical dressings applied by a physician are included as part of the professional service. Surgical dressings obtained by the patient to perform homecare as prescribed by the physician are covered.

A6262   Wound filler, dry form, per g, not otherwise specified

A6266   **Gauze, impregnated, other than water, normal saline, or zinc paste, sterile, any width, per linear yd**
Surgical dressings applied by a physician are included as part of the professional service. Surgical dressings obtained by the patient to perform homecare as prescribed by the physician are covered.

A6402   **Gauze, nonimpregnated, sterile, pad size 16 sq in or less, without adhesive border, each dressing**
Surgical dressings applied by a physician are included as part of the professional service. Surgical dressings obtained by the patient to perform homecare as prescribed by the physician are covered.

A6403   **Gauze, nonimpregnated, sterile, pad size more than 16 sq in, less than or equal to 48 sq in, without adhesive border, each dressing**
Surgical dressings applied by a physician are included as part of the professional service. Surgical dressings obtained by the patient to perform homecare as prescribed by the physician are covered.

A6404   Gauze, nonimpregnated, sterile, pad size more than 48 sq in, without adhesive border, each dressing

A6407   Packing strips, nonimpregnated, sterile, up to 2 in in width, per linear yd

A6410   Eye pad, sterile, each

A6411   Eye pad, nonsterile, each

A6412   Eye patch, occlusive, each

A6413   Adhesive bandage, first aid type, any size, each

A6441   Padding bandage, nonelastic, nonwoven/nonknitted, width greater than or equal to 3 in and less than 5 in, per yd

A6442   Conforming bandage, nonelastic, knitted/woven, nonsterile, width less than 3 in, per yd

A6443   Conforming bandage, nonelastic, knitted/woven, nonsterile, width greater than or equal to 3 in and less than 5 in, per yd

A6444   Conforming bandage, nonelastic, knitted/woven, nonsterile, width greater than or equal to 5 in, per yd

A6445   Conforming bandage, nonelastic, knitted/woven, sterile, width less than 3 in, per yd

A6446   Conforming bandage, nonelastic, knitted/woven, sterile, width greater than or equal to 3 in and less than 5 in, per yd

A6447   Conforming bandage, nonelastic, knitted/woven, sterile, width greater than or equal to 5 in, per yd

A6448   Light compression bandage, elastic, knitted/woven, width less than 3 in, per yd

A6449   Light compression bandage, elastic, knitted/woven, width greater than or equal to 3 in and less than 5 in, per yd

A6450   Light compression bandage, elastic, knitted/woven, width greater than or equal to 5 in, per yd

A6451   Moderate compression bandage, elastic, knitted/woven, load resistance of 1.25 to 1.34 ft lbs at 50% maximum stretch, width greater than or equal to 3 in and less than 5 in, per yd

A6452   High compression bandage, elastic, knitted/woven, load resistance greater than or equal to 1.35 ft lbs at 50% maximum stretch, width greater than or equal to 3 in and less than 5 in, per yd

A6453   Self-adherent bandage, elastic, nonknitted/nonwoven, width less than 3 in, per yd

A6454   Self-adherent bandage, elastic, nonknitted/nonwoven, width greater than or equal to 3 in and less than 5 in, per yd

A6455   Self-adherent bandage, elastic, nonknitted/nonwoven, width greater than or equal to 5 in, per yd

A6456   Zinc paste impregnated bandage, nonelastic, knitted/woven, width greater than or equal to 3 in and less than 5 in, per yd

A6457   Tubular dressing with or without elastic, any width, per linear yd

COMPRESSION GARMENTS

A6501 Compression burn garment, bodysuit (head to foot), custom fabricated

A6502 Compression burn garment, chin strap, custom fabricated

A6503 Compression burn garment, facial hood, custom fabricated

A6504 Compression burn garment, glove to wrist, custom fabricated

A6505 Compression burn garment, glove to elbow, custom fabricated

A6506 Compression burn garment, glove to axilla, custom fabricated

A6507 Compression burn garment, foot to knee length, custom fabricated

A6508 Compression burn garment, foot to thigh length, custom fabricated

A6509 Compression burn garment, upper trunk to waist including arm openings (vest), custom fabricated

A6510 Compression burn garment, trunk, including arms down to leg openings (leotard), custom fabricated

A6511 Compression burn garment, lower trunk including leg openings (panty), custom fabricated

A6512 Compression burn garment, not otherwise classified

A6513 Compression burn mask, face and/or neck, plastic or equal, custom fabricated

A6530 Gradient compression stocking, below knee, 18-30 mm Hg, each

A6531 Gradient compression stocking, below knee, 30-40 mm Hg, each

A6532 Gradient compression stocking, below knee, 40-50 mm Hg, each

A6533 Gradient compression stocking, thigh length, 18-30 mm Hg, each

A6534 Gradient compression stocking, thigh length, 30-40 mm Hg, each

A6535 Gradient compression stocking, thigh length, 40-50 mm Hg, each

A6536 Gradient compression stocking, full-length/chap style, 18-30 mm Hg, each

A6537 Gradient compression stocking, full-length/chap style, 30-40 mm Hg, each

A6538 Gradient compression stocking, full-length/chap style, 40-50 mm Hg, each

A6539 Gradient compression stocking, waist length, 18-30 mm Hg, each

A6540 Gradient compression stocking, waist length, 30-40 mm Hg, each

A6541 Gradient compression stocking, waist length, 40-50 mm Hg, each

A6544 Gradient compression stocking, garter belt

A6545 Gradient compression wrap, nonelastic, below knee, 30-50 mm Hg, each

A6549 Gradient compression stocking/sleeve, not otherwise specified

A6550 Wound care set, for negative pressure wound therapy electrical pump, includes all supplies and accessories
MED: 100-4,23,60.3

RESPIRATORY SUPPLIES

A7000 Canister, disposable, used with suction pump, each
MED: 100-4,23,60.3

A7001 Canister, nondisposable, used with suction pump, each

A7002 Tubing, used with suction pump, each

A7003 Administration set, with small volume nonfiltered pneumatic nebulizer, disposable

A7004 Small volume nonfiltered pneumatic nebulizer, disposable

A7005 Administration set, with small volume nonfiltered pneumatic nebulizer, nondisposable

A7006 Administration set, with small volume filtered pneumatic nebulizer

A7007 Large volume nebulizer, disposable, unfilled, used with aerosol compressor

A7008 Large volume nebulizer, disposable, prefilled, used with aerosol compressor

A7009 Reservoir bottle, nondisposable, used with large volume ultrasonic nebulizer

A7010 Corrugated tubing, disposable, used with large volume nebulizer, 100 ft

A7011 Corrugated tubing, nondisposable, used with large volume nebulizer, 10 ft

A7012 Water collection device, used with large volume nebulizer

A7013 Filter, disposable, used with aerosol compressor or ultrasonic generator

A7014 Filter, nondisposable, used with aerosol compressor or ultrasonic generator

A7015 Aerosol mask, used with DME nebulizer

A7016 Dome and mouthpiece, used with small volume ultrasonic nebulizer

A7017 Nebulizer, durable, glass or autoclavable plastic, bottle type, not used with oxygen

A7018 Water, distilled, used with large volume nebulizer, 1000 ml

A7020 Interface for cough stimulating device, includes all components, replacement only

A7025 High frequency chest wall oscillation system vest, replacement for use with patient-owned equipment, each

A7026 High frequency chest wall oscillation system hose, replacement for use with patient-owned equipment, each

A7027 Combination oral/nasal mask, used with continuous positive airway pressure device, each

A7028 Oral cushion for combination oral/nasal mask, replacement only, each

A7029 Nasal pillows for combination oral/nasal mask, replacement only, pair

A7030 Full face mask used with positive airway pressure device, each
MED: 100-4,23,60.3; 100-4,36,50.14

A7031 Face mask interface, replacement for full face mask, each

A7032 Cushion for use on nasal mask interface, replacement only, each
MED: 100-3,240.4

A7033 Pillow for use on nasal cannula type interface, replacement only, pair

A7034 Nasal interface (mask or cannula type) used with positive airway pressure device, with or without head strap

A7035 Headgear used with positive airway pressure device

A7036 Chinstrap used with positive airway pressure device

A7037 Tubing used with positive airway pressure device

A7038 Filter, disposable, used with positive airway pressure device

A7039 Filter, nondisposable, used with positive airway pressure device

A7040 One way chest drain valve

A7041 Water seal drainage container and tubing for use with implanted chest tube

A7042 Implanted pleural catheter, each

A7043 Vacuum drainage bottle and tubing for use with implanted catheter

A7044 Oral interface used with positive airway pressure device, each
MED: 100-3,240.4; 100-4,23,60.3; 100-4,36,50.14

A7045 Exhalation port with or without swivel used with accessories for positive airway devices, replacement only

A7046 Water chamber for humidifier, used with positive airway pressure device, replacement, each

A7047 Oral interface used with respiratory suction pump, each

TRACHEOSTOMY SUPPLIES

A7501 Tracheostoma valve, including diaphragm, each

A7502 Replacement diaphragm/faceplate for tracheostoma valve, each

A7503 Filter holder or filter cap, reusable, for use in a tracheostoma heat and moisture exchange system, each

A7504 Filter for use in a tracheostoma heat and moisture exchange system, each

A7505 Housing, reusable without adhesive, for use in a heat and moisture exchange system and/or with a tracheostoma valve, each

A7506 Adhesive disc for use in a heat and moisture exchange system and/or with tracheostoma valve, any type each

A7507 Filter holder and integrated filter without adhesive, for use in a tracheostoma heat and moisture exchange system, each

A7508 Housing and integrated adhesive, for use in a tracheostoma heat and moisture exchange system and/or with a tracheostoma valve, each

A7509 Filter holder and integrated filter housing, and adhesive, for use as a tracheostoma heat and moisture exchange system, each

A7520 Tracheostomy/laryngectomy tube, noncuffed, polyvinylchloride (PVC), silicone or equal, each
MED: 100-2,1,40

A7521 Tracheostomy/laryngectomy tube, cuffed, polyvinylchloride (PVC), silicone or equal, each
MED: 100-2,1,40

A7522 Tracheostomy/laryngectomy tube, stainless steel or equal (sterilizable and reusable), each
MED: 100-2,1,40

A7523 Tracheostomy shower protector, each

A7524 Tracheostoma stent/stud/button, each

A7525 Tracheostomy mask, each

A7526 Tracheostomy tube collar/holder, each

A7527 Tracheostomy/laryngectomy tube plug/stop, each

PROTECTIVE HELMET

A8000 Helmet, protective, soft, prefabricated, includes all components and accessories

A8001 Helmet, protective, hard, prefabricated, includes all components and accessories

A8002 Helmet, protective, soft, custom fabricated, includes all components and accessories

A8003 Helmet, protective, hard, custom fabricated, includes all components and accessories

A8004 Soft interface for helmet, replacement only

OTHER SUPPLIES AND DEVICES

A9150 Nonprescription drugs

A9152 Single vitamin/mineral/trace element, oral, per dose, not otherwise specified

A9153 Multiple vitamins, with or without minerals and trace elements, oral, per dose, not otherwise specified

A9155 Artificial saliva, 30 ml

A9180 Pediculosis (lice infestation) treatment, topical, for administration by patient/caretaker

A9270 Noncovered item or service
MED: 100-4,11,100.1

A9272 Wound suction, disposable, includes dressing, all accessories and components, any type, each

A9273 Hot water bottle, ice cap or collar, heat and/or cold wrap, any type

A9274 External ambulatory insulin delivery system, disposable, each, includes all supplies and accessories

A9275 Home glucose disposable monitor, includes test strips

A9276 Sensor; invasive (e.g., subcutaneous), disposable, for use with interstitial continuous glucose monitoring system, 1 unit = 1 day supply

A9277 Transmitter; external, for use with interstitial continuous glucose monitoring system

A9278 Receiver (monitor); external, for use with interstitial continuous glucose monitoring system

A9279 Monitoring feature/device, stand-alone or integrated, any type, includes all accessories, components and electronics, not otherwise classified

A9280 Alert or alarm device, not otherwise classified

A9281 Reaching/grabbing device, any type, any length, each

A9282 Wig, any type, each

A9283 Foot pressure off loading/supportive device, any type, each

A9284 Spirometer, nonelectronic, includes all accessories

A9300 Exercise equipment

RADIOPHARMACEUTICALS

A9500 Technetium Tc-99m sestamibi, diagnostic, per study dose
Use this code for Cardiolite.

A9501 Technetium Tc-99m teboroxime, diagnostic, per study dose

A9502 Technetium Tc-99m tetrofosmin, diagnostic, per study dose
Use this code for Myoview.

A9503 Technetium Tc-99m medronate, diagnostic, per study dose, up to 30 millicuries
Use this code for CIS-MDP, Draximage MDP-10, Draximage MDP-25, MDP-Bracco, Technetium Tc-99m MPI-MDP.
AHA: 2Q,'02,9

A9504 Technetium Tc-99m apcitide, diagnostic, per study dose, up to 20 millicuries
Use this code for Acutect.
AHA: 2Q,'02,9; 4Q,'01,5

A9505 Thallium Tl-201 thallous chloride, diagnostic, per millicurie
Use this code for MIBG, Thallous Chloride USP.
AHA: 2Q,'02,9

A9507 Indium In-111 capromab pendetide, diagnostic, per study dose, up to 10 millicuries
Use this code for Prostascint.

A9508 Iodine I-131 iobenguane sulfate, diagnostic, per 0.5 millicurie
Use this code for MIBG.
AHA: 2Q,'02,9

A9509 Iodine I-123 sodium iodide, diagnostic, per millicurie

A9510 Technetium Tc-99m disofenin, diagnostic, per study dose, up to 15 millicuries
Use this code for Hepatolite.

A9512 Technetium Tc-99m pertechnetate, diagnostic, per millicurie
Use this code for Technelite, Ultra-Technelow.

A9516 Iodine I-123 sodium iodide, diagnostic, per 100 microcuries, up to 999 microcuries

A9517 Iodine I-131 sodium iodide capsule(s), therapeutic, per millicurie

Medical and Surgical Supplies

A9520 — A9583

A9520 Technetium Tc-99m, tilmanocept, diagnostic, up to 0.5 millicuries

A9521 Technetium Tc-99m exametazime, diagnostic, per study dose, up to 25 millicuries
Use this code for Ceretec.

A9524 Iodine I-131 iodinated serum albumin, diagnostic, per 5 microcuries

A9526 Nitrogen N-13 ammonia, diagnostic, per study dose, up to 40 millicuries
MED: 100-4,13,60.3; 100-4,13,60.3.1; 100-4,13,60.3.2

A9527 Iodine I-125, sodium iodide solution, therapeutic, per millicurie

A9528 Iodine I-131 sodium iodide capsule(s), diagnostic, per millicurie

A9529 Iodine I-131 sodium iodide solution, diagnostic, per millicurie

A9530 Iodine I-131 sodium iodide solution, therapeutic, per millicurie

A9531 Iodine I-131 sodium iodide, diagnostic, per microcurie (up to 100 microcuries)

A9532 Iodine I-125 serum albumin, diagnostic, per 5 microcuries

A9536 Technetium Tc-99m depreotide, diagnostic, per study dose, up to 35 millicuries

A9537 Technetium Tc-99m mebrofenin, diagnostic, per study dose, up to 15 millicuries

A9538 Technetium Tc-99m pyrophosphate, diagnostic, per study dose, up to 25 millicuries
Use this code for CIS-PYRO, Phosphostec, Technescan Pyp Kit

A9539 Technetium Tc-99m pentetate, diagnostic, per study dose, up to 25 millicuries
Use this code for AN-DTPA, DTPA, MPI-DTPA Kit-Chelate, MPI Indium DTPA IN-111, Pentate Calcium Trisodium, Pentate Zinc Trisodium

A9540 Technetium Tc-99m macroaggregated albumin, diagnostic, per study dose, up to 10 millicuries

A9541 Technetium Tc-99m sulfur colloid, diagnostic, per study dose, up to 20 millicuries

A9542 Indium In-111 ibritumomab tiuxetan, diagnostic, per study dose, up to 5 millicuries
Use this code for Zevalin

A9543 Yttrium Y-90 ibritumomab tiuxetan, therapeutic, per treatment dose, up to 40 millicuries

A9544 Iodine I-131 tositumomab, diagnostic, per study dose

A9545 Iodine I-131 tositumomab, therapeutic, per treatment dose
Use this code for Bexxar.

A9546 Cobalt Co-57/58, cyanocobalamin, diagnostic, per study dose, up to 1 microcurie

A9547 Indium In-111 oxyquinoline, diagnostic, per 0.5 millicurie

A9548 Indium In-111 pentetate, diagnostic, per 0.5 millicurie

A9550 Technetium Tc-99m sodium gluceptate, diagnostic, per study dose, up to 25 millicurie

A9551 Technetium Tc-99m succimer, diagnostic, per study dose, up to 10 millicuries
Use this code for MPI-DMSA Kidney Reagent.

A9552 Fluorodeoxyglucose F-18 FDG, diagnostic, per study dose, up to 45 millicuries
MED: 100-3,220.6.13; 100-3,220.6.14; 100-3,220.6.17; 100-4,13,60.3.2

A9553 Chromium Cr-51 sodium chromate, diagnostic, per study dose, up to 250 microcuries
Use this code for Chromitope Sodium.

A9554 Iodine I-125 sodium iothalamate, diagnostic, per study dose, up to 10 microcuries
Use this code for Glofil-125.

A9555 Rubidium Rb-82, diagnostic, per study dose, up to 60 millicuries
Use this code for Cardiogen 82.
MED: 100-3,220.6.1; 100-4,13,60.3.2

A9556 Gallium Ga-67 citrate, diagnostic, per millicurie

A9557 Technetium Tc-99m bicisate, diagnostic, per study dose, up to 25 millicuries
Use this code for Neurolite.

A9558 Xenon Xe-133 gas, diagnostic, per 10 millicuries

A9559 Cobalt Co-57 cyanocobalamin, oral, diagnostic, per study dose, up to 1 microcurie

A9560 Technetium Tc-99m labeled red blood cells, diagnostic, per study dose, up to 30 millicuries

A9561 Technetium Tc-99m oxidronate, diagnostic, per study dose, up to 30 millicuries
Use this code for TechneScan.

A9562 Technetium Tc-99m mertiatide, diagnostic, per study dose, up to 15 millicuries
Use this code for TechneScan MAG-3.

A9563 Sodium phosphate P-32, therapeutic, per millicurie

A9564 Chromic phosphate P-32 suspension, therapeutic, per millicurie
Use this code for Phosphocol (P32).

A9566 Technetium Tc-99m fanolesomab, diagnostic, per study dose, up to 25 millicuries

A9567 Technetium Tc-99m pentetate, diagnostic, aerosol, per study dose, up to 75 millicuries
Use this code for AN-DTPA, DTPA, MPI-DTPA Kit-Chelate, MPI Indium DTPA IN-111, Pentate Calcium Trisodium, Pentate Zinc Trisodium.

A9568 Technetium Tc-99m arcitumomab, diagnostic, per study dose, up to 45 millicuries
Use this code for CEA Scan.

A9569 Technetium Tc-99m exametazime labeled autologous white blood cells, diagnostic, per study dose

A9570 Indium In-111 labeled autologous white blood cells, diagnostic, per study dose

A9571 Indium In-111 labeled autologous platelets, diagnostic, per study dose

A9572 Indium In-111 pentetreotide, diagnostic, per study dose, up to 6 millicuries
Use this code for Ostreoscan.

A9575 Injection, gadoterate meglumine, 0.1 ml
Use this code for Dotarem

A9576 Injection, gadoteridol, (ProHance multipack), per ml

A9577 Injection, gadobenate dimeglumine (MultiHance), per ml

A9578 Injection, gadobenate dimeglumine (MultiHance multipack), per ml

A9579 Injection, gadolinium-based magnetic resonance contrast agent, not otherwise specified (NOS), per ml
Use this code for Omniscan, Magnevist.

A9580 Sodium fluoride F-18, diagnostic, per study dose, up to 30 millicuries
MED: 100-3,220.6.19; 100-4,13,60.3.2; 100-4,13,60.18

A9581 Injection, gadoxetate disodium, 1 ml
Use this code for Eovist.

A9582 Iodine I-123 iobenguane, diagnostic, per study dose, up to 15 millicuries

A9583 Injection, gadofosveset trisodium, 1 ml
Use this code for Ablavar, Vasovist.

A9584   Iodine I-123 ioflupane, diagnostic, per study dose, up to 5 millicuries
Use this code for DaTscan.

A9585   Injection, gadobutrol, 0.1 ml
Use this code for Gadavist.

A9586   Florbetapir F18, diagnostic, per study dose, up to 10 millicuries
Use this code for Amyvid.

A9599   Radiopharmaceutical, diagnostic, for beta-amyloid positron emission tomography (PET) imaging, per study dose

A9600   Strontium Sr-89 chloride, therapeutic, per millicurie
Use this code for Metastron.

AHA: 2Q,'02,9

A9604   Samarium sm-153 lexidronam, therapeutic, per treatment dose, up to 150 millicuries
Use this code for Quadramet.

A9698   Nonradioactive contrast imaging material, not otherwise classified, per study

A9699   Radiopharmaceutical, therapeutic, not otherwise classified

A9700   Supply of injectable contrast material for use in echocardiography, per study
AHA: 4Q,'01,5

MISCELLANEOUS

A9900   Miscellaneous DME supply, accessory, and/or service component of another HCPCS code

A9901   DME delivery, set up, and/or dispensing service component of another HCPCS code

A9999   Miscellaneous DME supply or accessory, not otherwise specified

Enteral and Parenteral Therapy

B4034 — B4185

ENTERAL AND PARENTERAL THERAPY B4000-B9999

This section includes codes for supplies, formulae, nutritional solutions, and infusion pumps.

ENTERAL FORMULAE AND ENTERAL MEDICAL SUPPLIES

B4034 Enteral feeding supply kit; syringe fed, per day, includes but not limited to feeding/flushing syringe, administration set tubing, dressings, tape
MED: 100-4,23,60.3

B4035 Enteral feeding supply kit; pump fed, per day, includes but not limited to feeding/flushing syringe, administration set tubing, dressings, tape

B4036 Enteral feeding supply kit; gravity fed, per day, includes but not limited to feeding/flushing syringe, administration set tubing, dressings, tape

Many types of stylets are used. Some may be fitted with lights or optics. Others are used as guides

Detail of stylet

Stylet

Nasogastric tubing

Viewing piece

B4081 Nasogastric tubing with stylet
MED: 100-4,23,60.3

B4082 Nasogastric tubing without stylet

B4083 Stomach tube - Levine type

B4087 Gastrostomy/jejunostomy tube, standard, any material, any type, each

B4088 Gastrostomy/jejunostomy tube, low-profile, any material, any type, each

B4100 Food thickener, administered orally, per oz

B4102 Enteral formula, for adults, used to replace fluids and electrolytes (e.g., clear liquids), 500 ml = 1 unit

B4103 Enteral formula, for pediatrics, used to replace fluids and electrolytes (e.g., clear liquids), 500 ml = 1 unit

B4104 Additive for enteral formula (e.g., fiber)

B4149 Enteral formula, manufactured blenderized natural foods with intact nutrients, includes proteins, fats, carbohydrates, vitamins and minerals, may include fiber, administered through an enteral feeding tube, 100 calories = 1 unit
MED: 100-4,23,60.3

B4150 Enteral formula, nutritionally complete with intact nutrients, includes proteins, fats, carbohydrates, vitamins and minerals, may include fiber, administered through an enteral feeding tube, 100 calories = 1 unit
Use this code for Enrich, Ensure, Ensure HN, Ensure Powder, Isocal, Lonalac Powder, Meritene, Meritene Powder, Osmolite, Osmolite HN, Portagen Powder, Sustacal, Renu, Sustagen Powder, Travasorb.

B4152 Enteral formula, nutritionally complete, calorically dense (equal to or greater than 1.5 kcal/ml) with intact nutrients, includes proteins, fats, carbohydrates, vitamins and minerals, may include fiber, administered through an enteral feeding tube, 100 calories = 1 unit
Use this code for Magnacal, Isocal HCN, Sustacal HC, Ensure Plus, Ensure Plus HN.

B4153 Enteral formula, nutritionally complete, hydrolyzed proteins (amino acids and peptide chain), includes fats, carbohydrates, vitamins and minerals, may include fiber, administered through an enteral feeding tube, 100 calories = 1 unit
Use this code for Criticare HN, Vivonex t.e.n. (Total Enteral Nutrition), Vivonex HN, Vital (Vital HN), Travasorb HN, Isotein HN, Precision HN, Precision Isotonic.

B4154 Enteral formula, nutritionally complete, for special metabolic needs, excludes inherited disease of metabolism, includes altered composition of proteins, fats, carbohydrates, vitamins and/or minerals, may include fiber, administered through an enteral feeding tube, 100 calories = 1 unit
Use this code for Hepatic-aid, Travasorb Hepatic, Travasorb MCT, Travasorb Renal, Traum-aid, Tramacal, Aminaid.

B4155 Enteral formula, nutritionally incomplete/modular nutrients, includes specific nutrients, carbohydrates (e.g., glucose polymers), proteins/amino acids (e.g., glutamine, arginine), fat (e.g., medium chain triglycerides) or combination, administered through an enteral feeding tube, 100 calories = 1 unit
Use this code for Propac, Gerval Protein, Promix, Casec, Moducal, Controlyte, Polycose Liquid or Powder, Sumacal, Microlipids, MCT Oil, Nutri-source.

B4157 Enteral formula, nutritionally complete, for special metabolic needs for inherited disease of metabolism, includes proteins, fats, carbohydrates, vitamins and minerals, may include fiber, administered through an enteral feeding tube, 100 calories = 1 unit

B4158 Enteral formula, for pediatrics, nutritionally complete with intact nutrients, includes proteins, fats, carbohydrates, vitamins and minerals, may include fiber and/or iron, administered through an enteral feeding tube, 100 calories = 1 unit

B4159 Enteral formula, for pediatrics, nutritionally complete soy based with intact nutrients, includes proteins, fats, carbohydrates, vitamins and minerals, may include fiber and/or iron, administered through an enteral feeding tube, 100 calories = 1 unit

B4160 Enteral formula, for pediatrics, nutritionally complete calorically dense (equal to or greater than 0.7 kcal/ml) with intact nutrients, includes proteins, fats, carbohydrates, vitamins and minerals, may include fiber, administered through an enteral feeding tube, 100 calories = 1 unit

B4161 Enteral formula, for pediatrics, hydrolyzed/amino acids and peptide chain proteins, includes fats, carbohydrates, vitamins and minerals, may include fiber, administered through an enteral feeding tube, 100 calories = 1 unit

B4162 Enteral formula, for pediatrics, special metabolic needs for inherited disease of metabolism, includes proteins, fats, carbohydrates, vitamins and minerals, may include fiber, administered through an enteral feeding tube, 100 calories = 1 unit

PARENTERAL NUTRITION SOLUTIONS AND SUPPLIES

B4164 Parenteral nutrition solution: carbohydrates (dextrose), 50% or less (500 ml = 1 unit), home mix

B4168 Parenteral nutrition solution; amino acid, 3.5%, (500 ml = 1 unit) - home mix

B4172 Parenteral nutrition solution; amino acid, 5.5% through 7%, (500 ml = 1 unit) - home mix

B4176 Parenteral nutrition solution; amino acid, 7% through 8.5%, (500 ml = 1 unit) - home mix

B4178 Parenteral nutrition solution: amino acid, greater than 8.5% (500 ml = 1 unit), home mix

B4180 Parenteral nutrition solution: carbohydrates (dextrose), greater than 50% (500 ml = 1 unit), home mix

B4185 Parenteral nutrition solution, per 10 grams lipids

B4189   Parenteral nutrition solution: compounded amino acid and carbohydrates with electrolytes, trace elements, and vitamins, including preparation, any strength, 10 to 51 g of protein, premix

B4193   Parenteral nutrition solution: compounded amino acid and carbohydrates with electrolytes, trace elements, and vitamins, including preparation, any strength, 52 to 73 g of protein, premix

B4197   Parenteral nutrition solution; compounded amino acid and carbohydrates with electrolytes, trace elements and vitamins, including preparation, any strength, 74 to 100 grams of protein - premix

B4199   Parenteral nutrition solution; compounded amino acid and carbohydrates with electrolytes, trace elements and vitamins, including preparation, any strength, over 100 grams of protein - premix

B4216   Parenteral nutrition; additives (vitamins, trace elements, Heparin, electrolytes), home mix, per day

B4220   Parenteral nutrition supply kit; premix, per day

B4222   Parenteral nutrition supply kit; home mix, per day

B4224   Parenteral nutrition administration kit, per day

B5000   Parenteral nutrition solution: compounded amino acid and carbohydrates with electrolytes, trace elements, and vitamins, including preparation, any strength, renal - Amirosyn RF, NephrAmine, RenAmine - premix

     Use this code for Amirosyn-RF, NephrAmine, RenAmin.

B5100   Parenteral nutrition solution: compounded amino acid and carbohydrates with electrolytes, trace elements, and vitamins, including preparation, any strength, hepatic - FreAmine HBC, HepatAmine - premix

     Use this code for FreAmine HBC, HepatAmine.

B5200   Parenteral nutrition solution: compounded amino acid and carbohydrates with electrolytes, trace elements, and vitamins, including preparation, any strength, stress - branch chain amino acids - premix

ENTERAL AND PARENTERAL PUMPS

B9000   Enteral nutrition infusion pump - without alarm

     MED: 100-4,23,60.3

B9002   Enteral nutrition infusion pump - with alarm

B9004   Parenteral nutrition infusion pump, portable

B9006   Parenteral nutrition infusion pump, stationary

B9998   NOC for enteral supplies

B9999   NOC for parenteral supplies

     Determine if an alternative HCPCS Level II or a CPT code better describes the service being reported. This code should be used only if a more specific code is unavailable.

OUTPATIENT PPS C1300 - C9899

This section reports drug, biological, and device codes that must be used by OPPS hospitals. Non-OPPS hospitals, Critical Access Hospitals (CAHs), Indian Health Service Hospitals (HIS), hospitals located in American Samoa, Guam, Saipan, or the Virgin Islands, and Maryland waiver hospitals may report these codes at their discretion. The codes can only be reported for facility (technical) services.

The C series of HCPCS may include device catagories, new technology procedures, and drugs, biologicals and radiopharmaceuticals that do not have other HCPCS codes assigned. Some of these items and services are eligible for transitional pass-through payments for OPPS hospitals, have separate APC payments, or are items that are packaged. Hospitals are encouraged to report all appropriate C codes regardless of payment status.

C1300   Hyperbaric oxygen under pressure, full body chamber, per 30 minute interval
> MED: 100-4,32,30.1

C1713   Anchor/screw for opposing bone-to-bone or soft tissue-to-bone (implantable)
> AHA: 3Q,'02,5; 1Q,'01,5

C1714   Catheter, transluminal atherectomy, directional
> AHA: 4Q,'03,8; 3Q,'02,5; 1Q,'01,5

C1715   Brachytherapy needle
> AHA: 3Q,'02,5; 1Q,'01,5

C1716   Brachytherapy source, nonstranded, gold-198, per source
> AHA: 3Q,'02,5; 1Q,'01,5

C1717   Brachytherapy source, nonstranded, high dose rate iridium-192, per source
> AHA: 3Q,'02,5; 1Q,'01,5

C1719   Brachytherapy source, nonstranded, nonhigh dose rate iridium-192, per source
> AHA: 3Q,'02,5; 1Q,'01,5

C1721   Cardioverter-defibrillator, dual chamber (implantable)
> MED: 100-4,14,40.8
> AHA: 3Q,'02,5; 1Q,'01,5

C1722   Cardioverter-defibrillator, single chamber (implantable)
> AHA: 3Q,'02,5; 1Q,'01,5

C1724   Catheter, transluminal atherectomy, rotational
> AHA: 4Q,'03,8; 3Q,'02,5; 1Q,'01,5

C1725   Catheter, transluminal angioplasty, nonlaser (may include guidance, infusion/perfusion capability)
> AHA: 4Q,'03,8; 3Q,'02,5; 1Q,'01,5

C1726   Catheter, balloon dilatation, nonvascular
> AHA: 3Q,'02,5; 1Q,'01,5

C1727   Catheter, balloon tissue dissector, nonvascular (insertable)
> AHA: 3Q,'02,5; 1Q,'01,5

C1728   Catheter, brachytherapy seed administration
> AHA: 3Q,'02,5; 1Q,'01,5

C1729   Catheter, drainage
> AHA: 3Q,'02,5; 1Q,'01,5

C1730   Catheter, electrophysiology, diagnostic, other than 3D mapping (19 or fewer electrodes)
> AHA: 3Q,'02,5; 1Q,'01,5

C1731   Catheter, electrophysiology, diagnostic, other than 3D mapping (20 or more electrodes)
> AHA: 3Q,'02,5; 1Q,'01,5

C1732   Catheter, electrophysiology, diagnostic/ablation, 3D or vector mapping
> AHA: 1Q,'01,5

C1733   Catheter, electrophysiology, diagnostic/ablation, other than 3D or vector mapping, other than cool-tip
> AHA: 3Q,'02,5; 1Q,'01,5

C1749   Endoscope, retrograde imaging/illumination colonoscope device (implantable)

C1750   Catheter, hemodialysis/peritoneal, long-term
> AHA: 4Q,'03,8; 3Q,'02,5; 1Q,'01,5

C1751   Catheter, infusion, inserted peripherally, centrally or midline (other than hemodialysis)
> AHA: 4Q,'03,8; 3Q,'02,5; 3Q,'01,5

C1752   Catheter, hemodialysis/peritoneal, short-term
> AHA: 4Q,'03,8; 3Q,'02,5; 1Q,'01,5

C1753   Catheter, intravascular ultrasound
> AHA: 4Q,'03,8; 3Q,'02,5; 1Q,'01,5

C1754   Catheter, intradiscal
> AHA: 4Q,'03,8; 3Q,'02,5; 1Q,'01,5

C1755   Catheter, intraspinal
> AHA: 4Q,'03,8; 3Q,'02,5; 1Q,'01,5

C1756   Catheter, pacing, transesophageal
> AHA: 4Q,'03,8; 3Q,'02,5; 1Q,'01,5

C1757   Catheter, thrombectomy/embolectomy
> AHA: 4Q,'03,8; 3Q,'02,5; 1Q,'01,5

C1758   Catheter, ureteral
> AHA: 4Q,'03,8; 3Q,'02,5; 1Q,'01,6

C1759   Catheter, intracardiac echocardiography
> AHA: 4Q,'03,8; 3Q,'02,5; 1Q,'01,5; 3Q,'01,4

C1760   Closure device, vascular (implantable/insertable)
> AHA: 4Q,'03,8; 3Q,'02,5; 1Q,'01,6

C1762   Connective tissue, human (includes fascia lata)
> AHA: 3Q,'03,12; 4Q,'03,8; 3Q,'02,5; 1Q,'01,6

C1763   Connective tissue, nonhuman (includes synthetic)
> AHA: 3Q,'03,12; 4Q,'03,8; 3Q,'02,5; 1Q,'01,6

C1764   Event recorder, cardiac (implantable)
> MED: 100-4,14,40.8
> AHA: 4Q,'03,8; 3Q,'02,5; 1Q,'01,6

C1765   Adhesion barrier

C1766   Introducer/sheath, guiding, intracardiac electrophysiological, steerable, other than peel-away
> AHA: 3Q,'02,5; 3Q,'01,5

C1767   Generator, neurostimulator (implantable), nonrechargeable
> MED: 100-4,14,40.8; 100-4,32,40.1
> AHA: 4Q,'03,8; 1Q,'02,9; 3Q,'02,5

C1768   Graft, vascular
> AHA: 4Q,'03,8; 3Q,'02,5; 1Q,'01,6

C1769   Guide wire
> AHA: 4Q,'03,8; 3Q,'02,5; 1Q,'01,6; 3Q,'01,4

C1770   Imaging coil, magnetic resonance (insertable)
> AHA: 4Q,'03,8; 3Q,'02,5; 1Q,'01,6

C1771   Repair device, urinary, incontinence, with sling graft
> MED: 100-4,14,40.8
> AHA: 4Q,'03,8; 3Q,'02,5; 1Q,'01,6

C1772   Infusion pump, programmable (implantable)
> AHA: 3Q,'02,5; 1Q,'01,6

C1773   Retrieval device, insertable (used to retrieve fractured medical devices)
> AHA: 4Q,'03,8; 3Q,'02,5; 1Q,'01,6

C1776   Joint device (implantable)
> MED: 100-4,14,40.8
> AHA: 3Q,'02,5; 1Q,'01,6; 3Q,'01,5

C1777   Lead, cardioverter-defibrillator, endocardial single coil (implantable)
> AHA: 3Q,'02,5; 1Q,'01,6

C1778   Lead, neurostimulator (implantable)
> MED: 100-4,14,40.8; 100-4,32,40.1
> AHA: 1Q,'02,9; 3Q,'02,5

C1779   Lead, pacemaker, transvenous VDD single pass
> AHA: 3Q,'02,5; 1Q,'01,6

C1780   Lens, intraocular (new technology)
AHA: 3Q,'02,5; 1Q,'01,6

C1781   Mesh (implantable)
Use this code for OrthADAPT Bioimplant.
AHA: 3Q,'02,5; 1Q,'01,6

C1782   Morcellator
AHA: 3Q,'02,5; 1Q,'01,6

C1783   Ocular implant, aqueous drainage assist device

C1784   Ocular device, intraoperative, detached retina
AHA: 3Q,'02,5; 1Q,'01,6

C1785   Pacemaker, dual chamber, rate-responsive (implantable)
MED: 100-4,14,40.8
AHA: 4Q,'03,8; 3Q,'02,5; 1Q,'01,6

C1786   Pacemaker, single chamber, rate-responsive (implantable)
MED: 100-2,1,40
AHA: 4Q,'03,8; 3Q,'02,5; 1Q,'01,6

C1787   Patient programmer, neurostimulator
AHA: 4Q,'03,8; 3Q,'02,5; 1Q,'01,6

C1788   Port, indwelling (implantable)
AHA: 4Q,'03,8; 3Q,'02,5; 1Q,'01,6; 3Q,'01,4

C1789   Prosthesis, breast (implantable)
AHA: 4Q,'03,8; 3Q,'02,5; 1Q,'01,6

C1813   Prosthesis, penile, inflatable
MED: 100-4,14,40.8
AHA: 4Q,'03,8; 3Q,'02,5; 1Q,'01,6

C1814   Retinal tamponade device, silicone oil

C1815   Prosthesis, urinary sphincter (implantable)
MED: 100-4,14,40.8
AHA: 4Q,'03,8; 3Q,'02,5; 1Q,'01,6

C1816   Receiver and/or transmitter, neurostimulator (implantable)
AHA: 4Q,'03,8; 3Q,'02,5; 1Q,'01,6

C1817   Septal defect implant system, intracardiac
AHA: 4Q,'03,8; 3Q,'02,5; 1Q,'01,6

C1818   Integrated keratoprosthesis
AHA: 4Q,'03,4

C1819   Surgical tissue localization and excision device (implantable)

C1820   Generator, neurostimulator (implantable), with rechargeable battery and charging system
MED: 100-4,4,10.12; 100-4,14,40.8

C1821   Interspinous process distraction device (implantable)

C1830   Powered bone marrow biopsy needle

C1840   Lens, intraocular (telescopic)

C1841   Retinal prosthesis, includes all internal and external components

C1874   Stent, coated/covered, with delivery system
AHA: 4Q,'03,8; 1Q,'01,6

C1875   Stent, coated/covered, without delivery system
AHA: 4Q,'03,8; 1Q,'01,6

C1876   Stent, noncoated/noncovered, with delivery system
AHA: 4Q,'03,8; 3Q,'02,5; 1Q,'01,6; 3Q,'01,4

C1877   Stent, noncoated/noncovered, without delivery system
AHA: 4Q,'03,8; 3Q,'02,5; 1Q,'01,6; 3Q,'01,4

C1878   Material for vocal cord medialization, synthetic (implantable)
AHA: 3Q,'02,5; 1Q,'01,6

C1880   Vena cava filter
AHA: 4Q,'03,8; 3Q,'02,5; 1Q,'01,6

C1881   Dialysis access system (implantable)
MED: 100-4,14,40.8
AHA: 4Q,'03,8; 3Q,'02,5; 1Q,'01,6

C1882   Cardioverter-defibrillator, other than single or dual chamber (implantable)
AHA: 3Q,'02,5; 1Q,'01,5

C1883   Adaptor/extension, pacing lead or neurostimulator lead (implantable)
MED: 100-4,32,40.1
AHA: 1Q,'02,9; 3Q,'02,5; 1Q,'01,5

C1884   Embolization protective system

C1885   Catheter, transluminal angioplasty, laser
AHA: 4Q,'03,8; 3Q,'02,5; 1Q,'01,5

C1886   Catheter, extravascular tissue ablation, any modality (insertable)

C1887   Catheter, guiding (may include infusion/perfusion capability)
AHA: 3Q,'02,5; 1Q,'01,5

C1888   Catheter, ablation, noncardiac, endovascular (implantable)

C1891   Infusion pump, nonprogrammable, permanent (implantable)
MED: 100-4,14,40.8
AHA: 4Q,'03,8; 3Q,'02,5; 1Q,'01,6

C1892   Introducer/sheath, guiding, intracardiac electrophysiological, fixed-curve, peel-away
AHA: 3Q,'02,5; 1Q,'01,6

C1893   Introducer/sheath, guiding, intracardiac electrophysiological, fixed-curve, other than peel-away
AHA: 3Q,'02,5; 1Q,'01,6; 3Q,'01,4

C1894   Introducer/sheath, other than guiding, other than intracardiac electrophysiological, nonlaser
AHA: 3Q,'02,5

C1895   Lead, cardioverter-defibrillator, endocardial dual coil (implantable)
AHA: 3Q,'02,5; 1Q,'01,6

C1896   Lead, cardioverter-defibrillator, other than endocardial single or dual coil (implantable)
AHA: 3Q,'02,5; 1Q,'01,6

C1897   Lead, neurostimulator test kit (implantable)
MED: 100-4,14,40.8; 100-4,32,40.1
AHA: 1Q,'02,9; 3Q,'02,5; 1Q,'01,6

C1898   Lead, pacemaker, other than transvenous VDD single pass
AHA: 3Q,'01,4; 1Q,'01,6

C1899   Lead, pacemaker/cardioverter-defibrillator combination (implantable)
AHA: 3Q,'02,5; 1Q,'01,6

C1900   Lead, left ventricular coronary venous system
MED: 100-4,14,40.8

C2614   Probe, percutaneous lumbar discectomy

C2615   Sealant, pulmonary, liquid
AHA: 3Q,'02,5; 1Q,'01,6

C2616   Brachytherapy source, nonstranded, yttrium-90, per source
AHA: 3Q,'03,11; 3Q,'02,5

C2617   Stent, noncoronary, temporary, without delivery system
AHA: 4Q,'03,8; 3Q,'02,5; 1Q,'01,6

C2618   Probe/needle, cryoablation
AHA: 4Q,'03,8; 3Q,'02,5; 1Q,'01,6

C2619   Pacemaker, dual chamber, nonrate-responsive (implantable)
MED: 100-4,14,40.8
AHA: 3Q,'02,5; 1Q,'01,6; 3Q,'01,4

C2620   Pacemaker, single chamber, nonrate-responsive (implantable)
AHA: 4Q,'03,8; 3Q,'02,5; 1Q,'01,6

C2621   Pacemaker, other than single or dual chamber (implantable)
AHA: 4Q,'03,8; 1Q,'01,6

C2622   Prosthesis, penile, noninflatable
AHA: 4Q,'03,8; 3Q,'02,5; 1Q,'01,6

C2625   Stent, noncoronary, temporary, with delivery system
AHA: 4Q,'03,8; 3Q,'02,5; 1Q,'01,6

C2626   Infusion pump, nonprogrammable, temporary (implantable)
MED: 100-4,14,40.8
AHA: 3Q,'02,5; 1Q,'01,6

C2627 Catheter, suprapubic/cystoscopic

AHA: 4Q,'03,8; 3Q,'02,5; 1Q,'01,5

C2628 Catheter, occlusion

AHA: 4Q,'03,8; 3Q,'02,5; 1Q,'01,5

C2629 Introducer/sheath, other than guiding, other than intracardiac electrophysiological, laser

AHA: 3Q,'02,5; 1Q,'01,6

C2630 Catheter, electrophysiology, diagnostic/ablation, other than 3D or vector mapping, cool-tip

AHA: 3Q,'02,5; 1Q,'01,5

C2631 Repair device, urinary, incontinence, without sling graft

MED: 100-4,14,40.8

AHA: 4Q,'03,8; 3Q,'02,5; 1Q,'01,6

C2634 Brachytherapy source, nonstranded, high activity, iodine-125, greater than 1.01 mCi (NIST), per source

AHA: 2Q,'05,8

C2635 Brachytherapy source, nonstranded, high activity, palladium-103, greater than 2.2 mCi (NIST), per source

AHA: 2Q,'05,8

C2636 Brachytherapy linear source, nonstranded, palladium-103, per 1 mm

C2637 Brachytherapy source, nonstranded, ytterbium-169, per source

AHA: 3Q,'05,7

C2638 Brachytherapy source, stranded, iodine-125, per source

C2639 Brachytherapy source, nonstranded, iodine-125, per source

C2640 Brachytherapy source, stranded, palladium-103, per source

C2641 Brachytherapy source, nonstranded, palladium-103, per source

C2642 Brachytherapy source, stranded, cesium-131, per source

C2643 Brachytherapy source, nonstranded, cesium-131, per source

C2698 Brachytherapy source, stranded, not otherwise specified, per source

C2699 Brachytherapy source, nonstranded, not otherwise specified, per source

C5271 Application of low cost skin substitute graft to trunk, arms, legs, total wound surface area up to 100 sq cm; first 25 sq cm or less wound surface area

C5272 Application of low cost skin substitute graft to trunk, arms, legs, total wound surface area up to 100 sq cm; each additional 25 sq cm wound surface area, or part thereof (list separately in addition to code for primary procedure)

C5273 Application of low cost skin substitute graft to trunk, arms, legs, total wound surface area greater than or equal to 100 sq cm; first 100 sq cm wound surface area, or 1% of body area of infants and children

C5274 Application of low cost skin substitute graft to trunk, arms, legs, total wound surface area greater than or equal to 100 sq cm; each additional 100 sq cm wound surface area, or part thereof, or each additional 1% of body area of infants and children, or part thereof (list separately in addition to code for primary procedure)

C5275 Application of low cost skin substitute graft to face, scalp, eyelids, mouth, neck, ears, orbits, genitalia, hands, feet, and/or multiple digits, total wound surface area up to 100 sq cm; first 25 sq cm or less wound surface area

C5276 Application of low cost skin substitute graft to face, scalp, eyelids, mouth, neck, ears, orbits, genitalia, hands, feet, and/or multiple digits, total wound surface area up to 100 sq cm; each additional 25 sq cm wound surface area, or part thereof (list separately in addition to code for primary procedure)

C5277 Application of low cost skin substitute graft to face, scalp, eyelids, mouth, neck, ears, orbits, genitalia, hands, feet, and/or multiple digits, total wound surface area greater than or equal to 100 sq cm; first 100 sq cm wound surface area, or 1% of body area of infants and children

C5278 Application of low cost skin substitute graft to face, scalp, eyelids, mouth, neck, ears, orbits, genitalia, hands, feet, and/or multiple digits, total wound surface area greater than or equal to 100 sq cm; each additional 100 sq cm wound surface area, or part thereof, or each additional 1% of body area of infants and children, or part thereof (list separately in addition to code for primary procedure)

C8900 Magnetic resonance angiography with contrast, abdomen

MED: 100-4,13,40.1.2

C8901 Magnetic resonance angiography without contrast, abdomen

MED: 100-4,13,40.1.2

C8902 Magnetic resonance angiography without contrast followed by with contrast, abdomen

MED: 100-4,13,40.1.2

C8903 Magnetic resonance imaging with contrast, breast; unilateral

C8904 Magnetic resonance imaging without contrast, breast; unilateral

C8905 Magnetic resonance imaging without contrast followed by with contrast, breast; unilateral

C8906 Magnetic resonance imaging with contrast, breast; bilateral

C8907 Magnetic resonance imaging without contrast, breast; bilateral

C8908 Magnetic resonance imaging without contrast followed by with contrast, breast; bilateral

C8909 Magnetic resonance angiography with contrast, chest (excluding myocardium)

MED: 100-4,13,40.1.2

C8910 Magnetic resonance angiography without contrast, chest (excluding myocardium)

MED: 100-4,13,40.1.2

C8911 Magnetic resonance angiography without contrast followed by with contrast, chest (excluding myocardium)

MED: 100-4,13,40.1.2

C8912 Magnetic resonance angiography with contrast, lower extremity

MED: 100-4,13,40.1.2

C8913 Magnetic resonance angiography without contrast, lower extremity

MED: 100-4,13,40.1.2

C8914 Magnetic resonance angiography without contrast followed by with contrast, lower extremity

MED: 100-4,13,40.1.2

C8918 Magnetic resonance angiography with contrast, pelvis

MED: 100-4,13,40.1.2

AHA: 4Q,'03,4

C8919 Magnetic resonance angiography without contrast, pelvis

MED: 100-4,13,40.1.2

AHA: 4Q,'03,4

C8920 Magnetic resonance angiography without contrast followed by with contrast, pelvis

MED: 100-4,13,40.1.2

AHA: 4Q,'03,4

C8921 Transthoracic echocardiography with contrast, or without contrast followed by with contrast, for congenital cardiac anomalies; complete

MED: 100-4,4,200.7.2

C8922 Transthoracic echocardiography with contrast, or without contrast followed by with contrast, for congenital cardiac anomalies; follow-up or limited study

C8923 Transthoracic echocardiography with contrast, or without contrast followed by with contrast, real-time with image documentation (2D), includes M-mode recording, when performed, complete, without spectral or color doppler echocardiography

C8924 Transthoracic echocardiography with contrast, or without contrast followed by with contrast, real-time with image documentation (2D), includes M-mode recording when performed, follow-up or limited study

C8925 Transesophageal echocardiography (TEE) with contrast, or without contrast followed by with contrast, real time with image documentation (2D) (with or without M-mode recording); including probe placement, image acquisition, interpretation and report

C8926 Transesophageal echocardiography (TEE) with contrast, or without contrast followed by with contrast, for congenital cardiac anomalies; including probe placement, image acquisition, interpretation and report

C8927 Transesophageal echocardiography (TEE) with contrast, or without contrast followed by with contrast, for monitoring purposes, including probe placement, real time 2-dimensional image acquisition and interpretation leading to ongoing (continuous) assessment of (dynamically changing) cardiac pumping function and to therapeutic measures on an immediate time basis

C8928 Transthoracic echocardiography with contrast, or without contrast followed by with contrast, real-time with image documentation (2D), includes M-mode recording, when performed, during rest and cardiovascular stress test using treadmill, bicycle exercise and/or pharmacologically induced stress, with interpretation and report

C8929 Transthoracic echocardiography with contrast, or without contrast followed by with contrast, real-time with image documentation (2D), includes M-mode recording, when performed, complete, with spectral doppler echocardiography, and with color flow doppler echocardiography

C8930 Transthoracic echocardiography, with contrast, or without contrast followed by with contrast, real-time with image documentation (2D), includes M-mode recording, when performed, during rest and cardiovascular stress test using treadmill, bicycle exercise and/or pharmacologically induced stress, with interpretation and report; including performance of continuous electrocardiographic monitoring, with physician supervision

C8931 Magnetic resonance angiography with contrast, spinal canal and contents

C8932 Magnetic resonance angiography without contrast, spinal canal and contents

C8933 Magnetic resonance angiography without contrast followed by with contrast, spinal canal and contents

C8934 Magnetic resonance angiography with contrast, upper extremity

C8935 Magnetic resonance angiography without contrast, upper extremity

C8936 Magnetic resonance angiography without contrast followed by with contrast, upper extremity

C8957 Intravenous infusion for therapy/diagnosis; initiation of prolonged infusion (more than 8 hours), requiring use of portable or implantable pump
MED: 100-4,4,230.2; 100-4,4,230.2.1

C9113 Injection, pantoprazole sodium, per vial
Use this code for Protonix.

C9121 Injection, argatroban, per 5 mg

C9132 Prothrombin complex concentrate (human), Kcentra, per i.u. of Factor IX activity

C9133 Factor ix (antihemophilic factor, recombinant), Rixibus, per i.u.

C9248 Injection, clevidipine butyrate, 1 mg
Use this code for Cleviprex.

C9250 Human plasma fibrin sealant, vapor-heated, solvent-detergent (Artiss), 2 ml

C9254 Injection, lacosamide, 1 mg
Use this code for VIMPAT.

C9257 Injection, bevacizumab, 0.25 mg
Use this code for Avastin.

C9275 Injection, hexaminolevulinate HCl, 100 mg, per study dose
Use this code for Cysview.

C9285 Lidocaine 70 mg/tetracaine 70 mg, per patch
Use this code for SYNERA.

C9290 Injection, bupivacaine liposome, 1 mg
Use this code for EXPAREL.

C9293 Injection, glucarpidase, 10 units
Use this code for Voraxaze.

A synthetic "bridge" is affixed to each end of a severed nerve with sutures
This procedure is performed using an operating microscope

C9352 Microporous collagen implantable tube (NeuraGen Nerve Guide), per cm length

C9353 Microporous collagen implantable slit tube (NeuraWrap Nerve Protector), per cm length

C9354 Acellular pericardial tissue matrix of nonhuman origin (Veritas), per sq cm

C9355 Collagen nerve cuff (NeuroMatrix), per 0.5 cm length

C9356 Tendon, porous matrix of cross-linked collagen and glycosaminoglycan matrix (TenoGlide Tendon Protector Sheet), per sq cm

C9358 Dermal substitute, native, nondenatured collagen, fetal bovine origin (SurgiMend Collagen Matrix), per 0.5 sq cm

C9359 Porous purified collagen matrix bone void filler (Integra Mozaik Osteoconductive Scaffold Putty, Integra OS Osteoconductive Scaffold Putty), per 0.5 cc

C9360 Dermal substitute, native, nondenatured collagen, neonatal bovine origin (SurgiMend Collagen Matrix), per 0.5 sq cm

C9361 Collagen matrix nerve wrap (NeuroMend Collagen Nerve Wrap), per 0.5 cm length

C9362 Porous purified collagen matrix bone void filler (Integra Mozaik Osteoconductive Scaffold Strip), per 0.5 cc

C9363 Skin substitute (Integra Meshed Bilayer Wound Matrix), per square cm

C9364 Porcine implant, Permacol, per sq cm

C9399 Unclassified drugs or biologicals
MED: 100-4,17,90.3

C9441 Injection, ferric carboxymaltose, 1 mg

Outpatient PPS

C9497 — C9899

C9497 Loxapine, inhalation powder, 10 mg

C9600 Percutaneous transcatheter placement of drug eluting intracoronary stent(s), with coronary angioplasty when performed; single major coronary artery or branch

C9601 Percutaneous transcatheter placement of drug-eluting intracoronary stent(s), with coronary angioplasty when performed; each additional branch of a major coronary artery (list separately in addition to code for primary procedure)

C9602 Percutaneous transluminal coronary atherectomy, with drug eluting intracoronary stent, with coronary angioplasty when performed; single major coronary artery or branch

C9603 Percutaneous transluminal coronary atherectomy, with drug-eluting intracoronary stent, with coronary angioplasty when performed; each additional branch of a major coronary artery (list separately in addition to code for primary procedure)

C9604 Percutaneous transluminal revascularization of or through coronary artery bypass graft (internal mammary, free arterial, venous), any combination of drug-eluting intracoronary stent, atherectomy and angioplasty, including distal protection when performed; single vessel

C9605 Percutaneous transluminal revascularization of or through coronary artery bypass graft (internal mammary, free arterial, venous), any combination of drug-eluting intracoronary stent, atherectomy and angioplasty, including distal protection when performed; each additional branch subtended by the bypass graft (list separately in addition to code for primary procedure)

C9606 Percutaneous transluminal revascularization of acute total/subtotal occlusion during acute myocardial infarction, coronary artery or coronary artery bypass graft, any combination of drug-eluting intracoronary stent, atherectomy and angioplasty, including aspiration thrombectomy when performed, single vessel

C9607 Percutaneous transluminal revascularization of chronic total occlusion, coronary artery, coronary artery branch, or coronary artery bypass graft, any combination of drug-eluting intracoronary stent, atherectomy and angioplasty; single vessel

C9608 Percutaneous transluminal revascularization of chronic total occlusion, coronary artery, coronary artery branch, or coronary artery bypass graft, any combination of drug-eluting intracoronary stent, atherectomy and angioplasty; each additional coronary artery, coronary artery branch, or bypass graft (list separately in addition to code for primary procedure)

C9724 Endoscopic full-thickness plication of the stomach using endoscopic plication system (EPS); includes endoscopy

C9725 Placement of endorectal intracavitary applicator for high intensity brachytherapy

AHA: 3Q,'05,7

C9726 Placement and removal (if performed) of applicator into breast for intraoperative radiation therapy, add-on to primary breast procedure

C9727 Insertion of implants into the soft palate; minimum of 3 implants

C9728 Placement of interstitial device(s) for radiation therapy/surgery guidance (e.g., fiducial markers, dosimeter), for other than the following sites (any approach): abdomen, pelvis, prostate, retroperitoneum, thorax, single or multiple

C9733 Nonophthalmic fluorescent vascular angiography

C9734 Focused ultrasound ablation/therapeutic intervention, other than uterine leiomyomata, with magnetic resonance (MR) guidance

C9735 Anoscopy; with directed submucosal injection(s), any substance

C9737 Laparoscopy, surgical, esophageal sphincter augmentation with device (eg, magnetic band)

C9800 Dermal injection procedure(s) for facial lipodystrophy syndrome (LDS) and provision of Radiesse or Sculptra dermal filler, including all items and supplies

MED: 100-3,250.5; 100-4,32,260.1; 100-4,32,260.2.1

C9898 Radiolabeled product provided during a hospital inpatient stay

C9899 Implanted prosthetic device, payable only for inpatients who do not have inpatient coverage

DURABLE MEDICAL EQUIPMENT E0100-E9999

E codes include durable medical equipment such as canes, crutches, walkers, commodes, decubitus care, bath and toilet aids, hospital beds, oxygen and related respiratory equipment, monitoring equipment, pacemakers, patient lifts, safety equipment, restraints, traction equipment, fracture frames, wheelchairs, and artificial kidney machines.

CANES

E0100　Cane, includes canes of all materials, adjustable or fixed, with tip
White canes for the blind are not covered under Medicare.

E0105　Cane, quad or 3-prong, includes canes of all materials, adjustable or fixed, with tips

CRUTCHES

Forearm cuff

Axilla pad

Standard underarm crutch (E0112-E0117)

Hand grip

Hand grip

Adjustment

Standard forearm crutch (E0110-E0111)

E0110　Crutches, forearm, includes crutches of various materials, adjustable or fixed, pair, complete with tips and handgrips

E0111　Crutch, forearm, includes crutches of various materials, adjustable or fixed, each, with tip and handgrips

E0112　Crutches, underarm, wood, adjustable or fixed, pair, with pads, tips, and handgrips

E0113　Crutch, underarm, wood, adjustable or fixed, each, with pad, tip, and handgrip

E0114　Crutches, underarm, other than wood, adjustable or fixed, pair, with pads, tips, and handgrips

E0116　Crutch, underarm, other than wood, adjustable or fixed, with pad, tip, handgrip, with or without shock absorber, each

E0117　Crutch, underarm, articulating, spring assisted, each

E0118　Crutch substitute, lower leg platform, with or without wheels, each
Medicare covers walkers if patient's ambulation is impaired.

WALKERS

E0130　Walker, rigid (pickup), adjustable or fixed height
MED: 100-4,23,60.3; 100-4,36,50,15

E0135　Walker, folding (pickup), adjustable or fixed height
Medicare covers walkers if patient's ambulation is impaired.
MED: 100-4,36,50,15

E0140　Walker, with trunk support, adjustable or fixed height, any type
MED: 100-4,36,50,15

E0141　Walker, rigid, wheeled, adjustable or fixed height
Medicare covers walkers if patient's ambulation is impaired.

E0143　Walker, folding, wheeled, adjustable or fixed height
Medicare covers walkers if patient's ambulation is impaired.
MED: 100-4,36,50,15

E0144　Walker, enclosed, 4 sided framed, rigid or folding, wheeled with posterior seat

E0147　Walker, heavy-duty, multiple braking system, variable wheel resistance
Medicare covers safety roller walkers only in patients with severe neurological disorders or restricted use of one hand. In some cases, coverage will be extended to patients with a weight exceeding the limits of a standard wheeled walker.
MED: 100-4,36,50,15

E0148　Walker, heavy-duty, without wheels, rigid or folding, any type, each

E0149　Walker, heavy-duty, wheeled, rigid or folding, any type

ATTACHMENTS

E0153　Platform attachment, forearm crutch, each

E0154　Platform attachment, walker, each
MED: 100-4,23,60.3; 100-4,36,50.14; 100-4,36,50,15

E0155　Wheel attachment, rigid pick-up walker, per pair

E0156　Seat attachment, walker
MED: 100-4,36,50.14

E0157　Crutch attachment, walker, each

E0158　Leg extensions for walker, per set of 4

E0159　Brake attachment for wheeled walker, replacement, each

COMMODES

E0160　Sitz type bath or equipment, portable, used with or without commode
Medicare covers sitz baths if medical record indicates that the patient has an infection or injury of the perineal area and the sitz bath is prescribed by the physician.

E0161　Sitz type bath or equipment, portable, used with or without commode, with faucet attachment(s)
Medicare covers sitz baths if medical record indicates that the patient has an infection or injury of the perineal area and the sitz bath is prescribed by the physician.

E0162　Sitz bath chair
Medicare covers sitz baths if medical record indicates that the patient has an infection or injury of the perineal area and the sitz bath is prescribed by the physician.

E0163　Commode chair, mobile or stationary, with fixed arms
Medicare covers commodes for patients confined to their beds or rooms, for patients without indoor bathroom facilities, and to patients who cannot climb or descend the stairs necessary to reach the bathrooms in their homes.

E0165　Commode chair, mobile or stationary, with detachable arms
Medicare covers commodes for patients confined to their beds or rooms, for patients without indoor bathroom facilities, and to patients who cannot climb or descend the stairs necessary to reach the bathrooms in their homes.

E0167　Pail or pan for use with commode chair, replacement only
Medicare covers commodes for patients confined to their beds or rooms, for patients without indoor bathroom facilities, and to patients who cannot climb or descend the stairs necessary to reach the bathrooms in their homes.

E0168　Commode chair, extra wide and/or heavy-duty, stationary or mobile, with or without arms, any type, each

E0170　Commode chair with integrated seat lift mechanism, electric, any type

E0171　Commode chair with integrated seat lift mechanism, nonelectric, any type

E0172　Seat lift mechanism placed over or on top of toilet, any type

E0175 Footrest, for use with commode chair, each

DECUBITUS CARE EQUIPMENT

E0181 Powered pressure reducing mattress overlay/pad, alternating, with pump, includes heavy-duty
For Medicare coverage, a detailed written order must be received by the supplier before a claim is submitted.

E0182 Pump for alternating pressure pad, for replacement only
For Medicare coverage, a detailed written order must be received by the supplier before a claim is submitted.

E0184 Dry pressure mattress
For Medicare coverage, a detailed written order must be received by the supplier before a claim is submitted.

E0185 Gel or gel-like pressure pad for mattress, standard mattress length and width
For Medicare coverage, a detailed written order must be received by the supplier before a claim is submitted.

E0186 Air pressure mattress
For Medicare coverage, a detailed written order must be received by the supplier before a claim is submitted.

E0187 Water pressure mattress
For Medicare coverage, a detailed written order must be received by the supplier before a claim is submitted.

E0188 Synthetic sheepskin pad
For Medicare coverage, a detailed written order must be received by the supplier before a claim is submitted.

E0189 Lambswool sheepskin pad, any size
For Medicare coverage, a detailed written order must be received by the supplier before a claim is submitted.

E0190 Positioning cushion/pillow/wedge, any shape or size, includes all components and accessories

E0191 Heel or elbow protector, each

E0193 Powered air flotation bed (low air loss therapy)
MED: 100-4,23,60.3

E0194 Air fluidized bed
An air fluidized bed is covered by Medicare if the patient has a stage 3 or stage 4 pressure sore and, without the bed, would require institutionalization. For Medicare coverage, a detailed written order must be received by the supplier before a claim is submitted.

E0196 Gel pressure mattress
Medicare covers pads if physicians supervise their use in patients who have decubitus ulcers or susceptibility to them. For Medicare coverage, a detailed written order must be received by the supplier before a claim is submitted.

E0197 Air pressure pad for mattress, standard mattress length and width
Medicare covers pads if physicians supervise their use in patients who have decubitus ulcers or susceptibility to them. For Medicare coverage, a detailed written order must be received by the supplier before a claim is submitted.

E0198 Water pressure pad for mattress, standard mattress length and width
Medicare covers pads if physicians supervise their use in patients who have decubitus ulcers or susceptibility to them. For Medicare coverage, a detailed written order must be received by the supplier before a claim is submitted.

E0199 Dry pressure pad for mattress, standard mattress length and width
Medicare covers pads if physicians supervise their use in patients who have decubitus ulcers or susceptibility to them. For Medicare coverage, a detailed written order must be received by the supplier before a claim is submitted.

HEAT/COLD APPLICATION

E0200 Heat lamp, without stand (table model), includes bulb, or infrared element

E0202 Phototherapy (bilirubin) light with photometer

E0203 Therapeutic lightbox, minimum 10,000 lux, table top model

E0205 Heat lamp, with stand, includes bulb, or infrared element

E0210 Electric heat pad, standard

E0215 Electric heat pad, moist

E0217 Water circulating heat pad with pump

E0218 Water circulating cold pad with pump

E0221 Infrared heating pad system

E0225 Hydrocollator unit, includes pads
MED: 100-2,15,230

E0231 Noncontact wound-warming device (temperature control unit, AC adapter and power cord) for use with warming card and wound cover

E0232 Warming card for use with the noncontact wound-warming device and noncontact wound-warming wound cover

E0235 Paraffin bath unit, portable (see medical supply code A4265 for paraffin)
MED: 100-2,15,230

E0236 Pump for water circulating pad

E0239 Hydrocollator unit, portable
MED: 100-2,15,230

BATH AND TOILET AIDS

E0240 Bath/shower chair, with or without wheels, any size

E0241 Bathtub wall rail, each

E0242 Bathtub rail, floor base

E0243 Toilet rail, each

E0244 Raised toilet seat

E0245 Tub stool or bench

E0246 Transfer tub rail attachment

E0247 Transfer bench for tub or toilet with or without commode opening

E0248 Transfer bench, heavy-duty, for tub or toilet with or without commode opening

E0249 Pad for water circulating heat unit, for replacement only

HOSPITAL BEDS AND ACCESSORIES

E0250 Hospital bed, fixed height, with any type side rails, with mattress
MED: 100-4,23,60.3

E0251 Hospital bed, fixed height, with any type side rails, without mattress

E0255 Hospital bed, variable height, hi-lo, with any type side rails, with mattress

E0256 Hospital bed, variable height, hi-lo, with any type side rails, without mattress

E0260 Hospital bed, semi-electric (head and foot adjustment), with any type side rails, with mattress

E0261 Hospital bed, semi-electric (head and foot adjustment), with any type side rails, without mattress

E0265 Hospital bed, total electric (head, foot, and height adjustments), with any type side rails, with mattress

E0266 Hospital bed, total electric (head, foot, and height adjustments), with any type side rails, without mattress

E0270   Hospital bed, institutional type includes: oscillating, circulating and Stryker frame, with mattress

E0271   Mattress, innerspring
MED: 100-4,23,60.3; 100-4,36,50.14

E0272   Mattress, foam rubber

E0273   Bed board

E0274   Over-bed table

E0275   Bed pan, standard, metal or plastic
Reusable, autoclavable bedpans are covered by Medicare for bed-confined patients.

E0276   Bed pan, fracture, metal or plastic
Reusable, autoclavable bedpans are covered by Medicare for bed-confined patients.

E0277   Powered pressure-reducing air mattress
MED: 100-4,23,60.3

E0280   Bed cradle, any type
MED: 100-4,36,50.14

E0290   Hospital bed, fixed height, without side rails, with mattress

E0291   Hospital bed, fixed height, without side rails, without mattress

E0292   Hospital bed, variable height, hi-lo, without side rails, with mattress

E0293   Hospital bed, variable height, hi-lo, without side rails, without mattress

E0294   Hospital bed, semi-electric (head and foot adjustment), without side rails, with mattress

E0295   Hospital bed, semi-electric (head and foot adjustment), without side rails, without mattress

E0296   Hospital bed, total electric (head, foot, and height adjustments), without side rails, with mattress

E0297   Hospital bed, total electric (head, foot, and height adjustments), without side rails, without mattress

E0300   Pediatric crib, hospital grade, fully enclosed, with or without top enclosure

E0301   Hospital bed, heavy-duty, extra wide, with weight capacity greater than 350 pounds, but less than or equal to 600 pounds, with any type side rails, without mattress

E0302   Hospital bed, extra heavy-duty, extra wide, with weight capacity greater than 600 pounds, with any type side rails, without mattress

E0303   Hospital bed, heavy-duty, extra wide, with weight capacity greater than 350 pounds, but less than or equal to 600 pounds, with any type side rails, with mattress

E0304   Hospital bed, extra heavy-duty, extra wide, with weight capacity greater than 600 pounds, with any type side rails, with mattress

E0305   Bedside rails, half-length

E0310   Bedside rails, full-length
MED: 100-4,36,50.14

E0315   Bed accessory: board, table, or support device, any type

E0316   Safety enclosure frame/canopy for use with hospital bed, any type
MED: 100-4,23,60.3

E0325   Urinal; male, jug-type, any material

E0326   Urinal; female, jug-type, any material

E0328   Hospital bed, pediatric, manual, 360 degree side enclosures, top of headboard, footboard and side rails up to 24 in above the spring, includes mattress

E0329   Hospital bed, pediatric, electric or semi-electric, 360 degree side enclosures, top of headboard, footboard and side rails up to 24 in above the spring, includes mattress

E0350   Control unit for electronic bowel irrigation/evacuation system

E0352   Disposable pack (water reservoir bag, speculum, valving mechanism, and collection bag/box) for use with the electronic bowel irrigation/evacuation system

E0370   Air pressure elevator for heel

E0371   Nonpowered advanced pressure reducing overlay for mattress, standard mattress length and width
MED: 100-4,23,60.3

E0372   Powered air overlay for mattress, standard mattress length and width

E0373   Nonpowered advanced pressure reducing mattress

OXYGEN AND RELATED RESPIRATORY EQUIPMENT

E0424   Stationary compressed gaseous oxygen system, rental; includes container, contents, regulator, flowmeter, humidifier, nebulizer, cannula or mask, and tubing
For the first claim filed for home oxygen equipment or therapy, submit a certificate of medical necessity that includes the oxygen flow rate, anticipated frequency and duration of oxygen therapy, and physician signature. Medicare accepts oxygen therapy as medically necessary in cases documenting any of the following: erythocythemia with a hematocrit greater than 56 percent; a P pulmonale on EKG; or dependent edema consistent with congestive heart failure.
MED: 100-4,20,30.6

E0425   Stationary compressed gas system, purchase; includes regulator, flowmeter, humidifier, nebulizer, cannula or mask, and tubing

E0430   Portable gaseous oxygen system, purchase; includes regulator, flowmeter, humidifier, cannula or mask, and tubing

E0431   Portable gaseous oxygen system, rental; includes portable container, regulator, flowmeter, humidifier, cannula or mask, and tubing

E0433   Portable liquid oxygen system, rental; home liquefier used to fill portable liquid oxygen containers, includes portable containers, regulator, flowmeter, humidifier, cannula or mask and tubing, with or without supply reservoir and contents gauge

E0434   Portable liquid oxygen system, rental; includes portable container, supply reservoir, humidifier, flowmeter, refill adaptor, contents gauge, cannula or mask, and tubing

E0435   Portable liquid oxygen system, purchase; includes portable container, supply reservoir, flowmeter, humidifier, contents gauge, cannula or mask, tubing and refill adaptor

E0439   Stationary liquid oxygen system, rental; includes container, contents, regulator, flowmeter, humidifier, nebulizer, cannula or mask, & tubing

E0440   Stationary liquid oxygen system, purchase; includes use of reservoir, contents indicator, regulator, flowmeter, humidifier, nebulizer, cannula or mask, and tubing

E0441   Stationary oxygen contents, gaseous, 1 month's supply = 1 unit
MED: 100-4,20,30.6

E0442   Stationary oxygen contents, liquid, 1 month's supply = 1 unit

E0443   Portable oxygen contents, gaseous, 1 month's supply = 1 unit
MED: 100-4,20,30.6

E0444   Portable oxygen contents, liquid, 1 month's supply = 1 unit

E0445   Oximeter device for measuring blood oxygen levels noninvasively

E0446   Topical oxygen delivery system, not otherwise specified, includes all supplies and accessories

E0450   Volume control ventilator, without pressure support mode, may include pressure control mode, used with invasive interface (e.g., tracheostomy tube)

E0455   Oxygen tent, excluding croup or pediatric tents

E0457   Chest shell (cuirass)

E0459   Chest wrap

Durable Medical Equipment   **E0460 — E0627**

E0460 Negative pressure ventilator; portable or stationary

E0461 Volume control ventilator, without pressure support mode, may include pressure control mode, used with noninvasive interface (e.g., mask)

E0462 Rocking bed, with or without side rails

E0463 Pressure support ventilator with volume control mode, may include pressure control mode, used with invasive interface (e.g., tracheostomy tube)

E0464 Pressure support ventilator with volume control mode, may include pressure control mode, used with noninvasive interface (e.g., mask)

E0470 Respiratory assist device, bi-level pressure capability, without backup rate feature, used with noninvasive interface, e.g., nasal or facial mask (intermittent assist device with continuous positive airway pressure device)

MED: 100-3,240.4; 100-4,23,60.3

E0471 Respiratory assist device, bi-level pressure capability, with back-up rate feature, used with noninvasive interface, e.g., nasal or facial mask (intermittent assist device with continuous positive airway pressure device)

E0472 Respiratory assist device, bi-level pressure capability, with backup rate feature, used with invasive interface, e.g., tracheostomy tube (intermittent assist device with continuous positive airway pressure device)

E0480 Percussor, electric or pneumatic, home model

E0481 Intrapulmonary percussive ventilation system and related accessories

E0482 Cough stimulating device, alternating positive and negative airway pressure

E0483 High frequency chest wall oscillation air-pulse generator system, (includes hoses and vest), each

E0484 Oscillatory positive expiratory pressure device, nonelectric, any type, each

E0485 Oral device/appliance used to reduce upper airway collapsibility, adjustable or nonadjustable, prefabricated, includes fitting and adjustment

E0486 Oral device/appliance used to reduce upper airway collapsibility, adjustable or nonadjustable, custom fabricated, includes fitting and adjustment

E0487 Spirometer, electronic, includes all accessories

IPPB MACHINES

Battery pack and controls

Nebulizer

IPPB unit in use

Nebulizer reservoir

Oxygen supply tube

Intermittent Positive Pressure Breathing (IPPB) devices

E0500 IPPB machine, all types, with built-in nebulization; manual or automatic valves; internal or external power source

HUMIDIFIERS/COMPRESSORS/NEBULIZERS

E0550 Humidifier, durable for extensive supplemental humidification during IPPB treatments or oxygen delivery

E0555 Humidifier, durable, glass or autoclavable plastic bottle type, for use with regulator or flowmeter

E0560 Humidifier, durable for supplemental humidification during IPPB treatment or oxygen delivery

MED: 100-4,23,60.3

E0561 Humidifier, nonheated, used with positive airway pressure device

MED: 100-3,240.4; 100-4,36,50.14

E0562 Humidifier, heated, used with positive airway pressure device

E0565 Compressor, air power source for equipment which is not self-contained or cylinder driven

E0570 Nebulizer, with compressor

E0572 Aerosol compressor, adjustable pressure, light duty for intermittent use

E0574 Ultrasonic/electronic aerosol generator with small volume nebulizer

E0575 Nebulizer, ultrasonic, large volume

E0580 Nebulizer, durable, glass or autoclavable plastic, bottle type, for use with regulator or flowmeter

MED: 100-4,23,60.3

E0585 Nebulizer, with compressor and heater

PUMPS AND VAPORIZERS

E0600 Respiratory suction pump, home model, portable or stationary, electric

E0601 Continuous positive airway pressure (CPAP) device

MED: 100-3,240.4; 100-4,23,60.3

E0602 Breast pump, manual, any type

E0603 Breast pump, electric (AC and/or DC), any type

E0604 Breast pump, hospital grade, electric (AC and/or DC), any type

E0605 Vaporizer, room type

E0606 Postural drainage board

MONITORING DEVICES

E0607 Home blood glucose monitor

Medicare covers home blood testing devices for diabetic patients when the devices are prescribed by the patients' physicians. Many commercial payers provide this coverage to non-insulin dependent diabetics as well.

E0610 Pacemaker monitor, self-contained, (checks battery depletion, includes audible and visible check systems)

E0615 Pacemaker monitor, self-contained, checks battery depletion and other pacemaker components, includes digital/visible check systems

E0616 Implantable cardiac event recorder with memory, activator, and programmer

E0617 External defibrillator with integrated electrocardiogram analysis

E0618 Apnea monitor, without recording feature

E0619 Apnea monitor, with recording feature

E0620 Skin piercing device for collection of capillary blood, laser, each

PATIENT LIFTS

E0621 Sling or seat, patient lift, canvas or nylon

E0625 Patient lift, bathroom or toilet, not otherwise classified

E0627 Seat lift mechanism incorporated into a combination lift-chair mechanism

MED: 100-4,20,100; 100-4,20,130.2; 100-4,20,130.3; 100-4,20,130.4; 100-4,20,130.5

E0628 Separate seat lift mechanism for use with patient-owned furniture, electric
MED: 100-4,20,100; 100-4,20,130.2; 100-4,20,130.3; 100-4,20,130.4; 100-4,20,130.5

E0629 Separate seat lift mechanism for use with patient-owned furniture, nonelectric
MED: 100-4,20,100; 100-4,20,130.2; 100-4,20,130.3; 100-4,20,130.4; 100-4,20,130.5

E0630 Patient lift, hydraulic or mechanical, includes any seat, sling, strap(s), or pad(s)

E0635 Patient lift, electric, with seat or sling

E0636 Multipositional patient support system, with integrated lift, patient accessible controls

E0637 Combination sit-to-stand frame/table system, any size including pediatric, with seat lift feature, with or without wheels

E0638 Standing frame/table system, one position (e.g., upright, supine or prone stander), any size including pediatric, with or without wheels

E0639 Patient lift, moveable from room to room with disassembly and reassembly, includes all components/accessories

E0640 Patient lift, fixed system, includes all components/accessories

E0641 Standing frame/table system, multi-position (e.g., 3-way stander), any size including pediatric, with or without wheels

E0642 Standing frame/table system, mobile (dynamic stander), any size including pediatric

COMPRESSION DEVICES

E0650 Pneumatic compressor, nonsegmental home model

E0651 Pneumatic compressor, segmental home model without calibrated gradient pressure

E0652 Pneumatic compressor, segmental home model with calibrated gradient pressure

E0655 Nonsegmental pneumatic appliance for use with pneumatic compressor, half arm

E0656 Segmental pneumatic appliance for use with pneumatic compressor, trunk

E0657 Segmental pneumatic appliance for use with pneumatic compressor, chest

E0660 Nonsegmental pneumatic appliance for use with pneumatic compressor, full leg

E0665 Nonsegmental pneumatic appliance for use with pneumatic compressor, full arm

E0666 Nonsegmental pneumatic appliance for use with pneumatic compressor, half leg

E0667 Segmental pneumatic appliance for use with pneumatic compressor, full leg

E0668 Segmental pneumatic appliance for use with pneumatic compressor, full arm

E0669 Segmental pneumatic appliance for use with pneumatic compressor, half leg

E0670 Segmental pneumatic appliance for use with pneumatic compressor, integrated, 2 full legs and trunk

E0671 Segmental gradient pressure pneumatic appliance, full leg

E0672 Segmental gradient pressure pneumatic appliance, full arm

E0673 Segmental gradient pressure pneumatic appliance, half leg

E0675 Pneumatic compression device, high pressure, rapid inflation/deflation cycle, for arterial insufficiency (unilateral or bilateral system)

E0676 Intermittent limb compression device (includes all accessories), not otherwise specified

ULTRAVIOLET LIGHT

E0691 Ultraviolet light therapy system, includes bulbs/lamps, timer and eye protection; treatment area 2 sq ft or less

E0692 Ultraviolet light therapy system panel, includes bulbs/lamps, timer and eye protection, 4 ft panel

E0693 Ultraviolet light therapy system panel, includes bulbs/lamps, timer and eye protection, 6 ft panel

E0694 Ultraviolet multidirectional light therapy system in 6 ft cabinet, includes bulbs/lamps, timer, and eye protection

SAFETY EQUIPMENT

Fabric wrist restraint

Padded leather restraints may feature a locking device

Restraints (E0710)

Fabric gait belt for assistance in walking (E0700)

Body restraint

E0700 Safety equipment, device or accessory, any type

E0705 Transfer device, any type, each

E0710 Restraints, any type (body, chest, wrist, or ankle)

NERVE STIMULATORS AND DEVICES

E0720 Transcutaneous electrical nerve stimulation (TENS) device, 2 lead, localized stimulation
A Certificate of Medical Necessity is required for the purchase of a TENS. It is not required for rentals.
MED: 100-3,10.2; 100-3,160.7.1; 100-3,160.27; 100-4,20,30.1.2

E0730 Transcutaneous electrical nerve stimulation (TENS) device, 4 or more leads, for multiple nerve stimulation
A Certificate of Medical Necessity is required for the purchase of a TENS. It is not required for rentals.
MED: 100-3,10.2; 100-3,160.7.1; 100-3,160.27; 100-4,20,30.1.2

E0731 Form-fitting conductive garment for delivery of TENS or NMES (with conductive fibers separated from the patient's skin by layers of fabric)
MED: 100-3,10.2; 100-3,160.13

E0740 Incontinence treatment system, pelvic floor stimulator, monitor, sensor, and/or trainer

E0744 Neuromuscular stimulator for scoliosis

E0745 Neuromuscular stimulator, electronic shock unit

E0746 Electromyography (EMG), biofeedback device
Biofeedback therapy is covered by Medicare only for re-education of specific muscles or for treatment of incapacitating muscle spasm or weakness.

E0747 Osteogenesis stimulator, electrical, noninvasive, other than spinal applications
Medicare covers noninvasive osteogenic stimulation for nonunion of long bone fractures, failed fusion, or congenital pseudoarthroses.

Durable Medical Equipment

E0748 — E0961

E0748   Osteogenesis stimulator, electrical, noninvasive, spinal applications

Medicare covers noninvasive osteogenic stimulation as an adjunct to spinal fusion surgery for patients at high risk of pseudoarthroses due to previously failed spinal fusion, or for those undergoing fusion of three or more vertebrae.

E0749   Osteogenesis stimulator, electrical, surgically implanted

Medicare covers invasive osteogenic stimulation for nonunion of long bone fractures or as an adjunct to spinal fusion surgery for patients at high risk of pseudoarthroses due to previously failed spinal fusion, or for those undergoing fusion of three or more vertebrae.

MED: 100-4,4,190

E0755   Electronic salivary reflex stimulator (intraoral/noninvasive)

E0760   Osteogenesis stimulator, low intensity ultrasound, noninvasive

MED: 100-4,32,110.5

E0761   Nonthermal pulsed high frequency radiowaves, high peak power electromagnetic energy treatment device

E0762   Transcutaneous electrical joint stimulation device system, includes all accessories

E0764   Functional neuromuscular stimulation, transcutaneous stimulation of sequential muscle groups of ambulation with computer control, used for walking by spinal cord injured, entire system, after completion of training program

E0765   FDA approved nerve stimulator, with replaceable batteries, for treatment of nausea and vomiting

E0766   Electrical stimulation device used for cancer treatment, includes all accessories, any type

E0769   Electrical stimulation or electromagnetic wound treatment device, not otherwise classified

MED: 100-4,32,11.1

E0770   Functional electrical stimulator, transcutaneous stimulation of nerve and/or muscle groups, any type, complete system, not otherwise specified

INFUSION SUPPLIES

E0776   IV pole

MED: 100-4,23,60.3

E0779   Ambulatory infusion pump, mechanical, reusable, for infusion 8 hours or greater

E0780   Ambulatory infusion pump, mechanical, reusable, for infusion less than 8 hours

E0781   Ambulatory infusion pump, single or multiple channels, electric or battery operated, with administrative equipment, worn by patient

E0782   Infusion pump, implantable, nonprogrammable (includes all components, e.g., pump, catheter, connectors, etc.)

MED: 100-4,4,190

E0783   Infusion pump system, implantable, programmable (includes all components, e.g., pump, catheter, connectors, etc.)

MED: 100-4,4,190

E0784   External ambulatory infusion pump, insulin

Covered by some commercial payers with preauthorization.

E0785   Implantable intraspinal (epidural/intrathecal) catheter used with implantable infusion pump, replacement

MED: 100-4,4,190

E0786   Implantable programmable infusion pump, replacement (excludes implantable intraspinal catheter)

E0791   Parenteral infusion pump, stationary, single, or multichannel

TRACTION EQUIPMENT

E0830   Ambulatory traction device, all types, each

E0840   Traction frame, attached to headboard, cervical traction

E0849   Traction equipment, cervical, free-standing stand/frame, pneumatic, applying traction force to other than mandible

E0850   Traction stand, freestanding, cervical traction

E0855   Cervical traction equipment not requiring additional stand or frame

E0856   Cervical traction device, cervical collar with inflatable air bladder

E0860   Traction equipment, overdoor, cervical

E0870   Traction frame, attached to footboard, extremity traction (e.g., Buck's)

E0880   Traction stand, freestanding, extremity traction (e.g., Buck's)

E0890   Traction frame, attached to footboard, pelvic traction

E0900   Traction stand, freestanding, pelvic traction (e.g., Buck's)

ORTHOPEDIC DEVICES

E0910   Trapeze bars, also known as Patient Helper, attached to bed, with grab bar

MED: 100-4,23,60.3

E0911   Trapeze bar, heavy-duty, for patient weight capacity greater than 250 pounds, attached to bed, with grab bar

E0912   Trapeze bar, heavy-duty, for patient weight capacity greater than 250 pounds, freestanding, complete with grab bar

E0920   Fracture frame, attached to bed, includes weights

E0930   Fracture frame, freestanding, includes weights

E0935   Continuous passive motion exercise device for use on knee only

E0936   Continuous passive motion exercise device for use other than knee

E0940   Trapeze bar, freestanding, complete with grab bar

MED: 100-4,23,60.3

E0941   Gravity assisted traction device, any type

E0942   Cervical head harness/halter

E0944   Pelvic belt/harness/boot

E0945   Extremity belt/harness

E0946   Fracture, frame, dual with cross bars, attached to bed, (e.g., Balken, 4 Poster)

E0947   Fracture frame, attachments for complex pelvic traction

E0948   Fracture frame, attachments for complex cervical traction

WHEELCHAIR ACCESSORIES

E0950   Wheelchair accessory, tray, each

MED: 100-4,23,60.3

E0951   Heel loop/holder, any type, with or without ankle strap, each

E0952   Toe loop/holder, any type, each

E0955   Wheelchair accessory, headrest, cushioned, any type, including fixed mounting hardware, each

E0956   Wheelchair accessory, lateral trunk or hip support, any type, including fixed mounting hardware, each

E0957   Wheelchair accessory, medial thigh support, any type, including fixed mounting hardware, each

E0958   Manual wheelchair accessory, one-arm drive attachment, each

E0959   Manual wheelchair accessory, adapter for amputee, each

E0960   Wheelchair accessory, shoulder harness/straps or chest strap, including any type mounting hardware

MED: 100-4,23,60.3

E0961   Manual wheelchair accessory, wheel lock brake extension (handle), each

E0966   Manual wheelchair accessory, headrest extension, each

E0967   Manual wheelchair accessory, hand rim with projections, any type, each

E0968   Commode seat, wheelchair

E0969   Narrowing device, wheelchair

E0970   No. 2 footplates, except for elevating legrest
     See code(s): K0037, K0042

E0971   Manual wheelchair accessory, antitipping device, each

E0973   Wheelchair accessory, adjustable height, detachable armrest, complete assembly, each
     MED: 100-4,23,60.3

E0974   Manual wheelchair accessory, antirollback device, each

E0978   Wheelchair accessory, positioning belt/safety belt/pelvic strap, each
     MED: 100-4,23,60.3

E0980   Safety vest, wheelchair

E0981   Wheelchair accessory, seat upholstery, replacement only, each
     MED: 100-4,23,60.3

E0982   Wheelchair accessory, back upholstery, replacement only, each

E0983   Manual wheelchair accessory, power add-on to convert manual wheelchair to motorized wheelchair, joystick control

E0984   Manual wheelchair accessory, power add-on to convert manual wheelchair to motorized wheelchair, tiller control

E0985   Wheelchair accessory, seat lift mechanism

E0986   Manual wheelchair accessory, push activated power assist, each

E0988   Manual wheelchair accessory, lever-activated, wheel drive, pair

E0990   Wheelchair accessory, elevating legrest, complete assembly, each
     MED: 100-4,23,60.3

E0992   Manual wheelchair accessory, solid seat insert

E0994   Armrest, each

E0995   Wheelchair accessory, calf rest/pad, each
     MED: 100-4,23,60.3

E1002   Wheelchair accessory, power seating system, tilt only
     MED: 100-4,23,60.3

E1003   Wheelchair accessory, power seating system, recline only, without shear reduction

E1004   Wheelchair accessory, power seating system, recline only, with mechanical shear reduction

E1005   Wheelchair accessory, power seating system, recline only, with power shear reduction

E1006   Wheelchair accessory, power seating system, combination tilt and recline, without shear reduction

E1007   Wheelchair accessory, power seating system, combination tilt and recline, with mechanical shear reduction

E1008   Wheelchair accessory, power seating system, combination tilt and recline, with power shear reduction

E1009   Wheelchair accessory, addition to power seating system, mechanically linked leg elevation system, including pushrod and legrest, each

E1010   Wheelchair accessory, addition to power seating system, power leg elevation system, including legrest, pair

E1011   Modification to pediatric size wheelchair, width adjustment package (not to be dispensed with initial chair)

E1014   Reclining back, addition to pediatric size wheelchair

E1015   Shock absorber for manual wheelchair, each

E1016   Shock absorber for power wheelchair, each
     MED: 100-4,23,60.3

E1017   Heavy-duty shock absorber for heavy-duty or extra heavy-duty manual wheelchair, each

E1018   Heavy-duty shock absorber for heavy-duty or extra heavy-duty power wheelchair, each

E1020   Residual limb support system for wheelchair, any type
     MED: 100-4,23,60.3

E1028   Wheelchair accessory, manual swingaway, retractable or removable mounting hardware for joystick, other control interface or positioning accessory
     MED: 100-4,23,60.3; 100-4,23,60.3

E1029   Wheelchair accessory, ventilator tray, fixed

E1030   Wheelchair accessory, ventilator tray, gimbaled

E1031   Rollabout chair, any and all types with castors 5 in or greater

E1035   Multi-positional patient transfer system, with integrated seat, operated by care giver, patient weight capacity up to and including 300 lbs
     MED: 100-2,15,110

E1036   Multi-positional patient transfer system, extra-wide, with integrated seat, operated by caregiver, patient weight capacity greater than 300 lbs

E1037   Transport chair, pediatric size

E1038   Transport chair, adult size, patient weight capacity up to and including 300 pounds

E1039   Transport chair, adult size, heavy-duty, patient weight capacity greater than 300 pounds

WHEELCHAIRS

E1050   Fully-reclining wheelchair, fixed full-length arms, swing-away detachable elevating legrests

E1060   Fully-reclining wheelchair, detachable arms, desk or full-length, swing-away detachable elevating legrests

E1070   Fully-reclining wheelchair, detachable arms (desk or full-length) swing-away detachable footrest

E1083   Hemi-wheelchair, fixed full-length arms, swing-away detachable elevating legrest

E1084   Hemi-wheelchair, detachable arms desk or full-length arms, swing-away detachable elevating legrests

E1085   Hemi-wheelchair, fixed full-length arms, swing-away detachable footrests
     See code(s): K0002

E1086   Hemi-wheelchair, detachable arms, desk or full-length, swing-away detachable footrests
     See code(s): K0002

E1087   High strength lightweight wheelchair, fixed full-length arms, swing-away detachable elevating legrests

E1088   High strength lightweight wheelchair, detachable arms desk or full-length, swing-away detachable elevating legrests

E1089   High-strength lightweight wheelchair, fixed-length arms, swing-away detachable footrest
     See code(s): K0004

E1090   High-strength lightweight wheelchair, detachable arms, desk or full-length, swing-away detachable footrests
     See code(s): K0004

E1092   Wide heavy-duty wheel chair, detachable arms (desk or full-length), swing-away detachable elevating legrests

E1093   Wide heavy-duty wheelchair, detachable arms, desk or full-length arms, swing-away detachable footrests

E1100   Semi-reclining wheelchair, fixed full-length arms, swing-away detachable elevating legrests

Durable Medical Equipment

E1110 — E1405

E1110 Semi-reclining wheelchair, detachable arms (desk or full-length) elevating legrest

E1130 Standard wheelchair, fixed full-length arms, fixed or swing-away detachable footrests
See code(s): K0001

E1140 Wheelchair, detachable arms, desk or full-length, swing-away detachable footrests
See code(s): K0001

E1150 Wheelchair, detachable arms, desk or full-length swing-away detachable elevating legrests

E1160 Wheelchair, fixed full-length arms, swing-away detachable elevating legrests

E1161 Manual adult size wheelchair, includes tilt in space

E1170 Amputee wheelchair, fixed full-length arms, swing-away detachable elevating legrests

E1171 Amputee wheelchair, fixed full-length arms, without footrests or legrest

E1172 Amputee wheelchair, detachable arms (desk or full-length) without footrests or legrest

E1180 Amputee wheelchair, detachable arms (desk or full-length) swing-away detachable footrests

E1190 Amputee wheelchair, detachable arms (desk or full-length) swing-away detachable elevating legrests

E1195 Heavy-duty wheelchair, fixed full-length arms, swing-away detachable elevating legrests

E1200 Amputee wheelchair, fixed full-length arms, swing-away detachable footrest

E1220 Wheelchair; specially sized or constructed, (indicate brand name, model number, if any) and justification

E1221 Wheelchair with fixed arm, footrests

E1222 Wheelchair with fixed arm, elevating legrests

E1223 Wheelchair with detachable arms, footrests

E1224 Wheelchair with detachable arms, elevating legrests

E1225 Wheelchair accessory, manual semi-reclining back, (recline greater than 15 degrees, but less than 80 degrees), each

E1226 Wheelchair accessory, manual fully reclining back, (recline greater than 80 degrees), each
See also K0028

E1227 Special height arms for wheelchair

E1228 Special back height for wheelchair

E1229 Wheelchair, pediatric size, not otherwise specified

E1230 Power operated vehicle (3- or 4-wheel nonhighway), specify brand name and model number
Prior authorization is required by Medicare for this item.

E1231 Wheelchair, pediatric size, tilt-in-space, rigid, adjustable, with seating system

E1232 Wheelchair, pediatric size, tilt-in-space, folding, adjustable, with seating system

E1233 Wheelchair, pediatric size, tilt-in-space, rigid, adjustable, without seating system

E1234 Wheelchair, pediatric size, tilt-in-space, folding, adjustable, without seating system

E1235 Wheelchair, pediatric size, rigid, adjustable, with seating system

E1236 Wheelchair, pediatric size, folding, adjustable, with seating system

E1237 Wheelchair, pediatric size, rigid, adjustable, without seating system

E1238 Wheelchair, pediatric size, folding, adjustable, without seating system

E1239 Power wheelchair, pediatric size, not otherwise specified

E1240 Lightweight wheelchair, detachable arms, (desk or full-length) swing-away detachable, elevating legrest

E1250 Lightweight wheelchair, fixed full-length arms, swing-away detachable footrest
See code(s): K0003

E1260 Lightweight wheelchair, detachable arms (desk or full-length) swing-away detachable footrest
See code(s): K0003

E1270 Lightweight wheelchair, fixed full-length arms, swing-away detachable elevating legrests

E1280 Heavy-duty wheelchair, detachable arms (desk or full-length) elevating legrests

E1285 Heavy-duty wheelchair, fixed full-length arms, swing-away detachable footrest
See code(s): K0006

E1290 Heavy-duty wheelchair, detachable arms (desk or full-length) swing-away detachable footrest
See code(s): K0006

E1295 Heavy-duty wheelchair, fixed full-length arms, elevating legrest

E1296 Special wheelchair seat height from floor

E1297 Special wheelchair seat depth, by upholstery

E1298 Special wheelchair seat depth and/or width, by construction

WHIRLPOOL - EQUIPMENT

E1300 Whirlpool, portable (overtub type)

E1310 Whirlpool, nonportable (built-in type)

ADDITIONAL OXYGEN RELATED EQUIPMENT

E1352 Oxygen accessory, flow regulator capable of positive inspiratory pressure

E1353 Regulator
MED: 100-4,23,60.3

E1354 Oxygen accessory, wheeled cart for portable cylinder or portable concentrator, any type, replacement only, each

E1355 Stand/rack
MED: 100-4,23,60.3

E1356 Oxygen accessory, battery pack/cartridge for portable concentrator, any type, replacement only, each

E1357 Oxygen accessory, battery charger for portable concentrator, any type, replacement only, each

E1358 Oxygen accessory, DC power adapter for portable concentrator, any type, replacement only, each

E1372 Immersion external heater for nebulizer

E1390 Oxygen concentrator, single delivery port, capable of delivering 85 percent or greater oxygen concentration at the prescribed flow rate

E1391 Oxygen concentrator, dual delivery port, capable of delivering 85 percent or greater oxygen concentration at the prescribed flow rate, each

E1392 Portable oxygen concentrator, rental

E1399 Durable medical equipment, miscellaneous
MED: 100-4,32,110.5

E1405 Oxygen and water vapor enriching system with heated delivery
MED: 100-4,20,20; 100-4,20,20.4

E1406   Oxygen and water vapor enriching system without heated delivery
MED: 100-4,20,20; 100-4,20,20.4

ARTIFICIAL KIDNEY MACHINES AND ACCESSORIES

E1500   Centrifuge, for dialysis

E1510   Kidney, dialysate delivery system kidney machine, pump recirculating, air removal system, flowrate meter, power off, heater and temperature control with alarm, IV poles, pressure gauge, concentrate container

E1520   Heparin infusion pump for hemodialysis

E1530   Air bubble detector for hemodialysis, each, replacement

E1540   Pressure alarm for hemodialysis, each, replacement

E1550   Bath conductivity meter for hemodialysis, each

E1560   Blood leak detector for hemodialysis, each, replacement

E1570   Adjustable chair, for ESRD patients

E1575   Transducer protectors/fluid barriers, for hemodialysis, any size, per 10

E1580   Unipuncture control system for hemodialysis

E1590   Hemodialysis machine

E1592   Automatic intermittent peritoneal dialysis system

E1594   Cycler dialysis machine for peritoneal dialysis

E1600   Delivery and/or installation charges for hemodialysis equipment

E1610   Reverse osmosis water purification system, for hemodialysis

E1615   Deionizer water purification system, for hemodialysis

E1620   Blood pump for hemodialysis, replacement

E1625   Water softening system, for hemodialysis

E1630   Reciprocating peritoneal dialysis system

E1632   Wearable artificial kidney, each

E1634   Peritoneal dialysis clamps, each

E1635   Compact (portable) travel hemodialyzer system

E1636   Sorbent cartridges, for hemodialysis, per 10

E1637   Hemostats, each

E1639   Scale, each

E1699   Dialysis equipment, not otherwise specified

JAW MOTION REHABILITATION SYSTEM AND ACCESSORIES

E1700   Jaw motion rehabilitation system
Medicare jurisdiction: local contractor.

E1701   Replacement cushions for jaw motion rehabilitation system, package of 6
Medicare jurisdiction: local contractor.

E1702   Replacement measuring scales for jaw motion rehabilitation system, package of 200
Medicare jurisdiction: local contractor.

FLEXION/EXTENSION DEVICE

E1800   Dynamic adjustable elbow extension/flexion device, includes soft interface material

E1801   Static progressive stretch elbow device, extension and/or flexion, with or without range of motion adjustment, includes all components and accessories

E1802   Dynamic adjustable forearm pronation/supination device, includes soft interface material

E1805   Dynamic adjustable wrist extension/flexion device, includes soft interface material

E1806   Static progressive stretch wrist device, flexion and/or extension, with or without range of motion adjustment, includes all components and accessories

E1810   Dynamic adjustable knee extension/flexion device, includes soft interface material

E1811   Static progressive stretch knee device, extension and/or flexion, with or without range of motion adjustment, includes all components and accessories

E1812   Dynamic knee, extension/flexion device with active resistance control

E1815   Dynamic adjustable ankle extension/flexion device, includes soft interface material

E1816   Static progressive stretch ankle device, flexion and/or extension, with or without range of motion adjustment, includes all components and accessories

E1818   Static progressive stretch forearm pronation/supination device, with or without range of motion adjustment, includes all components and accessories

E1820   Replacement soft interface material, dynamic adjustable extension/flexion device

E1821   Replacement soft interface material/cuffs for bi-directional static progressive stretch device

E1825   Dynamic adjustable finger extension/flexion device, includes soft interface material

E1830   Dynamic adjustable toe extension/flexion device, includes soft interface material

E1831   Static progressive stretch toe device, extension and/or flexion, with or without range of motion adjustment, includes all components and accessories

E1840   Dynamic adjustable shoulder flexion/abduction/rotation device, includes soft interface material

E1841   Static progressive stretch shoulder device, with or without range of motion adjustment, includes all components and accessories

OTHER DEVICES

E1902   Communication board, nonelectronic augmentative or alternative communication device

E2000   Gastric suction pump, home model, portable or stationary, electric

E2100   Blood glucose monitor with integrated voice synthesizer

E2101   Blood glucose monitor with integrated lancing/blood sample

E2120   Pulse generator system for tympanic treatment of inner ear endolymphatic fluid

DME WHEELCHAIR ACCESSORY

E2201   Manual wheelchair accessory, nonstandard seat frame, width greater than or equal to 20 in and less than 24 in

E2202   Manual wheelchair accessory, nonstandard seat frame width, 24-27 in

E2203   Manual wheelchair accessory, nonstandard seat frame depth, 20 to less than 22 in

E2204   Manual wheelchair accessory, nonstandard seat frame depth, 22 to 25 in

E2205   Manual wheelchair accessory, handrim without projections (includes ergonomic or contoured), any type, replacement only, each

E2206   Manual wheelchair accessory, wheel Lock assembly, complete, each

E2207   Wheelchair accessory, crutch and cane holder, each

E2208   Wheelchair accessory, cylinder tank carrier, each
MED: 100-4,23,60.3

Durable Medical Equipment

E2209 — E2362

E2209   Accessory, arm trough, with or without hand support, each

E2210   Wheelchair accessory, bearings, any type, replacement only, each

E2211   Manual wheelchair accessory, pneumatic propulsion tire, any size, each

E2212   Manual wheelchair accessory, tube for pneumatic propulsion tire, any size, each

E2213   Manual wheelchair accessory, insert for pneumatic propulsion tire (removable), any type, any size, each

E2214   Manual wheelchair accessory, pneumatic caster tire, any size, each

E2215   Manual wheelchair accessory, tube for pneumatic caster tire, any size, each

E2216   Manual wheelchair accessory, foam filled propulsion tire, any size, each

E2217   Manual wheelchair accessory, foam filled caster tire, any size, each

E2218   Manual wheelchair accessory, foam propulsion tire, any size, each

E2219   Manual wheelchair accessory, foam caster tire, any size, each

E2220   Manual wheelchair accessory, solid (rubber/plastic) propulsion tire, any size, each

E2221   Manual wheelchair accessory, solid (rubber/plastic) caster tire (removable), any size, each

E2222   Manual wheelchair accessory, solid (rubber/plastic) caster tire with integrated wheel, any size, each

E2224   Manual wheelchair accessory, propulsion wheel excludes tire, any size, each

E2225   Manual wheelchair accessory, caster wheel excludes tire, any size, replacement only, each

E2226   Manual wheelchair accessory, caster fork, any size, replacement only, each

E2227   Manual wheelchair accessory, gear reduction drive wheel, each

E2228   Manual wheelchair accessory, wheel braking system and lock, complete, each

E2230   Manual wheelchair accessory, manual standing system

E2231   Manual wheelchair accessory, solid seat support base (replaces sling seat), includes any type mounting hardware

E2291   Back, planar, for pediatric size wheelchair including fixed attaching hardware

E2292   Seat, planar, for pediatric size wheelchair including fixed attaching hardware

E2293   Back, contoured, for pediatric size wheelchair including fixed attaching hardware

E2294   Seat, contoured, for pediatric size wheelchair including fixed attaching hardware

E2295   Manual wheelchair accessory, for pediatric size wheelchair, dynamic seating frame, allows coordinated movement of multiple positioning features

E2300   Wheelchair accessory, power seat elevation system, any type

E2301   Wheelchair accessory, power standing system, any type

E2310   Power wheelchair accessory, electronic connection between wheelchair controller and one power seating system motor, including all related electronics, indicator feature, mechanical function selection switch, and fixed mounting hardware

     MED: 100-4,23,60.3

E2311   Power wheelchair accessory, electronic connection between wheelchair controller and 2 or more power seating system motors, including all related electronics, indicator feature, mechanical function selection switch, and fixed mounting hardware

E2312   Power wheelchair accessory, hand or chin control interface, mini-proportional remote joystick, proportional, including fixed mounting hardware

E2313   Power wheelchair accessory, harness for upgrade to expandable controller, including all fasteners, connectors and mounting hardware, each

E2321   Power wheelchair accessory, hand control interface, remote joystick, nonproportional, including all related electronics, mechanical stop switch, and fixed mounting hardware

     MED: 100-4,23,60.3

E2322   Power wheelchair accessory, hand control interface, multiple mechanical switches, nonproportional, including all related electronics, mechanical stop switch, and fixed mounting hardware

E2323   Power wheelchair accessory, specialty joystick handle for hand control interface, prefabricated

E2324   Power wheelchair accessory, chin cup for chin control interface

E2325   Power wheelchair accessory, sip and puff interface, nonproportional, including all related electronics, mechanical stop switch, and manual swingaway mounting hardware

E2326   Power wheelchair accessory, breath tube kit for sip and puff interface

E2327   Power wheelchair accessory, head control interface, mechanical, proportional, including all related electronics, mechanical direction change switch, and fixed mounting hardware

E2328   Power wheelchair accessory, head control or extremity control interface, electronic, proportional, including all related electronics and fixed mounting hardware

E2329   Power wheelchair accessory, head control interface, contact switch mechanism, nonproportional, including all related electronics, mechanical stop switch, mechanical direction change switch, head array, and fixed mounting hardware

E2330   Power wheelchair accessory, head control interface, proximity switch mechanism, nonproportional, including all related electronics, mechanical stop switch, mechanical direction change switch, head array, and fixed mounting hardware

E2331   Power wheelchair accessory, attendant control, proportional, including all related electronics and fixed mounting hardware

E2340   Power wheelchair accessory, nonstandard seat frame width, 20-23 in

E2341   Power wheelchair accessory, nonstandard seat frame width, 24-27 in

E2342   Power wheelchair accessory, nonstandard seat frame depth, 20 or 21 in

E2343   Power wheelchair accessory, nonstandard seat frame depth, 22-25 in

E2351   Power wheelchair accessory, electronic interface to operate speech generating device using power wheelchair control interface

     MED: 100-4,23,60.3

E2358   Power wheelchair accessory, group 34 nonsealed lead acid battery, each

E2359   Power wheelchair accessory, group 34 sealed lead acid battery, each (e.g., gel cell, absorbed glass mat)

E2360   Power wheelchair accessory, 22 NF nonsealed lead acid battery, each

E2361   Power wheelchair accessory, 22 NF sealed lead acid battery, each (e.g., gel cell, absorbed glassmat)

     MED: 100-4,23,60.3

E2362   Power wheelchair accessory, group 24 nonsealed lead acid battery, each

E2363   Power wheelchair accessory, group 24 sealed lead acid battery, each (e.g., gel cell, absorbed glassmat)
MED: 100-4,23,60.3

E2364   Power wheelchair accessory, U-1 nonsealed lead acid battery, each

E2365   Power wheelchair accessory, U-1 sealed lead acid battery, each (e.g., gel cell, absorbed glassmat)
MED: 100-4,23,60.3

E2366   Power wheelchair accessory, battery charger, single mode, for use with only one battery type, sealed or nonsealed, each

E2367   Power wheelchair accessory, battery charger, dual mode, for use with either battery type, sealed or nonsealed, each

E2368   Power wheelchair component, drive wheel motor, replacement only

E2369   Power wheelchair component, drive wheel gear box, replacement only

E2370   Power wheelchair component, integrated drive wheel motor and gear box combination, replacement only

E2371   Power wheelchair accessory, group 27 sealed lead acid battery, (e.g., gel cell, absorbed glassmat), each

E2372   Power wheelchair accessory, group 27 nonsealed lead acid battery, each

E2373   Power wheelchair accessory, hand or chin control interface, compact remote joystick, proportional, including fixed mounting hardware
MED: 100-4,23,60.3

E2374   Power wheelchair accessory, hand or chin control interface, standard remote joystick (not including controller), proportional, including all related electronics and fixed mounting hardware, replacement only

E2375   Power wheelchair accessory, nonexpandable controller, including all related electronics and mounting hardware, replacement only

E2376   Power wheelchair accessory, expandable controller, including all related electronics and mounting hardware, replacement only

E2377   Power wheelchair accessory, expandable controller, including all related electronics and mounting hardware, upgrade provided at initial issue

E2378   Power wheelchair component, actuator, replacement only

E2381   Power wheelchair accessory, pneumatic drive wheel tire, any size, replacement only, each

E2382   Power wheelchair accessory, tube for pneumatic drive wheel tire, any size, replacement only, each

E2383   Power wheelchair accessory, insert for pneumatic drive wheel tire (removable), any type, any size, replacement only, each

E2384   Power wheelchair accessory, pneumatic caster tire, any size, replacement only, each

E2385   Power wheelchair accessory, tube for pneumatic caster tire, any size, replacement only, each

E2386   Power wheelchair accessory, foam filled drive wheel tire, any size, replacement only, each

E2387   Power wheelchair accessory, foam filled caster tire, any size, replacement only, each

E2388   Power wheelchair accessory, foam drive wheel tire, any size, replacement only, each

E2389   Power wheelchair accessory, foam caster tire, any size, replacement only, each

E2390   Power wheelchair accessory, solid (rubber/plastic) drive wheel tire, any size, replacement only, each

E2391   Power wheelchair accessory, solid (rubber/plastic) caster tire (removable), any size, replacement only, each

E2392   Power wheelchair accessory, solid (rubber/plastic) caster tire with integrated wheel, any size, replacement only, each

E2394   Power wheelchair accessory, drive wheel excludes tire, any size, replacement only, each

E2395   Power wheelchair accessory, caster wheel excludes tire, any size, replacement only, each

E2396   Power wheelchair accessory, caster fork, any size, replacement only, each

E2397   Power wheelchair accessory, lithium-based battery, each

WOUND THERAPY

E2402   Negative pressure wound therapy electrical pump, stationary or portable
MED: 100-4,23,60.3

SPEECH GENERATING DEVICE

E2500   Speech generating device, digitized speech, using prerecorded messages, less than or equal to 8 minutes recording time

E2502   Speech generating device, digitized speech, using prerecorded messages, greater than 8 minutes but less than or equal to 20 minutes recording time

E2504   Speech generating device, digitized speech, using prerecorded messages, greater than 20 minutes but less than or equal to 40 minutes recording time

E2506   Speech generating device, digitized speech, using prerecorded messages, greater than 40 minutes recording time

E2508   Speech generating device, synthesized speech, requiring message formulation by spelling and access by physical contact with the device

E2510   Speech generating device, synthesized speech, permitting multiple methods of message formulation and multiple methods of device access

E2511   Speech generating software program, for personal computer or personal digital assistant

E2512   Accessory for speech generating device, mounting system

E2599   Accessory for speech generating device, not otherwise classified

WHEELCHAIR CUSHION

E2601   General use wheelchair seat cushion, width less than 22 in, any depth
MED: 100-4,23,60.3

E2602   General use wheelchair seat cushion, width 22 in or greater, any depth

E2603   Skin protection wheelchair seat cushion, width less than 22 in, any depth

E2604   Skin protection wheelchair seat cushion, width 22 in or greater, any depth

E2605   Positioning wheelchair seat cushion, width less than 22 in, any depth

E2606   Positioning wheelchair seat cushion, width 22 in or greater, any depth

E2607   Skin protection and positioning wheelchair seat cushion, width less than 22 in, any depth

E2608   Skin protection and positioning wheelchair seat cushion, width 22 in or greater, any depth

E2609   Custom fabricated wheelchair seat cushion, any size

E2610   Wheelchair seat cushion, powered

E2611   General use wheelchair back cushion, width less than 22 in, any height, including any type mounting hardware
MED: 100-4,23,60.3

Durable Medical Equipment

E2612 — E8002

E2612   General use wheelchair back cushion, width 22 in or greater, any height, including any type mounting hardware

E2613   Positioning wheelchair back cushion, posterior, width less than 22 in, any height, including any type mounting hardware

E2614   Positioning wheelchair back cushion, posterior, width 22 in or greater, any height, including any type mounting hardware

E2615   Positioning wheelchair back cushion, posterior-lateral, width less than 22 in, any height, including any type mounting hardware

E2616   Positioning wheelchair back cushion, posterior-lateral, width 22 in or greater, any height, including any type mounting hardware

E2617   Custom fabricated wheelchair back cushion, any size, including any type mounting hardware

E2619   Replacement cover for wheelchair seat cushion or back cushion, each

     MED: 100-4,23,60.3

E2620   Positioning wheelchair back cushion, planar back with lateral supports, width less than 22 in, any height, including any type mounting hardware

E2621   Positioning wheelchair back cushion, planar back with lateral supports, width 22 in or greater, any height, including any type mounting hardware

E2622   Skin protection wheelchair seat cushion, adjustable, width less than 22 in, any depth

E2623   Skin protection wheelchair seat cushion, adjustable, width 22 in or greater, any depth

E2624   Skin protection and positioning wheelchair seat cushion, adjustable, width less than 22 in, any depth

E2625   Skin protection and positioning wheelchair seat cushion, adjustable, width 22 in or greater, any depth

WHEELCHAIR ARM SUPPORT

E2626   Wheelchair accessory, shoulder elbow, mobile arm support attached to wheelchair, balanced, adjustable

E2627   Wheelchair accessory, shoulder elbow, mobile arm support attached to wheelchair, balanced, adjustable Rancho type

E2628   Wheelchair accessory, shoulder elbow, mobile arm support attached to wheelchair, balanced, reclining

E2629   Wheelchair accessory, shoulder elbow, mobile arm support attached to wheelchair, balanced, friction arm support (friction dampening to proximal and distal joints)

E2630   Wheelchair accessory, shoulder elbow, mobile arm support, monosuspension arm and hand support, overhead elbow forearm hand sling support, yoke type suspension support

E2631   Wheelchair accessory, addition to mobile arm support, elevating proximal arm

E2632   Wheelchair accessory, addition to mobile arm support, offset or lateral rocker arm with elastic balance control

E2633   Wheelchair accessory, addition to mobile arm support, supinator

GAIT TRAINER

E8000   Gait trainer, pediatric size, posterior support, includes all accessories and components

E8001   Gait trainer, pediatric size, upright support, includes all accessories and components

E8002   Gait trainer, pediatric size, anterior support, includes all accessories and components

PROCEDURES/PROFESSIONAL SERVICES (TEMPORARY)
G0008-G9156

The G codes are used to identify professional health care procedures and services that would otherwise be coded in CPT but for which there are no CPT codes.

Please refer to your CPT book for possible alternate code(s).

IMMUNIZATION ADMINISTRATION

G0008 Administration of influenza virus vaccine

MED: 100-2,12,40.11; 100-4,18,10.2.1; 100-4,18,10.2.2.1; 100-4,18,10.2.2.1; 100-4,18,10.2.5.2; 100-4,18,10.3.1.1; 100-4,18,10.4; 100-4,18,10.4.1; 100-4,18,10.4.2; 100-4,18,10.4.3

G0009 Administration of pneumococcal vaccine

MED: 100-4,18,10.2.2.1; 100-4,18,10.4

G0010 Administration of hepatitis B vaccine

MED: 100-4,18,10.2.2.1; 100-4,18,10.4

SEMEN ANALYSIS

G0027 Semen analysis; presence and/or motility of sperm excluding Huhner

SCREENING SERVICES

G0101 Cervical or vaginal cancer screening; pelvic and clinical breast examination

G0101 can be reported with an E/M code when a separately identifiable E/M service was provided.

AHA: 4Q,'02,8; 3Q,'01,6

G0102 Prostate cancer screening; digital rectal examination

G0103 Prostate cancer screening; prostate specific antigen test (PSA)

G0104 Colorectal cancer screening; flexible sigmoidoscopy

Medicare covers colorectal screening for cancer via flexible sigmoidoscopy once every four years for patients 50 years or older.

MED: 100-4,18,60.1; 100-4,18,60.2; 100-4,18,60.6

G0105 Colorectal cancer screening; colonoscopy on individual at high risk

An individual with ulcerative enteritis or a history of a malignant neoplasm of the lower gastrointestinal tract is considered at high-risk for colorectal cancer, as defined by CMS.

MED: 100-4,18,60.1; 100-4,18,60.2; 100-4,18,60.6
AHA: 3Q,'01,6

G0106 Colorectal cancer screening; alternative to G0104, screening sigmoidoscopy, barium enema

MED: 100-4,18,60.1; 100-4,18,60.2; 100-4,18,60.6

G0108 Diabetes outpatient self-management training services, individual, per 30 minutes

MED: 100-2,15,270; 100-2,15,270.4.3; 100-2,15,300; 100-2,15,300.2; 100-2,15,300.3; 100-2,15,300.4; 100-4,4,300.6; 100-4,9,181; 100-4,12,190.3; 100-4,12,190.7; 100-4,18,120.1

G0109 Diabetes outpatient self-management training services, group session (2 or more), per 30 minutes

MED: 100-2,15,300.2; 100-4,4,300.6; 100-4,9,181

G0117 Glaucoma screening for high risk patients furnished by an optometrist or ophthalmologist

MED: 100-2,15,280.1
AHA: 1Q,'02,4; 3Q,'01,12

G0118 Glaucoma screening for high risk patient furnished under the direct supervision of an optometrist or ophthalmologist

MED: 100-2,15,280.1
AHA: 1Q,'02,4; 3Q,'01,12

G0120 Colorectal cancer screening; alternative to G0105, screening colonoscopy, barium enema

MED: 100-4,18,60.1; 100-4,18,60.2; 100-4,18,60.6

G0121 Colorectal cancer screening; colonoscopy on individual not meeting criteria for high risk

MED: 100-4,18,60.1; 100-4,18,60.2; 100-4,18,60.6
AHA: 1Q,'02,4; 3Q,'01,12

G0122 Colorectal cancer screening; barium enema

MED: 100-4,18,60.2; 100-4,18,60.6

G0123 Screening cytopathology, cervical or vaginal (any reporting system), collected in preservative fluid, automated thin layer preparation, screening by cytotechnologist under physician supervision
See also P3000-P3001.

G0124 Screening cytopathology, cervical or vaginal (any reporting system), collected in preservative fluid, automated thin layer preparation, requiring interpretation by physician
See also P3000-P3001.

MISCELLANEOUS SERVICES

G0127 Trimming of dystrophic nails, any number

MED: 100-2,15,290; 100-2,15,290

G0128 Direct (face-to-face with patient) skilled nursing services of a registered nurse provided in a comprehensive outpatient rehabilitation facility, each 10 minutes beyond the first 5 minutes

MED: 100-2,12,30.1; 100-2,12,40.8; 100-4,5,20.4; 100-4,5,100.3

G0129 Occupational therapy services requiring the skills of a qualified occupational therapist, furnished as a component of a partial hospitalization treatment program, per session (45 minutes or more)

G0130 Single energy x-ray absorptiometry (SEXA) bone density study, one or more sites; appendicular skeleton (peripheral) (e.g., radius, wrist, heel)

G0141 Screening cytopathology smears, cervical or vaginal, performed by automated system, with manual rescreening, requiring interpretation by physician

G0143 Screening cytopathology, cervical or vaginal (any reporting system), collected in preservative fluid, automated thin layer preparation, with manual screening and rescreening by cytotechnologist under physician supervision

G0144 Screening cytopathology, cervical or vaginal (any reporting system), collected in preservative fluid, automated thin layer preparation, with screening by automated system, under physician supervision

G0145 Screening cytopathology, cervical or vaginal (any reporting system), collected in preservative fluid, automated thin layer preparation, with screening by automated system and manual rescreening under physician supervision

G0147 Screening cytopathology smears, cervical or vaginal, performed by automated system under physician supervision

G0148 Screening cytopathology smears, cervical or vaginal, performed by automated system with manual rescreening

G0151 Services performed by a qualified physical therapist in the home health or hospice setting, each 15 minutes

MED: 100-4,10,40.2; 100-4,11,10; 100-4,11,30.3

G0152 Services performed by a qualified occupational therapist in the home health or hospice setting, each 15 minutes

G0153 Services performed by a qualified speech-language pathologist in the home health or hospice setting, each 15 minutes

G0154 Direct skilled nursing services of a licensed nurse (LPN or RN) in the home health or hospice setting, each 15 minutes

G0155 Services of clinical social worker in home health or hospice settings, each 15 minutes

G0156 Services of home health/hospice aide in home health or hospice settings, each 15 minutes

G0157 Services performed by a qualified physical therapist assistant in the home health or hospice setting, each 15 minutes

G0158 Services performed by a qualified occupational therapist assistant in the home health or hospice setting, each 15 minutes

G0159 Services performed by a qualified physical therapist, in the home health setting, in the establishment or delivery of a safe and effective physical therapy maintenance program, each 15 minutes

G0160 Services performed by a qualified occupational therapist, in the home health setting, in the establishment or delivery of a safe and effective occupational therapy maintenance program, each 15 minutes

    MED: 100-4,10,40.2

G0161 Services performed by a qualified speech-language pathologist, in the home health setting, in the establishment or delivery of a safe and effective speech-language pathology maintenance program, each 15 minutes

G0162 Skilled services by a registered nurse (RN) for management and evaluation of the plan of care; each 15 minutes (the patient's underlying condition or complication requires an RN to ensure that essential nonskilled care achieves its purpose in the home health or hospice setting)

    MED: 100-4,11,10

G0163 Skilled services of a licensed nurse (LPN or RN) for the observation and assessment of the patient's condition, each 15 minutes (the change in the patient's condition requires skilled nursing personnel to identify and evaluate the patient's need for possible modification of treatment in the home health or hospice setting)

G0164 Skilled services of a licensed nurse (LPN or RN), in the training and/or education of a patient or family member, in the home health or hospice setting, each 15 minutes

G0166 External counterpulsation, per treatment session

    MED: 100-4,32,130; 100-4,32,130.1

G0168 Wound closure utilizing tissue adhesive(s) only

    AHA: 4Q,'01,12; 3Q,'01,13

G0173 Linear accelerator based stereotactic radiosurgery, complete course of therapy in one session

    MED: 100-4,4,200.3.4; 100-4,4,200.3.4

G0175 Scheduled interdisciplinary team conference (minimum of 3 exclusive of patient care nursing staff) with patient present

G0176 Activity therapy, such as music, dance, art or play therapies not for recreation, related to the care and treatment of patient's disabling mental health problems, per session (45 minutes or more)

G0177 Training and educational services related to the care and treatment of patient's disabling mental health problems per session (45 minutes or more)

    MED: 100-1,3,30; 100-1,3,30.3

G0179 Physician re-certification for Medicare-covered home health services under a home health plan of care (patient not present), including contacts with home health agency and review of reports of patient status required by physicians to affirm the initial implementation of the plan of care that meets patient's needs, per re-certification period

    MED: 100-4,11,40.1.3.1; 100-4,12,180; 100-4,12,180.1

G0180 Physician certification for Medicare-covered home health services under a home health plan of care (patient not present), including contacts with home health agency and review of reports of patient status required by physicians to affirm the initial implementation of the plan of care that meets patient's needs, per certification period

    MED: 100-4,11,40.1.3.1; 100-4,12,180; 100-4,12,180.1

G0181 Physician supervision of a patient receiving Medicare-covered services provided by a participating home health agency (patient not present) requiring complex and multidisciplinary care modalities involving regular physician development and/or revision of care plans, review of subsequent reports of patient status, review of laboratory and other studies, communication (including telephone calls) with other health care professionals involved in the patient's care, integration of new information into the medical treatment plan and/or adjustment of medical therapy, within a calendar month, 30 minutes or more

    MED: 100-4,11,40.1.3.1; 100-4,12,180; 100-4,12,180.1

G0182 Physician supervision of a patient under a Medicare-approved hospice (patient not present) requiring complex and multidisciplinary care modalities involving regular physician development and/or revision of care plans, review of subsequent reports of patient status, review of laboratory and other studies, communication (including telephone calls) with other health care professionals involved in the patient's care, integration of new information into the medical treatment plan and/or adjustment of medical therapy, within a calendar month, 30 minutes or more

    MED: 100-4,11,40.1.3.1; 100-4,12,180; 100-4,12,180.1

G0186 Destruction of localized lesion of choroid (for example, choroidal neovascularization); photocoagulation, feeder vessel technique (one or more sessions)

G0202 Screening mammography, producing direct digital image, bilateral, all views

    MED: 100-4,18,20; 100-4,18,20.5

    AHA: 1Q,'02,3

G0204 Diagnostic mammography, producing direct digital image, bilateral, all views

    MED: 100-4,18,20; 100-4,18,20.4; 100-4,18,20.5

    AHA: 1Q,'03,7

G0206 Diagnostic mammography, producing direct digital image, unilateral, all views

    MED: 100-4,18,20; 100-4,18,20.4; 100-4,18,20.5

    AHA: 1Q,'03,7

G0219 PET imaging whole body; melanoma for noncovered indications

    MED: 100-3,220.6.3; 100-3,220.6.4; 100-3,220.6.6; 100-3,220.6.7; 100-3,220.6.10; 100-3,220.6.11; 100-3,220.6.12; 100-3,220.6.17; 100-4,13,60; 100-4,13,60.15; 100-4,13,60.16

    AHA: 1Q,'02,10

G0235 PET imaging, any site, not otherwise specified

    MED: 100-3,220.6.2; 100-3,220.6.3; 100-3,220.6.4; 100-3,220.6.5; 100-3,220.6.6; 100-3,220.6.7; 100-3,220.6.9; 100-3,220.6.10; 100-3,220.6.11; 100-3,220.6.12; 100-3,220.6.13; 100-3,220.6.17; 100-4,13,60; 100-4,13,60.13; 100-4,13,60.14; 100-4,13,60.15; 100-4,13,60.16; 100-4,13,60.17

G0237 Therapeutic procedures to increase strength or endurance of respiratory muscles, face-to-face, one-on-one, each 15 minutes (includes monitoring)

    MED: 100-2,12,30.1; 100-2,12,40.5

G0238 Therapeutic procedures to improve respiratory function, other than described by G0237, one-on-one, face-to-face, per 15 minutes (includes monitoring)

    MED: 100-2,12,40.5

G0239 Therapeutic procedures to improve respiratory function or increase strength or endurance of respiratory muscles, 2 or more individuals (includes monitoring)

    MED: 100-2,12,40.5

G0245 Initial physician evaluation and management of a diabetic patient with diabetic sensory neuropathy resulting in a loss of protective sensation (LOPS) which must include: (1) the diagnosis of LOPS, (2) a patient history, (3) a physical examination that consists of at least the following elements: (a) visual inspection of the forefoot, hindfoot, and toe web spaces, (b) evaluation of a protective sensation, (c) evaluation of foot structure and biomechanics, (d) evaluation of vascular status and skin integrity, and (e) evaluation and recommendation of footwear, and (4) patient education
  MED: 100-4,32,80.2; 100-4,32,80.8
  AHA: 4Q,'02,9

G0246 Follow-up physician evaluation and management of a diabetic patient with diabetic sensory neuropathy resulting in a loss of protective sensation (LOPS) to include at least the following: (1) a patient history, (2) a physical examination that includes: (a) visual inspection of the forefoot, hindfoot, and toe web spaces, (b) evaluation of protective sensation, (c) evaluation of foot structure and biomechanics, (d) evaluation of vascular status and skin integrity, and (e) evaluation and recommendation of footwear, and (3) patient education
  MED: 100-3,70.2.1; 100-4,32,80; 100-4,32,80.8
  AHA: 4Q,'02,9

G0247 Routine foot care by a physician of a diabetic patient with diabetic sensory neuropathy resulting in a loss of protective sensation (LOPS) to include the local care of superficial wounds (i.e., superficial to muscle and fascia) and at least the following, if present: (1) local care of superficial wounds, (2) debridement of corns and calluses, and (3) trimming and debridement of nails
  MED: 100-4,32,80.8
  AHA: 4Q,'02,9

G0248 Demonstration, prior to initiation of home INR monitoring, for patient with either mechanical heart valve(s), chronic atrial fibrillation, or venous thromboembolism who meets Medicare coverage criteria, under the direction of a physician; includes: face-to-face demonstration of use and care of the INR monitor, obtaining at least one blood sample, provision of instructions for reporting home INR test results, and documentation of patient's ability to perform testing and report results
  MED: 100-3,190.11; 100-4,32,60.4.1; 100-4,32,60.5.2
  AHA: 4Q,'02,9

G0249 Provision of test materials and equipment for home INR monitoring of patient with either mechanical heart valve(s), chronic atrial fibrillation, or venous thromboembolism who meets Medicare coverage criteria; includes: provision of materials for use in the home and reporting of test results to physician; testing not occurring more frequently than once a week; testing materials, billing units of service include 4 tests
  AHA: 4Q,'02,9

G0250 Physician review, interpretation, and patient management of home INR testing for patient with either mechanical heart valve(s), chronic atrial fibrillation, or venous thromboembolism who meets Medicare coverage criteria; testing not occurring more frequently than once a week; billing units of service include 4 tests
  AHA: 4Q,'02,9

G0251 Linear accelerator based stereotactic radiosurgery, delivery including collimator changes and custom plugging, fractionated treatment, all lesions, per session, maximum 5 sessions per course of treatment
  MED: 100-4,4,200.3.4; 100-4,4,200.3.4

G0252 PET imaging, full and partial-ring PET scanners only, for initial diagnosis of breast cancer and/or surgical planning for breast cancer (e.g., initial staging of axillary lymph nodes)
  MED: 100-3,220.6.3; 100-3,220.6.10; 100-4,13,60; 100-4,13,60.15; 100-4,13,60.16

G0255 Current perception threshold/sensory nerve conduction test, (SNCT) per limb, any nerve
  AHA: 4Q,'02,9

G0257 Unscheduled or emergency dialysis treatment for an ESRD patient in a hospital outpatient department that is not certified as an ESRD facility
  MED: 100-4,4,200.2; 100-4,8,60.4.7
  AHA: 1Q,'03,9; 4Q,'02,9

G0259 Injection procedure for sacroiliac joint; arthrography
  AHA: 4Q,'02,9

G0260 Injection procedure for sacroiliac joint; provision of anesthetic, steroid and/or other therapeutic agent, with or without arthrography
  AHA: 4Q,'02,9

G0268 Removal of impacted cerumen (one or both ears) by physician on same date of service as audiologic function testing
  AHA: 1Q,'03,12

G0269 Placement of occlusive device into either a venous or arterial access site, postsurgical or interventional procedure (e.g., angioseal plug, vascular plug)

G0270 Medical nutrition therapy; reassessment and subsequent intervention(s) following second referral in same year for change in diagnosis, medical condition or treatment regimen (including additional hours needed for renal disease), individual, face-to-face with the patient, each 15 minutes
  MED: 100-2,15,270; 100-2,15,270.2; 100-2,15,270.4; 100-4,9,182; 100-4,12,190.3; 100-4,12,190.3; 100-4,12,190.7

G0271 Medical nutrition therapy, reassessment and subsequent intervention(s) following second referral in same year for change in diagnosis, medical condition, or treatment regimen (including additional hours needed for renal disease), group (2 or more individuals), each 30 minutes
  MED: 100-4,9,182

G0278 Iliac and/or femoral artery angiography, nonselective, bilateral or ipsilateral to catheter insertion, performed at the same time as cardiac catheterization and/or coronary angiography, includes positioning or placement of the catheter in the distal aorta or ipsilateral femoral or iliac artery, injection of dye, production of permanent images, and radiologic supervision and interpretation (List separately in addition to primary procedure)

G0281 Electrical stimulation, (unattended), to one or more areas, for chronic Stage III and Stage IV pressure ulcers, arterial ulcers, diabetic ulcers, and venous stasis ulcers not demonstrating measurable signs of healing after 30 days of conventional care, as part of a therapy plan of care
  MED: 100-4,32,11.1
  AHA: 2Q,'03,7; 1Q,'03,7

G0282 Electrical stimulation, (unattended), to one or more areas, for wound care other than described in G0281
  MED: 100-4,32,11.1
  AHA: 2Q,'03,7; 1Q,'03,7

G0283 Electrical stimulation (unattended), to one or more areas for indication(s) other than wound care, as part of a therapy plan of care
  AHA: 2Q,'03,7; 1Q,'03,7

G0288 Reconstruction, computed tomographic angiography of aorta for surgical planning for vascular surgery

G0289 Arthroscopy, knee, surgical, for removal of loose body, foreign body, debridement/shaving of articular cartilage (chondroplasty) at the time of other surgical knee arthroscopy in a different compartment of the same knee

G0293 Noncovered surgical procedure(s) using conscious sedation, regional, general, or spinal anesthesia in a Medicare qualifying clinical trial, per day
  AHA: 4Q,'02,9

G0294 Noncovered procedure(s) using either no anesthesia or local anesthesia only, in a Medicare qualifying clinical trial, per day
  AHA: 4Q,'02,9

G0295 Electromagnetic therapy, to one or more areas, for wound care other than described in G0329 or for other uses
AHA: 1Q,'03,7

G0302 Preoperative pulmonary surgery services for preparation for LVRS, complete course of services, to include a minimum of 16 days of services

G0303 Preoperative pulmonary surgery services for preparation for LVRS, 10 to 15 days of services

G0304 Preoperative pulmonary surgery services for preparation for LVRS, 1 to 9 days of services

G0305 Postdischarge pulmonary surgery services after LVRS, minimum of 6 days of services

G0306 Complete CBC, automated (HgB, HCT, RBC, WBC, without platelet count) and automated WBC differential count

G0307 Complete (CBC), automated (HgB, Hct, RBC, WBC; without platelet count)

G0328 Colorectal cancer screening; fecal occult blood test, immunoassay, 1-3 simultaneous determinations
MED: 100-4,16,70.8; 100-4,18,60.1; 100-4,18,60.2; 100-4,18,60.6

G0329 Electromagnetic therapy, to one or more areas for chronic Stage III and Stage IV pressure ulcers, arterial ulcers, diabetic ulcers and venous stasis ulcers not demonstrating measurable signs of healing after 30 days of conventional care as part of a therapy plan of care
MED: 100-4,32,11.2

G0333 Pharmacy dispensing fee for inhalation drug(s); initial 30-day supply as a beneficiary

G0337 Hospice evaluation and counseling services, preelection
MED: 100-4,11,10; 100-4,11,10.1

G0339 Image guided robotic linear accelerator-based stereotactic radiosurgery, complete course of therapy in one session or first session of fractionated treatment
MED: 100-4,4,200.3.4; 100-4,4,200.3.4

G0340 Image guided robotic linear accelerator-based stereotactic radiosurgery, delivery including collimator changes and custom plugging, fractionated treatment, all lesions, per session, second through fifth sessions, maximum 5 sessions per course of treatment
MED: 100-4,4,200.3.4; 100-4,4,200.3.4

G0341 Percutaneous islet cell transplant, includes portal vein catheterization and infusion
MED: 100-4,32,70

G0342 Laparoscopy for islet cell transplant, includes portal vein catheterization and infusion
MED: 100-4,32,70

G0343 Laparotomy for islet cell transplant, includes portal vein catheterization and infusion
MED: 100-4,32,70

G0364 Bone marrow aspiration performed with bone marrow biopsy through the same incision on the same date of service

G0365 Vessel mapping of vessels for hemodialysis access (services for preoperative vessel mapping prior to creation of hemodialysis access using an autogenous hemodialysis conduit, including arterial inflow and venous outflow)

G0372 Physician service required to establish and document the need for a power mobility device
MED: 100-4,12,30.6.15.4

OBSERVATION/EMERGENCY DEPARTMENT SERVICES

G0378 Hospital observation service, per hour
MED: 100-2,6,20.6; 100-4,01,50.3.2; 100-4,4,290.1; 100-4,4,290.2.2; 100-4,4,290.4.1; 100-4,4,290.4.2; 100-4,4,290.4.3; 100-4,4,290.5.1; 100-4,4,290.5.2

G0379 Direct admission of patient for hospital observation care
MED: 100-2,6,20.6; 100-4,4,290.4.1; 100-4,4,290.4.2; 100-4,4,290.4.3; 100-4,4,290.5.1; 100-4,4,290.5.2

G0380 Level 1 hospital emergency department visit provided in a type B emergency department; (the ED must meet at least one of the following requirements: (1) it is licensed by the state in which it is located under applicable state law as an emergency room or emergency department; (2) it is held out to the public (by name, posted signs, advertising, or other means) as a place that provides care for emergency medical conditions on an urgent basis without requiring a previously scheduled appointment; or (3) during the calendar year immediately preceding the calendar year in which a determination under 42 CFR 489.24 is being made, based on a representative sample of patient visits that occurred during that calendar year, it provides at least one-third of all of its outpatient visits for the treatment of emergency medical conditions on an urgent basis without requiring a previously scheduled appointment)
MED: 100-4,4,160

G0381 Level 2 hospital emergency department visit provided in a type B emergency department; (the ED must meet at least one of the following requirements: (1) it is licensed by the state in which it is located under applicable state law as an emergency room or emergency department; (2) it is held out to the public (by name, posted signs, advertising, or other means) as a place that provides care for emergency medical conditions on an urgent basis without requiring a previously scheduled appointment; or (3) during the calendar year immediately preceding the calendar year in which a determination under 42 CFR 489.24 is being made, based on a representative sample of patient visits that occurred during that calendar year, it provides at least one-third of all of its outpatient visits for the treatment of emergency medical conditions on an urgent basis without requiring a previously scheduled appointment)
MED: 100-4,4,160

G0382 Level 3 hospital emergency department visit provided in a type B emergency department; (the ED must meet at least one of the following requirements: (1) it is licensed by the state in which it is located under applicable state law as an emergency room or emergency department; (2) it is held out to the public (by name, posted signs, advertising, or other means) as a place that provides care for emergency medical conditions on an urgent basis without requiring a previously scheduled appointment; or (3) during the calendar year immediately preceding the calendar year in which a determination under 42 CFR 489.24 is being made, based on a representative sample of patient visits that occurred during that calendar year, it provides at least one-third of all of its outpatient visits for the treatment of emergency medical conditions on an urgent basis without requiring a previously scheduled appointment)
MED: 100-4,4,160

G0383 Level 4 hospital emergency department visit provided in a type B emergency department; (the ED must meet at least one of the following requirements: (1) it is licensed by the state in which it is located under applicable state law as an emergency room or emergency department; (2) it is held out to the public (by name, posted signs, advertising, or other means) as a place that provides care for emergency medical conditions on an urgent basis without requiring a previously scheduled appointment; or (3) during the calendar year immediately preceding the calendar year in which a determination under 42 CFR 489.24 is being made, based on a representative sample of patient visits that occurred during that calendar year, it provides at least one-third of all of its outpatient visits for the treatment of emergency medical conditions on an urgent basis without requiring a previously scheduled appointment)
MED: 100-4,4,160

G0384   Level 5 hospital emergency department visit provided in a type B emergency department; (the ED must meet at least one of the following requirements: (1) it is licensed by the state in which it is located under applicable state law as an emergency room or emergency department; (2) it is held out to the public (by name, posted signs, advertising, or other means) as a place that provides care for emergency medical conditions on an urgent basis without requiring a previously scheduled appointment; or (3) during the calendar year immediately preceding the calendar year in which a determination under 42 CFR 489.24 is being made, based on a representative sample of patient visits that occurred during that calendar year, it provides at least one-third of all of its outpatient visits for the treatment of emergency medical conditions on an urgent basis without requiring a previously scheduled appointment)

    MED: 100-4,4,160; 100-4,4,290.5.1

OTHER SERVICES

G0389   Ultrasound B-scan and/or real time with image documentation; for abdominal aortic aneurysm (AAA) screening

    MED: 100-4,9,160

G0390   Trauma response team associated with hospital critical care service

    MED: 100-4,4,160.1

ALCOHOL OR SUBSTANCE ABUSE

G0396   Alcohol and/or substance (other than tobacco) abuse structured assessment (e.g., AUDIT, DAST), and brief intervention 15 to 30 minutes

    MED: 100-2,15,270; 100-2,15,270.2; 100-2,15,270.4; 100-4,4,200.6; 100-4,12,190.3; 100-4,12,190.7

G0397   Alcohol and/or substance (other than tobacco) abuse structured assessment (e.g., AUDIT, DAST), and intervention, greater than 30 minutes

    MED: 100-4,4,200.6

HOME SLEEP STUDY

G0398   Home sleep study test (HST) with type II portable monitor, unattended; minimum of 7 channels: EEG, EOG, EMG, ECG/heart rate, airflow, respiratory effort and oxygen saturation

    MED: 100-3,240.4

G0399   Home sleep test (HST) with type III portable monitor, unattended; minimum of 4 channels: 2 respiratory movement/airflow, 1 ECG/heart rate and 1 oxygen saturation

G0400   Home sleep test (HST) with type IV portable monitor, unattended; minimum of 3 channels

INITIAL PHYSICAL EXAM

G0402   Initial preventive physical examination; face-to-face visit, services limited to new beneficiary during the first 12 months of Medicare enrollment

    MED: 100-4,9,150; 100-4,12,80.1; 100-4,12,100.1.1; 100-4,18,80; 100-4,18,80.1; 100-4,18,80.2; 100-4,18,80.3.3; 100-4,18,80.3.3; 100-4,18,80.4; 100-4,18,140.6

G0403   Electrocardiogram, routine ECG with 12 leads; performed as a screening for the initial preventive physical examination with interpretation and report

G0404   Electrocardiogram, routine ECG with 12 leads; tracing only, without interpretation and report, performed as a screening for the initial preventive physical examination

    MED: 100-4,18,80.3.3

G0405   Electrocardiogram, routine ECG with 12 leads; interpretation and report only, performed as a screening for the initial preventive physical examination

FOLLOW-UP TELEHEALTH

G0406   Follow-up inpatient consultation, limited, physicians typically spend 15 minutes communicating with the patient via telehealth

    MED: 100-2,15,270; 100-2,15,270.2; 100-2,15,270.4; 100-4,12,190.3; 100-4,12,190.3; 100-4,12,190.3.1; 100-4,12,190.3.3; 100-4,12,190.7

G0407   Follow-up inpatient consultation, intermediate, physicians typically spend 25 minutes communicating with the patient via telehealth

G0408   Follow-up inpatient consultation, complex, physicians typically spend 35 minutes communicating with the patient via telehealth

PSYCHOLOGICAL SERVICES

G0409   Social work and psychological services, directly relating to and/or furthering the patient's rehabilitation goals, each 15 minutes, face-to-face; individual (services provided by a CORF qualified social worker or psychologist in a CORF)

    MED: 100-2,12,30.1; 100-4,5,100.4; 100-4,5,100.11

G0410   Group psychotherapy other than of a multiple-family group, in a partial hospitalization setting, approximately 45 to 50 minutes

G0411   Interactive group psychotherapy, in a partial hospitalization setting, approximately 45 to 50 minutes

FRACTURE CARE

G0412   Open treatment of iliac spine(s), tuberosity avulsion, or iliac wing fracture(s), unilateral or bilateral for pelvic bone fracture patterns which do not disrupt the pelvic ring, includes internal fixation, when performed

G0413   Percutaneous skeletal fixation of posterior pelvic bone fracture and/or dislocation, for fracture patterns which disrupt the pelvic ring, unilateral or bilateral, (includes ilium, sacroiliac joint and/or sacrum)

G0414   Open treatment of anterior pelvic bone fracture and/or dislocation for fracture patterns which disrupt the pelvic ring, unilateral or bilateral, includes internal fixation when performed (includes pubic symphysis and/or superior/inferior rami)

G0415   Open treatment of posterior pelvic bone fracture and/or dislocation, for fracture patterns which disrupt the pelvic ring, unilateral or bilateral, includes internal fixation, when performed (includes ilium, sacroiliac joint and/or sacrum)

SURGICAL PATHOLOGY

G0416   Surgical pathology, gross and microscopic examinations, for prostate needle biopsy, any method, 10-20 specimens

G0417   Surgical pathology, gross and microscopic examination, for prostate needle biopsy, any method, 21-40 specimens

G0418   Surgical pathology, gross and microscopic examination, for prostate needle biopsy, any method, 41-60 specimens

G0419   Surgical pathology, gross and microscopic examination, for prostate needle biopsy, any method, >60 specimens

EDUCATIONAL SERVICES

G0420   Face-to-face educational services related to the care of chronic kidney disease; individual, per session, per one hour

    MED: 100-2,15,270; 100-2,15,270.2; 100-2,15,270.4; 100-2,15,310; 100-2,15,310.1; 100-2,15,310.2; 100-2,15,310.3; 100-2,15,310.4; 100-2,15,310.5; 100-2,32,20.2; 100-4,12,190.3; 100-4,12,190.7

G0421   Face-to-face educational services related to the care of chronic kidney disease; group, per session, per one hour

CARDIAC AND PULMONARY REHABILITATION

G0422   Intensive cardiac rehabilitation; with or without continuous ECG monitoring with exercise, per session

    MED: 100-2,15,232; 100-4,32,140.2.2.1; 100-4,32,140.3; 100-4,32,140.3.1; 100-8,10,2.2.8

G0423 Intensive cardiac rehabilitation; with or without continuous ECG monitoring; without exercise, per session
MED: 100-4,32,140.3.1

G0424 Pulmonary rehabilitation, including exercise (includes monitoring), one hour, per session, up to 2 sessions per day
MED: 100-2,15,231; 100-4,32,140.4; 100-4,32,140.4; 100-4,32,140.4.1; 100-4,32,140.4.1

INPATIENT TELEHEALTH

G0425 Telehealth consultation, emergency department or initial inpatient, typically 30 minutes communicating with the patient via telehealth
MED: 100-2,15,270; 100-2,15,270.2; 100-2,15,270.4; 100-4,12,190.3; 100-4,12,190.3.1; 100-4,12,190.3.2; 100-4,12,190.7

G0426 Telehealth consultation, emergency department or initial inpatient, typically 50 minutes communicating with the patient via telehealth

G0427 Telehealth consultation, emergency department or initial inpatient, typically 70 minutes or more communicating with the patient via telehealth

DEFECT FILLERS

G0428 Collagen meniscus implant procedure for filling meniscal defects (e.g., CMI, collagen scaffold, Menaflex)
MED: 100-3,150.12

G0429 Dermal filler injection(s) for the treatment of facial lipodystrophy syndrome (LDS) (e.g., as a result of highly active antiretroviral therapy)
MED: 100-3,250.5; 100-4,32,260.1; 100-4,32,260.2.1; 100-4,32,260.2.2; 100-4,32,260.2.2

LABORATORY SERVICES

G0431 Drug screen, qualitative; multiple drug classes by high complexity test method (e.g., immunoassay, enzyme assay), per patient encounter

G0432 Infectious agent antibody detection by enzyme immunoassay (EIA) technique, HIV-1 and/or HIV-2, screening
MED: 100-3,190.14; 100-3,210.7; 100-4,18,130; 100-4,18,130.1; 100-4,18,130.4

G0433 Infectious agent antibody detection by enzyme-linked immunosorbent assay (ELISA) technique, HIV-1 and/or HIV-2, screening
MED: 100-3,210.7; 100-4,16,70.8; 100-4,18,130; 100-4,18,130.1; 100-4,18,130.4

G0434 Drug screen, other than chromatographic; any number of drug classes, by CLIA waived test or moderate complexity test, per patient encounter
MED: 100-4,16,70.8

G0435 Infectious agent antigen detection by rapid antibody test of oral mucosa transudate, HIV-1 or HIV-2, screening
MED: 100-3,210.7; 100-4,18,130; 100-4,18,130.1; 100-4,18,130.4

COUNSELING AND WELLNESS VISIT

G0436 Smoking and tobacco cessation counseling visit for the asymptomatic patient; intermediate, greater than 3 minutes, up to 10 minutes
MED: 100-2,15,270; 100-2,15,270.2; 100-2,15,270.4; 100-3,210.4; 100-4,12,190.3; 100-4,12,190.7; 100-4,18,150.2; 100-4,18,150.4

G0437 Smoking and tobacco cessation counseling visit for the asymptomatic patient; intermediate, greater than 10 minutes

G0438 Annual wellness visit; includes a personalized prevention plan of service (pps), initial visit
MED: 100-2,15,280.5; 100-2,15,280.5; 100-4,12,100.1.1; 100-4,18,140; 100-4,18,140.1; 100-4,18,140.5; 100-4,18,140.6

G0439 Annual wellness visit, includes a personalized prevention plan of service (pps), subsequent visit
MED: 100-2,15,280.5; 100-2,15,280.5; 100-4,18,140; 100-4,18,140.1; 100-4,18,140.5

OTHER SERVICES

G0442 Annual alcohol misuse screening, 15 minutes
MED: 100-2,15,270; 100-2,15,270.2; 100-2,15,270.4; 100-3,210.8; 100-4,12,190.3; 100-4,12,190.7; 100-4,18,180; 100-4,18,180.1; 100-4,18,180.2; 100-4,18,180.3; 100-4,18,180.4; 100-4,18,180.5; 100-4,32,180.4; 100-4,32,180.5

G0443 Brief face-to-face behavioral counseling for alcohol misuse, 15 minutes
MED: 100-4,18,180; 100-4,18,180.1; 100-4,18,180.2; 100-4,18,180.3; 100-4,18,180.4; 100-4,18,180.5

G0444 Annual depression screening, 15 minutes
MED: 100-4,18,190.0; 100-4,18,190.1; 100-4,18,190.2; 100-4,18,190.3

G0445 Semiannual high intensity behavioral counseling to prevent STIs, individual, face-to-face, includes education skills training & guidance on how to change sexual behavior
MED: 100-3,210.10; 100-4,18,170.1; 100-4,18,170.2; 100-4,18,170.3; 100-4,18,170.4; 100-4,18,170.4.1; 100-4,18,170.5

G0446 Annual, face-to-face intensive behavioral therapy for cardiovascular disease, individual, 15 minutes
MED: 100-3,210.11; 100-4,18,160; 100-4,18,160.1; 100-4,18,160.2.1; 100-4,18,160.2.2; 100-4,18,160.3; 100-4,18,160.4; 100-4,18,160.5

G0447 Face-to-face behavioral counseling for obesity, 15 minutes
MED: 100-3,210.12; 100-4,18,200; 100-4,18,200.1; 100-4,18,200.2; 100-4,18,200.3; 100-4,18,200.4; 100-4,18,200.5

G0448 Insertion or replacement of a permanent pacing cardioverter-defibrillator system with transvenous lead(s), single or dual chamber with insertion of pacing electrode, cardiac venous system, for left ventricular pacing

G0451 Development testing, with interpretation and report, per standardized instrument form
MED: 100-1,3,30; 100-1,3,30.3

MOLECULAR PATHOLOGY

G0452 Molecular pathology procedure; physician interpretation and report

NEUROPHYSIOLOGY MONITORING

G0453 Continuous intraoperative neurophysiology monitoring, from outside the operating room (remote or nearby), per patient, (attention directed exclusively to one patient) each 15 minutes (list in addition to primary procedure)

DOCUMENTATON AND PREPARATION

G0454 Physician documentation of face-to-face visit for durable medical equipment determination performed by nurse practitioner, physician assistant or clinical nurse specialist

G0455 Preparation with instillation of fecal microbiota by any method, including assessment of donor specimen

NEGATIVE WOUND PRESSURE THERAPY

G0456 Negative pressure wound therapy, (e.g. vacuum assisted drainage collection) using a mechanically-powered device, not durable medical equipment, including provision of cartridge and dressing(s), topical application(s), wound assessment, and instructions for ongoing care, per session; total wounds(s) surface area less than or equal to 50 sq cm

G0457 Negative pressure wound therapy, (e.g. vacuum assisted drainage collection) using a mechanically-powered device, not durable medical equipment, including provision of cartridge and dressing(s), topical application(s), wound assessment, and instructions for ongoing care, per session; total wounds(s) surface area greater than 50 sq cm

PROSTATE BRACHYTHERAPY

G0458 Low dose rate (LDR) prostate brachytherapy services, composite rate

QUALITY MEASURES

G0908 Most recent hemoglobin (HgB) level > 12.0 g/dl

G0909 Hemoglobin level measurement not documented, reason not given

G0910 Most recent hemoglobin level ≤ 12.0 g/dl

G0913 Improvement in visual function achieved within 90 days following cataract surgery

G0914 Patient care survey was not completed by patient

G0915 Improvement in visual function not achieved within 90 days following cataract surgery

G0916 Satisfaction with care achieved within 90 days following cataract surgery

G0917 Patient satisfaction survey was not completed by patient

G0918 Satisfaction with care not achieved within 90 days following cataract surgery

G0919 Influenza immunization ordered or recommended (to be given at alternate location or alternate provider); vaccine not available at time of visit

G0920 Type, anatomic location, and activity all documented

G0921 Documentation of patient reason(s) for not being able to assess (e.g., patient refuses endoscopic and/or radiologic assessment)

G0922 No documentation of disease type, anatomic location, and activity, reason not given

MEDICATION

G3001 Administration and supply of tositumomab, 450 mg

QUALITY MEASURES

G8126 Patient with a diagnosis of major depression documented as being treated with antidepressant medication during the entire 84 day (12 week) acute treatment phase

G8127 Patient with a diagnosis of major depression not documented as being treated with antidepressant medication during the entire 84 day (12 week) acute treatment phase

G8128 Clinician documented that patient was not an eligible candidate for antidepressant medication during the entire 12 week acute treatment phase measure

G8395 Left ventricular ejection fraction (LVEF) ≥ 40% or documentation as normal or mildly depressed left ventricular systolic function

G8396 Left ventricular ejection fraction (LVEF) not performed or documented

G8397 Dilated macular or fundus exam performed, including documentation of the presence or absence of macular edema and level of severity of retinopathy

G8398 Dilated macular or fundus exam not performed

G8399 Patient with central dual-energy x-ray absorptiometry (DXA) results documented or ordered or pharmacologic therapy (other than minerals/vitamins) for osteoporosis prescribed

G8400 Patient with central dual-energy x-ray absorptiometry (DXA) results not documented or not ordered or pharmacologic therapy (other than minerals/vitamins) for osteoporosis not prescribed, reason not given

G8401 Clinician documented that patient was not an eligible candidate for screening or therapy for osteoporosis for women measure

G8404 Lower extremity neurological exam performed and documented

G8405 Lower extremity neurological exam not performed

G8406 Clinician documented that patient was not an eligible candidate for lower extremity neurological exam measure

G8410 Footwear evaluation performed and documented

G8415 Footwear evaluation was not performed

G8416 Clinician documented that patient was not an eligible candidate for footwear evaluation measure

G8417 BMI is documented above normal parameters and a follow-up plan is documented

G8418 BMI is documented below normal parameters and a follow-up plan is documented

G8419 BMI documented outside normal parameters, no follow-up plan documented, no reason given

G8420 BMI is documented within normal parameters and no follow-up plan is required

G8421 BMI not documented and no reason is given

G8422 BMI not documented, documentation the patient is not eligible for BMI calculation

G8427 Eligible professional attests to documenting in the medical record they obtained, updated, or reviewed the patient's current medications

G8428 Current list of medications not documented as obtained, updated, or reviewed by the eligible professional, reason not given

G8430 Eligible professional attests to documenting in the medical record the patient is not eligible for a current list of medications being obtained, updated, or reviewed by the eligible professional

G8431 Screening for clinical depression is documented as being positive and a follow-up plan is documented

G8432 Clinical depression screening not documented, reason not given

G8433 Screening for clinical depression not documented, documentation stating the patient is not eligible

G8442 Pain assessment not documented as being performed, documentation the patient is not eligible for a pain assessment using a standardized tool

G8450 Beta-blocker therapy prescribed

G8451 Beta-blocker therapy for LVEF < 40% not prescribed for reasons documented by the clinician (e.g., low blood pressure, fluid overload, asthma, patients recently treated with an intravenous positive inotropic agent, allergy, intolerance, other medical reasons, patient declined, other patient reasons, or other reasons attributable to the healthcare system)

G8452 Beta-blocker therapy not prescribed

G8458 Clinician documented that patient is not an eligible candidate for genotype testing; patient not receiving antiviral treatment for hepatitis C

G8460 Clinician documented that patient is not an eligible candidate for quantitative RNA testing at week 12; patient not receiving antiviral treatment for hepatitis C

G8461 Patient receiving antiviral treatment for hepatitis C

G8464 Clinician documented that prostate cancer patient is not an eligible candidate for adjuvant hormonal therapy; low or intermediate risk of recurrence or risk of recurrence not determined

G8465 High risk of recurrence of prostate cancer

G8473 Angiotensin converting enzyme (ACE) inhibitor or angiotensin receptor blocker (ARB) therapy prescribed

G8474 Angiotensin converting enzyme (ACE) inhibitor or angiotensin receptor blocker (ARB) therapy not prescribed for reasons documented by the clinician

G8475 Angiotensin converting enzyme (ACE) inhibitor or angiotensin receptor blocker (ARB) therapy not prescribed, reason not given

G8476   Most recent blood pressure has a systolic measurement of < 130 mm Hg and a diastolic measurement of < 80 mm Hg

G8477   Most recent blood pressure has a systolic measurement of >= 130 mm Hg and/or a diastolic measurement of >= 80 mm Hg

G8478   Blood pressure measurement not performed or documented, reason not given

G8482   Influenza immunization administered or previously received

G8483   Influenza immunization was not ordered or administered for reasons documented by clinician (e.g., patient allergy or other medical reason, patient declined or other patient reasons, or other system reasons)

G8484   Influenza immunization was not ordered or administered, reason not given

G8485   I intend to report the diabetes mellitus (DM) measures group

G8486   I intend to report the preventive care measures group

G8487   I intend to report the chronic kidney disease (CKD) measures group

G8489   I intend to report the coronary artery disease (CAD) measures group

G8490   I intend to report the rheumatoid arthritis (RA) measures group

G8491   I intend to report the HIV/AIDS measures group

G8492   I intend to report the perioperative care measures group

G8493   I intend to report the back pain measures group

G8494   All quality actions for the applicable measures in the diabetes mellitus (DM) measures group have been performed for this patient

G8495   All quality actions for the applicable measures in the chronic kidney disease (CKD) measures group have been performed for this patient

G8496   All quality actions for the applicable measures in the preventive care measures group have been performed for this patient

G8497   All quality actions for the applicable measures in the coronary artery bypass graft (CABG) measures group have been performed for this patient

G8498   All quality actions for the applicable measures in the coronary artery disease (CAD) measures group have been performed for this patient

G8499   All quality actions for the applicable measures in the rheumatoid arthritis (RA) measures group have been performed for this patient

G8500   All quality actions for the applicable measures in the HIV/AIDS measures group have been performed for this patient

G8501   All quality actions for the applicable measures in the perioperative care measures group have been performed for this patient

G8502   All quality actions for the applicable measures in the back pain measures group have been performed for this patient

G8506   Patient receiving angiotensin converting enzyme (ACE) inhibitor or angiotensin receptor blocker (ARB) therapy

G8509   Pain assessment documented as positive using a standardized tool, follow-up plan not documented, reason not given

G8510   Screening for clinical depression is documented as negative, a follow-up plan is not required

G8511   Screening for clinical depression documented as positive, follow up plan not documented, reason not given

G8530   Autogenous AV fistula received

G8531   Clinician documented that patient was not an eligible candidate for autogenous AV fistula

G8532   Clinician documented that patient received vascular access other than autogenous AV fistula, reason not given

G8535   Elder maltreatment screen not documented; documentation that patient not eligible for the elder maltreatment screen

G8536   No documentation of an elder maltreatment screen, reason not given

G8539   Functional outcome assessment documented as positive using a standardized tool and a care plan based on identified deficiencies on the date of functional outcome assessment, is documented

G8540   Functional outcome assessment not documented as being performed, documentation the patient is not eligible for a functional outcome assessment using a standardized tool

G8541   Functional outcome assessment using a standardized tool, not documented, reason not given

G8542   Functional outcome assessment using a standardized tool is documented; no functional deficiencies identified, care plan not required

G8543   Documentation of a positive functional outcome assessment using a standardized tool; care plan not documented, reason not given

G8544   I intend to report the coronary artery bypass graft (CABG) measures group

G8545   I intend to report the hepatitis C measures group

G8547   I intend to report the ischemic vascular disease (IVD) measures group

G8548   I intend to report the heart failure (HF) measures group

G8549   All quality actions for the applicable measures in the hepatitis C measures group have been performed for this patient

G8551   All quality actions for the applicable measures in the heart failure (HF) measures group have been performed for this patient

G8552   All quality actions for the applicable measures in the ischemic vascular disease (IVD) measures group have been performed for this patient

G8559   Patient referred to a physician (preferably a physician with training in disorders of the ear) for an otologic evaluation

G8560   Patient has a history of active drainage from the ear within the previous 90 days

G8561   Patient is not eligible for the referral for otologic evaluation for patients with a history of active drainage measure

G8562   Patient does not have a history of active drainage from the ear within the previous 90 days

G8563   Patient not referred to a physician (preferably a physician with training in disorders of the ear) for an otologic evaluation, reason not given

G8564   Patient was referred to a physician (preferably a physician with training in disorders of the ear) for an otologic evaluation, reason not specified)

G8565   Verification and documentation of sudden or rapidly progressive hearing loss

G8566   Patient is not eligible for the "referral for otologic evaluation for sudden or rapidly progressive hearing loss" measure

G8567   Patient does not have verification and documentation of sudden or rapidly progressive hearing loss

G8568   Patient was not referred to a physician (preferably a physician with training in disorders of the ear) for an otologic evaluation, reason not given

G8569   Prolonged postoperative intubation (> 24 hrs) required

G8570   Prolonged postoperative intubation (> 24 hrs) not required

G8571   Development of deep sternal wound infection within 30 days postoperatively

G8572   No deep sternal wound infection

G8573   Stroke following isolated CABG surgery

G8574   No stroke following isolated CABG surgery

G8575 Developed postoperative renal failure or required dialysis

G8576 No postoperative renal failure/dialysis not required

G8577 Re-exploration required due to mediastinal bleeding with or without tamponade, graft occlusion, valve dysfunction or other cardiac reason

G8578 Re-exploration not required due to mediastinal bleeding with or without tamponade, graft occlusion, valve dysfunction or other cardiac reason

G8579 Antiplatelet medication at discharge

G8580 Antiplatelet medication contraindicated

G8581 No antiplatelet medication at discharge

G8582 Beta-blocker at discharge

G8583 Beta-blocker contraindicated

G8584 No beta-blocker at discharge

G8585 Antilipid treatment at discharge

G8586 Antilipid treatment contraindicated

G8587 No antilipid treatment at discharge

G8593 Lipid profile results documented and reviewed (must include total cholesterol, HDL-C, triglycerides and calculated LDL-C)

G8594 Lipid profile not performed, reason not given

G8595 Most recent LDL-C < 100 mg/dL

G8597 Most recent LDL-C ≥ 100 mg/dL

G8598 Aspirin or another antithrombotic therapy used

G8599 Aspirin or another antithrombotic therapy not used, reason not given

G8600 IV tPA initiated within 3 hours (≤ 180 minutes) of time last known well

G8601 IV tPA not initiated within 3 hours (≤ 180 minutes) of time last known well for reasons documented by clinician

G8602 IV tPA not initiated within 3 hours (<= 180 minutes) of time last known well, reason not given

G8627 Surgical procedure performed within 30 days following cataract surgery for major complications (e.g., retained nuclear fragments, endophthalmitis, dislocated or wrong power iol, retinal detachment, or wound dehiscence)

G8628 Surgical procedure not performed within 30 days following cataract surgery for major complications (e.g., retained nuclear fragments, endophthalmitis, dislocated or wrong power iol, retinal detachment, or wound dehiscence)

G8629 Documentation of order for prophylactic parenteral antibiotic to be given within one hour (if fluoroquinolone or vancomycin, 2 hours) prior to surgical incision (or start of procedure when no incision is required)

G8630 Documentation that administration of prophylactic parenteral antibiotics was initiated within one hour (if fluoroquinolone or vancomycin, 2 hours) prior to surgical incision (or start of procedure when no incision is required), as ordered

G8631 Clinician documented that patient was not an eligible candidate for ordering prophylactic parenteral antibiotics to be given within one hour (if fluoroquinolone or vancomycin, 2 hours) prior to surgical incision (or start of procedure when no incision is required)

G8632 Prophylactic parenteral antibiotics were not ordered to be given or given within one hour (if fluoroquinolone or vancomycin, 2 hours) prior to the surgical incision (or start of procedure when no incision is required), reason not given

G8633 Pharmacologic therapy (other than minerals/vitamins) for osteoporosis prescribed

G8634 Clinician documented patient not an eligible candidate to receive pharmacologic therapy for osteoporosis

G8635 Pharmacologic therapy for osteoporosis was not prescribed, reason not given

G8645 I intend to report the asthma measures group

G8646 All quality actions for the applicable measures in the asthma measures group have been performed for this patient

G8647 Risk-adjusted functional status change residual score for the knee successfully calculated and the score was equal to zero (0) or greater than zero (> 0)

G8648 Risk-adjusted functional status change residual score for the knee successfully calculated and the score was less than zero (< 0)

G8649 Risk-adjusted functional status change residual scores for the knee not measured because the patient did not complete FOTO's functional intake on admission and/or follow up status survey near discharge, patient not eligible/not appropriate

G8650 Risk-adjusted functional status change residual scores for the knee not measured because the patient did not complete FOTO's functional intake on admission and/or follow up status survey near discharge, reason not given

G8651 Risk-adjusted functional status change residual score for the hip successfully calculated and the score was equal to zero (0) or greater than zero (> 0)

G8652 Risk-adjusted functional status change residual score for the hip successfully calculated and the score was less than zero (< 0)

G8653 Risk-adjusted functional status change residual scores for the hip not measured because the patient did not complete FOTO's functional intake on admission and/or follow up status survey near discharge, patient not eligible/not appropriate

G8654 Risk-adjusted functional status change residual scores for the hip not measured because the patient did not complete FOTO's functional intake on admission and/or follow up status survey near discharge, reason not given

G8655 Risk-adjusted functional status change residual score for the lower leg, foot or ankle successfully calculated and the score was equal to zero (0) or greater than zero (> 0)

G8656 Risk-adjusted functional status change residual score for the lower leg, foot or ankle successfully calculated and the score was less than zero (< 0)

G8657 Risk-adjusted functional status change residual scores for the lower leg, foot or ankle not measured because the patient did not complete FOTO's functional intake on admission and/or follow up status survey near discharge, patient not eligible/not appropriate

G8658 Risk-adjusted functional status change residual scores for the lower leg, foot or ankle not measured because the patient did not complete FOTO's functional intake on admission and/or follow up status survey near discharge, reason not given

G8659 Risk-adjusted functional status change residual score for the lumbar spine successfully calculated and the score was equal to zero (0) or greater than zero (> 0)

G8660 Risk-adjusted functional status change residual score for the lumbar spine successfully calculated and the score was less than zero (< 0)

G8661 Risk-adjusted functional status change residual scores for the lumbar spine not measured because the patient did not complete FOTO's functional intake on admission and/or follow up status survey near discharge, patient not eligible/not appropriate

G8662 Risk-adjusted functional status change residual scores for the lumbar spine not measured because the patient did not complete FOTO's functional intake on admission and/or follow up status survey near discharge, reason not given

G8663 Risk-adjusted functional status change residual score for the shoulder successfully calculated and the score was equal to zero (0) or greater than zero (> 0)

Procedures/Professional Services (Temporary)

G8664 — G8736

G8664   Risk-adjusted functional status change residual score for the shoulder successfully calculated and the score was less than zero (< 0)

G8665   Risk-adjusted functional status change residual scores for the shoulder not measured because the patient did not complete FOTO's functional intake on admission and/or follow up status survey near discharge, patient not eligible/not appropriate

G8666   Risk-adjusted functional status change residual scores for the shoulder not measured because the patient did not complete FOTO's functional intake on admission and/or follow up status survey near discharge, reason not given

G8667   Risk-adjusted functional status change residual score for the elbow, wrist or hand successfully calculated and the score was equal to zero (0) or greater than zero (> 0)

G8668   Risk-adjusted functional status change residual score for the elbow, wrist or hand successfully calculated and the score was less than zero (< 0)

G8669   Risk-adjusted functional status change residual scores for the elbow, wrist or hand not measured because the patient did not complete FOTO's functional intake on admission and/or follow up status survey near discharge, patient not eligible/not appropriate

G8670   Risk-adjusted functional status change residual scores for the elbow, wrist or hand not measured because the patient did not complete FOTO's functional intake on admission and/or follow up status survey near discharge, reason not given

G8671   Risk-adjusted functional status change residual score for the neck, cranium, mandible, thoracic spine, ribs, or other general orthopedic impairment successfully calculated and the score was equal to zero (0) or greater than zero (> 0)

G8672   Risk-adjusted functional status change residual score for the neck, cranium, mandible, thoracic spine, ribs, or other general orthopedic impairment successfully calculated and the score was less than zero (< 0)

G8673   Risk-adjusted functional status change residual scores for the neck, cranium, mandible, thoracic spine, ribs, or other general orthopedic impairment not measured because the patient did not complete FOTO's functional intake on admission and/or follow up status survey near discharge, patient not eligible/not appropriate

G8674   Risk-adjusted functional status change residual scores for the neck, cranium, mandible, thoracic spine, ribs, or other general orthopedic impairment not measured because the patient did not complete FOTO's functional intake on admission and/or follow up status survey near discharge, reason not given

G8682   LVF testing documented as being performed prior to discharge or in the previous 12 months

G8683   LVF testing not performed prior to discharge or in the previous 12 months for a medical or patient documented reason

G8685   LVF testing not documented as being performed prior to discharge or in the previous 12 months, reason not given

G8694   Left ventricular ejection fraction (LVEF) < 40%

G8696   Antithrombotic therapy prescribed at discharge

G8697   Antithrombotic therapy not prescribed for documented reasons (e.g., patient admitted for performance of elective carotid intervention, patient had stroke during hospital stay, patient expired during inpatient stay, other medical reason(s)); (e.g., patient left against medical advice, other patient reason(s))

G8698   Antithrombotic therapy was not prescribed at discharge, reason not given

G8699   Rehabilitation services (occupational, physical or speech) ordered at or prior to discharge

G8700   Rehabilitation services (occupational, physical or speech) not indicated at or prior to discharge

G8701   Rehabilitation services were not ordered, reason not otherwise specified

G8702   Documentation that prophylactic antibiotics were given within 4 hours prior to surgical incision or intraoperatively

G8703   Documentation that prophylactic antibiotics were neither given within 4 hours prior to surgical incision nor intraoperatively

G8704   12-lead electrocardiogram (ECG) performed

G8705   Documentation of medical reason(s) for not performing a 12-lead electrocardiogram (ECG)

G8706   Documentation of patient reason(s) for not performing a 12-lead electrocardiogram (ECG)

G8707   12-lead electrocardiogram (ECG) not performed, reason not given

G8708   Patient not prescribed or dispensed antibiotic

G8709   Patient prescribed or dispensed antibiotic for documented medical reason(s) (e.g., intestinal infection, pertussis, bacterial infection, lyme disease, otitis media, acute sinusitis, acute pharyngitis, acute tonsillitis, chronic sinusitis, infection of the pharynx/larynx/tonsils/adenoids, prostatitis, cellulitis, mastoiditis, or bone infections, acute lymphadenitis, impetigo, skin staph infections, pneumonia/gonococcal infections, venereal disease (syphilis, chlamydia, inflammatory diseases (female reproductive organs)), infections of the kidney, cystitis or UTI, and acne)

G8710   Patient prescribed or dispensed antibiotic

G8711   Prescribed or dispensed antibiotic

G8712   Antibiotic not prescribed or dispensed

G8713   SpKt/V greater than or equal to 1.2 (single-pool clearance of urea [Kt] / volume V])

G8714   Hemodialysis treatment performed exactly 3 times per week > 90 days

G8717   SpKt/V less than 1.2 (single-pool clearance of urea [Kt] / volume V), reason not given

G8718   Total Kt/V greater than or equal to 1.7 per week (total clearance of urea [Kt] / volume V])

G8720   Total Kt/V less than 1.7 per week (total clearance of urea [Kt] / volume V), reason not given

G8721   pT category (primary tumor), pN category (regional lymph nodes), and histologic grade were documented in pathology report

G8722   Documentation of medical reason(s) for not including the PT category, the PN category or the histologic grade in the pathology report (e.g., re-excision without residual tumor; non-carcinomasanal canal)

G8723   Specimen site is other than anatomic location of primary tumor

G8724   pT category, pN category and histologic grade were not documented in the pathology report, reason not given

G8725   Fasting lipid profile performed (triglycerides, LDL-C, HDL-C and total cholesterol)

G8726   Clinician has documented reason for not performing fasting lipid profile (e.g., patient declined, other patient reasons)

G8728   Fasting lipid profile not performed, reason not given

G8730   Pain assessment documented as positive using a standardized tool and a follow-up plan is documented

G8731   Pain assessment using a standardized tool is documented as negative, no follow-up plan required

G8732   No documentation of pain assessment, reason not given

G8733   Elder maltreatment screen documented as positive and a follow-up plan is documented

G8734   Elder maltreatment screen documented as negative, no follow-up required

G8735   Elder maltreatment screen documented as positive, follow-up plan not documented, reason not given

G8736   Most current LDL-C < 100 mg/dL

G8737 Most current LDL-C ≥ 100 mg/dL

G8738 Left ventricular ejection fraction (LVEF) < 40% or documentation of severely or moderately depressed left ventricular systolic function

G8739 Left ventricular ejection fraction (LVEF) ≥ 40% or documentation as normal or mildly depressed left ventricular systolic function

G8740 Left ventricular ejection fraction (LVEF) not performed or assessed, reason not given

G8749 Absence of signs of melanoma (cough, dyspnea, tenderness, localized neurologic signs such as weakness, jaundice or any other sign suggesting systemic spread) or absence of symptoms of melanoma (pain, paresthesia, or any other symptom suggesting the possibility of systemic spread of melanoma)

G8751 Smoking status and exposure to secondhand smoke in the home not assessed, reason not given

G8752 Most recent systolic blood pressure < 140 mm Hg

G8753 Most recent systolic blood pressure ≥ 140 mm Hg

G8754 Most recent diastolic blood pressure < 90 mm Hg

G8755 Most recent diastolic blood pressure ≥ 90 mm Hg

G8756 No documentation of blood pressure measurement, reason not given

G8757 All quality actions for the applicable measures in the chronic obstructive pulmonary disease (COPD) measures group have been performed for this patient

G8758 All quality actions for the applicable measures in the inflammatory bowel disease (IBD) measures group have been performed for this patient

G8759 All quality actions for the applicable measures in the sleep apnea measures group have been performed for this patient

G8761 All quality actions for the applicable measures in the dementia measures group have been performed for this patient

G8762 All quality actions for the applicable measures in the Parkinson's disease measures group have been performed for this patient

G8763 All quality actions for the applicable measures in the hypertension (HTN) measures group have been performed for this patient

G8764 All quality actions for the applicable measures in the cardiovascular prevention measures group have been performed for this patient

G8765 All quality actions for the applicable measures in the cataract measures group have been performed for this patient

G8767 Lipid panel results documented and reviewed (must include total cholesterol, HDL-C, triglycerides and calculated LDL-C)

G8768 Documentation of medical reason(s) for not performing lipid profile (e.g., patients with palliative goals or for whom treatment of hypertension with standard treatment goals is not clinically appropriate)

G8769 Lipid profile not performed, reason not given

G8770 Urine protein test result documented and reviewed

G8771 Documentation of diagnosis of chronic kidney disease

G8772 Documentation of medical reason(s) for not performing urine protein test (e.g., patients with palliative goals or for whom treatment of hypertension with standard treatment goals is not clinically appropriate)

G8773 Urine protein test was not performed, reason not given

G8774 Serum creatinine test result documented and reviewed

G8775 Documentation of medical reason(s) for not performing serum creatinine test (e.g., patients with palliative goals or for whom treatment of hypertension with standard treatment goals is not clinically appropriate)

G8776 Serum creatinine test not performed, reason not gvien

G8777 Diabetes screening test performed

G8778 Documentation of medical reason(s) for not performing diabetes screening test (e.g., patients with a diagnosis of diabetes, or with palliative goals or for whom treatment of hypertension with standard treatment goals is not clinically appropriate)

G8779 Diabetes screening test not performed, reason not given

G8780 Counseling for diet and physical activity performed

G8781 Documentation of medical reason(s) for patient not receiving counseling for diet and physical activity (e.g., patients with palliative goals or for whom treatment of hypertension with standard treatment goals is not clinically appropriate)

G8782 Counseling for diet and physical activity not performed, reason not given

G8783 Normal blood pressure reading documented, follow-up not required

G8784 Blood pressure reading not documented, documentation the patient is not eligible

G8785 Blood pressure reading not documented, reason not given

G8797 Specimen site other than anatomic location of esophagus

G8798 Specimen site other than anatomic location of prostate

G8806 Performance of transabdominal or transvaginal ultrasound

G8807 Transabdominal or transvaginal ultrasound not performed for reasons documented by clinician (e.g., patient has visited the ED multiple times within 72 hours, patient has a documented intrauterine pregnancy (IUP)

G8808 Performance of trans-abdominal or trans-vaginal ultrasound not ordered, reason not given (e.g., patient has visited the ED multiple times with no documentation of a trans-abdominal or trans-vaginal ultrasound within ED or from referring eligible professional)

G8809 Rh immune globulin (RhoGam) ordered

G8810 Rh-immunoglobulin (RhoGAM) not ordered for reasons documented by clinician (e.g., patient had prior documented receipt of RhoGAM within 12 weeks, patient refusal)

G8811 Documentation Rh immunoglobulin (Rhogam) was not ordered, reason not specified

G8815 Statin therapy not prescribed for documented reasons (e.g., medical intolerance to statin, dealth of patient prior to discharge, transfer to care of another acute care or federal hospital, hospice admission, left against medical advice)

G8816 Statin medication prescribed at discharge

G8817 Statin therapy not prescribed at discharge, reason not given

G8818 Patient discharge to home no later than postoperative day #7

G8825 Patient not discharged to home by postoperative day #7

G8826 Patient discharged to home no later than postoperative day #2 following EVAR

G8833 Patient not discharged to home by postoperative day #2 following EVAR

G8834 Patient discharged to home no later than postoperative day #2 following CEA

G8838 Patient not discharged to home by postoperative day #2 following CEA

G8839 Sleep apnea symptoms assessed, including presence or absence of snoring and daytime sleepiness

G8840 Documentation of reason(s) for not performing an assessment of sleep symptoms (e.g., patient didn't have initial daytime sleepiness, patient visits between initial testing and initiation of therapy)

G8841 Sleep apnea symptoms not assessed, reason not given

G8842 Apnea hypopnea index (AHI) or respiratory disturbance index (RDI) measured at the time of initial diagnosis

G8843 Documentation of reason(s) for not measuring an apnea hypopnea index (AHI) or a respiratory disturbance index (RDI) at the time of initial diagnosis (e.g., abnormal anatomy, patient declined, financial, insurance coverage)

G8844 Apnea hypopna index (AHI) or respiratory disturbance index (RDI) not measured at the time of initial diagnosis, reason not given

G8845 Positive airway pressure therapy prescribed

G8846 Moderate or severe obstructive sleep apnea (apnea hypopnea index (AHI) or respiratory disturbance index (RDI) of 15 or greater)

G8848 Mild obstructive sleep apnea (apnea hypopnea index (AHI) or respiratory disturbance index (RDI) of less than 15)

G8849 Documentation of reason(s) for not prescribing positive airway pressure therapy (e.g., patient unable to tolerate, alternative therapies use, patient declined, financial, insurance coverage)

G8850 Positive airway pressure therapy not prescribed, reason not given

G8851 Objective measurement of adherence to positive airway pressure therapy, documented

G8852 Positive airway pressure therapy prescribed

G8853 Positive airway pressure therapy not prescribed

G8854 Documentation of reason(s) for not objectively measuring adherence to positive airway pressure therapy (e.g., patient did not bring data from continuous positive airway pressure (CPAP), therapy not yet initiated, not available on machine)

G8855 Objective measurement of adherence to positive airway pressure therapy not performed, reason not given

G8856 Referral to a physician for an otologic evaluation performed

G8857 Patient is not eligible for the referral for otologic evaluation measure (e.g., patients who are already under the care of a physician for acute or chronic dizziness)

G8858 Referral to a physician for an otologic evaluation not performed, reason not given

G8859 Patient receiving corticosteroids greater than or equal to 10 mg/day for 60 or greater consecutive days

G8860 Patients who have received dose of corticosteroids greater than or equal to 10 mg/day for 60 or greater consecutive days

G8861 Central dual-energy x-ray absorptiometry (DXA) ordered or documented, review of systems and medication history or pharmacologic therapy (other than minerals/vitamins) for osteoporosis prescribed

G8862 Patients not receiving corticosteroids greater than or equal to 10 mg/day for 60 or greater consecutive days

G8863 Patients not assessed for risk of bone loss, reason not given

G8864 Pneumococcal vaccine administered or previously received

G8865 Documentation of medical reason(s) for not administering or previously receiving pneumococcal vaccine (e.g., patient allergic reaction, potential adverse drug reaction)

G8866 Documentation of patient reason(s) for not administering or previously receiving pneumococcal vaccine (e.g., patient refusal)

G8867 Pneumococcal vaccine not administered or previously received, reason not given

G8868 Patients receiving a first course of anti-TNF therapy

G8869 Patient has documented immunity to hepatitis B and is receiving a first course of anti-TNF therapy

G8870 Hepatitis B vaccine injection administered or previously received and is receiving a first course of anti-TNF therapy

G8871 Patient not receiving a first course of anti-TNF therapy

G8872 Excised tissue evaluated by imaging intraoperatively to confirm successful inclusion of targeted lesion

G8873 Patients with needle localization specimens which are not amenable to intraoperative imaging such as MRI needle wire localization, or targets which are tentatively identified on mammogram or ultrasound which do not contain a biopsy marker but which can be verified on intraoperative inspection or pathology (e.g., needle biopsy site where the biopsy marker is remote from the actual biopsy site)

G8874 Excised tissue not evaluated by imaging intraoperatively to confirm successful inclusion of targeted lesion

G8875 Clinician diagnosed breast cancer preoperatively by a minimally invasive biopsy method

G8876 Documentation of reason(s) for not performing minimally invasive biopsy to diagnose breast cancer preoperatively (e.g., clinical and imaging findings consistent with a benign lesion, lesion too close to skin, implant, chest wall, etc., lesion could not be adequately visualized for needle biopsy, patient condition prevents needle biopsy weight, breast thickness, etc.), duct excision without imaging abnormality, prophylactic mastectomy, reduction mammoplasty, excisional biopsy performed by another physician

G8877 Clinician did not attempt to achieve the diagnosis of breast cancer preoperatively by a minimally invasive biopsy method, reason not given

G8878 Sentinel lymph node biopsy procedure performed

G8879 Clinically node negative (T1N0M0 or T2N0M0) invasive breast cancer

G8880 Documentation of reason(s) sentinel lymph node biopsy not performed (e.g., reasons could include but not limited to; non-invasive cancer, incidental discovery of breast cancer on prophylactic mastectomy, incidental discovery of breast cancer on reduction mammoplasty, pre-operative biopsy proven lymph node (LN) metastases, inflammatory carcinoma, stage 3 locally advanced cancer, recurrent invasive breast cancer, patient refusal after informed consent)

G8881 Stage of breast cancer is greater than T1N0M0 or T2N0M0

G8882 Sentinel lymph node biopsy procedure not performed, reason not given

G8883 Biopsy results reviewed, communicated, tracked and documented

G8884 Clinician documented reason that patient's biopsy results were not reviewed

G8885 Biopsy results not reviewed, communicated, tracked or documented

G8886 Most recent blood pressure under control

G8887 Documentation of medical reason(s) for most recent blood pressure not being under control (e.g., patients with palliative goals or for whom treatment of hypertension with standard treatment goals is not clinically appropriate)

G8888 Most recent blood pressure not under control, results documented and reviewed

G8889 No documentation of blood pressure measurement, reason not given

G8890 Most recent LDL-C under control, results documented and reviewed

G8891 Documentation of medical reason(s) for most recent LDL-C not under control (e.g., patients with palliative goals for for whom treatment of hypertension with standard treatment goals is not clinically appropriate)

G8892 Documentation of medical reason(s) for not performing LDL-C test (e.g., patients with palliative goals or for whom treatment of hypertension with standard treatment goals is not clinically appropriate)

G8893 Most recent LDL-C not under control, results documented and reviewed

G8894   LDL-C not performed, reason not given

G8895   Oral aspirin or other antithrombotic therapy prescribed

G8896   Documentation of medical reason(s) for not prescribing oral aspirin or other antithrombotic therapy (e.g., patient documented to be low risk or patient with terminal illness or treatment of hypertension with standard treatment goals is not clinically appropriate, or for whom risk of aspirin or other antithrombotic therapy exceeds potential benefits such as for individuals whose blood pressure is poorly controlled)

G8897   Oral aspirin or other antithrombotic therapy was not prescribed, reason not given

G8898   I intend to report the chronic obstructive pulmonary disease (COPD) measures group

G8899   I intend to report the inflammatory bowel disease (IBD) measures group

G8900   I intend to report the sleep apnea measures group

G8902   I intend to report the dementia measures group

G8903   I intend to report the Parkinson's disease measures group

G8904   I intend to report the hypertension (HTN) measures group

G8905   I intend to report the cardiovascular prevention measures group

G8906   I intend to report the cataract measures group

G8907   Patient documented not to have experienced any of the following events: a burn prior to discharge; a fall within the facility; wrong site/side/patient/procedure/implant event; or a hospital transfer or hospital admission upon discharge from the facility

G8908   Patient documented to have received a burn prior to discharge

G8909   Patient documented not to have received a burn prior to discharge

G8910   Patient documented to have experienced a fall within ASC

G8911   Patient documented not to have experienced a fall within ambulatory surgery center

G8912   Patient documented to have experienced a wrong site, wrong side, wrong patient, wrong procedure or wrong implant event

G8913   Patient documented not to have experienced a wrong site, wrong side, wrong patient, wrong procedure or wrong implant event

G8914   Patient documented to have experienced a hospital transfer or hospital admission upon discharge from ASC

G8915   Patient documented not to have experienced a hospital transfer or hospital admission upon discharge from ASC

G8916   Patient with preoperative order for IV antibiotic surgical site infection (SSI) prophylaxis, antibiotic initiated on time

G8917   Patient with preoperative order for IV antibiotic surgical site infection (SSI) prophylaxis, antibiotic not initiated on time

G8918   Patient without preoperative order for IV antibiotic surgical site infection (SSI) prophylaxis

G8923   Left ventricular ejection fraction (LVEF) < 40% or documentation of moderately or severely depressed left ventricular systolic function

G8924   Spirometry test results demonstrate FEV1/FVC < 60% with COPD symptoms (e.g., dyspnea, cough/sputum, wheezing)

G8925   Spirometry test results demonstrate FEV1/FVC >= 60% or patient does not have COPD symptoms

G8926   Spirometry test not performed or documented, reason not given

G8927   Adjuvant chemotherapy referred, prescribed or previously received for AJCC stage III, colon cancer

G8928   Adjuvant chemotherapy not prescribed or previously received for documented reasons (e.g., medical co-morbidities, diagnosis date more than 5 years prior to the current visit date, patient's cancer has metastasized, medical contraindication/allergy, poor performance status, other medical reasons, patient refusal, other patient reasons, patient is currently enrolled in a clinical trial that precludes prescription of chemotherapy, other system reasons)

G8929   Adjuvant chemotherapy not prescribed or previously received, reason not specified

G8930   Assessment of depression severity at the initial evaluation

G8931   Assessment of depression severity not documented, reason not given

G8932   Suicide risk assessed at the initial evaluation

G8933   Suicide risk not assessed at the initial evaluation, reason not given

G8934   Left ventricular ejection fraction (LVEF) < 40% or documentation of moderately or severely depressed left ventricular systolic function

G8935   Clinician prescribed angiotensin converting enzyme (ACE) inhibitor or angiotensin receptor blocker (ARB) therapy

G8936   Clinician documented that patient was not an eligible candidate for angiotensin converting enzyme (ACE) inhibitor or angiotensin receptor blocker (ARB) therapy

G8937   Clinician did not prescribe angiotensin converting enzyme (ACE) inhibitor or angiotensin receptor blocker (ARB) therapy, reason not given

G8938   BMI is documented as being outside of normal limits, follow-up plan is not documented, documentation the patient is not eligible

G8939   Pain assessment documented as positive, follow-up plan not documented, documentation the patient is not eligible

G8940   Screening for clinical depression documented as positive, a follow-up plan not documented, documentation stating the patient is not eligible

G8941   Elder maltreatment screen documented as positive, follow-up plan not documented, documentation the patient is not eligible

G8942   Functional outcomes assessment using a standardized tool is documented within the previous 30 days and care plan, based on identified deficiencies on the date of the functional outcome assessment, is documented

G8943   LDL-C result not present or not within 12 months prior

G8944   AJCC melanoma cancer stage 0 through IIC melanoma

G8946   Minimally invasive biopsy method attempted but not diagnostic of breast cancer (e.g., high risk lesion of breast such as atypical ductal hyperplasia, lobular neoplasia, atypical lobular hyperplasia, lobular carcinoma in situ, atypical columnar hyperplasica, flat epithelial atypia, radial scar, complex sclerosing lesion, papillary lesion, or any lesion with spindle cells)

G8947   One or more neuropsychiatric symptoms

G8948   No neuropsychiatric symptoms

G8949   Documentation of patient reason(s) for patient not receiving counseling for diet and physical activity (e.g., patient is not willing to discuss diet or exercise interventions to help control blood pressure, or the patient said he/she refused to make these changes)

G8950   Prehypertensive or hypertensive blood pressure reading documented, and the indicated follow-up is documented

G8951   Prehypertensive or hypertensive blood pressure reading documented, indicated follow-up not documented, documentation the patient is not eligible

G8952   Prehypertensive or hypertensive blood pressure reading documented, indicated follow-up not documented, reason not given

G8953   All quality actions for the applicable measures in the oncology measures group have been performed for this patient

G8955   Most recent assessment of adequacy of volume management

G8956   Patient receiving maintenance hemodialysis in an outpatient dialysis facility

G8957   Patient not receiving maintenance hemodialysis in an outpatient dialysis facility

G8958   Assessment of adequacy of volume management not documented, reason not given

G8959   Clinician treating major depressive disorder communicates to clinician treating comorbid condition

G8960   Clinician treating major depressive disorder did not communicate to clinician treating comorbid condition, reason not given

G8961   Cardiac stress imaging test primarily performed on low-risk surgery patient for preoperative evaluation within 30 days preceding this surgery

G8962   Cardiac stress imaging test performed on patient for any reason including those who did not have low risk surgery or test that was performed more than 30 days preceding low risk surgery

G8963   Cardiac stress imaging performed primarily for monitoring of asymptomatic patient who had PCI wihin 2 years

G8964   Cardiac stress imaging test performed primarily for any other reason than monitoring of asymptomatic patient who had PCI wthin 2 years (e.g., symptomatic patient, patient greater than 2 years since PCI, initial evaluation, etc.)

G8965   Cardiac stress imaging test primarily performed on low CHD risk patient for initial detection and risk assessment

G8966   Cardiac stress imaging test performed on symptomatic or higher than low CHD risk patient or for any reason other than initial detection and risk assessment

G8967   Warfarin or another oral anticoagulant that is FDA approved prescribed

G8968   Documentation of medical reason(s) for not prescribing warfarin or another oral anticoagulant that is FDA approved for the prevention of thromboembolism (e.g., patients with mitral stenosis or prosthetic heart valves, patients with transient or reversible causes of AF (e.g., pneumonia or hyperthyroidism), postoperative patients, patients who are pregnant, allergy, risk of bleeding, other medical reasons)

G8969   Documentation of patient reason(s) for not prescribing warfarin or another oral anticoagulant that is FDA approved (e.g., economic, social, and/or religious impediments, noncompliance patient refusal, other patient reasons)

G8970   No risk factors or one moderate risk factor for thromboembolism

G8971   Warfarin or another oral anticoagulant that is FDA approved not prescribed, reason not given

G8972   One or more high risk factors for thromboembolism or more than one moderate risk factor for thromboembolism

G8973   Most recent hemoglobin (HgB) level < 10 g/dl

G8974   Hemoglobin level measurement not documented, reason not given

G8975   Documentation of medical reason(s) for patient having a hemoglobin level < 10 g/dl (e.g., patients who have nonrenal etiologies of anemia [e.g., sickle cell anemia or other hemoglobinopathies, hypersplenism, primary bone marrow disease, anemia related to chemotherapy for diagnosis of malignancy, postoperative bleeding, active bloodstream or peritoneal infection], other medical reasons)

G8976   Most recent hemoglobin (HgB) level >= 10 g/dl

G8977   I intend to report the oncology measures group

FUNCTIONAL LIMITATION

G8978   Mobility: walking and moving around functional limitation, current status, at therapy episode outset and at reporting intervals
     MED: 100-4,5,10.6

G8979   Mobility: walking and moving around functional limitation, projected goal status, at therapy episode outset, at reporting intervals, and at discharge or to end reporting

G8980   Mobility: walking and moving around functional limitation, discharge status, at discharge from therapy or to end reporting

G8981   Changing and maintaining body position functional limitation, current status, at therapy episode outset and at reporting intervals

G8982   Changing and maintaining body position functional limitation, projected goal status, at therapy episode outset, at reporting intervals, and at discharge or to end reporting

G8983   Changing and maintaining body position functional limitation, discharge status, at discharge from therapy or to end reporting

G8984   Carrying, moving and handling objects functional limitation, current status, at therapy episode outset and at reporting intervals

G8985   Carrying, moving and handling objects, projected goal status, at therapy episode outset, at reporting intervals, and at discharge or to end reporting

G8986   Carrying, moving and handling objects functional limitation, discharge status, at discharge from therapy or to end reporting

G8987   Self care functional limitation, current status, at therapy episode outset and at reporting intervals

G8988   Self care functional limitation, projected goal status, at therapy episode outset, at reporting intervals, and at discharge or to end reporting

G8989   Self care functional limitation, discharge status, at discharge from therapy or to end reporting

G8990   Other physical or occupational therapy primary functional limitation, current status, at therapy episode outset and at reporting intervals

G8991   Other physical or occupational therapy primary functional limitation, projected goal status, at therapy episode outset, at reporting intervals, and at discharge or to end reporting

G8992   Other physical or occupational therapy primary functional limitation, discharge status, at discharge from therapy or to end reporting

G8993   Other physical or occupational therapy subsequent functional limitation, current status, at therapy episode outset and at reporting intervals

G8994   Other physical or occupational therapy subsequent functional limitation, projected goal status, at therapy episode outset, at reporting intervals, and at discharge or to end reporting

G8995   Other physical or occupational therapy subsequent functional limitation, discharge status, at discharge from therapy or to end reporting

G8996   Swallowing functional limitation, current status at therapy episode outset and at reporting intervals
     MED: 100-4,5,10.6

G8997   Swallowing functional limitation, projected goal status, at therapy episode outset, at reporting intervals, and at discharge or to end reporting

G8998   Swallowing functional limitation, discharge status, at discharge from therapy or to end reporting

G8999   Motor speech functional limitation, current status at therapy episode outset and at reporting intervals

COORDINATED CARE

G9001 Coordinated care fee, initial rate

G9002 Coordinated care fee (Level 1)

G9003 Coordinated care fee, risk adjusted high, initial

G9004 Coordinated care fee, risk adjusted low, initial

G9005 Coordinated care fee risk adjusted maintenance

G9006 Coordinated care fee, home monitoring

G9007 Coordinated care fee, scheduled team conference

G9008 Coordinated care fee, physician coordinated care oversight services

G9009 Coordinated care fee, risk adjusted maintenance, level 3

G9010 Coordinated care fee, risk adjusted maintenance, level 4

G9011 Coordinated care fee, risk adjusted maintenance, Level 5

G9012 Other specified case management service not elsewhere classified

DEMONSTRATION PROJECT

G9013 ESRD demo basic bundle Level I

G9014 ESRD demo expanded bundle including venous access and related services

G9016 Smoking cessation counseling, individual, in the absence of or in addition to any other evaluation and management service, per session (6-10 minutes) [demo project code only]

MED: 100-3,210.4

G9017 Amantadine HCl, oral, per 100 mg (for use in a Medicare-approved demonstration project)

G9018 Zanamivir, inhalation powder, administered through inhaler, per 10 mg (for use in a Medicare-approved demonstration project)

G9019 Oseltamivir phosphate, oral, per 75 mg (for use in a Medicare-approved demonstration project)

G9020 Rimantadine HCl, oral, per 100 mg (for use in a Medicare-approved demonstration project)

G9033 Amantadine HCl, oral brand, per 100 mg (for use in a Medicare-approved demonstration project)

G9034 Zanamivir, inhalation powder, administered through inhaler, brand, per 10 mg (for use in a Medicare-approved demonstration project)

G9035 Oseltamivir phosphate, oral, brand, per 75 mg (for use in a Medicare-approved demonstration project)

G9036 Rimantadine HCl, oral, brand, per 100 mg (for use in a Medicare-approved demonstration project)

G9050 Oncology; primary focus of visit; work-up, evaluation, or staging at the time of cancer diagnosis or recurrence (for use in a Medicare-approved demonstration project)

G9051 Oncology; primary focus of visit; treatment decision-making after disease is staged or restaged, discussion of treatment options, supervising/coordinating active cancer-directed therapy or managing consequences of cancer-directed therapy (for use in a Medicare-approved demonstration project)

G9052 Oncology; primary focus of visit; surveillance for disease recurrence for patient who has completed definitive cancer-directed therapy and currently lacks evidence of recurrent disease; cancer-directed therapy might be considered in the future (for use in a Medicare-approved demonstration project)

G9053 Oncology; primary focus of visit; expectant management of patient with evidence of cancer for whom no cancer-directed therapy is being administered or arranged at present; cancer-directed therapy might be considered in the future (for use in a Medicare-approved demonstration project)

G9054 Oncology; primary focus of visit; supervising, coordinating or managing care of patient with terminal cancer or for whom other medical illness prevents further cancer treatment; includes symptom management, end-of-life care planning, management of palliative therapies (for use in a Medicare-approved demonstration project)

G9055 Oncology; primary focus of visit; other, unspecified service not otherwise listed (for use in a Medicare-approved demonstration project)

G9056 Oncology; practice guidelines; management adheres to guidelines (for use in a Medicare-approved demonstration project)

G9057 Oncology; practice guidelines; management differs from guidelines as a result of patient enrollment in an institutional review board-approved clinical trial (for use in a Medicare-approved demonstration project)

G9058 Oncology; practice guidelines; management differs from guidelines because the treating physician disagrees with guideline recommendations (for use in a Medicare-approved demonstration project)

G9059 Oncology; practice guidelines; management differs from guidelines because the patient, after being offered treatment consistent with guidelines, has opted for alternative treatment or management, including no treatment (for use in a Medicare-approved demonstration project)

G9060 Oncology; practice guidelines; management differs from guidelines for reason(s) associated with patient comorbid illness or performance status not factored into guidelines (for use in a Medicare-approved demonstration project)

G9061 Oncology; practice guidelines; patient's condition not addressed by available guidelines (for use in a Medicare-approved demonstration project)

G9062 Oncology; practice guidelines; management differs from guidelines for other reason(s) not listed (for use in a Medicare-approved demonstration project)

G9063 Oncology; disease status; limited to nonsmall cell lung cancer; extent of disease initially established as Stage I (prior to neoadjuvant therapy, if any) with no evidence of disease progression, recurrence, or metastases (for use in a Medicare-approved demonstration project)

G9064 Oncology; disease status; limited to nonsmall cell lung cancer; extent of disease initially established as Stage II (prior to neoadjuvant therapy, if any) with no evidence of disease progression, recurrence, or metastases (for use in a Medicare-approved demonstration project)

G9065 Oncology; disease status; limited to nonsmall cell lung cancer; extent of disease initially established as Stage III a (prior to neoadjuvant therapy, if any) with no evidence of disease progression, recurrence, or metastases (for use in a Medicare-approved demonstration project)

G9066 Oncology; disease status; limited to nonsmall cell lung cancer; Stage III B-IV at diagnosis, metastatic, locally recurrent, or progressive (for use in a Medicare-approved demonstration project)

G9067 Oncology; disease status; limited to nonsmall cell lung cancer; extent of disease unknown, staging in progress, or not listed (for use in a Medicare-approved demonstration project)

G9068 Oncology; disease status; limited to small cell and combined small cell/nonsmall cell; extent of disease initially established as limited with no evidence of disease progression, recurrence, or metastases (for use in a Medicare-approved demonstration project)

G9069 Oncology; disease status; small cell lung cancer, limited to small cell and combined small cell/nonsmall cell; extensive Stage at diagnosis, metastatic, locally recurrent, or progressive (for use in a Medicare-approved demonstration project)

Procedures/Professional Services (Temporary)

G9070 — G9099

G9070   Oncology; disease status; small cell lung cancer, limited to small cell and combined small cell/nonsmall; extent of disease unknown, staging in progress, or not listed (for use in a Medicare-approved demonstration project)

G9071   Oncology; disease status; invasive female breast cancer (does not include ductal carcinoma in situ); adenocarcinoma as predominant cell type; stage I or stage IIA-IIB; or T3, N1, M0; and ER and/or PR positive; with no evidence of disease progression, recurrence, or metastases (for use in a Medicare-approved demonstration project)

G9072   Oncology; disease status; invasive female breast cancer (does not include ductal carcinoma in situ); adenocarcinoma as predominant cell type; stage I, or stage IIA-IIB; or T3, N1, M0; and ER and PR negative; with no evidence of disease progression, recurrence, or metastases (for use in a Medicare-approved demonstration project)

G9073   Oncology; disease status; invasive female breast cancer (does not include ductal carcinoma in situ); adenocarcinoma as predominant cell type; stage IIIA-IIIB; and not T3, N1, M0; and ER and/or PR positive; with no evidence of disease progression, recurrence, or metastases (for use in a Medicare-approved demonstration project)

G9074   Oncology; disease status; invasive female breast cancer (does not include ductal carcinoma in situ); adenocarcinoma as predominant cell type; stage IIIA-IIIB; and not T3, N1, M0; and ER and PR negative; with no evidence of disease progression, recurrence, or metastases (for use in a Medicare-approved demonstration project)

G9075   Oncology; disease status; invasive female breast cancer (does not include ductal carcinoma in situ); adenocarcinoma as predominant cell type; M1 at diagnosis, metastatic, locally recurrent, or progressive (for use in a Medicare-approved demonstration project)

G9077   Oncology; disease status; prostate cancer, limited to adenocarcinoma as predominant cell type; T1-T2C and Gleason 2-7 and PSA < or equal to 20 at diagnosis with no evidence of disease progression, recurrence, or metastases (for use in a Medicare-approved demonstration project)

G9078   Oncology; disease status; prostate cancer, limited to adenocarcinoma as predominant cell type; T2 or T3a Gleason 8-10 or PSA > 20 at diagnosis with no evidence of disease progression, recurrence, or metastases (for use in a Medicare-approved demonstration project)

G9079   Oncology; disease status; prostate cancer, limited to adenocarcinoma as predominant cell type; T3B-T4, any N; any T, N1 at diagnosis with no evidence of disease progression, recurrence, or metastases (for use in a Medicare-approved demonstration project)

G9080   Oncology; disease status; prostate cancer, limited to adenocarcinoma; after initial treatment with rising PSA or failure of PSA decline (for use in a Medicare-approved demonstration project)

G9083   Oncology; disease status; prostate cancer, limited to adenocarcinoma; extent of disease unknown, staging in progress, or not listed (for use in a Medicare-approved demonstration project)

G9084   Oncology; disease status; colon cancer, limited to invasive cancer, adenocarcinoma as predominant cell type; extent of disease initially established as T1-3, N0, M0 with no evidence of disease progression, recurrence or metastases (for use in a Medicare-approved demonstration project)

G9085   Oncology; disease status; colon cancer, limited to invasive cancer, adenocarcinoma as predominant cell type; extent of disease initially established as T4, N0, M0 with no evidence of disease progression, recurrence, or metastases (for use in a Medicare-approved demonstration project)

G9086   Oncology; disease status; colon cancer, limited to invasive cancer, adenocarcinoma as predominant cell type; extent of disease initially established as T1-4, N1-2, M0 with no evidence of disease progression, recurrence, or metastases (for use in a Medicare-approved demonstration project)

G9087   Oncology; disease status; colon cancer, limited to invasive cancer, adenocarcinoma as predominant cell type; M1 at diagnosis, metastatic, locally recurrent, or progressive with current clinical, radiologic, or biochemical evidence of disease (for use in a Medicare-approved demonstration project)

G9088   Oncology; disease status; colon cancer, limited to invasive cancer, adenocarcinoma as predominant cell type; M1 at diagnosis, metastatic, locally recurrent, or progressive without current clinical, radiologic, or biochemical evidence of disease (for use in a Medicare-approved demonstration project)

G9089   Oncology; disease status; colon cancer, limited to invasive cancer, adenocarcinoma as predominant cell type; extent of disease unknown, staging in progress or not listed (for use in a Medicare-approved demonstration project)

G9090   Oncology; disease status; rectal cancer, limited to invasive cancer, adenocarcinoma as predominant cell type; extent of disease initially established as T1-2, N0, M0 (prior to neoadjuvant therapy, if any) with no evidence of disease progression, recurrence, or metastases (for use in a Medicare-approved demonstration project)

G9091   Oncology; disease status; rectal cancer, limited to invasive cancer, adenocarcinoma as predominant cell type; extent of disease initially established as T3, N0, M0 (prior to neoadjuvant therapy, if any) with no evidence of disease progression, recurrence, or metastases (for use in a Medicare-approved demonstration project)

G9092   Oncology; disease status; rectal cancer, limited to invasive cancer, adenocarcinoma as predominant cell type; extent of disease initially established as T1-3, N1-2, M0 (prior to neoadjuvant therapy, if any) with no evidence of disease progression, recurrence or metastases (for use in a Medicare-approved demonstration project)

G9093   Oncology; disease status; rectal cancer, limited to invasive cancer, adenocarcinoma as predominant cell type; extent of disease initially established as T4, any N, M0 (prior to neoadjuvant therapy, if any) with no evidence of disease progression, recurrence, or metastases (for use in a Medicare-approved demonstration project)

G9094   Oncology; disease status; rectal cancer, limited to invasive cancer, adenocarcinoma as predominant cell type; M1 at diagnosis, metastatic, locally recurrent, or progressive (for use in a Medicare-approved demonstration project)

G9095   Oncology; disease status; rectal cancer, limited to invasive cancer, adenocarcinoma as predominant cell type; extent of disease unknown, staging in progress or not listed (for use in a Medicare-approved demonstration project)

G9096   Oncology; disease status; esophageal cancer, limited to adenocarcinoma or squamous cell carcinoma as predominant cell type; extent of disease initially established as T1-T3, N0-N1 or NX (prior to neoadjuvant therapy, if any) with no evidence of disease progression, recurrence, or metastases (for use in a Medicare-approved demonstration project)

G9097   Oncology; disease status; esophageal cancer, limited to adenocarcinoma or squamous cell carcinoma as predominant cell type; extent of disease initially established as T4, any N, M0 (prior to neoadjuvant therapy, if any) with no evidence of disease progression, recurrence, or metastases (for use in a Medicare-approved demonstration project)

G9098   Oncology; disease status; esophageal cancer, limited to adenocarcinoma or squamous cell carcinoma as predominant cell type; M1 at diagnosis, metastatic, locally recurrent, or progressive (for use in a Medicare-approved demonstration project)

G9099   Oncology; disease status; esophageal cancer, limited to adenocarcinoma or squamous cell carcinoma as predominant cell type; extent of disease unknown, staging in progress, or not listed (for use in a Medicare-approved demonstration project)

G9100 Oncology; disease status; gastric cancer, limited to adenocarcinoma as predominant cell type; post R0 resection (with or without neoadjuvant therapy) with no evidence of disease recurrence, progression, or metastases (for use in a Medicare-approved demonstration project)

G9101 Oncology; disease status; gastric cancer, limited to adenocarcinoma as predominant cell type; post R1 or R2 resection (with or without neoadjuvant therapy) with no evidence of disease progression, or metastases (for use in a Medicare-approved demonstration project)

G9102 Oncology; disease status; gastric cancer, limited to adenocarcinoma as predominant cell type; clinical or pathologic M0, unresectable with no evidence of disease progression, or metastases (for use in a Medicare-approved demonstration project)

G9103 Oncology; disease status; gastric cancer, limited to adenocarcinoma as predominant cell type; clinical or pathologic M1 at diagnosis, metastatic, locally recurrent, or progressive (for use in a Medicare-approved demonstration project)

G9104 Oncology; disease status; gastric cancer, limited to adenocarcinoma as predominant cell type; extent of disease unknown, staging in progress, or not listed (for use in a Medicare-approved demonstration project)

G9105 Oncology; disease status; pancreatic cancer, limited to adenocarcinoma as predominant cell type; post R0 resection without evidence of disease progression, recurrence, or metastases (for use in a Medicare-approved demonstration project)

G9106 Oncology; disease status; pancreatic cancer, limited to adenocarcinoma; post R1 or R2 resection with no evidence of disease progression, or metastases (for use in a Medicare-approved demonstration project)

G9107 Oncology; disease status; pancreatic cancer, limited to adenocarcinoma; unresectable at diagnosis, M1 at diagnosis, metastatic, locally recurrent, or progressive (for use in a Medicare-approved demonstration project)

G9108 Oncology; disease status; pancreatic cancer, limited to adenocarcinoma; extent of disease unknown, staging in progress, or not listed (for use in a Medicare-approved demonstration project)

G9109 Oncology; disease status; head and neck cancer, limited to cancers of oral cavity, pharynx and larynx with squamous cell as predominant cell type; extent of disease initially established as T1-T2 and N0, M0 (prior to neoadjuvant therapy, if any) with no evidence of disease progression, recurrence, or metastases (for use in a Medicare-approved demonstration project)

G9110 Oncology; disease status; head and neck cancer, limited to cancers of oral cavity, pharynx and larynx with squamous cell as predominant cell type; extent of disease initially established as T3-4 and/or N1-3, M0 (prior to neoadjuvant therapy, if any) with no evidence of disease progression, recurrence, or metastases (for use in a Medicare-approved demonstration project)

G9111 Oncology; disease status; head and neck cancer, limited to cancers of oral cavity, pharynx and larynx with squamous cell as predominant cell type; M1 at diagnosis, metastatic, locally recurrent, or progressive (for use in a Medicare-approved demonstration project)

G9112 Oncology; disease status; head and neck cancer, limited to cancers of oral cavity, pharynx and larynx with squamous cell as predominant cell type; extent of disease unknown, staging in progress, or not listed (for use in a Medicare-approved demonstration project)

G9113 Oncology; disease status; ovarian cancer, limited to epithelial cancer; pathologic stage 1A-B (Grade 1) without evidence of disease progression, recurrence, or metastases (for use in a Medicare-approved demonstration project)

G9114 Oncology; disease status; ovarian cancer, limited to epithelial cancer; pathologic stage IA-B (grade 2-3); or stage IC (all grades); or stage II; without evidence of disease progression, recurrence, or metastases (for use in a Medicare-approved demonstration project)

G9115 Oncology; disease status; ovarian cancer, limited to epithelial cancer; pathologic stage III-IV; without evidence of progression, recurrence, or metastases (for use in a Medicare-approved demonstration project)

G9116 Oncology; disease status; ovarian cancer, limited to epithelial cancer; evidence of disease progression, or recurrence, and/or platinum resistance (for use in a Medicare-approved demonstration project)

G9117 Oncology; disease status; ovarian cancer, limited to epithelial cancer; extent of disease unknown, staging in progress, or not listed (for use in a Medicare-approved demonstration project)

G9123 Oncology; disease status; chronic myelogenous leukemia, limited to Philadelphia chromosome positive and/or BCR-ABL positive; chronic phase not in hematologic, cytogenetic, or molecular remission (for use in a Medicare-approved demonstration project)

G9124 Oncology; disease status; chronic myelogenous leukemia, limited to Philadelphia chromosome positive and /or BCR-ABL positive; accelerated phase not in hematologic cytogenetic, or molecular remission (for use in a Medicare-approved demonstration project)

G9125 Oncology; disease status; chronic myelogenous leukemia, limited to Philadelphia chromosome positive and/or BCR-ABL positive; blast phase not in hematologic, cytogenetic, or molecular remission (for use in a Medicare-approved demonstration project)

G9126 Oncology; disease status; chronic myelogenous leukemia, limited to Philadelphia chromosome positive and/or BCR-ABL positive; in hematologic, cytogenetic, or molecular remission (for use in a Medicare-approved demonstration project)

G9128 Oncology; disease status; limited to multiple myeloma, systemic disease; smoldering, stage I (for use in a Medicare-approved demonstration project)

G9129 Oncology; disease status; limited to multiple myeloma, systemic disease; stage II or higher (for use in a Medicare-approved demonstration project)

G9130 Oncology; disease status; limited to multiple myeloma, systemic disease; extent of disease unknown, staging in progress, or not listed (for use in a Medicare-approved demonstration project)

G9131 Oncology; disease status; invasive female breast cancer (does not include ductal carcinoma in situ); adenocarcinoma as predominant cell type; extent of disease unknown, staging in progress, or not listed (for use in a Medicare-approved demonstration project)

G9132 Oncology; disease status; prostate cancer, limited to adenocarcinoma; hormone-refractory/androgen-independent (e.g., rising PSA on antiandrogen therapy or postorchiectomy); clinical metastases (for use in a Medicare-approved demonstration project)

G9133 Oncology; disease status; prostate cancer, limited to adenocarcinoma; hormone-responsive; clinical metastases or M1 at diagnosis (for use in a Medicare-approved demonstration project)

G9134 Oncology; disease status; non-Hodgkin's lymphoma, any cellular classification; Stage I, II at diagnosis, not relapsed, not refractory (for use in a Medicare-approved demonstration project)

G9135 Oncology; disease status; non-Hodgkin's lymphoma, any cellular classification; Stage III, IV, not relapsed, not refractory (for use in a Medicare-approved demonstration project)

G9136 Oncology; disease status; non-Hodgkin's lymphoma, transformed from original cellular diagnosis to a second cellular classification (for use in a medicare-approved demonstration project)

G9137   Oncology; disease status; non-Hodgkin's lymphoma, any cellular classification; relapsed/refractory (for use in a medicare-approved demonstration project)

G9138   Oncology; disease status; non-Hodgkin's lymphoma, any cellular classification; diagnostic evaluation, stage not determined, evaluation of possible relapse or nonresponse to therapy, or not listed (for use in a Medicare-approved demonstration project)

G9139   Oncology; disease status; chronic myelogenous leukemia, limited to Philadelphia chromosome positive and/or BCR-ABL positive; extent of disease unknown, staging in progress, not listed (for use in a Medicare-approved demonstration project)

G9140   Frontier extended stay clinic demonstration; for a patient stay in a clinic approved for the CMS demonstration project; the following measures should be present: the stay must be equal to or greater than 4 hours; weather or other conditions must prevent transfer or the case falls into a category of monitoring and observation cases that are permitted by the rules of the demonstration; there is a maximum frontier extended stay clinic (FESC) visit of 48 hours, except in the case when weather or other conditions prevent transfer; payment is made on each period up to 4 hours, after the first 4 hours

WARFARIN TESTING

G9143   Warfarin responsiveness testing by genetic technique using any method, any number of specimen(s)

     MED: 100-3,90.1; 100-4,32,250.1; 100-4,32,250.2

OUTPATIENT IV INSULIN TX

G9147   Outpatient Intravenous Insulin Treatment (OIVIT) either pulsatile or continuous, by any means, guided by the results of measurements for: respiratory quotient; and/or, urine urea nitrogen (UUN); and/or, arterial, venous or capillary glucose; and/or potassium concentration

     MED: 100-3,40.7; 100-4,4,320.1; 100-4,4,320.2

QUALITY ASSURANCE

G9148   National Committee for Quality Assurance-Level 1 medical home

G9149   National Committee for Quality Assurance-Level 2 medical home

G9150   National Committee for Quality Assurance-Level 3 medical home

G9151   MAPCP Demonstration-state provided services

G9152   MAPCP Demonstration-Community Health Teams

G9153   MAPCP Demonstration-Physician Incentive Pool

WHEELCHAIR EVALUATION

G9156   Evaluation for wheelchair requiring face-to-face visit with physician

MONITOR

G9157   Transesophageal Doppler used for cardiac monitoring

     MED: 100-4,32,310; 100-4,32,310.2; 100-4,32,310.10.3

FUNCTIONAL LIMITATION

G9158   Motor speech functional limitation, discharge status, at discharge from therapy or to end reporting

     MED: 100-4,5,10.6

G9159   Spoken language comprehension functional limitation, current status at therapy episode outset and at reporting intervals

G9160   Spoken language comprehension functional limitation, projected goal status at therapy episode outset, at reporting intervals, and at discharge from or to end reporting

G9161   Spoken language comprehension functional limitation, discharge status, at discharge from therapy or to end reporting

G9162   Spoken language expression functional limitation, current status at therapy episode outset and at reporting intervals

G9163   Spoken language expression functional limitation, projected goal status at therapy episode outset, at reporting intervals, and at discharge from or to end reporting

G9164   Spoken language expression functional limitation, discharge status at discharge from therapy or to end reporting

G9165   Attention functional limitation, current status at therapy episode outset and at reporting intervals

G9166   Attention functional limitation, projected goal status at therapy episode outset, at reporting intervals, and at discharge from or to end reporting

G9167   Attention functional limitation, discharge status at discharge from therapy or to end reporting

G9168   Memory functional limitation, current status at therapy episode outset and at reporting intervals

G9169   Memory functional limitation, projected goal status at therapy episode outset, at reporting intervals, and at discharge from or to end reporting

G9170   Memory functional limitation, discharge status at discharge from therapy or to end reporting

G9171   Voice functional limitation, current status at therapy episode outset and at reporting intervals

G9172   Voice functional limitation, projected goal status at therapy episode outset, at reporting intervals, and at discharge from or to end reporting

G9173   Voice functional limitation, discharge status at discharge from therapy or to end reporting

G9174   Other speech language pathology functional limitation, current status at therapy episode outset and at reporting intervals

G9175   Other speech language pathology functional limitation, projected goal status at therapy episode outset, at reporting intervals, and at discharge from or to end reporting

G9176   Other speech language pathology functional limitation, discharge status at discharge from therapy or to end reporting

G9186   Motor speech functional limitation, projected goal status at therapy episode outset, at reporting intervals, and at discharge from or to end reporting

     MED: 100-4,5,10.6

BPCI SERVICES

G9187   Bundled payments for care improvement initiative home visit for patient assessment performed by a qualified health care professional for individuals not considered homebound including, but not limited to, assessment of safety, falls, clinical status, fluid status, medication reconciliation/management, patient compliance with orders/plan of care, performance of activities of daily living, appropriateness of care setting; (for use only in the Medicare-approved bundled payments for care improvement initiative); may not be billed for a 30-day period covered by a transitional care management code

MISCELLANEOUS QUALITY MEASURES

G9188   Beta-blocker therapy not prescribed, reason not given

G9189   Beta-blocker therapy prescribed or currently being taken

G9190   Documentation of medical reason(s) for not prescribing beta-blocker therapy (e.g., allergy, intolerance, other medical reasons)

G9191   Documentation of patient reason(s) for not prescribing beta-blocker therapy (e.g., patient declined, other patient reasons)

G9192   Documentation of system reason(s) for not prescribing beta-blocker therapy (eg, other reasons attributable to the health care system)

G9193 Clinician documented that patient with a diagnosis of major depression was not an eligible candidate for antidepressant medication treatment or patient did not have a diagnosis of major depression

G9194 Patient with a diagnosis of major depression documented as being treated with antidepressant medication during the entire 180 day (6 month) continuation treatment phase

G9195 Patient with a diagnosis of major depression not documented as being treated with antidepressant medication during the entire 180 day (6 months) continuation treatment phase

G9196 Documentation of medical reason(s) for not ordering first or second generation cephalosporin for antimicrobial prophylaxis

G9197 Documentation of order for first or second generation cephalosporin for antimicrobial prophylaxis

G9198 Order for first or second generation cephalosporin for antimicrobial prophylaxis was not documented, reason not given

G9199 Venous thromboembolism (vte) prophylaxis not administered the day of or the day after hospital admission for documented reasons (eg, patient is ambulatory, patient expired during inpatient stay, patient already on warfarin or another anticoagulant, other medical reason(s) or eg, patient left against medical advice, other patient reason(s))

G9200 Venous thromboembolism (VTE) prophylaxis was not administered the day of or the day after hospital admission, reason not given

G9201 Venous thromboembolism (VTE) prophylaxis administered the day of or the day after hospital admission

G9202 Patients with a positive hepatitis C antibody test

G9203 RNA testing for hepatitis C documented as performed within 12 months prior to initiation of antiviral treatment for hepatitis C

G9204 RNA testing for hepatitis C was not documented as performed within 12 months prior to initiation of antiviral treatment for hepatitis C, reason not given

G9205 Patient starting antiviral treatment for hepatitis C during the measurement period

G9206 Patient starting antiviral treatment for hepatitis C during the measurement period

G9207 Hepatitis C genotype testing documented as performed within 12 months prior to initiation of antiviral treatment for hepatitis C

G9208 Hepatitis C genotype testing was not documented as performed within 12 months prior to initiation of antiviral treatment for hepatitis C, reason not given

G9209 Hepatitis C quantitative RNA testing documented as performed between 4-12 weeks after the initiation of antiviral treatment

G9210 Hepatitis C quantitative RNA testing not performed between 4-12 weeks after the initiation of antiviral treatment for reasons documented by clinician (e.g., patients whose treatment was discontinued during the testing period prior to testing, other medical reasons, patient declined, other patient reasons)

G9211 Hepatitis C quantitative RNA testing was not documented as performed between 4-12 weeks after the initiation of antiviral treatment, reason not given

G9212 DSM-IV TM criteria for major depressive disorder documented at the initial evaluation

G9213 DSM-IV-TR criteria for major depressive disorder not documented at the initial evaluation, reason not otherwise specified

G9214 CD4+ cell count or CD4+ cell percentage results documented

G9215 CD4+ cell count or percentage not documented as performed, reason not given

G9216 PCP prophylaxis was not prescribed at time of diagnosis of HIV, reason not given

G9217 PCP prophylaxis was not prescribed within 3 months of low CD4+ cell count below 200 cells/mm3, reason not given

G9218 PCP prophylaxis was not prescribed within 3 months of low CD4+ cell count below 500 cells/mm3 or a CD4 percentage below 15%, reason not given

G9219 Pneumocystis jiroveci pneumonia prophylaxis not prescribed within 3 months of low CD4+ cell count below 200 cells/mm3 for medical reason (i.e., patient's CD4+ cell count above threshold within 3 months after CD4+ cell count below threshold, indicating that the patient's CD4+ levels are within an acceptable range and the patient does not require PCP prophylaxis)

G9220 Pneumocystis jiroveci pneumonia prophylaxis not prescribed within 3 months of low CD4+ cell count below 500 cells/mm3 or a CD4 percentage below 15% for medical reason (i.e., patient's CD4+ cell count above threshold within 3 months after CD4+ cell count below threshold, indicating that the patient's CD4+ levels are within an acceptable range and the patient does not require PCP prophylaxis)

G9221 Pneumocystis jiroveci pneumonia prophylaxis prescribed

G9222 Pneumocystis jiroveci pneumonia prophylaxis prescribed wthin 3 months of low CD4+ cell count below 200 cells/mm3

G9223 Pneumocystis jiroveci pneumonia prophylaxis prescribed within 3 months of low CD4+ cell count below 500 cells/mm3 or a CD4 percentage below 15%

G9224 Documentation of medical reason for not performing foot exam (e.g., patient with bilateral foot/leg amputation)

G9225 Foot exam was not performed, reason not given

G9226 Foot examination performed (includes examination through visual inspection, sensory exam with monofilament, and pulse exam - report when all of the 3 components are completed)

G9227 Functional outcome assessment documented, care plan not documented, documented the patient is not eligible for a care plan

G9228 Chlamydia, gonorrhea and syphilis screening results documented (report when results are present for all of the 3 screenings)

G9229 Chlamydia, gonorrhea, and syphilis not screened, due to documented reason (patient refusal is the only allowed exclusion)

G9230 Chlamydia, gonorrhea, and syphilis not screened, reason not given

G9231 Documentation of end stage renal disease (ESRD), dialysis, renal transplant or pregnancy

G9232 Clinician treating major depressive disorder did not communicate to clinician treating comorbid condition for specified patient reason

G9233 All quality actions for the applicable measures in the total knee replacement measures group have been performed for this patient

G9234 I intend to report the total knee replacement measures group

G9235 All quality actions for the applicable measures in the general surgery measures group have been performed for this patient

G9236 All quality actions for the applicable measures in the optimizing patient exposure to ionizing radiation measures group have been performed for this patient

G9237 I intend to report the general surgery measures group

G9238 I intend to report the optimizing patient exposure to ionizing radiation measures group

G9239 Documentation of reasons for patient initiaiting maintenance hemodialysis with a catheter as the mode of vascular access (e.g., patient has a maturing avf/avg, time-limited trial of hemodialysis, patients undergoing palliative dialysis, other medical reasons, patient declined avf/avg, other patient reasons, patient followed by reporting nephrologist for fewer than 90 days, other system reasons)

G9240 Patient whose mode of vascular access is a catheter at the time maintenance hemodialysis is initiated

Procedures/Professional Services (Temporary)

G9241 — G9295

G9241   Patient whose mode of vascular access is not a catheter at the time maintenance hemodialysis is initiated

G9242   Documentation of viral load equal to or greater than 200 copies/ml

G9243   Documentation of viral load less than 200 copies/ml

G9244   Antiretroviral thereapy not prescribed

G9245   Antiretroviral therapy prescribed

G9246   Patient did not have at least one medical visit in each 6 month period of the 24 month measurement period, with a minimum of 60 days between medical visits

G9247   Patient had at least one medical visit in each 6 month period of the 24 month measurement period, with a minimum of 60 days between medical visits

G9248   Patient did not have a medical visit in the last 6 months

G9249   Patient had a medical visit in the last 6 months

G9250   Documentation of patient pain brought to a comfortable level within 48 hours from initial assessment

G9251   Documentation of patient with pain not brought to a comfortable level within 48 hours from initial assessment

G9252   Adenoma(s) or other neoplasm detected during screening colonoscopy

G9253   Adenoma(s) or other neoplasm not detected during screening colonoscopy

G9254   Documentation of patient discharged to home later than post-operative day 2 following CAS

G9255   Documentation of patient discharged to home no later than post operative day 2 following CAS

G9256   Documentation of patient death following CAS

G9257   Documentation of patient stroke following CAS

G9258   Documentation of patient stroke following CEA

G9259   Documentation of patient survival and absence of stroke following CAS

G9260   Documentation of patient death following CEA

G9261   Documentation of patient survival and absence of stroke following CEA

G9262   Documentation of patient death in the hospital following endovascular AAA repair

G9263   Documentation of patient survival in the hospital following endovascular AAA repair

G9264   Documentation of patient receiving maintenance hemodialysis for greater than or equal to 90 days with a catheter for documented reasons (e.g., patient is undergoing palliative dialysis with a catheter, patient approved by a qualified transplant program and scheduled to receive a living donor kidney transplant, other medical reasons, patient declined avf/avg, other patient reasons)

G9265   Patient receiving maintenance hemodialysis for greater than or equal to 90 days with a catheter as the mode of vascular access

G9266   Patient receiving maintenance hemodialysis for greater than or equal to 90 days without a catheter as the mode of vascular access

G9267   Documentation of patient with one or more complications or mortality within 30 days

G9268   Documentation of patient with one or more complications within 90 days

G9269   Documentation of patient without one or more complications and without mortality within 30 days

G9270   Documentation of patient without one or more complications within 90 days

G9271   LDL value < 100

G9272   LDL value >= 100

G9273   Blood pressure has a systolic value of < 140 and a diastolic value of < 90

G9274   Blood pressure has a systolic value of = 140 and a diastolic value of = 90 or systolic value < 140 and diastolic value = 90 or systolic value = 140 and diastolic value < 90

G9275   Documentation that patient is a current non-tobacco user

G9276   Documentation that patient is a current tobacco user

G9277   Documentation that the patient is on daily aspirin or has documentation of a valid contraindication to aspirin automatic contraindications include anti-coagulant use, allergy, and history of gastrointestinal bleed; additionally, any reason documented by the physician as a reason for not taking daily aspirin is acceptable (examples include non-steroidal anti-inflammatory agents, risk for drug interaction, or uncontrolled hypertension defined as > 180 systolic or > 110 diastolic)

G9278   Documentation that the patient is not on daily aspirin regimen

G9279   Pneumococcal screening performed and documentation of vaccination received prior to discharge

G9280   Pneumococcal vaccination not administered prior to discharge, reason not specified

G9281   Screening performed and documentation that vaccination not indicated/patient refusal

G9282   Documentation of medical reason(s) for not reporting the histological type or NSCLC-NOS classification with an explanation (e.g., biopsy taken for other purposes in a patient with a history of non-small cell lung cancer or other documented medical reasons)

G9283   Non small cell lung cancer biopsy and cytology specimen report documents classification into specific histologic type or classified as NSCLC-NOS with an explanation

G9284   Non small cell lung cancer biopsy and cytology specimen report does not document classification into specific histologic type or classified as NSCLC-NOS with an explanation

G9285   Specimen site other than anatomic location of lung or is not classified as non small cell lung cancer

G9286   Documentation of antibiotic regimen prescribed within 7 days of diagnosis or within 10 days after onset of symptoms

G9287   No antibiotic regimen prescribed within 7 days of diagnosis or within 10 days after onset of symptoms

G9288   Documentation of medical reason(s) for not reporting the histological type or nsclc-nos classification with an explanation (e.g., a solitary fibrous tumor in a person with a history of non-small cell carcinoma or other documented medical reasons)

G9289   Non small cell lung cancer biopsy and cytology specimen report documents classification into specific histologic type or classified as nsclc-nos with an explanation

G9290   Non small cell lung cancer biopsy and cytology specimen report does not document classification into specific histologic type or classified as nsclc-nos with an explanation

G9291   Specimen site other than anatomic location of lung, is not classified as non small cell lung cancer or classified as nsclc-nos

G9292   Documentation of medical reason(s) for not reporting pt category and a statement on thickness and ulceration and for pt1, mitotic rate (e.g., negative skin biopsies in a patient with a history of melanoma or other documented medical reasons)

G9293   Pathology report does not include the pt category and a statement on thickness and ulceration and for pt1, mitotic rate

G9294   Pathology report includes the pt category and a statement on thickness and ulceration and for pt1, mitotic rate

G9295   Specimen site other than anatomic cutaneous location

G9296 Patients with documented shared decision-making including discussion of conservative (non-surgical) therapy prior to the procedure

G9297 Shared decision-making including discussion of conservative (non-surgical) therapy prior to the procedure not documented, reason not given

G9298 Patients who are evaluated for venous thromboembolic and cardiovascular risk factors within 30 days prior to the procedure including history of dvt, pe, mi, arrhythmia and stroke

G9299 Patients who are not evaluated for venous thromboembolic and cardiovascular risk factors within 30 days prior to the procedure including history of dvt, pe, mi, arrhythmia and stroke, reason not given

G9300 Documentation of medical reason(s) for not completely infusing the prophylactic antibiotic prior to the inflation of the proximal tourniquet (e.g., a tourniquet was not used)

G9301 Patients who had the prophylactic antibiotic completely infused prior to the inflation of the proximal tourniquet

G9302 Prophylactic antibiotic not completely infused prior to the inflation of the proximal tourniquet, reason not given

G9303 Operative report does not identify the prosthetic implant specifications including the prosthetic implant manufacturer, the brand name of the prosthetic implant and the size of the prosthetic implant, reason not given

G9304 Operative report identifies the prosthetic implant specifications including the prosthetic implant manufacturer, the brand name of the prosthetic implant and the size of the prosthetic implant

G9305 Intervention for presence of leak of endoluminal contents through an anastomosis not required

G9306 Intervention for presence of leak of endoluminal contents through an anastomosis required

G9307 No return to the operating room for a surgical procedure, for any reason, within 30 days of the principal operative procedure

G9308 Unplanned return to the operating room for a surgical procedure, for any reason, within 30 days of the principal operative procedure

G9309 No unplanned hospital readmission within 30 days of principal procedure

G9310 Unplanned hospital readmission within 30 days of principal procedure

G9311 No surgical site infection

G9312 Surgical site infection

G9313 Amoxicillin, with or without clavulanate, not prescribed as first line antibiotic at the time of diagnosis for documented reason (e.g., cystic fibrosis, immotile cilia disorders, ciliary dyskinesia, immune deficiency, prior history of sinus surgery within the past 12 months, and anatomic abnormalities, such as deviated nasal septum, resistant organisms, allergy to medication, recurrent sinusitis, chronic sinusitis, or other reasons)

G9314 Amoxicillin, with or without clavulanate, not prescribed as first line antibiotic at the time of diagnosis, reason not given

G9315 Documentation amoxicillin, with or without clavulanate, prescribed as a first line antibiotic at the time of diagnosis

G9316 Documentation of patient-specific risk assessment with a risk calculator based on multi-institutional clinical data, the specific risk calculator used, and communication of risk assessment from risk calculator with the patient or family

G9317 Documentation of patient-specific risk assessment with a risk calculator based on multi-institutional clinical data, the specific risk calculator used, and communication of risk assessment from risk calculator with the patient or family not completed

G9318 Imaging study named according to standardized nomenclature

G9319 Imaging study not named according to standardized nomenclature, reason not given

G9320 Documentation of medical reason(s) for not naming CT studies according to a standardized nomenclature provided (e.g., CT studies performed for radiation treatment planning or image-guided radiation treatment delivery)

G9321 Count of previous CT (any type of CT) and cardiac nuclear medicine (myocardial perfusion) studies documented in the 12-month period prior to the current study

G9322 Count of previous CT and cardiac nuclear medicine (myocardial perfusion) studies not documented in the 12-month period prior to the current study, reason not given

G9323 Documentation of medical reason(s) for not counting previous CT and cardiac nuclear medicine (myocardial perfusion) studies (e.g., CT studies performed for radiation treatment planning or image-guided radiation treatment delivery)

G9324 All necessary data elements not included, reason not given

G9325 CT studies not reported to a radiation dose index registry due to medical reasons (e.g., CT studies performed for radiation treatment planning or image-guided radiation treatment delivery)

G9326 CT studies performed not reported to a radiation dose index registry, reason not given

G9327 CT studies performed reported to a radiation dose index registry with all necessary data elements

G9328 Dicom format image data availability not documented in final report due to medical reasons (e.g., CT studies performed for radiation treatment planning or image-guided radiation treatment delivery)

G9329 Dicom format image data available to non-affiliated external entities on a secure, media free, reciprocally searchable basis with patient authorization for at least a 12-month period after the study not documented in final report, reason not given

G9340 Final report documented that dicom format image data available to non-affiliated external entities on a secure, media free, reciprocally searchable basis with patient authorization for at least a 12-month period after the study

G9341 Search conducted for prior patient CT imaging studies completed at non-affiliated external entities within the past 12-months and are available through a secure, authorized, media-free, shared archive prior to an imaging study being performed

G9342 Search conducted for prior patient imaging studies completed at non-affiliated external entities within the past 12-months and are available through a secure, authorized, media-free, shared archive prior to an imaging study being performed not completed, reason not given

G9343 Search for prior patient completed dicom format images not completed due to medical reasons (e.g., CT studies performed for radiation treatment planning or image-guided radiation treatment delivery)

G9344 Search for prior patient completed dicom format images not completed due to system reasons (i.e., facility does not have archival abilities through a shared archival system)

G9345 Follow-up recommendations according to recommended guidelines for incidentally detected pulmonary nodules (e.g., follow-up CT imaging studies needed or that no follow-up is needed) based at a minimum on nodule size and patient risk factors documented

G9346 Follow-up recommendations according to recommended guidelines for incidentally detected pulmonary nodules not documented due to medical reasons (e.g., patients with known malignant disease, patients with unexplained fever, CT studied performed for radiation treatment planning or image-guided radiation treatment delivery)

G9347 Follow-up recommendations according to recommended guidelines for incidentally detected pulmonary nodules not documented, reason not given

G9348 CT scan of the paranasal sinuses ordered at the time of diagnosis for documented reasons (e.g., persons with sinusitis symptoms lasting at least 7 to 10 days, antibiotic resistance, immunocompromised, recurrent sinusitis, acute frontal sinusitis, acute sphenoid sinusitis, periorbital cellulitis, or other medical)

G9349 Documentation of a CT scan of the paranasal sinuses ordered at the time of diagnosis or received within 28 days after date of diagnosis

G9350 CT scan of the paranasal sinuses not ordered at the time of diagnosis or received within 28 days after date of diagnosis

G9351 More than one CT scan of the paranasal sinuses ordered or received within 90 days after diagnosis

G9352 More than one CT scan of the paranasal sinuses ordered or received within 90 days after the date of diagnosis, reason not given

G9353 More than one CT scan of the paranasal sinuses ordered or received within 90 days after the date of diagnosis for documented reasons (e.g., patients with complications, second CT obtained prior to surgery, other medical reasons)

G9354 More than one CT scan of the paranasal sinuses not ordered within 90 days after the date of diagnosis

G9355 Elective delivery or early induction not performed

G9356 Elective delivery or early induction performed

G9357 Post-partum screenings, evaluations and education performed

G9358 Post-partum screenings, evaluations and education not performed

G9359 Documentation of negative or managed positive TB screen with further evidence that TB is not active

G9360 No documentation of negative or managed positive TB screen

ALCOHOL AND DRUG ABUSE TREATMENT SERVICES
H0001-H2037

The H codes are used by those state Medicaid agencies that are mandated by state law to establish separate codes for identifying mental health services that include alcohol and drug treatment services.

H0001   Alcohol and/or drug assessment

H0002   Behavioral health screening to determine eligibility for admission to treatment program

H0003   Alcohol and/or drug screening; laboratory analysis of specimens for presence of alcohol and/or drugs

H0004   Behavioral health counseling and therapy, per 15 minutes

H0005   Alcohol and/or drug services; group counseling by a clinician

H0006   Alcohol and/or drug services; case management

H0007   Alcohol and/or drug services; crisis intervention (outpatient)

H0008   Alcohol and/or drug services; subacute detoxification (hospital inpatient)

H0009   Alcohol and/or drug services; acute detoxification (hospital inpatient)

H0010   Alcohol and/or drug services; subacute detoxification (residential addiction program inpatient)

H0011   Alcohol and/or drug services; acute detoxification (residential addiction program inpatient)

H0012   Alcohol and/or drug services; subacute detoxification (residential addiction program outpatient)

H0013   Alcohol and/or drug services; acute detoxification (residential addiction program outpatient)

H0014   Alcohol and/or drug services; ambulatory detoxification

H0015   Alcohol and/or drug services; intensive outpatient (treatment program that operates at least 3 hours/day and at least 3 days/week and is based on an individualized treatment plan), including assessment, counseling; crisis intervention, and activity therapies or education

H0016   Alcohol and/or drug services; medical/somatic (medical intervention in ambulatory setting)

H0017   Behavioral health; residential (hospital residential treatment program), without room and board, per diem

H0018   Behavioral health; short-term residential (nonhospital residential treatment program), without room and board, per diem

H0019   Behavioral health; long-term residential (nonmedical, nonacute care in a residential treatment program where stay is typically longer than 30 days), without room and board, per diem

H0020   Alcohol and/or drug services; methadone administration and/or service (provision of the drug by a licensed program)

H0021   Alcohol and/or drug training service (for staff and personnel not employed by providers)

H0022   Alcohol and/or drug intervention service (planned facilitation)

H0023   Behavioral health outreach service (planned approach to reach a targeted population)

H0024   Behavioral health prevention information dissemination service (one-way direct or nondirect contact with service audiences to affect knowledge and attitude)

H0025   Behavioral health prevention education service (delivery of services with target population to affect knowledge, attitude and/or behavior)

H0026   Alcohol and/or drug prevention process service, community-based (delivery of services to develop skills of impactors)

H0027   Alcohol and/or drug prevention environmental service (broad range of external activities geared toward modifying systems in order to mainstream prevention through policy and law)

H0028   Alcohol and/or drug prevention problem identification and referral service (e.g., student assistance and employee assistance programs), does not include assessment

H0029   Alcohol and/or drug prevention alternatives service (services for populations that exclude alcohol and other drug use e.g., alcohol free social events)

H0030   Behavioral health hotline service

H0031   Mental health assessment, by nonphysician

H0032   Mental health service plan development by nonphysician

H0033   Oral medication administration, direct observation

H0034   Medication training and support, per 15 minutes

H0035   Mental health partial hospitalization, treatment, less than 24 hours

H0036   Community psychiatric supportive treatment, face-to-face, per 15 minutes

H0037   Community psychiatric supportive treatment program, per diem

H0038   Self-help/peer services, per 15 minutes

H0039   Assertive community treatment, face-to-face, per 15 minutes

H0040   Assertive community treatment program, per diem

H0041   Foster care, child, nontherapeutic, per diem

H0042   Foster care, child, nontherapeutic, per month

H0043   Supported housing, per diem

H0044   Supported housing, per month

H0045   Respite care services, not in the home, per diem

H0046   Mental health services, not otherwise specified

H0047   Alcohol and/or other drug abuse services, not otherwise specified

H0048   Alcohol and/or other drug testing: collection and handling only, specimens other than blood

H0049   Alcohol and/or drug screening

H0050   Alcohol and/or drug services, brief intervention, per 15 minutes

H1000   Prenatal care, at-risk assessment

H1001   Prenatal care, at-risk enhanced service; antepartum management

H1002   Prenatal care, at risk enhanced service; care coordination

H1003   Prenatal care, at-risk enhanced service; education

H1004   Prenatal care, at-risk enhanced service; follow-up home visit

H1005   Prenatal care, at-risk enhanced service package (includes H1001-H1004)

H1010   Nonmedical family planning education, per session

H1011   Family assessment by licensed behavioral health professional for state defined purposes

H2000   Comprehensive multidisciplinary evaluation

H2001   Rehabilitation program, per 1/2 day

H2010   Comprehensive medication services, per 15 minutes

H2011   Crisis intervention service, per 15 minutes

H2012   Behavioral health day treatment, per hour

H2013   Psychiatric health facility service, per diem

H2014   Skills training and development, per 15 minutes

H2015   Comprehensive community support services, per 15 minutes

H2016   Comprehensive community support services, per diem

H2017   Psychosocial rehabilitation services, per 15 minutes

H2018   Psychosocial rehabilitation services, per diem

H2019   Therapeutic behavioral services, per 15 minutes

H2020   Therapeutic behavioral services, per diem

H2021   Community-based wrap-around services, per 15 minutes

Alcohol and Drug Abuse Treatment Services

H2022 — H2037

H2022   Community-based wrap-around services, per diem

H2023   Supported employment, per 15 minutes

H2024   Supported employment, per diem

H2025   Ongoing support to maintain employment, per 15 minutes

H2026   Ongoing support to maintain employment, per diem

H2027   Psychoeducational service, per 15 minutes

H2028   Sexual offender treatment service, per 15 minutes

H2029   Sexual offender treatment service, per diem

H2030   Mental health clubhouse services, per 15 minutes

H2031   Mental health clubhouse services, per diem

H2032   Activity therapy, per 15 minutes

H2033   Multisystemic therapy for juveniles, per 15 minutes

H2034   Alcohol and/or drug abuse halfway house services, per diem

H2035   Alcohol and/or other drug treatment program, per hour

H2036   Alcohol and/or other drug treatment program, per diem

H2037   Developmental delay prevention activities, dependent child of client, per 15 minutes

J CODES DRUGS J0120-J8499

J codes include drugs that ordinarily cannot be self-administered, chemotherapy drugs, immunosuppressive drugs, inhalation solutions, and other miscellaneous drugs and solutions

J0120   Injection, tetracycline, up to 250 mg

J0129   Injection, abatacept, 10 mg (code may be used for Medicare when drug administered under the direct supervision of a physician, not for use when drug is self-administered)
Use this code for Orencia

J0130   Injection abciximab, 10 mg
Use this code for ReoPro.

J0131   Injection, acetaminophen, 10 mg
Use this code for OFIRMEV.

J0132   Injection, acetylcysteine, 100 mg
Use this code for Acetadote.

J0133   Injection, acyclovir, 5 mg
Use this code for Zovirax

J0135   Injection, adalimumab, 20 mg
Use this code for Humira.

J0150   Injection, adenosine for therapeutic use, 6 mg (not to be used to report any adenosine phosphate compounds, instead use A9270)
Use this code for Adenocard.
AHA: 2Q,'02,10

J0151   Injection, adenosine for diagnostic use, 1 mg (not to be used to report any adenosine phosphate compounds, instead use A9270)
Use this code for Adenoscan

J0171   Injection, Adrenalin, epinephrine, 0.1 mg

J0178   Injection, aflibercept, 1 mg
Use this code for Eylea.

J0180   Injection, agalsidase beta, 1 mg
Use this code for Fabrazyme.

J0190   Injection, biperiden lactate, per 5 mg

J0200   Injection, alatrofloxacin mesylate, 100 mg
MED: 100-2,15,50.5

J0205   Injection, alglucerase, per 10 units
Use this code for Ceredase.

J0207   Injection, amifostine, 500 mg
Use this code for Ethyol.

J0210   Injection, methyldopa HCl, up to 250 mg
Use this code for Aldomet.

J0215   Injection, alefacept, 0.5 mg
Use this for Amevive.

J0220   Injection, alglucosidase alfa, 10 mg, not otherwise specified
Use this code for Myozyme.

J0221   Injection, alglucosidase alfa, (Lumizyme), 10 mg

J0256   Injection, alpha 1-proteinase inhibitor (human), not otherwise specified, 10 mg
Use this code for Aralast, Aralast NP, Prolastin C, Zemira.

J0257   Injection, alpha 1 proteinase inhibitor (human), (GLASSIA), 10 mg

J0270   Injection, alprostadil, 1.25 mcg (code may be used for Medicare when drug administered under the direct supervision of a physician, not for use when drug is self-administered)
Use this code for Alprostadil, Caverject, Edex, Prostin VR Pediatric.

J0275   Alprostadil urethral suppository (code may be used for Medicare when drug administered under the direct supervision of a physician, not for use when drug is self-administered)
Use this code for Muse.

J0278   Injection, amikacin sulfate, 100 mg
Use this code for Amikin.

J0280   Injection, aminophyllin, up to 250 mg

J0282   Injection, amiodarone HCl, 30 mg
Use this code for Cordarone IV.

J0285   Injection, amphotericin B, 50 mg
Use this for Amphocin, Fungizone

J0287   Injection, amphotericin B lipid complex, 10 mg
Use this code for Abelcet

J0288   Injection, amphotericin B cholesteryl sulfate complex, 10 mg
Use this code for Amphotec.

J0289   Injection, amphotericin B liposome, 10 mg
Use this code for Ambisome.

J0290   Injection, ampicillin sodium, 500 mg

J0295   Injection, ampicillin sodium/sulbactam sodium, per 1.5 g
Use this code for Unasyn.

J0300   Injection, amobarbital, up to 125 mg
Use this code for Amytal.

J0330   Injection, succinylcholine chloride, up to 20 mg
Use this code for Anectine, Quelicin.

J0348   Injection, anidulafungin, 1 mg
Use this code for Eraxis.

J0350   Injection, anistreplase, per 30 units
Use this code for Eminase.

J0360   Injection, hydralazine HCl, up to 20 mg

J0364   Injection, apomorphine HCl, 1 mg
Use this code for Apokyn.

J0365   Injection, aprotinin, 10,000 kiu
Use this code for Trasylol.

J0380   Injection, metaraminol bitartrate, per 10 mg
Use this code for Aramine.

J0390   Injection, chloroquine HCl, up to 250 mg
Use this code for Aralen.

J0395   Injection, arbutamine HCl, 1 mg

J0400   Injection, aripiprazole, intramuscular, 0.25 mg
Use this code for Abilify.

J0401   Injection, aripiprazole, extended release, 1 mg
Use this code for the Abilify Maintena kit

J0456   Injection, azithromycin, 500 mg
Use this code for Zithromax.
MED: 100-2,15,50.5

J0461   Injection, atropine sulfate, 0.01 mg
Use this code for AtroPen.

J0470   Injection, dimercaprol, per 100 mg
Use this code for BAL

J0475   Injection, baclofen, 10 mg
Use this code for Lioresal, Gablofen.

J0476   Injection, baclofen, 50 mcg for intrathecal trial
Use this code for Lioresal, Gablofen.

J0480   Injection, basiliximab, 20 mg
Use this code for Simulect.

J0485 Injection, belatacept, 1 mg
Use this code for Nulojix.

J0490 Injection, belimumab, 10 mg
Use this code for BENLYSTA.

J0500 Injection, dicyclomine HCl, up to 20 mg
Use this code for Bentyl.

J0515 Injection, benztropine mesylate, per 1 mg
Use this code for Cogentin.

J0520 Injection, bethanechol chloride, Myotonachol or Urecholine, up to 5 mg

J0558 Injection, penicillin G benzathine and penicillin G procaine, 100,000 units
Use this code for Bicillin CR, Bicillin CR 900/300, Bicillin CR Tubex.

J0561 Injection, penicillin G benzathine, 100,000 units

J0583 Injection, bivalirudin, 1 mg
Use this code for Angiomax.

J0585 Injection, onabotulinumtoxinA, 1 unit
Use this code for Botox, Botox Cosmetic.

J0586 Injection, abobotulinumtoxinA, 5 units
Use this code for Dysport.

J0587 Injection, rimabotulinumtoxinB, 100 units
Use this code for Myobloc.
AHA: 2Q,'02,8

J0588 Injection, incobotulinumtoxinA, 1 unit
Use this code for XEOMIN.

J0592 Injection, buprenorphine HCl, 0.1 mg
Use this code for Buprenex.

J0594 Injection, busulfan, 1 mg
Use this code for Busulfex.

J0595 Injection, butorphanol tartrate, 1 mg
Use this code for Stadol.

J0597 Injection, C-1 esterase inhibitor (human), Berinert, 10 units

J0598 Injection, C-1 esterase inhibitor (human), Cinryze, 10 units

J0600 Injection, edetate calcium disodium, up to 1,000 mg
Use this code for Calcium Disodium Versenate, Calcium EDTA.

J0610 Injection, calcium gluconate, per 10 ml

J0620 Injection, calcium glycerophosphate and calcium lactate, per 10 ml

J0630 Injection, calcitonin salmon, up to 400 units
Use this code for Calcimar, Miacalcin.
MED: 100-4,10,90.1

J0636 Injection, calcitriol, 0.1 mcg
Use this code for Calcijex.

J0637 Injection, caspofungin acetate, 5 mg
Use this code for Cancidas.

J0638 Injection, canakinumab, 1 mg
Use this code for ILARIS.

J0640 Injection, leucovorin calcium, per 50 mg

J0641 Injection, levoleucovorin calcium, 0.5 mg
Use this code for Fusilev.

J0670 Injection, mepivacaine HCl, per 10 ml
Use this code for Carbocaine, Polocaine, Isocaine HCl, Scandonest

J0690 Injection, cefazolin sodium, 500 mg
Use this code for Ancef, Kefzol

J0692 Injection, cefepime HCl, 500 mg
Use this code for Maxipime.

J0694 Injection, cefoxitin sodium, 1 g

J0696 Injection, ceftriaxone sodium, per 250 mg
Use this code for Rocephin.

J0697 Injection, sterile cefuroxime sodium, per 750 mg
Use this code for Zinacef.

J0698 Injection, cefotaxime sodium, per g
Use this code for Claforan.

J0702 Injection, betamethasone acetate 3 mg and betamethasone sodium phosphate 3 mg
Use this code for Celestone Soluspan.

J0706 Injection, caffeine citrate, 5 mg
Use this code for Cafcit.
AHA: 2Q,'02,8

J0710 Injection, cephapirin sodium, up to 1 g

J0712 Injection, ceftaroline fosamil, 10 mg
Use this code for Teflaro.

J0713 Injection, ceftazidime, per 500 mg
Use this code for Ceptaz, Fortaz, Tazicef

J0715 Injection, ceftizoxime sodium, per 500 mg
Use this code for Cefizox.

J0716 Injection, Centruroides immune f(ab)2, up to 120 mg
Use this code for Anascorp.

J0717 Injection, certolizumab pegol, 1 mg (code may be used for Medicare when drug administered under the direct supervision of a physician, not for use when drug is self administered)
Use this code for Cinzia

J0720 Injection, chloramphenicol sodium succinate, up to 1 g
Use this code for Chlormycetin.

J0725 Injection, chorionic gonadotropin, per 1,000 USP units

J0735 Injection, clonidine HCl, 1 mg
Use this code for Clorpres, Duraclon, Iopidine

J0740 Injection, cidofovir, 375 mg
Use this code for Vistide.

J0743 Injection, cilastatin sodium; imipenem, per 250 mg
Use this code for Primaxin I.M., Primaxin I.V.

J0744 Injection, ciprofloxacin for intravenous infusion, 200 mg
Use this code for Cipro.

J0745 Injection, codeine phosphate, per 30 mg

J0760 Injection, colchicine, per 1 mg

J0770 Injection, colistimethate sodium, up to 150 mg
Use this code for Coly-Mycin M.

J0775 Injection, collagenase, clostridium histolyticum, 0.01 mg
Use this code for XIAFLEX.

J0780 Injection, prochlorperazine, up to 10 mg
Use this code for Compazine, Ultrazine-10.

J0795 Injection, corticorelin ovine triflutate, 1 mcg
Use this code for Acthrel.

J0800 Injection, corticotropin, up to 40 units
Use this code for H.P. Acthar gel

J0833 Injection, cosyntropin, not otherwise specified, 0.25 mg
Use this code for Cortrosyn.

J0834 Injection, cosyntropin (Cortrosyn), 0.25 mg

J0840 Injection, crotalidae polyvalent immune fab (ovine), up to 1 g
Use this code for CroFab, FabAV.

J0850 Injection, cytomegalovirus immune globulin intravenous (human), per vial
Use this code for Cytogam.

J0878 Injection, daptomycin, 1 mg
Use this code for Cubicin.

J0881 Injection, darbepoetin alfa, 1 mcg (non-ESRD use)
Use this code for Aranesp.

J0882 Injection, darbepoetin alfa, 1 mcg (for ESRD on dialysis)
Use this code for Aranesp.
MED: 100-4,8,60.4; 100-4,8,60.4.1; 100-4,8,60.4.2; 100-4,8,60.4.5.1; 100-4,8,60.4.6.3; 100-4,8,60.4.6.4; 100-4,8,60.4.6.5; 100-4,8,60.7; 100-4,13,60.7.1

J0885 Injection, epoetin alfa, (for non-ESRD use), 1000 units
Use this code for Epogen/Procrit.

J0886 Injection, epoetin alfa, 1000 units (for ESRD on dialysis)
Use this code for Epogen/Procrit.
MED: 100-4,8,60.4; 100-4,8,60.4.1; 100-4,8,60.4.4; 100-4,8,60.4.4.1; 100-4,8,60.4.4.2; 100-4,8,60.4.5.1

J0890 Injection, peginesatide, 0.1 mg (for ESRD on dialysis)
Use this code for Omontys.
MED: 100-4,8,60.4; 100-4,8,60.4.1; 100-4,8,60.4.2; 100-4,8,60.4.5.1; 100-4,8,60.4.7

J0894 Injection, decitabine, 1 mg
Use this code for Dacogen.

J0895 Injection, deferoxamine mesylate, 500 mg
Use this code for Desferal.

J0897 Injection, denosumab, 1 mg
Use this code for XGEVA, Prolia.

J0900 Injection, testosterone enanthate and estradiol valerate, up to 1 cc

J0945 Injection, brompheniramine maleate, per 10 mg

J1000 Injection, depo-estradiol cypionate, up to 5 mg
Use this code for depGynogen, Depogen, Estradiol Cypionate.

J1020 Injection, methylprednisolone acetate, 20 mg
Use this code for Depo-Medrol.

J1030 Injection, methylprednisolone acetate, 40 mg
Use this code for DepoMedalone40, Depo-Medrol, Sano-Drol.

J1040 Injection, methylprednisolone acetate, 80 mg
Use this code for Cortimed, DepMedalone, DepoMedalone 80, Depo-Medrol, Duro Cort, Methylcotolone, Pri-Methylate, Sano-Drol.

J1050 Injection, medroxyprogesterone acetate, 1 mg

J1060 Injection, testosterone cypionate and estradiol cypionate, up to 1 ml
Use this code for Depo-Testadiol, Duo-Span, Duo-Span II.

J1070 Injection, testosterone cypionate, up to 100 mg
Use this code for Depo Testosterone Cypionate.

J1080 Injection, testosterone cypionate, 1 cc, 200 mg
Use this code for Depandrante, Depo-Testosterone, Virilon.

J1094 Injection, dexamethasone acetate, 1 mg
Use this code for Cortastat LA, Dalalone L.A., Dexamethasone Acetate Anhydrous, Dexone LA.

J1100 Injection, dexamethasone sodium phosphate, 1 mg
Use this code for Cortastat, Dalalone, Decaject, Dexone, Solurex, Adrenocort, Primethasone, Dexasone, Dexim, Medidex, Spectro-Dex.

J1110 Injection, dihydroergotamine mesylate, per 1 mg
Use this code for D.H.E. 45.

J1120 Injection, acetazolamide sodium, up to 500 mg
Use this code for Diamox.

J1160 Injection, digoxin, up to 0.5 mg
Use this code for Lanoxin.

J1162 Injection, digoxin immune fab (ovine), per vial
Use this code for Digibind, Digifab.

J1165 Injection, phenytoin sodium, per 50 mg
Use this code for Dilantin.

J1170 Injection, hydromorphone, up to 4 mg
Use this code for Dilaudid, Dilaudid-HP.

J1180 Injection, dyphylline, up to 500 mg

J1190 Injection, dexrazoxane HCl, per 250 mg
Use this code for Zinecard.

J1200 Injection, diphenhydramine HCl, up to 50 mg
Use this code for Benadryl, Benahist 10, Benahist 50, Benoject-10, Benoject-50, Bena-D 10, Bena-D 50, Nordryl, Dihydrex, Dimine, Diphenacen-50, Hyrexin-50, Truxadryl, Wehdryl.
AHA: 1Q,'02,2

J1205 Injection, chlorothiazide sodium, per 500 mg
Use this code for Diuril Sodium.

J1212 Injection, DMSO, dimethyl sulfoxide, 50%, 50 ml
Use this code for Rimso 50. DMSO is covered only as a treatment of interstitial cystitis.

J1230 Injection, methadone HCl, up to 10 mg
Use this code for Dolophine HCl.

J1240 Injection, dimenhydrinate, up to 50 mg
Use this code for Dramamine, Dinate, Dommanate, Dramanate, Dramilin, Dramocen, Dramoject, Dymenate, Hydrate, Marmine, Wehamine.

J1245 Injection, dipyridamole, per 10 mg
Use this code for Persantine IV.

J1250 Injection, Dobutamine HCl, per 250 mg

J1260 Injection, dolasetron mesylate, 10 mg
Use this code for Anzemet.

J1265 Injection, dopamine HCl, 40 mg

J1267 Injection, doripenem, 10 mg
Use this code for Doribax

J1270 Injection, doxercalciferol, 1 mcg
Use this code for Hectorol.

J1290 Injection, ecallantide, 1 mg
Use this code for KALBITOR.

J1300 Injection, eculizumab, 10 mg
Use this code for Soliris.

J1320 Injection, amitriptyline HCl, up to 20 mg
Use this code for Elavil

J1324 Injection, enfuvirtide, 1 mg
Use this code for Fuzeon.

J1325 Injection, epoprostenol, 0.5 mg
Use this code for Flolan. See K0455 for infusion pump for epoprosterol.

J1327 Injection, eptifibatide, 5 mg
Use this code for Integrilin.

J1330 Injection, ergonovine maleate, up to 0.2 mg
Medicare jurisdiction: local contractor. Use this code for Ergotrate Maleate.

J1335 Injection, ertapenem sodium, 500 mg
Use this code for Invanz.

J1364 Injection, erythromycin lactobionate, per 500 mg

J1380 Injection, estradiol valerate, up to 10 mg
Use this code for Delestrogen, Dioval, Dioval XX, Dioval 40, Duragen-10, Duragen-20, Duragen-40, Estradiol L.A., Estradiol L.A. 20, Estradiol L.A. 40, Gynogen L.A. 10, Gynogen L.A. 20, Gynogen L.A. 40, Valergen 10, Valergen 20, Valergen 40, Estra-L 20, Estra-L 40, L.A.E. 20.

J1410 Injection, estrogen conjugated, per 25 mg
Use this code for Natural Estrogenic Substance, Premarin Intravenous, Primestrin Aqueous.

J1430 Injection, ethanolamine oleate, 100 mg
Use this code for Ethamiolin.

J1435 Injection, estrone, per 1 mg
Use this code for Estone Aqueous, Estragyn, Estro-A, Estrone, Estronol, Theelin Aqueous, Estone 5, Kestrone 5.

J1436 Injection, etidronate disodium, per 300 mg
Use this code for Didronel.

J1438 Injection, etanercept, 25 mg (code may be used for Medicare when drug administered under the direct supervision of a physician, not for use when drug is self-administered)
Use this code for Enbrel.

J1442 Injection, filgrastim (G-CSF), 1 microgram
Use this code for Neupogen

J1446 Injection, TBO-filgrastim, 5 micrograms
Use this code for Granix

J1450 Injection, fluconazole, 200 mg
Use this code for Diflucan.
MED: 100-2,15,50.5

J1451 Injection, fomepizole, 15 mg
Use this code for Antizol.

J1452 Injection, fomivirsen sodium, intraocular, 1.65 mg
Use this code for Vitavene.
MED: 100-2,15,50.4.2

J1453 Injection, fosaprepitant, 1 mg
Use this code for Emend.

J1455 Injection, foscarnet sodium, per 1,000 mg
Use this code for Foscavir.

J1457 Injection, gallium nitrate, 1 mg
Use this code for Ganite.

J1458 Injection, galsulfase, 1 mg
Use this code for Naglazyme.

J1459 Injection, immune globulin (Privigen), intravenous, nonlyophilized (e.g., liquid), 500 mg

J1460 Injection, gamma globulin, intramuscular, 1 cc
Use this code for GamaSTAN SD.

J1556 Injection, immune globulin (bivigam), 500 mg
Use this code for Bivigam

J1557 Injection, immune globulin, (Gammaplex), intravenous, nonlyophilized (e.g., liquid), 500 mg

J1559 Injection, immune globulin (Hizentra), 100 mg

J1560 Injection, gamma globulin, intramuscular, over 10 cc
Use this code for GamaSTAN SD.

J1561 Injection, immune globulin, (Gamunex/Gamunex-C/Gammaked), nonlyophilized (e.g., liquid), 500 mg

J1562 Injection, immune globulin (Vivaglobin), 100 mg

J1566 Injection, immune globulin, intravenous, lyophilized (e.g., powder), not otherwise specified, 500 mg
Use this code for Carimune.

J1568 Injection, immune globulin, (Octagam), intravenous, nonlyophilized (e.g., liquid), 500 mg

J1569 Injection, immune globulin, (Gammagard liquid), nonlyophilized, (e.g., liquid), 500 mg

J1570 Injection, ganciclovir sodium, 500 mg
Use this code for Cytovene.

J1571 Injection, hepatitis B immune globulin (Hepagam B), intramuscular, 0.5 ml

J1572 Injection, immune globulin, (Flebogamma/Flebogamma Dif), intravenous, nonlyophilized (e.g., liquid), 500 mg

J1573 Injection, hepatitis B immune globulin (Hepagam B), intravenous, 0.5 ml

J1580 Injection, garamycin, gentamicin, up to 80 mg
Use this code for Gentamicin Sulfate, Jenamicin.

J1590 Injection, gatifloxacin, 10 mg
MED: 100-4,4,10.4

J1595 Injection, glatiramer acetate, 20 mg
Use this code for Copaxone.

J1599 Injection, immune globulin, intravenous, nonlyophilized (e.g., liquid), not otherwise specified, 500 mg

J1600 Injection, gold sodium thiomalate, up to 50 mg
Use this code for Myochrysine.
MED: 100-4,4,10.4

J1602 Injection, golimumab, 1 mg, for intravenous use
Use this code for Simponi

J1610 Injection, glucagon HCl, per 1 mg
Use this code for Glucagen.

J1620 Injection, gonadorelin HCl, per 100 mcg
Use this code for Factrel, Lutrepulse.

J1626 Injection, granisetron HCl, 100 mcg
Use this code for Kytril.
MED: 100-4,4,10.4

J1630 Injection, haloperidol, up to 5 mg
Use this code for Haldol.
MED: 100-4,4,10.4

J1631 Injection, haloperidol decanoate, per 50 mg
Use this code for Haldol Decanoate-50.

J1640 Injection, hemin, 1 mg
Use this code for Panhematin.

J1642 Injection, heparin sodium, (heparin lock flush), per 10 units
Use this code for Hep-Lock, Hep-Lock U/P, Hep-Pak, Lok-Pak.
MED: 100-4,4,10.4

J1644 Injection, Heparin sodium, per 1000 units
Use this code for Heparin Sodium, Liquaemin Sodium.
MED: 100-4,4,10.4

J1645 Injection, dalteparin sodium, per 2500 IU
Use this code for Fragmin.

J1650 Injection, enoxaparin sodium, 10 mg
Use this code for Lovenox.
MED: 100-4,4,10.4

J1652 Injection, fondaparinux sodium, 0.5 mg
Use this code for Atrixtra.

J1655 Injection, tinzaparin sodium, 1000 IU
Use this code for Innohep.
MED: 100-4,4,10.4

J1670 Injection, tetanus immune globulin, human, up to 250 units
Use this code for HyperTET SD.

J1675 Injection, histrelin acetate, 10 mcg
Use this code for Supprelin LA.

J1700 Injection, hydrocortisone acetate, up to 25 mg
Use this code for Hydrocortone Acetate.
MED: 100-4,4,10.4

J1710 Injection, hydrocortisone sodium phosphate, up to 50 mg
Use this code for Hydrocortone Phosphate.
MED: 100-4,4,10.4

J1720 Injection, hydrocortisone sodium succinate, up to 100 mg
Use this code for Solu-Cortef, A-Hydrocort.
MED: 100-4,4,10.4

J1725 Injection, hydroxyprogesterone caproate, 1 mg
Use this code for Makena.

J1730 Injection, diazoxide, up to 300 mg

J1740 Injection, ibandronate sodium, 1 mg
Use this code for Boniva.

J1741 Injection, ibuprofen, 100 mg
Use this code for Caldolor.

J1742 Injection, ibutilide fumarate, 1 mg
Use this code for Corvert.

J1743 Injection, idursulfase, 1 mg
Use this code for Elaprase.

J1744 Injection, icatibant, 1 mg
Use this code for Firazyr.

J1745 Injection infliximab, 10 mg
Use this code for Remicade.

J1750 Injection, iron dextran, 50 mg
Use this code for INFeD.

J1756 Injection, iron sucrose, 1 mg
Use this code for Venofer.

J1786 Injection, imiglucerase, 10 units
Use this code for Cerezyme.

J1790 Injection, droperidol, up to 5 mg
Use this code for Inapsine.
MED: 100-4,4,10.4

J1800 Injection, propranolol HCl, up to 1 mg
Use this code for Inderal.
MED: 100-4,4,10.4

J1810 Injection, droperidol and fentanyl citrate, up to 2 ml ampule
AHA: 2Q,'02,8

J1815 Injection, insulin, per 5 units
Use this code for Humalog, Humulin, Iletin, Insulin Lispo, Lantus, Levemir, NPH, Pork insulin, Regular insulin, Ultralente, Velosulin, Humulin R, Iletin II Regular Pork, Insulin Purified Pork, Relion, Lente Iletin I, Novolin R, Humulin R U-500.
MED: 100-4,4,10.4

J1817 Insulin for administration through DME (i.e., insulin pump) per 50 units
Use this code for Humalog, Humulin, Vesolin BR, Iletin II NPH Pork, Lispro-PFC, Novolin, Novolog, Novolog Flexpen, Novolog Mix, Relion Novolin.

J1826 Injection, interferon beta-1a, 30 mcg
Use this code for AVONEX, Rebif.

J1830 Injection interferon beta-1b, 0.25 mg (code may be used for Medicare when drug administered under the direct supervision of a physician, not for use when drug is self-administered)
Use this code for Betaseron.

J1835 Injection, itraconazole, 50 mg
Use this code for Sporonox IV.
MED: 100-4,4,10.4

J1840 Injection, kanamycin sulfate, up to 500 mg
Use this code for Kantrex
MED: 100-4,4,10.4

J1850 Injection, kanamycin sulfate, up to 75 mg
Use this code for Kantrex
MED: 100-4,4,10.4

J1885 Injection, ketorolac tromethamine, per 15 mg
Use this code for Toradol.
MED: 100-4,4,10.4

J1890 Injection, cephalothin sodium, up to 1 g
MED: 100-4,4,10.4

J1930 Injection, lanreotide, 1 mg
Use this code for Somatuline.

J1931 Injection, laronidase, 0.1 mg
Use this code for Aldurazyme.

J1940 Injection, furosemide, up to 20 mg
Use this code for Lasix
MED: 100-4,4,10.4

J1945 Injection, lepirudin, 50 mg
Use this code for Refludan.
This drug is used for patients with heparin induced thrombocytopenia.

J1950 Injection, leuprolide acetate (for depot suspension), per 3.75 mg
Use this code for Eligard, Lupron, Lupron-3, Lupron-4, Lupron Depot.

J1953 Injection, levetiracetam, 10 mg
Use this code for Keppra.

J1955 Injection, levocarnitine, per 1 g
Use this code for Carnitor

J1956 Injection, levofloxacin, 250 mg
Use this code for Levaquin.
MED: 100-4,4,10.4

J1960 Injection, levorphanol tartrate, up to 2 mg
Use this code for Levo-Dromoran.
MED: 100-4,4,10.4

J1980 Injection, hyoscyamine sulfate, up to 0.25 mg
Use this code for Levsin.
MED: 100-4,4,10.4

J1990 Injection, chlordiazepoxide HCl, up to 100 mg
Use this code for Librium.
MED: 100-4,4,10.4

J2001 Injection, lidocaine HCl for intravenous infusion, 10 mg
Use this code for Xylocaine.
MED: 100-4,4,10.4

J2010 Injection, lincomycin HCl, up to 300 mg
Use this code for Lincocin
MED: 100-4,4,10.4

J2020 Injection, linezolid, 200 mg
Use this code for Zyvok.
AHA: 2Q,'02,8

J2060 Injection, lorazepam, 2 mg
Use this code for Ativan.
MED: 100-4,4,10.4

J2150 Injection, mannitol, 25% in 50 ml
Use this code for Osmitrol.
MED: 100-4,4,10.4

J2170 Injection, mecasermin, 1 mg
Use this code for Iplex, Increlex.
MED: 100-4,4,10.4

J2175   Injection, meperidine HCl, per 100 mg
Use this code for Demerol.
MED: 100-4,4,10.4

J2180   Injection, meperidine and promethazine HCl, up to 50 mg
Use this code for Mepergan Injection.
MED: 100-4,4,10.4

J2185   Injection, meropenem, 100 mg
Use this code for Merrem.
MED: 100-4,4,10.4

J2210   Injection, methylergonovine maleate, up to 0.2 mg
Use this code for Methergine.
MED: 100-4,4,10.4

J2212   Injection, methylnaltrexone, 0.1 mg
Use this code for Relistor.

J2248   Injection, micafungin sodium, 1 mg
Use this code for Mycamine.

J2250   Injection, midazolam HCl, per 1 mg
Use this code for Versed.
MED: 100-4,4,10.4

J2260   Injection, milrinone lactate, 5 mg
Use this code for Primacor.
MED: 100-4,4,10.4

J2265   Injection, minocycline HCl, 1 mg
Use this code for MINOCIN.

J2270   Injection, morphine sulfate, up to 10 mg
Use this code for Depodur, Infumorph
MED: 100-4,4,10.4

J2271   Injection, morphine sulfate, 100 mg
Use this code for Depodur, Infumorph
MED: 100-4,4,10.4

J2275   Injection, morphine sulfate (preservative-free sterile solution), per 10 mg
Use this code for Astramorph PF, Duramorph, Infumorph.
MED: 100-4,4,10.4

J2278   Injection, ziconotide, 1 mcg
Use this code for Prialt.

J2280   Injection, moxifloxacin, 100 mg
Use this code for Avelox.
MED: 100-4,4,10.4

J2300   Injection, nalbuphine HCl, per 10 mg
Use this code for Nubain.
MED: 100-4,4,10.4

J2310   Injection, naloxone HCl, per 1 mg
Use this code for Narcan.

J2315   Injection, naltrexone, depot form, 1 mg
Use this code for Vivitrol.

J2320   Injection, nandrolone decanoate, up to 50 mg

J2323   Injection, natalizumab, 1 mg
Use this code for Tysabri.

J2325   Injection, nesiritide, 0.1 mg
Use this code for Natrecor.

J2353   Injection, octreotide, depot form for intramuscular injection, 1 mg
Use this code for Sandostatin LAR.

J2354   Injection, octreotide, nondepot form for subcutaneous or intravenous injection, 25 mcg
Use this code for Sandostatin.

J2355   Injection, oprelvekin, 5 mg
Use this code for Neumega.

J2357   Injection, omalizumab, 5 mg
Use this code for Xolair.

J2358   Injection, olanzapine, long-acting, 1 mg
Use this code for ZYPREXA RELPREVV.

J2360   Injection, orphenadrine citrate, up to 60 mg
Use this code for Norflex

J2370   Injection, phenylephrine HCl, up to 1 ml

J2400   Injection, chloroprocaine HCl, per 30 ml
Use this code for Nesacaine, Nesacaine-MPF.

J2405   Injection, ondansetron HCl, per 1 mg
Use this code for Zofran.

J2410   Injection, oxymorphone HCl, up to 1 mg
Use this code for Numorphan, Oxymorphone HCl.

J2425   Injection, palifermin, 50 mcg
Use this code for Kepivance.

J2426   Injection, paliperidone palmitate extended release, 1 mg
Use this code for INVEGA SUSTENNA.

J2430   Injection, pamidronate disodium, per 30 mg
Use this code for Aredia

J2440   Injection, papaverine HCl, up to 60 mg

J2460   Injection, oxytetracycline HCl, up to 50 mg
Use this code for Terramycin IM.

J2469   Injection, palonosetron HCl, 25 mcg
Use this code for Aloxi.

J2501   Injection, paricalcitol, 1 mcg
Use this code For Zemplar.

J2503   Injection, pegaptanib sodium, 0.3 mg
Use this code for Mucagen.

J2504   Injection, pegademase bovine, 25 IU
Use this code for Adagen.

J2505   Injection, pegfilgrastim, 6 mg
Use this code for Neulasta.

J2507   Injection, pegloticase, 1 mg
Use this code for KRYSTEXXA.

J2510   Injection, penicillin G procaine, aqueous, up to 600,000 units
Use this code for Wycillin, Duracillin A.S., Pfizerpen A.S., Crysticillin 300 A.S., Crysticillin 600 A.S.

J2513   Injection, pentastarch, 10% solution, 100 ml

J2515   Injection, pentobarbital sodium, per 50 mg
Use this code for Nembutal Sodium Solution.

J2540   Injection, penicillin G potassium, up to 600,000 units
Use this code for Pfizerpen.

J2543   Injection, piperacillin sodium/tazobactam sodium, 1 g/0.125 g (1.125 g)
Use this code for Zosyn.

J2545   Pentamidine isethionate, inhalation solution, FDA-approved final product, noncompounded, administered through DME, unit dose form, per 300 mg
Use this code for Nebupent, Pentam 300

J2550   Injection, promethazine HCl, up to 50 mg
Use this code for Phenergan

J2560   Injection, phenobarbital sodium, up to 120 mg

J2562   Injection, plerixafor, 1 mg
Use this code for Mozobil.

J2590 Injection, oxytocin, up to 10 units
Use this code for Pitocin, Syntocinon.

J2597 Injection, desmopressin acetate, per 1 mcg
Use this code for DDAVP.

J2650 Injection, prednisolone acetate, up to 1 ml

J2670 Injection, tolazoline HCl, up to 25 mg

J2675 Injection, progesterone, per 50 mg
Use this code for Gesterone, Gestrin.

J2680 Injection, fluphenazine decanoate, up to 25 mg

J2690 Injection, procainamide HCl, up to 1 g
Use this code for Pronestyl.

J2700 Injection, oxacillin sodium, up to 250 mg
Use this code for Bactocill

J2710 Injection, neostigmine methylsulfate, up to 0.5 mg
Use this code for Prostigmin.

J2720 Injection, protamine sulfate, per 10 mg

J2724 Injection, protein C concentrate, intravenous, human, 10 IU

J2725 Injection, protirelin, per 250 mcg
Use this code for Thyrel TRH

J2730 Injection, pralidoxime chloride, up to 1 g
Use this code for Protopam Chloride.

J2760 Injection, phentolamine mesylate, up to 5 mg
Use this code for Regitine.

J2765 Injection, metoclopramide HCl, up to 10 mg
Use this code for Reglan

J2770 Injection, quinupristin/dalfopristin, 500 mg (150/350)
Use this code for Synercid.

J2778 Injection, ranibizumab, 0.1 mg
Use this code for Lucentis.

J2780 Injection, ranitidine HCl, 25 mg
Use this code for Zantac.

J2783 Injection, rasburicase, 0.5 mg
Use this code for Elitek.

J2785 Injection, regadenoson, 0.1 mg
Use this code for Lexiscan.

J2788 Injection, Rho D immune globulin, human, minidose, 50 mcg (250 i.u.)
Use this code for RhoGam, MiCRhoGAM.

J2790 Injection, Rho D immune globulin, human, full dose, 300 mcg (1500 i.u.)
Use this code for RhoGam, HypRho SD.

J2791 Injection, Rho(D) immune globulin (human), (Rhophylac), intramuscular or intravenous, 100 IU
Use this for Rhophylac.

J2792 Injection, Rho D immune globulin, intravenous, human, solvent detergent, 100 IU
Use this code for WINRho SDF

J2793 Injection, rilonacept, 1 mg
Use this code for Arcalyst.

J2794 Injection, risperidone, long acting, 0.5 mg
Use this code for Risperidal Consta Long Acting.

J2795 Injection, ropivacaine HCl, 1 mg
Use this code for Naropin.

J2796 Injection, romiplostim, 10 mcg
Use this code for Nplate.

J2800 Injection, methocarbamol, up to 10 ml
Use this code for Robaxin

J2805 Injection, sincalide, 5 mcg
Use this code for Kinevac.

J2810 Injection, theophylline, per 40 mg

J2820 Injection, sargramostim (GM-CSF), 50 mcg
Use this code for Leukine

J2850 Injection, secretin, synthetic, human, 1 mcg

J2910 Injection, aurothioglucose, up to 50 mg
Use this code for Solganal.

J2916 Injection, sodium ferric gluconate complex in sucrose injection, 12.5 mg
MED: 100-3,110.10

J2920 Injection, methylprednisolone sodium succinate, up to 40 mg
Use this code for Solu-Medrol, A-methaPred.

J2930 Injection, methylprednisolone sodium succinate, up to 125 mg
Use this code for Solu-Medrol, A-methaPred.

J2940 Injection, somatrem, 1 mg
Use this code for Protropin.
AHA: 2Q,'02,8

J2941 Injection, somatropin, 1 mg
Use this code for Humatrope, Genotropin Nutropin, Biotropin, Genotropin, Genotropin Miniquick, Norditropin, Nutropin, Nutropin AQ, Saizen, Saizen Somatropin RDNA Origin, Serostim, Serostim RDNA Origin, Zorbtive.
AHA: 2Q,'02,8

J2950 Injection, promazine HCl, up to 25 mg
Use this code for Sparine, Prozine-50.

J2993 Injection, reteplase, 18.1 mg
Use this code for Retavase

J2995 Injection, streptokinase, per 250,000 IU
Use this code for Streptase

J2997 Injection, alteplase recombinant, 1 mg
Use this code for Activase, Cathflo.

J3000 Injection, streptomycin, up to 1 g
Use this code for Streptomycin Sulfate.

J3010 Injection, fentanyl citrate, 0.1 mg
Use this code for Sublimaze.

J3030 Injection, sumatriptan succinate, 6 mg (code may be used for Medicare when drug administered under the direct supervision of a physician, not for use when drug is self-administered)
Use this code for Imitrex.

J3060 Injection, taliglucerace alfa, 10 units
Use this code for Elelyso

J3070 Injection, pentazocine, 30 mg
Use this code for Talwin.

J3095 Injection, telavancin, 10 mg
Use this code for VIBATIV.

J3101 Injection, tenecteplase, 1 mg
Use this code for TNKase.

J3105 Injection, terbutaline sulfate, up to 1 mg
For terbutaline in inhalation solution, see K0525 and K0526.

J3110 Injection, teriparatide, 10 mcg
Use this code for Forteo.
MED: 100-4,10,90.1

J3120 Injection, testosterone enanthate, up to 100 mg
Use this code for Delatestryl.

Drugs Administered Other Than Oral Method

J3130 — J7131

J3130 Injection, testosterone enanthate, up to 200 mg
Use this code for Delatestryl.

J3140 Injection, testosterone suspension, up to 50 mg

J3150 Injection, testosterone propionate, up to 100 mg

J3230 Injection, chlorpromazine HCl, up to 50 mg
Use this code for Thorazine.

J3240 Injection, thyrotropin alpha, 0.9 mg, provided in 1.1 mg vial
Use this code for Thyrogen.

J3243 Injection, tigecycline, 1 mg
Use this code for Tygacil.

J3246 Injection, tirofiban HCl, 0.25 mg
Use this code for Aggrastat.

J3250 Injection, trimethobenzamide HCl, up to 200 mg
Use this code for Tigan, Tiject-20, Arrestin.

J3260 Injection, tobramycin sulfate, up to 80 mg
Use this code for Nebcin.

J3262 Injection, tocilizumab, 1 mg
Use this code for ACTEMRA.

J3265 Injection, torsemide, 10 mg/ml
Use this code for Demadex, Torsemide.

J3280 Injection, thiethylperazine maleate, up to 10 mg

J3285 Injection, treprostinil, 1 mg
Use this code for Remodulin.

J3300 Injection, triamcinolone acetonide, preservative free, 1 mg
Use this code for TRIVARIS, TRIESENCE

J3301 Injection, triamcinolone acetonide, not otherwise specified, 10 mg
Use this code for Kenalog-10, Kenalog-40, Tri-Kort, Kenaject-40, Cenacort A-40, Triam-A, Trilog.

J3302 Injection, triamcinolone diacetate, per 5 mg
Use this code for Aristocort, Aristocort Intralesional, Aristocort Forte, Amcort, Trilone, Cenacort Forte.

J3303 Injection, triamcinolone hexacetonide, per 5 mg
Use this code for Aristospan Intralesional, Aristospan Intra-articular.

J3305 Injection, trimetrexate glucuronate, per 25 mg
Use this code for Neutrexin.

J3310 Injection, perphenazine, up to 5 mg
Use this code for Trilafon.

J3315 Injection, triptorelin pamoate, 3.75 mg
Use this code for Trelstar Depot, Trelstar Depot Plus Debioclip Kit, Trelstar LA.

J3320 Injection, spectinomycin dihydrochloride, up to 2 g
Use this code for Trobicin.

J3350 Injection, urea, up to 40 g

J3355 Injection, urofollitropin, 75 IU
Use this code for Metrodin, Bravelle, Fertinex.

J3357 Injection, ustekinumab, 1 mg
Use this code for STELARA.

J3360 Injection, diazepam, up to 5 mg
Use this code for Diastat, Dizac, Valium.

J3364 Injection, urokinase, 5,000 IU vial
Use this code for Kinlytic.

J3365 Injection, IV, urokinase, 250,000 IU vial
Use this code for Kinlytic.

J3370 Injection, vancomycin HCl, 500 mg
Use this code for Vancocin.

J3385 Injection, velaglucerase alfa, 100 units
Use this code for VPRIV.

J3396 Injection, verteporfin, 0.1 mg
Use this code for Visudyne.

MED: 100-3,80.2; 100-3,80.2.1; 100-3,80.3; 100-3,80.3.1; 100-4,32,300; 100-4,32,300.1; 100-4,32,300.2

J3400 Injection, triflupromazine HCl, up to 20 mg

J3410 Injection, hydroxyzine HCl, up to 25 mg
Use this code for Vistaril, Vistaject-25, Hyzine, Hyzine-50.

J3411 Injection, thiamine HCl, 100 mg

J3415 Injection, pyridoxine HCl, 100 mg

J3420 Injection, vitamin B-12 cyanocobalamin, up to 1,000 mcg
Use this code for Sytobex, Redisol, Rubramin PC, Betalin 12, Berubigen, Cobex, Cobal, Crystal B12, Cyano, Cyanocobalamin, Hydroxocobalamin, Hydroxycobal, Nutri-Twelve.

J3430 Injection, phytonadione (vitamin K), per 1 mg
Use this code for AquaMephyton, Konakion, Menadione, Phytonadione.

J3465 Injection, voriconazole, 10 mg

J3470 Injection, hyaluronidase, up to 150 units

J3471 Injection, hyaluronidase, ovine, preservative free, per 1 USP unit (up to 999 USP units)

J3472 Injection, hyaluronidase, ovine, preservative free, per 1,000 USP units

J3473 Injection, hyaluronidase, recombinant, 1 USP unit

J3475 Injection, magnesium sulfate, per 500 mg
Use this code for Mag Sul, Sulfa Mag.

J3480 Injection, potassium chloride, per 2 mEq

J3485 Injection, zidovudine, 10 mg
Use this code for Retrovir, Zidovudine.

J3486 Injection, ziprasidone mesylate, 10 mg
Use this code for Geodon.

J3489 Injection, zoledronic acid, 1 mg
Use this code for Reclast and Zometa

J3490 Unclassified drugs

J3520 Edetate disodium, per 150 mg
Use this code for Endrate, Disotate, Meritate, Chealamide, E.D.T.A. This drug is used in chelation therapy, a treatment for atherosclerosis that is not covered by Medicare.

J3530 Nasal vaccine inhalation

J3535 Drug administered through a metered dose inhaler

J3570 Laetrile, amygdalin, vitamin B-17
The FDA has found Laetrile to have no safe or effective therapeutic purpose.

J3590 Unclassified biologics

J7030 Infusion, normal saline solution, 1,000 cc

J7040 Infusion, normal saline solution, sterile (500 ml=1 unit)

J7042 5% dextrose/normal saline (500 ml = 1 unit)

J7050 Infusion, normal saline solution, 250 cc

J7060 5% dextrose/water (500 ml = 1 unit)

J7070 Infusion, D-5-W, 1,000 cc

J7100 Infusion, dextran 40, 500 ml
Use this code for Gentran, 10% LMD, Rheomacrodex.

J7110 Infusion, dextran 75, 500 ml
Use this code for Gentran 75.

J7120 Ringers lactate infusion, up to 1,000 cc

J7131 Hypertonic saline solution, 1 ml

J7178   Injection, human fibrinogen concentrate, 1 mg
Use this code for RiaSTAP.

J7180   Injection, factor XIII (antihemophilic factor, human), 1 IU
Use this code for Corifact.

J7183   Injection, von Willebrand factor complex (human), Wilate, 1 IU
vWF:RCo

J7185   Injection, factor VIII (antihemophilic factor, recombinant) (XYNTHA), per IU
Use this code for Xyntha.

J7186   Injection, antihemophilic factor VIII/von Willebrand factor complex (human), per factor VIII i.u.
Use this code for Alphanate.
MED: 100-4,17,80.4.1

J7187   Injection, von Willebrand factor complex (Humate-P), per IU
VWF:RCO
MED: 100-4,17,80.4.1

J7189   Factor VIIa (antihemophilic factor, recombinant), per 1 mcg
MED: 100-4,17,80.4.1

J7190   Factor VIII (antihemophilic factor, human) per IU
Use this code for Koate-DVI, Monarc-M, Monoclate-P.

FACTOR VIII
Antihemophilic factor that is part of the intrinsic coagulation cascade used to treat Hemophilia A. The most common and oldest form of this is human derived factor concentrated from human plasma (HCPCS Level II code J7190). The Porcine variety (J7191) is supplied as lyophilized Factor VIII from concentrated pig's blood. Recombinant, purified factor VIII (J7192) without the albumin is produced by recombinant genes. May be sold under the brand names Hexilate, Kogenate.
MED: 100-4,17,80.4; 100-4,17,80.4.1

J7191   Factor VIII (antihemophilic factor (porcine)), per IU
FACTOR VIII
Antihemophilic factor that is part of the intrinsic coagulation cascade used to treat Hemophilia A. The most common and oldest form of this is human derived factor concentrated from human plasma (HCPCS Level II code J7190). The Porcine variety (J7191) is supplied as lyophilized Factor VIII from concentrated pig's blood. Recombinant, purified factor VIII (J7192) without the albumin is produced by recombinant genes. May be sold under the brand names Hexilate, Kogenate.
MED: 100-4,17,80.4; 100-4,17,80.4.1

J7192   Factor VIII (antihemophilic factor, recombinant) per IU, not otherwise specified
Use this code for Recombinate, Kogenate FS, Helixate FX, Advate rAHF-PFM, Antihemophilic Factor Human Method M Monoclonal Purified, Refacto.
FACTOR VIII
Antihemophilic factor that is part of the intrinsic coagulation cascade used to treat Hemophilia A. The most common and oldest form of this is human derived factor concentrated from human plasma (HCPCS Level II code J7190). The Porcine variety (J7191) is supplied as lyophilized Factor VIII from concentrated pig's blood. Recombinant, purified factor VIII (J7192) without the albumin is produced by recombinant genes. May be sold under the brand names Hexilate, Kogenate.
MED: 100-4,17,80.4; 100-4,17,80.4.1

J7193   Factor IX (antihemophilic factor, purified, nonrecombinant) per IU
Use this code for AlphaNine SD, Mononine.
MED: 100-4,17,80.4; 100-4,17,80.4.1
AHA: 2Q,'02,8

J7194   Factor IX complex, per IU
Use this code for Konyne-80, Profilnine SD, Proplex T, Proplex T, Bebulin VH, factor IX+ complex, Profilnine SD.
MED: 100-4,17,80.4; 100-4,17,80.4.1

J7195   Factor IX (antihemophilic factor, recombinant) per IU
Use this code for Benefix.
MED: 100-4,17,80.4; 100-4,17,80.4.1
AHA: 2Q,'02,8

J7196   Injection, antithrombin recombinant, 50 IU
Use this code for ATryn.

J7197   Antithrombin III (human), per IU
Use this code for Thrombate III, ATnativ.
MED: 100-4,17,80.4.1

J7198   Antiinhibitor, per IU
Medicare jurisdiction: local contractor. Use this code for Autoplex T, Feiba VH AICC.
MED: 100-3,110.3; 100-4,17,80.4; 100-4,17,80.4.1

J7199   Hemophilia clotting factor, not otherwise classified
Medicare jurisdiction: local contractor.
MED: 100-4,17,80.4; 100-4,17,80.4.1

J7300   Intrauterine copper contraceptive
Use this code for Paragard T380A.

J7301   Levonorgestrel-releasing intrauterine contraceptive system (Skyla), 13.5 mg
Use this code for Skyla

J7302   Levonorgestrel-releasing intrauterine contraceptive system, 52 mg
Use this code for Mirena.

J7303   Contraceptive supply, hormone containing vaginal ring, each
Use this code for Nuvaring Vaginal Ring.

J7304   Contraceptive supply, hormone containing patch, each

J7306   Levonorgestrel (contraceptive) implant system, including implants and supplies
Use this code for Norplant II.

J7307   Etonogestrel (contraceptive) implant system, including implant and supplies
Use this code for Implanon and Nexplanon

J7308   Aminolevulinic acid HCl for topical administration, 20%, single unit dosage form (354 mg)

J7309   Methyl aminolevulinate (MAL) for topical administration, 16.8%, 1 g
Use this code for Metvixia.

J7310   Ganciclovir, 4.5 mg, long-acting implant
Use this code for Vitrasert.

J7311   Fluocinolone acetonide, intravitreal implant
Use this code for Retisert.

J7312   Injection, dexamethasone, intravitreal implant, 0.1 mg
Use this code for OZURDEX.

J7315   Mitomycin, opthalmic, 0.2 mg
Use this code for Mitosol.

J7316   Injection, ocriplasmin, 0.125 mg
Use this code for Jetrea

J7321   Hyaluronan or derivative, Hyalgan or Supartz, for intra-articular injection, per dose

J7323   Hyaluronan or derivative, Euflexxa, for intra-articular injection, per dose

J7324   Hyaluronan or derivative, Orthovisc, for intra-articular injection, per dose

J7325   Hyaluronan or derivative, Synvisc or Synvisc-One, for intra-articular injection, 1 mg

J7326   Hyaluronan or derivative, Gel-One, for intra-articular injection, per dose

J7330   Autologous cultured chondrocytes, implant
Medicare jurisdiction: local contractor. Use this code for Carticel.

J7335   Capsaicin 8% patch, per 10 sq cm
Use this code for Qutenza.

J7500   Azathioprine, oral, 50 mg
Use this code for Azasan, Imuran.
MED: 100-2,15,50.5; 100-4,17,80.3

J7501   Azathioprine, parenteral, 100 mg
MED: 100-4,17,80.3

J7502   Cyclosporine, oral, 100 mg
Use this code for Neoral, Sandimmune, Gengraf, Sangcya
MED: 100-2,15,50.5; 100-4,17,80.3

J7504   Lymphocyte immune globulin, antithymocyte globulin, equine, parenteral, 250 mg
Use this code for Atgam.
MED: 100-4,17,80.3

J7505   Muromonab-CD3, parenteral, 5 mg
Use this code for Orthoclone OKT3.
MED: 100-4,17,80.3

J7506   Prednisone, oral, per 5 mg
MED: 100-2,15,50.5; 100-4,17,80.3

J7507   Tacrolimus, immediate release, oral, 1 mg
Use this code for Prograf.
MED: 100-2,15,50.5; 100-4,17,80.3

J7508   Tacrolimus, extended release, oral, 0.1 mg
Use this code for Astagraf XL

J7509   Methylprednisolone, oral, per 4 mg
Use this code for Medrol, Methylpred.
MED: 100-2,15,50.5; 100-4,17,80.3

J7510   Prednisolone, oral, per 5 mg
Use this code for Delta-Cortef, Cotolone, Pediapred, Prednoral, Prelone.
MED: 100-2,15,50.5; 100-4,17,80.3

J7511   Lymphocyte immune globulin, antithymocyte globulin, rabbit, parenteral, 25 mg
Use this code for Thymoglobulin.
MED: 100-4,17,80.3
AHA: 2Q,'02,8

J7513   Daclizumab, parenteral, 25 mg
Use this code for Zenapax.
MED: 100-2,15,50.5; 100-4,17,80.3

J7515   Cyclosporine, oral, 25 mg
Use this code for Neoral, Sandimmune, Gengraf, Sangcya.
MED: 100-4,17,80.3

J7516   Cyclosporine, parenteral, 250 mg
Use this code for Neoral, Sandimmune, Gengraf, Sangcya.
MED: 100-4,17,80.3

J7517   Mycophenolate mofetil, oral, 250 mg
Use this code for CellCept.
MED: 100-4,17,80.3

J7518   Mycophenolic acid, oral, 180 mg
Use this code for Myfortic Delayed Release.
MED: 100-4,17,80.3.1

J7520   Sirolimus, oral, 1 mg
Use this code for Rapamune.
MED: 100-2,15,50.5; 100-4,17,80.3

J7525   Tacrolimus, parenteral, 5 mg
Use this code for Prograf.
MED: 100-2,15,50.5; 100-4,17,80.3

J7527   Everolimus, oral, 0.25 mg
Use this code for Zortress, Afinitor.

J7599   Immunosuppressive drug, not otherwise classified
Determine if an alternative HCPCS Level II or a CPT code better describes the service being reported. This code should be used only if a more specific code is unavailable.
MED: 100-2,15,50.5; 100-4,17,80.3

INHALATION DRUGS

J7604   Acetylcysteine, inhalation solution, compounded product, administered through DME, unit dose form, per g

J7605   Arformoterol, inhalation solution, FDA approved final product, noncompounded, administered through DME, unit dose form, 15 mcg

J7606   Formoterol fumarate, inhalation solution, FDA approved final product, noncompounded, administered through DME, unit dose form, 20 mcg
Use this code for PERFOROMIST.

J7607   Levalbuterol, inhalation solution, compounded product, administered through DME, concentrated form, 0.5 mg

J7608   Acetylcysteine, inhalation solution, FDA-approved final product, noncompounded, administered through DME, unit dose form, per g
Use this code for Acetadote, Mucomyst, Mucosil.

J7609   Albuterol, inhalation solution, compounded product, administered through DME, unit dose, 1 mg

J7610   Albuterol, inhalation solution, compounded product, administered through DME, concentrated form, 1 mg

J7611   Albuterol, inhalation solution, FDA-approved final product, noncompounded, administered through DME, concentrated form, 1 mg
Use this code for Accuneb, Proventil, Respirol, Ventolin.

J7612   Levalbuterol, inhalation solution, FDA-approved final product, noncompounded, administered through DME, concentrated form, 0.5 mg
Use this code for Xopenex HFA.

J7613   Albuterol, inhalation solution, FDA-approved final product, noncompounded, administered through DME, unit dose, 1 mg
Use this code for Accuneb, Proventil, Respirol, Ventolin.

J7614   Levalbuterol, inhalation solution, FDA-approved final product, noncompounded, administered through DME, unit dose, 0.5 mg
Use this code for Xopenex.

J7615   Levalbuterol, inhalation solution, compounded product, administered through DME, unit dose, 0.5 mg

J7620   Albuterol, up to 2.5 mg and ipratropium bromide, up to 0.5 mg, FDA-approved final product, noncompounded, administered through DME

J7622   Beclomethasone, inhalation solution, compounded product, administered through DME, unit dose form, per mg
Use this code for Beclovent, Beconase.

J7624   Betamethasone, inhalation solution, compounded product, administered through DME, unit dose form, per mg

J7626   Budesonide, inhalation solution, FDA-approved final product, noncompounded, administered through DME, unit dose form, up to 0.5 mg
Use this code for Pulmicort, Pulmicort Flexhaler, Pulmicort Respules, Vanceril.

J7627   Budesonide, inhalation solution, compounded product, administered through DME, unit dose form, up to 0.5 mg

J7628   Bitolterol mesylate, inhalation solution, compounded product, administered through DME, concentrated form, per mg

J7629   Bitolterol mesylate, inhalation solution, compounded product, administered through DME, unit dose form, per mg

J7631   Cromolyn sodium, inhalation solution, FDA-approved final product, noncompounded, administered through DME, unit dose form, per 10 mg

    Use this code for Intal, Nasalcrom

J7632   Cromolyn sodium, inhalation solution, compounded product, administered through DME, unit dose form, per 10 mg

J7633   Budesonide, inhalation solution, FDA-approved final product, noncompounded, administered through DME, concentrated form, per 0.25 mg

    Use this code for Pulmicort, Pulmicort Flexhaler, Pulmicort Respules, Vanceril

J7634   Budesonide, inhalation solution, compounded product, administered through DME, concentrated form, per 0.25 mg

J7635   Atropine, inhalation solution, compounded product, administered through DME, concentrated form, per mg

J7636   Atropine, inhalation solution, compounded product, administered through DME, unit dose form, per mg

J7637   Dexamethasone, inhalation solution, compounded product, administered through DME, concentrated form, per mg

J7638   Dexamethasone, inhalation solution, compounded product, administered through DME, unit dose form, per mg

J7639   Dornase alfa, inhalation solution, FDA-approved final product, noncompounded, administered through DME, unit dose form, per mg

    Use this code for Pulmozyme.

J7640   Formoterol, inhalation solution, compounded product, administered through DME, unit dose form, 12 mcg

J7641   Flunisolide, inhalation solution, compounded product, administered through DME, unit dose, per mg

    Use this code for Aerobid, Flunisolide.

J7642   Glycopyrrolate, inhalation solution, compounded product, administered through DME, concentrated form, per mg

J7643   Glycopyrrolate, inhalation solution, compounded product, administered through DME, unit dose form, per mg

J7644   Ipratropium bromide, inhalation solution, FDA-approved final product, noncompounded, administered through DME, unit dose form, per mg

    Use this code for Atrovent.

J7645   Ipratropium bromide, inhalation solution, compounded product, administered through DME, unit dose form, per mg

J7647   Isoetharine HCl, inhalation solution, compounded product, administered through DME, concentrated form, per mg

J7648   Isoetharine HCl, inhalation solution, FDA-approved final product, noncompounded, administered through DME, concentrated form, per mg

    Use this code for Beta-2.

J7649   Isoetharine HCl, inhalation solution, FDA-approved final product, noncompounded, administered through DME, unit dose form, per mg

J7650   Isoetharine HCl, inhalation solution, compounded product, administered through DME, unit dose form, per mg

J7657   Isoproterenol HCl, inhalation solution, compounded product, administered through DME, concentrated form, per mg

J7658   Isoproterenol HCl, inhalation solution, FDA-approved final product, noncompounded, administered through DME, concentrated form, per mg

    Use this code for Isuprel HCl.

J7659   Isoproterenol HCl, inhalation solution, FDA-approved final product, noncompounded, administered through DME, unit dose form, per mg

    Use this code for Isuprel HCl

J7660   Isoproterenol HCl, inhalation solution, compounded product, administered through DME, unit dose form, per mg

J7665   Mannitol, administered through an inhaler, 5 mg

    Use this code for ARIDOL.

J7667   Metaproterenol sulfate, inhalation solution, compounded product, concentrated form, per 10 mg

J7668   Metaproterenol sulfate, inhalation solution, FDA-approved final product, noncompounded, administered through DME, concentrated form, per 10 mg

    Use this code for Alupent

J7669   Metaproterenol sulfate, inhalation solution, FDA-approved final product, noncompounded, administered through DME, unit dose form, per 10 mg

    Use this code for Alupent.

J7670   Metaproterenol sulfate, inhalation solution, compounded product, administered through DME, unit dose form, per 10 mg

J7674   Methacholine chloride administered as inhalation solution through a nebulizer, per 1 mg

J7676   Pentamidine isethionate, inhalation solution, compounded product, administered through DME, per 300 mg

J7680   Terbutaline sulfate, inhalation solution, compounded product, administered through DME, concentrated form, per mg

    Use this code for Brethine.

J7681   Terbutaline sulfate, inhalation solution, compounded product, administered through DME, per mg

    Use this code for Brethine.

J7682   Tobramycin, inhalation solution, FDA-approved final product, noncompounded, unit dose form, administered through DME, per 300 mg

    Use this code for Tobi.

J7683   Triamcinolone, inhalation solution, compounded product, administered through DME, concentrated form, per mg

    Use this code for Azmacort.

J7684   Triamcinolone, inhalation solution, compounded product, administered through DME, unit dose form, per mg

    Use this code for Azmacort.

J7685   Tobramycin, inhalation solution, compounded product, administered through DME, unit dose form, per 300 mg

J7686   Treprostinil, inhalation solution, FDA-approved final product, noncompounded, administered through DME, unit dose form, 1.74 mg

    Use this code for Tyvaso.

J7699   NOC drugs, inhalation solution administered through DME

J7799   NOC drugs, other than inhalation drugs, administered through DME

J8498   Antiemetic drug, rectal/suppository, not otherwise specified

J8499   Prescription drug, oral, nonchemotherapeutic, NOS

J CODES CHEMOTHERAPY DRUGS J8501-J9999

ORAL CHEMOTHERAPY DRUGS

J8501 Aprepitant, oral, 5 mg
Use this code for Emend.
MED: 100-4,17,80.2.1; 100-4,17,80.2.4

J8510 Busulfan, oral, 2 mg
Use this code for Busulfex, Myleran.
MED: 100-2,15,50.5; 100-4,17,80.1.1

J8515 Cabergoline, oral, 0.25 mg
Use this code for Dostinex.
MED: 100-2,15,50.5

J8520 Capecitabine, oral, 150 mg
Use this code for Xeloda.
MED: 100-2,15,50.5; 100-4,17,80.1.1

J8521 Capecitabine, oral, 500 mg
Use this code for Xeloda.
MED: 100-2,15,50.5; 100-4,17,80.1.1

J8530 Cyclophosphamide, oral, 25 mg
Use this code for Cytoxan.
MED: 100-2,15,50.5; 100-4,17,80.1.1

J8540 Dexamethasone, oral, 0.25 mg
Use this code for Decadron.

J8560 Etoposide, oral, 50 mg
Use this code for VePesid.
MED: 100-2,15,50.5; 100-4,17,80.1.1

J8562 Fludarabine phosphate, oral, 10 mg
Use this code for Oforta.

J8565 Gefitinib, oral, 250 mg
Use this code for Iressa.
MED: 100-4,17,80.1.1

J8597 Antiemetic drug, oral, not otherwise specified

J8600 Melphalan, oral, 2 mg
Use this code for Alkeran.
MED: 100-2,15,50.5; 100-4,17,80.1.1

J8610 Methotrexate, oral, 2.5 mg
Use this code for Trexall, RHEUMATREX.
MED: 100-2,15,50.5; 100-4,17,80.1.1

J8650 Nabilone, oral, 1 mg
Use this code for Cesamet

J8700 Temozolomide, oral, 5 mg
Use this code for Temodar.
MED: 100-2,15,50.5

J8705 Topotecan, oral, 0.25 mg
Use this code for Hycamtin.

J8999 Prescription drug, oral, chemotherapeutic, NOS
Determine if an alternative HCPCS Level II or a CPT code better describes the service being reported. This code should be used only if a more specific code is unavailable.
MED: 100-2,15,50.5; 100-4,17,80.1.1; 100-4,17,80.1.2

INJECTABLE CHEMOTHERAPY DRUGS

These codes cover the cost of the chemotherapy drug only, not the administration.

J9000 Injection, doxorubicin HCl, 10 mg
Use this code for Adriamycin PFS, Adriamycin RDF, Rubex.

J9010 Injection, alemtuzumab, 10 mg
Use this code for Campath.

J9015 Injection, aldesleukin, per single use vial
Use this code for Proleukin, IL-2, Interleukin.

J9017 Injection, arsenic trioxide, 1 mg
Use this code for Trisenox.
AHA: 2Q,'02,8

J9019 Injection, asparaginase (Erwinaze), 1,000 IU
Use this code for Erwinaze.

J9020 Injection, asparaginase, not otherwise specified, 10,000 units
Use this code for Elspar.

J9025 Injection, azacitidine, 1 mg
Use this code for Vidaza.

J9027 Injection, clofarabine, 1 mg
Use this code for Clolar.

J9031 BCG (intravesical) per instillation
Use this code for Tice BCG, PACIS BCG, TheraCys.

J9033 Injection, bendamustine HCl, 1 mg
Use this code for TREANDA.

J9035 Injection, bevacizumab, 10 mg
Use this code for Avastin.

J9040 Injection, bleomycin sulfate, 15 units
Use this code for Blenoxane.

J9041 Injection, bortezomib, 0.1 mg
Use this code for Velcade.

J9042 Injection, brentuximab vedotin, 1 mg
Use this code for Adcentris.

J9043 Injection, cabazitaxel, 1 mg
Use this code for Jevtana.

J9045 Injection, carboplatin, 50 mg
Use this code for Paraplatin.

J9047 Injection, carfilzomib, 1 mg
Use this code for Kyprolis

J9050 Injection, carmustine, 100 mg
Use this code for BiCNU.

J9055 Injection, cetuximab, 10 mg
Use this code for Erbitux.

J9060 Injection, cisplatin, powder or solution, 10 mg
Use this code for Plantinol AQ.

J9065 Injection, cladribine, per 1 mg
Use this code for Leustatin.

J9070 Cyclophosphamide, 100 mg
Use this code for Endoxan-Asta.

J9098 Injection, cytarabine liposome, 10 mg
Use this code for Depocyt.

J9100 Injection, cytarabine, 100 mg
Use this code for Cytosar-U, Ara-C, Tarabin CFS.

J9120 Injection, dactinomycin, 0.5 mg
Use this code for Cosmegen.

J9130 Dacarbazine, 100 mg
Use this code for DTIC-Dome.

J9150 Injection, daunorubicin, 10 mg
Use this code for Cerubidine.

J9151 Injection, daunorubicin citrate, liposomal formulation, 10 mg
Use this code for Daunoxome.

J9155 Injection, degarelix, 1 mg

J9160 Injection, denileukin diftitox, 300 mcg
Use this code for Ontak.

J9165 Injection, diethylstilbestrol diphosphate, 250 mg

J9171 Injection, docetaxel, 1 mg
Use this code for Taxotere.

J9175 Injection, Elliotts' B solution, 1 ml

J9178 Injection, epirubicin HCl, 2 mg
Use this code for Ellence.

J9179 Injection, eribulin mesylate, 0.1 mg
Use this code for Halaven.

J9181 Injection, etoposide, 10 mg
Use this code for VePesid, Toposar.

J9185 Injection, fludarabine phosphate, 50 mg
Use this code for Fludara.

J9190 Injection, fluorouracil, 500 mg
Use this code for Adrucil.

J9200 Injection, floxuridine, 500 mg
Use this code for FUDR.

J9201 Injection, gemcitabine HCl, 200 mg
Use this code for Gemzar.

J9202 Goserelin acetate implant, per 3.6 mg
Use this code for Zoladex.

J9206 Injection, irinotecan, 20 mg
Use this code for Camptosar.

J9207 Injection, ixabepilone, 1 mg
Use this code for IXEMPRA.

J9208 Injection, ifosfamide, 1 g
Use this code for IFEX, Mitoxana.

J9209 Injection, mesna, 200 mg
Use this code for Mesnex.

J9211 Injection, idarubicin HCl, 5 mg
Use this code for Idamycin.

J9212 Injection, interferon alfacon-1, recombinant, 1 mcg
Use this code for Infergen.

J9213 Injection, interferon, alfa-2a, recombinant, 3 million units
Use this code for Roferon-A.

J9214 Injection, interferon, alfa-2b, recombinant, 1 million units
Use this code for Intron A, Rebetron Kit.

J9215 Injection, interferon, alfa-N3, (human leukocyte derived), 250,000 IU
Use this code for Alferon N.

J9216 Injection, interferon, gamma 1-b, 3 million units
Use this code for Actimmune.

J9217 Leuprolide acetate (for depot suspension), 7.5 mg
Use this code for Lupron Depot, Eligard.

J9218 Leuprolide acetate, per 1 mg
Use this code for Lupron.

J9219 Leuprolide acetate implant, 65 mg
Use this code for Lupron Implant.
AHA: 4Q,'01,5

J9225 Histrelin implant (Vantas), 50 mg

J9226 Histrelin implant (Supprelin LA), 50 mg

J9228 Injection, ipilimumab, 1 mg
Use this code for YERVOY.

J9230 Injection, mechlorethamine HCl, (nitrogen mustard), 10 mg
Use this code for Mustargen.

J9245 Injection, melphalan HCl, 50 mg
Use this code for Alkeran, L-phenylalanine mustard.

J9250 Methotrexate sodium, 5 mg
Use this code for Folex, Folex PFS, Methotrexate LPF.

J9260 Methotrexate sodium, 50 mg
Use this code for Folex, Folex PFS, Methotrexate LPF.

J9261 Injection, nelarabine, 50 mg
Use this code for Arranon

J9262 Injection, omacetaxine mepesuccinate, 0.01 mg
Use this code for Synribo

J9263 Injection, oxaliplatin, 0.5 mg
Use this code for Eloxatin.

J9264 Injection, paclitaxel protein-bound particles, 1 mg
Use this code for Abraxane.

J9265 Injection, paclitaxel, 30 mg
Use this code for Taxol, Nov-Onxol.

J9266 Injection, pegaspargase, per single dose vial
Use this code for Oncaspar.
AHA: 2Q,'02,8

J9268 Injection, pentostatin, 10 mg
Use this code for Nipent.

J9270 Injection, plicamycin, 2.5 mg
Use this code for Mithacin.

J9280 Injection, mitomycin, 5 mg
Use this code for Mutamycin.

J9293 Injection, mitoxantrone HCl, per 5 mg
Use this code for Navantrone.

J9300 Injection, gemtuzumab ozogamicin, 5 mg
AHA: 2Q,'02,8

J9302 Injection, ofatumumab, 10 mg
Use this code for Arzerra.

J9303 Injection, panitumumab, 10 mg
Use this code for Vectibix.

J9305 Injection, pemetrexed, 10 mg
Use this code for Alimta.

J9306 Injection, pertuzumab, 1 mg
Use this code for Perjeta

J9307 Injection, pralatrexate, 1 mg
Use this code for FOLOTYN.

J9310 Injection, rituximab, 100 mg
Use this code for RituXan.

J9315 Injection, romidepsin, 1 mg
Use this code for ISTODAX.

J9320 Injection, streptozocin, 1 g
Use this code for Zanosar.

J9328 Injection, temozolomide, 1 mg
Use this code for Temodar.

J9330 Injection, temsirolimus, 1 mg
Use this code for TORISEL.

J9340 Injection, thiotepa, 15 mg
Use this code for Thioplex.

J9351 Injection, topotecan, 0.1 mg
Use this code for Hycamtin.

Chemotherapy Drugs

J9354 — J9999

J9354   Injection, ado-trastuzumab emtansine, 1 mg
     Use this code for Kadcyla

J9355   Injection, trastuzumab, 10 mg
     Use this code for Herceptin.

J9357   Injection, valrubicin, intravesical, 200 mg
     Use this code for Valstar.

J9360   Injection, vinblastine sulfate, 1 mg
     Use this code for Velban.

J9370   Vincristine sulfate, 1 mg
     Use this code for Oncovin, Vincasar PFS.

J9371   Injection, vincristine sulfate liposome, 1 mg
     Use this code for Marqibo kit

J9390   Injection, vinorelbine tartrate, 10 mg
     Use this code for Navelbine.

J9395   Injection, fulvestrant, 25 mg
     Use this code for Faslodex.

J9400   Injection, ziv-aflibercept, 1 mg
     Use this code for Zaltrap

J9600   Injection, porfimer sodium, 75 mg
     Use this code for Photofrin.

J9999   Not otherwise classified, antineoplastic drugs
     Determine if an alternative HCPCS Level II or a CPT code better describes the service being reported. This code should be used only if a more specific code is unavailable.

TEMPORARY CODES K0000-K9999

The K codes were established for use by the DME Medicare Administrative Contractors (DME MACs). The K codes are developed when the currently existing permanent national codes for supplies and certain product categories do not include the codes needed to implement a DME MAC medical review policy.

WHEELCHAIR AND WHEELCHAIR ACCESSORIES

K0001   Standard wheelchair

K0002   Standard hemi (low seat) wheelchair

K0003   Lightweight wheelchair

K0004   High strength, lightweight wheelchair

K0005   Ultralightweight wheelchair

K0006   Heavy-duty wheelchair

K0007   Extra heavy-duty wheelchair

K0008   Custom manual wheelchair/base

K0009   Other manual wheelchair/base

K0010   Standard-weight frame motorized/power wheelchair

K0011   Standard-weight frame motorized/power wheelchair with programmable control parameters for speed adjustment, tremor dampening, acceleration control and braking

K0012   Lightweight portable motorized/power wheelchair

K0013   Custom motorized/power wheelchair base

K0014   Other motorized/power wheelchair base

K0015   Detachable, nonadjustable height armrest, each
       MED: 100-4,23,60.3

K0017   Detachable, adjustable height armrest, base, each

K0018   Detachable, adjustable height armrest, upper portion, each

K0019   Arm pad, each

K0020   Fixed, adjustable height armrest, pair

K0037   High mount flip-up footrest, each

K0038   Leg strap, each

K0039   Leg strap, H style, each

K0040   Adjustable angle footplate, each

K0041   Large size footplate, each

K0042   Standard size footplate, each

K0043   Footrest, lower extension tube, each

K0044   Footrest, upper hanger bracket, each

K0045   Footrest, complete assembly

K0046   Elevating legrest, lower extension tube, each

K0047   Elevating legrest, upper hanger bracket, each

K0050   Ratchet assembly

K0051   Cam release assembly, footrest or legrest, each

K0052   Swingaway, detachable footrests, each

K0053   Elevating footrests, articulating (telescoping), each

K0056   Seat height less than 17 in or equal to or greater than 21 in for a high-strength, lightweight, or ultralightweight wheelchair

K0065   Spoke protectors, each

K0069   Rear wheel assembly, complete, with solid tire, spokes or molded, each

K0070   Rear wheel assembly, complete, with pneumatic tire, spokes or molded, each

K0071   Front caster assembly, complete, with pneumatic tire, each

K0072   Front caster assembly, complete, with semipneumatic tire, each

K0073   Caster pin lock, each

K0077   Front caster assembly, complete, with solid tire, each

K0098   Drive belt for power wheelchair
       MED: 100-4,23,60.3

K0105   IV hanger, each

K0108   Wheelchair component or accessory, not otherwise specified

K0195   Elevating legrests, pair (for use with capped rental wheelchair base)
       MED: 100-4,23,60.3

EQUIPMENT, REPLACEMENT, REPAIR, RENTAL

K0455   Infusion pump used for uninterrupted parenteral administration of medication, (e.g., epoprostenol or treprostinol)

K0462   Temporary replacement for patient-owned equipment being repaired, any type
       MED: 100-4,20,40.1

K0552   Supplies for external drug infusion pump, syringe type cartridge, sterile, each

K0601   Replacement battery for external infusion pump owned by patient, silver oxide, 1.5 volt, each
       AHA: 2Q,'03,7

K0602   Replacement battery for external infusion pump owned by patient, silver oxide, 3 volt, each
       AHA: 2Q,'03,7

K0603   Replacement battery for external infusion pump owned by patient, alkaline, 1.5 volt, each
       AHA: 2Q,'03,7

K0604   Replacement battery for external infusion pump owned by patient, lithium, 3.6 volt, each
       AHA: 2Q,'03,7

K0605   Replacement battery for external infusion pump owned by patient, lithium, 4.5 volt, each
       AHA: 2Q,'03,7

K0606   Automatic external defibrillator, with integrated electrocardiogram analysis, garment type
       AHA: 4Q,'03,4

K0607   Replacement battery for automated external defibrillator, garment type only, each
       AHA: 4Q,'03,4

K0608   Replacement garment for use with automated external defibrillator, each
       AHA: 4Q,'03,4

K0609   Replacement electrodes for use with automated external defibrillator, garment type only, each
       AHA: 4Q,'03,4

K0669   Wheelchair accessory, wheelchair seat or back cushion, does not meet specific code criteria or no written coding verification from DME PDAC

K0672   Addition to lower extremity orthotic, removable soft interface, all components, replacement only, each

K0730   Controlled dose inhalation drug delivery system

K0733   Power wheelchair accessory, 12 to 24 amp hour sealed lead acid battery, each (e.g., gel cell, absorbed glassmat)
       MED: 100-4,23,60.3

K0738   Portable gaseous oxygen system, rental; home compressor used to fill portable oxygen cylinders; includes portable containers, regulator, flowmeter, humidifier, cannula or mask, and tubing

K0739   Repair or nonroutine service for durable medical equipment other than oxygen equipment requiring the skill of a technician, labor component, per 15 minutes

K0740   Repair or nonroutine service for oxygen equipment requiring the skill of a technician, labor component, per 15 minutes

K0743   Suction pump, home model, portable, for use on wounds

K0744   Absorptive wound dressing for use with suction pump, home model, portable, pad size 16 sq in or less

K0745   Absorptive wound dressing for use with suction pump, home model, portable, pad size more than 16 sq in but less than or equal to 48 sq in

K0746   Absorptive wound dressing for use with suction pump, home model, portable, pad size greater than 48 sq in

POWER OPERATED VEHICLE AND ACCESSORIES

K0800   Power operated vehicle, group 1 standard, patient weight capacity up to and including 300 pounds
MED: 100-4,12,30.6.15.4; 100-4,23,60.3

K0801   Power operated vehicle, group 1 heavy-duty, patient weight capacity 301 to 450 pounds

K0802   Power operated vehicle, group 1 very heavy-duty, patient weight capacity 451 to 600 pounds

K0806   Power operated vehicle, group 2 standard, patient weight capacity up to and including 300 pounds

K0807   Power operated vehicle, group 2 heavy-duty, patient weight capacity 301 to 450 pounds

K0808   Power operated vehicle, group 2 very heavy-duty, patient weight capacity 451 to 600 pounds

K0812   Power operated vehicle, not otherwise classified

POWER WHEELCHAIRS

K0813   Power wheelchair, group 1 standard, portable, sling/solid seat and back, patient weight capacity up to and including 300 pounds
MED: 100-4,23,60.3

K0814   Power wheelchair, group 1 standard, portable, captain's chair, patient weight capacity up to and including 300 pounds

K0815   Power wheelchair, group 1 standard, sling/solid seat and back, patient weight capacity up to and including 300 pounds

K0816   Power wheelchair, group 1 standard, captain's chair, patient weight capacity up to and including 300 pounds

K0820   Power wheelchair, group 2 standard, portable, sling/solid seat/back, patient weight capacity up to and including 300 pounds

K0821   Power wheelchair, group 2 standard, portable, captain's chair, patient weight capacity up to and including 300 pounds

K0822   Power wheelchair, group 2 standard, sling/solid seat/back, patient weight capacity up to and including 300 pounds

K0823   Power wheelchair, group 2 standard, captain's chair, patient weight capacity up to and including 300 pounds

K0824   Power wheelchair, group 2 heavy-duty, sling/solid seat/back, patient weight capacity 301 to 450 pounds

K0825   Power wheelchair, group 2 heavy-duty, captain's chair, patient weight capacity 301 to 450 pounds

K0826   Power wheelchair, group 2 very heavy-duty, sling/solid seat/back, patient weight capacity 451 to 600 pounds

K0827   Power wheelchair, group 2 very heavy-duty, captain's chair, patient weight capacity 451 to 600 pounds

K0828   Power wheelchair, group 2 extra heavy-duty, sling/solid seat/back, patient weight capacity 601 pounds or more

K0829   Power wheelchair, group 2 extra heavy-duty, captain's chair, patient weight 601 pounds or more

K0830   Power wheelchair, group 2 standard, seat elevator, sling/solid seat/back, patient weight capacity up to and including 300 pounds

K0831   Power wheelchair, group 2 standard, seat elevator, captain's chair, patient weight capacity up to and including 300 pounds

K0835   Power wheelchair, group 2 standard, single power option, sling/solid seat/back, patient weight capacity up to and including 300 pounds
MED: 100-4,23,60.3

K0836   Power wheelchair, group 2 standard, single power option, captain's chair, patient weight capacity up to and including 300 pounds

K0837   Power wheelchair, group 2 heavy-duty, single power option, sling/solid seat/back, patient weight capacity 301 to 450 pounds

K0838   Power wheelchair, group 2 heavy-duty, single power option, captain's chair, patient weight capacity 301 to 450 pounds

K0839   Power wheelchair, group 2 very heavy-duty, single power option sling/solid seat/back, patient weight capacity 451 to 600 pounds

K0840   Power wheelchair, group 2 extra heavy-duty, single power option, sling/solid seat/back, patient weight capacity 601 pounds or more

K0841   Power wheelchair, group 2 standard, multiple power option, sling/solid seat/back, patient weight capacity up to and including 300 pounds

K0842   Power wheelchair, group 2 standard, multiple power option, captain's chair, patient weight capacity up to and including 300 pounds

K0843   Power wheelchair, group 2 heavy-duty, multiple power option, sling/solid seat/back, patient weight capacity 301 to 450 pounds

K0848   Power wheelchair, group 3 standard, sling/solid seat/back, patient weight capacity up to and including 300 pounds

K0849   Power wheelchair, group 3 standard, captain's chair, patient weight capacity up to and including 300 pounds

K0850   Power wheelchair, group 3 heavy-duty, sling/solid seat/back, patient weight capacity 301 to 450 pounds

K0851   Power wheelchair, group 3 heavy-duty, captain's chair, patient weight capacity 301 to 450 pounds

K0852   Power wheelchair, group 3 very heavy-duty, sling/solid seat/back, patient weight capacity 451 to 600 pounds

K0853   Power wheelchair, group 3 very heavy-duty, captain's chair, patient weight capacity 451 to 600 pounds

K0854   Power wheelchair, group 3 extra heavy-duty, sling/solid seat/back, patient weight capacity 601 pounds or more

K0855   Power wheelchair, group 3 extra heavy-duty, captain's chair, patient weight capacity 601 pounds or more

K0856   Power wheelchair, group 3 standard, single power option, sling/solid seat/back, patient weight capacity up to and including 300 pounds

K0857   Power wheelchair, group 3 standard, single power option, captain's chair, patient weight capacity up to and including 300 pounds

K0858   Power wheelchair, group 3 heavy-duty, single power option, sling/solid seat/back, patient weight 301 to 450 pounds

K0859   Power wheelchair, group 3 heavy-duty, single power option, captain's chair, patient weight capacity 301 to 450 pounds

K0860   Power wheelchair, group 3 very heavy-duty, single power option, sling/solid seat/back, patient weight capacity 451 to 600 pounds

K0861   Power wheelchair, group 3 standard, multiple power option, sling/solid seat/back, patient weight capacity up to and including 300 pounds

K0862   Power wheelchair, group 3 heavy-duty, multiple power option, sling/solid seat/back, patient weight capacity 301 to 450 pounds

K0863   Power wheelchair, group 3 very heavy-duty, multiple power option, sling/solid seat/back, patient weight capacity 451 to 600 pounds

K0864   Power wheelchair, group 3 extra heavy-duty, multiple power option, sling/solid seat/back, patient weight capacity 601 pounds or more

K0868   Power wheelchair, group 4 standard, sling/solid seat/back, patient weight capacity up to and including 300 pounds

K0869　Power wheelchair, group 4 standard, captain's chair, patient weight capacity up to and including 300 pounds

K0870　Power wheelchair, group 4 heavy-duty, sling/solid seat/back, patient weight capacity 301 to 450 pounds

K0871　Power wheelchair, group 4 very heavy-duty, sling/solid seat/back, patient weight capacity 451 to 600 pounds

K0877　Power wheelchair, group 4 standard, single power option, sling/solid seat/back, patient weight capacity up to and including 300 pounds

K0878　Power wheelchair, group 4 standard, single power option, captain's chair, patient weight capacity up to and including 300 pounds

K0879　Power wheelchair, group 4 heavy-duty, single power option, sling/solid seat/back, patient weight capacity 301 to 450 pounds

K0880　Power wheelchair, group 4 very heavy-duty, single power option, sling/solid seat/back, patient weight 451 to 600 pounds

K0884　Power wheelchair, group 4 standard, multiple power option, sling/solid seat/back, patient weight capacity up to and including 300 pounds

K0885　Power wheelchair, group 4 standard, multiple power option, captain's chair, patient weight capacity up to and including 300 pounds

K0886　Power wheelchair, group 4 heavy-duty, multiple power option, sling/solid seat/back, patient weight capacity 301 to 450 pounds

K0890　Power wheelchair, group 5 pediatric, single power option, sling/solid seat/back, patient weight capacity up to and including 125 pounds

K0891　Power wheelchair, group 5 pediatric, multiple power option, sling/solid seat/back, patient weight capacity up to and including 125 pounds

K0898　Power wheelchair, not otherwise classified

K0899　Power mobility device, not coded by DME PDAC or does not meet criteria

　　　MED: 100-4,12,30.6.15.4

K0900　Customized durable medical equipment, other than wheelchair

ORTHOTIC PROCEDURES AND DEVICES L0000-L4999

L codes include orthotic and prosthetic procedures and devices, as well as scoliosis equipment, orthopedic shoes, and prosthetic implants.

CERVICAL

L0112 Cranial cervical orthotic, congenital torticollis type, with or without soft interface material, adjustable range of motion joint, custom fabricated

L0113 Cranial cervical orthotic, torticollis type, with or without joint, with or without soft interface material, prefabricated, includes fitting and adjustment

L0120 Cervical, flexible, nonadjustable, prefabricated, off-the-shelf (foam collar)

L0130 Cervical, flexible, thermoplastic collar, molded to patient

L0140 Cervical, semi-rigid, adjustable (plastic collar)

L0150 Cervical, semi-rigid, adjustable molded chin cup (plastic collar with mandibular/occipital piece)

L0160 Cervical, semi-rigid, wire frame occipital/mandibular support, prefabricated, off-the-shelf

L0170 Cervical, collar, molded to patient model

L0172 Cervical, collar, semi-rigid thermoplastic foam, two-piece, prefabricated, off-the-shelf

L0174 Cervical, collar, semi-rigid, thermoplastic foam, two piece with thoracic extension, prefabricated, off-the-shelf

MULTIPLE POST COLLAR

L0180 Cervical, multiple post collar, occipital/mandibular supports, adjustable

L0190 Cervical, multiple post collar, occipital/mandibular supports, adjustable cervical bars (SOMI, Guilford, Taylor types)

L0200 Cervical, multiple post collar, occipital/mandibular supports, adjustable cervical bars, and thoracic extension

THORACIC

L0220 Thoracic, rib belt, custom fabricated

TLSO brace with adjustable straps and pads (L0450). The model at right and similar devices such as the Boston brace are molded polymer over foam and may be bivalve (front and back components)

Thoracic lumbar sacral orthosis (TLSO)

L0450 TLSO, flexible, provides trunk support, upper thoracic region, produces intracavitary pressure to reduce load on the intervertebral disks with rigid stays or panel(s), includes shoulder straps and closures, prefabricated, off-the-shelf

L0452 Thoracic-lumbar-sacral orthotic (TLSO), flexible, provides trunk support, upper thoracic region, produces intracavitary pressure to reduce load on the intervertebral disks with rigid stays or panel(s), includes shoulder straps and closures, custom fabricated

L0454 TLSO flexible, provides trunk support, extends from sacrococcygeal junction to above T-9 vertebra, restricts gross trunk motion in the sagittal plane, produces intracavitary pressure to reduce load on the intervertebral disks with rigid stays or panel(s), includes shoulder straps and closures, prefabricated item that has been trimmed, bent, molded, assembled, or otherwise customized to fit a specific patient by an individual with expertise

L0455 TLSO, flexible, provides trunk support, extends from sacrococcygeal junction to above T-9 vertebra, restricts gross trunk motion in the sagittal plane, produces intracavitary pressure to reduce load on the intervertebral disks with rigid stays or panel(s), includes shoulder straps and closures, prefabricated, off-the-shelf

L0456 TLSO, flexible, provides trunk support, thoracic region, rigid posterior panel and soft anterior apron, extends from the sacrococcygeal junction and terminates just inferior to the scapular spine, restricts gross trunk motion in the sagittal plane, produces intracavitary pressure to reduce load on the intervertebral disks, includes straps and closures, prefabricated item that has been trimmed, bent, molded, assembled, or otherwise customized to fit a specific patient by an individual with expertise

L0457 TLSO, flexible, provides trunk support, thoracic region, rigid posterior panel and soft anterior apron, extends from the sacrococcygeal junction and terminates just inferior to the scapular spine, restricts gross trunk motion in the sagittal plane, produces intracavitary pressure to reduce load on the intervertebral disks, includes straps and closures, prefabricated, off-the-shelf

L0458 Thoracic-lumbar-sacral orthotic (TLSO), triplanar control, modular segmented spinal system, 2 rigid plastic shells, posterior extends from the sacrococcygeal junction and terminates just inferior to the scapular spine, anterior extends from the symphysis pubis to the xiphoid, soft liner, restricts gross trunk motion in the sagittal, coronal, and transverse planes, lateral strength is provided by overlapping plastic and stabilizing closures, includes straps and closures, prefabricated, includes fitting and adjustment

L0460 TLSO, triplanar control, modular segmented spinal system, two rigid plastic shells, posterior extends from the sacrococcygeal junction and terminates just inferior to the scapular spine, anterior extends from the symphysis pubis to the sternal notch, soft liner, restricts gross trunk motion in the sagittal, coronal, and transverse planes, lateral strength is provided by overlapping plastic and stabilizing closures, includes straps and closures, prefabricated item that has been trimmed, bent, molded, assembled, or otherwise customized to fit a specific patient by an individual with expertise

L0462 Thoracic-lumbar-sacral orthotic (TLSO), triplanar control, modular segmented spinal system, 3 rigid plastic shells, posterior extends from the sacrococcygeal junction and terminates just inferior to the scapular spine, anterior extends from the symphysis pubis to the sternal notch, soft liner, restricts gross trunk motion in the sagittal, coronal, and transverse planes, lateral strength is provided by overlapping plastic and stabilizing closures, includes straps and closures, prefabricated, includes fitting and adjustment

L0464 Thoracic-lumbar-sacral orthotic (TLSO), triplanar control, modular segmented spinal system, 4 rigid plastic shells, posterior extends from sacrococcygeal junction and terminates just inferior to scapular spine, anterior extends from symphysis pubis to the sternal notch, soft liner, restricts gross trunk motion in sagittal, coronal, and transverse planes, lateral strength is provided by overlapping plastic and stabilizing closures, includes straps and closures, prefabricated, includes fitting and adjustment

L0466 TLSO, sagittal control, rigid posterior frame and flexible soft anterior apron with straps, closures and padding, restricts gross trunk motion in sagittal plane, produces intracavitary pressure to reduce load on intervertebral disks, prefabricated item that has been trimmed, bent, molded, or otherwise customized to fit a specific patient by an individual with expertise

L0467   TLSO, sagittal control, rigid posterior frame and flexible soft anterior apron with straps, closures and padding, restricts gross trunk motion in sagittal plane, produces intracavitary pressure to reduce load on intervertebral disks, prefabricated, off-the-shelf

L0468   TLSO, sagittal-coronal control, rigid posterior frame and flexible soft anterior apron with straps, closures and padding, extends from sacrococcygeal junction over scapulae, lateral strength provided by pelvic, thoracic, and lateral frame pieces, restricts gross trunk motion in sagittal, and coronal planes, produces intracavitary pressure to reduce load on intervertebral disks, prefabricated item that has been trimmed, bent, molded, assembled, or otherwise customized to fit a specific patient by an individual with expertise

L0469   TLSO, sagittal-coronal control, rigid posterior frame and flexible soft anterior apron with straps, closures and padding, extends from sacrococcygeal junction over scapulae, lateral strength provided by pelvic, thoracic, and lateral frame pieces, restricts gross trunk motion in sagittal and coronal planes, produces intracavitary pressure to reduce load on intervertebral disks, prefabricated, off-the-shelf

L0470   Thoracic-lumbar-sacral orthotic (TLSO), triplanar control, rigid posterior frame and flexible soft anterior apron with straps, closures and padding extends from sacrococcygeal junction to scapula, lateral strength provided by pelvic, thoracic, and lateral frame pieces, rotational strength provided by subclavicular extensions, restricts gross trunk motion in sagittal, coronal, and transverse planes, provides intracavitary pressure to reduce load on the intervertebral disks, includes fitting and shaping the frame, prefabricated, includes fitting and adjustment

L0472   Thoracic-lumbar-sacral orthotic (TLSO), triplanar control, hyperextension, rigid anterior and lateral frame extends from symphysis pubis to sternal notch with 2 anterior components (one pubic and one sternal), posterior and lateral pads with straps and closures, limits spinal flexion, restricts gross trunk motion in sagittal, coronal, and transverse planes, includes fitting and shaping the frame, prefabricated, includes fitting and adjustment

L0480   Thoracic-lumbar-sacral orthotic (TLSO), triplanar control, 1 piece rigid plastic shell without interface liner, with multiple straps and closures, posterior extends from sacrococcygeal junction and terminates just inferior to scapular spine, anterior extends from symphysis pubis to sternal notch, anterior or posterior opening, restricts gross trunk motion in sagittal, coronal, and transverse planes, includes a carved plaster or CAD-CAM model, custom fabricated

L0482   Thoracic-lumbar-sacral orthotic (TLSO), triplanar control, 1 piece rigid plastic shell with interface liner, multiple straps and closures, posterior extends from sacrococcygeal junction and terminates just inferior to scapular spine, anterior extends from symphysis pubis to sternal notch, anterior or posterior opening, restricts gross trunk motion in sagittal, coronal, and transverse planes, includes a carved plaster or CAD-CAM model, custom fabricated

L0484   Thoracic-lumbar-sacral orthotic (TLSO), triplanar control, 2 piece rigid plastic shell without interface liner, with multiple straps and closures, posterior extends from sacrococcygeal junction and terminates just inferior to scapular spine, anterior extends from symphysis pubis to sternal notch, lateral strength is enhanced by overlapping plastic, restricts gross trunk motion in the sagittal, coronal, and transverse planes, includes a carved plaster or CAD-CAM model, custom fabricated

L0486   Thoracic-lumbar-sacral orthotic (TLSO), triplanar control, 2 piece rigid plastic shell with interface liner, multiple straps and closures, posterior extends from sacrococcygeal junction and terminates just inferior to scapular spine, anterior extends from symphysis pubis to sternal notch, lateral strength is enhanced by overlapping plastic, restricts gross trunk motion in the sagittal, coronal, and transverse planes, includes a carved plaster or CAD-CAM model, custom fabricated

L0488   Thoracic-lumbar-sacral orthotic (TLSO), triplanar control, 1 piece rigid plastic shell with interface liner, multiple straps and closures, posterior extends from sacrococcygeal junction and terminates just inferior to scapular spine, anterior extends from symphysis pubis to sternal notch, anterior or posterior opening, restricts gross trunk motion in sagittal, coronal, and transverse planes, prefabricated, includes fitting and adjustment

L0490   Thoracic-lumbar-sacral orthotic (TLSO), sagittal-coronal control, 1 piece rigid plastic shell, with overlapping reinforced anterior, with multiple straps and closures, posterior extends from sacrococcygeal junction and terminates at or before the T-9 vertebra, anterior extends from symphysis pubis to xiphoid, anterior opening, restricts gross trunk motion in sagittal and coronal planes, prefabricated, includes fitting and adjustment

L0491   Thoracic-lumbar-sacral orthotic (TLSO), sagittal-coronal control, modular segmented spinal system, 2 rigid plastic shells, posterior extends from the sacrococcygeal junction and terminates just inferior to the scapular spine, anterior extends from the symphysis pubis to the xiphoid, soft liner, restricts gross trunk motion in the sagittal and coronal planes, lateral strength is provided by overlapping plastic and stabilizing closures, includes straps and closures, prefabricated, includes fitting and adjustment

L0492   Thoracic-lumbar-sacral orthotic (TLSO), sagittal-coronal control, modular segmented spinal system, 3 rigid plastic shells, posterior extends from the sacrococcygeal junction and terminates just inferior to the scapular spine, anterior extends from the symphysis pubis to the xiphoid, soft liner, restricts gross trunk motion in the sagittal and coronal planes, lateral strength is provided by overlapping plastic and stabilizing closures, includes straps and closures, prefabricated, includes fitting and adjustment

CERVICAL-THORACIC-LUMBAR-SACRAL ORTHOTIC

L0621   Sacroiliac orthosis, flexible, provides pelvic-sacral support, reduces motion about the sacroiliac joint, includes straps, closures, may include pendulous abdomen design, prefabricated, off-the-shelf

L0622   Sacroiliac orthotic, flexible, provides pelvic-sacral support, reduces motion about the sacroiliac joint, includes straps, closures, may include pendulous abdomen design, custom fabricated

L0623   Sacroiliac orthosis, provides pelvic-sacral support, with rigid or semi-rigid panels over the sacrum and abdomen, reduces motion about the sacroiliac joint, includes straps, closures, may include pendulous abdomen design, prefabricated, off-the-shelf

L0624   Sacroiliac orthotic, provides pelvic-sacral support, with rigid or semi-rigid panels placed over the sacrum and abdomen, reduces motion about the sacroiliac joint, includes straps, closures, may include pendulous abdomen design, custom fabricated

L0625   Lumbar orthosis, flexible, provides lumbar support, posterior extends from L-1 to below L-5 vertebra, produces intracavitary pressure to reduce load on the intervertebral discs, includes straps, closures, may include pendulous abdomen design, shoulder straps, stays, prefabricated, off-the-shelf

L0626   Lumbar orthosis, sagittal control, with rigid posterior panel(s), posterior extends from L-1 to below L-5 vertebra, produces intracavitary pressure to reduce load on the intervertebral discs, includes straps, closures, may include padding, stays, shoulder straps, pendulous abdomen design, prefabricated item that has been trimmed, bent, molded, assembled, or otherwise customized to fit a specific patient by an individual with expertise

L0627   Lumbar orthosis, sagittal control, with rigid anterior and posterior panels, posterior extends from L-1 to below L-5 vertebra, produces intracavitary pressure to reduce load on the intervertebral discs, includes straps, closures, may include padding, shoulder straps, pendulous abdomen design, prefabricated item that has been trimmed, bent, molded, assembled, or otherwise customized to fit a specific patient by an individual with expertise

L0628 Lumbar-sacral orthosis, flexible, provides lumbo-sacral support, posterior extends from sacrococcygeal junction to T-9 vertebra, produces intracavitary pressure to reduce load on the intervertebral discs, includes straps, closures, may include stays, shoulder straps, pendulous abdomen design, prefabricated, off-the-shelf

L0629 Lumbar-sacral orthotic, flexible, provides lumbo-sacral support, posterior extends from sacrococcygeal junction to T-9 vertebra, produces intracavitary pressure to reduce load on the intervertebral discs, includes straps, closures, may include stays, shoulder straps, pendulous abdomen design, custom fabricated

L0630 Lumbar-sacral orthosis, sagittal control, with rigid posterior panel(s), posterior extends from sacrococcygeal junction to T-9 vertebra, produces intracavitary pressure to reduce load on the intervertebral discs, includes straps, closures, may include padding, stays, shoulder straps, pendulous abdomen design, prefabricated item that has been trimmed, bent, molded, assembled, or otherwise customized to fit a specific patient by an individual with expertise

L0631 Lumbar-sacral orthosis, sagittal control, with rigid anterior and posterior panels, posterior extends from sacrococcygeal junction to T-9 vertebra, produces intracavitary pressure to reduce load on the intervertebral discs, includes straps, closures, may include padding, shoulder straps, pendulous abdomen design, prefabricated item that has been trimmed, bent, molded, assembled, or otherwise customized to fit a specific patient by an individual with expertise

L0632 Lumbar-sacral orthotic (LSO), sagittal control, with rigid anterior and posterior panels, posterior extends from sacrococcygeal junction to T-9 vertebra, produces intracavitary pressure to reduce load on the intervertebral discs, includes straps, closures, may include padding, shoulder straps, pendulous abdomen design, custom fabricated

L0633 Lumbar-sacral orthosis, sagittal-coronal control, with rigid posterior frame/panel(s), posterior extends from sacrococcygeal junction to T-9 vertebra, lateral strength provided by rigid lateral frame/panels, produces intracavitary pressure to reduce load on intervertebral discs, includes straps, closures, may include padding, stays, shoulder straps, pendulous abdomen design, prefabricated item that has been trimmed, bent, molded, assembled, or otherwise customized to fit a specific patient by an individual with expertise

L0634 Lumbar-sacral orthotic (LSO), sagittal-coronal control, with rigid posterior frame/panel(s), posterior extends from sacrococcygeal junction to T-9 vertebra, lateral strength provided by rigid lateral frame/panel(s), produces intracavitary pressure to reduce load on intervertebral discs, includes straps, closures, may include padding, stays, shoulder straps, pendulous abdomen design, custom fabricated

L0635 Lumbar-sacral orthotic (LSO), sagittal-coronal control, lumbar flexion, rigid posterior frame/panel(s), lateral articulating design to flex the lumbar spine, posterior extends from sacrococcygeal junction to T-9 vertebra, lateral strength provided by rigid lateral frame/panel(s), produces intracavitary pressure to reduce load on intervertebral discs, includes straps, closures, may include padding, anterior panel, pendulous abdomen design, prefabricated, includes fitting and adjustment

L0636 Lumbar-sacral orthotic (LSO), sagittal-coronal control, lumbar flexion, rigid posterior frame/panels, lateral articulating design to flex the lumbar spine, posterior extends from sacrococcygeal junction to T-9 vertebra, lateral strength provided by rigid lateral frame/panels, produces intracavitary pressure to reduce load on intervertebral discs, includes straps, closures, may include padding, anterior panel, pendulous abdomen design, custom fabricated

L0637 Lumbar-sacral orthosis, sagittal-coronal control, with rigid anterior and posterior frame/panels, posterior extends from sacrococcygeal junction to T-9 vertebra, lateral strength provided by rigid lateral frame/panels, produces intracavitary pressure to reduce load on intervertebral discs, includes straps, closures, may include padding, shoulder straps, pendulous abdomen design, prefabricated item that has been trimmed, bent, molded, assembled, or otherwise customized to fit a specific patient by an individual with expertise

L0638 Lumbar-sacral orthotic (LSO), sagittal-coronal control, with rigid anterior and posterior frame/panels, posterior extends from sacrococcygeal junction to T-9 vertebra, lateral strength provided by rigid lateral frame/panels, produces intracavitary pressure to reduce load on intervertebral discs, includes straps, closures, may include padding, shoulder straps, pendulous abdomen design, custom fabricated

L0639 Lumbar-sacral orthosis, sagittal-coronal control, rigid shell(s)/panel(s), posterior extends from sacrococcygeal junction to T-9 vertebra, anterior extends from symphysis pubis to xyphoid, produces intracavitary pressure to reduce load on the intervertebral discs, overall strength is provided by overlapping rigid material and stabilizing closures, includes straps, closures, may include soft interface, pendulous abdomen design, prefabricated item that has been trimmed, bent, molded, assembled, or otherwise customized to fit a specific patient by an individual with expertise

L0640 Lumbar-sacral orthotic (LSO), sagittal-coronal control, rigid shell(s)/panel(s), posterior extends from sacrococcygeal junction to T-9 vertebra, anterior extends from symphysis pubis to xyphoid, produces intracavitary pressure to reduce load on the intervertebral discs, overall strength is provided by overlapping rigid material and stabilizing closures, includes straps, closures, may include soft interface, pendulous abdomen design, custom fabricated

L0641 Lumbar orthosis, sagittal control, with rigid posterior panel(s), posterior extends from L-1 to below L-5 vertebra, produces intracavitary pressure to reduce load on the intervertebral discs, includes straps, closures, may include padding, stays, shoulder straps, pendulous abdomen design, prefabricated, off-the-shelf

L0642 Lumbar orthosis, sagittal control, with rigid anterior and posterior panels, posterior extends from L-1 to below L-5 vertebra, produces intracavitary pressure to reduce load on the intervertebral discs, includes straps, closures, may include padding, shoulder straps, pendulous abdomen design, prefabricated, off-the-shelf

L0643 Lumbar-sacral orthosis, sagittal control, with rigid posterior panel(s), posterior extends from sacrococcygeal junction to T-9 vertebra, produces intracavitary pressure to reduce load on the intervertebral discs, includes straps, closures, may include padding, stays, shoulder straps, pendulous abdomen design, prefabricated, off-the-shelf

L0648 Lumbar-sacral orthosis, sagittal control, with rigid anterior and posterior panels, posterior extends from sacrococcygeal junction to T-9 vertebra, produces intracavitary pressure to reduce load on the intervertebral discs, includes straps, closures, may include padding, shoulder straps, pendulous abdomen design, prefabricated, off-the-shelf

L0649 Lumbar-sacral orthosis, sagittal-coronal control, with rigid posterior frame/panel(s), posterior extends from sacrococcygeal junction to T-9 vertebra, lateral strength provided by rigid lateral frame/panels, produces intracavitary pressure to reduce load on intervertebral discs, includes straps, closures, may include padding, stays, shoulder straps, pendulous abdomen design, prefabricated, off-the-shelf

L0650 Lumbar-sacral orthosis, sagittal-coronal control, with rigid anterior and posterior frame/panel(s), posterior extends from sacrococcygeal junction to T-9 vertebra, lateral strength provided by rigid lateral frame/panel(s), produces intracavitary pressure to reduce load on intervertebral discs, includes straps, closures, may include padding, shoulder straps, pendulous abdomen design, prefabricated, off-the-shelf

L0651 Lumbar-sacral orthosis, sagittal-coronal control, rigid shell(s)/panel(s), posterior extends from sacrococcygeal junction to T-9 vertebra, anterior extends from symphysis pubis to xyphoid, produces intracavitary pressure to reduce load on the intervertebral discs, overall strength is provided by overlapping rigid material and stabilizing closures, includes straps, closures, may include soft interface, pendulous abdomen design, prefabricated, off-the-shelf

L0700 Cervical-thoracic-lumbar-sacral orthotic (CTLSO), anterior-posterior-lateral control, molded to patient model, (Minerva type)

L0710 Cervical-thoracic-lumbar-sacral orthotic (CTLSO), anterior-posterior-lateral-control, molded to patient model, with interface material, (Minerva type)

HALO PROCEDURE

L0810 Halo procedure, cervical halo incorporated into jacket vest

L0820 Halo procedure, cervical halo incorporated into plaster body jacket

L0830 Halo procedure, cervical halo incorporated into Milwaukee type orthotic

L0859 Addition to halo procedure, magnetic resonance image compatible systems, rings and pins, any material

L0861 Addition to halo procedure, replacement liner/interface material

ADDITIONS TO SPINAL ORTHOTIC

L0970 Thoracic-lumbar-sacral orthotic (TLSO), corset front

L0972 Lumbar-sacral orthotic (LSO), corset front

L0974 Thoracic-lumbar-sacral orthotic (TLSO), full corset

L0976 Lumbar-sacral orthotic (LSO), full corset

L0978 Axillary crutch extension

L0980 Peroneal straps, prefabricated, off-the-shelf, pair

L0982 Stocking supporter grips, prefabricated, off-the-shelf, set of four (4)

L0984 Protective body sock, prefabricated, off-the-shelf, each

L0999 Addition to spinal orthotic, not otherwise specified

Determine if an alternative HCPCS Level II or a CPT code better describes the service being reported. This code should be used only if a more specific code is unavailable.

ORTHOTIC DEVICES - SCOLIOSIS PROCEDURES

The orthotic care of scoliosis differs from other orthotic care in that the treatment is more dynamic in nature and uses continual modification of the orthosis to the patient's changing condition. This coding structure uses the proper names - or eponyms - of the procedures because they have historic and universal acceptance in the profession. It should be recognized that variations to the basic procedures described by the founders/developers are accepted in various medical and orthotic practices throughout the country. All procedures include model of patient when indicated.

Cervical component

A variety of configurations are available for the Milwaukee brace (L1000)

Thoracic component

Axilla sling (L1010)

Lumbar-sacral component

Milwaukee-style braces; cervical thoracic lumbar sacral orthosis (CTSLO)

L1000 Cervical-thoracic-lumbar-sacral orthotic (CTLSO) (Milwaukee), inclusive of furnishing initial orthotic, including model

L1001 Cervical-thoracic-lumbar-sacral orthotic (CTLSO), immobilizer, infant size, prefabricated, includes fitting and adjustment

L1005 Tension based scoliosis orthotic and accessory pads, includes fitting and adjustment

L1010 Addition to cervical-thoracic-lumbar-sacral orthotic (CTLSO) or scoliosis orthotic, axilla sling

L1020 Addition to cervical-thoracic-lumbar-sacral orthotic (CTLSO) or scoliosis orthotic, kyphosis pad

L1025 Addition to cervical-thoracic-lumbar-sacral orthotic (CTLSO) or scoliosis orthotic, kyphosis pad, floating

L1030 Addition to cervical-thoracic-lumbar-sacral orthotic (CTLSO) or scoliosis orthotic, lumbar bolster pad

L1040 Addition to cervical-thoracic-lumbar-sacral orthotic (CTLSO) or scoliosis orthotic, lumbar or lumbar rib pad

L1050 Addition to cervical-thoracic-lumbar-sacral orthotic (CTLSO) or scoliosis orthotic, sternal pad

L1060 Addition to cervical-thoracic-lumbar-sacral orthotic (CTLSO) or scoliosis orthotic, thoracic pad

L1070 Addition to cervical-thoracic-lumbar-sacral orthotic (CTLSO) or scoliosis orthotic, trapezius sling

L1080 Addition to cervical-thoracic-lumbar-sacral orthotic (CTLSO) or scoliosis orthotic, outrigger

L1085 Addition to cervical-thoracic-lumbar-sacral orthotic (CTLSO) or scoliosis orthotic, outrigger, bilateral with vertical extensions

L1090 Addition to cervical-thoracic-lumbar-sacral orthotic (CTLSO) or scoliosis orthotic, lumbar sling

L1100 Addition to cervical-thoracic-lumbar-sacral orthotic (CTLSO) or scoliosis orthotic, ring flange, plastic or leather

L1110 Addition to cervical-thoracic-lumbar-sacral orthotic (CTLSO) or scoliosis orthotic, ring flange, plastic or leather, molded to patient model

L1120 Addition to cervical-thoracic-lumbar-sacral orthotic (CTLSO), scoliosis orthotic, cover for upright, each

THORACIC-LUMBAR-SACRAL ORTHOTIC (TLSO) (LOW PROFILE)

L1200 Thoracic-lumbar-sacral orthotic (TLSO), inclusive of furnishing initial orthotic only

L1210 Addition to thoracic-lumbar-sacral orthotic (TLSO), (low profile), lateral thoracic extension

L1220 Addition to thoracic-lumbar-sacral orthotic (TLSO), (low profile), anterior thoracic extension

L1230 Addition to thoracic-lumbar-sacral orthotic (TLSO), (low profile), Milwaukee type superstructure

L1240 Addition to thoracic-lumbar-sacral orthotic (TLSO), (low profile), lumbar derotation pad

L1250 Addition to thoracic-lumbar-sacral orthotic (TLSO), (low profile), anterior ASIS pad

L1260 Addition to thoracic-lumbar-sacral orthotic (TLSO), (low profile), anterior thoracic derotation pad

L1270 Addition to thoracic-lumbar-sacral orthotic (TLSO), (low profile), abdominal pad

L1280 Addition to thoracic-lumbar-sacral orthotic (TLSO), (low profile), rib gusset (elastic), each

L1290 Addition to thoracic-lumbar-sacral orthotic (TLSO), (low profile), lateral trochanteric pad

OTHER SCOLIOSIS PROCEDURES

L1300 Other scoliosis procedure, body jacket molded to patient model

L1310 — L1907

Orthotic Devices and Procedures

L1310   Other scoliosis procedure, postoperative body jacket

L1499   Spinal orthotic, not otherwise specified

Determine if an alternative HCPCS Level II or a CPT code better describes the service being reported. This code should be used only if a more specific code is unavailable.

HIP ORTHOTIC (HO) - FLEXIBLE

L1600   Hip orthosis, abduction control of hip joints, flexible, Frejka type with cover, prefabricated item that has been trimmed, bent, molded, assembled, or otherwise customized to fit a specific patient by an inidividual with expertise

L1610   Hip orthosis, abduction control of hip joints, flexible, (Frejka cover only), prefabricated item that has been trimmed, bent, molded, assembled, or otherwise customized to fit a specific patient by an individual with expertise

L1620   Hip orthosis, abduction control of hip joints, flexible, (Pavlik harness), prefabricated item that has been trimmed, bent, molded, assembled, or otherwise customized to fit a specific patient by an individual with expertise

L1630   Hip orthotic (HO), abduction control of hip joints, semi-flexible (Von Rosen type), custom fabricated

L1640   Hip orthotic (HO), abduction control of hip joints, static, pelvic band or spreader bar, thigh cuffs, custom fabricated

L1650   Hip orthotic (HO), abduction control of hip joints, static, adjustable, (Ilfled type), prefabricated, includes fitting and adjustment

L1652   Hip orthotic, bilateral thigh cuffs with adjustable abductor spreader bar, adult size, prefabricated, includes fitting and adjustment, any type

L1660   Hip orthotic (HO), abduction control of hip joints, static, plastic, prefabricated, includes fitting and adjustment

L1680   Hip orthotic (HO), abduction control of hip joints, dynamic, pelvic control, adjustable hip motion control, thigh cuffs (Rancho hip action type), custom fabricated

L1685   Hip orthosis (HO), abduction control of hip joint, postoperative hip abduction type, custom fabricated

L1686   Hip orthotic (HO), abduction control of hip joint, postoperative hip abduction type, prefabricated, includes fitting and adjustment

L1690   Combination, bilateral, lumbo-sacral, hip, femur orthotic providing adduction and internal rotation control, prefabricated, includes fitting and adjustment

LEGG PERTHES

L1700   Legg Perthes orthotic, (Toronto type), custom fabricated

L1710   Legg Perthes orthotic, (Newington type), custom fabricated

L1720   Legg Perthes orthotic, trilateral, (Tachdijan type), custom fabricated

L1730   Legg Perthes orthotic, (Scottish Rite type), custom fabricated

L1755   Legg Perthes orthotic, (Patten bottom type), custom fabricated

KNEE ORTHOTIC

L1810   Knee orthosis, elastic with joints, prefabricated item that has been trimmed, bent, molded, assembled, or otherwise customized to fit a specific patient by an individual with expertise

L1812   Knee orthosis, elastic with joints, prefabricated, off-the-shelf

L1820   Knee orthotic, elastic with condylar pads and joints, with or without patellar control, prefabricated, includes fitting and adjustment

L1830   Knee orthosis, immobilizer, canvas longitudinal, prefabricated, off-the-shelf

L1831   Knee orthotic, locking knee joint(s), positional orthotic, prefabricated, includes fitting and adjustment

L1832   Knee orthosis, adjustable knee joints (unicentric or polycentric), positional orthosis, rigid support, prefabricated item that has been trimmed, bent, molded, assembled, or otherwise customized to fit a specific patient by an individual with expertise

L1833   Knee orthosis, adjustable knee joints (unicentric or polycentric), positional orthosis, rigid support, prefabricated, off-the shelf

L1834   Knee orthotic (KO), without knee joint, rigid, custom fabricated

L1836   Knee orthosis, rigid, without joint(s), includes soft interface material, prefabricated, off-the-shelf

L1840   Knee orthotic (KO), derotation, medial-lateral, anterior cruciate ligament, custom fabricated

L1843   Knee orthosis, single upright, thigh and calf, with adjustable flexion and extension joint (unicentric or polycentric), medial-lateral and rotation control, with or without varus/valgus adjustment, prefabricated item that has been trimmed, bent, molded, assembled, or otherwise customized to fit a specific patient by an individual with expertise

L1844   Knee orthotic (KO), single upright, thigh and calf, with adjustable flexion and extension joint (unicentric or polycentric), medial-lateral and rotation control, with or without varus/valgus adjustment, custom fabricated

L1845   Knee orthosis, double upright, thigh and calf, with adjustable flexion and extension joint (unicentric or polycentric), medial-lateral and rotation control, with or without varus/valgus adjustment, prefabricated item that has been trimmed, bent, molded, assembled, or otherwise customized to fit a specific patient by an individual with expertise

L1846   Knee orthotic, double upright, thigh and calf, with adjustable flexion and extension joint (unicentric or polycentric), medial-lateral and rotation control, with or without varus/valgus adjustment, custom fabricated

L1847   Knee orthosis, double upright with adjustable joint, with inflatable air support chamber(s), prefabricated item that has been trimmed, bent, molded, assembled, or otherwise customized to fit a specific patient by an individual with expertise

L1848   Knee orthosis, double upright with adjustable joint, with inflatable air support chamber(s), prefabricated, off-the-shelf

L1850   Knee orthosis, swedish type, prefabricated, off-the-shelf

L1860   Knee orthotic (KO), modification of supracondylar prosthetic socket, custom fabricated (SK)

ANKLE-FOOT ORTHOTIC (AFO)

L1900   Ankle-foot orthotic (AFO), spring wire, dorsiflexion assist calf band, custom fabricated

L1902   Ankle foot orthosis, ankle gauntlet, prefabricated, off-the-shelf

L1904   Ankle orthosis, ankle gauntlet, custom-fabricated

L1906   Ankle foot orthosis, multiligamentus ankle support, prefabricated, off-the-shelf

L1907   Ankle orthosis, supramalleolar with straps, with or without interface/pads, custom fabricated

Ankle foot orthotic (AFO), posterior bar (L1910)

Flexible carbon component

Foot component may fit inside shoe

L1910 Ankle-foot orthotic (AFO), posterior, single bar, clasp attachment to shoe counter, prefabricated, includes fitting and adjustment

L1920 Ankle-foot orthotic (AFO), single upright with static or adjustable stop (Phelps or Perlstein type), custom fabricated

L1930 Ankle-foot orthotic (AFO), plastic or other material, prefabricated, includes fitting and adjustment

L1932 Ankle-foot orthotic (AFO), rigid anterior tibial section, total carbon fiber or equal material, prefabricated, includes fitting and adjustment

L1940 Ankle-foot orthotic (AFO), plastic or other material, custom fabricated

Rigid tibial anterior floor reaction; ankle-foot orthosis (AFO) (L1945)

Spiral; ankle-foot orthosis (AFO) (L1950)

L1945 Ankle-foot orthotic (AFO), plastic, rigid anterior tibial section (floor reaction), custom fabricated

L1950 Ankle-foot orthotic (AFO), spiral, (Institute of Rehabilitative Medicine type), plastic, custom fabricated

L1951 Ankle-foot orthotic (AFO), spiral, (Institute of rehabilitative Medicine type), plastic or other material, prefabricated, includes fitting and adjustment

L1960 Ankle-foot orthotic (AFO), posterior solid ankle, plastic, custom fabricated

L1970 Ankle-foot orthotic (AFO), plastic with ankle joint, custom fabricated

L1971 Ankle-foot orthotic (AFO), plastic or other material with ankle joint, prefabricated, includes fitting and adjustment

L1980 Ankle-foot orthotic (AFO), single upright free plantar dorsiflexion, solid stirrup, calf band/cuff (single bar 'BK' orthotic), custom fabricated

L1990 Ankle-foot orthotic (AFO), double upright free plantar dorsiflexion, solid stirrup, calf band/cuff (double bar 'BK' orthotic), custom fabricated

KNEE-ANKLE-FOOT ORTHOTIC (KAFO) - OR ANY COMBINATION

L2000 Knee-ankle-foot orthotic (KAFO), single upright, free knee, free ankle, solid stirrup, thigh and calf bands/cuffs (single bar 'AK' orthotic), custom fabricated

L2005 Knee-ankle-foot orthotic (KAFO), any material, single or double upright, stance control, automatic lock and swing phase release, any type activation, includes ankle joint, any type, custom fabricated

L2010 Knee-ankle-foot orthotic (KAFO), single upright, free ankle, solid stirrup, thigh and calf bands/cuffs (single bar 'AK' orthotic), without knee joint, custom fabricated

L2020 Knee-ankle-foot orthotic (KAFO), double upright, free ankle, solid stirrup, thigh and calf bands/cuffs (double bar 'AK' orthotic), custom fabricated

L2030 Knee-ankle-foot orthotic (KAFO), double upright, free ankle, solid stirrup, thigh and calf bands/cuffs, (double bar 'AK' orthotic), without knee joint, custom fabricated

L2034 Knee-ankle-foot orthotic (KAFO), full plastic, single upright, with or without free motion knee, medial-lateral rotation control, with or without free motion ankle, custom fabricated

L2035 Knee-ankle-foot orthotic (KAFO), full plastic, static (pediatric size), without free motion ankle, prefabricated, includes fitting and adjustment

L2036 Knee-ankle-foot orthotic (KAFO), full plastic, double upright, with or without free motion knee, with or without free motion ankle, custom fabricated

L2037 Knee-ankle-foot orthotic (KAFO), full plastic, single upright, with or without free motion knee, with or without free motion ankle, custom fabricated

L2038 Knee-ankle-foot orthotic (KAFO), full plastic, with or without free motion knee, multi-axis ankle, custom fabricated

TORSION CONTROL: HIP-KNEE-ANKLE-FOOT ORTHOTIC (HKAFO)

L2040 Hip-knee-ankle-foot orthotic (HKAFO), torsion control, bilateral rotation straps, pelvic band/belt, custom fabricated

L2050 Hip-knee-ankle-foot orthotic (HKAFO), torsion control, bilateral torsion cables, hip joint, pelvic band/belt, custom fabricated

L2060 Hip-knee-ankle-foot orthotic (HKAFO), torsion control, bilateral torsion cables, ball bearing hip joint, pelvic band/ belt, custom fabricated

L2070 Hip-knee-ankle-foot orthotic (HKAFO), torsion control, unilateral rotation straps, pelvic band/belt, custom fabricated

L2080 Hip-knee-ankle-foot orthotic (HKAFO), torsion control, unilateral torsion cable, hip joint, pelvic band/belt, custom fabricated

L2090 Hip-knee-ankle-foot orthotic (HKAFO), torsion control, unilateral torsion cable, ball bearing hip joint, pelvic band/ belt, custom fabricated

L2106 Ankle-foot orthotic (AFO), fracture orthotic, tibial fracture cast orthotic, thermoplastic type casting material, custom fabricated

L2108 Ankle-foot orthotic (AFO), fracture orthotic, tibial fracture cast orthotic, custom fabricated

L2112 Ankle-foot orthotic (AFO), fracture orthotic, tibial fracture orthotic, soft, prefabricated, includes fitting and adjustment

L2114 Ankle-foot orthotic (AFO), fracture orthotic, tibial fracture orthotic, semi-rigid, prefabricated, includes fitting and adjustment

L2116 Ankle-foot orthotic (AFO), fracture orthotic, tibial fracture orthotic, rigid, prefabricated, includes fitting and adjustment

L2126 Knee-ankle-foot orthotic (KAFO), fracture orthotic, femoral fracture cast orthotic, thermoplastic type casting material, custom fabricated

L2128 Knee-ankle-foot orthotic (KAFO), fracture orthotic, femoral fracture cast orthotic, custom fabricated

L2132 Knee-ankle-foot orthotic (KAFO), fracture orthotic, femoral fracture cast orthotic, soft, prefabricated, includes fitting and adjustment

L2134 Knee-ankle-foot orthotic (KAFO), fracture orthotic, femoral fracture cast orthotic, semi-rigid, prefabricated, includes fitting and adjustment

L2136 Knee-ankle-foot orthotic (KAFO), fracture orthotic, femoral fracture cast orthotic, rigid, prefabricated, includes fitting and adjustment

ADDITIONS TO FRACTURE ORTHOTIC

L2180 Addition to lower extremity fracture orthotic, plastic shoe insert with ankle joints

L2182 Addition to lower extremity fracture orthotic, drop lock knee joint

L2184 Addition to lower extremity fracture orthotic, limited motion knee joint

L2186   Addition to lower extremity fracture orthotic, adjustable motion knee joint, Lerman type

L2188   Addition to lower extremity fracture orthotic, quadrilateral brim

L2190   Addition to lower extremity fracture orthotic, waist belt

L2192   Addition to lower extremity fracture orthotic, hip joint, pelvic band, thigh flange, and pelvic belt

ADDITIONS TO LOWER EXTREMITY ORTHOTIC: SHOE-ANKLE-SHIN-KNEE

L2200   Addition to lower extremity, limited ankle motion, each joint

L2210   Addition to lower extremity, dorsiflexion assist (plantar flexion resist), each joint

L2220   Addition to lower extremity, dorsiflexion and plantar flexion assist/resist, each joint

L2230   Addition to lower extremity, split flat caliper stirrups and plate attachment

L2232   Addition to lower extremity orthotic, rocker bottom for total contact ankle-foot orthotic (AFO), for custom fabricated orthotic only

L2240   Addition to lower extremity, round caliper and plate attachment

L2250   Addition to lower extremity, foot plate, molded to patient model, stirrup attachment

L2260   Addition to lower extremity, reinforced solid stirrup (Scott-Craig type)

L2265   Addition to lower extremity, long tongue stirrup

L2270   Addition to lower extremity, varus/valgus correction (T) strap, padded/lined or malleolus pad

L2275   Addition to lower extremity, varus/valgus correction, plastic modification, padded/lined

L2280   Addition to lower extremity, molded inner boot

L2300   Addition to lower extremity, abduction bar (bilateral hip involvement), jointed, adjustable

L2310   Addition to lower extremity, abduction bar, straight

L2320   Addition to lower extremity, nonmolded lacer, for custom fabricated orthotic only

L2330   Addition to lower extremity, lacer molded to patient model, for custom fabricated orthotic only

L2335   Addition to lower extremity, anterior swing band

L2340   Addition to lower extremity, pretibial shell, molded to patient model

L2350   Addition to lower extremity, prosthetic type, (BK) socket, molded to patient model, (used for PTB, AFO orthoses)

L2360   Addition to lower extremity, extended steel shank

L2370   Addition to lower extremity, Patten bottom

L2375   Addition to lower extremity, torsion control, ankle joint and half solid stirrup

L2380   Addition to lower extremity, torsion control, straight knee joint, each joint

L2385   Addition to lower extremity, straight knee joint, heavy-duty, each joint

L2387   Addition to lower extremity, polycentric knee joint, for custom fabricated knee-ankle-foot orthotic (KAFO), each joint

L2390   Addition to lower extremity, offset knee joint, each joint

L2395   Addition to lower extremity, offset knee joint, heavy-duty, each joint

L2397   Addition to lower extremity orthotic, suspension sleeve

ADDITIONS TO STRAIGHT KNEE OR OFFSET KNEE JOINTS

L2405   Addition to knee joint, drop lock, each

L2415   Addition to knee lock with integrated release mechanism (bail, cable, or equal), any material, each joint

L2425   Addition to knee joint, disc or dial lock for adjustable knee flexion, each joint

L2430   Addition to knee joint, ratchet lock for active and progressive knee extension, each joint

L2492   Addition to knee joint, lift loop for drop lock ring

ADDITIONS: THIGH/WEIGHT BEARING - GLUTEAL/ISCHIAL WEIGHT BEARING

L2500   Addition to lower extremity, thigh/weight bearing, gluteal/ischial weight bearing, ring

L2510   Addition to lower extremity, thigh/weight bearing, quadri-lateral brim, molded to patient model

L2520   Addition to lower extremity, thigh/weight bearing, quadri-lateral brim, custom fitted

L2525   Addition to lower extremity, thigh/weight bearing, ischial containment/narrow M-L brim molded to patient model

L2526   Addition to lower extremity, thigh/weight bearing, ischial containment/narrow M-L brim, custom fitted

L2530   Addition to lower extremity, thigh/weight bearing, lacer, nonmolded

L2540   Addition to lower extremity, thigh/weight bearing, lacer, molded to patient model

L2550   Addition to lower extremity, thigh/weight bearing, high roll cuff

ADDITIONS: PELVIC AND THORACIC CONTROL

L2570   Addition to lower extremity, pelvic control, hip joint, Clevis type 2 position joint, each

L2580   Addition to lower extremity, pelvic control, pelvic sling

L2600   Addition to lower extremity, pelvic control, hip joint, Clevis type, or thrust bearing, free, each

L2610   Addition to lower extremity, pelvic control, hip joint, Clevis or thrust bearing, lock, each

L2620   Addition to lower extremity, pelvic control, hip joint, heavy-duty, each

L2622   Addition to lower extremity, pelvic control, hip joint, adjustable flexion, each

L2624   Addition to lower extremity, pelvic control, hip joint, adjustable flexion, extension, abduction control, each

L2627   Addition to lower extremity, pelvic control, plastic, molded to patient model, reciprocating hip joint and cables

L2628   Addition to lower extremity, pelvic control, metal frame, reciprocating hip joint and cables

L2630   Addition to lower extremity, pelvic control, band and belt, unilateral

L2640   Addition to lower extremity, pelvic control, band and belt, bilateral

L2650   Addition to lower extremity, pelvic and thoracic control, gluteal pad, each

L2660   Addition to lower extremity, thoracic control, thoracic band

L2670   Addition to lower extremity, thoracic control, paraspinal uprights

L2680   Addition to lower extremity, thoracic control, lateral support uprights

ADDITIONS: GENERAL

L2750   Addition to lower extremity orthotic, plating chrome or nickel, per bar

L2755 Addition to lower extremity orthotic, high strength, lightweight material, all hybrid lamination/prepreg composite, per segment, for custom fabricated orthotic only

L2760 Addition to lower extremity orthotic, extension, per extension, per bar (for lineal adjustment for growth)

L2768 Orthotic side bar disconnect device, per bar

L2780 Addition to lower extremity orthotic, noncorrosive finish, per bar

L2785 Addition to lower extremity orthotic, drop lock retainer, each

L2795 Addition to lower extremity orthotic, knee control, full kneecap

L2800 Addition to lower extremity orthotic, knee control, knee cap, medial or lateral pull, for use with custom fabricated orthotic only

L2810 Addition to lower extremity orthotic, knee control, condylar pad

L2820 Addition to lower extremity orthotic, soft interface for molded plastic, below knee section

L2830 Addition to lower extremity orthotic, soft interface for molded plastic, above knee section

L2840 Addition to lower extremity orthotic, tibial length sock, fracture or equal, each

L2850 Addition to lower extremity orthotic, femoral length sock, fracture or equal, each

L2861 Addition to lower extremity joint, knee or ankle, concentric adjustable torsion style mechanism for custom fabricated orthotics only, each

L2999 Lower extremity orthotic, not otherwise specified
Determine if an alternative HCPCS Level II or a CPT code better describes the service being reported. This code should be used only if a more specific code is unavailable.

ORTHOPEDIC FOOTWEAR

INSERTS

L3000 Foot insert, removable, molded to patient model, UCB type, Berkeley shell, each
MED: 100-2,15,290

L3001 Foot, insert, removable, molded to patient model, Spenco, each
MED: 100-2,15,290

L3002 Foot insert, removable, molded to patient model, Plastazote or equal, each
MED: 100-2,15,290

L3003 Foot insert, removable, molded to patient model, silicone gel, each
MED: 100-2,15,290

L3010 Foot insert, removable, molded to patient model, longitudinal arch support, each
MED: 100-2,15,290

L3020 Foot insert, removable, molded to patient model, longitudinal/metatarsal support, each
MED: 100-2,15,290

L3030 Foot insert, removable, formed to patient foot, each
MED: 100-2,15,290

L3031 Foot, insert/plate, removable, addition to lower extremity orthotic, high strength, lightweight material, all hybrid lamination/prepreg composite, each

ARCH SUPPORT, REMOVABLE, PREMOLDED

L3040 Foot, arch support, removable, premolded, longitudinal, each
MED: 100-2,15,290

L3050 Foot, arch support, removable, premolded, metatarsal, each
MED: 100-2,15,290

L3060 Foot, arch support, removable, premolded, longitudinal/metatarsal, each
MED: 100-2,15,290

ARCH SUPPORT, NONREMOVABLE, ATTACHED TO SHOE

L3070 Foot, arch support, nonremovable, attached to shoe, longitudinal, each
MED: 100-2,15,290

L3080 Foot, arch support, nonremovable, attached to shoe, metatarsal, each
MED: 100-2,15,290

L3090 Foot, arch support, nonremovable, attached to shoe, longitudinal/metatarsal, each
MED: 100-2,15,290

L3100 Hallus-valgus night dynamic splint, prefabricated, off-the-shelf
MED: 100-2,15,290

ABDUCTION AND ROTATION BARS

A Denis-Browne style splint is a bar that can be applied by strapping or mounted on a shoe. This type of splint generally corrects congenital conditions such as genu varus

Denis-Browne splint

The angle may be adjusted on a plate on the sole of the shoe

L3140 Foot, abduction rotation bar, including shoes
MED: 100-2,15,290

L3150 Foot, abduction rotation bar, without shoes
MED: 100-2,15,290

L3160 Foot, adjustable shoe-styled positioning device

L3170 Foot, plastic, silicone or equal, heel stabilizer, prafabricated, off-the-shelf, each
MED: 100-2,15,290

ORTHOPEDIC SHOES AND BOOTS

L3201 Orthopedic shoe, Oxford with supinator or pronator, infant
MED: 100-2,15,290

L3202 Orthopedic shoe, Oxford with supinator or pronator, child
MED: 100-2,15,290

L3203 Orthopedic shoe, Oxford with supinator or pronator, junior
MED: 100-2,15,290

L3204 Orthopedic shoe, hightop with supinator or pronator, infant
MED: 100-2,15,290

L3206 Orthopedic shoe, hightop with supinator or pronator, child
MED: 100-2,15,290

L3207 Orthopedic shoe, hightop with supinator or pronator, junior
MED: 100-2,15,290

L3208 Surgical boot, each, infant

L3209 Surgical boot, each, child

L3211 Surgical boot, each, junior

L3212 Benesch boot, pair, infant

L3213 Benesch boot, pair, child

L3214 Benesch boot, pair, junior

L3215 Orthopedic footwear, ladies shoe, oxford, each

L3216 Orthopedic footwear, ladies shoe, depth inlay, each

Orthotic Devices and Procedures

L3217 — L3610

L3217   Orthopedic footwear, ladies shoe, hightop, depth inlay, each

L3219   Orthopedic footwear, mens shoe, oxford, each

L3221   Orthopedic footwear, mens shoe, depth inlay, each

L3222   Orthopedic footwear, mens shoe, hightop, depth inlay, each

L3224   Orthopedic footwear, woman's shoe, oxford, used as an integral part of a brace (orthotic)
MED: 100-2,15,290

L3225   Orthopedic footwear, man's shoe, oxford, used as an integral part of a brace (orthotic)
MED: 100-2,15,290

L3230   Orthopedic footwear, custom shoe, depth inlay, each
MED: 100-2,15,290

L3250   Orthopedic footwear, custom molded shoe, removable inner mold, prosthetic shoe, each
MED: 100-2,15,290

L3251   Foot, shoe molded to patient model, silicone shoe, each
MED: 100-2,15,290

L3252   Foot, shoe molded to patient model, Plastazote (or similar), custom fabricated, each
MED: 100-2,15,290

L3253   Foot, molded shoe, Plastazote (or similar), custom fitted, each
MED: 100-2,15,290

L3254   Nonstandard size or width
MED: 100-2,15,290

L3255   Nonstandard size or length
MED: 100-2,15,290

L3257   Orthopedic footwear, additional charge for split size
MED: 100-2,15,290

L3260   Surgical boot/shoe, each

L3265   Plastazote sandal, each

SHOE MODIFICATION - LIFTS

L3300   Lift, elevation, heel, tapered to metatarsals, per in
MED: 100-2,15,290

L3310   Lift, elevation, heel and sole, neoprene, per in
MED: 100-2,15,290

L3320   Lift, elevation, heel and sole, cork, per in
MED: 100-2,15,290

L3330   Lift, elevation, metal extension (skate)
MED: 100-2,15,290

L3332   Lift, elevation, inside shoe, tapered, up to one-half in
MED: 100-2,15,290

L3334   Lift, elevation, heel, per in
MED: 100-2,15,290

SHOE MODIFICATION - WEDGES

L3340   Heel wedge, SACH
MED: 100-2,15,290

L3350   Heel wedge
MED: 100-2,15,290

L3360   Sole wedge, outside sole
MED: 100-2,15,290

L3370   Sole wedge, between sole
MED: 100-2,15,290

L3380   Clubfoot wedge
MED: 100-2,15,290

L3390   Outflare wedge
MED: 100-2,15,290

L3400   Metatarsal bar wedge, rocker
MED: 100-2,290

L3410   Metatarsal bar wedge, between sole
MED: 100-2,15,290

L3420   Full sole and heel wedge, between sole
MED: 100-2,15,290

SHOE MODIFICATIONS - HEELS

L3430   Heel, counter, plastic reinforced
MED: 100-2,15,290

L3440   Heel, counter, leather reinforced
MED: 100-2,15,290

L3450   Heel, SACH cushion type
MED: 100-2,15,290

L3455   Heel, new leather, standard
MED: 100-2,15,290

L3460   Heel, new rubber, standard
MED: 100-2,15,290

L3465   Heel, Thomas with wedge
MED: 100-2,15,290

L3470   Heel, Thomas extended to ball
MED: 100-2,15,290

L3480   Heel, pad and depression for spur
MED: 100-2,15,290

L3485   Heel, pad, removable for spur
MED: 100-2,15,290

MISCELLANEOUS SHOE ADDITIONS

L3500   Orthopedic shoe addition, insole, leather
MED: 100-2,15,290

L3510   Orthopedic shoe addition, insole, rubber
MED: 100-2,15,290

L3520   Orthopedic shoe addition, insole, felt covered with leather
MED: 100-2,15,290

L3530   Orthopedic shoe addition, sole, half
MED: 100-2,15,290

L3540   Orthopedic shoe addition, sole, full
MED: 100-2,15,290

L3550   Orthopedic shoe addition, toe tap, standard
MED: 100-2,15,290

L3560   Orthopedic shoe addition, toe tap, horseshoe
MED: 100-2,15,290

L3570   Orthopedic shoe addition, special extension to instep (leather with eyelets)
MED: 100-2,15,290

L3580   Orthopedic shoe addition, convert instep to Velcro closure
MED: 100-2,15,290

L3590   Orthopedic shoe addition, convert firm shoe counter to soft counter
MED: 100-2,15,290

L3595   Orthopedic shoe addition, March bar
MED: 100-2,15,290

TRANSFER OR REPLACEMENT

L3600   Transfer of an orthotic from one shoe to another, caliper plate, existing
MED: 100-2,15,290

L3610   Transfer of an orthotic from one shoe to another, caliper plate, new
MED: 100-2,15,290

L3620 Transfer of an orthotic from one shoe to another, solid stirrup, existing

MED: 100-2,15,290

L3630 Transfer of an orthotic from one shoe to another, solid stirrup, new

MED: 100-2,15,290

L3640 Transfer of an orthotic from one shoe to another, Dennis Browne splint (Riveton), both shoes

MED: 100-2,15,290

L3649 Orthopedic shoe, modification, addition or transfer, not otherwise specified

Determine if an alternative HCPCS Level II or a CPT code better describes the service being reported. This code should be used only if a more specific code is unavailable.

MED: 100-2,15,290

SHOULDER ORTHOTIC (SO)

L3650 Shoulder orthosis, figure of eight design abduction restrainer, prefabricated, off-the-shelf

L3660 Shoulder orthosis, figure of eight design abduction restrainer, canvas and webbing, prefabricated, off-the-shelf

L3670 Shoulder orthosis, acromio/clavicular (canvas and webbing type), prefabricated, off-the-shelf

L3671 Shoulder orthotic (SO), shoulder joint design, without joints, may include soft interface, straps, custom fabricated, includes fitting and adjustment

L3674 Shoulder orthotic, abduction positioning (airplane design), thoracic component and support bar, with or without nontorsion joint/turnbuckle, may include soft interface, straps, custom fabricated, includes fitting and adjustment

L3675 Shoulder orthosis, vest type abduction restrainer, canvas webbing type or equal, prefabricated, off-the-shelf

L3677 Shoulder orthosis, shoulder joint design, without joints, may include soft interface, straps, prefabricated item that has been trimmed, bent, molded, assembled, or otherwise customized to fit a specific patient by an individual with expertise

L3678 Shoulder orthosis, shoulder joint design, without joints, may include soft interface, straps, prefabricated, off-the-shelf

ELBOW ORTHOTIC (EO)

L3702 Elbow orthotic (EO), without joints, may include soft interface, straps, custom fabricated, includes fitting and adjustment

L3710 Elbow orthosis, elastic with metal joints, prefabricated, off-the-shelf

L3720 Elbow orthotic (EO), double upright with forearm/arm cuffs, free motion, custom fabricated

L3730 Elbow orthotic (EO), double upright with forearm/arm cuffs, extension/flexion assist, custom fabricated

L3740 Elbow orthotic (EO), double upright with forearm/arm cuffs, adjustable position lock with active control, custom fabricated

L3760 Elbow orthotic (EO), with adjustable position locking joint(s), prefabricated, includes fitting and adjustments, any type

L3762 Elbow orthosis, rigid, without joints, includes soft interface material, prefabricated, off-the-shelf

L3763 Elbow-wrist-hand orthotic (EWHO), rigid, without joints, may include soft interface, straps, custom fabricated, includes fitting and adjustment

L3764 Elbow-wrist-hand orthotic (EWHO), includes one or more nontorsion joints, elastic bands, turnbuckles, may include soft interface, straps, custom fabricated, includes fitting and adjustment

L3765 Elbow-wrist-hand-finger orthotic (EWHFO), rigid, without joints, may include soft interface, straps, custom fabricated, includes fitting and adjustment

L3766 Elbow-wrist-hand-finger orthotic (EWHFO), includes one or more nontorsion joints, elastic bands, turnbuckles, may include soft interface, straps, custom fabricated, includes fitting and adjustment

WRIST-HAND-FINGER ORTHOTIC (WHFO)

L3806 Wrist-hand-finger orthotic (WHFO), includes one or more nontorsion joint(s), turnbuckles, elastic bands/springs, may include soft interface material, straps, custom fabricated, includes fitting and adjustment

L3807 Wrist hand finger orthosis, without joint(s), prefabricated item that has been trimmed, bent, molded, assembled, or otherwise customized to fit a specific patient by an individual with expertise

L3808 Wrist-hand-finger orthotic (WHFO), rigid without joints, may include soft interface material; straps, custom fabricated, includes fitting and adjustment

L3809 Wrist hand finger orthosis, without joint(s), prefabricated, off-the-shelf, any type

ADDITIONS TO UPPER EXTREMITY ORTHOTIC

L3891 Addition to upper extremity joint, wrist or elbow, concentric adjustable torsion style mechanism for custom fabricated orthotics only, each

DYNAMIC FLEXOR HINGE, RECIPROCAL WRIST EXTENSION/FLEXION, FINGER FLEXION/EXTENSION

L3900 Wrist-hand-finger orthotic (WHFO), dynamic flexor hinge, reciprocal wrist extension/flexion, finger flexion/extension, wrist or finger driven, custom fabricated

L3901 Wrist-hand-finger orthotic (WHFO), dynamic flexor hinge, reciprocal wrist extension/flexion, finger flexion/extension, cable driven, custom fabricated

EXTERNAL POWER

L3904 Wrist-hand-finger orthotic (WHFO), external powered, electric, custom fabricated

OTHER UPPER EXTREMITY ORTHOTICS

L3905 Wrist-hand orthotic (WHO), includes one or more nontorsion joints, elastic bands, turnbuckles, may include soft interface, straps, custom fabricated, includes fitting and adjustment

L3906 Wrist-hand orthosis (WHO), without joints, may include soft interface, straps, custom fabricated, includes fitting and adjustment

L3908 Wrist hand orthosis, wrist extension control cock-up, non molded, prefabricated, off-the-shelf

L3912 Hand finger orthosis (HFO), flexion glove with elastic finger control, prefabricated, off-the-shelf

L3913 Hand finger orthotic (HFO), without joints, may include soft interface, straps, custom fabricated, includes fitting and adjustment

L3915 Wrist hand orthosis, includes one or more nontorsion joint(s), elastic bands, turnbuckles, may include soft interface, straps, prefabricated item that has been trimmed, bent, molded, assembled, or otherwise customized to fit a specific patient by an individual with expertise

L3916 Wrist hand orthosis, includes one or more nontorsion joint(s), elastic bands, turnbuckles, may include soft interface, straps, prefabricated, off-the-shelf

Orthotic Devices and Procedures

L3917 — L4210

L3917 Hand orthosis, metacarpal fracture orthosis, prefabricated item that has been trimmed, bent, molded, assembled, or otherwise customized to fit a specific patient by an individual with expertise

L3918 Hand orthosis, metacarpal fracture orthosis, prefabricated, off-the-shelf

L3919 Hand orthotic (HO), without joints, may include soft interface, straps, custom fabricated, includes fitting and adjustment

L3921 Hand finger orthotic (HFO), includes one or more nontorsion joints, elastic bands, turnbuckles, may include soft interface, straps, custom fabricated, includes fitting and adjustment

L3923 Hand finger orthosis, without joints, may include soft interface, straps, prefabricated item that has been trimmed, bent, molded, assembled, or otherwise customized to fit a specific patient by an individual with expertise

L3924 Hand finger orthosis, without joints, may include soft interface, straps, prefabricated, off-the-shelf

L3925 Finger orthosis, proximal interphalangeal (PIP)/distal interphalangeal (DIP), non-torsion joint/spring, extension/flexion, may include soft interface material, prefabricated, off-the-shelf

L3927 Finger orthosis, proximal interphalangeal (PIP)/distal interphalangeal (DIP), without joint/spring, extension/flexion (e.g., static or ring type), may include soft interface material, prefabricated, off-the-shelf

L3929 Hand finger orthosis, includes one or more nontorsion joint(s), turnbuckles, elastic bands/springs, may include soft interface material, straps, prefabricated item that has been trimmed, bent, molded, assembled, or otherwise customized to fit a specific patient by an individual with expertise

L3930 Hand finger orthosis, includes one or more nontorsion joint(s), turnbuckles, elastic bands/springs, may include soft interface material, straps, prefabricated, off-the-shelf

L3931 Wrist-hand-finger orthotic (WHFO), includes one or more nontorsion joint(s), turnbuckles, elastic bands/springs, may include soft interface material, straps, prefabricated, includes fitting and adjustment

L3933 Finger orthotic (FO), without joints, may include soft interface, custom fabricated, includes fitting and adjustment

L3935 Finger orthotic, nontorsion joint, may include soft interface, custom fabricated, includes fitting and adjustment

L3956 Addition of joint to upper extremity orthotic, any material; per joint

SHOULDER, ELBOW, WRIST, HAND ORTHOTIC

L3960 Shoulder-elbow-wrist-hand orthotic (SEWHO), abduction positioning, airplane design, prefabricated, includes fitting and adjustment

L3961 Shoulder elbow wrist hand orthotic (SEWHO), shoulder cap design, without joints, may include soft interface, straps, custom fabricated, includes fitting and adjustment

L3962 Shoulder-elbow-wrist-hand orthotic (SEWHO), abduction positioning, Erb's palsy design, prefabricated, includes fitting and adjustment

L3967 Shoulder-elbow-wrist-hand orthotic (SEWHO), abduction positioning (airplane design), thoracic component and support bar, without joints, may include soft interface, straps, custom fabricated, includes fitting and adjustment

ADDITIONS TO MOBILE ARM SUPPORTS

L3971 Shoulder-elbow-wrist-hand orthotic (SEWHO), shoulder cap design, includes one or more nontorsion joints, elastic bands, turnbuckles, may include soft interface, straps, custom fabricated, includes fitting and adjustment

L3973 Shoulder-elbow-wrist-hand orthotic (SEWHO), abduction positioning (airplane design), thoracic component and support bar, includes one or more nontorsion joints, elastic bands, turnbuckles, may include soft interface, straps, custom fabricated, includes fitting and adjustment

L3975 Shoulder-elbow-wrist-hand-finger orthotic (SEWHO), shoulder cap design, without joints, may include soft interface, straps, custom fabricated, includes fitting and adjustment

L3976 Shoulder-elbow-wrist-hand-finger orthotic (SEWHO), abduction positioning (airplane design), thoracic component and support bar, without joints, may include soft interface, straps, custom fabricated, includes fitting and adjustment

L3977 Shoulder-elbow-wrist-hand-finger orthotic (SEWHO), shoulder cap design, includes one or more nontorsion joints, elastic bands, turnbuckles, may include soft interface, straps, custom fabricated, includes fitting and adjustment

L3978 Shoulder-elbow-wrist-hand-finger orthotic (SEWHO), abduction positioning (airplane design), thoracic component and support bar, includes one or more nontorsion joints, elastic bands, turnbuckles, may include soft interface, straps, custom fabricated, includes fitting and adjustment

FRACTURE ORTHOTIC

L3980 Upper extremity fracture orthotic, humeral, prefabricated, includes fitting and adjustment

L3982 Upper extremity fracture orthotic, radius/ulnar, prefabricated, includes fitting and adjustment

L3984 Upper extremity fracture orthotic, wrist, prefabricated, includes fitting and adjustment

L3995 Addition to upper extremity orthotic, sock, fracture or equal, each

L3999 Upper limb orthotic, not otherwise specified

REPAIRS

L4000 Replace girdle for spinal orthotic (cervical-thoracic-lumbar-sacral orthotic (CTLSO) or spinal orthotic SO)

L4002 Replacement strap, any orthotic, includes all components, any length, any type

L4010 Replace trilateral socket brim

L4020 Replace quadrilateral socket brim, molded to patient model

L4030 Replace quadrilateral socket brim, custom fitted

L4040 Replace molded thigh lacer, for custom fabricated orthotic only

L4045 Replace nonmolded thigh lacer, for custom fabricated orthotic only

L4050 Replace molded calf lacer, for custom fabricated orthotic only

L4055 Replace nonmolded calf lacer, for custom fabricated orthotic only

L4060 Replace high roll cuff

L4070 Replace proximal and distal upright for KAFO

L4080 Replace metal bands KAFO, proximal thigh

L4090 Replace metal bands KAFO-AFO, calf or distal thigh

L4100 Replace leather cuff KAFO, proximal thigh

L4110 Replace leather cuff KAFO-AFO, calf or distal thigh

L4130 Replace pretibial shell

L4205 Repair of orthotic device, labor component, per 15 minutes

L4210 Repair of orthotic device, repair or replace minor parts

MISCELLANEOUS LOWER LIMB SUPPORTS

L4350   Ankle control orthosis, stirrup style, rigid, includes any type interface (e.g., pneumatic, gel), prefabricated, off-the-shelf

L4360   Walking boot, pneumatic and/or vacuum, with or without joints, with or without interface material, prefabricated item that has been trimmed, bent, molded, assembled, or otherwise customized to fit a specific patient by an individual with expertise

L4361   Walking boot, pneumatic and/or vacuum, with or without joints, with or without interface material, prefabricated, off-the-shelf

L4370   Pneumatic full leg splint, prefabricated, off-the-shelf

L4386   Walking boot, non-pneumatic, with or without joints, with or without interface material, prefabricated item that has been trimmed, bent, molded, assembled, or otherwise customized to fit a specific patient by an individual with expertise

L4387   Walking boot, non-pneumatic, with or without joints, with or without interface material, prefabricated, off-the-shelf

L4392   Replacement, soft interface material, static AFO

L4394   Replace soft interface material, foot drop splint

L4396   Static or dynamic ankle foot orthosis, including soft interface material, adjustable for fit, for positioning, may be used for minimal ambulation, prefabricated item that has been trimmed, bent, molded, assembled, or otherwise customized to fit a specific patient by an individual with expertise

L4397   Static or dynamic ankle foot orthosis, including soft interface material, adjustable for fit, for positioning, may be used for minimal ambulation, prefabricated, off-the-shelf

L4398   Foot drop splint, recumbent positioning device, prefabricated, off-the-shelf

L4631   Ankle-foot orthotic, walking boot type, varus/valgus correction, rocker bottom, anterior tibial shell, soft interface, custom arch support, plastic or other material, includes straps and closures, custom fabricated

PROSTHETIC PROCEDURES L5000-L9999

The codes in this section are considered as "base" or "basic procedures or prosthetics" and may be modified by listing items/procedures or special materials from the "additions" sections and adding them to the base procedure.

PARTIAL FOOT

L5000   Partial foot, shoe insert with longitudinal arch, toe filler
     MED: 100-2,15,290

L5010   Partial foot, molded socket, ankle height, with toe filler
     MED: 100-2,15,290

L5020   Partial foot, molded socket, tibial tubercle height, with toe filler
     MED: 100-2,15,290

ANKLE

L5050   Ankle, Symes, molded socket, SACH foot

L5060   Ankle, Symes, metal frame, molded leather socket, articulated ankle/foot

BELOW KNEE

L5100   Below knee, molded socket, shin, SACH foot

L5105   Below knee, plastic socket, joints and thigh lacer, SACH foot

KNEE DISARTICULATION

L5150   Knee disarticulation (or through knee), molded socket, external knee joints, shin, SACH foot

L5160   Knee disarticulation (or through knee), molded socket, bent knee configuration, external knee joints, shin, SACH foot

ABOVE KNEE

L5200   Above knee, molded socket, single axis constant friction knee, shin, SACH foot

L5210   Above knee, short prosthesis, no knee joint (stubbies), with foot blocks, no ankle joints, each

L5220   Above knee, short prosthesis, no knee joint (stubbies), with articulated ankle/foot, dynamically aligned, each

L5230   Above knee, for proximal femoral focal deficiency, constant friction knee, shin, SACH foot

HIP DISARTICULATION

L5250   Hip disarticulation, Canadian type; molded socket, hip joint, single axis constant friction knee, shin, SACH foot

L5270   Hip disarticulation, tilt table type; molded socket, locking hip joint, single axis constant friction knee, shin, SACH foot

HEMIPELVECTOMY

L5280   Hemipelvectomy, Canadian type; molded socket, hip joint, single axis constant friction knee, shin, SACH foot

L5301   Below knee, molded socket, shin, SACH foot, endoskeletal system

L5312   Knee disarticulation (or through knee), molded socket, single axis knee, pylon, SACH foot, endoskeletal system

L5321   Above knee, molded socket, open end, SACH foot, endoskeletal system, single axis knee

L5331   Hip disarticulation, Canadian type, molded socket, endoskeletal system, hip joint, single axis knee, SACH foot

L5341   Hemipelvectomy, Canadian type, molded socket, endoskeletal system, hip joint, single axis knee, SACH foot

IMMEDIATE POSTSURGICAL OR EARLY FITTING PROCEDURES

Above-the-knee test socket

Below-the-knee early fitting rigid dressing (L5400)

Test sockets are often made of clear plastic so the prosthetist can visualize the fit against the residual limb

L5400   Immediate postsurgical or early fitting, application of initial rigid dressing, including fitting, alignment, suspension, and one cast change, below knee

L5410   Immediate postsurgical or early fitting, application of initial rigid dressing, including fitting, alignment and suspension, below knee, each additional cast change and realignment

L5420   Immediate postsurgical or early fitting, application of initial rigid dressing, including fitting, alignment and suspension and one cast change AK or knee disarticulation

L5430   Immediate postsurgical or early fitting, application of initial rigid dressing, including fitting, alignment and suspension, AK or knee disarticulation, each additional cast change and realignment

L5450   Immediate postsurgical or early fitting, application of nonweight bearing rigid dressing, below knee

L5460   Immediate postsurgical or early fitting, application of nonweight bearing rigid dressing, above knee

INITIAL PROSTHESIS

L5500   Initial, below knee PTB type socket, nonalignable system, pylon, no cover, SACH foot, plaster socket, direct formed

     MED: 100-2,1,40

L5505   Initial, above knee, knee disarticulation, ischial level socket, nonalignable system, pylon, no cover, SACH foot, plaster socket, direct formed

     MED: 100-2,1,40

PREPARATORY PROSTHESIS

L5510   Preparatory, below knee PTB type socket, nonalignable system, pylon, no cover, SACH foot, plaster socket, molded to model

L5520   Preparatory, below knee PTB type socket, nonalignable system, pylon, no cover, SACH foot, thermoplastic or equal, direct formed

L5530   Preparatory, below knee PTB type socket, nonalignable system, pylon, no cover, SACH foot, thermoplastic or equal, molded to model

L5535   Preparatory, below knee PTB type socket, nonalignable system, no cover, SACH foot, prefabricated, adjustable open end socket

L5540   Preparatory, below knee PTB type socket, nonalignable system, pylon, no cover, SACH foot, laminated socket, molded to model

L5560   Preparatory, above knee, knee disarticulation, ischial level socket, nonalignable system, pylon, no cover, SACH foot, plaster socket, molded to model

L5570   Preparatory, above knee - knee disarticulation, ischial level socket, nonalignable system, pylon, no cover, SACH foot, thermoplastic or equal, direct formed

L5580   Preparatory, above knee, knee disarticulation, ischial level socket, nonalignable system, pylon, no cover, SACH foot, thermoplastic or equal, molded to model

L5585   Preparatory, above knee - knee disarticulation, ischial level socket, nonalignable system, pylon, no cover, SACH foot, prefabricated adjustable open end socket

L5590   Preparatory, above knee, knee disarticulation, ischial level socket, nonalignable system, pylon, no cover, SACH foot, laminated socket, molded to model

L5595   Preparatory, hip disarticulation/hemipelvectomy, pylon, no cover, SACH foot, thermoplastic or equal, molded to patient model

L5600   Preparatory, hip disarticulation/hemipelvectomy, pylon, no cover, SACH foot, laminated socket, molded to patient model

ADDITIONS

ADDITIONS: LOWER EXTREMITY

L5610   Addition to lower extremity, endoskeletal system, above knee, hydracadence system

L5611   Addition to lower extremity, endoskeletal system, above knee, knee disarticulation, 4-bar linkage, with friction swing phase control

L5613   Addition to lower extremity, endoskeletal system, above knee, knee disarticulation, 4-bar linkage, with hydraulic swing phase control

L5614   Addition to lower extremity, exoskeletal system, above knee-knee disarticulation, 4 bar linkage, with pneumatic swing phase control

L5616   Addition to lower extremity, endoskeletal system, above knee, universal multiplex system, friction swing phase control

L5617   Addition to lower extremity, quick change self-aligning unit, above knee or below knee, each

ADDITIONS: TEST SOCKETS

L5618   Addition to lower extremity, test socket, Symes

L5620   Addition to lower extremity, test socket, below knee

L5622   Addition to lower extremity, test socket, knee disarticulation

L5624   Addition to lower extremity, test socket, above knee

L5626   Addition to lower extremity, test socket, hip disarticulation

L5628   Addition to lower extremity, test socket, hemipelvectomy

L5629   Addition to lower extremity, below knee, acrylic socket

ADDITIONS: SOCKET VARIATIONS

L5630   Addition to lower extremity, Symes type, expandable wall socket

L5631   Addition to lower extremity, above knee or knee disarticulation, acrylic socket

L5632   Addition to lower extremity, Symes type, PTB brim design socket

L5634   Addition to lower extremity, Symes type, posterior opening (Canadian) socket

L5636   Addition to lower extremity, Symes type, medial opening socket

L5637   Addition to lower extremity, below knee, total contact

L5638   Addition to lower extremity, below knee, leather socket

L5639   Addition to lower extremity, below knee, wood socket

L5640   Addition to lower extremity, knee disarticulation, leather socket

L5642   Addition to lower extremity, above knee, leather socket

L5643   Addition to lower extremity, hip disarticulation, flexible inner socket, external frame

L5644   Addition to lower extremity, above knee, wood socket

L5645   Addition to lower extremity, below knee, flexible inner socket, external frame

L5646   Addition to lower extremity, below knee, air, fluid, gel or equal, cushion socket

L5647   Addition to lower extremity, below knee, suction socket

L5648   Addition to lower extremity, above knee, air, fluid, gel or equal, cushion socket

L5649   Addition to lower extremity, ischial containment/narrow M-L socket

L5650   Additions to lower extremity, total contact, above knee or knee disarticulation socket

L5651   Addition to lower extremity, above knee, flexible inner socket, external frame

L5652   Addition to lower extremity, suction suspension, above knee or knee disarticulation socket

L5653   Addition to lower extremity, knee disarticulation, expandable wall socket

ADDITIONS: SOCKET INSERT AND SUSPENSION

L5654   Addition to lower extremity, socket insert, Symes, (Kemblo, Pelite, Aliplast, Plastazote or equal)

L5655   Addition to lower extremity, socket insert, below knee (Kemblo, Pelite, Aliplast, Plastazote or equal)

L5656   Addition to lower extremity, socket insert, knee disarticulation (Kemblo, Pelite, Aliplast, Plastazote or equal)

L5658   Addition to lower extremity, socket insert, above knee (Kemblo, Pelite, Aliplast, Plastazote or equal)

L5661   Addition to lower extremity, socket insert, multidurometer Symes

L5665   Addition to lower extremity, socket insert, multidurometer, below knee

L5666   Addition to lower extremity, below knee, cuff suspension

L5668 Addition to lower extremity, below knee, molded distal cushion

As the suspension sleeve is donned, air is driven out through a valve

Residual limb

Sealing membrane

Sleeve

Open valve

The valve is closed upon donning and a suction fit is formed around the residual limb

Closed valve

L5670 Addition to lower extremity, below knee, molded supracondylar suspension (PTS or similar)

L5671 Addition to lower extremity, below knee/above knee suspension locking mechanism (shuttle, lanyard, or equal), excludes socket insert

L5672 Addition to lower extremity, below knee, removable medial brim suspension

L5673 Addition to lower extremity, below knee/above knee, custom fabricated from existing mold or prefabricated, socket insert, silicone gel, elastomeric or equal, for use with locking mechanism

L5676 Additions to lower extremity, below knee, knee joints, single axis, pair

L5677 Additions to lower extremity, below knee, knee joints, polycentric, pair

L5678 Additions to lower extremity, below knee, joint covers, pair

L5679 Addition to lower extremity, below knee/above knee, custom fabricated from existing mold or prefabricated, socket insert, silicone gel, elastomeric or equal, not for use with locking mechanism

L5680 Addition to lower extremity, below knee, thigh lacer, nonmolded

L5681 Addition to lower extremity, below knee/above knee, custom fabricated socket insert for congenital or atypical traumatic amputee, silicone gel, elastomeric or equal, for use with or without locking mechanism, initial only (for other than initial, use code L5673 or L5679)

L5682 Addition to lower extremity, below knee, thigh lacer, gluteal/ischial, molded

L5683 Addition to lower extremity, below knee/above knee, custom fabricated socket insert for other than congenital or atypical traumatic amputee, silicone gel, elastomeric or equal, for use with or without locking mechanism, initial only (for other than initial, use code L5673 or L5679)

L5684 Addition to lower extremity, below knee, fork strap

L5685 Addition to lower extremity prosthesis, below knee, suspension/sealing sleeve, with or without valve, any material, each

L5686 Addition to lower extremity, below knee, back check (extension control)

L5688 Addition to lower extremity, below knee, waist belt, webbing

L5690 Addition to lower extremity, below knee, waist belt, padded and lined

L5692 Addition to lower extremity, above knee, pelvic control belt, light

L5694 Addition to lower extremity, above knee, pelvic control belt, padded and lined

L5695 Addition to lower extremity, above knee, pelvic control, sleeve suspension, neoprene or equal, each

L5696 Addition to lower extremity, above knee or knee disarticulation, pelvic joint

L5697 Addition to lower extremity, above knee or knee disarticulation, pelvic band

L5698 Addition to lower extremity, above knee or knee disarticulation, Silesian bandage

L5699 All lower extremity prostheses, shoulder harness

REPLACEMENTS

L5700 Replacement, socket, below knee, molded to patient model

L5701 Replacement, socket, above knee/knee disarticulation, including attachment plate, molded to patient model

L5702 Replacement, socket, hip disarticulation, including hip joint, molded to patient model

L5703 Ankle, Symes, molded to patient model, socket without solid ankle cushion heel (SACH) foot, replacement only

L5704 Custom shaped protective cover, below knee

L5705 Custom shaped protective cover, above knee

L5706 Custom shaped protective cover, knee disarticulation

L5707 Custom shaped protective cover, hip disarticulation

ADDITIONS: EXOSKELETAL KNEE-SHIN SYSTEM

L5710 Addition, exoskeletal knee-shin system, single axis, manual lock

L5711 Additions exoskeletal knee-shin system, single axis, manual lock, ultra-light material

L5712 Addition, exoskeletal knee-shin system, single axis, friction swing and stance phase control (safety knee)

L5714 Addition, exoskeletal knee-shin system, single axis, variable friction swing phase control

L5716 Addition, exoskeletal knee-shin system, polycentric, mechanical stance phase lock

L5718 Addition, exoskeletal knee-shin system, polycentric, friction swing and stance phase control

L5722 Addition, exoskeletal knee-shin system, single axis, pneumatic swing, friction stance phase control

L5724 Addition, exoskeletal knee-shin system, single axis, fluid swing phase control

L5726 Addition, exoskeletal knee-shin system, single axis, external joints, fluid swing phase control

L5728 Addition, exoskeletal knee-shin system, single axis, fluid swing and stance phase control

L5780 Addition, exoskeletal knee-shin system, single axis, pneumatic/hydra pneumatic swing phase control

L5781 Addition to lower limb prosthesis, vacuum pump, residual limb volume management and moisture evacuation system

L5782 Addition to lower limb prosthesis, vacuum pump, residual limb volume management and moisture evacuation system, heavy-duty

COMPONENT MODIFICATION

L5785 Addition, exoskeletal system, below knee, ultra-light material (titanium, carbon fiber or equal)

L5790 Addition, exoskeletal system, above knee, ultra-light material (titanium, carbon fiber or equal)

L5795 Addition, exoskeletal system, hip disarticulation, ultra-light material (titanium, carbon fiber or equal)

Prosthetic Devices and Procedures

L5810 — L5986

ADDITIONS: ENDOSKELETAL KNEE-SHIN SYSTEM

L5810   Addition, endoskeletal knee-shin system, single axis, manual lock

L5811   Addition, endoskeletal knee-shin system, single axis, manual lock, ultra-light material

L5812   Addition, endoskeletal knee-shin system, single axis, friction swing and stance phase control (safety knee)

L5814   Addition, endoskeletal knee-shin system, polycentric, hydraulic swing phase control, mechanical stance phase lock

L5816   Addition, endoskeletal knee-shin system, polycentric, mechanical stance phase lock

L5818   Addition, endoskeletal knee-shin system, polycentric, friction swing and stance phase control

L5822   Addition, endoskeletal knee-shin system, single axis, pneumatic swing, friction stance phase control

L5824   Addition, endoskeletal knee-shin system, single axis, fluid swing phase control

L5826   Addition, endoskeletal knee-shin system, single axis, hydraulic swing phase control, with miniature high activity frame

L5828   Addition, endoskeletal knee-shin system, single axis, fluid swing and stance phase control

L5830   Addition, endoskeletal knee-shin system, single axis, pneumatic/swing phase control

L5840   Addition, endoskeletal knee-shin system, 4-bar linkage or multiaxial, pneumatic swing phase control

L5845   Addition, endoskeletal knee-shin system, stance flexion feature, adjustable

L5848   Addition to endoskeletal knee-shin system, fluid stance extension, dampening feature, with or without adjustability

L5850   Addition, endoskeletal system, above knee or hip disarticulation, knee extension assist

L5855   Addition, endoskeletal system, hip disarticulation, mechanical hip extension assist

L5856   Addition to lower extremity prosthesis, endoskeletal knee-shin system, microprocessor control feature, swing and stance phase, includes electronic sensor(s), any type

L5857   Addition to lower extremity prosthesis, endoskeletal knee-shin system, microprocessor control feature, swing phase only, includes electronic sensor(s), any type

L5858   Addition to lower extremity prosthesis, endoskeletal knee shin system, microprocessor control feature, stance phase only, includes electronic sensor(s), any type

L5859   Addition to lower extremity prosthesis, endoskeletal knee-shin system, powered and programmable flexion/extension assist control, includes any type motor(s)

L5910   Addition, endoskeletal system, below knee, alignable system

L5920   Addition, endoskeletal system, above knee or hip disarticulation, alignable system

L5925   Addition, endoskeletal system, above knee, knee disarticulation or hip disarticulation, manual lock

L5930   Addition, endoskeletal system, high activity knee control frame

L5940   Addition, endoskeletal system, below knee, ultra-light material (titanium, carbon fiber or equal)

L5950   Addition, endoskeletal system, above knee, ultra-light material (titanium, carbon fiber or equal)

L5960   Addition, endoskeletal system, hip disarticulation, ultra-light material (titanium, carbon fiber or equal)

L5961   Addition, endoskeletal system, polycentric hip joint, pneumatic or hydraulic control, rotation control, with or without flexion and/or extension control

L5962   Addition, endoskeletal system, below knee, flexible protective outer surface covering system

L5964   Addition, endoskeletal system, above knee, flexible protective outer surface covering system

L5966   Addition, endoskeletal system, hip disarticulation, flexible protective outer surface covering system

L5968   Addition to lower limb prosthesis, multiaxial ankle with swing phase active dorsiflexion feature

L5969   Addition, endoskeletal ankle-foot or ankle system, power assist, includes any type motor(s)

L5970   All lower extremity prostheses, foot, external keel, SACH foot

L5971   All lower extremity prostheses, solid ankle cushion heel (SACH) foot, replacement only

L5972   All lower extremity prostheses, foot, flexible keel

L5973   Endoskeletal ankle foot system, microprocessor controlled feature, dorsiflexion and/or plantar flexion control, includes power source

Foot prosthesis
(L5974)

Energy storing foot
(L5976)

Carbon

L5974   All lower extremity prostheses, foot, single axis ankle/foot

L5975   All lower extremity prostheses, combination single axis ankle and flexible keel foot

L5976   All lower extremity prostheses, energy storing foot (Seattle Carbon Copy II or equal)

Foot prosthesis,
multi-axial ankle
(L5978)

L5978   All lower extremity prostheses, foot, multiaxial ankle/foot

L5979   All lower extremity prostheses, multiaxial ankle, dynamic response foot, one piece system

L5980   All lower extremity prostheses, flex-foot system

L5981   All lower extremity prostheses, flex-walk system or equal

L5982   All exoskeletal lower extremity prostheses, axial rotation unit

L5984   All endoskeletal lower extremity prostheses, axial rotation unit, with or without adjustability

L5985   All endoskeletal lower extremity prostheses, dynamic prosthetic pylon

L5986   All lower extremity prostheses, multiaxial rotation unit (MCP or equal)

L5987   All lower extremity prostheses, shank foot system with vertical loading pylon

L5988   Addition to lower limb prosthesis, vertical shock reducing pylon feature

L5990   Addition to lower extremity prosthesis, user adjustable heel height

L5999   Lower extremity prosthesis, not otherwise specified
Determine if an alternative HCPCS Level II or a CPT code better describes the service being reported. This code should be used only if a more specific code is unavailable.

PARTIAL HAND

L6000   Partial hand, thumb remaining

L6010   Partial hand, little and/or ring finger remaining

L6020   Partial hand, no finger remaining

L6025   Transcarpal/metacarpal or partial hand disarticulation prosthesis, external power, self-suspended, inner socket with removable forearm section, electrodes and cables, 2 batteries, charger, myoelectric control of terminal device

WRIST DISARTICULATION

L6050   Wrist disarticulation, molded socket, flexible elbow hinges, triceps pad

L6055   Wrist disarticulation, molded socket with expandable interface, flexible elbow hinges, triceps pad

BELOW ELBOW

L6100   Below elbow, molded socket, flexible elbow hinge, triceps pad

L6110   Below elbow, molded socket (Muenster or Northwestern suspension types)

L6120   Below elbow, molded double wall split socket, step-up hinges, half cuff

L6130   Below elbow, molded double wall split socket, stump activated locking hinge, half cuff

ELBOW DISARTICULATION

L6200   Elbow disarticulation, molded socket, outside locking hinge, forearm

L6205   Elbow disarticulation, molded socket with expandable interface, outside locking hinges, forearm

ABOVE ELBOW

L6250   Above elbow, molded double wall socket, internal locking elbow, forearm

SHOULDER DISARTICULATION

L6300   Shoulder disarticulation, molded socket, shoulder bulkhead, humeral section, internal locking elbow, forearm

L6310   Shoulder disarticulation, passive restoration (complete prosthesis)

L6320   Shoulder disarticulation, passive restoration (shoulder cap only)

INTERSCAPULAR THORACIC

L6350   Interscapular thoracic, molded socket, shoulder bulkhead, humeral section, internal locking elbow, forearm

L6360   Interscapular thoracic, passive restoration (complete prosthesis)

L6370   Interscapular thoracic, passive restoration (shoulder cap only)

IMMEDIATE AND EARLY POSTSURGICAL PROCEDURES

L6380   Immediate postsurgical or early fitting, application of initial rigid dressing, including fitting alignment and suspension of components, and one cast change, wrist disarticulation or below elbow

L6382   Immediate postsurgical or early fitting, application of initial rigid dressing including fitting alignment and suspension of components, and one cast change, elbow disarticulation or above elbow

L6384   Immediate postsurgical or early fitting, application of initial rigid dressing including fitting alignment and suspension of components, and one cast change, shoulder disarticulation or interscapular thoracic

L6386   Immediate postsurgical or early fitting, each additional cast change and realignment

L6388   Immediate postsurgical or early fitting, application of rigid dressing only

MOLDED SOCKET

L6400   Below elbow, molded socket, endoskeletal system, including soft prosthetic tissue shaping

L6450   Elbow disarticulation, molded socket, endoskeletal system, including soft prosthetic tissue shaping

L6500   Above elbow, molded socket, endoskeletal system, including soft prosthetic tissue shaping

L6550   Shoulder disarticulation, molded socket, endoskeletal system, including soft prosthetic tissue shaping

L6570   Interscapular thoracic, molded socket, endoskeletal system, including soft prosthetic tissue shaping

PREPARATORY SOCKET

L6580   Preparatory, wrist disarticulation or below elbow, single wall plastic socket, friction wrist, flexible elbow hinges, figure of eight harness, humeral cuff, Bowden cable control, USMC or equal pylon, no cover, molded to patient model

L6582   Preparatory, wrist disarticulation or below elbow, single wall socket, friction wrist, flexible elbow hinges, figure of eight harness, humeral cuff, Bowden cable control, USMC or equal pylon, no cover, direct formed

L6584   Preparatory, elbow disarticulation or above elbow, single wall plastic socket, friction wrist, locking elbow, figure of eight harness, fair lead cable control, USMC or equal pylon, no cover, molded to patient model

L6586   Preparatory, elbow disarticulation or above elbow, single wall socket, friction wrist, locking elbow, figure of eight harness, fair lead cable control, USMC or equal pylon, no cover, direct formed

L6588   Preparatory, shoulder disarticulation or interscapular thoracic, single wall plastic socket, shoulder joint, locking elbow, friction wrist, chest strap, fair lead cable control, USMC or equal pylon, no cover, molded to patient model

L6590   Preparatory, shoulder disarticulation or interscapular thoracic, single wall socket, shoulder joint, locking elbow, friction wrist, chest strap, fair lead cable control, USMC or equal pylon, no cover, direct formed

ADDITIONS: UPPER LIMB

The following procedures/modifications/components may be added to other base procedures. The items in this section should reflect the additional complexity of each modification procedure, in addition to the base procedure, at the time of the original order.

L6600   Upper extremity additions, polycentric hinge, pair

L6605   Upper extremity additions, single pivot hinge, pair

L6610   Upper extremity additions, flexible metal hinge, pair

Prosthetic Devices and Procedures

L6611 — L6810

L6611   Addition to upper extremity prosthesis, external powered, additional switch, any type

L6615   Upper extremity addition, disconnect locking wrist unit

L6616   Upper extremity addition, additional disconnect insert for locking wrist unit, each

L6620   Upper extremity addition, flexion/extension wrist unit, with or without friction

L6621   Upper extremity prosthesis addition, flexion/extension wrist with or without friction, for use with external powered terminal device

L6623   Upper extremity addition, spring assisted rotational wrist unit with latch release

L6624   Upper extremity addition, flexion/extension and rotation wrist unit

L6625   Upper extremity addition, rotation wrist unit with cable lock

L6628   Upper extremity addition, quick disconnect hook adapter, Otto Bock or equal

L6629   Upper extremity addition, quick disconnect lamination collar with coupling piece, Otto Bock or equal

L6630   Upper extremity addition, stainless steel, any wrist

L6632   Upper extremity addition, latex suspension sleeve, each

L6635   Upper extremity addition, lift assist for elbow

L6637   Upper extremity addition, nudge control elbow lock

L6638   Upper extremity addition to prosthesis, electric locking feature, only for use with manually powered elbow

L6640   Upper extremity additions, shoulder abduction joint, pair

L6641   Upper extremity addition, excursion amplifier, pulley type

L6642   Upper extremity addition, excursion amplifier, lever type

L6645   Upper extremity addition, shoulder flexion-abduction joint, each

L6646   Upper extremity addition, shoulder joint, multipositional locking, flexion, adjustable abduction friction control, for use with body powered or external powered system

L6647   Upper extremity addition, shoulder lock mechanism, body powered actuator

L6648   Upper extremity addition, shoulder lock mechanism, external powered actuator

L6650   Upper extremity addition, shoulder universal joint, each

L6655   Upper extremity addition, standard control cable, extra

L6660   Upper extremity addition, heavy-duty control cable

L6665   Upper extremity addition, Teflon, or equal, cable lining

L6670   Upper extremity addition, hook to hand, cable adapter

L6672   Upper extremity addition, harness, chest or shoulder, saddle type

L6675   Upper extremity addition, harness, (e.g., figure of eight type), single cable design

L6676   Upper extremity addition, harness, (e.g., figure of eight type), dual cable design

L6677   Upper extremity addition, harness, triple control, simultaneous operation of terminal device and elbow

L6680   Upper extremity addition, test socket, wrist disarticulation or below elbow

L6682   Upper extremity addition, test socket, elbow disarticulation or above elbow

L6684   Upper extremity addition, test socket, shoulder disarticulation or interscapular thoracic

L6686   Upper extremity addition, suction socket

L6687   Upper extremity addition, frame type socket, below elbow or wrist disarticulation

L6688   Upper extremity addition, frame type socket, above elbow or elbow disarticulation

L6689   Upper extremity addition, frame type socket, shoulder disarticulation

L6690   Upper extremity addition, frame type socket, interscapular-thoracic

L6691   Upper extremity addition, removable insert, each

L6692   Upper extremity addition, silicone gel insert or equal, each

L6693   Upper extremity addition, locking elbow, forearm counterbalance

L6694   Addition to upper extremity prosthesis, below elbow/above elbow, custom fabricated from existing mold or prefabricated, socket insert, silicone gel, elastomeric or equal, for use with locking mechanism

L6695   Addition to upper extremity prosthesis, below elbow/above elbow, custom fabricated from existing mold or prefabricated, socket insert, silicone gel, elastomeric or equal, not for use with locking mechanism

L6696   Addition to upper extremity prosthesis, below elbow/above elbow, custom fabricated socket insert for congenital or atypical traumatic amputee, silicone gel, elastomeric or equal, for use with or without locking mechanism, initial only (for other than initial, use code L6694 or L6695)

L6697   Addition to upper extremity prosthesis, below elbow/above elbow, custom fabricated socket insert for other than congenital or atypical traumatic amputee, silicone gel, elastomeric or equal, for use with or without locking mechanism, initial only (for other than initial, use code L6694 or L6695)

L6698   Addition to upper extremity prosthesis, below elbow/above elbow, lock mechanism, excludes socket insert

TERMINAL DEVICE

L6703   Terminal device, passive hand/mitt, any material, any size

L6704   Terminal device, sport/recreational/work attachment, any material, any size

L6706   Terminal device, hook, mechanical, voluntary opening, any material, any size, lined or unlined

L6707   Terminal device, hook, mechanical, voluntary closing, any material, any size, lined or unlined

L6708   Terminal device, hand, mechanical, voluntary opening, any material, any size

L6709   Terminal device, hand, mechanical, voluntary closing, any material, any size

L6711   Terminal device, hook, mechanical, voluntary opening, any material, any size, lined or unlined, pediatric

L6712   Terminal device, hook, mechanical, voluntary closing, any material, any size, lined or unlined, pediatric

L6713   Terminal device, hand, mechanical, voluntary opening, any material, any size, pediatric

L6714   Terminal device, hand, mechanical, voluntary closing, any material, any size, pediatric

L6715   Terminal device, multiple articulating digit, includes motor(s), initial issue or replacement

L6721   Terminal device, hook or hand, heavy-duty, mechanical, voluntary opening, any material, any size, lined or unlined

L6722   Terminal device, hook or hand, heavy-duty, mechanical, voluntary closing, any material, any size, lined or unlined

ADDITION TO TERMINAL DEVICE

L6805   Addition to terminal device, modifier wrist unit

L6810   Addition to terminal device, precision pinch device

L6880   Electric hand, switch or myoelectric controlled, independently articulating digits, any grasp pattern or combination of grasp patterns, includes motor(s)

L6881   Automatic grasp feature, addition to upper limb electric prosthetic terminal device

L6882   Microprocessor control feature, addition to upper limb prosthetic terminal device

REPLACEMENT SOCKET

L6883   Replacement socket, below elbow/wrist disarticulation, molded to patient model, for use with or without external power

L6884   Replacement socket, above elbow/elbow disarticulation, molded to patient model, for use with or without external power

L6885   Replacement socket, shoulder disarticulation/interscapular thoracic, molded to patient model, for use with or without external power

HAND RESTORATION

L6890   Addition to upper extremity prosthesis, glove for terminal device, any material, prefabricated, includes fitting and adjustment

L6895   Addition to upper extremity prosthesis, glove for terminal device, any material, custom fabricated

L6900   Hand restoration (casts, shading and measurements included), partial hand, with glove, thumb or one finger remaining

L6905   Hand restoration (casts, shading and measurements included), partial hand, with glove, multiple fingers remaining

L6910   Hand restoration (casts, shading and measurements included), partial hand, with glove, no fingers remaining

L6915   Hand restoration (shading and measurements included), replacement glove for above

EXTERNAL POWER

L6920   Wrist disarticulation, external power, self-suspended inner socket, removable forearm shell, Otto Bock or equal switch, cables, 2 batteries and 1 charger, switch control of terminal device

L6925   Wrist disarticulation, external power, self-suspended inner socket, removable forearm shell, Otto Bock or equal electrodes, cables, 2 batteries and one charger, myoelectronic control of terminal device

L6930   Below elbow, external power, self-suspended inner socket, removable forearm shell, Otto Bock or equal switch, cables, 2 batteries and one charger, switch control of terminal device

L6935   Below elbow, external power, self-suspended inner socket, removable forearm shell, Otto Bock or equal electrodes, cables, 2 batteries and one charger, myoelectronic control of terminal device

L6940   Elbow disarticulation, external power, molded inner socket, removable humeral shell, outside locking hinges, forearm, Otto Bock or equal switch, cables, 2 batteries and one charger, switch control of terminal device

L6945   Elbow disarticulation, external power, molded inner socket, removable humeral shell, outside locking hinges, forearm, Otto Bock or equal electrodes, cables, 2 batteries and one charger, myoelectronic control of terminal device

L6950   Above elbow, external power, molded inner socket, removable humeral shell, internal locking elbow, forearm, Otto Bock or equal switch, cables, 2 batteries and one charger, switch control of terminal device

L6955   Above elbow, external power, molded inner socket, removable humeral shell, internal locking elbow, forearm, Otto Bock or equal electrodes, cables, 2 batteries and one charger, myoelectronic control of terminal device

L6960   Shoulder disarticulation, external power, molded inner socket, removable shoulder shell, shoulder bulkhead, humeral section, mechanical elbow, forearm, Otto Bock or equal switch, cables, 2 batteries and one charger, switch control of terminal device

L6965   Shoulder disarticulation, external power, molded inner socket, removable shoulder shell, shoulder bulkhead, humeral section, mechanical elbow, forearm, Otto Bock or equal electrodes, cables, 2 batteries and one charger, myoelectronic control of terminal device

L6970   Interscapular-thoracic, external power, molded inner socket, removable shoulder shell, shoulder bulkhead, humeral section, mechanical elbow, forearm, Otto Bock or equal switch, cables, 2 batteries and one charger, switch control of terminal device

L6975   Interscapular-thoracic, external power, molded inner socket, removable shoulder shell, shoulder bulkhead, humeral section, mechanical elbow, forearm, Otto Bock or equal electrodes, cables, 2 batteries and one charger, myoelectronic control of terminal device

ELECTRIC HAND AND ACCESSORIES

L7007   Electric hand, switch or myoelectric controlled, adult

L7008   Electric hand, switch or myoelectric, controlled, pediatric

L7009   Electric hook, switch or myoelectric controlled, adult

L7040   Prehensile actuator, switch controlled

L7045   Electric hook, switch or myoelectric controlled, pediatric

ELECTRONIC ELBOW AND ACCESSORIES

L7170   Electronic elbow, Hosmer or equal, switch controlled

L7180   Electronic elbow, microprocessor sequential control of elbow and terminal device

L7181   Electronic elbow, microprocessor simultaneous control of elbow and terminal device

L7185   Electronic elbow, adolescent, Variety Village or equal, switch controlled

L7186   Electronic elbow, child, Variety Village or equal, switch controlled

L7190   Electronic elbow, adolescent, Variety Village or equal, myoelectronically controlled

L7191   Electronic elbow, child, Variety Village or equal, myoelectronically controlled

ELECTRONIC WRIST AND ACCESSORIES

L7260   Electronic wrist rotator, Otto Bock or equal

L7261   Electronic wrist rotator, for Utah arm

BATTERY COMPONENTS

L7360   Six volt battery, each

L7362   Battery charger, 6 volt, each

L7364   Twelve volt battery, each

L7366   Battery charger, twelve volt, each

L7367   Lithium ion battery, replacement

L7368   Lithium ion battery charger, replacement only

ADDITIONS TO UPPER EXTREMITY PROSTHESIS

L7400   Addition to upper extremity prosthesis, below elbow/wrist disarticulation, ultralight material (titanium, carbon fiber or equal)

L7401   Addition to upper extremity prosthesis, above elbow disarticulation, ultralight material (titanium, carbon fiber or equal)

L7402 Addition to upper extremity prosthesis, shoulder disarticulation/interscapular thoracic, ultralight material (titanium, carbon fiber or equal)

L7403 Addition to upper extremity prosthesis, below elbow/wrist disarticulation, acrylic material

L7404 Addition to upper extremity prosthesis, above elbow disarticulation, acrylic material

L7405 Addition to upper extremity prosthesis, shoulder disarticulation/interscapular thoracic, acrylic material

L7499 Upper extremity prosthesis, not otherwise specified

DONNING SLEEVE

L7600 Prosthetic donning sleeve, any material, each

REPAIRS

L7510 Repair of prosthetic device, repair or replace minor parts
Medicare jurisdiction: local contractor if repair of implanted prosthetic device.

L7520 Repair prosthetic device, labor component, per 15 minutes
Medicare jurisdiction: local contractor if repair of implanted prosthetic device.

MALE PROSTHETIC

L7900 Male vacuum erection system

L7902 Tension ring, for vacuum erection device, any type, replacement only, each

BREAST PROSTHESIS

L8000 Breast prosthesis, mastectomy bra, without integrated breast prosthesis form, any size, any type

L8001 Breast prosthesis, mastectomy bra, with integrated breast prosthesis form, unilateral, any size, any type

L8002 Breast prosthesis, mastectomy bra, with integrated breast prosthesis form, bilateral, any size, any type

L8010 Breast prosthesis, mastectomy sleeve

L8015 External breast prosthesis garment, with mastectomy form, post mastectomy

L8020 Breast prosthesis, mastectomy form

L8030 Breast prosthesis, silicone or equal, without integral adhesive

L8031 Breast prosthesis, silicone or equal, with integral adhesive

L8032 Nipple prosthesis, reusable, any type, each

L8035 Custom breast prosthesis, post mastectomy, molded to patient model

L8039 Breast prosthesis, not otherwise specified

FACE AND EAR PROSTHESIS

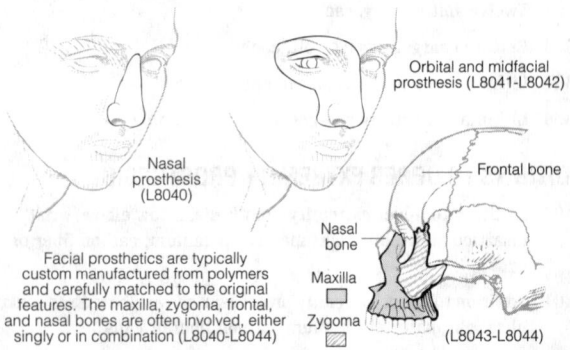

Nasal prosthesis (L8040)

Orbital and midfacial prosthesis (L8041-L8042)

Frontal bone

Nasal bone

Maxilla

Zygoma

(L8043-L8044)

Facial prosthetics are typically custom manufactured from polymers and carefully matched to the original features. The maxilla, zygoma, frontal, and nasal bones are often involved, either singly or in combination (L8040-L8044)

L8040 Nasal prosthesis, provided by a nonphysician

L8041 Midfacial prosthesis, provided by a nonphysician

L8042 Orbital prosthesis, provided by a nonphysician

L8043 Upper facial prosthesis, provided by a nonphysician

L8044 Hemi-facial prosthesis, provided by a nonphysician

L8045 Auricular prosthesis, provided by a nonphysician

L8046 Partial facial prosthesis, provided by a nonphysician

L8047 Nasal septal prosthesis, provided by a nonphysician

L8048 Unspecified maxillofacial prosthesis, by report, provided by a nonphysician

L8049 Repair or modification of maxillofacial prosthesis, labor component, 15 minute increments, provided by a nonphysician

TRUSSES

L8300 Truss, single with standard pad

L8310 Truss, double with standard pads

L8320 Truss, addition to standard pad, water pad

L8330 Truss, addition to standard pad, scrotal pad

PROSTHETIC SOCKS

L8400 Prosthetic sheath, below knee, each

L8410 Prosthetic sheath, above knee, each

L8415 Prosthetic sheath, upper limb, each

L8417 Prosthetic sheath/sock, including a gel cushion layer, below knee or above knee, each

L8420 Prosthetic sock, multiple ply, below knee, each

L8430 Prosthetic sock, multiple ply, above knee, each

L8435 Prosthetic sock, multiple ply, upper limb, each

L8440 Prosthetic shrinker, below knee, each

L8460 Prosthetic shrinker, above knee, each

L8465 Prosthetic shrinker, upper limb, each

L8470 Prosthetic sock, single ply, fitting, below knee, each

L8480 Prosthetic sock, single ply, fitting, above knee, each

L8485 Prosthetic sock, single ply, fitting, upper limb, each

L8499 Unlisted procedure for miscellaneous prosthetic services
Determine if an alternative HCPCS Level II or a CPT code better describes the service being reported. This code should be used only if a more specific code is unavailable.

LARYNX AND TRACHEA PROTHETICS AND ACCESSORIES

L8500 Artificial larynx, any type

L8501 Tracheostomy speaking valve

L8505 Artificial larynx replacement battery/accessory, any type

L8507 Tracheo-esophageal voice prosthesis, patient inserted, any type, each

L8509 Tracheo-esophageal voice prosthesis, inserted by a licensed health care provider, any type

L8510 Voice amplifier

L8511 Insert for indwelling tracheoesophageal prosthesis, with or without valve, replacement only, each

L8512 Gelatin capsules or equivalent, for use with tracheoesophageal voice prosthesis, replacement only, per 10

L8513 Cleaning device used with tracheoesophageal voice prosthesis, pipet, brush, or equal, replacement only, each

L8514 Tracheoesophageal puncture dilator, replacement only, each

L8515   Gelatin capsule, application device for use with tracheoesophageal voice prosthesis, each

BREAST IMPLANT

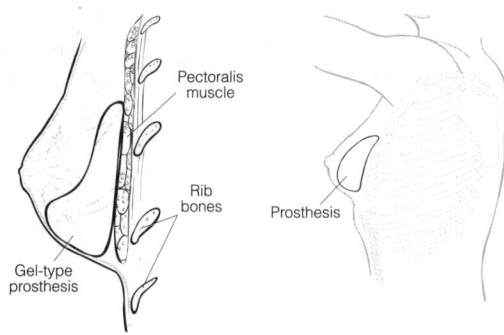

L8600   Implantable breast prosthesis, silicone or equal
Medicare covers implants inserted in post-mastectomy reconstruction in a breast cancer patient. Always report concurrent to the implant procedure.
MED: 100-4,4,190

URINARY BULKING AGENTS

L8603   Injectable bulking agent, collagen implant, urinary tract, 2.5 ml syringe, includes shipping and necessary supplies
MED: 100-4,4,190

L8604   Injectable bulking agent, dextranomer/hyaluronic acid copolymer implant, urinary tract, 1 ml, includes shipping and necessary supplies

L8605   Injectable bulking agent, dextranomer/hyaluronic acid copolymer implant, anal canal, 1 ml, includes shipping and necessary supplies

L8606   Injectable bulking agent, synthetic implant, urinary tract, 1 ml syringe, includes shipping and necessary supplies

EYE AND EAR IMPLANTS AND ACCESSORIES

L8609   Artificial cornea

L8610   Ocular implant
MED: 100-4,4,190

L8612   Aqueous shunt
MED: 100-4,4,190

L8613   Ossicula implant
MED: 100-4,4,190

L8614   Cochlear device, includes all internal and external components
A cochlear implant is covered by Medicare when the patient has bilateral sensorineural deafness.
MED: 100-4,4,190; 100-4,14,40.8
AHA: 4Q,'03,8; 3Q,'02,5

L8615   Headset/headpiece for use with cochlear implant device, replacement

L8616   Microphone for use with cochlear implant device, replacement

L8617   Transmitting coil for use with cochlear implant device, replacement

L8618   Transmitter cable for use with cochlear implant device, replacement

L8619   Cochlear implant, external speech processor and controller, integrated system, replacement
Medicare jurisdiction: local contractor.

L8621   Zinc air battery for use with cochlear implant device, replacement, each

L8622   Alkaline battery for use with cochlear implant device, any size, replacement, each

L8623   Lithium ion battery for use with cochlear implant device speech processor, other than ear level, replacement, each

L8624   Lithium ion battery for use with cochlear implant device speech processor, ear level, replacement, each

L8627   Cochlear implant, external speech processor, component, replacement

L8628   Cochlear implant, external controller component, replacement

L8629   Transmitting coil and cable, integrated, for use with cochlear implant device, replacement

UPPER EXTREMITY IMPLANTS

Bone is cut at the MP joint (arthroplasty)

Bone may be hollowed out in both metacarpal and phalangeal sides in preparation for a prosthesis

Prosthetic joint implant

Prosthesis in place

Metacarpophalangeal prosthetic implant

L8630   Metacarpophalangeal joint implant
MED: 100-4,4,190

L8631   Metacarpal phalangeal joint replacement, 2 or more pieces, metal (e.g., stainless steel or cobalt chrome), ceramic-like material (e.g., pyrocarbon), for surgical implantation (all sizes, includes entire system)

LOWER EXTREMITY IMPLANTS

L8641   Metatarsal joint implant
MED: 100-4,4,190

L8642   Hallux implant
MED: 100-4,4,190

INTERPHALANGEAL IMPLANTS

L8658   Interphalangeal joint spacer, silicone or equal, each
MED: 100-4,4,190

L8659   Interphalangeal finger joint replacement, 2 or more pieces, metal (e.g., stainless steel or cobalt chrome), ceramic-like material (e.g., pyrocarbon) for surgical implantation, any size

CARDIOVASCULAR IMPLANT

L8670   Vascular graft material, synthetic, implant
MED: 100-4,4,190

NEUROSTIMULATOR AND ACCESSORIES

L8679   Implantable neurostimulator, pulse generator, any type

L8680   Implantable neurostimulator electrode, each

L8681   Patient programmer (external) for use with implantable programmable neurostimulator pulse generator, replacement only

L8682   Implantable neurostimulator radiofrequency receiver

L8683   Radiofrequency transmitter (external) for use with implantable neurostimulator radiofrequency receiver

L8684   Radiofrequency transmitter (external) for use with implantable sacral root neurostimulator receiver for bowel and bladder management, replacement

L8685   Implantable neurostimulator pulse generator, single array, rechargeable, includes extension

L8686   Implantable neurostimulator pulse generator, single array, nonrechargeable, includes extension

L8687   Implantable neurostimulator pulse generator, dual array, rechargeable, includes extension

L8688   Implantable neurostimulator pulse generator, dual array, nonrechargeable, includes extension

L8689   External recharging system for battery (internal) for use with implantable neurostimulator, replacement only

MISCELLANEOUS PROSTHETICS AND ACCESSORIES

L8690   Auditory osseointegrated device, includes all internal and external components

MED: 100-4,14,40.8

L8691   Auditory osseointegrated device, external sound processor, replacement

L8692   Auditory osseointegrated device, external sound processor, used without osseointegration, body worn, includes headband or other means of external attachment

L8693   Auditory osseointegrated device abutment, any length, replacement only

L8695   External recharging system for battery (external) for use with implantable neurostimulator, replacement only

L8699   Prosthetic implant, not otherwise specified

Determine if an alternative HCPCS Level II or a CPT code better describes the service being reported. This code should be used only if a more specific code is unavailable.

MED: 100-4,4,190

L9900   Orthotic and prosthetic supply, accessory, and/or service component of another HCPCS L code

MEDICAL SERVICES M0000-M0301

OTHER MEDICAL SERVICES

M codes include office services, cellular therapy, prolotherapy, intragastric hypothermia, IV chelation therapy, and fabric wrapping of an abdominal aneurysm.

M0064 **Brief office visit for the sole purpose of monitoring or changing drug prescriptions used in the treatment of mental psychoneurotic and personality disorders**

MED: 100-1,3,30; 100-1,3,30.3; 100-4,12,210; 100-4,12,210.1

M0075 **Cellular therapy**

The therapeutic efficacy of injecting foreign proteins has not been established.

M0076 **Prolotherapy**

The therapeutic efficacy of prolotherapy and joint sclerotherapy has not been established.

M0100 **Intragastric hypothermia using gastric freezing**

Code with caution: This procedure is considered obsolete.

CARDIOVASCULAR SERVICES

M0300 **IV chelation therapy (chemical endarterectomy)**

Chelation therapy is considered experimental in the United States.

MED: 100-3,20.21; 100-3,20.22

M0301 **Fabric wrapping of abdominal aneurysm**

Code with caution: This procedure has largely been replaced with more effective treatment modalities. Submit documentation.

PATHOLOGY AND LABORATORY SERVICES P0000-P9999

P codes include chemistry, toxicology, and microbiology tests, screening Papanicolaou procedures, and various blood products.

CHEMISTRY AND TOXICOLOGY TESTS

P2028   Cephalin floculation, blood
> Code with caution: This test is considered obsolete. Submit documentation.

P2029   Congo red, blood
> Code with caution: This test is considered obsolete. Submit documentation.

P2031   Hair analysis (excluding arsenic)

P2033   Thymol turbidity, blood
> Code with caution: This test is considered obsolete. Submit documentation.

P2038   Mucoprotein, blood (seromucoid) (medical necessity procedure)
> Code with caution: This test is considered obsolete. Submit documentation.

PATHOLOGY SCREENING TESTS

P3000   Screening Papanicolaou smear, cervical or vaginal, up to 3 smears, by technician under physician supervision
> One Pap test is covered by Medicare every two years, unless the physician suspects cervical abnormalities and shortens the interval. See also G0123-G0124.

P3001   Screening Papanicolaou smear, cervical or vaginal, up to 3 smears, requiring interpretation by physician
> One Pap test is covered by Medicare every two years, unless the physician suspects cervical abnormalities and shortens the interval. See also G0123-G0124.

MICROBIOLOGY TESTS

P7001   Culture, bacterial, urine; quantitative, sensitivity study

MISCELLANEOUS

P9010   Blood (whole), for transfusion, per unit
> MED: 100-1,3,20.5; 100-1,3,20.5.2; 100-1,3,20.5.3; 100-2,1,10; 100-4,3,40.2.2

P9011   Blood, split unit
> MED: 100-1,3,20.5; 100-1,3,20.5.2; 100-1,3,20.5.3; 100-2,1,10; 100-4,3,40.2.2; 100-4,4,231.4

P9012   Cryoprecipitate, each unit
> MED: 100-2,1,10; 100-4,3,40.2.2

P9016   Red blood cells, leukocytes reduced, each unit
> MED: 100-2,1,10; 100-4,3,40.2.2

P9017   Fresh frozen plasma (single donor), frozen within 8 hours of collection, each unit
> MED: 100-2,1,10; 100-4,3,40.2.2

P9019   Platelets, each unit
> MED: 100-2,1,10; 100-4,3,40.2.2

P9020   Platelet rich plasma, each unit
> MED: 100-4,3,40.2.2

P9021   Red blood cells, each unit
> MED: 100-1,3,20.5; 100-1,3,20.5.2; 100-1,3,20.5.3; 100-2,1,10; 100-4,3,40.2.2

P9022   Red blood cells, washed, each unit
> MED: 100-1,3,20.5; 100-1,3,20.5.2; 100-1,3,20.5.3; 100-2,1,10; 100-4,3,40.2.2

P9023   Plasma, pooled multiple donor, solvent/detergent treated, frozen, each unit
> MED: 100-2,1,10; 100-4,3,40.2.2

P9031   Platelets, leukocytes reduced, each unit
> MED: 100-2,1,10; 100-4,3,40.2.2

P9032   Platelets, irradiated, each unit
> MED: 100-2,1,10; 100-4,3,40.2.2

P9033   Platelets, leukocytes reduced, irradiated, each unit
> MED: 100-2,1,10; 100-4,3,40.2.2

P9034   Platelets, pheresis, each unit
> MED: 100-2,1,10; 100-4,3,40.2.2

P9035   Platelets, pheresis, leukocytes reduced, each unit
> MED: 100-2,1,10; 100-4,3,40.2.2

P9036   Platelets, pheresis, irradiated, each unit
> MED: 100-2,1,10; 100-4,3,40.2.2

P9037   Platelets, pheresis, leukocytes reduced, irradiated, each unit
> MED: 100-2,1,10; 100-4,3,40.2.2

P9038   Red blood cells, irradiated, each unit
> MED: 100-1,3,20.5; 100-1,3,20.5.2; 100-1,3,20.5.3; 100-2,1,10; 100-4,3,40.2.2

P9039   Red blood cells, deglycerolized, each unit
> MED: 100-2,1,10; 100-4,3,40.2.2

P9040   Red blood cells, leukocytes reduced, irradiated, each unit
> MED: 100-2,1,10; 100-4,3,40.2.2

P9041   Infusion, albumin (human), 5%, 50 ml
> MED: 100-2,1,10; 100-4,3,40.2.2

P9043   Infusion, plasma protein fraction (human), 5%, 50 ml
> MED: 100-2,1,10; 100-4,3,40.2.2

P9044   Plasma, cryoprecipitate reduced, each unit
> MED: 100-2,1,10; 100-4,3,40.2.2

P9045   Infusion, albumin (human), 5%, 250 ml
> MED: 100-2,1,10; 100-4,3,40.2.2

P9046   Infusion, albumin (human), 25%, 20 ml
> MED: 100-2,1,10; 100-4,3,40.2.2

P9047   Infusion, albumin (human), 25%, 50 ml
> MED: 100-2,1,10; 100-4,3,40.2.2

P9048   Infusion, plasma protein fraction (human), 5%, 250 ml
> MED: 100-2,1,10; 100-4,3,40.2.2

P9050   Granulocytes, pheresis, each unit
> MED: 100-2,1,10; 100-4,3,40.2.2

P9051   Whole blood or red blood cells, leukocytes reduced, CMV-negative, each unit
> MED: 100-2,1,10; 100-4,3,40.2.2

P9052   Platelets, HLA-matched leukocytes reduced, apheresis/pheresis, each unit
> MED: 100-2,1,10; 100-4,3,40.2.2

P9053   Platelets, pheresis, leukocytes reduced, CMV-negative, irradiated, each unit
> MED: 100-2,1,10; 100-4,3,40.2.2

P9054   Whole blood or red blood cells, leukocytes reduced, frozen, deglycerol, washed, each unit
> MED: 100-2,1,10; 100-4,3,40.2.2

P9055   Platelets, leukocytes reduced, CMV-negative, apheresis/pheresis, each unit
> MED: 100-2,1,10; 100-4,3,40.2.2

P9056   Whole blood, leukocytes reduced, irradiated, each unit
> MED: 100-2,1,10; 100-4,3,40.2.2

P9057   Red blood cells, frozen/deglycerolized/washed, leukocytes reduced, irradiated, each unit
> MED: 100-2,1,10; 100-4,3,40.2.2

P9058   Red blood cells, leukocytes reduced, CMV-negative, irradiated, each unit
> MED: 100-2,1,10; 100-4,3,40.2.2

P9059 Fresh frozen plasma between 8-24 hours of collection, each unit
MED: 100-2,1,10; 100-4,3,40.2.2

P9060 Fresh frozen plasma, donor retested, each unit
MED: 100-2,1,10; 100-4,3,40.2.2

P9603 Travel allowance, one way in connection with medically necessary laboratory specimen collection drawn from homebound or nursing homebound patient; prorated miles actually travelled
MED: 100-4,16,60; 100-4,16,60.2

P9604 Travel allowance, one way in connection with medically necessary laboratory specimen collection drawn from homebound or nursing homebound patient; prorated trip charge
MED: 100-4,16,60; 100-4,16,60.2

P9612 Catheterization for collection of specimen, single patient, all places of service
MED: 100-4,16,60

P9615 Catheterization for collection of specimen(s) (multiple patients)
MED: 100-4,16,60; 100-4,16,60.1.4

Q CODES (TEMPORARY) Q0035 - Q9968

Temporary Q codes are used to pay health care providers for supplies, drugs, and biologicals to which no permanent code has been assigned.

Q0035 Cardiokymography

Covered only in conjunction with electrocardiographic stress testing in male patients with atypical angina or nonischemic chest pain, or female patients with angina.

Q0081 Infusion therapy, using other than chemotherapeutic drugs, per visit

AHA: 4Q,'02,7; 1Q,'02,7

Q0083 Chemotherapy administration by other than infusion technique only (e.g., subcutaneous, intramuscular, push), per visit

Q0084 Chemotherapy administration by infusion technique only, per visit

Q0085 Chemotherapy administration by both infusion technique and other technique(s) (e.g. subcutaneous, intramuscular, push), per visit

Q0091 Screening Papanicolaou smear; obtaining, preparing and conveyance of cervical or vaginal smear to laboratory

One pap test is covered by Medicare every two years for low risk patients and every one year for high risk patients. Q0091 can be reported with an E/M code when a separately identifiable E/M service is provided.

MED: 100-3, 190.2

AHA: 4Q,'02,8

Q0092 Set-up portable x-ray equipment

MED: 100-4,13,90.4

Q0111 Wet mounts, including preparations of vaginal, cervical or skin specimens

Q0112 All potassium hydroxide (KOH) preparations

Q0113 Pinworm examinations

Q0114 Fern test

Q0115 Postcoital direct, qualitative examinations of vaginal or cervical mucous

Q0138 Injection, ferumoxytol, for treatment of iron deficiency anemia, 1 mg (non-ESRD use)

Use this code for Feraheme.

Q0139 Injection, ferumoxytol, for treatment of iron deficiency anemia, 1 mg (for ESRD on dialysis)

Use this code for Feraheme.

Q0144 Azithromycin dihydrate, oral, capsules/powder, 1 g

Use this code for Zithromax, Zithromax Z-PAK.

Q0161 Chlorpromazine hydrochloride, 5 mg, oral, FDA approved prescription anti-emetic, for use as a complete therapeutic substitute for an IV anti-emetic at the time of chemotherapy treatment, not to exceed a 48 hour dosage regimen

Q0162 Ondansetron 1 mg, oral, FDA approved prescription antiemetic, for use as a complete therapeutic substitute for an IV antiemetic at the time of chemotherapy treatment, not to exceed a 48 hour dosage regimen

Use this code for Zofran, Zuplenz.

Q0163 Diphenhydramine HCl, 50 mg, oral, FDA approved prescription antiemetic, for use as a complete therapeutic substitute for an IV antiemetic at time of chemotherapy treatment not to exceed a 48-hour dosage regimen

See also J1200. Medicare covers at the time of chemotherapy if regimen doesn't exceed 48 hours. Submit on the same claim as the chemotherapy. Use this code for Truxadryl.

AHA: 1Q,'02,2

Q0164 Prochlorperazine maleate, 5 mg, oral, FDA approved prescription antiemetic, for use as a complete therapeutic substitute for an IV antiemetic at the time of chemotherapy treatment, not to exceed a 48-hour dosage regimen

Medicare covers at the time of chemotherapy if regimen doesn't exceed 48 hours. Submit on the same claim as the chemotherapy. Use this code for Compazine.

Q0166 Granisetron HCl, 1 mg, oral, FDA approved prescription antiemetic, for use as a complete therapeutic substitute for an IV antiemetic at the time of chemotherapy treatment, not to exceed a 24-hour dosage regimen

Medicare covers at the time of chemotherapy if regimen doesn't exceed 48 hours. Submit on the same claim as the chemotherapy. Use this code for Kytril.

Q0167 Dronabinol, 2.5 mg, oral, FDA approved prescription antiemetic, for use as a complete therapeutic substitute for an IV antiemetic at the time of chemotherapy treatment, not to exceed a 48-hour dosage regimen

Medicare covers at the time of chemotherapy if regimen doesn't exceed 48 hours. Submit on the same claim as the chemotherapy. Use this code for Marinol.

Q0169 Promethazine HCl, 12.5 mg, oral, FDA approved prescription antiemetic, for use as a complete therapeutic substitute for an IV antiemetic at the time of chemotherapy treatment, not to exceed a 48-hour dosage regimen

Medicare covers at the time of chemotherapy if regimen doesn't exceed 48 hours. Submit on the same claim as the chemotherapy. Use this code for Phenergan, Amergan.

Q0173 Trimethobenzamide HCl, 250 mg, oral, FDA approved prescription antiemetic, for use as a complete therapeutic substitute for an IV antiemetic at the time of chemotherapy treatment, not to exceed a 48-hour dosage regimen

Medicare covers at the time of chemotherapy if regimen doesn't exceed 48 hours. Submit on the same claim as the chemotherapy. Use this code for Tebamide, T-Gen, Ticon, Tigan, Triban, Thimazide.

Q0174 Thiethylperazine maleate, 10 mg, oral, FDA approved prescription antiemetic, for use as a complete therapeutic substitute for an IV antiemetic at the time of chemotherapy treatment, not to exceed a 48-hour dosage regimen

Medicare covers at the time of chemotherapy if regimen doesn't exceed 48 hours. Submit on the same claim as the chemotherapy.

Q0175 Perphenazine, 4 mg, oral, FDA approved prescription antiemetic, for use as a complete therapeutic substitute for an IV antiemetic at the time of chemotherapy treatment, not to exceed a 48 hour dosage regimen

Medicare covers at the time of chemotherapy if regimen doesn't exceed 48 hours. Submit on the same claim as the chemotherapy. Use this code for Trilifon.

Q0177 Hydroxyzine pamoate, 25 mg, oral, FDA approved prescription antiemetic, for use as a complete therapeutic substitute for an IV antiemetic at the time of chemotherapy treatment, not to exceed a 48-hour dosage regimen

Medicare covers at the time of chemotherapy if regimen doesn't exceed 48 hours. Submit on the same claim as the chemotherapy. Use this code for Vistaril.

Q0180 Dolasetron mesylate, 100 mg, oral, FDA approved prescription antiemetic, for use as a complete therapeutic substitute for an IV antiemetic at the time of chemotherapy treatment, not to exceed a 24-hour dosage regimen

Medicare covers at the time of chemotherapy if regimen doesn't exceed 24 hours. Submit on the same claim as the chemotherapy. Use this code for Anzemet.

Q0181   Unspecified oral dosage form, FDA approved prescription antiemetic, for use as a complete therapeutic substitute for an IV antiemetic at the time of chemotherapy treatment, not to exceed a 48-hour dosage regimen

Medicare covers at the time of chemotherapy if regimen doesn't exceed 48-hours. Submit on the same claim as the chemotherapy.

Q0478   Power adapter for use with electric or electric/pneumatic ventricular assist device, vehicle type

Q0479   Power module for use with electric or electric/pneumatic ventricular assist device, replacement only

Q0480   Driver for use with pneumatic ventricular assist device, replacement only

AHA: 3Q,'05,2

Q0481   Microprocessor control unit for use with electric ventricular assist device, replacement only

AHA: 3Q,'05,2

Q0482   Microprocessor control unit for use with electric/pneumatic combination ventricular assist device, replacement only

AHA: 3Q,'05,2

Q0483   Monitor/display module for use with electric ventricular assist device, replacement only

AHA: 3Q,'05,2

Q0484   Monitor/display module for use with electric or electric/pneumatic ventricular assist device, replacement only

AHA: 3Q,'05,2

Q0485   Monitor control cable for use with electric ventricular assist device, replacement only

AHA: 3Q,'05,2

Q0486   Monitor control cable for use with electric/pneumatic ventricular assist device, replacement only

AHA: 3Q,'05,2

Q0487   Leads (pneumatic/electrical) for use with any type electric/pneumatic ventricular assist device, replacement only

AHA: 3Q,'05,2

Q0488   Power pack base for use with electric ventricular assist device, replacement only

AHA: 3Q,'05,2

Q0489   Power pack base for use with electric/pneumatic ventricular assist device, replacement only

AHA: 3Q,'05,2

Q0490   Emergency power source for use with electric ventricular assist device, replacement only

AHA: 3Q,'05,2

Q0491   Emergency power source for use with electric/pneumatic ventricular assist device, replacement only

AHA: 3Q,'05,2

Q0492   Emergency power supply cable for use with electric ventricular assist device, replacement only

AHA: 3Q,'05,2

Q0493   Emergency power supply cable for use with electric/pneumatic ventricular assist device, replacement only

AHA: 3Q,'05,2

Q0494   Emergency hand pump for use with electric or electric/pneumatic ventricular assist device, replacement only

AHA: 3Q,'05,2

Q0495   Battery/power pack charger for use with electric or electric/pneumatic ventricular assist device, replacement only

AHA: 3Q,'05,2

Q0496   Battery, other than lithium-ion, for use with electric or electric/pneumatic ventricular assist device, replacement only

AHA: 3Q,'05,2

Q0497   Battery clips for use with electric or electric/pneumatic ventricular assist device, replacement only

AHA: 3Q,'05,2

Q0498   Holster for use with electric or electric/pneumatic ventricular assist device, replacement only

AHA: 3Q,'05,2

Q0499   Belt/vest/bag for use to carry external peripheral components of any type ventricular assist device, replacement only

AHA: 3Q,'05,2

Q0500   Filters for use with electric or electric/pneumatic ventricular assist device, replacement only

The base unit for this code is for each filter.

AHA: 3Q,'05,2

Q0501   Shower cover for use with electric or electric/pneumatic ventricular assist device, replacement only

AHA: 3Q,'05,2

Q0502   Mobility cart for pneumatic ventricular assist device, replacement only

AHA: 3Q,'05,2

Q0503   Battery for pneumatic ventricular assist device, replacement only, each

AHA: 3Q,'05,2

Q0504   Power adapter for pneumatic ventricular assist device, replacement only, vehicle type

AHA: 3Q,'05,2

Q0506   Battery, lithium-ion, for use with electric or electric/pneumatic ventricular assist device, replacement only

Q0507   Miscellaneous supply or accessory for use with an external ventricular assist device

Q0508   Miscellaneous supply or accessory for use with an implanted ventricular assist device

Q0509   Miscellaneous supply or accessory for use with any implanted ventricular assist device for which payment was not made under Medicare Part A

Q0510   Pharmacy supply fee for initial immunosuppressive drug(s), first month following transplant

Q0511   Pharmacy supply fee for oral anticancer, oral antiemetic, or immunosuppressive drug(s); for the first prescription in a 30-day period

Q0512   Pharmacy supply fee for oral anticancer, oral antiemetic, or immunosuppressive drug(s); for a subsequent prescription in a 30-day period

Q0513   Pharmacy dispensing fee for inhalation drug(s); per 30 days

Q0514   Pharmacy dispensing fee for inhalation drug(s); per 90 days

Q0515   Injection, sermorelin acetate, 1 mcg

Q1004   New technology, intraocular lens, category 4 as defined in Federal Register notice

Q1005   New technology, intraocular lens, category 5 as defined in Federal Register notice

Q2004   Irrigation solution for treatment of bladder calculi, for example renacidin, per 500 ml

Q2009   Injection, fosphenytoin, 50 mg phenytoin equivalent

Use this code for Cerebyx.

Q2017   Injection, teniposide, 50 mg

Use this code for Vumon.

Q2026   Injection, Radiesse, 0.1 ml

MED: 100-4,32,260.2.2

Q2028   Injection, sculptra, 0.5 mg

Q2034   Influenza virus vaccine, split virus, for intramuscular use (Agriflu)

Q2035   Influenza virus vaccine, split virus, when administered to individuals 3 years of age and older, for intramuscular use (AFLURIA)

MED: 100-2,15,50.4.4.2

Q2036 Influenza virus vaccine, split virus, when administered to individuals 3 years of age and older, for intramuscular use (FLULAVAL)

Q2037 Influenza virus vaccine, split virus, when administered to individuals 3 years of age and older, for intramuscular use (FLUVIRIN)

Q2038 Influenza virus vaccine, split virus, when administered to individuals 3 years of age and older, for intramuscular use (Fluzone)

Q2039 Influenza virus vaccine, split virus, when administered to individuals 3 years of age and older, for intramuscular use (not otherwise specified)

Q2043 Sipuleucel-T, minimum of 50 million autologous cd54+ cells activated with PAP-GM-CSF, including leukapheresis and all other preparatory procedures, per infusion
Use this code for PROVENGE.

Q2049 Injection, doxorubicin hydrochloride, liposomal, imported Lipodox, 10 mg

Q2050 Injection, doxorubicin hydrochloride, liposomal, not otherwise specified, 10 mg

Q2052 Services, supplies and accessories used in the home under the Medicare intravenous immune globulin (IVIG) demonstration

Q3001 Radioelements for brachytherapy, any type, each

Q3014 Telehealth originating site facility fee
MED: 100-4,12,190.6

Q3027 Injection, interferon beta-1a, 1 mcg for intramuscular use
Use this code for Avonex

Q3028 Injection, interferon beta-1a, 1 mcg for subcutaneous use
Use this code for Rebif

Q3031 Collagen skin test

Q4001 Casting supplies, body cast adult, with or without head, plaster
MED: 100-4,20,170

Q4002 Cast supplies, body cast adult, with or without head, fiberglass
MED: 100-4,20,170

Q4003 Cast supplies, shoulder cast, adult (11 years +), plaster
MED: 100-4,20,170

Q4004 Cast supplies, shoulder cast, adult (11 years +), fiberglass
MED: 100-4,20,170

Q4005 Cast supplies, long arm cast, adult (11 years +), plaster
MED: 100-4,20,170

Q4006 Cast supplies, long arm cast, adult (11 years +), fiberglass
MED: 100-4,20,170

Q4007 Cast supplies, long arm cast, pediatric (0-10 years), plaster
MED: 100-4,20,170

Q4008 Cast supplies, long arm cast, pediatric (0-10 years), fiberglass
MED: 100-4,20,170

Q4009 Cast supplies, short arm cast, adult (11 years +), plaster
MED: 100-4,20,170

Q4010 Cast supplies, short arm cast, adult (11 years +), fiberglass
MED: 100-4,20,170

Q4011 Cast supplies, short arm cast, pediatric (0-10 years), plaster
MED: 100-4,20,170

Q4012 Cast supplies, short arm cast, pediatric (0-10 years), fiberglass
MED: 100-4,20,170

Q4013 Cast supplies, gauntlet cast (includes lower forearm and hand), adult (11 years +), plaster
MED: 100-4,20,170

Q4014 Cast supplies, gauntlet cast (includes lower forearm and hand), adult (11 years +), fiberglass
MED: 100-4,20,170

Q4015 Cast supplies, gauntlet cast (includes lower forearm and hand), pediatric (0-10 years), plaster
MED: 100-4,20,170

Q4016 Cast supplies, gauntlet cast (includes lower forearm and hand), pediatric (0-10 years), fiberglass
MED: 100-4,20,170

Q4017 Cast supplies, long arm splint, adult (11 years +), plaster
MED: 100-4,20,170

Q4018 Cast supplies, long arm splint, adult (11 years +), fiberglass
MED: 100-4,20,170

Q4019 Cast supplies, long arm splint, pediatric (0-10 years), plaster
MED: 100-4,20,170

Q4020 Cast supplies, long arm splint, pediatric (0-10 years), fiberglass
MED: 100-4,20,170

Q4021 Cast supplies, short arm splint, adult (11 years +), plaster
MED: 100-4,20,170

Q4022 Cast supplies, short arm splint, adult (11 years +), fiberglass
MED: 100-4,20,170

Q4023 Cast supplies, short arm splint, pediatric (0-10 years), plaster
MED: 100-4,20,170

Q4024 Cast supplies, short arm splint, pediatric (0-10 years), fiberglass
MED: 100-4,20,170

Q4025 Cast supplies, hip spica (one or both legs), adult (11 years +), plaster
MED: 100-4,20,170

Q4026 Cast supplies, hip spica (one or both legs), adult (11 years +), fiberglass
MED: 100-4,20,170

Q4027 Cast supplies, hip spica (one or both legs), pediatric (0-10 years), plaster
MED: 100-4,20,170

Q4028 Cast supplies, hip spica (one or both legs), pediatric (0-10 years), fiberglass
MED: 100-4,20,170

Q4029 Cast supplies, long leg cast, adult (11 years +), plaster
MED: 100-4,20,170

Q4030 Cast supplies, long leg cast, adult (11 years +), fiberglass
MED: 100-4,20,170

Q4031 Cast supplies, long leg cast, pediatric (0-10 years), plaster
MED: 100-4,20,170

Q4032 Cast supplies, long leg cast, pediatric (0-10 years), fiberglass
MED: 100-4,20,170

Q4033 Cast supplies, long leg cylinder cast, adult (11 years +), plaster
MED: 100-4,20,170

Q4034 Cast supplies, long leg cylinder cast, adult (11 years +), fiberglass
MED: 100-4,20,170

Q4035 Cast supplies, long leg cylinder cast, pediatric (0-10 years), plaster
MED: 100-4,20,170

Q4036 Cast supplies, long leg cylinder cast, pediatric (0-10 years), fiberglass
MED: 100-4,20,170

Q4037 Cast supplies, short leg cast, adult (11 years +), plaster
MED: 100-4,20,170

Q4038 Cast supplies, short leg cast, adult (11 years +), fiberglass
MED: 100-4,20,170

Q4039 Cast supplies, short leg cast, pediatric (0-10 years), plaster
MED: 100-4,20,170

Q4040 Cast supplies, short leg cast, pediatric (0-10 years), fiberglass
MED: 100-4,20,170

Q4041 Cast supplies, long leg splint, adult (11 years +), plaster
MED: 100-4,20,170

Q4042 Cast supplies, long leg splint, adult (11 years +), fiberglass
MED: 100-4,20,170

Q4043 Cast supplies, long leg splint, pediatric (0-10 years), plaster
MED: 100-4,20,170

Q4044 Cast supplies, long leg splint, pediatric (0-10 years), fiberglass
MED: 100-4,20,170

Q4045 Cast supplies, short leg splint, adult (11 years +), plaster
MED: 100-4,20,170

Q4046 Cast supplies, short leg splint, adult (11 years +), fiberglass
MED: 100-4,20,170

Q4047 Cast supplies, short leg splint, pediatric (0-10 years), plaster
MED: 100-4,20,170

Q4048 Cast supplies, short leg splint, pediatric (0-10 years), fiberglass
MED: 100-4,20,170

Q4049 Finger splint, static
MED: 100-4,20,170

Q4050 Cast supplies, for unlisted types and materials of casts
MED: 100-4,20,170

Q4051 Splint supplies, miscellaneous (includes thermoplastics, strapping, fasteners, padding and other supplies)
MED: 100-4,20,170

Q4074 Iloprost, inhalation solution, FDA-approved final product, noncompounded, administered through DME, unit dose form, up to 20 mcg

Q4081 Injection, epoetin alfa, 100 units (for ESRD on dialysis)
MED: 100-4,8,60.4; 100-4,8,60.4.1; 100-4,8,60.4.2; 100-4,8,60.4.4; 100-4,8,60.4.4.1; 100-4,8,60.4.4.2; 100-4,8,60.4.5.1

Q4082 Drug or biological, not otherwise classified, Part B drug competitive acquisition program (CAP)

Q4100 Skin substitute, not otherwise specified

Q4101 Apligraf, per sq cm

Q4102 Oasis wound matrix, per sq cm

Q4103 Oasis burn matrix, per sq cm

Q4104 Integra bilayer matrix wound dressing (BMWD), per sq cm

Q4105 Integra dermal regeneration template (DRT), per sq cm

Q4106 Dermagraft, per sq cm

Q4107 GRAFTJACKET, per sq cm

Q4108 Integra matrix, per sq cm

Q4110 PriMatrix, per sq cm

Q4111 GammaGraft, per sq cm

Q4112 Cymetra, injectable, 1 cc

Q4113 GRAFTJACKET XPRESS, injectable, 1cc

Q4114 Integra flowable wound matrix, injectable, 1 cc

Q4115 AlloSkin, per sq cm

Q4116 AlloDerm, per sq cm

Q4117 HYALOMATRIX, per sq cm

Q4118 MatriStem micromatrix, 1 mg

Q4119 MatriStem Wound Matrix, PSMX, RS, or PSM, per sq cm

Q4120 MatriStem burn matrix, per sq cm

Q4121 TheraSkin, per sq cm

Q4122 DermACELL, per sq cm

Q4123 AlloSkin RT, per sq cm

Q4124 OASIS ultra tri-layer wound matrix, per sq cm

Q4125 Arthroflex, per sq cm

Q4126 MemoDerm, DermaSpan, TranZgraft or InteguPly, per sq cm

Q4127 Talymed, per sq cm

Q4128 FlexHD, AllopatchHD, or Matrix HD, per sq cm

Q4129 Unite biomatrix, per sq cm

Q4130 Strattice TM, per sq cm

Q4131 EpiFix, per sq cm

Q4132 Grafix core, per sq cm

Q4133 Grafix prime, per sq cm

Q4134 hMatrix, per sq cm

Q4135 Mediskin, per sq cm

Q4136 E-Z Derm, per sq cm

Q4137 Amnioexcel or biodexcel, per sq cm

Q4138 Biodfence dryflex, per sq cm

Q4139 Amniomatrix or biodmatrix, injectable, 1 cc

Q4140 Biodfence, per sq cm

Q4141 Alloskin AC, per sq cm

Q4142 XCM biologic tissue matrix, per sq cm

Q4143 Repriza, per sq cm

Q4145 Epifix, injectable, 1 mg

Q4146 Tensix, per sq cm

Q4147 Architect extracellular matrix, per sq cm

Q4148 Neox 1k, per sq cm

Q4149 Excellagen, 0.1 cc

Q5001 Hospice or home health care provided in patient's home/residence
MED: 100-4,10,40.2; 100-4,11,10; 100-4,11,30.3

Q5002 Hospice or home health care provided in assisted living facility

Q5003 Hospice care provided in nursing long-term care facility (LTC) or nonskilled nursing facility (NF)

Q5004 Hospice care provided in skilled nursing facility (SNF)

Q5005 Hospice care provided in inpatient hospital

Q5006 Hospice care provided in inpatient hospice facility

Q5007 Hospice care provided in long-term care facility

Q5008 Hospice care provided in inpatient psychiatric facility

Q5009 Hospice or home health care provided in place not otherwise specified (NOS)
MED: 100-4,10,40.2

Q5010 Hospice home care provided in a hospice facility

Q9951 Low osmolar contrast material, 400 or greater mg/ml iodine concentration, per ml
MED: 100-4,13,40

Q9953 Injection, iron-based magnetic resonance contrast agent, per ml

Q9954 Oral magnetic resonance contrast agent, per 100 ml

Q9955 Injection, perflexane lipid microspheres, per ml

Q9956 Injection, octafluoropropane microspheres, per ml
Use this code for Optison

Q9957 Injection, perflutren lipid microspheres, per ml
Use this code for Definity

Q9958 High osmolar contrast material, up to 149 mg/ml iodine concentration, per ml
MED: 100-4,13,40
AHA: 3Q,'05,7

Q Codes (Temporary)

Q9959 — Q9969

Q9959 High osmolar contrast material, 150-199 mg/ml iodine concentration, per ml

AHA: 3Q,'05,7

Q9960 High osmolar contrast material, 200-249 mg/ml iodine concentration, per ml

AHA: 3Q,'05,7

Q9961 High osmolar contrast material, 250-299 mg/ml iodine concentration, per ml

AHA: 3Q,'05,7

Q9962 High osmolar contrast material, 300-349 mg/ml iodine concentration, per ml

AHA: 3Q,'05,7

Q9963 High osmolar contrast material, 350-399 mg/ml iodine concentration, per ml

AHA: 3Q,'05,7

Q9964 High osmolar contrast material, 400 or greater mg/ml iodine concentration, per ml

AHA: 3Q,'05,7

Q9965 Low osmolar contrast material, 100-199 mg/ml iodine concentration, per ml

Use this code for Omnipaque 140, Omnipaque 180, Optiray 160, Optiray 140, ULTRAVIST 150

Q9966 Low osmolar contrast material, 200-299 mg/ml iodine concentration, per ml

Use this code for Omnipaque 240, Optiray 240, ULTRAVIST 240

Q9967 Low osmolar contrast material, 300-399 mg/ml iodine concentration, per ml

Use this code for Omnipaque 300, Omnipaque 350, Optiray, Optiray 300, Optiray 320, Oxilan 300, Oxilan 350, ULTRAVIST 300, ULTRAVIST 370

Q9968 Injection, nonradioactive, noncontrast, visualization adjunct (e.g., methylene blue, isosulfan blue), 1 mg

Q9969 Tc-99m from nonhighly enriched uranium source, full cost recovery add-on, per study dose

DIAGNOSTIC RADIOLOGY SERVICES R0000-R5999

R codes are used for the transportation of portable x-ray and/or EKG equipment.

R0070   **Transportation of portable x-ray equipment and personnel to home or nursing home, per trip to facility or location, one patient seen**

Only a single, reasonable transportation charge is allowed for each trip the portable x-ray supplier makes to a location. When more than one patient is x-rayed at the same location, prorate the single allowable transport charge among all patients.

MED: 100-4,13,90.3

R0075   **Transportation of portable x-ray equipment and personnel to home or nursing home, per trip to facility or location, more than one patient seen**

Only a single, reasonable transportation charge is allowed for each trip the portable x-ray supplier makes to a location. When more than one patient is x-rayed at the same location, prorate the single allowable transport charge among all patients.

MED: 100-4,13,90.3

R0076   **Transportation of portable EKG to facility or location, per patient**

Only a single, reasonable transportation charge is allowed for each trip the portable EKG supplier makes to a location. When more than one patient is tested at the same location, prorate the single allowable transport charge among all patients.

MED: 100-4,13,90.3

TEMPORARY NATIONAL CODES (NON-MEDICARE) S0000-S9999

The S codes are used by the Blue Cross/Blue Shield Association (BCBSA) and the Health Insurance Association of America (HIAA) to report drugs, services, and supplies for which there are no national codes but for which codes are needed by the private sector to implement policies, programs, or claims processing. They are for the purpose of meeting the particular needs of the private sector. These codes are also used by the Medicaid program, but they are not payable by Medicare.

S0012 Butorphanol tartrate, nasal spray, 25 mg
Use this code for Stadol NS.

S0014 Tacrine HCl, 10 mg
Use this code for Cognex.

S0017 Injection, aminocaproic acid, 5 g
Use this code for Amicar.

S0020 Injection, bupivicaine HCl, 30 ml
Use this code for Marcaine, Sensorcaine.

S0021 Injection, cefoperazone sodium, 1 g
Use this code for Cefobid.

S0023 Injection, cimetidine HCl, 300 mg
Use this code for Tagamet HCl.

S0028 Injection, famotidine, 20 mg
Use this code for Pepcid.

S0030 Injection, metronidazole, 500 mg
Use this code for Flagyl IV RTU.

S0032 Injection, nafcillin sodium, 2 g
Use this code for Nallpen, Unipen.

S0034 Injection, ofloxacin, 400 mg
Use this code for Floxin IV.

S0039 Injection, sulfamethoxazole and trimethoprim, 10 ml
Use this code for Bactrim IV, Septra IV, SMZ-TMP, Sulfutrim.

S0040 Injection, ticarcillin disodium and clavulanate potassium, 3.1 g
Use this code for Timentin.

S0073 Injection, aztreonam, 500 mg
Use this code for Azactam.

S0074 Injection, cefotetan disodium, 500 mg
Use this code for Cefotan.

S0077 Injection, clindamycin phosphate, 300 mg
Use this code for Cleocin Phosphate.

S0078 Injection, fosphenytoin sodium, 750 mg
Use this code for Cerebryx.

S0080 Injection, pentamidine isethionate, 300 mg
Use this code for NebuPent, Pentam 300, Pentacarinat. See also code J2545.

S0081 Injection, piperacillin sodium, 500 mg
Use this code for Pipracil.

S0088 Imatinib, 100 mg
Use this code for Gleevec.

S0090 Sildenafil citrate, 25 mg
Use this code for Viagra.

S0091 Granisetron HCl, 1 mg (for circumstances falling under the Medicare statute, use Q0166)
Use this code for Kytril.

S0092 Injection, hydromorphone HCl, 250 mg (loading dose for infusion pump)
Use this code for Dilaudid, Hydromorphone. See also J1170.

S0093 Injection, morphine sulfate, 500 mg (loading dose for infusion pump)
Use this code for Duramorph, MS Contin, Morphine Sulfate. See also J2270, J2271, J2275.

S0104 Zidovudine, oral, 100 mg
See also J3485 for Retrovir.

S0106 Bupropion HCl sustained release tablet, 150 mg, per bottle of 60 tablets
Use this code for Wellbutrin SR tablets.

S0108 Mercaptopurine, oral, 50 mg
Use this code for Purinethol oral.

S0109 Methadone, oral, 5 mg
Use this code for Dolophine.

S0117 Tretinoin, topical, 5 g

S0119 Ondansetron, oral, 4 mg (for circumstances falling under the Medicare statute, use HCPCS Q code)
Use this code for Zofran, Zuplenz.

S0122 Injection, menotropins, 75 IU
Use this code for Humegon, Pergonal, Repronex.

S0126 Injection, follitropin alfa, 75 IU
Use this code for Gonal-F.

S0128 Injection, follitropin beta, 75 IU
Use this code for Follistim.

S0132 Injection, ganirelix acetate, 250 mcg
Use this code for Antagon.

S0136 Clozapine, 25 mg
Use this code for Clozaril.

S0137 Didanosine (ddI), 25 mg
Use this code for Videx.

S0138 Finasteride, 5 mg
Use this code for Propecia (oral), Proscar (oral).

S0139 Minoxidil, 10 mg

S0140 Saquinavir, 200 mg
Use this code for Fortovase (oral), Invirase (oral).

S0142 Colistimethate sodium, inhalation solution administered through DME, concentrated form, per mg

S0145 Injection, pegylated interferon alfa-2a, 180 mcg per ml
Use this code for Pegasys.

S0148 Injection, pegylated interferon alfa-2B, 10 mcg

S0155 Sterile dilutant for epoprostenol, 50 ml
Use this code for Flolan.

S0156 Exemestane, 25 mg
Use this code for Aromasin.

S0157 Becaplermin gel 0.01%, 0.5 gm
Use this code for Regraex Gel.

S0160 Dextroamphetamine sulfate, 5 mg

S0164 Injection, pantoprazole sodium, 40 mg
Use this code for Protonix IV.

S0166 Injection, olanzapine, 2.5 mg
Use this code for Zyprexa.

S0169 Calcitrol, 0.25 mcg
Use this code for Calcijex.

S0170 Anastrozole, oral, 1 mg
Use this code for Arimidex.

S0171 Injection, bumetanide, 0.5 mg
Use this code for Bumex.

S0172 Chlorambucil, oral, 2 mg
Use this code for Leukeran.

S0174 Dolasetron mesylate, oral 50 mg (for circumstances falling under the Medicare statute, use Q0180)
Use this code for Anzemet.

S0175 Flutamide, oral, 125 mg
Use this code for Eulexin.

S0176 Hydroxyurea, oral, 500 mg
Use this code for Droxia, Hydrea, Mylocel.

S0177 Levamisole HCl, oral, 50 mg
Use this code for Ergamisol.

S0178 Lomustine, oral, 10 mg
Use this code for Ceenu.

S0179 Megestrol acetate, oral, 20 mg
Use this code for Megace.

S0182 Procarbazine HCl, oral, 50 mg
Use this code for Matulane.

S0183 Prochlorperazine maleate, oral, 5 mg (for circumstances falling under the Medicare statute, use Q0164-Q0165)
Use this code for Compazine.

S0187 Tamoxifen citrate, oral, 10 mg
Use this code for Nolvadex.

S0189 Testosterone pellet, 75 mg

S0190 Mifepristone, oral, 200 mg
Use this code for Mifoprex 200 mg oral.

S0191 Misoprostol, oral, 200 mcg

S0194 Dialysis/stress vitamin supplement, oral, 100 capsules

S0195 Pneumococcal conjugate vaccine, polyvalent, intramuscular, for children from 5 years to 9 years of age who have not previously received the vaccine
Use this code for Pneumovax II.

S0197 Prenatal vitamins, 30-day supply

S0199 Medically induced abortion by oral ingestion of medication including all associated services and supplies (e.g., patient counseling, office visits, confirmation of pregnancy by HCG, ultrasound to confirm duration of pregnancy, ultrasound to confirm completion of abortion) except drugs

S0201 Partial hospitalization services, less than 24 hours, per diem

S0207 Paramedic intercept, nonhospital-based ALS service (nonvoluntary), nontransport

S0208 Paramedic intercept, hospital-based ALS service (nonvoluntary), nontransport

S0209 Wheelchair van, mileage, per mile

S0215 Nonemergency transportation; mileage, per mile
See also codes A0021-A0999 for transportation.

S0220 Medical conference by a physician with interdisciplinary team of health professionals or representatives of community agencies to coordinate activities of patient care (patient is present); approximately 30 minutes

S0221 Medical conference by a physician with interdisciplinary team of health professionals or representatives of community agencies to coordinate activities of patient care (patient is present); approximately 60 minutes

S0250 Comprehensive geriatric assessment and treatment planning performed by assessment team

S0255 Hospice referral visit (advising patient and family of care options) performed by nurse, social worker, or other designated staff
MED: 100-4,11,10

S0257 Counseling and discussion regarding advance directives or end of life care planning and decisions, with patient and/or surrogate (list separately in addition to code for appropriate evaluation and management service)

S0260 History and physical (outpatient or office) related to surgical procedure (list separately in addition to code for appropriate evaluation and management service)

S0265 Genetic counseling, under physician supervision, each 15 minutes

S0270 Physician management of patient home care, standard monthly case rate (per 30 days)

S0271 Physician management of patient home care, hospice monthly case rate (per 30 days)

S0272 Physician management of patient home care, episodic care monthly case rate (per 30 days)

S0273 Physician visit at member's home, outside of a capitation arrangement

S0274 Nurse practitioner visit at member's home, outside of a capitation arrangement

S0280 Medical home program, comprehensive care coordination and planning, initial plan

S0281 Medical home program, comprehensive care coordination and planning, maintenance of plan

S0302 Completed early periodic screening diagnosis and treatment (EPSDT) service (list in addition to code for appropriate evaluation and management service)

S0310 Hospitalist services (list separately in addition to code for appropriate evaluation and management service)

S0315 Disease management program; initial assessment and initiation of the program

S0316 Disease management program, follow-up/reassessment

S0317 Disease management program; per diem

S0320 Telephone calls by a registered nurse to a disease management program member for monitoring purposes; per month

S0340 Lifestyle modification program for management of coronary artery disease, including all supportive services; first quarter/stage

S0341 Lifestyle modification program for management of coronary artery disease, including all supportive services; second or third quarter/stage

S0342 Lifestyle modification program for management of coronary artery disease, including all supportive services; 4th quarter / stage

S0353 Treatment planning and care coordination management for cancer initial treatment

S0354 Treatment planning and care coordination management for cancer established patient with a change of regimen

S0390 Routine foot care; removal and/or trimming of corns, calluses and/or nails and preventive maintenance in specific medical conditions (e.g., diabetes), per visit

S0395 Impression casting of a foot performed by a practitioner other than the manufacturer of the orthotic

S0400 Global fee for extracorporeal shock wave lithotripsy treatment of kidney stone(s)

S0500 Disposable contact lens, per lens

S0504 Single vision prescription lens (safety, athletic, or sunglass), per lens

S0506 Bifocal vision prescription lens (safety, athletic, or sunglass), per lens

S0508 Trifocal vision prescription lens (safety, athletic, or sunglass), per lens

S0510 Nonprescription lens (safety, athletic, or sunglass), per lens

S0512 Daily wear specialty contact lens, per lens

S0514 Color contact lens, per lens

S0515 Scleral lens, liquid bandage device, per lens

S0516 Safety eyeglass frames

S0518 Sunglasses frames

S0580 Polycarbonate lens (list this code in addition to the basic code for the lens)

S0581 Nonstandard lens (list this code in addition to the basic code for the lens)

S0590 Integral lens service, miscellaneous services reported separately

S0592 Comprehensive contact lens evaluation

S0595 Dispensing new spectacle lenses for patient supplied frame

S0596 Phakic intraocular lens for correction of refractive error

S0601 Screening proctoscopy

S0610 Annual gynecological examination, new patient

S0612 Annual gynecological examination, established patient

S0613 Annual gynecological examination; clinical breast examination without pelvic evaluation

S0618 Audiometry for hearing aid evaluation to determine the level and degree of hearing loss

S0620 Routine ophthalmological examination including refraction; new patient

S0621 Routine ophthalmological examination including refraction; established patient

S0622 Physical exam for college, new or established patient (list separately in addition to appropriate evaluation and management code)

S0630 Removal of sutures; by a physician other than the physician who originally closed the wound

S0800 Laser in situ keratomileusis (LASIK)

S0810 Photorefractive keratectomy (PRK)

S0812 Phototherapeutic keratectomy (PTK)

S1001 Deluxe item, patient aware (list in addition to code for basic item)

       MED: 100-2,1,10.1.4

S1002 Customized item (list in addition to code for basic item)

S1015 IV tubing extension set

S1016 Non-PVC (polyvinyl chloride) intravenous administration set, for use with drugs that are not stable in PVC e.g., Paclitaxel

S1030 Continuous noninvasive glucose monitoring device, purchase (for physician interpretation of data, use CPT code)

S1031 Continuous noninvasive glucose monitoring device, rental, including sensor, sensor replacement, and download to monitor (for physician interpretation of data, use CPT code)

S1040 Cranial remolding orthotic, pediatric, rigid, with soft interface material, custom fabricated, includes fitting and adjustment(s)

S1090 Mometasone furoate sinus implant, 370 micrograms

S2053 Transplantation of small intestine and liver allografts

S2054 Transplantation of multivisceral organs

S2055 Harvesting of donor multivisceral organs, with preparation and maintenance of allografts; from cadaver donor

S2060 Lobar lung transplantation

S2061 Donor lobectomy (lung) for transplantation, living donor

S2065 Simultaneous pancreas kidney transplantation

S2066 Breast reconstruction with gluteal artery perforator (GAP) flap, including harvesting of the flap, microvascular transfer, closure of donor site and shaping the flap into a breast, unilateral

S2067 Breast reconstruction of a single breast with "stacked" deep inferior epigastric perforator (DIEP) flap(s) and/or gluteal artery perforator (GAP) flap(s), including harvesting of the flap(s), microvascular transfer, closure of donor site(s) and shaping the flap into a breast, unilateral

S2068 Breast reconstruction with deep inferior epigastric perforator (DIEP) flap or superficial inferior epigastric artery (SIEA) flap, including harvesting of the flap, microvascular transfer, closure of donor site and shaping the flap into a breast, unilateral

S2070 Cystourethroscopy, with ureteroscopy and/or pyeloscopy; with endoscopic laser treatment of ureteral calculi (includes ureteral catheterization)

S2079 Laparoscopic esophagomyotomy (Heller type)

S2080 Laser-assisted uvulopalatoplasty (LAUP)

S2083 Adjustment of gastric band diameter via subcutaneous port by injection or aspiration of saline

S2095 Transcatheter occlusion or embolization for tumor destruction, percutaneous, any method, using yttrium-90 microspheres

S2102 Islet cell tissue transplant from pancreas; allogeneic

S2103 Adrenal tissue transplant to brain

S2107 Adoptive immunotherapy i.e. development of specific antitumor reactivity (e.g., tumor-infiltrating lymphocyte therapy) per course of treatment

S2112 Arthroscopy, knee, surgical for harvesting of cartilage (chondrocyte cells)

S2115 Osteotomy, periacetabular, with internal fixation

S2117 Arthroereisis, subtalar

S2118 Metal-on-metal total hip resurfacing, including acetabular and femoral components

S2120 Low density lipoprotein (LDL) apheresis using heparin-induced extracorporeal LDL precipitation

S2140 Cord blood harvesting for transplantation, allogeneic

S2142 Cord blood-derived stem-cell transplantation, allogeneic

S2150 Bone marrow or blood-derived stem cells (peripheral or umbilical), allogeneic or autologous, harvesting, transplantation, and related complications; including: pheresis and cell preparation/storage; marrow ablative therapy; drugs, supplies, hospitalization with outpatient follow-up; medical/surgical, diagnostic, emergency, and rehabilitative services; and the number of days of pre and post transplant care in the global definition

S2152 Solid organ(s), complete or segmental, single organ or combination of organs; deceased or living donor (s), procurement, transplantation, and related complications; including: drugs; supplies; hospitalization with outpatient follow-up; medical/surgical, diagnostic, emergency, and rehabilitative services, and the number of days of pre and posttransplant care in the global definition

S2202 Echosclerotherapy

S2205 Minimally invasive direct coronary artery bypass surgery involving mini-thoracotomy or mini-sternotomy surgery, performed under direct vision; using arterial graft(s), single coronary arterial graft

S2206 Minimally invasive direct coronary artery bypass surgery involving mini-thoracotomy or mini-sternotomy surgery, performed under direct vision; using arterial graft(s), 2 coronary arterial grafts

S2207 Minimally invasive direct coronary artery bypass surgery involving mini-thoracotomy or mini-sternotomy surgery, performed under direct vision; using venous graft only, single coronary venous graft

S2208 Minimally invasive direct coronary artery bypass surgery involving mini-thoracotomy or mini-sternotomy surgery, performed under direct vision; using single arterial and venous graft(s), single venous graft

S2209 Minimally invasive direct coronary artery bypass surgery involving mini-thoracotomy or mini-sternotomy surgery, performed under direct vision; using 2 arterial grafts and single venous graft

S2225 Myringotomy, laser-assisted

S2230 Implantation of magnetic component of semi-implantable hearing device on ossicles in middle ear

S2235 Implantation of auditory brain stem implant

S2260 Induced abortion, 17 to 24 weeks

S2265 Induced abortion, 25 to 28 weeks

S2266 Induced abortion, 29 to 31 weeks

S2267 Induced abortion, 32 weeks or greater

S2300 Arthroscopy, shoulder, surgical; with thermally-induced capsulorrhaphy

S2325 Hip core decompression

S2340 Chemodenervation of abductor muscle(s) of vocal cord

S2341 Chemodenervation of adductor muscle(s) of vocal cord

S2342 Nasal endoscopy for postoperative debridement following functional endoscopic sinus surgery, nasal and/or sinus cavity(s), unilateral or bilateral

S2348 Decompression procedure, percutaneous, of nucleus pulposus of intervertebral disc, using radiofrequency energy, single or multiple levels, lumbar

S2350 Diskectomy, anterior, with decompression of spinal cord and/or nerve root(s), including osteophytectomy; lumbar, single interspace

S2351 Diskectomy, anterior, with decompression of spinal cord and/or nerve root(s), including osteophytectomy; lumbar, each additional interspace (list separately in addition to code for primary procedure)

S2360 Percutaneous vertebroplasty, one vertebral body, unilateral or bilateral injection; cervical

S2361 Each additional cervical vertebral body (list separately in addition to code for primary procedure)

S2400 Repair, congenital diaphragmatic hernia in the fetus using temporary tracheal occlusion, procedure performed in utero

S2401 Repair, urinary tract obstruction in the fetus, procedure performed in utero

S2402 Repair, congenital cystic adenomatoid malformation in the fetus, procedure performed in utero

S2403 Repair, extralobar pulmonary sequestration in the fetus, procedure performed in utero

S2404 Repair, myelomeningocele in the fetus, procedure performed in utero

S2405 Repair of sacrococcygeal teratoma in the fetus, procedure performed in utero

S2409 Repair, congenital malformation of fetus, procedure performed in utero, not otherwise classified

S2411 Fetoscopic laser therapy for treatment of twin-to-twin transfusion syndrome

S2900 Surgical techniques requiring use of robotic surgical system (list separately in addition to code for primary procedure)

S3000 Diabetic indicator; retinal eye exam, dilated, bilateral

S3005 Performance measurement, evaluation of patient self assessment, depression

S3600 STAT laboratory request (situations other than S3601)

S3601 Emergency STAT laboratory charge for patient who is homebound or residing in a nursing facility

S3620 Newborn metabolic screening panel, includes test kit, postage and the laboratory tests specified by the state for inclusion in this panel (e.g., galactose; hemoglobin, electrophoresis; hydroxyprogesterone, 17-d; phenylanine (PKU); and thyroxine, total)

S3630 Eosinophil count, blood, direct

S3645 HIV-1 antibody testing of oral mucosal transudate

S3650 Saliva test, hormone level; during menopause

S3652 Saliva test, hormone level; to assess preterm labor risk

S3655 Antisperm antibodies test (immunobead)

S3708 Gastrointestinal fat absorption study

S3721 Prostate cancer antigen 3 (PCA3) testing

S3722 Dose optimization by area under the curve (AUC) analysis, for infusional 5-fluorouracil

S3800 Genetic testing for amyotrophic lateral sclerosis (ALS)

S3840 DNA analysis for germline mutations of the RET proto-oncogene for susceptibility to multiple endocrine neoplasia type 2

S3841 Genetic testing for retinoblastoma

S3842 Genetic testing for Von Hippel-Lindau disease

S3844 DNA analysis of the connexin 26 gene (GJB2) for susceptibility to congenital, profound deafness

S3845 Genetic testing for alpha-thalassemia

S3846 Genetic testing for hemoglobin E beta-thalassemia

S3849 Genetic testing for Niemann-Pick disease

S3850 Genetic testing for sickle cell anemia

S3852 DNA analysis for APOE epsilon 4 allele for susceptibility to Alzheimer's disease

S3853 Genetic testing for myotonic muscular dystrophy

S3854 Gene expression profiling panel for use in the management of breast cancer treatment

S3855 Genetic testing for detection of mutations in the presenilin - 1 gene

S3861 Genetic testing, sodium channel, voltage-gated, type V, alpha subunit (SCN5A) and variants for suspected Brugada Syndrome

S3865 Comprehensive gene sequence analysis for hypertrophic cardiomyopathy

S3866 Genetic analysis for a specific gene mutation for hypertrophic cardiomyopathy (HCM) in an individual with a known HCM mutation in the family

S3870 Comparative genomic hybridization (CGD) microarray testing for developmental delay, autism spectrum disorder and/or intellectual disability

S3890 DNA analysis, fecal, for colorectal cancer screening

S3900 Surface electromyography (EMG)

S3902 Ballistocardiogram

S3904 Masters 2 step

S4005 Interim labor facility global (labor occurring but not resulting in delivery)

S4011 In vitro fertilization; including but not limited to identification and incubation of mature oocytes, fertilization with sperm, incubation of embryo(s), and subsequent visualization for determination of development

S4013 Complete cycle, gamete intrafallopian transfer (GIFT), case rate

S4014 Complete cycle, zygote intrafallopian transfer (ZIFT), case rate

S4015 Complete in vitro fertilization cycle, not otherwise specified, case rate

S4016 Frozen in vitro fertilization cycle, case rate

S4017 Incomplete cycle, treatment cancelled prior to stimulation, case rate

S4018 Frozen embryo transfer procedure cancelled before transfer, case rate

S4020 In vitro fertilization procedure cancelled before aspiration, case rate

S4021 In vitro fertilization procedure cancelled after aspiration, case rate

S4022 Assisted oocyte fertilization, case rate

S4023 Donor egg cycle, incomplete, case rate

S4025 Donor services for in vitro fertilization (sperm or embryo), case rate

S4026 Procurement of donor sperm from sperm bank

S4027 Storage of previously frozen embryos

S4028 Microsurgical epididymal sperm aspiration (MESA)

S4030 Sperm procurement and cryopreservation services; initial visit

S4031 Sperm procurement and cryopreservation services; subsequent visit

S4035 Stimulated intrauterine insemination (IUI), case rate

S4037 Cryopreserved embryo transfer, case rate

S4040 Monitoring and storage of cryopreserved embryos, per 30 days

S4042 Management of ovulation induction (interpretation of diagnostic tests and studies, nonface-to-face medical management of the patient), per cycle

S4981 Insertion of levonorgestrel-releasing intrauterine system

S4989 Contraceptive intrauterine device (e.g., Progestacert IUD), including implants and supplies

S4990 Nicotine patches, legend

S4991 Nicotine patches, nonlegend

S4993 Contraceptive pills for birth control

S4995 Smoking cessation gum

S5000 Prescription drug, generic

S5001 Prescription drug, brand name

S5010 5% dextrose and 0.45% normal saline, 1000 ml

S5011 5% dextrose in lactated ringer's, 1000 ml

S5012 5% dextrose with potassium chloride, 1000 ml

S5013 5% dextrose/0.45% normal saline with potassium chloride and magnesium sulfate, 1000 ml

S5014 5% dextrose/0.45% normal saline with potassium chloride and magnesium sulfate, 1500 ml

S5035 Home infusion therapy, routine service of infusion device (e.g., pump maintenance)

S5036 Home infusion therapy, repair of infusion device (e.g., pump repair)

S5100 Day care services, adult; per 15 minutes

S5101 Day care services, adult; per half day

S5102 Day care services, adult; per diem

S5105 Day care services, center-based; services not included in program fee, per diem

S5108 Home care training to home care client, per 15 minutes

S5109 Home care training to home care client, per session

S5110 Home care training, family; per 15 minutes

S5111 Home care training, family; per session

S5115 Home care training, nonfamily; per 15 minutes

S5116 Home care training, nonfamily; per session

S5120 Chore services; per 15 minutes

S5121 Chore services; per diem

S5125 Attendant care services; per 15 minutes

S5126 Attendant care services; per diem

S5130 Homemaker service, NOS; per 15 minutes

S5131 Homemaker service, NOS; per diem

S5135 Companion care, adult (e.g., IADL/ADL); per 15 minutes

S5136 Companion care, adult (e.g., IADL/ADL); per diem

S5140 Foster care, adult; per diem

S5141 Foster care, adult; per month

S5145 Foster care, therapeutic, child; per diem

S5146 Foster care, therapeutic, child; per month

S5150 Unskilled respite care, not hospice; per 15 minutes

S5151 Unskilled respite care, not hospice; per diem

S5160 Emergency response system; installation and testing

S5161 Emergency response system; service fee, per month (excludes installation and testing)

S5162 Emergency response system; purchase only

S5165 Home modifications; per service

S5170 Home delivered meals, including preparation; per meal

S5175 Laundry service, external, professional; per order

S5180 Home health respiratory therapy, initial evaluation

S5181 Home health respiratory therapy, NOS, per diem

S5185 Medication reminder service, nonface-to-face; per month

S5190 Wellness assessment, performed by nonphysician

S5199 Personal care item, NOS, each

S5497 Home infusion therapy, catheter care/maintenance, not otherwise classified; includes administrative services, professional pharmacy services, care coordination, and all necessary supplies and equipment (drugs and nursing visits coded separately), per diem

S5498 Home infusion therapy, catheter care/maintenance, simple (single lumen), includes administrative services, professional pharmacy services, care coordination and all necessary supplies and equipment, (drugs and nursing visits coded separately), per diem

S5501 Home infusion therapy, catheter care/maintenance, complex (more than one lumen), includes administrative services, professional pharmacy services, care coordination, and all necessary supplies and equipment (drugs and nursing visits coded separately), per diem

S5502 Home infusion therapy, catheter care/maintenance, implanted access device, includes administrative services, professional pharmacy services, care coordination and all necessary supplies and equipment (drugs and nursing visits coded separately), per diem (use this code for interim maintenance of vascular access not currently in use)

S5517 Home infusion therapy, all supplies necessary for restoration of catheter patency or declotting

S5518 Home infusion therapy, all supplies necessary for catheter repair

S5520 Home infusion therapy, all supplies (including catheter) necessary for a peripherally inserted central venous catheter (PICC) line insertion

S5521 Home infusion therapy, all supplies (including catheter) necessary for a midline catheter insertion

S5522 Home infusion therapy, insertion of peripherally inserted central venous catheter (PICC), nursing services only (no supplies or catheter included)

S5523 Home infusion therapy, insertion of midline venous catheter, nursing services only (no supplies or catheter included)

Code	Description
S5550	Insulin, rapid onset, 5 units
S5551	Insulin, most rapid onset (Lispro or Aspart); 5 units
S5552	Insulin, intermediate acting (NPH or LENTE); 5 units
S5553	Insulin, long acting; 5 units
S5560	Insulin delivery device, reusable pen; 1.5 ml size
S5561	Insulin delivery device, reusable pen; 3 ml size
S5565	Insulin cartridge for use in insulin delivery device other than pump; 150 units
S5566	Insulin cartridge for use in insulin delivery device other than pump; 300 units
S5570	Insulin delivery device, disposable pen (including insulin); 1.5 ml size
S5571	Insulin delivery device, disposable pen (including insulin); 3 ml size
S8030	Scleral application of tantalum ring(s) for localization of lesions for proton beam therapy
S8035	Magnetic source imaging
S8037	Magnetic resonance cholangiopancreatography (MRCP)
S8040	Topographic brain mapping
S8042	Magnetic resonance imaging (MRI), low-field
S8055	Ultrasound guidance for multifetal pregnancy reduction(s), technical component (only to be used when the physician doing the reduction procedure does not perform the ultrasound, guidance is included in the CPT code for multifetal pregnancy reduction (59866)
S8080	Scintimammography (radioimmunoscintigraphy of the breast), unilateral, including supply of radiopharmaceutical
S8085	Fluorine-18 fluorodeoxyglucose (F-18 FDG) imaging using dual-head coincidence detection system (nondedicated PET scan)
S8092	Electron beam computed tomography (also known as ultrafast CT, cine CT)
S8096	Portable peak flow meter
S8097	Asthma kit (including but not limited to portable peak expiratory flow meter, instructional video, brochure, and/or spacer)
S8100	Holding chamber or spacer for use with an inhaler or nebulizer; without mask
S8101	Holding chamber or spacer for use with an inhaler or nebulizer; with mask
S8110	Peak expiratory flow rate (physician services)
S8120	Oxygen contents, gaseous, 1 unit equals 1 cubic foot
S8121	Oxygen contents, liquid, 1 unit equals 1 pound
S8130	Interferential current stimulator, 2 channel
S8131	Interferential current stimulator, 4 channel
S8185	Flutter device
S8186	Swivel adaptor
S8189	Tracheostomy supply, not otherwise classified
S8210	Mucus trap
S8262	Mandibular orthopedic repositioning device, each
S8265	Haberman feeder for cleft lip/palate
S8270	Enuresis alarm, using auditory buzzer and/or vibration device
S8301	Infection control supplies, not otherwise specified
S8415	Supplies for home delivery of infant
S8420	Gradient pressure aid (sleeve and glove combination), custom made
S8421	Gradient pressure aid (sleeve and glove combination), ready made
S8422	Gradient pressure aid (sleeve), custom made, medium weight

Code	Description
S8423	Gradient pressure aid (sleeve), custom made, heavy weight
S8424	Gradient pressure aid (sleeve), ready made
S8425	Gradient pressure aid (glove), custom made, medium weight
S8426	Gradient pressure aid (glove), custom made, heavy weight
S8427	Gradient pressure aid (glove), ready made
S8428	Gradient pressure aid (gauntlet), ready made
S8429	Gradient pressure exterior wrap
S8430	Padding for compression bandage, roll
S8431	Compression bandage, roll

Mobile dorsal splint
Static finger splint
Slip-on splint
Various types of digit splints (S8450)

Code	Description
S8450	Splint, prefabricated, digit (specify digit by use of modifier)
S8451	Splint, prefabricated, wrist or ankle
S8452	Splint, prefabricated, elbow
S8460	Camisole, postmastectomy
S8490	Insulin syringes (100 syringes, any size)
S8930	Electrical stimulation of auricular acupuncture points; each 15 minutes of personal one-on-one contact with patient
S8940	Equestrian/hippotherapy, per session
S8948	Application of a modality (requiring constant provider attendance) to one or more areas; low-level laser; each 15 minutes
S8950	Complex lymphedema therapy, each 15 minutes
S8990	Physical or manipulative therapy performed for maintenance rather than restoration
S8999	Resuscitation bag (for use by patient on artificial respiration during power failure or other catastrophic event)
S9001	Home uterine monitor with or without associated nursing services
S9007	Ultrafiltration monitor
S9015	Automated EEG monitoring
S9024	Paranasal sinus ultrasound
S9025	Omnicardiogram/cardiointegram
S9034	Extracorporeal shockwave lithotripsy for gall stones (if performed with ERCP, use 43265)
S9055	Procuren or other growth factor preparation to promote wound healing
S9056	Coma stimulation per diem
S9061	Home administration of aerosolized drug therapy (e.g., Pentamidine); administrative services, professional pharmacy services, care coordination, all necessary supplies and equipment (drugs and nursing visits coded separately), per diem
S9083	Global fee urgent care centers
S9088	Services provided in an urgent care center (list in addition to code for service)
S9090	Vertebral axial decompression, per session
S9097	Home visit for wound care

S9098 Home visit, phototherapy services (e.g., Bili-lite), including equipment rental, nursing services, blood draw, supplies, and other services, per diem

S9110 Telemonitoring of patient in their home, including all necessary equipment; computer system, connections, and software; maintenance; patient education and support; per month

S9117 Back school, per visit

S9122 Home health aide or certified nurse assistant, providing care in the home; per hour

S9123 Nursing care, in the home; by registered nurse, per hour (use for general nursing care only, not to be used when CPT codes 99500-99602 can be used)

S9124 Nursing care, in the home; by licensed practical nurse, per hour

S9125 Respite care, in the home, per diem

S9126 Hospice care, in the home, per diem
MED: 100-4,11,10

S9127 Social work visit, in the home, per diem

S9128 Speech therapy, in the home, per diem

S9129 Occupational therapy, in the home, per diem

S9131 Physical therapy; in the home, per diem

S9140 Diabetic management program, follow-up visit to non-MD provider

S9141 Diabetic management program, follow-up visit to MD provider

S9145 Insulin pump initiation, instruction in initial use of pump (pump not included)

S9150 Evaluation by ocularist

S9152 Speech therapy, re-evaluation

S9208 Home management of preterm labor, including administrative services, professional pharmacy services, care coordination, and all necessary supplies or equipment (drugs and nursing visits coded separately), per diem (do not use this code with any home infusion per diem code)

S9209 Home management of preterm premature rupture of membranes (PPROM), including administrative services, professional pharmacy services, care coordination, and all necessary supplies or equipment (drugs and nursing visits coded separately), per diem (do not use this code with any home infusion per diem code)

S9211 Home management of gestational hypertension, includes administrative services, professional pharmacy services, care coordination and all necessary supplies and equipment (drugs and nursing visits coded separately); per diem (do not use this code with any home infusion per diem code)

S9212 Home management of postpartum hypertension, includes administrative services, professional pharmacy services, care coordination, and all necessary supplies and equipment (drugs and nursing visits coded separately), per diem (do not use this code with any home infusion per diem code)

S9213 Home management of preeclampsia, includes administrative services, professional pharmacy services, care coordination, and all necessary supplies and equipment (drugs and nursing services coded separately); per diem (do not use this code with any home infusion per diem code)

S9214 Home management of gestational diabetes, includes administrative services, professional pharmacy services, care coordination, and all necessary supplies and equipment (drugs and nursing visits coded separately); per diem (do not use this code with any home infusion per diem code)

S9325 Home infusion therapy, pain management infusion; administrative services, professional pharmacy services, care coordination, and all necessary supplies and equipment, (drugs and nursing visits coded separately), per diem (do not use this code with S9326, S9327 or S9328)

S9326 Home infusion therapy, continuous (24 hours or more) pain management infusion; administrative services, professional pharmacy services, care coordination and all necessary supplies and equipment (drugs and nursing visits coded separately), per diem

S9327 Home infusion therapy, intermittent (less than 24 hours) pain management infusion; administrative services, professional pharmacy services, care coordination, and all necessary supplies and equipment (drugs and nursing visits coded separately), per diem

S9328 Home infusion therapy, implanted pump pain management infusion; administrative services, professional pharmacy services, care coordination, and all necessary supplies and equipment (drugs and nursing visits coded separately), per diem

S9329 Home infusion therapy, chemotherapy infusion; administrative services, professional pharmacy services, care coordination, and all necessary supplies and equipment (drugs and nursing visits coded separately), per diem (do not use this code with S9330 or S9331)

S9330 Home infusion therapy, continuous (24 hours or more) chemotherapy infusion; administrative services, professional pharmacy services, care coordination, and all necessary supplies and equipment (drugs and nursing visits coded separately), per diem

S9331 Home infusion therapy, intermittent (less than 24 hours) chemotherapy infusion; administrative services, professional pharmacy services, care coordination, and all necessary supplies and equipment (drugs and nursing visits coded separately), per diem

S9335 Home therapy, hemodialysis; administrative services, professional pharmacy services, care coordination, and all necessary supplies and equipment (drugs and nursing services coded separately), per diem

S9336 Home infusion therapy, continuous anticoagulant infusion therapy (e.g., Heparin), administrative services, professional pharmacy services, care coordination and all necessary supplies and equipment (drugs and nursing visits coded separately), per diem

S9338 Home infusion therapy, immunotherapy, administrative services, professional pharmacy services, care coordination, and all necessary supplies and equipment (drugs and nursing visits coded separately), per diem

S9339 Home therapy; peritoneal dialysis, administrative services, professional pharmacy services, care coordination and all necessary supplies and equipment (drugs and nursing visits coded separately), per diem

S9340 Home therapy; enteral nutrition; administrative services, professional pharmacy services, care coordination, and all necessary supplies and equipment (enteral formula and nursing visits coded separately), per diem

S9341 Home therapy; enteral nutrition via gravity; administrative services, professional pharmacy services, care coordination, and all necessary supplies and equipment (enteral formula and nursing visits coded separately), per diem

S9342 Home therapy; enteral nutrition via pump; administrative services, professional pharmacy services, care coordination, and all necessary supplies and equipment (enteral formula and nursing visits coded separately), per diem

S9343 Home therapy; enteral nutrition via bolus; administrative services, professional pharmacy services, care coordination, and all necessary supplies and equipment (enteral formula and nursing visits coded separately), per diem

S9345 Home infusion therapy, antihemophilic agent infusion therapy (e.g., factor VIII); administrative services, professional pharmacy services, care coordination, and all necessary supplies and equipment (drugs and nursing visits coded separately), per diem

S9346 Home infusion therapy, alpha-1-proteinase inhibitor (e.g., Prolastin); administrative services, professional pharmacy services, care coordination, and all necessary supplies and equipment (drugs and nursing visits coded separately), per diem

S9347 Home infusion therapy, uninterrupted, long-term, controlled rate intravenous or subcutaneous infusion therapy (e.g., epoprostenol); administrative services, professional pharmacy services, care coordination, and all necessary supplies and equipment (drugs and nursing visits coded separately), per diem

S9348 Home infusion therapy, sympathomimetic/inotropic agent infusion therapy (e.g., Dobutamine); administrative services, professional pharmacy services, care coordination, all necessary supplies and equipment (drugs and nursing visits coded separately), per diem

S9349 Home infusion therapy, tocolytic infusion therapy; administrative services, professional pharmacy services, care coordination, and all necessary supplies and equipment (drugs and nursing visits coded separately), per diem

S9351 Home infusion therapy, continuous or intermittent antiemetic infusion therapy; administrative services, professional pharmacy services, care coordination, and all necessary supplies and equipment (drugs and visits coded separately), per diem

S9353 Home infusion therapy, continuous insulin infusion therapy; administrative services, professional pharmacy services, care coordination, and all necessary supplies and equipment (drugs and nursing visits coded separately), per diem

S9355 Home infusion therapy, chelation therapy; administrative services, professional pharmacy services, care coordination, and all necessary supplies and equipment (drugs and nursing visits coded separately), per diem

S9357 Home infusion therapy, enzyme replacement intravenous therapy; (e.g., Imiglucerase); administrative services, professional pharmacy services, care coordination, and all necessary supplies and equipment (drugs and nursing visits coded separately), per diem

S9359 Home infusion therapy, antitumor necrosis factor intravenous therapy; (e.g., Infliximab); administrative services, professional pharmacy services, care coordination, and all necessary supplies and equipment (drugs and nursing visits coded separately), per diem

S9361 Home infusion therapy, diuretic intravenous therapy; administrative services, professional pharmacy services, care coordination, and all necessary supplies and equipment (drugs and nursing visits coded separately), per diem

S9363 Home infusion therapy, antispasmotic therapy; administrative services, professional pharmacy services, care coordination, and all necessary supplies and equipment (drugs and nursing visits coded separately), per diem

S9364 Home infusion therapy, total parenteral nutrition (TPN); administrative services, professional pharmacy services, care coordination, and all necessary supplies and equipment including standard TPN formula (lipids, specialty amino acid formulas, drugs other than in standard formula and nursing visits coded separately), per diem (do not use with home infusion codes S9365-S9368 using daily volume scales)

S9365 Home infusion therapy, total parenteral nutrition (TPN); 1 liter per day, administrative services, professional pharmacy services, care coordination, and all necessary supplies and equipment including standard TPN formula (lipids, specialty amino acid formulas, drugs other than in standard formula and nursing visits coded separately), per diem

S9366 Home infusion therapy, total parenteral nutrition (TPN); more than 1 liter but no more than 2 liters per day, administrative services, professional pharmacy services, care coordination, and all necessary supplies and equipment including standard TPN formula (lipids, specialty amino acid formulas, drugs other than in standard formula and nursing visits coded separately), per diem

S9367 Home infusion therapy, total parenteral nutrition (TPN); more than 2 liters but no more than 3 liters per day, administrative services, professional pharmacy services, care coordination, and all necessary supplies and equipment including standard TPN formula (lipids, specialty amino acid formulas, drugs other than in standard formula and nursing visits coded separately), per diem

S9368 Home infusion therapy, total parenteral nutrition (TPN); more than 3 liters per day, administrative services, professional pharmacy services, care coordination, and all necessary supplies and equipment including standard TPN formula (lipids, specialty amino acid formulas, drugs other than in standard formula and nursing visits coded separately), per diem

S9370 Home therapy, intermittent antiemetic injection therapy; administrative services, professional pharmacy services, care coordination, and all necessary supplies and equipment (drugs and nursing visits coded separately), per diem

S9372 Home therapy; intermittent anticoagulant injection therapy (e.g., Heparin); administrative services, professional pharmacy services, care coordination, and all necessary supplies and equipment (drugs and nursing visits coded separately), per diem (do not use this code for flushing of infusion devices with Heparin to maintain patency)

S9373 Home infusion therapy, hydration therapy; administrative services, professional pharmacy services, care coordination, and all necessary supplies and equipment (drugs and nursing visits coded separately), per diem (do not use with hydration therapy codes S9374-S9377 using daily volume scales)

S9374 Home infusion therapy, hydration therapy; 1 liter per day, administrative services, professional pharmacy services, care coordination, and all necessary supplies and equipment (drugs and nursing visits coded separately), per diem

S9375 Home infusion therapy, hydration therapy; more than 1 liter but no more than 2 liters per day, administrative services, professional pharmacy services, care coordination, and all necessary supplies and equipment (drugs and nursing visits coded separately), per diem

S9376 Home infusion therapy, hydration therapy; more than 2 liters but no more than 3 liters per day, administrative services, professional pharmacy services, care coordination, and all necessary supplies and equipment (drugs and nursing visits coded separately), per diem

S9377 Home infusion therapy, hydration therapy; more than 3 liters per day, administrative services, professional pharmacy services, care coordination, and all necessary supplies (drugs and nursing visits coded separately), per diem

S9379 Home infusion therapy, infusion therapy, not otherwise classified; administrative services, professional pharmacy services, care coordination, and all necessary supplies and equipment (drugs and nursing visits coded separately), per diem

S9381 Delivery or service to high risk areas requiring escort or extra protection, per visit

S9401 Anticoagulation clinic, inclusive of all services except laboratory tests, per session

S9430 Pharmacy compounding and dispensing services

S9433 Medical food nutritionally complete, administered orally, providing 100% of nutritional intake

S9434 Modified solid food supplements for inborn errors of metabolism

S9435 Medical foods for inborn errors of metabolism

S9436 Childbirth preparation/Lamaze classes, nonphysician provider, per session

S9437 Childbirth refresher classes, nonphysician provider, per session

S9438 Cesarean birth classes, nonphysician provider, per session

S9439 VBAC (vaginal birth after cesarean) classes, nonphysician provider, per session

S9441 Asthma education, nonphysician provider, per session

S9442 Birthing classes, nonphysician provider, per session

S9443 Lactation classes, nonphysician provider, per session

S9444 Parenting classes, nonphysician provider, per session

S9445 Patient education, not otherwise classified, nonphysician provider, individual, per session

S9446 Patient education, not otherwise classified, nonphysician provider, group, per session

S9447 Infant safety (including CPR) classes, nonphysician provider, per session

S9449 Weight management classes, nonphysician provider, per session

S9451 Exercise classes, nonphysician provider, per session

S9452 Nutrition classes, nonphysician provider, per session

S9453 Smoking cessation classes, nonphysician provider, per session

S9454 Stress management classes, nonphysician provider, per session

S9455 Diabetic management program, group session

S9460 Diabetic management program, nurse visit

S9465 Diabetic management program, dietitian visit

S9470 Nutritional counseling, dietitian visit

S9472 Cardiac rehabilitation program, nonphysician provider, per diem

S9473 Pulmonary rehabilitation program, nonphysician provider, per diem

S9474 Enterostomal therapy by a registered nurse certified in enterostomal therapy, per diem

S9475 Ambulatory setting substance abuse treatment or detoxification services, per diem

S9476 Vestibular rehabilitation program, nonphysician provider, per diem

S9480 Intensive outpatient psychiatric services, per diem

S9482 Family stabilization services, per 15 minutes

S9484 Crisis intervention mental health services, per hour

S9485 Crisis intervention mental health services, per diem

S9490 Home infusion therapy, corticosteroid infusion; administrative services, professional pharmacy services, care coordination, and all necessary supplies and equipment (drugs and nursing visits coded separately), per diem

S9494 Home infusion therapy, antibiotic, antiviral, or antifungal therapy; administrative services, professional pharmacy services, care coordination, and all necessary supplies and equipment (drugs and nursing visits coded separately), per diem (do not use this code with home infusion codes for hourly dosing schedules S9497-S9504)

S9497 Home infusion therapy, antibiotic, antiviral, or antifungal therapy; once every 3 hours; administrative services, professional pharmacy services, care coordination, and all necessary supplies and equipment (drugs and nursing visits coded separately), per diem

S9500 Home infusion therapy, antibiotic, antiviral, or antifungal therapy; once every 24 hours; administrative services, professional pharmacy services, care coordination, and all necessary supplies and equipment (drugs and nursing visits coded separately), per diem

S9501 Home infusion therapy, antibiotic, antiviral, or antifungal therapy; once every 12 hours; administrative services, professional pharmacy services, care coordination, and all necessary supplies and equipment (drugs and nursing visits coded separately), per diem

S9502 Home infusion therapy, antibiotic, antiviral, or antifungal therapy; once every 8 hours, administrative services, professional pharmacy services, care coordination, and all necessary supplies and equipment (drugs and nursing visits coded separately), per diem

S9503 Home infusion therapy, antibiotic, antiviral, or antifungal; once every 6 hours; administrative services, professional pharmacy services, care coordination, and all necessary supplies and equipment (drugs and nursing visits coded separately), per diem

S9504 Home infusion therapy, antibiotic, antiviral, or antifungal; once every 4 hours; administrative services, professional pharmacy services, care coordination, and all necessary supplies and equipment (drugs and nursing visits coded separately), per diem

S9529 Routine venipuncture for collection of specimen(s), single homebound, nursing home, or skilled nursing facility patient

S9537 Home therapy; hematopoietic hormone injection therapy (e.g., erythropoietin, G-CSF, GM-CSF); administrative services, professional pharmacy services, care coordination, and all necessary supplies and equipment (drugs and nursing visits coded separately), per diem

S9538 Home transfusion of blood product(s); administrative services, professional pharmacy services, care coordination and all necessary supplies and equipment (blood products, drugs, and nursing visits coded separately), per diem

S9542 Home injectable therapy, not otherwise classified, including administrative services, professional pharmacy services, care coordination, and all necessary supplies and equipment (drugs and nursing visits coded separately), per diem

S9558 Home injectable therapy; growth hormone, including administrative services, professional pharmacy services, care coordination, and all necessary supplies and equipment (drugs and nursing visits coded separately), per diem

S9559 Home injectable therapy, interferon, including administrative services, professional pharmacy services, care coordination, and all necessary supplies and equipment (drugs and nursing visits coded separately), per diem

S9560 Home injectable therapy; hormonal therapy (e.g., leuprolide, goserelin), including administrative services, professional pharmacy services, care coordination, and all necessary supplies and equipment (drugs and nursing visits coded separately), per diem

S9562 Home injectable therapy, palivizumab, including administrative services, professional pharmacy services, care coordination, and all necessary supplies and equipment (drugs and nursing visits coded separately), per diem

S9590 Home therapy, irrigation therapy (e.g., sterile irrigation of an organ or anatomical cavity); including administrative services, professional pharmacy services, care coordination, and all necessary supplies and equipment (drugs and nursing visits coded separately), per diem

S9810 Home therapy; professional pharmacy services for provision of infusion, specialty drug administration, and/or disease state management, not otherwise classified, per hour (do not use this code with any per diem code)

S9900 Services by a Journal-listed Christian Science practitioner for the purpose of healing, per diem

S9960 Ambulance service, conventional air services, nonemergency transport, one way (fixed wing)

S9961 Ambulance service, conventional air service, nonemergency transport, one way (rotary wing)

S9970 Health club membership, annual

S9975 Transplant related lodging, meals and transportation, per diem

S9976 Lodging, per diem, not otherwise classified

S9977 Meals, per diem, not otherwise specified

S9981 Medical records copying fee, administrative

S9982 Medical records copying fee, per page

S9986 Not medically necessary service (patient is aware that service not medically necessary)

S9988 Services provided as part of a Phase I clinical trial

S9989 Services provided outside of the United States of America (list in addition to code(s) for services(s))

S9990 Services provided as part of a Phase II clinical trial

S9991 Services provided as part of a Phase III clinical trial

S9992 Transportation costs to and from trial location and local transportation costs (e.g., fares for taxicab or bus) for clinical trial participant and one caregiver/companion

S9994 Lodging costs (e.g., hotel charges) for clinical trial participant and one caregiver/companion

S9996 Meals for clinical trial participant and one caregiver/companion

S9999 Sales tax

NATIONAL T CODES ESTABLISHED FOR STATE MEDICAID AGENCIES T1000-T9999

The T codes are designed for use by Medicaid state agencies to establish codes for items for which there are no permanent national codes but for which codes are necessary to administer the Medicaid program (T codes are not accepted by Medicare but can be used by private insurers). This range of codes describes nursing and home health-related services, substance abuse treatment, and certain training-related procedures.

T1000   Private duty/independent nursing service(s), licensed, up to 15 minutes

T1001   Nursing assessment/evaluation

T1002   RN services, up to 15 minutes

T1003   LPN/LVN services, up to 15 minutes

T1004   Services of a qualified nursing aide, up to 15 minutes

T1005   Respite care services, up to 15 minutes

T1006   Alcohol and/or substance abuse services, family/couple counseling

T1007   Alcohol and/or substance abuse services, treatment plan development and/or modification

T1009   Child sitting services for children of the individual receiving alcohol and/or substance abuse services

T1010   Meals for individuals receiving alcohol and/or substance abuse services (when meals not included in the program)

T1012   Alcohol and/or substance abuse services, skills development

T1013   Sign language or oral interpretive services, per 15 minutes

T1014   Telehealth transmission, per minute, professional services bill separately

T1015   Clinic visit/encounter, all-inclusive

T1016   Case management, each 15 minutes

T1017   Targeted case management, each 15 minutes

T1018   School-based individualized education program (IEP) services, bundled

T1019   Personal care services, per 15 minutes, not for an inpatient or resident of a hospital, nursing facility, ICF/MR or IMD, part of the individualized plan of treatment (code may not be used to identify services provided by home health aide or certified nurse assistant)

T1020   Personal care services, per diem, not for an inpatient or resident of a hospital, nursing facility, ICF/MR or IMD, part of the individualized plan of treatment (code may not be used to identify services provided by home health aide or certified nurse assistant)

T1021   Home health aide or certified nurse assistant, per visit

T1022   Contracted home health agency services, all services provided under contract, per day

T1023   Screening to determine the appropriateness of consideration of an individual for participation in a specified program, project or treatment protocol, per encounter

T1024   Evaluation and treatment by an integrated, specialty team contracted to provide coordinated care to multiple or severely handicapped children, per encounter

T1025   Intensive, extended multidisciplinary services provided in a clinic setting to children with complex medical, physical, mental and psychosocial impairments, per diem

T1026   Intensive, extended multidisciplinary services provided in a clinic setting to children with complex medical, physical, medical and psychosocial impairments, per hour

T1027   Family training and counseling for child development, per 15 minutes

T1028   Assessment of home, physical and family environment, to determine suitability to meet patient's medical needs

T1029   Comprehensive environmental lead investigation, not including laboratory analysis, per dwelling

T1030   Nursing care, in the home, by registered nurse, per diem

T1031   Nursing care, in the home, by licensed practical nurse, per diem

T1502   Administration of oral, intramuscular and/or subcutaneous medication by health care agency/professional, per visit

T1503   Administration of medication, other than oral and/or injectable, by a health care agency/professional, per visit

T1505   Electronic medication compliance management device, includes all components and accessories, not otherwise classified

T1999   Miscellaneous therapeutic items and supplies, retail purchases, not otherwise classified; identify product in "remarks"

T2001   Nonemergency transportation; patient attendant/escort

T2002   Nonemergency transportation; per diem

T2003   Nonemergency transportation; encounter/trip

T2004   Nonemergency transport; commercial carrier, multipass

T2005   Nonemergency transportation; stretcher van

T2007   Transportation waiting time, air ambulance and nonemergency vehicle, one-half (1/2) hour increments

T2010   Preadmission screening and resident review (PASRR) level I identification screening, per screen

T2011   Preadmission screening and resident review (PASRR) level II evaluation, per evaluation

T2012   Habilitation, educational; waiver, per diem

T2013   Habilitation, educational, waiver; per hour

T2014   Habilitation, prevocational, waiver; per diem

T2015   Habilitation, prevocational, waiver; per hour

T2016   Habilitation, residential, waiver; per diem

T2017   Habilitation, residential, waiver; 15 minutes

T2018   Habilitation, supported employment, waiver; per diem

T2019   Habilitation, supported employment, waiver; per 15 minutes

T2020   Day habilitation, waiver; per diem

T2021   Day habilitation, waiver; per 15 minutes

T2022   Case management, per month

T2023   Targeted case management; per month

T2024   Service assessment/plan of care development, waiver

T2025   Waiver services; not otherwise specified (NOS)

T2026   Specialized childcare, waiver; per diem

T2027   Specialized childcare, waiver; per 15 minutes

T2028   Specialized supply, not otherwise specified, waiver

T2029   Specialized medical equipment, not otherwise specified, waiver

T2030   Assisted living, waiver; per month

T2031   Assisted living; waiver, per diem

T2032   Residential care, not otherwise specified (NOS), waiver; per month

T2033   Residential care, not otherwise specified (NOS), waiver; per diem

T2034   Crisis intervention, waiver; per diem

T2035   Utility services to support medical equipment and assistive technology/devices, waiver

T2036   Therapeutic camping, overnight, waiver; each session

T2037   Therapeutic camping, day, waiver; each session

T2038   Community transition, waiver; per service

T2039　Vehicle modifications, waiver; per service

T2040　Financial management, self-directed, waiver; per 15 minutes

T2041　Supports brokerage, self-directed, waiver; per 15 minutes

T2042　Hospice routine home care; per diem
　　　　MED: 100-4,11,10

T2043　Hospice continuous home care; per hour

T2044　Hospice inpatient respite care; per diem

T2045　Hospice general inpatient care; per diem

T2046　Hospice long-term care, room and board only; per diem

T2048　Behavioral health; long-term care residential (nonacute care in a residential treatment program where stay is typically longer than 30 days), with room and board, per diem

T2049　Nonemergency transportation; stretcher van, mileage; per mile

T2101　Human breast milk processing, storage and distribution only

T4521　Adult sized disposable incontinence product, brief/diaper, small, each

T4522　Adult sized disposable incontinence product, brief/diaper, medium, each

T4523　Adult sized disposable incontinence product, brief/diaper, large, each

T4524　Adult sized disposable incontinence product, brief/diaper, extra large, each

T4525　Adult sized disposable incontinence product, protective underwear/pull-on, small size, each

T4526　Adult sized disposable incontinence product, protective underwear/pull-on, medium size, each

T4527　Adult sized disposable incontinence product, protective underwear/pull-on, large size, each

T4528　Adult sized disposable incontinence product, protective underwear/pull-on, extra large size, each

T4529　Pediatric sized disposable incontinence product, brief/diaper, small/medium size, each

T4530　Pediatric sized disposable incontinence product, brief/diaper, large size, each

T4531　Pediatric sized disposable incontinence product, protective underwear/pull-on, small/medium size, each

T4532　Pediatric sized disposable incontinence product, protective underwear/pull-on, large size, each

T4533　Youth sized disposable incontinence product, brief/diaper, each

T4534　Youth sized disposable incontinence product, protective underwear/pull-on, each

T4535　Disposable liner/shield/guard/pad/undergarment, for incontinence, each

T4536　Incontinence product, protective underwear/pull-on, reusable, any size, each

T4537　Incontinence product, protective underpad, reusable, bed size, each

T4538　Diaper service, reusable diaper, each diaper

T4539　Incontinence product, diaper/brief, reusable, any size, each

T4540　Incontinence product, protective underpad, reusable, chair size, each

T4541　Incontinence product, disposable underpad, large, each

T4542　Incontinence product, disposable underpad, small size, each

T4543　Adult sized disposable incontinence product, protective brief/diaper, above extra large, each

T4544　Adult sized disposable incontinence product, protective underwear/pull-on, above extra large, each

T5001　Positioning seat for persons with special orthopedic needs

T5999　Supply, not otherwise specified

Vision Services

V2020 — V2308

VISION SERVICES V0000-V2999

These V codes include vision-related supplies, including spectacles, lenses, contact lenses, prostheses, intraocular lenses, and miscellaneous lenses.

FRAMES

V2020 Frames, purchases

V2025 Deluxe frame
 MED: 100-4,1,30.3.5

SINGLE VISION, GLASS, OR PLASTIC

Monofocal spectacles (V2100-V2114)

Trifocal spectacles (V2300-V2314)

Low vision aids mounted to spectacles (V2610)

Telescopic or other compound lens fitted on spectacles as a low vision aid (V2615)

V2100 Sphere, single vision, plano to plus or minus 4.00, per lens

V2101 Sphere, single vision, plus or minus 4.12 to plus or minus 7.00d, per lens

V2102 Sphere, single vision, plus or minus 7.12 to plus or minus 20.00d, per lens

V2103 Spherocylinder, single vision, plano to plus or minus 4.00d sphere, 0.12 to 2.00d cylinder, per lens

V2104 Spherocylinder, single vision, plano to plus or minus 4.00d sphere, 2.12 to 4.00d cylinder, per lens

V2105 Spherocylinder, single vision, plano to plus or minus 4.00d sphere, 4.25 to 6.00d cylinder, per lens

V2106 Spherocylinder, single vision, plano to plus or minus 4.00d sphere, over 6.00d cylinder, per lens

V2107 Spherocylinder, single vision, plus or minus 4.25 to plus or minus 7.00 sphere, 0.12 to 2.00d cylinder, per lens

V2108 Spherocylinder, single vision, plus or minus 4.25d to plus or minus 7.00d sphere, 2.12 to 4.00d cylinder, per lens

V2109 Spherocylinder, single vision, plus or minus 4.25 to plus or minus 7.00d sphere, 4.25 to 6.00d cylinder, per lens

V2110 Spherocylinder, single vision, plus or minus 4.25 to 7.00d sphere, over 6.00d cylinder, per lens

V2111 Spherocylinder, single vision, plus or minus 7.25 to plus or minus 12.00d sphere, 0.25 to 2.25d cylinder, per lens

V2112 Spherocylinder, single vision, plus or minus 7.25 to plus or minus 12.00d sphere, 2.25d to 4.00d cylinder, per lens

V2113 Spherocylinder, single vision, plus or minus 7.25 to plus or minus 12.00d sphere, 4.25 to 6.00d cylinder, per lens

V2114 Spherocylinder, single vision, sphere over plus or minus 12.00d, per lens

V2115 Lenticular (myodisc), per lens, single vision

V2118 Aniseikonic lens, single vision

V2121 Lenticular lens, per lens, single

V2199 Not otherwise classified, single vision lens

BIFOCAL, GLASS, OR PLASTIC

V2200 Sphere, bifocal, plano to plus or minus 4.00d, per lens

V2201 Sphere, bifocal, plus or minus 4.12 to plus or minus 7.00d, per lens

V2202 Sphere, bifocal, plus or minus 7.12 to plus or minus 20.00d, per lens

V2203 Spherocylinder, bifocal, plano to plus or minus 4.00d sphere, 0.12 to 2.00d cylinder, per lens

V2204 Spherocylinder, bifocal, plano to plus or minus 4.00d sphere, 2.12 to 4.00d cylinder, per lens

V2205 Spherocylinder, bifocal, plano to plus or minus 4.00d sphere, 4.25 to 6.00d cylinder, per lens

V2206 Spherocylinder, bifocal, plano to plus or minus 4.00d sphere, over 6.00d cylinder, per lens

V2207 Spherocylinder, bifocal, plus or minus 4.25 to plus or minus 7.00d sphere, 0.12 to 2.00d cylinder, per lens

V2208 Spherocylinder, bifocal, plus or minus 4.25 to plus or minus 7.00d sphere, 2.12 to 4.00d cylinder, per lens

V2209 Spherocylinder, bifocal, plus or minus 4.25 to plus or minus 7.00d sphere, 4.25 to 6.00d cylinder, per lens

V2210 Spherocylinder, bifocal, plus or minus 4.25 to plus or minus 7.00d sphere, over 6.00d cylinder, per lens

V2211 Spherocylinder, bifocal, plus or minus 7.25 to plus or minus 12.00d sphere, 0.25 to 2.25d cylinder, per lens

V2212 Spherocylinder, bifocal, plus or minus 7.25 to plus or minus 12.00d sphere, 2.25 to 4.00d cylinder, per lens

V2213 Spherocylinder, bifocal, plus or minus 7.25 to plus or minus 12.00d sphere, 4.25 to 6.00d cylinder, per lens

V2214 Spherocylinder, bifocal, sphere over plus or minus 12.00d, per lens

V2215 Lenticular (myodisc), per lens, bifocal

V2218 Aniseikonic, per lens, bifocal

V2219 Bifocal seg width over 28mm

V2220 Bifocal add over 3.25d

V2221 Lenticular lens, per lens, bifocal

V2299 Specialty bifocal (by report)
 Pertinent documentation to evaluate medical appropriateness should be included when this code is reported.

TRIFOCAL, GLASS, OR PLASTIC

V2300 Sphere, trifocal, plano to plus or minus 4.00d, per lens

V2301 Sphere, trifocal, plus or minus 4.12 to plus or minus 7.00d per lens

V2302 Sphere, trifocal, plus or minus 7.12 to plus or minus 20.00, per lens

V2303 Spherocylinder, trifocal, plano to plus or minus 4.00d sphere, 0.12 to 2.00d cylinder, per lens

V2304 Spherocylinder, trifocal, plano to plus or minus 4.00d sphere, 2.25 to 4.00d cylinder, per lens

V2305 Spherocylinder, trifocal, plano to plus or minus 4.00d sphere, 4.25 to 6.00 cylinder, per lens

V2306 Spherocylinder, trifocal, plano to plus or minus 4.00d sphere, over 6.00d cylinder, per lens

V2307 Spherocylinder, trifocal, plus or minus 4.25 to plus or minus 7.00d sphere, 0.12 to 2.00d cylinder, per lens

V2308 Spherocylinder, trifocal, plus or minus 4.25 to plus or minus 7.00d sphere, 2.12 to 4.00d cylinder, per lens

Vision Services

V2309   Spherocylinder, trifocal, plus or minus 4.25 to plus or minus 7.00d sphere, 4.25 to 6.00d cylinder, per lens

V2310   Spherocylinder, trifocal, plus or minus 4.25 to plus or minus 7.00d sphere, over 6.00d cylinder, per lens

V2311   Spherocylinder, trifocal, plus or minus 7.25 to plus or minus 12.00d sphere, 0.25 to 2.25d cylinder, per lens

V2312   Spherocylinder, trifocal, plus or minus 7.25 to plus or minus 12.00d sphere, 2.25 to 4.00d cylinder, per lens

V2313   Spherocylinder, trifocal, plus or minus 7.25 to plus or minus 12.00d sphere, 4.25 to 6.00d cylinder, per lens

V2314   Spherocylinder, trifocal, sphere over plus or minus 12.00d, per lens

V2315   Lenticular, (myodisc), per lens, trifocal

V2318   Aniseikonic lens, trifocal

V2319   Trifocal seg width over 28 mm

V2320   Trifocal add over 3.25d

V2321   Lenticular lens, per lens, trifocal

V2399   Specialty trifocal (by report)
Pertinent documentation to evaluate medical appropriateness should be included when this code is reported.

VARIABLE ASPHERICITY LENS, GLASS, OR PLASTIC

V2410   Variable asphericity lens, single vision, full field, glass or plastic, per lens

V2430   Variable asphericity lens, bifocal, full field, glass or plastic, per lens

V2499   Variable sphericity lens, other type

CONTACT LENS

V2500   Contact lens, PMMA, spherical, per lens

V2501   Contact lens, PMMA, toric or prism ballast, per lens

V2502   Contact lens PMMA, bifocal, per lens

V2503   Contact lens, PMMA, color vision deficiency, per lens

V2510   Contact lens, gas permeable, spherical, per lens

V2511   Contact lens, gas permeable, toric, prism ballast, per lens

V2512   Contact lens, gas permeable, bifocal, per lens

V2513   Contact lens, gas permeable, extended wear, per lens

V2520   Contact lens, hydrophilic, spherical, per lens
Hydrophilic contact lenses are covered by Medicare only for aphakic patients. Local contractor if incident to physician services.

V2521   Contact lens, hydrophilic, toric, or prism ballast, per lens
Hydrophilic contact lenses are covered by Medicare only for aphakic patients. Local contractor if incident to physician services.

V2522   Contact lens, hydrophilic, bifocal, per lens
Hydrophilic contact lenses are covered by Medicare only for aphakic patients. Local contractor if incident to physician services.

V2523   Contact lens, hydrophilic, extended wear, per lens
Hydrophilic contact lenses are covered by Medicare only for aphakic patients.

V2530   Contact lens, scleral, gas impermeable, per lens (for contact lens modification, see 92325)

V2531   Contact lens, scleral, gas permeable, per lens (for contact lens modification, see 92325)

V2599   Contact lens, other type
Local contractor if incident to physician services.

VISION AIDS

V2600   Hand held low vision aids and other nonspectacle mounted aids

V2610   Single lens spectacle mounted low vision aids

V2615   Telescopic and other compound lens system, including distance vision telescopic, near vision telescopes and compound microscopic lens system

PROSTHETIC EYE

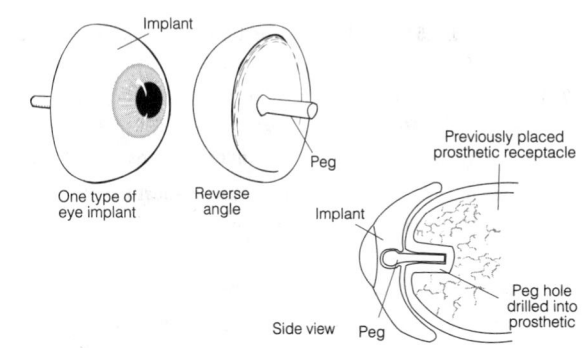

V2623   Prosthetic eye, plastic, custom

V2624   Polishing/resurfacing of ocular prosthesis

V2625   Enlargement of ocular prosthesis

V2626   Reduction of ocular prosthesis

V2627   Scleral cover shell
A scleral shell covers the cornea and the anterior sclera. Medicare covers a scleral shell when it is prescribed as an artificial support to a shrunken and sightless eye or as a barrier in the treatment of severe dry eye.

V2628   Fabrication and fitting of ocular conformer

V2629   Prosthetic eye, other type

INTRAOCULAR LENSES

V2630   Anterior chamber intraocular lens
The IOL must be FDA-approved for reimbursement. Medicare payment for an IOL is included in the payment for ASC facility services. Medicare jurisdiction: local contractor.

V2631   Iris supported intraocular lens
The IOL must be FDA-approved for reimbursement. Medicare payment for an IOL is included in the payment for ASC facility services. Medicare jurisdiction: local contractor.

V2632   Posterior chamber intraocular lens
The IOL must be FDA-approved for reimbursement. Medicare payment for an IOL is included in the payment for ASC facility services. Medicare jurisdiction: local contractor.
MED: 100-4,32,120.2

MISCELLANEOUS

V2700   Balance lens, per lens

V2702   Deluxe lens feature

V2710   Slab off prism, glass or plastic, per lens

V2715   Prism, per lens

V2718   Press-on lens, Fresnel prism, per lens

V2730   Special base curve, glass or plastic, per lens

V2744   Tint, photochromatic, per lens

V2745   Addition to lens; tint, any color, solid, gradient or equal, excludes photochromatic, any lens material, per lens

V2750   Antireflective coating, per lens

V2309 — V2750

Hearing Services

V2755 — V5272

V2755   U-V lens, per lens

V2756   Eye glass case

V2760   Scratch resistant coating, per lens

V2761   Mirror coating, any type, solid, gradient or equal, any lens material, per lens

V2762   Polarization, any lens material, per lens

V2770   Occluder lens, per lens

V2780   Oversize lens, per lens

V2781   Progressive lens, per lens

V2782   Lens, index 1.54 to 1.65 plastic or 1.60 to 1.79 glass, excludes polycarbonate, per lens

V2783   Lens, index greater than or equal to 1.66 plastic or greater than or equal to 1.80 glass, excludes polycarbonate, per lens

V2784   Lens, polycarbonate or equal, any index, per lens

V2785   Processing, preserving and transporting corneal tissue
Medicare jurisdiction: local contractor.
MED: 100-4,4,200.1

V2786   Specialty occupational multifocal lens, per lens

V2787   Astigmatism correcting function of intraocular lens
MED: 100-4,32,120.1; 100-4,32,120.2

V2788   Presbyopia correcting function of intraocular lens
MED: 100-4,32,120.1; 100-4,32,120.2

V2790   Amniotic membrane for surgical reconstruction, per procedure
Medicare jurisdiction: local contractor.
MED: 100-4,4,200.4

V2797   Vision supply, accessory and/or service component of another HCPCS vision code

V2799   Vision service, miscellaneous
Determine if an alternative HCPCS Level II or a CPT code better describes the service being reported. This code should be used only if a more specific code is unavailable.

HEARING SERVICES V5000-V5999

This range of codes describes hearing tests and related supplies and equipment, speech-language pathology screenings, and repair of augmentative communicative system.

HEARING SERVICES

V5008   Hearing screening

V5010   Assessment for hearing aid

V5011   Fitting/orientation/checking of hearing aid

V5014   Repair/modification of a hearing aid

V5020   Conformity evaluation

MONAURAL HEARING AID

V5030   Hearing aid, monaural, body worn, air conduction

V5040   Hearing aid, monaural, body worn, bone conduction

V5050   Hearing aid, monaural, in the ear

V5060   Hearing aid, monaural, behind the ear

OTHER HEARING SERVICES

V5070   Glasses, air conduction

V5080   Glasses, bone conduction

V5090   Dispensing fee, unspecified hearing aid

V5095   Semi-implantable middle ear hearing prosthesis

V5100   Hearing aid, bilateral, body worn

V5110   Dispensing fee, bilateral

HEARING AIDS, SERVICES, AND ACCESSORIES

V5120   Binaural, body

V5130   Binaural, in the ear

V5140   Binaural, behind the ear

V5150   Binaural, glasses

V5160   Dispensing fee, binaural

V5170   Hearing aid, CROS, in the ear

V5180   Hearing aid, CROS, behind the ear

V5190   Hearing aid, CROS, glasses

V5200   Dispensing fee, CROS

V5210   Hearing aid, BICROS, in the ear

V5220   Hearing aid, BICROS, behind the ear

V5230   Hearing aid, BICROS, glasses

V5240   Dispensing fee, BICROS

V5241   Dispensing fee, monaural hearing aid, any type

V5242   Hearing aid, analog, monaural, CIC (completely in the ear canal)

V5243   Hearing aid, analog, monaural, ITC (in the canal)

V5244   Hearing aid, digitally programmable analog, monaural, CIC

V5245   Hearing aid, digitally programmable, analog, monaural, ITC

V5246   Hearing aid, digitally programmable analog, monaural, ITE (in the ear)

V5247   Hearing aid, digitally programmable analog, monaural, BTE (behind the ear)

V5248   Hearing aid, analog, binaural, CIC

V5249   Hearing aid, analog, binaural, ITC

V5250   Hearing aid, digitally programmable analog, binaural, CIC

V5251   Hearing aid, digitally programmable analog, binaural, ITC

V5252   Hearing aid, digitally programmable, binaural, ITE

V5253   Hearing aid, digitally programmable, binaural, BTE

V5254   Hearing aid, digital, monaural, CIC

V5255   Hearing aid, digital, monaural, ITC

V5256   Hearing aid, digital, monaural, ITE

V5257   Hearing aid, digital, monaural, BTE

V5258   Hearing aid, digital, binaural, CIC

V5259   Hearing aid, digital, binaural, ITC

V5260   Hearing aid, digital, binaural, ITE

V5261   Hearing aid, digital, binaural, BTE

V5262   Hearing aid, disposable, any type, monaural

V5263   Hearing aid, disposable, any type, binaural

V5264   Ear mold/insert, not disposable, any type

V5265   Ear mold/insert, disposable, any type

V5266   Battery for use in hearing device

V5267   Hearing aid or assistive listening device/supplies/accessories, not otherwise specified

ASSISTIVE LISTENING DEVICE

V5268   Assistive listening device, telephone amplifier, any type

V5269   Assistive listening device, alerting, any type

V5270   Assistive listening device, television amplifier, any type

V5271   Assistive listening device, television caption decoder

V5272   Assistive listening device, TDD

V5273   Assistive listening device, for use with cochlear implant

V5274   Assistive listening device, not otherwise specified

MISCELLANEOUS HEARING SERVICES

V5275   Ear impression, each

V5281   Assistive listening device, personal FM/DM system, monaural (1 receiver, transmitter, microphone), any type

V5282   Assistive listening device, personal FM/DM system, binaural (2 receivers, transmitter, microphone), any type

V5283   Assistive listening device, personal FM/DM neck, loop induction receiver

V5284   Assistive listening device, personal FM/DM, ear level receiver

V5285   Assistive listening device, personal FM/DM, direct audio input receiver

V5286   Assistive listening device, personal blue tooth FM/DM receiver

V5287   Assistive listening device, personal FM/DM receiver, not otherwise specified

V5288   Assistive listening device, personal FM/DM transmitter assistive listening device

V5289   Assistive listening device, personal FM/DM adapter/boot coupling device for receiver, any type

V5290   Assistive listening device, transmitter microphone, any type

V5298   Hearing aid, not otherwise classified

V5299   Hearing service, miscellaneous
Determine if an alternative HCPCS Level II or a CPT code better describes the service being reported. This code should be used only if a more specific code is unavailable.

SPEECH-LANGUAGE PATHOLOGY SERVICES

V5336   Repair/modification of augmentative communicative system or device (excludes adaptive hearing aid)
Medicare jurisdiction: DME regional contractor.

V5362   Speech screening

V5363   Language screening

V5364   Dysphagia screening

APPENDIX 1 — TABLE OF DRUGS AND BIOLOGICALS

Introduction and Directions

The HCPCS 2013 Table of Drugs and Biologicals is designed to quickly and easily direct the user to drug names and their corresponding codes. Both generic and brand or trade names are alphabetically listed in the "Drug Name" column of the table. The associated A, C, J, K, Q, or S code is given only for the generic name of the drug. While we try to make the table comprehensive, it is not all-inclusive.

The "Unit Per" column lists the stated amount for the referenced generic drug as provided by CMS. "Up to" listings are inclusive of all quantities up to and including the listed amount. All other listings are for the amount of the drug as listed. The editors recognize that the availability of some drugs in the quantities listed is dependent on many variables beyond the control of the clinical ordering clerk. The availability in your area of regularly used drugs in the most cost-effective quantities should be relayed to your third-party payers.

The "Route of Administration" column addresses the most common methods of delivering the referenced generic drug as described in current pharmaceutical literature. The official definitions for Level II drug codes generally describe administration other than by oral method. Therefore, with a handful of exceptions, oral-delivered options for most drugs are omitted from the Route of Administration column.

Intravenous administration includes all methods, such as gravity infusion, injections, and timed pushes. When several routes of administration are listed, the first listing is simply the first, or most common, method as described in current reference literature. The "VAR" posting denotes various routes of administration and is used for drugs that are commonly administered into joints, cavities, tissues, or topical applications, in addition to other parenteral administrations. Listings posted with "OTH" alert the user to other administration methods, such as suppositories or catheter injections.

Please be reminded that the Table of Drugs, as well as all HCPCS Level II national definitions and listings, constitutes a post-treatment medical reference for billing purposes only. Although the editors have exercised all normal precautions to ensure the accuracy of the table and related material, the use of any of this information to select medical treatment is entirely inappropriate. Do not code directly from the table of drugs. Refer to the tabular section for complete information.

See Appendix 3 for abbreviations.

Drug Name	Unit Per	Route	Code
10% LMD	500 ML	IV	J7100
4-FACTOR PROTHROMBIN COMPLEX CONCENTRATE	1 IU	IV	C9132
5% DEXTROSE AND .45% NORMAL SALINE	1000 ML	IV	S5010
5% DEXTROSE IN LACTATED RINGER'S	1000 ML	IV	S5011
5% DEXTROSE WITH POTASSIUM CHLORIDE	1000 ML	IV	S5012
5% DEXTROSE/.45% NS WITH KCL AND MAG SULFATE	1500 ML	IV	S5014
5% DEXTROSE/.45% NS WITH KCL AND MAG SULFATE	1000ML	IV	S5013
5% DEXTROSE/NORMAL SALINE	5%	VAR	J7042
5% DEXTROSE/WATER	500 ML	IV	J7060
ABATACEPT	10 MG	IV	J0129
ABCIXIMAB	10 MG	IV	J0130
ABELCET	10 MG	IV	J0287
ABILIFY	0.25 MG	IM	J0400
ABILIFY MAINTENA KIT	1 MG	IM	J0401
ABLAVAR	1 ML	IV	A9583
ABOBOTULINUMTOXINA	5 UNITS	IM	J0586
ABRAXANE	1 MG	IV	J9264
ACCELULAR PERICARDIAL TISSUE MATRIX NONHUMAN	SQ CM	OTH	C9354
ACCUNEB NONCOMPOUNDED, CONCENTRATED	1 MG	INH	J7611
ACCUNEB NONCOMPOUNDED, UNIT DOSE	1 MG	INH	J7613
ACETADOTE	1 G	INH	J7608

Drug Name	Unit Per	Route	Code
ACETADOTE	100 MG	IV	J0132
ACETAMINOPHEN	10 MG	IV	J0131
ACETAZOLAMIDE SODIUM	500 MG	IM, IV	J1120
ACETYLCYSTEINE COMPOUNDED	PER G	INH	J7604
ACETYLCYSTEINE NONCOMPOUNDED	1 G	INH	J7608
ACTEMRA	1 MG	IV	J3262
ACTHREL	1 MCG	IV	J0795
ACTIMMUNE	3 MU	SC	J9216
ACTIVASE	1 MG	IV	J2997
ACUTECT	STUDY DOSE UP TO 20 MCI	IV	A9504
ACYCLOVIR	5 MG	IV	J0133
ADAGEN	25 IU	IM	J2504
ADALIMUMAB	20 MG	SC	J0135
ADCETRIS	1 MG	IV	J9042
ADENOCARD	6 MG	IV	J0150
ADENOSINE	6 MG	IV	J0150
ADENOSINE	1 MG	IV	J0151
ADENSOSCAN	1 MG	IV	J0151
ADO-TRASTUZUMAB EMTANSINE	1 MG	IV	J9354
ADRENALIN	0.1 MG	IM, IV, SC	J0171
ADRENOCORT	1 MG	IM, IV, OTH	J1100
ADRIAMYCIN	10 MG	IV	J9000
ADRUCIL	500 MG	IV	J9190
AEROBID	1 MG	INH	J7641
AFINITOR	0.25 MG	ORAL	J7527
AFLIBERCEPT	1 MG	OTH	J0178
AFLURIA	EA	IM	Q2035
AGALSIDASE BETA	1 MG	IV	J0180
AGGRASTAT	12.5 MG	IM, IV	J3246
AGRIFLU	UNKNOWN	IM	Q2034
A-HYDROCORT	100 MG	IV, IM, SC	J1720
ALATROFLOXACIN MESYLATE	100 MG	IV	J0200
ALBUTEROL AND IPRATROPIUM BROMIDE NONCOMPOUNDED	2.5MG/0.5 MG	INH	J7620
ALBUTEROL COMPOUNDED, CONCENTRATED	1 MG	INH	J7610
ALBUTEROL COMPOUNDED, UNIT DOSE	1 MG	INH	J7609
ALBUTEROL NONCOMPOUNDED, UNIT DOSE	1 MG	INH	J7613
ALBUTEROL, NONCOMPOUNDED, CONCENTRATED FORM	1 MG	INH	J7611
ALDESLEUKIN	1 VIAL	IV	J9015
ALDURAZYME	0.1 MG	IV	J1931
ALEFACEPT	0.5 MG	IV, IM	J0215
ALEMTUZUMAB	10 MG	IV	J9010
ALFERON N	250,000 IU	IM	J9215
ALGLUCERASE	10 U	IV	J0205
ALGLUCOSIDASE ALFA (LUMIZYME)	10 MG	IV	J0221
ALGLUCOSIDASE ALFA NOS	10 MG	IV	J0220
ALIMTA	10 MG	IV	J9305
ALKERAN	2 MG	ORAL	J8600
ALKERAN	50 MG	IV	J9245
ALLODERM	SQ CM	OTH	Q4116
ALLOGRAFT, CYMETRA	1 CC	INJ	Q4112
ALLOGRAFT, GRAFTJACKET EXPRESS	1 CC	INJ	Q4113
ALLOPATCHHD	SQ CM	OTH	Q4128
ALLOSKIN	SQ CM	OTH	Q4115

Drug Name	Unit Per	Route	Code
ALLOSKIN AC	SQ CM	OTH	Q4141
ALLOSKIN RT	SQ CM	OTH	Q4123
ALOXI	25 MCG	IV	J2469
ALPHA 1 - PROTEINASE INHIBITOR (HUMAN) NOS	10 MG	IV	J0256
ALPHA 1-PROTENIASE INHIBITOR (HUMAN) (GLASSIA)	10 MG	IV	J0257
ALPHANATE	PER FACTOR VIII IU	IV	J7186
ALPHANINE SD	1 IU	IV	J7193
ALPROSTADIL	1.25 MCG	IV	J0270
ALPROSTADIL	EA	OTH	J0275
ALTEPLASE RECOMBINANT	1 MG	IV	J2997
ALUPENT, NONCOMPOUNDED, CONCENTRATED	10 MG	INH	J7668
ALUPENT, NONCOMPOUNDED, UNIT DOSE	10 MG	INH	J7669
AMANTADINE HCL (DEMONSTRATION PROJECT)	100 MG	ORAL	G9017
AMANTADINE HYDROCHLORIDE (BRAND NAME) (DEMONSTRTION PROJECT)	100 MG	ORAL	G9033
AMANTADINE HYDROCHLORIDE (GENERIC)	100 MG	ORAL	G9017
AMBISOME	10 MG	IV	J0289
AMCORT	5 MG	IM	J3302
AMERGAN	12.5 MG	ORAL	Q0169
A-METHAPRED	40 MG	IM, IV	J2920
A-METHAPRED	125 MG	IM, IV	J2930
AMEVIVE	0.5 MG	IV, IM	J0215
AMICAR	5 G	IV	S0017
AMIFOSTINE	500 MG	IV	J0207
AMIKACIN SULFATE	100 MG	IM, IV	J0278
AMINOCAPRIOC ACID	5 G	IV	S0017
AMINOPHYLLINE	250 MG	IV	J0280
AMIODARONE HCL	30 MG	IV	J0282
AMITRIPTYLINE HCL	20 MG	IM	J1320
AMMONIA N-13	STUDY DOSE UP TO 40 MCI	IV	A9526
AMNIOEXCEL	SQ CM	OTH	Q4137
AMNIOMATRIX	1 CC	OTH	Q4139
AMOBARBITAL	125 MG	IM, IV	J0300
AMPHOCIN	50 MG	IV	J0285
AMPHOTEC	10 MG	IV	J0287
AMPHOTERICIN B	50 MG	IV	J0285
AMPHOTERICIN B CHOLESTERYL SULFATE COMPLEX	10 MG	IV	J0288
AMPHOTERICIN B LIPID COMPLEX	10 MG	IV	J0287
AMPHOTERICIN B LIPOSOME	10 MG	IV	J0289
AMPICILLIN SODIUM	500 MG	IM, IV	J0290
AMPICILLIN SODIUM/SULBACTAM SODIUM	1.5 G	IM, IV	J0295
AMYGDALIN	VAR	INJ	J3570
AMYTAL	125 MG	IM, IV	J0300
AMYVID	UP TO 10 MILLICUIRES	IV	A9586
ANASCORP	UP TO 120 MG	IV	J0716
ANASTROZOLE	1 MG	ORAL	S0170
ANCEF	500 MG	IM, IV	J0690
AN-DTPA DIAGNOSTIC	STUDY DOSE UP TO 25 MCI	IV	A9539

Drug Name	Unit Per	Route	Code
AN-DTPA THERAPEUTIC	STUDY DOSE UP TO 25 MCI	INH	A9567
ANECTINE	20 MG	IM, IV	J0330
ANGIOMAX	1 MG	IV	J0583
ANIDULAFUNGIN	1 MG	IV	J0348
ANISTREPLASE	30 U	IV	J0350
ANTAGON	250 MCG	SC	S0132
ANTIEMETIC NOC	VAR	ORAL	Q0181
ANTIEMETIC DRUG NOC	VAR	OTH	J8498
ANTIEMETIC DRUG NOS	VAR	ORAL	J8597
ANTIHEMOPHILIC FACTOR HUMAN METHOD M MONOCLONAL PURIFIED	1 IU	IV	J7192
ANTIHEMOPHILIC FACTOR PORCINE	1 IU	IV	J7191
ANTIHEMOPHILIC FACTOR VIII, XYNTHA, RECOMBINANT	1 IU	IV	J7185
ANTIHEMOPHILIC FACTOR VIII/VON WILLEBRAND FACTOR COMPLEX, HUMAN	PER FACTOR VIII IU	IV	J7186
ANTI-INHIBITOR	1 IU	IV	J7198
ANTITHROMBIN III	1 IU	IV	J7195
ANTITHROMBIN RECOMBINANT	50 IU	IV	J7196
ANTI-THYMOCYTE GLOBULIN, EQUINE	250 MG	OTH	J7504
ANTIZOL	15 MG	IV	J1451
ANZEMET	50 MG	ORAL	S0174
ANZEMET	10 MG	IV	J1260
ANZEMET	100 MG	ORAL	Q0180
APLIGRAF	SQ CM	OTH	Q4101
APOKYN	1 MG	SC	J0364
APOMORPHINE HYDROCHLORIDE	1 MG	SC	J0364
APREPITANT	5 MG	ORAL	J8501
APROTININ	10,000 KIU	IV	J0365
AQUAMEPHYTON	1 MG	IM, SC, IV	J3430
ARA-C	100 MG	SC, IV	J9100
ARALEN	UP TO 250 MG	IM, IV	J0390
ARAMINE	10 MG	IV, IM, SC	J0380
ARANESP, ESRD USE	1 MCG	SC, IV	J0882
ARANESP, NON-ESRD USE	1 MCG	SC, IV	J0881
ARBUTAMINE HCL	1 MG	IV	J0395
ARCALYST	1 MG	SC	J2793
ARCHITECT EXTRACELLULAR MATRIX	SQ CM	OTH	Q4147
AREDIA	30 MG	IV	J2430
ARFORMOTEROL	15 MCG	INH	J7605
ARIDOL	5 MG	INH	J7665
ARIMIDEX	1 MG	ORAL	S0170
ARIPIPRAZOLE	0.25 MG	IM	J0400
ARIPIPRAZOLE, EXTENDED RELEASE	1 MG	IM	J0401
ARISTOCORT	5 MG	IM	J3302
ARISTOCORTE FORTE	5 MG	IM	J3302
ARISTOCORTE INTRALESIONAL	5 MG	OTH	J3302
ARISTOSPAN	5 MG	VAR	J3303
ARIXTRA	0.5 MG	SC	J1652
AROMASIN	25 MG	ORAL	S0156
ARRANON	50 MG	IV	J9261
ARRESTIN	200 MG	IM	J3250
ARSENIC TRIOXIDE	1 MG	IV	J9017
ARTHROFLEX	SQ CM	OTH	Q4125
ARTISS FIBRIN SEALANT	2 ML	OTH	C9250
ARZERRA	10 MG	IV	J9302

Drug Name	Unit Per	Route	Code
ASPARAGINASE	10,000 U	IM, IV, SC	J9020
ASPARAGINASE	1,000 IU	IM,IV,SC	J9019
ASTAGRAF XL	0.1 MG	ORAL	J7508
ASTRAMORPH PF	10 MG	IM, IV, SC	J2275
ATGAM	250 MG	OTH	J7504
ATIVAN	2 MG	IM, IV	J2060
ATOPICLAIR	ANY SIZE	OTH	A6250
ATROPEN	0.01 MG	IM	J0461
ATROPINE SULFATE	0.01 MG	IM, IV, SC	J0461
ATROPINE, COMPOUNDED, CONCENTRATED	I MG	INH	J7635
ATROPINE, COMPOUNDED, UNIT DOSE	1 MG	INH	J7636
ATROVENT, NONCOMPOUNDED, UNIT DOSE	1 MG	INH	J7644
ATRYN	50 IU	IV	J7196
AUROTHIOGLUCOSE	50 MG	IM	J2910
AUTOPLEX T	1 IU	IV	J7198
AVASTIN	0.25 MG	IV	C9257
AVASTIN	10 MG	IV	J9035
AVELOX	100 MG	IV	J2280
AVONEX	30 MCG	IM	J1826
AVONEX	1 MCG	IM	Q3027
AZACITIDINE	1 MG	SC	J9025
AZACTAM	500 MG	IV	S0073
AZASAN	50 MG	ORAL	J7500
AZATHIOPRINE	100 MG	OTH	J7501
AZATHIOPRINE	50 MG	ORAL	J7500
AZITHROMYCIN	500 MG	IV	J0456
AZMACORT	PER MG	INH	J7684
AZMACORT CONCENTRATED	PER MG	INH	J7683
AZTREONAM	500 MG	IV, IM	S0073
BACLOFEN	50 MCG	IT	J0476
BACLOFEN	10 MG	IT	J0475
BACTOCILL	250 MG	IM, IV	J2700
BACTRIM IV	10 ML	IV	S0039
BAL	100 MG	IM	J0470
BASILIXIMAB	20 MG	IV	J0480
BCG INTRAVESICLE	VIAL	OTH	J9031
BEBULIN VH	1 IU	IV	J7194
BECAPLERMIN GEL 0.01%	0.5 G	OTH	S0157
BECLOMETHASONE COMPOUNDED	1 MG	INH	J7622
BECLOVENT COMPOUNDED	1 MG	INH	J7622
BECONASE COMPOUNDED	1 MG	INH	J7622
BELATACEPT	1 MG	IV	J0485
BELIMUMAB	10 MG	IV	J0490
BENA-D 10	50 MG	IV, IM	J1200
BENA-D 50	50 MG	IV, IM	J1200
BENADRYL	50 MG	IV, IM	J1200
BENAHIST 10	50 MG	IV, IM	J1200
BENAHIST 50	50 MG	IV, IM	J1200
BENDAMUSTINE HCL	1 MG	IV	J9033
BENEFIX	1 IU	IV	J7195
BENLYSTA	10 MG	IV	J0490
BENOJECT-10	50 MG	IV, IM	J1200
BENOJECT-50	50 MG	IV, IM	J1200
BENTYL	20 MG	IM	J0500
BENZTROPINE MESYLATE	1 MG	IM, IV	J0515

Drug Name	Unit Per	Route	Code
BERINERT	10 U	IV	J0597
BERUBIGEN	1,000 MCG	SC, IM	J3420
BETA-2	1 MG	INH	J7648
BETALIN 12	1,000 MCG	SC, IM	J3420
BETAMETHASONE ACETATE AND BETAMETHASONE SODIUM PHOSPHATE	3 MG, OF EACH	IM	J0702
BETAMETHASONE COMPOUNDED, UNIT DOSE	1 MG	INH	J7624
BETASERON	0.25 MG	SC	J1830
BETHANECHOL CHLORIDE, MYOTONACHOL OR URECHOLINE	5 MG	SC	J0520
BEVACIZUMAB	10 MG	IV	J9035
BEVACIZUMAB	0.25 MG	IV	C9257
BEXXAR THERAPEUTIC	TX DOSE	IV	A9545
BICILLIN CR	100,000 UNITS	IM	J0558
BICILLIN CR 900/300	100,000 UNITS	IM	J0558
BICILLIN CR TUBEX	100,000 UNITS	IM	J0558
BICILLIN LA	100,000 U	IM	J0561
BICNU	100 MG	IV	J9050
BIOCLATE	1 IU	IV	J7192
BIODEXCEL	SQ CM	OTH	Q4137
BIODFENCE	SQ CM	OTH	Q4140
BIODFENCE DRYFLEX	SQ CM	OTH	Q4138
BIODMATRIX	1 CC	OTH	Q4139
BIOTROPIN	1 MG	SC	J2941
BIPERIDEN LACTATE	5 MG	IM, IV	J0190
BITOLTEROL MESYLATE, COMPOUNDED CONCENTRATED	PER MG	INH	J7628
BITOLTEROL MESYLATE, COMPOUNDED UNIT DOSE	PER MG	INH	J7629
BIVALIRUDIN	1 MG	IV	J0583
BLENOXANE	15 U	IM, IV, SC	J9040
BLEOMYCIN LYOPHILLIZED	15 U	IM, IV, SC	J9040
BLEOMYCIN SULFATE	15 U	IM, IV, SC	J9040
BONIVA	1 MG	IV	J1740
BORTEZOMIB	0.1 MG	IV	J9041
BOTOX	1 UNIT	IM, OTH	J0585
BOTOX COSMETIC	1 UNIT	IM, OTH	J0585
BOTULINUM TOXIN TYPE A	1 UNIT	IM, OTH	J0585
BOTULINUM TOXIN TYPE B	100 U	OTH	J0587
BRAVELLE	75 IU	SC, IM	J3355
BRENTUXIMAB VENDOTIN	1 MG	IV	J9042
BRETHINE	PER MG	INH	J7681
BRETHINE CONCENTRATED	PER MG	INH	J7680
BRICANYL	PER MG	INH	J7681
BRICANYL CONCENTRATED	PER MG	INH	J7680
BROM-A-COT	10 MG	IM, SC, IV	J0945
BROMPHENIRAMINE MALEATE	10 MG	IM, SC, IV	J0945
BUDESONIDE COMPOUNDED, CONCETRATED	0.25 MG	INH	J7634
BUDESONIDE, COMPOUNDED, UNIT DOSE	0.5 MG	INH	J7627
BUDESONIDE, NONCOMPOUNDED, CONCENTRATED	0.25 MG	INH	J7633
BUDESONIDE, NONCOMPOUNDED, UNIT DOSE	0.5 MG	INH	J7626
BUMETANIDE	0.5 MG	IM, IV	S0171

Drug Name	Unit Per	Route	Code
BUPIVACAINE HCL	30 ML	VAR	S0020
BUPIVACAINE LIPOSOME	1 MG	VAR	C9290
BUPRENEX	0.1 MG	IM, IV	J0592
BUPRENORPHINE HCL	0.1 MG	IM, IV	J0592
BUPROPION HCL	150 MG	ORAL	S0106
BUSULFAN	2 MG	ORAL	J8510
BUSULFAN	1 MG	IV	J0594
BUSULFEX	2 MG	ORAL	J8510
BUTORPHANOL TARTRATE	25 MG	OTH	S0012
BUTORPHANOL TARTRATE	2 MG	IM, IV	J0595
C 1 ESTERASE INHIBITOR (HUMAN) (BERINERT)	10 UNITS	IV	J0597
C1 ESTERASE INHIBITOR (HUMAN) (CINRYZE)	10 UNITS	IV	J0598
CABAZITAXEL	1 MG	IV	J9043
CABERGOLINE	0.25 MG	ORAL	J8515
CAFCIT	5 MG	IV	J0706
CAFFEINE CITRATE	5 MG	IV	J0706
CALCIJEX	0.1 MCG	IM	J0636
CALCIJEX	0.25 MCG	INJ	S0169
CALCIMAR	UP TO 400 U	SC, IM	J0630
CALCITONIN SALMON	400 U	SC, IM	J0630
CALCITRIOL	0.1 MCG	IM	J0636
CALCITROL	0.25 MCG	IM	S0169
CALCIUM DISODIUM VERSENATE	1,000 MG	IV, SC, IM	J0600
CALCIUM GLUCONATE	10 ML	IV	J0610
CALCIUM GLYCEROPHOSPHATE AND CALCIUM LACTATE	10 ML	IM, SC	J0620
CALDOLOR	100 MG	IV	J1741
CAMPATH	10 MG	IV	J9010
CAMPTOSAR	20 MG	IV	J9206
CANAKINUMAB	1 MG	SC	J0638
CANCIDAS	5 MG	IV	J0637
CAPECITABINE	150 MG	ORAL	J8520
CAPROMAB PENDETIDE	STUDY DOSE UP TO 10 MCI	IV	A9507
CAPSAICIN 8% PATCH	10 SQ CM	OTH	J7335
CARBOCAINE	10 ML	VAR	J0670
CARBOPLATIN	50 MG	IV	J9045
CARDIOGEN 82	STUDY DOSE UP TO 60 MCI	IV	A9555
CARDIOLITE	STUDY DOSE	IV	A9500
CARFILZOMIB	1 MG	IV	J9047
CARIMUNE	500 MG	IV	J1566
CARMUSTINE	100 MG	IV	J9050
CARNITOR	1 G	IV	J1955
CARTICEL		OTH	J7330
CASPOFUNGIN ACETATE	5 MG	IV	J0637
CATAPRES	1 MG	OTH	J0735
CATHFLO	1 MG	IV	J2997
CAVERJECT	1.25 MCG	VAR	J0270
CEA SCAN	STUDY DOSE UP TO 45 MCI	IV	A9568
CEENU	10 MG	ORAL	S0178
CEFAZOLIN SODIUM	500 MG	IM, IV	J0690
CEFEPIME HCL	500 MG	IV	J0692
CEFIZOX	500 MG	IV, IM	J0715
CEFOBID	1 G	IV	S0021
CEFOPERAZONE SODIUM	1 G	IV	S0021

Drug Name	Unit Per	Route	Code
CEFOTAN	500 MG	IM, IV	S0074
CEFOTAXIME SODIUM	1 GM	IV, IM	J0698
CEFOTETAN DISODIUM	500 MG	IM. IV	S0074
CEFOXITIN SODIUM	1 GM	IV, IM	J0694
CEFTAROLINE FOSAMIL	10 MG	IV	J0712
CEFTAZIDIME	500 MG	IM, IV	J0713
CEFTIZOXIME SODIUM	500 MG	IV, IM	J0715
CEFTRIAXONE SODIUM	250 MG	IV, IM	J0696
CEFUROXIME	750 MG	IM, IV	J0697
CEFUROXIME SODIUM STERILE	750 MG	IM, IV	J0697
CELESTONE SOLUSPAN	3 MG	IM	J0702
CELLCEPT	250 MG	ORAL	J7517
CENACORT A-40	10 MG	IM	J3301
CENACORT FORTE	5 MG	IM	J3302
CENTRUROIDES (SCORPION) IMMUNE F(AB)2 (EQUINE)	UP TO 120 MG	IV	J0716
CEPHALOTHIN SODIUM	UP TO 1 G	INJ	J1890
CEPHAPIRIN SODIUM	1 G	IV	J0710
CEPTAZ	500 MG	IM, IV	J0713
CEREBRYX	750 MG	IM, IV	S0078
CEREBRYX	50 MG	IM, IV	Q2009
CEREDASE	10 U	IV	J0205
CERETEC	STUDY DOSE UP TO 25 MCI	IV	A9521
CEREZYME	10 U	IV	J1786
CERTOLIZUMAB PEGOL	1 MG	SC	J0717
CERUBIDINE	10 MG	IV	J9150
CESAMET	1 MG	ORAL	J8650
CETUXIMAB	10 MG	IV	J9055
CHEALAMIDE	150 MG	IV	J3520
CHLORAMBUCIL	2 MG	ORAL	S0172
CHLORAMPHENICOL SODIUM SUCCINATE	1 G	IV	J0720
CHLORDIAZEPOXIDE HCL	100 MG	IM, IV	J1990
CHLOROMYCETIN	1 G	IV	J0720
CHLOROPROCAINE HCL	30 ML	VAR	J2400
CHLOROQUINE HCL	UP TO 250 MG	IM, IV	J0390
CHLOROTHIAZIDE SODIUM	500 MG	IV	J1205
CHLORPROMAZINE HCL	50 MG	IM, IV	J3230
CHLORPROMAZINE HCL	5 MG	ORAL	Q0161
CHOLETEC	STUDY DOSE UP TO 15 MCI	IV	A9537
CHOREX	1000 USP	IM	J0725
CHORIONIC GONADOTROPIN	1,000 USP U	IM	J0725
CHROMIC PHOSPHATE P32 (THERAPEUTIC)	1 MCI	IV	A9564
CHROMITOPE SODIUM	STUDY DOSE UP TO 250 UCI	IV	A9553
CHROMIUM CR-51 SODIUM IOTHALAMATE, DIAGNOSTIC	STUDY DOSE UP TO 250 UCI	IV	A9553
CIDOFOVIR	375 MG	IV	J0740
CILASTATIN SODIUM	250 MG	IV, IM	J0743
CIMETIDINE HCL	300 MG	IM, IV	S0023
CIMZIA	1 MG	SC	J0717
CINRZYE	10 UNITS	IV	J0598
CIPRO	200 MG	IV	J0744

Drug Name	Unit Per	Route	Code
CIPROFLOXACIN FOR INTRAVENOUS INFUSION	200 MG	IV	J0744
CIS-MDP	STUDY DOSE UP TO 30 MCI	IV	A9503
CISPLATIN	10 MG	IV	J9060
CIS-PYRO	STUDY DOSE UP TO 25 MCI	IV	A9538
CLADRIBINE	1 MG	IV	J9065
CLAFORAN	1 GM	IV, IM	J0698
CLEOCIN PHOSPHATE	300 MG	IV	S0077
CLEVIDIPINE BUTYRATE	1 MG	IV	C9248
CLEVIPREX	1 MG	IV	C9248
CLINDAMYCIN PHOSPHATE	300 MG	IV	S0077
CLOFARABINE	1 MG	IV	J9027
CLOLAR	1 MG	IV	J9027
CLONIDINE HCL	1 MG	OTH	J0735
CLOZAPINE	25 MG	ORAL	S0136
CLOZARIL	25 MG	ORAL	S0136
COBAL	1,000 MCG	IM, SC	J3420
COBALT CO-57 CYNOCOBALAMIN, DIAGNOSTIC	STUDY DOSE UP TO 1 UCI	ORAL	A9559
COBATOPE 57	STUDY DOSE UP TO 1 UCI	ORAL	A9559
COBEX	1,000 MCG	SC, IM	J3420
CODEINE PHOSPHATE	30 MG	IM, IV, SC	J0745
COGENTIN	1 MG	IM, IV	J0515
COGNEX	10 MG	ORAL	S0014
COLCHICINE	1 MG	IV	J0760
COLHIST	10 MG	IM, SC, IV	J0945
COLISTIMETHATE SODIUM	1 MG	INH	S0142
COLISTIMETHATE SODIUM	150 MG	IM, IV	J0770
COLLAGEN BASED WOUND FILLER DRY FOAM	1 GM	OTH	A6010
COLLAGEN BASED WOUND FILLER, GEL/PASTE	1 GM	OTH	A6011
COLLAGEN MATRIX NERVE WRAP	0.5 CM	OTH	C9361
COLLAGEN NERVE CUFF	0.5 CM LENGTH	OTH	C9355
COLLAGENASE, CLOSTRIDIUM HISTOLYTICUM	0.01 MG	OTH	J0775
COLY-MYCIN M	150 MG	IM, IV	J0770
COMPAZINE	5 MG	ORAL	Q0164
COMPAZINE	5 MG	ORAL	S0183
COMPAZINE	10 MG	IM, IV	J0780
CONTRACEPTIVE SUPPLY, HORMONE CONTAINING PATCH	EACH	OTH	J7304
CONTRAST FOR ECHOCARDIOGRAM	STUDY	IV	A9700
COPAXONE	20 MG	SC	J1595
COPPER T MODEL TCU380A IUD COPPER WIRE/COPPER COLLAR	EA	OTH	J7300
CORDARONE	30 MG	IV	J0282
CORIFACT	1 IU	IV	J7180
CORTASTAT	1 MG	IM, IV, OTH	J1100
CORTASTAT LA	1 MG	IM	J1094
CORTICORELIN OVINE TRIFLUTATE	1 MCG	IV	J0795
CORTICOTROPIN	40 U	IV, IM, SC	J0800
CORTIMED	80 MG	IM	J1040
CORTROSYN	0.25 MG	IM, IV	J0834
CORVERT	1 MG	IV	J1742
COSMEGEN	0.5 MG	IV	J9120

Drug Name	Unit Per	Route	Code
COSYNTROPIN	0.25 MG	IM, IV	J0833
COTOLONE	5 MG	ORAL	J7510
CROFAB	UP TO 1 GM	IV	J0840
CROMOLYN SODIUM COMPOUNDED	PER 10 MG	INH	J7632
CROMOLYN SODIUM NONCOMPOUNDED	10 MG	INH	J7631
CROTALIDAE POLYVALENT IMMUNE FAB (OVINE)	UP TO 1 GM	IV	J0840
CRYSTAL B12	1,000 MCG	IM, SC	J3420
CRYSTICILLIN 300 A.S.	600,000 UNITS	IM, IV	J2510
CRYSTICILLIN 600 A.S.	600,000 UNITS	IM, IV	J2510
CUBICIN	1 MG	IV	J0878
CYANO	1,000 MCG	IM, SC	J3420
CYANOCOBALAMIN	1,000 MCG	IM, SC	J3420
CYANOCOBALAMIN COBALT 57/58	STUDY DOSE UP TO 1 UCI	IV	A9546
CYANOCOBALAMIN COBALT CO-57	STUDY DOSE UP TO 1 UCI	ORAL	A9559
CYCLOPHOSPHAMIDE	25 MG	ORAL	J8530
CYCLOPHOSPHAMIDE	100 MG	IV	J9070
CYCLOSPORINE	100 MG	ORAL	J7502
CYCLOSPORINE	250 MG	IV	J7516
CYCLOSPORINE	25 MG	ORAL	J7515
CYMETRA	1 CC	INJ	Q4112
CYSVIEW	STUDY DOSE	OTH	C9275
CYTARABINE	100 MG	SC, IV	J9100
CYTARABINE LIPOSOME	10 MG	IT	J9098
CYTOGAM	VIAL	IV	J0850
CYTOMEGALOVIRUS IMMUNE GLOB	VIAL	IV	J0850
CYTOSAR-U	100 MG	SC, IV	J9100
CYTOTEC	200 MCG	ORAL	S0191
CYTOVENE	500 MG	IV	J1570
CYTOXAN	100 MG	IV	J9070
CYTOXAN	25 MG	ORAL	J8530
D.H.E. 45	1 MG	IM, IV	J1110
DACARBAZINE	100 MG	IV	J9130
DACLIZUMAB	25 MG	OTH	J7513
DACOGEN	1 MG	IV	J0894
DACTINOMYCIN	0.5 MG	IV	J9120
DALALONE	1 MG	IM, IV, OTH	J1100
DALALONE LA	1 MG	IM	J1094
DALTEPARIN SODIUM	2,500 IU	SC	J1645
DAPTOMYCIN	1 MG	IV	J0878
DARBEPOETIN ALFA, ESRD USE	1 MCG	SC, IV	J0882
DARBEPOETIN ALFA, NON-ESRD USE	1 MCG	SC, IV	J0881
DATSCAN	STUDY DOSE	IV	A9584
DAUNORUBICIN	10 MG	IV	J9150
DAUNORUBICIN CITRATE, LIPOOSOMAL FORMULATION	10 MG	IV	J9151
DAUNOXOME	10 MG	IV	J9151
DDAVP	1 MCG	IV, SC	J2597
DECADRON	0.25 MG	ORAL	J8540
DECAJECT	1 MG	IM, IV, OTH	J1100
DECITABINE	1 MG	IV	J0894
DECOLONE-50	50 MG	IM	J2320
DEFEROXAMINE MESYLATE	500 MG	IM, SC, IV	J0895
DEGARELIX	1 MG	SC	J9155

Drug Name	Unit Per	Route	Code
DELATESTRYL	200 MG	IM	J3130
DELATESTRYL	100 MG	IM	J3120
DELESTROGEN	10 MG	IM	J1380
DELTA-CORTEF	5 MG	ORAL	J7510
DEMADEX	10 MG	IV	J3265
DEMEROL	100 MG	IM, IV, SC	J2175
DENILEUKIN DIFTITOX	300 MCG	IV	J9160
DENOSUMAB	1 MG	SC	J0897
DEPANDRATE	1 CC, 200 MG	IM	J1080
DEPANDROGYN	1 ML	IM	J1060
DEPGYNOGEN	UP TO 5 MG	IM	J1000
DEPHENACEN-50	50 MG	IM, IV	J1200
DEPMEDALONE	80 MG	IM	J1040
DEPMEDALONE	40 MG	IM	J1030
DEPOCYT	10 MG	IT	J9098
DEPODUR	UP TO 10 MG	IV	J2270
DEPODUR	100 MG	IV	J2271
DEPO-ESTRADIOL CYPIONATE	UP TO 5 MG	IM	J1000
DEPOGEN	UP TO 5 MG	IM	J1000
DEPO-MEDROL	40 MG	IM, OTH	J1030
DEPO-MEDROL	80 MG	IM, OTH	J1040
DEPO-MEDROL	20 MG	IM, OTH	J1020
DEPO-TESTADIOL	1 ML	IM	J1060
DEPO-TESTOSTERONE	UP TO 100 MG	IM	J1070
DEPO-TESTOSTERONE	200 MG	IM	J1080
DEPTESTROGEN	UP TO 100 MG	IM	J1070
DERMACELL	SQ CM	OTH	Q4122
DERMAGRAFT	SQ CM	OTH	Q4106
DERMAL SUBSTITUTE, NATIVE, NONDENATURED COLLAGEN, FETAL	0.5 SQ CM	OTH	C9358
DERMAL SUBSTITUTE, NATIVE, NONDENATURED COLLAGEN, NEONATAL	0.5 SQ CM	OTH	C9360
DESFERAL	500 MG	IM, SC, IV	J0895
DESMOPRESSIN ACETATE	1 MCG	IV, SC	J2597
DEXAMETHASONE	0.25 MG	ORAL	J8540
DEXAMETHASONE ACETATE	1 MG	IM	J1094
DEXAMETHASONE ACETATE ANHYDROUS	1 MG	IM	J1094
DEXAMETHASONE INTRAVITREAL IMPLANT	0.1 MG	OTH	J7312
DEXAMETHASONE SODIUM PHOSPHATE	1 MG	IM, IV, OTH	J1100
DEXAMETHASONE, COMPOUNDED, CONCENTRATED	1 MG	INH	J7637
DEXAMETHASONE, COMPOUNDED, UNIT DOSE	1 MG	INH	J7638
DEXASONE	1 MG	IM, IV, OTH	J1100
DEXEDRINE	5 MG	ORAL	S0160
DEXIM	1 MG	IM, IV, OTH	J1100
DEXONE	0.25 MG	ORAL	J8540
DEXONE	1 MG	IM, IV, OTH	J1100
DEXONE LA	1 MG	IM	J1094
DEXRAZOXANE HCL	250 MG	IV	J1190
DEXTRAN 40	500 ML	IV	J7100
DEXTROAMPHETAMINE SULFATE	5 MG	ORAL	S0160
DEXTROSE	500 ML	IV	J7060

Drug Name	Unit Per	Route	Code
DEXTROSE, STERILE WATER, AND/OR DEXTROSE DILUENT/FLUSH	10 ML	VAR	A4216
DEXTROSE/SODIUM CHLORIDE	5%	VAR	J7042
DEXTROSE/THEOPHYLLINE	40 MG	IV	J2810
DEXTROSTAT	5 MG	ORAL	S0160
DIALYSIS/STRESS VITAMINS	100 CAPS	ORAL	S0194
DIAMOX	500 MG	IM, IV	J1120
DIASTAT	5 MG	IV, IM	J3360
DIAZEPAM	5 MG	IV, IM	J3360
DIAZOXIDE	300 MG	IV	J1730
DIBENT	UP TO 20 MG	IM	J0500
DICYCLOMINE HCL	20 MG	IM	J0500
DIDANOSINE (DDI)	25 MG	ORAL	S0137
DIDRONEL	300 MG	IV	J1436
DIETHYLSTILBESTROL DIPHOSPHATE	250 MG	INJ	J9165
DIFLUCAN	200 MG	IV	J1450
DIGIBIND	VIAL	IV	J1162
DIGIFAB	VIAL	IV	J1162
DIGOXIN	0.5 MG	IM, IV	J1160
DIGOXIN IMMUNE FAB	VIAL	IV	J1162
DIHYDROERGOTAMINE MESYLATE	1 MG	IM, IV	J1110
DILANTIN	50 MG	IM, IV	J1165
DILAUDID	250 MG	OTH	S0092
DILAUDID	4 MG	SC, IM, IV	J1170
DIMENHYDRINATE	50 MG	IM, IV	J1240
DIMERCAPROL	100 MG	IM	J0470
DIMINE	50 MG	IV, IM	J1200
DINATE	50 MG	IM, IV	J1240
DIOVAL	10 MG	IM	J1380
DIOVAL 40	10 MG	IM	J1380
DIOVAL XX	10 MG	IM	J1380
DIPHENHYDRAMINE HCL	50 MG	ORAL	Q0163
DIPHENHYDRAMINE HCL	50 MG	IV, IM	J1200
DIPYRIDAMOLE	10 MG	IV	J1245
DISOTATE	150 MG	IV	J3520
DI-SPAZ	UP TO 20 MG	IM	J0500
DIURIL	500 MG	IV	J1205
DIURIL SODIUM	500 MG	IV	J1205
DIZAC	5 MG	IV, IM	J3360
DMSO, DIMETHYL SULFOXIDE	50%, 50 ML	OTH	J1212
DOBUTAMINE HCL	250 MG	IV	J1250
DOBUTREX	250 MG	IV	J1250
DOCETAXEL	1 MG	IV	J9171
DOLASETRON MESYLATE	50 MG	ORAL	S0174
DOLASETRON MESYLATE	10 MG	IV	J1260
DOLASETRON MESYLATE	100 MG	ORAL	Q0180
DOLOPHINE	5 MG	ORAL	S0109
DOLOPHINE HCL	10 MG	IM, SC	J1230
DOMMANATE	50 MG	IM, IV	J1240
DOPAMINE HCL	40 MG	IV	J1265
DORIBAX	10 MG	IV	J1267
DORIPENEM	10 MG	IV	J1267
DORNASE ALPHA, NONCOMPOUNDED, UNIT DOSE	1 MG	INH	J7639
DOSTINEX	0.25 MG	ORAL	J8515
DOTAREM	0.1 ML	IV	A9575
DOXERCALCIFEROL	1 MG	IV	J1270

Drug Name	Unit Per	Route	Code
DOXORUBICIN HCL	10 MG	IV	J9000
DOXORUBICIN HYDROCHLORIDE, LIPOSOMAL, IMPORTED LIPODOX	10 MG	IV	Q2049
DOXORUBICIN HYDROCHLORIDE, LIPOSOMAL, NOT OTHERWISE SPECIFIED, 10MG	10 MG	IV	Q2050
DRAMAMINE	50 MG	IM, IV	J1240
DRAMANATE	50 MG	IM, IV	J1240
DRAMILIN	50 MG	IM, IV	J1240
DRAMOCEN	50 MG	IM, IV	J1240
DRAMOJECT	50 MG	IM, IV	J1240
DRAXIMAGE MDP-10	STUDY DOSE UP TO 30 MCI	IV	A9503
DRAXIMAGE MDP-25	STUDY DOSE UP TO 30 MCI	IV	A9503
DRONABINAL	2.5 MG	ORAL	Q0167
DROPERIDOL	5 MG	IM, IV	J1790
DROPERIDOL AND FENTANYL CITRATE	2 ML	IM, IV	J1810
DROXIA	500 MG	ORAL	S0176
DTIC-DOME	100 MG	IV	J9130
DTPA	STUDY DOSE UP TO 25 MCI	IV	A9539
DTPA	STUDY DOSE UP TO 25 MCI	INH	A9567
DUO-SPAN	1 ML	IM	J1060
DUO-SPAN II	1 ML	IM	J1060
DURACILLIN A.S.	600,000 UNITS	IM, IV	J2510
DURACLON	1 MG	OTH	J0735
DURAGEN-10	10 MG	IM	J1380
DURAGEN-20	10 MG	IM	J1380
DURAGEN-40	10 MG	IM	J1380
DURAMORPH	500 MG	OTH	S0093
DURAMORPH	10 MG	IM, IV, SC	J2275
DURO CORT	80 MG	IM	J1040
DYMENATE	50 MG	IM, IV	J1240
DYPHYLLINE	500 MG	IM	J1180
DYSPORT	5 UNITS	IM	J0586
E.D.T.A	150 MG	IV	J3520
ECALLANTIDE	1 MG	SC	J1290
ECHOCARDIOGRAM IMAGE ENHANCER OCTAFLUOROPROPANE	1 ML	IV	Q9956
ECHOCARDIOGRAM IMAGE ENHANCER PERFLEXANE	1 ML	IV	Q9955
ECULIZUMAB	10 MG	IV	J1300
EDETATE CALCIUM DISODIUM	1,000 MG	IV, SC, IM	J0600
EDETATE DISODIUM	150 MG	IV	J3520
EDEX	1.25 MCG	VAR	J0270
ELAPRASE	1 MG	IV	J1743
ELAVIL	20 MG	IM	J1320
ELELYSO	10 U	IV	J3060
ELIGARD	7.5 MG	IM	J9217
ELIGARD	PER 3.75 MG	SC	J1950
ELITEK	50 MCG	IM	J2783
ELLENCE	2 MG	IV	J9178
ELLIOTTS B SOLUTION	1 ML	IV, IT	J9175
ELOXATIN	0.5 MG	IV	J9263
ELSPAR	10,000 U	IM, IV, SC	J9020
ELSPAR	1.000 IU	IM, IV, SC	J9019
EMEND	1 MG	IV	J1453

Drug Name	Unit Per	Route	Code
EMEND	5 MG	ORAL	J8501
EMINASE	30 U	IV	J0350
ENBREL	25 MG	IM, IV	J1438
ENDOXAN-ASTA	100 MG	IV	J9070
ENDRATE	150 MG	IV	J3520
ENFUVIRTIDE	1 MG	SC	J1324
ENOXAPARIN SODIUM	10 MG	SC	J1650
EOVIST	1 ML	IV	A9581
EPIFIX	PER SQ IN	OTH	Q4131
EPIFIX, INJECTABLE	1 MG	OTH	Q4145
EPINEPHRINE	0.1 MG	VAR	J0171
EPIRUBICIN HCL	2 MG	IV	J9178
EPOETIN ALFA FOR ESRD DIALYSIS	100 U	INJ	Q4081
EPOETIN ALFA, ESRD USE	1,000 U	SC, IV	J0886
EPOETIN ALFA, NON-ESRD USE	1,000 U	SC, IV	J0885
EPOGEN/ESRD	1,000 U	SC, IV	J0886
EPOGEN/NON-ESRD	1,000 U	SC, IV	J0885
EPOPROSTENOL	0.5 MG	IV	J1325
EPOPROSTENOL STERILE DILUTANT	50 ML	IV	S0155
EPTIFIBATIDE	5 MG	IM, IV	J1327
ERAXIS	1 MG	IV	J0348
ERBITUX	10 MG	IV	J9055
ERGAMISOL	50 MG	ORAL	S0177
ERGONOVINE MALEATE	0.2 MG	IM, IV	J1330
ERIBULIN MESYLATE	0.1 MG	IV	J9179
ERTAPENEM SODIUM	500 MG	IM, IV	J1335
ERYTHROCIN LACTOBIONATE	500 MG	IV	J1364
ESTONE AQUEOUS	1 MG	IM, IV	J1435
ESTRADIOL CYPIONATE	UP TO 5 MG	IM	J1000
ESTRADIOL L.A.	10 MG	IM	J1380
ESTRADIOL L.A. 20	10 MG	IM	J1380
ESTRADIOL L.A. 40	10 MG	IM	J1380
ESTRADIOL VALERATE	10 MG	IM	J1380
ESTRAGYN	1 MG	IV, IM	J1435
ESTRA-L 20	10 MG	IM	J1380
ESTRA-L 40	10 MG	IM	J1380
ESTRO-A	1 MG	IV, IM	J1435
ESTROGEN CONJUGATED	25 MG	IV, IM	J1410
ESTRONE	1 MG	IV, IM	J1435
ESTRONOL	1 MG	IM, IV	J1435
ETANERCEPT	25 MG	IM, IV	J1438
ETHAMOLIN	100 MG	IV	J1430
ETHANOLAMINE OLEATE	100 MG	IV	J1430
ETHYOL	500 MG	IV	J0207
ETIDRONATE DISODIUM	300 MG	IV	J1436
ETONOGESTREL	IMPLANT	OTH	J7307
ETOPOSIDE	50 MG	ORAL	J8560
ETOPOSIDE	10 MG	IV	J9181
EUFLEXXA	DOSE	OTH	J7323
EULEXIN	125 MG	ORAL	S0175
EVEROLIMUS	0.25 MG	ORAL	J7527
EXAMETAZIME LABELED AUTOLOGOUS WHITE BLOOD CELLS, TECHNETIUM TC-99M	STUDY DOSE	IV	A9569
EXCELLAGEN	0.1 CC	OTH	Q4149
EXMESTANE	25 MG	ORAL	S0156
EXPAREL	1 MG	VAR	C9290

Drug Name	Unit Per	Route	Code
EZ-DERM	PER SQ CM	OTH	Q4136
FABRAZYME	1 MG	IV	J0180
FACTOR IX (ANTIHEMOPHILIC FACTOR, RECOMBINANT), RIXIBUS, PER I.U.	IU	IV	C9133
FACTOR IX NON-RECOMBINANT	1 IU	IV	J7193
FACTOR IX RECOMBINANT	1 IU	IV	J7195
FACTOR IX+ COMPLEX	1 IU	IV	J7194
FACTOR VIIA RECOMBINANT	1 MCG	IV	J7189
FACTOR VIII PORCINE	1 IU	IV	J7191
FACTOR VIII RECOMBINANT	1 IU	IV	J7192
FACTOR VIII, HUMAN	1 IU	IV	J7190
FACTOR XIII (ANTIHEMOPHILIC FACTOR, HUMAN)	1 IU	IV	J7180
FACTREL	100 MCG	SC, IV	J1620
FAMOTIDINE	20 MG	IV	S0028
FASLODEX	25 MG	IM	J9395
FDG	STUDY DOSE UP TO 45 MCI	IV	A9552
FEIBA-VH AICC	1 IU	IV	J7198
FENTANYL CITRATE	0.1 MG	IM, IV	J3010
FERAHEME (FOR ESRD)	1 MG	IV	Q0139
FERAHEME (NON-ESRD)	1 MG	IV	Q0138
FERIDEX IV	1 ML	IV	Q9953
FERRIC CARBOXYMALTOSE	1 MG	IV	C9441
FERRLECIT	12.5 MG	IV	J2916
FERTINEX	75 IU	SC	J3355
FERUMOXYTOL (FOR ESRD)	1 MG	IV	Q0139
FERUMOXYTOL (NON-ESRD)	1 MG	IV	Q0138
FIBRIN SEALANT (HUMAN)	2ML	OTH	C9250
FILGRASTIM	1 MCG	SC, IV	J1442
FINASTERIDE	5 MG	ORAL	S0138
FIRAZYR	1 MG	SC	J1744
FLAGYL	500 MG	IV	S0030
FLEBOGAMMA	500 MG	IV	J1572
FLEXHD	SQ CM	OTH	Q4128
FLEXON	60 MG	IV, IM	J2360
FLOLAN	0.5 MG	IV	J1325
FLOXIN IV	400 MG	IV	S0034
FLOXURIDINE	500 MG	IV	J9200
FLUBLOK	0.5 ML	IM	Q2033
FLUCONAZOLE	200 MG	IV	J1450
FLUDARA	50 MG	IV	J9185
FLUDARABINE PHOSPHATE	50 MG	IV	J9185
FLUDARABINE PHOSPHATE	10 MG	ORAL	J8562
FLUDEOXYGLUCOSE F18	STUDY DOSE UP TO 45 MCI	IV	A9552
FLULAVAL	EA	IM	Q2036
FLUMADINE (DEMONSTATION PROJECT)	100 MG	ORAL	G9036
FLUNISOLIDE, COMPOUNDED, UNIT DOSE	1 MG	INH	J7641
FLUOCINOLONE ACETONIDE INTRAVITREAL	IMPLANT	OTH	J7311
FLUORODEOXYGLUCOSE F-18 FDG, DIAGNOSTIC	STUDY DOSE UP TO 45 MCI	IV	A9552
FLUOROURACIL	500 MG	IV	J9190
FLUPHENAZINE DECANOATE	25 MG	SC, IM	J2680
FLUTAMIDE	125 MG	ORAL	S0175
FLUVIRIN	EA	IM	Q2037

Drug Name	Unit Per	Route	Code
FLUZONE	EA	IM	Q2038
FOLEX	50 MG	IV, IM, IT, IA	J9260
FOLEX	5 MG	IV, IM, IT, IA	J9250
FOLEX PFS	50 MG	IV, IM, IT, IA	J9260
FOLEX PFS	5 MG	IV, IM, IT, IA	J9250
FOLLISTIM	75 IU	SC, IM	S0128
FOLLITROPIN ALFA	75 IU	SC	S0126
FOLLITROPIN BETA	75 IU	SC, IM	S0128
FOLOTYN	1 MG	IV	J9307
FOMEPIZOLE	15 MG	IV	J1451
FOMIVIRSEN SODIUM	1.65 MG	OTH	J1452
FONDAPARINUX SODIUM	0.5 MG	SC	J1652
FORMOTEROL FUMERATE NONCOMPOUNDED UNIT DOSE FORM	20 MCG	INH	J7606
FORMOTEROL, COMPOUNDED, UNIT DOSE	12 MCG	INH	J7640
FORTAZ	500 MG	IM, IV	J0713
FORTEO	10 MCG	SC	J3110
FORTOVASE	200 MG	ORAL	S0140
FOSAPREPITANT	1 MG	IV	J1453
FOSCARNET SODIUM	1,000 MG	IV	J1455
FOSCAVIR	1,000 MG	IV	J1455
FOSPHENYTOIN	50 MG	IM, IV	Q2009
FOSPHENYTOIN SODIUM	750 MG	IM, IV	S0078
FRAGMIN	2,500 IU	SC	J1645
FUDR	500 MG	IV	J9200
FULVESTRANT	25 MG	IM	J9395
FUNGIZONE	50 MG	IV	J0285
FUROSEMIDE	20 MG	IM, IV	J1940
FUSILEV	0.5 MG	IV	J0641
FUZEON	1 MG	SC	J1324
GABLOFEN	50 MCG	IT	J0476
GABLOFEN	10 MG	IT	J0475
GADAVIST	0.1 ML	IV	A9585
GADOBENATE DIMEGLUMINE (MULTIHANCE MULTIPACK)	1 ML	IV	A9577
GADOBUTROL	0.1 ML	IV	A9585
GADOFOSVESET TRISODIUM	1 ML	IV	A9583
GADOLINIUM -BASED CONTRAST NOS	1 ML	IV	A9579
GADOTERATE MEGLUMINE	0.1 ML	IV	A9575
GADOTERIDOL (PROHANCE MULTIPACK)	1 ML	IV	A9576
GADOXETATE DISODIUM	1 ML	IV	A9581
GALLIUM GA-67	1 MCI	IV	A9556
GALLIUM NITRATE	1 MG	IV	J1457
GALSULFASE	1 MG	IV	J1458
GAMASTAN	1 CC	IM	J1460
GAMASTAN	OVER 10 CC	IM	J1560
GAMASTAN SD	OVER 10 CC	IM	J1560
GAMASTAN SD	1 CC	IM	J1460
GAMMA GLOBULIN	OVER 10 CC	IM	J1560
GAMMA GLOBULIN	1 CC	IM	J1460
GAMMAGARD	500 MG	IV	J1569
GAMMAGRAFT	SQ CM	OTH	Q4111
GAMMAKED	500 MG	IV, SC	J1561
GAMMAPLEX	500 MG	IV	J1557
GAMUNEX	500 MG	IV, SQ	J1561
GAMUNEX-C	500 MG	IV, SC	J1561

Drug Name	Unit Per	Route	Code
GANCICLOVIR	4.5 MG	OTH	J7310
GANCICLOVIR SODIUM	500 MG	IV	J1570
GANIRELIX ACETATE	250 MCG	SC	S0132
GANITE	1 MG	IV	J1457
GARAMYCIN	80 MG	IM, IV	J1580
GASTROCROM	10 MG	INH	J7631
GASTROMARK	1 ML	ORAL	Q9954
GATIFLOXACIN	10 MG	IV	J1590
GEFITINIB	250 MG	ORAL	J8565
GEL-ONE	DOSE	OTH	J7326
GEMCITABINE HCL	200 MG	IV	J9201
GEMTUZUMAB OZOGAMICIN	5 MG	IV	J9300
GEMZAR	200 MG	IV	J9201
GENGRAF	25 MG	ORAL	J7515
GENGRAF	100 MG	ORAL	J7502
GENOTROPIN	1 MG	SC	J2941
GENOTROPIN MINIQUICK	1 MG	SC	J2941
GENOTROPIN NUTROPIN	1 MG	SC	J2941
GENTAMICIN	80 MG	IM, IV	J1580
GENTRAN	500 ML	IV	J7100
GENTRAN 75	500 ML	IV	J7110
GEODON	10 MG	IM	J3486
GEREF	1MCG	SC	Q0515
GLASSIA	10 MG	IV	J0257
GLATIRAMER ACETATE	20 MG	SC	J1595
GLEEVEC	100 MG	ORAL	S0088
GLOFIL-125	STUDY DOSE UP TO 10 UCI	IV	A9554
GLUCAGEN	1 MG	SC, IM, IV	J1610
GLUCAGON	1 MG	SC, IM, IV	J1610
GLUCOTOPE	STUDY DOSE UP TO 45 MCI	IV	A9552
GLYCOPYRROLATE, COMPOUNDED CONCENTRATED	PER MG	INH	J7642
GLYCOPYRROLATE, COMPOUNDED, UNIT DOSE	1 MG	INH	J7643
GOLD SODIUM THIOMALATE	50 MG	IM	J1600
GOLIMUMAB	1 MG	IV	J1602
GONADORELIN HCL	100 MCG	SC, IV	J1620
GONAL-F	75 IU	SC	S0126
GOSERELIN ACETATE	3.6 MG	SC	J9202
GRAFIX CORE	SQ CM	OTH	Q4132
GRAFIX PRIME	SQ CM	OTH	Q4133
GRAFTJACKET	SQ CM	OTH	Q4107
GRAFTJACKET EXPRESS	1 CC	INJ	Q4113
GRANISETRON HCL	1 MG	ORAL	Q0166
GRANISETRON HCL	1 MG	IV	S0091
GRANISETRON HCL	100 MCG	IV	J1626
GRANIX	5 MCG	SC	J1446
GYNOGEN L.A. 10	10 MG	IM	J1380
GYNOGEN L.A. 20	10 MG	IM	J1380
GYNOGEN L.A. 40	10 MG	IM	J1380
H.P. ACTHAR GEL	UP TO 40 UNITS	OTH	J0800
HALAVEN	0.1 MG	IV	J9179
HALDOL	5 MG	IM, IV	J1630
HALDOL DECANOATE	50 MG	IM	J1631
HALOPERIDOL	5 MG	IM, IV	J1630

Drug Name	Unit Per	Route	Code
HECTOROL	1 MG	IV	J1270
HELIXATE FS	1 IU	IV	J7192
HEMIN	1 MG	IV	J1640
HEMOFIL-M	1 IU	IV	J7190
HEMOPHILIA CLOTTING FACTOR, NOC	VAR	INJ	J7199
HEP LOCK	10 U	IV	J1642
HEPAGAM B	0.5 ML	IM	J1571
HEPAGAM B	0.5 ML	IV	J1573
HEPARIN SODIUM	10 U	IV	J1642
HEPARIN SODIUM	1,000 U	IV, SC	J1644
HEPATITIS B IMMUNE GLOBULIN	0.5 ML	IV	J1573
HEPATOLITE	STUDY DOSE UP TO 15 MCI	IV	A9510
HEP-PAK	10 UNITS	IV	J1642
HERCEPTIN	10 MG	IV	J9355
HEXADROL	0.25 MG	ORAL	J8540
HEXAMINOLEVULINATE	STUDY DOSE	OTH	C9275
HIGH OSMOLAR CONTRAST MATERIAL, UP TO 149 MG/ML IODINE CONCENTRATION	1 ML	IV	Q9958
HIGH OSMOLAR CONTRAST MATERIAL, UP TO 150-199 MG/ML IODINE CONCENTRATION	1 ML	IV	Q9959
HIGH OSMOLAR CONTRAST MATERIAL, UP TO 200-249 MG/ML IODINE CONCENTRATION	1 ML	IV	Q9960
HIGH OSMOLAR CONTRAST MATERIAL, UP TO 250-299 MG/ML IODINE CONCENTRATION	1 ML	IV	Q9961
HIGH OSMOLAR CONTRAST MATERIAL, UP TO 300-349 MG/ML IODINE CONCENTRATION	1 ML	IV	Q9962
HIGH OSMOLAR CONTRAST MATERIAL, UP TO 350-399 MG/ML IODINE CONCENTRATION	1 ML	IV	Q9963
HIGH OSMOLAR CONTRAST MATERIAL, UP TO 400 OR GREATER MG/ML IODINE CONCENTRATION	1 ML	IV	Q9964
HISTERLIN IMPLANT (VANTAS)	50 MG	OTH	J9225
HISTRELIN ACETATE	10 MG	INJ	J1675
HISTRELIN IMPLANT (SUPPRELIN LA)	50 MG	OTH	J9226
HIZENTRA	100 MG	SC	J1559
HMATRIX	PER SQ CM	OTH	Q4134
HUMALOG	50 U	SC	J1817
HUMALOG	5 U	SC	J1815
HUMAN FIGRINOGEN CONCENTRATE	1 MG	IV	J7178
HUMATE-P	1 IU	IV	J7187
HUMATROPE	1 MG	SC	J2941
HUMIRA	20 MG	SC	J0135
HUMULIN	5 U	SC	J1815
HUMULIN	50 U	SC	J1817
HUMULIN R	5 U	SC	J1815
HUMULIN R U-500	5 U	SC	J1815
HYALGAN	DOSE	OTH	J7321
HYALOMATRIX	SQ CM	OTH	Q4117
HYALURONAN OR DERITIVE, GEL-ONE	DOSE	OTH	J7326
HYALURONAN, EUFLEXXA	DOSE	OTH	J7323
HYALURONAN, HYALGAN OR SUPARTZ	DOSE	OTH	J7321
HYALURONAN, ORTHOVISC	DOSE	OTH	J7324
HYALURONAN, SYNVISC/SYNVISC-ONE	1 MG	OTH	J7325
HYALURONIDASE	150 UNITS	VAR	J3470

Drug Name	Unit Per	Route	Code
HYALURONIDASE RECOMBINANT	1 USP UNIT	SC	J3473
HYALURONIDASE, OVINE, PRESERVATIVE FREE	1 USP	OTH	J3471
HYALURONIDASE, OVINE, PRESERVATIVE FREE	1000 USP	OTH	J3472
HYCAMTIN	0.1 MG	IV	J9351
HYCAMTIN	0.25 MG	ORAL	J8705
HYDRALAZINE HCL	20 MG	IV, IM	J0360
HYDRATE	50 MG	IM, IV	J1240
HYDREA	500 MG	ORAL	S0176
HYDROCORTISONE ACETATE	25 MG	IV, IM, SC	J1700
HYDROCORTISONE SODIUM PHOSPHATE	50 MG	IV, IM, SC	J1710
HYDROCORTISONE SODIUM SUCCINATE	100 MG	IV, IM, SC	J1720
HYDROCORTONE PHOSPHATE	50 MG	SC, IM, IV	J1710
HYDROMORPHONE HCL	4 MG	SC, IM, IV	J1170
HYDROMORPHONE HCL	250 MG	OTH	S0092
HYDROXOCOBALAMIN	1,000 MCG	IM, SC	J3420
HYDROXYCOBAL	1,000 MCG	IM, SC	J3420
HYDROXYPROGESTERONE CAPROATE	1 MG	IM	J1725
HYDROXYUREA	500 MG	ORAL	S0176
HYDROXYZINE HCL	25 MG	IM	J3410
HYDROXYZINE PAMOATE	25 MG	ORAL	Q0177
HYOSCYAMINE SULFATE	0.25 MG	SC, IM, IV	J1980
HYPERRHO S/D	300 MCG	IV	J2790
HYPERTET SD	UP TO 250 MG	IM	J1670
HYPERTONIC SALINE SOLUTION	1 ML	VAR	J7131
HYREXIN	50 MG	IV, IM	J1200
HYZINE	25 MG	IM	J3410
HYZINE-50	25 MG	IM	J3410
I-131 TOSITUMOMAB DIAGNOSTIC	STUDY DOSE	IV	A9544
I-131 TOSITUMOMAB THERAPEUTIC	TX DOSE	IV	A9545
IBANDRONATE SODIUM	1 MG	IV	J1740
IBRITUMOMAB TUXETAN	STUDY DOSE UP TO 5 MCI	IV	A9542
IBUPROFEN	100 MG	IV	J1741
IBUTILIDE FUMARATE	1 MG	IV	J1742
ICATIBANT	1 MG	SC	J1744
IDAMYCIN	5 MG	IV	J9211
IDAMYCIN PFS	5 MG	IV	J9211
IDARUBICIN HCL	5 MG	IV	J9211
IDURSULFASE	1 MG	IV	J1743
IFEX	1 G	IV	J9208
IFOSFAMIDE	1 G	IV	J9208
IL-2	1 VIAL	IV	J9015
ILARIS	1 MG	SC	J0638
ILETIN	5 UNITS	SC	J1815
ILETIN II NPH PORK	50 U	SC	J1817
ILETIN II REGULAR PORK	5 U	SC	J1815
ILOPROST INHALATION SOLUTION	PER DOSE UP TO 20 MCG	INH	Q4074
IMAGENT	1 ML	IV	Q9955
IMATINIB	100 MG	ORAL	S0088
IMIGLUCERASE	10 U	IV	J1786
IMITREX	6 MG	SC	J3030
IMMUNE GLOBULIN	500 MG	IV	J1556
IMMUNE GLOBULIN (BIVIGAM)	500 MG	IV	J1556

Drug Name	Unit Per	Route	Code
IMMUNE GLOBULIN (FLEBOGAMMA, FLEBOGAMMA DIF	500 MG	IV	J1572
IMMUNE GLOBULIN (GAMMAGARD LIQUID)	500 MG	IV	J1569
IMMUNE GLOBULIN (GAMMAPLEX)	500 MG	IV	J1557
IMMUNE GLOBULIN (GAMUNEX)	500 MG	IV	J1561
IMMUNE GLOBULIN (HIZENTRA)	100 MG	SC	J1559
IMMUNE GLOBULIN (OCTAGAM)	500 MG	IV	J1568
IMMUNE GLOBULIN (PRIVIGEN) NONLYOPHILIZED	500 MG	IV	J1459
IMMUNE GLOBULIN (RHOPHYLAC)	100 IU	IM, IV	J2791
IMMUNE GLOBULIN LYOPHILIZED	500 MG	IV	J1566
IMMUNE GLOBULIN SUBCUTANEOUS	100 MG	SC	J1562
IMMUNE GLOBULIN, NONLYOPHILIZED (NOS)	500 MG	IV	J1599
IMPLANON	IMPLANT	OTH	J7307
IMURAN	50 MG	ORAL	J7500
IN-111 SATUMOMAB PENDETIDE	STUDY DOSE UP TO MCI	IV	A4642
INAPSINE	5 MG	IM, IV	J1790
INCOBUTULINUMTOXINA	1 UNIT	IM	J0588
INDERAL	1 MG	IV	J1800
INDIUM IN-111 IBRITUMOMAB TIUXETAN, DIAGNOSTIC	STUDY DOSE UP TO 5 MCI	IV	A9542
INDIUM IN-111 LABELED AUTOLOGOUS PLATELETS	STUDY DOSAGE	IV	A9571
INDIUM IN-111 LABELED AUTOLOGOUS WHITE BLOOD CELLS	STUDY DOSE	IV	A9570
INDIUM IN-111 OXYQUINOLINE	0.5 MCI	IV	A9547
INDIUM IN-111 PENTETREOTIDE	STUDY DOSE UP TO 6 MCI	IV	A9572
INDURSALFASE	1 MG	IV	J1743
INFED	50 MG	IM, IV	J1750
INFERGEN	1 MCG	SC	J9212
INFLIXIMAB	10 MG	IV	J1745
INFLUENZA VACCINE (FLUBLOK)	.05 ML	OM	Q2033
INFLUENZA VACCINE, AGRIFLU	UNKNOWN	IM	Q2034
INFLUENZA VIRUS VACCINE (AFLURIA)	EA	IM	Q2035
INFLUENZA VIRUS VACCINE (FLULAVAL)	EA	IM	Q2036
INFLUENZA VIRUS VACCINE (FLUVIRIN)	EA	IM	Q2037
INFLUENZA VIRUS VACCINE (FLUZONE)	EA	IM	Q2038
INFLUENZA VIRUS VACCINE, NOT OTHERWISE SPECIFIED	EA	IM	Q2039
INFUMORPH	10 MG	IM, IV, SC	J2270
INFUMORPH	10 MG	OTH	J2275
INFUMORPH PRESERVATIVE FREE	100 MG	IM, IV, SC	J2271
INNOHEP	1,000 IU	SC	J1655
INSULIN	5 U	SC	J1815
INSULIN	50 U	SC	J1817
INSULIN LISPRO	5 U	SC	S5551
INSULIN LISPRO	5 U	SC	J1815
INSULIN PURIFIED REGULAR PORK	5 U	SC	J1815
INTAL	10 MG	INH	J7631
INTEGRA BILAYER MATRIX DRESSING	SQ CM	OTH	Q4104
INTEGRA DERMAL REGENERATION TEMPLATE	SQ CM	OTH	Q4105
INTEGRA FLOWABLE WOUND MATRIX	1 CC	INJ	Q4114
INTEGRA MATRIX	SQ CM	OTH	Q4108

Drug Name	Unit Per	Route	Code
INTEGRA MOZAIK OSTEOCONDUCTIVE SCAFFOLD PUTTY	0.5 CC	OTH	C9359
INTEGRA MOZAIK OSTEOCONDUCTIVE SCAFFOLD STRIP	0.5 CC	OTH	C9362
INTEGRA OS OSTEOCONDUCTIVE SCAFFOLD PUTTY	0.5 CC	OTH	C9359
INTEGRILIN	5 MG	IM, IV	J1327
INTERFERON ALFA-2A	3,000,000 U	SC, IM	J9213
INTERFERON ALFA-2B	1,000,000 U	SC, IM	J9214
INTERFERON ALFACON-1	1 MCG	SC	J9212
INTERFERON ALFA-N3	250,000 IU	IM	J9215
INTERFERON BETA-1A	30 MCG	IM, SC	J1826
INTERFERON BETA-1A	1 MCG	SC	Q3028
INTERFERON BETA-1A	1 MCG	IM	Q3027
INTERFERON BETA-1B	0.25 MG	SC	J1830
INTERFERON, ALFA-2A, RECOMBINANT	3,000,000 U	SC, IM	J9213
INTERFERON, ALFA-2B, RECOMBINANT	1,000,000 U	SC, IM	J9214
INTERFERON, ALFA-N3, (HUMAN LEUKOCYTE DERIVED)	250,000 IU	IM	J9215
INTERFERON, GAMMA 1-B	3,000,000 U	SC	J9216
INTERLUEKIN	1 VIAL	IV	J9015
INTRON A	1,000,000 U	SC, IM	J9214
INVANZ	500 MG	IM, IV	J1335
INVEGA SUSTENNA	1 MG	IM	J2426
INVIRASE	200 MG	ORAL	S0140
IOBENGUANE SULFATE I-131	0.5 MCI	IV	A9508
IOBENGUANE, I-123, DIAGNOSTIC	PER STUDY DOSE UP TO 15 MCI	IV	A9582
IODINE I-123 IOBENGUANE, DIAGNOSTIC	15 MCI	IV	A9582
IODINE I-123 IOFLUPANE	STUDY DOSE UP TO 5 MCI	IV	A9584
IODINE I-123 SODIUM IODIDE CAPSULE(S), DIAGNOSTIC	100-9999 UCI	ORAL	A9516
IODINE I-123 SODIUM IODIDE, DIAGNOSTIC	1 MCI	IV	A9509
IODINE I-125 SERUM ALBUMIN, DIAGNOSTIC	5 UCI	IV	A9532
IODINE I-125 SODIUM IOTHALAMATE, DIAGNOSTIC	STUDY DOSE UP TO 10 UCI	IV	A9554
IODINE I-125, SODIUM IODIDE SOLUTION, THERAPEUTIC	1 MCI	ORAL	A9527
IODINE I-131 IOBENGUANE SULFATE, DIAGNOSTIC	0.5 MCI	IV	A9508
IODINE I-131 IODINATED SERUM ALBUMIN, DIAGNOSTIC	PER 5 UCI	IV	A9524
IODINE I-131 SODIUM IODIDE CAPSULE(S), DIAGNOSTIC	1 MCI	ORAL	A9528
IODINE I-131 SODIUM IODIDE CAPSULE(S), THERAPEUTIC	1 MCI	ORAL	A9517
IODINE I-131 SODIUM IODIDE SOLUTION, DIAGNOSTIC	1 MCI	ORAL	A9529
IODINE I-131 SODIUM IODIDE SOLUTION, THERAPEUTIC	1 MCI	ORAL	A9530
IODINE I-131 SODIUM IODIDE, DIAGNOSTIC	PER UCI UP TO 100 UCI	IV	A9531
IODINE I-131 TOSITUMOMAB, DIAGNOSTIC	STUDY DOSE	IV	A9544
IODINE I-131 TOSITUMOMAB, THERAPEUTIC	TX DOSE	IV	A9545
IODOTOPE THERAPEUTIC CAPSULE(S)	1 MCI	ORAL	A9517
IODOTOPE THERAPEUTIC SOLUTION	1 MCI	ORAL	A9530

Drug Name	Unit Per	Route	Code
IOFLUPANE	STUDY DOSE UP TO 5 MCI	IV	A9584
ION-BASED MAGNETIC RESONANCE CONTRAST AGENT	1 ML	IV	Q9953
IOTHALAMATE SODIUM I-125	STUDY DOSE UP TO 10 UCI	IV	A9554
IPILIMUMAB	1 MG	IV	J9228
IPLEX	1 MG	SC	J2170
IPRATROPIUM BROMIDE, NONCOMPOUNDED, UNIT DOSE	1 MG	INH	J7644
IPTRATROPIUM BROMIDE COMPOUNDED, UNIT DOSE	1 MG	INH	J7645
IRESSA	250 MG	ORAL	J8565
IRINOTECAN	20 MG	IV	J9206
IRON DEXTRAN, 50 MG	50 MG	IM, IV	J1750
IRON SUCROSE	1 MG	IV	J1756
ISOCAINE	10 ML	VAR	J0670
ISOETHARINE HCL COMPOUNDED, CONCENTRATED	1 MG	INH	J7647
ISOETHARINE HCL COMPOUNDED, UNIT DOSE	1 MG	INH	J7650
ISOETHARINE HCL, NONCOMPOUNDED CONCENTRATED	PER MG	INH	J7648
ISOETHARINE HCL, NONCOMPOUNDED, UNIT DOSE	1 MG	INH	J7649
ISOJEX	5 UCI	IV	A9532
ISOPROTERENOL HCL COMPOUNDED, CONCENTRATED	1 MG	INH	J7657
ISOPROTERENOL HCL COMPOUNDED, UNIT DOSE	1 MG	INH	J7660
ISOPROTERENOL HCL, NONCOMPOUNDED CONCENTRATED	1 MG	INH	J7658
ISOPROTERNOL HCL, NONCOMPOUNDED, UNIT DOSE	1MG	INH	J7659
ISOSULFAN BLUE	1 MG	SC	Q9968
ISTODAX	1 MG	IV	J9315
ISUPREL	1 MG	INH	J7658
ISUPREL	I MG	INH	J7659
ITRACONAZOLE	50 MG	IV	J1835
IVEEGAM	500 MG	IV	J1566
IXABEPILONE	1 MG	IV	J9207
IXEMPRA	1 MG	IV	J9207
JETREA	0.125 MG	OTH	J7316
JEVTANA	1 MG	IV	J9043
KADCYLA	1 MG	IV	J9354
KALBITOR	1 MG	SC	J1290
KANAMYCIN	500 MG	IM, IV	J1840
KANAMYCIN	75 MG	IM, IV	J1850
KANTREX	75 MG	IM, IV	J1850
KANTREX	500 MG	IM, IV	J1840
KCENTRA	PER I.U.	IV	C9132
KEFZOL	500 MG	IM, IV	J0690
KENAJECT-40	10 MG	IM	J3301
KENALOG-10	10 MG	IM	J3301
KEPIVANCE	50 MCG	IV	J2425
KEPPRA	10 MG	IV	J1953
KESTRONE	1 MG	IV, IM	J1435
KETOROLAC TROMETHAMINE	15 MG	IM, IV	J1885
KINEVAC	5 MCG	IV	J2805
KOATE-DVI	1 IU	IV	J7190
KOGENATE FS	1 IU	IV	J7192

Drug Name	Unit Per	Route	Code
KONAKION	1 MG	SC, IM, IV	J3430
KONYNE 80	1 IU	IV	J7194
KRYSTEXXA	1 MG	IV	J2507
KYPROLIS	1 MG	IV	J9047
KYTRIL	1 MG	ORAL	Q0166
KYTRIL	1 MG	IV	S0091
KYTRIL	100 MCG	IV	J1626
L.A.E. 20	10 MG	IM	J1380
LACOSAMIDE	1 MG	IV	C9254
LAETRILE	VAR	INJ	J3570
LANOXIN	0.5 MG	IM, IV	J1160
LANREOTIDE	1 MG	SC	J1930
LANTUS	5U	SC	J1815
LARONIDASE	0.1 MG	IV	J1931
LASIX	20 MG	IM, IV	J1940
LENTE ILETIN I	5 U	SC	J1815
LEPIRUDIN	50 MG	IV	J1945
LEUCOVORIN CALCIUM	50 MG	IM, IV	J0640
LEUKERAN	2 MG	ORAL	S0172
LEUKINE	50 MCG	IV	J2820
LEUPROLIDE ACETATE	7.5 MG	IM	J9217
LEUPROLIDE ACETATE	1 MG	IM	J9218
LEUPROLIDE ACETATE (FOR DEPOT SUSPENSION)	3.75 MG	IM	J1950
LEUPROLIDE ACETATE DEPOT	7.5 MG	IM	J9217
LEUPROLIDE ACETATE IMPLANT	65 MG	OTH	J9219
LEUSTATIN	1 MG	IV	J9065
LEVABUTEROL COMPOUNDED, UNIT DOSE	1 MG	INH	J7615
LEVABUTEROL, COMPOUNDED, CONCENTRATED	0.5 MG	INH	J7607
LEVALBUTEROL NONCOMPOUNDED, CONCENTRATED FORM	0.5 MG	INH	J7612
LEVALBUTEROL, NONCOMPOUNDED, UNIT DOSE	0.5 MG	INH	J7614
LEVAMISOLE HCL	50 MG	ORAL	S0177
LEVAQUIN	250 MG	IV	J1956
LEVEMIR	5 U	SC	J1815
LEVETIRACETAM	10 MG	IV	J1953
LEVOCARNITINE	1 G	IV	J1955
LEVO-DROMORAN	UP TO 2 MG	IV, IM	J1960
LEVOFLOXACIN	250 MG	IV	J1956
LEVOLEUCOVORIN CALCIUM	0.5 MG	IV	J0641
LEVONORGESTREL	52 MG	OTH	J7302
LEVONORGESTREL-RELEASING INTRAUTERINE CONTRACEPTIVE SYSTEM (SKYLA)	13.5 MG	OTH	J7301
LEVORPHANOL TARTRATE	2 MG	SC, IV, IM	J1960
LEVSIN	0.25 MG	SC, IM, IV	J1980
LEVULAN KERASTICK	354 MG	OTH	J7308
LEXISCAN	0.1 MG	IV	J2785
LIBRIUM	100 MG	IM, IV	J1990
LIDOCAINE 70 MG/TETRACAINE 70 MG	PATCH	OTH	C9285
LIDOCAINE HCL	10 MG	IV	J2001
LINCOCIN HCL	300 MG	IV	J2010
LINCOMYCIN HCL	300 MG	IM, IV	J2010
LINEZOLID	200 MG	IV	J2020
LIORESAL	10 MG	IT	J0475
LIORESAL INTRATHECAL REFILL	50 MCG	IT	J0476

Drug Name	Unit Per	Route	Code
LIPODOX	10 MG	IV	Q2049
LIQUAEMIN SODIUM	1,000 UNITS	SC, IV	J1644
LISPRO-PFC	50 U	SC	J1817
LOK-PAK	10 UNITS	IV	J1642
LOMUSTINE	10 MG	ORAL	S0178
LORAZEPAM	2 MG	IM, IV	J2060
LOVENOX	10 MG	SC	J1650
LOW OSMOLAR CONTRAST MATERIAL, 100-199 MG/ML IODINE CONCENTRATIONS	1 ML	IV	Q9965
LOW OSMOLAR CONTRAST MATERIAL, 200-299 MG/ML IODINE CONCENTRATION	1 ML	IV	Q9966
LOW OSMOLAR CONTRAST MATERIAL, 300-399 MG/ML IODINE CONCENTRATION	1 ML	IV	Q9967
LOW OSMOLAR CONTRAST MATERIAL, 400 OR GREATER MG/ML IODINE CONCENTRATION	1 ML	IV	Q9951
LOXAPINE, INHALATION POWDER	10 MG	OTH	C9497
L-PHENYLALANINE MUSTARD	50 MG	IV	J9245
LUCENTIS	0.1 MG	IV	J2778
LUMIZYME	10 MG	IV	J0221
LUPRON	1 MG	SC	J9218
LUPRON DEPOT	7.5 MG	IM	J9217
LUPRON DEPOT	PER 3.75 MG	IM	J1950
LUPRON IMPLANT	65 MG	OTH	J9219
LUTREPULSE	100 MCG	SC, IV	J1620
LYMPHAZURIN	1 MG	SC	Q9968
LYMPHOCYTE IMMUNE GLOBULIN, ANTITHYMOCYTE GLOBULIN, EQUINE	250 MG	OTH	J7504
LYMPHOCYTE IMMUNE GLOBULIN, ANTITHYMOCYTE GLOBULIN, RABBIT	25 MG	OTH	J7511
LYMPHOSEEK	0.5 MCI	SC, OTH	A9520
MACUGEN	0.3 MG	OTH	J2503
MAGNESIUM SULFATE	500 MG	IV	J3475
MAGNETIC RESONANCE CONTRAST AGENT	1 ML	ORAL	Q9954
MAGNEVIST	1 ML	IV	A9579
MAGROTEC	STUDY DOSE UP TO 10 MCI	IV	A9540
MAKENA	1 MG	IM	J1725
MANNITOL	25% IN 50 ML	IV	J2150
MANNITOL	5 MG	INH	J7665
MARCAINE HCL	30 ML	VAR	S0020
MARINOL	2.5 MG	ORAL	Q0167
MARMINE	50 MG	IM, IV	J1240
MARQIBO KIT	5 MG	IV	J9371
MATRISTEM BURN MATRIX	SQ CM	OTH	Q4120
MATRISTEM MICROMATRIX	1 MG	OTH	Q4118
MATRISTEM WOUND MATRIX	SQ CM	OTH	Q4119
MATULANE	50 MG	ORAL	S0182
MAXIPIME	500 MG	IV	J0692
MDP-BRACCO	STUDY DOSE UP TO 30 MCI	IV	A9503
MECASERMIN	1 MG	SC	J2170
MECHLORETHAMINE HCL (NITROGEN MUSTARD)	10 MG	IV	J9230
MEDIDEX	1 MG	IM, IV, OTH	J1100
MEDISKIN	PER SQ CM	OTH	Q4135
MEDROL	4 MG	ORAL	J7509

Drug Name	Unit Per	Route	Code
MEDROXYPROGESTERONE ACETATE	1 MG	IM	J1050
MEFOXIN	1 G	IV	J0694
MEGACE	20 MG	ORAL	S0179
MEGESTROL ACETATE	20 MG	ORAL	S0179
MELPHALAN HCL	50 MG	IV	J9245
MELPHALAN HCL	2 MG	ORAL	J8600
MEMETASONE SINUS IMPLANT	370 MCG	OTH	S1090
MEMODERM	SQ CM	OTH	Q4126
MENADIONE	1 MG	IM, SC, IV	J3430
MENOTROPINS	75 IU	SC, IM, IV	S0122
MEPERGAN	50 MG	IM, IV	J2180
MEPERIDINE AND PROMETHAZINE HCL	50 MG	IM, IV	J2180
MEPERIDINE HCL	100 MG	IM, IV, SC	J2175
MEPIVACAINE HCL	10 ML	VAR	J0670
MERCAPTOPURINE	50 MG	ORAL	S0108
MERITATE	150 MG	IV	J3520
MEROPENEM	100 MG	IV	J2185
MERREM	100 MG	IV	J2185
MESNA	200 MG	IV	J9209
MESNEX	200 MG	IV	J9209
METAPROTERENOL SULFATE COMPOUNDED, UNIT DOSE	10 MG	INH	J7670
METAPROTERENOL SULFATE, NONCOMPOUNDED, CONCENTRATED	10 MG	INH	J7668
METAPROTERENOL SULFATE, NONCOMPOUNDED, UNIT DOSE	10 MG	INH	J7669
METARAMINOL BITARTRATE	10 MG	IV, IM, SC	J0380
METASTRON STRONTIUM 89 CHLORIDE	1 MCI	IV	A9600
METATRACE	STUDY DOSE UP TO 45 MCI	IV	A9552
METHACHOLINE CHLORIDE	1 MG	INH	J7674
METHADONE	5 MG	ORAL	S0109
METHADONE HCL	10 MG	IM, SC	J1230
METHAPREL, COMPOUNDED, UNIT DOSE	10 MG	INH	J7670
METHAPREL, NONCOMPOUNDED, CONCENTRATED	10 MG	INH	J7668
METHAPREL, NONCOMPOUNDED, UNIT DOSE	10 MG	INH	J7669
METHERGINE	0.2 MG	IM, IV	J2210
METHOTREXATE	50 MG	IV, IM, IT, IA	J9260
METHOTREXATE	2.5 MG	ORAL	J8610
METHOTREXATE	5 MG	IV, IM, IT, IA	J9250
METHOTREXATE LPF	5 MG	IV, IM, IT, IA	J9250
METHOTREXATE LPF	50 MG	IV, IM, IT, IA	J9260
METHYL AMINOLEVULINATE 16.8%	1 G	OTH	J7309
METHYLCOTOLONE	80 MG	IM	J1040
METHYLDOPA HCL	UP TO 250 MG	IV	J0210
METHYLDOPATE HCL	UP TO 250 MG	IV	J0210
METHYLENE BLUE	1 MG	SC	Q9968
METHYLERGONOVINE MALEATE	0.2 MG	IM, IV	J2210
METHYLNALTREXONE	0.1 MG	SC	J2212
METHYLPRED	4 MG	ORAL	J7509
METHYLPREDNISOLONE	4 MG	ORAL	J7509
METHYLPREDNISOLONE	125 MG	IM, IV	J2930
METHYLPREDNISOLONE	UP TO 40 MG	IM, IV	J2920

Drug Name	Unit Per	Route	Code
METHYLPREDNISOLONE ACETATE	40 MG	IM	J1030
METHYLPREDNISOLONE ACETATE	20 MG	IM	J1020
METHYLPREDNISOLONE ACETATE	80 MG	IM	J1040
METOCLOPRAMIDE	10 MG	IV	J2765
METRONIDAZOLE	500 MG	IV	S0030
METVIXIA 16.8%	1 G	OTH	J7309
MIACALCIN	400 U	SC, IM	J0630
MIBG	0.5 MCI	IV	A9508
MICAFUNGIN SODIUM	1 MG	IV	J2248
MICRHOGAM	50 MCG	IV	J2788
MICROPOROUS COLLAGEN IMPLANTABLE SLIT TUBE	1 CM LENGTH	OTH	C9353
MICROPOROUS COLLAGEN IMPLANTABLE TUBE	1 CM LENGTH	OTH	C9352
MIDAZOLAM HCl	1 MG	IM, IV	J2250
MIFEPRISTONE	200 MG	ORAL	S0190
MILRINONE LACTATE	5 MG	IV	J2260
MINOCIN	1 MG	IV	J2265
MINOCYCLINE HCL	1 MG	IV	J2265
MINOXIDIL	10 MG	ORAL	S0139
MIRENA	52 MG	OTH	J7302
MISOPROSTOL	200 MG	ORAL	S0191
MITHRACIN	2.5 MG	IV	J9270
MITOMYCIN	5 MG	IV	J9280
MITOMYCIN	0.2 MG	OTH	J7315
MITOSOL	0.2 MG	OTH	J7315
MITOXANA	1 G	IV	J9208
MITOXANTRONE HCL	5 MG	IV	J9293
MONARC-M	1 IU	IV	J7190
MONOCLATE-P	1 IU	IV	J7190
MONONINE	1 IU	IV	J7193
MONOPUR	75 IU	SC, IM	S0122
MORPHINE SULFATE	100 MG	IM, IV, SC	J2271
MORPHINE SULFATE	10 MG	IM, IV, SC	J2270
MORPHINE SULFATE	500 MG	OTH	S0093
MORPHINE SULFATE, PRESERVATIVE FREE, STERILE SOLUTION	10 MG	VAR	J2275
MOXIFLOXACIN	100 MG	IV	J2280
MOZOBIL	1 MG	SC	J2562
MPI INDIUM DTPA	0.5 MCI	IV	A9548
MS CONTIN	500 MG	OTH	S0093
MUCOMYST	1 G	INH	J7608
MUCOSIL	1 G	INH	J7608
MULTIHANCE	1 ML	IV	A9577
MULTIHANCE MULTIPACK	1 ML	IV	A9578
MUROMONAB-CD3	5 MG	OTH	J7505
MUSE	EA	OTH	J0275
MUSTARGEN	10 MG	IV	J9230
MUTAMYCIN	5 MG	IV	J9280
MYCAMINE	1 MG	IV	J2248
MYCOPHENOLATE MOFETIL	250 MG	ORAL	J7517
MYCOPHENOLIC ACID	180 MG	ORAL	J7518
MYFORTIC DELAYED RELEASE	180 MG	ORAL	J7518
MYLERAN	2 MG	ORAL	J8510
MYLOCEL	500 MG	ORAL	S0176
MYOBLOC	100 U	IM	J0587
MYOCHRYSINE	50 MG	IM	J1600
MYOZYME	10 MG	IV	J0220

Drug Name	Unit Per	Route	Code
NABILONE	1 MG	ORAL	J8650
NAFCILLIN SODIUM	2 GM	IM, IV	S0032
NAGLAZYME	1 MG	IV	J1458
NALBUPHINE HCL	10 MG	IM, IV, SC	J2300
NALLPEN	2 GM	IM, IV	S0032
NALOXONE HCL	1 MG	IM, IV, SC	J2310
NALTREXONE, DEPOT FORM	1 MG	IM	J2315
NANDROLONE DECANOATE	50 MG	IM	J2320
NARCAN	1 MG	IM, IV, SC	J2310
NAROPIN	1 MG	VAR	J2795
NASALCROM	10 MG	INH	J7631
NATALIZUMAB	1 MG	IV	J2323
NATRECOR	0.1 MG	IV	J2325
NATURAL ESTROGENIC SUBSTANCE	1 MG	IM, IV	J1410
NAVELBINE	10 MG	IV	J9390
ND-STAT	10 MG	IM, SC, IV	J0945
NEBCIN	80 MG	IM, IV	J3260
NEBUPENT	300 MG	INH	J2545
NEBUPENT	300 MG	IM, IV	S0080
NELARABINE	50 MG	IV	J9261
NEMBUTAL SODIUM	50 MG	IM, IV, OTH	J2515
NEORAL	250 MG	ORAL	J7516
NEORAL	25 MG	ORAL	J7515
NEOSAR	100 MG	IV	J9070
NEOSCAN	1 MCI	IV	A9556
NEOSTIGMINE METHYLSULFATE	0.5 MG	IM, IV	J2710
NEOTECT	STUDY DOSE UP TO 35 MCI	IV	A9536
NEOX 1K	SQ CM	OTH	Q4148
NESACAINE	30 ML	VAR	J2400
NESACAINE-MPF	30 ML	VAR	J2400
NESIRITIDE	0.1 MG	IV	J2325
NEULASTA	6 MG	SC, SQ	J2505
NEUMEGA	5 MG	SC	J2355
NEUPOGEN	1 MCG	SC, IV	J1442
NEURAGEN NERVE GUIDE	1 CM LENGTH	OTH	C9352
NEUROLITE	STUDY DOSE UP TO 25 MCI	IV	A9557
NEUROMATRIX	0.5 CM LENGTH	OTH	C9355
NEUROMEND NERVE WRAP	0.5 CM	OTH	C9361
NEUROWRAP NERVE PROTECTOR	1 CM LENGTH	OTH	C9353
NEUTREXIN	25 MG	IV	J3305
NEUTROSPEC	STUDY DOSE UP TO 25 MCI	IV	A9566
NEXPLANON	IMPLANT	OTH	J7307
NIPENT	10 MG	IV	J9268
NITROGEN MUSTARD	10 MG	IV	J9230
NITROGEN N-13 AMMONIA, DIAGNOSTIC	STUDY DOSE UP TO 40 MCI	INJ	A9526
NOC DRUGS, INHALATION SOLUTION ADMINISTERED THROUGH DME	1 EA		J7699
NOLVADEX	10 MG	ORAL	S0187
NORDITROPIN	1 MG	SC	J2941
NORDYL	50 MG	IV, IM	J1200
NORFLEX	60 MG	IV, IM	J2360
NORMAL SALINE SOLUTION	500 ML	IV	J7040
NORMAL SALINE SOLUTION	250 CC	IV	J7050
NORMAL SALINE SOLUTION	1000 CC	IV	J7030

Drug Name	Unit Per	Route	Code
NORPLANT II	IMPLANT	OTH	J7306
NOT OTHERWISE CLASSIFIED, ANTINEOPLASTIC DRUGS			J9999
NOVANTRONE	5 MG	IV	J9293
NOVAREL	1,000 USP U	IM	J0725
NOVASTAN	5 MG	IV	C9121
NOVOLIN	50 U	SC	J1817
NOVOLIN R	5 U	SC	J1815
NOVOLOG	50 U	SC	J1817
NOV-ONXOL	30 MG	IV	J9265
NOVOSEVEN	1 MCG	IV	J7189
NPH	5 UNITS	SC	J1815
NPLATE	10 MCG	SC	J2796
NUBAIN	10 MG	IM, IV, SC	J2300
NULOJIX	1 MG	IV	J0485
NUMORPHAN	1 MG	IV, SC, IM	J2410
NUTRI-TWELVE	1,000 MCG	IM, SC	J3420
NUTROPIN	1 MG	SC	J2941
NUTROPIN A.Q.	1 MG	SC	J2941
NUVARING VAGINAL RING	EACH	OTH	J7303
OASIS BURN MATRIX	SQ CM	OTH	Q4103
OASIS ULTRA TRI-LAYER WOUND MATRIX	SQ CM	OTH	Q4124
OASIS WOUND MATRIX	SQ CM	OTH	Q4102
OCRIPLASMIN	0.125 MG	OTH	J7316
OCTAFLUOROPROPANE UCISPHERES	1 ML	IV	Q9956
OCTAGAM	500 MG	IV	J1568
OCTREOSCAN	STUDY DOSE UP TO 6 MCI	IV	A9572
OCTREOTIDE ACETATE DEPOT	1 MG	IM	J2353
OCTREOTIDE, NON-DEPOT FORM	25 MCG	SC, IV	J2354
OFATUMUMAB	10 MG	IV	J9302
OFIRMEV	10 MG	IV	J0131
OFLOXACIN	400 MG	IV	S0034
OFORTA	10 MG	ORAL	J8562
OLANZAPINE	2.5 MG	IM	S0166
OLANZAPINE LONG ACTING	1 MG	IM	J2358
OMACETAXINE MEPESUCCINATE	0.01 MG	SC	J9262
OMALIZUMAB	5 MG	SC	J2357
OMNIPAQUE 140	PER ML	IV	Q9965
OMNIPAQUE 180	PER ML	IV	Q9965
OMNIPAQUE 240	PER ML	IV	Q9966
OMNIPAQUE 300	PER ML	IV	Q9966
OMNIPAQUE 350	PER ML	IV	Q9967
OMNISCAN	1 ML	IV	A9579
OMONTYS (FOR ESRD ON DIALYSIS)	0.1 MG	SC, IV	J0890
ONABOTULINUMTOXINA	1 UNIT	IM, OTH	J0585
ONCASPAR	VIAL	IM, IV	J9266
ONCOSCINT	STUDY DOSE, UP TO 6 MCI	IV	A4642
ONDANSETRON	1 MG	ORAL	Q0162
ONDANSETRON	4 MG	ORAL	S0119
ONDANSETRON HYDROCHLORIDE	1 MG	IV	J2405
ONTAK	300 MCG	IV	J9160
ONXOL	30 MG	IV	J9265
OPRELVEKIN	5 MG	SC	J2355
OPTIRAY	PER ML	IV	Q9967
OPTIRAY 160	PER ML	IV	Q9965

Drug Name	Unit Per	Route	Code
OPTIRAY 240	PER ML	IV	Q9966
OPTIRAY 300	PER ML	IV	Q9967
OPTIRAY 320	PER ML	IV	Q9967
OPTISON	1 ML	IV	Q9956
ORAL MAGNETIC RESONANCE CONTRAST AGENT, PER 100 ML	100 ML	ORAL	Q9954
ORENCIA	10 MG	IV	J0129
ORPHENADRINE CITRATE	60 MG	IV, IM	J2360
ORTHADAPT BIOIMPLANT	SQ CM	OTH	C1781
ORTHOCLONE OKT3	5 MG	OTH	J7505
ORTHOVISC	DOSE	OTH	J7324
OSELTAMIVIR PHOSPHATE (BRAND NAME) (DEMONSTRATION PROJECT)	75 MG	ORAL	G9035
OSELTAMIVIR PHOSPHATE (GENERIC) (DEMONSTRATION PROJECT)	75 MG	ORAL	G9019
OSMITROL	25% IN 50 ML	IV	J2150
OXACILLIN SODIUM	250 MG	IM, IV	J2700
OXALIPLATIN	0.5 MG	IV	J9263
OXILAN 300	PER ML	IV	Q9967
OXILAN 350	PER ML	IV	Q9967
OXYMORPHONE HCL	1 MG	IV, SC, IM	J2410
OXYTETRACYCLINE HCL	50 MG	IM	J2460
OXYTOCIN	10 U	IV, IM	J2590
OZURDEX	0.1 MG	OTH	J7312
PACIS BCG	VIAL	OTH	J9031
PACLITAXEL	30 MG	IV	J9265
PACLITAXEL PROTEIN-BOUND PARTICLES	1 MG	IV	J9264
PALIFERMIN	50 MCG	IV	J2425
PALIPERIDONE PALMITATE EXTENDED RELEASED	1 MG	IM	J2426
PALONOSETRON HCL	25 MCG	IV	J2469
PAMIDRONATE DISODIUM	30 MG	IV	J2430
PANHEMATIN	1 MG	IV	J1640
PANITUMUMAB	10 MG	IV	J9303
PANTOPRAZOLE SODIUM	VIAL	IV	C9113
PANTOPRAZOLE SODIUM	40 MG	IV	S0164
PAPAVERINE HCL	60 MG	IV, IM	J2440
PARAGARD T380A	EA	OTH	J7300
PARAPLANTIN	50 MG	IV	J9045
PARICALCITOL	1 MCG	IV, IM	J2501
PEDIAPRED	5 MG	ORAL	J7510
PEGADEMASE BOVINE	25 IU	IM	J2504
PEGAPTANIB SODIUM	0.3 MG	OTH	J2503
PEGASPARGASE	VIAL	IM, IV	J9266
PEGFILGRASTIM	6 MG	SC	J2505
PEGINESATIDE (FOR ESRD ON DIALYSIS)	0.1 MG	SC, IV	J0890
PEGINTERFERON ALFA-2A	180 MCG	SC	S0145
PEG-INTRON	180 MCG	SC	S0145
PEGLOTICASE	1 MG	IV	J2507
PEGYLATED INTERFERON ALFA-2A	180 MCG	SC	S0145
PEGYLATED INTERFERON ALFA-2B	10 MCG	SC	S0148
PEMETREXED	10 MG	IV	J9305
PENICILLIN G BENZATHINE	100,000 U	IM	J0561
PENICILLIN G BENZATHINE AND PENICILLIN G PROCAINE	100,000 UNITS	IM	J0558
PENICILLIN G POTASSIUM	600,000 U	IM, IV	J2540
PENICILLIN G PROCAINE	600,000 U	IM, IV	J2510

Drug Name	Unit Per	Route	Code
PENTACARINAT	300 MG	INH	S0080
PENTAM	300 MG	IM, IV	J2545
PENTAM 300	300 MG	IM, IV	S0080
PENTAMIDINE ISETHIONATE	300 MG	IM, IV	S0080
PENTAMIDINE ISETHIONATE COMPOUNDED	PER 300 MG	INH	J7676
PENTAMIDINE ISETHIONATE NONCOMPOUNDED	300 MG	INH	J2545
PENTASPAN	100 ML	IV	J2513
PENTASTARCH 10% SOLUTION	100 ML	IV	J2513
PENTATE CALCIUM TRISODIUM	STUDY DOSE UP TO 25 MCI	IV	A9539
PENTATE CALCIUM TRISODIUM	STUDY DOSE UP TO 75 MCI	INH	A9567
PENTATE ZINC TRISODIUM	STUDY DOSE UP TO 75 MCI	INH	A9567
PENTATE ZINC TRISODIUM	STUDY DOSE UP TO 25 MCI	IV	A9539
PENTAZOCINE	30 MG	IM, SC, IV	J3070
PENTOBARBITAL SODIUM	50 MG	IM, IV, OTH	J2515
PENTOSTATIN	10 MG	IV	J9268
PEPCID	20 MG	IV	S0028
PERFLEXANE LIPID MICROSPHERE	1 ML	IV	Q9955
PERFLUTREN LIPID MICROSPHERE	1 ML	IV	Q9957
PERFOROMIST	20 MCG	INH	J7606
PERJETA	1 MG	IV	J9306
PERMACOL	SQ CM	OTH	C9364
PERPHENAZINE	4 MG	ORAL	Q0175
PERPHENAZINE	5 MG	IM, IV	J3310
PERSANTINE	10 MG	IV	J1245
PERTUZUMAB	1 MG	IV	J9306
PFIZERPEN A.S.	600,000 U	IM, IV	J2510
PHENERGAN	50 MG	IM, IV	J2550
PHENERGAN	12.5 MG	ORAL	Q0169
PHENOBARBITAL SODIUM	120 MG	IM, IV	J2560
PHENTOLAMINE MESYLATE	5 MG	IM, IV	J2760
PHENYLEPHRINE HCL	1 ML	SC, IM, IV	J2370
PHENYTOIN SODIUM	50 MG	IM, IV	J1165
PHOSPHOCOL	1 MCI	IV	A9563
PHOSPHOTEC	STUDY DOSE UP TO 25 MCI	IV	A9538
PHOTOFRIN	75 MG	IV	J9600
PHYTONADIONE	1 MG	IM, SC, IV	J3430
PIPERACILLIN SODIUM	500 MG	IM, IV	S0081
PIPERACILLIN SODIUM/TAZOBACTAM SODIUM	1 G/1.125 GM	IV	J2543
PITOCIN	10 U	IV, IM	J2590
PLATINOL AQ	10 MG	IV	J9060
PLERIXAFOR	1 MG	SC	J2562
PLICAMYCIN	2.5 MG	IV	J9270
PNEUMOCOCCAL CONJUGATE	EA	IM	S0195
PNEUMOVAX II	EA	IM	S0195
POLOCAINE	10 ML	VAR	J0670
POLYGAM	500 MG	IV	J1566
POLYGAM S/D	500 MG	IV	J1566
PORCINE IMPLANT, PERMACOL	SQ CM	OTH	C9364
PORFIMER SODIUM	75 MG	IV	J9600
PORK INSULIN	5 U	SC	J1815
POROUS PURIFIED COLLAGEN MATRIX BONE VOID FILLER	0.5 CC	OTH	C9362

Drug Name	Unit Per	Route	Code
POROUS PURIFIED COLLAGEN MATRIX BONE VOID FILLER, PUTTY	0.5 CC	OTH	C9359
POTASSIUM CHLORIDE	2 MEQ	IV	J3480
PRALATREXATE	1 MG	IV	J9307
PRALIDOXIME CHLORIDE	1 MG	IV, IM, SC	J2730
PREDNISOLONE	5 MG	ORAL	J7510
PREDNISOLONE ACETATE	1 ML	IM	J2650
PREDNISONE	5 MG	ORAL	J7506
PREDNORAL	5 MG	ORAL	J7510
PREGNYL	1,000 USP U	IM	J0725
PRELONE	5 MG	ORAL	J7510
PREMARIN	25 MG	IV, IM	J1410
PRENATAL VITAMINS	30 TABS	ORAL	S0197
PRIALT	1 MCG	OTH	J2278
PRIMACOR	5 MG	IV	J2260
PRIMATRIX	SQ CM	OTH	Q4110
PRIMAXIN	250 MG	IV, IM	J0743
PRIMESTRIN AQUEOUS	1 MG	IM, IV	J1410
PRIMETHASONE	1 MG	IM, IV, OTH	J1100
PRI-METHYLATE	80 MG	IM	J1040
PRIVIGEN	500 MG	IV	J1459
PROCAINAMIDE HCL	1 G	IM, IV	J2690
PROCARBAZINE HCL	50 MG	ORAL	S0182
PROCHLOPERAZINE MALEATE	5 MG	ORAL	S0183
PROCHLORPERAZINE	10 MG	IM, IV	J0780
PROCHLORPERAZINE MALEATE	5 MG	ORAL	Q0164
PROCRIT, ESRD USE	1,000 U	SC, IV	J0886
PROCRIT, NON-ESRD USE	1,000 U	SC, IV	J0885
PROFILNINE HEAT-TREATED	1 IU	IV	J7194
PROFILNINE SD	1 IU	IV	J7194
PROFONIX	VIAL	INJ	C9113
PROGESTERONE	50 MG	IM	J2675
PROGRAF	1 MG	ORAL	J7507
PROGRAF	5 MG	OTH	J7525
PROLASTIN	10 MG	IV	J0256
PROLEUKIN	1 VIAL	VAR	J9015
PROLIA	1 MG	SC	J0897
PROLIXIN DECANOATE	25 MG	SC, IM	J2680
PROMAZINE HCL	25 MG	IM	J2950
PROMETHAZINE HCL	50 MG	IM, IV	J2550
PROMETHAZINE HCL	12.5 MG	ORAL	Q0169
PRONESTYL	1 G	IM, IV	J2690
PROPECIA	5 MG	ORAL	S0138
PROPLEX SX-T	1 IU	IV	J7194
PROPLEX T	1 IU	IV	J7194
PROPRANOLOL HCL	1 MG	IV	J1800
PROREX	50 MG	IM, IV	J2550
PROSCAR	5 MG	ORAL	S0138
PROSTASCINT	STUDY DOSE UP TO 10 MCI	IV	A9507
PROSTIGMIN	0.5 MG	IM, IV	J2710
PROSTIN VR	1.25 MCG	INJ	J0270
PROTAMINE SULFATE	10 MG	IV	J2720
PROTEIN C CONCENTRATE	10 IU	IV	J2724
PROTEINASE INHIBITOR (HUMAN)	10 MG	IV	J0256
PROTIRELIN	250 MCG	IV	J2725
PROTONIX IV	VIAL	IV	C9113

Drug Name	Unit Per	Route	Code
PROTONIX IV	40 MG	IV	S0164
PROTOPAM CHLORIDE	1 G	SC, IM, IV	J2730
PROTROPIN	1 MG	SC, IM	J2940
PROVENGE	INFUSION	IV	Q2043
PROVENTIL NONCOMPOUNDED, CONCENTRATED	1 MG	INH	J7611
PROVENTIL NONCOMPOUNDED, UNIT DOSE	1 MG	INH	J7613
PROVOCHOLINE POWDER	1 MG	INH	J7674
PROZINE-50	25 MG	IM	J2950
PULMICORT	0.25 MG	INH	J7633
PULMICORT RESPULES	0.5 MG	INH	J7627
PULMICORT RESPULES NONCOMPOUNDED, CONCETRATED	0.25 MG	INH	J7626
PULMOZYME	1 MG	INH	J7639
PURINETHOL	50 MG	ORAL	S0108
PYRIDOXINE HCL	100 MG	IM, IV	J3415
QUADRAMET	PER DOSE UP TO 150 MCI	IV	A9604
QUELICIN	20 MG	IM, IV	J0330
QUINUPRISTIN/DALFOPRISTIN	500 MG	IV	J2770
QUTENZA	10 SQ CM	OTH	J7335
RADIESSE	0.1 ML	OTH	Q2026
RANIBIZUMAB	0.5 MG	OTH	J2778
RANITIDINE HCL	25 MG	INJ	J2780
RAPAMUNE	1 MG	ORAL	J7520
RASBURICASE	50 MCG	IM	J2783
REBETRON KIT	1,000,000 U	SC, IM	J9214
REBIF	1 MCG	SC	Q3028
REBIF	30 MCG	SC	J1826
RECLAST	1 MG	IV	J3489
RECOMBINATE	1 IU	IV	J7192
REDISOL	1,000 MCG	SC. IM	J3420
REFACTO	1 IU	IV	J7192
REFLUDAN	50 MG	IM, IV	J1945
REGADENOSON	0.1 MG	IV	J2785
REGITINE	5 MG	IM, IV	J2760
REGLAN	10 MG	IV	J2765
REGRANEX GEL	0.5 G	OTH	S0157
REGULAR INSULIN	5 UNITS	SC	J1815
RELAXIN	10 ML	IV, IM	J2800
RELENZA (DEMONSTRATION PROJECT)	10 MG	INH	G9034
RELION	5 U	SC	J1815
RELION NOVOLIN	50 U	SC	J1817
RELISTOR	0.1 MG	SC	J2212
REMICADE	10 MG	IV	J1745
REMODULIN	1 MG	SC	J3285
REODULIN	1 MG	SC	J3285
REOPRO	10 MG	IV	J0130
REPRIZA	SQ CM	OTH	Q4143
REPRONEX	75 IU	SC, IM, IV	S0122
RESPIROL NONCOMPOUNDED, CONCENTRATED	1 MG	INH	J7611
RESPIROL NONCOMPOUNDED, UNIT DOSE	1 MG	INH	J7613
RETAVASE	18.1 MG	IV	J2993
RETEPLASE	18.1 MG	IV	J2993
RETISERT	IMPLANT	OTH	J7311

Drug Name	Unit Per	Route	Code
RETROVIR	100 MG	ORAL	S0104
RETROVIR	10 MG	IV	J3485
RHEOMACRODEX	500 ML	IV	J7100
RHEUMATREX	2.5 MG	ORAL	J8610
RHEUMATREX DOSE PACK	2.5 MG	ORAL	J8610
RHO D IMMUNE GLOBULIN	300 MCG	IV	J2790
RHO D IMMUNE GLOBULIN (RHOPHYLAC)	100 IU	IM, IV	J2791
RHO D IMMUNE GLOBULIN MINIDOSE	50 MCG	IM	J2788
RHO D IMMUNE GLOBULIN SOLVENT DETERGENT	100 IU	IV	J2792
RHOGAM	50 MCG	IM	J2788
RHOGAM	300 MCG	IM	J2790
RHOPHYLAC	100 IU	IM, IV	J2791
RILONACEPT	1 MG	SC	J2793
RIMANTADINE HCL (DEMONSTRATION PROJECT)	100 MG	ORAL	G9020
RIMANTADINE HCL (DEMONSTRATION PROJECT)	100 MG	ORAL	G9036
RIMSO 50	50 ML	IV	J1212
RINGERS LACTATE INFUSION	UP TO 1000 CC	IV	J7120
RISPERDAL COSTA LONG ACTING	0.5 MG	IM	J2794
RISPERIDONE, LONG ACTING	0.5 MG	IM	J2794
RITUXAN	100 MG	IV	J9310
RITUXIMAB	100 MG	IV	J9310
ROBAXIN	10 ML	IV, IM	J2800
ROCEPHIN	250 MG	IV, IM	J0696
ROFERON-A	3,000,000 U	SC, IM	J9213
ROMIDEPSIN	1 MG	IV	J9315
ROMIPLOSTIM	10 MCG	SC	J2796
ROPIVACAINE HYDROCHLORIDE	1 MG	VAR	J2795
RUBEX	10 MG	IV	J9000
RUBIDIUM RB-82	STUDY DOSE UP TO 60 MCI	IV	A9555
RUBRAMIN PC	1,000 MCG	SC, IM	J3420
RUBRATOPE 57	STUDY DOSE UP TO 1 UCI	ORAL	A9559
SAIZEN	1 MG	SC	J2941
SAIZEN SOMATROPIN RDNA ORIGIN	1 MG	SC	J2941
SALINE OR STERILE WATER, METERED DOSE DISPENSER	10 ML	INH	A4218
SALINE, STERILE WATER, AND/OR DEXTROSE DILUENT/FLUSH	10 ML	VAR	A4216
SALINE/STERILE WATER	500 ML	VAR	A4217
SAMARIUM LEXIDRONAM	PER DOSE UP TO 150 MCI	IV	A9604
SANDIMMUNE	25 MG	ORAL	J7515
SANDIMMUNE	250 MG	IV	J7516
SANDIMMUNE	100 MG	ORAL	J7502
SANDOSTATIN	25 MCG	SC, IV	J2354
SANDOSTATIN LAR	1 MG	IM	J2353
SANGCYA	100 MG	ORAL	J7502
SANO-DROL	40 MG	IM	J1030
SANO-DROL	80 MG	IM	J1040
SAQUINAVIR	200 MG	ORAL	S0140
SARGRAMOSTIM (GM-CSF)	50 MCG	IV	J2820
SCANDONEST	PER 10 ML	IV	J0670
SCULPTRA	0.5 ML	OTH	Q2028
SECREFLO	1 MCG	IV	J2850

Drug Name	Unit Per	Route	Code
SECRETIN, SYNTHETIC, HUMAN	1 MCG	IV	J2850
SENSORCAINE	30 ML	VAR	S0020
SEPTRA IV	10 ML	IV	S0039
SERMORELIN ACETATE	1 MCG	IV	Q0515
SEROSTIM	1 MG	SC	J2941
SEROSTIM RDNA ORIGIN	1 MG	SC	J2941
SILDENAFIL CITRATE	25 MG	ORAL	S0090
SIMPONI	1 MG	IV	J1602
SIMULECT	20 MG	IV	J0480
SINCALIDE	5 MCG	IV	J2805
SIPULEUCEL-T	INFUSION	IV	Q2043
SIROLIMUS	1 MG	ORAL	J7520
SKIN SUBSTITUTE, ALLODERM	SQ CM	OTH	Q4116
SKIN SUBSTITUTE, ALLOSKIN	SQ CM	OTH	Q4115
SKIN SUBSTITUTE, APLIGRAF	SQ CM	OTH	Q4101
SKIN SUBSTITUTE, DERMAGRAFT	SQ CM	OTH	Q4106
SKIN SUBSTITUTE, GAMMAGRAFT	SQ CM	OTH	Q4111
SKIN SUBSTITUTE, GRAFTJACKET	SQ CM	OTH	Q4107
SKIN SUBSTITUTE, INTEGRA BILAYER MATRIX WOUND DRESSING	SQ CM	OTH	Q4104
SKIN SUBSTITUTE, INTEGRA DERMAL REGENERATION TEMPLATE	SQ CM	OTH	Q4105
SKIN SUBSTITUTE, INTEGRA MATRIX	SQ CM	OTH	Q4108
SKIN SUBSTITUTE, INTEGRA MESHED BILAYER WOUND MATRIX	SQ CM	OTH	C9363
SKIN SUBSTITUTE, OASIS BURN MATRIX	SQ CM	OTH	Q4103
SKIN SUBSTITUTE, OASIS WOUND MATRIX	SQ CM	OTH	Q4102
SKIN SUBSTITUTE, PRIMATRIX	SQ CM	OTH	Q4110
SKYLA	13.5 MG	OTH	J7301
SMZ-TMP	10 ML	IV	S0039
SODIUM FERRIC GLUCONATE COMPLEX IN SUCROSE	12.5 MG	IV	J2916
SODIUM FLUORIDE F-18, DIAGNOSTIC	STUDY DOSE UP TO 30 MCI	IV	A9580
SODIUM IODIDE I-131 CAPSULE DIAGNOSTIC	1 MCI	ORAL	A9528
SODIUM IODIDE I-131 CAPSULE THERAPEUTIC	1 MCI	ORAL	A9517
SODIUM IODIDE I-131 SOLUTION THERAPEUTIC	1 MCI	ORAL	A9530
SODIUM PHOSPHATE P32	1 MCI	IV	A9563
SOLGANAL	50 MG	IM	J2910
SOLIRIS	10 MG	IV	J1300
SOLTAMOX	10 MG	ORAL	S0187
SOLU-CORTEF	100 MG	IV, IM, SC	J1720
SOLU-MEDROL	125 MG	IM, IV	J2930
SOLU-MEDROL	40 MG	IM, IV	J2920
SOLUREX	1 MG	IM, IV, OTH	J1100
SOMATREM	1 MG	SC, IM	J2940
SOMATROPIN	1 MG	SC	J2941
SOMATULINE	1 MG	SC	J1930
SPECTINOMYCIN DIHYDROCHLORIDE	2 G	IM	J3320
SPECTRO-DEX	1 MG	IM, IV, OTH	J1100
SPORANOX	50 MG	IV	J1835
STADOL	1 MG	IM, IV	J0595
STADOL NS	25 MG	OTH	S0012
STELARA	1 MG	SC	J3357

Drug Name	Unit Per	Route	Code
STERILE WATER OR SALINE, METERED DOSE DISPENSER	10 ML	INH	A4218
STERILE WATER, SALINE, AND/OR DEXTROSE DILUENT/FLUSH	10 ML	VAR	A4216
STERILE WATER/SALINE	500 ML	VAR	A4217
STRATTICE TM	SQ CM	OTH	Q4130
STREPTASE	250,000 IU	IV	J2995
STREPTOKINASE	250,000 IU	IV	J2995
STREPTOMYCIN	1 G	IM	J3000
STREPTOZOCIN	1 G	IV	J9320
STRONTIUM 89 CHLORIDE	1 MCI	IV	A9600
SUBLIMAZE	0.1 MG	IM, IV	J3010
SUCCINYLCHOLINE CHLORIDE	20 MG	IM, IV	J0330
SULFAMETHOXAZOLE AND TRIMETHOPRIM	10 ML	IV	S0039
SULFUTRIM	10 ML	IV	S0039
SUMATRIPTAN SUCCINATE	6 MG	SC	J3030
SUPARTZ	DOSE	OTH	J7321
SUPPRELIN LA	10 MCG	OTH	J1675
SURGIMEND COLLAGEN MATRIX, FETAL	0.5 SQ CM	OTH	C9358
SURGIMEND COLLAGEN MATRIX, NEONATAL	0.5 SQ CM	OTH	C9360
SYMMETREL (DEMONSTRATION PROJECT)	100 MG	ORAL	G9033
SYNERA	70 MG/70 MG	OTH	C9285
SYNERCID	500 MG	IV	J2770
SYNRIBO	0.01 MG	SC	J9262
SYNTOCINON	10 UNITS	IV	J2590
SYNVISC/SYNVISC-ONE	1 MG	OTH	J7325
SYTOBEX	1,000 MCG	SC, IM	J3420
TACRINE HCL	10 MG	ORAL	S0014
TACROLIMUS	1 MG	ORAL	J7507
TACROLIMUS	5 MG	OTH	J7525
TACROLIMUS, EXTENDED RELEASE	0.1 MG	ORAL	J7508
TAGAMET HCL	300 MG	IM, IV	S0023
TALIGLUCERASE ALFA	10 U	IV	J3060
TALWIN	30 MG	IM, SC, IV	J3070
TALYMED	SQ CM	OTH	Q4127
TAMIFLU (DEMONSTRATION PROJECT)	75 MG	ORAL	G9019
TAMIFLU (DEMONSTRATION PROJECT)	75 MG	ORAL	G9035
TAMOXIFEN CITRATE	10 MG	ORAL	S0187
TAXOL	30 MG	IV	J9265
TAXOTERE	1 MG	IV	J9171
TAZICEF	500 MG	IM, IV	J0713
TBO-FILGRASTIM	5 MCG	SC	J1446
TC 99M TILOMANOCEPT	0.5 MCI	SC, OTH	A9520
TEBAMIDE	250 MG	ORAL	Q0173
TEBOROXIME TECHNETIUM TC 99	STUDY DOSE	IV	A9501
TEBOROXIME, TECHNETIUM	STUDY DOSE	IV	A9501
TECHNEPLEX	STUDY DOSE UP TO 25 MCI	IV	A9539
TECHNESCAN	STUDY DOSE UP TO 30 MCI	IV	A9561
TECHNESCAN FANOLESOMAB	STUDY DOSE UP TO 25 MCI	IV	A9566
TECHNESCAN MAA	STUDY DOSE UP TO 10 MCI	IV	A9540
TECHNESCAN MAG3	STUDY DOSE UP TO 15 MCI	IV	A9562

Drug Name	Unit Per	Route	Code
TECHNESCAN PYP	STUDY DOSE UP TO 25 MCI	IV	A9538
TECHNESCAN PYP KIT	STUDY DOSE UP TO 25 MCI	IV	A9538
TECHNETIUM SESTAMBI	STUDY DOSE	IV	A9500
TECHNETIUM TC 99M APCITIDE	STUDY DOES UP TO 20 MCI	IV	A9504
TECHNETIUM TC 99M ARCITUMOMAB, DIAGNOSTIC	STUDY DOSE UP TO 45 MCI	IV	A9568
TECHNETIUM TC 99M BICISATE	STUDY DOSE UP TO 25 MCI	IV	A9557
TECHNETIUM TC 99M DEPREOTIDE	STUDY DOSE UP TO 35 MCI	IV	A9536
TECHNETIUM TC 99M EXAMETAZIME	STUDY DOSE UP TO 25 MCI	IV	A9521
TECHNETIUM TC 99M FANOLESOMAB	STUDY DOSE UP TO 25 MCI	IV	A9566
TECHNETIUM TC 99M LABELED RED BLOOD CELLS	STUDY DOSE UP TO 30 MCI	IV	A9560
TECHNETIUM TC 99M MACROAGGREGATED ALBUMIN	STUDY DOSE UP TO 10 MCI	IV	A9540
TECHNETIUM TC 99M MDI-MDP	STUDY DOSE UP TO 30 MCI	IV	A9503
TECHNETIUM TC 99M MEBROFENIN	STUDY DOSE UP TO 15 MCI	IV	A9537
TECHNETIUM TC 99M MEDRONATE	STUDY DOSE UP TO 30 MCI	IV	A9503
TECHNETIUM TC 99M MERTIATIDE	STUDY DOSE UP TO 15 MCI	IV	A9562
TECHNETIUM TC 99M OXIDRONATE	STUDY DOSE UP TO 30 MCI	IV	A9561
TECHNETIUM TC 99M PENTETATE	STUDY DOSE UP TO 25 MCI	IV	A9539
TECHNETIUM TC 99M PYROPHOSPHATE	STUDY DOSE UP TO 25 MCI	IV	A9538
TECHNETIUM TC 99M SODIUM GLUCEPATATE	STUDY DOSE UP TO 25 MCI	IV	A9550
TECHNETIUM TC 99M SUCCIMER	STUDY DOSE UP TO 10 MCI	IV	A9551
TECHNETIUM TC 99M SULFUR COLLOID	STUDY DOSE UP TO 20 MCI	IV	A9541
TECHNETIUM TC 99M TETROFOSMIN, DIAGNOSTIC	STUDY DOSE	IV	A9502
TECHNETIUM TC-99M EXAMETAZIME LABELED AUTOLOGOUS WHITE BLOOD CELLS	STUDY DOSE	IV	A9569
TECHNETIUM TC-99M TEBOROXIME	STUDY DOSE	IV	A9501
TECHNILITE	1 MCI	IV	A9512
TEFLARO	10 MG	IV	J0712
TELAVANCIN	10 MG	IV	J3095
TEMODAR	1 MG	IV	J9328
TEMODAR	5 MG	ORAL	J8700
TEMOZOLOMIDE	1 MG	IV	J9328
TEMOZOLOMIDE	5 MG	ORAL	J8700
TEMSIROLIMUS	1 MG	IV	J9330
TENDON, POROUS MATRIX	SQ CM	OTH	C9356
TENDON, POROUS MATRIX CROSS-LINKED AND GLYCOSAMINOGLYCAN MATRIX	SQ CM	OTH	C9356
TENECTEPLASE	1 MG	IV	J3101
TENIPOSIDE	50 MG	IV	Q2017
TENOGLIDE TENDON PROTECTOR	SQ CM	OTH	C9356
TENOGLIDE TENDON PROTECTOR SHEET	SQ CM	OTH	C9356
TENSIX	SQ CM	OTH	Q4146

Drug Name	Unit Per	Route	Code
TEQUIN	10 MG	IV	J1590
TERBUTALINE SULFATE	1 MG	SC, IV	J3105
TERBUTALINE SULFATE, COMPOUNDED, CONCENTRATED	1 MG	INH	J7680
TERBUTALINE SULFATE, COMPOUNDED, UNIT DOSE	1 MG	INH	J7681
TERIPARATIDE	10 MCG	SC	J3110
TERRAMYCIN	50 MG	IM	J2460
TESTERONE	50 MG	IM	J3140
TESTOSTERONE CYPIONATE	1 CC, 200 MG	IM	J1080
TESTOSTERONE CYPIONATE	UP TO 100 MG	IM	J1070
TESTOSTERONE CYPIONATE & ESTRADIOL CYPIONATE	1 ML	IM	J1060
TESTOSTERONE ENANTHATE	200 MG	IM	J3130
TESTOSTERONE ENANTHATE	100 MG	IM	J3120
TESTOSTERONE ENANTHATE & ESTRADIOL VALERATE	1 CC	IM	J0900
TESTOSTERONE PELLET	75 MG	OTH	S0189
TESTOSTERONE PROPIONATE	100 MG	IM	J3150
TESTOSTERONE SUSPENSION	50 MG	IM	J3140
TESTRO AQ	50 MG	IM	J3140
TETANUS IMMUNE GLOBULIN	250 U	IM	J1670
TETRACYCLINE HCL	250 MG	IV	J0120
T-GEN	250 MG	ORAL	Q0173
THALLOUS CHLORIDE	1 MCI	IV	A9505
THALLOUS CHLORIDE TL-201	1 MCI	IV	A9505
THALLOUS CHLORIDE USP	1 MCI	IV	A9505
THEELIN AQUEOUS	1 MG	IM, IV	J1435
THEOPHYLLINE	40 MG	IV	J2810
THERACYS	VIAL	OTH	J9031
THERASKIN	SQ CM	OTH	Q4121
THIAMINE HCL	100 MG	INJ	J3411
THIETHYLPERAZINE MALEATE	10 MG	ORAL	Q0174
THIETHYLPERAZINE MALEATE	10 MG	IM	J3280
THIMAZIDE	250 MG	ORAL	Q0173
THIOTEPA	15 MG	IV	J9340
THORAZINE	50 MG	IM, IV	J3230
THROMBATE III	1 IU	IV	J7197
THYMOGLOBULIN	25 MG	OTH	J7511
THYROGEN	0.9 MG	IM, SC	J3240
THYROTROPIN ALPHA	0.9 MG	IM, SC	J3240
TICARCILLIN DISODIUM AND CLAVULANATE	3.1 G	IV	S0040
TICE BCG	VIAL	OTH	J9031
TICON	250 MG	IM	Q0173
TIGAN	200 MG	IM	J3250
TIGECYCLINE	1 MG	IV	J3243
TIJECT-20	200 MG	IM	J3250
TIMENTIN	3.1 G	IV	S0040
TINZAPARIN	1,000 IU	SC	J1655
TIROFIBAN HCL	0.25 MG	IM, IV	J3246
TNKASE	1 MG	IV	J3101
TOBI	300 MG	INH	J7682
TOBRAMYCIN COMPOUNDED, UNIT DOSE	300 MG	INH	J7685
TOBRAMYCIN SULFATE	80 MG	IM, IV	J3260
TOBRAMYCIN, NONCOMPOUNDED, UNIT DOSE	300 MG	INH	J7682

Drug Name	Unit Per	Route	Code
TOCILIZUMAB	1 MG	IV	J3262
TOLAZOLINE HCL	25 MG	IV	J2670
TOPOSAR	10 MG	IV	J9181
TOPOTECAN	0.25 MG	ORAL	J8705
TOPOTECAN	0.1 MG	IV	J9351
TORADOL	15 MG	IV	J1885
TORISEL	1 MG	IV	J9330
TORNALATE	PER MG	INH	J7629
TORNALATE CONCENTRATE	PER MG	INH	J7628
TORSEMIDE	10 MG	IV	J3265
TOSITUMOMAB	450 MG	IV	G3001
TOSITUMOMAB I-131 DIAGNOSTIC	STUDY DOSE	IV	A9544
TOSITUMOMAB I-131 THERAPEUTIC	TX DOSE	IV	A9545
TOTECT	PER 250 MG	IV	J1190
TRASTUZUMAB	10 MG	IV	J9355
TRASYLOL	10,000 KIU	IV	J0365
TREANDA	1 MG	IV	J9033
TRELSTAR DEPOT	3.75 MG	IM	J3315
TRELSTAR DEPOT PLUS DEBIOCLIP KIT	3.75 MG	IM	J3315
TRELSTAR LA	3.75 MG	IM	J3315
TREPROSTINIL	1 MG	SC	J3285
TREPROSTINIL, INHALATION SOLUTION	1.74 MG	INH	J7686
TRETINOIN	5 G	OTH	S0117
TRIAM-A	10 MG	IM	J3301
TRIAMCINOLONE ACETONIDE	10 MG	IM	J3301
TRIAMCINOLONE ACETONIDE, PRESERVATIVE FREE	1 MG	INJ	J3300
TRIAMCINOLONE DIACETATE	5 MG	IM	J3302
TRIAMCINOLONE HEXACETONIDE	5 MG	VAR	J3303
TRIAMCINOLONE, COMPOUNDED, CONCENTRATED	1 MG	INH	J7683
TRIAMCINOLONE, COMPOUNDED, UNIT DOSE	1 MG	INH	J7684
TRIBAN	250 MG	ORAL	Q0173
TRIESENCE	1 MG	OTH	J3300
TRIFLUPROMAZINE HCL	UP TO 20 MG	INJ	J3400
TRI-KORT	10 MG	IM	J3301
TRILIFON	4 MG	ORAL	Q0175
TRILOG	10 MG	IM	J3301
TRILONE	5 MG	IM	J3302
TRIMETHOBENZAMIDE HCL	200 MG	IM	J3250
TRIMETHOBENZAMIDE HCL	250 MG	ORAL	Q0173
TRIMETREXATE GLUCURONATE	25 MG	IV	J3305
TRIPTORELIN PAMOATE	3.75 MG	IM	J3315
TRISENOX	1 MG	IV	J9017
TRIVARIS	1 MG	VAR	J3300
TROBICIN	2 G	IM	J3320
TRUXADRYL	50 MG	IV, IM	J1200
TYGACIL	1 MG	IV	J3243
TYPE A BOTOX	1 UNIT	IM, OTH	J0585
TYSABRI	1 MG	IV	J2323
TYVASO	1.74 MG	INH	J7686
ULTRALENTE	5 U	SC	J1815
ULTRATAG	STUDY DOSE UP TO 30 MCI	IV	A9560
ULTRA-TECHNEKOW	1 MCI	IV	A9512
ULTRAVIST 150	1 ML	IV	Q9965

Drug Name	Unit Per	Route	Code
ULTRAVIST 240	1 ML	IV	Q9966
ULTRAVIST 300	1 ML	IV	Q9967
ULTRAVIST 370	1 ML	IV	Q9967
UNASYN	1.5 G	IM, IV	J0295
UNCLASSIFIED BIOLOGICS			J3590
UNCLASSIFIED DRUGS OR BIOLOGICALS	VAR	VAR	C9399
UNITE BIOMATRIX	SQ CM	OTH	Q4129
UREA	40 G	IV	J3350
URECHOLINE	UP TO 5 MG	SC	J0520
UROFOLLITROPIN	75 IU	SC, IM	J3355
UROKINASE	5,000 IU	IV	J3364
UROKINASE	250,000 IU	IV	J3365
USTEKINUMAB	1 MG	SC	J3357
VALERGEN	10 MG	IM	J1380
VALIUM	5 MG	IV, IM	J3360
VALRUBICIN INTRAVESICAL	200 MG	OTH	J9357
VALSTAR	200 MG	OTH	J9357
VANCOCIN	500 MG	IM, IV	J3370
VANCOMYCIN HCL	500 MG	IV, IM	J3370
VANTAS	50 MG	OTH	J9225
VECTIBIX	10 MG	IV	J9303
VELAGLUCERASE ALFA	100 U	IV	J3385
VELBAN	I MG	IV	J9360
VELCADE	0.1 MG	IV	J9041
VELOSULIN	5 U	SC	J1815
VELOSULIN BR	5 U	SC	J1815
VENOFER	1 MG	IV	J1756
VENTOLIN NONCOMPOUNDED, CONCENTRATED	1 MG	INH	J7611
VENTOLIN NONCOMPOUNDED, UNIT DOSE	1 MG	INH	J7613
VEPESID	10 MG	IV	J9181
VEPESID	50 MG	ORAL	J8560
VERITAS	SQ CM	OTH	C9354
VERSED	1 MG	IM, IV	J2250
VERTEPORFIN	0.1 MG	IV	J3396
VFEND	200 MG	IV	J3465
VIAGRA	25 MG	ORAL	S0090
VIBATIV	10 MG	IV	J3095
VIDAZA	1 MG	SC	J9025
VIDEX	25 MG	ORAL	S0137
VIMPAT	1 MG	IV, ORAL	C9254
VINBLASTINE SULFATE	1 MG	IV	J9360
VINCASCAR	1 MG	IV	J9370
VINCRISTINE SULFATE	1 MG	IV	J9370
VINCRISTINE SULFATE LIPOSOME	5 MG	IV	J9371
VINORELBINE TARTRATE	10 MG	IV	J9390
VIRILON	1 CC, 200 MG	IM	J1080
VISTAJECT-25	25 MG	IM	J3410
VISTARIL	25 MG	ORAL	Q0177
VISTARIL	25 MG	IM	J3410
VISTIDE	375 MG	IV	J0740
VISUDYNE	0.1 MG	IV	J3396
VITAMIN B-12 CYANOCOBALAMIN	1,000 MCG	IM, SC	J3420
VITAMIN B-17	VAR	INJ	J3570
VITRASE	1 USP	OTH	J3471
VITRASE	1,000 USP	OTH	J3472

Drug Name	Unit Per	Route	Code
VITRASERT	4.5 MG	OTH	J7310
VITRAVENE	1.65 MG	OTH	J1452
VIVITROL	1 MG	IM	J2315
VON WILLEBRAND FACTOR COMPLEX (HUMAN) (WILATE)	1 IU	IV	J7183
VON WILLEBRAND FACTOR COMPLEX, HUMATE-P	1 IU	IV	J7187
VON WILLEBRAND FACTOR VIII COMPLEX, HUMAN	PER FACTOR VIII IU	IV	J7186
VORAXAZE	10 UNITS	IV	C9293
VORICONAZOLE	200 MG	IV	J3465
VPRIV	100 U	IV	J3385
VUMON	50 MG	IV	Q2017
WEHAMINE	50 MG	IM, IV	J1240
WEHDRYL	50 MG	IM, IV	J1200
WELBUTRIN SR	150 MG	ORAL	S0106
WILATE	1 IU	IV	J7183
WINRHO SDF	100 IU	IV	J2792
WYCILLIN	600,000 U	IM, IV	J2510
XCM BIOLOGIC TISSUE MATRIX	SQ CM	OTH	Q4142
XELODA	500 MG	ORAL	J8521
XELODA	150 MG	ORAL	J8520
XENON XE-133	10 MCI	INH	A9558
XEOMIN	1 UNIT	IM	J0588
XGEVA	1 MG	SC	J0897
XIAFLEX	0.01 MG	OTH	J0775
XOLAIR	5 MG	SC	J2357
XYLOCAINE	10 MG	IV	J2001
XYNTHA	1 IU	IV	J7185
YERVOY	1 MG	IV	J9228
YTTRIUM 90 IBRITUMOMAB TIUXETAN	TX DOSE UP TO 40 MCI	IV	A9543
ZALTRAP	1 MG	IV	J9400
ZANAMIVIR (BRAND) (DEMONSTRATION PROJECT)	10 MG	INH	G9034
ZANAMIVIR (GENERIC) (DEMONSTRATION PROJECT)	10 MG	INH	G9018
ZANOSAR	1 GM	IV	J9320
ZANTAC	25 MG	INJ	J2780
ZEMAIRA	10 MG	IV	J0256
ZEMPLAR	1 MCG	IV, IM	J2501
ZENAPAX	25 MG	OTH	J7513
ZEVALIN	STUDY DOSE UP TO 5 MCI	IV	A9542
ZEVALIN DIAGNOSTIC	STUDY DOSE UP TO 5 MCI	IV	A9542
ZEVALIN THERAPEUTIC	TX DOSE UP TO 40 MCI	IV	A9543
ZICONOTIDE	1 MCG	IT	J2278
ZIDOVUDINE	100 MG	ORAL	S0104
ZIDOVUDINE	10 MG	IV	J3485
ZINACEFT	PER 750 MG	IM, IV	J0697
ZINECARD	250 MG	IV	J1190
ZIPRASIDONE MESYLATE	10 MG	IM	J3486
ZITHROMAX	1 G	ORAL	Q0144
ZITHROMAX	500 MG	IV	J0456
ZIV-AFLIBERCEPT	1 MG	IV	J9400
ZOFRAN	4 MG	ORAL	S0119
ZOFRAN	1 MG	IV	J2405
ZOFRAN	1 MG	ORAL	Q0162

Drug Name	Unit Per	Route	Code
ZOLADEX	3.6 MG	SC	J9202
ZOLEDRONIC ACID	1 MG	IV	J3489
ZOMETA	1 MG	IV	J3489
ZORBTIVE	1 MG	SC	J2941
ZORTRESS	0.25 MG	ORAL	J7527
ZOSYN	1 G/1.125 GM	IV	J2543
ZOVIRAX	5 MG	IV	J0133
ZUPLENZ	1 MG	ORAL	Q0162
ZUPLENZ	4 MG	ORAL	S0119
ZYPREXA	2.5 MG	IM	S0166
ZYPREXA RELPREVV	1 MG	IM	J2358
ZYVOX	200 MG	IV	J2020

NOT OTHERWISE CLASSIFIED DRUGS

Drug Name	Unit Per	Route	Code
ALFENTANIL	500 MCG	IV	J3490
ALLOPURINOL SODIUM	500 MG	IV	J3490
AMINOCAPROIC ACID	250 MG	IV	J3490
AZTREONAM	500 MG	IM, IV	J3490
AZTREONAM	500 MG	IV, IM	S0073
BUMETANIDE	0.25 MG	IM, IV	J3490
BUPIVACAINE, 0.25%	1 ML	OTH	J3490
BUPIVACAINE, 0.50%	1 ML	OTH	J3490
BUPIVACAINE, 0.75%	1 ML	OTH	J3490
CALCIUM CHLORIDE	100 MG	IV	J3490
CLAVULANTE POTASSIUM/TICARCILLIN DISODIUM	0.1-3 GM	IV	J3490
CLEVIDIPINE BUTYRATE	1 MG	IV	J3490
CLINDAMYCIN PHOSPHATE	150 MG	IV	J3490
COPPER SULFATE	0.4 MG	INJ	J3490

Drug Name	Unit Per	Route	Code
DILTIAZEM HCL	5 MG	IV	J3490
DOXAPRAM HCL	20 MG	IV	J3490
DOXYCYCLINE HYCLATE	100 MG	INJ	J3490
ENALAPRILAT	1.25 MG	IV	J3490
ESMOLOL HYDROCHLORIDE	10 MG	IV	J3490
ESOMEPRAZOLE SODIUM	20 MG	IV	J3490
ETOMIDATE	2 MG	IV	J3490
FAMOTIDINE	10 MG	IV	J3490
FLUMAZENIL	0.1 MG	IV	J3490
FOLIC ACID	5 MG	SC, IM, IV	J3490
FOSPROPOFOL DISODIUM	35 MG	IV	J3490
GLYCOPYRROLATE	0.2 MG	IM, IV	J3490
HEXAMINOLEVULINATE HCL	100 MG PER STUDY DOSE	IV	J3490
LABETALOL HCL	5 MG	INJ	J3490
METOPROLOL TARTRATE	1 MG	IV	J3490
METRONIDAZOLE INJ	500 MG	IV	J3490
MORRHUATE SODIUM	50 MG	OTH	J3490
NITROGLYCERIN	5 MG	IV	J3490
OLANZAPINE SHORT ACTING INTRAMUSCULAR INJECTION	0.5 MG	IM	J3490
PROPOFOL	10 MG	IV	J3490
RIFAMPIN	600 MG	IV	J3490
SODIUM ACETATE	2 MEQ	IV	J3490
SODIUM CHLORIDE, HYPERTONIC (3%-5% INFUSION)	250 CC	IV	J3490
SULFAMETHOXAZOLE-TRIMETHOPRIM	400-80 MG	IV	J3490
SURGIMEND	0.5 SQ CM	OTH	J3490
VASOPRESSIN	20 UNITS	SC, IM	J3490
VECURONIUM BROMIDE	1 MG	IV	J3490

APPENDIX 2 — MODIFIERS

A modifier is a two-position alpha or numeric code that is added to the end of a CPT code to clarify the services being billed. Modifiers provide a means by which a service can be altered without changing the procedure code. They add more information, such as the anatomical site, to the code. In addition, they help to eliminate the appearance of duplicate billing and unbundling. Modifiers are used to increase accuracy in reimbursement, coding consistency, editing, and to capture payment data.

A1	Dressing for one wound
A2	Dressing for 2 wounds
A3	Dressing for 3 wounds
A4	Dressing for 4 wounds
A5	Dressing for 5 wounds
A6	Dressing for 6 wounds
A7	Dressing for 7 wounds
A8	Dressing for 8 wounds
A9	Dressing for 9 or more wounds
AA	Anesthesia services performed personally by anesthesiologist
AD	Medical supervision by a physician: more than 4 concurrent anesthesia procedures
AE	Registered dietician
AF	Specialty physician
AG	Primary physician
AH	Clinical psychologist
AI	Principal physician of record
AJ	Clinical social worker
AK	Nonparticipating physician
AM	Physician, team member service
AO	Alternate payment method declined by provider of service
AP	Determination of refractive state was not performed in the course of diagnostic ophthalmological examination
AQ	Physician providing a service in an unlisted health professional shortage area (HPSA)
AR	Physician provider services in a physician scarcity area
AS	Physician assistant, nurse practitioner, or clinical nurse specialist services for assistant at surgery
AT	Acute treatment (this modifier should be used when reporting service 98940, 98941, 98942)
AU	Item furnished in conjunction with a urological, ostomy, or tracheostomy supply
AV	Item furnished in conjunction with a prosthetic device, prosthetic or orthotic
AW	Item furnished in conjunction with a surgical dressing
AX	Item furnished in conjunction with dialysis services
AY	Item or service furnished to an ESRD patient that is not for the treatment of ESRD
AZ	Physician providing a service in a dental health professional shortage area for the purpose of an electronic health record incentive payment
BA	Item furnished in conjunction with parenteral enteral nutrition (PEN) services
BL	Special acquisition of blood and blood products
BO	Orally administered nutrition, not by feeding tube
BP	The beneficiary has been informed of the purchase and rental options and has elected to purchase the item
BR	The beneficiary has been informed of the purchase and rental options and has elected to rent the item
BU	The beneficiary has been informed of the purchase and rental options and after 30 days has not informed the supplier of his/her decision
CA	Procedure payable only in the inpatient setting when performed emergently on an outpatient who expires prior to admission

CB	Service ordered by a renal dialysis facility (RDF) physician as part of the ESRD beneficiary's dialysis benefit, is not part of the composite rate, and is separately reimbursable
CC	Procedure code change (use CC when the procedure code submitted was changed either for administrative reasons or because an incorrect code was filed)
CD	AMCC test has been ordered by an ESRD facility or MCP physician that is part of the composite rate and is not separately billable
CE	AMCC test has been ordered by an ESRD facility or MCP physician that is a composite rate test but is beyond the normal frequency covered under the rate and is separately reimbursable based on medical necessity
CF	AMCC test has been ordered by an ESRD facility or MCP physician that is not part of the composite rate and is separately billable
CG	Policy criteria applied
CH	0 percent impaired, limited or restricted
CI	At least 1 percent but less than 20 percent impaired, limited or restricted
CJ	At least 20 percent but less than 40 percent impaired, limited or restricted
CK	At least 40 percent but less than 60 percent impaired, limited or restricted
CL	At least 60 percent but less than 80 percent impaired, limited or restricted
CM	At least 80 percent but less than 100 percent impaired, limited or restricted
CN	100 percent impaired, limited or restricted
CR	Catastrophe/Disaster related
CS	Item or service related, in whole or in part, to an illness, injury, or condition that was caused by or exacerbated by the effects, direct or indirect, of the 2010 oil spill in the gulf of Mexico, including but not limited to subsequent clean up activities
DA	Oral health assessment by a licensed health professional other than a dentist
E1	Upper left, eyelid
E2	Lower left, eyelid
E3	Upper right, eyelid
E4	Lower right, eyelid
EA	Erythropoetic stimulating agent (ESA) administered to treat anemia due to anticancer chemotherapy
EB	Erythropoetic stimulating agent (ESA) administered to treat anemia due to anticancer radiotherapy
EC	Erythropoetic stimulating agent (ESA) administered to treat anemia not due to anticancer radiotherapy or anticancer chemotherapy
ED	Hematocrit level has exceeded 39% (or hemoglobin level has exceeded 13.0 G/dl) for 3 or more consecutive billing cycles immediately prior to and including the current cycle
EE	Hematocrit level has not exceeded 39% (or hemoglobin level has not exceeded 13.0 G/dl) for 3 or more consecutive billing cycles immediately prior to and including the current cycle
EJ	Subsequent claims for a defined course of therapy, e.g., EPO, sodium hyaluronate, infliximab
EM	Emergency reserve supply (for ESRD benefit only)
EP	Service provided as part of Medicaid early periodic screening diagnosis and treatment (EPSDT) program
ET	Emergency services
EY	No physician or other licensed health care provider order for this item or service
F1	Left hand, 2nd digit
F2	Left hand, third digit
F3	Left hand, 4th digit
F4	Left hand, fifth digit
F5	Right hand, thumb
F6	Right hand, 2nd digit

F7	Right hand, third digit	GX	Notice of liability issued, voluntary under payer policy
F8	Right hand, 4th digit	GY	Item or service statutorily excluded, does not meet the definition of any Medicare benefit or for non-Medicare insurers, is not a contract benefit
F9	Right hand, 5th digit		
FA	Left hand, thumb	GZ	Item or service expected to be denied as not reasonable and necessary
FB	Item provided without cost to provider, supplier or practitioner, or full credit received for replaced device (examples, but not limited to, covered under warranty, replaced due to defect, free samples)	H9	Court-ordered
		HA	Child/adolescent program
FC	Partial credit received for replaced device	HB	Adult program, nongeriatric
FP	Service provided as part of family planning program	HC	Adult program, geriatric
G1	Most recent URR reading of less than 60	HD	Pregnant/parenting women's program
G2	Most recent URR reading of 60 to 64.9	HE	Mental health program
G3	Most recent URR reading of 65 to 69.9	HF	Substance abuse program
G4	Most recent URR reading of 70 to 74.9	HG	Opioid addiction treatment program
G5	Most recent URR reading of 75 or greater	HH	Integrated mental health/substance abuse program
G6	ESRD patient for whom less than 6 dialysis sessions have been provided in a month	HI	Integrated mental health and intellectual disability/developmental disabilities program
G7	Pregnancy resulted from rape or incest or pregnancy certified by physician as life threatening	HJ	Employee assistance program
G8	Monitored anesthesia care (MAC) for deep complex, complicated, or markedly invasive surgical procedure	HK	Specialized mental health programs for high-risk populations
		HL	Intern
G9	Monitored anesthesia care for patient who has history of severe cardiopulmonary condition	HM	Less than bachelor degree level
		HN	Bachelors degree level
GA	Waiver of liability statement issued as required by payer policy, individual case	HO	Masters degree level
		HP	Doctoral level
GB	Claim being resubmitted for payment because it is no longer covered under a global payment demonstration	HQ	Group setting
		HR	Family/couple with client present
GC	This service has been performed in part by a resident under the direction of a teaching physician	HS	Family/couple without client present
		HT	Multi-disciplinary team
GD	Units of service exceeds medically unlikely edit value and represents reasonable and necessary services	HU	Funded by child welfare agency
		HV	Funded state addictions agency
GE	This service has been performed by a resident without the presence of a teaching physician under the primary care exception	HW	Funded by state mental health agency
		HX	Funded by county/local agency
GF	Nonphysician (e.g., nurse practitioner (NP), certified registered nurse anesthetist (CRNA), certified registered nurse (CRN), clinical nurse specialist (CNS), physician assistant (PA)) services in a critical access hospital	HY	Funded by juvenile justice agency
		HZ	Funded by criminal justice agency
		J1	Competitive acquisition program no-pay submission for a prescription number
GG	Performance and payment of a screening mammogram and diagnostic mammogram on the same patient, same day	J2	Competitive acquisition program, restocking of emergency drugs after emergency administration
GH	Diagnostic mammogram converted from screening mammogram on same day	J3	Competitive acquisition program (CAP), drug not available through CAP as written, reimbursed under average sales price methodology
GJ	"Opt out" physician or practitioner emergency or urgent service		
GK	Reasonable and necessary item/service associated with GA or GZ modifier	J4	DMEPOS item subject to DMEPOS competitive bidding program that is furnished by a hospital upon discharge
GL	Medically unnecessary upgrade provided instead of nonupgraded item, no charge, no advance beneficiary notice (ABN)	JA	Administered intravenously
		JB	Administered subcutaneously
GM	Multiple patients on one ambulance trip	JC	Skin substitute used as a graft
GN	Services delivered under an outpatient speech language pathology plan of care	JD	Skin substitute not used as a graft
		JE	Administered via dialysate
GO	Services delivered under an outpatient occupational therapy plan of care	JW	Drug amount discarded/not administered to any patient
GP	Services delivered under an outpatient physical therapy plan of care	K0	Lower extremity prosthesis functional level 0-does not have the ability or potential to ambulate or transfer safely with or without assistance and a prosthesis does not enhance their quality of life or mobility
GQ	Via asynchronous telecommunications system		
GR	This service was performed in whole or in part by a resident in a department of veterans affairs medical center or clinic, supervised in accordance with VA policy	K1	Lower extremity prosthesis functional level 1 - has the ability or potential to use a prosthesis for transfers or ambulation on level surfaces at fixed cadence, typical of the limited and unlimited household ambulator.
GS	Dosage of erythropoietin stimulating agent has been reduced and maintained in response to hematocrit or hemoglobin level		
GT	Via interactive audio and video telecommunication systems	K2	Lower extremity prosthesis functional level 2 - has the ability or potential for ambulation with the ability to traverse low level environmental barriers such as curbs, stairs or uneven surfaces. typical of the limited community ambulator.
GU	Waiver of liability statement issued as required by payer policy, routine notice		
GV	Attending physician not employed or paid under arrangement by the patient's hospice provider		
GW	Service not related to the hospice patient's terminal condition		

K3	Lower extremity prosthesis functional level 3-has the ability or potential for ambulation with variable cadence, typical of the community ambulator who has the ability to traverse most environmental barriers and may have vocational, therapeutic, or exercise activity that demands prosthetic utilization beyond simple locomotion
K4	Lower extremity prosthesis functional level 4 - has the ability or potential for prosthetic ambulation that exceeds the basic ambulation skills, exhibiting high impact, stress, or energy levels, typical of the prosthetic demands of the child, active adult, or athlete.
KA	Add on option/accessory for wheelchair
KB	Beneficiary requested upgrade for ABN, more than 4 modifiers identified on claim
KC	Replacement of special power wheelchair interface
KD	Drug or biological infused through DME
KE	Bid under round one of the DMEPOS competitive bidding program for use with noncompetitive bid base equipment
KF	Item designated by FDA as class III device
KG	DMEPOS item subject to DMEPOS competitive bidding program number 1
KH	DMEPOS item, initial claim, purchase or first month rental
KI	DMEPOS item, 2nd or 3rd month rental
KJ	DMEPOS item, parenteral enteral nutrition (PEN) pump or capped rental, months 4 to 15
KK	DMEPOS item subject to DMEPOS competitive bidding program number 2
KL	DMEPOS item delivered via mail
KM	Replacement of facial prosthesis including new impression/moulage
KN	Replacement of facial prosthesis using previous master model
K0	Single drug unit dose formulation
KP	First drug of a multiple drug unit dose formulation
KQ	Second or subsequent drug of a multiple drug unit dose formulation
KR	Rental item, billing for partial month
KS	Glucose monitor supply for diabetic beneficiary not treated with insulin
KT	Beneficiary resides in a competitive bidding area and travels outside that competitive bidding area and receives a competitive bid item.
KU	DMEPOS item subject to DMEPOS competitive bidding program number 3
KV	DMEPOS item subject to DMEPOS competitive bidding program that is furnished as part of a professional service
KW	DMEPOS item subject to DMEPOS competitive bidding program number 4
KX	Requirements specified in the medical policy have been met
KY	DMEPOS item subject to DMEPOS competitive bidding program number 5
KZ	New coverage not implemented by managed care
LC	Left circumflex coronary artery
LD	Left anterior descending coronary artery
LL	Lease/rental (use the LL modifier when DME equipment rental is to be applied against the purchase price)
LM	Left main coronary artery
LR	Laboratory round trip
LS	FDA-monitored intraocular lens implant
LT	Left side (used to identify procedures performed on the left side of the body)
M2	Medicare secondary payer (MSP)
MS	Six month maintenance and servicing fee for reasonable and necessary parts and labor which are not covered under any manufacturer or supplier warranty
NB	Nebulizer system, any type, FDA-cleared for use with specific drug
NR	New when rented (use the NR modifier when DME which was new at the time of rental is subsequently purchased)
NU	New equipment
P1	A normal healthy patient
P2	A patient with mild systemic disease
P3	A patient with severe systemic disease
P4	A patient with severe systemic disease that is a constant threat to life
P5	A moribund patient who is not expected to survive without the operation
P6	A declared brain-dead patient whose organs are being removed for donor purposes
PA	Surgical or other invasive procedure on wrong body part
PB	Surgical or other invasive procedure on wrong patient
PC	Wrong surgery or other invasive procedure on patient
PD	Diagnostic or related non diagnostic item or service provided in a wholly owned or operated entity to a patient who is admitted as an inpatient within 3 days
PI	Positron emission tomography (PET) or PET/computed tomography (CT) to inform the initial treatment strategy of tumors that are biopsy proven or strongly suspected of being cancerous based on other diagnostic testing
PL	Progressive addition lenses
PM	Post mortem
PS	Positron emission tomography (PET) or PET/computed tomography (CT) to inform the subsequent treatment strategy of cancerous tumors when the beneficiary's treating physician determines that the PET study is needed to inform subsequent anti-tumor strategy
PT	Colorectal cancer screening test; converted to diagnostic test or other procedure
Q0	Investigational clinical service provided in a clinical research study that is in an approved clinical research study
Q1	Routine clinical service provided in a clinical research study that is in an approved clinical research study
Q2	HCFA/ORD demonstration project procedure/service
Q3	Live kidney donor surgery and related services
Q4	Service for ordering/referring physician qualifies as a service exemption
Q5	Service furnished by a substitute physician under a reciprocal billing arrangement
Q6	Service furnished by a locum tenens physician
Q7	One Class A finding
Q8	Two Class B findings
Q9	One class B and 2 class C findings
QC	Single channel monitoring
QD	Recording and storage in solid state memory by a digital recorder
QE	Prescribed amount of oxygen is less than 1 liter per minute (LPM)
QF	Prescribed amount of oxygen exceeds 4 liters per minute (LPM) and portable oxygen is prescribed
QG	Prescribed amount of oxygen is greater than 4 liters per minute (LPM)
QH	Oxygen conserving device is being used with an oxygen delivery system
QJ	Services/items provided to a prisoner or patient in state or local custody, however the state or local government, as applicable, meets the requirements in 42 CFR 411.4(B)
QK	Medical direction of 2, 3, or 4 concurrent anesthesia procedures involving qualified individuals
QL	Patient pronounced dead after ambulance called
QM	Ambulance service provided under arrangement by a provider of services
QN	Ambulance service furnished directly by a provider of services

QP	Documentation is on file showing that the laboratory test(s) was ordered individually or ordered as a CPT-recognized panel other than automated profile codes 80002-80019, G0058, G0059, and G0060
QS	Monitored anesthesia care service
QT	Recording and storage on tape by an analog tape recorder
QW	CLIA waived test
QX	CRNA service: with medical direction by a physician
QY	Medical direction of one certified registered nurse anesthetist (CRNA) by an anesthesiologist
QZ	CRNA service: without medical direction by a physician
RA	Replacement of a DME, orthotic or prosthetic item
RB	Replacement of a part of a DME, orthotic or prosthetic item furnished as part of a repair
RC	Right coronary artery
RD	Drug provided to beneficiary, but not administered "incident-to"
RE	Furnished in full compliance with FDA-mandated risk evaluation and mitigation strategy (REMS)
RI	Ramus intermedius coronary artery
RR	Rental (use the RR modifier when DME is to be rented)
RT	Right side (used to identify procedures performed on the right side of the body)
SA	Nurse practitioner rendering service in collaboration with a physician
SB	Nurse midwife
SC	Medically necessary service or supply
SD	Services provided by registered nurse with specialized, highly technical home infusion training
SE	State and/or federally-funded programs/services
SF	Second opinion ordered by a professional review organization (PRO) per section 9401, p.l. 99-272 (100% reimbursement - no Medicare deductible or coinsurance)
SG	Ambulatory surgical center (ASC) facility service
SH	Second concurrently administered infusion therapy
SJ	Third or more concurrently administered infusion therapy
SK	Member of high risk population (use only with codes for immunization)
SL	State supplied vaccine
SM	Second surgical opinion
SN	Third surgical opinion
SQ	Item ordered by home health
SS	Home infusion services provided in the infusion suite of the IV therapy provider
ST	Related to trauma or injury
SU	Procedure performed in physician's office (to denote use of facility and equipment)
SV	Pharmaceuticals delivered to patient's home but not utilized
SW	Services provided by a certified diabetic educator
SY	Persons who are in close contact with member of high-risk population (use only with codes for immunization)
T1	Left foot, 2nd digit
T2	Left foot, 3rd digit
T3	Left foot, 4th digit
T4	Left foot, 5th digit
T5	Right foot, great toe
T6	Right foot, 2nd digit
T7	Right foot, 3rd digit
T8	Right foot, 4th digit
T9	Right foot, 5th digit

TA	Left foot, great toe
TC	Technical component. Under certain circumstances, a charge may be made for the technical component alone. Under those circumstances the technical component charge is identified by adding modifier 'TC' to the usual procedure number. Technical component charges are institutional charges and not billed separately by physicians. However, portable x-ray suppliers only bill for technical component and should utilize modifier TC. The charge data from portable x-ray suppliers will then be used to build customary and prevailing profiles.
TD	RN
TE	LPN/LVN
TF	Intermediate level of care
TG	Complex/high tech level of care
TH	Obstetrical treatment/services, prenatal or postpartum
TJ	Program group, child and/or adolescent
TK	Extra patient or passenger, nonambulance
TL	Early intervention/individualized family service plan (IFSP)
TM	Individualized education program (IEP)
TN	Rural/outside providers' customary service area
TP	Medical transport, unloaded vehicle
TQ	Basic life support transport by a volunteer ambulance provider
TR	School-based individualized education program (IEP) services provided outside the public school district responsible for the student
TS	Follow-up service
TT	Individualized service provided to more than one patient in same setting
TU	Special payment rate, overtime
TV	Special payment rates, holidays/weekends
TW	Back-up equipment
U1	Medicaid level of care 1, as defined by each state
U2	Medicaid level of care 2, as defined by each state
U3	Medicaid level of care 3, as defined by each state
U4	Medicaid level of care 4, as defined by each state
U5	Medicaid level of care 5, as defined by each state
U6	Medicaid level of care 6, as defined by each state
U7	Medicaid level of care 7, as defined by each state
U8	Medicaid level of care 8, as defined by each state
U9	Medicaid level of care 9, as defined by each state
UA	Medicaid level of care 10, as defined by each state
UB	Medicaid level of care 11, as defined by each state
UC	Medicaid level of care 12, as defined by each state
UD	Medicaid level of care 13, as defined by each state
UE	Used durable medical equipment
UF	Services provided in the morning
UG	Services provided in the afternoon
UH	Services provided in the evening
UJ	Services provided at night
UK	Services provided on behalf of the client to someone other than the client (collateral relationship)
UN	2 patients served
UP	3 patients served
UQ	4 patients served
UR	5 patients served
US	6 or more patients served
V5	Vascular catheter (alone or with any other vascular access)

V6   Arteriovenous graft (or other vascular access not including a vascular catheter)

V7   Arteriovenous fistula only (in use with 2 needles)

VP   Aphakic patient

APPENDIX 3 — ABBREVIATIONS AND ACRONYMS

HCPCS Abbreviations and Acronyms

The following abbreviations and acronyms are used in the HCPCS descriptions:

/	or
<	less than
<=	less than equal to
>	greater than
>=	greater than equal to
AC	alternating current
AFO	ankle-foot orthosis
AICC	anti-inhibitor coagulant complex
AK	above the knee
AKA	above knee amputation
ALS	advanced life support
AMP	ampule
ART	artery
ART	Arterial
ASC	ambulatory surgery center
ATT	attached
A-V	Arteriovenous
AVF	arteriovenous fistula
BICROS	bilateral routing of signals
BK	below the knee
BLS	basic life support
BMI	body mass index
BP	blood pressure
BTE	behind the ear (hearing aid)
CAPD	continuous ambulatory peritoneal dialysis
Carb	carbohydrate
CBC	complete blood count
cc	cubic centimeter
CCPD	continuous cycling peritoneal analysis
CHF	congestive heart failure
CIC	completely in the canal (hearing aid)
CIM	Coverage Issue Manual
Clsd	closed
cm	centimeter
CMN	certificate of medical necessity
CMS	Centers for Medicare and Medicaid Services
CMV	Cytomegalovirus
Conc	concentrate
Conc	concentrated
Cont	continuous
CP	clinical psychologist
CPAP	continuous positive airway pressure
CPT	Current Procedural Terminology
CRF	chronic renal failure
CRNA	certified registered nurse anesthetist
CROS	contralateral routing of signals
CSW	clinical social worker
CT	computed tomography
CTLSO	cervical-thoracic-lumbar-sacral orthosis
cu	cubic
DC	direct current
DI	diurnal rhythm
Dx	diagnosis
DLI	donor leukocyte infusion
DME	durable medical equipment
DME MAC	durable medical equipment Medicare administrative contractor

DMEPOS	durable medical equipment, prosthestics, orthotics and other supplies
DMERC	durable medical equipment regional carrier
DR	diagnostic radiology
DX	diagnostic
e.g.	for example
Ea	each
ECF	extended care facility
EEG	electroencephalogram
EKG	electrocardiogram
EMG	electromyography
EO	elbow orthosis
EP	electrophysiologic
EPO	epoetin alfa
EPSDT	early periodic screening, diagnosis and treatment
ESRD	end-stage renal disease
Ex	extended
Exper	experimental
Ext	external
F	french
FDA	Food and Drug Administration
FDG-PET	Positron emission with tomography with 18 fluorodeoxyglucose
Fem	female
FO	finger orthosis
FPD	fixed partial denture
Fr	french
ft	foot
G-CSF	filgrastim (granulocyte colony-stimulating factor)
gm	gram (g)
H2O	water
HCl	hydrochloric acid, hydrochloride
HCPCS	Healthcare Common Procedural Coding System
HCT	hematocrit
HFO	hand-finger orthosis
HHA	home health agency
HI	high
HI-LO	high-low
HIT	home infusion therapy
HKAFO	hip-knee-ankle foot orthosis
HLA	human leukocyte antigen
HMES	heat and moisture exchange system
HNPCC	hereditary non-polyposis colorectal cancer
HO	hip orthosis
HPSA	health professional shortage area
HST	home sleep test
IA	intra-arterial administration
ip	interphalangeal
I-131	Iodine 131
ICF	intermediate care facility
ICU	intensive care unit
IM	intramuscular
in	inch
INF	infusion
INH	inhalation solution
INJ	injection
IOL	intraocular lens
IPD	intermittent peritoneal dialysis
IPPB	intermittent positive pressure breathing
IT	intrathecal administration
ITC	in the canal (hearing aid)
ITE	in the ear (hearing aid)
IU	international units

IV	intravenous		PHP	physician hospital plan
IVF	in vitro fertilization		PI	paramedic intercept
KAFO	knee-ankle-foot orthosis		PICC	peripherally inserted central venous catheter
KO	knee orthosis		PKR	photorefractive keratotomy
KOH	potassium hydroxide		Pow	powder
L	left		PQRS	Physician Quality Reporting System
LASIK	laser in situ keratomileusis		PRK	photoreactive keratectomy
LAUP	laser assisted uvulopalatoplasty		PRO	peer review organization
lbs	pounds		PSA	prostate specific antigen
LDL	low density lipoprotein		PTB	patellar tendon bearing
LDS	lipodystrophy syndrome		PTK	phototherapeutic keratectomy
Lo	low		PVC	polyvinyl chloride
LPM	liters per minute		R	right
LPN/LVN	Licensed Practical Nurse/Licensed Vocational Nurse		Repl	replace
LSO	lumbar-sacral orthosis		RN	registered nurse
MAC	Medicare administrative contractor		RP	retrograde pyelogram
mp	metacarpophalangeal		Rx	prescription
mcg	microgram		SACH	solid ankle, cushion heel
mCi	millicurie		SC	subcutaneous
MCM	Medicare Carriers Manual		SCT	specialty care transport
MCP	metacarparpophalangeal joint		SEO	shoulder-elbow orthosis
MCP	monthly capitation payment		SEWHO	shoulder-elbow-wrist-hand orthosis
mEq	milliequivalent		SEXA	single energy x-ray absorptiometry
MESA	microsurgical epididymal sperm aspiration		SGD	speech generating device
mg	milligram		SGD	sinus rhythm
mgs	milligrams		SM	samarium
MHT	megahertz		SNCT	sensory nerve conduction test
ml	milliliter		SNF	skilled nursing facility
mm	millimeter		SO	sacroilliac othrosis
mmHg	millimeters of Mercury		SO	shoulder orthosis
MRA	magnetic resonance angiography		Sol	solution
MRI	magnetic resonance imaging		SQ	square
NA	sodium		SR	screen
NCI	National Cancer Institute		ST	standard
NEC	not elsewhere classified		ST	sustained release
NG	nasogastric		Syr	syrup
NH	nursing home		TABS	tablets
NMES	neuromuscular electrical stimulation		Tc	technetium
NOC	not otherwise classified		Tc 99m	technetium isotope
NOS	not otherwise specified		TENS	transcutaneous electrical nerve stimulator
O2	oxygen		THKAO	thoracic-hip-knee-ankle orthosis
OBRA	Omnibus Budget Reconciliation Act		TLSO	thoracic-lumbar-sacral-orthosis
OMT	osteopathic manipulation therapy		TM	temporomandibular
OPPS	outpatient prospective payment system		TMJ	temporomandibular joint
ORAL	oral administration		TPN	total parenteral nutrition
OSA	obstructive sleep apnea		U	unit
Ost	ostomy		uCi	microcurie
OTH	other routes of administration		VAR	various routes of administration
oz	ounce		w	with
PA	physician's assistant		w/	with
PAR	parenteral		w/o	without
PCA	patient controlled analgesia		WAK	wearable artificial kidney
PCH	pouch		wc	wheelchair
PEN	parenteral and enteral nutrition		WHFO	wrist-hand-finger orthotic
PENS	percutaneous electrical nerve stimulation		Wk	week
PET	positron emission tomography		w/o	without
PHP	pre-paid health plan		Xe	xenon (isotope mass of xenon 133)

APPENDIX 4 — PUB 100 REFERENCES

The Centers for Medicare and Medicaid Services restructured its paper-based manual system as a web-based system on October 1, 2003. Called the online CMS manual system, it combines all of the various program instructions into internet-only manuals (IOMs), which are used by all CMS programs and contractors. In many instances, the references from the online manuals in appendix E contain a mention of the old paper manuals from which the current information was obtained when the manuals were converted. This information is shown in the header of the text, in the following format, when applicable, as A3-3101, HO-210, and B3-2049. Complete versions of all of the manuals can be found at http://www.cms.gov/manuals.

Effective with implementation of the IOMs, the former method of publishing program memoranda (PMs) to communicate program instructions was replaced by the following four templates:

- One-time notification
- Manual revisions
- Business requirements
- Confidential requirements

The web-based system has been organized by functional area (e.g., eligibility, entitlement, claims processing, benefit policy, program integrity) in an effort to eliminate redundancy within the manuals, simplify updating, and make CMS program instructions available more quickly. The web-based system contains the functional areas included below:

Pub. 100	Introduction
Pub. 100-1	Medicare General Information, Eligibility, and Entitlement Manual
Pub. 100-2	Medicare Benefit Policy Manual
Pub. 100-3	Medicare National Coverage Determinations (NCD) Manual
Pub. 100-4	Medicare Claims Processing Manual
Pub. 100-5	Medicare Secondary Payer Manual
Pub. 100-6	Medicare Financial Management Manual
Pub. 100-7	State Operations Manual
Pub. 100-8	Medicare Program Integrity Manual
Pub. 100-9	Medicare Contractor Beneficiary and Provider Communications Manual
Pub. 100-10	Quality Improvement Organization Manual
Pub. 100-11	Programs of All-Inclusive Care for the Elderly (PACE) Manual
Pub. 100-12	State Medicaid Manual (under development)
Pub. 100-13	Medicaid State Children's Health Insurance Program (under development)
Pub. 100-14	Medicare ESRD Network Organizations Manual
Pub. 100-15	Medicaid Integrity Program (MIP)
Pub. 100-16	Medicare Managed Care Manual
Pub. 100-17	CMS/Business Partners Systems Security Manual
Pub. 100-18	Medicare Prescription Drug Benefit Manual
Pub. 100-19	Demonstrations
Pub. 100-20	One-Time Notification
Pub. 100-21	Recurring Update Notification
Pub. 100-22	Medicare Quality Reporting Incentive Programs Manual
Pub. 100-24	State Buy-In Manual
Pub. 100-25	Information Security Acceptable Risk Safeguards Manual

A brief description of the Medicare manuals primarily used for *CPC Expert* follows:

The *National Coverage Determinations Manual* (NCD), is organized according to categories such as diagnostic services, supplies, and medical procedures. The table of contents lists each category and subject within that category. Revision transmittals identify any new or background material, recap the changes, and provide an effective date for the change.

When complete, the manual will contain two chapters. Chapter 1 currently includes a description of CMS's national coverage determinations. When available, chapter 2 will contain a list of HCPCS codes related to each coverage determination. The manual is organized in accordance with CPT category sequences.

The *Medicare Benefit Policy Manual* contains Medicare general coverage instructions that are not national coverage determinations. As a general rule, in the past these instructions have been found in chapter II of the *Medicare*

Carriers Manual, the *Medicare Intermediary Manual*, other provider manuals, and program memoranda.

The *Medicare Claims Processing Manual* contains instructions for processing claims for contractors and providers.

The *Medicare Program Integrity Manual* communicates the priorities and standards for the Medicare integrity programs.

100-1, 1, 10.1

Hospital Insurance (Part A) for Inpatient Hospital, Hospice, Home Health and Skilled Nursing Facility (SNF) Services - A Brief Description

Hospital insurance is designed to help patients defray the expenses incurred by hospitalization and related care. In addition to inpatient hospital benefits, hospital insurance covers post hospital extended care in SNFs and post hospital care furnished by a home health agency in the patient's home. Blood clotting factors, for hemophilia patients competent to use such factors to control bleeding without medical or other supervision, and items related to the administration of such factors, are also a Part A benefit for beneficiaries in a covered Part A stay. The purpose of these additional benefits is to provide continued treatment after hospitalization and to encourage the appropriate use of more economical alternatives to inpatient hospital care. Program payments for services rendered to beneficiaries by providers (i.e., hospitals, SNFs, and home health agencies) are generally made to the provider. In each benefit period, payment may be made for up to 90 inpatient hospital days, and 100 days of post hospital extended care services .Hospices also provide Part A hospital insurance services such as short-term inpatient care. In order to be eligible to elect hospice care under Medicare, an individual must be entitled to Part A of Medicare and be certified as being terminally ill. An individual is considered to be terminally ill if the individual has a medical prognosis that his or her life expectancy is 6 months or less if the illness runs its normal course.

100-1, 3, 20.5

Blood Deductibles (Part A and Part B)

Program payment may not be made for the first 3 pints of whole blood or equivalent units of packed red cells received under Part A and Part B combined in a calendar year. However, blood processing (e.g., administration, storage) is not subject to the deductible.

The blood deductibles are in addition to any other applicable deductible and coinsurance amounts for which the patient is responsible.

The deductible applies only to the first 3 pints of blood furnished in a calendar year, even if more than one provider furnished blood.

100-1, 3, 20.5.2

Part B Blood Deductible

Blood is furnished on an outpatient basis or is subject to the Part B blood deductible and is counted toward the combined limit. It should be noted that payment for blood may be made to the hospital under Part B only for blood furnished in an outpatient setting. Blood is not covered for inpatient Part B services.

100-1, 3, 20.5.3

Items Subject to Blood Deductibles

The blood deductibles apply only to whole blood and packed red cells. The term whole blood means human blood from which none of the liquid or cellular components have been removed. Where packed red cells are furnished, a unit of packed red cells is considered equivalent to a pint of whole blood. Other components of blood such as platelets, fibrinogen, plasma, gamma globulin, and serum albumin are not subject to the blood deductible. However, these components of blood are covered as biologicals.

Refer to Pub. 100-04, Medicare Claims Processing Manual, chapter 4, Sec.231 regarding billing for blood and blood products under the Hospital Outpatient Prospective Payment System (OPPS).

100-1, 3, 30

Outpatient Mental Health Treatment Limitation

Regardless of the actual expenses a beneficiary incurs in connection with the treatment of mental, psychoneurotic, and personality disorders while the beneficiary is not an inpatient of a hospital at the time such expenses are incurred, the amount of those expenses that may be recognized for Part B deductible and payment purposes is limited to 62.5 percent of the Medicare approved amount for those services. The limitation is called the outpatient mental health treatment limitation (the limitation). The 62.5 percent limitation has been in place since the inception of the Medicare Part B program and it will remain effective at this percentage amount until January 1, 2010. However, effective January 1, 2010, through January 1, 2014, the limitation will be phased out as follows:

- January 1, 2010–December 31, 2011, the limitation percentage is 68.75%. (Medicare pays 55% and the patient pays 45%).

- January 1, 2012–December 31, 2012, the limitation percentage is 75%. (Medicare pays 60% and the patient pays 40%).

- January 1, 2013–December 31, 2013, the limitation percentage is 81.25%. (Medicare pays 65% and the patient pays 35%).

- January 1, 2014–onward, the limitation percentage is 100%. (Medicare pays 80% and the patient pays 20%).

For additional details concerning the outpatient mental health treatment limitation, please see the Medicare Claims Processing Manual, Publication 100-04, chapter 9, section 60 and chapter 12, section 210.

100-1, 3, 30.1

Outpatient Mental Health Treatment Limitation

Regardless of the actual expenses a beneficiary incurs for treatment of mental, psychoneurotic, and personality disorders while the beneficiary is not an inpatient of a hospital at the time such expenses are incurred, the amount of those expenses that may be recognized for Part B deductible and payment purposes is limited to 62.5 percent of the Medicare allowed amount for these services. The limitation is called the outpatient mental health treatment limitation. Since Part B deductible also applies the program pays for about half of the allowed amount recognized for mental health therapy services.

Expenses for diagnostic services (e.g., psychiatric testing and evaluation to diagnose the patient's illness) are not subject to this limitation. This limitation applies only to therapeutic services and to services performed to evaluate the progress of a course of treatment for a diagnosed condition.

100-1, 3, 30.1

Disorders Subject to Mental Health Limitation

The term "mental, psychoneurotic, and personality disorders" is defined as the specific psychiatric conditions described in the American Psychiatric Association's Diagnostic and Statistical Manual of Mental Disorders, Third Edition - Revised (DSM-III-R).

If the treatment services rendered are for both a psychiatric condition and one or more nonpsychiatric conditions, the charges are separated to apply the limitation only to the mental health charge. Normally HCPCS code and diagnoses are used. Where HCPCS code is not available on the claim, revenue code is used.

If the service is primarily on the basis of a diagnosis of Alzheimer's Disease (coded 331.0 in the International Classification of Diseases, 9th Revision) or Alzheimer's or other disorders (coded 290.XX in DSM-III-R), treatment typically represents medical management of the patient's condition (rather than psychiatric treatment) and is not subject to the limitation.

100-1, 3, 30.3

Diagnostic Services

The mental health limitation does not apply to tests and evaluations performed to establish or confirm the patient's diagnosis. Diagnostic services include psychiatric or psychological tests and interpretations, diagnostic consultations, and initial evaluations. However, testing services performed to evaluate a patient's progress during treatment are considered part of treatment and are subject to the limitation.

100-1, 5, 90.2

Laboratory Defined

Laboratory means a facility for the biological, microbiological, serological, chemical, immuno-hematological, hematological, biophysical, cytological, pathological, or other examination of materials derived from the human body for the purpose of providing information for the diagnosis, prevention, or treatment of any disease or impairment of, or the assessment of the health of, human beings. These examinations also include procedures to determine, measure, or otherwise describe the presence or absence of various substances or organisms in the body. Facilities only collecting or preparing specimens (or both) or only serving as a mailing service and not performing testing are not considered laboratories.

100-2, 1, 10

Covered Inpatient Hospital Services Covered Under Part A
A3-3101, HO-210

Patients covered under hospital insurance are entitled to have payment made on their behalf for inpatient hospital services. (Inpatient hospital services do not include extended care services provided by hospitals pursuant to swing bed approvals. See Pub. 100-1, Chapter 8, Sec.10.1, "Hospital Providers of Extended Care Services."). However, both inpatient hospital and inpatient SNF benefits are provided under Part A - Hospital Insurance Benefits for the Aged and Disabled, of Title XVIII).

Additional information concerning the following topics can be found in the following manual chapters:

- Benefit periods is found in Chapter 3, "Duration of Covered Inpatient Services";

- Copayment days is found in Chapter 2, "Duration of Covered Inpatient Services";

- Lifetime reserve days is found in Chapter 5, "Lifetime Reserve Days";

- Related payment information is housed in the Provider Reimbursement Manual.

Blood must be furnished on a day which counts as a day of inpatient hospital services to be covered as a Part A service and to count toward the blood deductible. Thus, blood is not covered under Part A and does not count toward the Part A blood deductible when furnished to an inpatient after the inpatient has exhausted all benefit days in a benefit period, or where the individual has elected not to use lifetime reserve days. However, where the patient is discharged on their first day of entitlement or on the hospital's first day of participation, the hospital is permitted to submit a billing form with no accommodation charge, but with ancillary charges including blood.

The records for all Medicare hospital inpatient discharges are maintained in CMS for statistical analysis and use in determining future PPS DRG classifications and rates.

Non-PPS hospitals do not pay for noncovered services generally excluded from coverage in the Medicare Program. This may result in denial of a part of the billed charges or in denial of the entire admission, depending upon circumstance. In PPS hospitals, the following are also possible:

1. In appropriately admitted cases where a noncovered procedure was performed, denied services may result in payment of a different DRG (i.e., one which excludes payment for the noncovered procedure); or

2. In appropriately admitted cases that become cost outlier cases, denied services may lead to denial of some or all of an outlier payment.

The following examples illustrate this principle. If care is noncovered because a patient does not need to be hospitalized, the intermediary denies the admission and makes no Part A (i.e., PPS) payment unless paid under limitation on liability. Under limitation on liability, Medicare payment may be made when the provider and the beneficiary were not aware the services were not necessary and could not reasonably be expected to know that he services were not necessary. For detailed instructions, see the Medicare Claims Processing Manual, Chapter 30,"Limitation on Liability." If a patient is appropriately hospitalized but receives (beyond routine services) only noncovered care, the admission is denied.

NOTE: The intermediary does not deny an admission that includes covered care, even if noncovered care was also rendered. Under PPS, Medicare assumes that it is paying for only the covered care rendered whenever covered services needed to treat and/or diagnose the illness were in fact provided.

If a noncovered procedure is provided along with covered nonroutine care, a DRG change rather than an admission denial might occur. If noncovered procedures are elevating costs into the cost outlier category, outlier payment is denied in whole or in part.

When the hospital is included in PPS, most of the subsequent discussion regarding coverage of inpatient hospital services is relevant only in the context of determining the appropriateness of admissions, which DRG, if any, to pay, and the appropriateness of payment for any outlier cases.

If a patient receives items or services in excess of, or more expensive than, those for which payment can be made, payment is made only for the covered items or services or for only the appropriate prospective payment amount. This provision applies not only to inpatient services, but also to all hospital services under Parts A and B of the program. If the items or services were requested by the patient, the hospital may charge him the difference between the amount customarily charged for the services requested and the amount customarily charged for covered services.

An inpatient is a person who has been admitted to a hospital for bed occupancy for purposes of receiving inpatient hospital services. Generally, a patient is considered an inpatient if formally admitted as inpatient with the expectation that he or she will remain at least overnight and occupy a bed even though it later develops that the patient can be discharged or transferred to another hospital and not actually use a hospital bed overnight.

The physician or other practitioner responsible for a patient's care at the hospital is also responsible for deciding whether the patient should be admitted as an inpatient. Physicians should use a 24-hour period as a benchmark, i.e., they should order admission for patients who are expected to need hospital care for 24 hours or more, and treat other patients on an outpatient basis. However, the decision to admit a patient is a complex medical judgment which can be made only after the physician has considered a number of factors, including the patient's medical history and current medical needs, the types of facilities available to inpatients and to outpatients, the hospital's by-laws and admissions policies, and the relative appropriateness of treatment in each setting. Factors to be considered when making the decision to admit include such things as:

The severity of the signs and symptoms exhibited by the patient;

The medical predictability of something adverse happening to the patient;

The need for diagnostic studies that appropriately are outpatient services (i.e., their performance does not ordinarily require the patient to remain at the hospital for 24 hours or more) to assist in assessing whether the patient should be admitted; and

The availability of diagnostic procedures at the time when and at the location where the patient presents.

Admissions of particular patients are not covered or noncovered solely on the basis of the length of time the patient actually spends in the hospital. In certain specific situations coverage of services on an inpatient or outpatient basis is determined by the following rules:

Minor Surgery or Other Treatment - When patients with known diagnoses enter a hospital for a specific minor surgical procedure or other treatment that is expected to keep them in the hospital for only a few hours (less than 24), they are considered outpatients for coverage purposes regardless of: the hour they came to the hospital, whether they used a bed, and whether they remained in the hospital past midnight.

Renal Dialysis - Renal dialysis treatments are usually covered only as outpatient services but may under certain circumstances be covered as inpatient services depending on the patient's condition. Patients staying at home, who are ambulatory, whose conditions are stable and who come to the hospital for routine chronic dialysis treatments, and not for a diagnostic workup or a change in therapy, are considered outpatients. On the other hand, patients undergoing short-term dialysis until their kidneys recover from an acute illness (acute dialysis), or persons with borderline renal failure who develop acute renal failure every time they have an illness and require dialysis (episodic dialysis) are usually inpatients. A patient may begin dialysis as an inpatient and then progress to an outpatient status.

Under original Medicare, the Quality Improvement Organization (QIO), for each hospital is responsible for deciding, during review of inpatient admissions on a case-by-case basis, whether the admission was medically necessary. Medicare law authorizes the QIO to make these judgments, and the judgments are binding for purposes of Medicare coverage. In making these judgments, however, QIOs consider only the medical evidence which was available to the physician at the time an admission decision had to be made. They do not take into account other information (e.g., test results) which became available only after admission, except in cases where considering the post-admission information would support a finding that an admission was medically necessary.

Refer to Parts 4 and 7 of the QIO Manual with regard to initial determinations for these services. The QIO will review the swing bed services in these PPS hospitals as well.

NOTE: When patients requiring extended care services are admitted to beds in a hospital, they are considered inpatients of the hospital. In such cases, the services furnished in the hospital will not be considered extended care services, and payment may not be made under the program for such services unless the services are extended care services furnished pursuant to a swing bed agreement granted to the hospital by the Secretary of Health and Human Services.

100-2, 1, 10.1.4

Charges for Deluxe Private Room

A3-3101.1.D, HO-210.1.D

Beneficiaries found to need a private room (either because they need isolation for medical reasons or because they need immediate admission when no other accommodations are available) may be assigned to any of the provider's private rooms. They do not have the right to insist on the private room of their choice, but their preferences should be given the same consideration as if they were paying all provider charges themselves. The program does not, under any circumstances, pay for personal comfort items. Thus, the program does not pay for deluxe accommodations and/or services. These would include a suite, or a room substantially more spacious than is required for treatment, or specially equipped or decorated, or serviced for the comfort and convenience of persons willing to pay a differential for such amenities. If the beneficiary (or representative) requests such deluxe accommodations, the provider should advise that there will be a charge, not covered by Medicare, of a specified amount per day (not exceeding the differential defined in the next sentence); and may charge the beneficiary that amount for each day he/she occupies the deluxe accommodations. The maximum amount the provider may charge the beneficiary for such accommodations is the differential between the most prevalent private room rate at the time of admission and the customary charge for the room occupied. Beneficiaries may not be charged this differential if they (or their representative) do not request the deluxe accommodations.

The beneficiary may not be charged such a differential in private room rates if that differential is based on factors other than personal comfort items. Such factors might include differences between older and newer wings, proximity to lounge, elevators or nursing stations, desirable view, etc. Such rooms are standard 1-bed units and not deluxe rooms for purposes of these instructions, even though the provider may call them deluxe and have a higher customary charge for them. No additional charge may be imposed upon the beneficiary who is assigned to a room that may be somewhat more desirable because of these factors.

100-2, 1, 40

Supplies, Appliances, and Equipment

Supplies, appliances, and equipment, which are ordinarily furnished by the hospital for the care and treatment of the beneficiary solely during the inpatient hospital stay, are covered inpatient hospital services.

Under certain circumstances, supplies, appliances, and equipment used during the beneficiary's inpatient stay are covered under Part A even though the supplies, appliances and equipment leave the hospital with the patient upon discharge. These are circumstances in which it would be unreasonable or impossible from a medical standpoint to limit the patient's use of the item to the periods during which the individual is an inpatient. Examples of items covered under this rule are:

- Items permanently installed in or attached to the patient's body while an inpatient, such as cardiac valves, cardiac pacemakers, and artificial limbs; and

- Items which are temporarily installed in or attached to the patient's body while an inpatient, and which are also necessary to permit or facilitate the patient's release from the hospital, such as tracheotomy or drainage tubes.

Hospital "admission packs" containing primarily toilet articles, such as soap, toothbrushes, toothpaste, and combs, are covered under Part A if routinely furnished by the hospital to all its inpatients. If not routinely furnished to all patients, the packs are not covered. In that situation, the hospital may charge beneficiaries for the pack, but only if they request it with knowledge of what they are requesting and what the charge to them will be.

Supplies, appliances, and equipment furnished to an inpatient for use only outside the hospital are not, in general, covered as inpatient hospital services. However, a temporary or disposable item, which is medically necessary to permit or facilitate the patient's departure from the hospital and is required until the patient can obtain a continuing supply, is covered as an inpatient hospital service.

Oxygen furnished to hospital inpatients is covered under Part A as an inpatient supply.

100-2, 1, 70

Inpatient Services in Connection With Dental Services

A3-3101.7, HO-210.7

When a patient is hospitalized for a dental procedure and the dentist's service is covered under Part B, the inpatient hospital services furnished are covered under Part A. For example, both the professional services of the dentist and the inpatient hospital expenses are covered when the dentist reduces a jaw fracture of an inpatient at a participating hospital. In addition, hospital inpatient services, which are necessary because of the patient's underlying medical condition and clinical status or the severity of a noncovered dental procedure, are covered.

When the hospital services are covered, all ancillary services such as x-rays, administration of anesthesia, use of the operating room, etc., are covered.~Regardless of whether the inpatient hospital services are covered, the medical services of physicians furnished in connection with noncovered dental services are not covered. The services of an anesthesiologist, radiologist, or pathologist whose services are performed in connection with the care, treatment, filling, removal, or replacement of teeth or structures directly supporting teeth are not covered.

100-2, 6, 10

Medical and Other Health Services Furnished to Inpatients of Participating Hospitals

Payment may be made under Part B for physician services and for the nonphysician medical and other health services listed below when furnished by a participating hospital (either directly or under arrangements) to an inpatient of the hospital, but only if payment for these services cannot be made under Part A.

In PPS hospitals, this means that Part B payment could be made for these services if:

- No Part A prospective payment is made at all for the hospital stay because of patient exhaustion of benefit days before admission;

- The admission was disapproved as not reasonable and necessary (and waiver of liability payment was not made);

- The day or days of the otherwise covered stay during which the services were provided were not reasonable and necessary (and no payment was made under waiver of liability);

- The patient was not otherwise eligible for or entitled to coverage under Part A (See the Medicare Benefit Policy Manual, Chapter 1, Sec.150, for services received as a result of noncovered services); or

- No Part A day outlier payment is made (for discharges before October 1997) for one or more outlier days due to patient exhaustion of benefit days after admission but before the case's arrival at outlier status, or because outlier days are otherwise not covered and waiver of liability payment is not made.

However, if only day outlier payment is denied under Part A (discharges before October 1997), Part B payment may be made for only the services covered under Part B and furnished on the denied outlier days.

In non-PPS hospitals, Part B payment may be made for services on any day for which Part A payment is denied (i.e., benefit days are exhausted; services are not at the hospital level of care; or patient is not otherwise eligible or entitled to payment under Part A).

Services payable are:

- Diagnostic x-ray tests, diagnostic laboratory tests, and other diagnostic tests;

- X-ray, radium, and radioactive isotope therapy, including materials and services of technicians;

- Surgical dressings, and splints, casts, and other devices used for reduction of fractures and dislocations;

- Prosthetic devices (other than dental) which replace all or part of an internal body organ (including contiguous tissue), or all or part of the function of a permanently inoperative or malfunctioning internal body organ, including replacement or repairs of such devices;

- Leg, arm, back, and neck braces, trusses, and artificial legs, arms, and eyes including adjustments, repairs, and replacements required because of breakage, wear, loss, or a change in the patient's physical condition;

- Outpatient physical therapy, outpatient speech-language pathology services, and outpatient occupational therapy (see the Medicare Benefit Policy Manual, Chapter 15, "Covered Medical and Other Health Services," Sec.Sec.220 and 230);

- Screening mammography services;

- Screening pap smears;

- Influenza, pneumococcal pneumonia, and hepatitis B vaccines;

- Colorectal screening;

- Bone mass measurements;

- Diabetes self-management;

- Prostate screening;

- Ambulance services;

- Hemophilia clotting factors for hemophilia patients competent to use these factors without supervision);

- Immunosuppressive drugs;

- Oral anti-cancer drugs;

- Oral drug prescribed for use as an acute anti-emetic used as part of an anti-cancer chemotherapeutic regimen; and

- Epoetin Alfa (EPO).

Coverage rules for these services are described in the Medicare Benefit Policy Manual, Chapters: 11, "End Stage Renal Disease (ESRD);" 14, "Medical Devices;" or 15, "Medical and Other Health Services."

For services to be covered under Part A or Part B, a hospital must furnish nonphysician services to its inpatients directly or under arrangements. A nonphysician service is one which does not meet the criteria defining physicians' services specifically provided for in regulation at 42 CFR 415.102. Services "incident to" physicians' services (except for the services of nurse anesthetists employed by anesthesiologists) are nonphysician services for purposes of this provision. This provision is applicable to all hospitals participating in Medicare, including those paid under alternative arrangements such as State cost control systems, and to emergency hospital services furnished by nonparticipating hospitals.

In all hospitals, every service provided to a hospital inpatient other than those listed in the next paragraph must be treated as an inpatient hospital service to be paid for under Part A, if Part A coverage is available and the beneficiary is entitled to Part A. This is because every hospital must provide directly or arrange for any nonphysician service rendered to its inpatients, and a hospital can be paid under Part B for a service provided in this manner only if Part A coverage does not exist.

These services, when provided to a hospital inpatient, may be covered under Part B, even though the patient has Part A coverage for the hospital stay. This is because these services are covered under Part B and not covered under Part A. They are:

- Physicians' services (including the services of residents and interns in unapproved teaching programs);

- Influenza vaccine;

- Pneumoccocal vaccine and its administration;

- Hepatitis B vaccine and its administration;

- Screening mammography services;

- Screening pap smears and pelvic exams;

- Colorectal screening;

- Bone mass measurements;

- Diabetes self management training services; and

- Prostate screening.

However, note that in order to have any Medicare coverage at all (Part A or Part B), any nonphysician service rendered to a hospital inpatient must be provided directly or arranged for by the hospital.

100-2, 6, 20.6

Outpatient Observation Services

A. Outpatient Observation Services Defined

Observation care is a well-defined set of specific, clinically appropriate services, which include ongoing short term treatment, assessment, and reassessment before a decision can be made regarding whether patients will require further treatment as hospital inpatients or if they are able to be discharged from the hospital. Observation services are commonly ordered for patients who present to the emergency department and who then require a significant period of treatment or monitoring in order to make a decision concerning their admission or discharge.

Observation services are covered only when provided by the order of a physician or another individual authorized by State licensure law and hospital staff bylaws to admit patients to the hospital or to order outpatient tests. In the majority of cases, the decision whether to discharge a patient from the hospital following resolution of the reason for the observation care or to admit the patient as an inpatient can be made in less than 48 hours, usually in less than 24 hours. In only rare and exceptional cases do reasonable and necessary outpatient observation services span more than 48 hours.

Hospitals may bill for patients who are directly referred to the hospital for outpatient observation services. A direct referral occurs when a physician in the community refers a patient to the hospital for outpatient observation, bypassing the clinic or emergency department (ED) visit. Effective for services furnished on or after January 1, 2003, hospitals may bill for patients directly referred for observation services.

See Pub. 100-04,*Medicare Claims Processing Manual,*chapter 4, section 290, at http://www.cms.hhs.gov/manuals/downloads/clm104c04.pdf for billing and payment instructions for outpatient observation services.

Future updates will be issued in a Recurring Update Notification.

B. Coverage of Outpatient Observation Services

When a physician orders that a patient receive observation care, the patient's status is that of an outpatient. The purpose of observation is to determine the need for further treatment or for inpatient admission. Thus, a patient receiving observation services may improve and be released, or be admitted as an inpatient (see Pub. 100-02,*Medicare Benefit Policy Manual*, Chapter 1, Section 10 "Covered Inpatient Hospital Services Covered Under Part A" at http://www.cms.hhs.gov/manuals/Downloads/bp102c01.pdf). For more information on correct reporting of observation services, see Pub. 100-04,*Medicare Claims Processing Manual*, chapter 4, section 290.2.2.)

All hospital observation services, regardless of the duration of the observation care, that are medically reasonable and necessary are covered by Medicare.

Observation services are reported using HCPCS code G0378 (Hospital observation service, per hour). Beginning January 1, 2008, HCPCS code G0378 for hourly observation services is assigned status indicator N, signifying that its payment is always packaged. No separate payment is made for observation services reported with HCPCS code G0378. In most circumstances, observation services are supportive and ancillary to the other separately payable services provided to a patient. In certain circumstances when observation care is billed in conjunction with a high level clinic visit (Level 5), high level Type A emergency department visit (Level 4 or 5), high level Type B emergency department visit (Level 5), critical care services, or direct referral for observation services as an integral part of a patient's extended encounter of care, payment may be made for the entire extended care encounter through one of two composite APCs when certain criteria are met. For information about billing and payment methodology for observation services in years prior to CY 2008, see Pub. 100-04,*Medicare Claims Processing Manual*, Chapter 4, Sec.Sec.290.3-290.4. For information about payment for extended assessment and management under composite APCs, see Sec.290.5.

Payment for all reasonable and necessary observation services is packaged into the payments for other separately payable services provided to the patient in the same encounter. Observation services packaged through assignment of status indicator N are covered OPPS services. Since the payment for these services is included in the APC payment for other separately payable services on the claim, hospitals must not bill Medicare beneficiaries directly for the packaged services.

C. Services Not Covered by Medicare and Notification to the Beneficiary

In making the determination whether an ABN can be used to shift liability to a beneficiary for the cost of non-covered items or services related to an encounter that includes observation care, the provider should follow a two step process. First, the provider must decide whether the item or service meets either the definition of observation care or would be otherwise covered. If the item or service does not meet the definitional requirements of any Medicare-covered benefit under Part B, then the item or service is not covered by Medicare and an ABN is not required to shift the liability to the beneficiary. However, the provider may choose to provide voluntary notification for these items or services.

Second, if the item or service meets the definition of observation services or would be otherwise covered, then the provider must decide whether the item or service is "reasonable and necessary" for the beneficiary on the occasion in question, or if the item or service exceeds any frequency limitation for the particular benefit or falls outside of a timeframe for receipt of a particular benefit. In these cases, the ABN would be used to shift the liability to the beneficiary (see Pub. 100-04, *Medicare Claims Processing Manual*, Chapter 30, "Financial Liability Protections," Section 20, at http://www.cms.hhs.gov/manuals/downloads/clm104c30.pdf for information regarding Limitation On Liability (LOL) Under Sec.1879 Where Medicare Claims Are Disallowed).

If an ABN is not issued to the beneficiary, the provider may be held liable for the cost of the item or service unless the provider/supplier is able to demonstrate that they did not know and could not have reasonably been expected to know that Medicare would not pay for the item or service.

100-2, 10, 10.2.2

Reasonableness of the Ambulance Trip

Under the FS payment is made according to the level of medically necessary services actually furnished. That is, payment is based on the level of service furnished (provided they were medically necessary), not simply on the vehicle used. Even if a local government requires an ALS response for all calls, payment under the FS is made only for the level of service furnished, and then only when the service is medically necessary.

100-2, 10, 10.3.3

Separately Payable Ambulance Transport Under Part B versus Patient Transportation that is Covered Under a Packaged Hospital Service

Transportation of a beneficiary from his or her home, an accident scene, or any other point of origin is covered under Part B as an ambulance service only to the nearest hospital, critical access hospital (CAH), or skilled nursing facility (SNF) that is capable of furnishing the required level and type of care for the beneficiary's illness or injury and only if medical necessity and other program coverage criteria are met.

Medicare-covered ambulance services are paid either as separately billed services, in which case the entity furnishing the ambulance service bills Part B of the program, or as a packaged service, in which case the entity furnishing the ambulance service must seek payment from the provider who is responsible for the beneficiary's care. If either the origin or the destination of the ambulance transport is the beneficiary's home, then the ambulance transport is paid separately by Medicare Part B, and the entity that furnishes the ambulance transport may bill its Medicare carrier or intermediary directly. If both the origin and destination of the ambulance transport are providers, e.g., a hospital, critical access hospital (CAH), skilled nursing facility (SNF), then responsibility for payment for the ambulance transport is determined in accordance with the following sequential criteria.

NOTE: These criteria must be applied in sequence as a flow chart and not independently of one another.

1. Provider Numbers:

    If the Medicare-assigned provider numbers of the two providers are different, then the ambulance service is separately billable to the program. If the provider number of both providers is the same, then consider criterion 2, "campus".

2. Campus:

    Following criterion 1, if the campuses of the two providers (sharing the same provider numbers) are the same, then the transport is not separately billable to the program. In this case the provider is responsible for payment. If the campuses of the two providers are different, then consider criterion 3, "patient status." "Campus" means the physical area immediately adjacent to the provider's main buildings, other areas and structures that are not strictly contiguous to the main buildings, but are located within 250 yards of the main buildings, and any of the other areas determined on an individual case basis by the CMS regional office to be part of the provider's campus.

3. Patient Status: Inpatient vs. Outpatient

    Following criteria 1 and 2, if the patient is an inpatient at both providers (i.e., inpatient status both at the origin and at the destination, providers sharing the same provider number but located on different campuses), then the transport is not separately billable. In this case the provider is responsible for payment. All other combinations (i.e., outpatient-to-inpatient, inpatient-to-outpatient, outpatient-to-outpatient) are separately billable to the program.

In the case where the point of origin is not a provider, Part A coverage is not available because, at the time the beneficiary is being transported, the beneficiary is not an inpatient of any provider paid under Part A of the program and ambulance services are excluded from the 3-day preadmission payment window.

The transfer, i.e., the discharge of a beneficiary from one provider with a subsequent admission to another provider, is also payable as a Part B ambulance transport, provided all program coverage criteria are met, because, at the time that the beneficiary is in transit, the beneficiary is not a patient of either provider and not subject to either the inpatient preadmission payment window or outpatient payment packaging requirements. This includes an outpatient transfer from a remote, off-campus emergency department (ER) to becoming an inpatient or outpatient at the main campus hospital, even if the ER is owned and operated by the hospital.

Once a beneficiary is admitted to a hospital, CAH, or SNF, it may be necessary to transport the beneficiary to another hospital or other site temporarily for specialized care while the beneficiary maintains inpatient status with the original provider. This movement of the patient is considered "patient transportation" and is covered as an inpatient hospital or CAH service and as a SNF service when the SNF is furnishing it as a covered SNF service and payment is made under Part A for that service. (If the beneficiary is a resident of a SNF and must be transported by ambulance to receive dialysis or certain other high-end outpatient hospital services, the ambulance transport may be separately payable under Part B.) Because the service is covered and payable as a beneficiary transportation service under Part A, the service cannot be classified and paid for as an ambulance service under Part B. This includes intra-campus transfers between different departments of the same hospital, even where the departments are located in separate buildings. Such intra-campus transfers are not separately payable under the Part B ambulance benefit. Such costs are accounted for in the same manner as the costs of such a transfer within a single building.

100-2, 10, 20

Coverage Guidelines for Ambulance Service Claims.

Payment may be made for expenses incurred by a patient for ambulance service provided conditions I, 2, and 3 in the left-hand column have been met. The right-hand column indicates the documentation needed to establish that the condition has been met

Conditions	Review Action
1. Patient was transported by an approved supplier of ambulance services.	1. Ambulance suppliers are explained in greater detail in §10.1.3

Conditions	Review Action
2. The patient was suffering from an illness or injury, which contraindicated transportation by other means. (§10.2)	2. (a) The contractor presumes the requirement was met if the submitted documentation indicates that the patient: • Was transported in an emergency situation, e.g., as a result of an accident, injury or acute illness, or • Needed to be restrained to prevent injury to the beneficiary or others; or • Was unconscious or in shock; or • Required oxygen or other emergency treatment during transport to the nearest appropriate facility; or • Exhibits signs and symptoms of acute respiratory distress or cardiac distress such as shortness of breath or chest pain; or • Exhibits signs and symptoms that indicate the possibility of acute stroke; or • Had to remain immobile because of a fracture that had not been set or the possibility of a fracture; or • Was experiencing severe hemorrhage; or • Could be moved only by stretcher; or • Was bed-confined before and after the ambulance trip. (b) In the absence of any of the conditions listed in (a) above additional documentation should be obtained to establish medical need where the evidence indicates the existence of the circumstances listed below: (i) Patient's condition would not ordinarily require movement by stretcher, or (ii) The individual was not admitted as a hospital inpatient (except in accident cases), or (iii) The ambulance was used solely because other means of transportation were unavailable, or (iv) The individual merely needed assistance in getting from his room or home to a vehicle. (c) Where the information indicates a situation not listed in 2(a) or 2(b) above, refer the case to your supervisor.
3. The patient was transported from and to points listed below. (a) From patient's residence (or other place where need arose) to hospital or skilled nursing facility.	3. Claims should show the ZIP Code of the point of pickup. (a) i. Condition met if trip began within the institution's service area as shown in the carrier's locality guide. ii. Condition met where the trip began outside the institution's service area if the institution was the nearest one with appropriate facilities.

(b) Skilled nursing facility to a hospital or hospital to a skilled nursing facility.	(b) (i) Condition met if the ZIP Code of the pickup point is within the service area of the destination as shown in the carrier's locality guide. (ii) Condition met where the ZIP Code of the pickup point is outside the service area of the destination if the destination institution was the nearest appropriate facility.
(c) Hospital to hospital or skilled nursing facility to skilled nursing facility.	(c) Condition met if the discharging institution was not an appropriate facility and the admitting institution was the nearest appropriate facility.
(d) From a hospital or skilled nursing facility to patient's residence.	(d) (i) Condition met if patient's residence is within the institution's service area as shown in the carrier's locality guide. (ii) Condition met where the patient's residence is outside the institution's service area if the institution was the nearest appropriate facility.
(e) Round trip for hospital or participating skilled nursing facility inpatients to the nearest hospital or nonhospital treatment facility.	(e) Condition met if the reasonable and necessary diagnostic or therapeutic service required by patient's condition is not available at the institution where the beneficiary is an inpatient.

NOTE: Ambulance service to a physician's office or a physician-directed clinic is not covered. See §10.3.8 above, where a stop is made at a physician's office en route to a hospital and §10.3.3 for additional exceptions.)

4. Ambulance services involving hospital admissions in Canada or Mexico are covered (Medicare Claims Processing Manual, Chapter 1, "General Billing Requirements, "§10.1.3.) if the following conditions are met:	4. (a) The foreign hospitalization has been determined to be covered; and (b) The ambulance service meets the coverage requirements set forth in §§10-10.3. If the foreign hospitalization has been determined to be covered on the basis of emergency services (See the Medicare Claims Processing Manual, Chapter 1, "General Billing Requirements," §10.1.3), the necessity requirement (§10.2) and the destination requirement (§10.3) are considered met.
5. The carrier will make partial payment for otherwise covered ambulance service, which exceeded limits defined in item 6. The carrier will base the payment on the amount payable had the patient been transported:	5 & 6 (a) From the pickup point to the nearest appropriate facility, or 5 & 6 (b) From the nearest appropriate facility to the beneficiary's residence where he or she is being returned home from a distant institution.

100-2, 10, 30.1.1

Ground Ambulance Services:

Basic Life Support (BLS)

Definition: Basic life support (BLS) is transportation by ground ambulance vehicle and the provision of medically necessary supplies and services, including BLS ambulance services as defined by the State. The ambulance must be staffed by an individual who is qualified in accordance with State and local laws as an emergency medical technician-basic (EMT-Basic). These laws may vary from State to State or within a State. For example, only in some jurisdictions is an EMT-Basic permitted to operate limited equipment onboard the vehicle, assist more qualified personnel in performing assessments and interventions, and establish a peripheral intravenous (IV) line.

Basic Life Support (BLS) - Emergency

Definition: When medically necessary, the provision of BLS services, as specified above, in the context of an emergency response. An emergency response is one that, at the time the ambulance provider or supplier is called, it responds immediately. An immediate response is one in which the

NOTE: A Patient'sresidence is the place where he or she makes his/her home and dwells permanently, or for an extended period of time. A skilled nursing facility is one, which is listed in the Directory of Medical Facilities as a participating SNF or as an institution which meets §1861(j)(1) of the Act.

NOTE: A claim for ambulance service to a participating hospital or skilled nursing facility should not be denied on the grounds that there is a nearer nonparticipating institution having appropriate facilities.

ambulance provider/supplier begins as quickly as possible to take the steps necessary to respond to the call.

Application: The determination to respond emergently with a BLS ambulance must be in accord with the local 911 or equivalent service dispatch protocol. If the call came in directly to the ambulance provider/supplier, then the provider's/supplier's dispatch protocol must meet, at a minimum, the standards of the dispatch protocol of the local 911 or equivalent service. In areas that do not have a local 911 or equivalent service, then the protocol must meet, at a minimum, the standards of a dispatch protocol in another similar jurisdiction within the State or, if there is no similar jurisdiction within the State, then the standards of any other dispatch protocol within the State. Where the dispatch was inconsistent with this standard of protocol, including where no protocol was used, the beneficiary's condition (for example, symptoms) at the scene determines the appropriate level of payment.

Advanced Life Support, Level 1 (ALS1)
Definition: Advanced life support, level 1 (ALS1) is the transportation by ground ambulance vehicle and the provision of medically necessary supplies and services including the provision of an ALS assessment or at least one ALS intervention.

Advanced Life Support Assessment
Definition: An advanced life support (ALS) assessment is an assessment performed by an ALS crew as part of an emergency response that was necessary because the patient's reported condition at the time of dispatch was such that only an ALS crew was qualified to perform the assessment. An ALS assessment does not necessarily result in a determination that the patient requires an ALS level of service.

Application: The determination to respond emergently with an ALS ambulance must be in accord with the local 911 or equivalent service dispatch protocol. If the call came in directly to the ambulance provider/supplier, then the provider's/supplier's dispatch protocol must meet, at a minimum, the standards of the dispatch protocol of the local 911 or equivalent service. In areas that do not have a local 911 or equivalent service, then the protocol must meet, at a minimum, the standards of a dispatch protocol in another similar jurisdiction within the State or, if there is no similar jurisdiction within the State, then the standards of any other dispatch protocol within the State. Where the dispatch was inconsistent with this standard of protocol, including where no protocol was used, the beneficiary's condition (for example, symptoms) at the scene determines the appropriate level of payment.

Advanced Life Support Intervention
Definition: An advanced life support (ALS) intervention is a procedure that is in accordance with State and local laws, required to be done by an emergency medical technician-intermediate (EMT-Intermediate) or EMT-Paramedic.

Application: An ALS intervention must be medically necessary to qualify as an intervention for payment for an ALS level of service. An ALS intervention applies only to ground transports.

Advanced Life Support, Level 1 (ALS1) - Emergency
Definition: When medically necessary, the provision of ALS1 services, as specified above, in the context of an emergency response. An emergency response is one that, at the time the ambulance provider or supplier is called, it responds immediately. An immediate response is one in which the ambulance provider/supplier begins as quickly as possible to take the steps necessary to respond to the call.

Application: The determination to respond emergently with an ALS ambulance must be in accord with the local 911 or equivalent service dispatch protocol. If the call came in directly to the ambulance provider/supplier, then the provider's/supplier's dispatch protocol must meet, at a minimum, the standards of the dispatch protocol of the local 911 or equivalent service. In areas that do not have a local 911 or equivalent service, then the protocol must meet, at a minimum, the standards of a dispatch protocol in another similar jurisdiction within the State or, if there is no similar jurisdiction within the State, then the standards of any other dispatch protocol within the State. Where the dispatch was inconsistent with this standard of protocol, including where no protocol was used, the beneficiary's condition (for example, symptoms) at the scene determines the appropriate level of payment.

Advanced Life Support, Level 2 (ALS2)
Definition: Advanced life support, level 2 (ALS2) is the transportation by ground ambulance vehicle and the provision of medically necessary supplies and services including (1) at least three separate administrations of one or more medications by intravenous push/bolus or by continuous infusion (excluding crystalloid fluids) or (2) ground ambulance transport, medically necessary supplies and services, and the provision of at least one of the ALS2 procedures listed below:

a. Manual defibrillation/cardioversion;

b. Endotracheal intubation;

c. Central venous line;

d. Cardiac pacing;

e. Chest decompression;

f. Surgical airway; or

g. Intraosseous line.

Application: Crystalloid fluids include fluids such as 5 percent Dextrose in water, Saline and Lactated Ringer's. Medications that are administered by other means, for example: intramuscular/subcutaneous injection, oral, sublingually or nebulized, do not qualify to determine whether the ALS2 level rate is payable. However, this is not an all-inclusive list. Likewise, a single dose of medication administered fractionally (i.e., one-third of a single dose quantity) on three separate occasions does not qualify for the ALS2 payment rate. The criterion of multiple administrations of the same drug requires a suitable quantity and amount of time between administrations that is in accordance with standard medical practice guidelines. The fractional administration of a single dose (for this purpose meaning a standard or protocol dose) on three separate occasions does not qualify for ALS2 payment.

In other words, the administration of 1/3 of a qualifying dose 3 times does not equate to three qualifying doses for purposes of indicating ALS2 care. One-third of X given 3 times might = X (where X is a standard/protocol drug amount), but the same sequence does not equal 3 times X. Thus, if 3 administrations of the same drug are required to show that ALS2 care was given, each of those administrations must be in accord with local protocols. The run will not qualify on the basis of drug administration if that administration was not according to protocol.

An example of a single dose of medication administered fractionally on three separate occasions that would not qualify for the ALS2 payment rate would be the use of Intravenous (IV) Epinephrine in the treatment of pulseless Ventricular Tachycardia/Ventricular Fibrillation (VF/VT) in the adult patient. Administering this medication in increments of 0.25 mg, 0.25 mg, and 0.50 mg would not qualify for the ALS2 level of payment. This medication, according to the American Heart Association (AHA), Advanced Cardiac Life Support (ACLS) protocol, calls for Epinephrine to be administered in 1 mg increments every 3 to 5 minutes. Therefore, in order to receive payment for an ALS2 level of service, based in part on the administration of Epinephrine, three separate administrations of Epinephrine in 1 mg increments must be administered for the treatment of pulseless VF/VT.

A second example that would not qualify for the ALS2 payment level is the use of Adenosine in increments of 2 mg, 2 mg, and 2 mg for a total of 6 mg in the treatment of an adult patient with Paroxysmal Supraventricular Tachycardia (PSVT). According to ACLS guidelines, 6 mg of Adenosine should be given by rapid intravenous push (IVP) over 1 to 2 seconds. If the first dose does not result in the elimination of the supraventricular tachycardia within 1 to 2 minutes, 12 mg of Adenosine should be administered IVP. If the supraventricular tachycardia persists, a second 12 mg dose of Adenosine can be administered for a total of 30 mg of Adenosine. Three separate administrations of the drug Adenosine in the dosage amounts outlined in the later case would qualify for ALS2 payment.

Endotracheal intubation is one of the services that qualifies for the ALS2 level of payment; therefore, it is not necessary to consider medications administered by endotracheal intubation for the purpose of determining whether the ALS2 rate is payable. The monitoring and maintenance of an endotracheal tube that was previously inserted prior to transport also qualifies as an ALS2 procedure.

Advanced Life Support (ALS) Personnel
Definition: ALS personnel are individuals trained to the level of the emergency medical technician-intermediate (EMT-Intermediate) or paramedic.

Specialty Care Transport (SCT)
Definition: Specialty care transport (SCT) is the interfacility transportation of a critically injured or ill beneficiary by a ground ambulance vehicle, including the provision of medically necessary supplies and services, at a level of service beyond the scope of the EMT-Paramedic. SCT is necessary when a beneficiary's condition requires ongoing care that must be furnished by one or more health professionals in an appropriate specialty area, for example, emergency or critical care nursing, emergency medicine, respiratory care, cardiovascular care, or a paramedic with additional training.

Application: The EMT-Paramedic level of care is set by each State. SCT is necessary when a beneficiary's condition requires ongoing care that must be furnished by one or more health professionals in an appropriate specialty area. Care above that level that is medically necessary and that is furnished at a level of service above the EMT-Paramedic level of care is considered SCT. That is to say, if EMT-Paramedics - without specialty care certification or qualification - are permitted to furnish a given service in a State, then that service does not qualify for SCT. The phrase "EMT-Paramedic with additional training" recognizes that a State may permit a person who is not only certified as an EMT-Paramedic, but who also has successfully completed additional education as determined by the State in furnishing higher level medical services required by critically ill or critically injured patients, to furnish a level of service that otherwise would require a health professional in an appropriate specialty care area (for example, a nurse) to provide. "Additional training" means the specific additional training that a State requires a paramedic to complete in order to qualify to furnish specialty care to a critically ill or injured patient during an SCT.

Paramedic Intercept (PI)

Definition: Paramedic Intercept services are ALS services provided by an entity that does not provide the ambulance transport. This type of service is most often provided for an emergency ambulance transport in which a local volunteer ambulance that can provide only basic life support (BLS) level of service is dispatched to transport a patient. If the patient needs ALS services such as EKG monitoring, chest decompression, or I.V. therapy, another entity dispatches a paramedic to meet the BLS ambulance at the scene or once the ambulance is on the way to the hospital. The ALS paramedics then provide services to the patient.

This tiered approach to life saving is cost effective in many areas because most volunteer ambulances do not charge for their services and one paramedic service can cover many communities. Prior to March 1, 1999, Medicare payment could be made for these services, but only when the claim was submitted by the entity that actually furnished the ambulance transport. Payment could not be made directly to the intercept service provider. In those areas where State laws prohibit volunteer ambulances from billing Medicare and other health insurance, the intercept service could not receive payment for treating a Medicare beneficiary and was forced to bill the beneficiary for the entire service.

Paramedic intercept services furnished on or after March 1, 1999, may be payable separate from the ambulance transport, subject to the requirements specified below.

The intercept service(s) is:

- Furnished in a rural area;
- Furnished under a contract with one or more volunteer ambulance services; and,
- Medically necessary based on the condition of the beneficiary receiving the ambulance service.
- In addition, the volunteer ambulance service involved must:
- Meet the program's certification requirements for furnishing ambulance services;
- Furnish services only at the BLS level at the time of the intercept; and,
- Be prohibited by State law from billing anyone for any service.
- Finally, the entity furnishing the ALS paramedic intercept service must:
- Meet the program's certification requirements for furnishing ALS services, and,
- Bill all recipients who receive ALS paramedic intercept services from the entity, regardless of whether or not those recipients are Medicare beneficiaries.

For purposes of the paramedic intercept benefit, a rural area is an area that is designated as rural by a State law or regulation or any area outside of a Metropolitan Statistical Area or in New England, outside a New England County Metropolitan Area as defined by the Office of Management and Budget. The current list of these areas is periodically published in the Federal Register.

See the Medicare Claims Processing Manual, Chapter 15, "Ambulance," Sec.20.1.4 for payment of paramedic intercept services.

Services in a Rural Area

Definition: Services in a rural area are services that are furnished (1) in an area outside a Metropolitan Statistical Area (MSA); or, (2) in New England, outside a New England County Metropolitan Area (NECMA); or, (3) an area identified as rural using the Goldsmith modification even though the area is within an MSA.

Emergency Response

Definition: Emergency response is a BLS or ALS1 level of service that has been provided in immediate response to a 911 call or the equivalent. An immediate response is one in which the ambulance provider/supplier begins as quickly as possible to take the steps necessary to respond to the call.

Application: The phrase "911 call or equivalent" is intended to establish the standard that the nature of the call at the time of dispatch is the determining factor. Regardless of the medium by which the call is made (e.g., a radio call could be appropriate) the call is of an emergent nature when, based on the information available to the dispatcher at the time of the call, it is reasonable for the dispatcher to issue an emergency dispatch in light of accepted, standard dispatch protocol. An emergency call need not come through 911 even in areas where a 911 call system exists. However, the determination to respond emergently must be in accord with the local 911 or equivalent service dispatch protocol. If the call came in directly to the ambulance provider/supplier, then the provider's/supplier's dispatch protocol and the dispatcher's actions must meet, at a minimum, the standards of the dispatch protocol of the local 911 or equivalent service. In areas that do not have a local 911 or equivalent service, then both the protocol and the dispatcher's actions must meet, at a minimum, the standards of the dispatch protocol in another similar jurisdiction within the State, or if there is no similar jurisdiction, then the standards of any other dispatch protocol within the

State. Where the dispatch was inconsistent with this standard of protocol, including where no protocol was used, the beneficiary's condition (for example, symptoms) at the scene determines the appropriate level of payment.

EMT-Intermediate

Definition: EMT-Intermediate is an individual who is qualified, in accordance with State and local laws, as an EMT-Basic and who is also certified in accordance with State and local laws to perform essential advanced techniques and to administer a limited number of medications.

EMT-Paramedic

Definition: EMT-Paramedic possesses the qualifications of the EMT-Intermediate and, in accordance with State and local laws, has enhanced skills that include being able to administer additional interventions and medications.

Relative Value Units

Definition: Relative value units (RVUs) measure the value of ambulance services relative to the value of a base level ambulance service.

Application: The RVUs for the ambulance fee schedule are as follows:

Service Level RVUs

- BLS 1.00
- BLS - Emergency 1.60
- ALS1 1.20
- ALS1 - Emergency 1.90
- ALS2 2.75
- SCT 3.25
- PI 1.75
- RVUs are not applicable to FW and RW services

100-2, 12, 30.1

Rules for Payment of CORF Services

The payment basis for CORF services is 80 percent of the lesser of: (1) the actual charge for the service or (2) the physician fee schedule amount for the service when the physician fee schedule establishes a payment amount for such service. Payment for CORF services under the physician fee schedule is made for physical therapy, occupational therapy, speech-language pathology and respiratory therapy services, as well as the nursing and social and/or psychological services, which are a part of, or directly relate to, the rehabilitation plan of treatment.

Payment for covered durable medical equipment, orthotic and prosthetic (DMEPOS) devices and supplies provided by a CORF is based upon: the lesser of 80 percent of actual charges or the payment amount established under the DMEPOS fee schedule; or, the single payment amount established under the DMEPOS competitive bidding program, provided that payment for such an item is not included in the payment amount for other CORF services.

If there is no fee schedule amount for a covered CORF item or service, payment should be based on the lesser of 80 percent of the actual charge for the service provided or an amount determined by the local Medicare contractor.

Payment for CORF social and/or psychological services is made under the physician fee schedule only for HCPCS code G0409, as appropriate, and only when billed using revenue codes 0560, 0569, 0910, 0911, 0914 and 0919.

Payment for CORF respiratory therapy services is made under the physician fee schedule when provided by a respiratory therapist as defined at 42CFR485.70(j) and, only to the extent that these services support or are an adjunct to the rehabilitation plan of treatment, when billed using revenue codes 0410, 0412 and 0419. Separate payment is not made for diagnostic tests or for services related to physiologic monitoring services which are bundled into other respiratory therapy services appropriately performed by a respiratory therapist, such as Healthcare Common Procedure Coding System (HCPCS) codes G0237, G0238 and G0239.

Payment for CORF nursing services is made under the physician fee schedule only when provided by a registered nurse as defined at 42CFR485.70(h) for nursing services only to the extent that these services support or are an adjunct to the rehabilitation plan of treatment. In addition, payment for CORF nursing services is made only when provided by a registered nurse. HCPCS code G0128 is used to bill for these services and only with revenue codes 0550 and 0559.

For specific payment requirements for CORF, items and services see Pub. 100-04, Medicare Claims Processing Manual, Chapter 5, Part B Outpatient Rehabilitation and CORF/OPT Services.

100-2, 12, 40.5

Respiratory Therapy Services

A respiratory therapy plan of treatment is wholly established and signed by the referring physician before the respiratory therapist initiates the actual treatment.

A. Definition

Respiratory therapy services include only those services that can be appropriately provided to CORF patients by a qualified respiratory therapist, as defined at 42CFR485.70(j), under a physician-established respiratory therapy plan of treatment. The facility physician must be present in the facility for a sufficient time to provide, in accordance with accepted principles of medical practice, medical direction, medical care services and consultation. Respiratory therapy services include the physiological monitoring necessary to furnish these services. Payment for these services is bundled into the payment for respiratory therapy services and is not payable separately. Diagnostic and other medical services provided in the CORF setting are not considered CORF services, and therefore may not be included in a respiratory therapy plan of treatment because these are covered under separate benefit categories.

The respiratory therapist assesses the patient to determine the appropriateness of pursed lip breathing activity and may check the patient's oxygen saturation level (via pulse oximetry). If appropriate, the respiratory therapist then provides the initial training in order to ensure that the patient can accurately perform the activity. The respiratory therapist may again check the patient's oxygen saturation level, or perform peak respiratory flow, or check other respiratory parameters. These types of services are considered "physiological monitoring" and are bundled into the payment for HCPCS codes G0237, G0238 and G0239. Physiological monitoring also includes the provision of a 6-minute walk test that is typically conducted before the start of the patient's respiratory therapy activities. The time to provide this walk "test" assessment is included as part of the HCPCS code G0238. When provided as part of a CORF respiratory therapy plan of treatment, payment for these monitoring activities is bundled into the payment for other services provided by the respiratory therapist, such as the three respiratory therapy specific G-codes.

B. Guidelines for Applying Coverage Criteria

There are some conditions for which respiratory therapy services may be indicated. However, respiratory therapy performed as part of a standard protocol without regard to the individual patient's actual condition, capacity for improving, and the need for such services as established, is not reasonable and medically necessary. All respiratory therapy services must meet the test of being "reasonable and medically necessary" pursuant to Sec.1862(a)(1)(A) of the Act. Determinations of medical necessity are made based on local contractor decisions on a claim-by-claim basis.

The three HCPCS codes G0237, G0238, and G0239 are specific to services provided under the respiratory therapy plan of treatment and, as such, are not designated as subject to the therapy caps.

C. Patient Education Programs

Instructing a patient in the use of equipment, breathing exercises, etc. may be considered reasonable and necessary to the patient's respiratory therapy plan of treatment and can usually be given to a patient during the course of treatment by the respiratory therapist. These educational instructions are bundled into the covered service and separate payment is not made.

100-2, 12, 40.8

Nursing Services

CORF nursing services may only be provided by an individual meeting the qualifications of a registered nurse, as defined at 42CFR485.70(h). They must relate to, or be a part of, the rehabilitation plan of treatment.

CORF nursing services must be reasonable and medically necessary and are provided as an adjunct to the rehabilitation plan of treatment. For example, a registered nurse may perform or instruct a patient, as appropriate, in the proper procedure of "in and out" urethral catheterization, tracheostomy tube suctioning, or the cleaning for ileostomy or colostomy bags.

Nursing services may not substitute for or supplant the services of physical therapists, occupational therapists, speech-language pathologists and respiratory therapists, but instead must support or further the services and goals provided in the rehabilitation plan of treatment.

CORF nursing services must be provided by a registered nurse and may only be coded as HCPCS code G0128 indicating that CORF "nursing services" were provided.

100-2, 12, 40.11

Vaccines

A CORF may provide pneumococcal pneumonia, influenza virus, and hepatitis B vaccines to its patients. While not included as a service under the CORF benefit, Medicare will make payment to the CORF for certain vaccines and their administration provided to CORF patients (CY 2008 PFS Rule 72 FR 66293).

The following three vaccinations are covered in a CORF if a physician who is a doctor of medicine or osteopathy orders it for a CORF patient:

Pneumococcal pneumonia vaccine and its administration;

Hepatitis B vaccine and its administration furnished to a beneficiary who is at high or intermediate risk of contracting hepatitis B; and

Influenza virus vaccine and its administration

Payment for covered pneumococcal pneumonia, influenza virus, and hepatitis B vaccines provided in the CORF setting is based on 95 percent of the average wholesale price. The CORF registered nurse provides administration of any of these vaccines using HCPCS codes G0008, G0009 or G0010 with payment based on CPT code 90471.

100-2, 15, 50

Drugs and Biologicals

B3-2049, A3-3112.4.B, HO-230.4.B

The Medicare program provides limited benefits for outpatient drugs. The program covers drugs that are furnished "incident to" a physician's service provided that the drugs are not usually self-administered by the patients who take them.

Generally, drugs and biologicals are covered only if all of the following requirements are met:

- They meet the definition of drugs or biologicals (see Sec.50.1);

- They are of the type that are not usually self-administered. (see Sec.50.2);

- They meet all the general requirements for coverage of items as incident to a physician's services (see Sec.Sec.50.1 and 50.3);

- They are reasonable and necessary for the diagnosis or treatment of the illness or injury for which they are administered according to accepted standards of medical practice (see Sec.50.4);

- They are not excluded as noncovered immunizations (see Sec.50.4.4.2); and

- They have not been determined by the FDA to be less than effective. (See Sec.Sec.50.4.4).

Medicare Part B does generally not cover drugs that can be self-administered, such as those in pill form, or are used for self-injection. However, the statute provides for the coverage of some self-administered drugs. Examples of self-administered drugs that are covered include blood-clotting factors, drugs used in immunosuppressive therapy, erythropoietin for dialysis patients, osteoporosis drugs for certain homebound patients, and certain oral cancer drugs. (See Sec.110.3 for coverage of drugs, which are necessary to the effective use of Durable Medical Equipment (DME) or prosthetic devices.)

100-2, 15, 50.2

Determining Self-Administration of Drug or Biological

AB-02-072, AB-02-139, B3-2049.2

The Medicare program provides limited benefits for outpatient prescription drugs. The program covers drugs that are furnished "incident to" a physician's service provided that the drugs are not usually self-administered by the patients who take them. Section 112 of the Benefits, Improvements & Protection Act of 2000 (BIPA) amended sections 1861(s)(2)(A) and 1861(s)(2)(B) of the Act to redefine this exclusion. The prior statutory language referred to those drugs "which cannot be self-administered." Implementation of the BIPA provision requires interpretation of the phrase "not usually self-administered by the patient".

A. Policy

Fiscal intermediaries and carriers are instructed to follow the instructions below when applying the exclusion for drugs that are usually self-administered by the patient. Each individual contractor must make its own individual determination on each drug. Contractors must continue to apply the policy that not only the drug is medically reasonable and necessary for any individual claim, but also that the route of administration is medically reasonable and necessary. That is, if a drug is available in both oral and injectable forms, the injectable form of the drug must be medically reasonable and necessary as compared to using the oral form.

For certain injectable drugs, it will be apparent due to the nature of the condition(s) for which they are administered or the usual course of treatment for those conditions, they are, or are not, usually self-administered. For example, an injectable drug used to treat migraine headaches is usually self-administered. On the other hand, an injectable drug, administered at the same time as chemotherapy, used to treat anemia secondary to chemotherapy is not usually self-administered.

B. Administered

The term "administered" refers only to the physical process by which the drug enters the patient's body. It does not refer to whether the process is supervised by a medical professional (for example, to observe proper technique or side-effects of the drug). Only injectable (including intravenous) drugs are eligible for inclusion under the "incident to" benefit. Other routes of administration including, but not limited to, oral drugs, suppositories, topical medications are all considered to be usually self-administered by the patient.

C. Usually

For the purposes of applying this exclusion, the term "usually" means more than 50 percent of the time for all Medicare beneficiaries who use the drug. Therefore, if a drug is self-administered by more than 50 percent of Medicare beneficiaries, the drug is excluded from coverage and the contractor may not make any Medicare payment for it. In arriving at a single determination as to whether a drug is usually self-administered, contractors should make a separate determination for each indication for a drug as to whether that drug is usually self-administered.

After determining whether a drug is usually self-administered for each indication, contractors should determine the relative contribution of each indication to total use of the drug (i.e., weighted average) in order to make an overall determination as to whether the drug is usually self-administered. For example, if a drug has three indications, is not self-administered for the first indication, but is self administered for the second and third indications, and the first indication makes up 40 percent of total usage, the second indication makes up 30 percent of total usage, and the third indication makes up 30 percent of total usage, then the drug would be considered usually self-administered.

Reliable statistical information on the extent of self-administration by the patient may not always be available. Consequently, CMS offers the following guidance for each contractor's consideration in making this determination in the absence of such data:

1. Absent evidence to the contrary, presume that drugs delivered intravenously are not usually self-administered by the patient.

2. Absent evidence to the contrary, presume that drugs delivered by intramuscular injection are not usually self-administered by the patient. (Avonex, for example, is delivered by intramuscular injection, not usually self-administered by the patient.) The contractor may consider the depth and nature of the particular intramuscular injection in applying this presumption. In applying this presumption, contractors should examine the use of the particular drug and consider the following factors:

3. Absent evidence to the contrary, presume that drugs delivered by subcutaneous injection are self-administered by the patient. However, contractors should examine the use of the particular drug and consider the following factors:

   A. Acute Condition - Is the condition for which the drug is used an acute condition? If so, it is less likely that a patient would self-administer the drug. If the condition were longer term, it would be more likely that the patient would self-administer the drug.

   B. Frequency of Administration - How often is the injection given? For example, if the drug is administered once per month, it is less likely to be self-administered by the patient. However, if it is administered once or more per week, it is likely that the drug is self-administered by the patient. In some instances, carriers may have provided payment for one or perhaps several doses of a drug that would otherwise not be paid for because the drug is usually self-administered. Carriers may have exercised this discretion for limited coverage, for example, during a brief time when the patient is being trained under the supervision of a physician in the proper technique for self-administration. Medicare will no longer pay for such doses. In addition, contractors may no longer pay for any drug when it is administered on an outpatient emergency basis, if the drug is excluded because it is usually self-administered by the patient.

D. Definition of Acute Condition

For the purposes of determining whether a drug is usually self-administered, an acute condition means a condition that begins over a short time period, is likely to be of short duration and/or the expected course of treatment is for a short, finite interval. A course of treatment consisting of scheduled injections lasting less than two weeks, regardless of frequency or route of administration, is considered acute. Evidence to support this may include Food and Drug administration (FDA) approval language, package inserts, drug compendia, and other information.

E. By the Patient

The term "by the patient" means Medicare beneficiaries as a collective whole. The carrier includes only the patients themselves and not other individuals (that is, spouses, friends, or other care-givers are not considered the patient). The determination is based on whether the drug is self-administered by the patient a majority of the time that the drug is used on an outpatient basis by Medicare beneficiaries for medically necessary indications.

The carrier ignores all instances when the drug is administered on an inpatient basis. The carrier makes this determination on a drug-by-drug basis, not on a beneficiary-by-beneficiary basis. In evaluating whether beneficiaries as a collective whole self-administer, individual beneficiaries who do not have the capacity to self-administer any drug due to a condition other than the condition for which they are taking the drug in question are not considered. For example, an individual afflicted with paraplegia or advanced dementia would not have the capacity to self-administer any injectable drug, so such individuals would not be included in the population upon which the determination for self-administration by the patient was based. Note that some individuals afflicted with a less severe stage of an otherwise debilitating condition would be included in the population upon which the determination for "self-administered by the patient" was based; for example, an early onset of dementia.

F. Evidentiary Criteria

Contractors are only required to consider the following types of evidence: peer reviewed medical literature, standards of medical practice, evidence-based practice guidelines, FDA approved label, and package inserts. Contractors may also consider other evidence submitted by interested individuals or groups subject to their judgment.

Contractors should also use these evidentiary criteria when reviewing requests for making a determination as to whether a drug is usually self-administered, and requests for reconsideration of a pending or published determination.

Please note that prior to the August 1, 2002, one of the principal factors used to determine whether a drug was subject to the self-administered exclusion was whether the FDA label contained instructions for self-administration. However, CMS notes that under the new standard, the fact that the FDA label includes instructions for self-administration is not, by itself, a determining factor that a drug is subject to this exclusion.

G. Provider Notice of Noncovered Drugs

Contractors must describe on their Web site the process they will use to determine whether a drug is usually self-administered and thus does not meet the "incident to" benefit category. Contractors must publish a list of the injectable drugs that are subject to the self-administered exclusion on their Web site, including the data and rationale that led to the determination. Contractors will report the workload associated with developing new coverage statements in CAFM 21208.

Contractors must provide notice 45 days prior to the date that these drugs will not be covered. During the 45-day time period, contractors will maintain existing medical review and payment procedures. After the 45-day notice, contractors may deny payment for the drugs subject to the notice.

Contractors must not develop local medical review policies (LMRPs) for this purpose because further elaboration to describe drugs that do not meet the ‚Äòincident to' and the ‚Äònot usually self-administered' provisions of the statute are unnecessary. Current LMRPs based solely on these provisions must be withdrawn. LMRPs that address the self-administered exclusion and other information may be reissued absent the self-administered drug exclusion material. Contractors will report this workload in CAFM 21206. However, contractors may continue to use and write LMRPs to describe reasonable and necessary uses of drugs that are not usually self-administered. H. Conferences Between Contractors Contractors' Medical Directors may meet and discuss whether a drug is usually self-administered without reaching a formal consensus. Each contractor uses its discretion as to whether or not it will participate in such discussions. Each contractor must make its own individual determinations, except that fiscal intermediaries may, at their discretion, follow the determinations of the local carrier with respect to the self-administered exclusion.

I. Beneficiary Appeals

If a beneficiary's claim for a particular drug is denied because the drug is subject to the "self-administered drug" exclusion, the beneficiary may appeal the denial. Because it is a "benefit category" denial and not a denial based on medical necessity, an Advance Beneficiary Notice (ABN) is not required. A "benefit category" denial (i.e., a denial based on the fact that there is no benefit category under which the drug may be covered) does not trigger the financial liability protection provisions of Limitation On Liability (under Sec.1879 of the Act). Therefore, physicians or providers may charge the beneficiary for an excluded drug.

J. Provider and Physician Appeals

A physician accepting assignment may appeal a denial under the provisions found in Chapter 29 of the Medicare Claims Processing Manual.

K. Reasonable and Necessary

Carriers and fiscal intermediaries will make the determination of reasonable and necessary with respect to the medical appropriateness of a drug to treat the patient's condition. Contractors will continue to make the determination of whether the intravenous or injection form of a drug is appropriate as opposed to the oral form. Contractors will also continue to make the determination as to whether a physician's office visit was reasonable and necessary. However, contractors should not make a determination of whether it was reasonable and necessary for the patient to choose to have his or her drug administered in the physician's office or outpatient hospital setting. That is, while a physician's office visit may not be reasonable and necessary in a specific situation, in such a case an injection service would be payable.

L. Reporting Requirements

Each carrier and intermediary must report to CMS, every September 1 and March 1, its complete list of injectable drugs that the contractor has determined are excluded when furnished incident to a physician's service on the basis that the drug is usually self-administered. The CMS anticipates that contractors will review injectable drugs on a rolling basis and publish their list of excluded drugs as it is developed. For example, contractors should not wait to publish this list until every drug has been reviewed.

Contractors must send their exclusion list to the following e-mail address: drugdata@cms.hhs.gov a template that CMS will provide separately, consisting of the following data elements in order:

1. Carrier Name

2. State

3. Carrier ID#

4. HCPCS

5. Descriptor

6. Effective Date of Exclusion

7. End Date of Exclusion

8. Comments

Any exclusion list not provided in the CMS mandated format will be returned for correction. To view the presently mandated CMS format for this report, open the file located at: http://cms.hhs.gov/manuals/pm_trans/AB02_139a

100-2, 15, 50.4.2
Unlabeled Use of Drug
B3-2049.3

An unlabeled use of a drug is a use that is not included as an indication on the drug's label as approved by the FDA. FDA approved drugs used for indications other than what is indicated on the official label may be covered under Medicare if the carrier determines the use to be medically accepted, taking into consideration the major drug compendia, authoritative medical literature and/or accepted standards of medical practice. In the case of drugs used in an anti-cancer chemotherapeutic regimen, unlabeled uses are covered for a medically accepted indication as defined in Sec.50.5. These decisions are made by the contractor on a case-by-case basis.

100-2, 15, 50.4.4.2
Immunizations
Vaccinations or inoculations are excluded as immunizations unless they are directly related to the treatment of an injury or direct exposure to a disease or condition, such as anti-rabies treatment, tetanus antitoxin or booster vaccine, botulin antitoxin, antivenin sera, or immune globulin. In the absence of injury or direct exposure, preventive immunization (vaccination or inoculation) against such diseases as smallpox, polio, diphtheria, etc., is not covered. However, pneumococcal, hepatitis B, and influenza virus vaccines are exceptions to this rule. (See items A, B, and C below.) In cases where a vaccination or inoculation is excluded from coverage, related charges are also not covered.

A. Pneumococcal Pneumonia Vaccinations
Effective for services furnished on or after May 1, 1981, the Medicare Part B program covers pneumococcal pneumonia vaccine and its administration when furnished in compliance with any applicable State law by any provider of services or any entity or individual with a supplier number. This includes revaccination of patients at highest risk of pneumococcal infection. Typically, these vaccines are administered once in a lifetime except for persons at highest risk. Effective July 1, 2000, Medicare does not require for coverage purposes that a doctor of medicine or osteopathy order the vaccine. Therefore, the beneficiary may receive the vaccine upon request without a physician's order and without physician supervision.

An initial vaccine may be administered only to persons at high risk (see below) of pneumococcal disease. Revaccination may be administered only to persons at highest risk of serious pneumococcal infection and those likely to have a rapid decline in pneumococcal antibody levels, provided that at least 5 years have [passed since the previous dose of pneumococcal vaccine.

Persons at high risk for whom an initial vaccine may be administered include all people age 65 and older; immunocompetent adults who are at increased risk of pneumococcal disease or its complications because of chronic illness (e.g., cardiovascular disease, pulmonary disease, diabetes mellitus, alcoholism, cirrhosis, or cerebrospinal fluid leaks); and individuals with compromised immune

(e.g., splenic dysfunction or anatomic asplenia, Hodgkin's disease, lymphoma, multiple myeloma, chronic renal failure, HIV infection, nephrotic syndrome, sickle cell disease, or organ transplantation).

Persons at highest risk and those most likely to have rapid declines in antibody levels are those for whom revaccination may be appropriate. This group includes persons with functional or anatomic asplenia (e.g., sickle cell disease, splenectomy), HIV infection, leukemia, lymphoma, Hodgkin's disease, multiple myeloma, generalized malignancy, chronic renal failure, nephrotic syndrome, or other conditions associated with immunosuppression such as organ or bone marrow transplantation, and those receiving immunosuppressive chemotherapy. It is not appropriate for routine revaccination of people age 65 or older that are not at highest risk.

Those administering the vaccine should not require the patient to present an immunization record prior to administering the pneumococcal vaccine, nor should they feel compelled to review the patient's complete medical record if it is not available. Instead, provided that the patient is competent, it is acceptable to rely on the patient's verbal history to determine prior vaccination status. If the patient is uncertain about his or her vaccination history in the past 5 years, the vaccine should be given. However, if the patient is certain he/she was were vaccinated in the last 5 years, the vaccine should not be given. If the patient is certain that the vaccine was given more than 5 years ago, revaccination is covered only if the patient is at high risk.

B. Hepatitis B Vaccine
Effective for services furnished on or after September 1, 1984, P.L. 98-369 provides coverage under Part B for hepatitis B vaccine and its administration, furnished to a Medicare beneficiary who is at high or intermediate risk of contracting hepatitis B. This coverage is effective for services furnished on or after September 1, 1984. High-risk groups currently identified include (see exception below):

- ESRD patients;
- Hemophiliacs who receive Factor VIII or IX concentrates;
- Clients of institutions for the mentally retarded;
- Persons who live in the same household as a Hepatitis B Virus (HBV) carrier;
- Homosexual men; and
- Illicit injectable drug abusers; and
- Persons diagnosed with diabetes mellitus.

Intermediate risk groups currently identified include:

- Staff in institutions for the mentally retarded; and
- Workers in health care professions who have frequent contact with blood or blood-derived body fluids during routine work.

EXCEPTION: Persons in both of the above-listed groups in paragraph B, would not be considered at high or intermediate risk of contracting hepatitis B, however, if there were laboratory evidence positive for antibodies to hepatitis B. (ESRD patients are routinely tested for hepatitis B antibodies as part of their continuing monitoring and therapy.)

For Medicare program purposes, the vaccine may be administered upon the order of a doctor of medicine or osteopathy, by a doctor of medicine or osteopathy, or by home health agencies, skilled nursing facilities, ESRD facilities, hospital outpatient departments, and persons recognized under the incident to physicians' services provision of law.

A charge separate from the ESRD composite rate will be recognized and paid for administration of the vaccine to ESRD patients.

C. Influenza Virus Vaccine
Effective for services furnished on or after May 1, 1993, the Medicare Part B program covers influenza virus vaccine and its administration when furnished in compliance with any applicable State law by any provider of services or any entity or individual with a supplier number. Typically, these vaccines are administered once a flu season. Medicare does not require, for coverage purposes, that a doctor of medicine or osteopathy order the vaccine. Therefore, the beneficiary may receive the vaccine upon request without a physician's order and without physician supervision

100-2, 15, 100
Surgical Dressings, Splints, Casts, and Other Devices Used for Reductions of Fractures and Dislocations
B3-2079, A3-3110.3, HO-228.3

Surgical dressings are limited to primary and secondary dressings required for the treatment of a wound caused by, or treated by, a surgical procedure that has been performed by a physician or other health care professional to the extent permissible under State law. In addition, surgical dressings required after debridement of a wound are also covered, irrespective of the type of debridement, as long as the debridement was reasonable and necessary and was performed by a health care professional acting within the scope of his/her legal authority when performing this function. Surgical dressings are covered for as long as they are medically necessary. Primary dressings are therapeutic or protective coverings applied directly to wounds or lesions either on the skin or caused by an opening to the skin. Secondary dressing materials that serve a therapeutic or protective function and that are needed to secure a primary dressing are also covered. Items such as adhesive tape, roll gauze, bandages, and disposable compression material are examples of secondary dressings. Elastic stockings, support hose, foot coverings, leotards, knee supports, surgical leggings, gauntlets, and pressure garments for the arms and hands are examples of items that are not ordinarily covered as surgical dressings. Some items, such as transparent film, may be used as a primary or secondary dressing. If a physician, certified nurse midwife, physician assistant, nurse practitioner, or clinical nurse specialist applies surgical dressings as part of a professional service that is billed to Medicare, the surgical dressings are considered incident to the professional services of the health care practitioner. (See Sec. 60.1, 180, 190, 200, and 210.) When surgical dressings are not covered incident to the services of a health care practitioner and are obtained by the patient from a supplier (e.g., a drugstore, physician, or other health care practitioner that qualifies as a supplier) on an order from a physician or other health care professional authorized under State law or regulation to make such an order, the surgical dressings are covered separately under Part B. Splints and casts, and other devices used for reductions of fractures and dislocations are covered under Part B of Medicare. This includes dental splints.

100-2, 15, 110

Durable Medical Equipment - General

B3-2100, A3-3113, HO-235, HHA-220

Expenses incurred by a beneficiary for the rental or purchases of durable medical equipment (DME) are reimbursable if the following three requirements are met:

- The equipment meets the definition of DME (Sec.110.1);
- The equipment is necessary and reasonable for the treatment of the patient's illness or injury or to improve the functioning of his or her malformed body member (Sec.110.1); and
- The equipment is used in the patient's home. The decision whether to rent or purchase an item of equipment generally resides with the beneficiary, but the decision on how to pay rests with CMS. For some DME, program payment policy calls for lump sum payments and in others for periodic payment. Where covered DME is furnished to a beneficiary by a supplier of services other than a provider of services, the DMERC makes the reimbursement. If a provider of services furnishes the equipment, the intermediary makes the reimbursement. The payment method is identified in the annual fee schedule update furnished by CMS. The CMS issues quarterly updates to a fee schedule file that contains rates by HCPCS code and also identifies the classification of the HCPCS code within the following categories. Category Code Definition IN Inexpensive and Other Routinely Purchased Items FS Frequently Serviced Items CR Capped Rental Items OX Oxygen and Oxygen Equipment OS Ostomy, Tracheostomy & Urological Items SD Surgical Dressings PO Prosthetics & Orthotics SU Supplies TE Transcutaneous Electrical Nerve Stimulators The DMERCs, carriers, and intermediaries, where appropriate, use the CMS files to determine payment rules. See the Medicare Claims Processing Manual, Chapter 20, "Durable Medical Equipment, Surgical Dressings and Casts, Orthotics and Artificial Limbs, and Prosthetic Devices," for a detailed description of payment rules for each classification. Payment may also be made for repairs, maintenance, and delivery of equipment and for expendable and nonreusable items essential to the effective use of the equipment subject to the conditions in Sec.110.2. See the Medicare Benefit Policy Manual, Chapter 11, "End Stage Renal Disease," for hemodialysis equipment and supplies.

100-2, 15, 110.1

Definition of Durable Medical Equipment

B3-2100.1, A3-3113.1, HO-235.1, HHA-220.1, B3-2100.2, A3-3113.2, HO-235.2, HHA-220.2

- Durable medical equipment is equipment which:
- Can withstand repeated use;
- Is primarily and customarily used to serve a medical purpose;
- Generally is not useful to a person in the absence of an illness or injury; and
- Is appropriate for use in the home.

All requirements of the definition must be met before an item can be considered to be durable medical equipment. The following describes the underlying policies for determining whether an item meets the definition of DME and may be covered.

A. Durability

An item is considered durable if it can withstand repeated use, i.e., the type of item that could normally be rented. Medical supplies of an expendable nature, such as incontinent pads, lambs wool pads, catheters, ace bandages, elastic stockings, surgical facemasks, irrigating kits, sheets, and bags are not considered "durable" within the meaning of the definition. There are other items that, although durable in nature, may fall into other coverage categories such as supplies, braces, prosthetic devices, artificial arms, legs, and eyes.

B. Medical Equipment

Medical equipment is equipment primarily and customarily used for medical purposes and is not generally useful in the absence of illness or injury. In most instances, no development will be needed to determine whether a specific item of equipment is medical in nature. However, some cases will require development to determine whether the item constitutes medical equipment. This development would include the advice of local medical organizations (hospitals, medical schools, medical societies) and specialists in the field of physical medicine and rehabilitation. If the equipment is new on the market, it may be necessary, prior to seeking professional advice, to obtain information from the supplier or manufacturer explaining the design, purpose, effectiveness

and method of using the equipment in the home as well as the results of any tests or clinical studies that have been conducted.

1. Equipment Presumptively

    MedicalItems such as hospital beds, wheelchairs, hemodialysis equipment, iron lungs, respirators, intermittent positive pressure breathing machines, medical regulators, oxygen tents, crutches, canes, trapeze bars, walkers, inhalators, nebulizers, commodes, suction machines, and traction equipment presumptively constitute medical equipment. (Although hemodialysis equipment is covered as a prosthetic device (Sec.120), it also meets the definition of DME, and reimbursement for the rental or purchase of such equipment for use in the beneficiary's home will be made only under the provisions for payment applicable to DME. See the Medicare Benefit Policy Manual, Chapter 11, "End Stage Renal Disease," Sec.30.1, for coverage of home use of hemodialysis.) NOTE: There is a wide variety in types of respirators and suction machines. The DMERC's medical staff should determine whether the apparatus specified in the claim is appropriate for home use.

2. Equipment Presumptively Nonmedical

    Equipment which is primarily and customarily used for a nonmedical purpose may not be considered "medical" equipment for which payment can be made under the medical insurance program. This is true even though the item has some remote medically related use. For example, in the case of a cardiac patient, an air conditioner might possibly be used to lower room temperature to reduce fluid loss in the patient and to restore an environment conducive to maintenance of the proper fluid balance. Nevertheless, because the primary and customary use of an air conditioner is a nonmedical one, the air conditioner cannot be deemed to be medical equipment for which payment can be made. Other devices and equipment used for environmental control or to enhance the environmental setting in which the beneficiary is placed are not considered covered DME. These include, for example, room heaters, humidifiers, dehumidifiers, and electric air cleaners. Equipment which basically serves comfort or convenience functions or is primarily for the convenience of a person caring for the patient, such as elevators, stairway elevators, and posture chairs, do not constitute medical equipment. Similarly, physical fitness equipment (such as an exercycle), first-aid or precautionary-type equipment (such as preset portable oxygen units), self-help devices (such as safety grab bars), and training equipment (such as Braille training texts) are considered nonmedical in nature.

3. Special Exception Items

    Specified items of equipment may be covered under certain conditions even though they do not meet the definition of DME because they are not primarily and customarily used to serve a medical purpose and/or are generally useful in the absence of illness or injury. These items would be covered when it is clearly established that they serve a therapeutic purpose in an individual case and would include:

    a. Gel pads and pressure and water mattresses (which generally serve a preventive purpose) when prescribed for a patient who had bed sores or there is medical evidence indicating that they are highly susceptible to such ulceration; and

    b. Heat lamps for a medical rather than a soothing or cosmetic purpose, e.g., where the need for heat therapy has been established.

In establishing medical necessity for the above items, the evidence must show that the item is included in the physician's course of treatment and a physician is supervising its use.

NOTE: The above items represent special exceptions and no extension of coverage to other items should be inferred

C. Necessary and Reasonable

Although an item may be classified as DME, it may not be covered in every instance. Coverage in a particular case is subject to the requirement that the equipment be necessary and reasonable for treatment of an illness or injury, or to improve the functioning of a malformed body member. These considerations will bar payment for equipment which cannot reasonably be expected to perform a therapeutic function in an individual case or will permit only partial therapeutic function in an individual case or will permit only partial payment when the type of equipment furnished substantially exceeds that required for the treatment of the illness or injury involved. See the Medicare Claims Processing Manual, Chapter 1, "General Billing Requirements;" Sec.60, regarding the rules for providing advance beneficiary notices (ABNs) that advise beneficiaries, before items or services actually are furnished, when Medicare is likely to deny payment for them. ABNs allow beneficiaries to make an informed consumer decision about receiving items or services for which they may have to pay out-of-pocket and to be more active participants in their own health care treatment decisions.

1. Necessity for the Equipment

    Equipment is necessary when it can be expected to make a meaningful contribution to the treatment of the patient's illness or injury or to the improvement of his or her malformed body member. In most cases the physician's prescription for the equipment and other medical information available to the DMERC will be sufficient to establish that the equipment serves this purpose.

2. Reasonableness of the Equipment

   Even though an item of DME may serve a useful medical purpose, the DMERC or intermediary must also consider to what extent, if any, it would be reasonable for the Medicare program to pay for the item prescribed. The following considerations should enter into the determination of reasonableness:

   1. Would the expense of the item to the program be clearly disproportionate to the therapeutic benefits which could ordinarily be derived from use of the equipment?

   2. Is the item substantially more costly than a medically appropriate and realistically feasible alternative pattern of care?

   3. Does the item serve essentially the same purpose as equipment already available to the beneficiary?

3. Payment Consistent With What is Necessary and Reasonable

   Where a claim is filed for equipment containing features of an aesthetic nature or features of a medical nature which are not required by the patient's condition or where there exists a reasonably feasible and medically appropriate alternative pattern of care which is less costly than the equipment furnished, the amount payable is based on the rate for the equipment or alternative treatment which meets the patient's medical needs. The acceptance of an assignment binds the supplier-assignee to accept the payment for the medically required equipment or service as the full charge and the supplier-assignee cannot charge the beneficiary the differential attributable to the equipment actually furnished.

4. Establishing the Period of Medical Necessity

   Generally, the period of time an item of durable medical equipment will be considered to be medically necessary is based on the physician's estimate of the time that his or her patient will need the equipment. See the Medicare Program Integrity Manual, Chapters 5 and 6, for medical review guideline

D. Definition of a Beneficiary's Home

For purposes of rental and purchase of DME a beneficiary's home may be his/her own dwelling, an apartment, a relative's home, a home for the aged, or some other type of institution. However, an institution may not be considered a beneficiary's home if it:

- Meets at least the basic requirement in the definition of a hospital, i.e., it is primarily engaged in providing by or under the supervision of physicians, to inpatients, diagnostic and therapeutic services for medical diagnosis, treatment, and care of injured, disabled, and sick persons, or rehabilitation services for the rehabilitation of injured, disabled, or sick persons; or

- Meets at least the basic requirement in the definition of a skilled nursing facility, i.e., it is primarily engaged in providing to inpatients skilled nursing care and related services for patients who require medical or nursing care, or rehabilitation services for the rehabilitation of injured, disabled, or sick persons.

Thus, if an individual is a patient in an institution or distinct part of an institution which provides the services described in the bullets above, the individual is not entitled to have separate Part B payment made for rental or purchase of DME. This is because such an institution may not be considered the individual's home. The same concept applies even if the patient resides in a bed or portion of the institution not certified for Medicare.

If the patient is at home for part of a month and, for part of the same month is in an institution that cannot qualify as his or her home, or is outside the U.S., monthly payments may be made for the entire month. Similarly, if DME is returned to the provider before the end of a payment month because the beneficiary died in that month or because the equipment became unnecessary in that month, payment may be made for the entire month.

100-2, 15, 110.2

Repairs, Maintenance, Replacement, and Delivery

Under the circumstances specified below, payment may be made for repair, maintenance, and replacement of medically required DME, including equipment which had been in use before the user enrolled in Part B of the program. However, do not pay for repair, maintenance, or replacement of equipment in the frequent and substantial servicing or oxygen equipment payment categories. In addition, payments for repair and maintenance may not include payment for parts and labor covered under a manufacturer's or supplier's warranty.

A. Repairs

To repair means to fix or mend and to put the equipment back in good condition after damage or wear. Repairs to equipment which a beneficiary owns are covered when necessary to make the equipment serviceable. However, do not pay for repair of previously denied equipment or equipment in the frequent and substantial servicing or oxygen equipment payment categories. If the expense for repairs exceeds the estimated expense of purchasing or renting another item of

equipment for the remaining period of medical need, no payment can be made for the amount of the excess. (See subsection C where claims for repairs suggest malicious damage or culpable neglect.) Since renters of equipment recover from the rental charge the expenses they incur in maintaining in working order the equipment they rent out, separately itemized charges for repair of rented equipment are not covered. This includes items in the frequent and substantial servicing, oxygen equipment, capped rental, and inexpensive or routinely purchased payment categories which are being rented. A new Certificate of Medical Necessity (CMN) and/or physician's order is not needed for repairs. For replacement items, see Subsection C below.

B. Maintenance

Routine periodic servicing, such as testing, cleaning, regulating, and checking of the beneficiary's equipment, is not covered. The owner is expected to perform such routine maintenance rather than a retailer or some other person who charges the beneficiary. Normally, purchasers of DME are given operating manuals which describe the type of servicing an owner may perform to properly maintain the equipment. It is reasonable to expect that beneficiaries will perform this maintenance. Thus, hiring a third party to do such work is for the convenience of the beneficiary and is not covered. However, more extensive maintenance which, based on the manufacturers' recommendations, is to be performed by authorized technicians, is covered as repairs for medically necessary equipment which a beneficiary owns. This might include, for example, breaking down sealed components and performing tests which require specialized testing equipment not available to the beneficiary. Do not pay for maintenance of purchased items that require frequent and substantial servicing or oxygen equipment. Since renters of equipment recover from the rental charge the expenses they incur in maintaining in working order the equipment they rent out, separately itemized charges for maintenance of rented equipment are generally not covered. Payment may not be made for maintenance of rented equipment other than the maintenance and servicing fee established for capped rental items. For capped rental items which have reached the 15-month rental cap, contractors pay claims for maintenance and servicing fees after 6 months have passed from the end of the final paid rental month or from the end of the period the item is no longer covered under the supplier's or manufacturer's warranty, whichever is later. See the Medicare Claims Processing Manual, Chapter 20, "Durable Medical Equipment, Prosthetics and Orthotics, and Supplies (DMEPOS)," for additional instruction and an example. A new CMN and/or physician's order is not needed for covered maintenance.

C. Replacement

Replacement refers to the provision of an identical or nearly identical item. Situations involving the provision of a different item because of a change in medical condition are not addressed in this section.

Equipment which the beneficiary owns or is a capped rental item may be replaced in cases of loss or irreparable damage. Irreparable damage refers to a specific accident or to a natural disaster (e.g., fire, flood). A physician's order and/or new Certificate of Medical Necessity (CMN), when required, is needed to reaffirm the medical necessity of the item.

Irreparable wear refers to deterioration sustained from day-to-day usage over time and a specific event cannot be identified. Replacement of equipment due to irreparable wear takes into consideration the reasonable useful lifetime of the equipment. If the item of equipment has been in continuous use by the patient on either a rental or purchase basis for the equipment's useful lifetime, the beneficiary may elect to obtain a new piece of equipment. Replacement may be reimbursed when a new physician order and/or new CMN, when required, is needed to reaffirm the medical necessity of the item.

The reasonable useful lifetime of durable medical equipment is determined through program instructions. In the absence of program instructions, carriers may determine the reasonable useful lifetime of equipment, but in no case can it be less than 5 years. Computation of the useful lifetime is based on when the equipment is delivered to the beneficiary, not the age of the equipment. Replacement due to wear is not covered during the reasonable useful lifetime of the equipment. During the reasonable useful lifetime, Medicare does cover repair up to the cost of replacement (but not actual replacement) for medically necessary equipment owned by the beneficiary. (See subsection A.)

Charges for the replacement of oxygen equipment, items that require frequent and substantial servicing or inexpensive or routinely purchased items which are being rented are not covered. Cases suggesting malicious damage, culpable neglect, or wrongful disposition of equipment should be investigated and denied where the DMERC determines that it is unreasonable to make program payment under the circumstances. DMERCs refer such cases to the program integrity specialist in the RO.

D. Delivery

Payment for delivery of DME whether rented or purchased is generally included in the fee schedule allowance for the item. See Pub. 100-04, Medicare Claims Processing Manual, Chapter 20, "Durable Medical Equipment, Prosthetics and Orthotics, and Supplies (DMEPOS)," for the rules that apply to making reimbursement for exceptional cases.

100-2, 15, 110.3

Coverage of Supplies and Accessories

B3-2100.5, A3-3113.4, HO-235.4, HHA-220.5 B3-2100.5, A3-3113.4, HO-235.4, HHA-220.5

Payment may be made for supplies, e.g., oxygen, that are necessary for the effective use of durable medical equipment. Such supplies include those drugs and biologicals which must be put directly into the equipment in order to achieve the therapeutic benefit of the durable medical equipment or to assure the proper functioning of the equipment, e.g., tumor chemotherapy agents used with an infusion pump or heparin used with a home dialysis system. However, the coverage of such drugs or biologicals does not preclude the need for a determination that the drug or biological itself is reasonable and necessary for treatment of the illness or injury or to improve the functioning of a malformed body member. In the case of prescription drugs, other than oxygen, used in conjunction with durable medical equipment, prosthetic, orthotics, and supplies (DMEPOS) or prosthetic devices, the entity that dispenses the drug must furnish it directly to the patient for whom a prescription is written. The entity that dispenses the drugs must have a Medicare supplier number, must possess a current license to dispense prescription drugs in the State in which the drug is dispensed, and must bill and receive payment in its own name. A supplier that is not the entity that dispenses the drugs cannot purchase the drugs used in conjunction with DME for resale to the beneficiary. Reimbursement may be made for replacement of essential accessories such as hoses, tubes, mouthpieces, etc., for necessary DME, only if the beneficiary owns or is purchasing the equipment.Payment may be made for supplies, e.g., oxygen, that are necessary for the effective use of durable medical equipment. Such supplies include those drugs and biologicals which must be put directly into the equipment in order to achieve the therapeutic benefit of the durable medical equipment or to assure the proper functioning of the equipment, e.g., tumor chemotherapy agents used with an infusion pump or heparin used with a home dialysis system. However, the coverage of such drugs or biologicals does not preclude the need for a determination that the drug or biological itself is reasonable and necessary for treatment of the illness or injury or to improve the functioning of a malformed body member. In the case of prescription drugs, other than oxygen, used in conjunction with durable medical equipment, prosthetic, orthotics, and supplies (DMEPOS) or prosthetic devices, the entity that dispenses the drug must furnish it directly to the patient for whom a prescription is written. The entity that dispenses the drugs must have a Medicare supplier number, must possess a current license to dispense prescription drugs in the State in which the drug is dispensed, and must bill and receive payment in its own name. A supplier that is not the entity that dispenses the drugs cannot purchase the drugs used in conjunction with DME for resale to the beneficiary. Reimbursement may be made for replacement of essential accessories such as hoses, tubes, mouthpieces, etc., for necessary DME, only if the beneficiary owns or is purchasing the equipment.

100-2, 15, 120

Prosthetic Devices

B3-2130, A3-3110.4, HO-228.4, A3-3111, HO-229

A. General

Prosthetic devices (other than dental) which replace all or part of an internal body organ (including contiguous tissue), or replace all or part of the function of a permanently inoperative or malfunctioning internal body organ are covered when furnished on a physician's order. This does not require a determination that there is no possibility that the patient's condition may improve sometime in the future. If the medical record, including the judgment of the attending physician, indicates the condition is of long and indefinite duration, the test of permanence is considered met. (Such a device may also be covered under Sec.60.I as a supply when furnished incident to a physician's service.)

Examples of prosthetic devices include artificial limbs, parenteral and enteral (PEN) nutrition, cardiac pacemakers, prosthetic lenses (see subsection B), breast prostheses (including a surgical brassiere) for postmastectomy patients, maxillofacial devices, and devices which replace all or part of the ear or nose. A urinary collection and retention system with or without a tube is a prosthetic device replacing bladder function in case of permanent urinary incontinence. The foley catheter is also considered a prosthetic device when ordered for a patient with permanent urinary incontinence. However, chucks, diapers, rubber sheets, etc., are supplies that are not covered under this provision. Although hemodialysis equipment is a prosthetic device, payment for the rental or purchase of such equipment in the home is made only for use under the provisions for payment applicable to durable medical equipment.

An exception is that if payment cannot be made on an inpatient's behalf under Part A, hemodialysis equipment, supplies, and services required by such patient could be covered under Part B as a prosthetic device, which replaces the function of a kidney. See the Medicare Benefit Policy Manual, Chapter 11, "End Stage Renal Disease," for payment for hemodialysis equipment used in the home. See the Medicare Benefit Policy Manual, Chapter 1, "Inpatient Hospital Services," Sec.10, for additional instructions on hospitalization for renal dialysis.

NOTE: Medicare does not cover a prosthetic device dispensed to a patient prior to the time at which the patient undergoes the procedure that makes necessary the use of the device. For example, the carrier does not make a separate Part B payment for an intraocular lens (IOL) or pacemaker that a physician, during an office visit prior to the actual surgery, dispenses to the patient for his or her use. Dispensing a prosthetic device in this manner raises health and safety issues. Moreover, the need for the device cannot be clearly established until the procedure that makes its use possible is successfully performed. Therefore, dispensing a prosthetic device in this manner is not considered reasonable and necessary for the treatment of the patient's condition.

Colostomy (and other ostomy) bags and necessary accouterments required for attachment are covered as prosthetic devices. This coverage also includes irrigation and flushing equipment and other items and supplies directly related to ostomy care, whether the attachment of a bag is required.

Accessories and/or supplies which are used directly with an enteral or parenteral device to achieve the therapeutic benefit of the prosthesis or to assure the proper functioning of the device may also be covered under the prosthetic device benefit subject to the additional guidelines in the Medicare National Coverage Determinations Manual.

Covered items include catheters, filters, extension tubing, infusion bottles, pumps (either food or infusion), intravenous (I.V.) pole, needles, syringes, dressings, tape, Heparin Sodium (parenteral only), volumetric monitors (parenteral only), and parenteral and enteral nutrient solutions. Baby food and other regular grocery products that can be blenderized and used with the enteral system are not covered. Note that some of these items, e.g., a food pump and an I.V. pole, qualify as DME. Although coverage of the enteral and parenteral nutritional therapy systems is provided on the basis of the prosthetic device benefit, the payment rules relating to lump sum or monthly payment for DME apply to such items.

The coverage of prosthetic devices includes replacement of and repairs to such devices as explained in subsection D.

Finally, the Benefits Improvement and Protection Act of 2000 amended Sec.1834(h)(1) of the Act by adding a provision (1834 (h)(1)(G)(i)) that requires Medicare payment to be made for the replacement of prosthetic devices which are artificial limbs, or for the replacement of any part of such devices, without regard to continuous use or useful lifetime restrictions if an ordering physician determines that the replacement device, or replacement part of such a device, is necessary.

Payment may be made for the replacement of a prosthetic device that is an artificial limb, or replacement part of a device if the ordering physician determines that the replacement device or part is necessary because of any of the following:

1. A change in the physiological condition of the patient;

2. An irreparable change in the condition of the device, or in a part of the device; or

3. The condition of the device, or the part of the device, requires repairs and the cost of such repairs would be more than 60 percent of the cost of a replacement device, or, as the case may be, of the part being replaced.

This provision is effective for items replaced on or after April 1, 2001. It supersedes any rule that provided a 5-year or other replacement rule with regard to prosthetic devices.

B. Prosthetic Lenses

The term "internal body organ" includes the lens of an eye. Prostheses replacing the lens of an eye include post-surgical lenses customarily used during convalescence from eye surgery in which the lens of the eye was removed. In addition, permanent lenses are also covered when required by an individual lacking the organic lens of the eye because of surgical removal or congenital absence. Prosthetic lenses obtained on or after the beneficiary's date of entitlement to supplementary medical insurance benefits may be covered even though the surgical removal of the crystalline lens occurred before entitlement.

1. Prosthetic Cataract Lenses
   One of the following prosthetic lenses or combinations of prosthetic lenses furnished by a physician (see Sec.30.4 for coverage of prosthetic lenses prescribed by a doctor of optometry) may be covered when determined to be reasonable and necessary to restore essentially the vision provided by the crystalline lens of the eye:

   • Prosthetic bifocal lenses in frames;

   • Prosthetic lenses in frames for far vision, and prosthetic lenses in frames for near vision; or

   • When a prosthetic contact lens(es) for far vision is prescribed (including cases of binocular and monocular aphakia), make payment for the contact lens(es) and prosthetic lenses in frames for near vision to be worn at the same time as the contact lens(es), and prosthetic lenses in frames to be worn when the contacts have been removed.

   Lenses which have ultraviolet absorbing or reflecting properties may be covered, in lieu of payment for regular (untinted) lenses, if it has been determined that such lenses are medically reasonable and necessary for the individual patient. Medicare does not cover cataract sunglasses obtained in addition to the regular (untinted) prosthetic lenses since the sunglasses duplicate the restoration of vision function performed by the regular prosthetic lenses.

2. Payment for Intraocular Lenses (IOLs) Furnished in Ambulatory Surgical Centers (ASCs)
Effective for services furnished on or after March 12, 1990, payment for intraocular lenses (IOLs) inserted during or subsequent to cataract surgery in a Medicare certified ASC is included with the payment for facility services that are furnished in connection with the covered surgery. Refer to the Medicare Claims Processing Manual, Chapter 14, "Ambulatory Surgical Centers," for more information.

3. Limitation on Coverage of Conventional Lenses One pair of conventional eyeglasses or conventional contact lenses furnished after each cataract surgery with insertion of an IOL is covered.

C. Dentures

Dentures are excluded from coverage. However, when a denture or a portion of the denture is an integral part (built-in) of a covered prosthesis (e.g., an obturator to fill an opening in the palate), it is covered as part of that prosthesis.

D. Supplies, Repairs, Adjustments, and Replacement

Supplies are covered that are necessary for the effective use of a prosthetic device (e.g., the batteries needed to operate an artificial larynx). Adjustment of prosthetic devices required by wear or by a change in the patient's condition is covered when ordered by a physician. General provisions relating to the repair and replacement of durable medical equipment in Sec.110.2 for the repair and replacement of prosthetic devices are applicable. (See the Medicare Benefit Policy Manual, Chapter 16, "General Exclusions from Coverage," Sec.40.4, for payment for devices replaced under a warranty.) Replacement of conventional eyeglasses or contact lenses furnished in accordance with Sec.120.B.3 is not covered. Necessary supplies, adjustments, repairs, and replacements are covered even when the device had been in use before the user enrolled in Part B of the program, so long as the device continues to be medically required.

100-2, 15, 130

Leg, Arm, Back, and Neck Braces, Trusses, and Artificial Legs, Arms, and Eyes

B3-2133, A3-3110.5, HO-228.5, AB-01-06 dated 1/18/01

These appliances are covered under Part B when furnished incident to physicians' services or on a physician's order. A brace includes rigid and semi-rigid devices which are used for the purpose of supporting a weak or deformed body member or restricting or eliminating motion in a diseased or injured part of the body. Elastic stockings, garter belts, and similar devices do not come within the scope of the definition of a brace. Back braces include, but are not limited to, special corsets, e.g., sacroiliac, sacrolumbar, dorsolumbar corsets, and belts. A terminal device (e.g., hand or hook) is covered under this provision whether an artificial limb is required by the patient. Stump stockings and harnesses (including replacements) are also covered when these appliances are essential to the effective use of the artificial limb.

Adjustments to an artificial limb or other appliance required by wear or by a change in the patient's condition are covered when ordered by a physician.

Adjustments, repairs and replacements are covered even when the item had been in use before the user enrolled in Part B of the program so long as the device continues to be medically required.

100-2, 15, 140

Therapeutic Shoes for Individuals with Diabetes

B3-2134

Coverage of therapeutic shoes (depth or custom-molded) along with inserts for individuals with diabetes is available as of May 1, 1993. These diabetic shoes are covered if the requirements as specified in this section concerning certification and prescription are fulfilled. In addition, this benefit provides for a pair of diabetic shoes even if only one foot suffers from diabetic foot disease. Each shoe is equally equipped so that the affected limb, as well as the remaining limb, is protected. Claims for therapeutic shoes for diabetics are processed by the Durable Medical Equipment Regional Carriers (DMERCs). Therapeutic shoes for diabetics are not DME and are not considered DME nor orthotics, but a separate category of coverage under Medicare Part B. (See Sec.1861(s)(12) and Sec.1833(o) of the Act.)

A. Definitions

The following items may be covered under the diabetic shoe benefit:

1. Custom-Molded ShoesCustom-molded shoes are shoes that:

   - Are constructed over a positive model of the patient's foot;
   - Are made from leather or other suitable material of equal quality;
   - Have removable inserts that can be altered or replaced as the patient's condition warrants; and
   - Have some form of shoe closure.

2. Depth Shoes
Depth shoes are shoes that:

   - Have a full length, heel-to-toe filler that, when removed, provides a minimum of 3/16 inch of additional depth used to accommodate custom-molded or customized inserts;
   - Are made from leather or other suitable material of equal quality;
   - Have some form of shoe closure; and
   - Are available in full and half sizes with a minimum of three widths so that the sole is graded to the size and width of the upper portions of the shoes according to the American standard last sizing schedule or its equivalent. (The American standard last sizing schedule is the numerical shoe sizing system used for shoes sold in the United States.)

3. Inserts
Inserts are total contact, multiple density, removable inlays that are directly molded to the patient's foot or a model of the patient's foot and that are made of a suitable material with regard to the patient's condition.

B. Coverage

1. Limitations
For each individual, coverage of the footwear and inserts is limited to one of the following within one calendar year:

   - No more than one pair of custom-molded shoes (including inserts provided with such shoes) and two additional pairs of inserts; or
   - No more than one pair of depth shoes and three pairs of inserts (not including the noncustomized removable inserts provided with such shoes).

2. Coverage of Diabetic Shoes and Brace
Orthopedic shoes, as stated in the Medicare Claims Processing Manual, Chapter 20, "Durable Medical Equipment, Surgical Dressings and Casts, Orthotics and Artificial Limbs, and Prosthetic Devices," generally are not covered. This exclusion does not apply to orthopedic shoes that are an integral part of a leg brace. In situations in which an individual qualifies for both diabetic shoes and a leg brace, these items are covered separately. Thus, the diabetic shoes may be covered if the requirements for this section are met, while the brace may be covered if the requirements of Sec.130 are met.

3. Substitution of Modifications for Inserts
An individual may substitute modification(s) of custom-molded or depth shoes instead of obtaining a pair(s) of inserts in any combination. Payment for the modification(s) may not exceed the limit set for the inserts for which the individual is entitled. The following is a list of the most common shoe modifications available, but it is not meant as an exhaustive list of the modifications available for diabetic shoes:

Rigid Rocker Bottoms - These are exterior elevations with apex positions for 51 percent to 75 percent distance measured from the back end of the heel. The apex is a narrowed or pointed end of an anatomical structure. The apex must be positioned behind the metatarsal heads and tapered off sharply to the front tip of the sole. Apex height helps to eliminate pressure at the metatarsal heads. Rigidity is ensured by the steel in the shoe. The heel of the shoe tapers off in the back in order to cause the heel to strike in the middle of the heel;

   - Roller Bottoms (Sole or Bar) - These are the same as rocker bottoms, but the heel is tapered from the apex to the front tip of the sole;
   - Metatarsal Bars- An exterior bar is placed behind the metatarsal heads in order to remove pressure from the metatarsal heads. The bars are of various shapes, heights, and construction depending on the exact purpose;
   - Wedges (Posting) - Wedges are either of hind foot, fore foot, or both and may be in the middle or to the side. The function is to shift or transfer weight bearing upon standing or during ambulation to the opposite side for added support, stabilization, equalized weight distribution, or balance; and
   - Offset Heels- This is a heel flanged at its base either in the middle, to the side, or a combination, that is then extended upward to the shoe in order to stabilize extreme positions of the hind foot. Other modifications to diabetic shoes include, but are not limited to flared heels, Velcro closures, and inserts for missing toes.

4. Separate Inserts Inserts may be covered and dispensed independently of diabetic shoes if the supplier of the shoes verifies in writing that the patient has appropriate footwear into which the insert can be placed. This footwear must meet the definitions found above for depth shoes and custom-molded shoes.

C. Certification

The need for diabetic shoes must be certified by a physician who is a doctor of medicine or a doctor of osteopathy and who is responsible for diagnosing and treating the patient's diabetic systemic condition through a comprehensive plan of care. This managing physician must:

- Document in the patient's medical record that the patient has diabetes;

- Certify that the patient is being treated under a comprehensive plan of care for diabetes, and that the patient needs diabetic shoes; and

- Document in the patient's record that the patient has one or more of the following conditions:

- Peripheral neuropathy with evidence of callus formation;

  – History of pre-ulcerative calluses;

  – History of previous ulceration;

  – Foot deformity;

  – Previous amputation of the foot or part of the foot; or

  – Poor circulation.

D. Prescription

Following certification by the physician managing the patient's systemic diabetic condition, a podiatrist or other qualified physician who is knowledgeable in the fitting of diabetic shoes and inserts may prescribe the particular type of footwear necessary.

E. Furnishing

Footwear The footwear must be fitted and furnished by a podiatrist or other qualified individual such as a pedorthist, an orthotist, or a prosthetist. The certifying physician may not furnish the diabetic shoes unless the certifying physician is the only qualified individual in the area. It is left to the discretion of each carrier to determine the meaning of "in the area."

100-2, 15, 150

Dental Services

B3-2136

As indicated under the general exclusions from coverage, items and services in connection with the care, treatment, filling, removal, or replacement of teeth or structures directly supporting the teeth are not covered. "Structures directly supporting the teeth" means the periodontium, which includes the gingivae, dentogingival junction, periodontal membrane, cementum of the teeth, and alveolar process.

In addition to the following, see Pub 100-01, the Medicare General Information, Eligibility, and Entitlement Manual, Chapter 5, Definitions and Pub 3, the Medicare National Coverage Determinations Manual for specific services which may be covered when furnished by a dentist. If an otherwise noncovered procedure or service is performed by a dentist as incident to and as an integral part of a covered procedure or service performed by the dentist, the total service performed by the dentist on such an occasion is covered.

EXAMPLE 1: The reconstruction of a ridge performed primarily to prepare the mouth for dentures is a noncovered procedure. However, when the reconstruction of a ridge is performed as a result of and at the same time as the surgical removal of a tumor (for other than dental purposes), the totality of surgical procedures is a covered service.

EXAMPLE 2: Medicare makes payment for the wiring of teeth when this is done in connection with the reduction of a jaw fracture.

The extraction of teeth to prepare the jaw for radiation treatment of neoplastic disease is also covered. This is an exception to the requirement that to be covered, a noncovered procedure or service performed by a dentist must be an incident to and an integral part of a covered procedure or service performed by the dentist. Ordinarily, the dentist extracts the patient's teeth, but another physician, e.g., a radiologist, administers the radiation treatments.

When an excluded service is the primary procedure involved, it is not covered, regardless of its complexity or difficulty. For example, the extraction of an impacted tooth is not covered. Similarly, an alveoplasty (the surgical improvement of the shape and condition of the alveolar process) and a frenectomy are excluded from coverage when either of these procedures is performed in connection with an excluded service, e.g., the preparation of the mouth for dentures. In a like manner, the removal of a torus palatinus (a bony protuberance of the hard palate) may be a covered service. However, with rare exception, this surgery is performed in connection with an excluded service, i.e., the preparation of the mouth for dentures. Under such circumstances, Medicare does not pay for this procedure.

Dental splints used to treat a dental condition are excluded from coverage under 1862(a)(12) of the Act. On the other hand, if the treatment is determined to be a covered medical condition (i.e., dislocated upper/lower jaw joints), then the splint can be covered.

Whether such services as the administration of anesthesia, diagnostic x-rays, and other related procedures are covered depends upon whether the primary procedure being performed by the dentist is itself covered. Thus, an x-ray taken in connection with the reduction of a fracture of the jaw or facial bone is covered. However, a single x-ray or x-ray survey taken in connection with the care or treatment of teeth or the periodontium is not covered.

Medicare makes payment for a covered dental procedure no matter where the service is performed. The hospitalization or nonhospitalization of a patient has no direct bearing on the coverage or exclusion of a given dental procedure.

Payment may also be made for services and supplies furnished incident to covered dental services. For example, the services of a dental technician or nurse who is under the direct supervision of the dentist or physician are covered if the services are included in the dentist's or physician's bill.

100-2, 15, 150.1

Treatment of Temporomandibular Joint (TMJ) Syndrome

There are a wide variety of conditions that can be characterized as TMJ, and an equally wide variety of methods for treating these conditions. Many of the procedures fall within the Medicare program's statutory exclusion that prohibits payment for items and services that have not been demonstrated to be reasonable and necessary for the diagnosis and treatment of illness or injury (?1862(a)(1) of the Act). Other services and appliances used to treat TMJ fall within the Medicare program's statutory exclusion at 1862(a)(12), which prohibits payment "For services in connection with the care, treatment, filling, removal, or replacement of teeth or structures directly supporting teeth...." For these reasons, a diagnosis of TMJ on a claim is insufficient. The actual condition or symptom must be determined.

100-2, 15, 230

Practice of Physical Therapy, Occupational Therapy, and Speech-Language Pathology

A. Group Therapy Services.

Contractors pay for outpatient physical therapy services (which includes outpatient speech-language pathology services) and outpatient occupational therapy services provided simultaneously to two or more individuals by a practitioner as group therapy services (97150). The individuals can be, but need not be performing the same activity. The physician or therapist involved in group therapy services must be in constant attendance, but one-on-one patient contact is not required.

B. Therapy Students

1. General

   Only the services of the therapist can be billed and paid under Medicare Part B. The services performed by a student are not reimbursed even if provided under "line of sight" supervision of the therapist; however, the presence of the student "in the room" does not make the service unbillable. Pay for the direct (one-to-one) patient contact services of the physician or therapist provided to Medicare Part B patients. Group therapy services performed by a therapist or physician may be billed when a student is also present "in the room".

   EXAMPLES:

   Therapists may bill and be paid for the provision of services in the following scenarios:

   - The qualified practitioner is present and in the room for the entire session. The student participates in the delivery of services when the qualified practitioner is directing the service, making the skilled judgment, and is responsible for the assessment and treatment.

   - The qualified practitioner is present in the room guiding the student in service delivery when the therapy student and the therapy assistant student are participating in the provision of services, and the practitioner is not engaged in treating another patient or doing other tasks at the same time

   - The qualified practitioner is responsible for the services and as such, signs all documentation. (A student may, of course, also sign but it is not necessary since the Part B payment is for the clinician's service, not for the student's services.)

2. Therapy Assistants as Clinical Instructors

   Physical therapist assistants and occupational therapy assistants are not precluded from serving as clinical instructors for therapy students, while providing services within their scope of work and performed under the direction and supervision of a licensed physical or occupational therapist to a Medicare beneficiary.

3. Services Provided Under Part A and Part B

   The payment methodologies for Part A and B therapy services rendered by a student are different. Under the MPFS (Medicare Part B), Medicare pays for services provided by physicians and practitioners that are specifically authorized by statute. Students do not meet the definition of practitioners under Medicare Part B. Under SNF PPS, payments are based upon the case mix or Resource Utilization Group (RUG) category that describes the patient. In the rehabilitation groups, the number of therapy minutes delivered to the patient determines the RUG category. Payment levels for each category are based upon the costs of caring for patients in each group rather than providing pecific payment for each therapy service as is done in Medicare Part B.

100-2, 15, 231

Pulmonary Rehabilitation (PR) Program Services Furnished On or After January 1, 2010

A pulmonary rehabilitation (PR) program is typically a physician-supervised, multidisciplinary program individually tailored and designed to optimize physical and social performance and autonomy of care for patients with chronic respiratory impairment. The main goal is to empower the individuals' ability to exercise independently. Exercise is combined with other training and support mechanisms to encourage long-term adherence to the treatment plan. Effective January 1, 2010, Medicare Part B pays for PR programs and related items and services if specific criteria is met by the Medicare beneficiary, the PR program itself, the setting in which it is administered, and the physician administering the program, as outlined below:

PR Program Beneficiary Requirements:

- As specified in 42 CFR 410.47, Medicare covers PR items and services for patients with moderate to very severe chronic obstructive pulmonary disease (COPD) (defined as GOLD classification II, III, and IV), when referred by the physician treating the chronic respiratory disease. Additional medical indications for coverage for PR program services may be established through the national coverage determination process.

PR Program Component Requirements:

- Physician-prescribed exercise. This physical activity includes techniques such as exercise conditioning, breathing retraining, and step and strengthening exercises. Some aerobic exercise must be included in each PR session. Both low- and high- intensity exercise is recommended to produce clinical benefits and a combination of endurance and strength training should be conducted at least twice per week.

- Education or training. This should be closely and clearly related to the individual's care and treatment and tailored to the individual's needs, including information on respiratory problem management and, if appropriate, brief smoking cessation counseling. Any education or training must assist in achievement of individual goals towards independence in activities of daily living, adaptation to limitations, and improved quality of life (QoL).

- Psychosocial assessment. This assessment means a written evaluation of an individual's mental and emotional functioning as it relates to the individual's rehabilitation or respiratory condition. It should include: (1) an assessment of those aspects of the individual's family and home situation that affects the individual's rehabilitation treatment, and, (2) a psychological evaluation of the individual's response to, and rate of progress under, the treatment plan. Periodic re-evaluations are necessary to ensure the individual's psychosocial needs are being met.

- Outcomes assessment. These should include: (1) beginning and end evaluations based on patient-centered outcomes, which are conducted by the physician at the start and end of the program, and, (2) objective clinical measures of the effectiveness of the PR program for the individual patient, including exercise performance and self-reported measures of shortness of breath, and behavior. The assessments should include clinical measures such as the 6-minute walk, weight, exercise performance, self-reported dyspnea, behavioral measures (supplemental oxygen use, smoking status,) and a QoL assessment.

- An individualized treatment plan describing the individual's diagnosis and detailing how components are utilized for each patient. The plan must be established, reviewed, and signed by a physician every 30 days. The plan may initially be developed by the referring physician or the PR physician. If the plan is developed by the referring physician who is not the PR physician, the PR physician must also review and sign the plan prior to imitation of the PR program. It is expected that the supervising physician would have initial, direct contact with the individual prior to subsequent treatment by ancillary personnel, and also have at least one direct contact in each 30-day period. The plan must have written specificity with regards to the type, amount, frequency, and duration of PR items and services furnished to the individual, and specify the appropriate mix of services for the patient's needs. It must include measurable and expected outcomes and estimated timetables to achieve these outcomes.

As specified at 42 CFR 410.47(f), PR program sessions are limited to a maximum of 2 1-hour sessions per day for up to 36 sessions, with the option for an additional 36 sessions if medically necessary.

PR Program Setting Requirements:

PR items and services must be furnished in a physician's office or a hospital outpatient setting. The setting must have the necessary cardio-pulmonary, emergency, diagnostic, and therapeutic life-saving equipment accepted by the medical community as medically necessary (for example, oxygen , cardiopulmonary resuscitation equipment, and a defibrillator) to treat chronic respiratory disease. All settings must have a physician immediately available and accessible for medical consultations and emergencies at all times that the PR items and services are being furnished under the program. This provision is satisfied if the physician meets the requirements for direct supervision of physician office services as specified at 42 CFR 410.26, and for hospital outpatient therapeutic services as specified at 42 CFR 410.27.

PR Program Physician Requirements:

Medicare Part B pays for PR services supervised by a physician only if the physician meets all of the following requirements: (1) expertise in the management of individuals with respiratory pathophysiology, (2) licensed to practice medicine in the state in which the PR program is offered, (3) responsible and accountable for the PR program, and, (4) involved substantially, in consultation with staff, in directing the progress of the individual in the PR program.

(See Publication 100-04, Claims Processing Manual, chapter 32, section 140.4, for specific claims processing, coding, and billing requirements for PR program services.)

100-2, 15, 232

Cardiac Rehabilitation (CR) and Intensive Cardiac Rehabilitation (ICR) Services Furnished On or After January 1, 2010

Cardiac rehabilitation (CR) services mean a physician-supervised program that furnishes physician prescribed exercise, cardiac risk factor modification, including education, counseling, and behavioral intervention; psychosocial assessment, outcomes assessment, and other items/services as determined by the Secretary under certain conditions. Intensive cardiac rehabilitation (ICR) services mean a physician-supervised program that furnishes the same items/services under the same conditions as a CR program but must also demonstrate, as shown in peer-reviewed published research, that it improves patients' cardiovascular disease through specific outcome measurements described in 42 CFR 410.49(c). Effective January 1, 2010, Medicare Part B pays for CR/ICR programs and related items/services if specific criteria is met by the Medicare beneficiary, the CR/ICR program itself, the setting in which is it administered, and the physician administering the program, as outlined below:

CR/ICR Program Beneficiary Requirements:

- Medicare covers CR/ICR program services for beneficiaries who have experienced one or more of the following:

- Acute myocardial infarction within the preceding 12 months;

- Coronary artery bypass surgery;

- Current stable angina pectoris;

- Heart valve repair or replacement;

- Percutaneous transluminal coronary angioplasty (PTCA) or coronary stenting;

- Heart or heart-lung transplant.

For CR only, other cardiac conditions as specified through a national coverage determination (NCD).

CR/ICR Program Component Requirements:

Physician-prescribed exercise. This physical activity includes aerobic exercise combined with other types of exercise (i.e., strengthening, stretching) as determined to be appropriate for individual patients by a physician each day CR/ICR items/services are furnished.

Cardiac risk factor modification. This includes education, counseling, and behavioral intervention, tailored to the patients' individual needs.

Psychosocial assessment. This assessment means an evaluation of an individual's mental and emotional functioning as it relates to the individual's rehabilitation. It should include: (1) an assessment of those aspects of the individual's family and home situation that affects the individual's rehabilitation treatment, and, (2) a psychosocial evaluation of the individual's response to, and rate of progress under, the treatment plan.

Outcomes assessment. These should include: (i) minimally, assessments from the commencement and conclusion of CR/ICR, based on patient-centered outcomes which must be measured by the physician immediately at the beginning and end of the program, and, (ii) objective clinical measures of the effectiveness of the CR/ICR program for the individual patient, including exercise performance and self-reported measures of exertion and behavior.

Individualized treatment plan. This plan should be written and tailored to each individual patient and include (i) a description of the individual's diagnosis; (ii) the type, amount, frequency, and duration of the CR/ICR items/services furnished; and (iii) the goals set for the individual under the plan. The individualized treatment plan must be established, reviewed, and signed by a physician every 30 days.

As specified at 42 CFR 410.49(f)(1), CR sessions are limited to a maximum of 2 1-hour sessions per day for up to 36 sessions over up to 36 weeks with the option for an additional 36 sessions over an extended period of time if approved by the contractor under section 1862(a)(1)(A) of the Act. ICR sessions are limited to 72 1-hour sessions (as defined in section 1848(b)(5) of the Act), up to 6 sessions per day, over a period of up to 18 weeks.

CR/ICR Program Setting Requirements:

CR/ICR services must be furnished in a physician's office or a hospital outpatient setting (for ICR, the hospital outpatient setting must provide ICR using an approved ICR program). All settings must have a physician immediately available and accessible for medical consultations and emergencies at all times when items/services are being furnished under the program. This provision is satisfied if the physician meets the requirements for direct supervision of physician office services as specified at 42 CFR 410.26, and for hospital outpatient services as specified at 42 CFR 410.27.

ICR Program Approval Requirements:

All prospective ICR programs must be approved through the national coverage determination (NCD) process. To be approved as an ICR program, it must demonstrate through peer-reviewed, published research that it has accomplished one or more of the following for its patients: (i) positively affected the progression of coronary heart disease, (ii) reduced the need for coronary bypass surgery, or, (iii) reduced the need for percutaneous coronary interventions.

An ICR program must also demonstrate through peer-reviewed, published research that it accomplished a statistically significant reduction in five or more of the following measures for patients from their levels before CR services to after CR services: (i) low density lipoprotein, (ii) triglycerides, (iii) body mass index, (iv) systolic blood pressure, (v) diastolic blood pressure, and (vi) the need for cholesterol, blood pressure, and diabetes medications.

A list of approved ICR programs, identified through the NCD process, will be posted to the CMS Web site and listed in the Federal Register.

Once an ICR program is approved through the NCD process, all prospective ICR sites wishing to furnish ICR items/services via an approved ICR program may enroll with their local contractor to become an ICR program supplier using the designated forms as specified at 42 CFR 424.510, and report specialty code 31 to be identified as an enrolled ICR supplier. For purposes of appealing an adverse determination concerning site approval, an ICR site is considered a supplier (or prospective supplier) as defined in 42 CFR 498.2.

CR/ICR Program Physician Requirements:

Physicians responsible for CR/ICR programs are identified as medical directors who oversee or supervise the CR/ICR program at a particular site. The medical director, in consultation with staff, is involved in directing the progress of individuals in the program. The medical director, as well as physicians acting as the supervising physician, must possess all of the following: (1) expertise in the management of individuals with cardiac pathophysiology, (2) cardiopulmonary training in basic life support or advanced cardiac life support, and (3) licensed to practice medicine in the state in which the CR/ICR program is offered. Direct physician supervision may be provided by a supervising physician or the medical director.

(See Pub. 100-04, Medicare Claims Processing Manual, chapter 32, section 140.2, for specific claims processing, coding, and billing requirements for CR/ICR program services.)

100-2, 15, 270

Telehealth Services

Background

Section 223 of the Medicare, Medicaid and SCHIP Benefits Improvement and Protection Act of 2000 (BIPA) - Revision of Medicare Reimbursement for Telehealth Services amended §1834 of the Act to provide for an expansion of Medicare payment for telehealth services.

Effective October 1, 2001, coverage and payment for Medicare telehealth includes consultation, office visits, individual psychotherapy, and pharmacologic management delivered via a telecommunications system. Eligible geographic areas include rural health professional shortage areas (HPSA) and counties not classified as a metropolitan statistical area (MSA). Additionally, Federal telemedicine demonstration projects as of December 31, 2000, may serve as the originating site regardless of geographic location.

An interactive telecommunications system is required as a condition of payment; however, BIPA does allow the use of asynchronous "store and forward" technology in delivering these services when the originating site is a Federal telemedicine demonstration program in Alaska or Hawaii. BIPA does not require that a practitioner present the patient for interactive telehealth services.

With regard to payment amount, BIPA specified that payment for the professional service performed by the distant site practitioner (i.e., where the expert physician or practitioner is physically located at time of telemedicine encounter) is equal to what would have been paid without the use of telemedicine. Distant site practitioners include only a physician as described in §1861(r) of the Act and a medical practitioner as described in §1842(b)(18)(C) of the Act. BIPA also expanded payment under Medicare to include a $20 originating site facility fee (location of beneficiary).

Previously, the Balanced Budget Act of 1997 (BBA) limited the scope of Medicare telehealth coverage to consultation services and the implementing regulation prohibited the use of an asynchronous 'store and forward' telecommunications system. The BBA of 1997 also required the

professional fee to be shared between the referring and consulting practitioners, and prohibited Medicare payment for facility fees and line charges associated with the telemedicine encounter.

The BIPA required that Medicare Part B (Supplementary Medical Insurance) pay for this expansion of telehealth services beginning with services furnished on October 1, 2001.

Section 149 of the Medicare Improvements for Patients and Providers Act of 2008 (MIPPA) amended §1834(m) of the Act to add certain entities as originating sites for payment of telehealth services. Effective for services furnished on or after January 1, 2009, eligible originating sites include a hospital-based or critical access hospital-based renal dialysis center (including satellites); a skilled nursing facility (as defined in §1819(a) of the Act); and a community mental health center (as defined in §1861(ff)(3)(B) of the Act). MIPPA also amended§1888(e)(2)(A)(ii) of the Act to exclude telehealth services furnished under §1834(m)(4)(C)(ii)(VII) from the consolidated billing provisions of the skilled nursing facility prospective payment system (SNF PPS).

NOTE: MIPPA did not add independent renal dialysis facilities as originating sites for payment of telehealth services.

The telehealth provisions authorized by §1834(m) of the Act are implemented in 42 CFR 410.78 and 414.65.

100-2, 15, 270.2

List of Medicare Telehealth Services

The use of a telecommunications system may substitute for an in-person encounter for professional consultations, office visits, office psychiatry services, and a limited number of other physician fee schedule (PFS) services. These services are listed below.

- Consultations (Effective October 1, 2001- December 31, 2009)
- Telehealth consultations, emergency department or initial inpatient (Effective January 1, 2010)
- Follow-up inpatient telehealth consultations (Effective January 1, 2009)
- Office or other outpatient visits
- Subsequent hospital care services (with the limitation of one telehealth visit every 3 days) (Effective January 1, 2011)
- Subsequent nursing facility care services (with the limitation of one telehealth visit every 30 days) (Effective January 1, 2011)
- Individual psychotherapy
- Pharmacologic management (Effective March 1, 2003 – December 31, 2012)
- Psychiatric diagnostic interview examination (Effective March 1, 2003)
- End stage renal disease related services (Effective January 1, 2005)
- Individual and group medical nutrition therapy (Individual effective January 1, 2006; group effective January 1, 2011)
- Neurobehavioral status exam (Effective January 1, 2008)
- Individual and group health and behavior assessment and intervention (Individual effective January 1, 2010; group effective January 1, 2011)
- Individual and group kidney disease education (KDE) services (Effective January 1, 2011)
- Individual and group diabetes self-management training (DSMT) services (with a minimum of 1 hour of in-person instruction to be furnished in the initial year training period to ensure effective injection training) (Effective January 1, 2011)
- Smoking Cessation Services (Effective January 1, 2012)
- Alcohol and/or substance (other than tobacco) abuse structured assessment and intervention services (Effective January 1, 2013)
- Annual alcohol misuse screening (Effective January 1, 2013)
- Brief face-to-face behavioral counseling for alcohol misuse (Effective January 1, 2013).
- Annual Depression Screening (Effective January 1, 2013)
- High-intensity behavioral counseling to prevent sexually transmitted infections (Effective January 1, 2013)
- Annual, face-to-face Intensive behavioral therapy for cardiovascular disease (Effective January 1, 2013)
- Face-to-face behavioral counseling for obesity (Effective January 1, 2013)

NOTE: Beginning January 1, 2010, CMS eliminated the use of all consultation codes, except for inpatient telehealth consultation G-codes. CMS no longer recognizes office/outpatient or inpatient consultation CPT codes for payment of office/outpatient or inpatient visits. Instead, physicians and practitioners are instructed to bill a new or established patient office/outpatient visit CPT code or appropriate hospital or nursing facility care code, as appropriate to the particular patient, for all office/outpatient or inpatient visits. For detailed instructions regarding reporting these and other telehealth services, see Pub. 100-04, Medicare Claims Processing Manual, chapter 12, section 190.3.

The conditions of payment for Medicare telehealth services, including qualifying originating sites and the types of telecommunications systems recognized by Medicare, are subject to the provisions of 42 CFR 410.78. Payment for these services is subject to the provisions of 42 CFR 414.65.

100-2, 15, 270.4.3

Payment for Diabetes Self-Management Training (DSMT) as a Telehealth Service

Payment for Diabetes Self-Management Training (DSMT) as a Telehealth Service

Individual and group DSMT services may be paid as a Medicare telehealth service; however, at least 1 hour of the 10 hour benefit in the year following the initial DSMT service must be furnished in-person to allow for effective injection training. The injection training may be furnished through either individual or group DSMT services. By reporting the –GT or –GQ modifier with HCPCS code G0108 (Diabetes outpatient self-management training services, individual, per 30 minutes) or G0109 Diabetes outpatient self-management training services, group session (2 or more), per 30 minutes), the distant site practitioner certifies that the beneficiary has received or will receive 1 hour of in-person DSMT services for purposes of injection training during the year following the initial DSMT service.

As specified in 42 CFR 410.141(e) and stated in section 300.2 of this chapter, individual DSMT services may be furnished by a physician, individual, or entity that furnishes other services for which direct Medicare payment may be made and that submits necessary documentation to, and is accredited by, an accreditation organization approved by CMS. However, consistent with the statutory requirements of section 1834(m)(1) of the Act, as provided in 42 CFR 410.78(b)(1) and (b)(2) and stated in section 270.4 of this chapter, Medicare telehealth services, including individual DSMT services furnished as a telehealth service, could only be furnished by a licensed physician assistant (PA), nurse practitioner (NP), clinical nurse specialist (CNS), certified nurse-midwife (CNM), clinical psychologist, clinical social worker, or registered dietitian or nutrition professional.

100-2, 15, 280.1

Glaucoma Screening

A. Conditions of Coverage

The regulations implementing the Benefits Improvements and Protection Act of 2000, Sec.102, provide for annual coverage for glaucoma screening for beneficiaries in the following high risk categories:

- Individuals with diabetes mellitus;
- Individuals with a family history of glaucoma; or
- African-Americans age 50 and over. In addition, beginning with dates of service on or after January 1, 2006, 42 CFR 410.23(a)(2), revised, the definition of an eligible beneficiary in a high-risk category is expanded to include:
- Hispanic-Americans age 65 and over.

Medicare will pay for glaucoma screening examinations where they are furnished by or under the direct supervision in the office setting of an ophthalmologist or optometrist, who is legally authorized to perform the services under State law. Screening for glaucoma is defined to include:

- A dilated eye examination with an intraocular pressure measurement; and
- A direct ophthalmoscopy examination, or a slit-lamp biomicroscopic examination.

Payment may be made for a glaucoma screening examination that is performed on an eligible beneficiary after at least 11 months have passed following the month in which the last covered glaucoma screening examination was performed.

The following HCPCS codes apply for glaucoma screening:

G0117   Glaucoma screening for high-risk patients furnished by an optometrist or ophthalmologist; and

G0118   Glaucoma screening for high-risk patients furnished under the direct supervision of an optometrist or ophthalmologist.

The type of service for the above G codes is: TOS Q.

For providers who bill intermediaries, applicable types of bill for screening glaucoma services are 13X, 22X, 23X, 71X, 73X, 75X, and 85X. The following revenue codes should be reported when billing for screening glaucoma services:

- Comprehensive outpatient rehabilitation facilities (CORFs), critical access hospitals (CAHs), skilled nursing facilities (SNFs), independent and provider-based RHCs and free standing

and provider-based FQHCs bill for this service under revenue code 770. CAHs electing the optional method of payment for outpatient services report this service under revenue codes 96X, 97X, or 98X.

- Hospital outpatient departments bill for this service under any valid/appropriate revenue code. They are not required to report revenue code 770.

B. Calculating the Frequency

Once a beneficiary has received a covered glaucoma screening procedure, the beneficiary may receive another procedure after 11 full months have passed. To determine the 11-month period, start the count beginning with the month after the month in which the previous covered screening procedure was performed.

C. Diagnosis Coding Requirements

Providers bill glaucoma screening using screening ("V") code V80.1 (Special Screening for Neurological, Eye, and Ear Diseases, Glaucoma). Claims submitted without a screening diagnosis code may be returned to the provider as unprocessable.

D. Payment Methodology

1.   Carriers

    Contractors pay for glaucoma screening based on the Medicare physician fee schedule. Deductible and coinsurance apply. Claims from physicians or other providers where assignment was not taken are subject to the Medicare limiting charge (refer to the Medicare Claims Processing Manual, Chapter 12, "Physician/Non-physician Practitioners," for more information about the Medicare limiting charge).

2.   Intermediaries

    Payment is made for the facility expense as follows:

- Independent and provider-based RHC/free standing and provider-based FQHC - payment is made under the all inclusive rate for the screening glaucoma service based on the visit furnished to the RHC/FQHC patient;
- CAH - payment is made on a reasonable cost basis unless the CAH has elected the optional method of payment for outpatient services in which case, procedures outlined in the Medicare Claims Processing Manual, Chapter 3, Sec.30.1.1, should be followed;
- CORF - payment is made under the Medicare physician fee schedule;
- Hospital outpatient department - payment is made under outpatient prospective payment system (OPPS);
- Hospital inpatient Part B - payment is made under OPPS;
- SNF outpatient - payment is made under the Medicare physician fee schedule (MPFS); and
- SNF inpatient Part B - payment is made under MPFS. Deductible and coinsurance apply.

E. Special Billing Instructions for RHCs and FQHCs

Screening glaucoma services are considered RHC/FQHC services. RHCs and FQHCs bill the contractor under bill type 71X or 73X along with revenue code 770 and HCPCS codes G0117 or G0118 and RHC/FQHC revenue code 520 or 521 to report the related visit. Reporting of revenue code 770 and HCPCS codes G0117 and G0118 in addition to revenue code 520 or 521 is required for this service in order for CWF to perform frequency editing.

Payment should not be made for a screening glaucoma service unless the claim also contains a visit code for the service. Therefore, the contractor installs an edit in its system to assure payment is not made for revenue code 770 unless the claim also contains a visit revenue code (520 or 521).

100-2, 15, 280.5

Annual Wellness Visit (AWV) Providing Personalized Prevention Plan Services (PPPS)

A. General

Pursuant to section 4103 of the Affordable Care Act of 2010 (the ACA), the Centers for Medicare & Medicaid Services (CMS) amended section 411.15(a)(1) and 411.15(k)(15) of the Code of Federal Regulations (CFR)(list of examples of routine physical examinations excluded from coverage), effective for services furnished on or after January 1, 2011. This expanded coverage, as established at 42 CFR 410.15, is subject to certain eligibility and other limitations that allow payment for an annual wellness visit (AWV), providing personalized prevention plan services (PPPS), when performed by a qualified health professional (as defined in this section), for an individual who is no longer within 12 months after the effective date of his/her first Medicare Part B coverage period, and has not received either an initial preventive physical examination (IPPE) or an AWV within the past 12 months. Medicare coinsurance and Part B deductibles do not apply.

The AWV will include the establishment of, or update to, the individual's medical/family history, measurement of his/her height, weight, body-mass index (BMI) or waist circumference, and blood pressure (BP), with the goal of health promotion and disease detection and encouraging patients to obtain the screening and preventive services that may already be covered and paid for under Medicare Part B. Definitions relative to the AWV are included below.

Coverage is available for an AWV that meets the following requirements:

1. It is performed by a health professional; and,

2. It is furnished to an eligible beneficiary who is no longer within 12 months after the effective date of his/her first Medicare Part B coverage period, and he/she has not received either an IPPE or an AWV providing PPPS within the past 12 months.

Sections 4103 and 4104 of the ACA also provide for a waiver of the Medicare coinsurance and Part B deductible requirements for an AWV effective for services furnished on or after January 1, 2011.

B. Definitions Relative to the AWV:

Detection of any cognitive impairment: The assessment of an individual's cognitive function by direct observation, with due consideration of information obtained by way of patient reports, concerns raised by family members, friends, caretakers, or others.

Eligible beneficiary: An individual who is no longer within 12 months after the effective date of his/her first Medicare Part B coverage period and who has not received either an IPPE or an AWV providing PPPS within the past 12 months.

Establishment of, or an update to, the individual's medical/family history: At a minimum, the collection and documentation of the following:

a. Past medical and surgical history, including experiences with illnesses, hospital stays, operations, allergies, injuries, and treatments.

b. Use or exposure to medications and supplements, including calcium and vitamins.

c. Medical events in the beneficiary's parents and any siblings and children, including diseases that may be hereditary or place the individual at increased risk.

First AWV providing PPPS: The provision of the following services to an eligible beneficiary by a health professional that include, and take into account the results of, a health risk assessment as those terms are defined in this section:

a. Review (and administration if needed) of a health risk assessment (as defined in this section).

b. Establishment of an individual's medical/family history.

c. Establishment of a list of current providers and suppliers that are regularly involved in providing medical care to the individual.

d. Measurement of an individual's height, weight, BMI (or waist circumference, if appropriate), BP, and other routine measurements as deemed appropriate, based on the beneficiary's medical/family history.

e. Detection of any cognitive impairment that the individual may have as defined in this section.

f. Review of the individual's potential (risk factors) for depression, including current or past experiences with depression or other mood disorders, based on the use of an appropriate screening instrument for persons without a current diagnosis of depression, which the health professional may select from various available standardized screening tests designed for this purpose and recognized by national medical professional organizations.

g. Review of the individual's functional ability and level of safety based on direct observation, or the use of appropriate screening questions or a screening questionnaire, which the health professional may select from various available screening questions or standardized questionnaires designed for this purpose and recognized by national professional medical organizations.

h. Establishment of the following:

(1) A written screening schedule for the individual, such as a checklist for the next 5 to 10 years, as appropriate, based on recommendations of the United States Preventive Services Task Force (USPSTF) and the Advisory Committee on Immunization Practices (ACIP), and the individual's health risk assessment (as that term is defined in this section), the individual's health status, screening history, and age-appropriate preventive services covered by Medicare.

(2) A list of risk factors and conditions for which primary, secondary, or tertiary interventions are recommended or are underway for the individual, including any mental health conditions or any such risk factors or conditions that have been identified through an IPPE, and a list of treatment options and their associated risks and benefits.

i. Furnishing of personalized health advice to the individual and a referral, as appropriate, to health education or preventive counseling services or programs aimed at reducing identified risk factors and improving self-management, or community-based lifestyle interventions to reduce health risks and promote self-management and wellness, including weight loss, physical activity, smoking cessation, fall prevention, and nutrition.

j. Any other element determined appropriate through the National Coverage Determination (NCD) process.

Health professional:

a. A physician who is a doctor of medicine or osteopathy (as defined in section 1861(r)(1) of the Social Security Act (the Act); or,

b. A physician assistant, nurse practitioner, or clinical nurse specialist (as defined in section 1861(aa)(5) of the Act); or,

c. A medical professional (including a health educator, registered dietitian, or nutrition professional or other licensed practitioner) or a team of such medical professionals, working under the direct supervision (as defined in 42CFR 410.32(b)(3)(ii)) of a physician as defined in this section.

Health Risk Assessment means, for the purposes of the annual wellness visit, an evaluation tool that meets the following criteria:

a. collects self-reported information about the beneficiary.

b. can be administered independently by the beneficiary or administered by a health professional prior to or as part of the AWV encounter.

c. is appropriately tailored to and takes into account the communication needs of underserved populations, persons with limited English proficiency, and persons with health literacy needs.

d. takes no more than 20 minutes to complete.

e. addresses, at a minimum, the following topics:

1. demographic data, including but not limited to age, gender, race, and ethnicity.

2. self assessment of health status, frailty, and physical functioning.

3. psychosocial risks, including but not limited to, depression/life satisfaction, stress, anger, loneliness/social isolation, pain, and fatigue.

4. Behavioral risks, including but not limited to, tobacco use, physical activity, nutrition and oral health, alcohol consumption, sexual health, motor vehicle safety (seat belt use), and home safety.

5. Activities of daily living (ADLs), including but not limited to, dressing, feeding, toileting, grooming, physical ambulation (including balance/risk of falls), and bathing.

6. Instrumental activities of daily living (IADLs), including but not limited to, shopping, food preparation, using the telephone, housekeeping, laundry, mode of transportation, responsibility for own medications, and ability to handle finances.

Review of the individual's functional ability and level of safety: At a minimum, includes assessment of the following topics:

a. Hearing impairment,

b. Ability to successfully perform activities of daily living,

c. Fall risk, and, d. Home safety.

Subsequent AWV providing PPPS: The provision of the following services to an eligible beneficiary by a health professional that include, and take into account the results of an updated health risk assessment, as those terms are defined in this section:

a. Review (and administration if needed) of an updated health risk assessment (as defined in this section).

b. An update of the individual's medical/family history.

c. An update of the list of current providers and suppliers that are regularly involved in providing medical care to the individual, as that list was developed for the first AWV providing PPPS or the previous subsequent AWV providing PPPS.

d. Measurement of an individual's weight (or waist circumference), BP, and other routine measurements as deemed appropriate, based on the individual's medical/family history.

e. Detection of any cognitive impairment that the individual may have as defined in this section.

f. An update to the following:

(1) The written screening schedule for the individual as that schedule is defined in this section, that was developed at the first AWV providing PPPS, and,

(2) The list of risk factors and conditions for which primary, secondary, or tertiary interventions are recommended or are under way for the individual, as that list was

developed at the first AWV providing PPPS or the previous subsequent AWV providing PPPS.

g. Furnishing of personalized health advice to the individual and a referral, as appropriate, to health education or preventive counseling services or programs as that advice and related services are defined for the first AWV providing PPPS.

h. Any other element determined appropriate by the Secretary through the NCD process.

See Pub. 100-04, Medicare Claims Processing Manual, chapter 18, section 140, for detailed claims processing and billing instructions.

100-2, 15, 290
Foot Care

A. Treatment of Subluxation of Foot
Subluxations of the foot are defined as partial dislocations or displacements of joint surfaces, tendons ligaments, or muscles of the foot. Surgical or nonsurgical treatments undertaken for the sole purpose of correcting a subluxated structure in the foot as an isolated entity are not covered.

However, medical or surgical treatment of subluxation of the ankle joint (talo-crural joint) is covered. In addition, reasonable and necessary medical or surgical services, diagnosis, or treatment for medical conditions that have resulted from or are associated with partial displacement of structures is covered. For example, if a patient has osteoarthritis that has resulted in a partial displacement of joints in the foot, and the primary treatment is for the osteoarthritis, coverage is provided.

B. Exclusions from Coverage
The following foot care services are generally excluded from coverage under both Part A and Part B. (See Sec.290.F and Sec.290.G for instructions on applying foot care exclusions.)

1. Treatment of Flat Foot
   The term "flat foot" is defined as a condition in which one or more arches of the foot have flattened out. Services or devices directed toward the care or correction of such conditions, including the prescription of supportive devices, are not covered.

2. Routine Foot Care
   Except as provided above, routine foot care is excluded from coverage. Services that normally are considered routine and not covered by Medicare include the following:

   • The cutting or removal of corns and calluses;

   • The trimming, cutting, clipping, or debriding of nails; and

   • Other hygienic and preventive maintenance care, such as cleaning and soaking the feet, the use of skin creams to maintain skin tone of either ambulatory or bedfast patients, and any other service performed in the absence of localized illness, injury, or symptoms involving the foot.

3. Supportive Devices for Feet
   Orthopedic shoes and other supportive devices for the feet generally are not covered. However, this exclusion does not apply to such a shoe if it is an integral part of a leg brace, and its expense is included as part of the cost of the brace. Also, this exclusion does not apply to therapeutic shoes furnished to diabetics.

C. Exceptions to Routine Foot Care Exclusion
1. Necessary and Integral Part of Otherwise Covered Services
   In certain circumstances, services ordinarily considered to be routine may be covered if they are performed as a necessary and integral part of otherwise covered services, such as diagnosis and treatment of ulcers, wounds, or infections.

2. Treatment of Warts on Foot
   The treatment of warts (including plantar warts) on the foot is covered to the same extent as services provided for the treatment of warts located elsewhere on the body.

3. Presence of Systemic Condition
   The presence of a systemic condition such as metabolic, neurologic, or peripheral vascular disease may require scrupulous foot care by a professional that in the absence of such condition(s) would be considered routine (and, therefore, excluded from coverage). Accordingly, foot care that would otherwise be considered routine may be covered when systemic condition(s) result in severe circulatory embarrassment or areas of diminished sensation in the individual's legs or feet. (See subsection A.)

   In these instances, certain foot care procedures that otherwise are considered routine (e.g., cutting or removing corns and calluses, or trimming, cutting, clipping, or debriding nails) may pose a hazard when performed by a nonprofessional person on patients with such systemic conditions. (See Sec.290.G for procedural instructions.)

4. Mycotic Nails
   In the absence of a systemic condition, treatment of mycotic nails may be covered.

The treatment of mycotic nails for an ambulatory patient is covered only when the physician attending the patient's mycotic condition documents that (1) there is clinical evidence of mycosis of the toenail, and (2) the patient has marked limitation of ambulation, pain, or secondary infection resulting from the thickening and dystrophy of the infected toenail plate.

The treatment of mycotic nails for a nonambulatory patient is covered only when the physician attending the patient's mycotic condition documents that (1) there is clinical evidence of mycosis of the toenail, and (2) the patient suffers from pain or secondary infection resulting from the thickening and dystrophy of the infected toenail plate.

For the purpose of these requirements, documentation means any written information that is required by the carrier in order for services to be covered. Thus, the information submitted with claims must be substantiated by information found in the patient's medical record. Any information, including that contained in a form letter, used for documentation purposes is subject to carrier verification in order to ensure that the information adequately justifies coverage of the treatment of mycotic nails.

D. Systemic Conditions That Might Justify Coverage
Although not intended as a comprehensive list, the following metabolic, neurologic, and peripheral vascular diseases (with synonyms in parentheses) most commonly represent the underlying conditions that might justify coverage for routine foot care.

• Diabetes mellitus *

• Arteriosclerosis obliterans (A.S.O., arteriosclerosis of the extremities, occlusive peripheral arteriosclerosis)

• Buerger's disease (thromboangiitis obliterans)

• Chronic thrombophlebitis *

• Peripheral neuropathies involving the feet -

• Associated with malnutrition and vitamin deficiency *

   – Malnutrition (general, pellagra)

   – Alcoholism

   – Malabsorption (celiac disease, tropical sprue)

   – Pernicious anemia

• Associated with carcinoma *

• Associated with diabetes mellitus *

• Associated with drugs and toxins *

• Associated with multiple sclerosis *

• Associated with uremia (chronic renal disease) *

• Associated with traumatic injury

• Associated with leprosy or neurosyphilis

• Associated with hereditary disorders

• Hereditary sensory radicular neuropathy

• Angiokeratoma corporis diffusum (Fabry's)

• Amyloid neuropathy

When the patient's condition is one of those designated by an asterisk (*), routine procedures are covered only if the patient is under the active care of a doctor of medicine or osteopathy who documents the condition.

E. Supportive Devices for Feet
Orthopedic shoes and other supportive devices for the feet generally are not covered. However, this exclusion does not apply to such a shoe if it is an integral part of a leg brace, and its expense is included as part of the cost of the brace. Also, this exclusion does not apply to therapeutic shoes furnished to diabetics.

F. Presumption of Coverage
In evaluating whether the routine services can be reimbursed, a presumption of coverage may be made where the evidence available discloses certain physical and/or clinical findings consistent with the diagnosis and indicative of severe peripheral involvement. For purposes of applying this presumption the following findings are pertinent:

Class A Findings
   Nontraumatic amputation of foot or integral skeletal portion thereof.

Class B Findings
   Absent posterior tibial pulse;

Advanced trophic changes as: hair growth (decrease or absence) nail changes (thickening) pigmentary changes (discoloration) skin texture (thin, shiny) skin color (rubor or redness) (Three required); and

Absent dorsalis pedis pulse.

Class C Findings
Claudication;

Temperature changes (e.g., cold feet);

Edema;

Paresthesias (abnormal spontaneous sensations in the feet); and

Burning.

The presumption of coverage may be applied when the physician rendering the routine foot care has identified:

1. A Class A finding;

2. Two of the Class B findings; or

3. One Class B and two Class C findings.

Cases evidencing findings falling short of these alternatives may involve podiatric treatment that may constitute covered care and should be reviewed by the intermediary's medical staff and developed as necessary.

For purposes of applying the coverage presumption where the routine services have been rendered by a podiatrist, the contractor may deem the active care requirement met if the claim or other evidence available discloses that the patient has seen an M.D. or D.O. for treatment and/or evaluation of the complicating disease process during the 6-month period prior to the rendition of the routine-type services. The intermediary may also accept the podiatrist's statement that the diagnosing and treating M.D. or D.O. also concurs with the podiatrist's findings as to the severity of the peripheral involvement indicated.

Services ordinarily considered routine might also be covered if they are performed as a necessary and integral part of otherwise covered services, such as diagnosis and treatment of diabetic ulcers, wounds, and infections.

G. Application of Foot Care Exclusions to Physician's Services

The exclusion of foot care is determined by the nature of the service. Thus, payment for an excluded service should be denied whether performed by a podiatrist, osteopath, or a doctor of medicine, and without regard to the difficulty or complexity of the procedure.

When an itemized bill shows both covered services and noncovered services not integrally related to the covered service, the portion of charges attributable to the noncovered services should be denied. (For example, if an itemized bill shows surgery for an ingrown toenail and also removal of calluses not necessary for the performance of toe surgery, any additional charge attributable to removal of the calluses should be denied.)

In reviewing claims involving foot care, the carrier should be alert to the following exceptional situations:

1. Payment may be made for incidental noncovered services performed as a necessary and integral part of, and secondary to, a covered procedure. For example, if trimming of toenails is required for application of a cast to a fractured foot, the carrier need not allocate and deny a portion of the charge for the trimming of the nails. However, a separately itemized charge for such excluded service should be disallowed. When the primary procedure is covered the administration of anesthesia necessary for the performance of such procedure is also covered.

2. Payment may be made for initial diagnostic services performed in connection with a specific symptom or complaint if it seems likely that its treatment would be covered even though the resulting diagnosis may be one requiring only noncovered care.

The name of the M.D. or D.O. who diagnosed the complicating condition must be submitted with the claim. In those cases, where active care is required, the approximate date the beneficiary was last seen by such physician must also be indicated.

NOTE: Section 939 of P.L. 96-499 removed "warts" from the routine foot care exclusion effective July 1, 1981.

Relatively few claims for routine-type care are anticipated considering the severity of conditions contemplated as the basis for this exception. Claims for this type of foot care should not be paid in the absence of convincing evidence that nonprofessional performance of the service would have been hazardous for the beneficiary because of an underlying systemic disease. The mere statement of a diagnosis such as those mentioned in Sec.D above does not of itself indicate the severity of the condition. Where development is indicated to verify diagnosis and/or severity the carrier should follow existing claims processing practices which may include review of carrier's history and medical consultation as well as physician contacts.

The rules in Sec.290.F concerning presumption of coverage also apply.

Codes and policies for routine foot care and supportive devices for the feet are not exclusively for the use of podiatrists. These codes must be used to report foot care services regardless of the specialty of the physician who furnishes the services. Carriers must instruct physicians to use the most appropriate code available when billing for routine foot care.

100-2, 15, 300

Diabetes Self-Management Training Services

Section 4105 of the Balanced Budget Act of 1997 permits Medicare coverage of diabetes self-management training (DSMT) services when these services are furnished by a certified provider who meets certain quality standards. This program is intended to educate beneficiaries in the successful self-management of diabetes. The program includes instructions in self-monitoring of blood glucose; education about diet and exercise; an insulin treatment plan developed specifically for the patient who is insulin-dependent; and motivation for patients to use the skills for self-management.

Diabetes self-management training services may be covered by Medicare only if the treating physician or treating qualified non-physician practitioner who is managing the beneficiary's diabetic condition certifies that such services are needed. The referring physician or qualified non-physician practitioner must maintain the plan of care in the beneficiary's medical record and documentation substantiating the need for training on an individual basis when group training is typically covered, if so ordered. The order must also include a statement signed by the physician that the service is needed as well as the following:

- The number of initial or follow-up hours ordered (the physician can order less than 10 hours of training);

- The topics to be covered in training (initial training hours can be used for the full initial training program or specific areas such as nutrition or insulin training); and

- A determination that the beneficiary should receive individual or group training.

The provider of the service must maintain documentation in a file that includes the original order from the physician and any special conditions noted by the physician.

When the training under the order is changed, the training order/referral must be signed by the physician or qualified non-physician practitioner treating the beneficiary and maintained in the beneficiary's file in the DSMT's program records.

NOTE: All entities billing for DSMT under the fee-for-service payment system or other payment systems must meet all national coverage requirements.

100-2, 15, 300.2

Certified Providers

A designated certified provider bills for DSMT provided by an accredited DSMT program. Certified providers must submit a copy of their accreditation certificate to the contractor. The statute states that a "certified provider" is a physician or other individual or entity designated by the Secretary that, in addition to providing outpatient self-management training services, provides other items and services for which payment may be made under title XVIII, and meets certain quality standards. The CMS is designating all providers and suppliers that bill Medicare for other individual services such as hospital outpatient departments, renal dialysis facilities, physicians and durable medical equipment suppliers as certified. All suppliers/providers who may bill for other Medicare services or items and who represent a DSMT program that is accredited as meeting quality standards can bill and receive payment for the entire DSMT program. Registered dietitians are eligible to bill on behalf of an entire DSMT program on or after January 1, 2002, as long as the provider has obtained a Medicare provider number. A dietitian may not be the sole provider of the DSMT service. There is an exception for rural areas. In a rural area, an individual who is qualified as a registered dietitian and as a certified diabetic educator who is currently certified by an organization approved by CMS may furnish training and is deemed to meet the multidisciplinary team requirement.

The CMS will not reimburse services on a fee-for-service basis rendered to a beneficiary under Part A.

NOTE: While separate payment is not made for this service to Rural Health Clinics (RHCs), the service is covered but is considered included in the all-inclusive encounter rate. Effective January 1, 2006, payment for DSMT provided in a Federally Qualified Health Clinic (FQHC) that meets all of the requirements identified in Pub. 100-04, chapter 18, section 120 may be made in addition to one other visit the beneficiary had during the same day.

All DSMT programs must be accredited as meeting quality standards by a CMS approved national accreditation organization. Currently, CMS recognizes the American Diabetes Association, American Association of Diabetes Educators and the Indian Health Service as approved national accreditation organizations. Programs without accreditation by a CMS-approved national accreditation organization are not covered. Certified providers may be asked to submit updated accreditation documents at any time or to submit outcome data to an organization designated by CMS.

Enrollment of DMEPOS Suppliers

The DMEPOS suppliers are reimbursed for diabetes training through local carriers. In order to file claims for DSMT, a DMEPOS supplier must be enrolled in the Medicare program with the National Supplier Clearinghouse (NSC). The supplier must also meet the quality standards of a CMS-approved national accreditation organization as stated above. DMEPOS suppliers must obtain a provider number from the local carrier in order to bill for DSMT.

The carrier requires a completed Form CMS-855, along with an accreditation certificate as part of the provider application process. After it has been determined that the quality standards are met, a billing number is assigned to the supplier. Once a supplier has received a provider identification (PIN) number, the supplier can begin receiving reimbursement for this service.

Carriers should contact the National Supplier Clearinghouse (NSC) according to the instruction in Pub 100-08, the Medicare Program Integrity Manual, Chapter 10, "Healthcare Provider/Supplier Enrollment," to verify an applicant is currently enrolled and eligible to receive direct payment from the Medicare program.

The applicant is assigned specialty 87.

Any DMEPOS supplier that has its billing privileges deactivated or revoked by the NSC will also have the billing number deactivated by the carrier.

100-2, 15, 300.3

Frequency of Training

A - Initial Training

The initial year for DSMT is the 12 month period following the initial date.

Medicare will cover initial training that meets the following conditions:

- Is furnished to a beneficiary who has not previously received initial or follow-up training under HCPCS codes G0108 or G0109;

- Is furnished within a continuous 12-month period;

- Does not exceed a total of 10 hours* (the 10 hours of training can be done in any combination of 1/2 hour increments);

- With the exception of 1 hour of individual training, training is usually furnished in a group setting, which can contain other patients besides Medicare beneficiaries, and;

- One hour of individual training may be used for any part of the training including insulin training.

* When a claim contains a DSMT HCPCS code and the associated units cause the total time for the DSMT initial year to exceed '10' hours, a CWF error will set.

B - Follow-Up Training

Medicare covers follow-up training under the following conditions:

- No more than 2 hours individual or group training per beneficiary per year;

- Group training consists of 2 to 20 individuals who need not all be Medicare beneficiaries;

- Follow-up training for subsequent years is based on a 12 month calendar after completion of the full 10 hours of initial training;

- Follow-up training is furnished in increments of no less than one-half hour*; and

- The physician (or qualified non-physician practitioner) treating the beneficiary must document in the beneficiary's medical record that the beneficiary is a diabetic.

*When a claim contains a DSMT HCPCS code and the associated units cause the total time for any follow-up year to exceed 2 hours, a CWF error will set.

100-2, 15, 300.4

Coverage Requirements for Individual Training

Medicare covers training on an individual basis for a Medicare beneficiary under any of the following conditions:

- No group session is available within 2 months of the date the training is ordered;

- The beneficiary's physician (or qualified non-physician practitioner) documents in the beneficiary's medical record that the beneficiary has special needs resulting from conditions, such as severe vision, hearing or language limitations or other such special conditions as identified by the treating physician or non-physician practitioner, that will hinder effective participation in a group training session; or

- The physician orders additional insulin training.

The need for individual training must be identified by the physician or non-physician practitioner in the referral.

NOTE: If individual training has been provided to a Medicare beneficiary and subsequently the carrier or intermediary determines that training should have been provided in a group, carriers and intermediaries down-code the reimbursement from individual to the group level and provider education would be the appropriate actions instead of denying the service as billed.

100-2, 15, 310

Kidney Disease Patient Education Services

By definition, chronic kidney disease (CKD) is kidney damage for 3 months or longer, regardless of the cause of kidney damage. CKD typically evolves over a long period of time and patients may not have symptoms until significant, possibly irreversible, damage has been done. Complications can develop from kidneys that do not function properly, such as high blood pressure, anemia, and weak bones. When CKD progresses, it may lead to kidney failure, which requires artificial means to perform kidney functions (dialysis) or a kidney transplant to maintain life.

Patients can be classified into 5 stages based on their glomerular filtration rate (GFR, how quickly blood is filtered through the kidneys), with stage I having kidney damage with normal or increased GFR to stage V with kidney failure, also called end-stage renal disease (ESRD). Once patients with CKD are identified, treatment is available to help prevent complications of decreased kidney function, slow the progression of kidney disease, and reduce the risk of other diseases such as heart disease.

Beneficiaries with CKD may benefit from kidney disease education (KDE) interventions due to the large amount of medical information that could affect patient outcomes, including the increasing emphasis on self-care and patients' desire for informed, autonomous decision-making. Pre-dialysis education can help patients achieve better understanding of their illness, dialysis modality options, and may help delay the need for dialysis. Education interventions should be patient-centered, encourage collaboration, offer support to the patient, and be delivered consistently.

Effective for claims with dates of service on and after January 1, 2010, Section 152(b) of the Medicare Improvements for Patients and Providers Act of 2008 (MIPPA) covers KDE services under Medicare Part B. KDE services are designed to provide beneficiaries with Stage IV CKD comprehensive information regarding: the management of comorbidities, including delaying the need for dialysis; prevention of uremic complications; all therapeutic options (each option for renal replacement therapy, dialysis access options, and transplantation); ensuring that the beneficiary has opportunities to actively participate in his/her choice of therapy; and that the services be tailored to meet the beneficiary's needs.

Regulations for KDE services were established at 42 CFR 410.48. Claims processing instructions and billing requirements can be found in Pub. 100-04, Medicare Claims Processing Manual, Chapter 32 - Billing Requirements for Special Services, Section 20.

100-2, 15, 310.1

Beneficiaries Eligible for Coverage

Medicare Part B covers outpatient, face-to-face KDE services for a beneficiary that:

- is diagnosed with Stage IV CKD, using the Modification of Diet in Renal Disease (MDRD) Study formula (severe decrease in GFR, GFR value of 15-29 mL/min/1.73 m2), and

- obtains a referral from the physician managing the beneficiary's kidney condition. The referral should be documented in the beneficiary's medical records.

100-2, 15, 310.2

Qualified Person

Medicare Part B covers KDE services provided by a „Àòqualified person,' meaning a: physician (as defined in section 30 of this chapter), physician assistant, nurse practitioner, or clinical nurse specialist (as defined in sections 190, 200, and 210 of this chapter), hospital, critical access hospital (CAH), skilled nursing facility (SNF), comprehensive outpatient rehabilitation facility (CORF), home health agency (HHA), or hospice, if the KDE services are provided in a rural area (using the actual geographic location core based statistical area (CBSA) to identify facilities located in rural areas), or hospital or CAH that is treated as being rural (was reclassified from urban to rural status per 42 CFR 412.103).

NOTE: The "incident to" requirements at section 1861(s)(2)(A) of the Social Security Act (the Act) do not apply to KDE services.

The following providers are not „Àòqualified persons' and are excluded from furnishing KDE services:

- A hospital, CAH, SNF, CORF, HHA, or hospice located outside of a rural area (using the actual geographic location CBSA to identify facilities located outside of a rural area), unless the services are furnished by a hospital or CAH that is treated as being in a rural area; and

- Renal dialysis facilities.

100-2, 15, 310.3

Limitations for Coverage

Medicare Part B covers KDE services: Up to six (6) sessions as a beneficiary lifetime maximum. A session is 1 hour. In order to bill for a session, a session must be at least 31 minutes in duration. A session that lasts at least 31 minutes, but less than 1 hour still constitutes 1 session.

On an individual basis or in group settings; if the services are provided in a group setting, a group consists of 2 to 20 individuals who need not all be Medicare beneficiaries.

NOTE: Two HCPCS codes were created for this benefit and one or the other must be present, along with ICD-9-CM code 585.4 (chronic kidney disease, Stage IV (severe)), in order for a claim to be processed and paid correctly. They are: G0420: Face-to-face educational services related to the care of chronic kidney disease; individual, per session, per one hour G0421: Face-to-face educational services related to the care of chronic kidney disease; group, per session, per one hour

100-2, 15, 310.4

Standards for Content

Medicare Part B covers KDE services, provided by a qualified person, which provide comprehensive information regarding:

A. The management of comorbidities, including delaying the need for dialysis, which includes, but is not limited to, the following topics:

- Prevention and treatment of cardiovascular disease,
- Prevention and treatment of diabetes,
- Hypertension management,
- Anemia management,
- Bone disease and disorders of calcium and phosphorus metabolism management,
- Symptomatic neuropathy management, and
- Impairments in functioning and well-being.

B. Prevention of uremic complications, which includes, but is not limited to, the following topics:

- Information on how the kidneys work and what happens when the kidneys fail,
- Understanding if remaining kidney function can be protected, preventing disease progression, and realistic chances of survival,
- Diet and fluid restrictions, and
- Medication review, including how each medication works, possible side effects and minimization of side effects, the importance of compliance, and informed decision making if the patient decides not to take a specific drug.

C. Therapeutic options, treatment modalities and settings, advantages and disadvantages of each treatment option, and how the treatments replace the kidney, including, but not limited to, the following topics: Hemodialysis, both at home and in-facility;

- Peritoneal dialysis (PD), including intermittent PD, continuous ambulatory PD, and continuous cycling PD, both at home and in-facility;
- All dialysis access options for hemodialysis and peritoneal dialysis; and
- Transplantation.

D. Opportunities for beneficiaries to actively participate in the choice of therapy and be tailored to meet the needs of the individual beneficiary involved, which includes, but is not limited to, the following topics: Physical symptoms,

- Impact on family and social life,
- Exercise,
- The right to refuse treatment,
- Impact on work and finances,
- The meaning of test results, and
- Psychological impact.

100-2, 15, 310.5

Outcomes Assessment

Qualified persons that provide KDE services must develop outcomes assessments that are designed to measure beneficiary knowledge about CKD and its treatment. The assessment must be administered to the beneficiary during a KDE session, and be made available to the Centers for Medicare & Medicaid Services (CMS) upon request. The outcomes assessments serve to assist KDE educators and CMS in improving subsequent KDE programs, patient understanding, and assess program effectiveness of:

Preparing the beneficiary to make informed decisions about their healthcare options related to CKD, and

Meeting the communication needs of underserved populations, including persons with disabilities, persons with limited English proficiency, and persons with health literacy needs.

100-2, 16, 10

General Exclusions From Coverage

A3-3150, HO-260, HHA-232, B3-2300

No payment can be made under either the hospital insurance or supplementary medical insurance program for certain items and services, when the following conditions exist:

- Not reasonable and necessary (Sec.20);
- No legal obligation to pay for or provide (Sec.40);
- Paid for by a governmental entity (Sec.50);
- Not provided within United States (Sec.60);
- Resulting from war (Sec.70);
- Personal comfort (Sec.80);
- Routine services and appliances (Sec.90);
- Custodial care (Sec.110);
- Cosmetic surgery (Sec.120);
- Charges by immediate relatives or members of household (Sec.130);
- Dental services (Sec.140);
- Paid or expected to be paid under workers' compensation (Sec.150);
- Nonphysician services provided to a hospital inpatient that were not provided directly or arranged for by the hospital (Sec.170);
- Services Related to and Required as a Result of Services Which are not Covered Under Medicare (Sec.180);
- Excluded foot care services and supportive devices for feet (Sec.30); or
- Excluded investigational devices (See Chapter 14, Sec.30).

100-2, 16, 20

Services Not Reasonable and Necessary

A3-3151, HO-260.1, B3-2303, AB-00-52 - 6/00

Items and services which are not reasonable and necessary for the diagnosis or treatment of illness or injury or to improve the functioning of a malformed body member are not covered, e.g., payment cannot be made for the rental of a special hospital bed to be used by the patient in their home unless it was a reasonable and necessary part of the patient's treatment. See also Sec.80.

A health care item or service for the purpose of causing, or assisting to cause, the death of any individual (assisted suicide) is not covered. This prohibition does not apply to the provision of an item or service for the purpose of alleviating pain or discomfort, even if such use may increase the risk of death, so long as the item or service is not furnished for the specific purpose of causing death.

100-2, 16, 90

Routine Services and Appliances

A3-3157, HO-260.7, B3-2320, R-1797A3 - 5/00

Routine physical checkups; eyeglasses, contact lenses, and eye examinations for the purpose of prescribing, fitting, or changing eyeglasses; eye refractions by whatever practitioner and for whatever purpose performed; hearing aids and examinations for hearing aids; and immunizations are not covered.

The routine physical checkup exclusion applies to (a) examinations performed without relationship to treatment or diagnosis for a specific illness, symptom, complaint, or injury; and (b) examinations required by third parties such as insurance companies business establishments, or Government agencies.

If the claim is for a diagnostic test or examination performed solely for the purpose of establishing a claim under title IV of Public Law 91-173, "Black Lung Benefits," the service is not covered under Medicare and the claimant should be advised to contact their Social Security office regarding the filing of a claim for reimbursement under the "Black Lung" program.

The exclusions apply to eyeglasses or contact lenses, and eye examinations for the purpose of prescribing, fitting, or changing eyeglasses or contact lenses for refractive errors. The exclusions do not apply to physicians' services (and services incident to a physicians' service) performed in conjunction with an eye disease, as for example, glaucoma or cataracts, or to post-surgical prosthetic lenses which are customarily used during convalescence from eye surgery in which the lens of the eye was removed, or to permanent prosthetic lenses required by an individual lacking the organic lens of the eye whether by surgical removal or congenital disease. Such prosthetic lens is a replacement for an internal body organ - the lens of the eye. (See the Medicare Benefit Policy Manual, Chapter 15, "Covered Medical and Other Health Services," Sec.120). Expenses for all refractive procedures, whether performed by an ophthalmologist (or any other physician) or an optometrist and without regard to the reason for performance of the refraction, are excluded from coverage.

A. Immunizations

Vaccinations or inoculations are excluded as immunizations unless they are either

Directly related to the treatment of an injury or direct exposure to a disease or condition, such as antirabies treatment, tetanus antitoxin or booster vaccine, botulin antitoxin, antivenin sera, or immune globulin. (In the absence of injury or direct exposure, preventive immunization (vaccination or inoculation) against such diseases as smallpox, polio, diphtheria, etc., is not covered.); or

Specifically covered by statute, as described in the Medicare Benefit Policy Manual, Chapter 15, "Covered Medical and Other Health Services," Sec.50.

B. Antigens

Prior to the Omnibus Reconciliation Act of 1980, a physician who prepared an antigen for a patient could not be reimbursed for that service unless the physician also administered the antigen to the patient. Effective January 1, 1981, payment may be made for a reasonable supply of antigens that have been prepared for a particular patient even though they have not been administered to the patient by the same physician who prepared them if:

The antigens are prepared by a physician who is a doctor of medicine or osteopathy, and "The physician who prepared the antigens has examined the patient and has determined a plan of treatment and a dosage regimen.

A reasonable supply of antigens is considered to be not more than a 12-week supply of antigens that has been prepared for a particular patient at any one time. The purpose of the reasonable supply limitation is to assure that the antigens retain their potency and effectiveness over the period in which they are to be administered to the patient. (See the Medicare Benefit Policy Manual, Chapter 15, "Covered Medical and Other Health Services," Sec.50.4.4.2)

100-2, 16, 140

Dental Services Exclusion
A3-3162, HO-260.13, B3-2336

Items and services in connection with the care, treatment, filling, removal, or replacement of teeth, or structures directly supporting the teeth are not covered. Structures directly supporting the teeth mean the periodontium, which includes the gingivae, dentogingival junction, periodontal membrane, cementum, and alveolar process. However, payment may be made for certain other services of a dentist. (See the Medicare Benefit Policy Manual, Chapter 15, "Covered Medical and Other Health Services," Sec.150.)

The hospitalization or nonhospitalization of a patient has no direct bearing on the coverage or exclusion of a given dental procedure.

When an excluded service is the primary procedure involved, it is not covered regardless of its complexity or difficulty. For example, the extraction of an impacted tooth is not covered. Similarly, an alveoplasty (the surgical improvement of the shape and condition of the alveolar process) and a frenectomy are excluded from coverage when either of these procedures is performed in connection with an excluded service, e.g., the preparation of the mouth for dentures. In like manner, the removal of the torus palatinus (a bony protuberance of the hard palate) could be a covered service. However, with rare exception, this surgery is performed in connection with an excluded service, i.e., the preparation of the mouth for dentures. Under such circumstances, reimbursement is not made for this purpose.

The extraction of teeth to prepare the jaw for radiation treatments of neoplastic disease is also covered. This is an exception to the requirement that to be covered, a noncovered procedure or service performed by a dentist must be an incident to and an integral part of a covered procedure or service performed by the dentist. Ordinarily, the dentist extracts the patient's teeth, but another physician, e.g., a radiologist, administers the radiation treatments.

Whether such services as the administration of anesthesia, diagnostic x-rays, and other related procedures are covered depends upon whether the primary procedure being performed by the dentist is covered. Thus, an x-ray taken in connection with the reduction of a fracture of the jaw or facial bone is covered. However, a single x-ray or xray survey taken in connection with the care or treatment of teeth or the periodontium is not covered.

See also the Medicare Benefit Policy Manual, Chapter 1, "Inpatient Hospital Services, Sec.70, and Chapter 15, "Covered Medical and Other Health Services," Sec.150 for additional information on dental services.

100-2, 32, 20.2

Healthcare Common Procedure Coding System (HCPCS) Procedure Codes and Applicable Diagnosis Codes
Effective for services performed on and after January 1, 2010, the following new HCPCS codes have been created for KDE services when provided to patients with stage IV CKD.

G0420: Face-to-face educational services related to the care of chronic kidney disease; individual, per session, per one hour

G0421: Face-to-face educational services related to the care of chronic kidney disease; group, per session, per one hour

The following diagnosis code should be reported when billing for KDE services:

585.4 (chronic kidney disease, Stage IV (severe)).

NOTE: Claims with HCPCS codes G0420 or G0421 and ICD-9 code 585.4 that are billed for KDE services are not allowed on a professional and institutional claim on the same service date.

100-3, 10.2

The use of transcutaneous electrical nerve stimulation (TENS) for the relief of acute post-operative pain is covered under Medicare. TENS may be covered whether used as an adjunct to the use of drugs, or as an alternative to drugs, in the treatment of acute pain resulting from surgery.

The TENS devices, whether durable or disposable, may be used in furnishing this service. When used for the purpose of treating acute post-operative pain, TENS devices are considered supplies. As such they may be hospital supplies furnished inpatients covered under Part A, or supplies incident to a physician' service when furnished in connection with surgery done on an outpatient basis, and covered under Part B.

It is expected that TENS, when used for acute post-operative pain, will be necessary for relatively short periods of time, usually 30 days or less. In cases when TENS is used for longer periods, contractors should attempt to ascertain whether TENS is no longer being used for acute pain but rather for chronic pain, in which case the TENS device may be covered as durable medical equipment as described in §160.27.

Cross-references:
Medicare Benefit Policy Manual, Chapter 1, "Inpatient Hospital Services," ?40;

Medicare Benefit Policy Manual, Chapter 2, "Hospital Services Covered Under Part B," §?20, 20.4, and 80; Medicare Benefit Policy Manual, Chapter 15, "Covered Medical and other Health Services, §110."

100-3, 20.21

NCD for Chelation Therapy for Treatment of Atherosclerosis (20.21)
The application of chelation therapy using ethylenediamine-tetra-acetic acid (EDTA) for the treatment and prevention of atherosclerosis is controversial. There is no widely accepted rationale to explain the beneficial effects attributed to this therapy. Its safety is questioned and its clinical effectiveness has never been established by well designed, controlled clinical trials. It is not widely accepted and practiced by American physicians. EDTA chelation therapy for atherosclerosis is considered experimental. For these reasons, EDTA chelation therapy for the treatment or prevention of atherosclerosis is not covered.

Some practitioners refer to this therapy as chemoendarterectomy and may also show a diagnosis other than atherosclerosis, such as arteriosclerosis or calcinosis. Claims employing such variant terms should also be denied under this section.

100-3, 20.22

NCD for Ethylenediamine-Tetra-Acetic (EDTA) Chelation Therapy for Treatment of Atherosclerosis (20.22)
The use of EDTA as a chelating agent to treat atherosclerosis, arteriosclerosis, calcinosis, or similar generalized condition not listed by the FDA as an approved use is not covered. Any such use of EDTA is considered experimental.

100-3, 40.7

NCD for Outpatient Intravenous Insulin Treatment (40.7) (Effective December 23, 2009)

Indications and Limitations of Coverage

B. Nationally Covered Indications
N/A

C. Nationally Non-Covered Indications
Effective for claims with dates of service on and after December 23, 2009, the Centers for Medicare and Medicaid Services (CMS) determines that the evidence is adequate to conclude that OIVIT does not improve health outcomes in Medicare beneficiaries. Therefore, CMS determines that OIVIT is not reasonable and necessary for any indication under section 1862(a)(1)(A) of the Social Security Act. Services comprising an Outpatient Intravenous Insulin Therapy regimen are

nationally non-covered under Medicare when furnished pursuant to an OIVIT regimen (see subsection A. above).

D. Other

Individual components of OIVIT may have medical uses in conventional treatment regimens for diabetes and other conditions. Coverage for such other uses may be determined by other local or national Medicare determinations, and do not pertain to OIVIT. For example, see Pub. 100-03, NCD Manual, Section 40.2, Home Blood Glucose Monitors, Section 40.3, Closed-loop Blood Glucose Control Devices (CBGCD), Section 190.20, Blood Glucose Testing, and Section 280.14, Infusion Pumps, as well as Pub. 100-04, Claims Processing Manual, Chapter 18, Section 90, Diabetics Screening.

(This NCD last reviewed December 2009.)

100-3, 80.2

Photodynamic Therapy

Photodynamic therapy is a medical procedure which involves the infusion of a photosensitive (light-activated) drug with a very specific absorption peak. This drug is chemically designed to have a unique affinity for the diseased tissue intended for treatment. Once introduced to the body, the drug accumulates and is retained in diseased tissue to a greater degree than in normal tissue. Infusion is followed by the targeted irradiation of this tissue with a non-thermal laser, calibrated to emit light at a wavelength that corresponds to the drug? absorption peak. The drug then becomes active and locally treats the diseased tissue.

Ocular Photodynamic Therapy (OPT)

Ocular Photodynamic Therapy (OPT) is used in the treatment of ophthalmologic diseases. OPT is only covered when used in conjunction with verteporfin (see section 80.3, "Photosensitive Drugs").

- Classic Subfoveal Choroidal Neovascular (CNV) Lesions - OPT is covered with a diagnosis of neovascular age-related macular degeneration (AMD) with predominately classic subfoveal choroidal neovascular (CNV) lesions (where the area of classic CNV occupies = 50 percent of the area of the entire lesion) at the initial visit as determined by a fluorescein angiogram. Subsequent follow-up visits will require either an optical coherence tomography (OCT) or a fluorescein angiogram (FA) to access treatment response. There are no requirements regarding visual acuity, lesion size, and number of re-treatments.

- Occult Subfoveal Choroidal Neovascular (CNV) Lesions - OPT is noncovered for patients with a diagnosis of age-related macular degeneration (AMD) with occult and no classic CNV lesions.

- Other Conditions - Use of OPT with verteporfin for other types of AMD (e.g., patients with minimally classic CNV lesions, atrophic, or dry AMD) is noncovered. OPT with verteporfin for other ocular indications such as pathologic myopia or presumed ocular histoplasmosis syndrome, is eligible for coverage through individual contractor discretion.

100-3, 80.2.1

Ocular Photodynamic Therapy (OPT)- Effective April 3, 2013

A. General

Ocular Photodynamic Therapy (OPT) is used in the treatment of ophthalmologic diseases; specifically, for age-related macular degeneration (AMD), a common eye disease among the elderly. OPT involves the infusion of an intravenous photosensitizing drug called verteporfin followed by exposure to a laser. OPT is only covered when used in conjunction with verteporfin.

Effective July 1, 2001, OPT with verteporfin was approved for a diagnosis of neovascular AMD with predominately classic subfoveal choroidal neovascularization (CNV) lesions (where the area of classic CNV occupies = 50% of the area of the entire lesion) at the initial visit as determined by a fluorescein angiogram (FA).

On October 17, 2001, the Centers for Medicare & Medicaid Services (CMS) announced its "intent to cover" OPT with verteporfin for AMD patients with occult and no classic subfoveal CNV as determined by an FA. The October 17, 2001, decision was never implemented.

On March 28, 2002, after thorough review and reconsideration of the October 17, 2001, intent to cover policy, CMS determined that the current non-coverage policy for OPT for verteporfin for AMD patients with occult and no classic subfoveal CNV as determined by an FA should remain in effect.

Effective August 20, 2002, CMS issued a non-covered instruction for OPT with verteporfin for AMD patients with occult and no classic subfoveal CNV as determined by an FA.

B. Nationally Covered Indications

Effective April 1, 2004, OPT with verteporfin continues to be approved for a diagnosis of neovascular AMD with predominately classic subfoveal CNV lesions (where the area of classic CNV occupies = 50% of the area of the entire lesion) at the initial visit as determined by an FA. (CNV lesions are comprised of classic and/or occult components.) Subsequent follow-up visits require either an optical coherence tomography (OCT) (effective April 3. 2013) or an FA (effective April 1,

2004) to access treatment response. There are no requirements regarding visual acuity, lesion size, and number of re-treatments when treating predominantly classic lesions.

In addition, after thorough review and reconsideration of the August 20, 2002, non-coverage policy, CMS determines that the evidence is adequate to conclude that OPT with verteporfin is reasonable and necessary for treating:

1. Subfoveal occult with no classic CNV associated with AMD; and,

2. Subfoveal minimally classic CNV (where the area of classic CNV occupies <50% of the area of the entire lesion) associated with AMD.

The above 2 indications are considered reasonable and necessary only when:

1. The lesions are small (4 disk areas or less in size) at the time of initial treatment or within the 3 months prior to initial treatment; and,

2. The lesions have shown evidence of progression within the 3 months prior to initial treatment. Evidence of progression must be documented by deterioration of visual acuity (at least 5 letters on a standard eye examination chart), lesion growth (an increase in at least 1 disk area), or the appearance of blood associated with the lesion.

C. Nationally Non-Covered Indications

Other uses of OPT with verteporfin to treat AMD not already addressed by CMS will continue to be non-covered. These include, but are not limited to, the following AMD indications:

- Juxtafoveal or extrafoveal CNV lesions (lesions outside the fovea),
- Inability to obtain a fluorescein angiogram,
- Atrophic or "dry" AMD.

D. Other

The OPT with verteporfin for other ocular indications, such as pathologic myopia or presumed ocular histoplasmosis syndrome, continue to be eligible for local coverage determinations through individual contractor discretion.

100-3, 80.3

(NCD) for Photosensitive Drugs (80.3)

Photosensitive drugs are the light-sensitive agents used in photodynamic therapy. Once introduced into the body, these drugs selectively identify and adhere to diseased tissue. The drugs remain inactive until they are exposed to a specific wavelength of light, by means of a laser, that corresponds to their absorption peak. The activation of a photosensitive drug results in a photochemical reaction which treats the diseased tissue without affecting surrounding normal tissue.

Verteporfin

Verteporfin, a benzoporphyrin derivative, is an intravenous lipophilic photosensitive drug with an absorption peak of 690 nm. This drug was first approved by the Food and Drug Administration (FDA) on April 12, 2000, and subsequently, approved for inclusion in the United States Pharmacopoeia on July 18, 2000, meeting Medicare's definition of a drug when used in conjunction with ocular photodynamic therapy (OPT) (see section 80.2, "Photodynamic Therapy") when furnished intravenously incident to a physician? service. For patients with age-related macular degeneration (AMD), Verteporfin is only covered with a diagnosis of neovascular age-related macular degeneration with predominately classic subfoveal choroidal neovascular (CNV) lesions (where the area of classic CNV occupies = 50 percent of the area of the entire lesion) at the initial visit as determined by a fluorescein angiogram (FA). Subsequent follow-up visits will require either an optical coherence tomography (OCT) or an FA to access treatment response. OPT with verteporfin is covered for the above indication and will remain non-covered for all other indications related to AMD (see section 80.2). OPT with Verteporfin for use in non-AMD conditions is eligible for coverage through individual contractor discretion.

100-3, 80.3.1

Verteporfin-Effective April 3, 2013

A. General

Verteporfin, a benzoporphyrin derivative, is an intravenous lipophilic photosensitive drug with an absorption peak of 690 nm. Verteporfin was first approved by the Food and Drug Administration on April 12, 2000, and subsequently approved for inclusion in the United States Pharmacopoeia on July 18, 2000, meeting Medicare's definition of a drug as defined under Sec. 1861(t)(1) of the Social Security Act. Verteporfin is only covered when used in conjunction with ocular photodynamic therapy OPT) when furnished intravenously incident to a physician's service.

B. Nationally Covered Indications

Effective April 1, 2004, OPT with verteporfin is covered for patients with a diagnosis of neovascular age-related macular degeneration (AMD) with:

?Predominately classic subfoveal choroidal neovascularization (CNV) lesions (where the area of classic CNV occupies = 50 percent of the area of the entire lesion) at the initial visit as determined by a fluorescein angiogram. (CNV lesions are comprised of classic and/or occult components.) Subsequent follow-up visits require either an optical coherence tomography (OCT) (effective April 3, 2013) or a fluorescein angiogram (FA) (effective April 1, 2004) to access treatment response.

There are no requirements regarding visual acuity, lesion size, and number of retreatments when treating predominantly classic lesions.

- Subfoveal occult with no classic associated with AMD.
- Subfoveal minimally classic CNV CNV (where the area of classic CNV occupies <50% of the area of the entire lesion) associated with AMD.

The above 2 indications are considered reasonable and necessary only when:

1. The lesions are small (4 disk areas or less in size) at the time of initial treatment or within the 3 months prior to initial treatment; and,

2. The lesions have shown evidence of progression within the 3 months prior to initial treatment. Evidence of progression must be documented by deterioration of visual acuity (at least 5 letters on a standard eye examination chart), lesion growth (an increase in at least 1 disk area), or the appearance of blood associated with the lesion.

C. Nationally Non-Covered Indications
Other uses of OPT with verteporfin to treat AMD not already addressed by the Centers for Medicare & Medicaid Services will continue to be non-covered. These include, but are not limited to, the following AMD indications: juxtafoveal or extrafoveal CNV lesions (lesions outside the fovea), inability to obtain an FA, or atrophic or "dry" AMD.

D. Other
The OPT with verteporfin for other ocular indications, such as pathologic myopia or presumed ocular histoplasmosis syndrome, continue to be eligible for local coverage determinations through individual contractor discretion.

100-3, 90.1

Pharmacogenomic Testing to Predict Warfarin Responsiveness (Effective August 3, 2009)

A. General
Warfarin sodium is an orally administered anticoagulant drug that is marketed most commonly as Coumadin(R). (The Food and Drug Administration (FDA) approved labeling for Coumadin(R) includes a Black Box Warning dating back to 2007.) Anticoagulant drugs are sometimes referred to as blood thinners by the lay public. Warfarin affects the vitamin K-dependent clotting factors II, VII, IX, and X. Warfarin is thought to interfere with clotting factor synthesis by inhibition of the C1 subunit of the vitamin K epoxide reductase (VKORC1) enzyme complex, thereby reducing the regeneration of vitamin K1 epoxide. The elimination of warfarin is almost entirely by metabolic conversion to inactive metabolites by cytochrome P450 (CYP) enzymes in liver cells. CYP2C9 is the principal cytochrome P450 enzyme that modulates the anticoagulant activity of warfarin. From results of clinical studies, genetic variation in the CYP2C9 and/or VKORC1 genes can, in concert with clinical factors, predict how each individual responds to warfarin

Pharmacogenomics denotes the study of how an individual's genetic makeup, or genotype, affects the body's response to drugs. Pharmacogenomics as a science examines associations among variations in genes with individual responses to a drug or medication. In application, pharmacogenomic results (i.e., information on the patient's genetic variations) can contribute to predicting a patient's response to a given drug: good, bad, or none at all. Pharmacogenomic testing of CYP2C9 or VKORC1 alleles to predict a patient's response to warfarin occurs ideally prior to initiation of the drug. This would be an once-in-a-lifetime test, absent any reason to believe that the patient's personal genetic characteristics would change over time. Although such pharmacogenomic testing would be used to attempt to better approximate the best starting dose of warfarin, it would not eliminate the need for periodic PT/INR testing, a standard diagnostic test for coagulation activity and for assessing how a patient is reacting to a warfarin dose.

Nationally Covered Indications
Effective August 3, 2009, the Centers for Medicare & Medicaid Services (CMS) believes that the available evidence supports that coverage with evidence development (CED) under Sec.1862(a)(1)(E) of the Social Security Act (the Act) is appropriate for pharmacogenomic testing of CYP2C9 or VKORC1 alleles to predict warfarin responsiveness by any method, and is therefore covered only when provided to Medicare beneficiaries who are candidates for anticoagulation therapy with warfarin who:

1. Have not been previously tested for CYP2C9 or VKORC1 alleles; and

2. Have received fewer than five days of warfarin in the anticoagulation regimen for which the testing is ordered; and

3. Are enrolled in a prospective, randomized, controlled clinical study when that study meets the following standards. A clinical study seeking Medicare payment for pharmacogenomic testing of CYP2C9 or VKORC1 alleles to predict warfarin responsiveness provided to the Medicare

beneficiary who is a candidate for anticoagulation therapy with warfarin pursuant to CED must address one or more aspects of the following question:

Prospectively, in Medicare-aged subjects whose warfarin therapy management includes pharmacogenomic testing of CYP2C9 or VKORC1 alleles to predict warfarin response, what is the frequency and severity of the following outcomes, compared to subjects whose warfarin therapy management does not include pharmacogenomic testing?

Major hemorrhage

Minor hemorrhage

Thromboembolism related to the primary indication for anticoagulation

Other thromboembolic event

Mortality

The study must adhere to the following standards of scientific integrity and relevance to the Medicare population:

a. The principal purpose of the research study is to test whether a particular intervention potentially improves the participants' health outcomes.

b. The research study is well-supported by available scientific and medical information or it is intended to clarify or establish the health outcomes of interventions already in common clinical use.

c. The research study does not unjustifiably duplicate existing studies.

d. The research study design is appropriate to answer the research question being asked in the study.

e. The research study is sponsored by an organization or individual capable of executing the proposed study successfully.

f. The research study is in compliance with all applicable Federal regulations concerning the protection of human subjects found in the Code of Federal Regulations (CFR) at 45 CFR Part 46. If a study is regulated by the FDA, it also must be in compliance with 21 CFR Parts 50 and 56.

g. All aspects of the research study are conducted according to the appropriate standards of scientific integrity.

h. The research study has a written protocol that clearly addresses, or incorporates by reference, the Medicare standards.

i. The clinical research study is not designed to exclusively test toxicity or disease pathophysiology in healthy individuals. Trials of all medical technologies measuring therapeutic outcomes as one of the objectives meet this standard only if the disease or condition being studied is life-threatening as defined in 21 CFR Sec. 312.81(a) and the patient has no other viable treatment options.

j. The clinical research study is registered on the www.ClinicalTrials.gov website by the principal sponsor/investigator prior to the enrollment of the first study subject.

k. The research study protocol specifies the method and timing of public release of all pre-specified outcomes to be measured including release of outcomes if outcomes are negative or study is terminated early. The results must be made public within 24 months of the end of data collection. If a report is planned to be published in a peer-reviewed journal, then that initial release may be an abstract that meets the requirements of the International Committee of Medical Journal Editors. However, a full report of the outcomes must be made public no later than 3 years after the end of data collection.

l. The research study protocol must explicitly discuss subpopulations affected by the treatment under investigation, particularly traditionally underrepresented groups in clinical studies, how the inclusion and exclusion criteria affect enrollment of these populations, and a plan for the retention and reporting of said populations on the trial. If the inclusion and exclusion criteria are expected to have a negative effect on the recruitment or retention of underrepresented populations, the protocol must discuss why these criteria are necessary.

m. The research study protocol explicitly discusses how the results are or are not expected to be generalizable to the Medicare population to infer whether Medicare patients may benefit from the intervention. Separate discussions in the protocol may be necessary for populations eligible for Medicare due to age, disability or Medicaid eligibility. Consistent with section 1142 of the Act, the Agency for Healthcare Research and Quality (AHRQ) supports clinical research studies that CMS determines meet the above-listed standards and address the above-listed research questions.

B. Nationally Non-Covered Indications
The CMS believes that the available evidence does not demonstrate that pharmacogenomic testing of CYP2C9 or VKORC1 alleles to predict warfarin responsiveness improves health outcomes in

Medicare beneficiaries outside the context of CED, and is therefore not reasonable and necessary under Sec.1862(a)(1)(A) of the Act.

C. Other

This NCD does not determine coverage to identify CYP2C9 or VKORC1 alleles for other purposes, nor does it determine national coverage to identify other alleles to predict warfarin responsiveness.

(This NCD last reviewed August 2009.)

100-3,110.22

Autologous Cellular Immunotherapy Treatment (Effective June 30, 2011)

A. General

Prostate cancer is the most common non-cutaneous cancer in men in the United States. In 2009, an estimated 192,280 new cases of prostate cancer were diagnosed and an estimated 27,360 deaths were reported. The National Cancer Institute states that prostate cancer is predominantly a cancer of older men; the median age at diagnosis is 72 years. Once the patient has castration-resistant, metastatic prostate cancer the median survival is generally less than two years.

In 2010 the Food and Drug Administration (FDA) approved sipuleucel-T (PROVENGE®; APC8015), for patients with castration-resistant, metastatic prostate cancer. The posited mechanism of action, immunotherapy, is different from that of anti-cancer chemotherapy such as docetaxel. This is the first immunotherapy for prostate cancer to receive FDA approval.

The goal of immunotherapy is to stimulate the body's natural defenses (such as the white blood cells called dendritic cells, T-lymphocytes and mononuclear cells) in a specific manner so that they attack and destroy, or at least prevent, the proliferation of cancer cells. Specificity is attained by intentionally exposing a patient's white blood cells to a particular protein (called an antigen) associated with the prostate cancer. This exposure "trains" the white blood cells to target and attack the prostate cancer cells. Clinically, this is expected to result in a decrease in the size and/or number of cancer sites, an increase in the time to cancer progression, and/or an increase in survival of the patient.

Sipuleucel-T differs from other infused anti-cancer therapies. Most such anti-cancer therapies are manufactured and sold by a biopharmaceutical company and then purchased by and dispensed from a pharmacy. In contrast, once the decision is made to treat with sipuleucel-T, a multi-step process is used to produce sipuleucel-T. Sipuleucel-T is made individually for each patient with his own white blood cells. The patient's white blood cells are removed via a procedure called leukapheresis. In a laboratory the white blood cells are exposed to PA2024, which is a molecule created by linking prostatic acid phosphatase (PAP) with granulocyte/macrophage-colony stimulating factor (GM-CSF). PAP is an antigen specifically associated with prostate cancer cells; GM-CSF is a protein that targets a receptor on the surface of white blood cells. Hence, PAP serves to externally manipulate the immunological functioning of the patient's white blood cells while GM-CSF serves to stimulate the white blood cells into action. As noted in the FDA's clinical review, each dose of sipuleucel-T contains a minimum of 40 million treated white blood cells, however there is "high inherent variability" in the yield of sipuleucel-T from leukapheresis to leukapheresis in the same patient as well as from patient to patient. The treated white blood cells are then infused back into the same patient. The FDA-approved dosing regimen is three doses with each dose administered two weeks apart.

Indications and Limitations of Coverage

B. Nationally Covered Indications

Effective for services performed on or after June 30, 2011, The Centers for Medicare and Medicaid Services (CMS) proposes that the evidence is adequate to conclude that the use of autologous cellular immunotherapy treatment - sipuleucel-T; PROVENGE® improves health outcomes for Medicare beneficiaries with asymptomatic or minimally symptomatic metastatic castrate-resistant (hormone refractory) prostate cancer, and thus is reasonable and necessary for this on-label indication under 1862(a)(1)(A) of the Social Security Act.

C. Nationally Non-Covered Indications

N/A

D. Other

Effective for services performed on or after June 30, 2011, coverage of all off-label uses of autologous cellular immunotherapy treatment —sipuleucel-T; PROVENGE® for the treatment of prostate cancer is left to the discretion of the local Medicare Administrative Contractors.

(NCD last reviewed June 2011.)

100-3, 150.11

Thermal Intradiscal Procedures (TIPs)

A. General

Percutaneous thermal intradiscal procedures (TIPs) involve the insertion of a catheter(s)/probe(s) in the spinal disc under fluoroscopic guidance for the purpose of producing or applying heat and/or disruption within the disc to relieve low back pain.

The scope of this national coverage determination on TIPs includes percutaneous intradiscal techniques that employ the use of a radiofrequency energy source or electrothermal energy to apply or create heat and/or disruption within the disc for coagulation and/or decompression of disc material to treat symptomatic patients with annular disruption of a contained herniated disc, to seal annular tears or fissures, or destroy nociceptors for the purpose of relieving pain.

This includes techniques that use single or multiple probe(s)/catheter(s), which utilize a resistance coil or other delivery system technology, are flexible or rigid, and are placed within the nucleus, the nuclear-annular junction, or the annulus. Although not intended to be an all inclusive list, TIPs are commonly identified as intradiscal electrothermal therapy (IDET), intradiscal thermal annuloplasty (IDTA), percutaneous intradiscal radiofrequency thermocoagulation (PIRFT), radiofrequency annuloplasty (RA), intradiscal biacuplasty (IDB), percutaneous (or plasma) disc decompression (PDD) or coblation, or targeted disc decompression (TDD). At times, TIPs are identified or labeled based on the name of the catheter/probe that is used (e.g., SpineCath, discTRODE, SpineWand, Accutherm, or TransDiscal electrodes). Each technique or device has it own protocol for application of the therapy. Percutaneous disc decompression or nucleoplasty procedures that do not utilize a radiofrequency energy source or electrothermal energy (such as the disc decompressor procedure or laser procedure) are not within the scope of this NCD.

B. Nationally Covered Indications

N/A

C. Nationally Non-Covered Indications

Effective for services performed on or after September 29, 2008, the Centers for Medicare and Medicaid Services has determined that TIPs are not reasonable and necessary for the treatment of low back pain. Therefore, TIPs, which include procedures that employ the use of a radiofrequency energy source or electrothermal energy to apply or create heat and/or disruption within the disc for the treatment of low back pain, are noncovered.

D. Other

N/A

(This NCD last reviewed September 2008.)

100-3, 150.12

Collagen Meniscus Implant (Effective May 25, 2010)

A. General

The knee menisci are wedge-shaped, semi-lunar discs of fibrous tissue located in the knee joint between the ends of the femur and the tibia and fibula. There is a lateral and medial meniscus in each knee. It is known now that the menisci provide mechanical support, localized pressure distribution, and lubrication of the knee joint. Initially, meniscal tears were treated with total meniscectomy; however, as knowledge of the function of the menisci and the potential long term effects of total meniscectomy on the knee joint evolved, treatment of symptomatic meniscal tears gravitated to repair of the tear, when possible, or partial meniscectomy.

The collagen meniscus implant (also referred to as collagen scaffold (CS), CMI or MenaflexTM meniscus implant throughout the published literature) is used to fill meniscal defects that result from partial meniscectomy. The collagen meniscus implant is not intended to replace the entire meniscus at it requires a meniscal rim for attachment. The literature describes the placement of the collagen meniscus implant through an arthroscopic procedure with an additional incision for capture of the repair needles and tying of the sutures. After debridement of the damaged meniscus, the implant is trimmed to the size of meniscal defect and sutured into place. The collagen meniscus implant is described as a tissue engineered scaffold to support the generation of new meniscus-like tissue. The collagen meniscus implant is manufactured from bovine collagen and should not be confused with the meniscus transplant which involves the replacement of the meniscus with a transplant meniscus from a cadaver donor. The meniscus transplant is not addressed under this national coverage determination.

B. Nationally Covered Indications

N/A

C. Nationally Non-Covered Indications

Effective for claims with dates of service performed on or after May 25, 2010, the Centers for Medicare & Medicaid Services has determined that the evidence is adequate to conclude that the collagen meniscus implant does not improve health outcomes and, therefore, is not reasonable and necessary for the treatment of meniscal injury/tear under section 1862(a)(1)(A) of the Social Security Act. Thus, the collagen meniscus implant is non-covered by Medicare.

D. Other

N/A

(This NCD last reviewed May 2010.)

100-3, 160.13

NCD for Supplies Used in the Delivery of Transcutaneous Electrical Nerve Stimulation (TENS) and Neuromuscular Electrical Stimulation (NMES) (160.13)

Transcutaneous Electrical Nerve Stimulation (TENS) and/or Neuromuscular Electrical Stimulation (NMES) can ordinarily be delivered to patients through the use of conventional electrodes, adhesive tapes and lead wires. There may be times, however, where it might be medically necessary for certain patients receiving TENS or NMES treatment to use, as an alternative to conventional electrodes, adhesive tapes and lead wires, a form-fitting conductive garment (i.e., a garment with conductive fibers which are separated from the patients' skin by layers of fabric).

A form-fitting conductive garment (and medically necessary related supplies) may be covered under the program only when:

1. It has received permission or approval for marketing by the Food and Drug Administration;

2. It has been prescribed by a physician for use in delivering covered TENS or NMES treatment; and

3. One of the medical indications outlined below is met:

   • The patient cannot manage without the conductive garment because there is such a large area or so many sites to be stimulated and the stimulation would have to be delivered so frequently that it is not feasible to use conventional electrodes, adhesive tapes and lead wires;

   • The patient cannot manage without the conductive garment for the treatment of chronic intractable pain because the areas or sites to be stimulated are inaccessible with the use of conventional electrodes, adhesive tapes and lead wires;

   • The patient has a documented medical condition such as skin problems that preclude the application of conventional electrodes, adhesive tapes and lead wires;

   • The patient requires electrical stimulation beneath a cast either to treat disuse atrophy, where the nerve supply to the muscle is intact, or to treat chronic intractable pain; or

   • The patient has a medical need for rehabilitation strengthening (pursuant to a written plan of rehabilitation) following an injury where the nerve supply to the muscle is intact.

A conductive garment is not covered for use with a TENS device during the trial period specified in §160.3 unless:

4. The patient has a documented skin problem prior to the start of the trial period; and

5. The carrier's medical consultants are satisfied that use of such an item is medically necessary for the patient.

(See conditions for coverage of the use of TENS in the diagnosis and treatment of chronic intractable pain in §§160.3,160.13 and 160.27 and the use of NMES in the treatment of disuse atrophy in §150.4.)

100-3, 160.27

NCD for Transcutaneous Electrical Nerve Stimulation (TENS) for Chronic Low Back Pain (CLBP)

The TENS is a type of electrical nerve stimulator that is employed to treat chronic intractable pain. This stimulator is attached to the surface of the patient's skin over the peripheral nerve to be stimulated. It may be applied in a variety of settings (in the patient's home, a physician's office, or in an outpatient clinic). Payment for TENS may be made under the durable medical equipment benefit.

A. General

For the purposes of this decision chronic low back pain (CLBP) is defined as:

1. an episode of low back pain that has persisted for three months or longer; and

2. is not a manifestation of a clearly defined and generally recognizable primary disease entity. For example, there are cancers that, through metastatic spread to the spine or pelvis, may elicit pain in the lower back as a symptom; and certain systemic diseases such as rheumatoid arthritis and multiple sclerosis manifest many debilitating symptoms of which low back pain is not the primary focus. B. Nationally Covered Indications Effective June 8, 2012, the Centers for Medicare & Medicaid Services (CMS) will allow coverage for Transcutaneous Electrical Nerve Stimulation (TENS) for CLBP only when all of the following conditions are met:

In order to support additional research on the use of TENS for CLBP, we will cover this item under section 1862(a)(1)(E) of the Social Security Act (the Act) subject to all of the following conditions:

1. Coverage under this section expires three years after the publication of this decision on the CMS website.

2. The beneficiary is enrolled in an approved clinical study meeting all of the requirements below. The study must address one or more aspects of the following questions in a randomized, controlled design using validated and reliable instruments. This can include randomized crossover designs when the impact of prior TENS use is appropriately accounted for in the study protocol.

   i. Does the use of TENS provide clinically meaningful reduction in pain in Medicare beneficiaries with CLBP?

   ii. Does the use of TENS provide a clinically meaningful improvement of function in Medicare beneficiaries with CLBP?

   iii. Does the use of TENS impact the utilization of other medical treatments or services used in the medical management of CLBP?

These studies must be designed so that the patients in the control and comparison groups receive the same concurrent treatments and either sham (placebo) TENS or active TENS intervention.

The study must adhere to the following standards of scientific integrity and relevance to the Medicare population:

   a. The principal purpose of the research study is to test whether a particular intervention potentially improves the participants' health outcomes.

   b. The research study is well supported by available scientific and medical information or it is intended to clarify or establish the health outcomes of interventions already in common clinical use.

   c. The research study does not unjustifiably duplicate existing studies.

   d. The research study design is appropriate to answer the research question being asked in the study.

   e. The research study is sponsored by an organization or individual capable of executing the proposed study successfully. f. The research study is in compliance with all applicable Federal regulations concerning the protection of human subjects found at 45 CFR Part 46. If a study is regulated by the Food and Drug Administration (FDA), it must be in compliance with 21 CFR parts 50 and 56.

   g. All aspects of the research study are conducted according to appropriate standards of scientific integrity (see http://www.icmje.org).

   h. The research study has a written protocol that clearly addresses, or incorporates by reference, the standards listed here as Medicare requirements for CED coverage.

   i. The clinical research study is not designed to exclusively test toxicity or disease pathophysiology in healthy individuals. Trials of all medical technologies measuring therapeutic outcomes as one of the objectives meet this standard only if the disease or condition being studied is life threatening as defined in 21 CFR § 312.81(a) and the patient has no other viable treatment options.

   j. The clinical research study is registered on the ClinicalTrials.gov website by the principal sponsor/investigator prior to the enrollment of the first study subject.

   k. The research study protocol specifies the method and timing of public release of all prespecified outcomes to be measured including release of outcomes if outcomes are negative or study is terminated early. The results must be made public within 24 months of the end of data collection. If a report is planned to be published in a peer reviewed journal, then that initial release may be an abstract that meets the requirements of the International Committee of Medical Journal Editors (http://www.icmje.org).

   l. The research study protocol must explicitly discuss subpopulations affected by the treatment under investigation, particularly traditionally underrepresented groups in clinical studies, how the inclusion and exclusion criteria effect enrollment of these populations, and a plan for the retention and reporting of said populations on the trial. If the inclusion and exclusion criteria are expected to have a negative effect on the recruitment or retention of underrepresented populations, the protocol must discuss why these criteria are necessary

   m. The research study protocol explicitly discusses how the results are or are not expected to be generalizable to the Medicare population to infer whether Medicare patients may benefit from the intervention. Separate discussions in the protocol may be necessary for populations eligible for Medicare due to age, disability or Medicaid eligibility. .

C. Nationally Non-Covered Indications

TENS is not reasonable and necessary for the treatment of CLBP under section 1862(a)(1)(A) of the Act.

D. Other

See §160.13 for an explanation of coverage of medically necessary supplies for the effective use of TENS. See §160.7.1 for an explanation of coverage for assessing patients suitability for electrical nerve stimulation therapy. See §10.2 for an explanation of coverage of transcutaneous electrical nerve stimulation (TENS) for acute post-operative pain. Please note, §280.13Transcutaneous Electrical Nerve Stimulators (TENS) NCD has been removed from the NCD manual and incorporated into NCD 160.27.

(This NCD last reviewed June 2012

100-3,160.7.1

Assessing Patients Suitability for Electrical Nerve Stimulation Therapy

B. Percutaneous Electrical Nerve Stimulation (PENS)

This diagnostic procedure which involves stimulation of peripheral nerves by a needle electrode inserted through the skin is performed only in a physician's office, clinic, or hospital outpatient department. Therefore, it is covered only when performed by a physician or incident to physician's service. If pain is effectively controlled by percutaneous stimulation, implantation of electrodes is warranted.

As in the case of TENS (described in subsection A), generally the physician should be able to determine whether the patient is likely to derive a significant therapeutic benefit from continuing use of an implanted nerve stimulator within a trial period of 1 month. In a few cases, this determination may take longer to make. The medical necessity for such diagnostic services which are furnished beyond the first month must be documented.

NOTE: Electrical nerve stimulators do not prevent pain but only alleviate pain as it occurs. A patient can be taught how to employ the stimulator, and once this is done, can use it safely and effectively without direct physician supervision. Consequently, it is inappropriate for a patient to visit his/her physician, physical therapist, or an outpatient clinic on a continuing basis for treatment of pain with electrical nerve stimulation. Once it is determined that electrical nerve stimulation should be continued as therapy and the patient has been trained to use the stimulator, it is expected that a stimulator will be implanted or the patient will employ the TENS on a continual basis in his/her home. Electrical nerve stimulation treatments furnished by a physician in his/her office, by a physical therapist or outpatient clinic are excluded from coverage by §1862(a)(1) of the Act. (See §160.7 for an explanation of coverage of the therapeutic use of implanted peripheral nerve stimulators under the prosthetic devices benefit.) See §160.27 for an explanation of coverage of the therapeutic use of TENS under the durable medical equipment benefit.

100-3, 190.11

NCD for Home Prothrombin Time International Normalized Ratio (INR) Monitoring for Anticoagulation Management (190.11)

A. General

Use of the International Normalized Ratio (INR) or prothrombin time (PT) - standard measurement for reporting the blood's clotting time) - allows physicians to determine the level of anticoagulation in a patient independent of the laboratory reagents used. The INR is the ratio of the patient's PT (extrinsic or tissue-factor dependent coagulation pathway) compared to the mean PT for a group of normal individuals. Maintaining patients within his/her prescribed therapeutic range minimizes adverse events associated with inadequate or excessive anticoagulation such as serious bleeding or thromboembolic events. Patient self-testing and self-management through the use of a home INR monitor may be used to improve the time in therapeutic rate (TTR) for select groups of patients. Increased TTR leads to improved clinical outcomes and reductions in thromboembolic and hemorrhagic events.

Warfarin (also prescribed under other trade names, e.g., Coumadin(R)) is a self-administered, oral anticoagulant (blood thinner) medication that affects the vitamin K- dependent clotting factors II, VII, IX and X. It is widely used for various medical conditions, and has a narrow therapeutic index, meaning it is a drug with less than a 2-fold difference between median lethal dose and median effective dose. For this reason, since October 4, 2006, it falls under the category of a Food and Drug administration (FDA) "black-box" drug whose dosage must be closely monitored to avoid serious complications. A PT/INR monitoring system is a portable testing device that includes a finger-stick and an FDA-cleared meter that measures the time it takes for a person's blood plasma to clot.

B. Nationally Covered Indications

For services furnished on or after March 19, 2008, Medicare will cover the use of home PT/INR monitoring for chronic, oral anticoagulation management for patients with mechanical heart valves, chronic atrial fibrillation, or venous thromboembolism (inclusive of deep venous thrombosis and pulmonary embolism) on warfarin. The monitor and the home testing must be prescribed by a treating physician as provided at 42 CFR 410.32(a), and all of the following requirements must be met:

1. The patient must have been anticoagulated for at least 3 months prior to use of the home INR device; and,

2. The patient must undergo a face-to-face educational program on anticoagulation management and must have demonstrated the correct use of the device prior to its use in the home; and,

3. The patient continues to correctly use the device in the context of the management of the anticoagulation therapy following the initiation of home monitoring; and,

4. Self-testing with the device should not occur more frequently than once a week.

C. Nationally Non-Covered Indications
N/A

D. Other

1. All other indications for home PT/INR monitoring not indicated as nationally covered above remain at local Medicare contractor discretion.

2. This national coverage determination (NCD) is distinct from, and makes no changes to, the PT clinical laboratory NCD at section 190.17 of Publication 100-03 of the NCD Manual.

100-3,190.14

NCD for Human Immunodeficiency Virus (HIV) Testing (Diagnosis) (190.14)

Indications and Limitations of Coverage

Indications

Diagnostic testing to establish HIV infection may be indicated when there is a strong clinical suspicion supported by one or more of the following clinical findings:

The patient has a documented, otherwise unexplained, AIDS-defining or AIDS-associated opportunistic infection.

The patient has another documented sexually transmitted disease which identifies significant risk of exposure to HIV and the potential for an early or subclinical infection.

The patient has documented acute or chronic hepatitis B or C infection that identifies a significant risk of exposure to HIV and the potential for an early or subclinical infection.

The patient has a documented AIDS-defining or AIDS-associated neoplasm.

The patient has a documented AIDS-associated neurologic disorder or otherwise unexplained dementia.

The patient has another documented AIDS-defining clinical condition, or a history of other severe, recurrent, or persistent conditions which suggest an underlying immune deficiency (for example, cutaneous or mucosal disorders).

The patient has otherwise unexplained generalized signs and symptoms suggestive of a chronic process with an underlying immune deficiency (for example, fever, weight loss, malaise, fatigue, chronic diarrhea, failure to thrive, chronic cough, hemoptysis, shortness of breath, or lymphadenopathy).

The patient has otherwise unexplained laboratory evidence of a chronic disease process with an underlying immune deficiency (for example, anemia, leukopenia, pancytopenia, lymphopenia, or low CD4+ lymphocyte count).

The patient has signs and symptoms of acute retroviral syndrome with fever, malaise, lymphadenopathy, and skin rash.

The patient has documented exposure to blood or body fluids known to be capable of transmitting HIV (for example, needlesticks and other significant blood exposures) and antiviral therapy is initiated or anticipated to be initiated.

The patient is undergoing treatment for rape. (HIV testing is a part of the rape treatment protocol.)

Limitations

HIV antibody testing in the United States is usually performed using HIV-1 or HIV-¬¾ combination tests. HIV-2 testing is indicated if clinical circumstances suggest HIV-2 is likely (that is, compatible clinical findings and HIV-1 test negative). HIV-2 testing may also be indicated in areas of the country where there is greater prevalence of HIV-2 infections.

The Western Blot test should be performed only after documentation that the initial EIA tests are repeatedly positive or equivocal on a single sample.

The HIV antigen tests currently have no defined diagnostic usage.

Direct viral RNA detection may be performed in those situations where serologic

testing does not establish a diagnosis but strong clinical suspicion persists (for example, acute retroviral syndrome, nonspecific serologic evidence of HIV, or perinatal HIV infection).

If initial serologic tests confirm an HIV infection, repeat testing is not indicated.

If initial serologic tests are HIV EIA negative and there is no indication for confirmation of infection by viral RNA detection, the interval prior to retesting is 3-6 months.

Testing for evidence of HIV infection using serologic methods may be medically appropriate in situations where there is a risk of exposure to HIV. However, in the absence of a documented AIDS defining or HIV- associated disease, an HIV associated sign or symptom, or documented exposure to a known HIV-infected source, the testing is considered by Medicare to be screening and thus is not covered by Medicare (for example, history of multiple blood component transfusions, exposure to blood or body fluids not resulting in consideration of therapy, history of transplant, history of illicit drug use, multiple sexual partners, same-sex encounters, prostitution, or contact with prostitutes).

The CPT Editorial Panel has issued a number of codes for infectious agent detection by direct antigen or nucleic acid probe techniques that have not yet been developed or are only being used on an investigational basis. Laboratory providers are advised to remain current on FDA-approval status for these tests.

100-3, 210.3

Colorectal Cancer Screening Tests

A. General

Section 4104 of the Balanced Budget Act of 1997 provides for coverage of screening colorectal cancer procedures under Medicare Part B. Medicare currently covers: (1) annual fecal occult blood tests (FOBTs); (2) flexible sigmoidoscopy over 4 years; (3) screening colonoscopy for persons at average risk for colorectal cancer every 10 years, or for persons at high risk for colorectal cancer every 2 years; (4) barium enema every 4 years as an alternative to flexible sigmoidoscopy, or every 2 years as an alternative to colonoscopy for persons at high risk for colorectal cancer; and, (5) other procedures the Secretary finds appropriate based on consultation with appropriate experts and organizations.

Coverage of the above screening examinations was implemented in regulations through a final rule that was published on October 31, 1997 (62 FR 59079), and was effective January 1, 1998. At that time, based on consultation with appropriate experts and organizations, the definition of the term "FOBT" was defined in 42 CFR Sec.410.37(a)(2) of the regulation to mean a "guaiac-based test for peroxidase activity, testing two samples from each of three consecutive stools."

In the 2003 Physician Fee Schedule Final Rule (67 FR 79966) effective March 1, 2003, the Centers for Medicare & Medicaid Services (CMS) amended the FOBT screening test regulation definition to provide that it could include either: (1) a guaiac-based FOBT, or, (2) other tests determined by the Secretary through a national coverage determination.

B. Nationally Covered Indications
Fecal Occult Blood Tests (FOBT) (effective for services performed on or after January 1, 2004)

1. History

   The FOBTs are generally divided into two types: immunoassay and guaiac types. Immunoassay (or immunochemical) fecal occult blood tests (iFOBT) use "antibodies directed against human globin epitopes. While most iFOBTs use spatulas to collect stool samples, some use a brush to collect toilet water surrounding the stool. Most iFOBTs require laboratory processing.

   Guaiac fecal occult blood tests (gFOBT) use a peroxidase reaction to indicate presence of the heme portion of hemoglobin. Guaiac turns blue after oxidation by oxidants or peroxidases in the presence of an oxygen donor such as hydrogen peroxide. Most FOBTs use sticks to collect stool samples and may be developed in a physician's office or a laboratory. In 1998, Medicare began reimbursement for guaiac FOBTs, but not immunoassay type tests for colorectal cancer screening. Since the fundamental process is similar for other iFOBTs, CMS evaluated colorectal cancer screening using immunoassay FOBTs in general.

2. Expanded Coverage

   Medicare covers one screening FOBT per annum for the early detection of colorectal cancer. This means that Medicare will cover one guaiac-based (gFOBT) or one immunoassay-based (iFOBT) at a frequency of every 12 months; i.e., at least 11 months have passed following the month in which the last covered screening FOBT was performed, for beneficiaries aged 50 years and older. The beneficiary completes the existing gFOBT by taking samples from two different sites of three consecutive stools; the beneficiary completes the iFOBT by taking the appropriate number of stool samples according to the specific manufacturer's instructions. This screening requires a written order from the beneficiary's attending physician. ("Attending physician means a doctor of medicine or osteopathy (as defined in Sec.1861(r)(1) of the Social Security Act) who is fully knowledgeable about the beneficiary's medical condition, and who would be responsible for using the results of any examination performed in the overall management of the beneficiary's specific medical problem.)

C. Nationally Non-Covered Indications
All other indications for colorectal cancer screening not otherwise specified above remain non-covered. Non-coverage specifically includes:

1. Screening DNA (Deoxyribonucleic acid) stool tests, effective April 28, 2008, and,

2. Screening computed tomographic colonography (CTC), effective May 12, 2009.

D. Other
N/A

(This NCD last reviewed May 2009.)

100-3, 210.4

NCD for Smoking and Tobacco-Use Cessation Counseling (210.4)

A. General
Tobacco use continues to be the leading cause of preventable death in the United States. In 1964, the Surgeon General of the U.S. Public Health Service (PHS) issued the report of his Advisory Committee on Smoking and Health, officially recognizing that cigarette smoking is a cause of cancer and other serious diseases. Though smoking rates have significantly declined, 9.3% of the population age 65 and older smokes cigarettes. Approximately 440,000 people die annually from smoking related disease, with 68% (300,000) age 65 or older. Many more people of all ages suffer from serious illness caused from smoking, leading to disability and decreased quality of life. Reduction in smoking prevalence is a national objective in Healthy People 2010.

B. Nationally Covered Indications
Effective March 22, 2005, the Centers for Medicare and Medicaid Services (CMS) has determined that the evidence is adequate to conclude that smoking and tobacco use cessation counseling, based on the current PHS Guideline, is reasonable and necessary for a patient with a disease or an adverse health effect that has been found by the U.S. Surgeon General to be linked to tobacco use, or who is taking a therapeutic agent whose metabolism or dosing is affected by tobacco use as based on FDA-approved information.

Patients must be competent and alert at the time that services are provided. Minimal counseling is already covered at each evaluation and management (E&M) visit. Beyond that, Medicare will cover 2 cessation attempts per year. Each attempt may include a maximum of 4 intermediate or intensive sessions, with the total annual benefit covering up to 8 sessions in a 12-month period. The practitioner and patient have flexibility to choose between intermediate or intensive cessation strategies for each attempt.

Intermediate and intensive smoking cessation counseling services will be covered for outpatient and hospitalized beneficiaries who are smokers and who qualify as above, as long as those services are furnished by qualified physicians and other Medicare-recognized practitioners.

C. Nationally Non-Covered Indications
Inpatient hospital stays with the principal diagnosis of Tobacco Use Disorder are not reasonable and necessary for the effective delivery of tobacco cessation counseling services. Therefore, we will not cover tobacco cessation services if tobacco cessation is the primary reason for the patient's hospital stay.

D. Other
N/A

(This NCD last reviewed May 2005.)

100-3, 210.7

NCD for Screening for the Human Immunodeficiency Virus (HIV) Infection (210.7)

A. General
Infection with the human immunodeficiency virus (HIV) is a continuing, worldwide pandemic described by the World Health Organization as "the most serious infectious disease challenge to global public health". Acquired immunodeficiency syndrome (AIDS) is diagnosed when a HIV-infected person's immune system becomes severely compromised and/or a person becomes ill with a HIV-related opportunistic infection. Without treatment, AIDS usually develops within 8-10 years after a person's initial HIV infection. While there is presently no cure for HIV, an infected individual can be recognized by screening, and subsequent access to skilled care plus vigilant monitoring and adherence to continuous antiretroviral therapy may delay the onset of AIDS and increase quality of life for many years.

Significantly, more than half of new HIV infections are estimated to be sexually transmitted from infected individuals who are unaware of their HIV status. Consequently, improved secondary disease prevention and wider availability of screening linked to HIV care and treatment would not only delay disease progression and complications in untested or unaware older individuals, but could also decrease the spread of disease to those living with or partnered with HIV-infected individuals.

HIV antibody testing first became available in 1985. These commonly used, Food and Drug Administration (FDA)-approved HIV antibody screening tests – using serum or plasma from a venipuncture or blood draw – are known as EIA (enzyme immunoassay) or ELISA (enzyme-linked immunosorbent assay) tests.

Developed for point-of-care testing using alternative samples, six rapid HIV-1 and/or HIV-2 antibody tests – using fluid obtained from the oral cavity or using whole blood, serum, or plasma from a blood draw or fingerstick – were approved by the FDA from 2002-2006.

Effective January 1, 2009, the Centers for Medicare & Medicaid Services (CMS) is allowed to add coverage of "additional preventive services" through the national coverage determination (NCD) process if certain statutory requirements are met, as provided under section 101(a) of the Medicare Improvements for Patients and Providers Act. One of those requirements is that the service(s) be categorized as a grade A (strongly recommends) or grade B (recommends) rating by the US Preventive Services Task Force (USPSTF). The USPSTF strongly recommends screening for all adolescents and adults at risk for HIV infection, as well as all pregnant women.

B. Nationally Covered Indications
Effective for claims with dates of service on and after December 8, 2009, CMS determines that the evidence is adequate to conclude that screening for HIV infection is reasonable and necessary for early detection of HIV and is appropriate for individuals entitled to benefits under

Part A or enrolled under Part B. Therefore, CMS proposes to cover both standard and FDA-approved HIV rapid screening tests for:

1. A maximum of one, annual voluntary HIV screening of Medicare beneficiaries at increased risk for HIV infection per USPSTF guidelines as follows:

   • Men who have had sex with men after 1975

   • Men and women having unprotected sex with multiple [more than one] partners

   • Past or present injection drug users

   • Men and women who exchange sex for money or drugs, or have sex partners who do

   • Individuals whose past or present sex partners were HIV-infected, bisexual or injection drug users

   • Persons being treated for sexually transmitted diseases

   • Persons with a history of blood transfusion between 1978 and 1985

   • Persons who request an HIV test despite reporting no individual risk factors, since this group is likely to include individuals not willing to disclose high-risk behaviors; and,

2. A maximum of three, voluntary HIV screenings of pregnant Medicare beneficiaries: (1) when the diagnosis of pregnancy is known, (2) during the third trimester, and (3) at labor, if ordered by the woman's clinician.

C. Nationally Non-Covered Indications
Effective for claims with dates of service on and after December 8, 2009, Medicare beneficiaries with any known diagnosis of a HIV-related illness are not eligible for this screening test.

Medicare beneficiaries (other than those who are pregnant) who have had a prior HIV screening test within one year are not eligible (11 full months must have elapsed following the month in which the previous test was performed in order for the subsequent test to be covered).

Pregnant Medicare beneficiaries who have had three screening tests within their respective term of pregnancy are not eligible (beginning with the date of the first test).

D. Other
N/A

(This NCD last reviewed November 2009.)

100-3, 210.8

Screening and Behavioral Counseling Interventions in Primary Care to Reduce Alcohol Misuse (Effective October 14, 2011)

A. General
Based upon authority to cover "additional preventive services" for Medicare beneficiaries if certain statutory requirements are met, the Centers for Medicare & Medicaid Services (CMS) initiated a new national coverage analysis on annual screening and brief behavioral counseling in primary care to reduce alcohol misuse in adults, including pregnant women. Annual screening and behavioral counseling for alcohol misuse in adults is recommended with a grade of B by the U.S. Preventive Services Task Force (USPSTF) and is appropriate for individuals entitled to benefits under Part A and Part B.

CMS will cover annual alcohol screening and up to four, brief face-to-face behavioral counseling in primary care settings to reduce alcohol misuse. CMS does not identify specific alcohol misuse

screening tools. Rather, the decision to use a specific tool is at the discretion of the clinician in the primary care setting. Various screening tools are available for screening for alcohol misuse.

B. Nationally Covered Indications
Effective for claims with dates of service on or after October 14, 2011, CMS will cover annual alcohol screening, and for those that screen positive, up to four brief, face-to-face, behavioral counseling interventions per year for Medicare beneficiaries, including pregnant women:

   • Who misuse alcohol, but whose levels or patterns of alcohol consumption do not meet criteria for alcohol dependence (defined as at least three of the following: tolerance, withdrawal symptoms, impaired control, preoccupation with acquisition and/or use, persistent desire or unsuccessful efforts to quit, sustains social, occupational, or recreational disability, use continues despite adverse consequences); and

   • Who are competent and alert at the time that counseling is provided; and,

   • Whose counseling is furnished by qualified primary care physicians or other primary care practitioners in a primary care setting.

Each of the behavioral counseling interventions should be consistent with the 5A' approach that has been adopted by the USPSTF to describe such services. They are:

1. Assess: Ask about/assess behavioral health risk(s) and factors affecting choice of behavior change goals/methods.

2. Advise: Give clear, specific, and personalized behavior change advice, including information about personal health harms and benefits.

3. Agree: Collaboratively select appropriate treatment goals and methods based on the patient's interest in and willingness to change the behavior.

4. Assist: Using behavior change techniques (self-help and/or counseling), aid the patient in achieving agreed upon goals by acquiring the skills, confidence, and social/environmental supports for behavior change, supplemented with adjunctive medical treatments when appropriate.

5. Arrange: Schedule follow-up contacts (in person or by telephone) to provide ongoing assistance/support and to adjust the treatment plan as needed, including referral to more intensive or specialized treatment. For the purposes of this policy, a primary care setting is defined as one in which there is provision of integrated, accessible health care services by clinicians who are accountable for addressing a large majority of personal health care needs, developing a sustained partnership with patients, and practicing in the context of family and community. Emergency departments, inpatient hospital settings, ambulatory surgical centers, independent diagnostic testing facilities, skilled nursing facilities, inpatient rehabilitation facilities and hospices are not considered primary care settings under this definition.

For the purposes of this policy a "primary care physician" and "primary care practitioner" are to be defined based on two existing sections of the Social Security Act, §1833(u)(6), §1833(x)(2)(A)(i)(I) and §1833(x)(2)(A)(i)(II):

§1833(u)

(6)Physician Defined.—For purposes of this paragraph, the term "physician" means a physician described in section 1861(r)(1) and the term "primary care physician" means a physician who is identified in the available data as a general practitioner, family practice practitioner, general internist, or obstetrician or gynecologist.

§1833(x)(2)(A)(i)

(I) is a physician (as described in section 1861(r)(1)) who has a primary specialty designation of family medicine, internal medicine, geriatric medicine, or pediatric medicine; or

(II) is a nurse practitioner, clinical nurse specialist, or physician assistant (as those terms are defined in section 1861(aa)(5)).

C. Nationally Non-Covered Indications
1. Alcohol screening is non-covered when performed more than one time in a 12-month period.

2. Brief face-to-face behavioral counseling interventions are non-covered when performed more than once a day; that is, two counseling interventions on the same day are non-covered.

3. Brief face-to-face behavioral counseling interventions are non-covered when performed more than four times in a 12-month period

D. Other
Medicare coinsurance and Part B deductible are waived for this preventive service

(This NCD last reviewed October 2011.)

100-3, 210.10

Screening for Sexually Transmitted Infections (STIs) and High Intensity Behavioral Counseling (HIBC) to Prevent STIs

A. General

Sexually transmitted infections (STIs) are infections that are passed from one person to another through sexual contact. STIs remain an important cause of morbidity in the United States and have both health and economic consequences. Many of the complications of STIs are borne by women and children Often, STIs do not present any symptoms so can go untreated for long periods of time The presence of an STI during pregnancy may result in significant health complications for the woman and infant. In fact, any person who has an STI may develop health complications. Screening tests for the STIs in this national coverage determination (NCD) are laboratory tests.

Under §1861(ddd) of the Social Security Act (the Act), the Centers for Medicare & Medicaid Services (CMS) has the authority to add coverage of additional preventive services if certain statutory requirements are met. The regulations provide:

§410.64 Additional preventive services

(a) Medicare Part B pays for additional preventive services not described in paragraph (1) or (3) of the definition of "preventive services" under §410.2, that identify medical conditions or risk factors for individuals if the Secretary determines through the national coverage determination process (as defined in section 1869(f)(1)(B) of the Act) that these services are all of the following: (1) reasonable and necessary for the prevention or early detection of illness or disability.(2) recommended with a grade of A or B by the United States Preventive Services Task Force, (3) appropriate for individuals entitled to benefits under Part A or enrolled under Part B.

(b) In making determinations under paragraph (a) of this section regarding the coverage of a new preventive service, the Secretary may conduct an assessment of the relation between predicted outcomes and the expenditures for such services and may take into account the results of such an assessment in making such national coverage determinations.

The scope of the national coverage analysis for this NCD evaluated the evidence for the following STIs and high intensity behavioral counseling (HIBC) to prevent STIs for which the United States Preventive Services Task Force (USPSTF) has issued either an A or B recommendation:

- Screening for chlamydial infection for all sexually active non-pregnant young women aged 24 and younger and for older non-pregnant women who are at increased risk,
- Screening for chlamydial infection for all pregnant women aged 24 and younger and for older pregnant women who are at increased risk,
- Screening for gonorrhea infection in all sexually active women, including those who are pregnant, if they are at increased risk,
- Screening for syphilis infection for all pregnant women and for all persons at increased risk,
- Screening for hepatitis B virus (HBV) infection in pregnant women at their first prenatal visit,
- HIBC for the prevention of STIs for all sexually active adolescents, and for adults at increased risk for STIs.

B. Nationally Covered Indications

CMS has determined that the evidence is adequate to conclude that screening for chlamydia, gonorrhea, syphilis, and hepatitis B, as well as HIBC to prevent STIs, consistent with the grade A and B recommendations by the USPSTF, is reasonable and necessary for the early detection or prevention of an illness or disability and is appropriate for individuals entitled to benefits under Part A or enrolled under Part B.

Therefore, effective for claims with dates of services on or after November 8, 2011, CMS will cover screening for these USPSTF-indicated STIs with the appropriate Food and Drug Administration (FDA)-approved/cleared laboratory tests, used consistent with FDA-approved labeling, and in compliance with the Clinical Laboratory Improvement Act (CLIA) regulations, when ordered by the primary care physician or practitioner, and performed by an eligible Medicare provider for these services.

Screening for chlamydia and gonorrhea:

- Pregnant women who are 24 years old or younger when the diagnosis of pregnancy is known, and then repeat screening during the third trimester if high-risk sexual behavior has occurred since the initial screening test.
- Pregnant women who are at increased risk for STIs when the diagnosis of pregnancy is known, and then repeat screening during the third trimester if high-risk sexual behavior has occurred since the initial screening test.
- Women at increased risk for STIs annually.

Screening for syphilis:

- Pregnant women when the diagnosis of pregnancy is known, and then repeat screening during the third trimester and at delivery if high-risk sexual behavior has occurred since the previous screening test.
- Men and women at increased risk for STIs annually.

Screening for hepatitis B:

- Pregnant women at the first prenatal visit when the diagnosis of pregnancy is known, and then rescreening at time of delivery for those with new or continuing risk factors. In addition, effective for claims with dates of service on or after November 8, 2011, CMS will cover up to two individual 20- to 30-minute, face-to-face counseling sessions annually for Medicare beneficiaries for HIBC to prevent STIs, for all sexually active adolescents, and for adults at increased risk for STIs, if referred for this service by a primary care physician or practitioner, and provided by a Medicare eligible primary care provider in a primary care setting. Coverage of HIBC to prevent STIs is consistent with the USPSTF recommendation.

HIBC is defined as a program intended to promote sexual risk reduction or risk avoidance, which includes each of these broad topics, allowing flexibility for appropriate patient-focused elements:

- education,
- skills training,
- guidance on how to change sexual behavior.

The high/increased risk individual sexual behaviors, based on the USPSTF guidelines, include any of the following:

- Multiple sex partners
- Using barrier protection inconsistently
- Having sex under the influence of alcohol or drugs
- Having sex in exchange for money or drugs
- Age (24 years of age or younger and sexually active for women for chlamydia and gonorrhea)
- Having an STI within the past year
- IV drug use (for hepatitis B only)

In addition for men

- men having sex with men (MSM) and engaged in high risk sexual behavior, but no regard to age

In addition to individual risk factors, in concurrence with the USPSTF recommendations, community social factors such as high prevalence of STIs in the community populations should be considered in determining high/increased risk for chlamydia, gonorrhea, syphilis, and for recommending HIBC.

High/increased risk sexual behavior for STIs is determined by the primary care provider by assessing the patient's sexual history which is part of any complete medical history, typically part of an annual wellness visit or prenatal visit and considered in the development of a comprehensive prevention plan. The medical record should be a reflection of the service provided.

For the purposes of this NCD, a primary care setting is defined as the provision of integrated, accessible health care services by clinicians who are accountable for addressing a large majority of personal health care needs, developing a sustained partnership with patients, and practicing in the context of family and community. Emergency departments, inpatient hospital settings, ambulatory surgical centers, independent diagnostic testing facilities, skilled nursing facilities, inpatient rehabilitation facilities, clinics providing a limited focus of health care services, and hospice are examples of settings not considered primary care settings under this definition.

For the purposes of this NCD, a "primary care physician" and "primary care practitioner" will be defined based on existing sections of the Social Security Act (§1833(u)(6), §1833(x)(2)(A)(i)(I) and §1833(x)(2)(A)(i)(II)).

§1833(u)

(6) Physician Defined.?or purposes of this paragraph, the term "physician" means a physician described in section 1861(r)(1) and the term "primary care physician" means a physician who is identified in the available data as a general practitioner, family practice practitioner, general internist, or obstetrician or gynecologist.

§1833(x)(2)(A)(i)

(I) is a physician (as described in section 1861(r)(1)) who has a primary specialty designation of family medicine, internal medicine, geriatric medicine, or pediatric medicine; or

(II) is a nurse practitioner, clinical nurse specialist, or physician assistant (as those terms are defined in section 1861(aa)(5));

C. Nationally Non-Covered Indications

Unless specifically covered in this NCD, any other NCD, or in statute, preventive services are non-covered by Medicare.

D. Other

Medicare coinsurance and Part B deductible are waived for these preventive services.

HIBC to prevent STIs may be provided on the same date of services as an annual wellness visit, evaluation and management (E&M) service, or during the global billing period for obstetrical car, but only one HIBC may be provided on any one date of service. See the claims processing manual for further instructions on claims processing.

For services provided on an annual basis, this is defined as a 12-month period.

(This NCD last reviewed November 2011.)

100-3, 210.11

Intensive Behavioral Therapy for Cardiovascular Disease (CVD) (Effective November 8, 2011

A. General

Cardiovascular disease (CVD) is the leading cause of mortality in the United States. CVD, which is comprised of hypertension, coronary heart disease (such as myocardial infarction and angina pectoris), heart failure and stroke, is also the leading cause of hospitalizations. Although the overall adjusted mortality rate from heart disease has declined over the past decade, opportunities for improvement still exist. Risk factors for CVD include being overweight, obesity, physical inactivity, diabetes, cigarette smoking, high blood pressure, high blood cholesterol, family history of myocardial infarction, and older age.

Under §1861(ddd) of the Social Security Act (the Act), the Centers for Medicare & Medicaid Services (CMS) has the authority to add coverage of additional preventive services through the National Coverage Determination (NCD) process if certain statutory requirements are met. Following its review, CMS has determined that the evidence is adequate to conclude that intensive behavioral therapy for CVD is reasonable and necessary for the prevention or early detection of illness or disability, is appropriate for individuals entitled to benefits under Part A or enrolled under Part B, and is comprised of components that are recommended with a grade of A or B by the U.S. Preventive Services Task Force (USPSTF).

B. Nationally Covered Indications

Effective for claims with dates of service on or after November 8, 2011, CMS covers intensive behavioral therapy for CVD (referred to below as a CVD risk reduction visit), which consists of the following three components:

- encouraging aspirin use for the primary prevention of CVD when the benefits outweigh the risks for men age 45-79 years and women 55-79 years;

- screening for high blood pressure in adults age 18 years and older; and

- intensive behavioral counseling to promote a healthy diet for adults with hyperlipidemia, hypertension, advancing age, and other known risk factors for cardiovascular- and diet-related chronic disease.

We note that only a small proportion (about 4%) of the Medicare population is under 45 years (men) or 55 years (women), therefore the vast majority of beneficiaries should receive all three components. Intensive behavioral counseling to promote a healthy diet is broadly recommended to cover close to 100% of the population due to the prevalence of known risk factors.

Therefore, CMS covers one, face-to-face CVD risk reduction visit per year for Medicare beneficiaries who are competent and alert at the time that counseling is provided, and whose counseling is furnished by a qualified primary care physician or other primary care practitioner in a primary care setting.

The behavioral counseling intervention for aspirin use and healthy diet should be consistent with the Five As approach that has been adopted by the USPSTF to describe such services:

- Assess: Ask about/assess behavioral health risk(s) and factors affecting choice of behavior change goals/methods.

- Advise: Give clear, specific, and personalized behavior change advice, including information about personal health harms and benefits.

- Agree: Collaboratively select appropriate treatment goals and methods based on the patient's interest in and willingness to change the behavior.

- Assist: Using behavior change techniques (self-help and/or counseling), aid the patient in achieving agreed-upon goals by acquiring the skills, confidence, and social/environmental supports for behavior change, supplemented with adjunctive medical treatments when appropriate.

- Arrange: Schedule follow-up contacts (in person or by telephone) to provide ongoing assistance/support and to adjust the treatment plan as needed, including referral to more

intensive or specialized treatment. For the purpose of this NCD, a primary care setting is defined as the provision of integrated, accessible health care services by clinicians who are accountable for addressing a large majority of personal health care needs, developing a sustained partnership with patients, and practicing in the context of family and community. Emergency departments, inpatient hospital settings, ambulatory surgical centers, independent diagnostic testing facilities, skilled nursing facilities, inpatient rehabilitation facilities, and hospices are not considered primary care settings under this definition.

For the purpose of this NCD, a "primary care physician" and "primary care practitioner" are defined consistent with existing sections of the Act (§1833(u)(6), §1833(x)(2)(A)(i)(I) and §1833(x)(2)(A)(i)(II)).

§1833(u)

(6) Physician Defined.?or purposes of this paragraph, the term "physician" means a physician described in section 1861(r)(1) and the term "primary care physician" means a physician who is identified in the available data as a general practitioner, family practice practitioner, general internist, or obstetrician or gynecologist.

§1833(x)(2)

(A) Primary care practitioner. he term "primary care practitioner" means an individual—

(i) who—

(I) is a physician (as described in section 1861(r)(1)) who has a primary specialty designation of family medicine, internal medicine, geriatric medicine, or pediatric medicine; or

(II) is a nurse practitioner, clinical nurse specialist, or physician assistant (as those terms are defined in section 1861(aa)(5)).

C. Nationally Non-Covered Indications

Unless specifically covered in this NCD, any other NCD, or in statute, preventive services are non-covered by Medicare.

D. Other

Medicare coinsurance and Part B deductible are waived for this preventive service.

(This NCD last reviewed November 2011.)

100-3, 210.12

A. General

Based upon authority to cover "additional preventive services" for Medicare beneficiaries if certain statutory requirements are met, the Centers for Medicare & Medicaid Services (CMS) initiated a new national coverage analysis on intensive behavioral therapy for obesity. Screening for obesity in adults is recommended with a grade of B by the U.S. Preventive Services Task Force (USPSTF) and is appropriate for individuals entitled to benefits under Part A and Part B.

The Centers for Disease Control (CDC) reported that "obesity rates in the U.S. have increased dramatically over the last 30 years, and obesity is now epidemic in the United States." In the Medicare population over 30% of men and women are obese. Obesity is directly or indirectly associated with many chronic diseases including cardiovascular disease, musculoskeletal conditions and diabetes.

B. Nationally Covered Indications

Effective for claims with dates of service on or after November 29, 2011, CMS covers intensive behavioral therapy for obesity, defined as a body mass index (BMI) >= 30 kg/m2, for the prevention or early detection of illness or disability.

Intensive behavioral therapy for obesity consists of the following:

1. Screening for obesity in adults using measurement of BMI calculated by dividing weight in kilograms by the square of height in meters (expressed kg/m2);

2. Dietary (nutritional) assessment; and

3. Intensive behavioral counseling and behavioral therapy to promote sustained weight loss through high intensity interventions on diet and exercise.

The intensive behavioral intervention for obesity should be consistent with the 5-A framework that has been highlighted by the USPSTF:

1. Assess: Ask about/assess behavioral health risk(s) and factors affecting choice of behavior change goals/methods.

2. Advise: Give clear, specific, and personalized behavior change advice, including information about personal health harms and benefits.

3. Agree: Collaboratively select appropriate treatment goals and methods based on the patient's interest in and willingness to change the behavior.

4. Assist: Using behavior change techniques (self-help and/or counseling), aid the patient in achieving agreed-upon goals by acquiring the skills, confidence, and social/environmental

supports for behavior change, supplemented with adjunctive medical treatments when appropriate. 5. Arrange: Schedule follow-up contacts (in person or by telephone) to provide ongoing assistance/support and to adjust the treatment plan as needed, including referral to more intensive or specialized treatment. For Medicare beneficiaries with obesity, who are competent and alert at the time that counseling is provided and whose counseling is furnished by a qualified primary care physician or other primary care practitioner and in a primary care setting, CMS covers:

- One face-to-face visit every week for the first month;

- One face-to-face visit every other week for months 2-6;

- One face-to-face visit every month for months 7-12, if the beneficiary meets the 3kg weight loss requirement during the first six months as discussed below.

At the six month visit, a reassessment of obesity and a determination of the amount of weight loss must be performed. To be eligible for additional face-to-face visits occurring once a month for an additional six months, beneficiaries must have achieved a reduction in weight of at least 3kg over the course of the first six months of intensive therapy. This determination must be documented in the physician office records for applicable beneficiaries consistent with usual practice. For beneficiaries who do not achieve a weight loss of at least 3kg during the first six months of intensive therapy, a reassessment of their readiness to change and BMI is appropriate after an additional six month period.

For the purposes of this decision memorandum, a primary care setting is defined as one in which there is provision of integrated, accessible health care services by clinicians who are accountable for addressing a large majority of personal health care needs, developing a sustained partnership with patients, and practicing in the context of family and community. Emergency departments, inpatient hospital settings, ambulatory surgical centers, independent diagnostic testing facilities, skilled nursing facilities, inpatient rehabilitation facilities and hospices are not considered primary care settings under this definition.

For the purposes of this decision memorandum a "primary care physician" and "primary care practitioner" will be defined consistent with existing sections of the Social Security Act (§1833(u)(6), §1833(x)(2)(A)(i)(I) and §1833(x)(2)(A)(i)(II)).

§1833(u)

(6) Physician Defined.—For purposes of this paragraph, the term "physician" means a physician described in section 1861(r)(1) and the term "primary care physician" means a physician who is identified in the available data as a general practitioner, family practice practitioner, general internist, or obstetrician or gynecologist.

§1833(x)(2)(A)

Primary care practitioner—The term "primary care practitioner" means an individual—

(i) who—

(I) is a physician (as described in section 1861(r)(1)) who has a primary specialty designation of family medicine, internal medicine, geriatric medicine, or pediatric medicine; or

(II) is a nurse practitioner, clinical nurse specialist, or physician assistant (as those terms are defined in section 1861(aa)(5))

C. Nationally Non-Covered Indications
All other indications remain non-covered.

D. Other
Medicare coinsurance and Part B deductible are waived for this service

(This NCD last reviewed November 2011)

100-3, 220.6

NCD for Positron Emission Tomography (PET) Scans (220.6)

Item/Service Description
Positron Emission Tomography (PET) is a minimally invasive diagnostic imaging procedure used to evaluate metabolism in normal tissue as well as in diseased tissues in conditions such as cancer, ischemic heart disease, and some neurologic disorders. A radiopharmaceutical is injected into the patient that gives off sub-atomic particles, known as positrons, as it decays. PET uses a positron camera (tomograph) to measure the decay of the radiopharmaceutical. The rate of decay provides biochemical information on the metabolism of the tissue being studied.

(This NCD last reviewed March 2009.)

100-3, 220.6.1

NCD for PET for Perfusion of the Heart (220.6.1)

Indications and Limitations of Coverage
1. Rubidium 82 (Effective March 14, 1995)

Effective for services performed on or after March 14, 1995, PET scans performed at rest or with pharmacological stress used for noninvasive imaging of the perfusion of the heart for the diagnosis and management of patients with known or suspected coronary artery disease using the FDA-approved radiopharmaceutical Rubidium 82 (Rb 82) are covered, provided the requirements below are met:

The PET scan, whether at rest alone, or rest with stress, is performed in place of, but not in addition to, a single photon emission computed tomography (SPECT); or

The PET scan, whether at rest alone or rest with stress, is used following a SPECT that was found to be inconclusive. In these cases, the PET scan must have been considered necessary in order to determine what medical or surgical intervention is required to treat the patient. (For purposes of this requirement, an inconclusive test is a test(s) whose results are equivocal, technically uninterpretable, or discordant with a patient's other clinical data and must be documented in the beneficiary's file.)

For any PET scan for which Medicare payment is claimed for dates of services prior to July 1, 2001, the claimant must submit additional specified information on the claim form (including proper codes and/or modifiers), to indicate the results of the PET scan. The claimant must also include information on whether the PET scan was performed after an inconclusive noninvasive cardiac test. The information submitted with respect to the previous noninvasive cardiac test must specify the type of test performed prior to the PET scan and whether it was inconclusive or unsatisfactory. These explanations are in the form of special G codes used for billing PET scans using Rb 82. Beginning July 1, 2001, claims should be submitted with the appropriate codes.

2. Ammonia N-13 (Effective October 1, 2003)

Effective for services performed on or after October 1, 2003, PET scans performed at rest or with pharmacological stress used for noninvasive imaging of the perfusion of the heart for the diagnosis and management of patients with known or suspected coronary artery disease using the FDA-approved radiopharmaceutical ammonia N-13 are covered, provided the requirements below are met:

The PET scan, whether at rest alone, or rest with stress, is performed in place of, but not in addition to, a SPECT; or

The PET scan, whether at rest alone, or rest with stress, is used following a SPECT that was found to be inconclusive. In these cases, the PET scan must have been considered necessary in order to determine what medical or surgical intervention is required to treat the patient. (For purposes of this requirement, an inconclusive test is a test whose results are equivocal, technically uninterpretable, or discordant with a patient's other clinical data and must be documented in the beneficiary's file.)

(This NCD last reviewed March 2005.)

100-3, 220.6.17

Positron Emission Tomography (PET) (FDG) for Oncologic Conditions - (Various Effective Dates)

General
The Centers for Medicare and Medicaid Services (CMS) was asked to reconsider section 220.6, of the National Coverage Determinations (NCD) Manual, to end the prospective data collection requirements across all oncologic indications of FDG PET except for monitoring response to treatment. Section 220.6 of the NCD Manual, establishes the requirement for prospective data collection for FDG PET used in the diagnosis, staging, restaging, and monitoring response to treatment for brain, cervical, ovarian, pancreatic, small cell lung and testicular cancers, as well as for cancer indications not previously specified in section 220.6 in its entirety.

The CMS received public input indicating that the current coverage framework, which required cancer-by-cancer consideration of diagnosis, staging, restaging, and monitoring response to treatment should be replaced by a more omnibus consideration. Thus, CMS broadened the scope of this review through an announcement on the Web site and solicited additional public comment on the use of FDG PET imaging for solid tumors so that it could transparently consider this possibility.

1. Framework

Effective for claims with dates of service on and after April 3, 2009, CMS is adopting a coverage framework that replaces the four-part diagnosis, staging, restaging and monitoring response to treatment categories with a two-part framework that differentiates FDG PET imaging used to inform the initial antitumor treatment strategy from other uses related to guiding subsequent antitumor treatment strategies after the completion of initial treatment. CMS is making this change for all NCDs that address coverage of FDG PET for the specific oncologic conditions addressed in this decision.

2. Initial Anti-tumor Treatment Strategy

Effective for claims with dates of service on and after April 3, 2009, CMS has determined that the evidence is adequate to determine that the results of FDG PET imaging are useful in determining the appropriate initial treatment strategy for beneficiaries with suspected solid tumors and myeloma and improve health outcomes and thus are reasonable and necessary under Sec.1862(a)(1)(A) of the Social Security Act (the Act).

Therefore, CMS will cover only one FDG PET study for beneficiaries who have solid tumors that are biopsy proven or strongly suspected based on other diagnostic testing when the beneficiary's treating physician determines that the FDG PET study is needed to determine the location and/or extent of the tumor for the following therapeutic purposes related to the initial treatment strategy:

- To determine whether or not the beneficiary is an appropriate candidate for an invasive diagnostic or therapeutic procedure; or

- To determine the optimal anatomic location for an invasive procedure; or

- To determine the anatomic extent of tumor when the recommended anti-tumor treatment reasonably depends on the extent of the tumor.

As exceptions to the April 3, 2009, initial treatment strategy section above:

a. The CMS has reviewed evidence on the use of FDG PET imaging to determine initial anti-tumor treatment in patients with adenocarcinoma of the prostate. CMS has determined that the available evidence does not demonstrate that FDG PET imaging improves physician decision making in the determination of initial anti-tumor treatment strategy in Medicare beneficiaries who have adenocarcinoma of the prostate, does not improve health outcomes and is thus not reasonable and necessary under Sec.1862(a)(1)(A) of the Act. Therefore, FDG PET is nationally non-covered for this indication of this tumor type.

b. The CMS received no new evidence demonstrating a change was warranted with respect to the use of FDG PET imaging to determine initial anti-tumor treatment in breast cancer; thus CMS is not making any change to the current coverage policy for FDG PET in breast cancer. CMS is continuing to cover FDG PET imaging for the initial treatment strategy for male and female breast cancer only when used in staging distant metastasis. FDG PET imaging for diagnosis and initial staging of axillary nodes will remain non-covered.

c. The CMS received no new evidence demonstrating a change was warranted with respect to use of FDG PET imaging of regional lymph nodes in melanoma; thus CMS is not changing the current NCD for FDG PET in melanoma. CMS will continue non-coverage of FDG PET for the evaluation of regional lymph nodes in melanoma. Other uses to determine initial treatment strategy remain covered.

d. The CMS received no new evidence demonstrating a change was warranted with respect to use of FDG PET imaging in the initial treatment strategy for cervical cancer. CMS is continuing to cover FDG PET imaging as an adjunct test for the detection of pre-treatment metastasis (i.e., staging) in newly diagnosed cervical cancers following conventional imaging that is negative for extra-pelvic metastasis. All other uses of FDG PET for the initial treatment strategy for beneficiaries diagnosed with cervical cancer will continue to only be covered as research under Sec.1862(a)(1)(E) of the Act through Coverage with Evidence Development (CED). Therefore, CMS will cover one initial FDG PET study for newly diagnosed cervical cancer when not used as an adjunct test for the detection of pre-treatment metastases following conventional imaging that is negative for extra-pelvic metastasis only when the beneficiary's treating physician determines that the FDG PET study is needed to inform the initial anti-tumor treatment strategy and the beneficiary is enrolled in, and the FDG PET provider is participating in, the specific type of prospective clinical study outlined under subsequent treatment strategy below.

e. Effective November 10, 2009, as a result of a reconsideration request, CMS ended the prospective data collection requirements, or coverage with evidence development, for the use of FDG PET imaging in the initial staging of cervical cancer related to initial treatment strategy.

CMS is continuing to cover FDG PET imaging as an adjunct test for the detection of pre-treatment metastasis (i.e., staging) in newly diagnosed cervical cancers following conventional imaging that is negative for extra-pelvic metastasis.

Therefore, CMS will cover one initial FDG PET study for staging in beneficiaries who have biopsy-proven cervical cancer when the beneficiary's treating physician determines that the FDG PET study is needed to determine the location and/or extent of the tumor for the following therapeutic purposes related to initial treatment strategy:

- To determine whether or not the beneficiary is an appropriate candidate for an invasive diagnostic or therapeutic procedure; or

- To determine the optimal anatomic location for an invasive procedure; or

- To determine the anatomic extent of the tumor when the recommended anti-tumor treatment reasonably depends on the extent of the tumor.

Additionally, effective November 10, 2009, following a reconsideration request, CMS determines that there is no credible evidence that the results of FDG PET imaging are useful to make the initial diagnoses of cervical cancer, does not improve health outcomes, and is not reasonable and necessary under section 1862(a)(1)(A) of the Social Security Act. Therefore, CMS will non-cover FDG PET imaging for initial diagnosis of cervical cancer related to initial treatment strategy.

3. Subsequent Anti-tumor Treatment Strategy

As part of its April 3, 2009, NCD, the CMS reviewed evidence on the use of FDG PET in the subsequent treatment strategy for patients with tumor types other than those seven indications currently covered without exception (breast, colorectal, esophagus, head and neck (non-CNS/thyroid), lymphoma, melanoma, and non-small cell lung).

As a result, CMS determined that the available evidence is adequate to determine that FDG PET imaging also improves physician decision making in the determination of subsequent treatment strategy in Medicare beneficiaries who have ovarian cancer, cervical cancer, and myeloma, improves health outcomes, and is thus reasonable and necessary under Sec.1862(a)(1)(A) of the Act.

Therefore, effective for claims with dates of service on and after April 3, 2009, for tumor types other than breast, colorectal, esophagus, head and neck (non-CNS/thyroid), lymphoma, melanoma, non-small cell lung, ovarian, cervical, and myeloma, CMS has determined that the available evidence is not adequate to determine that FDG PET imaging improves physician decision making in the determination of subsequent anti-tumor treatment strategy or improves health outcomes in Medicare beneficiaries and thus is not reasonable and necessary under Sec.1862(a)(1)(A) of the Act.

However, CMS has determined that the available evidence is sufficient to determine that FDG PET imaging for subsequent anti-tumor treatment strategy for all other tumor types other than the 10 indications noted above may be covered as research under Sec.1862(a)(1)(E) of the Act through CED. Therefore, CMS will cover a subsequent FDG PET study for all other tumor types other than the 10 indications noted above, when the beneficiary's treating physician determines that the FDG PET study is needed to inform the subsequent anti-tumor treatment strategy and the beneficiary is enrolled in, and the FDG PET provider is participating in, the following type of prospective clinical study:

An FDG PET clinical study that is designed to collect additional information at the time of the scan to assist in patient management. Qualifying clinical studies must ensure that specific hypotheses are addressed; appropriate data elements are collected; hospitals and providers are qualified to provide the FDG PET scan and interpret the results; participating hospitals and providers accurately report data on all enrolled patients not included in other qualifying trials through adequate auditing mechanisms; and all patient confidentiality, privacy, and other Federal laws must be followed.

The clinical studies for which CMS will provide coverage must answer one or more of the following three questions:

Prospectively, in Medicare beneficiaries whose treating physician determines that the FDG PET study is needed to inform the subsequent anti-tumor treatment strategy, does the addition of FDG PET imaging lead to:

- A change in the likelihood of appropriate referrals for palliative care;

- Improved quality of life; or,

- Improved survival?

The study must adhere to the following standards of scientific integrity and relevance to the Medicare population:

a. The principal purpose of the research study is to test whether a particular intervention potentially improves the participants' health outcomes.

b. The research study is well-supported by available scientific and medical information or it is intended to clarify or establish the health outcomes of interventions already in common clinical use.

c. The research study does not unjustifiably duplicate existing studies.

d. The research study design is appropriate to answer the research question being asked in the study.

e. The research study is sponsored by an organization or individual capable of executing the proposed study successfully.

f. The research study is in compliance with all applicable Federal regulations concerning the protection of human subjects found in the Code of Federal Regulations (CFR) at 45 CFR Part 46.

If a study is regulated by the Food and Drug Administration (FDA), it also must be in compliance with 21 CFR Parts 50 and 56.

g. All aspects of the research study are conducted according to the appropriate standards of scientific integrity.

h. The research study has a written protocol that clearly addresses, or incorporates by reference, the Medicare standards.

i. The clinical research study is not designed to exclusively test toxicity or disease pathophysiology in healthy individuals. Trials of all medical technologies measuring therapeutic outcomes as one of the objectives meet this standard only if the disease or condition being studied is life-threatening as defined in 21 CFR 312.81(a) and the patient has no other viable treatment options.

j. The clinical research study is registered on the www.ClinicalTrials.gov Web site by the principal sponsor/investigator prior to the enrollment of the first study subject.

k. The research study protocol specifies the method and timing of public release of all pre-specified outcomes to be measured including release of outcomes if outcomes are negative or study is terminated early. The results must be made public within 24 months of the end of data collection. If a report is planned to be published in a peer-reviewed journal, then that initial release may be an abstract that meets the requirements of the International Committee of Medical Journal Editors. However, a full report of the outcomes must be made public no later than 3 years after the end of data collection.

l. The research study protocol must explicitly discuss subpopulations affected by the treatment under investigation, particularly traditionally underrepresented groups in clinical studies, how the inclusion and exclusion criteria affect enrollment of these populations, and a plan for the retention and reporting of said populations on the trial. If the inclusion and exclusion criteria are expected to have a negative effect on the recruitment or retention of underrepresented populations, the protocol must discuss why these criteria are necessary.

m. The research study protocol explicitly discusses how the results are or are not expected to be generalizable to the Medicare population to infer whether Medicare patients may benefit from the intervention. Separate discussions in the protocol may be necessary for populations eligible for Medicare due to age, disability or Medicaid eligibility.

Consistent with section 1142 of the Act, the Agency for Healthcare Research and Quality (AHRQ) supports clinical research studies that CMS determines meet the above-listed standards and address the above-listed research questions.

4. Synopsis of New Framework

Effective for claims with dates of service on and after April 3, 2009, the CMS transitioned the prior framework-diagnosis, staging, restaging, and monitoring response to treatment-into the initial treatment strategy and subsequent treatment strategy framework. The chart below summarizes FDG PET coverage as of November 10, 2009:

FDG PET Coverage for Solid Tumors and Myeloma

Tumor Type	Initial Treatment Strategy (formerly "diagnosis" & "staging")	Subsequent Treatment Strategy (formerly "restaging" & "monitoring response to treatment")
Colorectal	Cover	Cover
Esophagus	Cover	Cover
Head & Neck (not Thyroid, CNS)	Cover	Cover
Lymphoma	Cover	Cover
Non-Small Cell Lung	Cover	Cover
Ovary	Cover	Cover
Brain	Cover	CED
Cervix	Cover w/exception*	Cover
Small Cell Lung	Cover	CED
Soft Tissue Sarcoma	Cover	CED
Pancreas	Cover	CED
Testes	Cover	CED
Breast (female and male)	Cover w/exception*	Cover
Melanoma	Cover w/exception*	Cover
Prostate	Non-Cover	CED
Thyroid	Cover	Cover w/exception or CED*

Tumor Type	Initial Treatment Strategy (formerly "diagnosis" & "staging")	Subsequent Treatment Strategy (formerly "restaging" & "monitoring response to treatment")
All Other Solid Tumors	Cover	CED
Myeloma	Cover	Cover
All other cancers not listed	CED	CED

* Cervix: Non-covered for the initial diagnosis of cervical cancer related to initial treatment strategy. All other indications for initial treatment strategy are covered.

* Breast: Non-covered for initial diagnosis and/or staging of axillary lymph nodes. Covered for initial staging of metastatic disease. All other indications for initial treatment strategy are covered.

* Melanoma: Non-covered for initial staging of regional lymph nodes. All other indications for initial treatment strategy are covered.

* Thyroid: Covered for subsequent treatment strategy of recurrent or residual thyroid cancer of follicular cell origin previously treated by thyroidectomy and radioiodine ablation and have a serum thyroglobulin >10ng/ml and have a negative I-131 whole body scan. All other indications for subsequent treatment strategy are CED.

(This NCD last reviewed November 2009.)

100-3, 220.6.19

Positron Emission Tomography NaF-18 (NaF-18 PET) to Identify Bone Metastasis of Cancer (Effective February 26, 2010)

A. General

Positron Emission Tomography (PET) is a non-invasive, diagnostic imaging procedure that assesses the level of metabolic activity and perfusion in various organ systems of the body. A positron camera (tomograph) is used to produce cross-sectional tomographic images, which are obtained from positron-emitting radioactive tracer substances (radiopharmaceuticals) such as

F-18 sodium fluoride. NaF-18 PET has been recognized as an excellent technique for imaging areas of altered osteogenic activity in bone. The clinical value of detecting and assessing the initial extent of metastatic cancer in bone is attested by a number of professional guidelines for oncology. Imaging to detect bone metastases is also recommended when a patient, following completion of initial treatment, is symptomatic with bone pain suspicious for metastases from a known primary tumor.

B. Nationally Covered Indications

Effective February 26, 2010, the Centers for Medicare & Medicaid Services (CMS) will cover NaF-18 PET imaging when the beneficiary's treating physician determines that the NaF-18 PET study is needed to inform to inform the initial antitumor treatment strategy or to guide subsequent antitumor treatment strategy after the completion of initial treatment, and when the beneficiary is enrolled in, and the NaF-18 PET provider is participating in, the following type of prospective clinical study:

A NaF-18 PET clinical study that is designed to collect additional information at the time of the scan to assist in initial antitumor treatment planning or to guide subsequent treatment strategy by the identification, location and quantification of bone metastases in beneficiaries in whom bone metastases are strongly suspected based on clinical symptoms or the results of other diagnostic studies. Qualifying clinical studies must ensure that specific hypotheses are addressed; appropriate data elements are collected; hospitals and providers are qualified to provide the PET scan and interpret the results; participating hospitals and providers accurately report data on all enrolled patients not included in other qualifying trials through adequate auditing mechanisms; and all patient confidentiality, privacy, and other Federal laws must be followed.

The clinical studies for which Medicare will provide coverage must answer one or more of the following questions:

Prospectively, in Medicare beneficiaries whose treating physician determines that the NaF-18 PET study results are needed to inform the initial antitumor treatment strategy or to guide subsequent antitumor treatment strategy after the completion of initial treatment, does the addition of NaF-18 PET imaging lead to:

A change in patient management to more appropriate palliative care; or A change in patient management to more appropriate curative care; or Improved quality of life; or Improved survival?

The study must adhere to the following standards of scientific integrity and relevance to the Medicare population:

a. The principal purpose of the research study is to test whether a particular intervention potentially improves the participants' health outcomes.

b. The research study is well-supported by available scientific and medical information or it is intended to clarify or establish the health outcomes of interventions already in common clinical use.

c. The research study does not unjustifiably duplicate existing studies.

d. The research study design is appropriate to answer the research question being asked in the study.

e. The research study is sponsored by an organization or individual capable of executing the proposed study successfully.

f. The research study is in compliance with all applicable Federal regulations concerning the protection of human subjects found in the Code of Federal Regulations (CFR) at 45 CFR Part 46. If a study is regulated by the Food and Drug Administration (FDA), it also must be in compliance with 21 CFR Parts 50 and 56.

g. All aspects of the research study are conducted according to the appropriate standards of scientific integrity.

h. The research study has a written protocol that clearly addresses, or incorporates by reference, the Medicare standards.

i. The clinical research study is not designed to exclusively test toxicity or disease pathophysiology in healthy individuals. Trials of all medical technologies measuring therapeutic outcomes as one of the objectives meet this standard only if the disease or condition being studied is life-threatening as defined in 21 CFR Sec.312.81(a) and the patient has no other viable treatment options.

j. The clinical research study is registered on the www.ClinicalTrials.gov Web site by the principal sponsor/investigator prior to the enrollment of the first study subject.

k. The research study protocol specifies the method and timing of public release of all pre-specified outcomes to be measured including release of outcomes if outcomes are negative or study is terminated early. The results must be made public within 24 months of the end of data collection. If a report is planned to be published in a peer-reviewed journal, then that initial release may be an abstract that meets the requirements of the International Committee of Medical Journal Editors. However, a full report of the outcomes must be made public no later than three (3) years after the end of data collection.

l. The research study protocol must explicitly discuss subpopulations affected by the treatment under investigation, particularly traditionally underrepresented groups in clinical studies, how the inclusion and exclusion criteria affect enrollment of these populations, and a plan for the retention and reporting of said populations on the trial. If the inclusion and exclusion criteria are expected to have a negative effect on the recruitment or retention of underrepresented populations, the protocol must discuss why these criteria are necessary.

m. The research study protocol explicitly discusses how the results are or are not expected to be generalizable to the Medicare population to infer whether Medicare patients may benefit from the intervention. Separate discussions in the protocol may be necessary for populations eligible for Medicare due to age, disability or Medicaid eligibility.

Consistent with section 1142 of the Social Security Act (the Act), the Agency for Healthcare Research and Quality (AHRQ) supports clinical research studies that the Centers for Medicare and Medicaid Services (CMS) determines meet the above-listed standards and address the above-listed research questions.

C. Nationally Non-Covered Indications

Effective February 26, 2010, CMS determines that the evidence is not sufficient to determine that the results of NaF-18 PET imaging to identify bone metastases improve health outcomes of beneficiaries with cancer and is not reasonable and necessary under Sec.1862(a)(1)(A) of the Act unless it is to inform initial antitumor treatment strategy or to guide subsequent antitumor treatment strategy after completion of initial treatment, and then only under CED. All other uses and clinical indications of NaF-18 PET are nationally non-covered.

D. Other

The only radiopharmaceutical diagnostic imaging agents covered by Medicare for PET cancer imaging are 2-[F-18] Fluoro-D-Glucose (FDG) and NaF-18 (sodium fluoride-18). All other PET radiopharmaceutical diagnostic imaging agents are non-covered for this indication.

(This NCD was last reviewed in February 2010.)

100-3, 220.6.2
NCD for PET (FDG) for Lung Cancer (220.6.2)
220.6.2 - FDG PET for Lung Cancer (Replaced with Section 220.6.17)

100-3, 220.6.3
NCD for PET (FDG) for Esophageal Cancer (220.6.3)
220.6.3 - FDG PET for Esophageal Cancer (Replaced with Section 220.6.17)

100-3, 220.6.4
NCD for PET (FDG) for Colorectal Cancer (220.6.4)
220.6.4 - FDG PET for Colorectal Cancer (Replaced with Section 220.6.17

100-3, 220.6.5
NCD for PET (FDG) for Lymphoma (220.6.5)
220.6.5 - FDG PET for Lymphoma (Replaced with Section 220.6.17)

100-3, 220.6.6
NCD for PET (FDG) for Melanoma (220.6.6)
220.6.6 - FDG PET for Melanoma (Replaced with Section 220.6.17)

100-3, 220.6.7
NCD for PET (FDG) for Head and Neck Cancers (220.6.7)
220.6.7 - FDG PET for Head and Neck Cancers (Replaced with Section 220.6.17)

100-3, 220.6.9
FDG PET for Refractory Seizures (Effective July 1, 2001)
Beginning July 1, 2001, Medicare covers FDG PET for pre-surgical evaluation for the purpose of localization of a focus of refractory seizure activity.

Limitations: Covered only for pre-surgical evaluation.

Documentation that these conditions are met should be maintained by the referring physician in the beneficiary's medical record, as is normal business practice.

(This NCD last reviewed June 2001.)

100-3, 240.4
NCD for Continuous Positive Airway Pressure (CPAP) Therapy For Obstructive Sleep Apnea (OSA) (240.4)

B. Nationally Covered Indications
Effective for claims with dates of service on and after March 13, 2008, the Centers for Medicare & Medicaid Services (CMS) determines that CPAP therapy when used in adult patients with OSA is considered reasonable and necessary under the following situations:

1. The use of CPAP is covered under Medicare when used in adult patients with OSA. Coverage of CPAP is initially limited to a 12-week period to identify beneficiaries diagnosed with OSA as subsequently described who benefit from CPAP. CPAP is subsequently covered only for those beneficiaries diagnosed with OSA who benefit from CPAP during this 12-week period.

2. The provider of CPAP must conduct education of the beneficiary prior to the use of the CPAP device to ensure that the beneficiary has been educated in the proper use of the device. A caregiver, for example a family member, may be compensatory, if consistently available in the beneficiary's home and willing and able to safely operate the CPAP device.

3. A positive diagnosis of OSA for the coverage of CPAP must include a clinical evaluation and a positive:

   a. attended PSG performed in a sleep laboratory; or

   b. unattended HST with a Type II home sleep monitoring device; or

   c. unattended HST with a Type III home sleep monitoring device; or

   d. unattended HST with a Type IV home sleep monitoring device that measures at least 3 channels.

4. The sleep test must have been previously ordered by the beneficiaryÔø¾s treating physician and furnished under appropriate physician supervision.

5. An initial 12-week period of CPAP is covered in adult patients with OSA if either of the following criterion using the AHI or RDI are met:

   a. AHI or RDI greater than or equal to 15 events per hour, or

   b. AHI or RDI greater than or equal to 5 events and less than or equal to 14 events per hour with documented symptoms of excessive daytime sleepiness, impaired cognition, mood disorders or insomnia, or documented hypertension, ischemic heart disease, or history of stroke.

6. The AHI or RDI is calculated on the average number of events of per hour. If the AHI or RDI is calculated based on less than 2 hours of continuous recorded sleep, the total number of recorded events to calculate the AHI or RDI during sleep testing must be at a minimum the number of events that would have been required in a 2-hour period.

7. Apnea is defined as a cessation of airflow for at least 10 seconds. Hypopnea is defined as an abnormal respiratory event lasting at least 10 seconds with at least a 30% reduction in thoracoabdominal movement or airflow as compared to baseline, and with at least a 4% oxygen desaturation.

8. Coverage with Evidence Development (CED): Medicare provides the following limited coverage for CPAP in adult beneficiaries who do not qualify for CPAP coverage based on criteria 1-7

above. A clinical study seeking Medicare payment for CPAP provided to a beneficiary who is an enrolled subject in that study must address one or more of the following questions

a. In Medicare-aged subjects with clinically identified risk factors for OSA, how does the diagnostic accuracy of a clinical trial of CPAP compare with PSG and Type II, III & IV HST in identifying subjects with OSA who will respond to CPAP?

b. In Medicare-aged subjects with clinically identified risk factors for OSA who have not undergone confirmatory testing with PSG or Type II, III & IV HST, does CPAP cause clinically meaningful harm?

The study must meet the following additional standards:

c. The principal purpose of the research study is to test whether a particular intervention potentially improves the participantsÔø¾ health outcomes.

d. The research study is well-supported by available scientific and medical information or it is intended to clarify or establish the health outcomes of interventions already in common clinical use.

e. The research study does not unjustifiably duplicate existing studies.

f. The research study design is appropriate to answer the research question being asked in the study.

g. The research study is sponsored by an organization or individual capable of executing the proposed study successfully.

h. The research study is in compliance with all applicable Federal regulations concerning the protection of human subjects found in 45 CFR Part 46. If a study is Food and Drug Administration-regulated, it also must be in compliance with 21 CFR Parts 50 and 56.

i. All aspects of the research study are conducted according to the appropriate standards of scientific integrity.

j. The research study has a written protocol that clearly addresses, or incorporates by reference, the Medicare standards.

k. The clinical research study is not designed to exclusively test toxicity or disease pathophysiology in healthy individuals. Trials of all medical technologies measuring therapeutic outcomes as one of the objectives meet this standard only if the disease or condition being studied is life-threatening as defined in 21 CFR Ôø¾ 312.81(a) and the patient has no other viable treatment options.

l. The clinical research study is registered on the ClinicalTrials.gov Web site by the principal sponsor/investigator prior to the enrollment of the first study subject.

m. The research study protocol specifies the method and timing of public release of all pre-specified outcomes to be measured, including release of outcomes if outcomes are negative or study is terminated early. The results must be made public within 24 months of the end of data collection. If a report is planned for publication in a peer-reviewed journal, then that initial release may be an abstract that meets the requirements of the International Committee of Medical Journal Editors. However, a full report of the outcomes must be made public no later than 3 years after the end of data collection.

n. The research study protocol must explicitly discuss subpopulations affected by the treatment under investigation, particularly traditionally underrepresented groups in clinical studies, how the inclusion and exclusion criteria affect enrollment of these populations, and a plan for the retention and reporting of said populations in the trial. If the inclusion and exclusion criteria are expected to have a negative effect on the recruitment or retention of underrepresented populations, the protocol must discuss why these criteria are necessary.

o. The research study protocol explicitly discusses how the results are or are not expected to be generalizable to the Medicare population to infer whether Medicare patients may benefit from the intervention. Separate discussions in the protocol may be necessary for populations eligible for Medicare due to age, disability, or Medicaid eligibility.

C. Nationally Non-covered Indications

Effective for claims with dates of services on and after March 13, 2008, other diagnostic tests for the diagnosis of OSA, other than those noted above for prescribing CPAP, are not sufficient for the coverage of CPAP.

D. Other

N/A

(This NCD last reviewed March

100-3, 240.4.1

Sleep Testing for Obstructive Sleep Apnea (OSA) (Effective March 3, 2009)

A. General

Obstructive sleep apnea (OSA) is the collapse of the oropharyngeal walls and the obstruction of airflow occurring during sleep. Diagnostic tests for OSA have historically been classified into four types. The most comprehensive is designated Type I attended facility based polysomnography (PSG), which is considered the reference standard for diagnosing OSA. Attended facility based polysomnogram is a comprehensive diagnostic sleep test including at least electroencephalography (EEG), electro-oculography (EOG), electromyography (EMG), heart rate or electrocardiography (ECG), airflow, breathing/respiratory effort, and arterial oxygen saturation (SaO2) furnished in a sleep laboratory facility in which a technologist supervises the recording during sleep time and has the ability to intervene if needed. Overnight PSG is the conventional diagnostic test for OSA. The American Thoracic Society and the American Academy of Sleep Medicine have recommended supervised PSG in the sleep laboratory over 2 nights for the diagnosis of OSA and the initiation of continuous positive airway pressure (CPAP).

Three categories of portable monitors (used both in attended and unattended settings) have been developed for the diagnosis of OSA. Type II monitors have a minimum of 7 channels (e.g., EEG, EOG, EMG, ECG-heart rate, airflow, breathing/respiratory effort, SaO2)-this type of device monitors sleep staging, so AHI can be calculated). Type III monitors have a minimum of 4 monitored channels including ventilation or airflow (at least two channels of respiratory movement or respiratory movement and airflow), heart rate or ECG, and oxygen saturation. Type IV devices may measure one, two, three or more parameters but do not meet all the criteria of a higher category device. Some monitors use an actigraphy algorithm to identify periods of sleep and wakefulness.

B. Nationally Covered Indications

Effective for claims with dates of service on and after March 3, 2009, the Centers for Medicare & Medicaid Services finds that the evidence is sufficient to determine that the results of the sleep tests identified below can be used by a beneficiary's treating physician to diagnose OSA, that the use of such sleep testing technologies demonstrates improved health outcomes in Medicare beneficiaries who have OSA and receive the appropriate treatment, and that these tests are thus reasonable and necessary under section 1862(a)(1)(A) of the Social Security Act.

1. Type I PSG is covered when used to aid the diagnosis of OSA in beneficiaries who have clinical signs and symptoms indicative of OSA if performed attended in a sleep lab facility.

2. Type II or Type III sleep testing devices are covered when used to aid the diagnosis of OSA in beneficiaries who have clinical signs and symptoms indicative of OSA if performed unattended in or out of a sleep lab facility or attended in a sleep lab facility.

3. Type IV sleep testing devices measuring three or more channels, one of which is airflow, are covered when used to aid the diagnosis of OSA in beneficiaries who have signs and symptoms indicative of OSA if performed unattended in or out of a sleep lab facility or attended in a sleep lab facility.

4. Sleep testing devices measuring three or more channels that include actigraphy, oximetry, and peripheral arterial tone, are covered when used to aid the diagnosis of OSA in beneficiaries who have signs and symptoms indicative of OSA if performed unattended in or out of a sleep lab facility or attended in a sleep lab facility.

C. Nationally Non-Covered Indications

Effective for claims with dates of services on and after March 3, 2009, other diagnostic sleep tests for the diagnosis of OSA, other than those noted above for prescribing CPAP, are not sufficient for the coverage of CPAP and are not covered.

D. Other

N/A

(This NCD last reviewed March 2009.)

100-3, 250.5

Dermal Injections for the Treatment of Facial Lipodystrophy Syndrome (LDS) - Effective March 23, 2010

A. General

Treatment of persons infected with the human immunodeficiency virus (HIV) or persons who have Acquired Immune Deficiency Syndrome (AIDS) may include highly active antiretroviral therapy (HAART). Drug reactions commonly associated with long-term use of HAART include metabolic complications such as, lipid abnormalities, e.g., hyperlipidemia, hyperglycemia, diabetes, lipodystrophy, and heart disease. Lipodystrophy is characterized by abnormal fat distribution in the body.

The LDS is often characterized by a loss of fat that results in a facial abnormality such as severely sunken cheeks. The patient's physical appearance may contribute to psychological conditions (e.g., depression) or adversely impact a patient's adherence to antiretroviral regimens (therefore jeopardizing their health) and both of these are important health-related outcomes of interest in this population. Therefore, improving a patient's physical appearance through the use of dermal injections could improve these health-related outcomes.

B. Nationally Covered Indications
Effective for claims with dates of service on and after March 23, 2010, dermal injections for LDS are only reasonable and necessary using dermal fillers approved by the Food and Drug Administration (FDA) for this purpose, and then only in HIV-infected beneficiaries when LDS caused by antiretroviral HIV treatment is a significant contributor to their depression.

C. Nationally Non-Covered Indications
1. Dermal fillers that are not approved by the FDA for the treatment of LDS.
2. Dermal fillers that are used for any indication other than LDS in HIV-infected individuals who manifest depression as a result of their antiretroviral HIV treatments.

D. Other
N/A

(This NCD last reviewed March 2010.)

100-3, 260.6

Dental Examination Prior to Kidney Transplantation
Despite the "dental services exclusion" in §1862(a)(12) of the Act (see the Medicare Benefit Policy Manual, Chapter 16, "General Exclusions From Coverage," §140;), an oral or dental examination performed on an inpatient basis as part of a comprehensive workup prior to renal transplant surgery is a covered service. This is because the purpose of the examination is not for the care of the teeth or structures directly supporting the teeth. Rather, the examination is for the identification, prior to a complex surgical procedure, of existing medical problems where the increased possibility of infection would not only reduce the chances for successful surgery but would also expose the patient to additional risks in undergoing such surgery.

Such a dental or oral examination would be covered under Part A of the program if performed by a dentist on the hospital's staff, or under Part B if performed by a physician. (When performing a dental or oral examination, a dentist is not recognized as a physician under § 1861(r) of the Act.) (See the Medicare General Information, Eligibility, and Entitlement Manual, Chapter 5, "Definitions," § 70.2, and the Medicare Benefit and Entitlement Manual, Chapter 15, "Covered Medical and Other Health Services," § 150.)

100-3, 270.3

NCD for Blood-Derived Products for Chronic Non-Healing Wounds (270.3)

A. General
Wound healing is a dynamic, interactive process that involves multiple cells and proteins. There are three progressive stages of normal wound healing, and the typical wound healing duration is about 4 weeks. While cutaneous wounds are a disruption of the normal, anatomic structure and function of the skin, subcutaneous wounds involve tissue below the skin? surface. Wounds are categorized as either acute, in where the normal wound healing stages are not yet completed but it is presumed they will be, resulting in orderly and timely wound repair, or chronic, in where a wound has failed to progress through the normal wound healing stages and repair itself within a sufficient time period.

Platelet-rich plasma (PRP) is produced in an autologous or homologous manner. Autologous PRP is comprised of blood from the patient who will ultimately receive the PRP. Alternatively, homologous PRP is derived from blood from multiple donors.

Blood is donated by the patient and centrifuged to produce an autologous gel for treatment of chronic, non-healing cutaneous wounds that persists for 30 days or longer and fail to properly complete the healing process. Autologous blood derived products for chronic, non-healing wounds includes both: (1) platelet derived growth factor (PDGF) products (such as Procuren), and (2) PRP (such as AutoloGel).

The PRP is different from previous products in that it contains whole cells including white cells, red cells, plasma, platelets, fibrinogen, stem cells, macrophages, and fibroblasts.

The PRP is used by physicians in clinical settings in treating chronic, non-healing wounds, open, cutaneous wounds, soft tissue, and bone. Alternatively, PDGF does not contain cells and was previously marketed as a product to be used by patients at home.

B. Nationally Covered Indications
Effective August 2, 2012, upon reconsideration, The Centers for Medicare and Medicaid Services (CMS) has determined that platelet-rich plasma (PRP) ?an autologous blood-derived product, will be covered only for the treatment of chronic non-healing diabetic, venous and/or pressure wounds and only when the following conditions are met:

The patient is enrolled in a clinical trial that addresses the following questions using validated and reliable methods of evaluation. Clinical study applications for coverage pursuant to this National coverage Determination (NCD) must be received by August 2, 2014.

The clinical research study must meet the requirements specified below to assess the effect of PRP for the treatment of chronic non-healing diabetic, venous and/or pressure wounds. The clinical study must address:

Prospectively, do Medicare beneficiaries that have chronic non-healing diabetic, venous and/or pressure wounds who receive well-defined optimal usual care along with PRP therapy, experience clinically significant health outcomes compared to patients who receive well-defined optimal usual care for chronic non-healing diabetic, venous and/or pressure wounds as indicated by addressing at least one of the following:

a. Complete wound healing

b. Ability to return to previous function and resumption of normal activities

c. Reduction of wound size or healing trajectory which results in the patient's ability to return to previous function and resumption of normal activities

The required clinical trial of PRP must adhere to the following standards of scientific integrity and relevance to the Medicare population:

a. The principal purpose of the CLINICAL STUDY is to test whether PRP improves the participants?health outcomes.

b. The CLINICAL STUDY is well supported by available scientific and medical information or it is intended to clarify or establish the health outcomes of interventions already in common clinical use.

c. The CLINICAL STUDY does not unjustifiably duplicate existing studies.

d. The CLINICAL STUDY design is appropriate to answer the research question being asked in the study.

e. The CLINICAL STUDY is sponsored by an organization or individual capable of executing the proposed study successfully.

f. The CLINICAL STUDY is in compliance with all applicable Federal regulations concerning the protection of human subjects found at 45 CFR Part 46.

g. All aspects of the CLINICAL STUDY are conducted according to appropriate standards of scientific integrity set by the International Committee of Medical Journal Editors (http://www.icmje.org).

h. The CLINICAL STUDY has a written protocol that clearly addresses, or incorporates by reference, the standards listed here as Medicare requirements for coverage with evidence development (CED).

i. The CLINICAL STUDY is not designed to exclusively test toxicity or disease pathophysiology in healthy individuals. Trials of all medical technologies measuring therapeutic outcomes as one of the objectives meet this standard only if the disease or condition being studied is life threatening as defined in 21 CFR ?312.81(a) and the patient has no other viable treatment options.

j. The CLINICAL STUDY is registered on the ClinicalTrials.gov website by the principal sponsor/investigator prior to the enrollment of the first study subject.

k. The CLINICAL STUDY protocol specifies the method and timing of public release of all pre-specified outcomes to be measured including release of outcomes if outcomes are negative or study is terminated early. The results must be made public within 24 months of the end of data collection. If a report is planned to be published in a peer reviewed journal, then that initial release may be an abstract that meets the requirements of the International Committee of Medical Journal Editors (http://www.icmje.org). However a full report of the outcomes must be made public no later than three (3) years after the end of data collection.

l. The CLINICAL STUDY protocol must explicitly discuss subpopulations affected by the treatment under investigation, particularly traditionally underrepresented groups in clinical studies, how the inclusion and exclusion criteria effect enrollment of these populations, and a plan for the retention and reporting of said populations on the trial. If the inclusion and exclusion criteria are expected to have a negative effect on the recruitment or retention of underrepresented populations, the protocol must discuss why these criteria are necessary.

m. The CLINICAL STUDY protocol explicitly discusses how the results are or are not expected to be generalizable to the Medicare population to infer whether Medicare patients may benefit from the intervention. Separate discussions in the protocol may be necessary for populations eligible for Medicare due to age, disability or Medicaid eligibility. Consistent with ?1142 of the Social Security Act (the Act), the Agency for Healthcare Research and Quality (AHRQ) supports clinical research studies that CMS determines meet the above-listed standards and address the above-listed research questions.

Any clinical study undertaken pursuant to this NCD must be approved no later than August 2, 2014. If there are no approved clinical studies on or before August 2, 2014, this CED will expire. Any clinical study approved will adhere to the timeframe designated in the approved clinical study protocol.

C. Nationally Non-Covered Indications

1. Effective December 28, 1992, the Centers for Medicare & Medicaid Services (CMS) issued a national non-coverage determination for platelet-derived wound-healing formulas intended to treat patients with chronic, non-healing wounds. This decision was based on a lack of sufficient published data to determine safety and efficacy, and a public health service technology assessment.

100-4, 1, 10.1.4.1

Physician and Ambulance Services Furnished in Connection With Covered Foreign Inpatient Hospital Services

Payment is made for necessary physician and ambulance services that meet the other coverage requirements of the Medicare program, and are furnished in connection with and during a period of covered foreign hospitalization.

A. Coverage of Physician and Ambulance Services Furnished Outside the U.S.

Where inpatient services in a foreign hospital are covered, payment may also be made for

- Physicians' services furnished to the beneficiary while he/she is an inpatient,

- Physicians' services furnished to the beneficiary outside the hospital on the day of his/her admission as an inpatient, provided the services were for the same condition for which the beneficiary was hospitalized (including the services of a Canadian ship's physician who furnishes emergency services in Canadian waters on the day the patient is admitted to a Canadian hospital for a covered emergency stay and,

- Ambulance services, where necessary, for the trip to the hospital in conjunction with the beneficiary's admission as an inpatient. Return trips from a foreign hospital are not covered.

In cases involving foreign ambulance services, the general requirements in Chapter 15 are also applicable, subject to the following special rules:

- If the foreign hospitalization was determined to be covered on the basis of emergency services, the medical necessity requirements outlined in Chapter 15 are considered met.

- The definition of:

  – physician

  – for purposes of coverage of services furnished outside the U.S., is expanded to include a foreign practitioner, provided the practitioner is legally licensed to practice in the country in which the services are furnished.

- Only the enrollee can file for Part B benefits; the assignment method may not be used.

- Where the enrollee is deceased, the rules for settling Part B underpayments are applicable. Payment is made to the foreign physician or foreign ambulance company on an unpaid bill provided the physician or ambulance company accepts the payment as the full charge for the service, or payment an be made to a person who has agreed to assume legal liability to pay the physician or supplier. Where the bill is paid, payment may be made in accordance with Medicare regulations. The regular deductible and coinsurance requirements apply to physicians' and ambulance service

100-4, 1, 30.3.1

Mandatory Assignment on Carrier Claims

The following practitioners who provide services under the Medicare program are required to accept assignment for all Medicare claims for their services. This means that they must accept the Medicare allowed amount as payment in full for their practitioner services. The beneficiary's liability is limited to any applicable deductible plus the 20 percent coinsurance.

Assignment is mandated for the following claims:

- Clinical diagnostic laboratory services and physician lab services;

- Physician services to individuals dually entitled to Medicare and Medicaid;

Services of physician assistants, nurse practitioners, clinical nurse specialists, nurse midwives, certified registered nurse anesthetists, clinical psychologists, clinical social workers, registered dietitians/nutritionists, anesthesiologist assistants, and mass immunization roster billers.

NOTE: The provider type Mass Immunization Roster Biller can only bill for influenza and pneumococcal vaccinations and administrations. These services are not subject to the deductible or the 20 percent coinsurance.

- Ambulatory surgical center services; (No deductible and 25% coinsurance for colorectal cancer screening colonoscopies (G0105 and G0121) and effective for dates of service on or after January 1, 2008 G0104 also applies);

- Home dialysis supplies and equipment paid under Method II for dates of service prior to January 1, 2011. Refer to Section 30.3.8 for information regarding the elimination of Method II home dialysis for dates of service on and after January 1, 2011;

- Drugs and biologicals; and,

- Ambulance services

When these claims are inadvertently submitted as unassigned, carriers process them as assigned.

Note that, unlike physicians, practitioners, or suppliers bound by a participation agreement, practitioners/entities providing the services/supplies identified above are required to accept assignment only with respect to these services/supplies (unless they have signed participation agreements which blanket the full range of their services).

The carrier system must be able to identify (and update) the codes for those services subject to the assignment mandate.

For the practitioner services of physicians and independently practicing physical and occupational therapists, the acceptance of assignment is not mandatory. Nor is the acceptance of assignment mandatory for the suppliers of radiology services or diagnostic tests. However, these practitioners and suppliers may nevertheless voluntarily agree to participate to take advantage of the higher payment rate, in which case the participation status makes assignment mandatory for the term of the agreement. Such an agreement is known as the Medicare Participating Physician or Supplier Agreement. (See §30.3.12.2 Carrier Participation Agreement.) Physicians, practitioners, and suppliers who sign this agreement to participate are agreeing to accept assignment on all Medicare claims. The Medicare Participation Agreement and general instructions are on the CMS Web site.

Future updates to this section will be communicated in a Recurring Update Notification.

100-4, 1, 30.3.5

Effect of Assignment Upon Purchase of Cataract Glasses FromParticipating Physician or Supplier on Claims Submitted to Carriers

B3-3045.4

A pair of cataract glasses is comprised of two distinct products: a professional product (the prescribed lenses) and a retail commercial product (the frames). The frames serve not only as a holder of lenses but also as an article of personal apparel. As such, they are usually selected on the basis of personal taste and style. Although Medicare will pay only for standard frames, most patients want deluxe frames. Participating physicians and suppliers cannot profitably furnish such deluxe frames unless they can make an extra (noncovered) charge for the frames even though they accept assignment.

Therefore, a participating physician or supplier (whether an ophthalmologist, optometrist, or optician) who accepts assignment on cataract glasses with deluxe frames may charge the Medicare patient the difference between his/her usual charge to private pay patients for glasses with standard frames and his/her usual charge to such patients for glasses with deluxe frames, in addition to the applicable deductible and coinsurance on glasses with standard frames, if all of the following requirements are met:

A. The participating physician or supplier has standard frames available, offers them for saleto the patient, and issues and ABN to the patient that explains the price and other differences between standard and deluxe frames. Refer to Chapter 30.

B. The participating physician or supplier obtains from the patient (or his/her representative) and keeps on file the following signed and dated statement:

_____

Name of Patient   Medicare Claim Number

Having been informed that an extra charge is being made by the physician or supplier for deluxe frames, that this extra charge is not covered by Medicare, and that standard frames are available for purchase from the physician or supplier at no extra charge, I have chosen to purchase deluxe frames.

_____

Signature   Date

C. The participating physician or supplier itemizes on his/her claim his/her actual charge for the lenses, his/her actual charge for the standard frames, and his/her actual extra charge for the deluxe frames (charge differential). Once the assigned claim for deluxe frames has been processed, the carrier will follow the ABN instructions as described in Sec.60.

100-4, 1, 50.3.2

Policy and Billing Instructions for Condition Code 44

In cases where a hospital or a CAH's UR committee determines that an inpatient admission does not meet the hospital's inpatient criteria, the hospital or CAH may change the beneficiary's status from inpatient to outpatient and submit an outpatient claim (bill type 13x or 85x) for medically necessary Medicare Part B services that were furnished to the beneficiary, provided all of the following conditions are met:

1. The change in patient status from inpatient to outpatient is made prior to discharge or release, while the beneficiary is still a patient of the hospital;

2. The hospital has not submitted a claim to Medicare for the inpatient admission;

3. The practitioner responsible for the care of the patient and the UR committee concur with the decision; and

4. The concurrence of the practitioner responsible for the care of the patient and the UR committee is documented in the patient's medical record.

While typically the full UR committee makes the decision for the committee that a change in patient status under Condition Code 44 is warranted, in accordance with §482.30(d)(1) one physician member of the UR committee may make the decision for the committee, provided he or she is a different person from the concurring practitioner who is responsible for the care of the patient.

When the hospital has determined that it may submit an outpatient claim according to the conditions described above, the entire episode of care should be billed as an outpatient episode of care on a 13x or 85x bill type and outpatient services that were ordered and furnished should be billed as appropriate.

Refer to Pub. 100-04, Medicare Claims Processing Manual; Chapter 30, Financial Liability Protections; Section 20, Limitation On Liability (LOL) Under §1879 Where Medicare Claims Are Disallowed, for information regarding financial liability protections.

When the hospital submits a 13x or 85x bill for services furnished to a beneficiary whose status was changed from inpatient to outpatient, the hospital is required to report Condition Code 44 on the outpatient claim in one of Form Locators 24-30, or in the ANSI X12N 837 I in Loop 2300, HI segment, with qualifier BG, on the outpatient claim. Additional information may be found in Chapter 25 of this manual, (Completing and Processing the Form CMS-1450 Data Set). Condition Code 44 is used by CMS and QIOs to track and monitor these occurrences. The reporting of Condition Code 44 on a claim does not affect the amount of hospital outpatient payment that would otherwise be made for a hospital outpatient claim that did not require the reporting Condition Code 44.

One of the requirements for the use of Condition Code 44 is concurrence by the practitioner who is responsible for the care of the patient with the determination that an inpatient admission does not meet the hospital's admission criteria and that the patient should have been registered as an outpatient. This prerequisite for use of Condition Code 44 is consistent with the requirements in the CoP in §482.30 (d) of the regulations. This paragraph provides that the practitioner or practitioners responsible for the care of the patient must be consulted and allowed to present their views before the UR committee or QIO makes its determination that an admission is not medically necessary. It may also be appropriate to include the practitioner who admitted the patient if this is a different person than the practitioner responsible for the care of the patient.

If the conditions for use of Condition Code 44 are not met, the hospital may submit a 12x bill type for covered "Part B Only" services that were furnished to the inpatient. Medicare may still make payment for certain Part B services furnished to an inpatient of a hospital when payment cannot be made under Part A because an inpatient admission is determined not to be medically necessary. Information about "Part B Only" services is located in Pub. 100-02, Medicare Benefit Policy Manual, chapter 6, section 10. Examples of such services include, but are not limited to, diagnostic x-ray tests, diagnostic laboratory tests, surgical dressings and splints, prosthetic devices, and certain other services. The Medicare Benefit Policy Manual includes a complete list of the payable "Part B Only" services. See Pub. 100-04, Medicare Claims Processing Manual, chapter 4, section 10.12 for a discussion of the billing and payment rules regarding services furnished within the payment window for outpatient services treated as inpatient services.

Entries in the medical record cannot be expunged or deleted and must be retained in their original form. Therefore, all orders and all entries related to the inpatient admission must be retained in the record in their original form. If a patient's status changes in accordance with the requirements for use of Condition Code 44, the change must be fully documented in the medical record, complete with orders and notes that indicate why the change was made, the care that was furnished to the beneficiary, and the participants in making the decision to change the patient's status.

When Condition Code 44 is appropriately used, the hospital reports on the outpatient bill the services that were ordered and provided to the patient for the entire patient encounter. However, in accordance with the general Medicare requirements for services furnished to beneficiaries and billed to Medicare, even in Condition Code 44 situations, hospitals may not report observation services using HCPCS code G0378 (Hospital observation service, per hour) for observation services furnished during a hospital encounter prior to a physician's order for observation services. Medicare does not permit retroactive orders or the inference of physician orders. Like all hospital outpatient services, observation services must be ordered by a physician. The clock time begins at the time that observation services are initiated in accordance with a physician's order.

While hospitals may not report observation services under HCPCS code G0378 for the time period during the hospital encounter prior to a physician?s order for observation services, in Condition Code 44 situations, as for all other hospital outpatient encounters, hospitals may include charges on the outpatient claim for the costs of all hospital resources utilized in the care of the patient during the entire encounter. For example, a beneficiary is admitted as an inpatient and receives 12 hours of monitoring and nursing care, at which point the hospital changes the status of the beneficiary from inpatient to outpatient and the physician orders observation services, with all criteria for billing under Condition Code 44 being met. On the outpatient claim on an uncoded line with revenue code 0762, the hospital could bill for the 12 hours of monitoring and nursing care that were provided prior to the change in status and the physician order for observation services, in addition to billing HCPCS code G0378 for the observation services that followed the change in status and physician order for observation services. For other rules related to billing and payment of observation services, see chapter 4, section 290 of this manual, and Pub.100-02, Medicare Benefit Policy Manual, chapter 6, Section 20.6

100-4, 3, 10.4
Payment of Nonphysician Services for Inpatients

All items and nonphysician services furnished to inpatients must be furnished directly by the hospital or billed through the hospital under arrangements. This provision applies to all hospitals, regardless of whether they are subject to PPS.

Other Medical Items, Supplies, and Services the following medical items, supplies, and services furnished to inpatients are covered under Part A. Consequently, they are covered by the prospective payment rate or reimbursed as reasonable costs under Part A to hospitals excluded from PPS.

- Laboratory services (excluding anatomic pathology services and certain clinical pathology services);

- Pacemakers and other prosthetic devices including lenses, and artificial limbs, knees, and hips;

- Radiology services including computed tomography (CT) scans furnished to inpatients by a physician's office, other hospital, or radiology clinic;

- Total parenteral nutrition (TPN) services; and

- Transportation, including transportation by ambulance, to and from another hospital or freestanding facility to receive specialized diagnostic or therapeutic services not available at the facility where the patient is an inpatient.

The hospital must include the cost of these services in the appropriate ancillary service cost center, i.e., in the cost of the diagnostic or therapeutic service. It must not show them separately under revenue code 0540.

EXCEPTIONS

Pneumococcal Vaccine -is payable under Part B only and is billed by the hospital on the Form CMS-1450.

Ambulance Service For purposes of this section "hospital inpatient" means beneficiary who has been formally admitted it does not include a beneficiary who is in the process of being transferred from one hospital to another. Where the patient is transferred from one hospital to another, and is admitted as an inpatient to the second, the ambulance service is payable under only Part B. If transportation is by a hospital owned and operated ambulance, the hospital bills separately on Form CMS-1450 as appropriate. Similarly, if the hospital arranges for the ambulance transportation with an ambulance operator, including paying the ambulance operator, it bills separately. However, if the hospital does not assume any financial responsibility, the billing is to the carrier by the ambulance operator or beneficiary, as appropriate, if an ambulance is used for the transportation of a hospital inpatient to another facility for diagnostic tests or special treatment the ambulance trip is considered part of the DRG, and not separately billable, if the resident hospital is under PPS.

Part B Inpatient Services Where Part A benefits are not payable, payment maybe made to the hospital under Part B for certain medical and other health services. See Chapter 4 for a description of Part B inpatient services.

Anesthetist Services "Incident to" Physician Services

If a physician's practice was to employ anesthetists and to bill on a reasonable charge basis for these services and that practice was in effect as of the last day of the hospital's most recent 12-month cost reporting period ending before September 30, 1983, the physician may continue that practice through cost reporting periods beginning October 1, 1984. However, if the physician chooses to continue this practice, the hospital may not add costs of the anesthetist's service to its base period costs for purposes of its transition payment rates. If it is the existing or new practice of the physician to employ certified registered nurse anesthetists (CRNAs) and other qualified anesthetists and include charges for their services in the physician bills for anesthesiology services for the hospital's cost report periods beginning on or after October 1, 1984, and before October 1, 1987, the physician may continue to do so.

B. Exceptions/Waivers

These provisions were waived before cost reporting periods beginning on or after October 1, 1986, under certain circumstances. The basic criteria for waiver was that services furnished by outside suppliers are so extensive that a sudden change in billing practices would threaten the stability of patient care. Specific criteria for waiver and processing procedures are in Sec.2804 of the Provider Reimbursement Manual (CMS Pub. 15-1).

100-4, 3, 20.7.3

Payment for Blood Clotting Factor Administered to Hemophilia Patients

Section 6011 of Public Law (P.L.) 101-239 amended Sec.1886(a)(4) of the Social Security Act (the Act) to provide that prospective payment system (PPS) hospitals receive anadditional payment for the costs of administering blood clotting factor to Medicare hemophiliacs who are hospital inpatients. Section 6011(b) of P.L. 101.239 specified that the payment be based on a predetermined price per unit of clotting factor multiplied by the number of units provided. This add-on payment originally was effective for blood clotting factors furnished on or after June 19, 1990, and before December 19, 1991. Section 13505 of P. L. 103-66 amended Sec.6011 (d) of P.L. 101-239 to extend the period covered by the add-on payment for blood clotting factors administered to Medicare inpatients with hemophilia through September 30, 1994. Section 4452 of P.L. 105-33 amended Sec.6011(d) of P.L. 101-239 to reinstate the add-on payment for the costs of administering blood clotting factor to Medicare beneficiaries who have hemophilia and who are hospital inpatients for discharges occurring on or after October 1, 1998.

Local carriers shall process non-institutional blood clotting factor claims.

The FIs shall process institutional blood clotting factor claims payable under either Part A or Part B.

A. Inpatient Bills

Under the Inpatient Prospective Payment System (PPS), hospitals receive a special add-on payment for the costs of furnishing blood clotting factors to Medicare beneficiaries with hemophilia, admitted as inpatients of PPS hospitals. The clotting factor add-on payment is calculated using the number of units (as defined in the HCPCS code long descriptor) billed by the provider under special instructions for units of service.

The PPS Pricer software does not calculate the payment amount. The Fiscal Intermediary Standard System (FISS) calculates the payment amount and subtracts the charges from those submitted to Pricer so that the clotting factor charges are not included in cost outlier computations.

Blood clotting factors not paid on a cost or PPS basis are priced as a drug/biological under the Medicare Part B Drug Pricing File effective for the specific date of service. As of January 1, 2005, the average sales price (ASP) plus 6 percent shall be used.

If a beneficiary is in a covered Part A stay in a PPS hospital, the clotting factors are paid in addition to the DRG/HIPPS payment (For FY 2004, this payment is based on 95 percent of average wholesale price.) For a SNF subject to SNF/PPS, the payment is bundled into the SNF/PPS rate.

For SNF inpatient Part A, there is no add-on payment for blood clotting factors.

The codes for blood-clotting factors are found on the Medicare Part B Drug Pricing File. This file is distributed on a quarterly basis.

For discharges occurring on or after October 1, 2000, and before December 31, 2005, report HCPCS Q0187 based on 1 billing unit per 1.2 mg. Effective January 1, 2006, HCPCS code J7189 replaces Q0187 and is defined as 1 billing unit per 1 microgram (mcg).

The examples below include the HCPCS code and indicate the dosage amount specified in the descriptor of that code. Facilities use the units field as a multiplier to arrive at the dosage amount.

EXAMPLE 1

HCPCS	Drug	Dosage
J7189	Factor VIIa	1 mcg

Actual dosage: 13, 365 mcg

On the bill, the facility shows J7189 and 13, 365 in the units field (13, 365 mcg divided by 1 mcg = 13, 365 units).

NOTE:The process for dealing with one international unit (IU) is the same as the process of dealing with one microgram.

EXAMPLE 21

HCPCS	Drug	Dosage
J9355	Trastuzumab	10 mg

Actual dosage: 140 mg

On the bill, the facility shows J9355 and 14 in the units field (140 mg divided by 10mg = 14 units). When the dosage amount is greater than the amount indicated for the HCPCS code, the facility

rounds up to determine units. When the dosage amount is less than the amount indicated for the HCPCS code, use 1 as the unit of measure.

EXAMPLE 3

HCPCS	Drug	Dosage
J3100	Tenecteplase	50 mg

Actual Dosage: 40 mg

The provider would bill for 1 unit, even though less than 1 full unit was furnished.

At times, the facility provides less than the amount provided in a single use vial and there is waste, i.e.; some drugs may be available only in packaged amounts that exceed the needs of an individual patient. Once the drug is reconstituted in the hospital's pharmacy, it may have a limited shelf life. Since an individual patient may receive less than the fully reconstituted amount, we encourage hospitals to schedule patients in such a way that the hospital can use the drug most efficiently. However, if the hospital must discard the remainder of a vial after administering part of it to a Medicare patient, the provider may bill for the amount of drug discarded plus the amount administered.

Example 1:

Drug X is available only in a 100-unit size. A hospital schedules three Medicare patients to receive drug X on the same day within the designated shelf life of the product. An appropriate hospital staff member administers 30 units to each patient. The remaining 10 units are billed to Medicare on the account of the last patient. Therefore, 30 units are billed on behalf of the first patient seen and 30 units are billed on behalf of the second patient seen. Forty units are billed on behalf of the last patient seen because the hospital had to discard 10 units at that point.

Example 2:

An appropriate hospital staff member must administer 30 units of drug X to a Medicare patient, and it is not practical to schedule another patient who requires the same drug. For example, the hospital has only one patient who requires drug X, or the hospital sees the patient for the first time and did not know the patient's condition. The hospital bills for 100 units on behalf of the patient, and Medicare pays for 100 units.

When the number of units of blood clotting factor administered to hemophiliac inpatients exceeds 99, 999, the hospital reports the excess as a second line for revenue code 0636 and repeats the HCPCS code. One hundred thousand fifty (100,050) units are reported on one line as 99, 999, and another line shows 1,051.

Revenue Code 0636 is used. It requires HCPCS. Some other inpatient drugs continue to be billed without HCPCS codes under pharmacy.

No changes in beneficiary notices are required. Coverage is applicable to hospital Part A claims only. Coverage is also applicable to inpatient Part B services in SNFs and all types of hospitals, including CAHs. Separate payment is not made to SNFs for beneficiaries in an inpatient Part A stay.

B. FI Action

The FI is responsible for the following:

- It accepts HCPCS codes for inpatient services;

- It edits to require HCPCS codes with Revenue Code 0636. Multiple iterations of the revenue code are possible with the same or different HCPCS codes. It does not edit units except to ensure a numeric value;

- It reduces charges forwarded to Pricer by the charges for hemophilia clotting factors in revenue code 0636. It retains the charges and revenue and HCPCS codes for CWF; and

- It modifies data entry screens to accept HCPCS codes for hospital (including CAH) swing bed, and SNF inpatient claims (bill types 11X, 12X, 18x, 21x and, 22x).

The September 1, 1993, IPPS final rule (58 FR 46304) states that payment will be made for the blood clotting factor only if an ICD-9-CM diagnosis code for hemophilia is included on the bill.

Since inpatient blood-clotting factors are covered only for beneficiaries with hemophilia, the FI must ensure that one of the following hemophilia diagnosis codes is listed on the bill before payment is made:

- 286.0 Congenital factor VIII disorder

- 286.1 Congenital factor IX disorder

- 286.2 Congenital factor IX disorder

- 286.3 Congenital deficiency of other clotting factor

- 286.4 von Willebrands' disease

Effective for discharges on or after August 1, 2001, payment may also be made if one of the following diagnosis codes is reported:

- 286.5 Hemorrhagic disorder due to circulating anticoagulants
- 286.7 Acquired coagulation factor deficiency

C. Part A Remittance Advice

1. X12.835 Ver. 003030M

For remittance reporting PIP and/or non-PIP payments, the Hemophilia Add on will be reported in a claims level 2-090-CAS segment (CAS is the element identifier) exhibiting an "OA" Group Code and adjustment reason code "97" (payment is included in the allowance for the basic service/ procedure) followed by the associated dollar amount (POSITIVE) and units of service. For this version of the 835, "OA" group coded line level CAS segments are informational and are not included in the balancing routine. The Hemophilia Add On amount will always be included in the 2-010-CLP04 Claim Payment Amount.

For remittance reporting PIP payments, the Hemophilia Add On will also be reported in the provider level adjustment (element identifier PLB) segment with the provider level adjustment reason code "CA" (Manual claims adjustment) followed by the associated dollar amount (NEGATIVE).

NOTE: A data maintenance request will be submitted to ANSI ASC X12 for a new PLB adjustment reason code specifically for PIP payment Hemophilia Add On situations for future use. However, continue to use adjustment reason code "CA" until further notice.

The FIs enter MA103 (Hemophilia Add On) in an open MIA (element identifier) remark code data element. This will alert the provider that the reason code 97 and PLB code "CA" adjustments are related to the Hemophilia Add On.

2. X12.835 Ver. 003051

For remittances reporting PIP and/or non-PIP payments, Hemophilia Add On information will be reported in the claim level 2-062-AMT and 2-064-QTY segments. The 2-062-AMT01 element will carry a "ZK" (Federal Medicare claim MANDATE - Category 1) qualifier code followed by the total claim level Hemophilia Add On amount (POSITIVE). The 2-064QTY01 element will carry a "FL" (Units) qualifier code followed by the number of units approved for the Hemophilia Add On for the claim. The Hemophilia Add On amount will always be included in the 2-010-CLP04 Claim Payment Amount.

NOTE: A data maintenance request will be submitted to ANSI ASC X12 for a new AMT qualifier code specifically for the Hemophilia Add On for future use. However, continue to use adjustment reason code "ZK" until further notice.

For remittances reporting PIP payments, the Hemophilia Add On will be reported in the provider level adjustment PLB segment with the provider level adjustment reason "ZZ" followed by the associated dollar amount (NEGATIVE).

NOTE: A data maintenance request will be submitted to ANSI ASC X12 for a new PLB, adjustment reason code specifically for the Hemophilia Add On for future use. However, continue to use PLB adjustment reason code "ZZ" until further notice. The FIs enter MA103 (Hemophilia Add On) in an open MIA remark code data element. This will alert the provider that the ZK, FL and ZZ entries are related to the Hemophilia Add On. (Effective with version 4010 of the 835, report ZK in lieu of FL in the QTY segment.)

3. Standard Hard Copy Remittance Advice

For paper remittances reporting non-PIP payments involving Hemophilia Add On, add a "Hemophilia Add On" category to the end of the "Pass Thru Amounts" listings in the "Summary" section of the paper remittance. Enter the total of the Hemophilia Add On amounts due for the claims covered by this remittance next to the Hemophilia Add On heading.

The FIs add the Remark Code "MA103" (Hemophilia Add On) to the remittance advice under the REM column for those claims that qualify for Hemophilia Add On payments.

This will be the full extent of Hemophilia Add On reporting on paper remittance notices; providers wishing more detailed information must subscribe to the Medicare Part A specifications for the ANSI ASC X12N 835, where additional information is available.

See chapter 22, for detailed instructions and definitions.

100-4, 3, 40.2.2

Charges to Beneficiaries for Part A Services

The hospital submits a bill even where the patient is responsible for a deductible which covers the entire amount of the charges for non-PPS hospitals, or in PPS hospitals, where the DRG payment amount will be less than the deductible.

A hospital receiving payment for a covered hospital stay (or PPS hospital that includes at least one covered day, or one treated as covered under guarantee of payment or limitation on liability) may charge the beneficiary, or other person, for items and services furnished during the stay only as described in subsections A through H. If limitation of liability applies, a beneficiary's liability for payment is governed by the limitation on liability notification rules in Chapter 30 of this manual. For

related notices for inpatient hospitals, see CMS Transmittal 594, Change Request3903, dated June 24, 2005.

A. Deductible and Coinsurance

The hospital may charge the beneficiary or other person for applicable deductible and coinsurance amounts. The deductible is satisfied only by charges for covered services. The FI deducts the deductible and coinsurance first from the PPS payment. Where the deductible exceeds the PPS amount, the excess will be applied to a subsequent payment to the hospital. (See Chapter 3 of the Medicare General Information, Eligibility, and Entitlement Manual for specific policies.)

B. Blood Deductible

The Part A blood deductible provision applies to whole blood and red blood cells, and reporting of the number of pints is applicable to both PPS and non-PPS hospitals. (See Chapter 3 of the Medicare General Information, Eligibility, and Entitlement Manual for specific policies.) Hospitals shall report charges for red blood cells using revenue code 381, and charges for whole blood using revenue code 382.

C. Inpatient Care No Longer Required

The hospital may charge for services that are not reasonable and necessary or that constitute custodial care. Notification may be required under limitation of liability. See CMS Transmittal 594, Change Request3903, dated June 24, 2005, section V. of the attachment, for specific notification requirements. Note this transmittal will be placed in Chapter 30 of this manual at a future point. Chapter 1, section 150 of this manual also contains related billing information in addition to that provided below.

In general, after proper notification has occurred, and assuming an expedited decision is received from a Quality Improvement Organization (QIO), the following entries are required on the bill the hospital prepares:

- Occurrence code 31 (and date) to indicate the date the hospital notified the patient in accordance with the first bullet above;
- Occurrence span code 76 (and dates) to indicate the period of noncovered care for which it is charging the beneficiary;
- Occurrence span code 77 (and dates) to indicate the period of noncovered care for which the provider is liable, when it is aware of this prior to billing; and
- Value code 31 (and amount) to indicate the amount of charges it may bill the beneficiary for days for which inpatient care was no longer required. They are included as noncovered charges on the bill.

D. Change in the Beneficiary's Condition

If the beneficiary remains in the hospital after receiving notice as described in subsection C, and the hospital, the physician who concurred in the hospital's determination, or the QIO, subsequently determines that the beneficiary again requires inpatient hospital care, the hospital may not charge the beneficiary or other person for services furnished after the beneficiary again required inpatient hospital care until proper notification occurs (see subsection C).

If a patient who needs only a SNF level of care remains in the hospital after the SNF bed becomes available, and the bed ceases to be available, the hospital may continue to charge the beneficiary. It need not provide the beneficiary with another notice when the patient chose not to be discharged to the SNF bed.

E. Admission Denied

If the entire hospital admission is determined to be not reasonable or necessary, limitation of liability may apply. See 2005 CMS transmittal 594, section V. of the attachment, for specific notification requirements.

NOTE: This transmittal will be placed in Chapter 30 of this manual at a future point.

In such cases the following entries are required on the bill:

- Occurrence code 31 (and date) to indicate the date the hospital notified the beneficiary.
- Occurrence span code 76 (and dates) to indicate the period of noncovered care for which the hospital is charging the beneficiary.
- Occurrence span code 77 (and dates) to indicate any period of noncovered care for which the provider is liable (e.g., the period between issuing the notice and the time it may charge the beneficiary) when the provider is aware of this prior to billing.
- Value code 31 (and amount) to indicate the amount of charges the hospital may bill the beneficiary for hospitalization that was not necessary or reasonable. They are included as noncovered charges on the bill.

F. Procedures, Studies and Courses of Treatment That Are Not Reasonable or Necessary

If diagnostic procedures, studies, therapeutic studies and courses of treatment are excluded from coverage as not reasonable and necessary (even though the beneficiary requires inpatient hospital care) the hospital may charge the beneficiary or other person for the services or care according the procedures given in CMS Transmittal 594, Change Request3903, dated June 24, 2005.

The following bill entries apply to these circumstances:

- Occurrence code 32 (and date) to indicate the date the hospital provided the notice to the beneficiary.
- Value code 3l (and amount) to indicate the amount of such charges to be billed to the beneficiary. They are included as noncovered charges on the bill.

G. Nonentitlement Days and Days after Benefits Exhausted

If a hospital stay exceeds the day outlier threshold, the hospital may charge for some, or all, of the days on which the patient is not entitled to Medicare Part A, or after the Part A benefits are exhausted (i.e., the hospital may charge its customary charges for services furnished on those days). It may charge the beneficiary for the lesser of:

- The number of days on which the patient was not entitled to benefits or after the benefits were exhausted; or
- The number of outlier days. (Day outliers were discontinued at the end of FY 1997.)

If the number of outlier days exceeds the number of days on which the patient was not entitled to benefits, or after benefits were exhausted, the hospital may charge for all days on which the patient was not entitled to benefits or after benefits were exhausted. If the number of days on which the beneficiary was not entitled to benefits, or after benefits were exhausted, exceeds the number of outlier days, the hospital determines the days for which it may charge by starting with the last day of the stay (i.e., the day before the day of discharge) and identifying and counting off in reverse order, days on which the patient was not entitled to benefits or after the benefits were exhausted, until the number of days counted off equals the number of outlier days. The days counted off are the days for which the hospital may charge.

H. Contractual Exclusions

In addition to receiving the basic prospective payment, the hospital may charge the beneficiary for any services that are excluded from coverage for reasons other than, or in addition to, absence of medical necessity, provision of custodial care, non-entitlement to Part A, or exhaustion of benefits. For example, it may charge for most cosmetic and dental surgery.

I. Private Room Care

Payment for medically necessary private room care is included in the prospective payment. Where the beneficiary requests private room accommodations, the hospital must inform the beneficiary of the additional charge. (See the Medicare Benefit Policy Manual, Chapter 1.) When the beneficiary accepts the liability, the hospital will supply the service, and bill the beneficiary directly. If the beneficiary believes the private room was medically necessary, the beneficiary has a right to a determination and may initiate a Part A appeal.

J. Deluxe Item or Service

Where a beneficiary requests a deluxe item or service, i.e., an item or service which is more expensive than is medically required for the beneficiary's condition, the hospital may collect the additional charge if it informs the beneficiary of the additional charge. That charge is the difference between the customary charge for the item or service most commonly furnished by the hospital to private pay patients with the beneficiary's condition, and the charge for the more expensive item or service requested. If the beneficiary believes that the more expensive item or service was medically necessary, the beneficiary has a right to a determination and may initiate a Part A appeal.

K - Inpatient Acute Care Hospital Admission Followed By a Death or Discharge Prior To Room Assignment

A patient of an acute care hospital is considered an inpatient upon issuance of written doctor's orders to that effect. If a patient either dies or is discharged prior to being assigned and/or occupying a room, a hospital may enter an appropriate room and board charge on the claim. If a patient leaves of their own volition prior to being assigned and/or occupying a room, a hospital may enter an appropriate room and board charge on the claim as well as a patient status code 07 which indicates they left against medical advice. A hospital is not required to enter a room and board charge, but failure to do so may have a minimal impact on future DRG weight calculations.

100-4, 4, 10.4

Packaging

Under the OPPS, packaged services are items and services that are considered to be an integral part of another service that is paid under the OPPS. No separate payment is made for packaged services, because the cost of these items and services is included in the APC payment for the service of which they are an integral part. For example, routine supplies, anesthesia, recovery room use, and most drugs are considered to be an integral part of a surgical procedure so payment for these items is packaged into the APC payment for the surgical procedure.

A. Packaging for Claims Resulting in APC Payments

If a claim contains services that result in an APC payment but also contains packaged services, separate payment for the packaged services is not made since payment is included in the APC.

However, charges related to the packaged services are used for outlier and Transitional Corridor Payments (TOPs) as well as for future rate setting.

Therefore, it is extremely important that hospitals report all HCPCS codes and all charges for all services they furnish, whether payment for the services is made separately paid or is packaged.

B. Packaging for Claims Resulting in No APC Payments

If the claim contains only services payable under cost reimbursement, such as corneal tissue, and services that would be packaged services if an APC were payable, then the packaged services are not separately payable. In addition, these charges for the packaged services are not used to calculate TOPs.

If the claim contains only services payable under a fee schedule, such as clinical diagnostic laboratory tests, and also contains services that would be packaged services if an APC were payable, the packaged services are not separately payable. In addition, the charges are not used to calculate TOPs.

If a claim contains services payable under cost reimbursement, services payable under a fee schedule, and services that would be packaged services if an APC were payable, the packaged services are not separately payable. In addition, the charges are not used to calculate TOPs payments.

C. Packaging Types Under the OPPS

1. Unconditionally packaged services are services for which separate payment is never made because the payment for the service is always packaged into the payment for other services. Unconditionally packaged services are identified in the OPPS Addendum B with status indictor of N. See the OPPS Web site at http://www.cms.hhs.gov/HospitalOutpatientPPS/ for the most recent Addendum B (HCPCS codes with status indicators). In general, the charges for unconditionally packaged services are used to calculate outlier and TOPS payments when they appear on a claim with a service that is separately paid under the OPPS because the packaged service is considered to be part of the package of services for which payment is being made through the APC payment for the separately paid service.

2. STVX-packaged services are services for which separate payment is made only if there is no service with status indicator S, T, V or X reported with the same date of service on the same claim. If a claim includes a service that is assigned status indicator S, T, V, or X reported on the same date of service as the STVXpackaged service, the payment for the STVX-packaged service is packaged into the payment for the service(s) with status indicator S, T, V or X and no separate payment is made for the STVX-packaged service. STVX-packaged services are assigned status indicator Q. See the OPPS Webpage at http://www.cms.hhs.gov/HospitalOutpatientPPS/ for identification of STVXpackaged codes.

3. T-packaged services are services for which separate payment is made only if there is no service with status indicator T reported with the same date of service on the same claim. When there is a claim that includes a service that is assigned status indicator T reported on the same date of service as the T-packaged service, the payment for the T-packaged service is packaged into the payment for the service(s) with status indicator T and no separate payment is made for the T-packaged service. T-packaged services are assigned status indicator Q. See the OPPS Web site at http://www.cms.hhs.gov/HospitalOutpatientPPS/ for identification of T-packaged codes.

4. A service that is assigned to a composite APC is a major component of a single episode of care. The hospital receives one payment through a composite APC for multiple major separately identifiable services. Services mapped to composite APCs are assigned status indicator Q. See the discussion of composite APCs in section 10.2.1.

100-4, 4, 160

Clinic and Emergency Visits

CMS has acknowledged from the beginning of the OPPS that CMS believes that CPT Evaluation and Management (E/M) codes were designed to reflect the activities of physicians and do not describe well the range and mix of services provided by hospitals during visits of clinic and emergency department patients. While awaiting the development of a national set of facility-specific codes and guidelines, providers should continue to apply their current internal guidelines to the existing CPT codes. Each hospital's internal guidelines should follow the intent of the CPT code descriptors, in that the guidelines should be designed to reasonably relate the intensity of hospital resources to the different levels of effort represented by the codes. Hospitals should ensure that their guidelines accurately reflect resource distinctions between the five levels of codes.

Effective January 1, 2007, CMS is distinguishing between two types of emergency departments: Type A emergency departments and Type B emergency departments.

A Type A emergency department is defined as an emergency department that is available 24 hours a day, 7 days a week and is either licensed by the State in which it is located under applicable State law as an emergency room or emergency department or it is held out to the public (by name, posted signs, advertising, or other means) as a place that provides care for emergency medical conditions on an urgent basis without requiring a previously scheduled appointment.

A Type B emergency department is defined as an emergency department that meets the definition of a "dedicated emergency department" as defined in 42 CFR 489.24 under the EMTALA regulations. It must meet at least one of the following requirements: (1) It is licensed by the State in which it is located under applicable State law as an emergency room or emergency department; (2) It is held out to the public (by name, posted signs, advertising, or other means) as a place that provides care for emergency medical conditions on an urgent basis without requiring a previously scheduled appointment; or (3) During the calendar year immediately preceding the calendar year in which a determination under 42 CFR 489.24 is being made, based on a representative sample of patient visits that occurred during that calendar year, it provides at least one-third of all of its outpatient visits for the treatment of emergency medical conditions on an urgent basis without requiring a previously scheduled appointment.

Hospitals must bill for visits provided in Type A emergency departments using CPT emergency department E/M codes. Hospitals must bill for visits provided in Type B emergency departments using the G-codes that describe visits provided in Type B emergency departments.

Hospitals that will be billing the new Type B ED visit codes may need to update their internal guidelines to report these codes.

Emergency department and clinic visits are paid in some cases separately and in other cases as part of a composite APC payment. See section 10.2.1 of this chapter for further details.

100-4, 4, 160.1

Critical Care Services

Beginning January 1, 2007, critical care services will be paid at two levels, depending on the presence or absence of trauma activation. Providers will receive one payment rate for critical care without trauma activation and will receive additional payment when critical care is associated with trauma activation.

To determine whether trauma activation occurs, follow the National Uniform Billing Committee (NUBC) guidelines in the Claims Processing Manual, Pub 100-04, Chapter 25, Sec.75.4 related to the reporting of the trauma revenue codes in the 68x series. The revenue code series 68x can be used only by trauma centers/hospitals as licensed or designated by the state or local government authority authorized to do so, or as verified by the American College of Surgeons. Different subcategory revenue codes are reported by designated Level 1-4 hospital trauma centers. Only patients for whom there has been prehospital notification based on triage information from prehospital caregivers, who meet either local, state or American College of Surgeons field triage criteria, or are delivered by inter-hospital transfers, and are given the appropriate team response can be billed a trauma activation charge.

When critical care services are provided without trauma activation, the hospital may bill CPT code 99291, Critical care, evaluation and management of the critically ill or critically injured patient; first 30-74 minutes (and 99292, if appropriate). If trauma activation occurs under the circumstances described by the NUBC guidelines that would permit reporting a charge under 68x, the hospital may also bill one unit of code G0390, which describes trauma activation associated with hospital critical care services. Revenue code 68x must be reported on the same date of service. The OCE will edit to ensure that G0390 appears with revenue code 68x on the same date of service and that only one unit of G0390 is billed. CMS believes that trauma activation is a one-time occurrence in association with critical care services, and therefore, CMS will only pay for one unit of G0390 per day.

The CPT code 99291 is defined by CPT as the first 30-74 minutes of critical care. This 30 minute minimum has always applied under the OPPS. The CPT code 99292, Critical care, evaluation and management of the critically ill or critically injured patient; each additional 30 minutes, remains a packaged service under the OPPS, so that hospitals do not have the ongoing administrative burden of reporting precisely the time for each critical service provided. As the CPT guidelines indicate, hospitals that provide less than 30 minutes of critical care should bill for a visit, typically an emergency department visit, at a level consistent with their own internal guidelines.

Under the OPPS, the time that can be reported as critical care is the time spent by a physician and/or hospital staff engaged in active face-to-face critical care of a critically ill or critically injured patient. If the physician and hospital staff or multiple hospital staff members are simultaneously engaged in this active face-to-face care, the time involved can only be counted once.

In CY 2007 hospitals may continue to report a charge with RC 68x without any HCPCS code when trauma team activation occurs. In order to receive additional payment when critical care services are associated with trauma activation, the hospital must report G0390 on the same date of service as RC 68x, in addition to CPT code 99291 (or 99292, if appropriate.)

In CY 2007 hospitals should continue to report 99291 (and 99292 as appropriate) for critical care services furnished without trauma team activation. CPT 99291 maps to APC 0617 (Critical Care). (CPT 99292 is packaged and not paid separately, but should be reported if provided.)

Critical care services are paid in some cases separately and in other cases as part of a composite APC payment. See Section 10.2.1 of this chapter for further details.

100-4, 4, 200.1

Billing for Corneal Tissue

Corneal tissue will be paid on a cost basis, not under OPPS. To receive cost based reimbursement hospitals must bill charges for corneal tissue using HCPCS code V2785.

100-4, 4, 200.2

Hospital Dialysis Services For Patients with and without End Stage Renal Disease (ESRD)

Effective with claims with dates of service on or after August 1, 2000, hospital-based End Stage Renal Disease (ESRD) facilities must submit services covered under the ESRD benefit in 42 CFR 413.174 (maintenance dialysis and those items and services directly related to dialysis such as drugs, supplies) on a separate claim from services not covered under the ESRD benefit. Items and services not covered under the ESRD benefit must be billed by the hospital using the hospital bill type and be paid under the Outpatient Prospective Payment System (OPPS) (or to a CAH at reasonable cost). Services covered under the ESRD benefit in 42 CFR 413.174 must be billed on the ESRD bill type and must be paid under the ESRD PPS. This requirement is necessary to properly pay only unrelated ESRD services (those not covered under the ESRD benefit) under OPPS (or to a CAH at reasonable cost).

Medicare does not allow payment for routine or related dialysis treatments, which are covered and paid under the ESRD PPS, when furnished to ESRD patients in the outpatient department of a hospital. However, in certain medical situations in which the ESRD outpatient cannot obtain her or his regularly scheduled dialysis treatment at a certified ESRD facility, the OPPS rule for 2003 allows payment for non-routine dialysis treatments (which are not covered under the ESRD benefit) furnished to ESRD outpatients in the outpatient department of a hospital. Payment for unscheduled dialysis furnished to ESRD outpatients and paid under the OPPS is limited to the following circumstances:

- Dialysis performed following or in connection with a dialysis-related procedure such as vascular access procedure or blood transfusions;

- Dialysis performed following treatment for an unrelated medical emergency; e.g., if a patient goes to the emergency room for chest pains and misses a regularly scheduled dialysis treatment that cannot be rescheduled, CMS allows the hospital to provide and bill Medicare for the dialysis treatment; or

- Emergency dialysis for ESRD patients who would otherwise have to be admitted as inpatients in order for the hospital to receive payment.

In these situations, non-ESRD certified hospital outpatient facilities are to bill Medicare using the Healthcare Common Procedure Coding System (HCPCS) code G0257 (Unscheduled or emergency dialysis treatment for an ESRD patient in a hospital outpatient department that is not certified as an ESRD facility).

HCPCS code G0257 may only be reported on type of bill 13X (hospital outpatient service) or type of bill 85X (critical access hospital) because HCPCS code G0257 only reports services for hospital outpatients with ESRD and only these bill types are used to report services to hospital outpatients. Effective for services on and after October 1, 2012, claims containing HCPCS code G0257 will be returned to the provider for correction if G0257 is reported with a type of bill other than 13X or 85X (such as a 12x inpatient claim).

HCPCS code 90935 (Hemodialysis procedure with single physician evaluation) may be reported and paid only if one of the following two conditions is met:

1) The patient is a hospital inpatient with or without ESRD and has no coverage under Part A, but has Part B coverage. The charge for hemodialysis is a charge for the use of a prosthetic device. See Benefits Policy Manual 100-02 Chapter 15 section 120. A. The service must be reported on a type of bill 12X or type of bill 85X. See the Benefits Policy Manual 100-02 Chapter 6 section 10 (Medical and Other Health Services Furnished to Inpatients of Participating Hospitals) for the criteria that must be met for services to be paid when a hospital inpatient has Part B coverage but does not have coverage under Part A; or 2) A hospital outpatient does not have ESRD and is receiving hemodialysis in the hospital outpatient department. The service is reported on a type of bill 13X or type of bill 85X. CPT code 90945 (Dialysis procedure other than hemodialysis (e.g. peritoneal dialysis, hemofiltration, or other continuous replacement therapies)), with single physician evaluation, may be reported by a hospital paid under the OPPS or CAH method I or method II on type of bill 12X, 13X or 85X.

100-4, 4, 200.3.4

Billing for Linear Accelerator (Robotic Image-Guided and Non-Robotic Image-Guided) SRS Planning and Delivery

Effective for services furnished on or after January 1, 2006, hospitals must bill using existing CPT codes that most accurately describe the service furnished for both robotic and non-robotic image-guided SRS planning. For robotic image-guided SRS delivery, hospitals must bill using HCPCS code G0339 for the first session and HCPCS code G0340 for the second through the fifth sessions. For non-robotic image-guided SRS delivery, hospitals must bill G0173 for delivery if the delivery occurs in one session, and G0251 for delivery per session (not to exceed five sessions) if delivery occurs during multiple sessions.

Linear Accelerator-Based Robotic Image-Guided SRS	
Planning	Use existing CPT codes
Delivery	G0339 (complete, 1st session)
	G0340 (2nd – 5th session)

Linear Accelerator-Based Non-Robotic Image-Guided SRS	
Planning	Use existing CPT codes
Delivery	G0173 (single session)
	G0251 (multiple)

HCPCS Code	Long Descriptors
G0173	Linear accelerator based stereotactic radiosurgery, delivery including collimator changes and custom plugging, complete course of treatment in one session, all lesions.
G0251	Linear accelerator based stereotactic radiosurgery, delivery including collimator changes and custom plugging, fractionated treatment, all lesions, per session, maximum 5 sessions per course of treatment.
G0339	Image-guided robotic linear accelerator-based stereotactic radiosurgery, complete course of therapy in one session or first session of fractionated treatment.
G0340	Image-guided robotic linear accelerator-based stereotactic radiosurgery, delivery including collimator changes and custom plugging, fractionated treatment, all lesions, per session, second through fifth sessions, maximum five sessions per course of treatment

100-4, 4, 200.4

Billing for Amniotic Membrane

Hospitals should report HCPCS code V2790 (Amniotic membrane for surgical reconstruction, per procedure) to report amniotic membrane tissue when the tissue is used. A specific procedure code associated with use of amniotic membrane tissue is CPT code 65780 (Ocular surface reconstruction; amniotic membrane transplantation).

Payment for the amniotic membrane tissue is packaged into payment for CPT code 65780 or other procedures with which the amniotic membrane is used.

100-4, 4, 200.6

Billing and Payment for Alcohol and/or Substance Abuse Assessment and Intervention Services

For CY 2008, the CPT Editorial Panel has created two new Category I CPT codes for reporting alcohol and/or substance abuse screening and intervention services. They are CPT code 99408 (Alcohol and/or substance (other than tobacco) abuse structured screening (e.g., AUDIT, DAST), and brief intervention (SBI) services; 15 to 30 minutes); and CPT code 99409 (Alcohol and/or substance (other than tobacco) abuse structured screening (e.g., AUDIT, DAST), and brief intervention (SBI) services; greater than 30 minutes). However, screening services are not covered by Medicare without specific statutory authority, such as has been provided for mammography, diabetes, and colorectal cancer screening. Therefore, beginning January 1, 2008, the OPPS recognizes two parallel G-codes (HCPCS codes G0396 and G0397) to allow for appropriate reporting and payment of alcohol and substance abuse structured assessment and intervention services that are not provided as screening services, but that are performed in the context of the diagnosis or treatment of illness or injury.

Contractors shall make payment under the OPPS for HCPCS code G0396 (Alcohol and/or substance (other than tobacco) abuse structured assessment (e.g., AUDIT, DAST) and brief intervention, 15 to 30 minutes) and HCPCS code G0397, (Alcohol and/or substance(other than tobacco) abuse structured assessment (e.g., AUDIT, DAST) and intervention greater than 30 minutes), only when reasonable and necessary (i.e., when the service is provided to evaluate patients with signs/symptoms of illness or injury) as per section 1862(a)(1)(A) of the Act.

HCPCS codes G0396 and G0397 are to be used for structured alcohol and/or substance (other than tobacco) abuse assessment and intervention services that are distinct from other clinic and emergency department visit services performed during the same encounter. Hospital resources expended performing services described by HCPCS codes G0396 and G0397 may not be counted as resources for determining the level of a visit service and vice versa (i.e., hospitals may not double count the same facility resources in order to reach a higher level clinic or emergency department visit). However, alcohol and/or substance structured assessment or intervention services lasting less than 15 minutes should not be reported using these HCPCS codes, but the

hospital resources expended should be included in determining the level of the visit service reported.

100-4, 4, 200.7.2

Cardiac Echocardiography With Contrast

Hospitals are instructed to bill for echocardiograms with contrast using the applicable HCPCS code(s) included in Table 200.7.2 below. Hospitals should also report the appropriate units of the HCPCS codes for the contrast agents used in the performance of the echocardiograms.

Table 200.7.2 - HCPCS Codes For Echocardiograms With Contrast HCPCS Long Descriptor C8921 Transthoracic echocardiography with contrast for congenital cardiac anomalies; complete C8922 Transthoracic echocardiography with contrast for congenital cardiac anomalies; follow-up or limited study C8923 Transthoracic echocardiography with contrast, realtime with image documentation (2D) with or without HCPCS Long Descriptor M-mode recording; complete C8924 Transthoracic echocardiography with contrast, realtime with image documentation (2D) with or without M-mode recording; follow-up or limited study C8925 Transesophageal echocardiography (TEE) with contrast, real time with image documentation (2D) (with or without M-mode recording); including probe placement, image acquisition, interpretation and report C8926 Transesophageal echocardiography (TEE) with contrast for congenital cardiac anomalies; including probe placement, image acquisition, interpretation and report C8927 Transesophageal echocardiography (TEE) with contrast for monitoring purposes, including probe placement, real time 2-dimensional image acquisition and interpretation leading to ongoing (continuous) assessment of (dynamically changing) cardiac pumping function and to therapeutic measures on an immediate time basis C8928 Transthoracic echocardiography with contrast, realtime with image documentation (2D), with or without M-mode recording, during rest and cardiovascular stress test using treadmill, bicycle exercise and/or pharmacologically induced stress, with interpretation and report

100-4, 4, 230.2

Coding and Payment for Drug Administration

Coding and Payment for Drug Administration

A. Overview

Drug administration services furnished under the Hospital Outpatient Prospective Payment System (OPPS) during CY 2005 were reported using CPT codes 90780, 90781, and 96400-96459.

Effective January 1, 2006, some of these CPT codes were replaced with more detailed CPT codes incorporating specific procedural concepts, as defined and described by the CPT manual, such as initial, concurrent, and sequential.

Hospitals are instructed to use the full set of CPT codes, including those codes referencing concepts of initial, concurrent, and sequential, to bill for drug administration services furnished in the hospital outpatient department beginning January 1, 2007. In addition, hospitals are instructed to continue billing the HCPCS codes that most accurately describe the service(s) provided.

Hospitals are reminded to bill a separate Evaluation and Management code (with modifier 25) only if a significant, separately identifiable E/M service is performed in the same encounter with OPPS drug administration services.

B. Billing for Infusions and Injections

Beginning in CY 2007, hospitals were instructed to use the full set of drug administration CPT codes (90760-90779; 96401-96549), (96413-96523 beginning in CY 2008) (96360-96549 beginning in CY 2009) when billing for drug administration services provided in the hospital outpatient department. In addition, hospitals are to continue to bill HCPCS code C8957 (Intravenous infusion for therapy/diagnosis; initiation of prolonged infusion (more than 8 hours), requiring use of portable or implantable pump) when appropriate. Hospitals are expected to report all drug administration CPT codes in a manner consistent with their descriptors, CPT instructions, and correct coding principles. Hospitals should note the conceptual changes between CY 2006 drug administration codes effective under the OPPS and the CPT codes in effect beginning January 1, 2007, in order to ensure accurate billing under the OPPS. Hospitals should report all HCPCS codes that describe the drug administration services provided, regardless of whether or not those services are separately paid or their payment is packaged.

Medicare's general policy regarding physician supervision within hospital outpatient departments meets the physician supervision requirements for use of CPT codes 90760-90779, 96401-96549, (96413-96523 beginning in CY 2008). (Reference: Pub.100-02, Medicare Benefit Policy Manual, Chapter 6, §20.4.)

Drug administration services are to be reported with a line item date of service on the day they are provided. In addition, only one initial drug administration service is to be reported per vascular access site per encounter, including during an encounter where observation services span more than 1 calendar day.

C. Payments For Drug Administration Services

For CY 2007, OPPS drug administration APCs were restructured, resulting in a six-level hierarchy where active HCPCS codes have been assigned according to their clinical coherence and resource use. Contrary to the CY 2006 payment structure that bundled payment for several instances of a type of service (non-chemotherapy, chemotherapy by infusion, non-infusion chemotherapy) into a per-encounter APC payment, structure introduced in CY 2007 provides a separate APC payment for each reported unit of a separately payable HCPCS code.

Hospitals should note that the transition to the full set of CPT drug administration codes provides for conceptual differences when reporting, such as those noted below.

- In CY 2006, hospitals were instructed to bill for the first hour (and any additional hours) by each type of infusion service (non-chemotherapy, chemotherapy by infusion, non-infusion chemotherapy). Beginning in CY 2007, the first hour concept no longer exists. CPT codes in CY 2007 and beyond allow for only one initial service per encounter, for each vascular access site, no matter how many types of infusion services are provided; however, hospitals will receive an APC payment for the initial service and separate APC payment(s) for additional hours of infusion or other drug administration services provided that are separately payable.

- In CY 2006, hospitals providing infusion services of different types (non-chemotherapy, chemotherapy by infusion, non-infusion chemotherapy) received payment for the associated per-encounter infusion APC even if these infusions occurred during the same time period. Beginning in CY 2007, hospitals should report only one initial drug administration service, including infusion services, per encounter for each distinct vascular access site, with other services through the same vascular access site being reported via the sequential, concurrent or additional hour codes. Although new CPT guidance has been issued for reporting initial drug administration services, Medicare contractors shall continue to follow the guidance given in this manual.

(NOTE: This list above provides a brief overview of a limited number of the conceptual changes between CY 2006 OPPS drug administration codes and CY 2007 OPPS drug administration codes - this list is not comprehensive and does not include all items hospitals will need to consider during this transition)

For APC payment rates, refer to the most current quarterly version of Addendum B on the CMS Web site at http://www.cms.hhs.gov/HospitalOutpatientPPS/.

D. Infusions Started Outside the Hospital

Hospitals may receive Medicare beneficiaries for outpatient services who are in the process of receiving an infusion at their time of arrival at the hospital (e.g., a patient who arrives via ambulance with an ongoing intravenous infusion initiated by paramedics during transport). Hospitals are reminded to bill for all services provided using the HCPCS code(s) that most accurately describe the service(s) they provided. This includes hospitals reporting an initial hour of infusion, even if the hospital did not initiate the infusion, and additional HCPCS codes for additional or sequential infusion services if needed.

100-4, 4, 230.2.1

Administration of Drugs Via Implantable or Portable Pumps

for Implantable or Portable Pumps 2005 CPT Final CY 2006 OPPS 2005 CPT 2005 Description Code Description SI APC n/a n/a C8957 Intravenous infusion for therapy/diagnosis; initiation of prolonged infusion (more than 8 hours), requiring use of portable or implantable pump S 0120 96414 Chemotherapy administration, intravenous; infusion technique, initiation of prolonged infusion (more than 8 hours), requiring the use of a portable or implantable pump 96416 Chemotherapy administration, intravenous infusion technique; initiation of prolonged chemotherapy infusion (more than 8 hours), requiring use of portable or implantable pump S 0117 96425 Chemotherapy administration, infusion technique, initiation of prolonged infusion (more than 8 hours), requiring the use of a portable or implantable pump) 96425 Chemotherapy administration, intra-arterial; infusion technique, initiation of prolonged infusion (more than 8 hours), requiring the use of a portable or implantable pump S 0117 96520 Refilling and maintenance of portable pump 96521 Refilling and maintenance of portable pump T 0125 2005 CPT Final CY 2006 OPPS 2005 CPT 2005 Description Code Description SI APC 96530 Refilling and maintenance of implantable pump or reservoir for drug delivery, systemic [e.g. Intravenous, intra-arterial] 96522 Refilling and maintenance of implantable pump or reservoir for drug delivery, systemic (e.g., intravenous, intra-arterial) T 0125 n/a n/a 96523 Irrigation of implanted venous access device for drug delivery systems N - Hospitals are to report HCPCS code C8957 and CPT codes 96416 and 96425 to indicate the initiation of a prolonged infusion that requires the use of an implantable or portable pump. CPT codes 96521, 92522, and 96523 should be used by hospitals to indicate refilling and maintenance of drug delivery systems or irrigation of implanted venous access devices for such systems, and may be reported for the servicing of devices used for therapeutic drugs other than chemotherapy.

100-4, 4, 230.2.3

Non-Chemotherapy Drug Administration

Table 5: CY 2006 OPPS Non-Chemotherapy Drug Administration -Intravenous Infusion Technique

2005 CPT	Final CY 2006 OPPS	2005 CPT	2005 Description	Code	Desc	SI	APC
90780	Intravenous infusion for therapy/diagnosis, administered by physician or under direct supervision of physician; up to one hour\	C8950	Intravenous infusion for therapy/diagnosis; up to 1 hour	S	0120		
90781	Intravenous infusion for therapy/diagnosis, administered by physician or under direct supervision of physician; each additional hour, up to eight (8) hours (List separately in addition to code for primary procedure)	C8951	Intravenous infusion for therapy/diagnosis; each additional hour (List separately in addition to C8950)	N	-	n/a	n/a
		C8957	Intravenous infusion for therapy/diagnosis; initiation of prolonged infusion (more than 8 hours), requiring use of portable or implantable pump	S	120		

Hospitals are to report HCPCS code C8950 to indicate an infusion of drugs other than anti-neoplastic drugs furnished on or after January 1, 2006 (except as noted at 230.2.2(A) above). HCPCS code C8951 should be used to report all additional infusion hours, with no limit on the number of hours billed per line. Medically necessary separate therapeutic or diagnostic hydration services should be reported with C8950 and C8951, as these are considered intravenous infusions for therapy/diagnosis.

HCPCS codes C8950 and C8951 should not be reported when the infusion is a necessary and integral part of a separately payable OPPS procedure.

When more than one nonchemotherapy drug is infused, hospitals are to code HCPCS codes C8950 and C8951 (if necessary) to report the total duration of an infusion, regardless of the number of substances or drugs infused. Hospitals are reminded to bill separately for each drug infused, in addition to the drug administration services.

The OCE pays one APC for each encounter reported by HCPCS code C8950, and only pays one APC for C8950 per day (unless Modifier 59 is used). Payment for additional hours of infusion reported by HCPCS code C8951 is packaged into the payment for the initial infusion. While no separate payment will be made for units of HCPCS code C8951, hospitals are instructed to report all codes that appropriately describe the services provided and the corresponding charges so that CMS may capture specific historical hospital cost data for future payment rate setting activities.

OCE logic assumes that all services for non-chemotherapy infusions billed on the same date of service were provided during the same encounter. Where a beneficiary makes two separate visits to the hospital for non-chemotherapy infusions in the same day, hospitals are to report modifier 59 for non-chemotherapy infusion codes during the second encounter that were also furnished in the first encounter. The OCE identifies modifier 59 and pays up to a maximum number of units per day, as listed in Table 1.

EXAMPLE 1

A beneficiary receives infused drugs that are not anti-neoplastic drugs (including hydrating solutions) for 2 hours. The hospital reports one unit of HCPCS code C8950 and one unit of HCPCS code C8951. The OCE will pay one unit of APC 0120. Payment for the unit of HCPCS code C8951 is packaged into the payment for one unit of APC 0120. (NOTE: See 230.1 for drug billing instructions.)

EXAMPLE 2

A beneficiary receives infused drugs that are not anti-neoplastic drugs (including hydrating solutions) for 12 hours. The hospital reports one unit of HCPCS code C8950 and eleven units of HCPCS code C8951. The OCE will pay one unit of APC 0120. Payment for the 11 units of HCPCS code C8951 is packaged into the payment for one unit of APC 0120. (NOTE: See 230.1 for drug billing instructions.)

EXAMPLE 3

A beneficiary experiences multiple attempts to initiate an intravenous infusion before a successful infusion is started 20 minutes after the first attempt. Once started, the infusion lasts one hour. The hospital reports one unit of HCPCS code C8950 to identify the 1 hour of infusion time. The 20 minutes spent prior to the infusion attempting to establish an IV line are not separately billable in the OPPS. The OCE pays one unit of APC 0120. (NOTE: See 230.1 for drug billing instructions.)

B. Administration of Non-Chemotherapy Drugs by a Route Other Than Intravenous Infusion

Table 6: CY 2006 OPPS Non-Chemotherapy Drug Administration -Route Other Than Intravenous Infusion

2005 CPT	Final CY 2006 OPPS	2005 CPT	2005 Description	Code	Description	SI	APC
90784	Therapeutic, prophylactic or diagnostic injection (specify material injected); intravenous	C8952	Therapeutic, prophylactic or diagnostic injection; intravenous push	X	0359		
90782	Therapeutic, prophylactic or diagnostic injection (specify material injected); subcutaneous or intramuscular	90772	Therapeutic, prophylactic or diagnostic injection (specify substance or drug); subcutaneous or intramuscular	X	0353		
90783	Therapeutic, prophylactic or diagnostic injection (specify material injected); intra-arterial	90773	Therapeutic, prophylactic or diagnostic injection (specify substance or drug); intra-arterial	X	0359		
90779	Unlisted therapeutic, prophylactic or diagnostic intravenous or intra-arterial, injection or infusion	90779	Unlisted therapeutic, prophylactic or diagnostic intravenous or intra-arterial injection or infusion	X	0352		

100-4, 4, 231.4

Billing for Split Unit of Blood

HCPCS code P9011 was created to identify situations where one unit of blood or a blood product is split and some portion of the unit is transfused to one patient and the other portions are transfused to other patients or to the same patient at other times. When a patient receives a transfusion of a split unit of blood or blood product, OPPS providers should bill P9011 for the blood product transfused, as well as CPT 86985 (Splitting, blood products) for each splitting procedure performed to prepare the blood product for a specific patient.

Providers should bill split units of packed red cells and whole blood using Revenue Code 389 (Other blood), and should not use Revenue Codes 381 (Packed red cells) or 382 (Whole blood). Providers should bill split units of other blood products using the applicable revenue codes for the blood product type, such as 383 (Plasma) or 384 (Platelets), rather than 389. Reporting revenue codes according to these specifications will ensure the Medicare beneficiary's blood deductible is applied correctly.

EXAMPLE: OPPS provider splits off a 100cc aliquot from a 250 cc unit of leukocytereduced red blood cells for a transfusion to Patient X. The hospital then splits off an 80cc aliquot of the remaining unit for a transfusion to Patient Y. At a later time, the remaining 70cc from the unit is transfused to Patient Z.

In billing for the services for Patient X and Patient Y, the OPPS provider should report the charges by billing P9011 and 86985 in addition to the CPT code for the transfusion service, because a specific splitting service was required to prepare a split unit for transfusion to each of those patients. However, the OPPS provider should report only P9011 and the CPT code for the transfusion service for Patient Z because no additional splitting was necessary to prepare the split

unit for transfusion to Patient Z. The OPPS provider should bill Revenue Code 0389 for each split unit of the leukocyte-reduced red blood cells that was transfused.

100-4, 4, 240

Inpatient Part B Hospital Services

Inpatient Part B services which are paid under OPPS include:

- Diagnostic x-ray tests, and other diagnostic tests (excluding clinical diagnostic laboratory tests); X-ray, radium, and radioactive isotope therapy, including materials and services of technicians;

- Surgical dressings applied during an encounter at the hospital and splints, casts, and other devices used for reduction of fractures and dislocations (splints and casts, etc., include dental splints);

- Implantable prosthetic devices;

- Hepatitis B vaccine and its administration, and certain preventive screening services (pelvic exams, screening sigmoidoscopies, screening colonoscopies, bone mass measurements, and prostate screening.)

- Bone Mass measurements;

- Prostate screening;

- Immunosuppressive drugs;

- Oral anti-cancer drugs;

- Oral drug prescribed for use as an acute anti-emetic used as part of an anti-cancer chemotherapeutic regimen; and

- Epoetin Alfa (EPO)

When a hospital that is not paid under the OPPS furnishes an implantable prosthetic device that meets the criteria for coverage in Medicare Benefits Policy Manual, Pub.100-02, Chapter 6, Sec.10 to an inpatient who has coverage under Part B, payment for the implantable prosthetic device is made under the payment mechanism that applies to other hospital outpatient services (e.g. reasonable cost, all inclusive rate, waiver).

When a hospital that is paid under the OPPS furnishes an implantable prosthetic device to an inpatient who has coverage under Part B, but who does not have coverage of inpatient services on the date that the implanted prosthetic device is furnished, the hospital should report new HCPCS code, C9899, Implanted Prosthetic Device, Payable Only for Inpatients who do not Have Inpatient Coverage, that will be effective for services furnished on or after January 1, 2009. This code may be reported only on claims with TOB 12X when the prosthetic device is implanted on a day on which the beneficiary does not have coverage of the hospital inpatient services he or she is receiving. The line containing this new code will be rejected if it is reported on a claim that is not a TOB 12X or if it is reported with a line item date of service on which the beneficiary has coverage of inpatient hospital services. By reporting C9899, the hospital is reporting that all of the criteria for payment under Part B are met as specified in the

Medicare Benefits Policy Manual, Pub.100-02, Chapter 6, Sec.10, and that the item meets all Medicare criteria for coverage as an implantable prosthetic device as defined in that section.

Medicare contractors shall first determine that the item furnished meets the Medicare criteria for coverage as an implantable prosthetic device as specified in the *Medicare Benefits Policy Manual*, Pub. 100-02, Chapter 6, Sec.10. If the item does not meet the criteria for coverage as an implantable prosthetic device, the contractor shall deny payment on the basis that the item is outside the scope of the benefits for which there is coverage for Part B inpatients. The beneficiary is liable for the charges for the noncovered item when the item does not meet the criteria for coverage as an implanted prosthetic device as specified in the *Medicare Benefits Policy Manual*, Pub.100-02, Chapter 6, Sec.10.

If the contractor determines that the device is covered, the contractor shall determine if the device has pass through status under the OPPS. If so, the contractor shall establish the payment amount for the device at the product of the charge for the device and the hospital specific cost to charge ratio. Where the device does not have pass through status under the OPPS, the contractor shall establish the payment amount for the device at the amount for a comparable device in the DMEPOS fee schedule where there is such an amount. Payment under the DMEPOS fee schedule is made at the lesser of charges or the fee schedule amount and therefore if there is a fee for the specific item on the DMEPOS fee schedule, the payment amount for the item will be set at the lesser of the actual charges or the DMEPOS fee schedule amount. Where the item does not have pass through payment status and where there is no amount for a comparable device in the DMEPOS fee schedule, the contractor shall establish a payment amount that is specific to the particular implanted prosthetic device for the applicable calendar year. This amount (less applicable unpaid deductible and coinsurance) will be paid for that specific device for services furnished in the applicable calendar year unless the actual charge for the item is less than the established amount).

Where the actual charge is less than the established amount, the contractor will pay the actual charge for the item (less applicable unpaid deductible and coinsurance).

In setting a contractor established payment rate for the specific device, the contractor takes into account the cost information available at the time the payment rate is established. This information may include, but is not limited to, the amount of device cost that would be removed from an applicable APC payment for implantation of the device if the provider received a device without cost or a full credit for the cost of the device.

If the contractor chooses to use this amount, see www.cms.hhs.gov/HospitalOutpatientPPS/ for the amount of reduction to the APC payment that would apply in these cases. From the OPPS webpage, select "Device, Radiolabeled Product, and Procedure Edits" from the list on the left side of the page. Open the file "Procedure to Device edits" to determine the HCPCS code that best describes the procedure in which the device would be used. Then identify the APC to which that procedure code maps from the most recent Addenda B on the OPPS webpage and open the file "FB/FC Modifier Procedures and Devices". Select the applicable year's file of APCs subject to full and partial credit reductions (for example: CY 2008 APCs Subject to Full and Partial Credit Reduction Policy"). Select the "Full offset reduction amount" that pertains to the APC that is most applicable to the device described by C9899. It would be reasonable to set this amount as a payment for a device furnished to a Part B inpatient.

For example, if C9899 is reporting insertion of a single chamber pacemaker (C1786 or equivalent narrative description on the claim in "remarks") the file of procedure to device edits shows that a single chamber pacemaker is the dominant device for APC 0090 (APC 0089 is for insertion of both pacemaker and electrodes and therefore would not apply if electrodes are not also billed). The table of offset reduction amounts for CY 2008 shows that the estimated cost of a single chamber pacemaker for APC 0090 is $4881.77. It would therefore be reasonable for the contractor/MAC to set the payment rate for a single chamber pacemaker furnished to a Part B inpatient to $4881.77. In this case the coinsurance would be $936.75 (20 percent of $4881.77, which is less than the inpatient deductible).

The beneficiary coinsurance is 20 percent of the payment amount for the device (i.e. the pass through payment amount, the DMEPOS fee schedule amount, the contractor established amount, or the actual charge if less than the DMEPOS fee schedule amount or the contractor established amount for the specific device), not to exceed the Medicare inpatient deductible that is applicable to the year in which the implanted prosthetic device is furnished.

Inpatient Part B services paid under other payment methods include:

- Clinical diagnostic laboratory tests, prosthetic devices other than implantable ones and other than dental which replace all or part of an internal body organ (including contiguous tissue), or all or part of the function of a permanently inoperative or malfunctioning internal body organ, including replacement or repairs of such devices;

- Leg, arm, back and neck braces; trusses and artificial legs; arms and eyes including adjustments, repairs, and replacements required because of breakage, wear, loss, or a change in the patient's physical condition; take home surgical dressings; outpatient physical therapy; outpatient occupational therapy; and outpatient speech-language pathology services;

- Ambulance services;

- Screening pap smears, screening colorectal tests, and screening mammography;

- Influenza virus vaccine and its administration, pneumococcal vaccine and its administration;

- Diabetes self-management training;

- Hemophilia clotting factors for hemophilia patients competent to use these factors without supervision).

See Chapter 6 of the Medicare Benefit Policy Manual for a discussion of the circumstances under which the above services may be covered as Part B Inpatient services.

100-4, 4, 290.1

Observation Services Overview

Observation care is a well-defined set of specific, clinically appropriate services, which include ongoing short term treatment, assessment, and reassessment, that are furnished while a decision is being made regarding whether patients will require further treatment as hospital inpatients or if they are able to be discharged from the hospital. Observation status is commonly assigned to patients who present to the emergency department and who then require a significant period of treatment or monitoring in order to make a decision concerning their admission or discharge. Observation services are covered only when provided by the order of a physician or another individual authorized by State licensure law and hospital staff bylaws to admit patients to the hospital or to order outpatient services.

Observation services must also be reasonable and necessary to be covered by Medicare. In only rare and exceptional cases do reasonable and necessary outpatient observation services span more than 48 hours. In the majority of cases, the decision whether to discharge a patient from the hospital following resolution of the reason for the observation care or to admit the patient as an inpatient can be made in less than 48 hours, usually in less than 24 hours.

100-4, 4, 290.2.2

Reporting Hours of Observation

Observation time begins at the clock time documented in the patient's medical record, which coincides with the time the patient is placed in a bed for the purpose of initiating observation care in accordance with a physician's order. Hospitals should round to the nearest hour. For example, a patient who was placed in an observation bed at 3:03 p.m. according to the nurses' notes and discharged to home at 9:45 p.m. should have a "7" placed in the units field of the reported observation HCPCS code.

General standing orders for observation services following all outpatient surgery are not recognized. Hospitals should not report as observation care, services that are part of another Part B service, such as postoperative monitoring during a standard recovery period (e.g., 4-6 hours), which should be billed as recovery room services. Similarly, in the case of patients who undergo diagnostic testing in a hospital outpatient department, routine preparation services furnished prior to the testing and recovery afterwards are included in the payments for those diagnostic services. Observation services should not be billed concurrently with diagnostic or therapeutic services for which active monitoring is a part of the procedure (e.g., colonoscopy, chemotherapy). In situations where such a procedure interrupts observation services, hospitals would record for each period of observation services the beginning and ending times during the hospital outpatient encounter and add the length of time for the periods of observation services together to reach the total number of units reported on the claim for the hourly observation services HCPCS code G0378 (Hospital observation service, per hour).

Observation time ends when all medically necessary services related to observation care are completed. For example, this could be before discharge when the need for observation has ended, but other medically necessary services not meeting the definition of observation care are provided (in which case, the additional medically necessary services would be billed separately or included as part of the emergency department or clinic visit). Alternatively, the end time of observation services may coincide with the time the patient is actually discharged from the hospital or admitted as an inpatient.

Observation time may include medically necessary services and follow-up care provided after the time that the physician writes the discharge order, but before the patient is discharged. However, reported observation time would not include the time patients remain in the observation area after treatment is finished for reasons such as waiting for transportation home.

If a period of observation spans more than 1 calendar day, all of the hours for the entire period of observation must be included on a single line and the date of service for that line is the date that observation care begins.

100-4, 4, 290.4.1

Billing and Payment for All Hospital Observation Services Furnished Between January 1, 2006 and December 31, 2007

Since January 1, 2006, two G-codes have been used to report observation services and direct referral for observation care. For claims for dates of service January 1, 2006 through December 31, 2007, the Integrated Outpatient Code Editor (I/OCE) determines whether the observation care or direct referral services are packaged or separately payable. Thus, hospitals provide consistent coding and billing under all circumstances in which they deliver observation care.

Beginning January 1, 2006, hospitals should not report CPT codes 99217-99220 or 99234-99236 for observation services. In addition, the following HCPCS codes were discontinued as of January 1, 2006: G0244 (Observation care by facility to patient), G0263 (Direct Admission with congestive heart failure, chest pain or asthma), and G0264 (Assessment other than congestive heart failure, chest pain, or asthma).

The three discontinued G-codes and the CPT codes that were no longer recognized were replaced by two new G-codes to be used by hospitals to report all observation services, whether separately payable or packaged, and direct referral for observation care, whether separately payable or packaged:

G0378- Hospital observation service, per hour; and

G0379- Direct admission of patient for hospital observation care.

The I/OCE determines whether observation services billed as units of G0378 are separately payable under APC 0339 (Observation) or whether payment for observation services will be packaged into the payment for other services provided by the hospital in the same encounter. Therefore, hospitals should bill HCPCS code G0378 when observation services are ordered and provided to any patient regardless of the patient's condition. The units of service should equal the number of hours the patient receives observation services.

Hospitals should report G0379 when observation services are the result of a direct referral for observation care without an associated emergency room visit, hospital outpatient clinic visit, critical care service, or hospital outpatient surgical procedure (status indicator T procedure) on the day of initiation of observation services. Hospitals should only report HCPCS code G0379 when a patient is referred directly for observation care after being seen by a physician in the community (see Sec.290.4.2 below)

Some non-repetitive OPPS services provided on the same day by a hospital may be billed on different claims, provided that all charges associated with each procedure or service being reported are billed on the same claim with the HCPCS code which describes that service. See chapter 1, section 50.2.2 of this manual. It is vitally important that all of the charges that pertain to a non-repetitive, separately paid procedure or service be reported on the same claim with that procedure or service. It should also be emphasized that this relaxation of same day billing requirements for some non-repetitive services does not apply to non-repetitive services provided on the same day as either direct referral to observation care or observation services because the OCE claim-by-claim logic cannot function properly unless all services related to the episode of observation care, including diagnostic tests, lab services, hospital clinic visits, emergency department visits, critical care services, and status indicator T procedures, are reported on the same claim. Additional guidance can be found in chapter 1, section 50.2.2 of this manual.

100-4, 4, 290.4.2

Separate and Packaged Payment for Direct Admission to Observation
In order to receive separate payment for a direct referral for observation care (APC 0604), the claim must show:

1. Both HCPCS codes G0378 (Hourly Observation) and G0379 (Direct Admit to Observation) with the same date of service;

2. That no services with a status indicator T or V or Critical care (APC 0617) were provided on the same day of service as HCPCS code G0379; and

3. The observation care does not qualify for separate payment under APC 0339.

Only a direct referral for observation services billed on a 13X bill type may be considered for a separate APC payment.

Separate payment is not allowed for HCPCS code G0379, direct admission to observation care, when billed with the same date of service as a hospital clinic visit, emergency room visit, critical care service, or "T" status procedure.

If a bill for the direct referral for observation services does not meet the three requirements listed above, then payment for the direct referral service will be packaged into payments for other separately payable services provided to the beneficiary in the same encounter.

100-4, 4, 290.4.3

Separate and Packaged Payment for Observation Services Furnished Between January 1, 2006 and December 31, 2007
Separate payment may be made for observation services provided to a patient with congestive heart failure, chest pain, or asthma. The list of ICD-9-CM diagnosis codes eligible for separate payment is reviewed annually. Any changes in applicable ICD-9-CM diagnosis codes are included in the October quarterly update of the OPPS and also published in the annual OPPS Final Rule. The list of qualifying ICD-9-CM diagnosis codes is also published on the OPPS Web page.

All of the following requirements must be met in order for a hospital to receive a separate APC payment for observation services through APC 0339:

1. Diagnosis Requirements

   a. The beneficiary must have one of three medical conditions: congestive heart failure, chest pain, or asthma.

   b. Qualifying ICD-9-CM diagnosis codes must be reported in Form Locator (FL) 76, Patient Reason for Visit, or FL 67, principal diagnosis, or both in order for the hospital to receive separate payment for APC 0339. If a qualifying ICD-9-CM diagnosis code(s) is reported in the secondary diagnosis field, but is not reported in either the Patient Reason for Visit field (FL 76) or in the principal diagnosis field (FL 67), separate payment for APC 0339 is not allowed.

2. Observation Time

   a. Observation time must be documented in the medical record.

   b. Hospital billing for observation services begins at the clock time documented in the patient's medical record, which coincides with the time that observation services are initiated in accordance with a physician's order for observation services.

   c. A beneficiary's time receiving observation services (and hospital billing) ends when all clinical or medical interventions have been completed, including follow-up care furnished

by hospital staff and physicians that may take place after a physician has ordered the patient be released or admitted as an inpatient.

   d. The number of units reported with HCPCS code G0378 must equal or exceed 8 hours.

3. Additional Hospital Services

   a. The claim for observation services must include one of the following services in addition to the reported observation services. The additional services listed below must have a line item date of service on the same day or the day before the date reported for observation:

      An emergency department visit (APC 0609, 0613, 0614, 0615, 0616) or

      A clinic visit (APC 0604, 0605, 0606, 0607, 0608); or

      Critical care (APC 0617); or

      Direct referral for observation care reported with HCPCS code G0379 (APC 0604); must be reported on the same date of service as the date reported for observation services.

   b. No procedure with a T status indicator can be reported on the same day or day before observation care is provided.

4. Physician Evaluation

   a. The beneficiary must be in the care of a physician during the period of observation, as documented in the medical record by outpatient registration, discharge, and other appropriate progress notes that are timed, written, and signed by the physician.

   b. The medical record must include documentation that the physician explicitly assessed patient risk to determine that the beneficiary would benefit from observation care.

Only observation services that are billed on a 13X bill type may be considered for a separate APC payment.

Hospitals should bill all of the other services associated with the observation care, including direct referral for observation, hospital clinic visits, emergency room visits, critical care services, and T status procedures, on the same claim so that the claims processing logic may appropriately determine the payment status (either packaged or separately payable) of HCPCS codes G0378 and G0379.

If a bill for observation care does not meet all of the requirements listed above, then payment for the observation care will be packaged into payments for other separately payable services provided to the beneficiary in the same encounter.

100-4, 4, 290.5.1

Billing and Payment for Observation Services Beginning January 1, 2008
Observation services are reported using HCPCS code G0378 (Hospital observation service, per hour). Beginning January 1, 2008, HCPCS code G0378 for hourly observation services is assigned status indicator N, signifying that its payment is always packaged. No separate payment is made for observation services reported with HCPCS code G0378, and APC 0339 is deleted as of January 1, 2008. In most circumstances, observation services are supportive and ancillary to the other services provided to a patient. In certain circumstances when observation care is billed in conjunction with a high level clinic visit (Level 5), high level Type A emergency department visit (Level 4 or 5), high level Type B emergency department visit (Level 5), critical care services, or a direct referral as an integral part of a patient's extended encounter of care, payment may be made for the entire extended care encounter through one of two composite APCs when certain criteria are met. For information about payment for extended assessment and management composite APCs, see Sec.10.2.1 (Composite APCs) of this chapter.

APC 8002 (Level I Extended Assessment and Management Composite) describes an encounter for care provided to a patient that includes a high level (Level 5) clinic visit or direct referral for observation in conjunction with observation services of substantial duration (8 or more hours). APC 8003 (Level II Extended Assessment and Management Composite) describes an encounter for care provided to a patient that includes a high level (Level 4 or 5) emergency department visit or critical care services in conjunction with observation services of substantial duration. Beginning January 1, 2009, APC 8003 also includes high level (Level 5) Type B emergency department visits. There is no limitation on diagnosis for payment of these composite APCs; however, composite APC payment will not be made when observation services are reported in association with a surgical procedure (T status procedure) or the hours of observation care reported are less than 8. The I/OCE evaluates every claim received to determine if payment through a composite APC is appropriate. If payment through a composite APC is inappropriate, the I/OCE, in conjunction with the Pricer, determines the appropriate status indicator, APC, and payment for every code on a claim.

All of the following requirements must be met in order for a hospital to receive an APC payment for an extended assessment and management composite APC:

1. Observation Time

a. Observation time must be documented in the medical record.

b. Hospital billing for observation services begins at the clock time documented in the patient's medical record, which coincides with the time that observation services are initiated in accordance with a physician's order for observation services.

c. A beneficiary's time receiving observation services (and hospital billing) ends when all clinical or medical interventions have been completed, including follow-up care furnished by hospital staff and physicians that may take place after a physician has ordered the patient be released or admitted as an inpatient.

d. The number of units reported with HCPCS code G0378 must equal or exceed 8 hours.

2. Additional Hospital Services

a. The claim for observation services must include one of the following services in addition to the reported observation services. The additional services listed below must have a line item date of service on the same day or the day before the date reported for observation:

A Type A or B emergency department visit (CPT codes 99284 or 99285 or HCPCS code G0384); or

A clinic visit (CPT code 99205 or 99215); or

Critical care (CPT code 99291); or

Direct referral for observation care reported with HCPCS code G0379 (APC 0604) must be reported on the same date of service as the date reported for observation services.

b. No procedure with a T status indicator can be reported on the same day or day before observation care is provided.

3. Physician Evaluation

a. The beneficiary must be in the care of a physician during the period of observation, as documented in the medical record by outpatient registration, discharge, and other appropriate progress notes that are timed, written, and signed by the physician.

b. The medical record must include documentation that the physician explicitly assessed patient risk to determine that the beneficiary would benefit from observation care.

Criteria 1 and 3 related to observation care beginning and ending time and physician evaluation apply regardless of whether the hospital believes that the criteria will be met for payment of the extended encounter through extended assessment and management composite payment.

Only visits, critical care and observation services that are billed on a 13X bill type may be considered for a composite APC payment.

Non-repetitive services provided on the same day as either direct referral for observation care or observation services must be reported on the same claim because the OCE claim-by-claim logic cannot function properly unless all services related to the episode of observation care, including hospital clinic visits, emergency department visits, critical care services, and T status procedures, are reported on the same claim. Additional guidance can be found in chapter 1, section 50.2.2 of this manual.

If a claim for services provided during an extended assessment and management encounter including observation care does not meet all of the requirements listed above, then the usual APC logic will apply to separately payable items and services on the claim; the special logic for direct admission will apply, and payment for the observation care will be packaged into payments for other separately payable services provided to the beneficiary in the same encounter.

100-4, 4, 290.5.2

Billing and Payment for Direct Referral for Observation Care Furnished Beginning January 1, 2008

Direct referral for observation care continues to be reported using HCPCS code G0379 (Direct admission of patient for hospital observation care). Hospitals should report G0379 when observation services are the result of a direct referral for observation care without an associated emergency room visit, hospital outpatient clinic visit, or critical care service on the day of initiation of observation services. Hospitals should only report HCPCS code G0379 when a patient is referred directly to observation care after being seen by a physician in the community.

Payment for direct referral for observation care will be made either separately as a low level hospital clinic visit under APC 0604 or packaged into payment for composite APC 8002 (Level I Prolonged Assessment and Management Composite) or packaged into the payment for other separately payable services provided in the same encounter. For information about payment for extended assessment and management composite APCs, see, Sec.10.2.1 (Composite APCs) of this chapter.

The criteria for payment of HCPCS code G0379 under either APC 0604 or APC 8002 include:

1. Both HCPCS codes G0378 (Hospital observation services, per hr) and G0379 (Direct admission of patient for hospital observation care) are reported with the same date of service.

2. No service with a status indicator of T or V or Critical Care (APC 0617) is provided on the same day of service as HCPCS code G0379.

If either of the above criteria is not met, HCPCS code G0379 will be assigned status indicator N and will be packaged into payment for other separately payable services provided in the same encounter.

Only a direct referral for observation services billed on a 13X bill type may be considered for a composite APC payment.

100-4, 4, 300.6

Common Working File (CWF) Edits

The CWF edit will allow 3 hours of therapy for MNT in the initial calendar year. The edit will allow more than 3 hours of therapy if there is a change in the beneficiary's medical condition, diagnosis, or treatment regimen and this change must be documented in the beneficiary's medical record. Two new G codes have been created for use when a beneficiary receives a second referral in a calendar year that allows the beneficiary to receive more than 3 hours of therapy. Another edit will allow 2 hours of follow up MNT with another referral in subsequent years.

Advance Beneficiary Notice (ABN)

The beneficiary is liable for services denied over the limited number of hours with referrals for MNT. An ABN should be issued in these situations. In absence of evidence of a valid ABN, the provider will be held liable.

An ABN should not be issued for Medicare-covered services such as those provided by hospital dietitians or nutrition professionals who are qualified to render the service in their state but who have not obtained Medicare provider numbers.

Duplicate Edits

Although beneficiaries are allowed to receive training and therapy during the same time period Diabetes Self-Management and Training (DSMT) and Medical Nutrition Therapy (MNT) services may not be provided on the same day to the same beneficiary. Effective April 1, 2010 CWF shall implement a new duplicate crossover edit to identify and prevent claims for DSMT/MNT services from being billed with the same dates of services for the same beneficiaries submitted from institutional providers and from a professional provider.

100-4, 4, 320

Outpatient Intravenous Insulin Treatment (OIVIT)

Effective for claims with dates of service on and after December 23, 2009, the Centers for Medicare and Medicaid Services (CMS) determines that the evidence is adequate to conclude that OIVIT does not improve health outcomes in Medicare beneficiaries. Therefore, CMS determines that OIVIT is not reasonable and necessary for any indication under section 1862(a)(1)(A) of the Social Security Act, and services comprising an OIVIT regimen are nationally non-covered.

See Pub. 100-03, *Medicare National Coverage Determinations Manual*, Section 40.7, Outpatient Intravenous Insulin Treatment (Effective December 23, 2009), for general information and coverage indications.

100-4, 4, 320.1

HCPCS Coding for OIVIT

HCPCS code G9147, effective with the April IOCE and MPFSDB updates, is to be used on claims with dates of service on and after December 23, 2009, billing for non-covered OIVIT and any services comprising an OIVIT regimen.

NOTE: HCPCS codes 99199 or 94681(with or without diabetes related conditions 250.00-250.93) are not to be used on claims billing for non-covered OIVIT and any services comprising an OIVIT regimen when furnished pursuant to an OIVIT regimen. Claims billing for HCPCS codes 99199 and 94681 for non-covered OIVIT are to be returned to provider/returned as unprocessable.

100-4, 4, 320.2

Outpatient Intravenous Insulin Treatment (OIVIT)

Effective for claims with dates of service on and after December 23, 2009, the Centers for Medicare and Medicaid Services (CMS) determines that the evidence does not support a conclusion that OIVIT improves health outcomes in Medicare beneficiaries. Therefore, CMS has determined that OIVIT is not reasonable and necessary for any indication under section 1862(a)(1)(A) of the Social Security Act. Services comprising an OIVIT regimen are nationally non-covered under Medicare when furnished pursuant to an OIVIT regimen.

See Pub. 100-03, Medicare National Coverage Determinations Manual, Section 40.7, Outpatient Intravenous Insulin Treatment (Effective December 23, 2009), for general information and coverage indications.

100-4, 5, 10.2

A. Financial Limitation Prior to the Balanced Budget Refinement Act (BBRA)

Section 4541(a)(2) of the Balanced Budget Act (BBA) (P.L. 105-33) of 1997, which added ¬81834(k)(5) to the Act, required payment under a prospective payment system for outpatient rehabilitation services (except those furnished by or under arrangements with a hospital). Outpatient rehabilitation services include the following services:

- Physical therapy (which includes outpatient speech-language pathology); and

- Occupational therapy.

Section 4541(c) of the BBA required application of a financial limitation to all outpatient rehabilitation services (except those furnished by or under arrangements with a hospital). In 1999, an annual per beneficiary limit of $1,500 applied to all outpatient physical therapy services (including speech-language pathology services). A separate limit applied to all occupational therapy services. The limit is based on incurred expenses and includes applicable deductible and coinsurance. The BBA provided that the limits be indexed by the Medicare Economic Index (MEI) each year beginning in 2002.

The limitation is based on therapy services the Medicare beneficiary receives, not the type of practitioner who provides the service. Physical therapists, speech-language pathologists, occupational therapists as well as physicians and certain nonphysician practitioners could render a therapy service.

As a transitional measure, effective in 1999, providers/suppliers were instructed to keep track of the allowed incurred expenses. This process was put in place to assure providers/suppliers did not bill Medicare for patients who exceeded the annual limitations for physical therapy, and for occupational therapy services rendered by individual providers/suppliers. In 2003 and later, the limitation was applied through CMS systems.

B. Moratoria and Exceptions for Therapy Claims

Section 221 of the BBRA of 1999 placed a 2-year moratorium on the application of the financial limitation for claims for therapy services with dates of service January 1, 2000, through December 31, 2001.

Section 421 of the Medicare, Medicaid, and SCHIP Benefits Improvement and Protection Act (BIPA) of 2000, extended the moratorium on application of the financial limitation to claims for outpatient rehabilitation services with dates of service January 1, 2002, through December 31, 2002. Therefore, the moratorium was for a 3-year period and applied to outpatient rehabilitation claims with dates of service January 1, 2000, through December 31, 2002.

In 2003, there was not a moratorium on therapy caps. Implementation was delayed until September 1, 2003. Therapy caps were in effect for services rendered on September 1, 2003 through December 7, 2003.

Congress re-enacted a moratorium on financial limitations on outpatient therapy services on December 8, 2003 that extended through December 31, 2005. Caps were implemented again on January 1, 2006 and policies were modified to allow exceptions as directed by the Deficit Reduction Act of 2005 only for calendar year 2006. The Tax Relief and Health Care Act of 2006 extended the cap exceptions process through calendar year 2007. The Medicare, Medicaid, and SCHIP Extension Act of 2007 extended the cap exceptions process for services furnished through June 30, 2008.

Future exceptions. The cap exception for therapy services billed by outpatient hospitals was part of the original legislation and applies as long as caps are in effect. Exceptions to caps based on the medical necessity of the service are in effect only when Congress legislates the exceptions, as they did for 2007. References to the exceptions process in subsection C of this section apply only when the exceptions are in effect.

C. Application of Financial Limitations

Financial limitations on outpatient therapy services, as described above, began for therapy services rendered on or after on January 1, 2006. See C 1 to C 7 of this section when exceptions to therapy caps apply. The limits were $1740 in 2006 and $1780 in 2007. For 2008, the annual limit on the allowed amount for outpatient physical therapy and speech-language pathology combined is $1810; the limit for occupational therapy is $1810. Limits apply to outpatient Part B therapy services from all settings except outpatient hospital (place of service code 22 on carrier claims) and hospital emergency room (place of service code 23 on carrier claims). These excluded hospital services are reported on types of bill 12x or 13x on intermediary claims.

Contractors apply the financial limitations to the Medicare Physician Fee Schedule (MPFS) amount (or the amount charged if it is smaller) for therapy services for each beneficiary.

As with any Medicare payment, beneficiaries pay the coinsurance (20 percent) and any deductible that may apply. Medicare will pay the remaining 80 percent of the limit after the deductible is met. These amounts will change each calendar year. Medicare Contractors shall publish the financial limitation amount in educational articles. It is also available at 1-800-Medicare.

Medicare shall apply these financial limitations in order, according to the dates when the claims were received. When limitations apply, the Common Working File (CWF) tracks the limits. Shared System Maintainers are not responsible for tracking the dollar amounts of incurred expenses of rehabilitation services for each therapy limit.

In processing claims where Medicare is the secondary payer, the shared system takes the lowest secondary payment amount from MSPPAY and sends this amount on to CWF as the amount applied to therapy limits.

1. Exceptions to Therapy Caps - General
   The Tax Relief and Health Care Act of 2006 directed CMS to extend a process to allow for exceptions to the caps for services received in CY2007 in cases where continued therapy services are medically necessary. The following policies concerning exceptions to caps due to medical necessity apply only when the exceptions process is in effect. With the exception of the use of the KX modifier, the guidance in this section concerning medical necessity applies as well to services provided before caps are reached.

   Instructions for contractors to manage automatic process for exceptions will be found in the Program Integrity Manual, chapter 3, section 3.4.1.2. Provider and supplier information concerning exceptions is in this manual and in IOM Pub. 100-02, chapter 15, section 220.3. Exceptions shall be identified by a modifier on the claim and supported by documentation.

   Since the providers and suppliers will take an active role in obtaining an exception for a beneficiary, this manual section is written to address them as well as Medicare contractors.

   The beneficiary may qualify for use of the cap exceptions at any time during the episode when documented medically necessary services exceed caps. All covered and medically necessary services qualify for exceptions to caps.

   In 2006, the Exception Processes fell into two categories, Automatic Process Exceptions, and Manual Process Exceptions. Beginning January 1, 2007, there is no manual process for exceptions. All services that require exceptions to caps shall be processed using the automatic process. All requests for exception are in the form of a KX modifier added to claim lines. (See subsection C6 for use of the KX modifier.)

   Use of the automatic process for exceptions increases the responsibility of the provider/supplier for determining and documenting that services are appropriate.

   Also, use of the automatic process for exception does not exempt services from manual or other medical review processes as described in 100-08, Chapter 3, Section 3.4.1.1.1. Rather, atypical use of the automatic exception process may invite contractor scrutiny. Particular care should be taken to document improvement and avoid billing for services that do not meet the requirements for skilled services, or for services which are maintenance rather than rehabilitative treatment (See Pub. 100-02, chapter 15, sections 220.2, 220.3, and 230).

   The KX modifier, described in subsection C6, is added to claim lines to indicate that the clinician attests that services are medically necessary and justification is documented in the medical record.

2. Automatic Process Exceptions
   The term "automatic process exceptions" indicates that the claims processing for the exception is automatic, and not that the exception is automatic. An exception may be made when the patient's condition is justified by documentation indicating that the beneficiary requires continued skilled therapy, i.e., therapy beyond the amount payable under the therapy cap, to achieve their prior functional status or maximum expected functional status within a reasonable amount of time.

   No special documentation is submitted to the contractor for automatic process exceptions. The clinician is responsible for consulting guidance in the Medicare manuals and in the professional literature to determine if the beneficiary may qualify for the automatic process exception when documentation justifies medically necessary services above the caps. The clinician's opinion is not binding on the Medicare contractor who makes the final determination concerning whether the claim is payable.

   Documentation justifying the services shall be submitted in response to any Additional Documentation Request (ADR) for claims that are selected for medical review. Follow the documentation requirements in Pub. 100-02, chapter 15, section 220.3. If medical records are requested for review, clinicians may include, at their discretion, a summary that specifically addresses the justification for therapy cap exception.

   In making a decision about whether to utilize the automatic process exception, clinicians shall consider, for example, whether services are appropriate to--

   - The patient's condition including the diagnosis, complexities and severity (A list of the excepted evaluation codes are in C.2.a. A list of the ICD-9 codes for conditions and complexities that might qualify a beneficiary for exception to caps is in 10.2 C3. The list is a guideline and neither assures that services on the list will be excepted nor limits provision of covered and medically necessary services for conditions not on the list);

- The services provided including their type, frequency and duration;

- The interaction of current active conditions and complexities that directly and significantly influence the treatment such that it causes services to exceed caps.

In addition, the following should be considered before using the automatic exception process:

a. Exceptions for Services

Evaluation. The CMS will except therapy evaluations from caps after the therapy caps are reached when evaluation is necessary, e.g., to determine if the current status of the beneficiary requires therapy services. For example, the following evaluation procedures may be appropriate:

92506, 92597, 92607, 92608, 92610, 92611, 92612, 92614, 92616, 96105, 97001, 97002, 97003, 97004.

These codes will continue to be reported as outpatient therapy procedures as described in the Claims Processing Manual, Chapter 5, Section 20(B) "Applicable Outpatient Rehabilitation HCPCS Codes." They are not diagnostic tests. Definition of evaluations and documentation is found in Pub 100-02, sections 220 and 230.

Other Services. There are a number of sources that suggest the amount of certain services that may be typical, either per service, per episode, per condition, or per discipline. For example, see the CSC- Utilization and Edit Report, 2006, Appendices at www.cms.hhs.gov/TherapyServices (Studies and Reports). Professional literature and guidelines from professional associations also provide a basis on which to estimate whether the type, frequency and intensity of services are appropriate to an individual. Clinicians and contractors should utilize available evidence related to the patient's condition to justify provision of medically necessary services to individual beneficiaries, especially when they exceed caps. Contractors shall not limit medically necessary services that are justified by scientific research applicable to the beneficiary. Neither contractors nor clinicians shall utilize professional literature and scientific reports to justify payment for continued services after an individual's goals have been met earlier than is typical. Conversely, professional literature and scientific reports shall not be used as justification to deny payment to patients whose needs are greater than is typical or when the patient's condition is not represented by the literature.

b. Exceptions for Conditions or Complexities Identified by ICD-9 codes.

Clinicians may utilize the automatic process for exception for any diagnosis for which they can justify services exceeding the cap. Based upon analysis of claims data, research and evidence based practice guidelines, CMS has identified conditions and complexities represented by ICD-9 codes that may be more likely than others to require therapy services that exceed therapy caps. This list appears in 10.2 C3. Clinicians may use the automatic process of exception for beneficiaries who do not have a condition or complexity on this list when they justify the provision of therapy services that exceed caps for that patient's condition.

NOT ALL patients who have a condition or complexity on the list are "automatically" excepted from therapy caps. See Pub. 100-02, chapter 15, section 230.3 for documenting the patient's condition and complexities. Contractors may scrutinize claims from providers whose services exceed caps more frequently than is typical.

Regardless of the condition, the patient must also meet other requirements for coverage. For example, the patient must require skilled treatment for a covered, medically necessary service; the services must be appropriate in type, frequency and duration for the patient's condition and service must be documented appropriately. Guidelines for utilization of therapy services may be found in Medicare manuals, Local Coverage Determinations of Medicare contractors, and professional guidelines issued by associations and states.

Bill the most relevant diagnosis. As always, when billing for therapy services, the ICD-9 code that best relates to the reason for the treatment shall be on the claim, unless there is a compelling reason. For example, when a patient with diabetes is being treated for gait training due to amputation, the preferred diagnosis is abnormality of gait (which characterizes the treatment). Where it is possible in accordance with State and local laws and the contractors Local Coverage Determinations, avoid using vague or general diagnoses. When a claim includes several types of services, or where the physician/NPP must supply the diagnosis, it may not be possible to use the most relevant therapy code in the primary position. In that case, the relevant code should, if possible, be on the claim in another position.

Codes representing the medical condition that caused the treatment are used when there is no code representing the treatment. Complicating conditions are preferably used in non-primary positions on the claim and are billed in the primary position only in the rare circumstance that there is no more relevant code.

The condition or complexity that caused treatment to exceed caps must be related to the therapy goals and must either be the condition that is being treated or a complexity that directly and significantly impacts the rate of recovery of the condition being treated such that it is appropriate to exceed the caps. Codes marked as complexities represented by ICD-9 codes on the list below are unlikely to require therapy services that would exceed the caps unless they occur in a patient who also has another condition (either listed or not listed). Therefore, documentation for an exception should indicate how the complexity (or combination of complexities) directly and significantly affects treatment for a therapy condition. For example, if the condition underlying the reason for therapy is V43.64, hip replacement, the treatment may have a goal to ambulate 60' with stand-by assistance and a KX modifier may be appropriate for gait training (assuming the severity of the patient is such that the services exceed the cap). Alternatively, it would not be appropriate to use the KX modifier for a patient who recovered from hip replacement last year and is being treated this year for a sprain of a severity which does not justify extensive therapy exceeding caps.

3. ICD-9 Codes That are Likely to Qualify for the Automatic Process Therapy Cap Exception Based Upon Clinical Condition or Complexity

When using this table, refer to the ICD-9 code book for coding instructions. Some contractors' Local Coverage Determinations do not allow the use of some of the codes on this list in the primary diagnosis position on a claim. If the contractor has determined that these codes do not characterize patients who require medically necessary services, providers/suppliers may not use these codes, but must utilize a billable diagnosis code allowed by their contractor to describe the patient's condition. Contractors shall not apply therapy caps to services based on the patient's condition, but only on the medical necessity of the service for the condition. If a service would be payable before the cap is reached and is still medically necessary after the cap is reached, that service is excepted. Providers/suppliers may use the automatic process for exception for medically necessary services when the patient has a billable condition that is not on the list below. The diagnosis on the list below may be put in a secondary position on the claim and/or in the medical records, as the contractor directs.

When two codes are listed in the left cell in a row, all the codes between them are also eligible for exception. If one code is in the cell, only that one code is likely to qualify for exception. The descriptions in the table are not always identical to those in the ICD-9 code book, but may be summaries. Contact your contractor for interpretation if you are not sure that a condition or complexity is applicable for automatic process exception.

It is very important to recognize that most of the conditions on this list would not ordinarily result in services exceeding the cap. Use the KX modifier only in cases where the condition of the individual patient is such that services are APPROPRIATELY provided in an episode that exceeds the cap. In most cases, the severity of the condition, comorbidities, or complexities will contribute to the necessity of services exceeding the cap, and these should be documented. Routine use of the KX modifier for all patients with these conditions will likely show up on data analysis as aberrant and invite inquiry. Be sure that documentation is sufficiently detailed to support the use of the modifier.

The following ICD-9 codes describe the conditions (etiology or underlying medical conditions) that may result in excepted conditions (marked X) and complexities (marked *) that MIGHT cause medically necessary therapy services to qualify for the automatic process exception for each discipline separately. When the field corresponding to the therapy discipline treating and the diagnosis code is marked with a dash (¸Ì) services by that discipline are not appropriate for that diagnosis and, therefore, services do not qualify for exception to caps.

These codes are grouped only to facilitate reference to them. The codes may be used only when the code is applicable to the condition being actively treated. For example, an exception should not be claimed for a diagnosis of hip replacement when the service provided is for an unrelated dysphagia.

ICD-9 Cluster	ICD-9 (Cluster) Description	PT	OT	SLP
V43.61-V43.69	Joint Replacement	X	X	--
V45.4	Arthrodesis Status	*	*	--
V45.81-V45.82 and V45.89	Other Postprocedural Status	*	*	--
V49.61-V49.67	Upper Limb Amputation Status	X	X	--
V49.71-V49.77	Lower Limb Amputation Status	X	X	--
V54.10-V54.29	Aftercare for Healing Traumatic or Pathologic Fracture	X	X	--
V58.71-V58.78	Aftercare Following Surgery to Specified Body Systems, Not Elsewhere Classified	*	*	*

X   Amutomatic (only ICD-9 needed on claim)
*   Complexity (requires another ICD-9 on claim)
--   Does not serve as qualifying ICD-9 on claim

ICD-9 Cluster	ICD-9 (Cluster) Description	PT	OT	SLP
244.0-244.9	Acquired Hypothyroidism	*	*	*
250.00-251.9	Diabetes Mellitus and Other Disorders of Pancreatic Internal Secretion	*	*	*
276.0-276.9	Disorders of Fluid, Electrolyte, and Acid-Base Balance	*	*	*
278.00-278.01	Obesity and Morbid Obesity	*	*	*
280.0-289.9	Diseases of the blood and blood-forming organs	*	*	*
290.0-290.43	Dementias	*	*	*
294.0-294.9	Persistent Mental Disorders due to Conditions Classified Elsewhere	*	*	*
295.00-299.91	Other Psychoses	*	*	*
300.00-300.9	Anxiety, Disassociative and Somatoform Disorders	*	*	*
310.0-310.9	Specific Nonpsychotic Mental Disorders due to Brain Damage	*	*	*
311	Depressive Disorder, Not Elsewhere Classified	*	*	*
315.00-315.9	Specific delays in Development	*	*	*
317	Mild Mental Retardation	*	*	*
320.0-326	Inflammatory Diseases of the Central Nervous System	*	*	*
330.0-337.9	Hereditary and Degenerative Diseases of the Central Nervous System	X	X	X
340-345.91 and 348.0-349.9	Other Disorders of the Central Nervous System	X	X	X
353.0-359.9	Disorders of the Peripheral Nervous system	X	X	--
365.00-365.9	Glaucoma	*	*	*
369.00-369.9	Blindness and Low Vision	*	*	*
386.00-386.9	Vertiginous Syndromes and Other Disorders of Vestibular System	*	*	*
389.00-389.9	Hearing Loss	*	*	*
401.0-405.99	Hypertensive Disease	*	*	*
410.00-414.9	Ischemic Heart Disease	*	*	*
415.0-417.9	Diseases of Pulmonary Circulation	*	*	*
420.0-429.9	Other Forms of Heart Disease	*	*	*
430-438.9	Cerebrovascular Disease	X	X	X
440.0-448.9	Diseases of Arteries, Arterioles, and Capillaries	*	*	*
451.0-453.9 and 456.0-459.9	Diseases of Veins and Lymphatics, and Other Diseases of Circulatory System	*	*	*
465.0-466.19	Acute Respiratory Infections	*	*	*
478.30-478.5	Paralysis, Polyps, or Other Diseases of Vocal Cords	*	*	*
480.0-486	Pneumonia	*	*	*
490-496	Chronic Obstructive Pulmonary Disease and Allied Conditions	*	*	*
507.0-507.8	Pneumonitis due to solids and liquids	*	*	*
510.0-519.9	Other Diseases of Respiratory System	*	*	*
560.0-560.9	Intestinal Obstruction Without Mention of Hernia	*	*	*
578.0-578.9	Gastrointestinal Hemorrhage	*	*	*
584.5-586	Renal Failure and Chronic Kidney Disease	*	*	*
590.00-599.9	Other Diseases of Urinary System	*	*	*
682.0-682.8	Other Cellulitis and Abscess	*	*	--
707.00-707.9	Chronic Ulcer of Skin	*	*	--
710.0-710.9	Diffuse Diseases of Connective Tissue	*	*	*

ICD-9 Cluster	ICD-9 (Cluster) Description	PT	OT	SLP
711.00-711.99	Arthropathy Associated with Infections	*	*	--
712.10-713.8	Crystal Arthropathies and Arthropathy Associated with Other Disorders Classified Elsewhere	*	*	--
714.0-714.9	Rheumatoid Arthritis and Other Inflammatory Polyarthropathies	*	*	--
715.00-715.98	Osteoarthrosis and Allied Disorders (Complexity except as listed below)	*	*	--
715.09	Osteoarthritis and allied disorders, multiple sites	X	X	--
715.11	Osteoarthritis, localized, primary, shoulder region	X	X	--
715.15	Osteoarthritis, localized, primary, pelvic region and thigh	X	X	--
715.16	Osteoarthritis, localized, primary, lower leg	X	X	--
715.91	Osteoarthritis, unspecified id gen. or local, shoulder	X	X	--
715.96	Osteoarthritis, unspecified if gen. or local, lower leg	X	X	--
716.00-716.99	Other and Unspecified Arthropathies	*	*	--
717.0-717.9	Internal Derangement of Knee	*	*	--
718.00-718.99	Other Derangement of Joint (Complexity except as listed below)	*	*	--
718.49	Contracture of Joint, Multiple Sites	X	X	--
719.00-719.99	Other and Unspecified Disorders of Joint (Complexity except as listed below)	*	*	--
719.7	Difficulty Walking	X	X	--
720.0-724.9	Dorsopathies	*	*	--
725-729.9	Rheumatism, Excluding Back (Complexity except as listed below)	*	*	--
726.10-726.19	Rotator Cuff Disorder and Allied Syndromes	X	X	--
727.61-727.62	Rupture of Tendon, Nontraumatic	X	X	--
730.00-739.9	Osteopathies, Chondropathies, and Acquired Musculoskeletal Deformities (Complexity except as listed below)	*	*	--
733.00	Osteoporosis	X	X	--
741.00-742.9 and 745.0-748.9 and 754.0-756.9	Congenital Anomalies	*	*	*
780.31-780.39	Convulsions	*	*	*
780.71-780.79	Malaise and Fatigue	*	*	*
780.93	Memory Loss	*	*	*
781.0-781.99	Symptoms Involving Nervous and Musculoskeletal System (Complexity except as listed below)	*	*	*
781.2	Abnormality of Gait	X	X	--
781.3	Lack of Coordination	X	X	--
783.0-783.9	Symptoms Concerning Nutrition, Metabolism, and Development	*	*	*
784.3-784.69	Aphasia, Voice and Other Speech Disturbance, Other Symbolic Dysfunction	*	*	X
785.4	Gangrene	*	*	--
786.00-786.9	Symptoms involving Respiratory System and Other Chest Symptoms	*	*	*
787.2	Dysphagia	*	*	X
800.00-828.1	Fractures (Complexity except as listed below)	*	*	--

X   Amutomatic (only ICD-9 needed on claim)
*   Complexity (requires another ICD-9 on claim)
--   Does not serve as qualifying ICD-9 on claim

ICD-9 Cluster	ICD-9 (Cluster) Description	PT	OT	SLP
806.00-806.9	Fracture of Vertebral Column With Spinal Cord Injury	X	X	--
810.11-810.13	Fracture of Clavicle	X	X	--
811.00-811.19	Fracture of Scapula	X	X	--
812.00-812.59	Fracture of Humerus	X	X	--
813.00-813.93	Fracture of Radius and Ulna	X	X	--
820.00-820.9	Fracture of Neck of Femue	X	X	--
821.00-821.39	Fracture of Other and Unspecified Parts of Femur	X	X	--
828.0-828.1	Multiple Fractures Involving Both Lower Limbs, Lower with Upper Limb, and Lower Limb(s) with Rib(s) and Sternum	X	X	--
830.0-839.9	Dislocations	X	X	--
840.0-848.8	Sprains and Strains of Joints and Adjacent Muscles	*	*	--
851.00-854.19	Intracranial Injury, excluding those with Skull Fracture	X	X	X
888.00-884.2	Open Wound of Upper Limb	*	*	--
885.0-887.7	Traumatic Amputation, Thumb(s), Finger(s), Arm and Hand (complete)(partial)	X	X	--
890.0-894.2	Open Wound Lower Limb	*	*	--
895.0-897.7	Traumatic Amputation, Toe(s), Foot/Feet, Leg(s) (complete) (partial)			
905.0-905.9	Late Effects of Musculoskeletal and Connective Tissue Injuries	*	*	*
907.0-907.9	Late Effect of Injuries to the Nervous System	*	*	*
941.00-949.5	Burns	*	*	*
952.00-952.9	Spinal Cord Injury Without Evidence of Spinal Bone Injury	X	X	X
953.0-953.8	Injury to Nerve Roots and Spinal Plexus	X	X*	
959.01	Head Injury, Unspecified	X	X	X

X   Amutomatic (only ICD-9 needed on claim)
*   Complexity (requires another ICD-9 on claim)
--   Does not serve as qualifying ICD-9 on claim

100-4, 5, 10.6

Functional Reporting

A. General

Section 3005(g) of the Middle Class Tax Relief and Jobs Creation Act (MCTRJCA) amended Section 1833(g) of the Act to require a claims-based data collection system for outpatient therapy services, including physical therapy (PT), occupational therapy (OT) and speech-language pathology (SLP) services. 42 CFR 410.59, 410.60, 410.61, 410.62 and 410.105 implement this requirement. The system will collect data on beneficiary function during the course of therapy services in order to better understand beneficiary conditions, outcomes, and expenditures.

Beneficiary unction information is reported using 42 nonpayable functional G-codes and seven severity/complexity modifiers on claims for PT, OT, and SLP services. Functional reporting on one functional limitation at a time is required periodically throughout an entire PT, OT, or SLP therapy episode of care.

The nonpayable G-codes and severity modifiers provide information about the beneficiary's functional status at the outset of the therapy episode of care, including projected goal status, at specified points during treatment, and at the time of discharge. These G-codes, along with the associated modifiers, are required at specified intervals on all claims for outpatient therapy services — not just those over the cap.

B. Application of New Coding Requirements

This functional data reporting and collection system is effective for therapy services with dates of service on and after January 1, 2013. A testing period will be in effect from January 1, 2013, until July 1, 2013, to allow providers and practitioners to use the new coding requirements to assure that systems work. Claims for therapy services furnished on and after July 1, 2013, that do not contain the required functional G-code/modifier information will be returned or rejected, as applicable.

C. Services Affected

These requirements apply to all claims for services furnished under the Medicare Part B outpatient therapy benefit and the PT, OT, and SLP services furnished under the CORF benefit. They also apply to the therapy services furnished personally by and incident to the service of a physician or a nonphysician practitioner (NPP), including a nurse practitioner (NP), a certified nurse specialist (CNS), or a physician assistant (PA), as applicable.

D. Providers and Practitioners Affected.

The functional reporting requirements apply to the therapy services furnished by the following providers: hospitals, CAHs, SNFs, CORFs, rehabilitation agencies, and HHAs (when the beneficiary is not under a home health plan of care). It applies to the following practitioners: physical therapists, occupational therapists, and speech-language pathologists in private practice (TPPs), physicians, and NPPs as noted above. The term "clinician" is applied to these practitioners throughout this manual section. (See definition section of Pub. 100-02, chapter 15, section 220.)

E. Function-related G-codes

There are 42 functional G-codes, 14 sets of three codes each. Six of the G-code sets are generally for PT and OT functional limitations and eight sets of G-codes are for SLP functional limitations.

The following G-codes are for functional limitations typically seen in beneficiaries receiving PT or OT services. The first four of these sets describe categories of functional limitations and the final two sets describe "other" functional limitations, which are to be used for functional limitations not described by one of the four categories.

NONPAYABLE G-CODES FOR FUNCTIONAL LIMITATIONS

	Long Descriptor	Short Descriptor
Mobility G-code Set		
G8978	Mobility: walking & moving around functional limitation, current status, at therapy episode outset and at reporting intervals	Mobility current status
G8979	Mobility: walking & moving around functional limitation, projected goal status, at therapy episode outset, at reporting intervals, and at discharge or to end reporting	Mobility goal status
G8980	Mobility: walking & moving around functional limitation, discharge status, at discharge from therapy or to end reporting	Mobility D/C status
Changing & Maintaining Body Position G-code Set		
G8981	Changing & maintaining body position functional limitation, current status, at therapy episode outset and at reporting intervals	Body pos current status
G8982	Changing & maintaining body position functional limitation, projected goal status, at therapy episode outset, at reporting intervals, and at discharge or to end reporting	Body pos goal status
G8983	Changing & maintaining body position functional limitation, discharge status, at discharge from therapy or to end reporting	Body pos D/C status
Carrying, Moving & Handling Objects G-code Set		
G8984	Carrying, moving & handling objects functional limitation, current status, at therapy episode outset and at reporting intervals	Carry current status
G8985	Carrying, moving & handling objects functional limitation, projected goal status, at therapy episode outset, at reporting intervals, and at discharge or to end reporting	Carry goal status
G8986	Carrying, moving & handling objects functional limitation, discharge status, at discharge from therapy or to end reporting	Carry D/C status
Self Care G-code Set		
G8987	Self care functional limitation, current status, at therapy episode outset and at reporting intervals	Self care current status
G8988	Self care functional limitation, projected goal status, at therapy episode outset, at reporting intervals, and at discharge or to end reporting	Self care goal status
G8989	Self care functional limitation, discharge status, at discharge from therapy or to end reporting	Self care D/C status

The following "other PT/OT" functional G-codes are used to report:

- a beneficiary's functional limitation that is not defined by one of the above four categories;
- a beneficiary whose therapy services are not intended to treat a functional limitation;
- or a beneficiary's functional limitation when an overall, composite or other score from a functional assessment too is used and it does not clearly represent a functional limitation defined by one of the above four code sets.

	Long Descriptor	Short Descriptor
Other PT/OT Primary G-code Set		
G8990	Other physical or occupational therapy primary functional limitation, current status, at therapy episode outset and at reporting intervals	Other PT/OT current status
G8991	Other physical or occupational therapy primary functional limitation, projected goal status, at therapy episode outset, at reporting intervals, and at discharge or to end reporting	Other PT/OT goal status

	Long Descriptor	Short Descriptor
G8992	Other physical or occupational therapy primary functional limitation, discharge status, at discharge from therapy or to end reporting	Other PT/OT D/C status
Other PT/OT Subsequent G-code Set		
G8993	Other physical or occupational therapy subsequent functional limitation, current status, at therapy episode outset and at reporting intervals	Sub PT/OT current status
G8994	Other physical or occupational therapy subsequent functional limitation, projected goal status, at therapy episode outset, at reporting intervals, and at discharge or to end reporting	Sub PT/OT goal status

The following G-codes are for functional limitations typically seen in beneficiaries receiving SLP services. Seven are for specific functional communication measures, which are modeled after the National Outcomes Measurement System (NOMS), and one is for any "other" measure not described by one of the other seven.

	Long Descriptor	Short Descriptor
Swallowing G-code Set		
G8996	Swallowing functional limitation, current status, at therapy episode outset and at reporting intervals	Swallow current status
G8997	Swallowing functional limitation, projected goal status, at therapy episode outset, at reporting intervals, and at discharge or to end reporting	Swallow goal status
G8998	Swallowing functional limitation, discharge status, at discharge from therapy or to end reporting	Swallow D/C status
Motor Speech G-code Set (Note: These codes are not sequentially numbered)		
G8999	Motor speech functional limitation, current status, at therapy episode outset and at reporting intervals	Motor speech current status
G9186	Motor speech functional limitation, projected goal status at therapy episode outset, at reporting intervals, and at discharge or to end reporting	Motor speech goal status
G9158	Motor speech functional limitation, discharge status, at discharge from therapy or to end reporting	Motor speech D/C status
Spoken Language Comprehension G-code Set		
G9159	Spoken language comprehension functional limitation, current status, at therapy episode outset and at reporting intervals	Lang comp current status
G9160	Spoken language comprehension functional limitation, projected goal status, at therapy episode outset, at reporting intervals, and at discharge or to end reporting	Lang comp goal status
G9161	Spoken language comprehension functional limitation, discharge status, at discharge from therapy or to end reporting	Lang comp D/C status
Spoken Language Expressive G-code Set		
G9162	Spoken language expression functional limitation, current status, at therapy episode outset and at reporting intervals	Lang express current status
G9163	Spoken language expression functional limitation, projected goal status, at therapy episode outset, at reporting intervals, and at discharge or to end reporting	Lang press goal status
G9164	Spoken language expression functional limitation, discharge status, at discharge from therapy or to end reporting	Lang express D/C status

	Long Descriptor	Short Descriptor
Attention G-code Set		
G9165	Attention functional limitation, current status, at therapy episode outset and at reporting intervals	Atten current status
G9166	Attention functional limitation, projected goal status, at therapy episode outset, at reporting intervals, and at discharge or to end reporting	Atten goal status
G9167	Attention functional limitation, discharge status, at discharge from therapy or to end reporting intervals, and at discharge or to end reporting	Atten D/C status
Memory G-code Set		
G9168	Memory functional limitation, current status, at therapy episode outset and at reporting intervals	Memory current status
G9169	Memory functional limitation, projected goal status, at therapy episode outset, at reporting	Memory goal status
G9170	Memory functional limitation, discharge status, at discharge from therapy or to end reporting	Memory D/C status
Voice G-code Set		
G9171	Voice functional limitation, current status, at therapy episode outset and at reporting intervals	Voice current status
G9172	Voice functional limitation, projected goal status, at therapy episode outset, at reporting intervals, and at discharge or to end reporting	Voice goal status
G9173	Voice functional limitation, discharge status, at discharge from therapy or to end reporting	Voice D/C status

The following "other SLP" G-code set is used to report:

- on one of the other eight NOMS-defined functional measures not described by the above code sets; or
- to report an overall, composite or other score from assessment tool that does not clearly represent one of the above seven categorical SLP functional measures.

	Long Descriptor	Short Descriptor
Other Speech Language Pathology G-code Set		
G9174	Other speech language pathology functional limitation, current status, at therapy episode outset and at reporting intervals	Speech lang current status
G9175	Other speech language pathology functional limitation, projected goal status, at therapy episode outset, at reporting intervals, and at discharge or to end reporting	Speech lang goal status
G9176	Other speech language pathology functional limitation, discharge status, at discharge from therapy or to end reporting	Speech lang D/C status

F. Severity/Complexity Modifiers

For each nonpayable functional G-code, one of the modifiers listed below must be used to report the severity/complexity for that functional limitation.

Modifier	Impairment Limitation Restriction
CH	0 percent impaired, limited or restricted
CI	At least 1 percent but less than 20 percent impaired, limited or restricted
CJ	At least 20 percent but less than 40 percent impaired, limited or restricted
CK	At least 40 percent but less than 60 percent impaired, limited or restricted
CL	At least 60 percent but less than 80 percent impaired, limited or restricted
CM	At least 80 percent but less than 100 percent impaired, limited or restricted
CN	100 percent impaired, limited or restricted

The severity modifiers reflect the beneficiary's percentage of functional impairment as determined by the clinician furnishing the therapy services.

G. Required Reporting of Functional G-codes and Severity Modifiers

The functional G-codes and severity modifiers listed above are used in the required reporting on therapy claims at certain specified points during therapy episodes of care. Claims containing these functional G-codes must also contain another billable and separately payable (non-bundled) service. Only one functional limitation shall be reported at a given time for each related therapy plan of care (POC).

Functional reporting using the G-codes and corresponding severity modifiers is required reporting on specified therapy claims. Specifically, they are required on claims:

- At the outset of a therapy episode of care (i.e., on the claim for the date of service (DOS) of the initial therapy service);
- At least once every 10 treatment days, which corresponds with the progress reporting period;
- When an evaluative procedure, including a re-evaluative one, (HCPCS/CPT codes 92506, 92597, 92607, 92608, 92610, 92611, 92612, 92614, 92616, 96105, 96125, 97001, 97002, 97003, 97004) is furnished and billed;
- At the time of discharge from the therapy episode of care — i.e., on the date services related to the discharge [progress] report are furnished); and
- At the time reporting of a particular functional limitation is ended in cases where the need for further therapy is necessary.
- At the time reporting is begun for a new or different functional limitation within the same episode of care (i.e., after the reporting of the prior functional limitation is ended)

Functional reporting is required on claims throughout the entire episode of care. When the beneficiary has reached his or her goal or progress has been maximized on the initially selected functional limitation, but the need for treatment continues, reporting is required for a second functional limitation using another set of G-codes. In these situations two or more functional limitations will be reported for a beneficiary during the therapy episode of care. Thus, reporting on more than one functional limitation may be required for some beneficiaries but not simultaneously.

When the beneficiary stops coming to therapy prior to discharge, the clinician should report the functional information on the last claim. If the clinician is unaware that the beneficiary is not returning for therapy until after the last claim is submitted, the clinician cannot report the discharge status.

When functional reporting is required on a claim for therapy services, two G-codes will generally be required.

Two exceptions exist:

1. Therapy services under more than one therapy POC. Claims may contain more than two nonpayable functional G-codes when in cases where a beneficiary receives therapy services under multiple POCs (PT, OT, and/or SLP) from the same therapy provider.

2. One-Time Therapy Visit. When a beneficiary is seen and future therapy services are either not medically indicated or are going to be furnished by another provider, the clinician reports on the claim for the DOS of the visit, all three G-codes in the appropriate code set (current status, goal status and discharge status), along with corresponding severity modifiers.

Each reported functional G-code must also contain the following line of service information:

- Functional severity modifier
- Therapy modifier indicating the related discipline/POC -- GP, GO or GN -- for PT, OT, and SLP services, respectively
- Date of the related therapy service
- Nominal charge, e.g., a penny, for institutional claims submitted to the FIs and A/MACs. For professional claims, a zero charge is acceptable for the service line. If provider billing software requires an amount for professional claims, a nominal charge, e.g., a penny, may be included.

Note: The KX modifier is not required on the claim line for nonpayable G-codes, but would be required with the procedure code for medically necessary therapy services furnished once the beneficiary's annual cap has been reached.

The following example demonstrates how the G-codes and modifiers are used. In this example, the clinician determines that the beneficiary's mobility restriction is the most clinically relevant functional limitation and selects the Mobility G-code set (G8978 –G8980) to represent the beneficiary's functional limitation. The clinician also determines the severity/complexity of the beneficiary's functional limitation and selects the appropriate modifier. In this example, the clinician determines that the beneficiary has a 75 percent mobility restriction for which the CL modifier is applicable. The clinician expects that at the end of therapy the beneficiaries will have only a 15 percent mobility restriction for which the CI modifier is applicable. When the beneficiary attains the mobility goal, therapy continues to be medically necessary to addresss a functional limitation for which there is no categorical G-code. The clinician reports this using (G8990 –G8992).

At the outset of therapy. On the DOS for which the initial evaluative procedure is furnished or the initial treatment day of a therapy POC, the claim for the service will also include two G-codes as shown below.

- G8978-CL to report the functional limitation (Mobility with current mobility limitation of "at least 60 percent but less than 80 percent impaired, limited or restricted")

- G8979-CI to report the projected goal for a mobility restriction of "at least 1 percent but less than 20 percent impaired, limited or restricted."

At the end of each progress reporting period. On the claim for the DOS when the services related to the progress report (which must be done at least once each 10 treatment days) are furnished, the clinician will report the same two G-codes but the modifier for the current status may be different.

- G8978 with the appropriate modifier are reported to show the beneficiary's current status as of this DOS. So if thebeneficiary has made no progress, this claim will include G8978-CL. If the beneficiary made progress and now has a mobility restriction of 65 percent CL would still be the appropriate modifier for 65 percent, and G8978-CL would be reported in this case. If the beneficiary now has a mobility restriction of 45 percent, G8978-CK would be reported.

- G8979-CI would be reported to show the projected goal. This severity modifier would not change unless the clinician adjusts the beneficiary's goal.

This step is repeated as necessary and clinically appropriate, adjusting the current status modifier used as the beneficiary progresses through therapy.

At the time the beneficiary is discharged from the therapy episode. The final claim for therapy episode will include two G-codes.

- G8979-CI would be reported to show the projected goal. G8980-CI would be reported if the beneficiary attained the 15 percent mobility goal. Alternatively, if the beneficiary's mobility restriction only reached 25 percent; G8980-CJ would be reported.

To end reporting of one functional limitation. As noted above, functional reporting is required to continue throughout the entire episode of care. Accordingly, when further therapy is medically necessary after the beneficiary attains the goal for the first reported functional limitation, the clinician would end reporting of the first functional limitation by using the same G-codes and modifiers that would be used at the time of discharge. Using the mobility example, to end reporting of the mobility functional limitation, G8979-CI and G8980-CI would be reported on the same DOS that coincides with end of that progress reporting period.

To begin reporting of a second functional limitation. At the time reporting is begun for a new and different functional limitation, within the same episode of care (i.e., after the reporting of the prior functional limitation is ended). Reporting on the second functional limitation, however, is not begun until the DOS of the next treatment day -- which is day one of the new progress reporting period. When the next functional limitation to be reported is NOT defined by one of the other three PT/OT categorical codes, the G-code set (G8990 - G8992) for the "other PT/OT primary" functional limitation is used, rather than the G-code set for the "other PT/OT subsequent" ? because it is the first reported "other PT/OT" functional limitation. This reporting begins on the DOS of the first treatment day following the mobility "discharge" reporting, which is counted as the initial service for the "other PT/OT primary" functional limitation and the first treatment day of the new progress reporting period. In this case, G8990 and G8991, along with the corresponding modifiers, are reported on the claim for therapy services.

The table below illustrates when reporting is required using this example and what G-codes would be used.

Example of Required Reporting

Key: Reporting Period (RP)	Begin RP #1 for Mobility at Episode Outset	End RP#1for Mobility at Progress Report	Mobility RP #2 Begins Next Treatment Day	End RP#2 for Mobility at Progress Report	Mobility RP #3 Begins Next Treatment Day	D/C or End Reporting for \Mobility	Begin RP #1 for Other PT/OT Primary
Mobility: Walking & Moving Around							
G8978 – Current Status	X	X		X			
G 8979– Goal Status	X	X		X	-	X	
G8980 – Discharge Status						X	
Other PT/OT Primary							
G8990 – Current Status							X

G8991 – Goal Status						X
G8992 – Discharge Status						
No Functional Reporting Required			X		X	

H. Required Tracking and Documentation of Functional G-codes and Severity Modifiers

The clinician who furnishes the services must not only report the functional information on the therapy claim, but, he/she must track and document the G-codes and severity modifiers used for this reporting in the beneficiary's medical record of therapy services.

For details related to the documentation requirements, refer to Pub. 100-02, Medicare Benefit Policy Manual, chapter 15, section 220.3, subsection F - MCTRJCA-required Functional Reporting. For coverage rules related to MCTRJCA and therapy goals, refer to Pub. 100-02: a) for outpatient therapy services, see chapter 15, section 220.1.2 B and b) for instructions specific to PT, OT, and SLP services in the CORF, see chapter 12, section 10.

100-4, 5, 20

HCPCS Coding Requirement

A. Uniform Coding

Section 1834(k)(5) of the Act requires that all claims for outpatient rehabilitation therapy services and all comprehensive outpatient rehabilitation facility (CORF) services be reported using a uniform coding system. The current Healthcare Common Procedure Coding System/Current Procedural Terminology is used for the reporting of these services. The uniform coding requirement in the Act is specific to payment for all CORF services and outpatient rehabilitation therapy services - including physical therapy, occupational therapy, and speech-language pathology - that is provided and billed to carriers and fiscal intermediaries (FIs). The Medicare physician fee schedule (MPFS) is used to make payment for these therapy services at the nonfacility rate.

Effective for claims submitted on or after April 1, 1998, providers that had not previously reported HCPCS/CPT for outpatient rehabilitation and CORF services began using HCPCS to report these services. This requirement does not apply to outpatient rehabilitation services provided by:

- Critical access hospitals, which are paid on a cost basis, not MPFS;

- RHCs, and FQHCs for which therapy is included in the all-inclusive rate; or

- Providers that do not furnish therapy services.

The following "providers of services" must bill the FI for outpatient rehabilitation services using HCPCS codes:

- Hospitals (to outpatients and inpatients who are not in a covered Part A1 stay);

- Skilled nursing facilities (SNFs) (to residents not in a covered Part A1 stay and to nonresidents who receive outpatient rehabilitation services from the SNF);

- Home health agencies (HHAs) (to individuals who are not homebound or otherwise are not receiving services under a home health plan of care2 (POC);

- Comprehensive outpatient rehabilitation facilities (CORFs); and

- Providers of outpatient physical therapy and speech-language pathology services (OPTs), also known as rehabilitation agencies (previously termed outpatient physical therapy facilities in this instruction).

Note 1. The requirements for hospitals and SNFs apply to inpatient Part B and outpatient services only. Inpatient Part A services are bundled into the respective prospective payment system payment; no separate payment is made.

Note 2. For HHAs, HCPCS/CPT coding for outpatient rehabilitation services is required only when the HHA provides such service to individuals that are not homebound and, therefore, not under a home health plan of care.

The following practitioners must bill the carriers for outpatient rehabilitation therapy services using HCPCS/CPT codes:

- Physical therapists in private practice (PTPPs),

- Occupational therapists in private practice (OTPPs),

- Physicians, including MDs, DOs, podiatrists and optometrists, and

- Certain nonphysician practitioners (NPPs), acting within their State scope of practice, e.g., nurse practitioners and clinical nurse specialists.

Providers billing to intermediaries shall report:

- The date the therapy plan of care was either established or last reviewed (see Sec.220.1.3B) in Occurrence Code 17, 29, or 30.

- The first day of treatment in Occurrence Code 35, 44, or 45.

B. Applicable Outpatient Rehabilitation HCPCS Codes

The CMS identifies the following codes as therapy services, regardless of the presence of a financial limitation. Therapy services include only physical therapy, occupational therapy and speech-language pathology services. Therapist means only a physical therapist, occupational therapist or speech-language pathologist. Therapy modifiers are GP for physical therapy, GO for occupational therapy, and GN for speech-language pathology. Check the notes below the chart for details about each code.

When in effect, any financial limitation will also apply to services represented by the following codes, except as noted below

64550+	95834+	97032	97597+
90901+	95851+	97033	97598+ξ
92506■	95852+	97034	97602+****ξ
92507	95992+****	97035	97605+ξ
92508	96105+	97036	97606+ξ
92526	96110+✓	97039*✳	97750
92597	96111+✓	97110	97755
92605***	96125	97112	97760**
92606****	97001	97113	97761
92607	97002	97116	97762
92608	97003	97124	97799*
92609	97004	97139*	G0281
92610+	97010****	97140	G0283
92611+	97012	97150	G0329
92612+	97016	97530	0019T+***
92614+	97018	97532+	0029T+***
92616+	97022	97533	0183T+***E
95831+	97024	97535	
95832+	97026	97537	
95833+	97028	97542	

*   The code is priced by the carrier. Contact the carrier for appropriate fee schedule amount.
    Effective January 1, 2006, these codes will no longer be valued under the Medicare physician fee
    schedule (MPFS) and will be priced by the carriers.
    Effective January 1, 2006, the descriptors for these services have changed.
** CPT code 97760 should not be reported with CPT code 97116 for the same extremity.
*** Carrier priced codes.
**** Codes are bundled with any therapy codes. Regardless of whether they are billed alone or with another
    therapy code, separate payment will not be made for these codes.
    If billed by an outpatient hospital department, these are paid using the outpatient prospective payment
    system (OPPS).
U   Underlined codes designate therapy services, regardless of who performs them, and always require
    therapy modifiers (GP, GO, GN).
ξ   When billed by a hospital subject to OPPS for outpatient services, these codes (also indicated as
    "sometimes therapy" services) will be paid under the OPPS when the service is not performed by a
    qualified therapist and it is inappropriate to bill the service under a therapy plan of care. The
    requirements for other sometimes therapy codes, described below, apply.
+   Codes sometimes represent therapy services. These codes and all codes on the above list always
    represent therapy services when performed by therapists.

NOTE: Listing of the following codes does not imply that services are covered or applicable to all provider settings.

92526	92597	92605****	92606****	92607
92608	92609	92610+	92611+	92612+
92614+	92616+	95831+	95832+	95833+
95834+	95851+	95852+	95992****	96105+
96110+				

100-4, 5, 20.4

Coding Guidance for Certain CPT Codes - All Claims

The following provides guidance about the use of codes 96105, 97026, 97150, 97545, 97546, and G0128.

CPT Codes 96105, 97545, and 97546.

Providers report code 96105, assessment of aphasia with interpretation and report in 1-hour units. This code represents formal evaluation of aphasia with an instrument such as the Boston Diagnostic Aphasia Examination. If this formal assessment is performed during treatment, it is typically performed only once during treatment and its medical necessity should be documented.

If the test is repeated during treatment, the medical necessity of the repeat administration of the test must also be documented. It is common practice for regular assessment of a patient's progress in therapy to be documented in the chart, and this may be done using test items taken from the formal examinations. This is considered to be part of the treatment and should not be billed as 96105 unless a full, formal assessment is completed.

Other timed physical medicine codes are 97545 and 97546. The interval for code 97545 is 2 hours and for code 97546, 1 hour. These are specialized codes to be used in the context of rehabilitating a worker to return to a job. The expectation is that the entire time period specified in the codes 97545 or 97546 would be the treatment period, since a shorter period of treatment could be coded with another code such as codes 97110, 97112, or 97537. (Codes 97545 and 97546 were developed for reporting services to persons in the worker's compensation program, thus we do not expect to see them reported for Medicare patients except under very unusual circumstances. Further, we would not expect to see code 97546 without also seeing code 97545 on the same claim. Code 97546, when used, is used in conjunction with 97545.) CPT Code 97026 Effective for services performed on or after October 24, 2006, the Centers for Medicare & Medicaid Services announce a NCD stating the use of infrared and/or near-infrared light and/or heat, including monochromatic infrared energy (MIRE), is non-covered for the treatment, including symptoms such as pain arising from these conditions, of diabetic and/or non-diabetic peripheral sensory neuropathy, wounds and/or ulcers of the skin and/or subcutaneous tissues in Medicare beneficiaries. Further coverage guidelines can be found in the National Coverage Determination Manual (Publication 100-03), section 270.6.

Contractors shall deny claims with CPT 97026 (infrared therapy incident to or as a PT/OT benefit) and HCPCS E0221 or A4639, if the claim contains any of the following ICD-9 codes: 250.60-250.63 354.4, 354.5, 354.9 355.1-355.4 355.6-355.9 356.0, 356.2-356.4, 356.8-356.9 357.0-357.7 674.10, 674.12, 674.14, 674.20, 674.22, 674.24 707.00-707.07, 707.09-707.15, 707.19 870.0-879.9 880.00-887.7 890.0-897.7 998.31-998.32 Contractors can use the following messages when denying the service: Medicare Summary Notice # 21.11 "This service was not covered by Medicare at the time you received it." Reason Claim Adjustment Code #50 "These are noncovered services because this is not deemed a medical necessity by the payer." Advanced Beneficiary Notice (ABN): Physicians, physical therapists, occupational therapists, outpatient rehabilitation facilities (ORFs), comprehensive outpatient rehabilitation facilities (CORFs), home health agencies (HHA), and hospital outpatient departments are liable if the service is performed, unless the beneficiary signs an ABN.

Similarly, DME suppliers and HHA are liable for the devices when they are supplied, unless the beneficiary signs an ABN.

100-4,5,100.4

Outpatient Mental Health TreatmentLimitation

The Outpatient Mental Health Treatment Limitation (the limitation) is not applicable to CORF services because CORFs do not provide services to treat mental, psychoneurotic and personality disorders that are subject to the limitation in section 1833(c) of the Act. For dates of service on or after October 1, 2012, HCPCS code G0409 is the only code allowed for social work and psychological services furnished in a CORF. This service is not subject to the limitation because it is not a psychiatric mental health treatment service.

For additional information on the limitation, see Publication 100-01, Chapter 3, section 30 and Publication 100-02, Chapter 12, sections 50-50.5.

100-4,5,100.11

Billing for Social Work and Psychological Services in a CORF

The CORF providers shall only bill social work and psychological services with the following HCPCS code:

G0409 Social work and psychological services, directly relating to and/or the patient's rehabilitation goals, each 15 minutes, face-to-face; individual (services provided by a CORF-qualified social worker or psychologist in a CORF).

In addition, HCPCS code G0409 shall only be billed with revenue code 0569 or 0911.

100-4, 8, 60.2.1.1

Separately Billable ESRD Drugs

The following categories of drugs (including but not limited to) are separately billable when used to treat the patient's renal condition:

- Antibiotics;
- Analgesics;

- Anabolics;

- Hematinics;

- Muscle relaxants;

- Sedatives;

- Tranquilizers; and

- Thrombolytics: used to declot central venous catheters.

Note: Thrombolytics were removed from the separately billable drugs for claims with dates of service on or after January 1, 2013. For claims with dates of service on or after July 1, 2013, when these drugs are administered through the dialysate the provider must append the modifier JE (Administered via Dialysate).

These separately billable drugs may only be billed by an ESRD facility if they are actually administered in the facility by the facility staff. Staff time used to administer separately billable drugs is covered under the composite rate and may not be billed separately. However, the supplies used to administer these drugs may be billed in addition to the composite rate.

Effective January 1, 2011, section 153b of the MIPPA requires that all ESRD-related drugs and biologicals be billed by the renal dialysis facility. When a drug or biological is billed by providers other than the ESRD facility and the drug or biological furnished is designated as a drug or biological that is included in the ESRD PPS (ESRD-related), the claim will be rejected or denied. In the event that an ESRD-related drug or biological was furnished to an ESRD beneficiary for reasons other than for the treatment of ESRD, the provider may submit a claim for separate payment using modifier AY.

All drugs reported on the renal dialysis facility claim are considered included in the ESRD PPS. The list of drugs and biologicals for consolidated billing are designated as always ESRD-related and therefore not allowing separate payment to be made to ESRD facilities. However, CMS has determined that some of these drugs may warrant separate payment.

Exceptions to "Always ESRD Related" Drugs:
The following drugs have been approved for separate payment consideration when billed with the AY modifier attesting to the drug not being used for the treatment of ESRD. The ESRD facility is required to indicate (in accordance with ICD-9 guidelines) the diagnosis code for which the drug is indicated.

- Vancomycin, effective January 1, 2012

- Daptomycin, effective January 1, 2013

Items and services subject to the consolidated billing requirements for the ESRD PPS can be found on the CMS website at:
http://www.cms.gov/ESRDPayment/50_Consolidated_Billing.asp#TopOfPage.

Other drugs and biologicals may be considered separately payable to the dialysis facility if the drug was not for the treatment of ESRD. The facility must include the modifier AY to indicate it was not for the treatment of ESRD.

Drugs are assigned HCPCS codes. If no HCPCS code is listed for a drug (e.g., a new drug) the facility bills using HCPCS code J3490, "Unclassified Drugs," and submits documentation identifying the drug. To establish a code for the drug, the FI checks HCPCS to verify that there is no acceptable HCPCS code for billing and if a code is not found checks with the local carrier, which may have a code and price that is appropriate. If no code is found the drug is processed under HCPCS code J3490. See Chapter 17 for a complete description of drug pricing.

100-4, 8, 60.4
Erythropoietin Stimulating Agents (ESAs)
Coverage rules for ESAs are explained in the Medicare Benefit Policy Manual, Publication 100-02, chapter 11.

Fiscal intermediaries (FIs) pay for ESAs, to end-stage renal disease (ESRD) facilities as separately billable drugs to the composite rate. No additional payment is made to administer an ESA, whether in a facility or a home. Effective January 1, 2005, the cost of supplies to administer EPO may be billed to the FI. HCPCS A4657 and Revenue Code 270 should be used to capture the charges for syringes used in the administration of EPO.

ESAs and their administration supplies are included in the payment for the ESRD Prospective Payment System effective January 1, 2011. Providers must continue to report ESAs on the claim as ESAs are subject to a national claims monitoring program and are entitled to outlier payment consideration. The Medicare allowed payment (MAP) amount for outlier includes the ESA rate provided on the Average Sale Price (ASP) list, subject to reduction based on the ESA monitoring policy.

Medicare has an established national claims monitoring policy for erythropoietin stimulating agents for the in-facility dialysis population as outlined in the sections below.

100-4, 8, 60.4.1
ESA Claims Monitoring Policy
Effective for services provided on or after April 1, 2006, Medicare has implemented a national claims monitoring policy for ESAs administered in Medicare renal dialysis facilities. This policy does not apply to claims for ESAs for patients who receive their dialysis at home and self-administer their ESA.

While Medicare is not changing its coverage policy on erythropoietin use to maintain a target hematocrit level between 30% and 36%, we believe the variability in response to ESAs warrants postponing requiring monitoring until the hematocrit reaches higher levels. For dates of services April 1, 2006, and later, the Centers for Medicare & Medicaid Services (CMS) claims monitoring policy applies when the hematocrit level exceeds 39.0% or the hemoglobin level exceeds 13.0g/dL. This does not preclude the contractors from performing medical review at lower levels.

Effective for services provided on or after April 1, 2006, for claims reporting hematocrit or hemoglobin levels exceeding the monitoring threshold, the dose shall be reduced by 25% over the preceding month. Providers may report that a dose reduction did occur in response to the reported elevated hematocrit or hemoglobin level by adding a GS modifier on the claim. The definition of the GS modifier is defined as: "Dosage of ESA has been reduced and maintained in response to hematocrit or hemoglobin level." Thus, for claims reporting a hematocrit level or hemoglobin level exceeding the monitoring threshold without the GS modifier, CMS will reduce the covered dosage reported on the claim by 25%. The excess dosage is considered to be not reasonable and necessary. Providers are reminded that the patient's medical records should reflect hematocrit/hemoglobin levels and any dosage reduction reported on the claim during the same time period for which the claim is submitted.

Effective for dates of service provided on and after January 1, 2008, requests for payments or claims for ESAs for ESRD patients receiving dialysis in renal dialysis facilities reporting a hematocrit level exceeding 39.0% (or hemoglobin exceeding 13.0g/dL) shall also include modifier ED or EE. Claims reporting neither modifier or both modifiers will be returned to the provider for correction.

The definition of modifier ED is "The hematocrit level has exceeded 39.0% (or hemoglobin 1evel has exceeded 13.0g/dL) 3 or more consecutive billing cycles immediately prior to and including the current billing cycle." The definition of modifier EE is "The hematocrit level has exceeded 39.0% (or hemoglobin level has exceeded 13.0g/dL) less than 3 consecutive billing cycles immediately prior to and including the current billing cycle." The GS modifier continues to be defined as stated above.

Providers may continue to report the GS modifier when the reported hematocrit or hemoglobin levels exceed the monitoring threshold for less than 3 months and a dose reduction has occurred. When both modifiers GS and EE are included, no reduction in the covered dose will occur. Claims reporting a hematocrit or hemoglobin level exceeding the monitoring threshold and the ED modifier shall have an automatic 50% reduction in the covered dose applied, even if the claim also reports the GS modifier.

Below is a chart illustrating the resultant claim actions under all possible reporting scenarios:

Hct Exceeds 39.0% or Hgb Exceeds 13.0g/dL	ED Modifier? (Hct >39% or Hgb >13g/dL =3 cycles)	EE Modifier? Hct >39% or Hgb >13g/dL <3 cycles)	GS Modifier? (Dosage reduced and maintained)	Claim Action
No	N/A	N/A	N/A	Do not reduce reported dose.
Yes	No	No	No	Return to provider for correction. Claim must report either modifier ED or EE.
Yes	No	No	Yes	Return to provider for correction. Claim must report either modifier ED or EE.
Yes	No	Yes	Yes	Do not reduce reported dose.
Yes	No	Yes	No	Reduce reported dose 25%.
Yes	Yes	No	Yes	Reduce reported dose 50%.
Yes	Yes	No	No	Reduce reported dose 50%.

In some cases, physicians may believe there is medical justification to maintain a hematocrit above 39.0% or hemoglobin above 13.0g/dL. Beneficiaries, physicians, and/or renal facilities may submit additional medical documentation to justify this belief under the routine appeal process. You may reinstate any covered dosage reduction amounts under this first level appeal process when you believe the documentation supports a higher hematocrit/hemoglobin level.

Providers are reminded that, in accordance with FDA labeling, CMS expects that as the hematocrit approaches 36.0% (hemoglobin 12.0g/dL), a dosage reduction occurs. Providers are expected to maintain hematocrit levels between 30.0 to 36.0% (hemoglobin 10.0-12.0g/dL). Hematocrit levels that remain below 30.0% (hemoglobin levels below 10.0g/dL)) despite dosage increases, should have causative factors evaluated. The patient's medical record should reflect the clinical reason for dose changes and hematocrit levels outside the range of 30.0-36.0% (hemoglobin levels 10.0-12.0g/dL). Medicare contractors may review medical records to assure appropriate dose reductions are applied and maintained and hematological target ranges are maintained.

These hematocrit requirements apply only to ESAs furnished as an ESRD benefit under §1881(b) of the Social Security Act.

Medically Unlikely Edits (MUE)
For dates of service on and after January 1, 2008, the MUE for claims billing for Epogen® is reduced to 400,000 units from 500,000. The MUE for claims for Aranesp® is reduced to 1200 mcg from 1500 mcg.

For dates of service on and after April 1, 2013, the MUE for claims billing for peginesatide is applicable when units billed are equal to or greater than 26 mg.

It is likely that claims reporting doses exceeding the threshold reflect typographical errors and will be returned to providers for correction.

100-4, 8, 60.4.2

60.4.2 - Facility Billing Requirements for ESAs

Hematocrit and Hemoglobin Levels
Renal dialysis facilities are required to report hematocrit or hemoglobin levels for their Medicare patients receiving erythropoietin products. Hematocrit levels are reported in value code 49 and reflect the most recent reading taken before the start of the billing period. Hemoglobin readings before the start of the billing period are reported in value code 48.

To report a hemoglobin or hematocrit reading for a new patient on or after January 1, 2006, the provider should report the reading that prompted the treatment of epoetin alfa. The provider may use results documented on form CMS 2728 or the patient's medical records from a transferring facility.

Effective January 1, 2012, ESRD facilities are required to report hematocrit or hemoglobin levels on all ESRD claims. Reporting the value 99.99 is not permitted when billing for an ESA.

The revenue codes for reporting Epoetin Alfa are 0634 and 0635. All other ESAs are reported using revenue code 0636. The HCPCS code for the ESA must be included: HCPCS

HCPCS	HCPCS Description	Dates of Service
Q4055	Injection, Epoetin Alfa, 1,000 units (for ESRD on Dialysis)	1/1/2004 through 12/31/2005
J0886	Injection, Epoetin Alfa, 1,000 units (for ESRD on Dialysis)	1/1/2006 through 12/31/2006
Q4081	Injection, Epoetin alfa, 100 units (for ESRD on Dialysis)	1/1/2007 to present
Q4054	Injection, Darbepoetin Alfa, 1mcg (for ESRD on Dialysis)	1/1/2004 through 12/31/2005
J0882	Injection, Darbepoetin Alfa,	1/1/2006 to present

Each administration of an ESA is reported on a separate line item with the units reported used as a multiplier by the dosage description in the HCPCS to arrive at the dosage per administration.

Route of Administration Modifiers
Patients with end stage renal disease (ESRD) receiving administrations of erythropoiesis stimulating agents (ESA) for the treatment of anemia may receive intravenous administration or subcutaneous administrations of the ESA. Effective for claims with dates of services on or after January 1, 2012, all facilities billing for injections of ESA for ESRD beneficiaries must include the modifier JA on the claim to indicate an intravenous administration or modifier JB to indicate a subcutaneous administration. ESRD claims containing ESA administrations that are submitted without the route of administration modifiers will be returned to the provider for correction. Renal dialysis facilities claim including charges for administrations of the ESA by both methods must report separate lines to identify the number of administration provided using each method.

Effective July 1, 2013, providers must identify when a drug is administered via the dialysate by appending the modifier JE (administered via dialysate).

ESA Monitoring Policy Modifiers
Append modifiers ED, EE and GS as applicable, see instructions in section 60.4.1.

Maximum Allowable Administrations
The maximum number of administrations of EPO for a billing cycle is 13 times in 30 days and 14 times in 31 days.

The maximum number of administrations of Aranesp for a billing cycle is 5 times in 30/ 31days.

The maximum number of administrations of Peginesatide is 1 time in 30/ 31days.

100-4, 8, 60.4.4

Payment Amount for Epoetin Alfa (EPO)

~Dates of service prior to January 1, 2005, the Medicare contractor pays the facility $10 per 1,000 units of EPO administered, rounded to the nearest 100 units (i.e., $1.00 per 100 units). Effective January 1, 2005, EPO will be paid based on the ASP Pricing File. Also effective January 1, 2005, the cost of supplies to administer EPO may be billed to the Medicare contractor. HCPCS A4657 and Revenue Code 270 should be used to capture the charges for syringes used in the administration of EPO. Where EPO is furnished by a supplier that is not a facility, the DMERC pays at the same rate.

Physician payment is calculated through the drug payment methodology described in Chapter 17 of the Claims Processing Manual.

EXAMPLE: The billing period is 2/1/94 - 2/28/94.

The facility provides the following:

Date	Units	Date	Units
2/1	3000	2/15	2500
2/4	3000	2/18	2500
2/6	3000	2/20	2560
2/8	3000	2/22	2500
2/11	2500	2/25	2000
2/13	2500	2/27	2000

Total 31,060 units

For value code 68, the facility enters 31,060. The 31,100 are used to determine the rate payable. This is 31,060 rounded to the nearest 100 units. The amount payable is 31.1 x $10 =$311.00. In their systems, FIs have the option of setting up payment of $1.00 per 100 units. Effective January 1, 2005, EPO will be paid based on the ASP Pricing File.

Effective January 1, 2008, payment is calculated on a renal dialysis facility claim at the line level by multiplying the rate from the ASP pricing file by the number of units reported on the line billing for EPO.

EXAMPLE: 311 x $1.00 = $311.00

If an ESRD beneficiary requires 10,000 units or more of EPO per administration, special documentation must be made in the medical records. It must consist of a narrative report that addresses the following:

- Iron deficiency. Most patients need supplemental iron therapy while being treated, even if they do not start out iron deficient;
- Concomitant conditions such as infection, inflammation, or malignancy. These conditions must be addressed to assure that EPO has maximum effect;
- Unrecognized blood loss. Patients with kidney disease and anemia may easily have chronic blood loss (usually gastrointestinal) as a major cause of anemia. In those circumstances, EPO is limited in effectiveness;
- Concomitant hemolysis, bone morrow dysplasia, or refractory anemia for a reason other than renal disease, e.g., aluminum toxicity;
- Folic acid or vitamin B12 deficiencies;
- Circumstances in which the bone morrow is replaced with other tissue, e.g., malignancy or osteitis fibrosa cystica; and

Patient's weight, the current dose required, a historical record of the amount that has been given, and the hematocrit response to date.

Payment for ESRD-related EPO is included in the ESRD PPS for claims with dates of service on or after January 1, 2011.

100-4, 8, 60.4.4.1

Payment for Epoetin Alfa (EPO) in Other Settings

~With the implementation of the ESRD PPS, ESRD-related EPO is included in ESRD PPS payment amount and is not separately payable on Part B claims with dates of service on or after January 1, 2011 for other providers with the exception of a hospital billing for an emergency or unscheduled dialysis session.

In the hospital inpatient setting, payment under Part A is included in the DRG.

In the hospital inpatient setting, payment under Part B is made on bill type 12x. Hospitals report the drug units based on the units defined in the HCPCS description. Hospitals do not report value code 68 for units of EPO. For dates of service prior to April 1, 2006, report EPO under revenue code 0636. For dates of service from April 1, 2006 report EPO under the respective revenue code 0634 for EPO less than 10,000 units and revenue code 0635 for EPO over 10,000 units. Payment will be based on the ASP Pricing File.

In a skilled nursing facility (SNF), payment for EPO covered under the Part B EPO benefit is not included in the prospective payment rate for the resident's Medicare-covered SNF stay.

In a hospice, payment is included in the hospice per diem rate.

For a service furnished by a physician or incident to a physician's service, payment is made to the physician by the carrier in accordance with the rules for 'incident to" services. When EPO is administered in the renal facility, the service is not an "incident to" service and not under the "incident to" provision.

100-4, 8, 60.4.4.2

Epoetin Alfa (EPO) Provided in the Hospital Outpatient Departments
When ESRD patients come to the hospital for an unscheduled or emergency dialysis treatment they may also require the administration of EPO. Effective January 1, 2005, EPO will be paid based on the ASP Pricing File.

Hospitals use type of bill 13X (or 85X for Critical Access Hospitals) and report charges under the respective revenue code 0634 for EPO less than 10,000 units and revenue code 0635 for EPO over 10,000 units. Hospitals report the drug units based on the units defined in the HCPCS description. Hospitals do not report value code 68 for units of EPO. Value code 49 must be reported with the hematocrit value for the hospital outpatient visits prior to January 1, 2006, and for all claims with dates of service on or after January 1, 2008.

100-4, 8, 60.4.5.1

Self Administered ESA Supply
Initially, facilities may bill for up to a 2-month supply of an ESA for Method I beneficiaries who meet the criteria for selection for self-administration. After the initial two months' supply, the facility will bill for one month's supply at a time. Condition code 70 is used to indicate payment requested for a supply of an ESA furnished a beneficiary. Usually, revenue code 0635 would apply to EPO since the supply would be over 10,000 units. Facilities leave FL 46, Units of Service, blank since they are not administering the drug.

For claims with dates of service on or after January 1, 2008, supplies of an ESA for self administration should be billed according to the pre-determined plan of care schedule provided to the beneficiary. Submit a separate line item for each date an administration is expected to be performed with the expected dosage. In the event that the schedule was changed, the provider should note the changes in the medical record and bill according to the revised schedule. For patients beginning to self administer an ESA at home receiving an extra month supply of the drug, bill the one month reserve supply on one claim line and include modifier EM defined as "Emergency Reserve Supply (for ESRD benefit only)".

When billing for drug wastage in accordance with the policy in chapter 17 of this manual, section 40.1 the provider must show the wastage on a separate line item with the modifier JW. The line item date of service should be the date of the last covered administration according to the plan of care or if the patient dies use the date of death.

Condition code 70 should be reported on claims billing for home dialysis patients that self administer anemia management drugs including ESAs.

100-4, 8, 60.4.6.3

Payment Amount for Darbepoetin Alfa (Aranesp)
For Method I patients, the FI pays the facility per one mcg of Aranesp administered, in accordance with the MMA Drug Payment Limits Pricing File rounded up to the next highest whole mcg. Effective January 1, 2005, Aranesp will be paid based on the ASP Pricing File. Effective January 1, 2005, the cost of supplies to administer Aranesp may be billed to the FI. HCPCS A4657 and Revenue Code 270 should be used to capture the charges for syringes used in the administration of Aranesp.

Physician payment is calculated through the drug payment methodology described in Chapter 17, of the Claims Processing Manual.

The coinsurance and deductible are based on the Medicare allowance payable, not on the provider's charges. The provider may not charge the beneficiary more than 20 percent of the Medicare Aranesp allowance. This rule applies to independent and hospital based renal facilities.

Payment for ESRD-related Aranesp is included in the ESRD PPS for claims with dates of service on or after January 1, 2011.

100-4, 8, 60.4.6.4

Payment for Darbepoetin Alfa (Aranesp) in Other Settings
In the hospital inpatient setting, payment under Part A for Aranesp is included in the DRG.

In the hospital inpatient setting, payment under Part B is made on bill type 12x when billed with revenue code 0636. The total number of units as a multiple of 1mcg is placed in the unit field. Reimbursement is based on the payment allowance limit for Medicare Part B drugs as found in the ASP pricing file.

In a skilled nursing facility (SNF), payment for Aranesp covered under the Part B EPO benefit is not included in the prospective payment rate for the resident's Medicare-covered SNF stay.

In a hospice, payment is included in the hospice per diem rate.

For a service furnished by a physician or incident to a physician's service, payment is made to the physician by the carrier in accordance with the rules for 'incident to" services. When Aranesp is administered in the renal facility, the service is not an "incident to" service and not under the "incident to" provision.

With the implementation of the ESRD PPS, ESRD-related Aranesp is included in the ESRD PPS payment amount and is not separately payable on Part B claims with dates of service on or after January 1,2011 for other providers, with the exception of a hospital billing for an emergency or unscheduled dialysis session.

100-4, 8, 60.4.6.5

Payment for Darbepoetin Alfa (Aranesp) in the Hospital Outpatient Department
When ESRD patients come to the hospital for an unscheduled or emergency dialysis treatment they may also require the administration of Aranesp. For patients with ESRD who are on a regular course of dialysis, Aranesp administered in a hospital outpatient department is paid the MMA Drug Pricing File rate. Effective January 1, 2005, Aranesp will be paid based on the ASP Pricing File.

Hospitals use bill type 13X (or 85X for Critical Access Hospitals) and report charges under revenue code 0636. The total number of units as a multiple of 1mcg is placed in the unit field. Value code 49 must be reported with the hematocrit value for the hospital outpatient visits prior to January 1, 2006, and for all claims with dates of service on or after January 1, 2008.

100-4, 8, 60.4.7

Payment for Peginesatide in the Hospital Outpatient Department
When ESRD patients come to the hospital for an unscheduled or emergency dialysis treatment they may also require the administration of an ESA, such as peginesatide. When hospitals bill for an unscheduled or emergency outpatient dialysis session (G0257) they may include the administration of an ESA.

100-4, 8, 60.6

Vaccines Furnished to ESRD Patients
The Medicare program covers hepatitis B, influenza virus and Pneumococcal pneumonia virus (PPV) vaccines and their administration when furnished to eligible beneficiaries in accordance with coverage rules. Payment may be made for both the vaccine and the administration. The costs associated with the syringe and supplies are included in the administration fee: HCPCS code A4657 should not be billed for these vaccines.

Vaccines and their administration are reported using separate codes. See Chapter 18 of this manual for the codes required for billing vaccines and the administration of the vaccine.

Payment for vaccine administration (PPV, Influenza Virus, and Hepatitis B Virus) to freestanding RDFs is based on the Medicare Physician Fee Schedule (MPFS) according to the rate in the MPFS associated with code 90782 for services provided prior to March 1, 2003 and code 90471 for services provided March 1, 2005 and later and on reasonable cost for provider-based RDFs.

Vaccines remain separately payable under the ESRD PPS.

100-4, 8, 60.7

Darbepoetin Alfa (Aranesp) for ESRD Patients
Coverage rules for Aranesp® are explained in the Medicare Benefit Policy Manual, Publication 100-02, chapter 11. For an explanation of Method I and Method II reimbursement for patients dialyzing at home see section 40.1.

Fiscal intermediaries (FIs) pay for Aranesp® to end-stage renal disease (ESRD) facilities as a separately billable drug to the composite rate. No additional payment is made to administer Aranesp®, whether in a facility or a home. Effective January 1, 2005, the cost of supplies to administer Aranesp® may be billed to the FI. HCPCS A4657 and Revenue Code 270 should be used to capture the charges for syringes used in the administration of Aranesp®.

If the beneficiary obtains Aranesp® from a supplier for self-administration, the supplier bills the durable medical equipment regional carrier (DMERC), and the DMERC pays in accordance with MMA Drug Payment Limits Pricing File.

Program payment may not be made to a physician for self-administration of Aranesp®. When Aranesp® is furnished by a physician as "incident to services," the carrier processes the claim.

For ESRD patients on maintenance dialysis treated in a physician's office, code J0882, "injection, darbepoetin alfa, 1 mcg (for ESRD patients)," should continue to be used with the hematocrit included on the claim. (For ANSI 837 transactions, the hematocrit (HCT) value is reported in 2400 MEA03 with a qualifier of R2 in 2400 MEA02.) Claims without this information will be denied due to lack of documentation. Physicians who provide Aranesp® for ESRD patients on maintenance dialysis must bill using code J0882.

Darbepoetin Alfa Payment Methodology

Type of Provider	Separately Billable	DMERC Payment	No payment
In-facility freestanding and hospital-based ESRD facility	X		
Self-administer Home Method I	X		
Self-administer Home Method II		X	
Incident to physician in facility or for self-administration *			X

Medicare pays for a drug if self-administered by a dialysis patient. When Aranesp® is administered in a dialysis facility, the service is not an "incident to" service, and not under the "incident to" provision.

Renal dialysis facilities are required to report hematocrit or hemoglobin levels for their Medicare patients receiving erythropoietin products. Hematocrit levels are reported in value code 49 and reflect the most recent reading taken before the start of the billing period. Hemoglobin readings before the start of the billing period are reported in value code 48. See ?60.4.1.

Effective January 1, 2012, ESRD facilities are required to report hematocrit or hemoglobin levels on all ESRD claims irrespective of ESA administration. Reporting the value 99.99 is not permitted when billing for an ESA.

Effective January 1, 2012, renal dialysis facilities are required to report hematocrit or hemoglobin levels on all ESRD claims irrespective of ESA administration. Reporting the value 99.99 is not permitted when billing for an ESA.

Effective for services provided on or after April 1, 2006, Medicare has implemented a national claims monitoring policy for Aranesp® administered in Medicare renal dialysis facilities. This policy does not apply to claims for Aranesp® for patients who receive their dialysis at home and self-administer their Aranesp®.

While Medicare is not changing its coverage policy on erythropoietin use to maintain a target hematocrit level between 30% and 36%, we believe the variability in response to EPO warrants postponing requiring monitoring until the hematocrit reaches higher levels. For dates of services on and after April 1, 2006, the Centers for Medicare & Medicaid Services (CMS) will not initiate monitoring until the hematocrit level exceeds 39.0% or the hemoglobin level exceeds 13.0g/dL. This does not preclude the contractors from performing medical review at lower levels. The Food and Drug Administration (FDA) labeling for Aranesp® notes that as the hematocrit approaches a reading of 36.0% (or hemoglobin 12.0g/dL), the dose of the drug should be reduced by 25%.

Effective for dates of service provided on or after April 1, 2006, for claims reporting hematocrit or hemoglobin levels exceeding the monitoring threshold, the dose shall be reduced by 25% over the preceding month. Providers may report that a dose reduction did occur in response to the reported elevated hematocrit or hemoglobin level by adding a GS modifier on the claim. The definition of the GS modifier continues to be defined as: "Dosage of EPO or Darbepoetin Alfa has been reduced and maintained in response to hematocrit or hemoglobin level." Thus, for claims reporting a hematocrit level or hemoglobin level exceeding the monitoring threshold without the GS modifier, CMS shall reduce the dosage reported on the claim by 25%. The excess dosage is considered to be not reasonable and necessary. Providers are reminded that the patient? medical records should reflect hematocrit/hemoglobin levels and any dosage reduction reported on the claim during the same time period for which the claim is submitted.

Effective for dates of service provided on an after January 1, 2008, requests for payments or claims for Aranesp® for ESRD patients receiving dialysis in renal dialysis facilities reporting a hematocrit level exceeding 39.0% (or hemoglobin exceeding 13.0g/dL) shall also include modifier ED or EE. Claims reporting neither modifier or both modifiers will be returned to the provider for correction.

The definition of modifier ED is "The hematocrit level has exceeded 39.0% (or hemoglobin 1evel has exceeded 13.0g/dL) 3 or more consecutive billing cycles immediately prior to and including the current billing cycle." The definition of modifier EE is "The hematocrit level has exceeded 39.0% (or

hemoglobin level has exceeded 13.0g/dL) less than 3 consecutive billing cycles immediately prior to and including the current billing cycle." The GS modifier continues to be defined as stated above.

Providers may continue to report the GS modifier when the reported hematocrit or hemoglobin levels exceed the monitoring threshold for less than 3 months and a dose reduction has occurred. When both modifiers GS and EE are included, no reduction in the reported dose will occur. Claims reporting a hematocrit or hemoglobin level exceeding the monitoring threshold and the ED modifier shall have an automatic 50% reduction in the reported dose applied, even if the claim also reports the GS modifier.

Below is a chart illustrating the resultant claim actions under all possible reporting scenarios.

Hct Exceeds 39.0% or Hgb Exceeds 13.0g/dL	ED Modifier? (Hct >39% or Hgb >13g/dL =3 cycles)	EE Modifier? (Hct >39% or Hgb >13g/dL <3 cycles)	GS Modifier? (Dosage reduced and maintained)	Claim Action
No	N/A	N/A	N/A	Do not reduce reported dose.
Yes	No	No	No	Return to provider for correction. Claim must report either ED or EE.
Yes	No	No	Yes	Return to provider for correction. Claim must report either ED or EE.
Yes	No	Yes	Yes	Do not reduce reported dose.
Yes	No	Yes	No	Reduce reported dose 25%.
Yes	Yes	No	Yes	Reduce reported dose 50%.
Yes	Yes	No	No	Reduce reported dose 50%.

These hematocrit requirements apply only to Aranesp® furnished as an ESRD benefit under ?1881(b) of the Social Security Act. Aranesp® furnished incident to a physician? service is not included in this policy. Carriers have discretion for local policy for Aranesp® furnished as "incident to service."

100-4, 8, 60.7.3
Payment Amount for Darbepoetin Alfa (Aranesp)

For Method I patients, the FI pays the facility per one mcg of Aranesp administered, in accordance with the MMA Drug Payment Limits Pricing File rounded up to the next highest whole mcg. Effective January 1, 2005, Aranesp will be paid based on the ASP Pricing File. Effective January 1, 2005, the cost of supplies to administer Aranesp may be billed to the FI. HCPCS A4657 and Revenue Code 270 should be used to capture the charges for syringes used in the administration of Aranesp.

Physician payment is calculated through the drug payment methodology described in Chapter 17, of the Claims Processing Manual.

The coinsurance and deductible are based on the Medicare allowance payable, not on the provider‚Äüs charges. The provider may not charge the beneficiary more than 20 percent of the Medicare Aranesp allowance. This rule applies to independent and hospital based renal facilities.

Payment for ESRD-related Aranesp is included in the ESRD PPS for claims with dates of service on or after January 1, 2011.

100-4, 8, 60.7.4
Darbepoetin Alfa (Aranesp) Furnished to Home Patients

Medicare covers Aranesp for dialysis patients who use Aranesp in the home, when requirements for a patient care plan and patient selection as described in the Medicare Benefit Policy Manual, Chapter 11, are met.

When Aranesp is prescribed for a home patient, it may be either administered in a facility, e.g., the one shown on the Form CMS-382 (ESRD Beneficiary Method Selection Form) or furnished by a facility or Method II supplier for self-administration to a home patient determined to be competent to administer this drug. For Aranesp furnished for self-administration to Method I and Method II home patients determined to be competent, the renal facility bills its FI and the Method II supplier bills its DMERC. No additional payment is made for training a prospective self-administering patient or retraining an existing home patient to self-administer Aranesp.

Method II home patients who self-administer may obtain Aranesp only from either their Method II supplier or a Medicare-certified ESRD facility. In this case, the DMERC makes payment at the same rate that applies to facilities.

Program payment may not be made for Aranesp furnished by a physician to a patient for self-administration.

The DMERCs pay for Aranesp for Method II ESRD beneficiaries only. DMERCs shall deny claims for Aranesp where the beneficiary is not a Method II home dialysis patient.

When denying line items for patients that are not Method II, use the following message on the remittance advice:

The ANSI message 7011: Claim not covered by this payer contractor. You must send the claim to the correct payer contractor. When denying line items for patients that are not Method II, use the following message on the Medicare Summary Notice (MSN):

English: 8.59- Durable Medical Equipment Regional Carriers pay for Epoetin Alfa and Darbepoetin Alfa only for Method II End Stage Renal Disease home dialysis patients.

Spanish: 8.59- Las Empresas Regionales de Equipo Medico Duradero pagan por los medicamentos Epoetina Alfa y Darbepoetina Alfa sÐŠlo a pacientes del Metodo II de dialisis con enfermedad renal en etapa final que estan confinados al hogar.

100-4, 9, 150

Initial Preventive Physical Examination (IPPE)

Effective for services furnished on or after January 1, 2005, Section 611 of the Medicare Prescription Drug Improvement and Modernization Act of 2003 (MMA) provides for coverage under Part B of one initial preventive physical examination (IPPE) for new beneficiaries only, subject to certain eligibility and other limitations. For RHCs the Part B deductible for IPPE is waived for services provided on or after January 1, 2009. FQHC services are always exempt from the Part B deductible. Coinsurance is applicable.

Payment for the professional services will be made under the all-inclusive rate. Encounters with more than one health professional and multiple encounters with the same health professionals that take place on the same day and at a single location generally constitute a single visit. However, in rare circumstances an RHC/FQHC can receive a separate payment for an encounter in addition to the payment for the IPPE when they are performed on the same day.

RHCs and FQHCs must HCPCS code for IPPE for the following reasons:

- To avoid application of deductible (on RHC claims);
- To assure payment for this service in addition to another encounter on the same day if they are both separate, unrelated, and appropriate; and
- To update the CWF record to track this once in a lifetime benefit.

Beginning with dates of service on or after January 1, 2009 if an IPPE is provided in an RHC or FQHC, the professional portion of the service is billed to the FI or Part A MAC using TOBs 71X and 73X, respectively, and the appropriate site of service revenue code in the 052X revenue code series, and must include HCPCS G0402. Additional information on IPPE can be found in Chapter 18, section 80 of this manual. NOTE: The technical component of an EKG performed at a clinic/center is not a Medicare-covered RHC/FQHC service and is not billed by the independent RHC/FQHC. Rather, it is billed to Medicare carriers or Part B MACs on professional claims (Form CMS-1500 or 837P) under the practitioner's ID following instructions for submitting practitioner claims. Likewise, the technical component of the EKG performed at a provider-based clinic/center is not a Medicare-covered RHC/FQHC service and is not billed by the provider-based RHC\FQHC. Instead, it is billed on the applicable TOB and submitted to the FI or Part A MAC using the base provider's ID following instructions for submitting claims to the FI/Part A MAC from the base provider. For the professional component of the EKG, there is no separate payment and no separate billing of it. The IPPE is the only HCPCS for which the deductible is waived under this benefit. For more information on billing for a screening EKG see chapter 18 section 80 of this manual.

100-4, 9, 160

Ultrasound Screening for Abdominal Aortic Aneurysm (AAA)

Section 5112 of the Deficit Reduction Act of 2005 amended the Social Security Act to provide coverage under Part B of the Medicare program for a one-time ultrasound screening for abdominal aortic aneurysms (AAA). Payment for the professional services that meet all of the program requirements will be made under the all-inclusive rate. For RHCs the Part B deductible for screening AAA is waived for dates of service on or after January 1, 2007. FQHC services are always exempt from the Part B deductible. Coinsurance is applicable. Additional information on AAA can be found in Chapter 18, section 110 of this manual.

If the screening is provided in an RHC or FQHC, the professional portion of the service is billed to the FI or Part A MAC using TOBs 71X and 73X, respectively, and the appropriate site of service revenue code in the 052X revenue code series and must include HCPCS G0389.

If the AAA screening is provided in an independent RHC or freestanding FQHC, the technical component of the service can be billed by the practitioner to the carrier or Part B MAC under the practitioner's ID following instructions for submitting practitioner claims.

If the screening is provided in a provider-based RHC/FQHC, the technical component of the service can be billed by the base provider to the FI or Part A MAC under the base provider's ID, following instructions for submitting claims to the FI/Part A MAC from the base provider.

100-4, 9, 181

181 - Diabetes Self-Management Training (DSMT) Services Provided by RHCs and FQHCs

A - FQHCs Previously, DSMT type services rendered by qualified registered dietitians or nutrition professionals were considered incident to services under the FQHC benefit, if all relevant program requirements were met. Therefore, separate all-inclusive encounter rate payment could not be made for the provision of DSMT services. With passage of DRA, effective January 1, 2006, FQHCs are eligible for a separate payment under Part B for these services provided they meet all program requirements. See Pub. 100-04, chapter 18, section 120. Payment is made at the all-inclusive encounter rate to the FQHC. This payment can be in addition to payment for any other qualifying visit on the same date of service as the beneficiary received qualifying DSMT services.

For FQHCs to qualify for a separate visit payment for DSMT services, the services must be a one-on-one face-to-face encounter. Group sessions don't constitute a billable visit for any FQHC services. Rather, the cost of group sessions is included in the calculation of the all-inclusive FQHC visit rate. To receive separate payment for DSMT services, the DSMT services must be billed on TOB 73X with HCPCS code G0108 and the appropriate site of service revenue code in the 052X revenue code series. This payment can be in addition to payment for any other qualifying visit on the same date of service that the beneficiary received qualifying DSMT services as long as the claim for DSMT services contains the appropriate coding specified above. Additional information on DSMT can be found in Chapter 18, section 120 of this manual.

NOTE: DSMT is not a qualifying visit on the same day that MNT is provided.

Group services (G0109) do not meet the criteria for a separate qualifying encounter. All line items billed on TOBs 73x with HCPCS codes for DSMT services will be denied.

B - RHCs Separate payment to RHCs for these practitioners/services continues to be precluded as these services are not within the scope of Medicare-covered RHC benefits. Note that the provision of the services by registered dietitians or nutritional professionals, might be considered incident to services in the RHC setting, provided all applicable conditions are met. However, they do not constitute an RHC visit, in and of themselves. All line items billed on TOB 71x with HCPCS code G0108 or G0109 will be denied.

100-4, 9, 182

Medical Nutrition Therapy (MNT) Services

A - FQHCs

Previously, MNT type services were considered incident to services under the FQHC benefit, if all relevant program requirements were met. Therefore, separate all-inclusive encounter rate payment could not be made for the provision of MNT services. With passage of DRA, effective January 1, 2006, FQHCs are eligible for a separate payment under Part B for these services provided they meet all program requirements. Payment is made at the all-inclusive encounter rate to the FQHC. This payment can be in addition to payment for any other qualifying visit on the same date of service as the beneficiary received qualifying MNT services.

For FQHCs to qualify for a separate visit payment for MNT services, the services must be a one-on-one face-to-face encounter. Group sessions don't constitute a billable visit for any FQHC services. Rather, the cost of group sessions is included in the calculation of the all-inclusive FQHC visit rate. To receive payment for MNT services, the MNT services must be billed on TOB 73X with the appropriate individual MNT HCPCS code (codes 97802, 97803, or G0270) and with the appropriate site of service revenue code in the 052X revenue code series. This payment can be in addition to payment for any other qualifying visit on the same date of service as the beneficiary received qualifying MNT services as long as the claim for MNT services contain the appropriate coding specified above.

NOTE: MNT is not a qualifying visit on the same day that DSMT is provided.

Additional information on MNT can be found in Chapter 4, section 300 of this manual.

Group services (HCPCS 97804 or G0271) do not meet the criteria for a separate qualifying encounter. All line items billed on TOB 73x with HCPCS code 97804 or G0271 will be denied.

B - RHCs

Separate payment to RHCs for these practitioners/services continues to be precluded as these services are not within the scope of Medicare-covered RHC benefits. All line items billed on TOB 71x with HCPCS codes for MNT services will be denied.

100-4, 10, 40.2

HH PPS Claims

The following data elements are required to submit a claim under home health PPS. For billing of home health claims not under an HH plan of care (not under HH PPS), see §90. Home health services under a plan of care are paid based on a 60-day episode of care. Payment for this episode will usually be made in two parts. After an RAP has been paid and a 60-day episode has been completed, or the patient has been discharged, the HHA submits a claim to receive the balance of payment due for the episode.

HH PPS claims will be processed in Medicare claims processing systems as debit/credit adjustments against the record created by the RAP, except in the case of "No-RAP" LUPA claims (see §40.3). As the claim is processed the payment on the RAP will be reversed in full and the full payment due for the episode will be made on the claim. Both the debit and credit actions will be reflected on the remittance advice (RA) so the net payment on the claim can be easily understood. Detailed RA information is contained in chapter 22.

Billing Provider Name, Address, and Telephone Number

Required —The HHA— minimum entry is the agency's name, city, State, and ZIP Code. The post office box number or street name and number may be included. The State may be abbreviated using standard post office abbreviations. Five or nine-digit ZIP Codes are acceptable. Medicare contractors use this information in connection with the provider identifier to verify provider identity.

Patient Control Number and Medical/Health Record Number

Required - The patient's control number may be shown if the patient is assigned one and the number is needed for association and reference purposes.

The HHA may enter the number assigned to the patient's medical/health record. If this number is entered, the Medicare contractor must carry it through their system and return it on the remittance record.

Type of Bill

Required - This 3-digit alphanumeric code gives three specific pieces of information. The first digit identifies the type of facility. The second classifies the type of care. The third indicates the sequence of this bill in this particular episode of care. It is referred to as a "frequency" code. The types of bill accepted for HH PPS claims are any combination of the codes listed below:

Code Structure (only codes used to bill Medicare are shown).

Ist Digit-Type of Facility

3 - Home Health

2nd Digit-Bill Classification (Except Clinics and Special Facilities)

2 - Hospital Based or Inpatient (Part B) (includes HHA visits under a Part B plan of treatment).

NOTE: While the bill classification of 3, defined as "Outpatient (includes HHA visits under a Part A plan of treatment and use of HHA DME under a Part A plan of treatment)" may also be appropriate to an HH PPS claim, Medicare encourages HHAs to submit all claims with bill classification 2. Medicare claims systems determine whether an HH claim should be paid from the Part A or Part B trust fund and will change the bill classification digit on the electronic claim record as necessary to reflect this.

3rd Digit-Frequency - Definition

7 - Replacement of Prior Claim - HHAs use to correct a previously submitted bill. Apply this code for the corrected or "new" bill. These adjustment claims must be accepted at any point within the timely filing period after the payment of the original claim.

8 - Void/Cancel of a Prior Claim - HHAs use this code to indicate this bill is an exact duplicate of an incorrect bill previously submitted. A replacement RAP or claim must be submitted for the episode to be paid.

9 - Final Claim for an HH PPS Episode - This code indicates the HH bill should be processed as a debit/credit adjustment to the RAP. This code is specific to home health and does not replace frequency codes 7, or 8.

HHAs must submit HH PPS claims with the frequency of "9." These claims may be adjusted with frequency "7" or cancelled with frequency "8." Medicare contractors do not accept late charge bills, submitted with frequency "5," on HH PPS claims. To add services within the period of a paid HH claim, the HHA must submit an adjustment.

Statement Covers Period

Required - The beginning and ending dates of the period covered by this claim. The "from" date must match the date submitted on the RAP for the episode. For continuous care episodes, the "through" date must be 59 days after the "from" date. The patient status code must be 30 in these cases.

In cases where the beneficiary has been discharged or transferred within the 60-day episode period, HHAs will report the date of discharge in accordance with internal discharge procedures as the "through" date. If the beneficiary has died, the HHA reports the date of death in the "through date."

Any NUBC approved patient status code may be used in these cases. The HHA may submit claims for payment immediately after the claim "through" date. It is not required to hold claims until the end of the 60-day episode unless the beneficiary continues under care.

Patient Name/Identifier

Required —The HHA enters the patient's last name, first name, and middle initial.

Patient Address

Required - The HHA enters the patient's full mailing address, including street number and name, post office box number or RFD, City, State, and ZIP Code.

Patient Birth Date

Required - The HHA enters the month, day, and year of birth of patient. If the full correct date is not known, leave blank.

Patient Sex

Required - "M" for male or "F" for female must be present. This item is used in conjunction with diagnoses and surgical procedures to identify inconsistencies.

Admission/Start of Care Date

Required - The HHA enters the same date of admission that was submitted on the RAP for the episode.

Point of Origin for Admission or Visit

Required - The HHA enters the same point of origin code that was submitted on the RAP for the episode.

Patient Discharge Status

Required - The HHA enters the code that most accurately describes the patient's status as of the "Through" date of the billing period. Any applicable NUBC approved code may be used.

Patient status code 06 should be reported in all cases where the HHA is aware that the episode will be paid as a partial episode payment (PEP) adjustment. These are cases in which the agency is aware that the beneficiary has transferred to another HHA within the 60-day episode, or the agency is aware that the beneficiary was discharged with the goals of the original plan of care met and has been readmitted within the 60-day episode. Situations may occur in which the HHA is unaware at the time of billing the discharge that these circumstances exist. In these situations, Medicare claims processing systems will adjust the discharge claim automatically to reflect the PEP adjustment, changing the patient status code on the paid claims record to 06.

In cases where an HHA is changing the Medicare contractor to which they submit claims, the service dates on the claims must fall within the provider's effective dates at each contractor. To ensure this, RAPs for all episodes with "from" dates before the provider's termination date must be submitted to the contractor the provider is leaving. The resulting episode must be resolved by the provider submitting claims for shortened periods, with "through" dates on or before the termination date. The provider must indicate that these claims will be PEP adjustments by using patient status code 06. Billing for the beneficiary is being "transferred" to the new contractor.

In cases where the ownership of an HHA is changing and the CMS certification number (CCN) also changes, the service dates on the claims must fall within the effective dates of the terminating CCN. To ensure this, RAPs for all episodes with "from" dates before the termination date of the CCN must be resolved by the provider submitting claims for shortened periods, with "through" dates on or before the termination date. The provider must indicate that these claims will be PEP adjustments by using patient status 06. Billing for the beneficiary is being "transferred" to the new agency ownership. In changes of ownership which do not affect the CCN, billing for episodes is also unaffected.

In cases where an HHA is aware in advance that a beneficiary will become enrolled in a Medicare Advantage (MA) Organization as of a certain date, the provider should submit a claim for the shortened period prior to the MA Organization enrollment date. The claim should be coded with patient status 06. Payment responsibility for the beneficiary is being "transferred" from Medicare fee-for-service to MA Organization, since HH PPS applies only to Medicare fee-for-service.

If HHAs require guidance on OASIS assessment procedures in these cases, they should contact the appropriate state OASIS education coordinator.

Condition Codes

Conditional —The HHA enters any NUBC approved code to describe conditions that apply to the claim.

If the RAP is for an episode in which the patient has transferred from another HHA, the HHA enters condition code 47.

HHAs that are adjusting previously paid claims enter one of the condition codes representing Claim Change Reasons (code values D0 through E0). If adjusting the claim to correct a HIPPS code, HHAs use condition code D2 and enter "Remarks" indicating the reason for the HIPPS code change. HHAs use D9 if multiple changes are necessary.

When submitting a HH PPS claim as a demand bill, HHAs use condition code 20. See §50 for more detailed instructions regarding demand billing.

When submitting a HH PPS claim for a denial notice, HHAs use condition code 21. See §60 for more detailed instructions regarding no-payment billing.Required - If canceling the claim (TOB 3X8), HHAs report the condition codes D5 or D6 and enter "Remarks" indicating the reason for cancellation of the claim.

Occurrence Codes and Dates

Conditional - The HHA enters any NUBC approved code to describe occurrences that apply to the claim.

Occurrence Span Code and Dates

Conditional - The HHA enters any NUBC approved Occurrence Span code to describe occurrences that apply to the claim. Reporting of occurrence span code 74 is not required to show the dates of an inpatient admission during an episode.

Value Codes and Amounts

Required - Home health episode payments must be based upon the site at which the beneficiary is served. For episodes in which the beneficiary's site of service changes from one CBSA to another within the episode period, HHAs should submit the CBSA code corresponding to the site of service at the end of the episode on the claim.

NOTE: Contractor-entered value codes. The Medicare contractor enters codes 17 and 62 - 65 on the claim in processing. They may be visible in the Medicare contractor's online claim history and on remittances.

Code	Title	Definition
17	Outlier Amount	The amount of any outlier payment returned by the Pricer with this code. (Contractors always place condition code 61 on the claim along with this value code.)
61	Location Where Service is Furnished (HHA and Hospice)	HHAs report the MSA number or Core Based Statistical Area (CBSA) number (or rural state code) of the location where the home health or hospice service is delivered. The HHA reports the number in dollar portion of the form locator right justified to the left of the dollar/cents delimiter, add two zeros to the cents field if no cents.
62	HH Visits - Part A	The number of visits determined by Medicare to be payable from the Part A trust fund to reflect the shift of payments from the Part A to the Part B trust fund as mandated by §1812 (a)(3) of the Social Security Act.
63	HH Visits - Part B	The number of visits determined by Medicare to be payable from the Part B trust fund to reflect the shift of payments from the Part A to the Part B trust fund as mandated by §1812 (a)(3) of the Social Security Act.
64	HH Reimbursement - Part A	The dollar amounts determined to be associated with the HH visits identified in a value code 62 amount. This Part A payment reflects the shift of payments from the Part A to the Part B trust fund as mandated by §1812 (a)(3) of the Social Security Act.
65	HH Reimbursement - Part B	The dollar amounts determined to be associated with the HH visits identified in a value code 63 amount. This Part B payment reflects the shift of payments from the Part A to the Part B trust fund as mandated by §1812 (a)(3) of the Social Security Act.

If information returned from the Common Working File (CWF) indicates all visits on the claim are Part A, the shared system must place value codes 62 and 64 on the claim record, showing the total visits and total PPS payment amount as the values, change the TOB on the claim record to 33X, and send the claim to CWF with RIC code V.

If information returned from CWF indicates all visits on the claim are Part B, the shared system must place value codes 63 and 65 on the claim record, showing the total visits and total PPS payment amount as the values, change the TOB on the claim record to 32X, and send the claim to CWF with RIC code W.

If information returned from CWF indicates certain visits on the claim are payable from both Part A and Part B, the shared system must place value codes 62, 63, 64, and 65 on the claim record. The shared system also must populate the values for code 62 and 63 based on the numbers of visits returned from CWF and prorate the total PPS reimbursement amount based on the numbers of visits to determine the dollars amounts to be associated with value codes 64 and 65. The shared system will not change the TOB and will return the claim to CWF with RIC code U.

Revenue Code and Revenue Description

Required

HH PPS claims must report a 0023 revenue code line on which the first four positions of the HIPPS code match the code submitted on the RAP. The fifth position of the code represents the

non-routine supply (NRS) severity level. This fifth position may differ to allow the HHA to change a code that represents that supplies were provided to a code that represents that supplies were not provided, or vice versa. However, the fifth position may only change between the two values that represent the same NRS severity level. Section 10.1.9 of this chapter contains the pairs of corresponding values. If these criteria are not met, Medicare claims processing systems will return the claim.

HHAs enter only one 0023 revenue code per claim in all cases.

Unlike RAPs, claims must also report all services provided to the beneficiary within the episode. Each service must be reported in line item detail. Each service visit (revenue codes 042X, 043X, 044X, 055X, 056X and 057X) must be reported as a separate line. Any of the following revenue codes may be used:

027X	Medical/Surgical Supplies (Also see 062X, an extension of 027X)	
	Required detail: With the exception of revenue code 0274 (prosthetic and orthotic devices), only service units and a charge must be reported with this revenue code. If also reporting revenue code 0623 to separately identify specific wound care supplies, not just supplies for wound care patients, ensure that the charge amounts for revenue code 0623 lines are mutually exclusive from other lines for supply revenue codes reported on the claim. Report only nonroutine supply items in this revenue code or in 0623.	
	Revenue code 0274 requires an HCPCS code, the date of service units and a charge amount.	
	NOTE: Revenue Codes 0275 through 0278 are not used for Medicare billing on HH PPS types of bills	
042X	Physical Therapy	
	Required detail: One of the physical therapy HCPCS codes defined below in the instructions for the HCPCS code field, the date of service, service units which represent the number of 15 minute increments that comprised the visit, and a charge amount.	
043X	Occupational Therapy	
	Required detail: One of the occupational therapy HCPCS codes defined below in the instructions for the HCPCS code field, the date of service, service units which represent the number of 15 minute increments that comprised the visit, and a charge amount.	
044X	Speech-Language Pathology	
	Required detail: One of the speech-language pathology HCPCS codes defined below in the instructions for the HCPCS code field, the date of service, service units which represent the number of 15 minute increments that comprised the visit, and a charge amount.	
055X	Skilled Nursing	
	Required detail: One of the skilled nursing HCPCS codes defined below in the instructions for the HCPCS code field, the date of service, service units which represent the number of 15 minute increments that comprised the visit, and a charge amount.	
056X	Medical Social Services	
	Required detail: The medical social services HCPCS code defined below in the instructions for the HCPCS code field, the date of service, service units which represent the number of 15 minute increments that comprised the visit, and a charge amount.	

057X	Home Health Aide (Home Health)
	Required detail: The home health aide HCPCS code defined below in the instructions for the HCPCS code field, the date of service, service units which represent the number of 15 minute increments that comprised the visit, and a charge amount.

NOTE: Contractors do not accept revenue codes 058X or 059X when submitted with covered charges on Medicare home health claims under HH PPS. They also do not accept revenue code 0624, investigational devices, on HH claims under HH PPS.

029X	Durable Medical Equipment (DME) (Other Than Renal)
	Required detail: the applicable HCPCS code for the item, a date of service indicating the purchase date or the beginning date of a monthly rental, a number of service units, and a charge amount. Monthly rental items should be reported with a separate line for each month's rental and service units of one.
	Revenue code 0294 is used to bill drugs/supplies for the effective use of DME.

060X	Oxygen (Home Health)
	Required detail: the applicable HCPCS code for the item, a date of service, a number of service units, and a charge amount.

Revenue Codes for Optional Billing of DME

Billing of Durable Medical Equipment (DME) provided in the episode is not required on the HH PPS claim. Home health agencies retain the option to bill these services to their Medicare contractor processing home health claims or to have the services provided under arrangement with a supplier that bills these services to the DME MAC. Agencies that choose to bill DME services on their HH PPS claims must use the revenue codes below. These services will be paid separately in addition to the HH PPS amount, based on the applicable Medicare fee schedule. For additional instructions for billing DME services see chapter 20.

0274	Prosthetic/Orthotic Devices
	Required detail: the applicable HCPCS code for the item, a date of service, a number of service units, and a charge amount.

029X	Durable Medical Equipment (DME) (Other Than Renal)
	Required detail: the applicable HCPCS code for the item, a date of service indicating the purchase date or the beginning date of a monthly rental, a number of service units, and a charge amount. Monthly rental items should be reported with a separate line for each month's rental and service units of one.
	Revenue code 0294 is used to bill drugs/supplies for the effective use of DME.

060X	Oxygen (Home Health)
	Required detail: the applicable HCPCS code for the item, a date of service, a number of service units, and a charge amount.

Revenue Code for Optional Reporting of Wound Care Supplies

0623	Medical/Surgical Supplies - Extension of 027X
	Required detail: Only service units and a charge must be reported with this revenue code. If also reporting revenue code 027x to identify nonroutine supplies other than those used for wound care, the HHA must ensure that the charge amounts for the two revenue code lines are mutually exclusive.

HHAs may voluntarily report a separate revenue code line for charges for nonroutine wound care supplies, using revenue code 0623. Notwithstanding the standard abbreviation "surg dressings," HHAs use this code to report charges for ALL nonroutine wound care supplies, including but not limited to surgical dressings.

Pub. 100-02, Medicare Benefit Policy Manual, chapter 7, defines routine vs. nonroutine supplies. HHAs use that definition to determine whether any wound care supply item should be reported in this line because it is nonroutine.

HHAs can assist CMS—future refinement of payment rates if they consistently and accurately report their charges for nonroutine wound care supplies under revenue center code 0623. HHAs should ensure that charges reported under revenue code 027X for nonroutine supplies are also complete and accurate.

Validating Required Reporting of Supply Revenue Code

The HH PPS includes a separate case-mix adjustment for non-routine supplies. Non-routine supply severity levels are indicated on HH PPS claims through a code value in the 5th position of the HIPPS code. The 5th position of the HIPPS code can contain two sets of values. One set of codes (the letters S through X) indicate that supplies were provided. The second set of codes (the

numbers 1 through 6) indicate the HHA is intentionally reporting that they did not provide supplies during the episode. See section 10.1.9 for the complete composition of HIPPS under the HH PPS.

HHAs must ensure that if they are submitting a HIPPS code with a 5th position containing the letters S through X, the claim must also report a non-routine supply revenue with covered charges. This revenue code may be either revenue code 27x, excluding 274, or revenue code 623, consistent with the instructions for optional separate reporting of wound care supplies.

Medicare systems will return the claim to the HHA if the HIPPS code indicates non-routine supplies were provided and supply charges are not reported on the claim. When the HHA receives a claim returned for this reason, the HHA must review their records regarding the supplies provided to the beneficiary. The HHA may take one of the following actions, based on the review of their records:

- If non-routine supplies were provided, the supply charges must be added to the claim using the appropriate supply revenue code.

- If non-routine supplies were not provided, the HHA must indicate that on the claim by changing the 5th position of the HIPPS code to the appropriate numeric value in the range 1 through 6.

After completing one of these actions, the HHA may return the claim to the Medicare contractor for continued adjudication.

HCPCS/Accommodation Rates/HIPPS Rate Codes

Required - On the 0023 revenue code line, the HHA must report the HIPPS code that was reported on the RAP. The first four positions of the code must be identical to the value reported on the RAP. The fifth position may vary from the letter value reported on the RAP to the corresponding number which represents the same non-routine supply severity level but which reports that non-routine supplies were not provided.

HHAs enter only one HIPPS code per claim in all cases. Claims submitted with additional HIPPS codes will be returned to the provider.

For revenue code lines other than 0023, the HHA reports HCPCS codes as appropriate to that revenue code.

To report HH visits on episodes beginning before January 1, 2011, the HHA reports a single HCPCS code to represent each HH care discipline. These codes are:

G0151 Services of physical therapist in home health or hospice setting, each 15 minutes.

G0152 Services of an occupational therapist in home health or hospice setting, each 15 minutes.

G0153 Services of a speech language pathologist in home health or hospice setting, each 15 minutes.

G0154 Services of skilled nurse in the home health or hospice settings, each 15 minutes.

G0155 Services of a clinical social worker under a home health plan of care, each 15 minutes.

G0156 Services of a home health aide under a home health plan of care, each 15 minutes.

To report HH visits on episodes beginning on or after January 1, 2011, the HHA reports one of the following HCPCS code to represent each HH care discipline:

Physical Therapy (revenue code 042x)

G0151 Services performed by a qualified physical therapist in the home health or hospice setting, each 15 minutes.

G0157 Services performed by a qualified physical therapist assistant in the home health or hospice setting, each 15 minutes.

G0159 Services performed by a qualified physical therapist, in the home health setting, in the establishment or delivery of a safe and effective physical therapy maintenance program, each 15 minutes.

Occupational Therapy (revenue code 043x)

G0152 Services performed by a qualified occupational therapist in the home health or hospice setting, each 15 minutes.

G0158 Services performed by a qualified occupational therapist assistant in the home health or hospice setting, each 15 minutes.

G0160 Services performed by a qualified occupational therapist, in the home health setting, in the establishment or delivery of a safe and effective occupational therapy maintenance program, each 15 minutes.

Speech-Language Pathology (revenue code 044x)

G0153 Services performed by a qualified speech-language pathologist in the home health or hospice setting, each 15 minutes.

G0161 Services performed by a qualified speech-language pathologist, in the home health setting, in the establishment or delivery of a safe and effective speech-language pathology maintenance program, each 15 minutes.

Skilled Nursing (revenue code 055x)

G0154 Direct skilled services of a licensed nurse (LPN or RN) in the home health or hospice setting, each 15 minutes.

G0162 Skilled services by a licensed nurse (RN only) for management and evaluation of the plan of care, each 15 minutes (the patient's underlying condition or complication requires an RN to ensure that essential non-skilled care achieves its purpose in the home health or hospice setting).

G0163 Skilled services of a licensed nurse (LPN or RN) for the observation and assessment of the patient's condition, each 15 minutes (the change in the patient's condition requires skilled nursing personnel to identify and evaluate the patient's need for possible modification of treatment in the home health or hospice setting).

G0164 Skilled services of a licensed nurse (LPN or RN), in the training and/or education of a patient or family member, in the home health or hospice setting, each 15 minutes.

Medical Social Services (revenue code 056x)

G0155 Services of a clinical social worker under a home health plan of care, each 15 minutes.

Home Health Aide (revenue code 057x)

G0156 Services of a home health aide under a home health plan of care, each 15 minutes.

Regarding all skilled nursing and skilled therapy visits

In the course of a single visit, a nurse or qualified therapist may provide more than one of the nursing or therapy services reflected in the codes above. HHAs must not report more than one G-code for each visit regardless of the variety of services provided during the visit. In cases where more than one nursing or therapy service is provided in a visit, the HHA must report the G-code which reflects the service for which the clinician spent most of his/her time.

For instance, if direct skilled nursing services are provided, and the nurse also provides training/education of a patient or family member during that same visit, we would expect the HHA to report the G-code which reflects the service for which most of the time was spent during that visit. Similarly, if a qualified therapist is performing a therapy service and also establishes a maintenance program during the same visit, the HHA should report the G-code which reflects the service for which most of the time was spent during that visit. In all cases, however, the number of 15-minute increments reported for the visit should reflect the total time of the visit.

Service Date

Required - On the 0023 revenue code line, the HHA reports the date of the first service provided under the HIPPS code. For other line items detailing all services within the episode period, it reports service dates as appropriate to that revenue code. Coding detail for each revenue code under HH PPS is defined above under Revenue Codes. For service visits that begin in 1 calendar day and span into the next calendar day, report one visit using the date the visit ended as the service date.

Service Units

Required - Transaction standards require the reporting of a number greater than zero as the units on the 0023 revenue code line. However, Medicare systems will disregard the submitted units in processing the claim. For line items detailing all services within the episode period, the HHA reports units of service as appropriate to that revenue code. Coding detail for each revenue code under HH PPS is defined above under Revenue Codes.

For the revenue codes that represent home health visits (042X, 043X, 044X, 055X, 056X, and 057X), the HHA reports as service units a number of 15 minute increments that comprise the time spent treating the beneficiary. Time spent completing the OASIS assessment in the home as part of an otherwise covered and billable visit and time spent updating medical records in the home as part of such a visit may also be reported. Visits of any length are to be reported, rounding the time to the nearest 15-minute increment. Visits cannot be split into multiple lines. Report covered and noncovered increments of the same visit on the same line.

Total Charges

Required - The HHA must report zero charges on the 0023 revenue code line (the field must contain zero).

For line items detailing all services within the episode period, the HHA reports charges as appropriate to that revenue code. Coding detail for each revenue code under HH PPS is defined above under Revenue Codes. Charges may be reported in dollars and cents (i.e., charges are not required to be rounded to dollars and zero cents). Medicare claims processing systems will not make any payments based upon submitted charge amounts.

Non-covered Charges

Required —The HHA reports the total non-covered charges pertaining to the related revenue code here. Examples of non-covered charges on HH PPS claims may include:

- Visits provided exclusively to perform OASIS assessments
- Visits provided exclusively for supervisory or administrative purposes
- Therapy visits provided prior to the required re-assessments

Payer Name

Required - See chapter 25.

Release of Information Certification Indicator

Required - See chapter 25.

National Provider Identifier —Billing Provider

Required - The HHA enters their provider identifier.

Insured's Name

Required only if MSP involved. See Pub. 100-05, Medicare Secondary Payer Manual.

Patient's Relationship To Insured

Required only if MSP involved. See Pub. 100-05, Medicare Secondary Payer Manual.

Insured's Unique Identifier

Required only if MSP involved. See Pub. 100-05, Medicare Secondary Payer Manual.

Insured's Group Name

Required only if MSP involved. See Pub. 100-05, Medicare Secondary Payer Manual.

Insured's Group Number

Required only if MSP involved. See Pub. 100-05, Medicare Secondary Payer Manual.

Treatment Authorization Code

Required - The HHA enters the claim-OASIS matching key output by the Grouper software. This data element enables historical claims data to be linked to individual OASIS assessments supporting the payment of individual claims for research purposes. It is also used in recalculating payment group codes in the HH Pricer (see section 70).

The format of the treatment authorization code is shown here:

Position	Definition	Format
1-2	M0030 (Start-of-care date) —2 digit year	99
3-4	M0030 (Start-of-care date) —alpha code for date	XX
5-6	M0090 (Date assessment completed) —2 digit year	99
7-8	M0090 (Date assessment completed) —alpha code for date	XX
9	M0100 (Reason for assessment)	9
10	M0110 (Episode Timing) —Early = 1, Late = 2	9
11	Alpha code for Clinical severity points —under Equation 1	X
12	Alpha code for Functional severity points —under Equation 1	X
13	Alpha code for Clinical severity points —under Equation 2	X
14	Alpha code for Functional severity points —under Equation 2	X
15	Alpha code for Clinical severity points —under Equation 3	X
16	Alpha code for Functional severity points —under Equation 3	X
17	Alpha code for Clinical severity points —under Equation 4	X
18	Alpha code for Functional severity points —under Equation 4	X

NOTE: The dates in positions 3-4 and 7-8 are converted to 2 position alphabetic values using a hexavigesimal coding system. The 2 position numeric point scores in positions 11 –18 are converted to a single alphabetic code using the same system. Tables defining these conversions are included in the documentation for the Grouper software that is available on the CMS Web site.

This is an example of a treatment authorization code created using this format:

Position	Definition	Actual Value	Resulting Code
1-2	M0030 (Start-of-care date) —2 digit year	2007	07
3-4	M0030 (Start-of-care date) —code for date	09/01	JK
5-6	M0090 (Date assessment completed) —2 digit year	2008	08

Position	Definition	Actual Value	Resulting Code
7-8	M0090 (Date assessment completed) —code for date	01/01	AA
9	M0100 (Reason for assessment)	04	4
10	M0110 (Episode Timing)	01	1
11	Clinical severity points —under Equation 1	7	G
12	Functional severity points —under Equation 1	2	B
13	Clinical severity points —under Equation 2	13	M
14	Functional severity points —under Equation 2	4	D
15	Clinical severity points —under Equation 3	3	C
16	Functional severity points —under Equation 3	4	D
17	Clinical severity points —under Equation 4	12	L
18	Functional severity points —under Equation 4	7	G

The treatment authorization code that would appear on the claim would be, in this example: 07JK08AA41GBMDCDLG.

In cases of billing for denial notice, using condition code 21, this code may be filled with a placeholder value as defined in section 60.

The investigational device (IDE) revenue code, 0624, is not allowed on HH PPS claims. Therefore, treatment authorization codes associated with IDE items must never be submitted in this field.

The claims-OASIS matching key on the claim will match that submitted on the RAP.

Document Control Number (DCN)
Required - If submitting an adjustment (TOB 3X7) to a previously paid HH PPS claim, the HHA enters the control number assigned to the original HH PPS claim here.

Since HH PPS claims are processed as adjustments to the RAP, Medicare claims processing systems will match all HH PPS claims to their corresponding RAP and populate this field on the electronic claim record automatically. Providers do not need to submit a DCN on all HH PPS claims, only on adjustments to paid claims.

Employer Name
Required only if MSP involved. See Pub. 100-05, Medicare Secondary Payer Manual.

Principal Diagnosis Code
Required - The HHA enters the ICD-9-CM code for the principal diagnosis. The code must be reported according to Official ICD-9-CM Guidelines for Coding and Reporting, as required by the Health Insurance Portability and Accountability Act (HIPAA). The code may be the full ICD-9-CM diagnosis code, including all five digits where applicable. Where the proper code has fewer than five digits, the HHA does not fill it with zeros.

The ICD-9-CM code and principle diagnosis reported must match the primary diagnosis code reported on the OASIS form item M1020 (Primary Diagnosis).

The principal diagnosis code on the claim will match that submitted on the RAP.

Other Diagnosis Codes
Required - The HHA enters the full ICD-9-CM codes for up to eight additional conditions if they coexisted at the time of the establishment of the plan of care. These codes may not duplicate the principal diagnosis as an additional or secondary diagnosis.

For other diagnoses, the diagnoses and ICD-9-CM codes reported on the claim must match the additional diagnoses reported on the OASIS, form item M1022 (Other Diagnoses). In listing the diagnoses, the HHA places them in order to best reflect the seriousness of the patient's condition and to justify the disciplines and services provided in accordance with the Official ICD-9-CM Guidelines for Coding and Reporting. The sequence of codes should follow ICD-9-CM guidelines for reporting manifestation codes. Therefore, if a manifestation code is part of the primary diagnosis, the first two diagnoses should match and appear in the same sequence on both forms. Medicare does not have any additional requirements regarding the reporting or sequence of the codes beyond those contained in ICD-9-CM guidelines.

Diagnosis codes in OASIS form item M1024, which reports Payment Diagnoses, are not directly reported in any field of the claim form. If under ICD-9-CM coding guidelines the codes reported in these OASIS items must be reported as Other Diagnoses, the codes may be repeated in OASIS form item M1022 and will be reported on the claim. In other circumstances, the codes reported in payment diagnosis fields in OASIS may not appear on the claim form at all.

Attending Provider Name and Identifiers
Required - The HHA enters the name and provider identifier of the attending physician that has signed the plan of care.

Remarks
Conditional - Remarks are required only in cases where the claim is cancelled or adjusted.

100-4, 10, 90.1
Osteoporosis Injections as HHA Benefit

A - Billing Requirements
The administration of the drug is included in the charge for the skilled nursing visit billed under bill type 32X or 33X, as appropriate. The cost of the drug is billed under bill type 34X, using revenue code 0636. Drugs that have the ingredient calcitonin are billed using HCPCS code J0630. Drugs that have the ingredient teriparatide may be billed using HCPCS code J3110, if all existing guidelines for coverage under the home health benefit are met. All other osteoporosis drugs that are FDA approved and are awaiting an HCPCS code must use the miscellaneous code of J3490 until a specific HCPCS code is approved for use.

HCPCS code J0630 is defined as up to 400 units. Therefore, the provider must calculate units for the bill as follows:

Units Furnished During Billing Period	Units of Service Entry on Bill
100-400	1
401-800	2
801-1200	3
1201-1600	4
1601-2000	5
2001-2400	6

HCPCS code J3110 is defined as 10 mcg. Providers should report 1 unit for each 10 mcg dose provided during the billing period.

These codes are paid on a reasonable cost basis, using the provider's submitted charges to make initial payments, which are subject to annual cost settlement.

Coverage requirements for osteoporosis drugs are found in Pub. 100-02, Medicare Benefit Policy Manual, chapter 7, section 50.4.3. Coverage requirements for the home health benefit in general are found in Pub. 100-02, Medicare Benefit Policy Manual, chapter 7, section 30.

B - Denial Messages
If the claim for an osteoporosis drug is denied because it was not an injectable drug approved by the FDA, the Medicare contractor shall use the appropriate message below on the MSN:

MSN Message 6.2: "Drugs not specifically classified as effective by the Food and Drug Administration are not covered."

If the claim for an osteoporosis injection is denied because the patient did not meet the requirements for coverage, the Medicare contractor shall use:

MSN message 6.5, which reads, "Medicare cannot pay for this injection because one or more requirements for coverage were not met."

C - Edits
Medicare system edits require that the date of service on a 34X claim for covered osteoporosis drugs falls within the start and end dates of an existing home health PPS episode. Once the system ensures the service dates on the 34X claim fall within an HH PPS episode that is open for the beneficiary on CWF, CWF edits to assure that the provider number on the 34X claim matches the provider number on the episode file. This is to reflect that although the osteoporosis drug is paid separately from the HH PPS episode rate it is included in consolidated billing requirements (see Sec.10.1.25 regarding consolidated billing).

Claims are also edited to assure that the claim is an HH claim (type of bill 34X), the beneficiary is female and that the diagnosis code 733.01 (post-menopausal osteoporosis) is present.

100-4, 11, 10.1
Hospice Pre-Election Evaluation and Counseling Services
Effective January 1, 2005, Medicare allows payment to a hospice for specified hospice pre-election evaluation and counseling services when furnished by a physician who is either the medical director of or employee of the hospice.

Medicare covers a one- time only payment on behalf of a beneficiary who is terminally ill, (defined as having a prognosis of 6 months or less if the disease follows its normal course), has no previous hospice elections, and has not previously received hospice pre-election evaluation and counseling services.

HCPCS code G0337 "Hospice Pre-Election Evaluation and Counseling Services" is used to designate that these services have been provided by the medical director or a physician employed by the hospice. Hospice agencies bill their Medicare contractor with home health and hospice jurisdiction directly using HCPCS G0337 with Revenue Code 0657. No other revenue codes may appear on the claim.

Claims for "Hospice Pre-Election and Counseling Services", HCPCS code G0337, are not subject to the editing usually required on hospice claims to match the claim to an established hospice period. Further, contractors do not apply payments for hospice pre-election evaluation and counseling consultation services to the overall hospice cap amount.

Medicare must ensure that this counseling service occurs only one time per beneficiary by imposing safeguards to detect and prevent duplicate billing for similar services. If "new patient" physician services (HCPCS codes 99201-99205) are submitted by a Medicare contractor to CWF for payment authorization but HCPCS code G0337 (Hospice Pre-Election Evaluation and Counseling Services) has already been approved for a hospice claim for the same beneficiary, for the same date of service, by the same physician, the physician service will be rejected by CWF and the service shall be denied as a duplicate. Medicare contractors use the following messages in this case:

HCPCS code G0337 is only payable when billed on a hospice claim. Contractors shall not make payment for HCPCS code G0337 on professional claims. Contractors shall deny line items on professional claims for HCPCS code G0337 and use the following messages:

100-4, 11, 30.3
Data Required on the Institutional Claim to Medicare Contractor

See Pub. 100-02, Chapter 9, §§10 & 20.2 for coverage requirements for Hospice benefits. This section addresses only the submittal of claims. Before submitting claims, the hospice must submit a Notice of Election (NOE) to the Medicare contractor. See section 20, of this chapter for information on NOE transaction types.

The Social Security Act at §1862 (a)(22) requires that all claims for Medicare payment must be submitted in an electronic form specified by the Secretary of Health and Human Services, unless an exception described at §1862 (h) applies. The electronic form required for billing hospice services is the ANSI X12N 837 Institutional claim transaction. Since the data structure of the 837 transaction is difficult to express in narrative form and to provide assistance to small providers excepted from the electronic claim requirement, the instructions below are given relative to the data element names on the UB-04 (Form CMS-1450) hardcopy form. Each data element name is shown in bold type. Information regarding the form locator numbers that correspond to these data element names and a table to crosswalk UB-04 form locators to the 837 transaction is found in Chapter 25.

Because claim formats serve the needs of many payers, some data elements may not be needed by a particular payer. Detailed information is given only for items required for Medicare hospice claims. Items not listed need not be completed although hospices may complete them when billing multiple payers.

Provider Name, Address, and Telephone Number
The hospice enters this information for their agency.

Type of Bill
This three-digit alphanumeric code gives three specific pieces of information. The first digit identifies the type of facility. The second classifies the type of care. The third indicates the sequence of this bill in this particular benefit period. It is referred to as a "frequency" code.

Code Structure

1st Digit - Type of Facility
8 - Special facility (Hospice)

2nd Digit - Classification (Special Facility Only)
1 - Hospice (Nonhospital based)
2 - Hospice (Hospital based)

3rd Digit – Frequency	Definition
0 - Nonpayment/Zero Claims	Used when no payment from Medicare is anticipated.
I - Admit Through Discharge Claim	This code is used for a bill encompassing an entire course of hospice treatment for which the provider expects payment from the payer, i.e., no further bills will be submitted for this patient.
2 - Interim - First Claim	This code is used for the first of an expected series of payment bills for a hospice course of treatment.
3 - Interim - Continuing Claim	This code is used when a payment bill for a hospice course of treatment has already been submitted and further bills are expected to be submitted.

3rd Digit – Frequency	Definition
4 - Interim - Last Claim	This code is used for a payment bill that is the last of a series for a hospice course of treatment. The "Through" date of this bill is the discharge date, transfer date, or date of death.
5 - Late Charges	Use this code for late charges that need to be billed. Late charges can be submitted only for revenue codes not on the original bill.
	Effective April 1, 2012, hospice late charge claims are no longer accepted by Medicare. Providers should use type of bill frequency 7. See below.
7 - Replacement of Prior Claim	This code is used by the provider when it wants to correct a previously submitted bill. This is the code used on the corrected or "new" bill.
	For additional information on replacement bills see Chapter 3.
8 - Void/Cancel of a Prior Claim	This code is used to cancel a previously processed claim.
	For additional information on void/cancel bills see Chapter 3.

Statement Covers Period (From-Through)
The hospice shows the beginning and ending dates of the period covered by this bill in numeric fields (MM-DD-YY). The hospice does not show days before the patient? entitlement began. Since the 12-month hospice "cap period" (see §80.2) ends each year on October 31, hospices must submit separate bills for October and November.

Patient Name/Identifier
The hospice enters the beneficiary's name exactly as it appears on the Medicare card.

Patient Address
Patient Birth date
Patient Sex
The hospice enters the appropriate address, date of birth and gender information describing the beneficiary.

Admission/Start of Care Date
The hospice enters the admission date, which must be the same date as the effective date of the hospice election or change of election. The date of admission may not precede the physician's certification by more than 2 calendar days.

The admission date stays the same on all continuing claims for the same hospice election.

Patient Discharge Status
This code indicates the patient? status as of the 'Through' date of the billing period. The hospice enters the most appropriate National Uniform Billing Committee (NUBC) approved code.

Note that patient discharge status code 20 is not used on hospice claims. If the patient has died during the billing period, use codes 40, 41 or 42 as appropriate.

Medicare regulations at 42 CFR 418.26 define three reasons for discharge from hospice care:

1) The beneficiary moves out of the hospice's service area or transfers to another hospice,

2) The hospice determines that the beneficiary is no longer terminally ill or

3) The hospice determines the beneficiary meets their internal policy regarding discharge for cause.

Each of these discharge situations requires different coding on Medicare claims.

Reason 1: A beneficiary may move out of the hospice's service area either with, or without, a transfer to another hospice. In the case of a discharge when the beneficiary moves out of the hospice's service area without a transfer, the hospice uses the NUBC approved discharge status code that best describes the beneficiary's situation and appends condition code 52. The hospice does not report occurrence code 42 on their claim. This discharge claim will terminate the beneficiary's current hospice benefit period as of the 'Through' date on the claim. The beneficiary may re-elect the hospice benefit at any time as long they remain eligible for the benefit.

In the case of a discharge when the beneficiary moves out of the hospice's service area and transfers to another hospice, the hospice uses discharge status code 50 or 51, depending on whether the beneficiary is transferring to home hospice or hospice in a medical facility. The hospice does not report occurrence code 42 on their claim. This discharge claim does not terminate the beneficiary's current hospice benefit period. The admitting hospice submits a transfer Notice of Election (type of bill 8xC) after the transfer has occurred and the beneficiary's hospice benefit is not affected.

Reason 2: In the case of a discharge when the hospice determines the beneficiary is no longer terminally ill, the hospice uses the NUBC approved discharge status code that best describes the beneficiary's situation. The hospice does not report occurrence code 42 on their claim. This discharge claim will terminate the beneficiary's current hospice benefit period as of the "Through" date on the claim.

Reason 3: In the case of a discharge for cause, the hospice uses the NUBC approved discharge status code that best describes the beneficiary's situation. The hospice does not report occurrence code 42 on their claim. Instead, the hospice reports condition code H2 to indicate a discharge for cause. The effect of this discharge claim on the beneficiary's current hospice benefit period depends on the discharge status.

If the beneficiary is transferred to another hospice (discharge status codes 50 or 51) the claim does not terminate the beneficiary's current hospice benefit period. The admitting hospice submits a transfer Notice of Election (type of bill 8xC) after the transfer has occurred and the beneficiary's hospice benefit is not affected. If any other appropriate discharge status code is used, this discharge claim will terminate the beneficiary's current hospice benefit period as of the "Through" date on the claim. The beneficiary may re-elect the hospice benefit if they are certified as terminally ill and eligible for the benefit again in the future and are willing to be compliant with care.

If the beneficiary has chosen to revoke their hospice election, the provider uses the NUBC approved discharge patient status code and the occurrence code 42 indicating the date the beneficiary revoked the benefit. The beneficiary may re-elect the hospice benefit if they are certified as terminally ill and eligible for the benefit again in the future. Discharge Reason

Discharge Reason
Coding Required in Addition to Patient Status Code

Beneficiary Revokes
Occurrence Code 42

Beneficiary Transfers Hospices
Patient Status Code 50 or 51; no other indicator

Beneficiary No Longer Terminally Ill
No other indicator

Beneficiary Discharged for Cause
Condition code H2

Beneficiary Moves Out of Service Area
Condition code 52

Untimely Face-to-Face Encounters and Discharge
When a required face-to-face encounter occurs prior to, but no more than 30 calendar days prior to, the third benefit period recertification and every benefit period recertification thereafter, it is considered timely. A timely face-to-face encounter would be evident when examining the face-to-face attestation, which is part of the recertification, as that attestation includes the date of the encounter. If the required face-to-face encounter is not timely, the hospice would be unable to recertify the patient as being terminally ill, and the patient would cease to be eligible for the Medicare hospice benefit. In such instances, the hospice must discharge the patient from the Medicare hospice benefit because he or she is not considered terminally ill for Medicare purposes.

When a discharge from the Medicare hospice benefit occurs due to failure to perform a required face-to-face encounter timely, the claim should include the most appropriate patient discharge status code. The hospice can re-admit the patient to the Medicare hospice benefit once the required encounter occurs, provided the patient continues to meet all of the eligibility requirements and the patient (or representative) files an election statement in accordance with CMS regulations. Where the only reason the patient ceases to be eligible for the Medicare hospice benefit is the hospice's failure to meet the face-to-face requirement, we would expect the hospice to continue to care for the patient at its own expense until the required encounter occurs, enabling the hospice to re-establish Medicare eligibility.

Occurrence span code 77 does not apply to the above described situations when the face-to-face encounter has not occurred timely.

While the face-to-face encounter itself must occur no more than 30 calendar days prior to the start of the third benefit period recertification and each subsequent recertification, its accompanying attestation must be completed before the claim is submitted.

Condition Codes
The hospice enters any appropriate NUBC approved code(s) identifying conditions related to this bill that may affect processing.

Codes listed below are only those most frequently applicable to hospice claims. For a complete list of codes, see the NUBC manual.

| 07 | Treatment of Non-terminal Condition for Hospice | Code indicates the patient has elected hospice care but the provider is not treating the terminal condition, and is, therefore, requesting regular Medicare payment. |

| 20 | Beneficiary Requested Billing | Code indicates the provider realizes the services on this bill are at a noncovered level of care or otherwise excluded from coverage, but the beneficiary has requested a formal determination. |
| 21 | Billing for Denial Notice | Code indicates the provider realizes services are at a noncovered level of care or excluded, but requests a denial notice from Medicare in order to bill Medicaid or other insurers. |

Discharge by a Hospice Provider for Cause.
Note: Used by the provider to indicate the patient meets the hospice's documented policy addressing discharges for cause.

| 52 | Out of Hospice Service Area | Code indicates the patient is discharged for moving out of the hospice service area. This can include patients who relocate or who go on vacation outside of the hospice's service area, or patients who are admitted to a hospital or SNF that does not have contractual arrangements with the hospice. |

Occurrence Codes and Dates
The hospice enters any appropriate NUBC approved code(s) and associated date(s) defining specific event(s) relating to this billing period. Event codes are two numeric digits, and dates are six numeric digits (MM-DD-YY). If there are more occurrences than there are spaces on the form, use the occurrence span code fields to record additional occurrences and dates.

Codes listed below are only those most frequently applicable to hospice claims. For a complete list of codes, see the NUBC manual.

Code	Title	Definition
23	Cancellation of Hospice Election Period (Medicare contractor USE ONLY)	Code indicates date on which a hospice period of election is cancelled by a Medicare contractor as opposed to revocation by the beneficiary.
24	Date Insurance Denied	Code indicates the date of receipt of a denial of coverage by a higher priority payer.
27	Date of Hospice Certification or Re-Certification	Code indicates the date of certification or re-certification of the hospice benefit period, beginning with the first 2 initial benefit periods of 90 days each and the subsequent 60-day benefit periods.

Note regarding transfers from one hospice to another hospice: If a patient is in the first certification period when they transfer to another hospice, the receiving hospice would use the same certification date as the previous hospice until the next certification period. However, if they were in the next certification at the time of transfer, then they would enter that date in the Occurrence Code 27 and date.

Code	Title	Definition
42	Date of Termination of Hospice Benefit	Enter code to indicate the date on which beneficiary terminated his/her election to receive hospice benefits. This code can be used only when the beneficiary has revoked the benefit. It is not used in transfer situations.

Occurrence code 27 is reported on the claim for the billing period in which the certification or re-certification was obtained. When the re-certification is late and not obtained during the month it was due, the occurrence span code 77 should be reported with the through date of the span code equal to the through date of the claim.

Occurrence Span Code and Dates
The hospice enters any appropriate NUBC approved code(s) and associated beginning and ending date(s) defining a specific event relating to this billing period are shown. Event codes are two alphanumeric digits and dates are shown numerically as MM-DD-YY.

Codes listed below are only those most frequently applicable to hospice claims. For a complete list of codes, see the NUBC manual.

Code	Title	Definition
M2	Dates of Inpatient Respite Care	Code indicates From/Through dates of a period of inpatient respite care for hospice patients to differentiate separate respite periods of less than 5 days each. M2 is used when respite care is provided more than once during a benefit period.

Code	Title	Definition
77	Provider Liability ?tilization Charged	Code indicates From/Through dates for a period of non-covered hospice care for which the provider accepts payment liability (other than for medical necessity or custodial care).

Hospices must use occurrence span code 77 to identify days of care that are not covered by Medicare due to untimely physician recertification. This is particularly important when the non-covered days fall at the beginning of a billing period.

Value Codes and Amounts

The hospice enters any appropriate NUBC approved code(s) and the associated value amounts identifying numeric information related to this bill that may affect processing.

The most commonly used value codes on hospice claims are value codes 61 and G8, which are used to report the location of the site of hospice services. Otherwise, value codes are commonly used only to indicate Medicare is secondary to another payer. For detailed information on reporting Medicare secondary payer information, see the Medicare Secondary Payer Manual.

Code	Title	Definition
61	Place of Residence where Service is Furnished (Routine Home Care and Continuous Home Care)	MSA or Core-Based Statistical Area (CBSA) number (or rural State code) of the location where the hospice service is delivered.

A residence can be an inpatient facility if an individual uses that facility as a place of residence. It is the level of care that is required and not the location where hospice services are provided that determines payment. In other words, if an individual resides in a freestanding hospice facility and requires routine home care, then claims are submitted for routine home care.

Hospices must report value code 61 when billing revenue codes 0651 and 0652.

G8

Facility where Inpatient Hospice

MSA or Core Based Statistical Area (CBSA)

Service is Delivered (General Inpatient and Inpatient Respite Care).

number (or rural State code) of the facility where inpatient hospice services are delivered.

Hospices must report value code G8 when billing revenue codes 0655 and 0656.

If hospice services are provided to the beneficiary in more than one CBSA area during the billing period, the hospice reports the CBSA that applies at the end of the billing period. For routine home care and continuous home care (e.g., the beneficiary's residence changes between locations in different CBSAs), report the CBSA of the beneficiary's residence at the end of the billing period. For general inpatient and inpatient respite care (e.g., the beneficiary is served in inpatient facilities in different CBSAs), report the CBSA of the latest facility that served the beneficiary. If the beneficiary receives both home and inpatient care during the billing period, the latest home CBSA is reported with value code 61 and the latest facility CBSA is reported with value code G8.

Revenue Codes

The hospice assigns a revenue code for each type of service provided and enters the appropriate four-digit numeric revenue code to explain each charge.

For claims with dates of service before July 1, 2008, hospices only reported the revenue codes in the table below. Effective on claims with dates of service on or after January 1, 2008, additional revenue codes will be reported describing the visits provided under each level of care. However, Medicare payment will continue to be reflected only on claim lines with the revenue codes in this table.

Hospice claims are required to report separate line items for the level of care each time the level of care changes. This includes revenue codes 0651, 0655 and 0656. For example, if a patient begins the month receiving routine home care followed by a period of general inpatient care and then later returns to routine home care all in the same month, in addition to the one line reporting the general inpatient care days, there should be two separate line items for routine home care. Each routine home care line reports a line item date of service to indicate the first date that level of care began for that consecutive period. This will ensure visits and calls reported on the claim will be associated with the level of care being billed.

Code	Description	Standard Abbreviation
0651*	Routine Home Care	RTN Home
0652*	Continuous Home Care	CTNS Home
0655***	Inpatient Respite Care	IP Respite

A minimum of 8 hours of primarily nursing care within a 24-hour period. The 8-hours of care do not need to be continuous within the 24-hour period, but a need for an aggregate of 8 hours of primarily nursing care is required. Nursing care must be provided by a registered nurse or a licensed practical nurse. If skilled intervention is required for less than 8 aggregate hours (or less than 32 units) within a 24 hour period, then the care rendered would be covered as a routine home care day. Services provided by a nurse practitioner as the attending physician are not included in the CHC computation nor is care that is not directly related to the crisis included in the computation. CHC billing should reflect direct patient care during a period of crisis and should not reflect time related to staff working hours, time taken for meal breaks, time used for educating staff, time used to report etc.

Code	Description	Standard Abbreviation
0656***	General Inpatient Care	GNL IP
0657**	Physician Services	PHY SER (must be accompanied by a physician procedure code)

- * Reporting of value code 61 is required with these revenue codes.

-**Reporting of modifier GV is required with this revenue code when billing physician services performed by a nurse practitioner.

-***Reporting of value code G8 is required with these revenue codes.

NOTE: Hospices use revenue code 0657 to identify hospice charges for services furnished to patients by physician or nurse practitioner employees, or physicians or nurse practitioners receiving compensation from the hospice. Physician services performed by a nurse practitioner require the addition of the modifier GV in conjunction with revenue code 0657. Procedure codes are required in order for the Medicare contractor to determine the reimbursement rate for the physician services. Appropriate procedure codes are available from the Medicare contractor.

Effective on claims with dates of service on or after July 1, 2008, hospices must report the number of visits that were provided to the beneficiary in the course of delivering the hospice levels of care billed with the codes above. Charges for these codes will be reported on the appropriate level of care line. Total number of patient care visits is to be reported by the discipline (registered nurse, nurse practitioner, licensed nurse, home health aide (also known as a hospice aide), social worker, physician or nurse practitioner serving as the beneficiary's attending physician) for each week at each location of service. If visits are provided in multiple sites, a separate line for each site and for each discipline will be required. The total number of visits does not imply the total number of activities or interventions provided. If patient care visits in a particular discipline are not provided under a given level of care or service location, do not report a line for the corresponding revenue code.

To constitute a visit, the discipline, (as defined above) must have provided care to the beneficiary. Services provided by a social worker to the beneficiary's family also constitute a visit. For example, phone calls, documentation in the medical/clinical record, interdisciplinary group meetings, obtaining physician orders, rounds in a facility or any other activity that is not related to the provision of items or services to a beneficiary, do not count towards a visit to be placed on the claim. In addition, the visit must be reasonable and necessary for the palliation and management of the terminal illness and related conditions as described in the patient's plan of care.

Example 1: Week 1: A visit by the RN was made to the beneficiary's home on Monday and Wednesday where the nurse assessed the patient, verified effect of pain medications, provided patient teaching, obtained vital signs and documented in the medical record. A home health aide assisted the patient with a bath on Tuesday and Thursday. There were no social work or physician visits. Thus for that week there were 2 visits provided by the nurse and 2 by the home health aide. Since there were no visits by the social worker or by the physician, there would not be any line items for each of those disciplines.

Example 2: If a hospice patient is receiving routine home care while residing in a nursing home, the hospice would record visits for all of its physicians, nurses, social workers, and home health aides who visit the patient to provide care for the palliation and management of the terminal illness and related conditions, as described in the patient's plan of care. In this example the nursing home is acting as the patient's home. Only the patient care provided by the hospice staff constitutes a visit.

Hospices must enter the following visit revenue codes, when applicable as of July 1, 2008:

055x Skilled Nursing	Required detail: The earliest date of service this discipline was provided during the delivery of each level of care in each service location, service units which represent the number of visits provided in that location, and a charge amount.
056x Medical Social Services	Required detail: The earliest date of service this discipline was provided during the delivery of each level of care in each service location, service units which represent the number of visits provided in that location, and a charge amount.

| 057x Home Health Aide | | Required detail: The earliest date of service this discipline was provided during the delivery of each level of care in each service location, service units which represent the number of visits provided in that location, and a charge amount. |

For services provided on or after January 1, 2010, hospices report social worker phone calls and visits performed by hospice staff for other than General Inpatient (GIP) care in 15 minute increments using the following revenue codes and associated HCPCS:

Revenue Code	Required HCPCS	Required Detail
042x Physical Therapy	G0151	Required detail: Each visit is identified on a separate line item with the appropriate line item date of service and a charge amount. The units reported on the claim are the multiplier for the total time of the visit defined in the HCPCS description.
043x Occupational Therapy	G0152	Required detail: Each visit is identified on a separate line item with the appropriate line item date of service and a charge amount. The units reported on the claim are the multiplier for the total time of the visit defined in the HCPCS description.
044x Speech Therapy - Language Pathology	G0153	Required detail: Each visit is identified on a separate line item with the appropriate line item date of service and a charge amount. The units reported on the claim are the multiplier for the total time of the visit defined in the HCPCS description.
055x Skilled Nursing	G0154	Required detail: Each visit is identified on a separate line item with the appropriate line item date of service and a charge amount. The units reported on the claim are the multiplier for the total time of the visit defined in the HCPCS description.
056x Medical Social Services	G0155	Required detail: Each visit is identified on a separate line item with the appropriate line item date of service and a charge amount. The units reported on the claim are the multiplier for the total time of the visit defined in the HCPCS description.
0569 Other Medical Social Services	G0155	Required detail: Each social service phone call is identified on a separate line item with the appropriate line item date of service and a charge amount. The units reported on the claim are the multiplier for the total time of the call defined in the HCPCS description.
057x Aide	G0156	Required detail: Each visit is identified on a separate line item with the appropriate line item date of service and a charge amount. The units reported on the claim are the multiplier the total time of the visit defined in the HCPCS description

Visits by registered nurses, licensed vocational nurses and nurse practitioners (unless the nurse practitioner is acting as the beneficiary's attending physician) are reported under revenue code 055x.

All visits to provide care related to the palliation and management of the terminal illness or related conditions, whether provided by hospice employees or provided under arrangement, must be reported. The two exceptions are related to General Inpatient Care and Respite care. CMS is not requiring hospices to report visit data at this time for visits made by non-hospice staff providing General Inpatient Care or respite care in contract facilities. However, General Inpatient Care or respite care visits related to the palliation and management of the terminal illness or related conditions provided by hospice staff in contract facilities must be reported, and all General Inpatient Care and respite care visits related to the palliation and management of the terminal illness or related conditions provided in hospice-owned facilities must be reported.

Charges associated with the reported visits are covered under the hospice bundled payment and reflected in the payment for the level of care billed on the claim. No additional payment is made on the visit revenue lines. The visit charges will be identified on the provider remittance advice notice with remittance code 97 "Payment adjusted because the benefit for this service is included in the payment / allowance for another service/procedure that has already been adjudicated."

Effective January 1, 2010, Medicare will require hospices to report additional detail for visits on their claims. For all Routine Home Care (RHC), Continuous Home Care (CHC) and Respite care billing, Medicare hospice claims should report each visit performed by nurses, aides, and social

workers who are employed by the hospice, and their associated time per visit in the number of 15 minute increments, on a separate line. The visits should be reported using revenue codes 055x (nursing services), 057x (aide services), or 056x (medical social services), with the time reported using the associated HCPCS G-code in the range G0154 to G0156. Hospices should report in the unit field on the line level the units as a multiplier of the visit time defined in the HCPCS description.

Additionally, providers should begin reporting each RHC, CHC, and Respite visit performed by physical therapists, occupational therapists, and speech-language therapists and their associated time per visit in the number of 15 minute increments on a separate line. Providers should use existing revenue codes 042x for physical therapy, 043x for occupational therapy, and 044x for speech language therapy, in addition to the appropriate HCPCS G-code for recording of visit length in 15 minute increments. HCPCS G-codes G0151 to G0153 will be used to describe the therapy discipline and visit time reported on a particular line item. Hospices should report in the unit field on the line level the units as a multiplier of the visit time defined in the HCPCS description. If a hospice patient is receiving Respite care in a contract facility, visit and time data by non-hospice staff should not be reported.

Social worker phone calls made to the patient or the patient's family should be reported using revenue code 0569, and HCPCS G-code G0155 for the length of the call, with each call being a separate line item. Hospices should report in the unit field on the line level the units as a multiplier of the visit time defined in the HCPCS description. Only phone calls that are necessary for the palliation and management of the terminal illness and related conditions as described in the patient's plan of care (such as counseling, or speaking with a patient's family or arranging for a placement) should be reported. Report only social worker phone calls related to providing and or coordinating care to the patient and family and documented as such in the clinical records.

When recording any visit or social worker phone call time, providers should sum the time for each visit or call, rounding to the nearest 15 minute increment. Providers should not include travel time or documentation time in the time recorded for any visit or call. Additionally, hospices may not include interdisciplinary group time in time and visit reporting.

HCPCS/Accommodation Rates/HIPPS Rate Codes

For services provided on or before December 31, 2006, HCPCS codes are required only to report procedures on service lines for attending physician services (revenue 657). Level of care revenue codes (651, 652, 655 or 656) do not require HCPCS coding.

For services provided on or after January 1, 2007, hospices must also report a HCPCS code along with each level of care revenue code (651, 652, 655 and 656) to identify the type of service location where that level of care was provided.

The following HCPCS codes will be used to report the type of service location for hospice services:

HCPCS Code	Definition
Q5001	HOSPICE CARE PROVIDED IN PATIENT'S HOME/RESIDENCE
Q5002	HOSPICE CARE PROVIDED IN ASSISTED LIVING FACILITY
Q5003	HOSPICE CARE PROVIDED IN NURSING LONG TERM CARE FACILITY (LTC) OR NON-SKILLED NURSING FACILITY (NF)
Q5004	HOSPICE CARE PROVIDED IN SKILLED NURSING FACILITY (SNF)
Q5005	HOSPICE CARE PROVIDED IN INPATIENT HOSPITAL
Q5006	HOSPICE CARE PROVIDED IN INPATIENT HOSPICE FACILITY
Q5007	HOSPICE CARE PROVIDED IN LONG TERM CARE HOSPITAL (LTCH)
Q5008	HOSPICE CARE PROVIDED IN INPATIENT PSYCHIATRIC FACILITY
Q5009	HOSPICE CARE PROVIDED IN PLACE NOT OTHERWISE SPECIFIED (NOS)
Q5010	HOSPICE HOME CARE PROVIDED IN A HOSPICE FACILITY

If care is rendered at multiple locations, each location is to be identified on the claim with a corresponding HCPCS code. For example, routine home care may be provided for a portion of the billing period in the patient's residence and another portion in an assisted living facility. In this case, report one revenue code 651 line with HCPCS code Q5001 and the number of days of routine home care provided in the residence and another revenue code 651 line with HCPCS code Q5002 and the number of days of routine home care provided in the assisted living facility.

Q5003 is to be used for hospice patients in an unskilled nursing facility (NF) or hospice patients in the NF portion of a dually certified nursing facility, who are receiving unskilled care from the facility staff.

Q5004 is to be used for hospice patients in a skilled nursing facility (SNF), or hospice patients in the SNF portion of a dually certified nursing facility, who are receiving skilled care from the facility staff.

NOTE: Q5003 should be used for hospice patients located in a NF; many of these patients may also have Medicaid. Q5004 should be used when the hospice patient is in a SNF, and receiving skilled care from the facility staff, such as would occur in a GIP stay. For Q5004 to be used, the facility would have to be certified as a SNF. Some facilities are dually certified as a SNF and a NF; the hospice will have to determine what level of care the facility staff is providing (skilled or unskilled) in deciding which type of bed the patient is in, and therefore which code to use. When a patient is in the NF portion of a dually certified nursing facility, and receiving only unskilled care from the facility staff, Q5003 should be reported. Note that GIP care that is provided in a nursing facility can only be given in a SNF, because GIP requires a skilled level of care.

These service location HCPCS codes are not required on revenue code lines describing the visits provided under each level of care (e.g. 055X, 056X, 057X).

Service Date

The HIPAA standard 837 Institutional claim format requires line item dates of service for all outpatient claims. Medicare classifies hospice claims as outpatient claims (see Chapter 1, §60.4). For services provided on or before December 31, 2006, CMS allows hospices to satisfy the line item date of service requirement by placing any valid date within the Statement Covers Period dates on line items on hospice claims.

For services provided on or after January 1, 2007, service date reporting requirements will vary between continuous home care lines (revenue code 652) and other revenue code lines.

Revenue code 652 - report a separately dated line item for each day that continuous home care is provided, reporting the number of hours, or parts of hours rounded to 15-minute increments, of continuous home care that was provided on that date.

Other payment revenue codes - report a separate line for each level of care provided at each service location type, as described in the instructions for HCPCS coding reported above. Hospices report the earliest date that each level of care was provided at each service location. Attending physician services should be individually dated, reporting the date that each HCPCS code billed was delivered.

Non-payment service revenue codes - report dates as described in the table above under Revenue Codes.

For services provided on or after January 1, 2010, hospices report social worker phone calls and visits performed by hospice staff for other than GIP care as separate line items for each with the appropriate line item date of service. GIP visit reporting has not changed with the January 2010 update. GIP visits will continue to be reported as the number of visits per week.

For service visits that begin in one calendar day and span into the next calendar day, report one visit using the date the visit ended as the service date.

Service Units

The hospice enters the number of units for each type of service. Units are measured in days for revenue codes 651, 655, and 656, in hours for revenue code 652, and in procedures for revenue code 657. For services provided on or after January 1, 2007, hours for revenue code 652 are reported in 15-minute increments. For services provided on or after January 1, 2008, units for visit discipline revenue codes are measured by the number of visits.

For services provided on or after January 1, 2010, hospices report social worker phone calls and visits performed by hospice staff for other than GIP care as a separate line item with the appropriate line item date of service and the units as an increment of 15 minutes. GIP visit reporting has not changed with the January 2010 update. The units for visits under GIP level of care continue to reflect the number of visits per week.

Report in the unit field on the line level the units as a multiplier of the visit time defined in the HCPCS description.

Total Charges

The hospice enters the total charge for the service described on each revenue code line. This information is being collected for purposes of research and will not affect the amount of reimbursement.

Payer Name

The hospice identifies the appropriate payer(s) for the claim.

National Provider Identifier - Billing Provider

The hospice enters its own National Provider Identifier (NPI).

Principal Diagnosis Code

The hospice enters diagnosis coding as required by ICD-9-CM Coding Guidelines. Hospices may not report V-codes as the primary diagnosis on hospice claims. The principal diagnosis code describes the terminal illness of the hospice patient and V-codes do not describe terminal conditions.

Other Diagnosis Codes

The hospice enters diagnosis coding as required by ICD-9-CM Coding Guidelines.

Attending Provider Name and Identifiers

For claims with dates of service before January 1, 2010, the hospice enters the National Provider Identifier (NPI) and name of the physician currently responsible for certifying the terminal illness, and signing the individual's plan of care for medical care and treatment.

For claims with dates of service on or after January 1, 2010 the hospice shall enter the NPI and name of the attending physician designated by the patient as having the most significant role in the determination and delivery of the patient's medical care.

Other Provider Name and Identifiers

For claims with dates of service before January 1, 2010, if the attending physician is a nurse practitioner, the hospice enters the NPI and name of the nurse practitioner.

For claims with dates of service on or after January 1, 2010, the hospice enters the NPI and name of the hospice physician responsible for certifying that the patient is terminally ill, with a life expectancy of 6 months or less if the disease runs its normal course. Note: Both the attending physician and other physician fields should be completed unless the patient's designated attending physician is the same as the physician certifying the terminal illness. When the attending physician is also the physician certifying the terminal illness, only the attending physician is required to be reported.

Note: for electronic claims using version 5010 or later, this information is reported in Loop ID 2310F – Referring Provider Name.

100-4, 11, 40.1.3.1

Care Plan Oversight

Care plan oversight (CPO) exists where there is physician supervision of patients under care of hospices that require complex and multidisciplinary care modalities involving regular physician development and/or revision of care plans. Implicit in the concept of CPO is the expectation that the physician has coordinated an aspect of the patient's care with the hospice during the month for which CPO services were billed.

For a physician or NP employed by or under arrangement with a hospice agency, CPO functions are incorporated and are part of the hospice per diem payment and as such may not be separately billed.

For information on separately billable CPO services by the attending physician or nurse practitioner see Chapter 12, 180 of this manual.

100-4, 11, 100.1

Billing for Denial of Hospice Room and Board Charges

Hospice providers wishing to receive a line item denial for room and board charges may submit the charges as non-covered using revenue code 0659 with HCPCS A9270 and modifier GY on an otherwise covered hospice claim.

100-4, 12, 30.4

Cardiovascular System (Codes 92950-93799)

A. Echocardiography Contrast Agents

Effective October 1, 2000, physicians may separately bill for contrast agents used in echocardiography. Physicians should use HCPCS Code A9700 (Supply of Injectable Contrast Material for Use in Echocardiography, per study). The type of service code is 9. This code will be carrier-priced.

B. Electronic Analyses of Implantable Cardioverter-defibrillators and Pacemakers

The CPT codes 93731, 93734, 93741 and 93743 are used to report electronic analyses of single or dual chamber pacemakers and single or dual chamber implantable cardioverterdefibrillators. In the office, a physician uses a device called a programmer to obtain information about the status and performance of the device and to evaluate the patient's cardiac rhythm and response to the implanted device. Advances in information technology now enable physicians to evaluate patients with implanted cardiac devices without requiring the patient to be present in the physician's office. Using a manufacturer's specific monitor/transmitter, a patient can send complete device data and specific cardiac data to a distant receiving station or secure Internet server. The electronic analysis of cardiac device data that is remotely obtained provides immediate and long-term data on the device and clinical data on the patient's cardiac functioning equivalent to that obtained during an in-office evaluation. Physicians should report the electronic analysis of an implanted cardiac device using remotely obtained data as described above with CPT code 93731, 93734, 93741 or 93743, depending on the type of cardiac device implanted in the patient.

100-4, 12, 30.6.15.4

Power Mobility Devices (PMDs) (Code G0372)

Section 302(a)(2)(E)(iv) of the Medicare Prescription Drug, Improvement, and Modernization Act of 2003 (MMA) sets forth revised conditions for Medicare payment of Power Mobility Devices (PMDs). This section of the MMA states that payment for motorized or power wheelchairs may not be made unless a physician (as defined in §1861(r)(1) of the Act), a physician assistant, nurse practitioner, or a clinical nurse specialist (as those terms are defined in §1861(aa)(5)) has conducted a face-to-face examination of the beneficiary and written a prescription for the PMD.

Payment for the history and physical examination will be made through the appropriate evaluation and management (E&M) code corresponding to the history and physical examination of the patient. Due to the MMA requirement that the physician or treating practitioner create a written prescription and a regulatory requirement that the physician or treating practitioner prepare pertinent parts of the medical record for submission to the durable medical equipment supplier, code G0372 (physician service required to establish and document the need for a power mobility device)has been established to recognize additional physician services and resources required to establish and document the need for the PMD.

The G code indicates that all of the information necessary to document the PMD prescription is included in the medical record, and the prescription and supporting documentation is delivered to the PMD supplier within 30 days after the face-to-face examination.

Effective October 25, 2005, G0372 will be used to recognize additional physician services and resources required to establish and document the need for the PMD and will be added to the Medicare physician fee schedule.

100-4, 12, 60

Payment for Pathology Services
B3-15020, AB-01-47 (CR1499)

A. General Payment Rule
Payment may be made under the fee schedule for the professional component of physician laboratory or physician pathology services furnished to hospital inpatients or outpatients by hospital physicians or by independent laboratories, if they qualify as the reassignee for the physician service.. Payment may be made under the fee schedule, as noted below, for the technical component (TC) of pathology services furnished by an independent laboratory to hospital inpatients or outpatients. Payment may be made under the fee schedule for the technical component of physician pathology services furnished by an independent laboratory, or a hospital if it is acting as an independent laboratory, to non-hospital patients. The Medicare physician fee schedule identifies those physician laboratory or physician pathology services that have a technical component service.

CMS published a final regulation in 1999 that would no longer allow independent laboratories to bill under the physician fee schedule for the TC of physician pathology services. The implementation of this regulation was delayed by Section 542 of the Benefits and Improvement and Protection Act of 2000 (BIPA). Section 542 allows the Medicare carrier to continue to pay for the TC of physician pathology services when an independent laboratory furnishes this service to an inpatient or outpatient of a covered hospital. This provision is applicable to TC services furnished in 2001, 2002, 2003, 2004, 2005 or 2006.

For this provision, a covered hospital is a hospital that had an arrangement with an independent laboratory that was in effect as of July 22, 1999, under which a laboratory furnished the TC of physician pathology services to fee-for-service Medicare beneficiaries who were hospital inpatients or outpatients, and submitted claims for payment for the TC to a carrier. The TC could have been submitted separately or combined with the professional component and reported as a combined service.

The term, fee-for-service Medicare beneficiary, means an individual who:

- Is entitled to benefits under Part A or enrolled under Part B of title XVIII or both; and
- Is not enrolled in any of the following: A Medicare + Choice plan under Part C of such title; a plan offered by an eligible organization under 1876 of the Social Security Act; a program of all-inclusive care for the elderly under 1894; or a social health maintenance organization demonstration project established under Section 4108 of the Omnibus Budget Reconciliation Act of 1987.

In implementing Section 542, the carriers should consider as independent laboratories those entities that it has previously recognized as independent laboratories. An independent laboratory that has acquired another independent laboratory that had an arrangement of July 22, 1999, with a covered hospital, can bill the TC of physician pathology services for that hospital's inpatients and outpatients under the physician fee schedule.

An independent laboratory that furnishes the TC of physician pathology services to inpatients or outpatients of a hospital that is not a covered hospital may not bill the carrier for the TC of physician pathology services during the time 542 is in effect.

If the arrangement between the independent laboratory and the covered hospital limited the provision of TC physician pathology services to certain situations or at particular times, then the independent laboratory can bill the carrier only for these limited services.

The carrier shall require independent laboratories that had an arrangement, on or prior to July 22, 1999 with a covered hospital, to bill for the technical component of physician pathology services to provide a copy of this agreement, or other documentation substantiating that an arrangement was

in effect between the hospital and the independent laboratory as of this date. The independent laboratory must submit this documentation for each covered hospital that the independent laboratory services.

See Chapter 16 for additional instruction on laboratory services including clinical diagnostic laboratory services.

Physician laboratory and pathology services are limited to:

- Surgical pathology services;
- Specific cytopathology, hematology and blood banking services that have been identified to require performance by a physician and are listed below;
- Clinical consultation services that meet the requirements in subsection D below; and
- Clinical laboratory interpretation services that meet the requirements and which are specifically listed in subsection E below.

B. Surgical Pathology Services
Surgical pathology services include the gross and microscopic examination of organ tissue performed by a physician, except for autopsies, which are not covered by Medicare. Surgical pathology services paid under the physician fee schedule are reported under the following CPT codes:

88300, 88302, 88304, 88305, 88307, 88309, 88311, 88312, 88313, 88314, 88318, 88319, 88321, 88323, 88325, 88329, 88331, 88332, 88342, 88346, 88347, 88348, 88349, 88355, 88356, 88358, 88361, 88362, 88365, 88380.

Depending upon circumstances and the billing entity, the carriers may pay professional component, technical component or both.

C. Specific Hematology, Cytopathology and Blood Banking Services
Cytopathology services include the examination of cells from fluids, washings, brushings or smears, but generally excluding hematology. Examining cervical and vaginal smears are the most common service in cytopathology. Cervical and vaginal smears do not require interpretation by a physician unless the results are or appear to be abnormal. In such cases, a physician personally conducts a separate microscopic evaluation to determine the nature of an abnormality. This microscopic evaluation ordinarily does require performance by a physician. When medically necessary and when furnished by a physician, it is paid under the fee schedule.

These codes include 88104, 88106, 88107, 88108, 88112, 88125, 88141, 88160, 88161, 88162, 88172, 88173, 88180, 88182.

For services furnished prior to January 1, 1999, carriers pay separately under the physician fee schedule for the interpretation of an abnormal pap smear furnished to a hospital inpatient by a physician. They must pay under the clinical laboratory fee schedule for pap smears furnished in all other situations. This policy also applies to screening pap smears requiring a physician interpretation. For services furnished on or after January 1, 1999, carriers allow separate payment for a physician's interpretation of a pap smear to any patient (i.e., hospital or non-hospital) as long as: (1) the laboratory's screening personnel suspect an abnormality; and (2) the physician reviews and interprets the pap smear.

This policy also applies to screening pap smears requiring a physician interpretation and described in the National Coverage Determination Manual and Chapter 18. These services are reported under codes P3000 or P3001.

Physician hematology services include microscopic evaluation of bone marrow aspirations and biopsies. It also includes those limited number of peripheral blood smears which need to be referred to a physician to evaluate the nature of an apparent abnormality identified by the technologist. These codes include 85060, 38220, 85097, and 38221.

Carriers pay the professional component for the interpretation of an abnormal blood smear (code 85060) furnished to a hospital inpatient by a hospital physician or an independent laboratory.

For the other listed hematology codes, payment may be made for the professional component if the service is furnished to a patient by a hospital physician or independent laboratory. In addition, payment may be made for these services furnished to patients by an independent laboratory.

Codes 38220 and 85097 represent professional-only component services and have no technical component values.

Blood banking services of hematologists and pathologists are paid under the physician fee schedule when analyses are performed on donor and/or patient blood to determine compatible donor units for transfusion where cross matching is difficult or where contamination with transmissible disease of donor is suspected.

The blood banking codes are 86077, 86078, and 86079 and represent professional component only services. These codes do not have a technical component.

D. Clinical Consultation Services
- Clinical consultations are paid under the physician fee schedule only if they:

- Are requested by the patient's attending physician;

- Relate to a test result that lies outside the clinically significant normal or expected range in view of the condition of the patient;

- Result in a written narrative report included in the patient's medical record; and

- Require the exercise of medical judgment by the consultant physician.

Clinical consultations are professional component services only. There is no technical component. The clinical consultation codes are 80500 and 80502.

Routine conversations held between a laboratory director and an attending physician about test orders or results do not qualify as consultations unless all four requirements are met. Laboratory personnel, including the director, may from time to time contact attending physicians to report test results or to suggest additional testing or be contacted by attending physicians on similar matters. These contacts do not constitute clinical consultations. However, if in the course of such a contact, the attending physician requests a consultation from the pathologist, and if that consultation meets the other criteria and is properly documented, it is paid under the fee schedule.

EXAMPLE: A pathologist telephones a surgeon about a patient's suitability for surgery based on the results of clinical laboratory test results. During the course of their conversation, the surgeon ask the pathologist whether, based on test results, patient history and medical records, the patient is a candidate for surgery. The surgeon's request requires the pathologist to render a medical judgment and provide a consultation. The athologist follows up his/her oral advice with a written report and the surgeon notes in the patient's medical record that he/she requested a consultation. This consultation is paid under the fee schedule.

In any case, if the information could ordinarily be furnished by a nonphysician laboratory specialist, the service of the physician is not a consultation payable under the fee schedule.

See the Program Integrity Manual for guidelines for related data analysis to identify inappropriate patterns of billing for consultations.

E. Clinical Laboratory Interpretation Services

Only clinical laboratory interpretation services listed below and which meet the criteria in subsections D.1, D.3, and D.4 for clinical consultations and, as a result, are billable under the fee schedule. These services are reported under the clinical laboratory code with modifier 26. These services can be paid under the physician fee schedule if they are furnished to a patient by a hospital pathologist or an independent laboratory. Note that a hospital's standing order policy can be used as a substitute for the individual request by the patient's attending physician. Carriers are not allowed to revise CMS's list to accommodate local medical practice. The CMS periodically reviews this list and adds or deletes clinical laboratory codes as warranted.

Clinical Laboratory Interpretation Services

Code	Definition
83020	Hemoglobin; electrophoresis
83912	Nucleic acid probe, with electrophoresis, with examination and report
84165	Protein, total, serum; electrophoretic fractionation and quantitation
84181	Protein; Western Blot with interpretation and report, blood or other body fluid
84182	Protein; Western Blot, with interpretation and report, blood or other body fluid, immunological probe for band identification; each
85390	Fibrinolysin; screening
85576	Platelet; aggregation (in vitro), any agent
86255	Fluorescent antibody; screen
86256	Fluorescent antibody; titer
86320	Immunoelectrophoresis; serum, each specimen
86325	Immunoelectrophoresis; other fluids (e.g.urine) with concentration, each specimen
86327	Immunoelectrophoresis; crossed (2 dimensional assay)
86334	Immunofixation electrophoresis
87164	Dark field examination, any source (e.g. penile, vaginal, oral, skin); includes specimen collection
87207	Smear, primary source, with interpretation; special stain for inclusion bodies or intracellular parasites (e.g. malaria, kala azar, herpes)
88371	Protein analysis of tissue by Western Blot, with interpretation and report.
88372	Protein analysis of tissue by Western Blot, immunological probe for band identification, each
89060	Crystal identification by light microscopy with or without polarizing lens analysis, any body fluid (except urine)

100-4, 12, 80.1

Healthcare Common Procedure Coding System (HCPCS) Coding for the IPPE

The HCPCS codes listed below were developed for the IPPE benefit effective January 1, 2005, for individuals whose initial enrollment is on or after January 1, 2005.

G0344: Initial preventive physical examination; face-to-face visit, services limited to new beneficiary during the first 6 months of Medicare enrollment

    Short Descriptor: Initial Preventive Exam

G0366: Electrocardiogram, routine ECG with 12 leads; performed as a component of the initial preventive examination with interpretation and report

    Short Descriptor: EKG for initial prevent exam

G0367: tracing only, without interpretation and report, performed as a component of the initial preventive examination

    Short Descriptor: EKG tracing for initial prev

G0368: interpretation and report only, performed as a component of the initial preventive examination

    Short Descriptor: EKG interpret & report preve

The following new HCPCS codes were developed for the IPPE benefit effective January 1, 2009, and replaced codes G0344, G0366, G0367, and G0368 shown above beginning with dates of service on or after January 1, 2009:

G0402: Initial preventive physical examination; face-to-face visit, services limited to new beneficiary during the first 12 months of Medicare enrollment

    Short Descriptor: Initial Preventive exam

G0403: Electrocardiogram, routine ECG with 12 leads; performed as a screening for the initial preventive physical examination with interpretation and report

    Short Descriptor: EKG for initial prevent exam

G0404: Electrocardiogram, routine ECG with 12 leads; tracing only, without interpretation and report, performed as a screening for the initial preventive physical examination

    Short Descriptor: EKG tracing for initial prev

G0405: Electrocardiogram, routine ECG with 12 leads; interpretation and report only, performed as a screening for the initial preventive physical examination

    Short Descriptor: EKG interpret & report preve

100-4, 12, 100.1.1

Evaluation and Management (E/M) Services

A. General Documentation Instructions and Common Scenarios

Evaluation and Management (E/M) Services -- For a given encounter, the selection of the appropriate level of E/M service should be determined according to the code definitions in the American Medical Association's Current Procedural Terminology (CPT) and any applicable documentation guidelines.

For purposes of payment, E/M services billed by teaching physicians require that they personally document at least the following:

- That they performed the service or were physically present during the key or critical portions of the service when performed by the resident; and

- The participation of the teaching physician in the management of the patient.

When assigning codes to services billed by teaching physicians, reviewers will combine the documentation of both the resident and the teaching physician.

Documentation by the resident of the presence and participation of the teaching physician is not sufficient to establish the presence and participation of the teaching physician.

On medical review, the combined entries into the medical record by the teaching physician and the resident constitute the documentation for the service and together must support the medical necessity of the service.

Following are four common scenarios for teaching physicians providing E/M services:

Scenario 1:

The teaching physician personally performs all the required elements of an E/M service without a resident. In this scenario the resident may or may not have performed the E/M service independently.

In the absence of a note by a resident, the teaching physician must document as he/she would document an E/M service in a nonteaching setting.

Where a resident has written notes, the teaching physician's note may reference the resident's note. The teaching physician must document that he/she performed the critical or key portion(s) of the service, and that he/she was directly involved in the management of the patient. For payment, the composite of the teaching physician's entry and the resident's entry together must support the medical necessity of the billed service and the level of the service billed by the teaching physician.

Scenario 2:

The resident performs the elements required for an E/M service in the presence of, or jointly with, the teaching physician and the resident documents the service. In this case, the teaching physician must document that he/she was present during the performance of the critical or key portion(s) of the service and that he/she was directly involved in the

management of the patient. The teaching physician's note should reference the resident's note. For payment, the composite of the teaching physician's entry and the resident's entry together must support the medical necessity and the level of the service billed by the teaching physician.

Scenario 3:

The resident performs some or all of the required elements of the service in the absence of the teaching physician and documents his/her service. The teaching physician independently performs the critical or key portion(s) of the service with or without the resident present and, as appropriate, discusses the case with the resident. In this instance, the teaching physician must document that he/she personally saw the patient, personally performed critical or key portions of the service, and participated in the management of the patient. The teaching physician's note should reference the resident's note. For payment, the composite of the teaching physician's entry and the resident's entry together must support the medical necessity of the billed service and the level of the service billed by the teaching physician.

Scenario 4:

When a medical resident admits a patient to a hospital late at night and the teaching physician does not see the patient until later, including the next calendar day:

- The teaching physician must document that he/she personally saw the patient and participated in the management of the patient. The teaching physician may reference the resident's note in lieu of re-documenting the history of present illness, exam, medical decision-making, review of systems and/or past family/social history provided that the patient's condition has not changed, and the teaching physician agrees with the resident's note.

- The teaching physician's note must reflect changes in the patient's condition and clinical course that require that the resident's note be amended with further information to address the patient's condition and course at the time the patient is seen personally by the teaching physician.

- The teaching physician's bill must reflect the date of service he/she saw the patient and his/her personal work of obtaining a history, performing a physical, and participating in medical decision-making regardless of whether the combination of the teaching physician's and resident's documentation satisfies criteria for a higher level of service. For payment, the composite of the teaching physician's entry and the resident's entry together must support the medical necessity of the billed service and the level of the service billed by the teaching physician.

Following are examples of minimally acceptable documentation for each of these scenarios:

Scenario 1:

Admitting Note: "I performed a history and physical examination of the patient and discussed his management with the resident. I reviewed the resident's note and agree with the documented findings and plan of care."

Follow-up Visit: "Hospital Day #3. I saw and evaluated the patient. I agree with the findings and the plan of care as documented in the resident's note."

Follow-up Visit: "Hospital Day #5. I saw and examined the patient. I agree with the resident's note except the heart murmur is louder, so I will obtain an echo to evaluate."

(NOTE: In this scenario if there are no resident notes, the teaching physician must document as he/she would document an E/M service in a non-teaching setting.)

Scenario 2:

Initial or Follow-up Visit: "I was present with the resident during the history and exam. I discussed the case with the resident and agree with the findings and plan as documented in the resident's note."

Follow-up Visit: "I saw the patient with the resident and agree with the resident's findings and plan."

Scenarios 3 and 4:

Initial Visit: "I saw and evaluated the patient. I reviewed the resident's note and agree, except that picture is more consistent with pericarditis than myocardial ischemia. Will begin NSAIDs."

Initial or Follow-up Visit: "I saw and evaluated the patient. Discussed with resident and agree with resident's findings and plan as documented in the resident's note."

Follow-up Visit: "See resident's note for details. I saw and evaluated the patient and agree with the resident's finding and plans as written."

Follow-up Visit: "I saw and evaluated the patient. Agree with resident's note but lower extremities are weaker, now 3/5; MRI of L/S Spine today."

Following are examples of unacceptable documentation:

"Agree with above.", followed by legible countersignature or identity;

"Rounded, Reviewed, Agree.", followed by legible countersignature or identity;

"Discussed with resident. Agree.", followed by legible countersignature or identity;

"Seen and agree.", followed by legible countersignature or identity;

"Patient seen and evaluated.", followed by legible countersignature or identity; and

A legible countersignature or identity alone.

Such documentation is not acceptable, because the documentation does not make it possible to determine whether the teaching physician was present, evaluated the patient, and/or had any involvement with the plan of care.

B. E/M Service Documentation Provided By Students

Any contribution and participation of a student to the performance of a billable service (other than the review of systems and/or past family/social history which are not separately billable, but are taken as part of an E/M service) must be performed in the physical presence of a teaching physician or physical presence of a resident in a service meeting the requirements set forth in this section for teaching physician billing.

Students may document services in the medical record. However, the documentation of an E/M service by a student that may be referred to by the teaching physician is limited to documentation related to the review of systems and/or past family/social history. The teaching physician may not refer to a student's documentation of physical exam findings or medical decision making in his or her personal note. If the medical student documents E/M services, the teaching physician must verify and redocument the history of present illness as well as perform and redocument the physical exam and medical decision making activities of the service.

C. Exception for E/M Services Furnished in Certain Primary Care Centers

Teaching physicians providing E/M services with a GME program granted a primary care exception may bill Medicare for lower and mid-level E/M services provided by residents. For the E/M codes listed below, teaching physicians may submit claims for services furnished by residents in the absence of a teaching physician:

New Patient	Established Patient
99201	99211
99202	99212
99203	99213

Effective January 1, 2005, the following code is included under the primary care exception: HCPCS code G0402 (Initial preventive physical examination; face-to-face visit services limited to new beneficiary during the first 12 months of Medicare enrollment).

Effective January 1, 2011, the following codes are included under the primary care exception: HCPCS codes G0438 (Annual wellness visit, including personal preventive plan service, first visit) and G0439 (Annual wellness visit, including personal preventive plan service, subsequent visit).

If a service other than those listed above needs to be furnished, then the general teaching physician policy set forth in §100.1 applies. For this exception to apply, a center must attest in writing that all the following conditions are met for a particular residency program. Prior approval is not necessary, but centers exercising the primary care exception must maintain records demonstrating that they qualify for the exception.

The services must be furnished in a center located in the outpatient department of a hospital or another ambulatory care entity in which the time spent by residents in patient care activities is included in determining direct GME payments to a teaching hospital by the hospital's FI. This requirement is not met when the resident is assigned to a physician's office away from the center or makes home visits. In the case of a nonhospital entity, verify with the FI that the entity meets the requirements of a written agreement between the hospital and the entity set forth at 42 CFR 413.78(e)(3)(ii).

Under this exception, residents providing the billable patient care service without the physical presence of a teaching physician must have completed at least 6 months of a

GME approved residency program. Centers must maintain information under the provisions at 42 CFR 413.79(a)(6).

Teaching physicians submitting claims under this exception may not supervise more than four residents at any given time and must direct the care from such proximity as to constitute immediate availability. Teaching physicians may include residents with less than 6 months in a GME approved residency program in the mix of four residents under the teaching physician's supervision. However, the teaching physician must be physically present for the critical or key portions of services furnished by the residents with less than 6 months in a GME approved residency program. That is, the primary care exception does not apply in the case of residents with less than 6 months in a GME approved residency program.

Teaching physicians submitting claims under this exception must:

- Not have other responsibilities (including the supervision of other personnel) at the time the service was provided by the resident;

- Have the primary medical responsibility for patients cared for by the residents;

- Ensure that the care provided was reasonable and necessary;

- Review the care provided by the resident during or immediately after each visit. This must include a review of the patient's medical history, the resident's findings on physical examination, the patient's diagnosis, and treatment plan (i.e., record of tests and therapies); and

- Document the extent of his/her own participation in the review and direction of the services furnished to each patient.

Patients under this exception should consider the center to be their primary location for health care services. The residents must be expected to generally provide care to the same group of established patients during their residency training. The types of services furnished by residents under this exception include:

- Acute care for undifferentiated problems or chronic care for ongoing conditions including chronic mental illness;

- Coordination of care furnished by other physicians and providers; and,

- Comprehensive care not limited by organ system or diagnosis.

Residency programs most likely qualifying for this exception include family practice, general internal medicine, geriatric medicine, pediatrics, and obstetrics/gynecology.

Certain GME programs in psychiatry may qualify in special situations such as when the program furnishes comprehensive care for chronically mentally ill patients. These would be centers in which the range of services the residents are trained to furnish, and actually do furnish, include comprehensive medical care as well as psychiatric care. For example, antibiotics are being prescribed as well as psychotropic drugs.

100-4, 12, 180

Care Plan Oversight Services

The Medicare Benefit Policy Manual, Chapter 15, contains requirements for coverage for medical and other health services including those of physicians and non-physician practitioners.

Care plan oversight (CPO) is the physician supervision of a patient receiving complex and/or multidisciplinary care as part of Medicare-covered services provided by a participating home health agency or Medicare approved hospice.

CPO services require complex or multidisciplinary care modalities involving: Regular physician development and/or revision of care plans; Review of subsequent reports of patient status; Review of related laboratory and other studies; Communication with other health professionals not employed in the same practice who are involved in the patient's care; Integration of new information into the medical treatment plan; and/or Adjustment of medical therapy.

The CPO services require recurrent physician supervision of a patient involving 30 or more minutes of the physician's time per month. Services not countable toward the 30 minutes threshold that must be provided in order to bill for CPO include, but are not limited to: Time associated with discussions with the patient, his or her family or friends to adjust medication or treatment; Time spent by staff getting or filing charts; Travel time; and/or Physician's time spent telephoning prescriptions into the pharmacist unless the telephone conversation involves discussions of pharmaceutical therapies.

Implicit in the concept of CPO is the expectation that the physician has coordinated an aspect of the patient's care with the home health agency or hospice during the month for which CPO services were billed. The physician who bills for CPO must be the same physician who signs the plan of care.

Nurse practitioners, physician assistants, and clinical nurse specialists, practicing within the scope of State law, may bill for care plan oversight. These non-physician practitioners must have been providing ongoing care for the beneficiary through evaluation and management services. These non-physician practitioners may not bill for CPO if they have been involved only with the delivery of the Medicare-covered home health or hospice service.

A. Home Health CPO

Non-physician practitioners can perform CPO only if the physician signing the plan of care provides regular ongoing care under the same plan of care as does the NPP billing for CPO and either: The physician and NPP are part of the same group practice; or If the NPP is a nurse practitioner or clinical nurse specialist, the physician signing the plan of care also has a collaborative agreement with the NPP; or If the NPP is a physician assistant, the physician signing the plan of care is also the physician who provides general supervision of physician assistant services for the practice.

Billing may be made for care plan oversight services furnished by an NPP when: The NPP providing the care plan oversight has seen and examined the patient; The NPP providing care plan oversight is not functioning as a consultant whose participation is limited to a single medical condition rather than multidisciplinary coordination of care; and The NPP providing care plan oversight integrates his or her care with that of the physician who signed the plan of care.

NPPs may not certify the beneficiary for home health care.

B. Hospice CPO

The attending physician or nurse practitioner (who has been designated as the attending physician) may bill for hospice CPO when they are acting as an "attending physician".

An "attending physician" is one who has been identified by the individual, at the time he/she elects hospice coverage, as having the most significant role in the determination and delivery of their medical care. They are not employed nor paid by the hospice. The care plan oversight services are billed using Form CMS-1500 or electronic equivalent.

For additional information on hospice CPO, see Chapter 11, 40.1.3.1 of this manual.

100-4, 12, 180.1

Care Plan Oversight Billing Requirements

A. Codes for Which Separate Payment May Be Made

Effective January 1, 1995, separate payment may be made for CPO oversight services for 30 minutes or more if the requirements specified in the Medicare Benefits Policy Manual, Chapter 15 are met.

Providers billing for CPO must submit the claim with no other services billed on that claim and may bill only after the end of the month in which the CPO services were rendered. CPO services may not be billed across calendar months and should be submitted (and paid) only for one unit of service.

Physicians may bill and be paid separately for CPO services only if all the criteria in the Medicare Benefit Policy Manual, Chapter 15 are met.

B. Physician Certification and Recertification of Home Health Plans of Care

Effective 2001, two new HCPCS codes for the certification and recertification and development of plans of care for Medicare-covered home health services were created.

See the Medicare General Information, Eligibility, and Entitlement Manual, Pub. 100-01, Chapter 4, "Physician Certification and Recertification of Services," 10-60, and the Medicare Benefit Policy Manual, Pub. 100-02, Chapter 7, "Home Health Services", 30.

The home health agency certification code can be billed only when the patient has not received Medicare-covered home health services for at least 60 days. The home health agency recertification code is used after a patient has received services for at least 60 days (or one certification period) when the physician signs the certification after the initial certification period. The home health agency recertification code will be reported only once every 60 days, except in the rare situation when the patient starts a new episode before 60 days elapses and requires a new plan of care to start a new episode.

C. Provider Number of Home Health Agency (HHA) or Hospice

For claims for CPO submitted on or after January 1, 1997, physicians must enter on the Medicare claim form the 6-character Medicare provider number of the HHA or hospice providing Medicare-covered services to the beneficiary for the period during which CPO services was furnished and for which the physician signed the plan of care. Physicians are responsible for obtaining the HHA or hospice Medicare provider numbers.

Additionally, physicians should provide their UPIN to the HHA or hospice furnishing services to their patient.

NOTE: There is currently no place on the HIPAA standard ASC X12N 837 professional format to specifically include the HHA or hospice provider number required for a care plan oversight claim. For this reason, the requirement to include the HHA or hospice provider number on a care plan oversight claim is temporarily waived until a new version of this electronic standard format is adopted under HIPAA and includes a place to provide the HHA and hospice provider numbers for care plan oversight claims.

100-4,12,190.3

List of Medicare Telehealth Services

The use of a telecommunications system may substitute for an in-person encounter for professional consultations, office visits, office psychiatry services, and a limited number of other physician fee schedule (PFS) services. The various services and corresponding current procedure terminology (CPT) or Healthcare Common Procedure Coding System (HCPCS) codes are listed below.

- Consultations (CPT codes 99241 - 99275) - Effective October 1, 2001 – December 31, 2005;
- Consultations (CPT codes 99241 - 99255) - Effective January 1, 2006 – December 31, 2009;
- Telehealth consultations, emergency department or initial inpatient (HCPCS codes G0425 – G0427) - Effective January 1, 2010;
- Follow-up inpatient telehealth consultations (HCPCS codes G0406, G0407, and G0408) - Effective January 1, 2009;
- Office or other outpatient visits (CPT codes 99201 - 99215);
- Subsequent hospital care services, with the limitation of one telehealth visit every 3 days (CPT codes 99231, 99232, and 99233) – Effective January 1, 2011;
- Subsequent nursing facility care services, with the limitation of one telehealth visit every 30 days (CPT codes 99307, 99308, 99309, and 99310) – Effective January 1, 2011;
- Pharmacologic management (CPT code 90862) – Effective March 1, 2003 – December 31, 2012;
- Individual psychotherapy (CPT codes 90804 - 90809); Psychiatric diagnostic interview examination (CPT code 90801) – Effective March 1, 2003 – December 31, 2012;
- Individual psychotherapy (CPT codes 90832 – 90834, 90836 – 90838); Psychiatric diagnostic interview examination (CPT codes 90791 -- 90792) – Effective January 1, 2013.
- Neurobehavioral status exam (CPT code 96116) - Effective January 1, 2008;
- End Stage Renal Disease (ESRD) related services (HCPCS codes G0308, G0309, G0311, G0312, G0314, G0315, G0317, and G0318) – Effective January 1, 2005 – December 31, 2008;
- End Stage Renal Disease (ESRD) related services (CPT codes 90951, 90952, 90954, 90955, 90957, 90958, 90960, and 90961) – Effective January 1, 2009;
- Individual and group medical nutrition therapy (HCPCS codes G0270, 97802, 97803, and 97804) – Individual effective January 1, 2006; group effective January 1, 2011;
- Individual and group health and behavior assessment and intervention (CPT codes 96150 – 96154) – Individual effective January 1, 2010; group effective January 1, 2011.
- Individual and group kidney disease education (KDE) services (HCPCS codes G0420 and G0421) – Effective January 1, 2011; and
- Individual and group diabetes self-management training (DSMT) services, with a minimum of 1 hour of in-person instruction to be furnished in the initial year training period to ensure effective injection training (HCPCS codes G0108 and G0109) - Effective January 1, 2011.
- Smoking Cessation Services (CPT codes 99406 and 99407and HCPCS codes G0436 and G0437) – Effective January 1, 2012.
- Alcohol and/or substance (other than tobacco) abuse structured assessment and intervention services (HCPCS codes G0396 and G0397) – Effective January 1, 2013.
- Annual alcohol misuse screening (HCPCS code G0442) – Effective January 1, 2013.
- Brief face-to-face behavioral counseling for alcohol misuse (HCPCS code G0443) – Effective January 1, 2013.
- Annual Depression Screening (HCPCS code G0444) – Effective January 1, 2013.
- High-intensity behavioral counseling to prevent sexually transmitted infections (HCPCS code G0445) – Effective January 1, 2013.
- Annual, face-to-face Intensive behavioral therapy for cardiovascular disease (HCPCS code G0446) – Effective January 1, 2013.
- Face-to-face behavioral counseling for obesity (HCPCS code G0447) – Effective January 1, 2013.

NOTE: Beginning January 1, 2010, CMS eliminated the use of all consultation codes, except for inpatient telehealth consultation G-codes. CMS no longer recognizes office/outpatient or inpatient consultation CPT codes for payment of office/outpatient or inpatient visits. Instead, physicians and practitioners are instructed to bill a new or established patient office/outpatient visit CPT code or appropriate hospital or nursing facility care code, as appropriate to the particular patient, for all office/outpatient or inpatient visits.

100-4, 12, 190.3.1

Telehealth Consultation Services, Emergency Department or Initial Inpatient versus Inpatient Evaluation and Management (E/M) Visits

A consultation service is an evaluation and management (E/M) service furnished to evaluate and possibly treat a patient's problem(s). It can involve an opinion, advice, recommendation, suggestion, direction, or counsel from a physician or qualified nonphysician practitioner (NPP) at the request of another physician or appropriate source.

Section 1834(m) of the Social Security Act includes "professional consultations" in the definition of telehealth services. Inpatient or emergency department consultations furnished via telehealth can facilitate the provision of certain services and/or medical expertise that might not otherwise be available to a patient located at an originating site.

The use of a telecommunications system may substitute for an in-person encounter for emergency department or initial and follow-up inpatient consultations.

Medicare contractors pay for reasonable and medically necessary inpatient or emergency department telehealth consultation services furnished to beneficiaries in hospitals or SNFs when all of the following criteria for the use of a consultation code are met:

- An inpatient or emergency department consultation service is distinguished from other inpatient or emergency department evaluation and management (E/M) visits because it is provided by a physician or qualified nonphysician practitioner (NPP) whose opinion or advice regarding evaluation and/or management of a specific problem is requested by another physician or other appropriate source. The qualified NPP may perform consultation services within the scope of practice and licensure requirements for NPPs in the State in which he/she practices;
- A request for an inpatient or emergency department telehealth consultation from an appropriate source and the need for an inpatient or emergency department telehealth consultation (i.e., the reason for a consultation service) shall be documented by the consultant in the patient's medical record and included in the requesting physician or qualified NPP's plan of care in the patient's medical record; and
- After the inpatient or emergency department telehealth consultation is provided, the consultant shall prepare a written report of his/her findings and recommendations, which shall be provided to the referring physician.

The intent of an inpatient or emergency department telehealth consultation service is that a physician or qualified NPP or other appropriate source is asking another physician or qualified NPP for advice, opinion, a recommendation, suggestion, direction, or counsel, etc. in evaluating or treating a patient because that individual has expertise in a specific medical area beyond the requesting professional's knowledge.

Unlike inpatient or emergency department telehealth consultations, the majority of subsequent inpatient hospital, emergency department and nursing facility care services require in-person visits to facilitate the comprehensive, coordinated, and personal care that medically volatile, acutely ill patients require on an ongoing basis.

Subsequent hospital care services are limited to one telehealth visit every 3 days. Subsequent nursing facility care services are limited to one telehealth visit every 30 days.

100-4,12,190.3.2

Telehealth Consultation Services, Emergency Department or Initial Inpatient Defined

Emergency department or initial inpatient telehealth consultations are furnished to beneficiaries in hospitals or SNFs via telehealth at the request of the physician of record, the attending physician, or another appropriate source. The physician or practitioner who furnishes the emergency department or initial inpatient consultation via telehealth cannot be the physician of record or the attending physician, and the emergency department or initial inpatient telehealth consultation would be distinct from the care provided by the physician of record or the attending physician. Counseling and coordination of care with other providers or agencies is included as well, consistent with the nature of the problem(s) and the patient's needs. Emergency department or initial inpatient telehealth consultations are subject to the criteria for emergency department or initial inpatient telehealth consultation services, as described in section 190.3.1 of this chapter.

Payment for emergency department or initial inpatient telehealth consultations includes all consultation related services furnished before, during, and after communicating with the patient via telehealth. Pre-service activities would include, but would not be limited to, reviewing patient data (for example, diagnostic and imaging studies, interim labwork) and communicating with other professionals or family members. Intra-service activities must include the three key elements described below for each procedure code. Post-service activities would include, but would not be limited to, completing medical records or other documentation and communicating results of the consultation and further care plans to other health care professionals. No additional E/M service could be billed for work related to an emergency department or initial inpatient telehealth consultation.

Emergency department or initial inpatient telehealth consultations could be provided at various levels of complexity:

- Practitioners taking a problem focused history, conducting a problem focused examination, and engaging in medical decision making that is straightforward, would bill HCPCS code G0425 (Telehealth consultation, emergency department or initial inpatient, typically 30 minutes communicating with the patient via telehealth).

- Practitioners taking a detailed history, conducting a detailed examination, and engaging in medical decision making that is of moderate complexity, would bill HCPCS code G0426 (Telehealth consultation, emergency department or initial inpatient, typically 50 minutes communicating with the patient via telehealth).

- Practitioners taking a comprehensive history, conducting a comprehensive examination, and engaging in medical decision making that is of high complexity, would bill HCPCS code G0427 (Telehealth consultation, emergency department or initial inpatient, typically 70 minutes or more communicating with the patient via telehealth).

Although emergency department or initial inpatient telehealth consultations are specific to telehealth, these services must be billed with either the -GT or -GQ modifier to identify the telehealth technology used to provide the service. See section 190.6 of this chapter for instructions on how to use these modifiers.

100-4, 12, 190.3.3

Follow-Up Inpatient Telehealth Consultations Defined

Follow-up inpatient telehealth consultations are furnished to beneficiaries in hospitals or SNFs via telehealth to follow up on an initial consultation, or subsequent consultative visits requested by the attending physician. The initial inpatient consultation may have been provided in person or via telehealth.

Follow-up inpatient telehealth consultations include monitoring progress, recommending management modifications, or advising on a new plan of care in response to changes in the patient's status or no changes on the consulted health issue. Counseling and coordination of care with other providers or agencies is included as well, consistent with the nature of the problem(s) and the patient's needs.

The physician or practitioner who furnishes the inpatient follow-up consultation via telehealth cannot be the physician of record or the attending physician, and the follow-up inpatient consultation would be distinct from the follow-up care provided by the physician of record or the attending physician. If a physician consultant has initiated treatment at an initial consultation and participates thereafter in the patient's ongoing care management, such care would not be included in the definition of a follow-up inpatient consultation and is not appropriate for delivery via telehealth. Follow-up inpatient telehealth consultations are subject to the criteria for inpatient telehealth consultation services, as described in Sec.190.3.1

Payment for follow-up inpatient telehealth consultations includes all consultation related services furnished before, during, and after communicating with the patient via telehealth. Pre-service activities would include, but would not be limited to, reviewing patient data (for example, diagnostic and imaging studies, interim labwork) and communicating with other professionals or family members. Intra-service activities must include at least two of the three key elements described below for each procedure code. Post-service activities would include, but would not be limited to, completing medical records or other documentation and communicating results of the consultation and further care plans to other health care professionals. No additional evaluation and management service could be billed for work related to a follow-up inpatient telehealth consultation.

Follow-up inpatient telehealth consultations could be provided at various levels of complexity:

Practitioners taking a problem focused interval history, conducting a problem focused examination, and engaging in medical decision making that is straightforward or of low complexity, would bill a limited service, using HCPCS G0406, Follow-up inpatient telehealth consultation, limited. At this level of service, practitioners would typically spend 15 minutes communicating with the patient via telehealth.

Practitioners taking an expanded focused interval history, conducting an expanded problem focused examination, and engaging in medical decision making that is of moderate complexity, would bill an intermediate service using HCPCS G0407, Follow-up inpatient telehealth consultation, intermediate. At this level of service, practitioners would typically spend 25 minutes communicating with the patient via telehealth.

Practitioners taking a detailed interval history, conducting a detailed examination, and engaging in medical decision making that is of high complexity, would bill a complex service, using HCPCS G0408, Follow-up inpatient telehealth consultation, complex. At this level of service, practitioners would typically spend 35 minutes or more communicating with the patient via telehealth.

Although follow-up inpatient telehealth consultations are specific to telehealth, these services must be billed with either the "GT" or "GQ" modifier to identify the telehealth technology used to provide the service. (See Sec.190.6 et. al. for instructions on how to use these modifiers.)

100-4, 12, 190.6

1. Originating site defined

The term originating site means the location of an eligible Medicare beneficiary at the time the service being furnished via a telecommunications system occurs. For asynchronous, store and forward telecommunications technologies, an originating site is only a Federal telemedicine demonstration program conducted in Alaska or Hawaii.

2. Facility fee for originating site

The originating site facility fee is a separately billable Part B payment. The contractor pays it outside of other payment methodologies. This fee is subject to post payment verification.

For telehealth services furnished from October 1, 2001, through December 31, 2002, the originating site facility fee is the lesser of $20 or the actual charge. For services furnished on or after January 1 of each subsequent year, the originating site facility fee is updated by the Medicare Economic Index. The updated fee is included in the Medicare Physician Fee Schedule (MPFS) Final Rule, which is published by November 1 prior to the start of the calendar year for which it is effective. The updated fee for each calendar year is also issued annually in a Recurring Update Notification instruction for January of each year.

3. Payment amount:

The originating site facility fee is a separately billable Part B payment. The payment amount to the originating site is the lesser of 80 percent of the actual charge or 80 percent of the originating site facility fee, except CAHs. The beneficiary is responsible for any unmet deductible amount and Medicare coinsurance.

The originating site facility fee payment methodology for each type of facility is clarified below.

Hospital outpatient department. When the originating site is a hospital outpatient department, payment for the originating site facility fee must be made as described above and not under the outpatient prospective payment system (OPPS). Payment is not based on the OPPS payment methodology.

Hospital inpatient. For hospital inpatients, payment for the originating site facility fee must be made outside the diagnostic related group (DRG) payment, since this is a Part B benefit, similar to other services paid separately from the DRG payment, (e.g., hemophilia blood clotting factor).

Critical access hospitals. When the originating site is a critical access hospital, make payment separately from the cost-based reimbursement methodology. For CAH's, the payment amount is 80 percent of the originating site facility fee.

Federally qualified health centers (FQHCs) and rural health clinics (RHCs). The originating site facility fee for telehealth services is not an FQHC or RHC service. When an FQHC or RHC serves as the originating site, the originating site facility fee must be paid separately from the center or clinic all-inclusive rate.

Physicians' and practitioners' offices. When the originating site is a physician's or practitioner's office, the payment amount, in accordance with the law, is the lesser of 80 percent of the actual charge or 80 percent of the originating site facility fee, regardless of geographic location. The carrier shall not apply the geographic practice cost index (GPCI) to the originating site facility fee. This fee is statutorily set and is not subject to the geographic payment adjustments authorized under the MPFS.

Hospital-based or critical access-hospital based renal dialysis center (or their satellites). When a hospital-based or critical access hospital-based renal dialysis center (or their satellites) serves as the originating site, the originating site facility fee is covered in addition to any composite rate or MCP amount.

Skilled nursing facility (SNF). The originating site facility fee is outside the SNF prospective payment system bundle and, as such, is not subject to SNF consolidated billing. The originating site facility fee is a separately billable Part B payment.

Community Mental Health Center (CMHC). The originating site facility fee is not a partial hospitalization service. The originating site facility fee does not count towards the number of services used to determine payment for partial hospitalization services. The originating site facility fee is not bundled in the per diem payment for partial hospitalization. The originating site facility fee is a separately billable Part B payment.

To receive the originating facility site fee, the provider submits claims with HCPCS code "Q3014, telehealth originating site facility fee"; short description "telehealth facility fee." The type of service for the telehealth originating site facility fee is "9, other items and services." For carrier-processed claims, the "office" place of service (code 11) is the only payable setting for code Q3014. There is no participation payment differential for code Q3014. Deductible and coinsurance rules apply to Q3014. By submitting Q3014 HCPCS code, the originating site authenticates they are located in either a rural HPSA or non-MSA county.

This benefit may be billed on bill types 12X, 13X, 22X, 23X, 71X, 72X, 73X, 76X, and 85X. Unless otherwise applicable, report the originating site facility fee under revenue code 078X and include HCPCS code "Q3014, telehealth originating site facility fee."

Hospitals and critical access hospitals bill their intermediary for the originating site facility fee. Telehealth bills originating in inpatient hospitals must be submitted on a 12X TOB using the date of discharge as the line item date of service.

Independent and provider-based RHCs and FQHCs bill the appropriate intermediary using the RHC or FQHC bill type and billing number. HCPCS code Q3014 is the only non-RHC/FQHC service that is billed using the clinic/center bill type and provider number. All RHCs and FQHCs must use revenue code 078X when billing for the originating site facility fee. For all other non-RHC/FQHC services, provider based RHCs and FQHCs must bill using the base provider's bill type and billing number. Independent RHCs and FQHCs must bill the carrier for all other non-RHC/FQHC services. If an RHC/FQHC visit occurs on the same day as a telehealth service, the RHC/FQHC serving as an originating site must bill for HCPCS code Q3014 telehealth originating site facility fee on a separate revenue line from the RHC/FQHC visit using revenue code 078X.

Hospital-based or CAH-based renal dialysis centers (including satellites) bill their local FIs and/or Part A MACs for the originating site facility fee. Telehealth bills originating in renal dialysis centers must be submitted on a 72X TOB. All hospital-based or CAH-based renal dialysis centers (including satellites) must use revenue code 078X when billing for the originating site facility fee. The renal dialysis center serving as an originating site must bill for HCPCS code Q3014, telehealth originating site facility fee, on a separate revenue line from any other services provided to the beneficiary.

Skilled nursing facilities (SNFs) bill their local FIs and/or Part A MACs for the originating site facility fee. Telehealth bills originating in SNFs must be submitted on TOB 22X or 23X. For SNF inpatients in a covered Part A stay, the originating site facility fee must be submitted on a 22X TOB. All SNFs must use revenue code 078X when billing for the originating site facility fee. The SNF serving as an originating site must bill for HCPCS code Q3014, telehealth originating site facility fee, on a separate revenue line from any other services provided to the beneficiary.

Community mental health centers (CMHCs) bill their local FIs and/or Part A MACs for the originating site facility fee. Telehealth bills originating in CMHCs must be submitted on a 76X TOB. All CMHCs must use revenue code 078X when billing for the originating site facility fee. The CMHC serving as an originating site must bill for HCPCS code Q3014, telehealth originating site facility fee, on a separate revenue line from any other services provided to the beneficiary. Note that Q3014 does not count towards the number of services used to determine per diem payments for partial hospitalization services.

The beneficiary is responsible for any unmet deductible amount and Medicare coinsurance.

100-4, 12, 190.7

Contractor Editing of Telehealth Claims

Medicare telehealth services (as listed in section 190.3) are billed with either the "GT" or "GQ" modifier. The contractor shall approve covered telehealth services if the physician or practitioner is licensed under State law to provide the service. Contractors must familiarize themselves with licensure provisions of States for which they process claims and disallow telehealth services furnished by physicians or practitioners who are not authorized to furnish the applicable telehealth service under State law. For example, if a nurse practitioner is not licensed to provide individual psychotherapy under State law, he or she would not be permitted to receive payment for individual psychotherapy under Medicare. The contractor shall install edits to ensure that only properly licensed physicians and practitioners are paid for covered telehealth services.

If a contractor receives claims for professional telehealth services coded with the "GQ" modifier (representing "via asynchronous telecommunications system"), it shall approve/pay for these services only if the physician or practitioner is affiliated with a Federal telemedicine demonstration conducted in Alaska or Hawaii. The contractor may require the physician or practitioner at the distant site to document his or her participation in a Federal telemedicine demonstration program conducted in Alaska or Hawaii prior to paying for telehealth services provided via asynchronous, store and forward technologies.

If a contractor denies telehealth services because the physician or practitioner may not bill for them, the contractor uses MSN message 21.18: "This item or service is not covered when performed or ordered by this practitioner." The contractor uses remittance advice message 52 when denying the claim based upon MSN message 21.18.

If a service is billed with one of the telehealth modifiers and the procedure code is not designated as a covered telehealth service, the contractor denies the service using MSN message 9.4: "This item or service was denied because information required to make payment was incorrect." The remittance advice message depends on what is incorrect, e.g., B18 if procedure code or modifier is incorrect, 125 for submission billing errors, 4-12 for difference inconsistencies. The contractor uses B18 as the explanation for the denial of the claim.

The only claims from institutional facilities that FIs shall pay for telehealth services at the distant site, except for MNT services, are for physician or practitioner services when the distant site is located in a CAH that has elected Method II, and the physician or practitioner has reassigned his/her benefits to the CAH. The CAH bills its regular FI for the professional services provided at the distant site via a telecommunications system, in any of the revenue codes 096x, 097x or 098x. All requirements for billing distant site telehealth services apply.

Claims from hospitals or CAHs for MNT services are submitted to the hospital's or CAH's regular FI. Payment is based on the non-facility amount on the Medicare Physician Fee Schedule for the particular HCPCS codes.

100-4, 12, 210

Outpatient Mental Health Limitation

Regardless of the actual expenses a beneficiary incurs in connection with the treatment of mental, psychoneurotic, and personality disorders while the beneficiary is not an inpatient of a hospital at the time such expenses are incurred, the amount of those expenses that may be recognized for Part B deductible and payment purposes is limited to 62.5 percent of the Medicare approved amount for those services. This limitation is called the outpatient mental health treatment limitation (the limitation). The 62.5 percent limitation has been in place since the inception of the Medicare Part B program and it will remain effective at this percentage amount until January 1, 2010. However, effective January 1, 2010, through January 1, 2014, the limitation will be phased out as follows:

- January 1, 2010 –December 31, 2011, the limitation percentage is 68.75%. (Medicare pays 55% and the patient pays 45%).

- January 1, 2012–December 31, 2012, the limitation percentage is 75%. (Medicare pays 60% and the patient pays 40%).

- January 1, 2013–December 31, 2013, the limitation percentage is 81.25%. (Medicare pays 65% and the patient pays 35%).

- January 1, 2014 –onward, the limitation percentage is 100%. (Medicare pays 80% and the patient pays 20%).

For additional details concerning computation of the limitation, please see the examples under section 210.1 E.

100-4, 12, 210.1

Application of Limitation

A. Status of Patient

The limitation is applicable to expenses incurred in connection with the treatment of an individual who is not an inpatient of a hospital. Thus, the limitation applies to mental health services furnished to a person in a physician's office, in the patient's home, in a

skilled nursing facility, as an outpatient, and so forth. The term "hospital" in this context means an institution, which is primarily engaged in providing to inpatients, by or under the supervision of a physician(s):

- Diagnostic and therapeutic services for medical diagnosis, treatment and care of injured, disabled, or sick persons;

- Rehabilitation services for injured, disabled, or sick persons; or

- Psychiatric services for the diagnosis and treatment of mentally ill patients.

B. Disorders Subject to the Limitation

The term "mental, psychoneurotic, and personality disorders" is defined as the specific psychiatric diagnoses described in the International Classification of Diseases, 9th Revision (ICD-9), under the code range 290-319.

When the treatment services rendered are both for a psychiatric diagnosis as defined in the ICD-9 and one or more nonpsychiatric conditions, separate the expenses for the psychiatric aspects of treatment from the expenses for the nonpsychiatric aspects of treatment. However, in any case in which the psychiatric treatment component is not readily distinguishable from the nonpsychiatric treatment component, all of the expenses are allocated to whichever component constitutes the primary diagnosis.

1. Diagnosis Clearly Meets Definition - If the primary diagnosis reported for a particular service is the same as or equivalent to a condition described in the ICD-9 under the code range 290-319 that represents mental, psychoneurotic and personality disorders, the expense for the service is subject to the limitation except as described in subsection D.

2. Diagnosis Does Not Clearly Meet Definition - When it is not clear whether the primary diagnosis reported meets the definition of mental, psychoneurotic, and personality disorders, it may be necessary to contact the practitioner to clarify the diagnosis. In deciding whether contact is necessary in a given case, give consideration to such factors as the type of services rendered, the diagnosis, and the individual? previous utilization history.

C. Services Subject to the Limitation

Medicare Contractors must apply the limitation to claims for professional services that represent mental health treatment furnished to individuals who are not hospital inpatients by physicians, clinical psychologists, clinical social workers, nurse practitioners, clinical nurse specialists and physician assistants. Items and supplies furnished by physicians or other mental health practitioners in connection with treatment are also subject to the limitation.

Generally, Medicare Contractors must apply the limitation only to treatment services. However, diagnostic psychological and neuropsychological testing services performed to evaluate a patient's progress during treatment are considered part of treatment and are subject to the limitation.

D. Services Not Subject to the Limitation

1. Diagnosis of Alzheimer's Disease or Related Disorder - When the primary diagnosis reported for a particular service is Alzheimer's Disease or an Alzheimer's related disorder, Medicare Contractors must look to the nature of the service that has been rendered in determining whether it is subject to the limitation. Alzheimer's disease is coded 331.0 in the "International Classification of Diseases, 9th Revision", which is outside the code range 290-319 that represents mental, psychoneurotic and personality disorders. Additionally, Alzheimer's related disorders are identified by contractors under ICD-9 codes that are within the 290-319 code range (290.XX or others as contractors determine appropriate) or outside the 290-319 code range as determined appropriate by contractors. When the primary treatment rendered to a patient with a diagnosis of Alzheimer's disease or a related disorder is psychotherapy, it is subject to the limitation. However, typically, treatment provided to a patient with a diagnosis of Alzheimer's Disease or a related disorder represents medical management of the patient's condition (such as described under CPT code 90862 or any successor code) and is not subject to the limitation. CPT code 90862 describes pharmacologic management, including prescription, use, and review of medication with no more than minimal medical psychotherapy.

2. Brief Office Visits for Monitoring or Changing Drug Prescriptions - Brief office visits for the sole purpose of monitoring or changing drug prescriptions used in the treatment of mental, psychoneurotic and personality disorders are not subject to the limitation. These visits are reported using HCPCS code M0064 or any successor code (brief office visit for the sole purpose of monitoring or changing drug prescriptions used in the treatment of mental, psychoneurotic, and personality disorders). Claims where the diagnosis reported is a mental, psychoneurotic, or personality disorder (other than a diagnosis specified in subsection A) are subject to the limitation except for the procedure identified by HCPCS code M0064 or any successor code.

3. Diagnostic Services ?edicare Contractors do not apply the limitation to psychiatric diagnostic evaluations and diagnostic psychological and neuropsychological tests performed to establish or confirm the patient's diagnosis. Diagnostic services include psychiatric diagnostic evaluations billed under CPT codes 90801 or 90802 (or any successor codes) and, psychological and neuropsychological tests billed under CPT code range 96101-96118 (or any successor code range).

   An initial visit to a practitioner for professional services often combines diagnostic evaluation and the start of therapy. Such a visit is neither solely diagnostic nor solely therapeutic. Therefore, contractors must deem the initial visit to be diagnostic so that the limitation does not apply. Separating diagnostic and therapeutic components of a visit is not administratively feasible, unless the practitioner already has separately identified them on the bill. Determining the entire visit to be therapeutic is not justifiable since some diagnostic work must be done before even a tentative diagnosis can be made and certainly before therapy can be instituted. Moreover, the patient should not be disadvantaged because therapeutic as well as diagnostic services were provided in the initial visit. In the rare cases where a practitioner? diagnostic services take more than one visit, Medicare contractors must not apply the limitation to the additional visits. However, it is expected such cases are few. Therefore, when a practitioner bills for more than one visit for professional diagnostic services, Medicare contractors may find it necessary to request documentation to justify the reason for more than one diagnostic visit.

4. Partial Hospitalization Services Not Directly Provided by a Physician or a Practitioner - The limitation does not apply to partial hospitalization services that are not directly provided by a physician, clinical psychologist, nurse practitioner, clinical nurse specialist or a physician assistant. Partial hospitalization services are billed by hospital outpatient departments and community mental health centers (CMHCs) to Medicare Contractors. However, services furnished by physicians, clinical psychologists, nurse practitioners, clinical nurse specialists, and physician assistants to partial hospitalization patients are billed separately from the partial hospitalization program of services. Accordingly, these professional? mental health services to partial hospitalization patients are paid under the physician fee schedule by Medicare Contractors and may be subject to the limitation. (See chapter 4, section 260.1C).

E. Computation of Limitation

Medicare Contractors determine the Medicare approved payment amount for services subject to the limitation. They:

- Multiply the approved amount by the limitation percentage amount;
- Subtract any unsatisfied deductible; and,
- Multiply the remainder by 0.8 to obtain the amount of Medicare payment.

The beneficiary is responsible for the difference between the amount paid by Medicare and the full Medicare approved amount.

The following examples illustrate the application of the limitation in various circumstances as it is gradually reduced under section 102 of the Medicare Improvements for Patients and Providers Act (MIPPA). Please note that although the calendar year 2009 Part B deductible of $135 is used under these examples, the actual deductible amount for calendar year 2010 and future years is unknown and will be subject to change.

Example #1: In 2010, a clinical psychologist submits a claim for $200 for outpatient treatment of a patient's mental disorder. The Medicare-approved amount is $180. Since clinical psychologists must accept assignment, the patient is not liable for the $20 in

excess charges. The patient previously satisfied the $135 annual Part B deductible. The limitation reduces the amount of incurred expenses to 68 ? percent of the approved amount. Medicare pays 80 percent of the remaining incurred expenses. The Medicare payment and patient liability are computed as follows:

1. Actual charges..$200.00
2. Medicare-approved amount $180.00
3. Medicare incurred expenses (0.6875 x line 2).....................$123.75
4. Unmet deductible...0.00
5. Remainder after subtracting deductible (line 3 minus line 4) $123.75
6. Medicare payment (0.80 x line 5)......................................$99.00
7. Patient liability (line 2 minus line 6) $81.00

Example #2: In 2012, a clinical social worker submits a claim for $135 for outpatient treatment of a patient's mental disorder. The Medicare-approved amount is $120. Since clinical social workers must accept assignment, the patient is not liable for the $15 in excess charges. The limitation reduces the amount of incurred expenses to 75 percent of the approved amount. The patient previously satisfied $70 of the $135 annual Part B deductible, leaving $65 unmet. The Medicare payment and patient liability are computed as follows:

1. Actual charges..$135.00
2. Medicare-approved amount...$120.00
3. Medicare incurred expenses (0.75 x line 2)............................$90.00
4. Unmet deductible $65.00
5. Remainder after subtracting deductible (line 3 minus line 4) $25.00
6. Medicare payment (0.80 x line 5)......................................$20.00
7. Patient liability (line 2 minus line 6) $100.00

Example #3: In calendar year 2013, a physician who does not accept assignment submits a claim for $780 for services in connection with the treatment of a mental disorder that did not require inpatient hospitalization. The Medicare-approved amount is $750. Because the physician does not accept assignment, the patient is liable for the $30 in excess charges. The patient has not satisfied any of the $135 Part B annual deductible. The Medicare payment and patient liability are computed as follows:

1. Actual charges..$780.00
2. Medicare-approved amount...$750.00
3. Medicare incurred expenses (0.8125 x line 2).....................$609.38
4. Unmet deductible $135.00
5. Remainder after subtracting deductible (line 3 minus line 4) $474.38
6. Medicare payment (0.80 x line 5)....................................$379.50
7. Patient liability (line 1 minus line 6) 400.50

Example #4: A patient's Part B expenses during calendar year 2014 are for a physician's services in connection with the treatment of a mental disorder that initially required

inpatient hospitalization, with subsequent physician services furnished on an outpatient basis. The patient has not satisfied any of the $135 Part B deductible. The physician accepts assignment and submits a claim for $780. The Medicare-approved amount is $750. Since the limitation will be completely phased out as of January 1, 2014, the entire $750 Medicare-approved amount is recognized as the total incurred expenses because such expenses are no longer reduced. Also, there is no longer any distinction between mental health services the patient receives as an inpatient or outpatient. The Medicare payment and patient liability are computed as follows:

1. Actual charges $780.00
2. Medicare-approved amount...$750.00
3. Medicare incurred expenses (1.00 x line 2)...........................$750.00
4. Unmet deductible $135.00
5. Remainder after subtracting deductible (line 3 minus line 4) $615.00
6. Medicare payment (0.80 x line 5)..$492.00
7. Beneficiary liability (line 2 minus line 6) $258.00

100-4, 13, 40
Magnetic Resonance Imaging (MRI) Procedures
Effective September 28, 2009

The Centers for Medicare & Medicaid Services (CMS) finds that the non-coverage of magnetic resonance imaging (MRI) for blood flow determination is no longer supported by the available evidence. CMS is removing the phrase "blood flow measurement" and local Medicare contractors will have the discretion to cover (or not cover).

Consult Publication (Pub.) 100-03, National Coverage Determinations (NCD) Manual, chapter 1, section 220.2, for specific coverage and non-coverage indications associated with MRI and MRA (Magnetic Resonance Angiography).

Prior to January 1, 2007

Carriers do not make additional payments for three or more MRI sequences. The relative value units (RVUs) reflect payment levels for two sequences.

The technical component (TC) RVUs for MRI procedures that specify "with contrast" include payment for paramagnetic contrast media. Carriers do not make separate payment under code A4647.

A diagnostic technique has been developed under which an MRI of the brain or spine is first performed without contrast material, then another MRI is performed with a standard (0.1mmol/kg) dose of contrast material and, based on the need to achieve a better image, a third MRI is performed with an additional double dosage (0.2mmol/kg) of contrast material. When the high-dose contrast technique is utilized, carriers:

- Do not pay separately for the contrast material used in the second MRI procedure;
- Pay for the contrast material given for the third MRI procedure through supply code Q9952, the replacement code for A4643, when billed with Current Procedural Terminology (CPT) codes 70553, 72156, 72157, and 72158;
- Do not pay for the third MRI procedure. For example, in the case of an MRI of the brain, if CPT code 70553 (without contrast material, followed by with contrast material(s) and further sequences) is billed, make no payment for CPT code 70551 (without contrast material(s)), the additional procedure given for the purpose of administering the double dosage, furnished during the same session. Medicare does not pay for the third procedure (as distinguished from the contrast material) because the CPT definition of code 70553 includes all further sequences; and
- Do not apply the payment criteria for low osmolar contrast media in §30.1.2 to billings for code Q9952, the replacement code for A4643.

Effective January 1, 2007

With the implementation for calendar year 2007 of a bottom-up methodology, which utilizes the direct inputs to determine the practice expense (PE) relative value units (RVUs), the cost of the contrast media is not included in the PE RVUs. Therefore, a separate payment for the contrast media used in various imaging procedures is paid. In addition to the CPT code representing the imaging procedure, separately bill the appropriate HCPCS "Q" code (Q9945 – Q9954; Q9958-Q9964) for the contrast medium utilized in performing the service.

Effective February 24, 2011

Medicare will allow for coverage of MRI for beneficiaries with implanted PMs or cardioverter defibrillators (ICDs) for use in an MRI environment in a Medicare-approved clinical study as described in section 220.C.1 of the NCD manual.

Effective July 7, 2011

Medicare will allow for coverage of MRI for beneficiaries with implanted pacemakers (PMs) when the PMs are used according to the Food and Drug Administration (FDA)-approved labeling for use in an MRI environment as described in section 220.2.C.1 of the NCD Manual.

100-4, 13, 40.1.2
HCPCS Coding Requirements
Providers must report HCPCS codes when submitting claims for MRA of the chest, abdomen, head, neck or peripheral vessels of lower extremities. The following HCPCS codes should be used to report these services:

MRA of head	70544, 70544-26, 70544-TC
MRA of head	70545, 70545-26, 70545-TC
MRA of head	70546, 70546-26, 70546-TC
MRA of neck	70547, 70547-26, 70547-TC
MRA of neck	70548, 70548-26, 70548-TC
MRA of neck	70549, 70549-26, 70549-TC
MRA of chest	71555, 71555-26, 71555-TC
MRA of pelvis	72198, 72198-26, 72198-TC
MRA of abdomen (dates of service on or after July 1, 2003)—see below.	74185, 74185-26, 74185-TC
MRA of peripheral vessels of lower extremities	73725, 73725-26, 73725-TC

100-4, 13, 60
Positron Emission Tomography (PET) Scans - General Information
Positron emission tomography (PET) is a noninvasive imaging procedure that assesses perfusion and the level of metabolic activity in various organ systems of the human body. A positron camera (tomograph) is used to produce cross-sectional tomographic images which are obtained by detecting radioactivity from a radioactive tracer substance radiopharmaceutical) that emits a radioactive tracer substance (radiopharmaceutical FDG) such as 2 -[F-18] flouro-D-glucose FDG, that is administered intravenously to the patient.

The Medicare National Coverage Determinations (NCD) Manual, Chapter 1, Sec.220.6, contains additional coverage instructions to indicate the conditions under which a PET scan is performed.

A. Definitions
For all uses of PET, excluding Rubidium 82 for perfusion of the heart, myocardial viability and refractory seizures, the following definitions apply:

Diagnosis: PET is covered only in clinical situations in which the PET results may assist in avoiding an invasive diagnostic procedure, or in which the PET results may assist in determining the optimal anatomical location to perform an invasive diagnostic procedure. In general, for most solid tumors, a tissue diagnosis is made prior to the performance of PET scanning. PET scans following a tissue diagnosis are generally performed for the purpose of staging, rather than diagnosis. Therefore, the use of PET in the diagnosis of lymphoma, esophageal and colorectal cancers, as well as in melanoma, should be rare. PET is not covered for other diagnostic uses, and is not covered for screening (testing of patients without specific signs and symptoms of disease).

Staging: PET is covered in clinical situations in which (1) (a) the stage of the cancer remains in doubt after completion of a standard diagnostic workup, including conventional imaging (computed tomography, magnetic resonance imaging, or ultrasound) or, (b) the use of PET would also be considered reasonable and necessary if it could potentially replace one or more conventional imaging studies when it is expected that conventional study information is insufficient for the clinical management of the patient and, (2) clinical management of the patient would differ depending on the stage of the cancer identified.

NOTE: Effective for services on or after April 3, 2009, the terms "diagnosis" and "staging" will be replaced with "Initial Treatment Strategy." For further information on this new term, refer to Pub. 100-03, NCD Manual, section 220.6.17.

Restaging: PET will be covered for restaging: (1) after the completion of treatment for the purpose of detecting residual disease, (2) for detecting suspected recurrence, or metastasis, (3) to determine the extent of a known recurrence, or (4) if it could potentially replace one or more conventional imaging studies when it is expected that conventional study information is to determine the extent of a known recurrence, or if study information is insufficient for the clinical management of the patient. Restaging applies to testing after a course of treatment is completed and is covered subject to the conditions above.

Monitoring: Use of PET to monitor tumor response to treatment during the planned course of therapy (i.e., when a change in therapy is anticipated).

NOTE: Effective for services on or after April 3, 2009, the terms "restaging" and "monitoring" will be replaced with "Subsequent Treatment Strategy." For further information on this new term, refer to Pub. 100-03, NCD Manual, section 220.6.17.

B. Limitations

For staging and restaging: PET is covered in either/or both of the following circumstances:

The stage of the cancer remains in doubt after completion of a standard diagnostic workup, including conventional imaging (computed tomography, magnetic resonance imaging, or ultrasound); and/or

The clinical management of the patient would differ depending on the stage of the cancer identified. PET will be covered for restaging after the completion of treatment for the purpose of detecting residual disease, for detecting suspected recurrence, or to determine the extent of a known recurrence. Use of PET would also be considered reasonable and necessary if it could potentially replace one or more conventional imaging studies when it is expected that conventional study information is insufficient for the clinical management of the patient.

The PET is not covered for other diagnostic uses, and is not covered for screening (testing of patients without specific symptoms). Use of PET to monitor tumor response during the planned course of therapy (i.e. when no change in therapy is being contemplated) is not covered.

100-4, 13, 60.3

PET Scan Qualifying Conditions and HCPCS Code Chart

Below is a summary of all covered PET scan conditions, with effective dates.

NOTE: The G codes below except those a # can be used to bill for PET Scan services through January 27, 2005. Effective for dates of service on or after January 28, 2005, providers must bill for PET Scan services using the appropriate CPT codes. See section 60.3.1. The G codes with a # can continue to be used for billing after January 28, 2005 and these remain non-covered by Medicare. (NOTE: PET Scanners must be FDA-approved.)

Conditions	Coverage Effective Date	****HCPCS/CPT
*Myocardial perfusion imaging (following previous PET G0030-G0047) single study, rest or stress (exercise and/or pharmacologic)	3/14/95	G0030
*Myocardial perfusion imaging (following previous PET G0030-G0047) multiple studies, rest or stress (exercise and/or pharmacologic)	3/14/95	G0031
*Myocardial perfusion imaging (following rest SPECT, 78464); single study, rest or stress (exercise and/or pharmacologic)	3/14/95	G0032
*Myocardial perfusion imaging (following rest SPECT 78464); multiple studies, rest or stress (exercise and/or pharmacologic)	3/14/95	G0033
*Myocardial perfusion (following stress SPECT 78465); single study, rest or stress (exercise and/or pharmacologic)	3/14/95	G0034
*Myocardial Perfusion Imaging (following stress SPECT 78465); multiple studies, rest or stress (exercise and/or pharmacologic)	3/14/95	G0035
*Myocardial Perfusion Imaging (following coronary angiography 93510-93529); single study, rest or stress (exercise and/or pharmacologic)	3/14/95	G0036
*Myocardial Perfusion Imaging, (following coronary angiography), 93510-93529); multiple studies, rest or stress (exercise and/or pharmacologic)	3/14/95	G0037
*Myocardial Perfusion Imaging (following stress planar myocardial perfusion, 78460); single study, rest or stress (exercise and/or pharmacologic)	3/14/95	G0038
*Myocardial Perfusion Imaging (following stress planar myocardial perfusion, 78460); multiple studies, rest or stress (exercise and/or pharmacologic)	3/14/95	G0039
*Myocardial Perfusion Imaging (following stress echocardiogram 93350); single study, rest or stress (exercise and/or pharmacologic)	3/14/95	G0040

Conditions	Coverage Effective Date	****HCPCS/CPT
*Myocardial Perfusion Imaging (following stress echocardiogram, 93350); multiple studies, rest or stress (exercise and/or pharmacologic)	3/14/95	G0041
*Myocardial Perfusion Imaging (following stress nuclear ventriculogram 78481 or 78483); single study, rest or stress (exercise and/or pharmacologic)	3/14/95	G0042
*Myocardial Perfusion Imaging (following stress nuclear ventriculogram 78481 or 78483); multiple studies, rest or stress (exercise and/or pharmacologic)	3/14/95	G0043
*Myocardial Perfusion Imaging (following stress ECG, 93000); single study, rest or stress (exercise and/or pharmacologic)	3/14/95	G0044
*Myocardial perfusion (following stress ECG, 93000), multiple studies; rest or stress (exercise and/or pharmacologic)	3/14/95	G0045
*Myocardial perfusion (following stress ECG, 93015), single study; rest or stress (exercise and/or pharmacologic)	3/14/95	G0046
*Myocardial perfusion (following stress ECG, 93015); multiple studies, rest or stress (exercise and/or pharmacologic)	3/14/95	G0047
PET imaging regional or whole body; single pulmonary nodule	1/1/98	G0125
Lung cancer, non-small cell (PET imaging whole body) Diagnosis, Initial Staging, Restaging	7/1/01	G0210 G0211 G0212
Colorectal cancer (PET imaging whole body) Diagnosis, Initial Staging, Restaging	7/1/01	G0213 G0214 G0215
Melanoma (PET imaging whole body) Diagnosis, Initial Staging, Restaging	7/1/01	G0216 G0217 G0218
Melanoma for non-covered indications Lymphoma (PET imaging whole body)	7/1/01	#G0219
Diagnosis, Initial Staging, Restaging	7/1/01	G0220 G0221 G0222
Head and neck cancer; excluding thyroid and CNS cancers (PET imaging whole body or regional) Diagnosis, Initial Staging, Restaging	7/1/01	G0223 G0224 G0225

100-4, 13, 60.3.1

Appropriate CPT Codes Effective for PET Scans for Services Performed on or After January 28, 2005

NOTE: All PET scan services require the use of a radiopharmaceutical diagnostic imaging agent (tracer). The applicable tracer code should be billed when billing for a PET scan service. See section 60.3.2 below for applicable tracer codes.

CPT Code	Description
78459	Myocardial imaging, positron emission tomography (PET), metabolic evaluation
78491	Myocardial imaging, positron emission tomography (PET), perfusion, single study at rest or stress
78492	Myocardial imaging, positron emission tomography (PET), perfusion, multiple studies at rest and/or stress
78608	Brain imaging, positron emission tomography (PET); metabolic evaluation
78811	Tumor imaging, positron emission tomography (PET); limited area (eg, chest, head/neck)
78812	Tumor imaging, positron emission tomography (PET); skull base to mid-thigh
78813	Tumor imaging, positron emission tomography (PET); whole body

CPT Code	Description
78814	Tumor imaging, positron emission tomography (PET) with concurrently acquired computed tomography (CT) for attenuation correction and anatomical localization; limited area (eg, chest, head/neck)
78815	Tumor imaging, positron emission tomography (PET) with concurrently acquired computed tomography (CT) for attenuation correction and anatomical localization; skull base to mid-thigh
78816	Tumor imaging, positron emission tomography (PET) with concurrently acquired computed tomography (CT) for attenuation correction and anatomical localization; whole body

100-4, 13, 60.3.2

Tracer Codes Required for PET Scans

The following tracer codes are applicable only to CPT 78491 and 78492. They can not be reported with any other code.

Institutional providers billing the fiscal intermediary

HCPCS	Description
*A9555	Rubidium Rb-82, Diagnostic, Per study dose, Up To 60 Millicuries
* Q3000 (Deleted effective 12/31/05)	Supply of Radiopharmaceutical Diagnostic Imaging Agent, Rubidium Rb-82, per dose
A9526	Nitrogen N-13 Ammonia, Diagnostic, Per study dose, Up To 40 Millicuries

NOTE: For claims with dates of service prior to 1/01/06, providers report Q3000 for supply of radiopharmaceutical diagnostic imaging agent, Rubidium Rb-82. For claims with dates of service 1/01/06 and later, providers report A9555 for radiopharmaceutical diagnostic imaging agent, Rubidium Rb-82 in place of Q3000.

Physicians / practitioners billing the carrier:

*A4641	Supply of Radiopharmaceutical Diagnostic Imaging Agent, Not Otherwise Classified
A9526	Nitrogen N-13 Ammonia, Diagnostic, Per study dose, Up To 40 Millicuries
A9555	Rubidium Rb-82, Diagnostic, Per study dose, Up To 60 Millicuries

*   NOTE: Effective January 1, 2008, tracer code A4641 is not applicable for PET Scans.

The following tracer codes are applicable only to CPT 78459, 78608, 78811-78816. They can not be reported with any other code:

Institutional providers billing the fiscal intermediary:

* A9552	Fluorodeoxyglucose F18, FDG, Diagnostic, Per study dose, Up to 45 Millicuries
*C1775 (Deleted effective 12/31/05)	Supply of Radiopharmaceutical Diagnostic Imaging Agent, Fluorodeoxyglucose F18, (2-Deoxy-2-18F Fluoro-D-Glucose), Per dose (4-40 Mci/MI)
**A4641	Supply of Radiopharmaceutical Diagnostic Imaging Agent, Not Otherwise Classified
A9580	Sodium Fluoride F-18, Diagnostic, per study dose, up to 30 Millicuries

**   NOTE: Effective January 1, 2008, tracer code A4641 is not applicable for PET Scans.
*** NOTE: Effective for claims with dates of service February 26, 2010 and later, tracer code A9580 is applicable for PET Scans.

NOTE: For claims with dates of service prior to 1/01/06, OPPS hospitals report C1775 for supply of radiopharmaceutical diagnostic imaging agent, Fluorodeoxyglucose F18. For claims with dates of service January 1, 2006 and later, providers report A9552 for radiopharmaceutical diagnostic imaging agent, Fluorodeoxyglucose F18 in place of C1775.

Physicians / practitioners billing the carrier:

A9552	Fluorodeoxyglucose F18, FDG, Diagnostic, Per study dose, Up to 45 Millicuries

*   NOTE: Effective January 1, 2008, tracer code A4641 is not applicable for PET Scans.
*** NOTE: Effective for claims with dates of service February 26, 2010 and later, tracer code A9580 is applicable for PET Scans.

*A4641	Supply of Radiopharmaceutical Diagnostic Imaging Agent, Not Otherwise Classified
A9580	Sodium Fluoride F-18, Diagnostic, per study dose, up to 30 Millicuries

*   NOTE: Effective January 1, 2008, tracer code A4641 is not applicable for PET Scans.
*** NOTE: Effective for claims with dates of service February 26, 2010 and later, tracer code A9580 is applicable for PET Scans.

Positron Emission Tomography Reference Table

CPT	Short Descriptor	Tracer/Code	or	Tracer/Code	Comment
78459	Myocardial imaging, positron emission tomography (PET), metabolic imaging	FDG A9552	--	--	N/A
78491	Myocardial imaging, positron emission tomography (PET), perfusion; single study at rest or stress	N-13 A9526	or	Rb-82 A9555	N/A
78492	Myocardial imaging, positron emission tomography (PET), perfusion; multiple studies at rest and/or stress	N-13 A9526	or	Rb-82 A9555	N/A
78608	Brain imaging, positron emission tomography (PET); metabolic evaluation	FDG A9552	--	--	Covered indications: Alzheimer's disease/dementias, intractable seizures Note: This code is also covered for dedicated PET brain tumor imaging.
78609	Brain imaging, positron emission tomography (PET); perfusion evaluation	--	--	--	Nationally noncovered
78811	Positron emission tomography (PET) imaging; limited area (e.g, chest, head/neck)	FDG A9552	or	NaF-18 A9580	NaF-18 PET is covered only to identify bone metastasis of cancer.

100-4, 13, 60.7.1

Darbepoetin Alfa (Aranesp) Facility Billing Requirements

Revenue code 0636 is used to report Aranesp.

The HCPCS code for aranesp must be included: HCPCS HCPCS Description Dates of Service Q4054 Injection, darbepoetin alfa, 1mcg (for ESRD on Dialysis) 1/1/2004 through 12/31/2005 J0882 Injection, darbepoetin alfa, 1mcg (for ESRD on Dialysis) 1/1/2006 to present The hematocrit reading taken prior to the last administration of Aranesp during the billing period must also be reported on the UB-92/Form CMS-1450 with value code 49. For claims with dates of service on or after April 1, 2006, a hemoglobin reading may be reported on Aranesp claims using value code 48.

Effective January 1, 2006 the definition of value code 48 and 49 used to report the hemoglobin and hematocrit readings are changed to indicate the patient's most recent reading taken before the start of the billing period.

To report a hematocrit or hemoglobin reading for a new patient on or after January 1, 2006, the provider should report the reading that prompted the treatment of darbepoetin alfa. The provider may use results documented on form CMS 2728 or the patient's medical records from a transferring facility.

The payment allowance for Aranesp is the only allowance for the drug and its administration when used for ESRD patients. Effective January 1, 2005, the cost of supplies to administer Aranesp may be billed to the FI. HCPCS A4657 and Revenue Code 270 should be used to capture the charges for syringes used in the administration of Aranesp. The maximum number of administrations of Aranesp for a billing cycle is 5 times in 30/ 31days.

Format 100-4, 13, 60.13

Billing Requirements for PET Scans for Specific Indications of Cervical Cancer for Services Performed on or After January 28, 2005

Contractors shall accept claims for these services with the appropriate CPT code listed in section 60.3.1. Refer to Pub. 100-03, section 220.6.17, for complete coverage guidelines for this new PET oncology indication. The implementation date for these CPT codes will be April 18, 2005. Also see section 60.17, of this chapter for further claims processing instructions for cervical cancer indications.

100-4, 13, 60.14

Billing Requirements for PET Scans for Non-Covered Indications

For services performed on or after January 28, 2005, contractors shall accept claims with the following HCPCS code for non-covered PET indications: - G0235: PET imaging, any site not otherwise specified Short Descriptor: PET not otherwise specified Type of Service: 4

NOTE: This code is for a non-covered service.

100-4, 13, 60.15

Billing Requirements for CMS - Approved Clinical Trials and Coverage With Evidence Development Claims for PET Scans for Neurodegenerative Diseases, Previously Specified Cancer Indications, and All Other Cancer Indications Not Previously Specified

Carriers and FIs

Effective for services on or after January 28, 2005, contractors shall accept and pay for claims for PET scans for lung cancer, esophageal cancer, colorectal cancer, lymphoma, melanoma, head & neck cancer, breast cancer, thyroid cancer, soft tissue sarcoma, brain cancer, ovarian cancer, pancreatic cancer, small cell lung cancer, and testicular cancer, as well as for neurodegenerative diseases and all other cancer indications not previously mentioned in this chapter, if these scans were performed as part of a CMS-approved clinical trial. (See Pub. 100-03, NCD Manual, sections 220.6.13 and 220.6.17.)

Contractors shall also be aware that PET scans for all cancers not previously specified at Pub. 100-03, NCD Manual, section 220.6.17, remain nationally non-covered unless performed in conjunction with a CMS-approved clinical trial.

- Carriers Only

Carriers shall pay claims for PET scans for beneficiaries participating in a CMS-approved clinical trial submitted with an appropriate CPT code from section 60.3.1, of this chapter and the -QR (Item or Service Provided in a Medicare Specified Study) modifier.

- FIs Only

In order to pay claims for PET scans on behalf of beneficiaries participating in a CMS-approved clinical trial, FIs require providers to submit claims with ICD-9 code V70.7 in the second diagnosis position on the CMS-1450 (UB-04), or the electronic equivalent, with the appropriate principal diagnosis code and an appropriate CPT code from section 60.3.1. Effective for PET scan claims for dates of service on or after January 28, 2005, FIs shall accept claims with the -QR modifier on other than inpatient claims.

NOTE: Effective for services on or after January 1, 2008, -Q0 (investigational clinical service provided in a clinical research study that is in an approved clinical research study) replaces the -QR modifier.

100-4, 13, 60.16

Billing and Coverage Changes for PET Scans Effective for Services on or After April 3, 2009

A. Summary of Changes

Effective for services on or after April 3, 2009, Medicare will not cover the use of FDG PET imaging to determine initial treatment strategy in patients with adenocarcinoma of the prostate.

Medicare will also not cover FDG PET imaging for subsequent treatment strategy for tumor types other than breast, cervical, colorectal, esophagus, head and neck (non-CNS/thyroid), lymphoma, melanoma, myeloma, non-small cell lung, and ovarian, unless the FDG PET is provided under the coverage with evidence development (CED) paradigm (billed with modifier -Q0, see section 60.15 of this chapter).

Last, Medicare will cover FDG PET imaging for initial treatment strategy for myeloma.

For further information regarding the changes in coverage, refer to Pub.100-03, NCD Manual, section 220.6.17.

B. New Modifiers for PET Scans

Effective for claims with dates of service on or after April 3, 2009, the following modifiers have been created for use to inform for the initial treatment strategy of biopsy-proven or strongly suspected tumors or subsequent treatment strategy of cancerous tumors:

PI -Positron Emission Tomography (PET) or PET/Computed Tomography (CT) to inform the initial treatment strategy of tumors that are biopsy proven or strongly suspected of being cancerous based on other diagnostic testing.

Short descriptor: PET tumor init tx strat

PS - Positron Emission Tomography (PET) or PET/Computed Tomography (CT) to inform the subsequent treatment strategy of cancerous tumors when the beneficiary's treatment physician determines that the PET study is needed to inform subsequent anti-tumor strategy.

Short descriptor: PS - PET tumor subsq tx strategy

C. Billing Changes for A/B MACs, FIs and Carriers

Effective for claims with dates of service on or after April 3, 2009, contractors shall accept FDG PET claims billed to inform initial treatment strategy with the following CPT codes AND modifier - PI: 78608, 78811, 78812, 78813, 78814, 78815, 78816.

Effective for claims with dates of service on or after April 3, 2009, contractors shall accept FDG PET claims with modifier -PS for the subsequent treatment strategy for solid tumors using a CPT code above AND an ICD-9 cancer diagnosis code.

Contractors shall also accept FDG PET claims billed to inform initial treatment strategy or subsequent treatment strategy when performed under CED with one of the PET or PET/CT CPT codes above AND modifier -PI OR modifier -PS AND an ICD-9 cancer diagnosis code AND modifier -Q0 (Investigational clinical service provided in a clinical research study that is in an approved clinical research study).

NOTE: For institutional claims continue to use diagnosis code V70.7 and condition code 30 on the claim.

D. Medicare Summary Notices, Remittance Advice Remark Codes, and Claim Adjustment Reason Codes

Effective for dates of service on or after April 3, 2009, contractors shall return as unprocessable/return to provider claims that do not include the -PI modifier with one of the PET/PET/CT CPT codes listed in subsection C. above when billing for the initial treatment strategy for solid tumors in accordance with Pub.100-03, NCD Manual, section 220.6.17.

In addition, contractors shall return as unprocessable/return to provider claims that do not include the -PS modifier with one of the CPT codes listed in subsection C. above when billing for the subsequent treatment strategy for solid tumors in accordance with Pub.100-03, NCD Manual, section 220.6.17.

The following messages apply:

- Claim Adjustment Reason Code 4 - the procedure code is inconsistent with the modifier used or a required modifier is missing.

- Remittance Advice Remark Code MA-130 - Your claim contains incomplete and/or invalid information, and no appeal rights are afforded because the claim is unprocessable. Submit a new claim with the complete/correct information.

- Remittance Advice Remark Code M16 - Alert: See our Web site, mailings, or bulletins for more details concerning this policy/procedure/decision.

Also, effective for claims with dates of service on or after April 3, 2009, contractors shall return as unprocessable/return to provider FDG PET claims billed to inform initial treatment strategy or subsequent treatment strategy when performed under CED without one of the PET/PET/CT CPT codes listed in subsection C. above AND modifier -PI OR modifier -PS AND an ICD-9 cancer diagnosis code AND modifier -Q0.

The following messages apply to return as unprocessable claims:

- Claim Adjustment Reason Code 4 - the procedure code is inconsistent with the modifier used or a required modifier is missing.

- Remittance Advice Remark Code MA-130 - Your claim contains incomplete and/or invalid information, and no appeal rights are afforded because the claim is unprocessable. Submit a new claim with the complete/correct information.

- Remittance Advice Remark Code M16 - Alert: See our Web site, mailings, or bulletins for more details concerning this policy/procedure/decision.

Effective April 3, 2009, contractors shall deny claims with ICD-9 diagnosis code 185 for FDG PET imaging for the initial treatment strategy of patients with adenocarcinoma of the prostate.

Contractors shall also deny claims for FDG PET imaging for subsequent treatment strategy for tumor types other than breast, cervical, colorectal, esophagus, head and neck (non-CNS/thyroid), lymphoma, melanoma, myeloma, non-small cell lung, and ovarian, unless the FDG PET is provided under CED (submitted with the -Q0 modifier) and use the following messages:

- Medicare Summary Notice 15.4 - Medicare does not support the need for this service or item

- Claim Adjustment Reason Code 50 - These are non-covered services because this is not deemed a 'medical necessity' by the payer.

- Contractors shall use Group Code CO (Contractual Obligation)

If an ABN is provided with a GA modifier indicating there is a signed ABN on file, contractors shall use Group Code PR (Patient Responsibility) and the liability falls to the beneficiary.

If an ABN is provided with a GZ modifier indicating no ABN was provided, contractors shall use Group Code CO (Contractual Obligation) and the liability falls to the provider.

Format 100-4, 13, 60.17

Billing and Coverage Changes for PET Scans for Cervical Cancer Effective for Services on or After November 10, 2009

A. Billing Changes for A/B MACs, FIs, and Carriers

Effective for claims with dates of service on or after November 10, 2009, contractors shall accept FDG PET oncologic claims billed to inform initial treatment strategy; specifically for staging in beneficiaries who have biopsy-proven cervical cancer when the beneficiary's treating physician determines the FDG PET study is needed to determine the location and/or extent of the tumor as specified in Pub. 100-03, section 220.6.17.

EXCEPTION: CMS continues to non-cover FDG PET for initial diagnosis of cervical cancer related to initial treatment strategy.

NOTE: Effective for claims with dates of service on and after November 10, 2009, the ?0 modifier is no longer necessary for FDG PET for cervical cancer.

B. Medicare Summary Notices, Remittance Advice Remark Codes, and Claim Adjustment Reason Codes

Additionally, contractors shall return as unprocessable /return to provider for FDG PET for cervical cancer for initial treatment strategy billed without the following: one of the PET/PET/ CT CPT codes listed in 60.16 C above AND modifier ?I AND an ICD-9 cervical cancer diagnosis code.

Use the following messages:

- Claim Adjustment Reason Code 4 - the procedure code is inconsistent with the modifier used or a required modifier is missing.

- Remittance Advice Remark Code MA-130 - Your claim contains incomplete and/or invalid information, and no appeal rights are afforded because the claim is unprocessable. Submit a new claim with the complete/correct information.

- Remittance Advice Remark Code M16 - Alert: See our Web site, mailings, or bulletins for more details concerning this policy/procedure/decision.

100-4, 13, 60.18

Billing and Coverage Changes for PET (NaF-18) Scans to Identify Bone Metastasis of Cancer Effective for Claims With Dates of Services on or After February 26, 2010

A. Billing Changes for A/B MACs, FIs, and Carriers

Effective for claims with dates of service on and after February 26, 2010, contractors shall pay for NaF-18 PET oncologic claims to inform of initial treatment strategy (PI) or subsequent treatment strategy (PS) for suspected or biopsy proven bone metastasis ONLY in the context of a clinical study and as specified in Pub. 100-03, section 220.6. All other claims for NaF-18 PET oncology claims remain non-covered.

B. Medicare Summary Notices, Remittance Advice Remark Codes, and Claim Adjustment Reason Codes

Effective for claims with dates of service on or after February 26, 2010, contractors shall return as unprocessable NaF-18 PET oncologic claims billed with modifier TC or globally (for FIs modifier TC or globally does not apply) and HCPCS A9580 to inform the initial treatment strategy or subsequent treatment strategy for bone metastasis that do not include ALL of the following:

- PI or –PS modifier AND

- PET or PET/CT CPT code (78811, 78812, 78813, 78814, 78815, 78816) AND

- ICD-9 cancer diagnosis code AND

- Q0 modifier – Investigational clinical service provided in a clinical research study, are present on the claim.

NOTE: For institutional claims, continue to include diagnosis code V70.7 and condition code 30 to denote a clinical study.

Use the following messages:

- Claim Adjustment Reason Code 4 – The procedure code is inconsistent with the modifier used or a required modifier is missing. Note: Refer to the 835 Healthcare Policy Identification Segment (loop 2110 Service Payment Information REF), if present.

- Remittance Advice Remark Code MA-130 - Your claim contains incomplete and/or invalid information, and no appeal rights are afforded because the claim is unprocessable. Submit a new claim with the complete/correct information.

- Remittance Advice Remark Code M16 - Alert: See our Web site, mailings, or bulletins for more details concerning this policy/procedure/decision.

- Claim Adjustment Reason Code 167 – This (these) diagnosis(es) is (are) not covered.

Effective for claims with dates of service on or after February 26, 2010, contractors shall accept PET oncologic claims billed with modifier 26 and modifier KX to inform the initial treatment strategy or strategy or subsequent treatment strategy for bone metastasis that include the following:

- PI or –PS modifier AND

- PET or PET/CT CPT code (78811, 78812, 78813, 78814, 78815, 78816) AND

- ICD-9 cancer diagnosis code AND

- Q0 modifier – Investigational clinical service provided in a clinical research study, are present on the claim.

NOTE: If modifier KX is present on the professional component service, Contractors shall process the service as PET NaF-18 rather than PET with FDG.

Contractors shall also return as unprocessable NaF-18 PET oncologic professional component claims (i.e., claims billed with modifiers 26 and KX) to inform the initial treatment strategy or strategy or subsequent treatment strategy for bone metastasis billed with HCPCS A9580 and use the following message:

Claim Adjustment Reason Code 97 – The benefit for this service is included in the payment/allowance for another service/procedure that has already been adjudicated.

NOTE: Refer to the 835 Healthcare Policy identification Segment (loop 2110 Service Payment Information REF), if present.

100-4, 13, 140

Bone Mass Measurements (BMMs)

Sections H1861(s)(15)H and H(rr)(1)H of the Social Security Act (the Act) (as added by 4106 of the Balanced Budget Act (BBA) of 1997) standardize Medicare coverage of medically necessary bone mass measurements by providing for uniform coverage under Medicare Part B. This coverage is effective for claims with dates of service furnished on or after July 1, 1998.

Effective for dates of service on and after January 1, 2007, the CY 2007 Physician Fee Schedule final rule expanded the number of beneficiaries qualifying for BMM by reducing the dosage requirement for glucocorticoid (steroid) therapy from 7.5 mg of prednisone per day to 5.0 mg. It also changed the definition of BMM by removing coverage for a single-photon absorptiometry as it is not considered reasonable and necessary under section 1862 (a)(1)(A) of the Act. Finally, it required that in the case of monitoring and confirmatory baseline BMMs, they be performed with a dual-energy xray absorptiometry (axial) test.

Conditions of Coverage for BMMs are located in Pub.100-02, Medicare Benefit Policy Manual, chapter 15.

100-4, 14, 40.3

Payment for Intraocular Lens (IOL)

Prior to January 1, 2008, payment for facility services furnished by an ASC for IOL insertion during or subsequent to cataract surgery includes an allowance for the lens. The procedures that include insertion of an IOL are: Payment Group 6: CPT-4 Codes 66985 and 66986 Payment Group 8: CPT-4 Codes 66982, 66983 and 66984 Physicians or suppliers are not paid for an IOL furnished to a beneficiary in an ASC after July 1, 1988. Separate claims for IOLs furnished to ASC patients beginning March 12, 1990 are denied. Also, effective March 12, 1990, procedures 66983 and 66984 are treated as single procedures for payment purposes.

Beginning January 1, 2008, the Medicare payment for the IOL is included in the Medicare ASC payment for the associated surgical procedure. Consequently, no separate payment for the IOL is made, except for a payment adjustment for NTIOLs established according to the process outlined in 42 CFR 416.185. ASCs should not report separate charges for conventional IOLs because their payment is included in the Medicare payment for the associated surgical procedure. The ASC payment system logic that excluded $150 for IOLs for purposes of the multiple surgery reduction in cases of cataract surgery prior to January 1, 2008 no longer applies, effective for dates of service on or after January 1, 2008.

Effective for dates of service on and after February 27, 2006, through February 26, 2011, Medicare pays an additional $50 for specified Category 3 NTIOLs that are provided in association with a covered ASC surgical procedure. The list of Category 3 NTIOLS is available at: http://www.cms.hhs.gov/ASCPayment/08_NTIOLs.asp#TopOfPage.

ASCs should use HCPCS code Q1003 to bill for a Category 3 NTIOL. HCPCS code Q1003, along with one of the approved surgical procedure codes (CPT codes 66982, 66983, 66984, 66985, 66986) are to be used on all NTIOL Category 3 claims associated with reduced spherical aberration from February 27, 2006, through February 26, 2011. The payment adjustment for the NTIOL is subject to beneficiary coinsurance but is not wage-adjusted.

Any subsequent IOL recognized by CMS as having the same characteristics as the first NTIOL recognized by CMS for a payment adjustment as a Category III NTIOL (those of reduced spherical aberration) will receive the same adjustment for the remainder of the 5-year period established by the first recognized IOL.

100-4, 14, 40.8

40.8 - Payment When a Device is Furnished With No Cost or With Full or Partial Credit Beginning January 1, 2008

Contractors pay ASCs a reduced amount for certain specified procedures when a specified device is furnished without cost or for which either a partial or full credit is received (e.g., device recall). For specified procedure codes that include payment for a device, ASCs are required to include modifier -FB on the procedure code when a specified device is furnished without cost or for which full credit is received. If the ASC receives a partial credit of 50 percent or more of the cost of a specified device, the ASC is required to include modifier -FC on the procedure code if the procedure is on the list of specified procedures to which the -FC reduction applies. A single procedure code should not be submitted with both modifiers -FB and -FC. The pricing determination related to modifiers -FB and -FC is made prior to the application of multiple procedure payment reductions. Contractors adjust beneficiary coinsurance to reflect the reduced payment amount. Tables listing the procedures and devices to which the payment adjustments apply, and the full and partial adjustment amounts, are available on the CMS Web site.

In order to report that the receipt of a partial credit of 50 percent or more of the cost of a device, ASCs have the option of either: 1) Submitting the claim for the procedure to their Medicare contractor after the procedure's performance but prior to manufacturer acknowledgement of credit for a specified device, and subsequently contacting the contractor regarding a claims adjustment once the credit determination is made; or 2) holding the claim for the procedure until a determination is made by the manufacturer on the partial credit and submitting the claim with modifier -FC appended to the implantation procedure HCPCS code if the partial credit is 50 percent or more of the cost of the device. If choosing the first billing option, to request a claims adjustment once the credit determination is made, ASCs should keep in mind that the initial Medicare payment for the procedure involving the device is conditional and subject to adjustment.

100-4, 14, 40.9

Payment and Coding for Presbyopia Correcting IOLs (P-C IOLs) and Astigmatism Correcting IOLs (A-C IOLs) (CMS payment policies and recognition of P-C IOLs and A-C IOLs are contained in Transmittal 636 (CR3927) and Transmittal 1228 (CR5527) respectively.

Effective for dates of service on and after January 1, 2008, when inserting an approved A-C IOL in an ASC concurrent with cataract extraction, HCPCS code V2787 (Astigmatism-correcting function of intraocular lens) should be billed to report the non-covered charges for the A-C IOL functionality of the inserted intraocular lens. Additionally, note that HCPCS code V2788 (Presbyopia-correcting function of intraocular lens) is no longer valid to report non-covered charges associated with the A-C IOL. However, this code continues to be valid to report non-covered charges for a P-C IOL. The payment for the conventional lens portion of the A-C IOL and P-C IOL continues to be bundled with the ASC procedure payment.

Effective for services on and after January 1, 2010, ASCs are to bill for insertion of a Category 3 new technology intraocular lens (NTIOL) that is also an approved A-C IOL or P-C IOL, concurrent with cataract extraction, using three separate codes. ASCs shall use HCPCS code V2787 or V2788, as appropriate, to report charges associated with the non-covered functionality of the A-C IOL or P-C IOL, the appropriate HCPCS code 66982 (Extracapsular cataract removal with insertion of intraocular lens prosthesis (one stage procedure), manual or mechanical technique (e.g., irrigation and aspiration or phacoemulsification), complex, requiring devices or techniques not generally used in routine cataract surgery (e.g., iris expansion device, suture support for intraocular lens, or primary posterior capsulorrhexis) or performed on patients in the amblyogenic developmental stage); 66983 (Intracapsular cataract extraction with insertion of intraocular lens prosthesis (1 stage procedure)); or 66984 (Extracapsular cataract removal with insertion of intraocular lens prosthesis (1 stage procedure), manual or mechanical technique (e.g., irrigation and aspiration or phacoemulsification)), to report the covered cataract extraction and insertion procedure; and Q1003 (New technology, intraocular lens, category 3 (reduced spherical aberration) as defined in Federal Register notice, Vol. 65, dated May 3, 2000) to report the covered NTIOL aspect of the lens on claims for insertion of an A-C IOL or P-C IOL that is also designated as an NTIOL. Listings of the CMS-approved Category 3 NTIOLs, A-C IOLs, and P-C IOLs are available on the CMS web site.

100-4, 14, 60.1

60.1 - Applicable Messages for NTIOLs

Contractors shall return as unprocessable any claims for NTIOLs containing Q1003 alone or with a code other than one of the procedure codes listed in 40.3. Use the following messages for these returned claims:

- Claim Adjustment Reason Code 16 - Claim/service lacks information which is needed for adjudication. Additional information is supplied using remittance advice remark codes whenever appropriate.
- RA Remark Code M67 - Missing/Incomplete/Invalid other procedure codes.
- RA Remark Code MA130 - Your claim contains incomplete and/or invalid information, and no appeal rights are afforded because the claim is unprocessable. Please submit a new claim with the complete/correct information.

Contractors shall deny payment for Q1003 if services are furnished in a facility other than a Medicare-approved ASC. Use the following messages when denying these claims:

- MSN 16.2 - This service cannot be paid when provided in this location/facility.
- Claims Adjustment Reason Code 58 - Payment adjusted because treatment was deemed by the payer to have been rendered in an inappropriate or invalid place of service.

Contractors shall deny payment for Q1003 if billed by an entity other than a Medicare-approved ASC. Use the following messages when denying these claims:

- MSN 33.1 - The ambulatory surgical center must bill for this service.
- Claim Adjustment Reason Code 170 - Payment is denied when performed/billed by this type of provider.

Contractors shall deny payment for Q1003 if submitted for payment past the discontinued date (after the 5-year period, or after February 26, 2011). Use the following messages when denying these claims:

- MSN 21.11 - This service was not covered by Medicare at the time you received it.
- Claim Adjustment Reason Code 27 - Expenses incurred after coverage terminated.

Carriers shall deny payment for Q1003 if services are furnished in a facility other than a Medicare-approved ASC. Use the following messages when denying these claims:

- MSN 16.2 - This service cannot be paid when provided in this location/facility.
- Claims Adjustment Reason Code 58 - Payment adjusted because treatment was deemed by the payer to have been rendered in an inappropriate or invalid place of service.

Carriers shall deny payment for Q1003 if billed by an entity other than a Medicare-approved ASC. Use the following messages when denying these claims:

- MSN 33.1 - The ambulatory surgical center must bill for this service.
- Claim Adjustment Reason Code 170 - Payment is denied when performed/billed by this type of provider.

Carriers shall deny payment for Q1003 if submitted for payment past the discontinued date (after the 5-year period, or after February 26, 2011). Use the following messages when denying these claims:

MSN 21.11 - This service was not covered by Medicare at the time you received it.

- Claim Adjustment Reason Code 27 - Expenses incurred after coverage terminated.

100-4, 15, 20.1.4

Components of the Ambulance Fee Schedule

The mileage rates provided in this section are the base rates that are adjusted by the yearly ambulance inflation factor (AIF). The payment amount under the fee schedule is determined as follows:

- For ground ambulance services, the fee schedule amount includes:
  1. A money amount that serves as a nationally uniform base rate, called a "conversion factor" (CF), for all ground ambulance services;
  2. A relative value unit (RVU) assigned to each type of ground ambulance service;
  3. A geographic adjustment factor (GAF) for each ambulance fee schedule locality area (geographic practice cost index (GPCI));
  4. A nationally uniform loaded mileage rate;
  5. An additional amount for certain mileage for a rural point-of-pickup; and
  6. For specified temporary periods, certain additional payment amounts as described in section 20.1.4A, below.

- For air ambulance services, the fee schedule amount includes:

1. A nationally uniform base rate for fixed wing and a nationally uniform base rate for rotary wing;

2. A geographic adjustment factor (GAF) for each ambulance fee schedule locality area (GPCI);

3. A nationally uniform loaded mileage rate for each type of air service; and

4. A rural adjustment to the base rate and mileage for services furnished for a rural point-of-pickup.

A. Ground Ambulance Services

1. Conversion Factor

The conversion factor (CF) is a money amount used to develop a base rate for each category of ground ambulance service. The CF is updated annually by the ambulance inflation factor and for other reasons as necessary.

2. Relative Value Units

Relative value units (RVUs) set a numeric value for ambulance services relative to the value of a base level ambulance service. Since there are marked differences in resources necessary to furnish the various levels of ground ambulance services, different levels of payment are appropriate for the various levels of service. The different payment amounts are based on level of service. An RVU expresses the constant multiplier for a particular type of service (including, where appropriate, an emergency response). An RVU of 1.00 is assigned to the BLS of ground service, e.g., BLS has an RVU of 1; higher RVU values are assigned to the other types of ground ambulance services, which require more service than BLS.

The RVUs are as follows:

Service Level	RVU
BLS	1.00
BLS - Emergency	1.60
ALS1	1.20
ALS1 - Emergency	1.90
ALS2	2.75
SCT	3.25
PI	1.75

3. Geographic Adjustment Factor (GAF)

The GAF is one of two factors intended to address regional differences in the cost of furnishing ambulance services. The GAF for the ambulance FS uses the non-facility practice expense (PE) of the geographic practice cost index (GPCI) of the Medicare physician fee schedule to adjust payment to account for regional differences. Thus, the geographic areas applicable to the ambulance FS are the same as those used for the physician fee schedule.

The location where the beneficiary was put into the ambulance (POP) establishes which GPCI applies. For multiple vehicle transports, each leg of the transport is separately evaluated for the applicable GPCI. Thus, for the second (or any subsequent) leg of a transport, the POP establishes the applicable GPCI for that portion of the ambulance transport.

For ground ambulance services, the applicable GPCI is multiplied by 70 percent of the base rate. Again, the base rate for each category of ground ambulance services is the CF multiplied by the applicable RVU. The GPCI is not applied to the ground mileage rate.

4. Mileage

In the context of all payment instructions, the term "mileage" refers to loaded mileage. The ambulance FS provides a separate payment amount for mileage. The mileage rate per statute mile applies for all types of ground ambulance services, except Paramedic Intercept, and is provided to all Medicare contractors electronically by CMS as part of the ambulance FS. Providers and suppliers must report all medically necessary mileage, including the mileage subject to a rural adjustment, in a single line item.

5. Adjustment for Certain Ground Mileage for Rural Points of Pickup (POP)

The payment rate is greater for certain mileage where the POP is in a rural area to account for the higher costs per ambulance trip that are typical of rural operations where fewer trips are made in any given period.

If the POP is a rural ZIP Code, the following calculations should be used to determine the rural adjustment portion of the payment allowance. For loaded miles 1-17, the rural adjustment for ground mileage is 1.5 times the rural mileage allowance.

For services furnished during the period July 1, 2004 through December 31, 2008, a 25 percent increase is applied to the appropriate ambulance FS mileage rate to each mile of a transport (both urban and rural POP) that exceeds 50 miles (i.e., mile 51 and greater).

The following chart summarizes the above information:

Service	Dates of Service	Bonus	Calculation
Loaded miles 1-17, Rural POP	Beginning 4/1/02	50%	FS Rural mileage * 1.5
Loaded miles 18-50, Rural POP	4/1/02 – 12/31/03	25%	FS Rural mileage * 1.25
All loaded miles (Urban or Rural POP) 51+	7/1/04 – 12/31/08	25%	FS Urban or Rural mileage * 1.25

The POP, as identified by ZIP Code, establishes whether a rural adjustment applies to a particular service. Each leg of a multi-leg transport is separately evaluated for a rural adjustment application. Thus, for the second (or any subsequent) leg of a transport, the ZIP Code of the POP establishes whether a rural adjustment applies to such second (or subsequent) transport.

For the purpose of all categories of ground ambulance services except paramedic intercept, a rural area is defined as a U.S. Postal Service (USPS) ZIP Code that is located, in whole or in part, outside of either a Metropolitan Statistical Area (MSA) or in New England, a New England County Metropolitan Area (NECMA), or is an area wholly within an MSA or NECMA that has been identified as rural under the "Goldsmith modification." (The Goldsmith modification establishes an operational definition of rural areas within large counties that contain one or more metropolitan areas. The Goldsmith areas are so isolated by distance or physical features that they are more rural than urban in character and lack easy geographic access to health services.)

For Paramedic Intercept, an area is a rural area if:

- It is designated as a rural area by any law or regulation of a State;

- It is located outside of an MSA or NECMA; or

- It is located in a rural census tract of an MSA as determined under the most recent Goldsmith modification.

See IOM Pub. 100-02, Medicare Benefit Policy Manual, chapter 10 – Ambulance Services, section 30.1.1 – Ground Ambulance Services for coverage requirements for the Paramedic Intercept benefit. Presently, only the State of New York meets these requirements.

Although a transport with a POP located in a rural area is subject to a rural adjustment for mileage, Medicare still pays the lesser of the billed charge or the applicable FS amount for mileage. Thus, when rural mileage is involved, the contractor compares the calculated FS rural mileage payment rate to the provider's/supplier's actual charge for mileage and pays the lesser amount.

The CMS furnishes the ambulance FS files to claims processing contractors electronically. A version of the Ambulance Fee Schedule is also posted to the CMS website (http://www.cms.hhs.gov/AmbulanceFeeSchedule/02_afspuf.asp) for public consumption. To clarify whether a particular ZIP Code is rural or urban, please refer to the most recent version of the Medicare supplied ZIP Code file.

6. Regional Ambulance FS Payment Rate Floor for Ground Ambulance Transports

For services furnished during the period July 1, 2004 through December 31, 2009, the base rate portion of the payment under the ambulance FS for ground ambulance transports is subject to a minimum amount. This minimum amount depends upon the area of the country in which the service is furnished. The country is divided into 9 census divisions and each of the census divisions has a regional FS that is constructed using the same methodology as the national FS. Where the regional FS is greater than the national FS, the base rates for ground ambulance transports are determined by a blend of the national rate and the regional rate in accordance with the following schedule:

Year	National FS Percentage	Regional FS Percentage
7/1/04 - 12/31/04	20%	80%
CY 2005	40%	60%
CY 2006	60%	40%
CY 2007 – CY 2009	80%	20%
CY 2010 and thereafter	100%	0%

Where the regional FS is not greater than the national FS, there is no blending and only the national FS applies. Note that this provision affects only the FS portion of the blended transition payment rate. This floor amount is calculated by CMS centrally and is incorporated into the FS amount that appears in the FS file maintained by CMS and downloaded by CMS contractors. There is no calculation to be done by the Medicare B/MAC or A/MAC in order to implement this provision.

7. Adjustments for FS Payment Rate for Certain Rural Ground Ambulance Transports

For services furnished during the period July 1, 2004 through December 31, 2010, the base rate portion of the payment under the FS for ground ambulance transports furnished in certain rural areas is increased by a percentage amount determined by CMS . Section 3105 (c) and 10311 (c) of the Affordable Care Act amended section 1834 (1) (13) (A) of the Act to extend this rural bonus for an additional year through December 31, 2010. This increase applies if the POP is in a rural county (or Goldsmith area) that is comprised by the lowest quartile by population of all such rural areas arrayed by population density. CMS will determine this bonus amount and the designated POP rural ZIP Codes in which the bonus applies. Beginning on July 1, 2004, rural areas qualifying for the additional bonus amount will be identified with a "B" indicator on the national ZIP Code file. Contractors must apply the additional rural bonus amount as a multiplier to the base rate portion of the FS payment for all ground transports originating in the designated POP ZIP Codes.

Subsequently, section of 106 (c) of the MMEA again amended section 1843 (I) (13) (A) of the Act to extend the rural bonus an additional year, through December 31, 2011.

8. Adjustments for FS Payment Rates for Ground Ambulance Transports

The payment rates under the FS for ground ambulance transports (both the fee schedule base rates and the mileage amounts) are increased for services furnished during the period July 1, 2004 through December 31, 2006 as well as July 1, 2008 through December 31, 2010. For ground ambulance transport services furnished where the POP is urban, the rates are increased by 1 percent for claims with dates of service July 1, 2004 through December 31, 2006 in accordance with Section 414 of the Medicare Modernization Act (MMA) of 2004 and by 2 percent for claims with dates of service July 1, 2008 through December 31, 2010 in accordance with Section 146(a) of the Medicare Improvements for Patients and Providers Act of 2008 and Sections 3105(a) and 10311(a) of the Patient Protection and Affordable Care Act (ACA) of

2010. For ground ambulance transport services furnished where the POP is rural, the rates are increased by 2 percent for claims with dates of service July 1, 2004 through December 31, 2006 in accordance with Section 414 of the Medicare Modernization Act (MMA) of 2004 and by 3 percent for claims with dates of service July 1, 2008 through December 31, 2010 in accordance with Section 146(a) of the Medicare Improvements for Patients and Providers Act of 2008 and Sections 3105(a) and 10311(a) of the Patient Protection and Affordable Care Act (ACA) of 2010. Subsequently, section 106 (a) of the Medicare and Medicaid Extenders Act of 2010 (MMEA) again amended section 1834 (1) (12) (A) of the Act to extend the payment increases for an additional year, through December 31, 2011. These amounts are incorporated into the fee schedule amounts that appear in the Ambulance FS file maintained by CMS and downloaded by CMS contractors. There is no calculation to be done by the Medicare carrier or intermediary in order to implement this provision.

The following chart summarizes the Medicare Prescription Drug, Improvement, and Modernization Act (MMA) of 2003 payment changes for ground ambulance services that became effective on July 1, 2004 as well as the Medicare Improvement for Patients and Providers Act (MIPPA) of 2008 changes that became effective July 1, 2008 and were extended by the Patient Protection and Affordable Care Act of 2010 and the Medicare and Medicaid Extenders Act of 2010 (MMEA).

Summary Chart of Additional Payments for Ground Ambulance Services Provided by MMA, MIPPA and MMEA

Service	Effective Dates	Payment Increase*
All rural miles	7/1/04 - 12/31/06	2%
All rural miles	7/1/08 – 12/31/11	3%
Rural miles 51+	7/1/04 - 12/31/08	25% **
All urban miles	7/1/04 - 12/31/06	1%
All urban miles	7/1/08 – 12/31/11	2%
Urban miles 51+	7/1/04 - 12/31/08	25% **
All rural base rates	7/1/04 - 12/31/06	2%
All rural base rates	7/1/08 – 12/31/11	3%
Rural base rates (lowest quartile)	7/1/04 - 12/31/11	22.6 % **
All urban base rates	7/1/04 - 12/31/06	1%
All urban base rates	7/1/08 – 12/31/11	2%
All base rates (regional fee schedule blend)	7/1/04 - 12/31/09	Floor

NOTES: * All payments are percentage increases and all are cumulative.

**Contractor systems perform this calculation. All other increases are incorporated into the CMS Medicare Ambulance FS file.

B. Air Ambulance Services

1. Base Rates
   Each type of air ambulance service has a base rate. There is no conversion factor (CF) applicable to air ambulance services.

2. Geographic Adjustment Factor (GAF)
   The GAF, as described above for ground ambulance services, is also used for air ambulance services. However, for air ambulance services, the applicable GPCI is applied to 50 percent of each of the base rates (fixed and rotary wing).

3. Mileage
   The FS for air ambulance services provides a separate payment for mileage.

4. Adjustment for Services Furnished in Rural Areas
   The payment rates for air ambulance services where the POP is in a rural area are greater than in an urban area. For air ambulance services (fixed or rotary wing), the rural adjustment is an increase of 50 percent to the unadjusted FS amount, e.g., the applicable air service base rate multiplied by the GAF plus the mileage amount or, in other words, 1.5 times both the applicable air service base rate and the total mileage amount.

The basis for a rural adjustment for air ambulance services is determined in the same manner as for ground services. That is, whether the POP is within a rural ZIP Code as described above for ground services.

100-4, 15, 20.2

Payment for Mileage Charges
B3-5116.3, PM AB-00-131

Charges for mileage must be based on loaded mileage only, e.g., from the pickup of a patient to his/her arrival at destination. It is presumed that all unloaded mileage costs are taken into account when a supplier establishes his basic charge for ambulance services and his rate for loaded mileage. Suppliers should be notified that separate charges for unloaded mileage will be denied.

Instructions on billing mileage are found in Sec.30.

100-4, 15, 20.3

Air Ambulance
PHs AB-01-165, AB-02-036, and AB-02-131; B3-5116.5, B3-5205 partial

Refer to IOM Pub. 100-02, Medicare Benefit Policy Manual, chapter 10 - Ambulance Services, section 10.4 - Air Ambulance Services, for additional information on the coverage of air ambulance services. Under certain circumstances, transportation by airplane or helicopter may qualify as covered ambulance services. If the conditions of coverage are met, payment may be made for the air ambulance services.

Air ambulance services are paid at different rates according to two air ambulance categories:

- AIR ambulance service, conventional air services, transport, one way, fixed wing (FW) (HCPCS code A0430)

- AIR ambulance service, conventional air services, transport, one way, rotary wing (RW) (HCPCS code A0431)

Covered air ambulance mileage services are paid when the appropriate HCPCS code is reported on the claim:

HCPCS code A0435 identifies FIXED WING AIR MILEAGE

HCPCS code A0436 identifies ROTARY WING AIR MILEAGE

Air mileage must be reported in whole numbers of loaded statute miles flown. Contractors must ensure that the appropriate air transport code is used with the appropriate mileage code.

Air ambulance services may be paid only for ambulance services to a hospital. Other destinations e.g., skilled nursing facility, a physician's office, or a patient's home may not be paid air ambulance. The destination is identified by the use of an appropriate modifier as defined in Section 30(A) of this chapter.

Claims for air transports may account for all mileage from the point of pickup, including where applicable: ramp to taxiway, taxiway to runway, takeoff run, air miles, roll out upon landing, and taxiing after landing. Additional air mileage may be allowed by the contractor in situations where additional mileage is incurred, due to circumstances beyond the pilot's control. These circumstances include, but are not limited to, the following:

Military base and other restricted zones, air-defense zones, and similar FAA restrictions and prohibitions;

Hazardous weather; or

Variances in departure patterns and clearance routes required by an air traffic controller.

If the air transport meets the criteria for medical necessity, Medicare pays the actual miles flown for legitimate reasons as determined by the Medicare contractor, once the Medicare beneficiary is loaded onto the air ambulance.

IOM Pub. 100-08, Medicare Program Integrity Manual, chapter 6 - Intermediary MR Guidelines for Specific Services contains instructions for Medical Review of Air Ambulance Services.

100-4, 15, 20.6

Payment for Non-Emergency Trips to/from ESRD Facilities

Section 637 of the American Taxpayer Relief Act of 2012 requires that, effective for transports occurring on and after October 1, 2013, fee schedule payments for non-emergency basic life support (BLS) transports of individuals with end-stage renal disease (ESRD) to and from renal dialysis treatment be reduced by 10%. The payment reduction affects transports (base rate and mileage) to and from hospital-based and freestanding renal dialysis treatment facilities for dialysis services provided on a non-emergency basis. Non-emergency BLS ground transports are identified by Healthcare Common Procedure Code System (HCPCS) code A0428. Ambulance transports to and from renal dialysis treatment are identified by modifier codes "G" (hospital-based ESRD) and "J" (freestanding ESRD facility) in either the first position (origin code) or second position (destination code) within the two-digit ambulance modifier. (See Section 30 (A) for information regarding modifiers specific to ambulance.)

Effective for claims with dates of service on and after October 1, 2013, the 10% reduction will be calculated and applied to HCPCS code A0428 when billed with modifier code "G" or "J". The reduction will also be applied to any mileage billed in association with a non-emergency transport of a beneficiary with ESRD to and from renal dialysis treatment. BLS mileage is identified by HCPCS code A0425.

The 10% reduction will be taken after calculation of the normal fee schedule payment amount, including any add-on or bonus payments, and will apply to transports in rural and urban areas as well as areas designated as "super rural".

Payment for emergency transports is not affected by this reduction. Payment for non-emergency BLS transports to other destinations is also not affected. This reduction does not affect or change the Ambulance Fee Schedule.

Note: The 10% reduction applies to beneficiaries with ESRD that are receiving non-emergency BLS transport to and from renal dialysis treatment. While it is possible that a beneficiary who is not diagnosed with ESRD will require routine transport to and from renal dialysis treatment, it is highly unlikely. However, contractors have discretion to override or reverse the reduction on appeal if they deem it appropriate based on supporting documentation.

100-4, 15, 30.1.2

Coding Instructions for Paper and Electronic Claim Forms

Except as otherwise noted, beginning with dates of service on or after January 1, 2001, the following coding instructions must be used.

In item 23 of the CMS-1500 Form, billers shall code the 5-digit ZIP Code of the point of pickup.

Electronic billers using ANSI X12N 837 should refer to the Implementation Guide to determine how to report the origin information (e.g., the ZIP Code of the point of pickup).

Since the ZIP Code is used for pricing, more than one ambulance service may be reported on the same paper claim for a beneficiary if all points of pickup have the same ZIP Code. Suppliers must prepare a separate paper claim for each trip if the points of pickup are located in different ZIP Codes.

Claims without a ZIP Code in item 23 on CMS-1500 Form item 23, or with multiple ZIP Codes in item 23, must be returned as unprocessable. Carriers use message N53 on the remittance advice in conjunction with reason code 16.

ZIP Codes must be edited for validity.

The format for a ZIP Code is five numerics. If a nine-digit ZIP Code is submitted, the last four digits are ignored. If the data submitted in the required field does not match that format, the claim is rejected.

Generally, each ambulance trip will require two lines of coding, e.g., one line for the service and one line for the mileage. Suppliers who do not bill mileage would have one line of code for the service.

Beginning with dates of service on or after January 1, 2011, if mileage is billed it must be reported as fractional units in Item 24G of the Form CMS-1500 paper claim or the corresponding loop and segment of the ANSI X12N 837P electronic claim for trips totaling up to 100 covered miles. When reporting fractional mileage, suppliers must round the total miles up to the nearest tenth of a mile and report the resulting number

with the appropriate HCPCS code for ambulance mileage. The decimal must be used in the appropriate place (e.g., 99.9).

For trips totaling 100 covered miles and greater, suppliers must report mileage rounded up to the next whole number mile without the use of a decimal (e.g., 998.5 miles should be reported as 999).

For trips totaling less than 1 mile, enter a "0" before the decimal (e.g., 0.9).

Fractional mileage reporting applies only to ambulance services billed on a Form CMS-1500 paper claim, ANSI X12N 837P, or 837I electronic claims. It does not apply to providers billing on the Form CMS-1450.

For mileage HCPCS billed on a Form CMS-1500 or ANSI X12N 837P only, contractors shall automatically default to "0.1" units when the total mileage units are missing in Item 24G.

100-4, 15, 30.2

Intermediary Guidelines

For SNF Part A, the cost of transportation to receive most services included in the RUG rate is included in the cost for the service. This includes transportation in an ambulance. Payment for the SNF claim is based on the RUGs, and recalibration for future years takes into account the cost of transportation to receive the ancillary services.

If the services are excluded from the SNF PPS rate, the ambulance service may be billed separately as can the excluded service.

Refer to section 10.5, of chapter 3, of the Medicare Claims Processing Manual, for additional information on hospital inpatient bundling of ambulance services.

In general, the intermediary processes claims for Part B ambulance services provided by an ambulance supplier under arrangements with hospitals or SNFs. These providers bill intermediaries using only Method 2.

The provider must furnish the following data in accordance with intermediary instructions. The intermediary will make arrangements for the method and media for submitting the data: A detailed statement of the condition necessitating the ambulance service; A statement indicating whether the patient was admitted as an inpatient. If yes the name and address of the facility must be shown; Name and address of certifying physician; Name and address of physician ordering service if other than certifying physician; Point of pickup (identify place and completed address); Destination (identify place and complete address); Number of loaded miles (the number of miles traveled when the beneficiary was in the ambulance); Cost per mile; Mileage charge; Minimum or base charge; and Charge for special items or services. Explain.

A. General

The reasonable cost per trip of ambulance services furnished by a provider of services may not exceed the prior year's reasonable cost per trip updated by the ambulance inflation factor. This determination is effective with services furnished during Federal Fiscal Year (FFY) 1998 (between October 1, 1997, and September 30, 1998).

Providers are to bill for Part B ambulance services using the billing method of base rate including supplies, with mileage billed separately as described below.

The following instructions provide billing procedures implementing the above provisions.

B. Applicable Bill Types

The appropriate type of bill (13X, 22X, 23X, 83X, and 85X) must be reported. For SNFs, ambulance cannot be reported on a 21X type of bill.

C. Value Code Reporting

For claims with dates of service on or after January 1, 2001, providers must report on every Part B ambulance claim value code A0 (zero) and the related ZIP code of the geographic location from which the beneficiary was placed on board the ambulance in FLs 39-41 "Value Codes." The value code is defined as "ZIP Code of the location from which the beneficiary is initially placed on board the ambulance." Providers report the number in dollar portion of the form location right justified to the left to the dollar/cents delimiter. Providers utilizing the UB-92 flat file use Record Type 41 fields 16-39. On the X-12 institutional claims transactions, providers show HI*BE:A0:::12345, 2300 Loop, HI segment.

More than one ambulance trip may be reported on the same claim if the ZIP code of all points of pickup are the same. However, since billing requirements do not allow for value codes (ZIP codes) to be line item specific and only one ZIP code may be reported per claim, providers must prepare a separate claim for a beneficiary for each trip if the points of pickup are located in different ZIP codes.

D. Revenue Code/HCPCS Code Reporting

Providers must report revenue code 054X and, for services provided before January 1, 2001, one of the following CMS HCPCS codes in FL 44 "HCPCS/Rates" for each ambulance trip provided during the billing period: A0030 (discontinued 12/31/2000); A0040 (discontinued 12/31/2000); A0050 (discontinued 12/31/2000); A0320 (discontinued 12/31/2000); A0322 (discontinued 12/31/2000); A0324 (discontinued 12/31/2000); A0326 (discontinued 12/31/2000); A0328, (discontinued 12/31/2000); or A0330 (discontinued 12/31/2000).

In addition, providers report one of A0380 or A0390 for mileage HCPCS codes. No other HCPCS codes are acceptable for reporting ambulance services and mileage.

Providers report one of the following revenue codes: 0540; 0542; 0543; 0545; 0546; or 0548.

Do not report revenue codes 0541, 0544, or 0547.

For claims with dates of service on or after January 1, 2001, providers must report revenue code 540 and one of the following HCPCS codes in FL 44 "HCPCS/Rates" for each ambulance trip provided during the billing period: A0426; A0427; A0428; A0429; A0430; A0431; A0432; A0433; or A0434.

Providers using an ALS vehicle to furnish a BLS level of service report HCPCS code, A0426 (ALS1) or A0427 (ALS1 emergency), and are paid accordingly.

In addition, all providers report one of the following mileage HCPCS codes: A0380; A0390; A0435; or A0436.

Since billing requirements do not allow for more than one HCPCS code to be reported for per revenue code line, providers must report revenue code 0540 (ambulance) on two separate and consecutive lines to accommodate both the Part B ambulance service and the mileage HCPCS codes for each ambulance trip provided during the billing period. Each loaded (e.g., a patient is onboard) 1-way ambulance trip must be reported with a unique pair of revenue code lines on the claim. Unloaded trips and mileage are NOT reported.

However, in the case where the beneficiary was pronounced dead after the ambulance is called but before the ambulance arrives at the scene: Payment may be made for a BLS service if a ground vehicle is dispatched or at the fixed wing or rotary wing base rate, as applicable, if an air ambulance is dispatched. Neither mileage nor a rural adjustment would be paid. The blended rate amount will otherwise apply. Providers report the A0428 (BLS) HCPCS code. Providers report modifier QL (Patient pronounced dead after ambulance called) in Form Locator (FL) 44 "HCPCS/Rates" instead of the origin and destination modifier. In addition to the QL modifier, providers report modifier QM or QN.

E. Modifier Reporting
Providers must report an origin and destination modifier for each ambulance trip provided in FL 44 "HCPCS/Rates." Origin and destination modifiers used for ambulance services are created by combining two alpha characters. Each alpha character, with the exception of x, represents an origin code or a destination code. The pair of alpha codes creates one modifier. The first position alpha code equals origin; the second position alpha code equals destination. Origin and destination codes and their descriptions are listed below: D - Diagnostic or therapeutic site other than "P" or "H" when these are used as origin codes; E - Residential, Domiciliary, Custodial Facility (other than an 1819 facility); H - Hospital; I - Site of transfer (e.g. airport or helicopter pad) between modes of ambulance transport; J - Nonhospital based dialysis facility; N - Skilled Nursing Facility (SNF) (1819 facility); P - Physician's office (Includes HMO nonhospital facility, clinic, etc.); R - Residence; S - Scene of accident or acute event; or X - (Destination Code Only) intermediate stop at physician's office enroute to the hospital. (Includes HMO nonhospital facility, clinic, etc.) In addition, providers must report one of the following modifiers with every HCPCS code to describe whether the service was provided under arrangement or directly: QM - Ambulance service provided under arrangement by a provider of services; or QN - Ambulance service furnished directly by a provider of services.

F. Line-Item Dates of Service Reporting
Providers are required to report line-item dates of service per revenue code line. This means that they must report two separate revenue code lines for every ambulance trip provided during the billing period along with the date of each trip. This includes situations in which more than one ambulance service is provided to the same beneficiary on the same day. Line-item dates of service are reported on the hard copy UB-92 in FL 45 "Service Date" (MMDDYY), and on RT 61, field 13, "Date of Service" (YYYYMMDD) on the UB-92 flat file.

G. Service Units Reporting
For line items reflecting HCPCS code A0030, A0040, A0050, A0320, A0322, A0324, A0326, A0328, or A0330 (services before January 1, 2001) or code A0426, A0427, A0428, A0429, A0430, A0431, A0432, A0433, or A0434 (services on and after January 1, 2001), providers are required to report in FL 46 "Service Units" each ambulance trip provided during the billing period. Therefore, the service units for each occurrence of these HCPCS codes are always equal to one. In addition, for line items reflecting HCPCS code A0380 or A0390, the number of loaded miles must be reported. (See examples below.) Therefore, the service units for each occurrence of these HCPCS codes are always equal to one.

In addition, for line items reflecting HCPCS code A0380, A0390, A0435, or A0436, the number of loaded miles must be reported.

H. Total Charges Reporting
For line items reflecting HCPCS code: A0030, A0040, A0050, A0320, A0322, A0324, A0326, A0328, or A0330 (services before January 1, 2001); OR HCPCS code A0426, A0427, A0428, A0429, A0430, A0431, A0432, A0433, or A0434 (on or after January 1, 2001); Providers are required to report in FL 47 "Total Charges" the actual charge for the ambulance service including all supplies used for the ambulance trip but excluding the charge for mileage.

For line items reflecting HCPCS code A0380, A0390, A0435, or A0436, report the actual charge for mileage.

NOTE: There are instances where the provider does not incur any cost for mileage, e.g., if the beneficiary is pronounced dead after the ambulance is called but before the ambulance arrives at the scene. In these situations, providers report the base rate ambulance trip and mileage as separate revenue code lines. Providers report the base rate ambulance trip in accordance with current billing requirements. For purposes of reporting mileage, they must report the appropriate HCPCS code, modifiers, and units as a separate line item. For the related charges, providers report $1.00 in FL48 for noncovered charges. Intermediaries should assign ANSI Group Code OA to the $1.00 noncovered mileage line, which in turn informs the beneficiaries and providers that they each have no liability.

Prior to submitting the claim to CWF, the intermediary will remove the entire revenue code line containing the mileage amount reported in FL 48 "Noncovered Charges" to avoid nonacceptance of the claim.

EXAMPLES: The following provides examples of how bills for Part B ambulance services should be completed based on the reporting requirements above. These examples reflect ambulance services furnished directly by providers. Ambulance services provided under arrangement between the provider and an ambulance company are reported in the same manner except providers report a QM modifier instead of a QN modifier. The following examples are for claims submitted with dates of service on or after January 1, 2001.

EXAMPLE 1: Claim containing only one ambulance trip:

For the UB-92 Flat File, providers report as follows:

Modifier Record Type	Revenue Code	HCPCS Modifier	Date of Service	Units	Total Charges
61	0540	A0428RHQN	082701	1 (trip)	100.00
61	0540	A0380RHQN	082701	4 (mileage)	8.00

For the hard copy UB-92 (Form CMS-1450), providers report as follows:

Modifier Record Type	Revenue Code	HCPCS Modifier	Date of Service	Units	Total Charges
FL 42, FL 44 FL 45, FL 46 FL 47	0540	A0428RHQN	082701	1 (trip)	100.00
	0540	A0380RHQN	082701	4 (mileage)	8.00

EXAMPLE 2: Claim containing multiple ambulance trips:
For the UB-92 Flat File, providers report as follows:

Modifier Record Type	Revenue Code	HCPCS Code	Modifiers #1	#2	Date of Service	Units	Total Charges
61	0540	A0429	RH	QN	082801	1 (trip)	100.00
61	0540	A0380	RH	QN	082801	2 (mileage)	4.00
61	0540	A0330	RH	QN	082901	1 (trip)	400.00
61	0540	A0390	RH	QN	082901	3 (mileage)	6.00
61	0540	A0426	RH	QN	083001	1 (trip)	500.00
61	0540	A0390	RH	QN	083001	5 (mileage)	10.00
61	0540	A0390	RH	QN	082901	3 (mileage)	6.00
61	0540	A0426	RH	QN	083001	1 (trip)	500.00

For the hard copy UB-92 (Form CMS-1450), providers report as follows:

Modifier	Revenue Code	HCPCS Code	#1	#2	Date of Service	Units	Total Charges
FL42, FL 44, FL 45, FL 46, FL 47	0540	A0429	RH	QN	082801	1 (trip)	100.00
	0540	A0380	RH	QN	082801	2 (mileage)	4.00

EXAMPLE 3: Claim containing more than one ambulance trip provided on the same day: For the UB-92 Flat File, providers report as follows:

Modifier Record Type	Revenue Code	HCPCS Code	#1	#2	Date of Service	Units	Total Charges
61	0540	A0429	RH	QN	090201	1 (trip)	100.00
61	0540	A0380	RH	QN	090201	2 (mileage)	4.00
61	0540	A0429	HR	QN	090201	1 (trip)	100.00

Modifier Record Type	Revenue Code	HCPCS Code	#1	#2	Date of Service	Units	Total Charges
61	0540	A0380	HR	QN	090201	2 (mileage)	4.00

For the hard copy UB-92 (Form CMS-1450), providers report as follows:

Modifier	Revenue Code	HCPCS Code	#1	#2	Date of Service	Units	Total Charges
FL42,	0540	A0429	RH	QN	090201	1 (trip)	100.00
FL 44, FL 45,	0540	A0380	RH	QN	090201	2 (mileage)	4.00
FL 46,	0540	A0429	HR	QN	090201	1 (trip)	100.00
FL 47	0540	A0380	HR	QN	090201	2 (mileage)	4.00

I. Edits Intermediaries edit to assure proper reporting as follows:

For claims with dates of service before January 1, 2001, each pair of revenue codes 0540 must have one of the following ambulance trip HCPCS codes - A0030, A0040, A0050, A0320, A0322, A0324, A0326, A0328 or A0330; and one of the following mileage HCPCS codes - A0380 or A0390; For claims with dates of service on or after January 1, 2001, each pair of revenue codes 0540 must have one of the following ambulance HCPCS codes - A0426, A0427, A0428, A0429, A0430, A0431, A0432, A0433, or A0434; and one of the following mileage HCPCS codes - A0435, A0436 or for claims with dates of service before April 1, 2002, A0380, or A0390, or for claims with dates of service on or after April 1, 2002, A0425; For claims with dates of service on or after January 1, 2001, the presence of an origin and destination modifier and a QM or QN modifier for every line item containing revenue code 0540; The units field is completed for every line item containing revenue code 0540; For claims with dates of service on or after January 1, 2001, the units field is completed for every line item containing HCPCS codes A0030, A0040, A0050, A0320, A0322, A0324, A0326, A0328, A0330, A0426, A0427, A0428, A0429, A0430, A0431, A0432, A0433, or A0434 always equal "1" For claims with dates of service on or after July 1, 2001, each 1-way ambulance trip, line-item dates of service for the ambulance service, and corresponding mileage are equal.

100-4, 15, 30.2.1

A/MAC Bill Processing Guidelines Effective April 1, 2002, as a Result of Fee Schedule Implementation

For SNF Part A, the cost of medically necessary ambulance transportation to receive most services included in the RUG rate is included in the cost for the service. Payment for the SNF claim is based on the RUGs, which takes into account the cost of such transportation to receive the ancillary services.

Refer to IOM Pub. 100-04, Medicare Claims Processing Manual, chapter 6—SNF Inpatient Part A Billing, Section 20.3.1—Ambulance Services for additional information on SNF consolidated billing and ambulance transportation.

Refer to IOM Pub. 100-04, Medicare Claims Processing Manual, chapter 3—Inpatient Hospital Billing, section 10.5—Hospital Inpatient Bundling, for additional information on hospital inpatient bundling of ambulance services.

In general, the A/MAC processes claims for Part B ambulance services provided by an ambulance supplier under arrangements with hospitals or SNFs. These providers bill A/MACs using only Method 2.

The provider must furnish the following data in accordance with A/MAC instructions. The A/MAC will make arrangements for the method and media for submitting the data:

- A detailed statement of the condition necessitating the ambulance service;
- A statement indicating whether the patient was admitted as an inpatient. If yes the name and address of the facility must be shown;
- Name and address of certifying physician;
- Name and address of physician ordering service if other than certifying physician;
- Point of pickup (identify place and completed address);
- Destination (identify place and complete address);
- Number of loaded miles (the number of miles traveled when the beneficiary was in the ambulance);
- Cost per mile;
- Mileage charge;
- Minimum or base charge; and
- Charge for special items or services. Explain.

A. Revenue Code Reporting

Providers report ambulance services under revenue code 540 in FL 42 "Revenue Code."

B. HCPCS Codes Reporting

Providers report the HCPCS codes established for the ambulance fee schedule. No other HCPCS codes are acceptable for the reporting of ambulance services and mileage. The HCPCS code must be used to reflect the type of service the beneficiary received, not the type of vehicle used.

Providers must report one of the following HCPCS codes in FL 44 "HCPCS/Rates" for each base rate ambulance trip provided during the billing period:

A0426; A0427; A0428; A0429; A0430; A0431; A0432; A0433; or A0434.

These are the same codes required effective for services January 1, 2001.

In addition, providers must report one of HCPCS mileage codes:

A0425; A0435; or A0436.

Since billing requirements do not allow for more than one HCPCS code to be reported per revenue code line, providers must report revenue code 540 (ambulance) on two separate and consecutive line items to accommodate both the ambulance service and the mileage HCPCS codes for each ambulance trip provided during the billing period. Each loaded (e.g., a patient is onboard) 1-way ambulance trip must be reported with a unique pair of revenue code lines on the claim. Unloaded trips and mileage are NOT reported.

For UB-04 hard copy claims submission prior to August 1, 2011, providers code one mile for trips less than a mile. Miles must be entered as whole numbers. If a trip has a fraction of a mile, round up to the nearest whole number.

Beginning with dates of service on or after January 1, 2011, for UB-04 hard copy claims submissions August 1, 2011 and after, mileage must be reported as fractional units. When reporting fractional mileage, providers must round the total miles up to the nearest tenth of a mile and the decimal must be used in the appropriate place (e.g., 99.9).

For trips totaling less than 1 mile, enter a "0" before the decimal (e.g., 0.9).

For electronic claims submissions prior to January 1, 2011, providers code one mile for trips less than a mile. Miles must be entered as whole numbers. If a trip has a fraction of a mile, round up to the nearest whole number.

Beginning with dates of service on or after January 1, 2011, for electronic claim submissions only, mileage must be reported as fractional units in the ANSI X12N 837I element SV205 for trips totaling up to 100 covered miles. When reporting fractional mileage, providers must round the total miles up to the nearest tenth of a mile and the decimal must be used in the appropriate place (e.g., 99.9).

For trips totaling 100 covered miles and greater, providers must report mileage rounded up to the nearest whole number mile (e.g., 999) and not use a decimal when reporting whole number miles over 100 miles.

For trips totaling less than 1 mile, enter a "0" before the decimal (e.g., 0.9).

C. Modifier Reporting

Providers must report an origin and destination modifier for each ambulance trip provided and either a QM (Ambulance service provided under arrangement by a provider of services) or QN (Ambulance service furnished directly by a provider of services) modifier in FL 44 "HCPCS/Rates".

D. Service Units Reporting

For line items reflecting HCPCS codes A0426, A0427, A0428, A0429, A0430, A0431, A0432, A0433, or A0434, providers are required to report in FL 46 "Service Units" for each ambulance trip provided. Therefore, the service units for each occurrence of these HCPCS codes are always equal to one. In addition, for line items reflecting HCPCS code A0425, A0435, or A0436, providers must also report the number of loaded miles.

E. Total Charges Reporting

For line items reflecting HCPCS codes A0426, A0427, A0428, A0429, A0430, A0431, A0432, A0433, or A0434, providers are required to report in FL 47, "Total Charges," the actual charge for the ambulance service including all supplies used for the ambulance trip but excluding the charge for mileage. For line items reflecting HCPCS codes A0425, A0435, or A0436, providers are to report the actual charge for mileage.

NOTE: There are instances where the provider does not incur any cost for mileage, e.g., if the beneficiary is pronounced dead after the ambulance is called but before the ambulance arrives at the scene. In these situations, providers report the base rate ambulance trip and mileage as separate revenue code lines. Providers report the base rate ambulance trip in accordance with current billing requirements. For purposes of reporting mileage, they must report the appropriate HCPCS code, modifiers, and units. For the related charges, providers report $1.00 in non-covered charges. A/MACs should assign ANSI Group Code OA to the $1.00 non-covered mileage line, which in turn informs the beneficiaries and providers that they each have no liability.

F. Edits (A/MAC Claims with Dates of Service On or After 4/1/02)

For claims with dates of service on or after April 1, 2002, A/MACs perform the following edits to assure proper reporting:

Edit to assure each pair of revenue codes 540 have one of the following ambulance HCPCS codes - A0426, A0427, A0428, A0429, A0430, A0431, A0432, A0433, or A0434; and one of the following mileage HCPCS codes - A0425, A0435, or A0436.

Edit to assure the presence of an origin, destination modifier, and a QM or QN modifier for every line item containing revenue code 540;

Edit to assure that the unit's field is completed for every line item containing revenue code 540;

Edit to assure that service units for line items containing HCPCS codes A0426, A0427, A0428, A0429, A0430, A0431, A0432, A0433, or A0434 always equal "1"; and

Edit to assure on every claim that revenue code 540, a value code of A0 (zero), and a corresponding ZIP Code are reported. If the ZIP Code is not a valid ZIP Code in accordance with the USPS assigned ZIP Codes, intermediaries verify the ZIP Code to determine if the ZIP Code is a coding error on the claim or a new ZIP Code from the USPS not on the CMS supplied ZIP Code File.

Beginning with dates of service on or after April 1, 2012, edit to assure that only non-emergency trips (i.e., HCPCS A0426, A0428 [when A0428 is billed without modifier QL]) require an NPI in the Attending Physician field. Emergency trips do not require an NPI in the Attending Physician field (i.e., A0427, A0429, A0430, A0431, A0432, A0434 and A0428 [when A0428 is billed with modifier QL])

G. CWF (A/MACs)

A/MACs report the procedure codes in the financial data section (field 65a-65j). They include revenue code, HCPCS code, units, and covered charges in the record. Where more than one HCPCS code procedure is applicable to a single revenue code, the provider reports each HCPCS code and related charge on a separate line, and the A/MAC reports this to CWF. Report the payment amount before adjustment for beneficiary liability in field 65g "Rate" and the actual charge in field 65h, "Covered Charges."

100-4, 15, 30.2.4

30.2.4 - Non-covered Charges on Institutional Ambulance Claims

Medicare law contains a restriction that miles beyond the closest available facility cannot be billed to Medicare. Non-covered miles beyond the closest facility are billed with HCPCS procedure code A0888 ("non-covered ambulance mileage per mile, e.g., for miles traveled beyond the closest appropriate facility"). These non-covered line items can be billed on claims also containing covered charges. Ambulance claims may use the -GY modifier on line items for such non-covered mileage, and liability for the service will be assigned correctly to the beneficiary.

The method of billing all miles for the same trip, with covered and non-covered portions, on the same claim is preferable in this scenario. However, billing the non-covered mileage using condition code 21 claims is also permitted, if desired, as long as all line items on the claims are non-covered and the beneficiary is liable. Additionally, unless requested by the beneficiary or required by specific Medicare policy, services excluded by statute do not have to be billed to Medicare.

When the scenario is point of pick up outside the United States, including U.S. territories but excepting some points in Canada and Mexico in some cases, mileage is also statutorily excluded from Medicare coverage. Such billings are more likely to be submitted on entirely non-covered claims using condition code 21. This scenario requires the use of a different message on the Medicare Summary Notice (MSN) sent to beneficiaries.

Another scenario in which billing non-covered mileage to Medicare may occur is when the beneficiary dies after the ambulance has been called but before the ambulance arrives. The -QL modifier should be used on the base rate line in this scenario, in place of origin and destination modifiers, and the line is submitted with covered charges. The -QL modifier should also be used on the accompanying mileage line, if submitted, with non-covered charges. Submitting this non-covered mileage line is optional for providers.

Non-covered charges may also apply is if there is a subsidy of mileage charges that are never charged to Medicare. Because there are no charges for Medicare to share in, the only billing option is to submit non-covered charges, if the provider bills Medicare at all (it is not required in such cases). These non-covered charges are unallowable, and should not be considered in settlement of cost reports. However, there is a difference in billing if such charges are subsidized, but otherwise would normally be charged to Medicare as the primary payer. In this latter case, CMS examination of existing rules relating to grants policy since October 1983, supported by Federal regulations (42CFR 405.423), generally requires providers to reduce their costs by the amount of grants and gifts restricted to pay for such costs. Thereafter, section 405.423 was deleted from the regulations.

Thus, providers were no longer required to reduce their costs for restricted grants and gifts, and charges tied to such grants/gifts/subsidies should be submitted as covered charges. This is in keeping with Congress's intent to encourage hospital philanthropy, allowing the provider receiving the subsidy to use it, and also requiring Medicare to share in the unreduced cost. Treatment of subsidized charges as non-covered Medicare charges serves to reduce Medicare payment on the Medicare cost report contrary to the 1983 change in policy.

Medicare requires the use of the -TQ modifier so that CMS can track the instances of the subsidy scenario for non-covered charges. The -TQ should be used whether the subsidizing entity is governmental or voluntary. The -TQ modifier is not required in the case of covered charges submitted when a subsidy has been made, but charges are still normally made to Medicare as the primary payer.

If providers believe they have been significantly or materially penalized in the past by the failure of their cost reports to consider covered charges occurring in the subsidy case, since Medicare had previous billing instructions that stated all charges in the case of a subsidy, not just charges when the entity providing the subsidy never charges another entity/primary payer, should be submitted as non-covered charges, they may contact their FI about reopening the reports in question for which the time period in 42 CFR 405.1885 has not expired. FIs have the discretion to determine if the amount in question warrants reopening. The CMS does not expect many such cases to occur.

Billing requirements for all these situations, including the use of modifiers, are presented in the chart below:

Mileage Scenario	HCPCS	Modifiers*	Liability	Billing	Remit. Requirements	MSN Message
STATUTE: Miles beyond closest facility, OR **Pick up point outside of U.S.	A0888 on line item for the non-covered mileage	-QM or -QN, origin/destination modifier, and -GY unless condition code 21 claim used	Beneficiary	Bill mileage line item with A0888 -GY and other modifiers as needed to establish liability, line item will be denied; OR bill service on condition code 21 claim, no -GY required, claim will be denied	Group code PR, reason code 96	16.10 "Medicare does not pay for this item or service"; OR, "Medicare no paga por este artículo o servicio"
Beneficiary dies after ambulance is called	Most appropriate ambulance HCPCS mileage code (i.e., ground, air)	-QL unless condition code -21 claim	Provider	Bill mileage line item with -QL as non-covered, line item will be denied	Group Code CO, reason code 96	16.58 "The provider billed this charge as non-covered. You do not have to pay this amount."; OR, "El proveedor facuró este cargo como no cubierto. Usted no tiene que pagar ests cantidad."
Subsidy or government owned Ambulance, Medicare NEVER billed***	A0888 on line item for the non-covered mileage	-QM or -QN, origin/destination modifier, and -TQ must be used for policy purposes	Provider	Bill mileage line item with A0888, and modifiers as non-covered, line item will be denied	Group Code CO, reason code 96	16.58 "The provider billed this charge as non-covered. You do not have to pay this amount."; OR, "El proveedor facuró este cargo como no cubierto. Usted no tiene que pagar ests cantidad."

*   Current ambulance billing requirements state that either the -QM or -QN modifier must be used on services. The -QM is used when the "ambulance service is provided under arrangement by a provider of services," and the -QN when the "ambulance service is provided directly by a provider of services." Line items using either the -QM or -QN modifiers are not subject to the FISS edit associated with FISS reason code 31322 so that these lines items will process to completion. Origin/destination modifiers, also required by current instruction, combine two alpha characters: one for origin, one for destination, and are not non-covered by definition.

**   This is the one scenario where the base rate is not paid in addition to mileage, and there are certain exceptions in Canada and Mexico where mileage is covered as described in existing ambulance instructions.

*** If Medicare would normally have been billed, submit mileage charges as covered charges despite subsidies.

Medicare systems may return claims to the provider if they do not comply with the requirements in the table.

100-4, 15, 40
Medical Conditions List and Instructions

The following list is intended as primarily an educational guideline. This list was most recently updated by CMS Transmittal 1185, Change Request 5542 issued February 23, 2007. It will help ambulance providers and suppliers to communicate the patient's condition to Medicare contractors, as reported by the dispatch center and as observed by the ambulance crew. Use of the medical conditions list does not guarantee payment of the claim or payment for a certain level of service. Ambulance providers and suppliers must retain adequate documentation of dispatch instructions, patient's condition, other on-scene information, and details of the transport (e.g., medications administered, changes in the patient's condition, and miles traveled), all of which may be subject to medical review by the Medicare contractor or other oversight authority. Medicare contractors will rely on medical record documentation to justify coverage, not simply the HCPCS code or the condition code by themselves. All current Medicare ambulance policies remain in place.

The CMS issued the Medical Conditions List as guidance via a manual revision as a result of interest expressed in the ambulance industry for this tool. While the International Classification of Diseases, 9th Revision, Clinical Modification (ICD-9-CM) codes are not precluded from use on ambulance claims, they are currently not required (per Health Insurance Portability and Accountability Act (HIPAA)) on most ambulance claims, and these codes generally do not trigger a payment or a denial of a claim. Some carriers and fiscal intermediaries have Local Coverage Determinations (LCD) in place that cite ICD-9-CM that can be added to the claim to assist in documenting that the services are reasonable and necessary, but this is not common. Since ICD-9-CM codes are not required and are not consistently used, not all carriers or fiscal intermediaries edit on this field, and it is not possible to edit on the narrative field. The ICD-9-CM codes are generally not part of the edit process, although the Medical Conditions List is available for those who do find it helpful in justifying that services are reasonable and necessary.

The Medical Conditions List is set up with an initial column of primary ICD-9-CM codes, followed by an alternative column of ICD-9-CM codes. The primary ICD-9-CM code column contains general ICD-9-CM codes that fit the transport conditions as described in the subsequent columns. Ambulance crew or billing staff with limited knowledge of ICD-9-CM coding would be expected to choose the one or one of the two ICD-9-CM codes listed in this column to describe the appropriate ambulance transport and then place the ICD-9-CM code in the space on the claim form designated for an ICD-9-CM code. The option to include other information in the narrative field always exists and can be used whenever an ambulance provider or supplier believes that the information may be useful for claims processing purposes. If an ambulance crew or billing staff member has more comprehensive clinical knowledge, then that person may select an ICD-9-CM code from the alternative ICD-9-CM code column. These ICD-9-CM codes are more specific and detailed. An ICD-9-CM code does not need to be selected from both the primary column and the alternative column. However, in several instances in the alternative ICD-9-CM code column, there is a selection of codes and the word "PLUS." In these instances, the ambulance provider or supplier would select an ICD-9-CM code from the first part of the alternative listing (before the word "PLUS") and at least one other ICD-9-CM code from the second part of the alternative listing (after the word "PLUS"). The ambulance claim form does provide space for the use of multiple ICD-9-CM codes. Please see the example below:

The ambulance arrives on the scene. A beneficiary is experiencing the specific abnormal vital sign of elevated blood pressure; however, the beneficiary does not normally suffer from hypertension (ICD-9-CM code 796.2 (from the alternative column on the Medical Conditions List)). In addition, the beneficiary is extremely dizzy (ICD-9-CM code 780.4 (fits the "PLUS any other code" requirement when using the alternative list for this condition (abnormal vital signs)). The ambulance crew can list these two ICD-9-CM codes on the claim form, or the general ICD-9-CM code for this condition (796.4 - Other Abnormal Clinical Findings) would work just as well. None of these ICD-9-CM codes will determine whether or not this claim will be paid; they will only assist the contractor in making a medical review determination provided all other Medicare ambulance coverage policies have been followed.

While the medical conditions/ICD-9-CM code list is intended to be comprehensive, there may be unusual circumstances that warrant the need for ambulance services using ICD-9-CM codes not on this list. During the medical review process contractors may accept other relevant information from the providers or suppliers that will build the appropriate case that justifies the need for ambulance transport for a patient condition not found on the list.

Because it is critical to accurately communicate the condition of the patient during the ambulance transport, most claims will contain only the ICD-9-CM code that most closely informs the Medicare contractor why the patient required the ambulance transport. This code is intended to correspond to the description of the patient's symptoms and condition once the ambulance personnel are at the patient's side. For example, if an Advanced Life Support (ALS) ambulance responds to a condition on the medical conditions list that warrants an ALS-level response and the patient's

condition on-scene also corresponds to an ALS-level condition, the submitted claim need only include the code that most accurately reflects the on-scene condition of the patient as the reason for transport. (All claims are required to have HCPCS codes on them, and may have modifiers as well.) Similarly, if a Basic Life Support (BLS) ambulance responds to a condition on the medical conditions list that warrants a BLS-level response and the patient's condition on-scene also corresponds to a BLS-level condition, the submitted claim need only include the code that most accurately reflects the on-scene condition of the patient as the reason for transport.

When a request for service is received by ambulance dispatch personnel for a condition that necessitates the skilled assessment of an advanced life support paramedic based upon the medical conditions list, an ALS-level ambulance would be appropriately sent to the scene. If upon arrival of the ambulance the actual condition encountered by the crew corresponds to a BLS-level situation, this claim would require two separate condition codes from the medical condition list to be processed correctly. The first code would correspond to the "reason for transport" or the on-scene condition of the patient. Because in this example, this code corresponds to a BLS condition, a second code that corresponds to the dispatch information would be necessary for inclusion on the claim in order to support payment at the ALS level. In these cases, when MR is performed, the Medicare contractor will analyze all claim information (including both codes) and other supplemental medical documentation to support the level of service billed on the claim.

Contractors may have (or may develop) individual local policies that indicate that some codes are not appropriate for payment in some circumstances. These continue to remain in effect.

Information on appropriate use of transportation indicators:

When a claim is submitted for payment, an ICD-9-CM code from the medical conditions list that best describes the patient's condition and the medical necessity for the transport may be chosen. In addition to this code, one of the transportation indicators below may be included on the claim to indicate why it was necessary for the patient to be transported in a particular way or circumstance. The provider or supplier will place the transportation indicator in the "narrative" field on the claim.

- Air and Ground

- Transportation Indicator "C1": Transportation indicator "C1" indicates an interfacility transport (to a higher level of care) determined necessary by the originating facility based upon EMTALA regulations and guidelines. The patient's condition should also be reported on the claim with a code selected from either the emergency or non-emergency category on the list.

- Transportation Indicator "C2": Transportation indicator "C2" indicates a patient is being transported from one facility to another because a service or therapy required to treat the patient's condition is not available at the originating facility. The patient's condition should also be reported on the claim with a code selected from either the emergency or non-emergency category on the list. In addition, the information about what service the patient requires that was not available should be included in the narrative field of the claim.

- Transportation Indicator "C3": Transportation indicator "C3" may be included on claims as a secondary code where a response was made to a major incident or mechanism of injury. All such responses - regardless of the type of patient or patients found once on scene - are appropriately Advanced Level Service responses. A code that describes the patient's condition found on scene should also be included on the claim, but use of this modifier is intended to indicate that the highest level of service available response was medically justified. Some examples of these types of responses would include patient(s) trapped in machinery, explosions, a building fire with persons reported inside, major incidents involving aircraft, buses, subways, trains, watercraft and victims entrapped in vehicles.

- Transportation Indicator "C4": Transportation indicator "C4" indicates that an ambulance provided a medically necessary transport, but the number of miles on the claim form appear to be excessive. This should be used only if the facility is on divert status or a particular service is not available at the time of transport only. The provider or supplier must have documentation on file clearly showing why the beneficiary was not transported to the nearest facility and may include this information in the narrative field.

- Ground Only

- Transportation Indicator "C5": Transportation indicator "C5" has been added for situations where a patient with an ALS-level condition is encountered, treated and transported by a BLS-level ambulance with no ALS level involvement whatsoever. This situation would occur when ALS resources are not available to respond to the patient encounter for any number of reasons, but the ambulance service is informing you that although the patient transported had an ALS-level condition, the actual service rendered was through a BLS-level ambulance in a situation where an ALS-level ambulance was not available.

For example, a BLS ambulance is dispatched at the emergency level to pick up a 76-yearold beneficiary who has undergone cataract surgery at the Eye Surgery Center. The patient is weak and dizzy with a history of high blood pressure, myocardial infarction, and insulin-dependent diabetes mellitus. Therefore, the on-scene ICD-9-CM equivalent of the medical condition is 780.02 (unconscious, fainting, syncope, near syncope, weakness, or dizziness - ALS Emergency). In this case, the ICD-9-CM code 780.02 would be entered on the ambulance claim form as well as transportation indicator C5 to provide the further information that the BLS ambulance transported a patient with an ALS-level condition, but there was no intervention by an ALS service. This claim would be paid at the BLS level.

- Transportation Indicator "C6": Transportation indicator "C6" has been added for situations when an ALS-level ambulance would always be the appropriate resource chosen based upon medical dispatch protocols to respond to a request for service. If once on scene, the crew determines that the patient requiring transport has a BLS-level condition, this transportation indicator should be included on the claim to indicate why the ALS-level response was indicated based upon the information obtained in the operation's dispatch center. Claims including this transportation indicator should contain two primary codes. The first condition will indicate the BLS-level condition corresponding to the patient's condition found on-scene and during the transport. The second condition will indicate the ALS-level condition corresponding to the information at the time of dispatch that indicated the need for an ALS-level response based upon medically appropriate dispatch protocols.

- Transportation Indicator C7- Transportation indicator "C7" is for those circumstances where IV medications were required en route. C7 is appropriately used for patients requiring ALS level transport in a non-emergent situation primarily because the patient requires

monitoring of ongoing medications administered intravenously. Does not apply to self-administered medications. Does not include administration of crystalloid intravenous fluids (i.e., Normal Saline, Lactate Ringers, 5% Dextrose in Water, etc.). The patient's condition should also be reported on the claim with a code selected from the list.

- Air Only

- All "transportation indicators" imply a clinical benefit to the time saved with transporting a patient by an air ambulance versus a ground or water ambulance.

- D1 Long Distance - patient's condition requires rapid transportation over a long distance.

- D2 Under rare and exceptional circumstances, traffic patterns preclude ground transport at the time the response is required.

- D3 Time to get to the closest appropriate hospital due to the patient's condition precludes transport by ground ambulance. Unstable patient with need to minimize out-of-hospital time to maximize clinical benefits to the patient.

- D4 Pick up point not accessible by ground transportation.

Ambulance Fee Schedule - Medical Conditions List
(Rev. 1942; Issued: 04-02-10; Effective/Implementation Date: 05-03-10)

ICD 9 Primary Code	ICD9 Alternative Specific Code	Condition (General)	Condition (Specific)	Service Level	Comments and Examples (not all-inclusive)	HCPCS Crosswalk
Emergency Conditions - Non-Traumatic						
535.50	458.9, 780.2, 787.01, 787.02, 787.03, 789.01, 789.02, 789.03, 789.04, 789.05, 789.06, 789.07, 789.09, 789.60 through 789.69, or 789.40 through 789.49 PLUS any other code from 780 through 799 except 793, 794, and 795.	Severe abdominal pain	With other signs or symptoms	ALS	Nausea, vomiting, fainting, pulsatile mass, distention, rigid, tenderness on exam, guarding.	A0427/A0433
789.00	726.2, 789.01, 789.02, 789.03, 789.04, 789.05, 789.06, 789.07, or 789.09	Abdominal pain	Without other signs or symptoms	BLS		A0429
427.9	426.0, 426.3, 426.4, 426.6, 426.11, 426.13, 426.50, 426.53, 427.0, 427.1, 427.2, 427.31, 427.32, 427.41, 427.42, 427.5, 427.60, 427.61, 427.69, 427.81, 427.89, 785.0, 785.50, 785.51, 785.52, or 785.59.	Abnormal cardiac rhythm/Cardiac dysrhythmia.	Potentially life-threatening	ALS	Bradycardia, junctional and ventricular blocks, non-sinus tachycardias, PVC's >6, bi- and trigeminy, ventricular tachycardia, ventricular fibrillation, atrial flutter, PEA, asystole, AICD/AED fired	A0427/A0433
780.8	782.5 or 782.6	Abnormal skin signs		ALS	Diaphorhesis, cyanosis, delayed cap refill, poor turgor, mottled.	A0427/A0433
796.4	458.9, 780.6, 785.9, 796.2, or 796.3 PLUS any other code from 780 through 799	Abnormal vital signs (includes abnormal pulse oximetry)	With or without symptoms.	ALS		A0427/A0433
995.0	995.1, 995.2, 995.3, 995.4, 995.60, 995.61, 995.62, 995.63, 995.64, 995.65, 995.66, 995.67, 995.68, 995.69, or 995.7	Allergic reaction	Potentially life-threatening	ALS	Other emergency conditions, rapid progression of symptoms, prior history of anaphylaxis, wheezing, difficulty swallowing.	A0427/A0433
692.9	692.0, 692.1, 692.2, 692.3, 692.4, 692.5, 692.6, 692.70, 692.71, 692.72, 692.73, 692.74, 692.75, 692.76, 692.77, 692.79, 692.81, 692.82, 692.83, 692.89, 692.9, 693.0, 693.1, 693.8, 693.9, 695.9, 698.9, 708.9, 782.1.	Allergic reaction	Other	BLS	Hives, itching, rash, slow onset, local swelling, redness, erythema.	A0429
790.21	790.22, 250.02, or 250.03.	Blood glucose	Abnormal <80 or >250, with symptoms.	ALS	Altered mental status, vomiting, signs of dehydration.	A0427/A0433
799.1	786.02, 786.03, 786.04, or 786.09.	Respiratory arrest		ALS	Apnea, hypoventilation requiring ventilatory assistance and airway management.	A0427/A0433
786.05		Difficulty breathing		ALS		A0427/A0433
427.5		Cardiac arrest – resuscitation in progress		ALS		A0427/A0433

ICD 9 Primary Code	ICD9 Alternative Specific Code	Condition (General)	Condition (Specific)	Service Level	Comments and Examples (not all-inclusive)	HCPCS Crosswalk
786.50	786.51, 786.52, or 786.59.	Chest pain (non-traumatic)		ALS	Dull, severe, crushing, substernal, epigastric, left sided chest pain associated with pain of the jaw, left arm, neck, back, and nausea, vomiting, palpitations, pallor, diaphoresis, decreased LOC.	A0427/A0433
784.99	933.0 or 933.1.	Chocking episode	Airway obstructed or partially obstructed	ALS		A0427/A0433
991.6		Cold exposure	Potentially life or limb threatening	ALS	Temperature < 95F, deep frost bite, other emergency conditions.	A0427/A0433
991.9	991.0, 991.1, 991.2, 991.3, or 991.4.	Cold exposure	With symptoms	BLS	Shivering, superficial frost bite, and other emergency conditions	A0429
780.97	780.02, 780.03, or 780.09.	Altered level of consciousness (nontraumatic)		ALS	Acute condition with Glascow Coma Scale < 15.	A0427/A0433
780.39	345.00, 345.01, 345.2, 345.3, 345.10, 345.11, 345.40, 345.41, 345.50, 345.51, 345.60, 345.61, 345.70 , 345.71, 345.80, 345.81, 345.90, 345.91, or 780.31.	Convulsions, seizures	Seizing, immediate post-seizure, postictal, or at risk of seizure and requires medical monitoring/observation.	ALS		A0427/A0433
379.90	368.11, 368.12, or 379.91	Eye symptoms, non-traumatic	Acute vision loss and/or severe pain	BLS		A0429
437.9	784.0 PLUS 781.0, 781.1, 781.2, 781.3, 781.4, or 781.8.	Non-traumatic headache	With neurologic distress conditions or sudden severe onset	ALS		A0427/A0433
785.1		Cardiac symptoms other than chest pain.	Palpitations, skipped beats	ALS		A0472/A0433
536.2	787.01, 787.02, 787.03, 780.79, 786.8, or 786.52.	Cardiac symptoms other than chest pain.	Atypical pain or other symptoms	ALS	Persistent nausea and vomiting, weakness, hiccups, pleuritic pain, feeling of impending doom, and other emergency conditions.	A0427/A0433
992.5	992.0, 992.1, 992.3, 992.4, or 992.5.	Heat exposure	Potentially life-threatening	ALS	Hot and dry skin, Temp>105, neurologic distress, signs of heat stroke or heat exhaustion, orthostatic vitals, other emergency conditions.	A0427/A0433
992.2	992.6, 992.7, 992.8, or 992.9.	Heat exposure	With symptoms	BLS	Muscle cramps, profuse sweating, fatigue.	A0429
459.0	569.3, 578.0, 578.1, 578.9, 596.7, 596.8, 623.8, 626.9, 637.1, 634.1, 666.00, 666.02, 666.04, 666.10, 666.12, 666.14, 666.20, 666.22, 666.24, 674.30, 674.32, 674.34, 786.3, 784.7, or 998.11	Hemorrhage	Severe (quantity) and potentially life-threatening	ALS	Uncontrolled or significant signs of shock or other emergency conditions. Severe, active vaginal, rectal bleeding, hematemesis, hemoptysis, epistaxis, active post- surgical bleeding.	A0472/A0433
038.9	136.9, any other condition in the 001 through 139 code range which would require isolation.	Infectious diseases requiring isolation procedures / public health risk.		BLS		A0429
987.9	981, 982.0, 982.1, 982.2, 982.3, 982.4, 982.8, 983.0, 983.1, 983.2, 983.9, 984.0, 984.1, 984.8, 984.9, 985.0, 985.1, 985.2, 985.3, 985.4, 985.5, 985.6, 985.8, 985.9, 986, 987.0, 987.1, 987.2, 987.3, 987.4, 987.5, 987.6, 987.7, 987.8, 989.1, 989.2, 989.3, 989.4, 989.6, 989.7, 989.9, or 990.	Hazmat exposure		ALS	Toxic fume or liquid exposure via inhalation, absorption, oral, radiation, smoke inhalation.	A0472/A0433

ICD 9 Primary Code	ICD9 Alternative Specific Code	Condition (General)	Condition (Specific)	Service Level	Comments and Examples (not all-inclusive)	HCPCS Crosswalk
996.00	996.01, 996.02, 996.04, 996.09, 996.1, or 996.2.	Medical device failure	Life or limb threatening malfunction, failure, or complication.	ALS	Malfunction of ventilator, internal pacemaker, internal defibrillator, implanted drug delivery service.	A0427/A0433
996.30	996.31, 996.40, 996.41, 996.42, 996.43, 996.44, 996.45, 996.46, 996.47, 996.49, or 996.59.	Medical device failure	Health maintenance device failures that cannot be resolved on location.	BLS	Oxygen system supply malfunction, orthopedic device failure.	A0429
436	291.3, 293.82, 298.9, 344.9, 368.16, 369.9, 780.09, 780.4, 781.0, 781.2, 781.94, 781.99, 782.0, 784.3, 784.5, or 787.2.	Neurologic distress		Facial drooping; loss of vision; aphasia; difficulty swallowing; numbness, tingling extremity; stupor, delirium, confusion, hallucinations; paralysis, paresis (focal weakness); abnormal movements; vertigo; unsteady gait/balance; slurred speech, unable to speak	ALS	A0427/A0433
780.96		Pain, severe not otherwise specified in this list.	Acute onset, unable to ambulate or sit due to intensity of pain.	ALS	Pain is the reason for the transport. Use severity scale (7-10 for severe pain) or patient receiving pharmalogic intervention.	A0427/A0433
724.5	724.2 or 785.9	Back pain – non-traumatic (T and/or LS).	Suspect cardiac or vascular etiology	ALS	Other emergency conditions, absence of or decreased leg pulses, pulsatile abdominal mass, severe tearing abdominal pain.	A0427/A0433
724.9	724.2, 724.5, 847.1, or 847.2.	Back pain – non-traumatic (T and/or LS).	Sudden onset of new neurologic symptoms.	ALS	Neurologic distress list.	A0427/A0433
977.9	Any code from 960 through 979.	Poisons, ingested, injected, inhaled, absorbed.	Adverse drug reaction, poison exposure by inhalation, injection, or absorption.	ALS		A0427/A0433
305.0	303.00, 303.01, 303.02, 303.03, or any code from 960 through 979.	Alcohol intoxication or drug overdose (suspected).	Unable to care for self and unable to ambulate. No airway compromise.	BLS		A0429
977.3		Severe alcohol intoxication.	Airway may or may not be at risk. Pharmacological intervention or cardiac monitoring may be needed. Decreased level of consciousness resulting or potentially resulting in airway compromise.	ALS		A0427/A0433
998.9	674.10, 674.12, 674.14, 674.20, 674.22, 674.24, 997.69, 998.31, 998.32, or 998.83.	Post-operative procedure complications.	Major wound dehiscence, evisceration, or requires special handling for transport.	BLS	Non-life threatening	A0429
650	Any code from 630 through 679.	Pregnancy complication/childbirth/labor		ALS		A0427/A0433
292.9	291.0, 291.3, 291.81, 292.0, 292.81, 292.82, 292.83, 292.84, or 292.89.	Psychiatric/Behavioral	Abnormal mental status; drug withdrawal.	ALS	Disoriented, DTs, withdrawal symptoms.	A0427/A0433
298.9	300.9	Psychiatric/Behavioral	Threat to self or others, acute episode or exacerbation of paranoia, or disruptive behavior.	BLS	Suicidal, homicidal, or violent.	A0429
036.9	780.6 PLUS either 784.0 or 723.5.	Sick person – fever	Fever with associated symptoms (headache, stiff neck, etc.). Neurological changes.	BLS	Suspected spinal meningitis.	A0429

ICD 9 Primary Code	ICD9 Alternative Specific Code	Condition (General)	Condition (Specific)	Service Level	Comments and Examples (not all-inclusive)	HCPCS Crosswalk
787.01	787.02, 787.03, or 787.91.	Severe dehydration	Nausea and vomiting, diarrhea, severe and incapacitating resulting in severe side effects of dehydration.	ALS		A0427/A0433
780.02	780.2 or 780.4	Unconscious, fainting, syncope, near syncope, weakness, or dizziness.	Transient unconscious episode or found unconscious. Acute episode or exacerbation.	ALS		A0427/A0433

Emergency Conditions - Trauma

ICD 9 Primary Code	ICD9 Alternative Specific Code	Condition (General)	Condition (Specific)	Service Level	Comments and Examples (not all-inclusive)	HCPCS Crosswalk
959.8	800.00 through 804.99, 807.4, 807.6, 808.8, 808.9, 812.00 through 812.59, 813.00 through 813.93, 813.93, 820.00 through 821.39, 823.00 through 823.92, 851.00 through 866.13, 870.0 through 879.9, 880.00 through 887.7, or 890.0 through 897.7.	Major trauma	As defined by ACS Field Triage Decision Scheme. Trauma with one of the following: Glascow <14; systolic BP<90; RR<10 or >29; all penetrating injuries to head, neck, torso, extremities proximal to elbow or knee; flail chest; combination of trauma and burns; pelvic fracture; 2 or more long bone fractures; open or depressed skull fracture; paralysis; severe mechanism of injury including: ejection, death of another passenger in same patient compartment, falls >20", 20" deformity in vehicle or 12" deformity of patient compartment, auto pedestrian/bike, pedestrian thrown/run over, motorcycle accident at speeds >20 mph and rider separated from vehicle.	ALS	See "Condition (Specific)" column	A0427/A0433
518.5		Other trauma	Need to monitor or maintain airway	ALS	Decreased LOC, bleeding into airway, trauma to head, face or neck.	A0427/A0433
958.2	870.0 through 879.9, 880.00 through 887.7, 890.0 through 897.7, or 900.00 through 904.9.	Other trauma	Major bleeding	ALS	Uncontrolled or significant bleeding.	A0427/A0433
829.0	805.00, 810.00 through 819.1, or 820.00 through 829.1.	Other trauma	Suspected fracture/dislocation requiring splinting/immobilization for transport.	BLS	Spinal, long bones, and joints including shoulder elbow, wrist, hip, knee and ankle, deformity of bone or joint.	A0429
880.00	880.00 through 887.7 or 890.0 through 897.7	Other trauma	Penetrating extremity injuries	BLS	Isolated bleeding stopped and good CSM.	A0429
886.0 or 895.0	886.1 or 895.1	Other trauma	Amputation – digits	BLS		A0429
887.4 or 897.4	887.0, 887.1, 887.2, 887.3, 887.6, 887.7, 897.0, 897.1, 897.2, 897.3, 897.5, 897.6, or 897.7.	Other trauma	Amputation – all other	ALS		A0427/A0433
869.0 or 869.1	511.8, 512.8, 860.2, 860.3, 860.4, 860.5, 873.8, 873.9, or 959.01.	Other trauma	Suspected internal, head, chest, or abdominal injuries.	ALS	Signs of closed head injury, open head injury, pneumothorax, hemothorax, abdominal bruising, positive abdominal signs on exam, internal bleeding criteria, evisceration.	A0427/A0433

ICD 9 Primary Code	ICD9 Alternative Specific Code	Condition (General)	Condition (Specific)	Service Level	Comments and Examples (not all-inclusive)	HCPCS Crosswalk
949.3	941.30 through 941.39, 942.30 through 942.39, 943.30 through 943.39, 944.30 through 944.38, 945.30 through 945.39, or 949.3.	Burns	Major – per American Burn Association (ABA)	ALS	Partial thickness burns > 10% total body surface area (TBSA); involvement of face, hands, feet, genitalia, perineum, or major joints; third degree burns; electrical; chemical; inhalation; burns with preexisting medical disorders; burns and trauma	A0472/A0433
949.2	941.20 through 941.29, 942.20 through 942.29, 943.20 through 943.29, 944.20 through 944.28, 945.20 through 945.29, or 949.2.	Burns	Minor – per ABA	BLS	Other burns than listed above.	A0429
989.5		Animal bites, stings, envenomation.	Potentially life or limb-threatening.	ALS	Symptoms of specific envenomation, significant face, neck, trunk, and extremity involvement; other emergency conditions.	A0427/A0433
879.8	Any code from 870.0 through 897.7.	Animal bites/sting/envonmation.	Other	BLS	Local pain and swelling or special handling considerations (not related to obesity) and patient monitoring required.	A0429
994.0		Lightning		ALS		A0427/A0433
994.8		Electrocution		ALS		A0427/A0433
994.1		Near drowning	Airway compromised during near drowning event	ALS		A0427/A0433
921.9	870.0 through 870.9, 871.0, 871.1, 871.2, 871.3, 871.4, 871.5, 871.6, 871.7, 871.9, or 921.0 through 921.9.	Eye injuries	Acute vision loss or blurring, severe pain or chemical exposure, penetrating, severe lid lacerations.	BLS		A0429
995.83	995.53 or V71.5 PLUS any code from 925.1 through 929.9, 930.0 through 939.9, 958.0 through 958.8, or 959.01 through 959.9.	Sexual assault	With major injuries	ALS	Reference codes 959.8, 958.2, 869.0/869.1	A0427/A0433
995.80	995.53 or V71.5 PLUS any code from 910.0 through 919.9, 920 through 924.9, or 959.01 through 959.9.	Sexual assault	With minor or no injuries	BLS		

Non-Emergency

428.9		Cardiac/hemodynamic monitoring required en route.		ALS	Expectation monitoring is needed before and after transport.	A0426
518.81 or 518.89	V46.11 or V46.12.	Advanced airway management		ALS	Ventilator dependent, apnea monitor, possible intubation needed, deep suctioning.	A0426, A0434
293.0		Chemical restraint.		ALS		A0426
496	491.20, 491.21, 492.0 through 492.8, 493.20, 493.21, 493.22, 494.0, or 494.1.	Suctioning required en route, need for titrated O2 therapy or IV fluid management.		BLS	Per transfer instructions.	A0428
786.09		Airway control/positioning required en route.		BLS	Per transfer instructions.	A0428
492.8	491.20, 491.21, 492.0 through 492.8, 493.20, 493.21, 493.22, 494.0, or 494.1.	Third party assistance/attendant required to apply, administer, or regulate or adjust oxygen en route.		BLS	Does not apply to patient capable of self-administration of portable or home O2. Patient must require oxygen therapy and be so frail as to require assistance.	A0428

ICD 9 Primary Code	ICD9 Alternative Specific Code	Condition (General)	Condition (Specific)	Service Level	Comments and Examples (not all-inclusive)	HCPCS Crosswalk
298.9	Add 295.0 through 295.9 with 5th digits of 0, 1, 3, or 4, 296.00 or 299.90.	Patient safety: Danger to self or others – in restraints.		BLS	Refer to definition in 42 CFR Section 482.13(e).	A0428
293.1		Patient safety: Danger to self or others – monitoring.		BLS	Behavioral or cognitive risk such that patient requires monitoring for safety.	A0428
298.8	Add 295.0 through 295.9 with 5th digits of 0, 1, 3, or 4, 296.00 or 299.90	Patient safety: Danger to self or others – seclusion (flight risk).		BLS	Behavioral or cognitive risk such that patient requires attendant to assure patient does not try to exit the ambulance prematurely. Refer to 42 CFR Section 482.13(f) for definition.	A0428
781.3	Add 295.0 through 295.9 with 5th digits of 0, 1, 3, or 4, 296.00 or 299.90.	Patient safety: Risk of falling off wheelchair or stretcher while in motion (not related to obesity).		BLS	Patient's physical condition is such that patient risks injury during vehicle movement despite restraints. Indirect indicators include MDS criteria.	A0428
041.9		Special handling en route – isolation.		BLS	Includes patients with communicable diseases or hazardous material exposure who must be isolated from public or whose medical condition must be protected from public exposure; surgical drainage complications.	A0428
907.2		Special handling en route to reduce pain – orthopedic device.		BLS	Backboard, halotraction, use of pins and traction etc. Pain may be present.	A0428
719.45 or 719.49	718.40, 718.45, 718.49, or 907.2.	Special handling en route – positioning requires specialized handling.		BLS	Requires special handling to avoid further injury (such as with > grade 2 decubiti on buttocks). Generally does not apply to shorter transfers of < 1 hour. Positioning in wheelchair or standard car seat inappropriate due to contractures or recent extremity fractures – post-op hip as an example.	A0428

Transportation Indicators Air/Ground	Transportation Category	Transportation Indicator Description		Service Level	Comments and Examples (not all-inclusive)	HCPCS Crosswalk
Transportation Indicators						
C1	Inter-facility Transport	EMTALA-certified inter-facility transfer to a higher level of care.	Beneficiary requires higher level of care.	BLS, ALS, SCT, FW, RW	Excludes patient-requested EMTALA transfer.	A0428, A0429, A0426, A0427, A0433, A0434
C2	Inter-facility transport	Service not available at originating facility, and must meet one or more emergency or non-emergency conditions.		BLS, ALS, SCT, FW,RW		A0428, A0429, A0426, A0427, A0433, A0434
C3	Emergency Trauma Dispatch Condition Code	Major incident or mechanism of injury	Major Incident-This transportation indicator is to be used ONLY as a secondary code when the on-scene encounter is a BLS-level patient.	ALS	Trapped in machinery, close proximity to explosion, building fire with persons reported inside, major incident involving aircraft, bus, subway, metro, train and watercraft. Victim entrapped in vehicle.	A0427/A0433

Transportation Indicators Air/Ground	Transportation Category	Transportation Indicator Description		Service Level	Comments and Examples (not all-inclusive)	HCPCS Crosswalk
C4	Medically necessary transport but not to the nearest facility.	BLS or ALS response	Indicates to Carrier/Intermediary that an ambulance provided a medically necessary transport, but that the number of miles on the Medicare claim form may be excessive.	BLS/ALS	This should occur if the facility is on divert status or the particular service is not available at the time of transport only. In these instances the ambulance units should clearly document why the beneficiary was not transported to the nearest facility.	Based on transport level.
C5	BLS transport of ALS-level patient	ALS-level condition treated and transport by a BLS-level ambulance.	This transportation indicator is used for ALL situations where a BLS-level ambulance treats and transports a patient that presents an ALS-level condition. No ALS-level assessment or intervention occurs at all during the patient encounter.	BLS		A0429
C6	ALS-level response to BLS-level patient	ALS response required based upon appropriate dispatch protocols – BLS-level patient transport	Indicates to Carrier/Intermediary that an ALS-level ambulance responded appropriately based upon the information received at the time the call was received in dispatch and after a clinically appropriate ALS-assessment was performed on scene, it was determined that the condition of the patient was at a BLS level. These claims, properly documented, should be reimbursed at an ALS-1 level based upon coverage guidelines under the Medicare Ambulance Fee Schedule.	ALS		A0427
C7		IV meds required en route.	This transportation indicator is used for patients that require an ALS level transport in a non- emergent situation primarily because the patient requires monitoring of ongoing medications administered intravenously. Does not apply to self-administered medications. Does not include administration of crystalloid intravenous fluids (i.e., Normal Saline, Lactate Ringers, 5% Dextrose in Water, etc.). The patient's condition should also be reported on the claim with a code selected from the list	ALS	Does not apply to self-administered IV medications.	A0426

Air Ambulance Transportation Indicators	Transportation Indicator Description	Service Level	Comments and Examples (not all-inclusive)	HCPCS Crosswalk
Air Ambulance Transportation Indicators				
D1	Long Distance-patient's condition requires rapid transportation over a long distance	FW, RW	If the patient's condition warrants only.	A0430, A0431
D2	Under rare and exceptional circumstances, traffic patterns preclude ground transport at the time the response is required.	FW, RW	A0430, A0431	
D3	FW, RW	A0430, A0431		
D4	FW, RW	A0430, A0431		

Note: HCPCS Crosswalk to ALS1E (A0427) and ALS2 (A0433) would ultimately be determined by the number and type of ALS level services provided during transport. All medical condition codes can be cross walked to fixed wing and rotor wing HCPCS provided the air ambulance service has documented the medical necessity for air ambulance service versus ground or water ambulance. As a result, codes A0430 (Fixed Wing) and A0431 (Rotor Wing) can be included in Column 7 for each condition listed.

100-4, 16, 60.1.4

Coding Requirements for Specimen Collection

The following HCPCS codes and terminology must be used:

- 36415 Collection of venous blood by venipuncture.
- P9615 Catheterization for collection of specimen(s).

The allowed amount for specimen collection in each of the above circumstances is included in the laboratory fee schedule distributed annually by CMS.

100-4, 16, 60.2

Travel Allowance

In addition to a specimen collection fee allowed under Sec.60.1, Medicare, under Part B, covers a specimen collection fee and travel allowance for a laboratory technician to draw a specimen from either a nursing home patient or homebound patient under Sec.1833(h)(3) of the Act and payment is made based on the clinical laboratory fee schedule. The travel allowance is intended to cover the estimated travel costs of collecting a specimen and to reflect the technician's salary and travel costs.

The additional allowance can be made only where a specimen collection fee is also payable, i.e., no travel allowance is made where the technician merely performs a messenger service to pick up a specimen drawn by a physician or nursing home personnel. The travel allowance may not be paid to a physician unless the trip to the home, or to the nursing home was solely for the purpose of drawing a specimen. Otherwise travel costs are considered to be associated with the other purposes of the trip. The travel allowance is not distributed by CMS. Instead, the carrier must calculate the travel allowance for each claim using the following rules for the particular Code. The following HCPCS codes are used for travel allowances:

- Per Mile Travel Allowance (P9603)

- The minimum "per mile travel allowance" is $1.035. The per mile travel allowance is to be used in situations where the average trip to patients' homes is longer than 20 miles round trip, and is to be pro-rated in situations where specimens are drawn or picked up from non-Medicare patients in the same trip. - one way, in connection with medically necessary laboratory specimen collection drawn from homebound or nursing home bound patient; prorated miles actually traveled (carrier allowance on per mile basis); or

- The per mile allowance was computed using the Federal mileage rate plus an additional 45 cents a mile to cover the technician's time and travel costs. Contractors have the option of establishing a higher per mile rate in excess of the minimum (1.035 cents a mile in CY 2008) if local conditions warrant it. The minimum mileage rate will be reviewed and updated in conjunction with the clinical lab fee schedule as needed. At no time will the laboratory be allowed to bill for more miles than are reasonable or for miles not actually traveled by the laboratory technician.

Example 1: In CY 2008, a laboratory technician travels 60 miles round trip from a lab in a city to a remote rural location, and back to the lab to draw a single Medicare patient's blood. The total reimbursement would be $62.10 (60 miles x 1.035 cents a mile), plus the specimen collection fee.

Example 2: In CY 2008, a laboratory technician travels 40 miles from the lab to a

Medicare patient's home to draw blood, and then travels an additional 10 miles to a non- Medicare patient's home and then travels 30 miles to return to the lab. The total miles traveled would be 80 miles. The claim submitted would be for one half of the miles traveled or $41.40 (40 x 1.035), plus the specimen collection fee.

Flat Rate (P9604)

The CMS will pay a minimum of $9.55 one way flat rate travel allowance. The flat rate travel allowance is to be used in areas where average trips are less than 20 miles round trip. The flat rate travel fee is to be pro-rated for more than one blood drawn at the same address, and for stops at the homes of Medicare and non-Medicare patients. The laboratory does the pro-ration when the claim is submitted based on the number of patients seen on that trip. The specimen collection fee will be paid for each patient encounter.

This rate is based on an assumption that a trip is an average of 15 minutes and up to 10 miles one way. It uses the Federal mileage rate and a laboratory technician's time of $17.66 an hour, including overhead. Contractors have the option of establishing a flat rate in excess of the minimum of $9.55, if local conditions warrant it. The minimum national flat rate will be reviewed and updated in conjunction with the clinical laboratory fee schedule, as necessitated by adjustments in the Federal travel allowance and salaries.

The claimant identifies round trip travel by use of the LR modifier

Example 3: A laboratory technician travels from the laboratory to a single Medicare patient's home and returns to the laboratory without making any other stops. The flat rate would be calculated as follows: 2 x $9.55 for a total trip reimbursement of $19.10, plus the specimen collection fee.

Example 4: A laboratory technician travels from the laboratory to the homes of five patients to draw blood, four of the patients are Medicare patients and one is not. An additional flat rate would be charged to cover the 5 stops and the return trip to the lab (6 x $9.55 = $57.30). Each of the claims submitted would be for $11.46 ($57.30 /5 = $11.46). Since one of the patients is non-Medicare, four claims would be submitted for $11.46 each, plus the specimen collection fee for each.

Example 5: A laboratory technician travels from a laboratory to a nursing home and draws blood from 5 patients and returns to the laboratory. Four of the patients are on Medicare and one is not. The $9.55 flat rate is multiplied by two to cover the return trip to the laboratory (2 x $9.55 = $19.10) and then divided by five (1/5 of $19.10 = $3.82).

Since one of the patients is non-Medicare, four claims would be submitted for $3.82 each, plus the specimen collection fee.

If a carrier determines that it results in equitable payment, the carrier may extend the former payment allowances for additional travel (such as to a distant rural nursing home) to all

circumstances where travel is required. This might be appropriate, for example, if the carrier's former payment allowance was on a per mile basis. Otherwise, it should establish an appropriate allowance and inform the suppliers in its service area. If a carrier decides to establish a new allowance, one method is to consider developing a travel allowance consisting of:

- The current Federal mileage allowance for operating personal automobiles, plus a personnel allowance per mile to cover personnel costs based upon an estimate of average hourly wages and average driving speed.

Carriers must prorate travel allowance amounts claimed by suppliers by the number of patients (including Medicare and non-Medicare patients) from whom specimens were drawn on a given trip.

The carrier may determine that payment in addition to the routine travel allowance determined under this section is appropriate if:

- The patient from whom the specimen must be collected is in a nursing home or is homebound; and

- The clinical laboratory tests are needed on an emergency basis outside the general business hours of the laboratory making the collection.

Subsequent updated travel allowance amounts will be issued by CMS via Recurring Update Notification (RUN) on an annual basis.

100-4, 16, 70.8
Certificate of Waiver

Effective September 1, 1992, all laboratory testing sites (except as provided in 42 CFR 493.3(b)) must have either a CLIA certificate of waiver, certificate for provider-performed microscopy procedures, certificate of registration, certificate of compliance, or certificate of accreditation to legally perform clinical laboratory testing on specimens from individuals in the United States.

The Food and Drug Administration approves CLIA waived tests on a flow basis. The CMS identifies CLIA waived tests by providing an updated list of waived tests to the Medicare contractors on a quarterly basis via a Recurring Update Notification. To be recognized as a waived test, some CLIA waived tests have unique HCPCS procedure codes and some must have a QW modifier included with the HCPCS code.

For a list of specific HCPCS codes subject to CLIA see http://www.cms.hhs.gov/CLIA/downloads/waivetbl.pdf

100-4, 17, 80.4.1
Clotting Factor Furnishing Fee

Beginning January 1, 2005, a clotting factor furnishing fee is separately payable to entities that furnish clotting factor unless the costs associated with furnishing the clotting factor is paid through another payment system.

The clotting factor furnishing fee is updated each calendar year based on the percentage increase in the consumer price index (CPI) for medical care for the 12-month period ending with June of the previous year. The clotting factor furnishing fees applicable for dates of service in each calendar year (CY) are listed below:

CY 2005 - $0.140 per I.U.

CY 2006 - $0.146 per I.U.

CY 2007 - $0.152 per I.U.

CY 2008 - $0.158 per I.U.

CY 2009 - $0.164 per I.U.

CY 2010 - $0.170 per I.U.

CY 2011 - $0.176 per unit

Annual updates to the clotting factor furnishing fee are subsequently communicated by a Recurring Update Notification.

CMS includes this clotting factor furnishing fee in the nationally published payment limit for clotting factor billing codes. When the clotting factor is not included on the Average Sales Price (ASP) Medicare Part B Drug Pricing File or Not Otherwise Classified (NOC) Pricing File, the contractor must make payment for the clotting factor as well as make payment for the furnishing fee.

100-4, 17, 90.3
Hospital Outpatient Payment Under OPPS for New, Unclassified Drugs and Biologicals After FDA Approval But Before Assignment of a Product-Specific Drug or Biological HCPCS Code

Section 621(a) of the MMA amends Section 1833(t) of the Social Security Act by adding paragraph (15), Payment for New Drugs and Biologicals Until HCPCS Code Assigned. Under this provision, payment for an outpatient drug or biological that is furnished as part of covered outpatient department services for which a product-specific HCPCS code has not been assigned shall be paid an amount equal to 95 percent of average wholesale price (AWP). This provision applies only to payments under the hospital outpatient prospective payment system (OPPS).

Beginning January 1, 2004, hospital outpatient departments may bill for new drugs and biologicals that are approved by the FDA on or after January 1, 2004, for which a product-specific HCPCS code has not been assigned. Beginning on or after the date of FDA approval, hospitals may bill for the drug or biological using HCPCS code C9399, Unclassified drug or biological.

Hospitals report in the ANSI ASC X-12 837 I in specific locations, or in the "Remarks" section of the CMS 1450):

1. the National Drug Code (NDC),

2. the quantity of the drug that was administered, expressed in the unit of measure applicable to the drug or biological, and

3. the date the drug was furnished to the beneficiary. Contractors shall manually price the drug or biological at 95 percent of AWP. They shall pay hospitals 80 percent of the calculated price and shall bill beneficiaries 20 percent of the calculated price, after the deductible is met. Drugs and biologicals that are manually priced at 95 percent of AWP are not eligible for outlier payment.

HCPCS code C9399 is only to be reported for new drugs and biologicals that are approved by FDA on or after January 1, 2004, for which there is no HCPCS code that describes the drug.

100-4,18,10.1.2

Influenza Virus Vaccine

Effective for services furnished on or after May 1, 1993, the influenza virus vaccine and its administration is covered when furnished in compliance with any applicable State law. Typically, this vaccine is administered once a flu season. Medicare does not require for coverage purposes that a doctor of medicine or osteopathy order the vaccine. Therefore, the beneficiary may receive the vaccine upon request without a physician's order and without physician supervision. Since there is no yearly limit, contractors determine whether such services are reasonable and allow payment if appropriate.

See Pub. 100-02, Medicare Benefit Policy Manual, Chapter 15, Section 50.4.4.2 for additional coverage requirements for influenza virus vaccine.

Service	CPT/HCPCS Code	Long Descriptor	USPSTF Rating	Coins./ Deductible
Initial Preventive Physical Examination, IPPE	G0402	Initial preventive physical examination; face to face visits, services limited to new beneficiary during the first 12 months of Medicare enrollment	*Not Rated	WAIVED
	G0403	Electrocardiogram, routine ECG with 12 leads; performed as a screening for the initial preventive physical examination with interpretation and report		Not Waived
	G0404	Electrocardiogram, routine ECG with 12 leads; tracing only, without interpretation and report, performed as a screening for the initial preventive physical examination		Not Waived
	G0405	Electrocardiogram, routine ECG with 12 leads; interpretation and report only, performed as a screening for the initial preventive physical examination		Not Waived
Ultrasound Screening for Abdominal Aortic Aneurysm (AAA)	G0389	Ultrasound, B-scan and /or real time with image documentation; for abdominal aortic aneurysm (AAA) ultrasound screening	B	WAIVED
Cardiovascular Disease	80061	Lipid panel	A	WAIVED
	82465	Cholesterol, serum or whole blood, total		WAIVED

Service	CPT/HCPCS Code	Long Descriptor	USPSTF Rating	Coins./ Deductible
	83718	Lipoprotein, direct measurement; high density cholesterol (hdl cholesterol)		WAIVED
	84478	Triglycerides		WAIVED
Diabetes Screening Tests	82947	Glucose; quantitative, blood (except reagent strip)	B	WAIVED
	82950	Glucose; post glucose dose (includes glucose)		WAIVED
	82951	Glucose; tolerance test (gtt), three specimens (includes glucose)	*Not Rated	WAIVED
Diabetes Self-Management Training Services (DSMT)	G0108	Diabetes outpatient self-management training services, individual, per 30 minutes	*Not Rated	Not Waived
	G0109	Diabetes outpatient self-management training services, group session (2 or more), per 30 minutes		Not Waived
Medical Nutrition Therapy (MNT) Services	97802	Medical nutrition therapy; initial assessment and intervention, individual, face-to-face with the patient, each 15 minutes	B	WAIVED
	97803	Medical nutrition therapy; re-assessment and intervention, individual, face-to-face with the patient, each 15 minutes		WAIVED
	97804	Medical nutrition therapy; group (2 or more individual(s)), each 30 minutes		WAIVED
	G0270	Medical nutrition therapy; reassessment and subsequent intervention(s) following second referral in same year for change in diagnosis, medical condition or treatment regimen (including additional hours needed for renal disease), individual, face to face with the patient, each 15 minutes	B	WAIVED
	G0271	Medical nutrition therapy, reassessment and subsequent intervention(s) following second referral in same year for change in diagnosis, medical condition, or treatment regimen (including additional hours needed for renal disease), group (2 or more individuals), each 30 minutes		WAIVED
Screening Pap Test	G0123	Screening cytopathology, cervical or vaginal (any reporting system), collected in preservative fluid, automated thin layer preparation, screening by cytotechnologist under physician supervision	A	WAIVED
	G0124	Screening cytopathology, cervical or vaginal (any reporting system), collected in preservative fluid, automated thin layer preparation, requiring interpretation by physician		WAIVED

Service	CPT/HCPCS Code	Long Descriptor	USPSTF Rating	Coins./ Deductible
	G0141	Screening cytopathology smears, cervical or vaginal, performed by automated system, with manual rescreening, requiring interpretation by physician	A	WAIVED
	G0143	Screening cytopathology, cervical or vaginal (any reporting system), collected in preservative fluid, automated thin layer preparation, with manual screening and rescreening by cytotechnologist under physician supervision	A	WAIVED
	G0144	Screening cytopathology, cervical or vaginal (any reporting system), collected in preservative fluid, automated thin layer preparation, with screening by automated system, under physician supervision	A	WAIVED
	G0145	Screening cytopathology, cervical or vaginal (any reporting system), collected in preservative fluid, automated thin layer preparation, with screening by automated system and manual rescreening under physician supervision	A	WAIVED
	G0147	Screening cytopathology smears, cervical or vaginal, performed by automated system under physician supervision	A	WAIVED
	G0148	Screening cytopathology smears, cervical or vaginal, performed by automated system with manual rescreening	A	WAIVED
	P3000	Screening papanicolaou smear, cervical or vaginal, up to three smears, by technician under physician supervision		WAIVED
	P3001	Screening papanicolaou smear, cervical or vaginal, up to three smears, requiring interpretation by physician		WAIVED
	Q0091	Screening papanicolaou smear; obtaining, preparing and conveyance of cervical or vaginal smear to laboratory		WAIVED
Screening Pelvic Exam	G0101	Cervical or vaginal cancer screening; pelvic and clinical breast examination	A	WAIVED
Screening Mammography	77052	Computer-aided detection (computer algorithm analysis of digital image data for lesion detection) with further physician review for interpretation, with or without digitization of film radiographic images; screening mammography (list separately in addition to code for primary procedure)	B	WAIVED

Service	CPT/HCPCS Code	Long Descriptor	USPSTF Rating	Coins./ Deductible
	77057	Screening mammography, bilateral (2-view film study of each breast)	B	WAIVED
	G0202	Screening mammography, producing direct digital image, bilateral, all views		WAIVED
Bone Mass Measurement	G0130	Single energy x-ray absorptiometry (sexa) bone density study, one or more sites; appendicular skeleton (peripheral) (e.g., radius, wrist, heel)	B	WAIVED
	77078	Computed tomography, bone mineral density study, 1 or more sites; axial skeleton (e.g., hips, pelvis, spine)		WAIVED
	77079	Computed tomography, bone mineral density study, 1 or more sites; appendicular skeleton (peripheral) (e.g., radius, wrist, heel)		WAIVED
	77080	Dual-energy x-ray absorptiometry (dxa), bone density study, 1 or more sites; axial skeleton (e.g., hips, pelvis, spine)		WAIVED
	77081	Dual-energy x-ray absorptiometry (dxa), bone density study, 1 or more sites; appendicular skeleton (peripheral) (e.g., radius, wrist, heel)		WAIVED
	77083	Radiographic absorptiometry (e.g., photo densitometry, radiogrammetry), 1 or more sites		WAIVED
	76977	Ultrasound bone density measurement and interpretation, peripheral site(s), any method		WAIVED
Colorectal Cancer Screening	G0104	Colorectal cancer screening; flexible sigmoidoscopy	A	WAIVED
	G0105	Colorectal cancer screening; colonoscopy on individual at high risk		WAIVED
	G0106	Colorectal cancer screening; alternative to G0104, screening sigmoidoscopy, barium enema	*Not Rated	Coins. Applies & Ded. is waived
	G0120	Colorectal cancer screening; alternative to G0105, screening colonoscopy, barium enema.		Coins. Applies & Ded. is waived
	G0121	Colorectal cancer screening; colonoscopy on individual not meeting criteria for high risk	A	WAIVED
	82270	Blood, occult, by peroxidase activity (e.g., guaiac), qualitative; feces, consecutive		WAIVED
	G0328	Colorectal cancer screening; fecal occult blood test, immunoassay, 1-3 simultaneous		WAIVED

Service	CPT/HCPCS Code	Long Descriptor	USPSTF Rating	Coins./ Deductible
Prostate Cancer Screening	G0102	Prostate cancer screening; digital rectal examination	D	Not Waived
	G0103	Prostate cancer screening; prostate specific antigen test (PSA)		WAIVED
Glaucoma Screening	G0117	Glaucoma screening for high risk patients furnished by an optometrist or ophthalmologist	I	Not Waived
	G0118	Glaucoma screening for high risk patient furnished under the direct supervision of an optometrist or ophthalmologist		Not Waived
Influenza Virus Vaccine	90654	Influenza virus vaccine, split virus, preservative free, for intradermal use, for adults ages 18-64	B	WAIVED
	90654	Influenza virus vaccine, split virus, preservative free, for intradermal use, for adults ages 18-64	B	
	90655	Influenza virus vaccine, split virus, preservative free, when administered to children 6-35 months of age, for intramuscular use		WAIVED
	90656	Influenza virus vaccine, split virus, preservative free, when administered to individuals 3 years and older, for intramuscular use		WAIVED
	90657	Influenza virus vaccine, split virus, when administered to children 6-35 months of age, for intramuscular use		WAIVED
	90660	Influenza virus vaccine, live, for intranasal use		WAIVED
	90662	Influenza virus vaccine, split virus, preservative free, enhanced immunogenicity via increased antigen content, for intramuscular use		WAIVED
	Q2034	Influenza virus vaccine, split virus, for intramuscular use (Agriflu)		WAIVED
	Q2035	Influenza virus vaccine, split virus, when administered to individuals 3 years of age and older, for intramuscular use (afluria)		WAIVED
	Q2036	Influenza virus vaccine, split virus, when administered to individuals 3 years of age and older, for intramuscular use (flulaval)		WAIVED
	Q2037	Influenza virus vaccine, split virus when administered to individuals 3 years of age and older, for intramuscular use (fluvirin)		WAIVED

Service	CPT/HCPCS Code	Long Descriptor	USPSTF Rating	Coins./ Deductible
	Q2038	Influenza virus vaccine, split virus, when administered to individuals 3 years of age and older, for intramuscular use (fluzone)		WAIVED
	Q2039	Influenza virus vaccine, split virus, when administered to individuals 3 years of age and older, for intramuscular use (not otherwise specified)		WAIVED
	G0008	Administration of influenza virus vaccine		WAIVED
	G9141	Influenza A (H1N1) immunization administration (includes the physician counseling the patient/family)		WAIVED
	G9142	Influenza A (H1N1) Vaccine, any route of administration		WAIVED
Pneumococcal Vaccine	90669	Pneumococcal conjugate vaccine, polyvalent, when administered to children younger than 5 years, for intramuscular use	B	WAIVED
	90670	Pneumococcal conjugate vaccine, 13 valent, for intramuscular use.		WAIVED
	90732	Pneumococcal polysaccharide vaccine, 23-valent, adult or immunosuppressed patient dosage, when administered to individuals 2 years or older, for subcutaneous or intramuscular use		WAIVED
	G0009	Administration of pneumococcal vaccine		WAIVED
Hepatitis B Vaccine	90740	Hepatitis B vaccine, dialysis or immunosuppressed patient dosage (3 dose schedule), for intramuscular use	A	WAIVED
	90743	Hepatitis B vaccine, adolescent (2 dose schedule), for intramuscular use		WAIVED
	90744	Hepatitis B vaccine, pediatric/adolescent dosage (3 dose schedule), for intramuscular use		WAIVED
	90746	Hepatitis B vaccine, adult dosage, for intramuscular use		WAIVED
	90747	Hepatitis B vaccine, dialysis or immunosuppressed patient dosage (4 dose schedule), for intramuscular use		WAIVED
	G0010	Administration of hepatitis B vaccine	A	WAIVED
HIV Screening	G0432	Infectious agent antigen detection by enzyme immunoassay (EIA) technique, qualitative or semi-qualitative, multiple-step method, HIV-1 or HIV-2, screening	A	WAIVED

Service	CPT/HCPCS Code	Long Descriptor	USPSTF Rating	Coins./ Deductible
	G0433	Infectious agent antigen detection by enzyme-linked immunosorbent assay (ELISA) technique, antibody, HIV-1 or HIV-2, screening		WAIVED
	G0435	Infectious agent antigen detection by rapid antibody test of oral mucosa transudate, HIV-1 or HIV-2 , screening		WAIVED
Smoking Cessation	G0436	Smoking and tobacco cessation counseling visit for the asymptomatic patient; intermediate, greater than 3 minutes, up to 10 minutes	A	WAIVED
	G0437	Smoking and tobacco cessation counseling visit for the asymptomatic patient intensive, greater than 10 minutes		WAIVED
Annual Wellness Visit	G0438	Annual wellness visit, including PPPS, first visit	*Not Rated	WAIVED
	G0439	Annual wellness visit, including PPPS, subsequent visit		WAIVED

100-4,18,10.2.1

Healthcare Common Procedure Coding System (HCPCS) and Diagnosis Codes

Vaccines and their administration are reported using separate codes. The following codes are for reporting the vaccines only.

HCPCS	Definition
Q2034	Influenza virus vaccine, split virus, for intramuscular use (Agriflu)
90653	Influenza virus vaccine, inactivated, subunit, adjuvanted, for intramuscular use
90654	Influenza virus vaccine, split virus, preservative-free, for intradermal use, for adults ages 18-64;
90655	Influenza virus vaccine, split virus, preservative free, for children 6-35 months of age, for intramuscular use;
90656	Influenza virus vaccine, split virus, preservative free, for use in individuals 3 years and above, for intramuscular use;
90657	Influenza virus vaccine, split virus, for children 6-35 months of age, for intramuscular use;
90658	Influenza virus vaccine, split virus, for use in individuals 3 years of age and above, for intramuscular use;
90660	Influenza virus vaccine, live, for intranasal use;
90661	Influenza virus vaccine, derived from cell cultures, subunit, preservative and antibiotic free, for intramuscular use
90662	Influenza virus vaccine, split virus, preservative free, enhanced immunogenicity via increased antigen content, for intramuscular use
90669	Pneumococcal conjugate vaccine, polyvalent, for children under 5 years, for intramuscular use
90670	Pneumococcal conjugate vaccine, 13 valent, for intramuscular use
90672	Influenza virus vaccine, live, quadrivalent, for intranasal use
90685	Influenza virus vaccine, quadrivalent, split virus, preservative free, when administered to children 6-35 months of age, for intramuscular use
90686	Influenza virus vaccine, quadrivalent, split virus, preservative free, when administered to individuals 3 years of age and older, for intramuscular use
90687	Influenza virus vaccine, quadrivalent, split virus, when administered to children 6-35 months of age, for intramuscular use
90688	Influenza virus vaccine, quadrivalent, split virus, when administered to individuals 3 years of age and older, for intramuscular use

HCPCS	Definition
90732	Pneumococcal polysaccharide vaccine, 23-valent, adult or immunosuppressed patient dosage, for use in individuals 2 years or older, for subcutaneous or intramuscular use;
90739	Hepatitis B vaccine, adult dosage (2 dose schedule), for intramuscular use
90740	Hepatitis B vaccine, dialysis or immunosuppressed patient dosage (3 dose schedule), for intramuscular use;
90743	Hepatitis B vaccine, adolescent (2 dose schedule), for intramuscular use;
90744	Hepatitis B vaccine, pediatric/adolescent dosage (3 dose schedule), for intramuscular use;
90746	Hepatitis B vaccine, adult dosage, for intramuscular use; and
90747	Hepatitis B vaccine, dialysis or immunosuppressed patient dosage (4 dose schedule), for intramuscular use.

***Effective October 1, 2006, providers may report diagnosis code V06.6 on claims for pneumococcus and/or influenza virus vaccines when the purpose of the visit was to receive both vaccines.

If a diagnosis code for pneumococcus, hepatitis B, or influenza virus vaccination is not reported on a claim, contractors may not enter the diagnosis on the claim. Contractors must follow current resolution processes for claims with missing diagnosis codes.

If the diagnosis code and the narrative description are correct, but the HCPCS code is incorrect, the carrier or intermediary may correct the HCPCS code and pay the claim. For example, if the reported diagnosis code is V04.81 and the narrative description (if annotated on the claim) says "flu shot" but the HCPCS code is incorrect, contractors may change the HCPCS code and pay for the flu vaccine. Effective October 1, 2006, carriers/AB MACs should follow the instructions in Pub. 100-04, Chapter 1, Section 80.3.2.1.1 (Carrier Data Element Requirements) for claims submitted without a HCPCS code.

Claims for hepatitis B vaccinations must report the I.D. Number of the referring physician. In addition, if a doctor of medicine or osteopathy does not order the influenza virus vaccine, the intermediary claims require:

- UPIN code SLF000 to be reported on claims submitted prior to May 23, 2008, when Medicare began accepting NPIs, only
- The provider's own NPI to be reported in the NPI field for the attending physician on claims submitted on or after May 23, 2008, when NPI requirements were implemented.

100-4, 18, 10.2.2.1

FI/AB MAC Payment for Pneumococcal Pneumonia Virus, Influenza Virus, and Hepatitis B Virus Vaccines and Their Administration
Payment for Vaccines

Payment for all of these vaccines is on a reasonable cost basis for hospitals, home health agencies (HHAs), skilled nursing facilities (SNFs), critical access hospitals (CAHs), and hospital-based renal dialysis facilities (RDFs). Payment for comprehensive outpatient rehabilitation facilities (CORFs), Indian Health Service hospitals (IHS), IHS CAHs and independent RDFs is based on 95 percent of the average wholesale price (AWP). Section 10.2.4 of this chapter contains information on payment of these vaccines when provided by RDFs or hospices. See Sec.10.2.2.2 for payment to independent and provider- based Rural Health Centers and Federally Qualified Health Clinics.

Payment for these vaccines is as follows:

Facility	Type of Bill	Payment
Hospitals, other than Indian Health Service (IHS) Hospitals and Critical Access Hospitals (CAHs)	12x, 13x	Reasonable cost
IHS Hospitals	12x, 13x, 83x	95% of AWP
IHS CAHs	85x	95% of AWP
CAHs Method I and Method II	85x	Reasonable cost
Skilled Nursing Facilities	22x, 23x	Reasonable cost
Home Health Agencies	34x	Reasonable cost
Comprehensive Outpatient Rehabilitation Facilities	75x	95% of the AWP
Independent Renal Dialysis Facilities	72x	95% of the AWP
Hospital-based Renal Dialysis	72x	Reasonable cost

Facilities

Payment for Vaccine Administration

Payment for the administration of influenza virus and pneumococcal vaccines is as follows:

Facility	Type of Bill	Payment
Hospitals, other than IHS Hospitals and CAHs	12x, 13x	Outpatient Prospective Payment System (OPPS) for hospitals subject to OPPS
Reasonable cost for hospitals not subject to OPPS IHS Hospitals	12x, 13x, 83x	MPFS as indicated in guidelines below.
IHS CAHs	85x	MPFS as indicated in guidelines below.
CAHs Method I and II	85x	Reasonable cost
Skilled Nursing Facilities	22x, 23x	MPFS as indicated in the guidelines below
Home Health Agencies	34x	OPPS
Comprehensive Outpatient Rehabilitation Facilities	75x	MPFS as indicated in the guidelines below
Independent RDFs	72x	MPFS as indicated in the guidelines below
Hospital-based RDFs	72x	Reasonable cost

Guidelines for pricing pneumococcal and influenza virus vaccine administration under the MPFS.

Make reimbursement based on the rate in the MPFS associated with the CPT code 90782 or 90471 as follows:

HCPCS code	Effective prior to March 1, 2003	Effective on and after March 1, 2003
G0008	90782	90471
G0009	90782	90471

See Sec.10.2.2.2 for payment to independent and provider based Rural Health Centers and Federally Qualified Health Clinics.

Payment for the administration of hepatitis B vaccine is as follows:

Facility	Type of Bill	Payment
Hospitals other than IHS hospitals and CAHs	12x, 13x	Outpatient Prospective Payment System (OPPS) for hospitals subject to OPPS
Reasonable cost for hospitals not subject to OPPS IHS Hospitals	12x, 13x, 83x	MPFS as indicated in the guidelines below
CAHs Method I and II	85x	Reasonable cost
IHS CAHs	85x	MPFS as indicated in guidelines below.
Skilled Nursing Facilities	22x, 23x	MPFS as indicated in the chart below
Home Health Agencies	34x	OPPS
Comprehensive Outpatient Rehabilitation Facilities	75x	MPFS as indicated in the guidelines below
Independent RDFs	72x	MPFS as indicated in the chart below
Hospital-based RDFs	72x	Reasonable cost

Guidelines for pricing hepatitis B vaccine administration under the MPFS.

Make reimbursement based on the rate in the MPFS associated with the CPT code 90782 or 90471 as follows:

HCPCS code	Effective prior to March 1, 2003	Effective on and after March 1, 2003
G0010	90782	90471

See Sec.10.2.2.2 for payment to independent and provider based Rural Health Centers and Federally Qualified Health Clinics.

100-4, 18, 10.2.5.2

Carrier/AB MAC Payment Requirements

Payment for pneumococcal, influenza virus, and hepatitis B vaccines follows the same standard rules that are applicable to any injectable drug or biological. (See chapter 17 for procedures for determining the payment rates for pneumococcal and influenza virus vaccines.) Effective for claims with dates of service on or after February 1, 2001, Sec.114, of the Benefits Improvement and Protection Act of 2000 mandated that all drugs and biologicals be paid based on mandatory assignment. Therefore, all providers of influenza virus and pneumococcal vaccines must accept assignment for the vaccine.

Prior to March 1, 2003, the administration of pneumococcal, influenza virus, and hepatitis B vaccines, (HCPCS codes G0008, G0009, and G0010), though not reimbursed directly through the MPFS, were reimbursed at the same rate as HCPCS code 90782 on the MPFS for the year that corresponded to the date of service of the claim.

Prior to March 1, 2003, HCPCS codes G0008, G0009, and G0010 are reimbursed at the same rate as HCPCS code 90471. Assignment for the administration is not mandatory, but is applicable should the provider be enrolled as a provider type "Mass Immunization Roster Biller," submits roster bills, or participates in the centralized billing program.

Carriers/AB MACs may not apply the limiting charge provision for pneumococcal, influenza virus vaccine, or hepatitis B vaccine and their administration in accordance with Secs.1833(a)(1) and 1833(a)(10)(A) of the Social Security Act (the Act.) The administration of the influenza virus vaccine is covered in the influenza virus vaccine benefit under Sec.1861(s)(10)(A) of the Act, rather than under the physicians' services benefit. Therefore, it is not eligible for the 10 percent Health Professional Shortage Area (HPSA) incentive payment or the 5 percent Physician Scarcity Area (PSA) incentive payment.

No Legal Obligation to Pay Nongovernmental entities that provide immunizations free of charge to all patients, regardless of their ability to pay, must provide the immunizations free of charge to Medicare beneficiaries and may not bill Medicare. (See Pub. 100-02, Medicare Benefit Policy Manual, chapter 16.) Thus, for example, Medicare may not pay for influenza virus vaccinations administered to Medicare beneficiaries if a physician provides free vaccinations to all non-Medicare patients or where an employer offers free vaccinations to its employees. Physicians also may not charge Medicare beneficiaries more for a vaccine than they would charge non-Medicare patients. (See Sec.1128(b)(6)(A) of the Act.)

When an employer offers free vaccinations to its employees, it must also offer the free vaccination to an employee who is also a Medicare beneficiary. It does not have to offer free vaccinations to its non-Medicare employees.

Nongovernmental entities that do not charge patients who are unable to pay or reduce their charges for patients of limited means, yet expect to be paid if the patient has health insurance coverage for the services provided, may bill Medicare and expect payment.

Governmental entities (such as PHCs) may bill Medicare for pneumococcal, hepatitis B, and influenza virus vaccines administered to Medicare beneficiaries when services are rendered free of charge to non-Medicare beneficiaries.

100-4, 18, 10.3.1.1

Centralized Billing for Influenza Virus and Pneumococcal Vaccines to Medicare Carriers/AB MACs

The CMS currently authorizes a limited number of providers to centrally bill for influenza virus and pneumococcal immunization claims. Centralized billing is an optional program available to providers who qualify to enroll with Medicare as the

provider type "Mass Immunization Roster Biller," as well as to other individuals and entities that qualify to enroll as regular Medicare providers. Centralized billers must roster bill, must accept assignment, and must bill electronically.

To qualify for centralized billing, a mass immunizer must be operating in at least three payment localities for which there are three different contractors processing claims. Individuals and entities providing the vaccine and administration must be properly licensed in the State in which the immunizations are given and the contractor must verify this through the enrollment process.

Centralized billers must send all claims for influenza virus and pneumococcal immunizations to a single contractor for payment, regardless of the jurisdiction in which the vaccination was administered. (This does not include claims for the Railroad Retirement Board, United Mine Workers or Indian Health Services. These claims must continue to go to the appropriate processing entity.) Payment is made based on the payment locality where the service was provided. This process is only available for claims for the influenza virus and pneumococcal vaccines and their administration. The general coverage and coding rules still apply to these claims.

This section applies only to those individuals and entities that provide mass immunization services for influenza virus and pneumococcal vaccinations and that have been authorized by CMS to centrally bill. All other providers, including those individuals and entities that provide mass immunization services that are not authorized to centrally bill, must continue to bill for these claims to their regular carrier/AB MAC per the instructions in Sec.10.3.1 of this chapter.

The claims processing instructions in this section apply only to the designated processing contractor. However, all carriers/AB MACs must follow the instructions in Sec.10.3.1.1.J, below, "Provider Education Instructions for All Carriers/AB MACs." A. Processing Contractor Trailblazers Health Enterprises is designated as the sole contractor for the payment of influenza virus and pneumococcal claims for centralized billers from October 1, 2000, through the length of the contract. The CMS central office will notify centralized billers of the appropriate contractor to bill when they receive their notification of acceptance into the centralized billing program.

B. Request for Approval
Approval to participate in the CMS centralized billing program is a two part approval process. Individuals and corporations who wish to enroll as a CMS mass immunizer centralized biller must send their request in writing. CMS will complete Part 1 of the approval process by reviewing preliminary demographic information included in the request for participation letter. Completion of Part 1 is not approval to set up vaccination clinics, vaccinate beneficiaries, and bill Medicare for reimbursement. All new participants must complete Part 2 of the approval process (Form CMS-855 Application) before they may set up vaccination clinics, vaccinate Medicare beneficiaries, and bill Medicare for reimbursement. If an individual or entity's request is approved for centralized billing, the approval is limited to 12 months from September to August 31 of the next year. It is the responsibility of the centralized biller to reapply for approval each year. The designated contractor shall provide in writing to CMS and approved centralized billers notification of completion and approval of Part 2 of the approval process. The designated contractor may not process claims for any centralized biller who has not completed Parts 1 and 2 of the approval process. If claims are submitted by a provider who has not received approval of Parts 1 and 2 of the approval process to participate as a centralized biller, the contractor must return the claims to the provider to submit to the local carrier/AB MAC for payment.

C. Notification of Provider Participation to the Processing Contractor
Before September 1 of every year, CMS will provide the designated contractor with the names of the entities that are authorized to participate in centralized billing for the 12 month period beginning September 1 and ending August 31 of the next year.

D. Enrollment
Though centralized billers may already have a Medicare provider number, for purposes of centralized billing, they must also obtain a provider number from the processing contractor for centralized billing through completion of the Form CMS-855 (Provider Enrollment Application). Providers/suppliers are encouraged to apply to enroll as a centralized biller early as possible. Applicants who have not completed the entire enrollment process and received approval from CMS and the designated contractor to participate as a Medicare mass immunizer centralized biller will not be allowed to submit claims to Medicare for reimbursement.

Whether an entity enrolls as a provider type "Mass Immunization Roster Biller" or some other type of provider, all normal enrollment processes and procedures must be followed. Authorization from CMS to participate in centralized billing is dependent upon the entity's ability to qualify as some type of Medicare provider. In addition, as under normal enrollment procedures, the contractor must verify that the entity is fully qualified and certified per State requirements in each State in which they plan to operate.

The contractor will activate the provider number for the 12-month period from September 1 through August 31 of the following year. If the provider is authorized to participate in the centralized billing program the next year, the contractor will extend the activation of the provider number for another year. The entity need not re-enroll with the contractor every year. However, should there be changes in the States in which the entity plans to operate, the contractor will need to verify that the entity meets all State certification and licensure requirements in those new States.

E. Electronic Submission of Claims on Roster Bills
Centralized billers must agree to submit their claims on roster bills in an Electronic Media Claims standard format using the appropriate version of American National Standards Institute (ANSI) format. Contractors should refer to the appropriate ANSI Implementation Guide to determine the correct location for this information on electronic claims. The processing contractor must provide instructions on acceptable roster billing formats to the approved centralized billers. Paper claims will not be accepted.

F. Required Information on Roster Bills for Centralized Billing
In addition to the roster billing instructions found in Sec.10.3.1 of this chapter, centralized billers must complete on the electronic format the area that corresponds to Item 32 and 33 on Form CMS 1500 (08-05). The contractor must use the ZIP Code in Item 32 to determine the payment locality for the claim. Item 33 must be completed to report the provider of service/supplier's billing name, address, ZIP Code, and telephone number. In addition, the NPI of the billing provider or group must be appropriately reported.

For electronic claims, the name, address, and ZIP Code of the facility are reported in:

- The HIPAA compliant ANSI X12N 837: Claim level loop 2310D NM101=FA. When implemented, the facility (e.g., hospitals) NPI will be captured in the loop 2310D NM109 (NM108=XX) if one is available. Prior to NPI, enter the tax information in loop 2310D NM109 (NM108=24 or 34) and enter the Medicare legacy facility identifier in loop 2310D REF02 (REF01=1C). Report the address, city, state, and ZIP Code in loop 2310D N301 and N401, N402, and N403. Facility data is not required to be reported at the line level for centralized billing.

G. Payment Rates and Mandatory Assignment
The payment rates for the administration of the vaccinations are based on the Medicare Physician Fee Schedule (MPFS) for the appropriate year. Payment made through the MPFS is based on geographic locality. Therefore, payments vary based on the geographic locality where the service was performed.

The HCPCS codes G0008 and G0009 for the administration of the vaccines are not paid on the MPFS. However, prior to March 1, 2003, they must be paid at the same rate as HCPCS code 90782, which is on the MPFS. The designated contractor must pay per the correct MPFS file for each calendar year based on the date of service of the claim. Beginning March 1, 2003, HCPCS codes G0008, G0009, and G0010 are to be reimbursed at the same rate as HCPCS code 90471.

In order to pay claims correctly for centralized billers, the designated contractor must have the correct name and address, including ZIP Code, of the entity where the service was provided.

The following remittance advice and Medicare Summary Notice (MSN) messages apply:

- Claim adjustment reason code 16, "Claim/service lacks information which is needed for adjudication. At least one Remark Code must be provided (may be comprised of either the Remittance Advice Remark Code or NCPDP Reject Reason Code.)" and Remittance advice remark code MA114, "Missing/incomplete/invalid information on where the services were furnished." and MSN 9.4 - "This item or service was denied because information required to make payment was incorrect." The payment rates for the vaccines must be determined by the standard method used by Medicare for reimbursement of drugs and biologicals. (See chapter 17 for procedures for determining the payment rates for vaccines.) Effective for claims with dates of service on or after February 1, 2001, Sec.114, of the Benefits Improvement and Protection Act of 2000 mandated that all drugs and biologicals be paid based on mandatory assignment. Therefore, all providers of influenza virus and pneumococcal vaccines must accept assignment for the vaccine. In addition, as a requirement for both centralized billing and roster billing, providers must agree to accept assignment for the administration of the vaccines as well. This means that they must agree to accept the amount that Medicare pays for the vaccine and the administration. Also, since there is no coinsurance or deductible for the influenza virus and pneumococcal benefit, accepting assignment means that Medicare beneficiaries cannot be charged for the vaccination.

H. Common Working File Information
To identify these claims and to enable central office data collection on the project, special processing number 39 has been assigned. The number should be entered on the HUBC claim record to CWF in the field titled Demonstration Number.

I. Provider Education Instructions for the Processing Contractor
The processing contractor must fully educate the centralized billers on the processes for centralized billing as well as for roster billing. General information on influenza virus and pneumococcal coverage and billing instructions is available on the CMS Web site for providers.

J. Provider Education Instructions for All Carriers/AB MACs
By April 1 of every year, all carriers/AB MACs must publish in their bulletins and put on their Web sites the following notification to providers. Questions from interested providers should be forwarded to the central office address below. Carriers/AB MACs must enter the name of the assigned processing contractor where noted before sending.

NOTIFICATION TO PROVIDERS
Centralized billing is a process in which a provider, who provides mass immunization services for influenza virus and pneumococcal pneumonia virus (PPV) immunizations, can send all claims to a single contractor for payment regardless of the geographic locality in which the vaccination was administered. (This does not include claims for the Railroad Retirement Board, United Mine Workers or Indian Health Services. These claims must continue to go to the appropriate processing entity.) This process is only available for claims for the influenza virus and pneumococcal vaccines and their administration. The administration of the vaccinations is reimbursed at the assigned rate based on the Medicare physician fee schedule for the appropriate locality. The vaccines are reimbursed at the assigned rate using the Medicare standard method for reimbursement of drugs and biologicals.

Individuals and entities interested in centralized billing must contact CMS central office, in writing, at the following address by June 1 of the year they wish to begin centrally billing.

Center for Medicare & Medicaid Services Division of Practitioner Claims Processing Provider Billing and Education Group 7500 Security Boulevard Mail Stop C4-10-07 Baltimore, Maryland 21244 By agreeing to participate in the centralized billing program, providers agree to abide by the following criteria.

CRITERIA FOR CENTRALIZED BILLING

To qualify for centralized billing, an individual or entity providing mass immunization services for influenza virus and pneumococcal vaccinations must provide these services in at least three payment localities for which there are at least three different contractors processing claims.

Individuals and entities providing the vaccine and administration must be properly licensed in the State in which the immunizations are given.

Centralized billers must agree to accept assignment (i.e., they must agree to accept the amount that Medicare pays for the vaccine and the administration).

NOTE: The practice of requiring a beneficiary to pay for the vaccination upfront and to file their own claim for reimbursement is inappropriate. All Medicare providers are required to file claims on behalf of the beneficiary per Sec.1848(g)(4)(A) of the Social Security Act and centralized billers may not collect any payment.

The contractor assigned to process the claims for centralized billing is chosen at the discretion of CMS based on such considerations as workload, user-friendly software developed by the contractor for billing claims, and overall performance. The assigned contractor for this year is [Fill in name of contractor.]

The payment rates for the administration of the vaccinations are based on the Medicare physician fee schedule (MPFS) for the appropriate year. Payment made through the MPFS is based on geographic locality. Therefore, payments received may vary based on the geographic locality where the service was performed. Payment is made at the assigned rate.

The payment rates for the vaccines are determined by the standard method used by Medicare for reimbursement of drugs and biologicals. Payment is made at the assigned rate.

Centralized billers must submit their claims on roster bills in an approved Electronic Media Claims standard format. Paper claims will not be accepted.

Centralized billers must obtain certain information for each beneficiary including name, health insurance number, date of birth, sex, and signature. [Fill in name of contractor] must be contacted prior to the season for exact requirements. The responsibility lies with the centralized biller to submit correct beneficiary Medicare information (including the beneficiary's Medicare Health Insurance Claim Number) as the contractor will not be able to process incomplete or incorrect claims.

Centralized billers must obtain an address for each beneficiary so that a Medicare Summary Notice (MSN) can be sent to the beneficiary by the contractor. Beneficiaries are sometimes confused when they receive an MSN from a contractor other than the contractor that normally processes their claims which results in unnecessary beneficiary inquiries to the Medicare contractor. Therefore, centralized billers must provide every beneficiary receiving an influenza virus or pneumococcal vaccination with the name of the processing contractor. This notification must be in writing, in the form of a brochure or handout, and must be provided to each beneficiary at the time he or she receives the vaccination.

Centralized billers must retain roster bills with beneficiary signatures at their permanent location for a time period consistent with Medicare regulations. [Fill in name of contractor] can provide this information.

Though centralized billers may already have a Medicare provider number, for purposes of centralized billing, they must also obtain a provider number from [Fill in name of contractor]. This can be done by completing the Form CMS-855 (Provider Enrollment Application), which can be obtained from [Fill in name of contractor].

If an individual or entity's request for centralized billing is approved, the approval is limited to the 12 month period from September 1 through August 31 of the following year. It is the responsibility of the centralized biller to reapply to CMS CO for approval each year by June 1. Claims will not be processed for any centralized biller without permission from CMS.

Each year the centralized biller must contact [Fill in name of contractor] to verify understanding of the coverage policy for the administration of the pneumococcal vaccine, and for a copy of the warning language that is required on the roster bill.

The centralized biller is responsible for providing the beneficiary with a record of the pneumococcal vaccination.

The information in items 1 through 8 below must be included with the individual or entity's annual request to participate in centralized billing:

1. Estimates for the number of beneficiaries who will receive influenza virus vaccinations;
2. Estimates for the number of beneficiaries who will receive pneumococcal vaccinations;
3. The approximate dates for when the vaccinations will be given;
4. A list of the States in which influenza virus and pneumococcal clinics will be held;
5. The type of services generally provided by the corporation (e.g., ambulance, home health, or visiting nurse);

6. Whether the nurses who will administer the influenza virus and pneumococcal vaccinations are employees of the corporation or will be hired by the corporation specifically for the purpose of administering influenza virus and pneumococcal vaccinations;
7. Names and addresses of all entities operating under the corporation's application;
8. Contact information for designated contact person for centralized billing program.

100-4,18,10.4.1

CWF Edits on FI/AB MAC Claims

In order to prevent duplicate payment by the same FI/AB MAC, CWF edits by line item on the FI/AB MAC number, the beneficiary Health Insurance Claim (HIC) number, and the date of service, the influenza virus procedure codes Q2034, 90654,90655, 90656, 90657, 90658, 90660, or 90662 and the pneumococcal procedure codes 90669, 90670, or 90732, and the administration codes G0008 or G0009.

If CWF receives a claim with either HCPCS codes Q2034, 90654, 90655, 90656, 90657, 90658, 90660, or 90662 and it already has on record a claim with the same HIC number, same FI/AB MAC number, same date of service, and any one of those HCPCS codes, the second claim submitted to CWF rejects.

If CWF receives a claim with HCPCS codes 90669, 90670, or 90732 and it already has on record a claim with the same HIC number, same FI/AB MAC number, same date of service, and the same HCPCS code, the second claim submitted to CWF rejects when all four items match.

If CWF receives a claim with HCPCS administration codes G0008 or G0009 and it already has on record a claim with the same HIC number, same FI/AB MAC number, same date of service, and same procedure code, CWF rejects the second claim submitted when all four items match.

CWF returns to the FI/AB MAC a reject code "7262" for this edit. FIs/AB MACs must deny the second claim and use the same messages they currently use for the denial of duplicate claims.

100-4,18,10.4.2

CWF Edits on Carrier/AB MAC Claims

In order to prevent duplicate payment by the same carrier/AB MAC, CWF will edit by line item on the carrier/AB MAC number, the HIC number, the date of service, the influenza virus procedure codes Q2034, 90654, 90655, 90656, 90657, 90658, 90660, or 90662; the pneumococcal procedure codes 90669, 90670, or 90732; and the administration code G0008 or G0009.

If CWF receives a claim with either HCPCS codes Q2034, 90654, 90655, 90656, 90657, 90658, 90660, or 90662 and it already has on record a claim with the same HIC number, same carrier/AB MAC number, same date of service, and any one of those HCPCS codes, the second claim submitted to CWF will reject.

If CWF receives a claim with HCPCS codes 90669, 90670, or 90732 and it already has on record a claim with the same HIC number, same carrier/AB MAC number, same date of service, and the same HCPCS code, the second claim submitted to CWF will reject when all four items match.

If CWF receives a claim with HCPCS administration codes G0008 or G0009 and it already has on record a claim with the same HIC number, same carrier/AB MAC number, same date of service, and same procedure code, CWF will reject the second claim submitted.

CWF will return to the carrier/AB MAC a specific reject code for this edit. Carriers/AB MACs must deny the second claim and use the same messages they currently use for the denial of duplicate claims.

In order to prevent duplicate payment by the centralized billing contractor and local carrier/AB MAC, CWF will edit by line item for carrier number, same HIC number, same date of service, the influenza virus procedure codes Q2034, 90654, 90655, 90656, 90657, 90658, 90660, or 90662; the pneumococcal procedure codes 90669, 90670, or 90732; and the administration code G0008 or G0009.

If CWF receives a claim with either HCPCS codes Q2034, 90654, 90655, 90656, 90657, 90658, 90660, or 90662 and it already has on record a claim with a different carrier/AB MAC number, but same HIC number, same date of service, and any one of those same HCPCS codes, the second claim submitted to CWF will reject.

If CWF receives a claim with HCPCS codes 90669, 90670, or 90732 and it already has on record a claim with the same HIC number, different carrier/AB MAC number, same date of service, and the same HCPCS code, the second claim submitted to CWF will reject.

If CWF receives a claim with HCPCS administration codes G0008 or G0009 and it already has on record a claim with a different carrier/AB MAC number, but the same HIC number, same date of service, and same procedure code, CWF will reject the second claim submitted.

CWF will return a specific reject code for this edit. Carriers/AB MACs must deny the second claim. For the second edit, the reject code should automatically trigger the following Medicare Summary Notice (MSN) and Remittance Advice (RA) messages.

MSN: 7.2 —"This is a duplicate of a claim processed by another contractor. You should receive a Medicare Summary Notice from them."

Claim adjustment reason code 18 —duplicate claim or service

100-4, 18, 10.4.3

CWF A/B Crossover Edits for FI/AB MAC and Carrier/AB MAC Claims

When CWF receives a claim from the carrier/AB MAC, it will review Part B outpatient claims history to verify that a duplicate claim has not already been posted.

CWF will edit on the beneficiary HIC number; the date of service; the influenza virus procedure codes Q2043, 90654, 90655, 90656, 90657, 90658, 90660, or 90662; the pneumococcal procedure codes 90669, 90670, or 90732; and the administration code G0008 or G0009.

CWF will return a specific reject code for this edit. Contractors must deny the second claim and use the same messages they currently use for the denial of duplicate claims.

100-4, 18, 20

Mammography Services (Screening and Diagnostic)

A. Screening Mammography Beginning January 1, 1991, Medicare provides Part B coverage of screening mammographies for women. Screening mammographies are radiologic procedures for early detection of breast cancer and include a physician's interpretation of the results. A doctor's prescription or referral is not necessary for the procedure to be covered.~Whether payment can be made is determined by a woman's age and statutory frequency parameter. See Pub. 100-02, Medicare Benefit Policy Manual, chapter 15, section 280.3 for additional coverage information for a screening mammography.

Section 4101 of the Balanced Budget Act (BBA) of 1997 provides for annual screening mammographies for women over age 39 and waives the Part B deductible. Coverage applies as follows: Age Groups Screening Period Under age 35 No payment allowed for screening mammography.~35-39 Baseline (pay for only one screening mammography performed on a woman between her 35th and 40th birthday) Over age 39 Annual (11 full months have elapsed following the month of last screening NOTE:Count months between screening mammographies beginning the month after the date of the examination. For example, if Mrs. Smith received a screening mammography examination in January 2005, begin counting the next month (February 2005) until 11 months have elapsed. Payment can be made for another screening mammography in January 2006.~B. Diagnostic Mammography A diagnostic mammography is a radiological mammogram and is a covered diagnostic test under the following conditions: A patient has distinct signs and symptoms for which a mammogram is indicated; A patient has a history of breast cancer; or A patient is asymptomatic, but based on the patient's history and other factors the physician considers significant, the physician's judgment is that a mammogram is appropriate.~Beginning January 1, 2005, Medicare Prescription Drug, Improvement, and Modernization Act (MMA) of 2003, Sec. 644, Public Law 108-173 has changed the way Medicare pays for diagnostic mammography. Medicare will pay based on the MPFS in lieu of OPPS or the lower of the actual change.

100-4, 18, 20.4

Billing Requirements - FI/A/B MAC Claims

Contractors use the weekly-updated MQSA file to verify that the billing facility is certified by the FDA to perform mammography services, and has the appropriate certification to perform the type of mammogram billed (film and/or digital). (See Sec.20.1.) FIs/A/B MACs use the provider number submitted on the claim to identify the facility and use the MQSA data file to verify the facility's certification(s). FIs/A/B MACs complete the following activities in processing mammography claims:

If the provider number on the claim does not correspond with a certified mammography facility on the MQSA file, then intermediaries/A/B MACs deny the claim.

When a film mammography HCPCS code is on a claim, the claim is checked for a "1" film indicator.

If a film mammography HCPCS code comes in on a claim and the facility is certified for film mammography, the claim is paid if all other relevant Medicare criteria are met.

If a film mammography HCPCS code is on a claim and the facility is certified for digital mammography only, the claim is denied.

When a digital mammography HCPCS code is on a claim, the claim is checked for "2" digital indicator.

If a digital mammography HCPCS code is on a claim and the facility is certified for digital mammography, the claim is paid if all other relevant Medicare criteria are met.

If a digital mammography HCPCS code is on a claim and the facility is certified for film mammography only, the claim is denied.

NOTE: The Common Working File (CWF) no longer receives the mammography file for editing purposes.

Except as provided in the following sections for RHCs and FQHCs, the following procedures apply to billing for screening mammographies: The technical component portion of the screening mammography is billed on Form CMS-1450 under bill type 12X, 13X, 14X** , 22X, 23X or 85X using revenue code 0403 and HCPCS code 77057* (76092*).

The technical component portion of the diagnostic mammography is billed on Form CMS-1450 under bill type 12X, 13X, 14X** , 22X, 23X or 85X using revenue code 0401 and HCPCS code 77055* (76090*), 77056* (76091*), G0204 and G0206.

Separate bills are required for claims for screening mammographies with dates of service prior to January 1, 2002. Providers include on the bill only charges for the screening mammography. Separate bills are not required for claims for screening mammographies with dates of service on or after January 1, 2002.

See separate instructions below for rural health clinics (RHCs) and federally qualified health centers (FQHCs).

* For claims with dates of service prior to January 1, 2007, providers report CPT codes 76090, 76091, and 76092. For claims with dates of service January 1, 2007 and later, providers report CPT codes 77055, 77056, and 77057 respectively.

** For claims with dates of service April 1, 2005 and later, hospitals bill for all mammography services under the 13X type of bill or for dates of service April 1, 2007 and later, 12X or 13X as appropriate. The 14X type of bill is no longer applicable. Appropriate bill types for providers other than hospitals are 22X, 23X, and 85X.

In cases where screening mammography services are self-referred and as a result an attending physician NPI is not available, the provider shall duplicate their facility NPI in the attending physician identifier field on the claim.

100-4, 18, 60.1

Payment

Payment (contractor) is under the MPFS except as follows:

- Fecal occult blood tests (82270* (G0107*) and G0328) are paid under the clinical diagnostic lab fee schedule except reasonable cost is paid to all non-OPPS hospitals, including CAHs, but not IHS hospitals billing on TOB 83x. IHS hospitals billing on TOB 83x are paid the ASC payment amount. Other IHS hospitals (billing on TOB 13x) are paid the OMB approved AIR, or the facility specific per visit amount as applicable. Deductible and coinsurance do not apply for these tests. See section A below for payment to Maryland waiver on TOB 13X. Payment from all hospitals for non-patient laboratory specimens on TOB 14X will be based on the clinical diagnostic fee schedule, including CAHs and Maryland waiver hospitals

Flexible sigmoidoscopy (code G0104) is paid under OPPS for hospital outpatient departments and on a reasonable cost basis for CAHs; or current payment methodologies for hospitals not subject to OPPS.

Colonoscopies (G0105 and G0121) and barium enemas (G0106 and G0120) are paid under OPPS for hospital outpatient departments and on a reasonable costs basis for CAHs or current payment methodologies for hospitals not subject to OPPS. Also colonoscopies may be done in an Ambulatory Surgical Center (ASC) and when done in an ASC the ASC rate applies. The ASC rate is the same for diagnostic and screening colonoscopies. The ASC rate is paid to IHS hospitals when the service is billed on TOB 83x.

Prior to January 1, 2007, deductible and coinsurance apply to HCPCS codes G0104, G0105, G0106, G0120, and G0121. Beginning with services provided on or after January 1, 2007, Section 5113 of the Deficit Reduction Act of 2005 waives the requirement of the annual Part B deductible for these screening services. Coinsurance still applies. Coinsurance and deductible applies to the diagnostic colorectal service codes listed below.

The following screening codes must be paid at rates consistent with the diagnostic codes indicated.

Screening Code	Diagnostic Code
G0104	45330
G0105 and G0121	45378
G0106 and G0120	74280

A. Special Payment Instructions for TOB 13X Maryland Waiver Hospitals

For hospitals in Maryland under the jurisdiction of the Health Services Cost Review Commission, screening colorectal services HCPCS codes G0104, G0105, G0106, 82270* (G0107*), G0120, G0121 and G0328 are paid according to the terms of the waiver, that is 94% of submitted charges minus any unmet existing deductible, co-insurance and non-covered charges. Maryland Hospitals bill TOB 13X for outpatient colorectal cancer screenings.

B. Special Payment Instructions for Non-Patient Laboratory Specimen (TOB 14X) for all hospitals

Payment for colorectal cancer screenings (82270* (G0107*) and G0328) to a hospital for a non-patient laboratory specimen (TOB 14X), is the lesser of the actual charge, the fee schedule amount, or the National Limitation Amount (NLA), (including CAHs and Maryland Waiver hospitals). Part B deductible and coinsurance do not apply.

*NOTE: For claims with dates of service prior to January 1, 2007, physicians, suppliers, and providers report HCPCS code G0107. Effective January 1, 2007, code G0107 is discontinued and replaced with CPT code 82270.

100-4, 18, 60.2

HCPCS Codes, Frequency Requirements, and Age Requirements (If Applicable)

Effective for services furnished on or after January 1, 1998, the following codes are used for colorectal cancer screening services:

- 82270* (G0107*) - Colorectal cancer screening; fecal-occult blood tests, 1-3 simultaneous determinations;
- G0104 - Colorectal cancer screening; flexible sigmoidoscopy;
- G0105 - Colorectal cancer screening; colonoscopy on individual at high risk;
- G0106 - Colorectal cancer screening; barium enema; as an alternative to G0104, screening sigmoidoscopy;
- G0120 - Colorectal cancer screening; barium enema; as an alternative to G0105, screening colonoscopy.

Effective for services furnished on or after July 1, 2001, the following codes are used for colorectal cancer screening services:

- G0121 - Colorectal cancer screening; colonoscopy on individual not meeting criteria for high risk. Note that the description for this code has been revised to remove the term "noncovered."
- G0122 - Colorectal cancer screening; barium enema (noncovered).

Effective for services furnished on or after January 1, 2004, the following code is used for colorectal cancer screening services as an alternative to 82270* (G0107*):

- G0328 - Colorectal cancer screening; immunoassay, fecal-occult blood test, 1-3 simultaneous determinations

*NOTE: For claims with dates of service prior to January 1, 2007, physicians, suppliers, and providers report HCPCS code G0107. Effective January 1, 2007, code G0107 is discontinued and replaced with CPT code 82270.

- G0104 - Colorectal Cancer Screening; Flexible Sigmoidoscopy

Screening flexible sigmoidoscopies (code G0104) may be paid for beneficiaries who have attained age 50, when performed by a doctor of medicine or osteopathy at the frequencies noted below.

For claims with dates of service on or after January 1, 2002, contractors pay for screening flexible sigmoidoscopies (code G0104) for beneficiaries who have attained age 50 when these services were performed by a doctor of medicine or osteopathy, or by a physician assistant, nurse practitioner, or clinical nurse specialist (as defined in Sec.1861(aa)(5) of the Act and in the Code of Federal Regulations at42 CFR 410.74, 410.75, and410.76) at the frequencies noted above. For claims with dates of service prior to January 1, 2002, contractors pay for these services under the conditions noted only when a doctor of medicine or osteopathy performs them.

For services furnished from January 1, 1998, through June 30, 2001, inclusive:

- Once every 48 months (i.e., at least 47 months have passed following the month in which the last covered screening flexible sigmoidoscopy was done).
- For services furnished on or after July 1, 2001:
- Once every 48 months as calculated above unless the beneficiary does not meet the criteria for high risk of developing colorectal cancer (refer to Sec.60.3 of this chapter) and he/she has had a screening colonoscopy (code G0121) within the preceding 10 years. If such a beneficiary has had a screening colonoscopy within the preceding 10 years, then he or she can have covered a screening flexible sigmoidoscopy only after at least 119 months have passed following the month that he/she received the screening colonoscopy (code G0121).

NOTE:If during the course of a screening flexible sigmoidoscopy a lesion or growth is detected which results in a biopsy or removal of the growth; the appropriate diagnostic procedure classified as a flexible sigmoidoscopy with biopsy or removal should be billed and paid rather than code G0104.

G0105 - Colorectal Cancer Screening; Colonoscopy on Individual at High Risk

Screening colonoscopies (code G0105) may be paid when performed by a doctor of medicine or osteopathy at a frequency of once every 24 months for beneficiaries at high risk for developing colorectal cancer (i.e., at least 23 months have passed following the month in which the last covered G0105 screening colonoscopy was performed). Refer to Sec.60.3of this chapter for the criteria to use in determining whether or not an individual is at high risk for developing colorectal cancer.

NOTE:If during the course of the screening colonoscopy, a lesion or growth is detected which results in a biopsy or removal of the growth, the appropriate diagnostic procedure classified as a colonoscopy with biopsy or removal should be billed and paid rather than code G0105.

A. Colonoscopy Cannot be Completed Because of Extenuating Circumstances

1   FIs

When a covered colonoscopy is attempted but cannot be completed because of extenuating circumstances, Medicare will pay for the interrupted colonoscopy as long as the coverage conditions are met for the incomplete procedure. However, the frequency standards associated with screening colonoscopies will not be applied by CWF. When a covered colonoscopy is next attempted and completed, Medicare will pay for that colonoscopy according to its payment methodology for this procedure as long as coverage conditions are met, and the frequency standards will be applied by CWF. This policy is applied to both screening and diagnostic colonoscopies.

When submitting a facility claim for the interrupted colonoscopy, providers are to suffix the colonoscopy HCPCS codes with a modifier of "-73" or "-74" as appropriate to indicate that the procedure was interrupted. Payment for covered incomplete screening colonoscopies shall be consistent with payment methodologies currently in place for complete screening colonoscopies, including those contained in42 CFR 419.44(b). In situations where a critical access hospital (CAH) has elected payment Method II for CAH patients, payment shall be consistent with payment methodologies currently in place as outlined in Chapter 3. As such, instruct CAHs that elect Method II payment to use modifier "-53" to identify an incomplete screening colonoscopy (physician professional service(s) billed in revenue code 096X, 097X, and/or 098X). Such CAHs will also bill the technical or facility component of the interrupted colonoscopy in revenue code 075X (or other appropriate revenue code) using the "-73" or "-74" modifier as appropriate.Note that Medicare would expect the provider to maintain adequate information in the patient's medical record in case it is needed by the contractor to document the incomplete procedure.

2.   Carriers

When a covered colonoscopy is attempted but cannot be completed because of extenuating circumstances (see Chapter 12), Medicare will pay for the interrupted colonoscopy at a rate consistent with that of a flexible sigmoidoscopy as long as coverage conditions are met for the incomplete procedure. When a covered colonoscopy is next attempted and completed, Medicare will pay for that colonoscopy according to its payment methodology for this procedure as long as coverage conditions are met. This policy is applied to both screening and diagnostic colonoscopies.

When submitting a claim for the interrupted colonoscopy, professional providers are to suffix the colonoscopy code with a modifier of "-53" to indicate that the procedure was interrupted. When submitting a claim for the facility fee associated with this procedure, Ambulatory Surgical Centers (ASCs) are to suffix the colonoscopy code with "-73" or "-74" as appropriate. Payment for covered screening colonoscopies, including that for the associated ASC facility fee when applicable, shall be consistent with payment for diagnostic colonoscopies, whether the procedure is complete or incomplete.Note that Medicare would expect the provider to maintain adequate information in the patient's medical record in case it is needed by the contractor to document the incomplete procedure.

- G0106 - Colorectal Cancer Screening; Barium Enema; as an Alternative to G0104, Screening Sigmoidoscopy

Screening barium enema examinations may be paid as an alternative to a screening sigmoidoscopy (code G0104). The same frequency parameters for screening sigmoidoscopies (see those codes above) apply. In the case of an individual aged 50 or over, payment may be made for a screening barium enema examination (code G0106) performed after at least 47 months have passed following the month in which the last screening barium enema or screening flexible sigmoidoscopy was performed. For example, the beneficiary received a screening barium enema examination as an alternative to a screening flexible sigmoidoscopy in January 1999. Start counts beginning February 1999. The beneficiary is eligible for another screening barium enema in January 2003. The screening barium enema must be ordered in writing after a determination that the test is the appropriate screening test. Generally, it is expected that this will be a screening double contrast enema unless the individual is unable to withstand such an exam. This means that in the case of a particular individual, the attending physician must determine that the estimated screening potential for the barium enema is equal to or greater than the screening potential that has been estimated for a screening flexible sigmoidoscopy for the same individual. The screening single contrast barium enema also requires a written order from the beneficiary's attending physician in the same manner as described above for the screening double contrast barium enema examination.

- 82270* (G0107*) - Colorectal Cancer Screening; Fecal-Occult Blood Test, 1-3 Simultaneous Determinations

Effective for services furnished on or after January 1, 1998, screening FOBT (code 82270* (G0107*) may be paid for beneficiaries who have attained age 50, and at a frequency of once every 12 months (i.e., at least 11 months have passed following the month in which the last covered screening FOBT was performed). This screening FOBT means a guaiac-based test for peroxidase activity, in which the beneficiary completes it by taking samples from two different sites of three consecutive stools. This screening requires a written order from the beneficiary's attending physician. (The term "attending physician" is defined to mean a doctor of medicine or osteopathy (as defined in Sec.1861(r)(1)of the Act) who is fully knowledgeable about the beneficiary's medical condition, and who would be responsible for using the results of any examination performed in the overall management of the beneficiary's specific medical problem.)

Effective for services furnished on or after January 1, 2004, payment may be made for a immunoassay-based FOBT (G0328, described below) as an alternative to the guaiac-based FOBT, 82270* (G0107*). Medicare will pay for only one covered FOBT per year, either 82270* (G0107*) or G0328, but not both.

*NOTE: For claims with dates of service prior to January 1, 2007, physicians, suppliers, and providers report HCPCS code G0107. Effective January 1, 2007, code G0107 is discontinued and replaced with CPT code 82270.

- G0328 - Colorectal Cancer Screening; Immunoassay, Fecal-Occult Blood Test, 1-3 Simultaneous Determinations

Effective for services furnished on or after January 1, 2004, screening FOBT, (code G0328) may be paid as an alternative to 82270* (G0107*) for beneficiaries who have attained age 50. Medicare will pay for a covered FOBT (either 82270* (G0107*) or G0328, but not both) at a frequency of once every 12 months (i.e., at least 11 months have passed following the month in which the last covered screening FOBT was performed). Screening FOBT, immunoassay, includes the use of a spatula to collect the appropriate number of samples or the use of a special brush for the collection of samples, as determined by the individual manufacturer's instructions. This screening requires a written order from the beneficiary's attending physician. (The term "attending physician" is defined to mean a doctor of medicine or osteopathy (as defined in Sec.1861(r)(1) of the Act) who is fully knowledgeable about the beneficiary's medical condition, and who would be responsible for using the results of any examination performed in the overall management of the beneficiary's specific medical problem.)

- G0120 - Colorectal Cancer Screening; Barium Enema; as an Alternative to or G0105, Screening Colonoscopy

Screening barium enema examinations may be paid as an alternative to a screening colonoscopy (code G0105) examination. The same frequency parameters for screening colonoscopies (see those codes above) apply. In the case of an individual who is at high risk for colorectal cancer, payment may be made for a screening barium enema examination (code G0120) performed after at least 23 months have passed following the month in which the last screening barium enema or the last screening colonoscopy was performed. For example, a beneficiary at high risk for developing colorectal cancer received a screening barium enema examination (code G0120) as an alternative to a screening colonoscopy (code G0105) in January 2000. Start counts beginning February 2000. The beneficiary is eligible for another screening barium enema examination (code G0120) in January 2002. The screening barium enema must be ordered in writing after a determination that the test is the appropriate screening test. Generally, it is expected that this will be a screening double contrast enema unless the individual is unable to withstand such an exam. This means that in the case of a particular individual, the attending physician must determine that the estimated screening potential for the barium enema is equal to or greater than the screening potential that has been estimated for a screening colonoscopy, for the same individual. The screening single contrast barium enema also requires a written order from the beneficiary's attending physician in the same manner as described above for the screening double contrast barium enema examination.

- G0121 - Colorectal Screening; Colonoscopy on Individual Not Meeting Criteria for High Risk - Applicable On and After July 1, 2001

Effective for services furnished on or after July 1, 2001, screening colonoscopies (code G0121) performed on individuals not meeting the criteria for being at high risk for developing colorectal cancer (refer to Sec.60.3 of this chapter) may be paid under the following conditions:

- At a frequency of once every 10 years (i.e., at least 119 months have passed following the month in which the last covered G0121 screening colonoscopy was performed.)

If the individual would otherwise qualify to have covered a G0121 screening colonoscopy based on the above but has had a covered screening flexible sigmoidoscopy (code G0104), then he or she may have covered a G0121 screening colonoscopy only after at least 47 months have passed following the month in which the last covered G0104 flexible sigmoidoscopy was performed.

NOTE:If during the course of the screening colonoscopy, a lesion or growth is detected which results in a biopsy or removal of the growth, the appropriate diagnostic procedure classified as a colonoscopy with biopsy or removal should be billed and paid rather than code G0121.

- G0122 - Colorectal Cancer Screening; Barium Enema

The code is not covered by Medicare.

100-4, 18, 60.6

Billing Requirements for Claims Submitted to FIs

(Follow the general bill review instructions in Chapter 25. Hospitals use the ANSI X12N 837I to bill the FI or on the hardcopy Form CMS-1450. Hospitals bill revenue codes and HCPCS codes as follows:

Screening Test/Procedure	Revenue Code	HCPCS Code	TOB
Fecal Occult blood test	030X	82270*** (G0107***), G0328	12X, 13X, 14X**, 22X, 23X, 83X, 85X
Barium enema	032X	G0106, G0120, G0122	12X, 13X, 22X, 23X, 85X****
Flexible Sigmoidoscopy	*	G0104	12X, 13X, 22X, 23X, 83X, 85X****
Colonoscopy-high risk	*	G0105, G0121	12X, 13X, 22X, 23X, 83X, 85X****

* The appropriate revenue code when reporting any other surgical procedure.
** 14X is only applicable for non-patient laboratory specimens.
*** For claims with dates of service prior to January 1, 2007, physicians, suppliers, and providers report HCPCS code G0107. Effective January 1, 2007, code G0107, is discontinued and replaced with CPT code 82270.
**** CAHs that elect Method II bill revenue code 096X, 097X, and/or 098X for professional services and 075X (or other appropriate revenue code) for the technical or facility component.

Special Billing Instructions for Hospital Inpatients

When these tests/procedures are provided to inpatients of a hospital or when Part A benefits have been exhausted, they are covered under this benefit. However, the provider bills on bill type 12X using the discharge date of the hospital stay to avoid editing in the Common Working File (CWF) as a result of the hospital bundling rules.

100-4, 18, 80

Initial Preventive Physical Examination (IPPE)

(NOTE: For billing and payment requirements for the Annual Wellness Visit, see chapter 18, section 140, of this manual.)

Background: Effective for services furnished on or after January 1, 2005, Section 611 of the Medicare Prescription Drug Improvement and Modernization Act of 2003 (MMA) provides for coverage under Part B of one initial preventive physical examination (IPPE) for new beneficiaries only, subject to certain eligibility and other limitations. CMS amended §§411.15 (a)(1) and 411.15 (k)(11) of the Code of Federal Regulations (CFR) to permit payment for an IPPE as described at 42 CFR §410.16, added by 69 FR 66236, 66420 (November 15, 2004) not later than 6 months after the date the individual's first coverage period begins under Medicare Part B.

Under the MMA of 2003, the IPPE may be performed by a doctor of medicine or osteopathy as defined in section 1861 (r)(1) of the Social Security Act (the Act) or by a qualified mid-level nonphysician practitioner (NPP) (nurse practitioner, physician assistant or clinical nurse specialist), not later than 6 months after the date the individual's first coverage begins under Medicare Part B. (See section 80.3 for a list of bill types of facilities that can bill fiscal intermediaries (FIs) for this service.) This examination will include: (1) review of the individual's medical and social history with attention to modifiable risk factors for disease detection, (2) review of the individual's potential (risk factors) for depression or other mood disorders, (3) review of the individual's functional ability and level of safety; (4) a physical examination to include measurement of the individual's height, weight, blood pressure, a visual acuity screen, and other factors as deemed appropriate by the examining physician or qualified nonphysician practitioner (NPP), (5) performance and interpretation of an electrocardiogram (EKG); (6) education, counseling, and referral, as deemed appropriate, based on the results of the review and evaluation services described in the previous 5 elements, and (7) education, counseling, and referral including a brief written plan (e.g., a checklist or alternative) provided to the individual for obtaining the appropriate screening and other preventive services, which are separately covered under Medicare Part B benefits. The EKG performed as a component of the IPPE will be billed separately. Medicare will pay for only one IPPE per beneficiary per lifetime. The Common Working File (CWF) will edit for this benefit.

As required by statute under the MMA of 2003, the total IPPE service includes an EKG, but the EKG is billed with its own unique HCPCS code(s). The IPPE does not include other preventive services that are currently separately covered and paid under Section 1861 of the Act under Medicare Part B screening benefits. (That is, pneumococcal, influenza and hepatitis B vaccines and their administration, screening mammography, screening pap smear and screening pelvic examinations, prostate cancer screening tests, colorectal cancer screening tests, diabetes outpatient self-management training services, bone mass measurements, glaucoma screening, medical nutrition therapy for individuals with diabetes or renal disease, cardiovascular screening blood tests, and diabetes screening tests.)

Section 5112 of the Deficit Reduction Act of 2005 allows for one ultrasound screening for Abdominal Aortic Aneurysm (AAA) as a result of a referral from an IPPE effective January 1, 2007. For AAA physician/practitioner billing, correct coding, and payment policy information, refer to section 110 of this chapter.

Effective January 1, 2009, Section 101(b) of the Medicare Improvement for Patients and Providers Act (MIPPA) of 2008 updates the IPPE benefit described under the MMA of 2003. The MIPPA allows the IPPE to be performed not later than 12 months after the date the individual's first coverage period begins under Medicare Part B, requires the addition of the measurement of an individual's body mass index to the IPPE, adds end-of-life planning (upon an individual's consent) to the IPPE, and removes the screening EKG as a mandatory service of the IPPE. The screening EKG is optional effective January 1, 2009, and is permitted as a once-in-a-lifetime screening service as a result of a referral from an IPPE.

The MIPPA of 2008 allows for possible future payment for additional preventive services not otherwise described in Title XVIII of the Act that identify medical conditions or risk factors for eligible individuals if the Secretary determines through the national coverage determination (NCD) process (as defined in section 1869(f)(1)(B) of the Act) that they are: (1) reasonable and necessary for the prevention or early detection of illness or disability, (2) recommended with a grade of A or B by the United States Preventive Services Task Force, and, (3) appropriate for individuals entitled to benefits under Part A or enrolled under Part B, or both. MIPPA requires that there be education, counseling, and referral for additional preventive services, as appropriate, under the IPPE, if the Secretary determines in the future that such services are covered.

For the physician/practitioner billing correct coding and payment policy, refer to chapter 12, section 30.6.1.1, of this manual.

100-4, 18, 80.1

The HCPCS codes listed below were developed for the IPPE benefit effective January 1, 2005, for individuals whose initial enrollment is on or after January 1, 2005.

G0344: Initial preventive physical examination; face-to-face visit, services limited to new beneficiary during the first 6 months of Medicare enrollment

> Short Descriptor: Initial Preventive Exam

G0366: Electrocardiogram, routine ECG with 12 leads; performed as a component of the initial preventive examination with interpretation and report

> Short Descriptor: EKG for initial prevent exam

G0367: tracing only, without interpretation and report, performed as a component of the initial preventive examination

> Short Descriptor: EKG tracing for initial prev

> G0368: interpretation and report only, performed as a component of the initial preventive examination

Short Descriptor: EKG interpret & report preve

The following new HCPCS codes were developed for the IPPE benefit effective January 1, 2009, and replaced codes G0344, G0366, G0367, and G0368 shown above beginning with dates of service on or after January 1, 2009:

G0402: Initial preventive physical examination; face-to-face visit, services limited to new beneficiary during the first 12 months of Medicare enrollment

> Short Descriptor: Initial Preventive exam

G0403: Electrocardiogram, routine ECG with 12 leads; performed as a screening for the initial preventive physical examination with interpretation and report

> Short Descriptor: EKG for initial prevent exam

G0404: Electrocardiogram, routine ECG with 12 leads; tracing only, without interpretation and report, performed as a screening for the initial preventive physical examination

> Short Descriptor: EKG tracing for initial prev

G0405: Electrocardiogram, routine ECG with 12 leads; interpretation and report only, performed as a screening for the initial preventive physical examination

> Short Descriptor: EKG interpret & report preve

100-4, 18, 80.2

A/B Medicare Administrative Contractor (MAC) and Contractor Billing Requirements

Effective for dates of service on and after January 1, 2005, through December 31, 2008, contractors shall recognize the HCPCS codes G0344, G0366, G0367, and G0368 shown above in §80.1 for an IPPE. The type of service (TOS) for each of these codes is as follows:

> G0344: TOS = 1
>
> G0366: TOS = 5
>
> G0367: TOS = 5
>
> G0368: TOS = 5

Contractors shall pay physicians or qualified nonphysician practitioners for only one IPPE performed not later than 6 months after the date the individual's first coverage begins under Medicare Part B, but only if that coverage period begins on or after January 1, 2005.

Effective for dates of service on and after January 1, 2009, contractors shall recognize the HCPCS codes G0402, G0403, G0404, and G0405 shown above in §80.1 for an IPPE. The TOS for each of these codes is as follows:

> G0402: TOS = 1
>
> G0403: TOS = 5
>
> G0404: TOS = 5
>
> G0405: TOS = 5

Under the MIPPA of 2008, contractors shall pay physicians or qualified nonphysician practitioners for only one IPPE performed not later than 12 months after the date the individual's first coverage begins under Medicare Part B only if that coverage period begins on or after January 1, 2009.

Contractors shall allow payment for a medically necessary Evaluation and Management (E/M) service at the same visit as the IPPE when it is clinically appropriate. Physicians and qualified nonphysician practitioners shall use CPT codes 99201-99215 to report an E/M with CPT modifier 25 to indicate that the E/M is a significant, separately identifiable service from the IPPE code reported (G0344 or G0402, whichever applies based on the date the IPPE is performed). Refer to chapter 12, § 30.6.1.1, of this manual for the physician/practitioner billing correct coding and payment policy regarding E/M services.

If the EKG performed as a component of the IPPE is not performed by the primary physician or qualified NPP during the IPPE visit, another physician or entity may perform and/or interpret the EKG. The referring physician or qualified NPP needs to make sure that the performing physician or entity bills the appropriate G code for the screening EKG, and not a CPT code in the 93000 series. Both the IPPE and the EKG should be billed in order for the beneficiary to receive the complete IPPE service. Effective for dates of service on and after January 1, 2009, the screening EKG is optional and is no longer a mandated service of an IPPE if performed as a result of a referral from an IPPE.

Should the same physician or NPP need to perform an additional medically necessary EKG in the 93000 series on the same day as the IPPE, report the appropriate EKG CPT code(s) with modifier 59, indicating that the EKG is a distinct procedural service.

Physicians or qualified nonphysician practitioners shall bill the contractor the appropriate HCPCS codes for IPPE on the Form CMS-1500 claim or an approved electronic format. The HCPCS codes for an IPPE and screening EKG are paid under the Medicare Physician Fee Schedule (MPFS). The appropriate deductible and coinsurance applies to codes G0344, G0366, G0367, G0368, G0403, G0404, and G0405. The deductible is waived for code G0402 but the coinsurance still applies.

100-4, 18, 80.3.3

Outpatient Prospective Payment System (OPPS) Hospital Billing

Hospitals subject to OPPS (TOBs 12X and 13X) must use modifier -25 when billing the IPPE G0344 along with the technical component of the EKG, G0367, on the same claim. The same is true when billing IPPE code G0402 along with the technical component of the screening EKG, code G0404. This is due to an OPPS Outpatient Code Editor (OCE) which contains an edit that requires a modifier -25 on any evaluation and management (E/M) HCPCS code if there is also a status "S" or "T" HCPCS procedure code on the claim.

100-4, 18, 80.4

Coinsurance and Deductible

The Medicare deductible and coinsurance apply for the IPPE provided before January 1, 2009.

The Medicare deductible is waived effective for the IPPE provided on or after January 1, 2009. Coinsurance continues to apply for the IPPE provided on or after January 1, 2009.

As a result of the Affordable Care Act, effective for the IPPE provided on or after January 1, 2011, the Medicare deductible and coinsurance (for HCPCS code G0402 only) are waived.

100-4, 18, 120.1

Coding and Payment of DSMT Services

The following HCPCS codes are used to report DSMT: G0108 - Diabetes outpatient self-management training services, individual, per 30 minutes.

G0109 - Diabetes outpatient self-management training services, group session (2 or more), per 30 minutes.

The type of service for these codes is 1.

Type of Facility	Payment Method	Type of Bill
Physician (billed to the carrier)	MPFS	NA
Hospitals subject to OPPS	MPFS	12X, 13X
Method I and Method II Critical Access Hospitals (CAHs) (technical services)	101% of reasonable cost	12X and 85X
Indian Health Service (IHS) providers billing hospital outpatient Part B	OMB-approved outpatient per visit all inclusive rate (AIR)	13X
IHS providers billing inpatient Part B	All-inclusive inpatient ancillary per diem rate	12X
IHS CAHs billing outpatient Part B	101% of the all-inclusive facility specific per visit rate	85X
IHS CAHs billing inpatient Part B	101% of the all-inclusive facility specific per diem rate	12X
FQHCs*	All-inclusive encounter rate with other qualified services. Separate visit payment available with HCPCS.	73X
Skilled Nursing Facilities **	MPFS non-facility rate	22X, 23X
Maryland Hospitals under jurisdiction of the Health Services Cost Review Commission (HSCRC)	94% of provider submitted charges in accordance with the terms of the Maryland Waiver	12X, 13X
Home Health Agencies (can be billed only if the service is provided outside of the treatment plan)	MPFS non-facility rate	34X

 * Effective January 1, 2006, payment for DSMT provided in an FQHC that meets all of the requirements as above, may be made in addition to one other visit the beneficiary had during the same day, if this qualifying visit is billed to TOB 73X, with HCPCS G0108 or G0109, and revenue codes 0520, 0521, 0522, 0524, 0525, 0527, 0528, or 0900.

** The SNF consolidated billing provision allows separate part B payment for training services for beneficiaries that are in skilled Part A SNF stays, however, the SNF must submit these services on a 22 bill type. Training services provided by other provider types must be reimbursed by X the SNF.

NOTE: An ESRD facility is a reasonable site for this service, however, because it is required to provide dietician and nutritional services as part of the care covered in the composite rate, ESRD facilities are not allowed to bill for it separately and do not receive separate reimbursement. Likewise, an RHC is a reasonable site for this service, however it must be provided in an RHC with other qualifying services and paid at the all-inclusive encounter rate.

Deductible and co-insurance apply.

100-4, 18, 130

Healthcare Common Procedure Coding System (HCPCS) for HIV Screening Tests

Healthcare Common Procedure Coding System (HCPCS) for HIV Screening Tests

Effective for claims with dates of service on and after December 8, 2009, implemented with the April 5, 2010, IOCE, the following HCPCS codes are to be billed for HIV screening:

G0432   Infectious agent antibody detection by enzyme immunoassay (EIA) technique, HIV-1 and/or HIV-2, screening,

G0433   Infectious agent antibody detection by enzyme-linked immunosorbent assay (ELISA) technique, HIV-1 and/or HIV-2, screening, and,

G0435   Infectious agent antibody detection by rapid antibody test, HIV-1 and/or HIV-2, screening

100-4, 18, 130.1

Billing Requirements

Effective for dates of service December 8, 2009, and later, contractors shall recognize the above HCPCS codes for HIV screening.

Medicare contractors shall pay for voluntary HIV screening as follows in accordance with Pub. 100-03, Medicare National Coverage Determinations Manual, sections 190.14 and 210.7:

A maximum of once annually for beneficiaries at increased risk for HIV infection (11 full months must elapse following the month the previous test was performed in order for the subsequent test to be covered), and,

A maximum of three times per term of pregnancy for pregnant Medicare beneficiaries beginning with the date of the first test when ordered by the woman's clinician. Claims that are submitted for HIV screening shall be submitted in the following manner:

For beneficiaries reporting increased risk factors, claims shall contain HCPCS code G0432, G0433, or G0435 with diagnosis code V73.89 (Special screening for other specified viral disease) as primary, and V69.8 (Other problems related to lifestyle), as secondary.

For beneficiaries not reporting increased risk factors, claims shall contain HCPCS code G0432, G0433, or G0435 with diagnosis code V73.89 only.

For pregnant Medicare beneficiaries, claims shall contain HCPCS code G0432, G0433, or G0435 with diagnosis code V73.89 as primary, and one of the following ICD-9 diagnosis codes: V22.0 (Supervision of normal first pregnancy), V22.1 (Supervision of other normal pregnancy), or V23.9 (Supervision of unspecified high-risk pregnancy), as secondary.

100-4, 18, 130.4

Diagnosis Code Reporting

A claim that is submitted for HIV screening shall be submitted with one or more of the following diagnosis codes in the header and pointed to the line item:

a. For claims where increased risk factors are reported: V73.89 as primary and V69.8 as secondary.

b. For claims where increased risk factors are NOT reported: V73.89 as primary only.

c. For claims for pregnant Medicare beneficiaries, the following diagnosis codes shall be submitted in addition to V73.89 to allow for more frequent screening than once per 12-month period:

   V22.0 – Supervision of normal first pregnancy, or,

   V22.1 – Supervision of other normal pregnancy, or,

   V23.9 - Supervision of unspecified high-risk pregnancy).

100-4, 18, 140

Annual Wellness Visit (AWV)

Pursuant to section 4103 of the Affordable Care Act of 2010, the Centers for Medicare & Medicaid Services (CMS) amended section 411.15(a)(1) and 411.15(k)(15) of 42 CFR (list of examples of routine physical examinations excluded from coverage) effective for services furnished on or after January 1, 2011. This expanded coverage is subject to certain eligibility and other limitations that allow payment for an annual wellness visit (AWV), including personalized prevention plan services (PPPS), for an individual who is no longer within 12 months after the effective date of his or her first Medicare Part B coverage period, and has not received either an initial preventive physical examination (IPPE) or an AWV within the past 12 months.

The AWV will include the establishment of, or update to, the individual's medical/family history, measurement of his/her height, weight, body-mass index (BMI) or waist circumference, and blood pressure (BP), with the goal of health promotion and disease detection and encouraging patients to obtain the screening and preventive services that may already be covered and paid for under Medicare Part B. CMS amended 42 CFR §§411.15(a)(1) and 411.15(k)(15) to allow payment on or after January 1, 2011, for an AWV (as established at 42 CFR 410.15) when performed by qualified health professionals.

Coverage is available for an AWV that meets the following requirements:

1. It is performed by a health professional;

2. It is furnished to an eligible beneficiary who is no longer within 12 months after the effective date of his/her first Medicare Part B coverage period, and he/she has not received either an IPPE or an AWV providing PPPS within the past 12 months.

See Pub. 100-02, Medicare Benefit Policy Manual, chapter 15, section 280.5, for detailed policy regarding the AWV, including definitions of: (1) detection of cognitive impairment, (2) eligible beneficiary, (3) establishment of, or an update to, an individual's medical/family history, (4&5) first and subsequent AWVs providing PPPS, (6) health professional, and, (7) review of an individual's functional ability/level of safety.

100-4, 18, 140.1

Healthcare Common Procedure Coding System (HCPCS) Coding for the AWV

HCPCS codes listed below were developed for the AWV benefit effective January 1, 2011, for individuals whose initial enrollment is on or after January 1, 2011.

G0438 - Annual wellness visit; includes a personalized prevention plan of service (PPPS); first visit

G0439 – Annual wellness visit; includes a personalized prevention plan of service (PPPS); subsequent visit

100-4, 18, 140.5

Coinsurance and Deductible

Sections 4103 and 4104 of the Affordable Care Act provide for a waiver of Medicare coinsurance/copayment and Part B deductible requirements for the AWV effective for services furnished on or after January 1, 2011.

100-4,18,140.6

Common Working File (CWF) Edits

Effective for claims with dates of service on and after January 1, 2011, CWF shall reject:

- AWV claims for G0438 when a previous (first) AWV, HCPCS code G0438, is paid in history regardless of when it occurred.
- AWV claims when a previous AWV, G0438 or G0439, is paid in history within the previous 12 months.
- Beginning January 1, 2011, AWV claims when a previous IPPE, HCPCS code G0402, is paid in history within the previous 12 months.
- AWV claims (G0438 and G0439) billed for a date of service within 12 months after the effective date of a beneficiary's first Medicare Part B coverage period.

The following change shall be effective for claims processed on or after April 1, 2013. Typically, when a preventive service is posted to a beneficiary's utilization history, separate entries are posted for a "professional" service (the professional claim for the delivery of the service itself) and a "technical" service (the institutional claims for a facility fee). However, in the case of AWV services, since there is no separate payment for a facility fee, the AWV claim will be posted as the "professional" service only, regardless of whether it is paid on a professional claim or an institutional claim.

100-4, 18, 150

Counseling to Prevent Tobacco Use

Effective for claims with dates of service on and after August 25, 2010, the Centers for Medicare & Medicaid Services (CMS) will cover counseling to prevent tobacco use services for outpatient and hospitalized Medicare beneficiaries:

1. Who use tobacco, regardless of whether they have signs or symptoms of tobacco-related disease;
2. Who are competent and alert at the time that counseling is provided; and,
3. Whose counseling is furnished by a qualified physician or other Medicare-recognized practitioner. These individuals who do not have signs or symptoms of tobacco-related disease will be covered under Medicare Part B when the above conditions of coverage are met, subject to certain frequency and other limitations.

Conditions of Medicare Part A and Medicare Part B coverage for counseling to prevent tobacco use are located in the Medicare National Coverage Determinations (NCD) Manual, Publication 100-3, chapter 1, section 210.4.1.

100-4,18,150.1

Healthcare Common Procedure Coding System (HCPCS) and Diagnosis Coding

The CMS has created two new G codes for billing for tobacco cessation counseling services to prevent tobacco use for those individuals who use tobacco but do not have signs or symptoms of tobacco-related disease. These are in addition to the two CPT codes 99406 and 99407 that currently are used for smoking and tobacco-use cessation counseling for symptomatic individuals.

The following HCPCS codes should be reported when billing for counseling to prevent tobacco use effective January 1, 2011:

- G0436 - Smoking and tobacco cessation counseling visit for the asymptomatic patient; intermediate, greater than 3 minutes, up to 10 minutes

    Short descriptor: Tobacco-use counsel 3-10 min

- G0437 - Smoking and tobacco cessation counseling visit for the asymptomatic patient; intensive, greater than 10 minutes

    Short descriptor: Tobacco-use counsel >10min

NOTE: The above G codes will not be active in contractors' systems until January 1, 2011. Therefore, contractors shall advise non-outpatient perspective payment system (OPPS) providers to use unlisted code 99199 to bill for counseling to prevent tobacco use and tobacco-related disease services during the interim period of August 25, 2010, through December 31, 2010.

On January 3, 2011, contractor's systems will accept the new G codes for services performed on or after August 25, 2010.

Two new C codes have been created for facilities paid under OPPS when billing for counseling to prevent tobacco use and tobacco-related disease services during the interim period of August 25, 2010, through December 31, 2010:

- C9801 - Smoking and tobacco cessation counseling visit for the asymptomatic patient, intermediate, greater than 3 minutes, up to 10 minutes

    Short descriptor: Tobacco-use counsel 3-10 min

- C9802 - Smoking and tobacco cessation counseling visit for the asymptomatic patient, intensive, greater than 10 minutes

    Short descriptor: Tobacco-use counsel >10min

Claims for smoking and tobacco use cessation counseling services G0436 and G0437 shall be submitted with diagnosis code V15.82, history of tobacco use, or 305.1, non-dependent tobacco use disorder.

Contractors shall allow payment for a medically necessary E/M service on the same day as the smoking and tobacco-use cessation counseling service when it is clinically appropriate. Physicians and qualified non-physician practitioners shall use an appropriate HCPCS code to report an E/M service with modifier -25 to indicate that the E/M service is a separately identifiable service from G0436 or G0437.

100-4,18,150.2

Carrier Billing Requirements

Carriers shall pay for counseling to prevent tobacco use services billed with code G0436 or G0437 for dates of service on or after January 1, 2011. Carriers shall pay for counseling services billed with code 99199 for dates of service performed on or after August 25, 2010 through December 31, 2010. The type of service (TOS) for each of the new codes is 1.

Carriers pay for counseling services billed based on the Medicare Physician Fee Schedule (MPFS). Deductible and coinsurance apply for services performed on August 25, 2010, through December 31, 2010. For claims with dates of service on and after January 1, 2011, coinsurance and deductible do not apply on G0436 and G0437.

Physicians or qualified non-physician practitioners shall bill the carrier for counseling to prevent tobacco use services on Form CMS-1500 or an approved electronic format.

NOTE: The above G codes will not be active in contractors' systems until January 1, 2011. Therefore, contractors shall advise providers to use unlisted code 99199 to bill for counseling to prevent tobacco use services during the interim period of August 25, 2010, through December 31, 2010.

100-4,18,150.2.1

Fiscal Intermediary (FI) Billing Requirements

The FIs shall pay for counseling to prevent tobacco use services with codes G0436 and G0437 for dates of service on or after January 1, 2011. FIs shall pay for counseling services billed with code 99199 for dates of service performed on or after August 25, 2010, through December 31, 2010. For facilities paid under OPPS, FIs shall pay for counseling services billed with codes C9801 and C9802 for dates of service performed on or after August 25, 2010, through December 31, 2010.

Claims for counseling to prevent tobacco use services should be submitted on Form CMS-1450 or its electronic equivalent.

The applicable bill types are 12X, 13X, 22X, 23X, 34X, 71X, 77X, and 85X.

Payment for outpatient services is as follows:

- Type of Facility
- Method of Payment
- Rural Health Centers (RHCs) TOB 71X/Federally Qualified Health Centers (FQHCs)TOB 77X
- All-inclusive rate (AIR) for the encounter
- Hospitals TOBs 12X and 13X
- OPPS for hospitals subject to OPPS
- MPFS for hospitals not subject to OPPS
- Indian Health Services (IHS) Hospitals TOB 13X

- AIR for the encounter
- Skilled Nursing Facilities (SNFs) TOBs 22X and 23X
- Medicare Physician Fee Schedule (MPFS)
- Home Health Agencies (HHAs) TOB 34X
- MPFS
- Critical Access Hospitals (CAHs) TOB 85X
- Method I: Technical services are paid at 101% of reasonable cost. Method II: technical services are paid at 101% of reasonable cost, and Professional services are paid at 115% of the MPFS Data Base
- IHS CAHs TOB 85X
- Based on specific rate
- Maryland Hospitals

Payment is based according to the Health Services Cost Review Commission (HSCRC). That is 94% of submitted charges subject to any unmet deductible, coinsurance, and non-covered charges policies.

100-4, 18, 150.4

Common Working File (CWF)

The Common Working File (CWF) shall edit for the frequency of service limitations of counseling to prevent tobacco use sessions and smoking and tobacco-use cessation counseling services (G0436, G0437, 99406, 99407) rendered to a beneficiary for a combined total of 8 sessions within a 12-month period. The beneficiary may receive another 8 sessions during a second or subsequent year after 11 full months have passed since the first Medicare covered counseling session was performed. To start the count for the second or subsequent 12-month period, begin with the month after the month in which the first Medicare covered counseling session was performed and count until 11 full months have elapsed.

By entering the beneficiary's health insurance claim number (HICN), providers have the capability to view the number of sessions a beneficiary has received for this service via inquiry through CWF.

100-4,18,160

Intensive Behavioral Therapy (IBT) for Cardiovascular Disease (CVD)

For services furnished on or after November 8, 2011, the Centers for Medicare & Medicaid Services (CMS) covers intensive behavioral therapy (IBT) for cardiovascular disease (CVD). See National Coverage Determinations (NCD) Manual (Pub. 100-03) §210.11 for complete coverage guidelines.

100-4,18,160.1

Coding Requirements for IBT for CVD Furnished on or After November 8, 2011

The following is the applicable Healthcare Procedural Coding System (HCPCS) code for IBT for CVD:

G0446: Annual, face-to-face intensive behavioral therapy for cardiovascular disease, individual, 15 minutes

Contractors shall not apply deductibles or coinsurance to claim lines containing HCPCS code G0446.

100-4,18,160.2.1

Correct Place of Service (POS) Codes for IBT for CVD on Professional Claims

Contractors shall pay for IBT CVD, G0446 only when services are provided at the following POS:

- 11- Physician's Office
- 22-Outpatient Hospital
- 49- Independent Clinic
- 72-Rural Health Clinic

Claims not submitted with one of the POS codes above will be denied.

The following messages shall be used when Medicare contractors deny professional claims for incorrect POS:

Claim Adjustment Reason Code (CARC) 58: "Treatment was deemed by the payer to have been rendered in an inappropriate or invalid place of service." NOTE: Refer to the 835 Healthcare Policy Identification Segment (loop 2110 Service Payment Information REF), if present.

Remittance Advice Remark Code (RARC) N428: "Not covered when performed in this place of service."

Medicare Summary Notice (MSN) 21.25: "This service was denied because Medicare only covers this service in certain settings."

Spanish Version: El servicio fue denegado porque Medicare solamente lo cubre en ciertas situaciones."

Group Code PR (Patient Responsibility) assigning financial liability to the beneficiary, if a claim is received with a GA modifier indicating a signed ABN is on file.

Group Code CO (Contractual Obligation) assigning financial liability to the provider, if a claim is received with a GZ modifier indicating no signed ABN is on file.

100-4,18,160.2.2

Provider Specialty Edits for IBT for CVD on Professional Claims

Contractors shall pay claims for HCPCS code G0446 only when services are submitted by the following provider specialty types found on the provider? enrollment record:

- 01= General Practice
- 08 = Family Practice
- 11= Internal Medicine
- 16 = Obstetrics/Gynecology
- 37= Pediatric Medicine
- 38 = Geriatric Medicine
- 42= Certified Nurse Midwife
- 50 = Nurse Practitioner
- 89 = Certified Clinical Nurse Specialist
- 97= Physician Assistant

Contractors shall deny claim lines for HCPCS code G0446 performed by any other provider specialty type other than those listed above.

The following messages shall be used when Medicare contractors deny IBT for CVD claims billed with invalid provider specialty types:

CARC 185: "The rendering provider is not eligible to perform the service billed." NOTE: Refer to the 835 Healthcare Policy Identification Segment (loop 2110 Service Payment Information REF), if present.

RARC N95: "This provider type/provider specialty may not bill this service."

MSN 21.18: "This item or service is not covered when performed or ordered by this provider."

Spanish version: "Este servicio no esta cubierto cuando es ordenado o rendido por este proveedor."

Group Code PR (Patient Responsibility) assigning financial liability to the beneficiary, if a claim is received with a GA modifier indicating a signed ABN is on file.

Group Code CO (Contractual Obligation) assigning financial liability to the provider, if a claim is received with a GZ modifier indicating no signed ABN is on file.

100-4,18,160.3

Correct Types of Bill (TOB) for IBT for CVD on Institutional Claims

Effective for claims with dates of service on and after November 8, 2011, the following types of bill (TOB) may be used for IBT for CVD: 13X, 71X, 77X, or 85X. All other TOB codes shall be denied.

The following messages shall be used when Medicare contractors deny claims for G0446 when submitted on a TOB other than those listed above:

CARC 170: Payment is denied when performed/billed by this type of provider. Note: Refer to the 835 Healthcare Policy Identification Segment (loop 2110 Service Payment Information REF), if present.

RARC N428: Not covered when performed in this place of service."

MSN 21.25: "This service was denied because Medicare only covers this service in certain settings."

Spanish Version: El servicio fue denegado porque Medicare solamente lo cubre en ciertas situaciones."

Group Code PR (Patient Responsibility) assigning financial liability to the beneficiary, if a claim is received with a GA modifier indicating a signed ABN is on file.

Group Code CO (Contractual Obligation) assigning financial liability to the provider, if a claim is received with a GZ modifier indicating no signed ABN is on file.

100-4, 18, 160.4

Frequency Edits for IBT for CVD Claims

160.4-Frequency Edits for IBT for CVD Claims

(Rev. 2357, Issued: 11-23-11, Effective: 11-08-11, Implementation: 12-27-11 non-shared system edits, 04-02-12 shared system edits, 07-02-12 CWF/HICR/MCS MCDST)

Contractors shall allow claims for G0446 no more than once in a 12-month period.

NOTE: 11 full months must elapse following the month in which the last G0446 IBT for CVD took place.

Contractors shall deny claims IBT for CVD claims that exceed one (1) visit every 12 months.

Contractors shall allow one professional service and one facility fee claim for each visit.

The following messages shall be used when Medicare contractors deny IBT for CVD claims that exceed the frequency limit:

CARC 119: "Benefit maximum for this time period or occurrence has been reached."

RARC N362: "The number of days or units of service exceeds our acceptable maximum."

MSN 20.5: "These services cannot be paid because your benefits are exhausted at this time."

Spanish Version: "Estos servicios no pueden ser pagados porque sus beneficios se han agotado."

Group Code PR (Patient Responsibility) assigning financial liability to the beneficiary, if a claim is received with a GA modifier indicating a signed ABN is on file.

Group Code CO (Contractual Obligation) assigning financial liability to the provider, if a claim is received with a GZ modifier indicating no signed ABN is on file.

100-4, 18, 160.5

When applying frequency, CWF shall count 11 full months following the month of the last IBT for CVD, G0446 before allowing subsequent payment of another G0446 screening.

When applying frequency limitations to G0446, CWF shall allow both a claim for the professional service and a claim for the facility fee. CWF shall identify the following institutional claims as facility fee claims for screening services: TOB 13X, TOB85X when the revenue code is not 096X, 097X, or 098X. CWF shall identify all other claims as professional service claims for screening services. NOTE: This does not apply to RHCs and FQHCs.

100-4, 18, 170.1

Healthcare Common Procedure Coding System (HCPCS) Codes for Screening for STIs and HIBC to Prevent STIs

Effective for claims with dates of service on and after November 8, 2011, the claims processing instructions for payment of screening tests for STI will apply to the following HCPCS codes:

- Chlamydia: 86631, 86632, 87110, 87270, 87320, 87490, 87491, 87810, 87800 (used for combined chlamydia and gonorrhea testing)

- Gonorrhea: 87590, 87591, 87850, 87800 (used for combined chlamydia and gonorrhea testing)

- Syphilis: 86592, 86593, 86780

- Hepatitis B: (hepatitis B surface antigen): 87340, 87341

Effective for claims with dates of service on and after November 8, 2011, implemented with the January 2, 2012, IOCE, the following HCPCS code is to be billed for HIBC to prevent STIs:

G0445   high-intensity behavioral counseling to prevent sexually transmitted infections, face-to-face, individual, includes: education, skills training, and guidance on how to change sexual behavior, performed semi-annually, 30 minutes.

100-4, 18, 170.2

Diagnosis Code Reporting

A claim that is submitted for screening chlamydia, gonorrhea, syphilis, and/or hepatitis B shall be submitted with one or more of the following diagnosis codes in the header and pointed to the line item:

a. For claims for screening for chlamydia, gonorrhea, and syphilis in women at increased risk who are not pregnant use the following diagnosis codes:

- V74.5-Screening, bacterial ?sexually transmitted; and

- V69.8 -Other problems related to lifestyle as secondary (This diagnosis code is used to indicate high/increased risk for STIs).

b. For claims for screening for syphilis in men at increased risk use the following diagnosis codes:

- V74.5-Screening, bacterial ?sexually transmitted; and

- V69.8 -Other problems related to lifestyle as secondary. c. For claims for screening for chlamydia and gonorrhea in pregnant women at increased risk for STIs use the following diagnosis codes:

- Screening, bacterial ?sexually transmitted; and

- V69.8 - Other problems related to lifestyle, and,

- V22.0 -Supervision of normal first pregnancy, or

- V22.1 -Supervision of other normal pregnancy, or,

- V23.9-Supervision of unspecified high-risk pregnancy. d. For claims for screening for syphilis in pregnant women use the following diagnosis codes:

- V74.5-Screening, bacterial ?sexually transmitted; and

- V22.0 -Supervision of normal first pregnancy, or,

- V22.1-Supervision of other normal pregnancy, or,

- V23.9-Supervision of ?V74.5unspecified high-risk pregnancy.

e. For claims for screening for syphilis in pregnant women at increased risk for STIs use the following diagnosis codes:

- V74.5-Screening, bacterial ?sexually transmitted; and

- V69.8 -Other problems related to lifestyle, and,

- V22.0-Supervision of normal first pregnancy, or

- V22.1 -Supervision of other normal pregnancy, or,

- V23.9 -Supervision of unspecified high-risk pregnancy. f. For claims for screening for hepatitis B in pregnant women use the following diagnosis codes:

- V73.89-Screening, disease or disorder, viral, specified type NEC; and

- V22.0-Supervision of normal first pregnancy, or,

- V22.1-Supervision of other normal pregnancy, or,

- V23.9-Supervision of unspecified high-risk pregnancy.

g. For claims for screening for hepatitis B in pregnant women at increased risk for STIs use the following diagnosis codes:

- V73.89-Screening, disease or disorder, viral, specified type NEC; and

- V 69.8 -Other problems related to lifestyle, and,

- V22.0-Supervision of normal first pregnancy, or,

- V22.1-Supervision of other normal pregnancy, or,

- V23.9-Supervision of unspecified high-risk pregnancy.

ICD-10 Diagnosis Coding:

Contractors shall note the appropriate ICD-10 code(s) that are listed below for future implementation. Contractors shall track the ICD-10 codes and ensure that the updated edit is turned on as part of the ICD-10 implementation effective October 1, 2013.

ICD-10	Description
Z113	Encounter for screening for infections with a predominantly sexual mode of transmission
Z1159	Encounter for screening for other viral diseases
Z7289	Other problems related to lifestyle
Z3400	Encounter for supervision of normal first pregnancy, unspecified trimester
Z3480	Encounter for supervision of other normal pregnancy, unspecified trimester
O0990	Supervision of high risk pregnancy, unspecified, unspecified trimester

100-4, 18, 170.3

Billing Requirements

Effective for dates of service November 8, 2011, and later, contractors shall recognize HCPCS code G0445 for HIBC. Medicare shall cover up to two occurrences of G0445 when billed for HIBC to prevent STIs. A claim that is submitted with HCPCS code G0445 for HIBC shall be submitted with ICD-9 diagnosis code V69.8.

Medicare contractors shall pay for screening for chlamydia, gonorrhea, and syphilis (As indicated by the presence of ICD-9 diagnosis code V74.5); and/or hepatitis B (as indicated by the presence of ICD-9 diagnosis code V73.89) as follows:

- One annual occurrence of screening for chlamydia, gonorrhea, and syphilis (i.e., 1 per 12-month period) in women at increased risk who are not pregnant,

- One annual occurrence of screening for syphilis (i.e., 1 per 12-month period) in men at increased risk,

- Up to two occurrences per pregnancy of screening for chlamydia and gonorrhea in pregnant women who are at increased risk for STIs and continued increased risk for the second screening,

- One occurrence per pregnancy of screening for syphilis in pregnant women,

- Up to an additional two occurrences per pregnancy of screening for syphilis in pregnant women if the beneficiary is at continued increased risk for STIs,

- One occurrence per pregnancy of screening for hepatitis B in pregnant women, and,

- One additional occurrence per pregnancy of screening for hepatitis B in pregnant women who are at continued increased risk for STIs.

100-4, 18, 170.4

Types of Bill (TOBs) and Revenue Codes

The applicable types of bill (TOBs) for HIBC screening, HCPCS code G0445, are: 13X, 71X, 77X, and 85X.

On institutional claims, TOBs 71X and 77X, use revenue code 052X to ensure coinsurance and deductible are not applied.

Critical access hospitals (CAHs) electing the optional method of payment for outpatient services report this service under revenue codes 096X, 097X, or 098X.

100-4, 18, 170.4.1

Payment Method

Payment for HIBC is based on the all-inclusive payment rate for rural health clinics (TOBs 71X) and federally qualified health centers (TOB 77X). Hospital outpatient departments (TOB 13X) are paid based on the outpatient prospective payment system and CAHs (TOB 85X) are paid based on reasonable cost. CAHs electing the optional method of payment for outpatient services are paid based on 115% of the lesser of the Medicare Physician Fee Schedule (MPFS) amount or submitted charge.

Effective for dates of service on and after November 8, 2011, deductible and coinsurance do not apply to claim lines with G0445.

HCPCS code G0445 may be paid on the same date of service as an annual wellness visit, evaluation and management (E&M) code, or during the global billing period for obstetrical care, but only one G0445 may be paid on any one date of service. If billed on the same date of service with an E&M code, the E&M code should have a distinct diagnosis code other than the diagnosis code used to indicate high/increased risk for STIs for the G0445 service. An E&M code should not be billed when the sole reason for the visit is HIBC to prevent STIs.

For Medicare Part B physician and non-practitioner claims, payment for HIBC to prevent STIs is based on the MPFS amount for G0445.

100-4, 18, 170.5

Specialty Codes and Place of Service (POS)

Medicare provides coverage for screening for chlamydia, gonorrhea, syphilis, and/or hepatitis B and HIBC to prevent STIs only when ordered by a primary care practitioner (physician or non-physician) with any of the following specialty codes:

- 01-General Practice
- 08-Family Practice
- 11-Internal Medicine
- 16-Obstetrics/Gynecology
- 37-Pediatric Medicine
- 38-Geriatric Medicine
- 42-Certified Nurse Midwife
- 50-Nurse Practitioner
- 89-Certified Clinical Nurse Specialist
- 97-Physician Assistant

Medicare provides coverage for HIBC to prevent STIs only when provided by a primary care practitioner (physician or non-physician) with any of the specialty codes identified above.

Medicare provides coverage for HIBC to prevent STIs only when the POS billed is 11, 22, 49, or 71.

100-4, 18, 180

Alcohol Screening and Behavioral Counseling Interventions in Primary Care to Reduce Alcohol Misuse

~The United States Preventive Services Task Force (USPSTF) defines alcohol misuse as risky, hazardous, or harmful drinking which places an individual at risk for future problems with alcohol consumption. In the general adult population, alcohol consumption becomes risky or hazardous when consuming:

- Greater than 7 drinks per week or greater than 3drinks per occasion for women and persons greater than 65 years old.

- Greater than 14 drinks per week or greater than 4 drinks per occasion for men 65 years old and younger.

100-4, 18, 180.1

Policy

Claims with dates of service on and after October 14, 2011, the Centers for Medicare & Medicaid Services (CMS) will cover annual alcohol misuse screening (HCPCS code G0442) consisting of 1 screening session, and for those that screen positive, up to 4 brief, face-to-face behavioral counseling sessions (HCPCS code G0443) per 12-month period for Medicare beneficiaries, including pregnant women.

Medicare beneficiaries that may be identified as having a need for behavioral counseling sessions include those:

- Who misuse alcohol, but whose levels or patterns of alcohol consumption do not meet criteria for alcohol dependence (defined as at least three of the following: tolerance, withdrawal symptoms, impaired control, preoccupation with acquisition and/or use, persistent desire or unsuccessful efforts to quit, sustains social, occupational, or recreational disability, use continues despite adverse consequences); and,

- Who are competent and alert at the time that counseling is provided; and,

- Whose counseling is furnished by qualified primary care physicians or other primary care practitioners in a primary care setting.

Once a Medicare beneficiary has agreed to behavioral counseling sessions, the counseling sessions are to be completed based on the 5As approach adopted by the United States Preventive Services Task Force (USPSTF.) The steps to the 5As approach are listed below.

1. Assess: Ask about/assess behavioral health risk(s) and factors affecting choice of behavior change goals/methods.

2. Advise: Give clear, specific, and personalized behavior change advice, including information about personal health harms and benefits.

3. Agree: Collaboratively select appropriate treatment goals and methods based on the patient? interest in and willingness to change the behavior.

4. Assist: Using behavior change techniques (self-help and/or counseling), aid the patient in achieving agreed-upon goals by acquiring the skills, confidence, and social/environmental supports for behavior change, supplemented with adjunctive medical treatments when appropriate.

5. Arrange: Schedule follow-up contacts (in person or by telephone) to provide ongoing assistance/support and to adjust the treatment plan as needed, including referral to more intensive or specialized treatment.

100-4, 18, 180.2

For claims with dates of service on and after October 14, 2011, Medicare will allow coverage for annual alcohol misuse screening, 15 minutes, G0442, and brief, face-to-face behavioral counseling for alcohol misuse, 15 minutes, G0443 for:

- Rural Health Clinics (RHCs) - type of bill (TOB) 71X only -based on the all-inclusive payment rate

- Federally Qualified Health Centers (FQHCs) - TOB 77X only-based on the all-inclusive payment rate

- Outpatient hospitals ?TOB 13X - based on Outpatient Prospective Payment System (OPPS)- Critical Access Hospitals (CAHs) - TOB 85X-based on reasonable cost

- CAH Method II-TOB 85X - based on 115% of the lesser of the Medicare Physician Fee Schedule (MPFS) amount or actual charge as applicable with revenue codes 096X, 097X, or 098X.

For RHCs and FQHCs the alcohol screening/counseling is not separately payable with another face-to-face encounter on the same day. This does not apply to the Initial Preventive Physical Examination (IPPE), unrelated services denoted with modifier 59, and 77X claims containing

Diabetes Self Management Training (DSMT) and Medical Nutrition Therapy (MNT)services. DSMT and MNT apply to FQHCs only. However, the screening/counseling sessions alone when rendered as a face-to-face visit with a core practitioner do constitute an encounter and is paid based on the all-inclusive payment rate.

Note: For outpatient hospital settings, as in any other setting, services covered under this NCD must be provided by a primary care provider.

Claims submitted with alcohol misuse screening and behavioral counseling HCPCS codes G0442 and G0443 on a TOB other than 13X, 71X, 77X, and 85X will be denied.

Effective October 14, 2011, deductible and co-insurance should not be applied for line items on claims billed for alcohol misuse screening G0442 and behavioral counseling for alcohol misuse G0443.

100-4, 18, 180.3
Professional Billing Requirements
For claims with dates of service on or after October 14, 2011, CMS will allow coverage for annual alcohol misuse screening, 15 minutes, G0442, and behavioral counseling for alcohol misuse, 15 minutes, G0443, only when services are submitted by the following provider specialties found on the provider's enrollment record:

- 01 - General Practice
- 08 - Family Practice
- 11 - Internal Medicine
- 16 - Obstetrics/Gynecology
- 37 - Pediatric Medicine
- 38 - Geriatric Medicine
- 42 - Certified Nurse-Midwife
- 50 - Nurse Practitioner
- 89 - Certified Clinical Nurse Specialist
- 97 - Physician Assistant

Any claims that are not submitted from one of the provider specialty types noted above will be denied.

For claims with dates of service on and after October 14, 2011, CMS will allow coverage for annual alcohol misuse screening, 15 minutes, G0442, and behavioral counseling for alcohol misuse, 15 minutes, G0443, only when submitted with one of the following place of service (POS) codes:

- 11 - Physician's Office
- 22 - Outpatient Hospital
- 49 - Independent Clinic
- 71 - State or local public health clinic or

Any claims that are not submitted with one of the POS codes noted above will be denied.

The alcohol screening/counseling services are payable with another encounter/visit on the same day. This does not apply to RHCs and FQHCs.

100-4, 18, 180.4
Claim Adjustment Reason Codes, Remittance Advice Remark Codes, Group Codes, and Medicare Summary Not
Contractors shall use the appropriate claim adjustment reason codes (CARCs), remittance advice remark codes (RARCs), group codes, or Medicare summary notice (MSN) messages when denying payment for alcohol misuse screening and alcohol misuse behavioral counseling sessions:

- For RHC and FQHC claims that contain screening for alcohol misuse HCPCS code G0442 and alcohol misuse counseling HCPCS code G0443 with another encounter/visit with the same line item date of service, use group code CO and reason code:
  - Claim Adjustment Reason Code (CARC) 97-The benefit for this service is included in the payment/allowance for another service/procedure that has already been adjudicated. Note: Refer to the 835 Healthcare Policy Identification Segment (loop 2110 Service Payment Information REF) if present
- Denying claims containing HCPCS code G0442 and HCPCS code G0443 submitted on a TOB other than 13X, 71X, 77X, and 85X:
  - Claim Adjustment Reason Code (CARC) 5 - The procedure code/bill type is inconsistent with the place of service. Note: Refer to the 835 Healthcare Policy Identification Segment (loop 2110 Service Payment Information REF) if present

- Remittance Advice Remark Code (RARC) M77 -Missing/incomplete/invalid place of service
- Group Code PR (Patient Responsibility) assigning financial liability to the beneficiary, if a claim is received with a GA modifier indicating a signed ABN is on file.
- Group Code CO (Contractual Obligation) assigning financial liability to the provider, if a claim is received with a GZ modifier indicating no signed ABN is on file. NOTE: For modifier GZ, use CARC 50 and MSN 8.81 per instructions in CR 7228/TR 2148.

- Denying claims that contains more than one alcohol misuse behavioral counseling session G0443 on the same date of service:
  - Medicare Summary Notice (MSN) 15.6-The information provided does not support the need for this many services or items within this period of time.
  - Claim Adjustment Reason Code (CARC) 151-Payment adjusted because the payer deems the information submitted does not support this many/frequency of services.
  - Remittance Advice Remark Code (RARC) M86-Service denied because payment already made for same/similar procedure within set time frame.
  - Group Code PR (Patient Responsibility) assigning financial liability to the beneficiary, if a claim is received with a GA modifier indicating a signed ABN is on file.
  - Group Code CO (Contractual Obligation) assigning financial liability to the provider, if a claim is received with a GZ modifier indicating no signed ABN is on file. NOTE: For modifier GZ, use CARC 50 and MSN 8.81 per instructions in CR 7228/TR 2148.

- Denying claims that are not submitted from the appropriate provider specialties:
  - Medicare Summary Notice (MSN) 21.18-This item or service is not covered when performed or ordered by this provider.
  - Claim Adjustment Reason Code (CARC) 185 - The rendering provider is not eligible to perform the service billed. NOTE: Refer to the 835 Healthcare Policy Identification Segment (loop 2110 Service Payment Information REF), if present.
  - Remittance Advice Remark Code (RARC) N95 - This provider type/provider specialty may not bill this service.
  - Group Code PR (Patient Responsibility) assigning financial liability to the beneficiary, if a claim is received with a GA modifier indicating a signed ABN is on file.
  - Group Code CO (Contractual Obligation) assigning financial liability to the provider, if a claim is received with a GZ modifier indicating no signed ABN is on file. NOTE: For modifier GZ, use CARC 50 and MSN 8.81 per instructions in CR 7228/TR 2148.

- Denying claims without the appropriate POS code:
  - Medicare Summary Notice (MSN) 21.25-This service was denied because Medicare only covers this service in certain settings.
  - Claim Adjustment Reason Code (CARC) 58 -Treatment was deemed by the payer to have been rendered in an inappropriate or invalid place of service. Note: Refer to the 835 Healthcare Policy Identification Segment (loop 2110 Service Payment Information REF) if present.
  - Remittance Advice Remark Code (RARC) N428-Not covered when performed in this place of service.
  - Group Code PR (Patient Responsibility) assigning financial liability to the beneficiary, if a claim is received with a GA modifier indicating a signed ABN is on file.
  - Group Code CO (Contractual Obligation) assigning financial liability to the provider, if a claim is received with a GZ modifier indicating no signed ABN is on file. NOTE: For modifier GZ, use CARC 50 and MSN 8.81 per instructions in CR 7228/TR 2148.

- Denying claims for alcohol misuse screening HCPCS code G0442 more than once in a 12-month period, and denying alcohol misuse counseling sessions HCPCS code G0443 more than four times in the same 12-month period:
  - Medicare Summary Notice (MSN) 20.5-These services cannot be paid because your benefits are exhausted at this time.
  - Claim Adjustment Reason Code (CARC) 119-Benefit maximum for this time period or occurrence has been reached.
  - Remittance Advice Remark Code (RARC) N362-The number of Days or Units of service exceeds our acceptable maximum.
  - Group Code PR (Patient Responsibility) assigning financial liability to the beneficiary, if a claim is received with a GA modifier indicating a signed ABN is on file.
  - Group Code CO (Contractual Obligation) assigning financial liability to the provider, if a claim is received with a GZ modifier indicating no signed ABN is on file. NOTE: For modifier GZ, use CARC 50 and MSN 8.81 per instructions in CR 7228/TR 2148.

100-4, 18, 180.5

CWF Requirements

When applying frequency, CWF shall count 11 full months following the month of the last alcohol misuse screening visit, G0442, before allowing subsequent payment of another G0442 screening. Additionally, CWF shall create an edit to allow alcohol misuse brief behavioral counseling, HCPCS G0443, no more than 4 times in a 12-month period. CWF shall also count four alcohol misuse counseling sessions HCPCS G0443 in the same 12-month period used for G0442 counting from the date the G0442 screening session was billed.

When applying frequency limitations to G0442 screening on the same date of service as G0443 counseling, CWF shall allow both a claim for the professional service and a claim for a facility fee. CWF shall identify the following institutional claims as facility fee claims for screening services: TOB 13X, TOB 85X when the revenue code is not 096X, 097X, or 098X. CWF shall identify all other claims as professional service claims for screening services (professional claims, and institutional claims with TOB 71X, 77X, and 85X when the revenue code is 096X, 097X, or 098X). NOTE: This does not apply to RHCs and FQHCs.

100-4, 18, 190.0

Screening for Depression in Adults (Effective October 14, 2011)

A. Coverage Requirements

Effective October 14, 2011, the Centers for Medicare & Medicaid Services (CMS) will cover annual screening up to 15 minutes for Medicare beneficiaries in primary care settings that have staff-assisted depression care supports in place to assure accurate diagnosis, effective treatment, and follow-up. Various screening tools are available for screening for depression. CMS does not identify specific depression screening tools. Rather, the decision to use a specific tool is at the discretion of the clinician in the primary care setting. Screening for depression is non-covered when performed more than one time in a 12-month period. The Medicare coinsurance and Part B deductible are waived for this preventive service.

Additional information on this National Coverage Determination (NCD) for Screening for Depression in Adults can be found in Publication 100-3, NCD Manual, Section 210.9.

100-4, 18, 190.1

A/B MAC and Carrier Billing Requirements

Effective October 14, 2011, contractors shall recognize new HCPCS G0444, annual depression screening, 15 minutes.

100-4, 18, 190.2

Frequency

Medicare contractors shall pay for annual depression screening, G0444, no more than once in a 12-month period.

NOTE: 11 full months must elapse following the month in which the last annual depression screening took place.

100-4, 18, 190.3

Place of Service (POS)

Contractors shall pay for annual depression screening claims, G0444, only when services are provided at the following places of service (POS):

- 11–Office
- 22–Outpatient Hospital
- 49–Independent Clinic
- 71–State or Local Public Health Clinic

100-4, 18, 200

Intensive Behavioral Therapy for Obesity (Effective November 29, 2011)

The United States Preventive Services Task Force (USPSTF) found good evidence that body mass index (BMI) is a reliable and valid indicator for identifying adults at increased risk for mortality and morbidity due to overweight and obesity. It also good evidence that high intensity counseling combined with behavioral interventions in obese adults (as defined by a BMI =30 kg/m2) produces modest, sustained weight loss.

100-4, 18, 200.1

Policy

For services furnished on or after November 29, 2011, the Centers for Medicare & Medicaid Services (CMS) will cover Intensive Behavioral Therapy for Obesity. Medicare beneficiaries with obesity (BMI =30 kg/m2) who are competent and alert at the time that counseling is provided and whose counseling is furnished by a qualified primary care physician or other primary care practitioner in a primary care setting are eligible for:

- One face-to-face visit every week for the first month;
- One face-to-face visit every other week for months 2-6;
- One face-to-face visit every month for months 7-12, if the beneficiary meets the 3kg (6.6 lbs) weight loss requirement during the first six months as discussed below. The counseling sessions are to be completed based on the 5As approach adopted by the United States Preventive Services Task Force (USPSTF.) The steps to the 5As approach are listed below:

1. Assess: Ask about/assess behavioral health risk(s) and factors affecting choice of behavior change goals/methods.

2. Advise: Give clear, specific, and personalized behavior change advice, including information about personal health harms and benefits.

3. Agree: Collaboratively select appropriate treatment goals and methods based on the patient's interest in and willingness to change the behavior.

4. Assist: Using behavior change techniques (self-help and/or counseling), aid the patient in achieving agreed-upon goals by acquiring the skills, confidence, and social/environmental supports for behavior change, supplemented with adjunctive medical treatments when appropriate.

5. Arrange: Schedule follow-up contacts (in person or by telephone) to provide ongoing assistance/support and to adjust the treatment plan as needed, including referral to more intensive or specialized treatment.

Medicare will cover Face-to-Face Behavioral Counseling for Obesity, 15 minutes, G0447, along with 1 of the ICD-9 codes for BMI 30.0-BMI 70 (V85.30-V85.39 and V85.41-V85.45), up to 22 sessions in a 12-month period for Medicare beneficiaries. The Medicare coinsurance and Part B deductible are waived for this preventive service.

Contractors shall note the appropriate ICD-10 code(s) that are listed below for future implementation. Contractors shall track the ICD-10 codes and ensure that the updated edit is turned on as part of the ICD-10 implementation effective October 1, 2013.

ICD-10	Description
Z68.30	BMI 30.0-30.9, adult
Z68.31	BMI 31.0-31.9, adult
Z68.32	BMI 32.0-32.9, adult
Z68.33	BMI 33.0-33.9, adult
Z68.34	BMI 34.0-34.9, adult
Z68.35	BMI 35.0-35.9, adult
Z68.36	BMI 36.0-36.9, adult
Z68.37	BMI 37.0-37.9, adult
Z68.38	BMI 38.0-38.9, adult
Z68.39	BMI 39.0-39.9, adult
Z68.41	BMI 40.0-44.9, adult
Z68.42	BMI 45.0-49.9, adult
Z68.43	BMI 50.0-59.9, adult
Z68.44	BMI 60.0-69.9, adult
Z68.45	BMI 70 or greater, adult

See National Coverage Determinations (NCD) Manual (Pub. 100-03) §210.12 for complete coverage guidelines.

100-4, 18, 200.2

Institutional Billing Requirements

Effective for claims with dates of service on and after November 29, 2011, providers may use the following types of bill (TOB) when submitting HCPCS code G0447: 13x, 71X, 77X, or 85X. Service line items on other TOBs shall be denied.

The service shall be paid on the basis shown below:

- Rural Health Clinics (RHCs) - type of bill (TOB) 71X only —based on the all-inclusive payment rate
- Federally Qualified Health Centers (FQHCs) - TOB 77X only —based on the all-inclusive payment rate
- Outpatient hospitals —TOB 13X - based on Outpatient Prospective Payment System (OPPS)
- Critical Access Hospitals (CAHs) - TOB 85X —based on reasonable cost

• CAH Method II —TOB 85X - based on 115% of the lesser of the Medicare Physician Fee Schedule (MPFS) amount or actual charge as applicable with revenue codes 096X, 097X, or 098X.

For RHCs and FQHCs, obesity counseling is not separately payable with another face-to-face encounter on the same day. This does not apply to claims for the Initial Preventive Physical Examination (IPPE), claims with unrelated services denoted with modifier 59, and FQHC claims containing Diabetes Self Management Training (DSMT) and Medical Nutrition Therapy (MNT) services. However, the counseling sessions alone when rendered as a face-to-face visit with a core practitioner do constitute an encounter and are paid based on the all-inclusive payment rate.

Note: For outpatient hospital settings, as in any other setting, services covered under this NCD must be provided by a primary care provider.

100-4, 18, 200.3

Professional Billing Requirements

For claims with dates of service on or after November 29, 2011, CMS will allow coverage for Face-to-Face Behavioral Counseling for Obesity, 15 minutes, G0447, along with 1 of the ICD-9 codes for BMI 30.0-BMI 70 (V85.30-V85.39 and V85.41-V85.45), only when services are submitted by the following provider specialties found on the provider? enrollment record:

- 01 - General Practice
- 08 - Family Practice
- 11 - Internal Medicine
- 16 - Obstetrics/Gynecology
- 37 - Pediatric Medicine
- 38 - Geriatric Medicine
- 50 - Nurse Practitioner
- 89 - Certified Clinical Nurse Specialist
- 97 - Physician Assistant

Any claims that are not submitted from one of the provider specialty types noted above will be denied.

For claims with dates of service on or after November 29, 2011, CMS will allow coverage for Face-to-Face Behavioral Counseling for Obesity, 15 minutes, G0447, along with 1 of the ICD-9 codes for BMI 30.0-BMI 70 (V85.30-V85.39 and V85.41-V85.45), only when submitted with one of the following place of service (POS) codes:

- 11- Physician's Office
- 22- Outpatient Hospital
- 49- Independent Clinic
- 71- State or Local Public Health Clinic

Any claims that are not submitted with one of the POS codes noted above will be denied.

100-4, 18, 200.4

Claim Adjustment Reason Codes (CARCs), Remittance Advice Remark Codes (RARCs), Group Codes, and Medicare Summary Notice (MSN) Messages

Contractors shall use the appropriate claim adjustment reason codes (CARCs), remittance advice remark codes (RARCs), group codes, or Medicare summary notice (MSN) messages when denying payment for obesity counseling sessions:

- Denying services submitted on a TOB other than 13X, 71X, 77X, and 85X: CARC 5 - The procedure code/bill type is inconsistent with the place of service.

  – Note: Refer to the 835 Healthcare Policy Identification Segment (loop 2110 Service Payment Information REF), if present.

  – RARC M77 - Missing/incomplete/invalid place of service

  – MSN 21.25: "This service was denied because Medicare only covers this service in certain settings."

  – Group Code PR (Patient Responsibility) assigning financial responsibility to the beneficiary (if a claim is received with a GA modifier indicating a signed ABN is on file).

  – Group Code CO (Contractual Obligation) assigning financial liability to the provider (if a claim is received with a GZ modifier indicating no signed ABN is on file).

  – NOTE: For modifier GZ, use CARC 50 and MSN 8.81 per instructions in CR 7228/TR 2148.

• For RHC and FQHC services that contain HCPCS code G0447 with another encounter/visit with the same line item date of service: Claim Adjustment Reason Code (CARC) 97

  – The benefit for this service is included in the payment/allowance for another service/procedure that has already been adjudicated. Note: Refer to the 835 Healthcare Policy Identification Segment (loop 2110 Service Payment Information REF) if present

  – Group Code CO (Contractual Obligation)

• Denying services for obesity counseling sessions HCPCS code G0447 with 1 of the ICD-9 codes (V85.30-V85.39 or V85.41-V85.45) for more than 22 times in the same 12-month period:

  – CARC 119-Benefit maximum for this time period or occurrence has been reached.

  – RARC N362 - The number of days or units of service exceeds our acceptable maximum.

  – MSN 20.5 - These services cannot be paid because your benefits are exhausted at this time.

  – Group Code PR (Patient Responsibility) assigning financial responsibility to the beneficiary (if a claim is received with a GA modifier indicating a signed ABN is on file).

  – Group Code CO (Contractual Obligation) assigning financial liability to the provider (if a claim is received with a GZ modifier indicating no signed ABN is on file).

  – NOTE: For modifier GZ, use CARC 50 and MSN 8.81 per instructions in CR 7228/TR 2148. -

• Denying claim lines for obesity counseling sessions HCPCS code G0447 without 1 of the appropriate ICD-9 codes (V85.30-V85.39 or V85.41-V85.45):

  – CARC 167 - This (these) diagnosis(es) is (are) not covered.

  – Note: Refer to the 835 Healthcare Policy Identification Segment (loop 2110 Service Payment Information REF), if present.

  – RARC N386 -This decision was based on a National Coverage Determination (NCD). An NCD provides a coverage determination as to whether a particular item or service is covered. A copy of this policy is available at www.cms.gov/mcd/search.asp. If you do not have web access, you may contact the contractor to request a copy of the NCD.

  – MSN 14.9 - Medicare cannot pay for this service for the diagnosis shown on the claim.

  – Group Code PR (Patient Responsibility) assigning financial responsibility to the beneficiary (if a claim is received with a GA modifier indicating a signed ABN is on file).

  – Group Code CO (Contractual Obligation) assigning financial liability to the provider (if a claim is received with a GZ modifier indicating no signed ABN is on file).

  – NOTE: For modifier GZ, use CARC 50 and MSN 8.81 per instructions in CR 7228/TR 2148.

• Denying claim lines without the appropriate POS code: CARC 58 —Treatment was deemed by the payer to have been rendered in an inappropriate or invalid place of service. Note: Refer to the 835 Healthcare Policy Identification Segment (loop 2110 Service Payment Information REF), if present.

  – RARC N428 - Not covered when performed in certain settings.

  – MSN 21.25 - This service was denied because Medicare only covers this service in certain settings.

  – Group Code PR (Patient Responsibility) assigning financial responsibility to the beneficiary (if a claim is received with a GA modifier indicating a signed ABN is on file).

  – Group Code CO (Contractual Obligation) assigning financial liability to the provider (if a claim is received with a GZ modifier indicating no signed ABN is on file).

  – NOTE: For modifier GZ, use CARC 50 and MSN 8.81 per instructions in CR 7228/TR 2148.

• Denying claim lines that are not submitted from the appropriate provider specialties: CARC 185 - The rendering provider is not eligible to perform the service billed. NOTE: Refer to the 835 Healthcare Policy Identification Segment (loop 2110 Service Payment Information REF), if present.

  – RARC N95 - This provider type/provider specialty may not bill this service.

  – MSN 21.18 - This item or service is not covered when performed or ordered by this provider.

  – Group Code PR (Patient Responsibility) assigning financial responsibility to the beneficiary (if a claim is received with a GA modifier indicating a signed ABN is on file).

  – Group Code CO (Contractual Obligation) assigning financial liability to the provider (if a claim is received with a GZ modifier indicating no signed ABN is on file).

– NOTE: For modifier GZ, use CARC 50 and MSN 8.81 per instructions in CR 7228/TR 2148.

100-4, 18, 200.5

Common Working File (CWF) Edits

When applying frequency, CWF shall count 22 counseling sessions of G0447, along with 1 ICD-9 code from V85.30-V85.39 or V85.41-V85.45 in a 12-month period. When applying frequency limitations to G0447 counseling CWF shall allow both a claim for the professional service and a claim for a facility fee. CWF shall identify the following institutional claims as facility fee claims for this service: TOB 13X, TOB 85X when the revenue code is not 096X, 097X, or 098X. CWF shall identify all other claims as professional service claims. NOTE: This does not apply to RHCs and FQHCs.

100-4, 20, 30.1.2

Transcutaneous Electrical Nerve Stimulator (TENS)

In order to permit an attending physician time to determine whether the purchase of a TENS is medically appropriate for a particular patient, contractors pay 10 percent of the purchase price of the item for each of 2 months. The purchase price and payment for maintenance and servicing are determined under the same rules as any other frequently purchased item, except that there is no reduction in the allowed amount for purchase due to the two months rental.

Effective June 8, 2012, CMS will allow coverage for TENS use in the treatment of chronic low back pain (CLBP) only under specific conditions which are described in the NCD Manual, Pub. 100-03, chapter 1 Section 160.27.

100-4, 20, 100.2.2

Evidence of Medical Necessity for Parenteral and Enteral Nutrition (PEN) Therapy

The PEN coverage is determined by information provided by the treating physician and the PEN supplier. A completed certification of medical necessity (CMN) must accompany and support initial claims for PEN to establish whether coverage criteria are met and to ensure that the PEN therapy provided is consistent with the attending or ordering physician's prescription.

Contractors ensure that the CMN contains pertinent information from the treating physician. Uniform specific medical data facilitate the review and promote consistency in coverage determinations and timelier claims processing.The medical and prescription information on a PEN CMN can be most appropriatelycompleted by the treating physician or from information in the patient's records by an employee of the physician for the physician's review and signature.

Although PEN suppliers sometimes may assist in providing the PEN services, they cannot complete the CMN since they do not have the same access to patient information needed to properly enter medical or prescription information. Contractors use appropriate professional relations issuances, training sessions, and meetings to ensure that all persons and PEN suppliers are aware of this limitation of their role. When properly completed, the PEN CMN includes the elements of a prescription as well as other data needed to determine whether Medicare coverage is possible. This practice will facilitate prompt delivery of PEN services and timely submittal of the related claim.

100-4, 20, 160.1

Billing for Total Parenteral Nutrition and Enteral NutritionFurnished to Part B Inpatients

A3-3660.6, SNF-544, SNF-559, SNF-260.4, SNF-261, HHA-403, HO-438, HO-229

Inpatient Part A hospital or SNF care includes total parenteral nutrition (TPN) systems and enteral nutrition (EN).

For inpatients for whom Part A benefits are not payable (e.g., benefits are exhausted or the beneficiary is entitled to Part B only), total parenteral nutrition (TPN) systems and enteral nutrition (EN) delivery systems are covered by Medicare as prosthetic devices when the coverage criteria are met. When these criteria are met, the medical equipment and medical supplies (together with nutrients) being used comprise covered prosthetic devices for coverage purposes rather than durable medical equipment. However, reimbursement rules relating to DME continue to apply to such items.

When a facility supplies TPN or EN systems that meet the criteria for coverage as a prosthetic device to an inpatient whose care is not covered under Part A, the facility must bill one of the DMERCs. Additionally, HHAs, SNFs, and hospitals that provide PEN supplies, equipment and nutrients as a prosthetic device under Part B must use the CMS-1500 or the related NSF or ANSI ASC X12N 837 format to bill the appropriate DMERC. The DMERC is determined according to the residence of the beneficiary. Refer to Sec.10 for jurisdiction descriptions.

FIs return claims containing PEN charges for Part B services where the bill type is 12x,

13x, 22x, 23x, 32x, 33x, or 34x with instructions to the provider to bill the DMERC.

100-4, 23, 60.3

(Rev.2340, Issued: 11-04-11, Effective, 01-01-12, Implementation: 01-03-12)

The DME MACs and local carriers must gap-fill the DMEPOS fee schedule for items for which charge data were unavailable during the fee schedule data base year using the fee schedule amounts for comparable equipment, using properly calculated fee schedule amounts from a neighboring carrier, or using supplier price lists with prices in effect during the fee schedule data base year. Data base "year" refers to the time period mandated by the statute and/or regulations from which Medicare allowed charge data is to be extracted in order to compute the fee schedule amounts for the various DMEPOS payment categories. For example, the fee schedule base year for inexpensive or routinely purchased durable medical equipment is the 12 month period ending June 30, 1987. Mail order catalogs are particularly suitable sources of price information for items such as urological and ostomy supplies which require constant replacement. DME MACs will gap-fill based on current instructions released each year for implementing and updating the new year's payment amounts.

If the only available price information is from a period other than the base period, apply the deflation factors that are included in the current year implementation instructions against current pricing in order to approximate the base year price for gap-filling purposes.

The deflation factors for gap-filling purposes are:

Year*	OX	CR	PO	SD	PE
1987	0.965	0.971	0.974	n/a	n/a
1988	0.928	0.934	0.936	n/a	n/a
1989	0.882	0.888	0.890	n/a	n/a
1990	0.843	0.848	0.851	n/a	n/a
1991	0.805	0.810	0.813	n/a	n/a
1992	0.781	0.786	0.788	n/a	n/a
1993	0.758	0.763	0.765	0.971	n/a
1994	0.740	0.745	0.747	0.947	n/a
1995	0.718	0.723	0.725	0.919	n/a
1996	0.699	0.703	0.705	0.895	0.973
1997	0.683	0.687	0.689	0.875	0.951
1998	0.672	0.676	0.678	0.860	0.936
1999	0.659	0.663	0.665	0.844	0.918
2000	0.635	0.639	0.641	0.813	0.885
2001	0.615	0.619	0.621	0.788	0.857
2002	0.609	0.613	0.614	0.779	0.848
2003	0.596	0.600	0.602	0.763	0.830
2004	0.577	0.581	0.582	0.739	0.804
2005	0.563	0.567	0.568	0.721	0.784
2006	0.540	0.543	0.545	0.691	0.752
2007	0.525	0.529	0.530	0.673	0.732
2008	0.500	0.504	0.505	0.641	0.697
2009	0.508	0.511	0.512	0.650	0.707
2010	0.502	0.506	0.507	0.643	0.700
2011	0.485	0.488	0.490	0.621	0.676

* Year price in effect

Payment Category Key:

OX   Oxygen & oxygen equipment (DME)

CR   Capped rental (DME)

IN   Inexpensive/routinely purchased (DME)

FS   Frequently serviced (DME)

SU   DME supplies

PO   Prosthetics & orthotics

SD   Surgical dressings

OS   Ostomy, tracheostomy, and urological supplies

PE   Parental and enteral nutrition

TS   Therapeutic Shoes

After deflation, the result must be increased by 1.7 percent and by the cumulative covered item update to complete the gap-filling (e.g., an additional .6 percent for a 2002 DME fee).

Note that when gap-filling for capped rental items, it is necessary to first gap-fill the purchase price then compute the base period fee schedule at 10 percent of the base period purchase price.

For used equipment, establish fee schedule amounts at 75 percent of the fee schedule amount for new equipment.

When gap-filling, for those carrier areas where a sales tax was imposed in the base period, add the applicable sales tax, e.g., five percent, to the gap-filled amount where the gap-filled amount does not take into account the sales tax, e.g., where the gap-filled amount is computed from pre-tax price lists or from another carrier area without a sales tax. Likewise, if the gap-filled amount is calculated from another carrier? fees where a sales tax is imposed, adjust the gap-filled amount to reflect the applicable local sales tax circumstances.

DME MACs and local carriers send their gap-fill information to CMS. After receiving the gap-filled base fees each year, CMS develops national fee schedule floors and ceilings and new fee schedule amounts for these codes and releases them as part of the July update file each year and during the quarterly updates.

Attachment A 2012 Fees for Codes K0739, L4205, L7520

STATE	K0739	L4205	L7520	STATE	K0739	L4205	L7520
AK	$26.47	$30.16	$35.48	SC	$14.05	20.94	28.43
AL	14.05	20.94	28.43	SD	15.70	20.92	38.00
AR	14.05	20.94	28.43	TN	14.05	20.94	28.43
AZ	17.37	20.92	34.98	TX	14.05	20.94	28.43
CA	21.56	34.38	40.07	UT	14.09	20.92	44.27
CO	14.05	20.94	28.43	VA	14.05	20.92	28.43
CT	23.47	21.41	28.43	VI	14.05	20.94	28.43
DC	14.05	20.92	28.43	VT	15.08	20.92	28.43
DE	25.88	20.92	28.43	WA	22.39	30.69	36.45
FL	14.05	20.94	28.43	WI	14.05	20.92	28.43
GA	14.05	20.94	28.43	WV	14.05	20.92	28.43
HI	17.37	30.16	35.48	WY	19.59	27.91	39.64
IA	14.05	20.92	34.03				
ID	14.05	20.92	28.43				
IL	14.05	20.92	28.43				
IN	14.05	20.92	28.43				
KS	14.05	20.92	35.48				
KY	14.05	26.81	36.35				
LA	14.05	20.94	28.43				
MA	23.47	20.92	28.43				
MD	14.05	20.92	28.43				
ME	23.47	20.92	28.43				
MI	14.05	20.92	28.43				
MN	14.05	20.92	28.43				
MO	14.05	20.92	28.43				
MS	14.05	20.94	28.43				
MT	14.05	20.92	35.48				
NC	14.05	20.94	28.43				
ND	17.51	30.10	35.48				
NE	14.05	20.92	39.64				
NH	15.08	20.92	28.43				
NJ	18.96	20.92	28.43				
NM	14.05	20.94	28.43				
NV	22.39	20.92	38.75				
NY	25.88	20.94	28.43				
OH	14.05	20.92	28.43				

STATE	K0739	L4205	L7520	STATE	K0739	L4205	L7520
OK	14.05	20.94	28.43				
OR	14.05	20.92	40.88				
PA	15.08	21.54	28.43				
PR	14.05	20.94	28.43				
RI	16.75	21.56	28.43				

Attachment B

HCPCS Codes Selected for the Round One of the DMEPOS Competitive Bidding Program in 2008

PRODUCT CATEGORY 1

Oxygen Supplies and Equipment

E1390   OXYGEN CONCENTRATOR, SINGLE DELIVERY PORT, CAPABLE OF DELIVERING 85 PERCENT OR GREATER OXYGEN CONCENTRATION AT THE PRESCRIBED FLOW RATE

E1391   OXYGEN CONCENTRATOR, DUAL DELIVERY PORT, CAPABLE OF DELIVERING 85 PERCENT OR GREATER OXYGEN CONCENTRATION AT THE PRESCRIBED FLOW RATE, EACH

E0424   STATIONARY COMPRESSED GASEOUS OXYGEN SYSTEM, RENTAL; INCLUDES CONTAINER, CONTENTS, REGULATOR, FLOWMETER, HUMIDIFIER, NEBULIZER, CANNULA OR MASK, AND TUBING

E0439   STATIONARY LIQUID OXYGEN SYSTEM, RENTAL; INCLUDES CONTAINER, CONTENTS, REGULATOR, FLOWMETER, HUMIDIFIER, NEBULIZER, CANNULA OR MASK, & TUBING

E0431   PORTABLE GASEOUS OXYGEN SYSTEM, RENTAL; INCLUDES PORTABLE CONTAINER, REGULATOR, FLOWMETER, HUMIDIFIER, CANNULA OR MASK, AND TUBING

E0434   PORTABLE LIQUID OXYGEN SYSTEM, RENTAL; INCLUDES PORTABLE CONTAINER, SUPPLY RESERVOIR, HUMIDIFIER, FLOWMETER, REFILL ADAPTOR, CONTENTS GAUGE, CANNULA OR MASK, AND TUBING

A4608   TRANSTRACHEAL OXYGEN CATHETER, EACH

A4615   CANNULA, NASAL

A4616   TUBING (OXYGEN), PER FOOT

A4617   MOUTH PIECE

A4620   VARIABLE CONCENTRATION MASK

E0560   HUMIDIFIER, DURABLE FOR SUPPLEMENTAL HUMIDIFICATION DURING IPPB TREATMENT OR OXYGEN DELIVERY

E0580   NEBULIZER, DURABLE, GLASS OR AUTOCLAVABLE PLASTIC, BOTTLE TYPE, FOR USE WITH REGULATOR OR FLOWMETER

E1353   REGULATOR

E1355   STAND/RACK

PRODUCT CATEGORY 2

Standard Power Wheelchairs, Scooters, and Related Accessories

E0950   WHEELCHAIR ACCESSORY, TRAY, EACH

E0951   HEEL LOOP/HOLDER, ANY TYPE, WITH OR WITHOUT ANKLE STRAP,

PRODUCT CATEGORY 1

Oxygen Supplies and Equipment

E1390   OXYGEN CONCENTRATOR, SINGLE DELIVERY PORT, CAPABLE OF DELIVERING 85 PERCENT OR GREATER OXYGEN CONCENTRATION AT THE PRESCRIBED FLOW RATE

E1391   OXYGEN CONCENTRATOR, DUAL DELIVERY PORT, CAPABLE OF DELIVERING 85 PERCENT OR GREATER OXYGEN CONCENTRATION AT THE PRESCRIBED FLOW RATE, EACH

E0424   STATIONARY COMPRESSED GASEOUS OXYGEN SYSTEM, RENTAL; INCLUDES CONTAINER, CONTENTS, REGULATOR, FLOWMETER, HUMIDIFIER, NEBULIZER, CANNULA OR MASK, AND TUBING

E0439   STATIONARY LIQUID OXYGEN SYSTEM, RENTAL; INCLUDES CONTAINER, CONTENTS, REGULATOR, FLOWMETER, HUMIDIFIER, NEBULIZER, CANNULA OR MASK, & TUBING

E0431	PORTABLE GASEOUS OXYGEN SYSTEM, RENTAL; INCLUDES PORTABLE CONTAINER, REGULATOR, FLOWMETER, HUMIDIFIER, CANNULA OR MASK, AND TUBING
E0434	PORTABLE LIQUID OXYGEN SYSTEM, RENTAL; INCLUDES PORTABLE CONTAINER, SUPPLY RESERVOIR, HUMIDIFIER, FLOWMETER, REFILL ADAPTOR, CONTENTS GAUGE, CANNULA OR MASK, AND TUBING
A4608	TRANSTRACHEAL OXYGEN CATHETER, EACH
A4615	CANNULA, NASAL
A4616	TUBING (OXYGEN), PER FOOT
A4617	MOUTH PIECE
A4620	VARIABLE CONCENTRATION MASK
E0560	HUMIDIFIER, DURABLE FOR SUPPLEMENTAL HUMIDIFICATION DURING IPPB TREATMENT OR OXYGEN DELIVERY
E0580	NEBULIZER, DURABLE, GLASS OR AUTOCLAVABLE PLASTIC, BOTTLE TYPE, FOR USE WITH REGULATOR OR FLOWMETER
E1353	REGULATOR
E1355	STAND/RACK

PRODUCT CATEGORY 2

Standard Power Wheelchairs, Scooters, and Related Accessories

E0950	WHEELCHAIR ACCESSORY, TRAY, EACH
E0951	HEEL LOOP/HOLDER, ANY TYPE, WITH OR WITHOUT ANKLE STRAP, EACH
E0952	TOE LOOP/HOLDER, ANY TYPE, EACH
E0955	WHEELCHAIR ACCESSORY, HEADREST, CUSHIONED, ANY TYPE, INCLUDING FIXED MOUNTING HARDWARE, EACH
E0956	WHEELCHAIR ACCESSORY, LATERAL TRUNK OR HIP SUPPORT, ANY TYPE, INCLUDING FIXED MOUNTING HARDWARE, EACH
E0957	WHEELCHAIR ACCESSORY, MEDIAL THIGH SUPPORT, ANY TYPE, INCLUDING FIXED MOUNTING HARDWARE, EACH
E0960	WHEELCHAIR ACCESSORY, SHOULDER HARNESS/STRAPS OR CHEST STRAP, INCLUDING ANY TYPE MOUNTING HARDWARE
E0973	WHEELCHAIR ACCESSORY, ADJUSTABLE HEIGHT, DETACHABLE ARMREST, COMPLETE ASSEMBLY, EACH
E0978	WHEELCHAIR ACCESSORY, POSITIONING BELT/SAFETY BELT/PELVIC STRAP, EACH
E0981	WHEELCHAIR ACCESSORY, SEAT UPHOLSTERY, REPLACEMENT ONLY, EACH
E0982	WHEELCHAIR ACCESSORY, BACK UPHOLSTERY, REPLACEMENT ONLY, EACH
E0990	WHEELCHAIR ACCESSORY, ELEVATING LEG REST, COMPLETE ASSEMBLY, EACH
E0995	WHEELCHAIR ACCESSORY, CALF REST/PAD, EACH
E1016	SHOCK ABSORBER FOR POWER WHEELCHAIR, EACH
E1020	RESIDUAL LIMB SUPPORT SYSTEM FOR WHEELCHAIR
E1028	WHEELCHAIR ACCESSORY, MANUAL SWINGAWAY, RETRACTABLE OR REMOVABLE MOUNTING HARDWARE FOR JOYSTICK, OTHER CONTROL INTERFACE OR POSITIONING ACCESSORY
E2208	WHEELCHAIR ACCESSORY, CYLINDER TANK CARRIER, EACH
E2209	ACCESSORY, ARM TROUGH, WITH OR WITHOUT HAND SUPPORT, EACH
E2210	WHEELCHAIR ACCESSORY, BEARINGS, ANY TYPE, REPLACEMENT ONLY, EACH
E2361	POWER WHEELCHAIR ACCESSORY, 22NF SEALED LEAD ACID BATTERY, EACH, (E.G. GEL CELL, ABSORBED GLASSMAT)
E2363	POWER WHEELCHAIR ACCESSORY, GROUP 24 SEALED LEAD ACID BATTERY, EACH (E.G. GEL CELL, ABSORBED GLASSMAT)
E2365	POWER WHEELCHAIR ACCESSORY, U-1 SEALED LEAD ACID BATTERY, EACH (E.G. GEL CELL, ABSORBED GLASSMAT)
E2366	POWER WHEELCHAIR ACCESSORY, BATTERY CHARGER, SINGLE MODE, FOR USE WITH ONLY ONE BATTERY TYPE, SEALED OR NON-SEALED, EACH
E2367	POWER WHEELCHAIR ACCESSORY, BATTERY CHARGER, DUAL MODE, FOR USE WITH EITHER BATTERY TYPE, SEALED OR NON-SEALED, EACH

E2368	POWER WHEELCHAIR COMPONENT, MOTOR, REPLACEMENT ONLY
E2369	POWER WHEELCHAIR COMPONENT, GEAR BOX, REPLACEMENT ONLY
E2370	POWER WHEELCHAIR COMPONENT, MOTOR AND GEAR BOX COMBINATION, REPLACEMENT ONLY
E2371	POWER WHEELCHAIR ACCESSORY, GROUP 27 SEALED LEAD ACID BATTERY, (E.G. GEL CELL, ABSORBED GLASSMAT), EACH
E2381	POWER WHEELCHAIR ACCESSORY, PNEUMATIC DRIVE WHEEL TIRE, ANY SIZE, REPLACEMENT ONLY, EACH
E2382	POWER WHEELCHAIR ACCESSORY, TUBE FOR PNEUMATIC DRIVE WHEEL TIRE, ANY SIZE, REPLACEMENT ONLY, EACH
E2383	POWER WHEELCHAIR ACCESSORY, INSERT FOR PNEUMATIC DRIVE WHEEL TIRE (REMOVABLE), ANY TYPE, ANY SIZE, REPLACEMENT ONLY, EACH
E2384	POWER WHEELCHAIR ACCESSORY, PNEUMATIC CASTER TIRE, ANY SIZE, REPLACEMENT ONLY, EACH
E2385	POWER WHEELCHAIR ACCESSORY, TUBE FOR PNEUMATIC CASTER TIRE, ANY SIZE, REPLACEMENT ONLY, EACH
E2386	POWER WHEELCHAIR ACCESSORY, FOAM FILLED DRIVE WHEEL TIRE, ANY SIZE, REPLACEMENT ONLY, EACH
E2387	POWER WHEELCHAIR ACCESSORY, FOAM FILLED CASTER TIRE, ANY SIZE, REPLACEMENT ONLY, EACH
E2388	POWER WHEELCHAIR ACCESSORY, FOAM DRIVE WHEEL TIRE, ANY SIZE, REPLACEMENT ONLY, EACH
E2389	POWER WHEELCHAIR ACCESSORY, FOAM CASTER TIRE, ANY SIZE, REPLACEMENT ONLY, EACH
E2390	POWER WHEELCHAIR ACCESSORY, SOLID (RUBBER/PLASTIC) DRIVE WHEEL TIRE, ANY SIZE, REPLACEMENT ONLY, EACH
E2391	POWER WHEELCHAIR ACCESSORY, SOLID (RUBBER/PLASTIC) CASTER TIRE (REMOVABLE), ANY SIZE, REPLACEMENT ONLY, EACH
E2392	POWER WHEELCHAIR ACCESSORY, SOLID (RUBBER/PLASTIC) CASTER TIRE WITH INTEGRATED WHEEL, ANY SIZE, REPLACEMENT ONLY, EACH
E2394	POWER WHEELCHAIR ACCESSORY, DRIVE WHEEL EXCLUDES TIRE, ANY SIZE, REPLACEMENT ONLY, EACH
E2395	POWER WHEELCHAIR ACCESSORY, CASTER WHEEL EXCLUDES TIRE, ANY SIZE, REPLACEMENT ONLY, EACH
E2396	POWER WHEELCHAIR ACCESSORY, CASTER FORK, ANY SIZE, REPLACEMENT ONLY, EACH
E2601	GENERAL USE WHEELCHAIR SEAT CUSHION, WIDTH LESS THAN 22 INCHES, ANY DEPTH
E2602	GENERAL USE WHEELCHAIR SEAT CUSHION, WIDTH 22 INCHES OR GREATER, ANY DEPTH
E2603	SKIN PROTECTION WHEELCHAIR SEAT CUSHION, WIDTH LESS THAN 22 INCHES, ANY DEPTH
E2604	SKIN PROTECTION WHEELCHAIR SEAT CUSHION, WIDTH 22 INCHES OR GREATER, ANY DEPTH
E2605	POSITIONING WHEELCHAIR SEAT CUSHION, WIDTH LESS THAN 22 INCHES, ANY DEPTH
E2606	POSITIONING WHEELCHAIR SEAT CUSHION, WIDTH 22 INCHES OR GREATER, ANY DEPTH
E2607	SKIN PROTECTION AND POSITIONING WHEELCHAIR SEAT CUSHION, WIDTH LESS THAN 22 INCHES, ANY DEPTH
E2608	SKIN PROTECTION AND POSITIONING WHEELCHAIR SEAT CUSHION, WIDTH 22 INCHES OR GREATER, ANY DEPTH
E2611	GENERAL USE WHEELCHAIR BACK CUSHION, WIDTH LESS THAN 22 INCHES, ANY HEIGHT, INCLUDING ANY TYPE MOUNTING HARDWARE
E2612	GENERAL USE WHEELCHAIR BACK CUSHION, WIDTH 22 INCHES OR GREATER, ANY HEIGHT, INCLUDING ANY TYPE MOUNTING HARDWARE
E2613	POSITIONING WHEELCHAIR BACK CUSHION, POSTERIOR, WIDTH LESS THAN 22 INCHES, ANY HEIGHT, INCLUDING ANY TYPE MOUNTING HARDWARE

Code	Description
E2614	POSITIONING WHEELCHAIR BACK CUSHION, POSTERIOR, WIDTH 22 INCHES OR GREATER, ANY HEIGHT, INCLUDING ANY TYPE MOUNTING HARDWARE
E2615	POSITIONING WHEELCHAIR BACK CUSHION, POSTERIOR-LATERAL, WIDTH LESS THAN 22 INCHES, ANY HEIGHT, INCLUDING ANY TYPE MOUNTING HARDWARE
E2616	POSITIONING WHEELCHAIR BACK CUSHION, POSTERIOR-LATERAL, WIDTH 22 INCHES OR GREATER, ANY HEIGHT, INCLUDING ANY TYPE MOUNTING HARDWARE
E2619	REPLACEMENT COVER FOR WHEELCHAIR SEAT CUSHION OR BACK CUSHION, EACH
E2620	POSITIONING WHEELCHAIR BACK CUSHION, PLANAR BACK WITH LATERAL SUPPORTS, WIDTH LESS THAN 22 INCHES, ANY HEIGHT, INCLUDING ANY TYPE MOUNTING HARDWARE
E2621	POSITIONING WHEELCHAIR BACK CUSHION, PLANAR BACK WITH LATERAL SUPPORTS, WIDTH 22 INCHES OR GREATER, ANY HEIGHT, INCLUDING ANY TYPE MOUNTING HARDWARE
K0015	DETACHABLE, NON-ADJUSTABLE HEIGHT ARMREST, EACH
K0017	DETACHABLE, ADJUSTABLE HEIGHT ARMREST, BASE, EACH
K0018	DETACHABLE, ADJUSTABLE HEIGHT ARMREST, UPPER PORTION, EACH
K0019	ARM PAD, EACH
K0020	FIXED, ADJUSTABLE HEIGHT ARMREST, PAIR
K0037	HIGH MOUNT FLIP-UP FOOTREST, EACH
K0038	LEG STRAP, EACH
K0039	LEG STRAP, H STYLE, EACH
K0040	ADJUSTABLE ANGLE FOOTPLATE, EACH
K0041	LARGE SIZE FOOTPLATE, EACH
K0042	STANDARD SIZE FOOTPLATE, EACH
K0043	FOOTREST, LOWER EXTENSION TUBE, EACH
K0044	FOOTREST, UPPER HANGER BRACKET, EACH
K0045	FOOTREST, COMPLETE ASSEMBLY
K0046	ELEVATING LEGREST, LOWER EXTENSION TUBE, EACH
K0047	ELEVATING LEGREST, UPPER HANGER BRACKET, EACH
K0050	RATCHET ASSEMBLY
K0051	CAM RELEASE ASSEMBLY, FOOTREST OR LEGREST, EACH
K0052	SWINGAWAY, DETACHABLE FOOTRESTS, EACH
K0053	ELEVATING FOOTRESTS, ARTICULATING (TELESCOPING), EACH
K0098	DRIVE BELT FOR POWER WHEELCHAIR
K0195	ELEVATING LEG RESTS, PAIR (FOR USE WITH CAPPED RENTAL WHEELCHAIR BASE)
K0733	POWER WHEELCHAIR ACCESSORY, 12 TO 24 AMP HOUR SEALED LEAD ACID BATTERY, EACH (E.G., GEL CELL, ABSORBED GLASSMAT)
K0734	SKIN PROTECTION WHEELCHAIR SEAT CUSHION, ADJUSTABLE, WIDTH LESS THAN 22 INCHES, ANY DEPTH
K0735	SKIN PROTECTION WHEELCHAIR SEAT CUSHION, ADJUSTABLE, WIDTH 22 INCHES OR GREATER, ANY DEPTH
K0736	SKIN PROTECTION AND POSITIONING WHEELCHAIR SEAT CUSHION, ADJUSTABLE, WIDTH LESS THAN 22 INCHES, ANY DEPTH
K0737	SKIN PROTECTION AND POSITIONING WHEELCHAIR SEAT CUSHION, ADJUSTABLE, WIDTH 22 INCHES OR GREATER, ANY DEPTH
K0800	POWER OPERATED VEHICLE, GROUP 1 STANDARD
K0801	POWER OPERATED VEHICLE, GROUP 1 HEAVY DUTY
K0802	POWER OPERATED VEHICLE, GROUP 1 VERY HEAVY DUTY
K0806	POWER OPERATED VEHICLE, GROUP 2 STANDARD
K0807	POWER OPERATED VEHICLE, GROUP 2 HEAVY DUTY
K0808	POWER OPERATED VEHICLE, GROUP 2 VERY HEAVY DUTY

Code	Description
K0813	POWER WHEELCHAIR, GROUP 1 STANDARD, PORTABLE, SLING/SOLID SEAT AND BACK
K0814	POWER WHEELCHAIR, GROUP 1 STANDARD, PORTABLE, CAPTAINS CHAIR
K0815	POWER WHEELCHAIR, GROUP 1 STANDARD, SLING/SOLID SEAT AND BACK
K0816	POWER WHEELCHAIR, GROUP 1 STANDARD, CAPTAINS CHAIR
K0820	POWER WHEELCHAIR, GROUP 2 STANDARD, PORTABLE, SLING/SOLID SEAT/BACK
K0821	POWER WHEELCHAIR, GROUP 2 STANDARD, PORTABLE, CAPTAINS CHAIR
K0822	POWER WHEELCHAIR, GROUP 2 STANDARD, SLING/SOLID SEAT/BACK
K0823	POWER WHEELCHAIR, GROUP 2 STANDARD, CAPTAINS CHAIR
K0824	POWER WHEELCHAIR, GROUP 2 HEAVY DUTY, SLING/SOLID SEAT/BACK
K0825	POWER WHEELCHAIR, GROUP 2 HEAVY DUTY, CAPTAINS CHAIR
K0826	POWER WHEELCHAIR, GROUP 2 VERY HEAVY DUTY, SLING/SOLID SEAT/BACK
K0827	POWER WHEELCHAIR, GROUP 2 VERY HEAVY DUTY, CAPTAINS CHAIR
K0828	POWER WHEELCHAIR, GROUP 2 EXTRA HEAVY DUTY, SLING/SOLID SEAT/BACK
K0829	POWER WHEELCHAIR, GROUP 2 EXTRA HEAVY DUTY, CAPTAINS CHAIR

PRODUCT CATEGORY 3

Complex Rehabilitative Power Wheelchairs and Related Accessories

Code	Description
E0950	WHEELCHAIR ACCESSORY, TRAY, EACH
E0951	HEEL LOOP/HOLDER, ANY TYPE, WITH OR WITHOUT ANKLE STRAP, EACH
E0952	TOE LOOP/HOLDER, ANY TYPE, EACH
E0955	WHEELCHAIR ACCESSORY, HEADREST, CUSHIONED, ANY TYPE, INCLUDING FIXED MOUNTING HARDWARE, EACH
E0956	WHEELCHAIR ACCESSORY, LATERAL TRUNK OR HIP SUPPORT, ANY TYPE, INCLUDING FIXED MOUNTING HARDWARE, EACH
E0957	WHEELCHAIR ACCESSORY, MEDIAL THIGH SUPPORT, ANY TYPE, INCLUDING FIXED MOUNTING HARDWARE, EACH
E0960	WHEELCHAIR ACCESSORY, SHOULDER HARNESS/STRAPS OR CHEST STRAP, INCLUDING ANY TYPE MOUNTING HARDWARE
E0973	WHEELCHAIR ACCESSORY, ADJUSTABLE HEIGHT, DETACHABLE ARMREST, COMPLETE ASSEMBLY, EACH
E0978	WHEELCHAIR ACCESSORY, POSITIONING BELT/SAFETY BELT/PELVIC STRAP, EACH
E0981	WHEELCHAIR ACCESSORY, SEAT UPHOLSTERY, REPLACEMENT ONLY, EACH
E0982	WHEELCHAIR ACCESSORY, BACK UPHOLSTERY, REPLACEMENT ONLY, EACH
E0990	WHEELCHAIR ACCESSORY, ELEVATING LEG REST, COMPLETE ASSEMBLY, EACH
E0995	WHEELCHAIR ACCESSORY, CALF REST/PAD, EACH
E1002	WHEELCHAIR ACCESSORY, POWER SEATING SYSTEM, TILT ONLY
E1003	WHEELCHAIR ACCESSORY, POWER SEATING SYSTEM, RECLINE ONLY, WITHOUT SHEAR REDUCTION
E1004	WHEELCHAIR ACCESSORY, POWER SEATING SYSTEM, RECLINE ONLY, WITH MECHANICAL SHEAR REDUCTION
E1005	WHEELCHAIR ACCESSORY, POWER SEATNG SYSTEM, RECLINE ONLY, WITH POWER SHEAR REDUCTION
E1006	WHEELCHAIR ACCESSORY, POWER SEATING SYSTEM, COMBINATION TILT AND RECLINE, WITHOUT SHEAR REDUCTION
E1007	WHEELCHAIR ACCESSORY, POWER SEATING SYSTEM, COMBINATION TILT AND RECLINE, WITH MECHANICAL SHEAR REDUCTION
E1008	WHEELCHAIR ACCESSORY, POWER SEATING SYSTEM, COMBINATION TILT AND RECLINE, WITH POWER SHEAR REDUCTION
E1010	WHEELCHAIR ACCESSORY, ADDITION TO POWER SEATING SYSTEM, POWER LEG ELEVATION SYSTEM, INCLUDING LEG REST, PAIR
E1016	SHOCK ABSORBER FOR POWER WHEELCHAIR, EACH
E1020	RESIDUAL LIMB SUPPORT SYSTEM FOR WHEELCHAIR

E1028	WHEELCHAIR ACCESSORY, MANUAL SWINGAWAY, RETRACTABLE OR REMOVABLE MOUNTING HARDWARE FOR JOYSTICK, OTHER CONTROL INTERFACE OR POSITIONING ACCESSORY
E1029	WHEELCHAIR ACCESSORY, VENTILATOR TRAY, FIXED
E1030	WHEELCHAIR ACCESSORY, VENTILATOR TRAY, GIMBALED
E2208	WHEELCHAIR ACCESSORY, CYLINDER TANK CARRIER, EACH
E2209	ACCESSORY, ARM TROUGH, WITH OR WITHOUT HAND SUPPORT, EACH
E2210	WHEELCHAIR ACCESSORY, BEARINGS, ANY TYPE, REPLACEMENT ONLY, EACH
E2310	POWER WHEELCHAIR ACCESSORY, ELECTRONIC CONNECTION BETWEEN WHEELCHAIR CONTROLLER AND ONE POWER SEATING SYSTEM MOTOR, INCLUDING ALL RELATED ELECTRONICS, INDICATOR FEATURE, MECHANICAL FUNCTION SELECTION SWITCH, AND FIXED MOUNTING HARDWARE
E2311	POWER WHEELCHAIR ACCESSORY, ELECTRONIC CONNECTION BETWEEN WHEELCHAIR CONTROLLER AND TWO OR MORE POWER SEATING SYSTEM MOTORS, INCLUDING ALL RELATED ELECTRONICS, INDICATOR FEATURE, MECHANICAL FUNCTION SELECTION SWITCH, AND FIXED MOUNTING HARDWARE
E2321	POWER WHEELCHAIR ACCESSORY, HAND CONTROL INTERFACE, REMOTE JOYSTICK, NONPROPORTIONAL, INCLUDING ALL RELATED ELECTRONICS, MECHANICAL STOP SWITCH, AND FIXED MOUNTING HARDWARE
E2322	POWER WHEELCHAIR ACCESSORY, HAND CONTROL INTERFACE, MULTIPLE MECHANICAL SWITCHES, NONPROPORTIONAL, INCLUDING ALL RELATED ELECTRONICS, MECHANICAL STOP SWITCH, AND FIXED MOUNTING HARDWARE
E2323	POWER WHEELCHAIR ACCESSORY, SPECIALTY JOYSTICK HANDLE FOR HAND CONTROL INTERFACE, PREFABRICATED
E2324	POWER WHEELCHAIR ACCESSORY, CHIN CUP FOR CHIN CONTROL INTERFACE
E2325	POWER WHEELCHAIR ACCESSORY, SIP AND PUFF INTERFACE, NONPROPORTIONAL, INCLUDING ALL RELATED ELECTRONICS, MECHANICAL STOP SWITCH, AND MANUAL SWINGAWAY MOUNTING HARDWARE
E2326	POWER WHEELCHAIR ACCESSORY, BREATH TUBE KIT FOR SIP AND PUFF INTERFACE
E2327	POWER WHEELCHAIR ACCESSORY, HEAD CONTROL INTERFACE, MECHANICAL, PROPORTIONAL, INCLUDING ALL RELATED ELECTRONICS, MECHANICAL DIRECTION CHANGE SWITCH, AND FIXED MOUNTING HARDWARE
E2328	POWER WHEELCHAIR ACCESSORY, HEAD CONTROL OR EXTREMITY CONTROL INTERFACE, ELECTRONIC, PROPORTIONAL, INCLUDING ALL RELATED ELECTRONICS AND FIXED MOUNTING HARDWARE
E2329	POWER WHEELCHAIR ACCESSORY, HEAD CONTROL INTERFACE, CONTACT SWITCH MECHANISM, NONPROPORTIONAL, INCLUDING ALL RELATED ELECTRONICS, MECHANICAL STOP SWITCH, MECHANICAL DIRECTION CHANGE SWITCH, HEAD ARRAY, AND FIXED MOUNTING HARDWARE
E2330	POWER WHEELCHAIR ACCESSORY, HEAD CONTROL INTERFACE, PROXIMITY SWITCH MECHANISM, NONPROPORTIONAL, INCLUDING ALL RELATED ELECTRONICS, MECHANICAL STOP SWITCH, MECHANICAL DIRECTION CHANGE SWITCH, HEAD ARRAY, AND FIXED MOUNTING HARDWARE
E2351	POWER WHEELCHAIR ACCESSORY, ELECTRONIC INTERFACE TO OPERATE SPEECH GENERATING DEVICE USING POWER WHEELCHAIR CONTROL INTERFACE
E2361	POWER WHEELCHAIR ACCESSORY, 22NF SEALED LEAD ACID BATTERY, EACH, (E.G. GEL CELL, ABSORBED GLASSMAT)
E2363	POWER WHEELCHAIR ACCESSORY, GROUP 24 SEALED LEAD ACID BATTERY, EACH (E.G. GEL CELL, ABSORBED GLASSMAT)
E2365	POWER WHEELCHAIR ACCESSORY, U-1 SEALED LEAD ACID BATTERY, EACH (E.G. GEL CELL, ABSORBED GLASSMAT)
E2366	POWER WHEELCHAIR ACCESSORY, BATTERY CHARGER, SINGLE MODE, FOR USE WITH ONLY ONE BATTERY TYPE, SEALED OR NON-SEALED, EACH
E2367	POWER WHEELCHAIR ACCESSORY, BATTERY CHARGER, DUAL MODE, FOR USE WITH EITHER BATTERY TYPE, SEALED OR NON-SEALED, EACH
E2368	POWER WHEELCHAIR COMPONENT, MOTOR, REPLACEMENT ONLY
E2369	POWER WHEELCHAIR COMPONENT, GEAR BOX, REPLACEMENT ONLY
E2370	POWER WHEELCHAIR COMPONENT, MOTOR AND GEAR BOX COMBINATION, REPLACEMENT ONLY
E2371	POWER WHEELCHAIR ACCESSORY, GROUP 27 SEALED LEAD ACID BATTERY, (E.G. GEL CELL, ABSORBED GLASSMAT), EACH
E2373 KC	POWER WHEELCHAIR ACCESSORY, HAND OR CHIN CONTROL INTERFACE, COMPACT REMOTE JOYSTICK, PROPORTIONAL, INCLUDING FIXED MOUNTING HARDWARE
E2374	POWER WHEELCHAIR ACCESSORY, HAND OR CHIN CONTROL INTERFACE, STANDARD REMOTE JOYSTICK (NOT INCLUDING CONTROLLER), PROPORTIONAL, INCLUDING ALL RELATED ELECTRONICS AND FIXED MOUNTING HARDWARE, REPLACEMENT ONLY
E2375	POWER WHEELCHAIR ACCESSORY, NON-EXPANDABLE CONTROLLER, INCLUDING ALL RELATED ELECTRONICS AND MOUNTING HARDWARE, REPLACEMENT ONLY
E2376	POWER WHEELCHAIR ACCESSORY, EXPANDABLE CONTROLLER, INCLUDING ALL RELATED ELECTRONICS AND MOUNTING HARDWARE, REPLACEMENT ONLY
E2377	POWER WHEELCHAIR ACCESSORY, EXPANDABLE CONTROLLER, INCLUDING ALL RELATED ELECTRONICS AND MOUNTING HARDWARE, UPGRADE PROVIDED AT INITIAL ISSUE
E2381	POWER WHEELCHAIR ACCESSORY, PNEUMATIC DRIVE WHEEL TIRE, ANY SIZE, REPLACEMENT ONLY, EACH
E2382	POWER WHEELCHAIR ACCESSORY, TUBE FOR PNEUMATIC DRIVE WHEEL TIRE, ANY SIZE, REPLACEMENT ONLY, EACH
E2383	POWER WHEELCHAIR ACCESSORY, INSERT FOR PNEUMATIC DRIVE WHEEL TIRE (REMOVABLE), ANY TYPE, ANY SIZE, REPLACEMENT ONLY, EACH
E2384	POWER WHEELCHAIR ACCESSORY, PNEUMATIC CASTER TIRE, ANY SIZE, REPLACEMENT ONLY, EACH
E2385	POWER WHEELCHAIR ACCESSORY, TUBE FOR PNEUMATIC CASTER TIRE, ANY SIZE, REPLACEMENT ONLY, EACH
E2386	POWER WHEELCHAIR ACCESSORY, FOAM FILLED DRIVE WHEEL TIRE, ANY SIZE, REPLACEMENT ONLY, EACH
E2387	POWER WHEELCHAIR ACCESSORY, FOAM FILLED CASTER TIRE, ANY SIZE, REPLACEMENT ONLY, EACH
E2388	POWER WHEELCHAIR ACCESSORY, FOAM DRIVE WHEEL TIRE, ANY SIZE, REPLACEMENT ONLY, EACH
E2389	POWER WHEELCHAIR ACCESSORY, FOAM CASTER TIRE, ANY SIZE, REPLACEMENT ONLY, EACH
E2390	POWER WHEELCHAIR ACCESSORY, SOLID (RUBBER/PLASTIC) DRIVE WHEEL TIRE, ANY SIZE, REPLACEMENT ONLY, EACH
E2391	POWER WHEELCHAIR ACCESSORY, SOLID (RUBBER/PLASTIC) CASTER TIRE (REMOVABLE), ANY SIZE, REPLACEMENT ONLY, EACH
E2392	POWER WHEELCHAIR ACCESSORY, SOLID (RUBBER/PLASTIC) CASTER TIRE WITH INTEGRATED WHEEL, ANY SIZE, REPLACEMENT ONLY, EACH
E2394	POWER WHEELCHAIR ACCESSORY, DRIVE WHEEL EXCLUDES TIRE, ANY SIZE, REPLACEMENT ONLY, EACH
E2395	POWER WHEELCHAIR ACCESSORY, CASTER WHEEL EXCLUDES TIRE, ANY SIZE, REPLACEMENT ONLY, EACH
E2396	POWER WHEELCHAIR ACCESSORY, CASTER FORK, ANY SIZE, REPLACEMENT ONLY, EACH
E2601	GENERAL USE WHEELCHAIR SEAT CUSHION, WIDTH LESS THAN 22 INCHES, ANY DEPTH
E2602	GENERAL USE WHEELCHAIR SEAT CUSHION, WIDTH 22 INCHES OR GREATER, ANY DEPTH
E2603	SKIN PROTECTION WHEELCHAIR SEAT CUSHION, WIDTH LESS THAN 22 INCHES, ANY DEPTH
E2604	SKIN PROTECTION WHEELCHAIR SEAT CUSHION, WIDTH 22 INCHES OR GREATER, ANY DEPTH
E2605	POSITIONING WHEELCHAIR SEAT CUSHION, WIDTH LESS THAN 22 INCHES, ANY DEPTH

Code	Description
E2606	POSITIONING WHEELCHAIR SEAT CUSHION, WIDTH 22 INCHES OR GREATER, ANY DEPTH
E2607	SKIN PROTECTION AND POSITIONING WHEELCHAIR SEAT CUSHION, WIDTH LESS THAN 22 INCHES, ANY DEPTH
E2608	SKIN PROTECTION AND POSITIONING WHEELCHAIR SEAT CUSHION, WIDTH 22 INCHES OR GREATER, ANY DEPTH
E2611	GENERAL USE WHEELCHAIR BACK CUSHION, WIDTH LESS THAN 22 INCHES, ANY HEIGHT, INCLUDING ANY TYPE MOUNTING HARDWARE
E2612	GENERAL USE WHEELCHAIR BACK CUSHION, WIDTH 22 INCHES OR GREATER, ANY HEIGHT, INCLUDING ANY TYPE MOUNTING HARDWARE
E2613	POSITIONING WHEELCHAIR BACK CUSHION, POSTERIOR, WIDTH LESS THAN 22 INCHES, ANY HEIGHT, INCLUDING ANY TYPE MOUNTING HARDWARE
E2614	POSITIONING WHEELCHAIR BACK CUSHION, POSTERIOR, WIDTH 22 INCHES OR GREATER, ANY HEIGHT, INCLUDING ANY TYPE MOUNTING HARDWARE
E2615	POSITIONING WHEELCHAIR BACK CUSHION, POSTERIOR-LATERAL, WIDTH LESS THAN 22 INCHES, ANY HEIGHT, INCLUDING ANY TYPE MOUNTING HARDWARE
E2616	POSITIONING WHEELCHAIR BACK CUSHION, POSTERIOR-LATERAL, WIDTH 22 INCHES OR GREATER, ANY HEIGHT, INCLUDING ANY TYPE MOUNTING HARDWARE
E2619	REPLACEMENT COVER FOR WHEELCHAIR SEAT CUSHION OR BACK CUSHION, EACH
E2620	POSITIONING WHEELCHAIR BACK CUSHION, PLANAR BACK WITH LATERAL SUPPORTS, WIDTH LESS THAN 22 INCHES, ANY HEIGHT, INCLUDING ANY TYPE MOUNTING HARDWARE
E2621	POSITIONING WHEELCHAIR BACK CUSHION, PLANAR BACK WITH LATERAL SUPPORTS, WIDTH 22 INCHES OR GREATER, ANY HEIGHT, INCLUDING ANY TYPE MOUNTING HARDWARE
K0015	DETACHABLE, NON-ADJUSTABLE HEIGHT ARMREST, EACH
K0017	DETACHABLE, ADJUSTABLE HEIGHT ARMREST, BASE, EACH
K0018	DETACHABLE, ADJUSTABLE HEIGHT ARMREST, UPPER PORTION, EACH
K0019	ARM PAD, EACH
K0020	FIXED, ADJUSTABLE HEIGHT ARMREST, PAIR
K0037	HIGH MOUNT FLIP-UP FOOTREST, EACH
K0038	LEG STRAP, EACH
K0039	LEG STRAP, H STYLE, EACH
K0040	ADJUSTABLE ANGLE FOOTPLATE, EACH
K0041	LARGE SIZE FOOTPLATE, EACH
K0042	STANDARD SIZE FOOTPLATE, EACH
K0043	FOOTREST, LOWER EXTENSION TUBE, EACH
K0044	FOOTREST, UPPER HANGER BRACKET, EACH
K0045	FOOTREST, COMPLETE ASSEMBLY
K0046	ELEVATING LEGREST, LOWER EXTENSION TUBE, EACH
K0047	ELEVATING LEGREST, UPPER HANGER BRACKET, EACH
K0050	RATCHET ASSEMBLY
K0051	CAM RELEASE ASSEMBLY, FOOTREST OR LEGREST, EACH
K0052	SWINGAWAY, DETACHABLE FOOTRESTS, EACH
K0053	ELEVATING FOOTRESTS, ARTICULATING (TELESCOPING), EACH
K0098	DRIVE BELT FOR POWER WHEELCHAIR
K0195	ELEVATING LEG RESTS, PAIR (FOR USE WITH CAPPED RENTAL WHEELCHAIR BASE)
K0733	POWER WHEELCHAIR ACCESSORY, 12 TO 24 AMP HOUR SEALED LEAD ACID BATTERY, EACH (E.G., GEL CELL, ABSORBED GLASSMAT)
K0734	SKIN PROTECTION WHEELCHAIR SEAT CUSHION, ADJUSTABLE, WIDTH LESS THAN 22 INCHES, ANY DEPTH
K0735	SKIN PROTECTION WHEELCHAIR SEAT CUSHION, ADJUSTABLE, WIDTH 22 INCHES OR GREATER, ANY DEPTH
K0736	SKIN PROTECTION AND POSITIONING WHEELCHAIR SEAT CUSHION, ADJUSTABLE, WIDTH LESS THAN 22 INCHES, ANY DEPTH
K0737	SKIN PROTECTION AND POSITIONING WHEELCHAIR SEAT CUSHION, ADJUSTABLE, WIDTH 22 INCHES OR GREATER, ANY DEPTH
K0835	POWER WHEELCHAIR, GROUP 2 STANDARD, SINGLE POWER OPTION, SLING/SOLID SEAT/BACK, PATIENT WEIGHT CAPACITY UP TO AND INCLUDING 300 POUNDS
K0836	POWER WHEELCHAIR, GROUP 2 STANDARD, SINGLE POWER OPTION, CAPTAINS CHAIR, PATIENT WEIGHT CAPACITY UP TO AND INCLUDING 300 POUNDS
K0837	POWER WHEELCHAIR, GROUP 2 HEAVY DUTY, SINGLE POWER OPTION, SLING/SOLID SEAT/BACK, PATIENT WEIGHT CAPACITY 301 TO 450 POUNDS
K0838	POWER WHEELCHAIR, GROUP 2 HEAVY DUTY, SINGLE POWER OPTION, CAPTAINS CHAIR, PATIENT WEIGHT CAPACITY 301 TO 450 POUNDS
K0839	POWER WHEELCHAIR, GROUP 2 VERY HEAVY DUTY, SINGLE POWER OPTION SLING/SOLID SEAT/BACK, PATIENT WEIGHT CAPACITY 451 TO 600 POUNDS
K0840	POWER WHEELCHAIR, GROUP 2 EXTRA HEAVY DUTY, SINGLE POWER OPTION, SLING/SOLID SEAT/BACK, PATIENT WEIGHT CAPACITY 601 POUNDS OR MORE
K0841	POWER WHEELCHAIR, GROUP 2 STANDARD, MULTIPLE POWER OPTION, SLING/SOLID SEAT/BACK, PATIENT WEIGHT CAPACITY UP TO AND INCLUDING 300 POUNDS
K0842	POWER WHEELCHAIR, GROUP 2 STANDARD, MULTIPLE POWER OPTION, CAPTAINS CHAIR, PATIENT WEIGHT CAPACITY UP TO AND INCLUDING 300 POUNDS
K0843	POWER WHEELCHAIR, GROUP 2 HEAVY DUTY, MULTIPLE POWER OPTION, SLING/SOLID SEAT/BACK, PATIENT WEIGHT CAPACITY 301 TO 450 POUNDS
K0848	POWER WHEELCHAIR, GROUP 3 STANDARD, SLING/SOLID SEAT/BACK, PATIENT WEIGHT CAPACITY UP TO AND INCLUDING 300 POUNDS
K0849	POWER WHEELCHAIR, GROUP 3 STANDARD, CAPTAINS CHAIR, PATIENT WEIGHT CAPACITY UP TO AND INCLUDING 300 POUNDS
K0850	POWER WHEELCHAIR, GROUP 3 HEAVY DUTY, SLING/SOLID SEAT/BACK, PATIENT WEIGHT CAPACITY 301 TO 450 POUNDS
K0851	POWER WHEELCHAIR, GROUP 3 HEAVY DUTY, CAPTAINS CHAIR, PATIENT WEIGHT CAPACITY 301 TO 450 POUNDS
K0852	POWER WHEELCHAIR, GROUP 3 VERY HEAVY DUTY, SLING/SOLID SEAT/BACK, PATIENT WEIGHT CAPACITY 451 TO 600 POUNDS
K0853	POWER WHEELCHAIR, GROUP 3 VERY HEAVY DUTY, CAPTAINS CHAIR, PATIENT WEIGHT CAPACITY 451 TO 600 POUNDS
K0854	POWER WHEELCHAIR, GROUP 3 EXTRA HEAVY DUTY, SLING/SOLID SEAT/BACK, PATIENT WEIGHT CAPACITY 601 POUNDS OR MORE
K0855	POWER WHEELCHAIR, GROUP 3 EXTRA HEAVY DUTY, CAPTAINS CHAIR, PATIENT WEIGHT CAPACITY 601 POUNDS OR MORE
K0856	POWER WHEELCHAIR, GROUP 3 STANDARD, SINGLE POWER OPTION, SLING/SOLID SEAT/BACK, PATIENT WEIGHT CAPACITY UP TO AND INCLUDING 300 POUNDS
K0857	POWER WHEELCHAIR, GROUP 3 STANDARD, SINGLE POWER OPTION, CAPTAINS CHAIR, PATIENT WEIGHT CAPACITY UP TO AND INCLUDING 300 POUNDS
K0858	POWER WHEELCHAIR, GROUP 3 HEAVY DUTY, SINGLE POWER OPTION, SLING/SOLID SEAT/BACK, PATIENT WEIGHT 301 TO 450 POUNDS
K0859	POWER WHEELCHAIR, GROUP 3 HEAVY DUTY, SINGLE POWER OPTION, CAPTAINS CHAIR, PATIENT WEIGHT CAPACITY 301 TO 450 POUNDS
K0860	POWER WHEELCHAIR, GROUP 3 VERY HEAVY DUTY, SINGLE POWER OPTION, SLING/SOLID SEAT/BACK, PATIENT WEIGHT CAPACITY 451 TO 600 POUNDS
K0861	POWER WHEELCHAIR, GROUP 3 STANDARD, MULTIPLE POWER OPTION, SLING/SOLID SEAT/BACK, PATIENT WEIGHT CAPACITY UP TO AND INCLUDING 300 POUNDS
K0862	POWER WHEELCHAIR, GROUP 3 HEAVY DUTY, MULTIPLE POWER OPTION, SLING/SOLID SEAT/BACK, PATIENT WEIGHT CAPACITY 301 TO 450 POUNDS
K0863	POWER WHEELCHAIR, GROUP 3 VERY HEAVY DUTY, MULTIPLE POWER OPTION, SLING/SOLID SEAT/BACK, PATIENT WEIGHT CAPACITY 451 TO 600 POUNDS

K0864	POWER WHEELCHAIR, GROUP 3 EXTRA HEAVY DUTY, MULTIPLE POWER OPTION, SLING/SOLID SEAT/BACK, PATIENT WEIGHT CAPACITY 601 POUNDS OR MORE

PRODUCT CATEGORY 4

Mail-Order Diabetic Supplies

A4233 KL	REPLACEMENT BATTERY, ALKALINE (OTHER THAN J CELL), FOR USE WITH MEDICALLY NECESSARY HOME BLOOD GLUCOSE MONITOR OWNED BY PATIENT, EACH
A4234 KL	REPLACEMENT BATTERY, ALKALINE, J CELL, FOR USE WITH MEDICALLY NECESSARY HOME BLOOD GLUCOSE MONITOR OWNED BY PATIENT, EACH
A4235 KL	REPLACEMENT BATTERY, LITHIUM, FOR USE WITH MEDICALLY NECESSARY HOME BLOOD GLUCOSE MONITOR OWNED BY PATIENT, EACH
A4236 KL	REPLACEMENT BATTERY, SILVER OXIDE, FOR USE WITH MEDICALLY NECESSARY HOME BLOOD GLUCOSE MONITOR OWNED BY PATIENT, EACH
A4253 KL	BLOOD GLUCOSE TEST OR REAGENT STRIPS FOR HOME BLOOD GLUCOSE MONITOR, PER 50 STRIPS
A4256 KL	NORMAL, LOW AND HIGH CALIBRATOR SOLUTION / CHIPS
A4258 KL	SPRING-POWERED DEVICE FOR LANCET, EACH
A4259 KL	LANCETS, PER BOX OF 100

PRODUCT CATEGORY 5

Enteral Nutrients, Equipment, and Supplies

B4034	ENTERAL FEEDING SUPPLY KIT; SYRINGE FED, PER DAY
B4035	ENTERAL FEEDING SUPPLY KIT; PUMP FED, PER DAY
B4036	ENTERAL FEEDING SUPPLY KIT; GRAVITY FED, PER DAY
B4081	NASOGASTRIC TUBING WITH STYLET
B4082	NASOGASTRIC TUBING WITHOUT STYLET
B4083	STOMACH TUBE - LEVINE TYPE
B4087	GASTROSTOMY / JEJUNOSTOMY TUBE, ANY MATERIAL, ANY TYPE, (STANDARD), EACH
B4088	GASTROSTOMY / JEJUNOSTOMY TUBE, ANY MATERIAL, ANY TYPE, (LOW PROFILE), EACH
B4149	ENTERAL FORMULA, MANUFACTURED BLENDERIZED NATURAL FOODS WITH INTACT NUTRIENTS, INCLUDES PROTEINS, FATS, CARBOHYDRATES, VITAMINS AND MINERALS, MAY INCLUDE FIBER, ADMINISTERED THROUGH AN ENTERAL FEEDING TUBE, 100 CALORIES = 1 UNIT
B4150	ENTERAL FORMULA, NUTRITIONALLY COMPLETE WITH INTACT NUTRIENTS, INCLUDES PROTEINS, FATS, CARBOHYDRATES, VITAMINS AND MINERALS, MAY INCLUDE FIBER, ADMINISTERED THROUGH AN ENTERAL FEEDING TUBE, 100 CALORIES = 1 UNIT
B4152	ENTERAL FORMULA, NUTRITIONALLY COMPLETE, CALORICALLY DENSE (EQUAL TO OR GREATER THAN 1.5 KCAL/ML) WITH INTACT NUTRIENTS, INCLUDES PROTEINS, FATS, CARBOHYDRATES, VITAMINS AND MINERALS, MAY INCLUDE FIBER, ADMINISTERED THROUGH AN ENTERAL FEEDING TUBE, 100 CALORIES = 1 UNIT
B4153	ENTERAL FORMULA, NUTRITIONALLY COMPLETE, HYDROLYZED PROTEINS (AMINO ACIDS AND PEPTIDE CHAIN), INCLUDES FATS, CARBOHYDRATES, VITAMINS AND MINERALS, MAY INCLUDE FIBER, ADMINISTERED THROUGH AN ENTERAL FEEDING TUBE, 100 CALORIES = 1 UNIT
B4154	ENTERAL FORMULA, NUTRITIONALLY COMPLETE, FOR SPECIAL METABOLIC NEEDS, EXCLUDES INHERITED DISEASE OF METABOLISM, INCLUDES ALTERED COMPOSITION OF PROTEINS, FATS, CARBOHYDRATES, VITAMINS AND/OR MINERALS, MAY INCLUDE FIBER, ADMINISTERED THROUGH AN ENTERAL FEEDING TUBE, 100 CALORIES = 1 UNIT
B4155	ENTERAL FORMULA, NUTRITIONALLY INCOMPLETE/MODULAR NUTRIENTS, INCLUDES SPECIFIC NUTRIENTS, CARBOHYDRATES (E.G. GLUCOSE POLYMERS), PROTEINS/AMINO ACIDS (E.G. GLUTAMINE, ARGININE), FAT (E.G. MEDIUM CHAIN TRIGLYCERIDES) OR COMBINATON, ADMINISTERED THROUGH AN ENTERAL FEEDING TUBE, 100 CALORIES = 1 UNIT NOTE: (SEE J7060, J7070, J7042 FOR SOLUTION CODES FOR OTHER THAN PARENTERAL NUTRITION THERAPY USE)
B9000	ENTERAL NUTRITION INFUSION PUMP - WITHOUT ALARM
B9002	ENTERAL NUTRITION INFUSION PUMP - WITH ALARM
E0776	IV POLE

PRODUCT CATEGORY 6

Continuous Positive Airway Pressure Devices, Respiratory Assist Devices, and Related Supplies and Accessories

A4604	TUBING WITH INTEGRATED HEATING ELEMENT FOR USE WITH POSITIVE AIRWAY PRESSURE DEVICE
A7030	FULL FACE MASK USED WITH POSITIVE AIRWAY PRESSURE DEVICE, EACH
A7031	FACE MASK INTERFACE, REPLACEMENT FOR FULL FACE MASK, EACH
A7032	CUSHION FOR USE ON NASAL MASK INTERFACE, REPLACEMENT ONLY, EACH
A7033	PILLOW FOR USE ON NASAL CANNULA TYPE INTERFACE, REPLACEMENT ONLY, PAIR
A7034	NASAL INTERFACE (MASK OR CANNULA TYPE) USED WITH POSITIVE AIRWAY PRESSURE DEVICE, WITH OR WITHOUT HEAD STRAP
A7035	HEADGEAR USED WITH POSITIVE AIRWAY PRESSURE DEVICE
A7036	CHINSTRAP USED WITH POSITIVE AIRWAY PRESSURE DEVICE
A7037	TUBING USED WITH POSITIVE AIRWAY PRESSURE DEVICE
A7038	FILTER, DISPOSABLE, USED WITH POSITIVE AIRWAY PRESSURE DEVICE
A7039	FILTER, NON DISPOSABLE, USED WITH POSITIVE AIRWAY PRESSURE DEVICE
A7044	ORAL INTERFACE USED WITH POSITIVE AIRWAY PRESSURE DEVICE, EACH
A7045	EXHALATION PORT WITH OR WITHOUT SWIVEL USED WITH ACCESSORIES FOR POSITIVE AIRWAY DEVICES, REPLACEMENT ONLY
A7046	WATER CHAMBER FOR HUMIDIFIER, USED WITH POSITIVE AIRWAY PRESSURE DEVICE, REPLACEMENT, EACH
E0470	RESPIRATORY ASSIST DEVICE, BI-LEVEL PRESSURE CAPABILITY, WITHOUT BACKUP RATE FEATURE, USED WITH NONINVASIVE INTERFACE, E.G., NASAL OR FACIAL MASK (INTERMITTENT ASSIST DEVICE WITH CONTINUOUS POSITIVE AIRWAY PRESSURE DEVICE)
E0471	RESPIRATORY ASSIST DEVICE, BI-LEVEL PRESSURE CAPABILITY, WITH BACK-UP RATE FEATURE, USED WITH NONINVASIVE INTERFACE, E.G., NASAL OR FACIAL MASK (INTERMITTENT ASSIST DEVICE WITH CONTINUOUS POSITIVE AIRWAY PRESSURE DEVICE)
E0472	RESPIRATORY ASSIST DEVICE, BI-LEVEL PRESSURE CAPABILITY, WITH BACKUP RATE FEATURE, USED WITH INVASIVE INTERFACE, E.G., TRACHEOSTOMY TUBE (INTERMITTENT ASSIST DEVICE WITH CONTINUOUS POSITIVE AIRWAY PRESSURE DEVICE)
E0561	HUMIDIFIER, NON-HEATED, USED WITH POSITIVE AIRWAY PRESSURE DEVICE
E0562	HUMIDIFIER, HEATED, USED WITH POSITIVE AIRWAY PRESSURE DEVICE
E0601	CONTINUOUS AIRWAY PRESSURE (CPAP) DEVICE

PRODUCT CATEGORY 7

Hospital Beds and Related Supplies

E0250	HOSPITAL BED, FIXED HEIGHT, WITH ANY TYPE SIDE RAILS, WITH MATTRESS
E0251	HOSPITAL BED, FIXED HEIGHT, WITH ANY TYPE SIDE RAILS, WITHOUT MATTRESS
E0255	HOSPITAL BED, VARIABLE HEIGHT, HI-LO, WITH ANY TYPE SIDE RAILS, WITH MATTRESS
E0256	HOSPITAL BED, VARIABLE HEIGHT, HI-LO, WITH ANY TYPE SIDE RAILS, WITHOUT MATTRESS
E0260	HOSPITAL BED, SEMI-ELECTRIC (HEAD AND FOOT ADJUSTMENT), WITH ANY TYPE SIDE RAILS, WITH MATTRESS
E0261	HOSPITAL BED, SEMI-ELECTRIC (HEAD AND FOOT ADJUSTMENT), WITH ANY TYPE SIDE RAILS, WITHOUT MATTRESS
E0265	HOSPITAL BED, TOTAL ELECTRIC (HEAD, FOOT AND HEIGHT ADJUSTMENTS), WITH ANY TYPE SIDE RAILS, WITH MATTRESS
E0266	HOSPITAL BED, TOTAL ELECTRIC (HEAD, FOOT AND HEIGHT ADJUSTMENTS), WITH ANY TYPE SIDE RAILS, WITHOUT MATTRESS
E0271	MATTRESS, INNERSPRING

E0272	MATTRESS, FOAM RUBBER
E0280	BED CRADLE, ANY TYPE
E0290	HOSPITAL BED, FIXED HEIGHT, WITHOUT SIDE RAILS, WITH MATTRESS
E0291	HOSPITAL BED, FIXED HEIGHT, WITHOUT SIDE RAILS, WITHOUT MATTRESS
E0292	HOSPITAL BED, VARIABLE HEIGHT, HI-LO, WITHOUT SIDE RAILS, WITH MATTRESS
E0293	HOSPITAL BED, VARIABLE HEIGHT, HI-LO, WITHOUT SIDE RAILS, WITHOUT MATTRESS
E0294	HOSPITAL BED, SEMI-ELECTRIC (HEAD AND FOOT ADJUSTMENT), WITHOUT SIDE RAILS, WITH MATTRESS
E0295	HOSPITAL BED, SEMI-ELECTRIC (HEAD AND FOOT ADJUSTMENT), WITHOUT SIDE RAILS, WITHOUT MATTRESS
E0296	HOSPITAL BED, TOTAL ELECTRIC (HEAD, FOOT AND HEIGHT ADJUSTMENTS). WITHOUT SIDE RAILS, WITH MATTRESS
E0297	HOSPITAL BED, TOTAL ELECTRIC (HEAD, FOOT AND HEIGHT ADJUSTMENTS), WITHOUT SIDE RAILS, WITHOUT MATTRESS
E0300	PEDIATRIC CRIB, HOSPITAL GRADE, FULLY ENCLOSED
E0301	HOSPITAL BED, HEAVY DUTY, EXTRA WIDE, WITH WEIGHT CAPACITY GREATER THAN 350 POUNDS, BUT LESS THAN OR EQUAL TO 600 POUNDS, WITH ANY TYPE SIDE RAILS, WITHOUT MATTRESS
E0302	HOSPITAL BED, EXTRA HEAVY DUTY, EXTRA WIDE, WITH WEIGHT CAPACITY GREATER THAN 600 POUNDS, WITH ANY TYPE SIDE RAILS, WITHOUT MATTRESS
E0303	HOSPITAL BED, HEAVY DUTY, EXTRA WIDE, WITH WEIGHT CAPACITY GREATER THAN 350 POUNDS, BUT LESS THAN OR EQUAL TO 600 POUNDS, WITH ANY TYPE SIDE RAILS, WITH MATTRESS
E0304	HOSPITAL BED, EXTRA HEAVY DUTY, EXTRA WIDE, WITH WEIGHT CAPACITY GREATER THAN 600 POUNDS, WITH ANY TYPE SIDE RAILS, WITH MATTRESS
E0305	BED SIDE RAILS, HALF LENGTH
E0310	BED SIDE RAILS, FULL LENGTH
E0316	SAFETY ENCLOSURE FRAME/CANOPY FOR USE WITH HOSPITAL BED, ANY TYPE
E0910	TRAPEZE BARS, A/K/A PATIENT HELPER, ATTACHED TO BED, WITH GRAB BAR
E0911	TRAPEZE BAR, HEAVY DUTY, FOR PATIENT WEIGHT CAPACITY GREATER THAN 250 POUNDS, ATTACHED TO BED, WITH GRAB BAR
E0912	TRAPEZE BAR, HEAVY DUTY, FOR PATIENT WEIGHT CAPACITY GREATER THAN 250 POUNDS, FREE STANDING, COMPLETE WITH GRAB BAR
E0940	TRAPEZE BAR, FREE STANDING, COMPLETE WITH GRAB BAR

PRODUCT CATEGORY 8

Negative Pressure Wound Therapy Pumps and Related Supplies and Accessories

A6550	WOUND CARE SET, FOR NEGATIVE PRESSURE WOUND THERAPY ELECTRICAL PUMP, INCLUDES ALL SUPPLIES AND ACCESSORIES
A7000	CANISTER, DISPOSABLE, USED WITH SUCTION PUMP, EACH
E2402	NEGATIVE PRESSURE WOUND THERAPY ELECTRICAL PUMP, STATIONARY OR PORTABLE

PRODUCT CATEGORY 9

Walkers and Related Accessories

A4636	REPLACEMENT, HANDGRIP, CANE, CRUTCH, OR WALKER, EACH
A4637	REPLACEMENT, TIP, CANE, CRUTCH, WALKER, EACH.
E0130	WALKER, RIGID (PICKUP), ADJUSTABLE OR FIXED HEIGHT
E0135	WALKER, FOLDING (PICKUP), ADJUSTABLE OR FIXED HEIGHT
E0140	WALKER, WITH TRUNK SUPPORT, ADJUSTABLE OR FIXED HEIGHT, ANY TYPE
E0141	WALKER, RIGID, WHEELED, ADJUSTABLE OR FIXED HEIGHT
E0143	WALKER, FOLDING, WHEELED, ADJUSTABLE OR FIXED HEIGHT
E0144	WALKER, ENCLOSED, FOUR SIDED FRAMED, RIGID OR FOLDING, WHEELED WITH POSTERIOR SEAT
E0147	WALKER, HEAVY DUTY, MULTIPLE BRAKING SYSTEM, VARIABLE WHEEL RESISTANCE

E0148	WALKER, HEAVY DUTY, WITHOUT WHEELS, RIGID OR FOLDING, ANY TYPE, EACH
E0149	WALKER, HEAVY DUTY, WHEELED, RIGID OR FOLDING, ANY TYPE
E0154	PLATFORM ATTACHMENT, WALKER, EACH
E0155	WHEEL ATTACHMENT, RIGID PICK-UP WALKER, PER PAIR
E0156	SEAT ATTACHMENT, WALKER
E0157	CRUTCH ATTACHMENT, WALKER, EACH
E0158	LEG EXTENSIONS FOR WALKER, PER SET OF FOUR (4)
E0159	BRAKE ATTACHMENT FOR WHEELED WALKER, REPLACEMENT, EACH

PRODUCT CATEGORY 10

Support Surfaces

E0193	POWERED AIR FLOTATION BED (LOW AIR LOSS THERAPY)
E0277	POWERED PRESSURE-REDUCING AIR MATTRESS
E0371	NONPOWERED ADVANCED PRESSURE REDUCING OVERLAY FOR MATTRESS, STANDARD MATTRESS LENGTH AND WIDTH
E0372	POWERED AIR OVERLAY FOR MATTRESS, STANDARD MATTRESS LENGTH AND WIDTH
E0373	NONPOWERED ADVANCED PRESSURE REDUCING MATTRESS

100-4, 32, 11.1
Electrical Stimulation

A. Coding Applicable to Carriers & Fiscal Intermediaries (FIs)

Effective April 1, 2003, a National Coverage Decision was made to allow for Medicare coverage of Electrical Stimulation for the treatment of certain types of wounds. The type of wounds covered are chronic Stage III or Stage IV pressure ulcers, arterial ulcers, diabetic ulcers and venous stasis ulcers. All other uses of electrical stimulation for the treatment of wounds are not covered by Medicare. Electrical stimulation will not be covered as an initial treatment modality.

The use of electrical stimulation will only be covered after appropriate standard wound care has been tried for at least 30 days and there are no measurable signs of healing. If electrical stimulation is being used, wounds must be evaluated periodically by the treating physician but no less than every 30 days by a physician. Continued treatment with electrical stimulation is not covered if measurable signs of healing have not been demonstrated within any 30-day period of treatment. Additionally, electrical stimulation must be discontinued when the wound demonstrates a 100% epithelialzed wound bed.

Coverage policy can be found in Pub. 100-03, Medicare National Coverage Determinations Manual, Chapter 1, Section 270.1 (http://www.cms.hhs.gov/manuals/103_cov_determ/ncd103index.asp)

The applicable Healthcare Common Procedure Coding System (HCPCS) code for Electrical Stimulation and the covered effective date is as follows:

HCPCS	Definition	Effective Date
G0281	Electrical Stimulation, (unattended), to one or more areas for chronic Stage III and Stage IV pressure ulcers, arterial ulcers, diabetic ulcers and venous stasis ulcers not demonstrating measurable signs of healing after 30 days of conventional care as part of a therapy plan of care.	04/01/2003

Medicare will not cover the device used for the electrical stimulation for the treatment of wounds. However, Medicare will cover the service. Unsupervised home use of electrical stimulation will not be covered.

B. FI Billing Instructions

The applicable types of bills acceptable when billing for electrical stimulation services are 12X, 13X, 22X, 23X, 71X, 73X, 74X, 75X, and 85X. Chapter 25 of this manual provides general billing instructions that must be followed for bills submitted to FIs. FIs pay for electrical stimulation services under the Medicare Physician Fee Schedule for a hospital, Comprehensive Outpatient Rehabilitation Facility (CORF), Outpatient Rehabilitation Facility (ORF), Outpatient Physical Therapy (OPT) and Skilled Nursing Facility (SNF).

Payment methodology for independent Rural Health Clinic (RHC), provider-based RHCs, free-standing Federally Qualified Health Center (FQHC) and provider based FQHCs is made under the all-inclusive rate for the visit furnished to the RHC/FQHC patient to obtain the therapy service. Only one payment will be made for the visit furnished to the

RHC/FQHC patient to obtain the therapy service. As of April 1, 2005, RHCs/FQHCs are no longer required to report HCPCS codes when billing for these therapy services.

Payment Methodology for a Critical Access Hospital (CAH) is on a reasonable cost basis unless the CAH has elected the Optional Method and then the FI pays115% of the MPFS amount for the professional component of the HCPCS code in addition to the technical component.

In addition, the following revenues code must be used in conjunction with the HCPCS code identified:

Revenue Code	Description
420	Physical Therapy
430	Occupational Therapy
520	Federal Qualified Health Center *
521	Rural Health Center *
977, 978	Critical Access Hospital- method II CAH professional services only

* NOTE: As of April 1, 2005, RHCs/FQHCs are no longer required to report HCPCS codes when billing for these therapy services.

C. Carrier Claims

Carriers pay for Electrical Stimulation services billed with HCPCS codes G0281 based on the MPFS. Claims for Electrical Stimulation services must be billed on Form CMS-1500 or the electronic equivalent following instructions in chapter 12 of this manual (http://www.cms.hhs.gov/manuals/104_claims/clm104c12.pdf).

D. Coinsurance and Deductible

The Medicare contractor shall apply coinsurance and deductible to payments for these therapy services except for services billed to the FI by FQHCs. For FQHCs, only co-insurance applies.

100-4, 32, 11.2

Electromagnetic Therapy

A. HCPCS Coding Applicable to Carriers & Fiscal Intermediaries (FIs)

Effective July 1, 2004, a National Coverage Decision was made to allow for Medicare coverage of electromagnetic therapy for the treatment of certain types of wounds. The type of wounds covered are chronic Stage III or Stage IV pressure ulcers, arterial ulcers, diabetic ulcers and venous stasis ulcers. All other uses of electromagnetic therapy for the treatment of wounds are not covered by Medicare. Electromagnetic therapy will not be covered as an initial treatment modality.

The use of electromagnetic therapy will only be covered after appropriate standard wound care has been tried for at least 30 days and there are no measurable signs of healing. If electromagnetic therapy is being used, wounds must be evaluated periodically by the treating physician but no less than every 30 days by a physician. Continued treatment with electromagnetic therapy is not covered if measurable signs of healing have not been demonstrated within any 30-day period of treatment. Additionally, electromagnetic therapy must be discontinued when the wound demonstrates a 100% epithelialzed wound bed.

Coverage policy can be found in Pub. 100-03, Medicare National Coverage Determinations Manual, Chapter 1, Section 270.1. (www.cms.hhs.gov/manuals/103_cov_determ/ncd103index.asp)

The applicable Healthcare Common Procedure Coding System (HCPCS) code for Electrical Stimulation and the covered effective date is as follows:

HCPCS	Definition	Effective Date
G0329	ElectromagneticTherapy, to one or more areas for chronic Stage III and Stage IV pressure ulcers, arterial ulcers, diabetic ulcers and venous stasis ulcers not demonstrating measurable signs of healing after 30 days of conventional care as part of a therapy plan of care.	07/01/2004

Medicare will not cover the device used for the electromagnetic therapy for the treatment of wounds. However, Medicare will cover the service. Unsupervised home use of electromagnetic therapy will not be covered.

B. FI Billing Instructions

The applicable types of bills acceptable when billing for electromagnetic therapy services are 12X, 13X, 22X, 23X, 71X, 73X, 74X, 75X, and 85X. Chapter 25 of this manual provides general billing instructions that must be followed for bills submitted to FIs. FIs pay for electromagnetic therapy services under the Medicare Physician Fee Schedule for a hospital, CORF, ORF, and SNF.

Payment methodology for independent (RHC), provider-based RHCs, free-standing FQHC and provider based FQHCs is made under the all-inclusive rate for the visit furnished to the RHC/FQHC patient to obtain the therapy service. Only one payment will be made for the visit furnished to the

RHC/FQHC patient to obtain the therapy service. As of April 1, 2005, RHCs/FQHCs are no longer required to report HCPCS codes when billing for the therapy service.

Payment Methodology for a CAH is payment on a reasonable cost basis unless the CAH has elected the Optional Method and then the FI pays pay 115% of the MPFS amount for the professional component of the HCPCS code in addition to the technical component.

In addition, the following revenues code must be used in conjunction with the HCPCS code identified:

Revenue Code	Description
420	Physical Therapy
430	Occupational Therapy
520	Federal Qualified Health Center *
521	Rural Health Center *
977, 978	Critical Access Hospital- method II CAH professional services only

* NOTE: As of April 1, 2005, RHCs/FQHCs are no longer required to report HCPCS codes when billing for the therapy service.

C. Carrier Claims

Carriers pay for Electromagnetic Therapy services billed with HCPCS codes G0329 based on the MPFS. Claims for electromagnetic therapy services must be billed on Form CMS-1500 or the electronic equivalent following instructions in chapter 12 of this manual (www.cms.hhs.gov/manuals/104_claims/clm104index.asp).

Payment information for HCPCS code G0329 will be added to the July 2004 update of the Medicare Physician Fee Schedule Database (MPFSD).

D. Coinsurance and Deductible

The Medicare contractor shall apply coinsurance and deductible to payments for electromagnetic therapy services except for services billed to the FI by FQHCs. For FQHCs only co-insurance applies.

100-4, 32, 11.3.1

Policy

Effective for claims with dates of service on or after August 2, 2012, contractors shall accept and pay for autologous platelet-rich plasma (PRP) only for the treatment of chronic non-healing diabetic, venous and/or pressure wounds only in the context of an approved clinical study in accordance with the coverage criteria outlined in Pub 100-03, chapter 1, section 270.3, of the NCD Manual.

100-4, 32, 11.3.2

HCPCS Code

11.3.2—Healthcare Common Procedure Coding System (HCPCS) Codes and Diagnosis Coding

Effective for claims with dates of service on or after August 2, 2012 Medicare providers shall report HCPCS code G0460 for PRP services.

ICD-9 Diagnosis coding

For claims of service with dates of service on or after August 2, 2012, PRP, for the treatment of chronic non-healing diabetic, venous and/or pressure wounds only in the context of an approved clinical study must be billed using the following ICD-9 codes:

- =V70.7—ICD-9 code from the approved list of diagnosis codes maintained by the Medicare contractor

Additional billing requirement:

The following modifier and condition code shall be reported when billing for PRP services only in the context of an approved clinical study:

- Q0 modifier
- Condition code 30 (for institutional claims only)
- Value Code D4 with an 8-digit clinical trial number. NOTE: This is optional and only applies to Institutional claims.

100-4, 32, 11.3.3

The applicable TOBs for PRP services are: 12X, 13X, 22X, 23X, 71X, 75X, 77X, and 85X.

100-4, 32, 11.3.4

Payment Method

Payment for PRP services is as follows:

- Hospital outpatient departments TOBs 12X and 13X — based on OPPS
- SNFs TOBs 22X and 23X — based on MPFS

- TOB 71X — based on all-inclusive rate — TOB 75X — based on MPFS
- TOB 77X — based on all-inclusive rate
- TOB 85X — based on reasonable cost
- CAHs TOB 85X and revenue codes 096X, 097X, or 098X — based on MPFS

Contractors shall pay for PRP services for hospitals in Maryland under the jurisdiction of the Health Services Cost Review Commission (HSCRC) on an outpatient basis, TOB 13X, in accordance with the terms of the Maryland waiver.

100-4, 32, 11.3.5

Place of Service (POS) for Professional Claims
Effective for claims with dates of service on or after August 2, 2012, place of service codes 11, 22, and 49 shall be used for PRP services.

100-4, 32, 11.3.6

Medicare Summary Notices (MSNs), Remittance Advice Remark Codes (RARCs), Claim Adjustment Reason Codes (CARCs) and Group Codes
Contractors shall use the following messages when returning to provider/returning as unprocessable claims when required information is not included on claims for autologous platelet-rich plasma (PRP) only for the treatment of chronic non-healing diabetic, venous and/or pressure wounds only in the context of an approved clinical study:

CARC 16 - Claim/service lacks information which is needed for adjudication.

RARC M16 - Alert: See our Web site, mailings, or bulletins for more details concerning this policy/procedure/decision.

RARC MA130 — Your claim contains incomplete and/or invalid information, and no appeal rights are afforded because the claim is unprocessable. Please submit a new claim with the complete/correct information.

Contractors shall deny claims for RPR services, HCPCS code G0460, when services are provided on other than TOBs 12X, 13X, 22X, 23X, 71X, 75X, 77X, and 85X using:

MSN 21.25: "This service was denied because Medicare only covers this service in certain settings."

Spanish Version: "El servicio fue denegado porque Medicare solamente lo cubre en ciertas situaciones."

CARC 58: "Treatment was deemed by the payer to have been rendered in an inappropriate or invalid place of service. NOTE: Refer to the 832 Healthcare Policy Identification Segment (loop 2110 Service payment Information REF), if present.

RARC N428: "Service/procedure not covered when performed in this place of service."

Group Code — CO (Contractual Obligation)

Contractors shall deny claims for PRP services for POS other than 11, 22, or 49 using the following:

MSN 21.25: "This service was denied because Medicare only covers this service in certain settings."

Spanish Version: "El servicio fue denegado porque Medicare solamente lo cubre en ciertas situaciones."

CARC 58: "Treatment was deemed by the payer to have been rendered in an inappropriate or invalid place of service. NOTE; Refer to the 832 Healthcare Policy Identification Segment (loop 2110 Service payment Information REF), if present.

RARC N428: "Service/procedure not covered when performed in this place of service."

Group Code CO (Contractual Obligation)

100-4, 32, 30.1
Hyperbaric Oxygen Therapy is a modality in which the entire body is exposed to oxygen under increased atmospheric pressure. Effective April 1, 2003, a National Coverage Decision expanded the use of HBO therapy to include coverage for the treatment of diabetic wounds of the lower extremities. For specific coverage criteria for HBO Therapy, refer to the National Coverage Determinations Manual, chapter 1, section 20.29.

NOTE: Topical application of oxygen does not meet the definition of HBO therapy as stated above. Also, its clinical efficacy has not been established. Therefore, no Medicare reimbursement may be made for the topical application of oxygen.

I. Billing Requirements for Intermediaries
Claims for HBO therapy should be submitted on Form CMS-1450 or its electronic equivalent.

a. Applicable Bill Types
The applicable hospital bill types are 11X, 13X and 85X.

b. Procedural Coding
- 99183—Physician attendance and supervision of hyperbaric oxygen therapy, per session.
- C1300—Hyperbaric oxygen under pressure, full body chamber, per 30-minute interval.

NOTE: Code C1300 is not available for use other than in a hospital outpatient department. In skilled nursing facilities (SNFs), HBO therapy is part of the SNF PPS payment for beneficiaries in covered Part A stays.

For hospital inpatients and critical access hospitals (CAHs) not electing Method I, HBO therapy is reported under revenue code 940 without any HCPCS code. For inpatient services, show ICD-9-CM procedure code 93.59.

For CAHs electing Method I, HBO therapy is reported under revenue code 940 along with HCPCS code 99183.

c. Payment Requirements for Intermediaries
Payment is as follows:

Intermediary payment is allowed for HBO therapy for diabetic wounds of the lower extremities when performed as a physician service in a hospital outpatient setting and for inpatients. Payment is allowed for claims with valid diagnostic ICD-9 codes as shown above with dates of service on or after April 1, 2003. Those claims with invalid codes should be denied as not medically necessary.

For hospitals, payment will be based upon the Ambulatory Payment Classification (APC) or the inpatient Diagnosis Related Group (DRG). Deductible and coinsurance apply.

Payment to Critical Access Hospitals (electing Method I) is made under cost reimbursement. For Critical Access Hospitals electing Method II, the technical component is paid under cost reimbursement and the professional component is paid under the Physician Fee Schedule.

NOTE: Information regarding the form locator numbers that correspond to these data element names and a table to crosswalk UB-04 form locators to the 837 transaction is found in Chapter 25.

II. Carrier Billing Requirements
Claims for this service should be submitted on Form CMS-1500 or its electronic equivalent.

The following HCPCS code applies:

- 99183—Physician attendance and supervision of hyperbaric oxygen therapy, per session.

a. Payment Requirements for Carriers
Payment and pricing information will occur through updates to the Medicare Physician Fee Schedule Database (MPFSDB). Pay for this service on the basis of the MPFSDB. Deductible and coinsurance apply. Claims from physicians or other practitioners where assignment was not taken, are subject to the Medicare limiting charge.

III. Medicare Summary Notices (MSNs)
Use the following MSN Messages where appropriate:

In situations where the claim is being denied on the basis that the condition does not meet our coverage requirements, use one of the following MSN Messages:

"Medicare does not pay for this item or service for this condition." (MSN Message 16.48)

The Spanish version of the MSN message should read:

"Medicare no paga por este articulo o servicio para esta afeccion."

In situations where, based on the above utilization policy, medical review of the claim results in a determination that the service is not medically necessary, use the following MSN message:

"The information provided does not support the need for this service or item." (MSN Message 15.4)

The Spanish version of the MSN message should read:

"La informacion proporcionada no confirma la necesidad para este servicio o articulo."

IV. Remittance Advice Notices
Use appropriate existing remittance advice and reason codes at the line level to express the specific reason if you deny payment for HBO therapy for the treatment of diabetic wounds of lower extremities

100-4, 32, 40.1

Coverage Requirements
Effective January 1, 2002, sacral nerve stimulation is covered for the treatment of urinary urge incontinence, urgency-frequency syndrome and urinary retention. Sacral nerve stimulation involves both a temporary test stimulation to determine if an implantable stimulator would be effective and a permanent implantation in appropriate candidates. Both the test and the permanent implantation are covered.

The following limitations for coverage apply to all indications:

- Patient must be refractory to conventional therapy (documented behavioral, pharmacologic and/or surgical corrective therapy) and be an appropriate surgical candidate such that implantation with anesthesia can occur.

- Patients with stress incontinence, urinary obstruction, and specific neurologic diseases (e.g., diabetes with peripheral nerve involvement) that are associated with secondary manifestations of the above three indications are excluded.

- Patient must have had a successful test stimulation in order to support subsequent implantation. Before a patient is eligible for permanent implantation, he/she must demonstrate a 50% or greater improvement through test stimulation. Improvement is measured through voiding diaries.

- Patient must be able to demonstrate adequate ability to record voiding diary data such that clinical results of the implant procedure can be properly evaluated.

100-4, 32, 50

Deep Brain Stimulation for Essential Tremor and Parkinson's Disease

Deep brain stimulation (DBS) refers to high-frequency electrical stimulation of anatomic regions deep within the brain utilizing neurosurgically implanted electrodes. These DBS electrodes are stereotactically placed within targeted nuclei on one (unilateral) or both (bilateral) sides of the brain. There are currently three targets for DBS -- the thalamic ventralis intermedius nucleus (VIM), subthalamic nucleus (STN) and globus pallidus interna (GPi).

Essential tremor (ET) is a progressive, disabling tremor most often affecting the hands. ET may also affect the head, voice and legs. The precise pathogenesis of ET is unknown. While it may start at any age, ET usually peaks within the second and sixth decades. Beta-adrenergic blockers and anticonvulsant medications are usually the first line treatments for reducing the severity of tremor. Many patients, however, do not adequately respond or cannot tolerate these medications. In these medically refractory ET patients, thalamic VIM DBS may be helpful for symptomatic relief of tremor.

Parkinson's disease (PD) is an age-related progressive neurodegenerative disorder involving the loss of dopaminergic cells in the substantia nigra of the midbrain. The disease is characterized by tremor, rigidity, bradykinesia and progressive postural instability. Dopaminergic medication is typically used as a first line treatment for reducing the primary symptoms of PD. However, after prolonged use, medication can become less effective and can produce significant adverse events such as dyskinesias and other motor function complications. For patients who become unresponsive to medical treatments and/or have intolerable side effects from medications, DBS for symptom relief may be considere

100-4, 32, 60.4.1

Allowable Covered Diagnosis Codes

For services furnished on or after July 1, 2002, the applicable ICD-9-CM diagnosis code for this benefit is V43.3, organ or tissue replaced by other means; heart valve.

For services furnished on or after March 19, 2008, the applicable ICD-9-CM diagnosis codes for this benefit are:

V43.3 (organ or tissue replaced by other means; heart valve),

289.81 (primary hypercoagulable state),

451.0-451.9 (includes 451.11, 451.19, 451.2, 451.80-451.84, 451.89) (phlebitis & thrombophlebitis),

453.0-453.3 (other venous embolism & thrombosis),

453.40-453.49 (includes 453.40-453.42, 453.8-453.9) (venous embolism and thrombosis of the deep vessels of the lower extremity, and other specified veins/unspecified sites)

415.11-415.12, 415.19 (pulmonary embolism & infarction) or,

427.31 (atrial fibrillation (established) (paroxysmal)).

100-4, 32, 60.5.2

Applicable Diagnosis Codes for Carriers

For services furnished on or after July 1, 2002, the applicable ICD-9-CM diagnosis code for this benefit is V43.3, organ or tissue replaced by other means; heart valve.

For services furnished on or after March 19, 2008, the applicable ICD-9-CM diagnosis codes for this benefit are:

- V43.3 (organ or tissue replaced by other means; heart valve),

- 289.81 (primary hypercoagulable state),

- 451.0-451.9 (includes 451.11, 451.19, 451.2, 451.80-451.84, 451.89) (phlebitis & thrombophlebitis),

- 453.0-453.3 (other venous embolism & thrombosis),

- 453.40-453.49 (includes 453.40-453.42, 453.8-453.9) (venous embolism and thrombosis of the deep vessels of the lower extremity, and other specified veins/unspecified sites)

- 415.11-415.12, 415.19 (pulmonary embolism & infarction) or,

- 427.31 (atrial fibrillation (established) (paroxysmal)).

100-4, 32, 80

Billing of the Diagnosis and Treatment of Peripheral Neuropathy with Loss of Protective Sensation in People with Diabetes

Coverage Requirements - Peripheral neuropathy is the most common factor leading to amputation in people with diabetes. In diabetes, peripheral neuropathy is an anatomically diffuse process primarily affecting sensory and autonomic fibers; however, distal motor findings may be present in advanced cases. Long nerves are affected first, with symptoms typically beginning insidiously in the toes and then advancing proximally. This leads to loss of protective sensation (LOPS), whereby a person is unable to feel minor trauma from mechanical, thermal, or chemical sources. When foot lesions are present, the reduction in autonomic nerve functions may also inhibit wound healing.

Peripheral neuropathy with LOPS, secondary to diabetes, is a localized illness of the feet and falls within the regulation's exception to the general exclusionary rule (see 42 C.F.R. Sec.411.15(l)(l)(i)). Foot exams for people with diabetic peripheral neuropathy with LOPS are reasonable and necessary to allow for early intervention in serious complications that typically afflict diabetics with the disease.

Effective for services furnished on or after July 1, 2002, Medicare covers, as a physician service, an evaluation (examination and treatment) of the feet no more often than every 6 months for individuals with a documented diagnosis of diabetic sensory neuropathy and LOPS, as long as the beneficiary has not seen a foot care specialist for some other reason in the interim. LOPS shall be diagnosed through sensory testing with the 5.07 monofilament using established guidelines, such as those developed by the National Institute of Diabetes and Digestive and Kidney Diseases guidelines. Five sites should be tested on the plantar surface of each foot, according to the National Institute of Diabetes and Digestive and Kidney Diseases guidelines. The areas must be tested randomly since the loss of protective sensation may be patchy in distribution, and the patient may get clues if the test is done rhythmically. Heavily callused areas should be avoided. As suggested by the American Podiatric Medicine Association, an absence of sensation at two or more sites out of 5 tested on either foot when tested with the 5.07 Semmes-Weinstein monofilament must be present and documented to diagnose peripheral neuropathy with loss of protective sensation.

100-4, 32, 80.2

Applicable HCPCS Codes

G0245 - Initial physician evaluation and management of a diabetic patient with diabetic sensory neuropathy resulting in a loss of protective sensation (LOPS) which must include:

1. The diagnosis of LOPS;

2. A patient history;

3. A physical examination that consists of at least the following elements:

(a) visual inspection of the forefoot, hindfoot, and toe web spaces,

(b) evaluation of a protective sensation,

(c) evaluation of foot structure and biomechanics,

(d) evaluation of vascular status and skin integrity,

(e) evaluation and recommendation of footwear, and

4. Patient education.

G0246 - Follow-up physician evaluation and management of a diabetic patient with diabetic sensory neuropathy resulting in a loss of protective sensation (LOPS) to include at least the following:

1. a patient history;

2. a physical examination that includes:

(a) visual inspection of the forefoot, hindfoot, and toe web spaces,

(b) evaluation of protective sensation,

(c) evaluation of foot structure and biomechanics,

(d) evaluation of vascular status and skin integrity,

(e) evaluation and recommendation of footwear, and

3. patient education.

G0247 - Routine foot care by a physician of a diabetic patient with diabetic sensory neuropathy resulting in a LOPS to include if present, at least the following:

(1) local care of superficial (i.e., superficial to muscle and fascia) wounds;

(2) debridement of corns and calluses; and

(3) trimming and debridement of nails.

NOTE: Code G0247 must be billed on the same date of service with either G0245 or G0246 in order to be considered for payment.

The short descriptors for the above HCPCS codes are as follows:

G0245 - INITIAL FOOT EXAM PTLOPS

G0246 - FOLLOWUP EVAL OF FOOT PT LOP

G0247 - ROUTINE FOOTCARE PT W LOPS

100-4, 32, 80.8

CWF Utilization Edits

Edit 1 - Should CWF receive a claim from an FI for G0245 or G0246 and a second claim from a contractor for either G0245 or G0246 (or vice versa) and they are different dates of service and less than 6 months apart, the second claim will reject. CWF will edit to allow G0245 or G0246 to be paid no more than every 6 months for a particular beneficiary, regardless of who furnished the service. If G0245 has been paid, regardless of whether it was posted as a facility or professional claim, it must be 6 months before G0245 can be paid again or G0246 can be paid. If G0246 has been paid, regardless of whether it was posted as a facility or professional claim, it must be 6 months before G0246 can be paid again or G0245 can be paid. CWF will not impose limits on how many times each code can be paid for a beneficiary as long as there has been 6 months between each service.

The CWF will return a specific reject code for this edit to the contractors and FIs that will be identified in the CWF documentation. Based on the CWF reject code, the contractors and FIs must deny the claims and return the following messages:

MSN 18.4 -- This service is being denied because it has not been __ months since your last examination of this kind (NOTE: Insert 6 as the appropriate number of months.)

RA claim adjustment reason code 96 - Non-covered charges, along with remark code M86 - Service denied because payment already made for same/similar procedure within set time frame.

Edit 2

The CWF will edit to allow G0247 to pay only if either G0245 or G0246 has been submitted and accepted as payable on the same date of service. CWF will return a specific reject code for this edit to the contractors and FIs that will be identified in the CWF documentation. Based on this reject code, contractors and FIs will deny the claims and return the following messages:

MSN 21.21 - This service was denied because Medicare only covers this service under certain circumstances.

RA claim adjustment reason code 107 - The related or qualifying claim/service was not identified on this claim.

Edit 3

Once a beneficiary's condition has progressed to the point where routine foot care becomes a covered service, payment will no longer be made for LOPS evaluation and management services. Those services would be considered to be included in the regular exams and treatments afforded to the beneficiary on a routine basis. The physician or provider must then just bill the routine foot care codes, per Pub 100-02, Chapter 15, Sec.290.

The CWF will edit to reject LOPS codes G0245, G0246, and/or G0247 when on the beneficiary's record it shows that one of the following routine foot care codes were billed and paid within the prior 6 months: 11055, 11056, 11057, 11719, 11720, and/or 11721.

The CWF will return a specific reject code for this edit to the contractors and FIs that will be identified in the CWF documentation. Based on the CWF reject code, the contractors and FIs must deny the claims and return the following messages:

MSN 21.21 - This service was denied because Medicare only covers this service under certain circumstances.

The RA claim adjustment reason code 96 - Non-covered charges, along with remark code M86 - Service denied because payment already made for same/similar procedure within set time frame.

100-4, 32, 100

Billing Requirements for Expanded Coverage of Cochlear Implantation

Effective for dates of services on and after April 4, 2005, the Centers for Medicare & Medicaid Services (CMS) has expanded the coverage for cochlear implantation to cover moderate-to-profound hearing loss in individuals with hearing test scores equal to or less than 40% correct in the best aided listening condition on tape-recorded tests of open-set sentence recognition and who demonstrate limited benefit from amplification. (See Publication 100-03, chapter 1, section 50.3, for specific coverage criteria).

In addition CMS is covering cochlear implantation for individuals with open-set sentence recognition test scores of greater than 40% to less than or equal to 60% correct but only when the provider is participating in, and patients are enrolled in, either:

- A Food and Drug Administration (FDA)-approved category B investigational device exemption (IDE) clinical trial; or

- A trial under the CMS clinical trial policy (see Pub. 100-03, section 310.1); or

- A prospective, controlled comparative trial approved by CMS as consistent with the evidentiary requirements for national coverage analyses and meeting specific quality standards.

100-4, 32, 110.5

DMERC Billing Instructions

Effective for dates of service on or after April 27, 2005, DMERCs shall allow payment for ultrasonic osteogenic stimulators with the following HCPCS codes:

- E0760 for low intensity ultrasound (include modifier "KF"), or;

- E1399 for other ultrasound stimulation (include modifier "KF")

100-4, 32, 120.1

Payment for Services and Supplies

For an IOL inserted following removal of a cataract in a hospital, on either an outpatient or inpatient basis, that is paid under the hospital Outpatient Prospective Payment System (OPPS) or the Inpatient Prospective Payment System (IPPS), respectively; or in a Medicare-approved ambulatory surgical center (ASC) that is paid under the ASC fee schedule:

Medicare does not make separate payment to the hospital or ASC for an IOL inserted subsequent to extraction of a cataract. Payment for the IOL is packaged into the payment for the surgical cataract extraction/lens replacement procedure.

Any person or ASC, who presents or causes to be presented a bill or request for payment for an IOL inserted during or subsequent to cataract surgery for which payment is made under the ASC fee schedule, is subject to a civil money penalty.

For a P-C IOL or A-C IOL inserted subsequent to removal of a cataract in a hospital, on either an outpatient or inpatient basis, that is paid under the OPPS or the IPPS, respectively; or in a Medicare-approved ASC that is paid under the ASC fee schedule:

The facility shall bill for the removal of a cataract with insertion of a conventional IOL, regardless of whether a conventional, P-C IOL, or A-C IOL is inserted. When a beneficiary receives a P-C or A-C IOL following removal of a cataract, hospitals and ASCs shall report the same CPT code that is used to report removal of a cataract with insertion of a conventional IOL. Physicians, hospitals and ASCs may also report an additional HCPCS code, V2788, to indicate any additional charges that accrue when a P-C IOL or A-C IOL is inserted in lieu of a conventional IOL until Janaury 1, 2008. Effective for A-C IOL insertion services on or after January 1, 2008, physicians, hospitals and ASCs should use V2787 to report any additional charges that accrue. On or after January 1, 2008, physicians, hospitals, and ASCs should continue to report HCPCS code V2788 to indicate any additional charges that accrue for insertion of a P-C IOL. See Section 120.2 for coding guidelines.

There is no Medicare benefit category that allows payment of facility charges for services and supplies required to insert and adjust a P-C or A-C IOL following removal of a cataract that exceed the facility charges for services and supplies required for the insertion and adjustment of a conventional IOL.

There is no Medicare benefit category that allows payment of facility charges for subsequent treatments, services and supplies required to examine and monitor the beneficiary who receives a P-C or A-C IOL following removal of a cataract that exceeds the facility charges for subsequent treatments, services and supplies required to examine and monitor a beneficiary after cataract surgery followed by insertion of a conventional IOL.

A - For a P-C IOL or A-C IOL inserted in a physician's office

A physician shall bill for a conventional IOL, regardless of a whether a conventional, P-C IOL, or A-C IOL is inserted (see section 120.2, General Billing Requirements)

There is no Medicare benefit category that allows payment of physician charges for services and supplies required to insert and adjust a P-C or A-C IOL following removal of a cataract that exceed the physician charges for services and supplies for the insertion and adjustment of a conventional IOL.

There is no Medicare benefit category that allows payment of physician charges for subsequent treatments, service and supplies required to examine and monitor a beneficiary following removal of a cataract with insertion of a P-C or A-C IOL that exceed physician charges for services and supplies to examine and monitor a beneficiary following removal of a cataract with insertion of a conventional IOL.

B - For a P-C IOL or A-C IOL inserted in a hospital

A physician may not bill Medicare for a P-C or A-C IOL inserted during a cataract procedure performed in a hospital setting because the payment for the lens is included in the payment made to the facility for the surgical procedure.

There is no Medicare benefit category that allows payment of physician charges for services and supplies required to insert and adjust a P-C or A-C IOL following removal of a cataract that exceed the physician charges for services and supplies required for the insertion of a conventional IOL.

C - For a P-C IOL or A-C IOL inserted in an Ambulatory Surgical Center

Refer to Chapter 14, Section 40.3 for complete guidance on payment for P-C IOL or A-C IOL in Ambulatory Surgical Centers.

100-4, 32, 120.2

Coding and General Billing Requirements

Physicians and hospitals must report one of the following Current Procedural Terminology (CPT) codes on the claim:

- 66982 - Extracapsular cataract removal with insertion of intraocular lens prosthesis (one stage procedure), manual or mechanical technique (e.g., irrigation and aspiration or phacoemulsification), complex requiring devices or techniques not generally used in routine cataract surgery (e.g., iris expansion device, suture support for intraocular lens, or primary posterior capsulorrhexis) or performed on patients in the amblyogenic development stage.

- 66983 - Intracapsular cataract with insertion of intraocular lens prosthesis (one stage procedure)

- 66984 - Extracapsular cataract removal with insertion of intraocular lens prosthesis (one stage procedure), manual or mechanical technique (e.g., irrigation and aspiration or phacoemulsification)

- 66985 - Insertion of intraocular lens prosthesis (secondary implant), not associated with concurrent cataract extraction

- 66986 - Exchange of intraocular lens

In addition, physicians inserting a P-C IOL or A-C IOL in an office setting may bill code V2632 (posterior chamber intraocular lens) for the IOL. Medicare will make payment for the lens based on reasonable cost for a conventional IOL. Place of Service (POS) = 11.

Effective for dates of service on and after January 1, 2006, physician, hospitals and ASCs may also bill the non-covered charges related to the P-C function of the IOL using HCPCS code V2788. Effective for dates of service on and after January 22, 2007 through January 1, 2008, non-covered charges related to A-C function of the IOL can be billed using HCPCS code V2788. The type of service indicator for the non-covered billed charges is Q. (The type of service is applied by the Medicare carrier and not the provider). Effective for A-C IOL insertion services on or after January 1, 2008, physicians, hospitals and ASCs should use V2787 rather than V2788 to report any additional charges that accrue.

When denying the non-payable charges submitted with V2787 or V2788, contractors shall use an appropriate Medical Summary Notice (MSN) such as 16.10 (Medicare does not pay for this item or service) and an appropriate claim adjustment reason code such as 96 (non-covered charges) for claims submitted with the non-payable charges.

Hospitals and physicians may use the proper CPT code(s) to bill Medicare for evaluation and management services usually associated with services following cataract extraction surgery, if appropriate.

A - Applicable Bill Types

The hospital applicable bill types are 12X, 13X, 83X and 85X.

B - Other Special Requirements for Hospitals

Hospitals shall continue to pay CAHs method 2 claims under current payment methodologies for conditional IOLs.

100-4, 32, 130

External Counterpulsation (ECP) Therapy

Commonly referred to as enhanced external counterpulsation, is a non-invasive outpatient treatment for coronary artery disease refractory medical and/or surgical therapy. Effective for dates of service July 1, 1999, and after, Medicare will cover ECP when its use is in patients with stable angina (Class III or Class IV, Canadian Cardiovascular Society Classification or equivalent classification) who, in the opinion of a cardiologist or cardiothoracic surgeon, are not readily amenable to surgical intervention, such as PTCA or cardiac bypass, because:

- Their condition is inoperable, or at high risk of operative complications or post-operative failure;

- Their coronary anatomy is not readily amenable to such procedures; or

- They have co-morbid states that create excessive risk.

(Refer to Publication 100-03, section 20.20 for further coverage criteria.)

100-4, 32, 130.1

Billing and Payment Requirements

Effective for dates of service on or after January 1, 2000, use HCPCS code G0166 (External counterpulsation, per session) to report ECP services. The codes for external cardiac assist (92971), ECG rhythm strip and report (93040 or 93041), pulse oximetry (94760 or 94761) and plethysmography (93922 or 93923) or other monitoring tests for examining the effects of this treatment are not clinically necessary with this service and should not be paid on the same day, unless they occur in a clinical setting not connected with the delivery of the ECP. Daily evaluation and management service, e.g., 99201-99205, 99211-99215, 99217-99220, 99241-99245, cannot be billed with the ECP treatments. Any evaluation and management service must be justified with adequate documentation of the medical necessity of the visit. Deductible and coinsurance apply.

100-4, 32, 140.2.2.1

Correct Place of Service (POS) Code for CR and ICR Services on Professional Claims

Effective for claims with dates of service on and after January 1, 2010, place of service (POS) code 11 shall be used for CR and ICR services provided in a physician's office and POS 22 shall be used for services provided in a hospital outpatient setting. All other POS codes shall be denied. Contractors shall adjust their prepayment procedure edits as appropriate.

The following messages shall be used when contractors deny CR and ICR claims for POS:

Claim Adjustment Reason Code (CARC) 58 - Treatment was deemed by the payer to have been rendered in an inappropriate or invalid place of service.

NOTE: Refer to the 832 Healthcare Policy Identification Segment (loop 2110 Service payment Information REF), if present.

Remittance Advice Remark Code (RARC) N428 - Service/procedure not covered when performed in this place of service.

Medicare Summary Notice (MSN) 21.25 - This service was denied because Medicare only covers this service in certain settings.

Group Code PR (Patient Responsibility) - Where a claim is received with the GA modifier indicating that a signed ABN is on file.

Group Code CO (Contractor Responsibility) - Where a claim is received with the GZ modifier indicating that no signed ABN is on file.

100-4, 32, 140.3

Intensive Cardiac Rehabilitation Program Services Furnished On or After January 1, 2010

As specified at 42 CFR 410.49, Medicare covers intensive cardiac rehabilitation items and services for patients who have experienced one or more of the following: An acute myocardial infarction within the preceding 12 months; or A coronary artery bypass surgery; or Current stable angina pectoris; or Heart valve repair or replacement; or Percutaneous transluminal coronary angioplasty (PTCA) or coronary stenting; or A heart or heart-lung transplant.~Intensive cardiac rehabilitation programs must include the following components: Physician-prescribed exercise each day cardiac rehabilitation items and services are furnished; Cardiac risk factor modification, including education, counseling, and behavioral intervention at least once during the program, tailored to patients' individual needs; Psychosocial assessment; Outcomes assessment; and An individualized treatment plan detailing how components are utilized for each patient.~ Intensive cardiac rehabilitation programs must be approved by Medicare. In order to be approved, a program must demonstrate through peer-reviewed published research that it has accomplished one or more of the following for its patients: Positively affected the progression of coronary heart disease; Reduced the need for coronary bypass surgery; and Reduced the need for percutaneous coronary interventions.~An intensive cardiac rehabilitation program must also demonstrate through peer-reviewed published research that it accomplished a statistically significant reduction in 5 or more of the following measures for patients from their levels before cardiac rehabilitation services to after cardiac rehabilitation services: Low density lipoprotein; Triglycerides; Body mass index; Systolic blood pressure; Diastolic blood pressure; and The need for cholesterol, blood pressure, and diabetes medications.~Intensive cardiac rehabilitation items and services must be furnished in a physician's office or a hospital outpatient setting. All settings must have a physician immediately available and accessible for medical consultations and emergencies at all time items and services are being furnished under the program. This provision is satisfied if the physician meets the requirements for direct supervision of physician office services as specified at 42 CFR 410.26 and for hospital outpatient therapeutic services as specified at 42 CFR 410.27.~As specified at 42 CFR 410.49(f)(2), intensive cardiac rehabilitation program sessions are limited to 72 1-hour sessions, up to 6 sessions per day, over a period of up to 18 weeks.

100-4, 32, 140.3.1

Coding Requirements for Intensive Cardiac Rehabilitation Services Furnished On or After January 1, 2010

The following are the applicable HCPCS codes for intensive cardiac rehabilitation services:

G0422 (Intensive cardiac rehabilitation; with or without continuous ECG monitoring, with exercise, per hour, per session)

G0423 (Intensive cardiac rehabilitation; with or without continuous ECG monitoring, without exercise, per hour, per session)

Effective for dates of service on or after January 1, 2010, hospitals and practitioners may report a maximum of 6 1-hour sessions per day. In order to report one session of cardiac rehabilitation services in a day, the duration of treatment must be at least 31 minutes. Additional sessions of intensive cardiac rehabilitation services beyond the first session may only be reported in the same day if the duration of treatment is 31 minutes or greater beyond the hour increment. In other words, in order to report 6 sessions of intensive cardiac rehabilitation services on a given date of service, the first five sessions would account for 60 minutes each and the sixth session would account for at least 31 minutes. If several shorter periods of intensive cardiac rehabilitation services are furnished on a given day, the minutes of service during those periods must be added together for reporting in 1-hour session increments.

Example: If the patient receives 20 minutes of intensive cardiac rehabilitation services in the day, no intensive cardiac rehabilitation session may be reported because less than 31 minutes of services were furnished.

Example: If a patient receives 20 minutes of intensive cardiac rehabilitation services in the morning and 35 minutes of intensive cardiac rehabilitation services in the afternoon of a single day, the hospital or practitioner would report 1 session of intensive cardiac rehabilitation services under 1 unit of the appropriate HCPCS G-code for the total duration of 55 minutes of intensive cardiac rehabilitation services on that day.

Example: If the patient receives 70 minutes of intensive cardiac rehabilitation services in the morning and 25 minutes of intensive cardiac rehabilitation services in the afternoon of a single day, the hospital or practitioner would report two sessions of intensive cardiac rehabilitation services under the appropriate HCPCS G-code(s) because the total duration of intensive cardiac rehabilitation services on that day of 95 minutes exceeds 90 minutes.

Example: If the patient receives 70 minutes of intensive cardiac rehabilitation services in the morning and 85 minutes of intensive cardiac rehabilitation services in the afternoon of a single day, the hospital or practitioner would report three sessions of intensive cardiac rehabilitation services under the appropriate HCPCS G-code(s) because the total duration of intensive cardiac rehabilitation services on that day is 155 minutes, which exceeds 150 minutes and is less than 211 minutes.

100-4, 32, 140.4

Pulmonary Rehabilitation Program Services Furnished On or After January 1, 2010

As specified in 42 CFR 410.47, Medicare covers pulmonary rehabilitation items and services for patients with moderate to very severe COPD (defined as GOLD classification II, III and IV), when referred by the physician treating the chronic respiratory disease.

Pulmonary rehabilitation programs must include the following components:

- Physician-prescribed exercise. Some aerobic exercise must be included in each pulmonary rehabilitation session;

- Education or training closely and clearly related to the individual's care and treatment which is tailored to the individual's needs, including information on respiratory problem management and, if appropriate, brief smoking cessation counseling;

- Psychosocial assessment;

- Outcomes assessment; and,

- An individualized treatment plan detailing how components are utilized for each patient.

Pulmonary rehabilitation items and services must be furnished in a physician's office or a hospital outpatient setting. All settings must have a physician immediately available and accessible for medical consultations and emergencies at all time items and services are being furnished under the program. This provision is satisfied if the physician meets the requirements for direct supervision of physician office services as specified at 42 CFR 410.26 and for hospital outpatient therapeutic services as specified at 42 CFR 410.27.

As specified at 42 CFR 410.47(f), pulmonary rehabilitation program sessions are limited to a maximum of 2 1-hour sessions per day for up to 36 sessions, with the option for an additional 36 sessions if medically necessary. Contractors shall accept the inclusion of the KX modifier on the claim lines as an attestation by the provider of the service that documentation is on file verifying

that further treatment beyond the 36 sessions is medically necessary up to a total of 72 sessions for that beneficiary.

100-4, 32, 140.4.1

Coding Requirements for Pulmonary Rehabilitation Services Furnished On or After January 1, 2010

The following is the applicable HCPCS code for pulmonary rehabilitation services:

G0424 (Pulmonary rehabilitation, including exercise (includes monitoring), per hour, per session)

Effective for dates of service on or after January 1, 2010, hospitals and practitioners may report a maximum of 2 1-hour sessions per day. In order to report one session of pulmonary rehabilitation services in a day, the duration of treatment must be at least 31 minutes. Two sessions of pulmonary rehabilitation services may only be reported in the same day if the duration of treatment is at least 91 minutes. In other words, the first session would account for 60 minutes and the second session would account for at least 31 minutes, if two sessions are reported. If several shorter periods of pulmonary rehabilitation services are furnished on a given day, the minutes of service during those periods must be added together for reporting in 1-hour session increments.

Example: If the patient receives 20 minutes of pulmonary rehabilitation services in the day, no pulmonary rehabilitation session may be reported because less than 31 minutes of services were furnished.

Example: If a patient receives 20 minutes of pulmonary rehabilitation services in the morning and 35 minutes of pulmonary rehabilitation services in the afternoon of a single day, the hospital or practitioner would report 1 session of pulmonary rehabilitation services under 1 unit of the HCPCS G-code for the total duration of 55 minutes of pulmonary rehabilitation services on that day.

Example: If the patient receives 70 minutes of pulmonary rehabilitation services in the morning and 25 minutes of pulmonary rehabilitation services in the afternoon of a single day, the hospital or practitioner would report two sessions of pulmonary rehabilitation services under the HCPCS G-code because the total duration of pulmonary rehabilitation services on that day of 95 minutes exceeds 90 minutes.

Example: If the patient receives 70 minutes of pulmonary rehabilitation services in the morning and 85 minutes of pulmonary rehabilitation services in the afternoon of a single day, the hospital or practitioner would report two sessions of pulmonary rehabilitation services under the HCPCS G-code for the total duration of pulmonary rehabilitation services of 155 minutes. A maximum of two sessions per day may be reported, regardless of the total duration of pulmonary rehabilitation services.

100-4, 32, 250.1

Coverage Requirements

Effective August 3, 2009, pharmacogenomic testing to predict warfarin responsiveness is covered only when provided to Medicare beneficiaries who are candidates for anticoagulation therapy with warfarin; i.e., have not been previously tested for CYP2C9 or VKORC1 alleles; and have received fewer than five days of warfarin in the anticoagulation regimen for which the testing is ordered; and only then in the context of a prospective, randomized, controlled clinical study when that study meets certain criteria as outlined in Pub 100-03, section 90.1, of the NCD Manual.

NOTE: A new temporary HCPCS Level II code effective August 3, 2009, G9143, warfarin responsiveness testing by genetic technique using any method, any number of specimen(s), was developed to enable implementation of CED for this purpose.

100-4, 32, 250.2

Billing Requirements

Institutional clinical trial claims for pharmacogenomic testing for warfarin response are identified through the presence of all of the following elements:

Value Code D4 and 8-digit clinical trial number (when present on the claim) - Refer to Transmittal 310, Change Request 5790, dated January 18, 2008;

ICD-9 diagnosis code V70.7 - Refer to Transmittal 310, Change Request 5790, dated January 18, 2008;

Condition Code 30 - Refer to Transmittal 310, Change Request 5790, dated January 18, 2008;

HCPCS modifier Q0: outpatient claims only - Refer to Transmittal 1418, Change Request 5805, dated January 18, 2008; and,

HCPCS code G9143 (mandatory with the April 2010 Integrated Outpatient Code Editor (IOCE) and the January 2011 Clinical Laboratory Fee Schedule (CLFS) updates. Prior to these times, any trials should bill FIs for this test as they currently do absent these instructions, and the FIs should process and pay those claims accordingly.)

Practitioner clinical trial claims for pharmacogenomic testing for warfarin response are identified through the presence of all of the following elements:

ICD-9 diagnosis code V70.7;

8-digit clinical trial number(when present on the claim);

HCPCS modifier Q0; and HCPCS code G9143 (to be carrier priced for claims with dates of service on and after August 3, 2009, that are processed prior to the January 2011 CLFS update.)

100-4, 32, 260.1

Policy
The Centers for Medicare & Medicaid Services (CMS) received a request for national coverage of treatments for facial lipodystrophy syndrome (LDS) for human immunodeficiency virus (HIV)-infected Medicare beneficiaries. Facial LDS is often characterized by a loss of fat that results in a facial abnormality such as severely sunken cheeks. This fat loss can arise as a complication of HIV and/or highly active antiretroviral therapy. Due to their appearance and stigma of the condition, patients with facial LDS may become depressed, socially isolated, and in some cases may stop their HIV treatments in an attempt to halt or reverse this complication.

Effective for claims with dates of service on and after March 23, 2010, dermal injections for facial LDS are only reasonable and necessary using dermal fillers approved by the Food and Drug Administration for this purpose, and then only in HIV-infected beneficiaries who manifest depression secondary to the physical stigmata of HIV treatment.

100-4, 32, 260.2.1

Hospital Billing Instructions
For hospital outpatient claims, hospitals must bill covered dermal injections for treatment of facial LDS by having all of the required elements on the claim:

A line with HCPCS codes Q2026 or Q2027 with a Line Item Date of service (LIDOS) on or after March 23, 2010,

A line with HCPCS code G0429 with a LIDOS on or after March 23, 2010,

ICD-9-CM diagnosis codes 042 (HIV) and 272.6 (Lipodystrophy)

Note to Outpatient Prospective Payment System (OPPS) hospitals or Ambulatory Surgical Centers (ASCs): For line item dates of service on or after march 23, 2010, and until HCPCS codes Q2026 and Q2027 are billable, facial LDS claims shall contain a temporary HCPCS code C9800, instead of HCPCS G0429 and HCPCS Q2026/Q2027, as shown above.

For hospital inpatient claims, hospitals must bill covered dermal injections for treatment of facial LDS by having all of the required elements on the claim:

Discharge date on or after March 23, 2010, ICD-9-CM procedure code 86.99 (other operations on skin and subcutaneous tissue, i.e., injection of filler material),

ICD-9-CM diagnosis codes 042 (HIV) and 272.6 (Lipodystrophy).

Note on all hospital claims: An ICD-9-CM diagnosis code for a comorbidity of depression may also be required for coverage on an outpatient and/or inpatient basis as determined by the individual Medicare contractor's policy.

100-4, 32, 260.2.2

Practitioner Billing Instructions
Practitioners must bill covered claims for dermal injections for treatment of facial LDS by having all of the required elements on the claim:

Performed in a non-facility setting:

A line with HCPCS codes Q2026 or Q2027 with a LIDOS on or after March 23, 2010,

A line with HCPCS code G0429 with a LIDOS on or after March 23, 2010,

ICD-9-CM diagnosis codes 042 (HIV) and 272.6 (Lipodystrophy).

NOTE: An ICD-9-CM diagnosis code for a comorbidity of depression may also be required for coverage based on the individual Medicare contractor's policy.

Performed in a facility setting:

A line with HCPCS code G0429 with a LIDOS on or after March 23, 2010,

ICD-9-CM diagnosis codes 042 (HIV) and 272.6 (Lipodystrophy).

NOTE: An ICD-9-CM diagnosis code for a comorbidity of depression may also be required for coverage based on the individual Medicare contractor's policy.

100-4, 32, 280.1

Autologous Cellular Immunotherapy Treatment of Prostate Cancer
Effective for services furnished on or after June 30, 2011, a National Coverage Determination (NCD) provides coverage of sipuleucel-T (PROVENGE®) for patients with asymptomatic or minimally symptomatic metastatic, castrate-resistant (hormone refractory) prostate cancer.

Conditions of Medicare Part A and Medicare Part B coverage for sipuleucel-T are located in the Medicare NCD Manual, Publication 100-3, section 110.22.

100-4, 32, 280.2

Healthcare Common Procedure Coding System (HCPCS) Codes and Diagnosis Coding

HCPCS Codes
Effective for claims with dates of service on June 30, 2011, Medicare providers shall report one of the following HCPCS codes for PROVENGE®:

- C9273 - Sipuleucel-T, minimum of 50 million autologous CD54+ cells activated with PAP-GM-CSF, including leukapheresis and all other preparatory procedures, per infusion, or

- J3490 - Unclassified Drugs, or

- J3590 - Unclassified Biologics.

NOTE: Contractors shall continue to process claims for HCPCS code C9273, J3490, and J3590, with dates of service June 30, 2011, as they do currently.

Effective for claims with dates of service on and after July 1, 2011, Medicare providers shall report the following HCPCS code:

- Q2043 - Sipuleucel-T, minimum of 50 million autologous CD54+ cells activated with PAP-GM-CSF, including leukapheresis and all other preparatory procedures, per infusion; short descriptor, Sipuleucel-T auto CD54+.

ICD-9 Diagnosis Coding
For claims with dates of service on and after July 1, 2011, for PROVENGE®, the on-label indication of asymptomatic or minimally symptomatic metastatic, castrate-resistant (hormone refractory) prostate cancer, must be billed using ICD-9 code 185 (malignant neoplasm of prostate) and at least one of the following ICD-9 codes:

ICD-9 code	Description
196.1	Secondary and unspecified malignant neoplasm of intrathoracic lymph nodes
196.2	Secondary and unspecified malignant neoplasm of intra-abdominal lymph nodes
196.5	Secondary and unspecified malignant neoplasm of lymph nodes of inguinal region and lower limb
196.6	Secondary and unspecified malignant neoplasm of intrapelvic lymph nodes
196.8	Secondary and unspecified malignant neoplasm of lymph nodes of multiple sites
196.9	Secondary and unspecified malignant neoplasm of lymph node site unspecified – The spread of cancer to and establishment in the lymph nodes.
197.0	Secondary malignant neoplasm of lung – Cancer that has spread from the original (primary) tumor to the lung. The spread of cancer to the lung. This may be from a primary lung cancer, or from a cancer at a distant site.
197.7	Malignant neoplasm of liver secondary – Cancer that has spread from the original (primary) tumor to the liver. A malignant neoplasm that has spread to the liver from another (primary) anatomic site. Such malignant neoplasms may be carcinomas (e.g., breast, colon), lymphomas, melanomas, or sarcomas.
198.0	Secondary malignant neoplasm of kidney – The spread of the cancer to the kidney. This may be from a primary kidney cancer involving the opposite kidney, or from a cancer at a distant site.
198.1	Secondary malignant neoplasm of other urinary organs
198.5	Secondary malignant neoplasm of bone and bone marrow —Cancer that has spread from the original (primary) tumor to the bone. The spread of a malignant neoplasm from a primary site to the skeletal system. The majority of metastatic neoplasms to the bone are carcinomas.
198.7	Secondary malignant neoplasm of adrenal gland
198.82	Secondary malignant neoplasm of genital organs

Coding for Off-Label PROVENGE® Services
The use of PROVENGE® off-label for the treatment of prostate cancer is left to the discretion of the Medicare Administrative Contractors. Claims with dates of service on and after July 1, 2011, for PROVENGE® paid off-label for the treatment of prostate cancer must be billed using either ICD-9 code 233.4 (carcinoma in situ of prostate), or ICD-9 code 185 (malignant neoplasm of prostate) in addition to HCPCS Q2043. Effective with the implementation date for ICD-10 codes, off-label PROVENGE® services must be billed with either ICD-10 code D075(carcinoma in situ of prostate), or C61 (malignant neoplasm of prostate) in addition to HCPCS Q2043.

ICD-10 Diagnosis Coding

Contractors shall note the appropriate ICD-10 code(s) that are listed below for future implementation. Contractors shall track the ICD-10 codes and ensure that the updated edit is turned on as part of the ICD-10 implementation effective October 1, 2013.

ICD-10	Description
C61	Malignant neoplasm of prostate (for on-label or off-label indications)
D075	Carcinoma in situ of prostate (for off-label indications only)
C77.1	Secondary and unspecified malignant neoplasm of intrathoracic lymph nodes
C77.2	Secondary and unspecified malignant neoplasm of intra-abdominal lymph nodes
C77.4	Secondary and unspecified malignant neoplasm of inguinal and lower limb lymph nodes
C77.5	Secondary and unspecified malignant neoplasm of intrapelvic lymph nodes
C77.8	Secondary and unspecified malignant neoplasm of lymph nodes of multiple regions
C77.9	Secondary and unspecified malignant neoplasm of lymph node, unspecified
C78.00	Secondary malignant neoplasm of unspecified lung
C78.01	Secondary malignant neoplasm of right lung
C78.02	Secondary malignant neoplasm of left lung
C78.7	Secondary malignant neoplasm of liver
C79.00	Secondary malignant neoplasm of unspecified kidney and renal pelvis
C79.01	Secondary malignant neoplasm of right kidney and renal pelvis
C79.02	Secondary malignant neoplasm of left kidney and renal pelvis
C79.10	Secondary malignant neoplasm of unspecified urinary organs
C79.11	Secondary malignant neoplasm of bladder
C79.19	Secondary malignant neoplasm of other urinary organs
C79.51	Secondary malignant neoplasm of bone
C79.52	Secondary malignant neoplasm of bone marrow
C79.70	Secondary malignant neoplasm of unspecified adrenal gland
C79.71	Secondary malignant neoplasm of right adrenal gland
C79.72	Secondary malignant neoplasm of left adrenal gland
C79.82	Secondary malignant neoplasm of genital organs

100-4, 32, 280.4

Payment Method

Payment for PROVENGE® is as follows:

- TOBs 12X, 13X, 22X and 23X - based on the Average Sales Price (ASP) + 6%,
- TOB 85X – based on reasonable cost,
- TOBs 71X and 77X – based on all-inclusive rate.

For Medicare Part B practitioner claims, payment for PROVENGE® is based on ASP + 6%.

Contractors shall not pay separately for routine costs associated with PROVENGE®, HCPCS Q2043, except for the cost of administration. (Q2043 is all-inclusive and represents all routine costs except for its cost of administration).

100-4, 32, 280.5

Medicare Summary Notices (MSNs), Remittance Advice Remark Codes (RARCs), Claim Adjustment Reason Codes (CARCs), and Group Codes

Contractors shall use the following messages when denying claims for the on-label indication for PROVENGE®, HCPCS Q2043, submitted without ICD-9-CM diagnosis code 185 and at least one diagnosis code from the ICD-9 table in Section 280.2 above:

MSN 14.9 - Medicare cannot pay for this service for the diagnosis shown on the claim.

Spanish Version - Medicare no puede pagar por este servicio debido al diagn-tico indicado en la reclamaci.

RARC 167 - This (these) diagnosis (es) are not covered. Note: Refer to the 835 Healthcare Policy Identification segment (loop 2110 Service Payment Information REF), if present.

Group Code - Contractual Obligation (CO)

Contractors shall use the following messages when denying claims for the off-label indication for PROVENGE®, HCPCS Q2043, submitted without either ICD-9-CM diagnosis code 233.4 or ICD-9-CM diagnosis code 185:

MSN 14.9 - Medicare cannot pay for this service for the diagnosis shown on the claim.

Spanish Version - Medicare no puede pagar por este servicio debido al diagn?tico indicado en la reclamaci?.

RARC 167 - This (these) diagnosis (es) are not covered. Note: Refer to the 835 Healthcare Policy Identification segment (loop 2110 Service Payment Information REF), if present.

Group Code – CO.

100-4, 32, 300

Billing Requirements for Ocular Photodynamic Therapy (OPT) with Verteporfin

Ocular Photodynamic Therapy (OPT) is used in the treatment of ophthalmologic diseases; specifically, for age-related macular degeneration (AMD), a common eye disease among the elderly. OPT involves the infusion of an intravenous photosensitizing drug called Verteporfin, followed by exposure to a laser. For complete Medical coverage guidelines, see National Coverage Determinations (NCD) Manual (Pub 100-03) ? 80.2 through 80.3.1.

100-4, 32, 300.1

Coding Requirements for OPT with Verteporfin

The following are applicable Current Procedural Terminology (CPT) codes for OPT with Verteporfin:

67221- Destruction of localized lesion of choroid (e.g. choroidal neovascularization); photodynamic therapy (includes intravenous infusion)

67225- Destruction of localized lesion of choroid (e.g. choroidal neovascularization); photodynamic therapy, second eye, at single session (List separately in addition to code for primary eye treatment)

The following are applicable Healthcare Common Procedure Coding System (HCPCS) code for OPT with Verteporfin:

J3396- Injection, Verteporfin, 0.1 mg

100-4, 32, 300.2

Claims Processing Requirements for OPT with Verteporfin Services on Professional Claims and Outpatient Facility Claims

OPT with Verteporfin is a covered service when billed with ICD-9-CM code 362.52 (Exudative Senile Macular Degeneration of Retina (Wet)) or ICD-10-CM code H35.32 (Exudative Age-related Macular Degeneration).

Coverage is denied when billed with either ICD-9-CM code 362.50 (Macular Degeneration (Senile), Unspecified) or 362.51 (Non-exudative Senile Macular Degeneration) or their equivalent ICD-10-CM code H35.30 (Unspecified Macular Degeneration) or H35.31 (Non-exudative Age-Related Macular Degeneration).

OPT with Verteporfin for other ocular indications are eligible for local coverage determinations through individual contractor discretion.

Payment for OPT service (CPT code 67221/67225) must be billed on the same claim as the drug (J3396) for the same date of service.

Claims for OPT with Verteporfin for dates of service prior to April 3, 2013 are covered at the initial visit as determined by a fluorescein angiogram (FA) CPT code 92235 . Subsequent follow-up visits also require a FA prior to treatment.

For claims with dates of service on or after April 3, 2013, contractors shall accept and process claims for subsequent follow-up visits with either a FA, CPT code 92235, or optical coherence tomography (OCT), CPT codes 92133 or 92134, prior to treatment.

Regardless of the date of service of the claim, the FA or OCT is not required to be submitted on the claim for OPT and can be maintained in the patient? file for audit purposes.

100-4, 32, 310

Transesophageal Doppler Used for Cardiac Monitoring

Effective May 17, 2007, Transesophageal Doppler used for cardiac monitoring is covered for ventilated patients in the ICU and operative patients with a need for intra-operative fluid optimization was deemed reasonable and necessary. See National Coverage Determinations Manual (Pub. 100-03) ?220.5, for complete coverage guidelines.

A new Healthcare Common Procedure Coding System (HCPCS) code, G9157, Transesophageal Doppler used for cardiac monitoring, will be made effective for use for dates of service on or after January 1, 2013.

100-4, 32, 310.10.3

Correct Place of Service (POS) Code for Transesophageal Doppler Cardiac Monitoring Services on Professional Claims

Contractors shall pay for Transesophageal Doppler cardiac monitoring, G9157, only when services are provided at POS 21.

Contractors shall deny HCPCS G9157 when billed globally in any POS other than 21 for ventilated patients in the ICU or for operative patients with a need for intra-operative fluid optimization using the following messages:

CARC 58: "Treatment was deemed by the payer to have been rendered in an inappropriate or invalid place of service. Note: Refer to the 835 Healthcare Policy Identification Segment (loop 2110 Service Payment Information REF), if present.

MSN 16.2: This service cannot be paid when provided in this location/facility.

Group Code: CO

100-4, 32, 310.2

After January 1, 2013, the applicable HCPCS code for Transesophageal Doppler cardiac monitoring is:

HCPCS G9157: Transesophageal Doppler used for cardiac monitoring

Contractors shall allow HCPCS G9157 to be billed when services are provided in POS 21 for ventilated patients in the ICU or for operative patients with a need for intra-operative fluid optimization.

Contractors shall deny HCPCS 76999 when billed for Esophageal Doppler for ventilated patients in the ICU or for operative patients with a need for intra-operative fluid optimization using the following messages:

CARC 189: "'Not otherwise classified' or 'unlisted' procedure code (CPT/HCPCS) was billed when there is a specific procedure code for this procedure/service."

RARC M20: "Missing/incomplete/invalid HCPCS."

MSN 16.13: "The code(s) your provider used is/are not valid for the date of service billed."

(English version) or "El/los código(s) que usó su proveedor no es/son válido(s) en la fecha de servicio facturada." (Spanish version).

Group Code: Contractual Obligation (CO)

100-4, 36, 50.14

Purchased Accessories & Supplies for Use With Grandfathered Equipment

Purchased Accessories & Supplies for Use With Grandfathered Equipment

Purchased Accessories & Supplies for Use With Grandfathered Equipment

Non-contract grandfathered suppliers must use the KY modifier on claims for CBA-residing beneficiaries with dates of service on or after January 1, 2011, for purchased, covered accessories or supplies furnished for use with rented grandfathered equipment. The following HCPCS codes are the codes for which use of the KY modifier is authorized:

Continuous Positive Airway Pressure Devices, Respiratory Assistive Devices, and Related Supplies and Accessories – A4604, A7030, A7031, A7032, A7033, A7034, A7035, A7036, A7037, A7038, A7039, A7044, A7045, A7046, E0561, and E0562

Hospital Beds and Related Accessories – E0271, E0272, E0280, and E0310

Walkers and Related Accessories – E0154, E0156, E0157 and E0158 Grandfathered suppliers that submit claims for the payment of the aforementioned purchased accessories and supplies for use with grandfathered equipment should submit the applicable single payment amount for the accessory or supply as their submitted charge on the claim. Non-contract grandfathered suppliers should be aware that purchase claims submitted for these codes without the KY modifier will be denied. In addition, claims submitted with the KY modifier for HCPCS codes other than those listed above will be denied.

After the rental payment cap for the grandfathered equipment is reached, the beneficiary must obtain replacement supplies and accessories from a contract supplier. The supplier of the grandfathered equipment is no longer permitted to furnish the supplies and accessories once the rental payment cap is reached.

100-4, 36, 50, 15

Hospitals Providing Walkers and Related Accessories to Their Patients on the Date of Discharge

Hospitals may furnish walkers and related accessories to their own patients for use in the home during an admission or on the date of discharge and receive payment at the applicable single payment amount, regardless of whether the hospital is a contract supplier or not. Separate payment is not made for walkers furnished by a hospital for use in the hospital, as payment for these items is included in the Part A payment for inpatient hospital services.

To be paid for walkers as a non-contract supplier, the hospital must use the modifier J4 in combination with the following HCPCS codes: A4636; A4637; E0130; E0135; E0140; E0141; E0143; E0144; E0147; E0148; E0149; E0154; E0155; E0156; E0157; E0158; and E0159. Under this exception, hospitals are advised to submit the claim for the hospital stay before or on the same day that they submit the claim for the walker to ensure timely and accurate claims processing.

Hospitals that are located outside a CBA that furnish walkers and/or related accessories to travelling beneficiaries who live in a CBA must affix the J4 modifier to claims submitted for these items.

The J4 modifier should not be used by contract suppliers.

100-8, 10, 2.2.8

Cardiac Rehabilitation (CR) and Intensive Cardiac Rehabilitation (ICR)

A. General Background Information

Effective January 1, 2010, Medicare Part B covers Cardiac Rehabilitation (CR) and Intensive Cardiac Rehabilitation (ICR) program services for beneficiaries who have experienced one or more of the following:

- An acute myocardial infarction within the preceding 12 months;
- A coronary artery bypass surgery;
- Current stable angina pectoris;
- Heart valve repair or replacement;
- Percutaneous transluminal coronary angioplasty or coronary stenting;
- A heart or heart-lung transplant; or,
- Other cardiac conditions as specified through a national coverage determination (NCD) (CR only).

ICR programs must be approved by CMS through the national coverage determination (NCD) process and must meet certain criteria for approval. Individual sites wishing to provide ICR services via an approved ICR program must enroll with their local contractor or MAC as an ICR program supplier.

B. ICR Enrollment

In order to enroll as an ICR site, a supplier must complete a Form CMS-855B, with the supplier type of "Other" selected. Contractors shall verify that the ICR program is approved by CMS through the NCD process. A list of approved ICR programs will be identified through the NCD listings, the CMS Web site and the Federal Register. Contractors shall use one of these options to verify that the ICR program has met CMS approval.

ICR suppliers shall be enrolled using specialty code 31. ICR suppliers must separately enroll each of their practice locations. Therefore, each enrolling ICR supplier can only have one practice location on its CMS-855B enrollment application and shall receive its own PTAN.

Contractors shall only accept and process reassignments (855R's) to ICR suppliers for physicians defined in 1861(r)(1) of the Act.

C. Additional Information

For more information on ICR suppliers, refer to:

42 CFR Sec.410.49;

Pub. 100-04, Medicare Claims Processing Manual, chapter 32, sections 140.2.2 - 140.2.2.6; and

Pub. 100-02, Medicare Benefit Policy Manual. chapter 15, section 232.

ICD-9-CM Self Test Answer Key

PART I ICD-9-CM DIAGNOSIS

1. Code assignment:

   066.41   West Nile fever with encephalitis

   No additional code is necessary for describing the encephalomyelitis.

2. Code assignment:

   070.51   Acute hepatitis C without mention of hepatic coma

3. Code assignment:

   046.11   Variant Creutzfeld-Jakob disease

   294.11   Dementia in conditions classified elsewhere with behavioral disturbance

4. Code assignment:

   051.02   Vaccinia not from vaccination

   692.9   Contact dermatitis and other eczema, unspecified

5. Code assignment:

   258.02   Multiple endocrine neoplasia type IIA

   193   Malignant neoplasm of thyroid gland

   252.02   Secondary hyperparathyroidism, non-renal

   405.99   Secondary hypertension, unspecified

6. Code assignment:

   288.66   Bandemia

7. Code assignment:

   347.00   Narcolepsy without cataplexy

8. Code assignment:

   380.03   Chondritis of pinna

   041.7   Bacterial infection in conditions classified elsewhere, pseudomonas

9. Code assignment:

   434.91   Cerebral artery occlusion, unspecified, with cerebral infarction

10. Code assignment:

    453.41   Venous embolism and thrombosis of deep vessels of proximal lower extremity

11. Code assignment:

    209.72   Secondary neuroendocrine tumor of the liver

    209.14   Malignant carcinoid tumor of the transverse colon

12. Code assignment:

    491.22   Obstructive chronic bronchitis with acute bronchitis

13. Code assignment:

    521.01   Dental caries limited to enamel

    521.07   Dental caries of smooth surface

14. Code assignment:

    523.21   Gingival recession, minimal

15. Code assignment:

    996.82   Complications of transplanted organ, liver

    238.77   Post-transplant lymphoproliferative disorder

16. Code assignment:

    644.21   Early onset of delivery, delivered

    651.01   Multiple gestation, twins, delivered

    651.71   Multiple gestation following elective fetal reduction, delivered

    642.41   Mild pre-eclampsia, delivered

    V27.2   Outcome of delivery; twins, both liveborn

    V91.03   Twin gestation, dichorionic/diamniotic (two placentae, two amniotic sacs)

17. Code assignment:

    249.60   Secondary diabetes mellitus with neurological manifestation

    357.2   Polyneuropathy in diabetes

    E932.0   Drugs, medicinal and biological substances causing adverse effects in therapeutic use; adrenal cortical steroids

18. Code assignment:

    796.2   Elevated blood pressure reading without diagnosis of hypertension

    272.0   Pure hypercholesterolemia

    724.2   Lumbago

    338.29   Other chronic pain

19. Code assignment:

    274.03   Chronic gouty arthropathy with tophus (tophi)

20. Code assignment:

    250.50   Diabetes mellitus with ophthalmic manifestations, type II or unspecified type, not stated as uncontrolled

    362.07   Diabetic retinal edema

    362.06   Severe nonproliferative diabetic retinopathy

21. Code assignment:

    403.90   Hypertensive kidney disease, unspecified, with chronic kidney disease

    585.4   Chronic kidney disease, Stage IV (severe)

22. Code assignment:

    530.86   Infection of esophagostomy

    041.11   Methicillin-susceptible Staphylococcus aureus

    335.20   Amyotrophic lateral sclerosis

23. Code assignment:

    482.41   Methicillin resistant pneumonia due to Staphylococcus aureus

24. Code assignment:

    618.01   Cystocele, midline

    788.38   Overflow incontinence

25. Code assignment:

    202.82   Other lymphoma, intrathoracic lymph nodes

    511.81   Malignant pleural effusion

26. Code assignment:

584.9	Acute kidney failure, unspecified
277.88	Tumor lysis syndrome
E933.1	Adverse effects; antineoplastic and immunosuppressive drugs
202.40	Leukemic reticuloendotheliosis, unspecified site, extranodal and solid organ sites

27. Code assignment:

999.32	Bloodstream infection due to central nervous catheter
038.11	Staphylococcus aureus septicemia
995.91	Sepsis

28. Code assignment:

| 999.39 | Infection following other infusion, injection, transfusion or vaccination |

29. Code assignment:

| 569.44 | Dysplasia of anus |
| V08 | Asymptomatic human immunodeficiency virus [HIV] infection status |

30. Coding scenario:

707.05	Pressure ulcer, buttock
707.23	Pressure ulcer, stage III
290.40	Vascular dementia, uncomplicated

31. Code assignment:

| 518.7 | Transfusion related acute lung injury (TRALI) |
| 285.9 | Anemia, unspecified |

32. Code assignment:

695.11	Erythema multiform minor
695.51	Exfoliation due to erythematous condition involving 10-19 percent of body surface
382.9	Unspecified otitis media
E930.0	Drugs, medicinal and biological substances causing adverse effects in therapeutic use, Penicillins

33. Code assignment:

| 377.43 | Optic nerve hypoplasia |

34. Code assignment:

| 053.14 | Herpes zoster with other nervous system complications, herpes |

35. Code assignment:

692.6	Contact dermatitis and other eczema
372.30	Conjunctivitis, unspecified
462	Acute pharyngitis
E928.6	Environmental exposure to harmful algae and toxins
E002.0	Swimming

36. Code assignment:

| 345.41 | Localization-related (focal) (partial) epilepsy and epileptic syndromes with complex partial seizures, with intractable epilepsy |
| 348.81 | Temporal lobe sclerosis |

37. Code assignment:

| 996.74 | Other complications of internal (biological) (synthetic) prosthetic device, implant and graft, due to other vascular device, implant and graft |
| 453.85 | Acute venous embolism and thrombosis of subclavian veins |

38. Code assignment:

770.81	Primary apnea of newborn
779.81	Neonatal bradycardia
779.0	Convulsions in newborn
799.82	Apparent life-threatening event in infant

Code 799.82 should be assigned as an additional code if the event is documented in the medical record. However, it may be assigned as the principal diagnosis if no other diagnosis is documented.

39. Code assignment:

821.00	Fracture, Unspecified part of femur
518.82	Other pulmonary insufficiency, not elsewhere classified
276.61	Transfusion associated circulatory overload
427.31	Atrial fibrillation
V58.61	Long-term (current) use of anticoagulants

40. Code assignment:

278.03	Obesity hypoventilation syndrome
278.01	Morbid obesity
V85.42	Body Mass Index, 45.0-49.9
327.23	Obstructive sleep apnea (adult) (pediatric)

41. Code assignment:

| 488.01 | Influenza due to identified avian influenza virus with pneumonia |
| 480.1 | Pneumonia due to respiratory syncytial virus |

42. Code assignment:

| 752.33 | Unicornuate uterus |
| 752.43 | Cervical agenesis |

43. Code assignment:

784.92	Jaw pain
278.02	Overweight
V17.3	Family history, Ischemic heart disease

44. Code assignment:

999.62	ABO incompatibility with acute hemolytic transfusion reaction
282.60	Sickle cell disease, unspecified
E876.0	Mismatched in blood transfusion

45. Code assignment:

| 294.21 | Dementia, unspecified with behavioral disturbance |
| V40.31 | Wandering in diseases classified elsewhere |

46. Code assignment:

| 365.11 | Primary open angle glaucoma |
| 365.72 | Moderate stage glaucoma |

47. Code assignment:

| 162.5 | Malignant neoplasm of lower lobe, bronchus or lung |
| 512.82 | Secondary spontaneous pneumothorax |

48. Code assignment:

539.19   Other complications of gastric band procedure

537.89   Other specified disorders of stomach and duodenum (gastric stricture)

935.2   Foreign body in stomach (bezoar)

49. Code assignment:

759.89   Other specified anomalies, Other

745.5   Ostium secundum type atrial septal defect

746.84   Obstructive anomalies of heart, NEC

747.31   Pulmonary artery coarctation and atresia

50. Code assignment:

575.10   Cholecystitis, unspecified

998.2   Accidental puncture or laceration during a procedure

569.83   Perforation of intestine

V64.41   Laparoscopic surgical procedure converted to open procedure

PART II ICD-9-CM PROCEDURE CODING

1. Code assignment:

Diagnoses

414.00   Coronary atherosclerosis of unspecified type of vessel, native or graft

414.3   Coronary atherosclerosis due to lipid rich plaque

Procedure

38.23   Intravascular spectroscopy

2. Code assignment:

Diagnoses

038.40   Gram negative septicemia

995.92   Systemic inflammatory response syndrome due to infectious process with organ dysfunction

785.52   Septic shock

518.81   Acute respiratory failure

Procedure(s)

96.71   Continuous mechanical ventilation for less than 96 consecutive hours

00.17   Infusion of vasopressor agent

3. Code assignment:

Diagnosis

410.41   Acute myocardial infarction, of other inferior wall, initial episode of care

Procedure(s)

00.66   Percutaneous transluminal coronary angioplasty [PTCA]

17.55   Transluminal coronary atherectomy

36.07   Insertion of drug-eluting coronary artery stent(s)

00.40   Procedure on single vessel

00.45   Insertion of single vascular stent

37.22   Left heart cardiac catheterization

00.24   Intravascular imaging of coronary vessel

99.10   Injection or infusion of thrombolytic agent

4. Code assignment:

Diagnoses

820.09   Transcervical fracture of neck of femur, closed, other

E880.9   Fall on or from other stairs or steps

E849.0   Place of occurrence, home

Procedure(s)

81.51   Total hip replacement

00.31   Computer assisted surgery with CT/CTA

5. Code assignment:

Diagnosis

433.10   Occlusion and stenosis of precerebral arteries, carotid, without mention of cerebral infarction

Procedure(s)

00.61   Percutaneous angioplasty of precerebral (extracranial) vessel(s)

17.53   Percutaneous atherectomy of extracranial vessel(s)

00.63   Percutaneous insertion of carotid artery stent(s)

00.40   Procedure on single vessel

00.45   Insertion of single vascular stent

99.10   Injection or infusion of thrombolytic agent

6. Code assignment:

Diagnosis

492.8   Other emphysema

Procedure

33.72   Endoscopic pulmonary airway flow measurement

7. Code assignment:

Diagnoses

327.23   Obstructive sleep apnea (adult) (pediatric)

796.2   Elevated blood pressure reading without diagnosis of hypertension

Procedure(s)

29.4   Plastic repair on pharynx

27.69   Other plastic repair of palate

27.64   Insertion of palatal implant

8. Code assignment:

Diagnoses

402.01   Malignant hypertensive heart disease with heart failure

428.0   Congestive heart failure, unspecified

Procedure

37.66   Insertion of implantable heart assist system

9. Code assignment:

Diagnosis

553.1   Umbilical hernia without mention of obstruction or gangrene

Procedure

53.42   Laparoscopic repair of umbilical hernia with graft or prosthesis

10. Code assignment:

    Diagnoses

    736.81   Unequal leg length (acquired)

    905.4   Late effect of fracture of lower extremity

    Procedure(s)

    78.35   Limb lengthening procedure, femur

    84.53   Implantation of internal limb lengthening device with kinetic distraction

11. Code assignment:

    Diagnosis

    174.9   Malignant neoplasm of female breast, unspecified

    Procedure(s)

    85.21   Local excision of lesion of breast

    92.41   Intra-operative radiation therapy

12. Code assignment:

    Diagnoses

    V58.11   Encounter for antineoplastic chemotherapy

    191.8   Malignant neoplasm of brain, other parts of brain

    Procedure(s)

    00.19   Disruption of blood brain barrier via infusion [BBBD]

    99.25   Chemotherapy

13. Code assignment:

    Diagnoses

    745.69   Valgus deformities of feet; other

    343.9   Cerebral palsy, NOS

    Procedure

    81.18   Subtalar joint arthroereisis

14. Code assignment:

    Diagnosis

    823.00   Closed fracture, upper end, tibia alone

    Procedure(s)

    79.06   Closed reduction of fracture without internal fixation, tibia and fibula

    78.17   Application of external fixation device, tibia and fibula

    84.72   Application of external fixator device, ring system

15. Code assignment:

    Diagnosis

    722.52   Degeneration of lumbar or lumbosacral intervertebral disc

    Procedure

    80.53   Repair of the anulus fibrosus with graft or prosthesis

16. Code assignment:

    Diagnosis

    153.8   Malignant neoplasm of other specified sites of large intestine

    Procedure(s)

    45.82   Open total intra-abdominal colectomy

    48.69   Other resection of rectum, other

17. Code assignment:

    Diagnosis

    571.9   Other chronic nonalcoholic liver disease

    Procedure

    50.13   Transjugular liver biopsy

18. Code assignment:

    Diagnosis

    434.01   Cerebral thrombosis

    Procedure(s)

    39.74   Endovascular removal of obstruction from head and neck vessel(s)

    00.40   Procedure on single vessel

19. Code assignment:

    Diagnoses

    996.46   Articular bearing surface wear of prosthetic joint

    V43.64   Organ or tissue replaced by other means; hip

    Procedure(s)

    00.71   Revision of hip replacement, acetabular component only

    00.77   Hip bearing surface, ceramic-on-polyethylene

20. Code assignment:

    Diagnosis

    414.01   Coronary atherosclerosis of native coronary artery

    Procedure(s)

    00.66   Percutaneous transluminal coronary angioplasty [PTCA]

    36.07   Insertion of drug-eluting coronary artery stent(s)

    00.42   Procedure on three vessels

    00.47   Insertion of three vascular stents

    00.44   Procedure on bifurcated vessel

21. Code assignment:

    Diagnoses

    428.42   Chronic combined systolic and diastolic heart failure

    428.0   Congestive heart failure, unspecified

    V45.02   Automatic implantable cardiac defibrillator

    Procedure

    17.51   Implantation of rechargeable cardiac contractility modulation [CCM], total system

22. Code assignment:

    Diagnosis

    191.5   Malignant neoplasm of ventricles of brain

    Procedure

    17.61   Laser interstitial thermal therapy [LITT] of lesion or tissue of brain under guidance

23. Code assignment:

    Diagnosis

    560.9   Unspecified intestinal obstruction

    Procedure

    46.86   Endoscopic insertion of colonic stent(s)

24. Code assignment:

Diagnosis

440.20 Atherosclerosis of the extremities, unspecified

Procedure(s)

39.50 Angioplasty of other non-coronary vessels

00.60 Insertion of drug-eluting stent(s) of superficial femoral artery

00.40 Procedure on single vessel

00.45 Insertion of one vascular stent

25. Code assignment:

Diagnosis

345.41 Localization-related (focal) (partial) epilepsy and epileptic syndromes with complex partial seizures

Procedure(s)

01.20 Cranial implantation or replacement of neurostimulator pulse generator

02.93 Implantation or replacement of intracranial neurostimulator lead(s)

26. Code assignment:

Diagnoses

402.91 Hypertensive heart disease with heart failure

428.30 Diastolic heart failure, unspecified

Procedure

39.81 Implantation or replacement of carotid sinus baroreflex activation device, total system

27. Code assignment:

Diagnosis

331.4 Obstructive hydrocephalus

Procedure

02.22 Intracranial ventricular shunt or anastomosis

28. Code assignment:

Diagnosis

424.1 Aortic valve stenosis

Procedure

35.05 Endovascular replacement of aortic valve

29. Code assignment:

Diagnosis

218.1 Intramural leiomyoma of uterus

Procedure

68.25 Uterine artery embolization [UAE] without coils

30. Code assignment:

Diagnosis

174.4 Malignant neoplasm of female breast, upper-outer quadrant

Procedure

85.43 Unilateral simple extended mastectomy

31. Code assignment:

Diagnosis

823.00 Fracture of tibia and fibula, upper end, closed, tibia alone

Procedure

79.36 Open reduction of fracture with internal fixation, tibia and fibula

HCPCS Self Test Answer Key

1. b. A0431 Ambulance service, conventional air services, transport, one way (rotary wing) and A0436 Rotary wing air mileage, per statute mile

2. a. B4168, 2 units, Parenteral nutrition solution: amino acid, 3.5% (500 ml = 1 unit) –home mix

3. c. FIRAZYR is the trade name of icatibant, J1744 Injection, icatibant, 1 mg

4. c. G0410 Group psychotherapy other than of a multiple-family group, in a partial hospitalization setting, approximately 45 to 50 minutes.

5. d. Healthcare Common Procedure Coding System

    The term HCPCS (pronounced "hick-picks") is most accurately used as the acronym for the entire two level coding system.

6. b. CPT codes

    HCPCS level I is the American Medical Association's (AMA) *Physicians' Current Procedural Terminology*

7. Level II HCPCS refers to:

    a. HCPCS alphanumeric codes

    HCPCS is commonly used to specifically identify HCPCS level II national codes

8. b. Code from index

    Codes should never be assigned directly from the index. Once locating the term in the index, refer to the tabular section of the book to verify the code.

9. d. Drugs

10. a. A4550 Surgical tray

11. c. J0558 6 units, Injection, penicillin G benzathine and penicillin G procaine, 100,000 units

12. c. G0009 Administration of pneumococcal vaccine

13. This code is per 500 mg and should be reported with two units to report 1,000 mg.

14. a. J0897 x 60 Injection, denosumab, 1 mg

15. d. a and b

16. a. J0718 X 200 Injection, certolizumab pegol, 1 mg

    Cimzia is the brand name for the generic drug certolizumab pegol. This code is reported per milligram and will require 200 units in order to accurately represent the dosage given to the patient.

17. a. A6532-RT Gradient compression stocking, below knee, 40-50 mm Hg, each, right side

    Code A6532-RT describes gradient compression stocking 40–50 mm Hg. The code is for each stocking. RT modifier is for the right side.

18. d. G0379 Direct admission of patient for hospital observation care

    Code G0379 is for a direct admission to the hospital's observation unit.

19. d. A8001 Helmet, protective, hard, prefabricated, includes all components and accessories. A8001 includes the helmet and the chin strap.

20. d. Q5001, Hospice care provided in patient's home residence.

21. b. C8931 Magnetic resonance angiography without contrast followed by with contrast, spinal canal and contents

22. d. J0712 X 120, Injection, ceftaroline fosamil, 10 mg. Teflaro is the brand name for ceftaroline fosamil. The HCPCS code is in 10 mg units. The patient received a total of 1,200 mg over 24 hours (600 every 12 hours), which is 120 times the 10 mg of the code description.

23. b. C9286 X 400 Injection, belatacept, 1 mg. NULOJIX is the brand name for belatacept. Since the patient received 400 mg of the drug, units of 400 should be reported.

24. d. G9168 Memory functional limitation, current status at time of initial therapy treatment/episode outset and reporting intervals, with modifier CJ At least 20 percent but less than 40 percent impaired, limited or restricted.

NOTES

NOTES

NOTES

NOTES

NOTES